Cancer Nursing

Cancer Nursing

Principles and Practice

FIFTH EDITION

EDITED BY

Connie Henke Yarbro, RN, MS, FAAN

Clinical Associate Professor
Division of Hematology/Oncology
Adjunct Clinical Assistant Professor
Sinclair School of Nursing
Editor, *Seminars in Oncology Nursing*
University of Missouri–Columbia
Columbia, Missouri

Medical Advisory Board, CancerSource.com

Michelle Goodman, RN, MS

Oncology Clinical Nurse Specialist
Rush Cancer Institute
Assistant Professor of Nursing
Rush University College of Nursing
Rush-Presbyterian-St. Luke's Medical Center
Chicago, Illinois

Margaret Hansen Frogge, RN, MS

Vice President, Strategic Development
and System Integration
Riverside Health Care
Kankakee, Illinois

Assistant Professor of Nursing
Rush University College of Nursing
Rush-Presbyterian-St. Luke's Medical Center
Chicago, Illinois

Susan L. Groenwald, RN, MS

Assistant Professor of Nursing, Complemental
Department of Medical Nursing
Rush University College of Nursing
Rush-Presbyterian-St. Luke's Medical Center
Chicago, Illinois

JONES AND BARTLETT PUBLISHERS
Sudbury, Massachusetts
BOSTON   TORONTO   LONDON   SINGAPORE

World Headquarters
Jones and Bartlett Publishers
40 Tall Pine Drive
Sudbury, MA 01776
978-443-5000
info@jbpub.com
www.jbpub.com

Jones and Bartlett Publishers International
Barb House, Barb Mews
London W6 7PA
UK

Jones and Bartlett Publishers Canada
2406 Nikanna Road
Mississauga, ON L5C 2W6
CANADA

Copyright © 2000, 1997, 1993, 1990, 1987 by Jones and Bartlett Publishers, Inc.

Library of Congress Cataloging-in-Publication Data

Cancer nursing: principles and practice / edited by Connie Henke Yarbro . . . [et al.].—5th ed.
    p. cm.
    Includes bibliographical references and index.
    ISBN 0-7637-1164-0
    1. Cancer—Nursing. I. Yarbro, Connie Henke
    [DNLM: 1. Neoplasms—nursing. WY 156 C2197 2000]
  RC266.C356 2000
  610.73'698—DC21
                             99-086378

Acquisitions Editor: Greg Vis
Production Editor: Linda DeBruyn
Editorial/Production Assistant: Christine Tridente
Manufacturing Buyer: Therese Bräuer
Design/Editorial Production Service/Typesetting: Modern Graphics
Cover Design: Anne Spencer
Printing and Binding: Courier Westford

The selection and dosage of drugs presented in this book are in accord with standards accepted at the time of publication. The authors, editors, and publisher have made every effort to provide accurate information. However, research, clinical practice, and government regulations often change the accepted standard in this field. Before administering any drug, the reader is advised to check the manufacturer's product information sheet for the most up-to-date recommendations on dosage, precautions, and contraindications. This is especially important in the case of drugs that are new or seldom used.

Printed in the United States of America
03 02 01 00 10 9 8 7 6 5 4 3 2 1

Contents

Part VI   The Care of Individuals with Cancer   931

Preface

We welcome the new millenium with the Fifth Edition of *Cancer Nursing Principles and Practice*. The considerable progress in the science of oncology and oncology nursing has necessitated extensive revision of many chapters in this edition, which have been updated to include the latest developments in oncology nursing and cancer patient care. Over 35 new authors, all experts in their fields, contribute advanced knowledge and significant up to date information to our traditional chapter topics as well as newly designed chapters we feel will be of profound interest to our readers.

The basic science chapters in Part I have been reorganized and updated to reflect the massive increase in scientific knowledge that has occurred in the past few years, especially as it relates to genes and cancer. Several sections have been revised to make content more easily accessible to our readers. For example, the treatment modalities of radiation therapy and bone marrow transplantation have each been separated into three chapters that cover principles of the treatment modality, administration, and toxicity management. The topic of pain is now covered in separate chapters, one that covers the assessment of cancer pain, and another that covers the management of cancer pain. Gynecologic cancers and gastrointestinal malignancies are also each divided into individual chapters specific to the cancer site. We feel these changes will result in a more complete discussion of each cancer site and help the reader find information more easily and in a more timely fashion.

A new section on **Oncologic Emergencies,** including cardiac tamponade, disseminated intravascular coagulation, septic shock, spinal cord compression, superior vena cava syndrome, syndrome of inappropriate antidiuretic hormone, and tumor lysis syndrome, has been added to the 5th edition in response to requests from our readers. The section on **Issues in Delivery of Care** includes four new revised chapters addressing issues encountered by cancer nurses caring for patients in a hospital setting, ambulatory setting, at home, and in hospice. We feel this emphasis is especially appropriate considering the continued outpatient and ambulatory care focus of cancer care. As we enter the 21st century, a chapter on **Informatics** is especially appropriate because it provides a foundation of knowledge for cancer nurses regarding this important technology area. The **Cancer Nursing Resources** section has been extensively expanded, reformatted, and indexed so that the information can be more readily located. Every chapter has been updated with the latest references and research studies, and many include Web site addresses and resources. As with previous editions, *Cancer Nursing Principles and Practice* continues to present the most comprehensive information on oncology nursing from leading cancer nursing experts.

In the preparation of this edition there has been a major reassignment of the responsibilities among the editors and it is appropriate at this time to pay tribute to Susan L. Groenwald, who initiated the first edition of this text in 1981. Without her original vision and desire for excellence, this book would never have been possible.

The editors would also like to pay special tribute to our families, especially John, Jim, and Larry, and our colleagues who supported us through this lengthy, time-consuming process. We would like to thank the editorial staff at Jones and Bartlett Publishers, including Greg Vis, Linda DeBruyn, and John Danielowich; and Modern Graphics, especially Michael Granger, whose efforts have made possible the production of this edition. And, most importantly, we would like to extend our gratitude to those authors whose tireless review of the literature, and writing, revising, and updating of chapters have made this book possible. The dedication of these contributors and all involved with this 5th edition contributes to the quality of care provided to patients with cancer.

Connie Henke Yarbro
Margaret H. Frogge
Michelle Goodman

Contributors

Terri Ades, RN, CS, MS, AOCN (27)
Director, Health Content
American Cancer Society, Inc.
Atlanta, GA

Barbara A. Barhamand, RN, MS, AOCN (85)
Clinical Nurse Specialist/Practice Manager
Hematology Oncology Consultants, Ltd.
Naperville, IL

Andrea M. Barsevick, DNSc, RN, AOCN (69)
Director of Nursing Research and Education
Fox Chase Cancer Center
Philadelphia, PA

Linda Battiato, RN, MSN, OCN® (24)
Oncology/Cytokine Research Nurse
Indiana Cancer Pavilion
Indianapolis, IN

Susan M. Bauer, DNSc, RN (3)
Assistant Professor
Graduate School of Nursing and Division of Preventive &
  Behavorial Medicine
University of Massachusetts Worcester/University of
  Massachusetts Medical Center
Worcester, MA

Susan Weiss Behrend, RN, MSN (16)
Oncology Clinical Nurse Specialist
Fox Chase Center
Philadelphia, PA

Karen Belford, RN, MS, AOCN, CCRN (49)
Nurse Educator
Memorial Sloan-Kettering Cancer Center
Department of Nursing Education
New York, NY

Katherine McDermott Blackburn, RN, MPA, OCN® (83)
Senior Consultant
Ernst and Young
New York, NY

Catherine Bradley, PhD (70)
Faculty, Department of Medicine
Michigan State Univeristy
East Lansing, MI

Dawn Camp-Sorrell, RN, MSN, FNP, AOCN (20)
Oncology Nurse Practitioner
University of Alabama at Birmingham Hospital
Birmingham, AL

Dianne D. Chapman, RN, MS (48)
Coordinator
Comprehensive Breast Center
Chicago, IL

Rebecca F. Cohen, RN, MS, EdD, MPA, CPHQ (9)
Associate Professor
Rockford College, Department of Nursing
Rockford, IL

JoAnn Coleman, RN, MS, ACNP-CS, AOCN (55, 63)
Acute Care Nurse Practitioner
Pancreas and Biliary Surgery
Johns Hopkins Hospital
Baltimore, MD

Shawanna M. Cunning, RN, MSN, CCRN (14)
Clinical Nurse Specialist
Riverside Medical Center
Kankakee, IL

Mary L. Cunningham, RN, MS, AOCN (84)
Coordinator Pain and Palliative Care
Ellis Fischel Cancer Center
University of Missouri–Columbia
Columbia, MO

Diane Scott Dorsett, PhD, RN, FAAN (72)
Private Practice, Comprehensive Cancer Support Services
San Francisco, CA

Lynne M. Early, RN, MSN, CETN, OCN® (47)
Enterostomal Therapy Nurse
Los Angeles, CA

Heidi E. Ehrenberger, PhD, RN, OCN® (82)
Consultant, Health Information and Research Services
Adjunct Instructor, College of Nursing
University of Tennessee–Knoxville
Knoxville, TN

Jan Ellerhorst-Ryan, RN, MSN, CS (30)
Oncology–HIV Clinical Nurse Specialist
United Home Health
Cincinnati, OH

Coni Ellis, MS, RN-CS, C, OCN®, CWOCN (51)
Nursing Outreach Coordinator; Co-Director of the
    Wound, Ostomy, and Continence Nurse Education
    Program
The University of Texas M.D. Anderson Cancer Center
Houston, TX

Jayne Fernsler, DSN, RN, AOCN (6)
Professor
Department of Nursing
University of Delaware
Newark, DE

Carol Estwing Ferrans, PhD, RN, FAAN (12)
Associate Professor
Department of Medical-Surgical Nursing
College of Nursing
The University of Illinois at Chicago
Chicago, IL

Anne Marie Flaherty, RN, MSN, AOCN, CNSC (41)
Clinical Nurse Specialist
Hackensack University Medical Center, Adult Oncology
Hackensack, NJ

Ann T. Foltz, RN, DNS (33)
Consultant, ATF Quality Control
Leesburg, FL

Marilyn Frank-Stromborg, EdD, JD, NP, FAAN (9)
Chair and Presidential Research Professor
School of Nursing
Northern Illinois University
Dekalb, IL

Margaret Hansen Frogge, RN, MS (14)
Vice President, Strategic Development and System
    Integration
Riverside Health Care
Kankakee, IL
Assistant Professor of Nursing
Rush University College of Nursing
Rush-Presbyterian-St.Luke's Medical Center
Chicago, IL

Annette Galassi, RN, MA, CANP, AOCN (79)
Cancer Information Specialist
National Cancer Institute
Bethesda, MD

Barbara Given, PhD, RN, FAAN (70)
Professor of Nursing, College of Nursing
Associate Director, Institute for Managed Care
College of Human Medicine
Michigan State University
East Lansing, MI

Charles W. Given, PhD (70)
Professor
Department of Family Practice
College of Human Medicine
Michigan State University
East Lansing, MI

Barbara Holmes Gobel, RN, MS (31, 39)
Oncology Clinical Nurse Specialist
Gottlieb Memorial Hospital
Melrose Park, IL
Complementary Faculty
Rush University College of Nursing
Chicago, IL

Elizabeth Gomez, MSN, RN, AOCN (82)
Founder and Principal, Newtonnet Productions, LLC
Editor, ONS Online
Ridgefield, CT

Michelle Goodman, RN, MS (19, 48)
Assistant Professor of Nursing
Rush University College of Nursing
Oncology Clinical Nurse Specialist
Section of Medical Oncology
Rush Cancer Institute
Rush-Presbyterian-St. Luke's Medical Center
Chicago, IL

Jean Gribbon, RN, BSN (2)
Staff Nurse, Pediatrics
The University of Arizona Health Sciences Center
Tucson, AZ

Jill Griffin-Brown, RN, BSN, OCN® (11)
Nurse Manager
Bay Area Oncology
Tampa, FL

Carol Guarnieri, RN, MSN, AOCN (68)
Oncology Clinical Nurse Specialist
Samitivej Srinakarin Hospital
Bangkok, Thailand

Irene Stewart Haapoja, RN, MS, (35, 43)
Oncology Clinical Nurse Specialist
Section of Medical Oncology
Rush Cancer Institute
Rush-Presbyterian-St. Luke's Medical Center
Chicago, IL

Mel Haberman, PhD, RN, FAAN (80)
Associate Dean for Research and Professor
Washington State University College of Nursing
Spokane, WA

Gloria Hagopian, RN, EdD (78)
Professor
Adult Health Nursing Department
University of North Carolina at Charlotte
Charlotte, NC

Lenore L. Harris, RN, MSN, AOCN (56)
Study Development Coordinator
American College of Surgeons
Oncology Group
Chicago, IL

Pamela J. Haylock, RN, MA, ET (83)
Oncology Consultant
Medina, TX

Jeanne Held-Warmkessel, RN, MSN, CS, AOCN (64)
Clinical Nurse Specialist
Fox Chase Cancer Center
Philadelphia, PA

Wendy Hobbie, RN, MSN, CRNP (26)
Coordinator, Follow-up Program
Children's Hospital of Philadelphia
Associate Program Director
Pediatric Oncology Nurse Practitioner Program
Philadelphia, PA

Laura J. Hilderley, RN, MS (15) (Retired)
Clinical Nurse Specialist, Radiation Oncology
Radiation Oncology Services of Rhode Island
Warwick, RI

Rebecca J. Ingle, RN, MSN, CS, FNP (59)
Family Nurse Practitioner
Saint Thomas Hospital
Adjunct Instructor of Nursing
Vanderbuilt University School of Nursing
Nashville, TN

Joanne K. Itano, RN, PhD, OCN® (7)
Associate Professor
The University of Hawaii at Manoa
School of Nursing
Honolulu, HI

Roberta Kaplow, RN, PhD, CCNS, CCRN (38)
Nurse Educator, Critical Care
Memorial Sloan-Kettering Cancer Center
Deptartment of Nursing Education
New York, NY

Paula R. Klemm, RN, DNSc, OCN® (50, 68)
Associate Professor
University of Delaware, Department of Nursing
Newark, DE

Sharon L. Kozachik, RN, MSN (70)
Project Manager, Research Associate
Family Care Study, Walther Cancer Institute
Michigan State University
East Lansing, MI

Linda U. Krebs, RN, PhD, AOCN (37)
Nursing Oncology Program Leader and Senior Instructor
University of Colorado Cancer Center
University of Colorado School of Nursing
Denver, CO

Sharon Krumm, PhD, RN (74)
Administrator and Director of Nursing
The Johns Hopkins Oncology Center
Baltimore, MD

Dale Halsey Lea, RN, MPH (25)
Assistant Director, Southern Maine Genetics Services
Foundation for Blood Research
Scarborough, ME

Lois J. Loescher, PhDc, RN (2, 8)
Senior Research Specialist
Cancer Prevention and Control
Arizona Cancer Center
Tuscon, AZ

Jean Lydon, RN, MS, AOCN (44)
Manager Oncology Services
Christ Hospital
Oak Lawn, IL

Karen Maher, RN, MS, ANP, AOCN (17)
Adult Nurse Practitioner
Radiation Oncology
Legacy Health System
Portland, OR

Suzanne M. Mahon, RN, DNSc, AOCN (65)
Assistant Clinical Professor
St. Louis University, Division of Hematology and
  Oncology
St. Louis, MO

Virginia R. Martin, MSN, RN, AOCN (62, 75)
Clinical Director, Ambulatory Care
Fox Chase Cancer Center
Philadelphia, PA

Jeanne Marie Martinez, RN, MPH, CHPN (77)
Coordinator, Education & Research for Palliative Medical
Northwestern Memorial Hospice Program
Chicago, IL

Mary Maxwell, RN, PhD (36)
Clinical Specialist/Nurse Practitioner in Oncology
Portland, OR

Roxanne McDaniel, PhD, RN (32)
Associate Professor
Sinclair School of Nursing
University of Missouri–Columbia
Columbia, MO

Deborah B. McGuire, PhD, RN, FAAN (28, 29)
Associate Professor
Director, Oncology Advanced Practice Nursing Program
University of Pennsylvania, School of Nursing
Philadelphia, PA

Mary Ann Miller, PhD, RN (6)
Associate Professor
Department of Nursing
University of Delaware
Newark, DE

Ida M. (Ki) Moore, RN, DNS, FAAN (26)
Professor and Director
Division of Nursing Practice
College of Nursing
University of Arizona
Tucson, AZ

Judith Much, MSN, RN, CRNP, AOCN (69)
Nurse Practioner
The Cancer Institute of New Jersey
New Brunswick, NJ

Patricia G. Nedved, RN, MSN, ACRN (76)
Director of Clinical Services
Northwestern Memorial Home Health Care, Inc.
Chicago, IL

Susan A. O'Connell, MSN, RN, OCN® (23)
Oncology Clinical Nurse Specialist
Amgen, Inc.
Plymouth, MI

Katherine G. O'Connor, RN, MS, ANP (66)
Nurse Practitioner, Medical Oncology Units
Memorial Sloan-Kettering Cancer Center
New York, NY

James C. Pace, DSN, RN, MDiv, ANP-CS, (45)
Associate Professor of Adult and Elder Health Nursing
Nell Hodgson Woodruff School of Nursing
Emory University
Atalanta, GA

Lawrence F. Padberg, PhD (73)
Acting Vice President for Academic Affairs
Marymount University
Arlington, VA

Rose Mary Padberg, RN, MA (73)
Nurse Consultant/Program Director
Division of Cancer Prevention
National Cancer Institute
National Institutes of Health
Bethesda, MD
Nurse Consultant
Office of Associate Director
Early Detection & Community Oncology Division of
    Cancer Prevention National Cancer Inst.
Rockville, MD

Jennifer Petersen RN, MS, OCN® (40)
Oncology Clinical Nurse Specialist
Section of Medical Oncology
Rush Cancer Institute
Rush Presbyterian-St. Luke's Medical Center
Chicago, IL
Clinical Nurse Specialist
Rush Cancer Institute
Chicago, IL

Patricia Piasecki, RN, MS (46)
Clinical Coordinator Orthopedic Oncology
Chicago, IL

Shelley M. Poirier, MS, RN, OCN® (67)
Clinical Nurse Specialist GI Cancer Program
Indiana University Cancer Center
Indiana University School of Medicine
Indianapolis, IN

Rosemary Polomano, PhD, RN, FAAN (29)
Senior Nursing Research Specialist
Center for Patient Services Evaluation, Research and
    Informatics
Milton S. Hershey Medical Center
Hershey, PA

Rita M. Poquette, RN, MSN, FNP, CS (47)
Urology Nurse Practitioner
USC/Kenneth Norris Jr. Cancer Hospital
Los Angeles, CA

Kathy Price, RN, OCN® (22)
Clinical Research Specialist
Vanderbilt Cancer Center
Vanderbilt University
Nashville, TN

Susan M. Rawl, PhD, RN (67)
Postdoctoral Fellow
Indiana University School of Nursing
Indianapolis, IN

Anita M. Reedy, RN, MSN, OCN® (54)
Research Nurse
Johns Hopkins Oncology Center
Baltimore, MD

Mary E. Reid, PhD (5, 8)
Research Instructor
Co-Director, Cancer Prevention and Control Training
    Program
Arizona Cancer Center
Arizona College of Public Health
Tucson, AZ

Verna A. Rhodes, EdS, RN, FAAN (32)
Associate Professor Emeritus
Sinclair School of Nursing
University of Missouri–Columbia
Columbia, MO

Paula Trahan Rieger, RN, MSN, CS, AOCN, FAAN (10)
Nurse Practitioner
Human Clinical Cancer Genetics
Department of Clinical Cancer Prevention
The University of Texas M.D. Anderson Cancer Center
Houston, TX

Mary Roach, MS, RN, AOCN (21)
Hospice Nurse
Presbyterian Healthcare Services
Albuquerque, NM

Kimberly Rohan, MS, RN (52)
Edward Cancer Center
Naperville, IL

Jennifer Rychcik, MS, FNP, ACNP, CS, CETN, OCN® (58)
Acute Care Nurse Practitioner
Department of Surgical Nursing
The Johns Hopkins Hospital
Baltimore, MD

Delores Ann Hubbard Saddler, RN, MSN, CGRN (51)
Clinical Care Coordinator—GI Center
University of Texas
M.D. Anderson Cancer Center
Houston, TX

Vivian R. Scheidler, MS, RN (28, 29)
Senior Clinical Research Scientist
Glaxo Wellcome
Research Triangle Park, NC

Maria Serrano, RN, MSN, CS, NPC, AOCN
Radiation Oncology Nurse Practitioner
Montefiore Medical Center
Bronx, NY

Carol A. Sheridan, RN, MSN, AOCN (61)
Advanced Practice Nurse
Goldens Bridge, NY

Ellen Sitton RN, MSN, OCN® (42)
Advanced Practice Nurse, Radiation Oncology & Education
USC/Kenneth Norris Jr. Cancer Hospital
Los Angeles, CA

Carole Sweeney, MSN, RN, AOCN (69)
Research Assistant
Fox Chase Cancer Center
Philadelphia, PA

Karen N. Taoka, RN, MN, AOCN (7)
Clinical Nurse Specialist, Oncology
The Queen's Medical Center
Patient Care Consulting Services
Honolulu, HI

Elizabeth Johnston Taylor, PhD, RN (71)
Assistant Professor
University of Southern California
Los Angeles, CA

David C. Thomasma, PhD (81)
Director and Professor
Loyola University Chicago
Medical Humanities Program
Maywood, IL

Peter V. Tortorice, PharmD, BCOP (18)
Oncology Clinical Pharmacist
Illinois Masonic Cancer Center
Maywood, IL
Oncology Pharmacy Clinical Coordinator
Loyola University Medical Center
Cardinal Bernardin Cancer Center
Maywood, IL

Janet Ruth Walczak, RN, MSN, CRNP (53)
Nurse Practitioner
Breast Cancer Program
Johns Hopkins Oncology Center
Baltimore, MD

Steven Wagner, RN, BSN, CRNH (77)
Nurse Clinician
Northwestern Memorial Hospice Program
Chicago, IL

Marie Bakitas Whedon, MS, ARNP, FAAN (21)
Research Assistant Professor
Dartmouth Medical School
Palliative Care Nurse Practitioner
Norris Cotton Cancer Center
Lebanon, NH

Vera S. Wheeler, RN, MN, OCN® (24)
Consultant, Cancer Nursing and Biotherapy
Vancouver, WA

Rita Wickham, RN, PhD, AOCN (34, 52)
Associate Professor
Rush College of Nursing
Oncology Clinical Nurse Specialist
Rush-Presbyterian-St. Luke's Medical Center
Chicago, IL

Claire R. Works, RN, MN, ARNP (13, 36)
Nurse Practitioner
Fred Hutchinson Cancer Research Center
Seattle, WA

Debra Wujcik, RN, MSN, AOCN (22, 57)
Director, Clinical Trials Training and Outreach
Vanderbilt Ingram Cancer Center
Adjunct Instructor
Vanderbilt University School of Nursing
Nashville, TN

Deanna Xistris, APRN, MSN, AOCN (75)
Director of Nursing
Hematology Oncology
Carl and Dorothy Bennet Cancer Center
Stamford, CT

Susan G. Yackzan, RN, MSN, AOCN (65)
Oncology Clinical Nurse Specialist
Lexington, KY

Connie Henke Yarbro, RN, MS, FAAN (27, 60)
Clinical Associate Professor
Division of Hematology/Oncology
Adjunct Clinical Assistant Professor
Sinclair School of Nursing
Editors, *Seminars in Oncology Nursing*
University of Missouri–Columbia
Columbia, MO

John W. Yarbro MD, PhD (1,4)
Professor Emeritus, School of Medicine
University of Missouri–Columbia
Columbia, MO
Editor, *Seminars in Oncology*

Katherine A. Yeager, MS, RN (28)
Research Project Coordinator
Rollins School of Public Health
Emory University
Atlanta, GA

Connie Yuska, RN, MS, CORLN (76)
Vice President, Operations
Northwestern Memorial Home Health Care, Inc.
Chicago, IL

The Cancer Problem

CHAPTER 1

Milestones in Our Understanding of Cancer

John W. Yarbro, MD, PhD

Introduction

Cancer is such a fundamental biological problem that to begin to understand it requires a thorough understanding of biology. Multicellular life forms depend for their very existence on the meticulous balance and regulation of reproduction, growth, development, tissue repair, response to injury, and regeneration. Cancer results from an imbalance, a perversion really, of these mechanisms essential to life. It should be no surprise, then, that the historical milestones related to our understanding of cancer read very much like the significant events in the history of medicine.

Cancer has challenged physicians since antiquity. Early speculation as to its cause showed remarkable insight; for example, the relationship of nulliparity to breast cancer in nuns was first scrutinized in the 17th century, and of tobacco to nasal tumors only a few short decades after it was exported to London from the colonies. Some might be surprised to learn that the notion of a cancer research plan was not developed by the National Cancer Institute; rather, it was formulated in Europe two centuries ago.

Despite remarkable progress in the study of cancer over the years, only recently—within the last two decades—has a genuine understanding of the mechanisms of cancer been possible. With new technology came the ability to unravel and study in detail the genetic systems that lie at the heart of neoplastic growth. The story of our evolving knowledge is fascinating, even when limited to its barest outline, as is done here.

Cancer in the Ancient World

The earliest description of cancer appears in the Edwin Smith Papyrus from Egypt in the seventeenth century B.C. After providing the oldest written description of a patient with cancer, the physician advises, "Thou should say concerning him . . . 'There is no treatment.' "[1,p.21]

A thousand years later, Hippocrates, the Father of Medicine, formulated his rules for medical practice in a series of aphorisms. His cardinal aphorism, *Primum non nocere* ("First, do no harm"), is as valid today as it was in the fifth century B.C. It is widely believed that the Greek word for crab, *karkinos,* was first applied to cancer by Hippocrates. Aphorism number 38 states, "It is better not to apply any treatment in cases of occult cancer; for if treated, the patients die quickly; but if not treated, they hold out for a long time."[1,p.23] More times than we like to admit, this aphorism is forgotten today.

Celsus, the great first-century Roman physician, compiled an encyclopedia of medicine, *De medicina,* containing many accurate clinical descriptions of cancer. Careful distinctions were made between benign and malignant disease, along with treatment recommendations. His treatment was like that of Hippocrates. He noted:

After excision, even when a scar has formed, none the less the disease has returned, and caused death; while at the same time the majority of patients, though no violent measures are applied in the attempt to remove the tumor but only mild applications in order to soothe it, attain a ripe old age in spite of it.[1,p.26]

Galen, the second-century Roman physician, was the central medical authority for more than a thousand years because the Church preserved hundreds of his writings and endorsed his views. His influence on the practice of medicine was significant long after the medieval period. Galen viewed cancer much as Hippocrates did, and his views set the pattern for cancer management for centuries.

The Middle Ages saw little progress in Europe, although medicine flourished in Byzantium and Arabia, where civilization persisted after the fall of Rome. The approach to cancer treatment remained Hippocratic (or Galenic) for the most part. There are, however, descriptions of attempts at radical surgery, such as the following Byzantine procedure cited by Shimkin:

I personally am in the habit of operating for cancer arising in the breast thusly: I make the patient lie down; then I incise the healthy part of the breast beyond the cancerous area and I cauterize the incised parts until the blood ceases by the formation of a coating. Then I again incise and excise the breast from its depth and I again cauterize the incised areas. And I repeat this procedure often, first cutting then cauterizing until bleeding stops.[1,p.33]

There was, of course, no mention of anesthesia.

Beginning of Scientific Medicine

The advent of the Renaissance signaled the beginning of medical progress in Europe. With Galileo and Newton in the seventeenth century, there began what can legitimately be called the scientific method. William Harvey's *De Motu Cordis* in 1628, describing the circulation of the blood, provides the foundation for scientific cardiology. In 1761 Giovanni Morgagni of Padua was the first to correlate the clinical course of cancer to the gross pathological findings at autopsy, laying the groundwork for scientific oncology.

Finally, in the eighteenth century, the great Scot surgeon, John Hunter, provided descriptions of the surgery of cancer that would bring nods of approval from modern surgeons:

Great attention should be paid to the tumor, whether it is moveable or not, for as the disease is further extended so the parts are more united to the tumor. If the tumor is not only moveable but the part naturally so, then there is no impropriety in removing it. . . . [I]f any consequent cancers easy of extirpation are found, they may be safely removed also. But it requires very great caution to know if any of these consequent tumors are within proper reach, for we are apt to be deceived in regard to the lymphatic glands, which often appear moveable when, on extirpation, a chain of them is found to run far beyond out of our reach which renders the operation unsuccessful.[1,p.86]

A century was to pass before the development of anesthesia allowed the great surgeons of the nineteenth century to develop radical cancer operations such as the classic radical mastectomy, the principles of which can be recognized in the lectures of John Hunter.

Early Epidemiologists

The Egyptians blamed cancers on various gods. Hippocrates explained all diseases as resulting from an imbalance of the four humors, in the case of cancer an excess of black bile. For more than a thousand years, Galen and others echoed Hippocrates. Then, as Europe entered the Age of Reason, Bernardino Ramazzini, an Italian physician, noted the high incidence of breast cancer in nuns and hypothesized that this was in some way related to their celibate lifestyle.[1,p.92] The age of cancer epidemiology had begun.

John Hill of London was the first to recognize the dangers of tobacco.[1,p.93;2] In 1761, only a few decades after tobacco became popular in London, he published a description of his observations entitled, *Cautions Against the Immoderate Use of Snuff,* and subtitled, "Founded on the known Qualities of the Tobacco Plant and the Effects it must produce when this Way taken into the Body and Enforced by Instances of Persons who have perished miserably of Diseases, occasioned, or rendered incurable by its Use."[2,p.19]

The oft-cited description of scrotal cancer in chimney sweeps by Percival Pott of St Bartholomew's Hospital in London[3] was, according to Shimkin,[1,p.95] the third in a series of reports that launched the field of cancer epidemiology. It has remained the most frequently cited example and has dramatically influenced our view of cancer epidemiology and etiology. As we now know, however, it is the "immoderate use of snuff" that today is our major cancer problem.

The First Plan for the Scientific Study of Cancer

At the beginning of the nineteenth century a committee of English physicians and surgeons formed to investigate the nature of cancer formulated thirteen questions, the research significance of which would be instantly recognized by any cancer scientist today.[4] Many of these questions were quite profound:

> Are there premalignant lesions? If so, "though we are unable to cure cancer in an advanced stage, we might extinguish the disposition to it or suppress it completely in an early stage."

> "Are there any proofs of cancer being an hereditary disease?"

> Is cancer infectious? Do some diseases degenerate into cancer?

> "May cancer be regarded at any period or under any circumstances as merely a local disease?"

> "Are brute creatures subject to any disease resembling cancer in the human body?" If so, investigation of cancer in animals "may lead to much philosophical amusement and useful information; particularly it may teach us how far the prevalence or frequency of cancer may depend upon the manners and habits of life."

This systematic approach to cancer biology laid the foundation for scientific progress in the nineteenth century. For those of us who watched the National Cancer Plan evolve in the United States after passage of the National Cancer Act in 1971, such a systematic set of questions strikes a familiar cord, particularly because some of the questions asked in 1800 were asked again almost two centuries later.

Cancer Pathology and Ideas About Metastasis

The nineteenth century saw the birth of scientific oncology as the focus shifted from anatomy to pathology. Early in the century, a microscope of sufficient quality for research on tissues became available. The German physiologist Johannes Müller applied this instrument to cancer research and began to correlate cellular pathology with clinical symptoms. He established a cellular basis for tumor description. Subsequently, this work was carried on by the man usually described as the founder of cellular pathology, Rudolf Virchow of Berlin, who provided the scientific basis for the modern pathological study of cancer. As Morgagni had correlated the gross autopsy findings with the clinical history of illness, so now the microscopic findings were similarly correlated.

Rudolf Virchow established the microscopic basis for the characterization of cancer. But even Virchow failed to recognize the cellular nature of metastasis. He believed that circulating cancer cells in the blood would be trapped by the lungs, and he concluded:

> The manner in which the metastatic diffusion takes place seems, on the contrary, to render it probable that the transference takes place by means of certain fluids, and that these possess the power of producing an infection which disposes different parts to a reproduction of a mass of the same nature as that which originally existed. . . . There are, however, many facts, which speak but little in favor of the infection's taking place by means of really detached cells, for example, the circumstance that certain processes advance in a direction contrary to that of the current of lymph, so that after cancer of the breast, disease of the liver takes place whilst the lung remains unaffected. Here it seems pretty

probable that juices are taken up, which occasion a further propagation.[5,pp.219,460]

Wilhelm Waldeyer of Berlin did not agree that cancer metastases resulted from some kind of noncellular infectious substance; he believed that embolic transfer through the blood or lymph channels was the mechanism.[6] The pathologic basis of malignancy was gradually understood, and pathology began to replace anatomy as the key basic science.

The Century of the Surgeon 1846–1946 Begins

Soporific and narcotic agents had been used for centuries to control the pain of surgery. The effect of nitrous oxide (laughing gas) had been noted and led to its social use at parties in the nineteenth century. The suggestion that it might reduce surgical pain was not investigated. Hypnotism also had been used to control pain, but this practice was not accepted by the medical profession. Dr. Crawford Long of Georgia used sulfuric ether in 1842 but did not report his findings. Horace Wells, a dentist, attempted to demonstrate the anesthetic effect of laughing gas before a medical school class at Harvard, but the patient cried out and the dentist was summarily booed and hissed.[7]

Finally, in 1846 ether was definitively shown to control pain. John C. Warren, a Boston surgeon, trained under Astley Cooper in London, who had studied under the great Scot surgeon John Hunter, who had studied with Percival Pott. In 1846 Warren performed the first reported operation on a patient anesthetized with ether; dentist William Thomas Morton administered the ether. The absence of pain in his patient led Warren to observe, "Gentlemen, this is no humbug!"[7]

Oliver Wendell Holmes coined the term *anesthesia*. Prior to this time, the notion of anesthesia had bordered on quackery, and it was not widely accepted. The Calvinist church fathers in England decried its use for childbirth, citing the biblical admonition that women must bring forth children in pain. But Queen Victoria elected to use chloroform anesthesia during the birth of one of her many children, and this brought about general public acceptance.[7]

Anesthesia propelled surgery into the modern era. Prior to the discovery of anesthesia, there were great surgeons, among them John Hunter, Astley Cooper, and John Warren. But when anesthesia became available at mid-century, there emerged surgical giants whose work so rapidly advanced the art that the next hundred years became known as "the century of the surgeon."[8] Three surgeons stand out because of their contributions to the art of cancer surgery: Bilroth in Germany, Handley in London, and Halsted at Johns Hopkins. Their work led to the "cancer operation" designed to remove all of the tumor en bloc as well as the lymph nodes that normally drained the region where the tumor was located.

Nursing Becomes a Profession

Eight years after John Warren concluded that anesthesia was "no humbug," Florence Nightingale led a party of thirty-eight nurses on a mission of mercy to the Crimean War. When she returned to England in 1856, the care of the sick and the operation of hospitals were never to be the same again. She described nursing as the "finest of the fine arts,"[9,p.68] and she noted its uniqueness by observing that "nursing and medicine should never be mixed up. It spoils both."[9,p.68] She also demanded influence for nurses: "[D]octors are very liable to imagine they must have the control of the whole staff,"[9,p.54] and echoed Hippocrates' cardinal aphorism, relating it to hospitals: "[A] first requirement is that a hospital should do the sick no harm."[9,p.49] She advocated preventive medicine policies far ahead of her time when she said she wanted to "inoculate the country with the view of preventing instead of cure."[9,p.39]

Nursing is, of course, older than Florence Nightingale. There were many unnamed and unrecognized women (can we doubt that they were women?) who, from the beginning, gave to the sick that solicitude, understanding, and attention to the *human* response to illness that is the essence of nursing. But Florence Nightingale gave the hospital the professional nurse and began that tradition of scholarship and dedication that continues today in oncology nursing. She identified the uniqueness in the practice of nursing that was not the same as the practice of medicine, and she based the professionalism of nursing on that uniqueness.

The Dogma of the Anatomical Containment of Cancer

William Stewart Halsted, professor of surgery at Johns Hopkins University, developed the radical mastectomy during the last decade of the nineteenth century. His work was based in part on that of W. Sampson Handley, the London surgeon who believed that cancer spread centrifugally through the lymphatics in continuity with the original growth.[10] Halsted's concept of the natural history and biology of cancer and its treatment are best described in his own words:

> We believe with Handley that cancer of the breast in spreading centrifugally preserves in the main continuity with the original growth. . . . Although it undoubtedly occurs, I am not sure that I have observed from breast cancer, metastasis which seemed definitely to have been conveyed by way of the blood vessels. . . . [T]here comes to the surgeon an encouragement to greater endeavor. . . [W]e must remove not only a very large amount of skin and a much larger area of subcutaneous fat and fascia, but also strip the sheaths from the upper part of the rectus, the serratus magnus, the subscapularis, and at times from parts of the latissimus dorsi and teres major. Both pectoral muscles are, of course, removed. . . . It must be our endeavor to trace more definitely

the routes traveled in metastasis to bone, particularly the humerus, for it is even possible in cases of involvement of this bone that amputation of the shoulder joint plus a proper removal of the soft parts might eradicate the disease. So too it is conceivable that ultimately, when our knowledge of the lymphatics traversed in cases of femur involvement becomes sufficiently exact, amputation at the hip joint may seem indicated.[11,p.4]

The Halsted and Handley doctrine stated simply that cancer is contained within anatomical compartments and can be cured by radical resection en bloc of these compartments. This became the basis of the "cancer operation," the dogma that dominated cancer surgery for almost a century until it was called into question by the work of two twentieth-century surgeons.

Early Clinical Clues to Cancer Biology

At the same time Halsted and Handley were developing their radical operations based on their interpretation of the spread of breast cancer, another surgeon was asking, "What is it that decides which organs shall suffer in a case of disseminated cancer?" Stephen Paget wrote, "I have collected 735 fatal cases of cancer of the breast in each of which a necropsy was made and recorded," and he concluded that cancer cells spread by way of the bloodstream and, further, that the disproportion of metastases to certain organs "cannot be due to chance."[12,p.572] In a brilliant leap of logic Paget drew an analogy between cancer metastasis and seeds, which "are carried in all directions, but they can only live and grow if they fall on congenial soil."

Paget had concluded that cells from a primary tumor are able to grow in only certain other organs—not in any organ in which they happen to come to rest. This accurate but highly sophisticated hypothesis was confirmed by the techniques of modern molecular biology almost a hundred years later.[13] Paget, on the basis of careful pathological examination at hundreds of autopsies, drew the correct conclusion, whereas others viewing the same autopsy material, including Virchow and Halsted, drew the wrong conclusion. The implications for the treatment of cancer based on these findings are substantially different—indeed, in some ways quite the opposite. Paget's work contributed to the new biological understanding of cancer that is integral to the breast conservation surgery introduced in recent years.

First Endocrine Therapy of Cancer

The end of the nineteenth century saw publication of a second seminal but neglected paper. Thomas Beatson graduated from the University of Edinburgh in 1874 and developed an interest in lactation and ovarian function because he lived near a large sheep farm in rural Scotland. In 1878 he investigated the effect on the breasts of removing the ovaries of rabbits and found that lactation continued so long as the young were suckling, but that the breasts atrophied and became fatty after suckling ceased. He described his thoughts in a lecture to the Edinburgh Medico-Chirurgical Society in 1896:

> This fact seemed to me of great interest, for it pointed to one organ holding control over the secretion of another and separate organ. . . . I was struck by the local proliferation of epithelium seen in lactation. Here was the very thing characteristic of carcinoma of the breast, and indeed, of the cancerous process everywhere, but differing from it in that it was held in control by another organ.[14,p.105]

Because the breast was "held in control" by the ovaries, Beatson decided to test oophorectomy in advanced breast cancer. The first patient he treated presented with a massive local recurrence. Regression of the recurrent tumor began 5 weeks after the operation, and by 8 months "all vestiges of her previous cancerous disease had disappeared."[14,p.106] His second patient had a far-advanced inoperable primary breast cancer, and oophorectomy led to a good partial remission. His third patient, also having an advanced inoperable primary tumor, showed continued progression after oophorectomy.

These findings led Beatson to speculate that "the ovaries may be the exciting cause of carcinoma"[14,p.106] in women with breast cancer, an observation of particular note in view of our present large trials of tamoxifen as a preventive in breast cancer. Here, for the first time, was an experimental observation that illustrated the potential for systemic treatment of cancer.

A half century after Beatson, Charles Huggins, a urologist at the University of Chicago, reported dramatic regression of metastatic prostate cancer following castration.[15,16] In 1966 Huggins received the Nobel Prize.

Radiation Therapy for Cancer

In 1896, halfway through the century of the surgeon, a remarkable lecture was presented by Wilhelm Conrad Roentgen, a German physics professor from Würzburg. This lecture was to provide the clinician with a second modality of cancer therapy. Actually, the lecture was published before it was delivered because the editor of the journal recognized its major importance and rushed it into print. The paper was entitled, *Uber eine neue Art von Strahlen* ("Concerning a new kind of ray"), which Roentgen called the *x-ray*, "x" being the algebraic symbol for the unknown.[17]

There was immediate worldwide excitement. Roentgen's experiments were carefully confirmed and their significance widely recognized. Within months, systems were being devised to use x-rays for diagnosis and, remarkably, within 3 years radiation was used in the treatment of cancer. In 1901 Roentgen received the first Nobel Prize awarded in physics.

Radiation therapy began as brachytherapy with radium and as external beam therapy with relatively low-voltage diagnostic machines. It was in France that the major break-through took place when it was discovered that delivering radiation over a protracted period of time by use of daily fractions would greatly improve therapeutic response.[18]

Discovery of Radiation, Viral, and Chemical Carcinogenesis

The nineteenth century had begun with thirteen questions; the twentieth century opened with three important answers. In the short span of 13 years, radiation, viral, and chemical carcinogenesis were clearly demonstrated. These three discoveries changed the entire focus of cancer research.

Radiation was recognized as a carcinogen only 7 years after Roentgen's discovery of x-rays,[19] and a few years later a relationship to leukemia was recognized.[20] Early workers must have received massive doses of radiation for the clinical association between radiation and cancer to be noticed in such a short time. By comparison, the excess cancer deaths in the Hiroshima and Nagasaki populations were only about 8 percent, and leukemia was seen at an incidence of only about 1.5 cases per million people per year per rad of dose.[21]

In 1911 Peyton Rous, at the Rockefeller Institute, described a sarcoma in chickens caused by what later became known as the Rous sarcoma virus.[22] He ground up a tumor of chickens and passed it through a paper filter to remove the cells. He then injected this cell-free filtrate into chickens. "From a bit inoculated into the breast muscle of a susceptible fowl there develops rapidly a large firm growth; metastasis takes place to the viscera; and within four weeks the host dies."[22,p.1445] Since neither bacteria nor cells could pass through the filter, the idea that cancer might be caused by a virus was given firm experimental support. A half century later, the Rous virus was the source of the first well-characterized oncogene.

In 1915 cancer was induced in laboratory animals for the first time by coal tar applied to rabbit skin, at Tokyo University by Yamagiwa and Ichikawa.[23] The field of chemical carcinogenesis was launched with a firm scientific foundation and a research technique. This was a century and a half after the most destructive chemical carcinogen known to man, tobacco, was first identified by the astute clinician John Hill. The aniline dyes had been found to be related epidemiologically to bladder cancer in humans.[24] The first potent synthetic laboratory carcinogen, dibenzanthracene, was discovered in 1930.[25] It was to be many years until we "rediscovered" tobacco as a carcinogen.[26–28]

Cancer Treatment and Biology, 1900–1950

After Halsted, cancer surgery became synonymous with the radical resection of a cancer and its draining lymph node groups, in the hope of removing the tumor before it spread. The most welcome words a patient could hear after an operation were, "We got it all." Radiation therapy was viewed as a means of eradicating local and regional disease that was not resectable by the surgeon. Systemic therapy was virtually nonexistent. The "seed and soil" concept of Paget was forgotten.

Based on several good experiments, cancer was believed to be caused by chemicals or radiation. But the idea was widely held that a single change in the cell somehow transformed it to a malignant growth, and this clouded our thinking for many years until we learned that multiple genetic changes are required for transformation and that during this step by step process the cell evolves by natural selection through increasingly malignant phases of growth. Lymph nodes were thought to trap cancer cells, and the notion of regional spread and anatomic containment formed the basis for therapeutic strategy. The clinical behavior of cancer was well understood but not in modern terms. Progress was held back by the failure to understand multistage carcinogenesis and to grasp the relationship of clonal selection during progression to the metastasis of cancer. A key discovery was made by Peyton Rous.

In 1935 Peyton Rous, still at the Rockefeller Institute, was studying the manner in which a benign neoplasm, virus-induced rabbit papilloma, transformed into a malignant lesion. He reported:

> The early stages of the cancerous change cannot be comprehensively described without inclusion of the entire course of events in vigorous papillomas. These tend toward malignancy from the beginning and attain it by a continuous series of alterations. . . . Often the alterations which lead to carcinosis do not stop when malignancy has been achieved, but go further until a state of great anaplasia has been attained. The postcancerous changes appear to be no separate course of events, but only a continuation of what was long since begun. These facts might be taken to indicate that the virus is the immediate cause for the carcinosis; yet they are compatible with the assumption that it merely provides an essential, preliminary cell disturbance.[29,p.537]

In a subsequent paper, Rous reported his research with another model of carcinogenesis, the induction of skin cancers by the application of coal tar. It was in this paper that he most clearly defined the difference between what he termed *initiation* and *promotion*:

> Tarring provides them with the conditions needed for growth, but after it is discontinued the tumors all more or less gradually disappear unless some other aid is forthcoming. . . . Chloroform has a marked effect to cause latent neoplastic cells to form tumors, as we discovered by accident. Occasionally the external auditory canal of ears long previously painted with methylcholanthrene and still carrying growths became infested with mites. To kill them, chloroform was dropped into the canal and in several instances, through a technician's error, it was used for nearly two months and allowed to spread to the surface of the ear. There the skin became swollen and pink and many additional tumors arose and grew rapidly. . . . It seems certain that many agents and

influences which have no actual carcinogenicity will be found to stimulate the multiplication of latent neoplastic cells. . . . [T]his is distinct from carcinogenic power.[30,p.111]

These classic experiments, confirmed by Berenblum and Shubik[31] using croton oil as the promoter, formed the prototype for the way carcinogenesis was conceptualized. This led to the concept of *initiation* by one agent followed by *promotion* by another and finally *progression* of the tumor to a more malignant form. The initiator was viewed as a cancer-causing agent but only after a prolonged time. The promoter alone was viewed as not always capable of causing cancer but able to potentiate the effects of the initiator. The term *progression* was said by Rous to designate "the process by which tumors go from bad to worse."[32]

Foulds codified and expanded the concept of multistage carcinogenesis.[33] Progression to the metastatic phenotype has subsequently been well elucidated in modern biological terms by Fidler.[34] Evidence was obtained 20 years after Rous's work, indicating that the first stage, *initiation*, is characterized by damage to DNA, while the second stage, *promotion*, does not usually involve damage to DNA but, rather, stimulation of cellular proliferation. Promotion is reversible and exhibits a distinct dose response and measurable threshold that may be important in regard to environmental carcinogenesis. The third stage, *progression*, leads to morphological change and increased grades of malignant behavior, such as invasion, metastasis, and drug resistance. The highly malignant character that the cancer has attained at the time of diagnosis is the result of progression. In 1966, 55 years after his 1911 paper, Peyton Rous was awarded the Nobel Prize.

The simple sequence of initiation-promotion-progression formed the basis for numerous experiments that revealed the sequence was far more complex in humans than in the simple laboratory animal systems. Inactivation of multiple genes and activation of many other genes was shown to be necessary for cancer development, and occasionally the inheritance of a cancer susceptibility gene played a role. Nonetheless, the concepts of initiation and progression are useful in our conceptualization of the malignant process.

Beginning of Chemotherapy

The century of the surgeon began in 1846. Fifty years later, Roentgen presented his famous lecture on the x-ray. Exactly 100 years after the beginning of the century of the surgeon, the first anticancer activity of a chemical was reported, and an opportunity was provided for treatment that went beyond local and regional removal or destruction of tissue. Today the term *chemotherapy* is applied to cytotoxic agents used in the treatment of cancer. Nitrogen mustard was the first such agent.

Nitrogen mustard was developed by the chemical war-fare research division of the U.S. Army in the course of a search for agents more effective than the mustard gas used in World War I. Nitrogen mustard proved to have remarkable activity against the lymphomas; "[i]ndeed, the results were sometimes dramatic."[35] This agent served as the model for a long series of alkylating agents that killed rapidly proliferating cancer cells by damaging their DNA.

Two years later Sidney Farber of Boston reported the efficacy of aminopterin, the predecessor of methotrexate.[36] Subsequently, Hitchings and Elion developed the antimetabolite 6-mercaptopurine,[37] and Charles Heidelberger developed 5-fluorouracil.[38] The era of chemotherapy had begun. The first cure of metastatic cancer was obtained in 1956 by the use of methotrexate in choriocarcinoma.[39] In 1988 Hitchings and Elion received the Nobel Prize.

Research led to the discovery of many new chemotherapeutic agents, and the efficacy of multiagent chemotherapy was established. Fifty years of controlled clinical trials have now identified many cancers that are curable by chemotherapy alone or in combination with other modalities.

Discovery That Carcinogenesis Results from Mutations

It was not until 1944 that DNA was demonstrated to be the chemical mediator of heredity.[40] The Nobel Prize–winning discovery of the helical structure of DNA by Watson and Crick followed.[41] Classic work by the Millers had led to the understanding that covalent binding within the cell was essential for carcinogenic activity, and the active metabolites of carcinogens were later identified as electrophilic reactants that bind to DNA.[42] Carcinogens were found to be converted by a series of metabolic steps into free radicals, that is, compounds with a single unpaired electron that are highly reactive with molecules rich in electrons, such as DNA. Compounds called *antioxidants* inhibit carcinogenesis because they react with free radicals before the free radicals damage DNA.

A key discovery was made by Ames, who developed a classic assay system to measure carcinogens.[43] The assay, which employs bacteria, is based on the fact that most carcinogens are mutagens; that is, they damage DNA. The Ames system requires the addition of liver enzymes in order to convert the chemicals to be tested into their active form. The metabolism of a carcinogen leads to the final active chemical, called the *proximate carcinogen*, that reacts with the DNA.

The Ames assay, of course, only identifies mutagens. And whereas most carcinogens are mutagens, not *all* carcinogens are mutagens, and not all mutagens are carcinogens. To prove carcinogenicity, substantially more than merely a positive Ames assay is required. In smokers, for instance, it is possible to directly identify the carcinogen bound to DNA, the so-called *hydrocarbon adducts*.[44] The proximate carcinogen exerts its effect by binding to DNA and mutating it directly or by causing errors to be made when the host cell tries to repair the damaged DNA. However, many of the lesions produced by carcinogens are repaired. The best evidence for this is the extraordinary incidence of skin cancer in patients with xeroderma pigmentosum, a disease in which patients are unable to repair DNA damage from ultraviolet light.[45]

In the mid-twentieth century cancer biology was beginning to take form, but, as we shall see, the problems were exceedingly complex. An important next step was to correct the idea of anatomical containment, and this was done in the clinic rather than in the laboratory.

The New Biology of Cancer Challenges the Classic Dogma

Our recognition of the futility of radical surgery in the management of cancer began with randomized trials in breast cancer and malignant melanoma. Two surgeons, Fisher[46,47] and Veronesi,[48–50] led the way to the overthrow of the classic "cancer operation" by their demonstration that survival in breast cancer and melanoma is independent of the extent of surgical resection. The Halsted radical mastectomy was relegated to the ash heap of history, and the whole question of the "cancer operation" was thrown open to experimental trial. This not only forced a recognition that our treatment methods must change but also, and of greater importance, led to a reevaluation of our notion of the anatomic containment of cancer and to an understanding that it is our biology, not our anatomy, that restricts cancer spread.

This revolution was not easily accepted. I will always recall Dr. Bernard Fisher's calm response from the podium at a surgical society meeting when an irate questioner challenged his data by almost shouting, "You're saying we don't have to remove the lymph nodes to cure the cancer?" Dr. Fisher's answer: "I'm not saying it. The data are saying it."

What was not understood by those for whom anatomy was central to cancer spread was that cancer cells spread throughout the body from the time the first capillaries are attracted into the growing tumor by the angiogenesis factor secreted by the tumor cells. The initial capillary membranes growing into minute tumors are incomplete. Tumor cells spread into the bloodstream from the very beginning but are unable to establish metastatic deposits because the cells have not yet evolved the capacity to proliferate outside the site of the primary tumor. The most dramatic modern clinical example of this principle occurs when ovarian carcinomatosis is treated by shunting the ascitic fluid and cells into the jugular vein: There are no systemic metastases, even though ovarian cancer cells flow throughout the body in huge numbers.[51]

Rous had observed experimental tumor cells "going from bad to worse," and he recognized that it was this change that made metastasis possible, not the breakdown of some anatomic barrier. Time is indeed a factor, as simple clinical experience has long indicated; however, time is required not to overcome some anatomic containment but, rather, to allow evolution of the cells of the primary tumor into subclones capable of metastatic growth. This is a vitally important distinction because it has implications for alternate therapeutic strategies. Establishing the genetic basis of this biological behavior required elucidation of the genes that cause cancer, oncogenes.

Identification of Oncogenes, The Genes Mutated in Cancer

Researchers in chemical carcinogenesis identified mutagens, but the target genes of the mutagens were unknown. Virologists identified cancer-causing viruses, but their mechanism of carcinogenesis was obscure. These two separate lines of research would soon dramatically intersect.

A large number of oncogenic viruses were discovered in laboratory animal systems. They were originally called *type C viruses* and later *retroviruses;* the latter term applied because RNA viruses are converted to DNA by the enzyme reverse transcriptase. Retroviral DNA is then incorporated into the chromosomes of the infected cell; thus, retroviruses add their genes to the cell and in this way influence the cell's behavior.

Huebner and Todaro focused attention on the word *oncogene* in 1969 when they proposed that RNA viruses somehow placed viral genes in the human genome that were then genetically transmitted.[52] The idea that the targets of carcinogens were retroviral genes inserted into the genome was incorrect, except in the isolated cell systems. However, the notion of the oncogene as being the target of mutagens persisted.

Basic experiments in retroviral carcinogenesis used animal systems and cell-culture systems to demonstrate that the intact virus and isolated genes were able to induce malignant transformation. This facilitated the identification of *oncogenes,* the specific genes of oncogenic viruses that were capable of causing cancer. A host of retroviruses that caused animal cancers and transformed cells in culture were identified, and each was found to contain an essential cancer-causing gene that was named after the virus.

Genes are usually designated by a three-letter code in lowercase italics, sometimes preceded by a v- for viral gene or a c- for cellular gene. The abbreviation for the gene often relates to the system in which it was first discovered; for example, *ras* was discovered in a rat sarcoma, and *sis* was discovered in a simian sarcoma. Some genes such as *erb*B or H-*ras* have names that do not fit this system exactly.

It is customary to designate human genes using uppercase italic letters; for example, the human homologue of the animal gene *myc* is written *MYC*. Genes are also designated by letters describing the disease in which they were discovered: *RB* for retinoblastoma gene, *WT* for Wilms' tumor gene, *DCC* for deleted in colon cancer, and so on. Some writers use the term *proto-oncogene* to designate normal genes before they are modified (mutated) to become oncogenes. Other writers use the term *oncogene* as a general term for both the normal and the mutated gene. The protein product of a gene is often named after the gene but using only an initial capital letter: thus, the protein product of the gene *FAS* would be written Fas.

Two important discoveries led to the understanding that oncogenes were growth factor genes. It was found that the gene v-*sis* of the simian sarcoma virus coded for a protein that was very similar to platelet-derived growth factor (PDGF),[53,54] which is released by blood platelets in a clot to stimulate scar formation. Second, the gene v-*erb*B of the chicken erythroblastosis virus was found to be very similar to the gene coding for the epidermal growth factor (EGF) receptor.[55] These discoveries provided strong support for the hypothesis that the oncogenes found in retroviruses were the same as the growth factor and the growth factor receptor genes found in normal cells. Subsequently, other growth factor genes were discovered to be related to oncogenes in animal systems. These growth factor genes that when mutated form oncogenes are sometimes called *proto-oncogenes.*

It is now known that experimental retroviruses obtain their oncogenes by capture of normal genes from the host cell. The retroviral carcinogenesis experiments did not lead, as was first hoped, to identification of a large number of retroviruses that caused human cancer. Among the human retroviruses, human T-lymphotropic virus-1 (HTLV-1) has been clearly implicated in adult T-cell leukemia/lymphoma (ATLL), which is a malignancy of mature T4 lymphocytes endemic in Japan, the Caribbean, parts of Africa, and the southeastern United States.[57] Transmission of the virus is by sexual contact or through contaminated blood. The story on the retrovirus HIV in AIDS-related tumors is interesting but not yet complete.[58]

Retroviral oncogene research did, however, allow for the identification of many human oncogenes that code for normal growth-promoting substances and improved our understanding of the way in which oncogenes promote normal and neoplastic growth. Oncogenes have been identified for many cell signals in addition to growth factors and growth-factor receptors. These include signal amplification and transmission within the cell and signal reception within the nucleus.[58]

We now know that it is the human growth control genes, first identified as oncogenes in retroviruses, that are the long-sought-after targets of the mutating chemicals and radiation that contribute certain critical lesions leading to human cancer. But mutated proto-oncogenes alone are not sufficient to cause human malignancies. Fusing a cancer cell with a normal cell will lead to suppression of malignant growth,[59] indicating that there are genes that suppress growth. These suppressor genes were first demonstrated as the targets of the oncogene products of the DNA viruses.

Identification of Cancer Suppressor Genes ("Anti-Oncogenes")

The DNA viruses are involved in several tumors. Unlike the retroviruses, the oncogenes of DNA viruses are not recently captured cellular genes, and thus they do not have such a close structural relationship to human genes. Instead, their products react with the products of human genes. The first demonstration of this was the interaction of a protein of adenovirus with the *RB* gene product.[60]

The mechanisms of carcinogenesis by the DNA viruses are more complex than is the case for retroviruses. Three examples illustrate this complexity. The polyomavirus produces an oncogenic protein that binds to a cellular oncogene protein product (c-Src). This binding alters the c-Src protein so that it resembles that of the protein produced by the retroviral v-*src* of the Rous sarcoma virus. It would seem that the polyomavirus achieves the same end point as the Rous sarcoma virus, but by a somewhat different mechanism.

A second example is illustrated by the Epstein-Barr virus (EBV), a herpes virus. In patients with Burkitt lymphoma, a characteristic chromosomal translocation is seen that activates the *c-MYC* gene located on chromosome 8. This is the same proto-oncogene activated by the chicken myeloid leukemia retrovirus, but the mechanism of activation by the DNA virus is different from that of the retrovirus.

The third example involves three viruses (simian virus 40, papilloma, and adenovirus), all of which transform cells by producing oncogenic proteins that bind to normal cellular proteins and block their function. The function of the affected cellular proteins is to "turn off" cellular proliferation; they are of very special interest because they are the products of antioncogenes (cancer-suppressor genes).[61] Cancer-suppressor genes are as important as oncogenes in the biology of cancer

Whereas oncogenes code for proteins that induce malignant growth by "turning on" cell division, cancer-suppressor genes code for proteins with an opposite function, to "turn off" cell growth. Since the genes coding for these proteins had a function opposite to that of oncogenes, initially they were called *antioncogenes;* because they suppress malignant growth, now they are called *cancer-suppressor genes*. The absence of the protein product of one of these genes leads to a cell in which the effect of a growth-promoting factor goes unopposed. It is thought that most human cancers result from a combination of genetic changes that must include both the absence of the protein products of cancer-suppressor genes and the presence of abnormal products of oncogenes.

It is likely that for each "up-regulating" function coded by an oncogene there is a balancing "down-regulating" function coded by a cancer-suppressor gene. For example, to balance the protein kinases that activate molecules by phosphorylation, there exists a set of protein phosphorylases that inactivate the same molecule by dephosphorylation.[62-64] This down-regulating antioncogene system is at least as complicated as the up-regulating oncogene system, but it is only beginning to be understood.

The scientific basis for our understanding of this mechanism was laid and the first human cancer-suppressor gene was postulated in 1971 when Alfred Knudson argued, on the basis of a statistical model, that one of the two mutations required for the development of familial retinoblastoma was inherited and the second occurred in the retinal cells of the affected eye. In the nonheritable form, both mutations occurred in the same cell after birth, with neither mutation being inherited.[65] The gene has now been identified on chromosome 13 and named the *retinoblastoma gene (RB)*. The inheritance is dominant, but both copies of the gene must be absent or damaged for a cell to be transformed. We therefore know that the function of the gene is to prevent malignant growth; for example, when the retinoblastoma gene is introduced into cultured retinoblastoma cells, the malignant growth pattern is suppressed.[66]

Transcription factors are proteins that bind specifically to DNA and initiate expression of a set of genes controlled by the binding site. The *MYC* oncogene produces a transcription factor that stimulates cell division. The *RB* antioncogene product binds to the *MYC* oncogene product and blocks its action, which is presumed to be a normal physiologic control function because mutant RB protein does *not* bind MYC protein.[67] The conclusion is that the protein product of the *RB* antioncogene down-regulates cell division by binding to a growth-stimulating normal cellular protein.[68-70] In tumor cells, presumably, the failure of the mutant RB protein to bind the MYC or another transcription factor contributes to transformation. Interactions of this sort, up-regulation balanced by down-regulation, are present in large numbers and are responsible for the control of cell growth. Disruption of several of these interactions is necessary to transform a cell to malignant growth.

Retinoblastoma protein is regulated by the master cell cycle-control enzyme cdc2 kinase.[71] As a suppressor of cell division, the *RB* gene product competes with stimulating factors, such as cyclin A, for the same transcription factors.[72] When the *RB* gene is mutated, its normal suppression of cell division is absent, thus allowing for neoplastic growth.[73] The *RB* gene is commonly mutated in several human cancers, although it was first discovered in retinoblastoma.

Mutator Phenotype

As human cancers were being studied for mutations of the oncogenes and cancer-suppressor genes, it became clear that the number of such mutations was exceedingly large in all human tumors—too large, in fact, to be explained by the simple action of carcinogens on human cells. The spontaneous mutation rate in normal cells is simply not high enough to account for all the mutations seen in cancer cells.[74] This suggests that an early step in carcinogenesis is the induction of a mutator phenotype, a cell that mutates rapidly.

How is this mutator phenotype produced? Spontaneous mutations occur regularly in all cells. There are enzymes that repair these mutations, termed the "caretakers" of the genome.[75] By repairing damage to proto-oncogenes and cancer-suppressor genes these caretaker genes act indirectly to prevent cancer. Examples are the mismatch repair genes involved in hereditary nonpolyposis colorectal cancer, the gene associated with ataxia-telangiectasia, and the breast and ovarian cancer susceptibility gene *BRCA1*.[76] Inheritance of mutated repair genes, or spontaneous mutation of one of these genes, allows an increased mutation rate that may ultimately lead to malignant transformation.

Guardian of the Genome

One of the most important of the cancer-suppressor genes, and the one that appears to be the most commonly altered in human cancer, is the gene located at chromosome 17p13 that codes for a protein designated p53.[77] The *p53* gene is the most frequently mutated gene in human cancer, being altered in as many as half of the common neoplasms.[78] This gene codes for a transcription factor that, in the form of a dimer or tetramer, binds specifically[79] to DNA and mediates RNA synthesis. Originally identified in cells transformed by simian virus 40 and believed to be an oncogene product because mutant forms exerted a dominant transforming effect on cells, *p53* finally has been recognized as a cancer-suppressor gene product. Addition of the *p53* gene to cultures of prostate cancer suppresses malignant growth.[80]

The *p53* cancer-suppressor gene is the most important suppressor gene so far discovered. Not only is it the most frequently mutated, but when it is not mutated, as is the case in some sarcomas, there is another abnormal gene activated that blocks the p53 protein.[81]

What is the normal function of *p53*? Several observations provide clues. When cellular DNA is damaged by radiation or radiomimetic drugs, p53 protein accumulates and the cells are arrested in G1 so that they do not enter mitosis until the DNA is repaired.[82,83] When normal *p53* genes are inserted into cancer cells, they may induce apoptosis (programmed cell death).[84] There is a cancer family syndrome, the Li-Fraumeni syndrome, in which *p53* is inherited in mutant form, and a cancer-prone strain of mice has been developed with a mutated *p53* gene. Such patients and such mice develop normally, suggesting that *p53* has no role in normal cell development; but these patients and mice are at high risk of developing many different forms of cancer, and fibroblasts from pa-tients with the Li-Fraumeni syndrome are genetically un-stable.[85] These observations suggest that the protein product of *p53* is the guardian of the genome.[86] Its normal function may be to detect the presence of damaged DNA and arrest the cell cycle in G1 until the damage is repaired or, if not repaired, to induce apoptosis.

Programmed Cell Death

Apoptosis is cell suicide, better known as programmed cell death (PCD). It results from a specific set of genetically determined events leading to the death of the cell and its degeneration and resorption by surrounding cells. The concept of apoptosis is not new, but its importance in oncology has only recently been recognized. The term was derived a quarter century ago—from the Greek *apo,* meaning "apart," and *ptosis,* meaning "fallen"—to de-scribe a kind of cell death that is different from necrosis. There is no release of cell contents to excite inflamma-tion. Adjacent cells, not professional phagocytes, ingest the cell debris.[87]

Our understanding that multicellular life forms can live only if there is a proper balance between the different cell types of their bodies should, perhaps, have led us to the concept of apoptosis sooner. After all, the notion that some cells must die so that the whole organism can survive is hardly new. White blood cells sacrifice themselves in fighting infection; lymphocytes throw themselves against a foreign invader; skin cells protect for a few days and then are discarded. Programmed cell death evolved early and became an essential component of multicellular life forms. It is occasionally seen in some single-celled, social organisms when it offers an advantage to survival during a time of environmental stress.[88] Cells deficient in apoptosis are selected for growth in a hypoxic environment, the kind of environment typical of tumors.[89] The role of apoptosis in human disease has recently been reviewed.[90]

The sequential reactions of apoptosis are set in motion by a signal sent to the cell, or sometimes by the loss of a signal that is normally present. The cell, no longer needed by the body or perhaps dangerous to the body, then quietly dies. Drugs may induce apoptosis, as first observed when glucocorticoids were found to activate an endogenous endonuclease in thymocytes.[91]

When DNA is damaged beyond repair, the cell with the damage represents a danger to the host because it will have many, possibly hazardous, mutations. A system exists that checks the DNA to be sure it is undamaged before a cell is allowed to reproduce. This system involves the gene *p53,* the guardian of the genome described previously. When *p53* is mutated it cannot signal the cell to enter apoptosis, and the result is a proliferation of mutant cells, leading to malignant growth.

Another gene related to apoptosis is *BCL2,* first de-scribed in nodular lymphoma. This is one of a family of genes that control apoptosis. A protein called Bax directly initiates apoptosis in lymphocytes, and the protein prod-uct of *BCL2* exerts its antiapoptotic action by forming heterodimers with Bax.[92] Activation of the *BCL2* gene in lymphoma confers resistance to apoptosis, giving the lymphoma cells a kind of immortality. Further, because the cytotoxic killing of cells by chemotherapy depends on apoptosis of the cells whose DNA is damaged by the drugs, lymphocytes with activated *BCL2* genes are resis-tant to the chemotherapeutic agents commonly used in lymphoma.[93]

The progression of tumors to increasing degrees of malignant potential is related to the failure of apoptosis. As tumors grow, regions of hypoxia develop. Hypoxia normally induces apoptosis, but in the presence of a defective *p53* gene or if *BCL2* is activated, apoptosis is blocked. Thus, hypoxia acts to select cells with defective apoptosis and is a factor in tumor progression.[89]

It now appears that the primary mechanism by which most chemotherapeutic agents induce cell kill is by caus-ing cell damage, especially genetic damage, that results in the induction of apoptosis.[94] Resistance to apoptosis, therefore, represents the most potent form of tumor cell resistance to chemotherapy. In this light, then, the inacti-vation of *p53* as a late step in tumor progression takes on great significance, although pathways to apoptosis in-dependent of *p53* have been described.[95]

Discovery of the Immortality of the Cancer Cell

When grown in cell culture, cancer cells are immortal. All other cells of multicellular organisms, except germ cells, will grow old (*senescence*) and die. What is the mecha-nism of aging and death? Recently this has been eluci-dated, and there is an important relationship to cancer.

At the end of each chromosome is a structure known as the *telomere.* The telomere consists of a repeated code of DNA that serves as a biological clock.[96] Because of a peculiarity of DNA replication, each time the chromo-some is replicated a small sequence at the very end is not copied. Thus, the chromosomal DNA gets a little shorter each time it is copied. When it has been copied about thirty times, the DNA at the end is exposed in such a way that it appears damaged to the guardians of the genome. A signal is then sent out and the cell stops reproducing, ages, and dies by apoptosis. Germ cells, which are immortal, contain an enzyme called telomerase that copies the telomere and so the cell does not grow old. It should come as no surprise, then, that cancer cells have developed the capacity to produce the enzyme telomerase. This may serve as a marker of malignancy, and it also explains the immortality of the cancer cell. As this story continues to emerge it becomes more com-plex as new enzymes are discovered to be involved.[97] But the simple truth seems to be that if telomerase is intro-duced into normal human cells in culture, their life-span is extended.[98]

The discovery of the role of telomerase in cancer offers obvious diagnostic and therapeutic opportunities. The role of telomerase in the cell cycle in cancer cells is being elucidated and may contribute to our understanding of cancer.[99]

Conclusion

The story is far from complete, but the pieces are beginning to fit together in a pattern that allows an appreciation of how cancer violates the fundamental biological processes of multicellular life forms. In one sense, cancer can be viewed as a further step in evolution. Cells scheduled to die in the interest of the host evolve the capacity to escape host regulation and grow independently. Ultimately, of course, they die when they kill the host, but as they begin their mutant lives we recognize the biological control mechanisms that are circumvented as the cells attempt to avoid programmed cell death. Indeed, our understanding of many fundamental biological mechanisms has resulted from our study of cancer. The cell cycle itself, fundamental to all living cells, is likely the target of mutations in essentially every malignant growth.[100]

We can expect many new and exciting discoveries in the future in regard to the biology of cancer, and we can expect that this new biology will have important implications in the management of patients with cancer.[101,102] New targets for therapy are being identified, and there will likely be a number of significant milestones added to our story as we enter the new millennium.

References

1. Shimkin MB: *Contrary to Nature*. DHEW publication No. (NIH) 76-720. Washington, DC, 1977
2. Redmond DE Jr: Hill cautions against snuff in 1761. *N Engl J Med* 282:18–23, 1970
3. Pott P: *Chirurgical Observations Relative to the Cataract, ye Polypus of the Nose, the Cancer of the Scrotum, the Different Kinds of Ruptures, and the Mortification of the Toes and Feet*. London, Hawkes, Clarke, and Collins, 1775
4. Shimkin MB: Thirteen questions: Some historical outlines for cancer research. *J Natl Cancer Inst* 19:295–328, 1957
5. Virchow R: *Cellular Pathology*. Translated from the second edition by Frank Chance. London, John Churchill, 1860, pp 219, 460
6. Triolo VA: Nineteenth century foundations of cancer research: Advances in tumor pathology, nomenclature, and theories of oncogenesis. *Cancer Res* 25:75–106, 1965
7. Lyons AS, Petrucelli RJ: *Medicine, An Illustrated History*. New York, Abrams, 1978, pp 527–532
8. Thorwald J: *The Century of the Surgeon*. New York, Pantheon, 1956
9. Baly M: *As Miss Nightingale Said*. London, Scutari Press, 1991
10. Handley WS: The pathology of melanotic growths in relation to their operative treatment. *Lancet* 1:927–933, 1907
11. Halsted WS: The results of radical operations for the cure of carcinoma of the breast. *Ann Surg* 46:1–19, 1907
12. Paget S: The distribution of the secondary growths in cancer of the breast. *Lancet* 1:571–573, 1889
13. Fiddler IJ, Hart IR: Biological diversity in metastatic neoplasms: Origins and implications. *Science* 217:998–1003, 1982
14. Beatson GT: On the treatment of inoperable cases of carcinoma of the mamma: Suggestions for a new method of treatment with illustrative cases. *Lancet* 2:104–107, 1896
15. Huggins CB, Hodges CV: Studies on prostatic cancer: I. The effect of castration, of estrogen, and of androgen injection on serum phosphatase in metastatic carcinoma of the prostate. *Cancer Res* 1:293–297, 1941
16. Huggins CB: Endocrine-induced regression of cancers. *Science* 156:1050–1054, 1967
17. Roentgen WC: Uber eine neue Art von Strahlen. *Sitzungsber. phys.-med, Gesellsch. Wurzb* 132–141j, 1895
18. Coutard H: Roentgen therapy of epitheliomas of the tonsillar region, hypopharynx, and larynx from 1920 to 1926. *Am J Roentgenol* 28:313–331, 1932
19. Frieben A: Demonstration lines cancroids des rechten Handruckens, das sich nach langdauernder Einwirkung von Roentgenstrahlen entwichelt hatte. *Fortschr Geb Rontgenstr* 6:106, 1902
20. Von Jagic N, Scwarz G, von Siebenrock L: Blutbefunde bei Roentgenologon. *Berl Klin Wochenschr* 48:1220–1222, 1911
21. Preston DL, Kato H, Kopecky KJ, et al: Studies on the mortality of A-bomb survivors: 8. Cancer mortality, 1950–1982. *Radiat Res* 111:151–178, 1987
22. Rous P: Transmission of a malignant new growth by means of a cell free filtrate. *JAMA* 56:198, 1911 (reprinted *JAMA* 250:1445–1446, 1983)
23. Yamagiwa K, Ichikawa K: Experimentelle Studie uber die Pathogenese der Epitheliageschwulste. *Mitteilungen Med Facultat Kaiserl Univ Tokyo* 15:295, 1915
24. Rehn L: Blasengeschwulste bei Fuchsin-Arbeitern. *Arch Klin Chir* 50:588, 1895
25. Kennaway EL, Hieger I: Carcinogenic substances and their fluorescence spectra. *Br J Med* 1:1044, 1930
26. Wynder EL, Graham EA: Tobacco smoking as a possible etiologic factor in bronchiogenic carcinoma: A study of 684 proved cases. *JAMA* 143:329–336, 1950
27. Doll R, Hill AB: Smoking and carcinoma of the lung: Preliminary report. *Br Med J* 2:739–748, 1950
28. Levin ML, Goldstein H, Gerhardt PR: Cancer and tobacco smoking: A preliminary report. *JAMA* 143:336–338, 1950
29. Rous P, Beard JW: The progression to carcinoma of virus induced rabbit papillomas (Shope). *J Exp Med* 62:523–548, 1935
30. Friedewald WF, Rous P: The initiating and promoting elements in tumor production: An analysis of the effects of tar, benzpyrene, and methylcholanthrene on rabbit skin. *J Exp Med* 80:101–125, 1944
31. Berenblum I, Shubik P: The role of croton oil applications associated with a single painting of a carcinogen in tumor induction of the mouse's skin. *Br J Cancer* 1:379–382, 1947
32. Rous P, Kidd JG: Conditional neoplasms and subthreshold neoplastic states. *J Exp Med* 73:365–389, 1941
33. Foulds L: The experimental study of tumor progression: A review. *Cancer Res* 14:327–339, 1954
34. Fidler IJ: Critical factors in the biology of human metastasis. *Am Surg* 61:1065–1066, 1995

35. Goodman LS, Wintrobe MW, Dameshek W, et al: Nitrogen mustard therapy. *JAMA* 132:126–132, 1946 (reprinted *JAMA* 251:2255–2261, 1984)

36. Farber S, Diamond LK, Mercer RD, et al: Temporary remissions in acute leukemia in children produced by folic acid antagonist 4-aminopteroylglutamic acid (aminopterin). *N Engl J Med* 238:787–793, 1948

37. Elion GB: The purine path to chemotherapy. *Science* 244:41–47, 1989

38. Heidelberger C: Fluorinated pyrimidines, a new class of tumor inhibitory compounds. *Nature* 179:663–666, 1957

39. Li MC, Hertz R, Spencer DB: Effect of methotrexate therapy upon choriocarcinoma and chorioadenoma. *Proc Soc Exp Biol Med* 93:361–366, 1956

40. Avery OT, McCarty M, MacLeod CM: Studies on the chemical nature of the substance inducing transformation of pneumococcal types: Induction of transformation by desoxyribonucleic acid fraction from pneumococcus type III. *J Exp Med* 79:137–158, 1944

41. Watson JD, Crick FHC: Molecular structure of nucleic acids: A structure for deoxyribose nucleic acid. *Nature* 171:737–738, 1953

42. Miller EC: Some current perspectives on chemical carcinogenesis in humans and experimental animals: Presidential Address. *Cancer Res* 38:1479–1496, 1978

43. Ames BN, Durston WE, Yamasaki E, et al: Carcinogens are mutagens: A simple test system combining liver homogenates for activation and bacteria for detection. *Proc Natl Acad Sci U S A* 70:2281, 1973

44. Perera FP, Weinstein IB: Molecular epidemiology and carcinogen-DNA adduct detection: New approaches to studies of human cancer causation. *J Chronic Dis* 35:581–600, 1982

45. Hall EJ: Principles of carcinogenesis: Physical, in DeVita VT Jr, Hellman S, Rosenberg SA (eds): *Cancer: Principles and Practice of Oncology* (ed 4). Philadelphia, Lippincott, 1993, pp 213–227

46. Fisher B, Redmond C, Fisher ER, et al: Ten year results of a randomized clinical trial comparing radical mastectomy and total mastectomy with or without radiation. *N Engl J Med* 312:674–681, 1985

47. Fisher B, Bauer M, Margolese R, et al: Five year results of a randomized clinical trial comparing total mastectomy and segmental mastectomy with or without radiation in the treatment of breast cancer. *N Engl J Med* 312:665–673, 1985

48. Veronesi U, Valagussa P: Inefficacy of internal mammary node dissection in breast cancer surgery. *Cancer* 47:170–175, 1981

49. Veronesi U, Adamus J, Bandiera DC, et al: Inefficacy of immediate node dissection in stage 1 melanoma of the limbs. *N Engl J Med* 297:627–630, 1977

50. Veronesi U, Cascinelli N, Adamus J, et al: Thin stage I primary cutaneous malignant melanoma: Comparison of excision with margins of 1 or 3 cm. *N Engl J Med* 318:1159–1162, 1988

51. Tarin D, Vass AC, Kettlewell MG, et al: Absence of metastatic sequelae during long term treatment of malignant ascites by peritoneo-venous shunting. *Invasion Metastasis* 4:1–12, 1984

52. Huebner RJ, Todaro GJ: Oncogenes of RNA tumor viruses as determinants of cancer. *Proc Natl Acad Sci USA* 64:1087–1094, 1969

53. Waterfield MD, Scrace GT, Whittle N, et al: Platelet derived growth factor is structurally related to the putative transforming protein p28-sis of simian sarcoma virus. *Nature* 304:35–39, 1983

54. Doolittle RF, Hunkapiller MW, Hood LE, et al: Simian sarcoma virus onc gene *v-sis* is derived from the gene (or genes) encoding a platelet derived growth factor. *Science* 221:275–276, 1983

55. Xu YH, Ishii AJ, Clark M, et al: Human epidermal growth factor receptor cDNA is homologous to a variety of RNAs overproduced in A431 carcinoma cells. *Nature* 309:806–810, 1984

56. Poiesz BJ, Ruscetti FW, Gazdar AF, et al: Detection and isolation of type C retrovirus particles from fresh and cultured lymphocytes of a patient with cutaneous T-cell lymphoma. *Proc Natl Acad Sci USA* 77:7415–7419, 1980

57. Blattner WA: Human retroviruses and malignancy, in Brugge J, Curran T, Harlow E, McCormick F (eds): *Origins of Human Cancer.* Cold Spring Harbor, NY, Cold Spring Harbor Laboratory Press, 1991, pp 199–209

58. Weinberg RA: Growth factors and oncogenes, in RA Weinberg (ed): *Oncogenes and the Molecular Origins of Cancer.* Cold Spring Harbor, NY, Cold Spring Harbor Laboratory Press, 1989, pp 1–16

59. Pereira-Smith OM, Smith JR: Evidence for the recessive nature of cellular immortality. *Science* 221:964–966, 1983

60. Whyte P, Buchkovich KJ, Horowitz JM, et al: Association between an oncogene and an anti-oncogene: The adenovirus E1A proteins bind to the retinoblastoma gene product. *Nature* 334:124–129, 1988

61. Knudson AG: Hereditary cancer: Oncogenes and anti-oncogenes. *Cancer Res* 45:1437–1443, 1985

62. Hunter T: Protein-tyrosine phosphatases: The other side of the coin. *Cell* 58:1013–1016, 1989

63. Marx J: Biologists turn on to "off-enzymes." *Science* 251:744–746, 1991

64. Shen SH, Bastien L, Posner BI, et al: A protein tyrosine phosphatase with sequence similarity to the SH2 domain of the protein tyrosine kinases. *Nature* 352:736–739, 1991

65. Knudson A: Mutation and cancer: Statistical study of retinoblastoma. *Proc Natl Acad Sci USA* 68:820, 1971

66. Huang HJS, Yee JK, Shew JY, et al: Suppression of the neoplastic phenotype by replacement of the *RB* gene in human cancer cells. *Science* 242:1563–1566, 1988

67. Rustgi AK, Dyson N, Bernards R: Amino-terminal domains of c-myc and N-myc proteins mediate binding to the *retinoblastoma* gene product. *Nature* 352:541–544, 1991

68. Mihara K, Cao XR, Yen A, et al: Cell cycle dependent regulation of phosphorylation of the human *retinoblastoma* gene product. *Science* 246:1300–1303, 1989

69. Huang S, Lee WH, Lee EY: A cellular protein that competes with SV40 T antigen for binding to the *retinoblastoma* gene product. *Nature* 350:160–162, 1991

70. Bandara LR, La Thangue NB: Adenovirus Ela prevents the *retinoblastoma* gene product from complexing with a cellular transcription factor. *Nature* 351:494–497, 1991

71. Wagner S, Green MR: A transcriptional tryst. *Nature* 352:189–190, 1991

72. Bandara LR, Adamczewski JP, Hunt T, et al: Cyclin A and the *retinoblastoma* gene product complex with a common transcription factor. *Nature* 352:249–251, 1991

73. Marx J: The cell cycle: Spinning further afield. *Science* 252:1490–1492, 1991

74. Loeb LA: Transient expression of a mutator phenotype in cancer cells. *Science* 277:1449–1450, 1997

75. Kinzler KW, Vogelstein B: Landscaping the cancer terrain. *Science* 280:1036–1037, 1998

76. Gowen LC, Avrutskaya AV, Latour AM, et al: BRCA1 required for transcription-coupled repair of oxidative DNA damage. *Science* 281:1009–1012, 1998

77. Levine AJ, Momand J, Finlay CA: The *p53* tumour suppressor gene. *Nature* 351:453–456, 1991

78. Hollstein M, Sidransky D, Vogelstein B, et al: *p53* Mutations in human cancers. *Science* 253:49–53, 1991

79. Kern SE, Kinzler KW, Bruskin AM, et al: Identification of p53 as a sequence specific DNA binding protein. *Science* 252:1708–1711, 1991

80. Isaacs WB, Carter BS, Ewing CM: Wild type *p53* suppresses growth of human prostate cancer cells containing mutant *p53* alleles. *Cancer Res* 51:4716–4720, 1991

81. Oliner JD, Kinzler KW, Meltzer PS, et al: Amplification of a gene encoding a p53-associated protein in human sarcomas. *Nature* 358:80–83, 1992

82. Maltzman W, Czyzyk L: UV irradiation stimulates levels of *p53* cellular tumor antigen in nontransformed mouse cells. *Mol Cell Biol* 4:1689–1694, 1984

83. Kastan MB, Onyekwere O, Sidransky D, et al: Participation of p53 protein in the cellular response to DNA damage. *Cancer Res* 51:6304–6311, 1991

84. Shaw P, Bovey R, Tardy S, et al: Induction of apoptosis by wild-type *p53* in a human colon tumor-derived cell line. *Proc Natl Acad Sci USA* 89:4495–4499, 1992

85. Donehower LA, Harvey M, Slagle BL, et al: Mice deficient for *p53* are developmentally normal but susceptible to spontaneous tumours. *Nature* 356:215–221, 1992

86. Lane DP: *p53*, Guardian of the genome. *Science* 358:15–16, 1992

87. Kerr JFR, Wyllie AH, Currie AR: A basic biological phenomenon with wide-ranging implications in tissue kinetics. *Br J Cancer* 26:239–244, 1972

88. Ameisen JC: The origin of programmed cell death. *Science* 272:1278–1279, 1996

89. Graeber TG, Osmanian C, Jacks T, et al: Hypoxia-mediated selection of cells with diminished apoptotic potential in solid tumors. *Nature* 379:88–91, 1996

90. Hetts, SW: To die or not to die: An overview of apoptosis and its role in disease. *JAMA* 279:300–307, 1998

91. Wyllie AH: Glucocorticoid induced thymocyte apoptosis is associated with endogenous endonuclease activation. *Nature* 284:555–559, 1980

92. Yin XM, Oltvai ZN, Korsmeyer SJ: BH1 and BH2 domains of Bcl-2 are required for inhibition of apoptosis and heterodimerization with Bax. *Nature* 369:321–323, 1994

93. Miyashita T, Reed JC: Bcl-2 oncoprotein blocks chemotherapy induced apoptosis in a human leukemia cell line. *Blood* 81:151–157, 1993

94. Thompson CB: Apoptosis in the pathogenesis and treatment of disease. *Science* 267:1456–1462, 1995

95. Clarke AR, Pirdie CA, Harrison DJ, et al: Thymocyte apoptosis induced by *p53*-dependent and independent pathways. *Nature* 362:849–852, 1993

96. de Lange T: Telomeres and senescence: Ending the debate. *Science* 279:334–335, 1998

97. Pennisi E: A possible new partner for telomerase. *Science* 282:1395–1397, 1998

98. Bodnar AG, Ouellette M, Frolkis M, et al: Extension of life span by introduction of telomerase into normal human cells. *Science* 279:349–352, 1998

99. Shore D: Telomeres: The unsticky ends. *Science* 281:1818–1819, 1998

100. Clurman BE, Roberts JM: Cell cycle and cancer. *J Natl Cancer Inst* 87:1499–1501, 1995

101. Yarbro JW: Breast cancer: The new biology in conflict with the old dogma. *Semin Oncol Nurs* 1:157–162, 1985

102. Yarbro JW: The new biology of cancer: Future clinical applications. *Semin Oncol* 16:254–259, 1989

CHAPTER 2

Biology of Cancer

Jean Gribbon, RN, BSN
Lois J. Loescher, PhDc, RN

Introduction

In his now classic writings on the origin of cancer, Sir Richard Doll[1] proposed three potential causative factors underlying tumor development: (1) environmental factors, particularly diet, industrial pollution, and viruses; (2) systemic factors, including breakdowns in immunosurveillance; and (3) genetic factors, such as the degree of susceptibility to cancer. Since Doll's publications in the late 1970s, the biology underlying these proposed causative factors—which were drawn largely from epidemiologic studies—has been carefully scrutinized to determine the causes of cancer at the biochemical, cellular, and molecular levels. Because of the intensity of biological research and the rapid return of findings, we now know that cancer results from an interaction of factors at the cellular, genetic, immunologic, and environmental levels.

The fundamental goals of cancer research are to discern the mechanisms of cancer cell development, to determine how cancers grow and spread, and to discover the means to correct abnormal mechanisms and to eradicate or control cancer cell populations. This chapter reviews models of tumor development, genetic influences on cancer, cell growth and differentiation, and spread of cancer through various mechanisms of metastasis.

Theories and Research Models of Tumor Development

The rate-limiting step of cancer, genetic mutation, strongly suggests that cancer develops through multistep processes. Cancer is an accumulation of mutations that result from multiple events acting together and occurring through many series of pathways. The research models addressed in this section describe these multistep processes in greater detail.

Theory of Clonal Evolution

Nowell's theory of clonal evolution specifies that cells within a particular tumor all have the same genetic makeup;[2] that homogeneity is necessary or any one gene could not be identified. Even though a carcinogen may affect a large number of cells, the resultant tumor usually represents the progeny of only a single cell or of very few cells[2,3] (Figure 2-1). Initiation of clonal evolution may involve a stem cell that is already dividing, but in mitosis the proportion of daughter cells increases rather than proceeding to differentiation. Uncontrolled proliferation may be accompanied by morphological and biochemical changes or altered gene expression in early cancer cells. Eventually, proliferation may increase and show further evidence of escape from growth-control mechanisms. Nowell suggests that biological events in tumor progression represent the effects of acquired genetic instability.

A Genetic Model for Tumorigenesis

Fearon and Vogelstein expanded on the theory of clonal evolution when they proposed a model for the genetic basis of cancer.[4] These investigators studied colorectal cancers because (1) most colorectal tumors arise from preexisting benign tumors called *adenomas* or *adenomatous polyps;* (2) colorectal tumors in various stages of development (i.e., small adenomas to large metastatic lesions) can be easily accessed and removed for study; and (3) colorectal cancer shows both inherited and somatic muta-

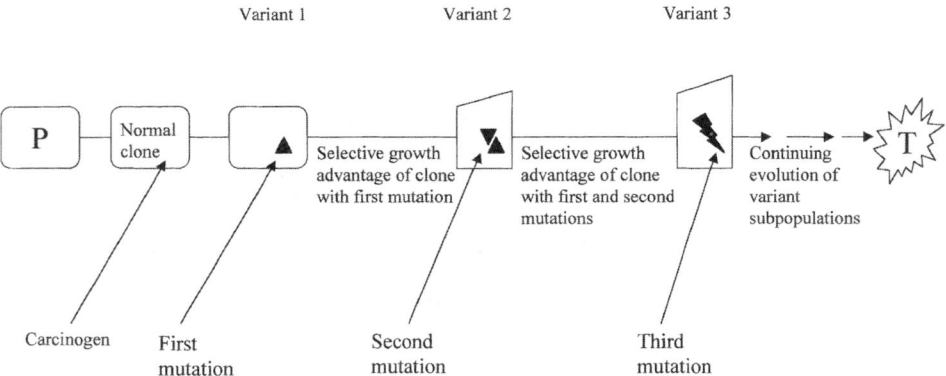

Figure 2-1 Clonal evolution in cancer. Specific genetic alterations in evolving tumors may range from gene mutations to major chromosomal aberrations (genetic instability). This figure illustrates a carcinogen-induced genetic change in a progenitor normal cell P, which produces a cell with selective growth advantage allowing clonal expansion to begin. In this case, gene mutations produce variant cells. Because they are at a disadvantage metabolically or immunologically, most variant cells are nonviable. If one variant has a selective advantage its progeny becomes the predominant subpopulation until another variant appears. The sequential selection of variant subpopulations in each tumor (T) differs because of genetic instability, which positively or negatively affects cell proliferation. (Adapted from Nowell,[2] and Strachan and Read.[3])

tions. Fearon and Vogelstein posited that colorectal cancers arise from mutational activation of oncogenes, coupled with the predominant mutational inactivation of tumor-suppressor genes (Figure 2-2). Mutations in at least four genes are necessary for colorectal tumor development. A key factor in tumorigenesis is that tumor formation reflects the total accumulation of mutations rather than their specific sequence of occurrence.[4]

Transformed Cell Models

Researchers can examine the various aspects of cell growth and development using stable, continuous cell lines from animals and, on occasion, from humans. There are several advantages of using cell lines, among them: (1) they can be developed from a single cell to provide a certain level of uniformity; (2) the culture environment can be defined and modified; and (3) they become continuous when they develop the ability to propagate indefinitely in tissue culture.[5]

Many normal cell lines cease proliferating and die after making a programmed or defined number of cell divisions (*senescence*). Occasionally, a cell line will continue to grow abnormally and indefinitely, often resembling neoplastic cells. These transformed cells can be studied experimentally; more practically, they represent a self-renewing population.[6]

Normal cells can be transformed to tumor cells by three general mechanisms: (1) spontaneous transformation to characteristics typical of cancer cells; (2) chemical/physical carcinogens and biological agents such as viruses; and (3) genetic manipulation. Normal cells typically grow in a continuous single layer in culture, stopping at the boundaries of the chamber; at that point the population stabilizes and cell loss approximates cell growth.

Conversely, transformed cells grow in multiple layers or clusters, reaching higher densities in culture.[6] Transformed cells can have characteristics of tumor cells (Table 2-1) but may or may not be tumorigenic.[7-11] The ultimate test for transformed cells is to inject them into compatible animal cells to see if tumors form.

Unless researchers have access to human tumor cells that successfully endure in culture, transformed cells provide the best opportunity for investigation of cellular processes and behavior, because they most closely approximate the nature of malignant cells. Nevertheless, extrapolation of data from cell culture to cells in vivo may be inaccurate or incomplete. For purposes of further discussion within this chapter, we assume that transformed cells and cancer cells are essentially identical.

Transgenic models

A transformed cell line represents one type of transgenic organism; another is an organism derived from a cell whose genome has been modified by the addition of exogenous, or foreign, DNA. This DNA may be a manipulated sequence from the same species or from another species that has some property desirable for a particular experiment. The operational gene in the exogenous DNA is called a *transgene*. In studies of cancer, transgenes are typically injected into cells.[12]

The gene of interest is injected into early mouse embryos. The foreign DNA integrates randomly, without preference for a particular chromosomal location. Three weeks after birth, the offspring are tested for presence of the transgene.[13]

There are many benefits for using transgenic adult mice to study cancer biology. Most important, this process allows the embryonic stem cells to be manipulated in vitro prior to injection into the embryo. Scientists then

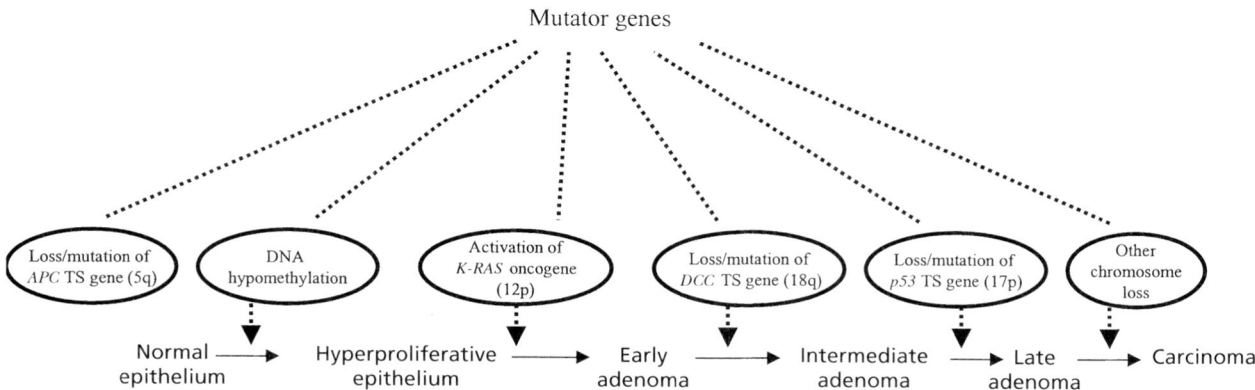

Figure 2-2   A conceptual genetic model for the development of colorectal cancer, illustrating multistep tumorigenesis. These alterations suggest a temporal sequence of genetic events. Not all alterations occur in individual tumors, and the order of alterations is variable. The accumulation of multiple genetic alterations in both oncogenes and tumor-suppressor (TS) genes is more important than the order of events. Mutator gene mutations do not play a direct role in the multistep pathway, but by increasing the overall mutation rate they make each individual transition more likely. *APC* = adenomatous polyposis coli gene; *DCC* = deleted in colorectal carcinoma gene. (Adapted from Strachan and Read;[3] Fearon and Vogelstein.[4])

Table 2-1   Properties of Transformed Cells

Property	Characteristics of Tumor Cells	Explanation
Cytological changes	Increased size and number of nucleoli	Reflects greater metabolic need and activity of tumor cell
	Increased nuclear/cytoplasmic ratio	Larger nucleus reflects more activity, more genetic information
	Formation of clusters and cords of cells	Transformed cells contain proteins present in normal cells; proteins are not polymerized, causing variable sizes and shapes (pleomorphism)
Altered cell growth	Immortality	Normal cells senesce (remain viable but do not divide)
		During a crisis, cells mutate, proliferate indefinitely, become "immortal"
		Telomeres (DNA segments at the ends of chromosomes) help limit the number of cell doublings. Telomeres shrink with each chromosomal replication until reaching a threshold, at which time they signal the cell to senesce. Telomere stability is critical for cancer progression. Many cancers contain an enzyme, *telomerase,* which enables the cell to replicate indefinitely.[7]
	Decreased density-dependent growth inhibition (contact inhibition)	Normal cells stop growing when they come in contact with other cells; crowding from contact compromises access to nutrients
		Transformed cells hold less firmly to each other, appear to move about more than normal cells, often have fewer requirements for growth substances in the surrounding media and therefore have different density-dependence than normal cells
	Decreased requirement for serum	Serum normally provides growth factors necessary for cell development and survival
		Typically the growth factor binds with a receptor on the cell surface, which in turn activates the intracytoplasmic portion of the receptor to send a message to the nucleus (signal transduction), where an effect on gene function occurs. Sometimes, an abnormal growth factor receptor on the surface of a transformed cell can activate the signal pathway spontaneously without exposure to a growth factor
		Transformed cell lines may grow in media without serum, suggesting that they can synthesize and secrete their own growth factors (autocrine stimulation)
	Loss of anchorage-dependent growth	Cells require substrate to grow; transformed cells do not grow on solid substrate
		Only tumor cells grow in soft agar (no anchorage); cell growth in soft agar highly correlates with tumorgenicity
	Loss of cell-cycle control	Cell does not progress normally through cell cycle pathways and checkpoints (see text)
	Reduced apoptosis	Normal cells lose ability to die a programmed death (see text)
Changes in cell membrane	New surface antigens	Transformed cells exhibit new molecules on the surface
		Viruses can transform and alter multiple cell surface antigens
		When cells are transformed by radiation or chemical carcinogens, the tumor antigens formed in these cells do not depend on the agent involved but vary with the cell type
	New or altered glycoproteins (proteins complexed with polysaccharides)	Transformed cells usually have profound changes in cell-surface glycoproteins
		Most changes reflect a lower protein content, e.g., transformed cells have low levels of fibronectin; low fibronectin levels change the cytoskeleton (cell-cell and cell-matrix adhesion)
		Glycoproteins that remain are altered, mostly by becoming simpler
		Mechanism by which polysaccharides are made and attached to proteins is deranged in transformed cells
	New or altered glycolipids	Content and complexity of glycolipids is reduced in transformed cell membranes
		Glycosphingolipid interacts with receptor proteins on the surface of normal cells to inhibit their responsiveness to growth factors.[8]
		Transformed cells have fewer and/or altered glycosphingolipids on their cell surfaces, thus increasing their responsiveness to growth factors. Glycosphingolipids also serve as components of surface markers involved in cell-cell recognition.

Table 2-1 Properties of Transformed Cells (continued)

Property	Characteristics of Tumor Cells	Explanation
Changes in cell membrane (cont.)	Tumor cells agglutinate in presence of lectins (polysaccharide glycoproteins derived from plants)	Tumor cells bind specifically to carbohydrates on cell surface; agglutination results from altered fluidity of membrane following a change in lipid balance[9]
	Changes in fluidity of cell membrane	Some new molecules appear, some molecules that normally appear are lost, and other molecules are changed.[10]
		Enhanced uptake of glucose, other sugars, amino acids; cyclic adenosine monophosphate (cAMP) regulates transport of nutrients in transformed cells.[11]

can produce mice with mutations in specific genes or replace a mutant gene with a wild-type (normal) gene.

Properties of Transformed Cells

Every somatic cell division provides the daughter cells with an exact copy of the human genome. Over time, different cells pursue various paths that facilitate organ development and a reserve pool of uncommitted cells, which may later develop into specific organs.

Embryonic cells are necessarily vigorous and possess certain characteristics that provide them with growth advantages over adult cells. Embryonic cells migrate extensively, secrete factors to develop a new blood supply, and release enzymes to break down tissue barriers. Adult cells that activate embryonic programs of gene expression or that inactivate portions of the adult program may behave like malignant tumor cells.[6]

Each human cell has the same DNA content, but only a portion of the total gene pool in a cell is expressed. As a cell assumes a distinct "personality," distinguishing it in structure and function from other cells, it becomes differentiated. A differentiated cell activates particular genes, leading to specific messenger RNA molecules that are translated into distinct proteins. These proteins determine the fate of the cell. As a cell becomes more differentiated, its activity may be more restricted and attuned to its organ of residence; it also may lose the ability to replicate.[6]

Cancer cells tend to be less differentiated than cells from surrounding normal tissue. Indeed, some cancer cells are so poorly differentiated (or *anaplastic*) that the tissue origin cannot be confirmed. Normal cells may undergo a gradual transition to malignancy, passing through the stages of *metaplasia* (the presence of a cell that appears mildly less differentiated), *dysplasia* (deranged cell growth with variable shape, size, and appearance), carcinoma in situ, and finally invasive cancer.[6,7,8] General properties of transformed cells are cytological changes, altered cell growth, and changes in the cell membrane[8-11] (see Table 2-1).

Genetic Influences Associated with Cancer

Chapter 1 provides an historical perspective and overview of how genes influence carcinogenesis. In this section, we expand the discussion to include DNA and chromosomes.

Mutations

A mutation is a permanent change in a DNA nucleotide sequence the order of bases adenine (A), cytosine (C), thymine (T), and guanine (G) along a gene. Mutations can alter both the structure of a gene and its regulatory sites. In humans, mutations occur at a rate of 1 in 1 million genes per cell generation. Since it takes as many as six independent mutations in specific genes to give rise to a tumor cell, the likelihood of a tumor developing is low, though everyone has cells that have mutations in at least one gene.[3] Most mutations are harmless. However, the mutation rate becomes a concern when mutations give rise to a clonal population of cells (see Figure 2-1) and when mutations affect cells that are particularly sensitive to mutation, for example, germ cells.[14] Usually mutations in somatic cells are only problematic when they (1) cause increases in cell proliferation; (2) occur early in embryogenesis, or (3) reduce genetic stability so as to increase the rate of mutation.

Germ-line mutations in genes that predispose to cancer comprise the strongest risk factors for cancer.[15] Germ-line mutations affect genes in the ova and sperm. During meiosis, each germ cell carries one of the two copies of mutated genes present in somatic cells, resulting in a 50% chance of a child inheriting a mutated gene from a parent. Such mutations are transmitted from generation to generation.

Causes of mutations

Mutations may be inherited, may arise spontaneously during DNA replication and recombination, or may be caused by mutagens such as environmental agents. DNA replication is a complex process resulting in the formation of DNA daughter strands with identical base pairing to the parent strand, i.e., replication of the genome. DNA replication errors are rare. More frequently, DNA rearranges itself by *recombination,* a process whereby DNA is either lost or inserted into the gene. Recombination may result in loss of control of gene expression or disrupt the coding sequence of the gene. Mutagens that damage DNA may be artificial (e.g., pesticides, organic chemicals, alkylating agents) or naturally occurring (e.g., plant toxins, viruses). Radiation can also damage DNA.

Types of mutations

Mutations commonly associated with cancer predisposition include point mutations, and insertion and deletion mutations (Figure 2-3).[16] These defects are often corrected by a process called *mismatch repair,* but defects in mismatch repair also constitute mutations.

Point mutations. The substitution of a single base with another base is termed a *point mutation.* Point mutations are the most common types of mutations. Point mutations that occur in DNA sequences encoding proteins are further classified as silent, missense, or nonsense mutations.

A *silent point mutation* is a base substitution in a codon (a section of three DNA nucleotides that codes for an amino acid) in which the amino acid does not change. In other words, the protein product of the gene is not altered.

Sometimes a base substitution results in generation of a codon that specifies a different amino acid, meaning that there will be an amino acid change in the sequence of the gene product. This change is termed a *missense point mutation.* A missense mutation may or may not result in a deleterious gene product, depending on the amino acid that has been substituted. If the structure and prop-

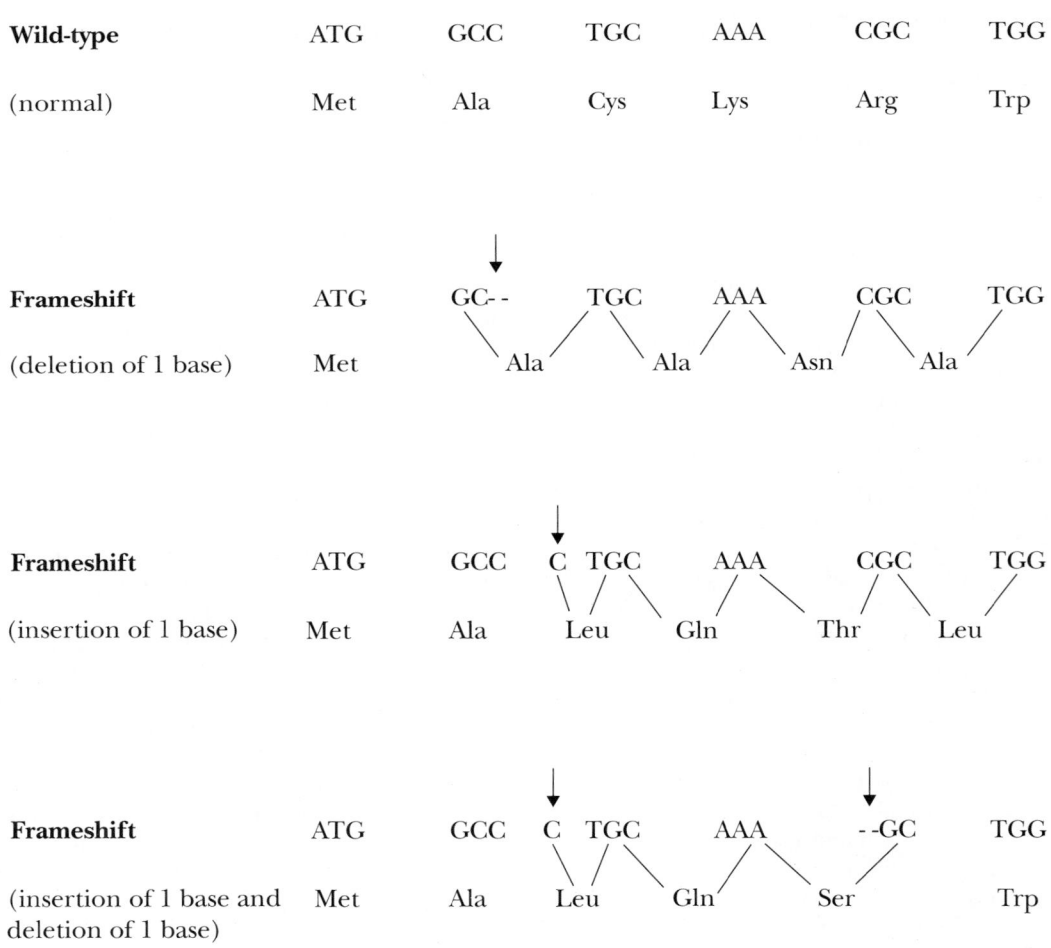

Figure 2-3 Frameshift mutations. Deletion and/or insertion of bases shifts the reading frame of the DNA sequence, thereby changing the expressed amino acids. Top rows in each set are DNA bases: A = adenine; T = thymine; C = cytosine; G = guanine. Bottom rows in each set are amino acids encoded by the bases: Ala = alanine; Arg = arginine; Asn = asparagine; Cys = cysteine; Gln = glutamine; Leu = leucine; Lys = lysine; Met = methionine; Ser = serine; Thr = threonine; Trp = tryptophan. (Used with permission from Loescher LJ: DNA testing for cancer predisposition. *Oncol Nurs Forum* 25:1320, 1998.)[16]

erties of the normal and substituted amino acids are similar, no deleterious gene products will result. If the structure and properties of the two amino acids are different, a deleterious gene product may result.

A *nonsense point mutation* occurs when a base substitution results in the generation of a stop codon, meaning that the gene product will be truncated and probably nonfunctional. Nonsense point mutations are deleterious mutations.

Deletions and insertions. A deletion occurs when one or more base pairs are lost from the DNA. This may result in a *frameshift mutation*. If one or two bases are deleted, the reading frame of the sequence is altered, usually resulting in a nonfunctional gene product. If three base pairs or a multiple of three base pairs are deleted, the reading frame is left intact but one or more amino acids are missing from the protein.

The insertion of additional base pairs may also lead to frameshift mutations, depending on whether multiples of three base pairs are inserted. Combinations of insertions and deletions are possible, and sometimes, an insertion mutation will restore the reading frame of a gene with a deletion mutation (and vice versa). Such a gene product would contain a garbled amino acid sequence between the insertion and deletion but would otherwise be correct (see Figure 2-3).

Defects in mismatch repair. During DNA-strand synthesis, if the wrong nucleotide incorporates into the strand the DNA's normal editing system fails to correct the error. This error results in a mismatched base pair. These mismatches, as well as single base insertions and deletions, are generally repaired by a mismatch-repair mechanism. This mechanism relies on a back-up signal within the DNA to distinguish between the parental strand and the daughter strand containing the replication error. A protein called MutS recognizes and binds the mismatched base pair. Protein MutL then binds to protein MutS. Bound to the mismatch, the MutL/MutS complex then links with protein MutH, which activates a process that unwinds DNA in the direction of the mismatch, degrades the DNA strand, and repairs the error. Defects in genes that encode the repair proteins have been associated with hereditary nonpolyposis colorectal cancer (HNPCC).[17]

Oncogenes

Oncogenes are genes that encode proteins (oncoproteins) whose action positively promotes cell proliferation. Oncogenes are the excessively or inappropriately active versions of normal cellular genes called *proto-oncogenes*. A mechanism for the overexpression of oncogenes is amplification. In *amplification,* the number of copies of a gene increases, resulting in overexpression of the gene product. The gene itself, however, remains unmodified. As tumor cells progress, they gain ability to amplify genes as they lose cell-cycle control (see below). Oncogenes

such as *MYC* and *HER/2NEU* often have amplified gene sequences, which may be related to tumor progression.[18]

Most proto-oncogenes participate in cellular signal transduction pathways, which can be visualized as molecular "bucket brigades" that relay growth-stimulating signals from the outside to the inside of the cell.[19] These complex signal transduction pathways control basic cell functions such as division, motility, and death, and therefore need to be highly regulated. Regulation occurs through alterations in the enzymatic activity of key components in the pathways and the assembly of large multimolecular signaling complexes within the cell.

The pathways play an important role in tumor development. The large number of components comprising the pathways provide many potential targets for oncogene activation and explain the large number of proto-oncogenes that have been identified. Also, the intrinsic redundancy and cross-talk within the pathways explain why human cancers rarely, if ever, result from aberrant activation of a single oncogene.[20]

Classification of oncogenes

Broad classes of oncogenes can be distinguished according to their overall function. A number of these genes encode growth factors, growth factor receptors, nonreceptor tyrosine kinases, G-proteins, serine/threonine protein kinases, and transcription factors.[18–20]

Growth factors. Growth factors are polypeptides that influence cell growth, differentiation, and survival positively and negatively by binding to specific receptors in the cell membrane and, consequently, activating intracellular signal transduction. To do this, however, growth factors must interact with a highly specific receptor. Growth factor activity results in transmission of a signal to the cell nucleus, where genes are turned off and on. The end result is change in expression (transcription into RNA) of certain genes.

Growth factors may be autocrine or paracrine. An *autocrine* growth factor is produced by the cell it stimulates. *Paracrine* growth factors stimulate adjacent or distant cells. Oncogenic growth factors can activate tumor cell proliferation by both forms of stimulation, but by themselves may not be sufficient to sustain the transformed cell.[19] For example, the oncogenes *FOS, JUN,* and *MYC* are early-response oncogenes that increase activity right after growth-factor stimulation. These genes play key roles in cell proliferation. The overexpression of *MYC* coupled with the addition of fibroblast growth factor (FGF) will cause DNA synthesis, whereas each alone may not. Similarly, when platelet-derived growth factor (PDGF) is combined with another growth factor such as epidermal growth factor (EGF), PDGF can stimulate cell division in cultures; it cannot accomplish this effect alone.

Overproduction of several growth factors is implicated in cancer development. *Epidermal growth factor* stimulates a variety of cells such as epidermal cells, glial cells, vascular endothelial cells, and many cancer cells. Epidermal growth factors produce a mitogenic response in cells that have the EGF receptor (EGFR). High levels of EGFRs are noted on many epithelial carcinomas, and mutant EGFRs have been found on high-grade glioblastomas.[21] *Transforming growth factor-alpha* (TGF-α) is a member of the EGF family. It tends to stimulate endothelial cell proliferation. *Transforming growth factor-beta* (TGF-β) tends to inhibit cell proliferation, largely through inhibition of cyclin-4 and cyclin-dependent kinase-4 (CDK4) in the cell cycle. *Platelet-derived growth factor* receptors are normally located on fibroblasts and smooth muscle cells and appear to play a role in the development and support of brain tumors.[22] *Fibroblast growth factor* stimulates the growth of fibroblasts and is released when a cell is damaged or dies, thereby stimulating surrounding tissue to proliferate. *Colony-stimulating growth factor* (CSF) is involved in the proliferation and differentiation of granulocytes and monocytes/macrophages.

Growth factor receptors. A second type of oncogene encodes altered growth factor receptors (GFRs), which release proliferative signals into the cell even in the absence of growth factors.[18] Most GFRs act through intrinsic tyrosine kinase activity, the ability to bond inorganic phosphate to the amino acid tyrosine. Increased tyrosine kinase activity leads to reactions that stimulate mitosis and can cause clonal expansion of cells. Point mutations may cause increased activity of tyrosine kinase. Nonmutation mechanisms for increasing tyrosine kinase activity include overexpression of GFR and autocrine stimulation.

When overproduced, EGFR is associated with poor prognosis for breast, bladder, colon, lung, and esophageal cancers.[23–26] Overexpression of *ERB-B2* is associated with poor prognosis for breast and ovarian cancers.[27,28] Together, EGFR and TGF-β serve as a prognostic marker for tumor relapse and survival. Increased expression of *HER/2NEU* receptors in breast carcinoma also increases the risk of recurrence.[25]

Nonreceptor tyrosine kinases. The normal cellular products of *src* proto-oncogenes have relatively low levels of tyrosine kinase activity. Although these proteins do not bind directly to growth factors, growth factors and other cellular activators may activate tyrosine kinases. For example, in platelets, thrombin activates tyrosine kinase. Platelet-derived growth factor activates *SRC* tyrosine kinase activity in fibroblasts. The *SRC* oncogene is activated in colorectal cancers and breast adenocarcinomas.

G-proteins. Guanine nucleotide-binding proteins (G-proteins) act as signal transducers for cell-surface growth factor receptors. An example of a G-protein is the *RAS* superfamily comprised of more than fifty members. The true *RAS* proteins (H *RAS*, K *RAS*, N *RAS*) act at the cell membrane to cause malignant transformation. Proteins encoded by unmutated *RAS* genes transmit stimulatory signals from other GFRs to other proteins. Mutated *RAS* genes cause activation of signaling pathways, even when unprompted by GFRs. Overall, *ras* activation occurs in two ways: (1) loss of guanosine 5′-triphosphate

activity (through point mutations that lead to transformation); and (2) increase in G-nucleotide exchange (point mutations lower affinity for G-nucleotide, leading to increased turn around of exchanges). Mutant *RAS* genes are found in several tumors, including cancers of the colon and lung and 90% of pancreatic cancers.[29]

Serine-threonine kinases. Another category of oncogenes is the cytoplasmic oncoprotein with serine-threonine protein-kinase activity. Serine-threonine kinases are centrally involved in cell-cycle progression. The prototype for the serine-threonine kinase category is the Raf-1 protein, which is activated by tyrosine kinase–associated receptors.[19] The Raf-1 protein acts as an intermediary in the signal transduction pathway between *RAS* and the cell nucleus by activating other kinases, mitogen-activated protein (MAP) kinases. These MAP kinases phosphorylate critical substrates regulating cell division. To be active, raf-1 must move to the cell membrane. Recruitment to the membrane is accomplished by active *RAS*, however, this interaction alone is not sufficient to cause transformation. Other protein kinases (e.g., protein kinase-C) are needed for transformation.[20]

Transcription factors. Transcription-factor proteins bind to DNA and cause changes in gene expression. In many tumors, mutated transcription factors that regulate genes involved in cell growth and survival spur transformation. Oncogenic transcription factors include proteins with activator protein-1 (AP-1) activity, such as Jun and Fos, which are part of signal-dependent processes that control cell growth.[30] The tumor-suppressor gene *p53* also acts as a transcription factor when it senses DNA damage and halts cell division by controlling expression of other genes that directly regulate the cell cycle. Oncogenic transcription factors have been associated with many kinds of human leukemias and Ewing's sarcoma.[31]

Tumor-Suppressor Genes

Tumor-suppressor genes normally suppress or negatively regulate cell proliferation by encoding proteins that block the action of growth-promoting proteins. Thus, the hallmark characteristic of a mutated tumor-suppressor gene is loss of function through loss of genetic material or information. Normally, tumor-suppressor genes suppress oncogenes.[32] Some normal tumor-suppressor gene products reside in the cell nucleus and also are considered to be transcription factors. Examples are the tumor suppressor genes *RB*, *MTS1*, and *p53* that are critical for operation of the cell cycle.

Tumor-suppressor genes are recessive in that both alleles (forms of the gene) of a pair must mutate for the gene to be inactivated. In other words, loss or mutation of both copies of the gene is required for tumorigenesis.[15] Inactivation of tumor-suppressor genes is most strongly associated with inherited cancers.

Loss of heterozygosity

Usually, the first (germ-line) mutation of a tumor-suppressor gene affects the actual gene. The second mutation involves loss of a whole chromosome or loss of part of a chromosome. In each case, there is loss of one allele of any the markers close to the tumor-suppressor gene. Thus, if a patient with cancer was heterozygous for a genetic marker located close to the tumor-suppressor gene, the tumor loses this heterozygosity. Most tumor specimens contain a mixture of tumor and nontumor tissue, indicating a decreased relative intensity of tumor, rather than total loss of genetic material from any one allele.[3,15]

Mutator Genes

Mutator genes control or regulate genetic instability to ensure integrity of genetic information. Mutator genes can be either oncogenes or tumor-suppressor genes. Mutations in these genes lead to inefficient replication or repair of DNA. Many times, these genes are characterized by microsatellite DNA—short stretches of DNA that have a simple repeating base sequence.[17,33] The length of microsatellite DNA repeats varies in tumors and normal tissue. Microsatellite instability has been found in colorectal, gastric, breast, bladder, and non-small cell lung cancers. Microsatellites provide clues to gene stability. For example, LOH studies of HNPCC using microsatellite markers showed that rather than lacking alleles in DNA, some tumors appeared to contain extra, novel alleles.[34]

Mutator genes in *Escherichia coli* and yeast encode an error-correction system that checks the DNA for mismatched base pairs. Because of DNA methylation, the system can identify the parent strand and selectively correct the newly synthesized daughter strand if it has not yet been methylated. Mismatches are excised and replaced. Mutations in genes that encode MutHLS error correction lead to a 100- to 1,000-fold general increase in mutations.[17,34]

Cytogenetic Abnormalities

Cancer cells typically have bizarre, unstable chromosomal structure, with many gains, losses, or rearrangements of chromosomes.

Translocations and deletions

Translocations are structural abnormalities in chromosomes that primarily affect oncogenes by causing overexpression and fusion at the points in the chromosome where abnormal breaks tend to occur (break points). In reciprocol translocations, exchange of genetic material occurs between two chromosomes or within the same chromosome. Leukemias and lymphomas typically involve translocations. For example, in chronic myelogenous leukemia, the reciprocal translocation between the q (long) arm of chromosome 9, band 34 and the q arm of chromosome 22, band 11 (9;22)(q34,q11), causes the *abl* proto-oncogene to be translocated to chromosome 22 (Philadelphia chromosome). This translocation produces a Bcr-Abl oncogenic protein with high tyrosine kinase activity. The translocation ultimately activates the *MYC* oncogene.[18,35]

Chromosomal deletions commonly involve deletions of specific gene sequences (i.e., loss of a chromosomal band or LOH of a specific allele).[18] Deletions are the hallmark of tumor suppressor genes, for example, retinoblastoma shows the deletion del(13)(q14q14).

Aneuploidy

Aneuploidy is an abnormal chromosome number, reflecting gain or loss of chromosomes. Aneuploidy usually is seen with malignant transformation, in that gross changes in chromosome number usually occur as tumorigenesis progresses. Aneuploidy can be random or nonrandom. In *random aneuploidy*, the change in chromosome number has no association with a tumor type; rather, it occurs late in tumorigenesis and reflects genetic instability of the tumor. *Nonrandom aneuploidy* involves a specific change in a given chromosome associated with a specific tumor. It tends to occur earlier in tumorigenesis than the random form.

The Cell Cycle

Cellular proliferation occurs as the result of two coordinated events: replication of DNA within the cell and mitosis (the division of the somatic cell into two daughter cells with identical complements of DNA). These two events make up what is known as the *cell cycle* (Figure 2-4). This complex molecular apparatus resides in the cell nucleus where it integrates the mix of growth-regulating signal received by the cell and makes the executive decision to allow the cell to pass through replication.[19]

Normal Function of the Cell Cycle

The cell cycle has four phases (see Figure 2-4). In the gap 1 (G1) phase, the cell enlarges and synthesizes proteins in preparation for copying its DNA. Late in G1 is a restriction point (R), the point at which the cell decides to commit itself to proceed with replication. Once the cell makes this decision, the cycle cannot be stopped. In the synthesis (S) phase, the cell replicates its DNA and duplicates its complement of chromosomes. Following chromosomal replication, the cell proceeds to gap 2 (G2), and prepares itself for mitosis. In the mitosis (M) phase, cytokinesis occurs: Equal divisions of chromosomes and cellular constituents apportion to two daughter cells; they immediately enter G1 again, where they can begin the cell cycle anew, or they may divert themselves into a resting or

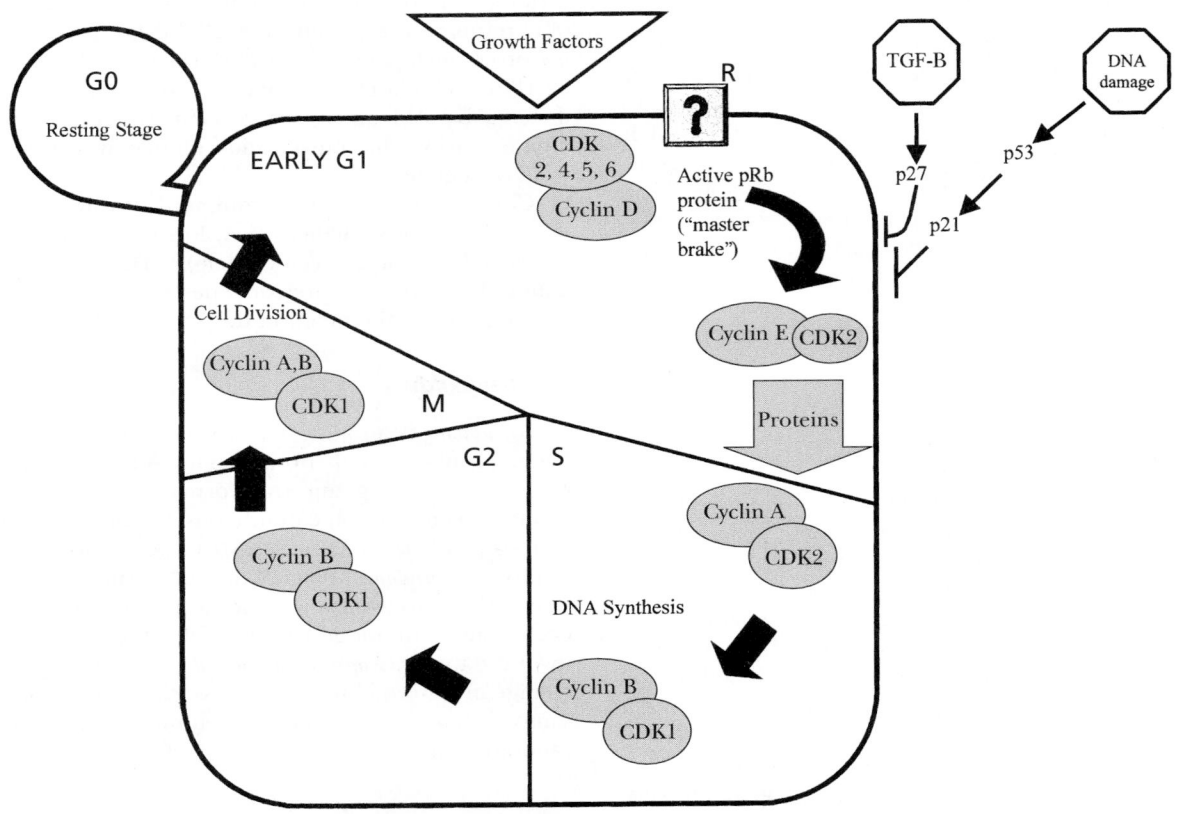

Figure 2-4 The cell cycle. The cell cycle consists of four stages (G1, S, G2, M) that are controlled by proteins called *cyclins*. The cyclins (D, E, A, B) are activated when complexed with enzymes called *cyclin-dependent kinases* (CDK). On activation, the cyclin-CDK complex allows the cell to progress through each specific cell-cycle stage. Present throughout the cell cycle, the cyclin-CDK complexes serve as checkpoints or monitors of the cell cycle. Inhibitory proteins prevent progression through the cell cycle if DNA damage is present or if nutrients or oxygen to support cellular proliferation is lacking. Examples of inhibitory proteins include p21, p27, and p53. The inhibitory proteins, in turn, are regulated by the presence of inhibitory growth factors and TGF-β. Once past R (the restriction point or "final decision" point), the cell cycle turns "on" and progression through the cell cycle is inevitable. Cyclin-CDK complexes and pRB (the "master brake") tightly regulate the R point. The stability of the inhibitory proteins and cyclin-CDK complexes are altered in cancer, thereby altering control of the cell cycle. Uncontrolled cellular proliferation prevails.

quiescent state called G0. Most of the cells in the adult body are in G0. Cells that are usually metabolically active, such as granulocytes and the epithelium of the gastrointestinal tract, are cycling cells.

The series of events that occurs in the cell cycle is tightly controlled by the cell-cycle clock, constituted by proteins called *cyclins,* which combine with and activate enzymes called CDKs. Activation of cyclins and CDKs occurs at specific points in the cell cycle (see Figure 2-4).

Situated at the R point in the cell cycle and acting as the master brake to prevent the cycle from proceeding further is the *Rb* protein (the product of the retinoblastoma gene). Certain cyclins begin a process that causes the normal braking action of Rb to stop and prevents the interaction of Rb with transcription factors, freeing them to promote expression of genes driving entry of cells into the S phase. Protein Rb then interacts with transcription factors to repress expression of target

genes.[19,36] Also contributing to deregulation of the cell cycle and excess proliferation is *MTS1*, which encodes protein p16.

Specific events in the cell cycle called *checkpoints* make certain that the cycle proceeds in correct sequence and that one event has been completed before another begins. For example, checkpoints exist at the decisions to enter S phase, mitosis (G2/M checkpoint), and to exit mitosis.[36] The checkpoint controlling entry into S phase prevents replication of damaged DNA.

The Cell Cycle and Cancer

Normal cells will often leave G1 and enter G0 at the restriction point if there is a shortage of nutrients or growth factors. Many cancer cells lack this degree of control, particularly if they have too little of the *Rb* protein.

Most likely, cancer cells have weak or deficient cell-cycle checkpoints.[19,33] Genetic instability in the G1/S checkpoint in human cancers currently is best understood. Loss of the G1/S checkpoint leads to instability of the human genome, survival of genetically damaged cells, and clonal evolution. For example, the *p53* gene is commonly mutated in several cancers, suggesting that abnormalities in the G1/S checkpoint are important in tumorigenesis.

logic stimuli that induce cell death in most cells and even less about the genes that mediate pathways to apoptosis.[37]

Characteristics of Cells Undergoing Apoptosis

Controlled autodigestion

Apoptotic cells activate endogenous proteases that digest the cell from the inside out and control degradation of the cell. The proteins involved in autodigestion are called *caspases*. Caspases are important and required components of apoptosis. The caspase cascade effects apoptotic changes in the nucleus, cell membrane, and cytoplasm. It may activate multiple members of the caspase family of proteases. Within a given cell type, different caspases are involved in different versions of apoptotic pathways. However, the specific substrates of these proteins are not known with certainty, nor is it known whether given caspases have specific, unique targets.[37,38]

Apoptosis

Apoptosis, often referred to as "programmed cell death," is a normal, active process by which cell death culminates from a distinct series of changes within the cell (Figure 2-5). The process is essential for the normal development of multicellular organisms; through apoptosis, an organism can remove old, dead, or unwanted cells. Apoptosis often requires gene activation and new protein synthesis, however, little is known about the physio-

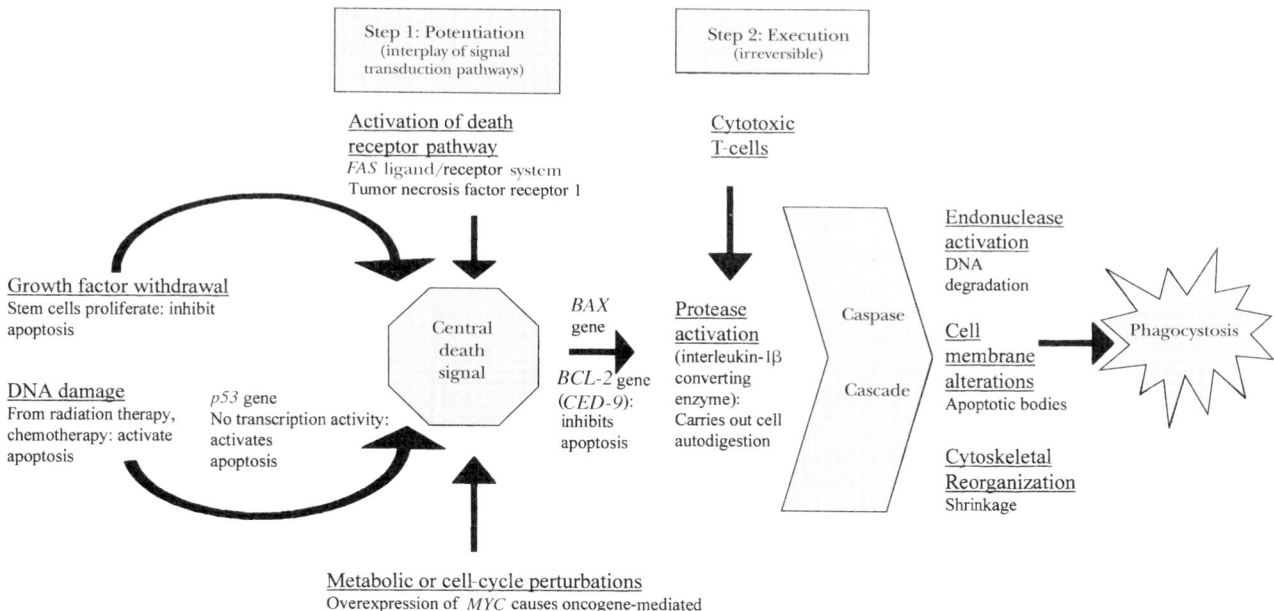

Figure 2-5 Apoptosis. Step 1: Potentiation is the interplay of signal transduction pathways. The best studied proteins described as sensors or triggers of apoptosis are the *p53* gene and the *FAS* ligand/receptor system: *p53* appears to accumulate following DNA damage. Wild-type (normal) *p53* function lowers the threshold for inducing apoptosis following genotoxic damage. However, DNA damage that alters *p53* may disable its transcription activity and activate apoptosis. The *FAS* ligand/receptor system, a cell-surface protein that is found predominantly on activated T cells, is a member of the tumor necrosis factor gene family. The *FAS* ligand triggers apoptosis in a variety of cells bearing *FAS* on their cell surface. Overexpression of the oncogene *MYC* causes cells to be more susceptible to apoptosis.

Genetic evidence in animals indicates that *ced-9/bcl*-2 belongs to an emerging family. A "ced" gene is a cell death gene. While *ced-9/bcl*-2 expression blocks apoptosis, other family members make cells more susceptible to apoptotic stimuli (e.g., *bax*). The *bax* and *bcl*-2 genes present together and the ratio of each fine-tunes the expression of apoptosis.

Step 2: Execution is irreversible. The binding of ligands to receptors leads to binding with other proteins, which initiates a cascade leading to cell death. When protease activation occurs, interleukin-1β converting enzyme (ICE; also called caspase 1 or *ced*-3) carries out cell degradation and activates the cascade of other caspases. The *ced*-3/ICE gene family proteases all appear to cause apoptosis when overexpressed in various cell types. Apoptotic cells demonstrate endonuclease activation (furthers DNA degradation), presence of apoptotic bodies (facilitate phagocytosis), and cytoskeletal reorganization and shrinking.

Structural changes

Blebbing and bubbling of the plasma membrane causes breakage into pieces called *apoptotic bodies*. Apoptotic bodies cause apoptotic cells to become phagocytized by neighboring cells that are not undergoing apoptosis. A cardinal feature of apoptosis is its ability to minimize leakage of cellular constituents from dying cells, i.e., to minimize an inflammatory response. This feature distinguishes apoptosis from necrosis, which usually results from trauma that causes injured cells to swell, lyse, and release cytoplasmic material that stimulates an inflammatory response.[39,40]

Apoptotic cells lose water, causing shrinkage or condensation of the cytoplasm. Large vacuoles also form in the cytoplasm. In the nucleus, margins of chromatin become concentrated at the inside of the nuclear membrane. The nucleus condenses into multiple fragments with an intact membrane.[39,40] The chromatin cleavage causes DNA degradation.

Genes and Gene Products Involved in Apoptosis

In animal studies, two genes, *ced-3* and *ced-4*, are thought to be required for cell death, and the presence of one gene, *ced-9/bcl-2*, can block the death-promoting effects of *ced-3* and *ced-4*.[41] The mammalian homolog protein BCL-2 appears localized to or associated with intracellular membranes of mitochondria, endoplasmic reticulum, and nuclei.[42] Although the mechanism of protein BCL-2 action is unknown, biochemical studies have shown that ecotopic expression of protein BCL-2 suppresses cell death induced by oxidizing agents.[43] Genetic evidence indicates that *ced-9/bcl-2* belongs to an emerging family of genes some of which can suppress apoptosis,[44] while other members make cells more susceptible to apoptotic stimuli.[44,45] Additionally, *bcl-2* family members suggest a model of regulation where cellular susceptibility or threshold for apoptosis is partly influenced by the level of *bcl-2* expression.[45]

Studies have identified several *ced-3* and its mammalian homolog interleukin-1β converting enzyme (ICE) gene-family proteases, all of which appear to cause apoptosis when overexpressed in various cell types.[46] Considerable research has focused on identifying the molecular sensors or triggers of apoptosis. In humans, these triggers are the *p53* tumor-suppressor gene and the *FAS* gene and its cognate receptor *FAS*, respectively.[47,48]

Impaired apoptosis may be a significant factor in the etiology of cancer. As a transcription factor, *p53* may have a role in DNA repair, because it appears to accumulate following DNA damage.[47] Studies using *p53* cell lines transfected with a temperature-sensitive mutant of *p53* have clearly shown that wild-type *p53* function lowers the threshold for inducing apoptosis following genotoxic damage.[49] Thus, *p53* may function as a sensor of DNA damage and has been called the "guardian" of the genome.[50]

Apoptosis may be exploited for therapeutic purposes. For example, triggering cell death might provide the means for eliminating unwanted cells, among them tumor cells. This might be accomplished by harnessing tumor necrosis factor (TNF), which triggers apoptosis in some target cells.

Metastasis

Metastasis is the major cause of cancer death.[51–53] Determining the presence of metastatic sites is an important cancer prognostic factor; unfortunately, in many cases metastases occur before the initial diagnosis of cancer.[51,52] The biology of the different steps involved in the process of metastasis comprises a fundamental area of cancer research. Currently, strategies are being developed to disrupt the metastatic process and thereby improve outcomes of cancer care.

Factors Contributing to Metastasis

Metastasis is the spread of tumor cells, via the bloodstream or lymphatic system, from the primary tumor site to a new target tissue in the body. Molecular mechanisms that contribute to the process of metastasis include angiogenesis, motility, alterations in cell adhesion, and secretion of proteolytic enzymes leading to barrier breakdown.[51–56] Further, once in circulation, metastatic tumor cells must escape immune surveillance, and angiogenesis must occur for the cells to establish themselves in a new tissue site.

Angiogenesis

When a tumor is larger than 2 mm^3 in size, its growth is limited unless it receives a new blood supply.[57] Formation of a new blood supply, a process termed *angiogenesis*, satisfies the nutrient and oxygen needs of tumor expansion. Angiogenesis involves the migration and proliferation of endothelial cells from existing vasculature near the tumor. Angiogenesis itself is invasive, as the new endothelial cells burrow their way into the tumor site, resembling steps of the metastatic cascade. Secreted matrix metalloproteinases (MMPs) and proliferation and migration of endothelial cells into the tumor site mediate degradation of the extracellular matrix (ECM). The newly formed blood vessels provide nutrition and oxygen to the growing tumor, as well as a potential route for metastatic tumor cells to exit the primary tumor site. The newly formed blood vessels tend to be "leaky," with loose cell-cell contacts, providing easy entrance for tumor cells into the bloodstream for potential transport to distant sites.

Both positive and negative regulators of angiogenesis exist. Tumor cells produce positive angiogenic factors such as vascular endothelial growth factor (VEGF), basic fibroblast growth factor (bFGF), TNF, and angiopoietin-

1, which serve as stimuli for the development of new capillaries. Angiogenic factors appear to stimulate locomotion and mitosis of vascular endothelium, and to release endothelial growth factors, thus stimulating capillary proliferation. Vascular endothelial growth factor, which promotes growth and chemotaxis of endothelial cells in vitro, is overexpressed in many tumors. Most important, VEGF may be the final pathway through which other angiogenic agents exert their influence.[58]

Negative regulators of angiogenesis are as important as the positive stimulatory agents and include TGF-β1, alfa-interferon, and angiostatin.[59] Of particular note, TGF-β1 inhibits the proteolysis necessary for the formation of viable and effective endothelial sprouts emanating from parent vessels. Use of alfa-interferon, the first antiangiogenic substance to be used in a clinical trial, evolved following its use in the treatment of a life-threatening angioma.[60] Angiostatin, a fragment of the plasminogen molecule, generally prevents proliferation of endothelial cells.[60] (The National Cancer Institute provides an online list of current clinical trials involving antiangiogenesis agents.[61])

The degree of angiogenesis in the primary tumor site correlates with metastatic potential and is a prognostic factor for breast cancer.[55,57] Clearly, increased blood vessels in the primary tumor site are associated with metastasis and have been determined to be the second most effective prognostic factor following lymph node status.[62]

Motility

A tumor cell must exhibit motile behavior to leave the primary tumor and circulate through the vasculature or lymphatic system. *Motogens,* or motility factors, stimulate tumor cell motility.[52] Motility factors are produced by tumor cells and tissue cells and include EGF and interleukins-1, -3, and -6.

It is widely accepted that cell shape and motility are interrelated because changes in the cytoskeleton are associated with increased motility of tumor cells.[63–66] The cytoskeleton is an internal supportive structure of a cell that consists of filamentous proteins including actin, keratin,

vimentin, and tubulin.[63] It appears that the coexpression and distribution of these filaments is associated with metastatic disease in some cancers.[65] Coexpression of vimentin and keratins 8 and 18 is associated with recurrent and metastatic melanoma.[64] There is also a strong correlation between keratin and vimentin coexpression and metastatic disease in breast cancer.[64–66]

Several antimotility factors are currently under investigation, particularly agents that target specific filamental structures of the cytoskeleton. Agents such as paclitaxol and colchicine work by altering microtubules. Cytochalasin D is associated with inhibition of cell motility following disruption of actin filaments.[52]

Cell adhesion

Cells express specific surface receptors that mediate both attachments to the ECM and cell-cell adhesion. The involvement of cell-cell and cell-matrix adhesion in the metastatic cascade necessitates the presence of large numbers of cell adhesion molecules. Cadherins and selectins are both families of adhesion molecules that mediate cell-cell adhesion. Tumor cells have an increased ability to downregulate E-cadherin, thereby increasing their ability to break off from the primary tumor.

The major components of the ECM include fibronectin, laminin, vitronectin, collagen type IV, and heparan sulfate proteoglycan. The ECM is the first barrier tumor cells encounter when attempting to leave the primary tumor site. Prior to degrading the ECM, tumor cells must first become adhesive to the ECM (Figure 2-6).

Integrins are a family of proteins that mediate cell-matrix adhesion. In contrast to cadherin expression, increased expression of integrins in tumor cells is associated with increased metastatic potential. Knowledge about these different molecules may enhance therapies aimed at modulating important adhesive steps in metastasis.

Proteolytic enzymes

To successfully metastasize, a tumor cell must cross a number of barriers including the basement membrane,

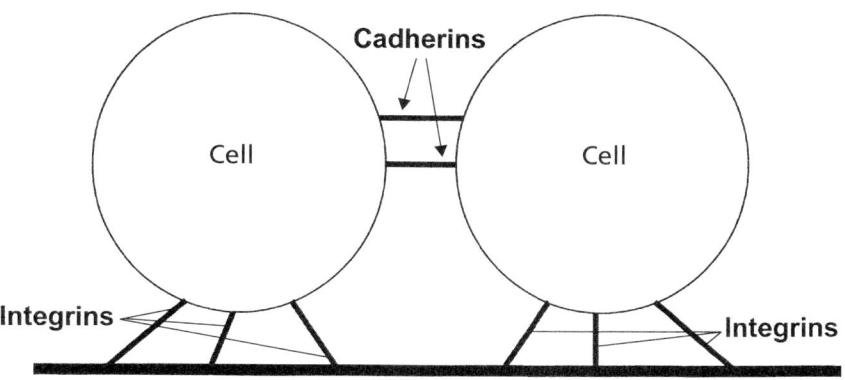

Figure 2-6 Cell adhesion. Cell adhesion molecules mediating cell-cell adhesion (cadherins) and cell-matrix adhesion (integrins) are important mediators of metastasis. Decreases in cell-cell adhesion and cell-matrix adhesion are necessary to allow detachment of tumor cells from the primary tumor site. Decreases in adhesion occur as specific adhesion molecules (cadherins and/or integrins) are down regulated via specific signaling pathways.

the ECM, connective tissue, and the endothelial barrier.[51,67] Tumor cells secrete a number of proteinases that assist with degradation of these barriers. Once secreted, the enzymes degrade the adjacent barrier and allow passage of the tumor cell either into circulation or into an underlying secondary tissue bed. Increased secretion of MMPs and urokinase-type plasminogen activator (uPA), for example, is associated with highly metastatic tumors.[51]

Tissue inhibitors of metalloproteinases (TIMPs) and plasminogen activator inhibitors (PAIs) represent the two most important families of metalloproteinase inhibitors.[68] The TIMP members are regulated by TGF-β and other cytokines, and they are made in endothelial cells and some tumor cells.[69] Of the TIMPs, TIMP-2 is able to bind to both latent and activated forms of type IV collagenase; this inhibitor essentially abolishes the hydrolytic activity of all members of the metalloproteinase family.[70] Additionally, TIMP-2 has the capability to inhibit growth factor-stimulated proliferation of transformed cells in culture.[71]

The ratio of proteolytic enzymes to their inhibitors determines tumor invasiveness. For example, a small tumor may remain noninvasive until it secretes a sufficient amount of proteolytic enzymes to overcome the inhibitors. This ratio has been used as a marker of metastasis for patients with breast cancer.[72]

Because neoplastic cells will invade all primary site tissue barriers, including the local endothelial basement membranes and the basement membranes of the target organ, an inhibitor of proteinase activity would be a likely candidate to interrupt metastasis.[73] Tumor-associated trypsin inhibitor (TATI) can inhibit the degradation of the ECM by tumor cells.[52] Leupeptin, a proteolytic enzyme inhibitor, also is an effective antimetastasis agent when combined with doxorubicin.[52] Despite knowledge of both general and specific inhibitors, it seems unlikely that a total blockade of the various degradative enzyme systems will be accomplished by one agent. Nevertheless, proteinase inhibitors will likely be studied clinically in the near future.[73]

Immunogenicity

Whether a tumor cell can elicit an immune response determines its ability to evade the immune system while in circulation. The theory of immune surveillance suggests that malignant cells develop randomly and often, but immune cells destroy cancer cells before they can gain the numbers or protection needed to survive. Cytotoxic T lymphocytes, activated macrophages, and natural killer (NK) cells are thought to be the predominant immune cells that defend against cancer and regulate metastasis.[51,74] For cytotoxic T-cell activation, the tumor antigen must be presented by an antigen-presenting cell (APC) to the T cell. Activation of the APC cell, in turn, depends on the presentation of tumor-associated antigens on the tumor cell surface.

Natural killer cells are large, granular lymphocytes that can naturally lyse a broad range of tumor-cell targets, even if there has been no prior exposure to the tumor cells. The exact mechanism of how NK cells recognize tumor cells is unclear. Natural killer cells do not require APC presentation of an antigen for spontaneous cytolytic activity.[51,74] Macrophages are the tissue-based counterparts to blood monocytes; they have a natural antitumor activity that is enhanced when they are "activated" by various substances. For example, interleukin-2 can heighten the antitumor actions of cytotoxic T cells and NK cells,[75] while gamma-interferon is a classic activator of macrophages.

Tumor cells evade or hide from the immune system in a multitude of ways. Many tumors downregulate MHC expression, escaping detection. Other tumors secrete immunosuppressive factors such as TGF-β, which decreases T-cell proliferation. Tumor cells can release soluble antigens or intracellular adhesion molecules that block T-cell interactions with APC. Tumor cells may also develop variants (in their tendency toward heterogeneity) with no recognizable antigenic structures.[76] Chemotherapy and radiation treatments may depress the immune system in general.

The Metastatic Cascade

The process of metastasis is complex and involves multiple steps called a *metastatic cascade.*[51] In the metastatic cascade (Figure 2-7), cells first break from the primary tumor, then motile cancer cells invade and enter the bloodstream or lymphatic vessels. If cancer cells are successful at evading the immune system, blood and lymph transport them to distant sites such as the bones, lungs, and liver. To invade normal tissues and establish metastatic colonies, the tumor cells again must penetrate the endothelium, degrade the underlying basement membrane, and induce angiogenesis. Many of the molecular mechanisms that tumor cells use facilitate this cascade of events.

Steps of the metastatic cascade

Detachment. Detachment from the primary tumor begins as a tumor cell grows and begins to press on the surrounding tissue and blood supply. Detachment is further accomplished by downregulation of cadherin-adhesion-molecule expression on the tumor surface. This decreases cell-cell contact, facilitating complete detachment from neighboring tumor cells.

Invasion. Tumor cells can invade the surrounding tissue, a lymphatic vessel, or a blood vessel. Direct extension into an adjacent tissue or lymphatic vessel is mediated by pressure that the enlarged tumor exerts on the tissue as well as by motility factors. Invasion is accomplished by secretion of proteolytic enzymes that are not overcome by local inhibitors. The secreted enzymes cause barrier breakdown and subsequent tumor invasion. If a tumor enters a vessel, the cells may localize at the entry site or disseminate to other destinations.

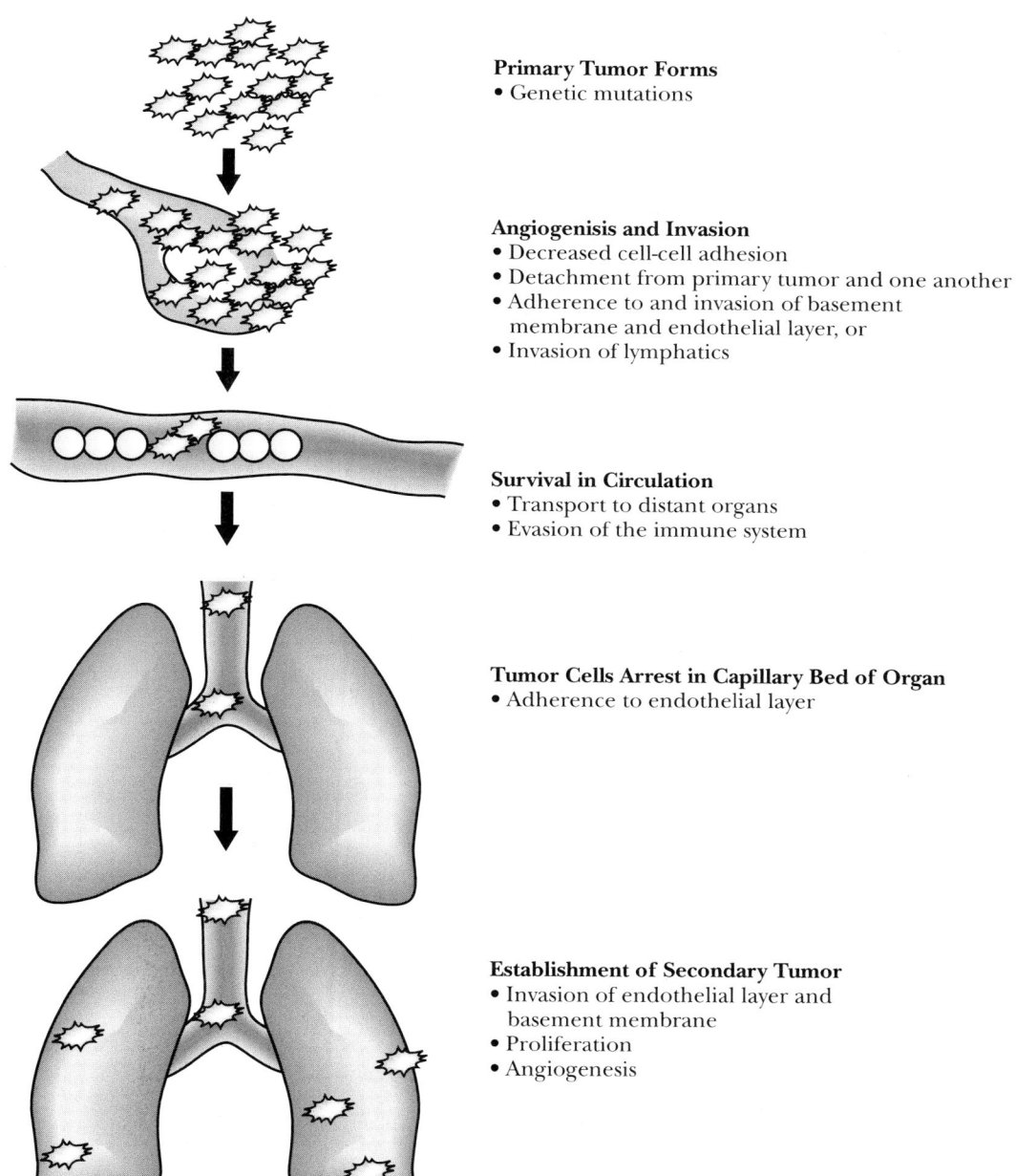

Primary Tumor Forms
• Genetic mutations

Angiogenisis and Invasion
• Decreased cell-cell adhesion
• Detachment from primary tumor and one another
• Adherence to and invasion of basement membrane and endothelial layer, or
• Invasion of lymphatics

Survival in Circulation
• Transport to distant organs
• Evasion of the immune system

Tumor Cells Arrest in Capillary Bed of Organ
• Adherence to endothelial layer

Establishment of Secondary Tumor
• Invasion of endothelial layer and basement membrane
• Proliferation
• Angiogenesis

Figure 2-7 The metastatic cascade. The multistep cascade begins when genetic events facilitate primary tumor formation. Angiogenesis (vascularization) increases proliferation of the growing tumor. Preceding invasion, there is a decrease in cell-cell contact and adherence to and invasion of the endothelial basement membrane. Once tumor cells have entered the lymphatic system or circulation, they are transported to distant sites. If the tumor cells are successful at evading the immune system, they eventually will arrest in a capillary bed of a distant organ. Establishment of a secondary site will follow once the tumor cells invade the endothelial barrier to gain entrance to the underlying organ tissue bed.

Survival in transport. In the bloodstream, tumor cells are at risk due to mechanical forces and attack by the immune system. Tumor cells rely on survival-enhancing mechanisms (see "Immunogenicity" in previous section) to evade the immune system.

Arrest in distant organ capillary bed. Arrest of tumor cells in an organ capillary bed requires that they adhere to the endothelial layer. To maximize the ability to adhere to a distant blood vessel, malignant cells may secrete substances that cause platelets to aggregate around them, resulting in a large, sticky mass. In turn, platelets secrete growth factors that favor continued survival of the adjoining tumor cells.[56]

Where circulating tumor cells adhere depends on certain factors that are not entirely clear. Yet, selective patterns of tumor spread do exist for different cancers. Cell-cell adhesion molecules expressed on the surface of tumor cells may influence what organs or sites certain tumors will favor, because corresponding adhesion molecules might be present in the microvasculature of distant organs.[56] This phenomenon helps explain why prostate carcinoma cells so often go to bone and ocular melanomas spread to the liver while typically sparing other organs.

In addition to selective target tissue adhesion, specific chemotactic factors or growth factors may lure circulating malignant cells to a particular site.[56] Neoplastic cells with higher affinity for laminin tend to metastasize to lung tissue, whereas other tumor cells with a higher affinity for fibronectin favor settlement in the liver.[56] Specific chemotactic substances have been isolated from various organ sources, including lung, brain, bone, and liver; for instance, melanoma cells that had metastasized to the brain were found to respond in culture preferentially to brain-derived chemotactic factors.[77]

Establishment of secondary tumor. The proteolytic process of degrading the endothelial basement membrane to enter the secondary site essentially mimics the process used by the tumor cell to gain initial entrance to the vascular system. Although the process must repeat in the secondary organ, the conditions in the new microenvironment may be very different. The tumor cell may have to adapt to changes in nutrients or to the presence of stimulatory growth factors. Additionally, the immune profiles of primary and secondary tumor sites may be quite different. For example, levels of interleukin-4 and TNF-α were found to be higher in the primary site of human colon carcinomas compared with metastatic sites.[78]

Treatment of Metastasis

The potential for success in interrupting the metastatic continuum seems brighter today than it has in the past. Despite a lack of knowledge regarding the biochemical mechanisms of metastasis, the mysteries of this process are quickly unraveling. It is inevitable that treatment options will include new agents to abrogate various steps in the metastatic cascade. Agents that inhibit tumor cell motility and invasiveness will have key roles as antimetastatic therapies. We still need to learn how to predict the metastatic potential of a tumor at the time of diagnosis, the degree of silent metastasis, and how to tell when a tumor is completely eradicated. We also need to better understand tumor cell heterogeneity.

Conclusion

The biology of cancer is a complex, continually evolving phenomenon, and one that is difficult to keep abreast of unless immersed in the basic sciences of cancer. Because cancer biology underlies every other aspect of cancer as a human disease, nurses need to have a basic understanding of cancer genetics, molecular and cell biology, immunology, and biochemistry. Establishing how these sciences interrelate will facilitate our ability to prevent and treat cancers based on knowledge of cancer development, growth, and metastasis.

References

1. Doll R: Introduction, in Hiatt HH, Watson JR, Winsten JA (eds): *Origins of Human Cancer.* Cold Spring Harbor, NY, Cold Spring Harbor Laboratory, 1977, pp 1–12
2. Nowell P: The clonal evolution of tumor cell populations. *Science* 194:23–28, 1976
3. Strachan TS, Read AD: *Human Molecular Genetics.* New York: Wiley-Liss, 1996
4. Fearon ER, Vogelstein B: A genetic model for colorectal carcinogenesis. *Cell* 61:759–767, 1990
5. Kupchella CE: *Dimensions of Cancer.* Belmont, CA, Wadsworth, 1987
6. LeMarbre PJ, Groenwald SL: Biology of cancer, in Groenwald SL, Frogge MH, Goodman M, Yarbro CH (eds): *Cancer Nursing Principles and Practice* (ed 4). Sudbury, MA: Jones and Bartlett, 1997, pp 17–37
7. Banks DA, Foessel M: Telomeres, cancer, and aging. *JAMA* 278:1345–1348, 1997
8. Hakomori S: Cancer-associated glycosphingolipid antigens: Their structure, organization, and function. *Acta Anatomica* 161:79–90, 1998
9. Singer S, Nicolson G: The fluid mosaic structure of cell membranes. *Science* 175:720–731, 1972
10. Nicolson GL: Transmembrane control of the receptors in normal and tumor cells: II. Surface changes associated with transformation and malignancy. *Biochem Biophys Acta* 458: 1–72, 1976
11. Ruchaud S, Lanotte M: cAMP and 'death signals' in a myeloid leukemia cell: From membrane receptors to nuclear responses: A review. *Biochem Soc Trans* 25:410–415, 1997
12. Griffiths JF, Miller JH, Suzuki DT, et al: *An Introduction to Genetic Analysis* (ed 6). New York, Freeman, 1996
13. Watson JD, Gilman M, Witkowski J, Zoller M: *Recombinant DNA* (ed 2). New York, Scientific American Books, 1992
14. Friend SH, Iggo R, Ishioka C, et al: Overcoming complexities in genetic screening for cancer susceptibility. *Cold Spring Harb Symp Quant Biol* 59:673–676, 1994
15. Knudson AG: Mutation and cancer: Statistical study of retinoblastoma. *Proc Natl Acad Sci USA* 68:820–823, 1971
16. Loescher LJ: DNA testing for cancer predisposition. *Oncol Nurs Forum* 25:1317–1327, 1998
17. Papadopoulos N, Nicolaides NC, Wei Y-F, et al: Mutation of a mutL homolog in hereditary colon cancer. *Science* 263: 1625–1629, 1994

18. Cooper GM: *Oncogenes.* Sudbury, MA; Jones and Bartlett, 1995

19. Weinberg RA: How cancer arises. *Sci Am* 275:62–70, 1996

20. Cantly LC, Auger KR, Carpenter C, et al: Oncogenes and signal transduction. *Cell* 64:281–302, 1991

21. Wong AJ, Ruppert JM, Bigner SH, et al: Structural alterations of the epidermal growth factor receptor gene in human gliomas. *Proc Natl Acad Sci USA* 89:2965–2969, 1992

22. Chin LS, Murray SF, Zitnay KM, et al: K252a inhibits proliferation of glioma cells by blocking platelet-derived growth factor signal transduction. *Clin Cancer Res* 3:771–776, 1997

23. Kitagawa Y, Ueda M, Ando N, et al. Further evidence for prognostic significance of epidermal growth factor receptor gene amplification in patients with esophageal squamous cell carcinoma. *Clin Cancer Res* 2:909–914, 1996

24. Radinsky R, Risin X, Fan X, et al: Level and function of epidermal growth factor receptor predict the metastatic potential of human colon carcinoma cells. *Clin Cancer Res* 1:19–31, 1995

25. Harris A, Nicholson S, Sainsbury J, et al: Epidermal growth factor receptor: A marker of early relapse in breast cancer and tumor stage progression in bladder cancer—interactions with NEU, in Furth M, Greaves M (eds): *The Molecular Diagnostics of Human Cancer,* vol 7. Cold Spring Harbor, NY, Cold Spring Harbor Laboratory Press, 1989, pp 353–357

26. De Luca A, Casamassimi A, Selvam MP, et al: EGF-related peptides are involved in the proliferation and survival of MDA-MB-468 human breast carcinoma cells. *Int J Cancer* 80:589–594, 1999

27. Naidu R, Yadav M, Nair S, et al.: Expression of c-erbB3 protein in primary breast carcinomas. *Br J Cancer* 78:1385–1390, 1998

28. Tsuda H, Sakamaki C, Tsugane S, et al: A prospective study of the significance of gene and chromosome alterations as prognostic indicators of breast cancer patients with lymph node metastases. *Breast Cancer Res Treat* 48:21–32, 1998

29. Kita K, Saito S, Morioka CY, et al: Growth inhibition of human pancreatic cancer cell lines by anti-sense oligonucleotides specific to mutated K-ras genes. *Int J Cancer* 80:553–558, 1999

30. Papavassiliou A: Transcription factors. *N Engl J Med* 332:45–47, 1995

31. Latchman DS: Transcription-factor mutations and disease. *N Engl J Med* 334:28–33, 1996

32. Weinberg RA: Oncogenes and tumor suppressor genes. *CA Cancer J Clin* 44:160–170, 1994

33. Orr-Weaver TL, Weinberg RA: A checkpoint on the road to cancer. *Nature* 392:223–224, 1998

34. Cama A, Genuardi M, Guanti G, et al: Molecular genetics of hereditary non-polyposis colorectal cancer (HNPCC). *Tumori* 82:122–135, 1996

35. Solomon E, Borrow J, Goddard AD: Chromosome aberrations and cancer. *Science* 254:1153–1160, 1991

36. Hartwell LH, Kastan MB: Cell cycle control and cancer. *Science* 266:1821–1828, 1994

37. Smith SW, Osborne BA: Private pathways to a common death. *J NIH Res* 9:33–37, 1997

38. Henkart PA: ICE family proteases: mediators of all apoptotic cell death? *Immun* 4:195–201, 1996

39. Steller H: Mechanisms and genes of cellular suicide. *Science* 267:1445–1449, 1995

40. Wyllie AH: Apoptosis: An overview. *Br Med Bull* 53:451–465, 1997

41. Ellis RE, Yuan JY, Horvitz HR: Mechanisms and function of cell death. *Annu Rev Cell Biol* 7:663–698, 1991

42. Reed JC: Bcl-2 family proteins. *Oncogene* 17:3225–3236, 1998

43. Chao DT, Korsmeyer SJ: BCL-2 family: Regulators of cell death. *Annu Rev Immunol* 16:395–419, 1998.

44. Minn AJ, Boise LH, Thompson CB: Bcl-x(S) antagonizes the protective effects of Bcl-x(L). *J Biol Chem* 271:6306–6312, 1996

45. Korsmeyer SJ, Shutter JR, Veis DJ, et al: Bcl-2/Bax: A rheostat that regulates an anti-oxidant pathway and cell death. *Semin Cancer Biol* 4:327–332, 1993

46. Martin SJ, Green DR: Protease activation during apoptosis: Death by a thousand cuts? *Cell* 82:349–352, 1995

47. Donehower LA: Effects of p53 mutation on tumor progression: Recent insights from mouse tumor models. *Biochim Biophys Acta* 1242:171–176, 1996

48. Nagata S: Fas-induced apoptosis. *Intern Med* 37:179–181, 1998

49. Lowe SW, Schmitt EM, Smith SW, et al: p53 is required for radiation-induced apoptosis in mouse thymocytes. *Nature* 362:847–849, 1993

50. Lane DP: Cancer: p53, guardian of the genome. *Nature* 358:15–16, 1992

51. Tannock I: Tumor progression and metastasis, in Tannock I, Hill R: *The Basic Science of Oncology* (ed 3). New York, McGraw-Hill, 1998, pp 219–262

52. Jiang W, Puntis C, Hallet M: Molecular and cellular basis of cancer invasion and metastasis: Implications for treatment. *Br J Surg* 81:1576–1590, 1994

53. Liotta L, Hoh E: Cancer invasion and metastasis. *JAMA* 263:1123–1126, 1990

54. Heppner G, Miller F: The cellular basis of tumor progression. *Int Rev Cytol* 177:1–56, 1998

55. Hart I, Saini A: Biology of tumor metastasis. *Lancet* 339:1453–1456, 1992

56. Ruoslahti E: How cancer spreads. *Sci Am* 275:72–77, 1996

57. Leek R, Harris A, Lewis C: Cytokine networks in solid tumors: Regulation of angiogenesis. *J Leukoc Biol* 56:423–435, 1994

58. Folkman J: What is the role of thymidine phosphorylase in tumor angiogenesis? *J Natl Cancer Inst* 88:1091–1092, 1996 (editorial)

59. Liotta L, Stetler-Stevenson W: Principles of molecular biology of cancer: Cancer metastasis, in DeVita VA, Hellman S, Rosenberg ST (eds): *Cancer: Principles and Practice of Oncology* (ed 4). Philadelphia, Lippincott, 1993, pp 134–149

60. Folkman J: Fighting cancer by attacking its blood supply. *Sci Am* 275:150–154, 1996

61. National Cancer Institute: Cancer trials. Anti-angiogenesis information. Available at: http://cancertrials.nci.nih.gov/ .Accessed 1999.

62. Weidner N, Semple J, Welch W, Folkman J: Tumor angiogenesis and metastasis: Correlation in invasive breast cancer. *N Engl J Med* 324:1–8, 1991

63. Kries T, Vale R: *Guidebook to the Cytoskeletal and Motor Proteins.* New York, Oxford University Press, 1993

64. Clarke R, Thompson E, Leonessa F, et al: Hormone resistance, invasiveness, and metastatic potential in breast cancer. *Breast Cancer Res Treat* 24:227–239, 1993

65. Hendrix M, Seftor E, Chu Y, et al: Role of intermediate filaments in migration, invasion and metastasis. *Cancer Metastasis Rev* 15:507–525, 1996

66. Strauli P, Haemmerli G: The role of cancer cell motility in invasion. *Cancer Metastasis Rev* 3:127–141, 1984

67. Chambers A, Matrisian L: Changing views of the role of matrix metalloproteinases in metastasis. *J Natl Cancer Inst* 89:1260–1270, 1997

68. Gottesman M: The role of proteases in cancer. *Semin Cancer Biol* 1:97–160, 1990

69. Boone T, Johnson M, DeClerck Y, et al: cDNA cloning and expression of a metalloproteinase inhibitor related to tissue inhibitor of metalloproteinases. *Proc Natl Acad Sci USA* 87: 2800–2804, 1990

70. Goldberg G, Marmer B, Grant G, et al: Human 72-kDA type IV collagenase forms a complex with a tissue inhibitor of metalloproteinase inhibitor. *Proc Natl Acad Sci USA* 86: 8207–8211, 1989

71. Corcoran M, Stetler-Stevenson W: Tissue inhibitor of metalloproteinase-2 stimulates fibroblast proliferation via a cAMP-dependent mechanism. *J Biol Chem* 270:13453–13459, 1995

72. Allesandro R, Kohn E: Molecular genetics of cancer-tumor invasion and angiogenesis. *Cancer* 76:1874–1877, 1995

73. DeClereck Y, Imren S: Protease inhibitors: Role and potential therapeutic use in human cancer. *Eur J Cancer* 30: 2170–2180, 1994

74. Brittenden J, Heys S, Ross J, et al: Natural killer cells and cancer. *Cancer* 77:1226–1265, 1996

75. Rosenberg S, Lotze M, Muul L, et al: A progress report on the treatment of 157 patients with advanced cancer using lymphokine-activated killer cells and interleukin-2 or high dose interleukin-2 alone. *N Engl J Med* 316:889–897, 1987

76. Nicholson G: Molecular mechanisms of cancer metastasis: Tumor and host properties and the role of oncogenes and suppressor genes. *Curr Opin Oncol* 3:75–92, 1991

77. Hujanen E, Terranova V: Migration of tumor cells to organ-derived chemoattractants. *Cancer Res* 45:3517–3521, 1985

78. Barth R, Camp B, Martuscello T, et al: The cytokine environment of human colon carcinoma. *Cancer* 78:1168–1178, 1996

Immunology

Susan M. Bauer, DNSc, RN

Introduction

Through understanding the immune system and factors that affect its function, oncology nurses can play an important role in promoting optimal immunologic responses and in preventing clinical complications in the patient with cancer. This chapter provides a basic review of immunology, including components of the immune system, key immunologic processes, and clinical implications. Cancer diagnosis and treatment are identified with changes in immune function. For example, suppressed or inadequate immune processes are associated with the development of some cancers, while chemotherapeutic drugs and radiation therapy used to treat cancer can induce immunosuppression. Other cancer therapies (e.g., biotherapies such as lymphokine-activated killer cells or monoclonal antibodies) can enhance the body's own immune system to fight off cancer. In addition, behavioral factors, such as nutrition, exercise, sleep, and stress, can also affect immunologic functioning.

Overview

The immune system provides the body's defense against infectious and malignant disease. It is a complex arrangement of cells, tissues, and soluble mediators. Two overall functions of the immune system are to recognize foreign substances (nonself) and to eliminate the foreign substances with restoration of homeostasis.[1,2] Foreign organisms that invade the body are called *antigens* and initiate immune responses.

Immune responses may be either innate or adaptive.[1,2] *Innate immunity,* referred to as the body's first line of defense, provides nonspecific responses to foreign substances. Inflammation and phagocytosis are examples of such nonspecific responses. Phagocytosis involves general recognition and engulfment of foreign organisms.

Adaptive, or acquired, immunity differs from innate immunity in that it is highly specific for particular antigens. This type of immunity has memory, referred to as *anamnesis,* meaning the responses improve with each successive encounter with the same antigen.[1,2] Humoral and cell-mediated immune responses are interdependent functional arms that fall within the domain of adaptive immunity. The specificity and memory associated with acquired immunity form the basis of vaccination to control certain diseases.

Immune responses can be characterized as appropriate, deficient, or overreactive. An *appropriate immune response* results in the elimination of antigen and the restoration of homeostasis with memory. *Immune deficiency* is an underreactivity of the immune processes, characterized by a pattern of repeated infections with a single organism. *Overreactive or inappropriate immune responses* are categorized three ways: (1) allergy, which involves inappropriate responses to innocuous foreign substances; (2) autoimmunity, which are responses to self-tissue antigens; and (3) graft rejection, as a result of transplanted organs.[1,2] Quality of immune responsiveness is quite variable and depends on myriad circumstances, such as genetics, age, medications, health behaviors, and environmental factors.

Components of the Immune System

Structures of the Immune System

Structures of the immune system are categorized as either primary or secondary lymphoid organs and tissues (Figure 3-1). The *primary lymphoid organs* are the anatomical locations in which lymphocytes develop immunocompetence: the bone marrow for B cells and the thymus for T cells.[1,2] *Secondary lymphoid organs* and tissues are where cellular and humoral responses take place: the spleen, lymph nodes, tonsils, Peyer's patches in the gastrointestinal tract, and the bone marrow are considered both a primary and secondary lymphoid organ. The spleen responds to predominantly blood-borne antigen; lymph nodes mount immune responses to antigens circulating in the lymph system; and tonsils and Peyer's patches respond to antigens that have penetrated the mucosal barriers.

Cells of the Immune System

The cells of the immune system, *leukocytes,* arise from the pluripotent hematopoietic stem cells of the bone marrow, which give rise to two identified cell lines: myeloid and lymphoid (Figure 3-2). Immune cells are distinguished from each other through the expression of different surface molecules, or markers, referred to as clusters of differentiation (CD). Different markers may be characteristic of different lineages, of different stages of cell maturation, or of the presence of cell activation. An immune cell may have more than one marker, or CD number, associated with it.[1,2]

The myeloid lineage

The myeloid lineage produces monocytes, polymorphonuclear leukocytes (neutrophils, eosinophils, and basophils/mast cells), and platelets.[1,2] *Monocytes* are circulating leukocytes that give rise to the mononuclear phagocyte system, which includes the following: Kupffer cells in the liver, intraglomerular mesangium of the kidney, alveolar macrophages in the lung, serosal macrophages, brain microglia, spleen sinus macrophages, and lymph node sinus macrophages. These cells play important roles in both innate and adaptive responses and have two main functions: (1) "professional" phagocytic macrophages remove particulate antigens; and (2) antigen-presenting cells (APCs) present antigen to lymphocytes.[1,2]

Polymorphonuclear granulocytes (polymorphs) make up

Figure 3-1 Primary and secondary lymphoid organs.

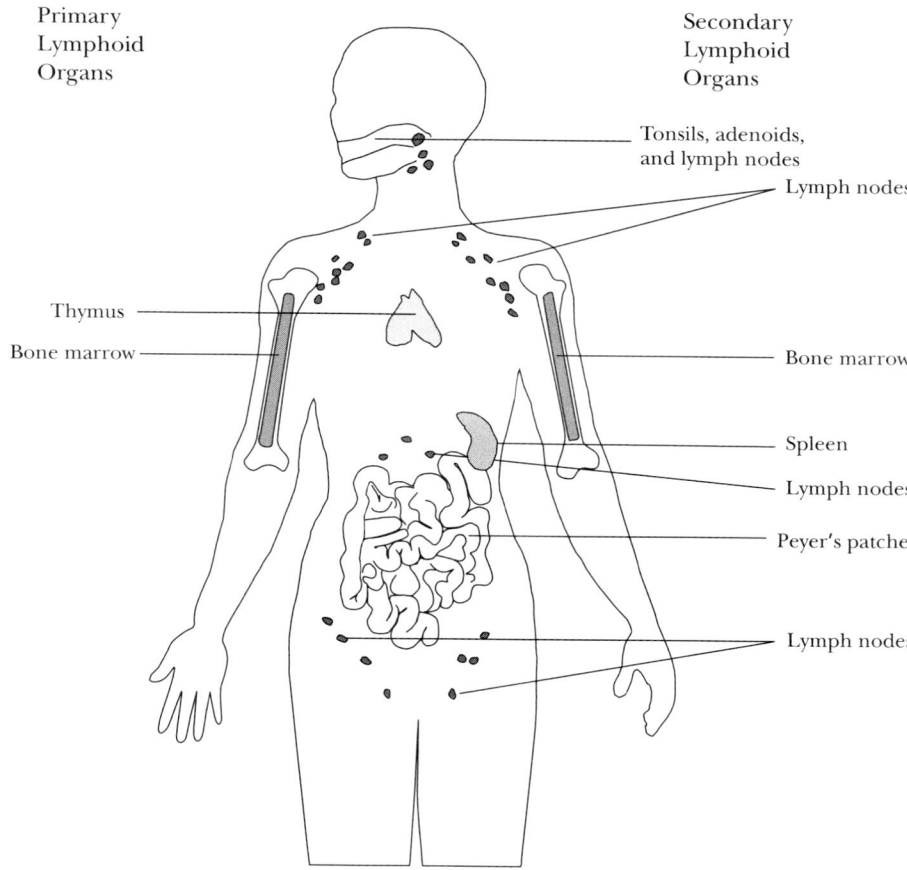

Primary Lymphoid Organs

Secondary Lymphoid Organs

Tonsils, adenoids, and lymph nodes

Lymph nodes

Thymus

Bone marrow

Bone marrow

Spleen

Lymph nodes

Peyer's patches

Lymph nodes

60%–70% of the total normal blood leukocytes but are also found in extravascular sites. They are rapidly produced in the bone marrow at a rate of about 80 million per minute and are relatively short lived (2–3 days) compared to monocytes/macrophages, which may live for months or years. *Neutrophils* constitute more than 90% of the circulating polymorphs. Their primary role is phagocytosis. Neutrophils are considered the cells for the body's first line of defense. Significant loss of neutrophils, or neutropenia, can be a serious threat to cancer patients receiving immunosuppressive therapies.

Eosinophils are polymorphs that constitute 2%–5% of blood leukocytes in healthy, nonallergic individuals. They play a role in dampening the inflammatory response but are also capable of phagocytosing and killing microorganisms. Eosinophils appear to play a specialized role in immunity to parasitic worms through a degranulating mechanism: adheres to worm larva and granules release a toxic protein substance.

Basophils constitute less than 0.2% of circulating leukocytes. *Mast cells* are indistinguishable from basophils, although resident only in body tissues (i.e., mucosal epithelia and in connective tissue). Basophils and mast cells play key roles in allergic responses through a degranulation process involving the release of histamine.

Although *platelets* are not leukocytes, they are derived from the myeloid lineage (megakaryocytes) and play im-

portant roles in various aspects of the immune response, in addition to a chief role in coagulation. Following damage to endothelial cells, platelets adhere to and aggregate at the surface of the damaged vascular tissue. They release mediators that increase permeability and activate complement, and therefore attract leukocytes.

The lymphoid lineage

The lymphoid lineage produces B lymphocytes (B cells), T lymphocytes (T cells), and large granular lymphocytes (LGL) called natural killer (NK) cells. *B cells*, so named because they were originally discovered in the bursa of birds, play a major role in the humoral arm of adaptive immunity through the production of antibodies, also called *immunoglobulins*.[1,2] On activation, B cells become antibody-secreting plasma cells. B cells have a less important role in the cell-mediated arm of adaptive immunity.

T cells, so named because they mature in the thymus, play the major role in cell-mediated immune responses and a less important role in humoral responses. Cell-mediated immunity provides defense against intracellular viruses, transplanted tissue, tumor cells, fungi, and protozoa. T cells recognize antigen not in its intact form, as it is recognized by B cells, but rather as peptide fragments that are bound to cell-surface molecules, called *major*

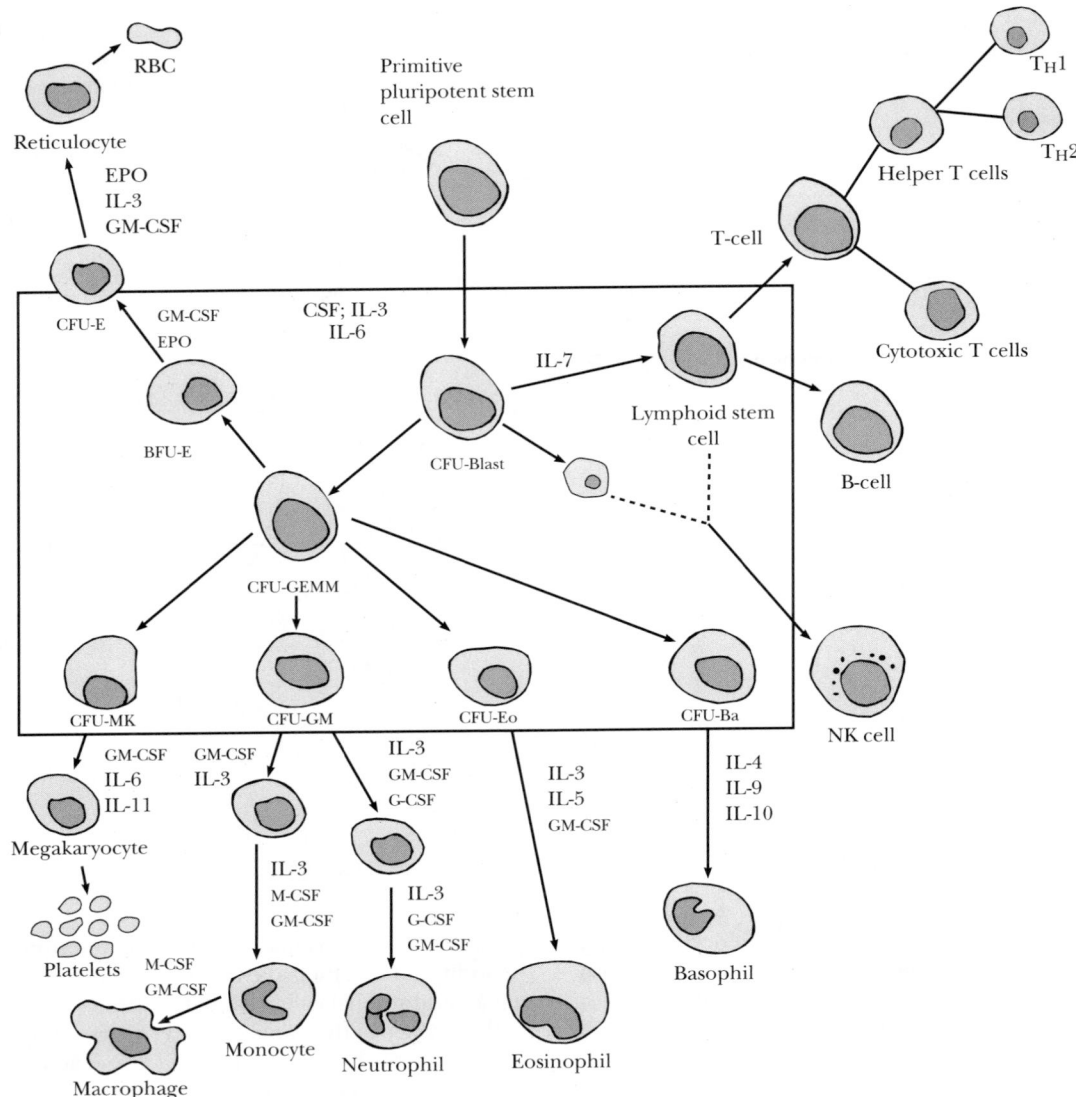

Figure 3-2 The hematologic cascade. Ba = basophil; BFU = burst-forming unit; CFU = colony-forming unit; CFU-GEMM = colony-forming unit-granulocyte/erythrocyte/monocyte/megakaryocyte; CSF = colony-stimulating factor; Eo = eosinophil; EPO = erythropoietin; G = granulocyte; GM = granulocyte/macrophage; M = macrophage; MK = megakaryocyte; NK = natural killer; RBC = red blood cells/erythrocytes; T_H = helper T cells.

histocompatibility complex (MHC) molecules.[1,2] T cells have specialized receptors that recognize the antigenic fragments bound to a MHC molecule. There are two different classes of the MHC molecule, MHC class I and MHC class II.

T cells (CD3+) are divided into three general subpopulations: helper T cells (T_H), suppressor T (T_S) cells, and cytotoxic T (T_C) cells. Helper T cells (CD4+), which are MHC class-II restricted, are differentiated into two types: T_H1 cells play a role in the enhancement of cell-mediated responses; T_H2 cells play a role in the enhancement of antibody production in humoral responses. Suppressor T cells, in general, act to shut off T_H2 when sufficient antibody has been produced. Cytotoxic T cells (CD8+),

which are MHC class-I restricted, are capable of recognizing and destroying specific target cells, usually virus-infected cells, through cell-cell contact.

Natural killer cells are considered LGL because of their morphologic characteristics: distinct granules in the cytoplasm, a kidney-shaped indented nucleus, high nuclear-cytoplasmic ratio, and low density.[3] These characteristics distinguish NK cells from other lymphocytes. Natural killer cells appear to arise from a stem cell other than the common lymphoid progenitor; however, this is not clear. Maturation of NK cells is dependent on intact bone marrow but not on thymus. Although expression of a number of surface molecules has been identified on NK cells, the major marker characteristics are CD16+, CD56+, and CD3⁻. Natural killer cells account for up to 15% of peripheral blood lymphocytes. In addition to circulating in the blood, other locations of human NK cells include the spleen, tonsils, interstitial lung space, intestinal mucosa, and liver; mature NK cells are virtually absent in bone marrow.

Natural killer cells were so named because of early identification of their activity of innate, non-MHC-restricted cytotoxicity of malignant and virally infected cells. In addition to their roles in tumor surveillance and natural resistance against certain microbial infections, NK cells have been found to be involved in many other important biologic activities.[3] Other regulatory functions of NK cells include involvement in hematopoiesis; adaptive immunity, with effects on both T-cell and B-cell responses; and allogeneic bone marrow transplantation, engraftment, and graft-versus-host reactions.

Dendritic cells, also called interdigitating reticular cells, are not lymphocytes per se, yet their activity and locations connect them to the lymphoid system. Dendritic cells are found in T-cell areas of lymphoid tissue and are the most potent stimulators of T-cell responses.[1,2]

Soluble Mediators of the Immune System

Cell-to-cell communication occurs due to the production and secretion of, and receptors for, various soluble mediators. Examples of soluble mediators include antibodies, cytokines, serum proteins, and prostaglandins.

Antibodies

Antibodies, also called immunoglobulins (Ig), are serum glycoproteins that have specificity to particular antigens. Each antibody is Y-shaped and consists of three fragments (Figure 3-3). Two identical fragments are for antigen-binding (Fab), and one crystalline fragment (Fc) is for nonspecific binding to other cells or soluble mediators of the immune system. The antibody molecule consists of four polypeptide chains: two identical light chains and two identical heavy chains. Both light and heavy chains are further divided into variable and constant regions. The sequencing of the amino acids, particularly with the heavy chains, determines the class of antibody, given here in decreasing order of abundance: IgG, IgA, IgM, IgE, IgD.[1,2]

IgG (γ) is the most abundant antibody, comprising approximately 75% of serum antibodies. It is the only antibody able to cross the placenta. IgG is the major antibody produced in a secondary immune response. It consists of four subclasses. IgG is involved in the activation of complement as well as in binding of phagocytes.

IgA (α) is present in both serum and seromucous secretions, playing a key role in secretory immunity. It comprises about 15%–20% of total serum antibody and consists of two subclasses.

IgM (μ) comprises approximately 10% of serum antibodies. It is the major antibody expressed on B cells and

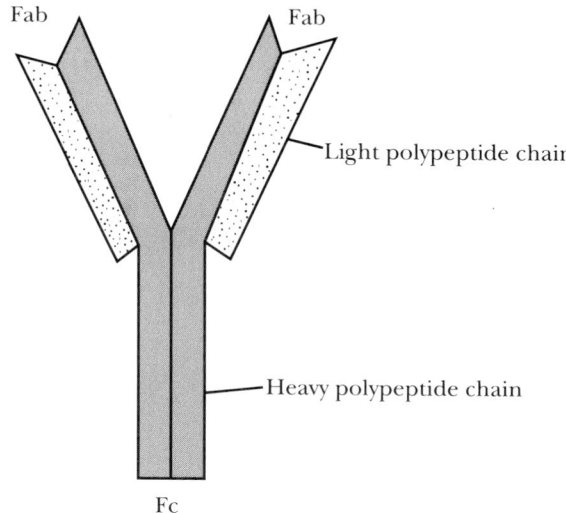

Figure 3-3 Basic antibody structure consists of a Y shape having two heavy and two light polypeptide chains, two antigen receptors (Fab), and one crystalline receptor (Fc) for binding to host cells or to soluble mediators.

is the chief antibody in primary immune responses. IgM is also considered to be the most efficient activator of complement.

IgE (ε) comprises less than 0.004% of serum antibodies. It binds to the Fc receptors on basophils and mast cells, playing the principal role in most hypersensitivity reactions.

IgD (δ) comprises less than 1% of serum antibodies. It is primarily expressed on B cells (along with IgM) and is a major B cell activator.

Cytokines

Cytokine is a general term for chemical (peptide) substances produced by a variety of different immune cells, which serve to mediate the activity of other cells.[1,2,4] Examples of types of cytokines are interleukins (IL), tumor necrosis factors (TNF), and colony stimulating factors (CSF). Table 3-1 provides an overview of the more common cytokines.

Serum proteins

Serum concentration levels of certain proteins increase during infection and are therefore called *acute-phase proteins.* Two key serum proteins are *C-reactive protein* (CRP) and *complement.*

C-reactive protein binds to and coats bacteria, while promoting the binding of complement and phagocytosis.[1,2] The complement system is a group of approximately twenty serum proteins whose overall function is to control inflammation. There are two mechanisms to activate the complement system: the alternate pathway and the classical pathway. The *alternate pathway,* described above with

Table 3-1 Cytokines: Sources and Main Functions

Type	Source	Major Functions
INTERLEUKINS (IL)		
IL-1 (α and β)	Predominantly macrophages	Activates T cells and B cells; inflammatory mediator; affects the neuroendocrine system w/ ↑glucocorticoids
IL-2 (T-cell growth factor [TCGF])	T_H1 cells, NK cells	↑ T-cell proliferation and differentiation; ↑ cytolytic activity of NK cells and production of LAK cells; activates B cells to ↑ Ig
IL-3 (multi-CSF)	Predominantly T_H1 and T_H2 cells	↑ production and differentiation of hematopoietic progenitor cells
IL-4 (B-cell growth factor)	T cells, macrophages, mast cells, B cells, basophils	Differentiation of T_H0 T_H2; induces proliferation and differentiation of B cells
IL-6	T_H2 cells, monocytes/macrophages, fibroblasts, hepatocytes, endothelial and neuronal cells	Activates hematopoietic progenitor cells; induces maturation and ↑ platelet number; ↑ growth and/or differentiation of various cells; ↑ acute phase protein release
IL-7	Bone marrow stromal cells, fetal liver cells	↑ proliferation and cytotoxic activity of T_C cells and LAK cells; support the growth of pre-B cells and proliferation of T cells
IL-8 (neutrophil chemotactic factor)	Monocytes, macrophages, endothelial cells	↑ chemotactic activity of neutrophils, T cells, and basophils; ↑ phagocytic activity of neutophils
IL-10 (cytokine synthesis inhibitory factor [CSIF])	T_H2, macrophages, B cells	↓ pro-inflammatory cytokine release of macrophages; inhibits T_H1; ↑ B-cell proliferation and Ig production
IL-12	Macrophages, B cells	Initiates cell-mediated immunity by inducing differentiation of $T_H0 \rightarrow T_H1$; ↑ growth and activity of NK and T_C cells
INTERFERON (IFN)		
IFN-α	T cells, B cells, macrophages	Antiviral activity; modulates class I and II MHC expression on various cells; ↓ B-cell proliferation, ↓ macrophage activity and production of IL-8
IFN-β	Fibroblasts, epithelial cells, macrophages	Antiviral activity; ↑ IL-6; ↓ IL-8
IFN-γ	T cells, NK cells	Activates NK cells; antiviral activity; ↑ class I and II MHC expression on macrophages; ↑ B-cell differentiation; ↑ macrophage activity
TUMOR NECROSIS FACTOR (TNF)		
TNF-α (cachectin)	Neutrophils, activated lymphocytes, NK cells, fibroblasts, endothelial cells, and malignant cells	↑ macrophage activity; ↑ cytokines from NK cells; mediates expression of genes for growth factors and cytokines, inflammatory mediators, acute phase proteins, and transcription factors
TNF-β (lymphotoxin)	T cells and malignant cells	Similar to TNF-α
COLONY-STIMULATING FACTORS (CSF)		
Granulocyte-CSF (G-CSF)	T cells, macrophages, neutrophils, endothelial cells, fibroblasts	↑ differentiation and activation of neutrophils
Granulocyte-macrophage-CSF (GM-CSF)	Macrophages, T cells, endothelial cells, polymorphs	↑ growth and differentiation of multipotential progenitor cells; stimulates all cells in myeloid lineage

Table 3-1 Cytokines: Sources and Main Functions (continued)

Type	Source	Major Functions
COLONY-STIMULATING FACTORS (CSF) (cont.)		
Macrophage-CSF (M-CSF)	T cells, macrophages, neutrophils, fibroblasts, endothelial cells	↑ growth and development of macrophage colonies; stimulates various functions of monocytes and macrophages
OTHERS		
Transforming growth factors (TGF) α and β	Macrophages, malignant cells, and other cells	Stimulates macrophages, ↑ fibroblasts, ↑ epithelial development and angiogenic activity, ↓ growth of various other cells
Stem cell factor (SCF)	Bone marrow stromal cells, epithelial cells, fibroblasts	Stimulates growth of myeloid, erythroid, and lymphoid progenitors; stimulates growth and proliferation of mast cells
Erythropoietin (EPO)	Liver, kidneys, macrophages	Stimulates growth and differentiation of erythroid progenitors; ↑ red blood cell production

↑ = increased; ↓ = decreased. See text for other abbreviations.

CRP, is an innate, nonspecific reaction leading to complement coating a microorganism and uptake by phagocytes. The *classical pathway* is a specific, adaptive response activated by antibodies. The major mechanisms of the classical complement pathway include the following: (1) opsonization (coating) of microorganisms for uptake by phagocytes; (2) chemotaxis, which is the attraction of phagocytes to sites of infection; (3) increased vascularity to the site of activation with increased permeability of capillaries to plasma molecules; and (4) damage to plasma membranes on cells or pathogens that have induced the activation, leading to lysis.[1,2]

Prostaglandins

Prostaglandins are important mediators involved in inflammation. They are major end products of arachidonic acid metabolism produced from inflammatory immune cells, such as monocytes/macrophages and basophils/mast cells.[1,2]

Mechanisms of Adaptive Immunity

Humoral and cell-mediated immune responses, involving both B cells and T cells, are interdependent functional arms that fall within the domain of adaptive immunity, as illustrated in Figure 3-4.

Humoral Immune Response

Humoral responses play important roles in defense against extracellular pathogens (bacteria and some viruses) as well as in certain hypersensitivity reactions.[1,2] The main mechanism in humoral immune responses in-

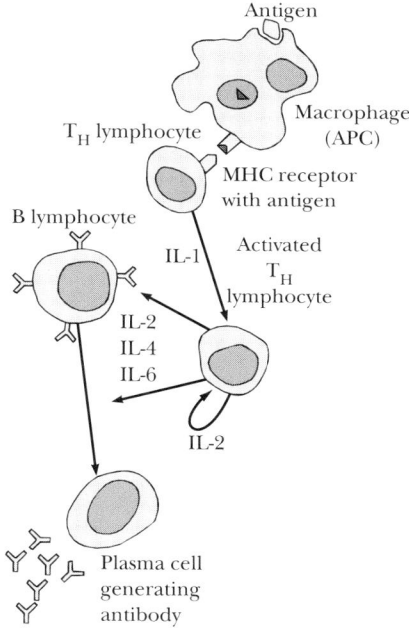

Figure 3-4 Major components of adaptive immune response. APC = antigen-presenting cell; T$_H$ = helper T lymphocyte.

volves the binding of antibodies to antigens. B cells play a key role in these processes through the production of antibodies.

Two proliferative steps take place before antibody production can occur: clonal diversity and clonal selection.[1,2] *Clonal diversity* takes place in the bone marrow and is antigen independent and hormonally driven. It results in the generation of immature but immunocompetent B cells, with plasma-membrane receptors that can recognize any antigenic molecule. *Clonal selection,* the second step, occurs in secondary lymphoid organs such as the spleen and lymph nodes. Antigens can stimulate B cells to become antibody-producing plasma cells either with or without the help of T cells; the latter are called *T-independent antigens.*

When a B cell encounters a specific antigen, it matures and proliferates into plasma cells and a set of memory B cells. Plasma cells are active during the primary immune response; IgM is the main antibody produced during this phase. Memory B cells are active in secondary responses that occur on future exposure to the antigen and are responsible for long-term immunity. Gamma-immunoglobulin is the predominant antibody in secondary responses. Class switching of antibodies from IgG to other classes or subclasses occurs with the help of cytokines released by a type of helper T cells (T_H2).[1,2]

Antibody-antigen processes

An antibody circulates in the blood, lymph fluid, or is suspended in body secretions until encountering and binding to its particular antigen. Binding of antigen (by antigenic-determinant sites) to the Fab portions of the antibody result in antigen-antibody complexes, also called *immune complexes.*[1,2] The class of antibody and specific characteristics of the antigen determine subsequent processes. Most humoral immune responses are polyclonal; however, monoclonal antibodies generated in laboratories are single antibodies of known specificity that play important roles in clinical therapeutics and diagnostics with cancer patients.

In general, antibodies function to target extracellular pathogens and their products for disposal by phagocytes, particularly macrophages and neutrophils. Three major roles of antibodies are as follows: (1) to neutralize bacterial and viral toxins; (2) to opsonize (or coat) bacteria; and (3) to activate complement.[1,2] *Neutralization* involves antibodies binding to and neutralizing toxins, which prevent interaction with host cells that can cause pathology. Unbound toxin can react with receptors on host cells, whereas antigen-antibody complexes cannot. These immune complexes are then typically scavenged and degraded by macrophages. *Opsonization* involves an antibody literally coating an antigen, rendering it recognizable as foreign by macrophages and polymorphonuclear leukocytes. These phagocytes then destroy and ingest the antibody-coated antigen complex. Finally, bound antibodies to antigens form a receptor to activate the first protein of the complement system, C3. This activation eventually forms a protein complex on the surface of the pathogen that favors its uptake and destruction by phagocytes.[1,2]

Cell-Mediated Immune Response

T cells are responsible for cell-mediated immunity, though interaction between both T cells and B cells often-times occurs. Maturation and initial proliferation of T cells take place in the thymus in processes similar to clonal diversity for B cells. While journeying through the thymus, lymphocytes destined to become T cells proliferate and develop the capacity to recognize a huge spectrum of antigens that the host will encounter throughout life. Antigen cluster differentiation on the plasma membrane of the T cells takes place in the thymus. On exiting the thymus through blood and lymph vessels, T cells mature and are antigenically committed. When these immunocompetent T cells encounter a recognizable antigen in the body, they proliferate.[1,2] This proliferation differs from that in the thymus: All T cells produced recognize the same antigen; proliferation is driven by antigen, not thymic hormones; and subpopulations of T cells are produced having different functions against the same antigen (cytotoxicity, memory, helper, or suppressor functions).

Naive CD8 cells leaving the thymus are predestined to become cytotoxic cells. The differentiation of CD4 cells is much more complex. Depending on the first encounter with antigen, CD4 cells can either become inflammatory (T_H1) or helper (T_H2) cells. Prior to this differentiation, they are thought to go through an intermediate stage, T_H0.[1,2,4]

Antigen processing, recognition, and presentation

After entering the host, an antigen flows through the bloodstream, is filtered through the spleen, and enters the lymphatics. Lymph nodes and other body tissues such as the skin and mucous membranes are lined with phagocytic cells, particularly macrophages, which ingest antigen. After its ingestion by a macrophage, the antigen is degraded. A portion of the degraded antigen is reexposed, or expressed, on the plasma membrane of the phagocyte, which "presents" it to B and T cells. This antigen-macrophage complex is referred to as APC and is necessary to induce most immune responses.[1,2] Three cell types that can serve as APCs are macrophages, dendritic cells, and B cells.

The only way a T cell can recognize antigen is when it is presented in the context of "self" material such as MHC molecules. To activate naive T cells, APCs must be capable of processing antigen from intracellular and extracellular pathogens and presenting it on MHC class-I and MHC class-II molecules. The particular MHC class determines which cell will respond to the presentation of antigen. Inflammatory CD4 cells (T_H1) and helper cells (T_H2) both express the CD4 coreceptor and recognize antigen displayed at the cell surface by MHC class-II molecules. On the other hand, T_C (CD8) cells kill target cells (particularly viruses) bound to MHC class-I molecules at the cell surface.

T-cell receptors (TCR) are the site on T cells where antigen-APC complexes bind. T-cell receptors are structurally similar to the Fab portion of an antibody and are antigen specific. There are two known types, TCR1 and TCR2, with each expressing different gene chains and binding patterns.[1,2]

Intercellular communication is dynamic during a cell-mediated immune response. Various cytokines and adhesion molecules on the surface of each cell (such as intercellular adhesion molecules [ICAMs]), play important roles. Examples of key cytokine activities are described as follows: Interleukin-1 (IL-1) is produced by the APC and helps the T cell respond. Interleukin-2 also plays a key role by facilitating maturation of a functional T_H1 cell. Interleukin-2 has an autocrine effect in that it binds to specific IL-2 receptors on the same cell that is producing it. This results in increased production of both IL-2 and IL-2 receptor, further differentiation and proliferation of the T_H1 cell, and the production of other cytokines.

Delayed-Type Hypersensitivity

Delayed-type hypersensitivity (DTH) reactions, also called type IV responses, are mediated by T cells.[1,2] Specifically in response to a previously responded pathogen, inflammatory (T_H1) CD4 cells recognize receptors on MHC class-II APC complexes. The T_H1 cells then release inflammatory cytokines, such as macrophage chemotactic factor (MCF), TNF-α, and γ-IFN, resulting in blood vessel permeability and fluid and protein accumulation into the tissue. This process evolves over 24 to 72 hours. Delayed-type hypersensitivity is often used as an in vivo measure of cell-mediated immunity.[5] The prototypic DTH reaction is the tuberculin skin test.

Cell-Mediated Cytotoxicity

Cell-mediated cytotoxicity is the recognition and lysis of target cells (which may be tumor cells or viruses) by either T_C cells or NK cells.[1-3] It may or may not be antibody-dependent (IgG). The mechanisms of action are quite similar regardless of the type of lymphocyte or involvement of IgG. The main difference lies in the different receptors and the binding of the cytotoxic cell to the target.

Cytotoxic T cells are antigen-specific and have MHC-restricted T-cell receptors. On the other hand, NK cells are not antigen-specific; rather, they recognize determinants expressed on neoplastic cells. Lymphokine-activated killer (LAK) cells are NK cells with enhanced cytotoxic activity due to stimulation with IL-2. Lyphokine-activated killer cells are used in the treatment of certain types of cancer by stimulating a patient's own NK cells with IL-2 in vitro, and then are returned to the patient.[6]

Antibody-mediated cytotoxicity involves the binding of an effector cell, referred to as a killer (K) cell, to antigen-bound IgG. Killer (K) cells are usually T_C cells; but may also be NK cells. The K cell has Fc receptors that can bind to the Fc region of antibody that has coated a target cell. Through these receptors, the K cell can adhere indirectly to and kill an IgG-coated target.

The mechanisms involved in the killing are similar whether T_C cells, NK cells, or K cells are the effectors, and no matter what receptor-target interaction is responsible (Figure 3-5). First, the effector cell recognizes and makes close contact with the target cell. On contact with the target cell, changes occur within the effector cell cytoplasm; specifically, the granule-containing vesicles of the Golgi apparatus fuse with the cell membrane. Through a calcium-dependent process, a protein substance called *perforin* is discharged from the vesicles.[7] This release of perforin causes the formation of pores on the target cell membrane, leading to an influx of water, electrolytes, and enzymes. Within minutes, the target cell swells and bursts. The effector cell survives this process, possibly because of a protective protein in the cell membrane called *protectin*, and continues to recognize and cause lysis of other target cells. Cytokines, particularly TNF (α and β) and γ-IFN, appear to play important roles in and are products of cell-mediated cytotoxicity.

NK cells and tumor surveillance

Clinical implications of NK cells' known ability to recognize and to lyse malignant cells include potential roles in cancer development, cancer recurrence, and overall survival from cancer. Although it is unclear if NK activity affects the development of cancer, there is much evidence to support the relationship between NK cytotoxicity and cancer recurrence and metastasis.[3,7-10]

Inverse relationships between NK activity and metastatic disease have been documented in studies of animals and humans. It has been observed that individuals with metastatic cancer have lower NK function compared with those with earlier stages of malignancy. Longitudinal studies with humans have observed low NK cytotoxicity at time of cancer diagnosis to be associated with subsequent cancer recurrence as well as diminished survival time.[8-10] This evidence supports the importance of NK function in individuals diagnosed with cancer, specifically in controlling metastases and perhaps in prolonging overall survival.

Tissue Destruction from Immune Responses

While attempting to rid the body of foreign organisms, products of certain immune processes have the potential to cause tissue damage. Specifically, neutrophils and macrophages produce toxins during inflammation and phagocytosis. For example, bacterial killing by neutrophils is done through an oxidative process with lysosomal release of such mediators as superoxide, hydrogen peroxide, and hydroxyl radical.[1,2] Fortunately, these free radicals are effective killers of pathogens. On the other hand, release of these chemicals affects surrounding cells, leading to damage of healthy cells. This is the basic mechanism to support the dietary intake of antioxidants.[11,12]

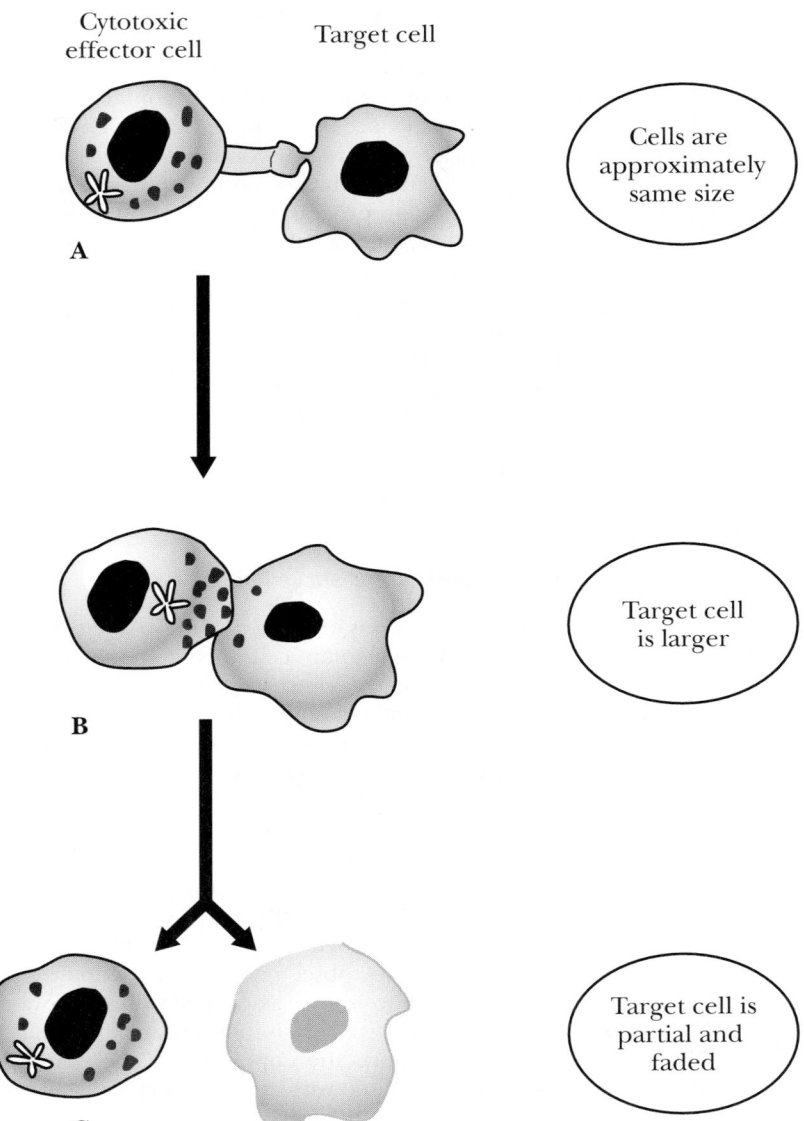

Cytotoxic effector cell

Target cell

Cells are approximately same size

A

Target cell is larger

B

Target cell is partial and faded

C

Figure 3-5 Cell-mediated cytotoxicity. **A.** Target cell (e.g., tumor cell) binds to effector cell (e.g., NK cell). **B.** Changes in the Golgi apparatus of the effector fuse with the cell membrane to release perforin, which forms pores on the target cell membrane. The target cell swells. **C.** The target cell bursts, while the effector remains intact and ready to lyse other targets.

Factors Affecting Immune Responses

Stress

Stress generally refers to demands placed on the body that threaten *homeostasis* (internal stability).[13] Stressful stimuli may be either external or internal. External stress is considered to be cognitive sensory stimuli because of its initial processing through the peripheral and central nervous systems; death of a loved one is an example of a cognitive stressor. Internal sensory input, or noncognitive stress, is received by the immune system and in turn relays this information to the neuroendocrine system; viral infection is an example of noncognitive stress. Regardless of the source, external or internal, stressful stimuli clearly

have systemic effects. The hypothalamus plays a key role mediating these processes (Figure 3-6).

Psychoneuroimmunology (PNI) is a scientific field involved in understanding the effects of stress on immune responses and related health outcomes.[14–16] The basis of PNI is the dynamic interplay and bidirectional communication between the neuroendocrine and immune systems. Substantial evidence supports interaction of the cells of these systems: (1) the immune system's interaction with the hypothalamic-pituitary-adrenal axis; (2) the innervation of lymphoid organs by the autonomic nervous system; and (3) the secretion of and receptors for identical soluble mediators such as cytokines, neuropeptides, and hormones.

The field of PNI has emerged over the last 30 years and involves interdisciplinary collaboration among

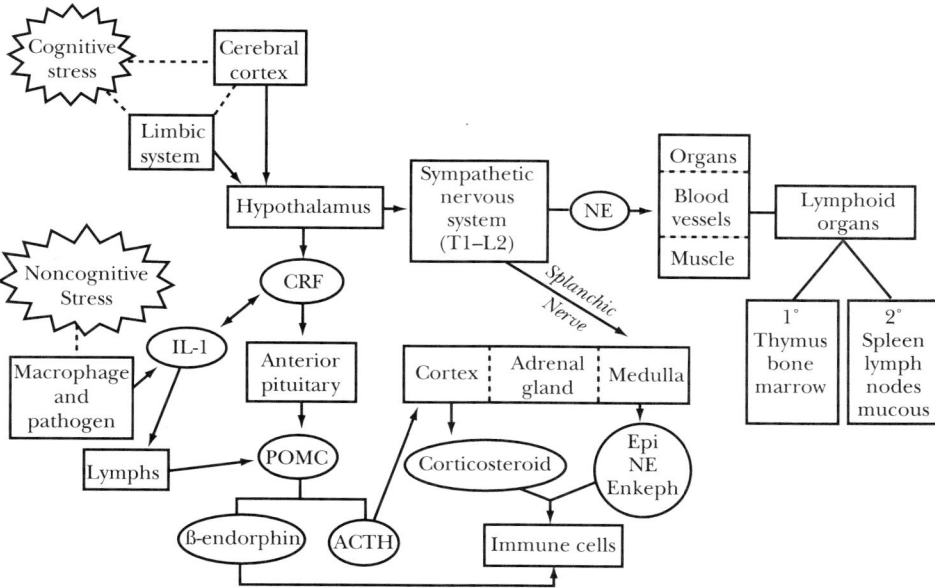

Figure 3-6 Major physiological mechanisms in response to stress: Focus on neuroendocrine and immune systems. CRF = corticotropin-releasing factor; POMC = pro-opiomelanocortin; ACTH = adrenocorticotropin hormone; Epi = epinephrine; NE = norepinephrine; Enkeph = enkephalin; T1 = thoracic spine, level 1; L2 = lumbar spine, level 2.

professionals of various basic science, social science, and clinical disciplines. Because of the substantial body of knowledge related to the negative impact of psychological stress on immune function,[14–16] clinical studies are evaluating and identifying the benefits of stress-reducing interventions. This is an area of particular interest to nurses, due to a knowledge base rooted in both basic and social sciences, and is reinforced by a holistic perspective that is at the core of the profession.[17]

Stress-reducing interventions

Cognitive-behavioral and other stress-reducing interventions have been associated with improvements in immune function as well as survival in cancer patients. Such interventions include progressive muscle relaxation, meditation, guided visual imagery, biofeedback, cognitive restructuring, and massage. Studies of these interventions have included a variety of populations: patients with cancer, patients who are HIV-positive, the elderly, caregivers, and healthy individuals.[17–21] For example, a well-controlled, experimental design, longitudinal study of patients with malignant melanoma found benefits associated with participation in a 6-week psycho-educational intervention. The intervention group had improvements in psychological and immunologic function, as well as lower recurrence and higher survival rates 6 years later.[22,23]

Aging

Advancing age is clearly associated with decline of immunologic functioning.[24] The thymus reaches its maximum size at about age 25, and then begins involuting. Thymic size is only 15% of its maximum by age 50. Although number of T cells may not decrease with age, T-cell func-tion does deteriorate. Older individuals, more than 60 years of age, generally exhibit diminished responsiveness with various T-cell-mediated activities. In addition, antibody activities can decrease or become dysfunctional with increasing age.

Female Reproductive Hormones

Variations in NK cytotoxicity have been observed in different phases of the menstrual cycle as well as during pregnancy, suggesting that female reproductive hormones have an impact on immune responses. Specifically, increased levels of estrogen and progesterone have been documented to have a negative effect on different immunologic functions.[25–27]

Behavioral Factors

Several behavioral factors have been identified as having the potential to influence immune function: nutrition, alcohol and other drugs, physical exercise, sleep, and cognitive-behavioral interventions. Because changes in these behaviors are often concurrent, it is difficult to fully comprehend the individual effects of these factors. For example, individuals who are distressed may be more likely to engage in self-destructive behaviors (e.g., increased smoking and alcohol/drug consumption) as well as experience changes in their appetite, energy level, and sleep pattern. Table 3-2 highlights the overall effect of behavioral as well as other factors that can influence immune function.

Nutrition

Nutritional status and dietary intake can influence immunocompetence and overall health function.

Table 3-2   Factors Affecting Immune Function

Factor	Effect on Immune Function*
Aging	Negative
Alcohol	Negative
Antioxidant vitamins	Positive
Caffeine	Negative
Female reproductive hormones	Negative
Marijuana	Negative
Physical exercise	Positive
Protein-calorie and zinc deficiencies	Negative
Sleep	Positive
Smoking	Negative
Stress (acute)	Positive
Stress (chronic)	Negative
Stress-reducing interventions	Positive

*Note: This is a general interpretation based on various research studies. More definitive studies on most of these factors are needed to make firm conclusions.

Protein-calorie and zinc deficiencies are associated with alterations in both innate and cell-mediated immune mechanisms,[28] while certain vitamins (A, C, and E) and micronutrients (e.g., selenium) play roles in the maintenance of healthy cells, most likely through elimination of free radicals. Soy proteins are also associated with immunologic function, cancer growth, and other physiologic processes and health outcomes; although the mechanisms of action are still unclear.[29]

Alcohol and other CNS drugs

Consumption of alcohol (ethanol) and other CNS-acting drugs can affect immune function.[30] Alcohol intake is associated with suppression of NK cytotoxicity in both animal models and humans.[31,32] The deleterious effects of marijuana on different mechanisms of immune function have also been documented.[33] Caffeine intake and smoking (nicotine) also affect immune function due to their associations with catecholamine and other neuroendocrine activities.[34]

Physical exercise

Changes in immune response to physical exercise have been recognized, with moderate aerobic exercise having a general positive effect.[35] Immune changes, specifically to NK cytotoxicity, has been identified in studies of aerobic activity in humans and animal models.[36,37] Different cytokines, including IL-2 and IL-1, as well as β-endorphins, have been identified in the mechanisms linking exercise and immune function.[38]

Sleep

Increasing evidence is clarifying the immunorestorative mechanisms of sleep.[39] Growth hormone and prolactin, known to be associated with enhanced immune function, are elevated during sleep; whereas levels of immunosuppressive corticosteroids and catecholamines are depressed. Of note, NK cytotoxicity has been found to be negatively correlated with sleep disturbances.[40]

Implications for Nursing Practice

Nursing professionals strive to improve quality-of-life and clinical outcomes, with an emphasis toward self-care and changing behaviors. Independent nursing interventions can be educational or supportive. Educational programs and individual or group counseling sessions can be aimed at changing behaviors such as diet, exercise, sleep habits, and stress reduction. These interventions and topics are germane to nursing and ripe areas for refinement and research.[17]

Conclusion

The immune system is a complex arrangement of cells, tissues, and soluble mediators, with two overall functions: (1) to recognize foreign substances and (2) to eliminate the foreign substances with restoration of homeostasis. Cancer diagnosis and treatment are identified with changes in immune function. The immune system dynamically communicates with other systems of the body, including the neuroendocrine system. A number of behavioral factors affect immunologic functioning. Nursing interventions that are educational and supportive in nature have the potential to impact immune responses and associated health outcomes.

References

1. Janeway CA, Travers P, Walport M, et al: *Immunobiology: The Immune System in Health and Disease* (ed 4). London, Elsevier Science/Garland, 1999
2. Roitt I: *Essential Immunology* (ed 9). Oxford UK, Blackwell Science 1997
3. Trinchieri G: Biology of natural killer cells. *Adv Immunol* 47:187–376, 1989
4. Curtsinger JM, Schmidt CS, Mondino A, et al: Inflammatory cytokines provide a third signal for activation of naïve CD4+ and CD8+ T cells. *J Immunol* 162:3256–3262, 1999
5. Chirstou NV, Boivert G, Broadhead M, et al: Two techniques of measurement of the delayed hypersensitivity skin test response for the assessment of bacterial host resistance. *World J Surg* 9:798–806, 1985
6. Dunbar PR, Chen JL, Chao D, et al: Cutting edge: Rapid cloning of tumor specific CTL suitable for adaptive immunotherapy of melanoma. *J Immunol* 162:6959–6962, 1999

7. Smyth MJ, Thia KYT, Creteney E, et al: Perforin is a major contributor to NK cell control of metastasis. *J Immunol* 162: 6658–6662, 1999

8. Barlozzari T, Leonhardt J, Wiltrout RH, et al: Direct evidence for the role of LGL in the inhibition of experimental tumor metastases. *J Immunol* 134:2783–2789, 1985

9. Page GG, Ben-Eliyahu S, Liebeskind JC: The role of LGL/NK cells in surgery-induced promotion of metastasis and its attenuation of morphine. *Brain Behav Immun* 8:241–250, 1994

10. Schantz SP, Brown BW, Lira E, et al: Evidence for the role of natural immunity in the control of metastatic spread of head and neck cancer. *Cancer Immunol Immunother* 25: 141–148, 1987

11. Eichholzer M, Stahelin HB, Gey KF, et al: Prediction of male cancer mortality by plasma levels of interacting vitamins: 17-year follow-up of the prospective Basel study. *Int J Cancer* 66:145–150, 1996

12. Schmidt K: Antioxidant vitamins and β-carotene: Effects on immunocompetence. *Am J Clin Nutr* 53:3835–3855, 1991

13. Glaser R, Kiecolt-Glaser J (eds): *Human Stress and Immunity.* San Diego, Academic Press, 1994

14. Ader R, Felten D, Cohen S (eds): *Psychoneuroimmunology* (ed 2). San Diego, Academic Press, 1991

15. Herbert TB, Cohen S: Stress and immunity in humans: A meta-analytic review. *Psychosom Med* 55:364–379, 1993

16. Buckingham JC, Gillies GE, Cowell A: *Stress, Stress Hormones and the Immune System.* West Suffix UK, John Wiley, 1997

17. Bauer SM: Psychoneuroimmunology and cancer: An integrated review. *J Adv Nurs* 19:1114–1120, 1994

18. Eller LS: Effects of two cognitive-behavioral interventions on immunity and symptoms in persons with HIV. *Ann Behav Med* 17:339–348, 1995

19. Kiecolt-Glaser JK, Glaser R, Williger D, et al: Psychosocial enhancement of immunocompetence in a geriatric population. *Health Psychol* 4:25–41, 1985

20. Zachariae R, Kristensen JS, Hokland P, et al: Effect of psychological intervention in the form of relaxation and guided imagery on cellular immune function in normal healthy subjects. *Psychother Psychosom* 54:32–39, 1990

21. Fawzy FI, Kemeny ME, Fawzy NW, et al: A structured psychiatric intervention for cancer patients: II. Changes over time in immunological measures. *Arch Gen Psych* 47:729–735, 1990

22. Fawzy FI, Cousins N, Fawzy NW, et al: A structured psychiatric intervention for cancer patients: I. Changes over time in methods of coping and affective disturbances. *Arch Gen Psychiatry* 47:720–725, 1990

23. Fawzy FI, Fawzy NW, Hyun C, et al: Malignant melanoma: Effects of an early structured psychiatric intervention, coping, and affective state on recurrence and survival six years later. *Arch Gen Psychiatry* 50:681–689, 1993

24. Gorczynski RM: Conditioned immunosuppression: Analysis of lymphocytes and host environment of young and aged mice, in Ader R, Felton D, Cohen S (eds): *Psychoneuroimmunology* (ed 2). 1991, pp 647–662

25. Sulke AN, Jones DB, Wood PJ: Variation in natural killer cell activity in peripheral blood during the menstrual cycle. *Br Med J* 290:884–886, 1985

26. Grossman CJ: Interactions between the gonadal steroids and the immune system. *Science* 227:257–261, 1985

27. Ochshorn-Adelson M, Bodner G, Toraker P, et al: Effects of ethanol on human natural killer activity: In vitro and acute, low-dose in vivo studies. *Alcohol Clin Exp Res* 18: 1361–1367, 1994

28. Zalewski PD: Zinc and immunity: Implications for growth, survival, and function of lymphoid cells *J Nutr Immunol* 4: 39–101, 1996

29. Tham D, Gardner CG, Haskell WL: Phytoestrogens and health: A review of the epidemiological, clinical and mechanistic evidence. *J Clin Endocrinol Metab* 83:2223–2235, 1998

30. Arbabi S, Garcia I, Baum GJ, et al: Alcohol (ethanol) inhibits IL-8 and TNF: Role of the p38 pathway. *J Immunol* 162: 7441–7445, 1999

31. Meadows GG, Wallendal M, Kosugi A, et al: Ethanol induces marked changes in lymphocyte populations and natural killer cell activity in mice. *Alcohol Clin Exp Res* 16:474–479, 1992

32. Ochshorn-Adelson M, Bodner G, Toraker P, et al: Effects of ethanol on human natural killer activity: In vitro and acute, low-dose in vivo studies. *Alcohol Clin Exp Res* 18: 1361–1367, 1994

33. Friedman H, Klein T, Specter S. Immunosuppression by marijuana and components, in Ader R, Felton D, Cohen N (eds): *Psychoneuroimmunology* (ed 2). San Diego, Academic Press, 1991, pp 931–954

34. Kiecolt-Glaser JK, Glaser R. Methodological issues in behavioral immunology research in humans. *Brain Behav Immun* 2:67–78, 1988

35. Nieman DD, Nehlsen-Cannarella SL: The immune response to exercise. *Semin Hematol* 31:166–179, 1994

36. Nieman DC, Henson DA, Gusewitch G, et al: Physical activity and immune function in elderly women. *Med Sci Sports Exerc* 25:823–831, 1993

37. MacNeil B, Hoffman-Goetz L: Chronic exercise enhances in vivo and in vitro cytotoxic mechanisms of natural immunity in mice. *J Appl Physiol* 74:388–395, 1993

38. Shepard RJ, Rhind S, Shek PN: Excercise and training: Influence on cytotoxicity, interleukin-1, interleukin-2 and receptor structures. *Intl J Sports Med* 15:154–166, 1994 (suppl 3)

39. Uthgenannt D, Schoolman D, Pietrowsky R, et al: Effects of sleep on the production of cytokines in humans. *Psychosom Med* 57:97–104, 1995

40. Cover H, Irwin M: Immunity and depression: Insomnia, retardation, and reduction of natural killer cell activity. *J Behav Med* 17:217–223, 1994

CHAPTER 4

Carcinogenesis

John W. Yarbro, MD, PhD

Introduction

Cancer represents the most fundamental biological challenge to a multicellular organism because it is the process by which some of the organism's cells attempt to destroy the organism itself. Normally, all of the body's cells are held under rigid growth control, except in the case of tissue repair and normal growth. Control of cell division is carefully maintained by two opposing sets of genes, one set promoting growth and the other inhibiting growth. Accidental damage to genes is carefully repaired by enzymes coded by DNA repair genes. When the damage to a cell cannot be repaired, that cell is destroyed by a process called *apoptosis*. The number of times a cell is allowed to replicate is limited by a biological clock, the telomere.

Growth regulatory genes were initially thought to be cancer genes, and their names reflect this: *Oncogenes* are growth-promoting genes, and *tumor-suppressor genes* are growth-inhibitory genes. *Carcinogenesis* is the process by which these genes are damaged to such an extent that clones of cells lose the normal control mechanisms of growth and proliferate out of control. For cancer to develop, oncogenes must be activated, tumor-suppressor genes and DNA repair genes must be inactivated, apoptosis must be blocked, and the biological clock must be turned off so that cells can become immortal.

Cancer develops and evolves by the process of *clonal selection*. Stated simply, an initial mutation in the genome of a cell may confer a survival advantage on that cell. If one of the progeny of that cell is hit by a second mutation that also confers a survival advantage, this new clone grows even more vigorously. A sequence of such events leads first to the selection of a clone with the characteristics of a neoplasm and later allows that neoplastic clone to progress to ever-greater stages of virulence characterized by invasion, metastatic spread, and drug resistance, among others, that ultimately lead to the death of the host. This is Darwinian evolution, or natural selection, on a clonal basis within a single organism. It is a perversion of the normal growth and repair mechanisms. Step-by-step, cancer overcomes a complex set of protective growth controls. The large number of mutations required to develop cancer indicates that genetic instability (an increased mutation rate) is an early change in the evolving cancer cell.

Damage to the genome may result from exposure to chemicals such as those in tobacco, radiation such as radon from natural sources or medical radiation, asbestos, or various types of infectious organisms. In all cases, the final common path of action of such agents is through oncogenes, tumor-suppressor genes, and DNA repair genes. Specifically, oncogenes must be mutated or relocated so as to be activated, and tumor-suppressor genes and DNA repair genes must be mutated or lost so as to be inactivated. Many times, though exactly how frequently is uncertain, an individual may inherit a defective tumor-suppressor gene or DNA repair gene from a parent. Oncogenes usually act as dominant genes; that is, only one gene of each pair needs to be mutated to have an effect. Tumor-suppressor genes and DNA repair genes usually act as recessive genes; that is, both genes of a pair must be mutated or lost to abolish their tumor-suppressor effect.

Cancer may be thought of as a defect in the control of the cell cycle that allows continuous operation of the cell cycle engine.[1] Normally, this engine is regulated by a series of enzymes, the cyclin-dependent kinases (CDKs), that associate with specific substrates, the cyclins, to form complexes that regulate the movement of the cell through a series of regulatory "checkpoints" in the cell cycle. Some cancer-suppressor genes code for proteins essential to the operation of these checkpoints. For example, the gene *ATM*, which is mutated in ataxia telangiectasia, codes for a protein that regulates two checkpoints; when this protein is absent, the patient is at increased risk for developing cancer.[2]

Cancer may also be thought of as being related to a defect in programmed cell death (apoptosis), which is a mechanism by which defective cells are disposed. Apoptosis is an ancient mechanism operative even in unicellular organisms.[3] Mutant cells with defective DNA are induced to undergo a process of cell death, however this process is defective in cancer cells. A cancer family syndrome, the Li-Fraumeni syndrome, has a defect in gene *p53*, which induces apoptosis in cells with severely mutated DNA. It is common for a tumor to grow faster than its blood supply and, therefore, for its center to become anoxic. Cells deficient in apoptosis do not die as readily under anoxic conditions as normal cells and are therefore selected for survival. Such evolution is a part of tumor progression.

The cancer cell is immortal for three reasons: (1) it reproduces in an uncontrolled manner; (2) it does not undergo normal programmed cell death; and (3) it seems to lack the normal "biological clocks," or telomeres, located at the ends of chromosomes that limit the number of times a chromosome may replicate. Telomeres are not completely copied when the chromosome is duplicated during cell division. The result is that, with age, the telomeres grow progressively shorter until the chromosome can no longer replicate. Only germ cells in the testis and ovary have telomerase, an enzyme that prevents aging by duplicating the telomeres. Cancer cells also develop telomerase, which contributes to their immortality.[4]

Discovery of new cancer-related genes has greatly accelerated in the past few years, and previously obscure molecular events in carcinogenesis are being elucidated in great detail. The genes associated with inherited cancer are being identified and are often the same genes damaged in the process of carcinogenesis. These discoveries offer the potential for identification of high-risk populations and improved cancer prevention.

Stages of Carcinogenesis

It has been customary in the past to divide carcinogenesis into three stages—initiation, promotion, and progression—based on the pioneering work of Peyton

Rous described in Chapter 1. Rous coined these terms based on a series of experiments in skin carcinogenesis.

1. *Initiation* indicates some primary change in the target produced by a carcinogen.
2. *Promotion* means some secondary effect of an agent (the promoter) that alone might not be able to induce a malignancy.
3. *Progression* designates "the process by which tumors go from bad to worse."[5-7]

Foulds codified and expanded this concept of multistage carcinogenesis.[8] Progression to the metastatic phenotype has subsequently been well-elucidated by Fidler.[9]

In humans, carcinogenesis is much more complex than in well-studied animal laboratory models. The distinction between the three stages is blurred, and there are many more steps. In addition, more than one type of initiating event is probably common. In some cases, it is likely that initiators act as their own promoters; that is, they are complete carcinogens. In other cases, an initiator may be a complete carcinogen for one organ and an incomplete carcinogen for another. The division between promotion and progression is indistinct. Even when we understand a great deal about a carcinogen, it may not seem to fit the laboratory model exactly. For example, in lung cancer, cigarette tars seem to act as both initiators and promoters, but unlike the laboratory model where initiation is irreversible, in humans the smoker who quits returns to the normal low-incidence pattern in 10–15 years. (These complexities are discussed in detail in an excellent review.[10])

Carcinogenesis is ordinarily classified as chemical, familial, physical, or viral, even though it is likely that human carcinogenesis involves a combination of factors. Carcinogenesis can also be classified as occupational, dietary, environmental, lifestyle, and so forth.

Chemical Carcinogenesis

In 1915 cancer was chemically induced in laboratory animals for the first time when coal tar was applied to rabbit skin at Tokyo University by Yamagiwa and Ichikawa.[11] Perhaps because the English physician Percival Pott had noted in 1775 that soot caused scrotal cancer in chimney sweeps, the chemical carcinogenesis theory became the leading theory of cancer causation. Preceding Pott's often-cited observation, the single most destructive chemical carcinogen yet to be found, tobacco, was identified by John Hill,[12] an astute clinician, only a few decades after it was introduced into common usage in London. From Hill's discovery in 1761 until 1950, when we "rediscovered" tobacco as a carcinogen,[13-15] the only other chemicals determined to be significant carcinogens in humans were the aniline dyes, which caused bladder cancer.[16] The first potent synthetic carcinogen, dibenzanthracene, was discovered in 1930.[17] Subsequently, many other chemicals were developed that caused cancer in various animal systems but not many in humans.

The large number of active chemicals discovered raised questions about how they caused cancer as they seemed to have no common chemical structure. Classic work by the Millers in 1951 led to the understanding that covalent binding within the cell was essential for carcinogenic activity; the active metabolite of the carcinogen was later identified to be an electrophilic reactant that bound to DNA.[18] Carcinogens are converted into *free radicals* (i.e., compounds with a single unpaired electron) by a series of metabolic steps. Free radicals are electrophilic—highly reactive with macromolecules, such as DNA, that are rich in electrons. Compounds called *antioxidants* inhibit carcinogenesis because they react with free radicals before the free radicals damage DNA.

Because different organisms have different metabolic systems, potential carcinogens are metabolized in one way in some organisms and in other ways in other organisms, with the result being that some chemicals are carcinogenic for one species but not for another. There may be as yet unidentified metabolic differences that render some people more sensitive than others to certain carcinogens. Ames developed a classic assay system to measure carcinogens. The assay employs bacteria and is based on the fact that most carcinogens are mutagens and damage DNA.[19] The Ames system requires the addition of liver microsomes in order to metabolize the chemicals to be tested into active carcinogens. The metabolism of a carcinogen leads to the final active chemical, called the *proximate carcinogen,* that reacts with DNA.

In smokers, it is possible to directly identify the carcinogen bound to DNA, the so-called *hydrocarbon adducts,* and even to identify selective binding at particular codons of genes involved in lung cancer (such as *p53*) that are known to be hot spots for mutations in lung cancer.[20] The proximate carcinogen exerts its effect by binding to DNA and mutating it directly or by causing errors to be made when the host cell tries to repair the damaged DNA. However, most of the lesions produced by carcinogens are repaired by enzymes coded for by DNA repair genes.

The specific targets of carcinogens are the oncogenes and cancer-suppressor genes—the "on" and "off" switches for cell growth—and the genes coding for DNA repair enzymes; these have been identified in some cancers. In systems in which known chemical carcinogens and radiation induce malignant transformation, it is possible to identify mutated cellular oncogenes.[21,22] Further, specific and consistent point mutations have been demonstrated in some human malignancies.[23] Movement of an oncogene to a different site on the same or another chromosome, which may cause activation, has also been demonstrated.[24] In a few cases, the specific structural change in the protein that leads to malfunction has been elucidated.[25]

Despite the vast array of chemicals discovered to cause cancer in animals, there exist few chemicals (other than tobacco) for which there is strong evidence of causation of the common cancers in humans. Occasional industrial chemicals have been documented as causing cancer, such as benzene, 2-naphthylamine, vinyl chloride, and some metals, but after extensive study the best estimate is that only 4% of all cancer deaths in the United States are due to occupational causes.[26] Cancer chemotherapeutic agents are carcinogenic, and cured cancer patients are at risk for leukemia and some other tumors.

Familial Carcinogenesis

A variety of sources estimate that up to 15% of all human cancers may have a hereditary component. Breast cancer, for example, is estimated to have a familial component in about 13% of cases.[27] The list of familial syndromes has begun to expand rapidly in recent years as the new techniques of molecular biology have been applied to the isolation of genes that when inherited increase the risk of cancer. In some cases, the syndromes have been known on a clinical basis for many years; in other cases, identification of genes from cancer patients has led to the description of new family syndromes.

A list of thirty-five familial cancer syndromes has been published.[28] Genes have now been isolated for several of the classic family cancer syndromes: *RB1* cancer-suppressor gene in retinoblastoma; *WT1* and *WT2* cancer-suppressor genes in Wilms' tumor; *NF1* and *NF2* in neurofibromatosis types 1 and 2; *APC* in familial polyposis associated with colon cancer; *hMLH1* and *hMSH2* DNA-repair genes in hereditary nonpolyposis colon cancer (HNPCC or the Lynch syndrome); *RET* in multiple endocrine neoplasias type 2 associated with tumors of the pituitary, parathyroid, and thyroid, and with pheochromocytoma and islet cell tumors; *VHL* proto-oncogene in the von Hipple-Lindau syndrome associated with hemangioblastoma, pheochromocytoma, and renal cell cancer; *ATM* in ataxia telangiectasia associated with leukemia and chronic lymphatic leukemia; *BLM* in Bloom syndrome associated with leukemia and several other tumors; *p53* cancer-suppressor gene in the Li-Fraumeni syndrome associated with multiple types of cancer; the *XPA* DNA repair gene group in xeroderma pigmentosum associated with skin cancer and leukemia; *HPC1* and *PRCA1* in prostate cancer; and *CDKN2* in the dysplastic nevus syndrome associated with melanoma.[28]

The long-recognized familial pattern in breast cancer has led to the isolation of *BRCA1*, associated with breast and ovarian cancer, and *BRCA2*,[28] associated with breast cancer. Isolation of these genes allows for identification of families at risk. Both genes are extremely large and have an extensive variety of mutations that makes screening difficult. *BRCA1* has been shown to function directly or indirectly in the repair of damaged DNA.[29]

Familial carcinogenesis is based in large part on a group of genes that when mutated cause cancer by their absence; that is, the genes seem to prevent cancer when they are functioning normally. The scientific basis for our understanding of familial cancer began in 1971 when

Alfred Knudson argued, on the basis of a statistical model, that one of the two mutations required for the development of familial retinoblastoma was inherited and that the second occurred in the retinal cells of the affected eye. In the nonheritable form, both mutations occurred in the same cell after birth, with neither mutation being inherited.[30] This model was derived from the observation that acquired retinoblastoma occurred as a single tumor, whereas children with hereditary retinoblastoma had multiple primary tumors, indicating an inherited genetic predisposition in all the cells of the retinal tissue. The gene has been identified and named the *retinoblastoma gene (RB1)*. The inheritance is dominant, but both copies of the gene must be absent or damaged for a cell to be transformed. When the retinoblastoma gene is introduced into cultures of retinoblastoma cells, the malignant growth pattern is suppressed.[31] This confirmed in humans the classic laboratory observation that fusing a cancer cell with a normal cell will lead to suppression of malignant growth.[32]

Subsequently, the mechanism discovered in retinoblastoma was found in other cancers such as Wilms' tumor. Of further interest, loss of the retinoblastoma gene was described in bladder cancer and breast cancer, which implied that genes associated with familial cancer might be a target for mutagens involved in nonhereditary cancers. For example, strong evidence has been presented for a role of the same tumor-suppressor gene associated with familial polyposis as the target for mutagenesis in a large proportion of colon cancer cases. Weinberg has reviewed the implications of the negative regulation exerted on cells by genes such as the retinoblastoma gene and has emphasized the importance of the loss of the normal copy of a gene by the process of mitotic recombination.[33] This is referred to as *loss of heterogeneity* or *reduction to homozygosity* because the cell becomes homozygous for the abnormal gene, thus losing its ability to prevent malignant growth. This process is important in carcinogenesis.

Up to 5% of colorectal cancers are due to the HNPCC syndrome, characterized by an early age onset of predominantly proximally located tumors.[34] This hereditary syndrome results from a defect in the DNA mismatch repair (MMR) system, a system that copyedits newly synthesized DNA and repairs any errors made at the time of synthesis. An inherited mutation of any one of four genes can lead to malfunction of the MMR system and the genomic instability that allows the mutations that transform the colonic mucosa. Some families with the syndrome have an excess only of colorectal cancers (Lynch syndrome I); others have an excess of endometrial adenocarcinoma and, to a lesser extent, cancers of the stomach, ovary, and other sites (Lynch syndrome II).[35]

Physical Carcinogenesis

Physical carcinogens are agents that damage the same oncogenes and cancer-suppressor genes that are attacked by chemicals, but they exert their action by physical rather than chemical means. In some cases, the nature of the reaction is known, as for example ionizing radiation, which releases sufficient energy to alter DNA. In other cases, the mechanism is obscure, as for example asbestos, which may act as a promoter by an as yet unknown method.

Radiation was recognized as a carcinogen just 4 years after Roentgen's discovery of x-rays.[36] Only a few years later, a relationship to leukemia was established.[37] Early workers in radiation must have received very large doses to make the association between radiation and cancer so obvious that it could be noticed in such a short time. The excess cancer deaths in the Hiroshima and Nagasaki populations were only about 8%, and leukemia was seen at an incidence of only about 1.5 cases per million people per year per rad of dose.[38]

There are two forms of radiation that induce cancer: ultraviolet radiation and ionizing radiation.

Ultraviolet Radiation

Ultraviolet radiation (UVR) from the sun induces a change in DNA, pyrimidine dimer formation, that if not properly repaired leads to malignant transformation. Basal cell and squamous cell carcinomas of the exposed areas of the skin result, and these tumors are quite common, with nearly half a million cases reported each year in the United States. Melanoma is also linked to ultraviolet exposure, though not as closely as basal and squamous cancers. The most active carcinogenic wavelength of UVR is 280–320 nm, which is referred to as ultraviolet B (UVB).

The most dramatic example of UVB carcinogenesis is seen in patients with xeroderma pigmentosum, an autosomal recessive disease in which DNA repair of UVR damage is defective.[39] These patients are hypersensitive to sunlight and have a high incidence of skin cancer, including melanoma.

Appropriate preventive techniques include avoidance of direct sunlight and the use of sunblocks that block out UVB radiation. That such measures will be effective is indicated by the protective effect of living in climates with low levels of sunlight, of skin pigmentation that blocks out UVB, and of occupations that minimize sun exposure.

Ionizing Radiation

Life evolved in an environment high in radiation; indeed, radiation-induced mutation no doubt accelerated evolution. There are effective mechanisms to repair the damage that results when high-energy radiation interacts with DNA. Ordinarily these mechanisms are extremely efficient. They are not perfect, however, and ionizing radiation leads to permanent mutations in DNA. When these mutations involve oncogenes, tumor-suppressor genes, or DNA repair genes, transformation of a cell to malignant

growth may occur. As with chemical carcinogenesis, multiple steps are involved. Furthermore, radiation and chemicals interact synergistically, and familial susceptibilities may play a role. In a hereditary melanoma syndrome, known as *familial dysplastic nevus syndrome* (FDNS), individuals have multiple nevi that have a strong tendency to evolve into melanoma. Cultured cells from these individuals have an increased sensitivity to radiation-induced genetic damage.[40]

In the United States, the average annual exposure of an individual to radiation from all sources is 360 mrem, 82% of which is from natural sources. Clearly, the largest portion of our radiation dose is unavoidable.[41] Women who as children received radiation therapy for Hodgkin's disease have a 75-fold increased risk for breast cancer.[42] The use of alkylating agents potentiates the carcinogenic effect of radiation, especially in the development of leukemia.

Recent interest has focused on the radon isotope, for which the home seems to be the major site of exposure. There are substantial geographic variations influencing radon dose. Basements may allow more radon to enter a home, and good insulation may prevent dispersal of radon into the atmosphere. At present, too little is known about radon effects to draw firm conclusions or to make useful recommendations for prevention, but one case-control study suggested that indoor radon exposure did not appear to be a significant cause of lung cancer.[43]

From the standpoint of prevention, little more can be done than is already being done: minimizing exposure to man-made radiation hazards. It is notable, however, that stopping smoking provides the greatest potential for prevention of radiation-induced cancer of the lung, as radon exposure acts synergistically with tobacco smoke. Smokers exposed to radon as miners had ten times the incidence of lung cancer as did nonsmokers because radiation acts synergistically with tobacco smoke.[44] The risk of medical radiation exposure has probably been exaggerated, except in the case of therapeutic radiation. The large unavoidable radiation doses from our natural environment dwarf the small medical exposure. Still, radiation is carcinogenic, and every attempt should be made to minimize our exposure consistent with effective diagnosis and therapy. Of particular public concern is exposure from mammography. This has undoubtedly been exaggerated, and the new techniques provide low exposures to the breast. Present recommendations of the American Cancer Society for mammography seem reasonable and are likely to save many more lives than are placed at risk by such a low level of radiation.

Asbestos

Asbestos, the major carcinogenic fiber, is believed to be related to about 2000 cases of mesothelioma annually[44] in the United States. Actually, asbestos causes more bronchogenic cancers than mesotheliomas, perhaps 6000, because of its synergism with tobacco smoke. Lung cancer is rare in asbestos workers who do not smoke. There is a long latent period between exposure and the onset of mesothelioma. Furthermore, the exposure may sometimes be so brief that the patient cannot remember when it occurred unless questioned closely. The mechanism of action of the asbestos fiber is unknown.

Data do not support an association between gastrointestinal cancer and asbestos, an observation of some importance since asbestos-lined cement pipes carry much of the U.S. water supply.[15] Physical properties such as crystal type and particle size play a major role in the physical carcinogenic properties of asbestos. Epidemiological studies indicate that only certain forms of asbestos increase the risk of mesothelioma.[45] Estimating the risk of exposure to asbestos is much more complicated than estimating risk from a soluble mutagenic carcinogen, and the linear dose-response model probably cannot be applied.

Viral Carcinogenesis

In 1911 Peyton Rous, at the Rockefeller Institute, described a sarcoma in chickens caused by what later became known as the Rous sarcoma virus (RSV).[46] This virus was the source of the first well-characterized oncogene. The work on possible cancer viruses in laboratory animals systems led to the discovery of human genes associated with cancer.

There is strong evidence in humans for a viral etiology of hepatoma, adult T-cell leukemia/lymphoma, Burkitt's lymphoma, nasopharyngeal cancer, lymphomas associated with immunodeficiency syndromes, and cervical cancer. Worldwide, perhaps one in seven human cancers are related to viruses.[47] It should be noted that in no case in humans, in contrast to animal and cell culture systems, has a viral infection directly produced a malignancy; in humans cancer is a multistep process.[48]

Among the human retroviruses, human T-cell leukemia virus type 1 (HTLV-1) has been clearly implicated in adult T-cell leukemia (ATL), a malignancy of mature T4 lymphocytes that is endemic in Japan, the Caribbean, parts of Africa, and the southeastern United States.[49] A small proportion of individuals with Sézary syndrome and mycosis fungoides also have evidence of HTLV-1. In ATL-endemic regions, only a small proportion of infected individuals, less than 1%, develop ATL. Transmission of the virus is by sexual contact, by mother's milk, and through contaminated blood, and the latency period between infection and ATL varies from a few years up to 40 years. The mechanism of carcinogenesis may be insertion of the virus into the host genome in such a way as to activate host proto-oncogenes; or, as is the case with human papillomavirus (HPV), there may be HTLV-coded proteins that interfere with the cell cycle.[50] Hairy-cell leukemia (HCL) is a disease of B lymphocytes for the most part, but a small portion of cases manifest T lympho-cytes. The HTLV-2 type has been isolated from the T-cell variety of HCL.

Hepatis B virus (HBV) is endemic in Asia and Africa where large numbers of people, as much as 10% of the population, are chronic carriers. Epidemiological studies have established HBV to be etiologic in hepatocellular carcinoma (HCC).[51] Hepatitis C virus may also induce hepatoma.[52] In China alone, between 500 thousand and 1 million cases of HCC occur annually; this may be the most common cancer in the world today. Hepatoma has almost doubled in incidence in the United States in the past 20 years, probably due to the increased incidence of hepatitis B and C secondary to contaminated needles in drug users.[53] Hepatitis B virus transforms the hepatocyte not because it has an oncogene, but because it integrates copies of itself into the host DNA at random sites and by chance may cause inappropriate activation of a proto-oncogene to initiate a clone of malignant cells. There is a mean duration of 35 years from the time of HBV infection to the onset of HCC.[53] Other factors may increase risk, though these are not proven. Hepatocellular carcinoma may be induced by a mechanism that does not involve HBV, such as the natural carcinogen aflatoxin.

Epstein-Barr virus (EBV), a double-stranded DNA virus of the herpes family, causes infectious mononucleosis in the United States and Burkitt's lymphoma in Africa. It infects B lymphocytes and stimulates their proliferation. If host immunity is intact, a T-lymphocyte response is generated against an EBV protein expressed on the B-cell membrane, and the proliferating B cells are brought under control. For some reason in Africa, perhaps because of the effect of chronic malaria on the immune system, a B-cell clone may emerge uncontrolled, and this leads to Burkitt's lymphoma, a monoclonal malignancy. Chromosome 8, which contains the *MYC* oncogene, exchanges genetic material with chromosome 14, or sometimes chromosome 2 or 22, where genes necessary for antibody synthesis are located. The presumption is that the *MYC* oncogene is activated when the immune genes are stimulated.

Burkitt's lymphoma is rare in Western countries; when it is seen, EBV is only occasionally present. An X-linked inherited immune deficiency has been described in which EBV induces a polyclonal lymphoma.[54] Individuals who have AIDS or those immunosuppressed for organ transplantation are also at risk for polyclonal lymphomas associated with EBV.[51,53]

The Chinese, no matter where they live, are at increased risk for nasopharyngeal carcinoma. Their tumors are associated with the EBV genome within the tumor cell. There are other causes of this tumor in other races, but the Chinese seem to have a unique association with EBV. The EBV genome is actively transcribed in these tumors in the same way as in latently infected lymphocytes,[55] providing strong evidence for an etiologic role.

Hodgkin's disease has been suspected of being related to EBV, but the data are conflicting. In some cases, the disease may be preceded by an altered antibody pattern against EBV.[56]

The human papillomaviruses (HPVs) are double-stranded circular DNA viruses that infect squamous epithelium. There are many strains, some of which cause the common human wart and the genital wart. These viruses are difficult to study because they cannot be grown in the laboratory. Two independent transforming oncogenes have been identified, and the protein product of one of these genes has been shown to bind specifically to the protein product of the retinoblastoma gene.[57] This provides strong support for the hypothesis that transformation results when the infecting HPV codes for a protein that blocks the product of a tumor-suppressor gene.

Cervical cancer is associated with sexual promiscuity. DNA from strains HPV-16 or HPV-18 is found in 93% of all cervical carcinomas, and the morphological changes of cervical dysplasia are linked to HPV infection.[58] Thus, there are strong data supporting an etiologic role for some strains of HPV in cervical cancer. To a lesser extent, there are associations of HPV with all genital cancers, including cancer of the penis and prostate.

Bacterial Carcinogenesis

One of the most exciting developments in the mechanism of carcinogenesis is the discovery of a relationship between the bacteria *Helicobacter pylori* and the B-cell lymphoma unique to the gastric mucosa, the mucosa-associated lymphoid tissue (MALT) lymphoma. *H. pylori* grows in the stomach and is responsible for gastric and duodenal ulcers. For many years it was suspected that there was some kind of relationship between chronic ulcer disease and the development of malignancy. A relationship between *H. pylori* and MALT lymphoma has now been noted,[59] and resolution of the lymphoma was observed[60] after treatment with antibiotics to eradicate the bacteria.

The pathogenesis of this unique mechanism of carcinogenesis seems to be an initial B-cell lymphoid proliferation driven by mucosal T-lymphocytes that are reacting to antigens from *H. pylori*. During this clonal expansion, mutations lead to a monoclonal population that is antigen-independent and able to proliferate autonomously.[61] Thus, the early proliferation is reversible by eradication of the bacteria with antibiotics, whereas the later tumor is not and requires conventional anticancer therapy, though eradication of *H. pylori* is still recommended. Polymerase chain reaction (PCR) analysis reveals that the monoclonal tumor cells are eradicated in some, though not all, patients after a complete remission of tumor is achieved with antibiotic therapy alone.[62] Late recurrences of disease occur, and the question of whether conventional chemotherapy and radiation therapy should follow complete remission induced by eradication of *H. pylori* is as yet unresolved.

This exciting observation provides a model for carcinogenesis by a mechanism that is initially reversible and later autonomous. It illustrates the potential for modification of the process of carcinogenesis when the precise molecular events are understood.

Chronic *H. pylori* gastritis has been associated with an increased risk of gastric carcinoma, and perhaps this is a result of an increase in mucosal cell proliferation with reduced apoptosis.[63]

Colon Cancer as a Model of Human Carcinogenesis

The work of many investigators, especially Vogelstein at Johns Hopkins, has provided the best insight so far into the pathogenesis of a common tumor, colon cancer.[64] These investigations reveal the complexity of the multistep process of carcinogenesis in humans and its relationship to the same genes identified in the familial cancer syndromes.

Adenomatosis polyposis coli, a familial syndrome, has long been known to be associated with such a high incidence of colorectal cancer that the treatment of choice is total colectomy. Recently, the gene *APC* has been shown to be mutated in all cases of this syndrome, providing a clue to the pathogenesis as the product of this gene seems to be involved in negatively regulating certain intracellular pathways associated with growth-stimulating signals, and especially with the oncogene *MYC*, the same oncogene known to be overactive in Burkitt's lymphoma.[65]

In HNPCC, a second form of familial colorectal cancer, four genes have now been identified that provide a better understanding of the mechanism of carcinogenesis.[65] The genes associated with HNPCC are directly related to the development of the high mutation rate known to be associated with the process of carcinogenesis because they function to proofread newly synthesized DNA and correct any mistakes that are made during synthesis. When mutated, these genes lead to a high mutation rate that promotes the sequence of events necessary for carcinogenesis to take place.[66] Why this inherited defect in DNA repair leads preferentially to colorectal tumors is not yet clear.

In nonfamilial colorectal cancer, the sequence of events required for carcinogenesis and progression has been worked out more completely than for any other neoplasm. The complete sequence involves more than a half dozen steps.[67] A gene at 5q21 is mutated in a substantial number of colorectal cancers.[67] The gene *APC* is located at this site and is mutated in a substantial number of spontaneous colorectal cancers, as it is in all individuals with familial polyposis.[68] This probably leads to lack of regulation of the growth-stimulating gene *MYC*. The next step is presumed to involve demethylation of DNA, a nongenetic change that alters DNA function. Subsequently, there is a mutation of the K-*ras* proto-oncogene on 12p. Next, there is a loss of a gene located on 18q.[69] The gene in this location has been called *deleted in colorectal cancer* (DCC), but its function is uncertain and it has not yet been firmly established to be the gene involved in colon cancer carcinogenesis. Finally, there is a mutation of the tumor-suppressor gene *p53*, located at 17p, leading to genetic instability and progression to frank malignancy with invasion and metastasis.[70] Addition of normal chromosomes 5 and 18 to colon cancer cell cultures reverses malignant growth.[71]

In colorectal cancer, then, several familial syndromes have been matched with their genes, and many of the genes mutated in the sporadic (nonhereditary) tumors have been identified. Genes associated with familial cancers are often mutated in sporadic cancers. Some of the functions of the involved genes have been elucidated and provide clues as to why there is loss of control of cell division. Specific chemical and physical agents that are etiologic have not been identified in colorectal cancer as is the case with bronchogenic cancer, but there are a few epidemiological associations that may be important in identifying the mutagens leading to colorectal cancer.

Controversies in Carcinogenesis

The cause of cancer is a popular media topic, and speculation based on preliminary or incomplete data has fueled many media "controversies." Most of these so-called controversies are not at all controversial from a scientific standpoint. But fear of cancer and the unavoidable scientific uncertainties prompt arguments that often spill over into the court of public opinion. Cancer clusters, for example, are almost always statistical outliers and not the result of some cancer-causing agent in a particular geographic region. Epidemiologic associations of various foods with cancer so frequently reported are almost always exaggerated or even totally false. Preventive effects often claimed for this or that herb or mineral are almost always unproven. Scientists who attempt to inject reality into these debates are frequently viewed with suspicion and their possible associations with vested interests questioned.

Several legitimate scientific controversies in the field of carcinogenesis do exist, however. These are important questions for which the answers are unknown or uncertain; several of these follow.

Estrogens and Carcinogenesis

One of the most controversial topics in carcinogenesis is the role of estrogens. Animal models and human studies have clearly shown that without estrogen, breast cancer will not develop. That estrogen is in some way related to breast cancer is not the issue. The central practical issues are two: First, does postmenopausal estrogen replacement therapy increase breast cancer risk? Second, does oral contraceptive use increase breast cancer risk?

A host of case-control studies have provided copious data to support either a yes or no answer to the first question. To date, there is no definitive answer to either question. Tamoxifen, an agent with antiestrogenic effects on the breast and estrogenic effect on the uterus, clearly reduces the incidence of breast cancer on a short-term basis.[72] In theory, this finding suggests that estrogen poses a risk. However, in view of the known benefits of postmenopausal estrogen in the prevention of osteoporosis and the reduction of cardiovascular risk by up to half,[73] any decision not to use estrogen based on a hypothetical or poorly documented breast cancer risk must be carefully evaluated. It is likely that cyclic replacement therapy has a weak effect, if any, and does not substantially alter breast cancer incidence, though an association with endometrial cancer seems well established.[74]

The role of contraceptives in breast cancer risk likewise is controversial and not clearly established, with most studies showing no relationship.[73,74] It is possible that long-term use before the first pregnancy may increase risk,[75] and because this is a frequent pattern of use it is obviously an important question to answer. At present the issue is unresolved, though the majority opinion is that contraceptives are safe.

Involuntary (Passive) Smoking

The question of the carcinogenic effect of passive, or "involuntary," smoking has been debated extensively. Numerous studies provided insufficient data from which to draw a firm conclusion. However, when many studies were pooled for analysis, the federal government issued a controversial statement indicating that environmental tobacco smoke increased the incidence of lung cancer. This conclusion, though hotly debated, justified measures restricting smoking.

Recently, a multicenter trial in Europe has reported no association between childhood exposure to environmental tobacco smoke and lung cancer risk, and only weak evidence of a dose-response relationship between lung cancer risk and spousal and workplace exposure.[76] This has led to a careful re-analysis of presently available data and the conclusion that the initial risk assessments were far too high.[77] A reasonable estimate for the increased risk of lung cancer in pack-a-day smokers is 15- to 20-fold (1500%–2000%), and these new data suggest the best estimate of the increase in risk after exposure to environmental tobacco smoke to be on the order of 1.2 (20%), substantially lower than our previous estimate. Although these new data lower the risk of passive smoking, they confirm that there is indeed a risk.

It is likely that this subject will remain controversial. It should be noted that all such estimates assume a linear relationship between carcinogen and risk, something which is as yet unproven.

Environmental Carcinogenesis

Perhaps the most popular subject for the lay press is environmental carcinogenesis. The term *environmental* is subject to a great deal of confusion. Its original use was intended to include all cancers that were not hereditary; that is, all cancers due to viruses, lifestyle, tobacco, diet, and a host of other causes. When the statement was made that "85% of cancer is environmental," this was misinterpreted in the lay press to mean contaminated air, water, and food. Often it has been further limited in the media to exclude natural carcinogens in our environment so that the focus has been on man-made chemicals. This has led to the mistaken notion that we can virtually eliminate cancer if we eliminate man-made cancer-causing chemicals from the air we breathe, the water we drink, and the food we eat.

Such a notion is incorrect. Ames has described what he considers the mistaken assumptions made by those who argue that environmental pollutants represent our highest priority in cancer prevention.[78] He points out the dangers of this approach. When we focus our attention on trivial or even nonexistent dangers, our attention is diverted from significant and real dangers. There are more than half a million deaths each year from tobacco, a number that dwarfs the insignificant number of deaths that result from the pollutants that receive so much emphasis in the media.

A preferred interpretation of the term *environmental* would focus on our personal environment or, in usual terminology, our lifestyle. It is the tobacco we abuse, the food we eat, and other lifestyle choices that have increased our risk of cancer more than everything else combined. The enemy is not the chemical plant down the street but ourselves. For example, the AIDS epidemic associated with lifestyle and intravenous drug use has led to substantial increases in a variety of cancers including non-Hodgkin's lymphoma, Kaposi's sarcoma, viral hepatitis–induced HCC, and other malignancies. Tobacco is directly related to more than 30% of cancer deaths. If these kinds of cancers are excluded, the death rate from cancer is actually decreasing.

Diet and Carcinogenesis

Doll and Peto have suggested that perhaps one-third of all cancers could be explained by dietary factors.[79] Such estimates are popular with the public. This would suggest that up to 50% of breast cancer and 90% of colon cancer in the United States could be prevented by a change in diet. Doll and Peto's estimated range was very wide (10%–70%), however. Although it may be true that there is a strong dietary relationship, radical changes would be required early in life to effect substantial reductions in incidence.

In Japan, cancer of the stomach is common and cancers of the colon and the breast uncommon. When Japanese move to the United States, they rapidly develop our pattern of common colon cancer and uncommon stomach cancer. Several generations later, they develop our pattern of common breast cancer. This has become a classic epidemiological observation, and most investigators assume the explanation is the change in diet. Willett has critically reviewed the data on dietary risk factors for colon and breast cancer.[80] He notes the striking correlation between the amount of fat a nation consumes and the incidence of colon cancer and breast cancer, as well as a similar correlation between meat consumption and colon cancer.

The notion that fat intake may be related to breast cancer has persisted, but there has been an inability to provide individual, as opposed to national, statistics relating breast cancer to fat intake. This has led to a wide acceptance that the relationship is not to fat but to total calories and especially to total calories consumed early in life. Willett has interpreted the correlation of height to breast cancer as supporting this hypothesis; in nations where malnutrition is present in some groups, breast cancer incidence is lower in short women; such a relationship is not seen in the United States and Scandinavia.[80] It has been suggested that the effect of dietary fat on breast cancer incidence is mediated through estrogen. Reduction in dietary fat may reduce serum estrogen levels, though the issue is complicated by other changes associated with dietary fat reduction.[81] However, the analysis of data from seven prospective studies in four countries showed no evidence of a positive association between total dietary fat and the risk of breast cancer.[82] Further, the delay in the development of increased breast cancer by several generations of Japanese immigrants suggests that the issue is more complex than diet alone.

The role of fat in colon cancer is supported by both the rapid change in incidence with dietary change and the potential relationship of fat consumption to bile acids, which are known to be mutagenic. In Japan, since 1945 the improved diet has been associated with an increase in colon cancer but not yet an increase in breast cancer.[80] The well-documented relationship of meat consumption to colon cancer likely reflects animal fat consumption. The role of fiber in colon cancer has repeatedly been postulated to relate to altered transit time, altered bacterial flora in the colon, and altered exposure of the colonic mucosa to potentially carcinogenic bacterially modified bile acids. Epidemiological studies have suggested an inverse relationship between dietary fiber and colon cancer, and animal studies suggest the type of fiber may be important.[83] Human studies have shown that wheat bran and cellulose, but not oat bran, are associated with lower stool mutagens by the Ames assay and reduced secondary bile acids.[84] Still, the relationship between fiber and colon cancer has yet to be firmly established.

Stomach cancer has been suggested to be related to the intake of food that is cured, smoked, pickled, salted, or otherwise preserved but not refrigerated. Some special methods of food preparation have also been incriminated. Long-term use of refrigeration seems particularly important in reducing the incidence of stomach cancer.[85]

The nature of the effect of fruits and vegetables is unclear. There has been speculation that the antioxidant effect of vitamin C might play a preventive role, but this has not been well established. Many food preservatives have an antioxidant effect and may actually antagonize possible carcinogens such as nitrites. Alcohol has been well documented as a risk factor in head and neck cancer and more recently has been incriminated in breast cancer,[86] although this observation is controversial.

Attempts to identify the specific components of the diet that are responsible for lowering cancer risk have been only modestly successful. Adequate folate and pyridoxine may reduce the risk of pancreatic cancer.[87] The antioxidant effects of lycopene, a carotenoid found in tomatoes, may explain the reduction in gastrointestinal tract, breast, and cervical cancer incidence.[88] Still, there is a remarkable paucity of specific data and a wealth of suggestive but weak relationships.

The actions to be taken on the basis of these observations are far from clear. The potential for substantial reduction in cancer incidence by dietary modification alone seems remote, given the extreme changes that may be required and the difficulty of changing the eating habits of most people. Even reduction in alcohol consumption may not be effective unless it takes place early in life. Nonetheless, a prudent diet, with at least minimum requirements of vitamins and minerals, that is rich in fruits, fiber, tomatoes, and cruciferous vegetables and low in animal fat is desirable for many health reasons and may perhaps reduce the risk of cancer.

Conclusion

Modern techniques of molecular biology have allowed replacement of the classic initiation-promotion-progression sequence of carcinogenesis with a detailed list of the genes that must be mutated to transform a normal tissue into a malignant neoplasm. There is a rapidly growing list of genes involved in this complex process, and their discovery has major implications for all aspects of cancer care, including identification of high-risk groups, genetic counseling, diagnosis and follow-up using tumor-specific markers, treatment targeted to unique genetically determined tumor characteristics, and primary prevention based on a better understanding of the steps in the process of carcinogenesis.

References

1. Clurman BE, Roberts JM: Cell cycle and cancer. *J Natl Cancer Inst* 87:1499–1501, 1995

2. Carr AM: Checkpoints take the next step. *Science* 271: 314–315, 1996

3. Ameisen JC: The origin of programmed cell death. *Science* 272:1278–1279, 1996

4. Rhyu MS: Telomeres, telomerase, and immortality. *J Natl Cancer Inst* 87:884–894, 1995

5. Rous P, Beard JW: The progression to carcinoma of virus induced rabbit papillomas (Shope). *J Exp Med* 62:523–548, 1935

6. Rous P, Kidd JG: Conditional neoplasms and subthreshold neoplastic states. *J Exp Med* 73:365–389, 1941

7. Friedewald WF, Rous P: The initiating and promoting elements in tumor production: An analysis of the effects of tar, benzpyrene, and methylcholanthrene in rabbit skin. *J Exp Med* 80:101–126, 1944

8. Foulds L: The experimental study of tumor progression: A review. *Cancer Res* 14:327–339, 1954

9. Fidler IJ: Critical factors in the biology of human cancer metastasis. *Am Surg* 61:1065–1066, 1995

10. Yuspa SH, Shields PG: Etiology of cancer: Chemical factors, in DeVita VT Jr, Hellman S, Rosenberg SA (eds): *Cancer: Principles and Practice of Oncology* (ed 5). Philadelphia, Lippincott-Raven, 1997, pp 185–202

11. Yamagiwa K, Ichikawa K: Experimentelle Studie uber die Pathogenese der Epitheliageschwulste. Tokyo, *Mitteilungen Med Facultat Kaiserl Univ Tokyo* 15:295, 1915

12. Redmond DE Jr: Hill cautions against snuff in 1761. *N Engl J Med* 282:18–23, 1970

13. Wynder EL, Graham EA: Tobacco smoking as a possible etiologic factor in bronchiogenic carcinoma: A study of 684 proved cases. *JAMA* 143:329–336, 1950

14. Doll R, Hill AB: Smoking and carcinoma of the lung: Preliminary report. *Br Med J* 2:739–748, 1950

15. Levin ML, Goldstein H, Gerhardt PR: Cancer and tobacco smoking: A preliminary report. *JAMA* 143:336–338, 1950

16. Rehn L: Blasengeschwulste bei Fuchsin-Arbeitern. *Arch Klin Chir* 50:588, 1895

17. Kennaway EL, Hieger I: Carcinogenic substances and their fluorescence spectra. *Br J Med* 1:1044, 1930

18. Miller EC: Some current perspectives on chemical carcinogenesis in humans and experimental animals: Presidential address. *Cancer Res* 38:1479–1496, 1978

19. Ames BN, Durston WE, Yamasaki E, et al: Carcinogens are mutagens: A simple test system combining liver homogenates for activation and bacteria for detection. *Proc Natl Acad Sci USA* 70:2281, 1973

20. Denissenko MF, Pao A, Tang M, et al: Preferential formation of benzo[a]pyrene adducts at lung cancer mutational hotspots in *P53*. *Science* 274:430–432, 1996

21. Sukumar S, Pulciani S, Doniger J, et al: A transforming *ras* gene in tumorigenic guinea pig cell lines initiated by diverse chemical carcinogens. *Science* 223:1197–1199, 1984

22. Guerrero I, Villasante A, Corces V, et al: Activation of a *c-K-ras* oncogene by somatic mutation in mouse lymphomas induced by gamma radiation. *Science* 225:1159–1162, 1984

23. Bos JL, Toksoz D, Marshall CJ, et al: Amino acid substitutions at codon 13 of the *N-ras* oncogene in human acute myeloid leukaemia. *Nature* 315:726–730, 1985

24. Dalla-Favera R, Martinotti S, Gallo RC, et al: Translocation and rearrangements of the *c-myc* oncogene locus in human undifferentiated B-cell lymphoma. *Science* 219:963–967, 1983

25. Tong L, de Vos AM, Milburn MV, et al: Structural differences between a *ras* oncogene protein and the normal protein. *Nature* 337:90–93, 1989

26. Doll R, Peto R: *The Causes of Cancer.* New York, Oxford University Press, 1981

27. Lynch HT, Albano WA, Heieck JJ: Genetic biomarkers and the control of breast cancer. *Cancer Genet Cytogenet* 13:43–92, 1984

28. Lindor NM, Greene MH, Mayo Familial Cancer Program: The concise handbook of family cancer syndromes. *J Natl Cancer Inst* 90:1039–1071, 1998

29. Gowan LC, Avrutskya AV, Latour AM, et al: BRCA1 required

for transcription coupled repair of oxidative DNA damage. *Science* 281:1009–1012, 1998

30. Knudson A: Mutation and cancer: Statistical study of retinoblastoma. *Proc Natl Acad Sci USA* 68:820, 1971

31. Huang HJS, Yee JK, Shew JY, et al: Suppression of the neoplastic phenotype by replacement of the *RB* gene in human cancer cells. *Science* 242:1563–1566, 1988

32. Pereira-Smith OM, Smith JR: Evidence for the recessive nature of cellular immortality. *Science* 221:964–966, 1983

33. Weinberg RA: The *RB* gene and the negative regulation of cell growth. *Blood* 74:529–532, 1989

34. Marra G, Boland CR: Hereditary nonpolyposis colorectal cancer: The syndrome, the genes, and historical perspectives. *J Natl Cancer Inst* 82:1114–1125, 1995

35. Boland CR, Troncale FJ: Familial colonic cancer without antecedent polyposis. *Ann Intern Med* 100:700–701, 1984

36. Frieben A: Demonstration lines cancroids des rechten Handruckens, das sich nach langdauernder Einwirkung von Roentgenstrahlen entwichelt hatte. *Fortschr Geb Rontgenstr* 6: 106, 1902

37. von Jagic N, Scwarz G, von Siebenrock L: Blutbefunde bei Roentgenologon. *Berl Klin Wochenschr* 48:1220–1222, 1911

38. Preston DL, Kato H, Kopecky KJ, et al: Studies on the mortality of A-bomb survivors: 8. Cancer mortality, 1950–1982. *Radiat Res* 111:151–178, 1987

39. Cleaver JE: Defective repair replication of DNA in xeroderma pigmentosum. *Nature* 218:652–656, 1968

40. Standford KK, Parshad R, Green MH, et al: Hypersensitivity to G_2 chromatid radiation damage in familial dysplastic nevus syndrome. *Lancet* 2:1111–1116, 1987

41. National Council on Radiation Protection Measurements (NRCP): *Ionizing Radiation Exposure of the Population of the United States.* NCRP Report No. 93. Bethesda, MD, NCRP, 1987

42. Bhatia S, Robison LL, Oberlin O, et al: Breast cancer and other second neoplasms after childhood Hodgkin's disease. *N Engl J Med* 334:745–751, 1996

43. Auvinen A, Makelainen I, Hakama M, et al: Indoor radon exposure and risk of lung cancer: A nested case control study in Finland. *J Natl Cancer Inst* 88:966–972, 1996

44. Nicholson WJ, Perbep G, Selikoff IJ: Occupational exposure to asbestos: Population at risk and projected mortality. *Am J Ind Med* 3:258–311, 1987

45. Mossman BT, Gee JBL: Asbestos related diseases. *N Engl J Med* 320:1721–1730, 1989

46. Rous P: Transmission of a malignant new growth by means of a cell free filtrate. *JAMA* 56:198, 1911

47. Poeschla EM, Wong-Staal F: Etiology of cancer: Viruses, in DeVita VT Jr, Hellman S, Rosenberg SA (eds): *Cancer: Principles and Practice of Oncology* (ed 5). Philadelphia, Lippincott-Raven, 1997, pp 153–167

48. Bishop JM: Retroviruses and oncogenes. *Biosci Rep* 10: 473–478, 1983

49. Poiesz BJ, Ruscetti FW, Gazdar AF, et al: Detection and isolation of type C retrovirus particles from fresh and cultured lymphocytes of a patient with cutaneous T-cell lymphoma. *Proc Natl Acad Sci USA* 77:7415–7419, 1980

50. Franchini G: Molecular mechanisms of human T-cell leukemia/lymphoma virus type I infection. *Blood* 86:3619–3639, 1995

51. Beasly RP, Linn CC, Hwang L, et al: Hepatocellular carcinoma and hepatitis B virus: A prospective study of 22,707 men in Taiwan. *Lancet* 2:1129–1133, 1981

52. Tanaka K, Ikematsu H, Kashiwagi S: Hepatitis C virus infection and risk of hepatocellular carcinoma among Japanese: Possible role of Type 1b(II) infection. *J Natl Cancer Inst* 88: 742–746, 1996

53. El-Serag HB, Mason AC: Rising incidence of hepatocellular carcinoma in the United States. *N Engl J Med* 340:745–750, 1999

54. Purtilo DT, Sakamoto K, Barnabai V, et al: Epstein-Barr virus induced diseases in boys with the X-linked lymphoproliferative syndrome (XLP): Updates on studies of the registry. *Am J Med* 73:49–56, 1982

55. Pagano JS: Epstein-Barr virus transcription in nasopharyngeal carcinoma. *J Virol* 48:580–590, 1983

56. Mueller N, Evans A, Harris NL, et al: Hodgkin's disease and Epstein-Barr virus: Altered antibody pattern before diagnosis. *N Engl J Med* 320:689–695, 1989

57. Dyson N, Howley PM, Munger K, et al: The human papilloma virus-16 E7 oncoprotein is able to bind to the retinoblastoma gene product. *Science* 243:934–936, 1989

58. Franco EL, Rohan TE, Villa LL: Epidemiologic evidence and human papillomavirus infection as a necessary cause of cervical cancer. *J Natl Cancer Inst* 91:506–511, 1999

59. Stolte M: *Helicobacter pylori* gastritis and gastric MALT lymphoma. *Lancet* 339:745–746, 1992

60. Wotherspoon AC, Doglioni C, Diss TC, et al: Regression of primary low-grade B-cell gastric lymphoma of mucosa associated lymphoid tissue type after eradication of *Helicobacter pylori*. *Lancet* 342:575–577, 1993

61. Roggero E, Zucca E, Cavalli F: Gastric musoca-associated lymphoid tissue lymphomas: More than a fascinating model. *J Natl Cancer Inst* 89:1328–1330, 1997

62. Neubauer A, Thiede C, Morgner A, et al: Cure of *Helicobacter pylori* infection and duration of remission of low grade gastric mucosa-associated lymphoid tissue lymphoma. *J Natl Cancer Inst* 89:1350–1355, 1997

63. Peek RM Jr, Moss SF, Tham KT, et al: *Helicobacter pylori* cagA$^+$ strains and dissociation of gastric epithelial cell proliferation from apoptosis. *J Natl Cancer Inst* 89:863–868, 1997

64. Vogelstein B: Cancer: A deadly inheritance. *Nature* 348: 681–682, 1990

65. He TC, Sparks AB, Rago C, et al: Identification of c-*MYC* as a target of the APC pathway. *Science* 281:1509–1512, 1998

66. Rhyu MS: Molecular mechanisms underlying hereditary nonpolyposis colorectal carcinoma. *J Natl Cancer Inst* 88: 240–251, 1996

67. Rosen N: Cancers of the gastrointestinal tract: Molecular biology of gastrointestinal cancers, in DeVita VT Jr, Hellman S, Rosenberg SA (eds): *Cancer: Principles and Practice of Oncology* (ed 5). Philadelphia, Lippincott-Raven, 1997, pp 971–979

68. Nishisho I, Nakamura Y, Miyoshi Y, et al: Mutations of chromosome 5q21 in FAP and colorectal cancer patients. *Science* 253:665–669, 1991

69. Fearon ER, Cho KR, Nigro JM, et al: Identification of a chromosome 18q gene that is altered in colorectal cancers. *Science* 247:49–56, 1990

70. Kern SE, Vogelstein B: Genetic alterations in colorectal tumors, in Brugge J, Curran T, Harlow E, McCormick F (eds): *Origins of Human Cancer*. Cold Spring Harbor, NY, Cold Spring Harbor Laboratory Press, 1991, pp 557–585

71. Tanaka K, Oshimura M, Kikuchi R, et al: Suppression of tumorigenicity in human colon carcinoma cells by introduction of normal chromosome 5 or 18. *Nature* 349:340–342, 1991

72. Fisher B, Costantino JP, Wickerham DL, et al: Tamoxifen

for prevention of breast cancer: Report of the National Surgical Adjuvant Breast and Bowel Project P-1 study. *J Natl Cancer Inst* 90:1371–1388, 1998

73. Barrett-Connor E: Postmenopausal estrogen replacement and breast cancer. *N Engl J Med* 321:319–320, 1989

74. Thomas DB: Do hormones cause breast cancer? *Cancer* 53: 595–604, 1984

75. Pike MC, Henderson BE, Casagrande JT, et al: Oral contraceptive use and early abortion as risk factors for breast cancer in young women. *Br J Cancer* 43:72–76, 1981

76. Boffetta P, Agudo A, Ahrens W, et al: Multicenter case-control study of exposure to environmental tobacco smoke and lung cancer in Europe. *J Natl Cancer Inst* 90:1440–1450, 1998

77. Blot WJ, McLaughlin JK: Passive smoking and lung cancer risk: What is the story now? *J Natl Cancer Inst* 90:1416–1417, 1998

78. Ames BN: What are the major carcinogens in the etiology of human cancer? Environmental pollution, natural carcinogens, and the causes of human cancer: Six errors, in DeVita VT, Hellman S, Rosenberg SA (eds): *Important Advances in Oncology* (ed 3). Philadelphia, Lippincott, 1989, pp 210–235

79. Doll R, Peto R: The causes of cancer: Quantitative estimates of available risks of cancer in the United States today. *J Natl Cancer Inst* 66:1191–1308, 1981

80. Willett W: The search for the causes of breast and colon cancer. *Nature* 338:389–394, 1989

81. Ballard-Barbash R, Forman MR, and Kipnis V: Dietary fat, serum estrogen levels, and breast cancer risk: A multifaceted story. *J Natl Cancer Inst* 91:492–494, 1999

82. Hunter DJ, Spiegelman D, Adami HO, et al: Cohort studies of fat intake and the risk of breast cancer: A pooled analysis. *N Engl J Med* 334:356–361, 1996

83. Wynder EL, Reddy BS: Dietary fat and fiber and colon cancer. *Semin Oncol* 10:264–272, 1983

84. Reddy B, Engle A, Katsifis S, et al: Biochemical epidemiology of colon cancer: Effect of types of dietary fiber on fecal mutagens, acid, and neutral sterols in healthy subjects. *Cancer Res* 49:4629–4635, 1989

85. Caggon D, Barker DJP, Cole RB, et al: Stomach cancer and food storage. *J Natl Cancer Inst* 81:1178–1182, 1989

86. Willett WC, Stampfer MJ, Colditz GA, et al: Moderate alcohol consumption and the risk of breast cancer. *N Engl J Med* 314:1174–1180, 1987

87. Stolzenberg-Soloman RZ, Albanes D, Nieto FJ, et al: Pancreatic cancer risk and nutrition related methyl-group availability indicators in male smokers. *J Natl Cancer Inst* 91:535–541, 1999

88. Giovannucci E: Tomatoes, tomato-based products, lycopene, and cancer: Review of the epidemiological literature. *J Natl Cancer Inst* 91:317–331, 1999

CHAPTER 5

Cancer Control and Epidemiology

Mary Reid, PhD

Introduction

Cancer epidemiology examines the frequency of cancer in populations, the role of certain risk factors that contribute to cancer rates, and the interrelationships or associations that exist between the host, the environment, and other conditions that may contribute to the development or inhibition of cancer.[1] The first section of this chapter reviews basic epidemiological concepts. These concepts will help you to better understand current clinical research, identify groups at higher risk for cancer development, review current medical literature, and develop relevant research hypotheses related to the field of cancer epidemiology. They also should serve as a basis for understanding the major issues involved in cancer research design, assessment, and estimation of cancer risks. A brief glossary of fundamental terms used in the field of epidemiology is given in Table 5-1. Table 5-2 includes rates and ratios frequently calculated in epidemiologic research.

Subsequent sections of the chapter discuss causes of cancer and host characteristics that influence cancer susceptibility, cancer control and related issues, and the application of epidemiologic principles and cancer prevention and control issues in nursing practice.

Table 5-1   Glossary of Epidemiological Terms

Association	*Statistical association* refers to the strength of the relationship between two variables. In epidemiological terms, association imitates the degree to which the rate of disease in persons with a specific exposure is either higher or lower than the rate of disease in persons without the exposure. The strength of this dependence is greater than what would be expected by chance.
	Causal association is a biological association between the occurrence of an exposure and presence of a disease. The available evidence indicates that the presence of the exposure increases the probability of the presence of the disease. Changes in the frequency or quality of an exposure or characteristic would result in a corresponding change in the frequency of the disease or outcome of interest.
Bias	*Selection bias* results from a systematic difference in the manner by which the case and the comparison groups are selected for participation in the study. This bias may produce spurious associations due to the differential inclusion or exclusion of subjects from the disease or exposure groups.
	Misclassification bias is a systematic error that occurs when the measurement of either the exposure (risk factor) or the disease condition is systematically different for the groups being compared (e.g., the disease outcome between the exposed and unexposed groups was evaluated by separate physicians using different criteria).
Confounding	The systematic overestimation or underestimation of the effect of an exposure because the influence of a disease risk factor has not been taken into account. A *confounding variable* is a risk factor for the disease being studied that is associated with the exposure being studied and is not an intermediate step between the exposure and the disease.[2]
Epidemiology	A field in medical science concerned with the study of the frequency and distribution of disease in the population, and which also explores the relationship between exposures and development of diseases.
Incidence	The number of *new* events or cases of disease that occur in a defined population at risk within a specified period of time. Incidence rates can be used to evaluate the changing patterns of disease frequency within a population and to assess the effectiveness of screening programs and treatment modalities on disease development.
Population	The number of persons in a defined group who are capable of developing the disease. Can also refer to the general population; a population specifically defined by geographic, physical, or social characteristics, or risk; the sampling population; and the study population.
Power	The probability that a study will have the statistical strength to detect relationships that exist between exposures and disease. The power of a study can be maximized by controlling factors such as sample sizes, measurement error, and bias.
Prevalence	The number of *new and existing* cases of a given disease or condition in a defined population within a specified period of time. *Point prevalence* refers to prevalence at one point in time. *Period prevalence* refers to prevalence between two points in time. Prevalence rates can be used to compare disease frequencies across populations and to assess the magnitude of effect of certain diseases on the health status of a population.
Rates and ratios	These calculations are used to compare the frequencies of diseases in a population. Commonly used rates and ratios are given in Table 5-2, which lists the rate names, the numerator and denominator values, and the population factor used to express the rate in a standard format.
Risk measures	*Attributable risk* is the arithmetic or absolute difference between the exposed group and the nonexposed group in the incidence rates or the death rates. It estimates the number of disease cases that can be attributed to or explained by the exposure (e.g., the majority of lung cancer cases can be attributed to exposure to cigarette smoking).
	The relative risk and the odds ratio are calculated using a standard 2 × 2 table that separates the exposed and nonexposed groups by disease status.

(continues)

Table 5-1 Glossary of Epidemiological Terms (continued)

Risk measures (cont.)	*Relative risk (RR)* is a ratio comparing the rates of a disease among the exposed group and the nonexposed group that serves as a measure of the association between the disease and the exposure. The RR is generally used in cohort studies. The formula for calculating it is:

$$\frac{a/(a\ +\ b)}{c/(c\ +\ d)}$$

Odds ratio (OR) approximates the relative risk by comparing the rates of disease among the exposed and nonexposed groups. The OR is generally used in case-control studies with smaller sample sizes. The formula for calculating it is:

$$\frac{ad}{cb}$$

Both the RR and the OR are expressed as ratios (e.g., an OR of 1.0 means the rate of disease among the exposed group equals that of the nonexposed group).

Sensitivity	Measures the probability that a screening test will correctly classify an individual as *positive* for a disease when he or she actually does have the disease.
Specificity	Measures the probability that a screening test will correctly classify an individual as *negative* for a disease when he or she actually does not have the disease.
Validity	*Internal validity* is the extent to which the subjects in an epidemiological study are truly comparable with respect to general characteristics (e.g., if most of the cases are from an urban setting and the controls are mainly from a rural setting, the two groups are not comparable; evaluation of the exposure-disease relationship may be affected by these differences). Internal validity is essential for the interpretability and reliability of a study.

External validity, or generalizability, is the extent to which the study population can be compared with a larger population (e.g., the general population). External validity must be assessed before study results can be applied to a broader population (e.g., a study that uses as its population a specific profession, such as nurses, may yield results that are not relevant to all women in that general population; while the study may have strong internal validity, the participating nurses may not be representative of the women in the general population or in the nursing profession).

Basic Considerations in Epidemiological Research

Six primary components are considered in evaluating an epidemiological research project:

1. Study design
2. Definition of the source and study population to be used in the study
3. Eligibility and exclusion criteria used to select study participants
4. Definitions of the disease and exposures related to the research hypothesis
5. Statistical plan measuring the association between the exposures and the disease
6. Identification of potential sources of bias and confounding

It is critical that the basic design of the protocol be established prior to initiating the project. It is equally important that the entire research team, including the principal investigator, study coordinator, data managers, and data collectors, understand the design of the project in order to provide constant direction and evaluation during the course of data collection and analysis.

Study Designs

Several standard study designs are used in epidemiologic research. Although the general features of these designs are discussed in this section, our primary emphasis is on those designs most commonly used in clinical cancer research: the case-control and clinical trial study designs. The major study designs are experimental, ecological, cross-sectional, case-control, cohort, and clinical trial studies.[2]

In selecting the appropriate study design, certain factors must be considered. These include:

- The frequency of the disease or the exposure in the general population and the defined population to be studied;

- The length of time the disease takes to develop;

- The anticipated size of the study sample (which may be dependent on the number of eligible subjects available or on funding limitations);

- The time allowed for subject recruitment; and

- The diagnostic characteristics of the disease and the measurability of the exposure.

Table 5-2   Rates and Ratios Commonly Used in Epidemiology

Rate Name	Rate Description	Population Factor
Crude birth rate	Number of live births / Average or midyear population	per 1000
Fertility rate	Number of live births / 15- to 41-year-old women at midyear	per 1000
Crude mortality rate	Total number of deaths / Total population at midyear	per 1000
Age-specific mortality rate	Deaths in specific age-group / Midyear population in age-group	per 100,000
Cause-specific mortality rate	Deaths from a specific cause / Total midyear population	per 100,000
Infant mortality rate	Deaths of children less than 1 year of age / Number of live births	per 1000
Neonatal mortality rate	Deaths in infants younger than 28 days / Number of live births	per 1000
Case fatality rate	Number of deaths from a disease in a given period of follow-up / Number of diagnosed cases of disease at start of follow-up period	per 1000
Proportional mortality rate	Number of deaths from a given cause / Number of deaths from all causes	per 1000
Morbidity rate	Number of cases of the disease that develop in a given period / Total population at midperiod	per 100,000

Experimental studies

The experimental study design is an attempt to control all variation in the host and in the environment, including the exposure of interest. These studies, which typically use animal models in laboratory settings, are often conducted during the development of a biological hypotheses. Animal models provide a group of genetically identical subjects and allow for strict control of the exposure. Once substantial and consistent evidence has accumulated from experimental studies, other study designs may be employed to further investigate the hypothesis in human populations. While experimental studies with animal models can provide information on the mechanisms of cancer development, the generalizability of these models to human subjects is limited.

Ecological studies

The next step in investigating a hypothesis is to conduct an ecological or correlational study. In this design, correlations in the distribution of a disease among humans across ecological or geographic areas are examined. The unit of measure is the geographic region and not individuals within the region. For example, cancer rates are often evaluated across different countries, or regions of a country, to investigate the effects of nutrient or natural environmental exposures. Examples of ecologic studies include the comparison of meat and fat consumption across the United States and Japan and the relative rates of colorectal cancer; the differences in county forage selenium levels across the United States and the corresponding rates of internal cancers; and the levels of radon exposure by neighborhood and the incidence of hematological cancers.

Cross-sectional studies

The cross-sectional study is another design that allows an investigator to assess the rates of disease and exposure in a population. In this study design, a onetime view of a population is taken; the rate of existing (prevalent) cases of the disease, the degree of exposure, and other demographic characteristics of interest are measured. While cross-sectional studies cannot establish a causal relationship between the exposure and the disease, they do provide descriptive statistics for the population and are often used as the preliminary step in establishing disease or exposure status in cohort studies. Cross-sectional studies can be nested at the baseline of cohort studies or clinical trials.

When performing a cross-sectional study nested in a phase III clinical trial, the entire population may have a common condition that made the subjects eligible for the study. For example, a phase III clinical trial on colorectal adenoma prevention may recruit subjects with a recent history of adenomas. Because everyone in the population has had an adenoma at baseline, you cannot evaluate the association of adenomas and dietary intake patterns, for example. However, in this case, you could describe the association of calcium intake and the location, size, or histology of the baseline adenomas. This is an example of a case-case analysis.

Case-control studies

The case-control study design should be considered if at least one of the following criteria is met:

- The disease is rare in the general or source population (such as most forms of cancer).

- The investigation is preliminary.

- Time and funding limitations prohibit the use of other, larger, more expensive study designs.

The information gained from case-control studies does not establish a causal relationship between the disease and the exposure, but it does explore the concurrent association between the two. If the strength of this association is significant and supported by other studies, this information can be used to justify the use of larger cohort studies or clinical trials that can investigate causative relationships.

Subjects in case-control studies are recruited on the basis of disease status. Cases of the disease in question can be either preexisting or newly developed. Generally, a strict definition of the disease is used to identify eligible subjects. For example, the stage or *histology* of a cancer can be used. The control subjects, or noncases, are defined as participants who do not have the disease at present but who, if the disease did develop, would have the same opportunity to be diagnosed as the case subjects. The selection of an appropriate control group is the major challenge of case-control studies and is often the source of selection bias introduced into the study.[3]

An example of the use of the case-control study design is a study examining the association between malignant melanoma and the use of sun beds and sunlamps.[4] The case group consisted of 583 individuals diagnosed with melanoma; the control group was composed of 608 subjects who did not have melanoma. The control subjects were randomly selected from property tax rolls. Each group was evaluated for exposure, which in this case was the use of sun beds or sunlamps. The calculated odds ratio, comparing the rate of exposure among the diseased group with that among the nondiseased, found that the exposed subjects, that is, those who reported using sun beds or sunlamps, had a 1.45- to 1.88-fold increase in the risk of developing melanoma. This difference was seen in both the male and the female subjects.

Demographic differences between case subjects and controls should be minimized. To make the two groups comparable, some investigators have used a technique called *matching*, in which certain demographic characteristics of the case subjects are matched to those of the controls. For example, if a case subject is female, 45 years old, white, and from a low-income household, a control subject would be selected with basically the same characteristics. The advantage of matching and analyzing the data in pairs of subjects is that fewer subjects are required in each group to see a relationship between the exposure and the disease, if such a relationship exists. This is useful when there are small numbers of case subjects with the disease available for study and when efficiency is a major issue.

Matching is also a means for controlling potential confounding introduced by the selection of the control group. The major disadvantage of matching is that any variable used in matching cannot be studied in relation to the disease. If little is actually known about the relationship between disease and exposure, the investigator may not want to limit the opportunities to study all possible variables. The melanoma study used matching to control the potential confounding variables of age, sex, and residence municipality.[4] The resulting groups contained similar proportions of each variable.

A commonly used alternative to matching is the recruitment of more than one control subject per case subject. For example, two to four control subjects may be recruited for each case subject. This technique affords an increase in statistical power without limiting the variables that can be investigated. In this scenario, the baseline characteristics of both groups would be assessed for comparability. Ideally, the age ranges, racial differences, socioeconomic status (SES), and other known potential confounding variables should not be significantly different between the groups. The association seen between an exposure and the disease can be clouded by extraneous variables that are poorly distributed between the case and control groups.

Another classic example of the case-control design is a study of endometrial cancer and the use of postmenopausal estrogens.[5] In this study, women with endometrial cancer constituted the case group, while women from the same hospital who had other gynecologic ailments were recruited into the control group. Matching was not implemented. The increase in risk of cancer related to exposure to the postmenopausal estrogens was dramatic (odds ratio [OR] = 11.28). Critics of the study stated that the two subject groups did not have comparable SES and that selection bias explained the elevated risk. The study was redesigned and a new control group recruited. The resulting odds ratios, after an attempt to control the selection bias, still showed that estrogens significantly increased a woman's risk of developing endometrial cancer (OR = 2.30–2.69).

Cohort studies

Once an association between a disease and an exposure has been established, a cohort study may be initiated to test the research hypothesis. The *cohort*, or group of subjects, that is included in this type of study design represents individuals who have a comparable risk of exposure and who do not have the disease of interest when recruited. An initial cross-sectional study or assessment of a population can identify and eliminate all active cases of the disease. Once the cohort is selected, the exposures of interest are assessed and the subjects monitored for a designated period of time to record development of the disease.

Cohort studies can be retrospective, prospective, or ambidirectional. *Retrospective studies* use a previously defined cohort, and, through the review of records, identify individuals who developed the disease and assess the level of exposure. While retrospective studies are often less time-consuming and less expensive than the other cohort designs, the quality of the information collected on the disease and exposure is constrained by the quality of the records available. Many occupational cohort studies are conducted retrospectively.

In *prospective studies*, a current population of disease-free individuals is selected and the exposure(s) measured. This study population is then followed into the future and evaluated for development of the disease. The rate of new cases is compared between levels of exposure to establish the disease-exposure relationship. While prospective studies often require several years of subject follow-up and are generally expensive to complete, they offer the opportunity to establish definitively a causative relationship between the exposure and the disease. In addition, the effect of multiple risk factors on disease development may be investigated.

The Framingham Heart Study is one of the best-known examples of this type of cohort design.[6] The residents of Framingham, Massachusetts, were selected for this prospective study, which examined the risk factors for cardiovascular disease. All eligible subjects were examined extensively for presence of heart disease, and potential risk factors were evaluated, such as family history, nutrition, exercise, smoking status, and alcohol consumption. Monitoring of these subjects for the development of heart disease and/or a cardiovascular-related event has continued to date and now includes a cohort of offspring of the original participants. Significant information on the multiple risk factors and treatment modalities of heart disease has been produced by this study.

The last type of cohort study is the *ambidirectional study*, which starts with a previously established cohort and continues subject follow-up into the future. This design carries the same advantages and disadvantages as the retrospective and prospective designs combined.

The study of the Vietnam veteran's postservice mortality is an example of the ambidirectional cohort design.[7] A cohort of Vietnam veterans was identified retrospectively from service records. The subjects were then followed prospectively through 1983 to determine the vital status and causes of deaths of the cohort. These rates were compared with mortality rates of veterans from World War II and the Korean War. While the death rates for Vietnam veterans were slightly elevated in the first five years following the end of active service, the overall death rates were not significantly different.

Clinical trials and intervention studies

The clinical trial or intervention study is the strongest study design used in human populations. This design tests the effect of an intervention on the rates of development or recurrence of the disease. At least two groups of subjects are created within the study population: a treatment group (receiving the treatment) and a control group (receiving the placebo or the current therapy). For example, to test the effect of a drug or nutritional supplement on the rates of cancer development, subjects are randomly assigned to one of the two groups and monitored over the time period of the study for the development or recurrence of the cancer. The design is called *double-blind* when the assignment of the treatment group is kept from the subject and the immediate clinical personnel. This controls the potential biasing effects on subject participation, disease diagnosis, and monitoring that can occur when participants and clinical staff know the group assignments.

A major benefit of a double-blind, placebo-controlled clinical trial is that the random assignment of treatment groups helps to distribute potential confounding variables evenly between the two groups, thus minimizing their effects on the measurement of the association between the exposure and the disease. If this control of confounding is successful and the primary difference between the two treatment groups is the intervention, then a clinical trial can definitively evaluate the efficacy of the intervention.

An example of a clinical trial is the Physicians' Health Study,[8] which randomized 22,071 licensed physicians into an expanded design to test the effectiveness of aspirin on decreasing the rates of heart attacks and the effect of beta-carotene on inhibiting the development of cancer. This was defined as a multifactorial design. After 5 years, the aspirin arm of the trial was stopped because a significantly lower risk of heart attack was observed among the subjects receiving aspirin. The beta-carotene arm of the trial was discontinued in December 1995; no effect of beta-carotene was observed on cancer incidence.[9]

A major limitation of the clinical trial design is that several years of subject follow-up may be required before significant changes in the rate of disease development are observed among treatment groups. The length of follow-up will depend on several factors, one of which is the strength of the effect the treatment has on the risk of the disease. Long-term studies raise patient management issues, such as maintaining active participation of subjects, monitoring subject deaths and adverse events, and tracking subjects who move from the study area. These factors, if unevenly distributed among the treatment groups, may confound the results of the project.

Defining the Population

In addition to defining the type of study design appropriate for testing a research hypothesis, the source population for study subjects and the actual study population must also be defined. This clarifies to whom the research results can be generalized (external validity), whether the study population represents the total population and the source population, and the overall characteristics of eligible subjects. The *source population* for the study is the larger group or population from which the study subjects are recruited. This might include, for instance, residents in a certain city or neighborhood, university students, or all subjects attending a particular hospital. The source population is usually a subgroup of the total population.

The *study population* is the group of subjects actually recruited into the project from the source population. Recruitment into the study population, based on the defined eligibility and exclusionary criteria, is planned to access all potential subjects within the source population. In reviewing sources of bias that may have been introduced into the study, it is important to review the type of subjects who were part of the source population but who were not eligible or not approached for recruitment. For example, if subjects were recruited from phone interviews, we could safely conclude that only subjects with telephones were eligible. Because the presence of a telephone in the household might be related to SES, it is possible that the study population might be biased toward subjects with a higher SES. With this selection bias and the recruitment of a homogeneous group of subjects with respect to SES, the relationship of SES to the disease may be impossible to evaluate and may affect the results of the study.

Eligibility and exclusion criteria

The selection of the study population is based on established eligibility criteria. These criteria are designed to gather a population of subjects with a sufficient prevalence of the disease to test the hypothesis efficiently and for whom the intervention is considered safe. Examples of commonly used eligibility criteria in cancer research are age ranges, race, gender-specific factors, disease stage, life expectancy, absence of other cancers or chronic diseases, exposure to certain drugs or treatments, and current health status. Examples of exclusion criteria include previous medical history; the presence of current, uncontrolled chronic conditions; and extreme dietary patterns or limitations on daily activities.

Defining the Disease and the Exposure

The disease should be defined as specifically as possible, including pathological criteria, specific blood chemistries, histological characteristics, specific test results, and physical symptoms according to current medical practice. Clear disease definition helps to limit the recruitment of subjects who are later found to be ineligible for the study. Even with a clear definition, good research practice requires that the disease status be confirmed with an external reviewer, further controlling bias.

Equally important as defining the disease is clarifying the definition of the exposure used in the study. An *exposure* is considered to be a subject's contact with the variable of interest, which may influence the development of or improvement in disease status. Exposures can include a broad range of variables, from environmental conditions, medications, nutrients, genetic influences, and health care accessibility to types of exercise. The characteristics of the exposure that are most important to clarify are the dose of the exposure, the duration or length of time of the exposure, and characteristics that are specific to the exposure, such as latency effects and effects that are synergistic with other exposures.

Dose refers to a standardized, measured amount of exposure issued (e.g., standard milligrams, as in the case of drugs, gray [Gy] for radiation, number of packs of cigarettes per year, drinks of alcohol per day, and so on). Be sure to assess whether the dose is constant throughout the exposure or whether certain variables or conditions have affected the dose over time.

Statistical Plan

In addition to calculating the rates and ratios of a disease as it develops in a population, epidemiological research affords the investigator the ability to examine the relationships of the disease to defined exposures. Epidemiological research strives to make inferences to a larger population based on information obtained from the study population. The external validity of these inferences (or *generalizability*) relies on the assumption that the study population is a representative sample of the larger group.

While risk estimates are useful, other statistical tests afford the opportunity to examine more closely the disease-exposure association. In the design stage of developing a research protocol, consult a biostatistician or epidemiologist to assist with estimating appropriate sample size and developing an analysis plan. The analysis plan assures in advance that you are collecting the right information, in the right format to actually answer the research question.

Potential Sources of Bias and Confounding

The potential sources of bias and confounding in a study must be evaluated. Bias, the result of how subjects were selected or how the exposure or disease were classified, can lead to spurious results. Bias is best controlled when it is anticipated in the design phase of the project. Reviewing your proposal with experienced researches and discussing the procedures for participant selection can help to minimize the effects of bias.

Confounding can also lead to a misinterpretation of the study results. When a variable is related both to the exposure and to the disease, confounding is present. The effects of confounding can be controlled in the analysis of data, often by stratifying on the confounding variable or including the confounder in the multivariate models. Again, seeking the advice of experienced researchers can help to minimize the effects of confounding on the conclusions drawn from the research study.

Textbooks, including basic epidemiologic texts,[10,11] basic biostatistical texts,[12,13] and summary texts on cancer prevention and genetic epidemiology,[14,15] are excellent resources for epidemiologic and statistical principles and practices.

Data Sources

In the United States, there are several data sources and systems relating to cancer and risk factors for cancer that can be accessed by investigators (Table 5-3). Such sources are frequently useful to gain preliminary data to formulate or support a hypothesis, as well as to provide a means of examining national, regional, or temporal differences in cancer or risk factors for cancer.

Environmental Factors Associated with Cancer Causation

How Do We Decide What Causes Cancer?

Inference regarding causality cannot be made from a single study but, rather, must be drawn from many sources. The criteria to be considered are:

- The magnitude of association between the exposure and the disease
- Consistency of findings from all studies
- Biological credibility
- Temporal association between the risk factor and the disease

Tobacco

Tobacco use is still the most prevalent known cause of cancer in the United States. Tobacco causes about 30%

Table 5-3   Data Sources for Epidemiological Research

Source	Description
National Health Interview Survey (NHIS)	Annual survey started in 1957. Household interviews are conducted in approximately 50,000 households representative of the civilian noninstitutionalized population. Provides data on the incidence of illness and accidental injuries, prevalence of chronic diseases and impairments, disability, physician visits, hospitalizations, and other health topics, and on the relationship between demographic and socioeconomic characteristics and health characteristics. The questionnaires change with time to focus on current health topics.
National Health and Nutrition Examination Survey (NHANES)	NHANES III was begun in 1988. Ultimately, 45,000 people representative of the U.S. population will be selected to participate. Participants undergo physical examinations and clinical and laboratory testing. For example, data are collected on blood pressure, serum cholesterol, and body measurements. Dietary assessment is also conducted as part of the survey.
Behavioral Risk Factor Surveillance System	Started in 1984, this system is coordinated by the Centers for Disease Control and Prevention (CDC), but the telephone interviews used as the survey methodology are conducted by the participating states—currently, 45 states and the District of Columbia. The survey's purpose is to collect information regarding the prevalence of self-reported health behaviors that relate to the ten leading causes of death, including cigarette smoking, hypertension, obesity, seat belt use, physical inactivity, and alcohol use. Several of these behaviors are risk factors for cancer. This system provides a means of assessing change in these behaviors over time or in response to an intervention.
National Vital Statistics System	This system provides data on births, deaths, marriages, and divorces. Annual data are produced for the United States, the individual states, counties, and other local areas. Cause of death is included in this system (e.g., breast cancer mortality rates can be compared for differing counties within a state, or over time within a specific location).
Surveillance, Epidemiology, and End Results (SEER) Program	This is the principal source of cancer incidence and survival data for the United States. The participating areas are Seattle (Puget Sound), Utah, San Francisco, New Mexico, Hawaii, Iowa, Detroit, Connecticut, and Atlanta (including ten rural counties), which include approximately 9.6% of the U.S. population. For each newly diagnosed cancer case, data collected include selected patient demographics, primary site, morphology, diagnostic confirmation, extent of disease, and first course of cancer-directed therapy. Active follow-up of all living patients is conducted to help ascertain survival time.
National Death Index	This system aids investigators in ascertaining mortality. A computerized database contains identifying information on all deaths reported by the state vital statistics offices. An investigator can determine if a study subject has died and, if relevant, where and how to obtain a copy of the death certificate.
Decennial Census	The goal of the 10-yearly census conducted in the United States is to count each person according to "usual place of residence." A limited amount of information is requested from each person; a sample of persons is then asked to complete a more detailed questionnaire. Detailed population numbers by age, sex, and ethnicity are important to the epidemiologist, because they are used in the denominator of calculations of population rates. The demographic data from the census can be used to give a population profile of areas of research interest.

of cancer deaths, and cigarette smoking causes 90% of lung cancers.[16]

Active tobacco use has been linked to many cancer types: lung, oropharyngeal, bladder, pancreatic, cervical, and kidney, and a clear linear relationship exists between the number of cigarettes smoked and the risk of lung and oropharyngeal cancers.[16,17]

There is a gradual decrease in the exsmoker's risk of dying from lung cancer; the risk decreases by approximately 50% after 5 years and 80% after 10 years.[18] The rate of decline of the risk after cessation of smoking is determined by the cumulative smoking exposure prior to cessation, the age when smoking began, and the degree of inhalation.

Study results regarding passive smoking as a risk factor for lung cancer are inconsistent, with some studies showing a positive relationship between lung cancer and exposure to sidestream smoke[19,20] and others showing no relationship.[21] Blot and Fraumeni combined data from existing studies and estimated an overall increase in risk for lung cancer of 30% for nonsmoking women married to smokers and an increased risk of 70% associated with heavy passive smoking.[22,23] A review of epidemiological studies supports the causal association between environmental tobacco smoke and lung cancer.[24]

The use of smokeless tobacco (chewing tobacco and snuff) is increasing among U.S. male youth, especially among whites.[25] This practice has been linked to both oral cancer and cancer of the tongue.[26]

The overall smoking prevalence is decreasing in the United States,[27] and this is reflected in declining lung cancer rates among men and rates that are beginning to slow and stabilize in women.[28] However, the decrease in smoking prevalence is not uniform among all groups within society. For the period 1974–1987, smoking prevalence in women aged 20 and over declined more slowly (31.5% to 26.8%) than for men (43.4% to 31.7%), with the smoking prevalence for women aged 20 to 24 years not changing significantly. Smoking prevalence declined from 1974 to 1985 in white adolescents, but no significant declines occurred during the period 1985–1991. In contrast, smoking prevalence declined through the entire 1974–1991 period in black adolescents. The reasons for these differences are unclear.[29]

Lung cancer mortality rate for white men in the United States likely has peaked, but the projected peak for mortality rates in women will not occur until the year 2010.[30,31] Similarly, lung cancer mortality for blacks is not expected to fall until after the year 2000.[31] However, even with the predicted declines in mortality rates, the absolute number of lung cancer deaths will continue to rise because of the increasing size of the population.[32]

Diet

Diet may be of great importance in cancer prevention, for it has been proposed as a contributing factor in 20%–70% of cancer deaths[33,34] and is a modifiable risk factor. Interest and research in the role of diet in cancer has flourished in recent years, with many micronutrients (vitamins and minerals) and some macronutrients (proteins, fats, carbohydrates) being investigated for adverse or protective effects against cancer, in both human (see Chapter 8 for description of some studies) and animal studies.[35] The impetus for many of these studies came from the results of ecological studies; for example, a high correlation was found between national per capita daily meat consumption and country-specific colon cancer incidence rates.[36]

Case-control and cohort studies of diet and cancer present several methodological problems:

1. Accurate assessment of dietary intake is very difficult, especially in large epidemiological studies. The two frequently used methods of dietary assessment are single or multiple 24-hour recall of dietary intake and the food-frequency questionnaire. In the latter method, subjects are asked how many times they ate numerous foods with reference to a given time period, such as the last year. The validity of these instruments varies with the nutrient of interest. Dietary assessment, including the previously described methods, has been thoroughly described by Willett[37] and Ocke.[38]

2. Dietary patterns correlate with socioeconomic and political characteristics.

3. Individual nutrients are often highly correlated because they are strongly related to caloric intake. This makes the assessment of the role of a single nutrient problematic. Statistical methods have been developed to adjust for caloric intake in an attempt to address this problem.[39]

4. Frequently, the range of nutrient intake within the study population is narrow, making it less likely that a nutrient effect will be observed. For example, this problem has been suggested as a possible reason for the lack of association between fat and breast cancer in the large Nurses' Health Study.[40]

5. The distribution of dietary components among individual foods varies greatly; the interactive roles of dietary components are not completely understood, particularly when several components are present in individual foods.

6. Recall bias may be present if dietary assessment is being conducted after the presentation of the disease, as in a case-control study. This means that individuals' recall of their past diet might be affected by their knowledge that they have the disease.[41]

To avoid the problems associated with self-reported dietary intake methods, direct assessment of some micronutrients has been developed, involving measuring the serum micronutrient levels.[34,42] However, this type of measurement has disadvantages; for example, in a case-control study the disease may affect blood micronutrient levels. Serum markers of intake of most macronutrients are not currently available, thus limiting this methodology. Some current issues regarding diet and cancer are discussed next.

Colon cancer and fat intake.   Ecological studies comparing many countries have shown a strong association between per capita meat consumption[36] or dietary fat[43] and incidence of colorectal cancer. However, a causal association cannot be assumed from such studies. Results from case-control and cohort studies generally have supported high fat intake as a risk factor for colon cancer.[44-47] Difficulties can arise in the interpretation of such results because it is often difficult to separate the effects of fat, protein, and total calories[46,47]—dietary factors that are generally highly correlated.

Colon cancer and fiber intake.   A majority of studies of differing epidemiological designs supports the hypothesis that high fiber intake is protective for colon cancer,[48] although not all studies are supportive. Vegetables as well as cereals are sources of fiber; in studies where the source of fiber has been examined, fiber from vegetables appears protective against colon cancer, whereas the data for cereal fiber are less supportive of a protective effect. The hypothesized mechanism is that fiber affects the bile acid content of the aqueous portion of stool. These differing results may be due to the difference in composition of fiber in cereals and vegetables or to the lack of a large range in cereal fiber intake, or they may indicate that some other chemical or nutrient in vegetables is protective against colon cancer.[48,49] Other studies have focused on the effects of fiber in the prevention of adenomatous polyps.[50]

Colon cancer and calcium intake.   A protective role of high calcium intake against colon cancer has been reported in several studies[51-54] but not in all.[45,55] Data from supportive studies suggest that to reduce the risk of colon cancer, calcium intake for females should be 1500 mg and for males 1800 mg.[56]

Breast cancer and fat intake.   Ecological studies that use data from many countries show a strong positive relationship between per capita fat intake and breast cancer mortality rates.[36] However, case-control and cohort studies give conflicting results. In a combined analysis of twelve case-control studies of dietary factors and breast cancer, Howe et al reported an association between high fat intake and breast cancer in postmenopausal women.[57]

Two of the largest cohort studies, the Nurses' Health Study[40] and the Iowa Women's Study,[58] show no relationship between dietary fat intake and breast cancer risk; however, some researchers suggest that this may be because the range of fat intake in such studies was too small. Current dietary recommendations are for women to reduce fat intake to less than 30% of calories. In Willett's study, the range of fat intake was 32%–44% of calories.[40]

Cancer, micronutrients, and intake of fruits and vegetables.   One of the most consistent dietary findings in analytic epidemiological studies with regard to cancer is the protective effect of fruits and vegetables.[59] What particu-lar nutrient, nonnutrient, or combination in fruits and vegetables is protective against cancer is still under investigation. Nonnutrient compounds that may have a protective effect have been summarized by Wattenberg.[60] The role of several micronutrients in cancer prevention, including the carotenoid beta-carotene, vitamin A, vitamin E, and selenium, has been extensively investigated (see Chapter 8). Relatively high levels of these four micronutrients have been found to be associated with lower cancer risk in many studies, although again not all study results are in agreement. The role of micronutrients in cancer prevention has been reviewed.[34,61] (See Chapter 8 for more information about cancer chemoprevention trials.)

Dietary intake has an impact not only on cancer but on many other chronic diseases as well, such as heart disease and diabetes, where its role is more fully understood. Even without proof of the role of a specific nutrient in cancer causation, there may be sufficient knowledge from a public health perspective to recommend that Americans change some aspect of their diet.[62] For example, the role of fat in breast cancer is still controversial, but there exists sufficient knowledge concerning the role of fat in obesity, heart disease, and colon cancer that recommendations to reduce fat intake have been made to the American public.

Several groups, such as the National Research Council, have published recommendations for an optimal diet. Their recommendations include eating at least five servings of fruit and vegetables a day, reducing fat intake to 30% or less of calories, maintaining protein intake at moderate levels, and balancing food intake and physical activity to maintain appropriate body weight.[63,64] The role of health professionals is to encourage patients to follow such guidelines and to help them avoid being influenced by published results of isolated studies of diet and its relationship to cancer.

Alcohol

Alcohol has been causally linked to cancers of the oral cavity, pharynx, larynx, esophagus, and liver, and may be linked to cancers of the breast and rectum.[65,66] For most cancer sites, alcohol appears to act synergistically with smoking.

Cancers at most sites do not appear to be associated with any particular type of alcohol. Rectal cancer is the exception, for it appears to be associated specifically with beer consumption.[67] Nitrosamines, which are found in beer, have been suggested as a possible cause of the association between rectal cancer and beer consumption.[68]

Studies regarding the relationship between alcohol and breast cancer suggest a positive but weak association. However, both the level of alcohol consumption required to significantly increase breast cancer risk[65] and the age at which exposure to alcohol is important[69] are unclear. If a causal association were shown, alcohol would present one of the only known avoidable causes of breast cancer. However, if increased risk of breast cancer is shown to be associated with moderate to low levels of alcohol intake, as some studies have shown, women will have to weigh the personal benefits of abstaining from alcohol to reduce breast cancer risk against the risk of increasing their risk of heart disease,[70] as moderate alcohol intake has been shown to be associated with a reduced risk of heart disease in women.[71]

Physical activity

Accurate measurement of physical activity in epidemiological studies has proved to be difficult, and many questionnaires have been developed in an attempt to improve assessment.[72] The close interrelationship of physical activity with obesity and diet, two factors associated with many cancers, also makes its role in relation to cancer risk more difficult to assess.[73] Increased physical activity consistently has been found to be protective for colon cancer[74-76] and precancerous colon polyps.[77,78] Mounting evidence suggests that increased physical activity is protective for breast cancer.[79,80] Intense physical activity at the age of usual menarche may be especially important, since it can cause a delay in onset of menarche.[81] Late onset of menarche is known to be protective against breast cancer.[82] Increased physical activity is known to be protective against heart disease, and a general increase in physical activity throughout the population would be beneficial for health.[83]

Occupational exposures

An estimated 4%–9% of cancer deaths can be attributed to exposure to occupational carcinogens. The lung is the most commonly affected site.[84] Reasons for conducting epidemiological studies of industrial populations include surveillance of groups to:

- Identify unusual disease patterns that might indicate exposure to previously unidentified hazards.

- Monitor and reevaluate "safe" levels of identified hazards.

- Monitor human exposure to complex mixtures of different chemicals or materials that probably have not been tested in animal experiments in the laboratory.

A summary of some occupational carcinogens that may cause cancer is found in Table 5-4.

Pollution

Epidemiological studies of pollution present a difficult methodological problem in the assessment of exposure—specifically, assessment of both how long a subject has been exposed and the level of exposure. Air pollution has been studied primarily in relation to risk for lung cancer. In heavily polluted areas, air pollution may contribute to lung cancer mortality; however, insufficient data are available to quantify the risk of pollution with lung cancer mortality.[85] Evidence is much stronger for the association of air pollution and increased mortality from respiratory diseases, showing the importance of air pollution as a health risk.

Table 5-4. Suspected Occupational Carcinogens

Carcinogen	Cancer
Aromatic compounds in soots, tar, some mineral oils	Skin
Arsenic compounds (pesticides, mining, smelting of metals)	Lung, skin
Asbestos	Lung, mesothelioma
Benzene	Leukemia
Benzidine	Bladder
Beryllium compounds	Lung
Bis(chloromethyl)ether and chloromethyl methyl ether	Lung
Cadmium compounds (battery manufacturing, alloying, plating, etc)	Lung
Formaldehyde	Nose and nasopharynx
Hair dressing	Bladder
Mustard gas	Lung, pharynx
2-naphthylamine (rubber, cable-making)	Bladder
Nickel compounds	Nasal sinuses and nose
Radon	Lung
Vinyl chloride	Liver
Wood dusts	Nasal sinuses

Data from Trichopoulos et al;[1] Searle, Teale.[84]

Associations between water pollution and site-specific cancer risk are also unproved. Arsenic in drinking water appeared to be associated with an increase of skin cancer in Taiwan[86] but not in the United States.[87] This observed difference might be due to a higher intensity of exposure in Taiwan. Trihalomethane, another more common pollutant of drinking water, may be linked to rectal and bladder cancer.[88] These compounds are produced by the action of chlorine on organic waste.

A type of pollution that may indirectly increase cancer risk is that of chlorofluorocarbons (CFCs), which are destroying the ozone layer in the stratosphere.[89] It is predicted that this destruction will increase the amount of ultraviolet light reaching the earth's surface, thereby increasing the risk for nonmelanoma and melanoma skin cancer. The Environmental Protection Agency (EPA) reports that for every 1% decrease in stratospheric ozone, there is a 2% increase in ultraviolet-B intensity, potentially increasing the incidence of skin cancer by 1%–3% each year that the condition of the deteriorating ozone exists.[90]

Reproductive factors and sexual behavior

Risk factors related to reproduction and sexual behavior have been identified only for cancers in women; these are summarized in Table 5-5. The risk factor patterns are

Table 5-5 Reproductive and Sexual Factors Associated with Female Cancers

Risk Factor	Breast	Cervical	Endometrial	Ovarian
Early menarche	X		X	X
Late menopause	X		X	X
Nulliparity	X		X	X
Late first pregnancy, >35 years old	X			
Obesity	X*		X	
Multiple sexual partners		X		

*Postmenopausal women only.

similar for breast, endometrial, and ovarian cancers. Pike discusses the reasons for these observed similarities, such as exposure to unopposed estrogen.[91] In contrast, cervical cancer has a very different risk factor pattern, with only multiple sexual partners being identified as a sexual behavioral risk factor. The number of sexual partners is a measure of the likelihood that an individual has been exposed to the human papillomavirus (HPV) which has been implicated as a cause of cervical dysplasia.[92]

In general, the reproductive risk factors associated with breast, endometrial, and ovarian cancers are unavoidable. Furthermore, there are no other proven risk factors for these cancers that can be avoided. Thus, early detection of these cancers is very important. Unfortunately, only breast cancer screening is available, although screening methods for ovarian cancer are being investigated. Nurses can play a strong role in encouraging all women to obtain mammography and in educating women regarding early signs of endometrial and ovarian cancer. (See Chapter 9 for more information on screening.)

Viruses and other biological agents

Viruses may contribute to approximately 15%–20% of human cancers throughout the world.[93,94] Well-known viruses thought to cause human cancers are Epstein-Barr virus (EBV), associated with Burkitt's lymphoma and nasopharyngeal cancer; hepatitis B and C viruses (HBV and HCV), associated with liver cancer; human HPV, particularly subtypes HPV16 and HPV18,[95] linked with cervical, penile, and some anal cancers; human T-lymphotropic virus types 1 and 2 (HTLV-1 and HTLV-2), associated with T-cell leukemia and lymphoma; and human immunodeficiency virus (HIV), associated with non-Hodgkin's lymphoma and Kaposi's sarcoma. Table 5-6 lists several putative human cancer viruses and their associated cancers. Epidemiological evidence for their role in cancer causation is relatively strong. Hepatitis B virus and HTLV-1 may be sufficient alone to cause cancer, whereas EBV alone is insufficient and requires the host to be immunodeficient.[94] Burkitt's lymphoma is seen primarily in Africa, where malarial infection causes the required immunodeficiency state.

Both cohort and case-control studies reveal an association between *Helicobacter pylori* infection and gastric cancer.[96–98] *Schistosoma haematobium*, a parasitic flatworm, is common in Iraq, Egypt, and southeast Africa; there is strong epidemiological evidence of its causative role in bladder cancer in these regions.[99]

Radiation

It is estimated that 20% of cancer deaths are due to natural sources of radiation, excluding occupational exposure.[1]

Ionizing radiation. For most of the earth's population, more than 80% of exposure to ionizing radiation is from natural sources, such as the food chain, air, water, minerals on or near the earth's crust, and cosmic rays. Man-made sources are x-rays (80% of exposure to man-made sources in the United States),[100] fallout from nuclear explosions, and emissions and waste from nuclear power stations.

Table 5-6 Cancer Types Associated with a Virus or Other Biological Agent

Virus or Biological Agent	Cancer
Hepatitis B virus	Hepatocellular carcinoma
Human papillomavirus (types 16 and 18)	Cervical cancer
Epstein-Barr virus	Burkitt's lymphoma
Human T-cell lymphotrophic virus type 1	Adult T-cell leukemia/lymphoma (ATLL)
Human immunodeficiency virus*	Kaposi's sarcoma; non-Hodgkin's lymphoma
Schistosoma	Bladder cancer
Helicobacter pylori	Gastric cancer

*The association may be due to immunosuppression caused by HIV, which places the individual at increased risk. But even HIV-seropositive patients with no measurable immunosuppression appear to be at higher risk.

Several populations have been studied to assess the cancer risk of ionizing radiation. These include survivors from Nagasaki and Hiroshima, people who received radiation therapy for medical reasons, and underground miners who were exposed to radon gas and decay products. There is no doubt that ionizing radiation causes many different cancer types, with the breast, thyroid, and bone marrow being particularly sensitive sites.[101,102] However, determining the effect of low-dose exposure, the level at which most such exposure occurs, is difficult. Dose extrapolation poses many problems. For example, attempting to extrapolate from the cancer risk of the high radon dose that miners receive to the relatively low dose that individuals living in a radon-contaminated house receive requires many assumptions regarding exposure to both the miners and the house's inhabitants.[103] Using extrapolated risk estimates, Lubin et al[103] calculated that in the United States 10% of all lung cancer deaths annually may be due to exposure to radon in the home, thus making radon exposure a great public health concern.

Occupational exposure to ionizing radiation is highest among underground uranium miners, commercial nuclear power plant workers, fuel fabricators, physicians, flight crews and attendants, industrial radiographers, and well loggers.[104]

Ultraviolet radiation. Ultraviolet radiation (UVR) is the major cause of nonmelanoma skin cancer, with cumulative exposure and number of lifetime sunburns being predictive of risk.[105,106] The relationship of UVR to melanoma skin cancer is not as clear, because the site of melanoma does not mimic the site of exposure, as happens in nonmelanoma skin cancer. However, it is thought that intense intermittent exposure to UVR, especially in childhood, is a risk factor for melanoma.[107] Individual exposure to UVR is dependent on latitude, altitude, humidity, and personal behaviors, such as wearing protective clothing, using sunscreens, and staying out of the sun as much as possible.

Nonionizing radiation. Nonionizing electromagnetic fields (EMF) are generated from a variety of electrical power, radar, and microwave sources[108] and have only recently been suspected of increasing cancer risk. Both occupational and residential exposures have been studied, and the results from some studies suggest that exposure to EMF is associated with increased cancer risk.[109] Early studies suggested that residential exposure is associated with an increased risk of leukemia and brain tumors in children and that occupational exposure is associated with increased leukemia risk in adults.[110] However, two large case-control studies found no detectable effect of residential magnetic field exposure on the development of brain tumors in children.[111,112]

The ubiquitous nature of EMF exposure makes its measurement difficult.[113] In addition, measurement of quantitative exposure to EMF is generally based on assumptions regarding the relationship of EMFs to the electrical wiring configuration of the home, which may not always be correct.

Drugs

The mechanism of action of many antineoplastic drugs is to damage cellular DNA, thereby killing the cell. However, because these drugs currently cannot be targeted to act specifically on tumor cells, normal cells also are damaged. A late effect of this damage can be the development of a second malignancy. Second tumors most frequently involve hematopoietic and lymphatic systems, but solid tumors also can occur. Single or combinations of antineoplastic drugs that have been implicated in the cause of second malignancies are discussed in Chapter 26.

Other drugs that have been associated with malignancies include the following:

- Phenacetin, associated with lower urinary tract cancers

- The immunosuppressive drugs azathioprine and cyclosporine, the former associated with an increase in non-Hodgkin's lymphoma and squamous cell cancer of the skin, the latter with an increased risk of lymphoma[114]

- 8-methoxypsoralen combined with UVR, used for the treatment of psoriasis and vitiligo, associated with an increased risk of squamous cell cancer of the skin[115]

Exogenous hormones

Exogenous hormones are prescribed most commonly for women, either as a contraceptive or as replacement therapy following natural or induced menopause. They are also used for disorders of the menstrual cycle and to control abnormal uterine bleeding. Progestins have been used in obstetrics to prevent premature labor and in the management of threatened abortions.

Diethylstilbestrol, a synthetic estrogen used in the past for the treatment of threatened abortions, has been associated with vaginal and cervical cancers in the daughters of treated women.[116] This is the only known carcinogen to act transplacentally.[114] The cancers occur 10–30 years after treatment.

In contrast, use of combined oral contraceptives has been associated with a decreased risk of endometrial and ovarian cancer. Five years of usage is associated with a 55% reduction of endometrial cancer and a 40% reduction of ovarian cancer, compared with nonusers.[117]

An increased risk of liver cancer in young women also has been associated with oral contraceptive use; because this is a rare tumor, however, the absolute number of cases is low.[118] Oral contraceptive use has been associated with an increased risk of breast cancer in women diagnosed at young ages.[119,120] The effect, if any, of oral contraceptive use on breast cancer risk in women diagnosed when older is still unclear.

Estrogen replacement therapy (ERT) in postmenopausal women has been shown to increase the risk of endometrial cancer. However, when estrogen is combined with progestin, the increased risk is eliminated.[121] A small increase in breast cancer risk has been associated with long-term ERT. Key and Pike estimate that 5 years of ERT is associated with a 10% increase in breast cancer when users are compared with nonusers.[122] In contrast, there is evidence that ERT is associated with a reduced risk of large bowel cancer.[123]

Host Characteristics Influencing Cancer Susceptibility

Age

Although cancer can occur at any age, it is very much a disease of the elderly, with those over age 65 being ten times more likely than those under 65 to develop cancer.[124] Increasing cancer incidence is not, however, uniform with advancing age for all cancer sites, and the leading cause of cancer deaths changes with age (Table 5-7).[28] Leukemia is the leading cause of death for children under 15 years of age but is no longer among the five leading causes of cancer death after age 40; in contrast, lung cancer is rarely a cause of death under the age of 39 but is the leading cause of death in males over the age of 40 and in females over the age of 60.[28]

Because age is such an important determinant of cancer risk, it is important in epidemiological studies to make adjustments for age in the statistical analysis, unless comparison groups have the same age distribution.

Table 5-7 Mortality for the Five Leading Cancer Sites by Age, United States, 1995

MALES

All Ages	Under 19	20–39	40–59	60–79	80+
All Sites **281,611**	**All Sites** **1341**	**All Sites** **5683**	**All Sites** **46,081**	**All Sites** **164,794**	**All Sites** **63,705**
Lung and bronchus 91,800	Leukemia 465	Non-Hodgkin's lymphoma 800	Lung and bronchus 15,606	Lung and bronchus 60,721	Prostate 15,657
Prostate 34,475	Brain and ONS 300	Leukemia 686	Colon and rectum 4275	Prostate 17,773	Lung and bronchus 14,892
Colon and rectum 28,409	Bones and joints 104	Brain and ONS 643	Non-Hodgkin's lymphoma 2370	Colon and rectum 16,306	Colon and rectum 7416
Pancreas 12,826	Endocrine system 102	Lung and bronchus 563	Pancreas 2347	Pancreas 7715	Urinary bladder 2752
Non-Hodgkin's lymphoma 11,597	Non-Hodgkin's lymphoma 102	Colon and rectum 399	Brain and ONS 1949	Non-Hodgkin's lymphoma 6012	Leukemia 2725

FEMALES

All Ages	Under 19	20–39	40–59	60–79	80+
All Sites **256,844**	**All Sites** **934**	**All Sites** **6452**	**All Sites** **44,963**	**All Sites** **133,588**	**All Sites** **70,896**
Lung and bronchus 59,304	Leukemia 305	Breast 1764	Breast 12,202	Lung and bronchus 37,426	Colon and rectum 11,720
Breast 43,844	Brain and ONS 220	Uterine cervix 637	Lung and bronchus 9937	Breast 20,083	Lung and bronchus 11,463
Colon and rectum 29,237	Endocrine system 77	Leukemia 500	Colon and rectum 3297	Colon and rectum 13,855	Breast 9793
Pancreas 13,940	Bones and joints 70	Lung and bronchus 467	Ovary 2757	Pancreas 7595	Pancreas 4730
Ovary 13,342	Soft tissue 50	Brain and ONS 401	Uterine cervix 1720	Ovary 7237	Non-Hodgkin's lymphoma 3501

ONS = other nervous system.
Note: All sites exclude basal and squamous cell skin cancers and in situ carcinomas except urinary bladder.
Data from Vital Statistics of the United States, 1998.

Sex

The distributions of cancer types in each sex are shown in Figure 5-1. Prostate cancer is the leading site for men, followed by lung and bronchus and colorectal cancer. The leading site of cancer in women is breast cancer, followed by lung and bronchus and colorectal cancer.[28]

Genetic Predisposition

Epidemiological investigation of genetic predisposition to cancer is growing as developments in molecular biology make it possible to study genetic markers in large populations. The ongoing Human Genome Project[125] is almost certain to accelerate this work by the discovery of

Estimated New Cancer Cases*
10 Leading Sites by Sex, United States, 1999

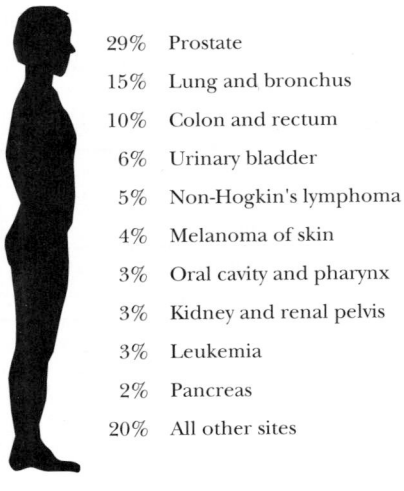

29%	Prostate
15%	Lung and bronchus
10%	Colon and rectum
6%	Urinary bladder
5%	Non-Hogkin's lymphoma
4%	Melanoma of skin
3%	Oral cavity and pharynx
3%	Kidney and renal pelvis
3%	Leukemia
2%	Pancreas
20%	All other sites

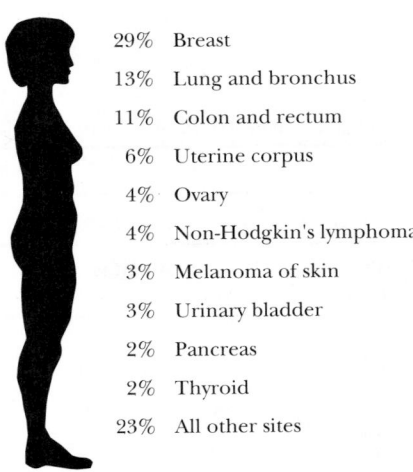

29%	Breast
13%	Lung and bronchus
11%	Colon and rectum
6%	Uterine corpus
4%	Ovary
4%	Non-Hodgkin's lymphoma
3%	Melanoma of skin
3%	Urinary bladder
2%	Pancreas
2%	Thyroid
23%	All other sites

Estimated Cancer Deaths*
10 Leading Sites by Sex, United States, 1999

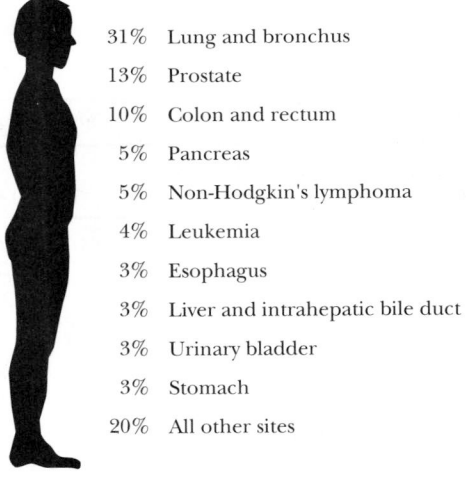

31%	Lung and bronchus
13%	Prostate
10%	Colon and rectum
5%	Pancreas
5%	Non-Hodgkin's lymphoma
4%	Leukemia
3%	Esophagus
3%	Liver and intrahepatic bile duct
3%	Urinary bladder
3%	Stomach
20%	All other sites

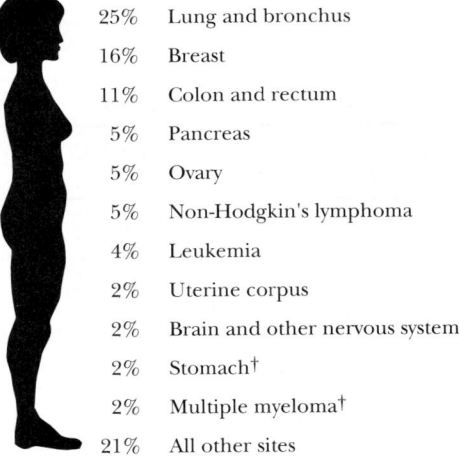

25%	Lung and bronchus
16%	Breast
11%	Colon and rectum
5%	Pancreas
5%	Ovary
5%	Non-Hodgkin's lymphoma
4%	Leukemia
2%	Uterine corpus
2%	Brain and other nervous system
2%	Stomach†
2%	Multiple myeloma†
21%	All other sites

*Excludes basal and squamous cell skin cancers and in situ carcinomas except urinary bladder.
†These two cancers both received a ranking of 10; they have the same number of deaths and contribute the same percentage.

Figure 5-1 Estimated cancer incidence and deaths by site and sex for 1999. (Data from Landis et al.[28])

new genes or gene markers associated with increased genetic predisposition for cancer.

Two genes have been discovered that are associated with susceptibility to breast cancer, *BRCA1*[126] and *BRCA2*.[127] The *BRCA1* gene is associated with increased susceptibility to both breast and ovarian cancer, whereas *BRCA2* is associated only with an increase in breast cancer. The genes are estimated to be involved in 5% of breast cancer cases and appear to be more strongly associated with breast cancer diagnosed at an early age. Much work remains to be done to further investigate the effects of these genes, including how other known risk factors for breast cancer modulate the risk conferred by the breast cancer genes.

Familial polyposis of the colon is an example of an autosomal dominant syndrome, where those with the syndrome develop colon cancer at a young age, in their thirties or forties, and have a high number of adenomatous polyps in the colon. The genetic steps required for the development of colon cancer have been studied in subjects with familial polyposis as well as in unaffected individuals who have adenomas or colon cancer. Vogelstein et al[128] reported that the steps include mutational activation of an oncogene, coupled with the loss of several genes that normally suppress tumorigenesis.[128] The mutation affecting individuals with familial polyposis, located on chromosome 5, represents one of these steps.

It has been observed for many years that cancer aggregates in some families. Such familial aggregation could be due to an inherited susceptibility or to common familial exposure(s), for example, diet. Most studies of this phenomenon have identified cancer familial aggregation for one cancer type, for example, colon cancer in relatives of individuals with colon cancer. However, Li and Fraumeni have identified an autosomal dominant syndrome from studying the kindred of children with rhabdomyosarcoma[129] in which the kindred have increased risk of developing cancers other than rhabdomyosarcoma. The genetic defect in these families may be a mutation in the suppressor gene *p53*.[130]

Some gene defects may increase a person's risk for cancer because the defects have an impact on carcinogen metabolism. It has been found that subjects who have slow acetylator status (i.e., the metabolism of aromatic amines by acetyltransferase is comparatively slow) are at higher risk for bladder cancer in certain occupational settings.[131] Acetylator status is genetically determined. Similarly, subjects who are slow metabolizers of the probe drug debrisoquine, due to a recessive Mendelian trait, appear to be at lower risk for lung cancer.[132]

Ethnicity and Race

Ethnicity and race can be important issues to assess in epidemiological research. However, several factors must be kept in mind when considering these points. First, ethnicity and race are both prone to misclassification. There is no accepted scientific definition for race. An individual may have grandparents from two or more ethnic or racial backgrounds and could be classified in many ways.

Second, ethnicity and race are often highly correlated with SES. Blacks, American Hispanics, and Native Americans generally have a lower SES than white non-Hispanics. Distinguishing an ethnic or racial effect from a socioeconomic effect may be difficult.

However, assessing biological or genetic differences, along with cultural differences, that may put an ethnic or racial group at increased or decreased risk of a specific cancer is important so that special attention can be given to high-risk groups. Racial or ethnic groups may also differ in attitudes to illness, care seeking, and prevention. It is important to identify such differences so that approaches can be tailored to each group to increase preventive health behavior. (See Chapter 7 for a detailed discussion on cultural diversity.)

Socioeconomic Factors

Socioeconomic status is usually assessed by data on income, education, or percent below the poverty level, and has been found to be associated with some cancers, independent of race.[133] Clearly, SES is not a cause of cancer but is a proxy measure for lifestyle characteristics that differ for cancer type and the particular situation under study. For example, cervical cancer has been associated with lower SES. In this case, SES may be a proxy for the number of partners the individual or her male spouse or partners have had; the larger the number, the greater the chance of the female partner's being HPV-positive. Alternatively, SES may be a proxy for Pap test frequency.

Socioeconomic status is now strongly associated with smoking prevalence, with low-income earners being more likely to smoke cigarettes.[134] Therefore, higher lung cancer rates in the lower SES group are likely to be due to this association.

Other Applications of Epidemiology in Oncology

Survival

Survival analysis is the calculation of the probability that an individual with a specific disease will be alive at a particular time point after diagnosis; 5 years is commonly used as this time point. For most cancers, the survival rate is greatly affected by the stage of cancer at diagnosis. For example, the 5-year survival rate for melanoma diagnosed as local disease is 87%; in comparison, the equivalent survival rate for metastatic melanoma is 11%. The histology of the cancer also affects survival time. For example, men with small-cell lung cancer have a 5-year survival rate of 4%, in comparison to other lung histologies, where the 5-year survival is 13%. Blacks have a lower survival rate for most cancer sites as compared with whites (Figure 5-2),[135] due in part to the distribution of stage at

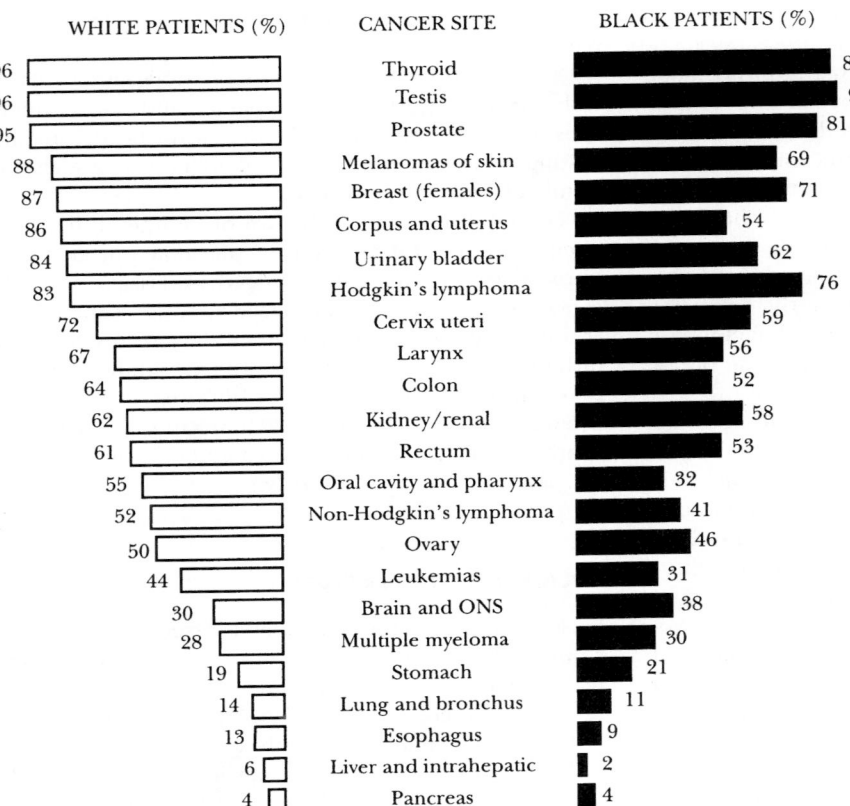

WHITE PATIENTS (%)	CANCER SITE	BLACK PATIENTS (%)
96	Thyroid	88
96	Testis	90
95	Prostate	81
88	Melanomas of skin	69
87	Breast (females)	71
86	Corpus and uterus	54
84	Urinary bladder	62
83	Hodgkin's lymphoma	76
72	Cervix uteri	59
67	Larynx	56
64	Colon	52
62	Kidney/renal	58
61	Rectum	53
55	Oral cavity and pharynx	32
52	Non-Hodgkin's lymphoma	41
50	Ovary	46
44	Leukemias	31
30	Brain and ONS	38
28	Multiple myeloma	30
19	Stomach	21
14	Lung and bronchus	11
13	Esophagus	9
6	Liver and intrahepatic	2
4	Pancreas	4

Figure 5-2 Five-year relative survival rates for white and black patients. Data from SEER Cancer Statistics Review 1973–1995, National Cancer Institute.[135]

diagnosis for the two groups. In turn, stage at diagnosis may be influenced by knowledge or attitudes about cancer (e.g., the importance of early diagnosis). Lack of access to care may also cause a delay in diagnosis.

Survival analysis is also used to assess the effectiveness of new treatment modalities for cancer, where survival following the new treatment is compared with survival following the standard treatment.

Cancer Control

Cancer control is an attempt to reduce cancer incidence, morbidity, and mortality through research on interventions and their impact in defined populations to the application of the research results.[136] In this definition, the term *cancer control* encompasses both cancer prevention and control. The term will be used similarly in the balance of this chapter. To help improve cancer control, Greenwald and Cullen[136] recommended the following phases of a model for cancer control research:

Phase I: Hypotheses are developed from basic biomedical research; for example, from the results of epidemiologic research.

Phase II: The necessary methods are developed; for example, the feasibility of an intervention is examined.

Phase III: The efficacy of the intervention is being determined in a group of subjects.

Phase IV: The impact of the intervention is tested using a sample representative of a large target population.

Phase V: An intervention that has been proved effective in phase IV is applied to a larger population, and the effect of the intervention in the population is evaluated.

In the Healthy People 2000 Study,[137] high-priority research needs for cancer control in the United States were identified. These needs reflect the numerous disciplines and areas of research involved in the field of cancer control. Some of the main areas of research involved in cancer control are discussed next.

Screening

Screening refers to the detection of disease by use of tests, examinations, or other procedures prior to the development of symptoms. Additional test(s) must follow a positive screening test to diagnose the disease. Epidemiology is an important aspect of developing and evaluating screening programs. During development, data must be available on the incidence, prevalence, distribution, and natural history of the disease. The distribution of the disease may influence the target population for screening and so improve the cost-benefit ratio of the screening program. Evaluation requires following an intervention (screened) population and a nonintervention (unscreened) population to assess the impact of screening on mortality. An implicit assumption regarding screening is that early detection will lead to a more favorable prognosis, because treatment begun early in the disease course will be more effective than later treatment. This has been shown to be the case for mammography and breast cancer mortality;[138] however, early detection of lung cancer using cytology or x-rays has proved to have no effect in reducing lung cancer mortality.[139]

Barriers to Participation in Screening Programs

General barriers to participation in screening programs include cost, availability, discrimination, time, and patient characteristics such as culture and knowledge. These factors can prevent individuals from benefiting from early detection of cancer. Studies show that females from minority groups or of low SES are less likely to seek mammography or Pap tests for screening.[140,141] In the study by Stein et al, specific barriers to receiving mammography included lack of knowledge, cost, embarrassment, and fear of radiation.[141] Interventions to increase screening compliance, especially among low-utilizer groups, must continue to be developed.

Behavioral change

Increasing public knowledge regarding a risk factor for cancer does not automatically result in a behavioral change within the at-risk group. Groups with differing characteristics, for example, demographics or risk behaviors, may require differing interventions to achieve behavioral change.

The Community Intervention Trial for Smoking Cessation (COMMIT) is an example of a program that incorporated several intervention strategies, the goal of which was to increase smoking cessation.[142] COMMIT incorporated many interventions that had been shown to be individually successful. In this trial, 22 communities were randomized to receive the intervention or to receive no intervention. The results of the trial showed that the multifaceted approach used in COMMIT had no effect on smoking cessation rates in heavy smokers (the primary target group) but had a significant effect in light to moderate smokers.[143] Such divergent results emphasize the importance of testing intervention approaches at the community level and measuring the effectiveness within different groups.

Government policy

National, state, and local governments have an impact on cancer control through legislation. Such legislation may directly affect cancer control. For example, in 1990 legislative action made screening mammography a covered benefit under Medicare.[144] Legislation may also indirectly affect cancer control. An example is recent legislation to mandate food labeling and to address the issue of health claims made by food companies.[145] This legislation will provide the public with information with which to select a healthier diet. Many state and local governments have restricted smoking in public places, effectively reducing the public's exposure to secondhand smoke.

Cancer control efforts are affected by the monies specifically appropriated by the government to cancer control in the National Institutes of Health budget. The government can influence advancement in this area by setting national goals for cancer control.

Application of Epidemiology to Nursing Practice

Nursing professionals play integral roles in all aspects of cancer prevention and cancer control. These involve the planning and implementation of cancer screening and educational programs, the design and coordination of cancer-related research projects, and clinical application of cancer-control treatments. These roles involve much more than data collection: Nurses function as principal investigators, as program directors, as educators, and as patient managers.

Within their roles in cancer prevention and control, nurses apply epidemiological data and research principles to three main phases of their work:[146]

1. *The development phase:* The epidemiological statistics of cancer incidence and mortality assist nursing professionals in identifying high-risk groups and individuals within their patient community. Changes in incidence and mortality rates over time, demographic characteristics of cancer patients, health-related behaviors, and environmental conditions associated with cancer promotion can be obtained through epidemiological data. These data can provide a basis for the development of research hypotheses and the theoretical foundation for program planning.

2. *The planning phases of research and prevention programs:* By using appropriate epidemiological research principles, nurses can design studies that are focused, valid, and ultimately important in the scientific and clinical communities. Program development and short- and long-term goals for cancer prevention and control can be based on epidemiological evidence from previous projects and new surveys that highlight changing cancer trends.

3. *The evaluation phase:* Via appropriate statistical methods, changes in cancer incidence and mortality rates, in stage of disease at diagnosis, in behavioral changes, and in survival time can be used to evaluate program effectiveness.

In all of these areas in which nurses are full participants, epidemiology supplies important information and the methodological foundation for the development, planning, and evaluation of cancer prevention and control programs.

References

1. Trichopoulos D, Lipworth L, Petridou E, et al: Epidemiology of Cancer, in DeVita VT, Hellman S, Rosenberg SA (eds): *Cancer Principles and Practice of Oncology*. Philadelphia, Lippincott-Raven, 1997, pp 231–257

2. Rothman KJ: *Modern Epidemiology*. Boston, Little, Brown, 1986, pp 51–76.

3. Hennekens CH, Buring JE: *Epidemiology in Medicine*. Boston, Little, Brown, 1987

4. Walter SD, Marrett LD, From L, et al: The association of cutaneous malignant melanoma with the use of sunbeds and sunlamps. *Am J Epidemiol* 131:232–243, 1990

5. Horowitz RL, Feinstein AR: Alternative analytic methods for case-control studies of estrogens and endometrial cancer. *N Engl J Med* 299:1089–1094, 1978

6. Dawber TR: *The Framingham Study: The Epidemiology of Atherosclerotic Disease*. Cambridge, MA, Harvard University Press, 1980

7. Postservice mortality among Vietnam veterans: The Centers for Disease Control Vietnam Experience Study. *JAMA* 257:790–795, 1987 ·

8. The Steering Committee of the Physicians' Health Study Research Group. Preliminary Report: Findings from the aspirin component of the ongoing physicians' health study. *N Engl J Med* 318:262–263, 1988

9. Hennekens CH, Buring JE, Manson JE, et al: Lack of effect of long-term supplementation with beta carotene on the incidence of malignant neoplasms and cardiovascular disease. *N Engl J Med* 334:1145–1149, 1996

10. Elwood M (ed): *Critical Appraisal of Epidemiological Studies and Clinical Trials*. Oxford, Oxford University Press, 1998

11. Kleinbaum DG, Kupper LL, Morgenstern H (eds): *Epidemiologic Research, Principles and Quantitative Methods*. New York, Reinhold, 1982

12. Selvin S (ed): *Statistical Analysis of Epidemiologic Data*. New York, Oxford University Press, 1991

13. Daniel WW (ed): *Biostatistics: A Foundation for Analysis in the Health Sciences*. New York, Wiley, 1991

14. Last JM, Wallace RB (eds): *Public Health and Preventive Medicine*. Norwalk, CT, Appleton and Lange, 1992

15. Lynch HT, Hirayama T (eds): *Genetic Epidemiology of Cancer*. Boca Raton, FL, CRC Press, 1989

16. Parkin DM, Pisani P, Lopez AD, et al: At least one in seven cases of cancer is caused by smoking: Global estimates for 1985. *Int J Cancer* 59:494–504, 1994

17. World Health Organization: *The World Health Report 1999*. Geneva, World Health Organization, 1999

18. U.S. Department of Health and Human Services: *The health benefits of smoking cessation: A report of the Surgeon General*. DHHS Publication no. (CDC) 90-8416. Washington, DC, U.S. Government Printing Office, 1990

19. Janerich DT, Thompson WD, Varela LR, et al: Lung cancer and exposure to tobacco smoke in the household. *N Engl J Med* 323:632–636, 1990

20. Fielding JE, Phenow KJ: Health effects of involuntary smoking. *N Engl J Med* 319:1452–1460, 1988

21. Ives JC, Buffler PA, Selwyn BJ, et al: Lung cancer mortality among women employed in high-risk industries and occupations in Harris County, Texas, 1977–1980. *Am J Epidemiol* 127:65–74, 1988

22. Blot WJ, Fraumeni JF: Passive smoking and lung cancer. *J Natl Cancer Inst* 77:993–1000, 1986

23. Blot WJ, Fraumeni JF: Passive smoking and cancer, in DeVita VT Jr, Hellman S, Rosenberg SA (eds): *Cancer Prevention*. Philadelphia, Lippincott, 1989, pp 1–10

24. Tredaniel J, Boffetta P, Saracci R, et al: Exposure to environmental tobacco smoke and risk of lung cancer: The epidemiological evidence. *Eur Respir J* 7:1877–1888, 1994

25. Rouse BA: Epidemiology of smokeless tobacco use: A national study. *NCI Monogr* 8:29–33, 1989

26. Mattson ME, Winn DM: Smokeless tobacco: Association with increased cancer risk. *NCI Monogr* 8:13–16, 1989

27. Parkin DM, Pisani P, Ferlay J: Global cancer statistics. *CA Cancer J Clin* 49:33–64, 1999

28. Landis SH, Murray T, Bolden S, et al: Cancer statistics, 1999. *CA Cancer J Clin* 49:8–31, 1999

29. Nelson DE, Giovino GA, Shopland DR, et al: Trends in cigarette smoking among US adolescents, 1974 through 1991. *JAMA* 85:34–40, 1995

30. Brown CC, Kessler LG: Projections of lung cancer mortality in the U.S. 1985–2025. *J Natl Cancer Inst* 80:43–51, 1988

31. Mahaney FX Jr: Lung cancer rates in white males leveling off. *J Natl Cancer Inst* 84:83–84, 1992

32. Novotny TE, Fiore MC, Hatziandreu EJ, et al: Trends in smoking by age and sex, United States, 1974–1987: The implications for disease impact. *Prev Med* 19:552–561, 1990

33. Doll R: Lifestyle: An overview. *Cancer Detect Prev* 14:589–594, 1990

34. Shatzkin A, et al: Diet and cancer: Future etiologic research. *Environ Health Perspect* 103:171–175, 1995 (suppl 8)

35. Bal DG, Foerster SB: Dietary strategies for cancer prevention. *Cancer* 72:1005–1010, 1993 (suppl 3)

36. Armstrong B, Doll R: Environmental factors and cancer incidence and mortality in different countries, with special reference to dietary practices. *Int J Cancer* 15:617–631, 1975

37. Willett WC (ed): *Nutritional Epidemiology*. New York, Oxford University Press, 1990

38. Ocke MC, Bueno de Mesquita HB, Feskens EJ, et al: Repeated measurements of vegetables, fruits, betacarotene and vitamins C and E in relation to lung cancer. The Zutphen study. *Am J Epidemiol* 145:358–365, 1997

39. Willett WC: Implications of total energy intake for epidemiologic analyses, in Willett WC (ed): *Nutritional Epidemiology*. New York, Oxford University Press, 1990, pp 245–271

40. Willett WC, Hunter DJ, Stampfer MJ, et al: Dietary fat and fiber in relation to risk of breast cancer: An 8-year follow-up. *JAMA* 268:2037–2044, 1992

41. Bueno de Mesquita HB, Smeets FW, Runia S, et al: The reproducibility of a food frequency questionnaire among control participants in a case-control study on cancer. *Nutr Cancer* 18:143–156, 1992

42. Hunter D: Biochemical indicators of dietary intake, in Willett W (ed): *Nutritional Epidemiology*. New York, Oxford University Press, 1990, pp 143–216

43. Wynder EL, Shigermatsu T: Environmental factors of cancer of the colon and rectum. *Cancer* 20:1520–1561, 1967

44. Whittemore AS, Wu-Williams AH, Lee M, et al: Diet, physical activity and colorectal cancer among Chinese in North America and China. *J Natl Cancer Inst* 82:915–926, 1990

45. Jain M, Cook GM, Davis FG, et al: A case-control study of diet and colorectal cancer. *Int J Cancer* 26:757–768, 1980

46. Lyon JL, Mahoney AW, West DW, et al: Energy intake: Its relationship to colon cancer risk. *J Natl Cancer Inst* 78:853–861, 1987

47. Potter JD, McMichael AJ: Diet and cancer of the colon and rectum: A case-control study. *J Natl Cancer Inst* 76:557–569, 1986

48. Trock B, Lanza E, Greenwald P: Dietary fiber, vegetables, and colon cancer: Critical review and meta-analyses of the epidemiologic evidence. *J Natl Cancer Inst* 82:650–651, 1990

49. Negri E, Franceschi S, Parpinel M, et al: Fiber intake and risk of colorectal cancer. *Cancer Epidemiol Biomarkers Prev* 7:667–671, 1998

50. Earnest DL, Sampliner RE, Roe DJ, et al: Progress report: The Arizona phase III study of the effect of wheat bran fiber on recurrence of adenomatous colon polyps. *Am J Med* 106:435–458, 1999

51. Slattery ML, Sorenson AW, Ford MH: Dietary calcium intake as a mitigating factor in colon cancer. *Am J Epidemiol* 128:504–514, 1988

52. Garland C, Shekell RB, Barrett-Connor E, et al: Dietary vitamin D and calcium, and risk of colorectal cancer: A 19-year prospective study in men. *Lancet* 1:307–309, 1985

53. Sorenson AW, Slattery ML, Ford MH: Calcium and colon cancer: A review. *Nutr Cancer* 11:135–145, 1988

54. Alberts DS, Einspahr J, Ritenbaugh C, et al: The effect of wheat bran fiber and calcium supplementation on rectal mucosal proliferation rates in patients with resected adenomatous colorectal polyps. *Cancer Epidemiol Biomarkers Prev* 6:161–169, 1997

55. Kune S, Kune GA, Watson LF: Case-control study of dietary etiological factors: The Melbourne Colorectal Cancer Study. *Nutr Cancer* 9:21–42, 1987

56. Newmark HL, Lipkin M: Calcium, vitamin D and colon cancer. *Cancer Res* 52:2067s–2070s, 1992

57. Howe GR, Hirohata T, Hislop TG, et al: Dietary factors and risk of breast cancer: Combined analysis of 12 case-control studies. *J Natl Cancer Inst* 82:561–569, 1990

58. Kushi L, Potter J, Drinkard C, et al: Dietary fat and risk of breast cancer according to hormone receptor status. *Cancer Epidemiol Biomarkers Prev* 4:9–11, 1995

59. Steinmetz KA, Potter JD: Vegetables, fruit and cancer: I. Epidemiology. *Cancer Causes Control* 2:325–327, 1991

60. Wattenberg LW: Inhibition of carcinogenesis by minor dietary constituents. *Cancer Res* 52:2085s–2091s, 1992

61. Moon TE, Micozzi MS: *Nutrition and Cancer Prevention: Investigating the Role of Micronutrients.* New York, Marcel Decker, 1989

62. Report of the Council of Scientific Affairs, Diet and Cancer: Where do matters stand? *Arch Intern Med* 153:50–56, 1993

63. *The Executive Summary in Diet and Health: Implications for Reducing Chronic Disease.* Washington, DC, National Academy Press, 3–22, 1989

64. Shike M: Diet and lifestyle in the prevention of colorectal cancer: An overview. *Am J Med* 106:11s–15s, 1999

65. Longnecker MP: Alcoholic beverage consumption in relation to risk of breast cancer: Meta-analysis and review. *Cancer Causes Control* 5:73–82, 1994

66. *Alcohol Drinking.* IARC Monographs on the Evaluation of Carcinogenic Risks of Chemicals to Humans, vol 44. Lyon, France, International Agency for Research on Cancer, 1988

67. Seitz HK, Simanowski UA: Alcohol and colorectal carcinogenesis, in Watson RR (ed): *Alcohol and Cancer.* Boca Raton, FL, CRC Press, 1992, pp 167–177

68. Spiegelhalder B, Eisenbrand G, Preussmann R: Contamination of beer with trace quantities of N-nitrosodimethylamine. *Food Cosmet Toxicol* 17:29–31, 1979

69. Longnecker MP, Newcomb PA, Mittendorf R, et al: Risk of breast cancer in relation to lifetime alcohol consumption. *J Natl Cancer Inst* 87:923–929, 1995

70. Byers T: Nutritional risk factors for breast cancer. *Cancer* 74:288–295, 1994

71. Colditz GA: A prospective assessment of moderate alcohol intake and major chronic diseases. *Ann Epidemiol* 1:167–177, 1990

72. Washburn RA, Montoye HJ: The assessment of physical activity by questionnaire. *Am J Epidemiol* 123:563–576, 1986

73. Gerber M, Corpet D: Energy balance and cancers. *Eur J Cancer Prev* 8:77–89, 1999

74. Slattery ML, Abd-Elghany N, Derber R, et al: Physical activity and colon cancer: A comparison of various indicators of physical activity to evaluate the association. *Epidemiology* 1:481–485, 1990

75. Gerhardsson De Verdier M, Steinbeck G, Hagman U, et al: Physical activity and colon cancer: A case-referent study in Stockholm. *Int J Cancer* 46:985–989, 1990

76. Albanes D, Blair A, Taylor PR: Physical activity and risk of cancer in NHANES 1 population. *Am J Public Health* 79:744–750, 1989

77. Kono S, Shinchi K, Ikeda N, et al: Physical activity, dietary habits and adenomatous polyps of the sigmoid colon: A study of self-defense officials in Japan. *J Clin Epidemiol* 44:1255–1261, 1991

78. Tavani A, Braga C, La Vecchia C, et al: Physical activity and the risk of cancers of the colon and rectum: an Italian case-control study. *Br J Cancer* 79:1912–1916, 1999

79. Bernstein L, Ross RK, Henderson B: Prospects for the primary prevention of breast cancer. *Am J Epidemiol* 135:142–152, 1992

80. Bernstein L, Henderson BE, Hanisch R, et al: Physical exercise and reduced risk of breast cancer in young women. *J Natl Cancer Inst* 86:1403–1408, 1994

81. Merzenick H, Boeing H, Wahrendorf J: Dietary fat and sports activity as determinants for age at menarche. *Am J Epidemiol* 138:217–224, 1993

82. McTiernan A, Ulrich C, Slate S, et al. Physical activity and cancer etiology: Associations and mechanisms. *Cancer Causes Control* 9:487–509, 1998

83. Kiningham RB: Physical activity and the primary prevention of cancer. *Prim Care* 25:515–536, 1998

84. Searle CE, Teale OJ: Occupational carcinogens, in Born GV, Cooper CS, Grover PL (eds): *Chemical Carcinogenesis and Mutagenesis 1: Handbook of Experimental Pharmacology,* vol 94/1. Berlin, Springer-Verlag, 1990, pp 103–151

85. Tomatis L (ed): Pollution, in *Cancer: Causes, Occurrence and Control.* Lyon, France, International Agency for Research on Cancer Scientific Publications, 1990, pp 229–239

86. Tseng WP: Effects and dose-response relationships of skin cancer and blackfoot disease with arsenic. *Environ Health Perspect* 19:109–119, 1977

87. Morton W, Starr G, Pohl D, et al: Skin cancer and water arsenic in Lane County, Oregon. *Cancer* 37:2523–2532, 1976

88. Morris RD, Audet A, Angelillo IF, et al: Chlorination, chlorination by-products and cancer: A meta analysis. *Am J Public Health* 82:955–963, 1992

89. McFarland M, Kaye J: Chlorofluorocarbons and ozone. *Photochem Photobiol* 55:911–929, 1992

90. National Institutes of Health Consensus Development Conference Statement: *Sunlight, Ultraviolet Radiation, and the Skin.* Bethesda, MD, U.S. Department of Health and Human Services, Public Health Service, National Institutes of Health, Office of Medical Applications of Research, 1989

91. Pike M: The prevention of breast, endometrial and ovarian cancer, in Fortner JG, Rhoads JE (eds): *Accomplishments in Cancer Research.* Philadelphia, Lippincott, 1989, pp 327–356

92. Ley C, Bauer HM, Reingold A, et al: Determinants of genital human papillomavirus infection in young women. *J Natl Cancer Inst* 83:997–1003, 1991

93. Zur Hausen H: Viruses in human cancers. *Science* 254: 1167–1173, 1991

94. Henderson BE: Establishment of an association between a virus and a human cancer. *J Natl Cancer Inst* 81:320–321, 1989

95. Schiffman MH, Bauer HM, Hoover RN, et al: Epidemiologic evidence showing that human papillomavirus infection causes most cervical intraepithelial neoplasia. *J Natl Cancer Inst* 85:958–964, 1993

96. Munoz N: Is Helicobacter pylori a cause of gastric cancer? An appraisal of the seroepidemiological evidence. *Epidemiol Biomarkers Prev* 3:445–451, 1994

97. IARC Monograph on the Evaluation of Carcinogenic Risks to Humans, vol 61. Schistosomes, liver flukes and *Helicobacter pylori.* Lyon, France, International Agency for Research on Cancer, 1994

98. Eurogast Study Group: An international association between *Helicobacter pylori* infection and gastric cancer. *Lancet* 342:1359–1362, 1993

99. Gentile JM: Schistosome-related cancers: A possible role for genotoxins. *Environ Mutagen* 7:775–785, 1985

100. Henderson BE, Ross RK, Pike MC: Toward the primary prevention of cancer. *Science* 254:1131–1138, 1991

101. Shigematsu I, Kagan A (eds): *Cancer in Atomic Bomb Survivors.* Japanese Cancer Association, GANN Monograph on Cancer Research 32. New York, Plenum Press, 1986

102. BEIR III, Committee on the Biological Effects of Ionizing Radiation: *The Effects on Populations of Exposure to Low Levels of Ionizing Radiation.* Washington, DC, National Academy Press, 1980

103. Lubin JH, Boice JD, Edling C, et al: Lung cancer in radon-exposed miners and estimation of risk from indoor exposure. *J Natl Cancer Inst* 87:817–826, 1995

104. *Exposure of the U.S. Population to Occupational Radiation.* NCRP report No. 101. Bethesda, MD, National Council on Radiation Protection and Measurements, 1989

105. Strickland PT, Vitasa BC, West SK, et al: Quantitative carcinogenesis in man: Solar ultraviolet B dose dependence of skin cancer in Maryland watermen. *J Natl Cancer Inst* 81: 1910–1913, 1989

106. Grodstein F, Speizer FE, Hunter DJ: A prospective study of incident squamous cell carcinoma of the skin in the Nurses' Health Study. *J Natl Cancer Inst* 87:1061–1066, 1995

107. Armstrong BK, English DR: Epidemiologic studies, in Balch CM, Houghton AN, Milton GW, et al (eds): *Cutaneous Melanoma* (ed 2). Philadelphia, Lippincott, 1992, pp 12–20

108. Adey WR: Joint actions of environmental nonionizing electromagnetic fields and chemical pollution in cancer promotion. *Environ Health Perspect* 86:297–305, 1990

109. Savitz DA, Pearce NE, Poole C: Methodological issues in the epidemiology of electromagnetic fields and cancer. *Epidemiol Rev* 131:763–773, 1990

110. London SJ, Bowman JD, Sobel E, et al: Exposure to magnetic fields among electrical workers in relationship to leukemia risk in Los Angeles County. *Am J Indust Med* 26: 47–60, 1994

111. Preston-Martin S, Navidi W, Thomas D, et al: Los Angeles study of residential magnetic fields and childhood brain tumors. *Am J Epidemiol* 143:105–119, 1996

112. Gurney JG, Mueller BA, Davis S, et al: Childhood brain tumor occurrence in relation to residential power line configurations, electric heating sources, and electric appliance use. *Am J Epidemiol* 143:120–128, 1996

113. Poole C: Invited commentary: Evolution of epidemiologic evidence on magnetic fields and childhood cancers. *Am J Epidemiol* 143:120–128, 1996

114. Tomatis L: Drugs and exogenous sex hormones, in *Cancer: Causes, Occurrence and Control.* Lyon, France, International Association for Research on Cancer Scientific Publications, 1990, pp 148–154

115. Stern RS, Thibodeau LA, Kleinerman RA, et al: Risk of cutaneous carcinoma in patients treated with oral methoxsalen photochemotherapy for psoriasis. *N Engl J Med* 300: 809–813, 1979

116. Herbst AL, Ulfelder H, Poskanzer DC: Adenocarcinoma of the vagina: Association of maternal stilbestrol therapy with tumor appearance in young women. *N Engl J Med* 284: 878–881, 1971

117. The WHO collaborative study of neoplasia and steroid contraceptives: Endometrial cancer and combined oral contraceptives. *Int J Epidemiol* 17:263–269, 1988

118. Henderson BE, Preston-Martin S, Edmonson HA, et al: Hepatocellular carcinoma and oral contraceptives. *Br J Cancer* 48:437–440, 1983

119. Briton LA, Daling JR, Liff JM, et al: Oral contraceptives and breast cancer risk among younger women. *J Natl Cancer Inst* 87:827–835, 1995

120. Rosenberg L, Palmer JR, Rao RS, et al: Case-control study of oral contraceptive use and risk of breast cancer. *Am J Epidemiol* 143:25–37, 1996

121. Lobo RO: Benefits and risks of estrogen replacement therapy. *Am J Obstet Gynecol* 173:982–989, 1995

122. Key TJA, Pike MC: The role of oestrogens and progestagens in the epidemiology and prevention of breast cancer. *Eur J Cancer Clin Oncol* 24:29–43, 1988

123. Newcomb PA, Storer BE: Postmenopausal hormone use and risk of large-bowel cancer. *J Natl Cancer Inst* 87: 1067–1071, 1995

124. Ries LAG, Hankey BF, Edwards BK (eds): *Cancer Statistics Review 1973–1987.* U.S. Department of Health and Human Services, NIH publication No. 90–2789, Bethesda, MD, 1991

125. The Human Genome Project: Implications for human genetics. *Am J Hum Genet* 49:687–691, 1991

126. Futreal PA, Liu Q, Shattuck-Eidens DE, et al: *BRCA1* mutations in primary breast and ovarian carcinomas. *Science* 266:120–122, 1994

127. Wooster R, Neuhausen SL, Mangion J, et al: Localization of a breast cancer susceptibility gene *BRCA2,* to chromosome 13q12-13. *Science* 265:2088–2090, 1994

128. Vogelstein B, Fearon ER, Hamilton SR, et al: Genetic alterations during colorectal-tumor development. *N Engl J Med* 319:525–532, 1988

129. Li FP, Fraumeni JF Jr: Rhabdomyosarcoma in children:

Epidemiologic study and identification of a familial cancer syndrome. *J Natl Cancer Inst* 43:1365–1373, 1969

130. Li FP, Fraumeni JF Jr, Mulvihill JJ, et al: A cancer family syndrome in twenty-four kindreds. *Cancer Res* 48:5358–5362, 1988

131. Cartwright RA, Glashan RW, Rogers HJ, et al: Role of N-acetyltransferase phenotypes in bladder carcinogenesis: A pharmacogenetic epidemiological approach to bladder cancer. *Lancet* 2:842–845, 1982

132. Ayesh R, Idle JR, Ritchie JC, et al: Metabolic oxidation phenotypes as markers for susceptibility to lung cancer. *Nature* 312:169–172, 1984

133. Baquet CR, Horm JW, Gibbs T, et al: Socioeconomic factors and cancer incidence among blacks and whites. *J Natl Cancer Inst* 83:551–557, 1991

134. Centers for Disease Control, Center for Chronic Disease Prevention and Health Promotion, Office on Smoking and Health: *Tobacco Use in 1986: Methods and Basic Tabulations from Adult Use of Tobacco Survey.* DHHS publication No. OM-90-2004. Rockville, MD, Centers for Disease Control, 1990

135. National Cancer Institute: *Seer Cancer Statistics Review 1973–1995.* Bethesda, MD, National Cancer Institute, 1999

136. Greenwald P, Cullen JW: The new emphasis in cancer control. *J Natl Cancer Inst* 74:543–551, 1985

137. *Healthy People 2000: National Health Promotion and Disease Prevention Objectives.* DHHS publication No. (PHS) 91-50212. Washington, DC, U.S. Government Printing Office, 1991

138. Feig SA: Follow-up studies of the Health Insurance Plan Study and the Breast Cancer Detection Demonstration Project Screening Trials in the U.S.A. *Recent Results Cancer Res* 119:39–52, 1988

139. Fontana RS, Sanderson DR, Woolner LB, et al: Screening for lung cancer: A critique of the Mayo Lung Project. *Cancer* 67:1155–1164, 1991

140. Peters RK, Moraye BB, Thomas D: Barriers to screening for cancer of the cervix. *Prev Med* 18:133–146, 1989

141. Stein JA, Fox SA, Murata PJ: The influence of ethnicity, socioeconomic status, and psychological barriers on use of mammography. *J Health Soc Behav* 32:101–113, 1991

142. COMMIT Research Group: Community Intervention Trial for Smoking Cessation (COMMIT): Summary of design and intervention. *J Natl Cancer Inst* 83:1620–1628, 1991

143. Community Intervention Trial for Smoking Cessation (COMMIT): I. Cohort results from a four-year community intervention. *Am J Public Health* 85:183–192, 1995

144. Oakar MR: Legislative effect of the 102nd Congress: Cancer prevention, detection, treatment, and research. *Cancer* 69:154–156, 1992

145. McNamara S: The brave new world of FDA nutrition regulation: Some thoughts about current trends and long-term effects. *Crit Rev Food Sci Nutr* 34:215–221, 1994

146. Rempusheski VF: Ask an expert. *Appl Nurs Res* 4:96–98, 1991

Prevention, Detection, and Diagnosis

CHAPTER 6

Factors Affecting Health Behavior

Jayne I. Fernsler, DSN, RN, AOCN
Mary Ann Miller, PhD, RN

Introduction

Promotion of positive health behavior has become a national initiative. The knowledge that unhealthful personal lifestyle choices account for a large proportion of both morbidity and mortality in the United States and recognition of the staggering subsequent cost of these choices to society have been the impetus for major policy and program development.

The health behavior initiative is an important component of cancer care. Personal choices with regard to diet, tobacco use, alcohol consumption, and sun exposure can have a powerful impact on cancer prevention. In addition, personal decisions about learning and performing routine self-examinations, participating in cancer screening activities, and seeking appropriate help when cancer signs and symptoms are noted are paramount to the early detection and potential cure of cancer. Also, behavior with regard to following a recommended treatment regimen and maintaining a healthful lifestyle while experiencing cancer may enhance both quantity and quality of life. Consequently, individual health behavior is a concern for health care professionals who interact with people at any phase of the cancer continuum.

The purpose of this chapter is to define "health behavior" and related terms, to identify national initiatives, and to describe factors that influence health behavior. Selected models and theories of health behavior are explained and their applications in research on cancer care are described. The implications of health behavior theory and research for nursing practice are discussed in the chapter's conclusion.

National Initiatives

The evolving body of knowledge about the association between personal behavior and cancer control has spurred activity in both the public and the private sectors. Major initiatives have included work by the National Cancer Institute (NCI), the American Cancer Society (ACS),[1] and the U.S. Department of Health and Human Services (DHHS).[2] The NCI's goal to reduce cancer mortality by 50% by the year 2000, the ACS's goal to reduce cancer mortality by 50% and cancer incidence by 25% by the year 2015, and the DHHS objectives for health promotion and cancer control all focus on influencing our health behavior. The behaviors of minority populations and people who are disadvantaged or at high risk for cancer are also a major target of these efforts.

Definitions

Health Behavior

Generally, *behavior* involves something that we do or refrain from doing, consciously or unconsciously, volun-

tarily or involuntarily.[3] A number of definitions of health behavior have been advanced by experts in the field. Gochman includes in his definition personal attributes, such as beliefs and values; personality characteristics; and behavior patterns related to health. All of these are influenced by a variety of family, societal, and cultural factors.

Health behavior encompasses actions taken by persons who believe they are healthy, and who have not experienced any signs or symptoms of illness, in order to remain disease free.[4] According to this definition, health behavior is confined to preventive actions. In 1979 Harris and Guten introduced the broader term *health protective behavior* to include both preventive and health-promoting activities. They define it as "any behavior performed by a person, regardless of his or her perceived or actual health status, in order to protect, promote or maintain his or her health, whether or not such behavior is objectively effective toward that end."[5,p.18]

Pender believes that a mixed model of promotion and protection may be the rule for most adults' health behaviors, while the promotion model is more likely to drive the health behavior of children for whom illness and injury are future events that lack immediate motivation potential.[6]

Illness Behavior

Kasl and Cobb define *illness behavior* as "any activity, undertaken by a person who feels ill, to define the state of his health and to discover a suitable remedy."[4,p.246] Thus, illness behavior refers to the perceptions and actions that result after we recognize bodily signs or symptoms, feel the need for advice, decide whether to seek it, and choose an adviser, whether it be relatives, friends, or lay or professional health care practitioners. We undertake illness behaviors to clarify the meaning of certain signs and symptoms. This may mean waiting to see if the symptoms will go away without therapy.

Sick-Role Behavior

Sick-role behavior is the activity taken by individuals who believe themselves (or whom others believe) to be ill in order to get well. It usually involves a range of dependent behaviors, includes accepting treatment, and leads to some neglect of one's usual duties.[4]

The distinctions made among these various types of health behaviors and their determinants should not be minimized.[3] Although their apparently common relationship to health unites them, more research is needed to confirm underlying commonalities among the categories and to uncover the variety of determinants to which each category is specifically related.[3]

Models and Theories of Health Behavior

A number of models and theories have been developed to address the complexities of health behavior and its determinants. An early review[7] of fourteen such models found the following general classes of explanatory variables:

- Attitudes toward health care benefits and health care quality

- Perception of symptoms and beliefs about susceptibility to illness

- Accessibility of health services,

- Knowledge about the disease/condition

- Social support characteristics

- Demographic variables, particularly social status, income, and education

A later review[8] of a similar body of work identified eight common primary determinants of behavior and behavior change: intention, environmental constraints, ability, anticipated outcomes, norms, self-standards, emotion, and self-efficacy.

The four models used most frequently are Social Cognitive Theory/Social Learning Theory, Health Belief Model, Self-Efficacy, and Theory of Reasoned Action.[9] Health care practitioners may be confused by the inconsistent definitions for similar variables across models and the lack of a single unifying theory on which the models are based. Therefore, practitioners and researchers often choose relevant components from several models in order to explain specific health behaviors and to suggest approaches to encourage behavior change. Predominant theories and models and their application to cancer care are presented in the following sections.

Social Cognitive Theory

Bandura's Social Cognitive Theory currently represents one of the most formally developed theories of behavior.[10] It provides an umbrella framework for analyzing health behavior in terms of a continuous, mutual interaction among cognitive, behavioral, and environmental determinants (reciprocal determinism). According to Bandura, adoptive behavior is determined primarily by stimulus inducements, anticipated satisfactions, observed benefits, experienced functional value, perceived risks, self-evaluative derivatives, and various social barriers and economic constraints.[11]

The environment is the source of social support that provides cues for reinforcement of behavior. The environment also provides the social and physical situation within which we must function. In so doing, it provides incentives and barriers for the performance of behavior (expectancies). We have the potential for self-control over our actions. In order to accomplish control, we must have a certain amount of knowledge and skill. We can anticipate certain events and outcomes and respond to them based on our past experiences or on the experiences of others whom we have observed. If all other things are equal, we

typically choose to perform an activity that maximizes a positive outcome or minimizes a negative one (principle of maximization).[10]

Sources of influence

Bandura views human behavior in terms of three interdependent sources of influence: antecedent determinants, consequent outcomes, and cognitive determinants.[11] Antecedent determinants stem from objects or events that precede behavior change. Cognitive factors partly determine which external events will be observed, how they will be perceived, and how information they convey will be organized for future use. In order to function effectively, we must anticipate the probable consequences of these different events and courses of action. We then regulate our behavior on the basis of such predictive antecedent events.

The more we believe that influences of past events remain viable, and the more severe the outcome we expect (e.g., their perceived susceptibility to ill effects due to a particular behavior), the stronger our anticipatory reaction will be. The failure of anticipated risks to materialize reinforces the expectation that the subsequent behaviors prevented negative consequences. Thus, most behavior is maintained by anticipated rather than by immediate consequences.[11]

Rewarding experiences are repeatedly associated with expressions of the interest and approval of others (their social support) and unrewarding experiences with their disapproval. These social reactions themselves become influential predictors of consequences and become incentives. Thus, the impact of rewards or punishments can be explained in terms of motivation. By representing foreseeable outcomes symbolically, we can convert future consequences into current motivations of behavior.[11]

Efficacy and outcome expectations

Bandura proposes that behavioral changes are generated from the common mechanisms of personal efficacy and outcome expectations.[11] An *outcome expectation* is defined as a personal belief that a given behavior will lead to certain outcomes. An *efficacy expectation* is the conviction that we can successfully execute a specific behavior required to produce a specific outcome.

Outcome and efficacy expectations are differentiated because we can believe that a certain course of action will produce certain outcomes and still question whether we can perform the required action. Both outcome and efficacy expectations reflect our beliefs about our capabilities and behavior-outcome links. Although self-efficacy and outcome expectations are conceptually distinct, the types of outcomes that we anticipate are strongly influenced by efficacy expectations, the most important prerequisite for behavior change.[10]

The strength of our belief in our own effectiveness determines whether we will even try to cope with difficult situations. Bandura speculates that perceived efficacy forms a mediating link between knowledge and behavior. Efficacy expectations determine how much effort we will expend and how long we will persist in the face of barriers and aversive experiences. In general, stronger efficacy expectations will produce more active and sustained efforts.

Perceptions of efficacy are usually acquired through direct environmental interaction or through social experiences such as personal experience, vicarious experience, verbal persuasion, and physiologic state.[11] The most dependable and powerful source of efficacy expectations is personal experience. Vicarious experience, that is, live or symbolic modeling or seeing what happens to others who perform activities with certain consequences, also contributes to efficacy expectations. Of the numerous cues that influence behavior, none is more common than the actions of others. Verbal persuasion also contributes to efficacy expectations, but the efficacy expectations that it generates are likely to be weak and of short duration. Lastly, our own physiological state or emotional arousal (anxiety, agitation, fatigue) in threatening situations contributes to efficacy expectations.[11]

Efficacy expectations vary greatly, depending on the particular task that confronts us. Individuals with low self-efficacy about a task may concentrate on personal deficiencies rather than thinking about accomplishing the task successfully. This can impede successful performance of the task.[12]

Application to cancer care

In the application of Social Cognitive Theory to analysis of health behavior, a major objective is determining what beliefs a person has developed about targeted health problems or behaviors. Taking the theoretical application one step further, we might conclude that when strong beliefs about health risks are combined with a strong sense of efficacy for avoiding them as well as a belief in the value of the avoidance behaviors, healthier outcomes can result.

The influence of self-efficacy has been studied in relation to general cancer prevention practices,[13] dietary cancer prevention practices,[14,15] smoking cessation,[16,17] testicular self-examination (TSE),[18] breast self-examination (BSE) and mammography screening,[19–24] compliance with screening for fecal occult blood,[25] skin cancer detection and prevention,[26,27] participation in prostate cancer screening,[28] and decision making regarding treatment.[29] Generally, a strong belief in our ability to carry out a required activity powerfully influences our decision to engage in healthy behavior.

Summary

Social Cognitive Theory as an umbrella framework addresses many of the constructs that are discussed in the models and theories that follow. Along with the Health Belief Model (HBM) and the Theory of Reasoned Action, it contains constructs that can be viewed as belonging to the larger family of expectancy-value theories. Outcome value has been a traditional component of these theories. While the HBM explicitly sets forth outcome benefits/barriers as a variable, Bandura suggests the construct of outcome value by emphasizing the role of rewarding outcomes in determining behavior.[11] The Theory of Reasoned Action includes evaluation of outcomes as a specific determinant of attitude toward behavior. This is another variable that is made explicit in the HBM. There is already a body of research to support the utility of both the concept of self-efficacy, as explained by Bandura,[11] and the variables of the HBM in studies of preventive health behavior.[30]

Another influential variable, social support, is alluded to in the reciprocal determinism of social cognitive theory, the environmental influence proposed by the HBM, and the variable of social norms in the Theory of Reasoned Action. Social support may be especially important for those of us who find it difficult to sustain a high level of motivation when pursuing a stressful course of action, such as trying to abstain from smoking. A high level of motivation is often contingent on the presence of "personal assets" or resources, including the presence of "important others" for emotional support.

Early Social Cognitive Theory also provided the foundation for current behavioral theories that include the variable of personal control. These include Locus of Control and Health Locus of Control. Control also appears as a variable in Attribution Theory.

Health Belief Model

The Health Belief Model was developed in the 1950s by Rosenstock and Hochbaum to explain preventive health behavior using psychosocial variables and psychological theories of decision making.[31] It evolved from a central tenet of Lewin's theory of goal setting: that behavior depends on the value that we attach to a given outcome and our expectation that a particular action will result in that outcome.[32] Translated to health behavior, the value becomes the desire to avoid illness or to get well, and the expectancy is the belief that a particular personal action will prevent or lessen the threat of illness. We will typically choose the behavior that we think will produce the maximum number of good outcomes and the minimum number of bad ones (principle of maximization).[10]

The HBM is based on the assumption that our subjective perception of the environment determines behavior.[33] Variables tested in current applications of the model are susceptibility, severity, benefits, barriers, and self-efficacy (Table 6-1). Research has shown that of the first four variables, perceived barriers is the most powerful single predictor of behavior, although perceived susceptibility and benefits are strong also. Perceived severity is the weakest predictor but appears to be strongly related to sick-role behaviors.[34]

The stimulus or cue to action may be internal, such

Table 6-1 Health Belief Model

Variable	Definition
Perceived susceptibility	Perception of vulnerability to a condition
Perceived severity	Perception of the seriousness of the consequences of developing a condition

Together these two variables constitute a perceived **Threat** and provide the individual with a psychological readiness to take action.

Benefits	Effectiveness of the action in reducing threat
Barriers	Psychological and other costs or negative aspects associated with the proposed action
Cue to action	Stimulus to behave in a certain manner
Self-efficacy	Conviction that one can successfully behave in the manner required to achieve a specific outcome
Modifying variables	
Demographic	Age, gender, etc.
Structural	Access
Attitudinal	Satisfaction
Interactional	Patient/practitioner relationship
Enabling	Social pressure

Data from Rosenstock,[33] Strecher and Rosenstock.[34]

as the perception of a symptom, or external, such as interaction with others or exposure to information sources such as billboards, TV, or radio.[31] Many researchers have found health care providers' recommendations to be a primary cue to action regarding cancer prevention and early detection.[35–38] The true role of such stimuli has been difficult to study because they may be only barely perceptible in our consciousness. If perceived susceptibility and severity are high, relatively insignificant stimuli may result in behavior change, but stronger stimuli may be required to effect change in the face of low perceptions of susceptibility and severity.[34]

A 1992 meta-analysis of sixteen studies that included all HBM variables revealed relatively weak relationships between these variables and health behaviors.[30] However, as long as research indicates that the dimensions of the HBM interact systematically in predicting health behavior, the model will continue to guide attempts to understand why we do what we do with regard to our health. The HBM has been identified as the most frequently cited model in research on health behavior and health education.[9]

It is believed that the addition of self-efficacy to the HBM has increased its explanatory power.[34] *Efficacy expectations*, or the belief that we can successfully execute the

particular behavior required to produce the desired outcome, are crucial in lifestyle behaviors requiring long-term changes, such as smoking. They affect how much effort we put into a given task and what levels of performance are attained. Repetition builds self-efficacy, which affects task persistence and endurance and thus promotes behavior change.

The HBM has been applied to all preventive health actions, illness behaviors, and sick-role behaviors. Underlying the ability of the model to explain health behavior is the assumption that we can accept the possibility that we may have a serious illness in the complete absence of symptoms. This may provide the impetus for many decisions to seek screening for health-related reasons. For example, the failure to believe in the possibility of asymptomatic illness may help to explain less-than-desirable responses to cancer screening programs.[34]

The HBM is based on the premise that health is a valued goal for most of us. As such, it can only account for as much of the variation in our health-related behaviors as can be explained by our attitudes and beliefs. People who value health are motivated to protect it.[39] Other forces also influence behavior. There is a habitual/addictive component to some behavior (e.g., smoking), and, in some cases, economic or environmental factors may prevent us from taking a preferred mode of action (e.g., residing in a city with high air pollution).[34,40]

Another limitation of the HBM is its inability to be quantified beyond an ordinal scale. The model's ability to measure beliefs specific to a given condition is an advantage as well as a limitation. Because there is no one generic instrument with proven reliability and validity that can be used by all researchers, a multitude of measures exist, each with different behaviors as targets.

Application to cancer care

The Health Belief Model has been used extensively as a framework to identify individuals who engage in behaviors relevant to primary and secondary cancer prevention. The HBM has been used to describe health beliefs of individuals who practice BSE,[22–24,41–51] skin cancer prevention,[39,52,53] and cancer risk reduction and early detection.[54,55] In addition, health beliefs have been studied in relation to participation in a diet intervention program,[56] mammographic screening for breast cancer,[22,35,37,41,45,46,49,57–62] Pap smear screening for cervical cancer,[63,64] and screening for prostate cancer.[65]

In general, health motivation and perceived barriers have been strong predictors of our intentions and behaviors where cancer prevention and screening activities are concerned. Perceived susceptibility has been associated positively with BSE, having a mammogram, and having a Pap test when perceived benefits are high. The relationship between beliefs about severity of a potential illness and health behavior has not been clearly established. However, the influence of health beliefs alone on our behaviors with regard to cancer prevention and screening activities is equivocal and may be modified by other factors. Consequently, several researchers have used the HBM in conjunction with other concepts and theories in an attempt to predict health behaviors.

Theory of Reasoned Action

Ajzen and Fishbein's Theory of Reasoned Action,[66] like the HBM, is a value-expectancy theory. It has been used to predict our intention to perform a behavior in a specific situation. The model is based on the assumption that intention to perform (or not to perform) a specific behavior is the immediate determinant of that behavior. For intention to predict behavior, the behavior must be under voluntary control, and the intention must be assessed close to the time of the behavior. The longer the time interval between statement of intention and the behavior, the more likely it is that events will occur that may change the intention.

Two factors contribute to the strength of the intention to perform a specific behavior: attitude toward the behavior and the influence of the social environment or general subjective norms on the behavior (Table 6-2). Attitude is determined by our belief that a specific outcome will occur if we perform the behavior (similar to outcome expectation) and by an evaluation of the outcome (cost/benefit analysis). Attitude toward the behavior (mammography screening) rather than attitude toward the target of the behavior (breast cancer) is a much better predictor of the behavior. The influence of norms stems from our feelings about what significant others believe we should do, weighted by our motivation to comply with their wishes (social pressure to perform). The model also emphasizes normative influences that might affect intention for *any* reason, health-related or otherwise, thus adding a cultural component to the prediction of behavior.[67] In addition, variables other than attitude or subjective norm can influence intention and behavior indirectly. For example, personality traits and demographic characteristics can affect intention and behavior through their influence on the attitudinal or subjective normative components.

When the Theory of Reasoned Action is used to explain health behavior, the effectiveness of interventions for change is greatly determined by the health professional's ability to identify major concerns and barriers that we will confront in the process. Through open-ended questions and interviews, data are generated that ultimately identify beliefs that can be changed. Though this method can systematically identify issues most salient to our desire to perform a specific behavior, it is possible that not all important variables will be discovered in the interview process. The Theory of Reasoned Action also involves a measurement technique that can be complicated, cumbersome, and time-consuming. Though well developed theoretically, the body of data on which to judge the predictive validity of this model is still evolving.[67]

Application to cancer care

The Theory of Reasoned Action has been used in research on perceptions about cancer detection in general;[68] BSE;[69] mammography screening;[62,70] women's beliefs, attitudes, and behaviors regarding Pap tests;[69,71] skin cancer protective behaviors;[27] and participation in chemotherapy clinical trials.[72] In a study of medically underserved African-American women, Burnett et al[69] supported the propositions of the Theory of Reasoned Action in relation to breast and cervical cancer screening and found no relationship between intentions and demographic variables.

Theory of Planned Behavior

The Theory of Reasoned Action was designed to apply to behaviors that are under complete volitional control. Its ability to predict behavior decreases when the behavior in question is one over which there is only limited control, such as access to health services. The Theory of Planned Behavior takes this phenomenon into account by broadening the Theory of Reasoned Action to include a dimension of perceived control determined by two variables: control beliefs and perceived power.[67] Perceived control reflects past experience as well as perceived ease or difficulty in achieving a behavioral goal (self-efficacy). It focuses on our control over factors that may influence a successful behavioral outcome, such as information, skills, willpower, time, and opportunity. Perceived control can affect behavior in several ways. It may motivate us to decide to behave in a certain way; it may directly affect our behavior to the extent that it realistically represents actual control over the behavior; or it may be used to predict behavior. The addition of this construct to the Theory of Reasoned Action has found support as a direct predictor of both intention and behavior.[73,74]

Application to cancer care

The Theory of Planned Behavior has been used to support research in the area of colorectal cancer. In these studies, the variable of perceived control not only enhanced prediction of intention to complete screening in

---

Table 6-2 Theory of Reasoned Action

I. *Behavior* is determined by *behavioral intention.*
II. Strength of *behavioral intention* depends on *attitude toward the behavior* and influence of the social environment or social norms.
   A. Attitude toward the behavior is determined by:
     1. Belief that a specific outcome will occur if the behavior is performed
     2. Evaluation of the outcome as positive or negative
   B. Social norm is determined by:
     1. The person's belief about what significant others think should be done
     2. The person's motivation to do what others wish

Data from Ajzen and Fishbein.[66]

low- and high-risk groups, but it also had a direct effect on screening behavior in the high-risk group.[75] Perceived behavioral control also was shown to be significantly related to BSE frequency,[76] adherence to a program of BSE or TSE in young adults,[77] cigarette smoking intention in teenage women,[78] and exercise during colorectal cancer treatment.[79]

Social Support

The field of relationships that we have with others in daily living has been called our *social* or *personal network.* Our social network comprises people on whom we can rely, who let us know that we are cared about, valued, and loved. Conceptual definitions of social support abound.[80,81] Kahn proposes that the components of supportive transactions include positive affect of one person toward another, endorsement (affirmation) of another's behavior or views, and giving some type of aid.[82] Affective support has been shown to have a consistent and strong relationship with good health and well-being.[83]

The precise mechanism of action linking social support and health is not known. Researchers have advanced a number of hypotheses,[80] among them that (1) social ties may provide a buffer against the effects of high stress; (2) social ties may increase the development of coping strategies, thereby facilitating adaptation to change; and (3) a perceived sense of support from others may lead to a person's more generalized sense of control and responsibility.

Social support, particularly that provided by a patient's family, has a positive influence on compliance with medical advice. The patient's family remains a largely untapped means for reminding, assisting, encouraging, and reinforcing therapeutic directions.

The lay (nonprofessional) network controls the flow of clients to practitioners. By conditioning accurate expectations about the type of help given by health professionals, the lay network can decrease the likelihood that patients will drop out of treatment. It can speed or delay use of professional services by involving patients in long or short periods of informal referral. It can contradict or concur with professionals' diagnoses of problems and improve or interfere with the patients' ability to follow the prescribed regimen.

Application to cancer care

The theory of social support has been used widely in the study of smoking behavior.[84,85] The support and smoking behavior of family members and close associates correlate with the smoking behavior of the subjects studied. Those subjects whose close social contacts were nonsmokers or former smokers were likely to be nonsmokers or successful abstainers. Social support also has been found to be influential in women's participation in screenings for breast cancer[86–91] and cervical cancer,[90,92] and in patients' coping with cancer treatment.[93,94]

Locus of Control/Health Locus of Control

Locus of control

When Rotter applied early social learning principles to clinical psychology in 1954, he developed the concepts of internal and external locus of control.[95] These concepts refer to the degree to which we perceive events in our lives as being consequences of our actions and thereby controllable (internal control), or as being unrelated to our own behavior and therefore beyond our control (external control). Rotter proposed that people who were more internally controlled were more likely to self-initiate change. Those who were externally controlled were more likely to be influenced by others.

Health locus of control

In 1978 Wallston and Wallston[96] developed a new construct, the *health locus of control,* a generalized expectation about whether health is controllable by our behavior or by external forces. The Wallstons considered this construct to be useful in health-related research because our sense of control often varies according to our particular health-related experiences. Still, the Wallstons' model does retain the concepts of internal and external locus of control; however, in their model the external locus is represented by *chance* (health determined by fate) and *powerful others* (health determined by externals such as health professionals).

The conviction that outcomes (good health) are determined by our actions can have an effect on behavior. If we consider health to be within our control but feel we lack the skills needed to carry out the behaviors that will result in good health (low self-efficacy) we might approach those activities with a sense of futility.[12]

Beliefs about internal locus of control, in combination with a high value placed on health, should predict our likelihood to engage in preventive health behaviors. However, if we hold such beliefs and do not value our health highly, there would seem to be no theoretical reason for us to perform health-relevant behaviors. Therefore, if these constructs are used to study health behavior, the interaction between health value and health locus of control must be examined. The fact that many investigators have not done this may explain why beliefs about health locus of control have not been linked consistently to the performance of a variety of preventive health behaviors.[97]

Oberle found that, generally, nursing studies related to locus of control have yielded little useful information for nursing practice.[98] However, disease-specific locus of control scales, including one for cancer, may provide more helpful data.[99,100]

Application to cancer care

The influence of beliefs about health locus of control has been examined in relation to BSE,[19,101,102] skin cancer prevention,[39] and adjustment to cancer.[103,104] In a study of elderly Hispanic women,[101] BSE was practiced more frequently by those who perceived an internal locus of control. Internal locus of control has also been associated with a more positive adjustment to cancer.[103]

Attribution Theory

Attribution Theory involves the explanations we use to make sense of our world, and the behavioral and emotional consequences of those explanations. According to the theory, we engage spontaneously in attributional activities, often asking "Why?" or "Why me?". Our search for answers is connected to the broader concept of personal or cognitive control.[105]

Ascribing causes can be especially relevant when our health is threatened, when symptoms or tensions are heightened, or when a catastrophic event takes place. If we can assign a cause, we can manage the situation more effectively and can plan future action.

Attributions can be used to predict behavior, feelings, and expectancies, and can serve to maintain self-esteem and reduce anxiety.[105] Attributions may be conscious and deliberate, or below the level of conscious awareness. There are four dimensions of causal attribution, and each is associated with certain consequences (Table 6-3).

Attributions have significant implications for our subsequent thoughts, feelings, and actions. Lewis and Daltroy speculate that there is an optimal set of attributions that best predict our health behaviors.[105] Attributions of success are usually related to stable, global, and internal causes. Therefore, the goal of the health professional is to offer support by attributing failure (e.g., failure to stop smoking) to unstable, specific, uncontrollable, and external causes. We can then move forward, recognizing that the desired behavior was not achievable at that time, that personal deficiency did not result in our failure, and that we can try again in the future. By obtaining information about our attributions, health professionals can begin to understand the motivations behind our behaviors and can appropriately tailor health interventions.[105] Research in the area of causal attributions is limited and does not reveal whether the dimensions of the attributions can be manipulated, in what manner, or by what method.

Application to cancer care

The influence of beliefs about attributions of the cause of cancer has been examined in relation to patients' adjustment behaviors.[106-111] Berckman and Austin found negative relationships between causal attributions and aspects of adjustment.[107] Although no clear association has been consistently validated,[108,110] Dirksen found that cancer survivors who searched for meaning as to why their cancer occurred reappraised their life situation positively.[111] Another study showed that making a causal attribution had no significant effect on women's adjustment to breast cancer, though attributing the cancer to an

Table 6-3 Attribution Theory

Dimensions of Attributions (Causes)	Consequences
Locus of Cause	
Internal to the person (*Example:* innate ability)	Can be associated with low self-esteem or depression or taking responsibility for one's treatment
External to the person (*Example:* chance, luck, environmental pollutants)	Can be associated with poorer long-term morbidity or better coping and adjustment
Controllability	
Controllable (*Example:* level of effort)	Usually results in increased effort, enhanced performance
Uncontrollable (*Example:* innate ability, task difficulty)	Offers little hope of influencing future outcomes
Stability	
Stable (*Example:* personal ability)	
Unstable (*Example:* attention span, mood)	Both stability and instability are important determinants of goal expectations and can be used to predict cognitive and motivational deficits
Globality	
Global (*Example:* innate intelligence)	Affects a wide variety of outcomes; can result in extensive performance deficits
Specific (*Example:* test anxiety)	Affects a limited set of outcomes in a given situation

Data from Lewis and Daltroy.[105]

uncontrollable cause was associated with information-seeking behavior.[109]

Transtheoretical Model of Change

The Transtheoretical Model of Change, developed by Prochaska and DiClemente,[112] is based on the assumption that a continuum of readiness to change applies to behavior. There are six stages in this process:

1. Precontemplation: Not considering change in the next 6 months and resistant to outside pressures to change
2. Contemplation: Starting to think about changing behavior within the next 6 months; more open to feedback and information; ambivalent about costs/benefits—can remain in this stage for years
3. Preparation: Taking some steps toward action and planning to change within the next month
4. Action: Initiating the new behavior and maintaining it for a minimal time

5. Maintenance: Sustaining the change for more than 6 months
6. Termination: Having no temptation and maximum self-efficacy[112]

The process of behavioral change is not linear and allows for cyclical relapses to an earlier point along the way to adoption of the new behavior.

The model also includes ten basic processes of change, overt and covert cognitive and behavioral strategies that we use to move through the six stages of the change continuum:

1. Consciousness-raising: Increased awareness and more accurate information processing
2. Self-liberation: Firm commitment to change
3. Social liberation: Notice of social changes that support personal changes
4. Self-reevaluation: Affective and cognitive assessment of self
5. Environmental reevaluation: Effect of personal behavior on our physical and social environment
6. Counter-conditioning: Substituting more positive behaviors for negative ones
7. Stimulus control: Restructuring our environment so that problem stimuli are less likely to occur
8. Contingency management: Reinforcement of positive behaviors and punishment of negative ones
9. Dramatic relief: Experiencing and releasing feelings
10. Helping relationships: Involving openness, caring, trust, empathy, and support for the behavior change

In general, cognitive, affective, and evaluative processes such as consciousness-raising and dramatic relief are used most frequently by individuals in the early stages of behavioral change, and helping relationships and contingency management in the later stages.[112,113] It is also possible that fewer change processes may be needed to progress to long-term maintenance, as in the infrequent behavior of a yearly mammogram.[112] Thus, interventions for behavioral change can emphasize processes that promote advancement to the next behavioral stage.[114]

In addition to the stage and process variables, the model highlights the concept of self-efficacy and elements of decision making. Decisional balance is achieved by a comparison of the perceived advantages of the new behavior (pros) with the perceived disadvantages of the behavior (cons). This variable has been operationalized in the Decisional Balance Scale.[115] The stages of behavioral adoption have been found to correspond to differences in the pros and cons separately and to the more general measure of decisional balance.[116] The model hypothesizes that individuals in the later stages of behavior adoption should have a decisional balance favoring the positive (pro) aspects of the target behavior; in the precontemplation stage, a balance favoring the negative (con) aspects of the behavior; and in the contemplation stage, a decisional balance somewhere between the two.

While the Transtheoretical Model does not focus directly on a particular psychological variable, its constructs draw heavily on those proposed by the Health Belief Model, the Theory of Reasoned Action, and Social Cognitive Theory, among others, and are integrated in a different and perhaps more comprehensive manner.

Application to cancer care

The Transtheoretical Model of Change has been applied extensively to smoking behavior.[117–120] Work by Rakowski et al has demonstrated the usefulness of stages of adoption and decisional balance as guides for designing specific interventions to increase mammography rates[116,121–123] and Pap testing.[123] Smoking cessation and mammography screening interventions that have been tailored to individuals' stages of behavioral change have been more successful than more traditional programs.[120,124]

Combined Theoretical Approaches to Health Behavior

In an attempt to enhance the explanatory power of the models described previously, many researchers have combined models or have elected to use variables from different models. To explain behavior related to cancer screening, the Health Belief Model has been combined with Social Cognitive Theory constructs;[22,24,42,125–128] Theory of Reasoned Action/Planned Behavior and Social Cognitive Theory;[23,62,129–133] Locus of Control;[39,49,64,134–136] the Transtheoretical Model of Change;[57] Transtheoretical Model of Change and Theory of Reasoned Action;[137] and Social Cognitive Theory, Transtheoretical Model of Change, and Social Support Theory.[138] When self-efficacy was added to the Theory of Planned Behavior to predict BSE or TSE, perceived control was a better predictor than self-efficacy.[77] The addition of facilitating conditions and perceived normative belief[139] or habit[140] to the constructs of the Theory of Reasoned Action increased the variance accounted for by the theory components alone in adherence to BSE in older women[139] and mammography participation.[140]

Related Factors

Sociodemographics

The influence of sociodemographics on health behavior is variable. In a large sample of men, Tingen et al found that participation in prostate cancer screening was significantly related to sociodemographic variables.[65] Significant predictors of participation included age (40–49 years), race (white), education (high school or higher), income ($9,601–$25,020 rather than below that amount), and marital status (married).

Knowledge and educational level

Because knowledge is often related to educational level, both factors are discussed in this section. Being knowledgeable about a specific cancer or a cancer detection or screening measure has been found to relate positively to health behaviors such as skin protective behavior,[26,36,39] dietary behavior,[15] having a mammogram,[126,141,142] practicing BSE,[21,24,38,130] having a Pap test,[92] and participating in prostate cancer screening.[28,65,143] Likewise, educational level has been found to relate positively to having a mammogram,[141] practicing BSE,[38,130] and having a Pap test.[144]

However, being knowledgeable or having a high level of education is not consistently associated with positive health behaviors.[43,52,64] Other factors, such as fear, may override the positive influence of knowledge on behavior. Still, fear messages can have a positive effect on a person whose fear level about a disease is not already overwhelming, and who believes that certain health behaviors will be helpful. If fear messages are used, they are likely to be most influential if they are given in the initial attempt to change behavior and if they contain advice that can be quickly and easily followed.[12]

Socioeconomic status

Educational level is sometimes used as an indicator of socioeconomic status (SES), another factor that has a strong association with health behavior. People of low SES have been found to be less likely than people of high SES to participate in screening for colorectal cancer,[145] cervical cancer,[64] breast cancer,[89,142] and prostate cancer.[65] However, the influence of SES on screening practices tends to diminish when factors such as cultural barriers and lack of social support are addressed.[146]

Age

Like educational level and SES, age is an important influence on health behavior. For example, perceived barriers to performing BSE vary among different age groups of women, though frequency of BSE has been shown to be no different.[43] Age also modifies the influence of health beliefs. Older women tend to believe that they no longer require Pap tests because they are no longer sexually active or bearing children. Also, they tend to have fewer close associates, such as spouses and friends, who would encourage them to have the test. In one study, age was significantly predictive of mammography screening, with women age 60 to 64 more likely to have a mammogram than younger or older women.[62] Others have found that younger women were more likely to be screened.[126,147] After an educational intervention, older adults (over age 65) have been reported to be significantly less compliant than younger people (ages 20–35) with skin protective measures.[148] In another study, however, older adults were found to be more compliant.[134] Confidence in our ability to carry out a task appears to be influential regardless of age.

Sociocultural Factors

Differences in cancer incidence, mortality, and survival rates among people of different sociocultural backgrounds have stimulated researchers to examine the health behaviors of these groups. The influence of sociocultural factors, exclusive of SES and education, is not evaluated easily. Many cancer risk factors, such as genetic predisposition, lifestyle, and environmental exposure, are socioculturally determined, as are our values and beliefs about cancer prevention and screening. For example, fatalism, a belief that death is inevitable when cancer is present, has been identified as a relevant barrier to screening behavior in blacks[149–151] and Hispanics.[152,153] (See Chapter 7 for a detailed discussion on cultural diversity).

Most research relating cultural and ethnic factors to health behaviors has been conducted with white, black, and Hispanic populations. McCoy et al found that compared to white men, black and Hispanic men were twice as likely to have never had a digital rectal examination for prostate cancer.[154] In a worksite study on skin cancer prevention, blacks and Hispanics reported that they would be less likely than whites to seek care for suspicious skin lesions.[155]

Perceived barriers to cancer prevention and cancer screening behaviors vary according to cultural orientation. Black women have been shown to have misbeliefs about breast cancer and BSE;[22] however, there is no clear evidence that they utilize mammography[61] or practice BSE less frequently than white women.[41,48] Embarrassment and shame associated with physical examinations repeatedly has surfaced as a deterrent for Hispanic women.[152,153,156] Acculturation and education positively influence the responses of Mexican American and other Hispanic/Latino women to cancer risk factors.[157,158] Language barriers and lack of trust in Western health care may influence cancer screening behaviors of Chinese women living in the United States. Hoeman et al found that early detection was not a clear concept for these women, as they did not believe themselves to be susceptible to diseases that are not a health priority in China.[159] Likewise, Egyptians may be doubtful of the benefits of cancer prevention and early detection practices;[160] they also believe that a diagnosis of cancer is God's will.[160,161]

Family ethnicity can be a powerful influence on health behavior. Some ethnic groups, such as Hispanics,[158] Chinese,[159] and Egyptians,[161] place great value on family involvement in decisions and care.

Women in the childbearing years are likely to access the health care system for obstetrical and child care services and may be more likely than older women to hear health-related messages directly from providers. These messages can influence health behaviors positively.[36,159] For example, in one study parents who received information frequently from health care providers practiced more sun protective measures for themselves and their children.[36]

Social support, social roles, and social stigma all influence our health behaviors with regard to cancer prevention, detection, and treatment. Social support has been found to have a positive influence on smoking cessation efforts.[84,85] Social roles, on the other hand, may influence health behavior either positively or negatively. Being married has been positively associated with women's having a mammogram,[68] practicing monthly BSE and having a yearly professional breast examination,[130] and getting a Pap smear.[162] Also, having support from a spouse has been associated with women's participation in a diet intervention program for breast cancer.[56] As alluded to previously, women in childbearing and child-rearing roles who may have more contact with the health care system are more likely than older women to practice BSE and participate in cancer-screening programs. Conversely, older women who are no longer sexually active often perceive that they do not need Pap tests.

Cancer is discussed relatively freely in the dominant culture of the United States. Media coverage of the diagnosis and treatment of cancer in both President[163] and Mrs. Reagan[164,165] had a positive influence on the information-seeking and cancer-screening behaviors of the public. Although health care professionals may not always agree with celebrities' treatment choices, such public disclosures do bring issues surrounding cancer prevention and screening to the public's attention.[166]

Institutional Factors

The organization of the health care delivery system influences people's health behavior. Services organized around care for the sick often include barriers for those people who seek prevention or screening services. Social priorities and, to some extent, the political system determine the allocation of resources to various health services. Cost reduction and follow-up reminders are two interventions that have been positively identified to increase women's participation in cervical screening[167] as well as breast cancer screening[168] in the United States. Current availability of at least some level of Medicaid reimbursement for Pap tests in most states and mammography in many states[169] should reduce the cost barrier for many disadvantaged women.

Health care providers influence people's health behavior in a number of ways. Individuals have reported that a health care provider's recommendation or reminder to have a cancer screening test was important in their decision to do so.[35–38,60,142,170–172] In a sample of elderly women, frequency of the practice of BSE was associated with having been taught BSE by health care providers.[38] Thus, it is unfortunate that the majority of nurses in one study rarely or only occasionally taught women about mammography.[173] Prompt, courteous, and competent examinations by health care providers have been associated with women's intention to engage in breast and cervical cancer screening.[69] Use of coaching and client navigators recently has been found to be effective in improving compliance in college women's practice of BSE[174] and in recruiting men's participation in prostate cancer screening.[65]

Implications for Nursing Practice

People's health behaviors are influenced by multiple interacting factors. Theories and models continue to evolve to identify and describe the interaction of these variables and to predict and prescribe health behavior. Nevertheless, human behavior is not totally predictable, and the totality of its complexity has not yet been described.

Health professionals may not recognize the powerful influence they can exert on patients' health behaviors. Nurses can apply some of the empirically validated concepts and propositions of health behavior by incorporating them into the nursing process. The models provide guidelines for assessment, nursing diagnosis, intervention, and evaluation. For example, health beliefs, self-efficacy, intentions, stages of readiness, and beliefs about control can be incorporated into all stages of the nursing process.

Considering the association between health behavior and demographics, nurses need to examine the latter. A thorough assessment of people's cultural beliefs and practices and the use of developmental and communication principles[175] are crucial to nurses' success in positively influencing people's health behaviors.

References

1. Blue Ribbon Advisory Group on Community Cancer Control: *American Cancer Society: Society-Wide Recommendations for Community Cancer Control. Report to the National Board of Directors.* Atlanta, American Cancer Society, 1997
2. U.S. Department of Health and Human Services: *Healthy People 2000, Midcourse Review and 1995 Revisions.* Sudbury, MA, Jones and Bartlett, 1996
3. Gochman D: Health behavior: Plural perspectives, in Gochman D (ed): *Health Behavior: Emerging Research Perspectives.* New York, Plenum, 1988, pp 3–17
4. Kasl S, Cobb S: Health behavior, illness behavior, and sick role behavior: I. Health and illness behavior. *Arch Environ Health* 12:246–266, 1966
5. Harris D, Guten S: Health protective behavior: An exploratory study. *J Health Soc Behav* 20:17–29, 1979
6. Pender, N: *Health Promotion in Nursing Practice* (ed 3). Stamford, CT, Appleton & Lange, 1996
7. Cummings K, Becker M, Maile M: Bringing the models together: An empirical approach to combining variables used to explain health actions. *J Behav Med* 3:123–145, 1980
8. Fishbein M, Bandura A, Triandis HC, et al: *Factors Influencing Behavior and Behavior Change: Final Report of Theorists' Workshop on AIDS-Related Behaviors.* Washington, DC, National Institute of Mental Health, 1991
9. Glanz K, Lewis FM, Rimer BK: Linking theory, research, and practice, in Glanz K, Lewis FM, Rimer BK (eds): *Health Behavior and Health Education* (ed 2). San Francisco, Jossey-Bass, 1997, pp 19–35

10. Baranowski T, Perry CL, Parcel GS: How individuals, environments, health behavior interact: Social cognitive theory, in Glanz K, Lewis FM, Rimer BK (eds): *Health Behavior and Health Education* (ed 2). San Francisco, Jossey-Bass, 1997, pp 153–178

11. Bandura A: *Social Foundations of Thought and Action: A Social Cognitive Theory.* Englewood Cliffs, NJ, Prentice-Hall, 1986

12. Becker M: Theoretical models of adherence and strategies for improving adherence, in Shumaker S, Schron E, Ockene J (eds): *The Handbook of Health Behavior Change.* New York, Springer-Verlag, 1990, pp 5–43

13. Lev EL: Bandura's theory of self-efficacy: Applications to oncology. *Sch Inquiry Nurs Pract* 11:21–37, 1997

14. Hertog JK, Finnegan JR, Rooney B, et al: Self-efficacy as a target population segmentation strategy in a diet and cancer risk reduction campaign. *Health Commun* 5:21–40, 1993

15. Harnack L, Block G, Subar A, et al: Association of cancer prevention-related nutrition knowledge, beliefs, and attitudes to cancer prevention dietary behavior. *J Am Diet Assoc* 97:957–965, 1997

16. Utz S, Shuster GF, Merwin E, et al: A community-based smoking-cessation program: Self-care behaviors and success. *Public Health Nurs* 11:291–299, 1994

17. Kowalski SD: Self-esteem and self-efficacy as predictors of success in smoking cessation. *J Holistic Nurs* 15:128–142, 1997

18. Brubaker RG, Fowler C: Encouraging college males to perform testicular self-examination: Evaluation of a persuasive message based on the revised Theory of Reasoned Action. *J Appl Soc Psychol* 20:1411–1422, 1990

19. Wehrwein TC, Eddy ME: Behaviors of midlife women. *J Holistic Nurs* 11:223–236, 1993

20. Chalmers KI, Luker KA: Breast self-care practices in women with primary relatives with breast cancer. *J Adv Nurs* 23:1212–1220, 1996

21. Adderley-Kelly B, Green PM: Breast cancer education, self-efficacy, and screening in older African American women. *J Natl Black Nurses Assoc* 9:45–57, 1997

22. Duke SS, Gordon-Sosby K, Reynolds KD, et al: A study of breast cancer detection practices and beliefs in black women attending public health clinics. *Health Educ Res* 9:331–342, 1994

23. Savage SA, Clarke VA: Factors associated with screening mammography and breast self-examination intentions. *Health Educ Res* 11:409–421, 1996

24. Persson K, Ek A, Svensson G: Factors affecting women to practise breast self-examination. *Scand J Caring Sci* 11:224–231, 1997

25. Myers RE, Ross E, Jepson C, et al: Modeling adherence to colorectal cancer screening. *Prev Med* 23:142–151, 1994

26. Friedman LC, Bruce S, Webb JA: Skin self-examination in a population at increased risk for skin cancer. *Am J Prev Med* 9:359–364, 1993

27. Keesling B, Friedman HS: Interventions to prevent skin cancer: Experimental evaluation of informational and fear appeals. *Psychol Health* 10:477–490, 1995

28. Boehm S, Coleman-Burns P, Schlenk EA, et al: Prostate cancer in African American men: Increasing knowledge and self-efficacy. *J Community Health Nurs* 12:161–169, 1995

29. Davison BJ, Degner LF: Empowerment of men newly diagnosed with prostate cancer. *Cancer Nurs* 20:187–196, 1996

30. Harrison JA, Mullen PD, Green LW: A meta-analysis of studies of the Health Belief Model with adults. *Health Educ Res* 7:107–116, 1992

31. Maiman L, Becker M: The Health Belief Model: Origins and correlates in psychological theory, in Becker M (ed): *The Health Belief Model and Personal Health Behavior.* Thorofare, NJ, Slack, 1974, pp 9–26

32. Lewin K: *A Dynamic Theory of Personality: Selected Papers.* New York, McGraw-Hill, 1935

33. Rosenstock I: Historical origins of the Health Belief Model, in Becker M (ed): *The Health Belief Model and Personal Health Behavior.* Thorofare, NJ, Slack, 1974, pp 1–8

34. Strecher VJ, Rosenstock I: The Health Belief Model, in Glanz K, Lewis F, Rimer B (eds): *Health Behavior and Health Education* (ed 2). San Francisco, Jossey-Bass, 1997, pp 41–59

35. Aiken LS, West SG, Woodward CK, et al: Health beliefs and compliance with mammography screening recommendations in asymptomatic women. *Health Psychol* 13:122–129, 1994

36. Buller DB, Callister MA, Reichert T: Skin cancer prevention by parents of young children: Health information sources, skin cancer knowledge, and sun-protection practices. *Oncol Nurs Forum* 22:1559–1566, 1995

37. Johnson JD, Meischke H: Factors associated with adoption of mammography screening: Results of a cross-sectional and longitudinal study. *J Womens Health* 3:97–105, 1994

38. Morrison C: Determining crucial correlates of breast self-examination in older women with low incomes. *Oncol Nurs Forum* 23:83–93, 1996

39. Carmel S, Shani E, Rosenberg L: Skin cancer protective behaviors among the elderly: Explaining their response to a health education program using the Health Belief Model. *Educ Gerontol* 22:651–668, 1996

40. Womeodu RJ, Bailey JE: Barriers to cancer screening. *Med Clin North Am* 80:115–133, 1996

41. Douglass M, Bartolucci A, Waterbor J, et al: Breast cancer early detection: Differences between African American and white women's health beliefs and detection practices. *Oncol Nurs Forum* 22:835–837, 1995

42. Lu ZJ: Variables associated with breast self-examination among Chinese women. *Cancer Nurs* 18:29–34, 1995

43. Sensiba ME, Stewart DS: Relationship of perceived barriers to breast self-examination in women of varying ages and levels of education. *Oncol Nurs Forum* 22:1265–1268, 1995

44. Sortet JP, Banks SR: Health beliefs of rural Appalachian women and the practice of breast self-examination. *Cancer Nurs* 20:231–235, 1997

45. Choudhry UK, Srivastava R, Fitch MI: Breast cancer detection practices of South Asian women: Knowledge, attitudes, and beliefs. *Oncol Nurs Forum* 25:1693–1701, 1998

46. Champion V, Menon U: Predicting mammography and breast self-examination in African American women. *Cancer Nurs* 20:315–322, 1997

47. Millar-Murray G: The effects of emotion on breast self-examination: Another look at the Health Belief Model. *Soc Behav Pers* 25:223–232, 1997

48. Foxall MJ, Barron CR, Houfek J: Ethnic differences in breast self-examination practice and health beliefs. *J Adv Nurs* 27:419–428, 1998

49. Erwin DO, Spatz TS, Stotts RC, et al: Increasing mammography and breast self-examination in African American women using the Witness Project Model. *J Cancer Educ* 11:210–215, 1996

50. Champion VL, Scott CR: Reliability and validity of breast cancer screening belief scales in African American women. *Nurs Res* 46:331–337, 1997

51. Barron CR, Houfek JF, Foxall MJ: Coping style, health beliefs, and breast self-examination. *Issues Ment Health Nurs* 18:331–350, 1997

52. Marlenga B: The health beliefs and skin cancer prevention practices of Wisconsin dairy farmers. *Oncol Nurs Forum* 22: 681–686, 1995

53. Gerbert B, Johnston K, Bleecker T, et al: Attitudes about skin cancer prevention: A qualitative study. *J Cancer Educ* 11:96–101, 1996

54. Sennott-Miller L: Using theory to plan appropriate interventions: Cancer prevention for older Hispanic and non-Hispanic white women. *J Adv Nurs* 20:809–814, 1994

55. Johnson JD: Factors distinguishing regular readers of breast cancer information in magazines. *Women Health* 26: 7–27, 1997

56. Naslund GK, Fredrikson M, Holm LE: Psychosocial factors associated with participation and nonparticipation in a diet intervention program. *J Psychosoc Oncol* 10:93–107, 1993

57. Champion VL: Beliefs about breast cancer and mammography by behavioral stage. *Oncol Nurs Forum* 21:1009–1014, 1994

58. Fischera SD, Frank DI: The Health Belief Model as a predictor of mammography screening. *Health Values* 18:3–9, 1994

59. Hyman RB, Baker S, Ephraim R, et al: Health Belief Model variables as predictors of screening mammography utilization. *J Behav Med* 17:391–406, 1994

60. Glanz K, Resch N, Lerman C, et al: Black-white differences in factors influencing mammography use among employed female health maintenance organization members. *Ethn Health* 1:207–220, 1996

61. Thomas LR, Fox SA, Leake BG, et al: The effects of health beliefs on screening mammography utilization among a diverse sample of older women. *Women Health* 24:77–94, 1996

62. Crane LA, Kaplan CP, Bastini R, et al: Determinants of adherence among health department patients referred for a mammogram. *Women Health* 24:43–64, 1996

63. Burak LJ, Myer M: Using the Health Belief Model to examine and predict college women's cervical cancer screening beliefs and behavior. *Health Care Women Int* 18:251–262, 1997

64. Beckmann CA, Beckmann CR, Lipscomb GH, et al: Pap smear screening: Determinants of patient compliance. *J Womens Health* 4:663–668, 1995

65. Tingen MS, Weinrich SP, Heydt DD, et al: Perceived benefits: A predictor of participation in prostate cancer screening. *Cancer Nurs* 21:349–357, 1998

66. Ajzen I, Fishbein M: *Understanding Attitudes and Predicting Social Behavior.* Englewood Cliffs, NJ, Prentice-Hall, 1980

67. Montano DE, Kasprzyk D, Taplin SH: The theory of reasoned action and the theory of planned behavior, in Glanz K, Lewis FM, Rimer BK (eds): *Health Behavior and Health Education* (ed 2). San Francisco, Jossey-Bass, 1997, pp 85–112

68. Nichols BS, Misra R, Alexy B: Cancer detection: How effective is public education? *Cancer Nurs* 19:98–103, 1996

69. Burnett CB, Steakley CS, Tefft MC: Barriers to breast and cervical cancer screening in underserved women of the District of Columbia. *Oncol Nurs Forum* 22:1551–1557, 1995

70. Crooks CE, Neutens JJ: Prediction and verification of a woman's intention to participate in a mammography screening program. *J Health Educ* 24:369–374, 1993

71. Barling NR, Moore SM: Prediction of cervical cancer screening using the Theory of Reasoned Action. *Psychol Rep* 79:77–78, 1996

72. Sutherland HJ, daCunha R, Lockwood GA, et al: What attitudes and beliefs underlie patients' decisions about participating in chemotherapy trials. *Med Decis Making* 18: 61–69, 1998

73. Ajzen I: The Theory of Planned Behavior. *Org Behav Hum Decis Process* 50:179–211, 1991

74. Madden TJ, Ellen PS, Ajzen I: A comparison of the Theory of Planned Behavior and the Theory of Reasoned Action. *Pers Soc Psychol Bull* 18:3–9, 1992

75. DeVellis BM, Blalock SJ, Sandler RS: Predicting participation in cancer screening: The role of perceived behavioral control. *J Appl Soc Psychol* 20:639–660, 1990

76. Lierman LM, Young HM, Powell-Cope G, et al: Effects of education and support on breast self-examination in older women. *Nurs Res* 43:158–163, 1994

77. McCaul KD, Sandgren AK, O'Neill HK, et al: The value of the Theory of Planned Behavior, perceived control, and self-efficacy expectations for predicting health-protective behaviors. *Basic Appl Soc Psychol* 14:231–252, 1993

78. Hanson MJ: The Theory of Planned Behavior applied to cigarette smoking in African-American, Puerto Rican, and non-Hispanic white teenage females. *Nurs Res* 46:155–162, 1997

79. Courneya KS, Friedenreich CM: Determinants of exercise during colorectal cancer treatment: An application of the Theory of Planned Behavior. *Oncol Nurs Forum* 24: 1715–1723, 1997

80. Heaney CA, Israel BA: Social networks and social support, in Glanz K, Lewis FM, Rimer BK (eds): *Health Behavior and Health Education* (ed 2). San Francisco, Jossey-Bass, 1997, pp. 179–205

81. Bottomly A, Jones L: Social support and the cancer patient. *Eur J Cancer Care* 6:117–123, 1997

82. House JS, Kahn RL: Measures and concepts of social support, in Cohen S, Syme L (eds): *Social Support and Health.* Orlando, FL, Academic Press, 1985, pp 83–108

83. Israel BA, Rounds KA: Social networks and social support: A synthesis for health educators. *Adv Health Educ Prom* 2: 311–351, 1987

84. Stewart MJ, Gillis A, Brosky G, et al: Smoking among disadvantaged women: Causes and cessation. *Can J Nurs Res* 28: 41–60, 1996

85. Pederson LL, Koval JJ, O'Connor K: Are psychosocial factors related to smoking in grade-6 students? *Addict Behav* 22:169–181, 1997

86. Kang SH, Bloom JR, Romano PS: Cancer screening among African-American women: Their use of tests and social support. *Am J Public Health* 84:101–103, 1994

87. McCance KL, Mooney KH, Field R, et al: Influence of others in motivating women to obtain breast cancer screening. *Cancer Pract* 4:141–146, 1996

88. Fite S, Frank DI, Curtin J: The relationship of social support to women's obtaining mammography screening. *J Am Acad Nurse Pract* 8:565–569, 1996

89. Maxwell CJ, Kozak JF, Desjardins-Denault MHK, et al: Factors important in promoting mammography screening among Canadian women. *Can J Public Health* 88:346–350, 1997

90. Gotay CC, Wilson ME: Social support and cancer screening in African American, Hispanic, and Native American women. *Cancer Pract* 6:31–37, 1998

91. Wagle A, Komorita NI, Lu ZJ: Social support and breast self-examination. *Cancer Nurs* 20:42–48, 1997

92. Crane LA: Social support and adherence behavior among women with abnormal Pap smears. *J Cancer Educ* 11: 164–173, 1996

93. Guidry JJ, Aday LA, Zhang D, et al: The role of informal

and formal support networks for patients with cancer. *Cancer Pract* 5:241–246, 1997

94. Steginga SK, Dunn J: Women's experiences following treatment for gynecologic cancer. *Oncol Nurs Forum* 24:1403–1408, 1997

95. Rotter J: Generalized expectancies for internal versus external control of reinforcement. *Psychol Med Monogr* 80:1–28, 1966

96. Wallston K, Wallston B: Locus of control and health. *Health Educ Monogr* 6:107–117, 1978

97. Lau R: Beliefs about control and health behavior, in Gochman D (ed): *Health Behavior: Emerging Research Perspectives.* New York, Plenum, 1988, pp 43–63

98. Oberle K: A decade of research in locus of control: What have we learned? *J Adv Nurs* 16:800–806, 1991

99. Dahnke GL, Garlick R, Kazoleas D: Testing a new disease-specific Health Locus of Control scale among cancer and aplastic anemia patients. *Health Commun* 6:37–53, 1994

100. Wallston KA, Stein MJ, Smith CA: Form C of the MHLC scales: A condition-specific measure of locus of control. *J Pers Assess* 63:534–553, 1994

101. Bundek NI, Marks G, Richardson JL: Role of Health Locus of Control beliefs in cancer screening of elderly Hispanic women. *Health Psychol* 12:193–199, 1993

102. Miller LY, Hailey BJ: Cancer anxiety and breast cancer screening in African American women: A preliminary study. *Womens Health Issues* 4:170–174, 1994

103. Blood GW, Kauffman SM, Dineen M, et al: Perceived control, adjustment, and communication problems in laryngeal cancer survivors. *Percept Mot Skills* 77:764–766, 1993

104. Greimel ER, Padilla GV, Grant MM: Self-care responses to illness of patients with various cancer diagnoses. *Acta Oncol* 36:141–150, 1997

105. Lewis F, Daltroy L: How causal explanations influence health behavior: Attribution Theory, in Glanz K, Lewis F, Rimer B (eds): *Health Behavior and Health Education.* San Francisco, Jossey-Bass, 1990, pp 92–114

106. Bearison DJ, Sadow AJ, Granowetter L, et al: Patients' and parents' causal attributions for childhood cancer. *J Psychosoc Oncol* 11:47–61, 1993

107. Berckman KL, Austin JK: Causal attributions, perceived control, and adjustments in patients with lung cancer. *Oncol Nurs Forum* 20:23–30, 1993

108. Eiser C, Havermans T, Eiser JR: Parents' attributions about childhood cancer: Implications for relationships with medical staff. *Child Care Health Dev* 21:31–42, 1994

109. Lavery JF, Clarke VA: Causal attributions, coping strategies, and adjustment to breast cancer. *Cancer Nurs* 19:20–28, 1996

110. Lowery BJ, Jacobsen BS, DuCette J: Causal attribution, control, and adjustment to breast cancer. *J Psychosoc Oncol* 10:37–53, 1993

111. Dirksen SR: Search for meaning in long-term cancer survivors. *J Adv Nurs* 21:628–633, 1995

112. Prochaska JO, Redding CA, Evers KE: The Transtheoretical Model and stages of change, in Glanz K, Lewis F, Rimer B (eds): *Health Behavior and Health Education* (ed 2). San Francisco, Jossey-Bass, 1997, pp 60–84

113. Prochaska JO, Redding CA, Harlow LL, et al: The Transtheoretical Model of Change and HIV prevention. A review. *Health Educ Q* 21:471–486, 1994

114. Hecht JP, Emmons KM, Brown RA, et al: Smoking interventions for patients with cancer: Guidelines for nursing practice. *Oncol Nurs Forum* 21:1657–1666, 1994

115. Prochaska JO, Velicer WF, Rossi JS, et al: Stages of change and decisional balance for 12 problem behaviors. *Health Psychol* 13:39–46, 1994

116. Rakowski W, Dube CE, Marcus BH, et al: Assessing elements of women's decisions about mammography. *Health Psychol* 11:111–118, 1992

117. DiClemente CC, Prochaska JO, Fairhurst S, et al: The process of smoking cessation: An analysis of precontemplation, contemplation and preparation stages of change. *J Consult Clin Psychol* 59:259–304, 1991

118. Prokhorov AV, Hudmon KS, Gritz ER: Promoting smoking cessation among cancer patients: A behavioral model. *Oncology* 11:1807–1813, 1997

119. Hudmon KS, Prokhorov AV, Koehly LM, et al: Psychometric properties of the Decisional Balance Scale and the Temptations to Try Smoking Inventory in adolescents. *J Child Adolesc Subst Abuse* 6:1–18, 1997

120. Prochaska JO, DiClemente CC, Velicer WF, et al: Standardized, individualized, interactive and personalized self-help programs for smoking cessation. *Health Psychol* 12:399–405, 1993

121. Rakowski W, Fulton JP: Feldman JP: Women's decision making about mammography: A replication of the relationship between stages of adoption and decisional balance. *Health Psychol* 12:209–214, 1993

122. Rakowski W, Ehrich B, Dube CE, et al: Screening mammography and constructs from the Transtheoretical Model: Associations using two definitions of the stage of adoption. *Ann Behav Med* 18:91–100, 1996

123. Rakowski W, Clark MA, Pearlman DN, et al: Integrating pros and cons for mammography and Pap testing: Extending the construct of decisional balance to two behaviors. *Prev Med* 26:664–673, 1997

124. Skinner CS, Strecher VJ, Hospers H: Physician recommendations for mammography: Do tailored messages make a difference? *Am J Public Health* 84:43–49, 1994

125. Friedman LC, Nelson DV, Webb JA, et al: Dispositional optimism, self-efficacy, and health beliefs as predictors of breast self-examination. *Am J Prev Med* 10:130–135, 1994

126. Glanz K, Resch N, Lerman C, et al: Factors associated with adherence to breast cancer screening among working women. *J Occup Med* 34:1071–1078, 1992

127. Kurtz ME, Given B, Given CW, et al: Relationships of barriers and facilitators to breast self-examination, mammography, and a clinical breast examination in a worksite population. *Cancer Nurs* 16:251–259, 1993

128. Marshburn J, Bradham DD, Studnicki J, et al: Mass mammography screening. *Cancer Pract* 2:146–153, 1994

129. Myers RE, Ross E, Jepson C, et al: Modeling adherence to colorectal cancer screening. *Prev Med* 23:142–151, 1994

130. Phillips JM, Wilbur J: Adherence to breast cancer screening guidelines among African-American women of differing employment status. *Cancer Nurs* 18:258–269, 1995

131. Lowe JB, Balanda KP, Gillespie AM, et al: Community perceptions of bowel cancer: A survey of Queenslanders. *Health Educ J* 54:331–339, 1995

132. Kreitler S, Kreitler H: Cognitive orientation and health-protective behaviors. *Int J Rehabil Health* 3:1–24, 1997

133. Bakker DA, Lightfoot NE, Steggles S, et al: The experience and satisfaction of women attending breast cancer screening. *Oncol Nurs Forum* 25:115–121, 1998

134. Carmel S, Shani E, Rosenberg L: The role of age and an expanded Health Belief Model in predicting skin cancer protective behavior. *Health Educ Res* 9:433–447, 1994

135. Funke BL, Nicholson ME: Factors affecting patient compli-

ance among women with abnormal Pap smears. *Patient Educ Counsel* 20:5–15, 1993

136. Murray M, McMillan C: Health beliefs, locus of control, emotional control and women's cancer screening behavior. *Br J Clin Psychol* 32:87–100, 1993

137. Beardall S, Edwards N: Social and cultural determinants of smoking behavior in selected immigrant groups: Results of key informant interviews. *Fam Community Health* 18:65–72, 1995

138. Glanz K, Kristal AR, Tilley BC, et al: Psychosocial correlates of healthful diets among male auto workers. *Cancer Epidemiol Biomarkers Prev* 7:119–126, 1998

139. Lierman LM, Kasprzyk D, Benoliel JQ: Understanding adherence to breast self-examination in older women. *West J Nurs Res* 13:46–66, 1991

140. Montano DE, Taplin SH: A test of an expanded Theory of Reasoned Action to predict mammography participation. *Soc Sci Med* 32:733–741, 1991

141. King E, Rimer BK, Balsheim A, et al: Mammography-related beliefs of older women. *J Aging Health* 5:82–100, 1993

142. Champion V, Miller AM: Recent mammography in women aged 35 and older: Predisposing variables. *Health Care Women Int* 17:233–245, 1996

143. Weinrich SP, Weinrich MC, Boyd MD, et al: The impact of prostate cancer knowledge on cancer screening. *Oncol Nurs Forum* 25:527–534, 1998

144. Sherman J, Abel E, Tavakoli A: Demographic predictors of clinical breast examination, mammography, and Pap test screening among older women. *J Am Acad Nurs Pract* 8:231–236, 1996

145. Neilson AR, Whynes DK: Determinants of compliance with screening for colorectal cancer. *Soc Sci Med* 41:365–374, 1995

146. Segnan N: Socioeconomic status and cancer screening. *IARC Sci Publications* 138:369–376, 1997

147. Blair KA: Cancer screening of older women. *Cancer Pract* 6:217–222, 1998

148. Robinson J: Behavior modification obtained by sun protection education coupled with removal of a skin cancer. *Arch Dermatol* 126:477–481, 1990

149. Jennings K: Getting Black women to screen for cancer: Incorporating health beliefs into practice. *J Am Acad Nurse Pract* 8:53–59, 1996

150. Powe BD: Cancer fatalism-Spiritual perspectives. *J Rel Health* 36:135–144, 1997

151. Powe BD, Johnson A: Fatalism as a barrier to cancer screening among African-Americans: Philosophical perspectives. *J Rel Health* 34:119–125, 1995

152. Lantz PM, Dupuis L, Reding D, et al: Peer discussions of cancer among Hispanic migrant farm workers. *Public Health Rep* 109:512–520, 1994

153. Jennings K: Getting a Pap smear: Focus group responses of African-American and Latina women. *Oncol Nurs Forum* 24:827–835, 1997

154. McCoy CB, Anwyl RS, Metsch LR, et al: Prostate cancer in Florida: Knowledge, attitudes, practices, and beliefs. *Cancer Pract* 3:88–93, 1995

155. Friedman LC, Bruce S, Weinberg AD, et al: Early detection of skin cancer: Racial/ethnic differences in behaviors and attitudes. *J Cancer Educ* 9:105–110, 1994

156. Salazar MK: Hispanic women's beliefs about breast cancer and mammography. *Cancer Nurs* 19:437–446, 1996

157. Balcazar H, Castro FG, Krull JL: Cancer risk reduction in Mexican American women: The role of acculturation, education and health risk factors. *Health Educ Q* 22:61–84, 1995

158. Suarez L: Pap smear and mammogram screening in Mexican-American women: The effects of acculturation. *Am J Public Health* 84:742–746, 1994

159. Hoeman SP, Ku YL, Ohl DR: Health beliefs and early detection among Chinese women. *West J Nurs Res* 18:518–533, 1996

160. Ali NS, Khalil H: Cancer prevention and early detection among Egyptians. *Cancer Nurs* 19:104–111, 1996

161. Ali NS: Providing culturally sensitive care to Egyptians with cancer. *Cancer Pract* 4:212–215, 1996

162. Yi JK: Acculturation and Pap smear screening practices among college-aged Vietnamese women in the United States. *Cancer Nurs* 21:335–341, 1998

163. Brown ML, Potosky AL: The presidential effect: The public health response to media coverage about Ronald Reagan's colon cancer episode. *Public Opin Q* 54:317–329, 1990

164. Lane DS, Polednak AP, Burg MA: The impact of media coverage of Nancy Reagan's experience on breast cancer screening. *Am J Public Health* 79:1551–1554, 1989

165. Stoddard A, Zapka J, Schoenfield S, et al: Effects of a news event on breast cancer screening survey responses. *Prog Clin Biol Res* 339:259–268, 1990

166. Nattinger AB, Hoffmann RG, Howell-Pelz A, et al: Effect of Nancy Reagan's mastectomy on choice of surgery by US women. *JAMA* 279:762–766, 1998

167. Lovejoy NC: Multinational approaches to cervical cancer screening: A review. *Cancer Nurs* 19:126–134, 1996

168. Lane DS, Polednak AP, Burg MA: Breast cancer screening practices among users of county-funded health centers vs women in the entire community. *Am J Public Health* 82:199–203, 1992

169. Boss LP, Guckes FH: Medicaid coverage of screening tests for breast and cervical cancer. *Am J Public Health* 82:252–253, 1992

170. Brown RL, Baumann LJ, Helberg CP, et al: The simultaneous analysis of patient, physician, and group practice influences on annual mammography performance. *Soc Sci Med* 43:315–324, 1996

171. Gulitz E, Bustillo-Hernandez M, Kent EB: Missed cancer screening opportunities among older women. *Cancer Pract* 6:289–295, 1998

172. Metch LR, McCoy CB, Pereyra M, et al: The role of the physician as an information source on mammography. *Cancer Pract* 6:229–236, 1998

173. Fischera S, Frank DI: Attitudes, practices, and role of nurses in the use of mammography. *Cancer Nurs* 17:223–228, 1994

174. Vietri V, Poskitt S, Slaninka SC: Enhancing breast cancer screening in the university setting. *Cancer Nurs* 20:323–329, 1997

175. Buller DB, Buller MK: Approaches to communicating preventive behaviors. *Semin Oncol Nurs* 7:53–63, 1991

CHAPTER 7

Cultural Diversity Among Individuals with Cancer

Karen N. Taoka, RN, MN, AOCN
Joanne K. Itano, RN, PhD, OCN®

Introduction

Culture is a fundamental element that uniquely shapes each individual. Cultural diversity encompasses more than just ethnic diversity. It is multifaceted and can include diversity in many forms such as sexual orientation, nontraditional lifestyle, age, socioeconomic status, and religious beliefs. In this chapter, the focus of cultural diversity is on ethnic diversity. (See Table 7-1 for definitions of selected terms.)

Overview

Historically, the United States has taken pride in its "melting pot," or multicultural composition of peoples from many nations. Until recently, however, this cultural diversity was largely limited to white immigrants from Europe who represented the majority of the population. In the twentieth century, immigration from areas such as southeast Asia, China, Japan, Korea, the Philippines, Mexico, and the Caribbean and long-overdue recognition of Native Americans as a people are factors that are rapidly redefining the population composition of the United States. This is clearly evident when comparing the population composition in the 1950s, when nine out of ten Americans were of European descent, with the composition in the 1990s, when one out of every four adults and one out of every three children are of African, Latin American, or Asian origin.[7]

Furthermore, current trends indicate that these ethnic minority populations are growing at rates that are surpassing the rest of the population. For example, Asian/Pacific Islanders (API) are the fastest growing minority in the United States. Between 1980 and 1990, the API population increased by 107.8 %.[8] Projections by the U.S. Census Bureau predict that by the year 2050, the U.S. population will include the following distribution: white 52.5%, Hispanic 22.5%, black 14.4%, API 9.7%, and Native American 0.9%. These projections reflect a steady decrease in the white population from 76% in 1990 to the projected 52.5% in 2050, as compared to steady growth in the minority populations.[9] In addition, ethnic minority populations will not be distributed uniformly across the United States. For example, it is projected that in 2020 nearly two-thirds (62%) of the API population will be concentrated in California, New York, Texas, Hawaii, and Washington.[10]

Unfortunately, this trend of growing ethnic minority populations is not matched in the composition of health care professionals. In particular, data from the 1990 census revealed the underrepresentation of ethnic minority registered nurses, where 3% of registered nurses were Hispanic, 4.4% API, and 8.1% black.[11] In 1994 the Institute of Medicine reported that minorities in the health professions were more underrepresented than 15 years prior.[7] Several reasons are identified for this underrepresentation and include inadequate math and science edu-

cation for minorities, a lack of scholarships, and a lack of qualified students.[7] Underrepresentation is of concern because health promotion activities and interventions for ethnic minorities are more successful when health care professionals of the same ethnic group are directly involved.

Table 7-1   Definition of Selected Terms

Acculturation:	Process by which an individual identifies with and adapts to another culture; often adopts the other culture's values but still retains a part of his/her original culture; occurs on a continuum; leads to biculturalism.
Culturally competent care:	Care that is provided with an awareness and appreciation of the cultural differences between the caregiver and patient; is individualized and respects the patient's cultural background.
Cultural relativity:	Refers to the attempt to view or interpret the behavior of culturally different individuals within the context of those individuals' cultures; acknowledges that behavior that is appropriate in one culture may not be acceptable in another culture.[1]
Culture:	"Culture refers to the learned, shared, and transmitted values, beliefs, norms, and lifeways of a particular group that guides their thinking, decisions, and actions in patterned ways."[2,p.47]
Enculturation:	"The process by which an individual assumes the traits and behaviors of a given culture, adapting to it, adopting its values, and taking on that particular cultural identity."[3,p.38] Generally refers to the culture into which an individual is born.
Ethnicity:	"A sense of identification associated with a cultural group's common social and cultural heritage. . . . A person is born into an ethnic group but . . . may also adopt characteristics of another ethnic group."[4,p.354] These characteristics include language, race, food preferences, religious faith, values, traditions, folklore, and many traits relevant to physical appearance.[4,5]
Ethnocentrism:	The tendency to view people unconsciously by using one's group and one's own customs as the standard for all judgments.[1]
Generalization:	Common patterns for beliefs and behaviors that are shared by a group; may be inaccurate when applied to specific individuals of that group.[6]
Race:	"A physical, not a cultural, differentiator based on a common heredity, using as identifiers characteristics such as skin color, head shape, and stature."[3,p.38]
Stereotype:	A fixed conception of a group allowing for no individuality; assumes all members of a group are alike.
Worldview:	"Refers to the way people tend to look out on the world or their universe to form a picture or a value stance about their life or world around them."[2,p.47]

Table 7-2 SEER Incidence Rates, 1988–1992, Selected Sites

Cancer Site	Alaska Native M	Alaska Native W	American Indian M	American Indian W	Black M	Black W	Chinese M	Chinese W	Filipino M	Filipino W	Hawaiian M	Hawaiian W
All sites	372.	348.	196.	180.	560.	326.	282.	213.	274.	224.	340.	321.
Brain and nervous system	*	*	*	*	4.5	3.4	3.1	2.1	3.6	2.8	*	*
Breast, invasive	*	78.9	*	31.6	1.2	95.4	*	55.0	*	73.1	*	105.6
Cervix uteri	—	15.8	—	9.9	—	13.2	—	7.3	—	9.6	—	9.3
Colon and rectum	79.7	67.4	18.6	15.3	60.7	45.5	44.8	33.6	35.4	20.9	42.4	30.5
Corpus uteri	—	*	—	10.7	—	14.4	—	11.6	—	12.1	—	23.9
Esophagus	*	*	*	*	15.0	4.4	5.3	*	2.9	*	9.4	*
Kidney and renal pelvis	*	*	15.6	*	12.8	6.0	4.6	2.3	5.8	2.8	9.8	*
Larynx	*	*	*	*	12.7	2.5	2.8	*	2.4	*	*	*
Leukemias	*	*	*	*	11.5	6.8	7.2	4.4	10.7	6.6	10.8	7.2
Liver and intrahepatic bile duct	*	*	*	*	6.9	2.4	20.8	5.3	10.5	3.4	*	*
Lung and bronchus	81.1	50.6	14.4	*	117.0	44.2	52.1	25.3	52.6	17.5	89.0	43.1
Lymphomas: Non-Hodgkin's lymphoma	*	*	*	*	13.2	7.6	12.4	6.8	12.9	9.0	12.5	*
Lymphomas: Hodgkin's disease	*	*	*	*	2.3	2.0	*	*	*	*	*	*
Melanoma of the skin	*	*	*	*	1.0	0.7	*	*	*	*	*	*
Multiple myeloma	*	*	*	*	11.3	7.4	2.3	1.8	4.8	2.6	*	*
Nasopharynx	*	*	*	*	1.0	*	10.8	3.9	3.9	*	*	*
Oral cavity (excluding nasopharynx)	*	*	*	*	20.4	5.8	5.3	2.3	5.4	5.3	11.7	*
Ovary	—	*	—	17.5	—	10.2	—	9.3	—	10.2	—	11.8
Pancreas	*	*	*	*	14.0	11.5	8.0	4.9	6.5	6.0	10.9	8.7
Prostate	46.1	—	52.5	—	180.6	—	46.0	—	69.8	—	57.2	—
Stomach	27.2	*	*	*	17.9	7.6	15.7	8.3	8.5	5.3	20.5	13.0
Testis	*	—	*	—	0.8	—	1.7	—	1.3	—	*	—
Thyroid	*	*	*	*	1.4	3.3	2.1	6.5	4.1	14.6	*	9.1
Urinary bladder	*	*	*	*	15.2	5.8	13.0	3.7	8.3	2.1	*	*

A fundamental challenge for health care providers is that the health care beliefs and practices of many ethnic groups may be incongruent with mainstream, Westernized medicine. The use of traditional healers and folk medicine, for example, often plays a major role in the provision of holistic care for blacks, API, Hispanics, and Native Americans.

This chapter provides an introduction to culture and cancer and the potential for oncology nurses to have a positive impact on the cancer experience of ethnic minority individuals and their families. Specific cultural information and nursing considerations for four ethnic minority groups (blacks, API, Hispanics, and Native Americans) are addressed. The discussion of these four ethnic minority groups is limited by several factors. Foremost is the diversity within each group. Blacks, API, Hispanics, and Native Americans are composed of several subgroups, each with its own subculture. For example,

the subgroups under the term Hispanic include Mexican American, Puerto Rican, Cuban American, and Central and South American. Added to the existence of subgroups and their unique cultures is the inherent heterogeneity due to intragroup differences, such as socioeconomic status, education attainment level, and degree of acculturation. Most important is the individual within the group. Although profiles of ethnic minority groups are provided in this chapter, each patient must be recognized as an individual with unique needs, regardless of cultural background.

Epidemiology

Blacks, on the whole, have higher cancer incidence and mortality rates than do whites.[12] Comparison data in other ethnic minority groups are limited because they only

Table 7-2 SEER Incidence Rates, 1988–1992, Selected Sites (continued)

Cancer Site	Japanese M	Japanese W	Korean M	Korean W	Vietnamese M	Vietnamese W	White M	White W	Hispanic† (Total) M	Hispanic† (Total) W
All sites	322	241	266	180	326	273	**469**	**346**	319	243
Brain and nervous system	2.1	*	*	*	*	*	**7.8**	**5.4**	**5.2**	**3.8**
Breast, invasive	*	82.3	*	28.5	*	37.5	0.9	**111.8**	0.6	69.8
Cervix uteri	—	5.8	—	15.2	—	**43.0**	—	8.7	—	**16.2**
Colon and rectum	**64.1**	**39.5**	31.7	21.9	30.5	27.1	56.3	38.3	38.3	24.7
Corpus uteri	—	**14.5**	—	3.8	—	8.4	—	**22.3**	—	13.7
Esophagus	**5.6**	*	*	*	*	*	5.4	**1.7**	4.4	**0.9**
Kidney and renal pelvis	7.3	2.3	6.3	*	*	*	**11.9**	**5.9**	10.0	**5.5**
Larynx	2.5	*	*	*	*	*	**7.5**	**1.5**	**5.1**	**0.7**
Leukemias	6.6	4.5	6.5	4.7	9.5	**8.3**	**13.5**	**7.9**	9.4	6.4
Liver and intrahepatic bile duct	6.3	**3.9**	**24.8**	**10.0**	**41.8**	*	3.7	1.5	6.7	2.6
Lung and bronchus	43.0	15.2	53.2	16.0	70.9	31.2	**76.0**	**41.5**	41.8	19.5
Lymphomas: Non-Hodgkin's lymphoma	11.6	7.8	5.8	6.0	**15.8**	*	**18.7**	**12.0**	**14.1**	**9.1**
Lymphomas: Hodgkin's disease	*	*	*	*	*	*	**3.3**	**2.6**	2.5	1.6
Melanoma of the skin	*	*	*	*	*	*	**14.5**	**10.1**	2.7	3.2
Multiple myeloma	1.6	*	*	*	*	*	**5.0**	**3.2**	4.2	**3.0**
Nasopharynx	*	*	*	*	**7.7**	*	0.6	0.2	0.6	*
Oral cavity (excluding nasopharynx)	7.0	**3.3**	*	*	11.6	*	**14.6**	**5.8**	8.9	2.7
Ovary	—	10.1	—	7.0	—	**13.8**	—	**15.8**	—	11.4
Pancreas	8.7	7.3	*	**7.6**	*	*	**9.8**	7.4	8.0	6.9
Prostate	88.0	—	24.2	—	40.0	—	**134.7**	—	**89.0**	—
Stomach	**30.5**	**15.3**	**48.9**	**19.1**	25.8	**25.8**	10.2	4.4	15.3	8.0
Testis	2.3	—	*	—	*	—	**5.0**	—	2.9	—
Thyroid	1.6	5.4	*	**7.8**	*	**10.5**	2.6	6.5	2.0	6.2
Urinary bladder	13.7	4.1	10.4	*	*	*	**31.7**	**7.8**	**15.8**	**4.3**

— = not applicable; * = rate not calculated when fewer than 25 cases; **numbers in boldface** = top three rates, as applicable.

†These figures are for **general comparison** only as this group may overlap the other ethnic populations in this table.

Note: Rates are "average annual" per 100,000 population, age-adjusted to 1970 U.S. standard.

Data from Miller, Kolonel, Bernstein, et al[14]

recently have been collected and then on a somewhat limited basis. Kagawa-Singer[13] reports that the National Cancer Institute Surveillance, Epidemiology, and End Results (SEER) tumor registry program has listed API only since 1978; however, initially only four out of sixty groups were coded: Chinese, Japanese, Filipino, and native Hawaiian. Recently, coding for Koreans and Vietnamese was initiated. In addition, aggregate data in the recent past combined major groups together, making it difficult to sift out specific information (e.g., data on Chinese were grouped with those reported for API).

There are obvious differences in cancer incidence, mortality, and survival rates when data are compared across all groups. Age-adjusted incidence rates (overall and selected cancer sites) for 1988–1992 are based on SEER data and are provided in Table 7-2.[14] These data represent 14% of the total U.S. population with the following percentages of the specific ethnic populations: native Hawaiian (78%), Japanese (60%), Filipino (49%), Chinese (43%), Korean (34%), Vietnamese (31%), American Indian (27%), and Hispanic (25%).[14] Mortality rates, age-adjusted for the same time period, are shown in Table 7-3 and are based on cancer deaths for the entire U.S. population, as provided by the National Center for Health Statistics.[14]

In reviewing the incidence tables, the reader is advised

Table 7-3 United States Cancer Mortality Rates, 1988–1992

Cancer Site	Alaska Native M	Alaska Native W	American Indian M	American Indian W	Black M	Black W	Chinese M	Chinese W	Filipino M	Filipino W	Hawaiian M	Hawaiian W
All sites	**225.**	**179.**	123.	99.	**319.**	**168.**	139.	86.	105.	63.	**239.**	**168.**
Brain and nervous system	*	*	*	*	**3.1**	**2.1**	2.1	1.4	1.6	1.4	*	*
Breast, invasive	*	*	*	*	0.4	**31.4**	*	11.2	*	11.9	*	**25.0**
Cervix uteri	—	*	—	*	—	**6.7**	—	2.6	—	2.4	—	*
Colon and rectum	**27.2**	**24.0**	*	*	**28.2**	20.4	15.7	10.5	11.4	5.8	**23.7**	11.4
Corpus uteri	—	*	—	*	—	**6.0**	—	2.2	—	1.3	—	**8.4**
Esophagus	*	*	*	*	**14.8**	**3.7**	4.2	*	2.2	*	*	*
Kidney and renal pelvis	*	*	*	*	**5.1**	**2.2**	1.3	0.9	1.9	*	*	*
Larynx	*	*	*	*	**5.6**	**0.9**	0.9	*	*	*	*	*
Leukemias	*	*	*	*	**8.0**	**4.6**	3.6	2.4	5.7	2.9	**7.8**	*
Liver and intrahepatic bile duct	*	*	*	*	6.6	2.7	**17.7**	**4.6**	**7.8**	2.3	**9.2**	*
Lung and bronchus	69.4	**45.3**	*	*	**105.6**	31.5	40.1	18.5	29.8	10.0	**88.9**	44.1
Lymphomas: Non-Hodgkin's lymphoma	*	*	*	*	**5.8**	**3.4**	5.2	2.3	5.0	3.0	**8.8**	*
Lymphomas: Hodgkin's disease	*	*	*	*	**0.7**	**0.4**	*	*	*	*	*	*
Melanoma of the skin	*	*	*	*	0.5	0.4	*	*	*	*	*	*
Multiple myeloma	*	*	*	*	7.3	5.0	1.2	1.3	2.2	1.0	*	*
Nasopharynx	*	*	*	*	0.6	0.2	**4.6**	**1.2**	1.7	*	*	*
Oral cavity (excluding nasopharynx)	*	*	*	*	**8.7**	**2.1**	1.6	0.7	1.2	**1.3**	*	*
Ovary	—	*	—	*	—	**6.6**	—	4.0	—	3.4	—	7.3
Pancreas	*	*	*	*	**14.4**	**10.4**	6.7	5.1	4.5	3.5	**12.8**	**9.1**
Prostate	*	—	16.2	—	**53.7**	—	6.6	—	13.5	—	**19.9**	—
Stomach	*	*	*	*	**13.6**	**5.6**	10.5	4.8	3.6	2.5	14.4	**12.8**
Testis	*	—	*	—	0.1	—	*	—	*	—	*	—
Thyroid	*	*	*	*	0.3	0.4	*	*	*	**1.1**	*	*
Urinary bladder	*	*	*	*	**4.8**	**2.4**	2.0	1.0	1.2	*	*	*

that there are limitations in the SEER data and to interpret these data cautiously because (1) SEER data do not reflect the total U.S. population; (2) cancer rates in smaller populations (e.g., native Hawaiian, Japanese, Vietnamese) are less precise than rates in larger populations (e.g., blacks, whites); (3) the Native American population is represented by two separate groups: Alaska native (composed of individuals who identified themselves as Aleut, Eskimo, or American Indian) and American Indian (New Mexico); and (4) individuals who classify themselves as being of Hispanic ethnicity may be of any race, resulting in some overlap between the Hispanic classification and the other ethnic groups. However, the SEER data are helpful in identifying general ethnic patterns of cancer. In the following paragraphs, several key cancer incidence, mortality, and survival data unique to each ethnic group are presented.

Blacks

Black men have the highest overall cancer incidence rates. The particular sites for which high incidence and mortality rates have been identified in both black men and women include esophagus (almost three times that of whites), prostate, uterine, cervix, liver, larynx, multiple myeloma, and stomach.[14] Their 5-year survival rate, based on data collected from blacks diagnosed with cancer from 1989–1993, was approximately 44% as compared to 60% for whites.[12]

Asian/Pacific Islanders

This group is composed of several diverse subgroups, including Chinese, Japanese, Filipino, Korean, Vietnamese, Laotian, Cambodian, Hmong, Thai, native Hawaiian,

Table 7-3   United States Cancer Mortality Rates, 1988–1992 (continued)

Cancer Site	Japanese M	Japanese W	White M	White W	Hispanic† (Total) M	Hispanic† (Total) W
All sites	133	88	213	140	129	85
Brain and nervous system	1.3	1.1	**5.4**	**3.7**	**3.0**	**2.0**
Breast, invasive	*	12.5	0.2	**27.0**	0.1	15.0
Cervix uteri	—	1.5	—	2.5	—	**3.4**
Colon and rectum	20.5	12.3	22.9	**15.3**	12.8	8.3
Corpus uteri	—	1.9	—	**3.2**	—	2.3
Esophagus	**4.8**	0.9	**5.3**	**1.2**	3.4	0.7
Kidney and renal pelvis	2.4	0.8	**5.0**	**2.3**	3.7	**1.7**
Larynx	*	*	**2.3**	**0.5**	1.9	**0.2**
Leukemias	4.4	2.2	**8.5**	**5.0**	5.1	**3.4**
Liver and intrahepatic bile duct	6.2	**4.0**	3.8	1.8	5.9	**2.8**
Lung and bronchus	32.4	12.9	**72.6**	**31.9**	32.4	10.8
Lymphomas: Non-Hodgkin's lymphoma	4.8	3.9	**8.1**	**5.3**	5.3	**3.6**
Lymphomas: Hodgkin's disease	*	*	**0.7**	**0.4**	0.6	0.3
Melanoma of the skin	*	*	**3.4**	**1.7**	0.8	0.5
Multiple myeloma	*	*	3.4	2.2	2.7	1.8
Nasopharynx	*	*	0.3	0.1	0.3	0.1
Oral cavity (excluding nasopharynx)	2.1	0.8	**3.8**	**1.5**	**2.7**	0.7
Ovary	—	5.0	—	**8.1**	—	**4.8**
Pancreas	8.5	6.7	**9.7**	**6.9**	7.1	5.2
Prostate	11.7	—	**24.1**	—	15.3	—
Stomach	**17.4**	**9.3**	6.1	2.8	8.4	4.2
Testis	*	—	0.3	—	0.2	—
Thyroid	*	*	0.3	0.3	0.2	0.5
Urinary bladder	2.0	**1.2**	**5.8**	**1.7**	**2.8**	0.9

— = not applicable; * = rate not calculated when fewer than 25 cases; **numbers in boldface** = top three rates, as applicable.

†These figures are for **general comparison** only as this group may overlap the other ethnic populations in this table.

Note: Rates are "average annual" per 100,000 population, age-adjusted to 1970 U.S. standard. No mortality data available for Korean and Vietnamese groups.

Data from Miller, Kolonel, Bernstein, et al[14]

Samoan, and Micronesian. The latest SEER data provide information only for the Chinese, Japanese, Filipino, native Hawaiian, Korean, and Vietnamese groups. Within these subgroups alone, the data are also very diverse. Native Hawaiians have the highest overall cancer incidence and mortality rates among the API. When compared to all other racial/ethnic groups, native Hawaiian women have the highest incidence rate for uterine cancer.[14] Japanese, Chinese, Filipinos, and Koreans, on the other hand, overall have lower incidence and mortality rates as compared to blacks, Alaskan natives, whites, and native Hawaiians. However, there are specific sites for which each of these subgroups have high incidence rates. For example, the Japanese have high incidence rates for stomach and colorectal cancers.[14,15] The Chinese have high incidence rates for oral cavity (in particular, nasopharyngeal cancer) and liver cancers.[8,14] Filipinos have the highest incidence rates for thyroid cancer.[14] However, Filipinos have the lowest cancer mortality rates and have among the lowest incidence rates along with Koreans and Native Americans (New Mexico). Vietnamese women have the highest incidence rates for cervical cancer, while Vietnamese men have the highest incidence rates for liver and intrahepatic bile duct cancers. Other sources similarly report a high incidence of liver cancer in Southeast Asian groups that has been attributed primarily to hepatitis B infection.[8,16]

Hispanics

Much like the API, several subgroups are included under the term Hispanics. Among these subgroups are the Mexican American, Cuban American, Puerto Rican American, and people from the Caribbean and South and Central America. The latest SEER data incidence rates that are available for Hispanic Americans primarily reflect Mexican Americans from the Los Angeles, San Francisco/Oakland, San Jose/Monterey, and New Mexico areas. Overall, Hispanics rank at the median for incidence and mortality rates when compared to other ethnic groups. However, Hispanics have high incidence rates for cervical, prostate, and urinary bladder cancers.[14]

Native Americans

Composed of many tribes and more than 400 federally recognized nations, Native Americans are yet another group that is made up of diverse subgroups. However, the SEER data is limited to only a portion of this group and, as mentioned earlier, reflects separate coding for Alaskan natives and American Indians living in New Mexico. Although Native Americans (New Mexico American Indians) have the lowest cancer incidence rates and rank mid to low in cancer mortality rates, they have the lowest 5-year relative survival rates.[14,17] Colon, rectum, and lung are high incidence cancer sites for Alaska natives, while cancers of the ovary and kidney and renal pelvis are high-incidence sites for the American Indians of New Mexico.[14]

Possible factors that contribute to these variations in cancer incidence and mortality in different ethnic groups include environmental and socioeconomic factors; access to health care; cultural values, beliefs, and health practices; and genetic predisposition. These factors are often interdependent and interrelated. An in-depth discussion of these factors can be found elsewhere.[13]

Transcultural Nursing and Assessment

Transcultural Nursing

The aim of transcultural nursing is to understand and assist diverse cultural groups and members of such groups with their nursing and health care needs. A thorough assessment of the cultural aspects of an individual's lifestyle, health beliefs, and health practices will enhance the nurse's decision making and judgment when providing care. Nursing interventions that are culturally relevant and sensitive to the needs of the patient decrease the possibility of stress or conflict arising from cultural misunderstandings.

There are often problems when individuals from two cultural backgrounds with conflicting values meet unless at least one is willing to recognize and adapt to the values of the other. One method to avoid such conflict is to sensitize nurses to their own cultural biases and behaviors as well as to those of their patients.[18]

Each individual is culturally unique. It is essential that nurses avoid stereotyping or projecting onto patients their own "cultural uniqueness" or "world views" if culturally appropriate care is to be provided. *Stereotyping* is a simplified, generally inflexible conception of the members of a group or subgroup. It is an end point in that no attempt is made to learn whether the individual in question fits the assumption.

Generalizations and stereotypes may appear similar but function differently. *Generalizations* are starting points. They indicate common trends, but further information is needed to ascertain whether the statement is appropriate to a particular individual. Generalizations are developed when looking for common patterns to beliefs and behaviors that are shared by a group. It is hoped that the nurse will use generalizations about specific ethnic minorities in planning culturally competent care. Regardless of the ethnic minority group, there are always differences among group members.

A nurse must carefully identify his or her personal cultural beliefs and values in order to separate them from the patient's beliefs and values. It is natural to view people unconsciously by using our own group and customs as the standard for all judgments. A nurse with this tendency will gather data only selectively in accordance with personal standards, values, and judgment, and may not be able to see what the patient has to offer or the different way in which the patient views the world. Such an ethnocentric view may limit the data the nurse gathers, distort the assessment of the patient's behavior, and lead to conflicts between the nurse and the patient. The nurse must also be aware of the Western health care culture of which she or he is a part.

Cultural relativity, the attempt to view or interpret the behavior of culturally different individuals within the context of their own culture, is the nurse's goal. This perspective acknowledges that behavior appropriate in one culture may not be so in another culture. It provides meaning to patient or family behaviors that caregivers might otherwise consider negative or confusing.[1]

Culturally competent care requires two things:

1. An understanding that caring is a universal phenomenon that varies only in form and manifestation. In other words, caring for others exists in all cultures, but the methods by which it is carried out and the meanings that caring conveys in different cultures are as diverse as the groups that define them.
2. An understanding that what is valued and judged as "good" care is culturally determined, culturally based, and culturally validated. That is, members of a cultural group can identify and define what is good care, but outsiders probably cannot do so in the same way. The

closer the nursing care matches the patients' values and expectations, the more likely that patients will accept it.

Thus, transcultural nursing is concerned with shared meanings and the degree to which the nurse and patient agree or disagree about the cultural symbols of health, healing, illness, disease, and caring. How cultural groups define and treat various illnesses, promote and maintain health, prevent illness, and structure their health care system are basic knowledge requirements for effective transcultural nursing care.[18]

Cultural Assessment

Nurses need knowledge in order to provide culturally competent care that is free of gender, race, or religious bias. Culturally appropriate care is based on an accurate assessment, a systematic appraisal or examination, of individuals, groups, and communities as to their cultural beliefs, values, and practices. Using this assessment, patient needs and nursing interventions are identified within the cultural context of the people being evaluated.

One useful assessment model is Giger and Davidhi-zar's Transcultural Assessment Model, outlined in Figure 7-1.[19] In this model, six essential cultural phenomena are identified that the nurse considers in providing culturally competent nursing care. These phenomena are evident in all cultural groups and include communication, space, social organization, time, environmental control, and biological variations.

The culturally unique individual is a significant component of this model. The model illustrates that each individual is a product of past experiences, cultural beliefs, and cultural norms and that there is diversity within cultural groups. However, knowledge of general baseline data relative to a specific cultural group is an excellent starting point to provide culturally appropriate care.

Communication

Communication is the means by which culture is transmitted and preserved. Culture influences how feelings are expressed and what verbal and nonverbal expressions are appropriate. Cultural patterns of communication are instilled early and are found in child-rearing practices.

Communication includes vocabulary, grammatical structure, voice qualities, intonation, rhythm, speed, pro-

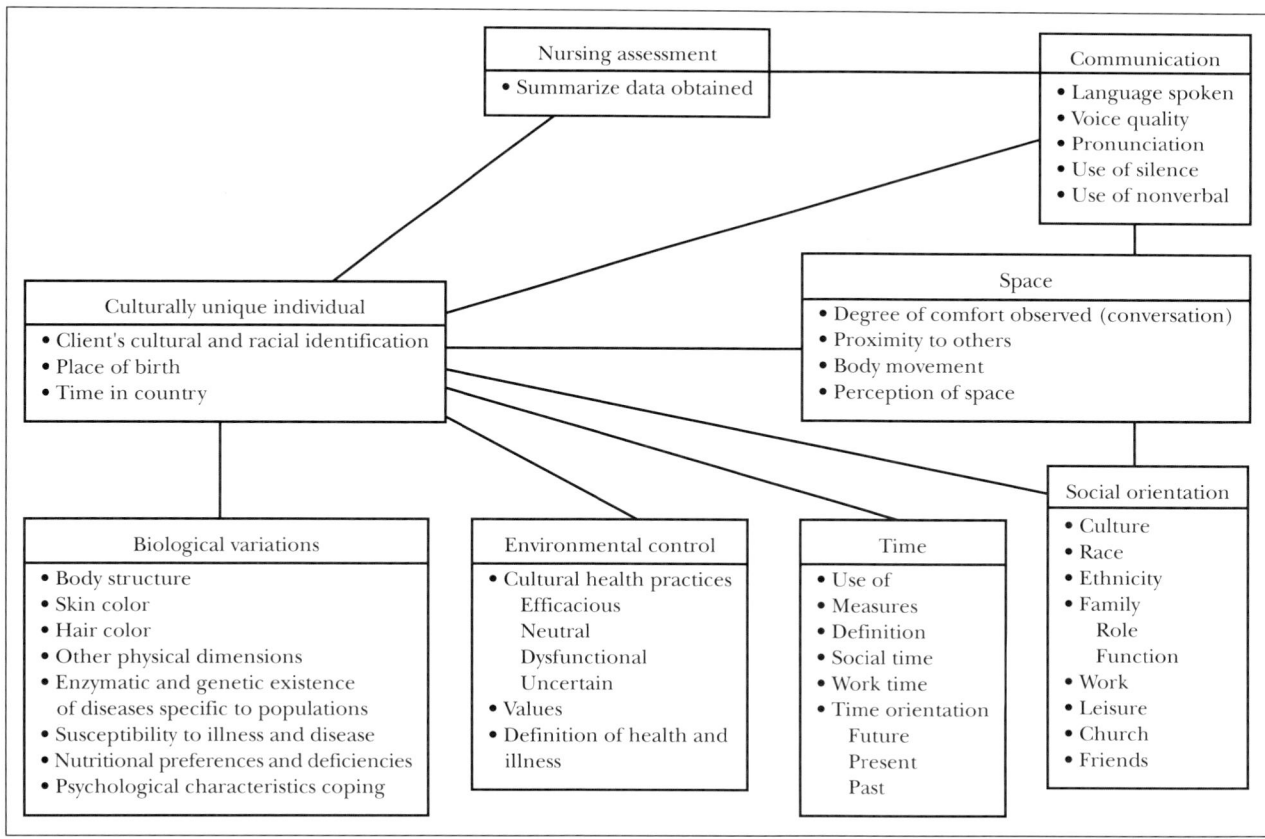

Figure 7-1 Giger and Davidhizar Transcultural Assessment Model. (Reprinted with permission from Giger JN, Davidhizar RE: Introduction to transcultural nursing, in Giger JN, Davidhizar RE (eds): *Transcultural Nursing: Assessment and Intervention* (ed 3). St. Louis, Mosby-Year Book, 1999, pp 3–19)[19]

nunciation, and use of silence. Language is basic to communication. Words are tools or symbols used to express ideas and feelings or to identify or describe objects. Words also shape experiences and influence cultural perceptions, convey interpretations, and influence relationships.

The most obvious cultural difference among people is language. If the nurse does not speak the patient's language, a translator may be necessary. More often, however, the patient speaks the nurse's language with limited ability or uses language with denotative or connotative meanings different from the nurse's meaning.

Nonverbal communication includes touch, facial expressions, eye movement, and body posture. Through body language or motions, an individual conveys what cannot or may not be said in words. For a message to be accurately communicated, not only must words be translated but also the meaning held by nuances, intonation patterns, and facial expressions. Just as verbal behavior may undo nonverbal behavior, nonverbal behavior may repeat, clarify, contradict, modify, emphasize, or regulate the flow of communication.[20]

To communicate effectively with culturally diverse patients, the nurse needs to be aware of what nonverbal behaviors mean to the patient and what specific nonverbal behaviors mean in the patient's culture. It is not wise to assign meaning to nonverbal behaviors without validating their meaning with the patient. Because communication is an essential part of establishing a relationship with a patient and family, strategies for effective communication are provided in Table 7-4.[20]

Space

Space is a relative concept that includes the individual, the body, the surrounding environment, and objects within that environment. The relationship between our body, objects, and people within a space is learned and influenced by our culture. In Western cultures, spatial distances are defined as the intimate zone, the personal zone, and the social and public zones. The intimate zone is the smallest area of space around the individual, while the public zone is the largest area. The size of these areas varies with specific cultures. Americans, Canadians, and the British require more personal space, while Latin Americans, Japanese, and Arabic individuals need the least amount of personal space and have a higher tolerance for crowding in public spaces.[21]

Territoriality is a state characterized by possessiveness, control, and authority over an area of physical space. For the needs of territoriality to be met, the individual must be in control of some space, be able to establish rules for the space, and be able to defend it against invasion or misuse by others.[22] The use of restraints may increase resistance by the patient, as they involve physical invasion of personal space.

Nurses move through all spatial zones. Thus, the nurse must be sensitive to patients' reactions to movement toward them. A patient may physically withdraw or back away if the nurse is perceived as being too close. Explaining why there is a need to be close and asking permission to do so are helpful interventions.[4]

Objects in the environment may affect communication differently in different cultures. For example, positioning chairs at a 90-degree angle can communicate a cooperative stance whereas a side-by-side arrangement of chairs can decrease communication with Americans.

Certain clothing or objects may be worn to reflect cultural beliefs. For example, a Native American patient may wish to wear a medicine bundle. Patients may also wish to arrange their space differently and control the placement of objects on their bedside cabinet or overbed table. These actions help patients establish personal space within which they feel a sense of control.

Social organization

Cultural behavior, or how one acts in certain situations, is socially acquired. Patterns of cultural behavior are learned through enculturation that involves acquiring knowledge and internalizing values. These patterns provide explanations for behavior related to life events (e.g., birth, illness, and death).

Significant components of social organization include knowledge of family structure and organization, religious values and beliefs, and how ethnicity and culture relate to role and role assignment within group settings.[23] The family is the basic unit of society. Cultural values can determine communication within the family, the norm for family size, and the roles of specific family members. Other aspects of social organization include the value placed on children and the elderly, gender roles, and the extent of the family's involvement in a hospitalized patient's care.

Religions have an influence on the lifestyles of most cultures and may affect health care practices. Most religions have rituals that mark important events like birth, the entrance into adulthood, marriage, and death. Religious practices may prohibit eating certain foods. Religion may influence a patient's perception of the cause of an illness, its severity, and the type of healer required. As always, it is important not to assume that membership in a particular ethnic or cultural group is equated with a specific religion.

Time

Time orientation refers to an individual's focus on the present or the future.[24] The American focus on time tends to be directed to the future, emphasizing planning and schedules. Long-range goals are important and health care measures in the present are often undertaken to prevent occurrence of illness in the future. Some African, Spanish, and southern European Americans are oriented more to the present than to the future. They may be late for appointments not because of their reluctance to make the appointment or lack of respect for the nurse, but because they are more concerned about the activity in

Table 7-4 Guidelines for Relating to Patients from Different Cultures

Goal	Specific Actions
Assess your personal beliefs surrounding patients from different cultures.	• Review your personal beliefs and past experiences. • Set aside any values, biases, ideas, and attitudes that are judgmental and may negatively affect care.
Assess communication variables from a cultural perspective.	• Determine the ethnic identity of the patient, including generation in America. • Use the patient as a source of information when possible. • Assess cultural factors that may affect your relationship with the patient and respond appropriately.
Plan care based on the communicated needs and cultural background.	• Learn as much as possible about the patient's cultural customs and beliefs. • Encourage the patient to reveal cultural interpretation of health, illness, and health care. • Be sensitive to the uniqueness of the patient. • Identify sources of discrepancy between the patient's and your own concepts of health and illness. • Communicate at the patient's personal level of functioning. • Evaluate effectiveness of nursing actions and modify nursing care plan when necessary.
Modify communication approaches to meet cultural needs.	• Be attentive to signs of fear, anxiety, and confusion in the patient. • Respond in a reassuring manner in keeping with the patient's cultural orientation. • Be aware that in some cultural groups discussion concerning the patient with others may be offensive and may impede the nursing process.
Understand that respect for the patient and communicated needs are central to the therapeutic relationship.	• Communicate respect by using a kind and attentive approach. • Learn how listening is communicated in the patient's culture. • Use appropriate active listening techniques. • Adopt an attitude of flexibility, respect, and interest to help bridge barriers imposed by culture.
Communicate in a nonthreatening manner.	• Conduct the interview in an unhurried manner. • Follow acceptable social and cultural amenities. • Ask general questions during the information-gathering stage. • Be patient with a respondent who gives information that may seem unrelated to the patient's health problem. • Develop a trusting relationship by listening carefully, allowing time, and giving the patient your full attention.
Use validating techniques in communication.	• Be alert for feedback that the patient is not understanding. • Do not assume meaning is interpreted without distortion.
Be considerate of reluctance to talk when the subject involves sexual matters.	• Be aware that in some cultures sexual matters are not discussed freely with members of the opposite sex.
Adopt special approaches when the patient speaks a different language.	• Use a caring tone of voice and facial expression to help alleviate the patient's fears. • Speak slowly and distinctly, but not loudly. • Use gestures, pictures, and play acting to help the patient understand. • Repeat the message in different ways if necessary. • Be alert to words the patient seems to understand and use them frequently. • Keep messages simple and repeat them frequently. • Avoid using medical terms and abbreviations that the patient may not understand. • Use an appropriate language dictionary.
Use interpreters to improve communication.	• Ask the interpreter to translate the message, not just the individual words. • Obtain feedback to confirm understanding. • Use an interpreter who is culturally sensitive.

Reprinted with permission from Giger JN, Davidhizar RE: Communication, in Giger JN, Davidhizar RE (eds): *Transcultural Nursing: Assessment and Intervention* (ed 3). St Louis, Mosby-Year Book, 1999, pp 21–43.[20]

which they are currently engaged than about planning ahead to be on time. The present-oriented perspective is that time is flexible and that events will begin when the person arrives.[4]

Environmental control

Environmental control refers to the ability of members of a particular cultural group to plan activities that control nature or direct environmental factors. Because health is a balance between the individual and the environment, beliefs about causes of illness, health behaviors, and actions taken when illness or disease occur are all influenced by our perception of the environment. This perception is in turn influenced by our culture.

Herberg describes three health belief views: magicoreligious, scientific, and holistic.[18]

- *Magicoreligious health belief view:* Health and illness are controlled by supernatural forces. Therefore, illness is seen as the result of being bad or of opposing God's will. Thus, getting well also may be viewed as being dependent on God's will. Some cultures believe magic can cause illness.

- *Scientific or biomedical health belief view:* Life and life processes are controlled by physical and biochemical processes that can be manipulated by humans.

- *Holistic health belief view:* The forces of nature must be in balance or harmony. When the natural balance is disturbed, illness results.

Folk medicine is defined as those beliefs and practices relating to illness, prevention, and health that derive from cultural traditions rather than from modern medicine's scientific base. Folk medicine is thought to be more humanistic. The consultation and treatment take place in the community of the recipient, often in the home of the healer. The healer typically prepares the treatment and, frequently, either the healer or the patient performs some ritual practice. Because folk healing is culturally based, patients often find it more comfortable and less frightening than traditional Western medicine.

Biological variations

Biological variations include differences in skin, eye, and hair color; facial characteristics; the amount of body hair; and body size and shape. Enzymatic and genetic variations may result in differences in the metabolism of drugs such as isoniazid, succinylcholine, caffeine, antihypertensives, and psychotropic drugs. Alcohol metabolism differs in European Americans and Asians because of different levels of the enzymes necessary for alcohol metabolism. The result in Asians is often facial flushing and palpitations after alcohol ingestion.

Some cultural groups are more susceptible to certain diseases. The increased or decreased incidence of a particular disease may be genetically determined. Nutritional preferences may also predispose certain cultural groups to particular diseases. Foods in various cultures have different status. For example, beef and lobster are considered high status in the United States. In many Native American tribes, corn is considered a status food.

Table 7-5 outlines a brief cultural assessment tool based on the Transcultural Assessment Model, which the nurse will find useful in gathering cultural data on patients and families.

Heritage Consistency

People tend to assume the characteristics of the dominant culture where they reside via schools, television, radio, and motion pictures. The values and beliefs of a Vietnamese adolescent raised in the United States may be less traditional than his parents who immigrated to the United States. The heritage consistency theory views acculturation on a continuum and aids in assessing the degree to which people identify with the dominant or traditional cultures. It is possible to assess health beliefs by determining an individual's ties to traditional beliefs and his or her stage of acculturation. A relationship exists between strong personal identity with either a person's heritage or his or her level of acculturation, and the individual's health beliefs.

Ethnicity and Cancer

Spector has summarized data for four major ethnic minority groups using the six cultural phenomena of the Transcultural Assessment Model (Table 7-6).[4,25] In this section, the impact of ethnicity on responses to the cancer experience is explored. For each of the four major ethnic groups, information about health beliefs and practices, healing practices, social organization, communication, space and time, death and dying, and biologic variations is presented. However, recall that this information provides only a guideline for practice; each person is culturally unique. Nursing interventions that consider the patient and family's cultural background must be based on a sound assessment and validation of the role culture plays in the life of the patient and family.

There are many subgroups within the four major ethnic groups (black, API, Hispanic, and Native American); however, it is beyond the scope of this chapter to provide an in-depth description of each subgroup's cultural beliefs and practices. Instead, relevant group characteristics regarding the cancer experience are presented. Various sources are available that further explore the individual subgroups.[26–33]

Blacks

Most blacks were brought to the United States as slaves between 1619 and 1860 from the west coast of Africa.

Table 7-5 Cultural Assessment Tool

Culturally unique individual	• Does the patient identify with a particular ethnic/racial/cultural group? • Where was the patient born? • How long has the patient lived in this country?
Communication	• What language is spoken? • Can the patient communicate in English? If yes, both spoken and written? • Does the patient speak for self or defer to another? • What nonverbal communication behaviors are observed (e.g., touching, eye contact)? What significance do these behaviors have for the nurse-patient interaction?
Space	• Observe the patient's proximity to other people and objects within the environment. • How does the patient react to the nurse's movement toward the patient? • Assess the patient's physical environment (especially important in home health nursing, community nursing, and long-term care nursing). • What cultural objects within the environment have importance for health promotion/health maintenance?
Social organization	• What are the patient's roles? Is the patient the primary decision-maker for health care behaviors? • Must the patient consult another to make health decisions? If yes, who? • What other family members are important to the patient's decision making? • Are there cultural or religious leaders who are important in the client's health decision making? • Is there a religious affiliation linked with cultural affiliation (e.g., Jewish, Latino Catholic)?
Time	• What is the patient's time orientation: past, present, or future? • What is the significance of time for the patient? • Does the patient talk about time in specifics, such as dates or times, or in generalities, such as "a long time" or "a short time"?
Environmental control	• How is health defined by the culture? • What does the patient believe to be the cause of the illness or health concern? • Has the patient used the services of cultural healers? • What healing practices has the patient used? Have folk healing behaviors been used? • Is the patient wearing or carrying any amulets or artifacts that are believed to have healing properties?
Biological variations	• Are there normal variations in anatomic characteristics (e.g., body structure or size, skin color, facial characteristics)? • What are the dietary preferences of the patient? Are the dietary preferences related to the patient's ethnicity? • Is the patient at risk for nutritional deficiencies because of ethnicity (e.g., pernicious anemia, lactose intolerance)? • Are there variations in physiologic functioning related to the patient's ethnicity or race (e.g., drug metabolism, alcohol metabolism)? • Are there illnesses or diseases that the patient is at risk for because of ethnicity or race (e.g., hypertension, diabetes mellitus, sickle-cell anemia)?

Reprinted with permission from *Fundamentals of Nursing,* Fifth Edition, by Barbara Kozier, Glenora Erb, and Kathleen Blais. Copyright © 1995 by Addison-Wesley Publishing Company.[21]

Many blacks have also immigrated to the United States from other African countries, the West Indies, the Dominican Republic, Haiti, and Jamaica.[4] Blacks constitute about one-tenth of the total U.S. population but are disproportionately represented among the poor. They represent about one-third of the population below poverty level, and one-fourth are unemployed. Individuals in a lower socioeconomic group are at greater risk for illness because seeking health care for early symptoms and preventive care generally are not priorities for those who struggle with day-to-day survival.

Many blacks worked or continue to work in occupations that place them at risk for certain cancers. Blacks were employed disproportionately in jobs involving coke ovens with greatest exposure to benzo[*a*]pyrene and other carcinogens. Years later, these workers had ten times the lung cancer rates, elevated skin cancer rates, and increased nonmalignant lung diseases. Compared to other races, more blacks worked in the rubber industry and developed increased rates of stomach, lung, blood, bladder, lymphatic, and prostate cancers.[34]

Health beliefs and practices

The health beliefs of blacks include a tendency to categorize events as either desirable or undesirable. Illness is just another undesirable event along with bad luck, poverty, and unemployment. Some believe illness results from their failure to live according to or to accept God's will. An individual may believe that cancer is an unnatural illness, caused by supernatural or sinful behavior, and that it cannot be treated by Western medicine.

For blacks, there is a strong relationship between faith and healing. All blessings come from God, and only God can heal the sick. Illness may be perceived as a natural occurrence resulting from disharmony and conflict in some aspect of an individual's life, generally falling into one of three main areas: divine punishment, impaired

Table 7-6   Cross-Cultural Examples of Cultural Phenomena That Have an Impact on Nursing Care

Nations of Origin	Environmental Control	Biological Variations*	Social Organization	Communication	Space	Time Orientation
Asian China Hawaii Philippines Korea Japan Southeast Asia (Laos, Cambodia, Vietnam)	Traditional health and illness beliefs Use of traditional medicines Traditional practitioners: Chinese doctors and herbalists	Liver cancer Stomach cancer Coccidioidomycosis Hypertension Lactose intolerance	Family: hierarchical structure, loyalty Devotion to tradition Many religions, including Taoism, Buddhism, Islam, and Christianity Community social organizations	National language preference Dialects, written characters Use of silence Nonverbal and contextual cuing	Noncontact	Present
African West Coast (as slaves) Many African countries West Indian Islands Dominican Republic Haiti Jamaica	Traditional health and illness beliefs Folk medicine tradition Traditional healer: root-worker	Sickle cell anemia Hypertension Cancer of the esophagus Stomach cancer Coccidioidomycosis Lactose intolerance	Family: many female, single parent Large, extended family networks Strong church affiliation within community Community social organizations	National languages Dialect: Pidgin, Creole, Spanish, and French	Close personal space	Present over future
Europe Germany England Italy Ireland Other European countries	Primary reliance on modern health care system Traditional health and illness beliefs Some remaining folk medicine tradition	Breast cancer Heart disease Diabetes mellitus Thalassemia	Nuclear families Extended families Judeo-Christian religions Community social organizations	National languages Many learn English immediately	Noncontact Aloof Distant Southern countries: closer contact and touch	Future over present
Native American 170 Native American Tribes Aleuts Eskimos	Traditional health and illness beliefs Folk medicine tradition Traditional healer: medicine man	Accidents Heart disease Cirrhosis of the liver Diabetes mellitus	Extremely family oriented Biological and extended families Children taught to respect traditions Community social organizations	Tribal languages Use of silence and body language	Space very important and has no boundaries	Present
Hispanic countries Spain Cuba Mexico Central and South America	Traditional health and illness beliefs Folk medicine tradition Traditional healers: *Curandero, Espiritista, Partera, Senora*	Diabetes mellitus Parasites Coccidioidomycosis Lactose intolerance	Nuclear family Extended families Compadrazgo: godparents Community social organizations	Spanish or Portuguese primary language	Tactile relationships Touch Handshakes Embracing Value physical presence	Present

*Indicates a high morbidity incidence

Adapted with permission from Spector RE: Cultural Diversity, in Potter PA, Perry AG (eds): *Fundamentals of Nursing: Concepts, Process, and Practice* (ed 4). St. Louis, Mosby-Year Book, 1997, pp 351–369. Modified from Giger JN, Davidhizar Re: *Transcultural nursing assessment and intervention* (ed 2). St. Louis, 1995, Mosby.[4]

social relationships, and environmental hazards. Divine punishment attributes illness to sin. An example of an impaired social relationship may be a spouse leaving or parents disowning a child. Environmental hazards include being struck by lightning or bitten by a snake.

Another belief among some blacks is that everything has an opposite. For every birth, there is a death; for every marriage, there is a divorce. Some may not distinguish between physical and mental illness and spiritual problems and may present themselves for treatment with a combination of somatic, psychological, and spiritual complaints. The nurse must acknowledge the patient's health belief system if the nurse expects the patient to participate in Western practices. Some blacks may respond to pain stoically out of a desire to be a perfect patient; others may view pain as God's will.

Blacks tend to be less knowledgeable about cancer than whites. They are less likely to see a physician when experiencing warning signs or symptoms and are less aware of the benefits of specific cancer screening methods. Blacks are often more fatalistic about cancer and are less likely to believe that early detection or treatment can make a difference in the outcome of the disease. These factors lead to diagnosis at a later stage of illness, a poorer prognosis, and higher mortality rates for cancer.[35]

Blacks are more likely than whites to prefer to remain ignorant of their own cancer diagnosis. They are also less likely than whites to regard surgery, chemotherapy, and radiation as effective cancer treatment measures and are less optimistic about the chances of surviving cancer. In one study, 64% of blacks believed that cancer was a death sentence, and 65% believed that treatment is worse than the disease. Eighty percent believed that cancer was spread by surgical treatment, and 20% indicated that they would rather not know that they had cancer.[36] Thus, nurses may find black patients unwilling, uncooperative, or what may appear to be noncompliant, partners in their treatment.[35]

Black attitudes about the U.S. health care system may be explained partially by history. During slavery, blacks received inconsistent and often barbaric health care treatment and developed a deep mistrust of their white master and his harsh remedies and prescriptions. Even after slavery was abolished, blacks often received poor health care and inferior treatment in hospitals and clinics, which only served to reinforce their negative view of Western medicine, and led to a high level of caution and mistrust.[37] Blacks may choose not to seek care if they perceive that their values will be compromised. To work effectively with black patients and families, the nurse will need to convey caring and understanding.

Healing practices

Different folk healers are used by some blacks. These healers are well-respected individuals and can be powerful resources for the health care team. The healers understand the beliefs and needs of the people they serve. Symptoms may be of minor importance. Cure may involve self-treatment, consultation with a neighbor knowledgeable in home remedies, a physician, or someone regarded to have unusual powers. Religion is incorporated as part of therapy and is a means to a cure. There is a lay referral system that services the health needs of the community, and determines whether Western practitioners can be trusted and incorporated into the treatment. Openness, acceptance, and cooperation with this referral system by health care professionals may enhance acceptance and use of Western health care providers by blacks.

Help may be sought from the "old lady," a woman in the community who acts as a local consultant. She is knowledgeable about different home remedies made from spices, herbs, and roots used to treat common illnesses. She also gives advice and makes appropriate referrals to another type of practitioner when an illness or a particular medical condition extends beyond her practice.[37] The spiritualist has received the gift from God for healing incurable diseases or solving personal problems. This practitioner combines rituals, spiritual beliefs, and herbal medicines and is the most prevalent and diverse type of folk practitioner. There is a root doctor who meets the needs for herbs, oils, candles, and ointments. The Voodoo priest/priestess may inherit this title only by birthright and is perceived to have a special gift. Voodoo, which combines African, Christian, and magical beliefs related to religion and health care, is practiced by some blacks. It is believed to cause, as well as prevent, the action of malevolent forces. Awareness of what home remedies have been used would help the nurse understand cultural practices and determine whether the remedies are helpful, harmful, or neutral.[35,38]

A treatment plan that is congruent with the patient's own beliefs has a better chance of being successful. Cultural health practices that are helpful should be encouraged. For example, use of herbal teas in place of water can serve both traditional and Western practices.

Social organization

The history of slavery likely contributes to the large number of female-headed households among blacks today. The number of female-headed households has doubled between 1950 and 1991 to represent 46% of all black families.[39] Thus, the wife or mother generally is charged with the responsibility for protecting the health of family members. Family members may enter the health care system at the advice of the matriarch of the family. The importance of the black woman in sharing information and helping the patient in decision making is important for the nurse to recognize.[38]

Some families have large social networks that are very supportive during times of illness. The added numbers may be helpful in provision of care and support but also may delay seeking help outside the network while consultation among the various members takes place. Including the members of the network in planning care may decrease the possibility of conflicting messages between the nurse and members of the network.[38]

The church plays an important role in the lives of blacks by championing their interests and providing tangible assistance during periods of economic and social instability. The church is also a source of social identity and allows escape from the harsh realities of life. It promotes self-esteem among its membership and serves as a curator for maintaining the cultures of many blacks. Given the importance of the church in the lives of many blacks, inclusion of the clergy in the health care team may be very helpful.

Communication

The dialect that is spoken by many blacks is sufficiently different from standard English in pronunciation, grammar, and syntax as to be classified as "black English." The use of standard English versus black English varies among blacks and is sometimes related to educational level and socioeconomic status. Black English is a unifying factor for blacks in maintaining their cultural and ethnic identity. It is not uncommon for some blacks to speak standard English when in a professional capacity or when socializing with whites and then revert to black English when in black settings. Some blacks who have not mastered standard English may become very quiet in settings in which they believe that standard English is required. This may be incorrectly interpreted as hostility, submissiveness, or agreement.[38]

For more effective communication, the nurse who works with blacks must understand as much of the context of the dialect as possible. Viewing black English as an unacceptable form of English may lead to labeling and stereotyping the patient. Chiding and correcting the speech of blacks may result in the patient becoming quiet, passive, aggressive, or hostile. On the other hand, attempting to use words common to the patient's vocabulary and mimicking the language may be interpreted as dehumanizing.

Slang also is used and may have different meanings among individuals and among cultural groups. Using words commonly understood by blacks in place of more sophisticated medical terms might make the patient more receptive to teaching and more cooperative. Examples of such words include "miseries" for pain, "tired or low blood" for anemia, "throw up" for vomit, and "pass water, tinkle, or peepee" for urinate.

When working with black patients, keep in mind that eye contact, nodding, and smiling do not necessarily mean that the black patient is paying attention. Validation of the message is very important in improving communication. Nurses may find it difficult to communicate with black patients who speak loudly and seem hostile and aggressive. However, it is the expressive quality of black English that is often responsible for this behavior.[40]

Space and time

Many blacks have a "today" or "present" health orientation, and their approach to the prevention of cancer may be to work out problems as they occur, rather than trying to prevent them from occurring. This approach is based on the belief that planning for the future is hopeless and is based on previous experiences with racism and discrimination.[41] In planning nursing care for individuals with such time orientation, explain when flexibility of time is acceptable and when a delay might result in a serious problem. Acceptance of lateness in appointments is helpful when possible.

Blacks are highly involved people who tend to have several activities going on at the same time. This may create conflict for the nurse, who, in an effort to complete nursing care, often may be interrupted by these activities. Negotiating with the patient and family to meet the needs of both the nurse and the patient may be helpful.

Death and dying issues

In the African language the primary time frames are past and present. No word exists for the distant future, as it has not yet happened. Consequently the future and the past are merged into the present. Life is viewed as cyclical in nature, and all events are given by God. Death is a natural part of the cycle of life and is unavoidable. It is familiar and near and evokes no great fear or awe.[42]

The strong family network of blacks is called into action when a family member is seriously ill. Care of the terminally ill is a public rather than a private undertaking, with neighbors and friends sharing resources. The family develops plans for the care of the patient, identifies tasks, and assigns family members to assume them. The home is usually viewed as the place for the ill person to spend his/her final days. Frequent visitors are common. The patient generally remains an active and vital force within the family until he or she can no longer do so. The decision as to whether to inform the patient of terminal illness is made on an individual basis.[42]

It is not uncommon for blacks to plan their funerals and purchase grave plots long before their own deaths. Public and communal grief are openly expressed at traditional black funerals, which are termed "home-goings." People in the congregation respond spontaneously and out loud to the sermon. There is a gradual increase in emotion as the funeral progresses, and many of those attending express deep emotion. Music provides a means of sending the deceased joyfully on to the next leg of his or her journey.[21,42,43]

Biological variations

A major biological variation in blacks is skin color. There is great variation in the darkness of skin color, and those who are fairer-skinned have a greater risk for developing skin cancers from sun exposure. A darker skin color makes the assessment of pallor, jaundice, ecchymosis, or erythema more difficult. Assessing areas of lighter melanin pigmentation such as the sclera, conjunctiva, soles of feet, and palms of the hands may be useful. The diet of many blacks contains little fresh produce, is highly seasoned, and includes frequent use of smoked and fatty meats as seasoning for vegetables and soups. Pork is often a staple meat. Thus, saturated fat intake may be high. In comparison to white women, black women are more likely to be obese, while black men are more likely to be underweight. The eating habits and compromised nutritional status of blacks could be a factor in the higher incidence and mortality rates from cancer.[35]

Lactose intolerance affects 75% of blacks. They lack the enzyme to convert lactose to glucose and galactose, resulting in gastrointestinal symptoms of bloating, cramping, and diarrhea after the ingestion of milk and other products containing lactose. The intolerance tends to occur primarily in infancy shortly after weaning and in the teen years or early twenties. Treatment is to avoid milk products. As milk products are often suggested to improve nutrition for patients with cancer, awareness of possible lactose intolerance in the black population is significant for the nurse in patient and family teaching.[38]

Alcoholism is a major health problem in the black community and a risk factor for cancers of the mouth, larynx, tongue, esophagus, lung, and liver. The factors associated with alcohol abuse include unemployment, the availability of the substance, peer pressure, escape from personal problems, and the prevalence of taverns as social centers in black communities. Thus, the causes are complex social issues and difficult to treat.[44]

Asian/Pacific Islanders

Asian/Pacific Islanders are the fastest growing ethnic minority group in the United States. A very heterogeneous group, API are composed of individuals "originating from 28 Asian countries and 25 identified Pacific Island cultures."[8] This marked ethnic diversity is further compounded by inherent variations within each subgroup, such as degree of acculturation and socioeconomic status. It was estimated in 1990 that approximately 74% of the total API population were foreign-born and were recent immigrants and refugees. Many have good incomes but approximately one out of eight API live in poverty. Similarly, many API have a college degree or postgraduate education, but there is a significant number who are functionally illiterate.[8,45]

Because approximately 95% of API are Asian Americans compared with 5% who are Pacific Islander Americans;[8] this discussion primarily addresses Asian Americans.

Health beliefs and practices

Common among API are the traditional health beliefs and practices that are carried out in varying degrees within each group. Nevertheless, because of the common influence of Chinese culture, there is much similarity in beliefs and practices among Asian groups. For example, one of the most common beliefs is that health is a state of harmony in body, mind, and spirit with nature and the universe.[4] Although native Hawaiians are not of Asian descent, harmony with nature is also an important health belief in this culture.[46]

Many API believe that a balance between hot and cold elements is essential for good health. In the Chinese, Japanese, and Korean cultures, in particular, this balance is defined as yin (cold) and yang (hot).[47–51] Yin and yang are life forces in which *yin* (cold) is characterized as female, dark, negative energy, and *yang* (hot) is male, light, positive energy. Illness is believed to result from an imbalance of these two forces. The Chinese believe that the human body, illnesses, and foods possess yin or yang characteristics, and treatment is aimed at reestablishing the balance.[48,49,52–54] For example, cancer is a yin or cold illness and would be treated with foods, herbs, and healing ceremonies that possess "hot" properties. The Filipino,[55] East Indian,[56] and Southeast Asian cultures[57,58] also have similar beliefs in hot and cold balance and health. Other explanations for illness include an imbalance of humoral elements, an obstruction of *chi* (an essential life energy), a curse by a spirit, spiritual imbalance, punishment for immoral behavior, or an imbalance in the body caused by exposure to wind or air.[48,56,59–61]

There exists a widespread belief among some API groups that suffering is part of life, a philosophy that may result in postponement in seeking medical treatment, either traditional or Western.[8,60] Fatalism is found in the Filipino culture where the attitude of *bahala na*—"It's in the hands of God"—exists, especially when illness and pain are seen as punishment.[61,62] In the Japanese culture, the term *shoganai* is used when misfortune strikes, such as an illness. Its translation, "It can't be helped," reflects an almost fatalistic view. Chinese Americans also have a fatalistic outlook on life in their belief that they lack control over nature.[49]

Many API believe that blood is a life force that cannot be replaced or, if taken, will disrupt the body's balance, causing weakness and even death.[56–58] Therefore, many API fear venipunctures. The Hmong may be reluctant to receive blood transfusions because their perception is that the donor's spirit may enter their body via the transfusion.[57] The Chinese and Vietnamese may not agree to surgery when organs or body parts are to be removed because of their belief that the human body must be intact at the time of death to avoid potential adverse consequences in the afterlife.[58,63] The Vietnamese also avoid surgery since it is perceived as a last resort and associated with death.[58] The Hmong may refuse surgery because of their belief that cutting into the body releases spirits, causing an imbalance.[57]

Healing practices

Included in their traditional health beliefs, API practice the use of herbal medications, seek traditional healers, and perform healing ceremonies. Because API often use herbal preparations concurrently with Western medicine, it is important to ascertain if, and what, herbal preparations are being used in order to anticipate possible drug interactions. For example, *ma huang* is a Chinese herb that contains ephedrine. Complications can arise if, in addition to the *ma huang,* the patient takes ephedrine via a Western practitioner's prescription.[63] Ginseng, another popular herb, is considered a stimulant and has hypertensive effects. Undesirable side effects can result if the patient takes ginseng in conjunction with Western antihypertensive medication.[49]

Traditional healers among API include shamans (Laotian, Hmong), Chinese herbalists, *kahuna la'au lapa'au* (native Hawaiian), and *Hilot* (Filipino). These healers are often consulted before Western medical practitioners. In some cases, the perceived cause of the illness determines who is consulted first. For example, if southeast Asians believe that an illness is organic in origin, they may seek a Western physician. However, if the cause of illness is thought to be supernatural, a traditional healer would be consulted. If the illness persists after consulting with traditional healers, then Western treatment might be sought.[60] At this point, however, the disease may be at an advanced stage and untreatable. Then, because Western medicine cannot cure the illness, it is seen as ineffective. This may reinforce the use of traditional healers. For many API, the Western health care system is foreign. There is comfort in consulting a healer who understands, with whom one can communicate, and whose practice is familiar to the patient. Additionally, healers are inexpensive and have a reputation for being effective for specific conditions.

Healing ceremonies or practices vary considerably across API groups. In the native Hawaiian culture, healing includes special rituals, prayers, and chants as well as the use of special herbs and plants.[64] Some other practices include moxibustion, cupping, acupuncture, massage, and skin scraping or coining.[49,54,59]

Moxibustion. This treatment, used to restore the yin-yang balance, involves a deeply penetrating heat. Small pellets or cones made of the herb *Artemesis vulgaris* (moxa) are placed at acupuncture points on the body and are then burned. The pellets or cones are removed when the patient feels the heat. This treatment leaves small, rounded or asymmetrical superficial burn marks. It is used in the treatment of ailments of the joints, muscles, bones, and back.[49,50]

Cupping. Like moxibustion, cupping uses heat but in a different fashion. A material, such as alcohol-soaked cotton, is placed in a special cup and set on fire to create a vacuum in the cup. When the flame is extinguished, the cup is then placed immediately on the treatment area of the body where suction is created. The cup is kept there for 15–20 minutes or until it is easily removed. Cupping is used to treat pain, body aches, and headaches. It is a painful procedure that leaves circular burn marks approximately 2 inches in diameter. These burn marks have been misinterpreted as child abuse in southeast Asian children who have been treated with cupping.[54,65]

Skin scraping or coining This treatment involves the application of a special menthol oil or ointment to the symptomatic area. With the edge of a coin, the area is then rubbed in a firm, downward motion.[48] This procedure is used to treat colds, heatstroke, headache, pain, vomiting, and indigestion.[65]

Social organization

Asian/Pacific Islanders have very strong, family-centered systems.[49,62,66] The family exerts an extremely powerful force in an individual's life, and the needs of the individual are often secondary to those of the larger group.[67,68] Health care decisions are often made by the family or social network.

In many API groups, patrilineal authority along with filial piety and respect for elders often means that the eldest son or male head of the clan is the spokesperson for the patient.[69] This individual is the designated family spokesperson with whom medical practitioners speak when information about the patient's condition is given or when treatment decisions need to be made.

Because of the strong value placed on the family, API family members are more likely to actively participate in the patient's daily care. Health care professionals need to be sensitive to these cultural needs and also must support the family to prevent caregiver exhaustion, especially if one family member is the sole caregiver.

Communication

In many API groups, communication patterns are influenced by values that emphasize politeness, respect for authority, and avoidance of shame. These values prevent many API from asking health professionals questions or challenging a proposed diagnostic workup or treatment plan.[53,60,62,67] Instead, an individual may nod his or her head, in what is interpreted as agreement. However, the patient may not necessarily agree or understand what the practitioner has said.[43,57] Thus, poor communication can occur between the API and the Western practitioner.

In communicating with some API groups, Western practitioners may need to avoid or limit engaging in direct eye contact, as such eye contact may be perceived as being rude, challenging, or just culturally unacceptable.[57,58,70] For example, in the Filipino culture, direct eye contact between an older man and a young woman usually implies seduction or anger.[62,66] In the East Indian culture, eye contact between a woman and a man other than her husband can have sexual significance.[71] Avoiding eye contact by the South Vietnamese is a sign of respect when talking with someone perceived to be of different rank in education, social status, age, or gender.[58]

Many API prefer limited or no physical contact.[49,58,67] In some API groups, the head is sacred and touching or patting the head is perceived as a rude gesture.[49,57] For some southeast Asians, crossing the legs and pointing the foot at the individual is also considered to be insulting.[60] Similarly, directing the sole of the shoe or foot toward Koreans is offensive to them.[70]

Many API do not speak English or have limited proficiency in English as their second language. Because of this language barrier, interpreters are often used. However, communication via a third party presents challenges in ensuring that the literal meaning of the conversation is translated correctly, along with the interpretation of nonverbal messages. When possible, use professional interpreters who can facilitate and ensure communication among the patient, family, and health professional.

In selecting an interpreter, first ascertain the specific dialect spoken by the patient and family. For example, there are several dialects spoken by Filipinos including Visayan, Tagalog, Ilocano, or Cebuano. Family interpreters are often used; however, the message relayed may not always be accurate.[72] For example, if the message is regarding a poor prognosis, the family member may modify it in an attempt to protect the patient. In addition, if interpreters are of the opposite sex, patients may not bring up symptoms or concerns that they perceive to be either embarrassing or culturally unacceptable to discuss in the presence of the opposite sex. The traditional hierarchy in many API families where power and influence run from elders to youths is another potential pitfall when using family interpreters. In some instances, especially with recent immigrants, children may be used as interpreters because they usually have a better command of English. However, this reverses the rank of the child in the family and may put undue stress on the family.[56,73]

Space and time

Asian/Pacific Islanders value privacy, and many are also very modest.[48,57,62,74] When physical examinations or procedures necessitate exposure of the body, exposure should be minimized by revealing only that part of the body that needs to be examined. Female API patients, such as East Indian and Chinese women, may feel more comfortable being examined by female practitioners.[56,75,76]

The concept of time varies among API groups. For example, the Japanese, who are present and future oriented, are usually prompt and adhere to fixed schedules.[67] On the other hand, Chinese are more present oriented, do not necessarily adhere to fixed schedules, and may be late for appointments.[49] Filipinos are past and present oriented and may disregard health-related matters. This time orientation is closely linked to their *bahala na* philosophy of leaving things in God's hands.[66]

Death and dying issues

There are many issues regarding death and dying in API groups. Bioethics, truth telling, patient's right to know, and advance directive decisions are based in Western culture. It is important to be aware that patient autonomy and self-determination in API groups may not be culturally acceptable or valued. As previously discussed, the family or family spokesperson frequently makes decisions about the patient's care rather than the patient.

The initiation and continuation of life-support measures also may vary from group to group. For example,

many Filipinos are Catholic and may view discontinuing life support as morally wrong.[69] A similar viewpoint is shared by many Koreans who consider stopping life support as interfering with God's will; however, the initiation of life support does not.[69]

Conflict may arise between the value in Western medicine of open disclosure of a terminal illness and the value shared by many API groups that "to tell someone he or she is dying is not only rude but dangerous."[77,p.325] For example, East Indians prefer not to tell patients the seriousness of their condition or the possibility of death. They believe that "speaking of possibilities may render them too real, and a traditional Indian does not speak lightly of death; . . . if a patient knows the gravity of the illness, he or she will give up hope and die."[56,p.269] This is also seen in the Hmong culture where the disclosure of prognosis to a terminally ill patient "is the same as wishing death upon that person and may in fact bring about that person's death."[78,p.426] Muller and Desmond further note that in many Asian groups,

> People fear that openly acknowledging an impending death is like casting a death curse upon the person; it will make the person despair and die even sooner. Thus, to engage in discussions of code status or the possibility of hospice care, interventions that can be seen as explicit preparation for death, is courting bad luck.[77,p.325]

On the other hand, although hospice care discussions may not always be encouraged, some APIs prefer to die at home rather than in the hospital.[63,69,70] This preference is due, in large part, to the value placed on the family and

> The belief that the unfortunate who die among strangers and away from their familiar dwelling are forever condemned to wander in pain, so-called orphan souls, endlessly searching in vain for the family and home they missed when they died.[79,p.24]

With the potential for conflict and frustration between the values of Western health care and the cultural values of various API groups, exploring life-support decisions with the patient and family is critical. Klessig suggests that information about the following be determined: sanctity of life, definition of death, religious background and extent of involvement, beliefs of causal agents in illness and how they relate to the dying process, social support system, and the family's decision maker.[69,p.321]

By facilitating communication about these issues between the patient and family and the health care team, oncology nurses can assist in narrowing the gap between these two value systems and support the patient and family through this phase of the cancer experience.

Biological variations

The incidence rate for liver cancer is exceptionally high in API groups, particularly the southeast Asian groups. This increased rate for liver cancer is linked to the high incidence of hepatitis B infection, largely due to the fact that these groups originate from areas where hepatitis B is endemic.

Japanese, Koreans, and Vietnamese all have high rates of stomach cancer.[14,47] This is attributed in part to genetic factors as well as to environmental factors, including the high ingestion of sodium, hot and spicy foods, and nitrates.[47]

Lactose intolerance is also common in API. Milk and cheese, common foods in the mainstream American diet, may therefore be unacceptable to this group. When providing oral supplements that are nonmilk containing but have the appearance of a milk product, the patient and family must be reassured that the supplement is not a milk product.

The physical characteristics of API may necessitate adjusting the dosage of certain medications. For example, Zhou et al reported that in Chinese men, the propranolol dose may need to be decreased due to the greater sensitivity among Chinese to the effects of propranolol on heart rate and blood pressure when compared to whites.[80] The exact mechanism for these effects has not been determined; however, decreased protein binding may play a role.

Many API also have the distinguishing yellow cast to their skin that ranges in tone. This yellow cast can make the recognition of jaundice more challenging. In order to assess for jaundice, the sclera and excreta need to be checked.

Although not a biological variation, the higher smoking rates among southeast Asian men as compared to the general population deserves mention.[8] This is a prime area for health promotion activities. Another area of concern is that API had the lowest self-reported rates for Pap tests within the past 2 years and for mammography and clinical breast exams.[81] Possible reasons for this low participation rate include lack of health education programs targeted specifically at this group, fatalism belief, and decreased access to health care.

Hispanics

Hispanics, in general, identify themselves as members of the same ethnic group—not by demographic characteristics but by their cultural values and language. *Hispanic* is the term that has been used by the U.S. federal government to classify individuals who claim ties to Spain in their heritage. The term *Latino* includes all Latin American individuals and describes immigrants from those Spanish-speaking countries where the integration of Spanish, indigenous people, and Africans has occurred. Whether an individual prefers to be called Hispanic or Latino is generally a matter of choice. Some have strong opinions; others do not. It may be helpful to use the name of the country of origin when referring to individuals or to a specific ethnic group. *Chicano* is another term used when discussing Hispanics, and it refers to all Americans of Mexican descent.

Generally, the cancer incidence rate among Hispanics ranks at the median when compared to other ethnic groups. The largest concentrated population of Hispanics in the United States lives in Los Angeles. In this group, there is a high risk of gallbladder, cervical, and stomach cancers; an intermediate risk of pancreatic and prostate cancers; and a low risk of melanoma and colorectal, lung, and reproductive cancers.[82]

There appears to be a genetic predisposition for and higher incidence of gallbladder cancer among Hispanic men and women in New Mexico. A similar pattern was found for biliary cancer in Hispanics in Los Angeles County.[83,84] Liver cancer rates after the age of 50 in Hispanic males and females increases dramatically.[85] A 1986 study found that Hispanic women with cervical cancer were younger, less educated, and had fewer sexual partners than white women with cervical cancer but were younger when they first had sex and had more children. They also had fewer visits to physicians and fewer Pap tests. These results may account for the advanced disease at diagnosis and the increased cervical cancer rates recorded.[86] Although the incidence rate of breast cancer is low, the mortality rate is high for Hispanic women. Cultural factors are thought to be responsible for delays in seeking health care and for larger, more advanced tumors at diagnosis of breast cancer in Hispanic women.[87]

Hispanic men and women are about two and half times more likely to report having no health insurance. This may be the result of the large number of Hispanics who are farm workers or in service occupations where health insurance is not a regular benefit. Interestingly, Hispanic women are as likely as non-Hispanic women to have had a recent Pap smear, mammogram, or a clinical breast exam. Chronic alcohol consumption and obesity are similar in Hispanic and non-Hispanic groups.[88-90]

Health beliefs and practices

For Hispanics, health often is believed to be the result of good luck or a reward from God for good behavior. The concept that a disease is God's will is widely accepted. Terminal illnesses especially are seen as the result of some indiscretion against God. Thus, health and illness in Hispanic groups have a strong religious association.

There is often a fatalistic belief that one is at the mercy of the environment and has little control over what happens. Personal efforts are unlikely to influence the outcome of a situation. Thus, Hispanics often do not believe that they are personally responsible for present or future successes or failures with regard to their health and otherwise.[91]

There are several categories of disease in the Hispanic culture. The concept of hot and cold imbalance resembles yin and yang in the Chinese culture. To ensure good health, it is believed that individuals must ingest both hot and cold foods.[92] Internal factors such as a change in body temperature and external factors such as the foods eaten can affect the hot-cold balance. Many of the disorders caused by hot and cold imbalances are digestive in nature. A stomach ulcer is a "hot illness" caused by eating too much hot food. Excesses of heat developed from within the body and extending outward are believed to be related to cancer, rheumatism, tuberculosis, and paralysis.

Another group of illnesses is believed to be caused by magical interventions. *Mal ojo,* or "evil eye," occurs when someone with a powerful glance looks improperly at a child; this is believed to be a manifestation of witchcraft and, as a result, the child is said to be affected by evil spirits. Treatment is a ceremonial ritual that includes passing an egg over the affected person's body while reciting prayers. *Susto,* or "sudden fright," occurs when an individual experiences a stressful event at some time prior to the onset of symptoms. The stressor may be the death of a significant person, a child's nightmare, or an inability to adequately fulfill social-role responsibilities. *Mal puesto* ("evil") is an illness caused by a hex bestowed by a *brujo* ("witch"), *curandero* ("folk healer"), or other person knowledgeable about witchcraft.[92]

There are two types of emotional diseases: mental and moral illnesses. Mental illness is seen as inevitable, and the affected person is viewed as a victim of consequence. Moral illness such as alcoholism is said to be caused by the individual, and treatment is the responsibility of family members.[93] The last category includes scientific diseases that cannot be treated by traditional health practices and must be diagnosed and treated by the Western health care system.

Hispanics commonly view cancer fatalistically as God's will, and they believe it goes against principle to treat the disease aggressively.[94] Family members with cancer, especially elders, often are not informed of their diagnosis, as it is believed such information will only worsen the illness because it is considered deadly and engenders great fear. Patients often say, "I deserve to suffer." Cancer is viewed by Hispanics as contagious and hard to prevent because it is caused by many things. Thus, going to see the doctor early serves no useful purpose. Many Hispanic patients believe that chemotherapy does not work, that radiation may cause cancer, and that cancer will remain even after surgery to remove it. Some believe that certain cancer treatments may have side effects that can be passed on to family members (e.g., that family members may become radioactive if the patient is receiving radiation therapy).[95]

Hispanic individuals may believe that there is no need to see a physician unless a person is very ill. Hospitals are seen as places where people die. Therefore, medical attention may be sought only after symptoms develop or when the individual is too ill to be cared for by the family.

One in four Hispanics lives at or below the poverty level. The cost of being sick includes not only the amount of money needed for care but also the loss of money in time missed from work.[96] Many Hispanics fear that because of their economic status and ethnicity, they may receive inferior care in the U.S. medical system.[97] Some Hispanics believe they should only receive health care that they can afford. So if they cannot afford to pay, some Hispanic individuals may not seek care.

In general, Hispanics are less likely than any other group to have medical insurance. In 1988, 13% of the U.S. population lacked health insurance: 10.2% white, 20% black, and 32% Hispanic.[98] The outcome in relation to cancer is late diagnosis and higher mortality rates despite the lower overall incidence of cancer in the Hispanic population.[95] The high percentage of Hispanics who are migrant farm workers also contributes to the overall decreased access to health care for that group.[99]

Individuals of Hispanic origin often believe that it is inappropriate to question those giving care, as they fear retaliation. Because some Hispanics believe that physical touch can promote healing, if Western providers do not touch Hispanic patients during their visit, the patients may believe that they did not derive any benefit from the visit.

Martaus offers six suggestions for assimilating Hispanic individuals to the U.S. health care system.[100]

1. Health care providers must communicate their acceptance of the person's value system to establish trust.
2. Providers should incorporate a culturally relevant interview in the admission process. This defines the individual's perception of illness and allows the health care provider to establish a workable treatment plan.
3. The treatment plan must include a family focus, as illness intensifies the need for family involvement.
4. Many Hispanics are very religious and may view treatment without prayer as ineffective.
5. Health care workers must take responsibility for finding common ground that incorporates traditional beliefs and modern health care.
6. Many Hispanics have a great fear of authority. They may believe that disease occurs because it is God's will and also may place great emphasis on treating doctors with respect.

Healing practices

For Hispanics, home remedies are the first line of treatment. To cure a hot or cold imbalance, the opposite quality of the causative agent is applied. For example, if the causative agent for a headache is thought to have a hot quality, cold herbs may be placed on the temples to absorb the heat. If the cause has a cold quality, hot herbs are applied.[101] If the stool is green or yellow, the diarrhea is hot and the remedy is cold tea. If the stool is white, the diarrhea is cold and the remedy is hot tea.

There is usually a family folk healer, someone respected for her knowledge of folk medicine. The healing practices are passed down in the family from mother to daughter. If home remedies do not work, Mexican Americans send for the *curandero* or *herbalista,* a traditional folk medicine healer. This person receives his or her skills through an apprenticeship or as a gift from God and is knowledgeable in the use of herbs, diet, massage, prayer, and ritual.[102] Puerto Ricans seek the *espiritismo,* a folk healer with the gift of contacting the spirit world and healing through the powers of spirits. They analyze dreams, foretell the future, and use medals, prayers, and amulets as part of their treatment approach.[92] The Cuban population may seek medical help from a *santero,* a medicine man who works with the spirits of good within a system to promote wellness. Animal sacrifices, rituals, chanting, and prayers are used to aid in healing.[102] A *jerbero* is a healer who uses herbs and spices for prevention of illness and for healing. A *brujo* uses witchcraft for healing illnesses that may be related to jealousy or envy (*envidia*). If these remedies fail, then Western physicians may be sought out for help.[103]

It is essential that the nurse demonstrate acceptance of the spiritual and folk basis of Hispanic people's health beliefs. Once this acceptance is conveyed, there is hope of influencing acceptance and understanding of the rationale for modern health care practices, thereby gaining the community's confidence.

Social organization

The nuclear family (parents and children) is the foundation of the Hispanic community. Men are the breadwinners, assume dominant roles in Hispanic families, and are considered to be big and strong (*macho*). The hesitancy of a woman or child to make a decision may be due to the need to inform and obtain approval of the husband and father.[92] In Hispanic culture, women have always been the primary caretakers. The extended family is valued, and the family's needs supersede those of the individual members. When a family member's illness is too serious for the wife and mother to handle alone, she may ask the extended family to help care for the sick individual. Family members may also speak for the patient. Because of the value of the family in the patient's treatment and recovery, the family should be used to help with the patient's care.

Roman Catholicism is the predominant religion of Hispanics. Because religion is such an important factor in the health beliefs of Hispanics, the patient may turn to religious practices, such as prayer, making special devotions, visiting shrines, or lighting a candle as an act of devotion and appeal to a patron saint, to help overcome the illness. Allowing time and providing privacy for the family to practice their religion during hospitalization will be helpful to many Hispanics.[103]

Communication

For Hispanics, Spanish is the primary language, though there are numerous dialectical differences. Many Hispanics are bilingual but have a strong preference for their native language; during times of illness, they often revert to it. There is some mistrust of whites and Western medicine, especially when the health care provider does not speak Spanish. Language may be a barrier, and Hispanics may not let the provider know that they do not understand. Translators may be necessary.

The traditional Hispanic approach to communication requires the use of much diplomacy and tactfulness. Concern and respect for another's feelings dictate that a screen always be provided to preserve the patient's dignity. The manner of expression is likely to be elaborate and indirect, to make a personal relationship at least appear harmonious, as respect of each person's individuality is important. Politeness and courtesy are highly regarded. Even if the Hispanic individual disagrees with another's point of view, direct argument or contradiction is considered rude and disrespectful. On the surface, he or she may seem agreeable, but only because manners dictate that his or her genuine opinions should not be openly expressed. This apparent agreement may lead to a false assumption on the part of the health care provider, that the patient understands and will follow through with whatever is proposed. In practice, this may not be true.

Body language may be dramatic when expressing pain or emotion. Hispanics in pain may moan and groan to let those around them know they are uncomfortable and suffering.[104]

Space and time

Adult Hispanics may be described as tactile in their relationships, but there also is a high degree of modesty. This is one reason why Hispanics do not enter the U.S. health care system. They generally do not like being touched by others or having to touch themselves and are not comfortable being examined by health care professionals of the opposite sex. Embarrassment is a common reaction to invasive procedures or body exposure during an examination.[95]

Despite the fact that Hispanics like consistent, close relationships and physical touching, female nurses should always assist a male physician when examining a female patient and, likewise, a male nurse should always assist a female physician when examining a male patient. Special care should be taken to guard against exposing body parts other than those that are the focus of the examination. Male patients may refuse a complete examination because of their modesty.

Hispanics generally have a relaxed concept of time—a present orientation—and may be late for appointments. The patient may be more concerned with a current activity than with the activity of planning ahead to be on time. Such a mindset suggests a belief that future-oriented activities can be recovered and that present-oriented activities cannot. The present time orientation helps explain why Hispanics often seek out the most accessible and affordable care first (folk healing and the folk practitioner). It is useful for the nurse to focus on short-term problems. For example, if a medication is not taken in a timely manner, the immediate effects should be emphasized.[91]

Death and dying issues

The afterlife of heaven and hell exists in the Hispanic culture. As many Hispanics are Catholic, religious practices like the sacrament of extreme unction, or anointing of the sick, are important.

The family serves as a supportive network for helping the terminally ill and later their survivors. Often, the patient is not told directly by the family of his or her condition but still demonstrates some awareness of death's likelihood. Though Hispanics typically prefer to remain at home to die, dying in a hospital is an acceptable alternative.[105] Public expression of grief is to be expected, especially among women.[106]

Biological variations

The traditional Hispanic diet is high in fiber and carbohydrates from staples such as rice, beans, and corn. It contains few leafy green vegetables. Beans are a source of protein and daily intake tends to be small. Use of lard and the common practice of frying foods contribute to the high fat content of the Hispanic diet.[95]

Among the high-risk behaviors in the Hispanic population are obesity, alcohol consumption, and sexual practices. Obesity is a common problem among Hispanics in the United States due to their diet and lack of physical activity. In general, the culture accepts obesity as part of the natural aging process and does not emphasize low body weight.[107] To older individuals, obesity may mean health and wealth. Obesity is a risk factor in cancers of the breast, colon/rectum, uterus, and prostate. Hispanic men tend to drink at younger ages and to consume larger amounts of alcohol and more frequently than do whites. Alcohol contributes to cancers of the esophagus and pancreas. Cigarette smoking is on the rise in Hispanic adolescents, although adult Hispanics smoke less than whites or blacks. There is a high risk for cervical cancer because of sexual promiscuity and infrequent use of condoms by males, predisposing females to sexually transmitted diseases. In addition, low socioeconomic status and low educational levels often result in infrequent Pap smears, infrequent use of barrier contraceptives, and lack of reporting of genital warts.[86]

Skin color in Hispanics can vary from a natural tan to dark brown. Those with lighter color have more Spanish ancestry, while darker-skinned individuals have more Indian ancestry.

Native Americans

The Native Americans include natives of the continental United States, Aleuts, and Alaskan Eskimos. They are a very diverse group consisting of many tribes and more than 400 federally recognized nations, each with its own traditions and cultural heritage. Until the 1800s, these native peoples lived in loosely formed, often nomadic bands and tribes and spoke more than 100 languages with countless dialects.[108] This section focuses on the natives of the continental United States.

There are approximately 2.1 million descendants of native North American residents that make up the smallest of the defined U.S. minority groups. There are 33 states with Indian reservations. The largest Native American tribes are the Navajo, Cherokee, Sioux, Chippewa, and Pueblo, with the greatest numbers living in Oklahoma, Arizona, California, New Mexico, and Alabama. The 1990 census shows a significant increase in the Native American population due to high birth rates, improved counting by the U.S. Bureau of the Census, and the increase in self-identification, particularly among urban Native Americans who have little connection to a tribal organization.[109,110]

Native Americans who live on reservations tend to lead a more isolated, rural type of existence. Reservations have a high percentage of very young members and a growing number of members over 55 years of age. Because reservation land cannot support a growing and increasingly concentrated population, poverty and welfare dependency are common. Native Americans who relocated from reservations tended to move to urban areas away from the secure network of their family, community, and tribal lifestyle. Although lured by greater opportunities and better jobs, many experienced culture shock at the significant differences in the environment. In the past 25 years, there has been a migration to urban areas and now nearly two-thirds of all Native Americans live in nonreservation communities.[111]

Cancer is ranked as the third leading cause of death among Native Americans, preceded by accidents and heart disease. Because of the heterogeneity of the Native American group, cancer rates likely vary among the tribes and between Native Americans of New Mexico and the Alaskan natives.

Mortality rates in 1988–1992 indicated that Alaskan native men died of lung, colon, and rectum cancers, while Native American men died of prostate cancer. For the latter, the number of deaths was fewer than 25 in other cancer sites, so no rates were reported. In Alaskan native women, lung, colon, and rectum cancers accounted for most of the deaths; there are no data for Native American women, as fewer than 25 deaths per site were reported for all cancer sites. Compared to women of other ethnic groups, the Alaskan native women's mortality rate for colon and rectum cancer was the highest.[14]

Gallbladder cancer and disease are high in Native American women. The reasons for these high rates are unknown, but diet and genetic factors are implicated.[112]

Cervical cancer occurs primarily among older Native American women.[113] Factors affecting the increased incidence of cervical cancer include infrequent or no history of Pap-smear screening and lack of follow-up for abnormal results. Barriers to screening and follow-up include poverty, significant unemployment, underfunded and overburdened health care services, lack of local treatment, use of the health care system for treatment of acute illness rather than for preventive care, and the belief that the test is unnecessary due to "good health."[114,115]

At least one-third of the Native American population lives in extreme poverty. The social condition of Native American communities such as limited educational levels, substandard housing, poor sanitation, malnutrition, and inadequate health services all contribute to the high incidence of death by accident, suicide, alcoholism, and cirrhosis of the liver. Native Americans are second only to Hispanics in their lack of health care coverage. It was estimated in 1991–1992, that 33.2% of Native American men and 24.8% of Native American women had no health care plan.[90]

The Indian Health Service, through the U.S. Public Health Service, provides inpatient facilities and outpatient clinics and serves Native Americans residing on reservations in 25 states as well as the Aleut and Eskimo residents of Alaska. Although health care is available, barriers preventing Native Americans from accessing it include poverty and lack of transportation. Native Americans believe in living day-to-day rather than in planning for the future and may not have savings or insurance to pay for health care. Many live long distances from health care facilities and are resistant to hospital treatment.[1,116]

Health beliefs and practices

Most tribes link health beliefs and religion. To the Native American, religion is something that surrounds an individual at all times and has a profound influence on the entire being.[117] Wellness is harmony in body, mind, and spirit as well as resilience, the ability to survive under exceedingly difficult circumstances. It is the patient's response or attitude toward circumstances that creates harmony.[118]

Native Americans believe that health reflects living in harmony with nature and that humans have an intimate relationship with nature. The earth is considered a living being, the body of a higher individual with a will and desire to be well. The earth is periodically healthy or ill just as humans are. A Native American is expected to treat both the physical body and the earth with respect. If an individual harms the earth, he or she harms him or herself and vice versa. Because of this relationship between humans and nature, Native Americans believe that humans should respect their bodies and nature through proper treatment.[119]

Unwellness is caused by the disharmony of mind, body, and spirit. Natural unwellness is caused by the violation of a sacred or tribal taboo. Taboos can be moral, religious, or cultural. Violations not only affect the offender but the family as well.[118]

Native Americans believe that illness may also be caused by witchcraft. Evil or negative energy comes from "one who is on the bad side" or "a person who walks at night." It can be premeditated or not, so Native Americans must be careful how they think or talk because bad thoughts can cause illness.[118] The Hopi Indians associate illness with evil spirits. The Navajos believe that witches are able to interact with evil spirits and can bring sickness and other unhappiness to those who annoy them. Traditionally, illness, disharmony, and sadness are seen by Navajos as the result

> of displeasing the holy people, annoying the elements, disturbing animal and plant life, neglecting the celestial bodies, misuse of a sacred Indian ceremony, or tampering with witches and witchcraft.[120,p.21]

The cause of disease, injury, damage to property, or continued misfortune of any kind can be traced back to an action that should not have been performed, such as breaking a taboo or contacting a ghost or witch. Thus, the treatment of illness must be focused on external causative factors and not on the illness or injury itself.[121]

All causes of illness or disease are believed to have supernatural aspects.[121] Treatment depends on whether the origins of bodily ailments are internal or external. Vogel states that external causes of illness are fractures, dislocations, wounds, and snake or insect bites.[122] If the cause is not apparent, then it is attributed to a supernatural agency. The belief that illnesses are caused by germs, a malfunctioning body part, or poor nutritional intake are foreign and unacceptable to Native Americans.

Sickness indicates a discord with the laws of nature and, according to Native Americans, is most often caused by sorcery or witchcraft, taboo violation, disease or object intrusion, spirit intrusion or being possessed by spirits, or loss of soul. Iroquois Indians also believe that unfulfilled dreams or desires can result in illness. Restriction violations are also thought to cause sickness. Most tribes have prescriptions and prohibitions governing behavior and daily activities, many of which pertain to the prevention of illness. For example, a Navajo boy was diagnosed as having urinary retention caused by his urinating on an ant hill. The boy caused the ants to suffer, and the ants' revenge came in the form of an illness. The boy was out of harmony with living entities that share the universe. The cure was a healing ceremony involving chants, prayers, and herbs administered by a medicine man.[111]

Diseases of *object intrusion* refer to the invasion of the body by a worm, snake, insect, or small animal. This may be a result of witchcraft. Navajos may orally suck out the foreign object using a hollow tube or bone. *Spirit intrusion* is being possessed by disease-causing spirits of humans and animals. The healing ceremony is an exorcism of the bad spirits.[122] *Soul loss* usually occurs during a dream when the soul leaves the body and travels about. Witches and evil spirits can steal a soul. It is believed that the individual is in danger of dying if the soul is not recovered.

Frequently, Native Americans use traditional medicine and Western medicine, either independently of each other or simultaneously. A Native American patient may consult both a medicine person and a Western doctor at the same time. One helps the individual heal himself by restoring harmony, while the other treats the physical disease. To treat the spirit and mind, a healer must understand why the disease occurred and begin to resolve the conflict occurring in mind, body, and spirit. In most instances, the two systems are complementary and should be encouraged.[123]

Preventive measures are generally practiced to ward off the effects of witchcraft, to reestablish harmony, or to prevent possession by an evil spirit. The medicine person may prescribe wearing a talisman, a buckskin, or cloth herbal bag that has preventive or curative powers. Removal of such items by the nurse without permission could result in serious consequences for the patient.[123]

Some tribes are not receptive to invasive bodily procedures and may reluctantly agree to surgery. Relatives may refuse to donate blood because they fear that if the recipient dies, they may die as well. Native Americans should be asked if they wish a body part back after surgery, as some tribes believe the body must be intact for burial or that body parts can be used as a means for spirits to enter the body and cause harm.[123]

Offering food to Native American patients during appointments may be helpful. This is referred to as "the give away," a celebration that meets basic needs and shows welcome, concern, caring, friendship, and neighborliness. Offering food is a tangible expression of the link in a relationship and serves as something always to be remembered about that individual.

Because of a history of inconsistent care and disrespectful treatment, Native Americans often are not comfortable with Western health care providers. Long waits in clinics, separation from their families, the unfamiliar routines of the hospital, and the often demanding and demeaning attitudes of nurses and physicians result in a variety of responses by the Native American patient that may include silence or even leaving never to return again.[116]

The pain threshold of Native Americans is often thought to be high, as stoicism is valued. This stems from Native Americans' tendency to look at things in totality, so that when sickness occurs it is viewed as an ailment of the whole body. Many will "grin and bear" fever and pain until the physical condition becomes disabling. Asking a Native American, "Where does it hurt?" might commonly be responded to with "All over." It may be more useful to have the patient point to where it hurts most. When treatment is sought, medication generally is expected. If none is given, the Native American may be disappointed, as his expectations for treatment were not met.[111]

Helpful interventions in working successfully with Native American patients include conveying acceptance without judgment of physical appearance, beliefs, or practices; recognition of unique cultural beliefs and behaviors; and making staff and services available when the need arises rather than by scheduling appointments. An unwillingness to accept traditional healing practices may discourage many Native Americans from using the Western health care system.

Healing practices

The traditional healer is the medicine person who is wise in the ways of the land and nature, and takes time to determine first the cause of the illness, the proper treatment, and often performs special ceremonies that may take several days.[116] These medicine men and women are "chosen," that is, divinely inspired. They are gifted with extrasensory perception that allows them to make mythological associations, and they seek spiritual causes of illness.[116] Medicine men and women spend many years learning their skills and serving as apprentices.

There are different types of medicine men and women having specific roles. They range from those who assume a purely positive role and whose focus is to maintain cultural integration at a time of great stress to the singer who is the medicine man and treats illnesses and disharmony.[121]

A cure often requires the involvement of several medicine men and women. Medicine people may use medicine bundles (*jists*) containing symbolic and sacred items or small jars of medicinal solutions; they may place red, grey, or black marks on the patient's skin; use tobacco; or burn cedar sage, grasses, or whatever is appropriate for that tribe. Bracelets of shells, seeds, beads, or arrowheads also may be used.

The goal of treatment is always to enhance total healing. If an herbalist treats a patient, prayers and songs are also offered for mental and spiritual renewal. An important component of the healing is the patient's motivation for recovery. Native Americans believe an individual gets back in equal proportion what he gives in words and actions to another.[111]

Healing ceremonies differ from tribe to tribe, with varying degrees of complexity. Most of these ceremonies take place in the home with the participation of family members and other tribal members. Supporting the use of healing ceremonies in the hospital and providing space and privacy is helpful for the Native American patient and family. Objects may be left in the room that were used in the ceremony. These objects are associated with elements identified with the cause of illness and should not be removed without the permission of the patient and his or her family.

Purification is often practiced to maintain harmony with nature and to cleanse the body and spirit. Many believe that for every natural disease, the earth provides a cure. Roots are often chewed to relieve pain, clear the mind, or treat a toothache. Herbs are viewed as being agents of nature.[116]

Traditional medicines include cedar incense for purification and corn pollen for blessings. A "seat" in a sweat lodge is a type of purging that is useful for preventing and treating illness. Monthly sweats may be used because it is believed that the body periodically builds up bad or negative spirits that block energy. Navajo women do not participate in sweats. Objects to guard against witchcraft may be carried by some tribes, especially at nonfamily gatherings.[122]

Western physicians are regarded by Native Americans as herbalists who can cure symptoms but cannot restore the patient's harmonious relationship with nature because they lack knowledge of the important rituals. Native Americans believe that a real medicine woman or man will know, without being told, what is wrong with a person. Western doctors ask many questions and often are unable to determine what is wrong. Some Native Americans believe that health care providers from the Indian Health Service come to the reservations to "practice."[116]

Social organization

As members of a matrilineal society, Native American patients may not give consent for anything until permission is obtained from the mother, grandmother, or aunt. Sometimes consent may be obtained only after a ceremony. If this cannot be done in the hospital, the patient may leave and return after the ceremony.[124]

The extended family is very important, especially during periods of crisis. When a family member is hospitalized, an assortment of relatives will come expecting to visit the relative. Limiting visitors to only close relatives is not relevant for Native Americans, as they do not distinguish between close and distant relatives. Family members may make great sacrifices traveling long distances to visit their family member. The hospitalized patient expects the family to visit, and the family expects to visit the patient.[123]

Communication

Older Native Americans may speak only their traditional language, and often there are no comparable medical terms in the tribal language. Although translators are needed, they must understand the nature of social, cultural, and familial lines of communication and respect. Some tribes believe that a discussion with one individual about another is a sign of disrespect and could break a cultural taboo, leaving the individual or family vulnerable to harm. For the Navajo, special emphasis is placed on individual rights. Each person speaks for himself or herself, and each individual's action should be self-initiated. In this case, trying to obtain information about another family member may be difficult. Limited ability to speak English may hamper the understanding of the patient. It is common for Native Americans to be silent rather than to admit to not understanding.

Making direct eye contact with a Native American may be considered as looking into his or her soul, which could result in its loss. Thus, Native Americans who do not look directly at care providers should not be labeled as "inattentive" or "uninterested." Prolonged eye contact is considered a sign of disrespect and pointing is viewed as insulting.

Interpersonal relationships are carefully spelled out among Native American tribes. Who one speaks to, when the speaking occurs, how one speaks, and the sequence of speaking are very important. For example, a mother-in-law cannot speak to her son-in-law or be in the same room with him.[125] Awareness of these relationships is helpful to the nurse who must communicate with Native American patients and families.

The importance of observing periods of silence is a cultural trait. Silence helps formulate one's thoughts so that the spoken words will have significance. An individual who interrupts, interjects, or hurries toward abrupt conclusions is perceived to be immature. Native Americans are very sensitive to body language. If a health care provider appears hurried, nervous, or impatient, Native Americans are quick to sense these cues, and blocks to communication may occur. Because Native Americans are comfortable with silence, they do not feel a need to talk constantly; therefore continual talking by a health care provider trying to obtain an adequate history may not be well received.[111]

Native Americans are private people who do not readily volunteer information. Patients may not understand a question or may give responses they think the nurse wishes to hear, particularly if the question is regarded as inappropriate. Making a declarative statement about an obvious symptom and allowing time for the patient to respond may be a better approach.

It is common for Native Americans to speak in a very soft voice. The listener is expected to be attentive in order to hear what is being said. Asking for a statement to be repeated is considered rude. Speak with a Native American patient in a quiet setting to improve communication.

Some Native Americans consider a firm handshake a sign of aggression. Navajos extend their hand and lightly touch the hand of the person they are greeting. Knocking on the door before entering the room and introducing oneself in the native language are often appreciated.

Using body language that is open without closing or crossing the arms is suggested. Loud speech may be viewed as rude or angry, and speaking slowly may be perceived as condescending. Note-taking is considered taboo for some Native Americans, as Indian history is passed on through verbal story telling.[116]

Initiating a visit with casual conversation about family, social functions, and about the tribe may be helpful because Native Americans are very private. This introductory period allows for a gradual easing into discussions about personal and family health. Never use second-person language when discussing risk factors (e.g., "If you don't stop smoking, you will get cancer,") as this may be perceived as putting a hex on the individual. For Native Americans, a direct address with the second person involves one's spirit. Some Native Americans may feel that talking with someone other than a family member about breasts, testicles, self-examination, and uterine bleeding is improper.

Space and time

Personal space is very important to some Native Americans who may have difficulty adapting to situations that place them in unfamiliar spaces such as clinics or hospitals. Hospitals may be considered a place to die, and Native Americans are hesitant to be admitted or put into a room where another person has died. Some tribes would welcome having the room ritually purified before they enter it.

Modesty is very significant to the Native American; limited exposure of body parts is suggested. Permission should be asked to perform a physical examination, and Native American women may prefer a female practitioner.

Native American time typically runs from 1 hour to a few days later than standard time.[126] Homes often have no clocks. For Native Americans, time is casual, present oriented, and relative to present needs that must be accomplished within a given time frame. A present time orientation may cause a Navajo patient to eat two meals today, four meals tomorrow, no meals the next day, and three the following day. This would create difficulty if the patient were instructed to take a medication three times a day with meals.

Death and dying issues

Existence is circular and continuous for most traditional Native Americans. They existed as spirit beings with the supreme creator before birth. At death, their spirit joins the creator and eventually returns to the physical world in another form.[118] Death consists of joining one's ancestors, and good or bad deeds have nothing to do with this reunion.

Attitudes and approaches to death and dying vary considerably among Native American tribes. Some are very accepting of death, and others view dying people and death with fear. Some prefer that their family members die at home, while others prefer the hospital. Suffering is a major value in the Native American culture, and dying and grief may be met with stoicism and silence. The opportunity to share feelings may be rejected by the patient or family.[127] The family, including children, should be with the dying person even though they often may avoid touching the dead person or articles associated with that person.[21]

Biological variations

There is a high incidence of obesity and alcohol abuse in Native Americans. Some believe that the disruption and subsequent loss caused by the European settlement of North America left many Native Americans feeling powerless and hopeless. These feelings may contribute to many of the social problems experienced today by Native Americans.

The Native American diet has changed over time. When they were nomadic, the diet was high in fiber and low in fat. Today, the diet is likely to be high in refined carbohydrates, fat, and sodium and low in fiber, meat, eggs, cheese, and milk. Obesity is a major problem. Many Native Americans are also lactose intolerant.

Nursing Issues

Cancer, Poverty, and Ethnicity

In the late 1970s the question of poverty's role in the differences in cancer incidence, mortality, and survival in different ethnic groups was first raised. It appeared

that poverty, not race, accounted for the 10%–15% lower survival rate from cancer in many ethnic groups. Baquet et al found that, when corrected for economic status, blacks had a slightly lower incidence and mortality than whites for a number of cancers.[128] The disproportionate number of blacks in the lower socioeconomic strata accounted for the increased incidence. Berg et al, in a study that included only whites who received the same level of care, found that indigent patients had poorer survival rates for each cancer type.[129] Page and Kuntz studied male Veteran's Administration patients with cancer and found similar survival rates between blacks and whites, except for cancer of the bladder.[130] All patients received the same treatment standard without regard to ability to pay for services. McWhorter et al analyzed SEER data from 1978–1982 and found that for cancers of the breast, cervix, esophagus, male lung, pancreas, and stomach, poverty accounted for most if not all of the ethnic differences.[131] However, consideration of poverty did not eliminate the differences in incidence rates for cancers of the bladder, prostate, uterus, and multiple myeloma.

Poverty's impact on cancer is felt most significantly in ethnic minorities in the United States. In 1990 a large percentage of API families were below the poverty level. In 1989, blacks comprised approximately one-third of America's poor, and 28.7% of all Hispanics were poor.[132,133]

The "culture of poverty" includes economic factors such as unemployment, unskilled occupations, no savings, no health insurance, and frequent daily food purchases in small amounts; social factors, such as crowded living quarters, women as single parents, low education, and critical attitudes toward the dominant class; and psychological factors such as feelings of helplessness, inferiority, fatalism and dependency, and a present time orientation with an inability to defer gratification. These increase cancer incidence and mortality by increasing the risk factors of chronic malnutrition; occupational exposure through unskilled jobs; early initiation into sex and multiple partners; and smoking and alcoholism, contributing to cancers of the lung, oral cavity, prostate, cervix, or esophagus.[132]

Secondary prevention may be absent because of a present orientation, where survival needs take precedence over screening and early detection. A critical attitude toward the middle class and a sense of fatalism may decrease participation in screening programs. Delayed tertiary prevention is due to a lack of insurance, inability to pay for service, or limited care access. Emergency rooms are often used inappropriately, and referral to clinics may result in fragmented care, impersonal service, long waiting hours, and transportation and child care problems.[134]

The recommendations made by the American Cancer Society report, *Cancer in the Economically Disadvantaged*, to reduce cancer incidence and mortality in the poor would be effective in many ethnic groups.[135] These recommendations seek to improve access by (1) establishing programs where the economically disadvantaged or ethnic minorities can gather in emergency rooms, neighborhood clinics, or churches; (2) developing culturally relevant educational materials that may be translated into different languages; and (3) recruiting and training health care providers and volunteers from the targeted groups in the special needs of the poor or of a particular ethnic group.

Strategies to Enhance Access to Health Care

A primary barrier to cancer care for many of the ethnic minority populations is access to health care, especially among the socioeconomically disadvantaged. Since 1989, when attention was directed to this particular need, several programs have been developed. Many of these programs focus on providing effective cancer screenings for ethnic minority populations by using culturally sensitive strategies, including (1) involvement of trusted and respected members of the community in the planning and delivery of health care services,[46] (2) provision of social support by women in the social network,[136] and (3) development of culturally sensitive patient education materials.[137]

One of these programs, The Witness Project, consists of African American women volunteers who are cancer survivors. By "witnessing" or talking about their cancer experience at churches and community centers, these volunteers help to increase breast and cervical cancer awareness and stress the importance of early detection among minority women in rural central and eastern Arkansas.[138]

Another program is the American Cancer Society's Harlem Education and Detection Project in New York City. The program uses the Patient Navigator Model to assist individuals in overcoming health care access barriers. This model "attempts to guide the individual around and through the labyrinth of the health care system, through many of the social, community, health, and attitudinal barriers to ensure that patients receive timely diagnosis and treatment."[139,p.97] In addition, the navigator provides education and support to the individual.

The Wai'anae Coast Cancer Control Project in Hawaii also uses the navigator model. This project emphasizes community-driven cancer control as a means of improving breast and cervical cancer screening practices among native Hawaiian women. The navigators in this project are community members who provide information on cancer and assist individuals in "navigating" the unfamiliar health care system by scheduling clinic appointments and patient follow-up services.[46]

Mujer a Mujer: Woman to Woman is an example of a successful, culturally sensitive patient education program targeting Hispanic women. It was developed to reduce the mortality from cervical cancer in this group.[137] Palos offers some of the culturally appropriate strategies used in the development of this and other effective cancer control programs:[137,p.112]

- Follow basic rules when initiating interpersonal communication, such as being courteous and respectful to establish trust or confidence.

- Use focus groups comprising grassroots (community) and professional individuals to validate promoters or barriers to attitudes, knowledge, and behavior related to cancer and its prevention.

- Use influential formal and informal leaders such as religious leaders, community gatekeepers, or opinion leaders.

- Integrate religious, cultural, and, when appropriate, traditional (folk) medicine and healing practices, beliefs, and taboos.

- Involve the family, friends, and members of other influential support systems.

- Determine a group's preferred communication process (verbal or nonverbal) as well as language preference.

- Determine an individual's degree of acculturation or assimilation, when appropriate.

- Involve paraprofessionals such as folk healers, when and if appropriate.

- Integrate cultural assessments into daily nursing practice.

The success of these culturally sensitive programs indicates that the targeted populations will use the services "if they are available, accessible, and acceptable" and are provided in a humane and caring manner.[140] In addition, the American Cancer Society identified several successful strategies including:[139,p.100]

- Hire outreach staff who are indigenous to the community.

- Piggyback onto other community program agendas.

- Avoid the "cancer only" approach.

- Develop materials that are culturally relevant and community specific.

- Keep educational messages simple.

- Fight fatalism by emphasizing the person's ability to affect health through action.

- Emphasize wellness and health, not cancer and fear.

Many other programs that target the socioeconomically disadvantaged and ethnic minority populations are reported in the literature.[77,141-144] However, this is just the beginning, and additional programs are needed to continue the outreach efforts to the socioeconomically disadvantaged ethnic minority populations.

Culturally Appropriate Public/Patient Education

Ethnic minority cancer patients are not much different from other cancer patients in their needs for basic cancer information and in their experiences of learning barriers such as anxiety and feelings of being overwhelmed about the disease and treatment. However, ethnic minorities present certain unique challenges such as communicating in a language other than English and cultural values, beliefs, and practices that can affect the teaching/learning process.

Strategies

Because of the challenges posed by ethnic minorities, several strategies have been identified to provide culturally sensitive patient education interventions. These strategies include:[72,137,139]

1. Developing culturally relevant and community-specific materials.
2. Keeping educational messages simple.
3. Determining the preferred language and learning process (e.g., video versus booklets; group versus one-on-one teaching).
4. Identifying the preferred communication style of the individual, such as how to address him or her and acceptable nonverbal communication. For example, as mentioned in the description of the different ethnic groups, the appropriateness and acceptance of direct eye contact varies among cultures.

In addition, determining decision-making patterns for the particular ethnic group is also important. An example of this is seen in many API groups where the family, instead of the patient, makes treatment decisions. In these situations, teaching solely the patient about a proposed chemotherapy treatment may not be appropriate if the educational effort needs to be directed to the family for subsequent decision making and consent to treatment.

Use of interpreters Language is a frequent barrier to effective patient education. The use of professional interpreters, if available, is the optimal choice. Family and friends may be used, but the correct or complete message may not be relayed. This distortion or omission of parts of the message may be due to the interpreter's own skill and fluency in the language, the interpreter's subjective censoring (e.g., to "protect" the patient), or the patient's comfort level in discussing personal issues in the presence of the family member or friend. Recommendations for using interpreters and what to do if there is no interpreter are listed in Table 7-7.[145,146]

Translating written materials Although there are translated cancer information materials now available, additional resources still are needed. Just as professional interpreters are desirable for clear, accurate communication, guidelines also exist for translating material. Translating material written in English into another language is not enough. To ensure that the content and tone is accurately captured and maintained throughout the translation, the newly translated material must be back-translated into English by independent translators.[147] After making any needed text corrections, it also

is helpful to pilot test the finished product with a sample of the target population for which the translated material was created.

Always assess the reading level of the original material before it is translated. Analyses of the reading levels of available cancer education materials have shown an average that is much higher than the reading level of the general population.[148,149] Thus, the reading level of the material to be translated may need to be adjusted before being translated. Just as literacy has been identified as a barrier to cancer patient education for the general population, literacy is also a challenge faced by many ethnic minority groups. As mentioned earlier, there are a significant number of API who are functionally illiterate.[8] In addition, the literacy level of ethnic minority groups will be influenced by whether they are literate in their native language. For example, the Hmong culture is primarily an oral culture, and many Hmong who immigrated to the United States are illiterate in Hmong.[150]

Preferred styles of learning Determining an individual's preferred style of learning is also important. The different styles include one-to-one versus group, oral tradition, story telling, peer educators, and receiving information from "powerful others."[72] Some cultural groups may have preferences for one or more learning styles. For example, in a survey of Spanish-speaking patients and family members, one-to-one teaching was preferred by the majority (79%) versus other strategies such as videos (37%), print materials (32%), and group classes (16%).[151]

In another example, knowing the learning style of the targeted ethnic minority population helped in the development of a culturally sensitive cancer education video. Because story telling is used by many Native Americans to relay information, one video, *Standing Strong Against the Cancer Enemy*, used the story format to convey its educational message on cancer prevention.[152]

Other successful educational strategies include the use of peer educators and "powerful others" to relay information. Enlisting fellow ethnic minorities to teach their peers is the basic principle behind the peer educator's strategy. The use of "powerful others" often involves the recruitment of respected community leaders who are recognized authorities people will listen to for information.[72]

Providing effective public and patient education for ethnic minority groups presents many challenges and opportunities for oncology nurses. Using the strategies presented here as well as knowledge of the individual's cultural background, can help oncology nurses develop and implement successful, culturally sensitive public and patient education interventions.

Clinical Trials and Cancer Research

Historically, there has been underrepresentation of minorities in clinical trials. Two major barriers that have

Table 7-7 Overcoming Language Barriers

USE OF AN INTERPRETER

- Before locating an interpreter, be sure that the language the patient speaks at home is known, since it may be different from the language spoken publicly (e.g., French is sometimes spoken by well-educated and upper-class members of certain Asian or Middle Eastern cultures).
- Avoid interpreters from a rival tribe, state, region, or nation (e.g., a Palestinian who knows Hebrew may not be the best interpreter for a Jewish client).
- Be aware of sex/gender differences between interpreter and patient. In general, same sex/gender is preferred.
- Be aware of age differences between interpreter and patient. In general, an older, more mature interpreter is preferred to a younger, less experienced one.
- Be aware of socioeconomic differences between interpreter and patient.
- Ask the interpreter to translate as closely to verbatim as possible.
- An interpreter who is a nonrelative may seek compensation for services rendered.

Recommendations for Institutions
- Maintain a computerized list of interpreters who may be contacted as needed.
- Network with area hospitals, colleges, universities, and other organizations that may serve as resources.
- Utilize the translation services provided by telephone companies (e.g., American Telephone and Telegraph Company).

WHAT TO DO WHEN THERE IS NO INTERPRETER

- Be polite and formal.
- Greet the person using the last or complete name. Gesture to yourself and say your name. Offer a handshake or nod. Smile.
- Proceed in an unhurried manner. Pay attention to any effort by the patient or family to communicate.
- Speak in a low, moderate voice. Avoid talking loudly. Remember that there is a tendency to raise the volume and pitch of your voice when the listener appears not to understand. The listener may perceive that the nurse is shouting and/or angry.
- Use any words known in the patient's language. This indicates that the nurse is aware of and respects the client's culture.
- Use simple words, such as *pain* instead of *discomfort*. Avoid medical jargon, idioms, and slang. Avoid using contractions. Use nouns repeatedly instead of pronouns. Example: Do *not* say, "He has been taking his medicine, hasn't he?" Do say, "Does Juan take medicine?"
- Pantomime words and simple actions while verbalizing them.
- Give instructions in the proper sequence. Example: Do *not* say, "Before you rinse the bottle, sterilize it," Do say, "First, wash the bottle. Second, rinse the bottle."
- Discuss one topic at a time. Avoid using conjunctions. Example: Do *not* say, "Are you cold and in pain?" Do say, "Are you cold [while pantomiming]? Are you in pain?"
- Validate if the patient understands by having him or her repeat instructions, demonstrate the procedure, or act out the meaning.
- Write out several short sentences in English, and determine the person's ability to read them.
- Try a third language. Many Indo-Chinese speak French. Europeans often know three or four languages. Try Latin words or phrases, if the nurse is familiar with the language.
- Ask who among the patient's family and friends could serve as an interpreter.
- Obtain phrase books from a library or bookstore, make or purchase flash cards, contact hospitals for a list of interpreters, and use both formal and informal networking to locate a suitable interpreter.

Reprinted with permission from Andrews MM, Herberg, P: Transcultural nursing care, in Andrews MM, Boyle JS (eds): *Transcultural Concepts in Nursing Care* (ed 3): Philadelphia, Lippincott, Williams & Wilkins, 1999, pp 23–77[145]

been identified are ethnic minorities' distrust of outsiders doing research in their communities (often referred to as "white-run research") and the lack of culturally sensitive and specific educational materials.

Brawley cites a number of additional barriers to accrual of ethnic minorities in clinical trials, including: difficulties in transportation, inconvenient clinic hours, lack of day care, differences in language, lack of understanding, fear of being denied care because of inadequate

financial support, fear that researchers will take advantage, and not understanding the value of the research to the participant.[138]

In response to this underrepresentation of minorities and to recruit more minorities to National Cancer Institute (NCI)-sponsored clinical trials, NCI developed the Minority-Based (MB) Community Clinical Oncology Program (CCOP). Since its inception in 1990, one of the fundamental factors that has facilitated the progress of this program is the health care providers' respect for, and increased understanding of, the unique cultures that they serve.[138]

Although progress has been made in accruing ethnic minority patients to cancer treatment trials, accrual to cancer prevention trials has not been as successful. For example, the number of ethnic minority patients enrolled in the NCI's breast and prostate cancer prevention trials is less than desired.[138] One of the reasons may be the disproportionate number of ethnic minorities who are socioeconomically disadvantaged. With immediate, day-to-day survival issues taking top priority, participating in a cancer prevention trial in which results may not be evident for years would probably be unattractive and even meaningless to these individuals.[138,153]

Whether the issue is accrual of ethnic minorities to cancer treatment or cancer prevention trials, continued efforts directed toward overcoming the identified barriers are needed. McCabe et al identified several factors that facilitate participation in clinical trials among ethnic minorities who are socioeconomically disadvantaged.[154] These factors include:[154,p.126]

- Adequate information and education about the risks, benefits, costs, and time commitment required.

- Peer group norms that are supportive of the goals of the trial.

- Endorsement of the goals of clinical trials by the church, the cultural or social group, and the employer.

- Improved access to the health care system and the specific location where the trial is being conducted.

- A perceived benefit to the individual from participation.

- Minimal actual cost to the individual in terms of time lost from work, transportation, and child care.

Research studies

Conducting research involving ethnic minorities presents several unique challenges: selection of the research sample, appropriate instruments and research methodology, and translation of research instruments.

Because of the heterogeneity of the major groups, study samples need to be selected carefully. For example, if the study sample were identified as Native Americans, knowing which subgroups were studied would make a difference in interpretation of the research findings and in determining for whom the data are generalizable.

Also, knowing which particular ethnic group will be studied while the research study is being planned can make a difference in the development of appropriate instruments and the chosen research methodology.[155] For example, Munet-Vilaro reports from personal experience that Latinos prefer to be interviewed rather than to take home a written test.[156] Based on the findings that several ethnic minority groups had difficulty in using Likert scales, a concern has also been raised about whether the Likert scale is culturally biased.[156,157] Flaskerud further proposes that

Problems in using Likert scales cross-culturally could be due to education, faulty translation, irrelevant content, lack of semantic equivalence, the differing character of social interactions in various groups, or the nature of the response required. It is also possible that the degree of variation Likert scales attempt to measure is meaningless in some cultural groups.[157,p.186]

Research instruments that are developed in English and translated into another language are also of particular concern. When such translation occurs, subtle cultural nuances and conceptual equivalency may be compromised, leading to difficulties in retaining the validity of the instrument.[156] Strategies to overcome these potential problems include translating newly translated materials back into the original language, the goal being to maintain the essence of the original meaning. Pilot testing the instrument with the appropriate population is also recommended to establish reliability.[156]

As the U.S. population becomes more culturally diverse, there is an obvious need for more cancer research involving ethnic minorities. Expertise is needed to incorporate cultural considerations when cancer research studies are developed and conducted.

Resources

In response to the increasing awareness of the needs of our culturally diverse populations and the health care professionals who care for them, specific resources have been created and new resources continue to be developed. These resources are available at the national and local levels, and include educational materials and professional organizations.

Three of the major resources available at the national level are the Office of Minority Health Resource Center (OMH-RC), the National Cancer Institute's Cancer Information Service (CIS), and the American Cancer Society (ACS). Information available at the federal, state, and local levels on health-related resources for blacks, APIs, Hispanics, and Native Americans are maintained by the OMH-RC.[36] The CIS and ACS provide information on cancer for the general public, cancer patients and families, and health care professionals. (See Chapter 85: Cancer Nursing Resources.)

Several professional organizations also exist to promote cultural awareness in nurses and to provide support for ethnic minority nurses. These include the Oncology Nursing Society (ONS) and its Transcultural Nursing Issues Special Interest Group (TNI SIG), and the Transcultural Nursing Society of Illinois. Professional nursing organizations that specifically target ethnic minority nurses include the Asian American/Pacific Islander Nurses' Association, the Association of Chicana/Latina Nurses, the Council of Black Nurses, the National Association of Hispanic Nurses, the National Black Nurses' Association, the National Center for the Advancement of Blacks in the Health Professions, and the Philippine Nurses' Association of America. National minority organizations such as the American Indian Health Care Association and the Intercultural Cancer Council (ICC) are other resources. Additional resources include Web sites such as DiversityRx (http://www.diversityrx.org), which promotes language and cultural competence to improve the quality of health care for minority, immigrant, and ethnically diverse communities; the Transcultural Nursing Society (http://www.tcns.org), which includes information about its journal, educational programs, bookstore and conferences; and the Intercultural Cancer Council (http://www.icc.bcm.tmc.edu), which describes the goal of ICC to work to reduce the higher incidence of suffering and death from cancer among minority, culturally diverse, and medically underserved populations. These Web sites also provide links to other sites.

These resources offer much-needed assistance to oncology nurses seeking to provide culturally competent care. As resource development continues at all levels in the United States, individuals with cancer, their families, and the health care professionals who serve them all will benefit.

Conclusion

Cultural diversity will remain a particular challenge, as the composition of the population of the United States continues to change. The impact of cultural diversity on cancer care is multilayered. At one level each ethnic group, with its unique values, health beliefs, and practices, responds to cancer somewhat differently. Additional factors such as degree of acculturation, socioeconomic status, and educational attainment add yet another layer of intergroup and intragroup diversity. A third level is an underlying, often negative perception among many ethnic minorities of the mainstream culture and Western medicine. This is primarily due to their history and experience with Western culture, that in turn influences their health behaviors, attitudes, and acceptance of mainstream health care.

In the midst of this diversity, there are also shared responses among the major cultural groups. Many of the ethnic minority groups believe in and practice folk healing, consult both traditional and Western practitioners, and use both traditional and Western medicine. Many groups also place a high value on the family. However, individual variations make it inappropriate to generalize certain group characteristics to all subgroups and each member of each group. Regardless of ethnicity, the individual must come first.

The heterogeneity and marked cultural diversity of our population presents many challenges for oncology nurses. Because of the inherent differences between mainstream and ethnic minority cultures and the potential for misunderstanding and conflict, continued efforts at increasing knowledge, appreciation, and understanding of each culture are needed. Our challenge is to facilitate these efforts within ourselves, among other health professionals, and in the community at large.

References

1. Barkauskas V, Stoltenberg-Allen K, Baumann L, et al: Cultural considerations in health assessment, in Barkauskas V, Stoltenberg-Allen K, Baumann L, et al (eds): *Health and Physical Assessment* (ed 2). St. Louis, Mosby-Year Book, 1998 pp 131–151
2. Leininger MM: The theory of culture care diversity and universality, in Leininger MM (ed): *Cultural Care Diversity and Universality: A Theory of Nursing.* New York, National League for Nursing Press, 1991, pp 5–68
3. Seidel HM, Ball JW, Dains JE, et al: Cultural awareness, in Seidel HM, Ball JW, Dains JE, et al (eds): *Mosby's Guide to Physical Examination* (ed 4). St. Louis, Mosby-Year Book, 1999, pp 36–46
4. Spector RE: Cultural Diversity, in Potter PA, Perry AG (eds): *Fundamentals of Nursing: Concepts, Process, and Practice* (ed 4). St. Louis, Mosby-Year Book, 1997, pp 351–369
5. Spector RE: Multicultural Nursing, in Potter PA, Perry AG (eds): *Basic Nursing: Theory and Practice* (ed 3). St. Louis, Mosby-Year Book, 1995, pp 402–418
6. Galanti G. *Caring for Patients from Different Cultures.* Philadelphia, University of Pennsylvania Press, 1991, pp 1–14
7. Lewin M, Rice B (eds): *Balancing the Scales of Opportunity: Ensuring Racial and Ethnic Diversity in the Health Professions.* Committee on Increasing Minority Participation in the Health Professions, Institute of Medicine. Washington, DC, National Academy Press, 1994
8. Lin-Fu JS: Asian and Pacific Islander Americans: An overview of demographic characteristics and health care issues. *Asia Am Pac Islander J Health* 1:20–36, 1993
9. Day JC: *Population Projections of the United States, by Age, Sex, Race, and Hispanic Origin: 1993 to 2050.* U.S. Bureau of the Census, Current Population Reports, P25-1104, Washington, DC, U.S. Government Printing Office, 1993
10. Campbell PR: *Population Projection for States, by Age, Race, Sex, and Hispanic Origin: 1993–2020.* U.S. Bureau of the Census, Current Population Reports, P25-111. Washington, DC, U.S. Government Printing Office, 1994
11. U.S. Dept. of Commerce, Bureau of the Census: *1990 Census of Population and Housing.* Equal Employment Opportunity File, Computer File, CD ROM. Washington, DC, Data User Services Division, 1993
12. American Cancer Society: *Cancer Facts & Figures—1999.* Atlanta, American Cancer Society, 1999
13. Kagawa-Singer M: Socioeconomic and cultural influences on cancer care of women. *Semin Oncol Nurs* 11:109–119, 1995
14. Miller BA, Kolonel LN, Bernstein L, et al (eds): *Racial/Ethnic Patterns of Cancer in the United States 1988–1992.* NIH Publication No. 96-4104. Bethesda, MD, National Cancer Institute, 1996
15. Frank-Stromborg M: Changing demographics in the United States: Implications for health professionals. *Cancer* 67:1772–1778, 1991 (suppl)
16. Chen MS: A 1993 status report on the health status of Asian Pacific Islander Americans: Comparisons with

Healthy People 2000 objectives. *Asia Am Pac Islander J Health* 1:37–55, 1993

17. American Cancer Society: *Cancer Facts and Figures for Minority Americans 1991.* Atlanta, American Cancer Society, 1991
18. Andrews MM: Theoretical foundations of transcultural nursing, in Andrews MM, Boyle JS (eds): *Transcultural Concepts in Nursing Care* (ed 3). Philadelphia, Lippincott Williams & Wilkins, 1999, pp 3–22
19. Giger JN, Davidhizar RE: Introduction to transcultural nursing, in Giger JN, Davidhizar RE (eds): *Transcultural Nursing: Assessment and Intervention* (ed 3). St. Louis, Mosby-Year Book, 1999, pp 3–19
20. Giger JN, Davidhizar RE: Communication, in Giger JN, Davidhizar RE (eds): *Transcultural Nursing: Assessment and Intervention* (ed 3). St Louis, Mosby-Year Book, 1999, pp 21–43
21. Kozier B, Erle G, Blais K, et al: Ethnicity and culture, in Kozier B, Erle G, Blais K, et al (eds): *Fundamentals of Nursing* (updated ed 5). Redwood City, CA, Addison-Wesley, 1998, pp 293–310
22. Giger JN, Davidhizar RE: Space, in Giger JN, Davidhizar RE (eds): *Transcultural Nursing: Assessment and Intervention* (ed 3). St Louis, Mosby-Year Book, 1999, pp 45–63
23. Giger JN, Davidhizar RE: Social organization, in Giger JN, Davidhizar RE (eds): *Transcultural Nursing: Assessment and Intervention* (ed 3). St Louis, Mosby-Year Book, 1999, pp 65–92
24. Galanti G: *Caring for Patients from Different Cultures.* Philadelphia, University of Pennsylvania Press, 1991, pp 15–33
25. Giger JN, Davidhizar RE (eds): *Transcultural Nursing: Assessment and Intervention.* St. Louis, Mosby-Year Book, 1991
26. Andrews MM, Boyle JE (eds): *Transcultural Concepts in Nursing Care* (ed 3). Philadelphia, Lippincott Williams & Wilkins, 1999
27. Frank-Stromborg M, Olsen SJ (eds): *Cancer Prevention in Minority Populations: Cultural Implications for Health Care Professionals.* St. Louis, Mosby-Year Book, 1993
28. Galanti G: *Caring for Patients from Different Cultures.* Philadelphia, University of Pennsylvania Press, 1991
29. Giger JN, Davidhizar RE (eds): *Transcultural Nursing: Assessment and Intervention* (ed 3). St. Louis, Mosby-Year Book, 1999
30. Lipson JG, Dibble SL, Minarik PA (eds): *Culture & Nursing Care: A Pocket Guide.* San Francisco, UCSF Nursing Press, 1996
31. Orque M, Bloch B, Monrrou LSA (eds): *Ethnic Nursing Care: A Multicultural Approach.* St. Louis, Mosby, 1983
32. Palafox N, Warren A (eds): *Cross-Cultural Caring: A Handbook for Health Care Professionals in Hawaii.* Honolulu, John A. Burns School of Medicine, 1980
33. Spector RE: *Cultural Diversity in Health and Illness* (ed 4). Stamford, CT, Appleton & Lange, 1996
34. Michaels D: Occupational cancer in the Black population: The health effects of job discrimination. *J Nat Med Assoc* 75:1014–1018, 1983
35. Kosary CL, Ries LAG, Miller BA, et al: *SEER Cancer Statistics Review, 1973–1992.* National Cancer Institute, NIH. Publication No. 95-2789. Bethesda, MD, 1995
36. Bloom JR, Hayes WA, Saunders F, et al: Physician induced and patient induced utilization of early cancer detection practices among Black Americans. *Adv Cancer Control Innov Res* 293:279–296, 1989
37. Winbush GB: African-American health care: Beliefs, practices and service issues, in Julia MC (ed.): *Multicultural Awareness in the Health Care Professions.* Boston: Allyn & Bacon, 1996, pp 8–22
38. Cherry B, Giger JN: African-Americans, in Giger JN, Davidhizar RE (eds): *Transcultural Nursing: Assessment and Intervention* (ed 3). St. Louis, Mosby-Year Book, 1999, pp 167–201
39. U.S. Dept. of Commerce, Bureau of the Census: *The Black Population in the United States, March 1991.* Washington, DC, U.S. Government Printing Office, 1992
40. Bloch B: Nursing care of black patients, in Orque M, Bloch B, Monrrou LSA (eds): *Ethnic Nursing Care: A Multicultural Approach.* St. Louis, Mosby, 1983, pp 81–114
41. Giger J, Davidhizar RE: Time, in Giger J, Davidhizar RE (eds): *Transcultural Nursing: Assessment and Intervention* (ed 3). St. Louis, Mosby-Year Book, 1999, pp 93–114
42. Brown JA: Social work practice with the terminally ill in the black community, in Parry JK (ed): *Social Work Practice With the Terminally Ill: A Transcultural Perspective.* Springfield, IL, Charles C Thomas, 1990, pp 67–82
43. Kemp C: *Terminal Illness: A Guide to Nursing Care.* Philadelphia, Lippincott, 1995
44. Ronan L: Alcohol-related health risks among Black Americans. *Alcohol Health Res World* 11:36–39, 1986
45. U.S. Bureau of the Census: *Current Population Reports, Population Characteristics: The Asian and Pacific Islander Population in the United States, March 1991 and 1990.* Washington, DC, U.S. Government Printing Office, pp 20–459, 1992
46. Hussey LOL, Itano JK, Taoka KN, et al: Cancer prevention and early detection in Native Hawaiians, in Frank-Stromborg M, Olsen SJ (eds): *Cancer Prevention in Minority Populations: Cultural Implications for Health Care Professionals.* St. Louis, Mosby, 1993, pp 113–138
47. Sawyers JE, Eaton L: Gastric cancer in the Korean-American: Cultural implications. *Oncol Nurs Forum* 19: 619–623, 1992
48. Gould-Martin K, Ngin C: Chinese Americans, in Harwood A (ed): *Ethnicity and Medical Care.* Cambridge, Harvard University Press, 1981, pp 130–171
49. Chang K: Chinese Americans, in Giger JN, Davidhizar RE (eds): *Transcultural Nursing: Assessment and Intervention* (ed 3). St. Louis, Mosby-Year Book, 1999, pp 385–401
50. Lee P, Takamura J: The Japanese Americans in Hawaii, in Palafox N, Warren A (eds): *Cross-Cultural Caring: A Handbook for Health Care Professionals in Hawaii.* Honolulu, John A. Burns School of Medicine, 1980, pp 105–135
51. Hashizume S, Takano J: Nursing care of Japanese American patients, in Orque M, Bloch B, Monrrou LSA (eds): *Ethnic Nursing Care: A Multicultural Approach.* St. Louis, Mosby, 1983, pp 219–243
52. Chin P: Chinese Americans, in Lipson JG, Dibble SL, Minarik PA (eds): *Culture & Nursing Care: A Pocket Guide,* San Francisco, UCSF Nursing Press, 1996, pp 74–81
53. Chen-Louie T: Nursing care of Chinese American patients, in Orque M, Block B, Monrrou LSA (eds): *Ethnic Nursing Care: A Multicultural Approach.* St. Louis, Mosby, 1983, pp 183–218
54. Buchwald D, Panwala S, Hooton TM: Use of traditional health practices by Southeast Asian refugees in a primary care clinic. *West J Med* 156:507–511, 1992
55. Anderson JN: Health and illness in Filipino immigrants. *West J Med* 139:811–819, 1983
56. Ramakrishna J, Weiss MG: Health, illness, and immigration—East Indians in the United States. *West J Med* 157: 265–270, 1992

57. Rairdan B, Higgs ZR: When your patient is a Hmong refugee. *Am J Nurs* 92:52–55, 1992

58. Stauffer RY: Vietnamese Americans, in Giger JN, Davidhizar RE (eds): *Transcultural Nursing: Assessment and Intervention* (ed 3). St. Louis, Mosby-Year Book, 1999, pp 427–457

59. Gilman SC, Justice J, Saepharn K, et al: Use of traditional and modern health services by Laotian refugees. *West J Med* 157:310–315, 1992

60. Uba L: Cultural barriers to health care for Southeast Asian refugees. *Public Health Rep* 107:544–548, 1992

61. Baysa E, Cabrera E, Camilon F, et al: The Filipinos, in Palafox N, Warren A (eds): *Cross-Cultural Caring: A Handbook for Health Care Professionals in Hawaii*. Honolulu, John A. Burns School of Medicine, 1980, pp 197–212

62. Orque MS: Nursing care of Filipino American patients, in Orque M, Bloch B, Monrrou LSA (eds): *Ethnic Nursing Care: A Multicultural Approach*. St. Louis, Mosby, 1983, pp 149–181

63. Kunz K, Lam C, Siu K, et al: The Chinese, in Palafox N, Warren A (eds): *Cross-Cultural Caring: A Handbook for Health Care Professionals in Hawaii*. Honolulu, John A. Burns School of Medicine, 1980, pp 26–50

64. Krauss BH: Medicine and medicinal herbs, in Krauss BH: *Plants in Hawaiian Culture*. Honolulu, University of Hawaii Press, 1993, pp 100–104

65. Andrews MM: Transcultural perspectives in the nursing care of children, in Andrews MM, Boyle JS (eds): *Transcultural Concepts in Nursing Care* (ed 3). Philadelphia, Lippincott Williams & Wilkins, 1999, pp 107–159

66. Vance AR: Filipino Americans, in Giger JN, Davidhizar RE (eds): *Transcultural Nursing: Assessment and Intervention* (ed 3). St. Louis, Mosby-Year Book, 1999, pp 403–425

67. Ishida D, Inouye J: Japanese Americans, in Giger JN, Davidhizar RE (eds): *Transcultural Nursing: Assessment and Intervention* (ed 3). St. Louis, Mosby-Year Book, 1999, pp 311–335

68. Lasky EM, Martz CH: The Asian/Pacific Islander population in the United States: Cultural perspectives and their relationship to cancer prevention and early detection, in Frank-Stromborg M, Olsen SJ (eds): *Cancer Prevention in Minority Populations: Cultural Implications for Health Care Professionals*. St. Louis, Mosby, 1993, pp 78–112

69. Klessig J: The effects of values and culture on life-support decisions. *West J Med* 157:316–322, 1992

70. Earp JB: Korean Americans, in Giger JN, Davidhizar RE (eds): *Transcultural Nursing: Assessment and Intervention* (ed 3). St. Louis, Mosby-Year Book, 1999, pp 535–549

71. Miller SW, Goodin JN: East Indian Hindu Americans, in Giger JN, Davidhizar RE (eds): *Transcultural Nursing: Assessment and Intervention* (ed 3). St. Louis, Mosby-Year Book, 1999, pp 459–481

72. Tripp-Reimer T, Afifi LA: Cross-cultural perspectives on patient teaching. *Nurs Clin North Am* 24:613–619, 1989

73. Haffner L: Translation is not enough—interpreting in a medical setting. *West J Med* 157:255–259, 1992

74. Jenkins CNH, McPhee SJ, Bird JA, et al: Cancer risks and prevention practices among Vietnamese refugees. *West J Med* 153:34–39, 1990

75. Mo B: Modesty, sexuality, and breast health in Chinese-American women. *West J Med* 157:260–264, 1992

76. Lovejoy NC, Jenkins C, Wu T, et al: Developing a breast cancer screening program for Chinese-American women. *Oncol Nurs Forum* 16:181–187, 1989

77. Muller JH, Desmond B: Ethical dilemmas in a cross-cultural context—a Chinese example. *West J Med* 157:323–327, 1992

78. Brotzman GL, Butler DJ: Cross-cultural issues in the disclosure of a terminal diagnosis: A case report. *J Fam Pract* 32: 426–427, 1991

79. Tung TM: Death, dying, and hospice: An Asian-American view. *Am J Hosp Palliat Care* 7:23–25, 1990

80. Zhou HH, Adeloyin A, Wilkinson GR: Differences in plasma binding of drugs between Caucasians and Chinese subjects. *Clin Pharmacol Ther* 48:10–7, 1990

81. Parker SL, Davis KJ, Wingo PA, et al: Cancer statistics by race and ethnicity. *CA Cancer J Clin* 48:31–48, 1998

82. Mack TM, Walker A, Mack W, et al: Cancer in Hispanics in Los Angeles County. *Monogr Natl Cancer Inst* 69:99–104, 1985

83. Devor EJ, Buechley RW: Gallbladder cancer in Hispanic New Mexicans: I. General population 1957–1977. *Cancer* 45:1705–1712, 1980

84. Menck HR, Mack TM: Incidence of biliary tract cancer in Los Angeles. *Monogr Natl Cancer Inst* 62:95–99, 1982

85. Suarez L, Martin J: Primary liver cancer mortality and incidence in Texas Mexican Americans 1969–1980. *Am J Public Health* 77:631–633, 1987

86. Peters RK, Thomas D, Hagan DG, et al: Risk factors in invasive cervical cancer among Latinas and non-Latinas in Los Angeles County. *J Natl Cancer Inst* 77:1063–1077, 1986

87. Daly MB, Clark GM, McGuire WL: Breast cancer prognosis in a mixed Caucasian Hispanic population. *J Natl Cancer Inst* 74:753–757, 1985

88. Centers for Disease Control and Prevention: Prevalence of selected risk factors for chronic disease by education level in racial/ethnic populations—United States, 1991–92. *MMWR Morb Mortal Wkly Rep 1994* 43:894–899, 1994

89. Freeman HE, Aiken LH, Blendon RJ et al: Uninsured working-age adults: Characteristics and consequences. *Health Serv Res* 24:811–823, 1990

90. Centers for Disease Control and Prevention: *Chronic Disease in Minority Populations: African Americans, American Indians and Alaskan Natives, Asian and Pacific Islanders, Hispanic Americans*. Atlanta, Centers for Disease Control and Prevention, 1994.

91. Kuipers J: Mexican-Americans, in Giger JN, Davidhizar RE (eds): *Transcultural Nursing: Assessment and Intervention* (ed 3). St. Louis, Mosby-Year Book, 1999, pp 203–235

92. Lassiter SM: *Multicultural Clients*. Westport, CT, Greenwood Press, 1995

93. Gonzales-Swafford MJ, Gutierrez MG: Ethnomedical beliefs and practices of Mexican Americans. *Nurs Pract* 8: 29–30, 32,34, 1983

94. Sugarek NJ, Deyo RA, Holmes BC: Locus of control and beliefs about cancer in a multi-ethnic clinic population. *Oncol Nurs Forum* 15:481–486, 1988

95. Cohen RJ, Rohaly JA: Cancer prevention and screening among Hispanic populations, in Frank-Stromborg M, Olsen SJ (eds): *Cancer Prevention in Minority Populations: Cultural Implications for Health Care Professionals*. St. Louis, Mosby-Year Book, 1993, pp 203–238

96. Rodriques J: Mexican Americans: Factors influencing health practices. *J Sch Health* 53:136–139, 1983

97. Mardiros M: A view toward hospitalization: The Mexican-American experience. *J Adv Nurs* 9:469–478, 1984

98. Estrada A, Trevino F, Ray L: Health care utilization barriers among Mexican Americans: Evidence from HHANES 1982–84. *Am J Public Health* 80:27–31, 1990 (suppl)

99. Kerr M, Ritchey D: Health promoting lifestyles of English-speaking and Spanish-speaking Mexican-American migrant farm workers. *Public Health Nurs* 7:80–87, 1990

100. Martaus TM: The health seeking process of Mexican-American migrant farm workers. *Home Health Care Nurse* 4:32–36, 1986

101. Ingham J: On Mexican folk medicine. *Am Anthropologist* 72:76–87, 1970

102. Gomez GE, Gomez EA: Folk healing among Hispanic Americans. *Public Health Nurs* 2:245–249, 1985

103. Burgos-Ocasio H: Understanding the Hispanic community, in Julia MC (ed): *Multicultural Awareness in the Health Care Professions*. Boston, Allyn & Bacon, 1996, pp 111–130

104. Murillo-Rohde I: Hispanic American patient care, in Henderson G, Primeaux M (eds): *Transcultural Health Care*. Menlo Park, CA, Addison-Wesley, 1981, pp 224–238

105. Kalish RA, Reynolds DK: Mexican-Americans, in Kalish RA, Reynolds DK (eds): *Death and Ethnicity: A Psychocultural Study*. Farmingdale, NY, Baywood, 1981, pp 155–184

106. Salcido RM: Mexican-Americans: Illness, death and bereavement, in Parry JK (ed): *Social Work with the Terminally Ill: A Transcultural Perspective*. Springfield, IL, Charles C Thomas, 1990, pp 113–127

107. National Coalition of Hispanic Health and Human Services Organizations: *Delivering Preventive Health Care to Hispanics: A Manual for Providers*. Washington, DC, The Coalition, 1988

108. Department of Health and Human Services, Healthy People 2000: *National Health Promotion and Disease Prevention Objectives—Full Report with Commentary*. Boston, Jones and Bartlett, 1992

109. U.S. Bureau of the Census: *Statistical Abstract of the United States: 1996* (ed 116). Washington, DC, 1996

110. Burhansstipanov L, Dresser CM: *Native American Monograph No. 1: Documentation of the Cancer Research Needs of American Indians and Alaskan Natives* (NIH Publication No. 93-3603, 1993) Bethesda, MD, National Institute of Health, 1993

111. Wilson UM: Nursing care of American Indian patients, in Orque M, Bloch B, Monrrou LSA (eds): *Ethnic Nursing Care: A Multicultural Approach*. St. Louis, Mosby, 1983, pp 271–295

112. Weiss KM, Ferrell RE, Hanis CL, et al: Genetics and epidemiology of gallbladder disease in new world native peoples. *Am J Hum Genet* 36:1259–1278, 1984

113. Bivens MD, Fleetwood HO: A ten year survey of cervical carcinoma in Indians of the southwest. *Obstet Gynecol* 32:11–16, 1968

114. Skubi D: Pap smear screening and cervical pathology in an American Indian population. *J Nurse Midwife* 33:203–207, 1988

115. Horner RD: Cancer mortality in Native Americans in North Carolina. *Am J Public Health* 80:940–944, 1990

116. Spector RE: Health and illness in the American Indian, Aleut, and Eskimo communities, in Spector RE (ed): *Cultural Diversity in Health and Illness* (ed 4). Stamford, CT, Appleton & Lange, 1996, pp 215–240

117. Hanley CE: Navajo Indians, in Giger J, Davidhizar RE (eds): *Transcultural Nursing: Assessment and Intervention* (ed. 3). St. Louis, Mosby-Year Book, 1999, pp 237–257

118. Locust CS: *American Indian Beliefs Concerning Health and Unwellness*. Native American Research and Training Center, Monograph Series. Tucson, AZ, University of Arizona, 1985

119. Boyd D: *Rolling Thunder*. New York, Random House, 1974

120. Bilagody H: An American Indian looks at health care, in Feldman R, Buch D (eds): *Ninth Annual Training Institute for Psychiatrist-Teachers of Practicing Physicians*. Boulder, CO, WICHE, 1969

121. Kluckhohn C, Leighton D: The supernatural: Power and danger, in Kluckhohn C, Leighton D (eds): *The Navajo* (rev ed). Garden City, NJ, Doubleday, 1962, pp 178–199

122. Vogel VJ: Indian theories of disease and shamanistic practices, in Vogel VJ (ed): *American Indian Medicine*. New York, Ballantine Books, 1979, pp 13–35

123. Primeaux M, Henderson G: American Indian patient care, in Henderson G, Primeaux M (eds): *Transcultural Health Care*. Menlo Park, CA, Addison-Wesley, 1981, pp 239–254

124. Antle A: Ethnic perspectives of cancer nursing: The American Indian. *Oncol Nurs Forum* 14:70–73, 1987

125. Lammers PK: How they view you, themselves, and disease. *AORN J* 45:1211–1216, 1987

126. Yuki T: Cultural responsiveness and social work practice: An Indian clinic's success. *Health Soc Work* 11:223–229, 1986

127. Lewis R: Death and dying among the American Indians, in Parry JK (ed): *Social Work Practice with the Terminally Ill: A Transcultural Perspective*. Springfield, IL, Charles C Thomas, 1990, pp 23–32

128. Baquet CR, Horm JW, Gibbs T, et al: Socioeconomic factors and cancer incidence among blacks and whites. *J Natl Cancer Inst* 83:551–557, 1991

129. Berg JW, Ross R, Latourette HB: Economic status and survival of cancer patients. *Cancer* 39:467–477, 1977

130. Page WF, Kuntz AJ: Racial and socioeconomic factors in cancer survival: A comparison of Veteran's Administration results with selected studies. *Cancer* 45:1029–1040, 1980

131. McWhorter WP, Schatzkin AG, Horm JW, et al: Contribution of socioeconomic status to black/white differences in cancer incidence. *Cancer* 63:982–987, 1989

132. Freeman HP: Cancer in the socioeconomically disadvantaged. *CA Cancer J Clin* 39:266–288, 1989

133. U.S. Bureau of the Census: *U.S. Bureau of the Census Statistics*. Washington, DC, Government Printing Office, 1991

134. Lewis O: The culture of poverty. *Sci Am* 215:19–25, 1966

135. American Cancer Society: *Cancer in the Economically Disadvantaged: A Special Report*. Atlanta, American Cancer Society, 1989

136. Wilkes G, Freeman H, Prout M: Cancer and poverty: Breaking the cycle. *Semin Oncol Nurs* 10:79–88, 1994

137. Palos G: Cultural heritage: Cancer screening and early detection. *Semin Oncol Nurs* 10:104–113, 1994

138. Brawley OW: Minority accrual and clinical trials. *Oncol Issues* 10:22–24, 1995

139. Black BL, Ades TB: American Cancer Society urban demonstration projects: Models for successful intervention. *Semin Oncol Nurs* 10:96–103, 1994

140. Black BL, Schweitzer R, Dezelsky T: Report on the American Cancer Society workshop on community cancer detection, education, and prevention demonstration projects for underserved populations. *CA Cancer J Clin* 43:226–233, 1993

141. Mack E, McGrath T, Pendleton D, et al: Reaching poor populations with cancer prevention and early detection programs. *Cancer Pract* 1:35–39, 1993

142. Eng E: The save our sisters project: A social network strategy for reaching rural Black women. *Cancer* 72:1071–1077, 1993

143. Dignan M, Sharp P, Blinson K, et al: Development of a cervical cancer education program for Native American women in North Carolina. *J Cancer Educ* 9:235–242, 1994

144. Robinson KD, Kimmel EA, Yasko JM: Reaching out to the African American community through innovative strategies. *Oncol Nurs Forum* 22:1383–1391, 1995

145. Andrews MM, Herberg, P: Transcultural nursing care, in Andrews MM, Boyle JS (eds): *Transcultural Concepts in Nurs-*

ing Care (ed 3): Philadelphia, Lippincott, Williams & Wilkins, 1999, pp 23–77

146. Jarvis C: *Physical Examination and Health Assessment* (ed 2). Philadelphia, Saunders, 1996, p 76

147. Marshall P: Cultural influences on perceived quality of life. *Semin Oncol Nurs* 6:278–284, 1990

148. Stephens ST: Patient education materials: Are they readable? *Oncol Nurs Forum* 19:83–85, 1992

149. Cooley ME, Moriarty H, Berger MS, et al: Patient literacy and the readability of written cancer educational materials. *Oncol Nurs Forum* 22:1345–1351, 1995

150. Shadick KM: Development of a transcultural health education program for the Hmong. *Clin Nurs Spec* 7:48–53, 1993

151. Villejo L: Patient education for Hispanic cancer patients, in Jones LA (ed): *Minorities and Cancer.* New York, Springer-Verlag, 1989, pp 295–300

152. Brant J: Video review: Standing strong against the cancer enemy. *Transcultural Nursing Issues Special Interest Group Newsletter* 4:3, 1994

153. Millon-Underwood S, Sander E, Davis M: Determinants of participation in state-of-the-art cancer prevention, early detection/screening, and treatment trials among African-Americans. *Cancer Nurs* 16:25–33, 1993

154. McCabe MS, Varricchio CG, Padberg RM: Efforts to recruit the economically disadvantaged to national clinical trials. *Semin Oncol Nurs* 10:123–129, 1994

155. Porter CP, Villarruel AM: Nursing research with African American and Hispanic people: Guidelines for action. *Nurs Outlook* 41:59–67, 1993

156. Munet-Vilaro F: Methodologic issues in the implementation of a Latino population. *Proceedings of the Third National Conference on Cancer Nursing Research.* Atlanta, American Cancer Society, 1994, pp 39–43

157. Flaskerud JH: Is the Likert scale format culturally biased? *Nurs Res* 37:185–186, 1988

CHAPTER 8

Dynamics of Cancer Prevention

Lois J. Loescher, PhDc, RN
Mary E. Reid, PhD

Introduction

Many believe that the best way to control cancer is to prevent it, specifically by reducing the risk of cancer.[1,2] The focus on cancer treatment and cure by clinicians, researchers, and funding agencies is slowly beginning to shift to cancer prevention. Since the passage of the National Cancer Act in 1971, cancer prevention and control activities have gradually been integrated into the National Cancer Program. Now, at the beginning of the twenty-first century, scientists in many disciplines, including nursing, are faced with the challenges of translating the findings of behavioral, epidemiological, clinical, and basic science research into specific interventions for preventing cancer.[3] This chapter presents a conceptual overview of cancer prevention as a component of cancer control. (For information about cancer risk, risk assessment, and specific screening activities, see Chapters 5, 9, and 10.)

Definitions of Cancer Prevention

Definitions of cancer prevention are evolving and often are unclear. In the past, nurses have generally used a stage-of-disease model[4] to define *prevention* as being all measures that limit the progression of disease at any time during its course. These prevention measures can occur anywhere along the health continuum. Three levels of prevention have been traditionally defined in the nursing literature:

1. *Primary prevention* decreases the vulnerability of a healthy individual or population to illness or dysfunction through health promotion strategies and specific protection recommendations.
2. *Secondary prevention* defines and identifies high-risk individuals and populations, including those with precursor lesions or syndromes, and consists of early diagnosis, early detection, screening, and treatment of early stages of disease.
3. *Tertiary prevention* minimizes morbidity resulting from permanent or irreversible disease by preventing complications.[5]

Although these traditional definitions of prevention, which encompasses the entire health continuum, have guided nursing science and practice for years, they do not reflect the evolving science or sentiment concerning cancer prevention.[6,7] Generally, cancer prevention is achieved when modulation or modification of self-care behaviors or exogenous factors results in reduced cancer risk.[7-9] This broadly covers preventive measures such as avoidance or reduction of exposure to carcinogens, use of chemopreventive agents, or surgical removal of precancerous lesions.[8] Byar and Freedman have suggested that primary prevention should relate to initiation, secondary prevention to promotion, and tertiary prevention to pro-

gression.[8] Thus, by these criteria, primary prevention is the avoidance of exposure to carcinogens (e.g., viruses, radiation, pollutants, chemicals), tobacco use, changes in diet, and the administration of specific agents (e.g., chemopreventives) to healthy individuals[7] to limit exposure to the carcinogens that initiate carcinogenesis. Secondary prevention is the prevention of promotion by smoking cessation, changes in diet, and administration of chemopreventive agents presumed to act on promotion. Mechanisms of prevention might be inhibiting the activation of proto-oncogenes or antagonizing the effects of oncogene expression.[10,11] Byar and Freedman state, "The term secondary prevention has often been used to describe screening activities. This usage should be discouraged because it is conceptually awkward to imagine preventing a lesion that is already present and that we wish to detect."[8,p.413] Tertiary prevention consists of arresting, removing, or reversing a premalignant lesion (e.g., with chemoprevention or surgery) to prevent recurrence or progression to cancer.[10] Not all investigators have adopted the definitions of Byar and Freedman.

The traditional definition of cancer prevention used in nursing now more aptly falls under the broad umbrella of cancer control, rather than cancer prevention per se.[6] The Division of Cancer Prevention and Control (DCPC) at the National Cancer Institute (NCI) defines cancer control as "the reduction of cancer incidence, morbidity, and mortality through an orderly sequence from research on interventions and their impact in defined populations to the broad, systematic application of the research results."[11,p.9]

Modern Approaches to Cancer Prevention

The multidisciplinary scientific community uses three main approaches to achieve primary, secondary, and tertiary prevention: (1) education and knowledge, (2) regulation, and (3) host modification.[13]

Education and Knowledge

Education focuses on changing lifestyle behaviors to reduce cancer incidence through translation of scientific findings into sensible and practical recommendations.[12,13] These recommendations may be based on objectives such as those proposed by the DCPC in its *Cancer Control Objectives for the Nation: 1985–2000.* These objectives target four areas of prevention (i.e., smoking, diet, sun exposure, counseling) that reflect an analysis and synthesis of current knowledge about cancer prevention (Table 8-1).[11] In addition to messages aimed at tobacco cessation, sun avoidance, and dietary changes, cancer prevention education consists primarily of modifying sexual practices and decreasing exposure to environmental and occupational carcinogens.[13]

Table 8-1 Cancer Control Healthy People 2000 Prevention Objectives

Factor	Year 2000 Objectives
Smoking	Reduce percent of adults who smoke to 15% or less
	Reduce percent of youths who smoke by age 20 to 15% or less
Diet	Reduce dietary fat to 30% of total calories or less.
	Reduce saturated fat to less than 10% of total calories (ages 2 and older)
	Increase complex carbohydrates and fiber in adult diets to 5 or more servings of fruit and 6 or more servings of grain products daily
Sun exposure	Increase to 60% or more people who limit sun exposure, use sunscreens and protective clothing when exposed to sunlight, and avoid artificial sources of ultraviolet light
Counseling	Increase to 75% or more primary care providers who routinely counsel patients about tobacco cessation, diet modification, and screening recommendations

Adapted from the Division of Cancer Prevention and Control: *'94 Annual Report.* Bethesda, MD, National Cancer Institute, 1994, p 13.

The U.S. Public Health Service, the NCI, state and local health care agencies, cancer centers, and voluntary health organizations such as the American Cancer Society and the American Lung Association have carried out prevention education. A large part of public health education has been facilitated by the lay media, particularly by newspapers, magazines, and television programs that learn about scientific discoveries and report the news in an audience-specific fashion to the public.[14,15]

Education alone, however, does not effect lifestyle change, and bridging the gap between acquiring knowledge and adopting or modifying lifestyle cancer preventive behaviors remains a critical and problematic issue. Several variables, including knowledge of the principles underlying prevention, perceived susceptibility to developing cancer, and perceived consequences of prevention and lack of prevention influence a person's decision to put knowledge into practice.[16] These and other variables critical for lifestyle changes aimed at preventing cancer are illustrated in Figure 8-1.

Educational efforts need to consider persuading people and populations to adopt preventive behaviors. Health care providers need to remember that persuasion is a nonlinear process and that lasting change is not achieved in a single encounter.[16] Persuasion depends on the following factors: (1) recipients of the information need to receive it from a source that is credible and is similar and attractive to the recipient; (2) the quality, quantity, and timing of messages are critical; (3) channels for communicating messages must maximize exposure or coverage of at-risk populations, speed of transmission, cost, and message function; and (4) the characteristics of the receiver (e.g., age, culture, ethnicity, developmental level, gender) must be considered.[16]

Regulation

Tobacco

Much of the regulations related to cancer prevention are a result of public demand. Both state and federal governments have attempted to regulate the production, sale, and consumption of tobacco products. All states have passed laws banning the sale of cigarettes to young people, and many states restrict or prohibit smoking at work sites.[17]

In 1995, the Food and Drug Administration (FDA) began efforts to regulate nicotine as a drug, and tobacco products as drug-delivery devices. The tobacco industry sued the FDA, but in 1997 a U.S. District Court ruled that the FDA was entitled to define nicotine as a drug, and tobacco products as drug-delivery devices.[17]

Representatives of the tobacco industry and a number of state attorneys general reached an agreement in 1997 that could dramatically change tobacco production, marketing, sales, and consumption in the United States. Under the settlement, tobacco manufacturers face restrictions on advertising and promotion of tobacco products and are subject to FDA regulation of their products. Cigarette retailers have to be licensed, are allowed to sell only to adults, and are subject to rules about where they place tobacco products in their outlets. Employers, fast-food restaurants, and some other establishments must create smoke-free environments. Despite these regulations, the rights of consumers to sue tobacco companies for past damages are severely limited.[17]

Other forms of regulation

Imposing and increasing excise taxes on alcohol products to reduce its accessibility is an important form of regulation. Additionally, regulation decreases or eliminates man-made environmental carcinogens (e.g., 2-naphthylamine, benzene) and prohibits the addition of carcinogens to food. Regulatory efforts monitor homes for radon and limit exposure to occupational carcinogens (e.g., asbestos).[13]

Unfortunately, the etiology for most cancers is unknown, thereby limiting the application of exposure-based regulatory strategies.[12] Additionally, the impact of regulatory efforts concerned with cancer prevention are difficult to evaluate. For example, it is still too early to evaluate the long-term gains from tobacco regulation.[13]

Host Modification

Host modification is the alteration of the body's internal environment to prevent initiation or progression of can-

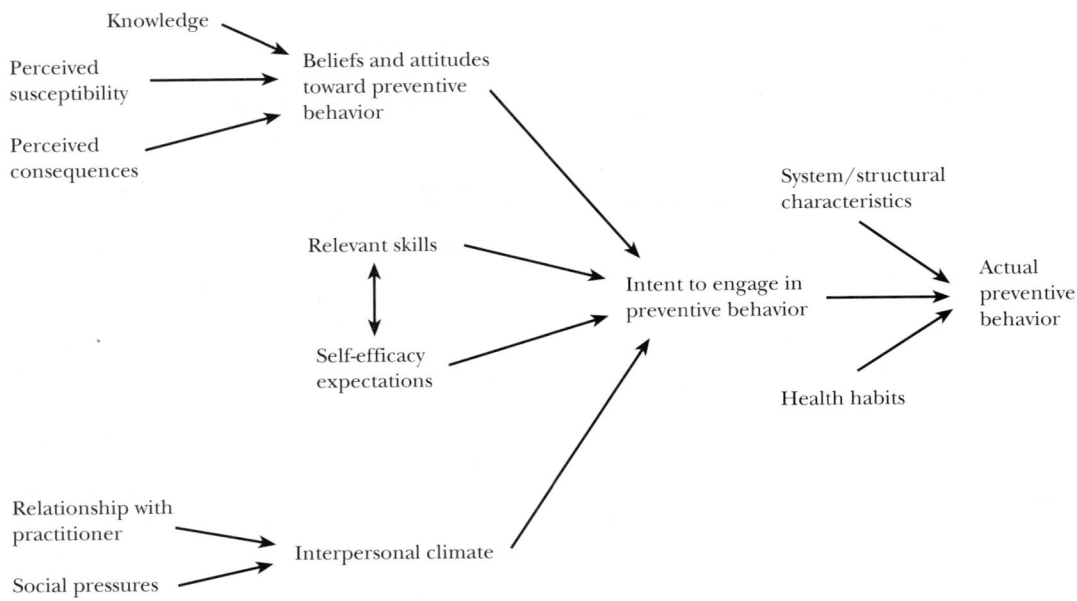

Figure 8-1 Factors affecting cancer prevention behavior. (Adapted with permission from Buller DB, Buller MK: Approaches to communicating preventive behaviors. *Semin Oncol Nurs* 7:53–63, 1991)[16]

cer. The principal methods are immunization and chemoprevention.[13]

Immunization

Tumor-associated viruses are probably necessary but alone are not sufficient to cause tumors. (Chapter 5 summarizes viruses that are implicated in cancer causation.) Generally, a cancer-causing virus is integrated into cellular DNA. A long latent period occurs between the initial infection and onset of cancer.[18] The discovery of cancer-causing viruses in humans shows some promise for cancer prevention in that similar viruses in animals have been eliminated by vaccines made from the attenuated (inactivated) viruses.[19] The current approach to vaccination in humans is to attenuate viruses and use them for immunostimulation.[20] Newer direct approaches to cancer vaccines are currently being explored or are in the planning stages. The direct approach uses two methods. In one, gene sequences of the desired antigen are delivered to the host by inserting the gene for the antigen via a nonreplicating plasmid vector. The gene coding for the desired protein is put into purified plasmid DNA, suspended in saline, and injected into the skin or muscle. The other method introduces the gene by bombarding the skin with a "gene gun" containing particles of the plasmid DNA.[20,21]

Researchers are optimistic that hepatomas related to hepatitis B virus (HBV) and hepatitis C virus (HCV) can be prevented by vaccination and screening of blood for transfusion.[22] Human papillomavirus and human T-lymphotropic virus (HTLV) vaccines are not ready for human trials. Two vaccines for human immunodeficiency virus are safe for phase I or II trials. Tumor antigen

vaccines against breast and pancreatic cancers are under development.[18,19] The Cancer Research Institute, a nonprofit organization that supports cancer immunology research, has established a cancer vaccine trial registry that will serve as a centralized source of information about all ongoing cancer vaccine trials.[21,23]

Chemoprevention

The most tested and promising form of host modification is *chemoprevention*, or the use of defined, noncytotoxic nutrients or pharmacologic agents to inhibit or reverse the process of carcinogenesis. Chemopreventive agents enhance the inactivation of carcinogens, modify the expression of oncogenes, or interfere with cell proliferation. Nutrient chemopreventives include dietary constituents (e.g., beta-carotene), vitamins (e.g., vitamins A, C, and E), and micronutrients (e.g., selenium). Examples of pharmacologic chemopreventives are synthetic retinoids (e.g., isotretinoin), antiestrogens (e.g., tamoxifen), and nonsteroidal anti-inflammatory drugs (NSAIDs).[24,25]

Chemoprevention and carcinogenesis. Knowledge of certain aspects of carcinogenesis is fundamental to understanding chemoprevention. (See Chapters 2 and 4 for a detailed explanation.) Multiple changes in cellular genetics occurring together, rather than a single event, are believed to initiate cancer.[11] During initiation, the DNA of a normal cell undergoes somatic mutation. If the cell repairs the DNA damage, cancer may not develop. However, after initiation, a mutation may remain dormant in an extended latency period. During this period, the multiple initiating events or promotion of a genetically altered cell required for tumor growth may begin.[12,25]

Proto-oncogenes, which code for proteins involved in normal cell growth and differentiation, most likely are involved in initiation and promotion of cancer.[26] Tumor-suppressor genes—genes that code for proteins that inhibit unregulated growth—also are involved. Genomic instability, which occurs through genetic mechanisms (e.g., translocation, gene amplification, point mutation), can convert proto-oncogenes to oncogenes. Genomic instability can be triggered by spontaneous somatic events or from exposure to carcinogens or mutagens.[11] Genomic mutations of a large number of oncogenes and tumor-suppressor genes may cause epithelial cells to undergo clonal expansion. Clonal expansion can be visualized in the context of intraepithelial neoplasia. That is, it is preinvasive, premalignant, precancer.[27]

Clonal expansion can occur by three basic mechanisms: (1) a mutational block in the differentiation pathway with continuing production of stem cells, (2) a mutational block in a proliferation-related signal pathway, and (3) a mutational block in apoptosis.[27] Thus, within this genetic framework, the theoretical disruption of carcinogenesis at several points provides the rationale for use of chemopreventive agents.[11,25]

Chemopreventive compounds generally are classified into three broad categories that reflect the point during carcinogenesis at which the agents are effective:

1. *Blocking agents* are compounds that block, or prevent, carcinogenesis. In essence, they function as barriers. For example, some blocking agents prevent activation of carcinogens or tumor promoters requiring metabolic activation. Others enhance detoxification systems. A third group of blocking agents trap carcinogens before they reach target sites. The drug oltipraz, which inhibits aflatoxin-induced carcinogenesis, is an example of a blocking agent.
2. *Chemopreventive agents that decrease tissue vulnerability to carcinogenesis* work by producing cellular maturation (e.g., decreasing vulnerability of the breast to neoplasia), decreased function or activity of cells (e.g., drug-induced castration to prevent cancer of sex hormone–dependent tissues), or decreased cell proliferation (e.g., evolution dietary changes).
3. *Suppressing agents* prevent the evolution of the neoplastic process in cells that otherwise would become cancerous. These agents can produce differentiation, suppress oncogene activation, or selectively inhibit proliferation of potentially malignant cells. Examples of suppressing agents are retinoids (e.g., vitamin A, beta-carotene), which can control expression of certain oncogenes and growth-factor receptors, thereby regulating cell differentiation and proliferation in most epithelia that are sites for cancer development.[26,28] Steroid hormones or analogues, such as tamoxifen (a synthetic antiestrogen) or finasteride (a synthetic antiandrogen), can bind to protein receptors in the cell nucleus and regulate translation. Anti-

inflammatory agents may inhibit the synthesis of prostaglandins, which reduce the formation of colon polyps.[11] Chemoprevention, therefore, has the potential for primary, secondary, and tertiary prevention.[10]

Intermediate end points of chemoprevention. A major limitation of chemoprevention is identification of end points that measure efficacy of the agent. Although detection of cancer is the definitive end point, it is not feasible because the time to cancer occurrence may be long, or the incidence uncommon, even in persons at high risk.[29] Thus, the current approach for assessing efficacy of chemoprevention consists of using intermediate markers as end points. Combinations of intermediate markers may most accurately predict the response to a chemopreventive agent.[30] Intermediate markers may be precursor lesions, including regression in atypia of sputum cytology of smokers, reduced recurrence of colon polyps following removal, regression of prostatic epithelial neoplasia in men at high risk of prostate cancer, and regression or abatement of oral leukoplakia in smokers or tobacco chewers.[31]

Intermediate markers also include prevention of disease recurrence or second primary cancers in people with a history of cancer, such as delayed appearance of second head and neck cancer primary lesions, and prostate-specific antigen (PSA) failure in men curatively treated for prostate cancer.[31]

Other intermediate markers are biological markers. These can be defined as "measurable markers of cellular or molecular events associated with specific stages of the multistep evolution and progression of carcinogenesis."[32,p.556] For chemoprevention to be feasible and cost-effective, biological markers must reveal earlier changes in carcinogenesis and more information about risk of transformation to cancer. Additionally, biological markers need to be sensitive, specific, quantitative, and reproducible.[32] Validation of a biological marker requires that its biological or biochemical properties correlate with the definitive end point—cancer.[24]

With the discovery of proto-oncogenes, oncogenes, and tumor-suppressor genes, use of biological genetic markers in clinical chemoprevention studies is feasible. For example, gene amplification or mutations in people at high risk for cancer and changes in expression during chemopreventive treatment may provide information on both treatment and the disease course.[30] Reports of DNA adducts (DNA damage following carcinogen exposure) and micronuclei (chromosomal fragments created in proliferating cells during carcinogenic damage to DNA) as sole intermediate end-point markers remain inconclusive.[29,30,32]

As biological proliferation markers, precancerous lesions can show regression to a lower degree of precancer, progression to a higher degree, and the status of surrounding unaffected tissue and its relation to the precancer (field-cancerization effect).[29,32] Measures of cellular proliferation using mitotic index, thymidine labeling, proliferating cell nuclear antigen (PCNA), and Ki 67 antigen have been impressive biomarkers of chemoprevention activity.[29,32]

Biological differentiation markers include growth factors and epithelial markers such as cytokeratins, involucrin, and certain blood-related antigens of epithelial cells. Growth factors are promising intermediate end-point markers of differentiation because of their postulated link to oncogenes.[30] *Cytokeratins* are epithelial intracellular filaments comprising keratin-like proteins that are expressed in different epithelia in different patterns. As epithelial cells undergo differentiation, the patterns change. *Involucrin*, a protein component synthesized by human epithelial cells, reflects epithelial differentiation. Expression of Lewis blood antigens has been correlated with histologic type and degree of colonic epithelial cell dysplasia.[30]

Ornithine decarboxylase (ODC), the rate-limiting enzyme in polyamine synthesis (which has an essential role in cell proliferation), has been established as a biochemical marker for chemopreventive activity in people with Barrett's esophagus, familial polyposis of the colon, and adenomatous colon polyps. Epidermal transglutamase serves as a marker of squamous cell differentiation of epithelial tissue. Immunologic markers are not well understood but may reflect changes in cellular or hormonal immunity or identify cellular and molecular alterations in incipient tumor cells.[24]

Examples of micronutrient markers are serum levels of micronutrients, such as vitamins and trace elements that can serve as useful intermediate markers of intake and tissue distribution.[29,30] Effects of the chemopreventive agent directly on the target tissue also serve as intermediate tissue markers of efficacy, but correlations with the definitive end point (e.g., changes in precancers, cancer occurrence) could take some time.[29]

Challenges of Conducting Cancer Prevention Trials

The overall goal of cancer prevention research is to identify the preventable causes of cancer and to reduce cancer incidence by effectively applying prevention strategies in specific populations.[33]

Comparisons of Prevention and Treatment Trials

Although cancer prevention trials resemble cancer treatment trials in that they commonly use prospective design, random assignment of participants, control groups, blinding when feasible, and rigorous statistical analyses, cancer prevention trials do have some unique features.[34,35] Cancer prevention trials commonly involve more collaboration with biology, epidemiology, and behavioral sciences than do treatment trials.[36] The specific goals of cancer chemoprevention trials are safety and efficacy.

Safety is important because cancer prevention trials usually involve an essentially healthy rather than an ailing population and therefore should not expose participants to undue risk. Efficacy of a selected agent establishes its cancer prevention effect.[37]

Similar to cancer treatment trials, clinical cancer chemoprevention trials have specific phases. Phase I trials develop pharmacokinetic safety and toxicity profiles on potential chemopreventive agents. Phase II trials demonstrate efficacy and develop biomarkers of efficacy. Phase III trials demonstrate modulation of surrogate end points of cancer or demonstrate cancer incidence reduction.[12,25] Table 8-2 further compares cancer prevention and cancer treatment trials.

Design

Cancer prevention trials usually are randomized single- or double-blinded studies. Generally a high-risk population selected for study is one with a risk for a particular cancer that exceeds the risk of the general population by a factor of at least two.[8] Usual eligibility criteria include age, family history of the same cancer or related cancers, abnormalities of specific laboratory tests, carcinogen exposure, and the presence of other risk factors identified in epidemiologic studies.[8] A study with simple, straightforward objectives and end points based on a clearly defined rationale and hypothesis has a greater chance of meeting its recruitment goals.[38] Depending on the statistical power (the probability that the study will detect a statistically significant benefit), the recruitment pool can range from hundreds to thousands of people. This very large sample size presents a major methodological problem of chemoprevention trials.[31]

Selection of the intervention used in a cancer prevention trial, particularly a chemoprevention trial, may be influenced by the identification of human carcinogenic exposures to determine high-risk study participants, the availability of intermediate markers to assess risk status of participants or to efficiently serve as end points, and the interest and ability of potential study participants to adopt and adhere to behaviors specified in the trial.[3] Prevention trial interventions usually contain many dimensions beyond the participant, such as family, social network, school, work site, health care system, and the mass media. Chemoprevention trials generally combine the chemopreventive agent or placebo with corresponding behavioral interventions (e.g., smoking cessation, dietary modification, avoidance of sun exposure).[3] Other factors considered in the design of a cancer prevention trial include the number of study groups, the unit of randomization, end points (e.g., death, cancer diagnosis, changes in a precancerous lesion, or targets of a biological marker), and the duration. Other independent variables may include behavioral changes and quality-of-life measures.[39] Analysis of the trials may be affected by factors such as nonadherence, delays in the effect of the intervention, and available statistical methods.

Table 8-2 Features of Cancer Prevention Trials versus Cancer Treatment Trials

Variable	Prevention Trial	Treatment Trial
Goals	Decrease incidence/mortality	Increase cancer cure/remission rates
	Prevent/ameliorate precancerous lesions or markers of cancer risk Prevent second primary cancer	Decrease cancer morbidity/mortality
Study population	People without cancer 　General population 　High-risk population 　People with precancerous lesions 　Disease-free cancer survivors	People with confirmed diagnosis of cancer
Toxicity of agent	None to moderate, acceptable	Moderate to severe, acceptable
Study protocol	Design 　Simple (dichotomy) 　Intervention *vs* placebo 　Factorial 　Intervention A *vs* intervention B versus 　　intervention AB *vs* placebo 　Multiple simultaneous interventions, including 　　interactions 　Large scale (thousands of subjects) Pilot study usually required Placebo run-in useful Study may require 5–10+ years of intervention and 　follow-up	Design 　Simple (dichotomy or multiagent) 　Therapy *vs* placebo 　Therapy A *vs* therapy B 　Therapy A *vs* therapy B versus therapy C 　Small scale (hundreds of subjects) Pilot study rarely needed Run-in inappropriate Study length may be short for aggressive cancers, longer 　for slower-growing cancers or adjuvant studies
Adherence	Adherence to protocol may be difficult to maintain, i.e., 　subject-dependent	Adherence to protocol easier to maintain, i.e., physician- 　dependent

Adapted with permission from Greenwald P, Nixon DW, Malone W, et al: Concepts in chemoprevention research. *Cancer* 65:1487, 1990.[12]

Recruitment

Finding people at high risk for a certain cancer is much more challenging than finding people at ordinary risk.[8,38] Recruitment also is made more difficult by the fact that only 10%–25% of eligible subjects will choose to enroll in a chemoprevention trial.[10] A delay in recruitment increases both the cost and length of the study while reducing the power of the study because of fewer patient-years of observation.[38] Recruitment to chemoprevention trials, therefore, requires considerable cost, time, and effort on the part of study personnel.

The pool of potential subjects for cancer chemoprevention trials emanates from a variety of sources. Referrals from health care providers who care for the population under study (e.g., people with premalignant conditions) constitute the major recruitment source. Care must be taken to respect the health care providers' role as "gatekeeper" and not to interfere with the provider-patient relationship. Supplying providers with sufficient resources to help with patient inconvenience, excessive provider time requirements, and lack of support for follow-up could enhance enrollment. Health care providers who do not believe in the scientific rationale underlying a protocol may serve as barriers to recruitment, as will a provider whose main allegiance is to the individual patient, rather than aggregate or future patients.[38]

Other recruitment sources include public relation campaigns,[10] screening clinics, tumor registries, pathology databases, behavioral instruments that assess lifestyle, genetic and hereditary cancer screening, and cancer survivors who are at high risk for a second malignancy.[3] Also influencing recruitment are a potential participant's motivation to maintain personal autonomy or be altruistic in terms of contribution to medical knowledge. Other characteristics increasing the likelihood of enrollment are younger age, higher socioeconomic status, higher education, higher occupational status, and prior experience with a clinical study.[38]

Criteria for trial eligibility or ineligibility may pose some barriers to recruitment. These criteria vary according to the design of the trial, the cancer under study, and the agent being tested. To be eligible for a trial, potential participants may be asked to cease taking certain medications that they have been using for general health maintenance. For example, the completed Breast Cancer Prevention Trial (BCPT) required women to discontinue estrogen they may have taken for years to control symptoms of menopause. In general, women who are pregnant or who intend to become pregnant are not candidates for chemoprevention studies because of actual or potential teratogenic effects of the intervention. Other potential barriers to recruitment include psychosocial factors such as fear of risk, desire for privacy, and lack of family support; and practical issues like transportation, time off from work, waiting time, time for venipunctures, or unwillingness to tolerate toxicity.[38]

In most chemoprevention trials, participants are randomly assigned to either an intervention (treatment) arm using a chemopreventive agent or to a placebo arm. Thus, the informed consent process involves informing potential participants before they enroll in a trial about the short- and long-term toxicities of the chemopreventive agents under study. Learning all the known potential side effects of the intervention may be sufficiently daunting to dampen the person's desire to enroll in the trial. Additionally, people who suspect they might be assigned to the placebo arm may choose not to enroll in the trial because they desire the chemopreventive agent. If a compound that is easily available over-the-counter, such as a vitamin or a mineral, is being used as a study agent, potential participants may choose not to enroll in the study and subsequently self-prescribe their own treatment. Thus, health care providers are responsible for educating potential participants and reinforcing teaching of the possible hazards involved in self-treatment.[40] The NCI has published a patient education booklet that discusses some of these issues and provides general information about chemoprevention trials for potential participants.[41]

Enrollment

Toxicity monitoring

Once a person provides written, informed consent to enroll in a trial and is randomly assigned to the intervention or control arm, study personnel are responsible for several important tasks to ensure the participant's safety. Early identification of toxicity is critical and entails carefully following the trial protocol and seeing that participants undergo proper testing (e.g., laboratory tests, radiographs) to evaluate toxicity. However, one methodological problem with chemoprevention trials is that dose levels of the chemopreventive agent must be so low that the risk of adverse side effects is virtually nil.[31] Maintaining a current record of concomitant prescription and over-the-counter medications is also important because some compounds interfere with chemopreventive agents.

Adherence

Study personnel also monitor and promote short- and long-term adherence to the assigned regimen. This is a challenging task in that most chemoprevention trials last between 5 and 10 years and ideally incorporate long-term follow-up after completion of the intervention. Several trials also incorporate lifestyle changes, and adherence to these changes is considerably more difficult than adherence to taking a medication.[8]

Some trials build a run-in period into the design to assess likely adherence. During this period, study personnel ask potential participants to adhere to similar tasks (e.g., taking a pill, eating a certain diet) that will be required of them following randomization. If their adherence is unacceptable during the run-in period, the potential participants are not enrolled in the trial.[7]

Other strategies to promote adherence include keeping the study regimen as simple as possible, and whenever possible tailoring it to the convenience and lifestyle of the participant; packaging the chemopreventive agent in calendar packs; and fostering a positive relationship between participants and study personnel.[38] Maintaining adherence among different ethnic groups requires sensitivity to their ethnocultural views on health, access to health care resources, and other cultural and economic barriers to continued participation.

Enrolled participants who are assigned to the intervention group and fail to adhere to the regimen are called *drop-outs,* whereas participants in the control group who adopt the intervention are called *drop-ins.*[8] These forms of nonadherence may be influenced by the media, advice from other health care providers not involved in or knowledgeable about the trial, health fads, alternative therapies, or family. Unfortunately, information gleaned from these sources may not always be accurate or based on well-designed scientific research. Study personnel must therefore be continually aware of media and scientific developments in the area of cancer prevention and must educate subjects appropriately. Study personnel need to develop a relationship based on honesty and trust with each participant in order to facilitate exchange of accurate information and promote adherence.[37,40]

Chemoprevention Research

Chemoprevention research at the NCI began in the late 1970s. In 1982 the NCI established the Chemoprevention Research Program, which is divided into two broad categories: chemoprevention, and diet and nutrition. These areas of research are pursued through extramural and intramural funding to identify and evaluate the efficacy of specific micronutrients, natural compounds, and drugs in reducing cancer incidence.[11,12]

Chemoprevention Trials

Table 8-3 provides a summary of representative phase II and phase III chemoprevention trials sponsored by the NCI. Recent, high-priority trials sponsored by the NCI include the Study of Tamoxifen and Raloxifine (STAR) and the Prostate Cancer Prevention Trial (PCPT).

Study of Tamoxifen and Raloxifine

The National Surgical Adjuvant Breast and Bowel Project (NSABP) has selected 193 institutions to participate in STAR, which began in early 1999. STAR is examining whether raloxifine, a drug similar to tamoxifen, used in

Table 8-3 Current Phase II and III Clinical Cancer Chemoprevention Trials Sponsored by the National Cancer Institute*

Target Cancer	Study Title	Institution/Group	Agent and Schedule
Bladder	Phase IIB randomized, double-blind chemoprevention study of fenretinide vs. placebo in patients with resected transitional cell carcinoma of the bladder at high risk of recurrence	Southwest Oncology Group	Intravesical BCG weekly × 6 wk, then 6-wk rest; BCG weekly × 3 wk if NED; then randomized to oral fenretinide or placebo qd × 11 days and 3-day rest. Repeat q14 days × 52-wk total.
Bladder	Phase III randomized study of high-dose multivitamins as chemoprevention of stage 0 and I resected transitional cell carcinoma of the bladder	North Central Cancer Treatment Group	Oral multivitamins or placebo qd × 3 yr
Breast	Phase II study of difluoromethylornithine (DFMO) in breast dysplasia with biomarker abnormalities	University of Kansas Medical Center	Randomized to oral DFMO or placebo qd × 6 mo
Breast	Phase II study of raloxifine as a chemopreventive agent for premenopausal women at high risk for developing invasive breast cancer	NCI, Division of Clinical Sciences	2 cohorts treated with different doses of oral raloxifine 2 tabs qd × 2 yr
Cervix	Phase II study of a carotenoid rich diet to reverse cervical intraepithelial neoplasia (CIN I and II)	University of California San Diego Cancer Center	Randomized to dietary counseling and eat 5–10 servings of carotenoid rich fruit and vegetables qd × 1 yr vs. no counseling and regular diet
Cervix	Phase III randomized, double-blind placebo-controlled study of fenretinide in patients with CIN grade 2–3	University of Texas MD Anderson Cancer Center	Oral fenretinide vs. placebo qd × 6 mo; 3 days of rest each mo; 1 yr total
Colon	Phase II clinical trial of sulindac, a nonsteroidal anti-inflammatory agent, for chemoprevention of colorectal neoplasia	Herbert Irving Comprehensive Cancer Center	Randomized to oral sulindac vs. placebo bid × 6 mo
Colon	Phase I/II randomized study of celecoxib for hereditary nonpolyposis colorectal cancer patients and gene carriers	NCI, Division of Clinical Sciences	Oral celecoxib or placebo bid × 1 year. Randomized to 3 treatment arms: Arms I and II receive 1 of 2 dose levels of celecoxib; arm III receives placebo
Colon	Phase II double-blind, randomized placebo-controlled chemoprevention study of calcium carbonate in combination with vitamin D vs. placebo in patients with colorectal polyp growth	Herbert Irving Comprehensive Cancer Center	Arm I: oral calcium carbonate tid and oral vitamin D as single capsule qd × 6 mo; arm II: oral placebo tid qd × 6 mo
Colon	Phase II randomized, double-blind, placebo-controlled study of high-dose folic acid for the prevention of colorectal cancer in patients with resected adenomatous polyps	Eastern Cooperative Oncology Group	Arm I: oral folic acid; arm II: oral placebo
Colon	Pilot randomized study of calcium for chemoprevention of colorectal adenomas and new primary carcinomas in surgically treated patients	Southwest Oncology Group	Arm I: oral calcium carbonate; arm II: oral placebo. About 25% of patients registered separately for study of intermediate biomarkers
Colon	Phase III randomized chemoprevention study of aspirin in patients with curatively treated Duke's stage A/B1/B2/C colorectal cancer	Cancer and Leukemia Group B	Arm I: oral, enteric-coated aspirin; arm II: oral placebo
Colon	Phase II study of the effects of ursodeoxycholic acid (URSO) on adenomatous polyp recurrence, bile acid concentration in blood and feces, and rectal mucosal proliferation rates in persons with adenomatous colon polyps	University of Arizona Cancer Center	Oral URSO (8–10 mg/kg/day) vs. placebo
Endometrium	Two part study of atypical endometrial hyperplasia: prospective study of immediate hysterectomy and phase II randomized study of medroxyprogesterone acetate (Provera) vs. depot-medroxyprogesterone (Depo-Provera) prior to hysterectomy	Gynecologic Oncology Group	Part A: immediate hysterectomy; Part B: randomized to oral Provera qd × 3 mo or 3 monthly injections of Depo-Provera on days 1, 31, and 62; then hysterectomy

(continued)

Table 8-3 Current Phase II and III Clinical Cancer Chemoprevention Trials Sponsored by the National Cancer Institute*
(continued)

Target Cancer	Study Title	Institution/Group	Agent and Schedule
Esophagus	Phase IIB chemoprevention study of eflornithine (DFMO) in patients with intestinal-type Barrett's esophagus	University of Michigan Comprehensive Cancer Center	Randomized to oral DFMO or placebo qd × 26 wk
Head and Neck	Phase II randomized study of eflornithine vs. placebo for the treatment of leukoplakic dysplasia	Fox Chase Cancer Center	Placebo × 4 wk then randomized to DFMO vs. placebo qd × 6 mo
Head and Neck	Phase II randomized, double-blind study of isotretinoin vs. placebo for oral dysplastic leukoplakia	University of Alabama Comprehensive Cancer Center	Oral placebo × 1 mo then randomized to isotretinoin at higher dose × 3 mo then lower dose × 9 mo vs. oral placebo × 12 mo
Head and Neck	Phase II study of fenretinide in patients with oral mucosal intraepithelial neoplasia	Southwest Oncology Group	Oral fenretinide days 1–25 q28 days for maximum of 6 courses
Head and Neck	Phase IIB randomized chemoprevention study of ketorolac mouth rinse in patients with oropharyngeal leukoplakia	NCI Division of Clinical Sciences	Randomized to mouth rinse containing ketorolac or placebo bid × 3 mo
Head and Neck	Phase III double-blind, randomized study of low-dose 13-CRA on prevention of second primary tumors in patients with totally resected stage I/II squamous cell carcinoma of the head and neck	Eastern Cooperative Oncology Group	Arm I: isotretinoin; arm II: oral placebo
Head and Neck	Phase III chemoprevention study of low-dose 13-cis-retinoic acid for second primary tumors in patients with head and neck cancer	Radiation Therapy Oncology Group	Arm I: low-dose isotretinoin; arm II: oral placebo
Lung	Phase II study of anetholtrithione as a chemoprevention agent in current or former chronic smokers with bronchial dysplasia	Vancouver Cancer Center	Randomized to oral anetholtrithione vs. placebo tid × 6 mo
Lung	Phase II randomized double-blind study of fenretinide vs. placebo in chronic smokers with squamous metaplasia/dysplasia in the bronchial epithelium	University of Texas MD Anderson Cancer Center	Oral fenretinide or placebo vs. × 6 mo
Lung	Phase II study of oltipraz as a chemopreventive agent in patients with bronchial lung dysplasia	Fox Chase Cancer Center	Randomized to oral oltipraz vs. placebo twice weekly × 6 mo
Skin	Phase II study of low-fat dietary intervention for skin cancer prevention (nonmelanoma)	Baylor College of Medicine	Randomized to dietary intervention (assessment of eating habits, low-fat balanced diet) or nonintervention group (assessment of eating habits) × 2 yr
Skin	Randomized study of acitretin in patients with multiple prior skin cancers who received solid organ transplantation	North Central Cancer Treatment Group	Oral acitretin vs. placebo qd × 2 yr
Skin	Phase II randomized chemoprevention study of topical tretinoin with or without oral fenretinide in patients with dysplastic nevus syndrome	Eastern Cooperative Oncology Group	Topical tretinoin bid and oral fenretinide qd × 12 mo vs. topical tretinoin bid and oral placebo qd × 12 mo

BCG = bacille Calmette-Guérin; NED = no evidence of disease; 13-CRA = 13 cis-retinoic acid.
*Listed alphabetically by target cancer site.
Data from PDQ® Clinical Trials Search Form. Trial type: prevention available at http://cancertrials.nci.nih.gov.

the first breast cancer chemoprevention trial[42] (see Table 8-4), prevents breast cancer in high-risk women. Benefits of raloxifine over tamoxifen also are being assessed. STAR is a randomized, double-blind study that will enroll 22,000 postmenopausal women aged 35 or older who are at increased risk for developing cancer. Women will be randomly assigned to receive 20 mg of tamoxifen or 60 mg of raloxifine daily for 5 years. They will be followed for 7 years.[43]

Prostate Cancer Prevention Trial

Initiated in 1993, the PCPT is a double-blind, randomized intergroup trial testing the ability of finasteride to

Table 8-4 Selected Completed Chemoprevention Trials*

Trial Name/Dates	Prevention Target	Regimen	Approximate Sample Size	Results
Alpha-Tocopherol, Beta-Carotene Lung Cancer Prevention Study (ATBC) (1992–1996)[46–49]	Lung cancer in male cigarette smokers	Oral alpha-tocopherol (vitamin E) (50 mg), beta-carotene (20 mg) qd	29,133	No reduction in lung cancer incidence with alpha-tocopherol; 18% higher incidence of lung cancer with beta-carotene
	Secondary analysis: prostate cancer in male cigarette smokers			Alpha-tocopherol reduced prostate cancer incidence in men (age 50–60 years) by 32% and prostate cancer deaths by 41%
Breast Cancer Prevention Trial (BCPT) (1992–1998)[42,50]	Breast cancer in high-risk women	Oral tamoxifen (20 mg) qd vs. placebo	13,388	49% reduced incidence of invasive breast cancer with tamoxifen
Carotenoid & Retinoid Efficacy Trial (CARET) (1992–1996)[51]	Lung cancer in high-risk groups	Oral beta-carotene (30 mg) and retinol (25,000 units) qd vs. placebo	18,314	28% more lung cancers diagnosed and 17% more deaths in beta-carotene and retinol group than in placebo group
Nutritional Intervention Studies of Esophageal Cancer (1986–1991)[52]	Esophageal cancer in China	4 arms: (1) vitamin C/molybdenum; (2) beta-carotene, vitamin E, selenium; (3) retinol, zinc; (4) riboflavin, niacin	30,000	Beta-carotene, vitamin E, selenium group had lower cancer incidence and significantly reduced mortality, particularly stomach cancer
Nutritional Prevention of Cancer (1990–1996)[53]	Secondary cancers in people with a history of skin cancer	Oral selenium (200 μg) vs. placebo qd	1,312	Total cancers and prostate, colorectal, lung cancers lower in selenium group; selenium group had 17% fewer cancers overall and fewer lung cancer deaths
Physicians Health Study (1983–1995)[54]	All cancers	Beta-carotene (50 mg) qod or placebo	22,071	Beta-carotene produced neither benefit nor harm for cancer incidence or deaths

*Chemoprevention trials are listed alphabetically by trial name.

prevent prostate cancer in healthy men aged 55 and older. Enrollment of the 18,000 men was completed in the fall of 1995. The men were randomly assigned to oral finasteride (5 mg per day) or placebo. Participants are still being followed, and trial results can be expected in 2003. The primary end point of the study is a prostate biopsy that is negative for cancer. Secondary objectives include evaluating side effects and toxicity, and determining grade and stage of prostate and other cancers, cancer mortality, incidence of benign prostatic hypertrophy, effectiveness of prostate-specific antigen screening and digital rectal examination, and quality of life.[44,45]

Completed Phase III Chemoprevention Trials

Alberts and Garcia critically reviewed results of several positive phase III chemoprevention studies reported in the literature.[25] In brief, patients with non-small cell lung cancer who received retinol developed fewer second primary lung cancers than did controls. Synthetic retinoids (isotretinoin and 4-hydroxyphenyl retinamide) provide significant clinical improvement and reduction in relapse for oral leukoplakia. Patients with familial adenomatous polyposis who took a wheat-bran fiber supplement had a significant inverse correlation between the number of polyps and amount of ingested prescribed fiber. Another study of familial polyposis showed that sulindac significantly decreased the number of polyps.

Table 8-4 summarizes selected completed chemoprevention trials that advanced knowledge of chemoprevention. These trials include the Alpha-Tocopherol, Beta-Carotene Lung Cancer Prevention Study (ATBC),[46–49] Breast Cancer Prevention Trial (BCPT),[42,50] Carotenoid and Retinoid Efficacy Trial (CARET),[51] Nutritional Intervention Studies of Esophageal Cancer,[52] Nutritional Prevention of Cancer,[53] and the Physicians Health Study.[54]

Diet and Nutrition Research

The NCI is sponsoring several studies targeting diet and nutrition in cancer prevention. These include (1) physiochemical effects of dietary fiber on transit time, stool weight, pH, bile acids, serum lipids, mineral absorption, and intestinal flora; (2) retinoids and carotenoids (object is to identify mechanisms that control absorption of vitamin A and carotenoids, evaluate conversion of carotenoids to retinol, and evaluate storage in tissues); (3) nutritive and nonnutritive constituents of fruits and vegetables (goal is to develop analytic methods for identifying and quantifying these constituents and determine their biological activity, absorption, metabolism, and mechanisms of action); and (4) biomarkers for monitoring dietary changes.[12]

The goal of other cancer prevention trials involving diet is to change the intake of a macronutrient in the intervention arm while having minimal effect on the nonintervention arm. Two examples of such ongoing trials are the Women's Health Initiative (WHI)[55,56] and the Wheat Bran Fiber Study.[57] The WHI to date is the largest community-based clinical prevention and intervention trial ever conducted in the United States.[56] It has a complex trial design that involves an intervention in which women lower their fat intake to less than 20% of total calories. Other interventions include hormone replacement therapy and calcium/vitamin D supplementation. Among the outcomes to be assessed are breast cancer and colon cancer. In the Wheat Bran Fiber Study, participants who have had a history of adenomatous polyps, a precancerous lesion of the colon, are randomized to either receive a daily high-bran (13.5-g) supplement or a lower dose (2 g). Trial outcomes are adenoma recurrence, intermediate markers of epithelial cell proliferation and fecal bile acid concentrations, and protein kinase C expression.

Cancer Prevention Controversies and Dilemmas

Incomplete Knowledge

Epidemiological reports of cancer prevention and detection may use statistical analyses to group associated risk factors of certain cancers. Although these risk factors may be confounded either with each other or with their reputed effects, interventions aimed at reducing risks often are implemented before the relationship among the factors is known.[58] The controversy surrounding the role of diet and cancer illustrates this dilemma.

Diet can be considered a lifestyle factor or a carcinogenic risk factor. The current dietary recommendations for preventing cancer (see Table 8-1) are based largely on epidemiological research. However, countless variables (see Chapter 5) interfere with the interpretation of some epidemiological dietary studies. The uncertainty of the period of life during which dietary intake most affects carcinogenesis also affects interpretation of these studies.[12,31,59] Publication bias may come into play if more "positive" dietary findings than "negative" dietary findings are printed.[59] Proponents of dietary guidelines for cancer prevention argue that the recommended diet is healthful even if it does not reduce cancer incidence and mortality.[58]

Kottke suggests that lack of evidence from randomized, controlled trials for an intervention's efficacy should not prevent us from recommending the intervention if other evidence is compelling, and that equal weight should not be assigned to all classes of evidence.[60] In his own words, "We should not be embarrassed to admit that a recommendation must be based on a 'best guess' because of inadequate information."[60,p.902] Kottke recommends using the consensus process to summarize and simplify knowledge that may be difficult to interpret. This process also can facilitate action by minimizing the appearance of tentativeness and minimizing potential contradictory messages by individuals or organizations.

Overselling Prevention

Goodman and Goodman commented that, in their enthusiasm to move from tentative hypotheses to implementing programs, health care organizations and industries, such as the food industry, acknowledge the caveats and qualifications of science but use more of a marketing approach than an educational approach to disseminating information.[58] For example, when the ACS published its dietary guidelines a decade ago, it also mobilized millions of volunteers to promote them.[58]

The public education sponsored by many cancer organizations is a noble focus. However, these campaigns, which may cost thousands of dollars and be disseminated to thousands of people, often are not rigorously evaluated for their effectiveness in terms of efficacy, outcomes, economic impact, and benefit. If a campaign is not evaluated for its ability to change a certain behavior, for example, one could question the logic and underlying motivation for conducting the campaign. Is it being conducted purely to enhance knowledge, even though this outcome was not determined via evaluation? To provide visibility for the sponsor? Many organizations keep statistics to document the number of people reached with a certain prevention message (e.g., numbers of brochures distributed). These numbers do not constitute an evaluation of a campaign. The earnestness and vigor of these organizations cannot be discounted, because in the minds of many, one life saved is worth the cost of the campaign. However, these groups need to take care not to eclipse known information about cancer with notions of cancer prevention, particularly in this era of budget cutting and cost containment. Teutsch recommends that prevention campaigns also be evaluated for their ability to determine the potential and practical consequences of prevention strategies, including social, legal, and ethical factors.

From the standpoint of the media's role in selling prevention, Brody believes that health care professionals must provide the mass media with "sound scientific information and well-considered comments based on real evidence, not speculation or hysteria-mongering possibilities."[15,p.164] She recommends that cancer prevention messages avoid a "quick-fix" mentality, emphasize that healthful living is not an all-or-nothing phenomenon, and encourage moderation of lifestyle behaviors.

Attribution of Responsibility

The ongoing discoveries of carcinogens and cancer genes generate skepticism, making people indifferent to changing or adopting behaviors aimed at preventing cancer.[13] People also are reluctant to give up behaviors such as suntanning or cigarette smoking in order to gain health.[5] However, after developing cancer, it is natural to seek an explanation for why the event happened. In all human societies, morality may be a frame of reference for that explanation; that is, something may have been done incorrectly or not at all. When an illness such as cancer occurs, solace and exoneration are found in assigning blame for the disease to someone or something.[58]

At the same time, cancer prevention programs must take care not to impart a false sense of security. The person who faithfully adheres to prevention and screening guidelines may still develop cancer. Participants in prevention and screening campaigns need to be reminded that observance of guidelines does not guarantee a cancer-free existence, particularly when guidelines are based on incomplete knowledge.

The focus on the individual's role in preventing cancer may also serve to shift responsibility for health away from other bodies, such as the federal government. Goodman and Goodman note that "recognizing the role of individual choice and discipline [in practicing preventive behaviors] is no substitute for health insurance, research, therapy, or exercising responsibility for the environment."[58,p.36]

Cancer Prevention and Changes in Health Care

The role of prevention has been overshadowed by more dramatic advances in medical science.[61] For cancer prevention to be successful, the health care community and policy makers need first to change the existing treatment-oriented model to one that is prevention-oriented.[14,62] They also need to recognize the importance of intervening before carcinogenesis or during initiation or promotion, when the process may be halted, slowed, or reversed. This concept of early intervention parallels that used in cardiovascular disease, which is now accepted by the health care community and health insurers alike. As with cardiovascular disease, the health care community must be aware of the biological significance of precancerous lesions and the importance of early detection of these lesions, so as to treat them with effective agents to prevent progression to cancer.[26] Still, focusing on opportunities for prevention is a daunting task because it involves a long-term commitment by the patient, health care provider, and society at large.[63]

Historically in the United States, payers at all levels have not reimbursed cancer prevention services. Most private health insurance plans do not pay for prevention counseling and testing. They may only pay for counseling that is incidental to the problem (e.g., reimbursing for tobacco cessation counseling of a patient with lung cancer but not reimbursing for identical counseling of a healthy individual).[64] The growth of managed care and capitation, and the increasing use of primary health care providers as gatekeepers are driving the coverage of preventive services. Quality-control efforts by health plans carefully monitor whether patients received necessary preventive services.[62] However, funding for preventive services remains inadequate, even in prepaid health systems. These plans may need to earmark revenues (e.g., a percentage of capitation dues) to be devoted to prevention.[65]

Effective cancer prevention counseling and intervention often require additional time spent with the patient (e.g., to conduct a complete risk assessment, explain available clinical prevention trials) and repeated visits or examinations that may be necessary to establish eligibility for clinical prevention trials. Managed-care groups generally will not reimburse health care providers for these efforts, a decision that could have two main effects: (1) health care providers will choose to spend less time counseling and educating patients about cancer prevention, and (2) the successful implementation of clinical cancer prevention trials may be compromised. However, cancer prevention guidelines and programs disseminated to even a portion of managed-care groups can reach thousands of health care professionals who can serve as conduits to millions of people.[62]

The health care community must recognize that no individual or single public or private agency can achieve the goal of prevention.[62] People will have to be actively involved in their own health care and in the management of their health.[65] Partnerships of public health agencies at all levels with professional, voluntary, and community organizations; health care organizations; academic institutions; philanthropic foundations; industry and labor; and schools, churches, and other local institutions will be needed for prevention to be achieved.[62,66]

Commitment to research needs to be expanded and private organizations should consider following existing prevention research models (e.g., NCI-DCPC). This would enhance efforts to validate efficacy of preventive strategies in clinical settings. Such a commitment by private organizations also would encourage new development of chemopreventive agents.[63]

Implications for Nursing

Nurses play a key role in cancer prevention. They perform valuable, traditional services such as identifying people at high risk and counseling and educating patients about cancer prevention.[5] Additionally, nurses must strive to keep pace with the science of cancer prevention. For example, in the near future, individual risk profiles based on genetic factors, lifestyle behaviors, environmental exposure, history of precursor lesions, or any combination of these will define specific interventions, such as chemoprevention, for modulating cancer risk.[26,67] With sophisticated molecular biology techniques, it also may be possible to identify early damage to key proto-oncogenes in individuals at high risk.[24] Another future preventive strategy, gene transfer technology, may replace deficient genes prior to cancer development.[14] This could involve inserting intact genes into precancerous cells or into hereditary cancer-prone persons.[22]

To understand and participate in these advances in cancer prevention, nursing education, clinical practice, and research will need to have a strong foundation in genetics, carcinogenesis, bioethics, behavioral change strategies, health policy, and environmental health.[5,63,68] Oncology nurse educators bear much of the responsibility for preparing nurses with knowledge and skills to participate in cancer prevention. Educators need to continually assess and update cancer prevention information in nursing program curricula at all levels.[9] This is no small task in light of the rapid changes in cancer prevention. Similarly, health care administrators should allow nurses time to plan and implement cancer prevention services. Given the opportunity, nurses can be instrumental in developing cancer prevention standards of care along with developing, supporting, and steering health policies related to cancer prevention. By being actively involved in collaborative, multidisciplinary research, nurses have a key opportunity to influence prevention interventions and outcomes. Oncology nurses are particularly well positioned to conduct cancer prevention research in socioeconomically disadvantaged populations. Engelking strongly stated the onus for oncology nurses: To meet the challenges of cancer prevention, nurses must prepare proactively, not reactively.[69]

Acknowledgments

The authors thank David S. Alberts, MD, for scientific review of this chapter.

References

1. Garfinkel L: Perspectives on cancer prevention. *CA Cancer J Clin* 45:5–7, 1995 (editorial)
2. Meyskens FL Jr: Coming of age: The chemoprevention of cancer. *N Engl J Med* 323:825–827, 1990 (editorial)
3. Gritz ER, Moon TE: The new cancer prevention and control. *Cancer Epidemiol Biomarkers Prev* 1:163–165, 1992
4. Teutsch SM: A framework for assessing the effectiveness of disease and injury prevention. *MMWR Morb Mortal Wkly Rep* 41(RR-3):1–12, 1992
5. Frank-Stromborg M, Cohen R: Assessment and interventions for cancer prevention and detection, in Groenwald SL, Frogge MH, Goodman M, Yarbro CH (eds): *Cancer Nursing: Principles and Practice* (ed 4). Boston, Jones and Bartlett, 1997, pp 133–174
6. Loescher LJ: Commentary: Expanding our horizons with an alternative approach to cancer prevention and detection. *Semin Oncol Nurs* 9:147–149, 1993
7. DeFlora S: Mechanisms of inhibitors of mutagenesis and carcinogenesis. *Mutat Res* 402:151–158, 1998
8. Byar DP, Freedman LS: The importance and nature of cancer prevention trials. *Semin Oncol* 17:413–424, 1990
9. McMillan SC: Nurses' compliance with American Cancer Society Guidelines for Cancer Prevention and Detection. *Oncol Nurs Forum* 17:721–727, 1990
10. Bertram JS, Kolonel LN, Meyskens FL Jr: Rationale and strategies for chemoprevention of cancer in humans. *Cancer Res* 47:3012–3031, 1987
11. Division of Cancer Prevention and Control: *1994 Annual Report.* Bethesda, MD, National Institutes of Health/National Cancer Institute, 1994
12. Greenwald P, Nixon DW, Malone W, et al: Concepts in chemoprevention research. *Cancer* 65:1483–1490, 1990
13. Cole P, Amoateng-Adjepong Y: Cancer prevention: Accomplishments and prospects. *Am J Public Health* 84:8–10, 1994 (editorial)
14. Terris M: Healthy lifestyles: The perspective of epidemiology. *J Public Health Policy* 13:186–194, 1992
15. Brody JE: Communicating cancer-prevention information. *J Natl Cancer Inst Monogr* 12:163–164, 1992
16. Buller DB, Buller MK: Approaches to communicating preventive behaviors. *Semin Oncol Nurs* 7:53–63, 1991
17. Studies and Reports, Health and Human Resources: The proposed tobacco settlement: Issues from a federal perspective. Available at: http://www.cbo.gov/, April 1998. Accessed 9/28/99
18. Dalgleish AG: Viruses and cancer. *Br Med Bull* 47:21–46, 1991
19. Fischinger PJ: Prospects for reducing virus-associated human cancers by antiviral vaccines. *J Natl Cancer Inst Monogr* 12:109–114, 1992
20. Marwick C: Exciting potential of DNA vaccines explored. *JAMA* 273:1403–1404, 1995
21. Skolnick AA: Essential components now in place for clinical testing of cancer vaccine strategies, experts say. *JAMA* 273:528–530, 1995
22. Sugimura T: Cancer prevention: Past, present, future. *Mutat Res* 402:7–14, 1998
23. Cancer Research Institute. Available at: http://www.cancerresearch.org/index.html. Accessed 9/28/99
24. Meyskens FL Jr: Chemoprevention of cancer in humans 1990: Where do we go from here?, in Pastorino U, Hong WK (eds): Chemoimmuno Prevention of Cancer: Proceedings of the First International Conference, Vienna, Austria. New York, Thieme Medical Publishers, 1991, pp 245–252
25. Alberts DS, Garcia D: An overview of clinical cancer chemoprevention studies with emphasis on positive phase III studies. *J Nutr* 125:692S–697S, 1995

26. Greenwald P, Kelloff G, Burch-Whitman C, et al: Chemo-prevention. *CA Cancer J Clin* 45:31–49, 1995

27. Boone CW, Bacus JW, Bacus JV, et al: Properties of intraepithelial neoplasia relevant to cancer chemoprevention and to the development of surrogate end points for clinical trials. *Proc Soc Exp Biol Medi*, 216:151–165, 1997

28. Wattenberg LW: An overview of chemoprevention: Current status and future prospects. *Proc Soc Exp Biol Medi* 216:133–141, 1997

29. Meyskens FL Jr: Biomarkers as intermediate endpoints and cancer prevention. *J Natl Cancer Inst Monogr* 13:177–181, 1992

30. Pillai R, Garewal HS, Wood S, et al: Biological monitoring of cancer chemoprevention. *J Surg Oncol* 51:195–202, 1992

31. Mettlin C: Chemoprevention: Will it work? *Int J Cancer* 10:18–21, 1997 (suppl)

32. Lippman SM, Lee JS, Lotan R, et al: Biomarkers as intermediate end points in chemoprevention trials. *J Natl Cancer Inst* 82:555–560, 1990

33. Greenwald P, Sondik E, Lynch BS: Diet and chemoprevention in NCI's research strategy to achieve national cancer control objectives. *Annu Rev Public Health* 7:267–291, 1986

34. Hennekens CH: Issues in the design and conduct of clinical trials. *J Natl Cancer Inst* 73:1473–1476, 1984

35. Nixon DW: Special aspects of chemoprevention trials. *Cancer* 74:2683–2686, 1994 (suppl)

36. Meyskens FL Jr: Commentary: Thinking about cancer causality and chemoprevention. *J Natl Cancer Inst* 80:1278–1281, 1988

37. Padberg RM: Chemoprevention trials. *Cancer Pract* 2:154–156, 1994

38. Tangrea JA: Patient participation and compliance in cancer chemoprevention trials: Issues and concerns. *Proc Soc Exp Biol Medi* 216:260–265, 1997.

39. Moon TE: Planning the analysis of a breast cancer prevention trial. *Prev Med* 20:109–118, 1991

40. Loescher LJ: Chemoprevention of human skin cancers. *Semin Oncol Nurs* 7:45–52, 1991

41. National Cancer Institute: *What Are Chemoprevention Clinical Trials?* NIH publication No. 93-3595. Bethesda, MD, National Cancer Institute, 1992

42. National Surgical Adjuvant Breast and Bowel Project. Protocol P-1. A clinical trial to determine the worth of tamoxifen for preventing breast cancer. Pittsburgh, NSABP, 1992

43. National Surgical Adjuvant Breast and Bowel Project. General Information. Study of Tamoxifen and Raloxifine. Available at: http://www.nsabp.pitt.edu. Accessed 9/28/99

44. Thompson I, Brawer M, Crawford ED, et al: Chemoprevention of prostate cancer with finasteride (Proscar). Protocol no. 9217. San Antonio, Southwest Oncology Group, 1993

45. Prostate Cancer Prevention Trial recruitment of 18,000 men completed. Available at: http://cancernet.nci.nih.gov/clinpdq/prevention.html. Accessed 9/28/99

46. The Alpha-Tocopherol, Beta Carotene Cancer Prevention Study Group: The effect of vitamin E and beta carotene on the incidence of lung cancer and other cancers in male smokers. *N Engl J Med* 330:1029–1035, 1994

47. Omenn GS, Goodman GE, Thornquist MD, et al: Effects of a combination of beta carotene and vitamin A on lung cancer and cardiovascular disease. *N Engl J Med* 334:1150–1155, 1996

48. Albanes D, Heinonen OP, Taylor PR, et al: Alpha-tocopherol and beta-carotene supplements and lung cancer incidence in the alpha-tocopherol, beta-carotene cancer prevention study: Effects of base-line characteristics and study compliance. *J Natl Cancer Inst* 88:1560–1570, 1996

49. Heinonen OP, Albanes D, Virtamo J, et al: Prostate cancer and supplementation with alpha-tocopherol and beta-carotene. Incidence and mortality in a controlled trial. *J Natl Cancer Inst* 90:440–446, 1998.

50. Breast Cancer Prevention Studies. Available at: http://cancernet.nci.nih.gov/clinpdq/prevention.html. Accessed 9/28/99

51. Goodman GE: The clinical evaluation of cancer prevention agents. *Proc Soc Exp Biol Medi* 216:253–259, 1997

52. Blot WJ, Li J-Y, Taylor PR, et al: Nutrition intervention trials in Linxian, China: Supplementation with specific vitamin/mineral combinations, cancer incidence, and disease-specific mortality in the general population. *J Natl Cancer Inst* 85:1483–1492, 1993

53. Clark LC, Combs GF, Turnbull BW, et al: For the Nutritional Prevention of Cancer Study Group: Effect of selenium supplementation for cancer prevention of carcinoma of the skin: A randomized controlled trial. *JAMA* 276:1957–1963, 1996

54. Hennekens CH, Buring JE, Manson JE, et al: Lack of effect of long-term supplementation with beta carotene on the incidence of malignant neoplasms and cardiovascular disease. *N Engl J Med* 334:1145–1149, 1996

55. Freedman LS, Prentice RL, Clifford C, et al: Dietary fat and breast cancer: Where are we? *J Natl Cancer Inst* 85:764–765, 1993

56. Highlights of NCIs Cancer Prevention and Control Programs. Available at: http://cancernet.nci.nih.gov/clinpdq/prevention.html. Accessed 9/28/99

57. Alberts D, Ritenbaugh C, Story J, et al: Randomized, double-blinded, placebo-controlled study of effect of wheat bran fiber and calcium on fecal bile acids in patients with resected adenomatous colon polyps. *J Natl Cancer Inst* 88:81–92, 1996

58. Goodman LE, Goodman MJ: Prevention: How misuse of a concept undercuts its worth. *Hastings Cent Rep* 16(2):26–38, 1986

59. Modan B: Diet and cancer: Causal relation or just wishful thinking? *Lancet* 340:162–164, 1992.

60. Kottke TE: Clinical preventive services: How should we define the indications? *Mayo Clin Proc* 65:899–902, 1990

61. Sutchfield FD, Hartman KT: Physicians and preventive medicine. *JAMA* 273:1150–1151, 1995

62. Satcher D, Hull F: The weight of an ounce. *JAMA* 273:1149–1159, 1995 (editorial)

63. Rustgi AK: Rethinking the approach to cancer: The power of prevention. *Gastroenterology* 115:523, 1998 (editorial)

64. Fogle S: Bench notes special report. Pitching prevention: Will doctors listen? *J Natl Inst Health Res* 3:90–92, 1991

65. Thompson RS, Taplin SH, McAfee TA, et al: Primary and secondary prevention services in clinical practice: Twenty years' experience in development, implementation, and evaluation. *JAMA* 273:1130–1135, 1995

66. Baker EL, Melton RH, Stange PV, et al: Health reform and the health of the public: Forging community health partnerships. *JAMA* 272:1276–1282, 1994

67. Greenwald P: Keynote address: Cancer prevention. *J Natl Cancer Inst Monogr* 12:9–14, 1992

68. Loescher LJ: Genetics in cancer prediction, screening and counseling: Part 1. Genetics in cancer prediction and screening. *Oncol Nurs Forum* 22:10–15, 1995 (suppl)

69. Engelking C: New approaches: Innovations in cancer prevention, diagnosis, treatment, and support. *Oncol Nurs Forum* 21:62–71, 1994

CHAPTER 9

Assessment and Interventions for Cancer Detection

Marilyn Frank-Stromborg, EdD, JD, NP, FAAN
Rebecca F. Cohen, RN, MS, EdD, MPA, CPHQ

Introduction

Focus on Cancer Prevention, Early Detection, and Cancer Screening

In the past, the focus of health care providers was primarily on providing more technology and services for individuals with symptomatic conditions. Prevention and early intervention received little attention in the fight against disease, particularly cancer. However, the shift in health care policy and priorities has caused the focus of care to change, due in part to economics and an aging population. The American Cancer Society notes that the development of financial incentives for providers and third-party payers to prevent disease or detect it early has been a major driving force in creating this shift in focus.[1] In addition, recent evidence leads to the inescapable conclusion that cancer is not entirely inevitable and that individual lifestyles may influence its occurrence. Lifestyle habits of tobacco use, diet and nutrition, and sexual practices have been found to influence the frequency of cancer.[2] Therefore, to reduce the morbidity and mortality rates from cancer, and to enhance the financial benefits of prevention and early detection, programs must include an educational component to help individuals adopt healthy lifestyles and change harmful behaviors. According to several sources, a comprehensive program of controlling cancer must include interventions at the primary, secondary, and tertiary levels with a focus on cancer prevention, risk assessment, screening for preclinical disease, early detection of disease or surveillance, and education, regulation, and host modification components.[2–9]

It was this recognition of the need to focus on protecting, maintaining, and restoring the health of individuals and the population at large that led to the creation of *The Healthy People 1990 Report* by the U.S. Department of Health and Human Services in 1979. The first revision, *The Healthy People 2000 Report*, identifies three targets for the health of the people in the United States:

1. **To increase the span of healthy life for Americans.** This goal represents a shift in focus from primarily being concerned with length of life to a clear emphasis on quality of life.
2. **To reduce health disparities among Americans.** This goal addresses the greatest failures of the 1990 objectives, which were those for improving the health of disadvantaged populations. Groups at particular risk include those with low income, blacks, Hispanic Americans, Asian/Pacific Islander Americans, Native Americans and Alaska Natives, and people with disabilities.
3. **To achieve preventive services for all Americans.** This goal makes a commitment to universal access to the basic primary care services essential to ensuring the availability of clinical preventive services.[4,10,11] As McGinnis et al emphasize, "It is an acknowledgment that the human and economic costs of illness are too great for the nation not to provide such vital health services."[11,p.2551]

To accomplish its goals, *The Healthy People 2000 Report* is divided into three areas: health promotion, health protection, and disease prevention. Health promotion has eight subcategories: physical activity and fitness, nutrition, tobacco use, alcohol and other drug use, family planning, mental health and mental disorders, violent and abusive behavior, and education and community-based programs. Health protection has five subcategories: unintentional injuries, occupational safety and health, environmental health, food and drug safety, and oral health. Disease prevention has eight subcategories: maternal and infant health, heart disease and stroke, cancer, diabetes and chronic disabling conditions, HIV infection, sexually transmitted diseases, immunologic and infectious diseases, and clinical preventive services.[4,10,11]

An analysis of the success of *The Healthy People 2000* objectives was done in 1995 by the U.S. Department of Health and Human Services. The analysis appears to indicate that, although the health of Americans is improving, much work remains to be done in meeting the goals of the report. Of the 17 objectives listed for the health promotion subcategories, change is occurring in the right direction for 10, no data are available for 2, no change has been observed for 1, and change in the wrong direction has been observed for 4. Of the 10 objectives listed for the health protection subcategories, positive change is occurring in all except in the area of reducing work-related injuries. The 19 sentinel objectives for disease prevention indicate:

- Change in the right direction has been achieved for 13 (including all four of the cancer objectives directed toward achieving a decrease in cancer deaths, an increase in screening for breast cancer for women over 50 and cervical cancer for women over 18, and an increase in fecal occult blood testing for everyone over age 50)

- No data are available for one (to have a slower increase in HIV infections/100,000)

- No change has been observed for another (to decrease diabetes related deaths/100,000)

- Change is occurring in the wrong direction for four (to have fewer newborns with low birth weight, to have fewer persons disabled by chronic conditions, to have fewer pneumonia and influenza deaths per 100,000 persons, and to have no financial barriers to recommended preventive services).[4,10,11]

The U.S. Public Health Service reports that, as a result of studying the success of the 1990 and year 2000 objectives in 1995, many lessons were learned about developing national health objectives and measuring outcomes.[10] Setting specific surveillance and evaluation targets has proved to be a valid monitoring method to measure health progress. A combination of education (promotion), service provision (services), and regulation (protection) has been demonstrated to help save lives when specific health risks can be identified and when acceptable and cost-effective interventions are available. Also, assessing the outcomes of *The Healthy People 2000* objectives has helped to identify revisions that need to be made in *The Healthy People 2010* objectives: (1) target revisions based on technical baseline revisions or the achievement of certain targets; (2) where disparities or differing trends in health status exist, add special population targets; and (3) modify language to clarify the meaning and intent of objectives or to integrate objectives with current data sources.

The areas of health promotion, health protection, and disease prevention not only provide three ways to accomplish the *Healthy People 2000* objectives, but also are vital in achieving the *Cancer Control Objectives for the Nation: 1985–2000* developed by the National Cancer Institute.[3] The cancer control objectives established screening recommendations directed at reducing the cancer mortality rate in the United States by 50% by the year 2000. These reductions are to be achieved by smoking cessation, diet modification, early detection through cancer screening programs, and state-of-the-art cancer treatments. Prevention and early detection of all cancers becomes increasingly important as evidence shows that treatment modalities do not always produce the desired goal of a cure.[12]

It is important to differentiate screening from early detection. The term *screening* is often used synonymously with "early detection" or "secondary prevention," however a fundamental distinction must be drawn. *Early detection* refers to an attempt to diagnose cancer in a curable stage, whereas cancer screening is just one of the strategies used to achieve this goal.[3] Thus, *detection* is the early identification of cancers in asymptomatic or symptomatic individuals through tests, examinations, and observations; *screening* is an organized effort conducted at specific time intervals to detect cancer early in asymptomatic and high-risk persons.[12] Efforts at detection are a continuous process. Individuals must take responsibility for their own self-care and pay attention to symptoms in order to seek prompt help if anything unusual is detected. Cancer screening involves the use of examinations and tests and is done periodically by a health care professional to search for and identify disease in an asymptomatic person. A person is asymptomatic if he or she is not aware of any signs or symptoms of cancer.[3] A vital part of successful detection and screening is ready access to medical facilities for diagnosis and treatment.

Early attempts to identify existing cancer prevention, screening, and early detection efforts focused primarily on primary care physicians. Few studies assessed the practices of nurses and those that did considered nurse practitioners who had advanced preparation. A study of 673 nurses in North Carolina found that the majority of nurse respondents in primary care practice settings were routinely engaged in cancer prevention, screening, and early detection efforts that included teaching, counseling, and distribution of educational materials.[7] More than half of the nurse respondents served predominantly low-income populations. Thus, Germino suggests that it is within the scope of nursing practice to engage in cancer prevention counseling, education, and many cancer screening procedures.[7] Nurse practitioners also can routinely carry out many of the more complex procedures in their practices. The field of nursing has always considered patient education to be an integral part of the nurse's role in health care, and the combination of knowledge and skills offered by nurses in the primary care setting is a potential contribution that cannot be ignored. Also, with increasing efforts to target the socioeconomically disadvantaged, materials and continuing education programs must be developed to increase the awareness, knowledge, and skill of nurse practitioners already serving the populations of interest. Of particular interest is involving nurses in the resolution of early detection issues that influence whether individuals access screening programs or follow-up once they experience symptoms or have a positive screening test. Early detection issues include the following:

- An individual may delay reporting symptom(s) or follow-up on a positive test

- Lack of knowledge of the early warning signs of cancer by the public and health care professionals may cause a delay in receiving immediate attention for a particular symptom

- Individual personality characteristics may create barriers to accessing screening programs or early detection and include low self-esteem, denial, fear, or embarrassment

- Lack of confidence in the value of early detection may cause a decrease in participation in screening programs

- Negative health beliefs concerning preventive health practices and cancer may cause an individual not to participate in early detection or screening programs

- Lower socioeconomic status is often associated with a decreased level of reporting suspicious symptoms, participation in screening programs, access to care, and survival rate

- The elderly tend to have decreased levels of participation in screening programs, less access to care, and report suspicious symptoms less frequently

- Race/ethnicity affects knowledge about cancer, reporting of suspicious symptoms, health beliefs, language barriers[13,pp.48-49]

Several other issues have been identified that create barriers to the process of early detection and screening for cancer.[4] First among them is identifying clear lines of responsibility for health promotion, protection, and disease prevention. Barton believes that it is easy to make individuals responsible for their own health status but questions the appropriateness of this practice if individuals lack the competency and self-efficacy to make informed decisions.[4] Placing all responsibility on the individual may result in "victim blaming"; therefore, Barton believes it may be more appropriate to have provider, client, and society all share responsibility for health promotion, protection, and disease prevention, as well as for the development of effective strategies to improve health. Three other factors that affect the way we view health promotion, protection, and disease prevention are (1) the transition from a focus on contagious and communicable diseases to the lifestyle diseases threatening the modern world; (2) a reorientation toward primary care; and (3) technologic advances that affect the diagnosis, treatment, and prevention of disease. In addition, an individual's managed care plan and insurance coverage greatly affect the extent and duration of health promotion, protection, and prevention services received. Finally, what level of intervention should be used to resolve specific health problems? Should the focus of programs and monies be directed toward the individual, the community, or a combination of the two?

The involvement of nurses in cancer prevention and early detection has primarily centered on breast, cervical, and lung cancer.[5] Nursing participation in the prevention and early detection of other cancers, such as testicular, gastric, esophageal, oral, prostatic, colorectal, and skin, has been less extensive. If the National Cancer Institute year 2000 goal of reducing cancer mortality by 50% is to be attained, involvement of the nursing profession as a whole must be expanded to include cancers that affect both men and women. Moreover, we must recognize that a large percentage of nurses serve predominantly low-income populations. With the increasing need to promote early detection efforts in socioeconomically disadvantaged communities, nurse practitioners already serving these populations must be involved. Primary and secondary prevention of cancer are efforts in which nurses can and should actively participate.

Detection of Major Cancer Sites

Physical assessment has become a vital part of the nursing role, regardless of the nurse's setting. Physical assessment is now routinely taught in all undergraduate nursing programs, with the expectation that nursing students will incorporate the four cardinal techniques (i.e., inspection, palpation, percussion, and auscultation) into their daily clinical practice. These techniques enable the nurse to assume an active role in the early detection of cancer.

Cancers of the lung, breast, cervix, colon/rectum, and prostate are among the cancers that result in the highest morbidity and mortality rates in the United States.[14] The nursing interventions for these five cancers and for skin, testicular, head and neck, and other gynecologic cancers will be discussed. Each of the following sections presents the nursing role in terms of obtaining the health history, conducting the physical examination, using screening tests for asymptomatic individuals, and initiating patient education for primary and secondary prevention of the cancer.

Lung Cancer

It is estimated that in 1999 171,600 Americans will be diagnosed with lung cancer.[15] It is the leading cause of death from cancer in men and women over 35 years of age. Once considered a male disease, lung cancer has replaced breast cancer as the chief cause of cancer deaths among women since the late 1980s. Of all the known risk factors for lung cancer, the most important is cigarette smoking. Cigarette smoking is the largest single preventable cause of premature death and disability and the major single cause of cancer mortality.[16]

History assessment

When obtaining the history, the nurse should inquire about smoking habits, including marijuana use, occupational history, and the general respiratory environment of both the workplace and the home. Individuals at high risk for lung cancer are those exposed to high levels of respiratory carcinogens in their workplace, in their general environment, and in their homes. Because of the risks of passive smoking, a detailed history should be taken of the number of smokers in the home and the length of time the individual has been exposed to the smoke environment.[17,18] Exposure to passive smoking, particularly during childhood, has been shown to increase the risk of female lung cancer.[19]

Although obtaining a detailed, lifetime occupational history is time consuming, it is strongly recommended for anyone who has worked in shipyards or who is believed to have been exposed to asbestos; significant exposures may have been as brief as 1 month and may have occurred many years ago, even during World War II. Because the World War II workforce was composed of women as well as men, the female patient should not be overlooked in this regard. The latest research indicates that the risk of lung cancer following exposure to asbestos may be limited to occupational exposure rather than environmental exposure (i.e., working with asbestos vs. living in an asbestos mining region).[20] The same type of detailed, lifetime occupational history should be obtained if exposure to other known carcinogenic respiratory agents, such as those found in the following occupations, is suspected: clothing and textile workers, laundry workers, meat wrappers and cutters, hairdressers, agricultural workers, chemical workers, electrical machinery manufacturers, and health care workers.[21] In the assessment of elderly individuals, prior employment in settings unregulated by the National Institute of Occupational Safety and Health, the Occupational Safety and Health Act of 1970, or the Toxic Substances Control Act of 1976 must be considered because of possible exposure to toxic chemicals or carcinogens that are no longer manufactured or permitted in unsupervised occupational settings.

An occupational history includes dates of employment, a list of current and longest-held jobs, average hours worked per week, exposure to potential hazards in the workplace, common illness in coworkers, and personal protective equipment worn on the job. In any occupational history, the mode of entry of any suspected chemical should be ascertained (i.e., ingestion, skin absorption, or inhalation).

Questions that should be included in the history and review of systems for lung cancer are the following:

1. When was your last chest x-ray film?
2. When was your last tuberculin skin test? If positive, what was the treatment?
3. Do you presently smoke? How many packs a day and for how many years? (*Pack-years* equal packs per day times years of smoking.) What do you smoke? Are they filtered? What's your style of smoking? Have you ever tried to stop smoking? What happened? Do you have a "smoker's" cough? Who else in the home smokes, and how much do they tend to smoke a day? Are you exposed to smoking in your work setting?
4. Has your home ever been tested for radon? Have homes around you been tested for radon and found to have high levels? If you tested your home for radon, was it high or low? If high, what did you do to remedy the situation?
5. Do you have bronchitis or asthma?
6. Have you ever had pneumonia?
7. Do you get short of breath when walking? climbing stairs? while resting? with exercise?
8. Have you ever been told you have emphysema?
9. How many pillows do you sleep on? What happens if you don't use pillows?
10. Do you ever spit or cough up blood?
11. *Smokers:* What color is the sputum you cough up? Does it have a smell? How much is routinely coughed up in the morning?
12. What occupations have you had?
13. *Chronic obstructive pulmonary disease:* How often do you get flu shots? Have you been taught ways to drain the secretions from your lungs?
14. Have you ever had a pulmonary function test? What were the results?
15. Do you ever wheeze?
16. Do you cough a lot?
17. Do you have any skeletal deformities? Or were you born with any skeletal conditions?
18. Have you had any broken ribs?
19. Do you have to purse your lips to breathe?
20. Are you aware of any sounds when you breathe?
21. Have you noticed any color changes of your lips or nails?
22. Are you now (or have you been at some time in the past) exposed to fumes, chemicals, dust, or radiation?

The majority of patients have no profound early symptoms, but most have some combination of cough, chest pain, weight loss, dyspnea, fever, fatigue, and transient hemoptysis. Because these symptoms are general in nature, they usually cause no alarm and delay diagnosis. The most frequently reported symptom of lung cancer is a cough that is productive and often associated with hemoptysis or chest pain.[22] Cough may be the primary or only complaint in such varied diseases as congestive heart failure, asthma, upper respiratory infection, pneumonia, and bronchitis. The irritative cough may occur at night, accompanied by mucoid expectoration. However, if the lung cancer is centrally located or if only the main carina is involved, the cough is nonproductive.

Late symptoms are increased frequency of early symptoms and some combination of wheezes; pleuritic pain; hoarseness; nerve disorders from local invasion; edema of head, neck, or arms; and dysphagia. There is a high index of suspicion in anyone with a history of smoking or exposure to carcinogenic agents who complains of pneumonitis that persists longer than 2 weeks despite antibiotic therapy. Unfortunately, the first symptoms of lung cancer are usually not alarming and therefore tend to be considered lightly by health professionals. Because elderly individuals experience changes in respiratory structure and function, their initial vague respiratory complaints go unnoticed or are attributed to the aging process or chronic illnesses (e.g., congestive heart failure).

Physical examination

Inspection. On inspection there may be many systemic as well as localized signs that will alert the practitioner to the possibility of lung cancer.

Finger clubbing. This may be either an early or a late sign of thoracic disease, and it may be absent even in the presence of advanced disease. Approximately 5%–12% of patients with carcinoma of the lung will have clubbing of the fingers. It also may be seen in other diseases such as industrial lung disease (e.g., asbestosis).[22] It is important to inspect the nails closely and to palpate them for sponginess. With clubbing, the nail bed becomes thickened and boggy, which is first observed by palpating the nail bed to elicit fluctuation. Clubbing usually occurs first in the thumb and the index finger and then spreads to the other fingers.

The changes associated with clubbing usually occur gradually over many weeks, months, and years. However, they have been noted to appear within a week of the onset of lung cancer. Clubbing is best assessed by viewing the finger from the side. A normal finger viewed from this direction has an angle of about 160 degrees between the base of the nail and the skin next to the cuticle (Figure 9-1). In clubbing, this base angle is obliterated and becomes 180 degrees or more.[23]

Barrel chest. This is characterized by prominence of the sternum and a barrel-shaped configuration of the chest that appears to be held in a state of full inspiration. This finding is associated with pulmonary emphysema or normal aging. Emphysema can be inherited, but the vast majority of individuals with this disease have acquired it from a lifetime of smoking. Those with emphysema are at high risk for lung cancer. Typical physical findings of emphysema are pursed lips during breathing, retraction

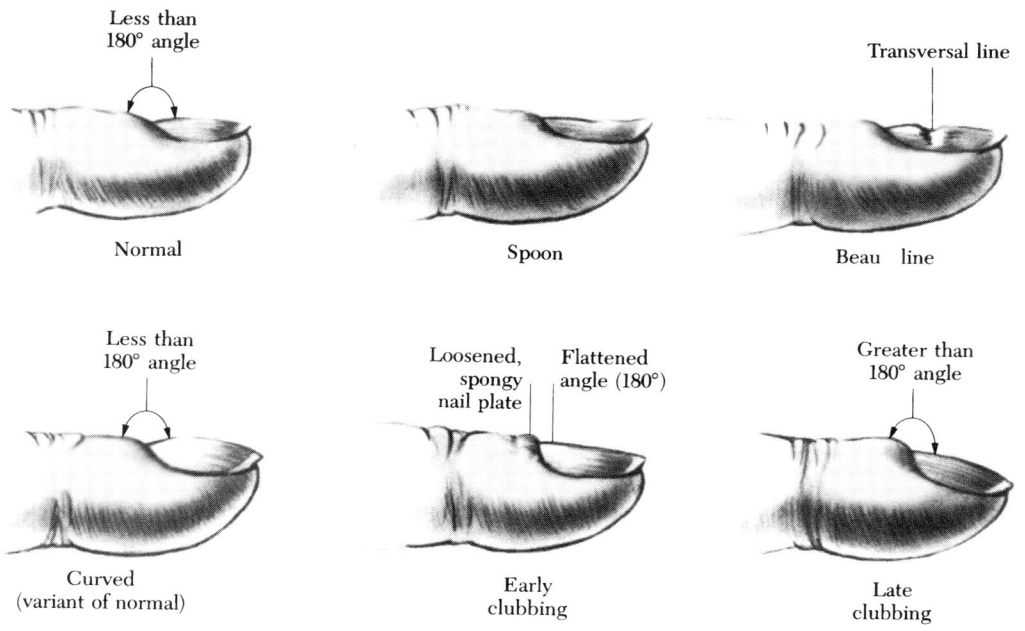

Figure 9-1   Normal and abnormal nails (Grimes J, Burns E (eds): *Health Assessment in Nursing Practice* [ed 2]. Sudbury, MA, Jones and Bartlett, 1987)

of the intercostal spaces during inspiration, use of accessory muscles during quiet respirations, and audible wheezes.

Abnormal breathing.   With obstructive types of pulmonary disease, expiration is prolonged and inspiration is gasping and may require the use of the accessory muscles of respiration in the neck and about the shoulder girdle.[24] Figure 9-2 shows the stance taken by individuals with pulmonary obstruction. This stance is called the *professorial attitude* because it resembles a professor lecturing.

Bulges on the thorax.   With the use of indirect lighting, the practitioner may observe a bulge on the chest. Neoplasm of the ribs may protrude and will be visible on inspection.

Breathlessness.   The patient's breathlessness during the history taking may indicate obstruction of the lungs.

Skin.   Inspection of the skin of a heavy smoker may reveal premature wrinkling. Heavy cigarette smokers (50 pack-years) are 4.7 times more likely to be wrinkled than nonsmokers.[25]

Superior vena cava obstruction.   Obstruction of the superior vena cava is a common complication of malignant disease, with the majority of cases caused by lung cancer.[26] Dyspnea, facial edema, and cough are the most common symptoms. The clinical picture is described by Buckingham:

> Edema of both eyelids, arms, and hands develops and will "pit" on pressure; . . . the face is a dusky blue color, the lips are deeply cyanotic; and the swollen, blue head sits on

a thick "bull neck" which is distended by many large tense collateral veins. The shoulders, chest, and upper abdomen are covered with a lacy collateral venous pattern.[24]

Palpation.   Palpation of the thorax includes testing for vocal fremitus, respiratory excursion and compression, and ascertaining the position and movability of the trachea. The following discussion presents physical signs on palpation that may indicate lung cancer.

Deviation and fixed trachea.   Normally the trachea is located in the midline and is freely movable. Localized disease may produce tracheal shift, or the trachea may be fixed by disease in the surrounding structures. Carcinoma of the lung rarely causes displacement, except by producing atelectasis.[27]

Thoracic wall.   Palpation of the thoracic wall reveals masses.

Vocal fremitus.   Decreased or absent vocal fremitus indicates local bronchial obstruction from bronchial carcinomas, adenomas, or foreign bodies. Sound transmission through the bronchus is interrupted, causing the change in fremitus. Absent vocal fremitus also may indicate pleural effusions. Lung tumors immediately adjacent to the visceral pleura often cause early, insidious formation of pleural effusion that is responsible for the initial complaint of dyspnea.

Percussion and auscultation.   These may provide the final clues to assessment of the individual who is at high risk for lung cancer. Auscultation is best done with the

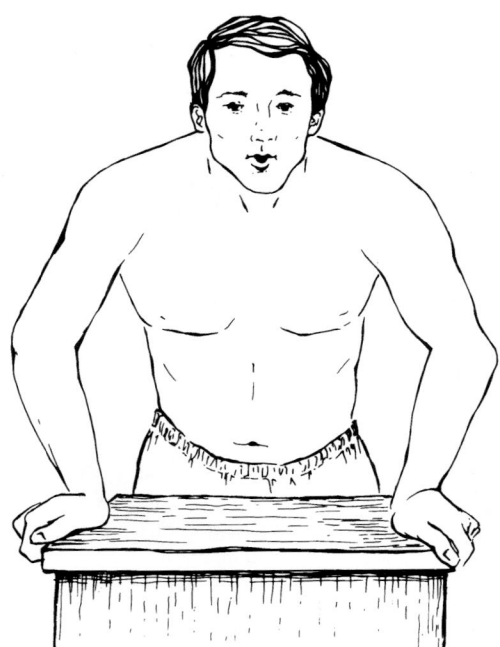

Figure 9-2 Patient fixes the arms and leans forward to use pectoral muscles as accessory inspiratory muscles for obstructed breathing.

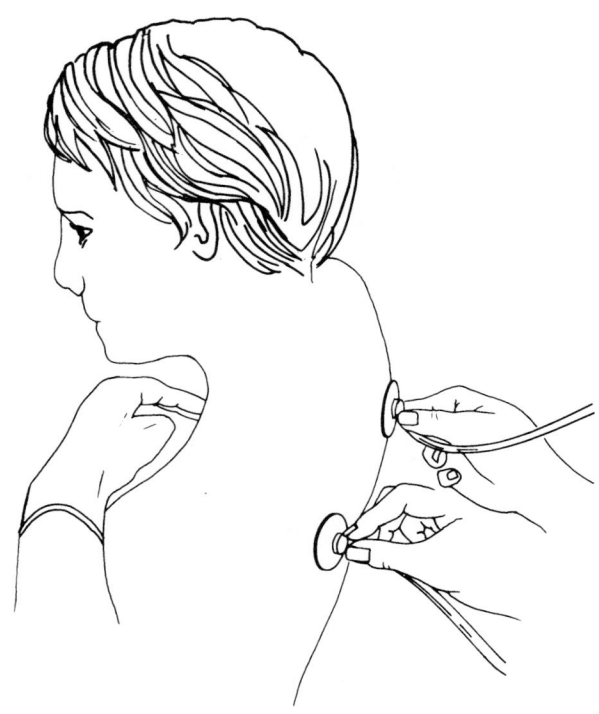

Figure 9-3 Auscultatory-percussion technique

diaphragm of the stethoscope in a slow, methodical sequence of upper, middle, and lower zones and front, sides, and back. Physical signs that would require referral to a physician are discussed next.

Dullness. In the normal chest, the sound on auscultatory percussion is resonance. If any pathologic condition exists between the sound source (manubrium) and the reception point (stethoscope), the sound produced is a duller tone than normal.

An excellent technique for assessing dullness in the thorax is the auscultatory-percussion technique. This technique is accomplished by having the examiner lightly percuss the patient's manubrium while listening with the diaphragm piece on the posterior chest wall[28] (Figure 9-3). This technique enables the examiner to detect small, deep areas of pathologic disease.

Dullness on percussion indicates either pleural effusion or a consolidated lung. Lung cancer is the most common cause of hemorrhagic pleural effusion in middle-aged and elderly male smokers. The early production of pleural fluid by most tumors produces the classic signs of pleural effusion: flatness, absence of fremitus, and breath sounds.[27]

Decreased or absent breath sounds. Breath sounds are decreased or absent when air flow is decreased or when fluid or tissue separates the air passages from the stethoscope.

Unilateral wheezing and the bagpipe sign. Tumors in the main bronchus may cause a localized expiratory and/

or inspiratory wheeze, or "honk," which sometimes is reproduced only when the individual lies on the affected side. When a continuous wheeze is heard at the end of expiration as air continues to whistle out past a partial obstruction, this is known as the *bagpipe sign.*

Presence of whispered pectoriloquy, bronchophony, and egophony. When the lungs are normal, whispered test words are faint and their syllables are not distinct when the examiner listens with a stethoscope over the lungs. When a lung is consolidated or compressed by a pleural effusion, transmission of voice sounds is altered. The sounds are louder, clearer than usual, and sometimes changed in quality. These three criteria are assessed as follows:

1. *Whispered pectoriloquy.* The patient whispers numerals (e.g., one, two, and three). Normally these sounds are muffled; in consolidation they are clearly transmitted.[29]
2. *Bronchophony.* When the patient says a number (e.g., 99), the sound normally is muffled. When the sound transmitted is a clear sound of the vocalized numerals, it is created by mucus- or fluid-filled alveoli or by cellular mass replacing alveolar tissue.[30]
3. *Egophony.* The patient says *e*, which normally results in a muffled, indistinct sound. In pleural effusion the *e* sound is heard as a nasal-sounding *a*.

Figure 9-4 presents a synopsis of the physical findings commonly seen with tumors of different anatomic sites in the lungs. The majority of physical signs discussed previously are found in late or advanced lung cancer.

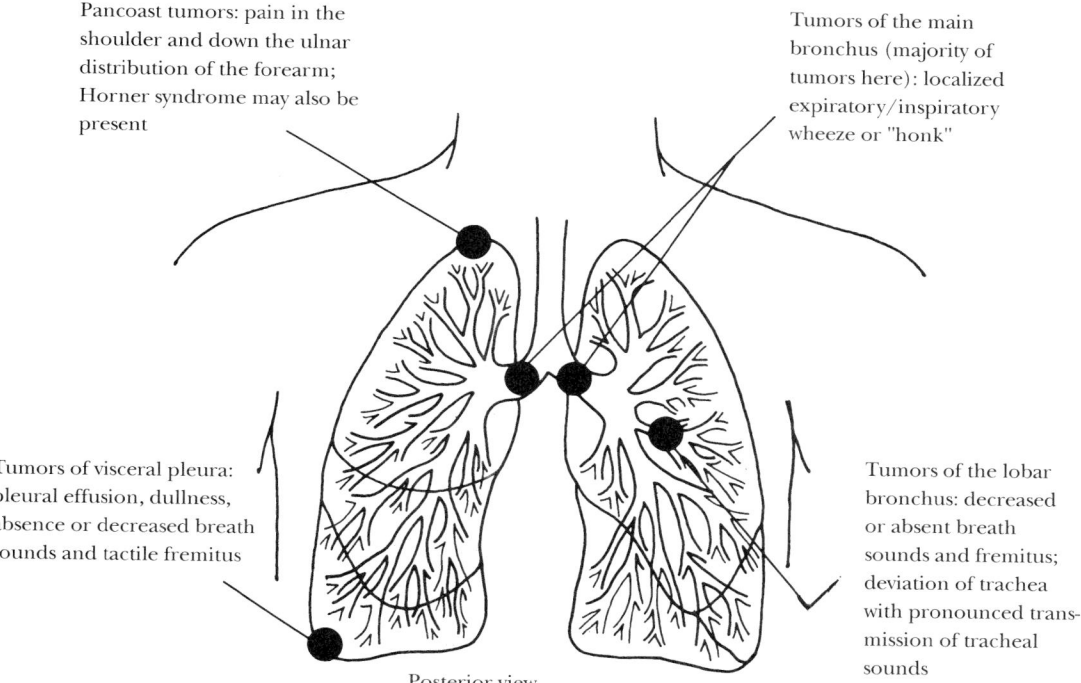

Pancoast tumors: pain in the shoulder and down the ulnar distribution of the forearm; Horner syndrome may also be present

Tumors of the main bronchus (majority of tumors here): localized expiratory/inspiratory wheeze or "honk"

Tumors of visceral pleura: pleural effusion, dullness, absence or decreased breath sounds and tactile fremitus

Tumors of the lobar bronchus: decreased or absent breath sounds and fremitus; deviation of trachea with pronounced trans-mission of tracheal sounds

Posterior view

Figure 9-4 Synopsis of physical findings of lung cancer

The *only early* physical finding that most strongly suggests lung cancer is wheezing localized to a single lobe of the lung in an elderly person with a long history of smoking.

Screening tests for asymptomatic individuals

There are no recommended screening programs or tests for lung cancer because studies have not shown any evidence of a significant reduction in mortality from these programs. Recent research has indicated that molecular genetics may hold promise for the detection of early lung cancer. Mao et al were able to follow the development of clinical lesions after sputum collection, indicating that these gene mutations may be detected with significant lead time prior to clinical diagnosis.[31] The American Cancer Society (ACS) focuses on primary prevention: helping smokers to stop and keeping nonsmokers from starting.

Smoking cessation

The greatest reduction in mortality can be achieved by cessation of smoking. Between 80% and 85% of deaths from lung cancer are directly attributable to smoking, thus making smoking the leading cause of cancer mortality in the United States.[32] Smoking in the United States is on the decline. Per capita cigarette consumption among adults fell from 4141 in 1974 to 3196 in 1987, and this is the lowest per capita consumption since 1944.[33] In general, smoking prevalence is decreasing across all race-gender groups, although at a slower rate for women than

men.[34] However, smoking prevalence has increased among American teens and college students.[35] Thus, adult smokers who quit or die are being replaced by children and young adults who are taking up the habit despite all the information on television, radio, and in print media pointing out the dangers of smoking. The latest data collected by the National Health Interview Surveys indicate that educational level is the major demographic predictor of whether an individual will smoke cigarettes. Regardless of gender, a person who does not attend college is more than twice as likely to start smoking than the person who does. In addition, smoking cessation occurs more frequently in groups with higher levels of education than in groups with less education, and the gap is widening over time.[34]

Cigarette advertising campaigns have been directed to groups that tend to smoke (youth, women, minorities, and blue-collar workers) in order to recruit new smokers or to increase cigarette consumption among smokers.[36] Knowing the groups that tend to smoke and that are being targeted by the tobacco industry should assist health professionals in identifying and predicting patterns of cigarette use and in developing health promotion materials specifically designed for these high-risk groups. Chapter 85 of this text provides a list of smoking cessation materials specifically written for blue-collar workers, minorities, and women.

Obviously, the nurse wants to monitor most aggressively those who smoke, who have had a history of heavy smoking, or who were employed in high-risk occupations.

These individuals should have (1) a complete baseline respiratory assessment, (2) a thorough assessment of respiratory symptoms, and (3) physical assessment of their respiratory system at periodic intervals. Deviations from normal merit referral for chest x-ray studies and/or sputum cytologic findings. In this high-risk population, a cold that lingers or "smoker's cough" that is accompanied by fatigue and weight loss should not be ignored.

One fallacy commonly heard about individuals who smoke is that because they have smoked for years, "what harm is there in letting them continue?" Nothing could be further from the truth or more detrimental to their health. Continual smoking damages not only their already compromised respiratory system but their cardiovascular system as well. Research clearly documents that smoking cessation results in improved sensory, respiratory, and cardiovascular status.[37] Fielding noted that a British physician study reported that exsmokers who had not smoked for 5 years had a lung cancer mortality rate approximately 40% that of a current smoker.[38] After 15 years without smoking, the mortality rate of exsmokers was only slightly greater than that of nonsmokers. No one is ever too old or has smoked too long to *stop* smoking.

The nurse should take a nonjudgmental approach with those who refuse or are unable to stop smoking. The 1988 surgeon general's report stated that nicotine is the drug in tobacco that causes addiction and that the processes of tobacco addiction are similar to those that determine addiction to drugs such as heroin and cocaine.[34] Because of the addicting qualities of nicotine, many exsmokers are not able to give up the habit on the first attempt but must try three or more times before finally succeeding.[39] In the hope of reducing the adverse health consequences of smoking, health professionals frequently advise individuals who cannot quit to smoke fewer cigarettes, to smoke cigarettes with less than 10 mg of tar, to smoke filtered cigarettes, and to smoke only half of each cigarette. However, habitual smokers may compensate for the reduced number of cigarettes by taking in more smoke per cigarette ("oversmoking").[40] The current preferred strategy is to urge smokers to establish a quit day and "quit cold turkey," rather than tapering off.

It is the nurse's responsibility to disseminate information actively and assertively on the disease potential of smoking whenever possible. Every assistance should be afforded to those who want to stop smoking. Nurses who smoke are less likely to discuss the need to stop smoking or the various smoking cessation methods that can be employed. It is essential that nurses act as role models by not smoking and by actively working at creating nonsmoking environments in both their employment and their home settings.

Nurses have frequent opportunities to advise smokers to quit, either in health care settings or in the community. The importance of counseling smokers to quit is underscored by the research of Anda et al.[41] In their study of 5875 Michigan adults who smoked, of those who had seen a physician in the previous year, only 44% reported being told to quit smoking by a physician. In general,

most smokers did not perceive physicians to be even minimally involved in their efforts to quit. In fairness to physicians, there may be a tendency for smokers to hear only what they want to hear.[42] For this reason, the U.S. Preventive Services Task Force recommends that smokers be exposed to a variety of intervention techniques on multiple occasions delivered by both physicians and nonphysicians to improve smoking cessation rates.[43] Kottke et al also found that the best method for helping smokers quit was to use a team of physicians and nonphysicians that employed multiple intervention modalities to deliver individualized advice on multiple occasions.[44] The U.S. Agency for Health Care Policy and Research's *Smoking Cessation Clinical Practice Guidelines* provides recommendations for primary care clinicians, smoking cessation specialists, health care administrators, insurers, and purchasers on the treatment of tobacco addiction.[43] The multiple smoking cessation interventions suggested by all authorities include the following:

- Direct, face-to-face advice and suggestions on smoking cessation

- Smoking cessation self-help materials that are culturally and educationally relevant to the individual person

- Referral to community smoking cessation programs

- Drug therapy when appropriate (e.g., nicotine gum, nicotine patch, antidepressant)

- Scheduled reinforcement with the smoker

Table 9-1 presents the process the nurse should follow to successfully assist the smoker in quitting. When individuals are referred to smoking cessation programs, it is advised that cost effectiveness be considered in the selection. Altman et al found that self-help programs not only had the lowest total cost and lowest time requirement for participants, but that their quit rate percentage was also the lowest.[45] In contrast, smoking cessation classes were expensive but had the most success in getting individuals to stop smoking.

A new development to assist smokers in quitting is the nicotine patch. These can be purchased over-the-counter and do not require a physician's prescription. These patches are available in three sizes that deliver 21 mg, 14 mg, or 7 mg of nicotine over 16–24 hours. The nicotine is either directly released through the skin or through a membrane system in contact with the skin. Side effects are minimal and include mild-to-moderate sleep disturbances; skin reactions including transient itching, burning, and erythema; poorly defined body aches; and increased cough. Nicotine gum is also available to assist the smoker in quitting. Smokers are advised to chew 1–2 pieces per hour and to use 20 mg if they smoke fewer than 25 cigarettes per day (4 mg if more than 25 cigarettes per day).[46,47] Other new nicotine delivery methods that may hold promise are the nicotine nasal spray and nicotine inhaler. The latest recommendations are to use a

Table 9-1   Smoking Cessation Strategies

1. ASK
    Screen every patient for tobacco use
    Identify patient's smoking behavior
    Review smoking history
    Provide risk-benefit information, personalizing when possible
    Assess health beliefs about smoking
2. ADVISE
    Urge smokers to quit
3. ASSESS
    Determine interest in smoking cessation
    Determine patient's readiness to quit in terms of motivation, intention, and self-efficacy
4. ASSIST
    Aid patient in quitting
    Set the target quit-date
    Pick a realistic calendar quit-date
    Stop smoking "cold turkey"
    Encourage nicotine replacement therapy as appropriate
        Provide education on use of nicotine gum and/or nicotine patch, which can be obtained over-the-counter
        Provide education on the use of antidepressant, which can be used with nicotine replacement therapy
        Secure prescription for slow-release antidepressant (bupropion)
        Discuss known side effects of nicotine-replacement therapy
    Describe preparatory techniques
        List reasons for quitting
        Review previous quit attempts
        Become aware of smoking-related situations
        Seek social support
        Reduce number of cigarettes and/or amount of nicotine
        Replace cigarettes with gum or food (preference low-fat, low-calorie)
        Eliminate environmental cues, alcohol
        Avoid, distract, delay
    Discuss withdrawal symptoms
    Review cognitive and behavioral strategies to use in high-risk situations—social, relaxation, work, and upsetting situations
5. FOLLOW-UP
    Contact during the first week and again within first month
    Congratulate success
    Encourage the maintenance of successful abstinence and discuss "slips"
    Review relapse and refer to more specialized program
        Review benefits of quitting
        Review patient's success in quitting
        Anticipate problems and counsel
    Assess nicotine-replacement therapy use and problems

Data from A Systems Approach: Clinical Practice Guideline, Number 18. AHCPR Publication No. 97-0698. Rockville, MD, Agency for Health Care Policy and Research, April 1997. *http://www.ahcpr.gov/clinic/smokesys.htm*

sustained-release antidepressant (bupropion) along with a nicotine patch for the highest quit rates. A combination of the nicotine patch with gum or patch with bupropion may increase the quit rate compared with any single treatment.[46]

Chemoprevention efforts aimed at the prevention of lung cancer in smokers have not proved to be effective.[48,49] (See Chapter 8 for an in-depth discussion.)

Significant changes in the U.S. social and work-related environments have resulted in less tolerance of smoking and have made smokers more receptive to the antismoking messages of health professionals. The 1987 Bureau of National Affairs survey of 623 large corporations found that 54% had adopted some type of plan to restrict employee smoking. This was a 36% increase from a similar survey the previous year.[50] In the health care field, the Joint Commission on Accreditation of Healthcare Organizations, which accredits about 80% of all U.S. hospitals, has mandated a ban on smoking in hospitals.[51] In addition, many states have passed laws that place limitations on smoking. These antismoking policies appear to have a dramatic effect on the nation's smoking habits. Theoretically, they will encourage people to quit smoking by increasing the social pressure against it and by restricting the time available for it.

Gastrointestinal Cancer

Colorectal cancer incidence and mortality in the United States are second only to those of lung cancer. It is estimated that in 1999, 129,400 new colorectal cases will be diagnosed, and 56,600 people will die of this cancer. In both men and women 35 years of age and older, colorectal cancer is one of the leading causes of deaths from cancer.[15]

History assessment

Several conditions and health practices must be questioned to obtain a realistic picture of the patient's gastrointestinal system. For example, after the age of 50 years, approximately 25% of the population has demonstrable diverticulosis, and by age 80 years the proportion is 70%.[52] Slight rectal bleeding commonly is found with this disorder. Another condition that causes symptoms that mimic gastrointestinal cancer is depression. Depression is more common in the elderly than in the young because of increasing losses and limitations that accompany the aging process.[52] Some of the cardinal manifestations of depression are anorexia, constipation, and somatic pains. In addition, weight loss in the elderly may be due to nutritional disturbances rather than a malignancy. Loss of income, depression, decreased sensation of taste, loss of teeth, and difficulty swallowing all contribute to decreased food intake. Another important part of the nursing assessment is a thorough history of drug intake. The elderly tend to use aspirin frequently for the pain of arthritis and to abuse laxatives. Considering these factors, the history and review of systems should include the following questions:

1. Do you have a history of cancer of the bowel or ulcerative colitis?
2. Have you ever been told you have polyps of the bowel? Gardner syndrome? Have you had any polyps removed?
3. Do any of your relatives have (or have any had) bowel cancer?
4. Would you characterize your diet as consisting of more red meat than fish, veal, and poultry? Has your diet usually consisted of more starches and sweets than vegetables and fruits? Would you characterize your diet as being high in fats?
5. Do you take laxatives? If so, what kind, how often, and what amount? How long have you taken laxatives?
6. Have you noticed a difference in your bowel habits? Do you have more constipation, more diarrhea? Do these two conditions seem to alternate?
7. What is your usual bowel habit? Has this changed in the last few years? Has the shape of your bowel movements changed recently?
8. Have you ever been told you have diverticulosis? ulcers? nervous stomach?
9. Have you had gastrointestinal x-ray studies within the last 2–3 years? Have you had a barium enema, proctoscopy, or related procedure to examine your rectum and colon in the last 2–3 years? If you did, why was the test done and what were the results?
10. Do you take aspirin? How often and how much? What other medications (antacids, stool softeners, antispasmodics) are you now taking?
11. Are you familiar with at-home stool guaiac testing? Have you ever used this?
12. Do you have hemorrhoids or anal fissures?
13. Have you noticed any change in appetite? Are you experiencing nausea or vomiting?
14. Have you experienced any weight loss recently?
15. Do you have excessive gas? feelings of being bloated? abdominal pain?
16. Do you have the feeling after you have a bowel movement that you still have to go to the bathroom and expel more stool? Do you experience pain before, with, or after defecation?

The signs and symptoms of cancers of the colon and rectum often are related to the portion of intestine involved. Figure 9-5 identifies the most frequent presenting signs and symptoms of each area of the intestinal tract affected by cancer.

Physical examination

Inspection. The assessment of the gastrointestinal system begins with inspection. The findings that may suggest cancer of the gastrointestinal system include the following:

- Nodular umbilicus. Abdominal carcinoma, especially gastric, may metastasize to the navel. This is called Sister Joseph nodule.

- Masses that distort the abdominal profile and indicate organomegaly.

- Subcutaneous nodules under the skin that are visible with tangential lighting.

- Distention. The abdominal profile should be inspected because neoplasms can distort the profile. The examiner may see distention of the lower half, lower third, or upper half of the abdomen.

- Venous distention caused by blockage of the inferior vena cava, which can occur from spread of cancer. In this condition there is edema of the eyelids, a bluish face and lips, prominent neck veins, and pitting edema of the arms and large veins over the upper portions of the chest and shoulders.

- Visible peristaltic waves, which may appear in normal individuals with thin abdomens and may be accentuated in patients with obstruction to the forward passage of gastrointestinal contents. Small bowel obstruction gives rise to a condition resembling a "bag of worms" or a "stepladder." Numerous segments of small bowel contract and relax in an irregular manner, and the peristalsis has no recognizable pattern.

- Bulging of the flanks may signal intraabdominal fluid.

Auscultation. After a thorough inspection of the abdomen is performed with the use of tangential lighting, the abdomen should be auscultated. Bowel sounds that are heard without the use of a stethoscope are called

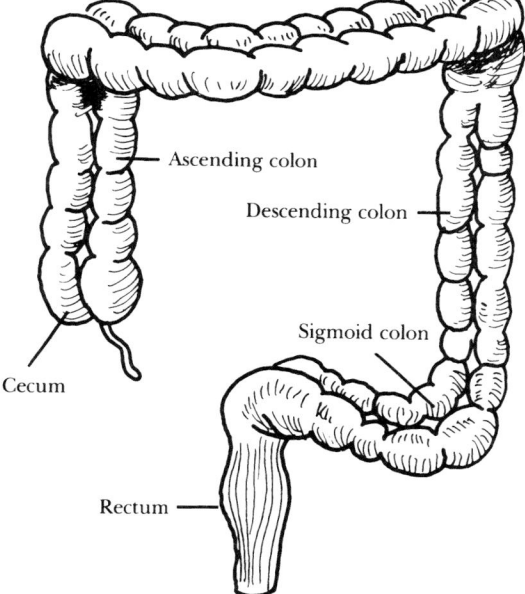

Transverse colon
10% of GI cancers are in this area; presenting signs and symptoms: Change in bowel habits and blood in stool

Right side of the cecum and ascending colon
15% of GI cancers are in this area; presenting signs and symptoms:

Anemia
GI tract bleeding
Vague pain
Weight loss and anorexia
Palpable mass

Ascending colon

Descending colon

Sigmoid colon

Cecum

Rectum

Descending colon, rectosigmoid, rectum
75% of all GI cancers are in this area; may obstruct the movement of more solid fecal material; presenting signs and symptoms:

Abdominal pain
Change in bowel habits
Increased use of laxatives
Decrease in caliber of stools
Bright red blood coating surface of stools
Nausea and vomiting

Rectal presenting signs and symptoms:

Rectal pain
Gross blood per rectal tenesmus
Sense of incomplete evacuation
Constipation

Figure 9-5   Presenting signs and symptoms of colorectal cancers based on location in the intestinal tract

borborygmi. Bowel sounds heard with the stethoscope bell range from absent to frequent. Significant types of bowel sounds include the following:

- High-pitched, long, intense peristaltic rushes occur with any hypermotile state such as partial obstruction.

- High-pitched "tingling" sounds indicate a more complete mechanical intestinal obstruction.

- Extremely weak or infrequent sounds may also indicate bowel immobility.

- Absent bowel sounds, determined by listening to the bowel for at least *5 minutes,* may indicate advanced intestinal obstruction.

Another sound that may signal obstruction of the small intestines is a *succussion splash.* Succussion splash is produced by a combination of air and fluid in the gut when the examiner shakes the stomach or vigorously moves the abdomen. The sound resembles loud splashes.

Some abdominal circulatory sounds also signal cancer. A bruit heard over the liver with the bell of the stethoscope when the patient takes a deep breath may indicate a hepatoma with arteriovenous shunting. In addition, a hepatic friction rub heard with the bell of the stethoscope may indicate a hepatoma. A bruit heard over the pancreas may indicate pancreatic carcinoma. A murmur over the left hypochondrium is one of the rare physical signs that suggests an early carcinoma of the body of the pancreas.

Thus, auscultation of the abdomen may indicate a bowel obstruction, a hepatoma, or pancreatic carcinoma.

Palpation and percussion.   The information obtained from inspection and auscultation should alert the examiner to expected findings during palpation and percussion of the abdomen. On palpation of the abdomen the organs that are normally palpated are the abdominal aorta, the edge of the liver, the lower pole of the right kidney, the descending colon and the sigmoid, and the ascending colon. The following findings on palpation and percussion merit further attention and may signal colorectal cancer.

Hepatomegaly.   Total liver span is the best estimate of liver size because liver height cannot be determined by feeling only the edge. Palpation alone detects the inferior portion as it descends below the costal margin. A normal liver at the midclavicular line is 10–12 cm in span. Nodules on the liver or an irregular edge suggest malignancy.

Splenomegaly.   Because the normal spleen is rarely palpable, a spleen that descends below the left costal margin on deep inspiration is enlarged. Cancer conditions that enlarge the spleen are leukemias and lymphomas.

Enlargement of the colon.   Carcinoma of the colon may produce a palpable mass anywhere along the course of the colon.

Fluid.   Several tests can be used to determine if there is free fluid in the abdomen. The presence of intraperitoneal fluid is suspected when there is abdominal distention with bulging flanks and possibly an everted umbilicus. *Shifting dullness* and *fluid wave* are two tests frequently used to detect fluid in the abdomen. The *puddle sign* has the advantage of detecting small amounts of intraabdominal fluid. After the patient has been on hands and knees for several minutes, the examiner percusses the periumbilical area to detect a line between fluid and air, as in the determination of shifting dullness. As little as several hundred milliliters of ascitic fluid can be detected by this method.[27]

Rectal examination. Half the cancers that occur in the rectum and colon are within reach of the examining finger. Lesions high in the rectum are sometimes felt more readily when the patient bears down as if having a bowel movement. On palpation the examiner may feel a *rectal shelf,* which, in men, is a stony hard mass above the prostate on the anterior rectal wall. In women, it is felt as a stony hard mass in the cul-de-sac. The shelf indicates a carcinoma that has metastasized to the pelvic floor and therefore is a sign of advanced malignancy. Carcinoma of the rectum causes plateaulike, nodular, annular, and cauliflower masses in the rectum.[24]

Other physical findings. Several physical findings in other parts of the body, which are not revealed in the abdominal examination, are typical in abdominal carcinoma. For instance, enlargement of a single node, usually in the left supraclavicular group, is a sign of carcinomatous metastasis from a primary lesion in the upper portion of the abdomen. This node, called *Virchow node,* is frequently behind the clavicular head of the left supraclavicular group. The Valsalva maneuver causes the node to rise, which enables the nurse to palpate the node.

Another physical finding associated with abdominal carcinoma is *acanthosis nigricans,* a skin lesion. Acanthosis nigricans is probably the most well-known cutaneous syndrome of intestinal malignancy. It is a velvety, brownish skin eruption that strongly suggests an intestinal malignancy when it occurs in patients older than 40 years of age.[53]

Another systemic finding related to pathology of the gastrointestinal system is jaundice. Jaundice and accompanying steady pain may indicate hepatic or pancreatic lesions. Although painless obstructive jaundice is said to be a feature of carcinoma of the head of the pancreas, the majority of individuals with pancreatic cancer have some degree of anterior abdominal or back pain. By means of daylight or fluorescent light the sclerae, the undersurface of the tongue, and the frenulum of the tongue should be examined for jaundice.

Although there are many physical findings that suggest cancer of the gastrointestinal system, the findings that most strongly suggest cancer of the colorectal area are (1) a mass palpated in the rectum, (2) a palpable mass in the abdomen, and (3) evidence of blood in the feces. Nurses who work with the elderly or high-risk individuals in nursing homes, residential settings, acute-care institutions, and physicians' offices are encouraged to take the time to thoroughly assess an individual's gastrointestinal complaints. Often the elderly will share their complaints with the nurse rather than the physician because they hesitate to bother the doctor with "trivial" problems.

Screening tests for asymptomatic individuals

The two most important screening tests for asymptomatic individuals are examination of the feces for occult blood and the digital rectal examination.[54] Debate about the use of occult blood tests has been laid to rest with the results of several recent clinical trials. The results from the only true randomized controlled study in the United States that assessed the effect of occult blood screening on colorectal cancer mortality has thus far shown a 33% decrease in the 13-year cumulative mortality from colorectal cancer.[55,56] This study made extensive use of rehydration of fecal occult blood testing (Hemoccult) slides, a process that makes detection of blood more likely.[57] There are researchers who argue against the use of rehydrated slides because of the possibility of more positive test results. However, researchers in Italy who have been rehydrating Hemoccult slides since 1982 recommend this procedure and conclude that rehydrated Hemoccult slides should be introduced as the standard test for screening in order to increase sensitivity for colorectal cancer and adenomas. A randomized trial conducted in Sweden using rehydration of Hemoccult slides[58] found that the cancers detected in this randomized trial were at a less advanced stage than in the control group. The debate on whether or not to rehydrate Hemoccult slides continues. However, the latest evidence from these three randomized, controlled trials indicates that screening with fecal occult blood tests reduces mortality rates associated with colorectal cancer. Mortality rates associated with colorectal cancer can be reduced by about 15%–35% by screening with fecal occult blood tests.[59]

One problem with occult blood tests is the number of false-positive results that necessitates additional tests. It is argued that although the test itself is inexpensive, the recommended follow-up diagnostic procedure is expensive. For instance, if one million people were screened, about 100,000 of them (10%) would show positive findings and the costs of the follow-up tests would be $50 million for the detection of 2300 colorectal cancers.[60] In a review of all the articles published on colorectal cancer screening from 1989 and 1993, the Canadian Task Force on the Periodic Health Examination concluded that insufficient evidence existed to support screening with colonoscopy.[61]

Because the role of fecal occult blood tests in the early detection of colorectal cancer has been validated, the nurse should be aware of the following specific recommendations that will increase the accuracy of the test:

1. Duplicate samples should be taken from different parts of the feces each day for 3 consecutive days while the patient follows a meat-free diet. It is important for the nurse to encourage the patient to collect stool for

3 consecutive days because not all bowel cancers bleed, and occult blood is not always uniformly distributed in feces. Increasing the number of tests may therefore address these two causes of false-negative tests.[59,60] Presently no scientific validation exists for a high-residue diet during the 3 days of stool specimen collection.

2. During the 3 days of stool collection, patients should avoid:
   a. Aspirin-containing compounds in dosages greater than 325 mg/day (cause false-positive reaction)
   b. Antibiotics (cause false-positive reaction)
   c. Anti-inflammatory drugs (cause false-positive reaction)
   d. Ascorbic acid (cause false-negative reaction)
   e. Foods high in peroxidase—broccoli, cabbage, potatoes, cantaloupe, turnips, apricots, apples, pears, horseradish (cause false-positive reaction)
   f. Oral iron compounds (cause false-positive reactions)
3. The stool specimens should be read within 6 days of collection because delay contributes to false-negative results.

Because of the false-positive and false-negative results frequently obtained with the current tests for occult stool by means of guaiac-impregnated cards, alternate methods to detect colorectal cancer are being sought. Several researchers have published preliminary data on immuno-chemical tests that do not rely on blood loss to detect gastrointestinal changes caused by cancer.[62,63] Nakama and Kamijo conducted a mass screening for colorectal cancer using immunologic fecal occult blood testing and reported higher accuracy than that achieved by chemical occult testing.[62]

Dietary restrictions have been reported to decrease compliance, and self-administered fecal occult blood tests have not been found to increase compliance either.[64] Those who are most likely to be helped by screening (e.g., the elderly) are less likely to cooperate. Those studies that report good compliance usually deal with a highly motivated or selected group of volunteers.

The ACS recommends that asymptomatic individuals at average risk should begin screening by age 50 with an annual fecal occult blood test plus either sigmoidoscopic (preferably flexible) examination (every 5 years) or a total colon examination either by colonoscopy (every 10 years) or by double-contrast barium enema (every five to 10 years). They recommend that the digital rectal examination should be performed at the time of the sigmoidoscopy or the total colon exam. For individuals at moderate risk, those with adenomatous polyps, they should have a colonoscopy at the time of diagnosis and total colon examination within 3 years of polyp removal. Individuals with a family history of adenomatous polyposis or nonpolyposis colon cancer should have intensive supervision at an earlier age.[65] First-degree relatives of individuals with newly diagnosed adenomas, particularly if they are 50 years of age or younger at diagnosis, are at

increased risk for colorectal cancer and should undergo screening similar to the recommendations for relatives of patients with colorectal cancer.[66,67]

Additional nursing interventions

Nurses have a variety of roles in colorectal cancer detection. One of the most important roles the nurse assumes is that of educator. As educators, nurses can (1) inform the general public about colorectal cancer and the value of early detection, as well as make a special effort to inform the elderly and other high-risk groups; (2) encourage the participation of the general public and high-risk groups in early detection of the disease through the use of a stool guaiac slide test, digital rectal examination, and, after 50 years of age, proctosigmoidoscopic examination; and (3) emphasize the effectiveness of the stool guaiac test, stressing that it is painless and convenient (it can be administered in the privacy of one's home).

Nurses who work in community organizations, clinics, nursing homes, retirement centers, geriatric day care centers, and hospitals are in ideal settings to provide education and to plan and participate in colorectal screening programs. These screening programs could be conducted by community organizations such as the ACS, local service groups, and community religious groups, with the nurse coordinating the efforts.

Another role for the nurse as educator is to promote the following seven dietary recommendations of the ACS and the National Cancer Institutes to lower overall cancer risk including colorectal cancer:

1. Avoid obesity.
2. Decrease total fat intake. It is recommended that fat be only 30% of total calories. The year 2000 cancer control objective is to reduce average consumption of fat from 40% to 25% or less of total calories. There are many simple methods to reduce dietary fat in the diet. For example, (1) use low-fat cottage cheese instead of sour cream for dips; (2) use baked potatoes instead of french fries; (3) use nonstick pans or a cooking spray for grilling sandwiches instead of grilling them in oil; and (4) select bagels or whole wheat bread for breakfast instead of doughnuts, rolls, or croissants.
3. Consume more high-fiber foods, such as whole grain cereals, fruits, and vegetables. The year 2000 cancer control objective is to increase the average consumption of fiber from 8–12 g/day to 20–30 g/day.
4. Include foods rich in vitamins A and C in the daily diet. Foods rich in carotene, a form of vitamin A, are carrots, tomatoes, spinach, apricots, peaches, and cantaloupes. In general, dark green and deep yellow vegetables are rich in vitamin A.
5. Be moderate in the consumption of alcoholic beverages.
6. Be moderate in the consumption of salt-cured, smoked, and nitrite-cured foods.

7. Include cruciferous vegetables in the diet, such as cabbage, broccoli, brussels sprouts, kohlrabi, and cauliflower.[68–70]

Research supports the assumption that Americans will change their diet in an effort to be healthier. A survey in Illinois, conducted in 1982 and in 1986, found that 42% of the 46,830 subjects reported a major change in their diet since the first survey. Subjects reported eating less meat and pork and more fish and chicken, and there was a shift toward whole grains from refined grains and an increase in the number of times per week that subjects ate cruciferous vegetables.[71]

In the role of researcher, it is extremely important that a nurse be knowledgeable about emerging information on the relationship between diet and colorectal cancer. Future research may establish definitive relationships, as well as additional relationships not presently known. Nurses also should be able to evaluate research findings. Those reports that are based on sound, ethical research principles may be judged appropriate for inclusion in patient education. Because of debate about the use of guaiac tests vs. immunological fecal occult blood tests in screening programs in terms of lowering mortality from colorectal cancer, nurses need to remain alert to new research that either supports or refutes the use of one type of test over the other. Nurses also can plan or participate in the wide range of research projects related to colorectal cancer such as health behaviors, dietary habits, motives that facilitate early detection and dietary changes, and effective educational approaches for changing dietary patterns. Results certainly would benefit existing nursing practice as it relates to the prevention and early detection of colorectal cancer.

As practitioners, nurses are urged to use their physical assessment skills when they deal with individuals who have gastrointestinal complaints. Geriatric patients often share their symptoms first with a sympathetic nurse. Thus, the nurse is in the ideal position to detect colorectal cancer in its initial stages. Physical assessment of the abdomen may reveal subtle clues of a pathologic condition that merits referral, one that otherwise might be overlooked by an elderly patient. Hospital-based nurses are cautioned not to assume that elderly patients must have had a thorough physical examination because they are in the hospital. If the primary complaints are not related to the gastrointestinal system, that system may not have been thoroughly assessed.

Prostate Cancer

Prostate cancer is currently the second most common cancer in American men. In men older than 75 years of age, it is estimated that the prevalence of prostate cancer is 500/100,000. The ACS estimates that in 1999 there will be 179,300 new cases of prostate cancer and 37,000 deaths caused by this cancer.[15] A large percentage of men have advanced disease at the time of diagnosis; approximately 35% have metastases to the bones or lymph nodes, and another 40% have extracapsular invasion.[15] Black men have the highest incidence of prostate cancer in the world. Between 1937 and 1985 the incidence of prostate cancer increased 53.5% among white men and more than 100% in black men.[72] Prostate cancer increases in incidence with age more rapidly than any other cancer.

History assessment

There are no real symptoms of early, probably curable, disease. Most symptoms are related to late complications of stage III or IV prostate cancer. Because many of the initial symptoms may be related to carcinomatous obstruction of the prostatic urethra, the inquiries made during the history should be about nonspecific urinary symptoms. The following questions are recommended:

1. Do you have to wait for your stream to begin?
2. Does your stream stop while you still have the urge to void?
3. Do you have to strain to urinate?
4. Does your stream seem weak to you?
5. Do you have the urge to urinate but find you can't?
6. Have you noticed blood in your urine? Has your urine changed in color or smell at all?
7. Does the blood seem to come at the beginning or end of your stream?
8. Do you dribble after urinating?
9. Do you find you have to urinate more than you used to?
10. Do you have pain on urination?
11. Do you ever wet your pants?
12. How often do you urinate during the day? Do you get up at night to urinate? How often?
13. When was your last rectal examination? Why was this done? What was found?

Symptoms that suggest prostatic cancer are urinary difficulty manifested by a decrease in urinary stream and a frequency and urgency to urinate, often associated with pain. These symptoms also are found with prostatic enlargement (benign prostatic hypertrophy) that is common in older men. The most frequent initial symptoms of prostate cancer are frequency of urination, difficult or painful urination, pain, complete urinary retention, and hematuria.

Physical examination

An early diagnosis of prostate cancer can be done only by digital rectal palpation of the prostate (Figure 9-6). It is recommended that the examiner flex the distal finger joint 2–3 mm into the gland substance rather than keep the finger straight (Figure 9-7). Having the patient perform the Valsalva maneuver during the rectal examination will bring the prostate gland closer to the examining finger. Early prostatic carcinoma is a nodule *within*, not *on*, the gland. Simply rubbing the gland is not effective for early detection of prostate cancer.[73]

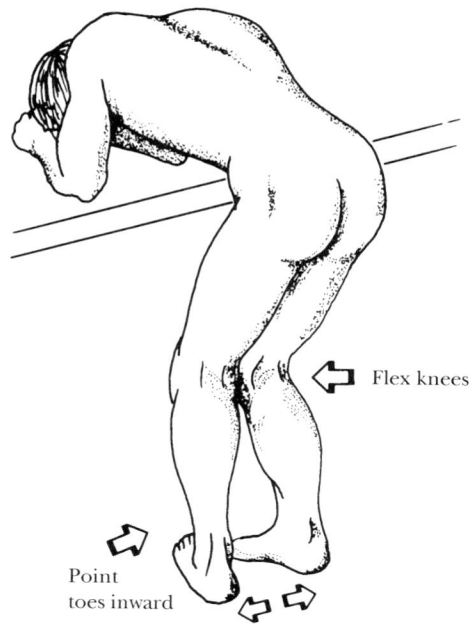

Flex knees

Point
toes inward

For better exposure of the anus, instruct the patient to
point his toes inward and flex his knees to help you to
better assess the seminal vesicles.

Figure 9-6 Recommended position for digital rectal
examination

The normal prostate on palpation is usually a rounded
structure about 4 cm in diameter, feels firm rather than
boggy, soft, or rock hard, and usually is not tender. Some
examiners describe the consistency of the normal prostate as that of a pencil eraser. Cancer of the prostate
typically appears as a stony-hard nodule, whereas benign
prostatic hypertrophy usually results in a diffuse enlargement of the prostate without masses.

It is common to find in older men a diffusely enlarged
prostate gland without masses (benign prostatic hypertrophy). Carcinoma of the prostate is manifested by a palpable hard nodule near the posterior surface of the prostate. As the carcinoma grows, the entire gland may become stony hard, or there may be several hard nodules.[27]

Screening tests for asymptomatic individuals

There is national and international debate over the
issue of screening asymptomatic men for prostate cancer.[74–79] The debate involves multiple factors including
the low percentage of localized cancers diagnosed by
conventional methods, lack of evidence that early treatment reduces the probability of dying of prostate cancer,
and the development of serum prostate-specific antigen
(PSA) assay, which improves the early detection of prostate cancer. Because of these factors, the Canadian Task
Force on the Periodic Health Examination concluded

that there is insufficient evidence to promote screening
for prostate cancer among asymptomatic men.[76] The U.S.
Preventive Services Task Force also does not recommend
screening for prostate cancer among asymptomatic
men.[75] In contrast, the ACS and the American Urological
Association recommend that men older than 50 years be
tested annually using digital rectal examination and PSA.
The ACS recommends that men be screened who have
at least a 10-year life expectancy. Another change in the
new ACS guidelines for prostate cancer screening is the
recognition that some groups of men may be at higher
risk of developing prostate cancer, including those that
have a strong familial predisposition to the disease and
black men. The major argument against screening for
prostate cancer revolves around the absence of any randomized clinical trials documenting that screening reduces mortality or increases life expectancy. Two such
studies, the Prostate Cancer Intervention Versus Observation Trial (PIVOT) and the National Cancer Institute
Prostate, Lung, Colon, Ovarian Cancer (PLCO) screening project, have been launched in the United States
and should answer many questions and doubts about
screening for prostate cancer.[80] Unfortunately, it will take
about 10 to 15 years before these trials are completed.
Until mortality and morbidity benefits are known, it is
recommended that screening be limited to men with life
expectancies greater than 10 years.

While morbidity and mortality issues affect the practicality of screening for prostate cancer, cost considerations
are also a significant barrier to the use of PSA and
transrectal ultrasound in screening for this cancer. Handley and Stuart investigated the routine use of PSA as a
screening test in a managed care organization.[81] They
concluded that use of PSA to screen for prostate cancer
did not meet the criteria for an effective screening program and if PSA screening had continued, there would
have been $4,800,000 in increased costs (400,000 pa-
tients). While there has been enthusiasm for the use
of PSA screening and aggressive treatment of localized
disease, there is no evidence that PSA can distinguish
between indolent and aggressive cancer, that aggressive
treatment of localized cancer decreases disease-specific
mortality, or that PSA screening decreases disease-specific
mortality for a population.

Krahn et al used a cost-utility analysis to compare
three screening strategies (PSA, digital rectal examination [DRE], transrectal ultrasound [TRUS]) with a strategy of not screening.[82] Transrectal ultrasound consists of
a probe that is inserted into the rectum and ultrasound
images of the prostate are recorded on film. It is considered by most men to be less uncomfortable than a digital
examination. Two questions guided their research: (1)
given the available evidence, what is the net clinical benefit of screening for prostate cancer, and (2) what is the
economic burden of screening for this cancer? Their
analysis did not support using PSA, TRUS, or DRE to
screen asymptomatic men for prostate cancer. Furthermore, they do not advocate selecting high-prevalence
populations because to do so would not improve the

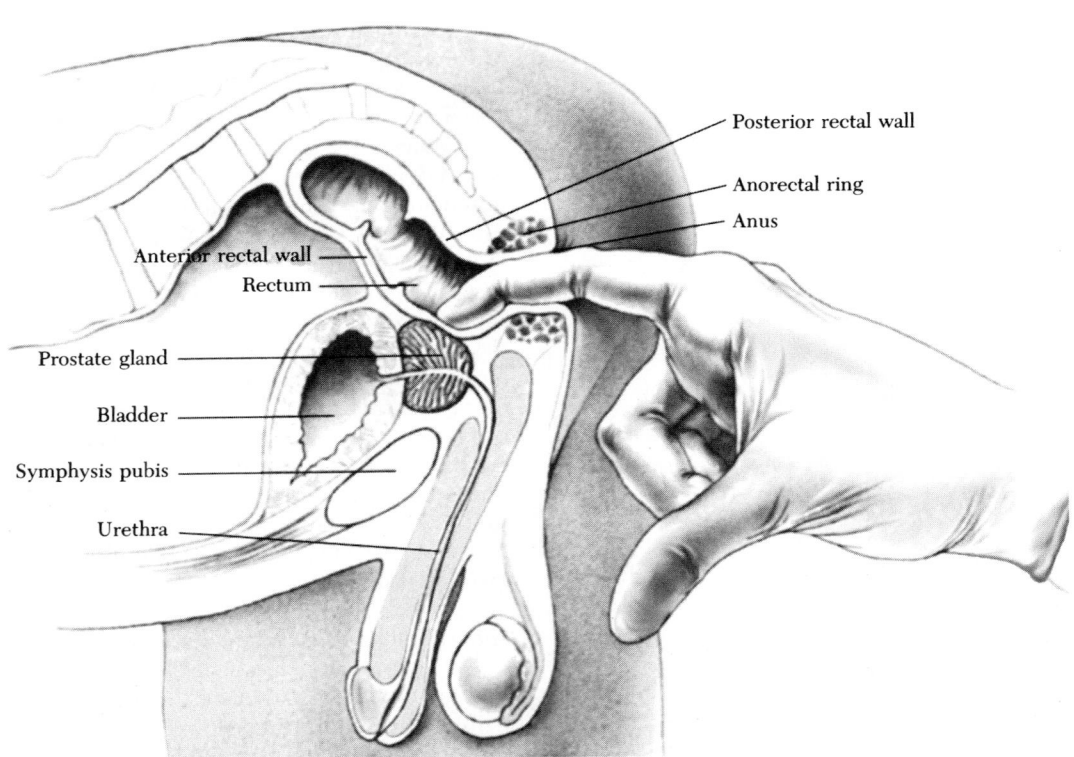

Labels in figure: Posterior rectal wall, Anorectal ring, Anus, Anterior rectal wall, Rectum, Prostate gland, Bladder, Symphysis pubis, Urethra

Figure 9-7 Technique for palpation of the prostate gland (Grimes J, Burns E [eds]: *Health Assessment in Nursing Practice* [ed 2]. Sudbury, MA, Jones and Bartlett, 1987)

benefit of screening. The recommendation not to screen for prostate cancer centered on cost considerations and poor health outcomes of treatment.

Prostate-specific antigen is a tumor marker that the Food and Drug Administration approved in 1994 for use with digital rectal examination for early detection of prostate cancer. As discussed earlier, the use of this tumor marker has resulted in unnecessary biopsies (low specificity) due to the test's lack of discrimination between prostate cancer and benign conditions that elevate PSA. However, two developments have dramatically improved the specificity of the test. In a refinement of the test for serum PSA values, the relative percentage of free PSA and PSA that binds to serum proteins (bound PSA) is determined. Men with a higher ratio of bound to free PSA are more likely to have prostate cancer seen on examination of biopsy specimens regardless of total serum PSA level.[83] The other refinement is the development of age-specific reference ranges. The ultimate value of this approach is that it decreases the number of biopsies in older patients with PSA values greater than 4 ng/mL and that it may increase the rate of cancer detection in younger men with PSA values less than 4 ng/mL.[83] It is suggested that normal ranges of PSA for men aged 50–59 is 0.0–3.5, for 60–69 years of age is 0.0–4.5, and for men aged 70–79 is 0.0–6.5 ng/mL. These two refinements of PSA address the recommendation of the ACS-National Prostate Cancer Detection Project that

"more specific PSA assay needs to be highly encouraged" to lower net detection costs.[84]

What has added further to the debate over the screening of prostate cancer is the study of U.S. male physicians who participated in the Physicians' Health Study, which started in 1982.[85] Before the physicians were randomized in the double-blind trial, they sent blood samples (n = 14,916). Gann et al examined and conducted PSA analysis on a smaller sample of the blood samples. The researchers found that a single PSA level would have detected nearly 80% of all aggressive cancers diagnosed within 5 years and about 5% of aggressive cancers as much as 9 or 10 years later. Specificity of the single PSA measurement was also high—only 96 of 1098 men who remained free of a prostate cancer diagnosis through 10 years had a false-positive test result. The final recommendation of this study echoed that of the ACS-National Prostate Cancer Detection Project. These results support the conclusion that PSA has the highest validity of any circulating cancer screening marker discovered thus far. Intensive efforts to identify cost-effective screening strategies incorporating PSA testing is warranted.

One of the most important roles the nurse can assume in the detection of early prostate cancer is that of educator. All men older than 40 years of age, especially black men, should be informed of the importance and rationale for yearly or biannual rectal examinations. Men with strong family histories of prostate cancer should be urged to *request* and *expect* rectal examinations and a PSA blood test at their annual physical. Men need to be encouraged to discuss the risk-benefits of early detection of prostate cancer with their primary health care provider. In some managed care settings, the man may be asked to pay for the PSA blood test if the health care plan does not follow ACS recommendations.

In some communities it may be necessary for the nurse to conduct the physical examination that includes the rectal examination for prostate as well as colorectal cancer. Female nurses who conduct physical examinations but omit the rectal assessment because of their embarrassment or the patient's discomfort must request a male physician or nurse practitioner to complete this portion of the examination rather than omitting it. In other settings it may be possible to develop a once-a-year volunteer transportation program that will enable infirm or geographically isolated elderly men to have the recommended yearly examination. The development of a prostate screening program for each isolated, poor, or infirm elderly man is a problem all nurses should attempt to solve. At the very least, the nurse should question all hospitalized elderly men about their last rectal examination and contact the physician about those men who have not had one within the last year (or who have "deferred" written on their chart next to "rectal examination").

Breast Cancer

Breast cancer is the most common cancer in women in the Western world.[86] It is the leading cause of cancer deaths in American women aged 40–55 and the second cause of cancer deaths in women older than 55 years of age.[15] It was estimated that in 1999, 176,300 women will be diagnosed with invasive breast cancer and 43,700 will die of the disease.[15] The probability that breast cancer will develop in a woman's lifetime is 12.6% or one in eight.[87] At age 20, women have only a one in 2500 chance of having the disease. By the age of 50, the rate jumps to one in 41.[88]

History assessment

Questions that may be asked during the history include the following:

1. Do you practice breast self-examination (BSE)?
   a. *"Yes" response:* How often do you do BSE? Where did you learn to do this? Do you feel comfortable doing BSE, or would you like me to go over it with you?
   b. *"No" response:* Have you ever been shown BSE? Would you be interested in learning BSE? Some women don't examine their breasts because they feel unsure, embarrassed, or frightened about doing it. Do you feel this way about BSE?
2. Have you ever been advised to have a mammogram? If you have had a mammogram, what were the results?
3. Do you experience sore breasts?
4. Have you ever been told you had "lumpy" or "cystic breasts"?
5. Have you noticed any color or temperature change on your breasts? Do you have trouble with scaly, itching nipples?
6. Have you ever had breast infections?
7. Have you ever had breast surgery or cosmetic surgery on your breasts? Tell me about the surgery that was done.
8. Do you have any sores or open wounds on your breasts?
9. Have you noticed any "dimpling" of your breasts?
10. Have you noticed any change in your nipples or discharge?
11. Have you ever been told that you had cancer of the breast?
12. Do you have or have you discovered any breast lumps?
13. Is there anyone in your family—grandparents, siblings, cousins, parents, aunts, and uncles—who have or had cancer? Breast cancer? Can you remember how old your _____ was when she first was diagnosed as having breast cancer?
14. At what age (or grade in school) did you start menstruating? At what age did you stop menstruating?

The *most common* presenting complaint of women with breast cancer is a painless lump or mass in the breast. It is estimated that 90% of all palpable breast tumors are discovered by women themselves either accidentally or through planned self-examination.[89]

Physical examination

Inspection. The physical examination begins with inspection of the breast with the woman sitting relaxed with arms at side, then sitting with arms at side pressed against body, hands on waist pressed against body, and then sitting with arms overhead (Figure 9-8).[90] Visible signs of cancer of the breast include the following:

- *Dimpling of the breast* results from a shortening of Cooper ligaments as the tumor spreads in the breast.

- *Unilateral flattening of the nipple* is caused by fibrosis and contraction of this fibrotic tissue, thus producing retraction signs, including flattening or deviation of the nipple.[27]

- *Abnormal contours or flattening* becomes apparent as the woman changes positions. It is important to compare one breast with the other. An excellent position for observing this is when the woman leans forward.

- *Peau d'orange,* orange peel skin, is caused by interference with the lymphatic drainage of the skin.

- *Increased venous prominence* usually is unilateral. Carcinomas demand an increased blood flow; thus the dilated venous channels will be obvious on inspection.

- *Scaling or eczematoid lesions* of the nipple indicate Paget's disease, a slow-growing intraductal carcinoma.

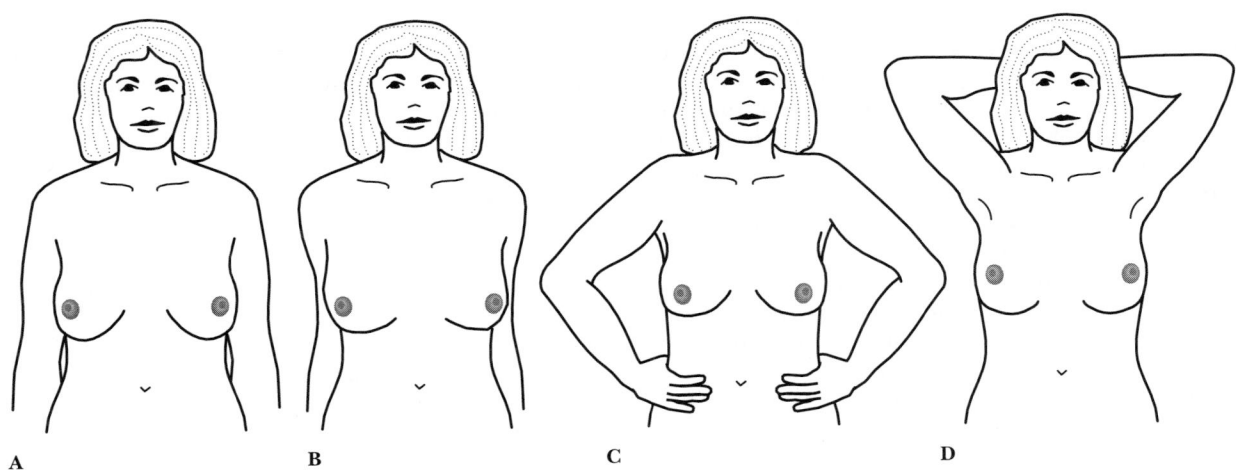

Figure 9-8   Positions for inspection of the breast. **A.** Arms at side with woman relaxed. **B.** Arms at side pressed against body. **C.** Hands on waist pressed against body. **D.** Arms over head.

It is essential that good lighting (e.g., use of a goose-neck lamp) be used for examination of the woman so that subtle contours will be detected by the examiner. The initial inspection *must* include all positions shown in Figure 9-8 and having the woman lean forward to observe abnormal contours; omitting a position may cause the nurse to miss important pathologic findings.

Palpation.   After inspection, the entire breast should be lightly palpated for thickening. This is accomplished by using the pads of your fingers. Palpation for thickening is done lightly and slowly toward the nipple enabling the nurse to detect subtle differences in consistency in the breasts. It should be viewed as a "scouting expedition" before palpation for masses is begun. If the woman complains of a lump, she should find it for the examiner. It is best to first palpate the normal breast. Cancer occurs as a hard, poorly circumscribed nodule, fixed to the skin or underlying tissue.

If cancer is suspected, the breast should be gently moved or compressed and observed for dimpling. A malignant tumor that may be attached to the deep fascia will limit the mobility of the breast on the chest wall. The examiner checks for such a lump by having the patient place her hands on her hip; then the examiner moves the breast medially and laterally with the muscles relaxed and then with the muscles under tension by forced adduction.

The breasts need to be thoroughly palpated while the woman is supine with her arms above her head. Powder on the breasts may be useful to establish a frictionless surface. Palpation should be done with the flat part of the tips of three fingers. Using a spiral motion, rotate the fingers in small circles. It is recommended that the nurse start at the areolar margin and examine the breast by palpation in ever-widening concentric circles. Any mass

that is felt should be charted as to its location, size, shape, consistency, discreteness, mobility, tenderness, erythema, and dimpling over the mass. Location of a nodule should be charted in terms of the quadrant, that is, right upper, left outer, and so forth. Special attention should be paid to the breast tissue along the inframammary crease. In its early stage cancer in this area may be hidden under the overlying breast tissue, and the normal induration of the inframammary crease can be confusing.[91] A device called a *Sensorpad* may be used to conduct physical palpation of the breasts. The Sensorpad consists of two thin round sheets of plastic that have liquid silicone sealed between them, allowing the two sheets of plastic to slide easily over each other. The Sensorpad increases the ability to detect breast lesions because it reduces friction between the woman's fingers and her breast during BSE. The device, made by Inventive Products, Inc. (Decatur, IL), has received FDA clearance for marketing.

Heymann recommends that physical examination of a woman's breasts include right and left semilateral decubitus positions[92] (Figure 9-9). The rationale for this is as follows: Lesions deep within the medial aspects, upper outer quadrants, or axillary tail, especially in large breasts, may be hidden within dense parenchyma or a thick layer of fat or may sink between ribs onto intercostal muscles when they are examined in the usual erect and supine positions (Figure 9-9A). By means of the right and left semilateral decubitus positions with both of the patient's arms elevated (Figure 9-9B), both breasts will fall dependently, thereby thinning the lateral aspects, upper outer quadrant, and axillary tail of the upper portion of the breasts and the medial aspect of the lower portion of the breast[93] (Figure 9-9C).

Next, the examiner needs to check for nipple discharge. Because the ducts are like spokes of a wheel, a discharge from the ten o'clock position indicates trouble

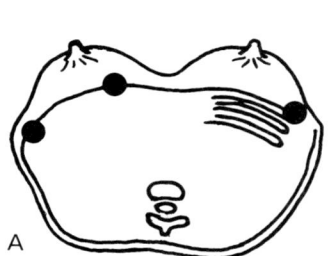 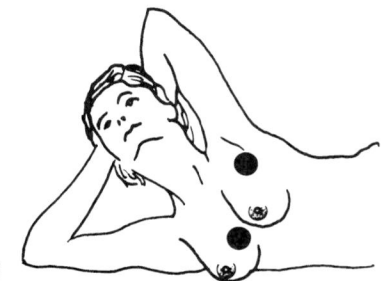 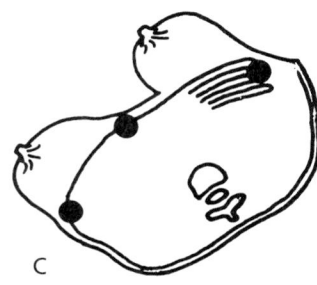

Figure 9-9 Semilateral decubitus breast examination. **A.** Small masses obscured by breast parenchyma or ribs when breast is examined in upright or supine position. **B.** Semilateral decubitus position. **C.** Thinning of parenchyma with clarification of obscured masses when patient is in semilateral decubitus position. (Adapted from Heymann A: Semilateral decubitus breast examination. *JAMA* 243:1713, 1980)[92]

in the upper inner quadrant, and so forth. The nipple should be gently compressed in *all* directions for the presence of discharge. Smears should be taken for cytologic examination of any suspicious discharge.

Because carcinoma of the breast may metastasize to regional lymph nodes, a careful palpation of the axillae and the supraclavicular regions is necessary. Most clinicians believe that the axilla is best palpated with the patient sitting erect and at a higher level than the examiner. Hard, fixed nodes palpated in the axillae or the supraclavicular region raise the suspicion of cancer. Normally, lymph nodes are felt as soft, movable structures.

When the clinician examines the breasts of an older woman, it should be kept in mind that the physiologic changes that normally occur with aging may simulate cancer of the breast. As a woman ages, there is atrophy of glandular elements that accentuates anatomic landmarks and reduces the amount of palpable tissue. Shrinkage and fibrotic changes of the breast may cause retraction of the nipple, and the terminal ducts are more visible. Both these changes may cause the examiner to suspect cancer. Because of the high incidence of breast cancer in elderly women, it is best to refer all suspicious findings rather than assume they are due to aging.

In conclusion, the physical signs that most strongly suggest cancer of the breast are dimpling; peau d'orange; abnormal contours of the breast; flattening of the nipple; palpable hard, poorly circumscribed nodules that are fixed to the skin or underlying tissue; and palpable hard, fixed nodes in the axillae or supraclavicular region.

Screening tests for asymptomatic individuals

Three methods used in screening for breast cancer are physical examination of the breast by the health professional, teaching the woman BSE, and mammography.

The ACS's revised recommendations for screening for breast cancer are as follows:

1. All women from age 20 years should perform BSE monthly.

2. Women 20–39 years of age should have a breast physical examination every 3 years, and women older than 40 years should have a breast physical examination by a health professional every year

3. Screening mammography should begin by age 40 and be done every year.[93,94]

Mammography allows visualization of the internal structure of the breast; it has a sensitivity that is higher than that of the clinical breast examination or the BSE.[87] Despite improvements in the ability to detect breast cancer through mammography, mammography screening may miss 10%–15% of breast cancers due to increased density of breast tissue in younger women.[95] Therefore, it is essential that a clinical examination be performed by a trained health care professional in combination with mammography.

However, there is a continuing national debate about the age that women should start having screening mammograms and conflicting national recommendations on this issue. One of the issues is the number of false-positive screening mammograms that result when screening large numbers of women. Elmore et al report that over a 10-year period of time, one-third of the women screened had abnormal test results requiring additional evaluation, even though no breast cancer was present.[96] It would appear that periodic screening invites repeated exposure to the possibility of a false-positive result, as occurs in fecal occult-blood testing for colorectal cancer.[97]

The debate about the age women should start to be screened centers on the results from clinical trials that show that women 50–74 years of age benefit from participating in screening. Specifically, mammography reduces the risk of dying of breast cancer by 26%.[98] In contrast, the benefit of breast cancer screening remains unclear in women 40–49 years of age. Eight randomized controlled trials reported no statistically significant reduction in breast cancer mortality among women age 40–49 years after 7–9 years from the initiation of screening. After 10–12 years from the initiation of screening, there is a trend toward a reduction in breast cancer mortality that appears to be smaller than that observed in women age 50 and older.[99] Because of the lack of evidence documenting the benefits of screening for women 40–48 years, many national organizations do not recommend mammography for this age group. Organizations not recommending screening for this age group include: American College of Physicians, U.S. Preventive Services Task Force, National Cancer Institute, Canadian Task Force on the Periodic Health Exam, and American Academy of Family Practice. Those organizations recommending screening for women 40–49 years of age are: American College of Obstetrics and Gynecology, American College of Radiology, and American Medical Association.[99] There is evidence that screening younger women will detect ductal carcinoma in situ, which occurs more often in the 40–49 year age group and improves survival.[100] Because of the conflicting evidence, the National Institutes of Health Consensus Development Conference concluded that the data did not warrant a universal recommendation for mammography for all women in their forties.[97]

Breast self-examination. The importance of BSE is based on the fact that approximately 95% of breast cancers are self-discovered either accidentally or through planned examination. Because approximately 10% of cancers termed *interim cancers* will become apparent within a year of an examination with negative results, reliance has been placed on BSE to find these lesions. There has been considerable debate about the value of BSE in reducing mortality and increasing survival rates.[101–103] The problem to date is that the efficacy of BSE in reducing the rate of death from this disease is still uncertain. Because BSE results in both false-positive and false-negative results, the practice does carry costs and risks. If BSE leads to earlier detection without affecting rates of death due to breast cancer, it results only in an extension of the time a woman is aware of the disease. Definitive studies of the efficacy of BSE are still lacking. Over the last 20 years, descriptive, case-control, and cohort studies have yielded contradictory results, but randomized controlled trials now under way in China and Russia should assist in answering whether or not BSE reduces mortality from breast cancer.[104,105] Preliminary results from the first 5 years of the studies in China showed neither lower death rates nor a shift toward the diagnosis of less advanced disease among the women practicing BSE.[104]

Holmberg et al studied a cohort of 450,000 women and found that self-reported monthly practice of BSE did not reduce the rate of death from breast cancer.[106] However, researchers have found that a thorough and careful technique was associated with the detection of tumors at a less advanced stage.[103,106,107] Using prospectively collected data, Harvey et al[103] conducted a case-control study of BSE involving women in the Canadian National Breast Screening Study to measure the effect of doing BSE on the risk of death due to breast cancer. The researchers found that women who left out one of the components of their BSE technique were almost twice as

likely to die from breast cancer or to have distant metastatic disease compared to women who included all three components. Leaving out two of the three components more than doubled the odds of dying compared to when all three components were included. Those women who do practice BSE do not always adhere to the published recommendations. One study found that adherence to all three position types when doing BSE was obtained in only 40% of the examinations done by the sample of women. In fact, 42% of the BSE examinations included only one position.[108]

Because BSE has not been studied in a prospective, controlled trial with mortality as an outcome, the U.S. Preventive Services Task Force does not make a recommendation about the inclusion or exclusion of teaching BSE during the periodic health examination.[102] The American Society of Clinical Oncology recommends that women practice BSE monthly although they note that there is little or no systematic empirical evidence for this recommendation.[109] In addition, the World Health Organization does not recommend BSE screening programs as public health policy, although there is insufficient evidence to change them where they already exist. The ACS recommends that all women over the age of 20 years examine their breasts once a month.[110]

Although there probably is not sufficient evidence to justify BSE as a large-scale, community-based intervention, many authorities believe it should be encouraged as part of a woman's regular medical care.[111] A study of 2093 women with breast cancer found that self-examiners tended to seek medical care more rapidly and to have earlier stages of disease at diagnosis than nonself-examiners.[112] Five years after diagnosis the cumulative observed survival rates in breast cancer were 76.7% among self-examiners and 60.9% among nonself-examiners ($p < 0.0001$). The researchers acknowledge that the observed survival advantage may be due to characteristics of the self-examiners other than BSE per se; however, they encourage BSE as an adjunctive technique for the early detection of breast cancer.[112]

In any discussion of BSE it must be remembered that the majority of women do not practice monthly BSE. Although nearly all women are aware of this early detection practice, only 15%–40% perform BSE monthly.[113] A recent study conducted in 20 European countries with over 9000 women found that 54% of the women had never practiced BSE, and regular practice (monthly) was done by only 8% of the sample.[114] Researchers in the United States also report low frequency of practice among women with and without a family history of breast cancer.[109] Bennett et al interviewed 616 women and found that women who were more likely to practice BSE on a frequent basis were living with their sexual partner, had a maternal history of breast disease, had been shown how to perform BSE, and were confident in their examination technique.[115] They found no association between monthly BSE practice and formal education. Studies consistently have shown that lack of knowledge and low confidence are related to low rates of practice or no practice at all.

Knowledge of how it should be done and confidence in one's ability are characteristics that differentiate frequent from less frequent practitioners of BSE.[116] A prospective study of adherence to mammography, clinical breast examination, and BSE in a group of women over a 3-year period of time found that women who perform BSE regularly over time were more likely to adhere to the other breast cancer screening guidelines.[117]

Personal instruction results in more frequent BSE than do films, pamphlets, or lectures. It also has been shown that individual contact is successful in bringing both low users of health services and women at high risk for cancer into cancer screening programs.[115] Self-instruction includes teaching a woman to do BSE by using her own hand on her breast under the direct guidance of a professional. Because women can be taught to detect lesions of 1 cm or less in their own breasts, those who practice regular BSE will detect tumors within a size range that will maximize chances for survival and minimize chances for axillary node involvement.[103] When teaching BSE, the nurse should stress the importance of a yearly physical examination by a health professional and mammographic examination at intervals determined by the woman's age.

Because a high percentage of cancerous lesions are potentially palpable, it is important for nurses to include one-on-one instruction in BSE techniques whenever possible. Research documents the effectiveness of registered nurses teaching BSE to women in their place of employment. In the BSE program reported by Styrd, more than 60% of the eligible female employees participated in the program, and 1 year later 80% reported performing BSE some time during the 3 months before being surveyed.[118] In addition, the proportion of employees who indicated they had performed BSE on a monthly basis increased significantly after the program.

Primary nursing, as well as public health and occupational health nursing, afford the nurse excellent opportunities for BSE education. To date, there is some empirical evidence that supports nurses' ability to promote the practice of BSE in the acute care setting. Shamian and Edgar studied the knowledge and the frequency pattern of 223 women taught BSE by nurse clinicians.[119] They concluded that nurses influence positively the factual and proficiency knowledge base and the frequency of BSE practice. To reinforce personal instruction in BSE there could be posters, multimedia events such as videos and films, and educational panels portraying the techniques of BSE. These methods, however, should reinforce, *not* replace, personal instruction.

Testicular Cancer

Although testicular cancer is relatively rare (1% of all cancers), it is the most common solid tumor in young men between 15 and 34 years of age.[120] A lesser peak occurs in early childhood. Testicular cancer, which is uncommon after 40 years of age, affects white men more than black men. It is estimated that in 1999, 7400 men will be diagnosed with this cancer and 300 will die from it.[15]

History assessment

When obtaining the health history, the nurse should inquire about the following:

1. Do you have a history of undescended testicles? Was this surgically corrected? At what age?
2. Is there a history of mumps, orchitis, or testicular cancer in the family?[121] History of inguinal hernia?
3. Did your mother take any type of hormones while she was pregnant with you?
4. Are you aware of any lumps in your scrotum?
5. Were there signs of early puberty as a child?
6. Have you noticed any changes in your genital organs or interest in sex?
7. Are you aware of any scrotal heaviness or heavy discomfort in the scrotum or lower portion of the abdomen and groin?
8. Are you aware of any breast swelling or nipple tenderness?
9. Do you practice testicular self-examination (TSE)? If not, have you ever been shown?
10. Are you aware of any recent trauma to the genital organs?

Although there is no direct proof that trauma causes testicular cancer, many men link swelling or a lump to a recent trauma. The most common presenting complaint is a painless enlargement of the testis, or "heaviness," which is noticed by about two-thirds of men.[122] Nodules in the testes are typically small, hard, and usually painless, and they are slightly more common in the right testis (52.3%) than in the left (47.7%).[123]

The major obstacle to early detection of testicular cancer is the delay that commonly occurs between initial detection of the lesion in the testis to the time of treatment. Approximately 6 months will elapse before treatment is either sought by the patient or begun by the physician.[123] The uninformed young man may ignore the unilateral enlargement for quite some time for the following reasons: (1) the man may hope that the testis will spontaneously revert to normal; (2) he may feel a certain pride in his enlarging sexual organ; (3) he may perceive the tumor as punishment for past sexual sins; (4) he may perceive the lack of pain as an indication that the lump is innocent; and (5) he may fear it is cancer.[124]

In 1978 Conklin et al explored the need for and the interest in a health education program about TSE at the University of Vermont.[125] Although 58% of the 90 students interviewed had taken a health-related course in the previous 2 years, 75% had never heard of testicular cancer. None knew how to examine their testes correctly, and only one knew what to palpate for. In 1986 Blesch[126] surveyed a random sample of 233 professional men about their knowledge and perceptions of testicular cancer and TSE and found the same lack of knowledge about TSE as Conklin et al. Of 129 responses, only 31% of the sample subjects were aware of TSE and only 9.5% practiced TSE. Although more than half the sample (61%) were aware of testicular cancer, four out of nine men with a personal history of undescended testis (a significant risk factor) had not heard of testicular cancer.[126] A similar study conducted in 1994 by Wardle et al in Europe found that in a sample of more than 16,000 men the majority were unaware of the value of TSE, 89% had never practiced TSE, and only 3% practiced TSE monthly.[127] Wardle makes the point that this was a highly educated group and if this "at-risk" group was not carrying out the recommendations, it is unlikely that there are higher levels of compliance in other groups.

Because the effectiveness of TSE in lowering mortality has not been documented, there is debate about recommending this practice for men in screening programs.[124,128] The ACS and the National Cancer Institute recommend annual clinical examinations and monthly TSEs be started during puberty.[123] The U.S. Preventive Services Task Force found that there was insufficient evidence of clinical benefit or harm to recommend for or against routine screening of asymptomatic men for testicular cancer but that clinicians should advise adolescent and young adult males to seek prompt medical attention for testicular symptoms.[129]

Physical examination

The examination begins with inspection of the scrotum. Cancer of the testes may be manifested by asymmetry of the scrotum. In most men the left side of the scrotal sac descends lower than the right because of the greater length of the left spermatic cord.[130] Another clue to the presence of a tumor in the scrotum is scrotal skin that appears stretched and thin over the tumor.

Palpation of the scrotal contents can be done with the man standing or in a recumbent position; however, the examination should be thorough and gentle because the testes are exquisitely tender to physical pressure.[131] The examiner must conduct the palpation as gently as possible to avoid eliciting the cremasteric reflex. Stimulation of the scrotum or inner thigh may elicit this reflex and cause the testes to be retracted into the inguinal canal (migratory testis). Several procedures are recommended for palpating the testes. Some authors advocate that the examiner palpate the scrotal contents with both hands to help differentiate the testicles from the other scrotal structures—epididymis, vas deferens, and spermatic cord. Palpating bimanually also improves the chances of detecting any weight differential between the testicles, an important clue to malignancy.[132] The bimanual procedure of using index and middle fingers to separate testes and scrotum so that the right testis and epididymis can be examined with left hand and vice versa is illustrated in Figure 9-10. DeGowin recommends comparing both testes simultaneously by grasping one with each hand, using the thumb and forefinger.[27] As is true with breast lesions, if the man has symptoms, the uninvolved testis should be examined first to provide a baseline comparison.[133]

A normal testicle has a somewhat rubbery, spongy consistency, and the consistency is uniform throughout, with a surface free of lumps or indurations. Diffuse induration of the testis in the absence of discrete nodularity also may be the initial abnormality.[134] The most common sites for tumors are on the testicular anterior and lateral surfaces.[135] In the young male, the testis is apt to feel firm and smooth, whereas in the elderly male it may be very soft, almost mushy.[129] Even though the testes feel normal, each should be transilluminated. One may be atrophied and the normal size attained by a hydrocele.[27] Transillumination is helpful in distinguishing cystic from solid masses. Transillumination can be accomplished by aiming a small flashlight behind or on the side of the scrotum in a darkened room. It should be remembered that hydroceles may develop as a result of a tumor.[136] Testicular tumors tend to remain ovoid, being limited by the tough tunica albuginea. Spread to the epididymis may occur in 10%–15% of men.[131] Typically, a testicular tumor occurs as a painless scrotal mass that does not transilluminate. The size may range from less than 1 cm to 10 cm in diameter. The examiner needs to be aware that the scrotal skin overlying the tumor is rarely attached, although attachment may exist in lymphomatous involvement of the testis.[130]

Other areas should be checked to ascertain if there has been metastasis; for example, a mass in the epigastrium or an enlarged left supraclavicular node (Virchow node) may be palpable. The examiner also should palpate the abdomen for retroperitoneal lymph node involvement. To feel any metastatic nodes the examiner will have to palpate the abdomen fairly deeply. Metastatic nodes usually lie at the level of, or slightly caudal to, the umbilicus. Ultrasonographic examination is often useful in further defining an abnormality of the testicular parenchyma.[134]

Education: Testicular self-examination

There is a need for nurses to educate themselves, their colleagues, and their patients about testicular cancer and TSE. Unfortunately health care professionals are not teaching young men about the importance of the health practice TSE. Misener and Fuller found that few primary care providers included TSE instruction in contrast to a high percentage who included BSE instruction in the annual physical examination.[137] Only 29% of the primary care physicians taught men about TSE while 86% taught BSE to women. The major deterrent to early detection and treatment is young men's lack of knowledge of the great danger of testicular cancer and the lack of awareness of the need for regular self-examination.[138] Because the prognosis is good when the tumor is treated early, there is a vital need to educate the public about early detection and treatment. The majority of men discover the changes in the testes while bathing or showering, or it is found by their sexual partners. Only 4% of tumors are detected by clinicians doing a work-up for infertility.[139]

Pediatric hospital and office-based nurses, pediatric nurse practitioners, and school nurses must instruct the parents of high-risk boys and adolescents—those who

Figure 9-10 Palpation of the scrotum. Bimanual procedure of using the index and middle fingers to separate the testes and scrotum so that the right testes and epididymis can be examined with the left hand and vice versa. (Grimes J, Burns E [eds]: *Health Assessment in Nursing Practice* [ed 2]. Sudbury, MA, Jones and Bartlett, 1987)

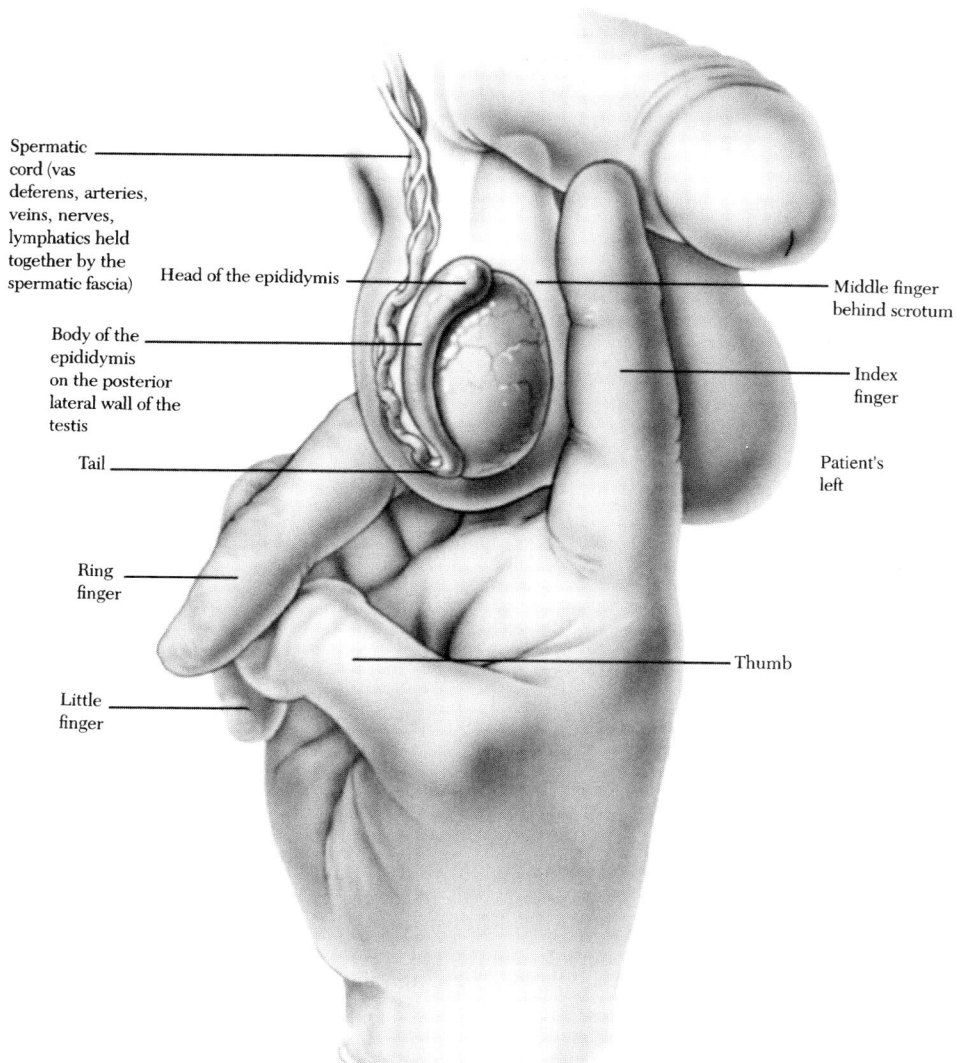

Spermatic cord (vas deferens, arteries, veins, nerves, lymphatics held together by the spermatic fascia)

Head of the epididymis

Body of the epididymis on the posterior lateral wall of the testis

Tail

Ring finger

Little finger

Middle finger behind scrotum

Index finger

Patient's left

Thumb

have or have had undescended testes—how to correctly palpate the scrotum and what physical findings are significant. These same children should be instructed in TSE as they mature. Testicular self-examination techniques should be included in health education classes just as BSE is now routinely included in these classes. Education should emphasize the importance of reporting abnormal findings immediately because delay in reporting testicular lesions is common. Table 9-2 summarizes what should be taught during TSE.

Nurses who work in the military, in occupational health settings, in physicians' offices, in public health departments, in clinics for sexually transmitted diseases, and in educational settings are in ideal clinical settings for teaching TSE and providing education that will dispel the myths that contribute to delay once a testicular lump is found.[138,139] Teaching TSE should be incorporated into routine physical examinations by the examining health professional. A nursing assessment of any male younger

Table 9-2 Testicular Self-Examination (TSE)*

- Stand in front of mirror and look for any swelling on the skin of the scrotum.

- Examine each testicle gently with both hands. The index and middle fingers should be placed underneath the testicle while the thumbs are placed on the top. Roll the testicle gently between the thumbs and fingers. It is normal if one testicle is larger than the other.

- Find the epididymis, which is a cord-like structure on the top and back of the testicle that stores and transports the sperm. Do not mistake the epididymis for an abnormal lump.

- Feel for any abnormal lumps (about the size of a pea) on the front or the side of the testicle. These lumps are usually painless.

- If you do find a lump, you should contact your doctor right away.

*Note: Self-examination of the testicles is best performed when the scrotum is relaxed, after a warm bath or shower. This will also allow the testicles to drop down.

than 40 years of age should include a health history to elicit any subjective symptoms and established risk factors for testicular cancer. A man who complains of vague scrotal symptoms should be referred for a careful genital examination, and those men identified as being at high risk for testicular cancer should be instructed in TSE.

The best defense against testicular cancer is a well-educated male population that practices TSE and understands the importance of seeking medical attention when a "lump" is discovered. Much progress has been made in the last 10 years in discussing and promoting BSE among women. The time has come for nurses to address the issue of testicular cancer in the same forthright, open manner that breast cancer has been discussed so that men will incorporate this health practice into their lives.

Skin Cancer

Cancers of the skin are the most common cancers in humans. In 1999, it is estimated that 44,200 people in the United States will be diagnosed with melanoma and 9200 will die of skin cancer.[15] The incidence rate of melanoma is increasing approximately 4% per year.[140] Today, the lifetime risk of developing invasive melanoma is 1 in 90. However, this is projected to increase to 1 in 75 by the year 2000.[140]

Malignant melanoma accounts for about 74% of all deaths that result from cutaneous cancers.[141] The mortality rate from malignant melanoma is increasing faster than that of any other cancer except lung cancer. Today, the majority of individuals with malignant melanoma are relatively young: the median age at diagnosis is 45 years, and it is the most common cancer in women between the ages of 25 and 35.[142,143] The incidence of malignant melanoma has doubled in the last decade.[142]

History assessment

When obtaining the health history, the nurse should inquire about the following:

1. Have you noticed any changes in any of your moles in terms of color, size, surface characteristics, sensation, areas around the mole, and elevation of the mole?
2. Are you aware of any skin lesions on your body that are new or don't seem to "go away"?
3. Are you aware of the development of any new moles?
4. Have you ever been told you should have a mole removed? Why were you told this?
5. Have you (or any members of your family) ever been told you have dysplastic nevi? Have you (or any members of your family) ever had skin cancer? melanoma? If yes, where was the cancer?
6. Do you feel you have a lot of moles? Where are the majority of these moles?
7. Do you sunbathe? How often? Do you use sunscreen?
8. Do you go to a tanning salon or use a tanning bed? How often?

9. Does your skin generally burn when in the sun or tan?
10. What is your occupation? Have you ever worked in a position in which you were outside for long periods of time? How long did you hold that job?
11. Have you ever worked in occupations in which you were exposed to tar and pitch, oils, paraffins, arsenic, x-rays, or radium?
12. Were you ever burned, or do you have scarring from corrosive or thermal damage?
13. Do you have any outdoor recreational habits or hobbies that you consistently engage in?

When obtaining a health history, the nurse must inquire whether any of the aforementioned changes in moles have occurred. A history of change, often extending over a period of weeks or months, in a preexisting mole or the development of a new mole in an adult is of great importance and requires inspection. The nurse needs to be aware that almost half the melanomas arise in moles or pigmented areas; thus, there should be a high index of suspicion in any mole that is changing or enlarging.[144]

Physical examination

It is essential that the entire integument be inspected during the examination of a patient. Skin assessment includes inspection of the inner lip mucosa, the axillae, the nail beds, the external genitalia, the webs between the toes, the soles of the feet, and the areas in skin folds.[145] This is best accomplished in a setting with good lighting (e.g., a gooseneck lamp) that enables the nurse to project the light obliquely across the body surface. A pen light can be used instead of a gooseneck lamp. A magnifying glass also allows closer inspection of minute details.

All areas that are chronically exposed to the sun should be meticulously assessed, including the neck, ears, shoulders, face, scalp, arms, and hands. Areas that have been chronically exposed to sunlight are common sites for basal cell and squamous cell carcinomas. However, melanomas are found on head, neck, and trunk, which may or may not be exposed to sun, and on the legs in women; occurrence of malignant melanoma is infrequent in rarely exposed or unexposed areas (breasts and bathing suit area of women and bathing trunk area of men).[145] The surface distribution of melanomas in blacks differs from that in whites; the relatively depigmented palms, soles, nail beds, and mucous membranes are primary sites in almost all black patients.[146]

It is recommended that the entire posterior and anterior aspect of the body be viewed and the location of moles be mapped to serve as baseline data for future skin assessments. If a skin lesion is detected, the nurse has three responsibilities: accurate documentation (size, location, description of the lesion), referral of the patient to a physician for diagnosis, and follow-up for recurrent disease.[145]

There are three types of skin cancer: basal cell carcinoma, squamous cell carcinoma, and melanoma. The nurse should be aware of the following precancerous skin lesions: leukoplakia (found in the oral mucosa), senile and actinic keratoses, and dysplastic nevi. Table 9-3[141,145,146] lists the incidence, clinical characteristics, and common sites of actinic keratoses and basal cell and squamous cell skin cancer.

Education

Of all the known risk factors, ultraviolet radiation from the sun is the leading cause of skin cancer. Exposure to solar radiation is increasing worldwide because the protective ozone layer is thinning.[142] It was previously advocated by all leading medical organizations that sunscreens would protect the individual from the most carcinogenic of the ultraviolet wavelengths and thus provide protection from skin cancer.[142,143,147] Sunscreens are rated according to *sun protection factor* (SPF), on a scale currently ranging from 2 to 35. An SPF of 2 in a sunscreen means that proper application allows users to stay in the sun twice as long as they could without any protection at all. Sunbathing should be avoided during the 2-hour period around noon, because two-thirds of the day's ultraviolet light comes through during that time. Skin types are similarly rated from 1 to 6 according to intensity of sunburn in the first 30–45 minutes of unprotected exposure to the sun after a period of no exposure. Skin type 1 burns easily and never tans, whereas skin types 5 and 6 rarely burn and tan well.

Several national organizations, American College of Preventive Medicine and the American Academy of Der-matology, are questioning the use of sunscreens for protection against skin cancer. The American College of Preventive Medicine states that animal studies have been unable to show that sunscreen protects against malignant melanoma, and case-control and clinical trials have shown no reduction or an increase in malignant melanoma incidence with broad-spectrum sunscreen use.[142] The argument is that recommending sunscreen gives people a false sense of security, causing them to increase hours of sun exposure. In contrast, the ACS recommends that until further evidence exists to the contrary and is supported by unbiased scientific data, sunscreens continue to be part of a program for the prevention of cutaneous melanoma in a high-risk population.[143]

The following information about decreasing or eliminating skin cancer risks should be discussed with each patient:

- Ultraviolet rays can penetrate thin clothing like cotton T-shirts; those who desire protective clothing should select hats, long-sleeved shirts, and beach robes rather than rely on T-shirts.

- Individuals with skin types 1 and 2 should avoid sunbathing.

- People who live or vacation in areas of higher altitudes need to be aware that there is less atmosphere to filter out ultraviolet rays so that the sun's effects are more intense.

- Individuals need to be informed that the sun's rays are reflected off snow, sand, and water and that signifi-

Table 9-3   Incidence, Clinical Characteristics, and Common Sites of Premalignant Skin Cancers and Skin Cancer

Skin Carcinoma	Incidence	Clinical Characteristics	Common Sites
Actinic keratoses (senile keratoses, solar keratoses)	Most common premalignant keratoses; develop in persons with fair complexions as result of excessive exposure to light; located on sun-exposed areas	Appear as circumscribed dry patches with adherent scales on slightly red, inflamed skin	Most commonly found on the face and the backs of hands; 20% of cases lead to squamous cell carcinoma
Basal cell carcinoma	Most common form of skin cancer; occurs primarily in persons exposed to intense sunlight, especially fair-complexioned white persons with light eyes and hair	*Nodular basal cell carcinoma:* Elevated papule to lesions with an ulcerated center, raised margin, and waxy or "pearly" border; firm *Superficial basal cell carcinoma:* Plaque, usually with a crusted and erythematous center, flat, and defined margins	Commonly found on the nose, eyelids, cheeks, and neck Commonly found on trunk and extremities
Squamous cell carcinoma	Less common than basal cell carcinoma; occurs primarily on areas exposed to actinic or ultraviolet (UV) radiation	Appearance varies from an elevated nodular mass to a punched-out ulcerated lesion or a large fungating mass. Unlike basal cell carcinoma, squamous cell tumors are opaque and aggressive	Commonly found on head and hands

Data from Friedman et al[141]; Daniel et al[145]; Edwards et al.[146]

cant sun exposure can result from activities on these surfaces.

- As the ozone layer of the earth changes, people need to be aware that this significantly alters the amount of ultraviolet radiation that reaches the earth.

Routine self-examination of the skin is the best defense against skin cancer, especially malignant melanoma. It is inexpensive, noninvasive, and totally free of danger. Periodic self-examination for melanoma and examination by others may result in improved survival.[145] It is recommended that individuals older than 30 years of age who have fair skin and are subject to heavy sun exposures be taught skin self-assessment. Those with dysplastic nevus syndrome (DNS) or a history of melanoma in a first-degree relative also should have regular medical examinations that include measurement and charting of location of unusual pigmented lesions.[141] It also is recommended that patients be given copies of blank body charts so that they can chart lesions found during self-skin assessment. Figure 9-11 illustrates the correct procedure for self-assessment of skin.

Along with self-assessment of the skin, patients should be instructed about the changes in moles that merit immediate medical attention: size, color, elevation, surface characteristics, and sensation. Melanoma is more likely to develop in individuals and families with a history of dysplastic nevus syndrome than it is in most people.[148] The initial diagnosis is based on a physical examination and confirmed by the removal and biopsy of several moles. Individuals with familial DNS should visit their clinician or dermatologist twice a year for assessment and follow-up. They also should conduct self-assessments of the skin on a monthly basis. Assistance usually is necessary because many of the nevi are present in areas such as the scalp or back that are difficult for the individual to inspect.

The elderly constitute the highest-risk group for skin cancer because of the number of years of exposure to the sun. It is estimated that 40%–50% of all those who live to be 65 years of age will have at least one skin cancer during their lifetime.[149] Changes normally occur in the skin with age, which increase the risk of skin cancer. Keratoses, lentigines, and pigmented alterations develop with aging and in areas of chronic solar exposure. Elderly persons should be taught skin self-assessment and the importance of having a health professional examine any new lesions or changing lesions. Any setting where older adults congregate offers the nurse an excellent opportunity to provide an educational program on skin self-examination and early detection for skin cancer. Any areas that have been chronically exposed to the sun should be meticulously screened.

Oral Cancer

It is estimated that in 1999 there will be 29,800 new cases of oral cancer in the United States. The majority of these cancers (11,300) will be cancers of the mouth. There will be 8100 deaths from oral cancer.[15] These figures indicate that oral cancer incidence is not declining nationally and that we have not made significant headway in treatment during the last decade.[150] Approximately 95% of all oral malignancies begin in the surface mucosa. Although the surface of the oral mucosa is easily inspected and palpated, by the time of diagnosis more than 60% of oral cancers have spread to the lymph nodes. Oral and oropharyngeal carcinoma is predominately a disease of men aged 50 to 70 years and women aged 60 to 80 years.[150]

History assessment

When the nurse obtains the health history, it is important to ask the following questions:

1. Do you smoke? How much do you smoke, and how many years have you smoked (pack-years)?
2. Do you chew tobacco or dip snuff? How long have you done this? How much tobacco do you use in a day? Can you describe where you place the tobacco in your mouth?
3. Do you smoke a pipe? How long have you smoked a pipe? Do you smoke cigars?
4. Do you drink alcohol? Approximately how much alcohol do you drink in a day? What type of alcohol do you consume?
5. For the patient from Southeast Asia or Central Asia: Do you chew *betel quid*? Do you use betel quid with any form of tobacco (chewing or smoking)?[151]
6. Do you wear dentures? Do you have any sore spots in your mouth from your dentures? Do you inspect under your dentures at least weekly?
7. When was your last dental examination?
8. How often do you brush your teeth? floss your teeth?
9. Have you ever been in an occupation in which you spent a lot of time outside? Do you have any hobbies or sports interests that involve spending a great deal of time outdoors? Do you wear lip balm when outdoors to protect your lips?
10. Have you noticed any white or red sores in your mouth for longer than a month? any lumps, swelling, or rough spots?
11. Have you been aware of any limitation of tongue or jaw movement?
12. Have you noticed taste changes, dry mouth, speech changes, hoarseness, or chronic cough?
13. Are you aware of any sores or crusts on your lips?
14. Are you aware of any lumps or growing "bumps" in your neck or face?
15. Do you have problems with persistent halitosis that does not seem to respond to any home remedies?

Physical examination

The majority of oral cancers cause no symptoms in their early stages. Most individuals who notice a white or bright red spot, "sore," or a swelling in their mouth

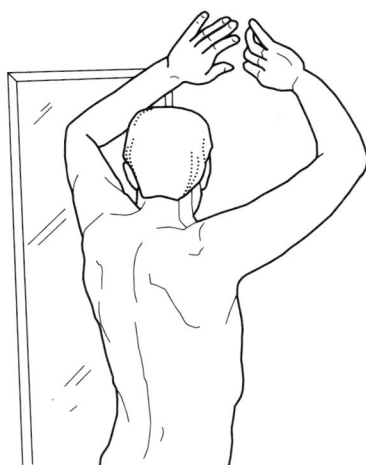

A. Examine the front and back of your body in the mirror. Raise your arms and look at right and left sides.

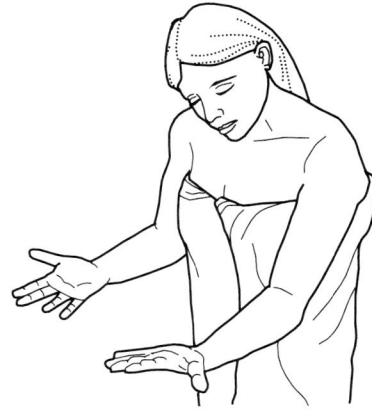

B. Bend elbows, look carefully at forearms, back of upper arms, and palms of your hands.

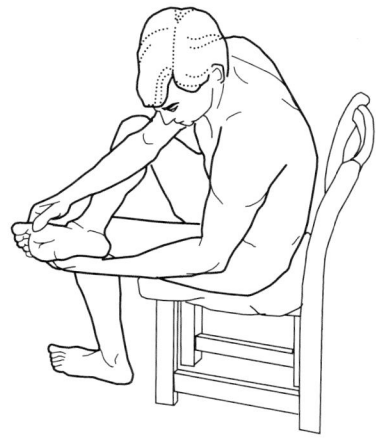

C. Sit down and draw up leg. Look at backs of legs and examine your feet including the spaces between your toes and the skin on the soles.

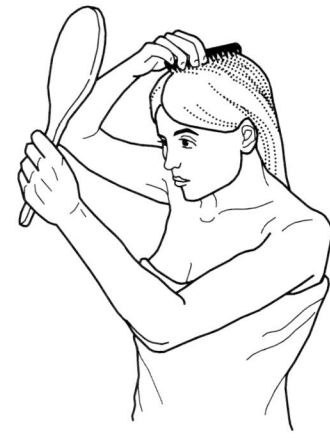

D. Examine back of neck and scalp with a hand mirror. Use a comb or hair dryer to part hair so you can see your scalp better

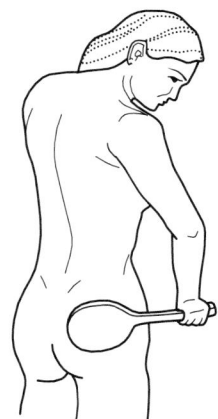

E. Check your neck, back, and buttocks with a hand mirror.

Figure 9-11   Self-examination of the skin. To perform self-examination of the skin you need a full-length mirror, a hand mirror, and a brightly lit room.

attribute it to their teeth or dentures and thus seek the consultation of a dentist.

Physical examination of the mouth includes inspection, digital palpation, and olfaction of the oral cavity. The following maneuvers should be performed during the oral examination:

1. Have the patient extend the tongue and move it from side to side. The patient also should be asked to move the jaw from side to side and up and down. Limitation of normal movement could indicate that a tumor is interfering with muscle action.

2. Palpate the tongue with a gloved hand. Palpation may reveal a lesion not otherwise visible. Palpation of a hard lesion should be referred for biopsy to establish the diagnosis.[152]

3. Inspect the anterior two-thirds of the tongue by grasping the tip of the tongue with a piece of gauze and gently pulling the tongue forward and to each side. Lesions of the base of the tongue are most often overlooked and must be both inspected and palpated. The nurse should be aware that most tongue cancers appear on the lateral surfaces.

4. The floor of the mouth should be inspected by having the patient place the tongue on the hard palate. Squamous cell carcinomas frequently are found on the floor of the mouth. The floor of the mouth should be palpated bimanually, with the fingers of one hand in the floor of the mouth and the fingers of the other hand placed on the skin under the right side of the jaw.

5. Inspection of the mouth may reveal snuff keratosis from the use of snuff in one spot in the mouth and nicotine stomatitis from cigar or pipe smoking. Nicotine stomatitis is a diffuse white condition that contains numerous red dots. This lesion usually covers the entire hard palate and is almost always associated with pipe smoking and has minimal or no malignant potential. Complete resolution should occur with cessation of smoking.

6. While inspecting the lips, observe them for any skin changes, such as keratosis of the lips from excessive sun exposure and pipe smoking. Solar keratoses occur on sun-exposed surfaces and are flat, reddish-to-tan plaques that are usually scaly. In the earliest stages a cancerous lesion may appear as a small swelling or induration that may be difficult to see but that can be palpated. An area of roughness, induration, or granularity often is the best clue to the diagnosis of early carcinoma. The upper lip should be grasped between the index finger and the thumb and bidigitally palpated along its complete length to discover masses that may be located deep under the surface.[152]

7. Olfaction of the breath. An odor of sourness may indicate obstruction and fermentation, whereas fetid and foul odors may signal necrotic neoplasms indicative of advanced disease. All large, fungating oral cancers produce a marked halitosis; however, small oral cancers are not particularly associated with mouth odor.[153] Referral to a dentist may be necessary if the breath odors indicate advanced dental decay and poor oral hygiene.

8. Palpate the parotid, submandibular, and submental areas and the cervical lymph nodes.

Other physical findings. Individuals who use smokeless tobacco may develop leukoplakias in the exact region where they hold the quid. The leukoplakia may vary from a mild whiteness, which may be difficult to see, to an obvious white lesion.[153,154] When a white oral lesion is found, the area should be rubbed to see if it can be removed. White lesions that adhere to the surface are classified as keratotic and have a greater probability of malignancy. Leukoplakia occurs in men more commonly than in women, and the vast majority are seen in individuals older than 40 years of age. When documenting the examination, clinicians are urged to use descriptive adjectives instead of the broad term leukoplakia (e.g., red, white, yellow, speckled, mixed, granular).[153]

In erythroplakia, also considered premalignant, a red plaque or well-defined red patches have a velvety consistency and often have tiny areas of ulceration. These lesions are the earliest and most consistent clinical presentation of carcinoma of the oral cavity in the industrialized Western world. Erythroplakia lesions usually have a more malignant histologic component than does leukoplakia.[152] Erythroplakia patches are characteristically painless and occur with about equal frequency in men and women who usually are older than 50 years of age.

The topical application of toluidine blue to suspicious lesions serves as a diagnostic "control" over the clinician's subjective impression. Lesions not detected during a visual examination may therefore be revealed by the stain. If an entire lesion or portion of a lesion stains dark blue in a solid or strippled pattern, malignancy must be considered. Normal tissue does not absorb stain, but small areas of intense, mechanically retained stain may be observed. (See the Mashberg and Samit[153] article for specific details on this procedure and follow-up questions and answers on this article in *CA Cancer J Clin* 46:126–128, 1996.)

Screening

Because alcoholics who smoke constitute the largest risk group for oral cancers, screening programs should be geared to this population. Any screening programs would have to be conducted in settings in which alcoholics could be approached as a group, such as in reform organizations, Salvation Army facilities for this population, shelters for the homeless, or alcoholic rehabilitation units. Although primary prevention by limiting alcohol intake and cessation of smoking is a more desirable goal, many alcoholics cannot be reached by these types of programs. Thus, the more realistic approach with this group is to encourage periodic oral examinations so that cancer can be detected in the early stages.

It is important for the nurse to explain to individuals

40 years of age and older that it is necessary to have a complete oral and dental examination on a periodic basis to detect serious lesions.[154] Individuals with complete dentures frequently believe they no longer require periodic oral examinations because of their loss of natural teeth.[155] Unfortunately, few people have examinations for oral cancer. The Center for Disease Control analyzed data from the 1992 National Health Interview Survey-Cancer Control and found that only 14% of the respondents had ever been examined for oral cancer. People who were older, poorer, less educated, and smoked were less likely to have had an examination.[156]

The use of smokeless tobacco (e.g., snuff and chewing tobacco) has risen dramatically in the last 10 years. The increase in the sales of smokeless tobacco, predominantly snuff, since the early 1970s has been estimated at 11% per year, representing an estimated 7–12 million users.[157] In the early 1970s a majority of users were men 50 years of age and older; now most are young men between 16 and 29 years of age. Nurses need to stress that smokeless tobacco is *not* a safe substitute for smoking. Long-term use of smokeless tobacco increases the risk of gingival and buccal carcinomas nearly 50-fold.[158] Many young people are not aware that smokeless tobacco is as addicting as cigarette smoking.[157] Information about the health hazards of smokeless tobacco should be shared with young people. Because so many users are young children, it is advocated that education on the dangers of smokeless tobacco begin with children as young as 6 and 7 years of age.[158] School nurses and nurses who work in settings with young people need to actively initiate educational programs on this subject or make sure that whenever smoking is discussed in health and science classes that the issue of smokeless tobacco also is addressed. In addition, parents, teachers, and athletic coaches should not neglect the powerful influence they can have as positive role models. Youngsters perceive the use of smokeless tobacco as "macho," and athletic coaches can have a tremendous influence in dispelling this myth. (Chapter 85 provides a list of sources for obtaining patient education materials on smokeless tobacco.)

In summary, education first begins with the identification of individuals at high risk for oral cancer. Depending on the risk factors identified, the individual could be referred to a physician or a dentist or taught oral self-examination for the early signs of cancer, or the nurse could conduct the oral examination at predetermined intervals. It is advocated that oral self-examination techniques need to be popularized in the same manner as BSE techniques.

The goal to increase national awareness and screening for oral cancer will be difficult to achieve in the near future since the American public is ill-informed about the risk factors and signs and symptoms of oral cancers. Not only is the American public ill-informed about this cancer, but few U.S. adults have ever had an oral cancer examination.[159] One of the primary reasons for the lack of knowledge is that there is a lack of coverage about oral cancer in the popular press.[160] In response to this national problem, the federal government convened a national conference to develop strategies for preventing and controlling oral and pharyngeal cancer in the United States. The result of this conference was the development of strategies to reduce this cancer including: (1) encouraging Medicaid, Medicare, traditional insurance plans, and managed-care entities to consider making oral cancer examinations an integral part of comprehensive physical and oral examinations; (2) developing and conducting a national promotional campaign to raise public awareness of oral cancer and its link to tobacco use and heavy alcohol consumption; and (3) developing health care curricula that require competency in prevention, diagnosis, and multidisciplinary management of oral and pharyngeal cancer.[158] Whenever possible, nurses need to join in promoting and participating in these national strategies.

Gynecologic Cancer

It is estimated that in 1999 there will be 37,400 cases of endometrial cancers and 12,800 cases of cervical cancers in the United States. The anticipated mortality rates in this same period are expected to be 4800 deaths from cervical cancer and 6400 deaths from endometrial cancer.[15] The risk of endometrial cancer is age related; the disease usually occurs in women 50–60 years old.

In stark contrast are the incidence and mortality rates for ovarian cancer. It is estimated that in 1999, 25,200 U.S. women will be diagnosed with this cancer and 14,500 will die of the disease. Ovarian cancer accounts for about 26% of all gynecologic cancer and about 52% of all genital cancer deaths. The greatest number of cases of ovarian cancer are found in the age group of 55- to 74-year-old women.

History assessment

The health history should include questions that will elicit an accurate menstrual, obstetric, gynecologic, and sexual history. The majority of women at risk for cancer of the reproductive organs can be identified only after a thorough and complete gynecologic history has been obtained. The following questions will help identify high-risk women:

1. When was your last Pap smear? Do you remember the results? Was any follow-up done or recommended?
2. Have you ever been told that you have herpes? genital warts? Were the genital warts treated? What type of treatment was done for the genital warts? Have you been treated for pelvic inflammatory disease or any other sexually transmitted diseases?
3. Do you have any vaginal bleeding or discharge not connected with menses?
4. Do you have spotting between menstrual periods?
5. Do you have bleeding or spotting although you no longer have menstrual periods?
6. Do you have bleeding after intercourse or douching?

7. At what age did you start sexual activity?
8. Have you had a consistent sexual partner since beginning sexual activity, or have you had different partners?
9. What is the approximate number of sexual partners you have had?
10. What age did you start menstruation?
11. What age did you start menopause? When was your last period?
12. How many pregnancies have you had? How many live births? miscarriages? elective abortions?
13. Have you ever taken birth control pills? How long did you take birth control pills? Do you remember the name of the pill that you took?
14. Have you ever taken estrogens? How long did you take these? What was the dose that you were given? What follow-up tests were recommended for you while taking estrogens?
15. Have you ever had infertility problems? Have you ever had endometriosis? polycystic ovaries? Stein-Leventhal syndrome? uterine fibroids?
16. Are you aware of abdominal distention or vague abdominal discomfort?
17. Are you aware if your mother received diethylstilbestrol (DES) when she was pregnant with you?
18. Have you had any gynecologic surgery—hysterectomy, tubal pregnancy, sterilization, ovarian cysts, cancer?
19. Have you ever had office procedures for a gynecologic problem, such as cervical cautery and colposcopic examination?
20. Has your present sexual partner ever had a sexual partner who had cervical cancer?
21. Have any women in your family had ovarian cancer? Who?
22. Have you ever been treated for infertility? Taken ovulation-inducing medications?[161]

Physical examination

The early signs and symptoms of gynecologic cancer are as follows. Ovarian cancer usually has no early manifestations. There may be vague abdominal discomfort, dyspepsia, indigestion, gas with constant distention, flatulence, eructation, a feeling of fullness after a light meal, or slight loss of appetite. The majority of patients with endometrial cancer have unexplained bleeding. In postmenopausal women, abnormal bleeding takes the form of intermittent spotting or bleeding that the patient describes as a "very light period." A malodorous watery discharge may be noticed as an early sign. The symptoms of cervical cancer typically are abnormal vaginal discharge, irregular bleeding, elongation of menstrual period, or bleeding that may occur after douching or intercourse.

The gynecologic examination includes *inspection* and *palpation*. The nurse should be aware of the following maneuvers performed during the gynecologic examination and related signs that indicate cancer.

Abdomen. The abdomen must be thoroughly and slowly palpated to detect any masses, areas of tenderness, or inguinal adenopathy. A mass in the upper portion of the abdomen may suggest the presence of omental cake, the solid mass formed when the omentum is infiltrated with cancer, which is a sign of advanced ovarian disease. It may be palpated or detected by ballottement during the abdominal examination. Other signs of advanced ovarian cancer are abdominal distention and ascites.

Vulva. The vulva should be inspected and palpated for signs of cancer of the vulva: excoriation of skin because of pruritus, ulcers, lumps, leukoplakia, bleeding, atrophy of the labia, and narrowing of the introitus.

Infection with human papillomavirus (HPV) may produce the typically raised exophytic tumors (warts) that can be seen with simple inspection of the vulva. There is, however, a variety of anogenital warts known as "flat" or "noncondylomatous" warts that may be invisible before the application of acetic acid. Several gauze pads (4-in. diameter) that are soaked in 3%–5% acetic acid should be compressed on the vulva and left in place for 10 minutes. After the compress is removed, the area should be inspected with a high-quality magnification lens for the *acetowhite reaction*. Acetic acid will cause the surface of both flat and exophytic warts to turn white.[162] Colposcopic examination also can be used to inspect lesions after acetic acid application. Further, carcinoma in situ also may appear as a hyperpigmented lesion. In addition, HPV can infect the entire lower female genital tract—the vagina and cervix. Patients with vulvar HPV lesions should have a thorough examination of the vagina, cervix, and perirectal epithelium with the use of an acetic acid compress application and a colposcopic examination.[162] Change to an invasive cancer can occur within 1 year of infection with HPV, but averages between 3–5 years. However, the majority of those infected do not develop malignancies, suggesting that HPV infection alone is not enough to cause cancer. Other cofactors may be required before cancer can occur.[163,164]

Vagina. The vagina should be inspected and palpated for cancer—masses, vaginal bands, texture changes, ulcers, erosions, leukoplakia, pink blush, induration, telangiectasis, and erythematosus. Induration and nodulation may indicate submucosal vaginal lesions. Most squamous cell carcinomas are found in the posterior vaginal wall, but 25% involve the anterior wall and at least 15% arise from the lateral walls.[165] The majority of lesions occur in the upper third of the vagina.

The nurse may elect to do a Schiller test on any suspicious area of the vagina or cervix. The mucosa is painted with an iodine solution (Lugol solution), and the normal mucosa becomes brown, whereas areas of abnormal epithelium remain uncolored. This test is merely an adjunctive aid to colposcopic examination or used when colposcopy is not available.

Cervix. The cervix should be inspected and palpated, and a Pap smear should be taken for cytologic examination. To avoid contamination of the cell sample with foreign material, vaginal jelly should not be used before Pap smears are obtained. The cervical sample should contain cells from the squamous epithelium of the vaginal portion of the cervix, from the squamocolumnar junction (also known as the transformation zone), and from the endocervical epithelium.[166] With aging, the transformation zone becomes increasingly invisible as it moves into the endocervical canal. In women during and after menopause, a sample of the vaginal pool cells is obtained, in addition to the cervical smear, to identify cancer cells from the endometrium, tubes, and ovaries.[167]

The nurse should inspect and palpate the cervix for position, shape, consistency, regularity, mobility, friability, and tenderness. The cervix is freely movable, firm, and smooth, and if it has been invaded by cancer, it becomes hard and immobile. In addition to rendering the cervix much harder than normal, malignancy produces a rough, granular surface and is likened to both the feel and appearance of cauliflower.[130] However, the nurse needs to be cognizant of the fact that early carcinoma has an appearance that cannot be well differentiated visually from erosion. Cancer arising within the cervical canal may cause no abnormal appearance of the cervix.

Several physical changes may be apparent in the cervix that indicate possible patient exposure to DES in utero. Cervical ectropion, or cervical bumps or ridges ("cockscombs," "hoods," or "collars"), and other non-neoplastic changes are immediate clues to DES exposure. These physical signs merit referral to a physician.

The conventional Pap smear, taken in the usual manner for cervix cancer screening, is inaccurate for a diagnosis of endometrial lesions.[168] For this reason an annual suction curettage is recommended for menopausal women and women who have taken estrogen without progestational modification for a prolonged period after menopause. Suction curettage can provide an excellent sample and in most cases can be done in the office without need for anesthesia. Monitoring of women who have received long-term estrogen therapy will detect those whose endometrium is overstimulated (adenomatous hyperplasia), and appropriate referrals can be made.

Uterus and adnexa. A bimanual examination of the uterus and adnexa should be done. The nurse should note the size, shape, mobility, position, tenderness, and consistency of the uterus. Uterine tenderness, immobility, or enlargement merits further investigation and appropriate referrals. An enlarged boggy uterus is an indication of advanced disease.

Ovaries. Palpation of the ovaries in prepubertal girls or postmenopausal women also merits investigation because (1) normal ovaries and tubes are usually not palpable, (2) ovaries in these two groups of women are smaller than the usual ovarian size of 4 cm in its largest dimension, and (3) 3–5 years after menopause the ovaries usually have atrophied and are no longer palpable. In actively menstruating women, any ovarian enlargement that persists or increases requires prompt referral. In general, the findings on the pelvic examination that can alert the nurse to a possible ovarian cancer are adnexal enlargement, fixation or immobility, bilateral irregularity or nodulation and masses, relative insensitivity of the mass, and bilaterality of the mass.

Rectovaginal palpation. Rectovaginal palpation, as well as rectal palpation, should be done. It is extremely important that the anterior rectal wall in the region of the peritoneal rectovaginal pouch, or Douglas cul-de-sac, be palpated. Thickening of this area occurs from spread of cervical carcinoma, whereas spread from ovarian cancer may be felt as a shelf, nodule, or "handful-of-knuckles" on rectal palpation.

Screening of asymptomatic individuals

The United States Preventive Services Task Force, The American College of Physicians, the ACS, the American College of Obstetricians and Gynecologists, the National Cancer Institute, the American Medical Association, and the American Academy of Family Physicians recommend that all women who are or who have been sexually active or who have reached the age of 18 should undergo an annual Pap test and pelvic examination. After a woman has had three or more consecutive normal Pap smears, this test may be performed less frequently in a low-risk woman at the discretion of her physician. When a low-risk woman has a new sexual contact, she needs to have a repeat Pap smear.[169,170]

Screening for ovarian cancer is not recommended by any national organization.[171,172] A National Institutes of Health Consensus Conference on Ovarian Cancer recommends taking a careful family history and performing an annual pelvic examination in all women; screening procedures such as CA 125 testing and ultrasonography are recommended only for women with a presumed hereditary cancer syndrome.[173]

Cervical smears Because of the Pap test, the death rate from invasive cervical cancer has decreased over the last 40 years. However, 15%–20% of American women do not have regular Pap testing.[174] The majority of women in whom cervical cancer develops have not had the test on a regular basis.

The importance of regular Pap smears was documented by Stenkvist et al who studied 207,455 women for 10 years and found that when women were screened at least once, the incidence of cervical cancer dropped from 32/100,000 to 10/100,000 (a 75% decrease in invasive cervical cancer incidence among women who had smears taken at least once during the 10-year period).[175] Among women with at least one normal smear, the incidence drops still lower, to 7/100,000. Because elderly women will constitute 17.3% of the adult population by the year 2020, screening programs for older, high-risk women will be needed.

In the past 20 years, the screening rate in older women has been low, with up to 62% of women older than the age of 65 reporting that they never had a Pap smear. This is of concern because older women comprise 25% of patients with carcinoma of the cervix but 40% of the deaths. A disproportionate number of older women present with locally advanced massive cancer of the cervix, which explains the poor survival of these women.[176]

Mandelblatt and Fahs conducted a study of the cost-effectiveness of a cervical cancer screening program for infrequently screened elderly women.[177] The results of the Pap smears were abnormal in 11/816 women screened. This early detection of cervical neoplasia saved $5907 and 3.7 years of life per 100 Pap tests. The average medical costs per year of life extended by screening were included, and the program cost $2874 per year of life saved. The researchers concluded that the benefits from cervical cancer screening for elderly women can offset the costs of these programs.

Several factors contribute to false-negative results from Pap smears and other errors.

Patient error. Patient error consists of women failing to have follow-up annual examinations, delay in seeing a physician while symptoms are present, and refusal to undergo diagnostic measures.

Physician error. Physician error consists of failure to act on reports of abnormal cytologic findings, failure to perform a pelvic examination with a Pap smear, reading of Pap smears by untrained physicians, and diagnosis of "dysplasia," which is considered inconsequential by uninformed physicians.

Laboratory error. Koss reports in his excellent review article that studies have found a false-negative laboratory rate for invasive cancer of approximately 50%.[178] The rate of screening errors for precancerous lesions was at least 28%.

Although nurses generally do not have control over laboratory errors, they can play a significant role in decreasing patient and physician error by:

- Educating women about the early symptoms of gynecologic cancer and the necessity of seeking medical advice with these early symptoms

- Educating women about the recommended intervals for Pap smears

- Educating women, particularly older women, to the necessity of asking for a Pap smear when they have a physical examination

- Educating women to request information about the mechanism used by the health care setting to inform them about the results of their Pap smears: Women with a history of abnormal or questionable Pap smear results should be encouraged to personally call about their results rather than rely on the health professional to alert them

- Educating women about the importance of receiving additional medical care with an abnormal or a questionable Pap smear finding

- Performing Pap smears only after they are thoroughly versed in the proper procedures for obtaining a smear.

Improperly done smears probably contribute to at least half of the 10%–35% false-negative rate generally reported for Pap smears.[179] Errors made by cytotechnologists may be minimized in the future by new techniques that measure the DNA content of standard Pap smears. Researchers are investigating the feasibility of automating the procedure of reading Pap smears on the basis of optical density of the specimens or DNA content of cell nuclei.[180,181]

Several new techniques to reduce the false-negative reporting rates of Pap smears have been developed and approved by the U.S. Food and Drug Administration. Two instruments, the Papnet (Neuromedical Systems Inc, Suffern, NY) and AutoPap 300 QC (NeoPath Inc, Redmond, WA), are approved for use as adjuncts to manual screening. Cytyc ThinPrep 2000 (Cytyc-Sands, Boxborough, MA) has also been approved as an alternative preparation method to conventional gynecologic smear. The Papnet and AutoPap 300 QC systems combine automated microscopy and computerized analysis to reduce screening error—the failure to identify abnormalities on the slide—by detecting abnormal cells overlooked on initial examination.[182-187] Cytyc ThinPrep 2000 is an improved slide preparation method for cervical cytologic testing. It is a semiautomated, liquid-based slide preparation system. All three technologies increase the cost per slide screened and thus are recommended for infrequent screening not annual screening.[182]

Two classification methods are used to identify abnormal changes in the Pap smear. One method is the classification system accepted by the World Health Organization. This system identified two types of lesions, dysplasia and carcinoma in situ. The dysplasias are subdivided into very mild, mild, moderate, and severe grades, depending on the extent of involvement of the epithelium. Another classification method is the cervical intraepithelial neoplasia (CIN) nomenclature. CIN is a continuum of change and generally begins as a well-differentiated lesion (CIN 1, or mild dysplasia), passes through a less well-differentiated phase (CIN 2, or moderate dysplasia), and leads to an undifferentiated intraepithelial lesion (CIN 3). CIN 3 is the severe dysplasia/carcinoma in situ in the World Health Organization system.

The most recent attempt to standardize cytologic terminology involves the Bethesda System instituted in 1988. The Bethesda System of reporting Pap smears was instituted to replace other classification systems and to improve interpretation among health care professionals. The Bethesda System offers a more specific and precise diagnosis than the other classification systems. This system separates the report into three main categories: (1) a statement of adequacy of the specimen, (2) a general categorization of normal or abnormal, and (3) descriptive diagnoses.[187,188] It separates squamous intraepithelial lesions into two categories: low- and high-grade squamous intraepithelial lesions. It thus encompasses many of the former categories of the CIN system, but it divides the squamous intraepithelial lesions into low and high grade. The Bethesda System also provides information about changes consistent with cervical and vaginal infection and a statement on the adequacy of the sample. (The reader is referred to Table 50-1 in the chapter on cervical cancer, which lists the Bethesda classification of cervical cytology.)

Colposcopic examination is an accurate and reliable method for evaluating the cervix and vagina of a woman with an abnormality revealed by Pap smear. This modality (a well-illuminated binocular microscope) not only provides visualization of the cervical transformation zone but also allows directed biopsy of specific areas of the epithelium, removing only small amounts of tissue.

Additional nursing interventions

Reaching those women who are at high risk for gynecologic cancer is one of the most challenging roles for nurses. Patient acceptance and increasing the availability of screening are areas that require major effort on the part of nurses if the entire population at greatest risk is to be reached. Because cytologic screening is closely tied to obstetric care and contraceptive services, a higher proportion of women are screened among the groups that require such attention than among those that do not. This is effective for screening for cervical and vaginal cancer in the reproductive years but does not reach the postmenopausal women who are at risk for ovarian and endometrial malignancies. Nurses who work in retirement centers, extended care facilities, physicians' offices, factories, public health agencies, and ambulatory care settings are urged to provide health education programs that include the early signs and symptoms of ovarian, cervical, and endometrial cancer and to stress the need for gynecologic examinations after menopause as well as during the reproductive years. Female patients being followed routinely for chronic problems (such as hypertension, diabetes, heart condition, or chronic lung disease) should be asked when they had their last pelvic examination.

When appropriate, nurses should discuss the myths about menopause with women who are in their late 30s and early 40s. There are several significant barriers to early detection of gynecologic cancer in older women. Many women have the mistaken belief that once they are past childbearing years and/or are sexually inactive, they no longer need pelvic examinations. There are also physical changes that occur that make the gynecologic examination difficult for older women. There is decreased mobility of the femoropelvic structure, which leads to pain when the woman is put in the lithotomy position for a gynecologic examination. Nurses need to be aware of this physical barrier and suggest the use of the left lateral Sims position instead of the traditional lithotomy position. Because the vaginal orifice may have narrowed with age, the insertion of the traditional speculum may cause discomfort or admit only the passage of one finger.

Nurses must conduct educational programs in community settings that dispel these myths that surround menopause and aging and provide factual information on the early signs and symptoms of the common gynecologic cancers in older women, as well as discuss methods to make the gynecologic examination more comfortable for the woman. Women taking estrogens should be advised that they should be routinely monitored by their physician in terms of an examination to detect endometrial cancer.[189,190]

Nurses need to be aware that older women are at high risk for endometrial, vulvar, vaginal, and ovarian cancer. Several premalignant conditions commonly found in elderly women predispose them to gynecologic cancers. These premalignant conditions are leukoplakic vulvitis, which precedes epidermoid carcinoma; lichen sclerosus et atrophicus, which precedes epidermoid carcinoma; and endometrial adenoma, which precedes hyperplastic lesions. Normal changes that occur with aging frequently obscure the early symptoms of cancer. The vaginal mucosa thins with aging, and there is a decrease in vaginal/cervical lubrication. Bleeding that results from endometrial or vaginal cancer is shrugged off as normal "postmenopausal bleeding" or attributed by health professionals to atrophic vaginitis and often is not followed up.[168]

Young women who have had venereal disease (syphilis, gonorrhea, genital herpes, or human papillomavirus [HPV] infection) must be alert to the necessity of having regular Pap smears. Women with vulvar condyloma acuminatum should be referred for a thorough examination of the vagina, cervix, and perirectal epithelium with the use of acetic acid compress application, a colposcopic examination, and a Pap smear. It also is recommended that these women (and infected male partners) have frequent follow-up examinations to detect precancerous conditions caused by a latent virus in clinically and histologically normal tissue.[162] Infection of the genital tract by HPV is a common disease and often encountered in clinics for family planning, prenatal care, and sexually transmitted diseases. Women whose Pap smears indicate the presence of warty infections such as koilocytotic cells or who show cells consistent with squamous papilloma or warty atypia also should be referred to a physician for further evaluation.[191]

Nurses are urged to acquire physical assessment skills that will enable them to perform pelvic examinations. It has been documented that nurses who perform pelvic examinations can detect gynecologic malignancies, that patient acceptance and satisfaction are high, and that pelvic examinations done by nurses are cost-effective.[192]

Nurses trained to conduct gynecologic examinations are in an ideal position to reach those women who are at highest risk for the development of various types of gynecologic cancers but who are least likely to use conventional screening programs or have routine health examinations, such as older women in residential settings or older poor women in the community. Nurses actively involved in conducting pelvic examinations would increase the availability of screening programs and thus reach more women.[1]

References

1. Heusinkveld K: Cancer prevention and risk assessment, in Varricchio C (ed): *A Cancer Source Book for Nurses* (ed 7). Sudbury, MA, Jones and Bartlett, 1997, pp 35–42

2. Heusinkveld K: Clinical detection and support: Preventive oncology, in Baird S, McCorkle R, Grant M: *Cancer Nursing: A Comprehensive Textbook*. Philadelphia, Saunders, 1991, pp 143–154

3. Olsen S, Frank-Stromborg M: Cancer screening and early detection. In McCorkle R, Grant M, Frank-Stromborg M, Baird S: *Cancer Nursing: A Comprehensive Textbook* (ed 2). Philadelphia, Saunders, 1996, pp 265–297

4. Barton P: *Understanding the U.S. Health Services System*. Chicago, Health Administration Press, 1999

5. Frank-Stromborg M, Rohan K: Nursing's involvement in the primary and secondary prevention of cancer: Nationally and internationally. *Cancer Nurs* 15:79–108, 1992

6. Mettlin C: Research in cancer prevention and detection, in Hubbard S, Greene P, Knobf M (eds): *Current Issues in Cancer Nursing Practice Updates*. Philadelphia, Lippincott, 1: 1–10, 1992

7. Germino B: Cancer prevention and detection: A role for all nurses, in *Cancer Prevention, Early Detection and Screening: Proceedings of the Sixth National Conference on Cancer Nursing*. Atlanta, American Cancer Society, 1992, pp 2–14

8. Sobel J, Curtin A, Fell D: The Oregon Breast Cancer Detection and Awareness Project: The legacy of a mammogram screening campaign. *Health Values* 15:3–8, 1991

9. NCI Breast Cancer Screening Consortium: Screening mammography: A missed clinical opportunity? Results of the NCI Breast Cancer Screening Consortium and National Health Interview Survey Studies. *JAMA* 264:54–58, 1990

10. U.S. Public Health Service: *Prevention Report*. Washington, DC, Office of Disease Prevention and Health Promotion, Fall 1995, pp 1–9

11. McGinnis J, Richmond J, Brandt E, et al: Health Progress in the United States: Results of the 1990 Objectives for the Nation. *JAMA* 268:2545–2552, 1992

12. Carlson J: Prevention, screening and detection, in Otto S (ed): *Oncology Nursing*. St. Louis, Mosby-Year Book, 1991, pp 28–37

13. Frank-Stromborg M: Cancer screening and early detection, in Varricchio C (ed): *A Cancer Source Book for Nurses* (ed 7). Sudbury, MA, Jones and Bartlett, 1997, pp 43–55

14. Hospital discharge rates for four major cancers—United States, 1970–1986. *JAMA* 260:3412–3416, 1988

15. Landis SH, Murray T, Bolden S, et al: Cancer statistics, 1999. *CA Cancer J Clin* 49:8–31, 1999

16. Bartecchi C, MacKenzie T, Schrier R: The human costs of tobacco use. *N Engl J Med* 330:907–912, 1994

17. Fontham ET, Correa P, Reynolds P, et al: Environmental tobacco smoke and lung cancer in nonsmoking women. *JAMA* 271:1752–1759, 1994

18. Celermajer DS, Adams MR, Clarkson P, et al: Passive smoking and impaired endothelium-dependent arterial dilatations in healthy young adults. *N Engl J Med* 334:150–154, 1996

19. Wang F, Love EJ, Liu N, et al: Childhood and adolescent passive smoking and the risk of female lung cancer. *Int J Epididemiol* 23:223–230, 1994

20. Camus M, Siemiatycki J, Meek B: Nonoccupational exposure to chrysotile asbestos and the risk of lung cancer. *N Engl J Med* 338:1565–1571, 1998

21. Coultas DB, Samet JM: Occupational lung cancer. *Clin Chest Med* 13:341–354, 1992

22. Patel AM, Peters SG: Clinical manifestations of lung cancer. *Mayo Clin Proc* 68:273–277, 1993

23. Grimes J, Burns E (eds): *Health Assessment in Nursing Practice* (ed 2). Sudbury, MA, Jones and Bartlett, 1987

24. Buckingham W: *A Primer of Clinical Diagnosis* (ed 2). New York, Harper & Row, 1979

25. Kadunce DP, Burr R, Gress R, et al: Cigarette smoking: Risk factor for premature facial wrinkling. *Ann Intern Med* 114:840–844, 1991

26. Yahalom J: Superior vena cava syndrome, in DeVita VT, Hellman S, Rosenberg SA (eds): *Cancer Principles and Practice of Oncology* (ed 5). Philadelphia, Lippincott, 1997, pp 2469–2476

27. DeGowin E: *Bedside Diagnostic Examination* (ed 6). New York, Macmillan, 1994

28. Guarino JR: Auscultatory percussion of the chest. *Lancet* 1:1332–1334, 1980

29. Bates B: *A Guide to Physical Examination and History Taking* (ed 6). Philadelphia, Lippincott, 1995

30. Swartz M: *Textbook of Physical Diagnosis* (ed 3). Philadelphia, Saunders, 1998

31. Mao L, Hruban R, Boyle J, et al: Detection of oncogene mutations in sputum precedes diagnosis of lung cancer. *Cancer Res* 54:1634–1637, 1994

32. Beckett WS: Epidemiology and etiology of lung cancer. *Clin Chest Med* 14:1–15, 1993

33. Fiore M, Novotny R, Pierce J, et al: Trends in cigarette smoking in the United States: The changing influence of gender and race. *JAMA* 261:49–55, 1989

34. Cinciripini PM, Hecht SS, Henningfield JE, et al: Tobacco addiction: Implications for treatment and cancer prevention. *J Natl Cancer Inst* 89:1852–1866, 1997

35. Wechsler H, Rigotti NA, Gledhill-Hoyt J, et al: Increased levels of cigarette use among college students. *JAMA* 280: 1673–1678, 1998

36. Bartecchi CE, MacKenzie TD, Schrier RW: The global tobacco epidemic. *Sci Am* 272:44–51, 1995

37. Hermanson B, Omenn G, Kronmal R, et al: Participants in the Coronary Artery Surgery Study: Beneficial six-year outcome of smoking cessation in older men and women with coronary artery disease. *N Engl J Med* 319:1365–1369, 1988

38. Fielding J: Smoking: Health effects and control. *N Engl J Med* 313:491–498, 1985

39. Novello AC, Davis RM, Giovino GA: The slowing of the lung cancer epidemic and the need for continued vigilance. *CA Cancer J Clin* 41:133–136, 1991

40. Benowitz N, Jacob P, Kozlowski L, et al: Influence of smoking fewer cigarettes on exposure to tar, nicotine, and carbon monoxide. *N Engl J Med* 315:1310–1313, 1986

41. Anda R, Remington P, Sienko D, et al: Are physicians advising smokers to quit? The patient's perspective. *JAMA* 257:1916–1919, 1987

42. Ayanian JZ, Cleary PD: Perceived risks of heart disease and cancer among cigarette smokers. *JAMA* 281:1019–1021, 1999

43. Clinical Practice Guideline on Smoking Cessation. Agency

for Health Care Policy and Research. Available at: http://www.ahcpr.gov/clinic/smokepcc.htm. Accessed 9/29/99

44. Kottke T, Battista R, Defriese G, et al: Attributes of successful smoking cessation interventions in medical practice: A meta-analysis of 39 controlled trials. *JAMA* 259:2883–2889, 1988

45. Altman D, Flora J, Fortmann S, et al: The cost-effectiveness of three smoking cessation programs. *Am J Public Health* 77:162–165, 1987

46. Hughes JR, Goldstein MG, Hurt RD, et al: Recent advances in the pharmacotherapy of smoking. *JAMA* 281:72–76, 1999

47. Jorenby DE, Leischow SJ, Nides MA, et al: A controlled trial of sustained-release Bupropion, a nicotine patch, or both for smoking cessation. *N Engl J Med* 340:685–691, 1999

48. Leo MA, Lieber CS: Re: Risk factors for lung cancer and for intervention effects in CARET, the Beta-carotene and Retinol efficacy trial. *J Natl Cancer Inst* 89:1722–1723, 1997

49. Lotan R: Lung cancer promotion by beta-carotene and tobacco smoke: Relationship to suppression of retinoic acid receptor beta and increased activator protein-1? *J Natl Cancer Inst* 91:7–9, 1999

50. New rules extinguish "smoking lamp" in growing number of public places. *JAMA* 259: 2809, 1988

51. Longo DR, Brownson RC, Johnson JC, et al: Hospital smoking bans and employee smoking behavior: Results of a national survey. *JAMA* 275:1252–1257, 1996

52. Shamburek RD, Farrar JT: Disorders of the digestive system in the elderly. *N Engl J Med* 322:438–443, 1990

53. Bunn PA, Ridgway EC: Paraneoplastic syndromes, in DeVita VT, Hellman S, Rosenberg SA (eds): *Cancer: Principles and Practice of Oncology* (ed 4). Philadelphia, Lippincott, 1993, pp 2026–2071

54. DeCosse JJ, Tsioulias GJ, Jacobson JS: Colorectal cancer: Detection, treatment, and rehabilitation. *CA Cancer J Clin* 44:27–42, 1994

55. Mandel JS, Bond JH, Church TR, et al: Reducing mortality from colorectal cancer by screening for fecal occult blood. *N Engl J Med* 328:1365–1371, 1993 [Erratum *N Engl J Med* 329:329, 672, 1993]

56. Mandel JS: Screening for colorectal cancer will reduce mortality. *Clin Geriatr* 5:19–33, 1997

57. Castiglione G, Biangini M, Barchielli A, et al: Effect of rehydration on guaiac-based fecal occult blood testing in colorectal cancer screening. *Br J Cancer* 67:1142–1144, 1993

58. Reiventer J, Brevinge H, Engarás B, et al: Results of screening, rescreening, and follow-up in a prospective randomized study of colorectal cancer by fecal occult blood test. *Scand J Gastroenterol* 29:468–473, 1994

59. American College of Physicians: Clinical Guideline: Part I. Suggested technique for fecal occult blood testing and interpretation in colorectal cancer screening. *Ann Intern Med* 126:808–810, 1997

60. Ransohoff DF, Lang CA: Clinical Guideline II: Part II. Screening for colorectal cancer with the fecal occult blood test: A background paper. *Ann Intern Med* 126:811–822, 1997

61. Solomon MJ, McLeod RS: Periodic health examination, 1994 update: 2. Screening strategies for colorectal cancer. Canadian Task Force on the Periodic Health Examination. *CMAJ* 150:1961–1970, 1994

62. Nakama H, Kamijo N: Accuracy of immunological fecal occult blood testing for colorectal cancer screening. *Prev Med* 23:309–313, 1994

63. Allison JE, Tekawa IS, Ransom LJ, et al: A comparison of fecal occult-blood tests for colorectal-cancer screening. *N Engl J Med* 334:155–159, 1996

64. Robinson M, Pye G, Thomas J, et al: Haemoccult screening for colorectal cancer: The effect of dietary restriction on compliance. *Eur J Surg Oncol* 20:545–548, 1994

65. ACS announces revised colorectal screening guidelines. *Oncology News Int* 6:20, 1997

66. Ahsan H, Neugut AI, Garbowski GC, et al: Family history of colorectal adenomatous polyps and increased risk for colorectal cancer. *Ann Intern Med* 128:900–905, 1998

67. Jessup JM, Menck HR, Fremgen A, et al: Diagnosing colorectal carcinoma: Clinical and molecular approaches. *CA Cancer J Clin* 47:70–92, 1997

68. Kritchevsky D: Diet and cancer. *CA Cancer J Clin* 41:328–333, 1991

69. The Work Study Group on Diet, Nutrition, and Cancer: American Cancer Society Guidelines on diet, nutrition, and cancer. *CA Cancer J Clin* 41:334–338, 1991

70. The American Cancer Society 1996 Dietary Guidelines Advisory Committee: *Guidelines on Diet, Nutrition, and Cancer Prevention: Reducing the Risk of Cancer with Healthy Food Choices and Physical Activity*. Atlanta, American Cancer Society, 1999

71. The changing diet: Illinois 1982–1986. *Am Cancer Soc Cancer Prev Study II Newsletter* 5:3, 1987

72. National Cancer Institute: *Cancer Among Blacks and Other Minorities: Statistical Profiles*. NIH publication No. 86-2785. Washington, DC, National Cancer Institute, 1986

73. American College of Physicians: Clinical guideline: Part III. Screening for prostate cancer. *Ann Intern Med* 126:480–484, 1997

74. Chodak G: Screening for prostate cancer: The debate continues. *JAMA* 272:813–814, 1994

75. Sox H: Preventative health services in adults. *N Engl J Med* 330:1589–1595, 1994

76. Feightner J: The early detection and treatment of prostate cancer: The perspective of the Canadian Task Force on the Periodic Health Examination. *J Urol* 152:1682–1684, 1994

77. Middleton RG: Prostate cancer: Are we screening and treating too much? *Ann Intern Med* 126:465–467, 1997

78. Coley CM, Barry MJ, Fleming C, et al: Early detection of prostate cancer. Part I: Prior probability and effectiveness of tests. *Ann Intern Med* 126:394–406, 1997

79. Coley CM, Barry MJ, Fleming C, et al: Early detection of prostate cancer. Part II: Estimating the risks, benefits, and costs. *Ann Intern Med* 126:468–479, 1997

80. Lange P: New information about prostate-specific antigen and the paradoxes of prostate cancer. *JAMA* 273:336–337, 1995

81. Handley M, Stuart M: The use of prostate-specific antigen for prostate cancer screening: A managed care perspective. *J Urol* 152:1689–1692, 1994

82. Krahn M, Mahoney J, Eckman M, et al: Screening for prostate cancer: A decision analytic view. *JAMA* 272:773–780, 1994

83. Garnick M, Fair W: Prostate cancer: Emerging concepts. Part I. *Ann Intern Med* 125:118–125, 1996

84. Littrup P, Goodman A, Mettlin C: The Investigators of the American Cancer Society–National Prostate Cancer Detection Project: The benefit and cost of prostate cancer early detection. *CA Cancer J Clin* 43:134–149, 1993

85. Gann P, Hennekens C, Stampfer M: A prospective evalua-

tion of plasma prostate-specific antigen for detection of prostate cancer. *JAMA* 273:289–294, 1995

86. Henderson IC: Breast cancer, in Murphy GP, Lawrence W, Lenhard RE (eds): *American Cancer Society Textbook of Oncology.* Atlanta, GA, American Cancer Society, 1995, pp 198–219

87. American Cancer Society: *Breast Cancer Facts and Figures 1996.* Atlanta, American Cancer Society, 1996

88. Self-exams are crucial in detecting breast cancer. *Detroit Free Press,* October 14, 1997

89. Barton MB, Elmore JG, Fletcher SW: Breast symptoms among women enrolled in a health maintenance organization: Frequency, evaluation, and outcome. *Ann Intern Med* 130:651–657, 1999

90. Olsen S: *Examinations for Detecting Breast Cancer.* Cancer Prevention Program, Wisconsin Clinical Cancer Center, 1300 University Ave-7C, Medical Science Center, Madison, WI 53706

91. Scanlon E: A photo checklist for a better breast palpation. *Prim Care Cancer* 7:13–20, 1987

92. Heymann A: Semilateral decubitus breast examination. *JAMA* 243:1713, 1980

93. The Breast Cancer Resource Center, American Cancer Society: Breast cancer: Detection and symptoms. Available at http://www3.cancer.org/cancerinfo/main_cont.asp?st=ds&ct=5. Accessed 7/2/99

94. Update January 1992: The American Cancer Society guidelines for the cancer-related checkup. *CA Cancer J Clin* 42:44–45, 1992

95. American Cancer Society: *Breast Cancer Facts and Figures 1997.* Atlanta, American Cancer Society, 1997

96. Elmore JG, Barton MB, Moceri VM, et al: Ten-year risk of false positive screening mammograms and clinical breast examinations. *N Engl J Med* 338:1089–1096, 1998

97. Sox HC: Benefit and harm associated with screening for breast cancer. *N Engl J Med* 338:1145–1146, 1998

98. Nystrom L, Rutquist LE, Wall S, et al: Breast cancer screening with mammography: Overview of Swedish randomised trials. *Lancet* 341:973–978, 1993

99. Esserman L, Kerlikowske K: Should we recommend screening mammography for women aged 40 to 49? *Oncology* 10:357–364, 1996

100. New evidence supports screening in younger women. *Oncol News* 6:29–33, 1997

101. Hislop TG: Is breast self-examination still necessary? *CMAJ* 157:1225–1226, 1997

102. Morrison BJ: Screening for breast cancer, in Canadian Task Force on the Periodic Health Examination, Canadian Guide to Clinical Preventive Health Care. Ottawa: Health Canada, 1994, pp 788–795

103. Harvey BJ, Miller AB, Baines CJ, et al: Effect of breast self-examination techniques on the risk of death from breast cancer. *CMAJ* 157:1205–1212, 1997

104. Thomas DB, Gao DL, Self SG, et al: Randomized trial of breast self-examination in Shanghai: Methodology and preliminary results. *J Natl Cancer Inst* 89:355–365, 1997

105. Semiglazov VF, Sagaidak VN, Moiseyenko VM, et al: Study of the role of breast self-examination in the reduction of mortality from breast cancer: The Russian Federation/World Health Organization Study. *Eur J Cancer* 29A:2039–2046, 1993

106. Holmberg L, Ekbom A, Calle E, et al: Breast cancer mortality in relation to self-reported use of breast self-examination: A cohort study of 450,000 women. *Breast Cancer Res Treat* 43:137–140, 1997

107. Newcomb PA, Weiss NS, Storer BE, et al: Breast self-examination in relation to the occurrence of advanced breast cancer. *J Natl Cancer Inst* 83: 260–265, 1991

108. Stevens VM, Hatcher JW, Bruce BK: How compliant is compliant? Evaluating adherence with breast self-exam positions. *J Behav Med* 17:523–534, 1994

109. Smith TJ, Davidson NE, Schapira DV, et al: American Society of Clinical Oncology 1998 update of recommended breast cancer surveillance guidelines. *J Clin Oncol* 17: 1080–1082, 1999

110. Stefanek ME, Wilcox P: Breast self examination among women at increased risk: Assessment proficiency. *Cancer Prev* 1:79–83, 1990

111. Feldman J: Breast self-examination—A practice whose time has come? *NY State J Med* 85:482–483, 1985

112. Huguley C, Brown R, Greenberg R, et al: Breast self-examination and survival from breast cancer. *Cancer* 62:1389–1396, 1988

113. O'Malley M, Fletcher S: Screening for breast cancer with breast self-examination. A critical review. *JAMA* 257:2197–2203, 1987

114. Wardle J, Steptoe A, Smith H, et al: Breast self-examination: Attitudes and practices among young women in Europe. *Eur J Cancer Prev* 4: 61–68, 1995

115. Bennett S, Lawrence R, Fleischmann K, et al: Profile of women practicing breast self-examination. *JAMA* 249:488–491, 1983

116. Kegeles S: Education for breast self-examination: Why, who, what, and how? *Prev Med* 14:702–720, 1985

117. Solomon LJ, Mickey RM, Rairikar CJ, et al: Three-year prospective adherence to three breast cancer screening modalities. *Prev Med* 27:781–786, 1998

118. Styrd A: A breast self-examination program in an occupational health setting. *Occup Health Nurs* 30:33–35, 1982

119. Shamian J, Edgar L: Nurses as agents for change in teaching breast self-examination. *Public Health* 4:29–34, 1987

120. Kassabian VS, Graham SD: Urologic and male genital cancers, in Murphy GP, Lawrence W, Lenhard RE (eds): *American Cancer Society Textbook of Oncology.* Atlanta, American Cancer Society, 1995, pp 311–329

121. Patel SR, Kvols LK, Richardson RL: Familial testicular cancer: Report of six cases and review of the literature. *Mayo Clin Proc* 65:804–808, 1990

122. Kinkade S: Testicular cancer. *Am Fam Physician* 59:2539–2544, 2549–2550, 1999

123. American Cancer Society: Testicular cancer: Detection and symptoms. Available at: http://www3.cancer.org/cancerinfo/main_cont.asp?st=ds&ct=41. Accessed 9/29/99

124. Hawkins C, Miaskowski C: Testicular cancer: A review. *Oncol Nurs Forum* 23:1203–1211, 1996

125. Conklin M, Klint K, Morway A, et al: Should health teaching include self-examination of the testis? *Am J Nurs* 78:2073–2074, 1978

126. Blesch K: Health beliefs about testicular cancer and self-examination among professional men. *Oncol Nurs Forum* 13:29–33, 1986

127. Wardle J, Steptoe A, Burckhardt R, et al: Testicular self-examination: Attitudes and practices among young men in Europe. *Prev Med* 23: 206–210, 1994

128. Sladden M, Dickinson J: Testicular cancer. How effective is screening? *Aust Fam Physician* 22:1350–1356, 1993

129. U.S. Preventive Services Task Force: *Guide to Clinical Preventive Services: An Assessment of the Effectiveness of 169 Interventions.* Baltimore, Williams & Wilkins, 1989, pp 77–80

130. Smith J, Hollenbeck Z: Genitalia, in Prior J, Silberstein J, Stang J (eds): *Physical Diagnosis: The History and Examination of the Patient.* St. Louis, Mosby, 1981, pp 330–364

131. Richie J: Detection and treatment of testicular cancer. *CA Cancer J Clin* 43:151–175, 1993

132. Boyd J (ed): Office urology: When your patient fears testicular cancer. *Patient Care* 9:102, 1975

133. Frank-Stromborg M: The role of the nurse in cancer detection and screening. *Semin Oncol Nurs* 2:191–199, 1986

134. Garnick M: Urologic cancer, in Rubenstein E, Federman D (eds): *Oncology*, vol. 9. New York, Scientific American Medicine, 1988, pp 1–17

135. Henkel J: Testicular cancer: Survival high with early treatment. U.S. Food and Drug Administration. Available at: http://www.fda.gov/fdac/features/196__test.html. Accessed 9/29/99

136. Malasanos L, Barkauskas V, Moss M, et al: *Health Assessment*. St. Louis, Mosby, 1986, pp 401–414

137. Misener TR, Fuller SG: Testicular versus breast and colorectal cancer screening: Early detection practices of primary care physicians. *Cancer Pract* 3:310–316, 1995

138. Peate I: Testicular cancer: Importance of effective health education. *Br J Nurs* 6:311–316, 1997

139. Carlin P: Testicular self-examination: A public awareness program *Public Health Rep* 101:98–102, 1986

140. Rigel DS: Malignant melanoma: Perspectives on incidence and its effects on awareness, diagnosis, and treatment. *CA Cancer J Clin* 46:195–198, 1996

141. Friedman RJ, Rigel DS, Silverman MK, et al: Malignant melanoma in the 1990s: The continued importance of early detection and the role of physician examination and self-examination of the skin. *CA Cancer J Clin* 41:201–226, 1991

142. Hill L, Ferrini RL: Skin cancer prevention and screening: Summary of the American College of Preventive Medicine's practice policy statements. *CA Cancer J Clin* 48:232–235, 1998

143. McDonald CJ: American Cancer Society perspective on the American College of Preventive Medicne's policy statements on skin cancer prevention and screening. *CA Cancer J Clin* 48:229–231, 1998

144. Marks R: Prevention and control of melanoma: The public health approach. *CA Cancer J Clin* 46:199–216, 1996

145. Daniel CR, Dolan NC, Wheeland RG: Don't overlook skin surveillance. *Patient Care* 15:90–107, 1996

146. Edwards L, Glass LF, Levine N, et al: Melanoma. A strategy for detection and treatment. *Patient Care* 15:126–153, 1996

147. Rigel DS: Is the ounce of screening and prevention for skin cancer worth the pound of cure? *CA Cancer J Clin* 46:236–238, 1996

148. Loescher LJ, Ketcham MA: Skin cancers, in Groenwald SL, Frogge MH, Goodman M, Yarbro CH (eds): *Cancer Nursing: Principles and Practice* (ed 4). Boston, Jones and Bartlett, 1997, pp 1355–1373

149. Diekmann J: Cancer in the elderly: Systems overview. *Semin Oncol Nurs* 4:169–177, 1988

150. Salisbury PL: Diagnosis and patient management of oral cancer. *Dent Clin North Am* 41:891–914, 1997

151. Ship J, Chavez E, Gould K, Henson B, et al: Evaluation and management of oral cancer. *Home Health Care Consult* 6:2–12, 1999

152. National Institute of Dental Research: *Detecting oral cancer: A guide for dentists*. Bethesda, National Institute of Dental Research, 1994

153. Mashberg A, Samit A: Early detection of asymptomatic oral and oropharyngeal squamous cancers. *CA Cancer J Clin* 45:328–351, 1995

154. American Cancer Society: Oral cavity & oropharyngeal cancer. Available at: http://www3.cancer.org/cancerinfo/main__cont.asp?st=pr&ct=60. Accessed 9/29/99

155. Kabot T, Heffez L, Bergschneider J: Prevention, detection and referral. Responsibility of the dental team: Prevention and patient education. *Ill Dental J* 57:324–325, 1988

156. Current trends examinations for oral cancer-United States, 1992. *MMWR Morb Mortal Wkly Rep* 43:198–200, 1994

157. Lewin F, Norell SE, Johansson H, et al: Smoking tobacco, oral snuff, and alcohol in the etiology of squamous cell carcinoma of the head and neck: A population-based case-referent study in Sweden. *Cancer* 82:1367–1375, 1998

158. Ernster VL, Grady DG, Greene JG, et al: Smokeless tobacco use and health effects among baseball players. *JAMA* 264:218–224, 1990

159. Horowitz AM, Goodman HS, Yellowitz JA, et al: The need for health promotion in oral cancer prevention and early detection. *J Public Health Dent* 56:319–330, 1996

160. Canto MT, Kawaguchi Y, Horowitz AM: Coverage and quality of oral cancer information in the popular press. *J Public Health Dent* 58:241–247, 1998

161. Rossing MA, Daling JR, Weiss NE, et al: Ovarian tumors in a cohort of infertile women. *N Engl J Med* 331:771–776, 1994

162. Mitchell MF, Sandella JA, White LN: Cervical cancer: The role of the human papillomavirus, in Hubbard SM, Greene PE, Knobf MT (eds): *Current Issues in Cancer Nursing Practice Updates*. Philadelphia, Lippincott, 1992, pp 1–9

163. Lungu O, Sun XW, Felix J, et al: Relationship of human papillomavirus type to grade of cervical intraepithelial neoplasia. *JAMA* 267:2493–2496, 1992

164. Beutner KR, Tyring S: Human papillomavirus and human disease. *Am J Med* 102: 9–12, 1997

165. Noller KL: Screening for vaginal cancer. *N Engl J Med* 335:1599–1600, 1996

166. Harrison DD, Hernandez E, Dunton CJ: Endocervical brush versus cotton swab for obtaining cervical smears at a clinic: A cost comparison. *J Reprod Med* 38:285–288, 1993

167. Brooks SE: Cervical cancer screening and the older woman: Obstacles and opportunities. *Cancer Pract* 4:125–134, 1996

168. Persky V, Davis F, Barrett R, et al: Recent time trends in uterine cancer. *Am J Pub Health* 80:935–939, 1990

169. Committee on Gynecologic Practice. *Recommendations on frequency of Pap test screening*. Washington DC. American College of Obstetrics and Gynecologists Committee Opinion 1995

170. American Cancer Society: *Guidelines for the cancer-related checkup: An update*. Atlanta, American Cancer Society, 1993

171. NIH Consensus Development Panel on Ovarian Cancer. Ovarian cancer: Screening, treatment, and follow-up. *JAMA* 273: 491–497, 1995

172. US Preventive Services Task Force. *Guide to Clinical Preventive Services*, (ed 2). Baltimore, Williams & Wilkins, 1996, p 159

173. Carlson KJ, Skates SJ, Singer DE: Screening for ovarian cancer. *Ann Intern Med* 121:124–132, 1994

174. Fink D: Change in American Cancer Society checkup guidelines for detection of cervical cancer. *CA Cancer J Clin* 38:127–128, 1988

175. Stenkvist B, Bergstrom R, Eklund G, et al: Papanicolaou smear screening and cervical cancer: What can you expect? *JAMA* 252:1423–1426, 1984

176. Brooks S: Cervical cancer screening and the older woman. *Cancer Pract* 4:125–129, 1996

177. Mandelblatt J, Fahs M: The cost-effectiveness of cervical

cancer screening for low-income elderly women. *JAMA* 259:2409–2413, 1988

178. Koss L: The Papanicolaou test for cervical cancer detection: A triumph and a tragedy. *JAMA* 261:737–743, 1989

179. Eddy DM: Screening for cervical cancer. *Ann Intern Med* 113:214–226, 1990

180. Diagnosing cervical cancer by measuring DNA content. *Primary Care Cancer* 2:29, 1988

181. Jones G: Densitometric screening found accurate for detecting cervical cancer. *Oncol Biotechnol News* 2:3, 1988

182. Brown AD, Garber AM: Cost-effectiveness of 3 methods to enhance the sensitivity of Papanicolaou testing. *JAMA* 281:347–353, 1999

183. Koss LG, Lin E, Schreiber K, et al: Evaluation of the PAP-NET cytologic screening system for quality control of cervical smears. *Am J Clin Pathol* 101: 220–229, 1994

184. Birdsong GG: Automated rescreening of Papanicolaou smears: What are the implications? *Diagn Cytopathol* 13: 283–286, 1995

185. Colgan RTJ, Patten SF, Lee JS: A clinical trial of the Auto-Pap 300 QC system for quality control of cervicovaginal cytology in the clinical laboratory. *Acta Cytol* 39:1191–1198, 1992

186. Lovejoy N: Precancerous lesions of the cervix: Personal risk factors. *Cancer Nurs* 10:2–14, 1987

187. McCauley K, Oi R: Evaluating the Papanicolaou smear: Part I. *Consultant* 29:31–40, 1988

188. Yoder L, Rubin M: The epidemiology of cervical cancer and its precursors. *Oncol Nurs Forum* 19:485–493, 1992

189. Braunstein G: The benefits of estrogen to the menopausal woman outweigh the risks of developing endometrial cancer [Opinion: Pro]. *CA Cancer J Clin* 34:210–219, 1984

190. Morrow C: The benefits of estrogen to the menopausal woman outweigh the risks of developing endometrial cancer [Opinion: Con]. *CA Cancer J Clin* 34:220–231, 1984

191. Jones W, Saigo P: The "atypical" Papanicolaou smear. *CA Cancer J Clin* 36:237–242, 1986

192. Stromborg M, Nord S: A cancer detection clinic: Patient motivation and satisfaction. *Nurse Pract* 4:10–14, 1979

CHAPTER 10

Counseling on Genetic Risk for Cancer

Paula Trahan Rieger, RN, MSN, CS, AOCN, FAAN

Introduction

An important component of cancer prevention is risk assessment. The ability to identify individuals who are at increased risk for developing cancer will allow intensive screening programs and prevention strategies to be targeted to those individuals most in need. Advances in the understanding of cancer biology and of the role of genetics in the development of cancer are dramatically changing the field of cancer care. This chapter focuses on how this new knowledge is being applied in the field of risk assessment.

The discovery of genes that, when altered, confer an increased risk for cancer development will have a profound effect on cancer care. It is currently estimated that 5%–10% of cancers arise in individuals who inherit one of these altered genes and are members of a family in which multiple individuals have an increased risk for developing certain types of cancer. The identification of affected members of these families is now possible. Predisposition genetic testing is having and will continue to have a significant impact on health care, even though many ethical, legal, financial, and psychosocial issues associated with testing remain unresolved.

In the coming years, it will be important for health care professionals to understand how advances in genetics can be integrated into cancer care. All nurses involved in cancer care will ultimately need to be knowledgeable about hereditary cancer syndromes, how to recognize characteristics that may indicate the presence of such a syndrome in a family, and how to initiate appropriate referrals for risk management in members of such families.

Human Genome Project

Errors in genes are known to be responsible for thousands of hereditary diseases such as cystic fibrosis, sickle cell anemia, and Huntington's disease. In addition, altered genes are known to influence the development of multifactorial diseases such as cancer, heart disease, and diabetes; these diseases result from the interaction of genes and environmental factors.[1-4] Advances in technology are making possible discoveries and achievements that were only dreamed of a few years ago. We are on the verge of identifying the genetic changes responsible for a multitude of diseases. A major reason for these achievements is knowledge and technology generated from a landmark project, the Human Genome Project. This project is an international research program established in 1990 through a collaboration between the National Institutes of Health and the U.S. Department of Energy. The project is administered by the National Center for Human Genome Research, an institute of the National Institutes of Health. Scientists from around the world seek to analyze the structure of human DNA and to determine the loca-

tions and sequences of an upward estimate of 100,000 human genes. Understanding the complete set of genes within the human genome will have a profound impact on the management of disease. The initial major goals of the project included development of maps to assist in pinpointing the location of genes and the decoding of the sequences of all nucleotide bases within the genome and thus the identification of specific genes. By identifying a gene's sequence, the protein product of that gene and its normal function in the body can be determined.[1,3,4] In 1998, a new 5-year plan was published in which human DNA sequencing will be the major emphasis. An ambitious schedule has been set to complete the full sequence by the end of 2003, 2 years ahead of previous projections.[2]

The pace of progress often surpasses society's ability to manage the changes that progress brings. To address these changes, the Ethical, Legal, and Social Implications (ELSI) Program was established as part of the project to investigate four areas: (1) ethical issues of genetics research; (2) responsible clinical integration of new genetic technologies; (3) privacy issues and fair use of genetic information by employers, insurers, and others; and (4) professional and public education. To date, the ELSI office has sponsored conferences, courses, and research grants for studies evaluating the implications of this new knowledge.[5] Despite concerns, the Human Genome Project ultimately holds the promise of initiating a new chapter in medicine, that of molecular medicine, that will transform the diagnosis, treatment, and prevention of diseases.

Cancer Risk Assessment

The assessment of risk for developing cancer is an important component of oncology nursing practice and should include obtaining from the patient information about risk factors associated with the development of cancer (e.g., exposure to carcinogens), medical history, and a detailed family history. A *risk factor* is defined broadly as any event or characteristic associated with an increased probability of disease. A major requisite of fully using *primary prevention* (i.e., intervention before pathological changes have begun) as a means of cancer control is the ability to identify carcinogenic agents and host factors that make individuals susceptible to developing cancer. Cancer epidemiology is the field that studies the frequencies, patterns of distribution, and determinants of tumor occurrence in humans.[6] Both environmental and host factors (e.g., genetic predisposition) are examined in an effort to determine causal relationships. The identification of etiologic influences can facilitate prevention, especially in individuals at increased risk, and detection of cancer at an early stage when cure is a realistic expectation.

Advances in technology are also influencing the field of epidemiology. An emerging field is *molecular epidemiology,* which combines the standard tools of epidemiology (case histories, questionnaires, and monitoring of exposure) with sensitive molecular biology laboratory techniques. The goal is to uncover critical precancerous events taking place inside the body and to identify measurable biological flags or markers signaling their occurrence. These biological markers may ultimately be used to more precisely determine exposure to carcinogenic agents and resultant increased risk.[7]

An understanding of how individuals perceive their risk for developing cancer is crucial and will assist the health care professional when providing specific information about risks and prevention and screening recommendations. Research has demonstrated that many individuals tend to overestimate their risk for developing cancer.[8,9] This perception can be influenced by many factors such as family history, life experiences (e.g., losing a parent to cancer at a young age), and understanding of information presented in the media. It is important that individuals understand that the presence of a particular risk factor or trait does not mean that a person will develop a specific cancer and that the absence of a risk factor does not ensure that a person will not develop cancer. For example, a majority of women who develop breast cancer do not have any of the known risk factors.[10,11]

The goals of risk assessment are to understand an individual's perception and concern related to risk for developing cancer, to provide information regarding that risk, to outline recommendations for primary and secondary prevention (i.e., detect disease at its earliest stage and treat it promptly), and to offer psychosocial support so that an individual may better cope with information related to risk and adhere to the recommendations for prevention and screening.[12]

Medical History

A review of the individual's medical and lifestyle history will provide information related to risk for developing cancer. Specific information should be obtained about any previous diagnosis of cancer, the age at diagnosis, and the treatments for that cancer as well as about any preneoplastic lesions such as polyps or breast lesions. For women, information related to reproductive history should also be obtained (e.g., age at menarche, age at menopause, number of children and age at first live birth, hormone history, and sexual history). Information about exposure to carcinogens can be obtained by asking questions about occupation and lifestyle (e.g., smoking, alcohol use, sunlight exposure, dietary practices, and exposure to chemicals).

Family History

A review of family history is important to determine risk and whether characteristics indicative of a hereditary cancer syndrome may be present. Visual representation of

the family history in a pedigree is often helpful (Figure 10-1). While it is desirable to obtain complete information on three generations of the family, both affected (i.e., those with a cancer diagnosis) and unaffected individuals, this is often not realistic in clinical practice. At minimum, information related to parents, siblings, and both maternal and paternal grandparents and aunts and uncles should be obtained. Specific details related to cancers present, age at diagnosis, bilaterality of disease (e.g., bilateral breast cancer), presence of more than one primary tumor, preneoplastic lesions, and prophylactic surgeries will aid in the identification of individuals at an increased risk for cancer and those who should be referred for cancer genetic counseling because of the potential presence of a hereditary cancer syndrome.[13–16] Confirmation of the cancer diagnoses through pathology reports or death certificates is critical for accurate interpretation of risk in high-risk clinics as recall of cancer diagnoses by family members may be inaccurate.

Models for Determining Risk

Models have been developed for determining risk in some cancers. In breast cancer, two tools are currently available for calculating risk. These tools, or models, use data derived from different epidemiological studies. Tabular data, compiled by Claus et al using information from the Cancer and Steroid Hormone Study, is especially useful for evaluating family history because it takes into account the age of affected relatives at cancer onset.[17] The second tool is the Gail Model, based on information gathered from the Breast Cancer Detection and Demonstration Project. The Gail Model uses five variables to calculate risk ratios: current age, age at first live birth, age at menarche, number of first-degree relatives with breast cancer, and number of breast biopsies. With respect to breast biopsies, high-risk indicators such as atypical ductal hyperplasia and lobular neoplasia are also factored in.[11,18] Tables and computer programs are available to estimate individualized age-specific risk based on this model; a program disk is available from the National Cancer Institute. The Gail Model was used to determine eligibility for participation in the breast cancer prevention trial that led to the approval in 1998 of tamoxifen for chemoprevention in women at increased risk for breast cancer.

While these models are useful, they both have limitations. Data were acquired primarily from white women, and thus the models may not apply to women of other races. In addition, both models were developed prior to the discovery of genes associated with hereditary cancer syndromes. Thus, the models tend to underestimate the risk for individuals from families with hereditary breast cancer while overestimating the risk in others. The Gail Model also fails to factor in the powerful indicator of ovarian cancer in a close relative. To date, models are not yet available for use in estimating risk for the development of other types of cancers such as colorectal or prostate cancer.

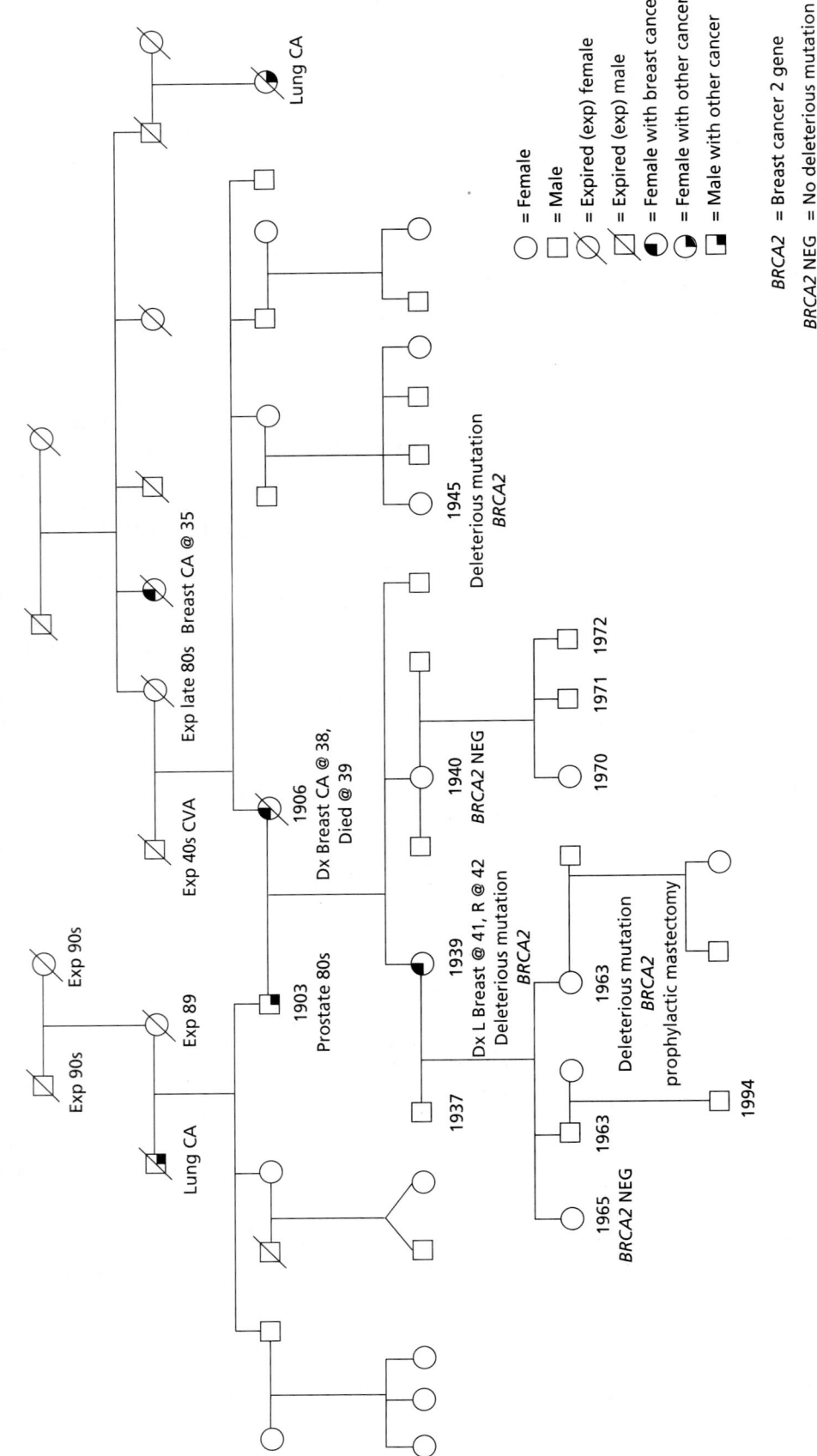

Figure 10-1 Example of a pedigree from a family with known mutation in *BRCA2*.

Hereditary Cancer Syndromes

Many individuals voice the sentiment, "Everyone in my family has cancer." Cancer is a common disease affecting an estimated one in three individuals, contributing to a misconception of increased incidence within families. Aggregation of cancers in a family may occur because of shared cultural, lifestyle, and environmental factors, hereditary influences, chance, or a combination of these factors. Since the eighteenth century, it has been observed that certain types of cancers tend to cluster within some families at a higher rate than would be expected by chance alone. Although many believed that some cancers were hereditary, until recently no genetic basis had been elucidated. Today, as a result of advances in molecular biology and research efforts such as the Human Genome Project,[1,19] the genes associated with hereditary cancer syndromes are rapidly being identified (Table 10-1).[15,20–23] To date, more than 50 cancer-linked genes have been identified.[15,20,24]

Today, it is accepted that all cancer is "genetic," that is, that cancer occurs because of a series of stepwise mutations in genes that control important cellular processes such as cell growth, differentiation, DNA repair, and death. Most cancers are sporadic, resulting from a series of mutations in somatic, or body, cells. It is estimated that only 5%–10% of cancers are due to inheritance of a highly penetrant, rare cancer predisposition gene.[24] Mutated genes associated with hereditary cancer syndromes are

Table 10-1 Overview of Hereditary Cancer Syndromes

Hereditary Cancer Syndromes	Gene/Chromosome Locus	Type of Gene	Inherited Tumor(s)	Recommendations for Testing*
Ataxia telangiectasia	ATM/11q22-23	DNA damage response	Lymphoid leukemias, lymphomas account for majority of tumors; breast cancer and possibly stomach and other cancers	Significance of detection of a germline mutation is not clear; germline mutations have been identified in only a small number of families; medical benefit of identification of carrier not established
Breast/ovarian cancer	BRCA1/17q21	Tumor-suppressor (potential interactions with RAD51 DNA repair genes)	Early-onset breast, ovarian; possibly colon and prostate	High probability of linkage to known cancer susceptibility genes, and for which the medical benefit of the identification of carriers is presumed but not established; potential clinical value and reliability of test are based on research studies
	BRCA2/13q12-13	Tumor-suppressor (potential interactions with RAD51 DNA repair genes)	Early-onset breast, ovarian, male breast cancer, pancreatic cancer, and possibly other cancers	
Cowden's disease	PTEN/MMAC1/10q23	Tumor-suppressor	Breast, thyroid, and colon cancer Associated with other clinical features such as hamartomatous polyps of the colon, breast, thyroid, skin, and mucous membranes; facial trichilemmomas, subcutaneous lipomas, and palmar pits	Not included in original guidelines Germline mutations have been identified in only a small number of families; medical benefit of identification of carrier not well established
Colon cancer Hereditary nonpolyposis colorectal cancer (HNPCC)	hMSH2/2p16 hMLH1/3p21 hPMS1/2q32 hPMS2/7p22 hMSH6/2p16	DNA damage response genes; also termed mismatch repair genes	Colorectal carcinoma, gastric, endometrial, ovarian carcinoma hMSH2 accounts for about 50% of HNPCC hMLH1 accounts for about 30% of HNPCC hPMS1 accounts for <5% of HNPCC hPMS2 accounts for <5% of HNPCC Variant: Muir-Torre syndrome (hMSH2)—Colon, gastric, and larynx tumors; sebaceous skin tumors, keratocanthomata of skin	High probability of linkage to known cancer susceptibility genes, and for which the medical benefit of the identification of carriers is presumed but not established; the potential clinical value and reliability of the test are based on research studies

(continued)

Table 10-1   Overview of Hereditary Cancer Syndromes (continued)

Hereditary Cancer Syndromes	Gene/Chromosome Locus	Type of Gene	Inherited Tumor(s)	Recommendations for Testing*
Peutz-Jeghers	STK11/19p	Tumor-suppressor	Breast, pancreas carcinomas, benign ovarian tumors, testicular cancer; mucocutaneous pigmentation, polyps in the GI tract (especially jejunal polyps), bladder, and renal pelvis	Not included in original guidelines. Germline mutations have been identified in only a small number of families; medical benefit of identification of carrier not established
Familial adenomatous polyposis (FAP)	APC/5q21	Tumor-suppressor	Colorectal cancer: Characterized by multiple (hundreds) adenomatous polyps occurring in the colon and rectum; polyps may be found throughout the GI tract. Nonmalignant features include epidermoid cysts, osteomas, desmoid tumors, and congenital hypertrophy of the retinal pigment epithelium (CHRPE) Variant: Turcot syndrome—polyps in association with brain tumor. In this syndrome, mutations have also been found in HNPCC associated genes	Test used for families with well-defined hereditary syndromes for which either a positive or negative result will change medical care and for which genetic testing may be considered part of the standard management of affected families
Li-Fraumeni syndrome	p53/17p13	Tumor-suppressor	Early-onset breast cancer, childhood bone and soft-tissue sarcomas, brain tumors, childhood leukemias, adrenocortical carcinoma	High probability of linkage to known cancer susceptibility genes, and for which the medical benefit of the identification of carriers is presumed but not established; potential clinical value and reliability of test are based on research studies
Malignant melanoma	CDKN2A (also termed p16, MTS1)/9p	Tumor-suppressor	Cutaneous melanomas; possibly pancreatic cancer and other GI cancers	Significance of detection of a germline mutation is not clear; germline mutations have been identified in only a small number of families; medical benefit of identification of carrier not established
	CDK4/12q14	Oncogene	CDKN2: About 20%–25% of melanoma-prone kindreds	
Multiple endocrine neoplasia (MEN) type 1	MEN1/11q13	Function unknown	Adenomas of the pituitary, parathyroid, pancreas, thyroid, and adrenal cortex; carcinoid tumors of the thyroid, intestine, and bronchus in some cases. Characterized by a high frequency of peptic ulcer disease and endocrine abnormalities	Not included in original guidelines. Germline mutations have been identified in only a small number of families; medical benefit of identification of carrier not well established
Multiple endocrine neoplasia type 2	RET/10q11.2	Oncogene	Pheochromocytoma and medullary thyroid carcinomas; parathyroid tumors and neurofibromas in some cases MEN2A: Characterized by mutations in exons 10 and 11 of RET MEN2B: Characterized by a single mutation in codon 918 (exon 16)	Test used for families with well-defined hereditary syndromes for which either a positive or negative result will change medical care and for which genetic testing may be considered part of the standard management of affected families

Table 10-1   Overview of Hereditary Cancer Syndromes (continued)

Hereditary Cancer Syndromes	Gene/Chromosome Locus	Type of Gene	Inherited Tumor(s)	Recommendations for Testing*
Nevoid basal cell carcinoma syndrome (Gorlin syndrome)	Patched/*PTCH*/9q22	Transmembrane receptor	Multiple basal cell carcinomas (one before age 30); medulloblastoma (5% affected individuals); ovarian carcinomas, fibrosarcomas. Benign neoplasms include jaw cysts, palmar or plantar pits, cutaneous keratocysts and milia, ovarian fibromas, cardiac fibromas, and hamartomatous polyps of the stomach	Not included in original guidelines. Germline mutations have been identified in only a small number of families; medical benefit of identification of carrier not well established
Retinoblastoma	*RB*/13q14	Tumor-suppressor Negative regulators of cell growth	Retinoblastoma; second primary sarcomas such as osteosarcoma of the leg and radiogenic sarcoma of the orbit; cutaneous melanoma	Test used for families with well-defined hereditary syndromes for which either a positive or negative result will change medical care and for which genetic testing may be considered part of the standard management of affected families
von Hippel-Lindau disease	*VHL*/3p25	Tumor-suppressor	Renal cell carcinoma, pheochromocytoma (seen with or without renal cell cancer); additional features include hemangioblastoma; retinal angiomata; pancreatic, renal, and liver hemangiomas; subarachnoid hemorrhage	Test used for families with well-defined hereditary syndromes for which either a positive or negative result will change medical care and for which genetic testing may be considered a part of the standard management of affected families

Data from Fraser[15]; National Cancer Institute[20]; Mills et al[22]; Lindor, Greene.[23]

*Recommendations based on American Society of Clinical Oncology.[60]

carried in the germline cells, the cells responsible for reproduction; these genes have the potential to be passed from generation to generation and confer an inheritable predisposition for cancer development (Figure 10-2).[25] This means that a person who inherits a mutated gene known to cause cancer has an increased likelihood of developing cancer, although for a cancer to develop, other genetic mutations must also occur. In addition, the effects of environment, lifestyle, and other genetic factors on the development of cancer are currently not known. Thus, although cancer predisposition genes increase the likelihood of developing cancer, cancer is not an inevitable outcome. This concept is critically important for genetic counseling and as an underpinning for cancer prevention.

Patterns of Inheritance

The monk Gregor Mendel described the basic modes of inheritance in his pea garden in the 1850s. Different forms (alleles) of a gene may occupy a given genetic locus, or position on the chromosome. Each individual has two copies (alleles) of each gene. The two alleles may be identical or different; together they determine a disease or physical trait. The genetic constitution of an individual is referred to as the *genotype*, whereas the physical, biochemical, or clinical characteristics of the trait are referred to as the *phenotype*.

For diseases produced by dominant genes, only one altered allele is required to produce the disease. Genes that predispose for the development of cancer are generally transmitted in an *autosomal dominant* fashion, meaning that individuals who harbor a mutated gene have a 50% chance of passing the mutated gene on to their children. Inheritance of the altered gene confers an increased risk for developing cancer. The pattern of transmission seen with cancer susceptibility genes is usually vertical (successive generations are affected), and depending on the disease, males and females are generally equally affected (Figure 10-3).[26,27] In classic autosomal dominant inheritance, every affected person in a pedigree has an affected parent. However, this may not be the case in hereditary cancer kindreds for several reasons. First, cancer is a multifactorial disease. The factors that influence the *penetrance*, or expression of a gene that

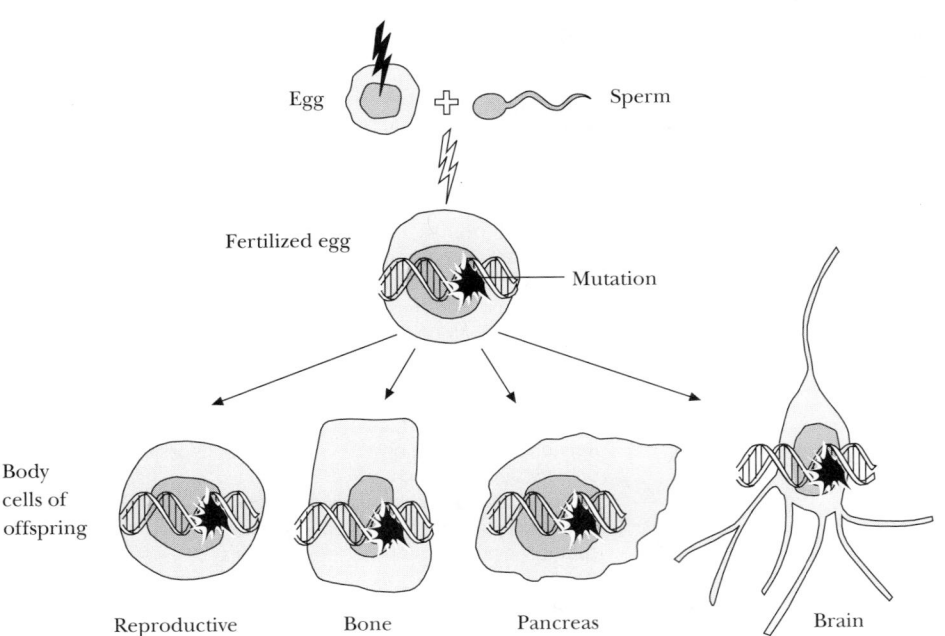

Figure 10-2 Hereditary mutations are carried in the DNA of the reproductive cells. When reproductive cells containing mutations combine to produce offspring, the mutation will be present in all of the offspring's body cells. (Reprinted from the National Institutes of Health and National Cancer Institute, *Understanding Gene Testing*. [NIH pub. no. 96-3905]. Washington, DC, U.S. Department of Health and Human Services, 1995[25])

predisposes for the development of cancer, have not been well elucidated. Thus, within a family, individuals may inherit a gene alteration that predisposes for the development of cancer yet never develop a cancer. Furthermore, the type of cancer usually caused by a specific gene alteration may not be equally expressed in males and females. For example, breast cancer 1 (*BRCA1*), the altered gene associated with hereditary breast and ovarian cancer, may be carried by a male yet not expressed. Males cannot develop ovarian cancer and generally do not develop breast cancer as a consequence of mutations in *BRCA1*. Thus, skipped generations may be seen in families with a hereditary cancer syndrome.

Characteristics of Hereditary Cancer Syndromes

Table 10-1 reviews the most common hereditary cancer syndromes and the associated genes, that when altered, predispose for the development of cancers associated with that syndrome. There are also many syndromes that include an increased susceptibility to cancer in addition to other abnormalities or diseases. However, most of these syndromes, such as Cowden's disease, are quite rare. (Table 10-1 lists some of these syndromes and their other associated clinical features.)

Several common characteristics are seen in families with a hereditary cancer syndrome:

- The occurrence of multiple cases of cancer, especially cancers of the same type (e.g., melanomas or colorectal cancers) or types related to a specific syndrome (e.g., breast and ovary; bowel and endometrium; leu-

kemia and sarcoma) within a single lineage (i.e., the maternal side or the paternal side)

- A diagnosis of cancer at an earlier age than is seen in the general population (e.g., breast cancer before age 50 years)

- The occurrence of multiple cancers in one person (e.g., a person with both colon and uterine cancer)

- The presence of rare tumors, such as retinoblastomas or brain tumors

- Cancer in paired organs (i.e., both breasts or both kidneys)

- Nonmalignant manifestations of a hereditary cancer syndrome (e.g., hamartomas of the skin and mucous membranes and palmar pits, as seen in Cowden disease)

When any of these conditions is present alone or in combination, the possibility of a hereditary cancer syndrome should be considered. During risk assessment, these criteria can serve as "flags" to identify individuals who should be referred for more intensive cancer genetic counseling. Following is a brief review of the hereditary cancer syndromes most commonly seen in clinical practice.

Hereditary Breast and Ovarian Cancer Syndromes

Syndromes of breast cancer susceptibility have been linked to mutations in several genes, including *BRCA1* and breast cancer 2 (*BRCA2*). The precise functions of the *BRCA1* and *BRCA2* genes remain unknown; however, they are both believed to be tumor-suppressor genes.

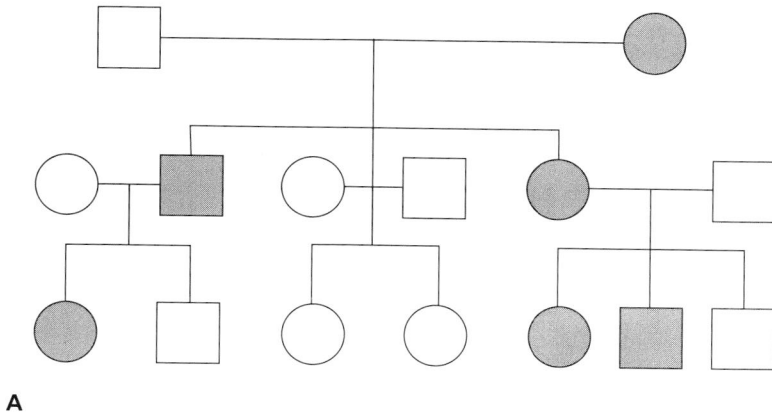

Figure 10-3 Autosomal-dominant inheritance. **A.** A pedigree with affected family members. **B.** How an altered gene is passed. Reprinted with permission from Lea, DH; Jenkins, JL & Francoman O, 1998. *Genetics in Clinical Practice, New Directions for Nursing and Health Care.* Sudbury, MA, Jones & Bartlett, p. 45.

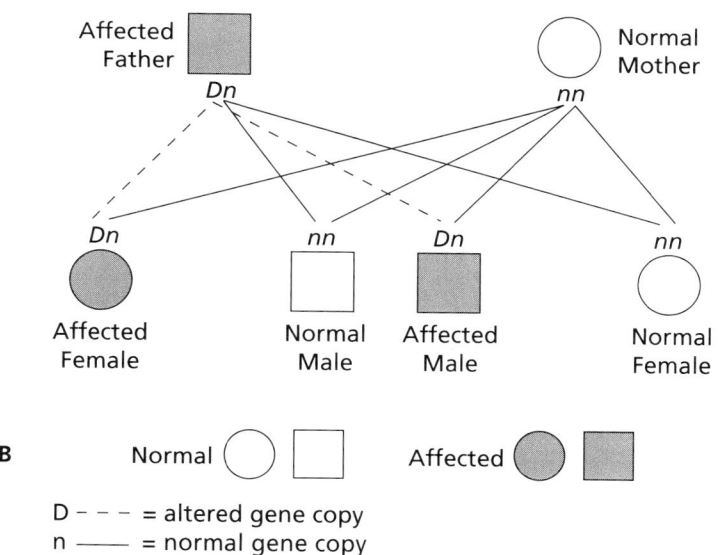

Their most likely function is in transcriptional regulation and DNA repair.[28] The traditional approach to identifying genes that predispose to cancer has been to localize the gene to a particular chromosome by using a technique known as *linkage analysis*. In this approach, DNA from multiple family members is studied, and the gene is localized to a particular chromosome according to how it segregates with identified markers on the chromosome during the meiotic phase of cell division. This was accomplished for *BRCA1* in 1990[29,30] and for *BRCA2* in 1994.[31]

The sequence of nucleotide bases in a gene codes for the production of a protein. Once a gene has been localized to a particular chromosome, the next step is to identify the gene and determine the precise sequence of nucleotide bases for that gene. This was accomplished for *BRCA1* in 1994[32] and for *BRCA2* in 1995.[33] *BRCA1* is located on chromosome 17q (long arm) and is thought to account for 30%–45% of breast cancer cases in families with a high incidence of early-onset breast and ovarian cancer. *BRCA2* is located on chromosome 13q and appears to account for about 35% of families with early-onset breast cancer. Thus, while *BRCA1* and *BRCA2* mutations account for a significant percentage of hereditary breast cancer, it is believed that other, as yet undiscovered genes such as breast cancer 3 (*BRCA3*) may also increase susceptibility to breast and other cancers. In contrast, it is believed that *BRCA1* and *BRCA2* mutations account for the majority of familial ovarian cancers.

With respect to certain hereditary cancer syndromes, the concept of a *founder effect* is important. This effect is defined as an unusual prevalence of specific genotypes in a population and produces a greater-than-expected frequency of a specific mutation in common descendants of an ancestor. Founder effects frequently occur due to migration, a limited number of ancestors, and catastrophes. Founder effects have been seen in several hereditary cancer syndromes. For example, in *BRCA1* and *BRCA2* families, specific mutations are commonly seen in those of Ashkenazi Jewish, French-Canadian, Dutch, and Icelandic heritage. Thus, it is always important to inquire about an individual's heritage.

The lifetime risk for developing breast cancer in *BRCA1*-linked families is relatively high. In the general population, the cumulative incidence for breast cancer by age 50 is 2%, whereas in women with an alteration in *BRCA1*, the risk may be as high as 50%. Some mutations may carry a lower penetrance than others; thus, lifetime risk for breast cancer may range from 60% to as high as 85% in some families. In the general population, the lifetime risk for ovarian cancer is in the range of 1%–2%. In those women with an alteration in *BRCA1*, the lifetime risk may range from 20%–60%. There may also be a small but significant increased risk for prostate cancer in men and colon cancer in men and women with *BRCA1* mutations.[34–36]

A lifetime risk of breast cancer similar to that in families with *BRCA1* mutations is seen in families with *BRCA2* alterations, although some data indicate that the onset of breast cancer may be at an older age. Ovarian cancer is also seen in women carrying mutations in *BRCA2* although to a lesser extent than with *BRCA1*. Estimates for the lifetime risk of ovarian cancer range from 10%–20% in women with *BRCA2* mutations. Other cancers that may be associated with *BRCA2* mutations include pancreatic, fallopian tube, laryngeal, uterine, and male breast cancers as well as leukemia. The estimated lifetime risk of breast cancer for male carriers of *BRCA2* mutations is roughly 6%.[21,34,37–40]

Hereditary Colon Cancers

About 1 in 18 individuals will be diagnosed with colorectal cancer in their lifetime. Highly penetrant cancer susceptibility syndromes account for about 5% of colorectal cancers. The most common syndrome is hereditary nonpolyposis colon cancer (HNPCC), with familial adenomatous polyposis (FAP) being much less frequent.

Hereditary nonpolyposis colon cancer

This cancer is evidenced by early-onset colorectal cancer (diagnosis before the age of 50 years), and extracolonic tumors such as uterine, ovarian, stomach, and small intestine tumors, and transitional cell tumors of the renal pelvis and ureter. Individuals who have HNPCC have inherited a germline mutation in one of the several genes responsible for repairing DNA mismatches. These genes have been termed *spell checker genes*. Mismatch repair genes allow for accurate transmission of genetic information from a cell to its progeny by recognizing abnormal base pairs and correcting the sequence on one strand to restore normal base pairing. Mutations in the following genes have been found to cause HNPCC: *hMSH2* (found on chromosome 2p [short arm]), *hMLH1* (found on chromosome 3p), *hPMS1* (found on chromosome 2p), *hPMS2* (found on chromosome 7p), and *hMSH6* (found on chromosome 2p). *Microsatellites* are stable stretches

of DNA throughout the genome that are repetitive and usually do not encode for proteins. Most cancers in patients with HNPCC show a high degree of microsatellite instability. Microsatellite instability provided clues for the discovery of genes associated with this syndrome in the early 1990s.[41–43]

Individuals inheriting one of these genes can anticipate a 70%–75% risk of developing colorectal cancer by age 65 years. In some families, the penetrance may range as high as 90%. The median age at diagnosis is less than 50 years. In many families, *synchronous cancers* of the colon (several tumors presenting at the same time) and *metachronous tumors* (several tumors presenting at different times) have been documented. The risk for endometrial cancer ranges from 20%–30% by age 70 years as compared to a populational risk of 3%.[21,39]

The International Collaborative Group on HNPCC defined criteria for identifying the syndrome at a meeting in Amsterdam in 1991. These criteria are known as the *Amsterdam criteria* and define the syndrome as histologically verified colorectal cancer in three or more relatives, one of whom is a first-degree relative of the other two; colorectal cancer involving at least two generations; and one or more colorectal cancer cases diagnosed before 50 years of age. A limitation of these criteria has been the omission of endometrial and other extracolonic tumors. A subsequent meeting developed the Bethesda criteria for HNPCC, which includes the Amsterdam criteria, pedigrees with a colon cancer case before 40 years, and pedigrees with a high incidence of noncolonic tumors associated with HNPCC.[44] A National Cancer Institute workshop was held in December 1997 to review and unify the field and develop recommendations on microsatellite instability and its use for cancer detection and identification of familial predisposition. At this meeting, the Bethesda guidelines were endorsed.[45]

Familial adenomatous polyposis

This is a rare syndrome characterized by hundreds to thousands of polyps carpeting the colon that inevitably progress to colon cancer. Polyps usually begin to appear in an affected person's late teens and twenties, and if untreated (generally by prophylactic colectomy), death from colon cancer will occur in virtually all cases by age 50 years. Congenital hypertrophy of the retinal pigment epithelium is a useful diagnostic marker for the syndrome and consists of pigmented lesions in the retina that can be detected by funduscopic examination. Individuals with a variant form of FAP known as Gardner's syndrome also exhibit sebaceous cysts, lipomas, desmoid tumors, fibromas, facial bone osteomas, and impacted or supernumerary teeth.

The *APC* gene is associated with FAP. As are most genes associated with hereditary cancer syndromes, the *APC* gene is large, and a wide spectrum of mutations have been observed. However, genotype-phenotype correlations have begun to be identified. Most mutations in *APC* have been observed in the 5′ half of the gene, with a large number in a defined region within exon 15.[21,46,47]

Cancer Genetic Counseling

A variety of health care professionals with specialized training such as oncologists, oncology nurses, genetic counselors, and clinical geneticists now provide cancer genetic counseling. It is helpful for the practicing oncology nurse to understand the process of cancer genetic counseling and genetic testing so that when individuals are referred for these specialized services, the nurse will be knowledgeable regarding the type and scope of services that should be provided. Table 10-2 provides an overview of the cancer genetic counseling process.[12,26]

Definition

Genetic counseling is a risk assessment, communication and educational process by which individuals and family members receive information about the nature and limitations of genetic tests, benefits, risks, costs, and meaning of test results. Counseling and support concerning the implications of information gained from testing are a vital component of this process.[21,48,49] Regardless of the setting in which cancer predisposition genetic testing is offered (e.g., within the context of a clinical trial or as a commercially available test), individuals must receive adequate information to make an informed decision concerning their health and give informed consent to undergo testing. Genetic testing must be conducted only in conjunction with genetic counseling to assure that this process occurs.

Services Provided

Comprehensive services should include determinations of the individual's reasons for seeking cancer risk counseling; data collection that provides an in-depth review of the family history (a minimum of three complete generations) and patterns of transmission of cancers within the family; risk assessment as outlined above; determination of the client's level of knowledge regarding hereditary cancer syndromes and cancer genetics, self-perception of risk for developing cancer, and the motivation for seeking predisposition genetic testing; recommendations for management of risk (i.e., surveillance, chemoprevention, prophylactic surgery); evaluation of the appropriateness of testing; education regarding the testing process and the benefits, risks, limitations, costs, and potential outcomes that may result from testing; and disclosure of test results and their implications. All counseling should

---

Table 10-2 The Cancer Genetic Counseling Process

Clinical Activity	Information To Be Discussed
Assessment and information gathering	
Reason for referral	Patient concerns and questions Physician recommendation
Information gathering	
Family history	Collect information on 3 generations when possible Minimum: parents, siblings, aunts, uncles, grandparents Cancers in the family: age at diagnosis, bilaterality in paired organs, more than one primary tumor Relevant genetic testing results Verification by pathology report or death certificates of cancers in the family is critical
Personal history	Past medical history and screening practices History relevant to cancer risk assessment (e.g., gynecologic history for breast/ovarian cancer) Lifestyle factors (e.g., smoking, alcohol, carcinogen exposure)
Patient perception of risk for cancer	Beliefs about cancer and its causation Patient perception of lifetime risk for developing cancer and probability of altered gene in the family that is "responsible" for cancer
Social, emotional, and cultural concerns	Cultural beliefs Support systems Economic factors
Evaluation and analysis of data	
Family history	Assess family for characteristics seen with hereditary cancer syndromes Estimate of probability that family would test positive for alteration in cancer predisposition gene
Focused physical examination	Dependent on syndrome present in the family (e.g., eye exam for FAP)
Laboratory testing	Dependent on syndrome present in the family

(continued)

Table 10-2 The Cancer Genetic Counseling Process (continued)

Clinical Activity	Information To Be Discussed
Communication of genetic and risk information	
Natural history of condition	Discussion of types of cancer seen in the family Explanation of suspected hereditary cancer syndrome
Inheritance patterns	Review of autosomal dominant transmission of cancer predisposition genes
Discussion of risk for developing cancer	Populational risk and estimated risk for patient Review in terms of several types of risk (e.g., in terms of relative risk, lifetime risk)
Ramifications and appropriateness of cancer predisposition genetic testing	Benefits, risks, limitations, costs of testing Potential answers that may be obtained Who in the family is best to test
Strategies for managing risk	Lifestyle changes Options for screening and detection Signs and symptoms of cancer Chemoprevention Prophylactic surgery
Supportive counseling	
Discussion of patient and family questions and concerns	Common concerns include potential risk for children, potential for discrimination due to cancer predisposition genetic testing
Providing emotional and social support	Determination of existing coping patterns and support systems Teaching new coping strategies as required Assisting patient in discussing genetic testing results with family Allow patient and family to voice fears and concerns Discussion of how to communicate results to relatives
Referral for additional counseling and support as needed	Available support systems for patients with extreme anxiety and distress
Follow-up counseling	
Further discussion of genetic testing results (if performed) and risk for developing cancer	Review patient questions and concerns Review strategies for managing increased risk Discuss availability of clinical trials for long-term follow-up, chemoprevention, new screening technologies
Written summary and follow-up letter	Summary of discussion of family history, assessment of risk for developing cancer, probability of gene in the family, issues related to genetic testing, and strategies for managing risk
Coordination of care with other health care providers such as oncologist, primary care provider	Obtain permission from patient for release to other health care providers
Discussion with relatives about implications of results	Obtain permission from patients for release of information to relatives who may wish to come for cancer genetic counseling

Data from Mahon[12]; Lea et al.[26]

include an evaluation of the patient's psychosocial status, support systems, ability to receive and cope with test results, and referrals as appropriate for medical or surgical means of early detection or prevention of cancer.[16,21,50,51] It is considered mandatory, and is often standard practice in many centers that provide cancer genetic counseling, that individuals receive a follow-up letter after counseling that documents clearly the information provided regarding family history, risk assessment, implications of testing and/or known results, and recommendations for management of risks. It is also critically important to attempt to obtain documentation of the cancers in the family through securing pathology records or death certificates.

Health Care Professionals Involved in Cancer Genetic Counseling

Cancer genetic counseling services are generally provided using a multidisciplinary approach. Most counseling is provided by advanced practice oncology nurses with specialized training in cancer genetics or by genetic counselors with specialized training in the field of oncology in collaboration with medical oncologists or clinical geneticists. Traditionally, the nondirective provision of information was used as a guiding principle in genetic counseling to enable individuals to make their own decisions. This approach was applied to all components of the process, including discussion of the use of genetic testing to identify disease or a predisposition for disease, and discussion of the specific features or management of the genetic condition. In essence, counselors did not make recommendations one way or the other as to which decision would be the "best."

With respect to cancer genetic counseling, however, this philosophy has been questioned because occasionally, clear medical recommendations can be made about managing genetic risk. For example, effective surgical options exist for managing individuals at increased risk for developing colorectal cancer. The health care provider is obligated to recommend such options. Nevertheless, the ultimate goal is the provision of balanced and complete information so that an individual may make an informed decision concerning his or her health. Those providing counseling should be aware of their own biases and philosophy toward testing so that their opinions do not inadvertently influence an individual's decisions.

Patient Education

During the process of cancer genetic counseling, information that is often technically complex and emotionally laden must be presented to individuals. Oncology nurses are well versed in the provision of patient education, and the fundamentals for providing quality education can be applied to the counseling process. Assessment of an individual for any barriers to learning, such as hearing problems, decreased visual acuity, primary language other than English, low literacy level, or changes in emotional status (extreme anxiety, distress, or distrust), is important to guide both choice and adjustment of teaching and counseling methodologies. A variety of teaching methodologies, such as face-to-face communication, and video, audio, and written materials, can be used to present information in a manner that best suits the person seeking consultation. The individual's understanding of the information given should be assessed periodically during the counseling session, and an opportunity for questions should be provided.[52-54]

Problems and Issues Related to Cancer Genetic Counseling and Genetic Testing

Predisposition genetic testing is new, and there are many issues surrounding its use. The major topics that must be addressed during the process of cancer genetic counseling include the setting for testing, informed consent, discussion of the accuracy of the test and interpretation of test results, psychosocial issues, and management of risk.

Setting for Testing

Controversy exists over whether cancer predisposition genetic testing should be offered to patients outside of a research setting as such testing has not been integrated into medical decision making for the majority of cancers.[55-58] Predisposition testing is commercially available for numerous cancers, so it may not always be offered within the context of clinical research or even with cancer genetic counseling. However, some groups contend that all cancer predisposition testing should be conducted within the context of research because many unanswered questions remain regarding genetic testing for hereditary cancer syndromes and management of individuals who are at increased risk for developing cancer. If all testing is done within a clinical trial, answers to these questions can be obtained more rapidly.[59] Examples of clinical trials focused on predisposition genetic testing would be those designed to answer questions related to management of risk, to determine psychological responses to genetic information, or to search for additional genes that, when altered, are associated with hereditary cancer syndromes. The American Society of Clinical Oncology has set forth guidelines for cancer predisposition testing.[60] The provision of cancer genetic counseling may be impacted by many factors. Table 10-3 outlines individual, family, cultural, ethnic, and structural factors that must be considered when providing services.[61]

Table 10-3 Factors Influencing Cancer Genetic Counseling

Individual frame of reference
  Personal philosophy about cancer
  Life experience with cancer
  Self-perception of risk
  Anxiety over cancer risk
  Opinions about obtaining genetic information

Family considerations
  Differing opinions about obtaining genetic information
  Presence of family members during counseling

Cultural and ethnic considerations
  Views on cancer as a disease
  Views on genetics and genetic testing
  Decision-making process within the family

Structural considerations
  Health care providers
    Multidisciplinary team providing counseling and expertise in cancer care
  Setting
    Wellness setting (e.g., prevention center)
    Illness setting (e.g., within cancer treatment center)
  Payment for counseling services
  Payment for genetic testing
  Timing (e.g., near recent diagnosis of cancer, near recent death in the family from cancer)
  Record keeping
    Documentation of services
    Communication with other health care professionals

Data from Rieger, Pentz.[61]

Informed Consent

A principal concern about predisposition genetic testing is that individuals receive adequate information to give informed consent.[61-63] Many believe that performing predisposition testing within the context of a clinical trial will assure that adequate information is provided to individuals because of the requirement for written informed consent for participants in research. Numerous position statements have been published concerning the process of genetic testing and counseling [60,63-68] (Table 10-4),[59,60,64-73] and although the majority speak to the necessity of informed consent, most do not mandate that all genetic testing be conducted within clinical trials. The Task Force on Genetic Testing strongly advocates written informed consent and states that respect for personal autonomy is paramount.[74] Table 10-5 reviews topics that should be discussed during the informed-consent process.[26,61]

Accuracy of the Test and Interpretation of Results

Information about cancer predisposition genetic testing abounds in the lay media and on the Internet; thus, individuals frequently seek predisposition genetic testing with unrealistic expectations of what testing can provide. During cancer genetic counseling, the counselor must review how the test is performed, the type of test to be used (e.g., protein truncation versus full-sequencing of the gene), the sensitivity and specificity of the test, who

in the family is the best person to test, potential answers that may be obtained, and the meaning of each answer.

In the broadest sense, genetic tests are defined as the analysis of human DNA, RNA, chromosomes, proteins, and other gene products to detect disease-related genotypes, mutations, phenotypes, or karyotypes.[73] The tests may be helpful in identifying those at risk of getting the disease in question, identifying carriers of mutated genes, establishing diagnoses or prognoses, and establishing genetic identity (paternity). Commercially available genetic tests are based on a variety of techniques such as protein truncation assays, heteroduplex analysis, versions of single-strand conformational polymorphism (SSCP) analysis, and direct sequencing of the gene of interest. The first three techniques involve the use of gels to detect changes in mobility patterns of either proteins or single strands of DNA (SSCP) or double strands of DNA (heteroduplex analysis). The most sensitive technique to date, considered the gold standard, is the test done to determine the DNA sequence of both copies of the gene. Although highly accurate, sequencing is both expensive and labor intensive. It can be likened to trying to find a spelling error in one word in an article that is several thousand words long. The cost of commercial predisposition genetic testing may range from several hundred dollars (e.g., when confirming a known mutation that has been found in another family member or when using panels that assess for several mutations commonly seen in those of a specific heritage) to several thousand dollars for full sequencing of large genes such as *BRCA1* or *BRCA2*. Depending on the test being performed and the

Table 10-4   Position Statements on Genetic Testing

Organization	Position Statement
American Society of Clinical Oncology (ASCO)	Genetic Testing for Cancer Susceptibility
	Cancer Genetics and Cancer Predisposition Testing Curriculum Guidelines
American Society of Human Genetics	Statement on Informed Consent for Genetic Research
	Statement on Disclosure of Familial Genetic Information
	Breast/Ovarian Cancer Predisposition
American Society of Human Genetics and American College of Medical Genetics	Points to Consider: Ethical, Legal, and Psychosocial Implications of Genetic Testing in Children and Adolescents
Cancer Genetic Studies Consortium (Task Force on Informed Consent)	Genetic Testing for Susceptibility to Adult-Onset Cancer: The Process and Content of Informed Consent
National Advisory Council for Human Genome Research	Statement on the Use of DNA Testing for Presymptomatic Identification of Cancer Risk
National Breast Cancer Coalition	Presymptomatic Genetic Testing for Heritable Breast Cancer Risk
National Society of Genetic Counselors	Predisposition Genetic Testing
Oncology Nursing Society	The Role of the Oncology Nurse in Cancer Genetic Counseling
	Cancer Genetic Testing and Risk Assessment Counseling

Data from American Society of Human Genetics ad Hoc Committe,[59] American Society of Clinical oncology,[60] American Society of Human Genetics,[64] National Advisory Council for Human Genome Research,[65] National Breast Cancer Coalition,[66] National Society of Genetic Counselors I,[67] Oncology Nursing Society,[68] American Society of Clinical Oncology,[69] American Society of Human Genetics,[70] College of Medical Genetics, American Society of Human Genetics,[71] Oncology Nursing Society,[72] Task Force on Genetic Testing.[73]

Table 10-5   Topics To Be Discussed During the Informed Consent Process

Purpose of the genetic test

Reason for offering testing

Type and nature of genetic condition being tested for

Accuracy of genetic test

Benefits of participating in testing

Risks associated with genetic testing, including unexpected results

Other available testing options

Available treatment and intervention options

Further decision making that may be needed on receipt of test results

Consent to use patient's DNA for further research purposes

Availability of additional counseling and support services

Acknowledgment of the right to refuse testing

Reprinted with permission from Lea D, Jenkins JF, Francomano C: *Genetics in Clinical Practice: New Directions for Nursing and Health Care.* Sudbury, MA, Jones and Bartlett, p 85, 1998.[26]

approach used, it often requires 4–6 weeks to obtain results.[34,37,75–77]

The meaning and likelihood of each genetic test result (positive, negative, or inconclusive) must be reviewed in detail. If a deleterious mutation is found (positive test result), the individual must clearly understand that this denotes a predisposition for the development of cancer, not a diagnosis or even inevitability of cancer development. Information related to the penetrance of the mutation must be reviewed. Because cancer susceptibility genes were only recently discovered, knowledge in this field continues to evolve. With some genes, such as the *APC* gene associated with FAP, penetrance is near 100%, and medical management is well defined; while with others, such as the *BRCA1* gene, penetrance is less, and medical management is not yet clearly defined.[21,60,78] When there is a known mutation in the family and an individual's test is negative for that mutation, it is important for the individual to realize that he or she still has the general populational risk for the development of cancer.

Some answers from testing may provide no additional information for an individual or the family. A negative test result is often difficult to interpret when no known mutation has yet been detected in a family. Negative test results may be obtained because the test missed something (i.e., a false-negative because of technical difficulties or the location of a mutation in a region of the gene not tested, such as promoter, enhancer, or intronic regions), because there is an as yet undiscovered gene responsible for the constellation of cancers seen in the family, or because the cancers may have resulted purely from chance. Results are considered inconclusive if sequence changes are found about which insufficient information currently exists to determine whether the changes are deleterious or simply a harmless genetic variation within the population (polymorphism). In such cases, it remains difficult to determine cancer risk. Depending

on the family history, in many instances the individual would still be considered at high risk.

To provide the most information for a family, it is best to test an affected individual (e.g., one who has already developed cancer). However, even this carries with it the risk of testing a person who developed a sporadic cancer within a family that has a specific genetic alteration. Many centers will *only* test affected individuals. In many families, however, this may not be possible or practical. Therefore, when an unaffected individual is tested, it is important to reinforce the limitations of this approach and how results will ultimately be interpreted within the context of the family. A positive test result for a known deleterious mutation will provide information for the family. However, depending on the syndrome, a negative test result—one that finds no evidence of a mutation—may provide no information for the family. It provides information solely for the individual being tested. Thus, individuals must realize that testing for many hereditary cancer syndromes is new and may provide no additional information concerning risk for developing cancer.

Psychosocial Issues

Predisposition genetic testing for susceptibility to cancer carries with it unique psychosocial implications of which oncology nurses and those providing cancer risk counseling services must be aware and able to discuss openly with patients. Because the ability to perform predisposition genetic tests is new, assessing the psychological impact of test results remains an important area of research. Studies are just beginning to evaluate the reasons persons seek to be tested and the factors that influence their desire to receive results. Most published studies on psychosocial issues have evaluated high-risk families who participated in the original research studies attempting to identify cancer predisposition genes. To prevent and manage a patient's potential adverse reactions to the disclosure of genetic status, health care professionals who provide cancer risk assessment and counseling services must be sure the patient understands the benefits, risks, and limitations of testing prior to cancer susceptibility testing and once again before results are disclosed. The health care provider must evaluate family dynamics and the patient's cultural and health care beliefs, reinforce the patient's existing coping skills and teach new ones for handling the information provided, facilitate the patient's decision-making through nondirective counseling, and identify patients who may need referral to a mental health professional.[79–83] Table 10-6 outlines some of the benefits and risks that are related to cancer predisposition genetic testing.

The confidentiality of results remains an area of question and concern. Many individuals harbor concerns over misuse of information or negative sequelae that may result from release of test results, such as discrimination with respect to employment opportunities, or health, life, disability, or mortgage insurance coverage.[84–86] At a workshop jointly sponsored by the ELSI Working Group and the National Action Plan on Breast Cancer, a public-

Table 10-6 Benefits and Risks of Cancer Genetic Testing

Positive Results	Inconclusive Results	Negative Results*
BENEFITS		
Ability to tailor more aggressive cancer screening and detection measures to those individuals carrying the highest risk	May provide feeling of empowerment, i.e., something was done to look for cause of multiple cancers within the family	Extra surveillance unnecessary as cancer risk would be the same as for the general population
Reduction of uncertainty and anxiety		Relief that children cannot inherit the altered gene
Ability to test other family members for known mutation within the family		Financial savings from decreased surveillance
Reason as to "why" cancer developed		Decreased anxiety about ability to plan for the future
		Relief over not having greatly increased risk for developing cancer
RISKS		
Anxiety and depression over increased cancer risk	Anxiety and depression over uncertain results	Delay in seeking recommended cancer screening measures
Fear that "nothing can be done" to minimize risk for developing cancer	Family continues to be monitored as high-risk family	Survivor guilt
Lowered life goals	"No news"	Depression because increased cancer risks can no longer serve as cause of problems
Strained relationships with family (e.g., guilt over passing mutation to children)	Current testing techniques and state of knowledge cannot classify all mutations as positive (deleterious) or negative	Strained relationships within the family
Potential for discrimination by employers, insurers, and state licensing agencies		
Financial costs of cancer screening and detection		
Positive tests predict risk of developing disease, not occurrence of cancer; age or time of developing cancer unknown		

*when there is a known mutation within the family
Data from Rieger[16]; Lea et al[26]; Loescher.[77]

private partnership created to eliminate breast cancer, issues related to genetic discrimination and health insurance were discussed and recommendations formulated for state and federal policy-makers to protect against genetic discrimination.[84] Several states have enacted legislation prohibiting discrimination by health insurers and, in some cases, employers. Federal legislation passed in 1996, the Kennedy-Kassebaum bill,[87] includes safeguards against discrimination based on genetic information, but its effectiveness in protecting consumers has yet to be tested in the courts. It is anticipated that in the future, additional federal and state bills will be enacted to address these concerns. To date, few if any cases of overt discrimination related to cancer genetic testing have been documented. Nevertheless, individuals' fears of discrimination have a direct impact on patients' willingness to seek genetic counseling and testing and on the practice of health care professionals. Serious consideration must be given to how results are documented, communicated, and managed to ensure confidentiality. Many institutions do not place results obtained from cancer predisposition genetic testing in the patient's medical record, and in addition they may require signed consent from the individual who has been tested to release or discuss results with family members, insurers, or other health care professionals. See Table 10-7 for questions patients should ask genetic testing providers.[77]

Management of Risk

The field of cancer prevention is changing rapidly as information gleaned through an understanding of cancer at the molecular level and an ability to target those at the highest risk of developing cancer are integrated into new prevention and detection strategies. Because of the high lifetime risk for developing cancer associated with mutations in cancer predisposition genes, measures to manage risk for those carrying a mutation is of pressing importance. Options fall into three basic categories: (1) chemoprevention, (2) prophylactic surgery, and (3) screening and detection measures.

Table 10-7   Questions for Patients To Ask During Cancer Genetic Counseling

Questions for Providers of Commercial Testing	Questions for Providers of Testing Performed as Research
• How much does the test cost?	• If the cost of testing is covered under the research protocol, what additional costs are borne by participants?
• Is payment for the test required at the time of testing?	• What is the turnaround time for receiving test results?
• What are the informed consent procedures for the test?	• Is the testing protocol approved by an IRB? Which IRB?
• Has the consent been approved by an institutional review board (IRB)?	• What are the informed consent procedures for the test? Have these been approved by an IRB?
• Is there established clinical/analytical validity of the test?	• Are protocols of tests in developmental phases being conducted in a laboratory certified under CLIA?
• Does the testing laboratory participate in internal or external (e.g., College of American Pathology molecular oncology program or American College of Medical Genetics medical genetics proficiency program) monitoring of procedures?	• Has a pilot phase been conducted verifying that all steps in the testing process are operating appropriately?
• Do laboratory personnel have formal training in human and medical genetics? Cancer genetics?	• Does the testing laboratory participate in internal or external monitoring of procedures?
• What types of follow-up data are/have been collected after marketing of the test?	• Do laboratory personnel have formal training in human and medical genetics? Cancer genetics?
• How is confidentiality maintained?	• How is confidentiality of results maintained?
• What are the qualifications of the personnel providing cancer genetic counseling?	• What are the qualifications of the personnel providing cancer genetic counseling?
• What type of support services are available?	• What type of support services are available?
• Are Clinical Laboratory Improvement Act (CLIA) regulations followed?	

Adapted with permission from Loescher LJ: DNA testing for coancer predisposition. *Oncol Nurs Forum* 25:1317–1327, 1998.[77]

Chemoprevention

Preventive measures for those at high risk of developing cancer are only beginning to be evaluated. *Chemoprevention* is defined as the use of natural or synthetic chemical agents to reverse, suppress, or prevent carcinogenic progression to invasive cancer.[88] As more is understood about the nature of carcinogenesis, the ability to intervene at the earliest stages is becoming a greater possibility. Recognition of dysplastic lesions as biologically significant at their preinvasive stage is a paradigm shift that may lead to the design of effective prevention measures. In addition, study of the intrinsic biological mechanisms that may prevent these lesions from becoming invasive and metastatic can also offer insight into the design of new, effective therapeutic strategies.[89,90]

Conceptually, chemoprevention agents may be classified into two categories: agents that prevent initiation of the carcinogenic process (blocking agents) and those that prevent further promotion or progression of lesions that have already been established (suppressing agents). In reality, the distinction between these categories is often artificial. Over the last 20 years, there have been numerous trials to evaluate the effectiveness of various agents in the chemoprevention of cancer. For a complete review of chemoprevention trials and major categories of agents used in the chemoprevention of cancer, see Chapter 8.[90–92]

An example of how chemoprevention may potentially be applied to high-risk populations is the use of nonsteroidal anti-inflammatory drugs (NSAIDs) for the prevention

of colorectal cancer. Several large, observational, epidemiological studies for those who self-elect to take NSAIDs have demonstrated a lowering of the risk for colorectal cancer. Limitations of these studies are difficulty in controlling for confounding variables and lack of randomization. However, based on these findings and those from basic research, the rationale for the use of NSAIDs in preventing colorectal cancer is supported.[93] The National Cancer Institute has sponsored several chemoprevention trials using NSAIDs for the prevention of adenomas in those at high risk for developing colorectal cancer due to an inherited predisposition (FAP or HNPCC).

The finding of a decrease in contralateral breast cancer incidence following tamoxifen administration for adjuvant breast cancer therapy led to the concept that the drug might play a role in breast cancer prevention. To test this hypothesis, the National Surgical Adjuvant Breast and Bowel Project initiated the Breast Cancer Prevention Trial (BCPT) in 1992. Women at increased risk for breast cancer because they were (1) 60 years of age or older, (2) 35–59 years of age with a 5-year predicted risk for breast cancer of at least 1.67%, or (3) had a history of lobular carcinoma in situ were randomly assigned to receive placebo or tamoxifen 20 mg/day for 5 years. The Gail Model, based on a multivariate logistic regression model using combinations of risk factors, was used to estimate the probability (risk) of occurrence of breast cancer over time.

Results from the trial were publicly released in 1998. Tamoxifen reduced the risk of invasive breast cancer by

49%, with cumulative incidences through 69 months of follow-up of 43.4 and 22.0 per 1000 women in the placebo and tamoxifen groups, respectively. Risk was decreased 44% in women aged 49 years or younger, 51% in those aged 50–59 years, and 55% in those 60 years or older. Risk was also reduced 56% in women with a history of lobular carcinoma in situ and 86% in those with a history of atypical hyperplasia. In fact, risk was reduced in women in all risk categories. Tamoxifen reduced the risk of non-invasive breast cancer by 50% and the occurrence of estrogen receptor–positive tumors by 69%, but no difference in the occurrence of estrogen receptor–negative tumors was seen.[94] Although two small European trials failed to confirm the observations from the BCPT trial, tamoxifen received regulatory approval for use in women at increased risk for developing breast cancer in 1998. Differences between these trials may result from reduced power in the smaller trials and different selection criteria. The implications of these results for women who may be carriers of mutations in *BRCA1* or *BRCA2* were not addressed in the trial but are currently being analyzed.

Oral contraceptives have been proven to protect against ovarian cancer in general, but it is not known whether they also protect against hereditary forms of ovarian cancer. Narod et al enrolled 207 women with hereditary ovarian cancer and 161 of their sisters as controls in a case-control study.[95] Lifetime histories of oral contraceptive use were obtained by interview or by written questionnaire and were compared between patients and control women, after adjustment for year of birth and parity. Their results demonstrated that risk for developing ovarian cancer decreased with increasing duration of use of oral contraceptives. They concluded that oral contraceptive use may reduce the risk of ovarian cancer in women with pathogenic mutations in the *BRCA1* or *BRCA2* gene.[95]

Prophylactic surgery

Many individuals faced with a high lifetime risk of developing cancer consider the option of prophylactic surgery as a means to manage their risk. The effectiveness of prophylactic surgery must be evaluated in the context of clinical trials, and currently few data exist on the effectiveness of this intervention. For some conditions, such as FAP or hereditary medullary thyroid cancer, prophylactic surgery is accepted practice.[47,96,97] In other situations, such as hereditary breast and ovarian cancer, prophylactic surgery is more controversial. Although it is often assumed that prophylactic mastectomy will greatly decrease the risk of breast cancer, not all breast cells can realistically be removed. The precise degree of risk reduction associated with prophylactic mastectomy or oophorectomy has not yet been determined for individuals who carry a mutation that predisposes for breast or ovarian cancer. Individuals that choose the option of prophylactic mastectomy must realize that some risk remains. Hartmann et al published results from a retrospective study of all women with a family history of breast cancer who underwent bilateral

prophylactic mastectomy at the Mayo Clinic between 1960 and 1993.[98] The women were divided into two groups—high risk and moderate risk—on the basis of family history. A control study of the sisters of the high-risk probands and the Gail Model were used to predict the number of breast cancers expected in these two groups in the absence of prophylactic mastectomy. The study included 639 women with a family history of breast cancer who had undergone bilateral prophylactic mastectomy: 214 at high risk and 425 at moderate risk. The median length of follow-up was 14 years. The median age at prophylactic mastectomy was 42 years. According to the Gail Model, 37.4 breast cancers were expected in the moderate-risk group; 4 breast cancers occurred (reduction in risk, 89.5%; *P*<.001). Hartmann et al also compared the numbers of breast cancers among the 214 high-risk probands with the numbers among their 403 sisters who had not undergone prophylactic mastectomy. Of these sisters, 38.7% (156) had been given a diagnosis of breast cancer (115 cases were diagnosed before the respective proband's prophylactic mastectomy, 38 were diagnosed afterward, and the time of the diagnosis was unknown in 3 cases). By contrast, breast cancer was diagnosed in 1.4% (3 of 214) of the probands. Thus, prophylactic mastectomy was associated with a reduction in the incidence of breast cancer of at least 90%. The authors concluded that in women with a high risk of breast cancer on the basis of family history, prophylactic mastectomy can significantly reduce the incidence of breast cancer. A limitation of this study was that cancer predisposition genetic testing was not done, thus it is unknown whether the high-risk women were carriers of mutations in either *BRCA1* or *BRCA2*.[98,99]

Screening and detection

Another option for risk management is more aggressive cancer screening beginning at an earlier age and at more frequent intervals for those at an increased risk for cancer due to inheritance of a mutated cancer predisposition gene. A task force of the Cancer Genetics Studies Consortium, a group of researchers investigating the psychosocial implications of cancer susceptibility testing, has published follow-up recommendations for individuals at high risk for developing cancer[100,101] (Tables 10-8[21,22,100] and 10-9[21,22,101,102]). Clinical trials to determine the most appropriate surveillance measures for those carrying mutated cancer susceptibility genes and the development of newer and more sensitive screening tests remain a high priority.

Models for Cancer Risk Counseling Programs

As the integration of genetic information into the management of patients with cancer continues, there will be an increasing need for the provision of clinical services

Table 10-8   Options for Cancer Prevention/Detection in Carriers of *BRCA1* and *BRCA2* Mutations

Chemoprevention

No known chemoprevention methods

Discuss option of entrance into chemoprevention trials
  Data indicates that oral contraceptive pills may decrease the risk of ovarian cancer; the impact on breast cancer is unclear
  Data pending on efficacy of tamoxifen in decreasing risk for developing breast cancer

Prophylactic surgery

Discuss options and limitations of prophylactic mastectomy

Discuss options and limitations of prophylactic oophorectomy

Screening

Instruction in breast self-exam
  Perform monthly beginning at age 18 years

Clinical breast exam
  Annual or semiannual beginning at age 25 years

Mammography
  Annual beginning at age 25 years

Pelvic examination
  Annual beginning at age 25 years

CA-125 blood level
  Annual or semiannual beginning at age 25–35 years

Transvaginal ultrasound
  Annual or semiannual beginning at age 25–35 years

Data from Offit[21]; Mills et al[22]; Burke et al.[100]

Table 10-9   Options for Cancer Prevention/Detection in Carriers of Mutations Causing HNPCC

Chemoprevention

No known chemoprevention methods

Discuss option of entrance into chemoprevention trials
  Preliminary data indicates that use of nonsteroidal anti-inflammatory agents may decrease risk of cancer and formation of polyps

Prophylactic surgery

Discuss options of prophylactic colectomy
  Generally discussed following diagnosis of cancer or detection of ardenomas

Discuss options of prophylactic hysterectomy/oophorectomy

Screening

Colonoscopy
  Every 1–3 years beginning at age 20–25 years

Pelvic examination
  Annual beginning at age 25 years

CA-125 blood level
  Annual or semiannual beginning at age 25–35 years

Transvaginal ultrasound
  Annual or semiannual beginning at age 25–35 years

HNPCC = hereditary nonpolyposis colon cancer.
Data from Offit[21]; Mills et al[22]; Burke et al[101]; NCCN.[102]

that provide cancer genetic counseling and address issues related to predisposition genetic testing for cancer susceptibility genes. There exists no standard model of a cancer risk evaluation program that specifically addresses the unique issues associated with genetic testing. An effective program would include clinical and psychosocial assessment, education, individualized cancer risk analysis, and genetic counseling, in addition to long-term screening and surveillance for cancer, preferably within the context of a strong prevention program. Large academic centers should provide a forum for ongoing genetic and clinical research. In many institutions, centers providing cancer genetic counseling services are housed within prevention centers, as opposed to disease site centers. As described above, cancer predisposition genes predispose to patterns of cancer that often do not respect current disease site boundaries. For example, women with HNPCC syndrome followed in a gastrointestinal clinic may not receive adequate surveillance for gynecologic cancers, such as endometrial and ovarian cancer, and vice versa. A multidisciplinary mix of health care professionals is important so that individuals seen will have full access to a range of professional services and skills.[21,103,104]

The National Comprehensive Cancer Network (NCCN), a not-for-profit, tax-exempt corporation, is an alliance of 17 of the world's leading cancer centers located throughout the United States. Network member institutions provide superior cancer care and seek to continuously improve this care through the implementation of oncology practice guidelines and through performance measurement. In 1997, an article reviewed the challenges inherent in creating guidelines for cancer susceptibility testing.[104] Six aspects of testing that could potentially be encompassed within practice guidelines were identified: (1) the process of informed consent, (2) the need for counseling on nonmedical issues, (3) a process for ensuring the use of current information to guide medical decision-making, (4) detailed training for those providing counseling, (5) mandatory follow-up, and (6) the value of participating in research.[104] Practice guidelines for these areas were presented at the annual NCCN conference in February 1999.

Implications for Oncology Nurses

As advances in technology continue to yield new methods of prevention, diagnosis, detection, and treatment of cancer, part of our professional responsibility as nurses is to expand our level of knowledge. Additionally, the abundance of information available to patients through the media and newer resources such as the Internet challenge us more than ever to keep up the pace of learning. All licensed registered nurses, regardless of their practice setting, will have a role in the delivery of genetic services and the management of genetic information. Nurses will require genetic knowledge to identify, refer, support, and care for persons affected by or at risk for manifesting or transmitting genetic conditions.[48]

As part of the nursing assessment, the family history should always be evaluated. Determination of the number of affected relatives and the age at diagnosis of cancer may provide clues to the possible existence of a hereditary cancer syndrome. How many first-degree relatives (e.g., mother, sibling, father) and second-degree relatives (e.g., aunt, cousin, grandmother) are affected with cancer or, more specifically, cancers that are part of a known syndrome? Are there characteristics of a hereditary cancer syndrome in the family? Not all oncology nurses will be experts in this new area. However, knowledge and awareness of hereditary cancer syndromes will help in the identification of patients who should be referred to a specialized cancer risk assessment clinic for further evaluation and counseling. As a general rule, patients should be referred for further evaluation if they:

- Have more than two first-degree relatives affected by like cancers.

- Are from families with a high rate of cancer.

- Have features of hereditary cancers (e.g., young age at onset).

- Have relatives with rare cancers, such as retinoblastoma.

- Have relatives with a known mutation in a cancer susceptibility gene.

Knowing that tests are now available to identify some of the genes that predispose to the development of cancer can be useful in answering questions and referring individuals to appropriate resources for more specific information.

We are living in the age of information, in which knowledge multiplies exponentially. It is impossible to remain an expert in all areas of cancer care. One of an oncology nurse's greatest assets, therefore, is awareness of available resources. We may not have all the answers to questions raised by individuals who seek health care services, but we can direct them to the person, clinic, or source who will be able to answer their questions. In cancer genetics, we might begin by identifying experts in our institution, city, county, or state who provide cancer risk assessment and counseling. The National Cancer Institute's Web site provides an on-line resource for the identification of professionals who provide cancer genetic counseling services across the United States. Nurses who specialize in the provision of cancer genetic counseling services can be identified through professional organizations such as the Oncology Nursing Society, which has a special interest group in cancer genetics, or the International Society of Nurses in Genetics. These societies also serve as resources for information and continuing education.[14,16,21,105,106] Table 10-10 shows a partial list of current Web sites that address questions related to inherited can-

Table 10-10 Genetic Resources for Health Care Professionals

Societies

International Society of Nurses in Genetics (ISONG)
ISONG c/o Eileen Rawnsley, Executive Director
7 Haskins Road
Hanover, NH 03775
603-643-5706
erawn@valley.net
http://nursing.creighton.edu/isong

Oncology Nursing Society
Cancer Genetics Special Interest Group
  Position Statements
501 Holiday Drive
Pittsburgh, PA 15520-2749
412-921-7373
http://www.ons.org

Council of Regional Genetics Networks
Cornell University Medical Center
Genetics Box 53
New York, NY 10021-4885
212-746-3475
http://www.cc.emory.edu/PEDIATRICS/corn/corn.htm

Web sites

GeneTests™: A national directory of DNA diagnostic laboratories; designed for health care providers; computerized directory of laboratories providing DNA diagnosis for clinical services and research. Requires registration.
  http://www.genetests.org/

Genetics Education Center, University of Kansas Medical Center
  http://www.kumc.edu/gec/

Blazing A Genetic Trail: on-line tutorial on human genetics
  http://www.hhmi.org/genetictrail/

National Human Genome Research Institute
  http://www.nhgri.nih.gov

National Cancer Institute
  http://www.nci.nih.gov

CancerNet
  http://cancernet.nci.nih.gov

Search for genetic counselors
  http://cancernet.nci.nih.gov/www.prot/genetic/genersrch.shtml

Oncolink
  http://www.oncolink.upenn.edu

Cancer Information Network
  http://www.cancernetwork.com/

Stanford Human Genome Center
  http://www-shgc.stanford.edu/

Understanding Gene Testing Book: on-line
  http://www.gene.com/ae/AE/AEPC/NIH/index.html

cers and genetic testing. Additionally, an excellent starting point is the National Cancer Institute's Information line, 1-800-4CANCER.

Following evaluation at a specialized center, patients may return to a primary care provider or be referred to an oncologist for cancer screening and detection services. Nurse practitioners can provide physical assessments, coordinate and evaluate cancer screening examinations based on an individual's level of risk, and serve as a source of psychosocial support for those patients found to be carriers of a mutated cancer susceptibility gene. Both basic and advanced practice nurses can encourage and support patients in health-promoting behaviors and cancer screening and detection practices.

A new role for oncology nurses in the future will be to participate in the provision of cancer genetic counseling. Genetic counselors are health care professionals who provide information and support to families who may be at risk for a variety of inherited conditions.[107] Traditionally, genetic counselors have focused on prenatal counseling and, until recently, few have specialized in cancer risk assessment and counseling. The anticipated need for qualified health care professionals who can provide genetic counseling services, especially in cancer care, is expected to far exceed the number of genetic counselors qualified and trained to provide these services.[108] Oncology nurses, because of their extensive background in cancer care and complement of professional skills, are well suited to assume these roles with appropriate specialized training and to participate fully as members of the multidisciplinary team providing cancer risk assessment and counseling services. It is the position of both the Oncology Nursing Society and The International Society of Nurses in Genetics that counseling be provided by advanced practice nurses with a Master's degree or higher.[48,69] Oncology nurses with additional training in cancer genetics could also provide services at the basic level for individuals at increased risk for developing cancer and work closely with advanced practice nurses and physicians. The critical elements that distinguish advanced from basic level genetics nursing practice are the complexity of decision-making, leadership, the ability to negotiate complex organizations, and expanded practice skills and knowledge in nursing and genetics.[48] Specialized practitioners at both the basic and the advanced levels would serve as professional resources and educators to both nursing colleagues and other health care professionals.

Future Directions

The rapid pace of the acquisition of knowledge related to cancer biology and causation and cancer genetics shows no signs of slowing. Several global issues that relate to cancer risk assessment and counseling include improvement in testing technology, populational screening, management of information, timing of testing, and training of health care professionals to provide cancer genetic counseling services.

New Technology for Testing

New technologies are being developed that will provide more accurate results in a shorter period of time, test for multiple genes at once, and cost less. One exciting area of research is DNA chip technology. DNA chips are similar in construction and concept to the chips used in computers. The minute chips are filled with dense grids of DNA probes (i.e., short stretches of DNA). Extracts from cells are incubated with the chips so that gene fragments will bind to the DNA probes on the chips. The probes on the chips can be thought of as "molecular tweezers," picking out gene fragments for which they are tailored or matched. Probes could be designed to pick out known alterations in genes associated with hereditary cancer syndromes or other diseases. Currently, a DNA chip is being marketed to detect *p53* mutations, the most common genetic mutation in human cancers; chips to detect *BRCA1* and *BRCA2* mutations are also being evaluated. In the future, DNA from a few cells might be placed in a DNA gene chip scanner and quickly analyzed to determine a person's risk for development of numerous diseases. Other areas of research include customizing cancer therapy for individuals by "profiling" them to identify all the genetic defects present and designing gene therapy to correct defects.[77,109,110]

Populational Screening

Genetic screening is the application of genetic testing to specific populations, independent of a family history of a disorder. Identification of individuals with a genetic condition, prior to the onset of symptoms, can allow for more effective treatment planning. This currently occurs for some diseases such as phenylketonuria. As the relationship between genes and disease continues to unfold, a determination must be made as to which diseases require genetic screening. Hence, discussions of genetics will become part of public policy debates. The ability of decision makers to balance such factors as benefits, costs, privacy, and other ethical considerations, as well as management of those found to be at risk for disease will be paramount. Genetic screening may become possible for a multitude of single-gene diseases and multifactorial diseases such as cancer and heart disease. Nurses in a variety of settings may participate in discussions of relevant information that will allow individuals to make informed decisions and so should participate in the establishment of public policy.[26,111]

Information Management

How to manage information obtained from genetic testing will remain a relevant issue in the near future. Who should have access to results will continue to be debated. Until individual fears related to potential discrimination when attempting to obtain health, life, mortgage, or disability insurance because of information obtained from genetic testing are addressed and conquered, appropriate handling of genetic information will remain an issue. While no cases of genetic testing–related discrimination with respect to health insurance have yet been documented in the United States, in some countries genetic information is being used to guide decisions regarding life insurance.[112]

Timing of Testing

The question of when to test for genes that predispose for the development of cancer will continue to be posed. Should children be tested for adult-onset disease? Is it ethical to test for genes that predispose for cancer in the prenatal setting? Should adoptive parents be allowed to request genetic testing on children they are considering adopting? Predictive genetic testing of apparently healthy children has been urged as a way to generate information about children's future health and assisting families in deciding whether to adopt.[113] In some diseases, such as multiple endocrine neoplasia type 2A and 2B and FAP, children are tested so that preventive measures such as prophylactic surgery can be instituted at a young age.[114-117] However, at which point testing should occur (e.g., on diagnosis of a disease such as medullary thyroid cancer, at birth, or some other time prior to diagnosis of a disease) has yet to be determined. Genetic tests may offer medical or psychological benefits but may also create harm. Potential risks include stigmatization and alteration of the child's self-concept or of parent-child bonds.

Training of Health Care Professionals

The need exists to train health care professionals concerning genetics and the integration of genetic information into practice. Few nurses have received education in basic genetic concepts during their training. A study funded by the Human Genome Project assessed the ways in which nurses in the United States are currently managing genetic information. Less than 10% of nurses had a course in basic genetics during their basic nursing education, while almost 70% thought a course in human genetics should be required.[118] A future challenge will be integrating not only basic genetics into nursing programs but educating the millions of nurses currently practicing.

With respect to cancer genetics, debate continues as to the amount and type of education required to provide cancer genetic counseling services. There currently exists no specially trained health care professional to provide these services. While most oncology specialists (e.g., nurses and physicians) are knowledgeable in the field of oncology, few have received formal genetic education during their training. Few genetic counselors or clinical geneticists have received specialized training in oncology. The majority of professionals who currently practice in the field of cancer genetic counseling have acquired specific components of the required expertise through additional training, education, and clinical practice. Still undetermined are the amount of additional training required for each discipline and how to certify "competence." Several initiatives are under way to address issues specific to cancer genetics and global genetic issues related to medical and nursing practice.

The National Coalition for Health Professional Education in Genetics (NCHPEG) is a consortium of leaders from approximately 100 diverse health care professional organizations, consumer and volunteer groups, government agencies, industry, managed care organizations, and genetics professional organizations. The idea for NCHPEG was catalyzed by the American Medical Association, the American Nurses Association, and the National Human Genome Research Institute in an effort to provide an organized, systematic, and national approach to the provision of genetics education to all health care professionals. The coalition's mission is to ensure that our nation's health care providers have the knowledge, skills, and resources needed to effectively and responsibly integrate new genetic knowledge and technologies into the prevention, diagnosis, and management of disease.[119] Grants to develop a Web site that will provide resources, content, and commentary related to health professional education has been obtained by NCHPEG. Several work groups within the coalition are addressing concerns related to development of a core curriculum that can be modified according to discipline and to provision of incentives (such as integration of genetics questions into certification and licensure exams) for learning about genetics.

Both the Oncology Nursing Society and the American Society of Clinical Oncology have initiatives targeted toward cancer genetics. The American Society of Clinical Oncology has developed a slide set and CD-ROM as educational materials on cancer genetics. The Oncology Nursing Society held a think tank on cancer genetics in fall of 1996 to review the impact of advances in cancer genetics on oncology nursing and to develop strategies to address issues related to genetic testing in patients with cancer, ranging from basic education of Society members to ethics. The report from this group outlined strategies, such as the development of a core curriculum in genetics, that will guide future initiatives.

Conclusion

The Human Genome Project continues its progress at a phenomenal rate, and it is now anticipated that the goal of sequencing all human DNA will be completed by 2003 instead of 2005, as was originally projected. Those in health care can anticipate that discoveries that influence the provision of cancer care will continue at an ever-increasing pace. Although these discoveries often raise difficult questions, they challenge us to find ways to rapidly, efficiently, and ethically apply the information to clinical practice. Genetic tests to identify persons at highest risk of developing cancer were impossible 10 years ago but will likely be an integral component of cancer care in the near future. While not all oncology nurses will assume new specialized roles in this area, nurses must be aware of the changes and discoveries being made. The oncology nurse of the future will use this new knowledge to assess patients for a history of cancer within the family, to refer patients to appropriate resources and care centers, to support individuals who are found to be at increased risk for developing cancer, and to educate patients about the application of genetics to cancer care. Ultimately, the integration of genetics into cancer care will guide all aspects of the management of cancer: risk assessment, prevention, detection, prognostics, and treatment.[120,121] Today, we stand on the verge of a new era in cancer care.

References

1. Collins FS, Jenkins JF: Implications of the human genome project for the nursing profession, in Lashley FR (ed): *The Genetic Revolution: Implications for Nursing.* Washington, DC, American Academy of Nursing, 1997, pp 9–13
2. Collins FS, Patrino A, Jordan E, et al: New goals for the Human Genome Project 1998–2003. *Science* 282:682–689, 1998
3. Drlica KA: *Double-Edged Sword: The Promises and Risks of the Genetic Revolution.* Reading, MA, Helix/Addison-Wesley, 1994
4. National Center for Human Genome Research. *The Human Genome Project: From Maps to Medicine.* NIH Pub no 96-3897. Bethesda, MD, Department of Health and Human Services, Public Health Service, National Institutes of Health, 1995
5. National Center for Human Genome Research and National Institutes of Health. *Review of the Ethical, Legal, and Social Implications Research Program and Related Activities 1990–1995.* Washington, DC, U.S. Department of Health and Human Services, Public Health Service, National Institutes of Health, National Center for Human Genome Research, 1996
6. Li FP, Kantor AF: Cancer epidemiology, in Holland JF, Bast RC, Morton DL, et al (eds): *Cancer Medicine.* Baltimore, MD, Williams & Wilkins, 1997, pp 401–420
7. Perera FP: Uncovering new clues to cancer risk. *Sci Am* 274:54–62, 1996
8. Iglehart JD, Miron A, Rimer BK, et al: Overestimation of hereditary breast cancer risk. *Ann Surg* 228:375–384, 1998
9. Smith BL, Gadd MA, Lawler C, et al: Perception of breast cancer risk among women in breast center and primary care settings: Correlation with age and family history of breast cancer. *Surgery* 120:297–303, 1996
10. Madigan MP, Ziegler RG, Benichou J, et al: Proportion of breast cancer cases in the United States explained by well-established risk factors. *J Natl Cancer Inst* 87:1681–1685, 1995
11. Vogel VG: Breast cancer risk factors and preventive approaches to breast cancer, in Kavanagh JJ, Singletary SE, Einhorn N, DePetrillo AD (eds): *Cancer in Women.* Malden, MA, Blackwell Science, 1998, pp 58–91
12. Mahon SM: Cancer risk assessment: Conceptual considerations for clinical practice. *Oncol Nurs Forum* 25:1535–1547, 1998
13. Loescher LJ: The family history component of cancer genetic risk counseling. *Cancer Nurs* 22:96–102, 1999
14. Dimond E, Calzone KA, Davis J, Jenkins JF: The role of the nurse in cancer genetics. *Cancer Nurs* 21:57–75, 1998
15. Fraser MC, Calzone KA, Goldstein AM: Familial cancers: Evolving challenges for nursing practice. *Oncol Nurs Updates* 4(3), 1–18, 1997
16. Rieger PT: Overview of Cancer and Genetics: Implications for Nurse Practitioners. *Nurse Pract Forum* 9:122–133, 1998
17. Claus EB, Risch N, Thompson WD: Autosomal dominant inheritance of early-onset breast cancer: Implications for risk prediction. *Cancer* 73:643–651, 1994
18. Benichou J, Gail MH, Mulvihill JJ: Graphs to estimate an individualized risk of breast cancer. *J Clin Oncol* 14:103–110, 1996
19. Goldspiel BR: Future cancer therapies. *Highlights Oncol Pract* 16:1–2, 1998
20. National Cancer Institute. *The Nation's Investment in Cancer Research: A Budget Proposal for Fiscal Years 1997/1998.* Bethesda, MD, National Institute of Health, National Cancer Institute, 1996
21. Offit K: *Clinical Cancer Genetics: Risk Counseling and Management.* New York, Wiley-Liss, 1998
22. Mills GB, Rieger PT, Watt MA, et al: Genetic predisposition to cancer. In Pollock R, *Manual of Clinical Oncology* (ed 7). Springer Verlag, Berlin, (in press)
23. Lindor NM, Greene MH: The concise handbook of family cancer syndromes. Mayo Familial Cancer Program. *J Natl Cancer Inst* 90:1039–1071, 1998
24. Knudson A: Hereditary cancer: Theme and variations. *J Clin Oncol* 15:3280–3287, 1997
25. National Institutes of Health and National Cancer Institute: *Understanding Gene Testing.* NIH Pub no 96–3905. Washington, DC: US Department of Health and Human Services, 1995
26. Lea D, Jenkins JF, Francomano C: *Genetics in Clinical Practice: New Directions for Nursing and Health Care.* Sudbury, MA, Jones and Bartlett, 1998
27. Thompson MW, McInnes RR, Willard HF: *Genetics in Medicine.* Philadelphia, Saunders, 1991
28. Bertwistle D, Ashworth A: Functions of the BRCA1 and BRCA2 genes. *Curr Opin Genet Dev* 8:14–20, 1998
29. Hall JM, Lee MK, Newman B, et al: Linkage of early-onset familial breast cancer to chromosome 17q21. *Science* 250:1684–1689, 1990
30. Narod SA, Feunteun J, Lynch HT, et al: Familial breast-ovarian cancer locus on chromosome 17q12-q23. *Lancet* 338:82–83, 1991
31. Wooster R, Neuhausen SL, Mangion J, et al: Localization of a breast cancer susceptibility gene, BRCA2, to chromosome 13q12-13. *Science* 265:2088–2090, 1994
32. Miki Y, Swensen J, Shattuck-Eidens D, et al: Isolation of BRCA1, the 17q-linked breast and ovarian cancer susceptibility gene. *Science* 266:66–71, 1994
33. Wooster R, Bignell G, Lancaster J, et al: Identification of the breast cancer susceptibility gene BRCA2. *Nature* 378:789–792, 1995
34. Cummings S, Olopade OI: Predisposition testing for breast cancer. *Oncology* 12:1227–1242, 1998
35. Easton DF, Ford D, Bishop T, et al: Breast and ovarian cancer incidence in BRCA1-mutation carriers. *Am J Hum Genet* 56:2265–2271, 1995
36. Streuwing JP, Hartge P, Wacholder S, et al: The risk of cancer associated with specific mutations of BRCA1 and BRCA2 among Ashkenazi Jews. *N Engl J Med* 336:1401–1408, 1997
37. Blackwood A, Weber BL: Biology of neoplasia BRCA1 and

BRCA2: From molecular genetics to clinical medicine. *J Clin Oncol* 16:1969–1977, 1998

38. Calzone KA: Predictive testing for breast and ovarian cancer susceptibility. *Semin Oncol Nurs* 13:82–90, 1997

39. de la Chapelle A, Peltomaki P: The genetics of hereditary common cancers. *Curr Opin Genet Dev* 8:298–303, 1998

40. Frank TS, Manley SA, Olopade OI, et al: Sequence analysis of BRCA1 and BRCA2: Correlation of mutations with family history and ovarian cancer risk. *J Clin Oncol* 16:2417–2425, 1998

41. Bronner CE, Baker SM, Morrison PT, et al: Mutation in the DNA mismatch repair gene homologue hMLH1 is associated with hereditary nonpolyposis colon cancer. *Nature* 368:258–261, 1994

42. Liu B, Parson RE, Hamilton ST, et al: hMSH2 mutations in hereditary nonpolyposis colorectal cancer kindreds. *Cancer Res* 54:4590–4594, 1994

43. Nicolaides NC, Papadopoulos N, Liu B, et al: Mutations of two PMS homologues in hereditary nonpolyposis colorectal cancer kindreds. *Nature* 371:75–80, 1994

44. Rodriguez-Bigas MA, Boland CR, Hamilton SR, et al: A National Cancer Institute Workshop on Hereditary Nonpolyposis Colorectal Cancer Syndrome: Meeting highlights and Bethesda guidelines. *J Natl Cancer Inst* 89:1758–1762, 1997

45. Boland CR, Thibodeau SN, Hamilton SR, et al: A National Cancer Institute Workshop on Microsatellite Instability for cancer detection and familial predisposition: Development of international criteria for the determination of microsatellite instability in colorectal cancer. *Cancer Res* 58:5248–5257, 1998

46. Peterson GM, Boyd PA: Gene tests and counseling for colorectal cancer risk: Lessons from familial polyposis. *J Natl Cancer Inst Monogr* 17:67–71, 1995

47. Peterson GM, Brensinger JP: Genetic testing and counseling in familial adenomatous polyposis. *Oncology* 10:89–94, 1996

48. International Society of Nurses in Genetics, American Nurses Association: *Statement on the Scope and Standards of Genetics Clinical Nursing Practice.* Washington, DC, American Nurses Publishing, 1998

49. Peters JA, Stopfer JE: Role of the genetic counselor in familial cancer risk. *Oncology* 10:159–175, 1996

50. Calzone KA: Genetic predisposition testing: Clinical implications for oncology nurses. *Oncol Nurs Forum* 24:712–718, 1997

51. MacDonald DJ: The oncology nurse's role in cancer risk assessment and counseling. *Semin Oncol Nurs* 13:123–128, 1997

52. Cooley ME, Moriarty H, Berger MS: Patient literacy and the readability of written cancer educational materials. *Oncol Nurs Forum* 22:1345–1351, 1995

53. Doak CC, Doak LG, Friedell GH, et al: Improving comprehension for cancer patients with low literacy skills: Strategies for clinicians. *CA Cancer J Clin* 48:151–162, 1998

54. Morra ME, Grant M: Cancer patient education. *Semin Oncol Nurs* 7:77–145, 1991

55. Garber JE, Schrag D: Testing for inherited cancer susceptibility (editorial). *JAMA* 2275:1928–1929, 1996

56. Healy B: BRCA genes—Bookmaking, fortunetelling and medical care. *N Engl J Med* 366:1448–1450, 1997

57. Ponder B: Genetic testing for cancer risk. *Science* 278:1050–1054, 1997

58. Olopade OI, Offit K, and Garber JE: Genetic for susceptibility to cancer. *JAMA* 279:1612–1613. 1998

59. American Society of Human Genetics, Ad Hoc Committee on Breast and Ovarian Cancer Screening. Statement of the American Society of Human Genetics on genetic testing for breast and ovarian cancer predispostion. *Am J Hum Genet* 55:i–iv, 1994

60. American Society of Clinical Oncology. Statement of the American Society of Clinical Oncology: Genetic testing for cancer susceptibility. *J Clin Oncol* 14:1730–1736, 1996

61. Rieger PT, Pentz RB: Genetic testing and informed consent. *Semin Oncol Nurs* 15:104–115, 1999

62. Bove C, Fry ST, MacDonald DJ: Presymptomatic and predisposition genetic testing: Ethical and social considerations. *Semin Oncol Nurs* 13:135–140, 1997

63. Geller G, Botkin JR, Green MJ, et al: Genetic testing for susceptibility to adult-onset cancer: The process and content of informed consent. *JAMA* 277:1471–1474, 1997

64. American Society of Human Genetics Social Issues Subcommittee on Familial Disclosure: ASHG Statement Professional Disclosure of Familial Genetic Information. *Am J Hum Genet* 62:474–483, 1998

65. National Advisory Council for Human Genome Research: Statement on use of DNA testing for presymptomatic identification of cancer risk. *JAMA* 271:785, 1994

66. National Breast Cancer Coalition: Presymptomatic genetic testing for heritable breast cancer risk. Press Release. September 28, 1995

67. National Society of Genetic Counselors I: Predisposition genetic testing for late-onset disorders in adults. *JAMA* 278:1217–1220, 1997

68. Oncology Nursing Society: ONS Position: The role of the oncology nurse in cancer genetic counseling. *Oncol Nurs Forum* 25:463, 1998

69. American Society of Clinical Oncology: Resource document for curriculum development in cancer genetics education. *J Clin Oncol* 15:2157–2169, 1997

70. American Society of Human Genetics, American College of Medical Genetics: Points to consider: Ethical, legal, and psychosocial implications of genetic testing in children and adolescents. *Am J Hum Genet* 57:1233–1241, 1995

71. American Society of Human Genetics. Statement on informed consent for genetic research. *Am J Hum Genet* 59:471–474, 1996

72. Oncology Nursing Society: ONS Position Statement: Cancer genetic testing and risk assessment counseling. *Oncol Nurs Forum* 25:464 1998

73. Task Force on Genetic Testing. *Interim Principles of the Task Force on Genetic Testing, 1996.* Available at http://www.infonet.welch.jhu.edu/policy/genetics/intro.html. Accessed 10/11/99

74. Holtzman NA, Watson MS. *Promoting Safe and Effective Genetic Testing in the United States.* Task Force on Genetic Testing, 1997. Available at http://www.nhgri.nih.gov/ELSI/TFGT__Final/ Accessed 10/11/99

75. Biesecker B: Genetic testing for cancer predisposition. *Cancer Nurs* 20:285–296, 1997

76. Jacobs LA: Hereditary nonpolyposis colon cancer: Genetic basis, testing, and patient-care issues. *Oncol Nurs Forum* 25:719–725, 1998

77. Loescher LJ: DNA testing for cancer predisposition. *Oncol Nurs Forum* 25:1317–1327, 1998

78. Weber W, Mulvihill JJ, Narod SA: *Familial Cancer Management.* Boca Raton, FL, CRC Press, 1996

79. Biesecker BB: Psychological issues in cancer genetics. *Semin Oncol Nurs* 13:129–134, 1997

80. Lerman C, Croyle RT: Emotional and behavioral responses

to genetic testing for susceptibility to cancer. *Oncology* 10: 191–199, 1996

81. Lerman C, Croyle RT. Genetic testing for cancer predisposition: Behavioral science issues. *J Natl Cancer Inst Monogr* 17: 63–66, 1995

82. Mahon SM, Casperson DS: Hereditary cancer syndrome. Part 2. Psychosocial issues, concerns, and screening—results of a qualitative study. *Oncol Nurs Forum* 22:775–782, 1995

83. Malkin D, Knoppers BM: Genetic predisposition to cancer—issue to consider. *Cancer Biol* 7:49–53, 1996

84. Hudson KL, Rothenberg KH, Andrews LB, et al: Genetic discrimination and health insurance: An urgent need for reform. *Science* 270:391–393, 1995

85. Jacobs LA: At-risk for cancer: Genetic discrimination in the workplace. *Oncol Nurs Forum* 25:475–480, 1998

86. Rothenberg K, Fuller B, Rothstein M, et al: Genetic information and the workplace: Legislative approaches and policy challenges. *Science* 275:1755–1757, 1997

87. Holtzman D: Health insurance bill provides first step toward tackling genetic discrimination. *J Natl Cancer Inst* 88: 1521–1523, 1996

88. Sporn MB, Dunlop NM, Newton DL, et al: Prevention of chemical carcinogenesis by vitamin A and its synthetic analogs (retinoids). *Fed Proc* 35:1332–1338, 1976

89. Sporn MB, Lippmann SM: Chemoprevention of cancer, in Holland JF, Bast RC, Morton DL, et al (eds): *Cancer Medicine*. Baltimore, MD, Williams & Wilkins, 1997, pp 495–508

90. Singh DK, Lippman SM: Cancer chemoprevention. Part I: Retinoids and carotenoids and other classic antioxidants. *Oncology* 12:1643–1658, 1998

91. Swan DK, Ford B: Chemoprevention of cancer: Review of the literature. *Oncol Nurs Forum* 24:719–727, 1997

92. Greenwald P, Kelloff G, Burch-Whitman C, Kramer B: Chemoprevention. *CA Cancer J Clin* 45:31–49, 1995

93. Lee IM, Hennekens CH, Buring JE: Use of aspirin and other nonsteroidal antiinflammatory drugs and the risk of cancer development, in Devita VT, Hellman S, Rosenberg SA (eds): *Cancer: Principles and Practice of Oncology.* (5 ed) Philadelphia, Lippincott-Raven, 1997, pp 599–607

94. Fisher B, Costantino JP, Wickerham DL, et al: Tamoxifen for prevention of breast cancer: report of the National Surgical Adjuvant Breast and Bowel Project P-1 Study. *J Natl Cancer Inst* 90:1371–1388, 1998

95. Narod SA, Risch H, Moslehi R, et al: Oral contraceptives and the risk of hereditary ovarian cancer. Hereditary Ovarian Cancer Clinical Study Group. *N Engl J Med* 339:424–428, 1998

96. Chi DD, Moley JF: Medullary thyroid carcinoma: Genetic advances, treatment recommendations, and the approach to the patient with persistent hypercalcitoninemia. *Surg Oncol Clin N Am* 7:681–706, 1998

97. Giarelli E: Medullary thyroid carcinoma: One component of the inherited disorder multiple endocrine neoplasia type 2A. *Oncol Nurs Forum* 24:1007–1020, 1997

98. Hartmann LC, Schaid DJ, Woods JE, et al: Efficacy of bilateral prophylactic mastectomy in women with a family history of breast cancer. *N Engl J Med* 340:77–84, 1999

99. Eisen A, Weber BL: Prophylactic mastectomy—the price of fear. *N Engl J Med* 340:137–138, 1999

100. Burke W, Daly M, Garber JE, et al: Recommendations for follow-up care of individuals with an inherited predisposition to cancer. II. BRCA1 and BRCA2. *JAMA* 277:997–1003, 1997

101. Burke W, Peterson G, Lynch P, et al: Recommendations for follow-up care of individuals with an inherited predisposition to cancer. I. Hereditary nonpolyposis colon cancer. *JAMA* 277:915–917, 1997

102. National Comprehensive Cancer Network: NCCN colorectal cancer screening practice guidelines. *Oncology* 13: 152–178, 1999

103. Calzone KA, Stopfer J, Blackwood A, et al: Establishing a cancer risk evaluation program. *Cancer Pract* 5:228–233, 1997

104. Greely JD: Genetic testing for cancer susceptibility: Challenges for creators of practice guidelines. *Oncology* 11: 171–176, 1997

105. Calzone KA: Where to look for information about cancer genetics and genetic testing. *Cancer Pract* 4:346–349, 1996

106. Fineman RM, Francomano CA, Ribble JA: Accessing genetic resources. *Patient Care Nurse Pract* 1:39–48, 1998

107. National Society of Genetic Counselors, Inc. *National Society of Genetic Counselors Pamphlet.* Wallingford, PA, National Society of Genetic Counselors, 1994

108. Loescher LJ: Genetics in cancer prediction, screening, and counseling. Part II. The nurse's role in genetic counseling. *Oncol Nurs Forum* 22:16–19, 1995 (suppl)

109. Affymetrix. Gene Chip System. Available at http://www.affymetrix.com/products/system.html. Accessed 10/11/99. 1998

110. Stipp D. Gene chip breakthrough. *Fortune* 135:56–73, 1997

111. Penticuff JH: Ethical dimensions in genetic screening: A look into the future. *J Obstet Gynecol Neonatal Nurs* 25: 785–789, 1996

112. Wilkie T: Genetics and insurance in Britain: Why more than just the Atlantic divides the English-speaking nations. *Nat Genet* 20:119–121, 1998

113. Freundlich MD: The case against preadoption genetic testing. *Child Welfare* 77:663–679, 1998

114. Kinder BK: Genetic and biochemical screening for endocrine disease: II. Ethical issues. *World J Surg* 22:1208–1211, 1998

115. Goretzki PE, Hoppner W, Dotzenrath C, et al: Genetic and biochemical screening for endocrine disease. *World J Surg* 22:1202–1207, 1998

116. Wertz DC, Reilly PR: Laboratory policies and practices for the genetic testing of children: A survey of the Helix network. *Am J Hum Genet* 61:1163–1168, 1997

117. Lessick M, Faux S: Implications of genetic testing of children and adolescents. *Holist Nurs Pract* 12:38–46, 1998

118. Scanlon C, Fibison W: *Managing Genetic Information: Implications for Nursing Practice.* Washington, DC, American Nurses Association, 1995

119. National Coalition for Health Professional Education in Genetics. Available at http://www.nchpeg.org/ Accessed 10/11/99

120. Li FP: Cancer control in susceptible groups: Opportunities and challenges. *J Clin Oncol* 17:719–725, 1999

121. Collins FS: Shattuck lecture—medical and societal consequences of the Human Genome Project. *N Engl J Med* 341: 28–37, 1999

CHAPTER 11

Diagnostic Evaluation, Classification, and Staging

Jill Griffin-Brown, RN, BSN, OCN®

Diagnostic Evaluation

Factors Affecting the Diagnostic Approach

Cancer is a significant health care problem in the United States. The etiology of most cancers remains unknown, and cancer prevention measures are complicated by multiple economic, behavioral, social, and cultural factors. Early detection efforts and comprehensive diagnostic evaluations hold the most promise for controlling the associated morbidity and cost of cancer. This chapter focuses on the process of diagnostic evaluation, classification, and staging when a suspicion of cancer exists for an individual.

The major goals of the diagnostic evaluation for a suspected cancer are to determine the tissue type of the malignancy, the primary site of the malignancy, the extent of disease within the body, and the tumor's potential to recur in the future. This information comprises the critical first step in planning the therapeutic management. The approach to the diagnostic evaluation depends on:

- Presenting signs and symptoms

- Clinical status and ability to tolerate invasive procedures

- Anticipated goal of treatment when diagnosis is made

- Biological characteristics of the suspected malignancy

- Diagnostic equipment available in the community

- Third-party payer approval of diagnostic procedures

The diagnosis and staging of cancer have been affected by rapidly changing technology in imaging modalities and biochemical analysis. Historically, there has been a progression from the gross evaluation of a tumor mass at surgery to the assessment of genetic expression and structure of tumor cells to diagnose and predict the natural history of the disease.

Even with the most sophisticated technology and resources presently available for cancer diagnosis, the key to survival continues to be early detection of disease. The discovery of a precancerous lesion or a malignant neoplasm at its earliest stage affords the very best opportunity for cure, extended survival, and less extensive treatment. For example, the nonpalpable breast mass found on a screening mammogram or the isolated tumor found incidentally on a chest film is more likely to be diagnosed as localized disease amenable to treatment and cure. More typically, the tumor goes undetected until specific signs or symptoms become apparent and prompt the person to consult a health professional.

Frequently, these symptoms include the complaints of weight loss, persistent pain, unexplained fever, fatigue, or one of the seven warning signals that have brought the early detection of cancer into public awareness.[1] A patient's attitude and behavior influence when medical attention is sought, as does cultural makeup, geographic location, and socioeconomic background. Changes in the framework of health care make it a priority to identify, address, and eliminate these potential barriers.

Those at highest risk for developing cancer are the poor, the elderly, minorities, and those with a low-level education. Unfortunately, many of the people at greatest risk for developing cancer have an inadequate understanding of the importance of early attention to symptoms and may lack accessibility to available resources. A study of cancer knowledge among the elderly revealed that most respondents were uncertain about the seven warning signals of cancer and lacked awareness of their increased cancer risk.[2] Nurses need to make a concerted effort to gather information, analyze the data, and then identify ways to reduce the threat of cancer in these individuals. Table 11-1 identifies the most common warning signals of cancer, the significance of each signal or symptom, and the persons at greatest risk for developing an associated malignancy.[1,3,4]

The worst prognosis can be expected in those people who delay seeking medical evaluation at the onset of their symptoms, in those cancers for which technologic methods are unavailable to make an early diagnosis, and in people for whom the primary lesion cannot be found. For the person who presents with widespread extensive disease, the palliative goal of treatment may direct and abbreviate an otherwise exhaustive and expensive diagnostic workup.

An effective clinical evaluation of the person with a suspected malignancy includes a comprehensive history with the identification of risk factors, a thorough physical examination, laboratory and imaging tests, and perhaps most importantly a histologic verification of the malignancy. Known biological characteristics of the suspected malignancy and the typical routes of regional and distant metastases will direct the approach of further diagnostic and staging procedures. In some situations, extensive laboratory and imaging examinations precede tissue biopsy in an attempt to locate the primary tumor or an accessible tumor. In other patients, results of a biopsy specimen that confirm the presence of malignancy direct further testing that will be done to accurately stage the extent of disease. Those tests that are the least taxing to the individual, that are cost effective, and that yield the information necessary for treatment planning are considered.

In the present era of cost containment in health care, the judicious selection and sequencing of diagnostic studies are stressed. The proper test is one that yields information on the suspicious site of malignancy and complements rather than merely confirms known information. The increased availability of sophisticated equipment, the fear of litigation, and pressure from patients and families all are factors that may influence the physician to potentially overinvestigate.

It is apparent that third-party payers, prospective payment systems, and managed care networks also play important roles as gatekeepers in the diagnostic evaluation.

Table 11-1 Seven Warning Signals of Cancer and Their Significance

Warning Signals	Significance of Warning Signal	Persons at Greatest Risk
Change in bowel or bladder habits	Changes in stool caliber and regular bowel function are frequent signs of colorectal cancer; dependent on the area of intestine involved. A change in bladder function, frequency, dysuria, retention, or hematuria may indicate prostate or bladder cancer.	*Colorectal cancer:* Over age 40, personal or family history of polyps or colorectal cancer, family history of polyposis syndromes, inflammatory bowel disease *Prostate cancer:* Over age 65, black males *Bladder cancer:* Smokers, males, chemical exposure
Unusual bleeding or discharge	Any unusual bleeding or discharge can signify malignancy. Occult or bright red blood may be seen with colorectal cancer. Abnormal vaginal bleeding is the most frequent sign of endometrial or cervical cancer. A clear, milky, or bloody discharge from the nipple is the second-most common symptom of breast cancer. Hemoptysis is a sign of lung cancer. Hematuria is the most frequent sign of bladder cancer and is also seen in renal and prostate cancer.	*Endometrial cancer:* Postmenopausal women over age 50, family history of endometrial cancer, obesity, diabetes, hypertension, prolonged estrogen administration, nulliparity *Cervix cancer:* First vaginal intercourse at early age, multiple sexual partners, genital human papillomavirus, smokers, low socioeconomic status
A sore that does not heal	Delayed healing of a sore or a change in a skin lesion's size, color, or shape, particularly on a surface exposed to ultraviolet light, can represent basal cell or squamous cell cancer. Oral lesions and leukoplakia, particularly in tobacco or alcohol users, need careful follow-up. Persistent sores or itching of the vulva can indicate a preinvasive or malignant lesion.	*Skin cancer (nonmelanoma):* Exposure to UV radiation, psoralens, and UV light, or chemical carcinogens; fair-skinned whites, family history *Oral cancer:* Males, over age 40, tobacco users (chewed or smoked), pipe smokers, combined tobacco and alcohol use, excessive sun exposure (lip lesions)
Obvious change in wart or mole	A change in a mole's color and pigmentation pattern, irregularities in border or surface topography, or increasing size causes suspicion of malignancy. Occurs in areas protected from or exposed to the sun.	*Melanoma:* Fair-skinned whites with history of sun exposure, family or personal history of melanoma or dysplastic nevi, large congenital moles
Thickening or lump in breast or elsewhere	A painless lump or mass is the most common presenting sign in cancer of the breast, testis, and soft-tissue sarcoma. Persistent enlarged lymph nodes can signify lymphoma or metastatic nodal disease.	*Breast cancer:* All women, particularly over age 50, endogenous hormonal factors, personal history or family history of breast cancer (mutations of specific breast genes), nulliparity or first child after age 30, history of early menses *Testis cancer:* Males aged 20–35, undescended testes
Nagging cough or hoarseness	Persistent, productive cough is the most frequently reported symptom of lung cancer. Hoarseness may indicate lung, laryngeal, or thyroid cancer.	*Lung cancer:* All smokers, black males, history of asbestos exposure *Larynx cancer:* Males over age 60, combined tobacco and alcohol use
Indigestion or difficulty in swallowing	Indigestion, gastroesophageal reflux, painful "spasms" after eating, or difficulty swallowing can be symptoms of cancer of the esophagus, stomach, or pharynx.	*Stomach cancer:* Males over age 50, Japanese emigrants, history of pernicious anemia, atrophic gastritis, tobacco use, and alcohol consumption *Esophagus cancer:* Males over age 60, history of Barrett's esophagus, achalasia, caustic injury to esophagus, tobacco use, and heavy alcohol consumption

Blue Cross of California is an example of a health insurance provider with published practice guidelines for breast cancer screening, diagnosis, staging, and treatment.[5] Due to cost-containment and insurance directives, many diagnostic evaluations are now being completed in ambulatory or outpatient facilities, unless patients are acutely ill and require hospitalization.

Nursing Implications

Many opportunities exist for nurses to promote the early detection and diagnosis of cancer. Serving as role models by incorporating early detection practices in their own personal health care is a starting point. As respected members of the health care profession, nurses are consulted formally and informally about perceived signs and symptoms of cancer. Through communication, education, and intervention, nurses can increase public awareness about cancer.

Nurses have the necessary skills and opportunities to assess and teach patients about the importance of early detection. Nurses also can facilitate entry into the health care system by encouraging appropriate follow-up without delay, providing accurate information on cancer detection and diagnostic procedures, clarifying misconceptions, and referring individuals to trusted health care providers or community programs. Nurses must explain risk assessment clearly to help patients understand which risk factors may be applicable and are of highest priority.[6] (See Chapters 8 and 9 for an extensive review of nursing involvement in cancer prevention and early detection, especially in the areas of breast, cervical, and lung cancer.[7])

Table 11-1 presents information on the significance of the early warning signals of cancer and can be used to design community education programs that target individuals who are at higher risk for developing a malignancy and who are most likely to delay seeking medical attention. The program content should stress the importance of recognizing symptoms early to improve survival. In addition, the rationale for participating in screening or annual physical examinations that include rectal and pelvic examinations should be given. Nurses proficient in physical assessment and screening techniques can perform early detection examinations, including digital rectal examinations, pelvic examinations, Papanicolaou tests, and testicular and breast examinations.[8] Integrating instruction on breast self-examination, testicular self-examination, or skin self-examination in community education programs can be done by nurses in most practice settings. Displaying posters and making available pamphlets from the American Cancer Society that identify warning signals and recommendations for a cancer-related checkup are effective ways to reach many people. Educational programs are most accessible and acceptable if they are based in the local church, work site, shopping center, health fair, senior center, or wherever participation can be maximized. Successful examples of community-based programs include a testicular and prostate cancer awareness program presented to 3000 men at their work site, and a breast cancer screening and awareness program coordinated by nursing students for low-income and ethnically diverse communities.[9,10]

Nurses are integral members of the professional team, providing support to individuals facing the potential threat of cancer. The time elapsed between the discovery of a suspicious symptom, such as a breast lump, the seeking of medical attention, and the completion of diagnostic evaluation varies for every person and for many reasons. However, the potential for stress, disruption, anxiety, and fear always exists for individuals suspected of having cancer and their family members.

During the prediagnostic period, a delay in seeking attention can be attributed to the perceived threat or "importance" of the symptom, the severity of the symptom, personal beliefs about cancer and treatment, and personal and financial resources. Once the individual acts on his or her concerns and seeks medical attention, the diagnostic period begins. Anxiety about the results of examinations and fear and curiosity regarding the technology used in procedures are common.[11] Psychological responses after receiving a diagnosis of cancer are individualized and range from suspicion, shock, denial, grief, and helplessness to loss and fear of death.[12] Guilt feelings may be apparent if the patient did not seek attention early or if lifestyle may have contributed to the cancer.[4] In such situations, professional nurses can intervene by taking time to listen to concerns, responding to questions, and providing support. Projecting optimism and hope helps to counter the worst-case scenarios often assumed by the patient and family.

Oncology nurses play a key role in providing information and support to reduce the stress of going through a diagnostic evaluation for a suspected malignancy. An accurate assessment of the individual's and family's desire to know, in addition to their ability to understand, is the first step in providing this much-needed support. Educational preparation for an examination should include an explanation of the procedure and a description of any physical sensations that might be expected, such as pain, discomfort, and facial flushing. The purpose of the examination, what information can and cannot be gleaned from the examination, and when and from whom the results can be expected should be explained. Reinforcing verbal information with written materials has proved helpful.[13] Scheduling of the procedure should be done in a timely manner to help decrease the patient's stress level.

Nurses also must be cognizant of any potential for complications during or after a procedure, including reactions to contrast agents, bleeding, vasovagal response, and the need for intravenous analgesia or conscious sedation. Nurses may assist with a procedure, perform the procedure, or provide postprocedure care.

Including the family members in all aspects of the diagnostic evaluation benefits the individual, the family, and the health care team. Families can reinforce instructions and information, assist with preparation for an examination, observe for untoward effects from procedures, and provide emotional support to the patient. An assessment of the family's ability to cope with the cancer diagnosis may prompt referrals to a variety of support services including social services, psycho-oncology support groups, and home care agencies.

Laboratory Techniques

Laboratory studies are performed to help formulate or confirm a clinical diagnosis and to monitor the patient's response to or relapse from a specific therapy. The data provide information on the functioning of specific organs and metabolic processes that may be altered by disease or a malignant process.

Biochemical analysis of blood, serum, urine, and other body fluids identifies chemical and hematologic values outside the narrow, homeostatic range. Specific malignancies characteristically alter chemical composition of the blood, but no single value is diagnostic for a malignancy. For example, elevated serum levels of bilirubin, alkaline phosphatase, and glutamic-oxaloacetic transaminase are seen in approximately 50% of individuals presenting with liver cancer, and these abnormalities are significant in their correlation with shorter survival. Nonspecific changes such as anemia, leukocytosis or leukopenia, and thrombocytosis or thrombocytopenia also may contribute to the diagnostic evaluation.

Tumor markers are proteins, antigens, genes, ectopically produced hormones, and enzymes that are *tumor derived* (expressed by the tumor) or *tumor associated* (produced by normal tissue in response to the tumor). Markers have been recognized in serum and body fluids, in tissue, and—with recent technologies like flow cytometry—at the cellular and genetic levels.

The accuracy of a particular laboratory study or imaging technique often is reported in terms of sensitivity or specificity. *Sensitivity* establishes the percentage of people with cancer who will have positive (abnormal) test results, known as *true-positive* results. Test results of people with cancer that are negative (normal) are *false-negative* findings. *Specificity* establishes the percentage of people without cancer who will have negative (normal) test results, known as *true-negative* results. People who are free of disease and show positive (abnormal) results are considered to have *false-positive* results. A clinically useful test will detect a malignant abnormality early in its development (sensitivity) and exclude nonmalignant sources for the abnormality (specificity). In reality, many tests are highly sensitive but not very specific. The *predictive value* of a test establishes the probability that a test result correctly predicts the actual disease status.

An increase or decrease in a tumor marker can indicate whether a patient is responding to a certain therapy, to locate the tumor's origin, or to determine recurrence. One of the best detectors for certain tumors is the tumor marker human chorionic gonadotropin (HCG).[14] Several other markers are clinically useful in monitoring tumor activity during treatment and in detecting recurrent cancer but lack the specificity required to be good screening tools. The carcinoembryonic antigen (CEA), although less specific, is a marker widely used as a prognostic factor in colon cancer, reflecting tumor burden, and used to monitor other disease sites such as breast and lung.[15,16] Carcinoembryonic antigen lacks specificity because the antigen is expressed by benign as well as many different malignant cells. Table 11-2 identifies several tumor markers and their clinical significance in the diagnosis and monitoring of cancer.[16–21]

Recent technological advances in monoclonal antibody production, radioimmunoassay, and flow cytometry have provided diagnostic and prognostic information in a variety of cancers. Techniques to produce monoclonal antibodies that detect specific tumor antigens have been important to the diagnosis, classification, localization, and treatment of several solid tumors, T- and B-cell lymphomas, and leukemia. Identified tumor antigens include surface immunoglobulins (cytoplasmic membranes), surface epitopes (antigen sites), antigens in various stages of cell differentiation, and enzymes.[19]

Radioimmunoassay, an important technique in the measurement of tumor markers, determines the amount of tumor antigen in a serum sample. A known amount of radiolabeled antigen, combined with antibody, is added to a serum sample. The individual's unlabeled antigen displaces the radiolabeled antigen, which permits quantification.

Flow cytometry rapidly measures and identifies DNA characteristics and cell-surface markers that correlate with patient prognosis and are useful in diagnosing a malignancy and monitoring response to therapy. A *cell sorter* measures fluorescence and light scatter as cells flow past an excitation source. In hematologic and lymphoid malignancies, fluorescent-marked antibodies directed against specific cell surface antigens (T-cell antigens, common acute lymphocytic leukemia antigen) help to differentiate hematopoietic cell lines. The primary application of flow cytometry analysis in solid tumors has been to determine DNA content (ploidy) and the percentage of cells synthesizing DNA (the S-phase fraction). Normal DNA is characterized as diploid and contrasts with abnormal, disorganized DNA, which is aneuploid. The proliferative potential of a tumor is measured by the percentage of cells in the synthesis phase of the cell cycle. Both of these factors—aneuploidy and high S-phase fraction—correlate with the biological aggressiveness of several tumors.[22,23] Breast cancer is a tumor in which DNA aneuploidy and high S-phase appear to be predictors of poor prognosis for women, regardless of their node-negative or node-positive status. Although no standard for treatment has been established, some physicians and research protocols are incorporating this information into adjuvant treatment decisions.[24]

Over the last decade substantial progress has been made in cancer genetics. A great deal of this progress stems from the Human Genome Project (HGP) due to complete its research in the next decade.[25] Researchers have already unlocked the key to the genetic puzzle of many cancers.

As a result of the rapid advancement in this area, patients and their families are ready to pursue genetic analysis and therapy. Unfortunately, along with this willingness and potential need for testing comes heightened expectation and anxiety on the part of patients and families.

It is well known that there are a significant number of ongoing clinical trials studying gene therapy and its relationship to the treatment of cancer. One such study involves the suppression of the Her-2/neu protein or receptor, which, when overexpressed, appears to make breast cancer more aggressive.[26,27] Practicing oncologists are now able to test patients diagnosed with breast cancer for Her-2/neu, enabling them to determine appropriate therapies.

Genetic testing for breast, ovarian, colon cancers, and melanoma has only recently become available. Inheritance of the mutated form of the genes *BRCA1* and *BRCA2* place women at a 90% risk for developing breast cancer and a 60% risk for developing ovarian cancer at a significantly young age.[25] Mutation in the adenomatous polyposis coli gene leads to the colon cancer adenomatous familial polyposis that affects patients early in life. Chromosome abnormalities have also been documented in hereditary nonpolyposis colorectal cancer (HNPCC).[25]

Although genetic testing assists in the prediction of disease risk, it brings with it complex social, legal, and

Table 11-2 Selected Markers in the Diagnosis and Monitoring of Malignant Disease

Laboratory Test	Associated Malignancy	Comments
ENZYMES		
Lactic dehydrogenase (LDH)	Lymphoma, seminoma, acute leukemia, metastatic carcinoma	Elevated in 50% of patients with advanced disease; also in hepatitis and myocardial infarction
Prostatic acid phosphatase (PAP)	Metastatic cancer of prostate, myeloma, lung cancer, osteogenic sarcoma	Elevated in 80% of patients with bone metastases from prostate cancer; also in prostatitis, nodular prostatic hypertrophy
Placental alkaline phosphatase (PLAP)	Seminoma, lung, ovary, uterus	Elevated in pregnancy
Neuron-specific enolase (NSE)	Small cell lung cancer, neuroendocrine tumors, neuroblastoma, medullary thyroid cancer	
Creatine kinase-BB (CK-BB)	Breast, colon, ovary, prostate cancers, small-cell lung cancer	Elevated in bowel infarction, renal failure, stroke
Terminal deoxynucleotidal transferase (TdT)	Lymphoblastic malignancy	Helpful in differentiating between AML and ALL
HORMONES		
Parathyroid hormone (PTH)	Ectopic hyperparathyroidism from cancer of the kidney, lung (squamous cell), pancreas, ovary, myeloma	Elevated in primary hyperparathyroidism
Calcitonin	Medullary thyroid, small cell lung, breast cancer, and carcinoid	
Antidiuretic hormone (ADH)	Small cell lung cancer, adenocarcinomas	Inappropriate secretion associated with pneumonia, porphyria, CNS disease, various drugs, and endocrinopathies
Adrenocorticotropic hormone (ACTH)	Lung, prostate, gastrointestinal cancers, neuroendocrine tumors	Elevated in Cushing's disease
Human chorionic gonadotropin, beta subunit (B-HCG)	Germ cell tumors of testicle and ovary; ectopic production in cancer of stomach, pancreas, lung, colon, liver	Elevated in almost all choriocarcinoma, 60% of testicular cancer; also in pregnancy
METABOLIC PRODUCTS		
5-Hydroxyindoleacetic acid (5-HIAA)	Carcinoid, lung	Drugs and diet interfere with test
Vanillylmandelic acid (VMA)	Neuroblastoma	Drugs and diet interfere with test; detected in ganglioneuroma
PROTEINS		
Protein electrophoresis (urine—Bence Jones) (serum—immunoglobulins)	Myeloma, lymphoma	Elevated in connective tissue disease, benign monoclonal gammopathy, chronic renal failure
IgG	IgG myeloma	
IgA	IgA myeloma	
IgM	Waldenström's macroglobulinemia	
IgD	IgD myeloma	
IgE	IgE myeloma	
	Advanced neoplasms	
Beta-2 microglobulin	Myeloma, lymphoma	Invalid if patient received radioactive dyes 1 week prior to test
ANTIGENS		
Alpha-fetoprotein (AFP)	Nonseminomatous germ cell testicular cancer, choriocarcinoma, gonadal teratoblastoma in children, cancer of the pancreas, colon, lung, stomach, biliary system, liver	Elevated in 80% of hepatocellular cancer, 60% of nonseminomatous germ cell cancer; also in cirrhosis, hepatitis, toxic liver injury

Table 11-2 Selected Markers in the Diagnosis and Monitoring of Malignant Disease (continued)

Laboratory Test	Associated Malignancy	Comments
ANTIGENS (cont.)		
Carcinoembryonic antigen (CEA)	Cancer of the colon-rectum, stomach, pancreas, prostate, lungs, breast	Elevated in smokers, chronic obstructive pulmonary disease, pancreatitis, hepatitis, inflammatory bowel disease
Prostate-specific antigen (PSA)	Prostate cancer	Elevated in prostatitis, nodular prostatic hyperplasia
Tissue polypeptide antigen (TPA)	Breast, colon, lung, pancreas cancer	Marker for cell proliferation in benign or malignant disease
CA-125	Ovary (epithelial), pancreas, breast, colon, lung, liver cancer	Elevated in >85% of ovarian cancer; also in endometriosis, pelvic inflammatory disease, peritonitis
CA-19-9	Pancreas, colon, gastric cancer	Differentiates benign from malignant pancreatobiliary disease
CA-15-3	Breast cancer	
CA-27.29	Breast cancer	
CA-72-4	Gastric cancer	
OTHER		
Lipid-associated sialic acid (LSA)	Leukemia, lymphoma, melanoma, most solid tumors	
Chromosome rearrangements (deletion, translocation, inversion)	Melanoma, small cell lung, renal, testicular cancers, liposarcoma, neuroblastoma, lymphoma, leukemia, and others	
Amplified oncogenes		
MYC	Neuroblastoma, small cell lung cancer, lymphoma, breast cancer	
EP1B-B	Glioblastoma, squamous cell carcinomas, breast, gastric, esophagus cancers	
C-ERB-B2 (HER-2)	Breast and ovarian cancers, adenocarcinomas	

ethical implications. The advent of genetic analysis finds health professionals fielding a wide variety of questions on this topic. Oncology nurses are now being called on to interpret and integrate this new genetic information into patient education.

The American Society of Clinical Oncology recommends that physicians offering genetic testing be able to explain the risks, benefits, and limitations of the testing procedure.[28] Once the test results become available, the physician should then discuss treatment options based on those results with the patient and family.

Technological advancements in genetic analysis are bound to continue. The challenge of problem solving and knowledge application in genetic risk assessment requires that the health professional seek continued education in this area.

Tumor Imaging

Many diagnostic procedures are available to ascertain the presence of a tumor mass, localize the mass for biopsy, provide tissue characterization, and further assess or stage the anatomical extent of disease. Although diagnostic imaging has benefited from the technology that produced computerized tomography (CT) and magnetic resonance imaging (MRI), an important role remains for the conventional diagnostic procedures. Examinations are selected that are efficient in detecting suspicious lesions and that also result in the least risk, discomfort, and expense for the patient. Table 11-3 identifies preferred imaging procedures for tumor definition and staging in several organ sites.[29-38] Table 11-4 elaborates on patient preparation and education for select examinations.[39]

Radiographic techniques

Radiographic studies, or x-ray films, allow for visualization of internal structures of the body. Distinction is made between normal and abnormal structure and function. X-rays, or gamma rays, are passed through the body and are absorbed variably by tissues of differing densities; they react on specially sensitized film or fluoroscopic screens. Radiographs may be site specific, such as the standard

Table 11-3   Preferred Imaging Procedures for Tumor Definition and Staging

Site	Imaging Techniques	Comments
Central nervous system	Positron emission tomography (PET)	Useful as a guidance tool in biopsy of lesions Ability to determine grade of tumor due to metabolic uptake
	Magnetic resonance imaging (MRI) with contrast	Superior to CT due to exquisite sensitivity of lesions <1 cm and lack of bone artifact in posterior fossa imaging
Head and neck	PET	Superior to CT in determining tumor necrosis versus tumor recurrence after radiotherapy
	Computerized axial tomography (CT)	Best for osseous change
	MRI	Superior for soft-tissue lesions, tumor-tissue interface, parapharyngeal spaces
Lung	PET	Detects benign versus malignant in solitary pulmonary modules Aids in staging of non–small cell lesions due to high sensitivity in depicting mediastinal involvement
	Chest x-ray (CXR)	Good for detection of peripheral lesions
	CT	Preferred for parenchyma and mediastinal nodes
	MRI	Advantage over CT in chest wall, hilum, and mediastinal vascular invasion
Esophagus	Esophagram with contrast	Preferred for measuring lesion length, necessary for staging
	Endoscopic ultrasound (EUS) CT	Superior to CT (except with severe stenosis) for depth of tumor invasion and lymph node assessment
Stomach	Barium studies with double contrast	Good for detection
	EUS	Preferred over CT for staging due to better detection of small nodes
Colon	PET	More sensitive than CT in diagnosing liver metastases and lymph node involvement with recurrent disease
	Barium enema with double contrast	Most tumors originate in mucosa, where barium studies will detect 90% of lesions >1 cm
Liver	Ultrasound (US)	Preferred for differentiating biliary obstruction from hepatic parenchymal disease
	CT or MRI with contrast	CT has been preferred for imaging, but MRI with contrast may be equivalent
Bladder	Intravenous pyelogram (IVP)	Detects lesions >1.5–2 cm
	MRI or CT	MRI preferred for bladder wall invasion, identifying large nodes, and separating them from vessels
Kidney	IVP	Preferred for detection
	CT	CT with contrast provides 90% accuracy for staging
Musculoskeletal	X-ray	For initial detection
	Bone scan	More sensitive than x-ray in identifying metastatic bone lesions (except multiple myeloma)
	CT or MRI	CT preferred for intraosseous lesion; MRI preferred for extraosseous lesion or intraosseous lesion extending into bone
Breast	Mammogram	Mammography provides the standard for breast imaging; sensitivity rate of >80% for screening purposes
Prostate	Transrectal ultrasound (TRUS)	Continues to be evaluated as a screening tool; detects extracapsular lesion extension Used as guidance tool for biopsy
	MRI or CT	MRI preferred for staging seminal vesicle invasion
Endometrium	MRI	Primary staging is by surgery; MRI assists with staging of local and nodal disease
Ovary	US (transvaginal and transabdominal) or CT	Tumor mass >1 cm can be defined by US or CT; primary staging is by surgery
Lymphoma and Hodgkin's disease	CXR CT of chest and abdomen	Required CT replacing need for lymphangiogram (LAG) in non-Hodgkin's lymphoma; CT of abdomen images upper retroperitoneal and mesenteric nodes, liver, and spleen

Table 11-4   Several Tumor Imaging Techniques with Instructions for Preparing the Patient

Tumor Imaging Examination	Patient Instructions	Comments
Barium studies	• Restriction of diet, smoking, and most medication before examination • Laxatives and enemas to cleanse bowel before colon examination • Will lie on tilting x-ray table, secured • Barium will taste chalky, milkshake consistency • Barium enema (BE) will feel cool, may cause cramping • Laxatives to clear barium after UGI • *Time:* 30–60 min	Bowel cleansing and procedure are exhausting for elderly patients. BE must precede UGI and small-bowel series. BE should follow other imaging examinations. Average cost for BE = $470. Single contrast preferred for elderly. Double contrast requires full patient cooperation due to time frame.
Computerized tomography	• Diet restrictions before examination • Will lie still on adjustable table; x-ray tube rotates around patient to take many pictures • Machinery noisy • Test painless • May receive intravenous contrast dye; may feel burning sensation as injected • May report feelings of nausea, vomiting, flushing, itching, bitter taste • Drink fluids after examination to eliminate dye • *Time:* 30–90 min	Careful history required to determine prior adverse reaction to contrast. Average cost for CT of abdomen and pelvis = $1800; cost depends on use of contrast and radiologist's interpretation. Discontinue Gluiophage for 3 days prior to CT scan because it is incompatible with IV contrastdye.
Angiogram	• Diet restriction before examination • May receive sedative just before examination • Will lie still on x-ray table • Skin over selected artery site cleansed and anesthetized • Cannula passed into artery or vein • Contrast die rapidly injected, may feel burning sensation as injected • Several x-ray films taken • May report feelings of nausea, vomiting, flushing, itching, bitter or salty taste • Cannula removed after examination, pressure applied, limb immobilized • *Time:* 1–3 hr	Decreased use as diagnostic procedure. Being replaced by percutaneous procedures. Useful in preoperative planning and therapeutic embolization.
Positron emission tomography	• Diet restriction before exam to optimize sensitivity • Must lie still during exam • Receives injection of glucose-tagged radioisotopes with no adverse effect • Radiation exposure is minimal • Must refrain from excessive physical activity for minimum of 24 hours prior to test • A glucose level may be drawn prior to testing • *Time:* 4 hr	Substances that alter metabolism such as ETOH, caffeine, and nicotine should be avoided. Use of sedatives may decrease test sensitivity. Average cost = $1900.

(continued)

Table 11-4 Several Tumor Imaging Techniques with Instructions for Preparing the Patient (continued)

Tumor Imaging Examination	Patient Instructions	Comments
Magnetic resonance imaging	• No diet restriction • Remove anything affected by a magnet • Lie still on table, secured with Velcro straps • Table will move into narrow magnet opening • Knocking or beating sound in machinery is normal • Painless • May receive intravenous contrast dye • May report nausea, vomiting, itching if given contrast dye • *Time:* 45–60 min	Difficult to titrate medication for comfort and sedation during lengthy procedures. Average cost of MRI of brain with gadolinium = $1050–$1250. May need sedation if claustrophobic.
Ultrasonogram	• Diet restriction before examination • Full bladder for pelvic ultrasound • Will lie on exam table • Ultrasound gel applied over skin of area to be examined • Transducer passes over skin • May feel pressure; no pain • No radiation involved • *Time:* 30 min	Increased use of probes introduced into the body (transrectal, transvaginal) for detection of cancer. Also has intraoperative use for intracranial and intraabdominal tumor localization. Average cost for abdominal ultrasound = $300.
Bone scan	• No diet restriction • Radioisotope injected before exam • Must void before scan to decrease tracer activity • Will lie on scanner table • Scanner moves back and forth, taking several pictures, emitting a clicking sound • Procedure painless • Radioisotope harmless • Patient instructed to drink water over 1–3 hr to aid renal clearance of radioisotope • *Time:*	Increased use of radioimmunoimaging using radio-labeled monoclonal antibodies. Highly sensitive over routine x-ray in detecting metastatic disease to bone. Average cost for whole body bone scan = $1100.
Endoscopy	• Diet restriction before examination • Mild sedation before procedure, but patient remains conscious • Intravenous infusion for medications and hydration *Oral:* • Local anesthetic sprayed in mouth • Flexible tube passed through mouth to level to be examined • Tongue and throat feel swollen; difficult to swallow • May feel pressure and fullness if scope in stomach	Screening sigmoidoscopy is recommended every 3–5 yr, beginning at age 50. Average cost range = $400–$700. Medicare does not pay for screening procedure. Colonoscopy requires more extensive preparation. Average cost range = $900–$1000.

(continued)

Table 11-4 Several Tumor Imaging Techniques with Instructions for Preparing the Patient (continued)

Tumor Imaging Examination	Patient Instructions	Comments
Endoscopy (cont.)	*Rectal:* • Prepared for exam with laxatives, enemas • Lubricated endoscope inserted anally • Feels cold, urge to defecate • May need to change positions during examination as scope is advanced • *Time:* 30–60 min	
Mammogram	• Breast is compressed between 2 plates on x-ray cassette • Compression may feel tight, but not painful • Radiation exposure is minimal and safe *Screening:* • Two views are taken of each breast: one view from head to foot (craniocaudal), the other lateral • *Time:* 15 min *Diagnostic:* • Three views taken of breast; craniocaudal, lateral, oblique • Spot compression and magnification films • *Time:* 30 min	Clinical breast exam and instruction on breast self-examination should be included. Average cost for screening mammogram = $50–$100. Covered by Medicare. Average cost for diagnostic mammogram = $85–$175.

chest film or mammogram, or they may view the dynamic function of an entire organ system. For example, in a gastrointestinal series, a continuous flow of x-rays passes through the digestive tract to assess the action of peristalsis, to detect displacement of structures, and to visualize mucosal abnormalities.

Mammographic examination is performed primarily in radiology suites dedicated solely to this procedure. These units are distinguished by the incorporation of a tissue compression device or cone that improves the quality of the image and reduces the amount of primary and scatter radiation. Informing women that this examination offers a safe, low dose of radiation and a high-quality mammographic image that is sensitive to abnormalities has been necessary to promote participation in screening efforts. Since 1987, the American College of Radiology (ACR) has provided accreditation of mammography facilities, which has resulted in a standard of quality assurance.[40] Additionally, many states have passed legislation or regulation to monitor the quality of mammography. In an attempt to establish national uniform quality standards, Congress enacted the Mammography Quality Standards Act in 1992. As of October 1994, every mammography facility, except for those in the Department of Veteran's Affairs, must be certified by the Food and Drug Administration and accredited by an approved accrediting body. In addition, each facility undergoes annual inspection and meets standards for personnel, equipment, equipment performance, and quality-control practices.[41] A list of qualified facilities can be obtained from a local American Cancer Society office, the ACR, or the National Cancer Institute.

Diagnostic mammography is indicated when symptoms or clinical findings exist that suggest an abnormality. The examination requires that more views be taken than for the standard two-view screening mammogram, as well as spot compression and magnification views of suspicious spots. Ultrasound may also be used for clarification purposes as an adjunct to the mammogram. Frequently, mammography is used to guide the placement of a wire, needle, dye, or catheter near a suspicious lesion in preparation for biopsy or surgery. Figure 11-1 shows a mammographically guided needle localization of a nonpalpable breast lesion. The localizer penetrates and extends beyond the lesion for more reliable surgical excision.

Tomography provides a radiographic image of a selected layer or plane of the body that would otherwise be obscured by shadows of other structures. Tomograms are particularly helpful in evaluating small calcified or cavitated lesions in the chest as well as hilar adenopathy and mediastinal abnormalities.

Computerized tomography also provides sectional (axial, coronal, or sagittal) views of structures in the body. After serial x-ray exposures are taken through different angles of the body, a computer analyzes the information and provides a three-dimensional, reconstructed picture of the area studied. Computerized tomography has become one of the most useful, informative, and available tests in the diagnosis and staging of malignancies. Due to its profound spatial resolution, it is the diagnostic tool

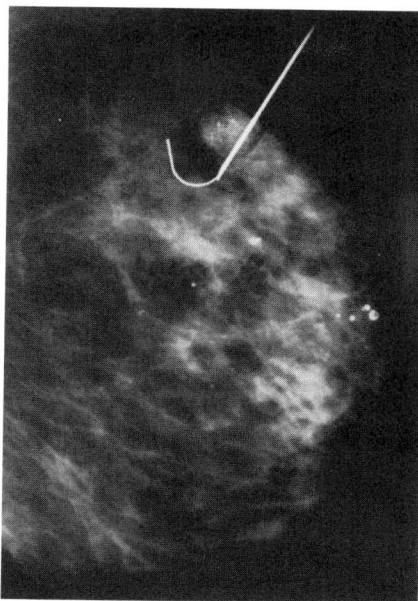

Figure 11-1 Mammographically guided hook-wire needle localization of nonpalpable breast lesion with multiple pathologic microcalcifications. (Courtesy of Scripps Memorial Hospital, Department of Radiology, La Jolla, CA.)

of choice for evaluation of the thorax, as it is capable of visualizing small lung nodules much earlier than standard imaging tests.[42] A CT scan is able to detect minor differences between tissue densities in any area of the body. The major drawback is its production of artifact in areas of cortical bone content. The MRI is the dominant imaging study over CT when evaluating musculoskeletal tumors.[43] Computerized tomography may be completed with or without radioiodinated contrast agents. Figure 11-2 demonstrates two different tumors imaged by CT with intravenous contrast. Computerized tomography frequently is used to direct a needle to a tumor site for percutaneous biopsy.

Several radiographic examinations rely on contrast materials to enhance or outline the structures to be visualized. Angiography, venography, cholangiography, and urography, in addition to CT, all rely on the intravascular administration of iodinated contrast agents for optimal visualization of body structure and function. An example is the excretory radiograph, also known as the intravenous pyelogram (IVP), which is used in the initial diagnostic evaluation of renal masses.

Patients who undergo studies requiring iodinated contrast material can experience minor, to intermediate, to life-threatening anaphylactoid reactions.[44] A metallic or bitter taste, becoming flushed, and a feeling of warmth all are common and transient sensations experienced

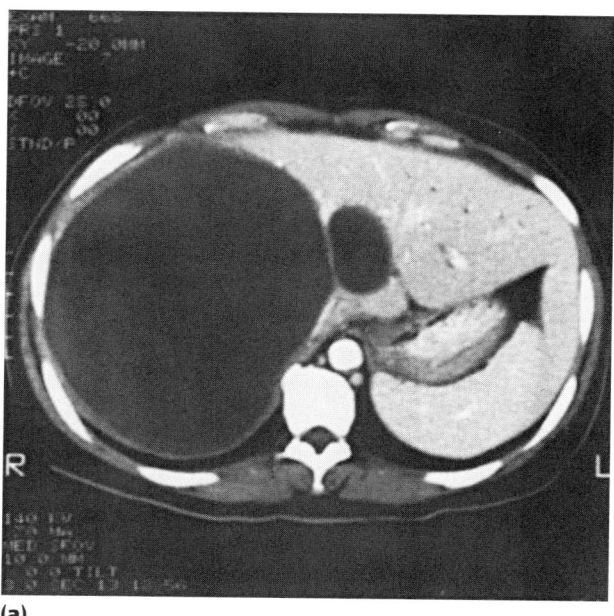

(a)

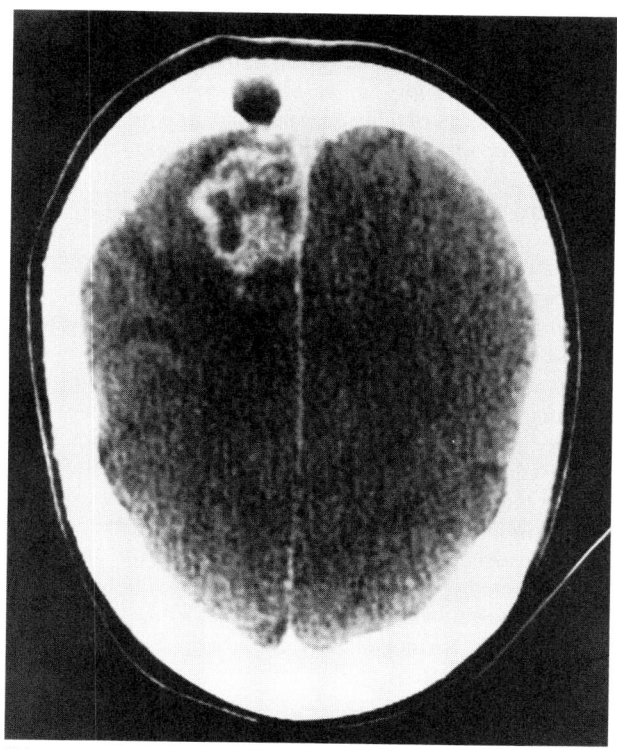

(b)

Figure 11-2 Examples of contrast-enhanced CT: CT abdominal scan revealing huge cystadenocarcinoma involving most of the liver (a), and CT head scan demonstrating lobular glioblastoma with peripheral rim enhancement (b). (Courtesy of Scripps Memorial Hospital, Department of Radiology, La Jolla, CA.)

during injection of contrast material. Vesicular reactions such as itching, angioedema, and mild urticaria may occur from a few minutes to several hours after contrast injection;[44] these symptoms do not require treatment and will not progress to life-threatening reactions. The incidence of a severe reaction such as cardiopulmonary arrest or seizure is extremely uncommon, occurring in only 1 of 5000 patients.[45] There is no good predictor for severe reactions; however, patients with a history of allergic response should be considered high risk, closely monitored, and premedicated. Those considered to be at risk for adverse reaction can receive a test dose of the contrast agent and should be premedicated with diphenhydramine, steroids, or epinephrine. Delayed reactions in patients have been noted from 2 to 6 hours after testing.[45] On completion of an iodinated contrast examination, patients should be instructed to drink a minimum of 8 glasses of fluid in 24 hours to prevent renal toxicity. Nonionic contrast agents are available, at considerable expense, for use with patients who have had serious reactions in the past.

Intrathecal contrast agents are used in myelography and in CT. Radiographs of the subarachnoid space are taken after the injection of either an oily or a water-soluble contrast agent. The contrast agent flows only to the point of obstruction, and more than one injection may be required. The specificity of MRI is one reason it has become the superior examination for detection of spinal cord compression and for skeletal metastatic deposits.

Barium sulfate is a nonabsorbable, radiopaque agent used to enhance the contrast between the lumen of the gastrointestinal tract and adjacent soft tissues. Studies that use barium include esophagography, upper gastrointestinal (UGI) series, small-bowel series, barium enema, and hypotonic duodenography. Barium is ingested or introduced into the gastrointestinal tract and allowed to coat the intraluminal surfaces. Radiographs are taken that can detect primary malignancies of the gastrointestinal organs or extrinsic compression from other tumor sites. Figure 11-3 presents a classic annular lesion of the colon imaged with radiopaque contrast. By combining barium and air, a double-contrast study is performed that is more sensitive than barium alone in detecting cancers larger than 1 cm, with a sensitivity rate of greater than 90%.[46] Complications seldom result from this examination unless there is an obstruction or a perforation of the digestive tract. Retention of the barium may cause fecal impaction and discomfort in some patients. The administration of a laxative or an enema may be necessary to assist with bowel evacuation.

Nuclear medicine techniques

Nuclear medicine imaging involves the intravenous injection or the ingestion of radioisotope compounds followed by camera imaging of those organs or tissues that have concentrated the radioisotopes. Nuclear medicine studies are extremely sensitive and often will detect sites of

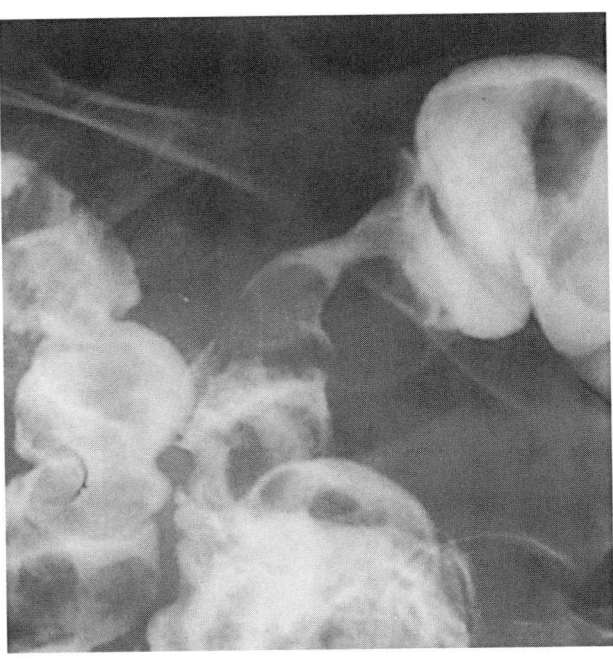

Figure 11-3 Barium enema visualizes annular, "apple core" lesion that is constricting the colon. (Courtesy of Scripps Memorial Hospital, Department of Radiology, La Jolla, CA.)

abnormal metabolism or early malignancy several months before changes are seen on a radiograph. Scans of the bones, liver and spleen, brain, thyroid, and kidneys are useful in the detection of malignancy. Figure 11-4 shows an abnormal bone scan suggestive of widespread metastasis from prostate cancer. Gallium scans are particularly sensitive in detecting bronchogenic carcinomas and lymphomas. However, many radioisotope examinations are being replaced by CT because of its sensitivity and ease of administration.

Positron emission tomography (PET) is an imaging modality that provides information based on the biochemical and metabolic activity of tissue. Infused biochemical compounds such as glucose are tagged with radioactive particles that emit positrons detectable by gamma camera tomography. F-18 fluorodeoxyglucose (FDG) is the most widely used radiopharmaceutical. Tumors have a higher rate of glycolysis, thus FDG is able to trace glucose metabolism in cancerous tissues, unlike other diagnostic tests that examine only structural changes.[4,47] Figure 11-5 is a PET image demonstrating a large lung tumor. In order to allow maximum accumulation of FDG in cancerous tissue, patients must fast for at least 8 hours prior to the examination.

Previously used for cardiac and neurologic disorders, the PET scan has demonstrated accuracy in a variety of cancers such as those of the head and neck, breast, and lung, as well as gastrointestinal malignancies, lymphomas, and melanoma.[48] The most extensive application of PET in clinical oncology has been in brain imaging. Many

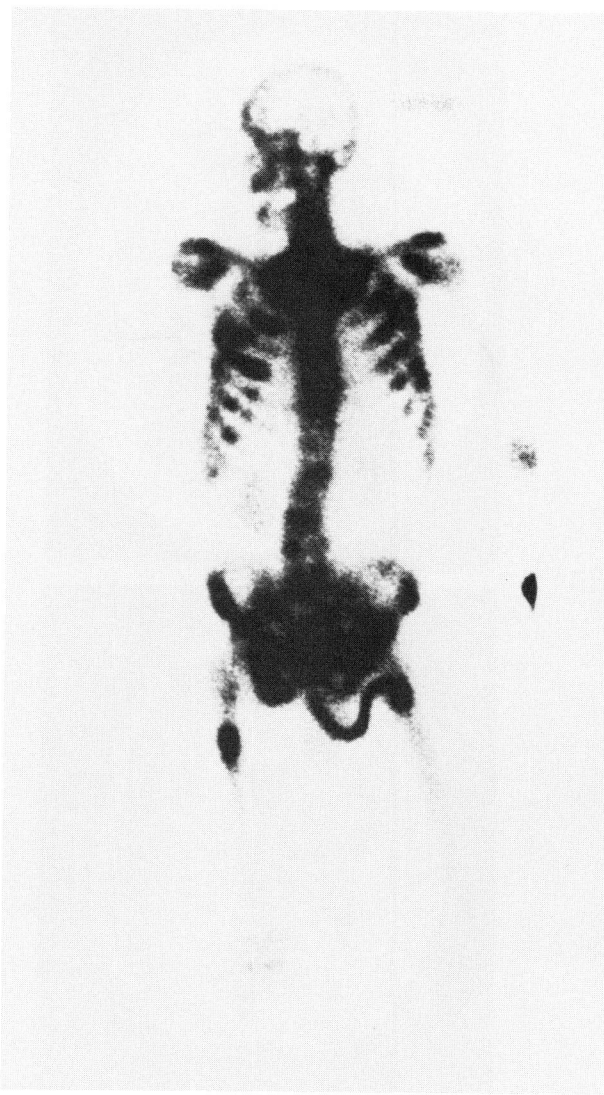

Figure 11-4 Abnormal bone scan suggesting widespread bony metastasis in central axial skeleton, pelvis, hips, and right proximal femur. (Courtesy of Scripps Memorial Hospital, Department of Radiology, La Jolla, CA.)

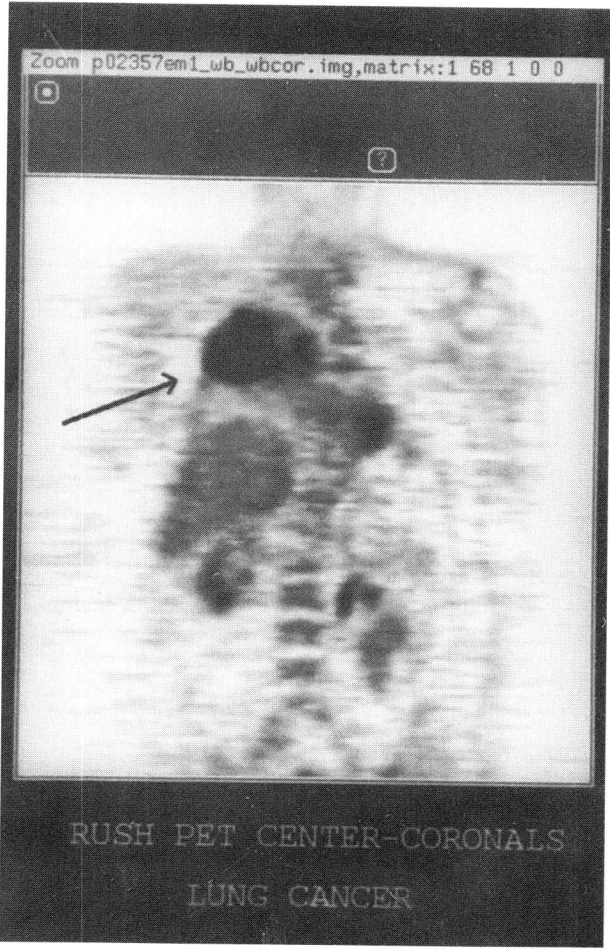

Figure 11-5 PET Scan of Lung Courtesy Rush PET Center

insurers have accepted this technology for imaging brain tumors, offering reimbursement, while other insurance carriers question this exam versus MRI and CT.

The PET-FDG test is particularly useful in differentiating low-grade from high-grade tumors and in distinguishing treatment-induced tissue necrosis from recurrent tumor. It has proved highly effective when evaluating patients for metastatic disease. In a study done by Delbeke et al,[49] fifty-two patients diagnosed with colon cancer were evaluated for recurrent disease to the liver using both PET and CT scans. The PET scan proved more accurate than CT in diagnosing liver metastases and extrahepatic metastases. Surgical evaluation for restaging was also avoided because of the accuracy of the PET scan.

Limitations of this modality are its expense, the need for a cyclotron to produce the isotopes, and fasting protocols that patients must undergo to allow for maximum tissue uptake of FDG.[47,48,50–52] The PET scan will continue to be investigated as a diagnostic tool for cancer or as an adjunct with other imaging studies to obtain additional information. Thus far, it has shown great promise and plays a key role in the management and staging of cancer.

Nuclear imaging with radiolabeled monoclonal antibodies visualizes microscopic sites of metastasis or suspected malignancy. This technique requires that a monoclonal antibody targeted against a specific tumor antigen be combined with trace amounts of radioactivity. After intravenous injection, the antibody binds to antigen on the tumor. Tumor sites then "light up" with imaging scanners. CYT-103 (OncoSCINT OV/CR) is the first FDA-approved radiolabeled monoclonal antibody for diagnostic use in cancer. The indium-111–labeled antibody targets the tumor-associated glycoprotein (TAG-72) found in mucin-producing adenocarcinomas.[53] Although data remains limited, its imaging is approved for colon and ovarian cancer and plays a role in occult recurrent disease.[54]

Ultrasonography

Ultrasonography (US) is a nonradiographic and non-invasive technique of imaging deep soft-tissue structures within the body. The reflecting echoes of high-frequency sound waves directed into specific tissues are recorded on an imaging screen. The echoes are variable, depending on the tissue density, and can be used to discriminate masses. A limitation of the examination is its inability to visualize through bone or air. Ultrasonography is most applicable in detecting ascites, renal or biliary obstruction, or tumors within the pelvis of patients with cancer.[55] Masses greater than 2 cm in diameter can be detected and localized for possible percutaneous biopsy. Transrectal ultrasound is useful in guiding a needle biopsy of suspicious prostate lesions but has not proved to be an effective screening tool. In the diagnosis of breast cancer, ultrasound is an important adjunct to mammography for distinguishing cysts from solid lesions with 98%–100% accuracy.

Magnetic resonance imaging

Magnetic resonance imaging creates sectional images of the body, similar to CT, but does not expose the patient to ionizing radiation. Images are created by placing the individual within a powerful magnetic field that aligns the body's hydrogen nuclei in one direction. Radiofrequency pulses are used to excite the magnetized nuclei and change their alignment. Between radiofrequency pulses, the nuclei return to a state of relaxation, and variable signals are transmitted on the basis of tissue characteristics. These signals are analyzed by the computer, and multiplaner (sagittal, coronal, and axial) images are produced with exquisite clarity. Magnetic resonance imaging can be enhanced with the intravenous paramagnetic contrast agents gadolinium diethylenetriamine pentaacetic acid (DTPA) and gadotetrate meglumine (DOTA).[56] These agents work by reducing tissue relaxation time, thus increasing signal intensity and image production. Adverse reactions to gadolinium DTPA, which are rare, include nausea, pain localized to the injection site, and headache occurring several hours after the examination. Anaphylactoid reactions to the contrast agent have also been reported.[57]

Magnetic resonance imaging is most applicable in the detection, localization, and staging of malignant disease in the central nervous system, spine, head and neck, and musculoskeletal system. At present, MRI enhanced with gadolinium and used for the detection of brain metastasis stands alone, continuing to be the best diagnostic tool for this diagnosis (Figure 11-6).[58]

Significant limitations do exist in the use of MRI. Persons with aneurysm or surgical clips, pacemakers, implanted pumps, tattooed eyeliner, or any ferromagnetic

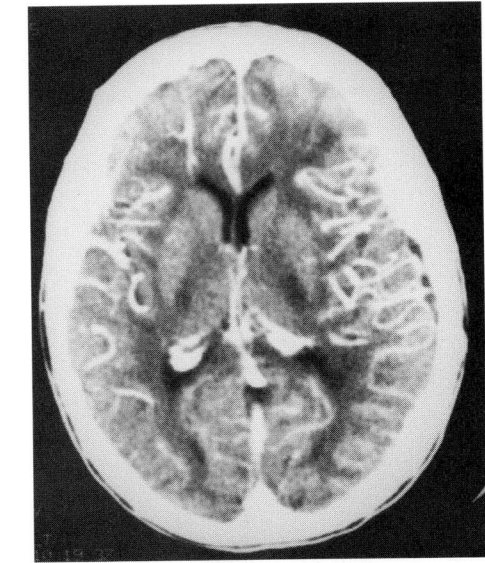

(a)

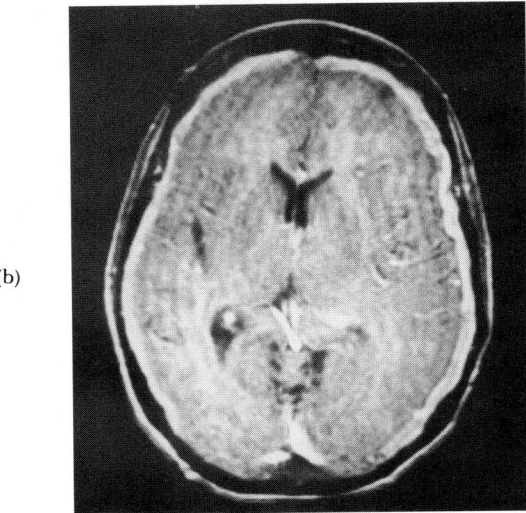

(b)

Figure 11-6 Contrast-enhanced CT (a) and contrast-enhanced MRI (b) of metastatic intracranial tumor. MRI shows "rind" of metastatic deposit around brain that was invisible on CT due to bone artifact. (Courtesy of Scripps Memorial Hospital, Department of Radiology, La Jolla, CA.)

metallic implant cannot undergo MRI examination. The magnetic pull of the MRI is capable of dislodging the implant, interfering with its operation, or removing the object from the person's body. This excludes the MRI examination from use in acutely ill patients with life-support or monitoring devices. Nonferrous metallic implants may produce artifacts that distort the MRI image but are generally safe for the patient. Implanted ports, frequently used in cancer patients to provide vascular, peritoneal, and epidural access, are made from many different materials. Shellock provides a list of ports that do not move or deflect during exposure to magnetic scanning.[59] Camp-Sorrell identifies ports causing the least artifact but concludes that attention must be paid to the manufacturer's recommendations as materials change and new ports are developed.[60] High-grade titanium and nonmetal ports produce the least amount of or no artifact.

Claustrophobic individuals may require sedation if they are to undergo an MRI scan, but they also benefit from explanations prior to the procedure, a support person nearby, verbal contact, MRI-compatible headphones, prisms or mirrors to allow a view outside of the tube, and relaxation techniques.[59] Free-standing, open MRI facilities offer a welcome alternative for individuals who are claustrophobic. The cost of the MRI and length of the examination (1 to 2 hours for a total scan of the spine) are disadvantages.

After many years of rapid growth, diagnostic imaging technology is now being intensely scrutinized by health care providers. Hospitals and free-standing radiology centers are considered cost environments, and insurance carriers require authorization or certification for all diagnostic studies. In the recent past, many studies were automatically added to clinical practice without considering whether it would be money well spent.[61]

High-tech studies such as the PET scan, OncoSCINT, and OctreoSCAN (OctreoSCAN, Mallinskrodt Medical Inc., also known as Octreotide scan) are just some of the diagnostic modalities that continue to be developed due to their greater sensitivity in detecting and distinguishing benign from malignant tumors; however, the efficacy of these modalities is questioned due to cost and availability. The nurse's role is one of teacher, educating the patient about the testing procedure, and offering guidance and reassurance. Serving also as a liaison between physician and insurance carrier, the nurse will be called on to explain the procedure and purpose behind the diagnostic study.

Invasive Diagnostic Techniques

Endoscopy

Endoscopy is a method to directly visualize the interior of a hollow viscus by the insertion of an endoscope into a body cavity or opening. The endoscope contains fiberoptic glass bundles that transmit light and then return an image to the optical head of the endoscope. The instrument may be rigid or flexible. Visual inspection, tissue biopsy, cytologic aspiration, staging the extent of disease, and excision of pathologic processes are possible through the endoscope.

By passing a flexible scope through the mouth, endoscopic examinations can visualize directly the larynx, the upper airway passages and the bronchial tree, the esophagus, the stomach, and the upper duodenum. Visualization of the distal sigmoid colon, the rectum, and the anal canal is performed by means of a rigid scope. The entire large intestine can be viewed with a flexible colonoscope that is inserted anally. Endoscopic retrograde cholangio-

pancreatography (ERCP) combines the diagnostic procedures of endoscopy and contrast-enhanced radiography to evaluate biliary tract obstruction and pancreatic masses.

The endoscopic ultrasound (EUS) may prove superior to other imaging modalities for assessing direct depth of tumor invasion and local lymph node status for esophageal, gastric, and colon malignancy. Where available, EUS is indicated to distinguish benign from malignant lesions, to stage neoplasms, to establish operability and surgical approach, and to determine response or recurrence.[62]

The cervix and vagina are visualized with the magnification lens of the colposcope. Peritoneoscopy or laparoscopy permits assessment of surfaces within the peritoneal cavity by the insertion of a peritoneoscope through a small incision below the umbilicus. Thoracoscopy allows visualization of the visceral and parietal pleura, the mediastinum, and the diaphragm by means of a thoracoscope passed through an incision in the midaxillary line of the sixth to the eighth intercostal space. The direct visualization of the tissues and organs of the mediastinum is performed by passing an endoscope into the mediastinum through a small incision above the manubrium.

Biopsy

The importance of obtaining accurate histologic or cytologic proof of malignancy cannot be overstated. Treatment decisions for cancers arising within the same organ differ on the basis of the histopathology report. An example is the very different treatment regimens for small-cell cancer of the lung and adenocarcinoma of the lung. Exactly what tissue is to be biopsied depends on several factors: the clinical status of the person, the person's willingness to undergo invasive procedures, the size and location of the identified tumor, and the amount of tissue needed by the pathologist for analysis.[63]

The cytologic examination of aspirated fluid, secretions, scrapings, or washings of body cavities may reveal malignant cells that have exfoliated from a primary or metastatic tumor. Tissue will not be obtained by this method, and the pathologist's ability to establish the primary site of the malignancy may be limited. Cancer of the cervix is one example of a malignancy that is successfully detected by the cytologic examination of cells acquired from a Papanicolaou smear.

The fine-needle aspiration biopsy, guided by palpation or an imaging technique, is extensively used and is available in the ambulatory setting. It provides not only cytologic information but also microhistologic information if adequate tissue fragments are obtained. Table 11-5 provides general instructions for preparing the patient for an image-guided fine-needle aspiration biopsy.[64]

Stereotactic localization is another diagnostic tool that utilizes CT or MRI to establish the coordinates of a lesion and accurately position a needle for the tissue biopsy. Stereotactic breast biopsy of nonpalpable lesions is comparable to conventional needle-localization surgical biopsy, with a sensitivity of 90%–95% for breast cancer

Table 11-5   Instructions for Preparing the Patient for Image-Guided Fine-Needle Aspiration Biopsy

- Contrast agent may be required—intravenous or oral.
- Intravenous line established as a precaution or for sedation.
- Sedatives may be offered.
- Vital signs and oximetry will be monitored if intravenous sedation is used.
- Some pain may be experienced; local anesthetic is used.
- Skin at biopsy site is cleansed, and the needle inserted.
- Needle position is established by an imaging technique (e.g., CT, ultrasound, or chest fluoroscopy).
- Syringe is attached to the needle, and the fluid and tissue are aspirated.
- Patient is observed for infection, bleeding, or increase in pain.

detection.[65] Figure 11-7 demonstrates stereotactic images of a breast nodule and the accurate placement of a needle for biopsy. Stereotactic brain biopsy of suspicious lesions is a relatively safe and quick procedure. A stereotactic head frame is fixed to the skull under local anesthesia, the lesion is scanned for localizing landmarks (including the location of arteries and vessels), a small hole is made in the skull, and the biopsy is then directed by an instrument attached to the frame.

Cooperation and skill are required of the surgeon, pathologist, and the affiliated pathology lab to ensure that an accurate diagnosis is made. Local or topical anesthesia is commonly used. Table 11-6 lists specific details of each type of needle biopsy: (1) aspiration needles, (2) cutting or core needles, (3) large cutting needles, and (4) automated biopsy systems (biopsy guns). Some needles have carriers that shield and guide the actual biopsy needle, cup, or punch used to obtain the specimen. The carrier reduces the possibility of contaminating the needle tract with tumor cells from the specimen as the needle is withdrawn. An unfortunate limitation of either needle aspiration or core biopsy is the possibility that the tumor will be missed; therefore, only a positive finding of malignancy is diagnostically significant.[66–69]

The biopsy needles are small bore, usually 20- to 23-gauge. Fine-needle biopsies are well tolerated by the patient, result in limited trauma to tissue, and cause minimal manipulation of the tumor. Hematoma and infection are potential complications.

Fluoroscopy, ultrasound, or CT is often used to guide the clinician during core biopsy procedures. Local anesthesia is used. Hematoma, infection, and pain are postbiopsy considerations.

Regional biopsy is performed using a variety of approaches and needles. Regional biopsy involves obtaining several samples of tissue from different locations within a tumor or within a diseased organ. Regional biopsies are used to diagnose metastatic disease in a defined, but not localized, region of the body. Regional biopsies also are used to sample diffuse disease within an organ or to sample multiple nodes within a region. Examples include transthoracic, pancreatic adrenal gland, liver, pelvic mass, prostate, renal, breast, thyroid, and bone regional biopsies.

For a definitive diagnosis of malignancy, it is imperative that the pathologist receive an adequate, representative, and well-preserved tissue specimen. A cytologic or

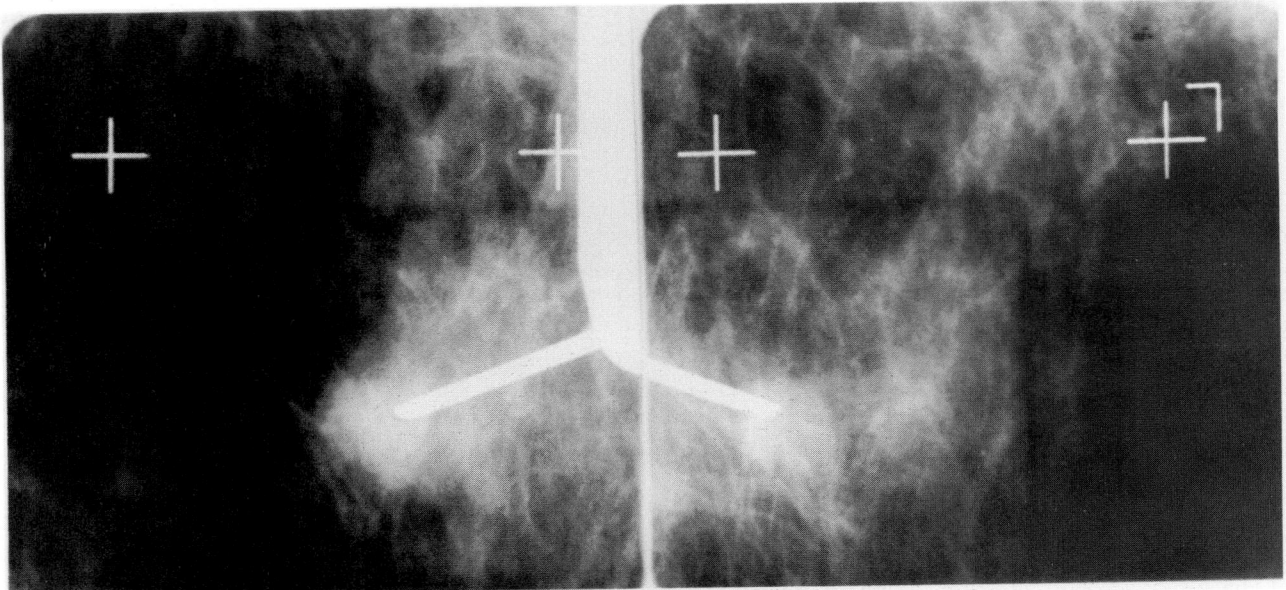

Figure 11-7   Pair of images confirming accurate placement of needle at the margin of a breast nodule for stereotactic core biopsy. (Courtesy of Scripps Memorial Hospital, Department of Radiology, La Jolla, CA.)

Table 11-6 Approaches for Biopsy

Type	What Used For	Where Done	Rationale
Needle biopsy			
Fine-needle aspiration (21–22 g needle 5-cc syringe): Local anesthesia	Solid, palpable lesion (i.e., breast mass, thyroid nodule)	Outpatient setting Operating room	Involves only small amount of trauma to tissue, so if positive then surgical procedure is avoided. Used when there is a high level of suspicion of malignancy.
Sterotaxic fine-needle aspiration (21–22 g needle, sterotaxic equipment): Local anesthesia	Solid, nonpalpable lesion (i.e., mammographic abnormality)	Outpatient setting Radiology center	Same as for fine-needle aspiration, but able to sample small, *nonpalpable* lesions
Core needle biopsy (special cutting needle): Local anesthesia; can use ultrasound to help guide	Solid, accessible tumor	Outpatient setting	Removes larger amount of tissue than fine-needle aspiration; may allow for more information (i.e., hormone receptor tests)
Surgical biopsy			
Excisional biopsy: Usually local anesthesia	Solid, palpable mass (i.e., melanoma, breast mass)	Day surgery	Attempt is made to remove the whole mass only, without regard to clear margin. Result should be cosmetically acceptable.
Incisional biopsy: Usually local anesthesia	Solid, palpable large mass (i.e., large, ulcerating or bleeding mass)	Day surgery	Biopsy is for diagnosis; mass is too large to remove without major surgery. May bleed profusely.
Endoscopy (special endoscope): May use sedation	Solid mass in an accessible lumen (i.e., colon, esophagus)	Outpatient setting Day surgery	May be for diagnosis or treatment. Avoids surgical trauma.

histologic report that is negative for malignancy may suggest a specimen inadequate for diagnostic evaluation, thus necessitating repeat biopsy. Only a complete excisional biopsy can exclude malignancy with certainty. When the results of a biopsy are equivocal, the specimen should be sent to an outside source for a second evaluation. The Armed Forces Institute of Pathology in Washington, DC, is used by pathologists worldwide as a reference and for review.

Not infrequently, the biopsied tissue will confirm malignancy, but the primary site or tissue of origin cannot be established by the pathologist or the clinician. An example is the individual who undergoes biopsy of a cervical node and is diagnosed with squamous cell carcinoma but for whom a thorough examination of the chest and head and neck area fails to yield the source of the malignancy. The goals for pursuing the primary site in this situation are discussed later in this chapter under "Tumors of Unknown Origin."

Surgical biopsy techniques

In some cases, such as tumors of the lip, nose, ear, or breast, excisional biopsy alone will be definitive therapy. The pathologist and the surgeon will determine whether the extent of the excisional biopsy is sufficient to eliminate the possibility of residual disease or whether more extensive surgery is indicated. The tissue is covered with

ink, sliced, and then put on the slide for microscopic evaluation.

Incisional biopsies are generally selected for the diagnosis of large tumors that will require major surgery for complete removal. A portion of the mass is removed by incisional biopsy for pathologic examination. Incisional biopsy should be positioned in such a way that the biopsy site will be totally excised with subsequent definitive surgery.

Endoscopy is a surgical technique used to obtain biopsy specimens for diagnosis of tumors in accessible lumens.[70] Tumors of the gastrointestinal, genitourinary, or pulmonary system, and, more recently, the ductal system of the breast can be diagnosed by inserting an optical instrument into the lumen to examine the area and to secure a biopsy for analysis or secretions for cytologic examination. Flexible instruments have made endoscopy more tolerable for the patient and more functional for the clinician. Bleeding and infection are potential problems.

Laparoscopy

During the last decade, laparoscopy has been increasingly used for the detection, staging, and treatment of cancer, thereby legitimizing it as an acceptable surgical procedure. The development of high-resolution monitors and instrumentation as well as surgical experience have made this possible.[71]

Laparoscopy has been used to diagnose and treat a wide variety of cancers, including lymphoma and gastrointestinal, urologic, and gynecologic malignancies.[72] It has a distinct advantage over other diagnostic procedures in visualizing the abdominal cavity and lesions, and in evaluating adenopathy and liver abnormalities. Laparoscopy also offers the opportunity to visualize the diaphragm and peritoneal surfaces.

Patients facing a diagnosis of cancer of the pancreas, stomach, or esophagus have benefited by laparoscopy rather than CT and US to determine resectability and nodal status. Surgical approach using this method decreases the need for and may prevent putting the patient through an unnecessary laparotomy. Accurate diagnosis and staging of Hodgkin's lymphoma can now be done because of current laparoscopic capabilities. Staging laparotomies have decreased by 70% in these patients due to the advent of laparoscopic liver and spleen biopsies.[72]

Many gynecologic oncologists are now using laparoscopy to manage patients with cervical, endometrial, and ovarian cancers, although its exact role continues to be evaluated. It is important to note that with laparoscopy metastatic disease in all three of these cancers is diagnosed at a rate similar to that of a laparotomy procedure.[73] Unavailable survival data, lack of direct tactile palpation, longer initial operative time, and inability to visualize behind the liver are just some of the disadvantages of laparoscopy.[65] Further development of this technique for gynecologic cancers along with clinical trials is needed.

Overall, for some patients who face the diagnosis of cancer there may be an advantage to using laparoscopy as a diagnostic tool. A shorter hospital stay and recovery time that lowers cost along with decreased pain and a quicker return to activities of daily living have a definite impact on the patient's quality of life. The future of laparoscopy holds promise, but emphasis must be placed on proper surgical training, gathering of scientific data, and evaluation of this procedure if patients are to benefit.

Classification and Nomenclature

Basic Terminology

The terms *cancer* and *tumor* often are used interchangeably and inappropriately and can be misleading for patients, families, and professionals. A *tumor* is a swelling or mass of tissue that may be benign or malignant. *Cancer,* synonymous with *malignant neoplasm,* is an uncontrolled "new growth" capable of metastasis and invasion that threatens host survival.

The term *primary tumor* is used to describe the original histologic site of tumorigenesis. A *secondary,* or metastatic, *tumor* resembles the primary tumor histologically but sometimes may be so anaplastic as to obscure the cell of origin. A *second primary lesion* refers to an additional, histologically separate malignant neoplasm in the same patient. Although this is a relatively unusual occurrence,

it must be excluded at the time of an apparent recurrence. Tables of probability for recurrence exist to guide the clinician in these determinations. A general rule is always to biopsy the first recurrence, because it may actually represent a new, curable or treatable malignancy; for example, a patient with a history of breast cancer who presents with suspicious lymph nodes and is found on biopsy to have lymphoma. Unfortunately, some recurrences present in sites where the morbidity from biopsy is so significant that the lesion is treated without tissue confirmation; for example, a woman with breast cancer who presents with a vertebral pedicle lesion.

Benign and Malignant Tumor Characteristics

Certain biological, histologic, and cytologic characteristics distinguish a benign tumor from a malignant tumor. However, with the exception of the properties of invasion and metastasis, which are found only in cancer, the differences between a benign process and a malignant process are relative. In some circumstances, a definitive diagnosis of benign tumor versus malignant tumor cannot be made. For example, a well-differentiated follicular carcinoma of the thyroid may be solitary and encapsulated and may mimic a benign adenoma of the thyroid. Occasionally, a benign tumor will transform into a malignant tumor over time. An adenomatous polyp of the colon is an example of a relatively benign process that can transform into cancer of the colon if left untreated.

In general, the following features distinguish benign tumors from those that are malignant. The *benign tumor* is relatively slow-growing. Tumor stasis or regression may occur. Growth occurs as the tumor expands locally within a capsule of fibrous tissue. Benign tumors do not invade adjacent tissues, destroy normal tissue, or metastasize elsewhere in the body. Although death from a benign tumor is rare, distressing symptoms may result from a tumor's pressure on vital organs or from ectopic hormone production. Cytologic examination reveals uniform, well-differentiated cells that resemble those of the adult tissue of origin and demonstrate little or no anaplasia and rare mitoses.

In contrast, the *malignant tumor* is characterized by its generally high mitotic rate, rapid growth, and disregard for normal growth limitations. Malignant tumors are almost never encapsulated. The malignant cells invade surrounding tissue, lymphatic vessels, and blood vessels and metastasize to distant sites. Malignant tumor cells are anaplastic, vary in morphologic characteristics within the same tumor, are poorly differentiated, and have abnormal and inconstant numbers of chromosomes.

Tumor Classification System

The most relevant classification systems will universally communicate clinical and prognostic information. Tumors may be classified not only by their biological behavior (benign versus malignant), but also by their tissue of origin.

To understand the nomenclature of tumors, it is useful to review normal cell differentiation in the embryonic state. An early occurrence in the life of the embryo is the development of three primary germ layers: the ectoderm, the mesoderm, and the endoderm. The cells within these layers divide, specialize, and give rise to all cells, tissues, and organs within the body. The ectoderm differentiates into the skin and nervous system. The mesoderm differentiates into organs and connective tissue, bones, blood, cartilage, fat, fibrous tissue, muscle, and blood and lymph vessels. The endoderm differentiates into the lining of the digestive and respiratory tracts, the bladder, and the urethra.

Virtually every cell type in the body is capable of transforming into a malignant cell. It is fairly well accepted that the malignant cell derives from a postembryonic cell that is arrested in the process of differentiation. Most tumors retain sufficient characteristics—such as function and structure of the normal, differentiated cell—to allow recognition of the type of tissue from which they were derived, which is the basis for the classification of human tumors by tissue type (Table 11-7).[74] Specific nomenclature provides information on characteristics of the neoplasm. A suffix is added to the name of the tissue or cell type under pathologic study to designate its benign or malignant nature. Benign tumors usually end in the suffix *-oma,* the Greek root for "tumor." Most malignant tumors end in either the suffix *-sarcoma* or the suffix *-carcinoma,* depending on the tissues from which they arise. For example, lipoma is a benign tumor of fat tissue, and liposarcoma is a malignancy of fat tissue. *Sarcoma* specifies a malignant tumor of the connective tissues, that is, those tissues originating from the mesodermal embryonic layer. *Carcinoma* specifies a malignant tumor arising from epithelial tissues. Epithelium covers or lines surfaces in the body and arises from the ectodermal, mesodermal, or endodermal embryonic layers.

Carcinomas are further delineated by the prefixes *adeno-,* for tumors that arise from glandular epithelial tissue, and *squamous,* for tumors that originate from squamous epithelial tissues. Descriptive terms such as *cystic, follicular, papillary, medullary, exophytic,* and *polypoid* are added to further define histologic characteristics.

The suffix that describes malignant tumors resembling the primitive blastula phase in embryonic development is *-blastoma.* Examples are neuroblastoma and retinoblastoma.

Mixed tumors, such as adenosquamous carcinoma of the bronchi, represent tumors with mixed squamous and glandular elements that arise from the same germ layer and tissue. Some tumors, although rare and highly malignant, have such primitive differentiation that they may be classified by the appearance of the neoplastic cell.[75]

Teratoma and its malignant counterpart, teratocarcinoma, arise from tissue of all three germ layers and are not limited to those tissues present in the area of origin.[76]

Several exceptions exist to the classification system just described. For instance, lymphoma, melanoma, and hepatoma are malignant tumors with the *-oma* suffix. In addition, some malignancies are named after the person who characterized them. Hodgkin's disease, Ewing's sarcoma, and Wilms' tumor are examples. The hematopoietic malignancies are classified separately by predominant cell type and their acute versus chronic nature.

Tumors of Unknown Origin

Five to ten percent of patients diagnosed with cancer each year are found to have a malignancy from an unknown primary site.[77] Most frequently, the histologic classification will be adenocarcinoma, but the site of origin may never be determined, even on autopsy. The prognosis is poor, with an overall median survival of 3 to 4 months.[78] The goal of proceeding with a diagnostic investigation in this situation is to identify those malignancies, even if they are disseminated, that are potentially curable or palliated with known, effective treatment. For example, lymphomas and germ cell tumors are potentially curable with systemic chemotherapy. Lesions in the nasopharynx may be cured with radiation. Local complications such as bowel obstruction, spinal cord compression, and pathologic fractures can be palliated with surgery or radiation treatment, even when the primary site of malignancy is unknown. Hormonal therapy may be recommended if the presumptive diagnosis, based on tumor markers or hormone receptor analysis, is breast, prostate, or endometrial malignancy.

Patients and their families who are facing cancer from an unknown source present unique challenges for the nurse. Not only do they need information and preparation for extensive imaging and laboratory testing, but they also need support when these tests fail to yield a definitive diagnosis. It is often hoped, though not necessarily true, that a known primary source of malignancy will be more treatable or curable than an unknown primary source. Coping with any cancer diagnosis is difficult. Coping with an "unknown" cancer accentuates the feelings of loss of control, anxiety, and frustration. The involved nurse can be most helpful by identifying psychosocial concerns and available support systems early in the diagnostic period, clarifying and reinforcing known information and the rationale for extensive testing, and providing hope and reassurance that treatment is offered for the most probable and most treatable source of malignancy.[79]

Staging and Grading Classifications

Staging the Extent of the Disease

The staging process is a method of classifying a malignancy by the extent of its spread within the body. It is a clinical and histologic determination that depends on the natural course of each particular type of cancer. Staging is

Table 11-7 Select Benign and Malignant Neoplasms Listed by Histogenetic Classification

Tissue of Origin	Benign Neoplasm	Malignant Neoplasm
Epithelial (Endodermal)		
Squamous	Squamous cell papilloma	Squamous cell or epidermoid carcinoma
Glandular	Adenoma	Adenocarcinoma
	Papilloma	Papillary carcinoma
	Cystadenoma	Cystadenocarcinoma
Respiratory tract		Bronchogenic carcinoma
Renal epithelium	Renal tubular adenoma	Renal cell carcinoma (hypernephroma)
Urinary tract	Transitional cell papilloma	Transitional cell carcinoma
Placental epithelium	Hydatidiform mole	Choriocarcinoma
Testicular epithelium		Seminoma
		Embryonal carcinoma
Liver	Liver cell adenoma	Hepatocellular carcinoma (hepatoma)
Biliary tree	Cholangioma	Cholangiocarcinoma
Stomach	Gastric polyp	Gastric carcinoma
Colon	Colonic polyp	Adenocarcinoma of the colon
Mesenchymal (Mesodermal)		
Connective		
Fibrous tissue	Fibroma	Fibrosarcoma
Adipose tissue	Lipoma	Liposarcoma
Cartilage	Chondroma	Chondrosarcoma
Bone	Osteoma	Osteosarcoma
Muscle		
Smooth muscle	Leiomyoma	Leiomyosarcoma
Striated muscle	Rhabdomyoma	Rhabdomyosarcoma
Endothelial		
Blood vessels	Hemangioma	Hemangiosarcoma
Lymphatic vessels	Lymphangioma	Lymphangiosarcoma
Hematopoietic and lymphoreticular		
Hematopoietic cells		Leukemias
Lymphoid tissue		Lymphomas
		Hodgkin's disease
Plasma cells		Plasmacytoma (multiple myeloma)
Neural (Ectodermal)		
Meninges	Meningioma	Meningeal sarcoma
Glia	Astrocytoma	Glioblastoma multiforme
Nerve cells	Ganglioneuroma	Neuroblastoma
		Medulloblastoma
Melanocytes	Nevus	Malignant melanoma
Mixed Tissues		
Kidney		Wilms' tumor
Salivary gland	Mixed tumor of salivary gland (pleomorphic adenoma)	Malignant mixed tumor of salivary gland

based on the premise that cancers with similar histologic features and sites of origin will extend and metastasize in a predictable manner. Although most staging classifications are based on the anatomic extent of disease, other criteria are included for specific malignancies. For thyroid cancer, the age of the patient and the histologic diagnosis (papillary, follicular, medullary, or anaplastic) are included in the staging system. In the staging of prostate cancer, soft-tissue sarcomas, primary malignant tumors of the bone, and brain tumors, the histopathologic grade of the tumor is significant.

There are multiple objectives of solid-tumor staging, but the most important is to provide the necessary infor-mation for individual treatment planning. Other reasons for using a uniform staging system include to give prognostic information, to assist in treatment evaluation, to facilitate the exchange of information and comparative statistics among treatment centers, and to stratify individuals who may be eligible for clinical trials.[80]

With the goal of developing an internationally consistent system of staging solid-tumor malignancy, the TNM committee of the International Union Against Cancer (UICC) and the American Joint Committee on Cancer (AJCC) have agreed on the TNM staging system. The TNM staging system classifies solid tumors by the anatomic extent of disease, as determined clinically and histologically. Three categories are quantified, with gradations representing progressive tumor size or involvement. The extent of the primary tumor (T) is evaluated on the basis of depth of invasion, surface spread, and tumor size. Secondly, the absence or presence and extent of regional lymph node (N) metastasis are considered, with attention to the size and location of the nodes. Thirdly, the absence or presence of distant metastasis (M) is assessed. A three-letter abbreviation may specify the site of metastasis. For example, M1 PUL denotes pulmonary metastasis. The TNM system is further classified by whether the assessment is obtained clinically (cTNM or TNM), after pathologic review (pTNM), at the time of retreatment (rTNM), or on autopsy (aTNM). For reporting purposes, the TNM stage classification remains constant throughout the disease process. Progression of disease does not change the initial stage of disease. Table 11-8 presents the nomenclature of the TNM system for classification.[80]

It is important to distinguish the cTNM, based on a clinical exam, from the pTNM, which is determined after surgery when the true extent of the disease is known and treatment decisions can be made. This is particularly true in breast cancer, where the lymph node status (pN) is the most precise prognostic indicator and directs adjuvant therapy decisions. Surgical nurses are well aware of the support needed by the woman with breast cancer in the first 24–48 hours after lymphadenectomy while she is awaiting the pathologist's review of lymph nodes. Another example occurs in the treatment of prostate cancer when the discovery of tumor in the pelvic lymph nodes (pN) at the time of surgery precludes the anticipated radical prostatectomy.

After numerical values are assigned to the T, N, and M categories, they are clustered into one of four stages (I through IV), or stage 0 for carcinoma in situ. Stage IV consistently includes distant metastases (M1) and predicts the worst prognosis. All tumor sites are grouped differently on the basis of characteristics of the disease.

Several established and accepted staging classifications other than TNM exist for particular malignancies. Melanomas have been staged not only by the level of invasion of the primary lesion but by lesion thickness—both major determinants of prognosis. The Clark levels of invasion along with Breslow's measurement of vertical thickness are universal staging systems. The TNM system, which is now in use and highly valued in clinical practice, encompasses four stages utilizing both microstaging classifications for tumor assessment. For many years, the staging system of choice for colorectal cancer had been the Duke's system, which classifies tumors by their depth of invasion and presence of nodal metastasis. Only recently has the TNM system become widely accepted and incorporated into the medical arena. The issue of what is the preferred staging system remains open. The International Federation of Gynecology and Obstetrics has an accepted staging system for cervical and endometrial cancers. Hodgkin's disease and non-Hodgkin's lymphoma are standardly described by the Ann Arbor classification, which recognizes disease distribution and symptoms. Can-

Table 11-8 TNM Classification System for Describing the Anatomic Extent of Disease

TNM Definitions

(T)	Primary tumor	
	TX	Primary tumor cannot be assessed
	T0	No evidence of primary tumor
	Tis	Carcinoma in situ
	T1, T2, T3, T4	Increasing size and/or local extent of the primary tumor
(N)	Regional lymph nodes	
	NX	Regional lymph nodes cannot be assessed
	N0	No regional lymph node metastasis
	N1, N2, N3	Increasing involvement of regional lymph nodes
(M)	Distant metastasis	
	MX	Presence of distant metastasis cannot be assessed
	M0	No distant metastasis
	M1	Distant metastasis

TNM Classifications

cTNM or TNM	*Clinical Classification:* Based on information obtained from the physical examination, laboratory and imaging studies, endoscopy, biopsy, and surgical exploration. Clinical staging uses all information available before the initiation of definitive treatment.
pTNM	*Pathologic Classification:* Based on information acquired before treatment, supplemented or modified by information from surgery and the pathologic examination of a resected specimen. This includes resected tumor (pT), lymph nodes (pN), and distant metastasis (pM).
rTNM	*Retreatment Classification:* Based on all information available after a disease-free interval or at the time of a second-look surgery. The extent or absence of disease recurrence is documented before retreatment planning is begun.
aTNM	*Autopsy Classification:* Based on all information available at the time of a postmortem examination. It is helpful in answering questions about the tumor's response to treatment, recurrence patterns, and the extent of disease at the time of death.

cers of the brain are not entirely suited to the TNM system because there are no lymphatic structures to categorize nodal (N) involvement.

The nonsolid tumors do not conform to solid-tumor staging principles because of their disseminated nature. Leukemias are best classified according to their predominant cell types (i.e., lymphocytic or nonlymphocytic), cell maturation, and acute or chronic nature. Clinical, morphologic, histochemical, and immunologic findings help to define favorable or unfavorable prognostic categories in acute lymphoblastic leukemia. The French-American-British classification has clinical and prognostic significance in acute myeloblastic leukemia but is not a staging system. In chronic lymphocytic leukemia, there are two staging systems that exist: the Rai classification and the Binet classification system. For patients with myeloma, there is a three-stage classification system that correlates M proteins with myeloma cell mass to provide prognostic information.[81] The AJCC, with the UICC, continues to work on the development of staging systems for malignancies not yet classified by the TNM system. These include cancers of the small intestine, mesothelioma, spinal cord, carcinoid, and Kaposi's sarcoma. Additionally, they are likely to incorporate tumor markers into the present anatomic staging to produce a system with better prognostic indexes.[82] This has important implications for patients with early-stage disease (based on anatomic staging) but who are actually at risk for recurrence based on other measurements of malignant potential and who will need further treatment. The 30% of women with node-negative breast cancer who eventually experience a recurrence are a subset of people with early stage disease who have a less favorable prognosis. The staging system of the future will be an estimation of risk (of local extension and distant metastases) based on the sum of risks associated with anatomic stage, morphologic grade, biological grade, and genetic potential.[83] In breast cancer, this could include the TNM stage, degree of morphologic anaplasia, estrogen and progesterone receptor status, S-phase fraction and DNA ploidy, epidermal growth factor receptors, *HER-2 or ERB-2*, and *MYC* oncogene expression.[83]

Patient Performance Classification

There are a multitude of factors that affect treatment decisions at the time of diagnosis, with the patient's physical condition being a primary component. Patients who are bedridden are much less likely to respond to treatment than are those who are asymptomatic and able to maintain the activities of daily living. Performance scales that measure a person's functional status are used frequently in the eligibility criteria for cooperative group clinical trials and also periodically to evaluate the effects of treatment and disease. It is important to assess whether aggressive, toxic treatment protocols actually will permit people to feel better and to maintain their optimum functional status. The most prevalent performance scales are the Karnofsky Performance Status scale, the Eastern Cooperative Oncology Group (ECOG) scale, and the World Health Organization (WHO) scale.[84–86] The three scales are compared in Table 11-9. Nurses need to be familiar with the scoring systems, for they may be able to contribute the most accurate information to a primarily subjective rating.

Table 11-9 Comparison of Frequently Used Performance Status Scales

Karnofsky Scale		ECOG Scale		WHO Scale	
% Score	**Status**	**Score**	**Status**	**Score**	**Status**
100%	Normal; no complaints; no evidence of disease	0	Asymptomatic	0	Fully active, able to carry out all predisease activities without restriction
90	Able to carry on normal activity; minor signs or symptoms of disease	1	Symptomatic; fully ambulatory	1	Restricted in strenuous activity but ambulatory and able to carry out light work or pursue sedentary occupation
80	Normal activity with effort; some signs or symptoms of disease				
70	Cares for self; unable to carry on normal activity or to do active work	2	Symptomatic; in bed less than 50% of day	2	Ambulatory and capable of all self-care but unable to do any light work; up and about more than 50% of waking hours
60	Requires occasional assistance, but able to care for most needs				
50	Requires considerable assistance and frequent medical care	3	Symptomatic; in bed more than 50% of day but not bedridden	3	Capable of only limited self-care; confined to bed or chair more than 50% of waking hours
40	Disabled; requires special care and assistance				
30	Severely disabled; hospitalization indicated, although death not imminent	4	Bedridden	4	Completely disabled; unable to carry out any self-care and confined totally to bed or chair
20	Very sick; hospitalization necessary; active supportive treatment necessary				
10	Moribund; fatal processes progressing rapidly				
0	Dead				

Grading

Grading a malignant neoplasm is a method of classification based on histopathologic characteristics of the tissue. The pathologist assesses the aggressiveness or degree of malignancy of tumor cells by comparing the cellular anaplasia, differentiation, and mitotic activity with normal counterparts. Specific characteristics vary with each type of cancer.

The objective of grading a tumor is to quantify information to assist with treatment planning and prognostic determinations. For selected tumors, the grade is considered more significant than anatomic staging in terms of prognostic value and treatment. In cancer of the prostate, a well-differentiated T1a tumor requires no specific therapy other than close observation; however, a poorly differentiated T1 tumor needs to be treated aggressively with radiation or radical prostatectomy if the lymph nodes are negative for disease.[87] In soft tissue sarcomas, the grade is the primary determinant of stage of disease and of prognosis. In other tumors, such as melanoma of the skin, testicular and thyroid cancer, and neuroblastoma, histologic grading has no useful application.

Two grading systems are commonly seen. One descriptively identifies the tumor as well differentiated (i.e., retaining most of the morphologic features and behavior of the normal cell of the tissue of origin), moderately well differentiated, poorly differentiated, or undifferentiated. The other system numerically grades from 1 to 3 or 4, with 1 being the most differentiated and 3 and 4 being the least well differentiated; grade 4 applies to tumors with no specific differentiation. It is important to remember that the grade 1, well-differentiated tumor implies the best prognosis for the patient. The AJCC recommends the following grading classification[80]:

GX   Grade cannot be assessed

G1   Well-differentiated

G2   Moderately well-differentiated

G3   Poorly differentiated

G4   Undifferentiated

Certain problems exist with grading classifications; most notably, a tumor's level of differentiation may vary with time. Several grades of malignancy may exist within one tumor, in which case the tumor should be labeled as the least favorable level of differentiation. It is essential that an adequate and representative biopsy specimen be obtained for a valid interpretation by the pathologist. Nurses aware of the significance of a malignant tumor's grade and stage, as well as new prognostic, molecular markers, will be able to respond realistically to the patient's questions about treatment and prognosis.

Conclusion

The diagnostic phase of a cancer illness is a time of adjustment, learning, anxiety, and uncertainty for both patient and family. With adequate knowledge of the symptoms of disease and of the diagnostic process required for evaluation, nurses can help prepare patients, thereby easing the anxiety associated with the unknown. During this time, nurses will interact with the individual in several health care settings—primary clinics, inpatient and outpatient units, and extended care units—as well as in the community. Oncology nurses have used their expertise to

1. Facilitate early diagnosis of cancer by promoting awareness of "warning signals" of cancer and conducting screening programs
2. Educate and prepare individuals for a diagnostic evaluation of suspicious signs or symptoms
3. Perform or assist with diagnostic procedures and interpret or clarify results
4. Counsel and support the individual and family in a therapeutic relationship
5. Prepare the individual for the possible treatment options once a definitive diagnosis is made

Nurses have the power to promote the detection of cancer at the earliest possible stage and to assist the individual and family to regain hope, control, and quality of life once the diagnosis of cancer has been determined.

References

1. *Cancer Facts and Figures.* Atlanta, American Cancer Society, 1998
2. Fitch MI, Greenberg M, Levstein L, et al: Health promotion and early detection of cancer in older adults: Assessing knowledge about cancer. *Oncol Nurs Forum* 24:1743–1748, 1997
3. Fink DJ, Mettlin CJ: Cancer detection: The cancer-related checkup guidelines, in Murphy GP, Lawrence W, Lenhard RE (eds): *American Cancer Society Textbook of Clinical Oncology* (ed 2). Atlanta, American Cancer Society, 1995, pp 178–193
4. Luckmann J: *Saunders Manual of Nursing Care.* Philadelphia, Saunders, 1997
5. Blue Cross of California Presents: *Breast Cancer Practice Guidelines.* Woodland Hills, Blue Cross of California, 1995
6. Mahon SM: Cancer risk assessment conceptual considerations for clinical practice. *Oncol Nurs Forum* 25:1535–1547, 1998
7. Frank-Stromborg M, Rohan K: Nursing's involvement in the primary and secondary prevention of cancer. *Cancer Nurs* 15:79–108, 1992
8. Perry AG, Potter PA: *Clinical Nursing Skill Techniques* (ed 4). St. Louis, Mosby, 1998
9. Martin J: Male cancer awareness: Impact of an employee education program. *Oncol Nurs Forum* 17:59–64, 1990
10. Bailey S, Bennett P, Hicks J, et al: Cancer detection activities coordinated by nursing students in community health. *Cancer Nurs* 19:348–352, 1996
11. Peteet JR, Stomper PC, Ross DM, et al: Emotional support for patients with cancer who are undergoing CT: Semistruc-

tured interviews of patients at a cancer institute. *Radiology* 182:99–102, 1992

12. McCray ND: Psychosocial and quality of life issues, in Otto SE (ed): *Oncology Nursing* (ed 3). St. Louis, Mosby, 1997

13. Mahon SM, Casperson D: Teaching women about mammography through use of a brochure. *Oncol Nurs Forum* 18:1375–1378, 1991

14. McCance KL, Roberts LK: Biology of cancer, in McCance KL, Huether SE (eds): *Pathophysiology: The Biologic Basis for Disease in Adults and Children* (ed 3). St. Louis, Mosby, 1998, pp 304–349

15. Bast RC Jr, Mills GB, Gibson S, et al: Tumor immunology, in Holland JF, Bast RC Jr, Morton DL, et al (eds): *Cancer Medicine* (ed 4). Baltimore, Williams & Wilkins, 1997, pp 207–242

16. Wallach J: *Interpretation of Diagnostic Tests: A Synopsis of Laboratory Medicine* (ed 5). Boston, Little, Brown, 1992, pp. 694–714

17. Tietz NW: *Clinical Guide to Laboratory Tests* (ed 3). Philadelphia, Saunders, 1995

18. Perkins AS, Stern DF: Molecular biology of cancer: Oncogenes, in DeVita VT, Hellman S, Rosenberg SA (eds): *Cancer Principles and Practice of Oncology* (ed 5). Philadelphia, Lippincott, 1997, pp 79–102

19. Ravel R: *Clinical Laboratory Medicine: Clinical Application of Laboratory Data* (ed 6). St. Louis, Mosby, 1995

20. Rodriquez De Paterna L, Arnaiz F, Estenoz J, et al: Study of serum tumor markers CEA, CA 15.3 and CA 27.29 as diagnostic parameters in patients with breast carcinoma. *Int J Biol Markers* 10:24–29, 1995

21. Chernecky CC, Krech RL, Berger BJ: *Laboratory Tests and Diagnostic Procedures.* Philadelphia, Saunders, 1993

22. Madeya ML, Pfab-Tokarsky JM: Flow cytometry: An overview. *Oncol Nurs Forum* 19:459–463, 1992

23. Williams NN, Daly JM: Flow cytometry and prognostic implications in patients with solid tumors. *Surg Gynecol Obstet* 171:257–266, 1990

24. Collins-Hattery AM, Blumberg BD: S phase index and ploidy prognostic markers in node negative breast cancer: Information for nurses. *Oncol Nurs Forum* 18:59–62, 1991

25. Gould RL: *Cancer and Genetics: Answering Your Patient's Questions.* New York, American Cancer Society and PRR, Inc., 1997

26. Lea DH: Gene therapy: Current and future implications for oncology nursing practice. *Semin Oncol Nurs* 13:115–122, 1997

27. Albain KS, Hortobagyi G, Ravdin P (eds): HER2 overexpression in breast cancer, in *Genetech Biology.* San Francisco, Genetech, Inc., 1998

28. Statement of the American Society of Clinical Oncology: Genetic testing for cancer susceptibility. *J Clin Oncol* 4:1730–1736, 1996

29. Dillon WP, Harnsberger HR: The impact of radiologic imaging on staging of cancer of the head and neck. *Semin Oncol* 18:64–79, 1991

30. Bragg DG: The application of imaging in lung cancer. *Cancer* 67:1150–1154, 1991 (suppl)

31. McClennan BL: Oncologic imaging, staging, and follow-up of renal and adrenal carcinoma. *Cancer* 67:1199–1208, 1991 (suppl)

32. Hricak H: Role of imaging in the evaluation of pelvic cancer, in DeVita VT, Hellman S, Rosenberg SA (eds): *Important Advances in Oncology 1991.* Philadelphia, Lippincott, 1991, pp 103–131

33. Castellino RA: Diagnostic imaging evaluation of Hodgkin's disease and non-Hodgkin's lymphoma. *Cancer* 67:1177–1180, 1991 (suppl)

34. Shaha AR, Strong EW: Cancer of the head and neck, in Murphy GP, Lawrence W, Lenhard RE (eds): *American Cancer Society Textbook of Oncology* (ed 2). Atlanta, American Cancer Society, 1995, pp 355–377

35. Rubin P, Bragg DG, O'Mara RE: Principles of oncologic imaging and tumor imaging strategies, in Rubin P (ed): *Clinical Oncology: A Multidisciplinary Approach for Physicians and Students* (ed 7). Philadelphia, Saunders, 1993, pp 169–176

36. Clark RA: Imaging of breast cancer, in Berman CG, Brodsky NJ, Clark RA (eds): *Oncologic Imaging.* New York, McGraw-Hill, 1998, pp 133–145

37. Skarin AT: *Atlas of Diagnostic Oncology* (ed 2). London, Mosby-Wolfe, 1996

38. Miaskowski C: *Oncology Nursing: An Essential Guide for Patient Care.* Philadelphia, Saunders, 1997, pp 1–68

39. Belcher AE: *Cancer Nursing.* St. Louis, Mosby, 1992, pp 27–54

40. McLelland R, Hendrick RE, Zinninger MD, et al: The American College of Radiology Mammography Accreditation Program. *Am J Radiology* 157:473–479, 1991

41. *Mammography Quality Control Standards Act of 1992.* 102nd Cong., 2nd sess. (1 October 1992): S.R. 102–448

42. Clark RA: Imaging of lung cancer, in Berman CG, Brodsky NJ, Clark RA (eds): *Oncologic Imaging.* New York, McGraw-Hill, 1998, pp 119–132

43. Fishman EK: Computed tomography, in DeVita VT, Hellman S, Rosenberg SA (eds): *Cancer Principles and Practice of Oncology* (ed 5). Philadelphia, Lippincott, 1997, pp 643–654

44. Bittengle JR, Davis DC: Preventative care and emergency response to contrast media, in Tortorici M (ed): *Administration of Imaging Pharmaceuticals.* Philadelphia, Saunders, 1996, pp 71–86

45. Pagana KD, Pagana TJ: *Mosby's Manual of Diagnostic and Laboratory Tests.* St. Louis, Mosby, 1998

46. Ferucci JT: Screening for colon cancer. *Radiol Clin North Am* 31:1189–1195, 1993

47. Metler FA, Guiberteau MJ: *Essentials of Nuclear Medicine Imaging* (ed 4). Philadelphia, Saunders, 1998

48. Hawkins RA: Radionucleotide imaging, in Holland JF, Bast RC Jr, Morton DL, et al (eds): *Cancer Medicine.* Baltimore, Williams & Wilkins, 1997, pp 603–609

49. Delbeke D, Vitola JV, Sandler MP, et al: Staging recurrent metastatic colorectal carcinoma with PET. *J Nucl Med* 38:1196–1201, 1996

50. Shafer K: Radiographic evaluation of cancer, in Skarin AT (ed): *Diagnostic Imaging.* London, Mosby-Wolfe, 1996

51. Gupta NC, Frick MP: Clinical applications of positron-emission tomography in cancer. *CA Cancer J Clin* 43:235–254, 1993

52. Wahl RD, Hawkins RA, Larson SM, et al: Proceedings of a National Cancer Institute workshop: PET in oncology—a clinical research agenda. *Radiology* 193:604–606, 1994

53. Harrison KA, Tempero MA: Diagnostic use of radiolabeled antibodies for cancer. *Oncology* 9:625–631, 1995

54. Berman CG, Brodsky NJ: Newer imaging modalities, in Berman CG, Brodsky NJ, Clark RA (eds): *Oncologic Imaging.* New York, McGraw-Hill, 1998, pp 367–381

55. Jeffrey RB Jr: Imaging techniques in cancer management, in DeVita VT, Hellman S, Rosenberg SA (eds): *Cancer Principles and Practice of Oncology* (ed 5). Philadelphia, Lippincott, 1997, pp 669–672

56. Watson AD, Rocklage SM: Theory and mechanisms of contrast enhancing agents, in Higgins CB, Hricak H, Helms

CA (eds): *Magnetic Resonance Imaging of the Body*. New York, Raven, 1992, pp 1257–1287.

57. Lufkin RB: Severe anaphylactoid reaction to GD-DTPA. *Radiology* 176:879, 1990

58. Loeffler JS, Patcheu RA, Sawaya R: Treatment of metastatic cancer, in DeVita VT, Hellman S, Rosenberg SA (eds): *Cancer Principles and Practice of Oncology* (ed 5). Philadelphia, Lippincott, 1997, pp 2523–2536

59. Shellock FG: MRI biologic effects and safety considerations, in Higgins CB, Hricak H, Helms CA (eds): *Magnetic Resonance Imaging of the Body*. New York, Raven, 1992, pp 233–265

60. Camp-Sorrell D: Magnetic resonance imaging and the implantable port. *Oncol Nurs Forum* 17:197–199, 1990

61. Hogstrom B, Sverre JM: Health economics in diagnostic imaging. *J Magn Reson Imaging* 1:26–32, 1996

62. Nickl NJ, Cotton PB: Clinical application of endoscopic ultrasonography. *Am J Gastroenterol* 85:675–682, 1990

63. Neiman RS, Smith TJ: Biopsy principles, pathologic evaluation of specimens and staging, in *Cancer Manual* (ed 8). Boston, American Cancer Society, Massachusetts Division, 1990, pp 70–77

64. Ell SR: Imaging techniques: Fine-needle aspiration of various organs and body sites, in Bibbo M (ed): *Comprehensive Cytopathology*. Philadelphia, Saunders, 1997, pp 615–620

65. Schmidt RA: Stereotactic breast biopsy. *CA Cancer J Clin* 44: 172–191, 1994

66. Balch CM, Pellis NR, Morton DL, et al: Oncology, in Swartz SI, Shires GT, Spencer FC (eds): *Principles of Surgery* (ed 6). New York, McGraw-Hill, 1994, pp 305–385

67. Moffat FL, Ketcham AS: Surgery for malignant neoplasia: The evolution of oncologic surgery and its role in the management of cancer patients, in McKenna RJ, Murphy GP (eds): *Cancer Surgery*. Philadelphia, Lippincott, 1994, pp 1–20

68. Bibbo M, Underhill S: Cytology of fine-needle aspiration, in Harris JR, Hellman S, Henderson IC, Kinne D (eds): *Breast Diseases*. Philadelphia, Lippincott, 1991, pp 297–300

69. Flynn MB, Wolfson SE, Thomas S, et al: Fine needle aspiration biopsy in cinical management of head and neck tumors. *J Surg Oncol* 44:214–217, 1990

70. Turner AF: Radiographically guided techniques of biopsy, in McKenna RJ, Murphy GP (eds): *Cancer Surgery*. Philadelphia, Lippincott, 1994, pp 21–34

71. Ramshaw BJ: Laparoscopic surgery for cancer patients. *CA Cancer J Clin* 47:327–350, 1997

72. Edye M, Salky B, Keller SM, et al: Minimal invasive surgery,

in Holland JF, Bast RC Jr, Morton DC, et al (eds): *Cancer Medicine* (ed 4). Baltimore, Williams and Wilkins, 1997, 675–682

73. Childers JM, Surwit EA: The role of operative laparoscopy in gynecologic oncology, in Hulka JF, Reich H (eds): *Textbook of Laparoscopy* (ed 3). Philadelphia, Saunders, 1998, pp 431–441

74. Ruddon RW: *Cancer Biology* (ed 3). New York, Oxford University Press, 1995, pp 3–18

75. Walter JB, Talbot C: *General Pathology* (ed 7). New York, Churchill-Livingstone, 1996, pp 471–487

76. Chandrasoma P, Taylor CL: *Concise Pathology* (ed 3). Stamford, CT, Appleton and Lange, 1998, pp 260–274

77. Greco FA, Hainsworth JD: Cancer of unknown primary site, in DeVita VT, Hellman S, Rosenberg SA (eds): *Cancer Principles and Practice in Oncology* (ed 5). Philadelphia, Lippincott, 1997, pp 2423–2443

78. Hainsworth JD, Greco A: Neoplasms of unknown primary site, in Holland JF, Bast RC Jr, Morton DL, et al (eds): *Cancer Medicine* (ed 4). Baltimore, Williams & Wilkins, 1997, pp 2869–2881

79. Yeomans AC, Washington JB: Occult primary malignancies. *Oncol Nurs Forum* 18:539–544, 1991

80. Beahrs OH, Henson DE, Hutter RVP, et al: *American Joint Committee on Cancer: Manual for Staging of Cancer* (ed 5). Philadelphia, Lippincott, 1997

81. Durie BGM, Salmon SE: A clinical staging system for multiple myeloma correlation of measured myeloma cell mass with presenting clinical features, response to treatment and survival. *Cancer* 36:842–854, 1975

82. Henson DE: Future directions for the American Joint Committee on Cancer. *Cancer* 69:1639–1644, 1992 (suppl)

83. Preisler HD, Raza A: The role of emerging technologies in the diagnosis and staging of neoplastic diseases. *Cancer* 69: 1520–1526, 1992 (suppl)

84. Karnofsky DA, Abelmann WH, Craver LF, et al: The use of the nitrogen mustards in the palliative treatment of carcinoma. *Cancer* 1:634–656, 1948

85. Oken MM, Creech RH, Tormey DC, et al: Toxicity and response criteria of the Eastern Cooperative Oncology Group. *Am J Clin Oncol* 5:649–655, 1982

86. World Health Organization: *World Handbook for Reporting Results of Cancer Treatment*. Geneva, WHO, 1979

87. Shipley WU, Meares EM, Schwartz JH, et al: Cancer of the prostate, in *Cancer Manual* (ed 8). Boston, American Cancer Society, Massachusetts Division, 1990, pp 284–294

PART III

Treatment

CHAPTER 12

Quality of Life as an Outcome of Cancer Care

Carol Estwing Ferrans, PhD, RN, FAAN

Introduction

Quality of life has become a relevant gauge with which to evaluate health care outcomes. Over the past 30 years, it has grown into a respected measure of efficacy of treatment. Providers of cancer care have been front-runners in the evaluation of quality of life, recognizing the need to assess outcomes more broadly than tumor response and length of survival. Although these end points remain important, the impact of cancer and treatment on the patient is also crucial. New anticancer drugs are required to show quality-of-life benefit in order to obtain approval from the U.S. Food and Drug Administration.[1] The highest priority of the Cancer Therapy Evaluation Program (CTEP) of the National Cancer Institute is research aimed at improving survival and quality of life for persons with cancer.[2] Increasingly, clinical trials have been designed with quality-of-life components, and the major clinical trial cooperative groups in the United States all have significant quality-of-life evaluations under way. In Canada, the National Cancer Institute now requires the use of quality-of-life end points in all of its phase III clinical trials.[3] Quality-of-life issues are not limited to clinical trials, however. Evaluation of quality of life is appropriate for the entire spectrum of care for cancer patients, including palliative care, end-of-life care, and long-term survivorship issues.

The concept of quality of life is particularly salient for oncology nursing, because nurses traditionally have viewed patients from a holistic perspective, focusing on the quality of survival as well as length of survival. The holistic perspective encompasses all aspects of life affected by cancer and treatment, such as physical symptoms, treatment toxicities, mental and physical functioning, body image, psychological state, work and role responsibilities, social and family life, and spiritual concerns. Because the concept of quality of life is a multidimensional construct that encompasses the whole of life, it is congruent with the holistic perspective, and thus can provide a useful appraisal of outcomes important in oncology nursing.

Treatment Decisions

Information about quality-of-life outcomes is important both for treatment decision making and the provision of supportive care. Table 12-1 lists clinical situations in which information about quality of life is particularly valuable for decision making. Oncology nurses play a critical role in providing this information to patients, so that they can evaluate the balance of risks and benefits associated with therapeutic regimens. As early as 1984, Schipper et al suggested that information about quality-of-life outcomes should be provided to patients, in addition to survival statistics, to enable them to make decisions about their treatment.[8] Subsequently, others have argued that fully

Table 12-1 Situations in Which Quality-of-Life Information Is Useful for Treatment Decisions

- Two treatments are similar in terms of survival but differ in toxicities or sequelae
- One treatment produces better survival rates than another but is more toxic, particularly when survival time is short
- Different intensities (doses or time periods of administration) can be used for the same therapeutic agent
- Treatment is expected to have only a small impact on length of survival
- Adjuvant therapy is used to try to prevent cancer recurrence

Compiled in part from: Gallup and Cella,[4] Gotay et al,[5] Moinpour et al,[6] Nayfield et al[7]

informed choices cannot be made without this information.[9] For patients to give informed consent, they must be able to decide whether the likelihood of longer life is worth the additional morbidity caused by treatment.[10]

Unfortunately, clinicians have only limited information regarding the impact of various therapeutic regimens on quality of life at present. Despite the expanding interest in quality-of-life outcomes, the number of completed studies is relatively small, due to the complexity of conducting such studies and the limited funding resources available.[11] Examples of quality-of-life studies that have contributed to treatment decision making and the provision of supportive care are addressed in the following sections.

Treatments with Similar Survival Outcomes

When two treatments produce similar outcomes in survival, information about differences in quality-of-life outcomes can help determine the best choice. An example of this can be found in treatment for localized prostate cancer, which has equivalent survival rates for patients treated by radical prostatectomy or radiation therapy.[12,13] Yarbro and Ferrans compared quality-of-life outcomes for men receiving radical prostatectomy or radiation therapy and found that those treated by surgery had significantly worse urinary and sexual functioning.[14] Protective pads or adult diapers were worn daily by 32% of the men in the surgical group, as compared with only 6% of the radiation group. Ability to have an erection was reported to be very poor for 88% of the surgical group and for only 46% of the radiation group. In contrast, the radiation group had worse bowel functioning due to radiation damage to the rectal mucosa, although the differences between groups were smaller in this area. Diarrhea and cramping pain were problems for only a few men. Similar findings have been reported in other studies,[15–17] which increases confidence that these results are generalizable. These studies indicate that radiation therapy produces more favorable outcomes regarding long-term sequelae, which is an important consideration for men when deciding between these treatments.

Modified radical mastectomy and breast-conserving treatment for breast cancer also produce similar survival rates but different quality-of-life outcomes. It would be expected that women receiving breast-conserving treatment would have fewer problems in terms of body image, lymphedema, and surgery-related numbness and pain, which has been found in studies comparing the two treatment approaches.[18,19] However, quality-of-life studies also have found that women with breast-conserving treatment experience psychological distress that is as severe as that experienced by women with mastectomies.[18,20,21] Both groups are faced with a life-threatening disease and the disruption of surgery. Although lumpectomy or segmental resection removes only part of the breast, the disfigurement is often significant and disturbing. In fact, women with breast-conserving treatment were found to have greater distress 1 month after surgery than those with mastectomies, which was related to the added burden of radiation therapy.[18] These results indicate that women with breast-conserving treatment also require support and psychosocial intervention in the postoperative period. These findings demonstrate the usefulness of quality-of-life outcomes in identifying the need for supportive care, as well as in making treatment decisions.

The treatment of soft-tissue sarcoma also is a case in point. In an early study, Sugarbaker et al compared patients who underwent amputation versus patients who had a limb-sparing regimen that entailed surgery and radiation; both treatments produced similar survival outcomes.[22] It was expected that the limb-sparing group would experience a better quality of life. Surprisingly, patients with amputation were found to have less impairment in terms of functional status, emotional disturbance, and sexual relationships. Subsequent studies revealed similar difficulties associated with multimodal limb-sparing treatment, as well as employment and financial problems.[23,24] Contributing to these problems was an increased incidence of joint contracture found in patients receiving a combination of chemotherapy and radiation therapy.[23] Thus, in this example, unanticipated problems were identified through the exploration of quality-of-life outcomes, which contribute to informed choice of treatment.

Therapies with Different Survival Outcomes

Information about quality-of-life outcomes also can provide useful information for decision making when two treatments produce different survival outcomes, particularly when one has significantly greater toxicity and survival time is short. Patients may choose to risk a shorter lifespan in order to enjoy a better quality of life for the time they have left, without the disabling toxicities of therapy. However, a more toxic therapy can sometimes produce a better quality of life during treatment by reducing disease symptoms. In an early study of advanced breast cancer, women were treated either with chemotherapy or endocrine therapy.[25] Although the chemotherapy group experienced greater toxic effects, such as nausea, vomiting, constipation, and alopecia, their quality of life was better than that of the endocrine group. At 11 weeks into treatment, the chemotherapy group reported improvements in functional status, pain, anorexia, depression, ability to sleep, and well-being, all of which were related to disease remission.

Different Intensities of Therapeutic Agents

Information about quality-of-life outcomes can contribute to the evaluation of variations in dose and timing of administration of therapeutic agents. In an early study, Coates et al compared intermittent and continuous chemotherapy to treat metastatic breast cancer.[26] The group receiving intermittent chemotherapy was given only three cycles, then therapy was stopped until there was evidence of disease progression. The group receiving continuous chemotherapy was given chemotherapy every 3 weeks without stopping. It was expected that the quality of life of the intermittent group would be better because, though they would experience side effects of treatment, the side effects would last for a shorter period. In contrast, after the three cycles were completed, the continuous group had better physical status, mood, and overall quality of life, which were thought to be related to better tumor response, disease progression, and length of survival. The findings of the study indicated that the side effects of therapy were offset by disease regression for the continuous therapy group, so that the more aggressive therapy produced a better quality of life.

More aggressive therapy does not always result in such improvement, however. Another study of advanced breast cancer compared chemotherapy administered every 3 weeks to the same chemotherapy administered every week.[27] The group who received weekly chemotherapy experienced worse quality-of-life outcomes in terms of nausea, malaise, and psychological distress, which were not related to disease response.

Citron et al compared the pain relief provided by morphine administered through continuous intravenous infusion versus patient-controlled analgesia (PCA).[28] The PCA group reported greater pain intensity than the intravenous group. Nevertheless, the PCA group experienced equivalent pain relief, even though they used significantly less morphine. In addition, the PCA group reported better quality-of-life outcomes, experiencing less sedation and psychological distress. Therefore, timing of administration can also affect quality of life.

Limited Impact of Treatment on Survival

Quality-of-life outcomes become particularly salient when the impact of treatment on survival is expected to be limited. For instance, for men diagnosed with early-stage prostate cancer who are aged 70 years and older, aggressive therapy has not been shown to prolong survival or reduce mortality rates.[29,30] Prostate cancer typically progresses slowly in these men, and it is assumed that comorbid conditions will cause their death, resulting in death with the cancer rather than because of it. Prostatectomy and radiation therapy are associated with long-term detrimental effects on urinary, sexual, and bowel functioning.[14] Because of the impact on quality of life, some clinicians practice "watchful waiting," observing the status of the prostate cancer rather than treating it.

Adjuvant Therapy to Prevent Recurrence

When adjuvant therapy has been used to prevent cancer recurrence, quality-of-life concerns regarding toxicity and long-term disability have led to changes in practice. For example, cranial radiation has been used for central nervous system prophylaxis for acute lymphoblastic leukemia (ALL) in children. An early study found that these children had deficits in attention and overall intellectual functioning.[31] A later study of long-term survivors of childhood ALL (aged 18–33 years) corroborated the association between learning disabilities and childhood cranial radiation, with the incidence increasing with higher doses.[32] In addition, researchers found that those who had been treated with 24 Gy and those who were treated when younger than 6 years of age were less likely to enter college. The survivors also experienced more anxiety and depression than sibling controls.[33]

Yet another study supported the conclusion that these problems were related to cranial radiation rather than to some other aspect of ALL and treatment.[34] Two groups of survivors of childhood ALL were compared: one group had been treated with 24 Gy of cranial radiation and intrathecal methotrexate, the other with systemic and intrathecal methotrexate but no cranial radiation. The group who had received cranial radiation had significantly worse academic achievement and greater psychological distress. As a result of these quality-of-life concerns, intensive efforts have been made to find effective alternatives to cranial radiotherapy to prevent relapse, such as high-dose systemic chemotherapy and intensive intrathecal therapy.[35]

Supportive Care

Quality-of-life information also can play an important role in revealing needs for supportive care, both during treatment and afterward. Many of the problems caused by cancer and treatment can be anticipated intuitively, such as body image disruptions caused by mastectomy. However, quality-of-life studies have identified some needs of patients that would not necessarily be expected. For example, although treatment for Hodgkin's disease does not commonly cause changes in appearance, one study reported that 26% of survivors believed that they were less physically attractive because of their cancer, and this belief was associated with depression and decreased

sexual activity.[36] Another study found that 22% were experiencing psychological distress severe enough to meet the criterion suggested for psychiatric diagnosis.[37] In addition, 39% still experienced conditioned nausea triggered by smells and sights that reminded them of chemotherapy. They reported problems with sex life, employment, income, education, and denial of health and life insurance. Because of these findings, an intervention was implemented at the completion of treatment to facilitate adaptation by providing counseling via telephone.[38]

Other interventions also have been instituted based on quality-of-life outcomes. For example, through a standardized interview breast cancer patients undergoing mastectomy were found to have significant psychological distress, which previously was not recognized.[39] As a result, an intervention was put into place, whereby a nurse provided information and emotional support after surgery. The intervention was effective, as patients who received the counseling had significantly less psychiatric morbidity at 12 months postmastectomy.

Quality-of-life data also can help to identify patients who may be at greater risk, over and above what would be expected based on their disease status. In a study of patients undergoing treatment for primary brain tumors, Weitzner et al found outcomes that would be expected, such as a poorer quality of life for patients who had bilateral tumor involvement, poorer functional status, or more aggressive treatment.[40] However, they also found that patients who were female, divorced, or unable to work were at greatest risk for poorer quality of life while undergoing treatment. Similarly, based on an extensive review of studies of cancer survivors, Kornblith concluded that patients were at highest risk who had (1) less social support to buffer stress, (2) poorer prediagnosis psychological adjustment, and (3) fewer economic resources, as well as having greater cancer-related physical problems and comorbidities.[41] Length of time since completion of treatment also played a role, in that adjustment tended to improve over time.

Still, not all problems resolved with the passage of time, even for long-term survivors who were free of disease. For instance, some breast cancer survivors, particularly those with mastectomies, were found to have significant problems with body image, sex life, and depression years after treatment.[19–21] In addition, long-term survivors of various cancers have been found to experience common problems, such as chronic fatigue, fear of recurrence and death, infertility, issues of control and independence, altered meaning of health, and uncertainty about the future.[42] To help cancer patients cope with the array of problems presented by the experience of cancer, Kornblith has recommended provision of both educational and counseling programs that are comprehensive in nature, provided either in groups or individually, to address these needs.[41]

As well as identifying problems, quality-of-life studies of long-term cancer survivors have revealed positive outcomes that can be used to encourage patients. For example, a large study found that the overall quality of life of breast cancer survivors was as good as or better than that of healthy aged-matched women, even though cancer survivors reported higher rates of physical symptoms.[43] In addition, many studies have reported positive changes in people's lives because of their experience with cancer.[20,41–44] Survivors have reported that they have become better people, understand life better, have reassessed their values and priorities, and are proud of their accomplishments. They characterize their lives as fuller and more meaningful, and have a greater appreciation for life and the other people in their lives. They also have reported a strengthening of spirituality and faith in God, as well as a more optimistic outlook and decreased fear of death.

Quality of Life as a Prognostic Indicator

There is some evidence that patients' ratings of their quality of life before treatment are predictive of survival. Studies reporting findings such as these have all been clinical trials of patients with advanced disease, primarily lung cancer[45–48] and breast cancer.[49] These findings are particularly interesting, because the studies used different instruments to measure quality of life, and the clinical trials were of different treatment regimens, which provides greater confidence that a relationship between pretreatment quality of life and survival actually exists. What is not entirely clear, however, is whether patient ratings of quality of life provide predictive power beyond traditional clinical factors. Herndon et al explored this question in a study of 206 advanced non–small cell lung cancer patients treated on a clinical trial.[47] Survival was predicted by baseline scores of a quality-of-life instrument for pain, appetite loss, fatigue, lung cancer symptoms, physical functioning, and overall quality of life. However, when clinical factors such as histology, weight loss, dyspnea, and other factors were taken into account by statistical analysis, only one score from the quality-of-life instrument was still predictive. Self-rated pain was a predictor for survival, over and above the clinical factors. Ruckdeschel et al also found that self-rated quality of life was predictive of survival, independent of cancer stage, histology, and physical performance status.[48] Based on the findings of these studies, it has been recommended that patient-rated quality-of-life assessment should be obtained as an integral part of cancer management as a guide to patient needs, as an outcome measure, and as a prognostic variable for survival time.[46] Osoba has even suggested that pretreatment quality-of-life ratings could be used as an eligibility criterion and stratification variable in clinical trials.[50]

Definitions of Quality of Life

A major challenge confronted when using quality of life to assess outcomes is its definition. There is no general agreement regarding definition of quality of life, nor is there a gold standard for measurement to provide an operational definition. The term *quality of life* is used to mean a wide variety of things, which makes comparisons among studies difficult if not impossible. Clarity about what is meant by quality of life is extremely important, because differences in meaning can lead to significant differences in outcomes. For instance, a case description of an elderly man with chronic pulmonary disease was presented to 205 family and internal medicine physicians, each of whom made decisions regarding treatment based on their own personal definitions of quality of life.[51] Their judgments of the patient's quality of life varied so widely that many arrived at opposing conclusions as to whether treatment should be given or withheld.

Quality of life is rarely defined explicitly, which has led to a great deal of confusion about what the term actually means. In most cases, what is meant by quality of life must be construed from the instruments used to measure it. Attempts have been made to characterize the wide variety of conceptualizations of quality of life in health care,[52–54] which have helped to clarify differences among various approaches. Over the past few decades, there has been substantial development of the concept. Early determinations of quality of life included evaluations of social utility, which essentially meant that quality of life was assessed in terms of the contributions (or potential contributions) that the person made to society. For example, in the early days of hemodialysis before 1972, when access was quite limited, decisions regarding who would be given dialysis were commonly made based on quality of life as defined by social utility.[55] Social utility definitions now have largely been abandoned, although they have not disappeared entirely.

The definitions that are most commonly used in health care today can be classified into two broad groups, the first focusing on level of function in a variety of domains and the second on patient satisfaction with those domains. Gotay et al fuse both into the following definition:

> Quality of life is a state of well-being that is a composite of two components: (1) the ability to *perform* everyday activities that reflect physical, psychological, and social well-being and (2) patient *satisfaction* with levels of functioning and the control of disease and/or treatment-related symptoms.[5, p. 576]

Gotay et al argue that both components are important measures of outcomes in cancer care, as the first provides information about the actual levels of functioning and the second patient evaluations of quality of life. Each component provides different information because evaluations of functional ability can differ from patients' evaluations of their lives. For example, individuals can consider their quality of life to be good even when they have severe physical limitations.[56] This notion is particularly important in long-term illness, because individuals make adjustments to compensate for functional disability, which can preserve life satisfaction.[56] For palliative care in particular, satisfaction is an important outcome, as it can be used as a nonintrusive indicator of the humaneness of care.[57] Cohen et al pointed out that physical status alone is insufficient to assess quality of life among those with terminal illness, because in many cases their performance scores are uniformly low.[58] In addition, measures are needed to tap existential concerns, such as spirituality or personal meaning, as well as positive contributions to quality of life, all of which are important to patients at the end of life.[58]

A number of definitions of both types can be found in the literature. An example of a definition of quality of life that focuses primarily on health and functioning is provided by Cella, who stated that quality-of-life assessment should entail an evaluation of functional status as perceived by the patient.[59] He defines health-related quality of life as "the extent to which one's usual or expected physical, emotional, and social well-being are affected by a medical condition or its treatment."[60,p.73] This definition is similar to the World Health Organization's (WHO) definition of health, which is commonly used for quality of life: "Health is a state of complete physical, mental, and social well-being and not merely the absence of disease or infirmity."[61,p.1] A quality-of-life definition that focuses primarily on satisfaction is provided by Ferrans: "[Quality of life is] a person's sense of well-being that stems from satisfaction or dissatisfaction with the areas of life that are important to him/her."[62,p.15]

Health-Related Quality of Life

When defining quality of life as it applies to health care, the term *health-related* commonly is used to focus on the effects of illness or treatment on quality of life and to distinguish these from aspects beyond the realm of health care, such as education, income, and quality of the environment. Although social and economic problems can affect health adversely, it is argued that these problems are distant from the concerns of health care providers.[63] However, it also has been pointed out that illness can make almost all aspects of life "health-related."[63] Leplege and Hunt have argued against the use of the term, stating that it fails to acknowledge the interconnectedness of health with other aspects of life.[56] It is interesting to note that the WHO has chosen to define quality of life in a comprehensive manner, as:

> [An] individual's perception of their position in life in the context of the culture and value systems in which they live and in relation to their goals, expectations, standards, and concerns. It is a broad-ranging concept affected in a complex way by the person's physical health, psychological state, level of independence, social relationships, and their relationship to salient features of their environment."[64,p.1570]

Domains of Quality of Life

Regardless of the approach that is chosen to define quality of life, there is general agreement that quality of life is a multidimensional construct.[7,50] Quality of life is more than physical health status, clinical symptoms, or functional ability. Although there is variability among researchers as to the number of domains that constitute quality of life, there is general consensus that body, mind, and spirit need to be included.[65] However, Leplege and Hunt have criticized many of the models developed to characterize the domains of quality of life, because, they assert, insufficient attention has been paid to the closeness of fit between domains and patients' viewpoints.[56] They advocate transforming qualitative information about the concerns of individuals into the common elements constituting quality of life.

The two models of quality of life presented here are based on qualitative analysis of patients' perspectives; the models were validated with additional patient data. One model was developed by Ferrell et al (Figure 12-1) and the other by Ferrans et al (Figure 12-2 and Table 12-2). Both models are quite similar in terms of the domains identified. Both contain domains for physical health and functioning, and social, psychological, and spiritual domains. Additionally, the Ferrans model addresses economic elements and has a separate family domain. Because the two models were developed independently and simultaneously based on different patient data, the close match between the two models provides mutual validation. The Ferrell et al model was based on qualitative data from cancer patients with pain.[66,67] Subsequently, it was developed and validated further for patients with breast cancer, bone marrow transplantation, and cancer survivors.[68–71] The Ferrans model was based on descriptions of the components of a satisfying life given by dialysis patients.[72,73] It then was modified to include cancer patients[62] and later was validated using information from patients with breast cancer, sarcoma, bone marrow transplant, and other chronic illnesses.[24,44,73–78] By identifying the range of domains, both of these models guide the assessment of quality of life for research and clinical practice. When instruments are chosen to measure quality of life, care should be taken so that the entire concept is represented. One instrument or a battery of instruments may be needed to capture the broad nature of the concept.

Measuring Quality of Life

Choosing Instruments to Measure Quality of Life

There are myriad quality-of-life instruments from which to choose. A number of excellent reviews are available that can assist in narrowing the choice of quality-of-life instruments (Table 12-3). Evidence of reliability, validity, and sensitivity are prerequisites for the choice of an instrument, as they provide assurance that the instrument is reasonably free of random error, measures what it was intended to, and is sufficiently sensitive to detect change

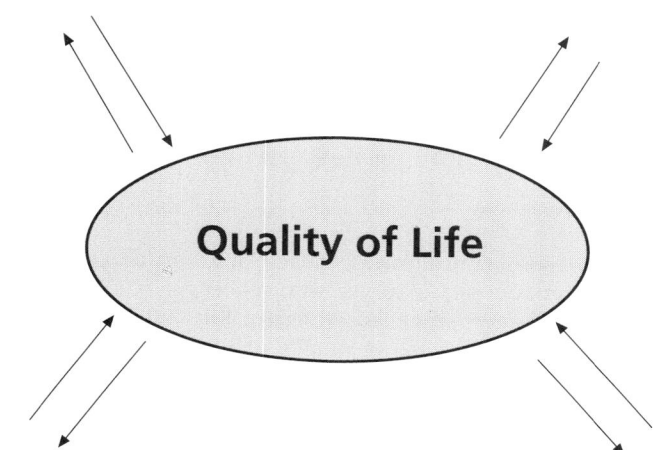

Figure 12-1 Ferrell and Grant conceptual model for quality of life. (Reprinted with permission by BR Ferrell).

in quality of life. However, no one instrument is ideal for all situations in which quality-of-life outcomes can be assessed. Each instrument is different in terms of the nature of the domains covered and the conceptual approach used. When choosing instruments, clinicians and researchers need to consider the purpose of the evaluation, the nature of specific disease and treatment, and the characteristics of the patient population that will be assessed.[5,7] In light of these considerations, instruments should be examined to determine which ones provide the best fit. Gill and Feinstein recommend this sort of instrument evaluation, calling it "the application of en-

lightened common sense, which is a mixture of ordinary common sense plus a reasonable knowledge of pathophysiology and clinical reality."[85,p.620]

One or more instruments may be used to measure quality of life for a particular study or clinical situation. Because quality of life is a multidimensional construct, the use of a unidimensional instrument alone is not adequate to measure it. For example, the Karnofsky Performance Status is a unidimensional indicator of the ability to carry on normal activity and so is not a measure of quality of life, nor was it originally intended to be one.[86]

Table 12-4 presents examples of multidimensional in-

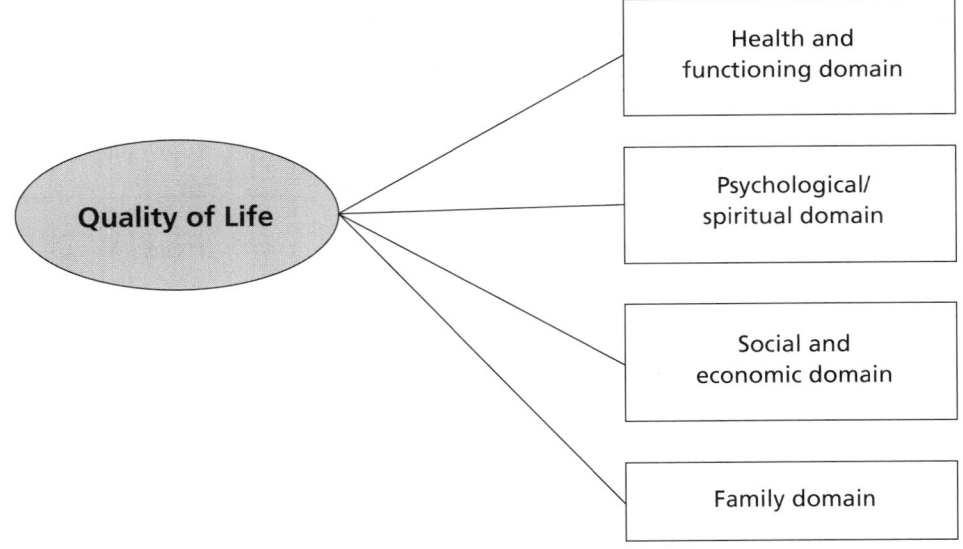

Figure 12-2 Ferrans conceptual model for quality of life.

struments that are used to measure quality of life. All of the instruments listed were developed for use with cancer patients, except for the SF-36,[94] which was designed for the general population. The domains of quality of life that each instrument measures listed, as well as whether they provide a score for overall quality of life, which is usually a composite score for the instrument.

In addition to domains, consideration should be given to the conceptual approach taken to measure quality of life. Some instruments measure similar domains, but use different conceptual approaches, which results in evaluation of different aspects of quality of life. For example, although the Functional Assessment of Cancer Therapy (FACT) scale[89,90] and the Ferrans and Powers Quality of Life Index—Cancer Version (QLI)[61] measure many of the same domains, Weitzner et al[40] found that the correlation between the two was only .41 in a sample of patients with primary brain cancer. Both instruments are well-established, valid measures of quality of life. However, the FACT primarily assesses functioning, whereas the QLI measures satisfaction, so they yield different information. To provide a comprehensive evaluation of quality of life, Gotay et al recommended collecting data on both functioning and satisfaction in quality-of-

---

Table 12-2   Elements of the Ferrans Conceptual Model for Quality of Life

Health and Functioning Domain
Your health
Pain
Energy (fatigue)
Ability to take care of yourself without help
Ability to take care of family responsibilities
Usefulness to others
Worries
Control over life
Chances of living as long as you would like
Chances for a happy future
Sex life
Leisure-time activities
Health care

Family Domain
Family happiness
Spouse, lover, or partner
Children
Emotional support from family
Family health

Psychological/Spiritual Domain
Satisfaction with life
Happinesss in general
Achievement of personal goals
Peace of mind
Faith in God
Personal appearance
Satisfaction with self

Social and Economic Domain
Friends
Emotional support from friends
Home (house, apartment)
Neighborhood
Job/unemployment
Ability to take care of financial needs
Education

Table 12-3   Reviews of Quality-of-Life Instruments

Author	Title
Anderson, Aaronson, and Wilkin[79]	Critical review of the international assessments of health-related quality of life
Cella and Bonomi[59]	Measuring quality of life: 1995 update
Dean[10]	Multiple instruments for measuring quality of life
Litwin[80]	Measuring health-related quality of life in men with prostate cancer
McDowell and Newell[81]	*Measuring health: A Guide to Rating Scales and Questionnaires*
Moinpour, Feigl, Metch, et al[6]	Quality of life end points in cancer clinical trials: Review and recommendations
Padilla and Frank-Stromborg[65]	Single instruments for measuring quality of life
Spilker[82]	*Quality of Life and Pharmacoeconomics in Clinical Trials*
Tchekmedyian, Cella, and Winn[83]	Economic and quality-of-life outcomes in oncology

Note: An extensive collection of quality-of-life instruments can be viewed in their entirety at http://www.QLMed.org/[84]

life research.[5] Some instruments measure either functioning or satisfaction, and others provide some combination of the two. For example, most instruments include an item that asks patients to rate their overall quality of life, which allows patients to express their general level of satisfaction.[5]

Generic versus disease-specific instruments

Another distinction made among quality-of-life measures is whether the instrument is generic or disease specific. Generic instruments produce scores for all domains of quality of life, whereas disease-specific instruments focus on concerns that are most relevant to a specific illness and treatment. Some disease-specific instruments are so general in content that they bridge the gap between the two categories.[61] For example, the SF-36 Health Survey is a generic instrument that was developed for the general population but has been used widely in cancer studies.[94] The other instruments listed in Table 12-4 are disease specific, although many of them bridge the gap between generic and disease specific because of their broad coverage of domains.

There are advantages and disadvantages for both types of instruments. Generic instruments are useful for making comparisons with the general population, which is particularly helpful for the interpretation of results. They also can be used across treatment groups and illness populations, making it possible to evaluate the relative impact of therapies and health care programs.[63,80] In addition, they can be used to put symptoms in the context of overall quality of life, which can help make clear the impact of treatment.[9] They are particularly useful for documenting the range of treatment effects, which may help to identify unanticipated adverse effects.[63] The major disadvantage of generic instruments is that because they are so broad, they tend to cover each area superficially and may not even address the primary symptoms.[9] Disease-specific instruments tend to be much more powerful in detecting treatment effects and are more responsive to changes in specific conditions.[9,63] However, disease-specific instruments are limited in scope and so may miss critical aspects of quality of life.[6] For these reasons, there is general

agreement that both types of measures should be used, even in clinical trials.[5,7,61]

Measurement of values

Quality of life has been described as a uniquely personal perception.[85] As early as 1976, Campbell et al characterized quality of life as something that depends on the person's own judgment of the experience of life.[97] The individual's judgment is essential, because different people value different things. A disability that makes life not worth living for one person may be only a bother for another. Even people with the same illness often vary markedly in the problems they experience and in the importance they place on them.[9] A number of studies have provided evidence that people vary in the values they place on different aspects of life, particularly among ages and genders.[97–100] In addition, people also change over time in response to life events. For example, many studies have reported that cancer survivors experience changes in values as a result of the experience of cancer and treatment.[20,42,44,67,101–104]

Gill and Feinstein have argued that it is the incorporation of patients' values that sets quality of life assessment apart from all other measures of health.[85] They state that researchers may measure health status, but if patients' values and preferences are not included, researchers are not measuring quality of life. Supporting this idea is the finding of Blalock et al that psychological distress was affected more by satisfaction with abilities than by the actual state of those abilities, and then only for abilities considered to be very important by patients.[99]

Assessment of importance

Traditionally, quality-of-life instruments have presumed that different people perceive conditions in the same way by using the same criteria.[40] However, in 1990 a workshop sponsored by the National Cancer Institute recommended that research be done to develop methods to determine the importance of aspects of life for individual patients and to incorporate these weights into quality-of-life assessment.[7] *Weighting* is based on the idea that

Table 12-4 Multidimensional Instruments Used to Measure Quality of Life (QOL)

Cancer Rehabilitation Evaluation System (CARES)—Short Form[87]
   Physical
   Psychosocial
   Marital
   Sexual
   Medical interaction
   Overall QOL
	Functional Living Index—Cancer (FLIC)[8,91,92]
	   Physical well-being and ability
	   Nausea
	   Hardship due to cancer
	   Psychological well-being
	   Social well-being
	   Overall QOL

EORTC Quality-of-Life Questionnaire (EORTC QLQ-C30)[88]
   Physical functioning
   Pain
   Fatigue
   Nausea and vomiting
   Overall symptoms
   Role functioning
   Cognitive ability
   Psychological functioning
   Social interaction
   Finances
	McGill Quality-of-Life Questionnaire[58]
	   Physical symptoms
	   Psychological symptoms
	   Outlook on life
	   Meaningful existence
	   Overall QOL

Ferrans and Powers Quality-of-Life Index—Cancer Version (QLI)[61,72,74]
   Health and functioning
   Psychological/spiritual
   Social and economic
   Family
   Overall QOL
	Quality-of-Life Scale for Cancer (QOL-CA)[71,93]
	   Physical well-being
	   Psychological well-being
	   Spiritual well-being
	   Social well-being
	   Overall QOL

Functional Assessment of Cancer Therapy (FACT)[89,90]
   Physical well-being
   Social/family well-being
   Emotional well-being
   Functional well-being
   Overall QOL
	SF-36 Health Survey[94,95]
	   Physical function
	   Physical role function
	   Vitality
	   Bodily pain
	   Mental health
	   Emotional role function
	   Social function
	   General health perceptions

	Spitzer Quality-of-Life Index (QL-Index)[96]
	   Health
	   Activity
	   Daily living
	   Support
	   Outlook
	   Overall QOL

Note: All the instruments listed were developed for use with patients with cancer, except for the SF-36, which was designed for the general population.

highly valued areas of life have greater influence on quality of life than areas of less importance. A number of quality-of-life instruments have been developed that measure importance in a structured manner. They use a variety of terms to elicit information regarding values. For example, patients may be asked to rate importance, distress, bother, or effect on quality of life. Some instruments use ratings of importance of individual aspects of life as weights to produce scores, such as the Quality of Life Inventory (QOLI)[105] and the Ferrans and Powers QLI.[62,72,74] Other instruments ask respondents to rate the importance of an entire domain, but do not use the information in a weighting scheme. Examples are the FACT,[89,90] the WHOQOL-100 instrument,[64] and the Prostate Cancer Index (PCI).[17]

Global ratings

In addition to measuring importance in a structured manner, values can be described through a global rating, in which patients rate their quality of life on a one-item scale, for example, ranging from excellent to poor.[85] Cantril's Self-Anchoring Scale has been used successfully to produce a global rating.[106] Respondents rate their quality of life on a 10-point scale, which has as its end points the best and worst lives they can imagine. Measures such as these implicitly take the individual's values into consideration.

Utilities

Measurement of utilities focuses on the relative value of various health states or the strength of a person's preference for a healthy outcome.[107] An example of a utility measure is the Quality Adjusted Life Year (QALY),[108] in which a year of perfect health is compared to a year with an illness or disability, on a scale ranging from 0 (death) to 1 (perfect health). For instance, in one study the value of a year of life with a mastectomy was determined to be

0.5 using the QALY scale, which meant it was worth only half a year of healthy life.[109] The values or preferences expressed may be the patient's or, alternatively, may be the general population's, depending on the purpose of the assessment. A patient's values may be elicited to assist in decisions about treatment, whereas the general population's values may be assessed to determine what health care will be paid for by the public. For instance, for the Oregon Health Care Initiative the values of the public were used to determine the health care services that would be provided to Medicaid patients.[110,111] However, the use of utilities for quality-of-life assessment is controversial. (For a detailed discussion, see Avorn[112] and Harris[113]). In most cases, utility ratings are made by health care providers or the general population, however, these raters may not be sufficiently knowledgeable to provide valid judgments.[107] This is evidenced by the findings that QALY ratings assigned by physicians and healthy people are typically lower than those given by people experiencing the particular health state.[114]

A utility measure that was developed specifically for cancer care is Q-TWiST (Quality-Adjusted Time Without Symptoms and Toxicity).[115] It was developed to evaluate adjuvant therapies for early-stage breast cancer. Survival time is discounted to take into consideration the effect of treatment side effects and disease symptoms, using a utility weight ranging from 0 to 1. The utility weights, which reflect preferences, were determined by the investigators themselves, rather than by asking patients with breast cancer. However, there is no theoretical reason that patients' preferences could not be used for Q-TWiST or any other utility measure.[116] Utility measures such as Q-TWiST provide a single summary score that reflects both the health state and the value of that health state.[63] They could be used to determine whether patients are better off as a result of treatment, by providing an idea of the balance between the gains of treatment and the burdens of toxicity.[63] Nevertheless, they do not provide information pinpointing the areas in which patients improved or worsened.[63] Because of this, Guyatt et al[63] have suggested that disease-specific instruments be used simultaneously with utility measures to provide this information.

Who Should Evaluate Quality of Life?

The term *quality of life* conveys the idea of a value judgment about a person's life requiring some kind of rating, such as good/bad, high/low, or best/worst. It makes a difference who does the rating, because people use their own internal standards for what they consider a desirable or undesirable quality of life.[50] There is general agreement that quality of life is best evaluated by the patient, rather than by an outside observer.[7,50] Quality of life is commonly viewed as a subjective evaluation of the experience of life and, as such, is dependent on the individual's own perspective, expectations, and values.

Subjective versus objective assessment

A distinction between subjective and objective measures has been made historically in quality-of-life assessment. Subjective indicators rely on individuals' own evaluations of their quality of life. In contrast, objective indicators do not require such an evaluation but are directly measurable, such as blood pressure, hemoglobin levels, tumor size, income, or years of education. Moreover, Schipper points out that within the realm of health care, objective indicators are frequently externally observable by a third party.[117]

Occasionally, there is a mistaken notion that all patient-reported data is subjective, and all data reported by an outside observer is objective. However, it is the nature of the information, rather than who reports it, that is the distinguishing characteristic. Information concerning objective indicators can be reported by patients, but they still remain objective. Similarly, an outside observer can make a subjective judgment about another individual.

Proxy ratings

Although the patient's own evaluation of quality of life is acknowledged to be the gold standard, there are situations in which such evaluations cannot be obtained. Patients may be unable or unwilling to answer questions because of cognitive impairment, debilitating fatigue, severe nausea, pain, or other symptoms. These are times when quality-of-life information is most needed, which makes the use of proxy raters appealing. A proxy rater is anyone other than the patient who would evaluate the patient's quality of life. However, because patients' own perspectives differ from those of outside observers, ratings assigned by proxies may be quite different from what patients would give themselves.[50] The accuracy of the resulting outcome will vary depending on whose perspective is reflected in the quality-of-life assessment. These differences have been demonstrated in studies comparing patients' ratings with those of physicians, nurses, and significant others (spouse, family, friends), as seen in a review of 49 studies.[118] In general, the quality-of-life ratings provided by patients and proxies had only modest agreement, with proxies tending to underestimate quality of life. For example, one study reported that correlations between quality-of-life ratings by patients and physicians ranged only from .26 to .45, and that patient and nurse correlations were no better, ranging from .19 to .47.[119]

This does not mean that the proxies' opinions are invalid, but rather that they are valid only as their points of view.[50] Therefore, it is important to examine the three circumstances in which proxies have historically provided the best possible information. First, information from proxies has been found to be more accurate when they live in the same household as the patient.[118] However, if the proxies are caregivers, the information provided may be biased to reflect favorably on themselves and the care they have provided. Second, proxies have been found to provide more accurate information when they assess things that are concrete and observable,[118] such as functional status,[118] cigarette smoking,[120] and consumption of food, coffee, and alcohol.[121,122] Proxies provide less accurate information when they assess things that are subjective and unobservable,[118] such as the patient's satisfaction,[123] level of pain,[124] cognitive functioning,[125] depression,[125] or psychosocial adjustment to cancer.[126] For example, correlations between cancer patients and their oncologists on measures of anxiety and depression ranged from only .21 to .33,[127] and correlations between patients and nurses on ratings of pain severity ranged only from .28 to .50.[128] Another study found that the least accurate assessments were made for cancer patients who experienced the most severe pain. Nurses, house officers, and oncology fellows correctly assessed pain only 7%, 20%, and 27% of the time, respectively, for patients who reported pain in the upper third of the scale.[129] Third, whenever possible, the level of agreement between patients and the proxies should be determined when patients are still able to answer questions. Later, when patients are no longer able to provide information, the proxy ratings can be interpreted in light of the concordance found previously between proxy and patient.[116,118]

Populations Presenting Special Challenges

Because their concerns differ from those of target populations for which most quality-of-life instruments were developed, some populations present special challenges in assessment of quality-of-life outcomes. This has meant that many instruments are inappropriate for use with these populations in their original forms. Examples of these populations are children, people at the end of life, and different cultural groups.

Children

The assessment of quality of life in children is made difficult by the wide span of developmental stages that are affected by the experience of cancer.[35,130] Hinds believes that quality of life for children is determined by the closeness of fit between their desires and hopes and what is actually happening in their lives.[131] She points out that a child's sense of well-being is highly variable, fluctuating in response to daily events and chronic problems. It also is affected by developing cognitive ability and personality styles.[131] This complexity has made the development of quality-of-life measures a very difficult task in pediatric oncology. Adding to the challenge is the need for proxies for very young children and consideration of the family context.[35,130] Because of these issues, quality-of-life assessment for children is in an earlier phase of development than for adults. Outcomes have only rarely been included in cancer clinical trials for children. However, concerted efforts have been made in recent years to include these outcomes in studies conducted by the national clinical trials groups for pediatric oncology.[130]

End of life

Quality-of-life assessment at the end of life also presents unique challenges, because the traditional outcomes of cancer treatment are less relevant. Palliative care focuses primarily on symptom relief, rather than on survival time and tumor response.[57] Still, measurement of outcomes in terms of quality of life is essential, because enhancement of quality of life is the very reason for every intervention in palliative care.[58] Assessment of changes in physical function and activities of daily living are important,[116] but care must be taken to tap existential concerns and positive contributions to quality of life as well.[58] Because physical status deteriorates as disease progresses, at some point measures of physical function no longer provide discrimination, because scores will all be low.[58] To address these concerns, the McGill Quality-of-Life Questionnaire was developed specifically for palliative care in advanced disease.[58] The instrument measures sense of meaning in life and outlook on life, as well as physical and psychological symptoms (see Table 12-4).

Different cultural groups

It has been well-documented that there are significant cross-cultural differences in the meaning of quality of life.[78,132-136] However, development of instruments for use with different cultural groups has focused primarily on language issues, such as linguistic equivalence of translated versions.[79] Anderson et al provide an excellent review of national and linguistic comparisons for a variety of instruments used to measure quality of life.[79] However, they also point out that these comparisons do not provide information on cultural differences in quality of life, which have only begun to be addressed. Continued work in this area is needed to provide assurance that quality of life is assessed validly for various cultural groups. Differences between and within nations, among broad cultural and language groups, must be examined.[79] This information then can be used to modify existing instruments. In addition, efforts are under way to develop new instruments expressly for cross-cultural international use. Notable examples are the Quality of Life Questionnaire of the EuroQol (EuroQol)[137] and the WHOQOL-100.[64]

Conclusion

Quality of life has become a respected outcome for cancer care. Increasingly, it is recognized as a valuable supplement to tumor response and survival data, providing information about the positive and negative impact of therapy from the patient's perspective.[6] It is helpful in determining the trade-offs between toxicity and quality of life, and in evaluating whether small gains in life span come at too high a cost.[9] Although interest in quality-of-life outcomes is expanding, there are fewer studies with quality-of-life end points than might be hoped. This is largely due to the complexity of conducting these studies and limited funding resources.[11] Assessment of quality of life in research and clinical practice is still relatively new, and there is significant work yet to be done. Much more information about quality-of-life outcomes is needed for clinical decision making, provision of supportive services, and health policy for cancer care.

References

1. Johnson JR, Temple R: Food and Drug Administration requirements for approval of new anticancer drugs. *Cancer Treat Reps* 69:1155–1157, 1985

2. Clinical Trials Cooperative Group Program, *Cancer Therapy Evaluation Program: Guidelines*. Bethesda, MD, Division of Cancer Treatment, National Cancer Institute, February 29, 1988

3. Osoba D. The Quality of Life Committee of the Clinical Trials Group of the National Cancer Institute of Canada: Organization and functions. *Qual Life Res* 1:211–218, 1992

4. Gallup DG, Cella DF: Gynecologic Oncology Group (GOG). *J Natl Cancer Inst Monogr* 20:77–78, 1996

5. Gotay CC, Korn EL, McCabe MS, et al: Quality-of-life assessment in cancer treatment protocols: Research issues in protocol development. *J Natl Cancer Inst* 84:575–579, 1992

6. Moinpour CM, Feigl P, Metch B, et al: Quality of life end points in cancer clinical trials: Review and recommendations. *J Natl Cancer Inst* 81:485–495, 1989

7. Nayfield SG, Ganz PA, Moinpour CM, et al: Report from a National Cancer Institute (USA) workshop on quality of life assessment in cancer clinical trials. *Qual Life Res* 1:203–210, 1992

8. Schipper H, Clinch JJ, McMurray A, et al: Measuring the quality of life of cancer patients: The Functional Living Index—Cancer: Development and validation. *J Clin Oncol* 2:472–483, 1984

9. Guyatt GH, Naylor CD, Juniper EF, et al: Users' guide to the medical literature: XII. How to use articles about health-related quality of life. *JAMA* 277:1232–1237, 1997

10. Dean H: Multiple instruments for measuring quality of life, in Frank-Stromborg M, Olsen SJ (eds): *Instruments for Clinical Health-Care Research* (ed 2). Sudbury, MA, Jones and Bartlett, 1997, pp 135–148

11. Ganz PA: Impact of quality of life outcomes on clinical practice. *Oncology* 9:61–65, 1995

12. Hanks G: External beam radiation treatment for prostate cancer: Still the gold standard? *Oncology* 6:79, 1992

13. Walsh PG, Partin A: Treatment of early stage prostate cancer: Radical prostatectomy, in DeVita VT Jr, Hellman S, Rosenberg SA (eds): *Important Advances in Oncology*. Philadelphia, Lippincott, 1994, pp 211–223

14. Yarbro CH, Ferrans CE: Quality of life of patients with prostate cancer treated with surgery or radiation therapy. *Oncol Nurs Forum* 25:685–693, 1998

15. Fowler FJ, Barry MJ, Lu-Yao G, et al: Outcomes of external-beam radiation therapy for prostate cancer: A study of Medicare beneficiaries in three surveillance, epidemiology, and end results areas. *J Clin Oncol* 14:2258–2265, 1996

16. Lim AJ, Brandon AH, Fiedler J, et al: Quality of life: Radical prostatectomy versus radiation therapy for prostate cancer. *J Urol* 154:1420–1425, 1995

17. Litwin MS, Hays RD, Fink A, et al: Quality-of-life outcomes in men treated for localized prostate cancer. *JAMA* 273:129–135, 1995

18. Ganz PA, Schag CAC, Lee JJ, et al: Breast conservation versus mastectomy. *Cancer* 69:1729–1738, 1992

19. Polinsky M: Functional status of long-term breast cancer survivors: Demonstrating chronicity. *Health Soc Work* 19:165–173, 1994

20. Ferrans CE: Quality of life through the eyes of survivors of breast cancer. *Oncol Nurs Forum* 21:1645–1651, 1994

21. Lasry JC, Margolese RG, Poisson R, et al: Depression and body image following mastectomy and lumpectomy. *J Chronic Dis* 40:529–534, 1987

22. Sugarbaker PH, Barofsky I, Rosenberg SA, et al: Quality of life assessment of patients in extremity sarcoma clinical trials. *Surgery* 9:17–23, 1981

23. Chang AE, Steinberg SM, Culnane M, et al: Functional and psychosocial effects of multimodality limb-sparing therapy in patients with soft tissue sarcomas. *J Clin Oncol*, 7:1217–1228, 1989

24. Arzouman JMR, Dudas S, Ferrans CE, et al: Quality of life of patients with sarcoma post-chemotherapy. *Oncol Nurs Forum* 18:889–894, 1991

25. Priestman T, Baum M: Evaluation of quality of life in patients receiving treatment for advanced breast cancer. *Lancet* 1:899–901, 1976

26. Coates A, Gebski V, Bishop JF, et al: Improving the quality of life during chemotherapy for advanced breast cancer: A comparison of intermittent and continuous treatment strategies. *N Engl J Med* 317:1490–1495, 1987

27. Richards MA, Hopwood P, Ramirez AJ, et al: Doxorubicin in advanced breast cancer: Influence of schedule on response, survival, and quality of life. *Eur J Cancer* 28A:1023–1028, 1992

28. Citron M, Conaway M, Zhukovsky D, et al: Efficacy of patient-controlled analgesia (PCA) vs. continuous intravenous morphine (CIVM) for the treatment of severe cancer pain: CALGB 8872. *Proc Am Soc Clin Oncol* 12:433, 1993 (abstr)

29. Chodak G: Treatment of early stage prostate cancer: Conservative management—delayed therapy, in DeVita VT Jr, Hellman S, Rosenberg SA (eds): *Important Advances in Oncology*. Philadelphia: Lippincott, 1994, pp 241–244

30. Garnick M: The dilemmas of prostate cancer. *Sci Am* 27:72–81, 1994

31. Rowland JH, Glidewell OJ, Sibley RF, et al: Effects of different forms of central nervous system prophylaxis on neuropsychologic function in childhood leukemia. *J Clin Oncol* 2:1327–1335, 1984

32. Haupt R, Fears TR, Robison LL, et al: Educational attainment in long-term survivors of childhood acute lymphoblastic leukemia. *JAMA* 272:1427–1432, 1994

33. Zeltzer LK, Zhang F, Stuber M, et al: Psychological sequelea in adult survivors of childhood acute lymphoblastic leukemia. *Med Pediatr Oncol* 23:169, 1994 (abstr)

34. Hill JM, Kornblith AB, Jones D, et al: A comparative study of the long term psychosocial functioning of childhood acute lymphoblastic leukemia survivors treated by intrathecal methotrexate with or without cranial radiation. *Cancer* 82:208–218, 1998

35. MacLean W: Childrens Cancer Group (CCG). *J Natl Cancer Inst Monogr* 20:87–88, 1996

36. Fobair P, Hoppe RT, Bloom J, et al: Psychosocial problems among survivors of Hodgkin's disease. *J Clin Oncol* 4: 805–814, 1986

37. Kornblith AB, Anderson J, Cella DF, et al: Hodgkin disease survivors at increased risk for problems in psychosocial adaptation. *Cancer* 70:2214–2224, 1992

38. Kornblith AB: Cancer and Leukemia Group B (CALGB). *J Natl Cancer Inst Monogr* 20:67–71, 1996

39. Maguire P: Using measures of psychological impact of disease to inform clinical practice, in Ventafridda V, van Dam F, Yancik R, et al (eds): *Proceedings of the International Workshop on Quality of Life Assessment and Cancer Treatment.* Amsterdam: Excerpta Medica, 1986, pp 119–126

40. Weitzner MA, Meyers CA, Byrne KS: Psychosocial functioning and quality of life in patients with primary brain tumors. *J Neurosurg* 84:29–34, 1996

41. Kornblith AB: Psychosocial adaptation of cancer survivors, in Holland J (ed): *Psycho-oncology* New York; Oxford University Press, 1998, pp 223–254

42. Dow KH, Ferrell BR, Haberman MR, et al: The meaning of quality of life in cancer survivorship. *Oncol Nurs Forum* 26:519–528, 1999

43. Ganz PA, Rowland JH, Desmond K, et al: Life after breast cancer: Understanding women's health-related quality of life and sexual functioning. *J Clin Oncol* 16:501–514, 1998

44. Belec RH: Quality of life: Perceptions of long-term survivors of bone marrow transplantation. *Oncol Nurs Forum* 19: 31–37, 1992

45. Cella DF: Changes in quality of life predict survival in NSCLC. *Oncol News Int* 6:19, 1997 (suppl 2)

46. Ganz PA, Lee JJ, Siau J: Quality of life assessment: An independent prognostic variable for survival in lung cancer. *Cancer* 67:3131–3135, 1991

47. Herndon JE, Fleishman S, Kornblith AB, et al: Is quality of life predictive of survival among patients with advanced non-small cell lung cancer? *Cancer* 85:333–340, 1999

48. Ruckdeschel J, Piantadosi S: The Lung Cancer Study Group: Quality of life assessment in lung surgery for bronchogenic carcinoma. *J Thorac Surg* 6:201–205, 1991

49. Coates A, Gebski V, Signorini D, et al: Prognostic value of quality of life scores during chemotherapy for advanced breast cancer. *J Clin Oncol* 10:1833–1838, 1992

50. Osoba D: Lessons learned from measuring health-related quality of life in oncology. *J Clin Oncol* 12:608–616, 1994

51. Pearlman R, Jonsen A: The use of quality of life considerations in medical decision making. *J Am Geriatr Soc* 33: 344–352, 1985

52. Edlund M, Tancredi L: Quality of life: An ideological critique. *Perspect Biol Med* 28:591–607, 1985

53. Ferrans CE: Quality of life: Conceptual issues. *Semin Oncol Nurs* 6:248–254, 1990

54. Ferrans CE: Conceptualizations of quality of life in cardiovascular research. *Prog Cardiovasc Nurs* 7:2–6, 1992

55. Ferrans CE: Quality of life as a criterion for allocation of life sustaining treatment, in Anderson G, Glesnes-Anderson V (eds): *Health Care Ethics.* Rockville, MD, Aspen, 1987, pp 109–124

56. Leplege A, Hunt S: The problem of quality of life in medicine. *JAMA* 278:47–50, 1997

57. Rinck GC, van den Bos GAM, Kleijnen J, et al: Methodologic issues in effectiveness research on palliative cancer care: A systematic review. *J Clin Oncol* 15:1697–1707, 1997

58. Cohen SR, Mount BM, Strobel MG, et al: The McGill Quality of Life Questionnaire: A measure of quality of life appropriate for people with advanced disease. *Palliat Med* 9:207–219, 1995

59. Cella DF, Bonomi AE: Measuring quality of life: 1995 update. *Oncology* 9:47–48, 1995

60. Cella DF: Measuring quality of life in palliative care. *Sem Oncol* 22:73–81, 1995

61. Spilker B: Introduction, in Spilker B (ed): *Quality of Life and Pharmacoeconomics in Clinical Trials* (ed 2). Philadelphia, Lippincott-Raven 1996, pp 1–10

62. Ferrans CE: Development of a quality of life index for patients with cancer. *Oncol Nurs Forum* 17:15–19, 1990

63. Guyatt GH, Jaeschke R, Feeny DH, et al: Measurements in clinical trials: Choosing the right approach, in Spilker B (ed), *Quality of Life and Pharmacoeconomics in Clinical Trials* (ed 2). Philadelphia, Lippincott-Raven, 1996, pp 41–48

64. WHOQOL Group: The World Health Organization Quality of Life Assessment (WHOQOL): Development and general psychometric properties. *Soc Sci Med* 46:1569–1585, 1998

65. Padilla GV, Frank-Stromborg M: Single instruments for measuring quality of life, In Frank-Stromborg M, Olsen S, (eds): *Instruments for Clinical Health-Care Research* (ed 2). Sudbury, MA: Jones and Bartlett, 1997, pp 114–134

66. Ferrell BR, Wisdom C, Wenzl C: QOL as an outcome variable in the management of cancer pain. *Cancer* 63: 2321–2327, 1989

67. Padilla GV, Ferrell BR, Grant MM, et al: Defining the content domain of quality of life for cancer patients with pain. *Cancer Nurs* 13:108–115, 1990

68. Ferrell B, Grant M, Padilla G, et al: Experience of pain and perceptions of quality of life: Validation of a conceptual model. *Hospice J* 7:9–24, 1991

69. Ferrell BR, Grant MM, Schmidt GM, et al: The meaning of quality of life for bone marrow transplant survivors. Part 1: The impact of bone marrow transplant on QOL. *Cancer Nurs* 15:153–160, 1992

70. Ferrell BR, Dow K, Leigh S, et al: Quality of life in long term cancer survivors. *Oncol Nurs Forum* 22:915–922, 1995

71. Grant MM, Ferrell BR, Schmidt GM, et al: Measurement of quality of life in bone marrow transplantation survivors. *Qual Life Res* 1:375–384, 1992

72. Ferrans CE, Powers MJ: Quality of Life Index: Development and psychometric properties. *Adv Nurs Sci* 8:15–24, 1985

73. Ferrans CE: Development of a conceptual model of quality of life. *Schol Inq Nurs Pract Int J* 10:293–304, 1996

74. Ferrans CE, Powers MJ: Psychometric assessment of the Quality of Life Index. *Res Nurs Health* 15:29–38, 1992

75. Ferrans CE, Powers MJ: Quality of life of hemodialysis patients. *Am Nephrol Nurses Assoc J* 20:575–581, 1993.

76. Ferrans CE, Cohen FL, Smith K: Quality of life of persons with narcolepsy. *Grief Loss Care* 5:23–32, 1992

77. Anderson J, Ferrans CE: The quality of life of persons with chronic fatigue syndrome. *J Nerv Ment Dis* 106:359–367, 1997

78. Warnecke RB, Ferrans CE, Johnson TP, et al: Measuring quality of life in culturally diverse populations. *J Natl Cancer Inst Monogr* 20:29–38, 1996

79. Anderson RT, Aaronson NK, Wilkin D: Critical review of the international assessments of health-related quality of life. *Qual Life Res* 2:369–395, 1993

80. Litwin MS: Measuring health-related quality of life in men with prostate cancer. *J Urol* 152:1882–1887, 1994

81. McDowell I, Newell C: *Measuring Health: A Guide to Rating Scales and Questionnaires.* New York: Oxford University Press, 1987

82. Spilker B (ed): *Quality of Life and Pharmacoeconomics in Clinical Trials,* (ed 2) Philadelphia, Lippincott-Raven, 1996

83. Tchekmedyian SD, Cella DF, Winn RJ: Economic and qual-

ity of life outcomes in oncology. *Oncology* 9:1–216, 1995 (suppl)

84. Tamburini M: Clinician's Computer-Assisted Guide to the Choice of Instruments for Quality of Life Assessment in Medicine. Available at: http://www.QLMed.org/. Accessed 10/5/1999

85. Gill TM, Feinstein AR: A critical appraisal of the quality of quality-of-life measurements. *JAMA* 272:619–626, 1994

86. Karnofsky D, Abelman W, Craver L, et al: The use of nitrogen mustards in the palliative treatment of carcinoma with particular reference to bronchogenic carcinoma. *Cancer* 1:634–656, 1948

87. Shag C, Ganz PA, Heinrich R: Cancer Rehabilitation Evaluation System-Short Form (CARES-SF). *Cancer* 68:1406–1413, 1991

88. Aaronson NK, Ahmedzai S, Bergman G, et al: The European Organization for the Research and Treatment of Cancer: A quality of life instrument for use in international clinical trials in oncology. *J Natl Cancer Inst* 85:365–376, 1993

89. Cella DF, Tulsky D, Gray G, et al: The Functional Assessment of Cancer Therapy (FACT) Scale: Development and validation of the general version. *J Clin Oncol* 11:570–579, 1993

90. Cella DF, Bonomi AE, Lloyd S, et al: Reliability and validity of the Functional Assessment of Cancer Therapy-Lung (FACT-L) quality of life instrument. *Lung Cancer* 12:199–220, 1995

91. Morrow G, Lindke J, Black P: Measurement of quality of life in patients: Psychometric analysis of the Functional Living Index—Cancer (FLIC). *Qual Life Res* 1:287–296, 1992

92. Clinch J: The Functional Living Index—Cancer: Ten years later, in Spilker B (ed): *Quality of Life and Pharmacoeconomics in Clinical Trials* (ed 2). Philadelphia, Lippincott-Raven, pp 215–225

93. Padilla GV, Grant M, Lipsett J, et al: Health quality of life and colorectal cancer. *Cancer* 70:1450–1456, 1992(suppl)

94. Ware J, Sherbourne C: The MOS 36-Item Short-Form Health Survey (SF-36). *Med Care* 30:473–483, 1992

95. Stewart A, Hays R, Ware J: The MOS Short-Form General Health Survey. *Med Care* 26:724–735, 1988

96. Spitzer WO, Dobson AJ, Hall J, et al: Measuring the quality of life of cancer patients: A concise QL-Index for use by physicians. *J Chronic Dis* 34:585–597, 1981

97. Campbell A, Converse P, Rodgers W: *The Quality of American Life*. New York, Russell Sage, 1976

98. Guyatt GH, Berman LB, Townsend M, et al: A measure of quality of life for clinical trials in chronic lung disease. *Thorax* 42:773–778, 1987

99. Blalock SJ, DeVellis BM, DeVellis RF, et al: Psychological well-being among people with recently diagnosed rheumatoid arthritis. *Arthritis Rheum* 35:1267–1272, 1992

100. Flanagan JC: Measurement of quality of life: Current state of the art. *Arch Phys Med Rehabil* 63:56–59, 1982

101. Carter BJ: Long-term survivors of breast cancer. A qualitative descriptive study. *Cancer Nurs* 16:354–361, 1993

102. Loescher LJ, Clark L, Atwood JR, et al: The impact of the cancer experience on long-term survivors. *Oncol Nurs Forum* 17:223–229, 1990

103. Wyatt G, Kurtz ME, Liken M: Breast cancer survivors: An exploration of quality of life issues. *Cancer Nurs* 16:440–448, 1993

104. Zemore R, Shepel L: Effects of breast cancer and mastectomy on emotional support and adjustment. *Soc Sci Med* 28:19–27, 1989

105. Frisch MB: The Quality of Life Inventory: A cognitive-behavioral tool for complete problem assessment, treatment planning, and outcome evaluation. *Behav Ther* 16:42–44, 1993

106. Cantril H: *The Patterns of Human Concerns*. New Bruswick, NJ, Rutgers University Press, 1965

107. Weeks J: Measurement of utilities and quality-adjusted survival. *Oncology* 9:67–70, 1995

108. Schelling T: The life you save may be your own, in Chase S (ed): *Problems in Public Expenditure Analysis*. Washington, DC, Brookings Institution, 1968, pp. 127–176

109. Sackett D, Torrance G: The utility of different health states as perceived by the general public. *J Chronic Dis* 31:697–704, 1978

110. Hadorn D: The Oregon priority-setting exercise: Quality of life and public policy. *Hastings Cent Rep* 21:11–16, 1991

111. Steinbrook R, Lo B: The Oregon medicaid demonstration project—Will it provide adequate medical care? *N Engl J Med* 326:340–344, 1992

112. Avorn J: Benefit and cost analysis in geriatric care: Turning age discrimination into health policy. *N Engl J Med* 310:1294–1301, 1984

113. Harris J: QALYfying the value of life. *J Med Ethics* 13:117–123, 1987

114. Boyd NF, Sutherland HJ, Heasman KZ, et al: Whose utilities for decision analysis? *Med Decis Making* 10:58–67, 1990

115. Gelber RP, Goldhirsch A, Cavelli F: Quality-of-life-adjusted evaluation of adjuvant therapies for operable breast cancer. *Ann Intern Med* 114:621–628, 1991

116. Cella DF: Measuring quality of life in palliative care. *Semin Oncol* 22:73–81, 1995

117. Schipper H, Clinch JJ, Olweny CLM: Quality of life studies: Definitions and conceptual issues, in Spilker B (ed): *Quality of Life and Pharmacoeconomics in Clinical Trials* (ed 2). Philadelphia, Lippincott-Raven, 1996, pp 11–23

118. Sprangers MA, Aaronson NK: The role of health care providers and significant others in evaluating the quality of life of patients with chronic disease: A review. *J Clin Epidemiol* 45:743–760, 1992

119. Molzahn AE, Northcott HC, Dossetor JB: Quality of life of individuals with end stage renal disease: Perceptions of patients, nurses, and physicians. *ANNA J* 24:325–333, 1997

120. McLaughlin JK, Dietz MS, Mehl ES, et al: Reliability of surrogate information on cigarette smoking by type of informant. *Am J Epidemiol* 12:144–146, 1987

121. McLaughlin JK, Mandel J, Mehl ES, et al: The ability of next-of-kin and self-respondents for cigarette, coffee, and alcohol consumption. *Epidemiol* 1:408–412, 1990

122. Samet J: Surrogate sources of dietary information, in Willett W (ed): *Nutritional Epidemiology*. New York, Oxford University Press, 1990, pp 133–142

123. Epstein AM, Hall JA, Tognetti J, et al: Using proxies to evaluate quality of life: Can they provide valid information about patients' health status and satisfaction with medical care? *Med Care* 27:91–98, 1989 (suppl)

124. O'Brien J, Francis A: The use of next-of-kin to estimate pain in cancer patients. *Pain* 35:171–178, 1988

125. Rozenbilds UY, Goldney RD, Gilchrist PN, et al: Assessment by relatives of elderly patients with psychiatric illness. *Psychol Rep* 58:795–801, 1986

126. Watson M, Greer S, Young J, et al: Development of a questionnaire measure of adjustment to cancer: The MAC Scale. *Psychol Med* 18:203–209, 1988

127. Sensky T, Dennehy M, Gilbert A, et al: Physicians' perceptions of anxiety and depression among their outpatients. *J R Coll Physicians Lond* 23:33–38, 1989

128. Teske K, Daut RL, Cleeland CS. Relationships between nurses' observations and patients' self-reports of pain. *Pain* 16:289–296, 1983

129. Grossman SA, Sheidler VR, Swedeen K, et al: Correlation of patient and caregiver ratings of cancer pain. *J Pain Symp Manage* 6:53–57, 1991

130. Bradlyn AS, Pollock BH: Pediatric Oncology Group (POG). *J Natl Cancer Inst Monogr* 20:89–90, 1996

131. Hinds PS: Quality of life in children and adolescents with cancer. *Semin Oncol Nurs* 6:285–291, 1990

132. Rogler LH: The meaning of culturally sensitive research in mental health. *Am J Psych* 146:296–303, 1989

133. Vaughan D, Kashner J, Stork W, et al: A structural model of subjective well-being. *Soc Indicators Res* 16:315–332, 1985

134. Mukherjee R: On the quality of life in India. *Soc Indicators Res* 9:455–476, 1981

135. Mastekassa A, Moum T: The perceived quality of life in Norway. *Soc Indicators Res* 14:385–420, 1984

136. Meyerowitz B, Richardson J, Hudson S, et al: Ethnicity and cancer outcomes: Behavioral and psychosocial considerations. *Psychol Bull* 123:47–70, 1998

137. EuroQol Group: EuroQol—a new facility for the measurement of health-related quality of life. *Health Policy* 16:199–208, 1990

CHAPTER 13

Principles of Treatment Planning and Clinical Research

Claire R. Works, RN, MN, ARNP

Introduction

Cancer is not just one disease; it comprises more than 100 different disease entities. It has been referred to as a "chaotic" disease that can occur at any age and involve virtually any organ of the body.[1] In many cases, cancer is a chronic illness, with manifestations that change over time. Because of this complexity, treatment decisions in oncology involve many factors.

Oncology nurses need to understand the principles involved in establishing a treatment plan, the rationale for continuing with a therapy despite serious toxicity, and how response to treatment is measured. This enables nurses to support and educate patients throughout cancer treatment and to contribute to the multidisciplinary cancer team. The first and second section of this chapter address the factors involved in planning therapy throughout the disease continuum: treatment aimed at cure or complete response, treatment to control disease and prolong life, and treatment for palliation. The third section of the chapter discusses the conduct of clinical trials.

Factors Involved in Treatment Planning

Treatment Goals

Treatment of cancer is intended to achieve one of three outcomes: cure, control and prolongation of life, or palliation of symptoms. These goals can overlap: Treatment may begin with curative intent, then shift to controlling disseminated disease, as illustrated in Figure 13-1.[2] An individual could initially undergo potentially curative treatment, then require additional therapy years later for recurrent disease, and, ultimately, treatment for palliation.

In most cases, there are many treatment options available. The oncologist and the individual needing treatment must decide on a goal and the best therapeutic plan to meet the goal. In setting broad goals (whether to treat for cure, control, or palliation), survival statistics are considered. Five-year relative survival rates by race (white and black) and stage are known for most tumor types.[3] Cancers with a 5-year survival in the range of 1%–5% are considered to have no or minimal chance for cure. This poor prognosis dictates that the goal is prolonging life or palliating symptoms. Treatment is

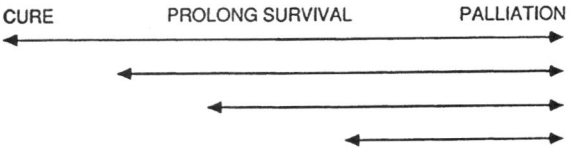

Figure 13-1 The continuum of cancer care. The goals of treatment are dynamic and interrelated. (Reprinted with permission from Olweny CLM: Goals and rationale of cancer treatment. *Med J Aust* 155:187–192, 1991.[2])

sometimes viewed as a "bridge" to assist a person to live until a better therapy is developed.

In cases with more optimistic 5-year survival rates, cure or control of disease is a realistic goal. Cancers can be divided into three categories: (1) those that are known to be curable by conventional treatment methods; (2) those that may be curable in the context of a research protocol; (3) those for which no cure is currently known.

The responsibility of the oncologist and oncology nurse is to help the individual understand the survival statistics and how to apply this information to his or her own specific situation. The survival statistics indicate the percentage of people with a given disease who live 5 years or more. There is no way to predict with certainty how a particular individual will fare. An individual's tumor may respond very well or very poorly to treatment. The person who is cured by treatment experiences 100% benefit from that treatment, no matter what the 5-year survival statistic indicates.[1] The oncologist and nurse help an individual understand what is possible and what is likely to be the expected or probable outcome.

A correct determination of whether to treat for cure is one of the most important decisions that an oncologist must make. The basic principle of cancer therapy is to cure if possible while causing minimal structural and functional impairment. Cancer treatment often results in some degree of temporary or permanent impairment; risks and benefits must be weighed carefully. An aggressive approach to treatment can expose individuals who are incurable to needless morbidity and prolonged and expensive treatment. On the other hand, therapeutic decisions that are too pessimistic or overly conservative may deprive a person who has a small but significant opportunity for cure the chance to live out the rest of life.

The patient's feelings and values are crucial to the treatment decision. Some people, even knowing they have only a small chance for cure, will prefer an aggressive plan of action and accept the accompanying side effects. Others will make it clear that they prefer to avoid challenging such odds and will opt to maximize quality of life despite less time.

Treatment Planning Variables

Factors relating to the tumor, the treatment, and the person needing treatment all contribute to determination of the therapeutic plan. The following variables must be analyzed: (1) the tumor's aggressiveness and potential for early dissemination; (2) the effectiveness and morbidity and mortality of available treatments; (3) the individual's performance status and comorbidities. Careful consideration of each of these factors assists the clinician and the patient in setting a goal and selecting the most appropriate treatment plan.

Tumor factors

The tumor's histopathologic classification and stage are key factors in predicting how aggressively the tumor will behave. In addition, staging information provides the most accurate means of predicting the potential success of a treatment under consideration.[1] Accurate staging also provides baseline data to help measure subsequent response to therapy. (See Chapter 11 for a detailed discussion of the staging process.)

Prognostic factors and risk factors are considered in the decision-making process. For example, in non-Hodgkin's lymphoma, risk factors of age, performance status, LDH level, stage, and extranodal involvement help to predict 5-year survival rate.[4] Based on these risk factors, individuals expected to have a low relapse rate are guided toward standard therapy, while those with higher risk disease may be guided toward treatment in clinical trials.

Treatment factors

Once the goal of treatment is determined, the next decision involves choosing the optimal treatment plan. To find the treatment plan with the greatest possibility of meeting the desired goal for the newly diagnosed person, the oncologist examines what is known about treatments used in similar situations (e.g., tumors of the same histopathologic grade and stage, patients of similar age and performance status). The "track record" of a treatment is collected by the tumor registrars and research data specialists. For rare tumors, there is not as much data available, and the oncologist searches the literature for case reports addressing this unusual situation. Often, the oncologist will consult with other cancer specialists. Individual cases are presented at meetings of the tumor board for input by medical, surgical, and radiation oncologists regarding the risks and benefits of the available treatment options. In some instances, enrollment in a clinical trial may offer the latest advances in therapy.

The oncologist matches the patient with a therapy that has known activity for a particular tumor. The morbidity and mortality associated with the treatment are weighed against its potential benefit. Treatment benefit is assessed by the response of the tumor to chemotherapy and/or radiation therapy. A *complete response* is defined as the disappearance of all signs of cancer for two or more evaluations separated by 4 weeks or more.[5] In advanced cancer, cure is impossible without first achieving a complete response. Thus, DeVita asserts that a complete response rate is by far the best indicator to evaluate the efficacy of a chemotherapeutic regimen.[6]

Another measure, *partial response*, refers to at least a 50% reduction in the size of the tumor mass for 4 weeks or more, with no new lesions appearing. Partial responses are often brief and, therefore, are of limited value in treatment planning.[6]

Patient factors

As mentioned earlier, an individual's general health, age, performance status, and personal preferences and values influence choice of therapy. For example,

- Concomitant disease or illness may require adjustment of the treatment plan.

- Performance status helps predict how well a person will tolerate treatment.

- Individual patient preferences regarding how aggressively to seek cure and acceptable level of risk or toxicity vary widely.

- Age is an important factor if growth is still occurring, if fertility or hormonal status will be affected by treatment, or if age has affected performance status.

Interaction of the factors

Treatment selection is based on a full evaluation of the many factors previously mentioned and knowledge of the current cutting-edge treatment approaches. Chronic myelogenous leukemia (CML) provides an example of the interplay between the various factors considered in choosing a treatment plan. Initial therapy for a newly diagnosed patient with CML is either alfa-interferon or allogeneic bone marrow transplant.[7] The oncologist must determine which option will offer the best chance of prolonged survival and help the patient choose between the two treatments. Interferon therapy slows disease progression but has significant side effects and is not curative. Bone marrow transplant offers a potential cure but produces greater toxicity and potential morbidity.

Cancer therapies have the greatest chance of success if treatment is initiated early in the course of the disease. It can be difficult for newly diagnosed individuals (who are sometimes asymptomatic or have mild symptoms) to commit to a treatment that may involve significant side effects (interferon) or is potentially life threatening (bone marrow transplant).

Age can influence the choice of treatment in CML. Young patients, less than 40 years of age, are encouraged to have the allogeneic transplant. In middle-aged individuals, the recommendation is based on the availability of a related matched donor versus an unrelated matched marrow donor. Those who have a related matched donor are encouraged to undergo bone marrow transplant within the first year after diagnosis, as this provides the longest life expectancy. If only an unrelated matched donor is available, tumor factors (e.g., spleen size, platelet count, and percentage of blasts in peripheral blood) are considered.[7]

Treatment Planning Throughout the Disease Continuum

Treatment Aimed at Cure or Complete Response

Most often curative therapy is undertaken for localized or early stage disease, but some advanced stage cancers (testicular cancer, osteogenic sarcoma, Hodgkin's disease, intermediate- and high-grade non-Hodgkin's lymphoma, and gestational trophoblastic cancers) can also be cured.[1] Accurate staging information is critical, as generally the chance of cure decreases dramatically if there is any metastatic disease.[1]

Treatment for cure must be aggressive

If a cure is the goal, then treatment must be aggressive. The initial treatment is the best and often the only opportunity to achieve a cure.[1] Surgery must be adequate to eradicate the tumor mass. Chemotherapy or radiation therapy must be administered at full dosage with short treatment intervals. Dose reductions or delays in treatment are to be avoided, because most tumors respond well to maximum doses of chemotherapy or radiation therapy. It is much more difficult to achieve an adequate response when treatment is attenuated. Toxicities of aggressive therapy must also be weighed against the consequence of treatment failure, which is most likely death from the disease.[1] Some curative treatment protocols can induce significant side effects that require close monitoring and management.

Treatment Modalities

The three main modalities of cancer treatment are chemotherapy (including biologic therapy), radiation therapy, and surgery. These treatments can be used alone or in combination. In the past, single-modality treatment was the rule. Current cancer therapy is most often multimodal, combining two or three different treatment modalities.[8,9] Treatment decisions are commonly made by a multidisciplinary tumor board composed of specialists in medical, surgical, and radiation oncology. Other team members include oncology nurses, social workers, psychologists, dietitians, and physical therapists. The team determines which therapeutic modalities are appropriate and in what sequence.

Early consultation among all disciplines can prevent potential treatment errors and maximize the likelihood of effective treatment.[8] For example, early collaboration and planning would likely result in surgical anastomosis being placed to avoid an upcoming radiation field. Radiation can then be delivered with maximal effectiveness and minimal organ toxicity based on the radiation oncologist's thorough knowledge of the operative findings. In some cases, the radiation oncologist is present during the operation.[8]

Standard treatment for specific cancers versus entering the patient into a clinical research trial must also be considered.[10] The patient may have already explored the clinical trials available for his or her particular tumor type or, conversely, the possibility of enrollment in a clinical trial may be a completely new concept for the patient. Research versus traditional therapy is a difficult decision for a patient to make without an adequate discussion with the oncologist. The oncologist and nurse need to ensure that the patient is fully informed and has every opportunity to access the latest treatment.

Surgery aimed at cure

Surgery is the primary means of curing solid tumors confined to the anatomic site of origin. Localized non–small cell lung carcinoma, malignant melanoma, and cancers of the endometrium, breast, and colon are examples of tumors that may be cured with surgery alone.[11-14] The surgeon must decide how extensive a resection is needed. The morbidity and mortality of the surgical procedure are weighed against the potential benefit. Surgeons should be knowledgeable about the efficacy of chemotherapy and radiation therapy for a given malignancy. Often, a second or third treatment modality is added in early stage disease treatment; this added therapy is referred to as *adjuvant therapy*. In some instances, chemotherapy or radiation therapy may be administered prior to surgery. This presurgery sequence of combined therapy is referred to as primary or *neoadjuvant therapy*.

Adjuvant therapy. Surgery is essentially a macroscopic treatment modality, yet cancer typically spreads microscopically. For many localized cancers, adjuvant (aiding or assisting) therapy is given in combination with surgery to decrease the likelihood of recurrence. Adjuvant therapy seeks to eliminate both local residual disease and distant micrometastases. Adjuvant therapy consists of either chemotherapy or radiation therapy administered after surgery. Adjuvant radiation therapy reduces local recurrence by destroying any microscopic tumor remaining in the surgical site or regional lymph nodes. Adjuvant chemotherapy is given for the same reasons as radiation therapy, as well as to eliminate any systemic micrometastases. Adjuvant chemotherapy and radiation are commonly used in the treatment of breast cancer,[15,16] colorectal cancer,[17,18] and ovarian cancer.[19]

Adjuvant therapy has two major theoretical advantages.[9] By eliminating potential micrometastases, adjuvant therapy increases the chances that an early-stage cancer may be cured. In some cases, adjuvant therapy can enable a less radical surgical procedure to be performed.

The use of adjuvant therapy requires careful evaluation of the risks and benefits. Early stage cancers may be cured by surgery alone, hence adjuvant therapy may expose the individual to additional toxicity and costs. Two conditions should be met to justify using adjuvant therapy.[1] First, the risk of recurrence must be greater than the risk of death or serious disability caused by the adjuvant therapy. Second, clinical trials must have demonstrated that the adjuvant therapy increases survival in similar cases.

Primary or neoadjuvant therapy. *Primary* or *neoadjuvant therapy* refers to chemotherapy or radiation therapy given *before* other modalities. Neoadjuvant therapy is used with colorectal, esophageal, lung, head and neck cancers, and early stage breast cancer.[9,17] The purpose of neoadjuvant therapy is to shrink the primary tumor and control local disease and micrometastases prior to surgery. Like adjuvant therapy, neoadjuvant therapy has advantages and disadvantages.[9,17] Neoadjuvant chemotherapy provides valuable information regarding the tumor's sensitivity to a particular drug regimen.[9] As a result of effective neoadjuvant treatment, a previously unresectable tumor may be reduced to become resectable.[9] Neoadjuvant therapy also may reduce the tumor size to allow for a less disfiguring surgery.[9] Another advantage of neoadjuvant chemotherapy is that there is no delay in exposing the tumor (and possibly distant metastases) to the cytotoxic impact of chemotherapy.[20,21] Tumors are believed to be more sensitive to chemotherapy early in their growth cycle and when the tumor mass is small.[9]

However, there are three serious drawbacks to the use of neoadjuvant therapy.[9] First, there is a possibility that the tumor may be unresponsive to the radiation therapy or chemotherapy. In such a case, potentially curative surgery will have been delayed while the tumor has had an opportunity to grow. Second, successful neoadjuvant therapy can obscure the actual stage of the tumor. The tumor margins may regress and lymph node status may convert from histologically positive to negative. Uncertainty regarding the true stage of the disease complicates treatment planning. Aggregate results of treatment with a particular regimen are difficult to interpret because the clinician cannot be sure that the individual tumors treated were really a homogeneous group. Third, successful neoadjuvant therapy may lead to a decision to perform an inappropriately conservative surgery or may cause the patient to reject a recommended treatment. Conservative decisions could contribute to cancer recurrence in an individual whose best chance of cure is early, aggressive treatment.

Chemotherapy or radiation therapy alone

Either chemotherapy or radiation therapy alone may be used to cure malignancies. Chemotherapy is typically used with curative intent for high-grade non-Hodgkin's lymphoma, germ-cell testicular cancer, acute lymphoid leukemia, and Hodgkin's disease.[9] One advantage of initial treatment with chemotherapy is the ability to evaluate the sensitivity of the tumor to a particular chemotherapeutic regimen.

Radiation therapy alone is effective in curing certain cancers. Hodgkin's disease, some gynecologic tumors, many head and neck cancers, and medulloblastoma are examples of malignancies that may be cured by radiation therapy alone.[8]

Combined chemotherapy and radiation therapy

Chemotherapy combined with radiation therapy provides control of both systemic and local disease. For example, advanced non-Hodgkin's lymphoma is a chemo-sensitive tumor that tends to recur at the original site of bulky disease. It is thought that the original tumor site may contain too many tumor cells for the chemotherapy to eliminate, which eventually leads to recurrence. Radiation therapy can be effectively targeted to these original tumor sites.[8]

Chemotherapy may be used to sensitize tumors to the effects of radiation therapy[22] and to overcome tumor resistance to radiation therapy.[9] Such strategies to enhance treatment are commonly used in treating head and neck cancer.

When combining radiation therapy and chemotherapy, care must be taken to select effective doses and to monitor the additive toxicities possible from combined therapy. Toxicities can lead to dose reductions or treatment delays that may compromise the effectiveness of the treatment.[9] For example, mucositis can be a dose-limiting toxicity in treating head and neck cancers with both radiation and chemotherapy. Thus, cisplatin is commonly used in combination with radiation to treat head and neck cancer, due both to the efficacy of cisplatin and its lack of mucosal toxicity.[22]

Multimodality therapy may be scheduled sequentially, alternately, or concurrently. Based on clinical research and collective knowledge, the most effective sequence and schedule for multimodality therapy can be determined prior to initiation of therapy.

Treatment for Advanced or Recurrent Disease

Prolonging survival and possibly providing cure are realistic treatment goals in recurrent or advanced cancer. Many advanced cancers are incurable, but a few types (testicular cancer, osteogenic sarcoma, Hodgkin's disease, some non-Hodgkin's lymphomas) may be cured even in an advanced stage.[1] Chemotherapy, radiation therapy, and surgery are used to control locally advanced or disseminated disease. Some individuals with advanced cancer may have long symptom-free periods.

An example of the decision-making process involved in treating metastatic breast cancer is shown in Figure 13-2.[23] The figure clearly illustrates that there are multiple levels of treatment and options to consider at all stages of the disease. Accurate staging is important in recurrent disease. Knowing the extent of disease assists the team in selecting the appropriate treatment. Histopathologic verification of recurrence should be obtained to rule out a second primary tumor or fibrosis mimicking residual disease.[1]

Surgical resection can result in a period of remission when the recurrent tumor is slow growing.[24] In the case of metastases to a single site (lung, liver, or brain), surgical removal of the metastatic disease may be curative when combined with successful treatment of the primary tumor.[11] Debulking of large tumors can enhance the effectiveness of chemotherapy against the residual disease.[24,25] Regression of distant metastases has been noted following surgical resection of the primary tumor.[25]

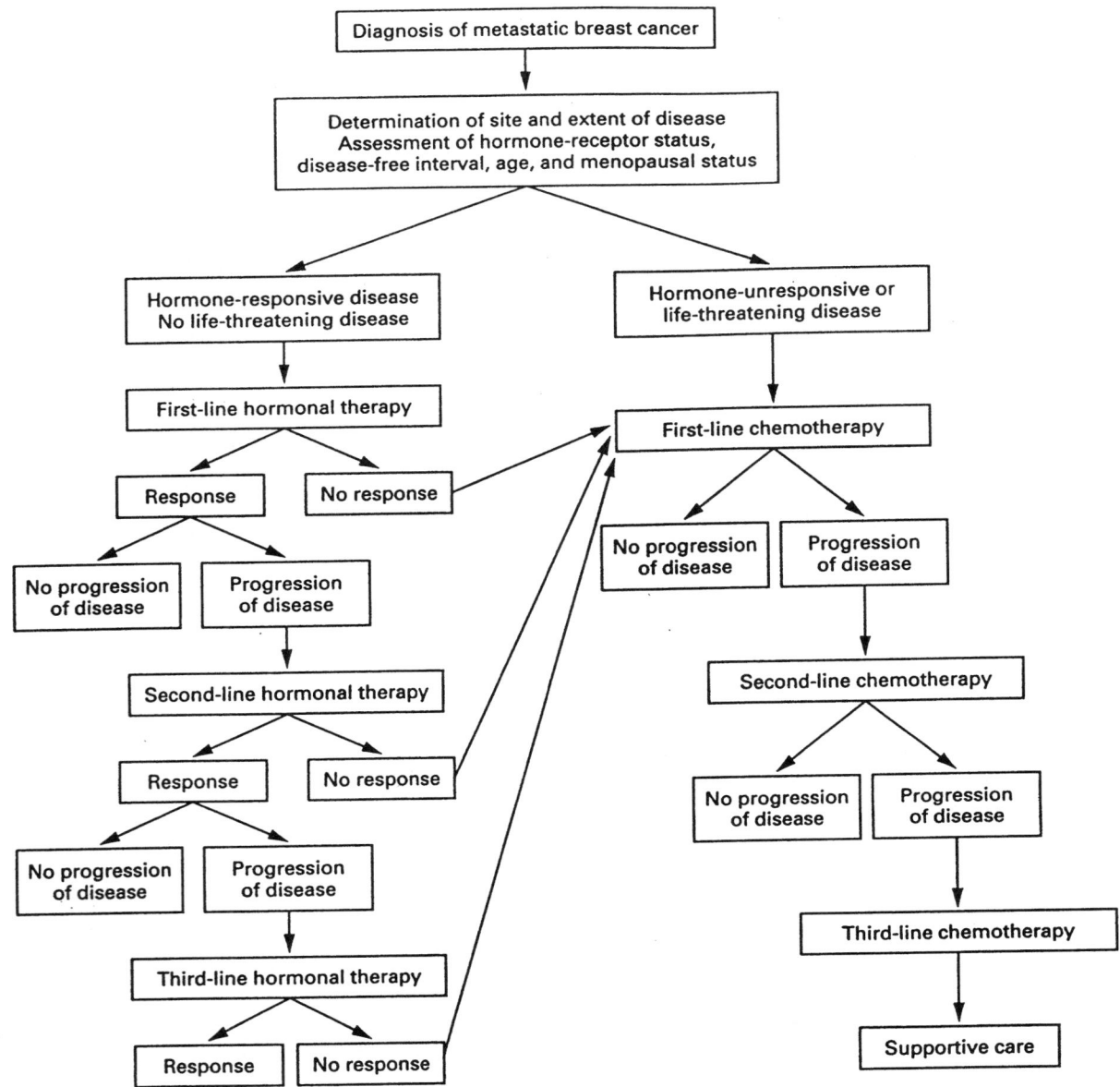

Figure 13-2 Optimal palliative therapy for women with metastatic breast cancer. (Reprinted with permission from Hortobagyi GN: Treatment of breast cancer. *N Engl J Med* 339:979, 1998.[23])

Palliative Treatment

When prolonging life is no longer realistic, the goal of treatment becomes palliative. Palliative treatment may involve any single or combined treatment modality. For example, a painful bowel obstruction may be relieved surgically. Radiation therapy can be used to control bleeding and pain or to prevent pathologic fractures. Chemotherapy can be used palliatively for control of symptoms such as pain, nausea, vomiting, or weight loss.

Palliative treatment should be used with discretion and have a specific objective based on sound clinical indications. Palliative therapy should minimize cost, in-

convenience, discomfort, and risks, as well as be completed in the shortest possible time frame. Palliative measures may sometimes be used for people who are asymptomatic but in whom the impending development of a catastrophic problem can be reasonably anticipated. Problems benefiting from palliative interventions include impending obstruction of the superior vena cava, or obstruction of major bronchus, or potential collapse of a vertebral body. However, palliative treatment of patients who are asymptomatic and incurable is usually deferred until there is a definitive appearance of specific problems. People with such impending complications should be followed closely and offered emotional support and reassurance that appropriate palliative therapy will be initiated immediately if the need arises. It is critical to avoid the perception that the health care team is no longer interested in the patient when the stage of active treatment is completed and goals have shifted.

Continuity of Care

A person with cancer usually interacts sequentially or concurrently with multiple physicians and nurses who specialize in various aspects of oncology. Throughout the course of the disease, there may be inpatient admission for surgery and then outpatient radiation or chemotherapy, each phase of treatment occurring in a separate office with separate staff. Even complex and technical treatments are becoming available in home care and hospice settings, which introduces yet another group of caregivers. Patients and providers alike are challenged to overcome and avoid any negative consequences resulting from lack of continuity. Two major areas potentially affected by lack of continuity are relationships and communication.

Disruption of relationships

A change in the focus of treatment, such as switching from active treatment to palliative care, usually means that the patients will receive care from an entirely new team. The patients must form new bonds at a particularly difficult time. In leaving the team they have trusted, the patients may feel that they must now receive care from "strangers" during the final stage of their lives. Likewise, the team who has cared for the patients becomes stressed by the loss of a close relationship.

Contacting the forthcoming care team and offering to discuss issues known to provide patient comfort and support help to ensure continuity of care. If the new team has a nurse contact who can speak with the patients knowledgeably about their prior experiences, the feelings of disruption will be lessened.

Communication

The various specialists involved in the care of a person with cancer may or may not be part of the same health care organization. Even within one institution, medical records and information are not always shared or communicated between different departments.[26] This gap in communication can result in the same questions constantly being asked of the patient. Apparently lacking essential information, the providers' ability to coordinate and maximize patient care may be questioned.

It is not uncommon for people undergoing treatment for cancer to feel that information from one health care provider conflicts with information provided by another source. Individual health care professionals may present similar information in somewhat different ways. This can be confusing for the patient. In other instances, there may actually be a difference of opinion as to the optimum treatment plan. It can be difficult for patients to understand that there may be some uncertainty among the clinicians as to which treatment course is best. The nurse often can ease this uncertainty by discussing the treatment decision process with the patient in a relaxed, nonstressful conversation where no decisions are being made.

Teaching hospitals, where resident medical staffs typically rotate each month, present additional challenges to coordination, communication, and continuity. Negative information about treatment, disease progression, or recurrence should be communicated to the patient by someone with whom the patient has an established relationship. Delivering such information is stressful for the caregiver as well.

Measures to increase the continuity of care

There is widespread endorsement of efforts to improve continuity and collaboration in cancer care.[26–30] Coordination of services is recognized as an important goal. The need for increased continuity of cancer care has led to the development of new roles. In some settings, nurses and social workers help to coordinate care.[28,30] The challenge for the future is to focus not only on coordinated care but on care that is truly integrated.[26]

Principles of Clinical Research

Although modern oncology practice advances from empiricism to therapy by clinical trial and treatment design, many questions about the best treatment approach remain unanswered. No curative treatment exists for some cancers, such as multiple myeloma. The search for more effective and better tolerated chemotherapeutic agents and regimens is ongoing. In surgical oncology, questions exist regarding radical versus limited procedures and what method of node sampling is most informative. The optimal sequencing of adjuvant therapy and who will benefit from adjuvant treatment remains uncertain in some cases. Questions such as these are best answered through clinical trials.

This section describes the principles of clinical research in the areas of medical, surgical, and radiation oncology. General research principles that apply to all three treatment specialties (chemotherapy, surgery, radiation therapy) are discussed, as well as aspects of research that pertain specifically to each specialty area. Ethical aspects of clinical research are also addressed. First, it is important to be aware of the various groups and agencies that conduct and fund clinical trials.

Who Conducts and Funds Clinical Trials?

Cooperative groups

The National Cancer Institute (NCI) sponsors the Clinical Trials Cooperative Group Program. Cooperative groups consist of academic institutions and cancer treatment centers throughout the United States, Canada, and Europe. These groups design and conduct multi-institutional clinical trials of new drug treatment techniques, such as a new surgical procedure, or a method of delivering radiation therapy. The clinical trials they conduct are funded in part or whole by NCI grants. Some cooperative groups focus only on one type of cancer, other groups focus on a single treatment modality, and still others may focus on a broad range of cancers. The major cooperative groups involved in cancer clinical trials are listed in Table 13-1.

Comprehensive cancer centers

A treatment center that performs basic and clinical cancer research and meets specific NCI criteria may be designated by the NCI as a Comprehensive Cancer Center. These centers conduct independent cancer clinical trials and participate in cooperative group trials. Though some comprehensive centers opt not to have NCI designation, most seek to achieve this specific level of recognition.

Community clinical oncology programs

In order to increase the availability of cancer research to those in community settings, the NCI established the Community Clinical Oncology Program (CCOP). This program consists of community-based physicians who affiliate with either a cooperative group or a comprehensive cancer center to carry out cancer clinical trials. There are certain CCOPs that specifically serve low-income or minority populations. Many community cancer programs are affiliated with university cancer programs and will conduct clinical trials as satellite sites for the university program. The community programs have been instrumental in providing a broader base of patients to accrue for clinical trials.

Pharmaceutical companies

A pharmaceutical company may carry out its own clinical research trials and also help to fund trials being performed by the cooperative groups and cancer centers. In some cases, pharmaceutical companies provide the drugs without charge for the patients enrolled in these clinical studies. Pharmaceutical company clinical research trials are regulated and approved by the Food and Drug Administration (FDA).

Innovative partnerships. Pharmaceutical and biotech companies have used the services of contract research organizations (CROs) to carry out various phases of research, from preclinical studies, consulting, and management of clinical trials through drug marketing. Some CROs have merged with related companies, such as physician practice management organizations, increasing their ability to design relevant trials and to accrue more patients to clinical trials.[31] There has recently been growth of services offered by a related field, referred to as *site management organizations* (SMOs). These management companies provide oversight and support for clinical trials, with an emphasis on streamlining studies and cost reduction.

Overall Principles of Research

Clinical trials are highly controlled research experiments that require careful planning and rigorous conduct. The purpose of clinical trials is to provide "definitive answers to well-defined questions."[32] The consequence of a clinical trial that is poorly designed could be the incorrect rejection of a useful therapy or misguided acceptance of an ineffective treatment.

The elements of a well-designed study are listed in Table 13-2.[33] A thoughtful hypothesis is essential to the success of the study.[34] The hypothesis, the critical question under study, helps to convince clinicians and potential patient participants that the research has value. A carefully developed hypothesis facilitates subject recruitment and timely completion of the study.

The research plan is delineated in a written study protocol. The protocol describes the target patient population and the specifics of the treatment plan. The proto-

---

Table 13-1 Examples of Cooperative Research Groups

Southwest Oncology Group (SWOG)

Radiation Therapy Oncology Group (RTOG)

National Surgical Adjuvant Breast and Bowel Project (NSABP)

Eastern Cooperative Study Group (ECOG)

Gynecology Oncology Group (GOG)

Lung Cancer Study Group

Children's Oncology Group

Brain Tumor Study Group

European Organization for Research on Treatment for Cancer (EORTC)

Table 13-2 Essential Elements in the Design of a Clinical Trial

Clearly stated testable hypothesis

Well-defined primary end point

Appropriate trial design

Adequate power to answer the study question

Accrual of adequate number of patients to complete the study in a reasonable amount of time

Appropriate statistical analysis of predetermined trial end points

Conclusions drawn directly from the data

col defines the goals of the study and provides evidence that the study design is adequate to meet the goals. All clinical research protocols contain certain elements; sample protocol elements are shown in Table 13-3.[32]

Clinical Trials of New Chemotherapeutic Agents

The clinical evaluation of new chemotherapeutic agents is divided into four phases: phase I, phase II, phase III, and phase IV. Drugs are studied through at least the first three phases before the FDA grants final approval for widespread use. Phase I trials are the earliest human trials and are designed to determine the toxicities and the maximum tolerated dose of the new agent. Using the facts established in phase I, the goal of phase II trials is to establish whether the drug has sufficient antitumor efficacy to warrant further testing. Next, in phase III trials, both the efficacy and toxicities of the new drug alone and in combination with other drugs are compared to those of existing established treatments to determine which approach is most effective. Phase IV trials, called postmarketing trials, are used to learn more about the long-term use of the drugs.

Phase I trials

Phase I trials are intended to establish the maximum tolerated dose (MTD) and the dose-limiting toxicities of a new drug. These trials determine the dose that will be used in phase II studies of the drug.

Patient selection. Eligibility requirements for phase I trials are broad. Patients must have proven neoplastic disease for which no effective treatment currently exists. Eligibility is not usually restricted to patients with a particular tumor type. Because response to treatment is not

being evaluated in a phase I study, it is not necessary that participants have a measurable tumor mass. New drugs are always tested first in adults; pediatric trials follow the determination of the adult MTD.[35] Patients with acute leukemia are usually not included in phase I studies, because hematologic toxicity would be difficult to evaluate in individuals with already severely compromised bone marrow function.[35] Patients eligible for phase I trials have often been extensively treated before entering the study. At least 1 month should have elapsed since receiving other cancer therapy, so that the toxicity attributed to the drug under investigation may be distinguished from that of prior treatment. Study participants must be expected to live at least 1 to 2 months, as this time is considered to be the minimum period required to observe toxic drug effects. The difficulty in distinguishing treatment-related mortality from that of advanced disease may eventually lead to a requirement for a longer life expectancy for participants in phase I trials.[36] Major organ function must be adequate so that the drug will be metabolized normally. This helps ensure that evaluation of major organ toxicity is accurate and that patients will not be knowingly subjected to unduly severe toxicity.

Starting dose and dose escalation. Phase I trials usually involve a drug that has never been administered to humans. The dose given to the initial group of patients is low enough that it is not expected to cause serious toxicity. The starting dose level in a clinical trial is usually one-tenth of the dose that was found to be lethal for 10% of the mice in preclinical testing.[36] The initial dose must be set low, as animal models are not perfect predictors of toxicity in humans.[33,35] Cohorts of three to six patients receive each dose level.[32]

The dose is then increased for each subsequent group of patients. Dose escalation is done only after at least 1 week has passed to observe the initial group for acute toxicities.[36] The most common plan for dose escalation is the "modified Fibonacci" scheme.[33,36] This sets the second dose level at double the initial dose; the third level is 67% higher than the second; the fourth is 50% higher than the third; and each subsequent level is increased by 33%. The goal is to avoid the problems of escalating too rapidly (potential exposure of patients to severe toxicity), or too slowly (depriving participants of potential benefit through administration of subtherapeutic doses).[35]

The dose that is found to cause moderate, reversible toxicity in the majority of patients is recommended for further study in a phase II trial.[36] The maximum acceptable dose tends to be pushed upward with time, as advances in transfusion support and pharmacologic rescue techniques increase our ability to support patients through what were once dose-limiting side effects.[35]

Phase II trials

The goal of phase II trials is to prove the new drug's effectiveness against specific tumors. Phase II testing determines whether the drug should undergo further evalu-

---

Table 13-3 Subject Headings for a Protocol

1. Introduction and scientific background
2. Objectives
3. Selection of patients
4. Design of study (including schematic diagram)
5. Treatment plan
6. Drug information
7. Toxicities to be monitored and dosage modifications
8. Required clinical and laboratory data and study calendar
9. Critieria for evaluating the effect of treatment and end-point definition
10. Statistical considerations
11. Informed consent and regulatory considerations
12. Data forms
13. References
14. Study chairperson, collaborating participants, addresses, and telephone numbers

Reprinted with permission from Simon RM: Clinical trials in cancer, in DeVita VT Jr, Hellman S, Rosenberg SA (eds): *Cancer: Principles and Practice of Oncology* (ed 5). Philadelphia, Lippincott-Raven, 1997, p 514.[32]

ation. Careful selection of the patient population to be studied is key in ensuring that the trial results will be meaningful.[33]

Patient selection. Phase II trials evaluate the response of the tumor to the new drug, so participants must have a specific diagnosis and measurable tumor. Certain representative tumor types, called "signal tumors," have been selected by the NCI for study in phase II trials. These include breast, colorectal, and lung cancers, melanoma, acute leukemia, and lymphoma.[36] Subjects in phase II trials should be individuals likely to benefit from the new treatment and for whom no effective therapy currently exists. They should have good performance status and minimal prior exposure to chemotherapy. One or, at most, two prior chemotherapy regimens are acceptable. In patients heavily pretreated with chemotherapy, a drug may not demonstrate its true activity (a type II error).[32,33] The inherent problem in phase II trials is that individuals who have failed conventional treatment may be the least likely to provide a satisfactory evaluation of the new therapy.[37] Subjects must have adequate organ function and a life expectancy of at least 12 weeks to participate. Phase II studies usually enroll fourteen to twenty patients in a cohort group.[33]

Considerations in phase II trials. Drawing conclusions regarding treatment benefit from a phase II single-agent trial is complex. The usual measure of a drug's antitumor activity in a phase II trial is response rate.[32,38] While this answers the basic question posed by the trial, partial responses do not necessarily indicate patient benefit. A partial response (50% reduction in tumor mass) may be brief and complicated by treatment toxicity. Additionally, if responders live longer than nonresponders, this is not proof that the treatment caused the longer survival.[32] Typically, multiple follow-up studies are done to duplicate and refine results of phase II trials that demonstrate treatment benefit.[36]

Phase II trials are also used to evaluate the practicality and tolerability of combination chemotherapy regimens. Results of this type of study are difficult to interpret.[32] Often, the drugs under study are known to be of some benefit as single agents. The combination of drugs has to demonstrate greater activity than its most active component or than another combination. Often, this comparison is not taken into account, and drug combinations are reported to be as effective when they have not been held to a sufficiently high standard.[32]

A phase II trial in which participants are randomized to treatment groups avoids some of these difficulties. However, this requires simultaneous testing of two or more therapies and the availability of a large number of participants. For these reasons, randomized phase II studies are rare.[33]

Phase III trials

In a phase III trial, a new treatment is compared to standard therapy. A new drug enters phase III testing if it has demonstrated significant efficacy in phase II trials. A drug may be tested as single-agent therapy, or as part of a drug combination, or comparing combined modality treatment with single modality. Phase III trials require hundreds of participants and are most often carried out by multiple institutions, linked through NCI clinical cooperative groups.

Patient selection. The requirements for participation in phase III trials are similar to those in phase II. Patients must have measurable disease, adequate major organ function, good performance status, and little or no prior anticancer therapy. There is debate regarding how narrow the eligibility criteria in phase III trials should be.[32,39] Narrow eligibility criteria limit the generalizability of the results.

Trial design. The preferred design for a phase III trial is a prospective, randomized trial.[32,36,37] Randomization means that participants are assigned randomly to one or the other of the chemotherapy treatments being evaluated. The assignment is not biased by knowledge of specific individual characteristics. Randomization does not mean that the two groups are medically equivalent. Rather, it means that both known and unknown prognostic factors of participants are distributed randomly. This allows results to be interpreted as due to the treatment, not due to nonrandom variation in the distribution of unknown prognostic factors.[32] A randomized design is necessary to detect small but significant differences between treatments.[1,32]

Phase IV trials

Following the FDA approval of a chemotherapy agent or drug regimen, additional studies, usually considered postmarketing studies, can be conducted. Not all new drugs will be followed with phase IV trials. The purpose of phase IV trials is to accrue new information about any risks or side effects not previously identified. Phase IV trials have proved extremely useful for identifying potential issues with the drug that were not discovered during the early-phase trials. Some refer to phase IV trials as long-term experiential trials. Though not required, these trials prove to be useful, facilitating even more effective use of the drugs.

Research Principles in Surgical Oncology

Clinical trials in surgical oncology evaluate the effect of an intervention, such as a modification in surgical technique, or a new form of adjuvant therapy on patient outcome. Most aspects (e.g., randomization, exclusion criteria, number of participants) of surgical oncology trials are quite similar to trials of chemotherapeutic agents. However, there are some unique challenges in surgical oncology trials.

The success of a new surgical technique may depend heavily on the skill of the individual surgeon. Certain surgical techniques may be developed by or become individualized to specific surgeons or institutions.[40] In trials evaluating a new operative procedure, the surgeons' technique must be uniform. This can be accomplished by standardized training of all participating surgeons,[41] or written and videotaped descriptions of the procedure.[42]

When comparing two similar surgeries, creativity is required to eliminate patient or caregiver bias. Individual clinicians may use differing wound-care techniques that could affect outcomes such as infection, disease, or healing. In some cases, it is possible to "blind" the identity of the caregivers by using prepared identical surgical dressings on all patients.[43]

Another challenge with surgical trials is the irreversibility of surgery. If one type of surgery proves to be more effective, patients who have already received a different procedure cannot be "crossed over" to the more effective treatment.[44] Advances in surgical oncology tend to emanate from retrospective case analysis rather than prospective trials.

Research Principles in Radiation Oncology

A striking difference occurs with radiation clinical trials because radiation therapy is known to be effective in treating malignancies. In radiation therapy trials, tumor response is expected and the challenge is to discover the most effective treatment. Radiation therapy trials typically compare radiation delivery methods, schedules, or different combinations of adjuvant therapies.

Radiation therapy trials measure both initial tumor response and locoregional control. Initial tumor response may be evaluated early in the trial. Locoregional control, the more meaningful outcome, requires longer follow-up. Because of the longer duration to definitive outcomes, radiation therapy trials sometimes combine phases I and II.[45] Longer follow-up also necessitates a significantly larger sample size than is usually accrued in chemotherapy trials. Since some patients will not survive for the entire follow-up period, radiation trials may need to accrue two or three times more participants than a chemotherapy trial.[45]

Issues in Oncology Clinical Trials

In the United States, the process of approval for new medical techniques, drugs, and equipment is a rigorous, peer-reviewed research process. This highly regulated process of approval results in significant challenges to both the clinicians and the patients. There are instances where a new drug or technique quickly becomes headline news and the patients become understandably anxious for access to this breakthrough. The rigorous scientific research process is specifically designed to assure maximum safety and efficacy before general application is possible. With any research process, there are some significant issues that can develop.

Exclusion criteria

All clinical trials have specific exclusion criteria. Phase III trials, in particular, have restrictive eligibility requirements. These criteria form the "gateway" for participation in the study and provide a homogenous sample to study and determine conclusions.

Patient perspective

Individuals with cancer may feel that entering a clinical trial is the best hope for cure or prolonged life. Many of those who are faced with a disease for which there currently is no effective treatment are willing to try almost anything that might help. These individuals are looking for a means of prolonging their life until a better treatment is developed. They often are motivated by a desire to contribute to medical knowledge in order to benefit others with the disease. It can be devastating to learn that one does not meet the requirements for participation in a trial.

The increased knowledge that is easily accessible today via the Internet and mass media has heightened awareness and created a need for more information. Patients and their families will search available resources and have challenging questions for clinicians about their potential for entering a clinical trial. Patients and families come prepared with entire reviews of current clinical trials. This knowledge must be handled with forthright and open discussion about eligibility, prognosis, potential outcomes, and a strong orientation toward hope.

Clinical perspective

From a scientific standpoint, participation in a clinical trial must be limited to subjects who can help answer the question or hypothesis posed by the trial. Obviously, participants must have a specific diagnosis and stage of disease. Eligibility requirements are designed to include individuals most likely to benefit from the therapy being studied and to exclude those less likely to benefit.[39] In addition, participants must not be exposed to excessive risk. For instance, patients with poor pulmonary function are not allowed to participate in trials involving treatments that cause pulmonary toxicity.

It has been argued that eligibility requirements should be relaxed.[39] Restrictive exclusion criteria limit the generalizability of the trial results.[32] Individuals who meet the eligibility requirements may not be representative of the majority of people with that disease.[39] Strict exclusion criteria also necessitate lengthy, expensive evaluations to determine eligibility. Greater time is required to accrue enough patients to complete the trial. Debate regarding restrictive versus relaxed exclusion criteria is ongoing.

Ethics of randomization

Some clinicians feel that randomized trials create a conflict of interest between the physician's dual roles as doctor and as clinical investigator. The conflict arises if the physician believes that one arm of a randomized trial would be better for a particular patient. This argument maintains that randomization treats the patient as an interchangeable unit, rather than as an individual.[46]

On the other hand, some argue that oncologists are often in the position of making educated guesses about what is best for their patients.[47,48] When one does not know for certain which treatment is superior, randomization provides the patient with the greatest possibility of getting effective treatment. It may be more honest and ethical to admit that there is uncertainty regarding treatment in some situations. There is widespread agreement that when the physician truly does not know which treatment is best, treating within a randomized trial is acceptable and perhaps mandatory.[33,46]

Economic issues

The economic issue of clinical trial participation is one of the toughest challenges facing oncology clinicians today. Insurance companies often have very restrictive views of clinical research and may deny payment or be reluctant to approve payment for participation in cancer clinical trials. Patients must understand that the reimbursement for clinical trials must be secured before the decision to enter the trial is complete. The potential out-of-pocket costs could be substantial for someone whose insurance carrier denies payment for the research trial. Even in cases where the drugs given during the trial are free, the accompanying tests and visits may be denied for reimbursement. It is incumbent on the clinical staff to determine the entire financial situation and also to discuss this with the patient family prior to any final decision about the trial under consideration. Most oncology clinicians have become skilled at negotiating for the inclusion of patients in clinical trials. This process is extremely time-consuming and has added a new dimension of uncertainty into the clinical decision-making process. Informed consent has been broadened to include the patient understanding not only the medical aspects of care but also the financial responsibilities.

Conclusion

The treatment plan for each cancer patient is selected based on a compendium of factors, including tumor characteristics, stage, patient condition, and clinician expertise. The basic science and clinical application research that has built the framework for cancer treatment plans is a complex intermingling of scientific knowledge. For years, teams of cancer specialists have used interdisciplinary collaboration as a way to assure that cancer patients receive the most efficacious and carefully planned care possible. Oncology nurses with specialized patient management and support skills have added significant research and knowledge to the treatment process.

References

1. Weiss GR: Diagnosis and management of early and advanced cancer, in Weiss GR (ed): *Clinical Oncology.* East Norwalk, CT, Appleton & Lange, 1993, pp 29–34
2. Olweny CLM: Goals and rationale of cancer treatment. *Med J Austr* 155:187–192, 1991
3. Landis SH, Murray T, Bolden S, et al: Cancer statistics, 1998. *CA Cancer J Clin* 48:6–29, 1998
4. Skarkin AT, Dorfman DM: Non-Hodgkin's lymphomas: Current classification and management. *CA Cancer J Clin* 47: 351–372, 1997
5. Skeel RT, Ganz PA: Systematic assessment of the patient with cancer and long-term medical complications of treatment, in Skeel RT, Lachant NA (eds): *Handbook of Cancer Chemotherapy* (ed 5). Boston, Little, Brown, 1995, pp 95–115
6. DeVita VT: Principles of cancer management: Chemotherapy, in DeVita VT Jr, Hellman S, Rosenberg SA (eds): *Cancer: Principles and Practice of Oncology.* Philadelphia, Lippincott-Raven, 1997, pp 333–347
7. Lee SJ, Anasetti C, Horowitz MM, et al: Initial therapy for chronic myelogenous leukemia: Playing the odds. *J Clin Oncol* 16:2897–2903, 1998 (editorial)
8. Dobelbower RR: Principles and practical aspects of radiation therapy, in Skeel RT, Lachant NA (eds): *Handbook of Cancer Chemotherapy* (ed 4). Boston, Little, Brown, 1995, pp 52–70
9. Lichter AS, Abeloff MD, Armitage JO, et al: Multimodality therapy, in Abeloff MD, Armitage JO, Lichter AS, et al (eds): *Clinical Oncology.* New York, Churchill Livingstone, 1995, pp 307–314
10. Donehower RC, Abeloff MD, Perry MC: Chemotherapy, in Abeloff MD, Armitage JO, Lichter AS, et al (eds): *Clinical Oncology.* New York, Churchill Livingstone, 1995, pp 201–218
11. Rosenberg SA: Principles of cancer management: Surgical oncology, in DeVita VT Jr, Hellman S, Rosenberg SA (eds): *Cancer: Principles and Practice of Oncology* (ed 5). Philadelphia, Lippincott-Raven, 1997, pp 295–306
12. Langmuir VK, Poulter CA, Qazi R, et al: Breast cancer, in Rubin P (ed): *Clinical Oncology: A Multidisciplinary Approach for Physicians and Students* (ed 7). Philadelphia, Saunders, 1993, pp 187–215
13. DuBeshter B, Lin J, Angel C, et al: Gynecologic tumors, in Rubin P (ed): *Clinical Oncology: A Multidisciplinary Approach for Physicians and Students* (ed 7). Philadelphia, Saunders, 1993, pp 363–418
14. Salazar OM, McCune CS, Rubin P, et al: Lung cancer, in Rubin P (ed): *Clinical Oncology: A Multidisciplinary Approach for Physicians and Students* (ed 7). Philadelphia, Saunders, 1993, pp 645–665
15. Overgaard M, Hansen PS, Overgaard J, et al: Postoperative radiotherapy in high-risk premenopausal women with breast cancer who receive adjuvant chemotherapy. *N Engl J Med* 337:949–955, 1997
16. Ragaz J, Jackson SM, Le N, et al: Adjuvant radiotherapy and chemotherapy in node-positive premenopausal women with breast cancer. *N Engl J Med* 337:956–962, 1997
17. Minsky BD: The role of adjuvant radiation therapy in the treatment of colorectal cancer. *Hematol Oncol Clin North Am* 11:679–697, 1997
18. Vaughn DJ, Haller DG: The role of adjuvant chemotherapy in the treatment of colorectal cancer. *Hematol Oncol Clin North Am* 11:699–719, 1997
19. Granai CO, Gajewski WH: Gynecologic cancer, in Skeel RT,

Lachant NA (eds): *Handbook of Cancer Chemotherapy* (ed 4). Boston, Little, Brown, 1995, pp 288–317

20. Havlin KA: Sarcomas of soft tissue and bone, in Weiss GR (ed): *Clinical Oncology*. East Norwalk, CT, Appleton & Lange, 1993, pp 264–271

21. Leventhal BG, Wittes RE: Combined modality therapy, in Leventhal BG, Wittes RE: *Research Methods in Clinical Oncology*. New York, Raven, 1988, pp 150–170

22. DeConti RC: Carcinomas of the head and neck, in Skeel RT, Lachant NA (eds): *Handbook of Cancer Chemotherapy* (ed 5). Boston, Little, Brown, 1995, pp 201–220

23. Hortobagyi GN: Treatment of breast cancer. *N Engl J Med* 339:974–984, 1998

24. Morton DL: Principles of surgical oncology, in Holland JF, Frei E, Bast RC, et al (eds): *Cancer Medicine*, vol 1 (ed 3). Philadelphia, Lea & Febiger, 1993, pp 523–538

25. Sindelar WF, Ketcham AS: Regression of cancer following surgery, in Lewison EF (ed): *Conference on Spontaneous Regression of Cancer*. DHEW Publication No. (NIH) 76-1038, Bethesda, National Cancer Institute, 1976, pp 81–84

26. Beddar SM, Aikin JL: Continuity of care: A challenge for ambulatory oncology nursing. *Semin Oncol Nurs* 10:254–263, 1994

27. American Federation of Clinical Oncologic Societies: Access to quality cancer care: Consensus statement. *J Clin Oncol* 16: 1628–1630, 1998

28. Benninger MS: Medical liaisons for continuity of head and neck cancer care. *Head & Neck* 14:28–32, 1992

29. Hange-Dickerson PA: Oncology nurse practitioner provides continuity of care. *Nurse Pract* 17:14, 1992 (letter)

30. Lauria MM: Continuity of cancer care. *Cancer* 67:1759–1766, 1991

31. Dutton G: Mergers and growth of CROs leading to full-service, multinational companies. *Genet Eng News* Sept 1, 1997, pp 17–21.

32. Simon RM: Clinical trials in cancer, in DeVita VT Jr, Hellman S, Rosenberg SA (eds): *Cancer: Principles and Practice of Oncology* (ed 5). Philadelphia, Lippincott-Raven, 1997, pp 513–542

33. Rothenberg ML, Chabner BA: The goals of clinical cancer trials, in Niederhuber JE (ed): *Current Therapy in Oncology*. St. Louis, Mosby-Year Book, 1993, pp 22–27

34. Rew DA: The (continued) importance of the hypothesis in surgical oncology research. *Eur J Surg Oncol* 24(1):67–72, 1998

35. Leventhal BG, Wittes RE: Phase I trials, in Leventhal BG, Wittes RE: *Research Methods in Clinical Oncology*. New York, Raven Press, 1988, pp 41–59

36. Carter SK, Schein PS: Clinical evaluation of new anticancer agents, in Calabresi P, Schein PS (eds): *Medical Oncology: Basic Principles and Clinical Management of Cancer*. New York, McGraw Hill, 1993, pp 371–382

37. Zelen M: Theory and practice of clinical trials, in Holland JF, Frei E, Bast RC, et al (eds): *Cancer Medicine*, vol 1 (ed 3). Philadelphia, Lea & Febiger, 1993, pp 340–360

38. Thiesse P, Ollivier L, Di Stefano-Louineau D, et al: Response rate accuracy in oncology trials: Reasons for interobserver variability. *J Clin Oncol* 15:3507–3514, 1997

39. George SL: Reducing patient eligibility criteria in cancer clinical trials. *J Clin Oncol* 14:1364–1370, 1996

40. Piantadosi S: Clinical trials as experimental designs, in Piantadosi S: *Clinical Trials: A methodologic perspective*. New York, John Wiley & Sons, 1997, pp 61–105

41. Krag D, Weaver D, Ashikaga T, et al: The sentinel node in breast cancer. *N Engl J Med* 339:941–946, 1998

42. Cushieri A, Fayers P, Fielding J, et al: Postoperative morbidity and mortality after D_1 and D_2 resections for gastric cancer: Preliminary results of the MRC randomised controlled surgical trial. *Lancet* 347:995–999, 1996

43. Majeed AW, Troy G, Nicholl JP, et al: Randomised, prospective, single-blind comparison of laparoscopic versus small-incision cholecystectomy. *Lancet* 347:989–994, 1996

44. Solomon MJ, Laxamana A, Devore L, et al: Randomized controlled trials in surgery. *Surgery* 115:707–712, 1994

45. Pajak TF: Methodology of clinical trials, in Perez CA, Brady LW (eds): *Principles and Practice of Radiation Oncology* (ed 2). Philadelphia, Lippincott, 1997, pp 173–182

46. Emanuel EJ, Patterson WB (eds): Ethics of randomized clinical trials. *J Clin Oncol* 16:365–371, 1998

47. Buyse M: Randomized clinical trials in surgical oncology. *Eur J Surg Oncol* 17:421–428, 1991

48. Leventhal BG, Wittes RE: Protection of human subjects, in Leventhal BG, Wittes RE: *Research Methods in Clinical Oncology*. New York, Raven, 1988, pp 206–216

CHAPTER 14

Surgical Therapy

Margaret Hansen Frogge, RN, MS
Shawnna M. Cunning, RN, MSN, CCRN

Introduction

Surgical therapy is the most frequently used and most successful cancer therapy available today. More patients are cured of cancer by surgery than any other single therapeutic method. However, surgery is generally curative only for patients who have localized disease confined to the primary site and regional nodes. The natural history of cancer is such that the initial treatment approach, whether single therapy or combination therapy, is the critical opportunity to cure a patient with cancer. Once disease recurs or metastasizes, cure is less likely.

Although surgery is the treatment of choice for many tumors, current understanding of tumor responses and advances in interdisciplinary cancer management have altered the reliance on surgery. Practitioners have reevaluated the magnitude of surgical resections needed to effect desired outcomes of treatment. Surgery and radiation therapy are the most common methods used to treat localized or regionally localized primary cancer.[1] By using combinations of surgery, chemotherapy, radiation therapy, or biotherapy, disease-free intervals have been significantly lengthened and survival advantages have been realized.[2] Surgery can be used for prevention, diagnosis, definitive treatment, rehabilitation, or palliation with a variety of cancers.

This chapter reviews the role of surgery in the treatment of cancer, and the multitude of physical, psychological, and personal aspects that surgical cancer treatment involves. Additionally, this chapter highlights areas of nursing practice specific to caring for individuals with cancer who will undergo surgical intervention.

Factors Influencing Surgical Oncology

Ambulatory Surgery

It is estimated that by the year 2000, nearly 75% of the surgical procedures performed in the United States will occur within the ambulatory setting.[3] Ambulatory surgical services are provided in hospitals, freestanding ambulatory surgery centers, physician offices, or mobile units. Technological and scientific advances in surgery and anesthesia have enabled this change in venue to include a broad array of delivery sites for ambulatory surgery. Economic pressures and, likewise, economic opportunities have had a significant influence on the rapid change to ambulatory surgery.

Most often, an ambulatory surgical procedure is performed and the patient is discharged to home care or to family care in less than 23 hours following surgery. Educating the patient and family in self-care following surgery is a significant challenge to surgical nurses, office staff, and family members providing supportive care. Educational materials are needed to supplement verbal instruction. Because the average American reads at an eighth-grade level, with more than 20% of adults reading at or below a fifth-grade level (ABC Project), written educational materials must be carefully selected in order for maximum benefit to be derived.[4] It is estimated that 20% of the U.S. population has a serious literacy problem, thus visuals and demonstrations or videos can be useful adjuncts to written materials.

Individuals with cancer who have an ambulatory procedure for treatment or diagnosis, such as breast lumpectomy or prostate biopsy, are usually in need of additional support and education beyond what can be provided in such a brief period. Thus, support groups, follow-up phone checks, individual consultation, and educational sessions can be used to assist patients and families to understand the disease and any necessary follow-up care. (See Chapter 73 for more information about effective patient teaching.)

Technological Advances

Lasers, laparoscopes, endoscopes, stereotaxis, conscious sedation, and new anesthetic agents are among the leading approaches in the field of ambulatory surgical care. Patients are quite accepting of less invasive ambulatory surgical procedures because there are fewer surgical risks, less pain, and a less extensive recovery period.[5] These minimally invasive procedures cost less overall and allow the patient to resume daily activities sooner than with invasive procedures.

As an example, laparoscopes and endoscopes can be used to perform splenectomy, adrenelectomy, pelvic biopsy, mediastinal biopsy, and colon resection.[6–10] Previously, these types of surgical procedures were performed via open technique, required longer recovery periods, and posed a greater risk for bleeding and infection. Surgical staging and a variety of palliative procedures can also be performed in the ambulatory setting via laparoscope or endoscope. However, before a minimally invasive approach is selected, the surgeon must be reasonably certain that the disease can be fully resected, with adequate margins, using the minimally invasive surgical method. Though minimally invasive surgical procedures are generally less costly and easier for the patient to tolerate, if an open surgical approach should become necessary during the course of the minimally invasive surgical procedure, then the overall cost and the patient variables change significantly.[11]

Minimally invasive surgical techniques of microvascular surgery, radiosurgery, laser surgery, and cryosurgery result in less blood loss, which has reduced operative mortality. Laser vaporization with a variety of laser beam sources is used in the treatment of small, early lesions. *Cryosurgery*, or thermal surgery through extreme cooling, can be used for gastrointestinal, gynecologic, and neurologic surgeries. The extreme temperature results in cryogenic necrosis of the surrounding tissues, capillaries, and venules.[12,13] Anesthesia, intraoperative monitoring, and postoperative management techniques for ambulatory surgery continue to be refined and enable more procedures to be performed in the ambulatory setting.

Economic Forces

Economic forces and managed care plans have precipitated the development of aggressive measures to reduce lengthy and costly hospital stays. Preoperative preparation, surgical management, and postoperative care all are scrutinized closely for ways to decrease utilization of ancillary drugs and tests and to reduce the direct costs of surgical care. Ambulatory surgery, increased efficiency, clinical pathways, algorithms, and changes in medical education are a few of the measures that have been taken to reduce the cost of surgical care. Despite these advances, from the patient's perspective, the health care system has become more difficult to manage and understand. The individual with cancer who is approaching an ambulatory surgical procedure may need help navigating the fragmented and cumbersome course of precertification, preprocedure testing, same-day admission, and multiple sites for follow-up care. In many settings, nurses act as case managers to assist the patient and family in the complex negotiations that are often necessary in the continuum of cancer care. Additionally, case managers can help coordinate patient education, discharge planning, and home care, which take on greater importance in achieving the desired outcomes with ambulatory cancer surgery.

Factors Influencing Treatment Decisions

Tumor Cell Kinetics

An understanding of the biology and natural history of individual tumors is fundamental to the surgical treatment of cancer.[14] Historically, it was thought that cancer was essentially a mass of uncontrolled, rapidly proliferating cells that extended into surrounding tissues and lymph nodes and inevitably reached the circulatory system. With this in mind, surgeons felt that time was of the essence in curing cancer and that the lymph nodes had to be included in any resection because metastatic extensions would rest there. With these ideas guiding surgeons to extend the surgical margin and resect more tissue, extensive radical procedures such as hemicorporectomies and radical mastectomies were performed, still with disappointing long-term results. Research has definitively demonstrated that these types of extended radical procedures fail to significantly increase cure rates.[15–17]

The goal of all cancer therapy is to completely eradicate the tumor with the least amount of disruption or damage to normal tissue and organ function as possible. Thus, decisions about the extent of surgical resection are guided by the characteristics of the tumor cells. Interdisciplinary collaboration and treatment planning are necessary to select the most effective treatment method for cancer.[14,18] Oncology practitioners must understand the potential of surgery, chemotherapy, radiation therapy, and biotherapy in order to select the most effective course of therapy. The factors that affect the decision of whether an individual with cancer should be treated by surgery are discussed in the following sections.

Growth rate

Growth rate, measured as volume-doubling time, is the time it takes for a tumor mass to double in size. Growth rate depends on the cell-cycle activity of proliferating cells within the tumor; the *growth fraction*, or number of cells proliferating in the tumor; and the rate of cell loss from the tumor. In general, tumors that are slow growing and that consist of cells with prolonged cell cycles lend themselves best to surgical treatment, because these types of tumors are more likely to be confined locally.[19]

Invasiveness

Cancer can be insidious and progress as an asymptomatic lesion too small to be detected for long periods of time. Any cancer cell remaining after treatment constitutes a potential risk for recurrence or metastasis if that cell is capable of proliferating. Therefore, a surgical procedure intended to be curative must involve resection of the entire tumor mass and normal tissue surrounding the tumor to ensure a margin of safety for removal of all cancer cells. Some cancers (e.g., melanomas) invade deeply into adjacent tissues, either requiring an extensive surgical procedure to remove the tumor mass or making surgery an impractical treatment option. Other tumors, such as basal cell carcinoma and chrondrosarcoma, are highly cohesive and are more amenable to complete surgical excision. Local, less invasive surgical procedures are performed for those particular tumors where research has demonstrated an equally effective result compared with radical surgery.[20–23]

Metastatic potential

The initial operation performed for removal of a cancer has a better chance for success than a subsequent operation performed for a recurrence. Some tumors metastasize late or not at all. Other tumors predictably metastasize to local or regional sites, and cure may be achieved by a procedure that involves removal of the primary tumor-bearing organ and the involved adjacent tumor sites or lymph nodes. Some tumors are known to metastasize early. In such cases, surgery may be used to remove all visible tumor in preparation for adjuvant system therapy (e.g., testicular cancer).[20–23]

It is thought that micrometastases are present in 60% of individuals by the time a tumor is large enough to be detected clinically.[24] When surgery has been the only treatment used, subclinical metastasis or occult disease is usually responsible for recurrences. Thus, it is clear that interdisciplinary planning and selection of the most appropriate treatment methods are vital for improving survival and lowering an individual's risk of systemic metastasis.

Usually, the site of origin or primary area for a metastasis is known. However, a metastatic lesion can be found at a great distance from its primary lesion (Table 14-1). In some cases, the metastasis may have mutated so far from the primary tumor that the primary pathology is never found. However, surgical resection of the metastatic lesions can result in long-term cure without the primary source ever being discovered.[1]

Tumor Location

Once the location and extent of the tumor are determined through diagnostic and staging procedures, the clinician assesses the structural and functional changes that can be expected as a result of the surgical procedure. This assessment will assist the clinician, patient, and family in weighing the benefits and risks involved in treatment. In some cases, the decision to treat an individual's cancer with surgery may rest solely on whether the tumor involves vital structures. Superficial and encapsulated tumors are more easily resected than those that are embedded in inaccessible or delicate tissues or those that have invaded tissues in multiple directions. New methods of gaining access to tumors previously in inoperable locations are being developed using stereotaxis. *Stereotaxis* is a procedure that precisely locates a specific target point based on three-dimensional coordinates. Through computer mapping using a series of magnetic resonance images (MRIs) and computed tomography (CT) scans, the point of intersection of all three coordinates identifies the target tissue. This precision is then utilized with a stereotaxic frame and instrumentation to directly localize deep lesions. Stereotaxis is used frequently in neurosurgery to locate deep brain lesions for surgical biopsy and removal.

Physical Status

Careful preoperative assessment is critical for evaluating the significant factors that would potentially increase the risk of surgical morbidity and mortality. Evaluation of respiratory, cardiovascular, nutritional, immunologic, renal, and central nervous system (CNS) status are important.[25] The severity of the underlying illness and comorbid conditions are considered in the decision regarding surgical therapy. Some patients are not surgical candidates due to underlying cardiac, pulmonary, hematologic, or renal problems. The health care team assesses the patient's rehabilitation potential, particularly if the intended surgery will significantly alter normal physiological function. In some cases, the intended surgical procedure may produce physiological alterations that are beyond that particular individual's capabilities. Because cancer incidence is much greater in elderly patients, age

Table 14-1 Most Frequent Sites of Metastatic Neoplasms

Cervix
Supraclavicular lymph nodes
Lungs
Liver
Bones
Brain

can be a consideration in the treatment decision. In general, elderly individuals have a higher surgical risk than younger individuals. However, the elderly individual should be treated as aggressively as possible but may require additional preoperative support (e.g., hyperalimentation and/or blood products). Elderly individuals with cancer do not appear to have a higher risk or complication rate than their age-matched cohorts.[26,27]

Quality of Life

The goal of therapy for the patient with cancer varies according to the stage of disease. In some instances, surgery is a cure; in others it is only palliative. Selection of the treatment approach includes consideration of the quality of the individual's life when treatment is complete. Research has shown that some radical surgical procedures are not warranted, either because they do not improve the end result or because they interfere unduly with the individual's functional or psychological well-being. Multidisciplinary planning that includes the individual with cancer and significant others will facilitate the selection of a treatment plan tailored to that individual's unique needs and desires.

It is important for health care professionals to make the patient and their family members aware of all treatment options. They must also know that they have a right to refuse any treatments proposed if they do not feel it will be beneficial or do not like the risks involved. Decisions should be made by the patient and their family members, after a thorough explanation of the proposed procedure, its benefits and risks, and other possible treatments available.

Preventing Cancer Using Surgical Procedures

Certain conditions, diseases, and genetic or congenital traits are known to be associated with a higher risk of developing cancer. In some instances, surgical removal of nonvital benign tissue or an organ that is responsible for predisposing the individual to higher risk can lower incidence and possibly prevent occurrence of cancer.

Polyposis is a clear example of a condition that increases the individual's risk for developing colon cancer. Surgical excision of colon polyps is a relatively simple preventive procedure to reduce the risk of developing colon cancer.[28]

Another, more complex situation is that of women who have a high risk for breast cancer. After careful review and thorough explanation, some women may elect to undergo prophylactic bilateral mastectomy to lower the risk of breast cancer.[29,30] At this time, prophylactic mastectomy is highly controversial. The role of surgery in cancer prevention is somewhat limited; however, epidemiological and etiologic findings may indicate a more definitive role for surgery in the future. Genetic testing and chemoprevention will undoubtedly influence the use of surgery in the prevention of cancer in the future.

An important component of cancer prevention using surgical techniques or other modalities is patient teaching. Patients can assess their body changes better than anyone else. Knowledge of a change or problem can alert a patient to get treatment early and prevent further complications. Such signs include a change in bowel or bladder habits; unusual bleeding or discharge; a harsh nagging cough or hoarseness; indigestion or difficulty swallowing; thickening or lump in tissue, breast, or elsewhere; temperature greater than 100.4° F; and weight loss.

Diagnosing Cancer Using Surgical Techniques

Each type of cancer responds differently to therapy; therefore, a histological diagnosis is crucial to selecting effective treatment. Surgical diagnostic techniques such as endoscopy, needle aspiration, incisional biopsy, excisional biopsy, and core needle biopsy are commonly used to procure cells or tissue specimens for histopathologic examination.

An adequate biopsy requires careful planning by the physician. The biopsy specimen should contain both normal cells and tumor cells for comparison; it should be intact and not crushed or contaminated; and it should be labeled and preserved properly for complete evaluation. An important principle to note in the diagnosis of cancer is that only positive biopsy findings are definitive. A negative biopsy finding can mean no cancer, but it can also mean that the biopsy specimen was not representative of the tumor. If a high index of suspicion for cancer exists, another biopsy technique may be in order.

Before selecting the most appropriate biopsy technique, the surgeon considers the possible treatment approaches to be used if cancer is diagnosed. The placement and orientation of the biopsy incision should facilitate any further surgical resections deemed necessary. Because tumor cells can contaminate the biopsy site, the biopsy site should be located so it will be removed during subsequent, more definitive surgery. If more extensive surgery is not planned, then the initial biopsy should contain the tumor in toto.[31] The goal is to have minimum disruption or disturbance to the tumor mass, while achieving an adequate biopsy specimen. This requires careful planning and consideration prior to biopsy. Aesthetic results are also considered, so that incision lines and subsequent incisions will be located in cosmetically acceptable areas or folds, if possible.

Important principles of biopsy include minimizing dissection as much as possible and maintaining adequate hemostasis to avoid inadvertent tumor spread. Use of incisional, excisional, aspiration, or core biopsy depends on tumor size, location, and growth characteristics.[32] Possible complications following any biopsy are pain, bleeding, hematoma, infection, dehiscence, and tumor cell seeding.

Individuals should be instructed about biopsy site care and possible complications. Individuals should also know in advance when the biopsy results will be available and how the physician will give the results (e.g., by phone call or in person). To prevent anxiety, the individual should be informed as to whether the result will be known immediately (frozen section result) or whether the physician prefers to wait until the permanent sections have been prepared and interpreted, usually between 2 and 5 days later. The most common surgical biopsy techniques used are needle biopsy and open surgical biopsy. [1,31–34]

Needle biopsies are usually performed in an outpatient or office setting, as they do not require extensive surgical support and are simple and safe for the patient. Local or topical anesthesia is commonly used. Fine-needle aspiration or biopsy is the procedure of choice when there is a high index of suspicion for malignancy and the lesion is both accessible and solid. Needle biopsies are well tolerated by the patient, result in a small amount of trauma to tissue, and cause minimal manipulation of the tumor. This method is used for biopsy of subcutaneous masses, muscular masses, and internal organ tissues, such as liver, kidney, and pancreas. Hematoma and infection are potential complications.

Core biopsies are usually indicated when there is a need to confirm malignancy, yet there is clinical and diagnostic evidence that the disease will be treated with nonsurgical approaches. If surgery is likely, the biopsy approach selected is often the fine-needle rather than the core biopsy. Regional biopsy involves obtaining several samples of tissue from different locations within a tumor or within a diseased organ. Regional biopsies are used to diagnose metastatic disease in a defined, but not localized, region of the body.[35] Stereotactic biopsy uses radiographic images to create three-dimensional images of a suspected neoplasm.

Surgical biopsies are performed to secure a piece of tumor tissue larger than is possible with a needle. Excisional biopsy is performed on small, discrete, accessible tumors to remove the entire suspected mass, with little or no margin of surrounding normal tissue included in the biopsy specimen. In some cases, such as tumors of the lip, nose, ear, or breast, excisional biopsy alone will be definitive surgical therapy. Incisional biopsies are generally selected for the diagnosis of large tumors that will likely require major surgery for complete removal, thus only a portion of the mass is removed by incisional biopsy for pathological examination.

A new option of biopsy for breast cancer is sentinel node biopsy. The sentinel node, the node nearest the tumor, is located through injection of blue dye or a radioactive substance and then biopsied. If the sentinel node is determined to have no cancer, then no other nodes are removed. This prevents the removal of unaffected nodes, and facilitates faster recovery with less pain and less cost.[20]

Staging Cancer Using Surgical Procedures

Surgical procedures are selected for the precise diagnosis of cancer and for defining the stage of the disease. For example, staging laparotomy is an important diagnostic measure for the pathological staging of Hodgkin's disease. Exploratory surgical procedures can be done to diagnose most intracavitary tumors or to define the extent of tumor growth, size, nodal involvement, implants, or multiorgan involvement.

Before recommending a surgical resection of the tumor for cure, the physician undertakes a search for evidence of distant metastasis. If distant metastases are present, surgery may not be the treatment of choice to achieve control, and the focus of treatment then shifts to systemic treatment or palliation. A debulking surgical procedure can be used to reduce tumor burden prior to initiating systemic therapy.

During the diagnostic phase, including the biopsy and surgical staging, the patient with cancer and his or her family can experience profound anxiety that can be alleviated or reduced to some extent. It is important to assess the factors that could contribute to anxiety, such as previous hospitalizations, experience with other individuals with cancer, influence of the mass media, formal and informal sources of information, and the patient's developmental stage. The nurse should carefully assess the patient's understanding of the diagnostic procedures and the significance of the findings. Emotional support is also very important at this stage, to assist patient and family in making informed, rational decisions regarding treatment.

Surgery for Treatment of Cancer

After diagnosis, staging, and classification of the tumor, the interdisciplinary oncology team will propose the most appropriate plan and sequence of therapy. The goal of therapy is based on the patient's desires, general condition, and tumor stage and classification.

The decision-making process for creating a treatment plan requires the integration of all gathered subjective and clinical data. The ultimate decision of which type of intervention to choose depends essentially on four factors: (1) natural history of the disease by histologic type, (2) the clinical stage of the cancer, (3) goals of treatment, and (4) indications and risks for all choices of treatments or combination of treatments (based on results of clinical trials).[1]

The most important questions at this point are, Is the patient curable? and, What does the patient desire from treatment? The sequence and methods of treatment used will be guided by this information and the most effective treatment protocols available for the particular tumor type. Surgical intervention may be the definitive treatment or may be part of a sequence of combined treatment modalities.

Preoperative considerations include a thorough patient and family history and physical examination. Assessments are made of lifestyle, concomitant disease, general physical condition, nutritional status, hematologic status, and pulmonary status. Measures to improve the patient's overall health status are initiated before surgery whenever possible.[25] In addition, an assessment of the patient's understanding of the surgery and rehabilitation should be completed. Involving the individual's significant others in preoperative teaching can often facilitate understanding and reduce anxiety.

During the preoperative period, the nurse instructs the individual on what to expect throughout the surgical course. It is important that the individual understand the anticipated outcomes of surgical therapy, as well as how surgery fits in the overall plan of therapy. Very often, the patient and significant others have many questions and need information repeated and validated. Encouraging dialogue and allowing adequate time for instruction and verbalization of feelings and fears during the preoperative period can enhance adjustment and acceptance of the surgery and its effects.

Surgery Aimed at Cure

Advances in our understanding of cancer biology have changed the surgical approach for cure from "more is better" to an approach that focuses on tissue and functional preservation and that relies on effective use of radiation therapy, chemotherapy, and biotherapy. Tumors that are solid, accessible, have relatively well-defined margins, and are without evidence of spread can generally be surgically excised with a goal of eradicating the tumor.

The decision-making process for creating a treatment plan for a patient with cancer is based on the integration of four key elements: (1) the natural history of the disease based on histological type, (2) clinical staging, (3) goals of the treatment (palliative or cure), and (4) indications and risks for each treatment or combinations of treatments.

Resection—local and radical

The type of surgical procedure selected for curative treatment of a primary tumor depends on the specific tumor cell characteristics, site, and extent of involvement. In the preoperative period, the surgeon is challenged to identify those patients who will best be treated by limited or extensive surgery and to select the adjuvant therapies that will control local and distant disease.[1]

The magnitude of the surgical excision for many tumors has been greatly modified in recent years. There is a limit beyond which larger excisions fail to yield improved long-term outcomes.[36] A better understanding of the biology and natural history of specific cancers, combined with advances in adjuvant treatment, has led to less radical surgery for some cancers. Breast cancer is probably the best example of a tumor that is approached much differently now because of our understanding of tumor biology.[37]

Local resection is used for small lesions if the entire tumor and an adequate margin of tumor-free tissue can be encompassed in the excision. Tumors of the ear, skin, or lip are typical lesions where local excision can be used as definitive therapy for cure. Hemostasis and infection are the major postoperative concerns.

Radical surgical resections are performed when the tumor is surgically accessible and there is hope that the tumor can be resected en bloc, along with the necessary local or regional tissues and lymphatics. If possible, it is desirable to include a wide margin of normal tissue to assure complete resection of the tumor.

Depending on the characteristic pattern of spread of the tumor involved, a radical resection may include the primary tumor and the regional lymph nodes surrounding the area. The surgeon must carefully identify the collecting nodes and lymphatic channels to include in this type of resection. The en bloc regional lymph node dissection is critical to preventing local tumor recurrence.[1] Extensive surgery may be needed if the disease is to be eradicated and the patient is to be given the chance to live a normal life span. Surgical resections can greatly alter an individual's body image as well as the structure and function of his or her body. There are obvious trade-offs and concessions that an individual with cancer must consider. Striking a balance between length of life and quality of life is a major challenge in surgical oncology.

Extensive radical resections or supraradical procedures are not used often, but they can provide a chance for cure for a limited set of individuals with cancer. Indications for extensive radical surgery include primary tumors that grow slowly, have wide local infiltration, and are large. The entire spectrum of care for an extended radical procedure is best handled by a highly experienced team of clinicians. Examples of these procedures are hemipelvectomy, forequarter amputation, and pelvic exenteration. The emotional and adaptive challenges to the patient receiving this type of surgery must be carefully assessed and evaluated before electing to proceed with the procedure.

Surgery and adjuvant therapies

Surgery is local therapy and thus is limited in what it can achieve as a treatment modality for cancer. Surgery was once the sole therapy for many solid tumors, such as carcinoma of the breast, colon, and head and neck. Survival rates for these cancers and others have not been satisfactory with surgery alone.[2] For this reason, combination or adjuvant therapies are used to improve the rates of cure and disease-free survival. Adjuvant therapy can be initiated preoperatively, intraoperatively, or postoperatively. Surgery may be combined with radiation therapy for local and regional tumor control. Chemotherapy is given to provide systemic control of micrometastases and distant metastases.

In some situations, surgery, called *cytoreductive surgery*, is used to debulk or reduce the tumor mass to a size in which combination therapy can be most effective.[38] Ovarian cancer is usually spread throughout the peritoneum by the time of diagnosis, and clinicians have found that cytoreductive surgery followed by aggressive chemotherapy has resulted in significantly improved survival rates.[38] The individual may undergo definitive therapy for months or even years. Other examples of tumors in which debulking procedures have been used are Burkitt's lymphoma, rhabdomyosarcoma, chordoma, glioblastoma multiforme, and some neoplastic syndromes. This adjuvant approach to the treatment of the person with cancer requires a multidisciplinary team effort.

Excision of metastatic lesions

Surgery also may be used to resect a metastatic lesion if the primary tumor is believed to be eradicated, if the metastatic site is solitary, and if the patient can undergo surgery without significant morbidity. Resection of the metastatic lesion is not indicated if there is evidence of additional metastatic disease or if the metastatic lesion is particularly aggressive or inaccessible. A solitary pulmonary lesion, a liver lesion, and a cerebral mass are examples of metastatic sites that may be amenable to resection with a curative intent.[1,39]

Surgery Aimed at Palliation

Surgical procedures are commonly performed for the palliation of the debilitating manifestations of cancer. These procedures are aimed at controlling the cancer and improving the quality of life for the individual with cancer, even when all the cancer cannot be removed. If the quality of the individual's life cannot be improved as a result of the surgery, then surgery is not warranted. If the surgery carries an unnecessary risk of morbidity or mortality, it is not indicated.

Issues such as biological pace of the disease, the patient's life expectancy, and expected outcome of the palliative procedure all require careful consideration if the patient is to benefit from the procedure. Open communication among the patient, the family, and the physician is of paramount importance. The patient must know the goals and risks of the procedure and realistically understand the expected outcome. If the patient's hope is unrealistic, the potential disappointment experienced postoperatively can be devastating. For instance, consider the individual experiencing chronic pain who is offered a surgical procedure that can possibly alleviate suffering. It is more compassionate to ensure that the individual understands and accepts that the pain may be relieved only temporarily rather than indefinitely. The patient who lives with cancer knows well the meaning of palliation. Clinicians should always respect the strength and will of the individual with uncontrolled cancer and promote his or her active participation in the plan of care.

The goal of palliative surgery is to relieve suffering and minimize the symptoms of the disease. For example, palliative surgery may involve removal of a tumor that has become ulcerative and a likely source of infection or may involve the amputation of a nonfunctioning, painful limb with sarcoma. Some tumors are slow growing and, although metastatic sites are evident and the patient is technically incurable, resection of the primary tumor is warranted to prevent future complications such as bleeding or obstruction. Several surgical techniques are used for palliation of cancer: fulgeration, electrocoagulation, lasers, photodynamic therapy, shunts, and bone stabilization procedures.[39,40]

Palliative procedures are not undertaken unless the clinician is reasonably confident that the wound will heal. For example, surgery is contraindicated for the patient who has a local recurrence and lung metastasis following radiation therapy to an oropharyngeal lesion. In this case, a surgical wound would probably not heal without extensive skin-flap reconstruction, which would not be warranted in view of the distant metastasis. The patient must also tolerate anesthesia.

Palliative surgery is particularly useful in relieving suffering caused by an obstructive process. Obstruction occurs in the respiratory, gastrointestinal, or urinary system. Surgical intervention such as a tracheostomy restores airway patency, and a gastrostomy tube facilitates adequate nutrition. Through palliative procedures, the individual can be supported while therapy is initiated to control the primary disease. Surgery may also be used to decompress vital structures (i.e., laminectomy) or to help in the control of pain.

Surgery for Rehabilitation

Although surgical procedures have long been used to treat cancer, their use in the rehabilitation of individuals with cancer is underemphasized. Today, significant value is placed on the quality of life for the individual with cancer. With this emphasis has come an effort to develop techniques to restore an individual to as near a normal life as possible following surgery for cancer. Cosmetic and functional success have been achieved through procedures such as breast reconstruction following mastec-

tomy, facial reconstruction after head and neck surgery, and skin grafting following major resections for melanoma.[1] The development of various implants, microvascular surgery, allografts, and autogenous reconstructive techniques has enlarged the scope of reconstructive surgery.[31] Reconstructive procedures can be done immediately following resection or can be delayed several days or years.[41]

Rehabilitation potential is considered before initiation of primary therapy. Careful interdisciplinary planning assists the clinician in preparing the patient emotionally and physically for both the primary treatment and subsequent rehabilitation. In preparing an individual for rehabilitation, the clinician strikes a fine balance between optimism and realism. Rehabilitative teaching and counseling generally are begun before primary surgical therapy is initiated. Some people fear that their desire for rehabilitative surgical procedures will be interpreted as valuing their physical appearance or function more than the length of their life. Nurses can assist the patient to see that rehabilitation is desirable and sometimes necessary for achieving the highest possible level of functioning.

Success of surgery for rehabilitation purposes is measured not only by aesthetic improvement but also by improvements in function and self-esteem. As surgical techniques improve, more people with cancer will select and enjoy the benefits of surgical rehabilitation.

Special Considerations for Nursing Care

Nursing care of the patient with cancer who is undergoing surgery follows many of the same principles as care for an individual undergoing non-cancer-related surgery. The nurse's role in coordination, education, and communication within the health care team is of utmost importance because surgical procedures are complex, surgical stays are short, and patients receive several forms of cancer therapy in a short amount of time.

Surgical Setting and Length of Stay

Historically, surgical procedures were performed in an inpatient hospital setting, with a generous amount of time allowed for recuperation in the hospital before discharge. Today, more surgical procedures are done in an ambulatory setting as a result of the many advances in surgical and anesthetic technique and the multiple measures to contain costs.[42,43] This change in the method of delivery of surgical care challenges ambulatory nurses to ensure that adequate information is given and surgical complications are minimized. Innovative ambulatory surgical programs are providing extensive education prior to the day of surgery in order to assure that the patient and family are well prepared for the surgical procedure and care afterward.[44] Patients identify their most important concerns as the effectiveness of treatment, the options for treatment, the effects of therapy on life expectancy, and how to manage the effects of treatment.[44] Many educational strategies can be used to support patients; however, because the period of contact with health care professionals during surgical care is of such short duration, it is most important for patients and their families to know whom to contact and how to do so when they need help or further information.

General Surgical Care and Oncologic Emergencies

Surgical teams are well acquainted with typical surgical complications of pulmonary problems, sepsis, perforation, and hemorrhage. (The nursing care issues and considerations for care are summarized in Table 14-2.) The

Table 14-2 Potential Nursing Care Issues in Surgical Oncology Patients

Potential/Actual Complication	Contributing Factors
ARDS	Hemorrhage Aspiration Prolonged atelectasis Infection Pulmonary edema Deposition of platelets Trauma to lung parenchyma Cardiopulmonary bypass Pulmonary emboli
Aspiration pneumonia	Difficulty in swallowing Mechanical obstruction from cancer Excessive sedation
Infection	Myelosuppression Radiation therapy Chemotherapy Malnutrition
Bleeding	Hypothermia Prolonged cardiopulmonary bypass Medications
Poor wound healing	Prior radiation therapy Steroid therapy Chemotherapy Local tumor invasion Malnutrition Immune dysfunction Neutropenia
Stomatitis	Antimetabolite chemotherapeutic agents Bleomycin Head and neck radiation Dehydration

Adapted with permission from Polomano R, Weintraub FN, Wurster A: Surgical critical care for cancer patients. *Semin Oncol Nurs* 10:165–176, 1994.[45]

current challenges in surgical care are rapidly changing as the technology of surgical instrumentation (lasers, laparoscopes, endoscopes) and the role of adjuvant therapies advance. Particularly challenging is the patient with concomitant diseases (cardiac, pulmonary, renal, endocrine) who will receive aggressive treatment for the cancer because of advances made in the management and supportive therapies available today. Antibiotic therapy, hematopoietic growth factors, implantable pumps, high-tech infusion equipment, and transplantation are a few of the overall advances that contribute to the challenging care of today's surgical oncology patient.

The effects of the disease and the treatments can lead to clinical situations that are categorized as oncologic emergencies. The surgical patient may experience a complex set of reactions and responses to therapy that may be precipitated by the concomitant therapies or the complications of the underlying disease process itself. Beyond classic surgical complications and emergencies, the surgical team and nursing staff should be aware of the most common oncologic emergencies that can occur.[45]

Autologous Blood Donation

Autologous blood donation is common when the surgical procedure is not emergent and the patient is hemodynamically stable and can donate blood. Some hospitals have autologous donation programs; others use the services of external agencies such as the American Red Cross Autologous Donor Program. It is important to schedule this autologous blood donation well in advance of surgery. Nonanemic patients can donate up to 6 units of blood prior to surgery. Blood usually can be donated from 42 days to 72 hours prior to surgery. Because of the small but real risk of infection or reactions from homologous blood transfusions, most individuals are eager to donate their own blood.[46,47]

However, in many instances, the cancer patient may experience cancer-related anemia and will not be able to donate blood prior to surgery. In some instances, an anemic patient may receive aggressive treatment of the anemia in order to enable autologous blood donation for surgery. Regular administration of epoetin alfa is one treatment approach being studied in clinical trials to determine its role, particularly in orthopedic oncology cases where autologous blood donation is highly desirable.[47]

Anxiety and Pain Control

Anxiety relief and pain control should be addressed prior to surgery to allow patients to verbalize fears, discuss previous experiences, and be made aware of advances in pharmacological methods of pain relief as well as the advantages of behavioral methods of pain control and relaxation techniques. In the preoperative period, Carr et al recommend discussions of expectations of pain and its relief, including dosing of analgesic medicine, availability of patient-controlled analgesia (PCA) units, use of rating scales to measure pain, and nonpharmacological maneuvers to decrease pain and anxiety (Table 14-3).[48,49] (See Chapters 28 and 29 for additional information.)

Relaxation, deep breathing, visualization, guided imagery, and self-hypnosis are techniques to help patients decrease anxiety and pain during painful procedures (i.e., bone marrow biopsy, needle localization, breast biopsy) as well as during the postoperative period.[50-52] Health care professionals should make it a priority to encourage and teach methods of reducing anxiety and providing pain relief to individuals anticipating a surgical procedure.[52] Anxiety and pain may also be signaling an underlying and unresolved pathology. Nurses should be acutely aware of problems that can occur as a result of the cancer disease process itself, as well as anticipating possible postoperative complications.

Nutritional Support

Certain surgical procedures can alter the body's ability to achieve adequate nutrition. The most common nutrition-related alterations occur with surgeries for cancer of the gastrointestinal tract or head and neck neoplasms. Both the scope of the surgical excision and the resultant organ dysfunction must be factored into an aggressive, proactive nutrition plan. Most alterations can be handled with enzyme replacements, dietary modification, and close monitoring. If swallowing is altered, reconstruction and rehabilitation can take several weeks. Enteral and parenteral feedings may become necessary.

Surgery can accelerate basic energy requirements up to 1.5 times normal. Loss of appetite or diminished appetite is a common problem for cancer patients, and is heightened in the surgical patient by the demands of surgical healing. Protein-calorie malnutrition is a common occurrence among cancer patients, especially those with advanced disease. Most chemotherapy agents act by interfering with protein synthesis, further depleting protein stores. The nutritionally debilitated individual with cancer is a poor surgical candidate. These patients will likely experience severe postoperative complications unless their nutritional status is fully assessed and an aggressive plan of support is developed and initiated preoperatively. Complications of surgery associated with

Table 14-3 Nonpharmacologic Interventions for Pain Control[48]

Intervention*		Type of Evidence†	Comments
Simple relaxation (begin preoperatively)	Jaw relaxation	Ia, IIa, IIb, IV	Effective in reducing mild to moderate pain and as an adjunct to analgesic drugs for severe pain. Use when patients express an interest in relaxation. Requires 3–5 minutes of staff time for instructions.
	Progressive muscle relaxation		
	Simple imagery		
	Music	Ib, IIa, IV	Both patient-preferred and "easy listening" music are effective in reducing mild to moderate pain.
Complex relaxation (begin preoperatively)	Biofeedback	Ib, IIa, IIb, IV	Effective in reducing mild to moderate pain and operative site muscle tension. Requires skilled personnel and special equipment.
	Imagery	Ib, IIa, IV	Effective for reduction of mild to moderate pain. Requires skilled personnel.
Education/instruction (begin preoperatively)		Ia, IIa, IIb, IV	Effective for reduction of pain. Should include sensory and procedural information and instruction aimed at reducing activity-related pain. Requires 5–15 minutes of staff time.
TENS		Ia, IIa, III, IV	Effective in reducing pain and improving physical function. Requires skilled personnel and special equipment. May be useful as an adjunct to drug therapy.

*Selected references are included in this Clinical Practice Guideline. For more complete references, see: Acute Pain Management Guideline Panel: *Acute Pain Management: Operative or Medical Procedures and Trauma. Guideline Report.* AHCPR Pub. No. 92-0022. Rockville, MD: Agency for Health Care Policy and Research, Public Health Service, U.S. Department of Health and Human Services, 1992.

†Insufficient scientific evidence is available to provide specific recommendations regarding the use of hypnosis, acupuncture, and other physical modalities for relief of postoperative pain.

†**Key to Type of Evidence**
Ia Evidence obtained from meta-analysis of randomized controlled trials
b   Evidence obtained from at least one randomized controlled trial
IIa Evidence obtained from at least one well-designed controlled study without randomization
b   Evidence obtained from at least one other type of well-designed quasi-experimental study
III Evidence obtained from well-designed nonexperimental studies, such as comparative studies, correlational studies, and case studies
IV Evidence obtained from expert committee reports or opinions and/or clinical experiences of respected authorities

malnutrition include pneumonia, ileus, sepsis, wound dehiscence, and diminished tolerance of subsequent antineoplastic therapies.

When subjected to a major stress, such as surgical trauma or infection, the cancer patient who is malnourished will not mount the usual defense of conserving lean body mass. The catabolism of body mass that accompanies cancer is persistent and somewhat refractory to nutritional therapy. The challenge of supporting the surgical patient with nutritional therapy requires a knowledgeable and comprehensive team approach because the simple approach of increased caloric intake by whatever route possible will not likely produce adequate results to avoid significant morbidity.[53–55]

There are special indications for the use of total parenteral nutrition (TPN) with surgical patients. Patients with enterocutaneous fistulas are not able to use the enteral route for nutrition because oral intake stimulates fistula output and can lead to metabolic and electrolyte disturbances. The fistula may close more rapidly if the person is nutritionally well supported. Hepatic failure due to chemotherapy or major surgery, acute renal failure, prolonged ileus, and acute radiation enteritis are all clinical situations that may benefit from the addition of TPN to the treatment plan. The nutrition plan should be individualized and aggressive. (See Chapter 33 for specific nursing measures to improve the nutritional status of patients.)

Hemostasis

Another common manifestation of cancer that can significantly increase the risk of postoperative complications is altered hemostasis, particularly hypercoagulability and thrombosis. Elevated clotting factors and shortened partial thromboplastin and prothrombin times have been noted to occur in individuals with cancer. The individual with cancer therefore is highly susceptible to minor changes in the hemostatic process. Thus, an individual with cancer is more likely to develop postoperative thrombophlebitis than is an individual without cancer.

The nursing management of the individual with cancer undergoing surgery is based on accurate assessment of hemodynamic parameters and an understanding of the implications of abnormalities in clotting factors that can result in bleeding tendencies and hemorrhage. The importance of early postoperative ambulation cannot be overemphasized. Because these individuals are at high risk for deep-vein thrombosis, the nurse observes the patient for signs and symptoms of this disorder. (See Chapter 31 for more on bleeding abnormalities in individuals with cancer.)

Combination Therapy

Combination therapy, or combined treatment modality, has introduced a new set of challenges for health care providers. Chemotherapy, radiation therapy, and biotherapy are being given for certain tumors in varied sequences according to the most effective protocol, including preoperative, intraoperative, and postoperative treatment. The synergistic effects of combination therapies can produce postoperative reactions and complications that may be difficult to manage. In addition to the expected side effects produced by the treatments, fatigue is a variable that causes a significant change in the quality of life for many patients. Innovative measures to reduce and manage fatigue include fatigue diaries, napping frequently, and timing activities during peak energy levels.[56–58]

Preoperative chemotherapy or radiation therapy, alone or in combination, is used with particular tumors that have better response rates when combination therapy is sequenced in this manner. The timing and extent of surgery may require modification following radiation or chemotherapy, depending on the type of treatment, the individual's response to therapy, and the side effects experienced.

Surgical procedures sometimes become necessary during active radiation or chemotherapy treatment cycles, such as inserting a vascular access device, relieving an obstruction, or repairing a perforation. Preoperative assessment of the patient who is actively receiving combination therapy is specifically focused on those body systems and organs that are being affected by the current therapy. For example, if a patient has been receiving anthracycline chemotherapy (doxorubicin, bleomycin, mitomycin C, or mithramycin), there are known cardiac and pulmonary toxicities that require special attention during any operative and postoperative period.[59]

Intraoperative radiation therapy and intraoperative chemotherapy are being researched for their potential to decrease recurrence and metastases. Radiation therapy or chemotherapy given intraoperatively involves the delivery of a single, high dose directly to the surgically exposed tumor or tumor bed. Intraoperative therapy requires extensive multidisciplinary collaboration. Patient and staff safety are carefully considered in making the decision to use these agents.[60] Potential side effects of intraoperative therapy are not yet fully known but appear to be similar to those of traditional delivery methods. These intraoperative treatments, used predominantly in major cancer centers, are administered for locally advanced abdominal and pelvic malignancies. Gastric, pancreatic, ovarian, bladder, and colorectal are a few of the tumor types being treated with intraoperative radiation therapy.[60,61]

A major challenge in caring for a patient who has received combination therapy is wound healing. If the patient was previously treated with radiation to the surgical site, there may be long-term damage to the underlying tissues, such as fibrosis and obliteration of lymphatic and vascular channels.[62] Once the integrity of the tissue is damaged by radiation, additional trauma is not tolerated well. Postoperative wound dehiscence, infection, tissue necrosis, and bone necrosis are potential complications of surgery performed on previously irradiated tissue. It is also known that radiation itself will interfere with healing if it is administered in the early postoperative period.

In some cases, it becomes necessary or highly desirable to initiate chemotherapy early in the postoperative period. There are many unanswered questions regarding the appropriate timing and effects of specific chemotherapeutic agents on wound healing.[63] Certain chemotherapeutic agents are toxic to specific organ systems, resulting in long-term side effects that can increase the individual's risk of surgical complications.[64]

Most chemotherapy agents act by interfering with protein synthesis. Because of this interference, it follows that wound healing could be disrupted by the administration of most chemotherapeutic agents in the early phases of wound healing. Research studies on humans to test this deduction are limited, but animal studies have been conducted that indicate that the immediate and early postoperative period are times when wound healing could be adversely affected or delayed by the administration of chemotherapy. Typical patterns of care allow a period of recovery before combination therapy is initiated.

The nurse needs to be aware of these effects and focus assessments and nursing care toward early identification and measures to minimize complications. As new therapies become available and are used aggressively in an attempt to eradicate malignancies, the potential exists for different and more severe complications to occur.

Conclusion

Surgery is the oldest form of cancer therapy still in use; however, there have been progressive advances and changes in the scope and role of surgical therapy. Most individuals with cancer have some sort of surgical procedure as part of their treatment plan. Current understanding of cancer biology and the natural history and progression of certain tumors has caused the role of surgery to be questioned and modified in many instances. Radical surgery is still a reasonable and valid approach for several tumor types, but not for others. Breast cancer is the most profound example of a less radical surgical approach that can achieve control and survival equivalent to the radical procedure.

Nursing care of individuals with cancer is multidisciplinary. Patients undergoing surgery for cancer require nursing support from oncology, surgery, and various other settings for total care. A holistic, collaborative approach best provides for thorough patient care, patient and family education, and emotional support. These patients are challenging, as they require nurses to pull together knowledge from an array of concepts and fields, while dealing with rapidly changing physical and psychological needs.

Prospective clinical research, both physiological and psychological, that includes active participation of surgical practitioners will continue to be needed. Effective surgical cancer therapy depends on a solid integration of the biological and clinical sciences of cancer. Clinicians have learned a great deal about the educational, psychological, social, and rehabilitative needs of individuals who are undergoing surgical procedures for cancer therapy.[65,66] Nursing and medical practitioners will continue to make strides toward cancer treatment and palliative therapy into the next millennium.

References

1. Balch CM, Pellis NR, Morton DL, et al: Oncology, in Schwartz SI, Shires GT, Spencer FC (eds): *Principles of Surgery* (ed 6). New York, McGraw-Hill, 1994, pp 305–385
2. DeVita VT: Principles of chemotherapy, in DeVita VT, Hellman S, Rosenberg SA (eds): *Cancer: Principles and Practice of Oncology* (ed 5). Philadelphia, Lippincott-Raven, 1997, pp 333–348
3. Stone MD, Doyle J: The influence of surgical training on the practice of surgery. *Surg Clin North Am* 76:1–10, 1996
4. Doak LG, Doak CC, Meade CD: Strategies to improve cancer educational materials. *Oncol Nurs Forum* 23:1305–1312, 1996
5. Covera CU, Kirkwood KS: General surgery: Recent advances. *BMJ* 315: 586–900, 1997
6. Rosenberg SA: Principles of surgical oncology, in DeVita VT, Hellman S, Rosenberg SA (eds): *Cancer: Principles and Practice of Oncology* (ed 5). Philadelphia, Lippincott-Raven, 1997, pp 295–306
7. Gagner M: Laparoscopic adrenalectomy. *Surg Clin North Am* 76:523–538, 1996
8. Chi DS, Curtin JP: Gynecologic cancer and laparoscopy. *Obstet Gynecol Clin North Am* 26:201–215, 1999
9. Dargent DF: Laparoscopic techniques for gynecologic cancer: Description and indications. *Hematol Oncol Clin North Am* 13:1–19, 1999
10. Schirmer BD: Laparoscopic colon resection. *Surg Clin North Am* 76:571–584, 1996
11. Traverso LW: The laparoscopic surgical value package and how surgeons can influence costs. *Surg Clin North Am* 76: 631–640, 1996
12. Weaver ML: Treatment of colorectal liver metastases by cryotherapy. *Semin Surg Oncol* 14:163–170, 1998
13. Zhou XD: Cryotherapy for primary liver cancer. *Semin Surg Oncol* 14:171–174, 1998
14. Preisler HD, Taza A: The role of emerging technologies in the diagnosis and staging of neoplastic diseases. *Cancer* 9: 1520–1525, 1992 (suppl)
15. Herrera L, Luna P, Villarreal J: Perspectives in colorectal cancer. *J Surg Oncol* 2:92–103, 1991 (suppl)
16. Mintzer D: The changing role of surgery in the diagnosis and treatment of cancer. *Am J Med* 6:1–2, 1999
17. Kim DH, Moon JS: Laparoscopic radical hysterectomy with pelvis lymphadenectomy for early, invasive cervical carcinoma. *J Am Assoc Gynecol Laparosc* 5:82–91, 1998
18. Steele G, Cady B: The surgical oncologist as the patient manager, in Steele G, Cady B (eds): *General Surgical Oncology.* Philadelphia, Saunders, 1992, pp 18–21
19. Fidler IJ: Molecular biology of cancer: Invasion and metastases, in DeVita VT, Hellman S, Rosenberg S (eds): *Cancer: Principles and Practice of Oncology* (ed 5). Philadelphia, Lippincott-Raven, 1997, pp 135–152
20. Veronesi U, Paganelli G, Viale G, et al: Sentinel node biopsy

and axillary dissection in breast cancer: Results of a large series. *J Natl Cancer Inst* 91:368–373, 1999

21. Schuller DE, Laramore G, Al-Sarraf M, et al: Combined therapy for resectable head and neck cancer. *Arch Otolaryngol Head Neck Surg* 115:364–368, 1989

22. Shepard FA, Ginsberg RJ, Patterson GA, et al: A prospective study of adjuvant surgical resection after chemotherapy for limited small cell lung cancer. *J Thorac Cardiovasc Surg* 97: 177–186, 1989

23. Siegel B, Mayzel K, Love S: Level I and II axillary dissection in the treatment of early-stage breast cancer. *Arch Surg* 25: 1144–1147, 1990

24. Castellino RA: Imaging techniques in cancer management, in DeVita VT, Hellman S, Rosenberg SA (eds): *Cancer Principles and Practice of Oncology* (ed 5). Philadelphia, Lippincott-Raven, 1997, pp 633–654

25. Ewer M, Ali MK: Surgical treatment of the cancer patient: Preoperative assessment and perioperative medical management. *J Surg Oncol* 44:185–190, 1990

26. Patterson WB: Surgical issues in geriatric oncology. *Semin Oncol* 16:57–65, 1989

27. Law TM, Hesketh PJ, Porter KA, et al: Breast cancer in elderly women: Presentation, survival, and treatment options. *Surg Clin North Am* 76:289–308, 1996

28. Ravikumar TS, Steele G: Colon cancer, in Steele G, Cady B (eds): *General Surgical Oncology*. Philadelphia, Saunders, 1992, pp 149–169

29. Wapnir IL, Rabinowitz B: A reappraisal of prophylactic mastectomy. *Surg Gynecol Obstet* 171:171–181, 1990

30. Lopez MJ, Porter KA: The current role of prophylactic mastectomy. *Surg Clin North Am* 76:231–242, 1996

31. Moffat FL, Ketcham AS: Surgery for malignant neoplasia: The evolution of oncologic surgery and its role in the management of cancer patients, in McKenna RJ, Murphy GP (eds): *Cancer Surgery*. Philadelphia, Lippincott, 1994, pp 1–20

32. Love S: *Dr. Susan Love's Breast Book* (ed 2). Reading, MA, Addison-Wesley, 1995, pp 23–79

33. Iglehart JD: The breast, in Sabiston DC, Lyerly HK (eds): *Textbook of Surgery* (ed 15). Philadelphia, Saunders, 1997, pp 555–598

34. Flynn MB, Wolfson SE, Thomas S, et al: Fine needle aspiration biopsy in clinical management of head and neck tumors. *J Surg Oncol* 44:214–217, 1990

35. Turner AF: Radiographically guided techniques of biopsy, in McKenna RJ, Murphy GP (eds): *Cancer Surgery*. Philadelphia, Lippincott, 1994, pp 21–34

36. Greene FL, Williams RB: Endoscopic management of gastrointestinal malignancy, in McKenna RT, Murphy GP (eds): *Cancer Surgery*. Philadelphia, Lippincott, 1994, pp 35–46

37. Kalinowski BH: Local therapy for breast cancer; Treatment choices and decision making. *Semin Oncol Nurs* 7:187–193, 1991

38. Ozols RF, Schwartz PE, Eifel PJ: Cancer of the ovary, in DeVita VT, Hellman S, Rosenberg SA (eds): *Cancer: Principles and Practice of Oncology* (ed 5). Philadelphia, Lippincott-Raven, 1997, pp 1502–1540

39. Steele G, Ravikumar TS, Benotti PN: New surgical treatments for recurrent colorectal cancer. *Cancer* 65:723–730, 1990

40. Dyck S: Surgical instrumentation as a palliative treatment for spinal cord compression. *Oncol Nurs Forum* 18:515–521, 1991

41. Corral CJ, Mustoe TA: Controversy in breast reconstruction. *Surg Clin North Am* 76:309–326, 1996

42. Moskowitz AJ, Reemtsma K, Rose EA: Clinical outcomes in surgery, in Sabiston DC, Lyerly HK (eds): *Textbook of Surgery* (ed 15). Philadelphia, Saunders, 1997, pp. 36–54

43. Clyne ME, Forlenza M: Consumer-focused preadmission testing: A paradigm shift. *J Nurs Qual* 11:9–16, 1997

44. Griffiths M, Leek C: Patient education needs: Opinions of oncology nurses and their patients. *Oncol Nurs Forum* 22: 139–144, 1995

45. Polomano R, Weintraub FN, Wurster A: Surgical critical care for cancer patients. *Semin Oncol Nurs* 10:165–176, 1994

46. Lichtiger B, Huh YO, Armintor M, et al: Autologous transfusions for cancer patients undergoing elective ablative surgery. *J Surg Oncol* 43:19–23, 1990

47. Jaffe K: Blood management challenges in orthopedic oncology. *Orthopedics* 22:161–163, 1999 (1 suppl)

48. Carr DB, Jacox A, Payne R, et al: *Management of Cancer Pain. Clinical Practice Guideline*. Agency for Health Care Policy and Research, publication No. 94-0592. Rockville, MD, U.S. Department of Health and Human Services, 1994

49. Jacox A, Carr DB, Chapman CR, et al: *Acute Pain Management: Operative or Medical Procedures and Trauma*. Agency for Health Care Policy and Research, publication No. 92-0032. Rockville, MD, U.S. Department of Health and Human Services, 1992

50. Gobel BH: Grief, in Yarbro CH, Frogge MH, Goodman M (eds): *Cancer Symptom Management* (ed 2). Sudbury, MA, Jones and Bartlett, 1999, pp 580–593

51. Syrjala KL, Donaldson GW, Davis MW, et al: Relaxation and imagery and cognitive-behavioral training reduce pain during cancer treatment: A controlled clinical trial. *Pain* 63:189–198, 1995

52. Paice JA: Pain, in Yarbro CH, Frogge MH, Goodman M (eds): *Cancer Symptom Management* (ed 2). Sudbury, MA, Jones and Bartlett, 1999, pp 118–148.

53. Sarantos P, Copeland EM, Souba WW: Nutritional support of the surgical oncology patient, in McKenna RJ, Murphy GP (eds): *Cancer Surgery*. Philadelphia, Lippincott, 1994, pp 761–772

54. Falcone RE, Nappi JF: Chemotherapy and wound healing. *Surg Clin North Am* 64:779–794, 1984

55. Ehrlichman RJ, Seckel Br, Bryan DJ, et al: Common complications of wound healing. *Surg Clin North Am* 71:1323–1351, 1991

56. Munro AJ, Potter S: A quantitative approach to the distress caused by symptoms in patients treated with radical radiotherapy. *Cancer Nurs* 21:127–135, 1998

57. Irvine DM, Vincent L, Graydon JE: Fatigue in women with breast cancer receiving radiation therapy. *Cancer Nurs* 21: 127–135, 1998

58. Broeckel JA, Jacobsen PB, Horton J, et al: Characteristics and correlates of fatigue after chemotherapy for breast cancer. *J Clin Oncol* 16:1689–1696, 1998

59. Mathes DD, Bogdonoff DL: Preoperative evaluation of the cancer patient, in Lefor AT (ed): *Surgical Problems Affecting the Patient with Cancer: Interdisciplinary Management*. Philadelphia, Lippincott-Raven, 1996, pp 273–304

60. Smith R: Intraoperative radiation therapy, in Dow KH, Bucholtz JD, Iwamoto R, et al (eds): *Nursing Care in Radiation Oncology* (ed 2). Philadelphia, Saunders, 1997, 178–196

61. Haibeck SV: Intraoperative radiation therapy. *Oncol Nurs Forum* 15:143–147, 1988

62. Calvo FA, Santos M, Azinovic I: Intraoperative radiotherapy. *Rays* 23:439–461, 1998

63. Schaffer M, Barbul A: Chemotherapy and wound healing, in Lefor AT (ed): *Surgical Problems Affecting the Patient with*

Cancer: Interdisciplinary Management. Philadelphia, Lippincott-Raven, 1996, pp 305–320

64. Ratain MJ: Pharmacology of cancer chemotherapy, in DeVita VT, Hellman S, Rosenberg SA (eds): *Cancer: Principles and Practice of Oncology* (ed 5). Philadelphia, Lippincott-Raven, 1997, pp 375–384

65. Thorne SE: Helpful and unhelpful communication in cancer care: The patient perspective. *Oncol Nurs Forum* 15: 167–172, 1988

66. Dodd MJ: Self-care and patient/family teaching, in Yarbro CH, Frogge MH, Goodman M (eds): *Cancer Symptom Management* (ed 2). Sudbury, MA, Jones and Bartlett, 1999, pp. 20–32

CHAPTER 15

Principles of Radiation Therapy

Laura J. Hilderley, RN, MS

Introduction

Radiation therapy has been used in the treatment of cancer since the early 1900s. Roentgen's discovery of the x-ray in 1895, and Marie and Pierre Curie's investigation of radioactive sources during the late 19th and early 20th century led to recognition of the ionizing property of radiation and its effect on living matter. Through many years of trial and discovery, the science of radiation oncology has evolved to its current place as a primary cancer treatment modality.

Radiation therapy often is combined with surgery or chemotherapy and immunotherapy, and can be the sole treatment for cancer in some instances. For example, stage IIB adenocarcinoma of the endometrium is usually treated with postoperative adjuvant radiation, whereas stage IIB squamous cell carcinoma of the cervix is treated with radiation alone.

Goals of Treatment Approaches

The goal of radiation therapy in early-stage cancers is curative, as in the treatment of skin cancer, carcinoma of the cervix, Hodgkin's disease, or seminoma. Treatment is vigorous and often lengthy, but the prognosis and probability of long-term survival make such an effort worthwhile.

For certain types of cancer and those in later stages, cure or eradication is not possible, and control of the cancer with radiation therapy for periods ranging from months to years may be the goal. Recurrent breast cancer, some soft-tissue sarcomas, and lung cancer are examples of cancers controlled by radiation therapy in combination with surgery or chemotherapy.

Palliation may be another goal of radiation therapy. Relief of pain, prevention of pathological fractures, and return of mobility can be achieved with radiation to metastatic bone lesions from primary sites such as breast, lung, and prostate. Pain relief often is dramatic, and it is not uncommon for one individual to receive multiple palliative courses to different bony structures over the course of several years. Radiation therapy contributes significantly to improved quality of life for the person with bone metastases. Palliative radiation therapy also is given for the relief of central nervous system (CNS) symptoms caused by brain metastasis or spinal cord compression. Hemorrhage, ulceration, and fungating lesions can be effectively reduced and in some instances eliminated by palliative radiation therapy.

"Anticipatory" palliation is a useful application of radiation therapy in treating potentially symptomatic lesions before they become problematic. Examples of anticipatory palliation include treatment of a mediastinal mass that threatens to produce a superior vena caval syndrome and treatment to a vertebral lesion when spinal cord compression is impending.

Although treatment techniques and equipment may vary, the fundamental principles of radiobiology and radiation physics form the basis on which a course of treatment is selected and designed for each patient. Understanding these principles enables the oncology nurse to support and care for the patient receiving radiation therapy—attending to the emotional and physical needs that result from the disease and the therapy.

Applied Radiation Physics

The use of ionizing radiation in the treatment of cancer is based on the ability of radiation to interact with the atoms and molecules of the tumor cells to produce specific harmful biological effects. Ionization affects either the molecules of the cell or the cell environment.

An understanding of atomic structure is essential to understanding the ionizing effects of radiation. The atom, the basic unit of molecular structure, has two parts: (1) the nucleus, containing positively charged protons and neutrons that have mass but no charge; and (2) the shells (orbits), containing electrons (equivalent to the number of protons), each of which has a negative charge. Each shell can accommodate only a certain number of electrons; if this number is exceeded, a second or third shell is established more distant from the nucleus (Figure 15-1). The negatively charged electrons orbit the nucleus and are held in place by the attractive force of the positive protons in the nucleus; thus, a stable state is maintained. Certain atoms are known to be unstable, however, and it is in this process of decay or breakdown into a more stable state that alpha, beta, or gamma rays may be emitted. Radium, radon, and uranium are examples of unstable atoms that produce ionizing radiation.

Stable atoms also may be made to produce ionizing radiation through excitation, ionization, and nuclear disintegration. Radiation produced by these processes can be classified as electromagnetic radiation or particulate radiation. The electromagnetic spectrum can be further divided into five levels of decreasing wavelength: (1) radio waves, (2) infrared radiation, (3) visible light, (4) ultraviolet radiation, and (5) ionizing radiation.

Ionizing radiation has the shortest wavelength and the greatest energy of the electromagnetic spectrum and is therefore the form of energy used in radiation therapy. A classification system for ionizing radiation is shown in Figure 15-2. As seen in the figure, the terms *x-ray* and *gamma ray* both describe ionizing electromagnetic radiation and differ only in their means of production. That is, x-rays are produced by specially designed equipment, and gamma rays are emitted by radioactive materials such as ^{60}Co undergoing nuclear transition. Both x-rays and gamma rays have no mass; rather, they are packets of available energy ready to be released on collision with a substance. Because they have no mass, x-rays and gamma rays can penetrate more deeply into tissue before releasing their energy.

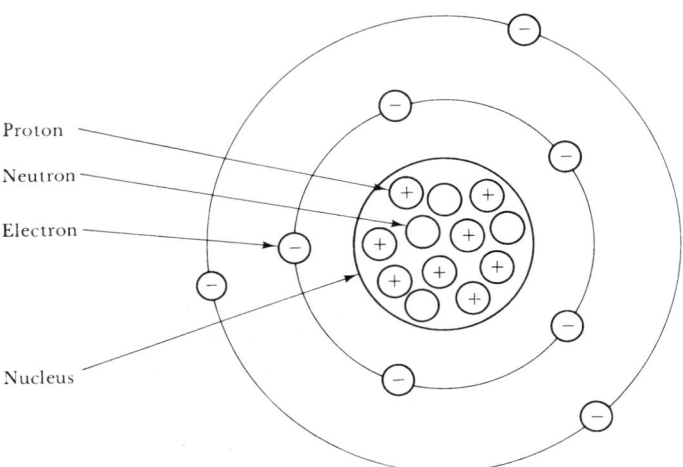

Figure 15-1 Basic structure of an atom. Protons, which are positively charged, and neutrons, which have no electrical charge, are the major components of the nucleus of an atom. The number of protons is equal to the number of negatively charged electrons orbiting the nucleus. Atoms of any given element may have different numbers of neutrons in the nucleus, thus giving atoms of the same element different atomic weights. An atom of a given element that differs only in its atomic weight is called an *isotope*.

Labels: Proton, Neutron, Electron, Nucleus

Particulate radiation, on the other hand, is composed of alpha and beta particles, as well as electrons and neutrons, which have mass. The relatively large size of alpha particles allows them to penetrate only a short distance into tissue before collision and energy release take place; beta particles, which are smaller than alpha particles, penetrate more deeply but, because of their mass, do not have the ability to reach as deeply into tissues as do x-rays and gamma rays. The significance of these variations in ability to penetrate tissue will become obvious when treatment beams and equipment are discussed in Chapter 16.

X-rays are produced when a stream of fast-moving electrons, accelerated by the application of high voltage (between the filament and the target), strikes the target, and the electrons give up their energy. This radiation loss occurs because the electron is attracted to and slowed

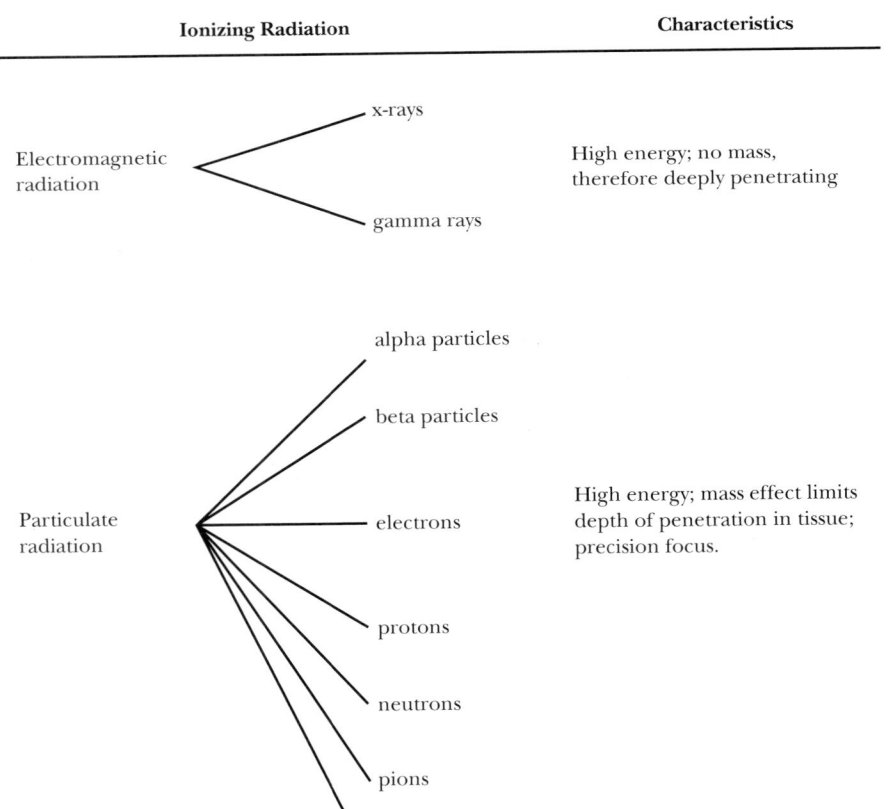

Ionizing Radiation   **Characteristics**

Figure 15-2 Characteristics of ionizing radiations.

Electromagnetic radiation — x-rays, gamma rays: High energy; no mass, therefore deeply penetrating

Particulate radiation — alpha particles, beta particles, electrons, protons, neutrons, pions, heavy ions: High energy; mass effect limits depth of penetration in tissue; precision focus.

down by the nucleus of the tungsten (target) atom. Figure 15-3 illustrates the basic structure of an x-ray tube.

In addition to x-rays, some treatment machines (beta-tron, linear accelerator) are equipped to produce particle irradiation in the form of electrons. Electron energy is produced in an x-ray tube by bypassing one of the steps used to produce x-rays (Figure 15-3). Electrons from the heated tungsten filament are injected into the vacuum tube and accelerated at a high velocity; they then emerge from a window in the vacuum tube, thus bypassing the tungsten target and emerging as electron particles suitable for treating surface lesions and those located a few centimeters below the skin.

Electromagnetic and particulate radiations also are produced through the process of decay of radioactive elements and radioactive isotopes. This process, which produces radiation in the form of alpha, beta, or gamma rays, is illustrated as follows:

$$\text{atom} \xrightarrow{\text{radioactive decay}} \text{atom } y + \text{radiation}$$

The time required for half of the radioactive atoms present at any time to decay is known as the *half-life* of that radioactive element or isotope.

Because most radioisotopes are produced by neutron bombardment of stable elements (^{60}Co, ^{32}P, ^{182}Ta, ^{198}Au) or by nuclear fission of uranium in a nuclear reactor (^{90}SR, ^{137}Cs), they are referred to as *artificial isotopes* to distinguish them from naturally occurring radioisotopes such as ^{226}Ra and ^{222}Rn. Radioactive isotopes are listed in Table 15-1.

High Linear Energy Transfer and Charged Particle Radiation Therapy

One of the important physical properties of ionizing radiation is linear energy transfer (LET). *Linear energy transfer* describes the rate at which energy is deposited as radiation travels through matter. Electromagnetic radiation has no mass or charge and is therefore sparsely ionizing as it penetrates matter. X-rays, gamma rays, and electrons are electromagnetic and low LET sources.

By contrast, the number of ionizing events produced by molecules of high LET radiation is significant because of their considerable mass and charge. High LET radiation, which includes neutron beams, heavy ions, and negative pi-mesons (pions), loses energy rapidly as it passes through matter. Multiple ionizing events occur in a relatively short distance with high LET radiation. Figure 15-4 illustrates the physics of LET.[1] High LET radiation facilities are limited in the United States and elsewhere. Years of research have shown that there are distinct advantages to

Figure 15-3 Basic structure of an x-ray tube. Electrons emitted from a heated tungsten filament are accelerated across a high-voltage source. These high-speed electrons then strike a positively charged tungsten target, producing x-rays. The primary beam of radiation thus produced penetrates tissues. The greater the voltage, the greater the penetrating power of the beam.

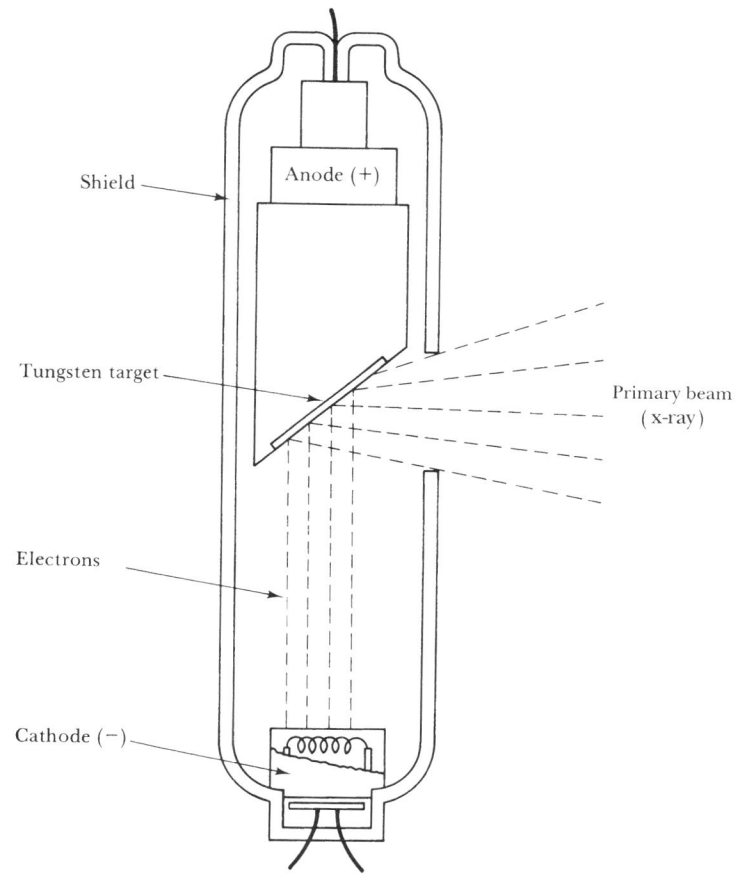

Table 15-1 Radioactive Isotopes Used in Radiation Therapy

Isotope	Symbol	Half-Life	Alpha	Beta	Gamma
			Emissions		
Cesium	^{137}Cs	30 years			X
Cobalt	^{60}Co	5.3 years		X	X
Gold	^{198}Au	2.69 days		X	X
Iodine	^{131}I	8.0 days		X	X
Iridium	^{192}Ir	74.5 days		X	X
Phosphorus	^{32}P	14.3 days		X	
Radium	^{226}Ra	1622 years	X	X	X
Radon	^{222}Rn	3.83 days	X	X	X
Strontium	^{90}Sr	28 years		X	
Tantalum	^{182}Ta	118 days		X	X
Yttrium	^{90}Y	64 hours		X	

this form of therapy, yet the cost of such facilities and the technological sophistication needed for their operation have meant that they function primarily as referral centers for carefully selected individuals with cancer.[2]

Still, high LET radiation has several advantages over low LET radiation:

- Greater relative biological effectiveness (RBE)

- Reduced relative radioresistance of hypoxic cells in tumors (low oxygen enhancement ratio [OER])

- Less intertreatment recovery of tumor cells in fractionated dosage

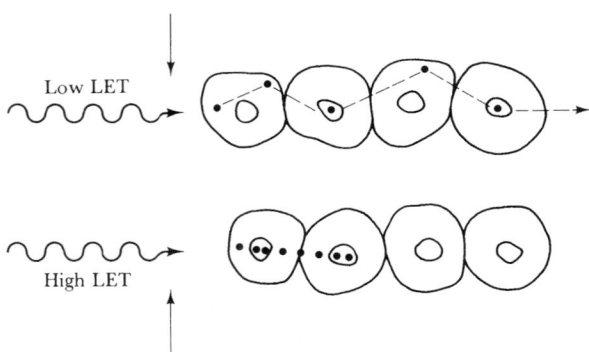

Figure 15-4 Comparison of the effects of low- and high-linear energy transfer (LET) radiations on a population of cells. Notice the irregular path of the low-LET radiation, interacting with four cells, compared with the relatively straight path of the high-LET radiation, which is interacting with only two cells. However, the low-LET radiation produces only *one* hit in two nuclei, whereas the high-LET radiation produces *two* hits in two nuclei. (Travis EL: *Primer of Medical Radiobiology.* Chicago, Year Book Medical Publishers, 1975, p 71. © 1975 Year Book Medical Publishers. Reproduced with permission.)

Neutron Beam Therapy

Fast neutrons are produced by a *cyclotron*, equipment in which high-energy neutrons bombard targets of either beryllium or tritium. Neutron therapy is less expensive than other high LET energy producers; however, technological problems and the low dose rate (5–6 cGy/min) are among the disadvantages to this form of therapy.

Heavy Charged Particle Therapy

Heavy ions, such as protons, helium, and nitrogen, are mainly useful for small tumors, because the dose distribution is best for treating a small volume. As the tumor size increases, treatment volume and OER also increase.

Negative Pi-meson Therapy

Negative pi-mesons (pions) are small, negatively charged particles found in the nuclei of atoms that "cement" protons and neutrons together. Pions are produced when protons are accelerated at approximately 131,000 miles/sec before striking a carbon target. The pions are then collected by a system of magnets, and the beam of high LET energy is directed at the target tissue. The first application of this form of treatment for humans took place at the Los Alamos Meson Physics Facility in Los Alamos, New Mexico, in 1974. The advantage of pion therapy, like other forms of high LET radiation, is that the beam can be shaped to fit the tumor precisely, thus minimizing the amount of radiation to surrounding normal structures. Pions can be aimed and stopped at a specific target site by adjusting the momentum of the particles.

At Los Alamos, a number of tumor sites and histologies were treated with good local cure rates and minimal morbidity, particularly in cancers of the head and neck, lung, bladder, cervix, and prostate gland. Tumors of the large bowel, pancreas, and brain did not respond as well. The Los Alamos program was terminated in 1981, however, because overall results were not impressive and costs were prohibitive.

A second pion facility opened in 1979 in Vancouver, British Columbia, and a third in Villigen, Switzerland, in 1980. Approximately 500 patients were treated at Villigen, with a high incidence of long-term toxicities noted. The severity of late effects was attributed to the use of treatment volumes nearly three times that used by the Vancouver group. The program at Villigen was discontinued in 1993.

The Vancouver pion group completed two randomized trials in late 1995, comparing photon and pion irradiation for high-grade gliomas and advanced prostate cancers. The glioma study found no difference between the two treatment groups in overall survival, time to recurrence, toxicity, and quality of life. Acute effects of pion therapy were increased over photon therapy; however, late toxicity was reduced in pion treatment.

Raju concludes that clinical results with pions appear to be about equal to photons for all sites investigated, except for the bladder.[3] Because of the cost and complexity of building and operating pion facilities, Raju also concludes that pion radiation will not likely be pursued in the future.

Radiobiology

The biological effects of radiation on humans are the result of a sequence of events that follows the absorption of energy from ionizing radiation and the organism's attempts to compensate for this assault. Radiation effect takes place at the cellular level, with consequences in tissues, organs, and the entire body.

Cellular Response to Radiation

Target theory

Radiation effect at the cellular level may be either direct or indirect, according to the target theory.[4] A direct hit occurs when any of the key molecules within the cell, such as DNA or RNA, are damaged. After high-dose radiation of DNA molecules in vitro, the types of damage observed are (1) change or loss of a base (thymine, adenine, guanine, or cytosine), (2) breakage of the hydrogen bond between the two chains of the DNA molecule, (3) breaks in one or both chains of the DNA molecule, and (4) cross-linking of the chains after breakage. Such unrepaired breaks or alterations in the base lead to mutations that result in impaired cellular function or cell death.

An indirect hit, according to target theory, occurs when ionization takes place in the medium (mostly water) surrounding the molecular structures within the cell. Ra-

diation absorbed by the water molecules results in the formation of a free radical when an electron is literally knocked out of orbit surrounding the ion. These free radicals may trigger a variety of chemical reactions, producing new compounds that are toxic to the cell. Figure 15-5 illustrates the ionizing effect of radiation on the water contained within a cell.

It generally is agreed that a direct hit (i.e., DNA damage and chromosomal aberrations) accounts for the most effective and lethal injury produced by ionizing radiation.[1,4] However, because of the relative proportion of water to DNA in a single cell, the probability of indirect damage through ionization of intracellular water is much greater than the probability of damage from a direct hit.

In addition to the damage produced by a direct or indirect hit, experimental evidence shows that radiation can cause damage to proteins, carbohydrates, and enzymes within the cell. Damage to these additional molecules, as well as alterations in the permeability of the cell membrane, may contribute to the ultimate effect of radiation at the cellular level.

Cell cycle and radiosensitivity

According to Hall and Cox, radiosensitivity appears to maximize during the M and G_2 phases of the cell cycle

---

The final products of the ionization of water molecules (HOH) by radiation are an ion pair (H^+, OH^-) and free radicals ($H^{\cdot}$, $OH^{\cdot}$), which are capable of damaging the cell. The ionization of water is shown in the following steps:

$$HOH \xrightarrow{\text{radiation}} HOH^+ + e^-$$

The free electron (e^-) is then captured by another available water molecule and, as shown in the next step, forms the second ion:

$$HOH + e^- \rightarrow HOH^-$$

Because the two ions (HOH^+, HOH^-) produced by these reactions are unstable, rapid breakdown occurs (in the presence of other, normal water molecules), forming yet another ion and a free radical as follows:

$$HOH^+ \rightarrow H^+ + OH^{\cdot}$$
$$HOH^- \rightarrow OH^- + H^{\cdot}$$

Although the resulting pair of ions (H^+, OH^-) have some potential for cellular damage through chemical reactions, they are more likely to recombine and form water (HOH). The free radicals ($H^{\cdot}$, $OH^{\cdot}$) are extremely reactive, and they too may simply recombine to form water. However, free radicals appear to be more likely to undergo chemical interactions with other free radicals, forming cytotoxic agents, as shown in this reaction:

$$OH^{\cdot} + OH^{\cdot} \rightarrow H_2O_2 \text{ (hydrogen peroxide)}$$

Free radicals that result from the interaction of radiation with water are capable of triggering a variety of chemical reactions within the cell and are therefore believed to be a major factor in the production of damage in the cell.

Figure 15-5   The effect of ionizing radiation on water molecules.

(Figure 15-6).[5] Thus, the maximum effect from radiation should occur just before and during actual cell division. In early research, Bergonie and Tribondeau formulated a law stating that the sensitivity of cells to irradiation is in direct proportion to their reproductive activity and inversely proportional to their degree of differentiation.[6] A differentiated cell is one that is morphologically or functionally specialized (such as the erythrocyte) and does not undergo mitosis. An undifferentiated cell (such as the red blood cell stem cell or erythroblast) has few specialized morphological or functional characteristics, and its primary purpose is to divide and provide new cells to maintain its own population. Because the effect of radiation is known to be greatest during mitosis, undifferentiated cell populations generally are most sensitive to radiation. In contrast, well-differentiated cells are relatively radioresistant.

Changes in mitotic activity due to radiation can be classified as either delayed onset or complete inhibition. *Delayed onset of mitosis* indicates that although damage occurred at some point during prophase, repair was accomplished and division occurred. *Complete inhibition of mitosis,* or cell sterilization, renders the cell incapable of division, although it may continue to live in a nonreproducing state.

Cell death

There are three types of cell death: (1) mitotic (or genetic), (2) interphase, and (3) instant. *Mitotic death* occurs after one or more cell divisions and usually with much smaller radiation doses than those required to produce interphase death. *Interphase death* occurs many hours after irradiation and before the cell begins the mitotic process. *Instant death* occurs following extremely high doses of radiation and would take place only in the experimental laboratory or in the event of a nuclear accident.

Contributing biological factors

A number of additional factors directly affect the biological response to radiation and ultimately the treatment outcome. Among these are the oxygen effect, LET, relative biological effectiveness, dose rate, radiosensitivity, and fractionation.

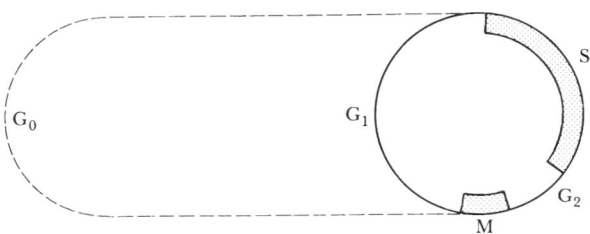

Figure 15-6 Stages in cell replication cycle: S = DNA synthesis; G_2 = the gap between DNA synthesis and mitosis; M = mitosis; G_1 = the gap between the end of mitosis and the start of DNA synthesis.

Oxygen effect.   Well-oxygenated tumors show a much greater response to radiation; that is, they are more radiosensitive than poorly oxygenated tumors. Extensive laboratory and clinical research has shown that the existence of oxygen tension from 20–40 mm Hg at time of radiation greatly enhances the radiosensitivity of the cells.[4,7] Theoretically, the mechanism of the oxygen effect is related to the ability of oxygen to combine with the free radicals formed during ionization, producing new and toxic combinations. A second theory holds that the presence of oxygen at the time of irradiation prevents the reversal (and thus the repair) of some of the chemical changes that occur as the result of ionization. The clinical significance of the *oxygen effect* is that oxygen modifies the dose of radiation needed to produce a given degree of biological damage. The magnitude of the oxygen effect is expressed as the oxygen enhancement ratio (OER). The OER is the ratio of radiation dose in the absence of oxygen (or hypoxia) to the radiation dose in the presence of oxygen required for the same biological effect.

Linear energy transfer.   *Linear energy transfer* describes the rate at which energy is lost from different types of radiation while traveling through matter. Low-LET radiations (x-rays and gamma rays) are sparsely ionizing, having a random pathway that results in few direct hits within the cell nucleus. Radiation of higher LET (alpha particles, neutrons, and negative pions) has a greater probability of interacting with matter and producing more direct hits within the cell (see Figure 15-4).[1]

Relative biological effectiveness.   Because different radiations have varying rates of energy loss, the biological response likewise will be different. Therefore, RBE is used to compare a dose of test radiation with a dose of standard radiation that produces the same biological response. The following formula is used to express RBE:

$$RBE = \frac{\textit{Dose of reference radiation to produce a given biological effect}}{\textit{Dose of test radiation to produce the same biological effect}}$$

Dose rate.   *Dose rate* refers to the rate at which a given dose is delivered by a treatment machine or equipment. Dose rate becomes particularly significant when a course of therapy is fractionated over many days and weeks, as it is in standard external beam teletherapy. Studies have shown low dose rates to be much less effective in producing lethal cell damage than high dose rates, primarily because low dose rates permit cell repair to occur before the lethal dose has been reached in fractionated teletherapy.

Radiosensitivity.   According to Bergonie and Tribondeau's law, ionizing radiation is most effective on cells that are undifferentiated and undergoing active mitosis.[6] Laboratory and clinical experience has shown this to be true in most tissues.

Fractionation. *Fractionation*, or the dividing of a total dose of radiation into a number of equal fractions, is based on four important factors: repair, redistribution, repopulation, and reoxygenation,[1,4,8] commonly referred to as the four Rs of radiobiology.[9]

The Four Rs of Radiobiology.

Repair. Repair of intracellular sublethal damage by normal cells between daily-dose fractions is one benefit of fractionation. The goal of fractionation is to deliver a dose sufficient to prevent tumor cells from being repaired while allowing normal cells to recover before the next dose is given. Although some tumor cells may be repaired between daily doses, they also may reoxygenate, rendering them more radiosensitive when the next dose is given. Thus, though some degree of repair of tumor cells is possible between fractionated doses, repeated daily doses ultimately would lead to tumor control.

Redistribution. Redistribution of cell age (within the cell cycle) as a result of daily radiation is advantageous because more tumor cells are made radiosensitive. Theoretically, with succeeding daily doses of radiation, more and more tumor cells would be delayed in cycle and reach the mitotic phase as the next dose is given, thus increasing the cell kill. Certain chemotherapeutic agents, such as methotrexate and hydroxyurea, are being used in combination with radiation to take advantage of this synchronization in the cell cycle.

Repopulation. Repopulation of normal tissues takes place through cell division at some time during a multifraction treatment course. Fractionation of dose allows this repopulation in normal tissues, sparing them from some of the late consequences that might occur if repopulation (new growth) was inhibited. On the other hand, those tumor cells that succeed in dividing while undergoing a fractionated course of radiation therapy are usually incapable of surviving because of the radiation effect. Thus, fractionation favors normal tissue while still eradicating tumor.

Reoxygenation. Reoxygenation is the fourth consideration favoring fractionation of the radiation dose. Whereas normal tissues usually are well oxygenated, tumors characteristically range from normal to hypoxic to anoxic. As discussed earlier, radiosensitivity is closely related to oxygen tension in the tumor cell; hypoxic or anoxic cells generally are radioresistant, whereas oxygenated cells are radiosensitive. Fractionating the dose allows time between treatments for the tumor to reoxygenate.

Tissue and organ response to radiation is based on the sensitivity of cellular components. It is important to note that tissues and organs are composed of more than one cell category, each cell category having different degrees of radiosensitivity. A second factor in determining tissue response is related to the parenchymal versus stromal substance found in that tissue. The parenchyma is composed of cells characteristic of the tissue or organ, and if those cells are radiosensitive (e.g., the testis), ioniz-

ing radiation has its greatest impact on the parenchyma. However, if parenchymal tissue is relatively radioresistant (e.g., the spinal cord), radiation response in that organ is due to the indirect effects on the stromal components (especially the vasculature) that support the parenchyma. Table 15-2 lists various organs according to their degree of radiosensitivity as measured by parenchymal hypoplasia.

Apoptosis. A major focus of research in radiobiology is currently directed toward the study of various mechanisms regulating apoptosis. *Apoptosis*, or programmed cell death, occurs in both normal and malignant cells in a process that is distinct from cellular death due to hypoxia. Failure of the normal apoptotic process results in survival and uncontrolled proliferation of malignant cells.

As described earlier, repair of radiation injury (sublethal damage repair) takes place in healthy tissues but may also occur in the targeted malignancy, thus reducing radioresponsiveness and the likelihood of potential cure. Ionization and direct damage to DNA accounts for the death during mitosis of most irradiated cells. It has been demonstrated that the process of apoptosis is also accelerated by radiation, particularly in lymphocytes, small bowel crypt cells, salivary gland cells, and germ cells.[10]

The role of certain genetic, molecular, and biochemical substances (*p53, BCL-2*), basic fibroblast growth factors (bFGF), and protein kinase C (PKC) inhibitors, among others, at the time of irradiation is thought to be significant in radiation-induced apoptosis.[10,11] The presence or absence of these substances and many others could enhance radioresponsiveness in various cell lines. Intensive research to identify the pathways that ultimately lead to apoptosis is under way. Manipulating these pathways may hold the key to increasing the therapeutic benefit ratio in radiation oncology.[12]

Radiobiology of Brachytherapy

The basic radiobiologic mechanism of cell kill in brachytherapy and teletherapy is the same, as the principles described previously as the 4 Rs (i.e., repair, redistribu-

Table 15-2 Degree of Radiosensitivity of Various Organs Based on Parenchymal Hypoplasia

Organ	Radiosensitivity
Lymphoid organs, bone marrow, blood, testes, ovaries, intestines	High
Skin, cornea, oral cavity, esophagus, rectum, bladder, vagina, cervix, ureters	Fairly high
Optic lens, stomach, growing cartilage, fine vasculature, growing bone	Medium
Mature cartilage or bone, salivary glands, respiratory organs, kidneys, liver, pancreas, thyroid, adrenals, pituitary gland	Fairly low
Muscle, brain, spinal cord	Low

tion, repopulation, reoxygenation) apply to both forms of radiation delivery. However, the temporal and spatial principles of physics are what account for the effectiveness of both brachytherapy and teletherapy.[13] Standard brachytherapy delivers continuous radiation at a low dose rate over a period of several days. Standard teletherapy delivers low dose rate radiation in higher doses, given in daily fractions over a number of weeks.

Brachytherapy, the use of implanted or injected radioactive sources, capitalizes on the effects of continuous rather than fractionated irradiation. These differences in effect occur when the dose rate is less than 5 cGy per minute.

Low dose rate brachytherapy

Low dose rate (LDR) brachytherapy, commonly used for gynecologic and head and neck cancers, delivers a continuous dose of radiation for as long as the source remains in place within the patient. This is in contrast to the intermittent dosing that takes place when treating with fractionated external-beam teletherapy. Following doses of fractionated teletherapy, cellular sublethal damage repair (SLD-R) occurs within 1 to 4 hours following treatment, producing the initial portion of the cell-survival curve referred to as the *shoulder*. Recall that cells are most radiosensitive during M and G_2 portions of the cell cycle. Low dose rate brachytherapy increases the effectiveness of radiation by redistributing an even greater proportion of cells into the G_2 phase when compared with fractionated treatment. Irradiated cells that manage to divide are blocked in the G_2 phase by continuous LDR brachytherapy.

Hypoxia in a tumor being treated with LDR brachytherapy is a less significant negative factor than it is in teletherapy. Low dose rates reduce the OER, and SLD-R is inhibited under prolonged hypoxic conditions. Low dose rate brachytherapy, therefore, enhances radiation effect by taking advantage of repair, redistribution, and repopulation principles even in poorly oxygenated tissue.

High dose rate brachytherapy

High dose rate brachytherapy (HDR) is the newest delivery method for brachytherapy. High dose rate sources deliver more than 1200 cGy per hour, administered as single, repeated fractions rather than continuously as in LDR treatments. High dose rate equipment is highly sophisticated, with computer optimization of dose distribution and sparing of normal tissues. In addition to the advantages of outpatient treatment and reduced staff exposure to radioactivity, HDR brachytherapy has shown a lower complication rate in treatment of cervix cancer than LDR therapy, without any decrease in local control.[14]

Capitalizing on Immunobiology: Radiolabeled Antibody Therapy

Radiolabeled antibody therapy has been the subject of considerable interest and effort since the 1970s.[15] This treatment technique is based on the information acquired in recent years regarding immunobiology and the isolation of many tumor-specific monoclonal and polyclonal antibodies. Among the numerous radioactive isotopes that have been used therapeutically, ^{131}I and ^{90}Y in particular have been adopted for use in radiolabeled antibody therapy.

The underlying biologic principle of radiolabeled antibody therapy involves attachment of a radioactive isotope to the tumor-specific antibody, which is then administered intravenously. Next, the circulating antibody is taken up by the targeted organ, delivering therapeutic radiation directly to the tumor. Theoretically, this technique avoids prolonged radiation exposure to healthy cells while delivering lethal or sublethal doses to the tumor. Among numerous phase I, II, and III clinical trials over the past two decades, some of the more significant results have been achieved in the treatment of hepatoma.[16]

A major problem in delivering the intended dose of radiation to the target site is the fact that the radiolabeled antibody is rapidly cleared from the target organ by the normal blood flow, thus limiting the time of contact with the tumor target. A new delivery method has been developed and patented (US Patent No. 5,424,288) that uses macroaggregated proteins injected into the organ site directly to block the rapid clearance of the radioactive substance.[17,18] This procedure, called *infusional brachytherapy*, is being used for a number of different advanced cancers, with the most extensive application in pancreatic adenocarcinoma.[18] Phase II multicenter trials have been initiated in the United States and in Europe, using macroaggregated albumin (MAA) as the blocking agent and P32 (chromic phosphate) as the radioactive source for treatment of pancreatic cancer.[17,18]

Chemical and Thermal Modifiers of Radiation

Radiosensitizers and Radioprotectors

The goal of radiation therapy is to achieve maximum tumor cell kill while minimizing injury to normal tissues (therapeutic ratio). Efforts to improve the therapeutic ratio have resulted in the development of certain compounds that act to increase the radiosensitivity of tumor cells or to protect normal cells from radiation effect. Combined modality therapy, using both radiation and certain chemotherapeutic agents, also takes advantage of enhanced tumor cell kill. Drugs such as doxorubicin, actinomycin-D, cyclophosphamide, bleomycin, cisplatin, and taxotere often are used along with radiation to achieve greater cell kill than either therapy could achieve alone.[19] When used independently, however, chemical modifiers of radiation therapy (*radiosensitizers*) are not generally cytotoxic like the chemotherapeutic agents.

Phillips proposed several definitions useful in describing the various interactions of radiation with other agents.[20] *Enhancement* or *potentiation* describes any radiation effect that is greater in the presence of the chemical than in its absence. When the effect is less than that caused by the most active agent in the combination, it is known as *interference*. *Antagonism* is the term used to describe an outcome less than that of the least effective agent in a given combination. In clinical radiation therapy, enhancement by noncytotoxic sensitizers is called *radiosensitization*. Antagonism by protective compounds is called *radioprotection*.

Radiosensitizers are compounds that apparently promote fixation of the free radicals produced by radiation damage at the molecular level. The mechanism of this action is similar to the oxygen effect described previously, in which biochemical reactions in the damaged molecules prevent repair of the cellular radiation damage. Free radicals (such as OH^+) are captured by the electron affinity of the radiosensitizers, rendering the molecules incapable of repair.

The two most biologically active radiosensitizing compounds first tested in phase II and III studies were metronidazole (Flagyl) and misonidazole (RO-07-0582). Major side effects are neurotoxicity, including peripheral neuropathies, somnolence, confusion, and transient coma. Nausea and vomiting are also frequent side effects that seem to be dose related.

Early clinical trials using misonidazole as a radiosensitizer indicated some degree of effectiveness in treatment of squamous carcinoma of the head and neck and of the uterine cervix. Overall results were disappointing, however, due to severe toxicity and only marginal improvement in tumor control.[21] Misonidazole is the only such substance to have undergone extensive clinical trial evaluation. Misonidazole has been shown to increase the cytotoxicity of alkylating agents, nitrosoureas, 5-fluorouracil (5-FU), cyclophosphamide, and melphalan. However, the side effects commonly experienced with these agents also are apparently enhanced by the addition of misonidazole. This nonselective enhancement significantly detracts from the potential benefits to be gained.

The compound SR-2508 (etanidazole) has been tested, with encouraging results in early phase II and III trials. This member of the nitroimidazole group of compounds appears to be less toxic to the CNS tissue than misonidazole and also has been shown to cross the blood-brain barrier in limited quantity. However, a recent phase I study of etanidazole and radiation therapy for patients with malignant glioma failed to show improvement over those treated with conventional therapy.[22]

Early studies with nitroimidazoles used in vitro showed that these radiosensitizers are also capable of cytotoxic activity in hypoxic cells after periods of long exposure.[23] The high doses required to achieve actual cell kill in vitro have prohibited their use in vivo for this purpose.

The established basis for use of chemical radiosensitizers is the result of extensive laboratory research. However, clinical trials thus far have failed to establish the overall efficacy of radiosensitizers as routine adjuncts to radiation therapy in the clinical setting.[24]

Radioprotectors are compounds that can protect oxygenated (nontumor) cells while having a limited effect on hypoxic (tumor) cells. This selective action serves to increase the therapeutic ratio by promoting the repair of irradiated normal tissues. Repair or return to a nondamaged state takes place through the chemical process of reduction. Free electrons are captured by the radioprotective substance and thus are unavailable to participate in further chemical reactions that lead to cellular damage. This process can be viewed as the opposite of what occurs when radiosensitizers are used.

The sulfhydryl groups contained in the nonprotein fraction of most cells aid in the reduction process following radiation damage. Thiophosphate compounds (such as cysteine and cysteamine) containing sulfhydryl and aminopropyl groups were among the earliest radioprotectors synthesized. The compound that has been most widely investigated is designated WR-2721.[25]

The study of radiosensitizers and radioprotectors in phase II and phase III clinical trials continues in an effort to achieve better results with radiation therapy. With combined therapy, toxicity is often increased and patient comfort may be compromised.

Combined Modality Therapy

Treatment of cancer with any single modality (surgery, chemotherapy, or radiation) does not always produce the desired effect of tumor eradication. Chemotherapy and radiation therapy produce dose-limiting side effects that govern the extent of single modality treatment. In order to increase or improve the therapeutic index (ratio of tumor control versus normal tissue damage), various combinations of chemotherapy and radiation have been studied.[26,27]

Ideally, a chemotherapeutic agent (or combination of agents) will shrink a tumor when given prior to local radiation (*neoadjuvant chemotherapy*); enhance or increase radiation cell kill when given during radiation (*concomitant therapy*); or control micrometastases and subclinical disease after a course of radiation (*adjuvant therapy*). Radiation and chemotherapy sometimes are given on a planned, alternating schedule using the so-called sandwich technique. This approach utilizes a split course of radiation in which the patient is treated with chemotherapy during a planned break in the total course of radiation therapy.

Combined modality therapy is being used in the treatment of a variety of cancer types, including squamous cell cancer of the cervix, anus, head and neck, and lung. Cancers of the bladder, esophagus, pancreas, and stomach frequently are treated with both chemotherapy and radiation therapy in varying schedules. Vigorous combined-modality therapy has allowed organ preservation for some individuals with carcinoma of the larynx, bladder, or anus.[26,28]

Some of the chemotherapeutic agents in common use for their radiosensitizing effect include cisplatin, methotrexate, doxorubicin, vinblastin VP-16, mitomycin C, 5-fluorouracil, actinomycin D, bleomycin, and taxotere. As would be expected, combined modality therapy has the potential for enhanced side effects as well as enhanced tumor effect. Organ systems at greatest risk for toxicity are the gastrointestinal, integumentary, and myeloproliferative systems.

Hyperthermia

The use of hyperthermia to achieve a synergistic effect with radiation therapy has been studied and applied in clinical situations with considerable enthusiasm. Although it is technically arguable whether hyperthermia actually sensitizes tumor cells to radiation effect or simply combines with it to produce a greater effect than either modality can achieve alone, it is generally agreed that this combined technique is warranted, and research continues.[29-32]

The biological basis for combining hyperthermia with radiation involves several factors. Heat is cytotoxic to cancer cells but is also destructive to healthy tissue if applied in excess of tolerable ranges. Controlled hyperthermia combined with radiation achieves tumor cell kill without excess toxicity.

Tumor cells are least radiosensitive during S phase; hyperthermia is most effective during S phase. Therefore, the combined effect of radiation and hyperthermia on a tumor produces greater cell kill than either does alone. Similarly, hypoxic cells, which are generally radioresistant, have been found to be quite thermosensitive. Heat is also known to inhibit the repair of radiation damage, thus increasing the therapeutic ratio.

There are a number of important physical and biological parameters that may influence tumor response to combined hyperthermia and radiation therapy. Pretreatment parameters include tumor size, histological findings, and disease site. Treatment parameters include total dose of radiation and dose per fraction, thermal dose, total and weekly number of hyperthermia sessions, and, finally, the sequencing of hyperthermia and radiation.

Incidental and Accidental Radiation Exposure

Chronic Low-Dose Exposure

Chronic low-dose radiation exposure occurs to all individuals, due to background radiation from naturally occurring radioactive substances and cosmic rays.[33] Such exposure is largely unavoidable and is considered to be within safe limits as defined by federal regulations. Radiation workers are exposed to a somewhat higher level of ionizing radiation, but the allowable limit is well below that which is known to produce ill effects.

Total Body Radiation Syndrome

Total body radiation syndrome refers to the effects of acute exposure of an organism to doses of radiation received in a matter of minutes rather than hours or days. Acute exposure of human beings has been studied through data obtained from industrial and laboratory accidents, individuals exposed at Hiroshima and Nagasaki, Pacific Testing Grounds fallout exposure, and medical treatment procedures.[34,35] Doses of 150–2000 cGy delivered to the whole body in a short time produce life-shortening or lethal damage through effects on the hematopoietic, gastrointestinal, and central nervous systems. The April 1986 nuclear accident in Chernobyl, Ukraine, has yielded additional significant information about the somatic effects of exposure to high levels of radioactivity. Total body syndrome is manifested by the critical effects seen in the hematopoietic, gastrointestinal, and cerebrovascular systems.

Hematopoietic syndrome

Total body radiation exposure in a single dose ranging from 300cGy to 800cGy leads to hematopoietic failure. Stem cells are most susceptible and are sterilized almost immediately on exposure. When the circulating cells begin to die off in a matter of a few weeks, and marrow replacement is insufficient, the crisis and symptoms appear. Generally, within 3 weeks after exposure, the patient experiences chills, fever, fatigue, petechiae, and mouth ulcerations, all symptoms of depressed blood components. Death ensues unless marrow recovery or successful transplantation occurs.

Gastrointestinal syndrome

Following total body exposure of 10 Gy or more, death occurs within a few days to 2 weeks due to the severity of gastrointestinal damage. The highly radiosensitive intestinal epithelium is essentially denuded of villi, with total loss of the normal cell-renewal mechanism. The patient suffers nausea, anorexia, vomiting, lethargy, and severe, prolonged diarrhea leading to death.

Cerebrovascular syndrome

No human has survived accidental total body exposure of more than 10 Gy. At this dosage level, death is due to the cerebrovascular consequences. Although the exact mechanism of cerebrovascular death is not clear, symptoms include disorientation, incoordination, seizures, visual impairment, hypotension, renal failure, and coma. At this high-dose exposure level (10 Gy total body), gastrointestinal symptoms also occur almost immediately, and death due to neurovascular failure occurs in a matter of hours to a few days. (For case descriptions of total body radiation syndrome, see Hall,[4] Kato and Schull,[34] and Schull.[35]

Radiation Effects on the Embryo and Fetus

Data regarding fetal and embryonic response to radiation has been obtained primarily from laboratory animals for the obvious reason that human experimentation is unethical. Information that has become available on human fetal exposure has been acquired from studies of the surviving children who were in utero at the time of the atomic explosions in Nagasaki and Hiroshima.[36,37] Information has also come from medical radiation exposure in the early twentieth century before fetal dangers were known.

Three critical periods in gestation have been identified in laboratory animals, preimplantation, organogenesis, and the fetal period.[4] During preimplantation or shortly afterward, radiation is almost always lethal. Surprisingly, a surviving embryo progresses to normal growth because, at this point in gestation, the only task of the cells is division, not differentiation.

During the next phase, organogenesis, the embryo is at greatest danger of developing malformations. Neonatal death is common, as multiple abnormalities that result from the radiation exposure are incompatible with life. When radiation exposure occurs during the growth or fetal period (after 6 weeks in humans), the most common effects are overall growth retardation, microcephaly, and mental retardation.[38] Other reported abnormalities in humans include spina bifida, hydrocephalus, blindness, clubfoot, and scalp alopecia.[39]

Radiation-Induced Malignancies

The carcinogenic effects of radiation, from both chronic low-dose exposure and therapeutic radiation, are of particular interest and concern to the nurse, especially in providing support to the individual who is hesitant about accepting treatment. The key to understanding lies in the fact that acute exposure occurring in radiation accidents is rare, and chronic low-dose occupational or environmental exposure is the exception. The therapeutic doses usually prescribed (in the range of 2500–6500 cGy) are believed to be less carcinogenic than lower doses given over a much longer time period. Theoretically, a cell that has survived in a damaged or altered state after low-dose irradiation may undergo carcinogenic mutation in the presence of other conditional factors. At the same time, a cell that has been sterilized or destroyed by therapeutic doses of radiation should be incapable of malignant changes.

Malignancies that have been associated with radiation exposure are skin carcinoma, leukemia, sarcoma, thyroid carcinoma, and lung cancer.[33,40] Other reports have suggested the possibility of inducing breast cancer in females by frequent radiographic exposure for screening for tuberculosis, lung disease, and breast cancer itself.[33,41,42]

Radiation carcinogenesis depends on a number of variables.[43] These include a latent period of 1 to 30 years, radiation dose, concomitant factors in the radiated organism's environment, and the actual fate of the cell as it responds to radiation injury. (For a more comprehensive review of radiation carcinogenesis, see Hall[4] and Bucholtz.[44])

Conclusion

The science of radiobiology has accelerated continuously from the 1950s, when basic research in radiation biology was at last recognized as fundamental in advancing cancer treatment. The biologic effects of radiation therapy had long been observed, recognized, and acknowledged, but not well understood. Scientific effort had been focused primarily on the development of treatment equipment such as the cobalt machine and linear accelerator. Henry Kaplan, the preeminent radiation oncologist at Stanford University, was quoted in 1952 as saying, "The time has come when we must face up squarely to the fact that the mere construction and installation of very elaborate equipment . . . is not going to scare cancers into submission."[45]

It is the recognition and pursuit of both basic and clinical radiobiologic research that has led to today's emphasis on maximizing treatment outcome while minimizing both early and late effects of treatment. This is being achieved with combined-modality therapy, altered fractionation schedules, reduction in treatment volume and dose, and ever more sophisticated treatment planning and techniques of delivery.

Knowledge of radiobiologic effect also has led to the expansion of radiation therapy for some nonmalignant conditions. Nonmalignant treatment indications being explored include cardiac and lung allograft rejection,[46,47] macular degeneration,[48,49] and endovascular brachytherapy for arterial restenosis following angioplasty.[50,51,52] Research in molecular and cellular biology will continue to be of primary importance in radiation oncology and improved cancer treatment.

References

1. Travis E: *Primer of Medical Radiobiology.* Chicago, Year Book, 1975
2. Munzenrider JE, Crowell C: Charged particles, in Mauch PM, Loeffler JS (eds): *Radiation Oncology, Technology and Biology.* Philadelphia, Saunders, 1994, pp 34–55
3. Raju MR: Particle radiotherapy: Historical developments and current status. *Radiat Res* 145:391–407, 1996
4. Hall EJ: *Radiobiology for the Radiologist* (ed 4). Philadelphia, Lippincott, 1994
5. Hall EJ, Cox JD: Physical and biologic basis of radiation

therapy, in Cox JD (ed): *Moss' Radiation Oncology: Rationale, Technique, Results* (ed 7). St. Louis, Mosby-Year Book, 1994, pp 3–66

6. Bergonie J, Tribondeau L: Interpretation of some results of radiotherapy and an attempt at determining a logical technique of treatment. *Radiat Res* II:587, 1959

7. Gray LH: Radiobiologic basis of oxygen as a modifying factor in radiation therapy. *Am J Roentgenol* 85:805, 1961

8. Ritter MA: Cell proliferation, in Mauch PM, Loeffler JS (eds): *Radiation Oncology, Technology and Biology*. Philadelphia, Saunders, 1994, pp 525–544

9. Withers HR: Biologic basis of radiation therapy, in Perez CA, Brady LW (eds): *Principles and Practice of Radiation Oncology* (ed 2). Philadelphia, Lippincott, 1992, pp 64–96

10. Dewey WC, Ling CC, Meyn RE: Radiation-induced apoptosis: Relevance to radiotherapy. *Int J Radiat Oncol Biol Phys* 33:781–796, 1995

11. Fuks Z, Haimovitz-Friedman A, Kolesnick RN: The role of the sphyngomyelin pathway and protein kinase C in radiation-induced cell kill, in DeVita VT, Hellman S, Rosenberg SA (eds): *Important Advances in Oncology 1995*. Philadelphia, Lippincott, 1995, pp 19–31

12. Kim HE, Han JS, Kasza T, et al: Platelet-derived growth factor (PDGF)–signaling mediates radiation-induced apoptosis in human prostate cancer cells with loss of p53 function. *Int J Radiat Oncol Biol Phys* 39:731–736, 1997

13. Orton C: Radiobiology in brachytherapy: Biologic aspects and practical applications, in Nag S (ed): *Principles and Practice of Brachytherapy*. Armonk, NY, Futura, 1997, pp 51–65

14. Patel FD, Sharma SC, Negi PS , et al: Low dose rate vs high dose rate brachytherapy in treatment of carcinoma of the uterine cervix: A clinical trial. *Int J Radiat Oncol Biol Phys* 28:335–341, 1994

15. Bucholtz J: Radiolabeled antibody therapy, in Hassey-Dow K, Hilderley L (eds): *Nursing Care in Radiation Oncology*. Philadelphia, Saunders, 1992, pp 275–284

16. Macklis R: Radioimmunoconjugates and other target-selective therapeutic radiopharmaceuticals, in Mauch PM, Loeffler JS (eds): *Radiation Oncology, Technology and Biology*. Philadelphia, Saunders, 1994, pp 357–381

17. Order SE, Seigel JA, Lustig RA, et al: Infusional brachytherapy in the treatment of non-resectable pancreatic cancer: A new radiation modality (Preliminary report of the Phase I study). *Antib Immunoconj Radiopharm* 7:11–27, 1994

18. Westlin JE, Anderson-Forsman C, Garske U, et al: Objective responses after fractionated infusional brachytherapy of unresectable pancreatic adenocarcinomas. *Cancer* 80:2743–2748, 1997 (suppl)

19. Lederman G, Arbit E, Odaimi M, et al: Fractionated stereotactic radiosurgery and concurrent taxol in recurrent glioblastoma multiforme: A preliminary report. *Int J Radiat Oncol Biol Phys* 40:661–666, 1998

20. Phillips TL. Biochemical modifiers: Drug-radiation interactions, in Mauch PM, Loeffler JS (eds): *Radiation Oncology, Technology and Biology*. Philadelphia, Saunders, 1994, pp 113–151

21. Brown JM: Hypoxic cell radiosensitizers: Where next? *Int J Radiat Oncol Biol Phys* 16:987–993, 1989

22. Chang EL, Loeffler JS, Reise NE, et al: Survival results from a phase I study of etanidazole (SR2508) and radiotherapy in patients with malignant glioma. *Int J Radiat Oncol Biol Phys* 40:65–70, 1998

23. Hall EJ, Miller R, Astor M, et al: The nitroimidazoles as radiosensitizers and cytotoxic agents. *Br J Cancer* 37:120, 1978 (suppl 3)

24. Prados MD, Scott CB, Rotman M, et al: Influence of bromodeoxyuridine radiosensitization on malignant glioma patient survival: A retrospective comparison of survival data from the Northern California Oncology Group (RTOG) Trials for glioblastoma multiforme and anaplastic astrocytoma. *Int J Radiat Oncol Biol Phys* 40:653–659, 1998

25. Fleming ID, Brady LW, Mieszkalski GB, et al: Basis for major current therapies for cancer, in Murphy GP, Lawrence Jr. W, Lenhard RE (eds): *American Cancer Society Textbook of Clinical Oncology* (ed 2). Atlanta, GA, American Cancer Society, 1995, pp 96–134

26. Marks L, Carroll P, Dugan T, et al: The response of the urinary bladder, urethra and ureter to radiation and chemotherapy. *Int J Radiat Oncol Biol Phys* 31:1257–1280, 1995

27. Komaki R: Combined chemotherapy and radiation therapy in surgically unresectable regionally advanced non–small cell lung cancer. *Semin Radiat Oncol* 6:86–91, 1996

28. Cummings BJ, Keane TJ, O'Sullivan B, et al: Epidermoid anal cancer: Treatment by radiation alone or by radiation and 5-fluorouracil with and without Mitomycin-C. *Int J Radiat Oncol Biol Phys* 21:1115–1125, 1991

29. Coughlin CT, Wong TZ, Ryan TP, et al: Interstitial microwave-induced hyperthermia and iridium brachytherapy for the treatment of obstructing biliary carcinoma. *Int J Hyperthermia* 8:157–171, 1992

30. Kapp KS, Kapp DS, Stuecklschweiger G, et al: Interstitial hyperthermia and high-dose rate brachytherapy in the treatment of anal cancer: A phase I-II study (Review). *Int J Radiat Oncol Biol Phys* 28:189–199, 1994

31. Seegenschmiedt MH, Martus P, Fietkau R, et al: Multivariate analysis of prognostic parameters using interstitial thermoradiotherapy (IHT-IRT): Tumor and treatment variables predict outcome. *Int J Radiat Oncol Biol Phys* 29:1049–1063, 1994

32. Moros EG, Straube WL, Klein EE, et al: Clinical system for simultaneous external superficial microwave hyperthermia and cobalt-60 radiation. *Int J Hyperthermia* 11:11–26, 1995

33. Mettler FA, Upton AC: *Medical Effects of Ionizing Radiation* (ed 2). Philadelphia, Saunders, 1995, pp 73–112

34. Kato H, Schull WJ: Studies of the mortality of A-bomb survivors. Mortality, 1950–78. I. Cancer mortality. *Radiat Res* 90: 395–432, 1982

35. Schull WJ: *Effects of Atomic Radiation: A Half Century of Studies from Hiroshima and Nagasaki*. New York, Wiley-Liss, 1995

36. Wood JW, Johnson KG, Omori Y: In utero exposure to the Hiroshima atomic bomb: Follow up at 20 years. *Pediatrics* 39: 385–392, 1967

37. Otake M, Schull WJ: In utero exposure to A-bomb radiation and mental retardation: A reassessment. *Br J Radiol* 57: 409–414, 1984

38. Miller RW: Effects of prenatal exposure to ionizing radiation. *Health Phys* 59:57–61, 1990

39. Dekaban AS: Abnormalities in children exposed to x-radiation during various stages of gestation: Tentative timetable of radiation to the human fetus. *Int J Nucl Med* 9:471–477, 1968

40. March HC: Leukemia in radiologists in a twenty-year period. *Am J Med Sci* 220:282, 1950

41. MacKenzie I: Breast cancer following multiple fluoroscopies. *Br J Cancer* 19:1–8, 1965

42. Myrden JA, Hiltz JE: Breast cancer following multiple fluoroscopies during artificial pneumothorax treatment of pulmonary tuberculosis. *Can Med Assoc J* 100:1032–1034, 1969

43. Rubin P, Costine L, Fajardo LF: Overview: Late effects of

normal tissue (LENT) scoring system. *Int J Radiat Oncol Biol Phys* 31:1041–1042, 1995

44. Bucholtz JD: Radiation carcinogenesis, in Hassey-Dow K, Bucholtz JD, Iwamoto R, et al (eds): *Nursing Care in Radiation Oncology* (ed 2). Philadelphia, Saunders, 1997, pp 57–68

45. Stein JJ: Some observations of the history of radiation therapy. *Endocurie Hypertherm Oncol* 1:59–65, 1985

46. Wolden SL, Tate DJ, Hunt SA, et al: Long-term results of total lymphoid irradiation in the treatment of cardiac allograft rejection. *Int J Radiat Oncol Biol Phys* 39:953–960, 1997

47. Diamond DA, Michalski JM, Lynch JP, et al: Efficacy of total lymphoid irradiation for chronic allograft rejection following bilateral lung transplantation. *Int J Radiat Oncol Biol Phys* 41:795–800, 1998

48. Akmansu M, Dirican B, Ozturk B, et al: External radiotherapy in macular degeneration: Our technique, dosimetric calculation, and preliminary results. *Int J Radiat Oncol Biol Phys* 40:923–927, 1998

49. Archambeau JO, Mao XW, Yonemoto LT, et al: What is the role of radiation in the treatment of subfoveal membranes: Review of radiobiologic, pathologic and other considerations to initiate a multimodality discussion. *Int J Radiat Oncol Biol Phys* 40:1125–1136, 1998

50. Carter AJ, Fischell TA: Current status of radioactive stents for the prevention of in-stent restenosis. *Int J Radiat Oncol Biol Phys* 41:127–133, 1998

51. Fajardo LF: The nature of arterial restenosis after angioplasty. *Int J Radiat Oncol Biol Phys* 40:761–763, 1998

52. Rubin P, Williams JP, Riggs PN, et al: Cellular and molecular mechanisms of radiation inhibition of restenosis. Part I: Role of the macrophage and platelet-derived growth factor. *In J Radiat Oncol Biol Phys* 40:929–941, 1998

CHAPTER 16

Radiation Therapy Treatment Planning

Susan Weiss Behrend, RN, MSN

Introduction

Radiation oncology nurses are challenged to understand the scientific framework of treatment and the equipment used to plan and deliver radiation treatment. Radiation Therapy Centers include both technological and clinical components. Patient management issues are fundamental to the nursing process and evolve naturally during the course of treatment. This information needs to be supplemented and supported by the expertise of the multidisciplinary team, including radiation oncologists, nurses, medical physicists, dosimetrists, engineers, and radiation therapists.

Treatment Planning and Simulation Processes

Receiving radiation therapy is a multifaceted process. Initially, a thorough consultation must occur in which the patient and family are introduced to the radiation oncologist and the radiation oncology nurse. Later, the patient meets other members of the multidisciplinary team—dosimetrists, therapists, social workers, and administrative support staff. The initial consultation includes a thorough review of the patient's history, physical and psychosocial assessment, histologic reconfirmation of the cancer diagnosis, discussion of treatment options, and educational informed consent. Treatment recommendations are based on potential for disease response and risk of acute and long-term toxicity. A variety of radiation treatment modalities may be offered, including external beam alone or a combined regimen with internal radiation. The type and length of treatment varies according to diagnosis, radiation sensitivity of the tumor, and patient performance status. Once these parameters are considered, the patient is offered a therapeutic plan. The radiation oncologist, in conjunction with medical physicists, develops the radiation prescription. Treatment planning is a detailed and precise process that involves obtaining a series of radiographic studies to identify tumor type, size, and location. Simulation involves a series of fluoroscopic films that, combined with a computerized planning program, circumscribe the tumor and vital organs and tissues in the area. This information is used to determine the exact dose required for the target volume and surrounding normal tissues.

At the first appointment, the simulation procedure may require 1–2 hours, thus in order to allay anxiety the patient should be prepared for an extended visit. At this time, the treatment field is identified and measured. Indelible small tattoos are injected on the patient's skin to mark the treatment area and enable daily replication of the target treatment field. Patients should be aware that they will be partially disrobed during the simulation and daily treatments. The patient may be required to drink radio-opaque contrast or have intravenous contrast injected to enhance visualization of the tumor. Additionally, mold-room technicians will create customized blocks and immobilization devices to shield vital organs from scatter radiation and to safely secure the patient. At this time, the physician will obtain final informed consent. Depending on the facility policy, the patient may be required to return for a treatment setup prior to the initial dose so the plan can be checked methodically before actual administration. The aforementioned events can create tremendous anxiety for patients and families,[1] hence it is incumbent on the professional radiation oncology nurse to provide an environment where patients feel physically comfortable and psychosocially supported.

During the initial consultation, the patient and family learn about the treatment process. The patient is required to maintain the same position throughout the treatment session. The machinery (typically a linear accelerator) rotates around the patient, and average treatment time varies between 10–15 minutes. The radiation beam is odorless, colorless, and painless. The patient is comfortably situated alone in the treatment room and is monitored at the therapist's control station with audiovisual cameras. Patients may require pretreatment medication with antiemetics, steroids, or analgesics. Pediatric patients may need sedation or anesthesia in order to diminish risk of movement during the treatment session.[2] The typical treatment course is daily for 5 days and varies in the total number of weeks. Weekly planning films to monitor beam placement are checked by the radiation oncologist. Weekly appointments are scheduled for all patients on treatment so that the radiation oncology nurse and the radiation oncologist can assess the patient for development of acute toxicities and overall status.

The planning and simulation processes depend on highly accurate measurements of patient characteristics to provide for differences in dose distribution. Dosimetric planning requires expert medical physicists, dosimetrists, and equipment. The data required by the physicists to plan treatment include body contour, outline and depth of internal structures, and location and size of the target.[3] Patient contours can be determined by mechanical, optical, ultrasonic, and computerized tomography (CT) equipment. The patient's contour must be assessed in the same position as the one proposed for actual treatment. Additionally, the tabletop should be included in the contour as a reference for beam angles, and bony landmarks and beam entry points should be indicated. Body contour should be continuously checked throughout treatment in anticipation of changes due to tumor response or weight change.

Internal structure identification provides vital information about the size and location of critical organs. This quantitative data complements qualitative diagnostic radiographic findings that are essential for the identification of realistic contours. Several techniques and devices are used for localizing internal structures to facilitate treatment planning: Transverse tomography, CT, ultrasound, treatment simulators, and port films are examples.

The characteristics of treatment simulators and port films are explained below.

Treatment Simulators

A treatment simulator is an x-ray machine that has the ability to duplicate the geometry and mechanics of radiation treatment machines (Figure 16-1). Pretreatment CT scans are often required to identify the target tumor and surrounding anatomical structures, and to guide the fluoroscopic simulation of the treatment position. The treatment simulator displays the treatment fields, ensuring the location of the target volume and identifying the surrounding normal tissues, thereby protecting them from excessive radiation. Radiographs are taken of the treatment field, and customized block templates are drawn on these films by the radiation oncologists. Mold-room technicians use these films to create customized lead blocks to protect normal tissues from the radiation beams.[4] Once the treatment field is confirmed, the fields are indicated on the skin surface with indelible marks that serve as guides for treatment field placement and as permanent records if future radiation treatment should be required. Patients must assume and maintain the same exact position throughout the course of treatment. In order to facilitate this degree of precision, polystyrene plastic casts are created that conform to the body contours and help the patient to maintain the same position over the course of treatment. Additionally, laser lights are used to align patient position on the treatment machines.

Simulators have improved the precision of the delivery of radiation therapy. The need to use simulators evolved for the following reasons: (1) the relationship between the radiation beam and external and internal anatomy cannot be assessed by diagnostic radiology; (2) the radiographic quality of the treatment machines is not sophisticated enough to be used for precise field localization; and (3) the use of a treatment machine for field localization is impractical and creates time constraints. Potential problems with patient treatment setup can be identified and solved during simulation. Anatomical contours and thickness relating to tissue compensators or bolus designs can be obtained during simulation. The simulator can determine the adequacy of the fabrication of shielding blocks. Laser lights, contour makers, and shadow trays are equipment accessories of simulators that facilitate these functions.[3]

Port Films

Port films are radiographic images taken by linear accelerators to verify treatment fields. These high beam energies do not produce images as detailed as standard diagnostic radiographs, however, they provide information about treatment accuracy and quality.[4] Weekly port films should be considered mandatory to ensure departmental quality assurance. Patients frequently ask the radiation oncology nurse about the results of the "x-rays," or the port films. Nurses need to educate patients and families about the specific purpose of the port films, explaining that tumor filming for diagnostic and staging purposes usually occurs at the completion of treatment and beyond.

The Treatment Plan

Appropriate, effective radiation dose distribution is determined by the medical physicist and dosimetrists using

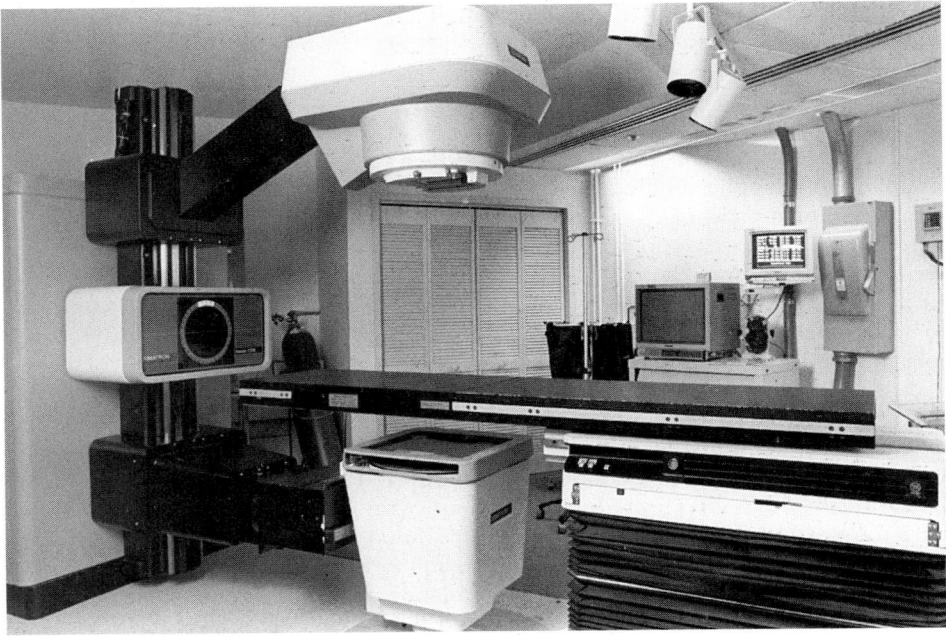

Figure 16-1 The treatment simulator is a conventional radiation treatment planning unit. This includes a fluroscopy unit that geometrically duplicates an actual radiation treatment machine. (Photo courtesy of Fox Chase Cancer Center.)

the information from pretreatment CT scans and the simulation. All of these calculations are computerized and include depth of beam dose and beam profile. The usual numbers of beams are two to four and are determined by the medical physicist in conjunction with the radiation oncologist. The goal of treatment and appropriate dosing always remains constant: Maximize the tumor dose and minimize surrounding normal tissue exposure. The radiation oncologist is usually given a choice of several treatment plans, and the one that provides the most optimal dose is chosen. Specific planning computers calculate the amount of time that each beam is on during treatment. The details of the treatment planning, including beam time, beam angles, compensators, casts, tattoos, lasers, and blocks, are documented in the patient's chart, which resides at the treatment machine. Therapists administering the treatment use the patient record to set up the patient each day.[4]

Delivery of Radiation Therapy: Machines and Complementary Equipment

Linear Accelerator

Linear accelerators (LINAC) deliver high-energy radiation to tumors (Figure 16-2). They use high-frequency electromagnetic waves to accelerate charged particles like electrons to high energies through a linear tube. When a beam of electrons is generated and accelerated by the LINAC, the energy increases. The electron volt (eV) is the basic unit of energy used in radiation oncology, and the escalating energy levels are kilovolts (10^3 eV = 1 kV)

and megavolts (10^6 eV = 1 MeV). The electrons produced by the LINAC strike a target and produce x-rays of varying energies in the 10- to 30-kV range; superficial units are between 30–125 kV, and orthovoltage units produce x-rays from 125–500 kV. The charged electrons of the LINAC can be used to treat surface lesions as well as deep tumor targets.[4]

In lower energy LINAC machines (6 MeV), the electrons proceed straight down a short accelerator tube to strike a target and produce x-rays. In higher energy LINAC machines (18 MeV), the accelerator structure is longer and therefore must be angled to bend the electrons before striking the target.[5] An elaborate beam transport system made of specific bending magnets and focusing coils is responsible for directing the highly charged angled electrons. The LINAC treatment head is made of a thick shell of shielding material to provide protection from the danger of radiation leakage.[3]

Collimation

Collimation refers to the treatment administration technique of shaping the radiation beam to the desired target. The collimator is located in the head of the LINAC. The high atomic number collimators can vary the treatment field size from 4 × 4 cm to 40 × 40 cm.[4] Electrons disperse easily in air and, therefore, the beam collimator must be approximated to the patient; 80–100 cm is the most common distance. The collimation system basically consists of a primary fixed collimator situated beyond the target in the direction of the beam, and secondary movable collimators that shape the beam into square or rectangular fields. The two pairs of leaves in the secondary collimator can be

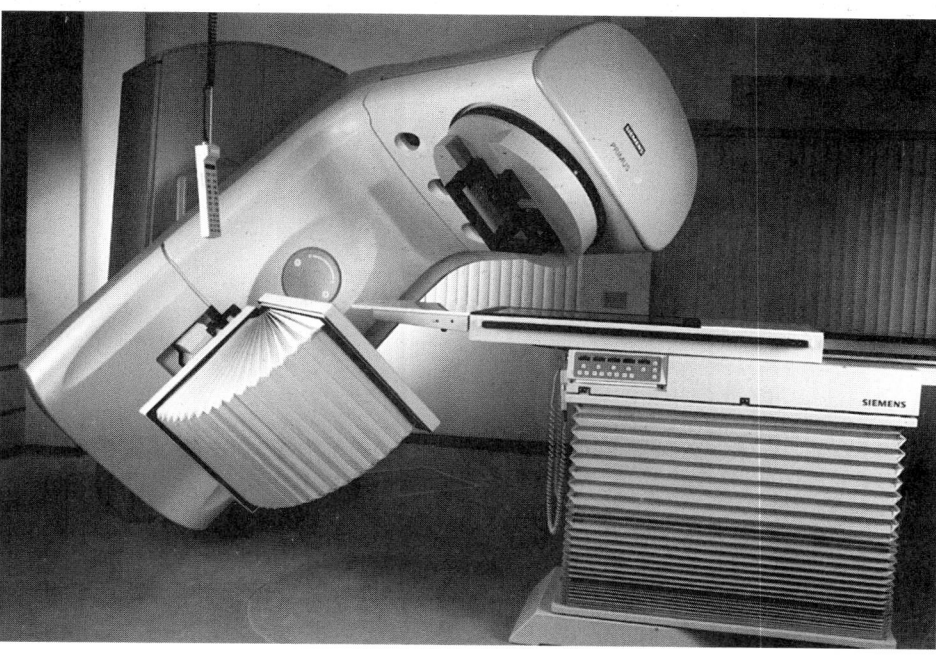

Figure 16-2   The linear accelerator (LINAC) is the most frequently used contemporary radiation therapy delivery unit. (Photo courtesy of Siemens Corporation.)

moved in and out from the beam to increase or decrease the size of the treatment field. The leaves also can be closed or opened to provide the widest treatment field necessary.[5] Various sizes of cones are attached to the collimators and extend to the skin surface of the patient. Lead cutouts at the end of the electron cone can provide additional beam shaping. Collimation is required for each treatment setup.[5]

The recent introduction of multileaf collimators (Figure 16-3) installed in the gantry of the LINAC, directly in the path of the beam, has revolutionized treatment field shaping. The treatment fields produced by the multileaf collimator have rough edges compared with the well-circumscribed fields from custom beam-shaping blocks.[5] Multileaf collimators have been useful in providing computerized customized blocking that does not require the physical creation of a new block for each field. This has lessened the workload of the mold-room technicians and has minimized the amount of time required for treatment planning and administration. The multileaf collimator can be programmed to change the shape of the beam to match the target shape as the beam moves around the target. This is called *dynamic beam shaping*.[3] The process is considered to be clinically superior because of enhanced tissue sparing.

The multifaceted radiation oncology nurse role demands that the nurse develop an expanded knowledge base beyond clinical management issues. It is important for the radiation oncology nurse to understand the intricacies of treatment machine options, the associated costs, maintenance requirements, and pertinent information for patient education. This knowledge will provide a more comprehensive approach to patient care.

Orthovoltage Units

Orthovoltage units are x-ray machines that operate in the range of 150–500 peak kilovoltage (kV[p]). Filters are used to harden the x-ray beam and facilitate the limited penetration of these superficial x-rays. The degree of hardening depends on the generated energy of the beam and the thickness of the filter. This event is known as the half-value thickness (HVT).[3] Many combinations of filters are used in orthovoltage units to achieve desired therapeutic ranges of HVT. Orthovoltage machines operate at source surface distance (SSD) of 50–70 cm. Some of these machines have lead shields installed in the head that define the square and rectangular field sizes. Often, lead shields can be fashioned and placed directly on the patient. Only minimal lead thickness is required to shield the dose.[3,5] The maximum dose of the orthovoltage machine occurs very close to the skin surface and diminishes by 90% at about 2 cm of depth. Because the maximum dose from this low-energy unit is found on the surface of the patient, the skin becomes the dose-limiting organ.[4] It is therefore essential to protect the overlying skin from excessive radiation and to avoid treating deeper lesions. Backscatter is significant in the orthovoltage treatment range and increases proportionately as the size of the field increases. Dose rates are low due to the long SSD and due to the filtration of the beam.[5]

Orthovoltage machines continue to be used at radiation oncology centers to treat superficial skin lesions. However, the use of electron therapy to treat superficial cancers has made orthovoltage equipment obsolete. Therefore, as these units require repair and maintenance they are being replaced.

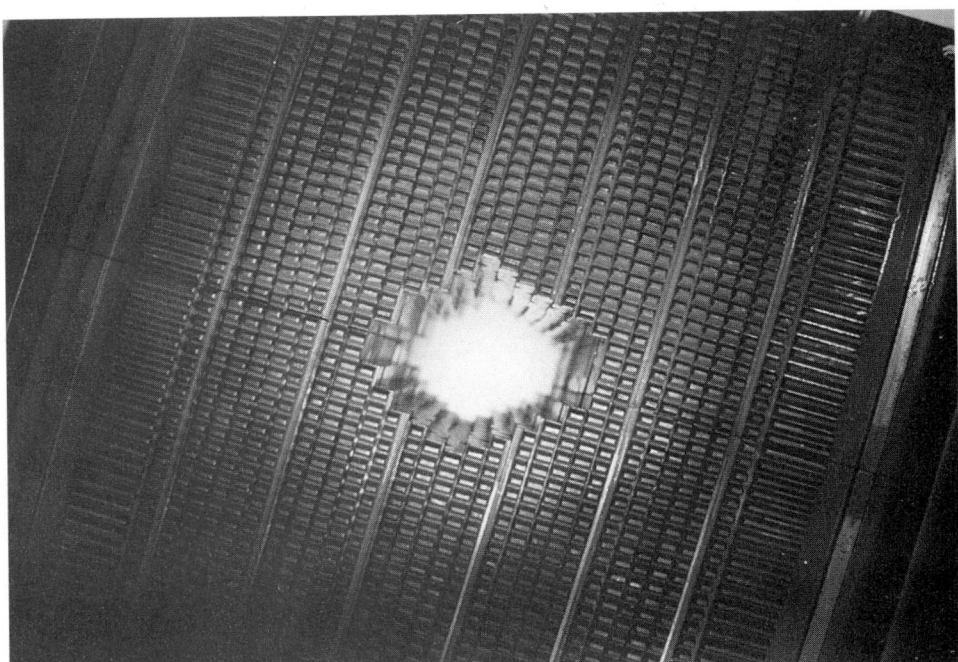

Figure 16-3 The multileaf collimator is used to define the treatment field configuration while shielding local and regional normal tissues. (Photo courtesy of Siemens Corporation.)

Megavoltage Units

During the past few decades the megavoltage linear accelerator has been the contemporary machine of choice used to deliver radiation treatment. The production of x-rays is exactly similar to the lower voltage machines. The energy range of the megavoltage machines is broad and ranges from 4–20 MeV. The depth of the maximum dose ranges from 1.5–3.5 cm. The skin dose is 30%–40% of the delivered dose. The electron beam capabilities of the megavoltage machines range from 5–20 MeV. An electron beam is produced by the removal of the tungsten target from the path of the beam. This electron beam is used for treatment purposes. The electron skin dose is high from megavoltage machines, about 80%–95% of the delivered dose. A standard formula relating to the depth of electron penetration is that 80% of the dose is delivered (in cm) at a depth corresponding to one-third of the electron energy in MeV. For example, a 12-MeV beam will deliver 80% of the dose at a depth of 4 cm.[4]

Machine Design

The treatment machines are built to accommodate continual daily use for large cohorts of patients. The machines are compact and have a rotating feature that allows for 360-degree movement around the patient. This rotation offers a variety of options for beam angles to reach the target site. Distance must be provided between the patient and the beam-defining structures to allow for a safe rotation and to avoid collision with the patient and the treatment table or couch (Figure 16-4). The couch must be positioned to avoid potential interference of the beam by bars or rails. Treatment couches typically have removable sections that can be replaced either by thin polyester-film sheeting or a meshlike insert to support the patient. The removable sections provide two different options for patient treatment. Removable side sections with a center spine for a continuous surface provides treatment of posterior oblique fields without side rail interference. A large removable center couch section allows for the treatment of a wide posterior field. Side rails are the link to support the segments of the couch, which are separated.[5] Patient safety and comfort are priorities when treatment positioning occurs. The radiation therapists, together with the radiation nurses, must develop thorough preparatory information to ease patient fears and to ensure that a secure environment is provided throughout the treatment course. It may be appropriate to invite the patient and family to visit the treatment room to see the machines and associated equipment early in the process so that questions and concerns can be addressed prior to the actual planning and treatment sessions. Concerns about an unfamiliar environment, coupled with the multitude of anxieties associated with the entire cancer experience, can be alleviated by providing a personal introduction and tour.

Principles of External Beam Radiation Dosing/Dosimetry

Radiation dosing is a complex process that requires a strong background in physics. For purposes of this chapter, general definitions and key concepts are provided to serve as an adjunct to the radiation oncology nurse's clinical knowledge. Dose measurements of radiation are

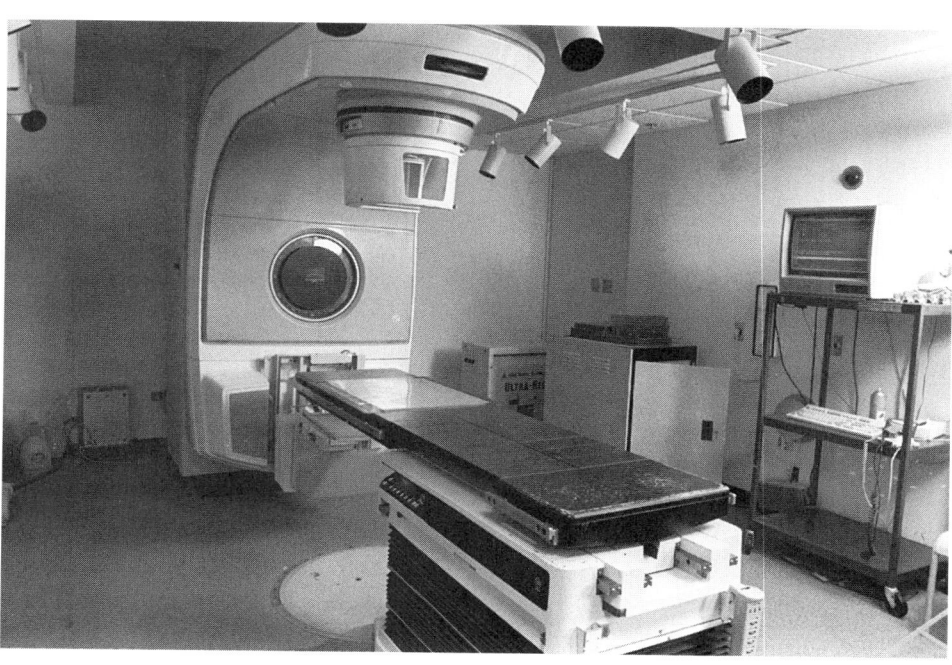

Figure 16-4 The treatment couch is used to position the patient for radiation treatment delivery. (Photo courtesy of Fox Chase Cancer Center.)

determined when the radiation beam hits the target (i.e., the patient). These measurements are dependent on the depth of the calculation point below the point of entry (depth), the penetrating power of the beam (energy), the tissue type that must be penetrated (density), the distance from the radiation source to the skin surface (SSD), the size of the field on the skin surface (field size), and the type and design of the collimator.

Measured data tables are created for each treatment machine and are planned using anthropomorphic phantoms, which are commercial systems that simulate various body tissues and are also used to determine dose distribution. Frequently, water is used as the phantom material because it absorbs radiation similarly to human soft tissue. Sheets of varied tissue-equivalent plastics are also used for convenience. These measured data tables are referred to as *dosimeters* and are used by dosimetrists to quantify radiation dose distributions within phantom substances. These measurements are then used as patient controls for dose.[5]

The dose calculation must adhere to a strict check-and-balance system to ensure the utmost precision of the derived values. The components of dosing must include consistency of all aspects of the treatment machine and the data tables in order to avoid fatalities associated with either overdosing or underdosing. The radiation physics team is responsible for documenting congruence of machine settings with treatment plans on a daily basis. Occasionally, dosimeters may be placed inside patient tissues to measure the actual dose delivered. This information can then be correlated with the treatment dose prescribed. Dose calculations are often written to four significant figures, however in practice the exact dose cannot be known with this degree of certainty. Although computers have enabled radiation treatment planners to carry dose calculations to large numbers, such large numbers do not ensure increased accuracy. Typically, medical physicists and dosimetrists round the numbers to the nearest whole number derived for dosing. This practice can be done with confidence, as it is not clinically possible to set treatment machines to fractions of dosing units.[5]

The *absorbed dose* of radiation is the energy deposited in a small fixed weight of the material (tissue) surrounding the point in question. The unit of dose measurement is the rad (radiation absorbed dose) that is considered a dose or energy-deposition of 100 erg per gram. In clinical practice, the rad is being replaced by the gray (Gy), which is 100 times larger (1 Gy = 100 rad). One rad is therefore the same as one hundredth of a gray, or 1 centigray, usually written cGy:

$$1 \text{ rad} = 1/100 \text{ Gy} = 1 \text{ cGy}$$

Dose Delivery of Radiation

Dose delivery of radiation involves two major components. The first determination is to identify the output of the treatment machines from a specified point in the beam, to the specific distance from the target, and through a specific medium. The second aspect of dosing is the determination of the actual absorbed dose within the medium. Both of these dose delivery concepts require precise calculations, thorough knowledge of the irradiated material, and a geometric relationship with the proposed beam, and the size of the irradiated field.[3]

Secondary electrons are set in motion when high-energy photon beams strike a medium. These secondary electrons have the ability to penetrate to a depth that depends on the photon energy and the composition of the medium. When the electron equilibrium is reached at this depth, the maximum dose is achieved. The maximum depth is referred to and written as *Dmax*; the maximum dose is also referred to and written as *Dmax*. These abbreviations are used interchangeably. The Dmax is the point of build-up of peak radiation dose in tissue. As the x-ray energy increases, the Dmax extends more deeply in the tissue. This is a significant measurement due to the increased skin-sparing abilities of high-energy LINAC. The *build-up region* is the difference between the surface and this depth. The dose in the build-up region increases as the electrons add to the total dose administered. This is the premise for skin-sparing capabilities. The surface layer receives a smaller dose than layers between the surface and Dmax. If mechanical devices from the machines or if the patient's clothing intercepts the beam within a few centimeters of the skin surface, the skin-sparing effect is diminished or lost. More efficient skin sparing occurs with the use of higher energies, through which the Dmax increases. The beam dose falls gradually off at higher energies due to the combination of a smaller photon supply and increased distance from the target.

The *percent depth dose* (%DD) is the absorbed dose at a given depth expressed as a percentage of the absorbed dose at a reference depth. This value varies according to energy, field size, SSD, and by change in medium. The %DD falls less rapidly with higher energy.[3,5] The %DD can be measured and plotted to form a %DD curve. As energy increases, the penetrative ability of the beam increases and the skin dose decreases (Table 16-1).

The *inverse square law of radiation* states that the intensity of a radiation beam is inversely proportional to the distance from the source squared. For example, the radiation dose at 2 cm will be one-fourth the dose at 1 cm. The inverse square law governs the theory of the intensity of an x-ray beam. Collimators and other scattering devices may cause deviation from the inverse square law. The inverse square law must be checked for completion and accuracy in order to avoid serious error in dosing.

The radiation beam must pass through tissues of different densities. The variance in lung, bone, fat, muscle, and air affects the beam penetration and amount of scatter. The overall effect on the dose depends on the size of the treatment volume, on the amount of density, and on the beam energy. The variability of irradiated mediums requires complicated changes in dosimetry. The dose effect near the interface between layers of different densities is complex. Historic difficulties outlining treatment

Table 16-1 Dose Determination Measurements and Techniques for External Beam Radiation

Acronym	Term Defined
HVT	Half-value thickness: Penetration or quality or hardness of beam. The thickness of the material that reduces the intensity of the beam to half its original value. Low-energy beams and photon beams are described in terms of HVT.
SSD	Source surface distance: Measure of radiation dose in the absence of a scattering phantom. Sometimes referred to as "in air" measure.
SAD	Source axis distance: Measurements of radiation beam in air.
Dmax	The point of build-up of peak radiation dose in tissue.
%DD	The absorbed dose at a given depth expressed as a percentage of the absorbed dose at a reference depth.
TAR	Tissue air ratio: Calculates radiation dose in rotation therapy; when source of radiation moves in a circle around the axis of the gantry rotation, TAR is the ratio of the dose at a given point in a medium to the dose at the same point in free space. $$TAR = \frac{\text{Dose in tissue}}{\text{Dose in air}}$$
TPR	Tissue phantom ratio: Used in dosimetry of high-energy beams; eliminates unreliable in-air measurements. The ratio of dose at a specified point in tissue or in a phantom to the dose at the same distance in the beam at a reference depth of 5 cm. $$TPR = \frac{\text{Dose in tissue}}{\text{Dose in phantom}}$$
TMR	Tissue maximum ratio: A special case of TPR; reference depth is at Dmax. TMR is the ratio of the dose at a specified point in tissue or in a phantom to the dose when it is at the depth of maximum dose. $$TMR = \frac{\text{Dose in tissue}}{\text{Dose in phantom Dmax}}$$
SAR	Scatter air ratio: The ratio of the scattered dose at a given point in a medium to the dose in air at the same point. Used for calculating scattered dose in a medium.
Isocentric technique	Known as fixed source-axis technique to distance (SAD). Occurs when the axis of machine rotation (the isocenter) is placed in the target volume. Spares tissue around the target by limiting tissue exposure to the radiation beam.
Penumbra	Region near the edge of the field where dose rapidly falls.

Data from Bentel.[5]

borders had created tremendous problems when calculating a dose from beams that crossed inhomogeneous volumes. The contemporary use of CT to provide detailed outline of irregularities and information about the density of the target medium has improved dosing capabilities.

Radiation doses must be measured through different mediums to accurately determine patient dose. Dosimetrists measure ionization of the radiation beam in air and identify this quantity as the degree of exposure. The next steps in the process involve correcting for the presence of soft tissue in air, and the absorbed dose is derived in grays.

Identifying dose variations within a field at prescribed depths is an essential component of radiation dosing techniques. The variety of clinical presentations requires that radiation treatment planning and dosing provide the capabilities to achieve a standard of safe, effective, and methodically planned treatment to targets while sparing surrounding anatomic structures. This treatment must also be reproducible on a daily basis to an exact standard, and concomitant accuracy checks and balances must be provided. Radiation oncology nurses benefit from understanding the conceptual framework that guides dosimetric treatment planning so that technical and clinical patient queries can be appropriately answered or referred.

Field-Modifying Instruments

Beam-modifying absorbers known as *filters* or *wedges* can be placed in the path of a beam. A typical beam-modifying filter is a wedge-shaped device made of dense material such as lead that progressively extends the beam across the field. The wedge has a thick and a thin side, which creates tilted isodose curves. The angle of the wedge is the angle through which an isodose curve is tilted at the central axis of the beam and at a specific depth. The degree of tilt changes with the depth, therefore the predetermined depth is critical. The reference depth may vary, however, the wedge angle is commonly defined at the intersection of the central axis of the beam and the 50% isodose curve. The *wedge angle* refers to the tilt of the isodose curve, not the angle of the wedge filter. The wedge angle or tilt produced by a wedge has a different angle than the wedge material. Some wedge filters with standard isodose curves are prefabricated; others can be customized by technicians[5] (Table 16-2).

Tissue Compensation

When a radiation beam is projected along an irregular or sloping surface, this causes bending of the isodose curves. Such distortion may be responsible for unacceptable nonuniformity of dose within the target and also has the potential to cause excessive irradiation of sensitive structures such as the spinal cord. Several techniques are used to preempt this problem, such as the use of wedges and the addition of bolus material or compensators. Treatment fields with thinner tissue planes can be blocked for the last few treatments to reduce radiation dose.[3]

Bolus is a tissue-equivalent material that is put directly on the patient's skin to even the irregular contours and to create a flat surface that normalizes the radiation beam

Table 16-2 Field-Modifying Instruments, Glossary

Instrument	Definition
Wedge transmission factor	Ratio of the dose rated on the central axis with and without the wedge. Must be included in the dose calculation to account for progressive attenuation of the beam by the wedge.
Universal wedge	A given angle, fixed in the beam and applied to all beam widths up to a specific limit; creates uniform attenuation across the field.
Individualized wedge system	Multiple wedges designed for a particular field width. Beam passes through minimal material and slightly reduces the dose.
Dynamic wedging	Wedge effect by driving a collimator leaf across the field to increase the field size. Starting position of moving leaf receives higher dose, then final position.

Data from Bentel.[5]

(Figure 16-5). The use of a bolus differs from the application of a bolus layer, which is sufficiently thick to provide adequate dose build-up over the skin surface. The bolus layer is often referred to as the *build-up bolus*. When orthovoltage energy is administered, placing bolus directly on the skin surface is an appropriate treatment administration technique. When higher energy beams are used, bolus application on the skin surface creates a loss of the skin-sparing advantage. In this instance, compensating filters are used that approximate the effect of the bolus and also preserve the skin-sparing effect.

Compensators are designed to provide the required beam arrangement that occurs in the "missing" tissue when the body surface is irregular. The compensator is positioned at a distance from the target (15–20 cm away from the skin) in order to preserve the skin-sparing effect of the megavoltage machines. Compensators should have adjustable dimensions and shapes. The compensator must account for beam divergence, linear attenuation coefficients of the filter material and soft tissues, and the reduction in scatter at different depths. Compensators are constructed of various materials in order to accomplish their objectives. Compensating wedges (C-wedges) are used for oblique beam incidence or curved surfaces and are made from various metals such as copper, brass, or lead. Their function is to compensate for a missing wedge of tissue in the treatment field.[3,5]

The difference between a wedge filter (Figure 16-6) and a C-wedge is as follows: Wedge filters can be used as compensators but are primarily used for tilting the standard isodose curves through a certain wedge angle in conjunction with the wedge-pair technique. The C-wedge is used *only* as a compensator that enables the use of the standard isodose charts without modification. As such, C-wedges are more clinically practical than wedge filters as compensators because they can be used for partial-field compensation. The C-wedge is used to compensate only a portion of the irregularly shaped con-

Figure 16-5 A bolus is a tissue-equivalent material placed in path of beam directly on the target surface. It modifies beam interaction with target surface. (Photo courtesy of Fox Chase Cancer Center.)

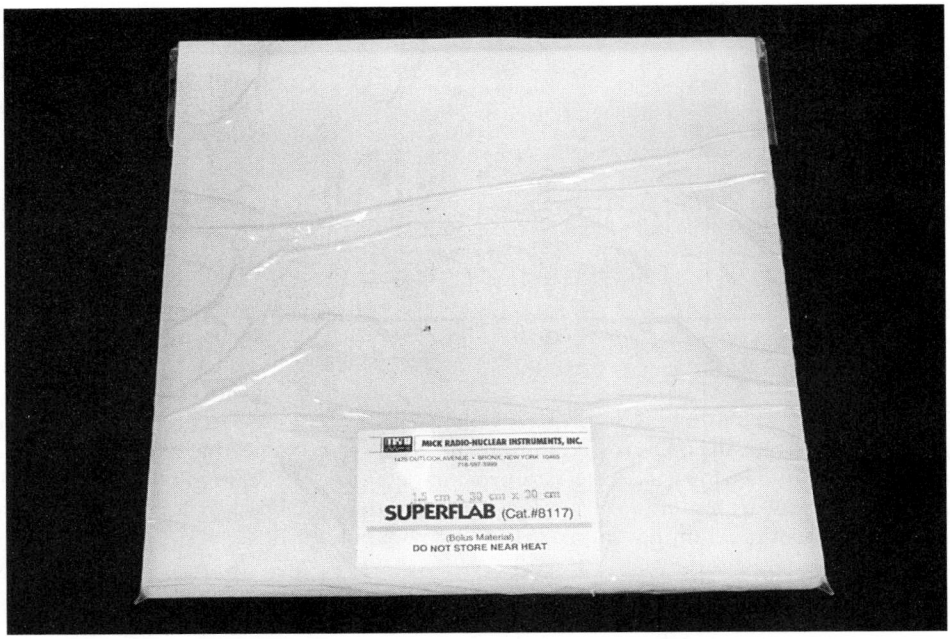

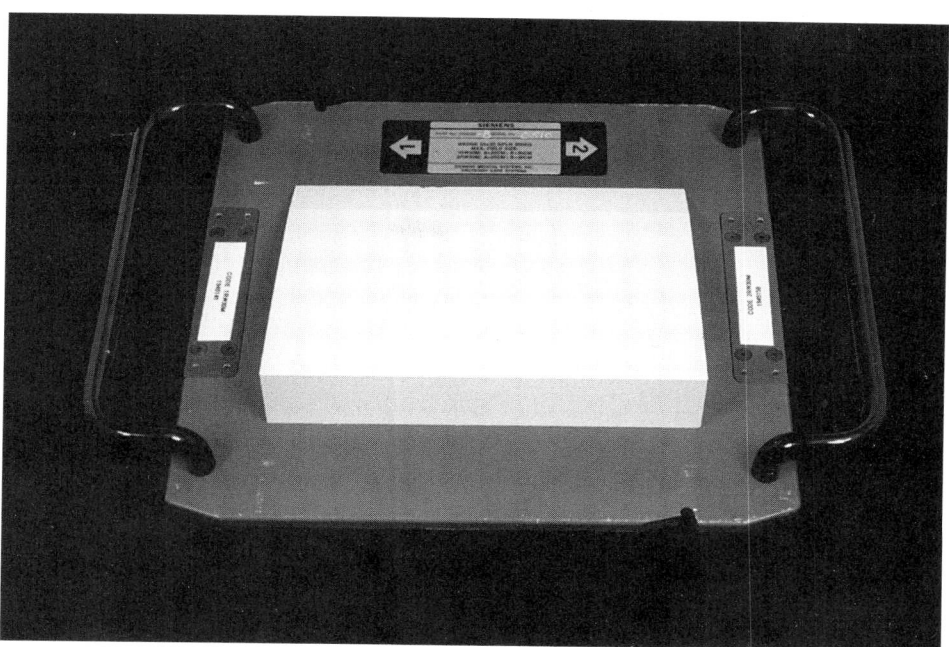

Figure 16-6 A wedge filter is placed in the path of radiation beam at a distance from the target and modifies radiation beam characteristics. (Photo courtesy of Fox Chase Cancer Center.)

tour. A wedge filter is designed to be placed in the field in a fixed position and therefore cannot partially compensate the treatment field. Additional applications of compensating filters include compensators for tissue heterogeneity (for total body irradiation), and improvement of dose uniformity in fields where nonuniformity of the dose arises from sources other than contour irregularity, such as with large-mantle fields.[3,5]

Patient Positioning and Immobilization Techniques

Patient positioning and immobilization are critical components of radiation treatment delivery. In order to achieve the goals of tumor kill and preservation of normal organs and tissues, it is mandatory that daily treatment be reproducible and accurate. If patient positioning is not exact and if immobilization devices are inadequate, lethal consequences could occur. Accuracy of radiation treatment depends on both dosimetric and geometric exactness. This section focuses on the elements necessary to achieve *geometric accuracy*, which refers to issues of patient positioning and immobilization.

Patients must be positioned so that the target is at the isocenter.[6] The advantage of isocentric technique over SSD is that the patient is not moved between fields. If the patient is supine on a horizontal treatment couch, a single skin mark (such as a tattoo or permanent ink) will locate the center of the target volume that imaging has shown to be at a certain depth (d) beneath the surface. Table 16-3 describes steps for treatment setup for isocentric radiation therapy plans.[6]

In order to achieve treatment setup accuracy, it is

essential that continuous evaluation by the team of radiation oncology professionals occur. Patients must also be assessed for safety and comfort. Patients will move if they are uncomfortable, and initially tense muscles may relax during the treatment process. Using wedges, pillows, and head cups can avoid this unintentional patient movement. The laser crosshair system is useful for providing additional markings for treatment setup guides that can ensure the patient is in the same position each day. Extending the skin markings as far superior and inferior to the central treatment plane will improve reproducibility of beams. External anatomical landmarks should always

Table 16-3 Steps for Treatment Setup for Isocentric External Beam Radiation Therapy

1. Patient is positioned on the treatment couch in either a supine or prone position, with or without bolsters, wedges, or immobilization apparatus.
2. Treatment couch is raised to the required height to align patient coordinate system with the room coordinate system. Verification occurs by superpositioning of the orthogonal room lasers with the skin marks.
3. Gantry points straight down and secondary confirmation checks are made of the target-to-surface distance (TSD) using the optical distance indicator (ODI). This is identified as the proper treatment setup position.
4. Treatment plan is implemented for each field by proper rotation of the gantry and collimator as well as by choice of field and size beam modifiers. Before treatment, a secondary check of TSD should be made for each identified treatment field.
5. Complex treatment planning (multiple isocenters) may require further delineation of the patient coordinate system in relationship to the room and beam coordinate systems.

Data adapted from Reinstein.[6]

be referred to during daily treatment setup. Distance between several visible landmarks should be done in order to determine accuracy of position. Immobilization devices should be used when appropriate. These devices begin as soft, flexible materials and then become rigid sanctuaries of comfort and security for patients during daily treatment.

Immobilization Devices

Immobilization devices help keep patients in a stationary position for daily treatment. These devices also help to minimize the potential for treatment setup errors, reduce the amount of radiation of normal tissues, and ensure appropriate treatment to the target volume. Patient immobilization equipment varies in construction materials and styles. Some are fabricated on-site and some are available from commercial suppliers. Before implementing an immobilization system, it may be helpful to assess and evaluate the individual patient and treatment objectives. This inquiry can guide the radiation oncology team in creating a safe and comfortable physical environment for patients.

The assessment begins by observing the patient's physical comfort and degree of relaxation. If the immobilization device touches the patient, it can serve as a reminder of how the position feels to the patient and therefore can be used to direct the therapists in replicating the setup. The patient must be secured in such a way as to preclude any movement. The immobilization equipment should be contoured to the patient's body surface. The equipment must fit the patient's anatomy properly and allow for variance in symmetry, body fat, and target location. The device should be able to position the patient in such a way as to minimize normal tissue complications. The immobilization equipment also should allow for unobstructed radiation beams and not interfere with the treatment plan. The material used to construct the devices should be radiotransparent, rigid, and able to be trimmed to remove sections. The devices must not cause mechanical obstruction by interfering with the LINAC gantry during beam rotation. Devices must be useable with all treatment planning systems in order to establish consistency for patient setup and treatment. If the radiation beam passes through the device, the effect on surface dose must be considered. An accumulation of surface build-up may be small, however it must be documented.[6]

The immobilization device must allow sufficient space for reference marks to be seen so patient setup can be reproduced. The immobilization device defines the patient coordinate system, which must be aligned with the room coordinate system using reference marks. This alignment occurs through the use of treatment tables and specialized adapters.[6] The immobilization device must be rigid and maintain its shape over time. If the device loosens over time, the patient may move within it, which could potentially flaw the setup. Radiation therapists should assess the fit of the device daily, and determine normal wear and tear as well as changes in the patient's weight and environmental factors that may affect the required fit.

Every aspect of medical care has become subject to cost analysis. The costs of using complex immobilization systems must be evaluated in terms of the benefit of the clinical outcome. The factors contributing to cost of an immobilization system include materials, staff time for construction and setup, supplies, potential for recycling of materials and available storage space.[6] Overall, immobilization devices have been identified as being beneficial and serve to enhance the administration of radiation treatments. Properly constructed immobilization devices can reduce daily setup times, and increase efficiency and reduce overall costs of treatment. Comfortable, well-fitting immobilization devices can reduce patient's fear and minimize misconceptions of treatment.

Immobilization devices have been identified by category. Following are the most common.

Hook-and-loop tape and straps

Many types of adhesive tape have been used in the past to secure patient position during treatment. Currently, straps with hook-and-loop backing are used to assist patient setup. Hook-and-loop tape can be affixed to the side rails of the treatment couch and then wrapped around the patient and attached to the side rail hooks. These hook-and-loop straps are padded, reusable, and much more comfortable than adhesive tape. The hook-and-loop tapes can keep both of the extremities aligned and support the chin and head and neck region.

Generic body supports

This group of devices includes foam rubber wedges and supports, plastic head cups, neck rolls, knee and lumbar supports, thigh and heel stirrups, and prone face holders. This equipment provides comfort and stability during treatment. Indexed supports are a type of body support that are indexed by size, shape, and elevation above the treatment couch. These devices provide head and neck body support as well as height and angle information for setup duplication.

Body casts

Methods and materials used to make effective body casts have evolved over the past two decades due to a need to reduce patient setup errors and to allow for three-dimensional (3-D) conformal therapy treatment methods. Many of these materials are based on the specialties of orthopedics and dentistry and use modern packaging systems. The Alpha Cradle (Smithers Medical Products, Inc., North Canton, OH) is a polyurethane foam cast that is created by placing the patient in the treatment position on a plastic bag that is within a specialized form. The form is constructed of rigid polystyrene plastic blocks. When a combination of two chemicals known as Alpha

Cradle Foaming agent is combined in the bag it expands into a polyurethane foam. The foam rises, and the patient's anatomical structures are supported. When the foam hardens, the cast is ready to use. Alpha Cradles are effectively used for a variety of disease sites. They are rigid, radiolucent, and fit snugly and comfortably to the patient's contours. However, they are unable to prevent patient movement and rotation and therefore must be used in combination with other immobilization devices. Additional methods and materials used to create body casts are vacuum bags and thermoplastics (Figure 16-7).

Positioning Devices

Positioning devices secure patients in nontraditional positions for treatment. These devices are necessary to improve the therapeutic ratio and enhance patient comfort. Varied anatomical features coupled with nonrigid human body contours require the use of positioning devices to provide stability. Neck rolls, foam wedges, head holders, and Timo, a head and neck support (Bionix, Toledo, OH) are used to arrange body parts away from the path of the radiation beam and to improve positioning.

Arm boards, knee saddles, and thigh stirrups are additional appliances used to position the extremities comfortably. Treating soft-tissue sarcomas of the limbs often requires careful positioning of the extremities. Handgrips, overhead arm positioners, and shoulder retractors are also used to place extremities out of the path of critical treatment regions. Arms can be placed above the head or at the sides in reproducible locations with couch rail–mounted or tilt board–mounted handgrips and arm supports or with overhead arm positioners.

Patient elevation systems include tilt boards, slant boards, and breast boards. Patients required to maintain supine treatment positions are often placed on tilting or slanting rigid plastic boards. These positioning devices can assist individuals who have difficulty lying supine. Tilt boards have built-in handgrips that provide comfort for arms-up treatment setups. The breast board is used most commonly for the treatment of breast cancer with parallel-opposed tangential fields. The breast board allows for arm support above the shoulders and away from the lateral field. Additionally, it allows for unobstructed access to the breast by the lateral field, places the chest wall position horizontal to avoid angulation of the collimator, and by gravity pulls the large breast down for an improved treatment position. Several clinical circumstances must be considered when treating breast patients, such as stabilizing large pendulous breasts and minimizing skin reaction in the inframammary crease.

Belly boards are specialized positioning devices used to support patients in prone positions with a window cutout for the patient's abdomen. This equipment provides comfort and stability for obese patients and minimizes the amount of intestine in the field. The treatment chair is a positioning device that is mounted on the treatment couch. The chair has head and neck supports and can provide a variety of arm positions. The treatment chair is used for patients with respiratory compromise and for mediastinal disease, as the position minimizes the amount of irradiated normal tissue.

Head fixation devices are used for immobilization during stereotactic radiosurgery and for treatment of head and neck cancer. Stereotactic radiosurgery requires the use of a frame that is bolted to the patient's skull before target localization. Metal stereotactic frames are not comfortable and are used for single fraction administration only. New noninvasive, relocatable frames are now

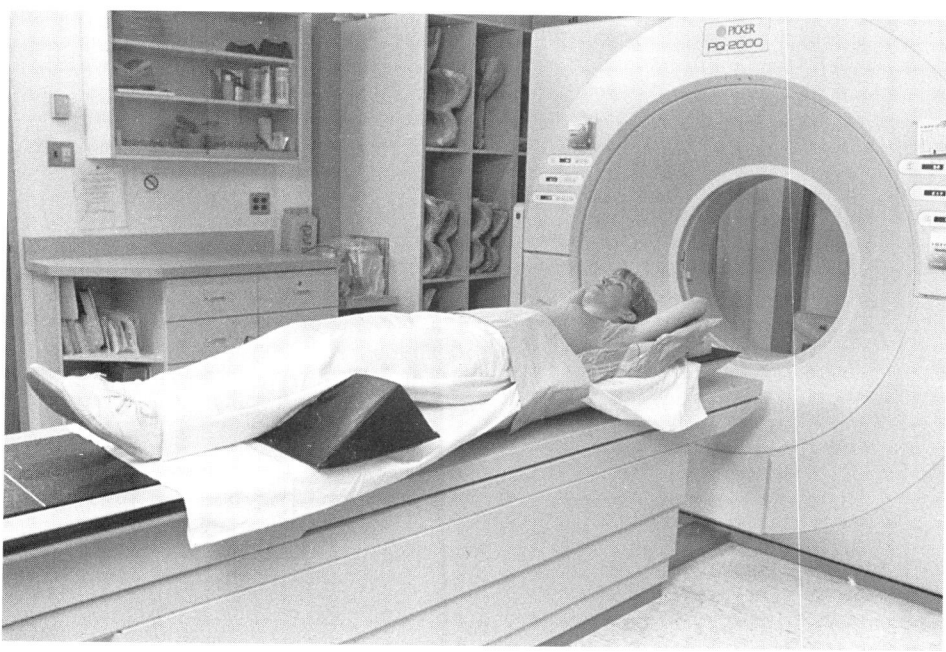

Figure 16-7 Various immobilization devices are used to maintain daily accurate reproducible patient positioning. Examples are the angle-wedged foam behind the knees and the custom-molded alpha cradle to support the head and torso. (Photo courtesy of Fox Chase Cancer Center.)

available that facilitate patient comfort and precise treatment planning. Nonstereotactic head immobilization is commonly used during treatment of head and neck regions. This device is commonly made of precut thermoplastic mesh sheets that are attached to a rigid frame. Warm water softens this system and enables the thermoplastic masks to be pulled down over the patient's face, molding to the facial contours; the masks are then attached to a base plate. Bite blocks use a dental impression mouthpiece supported by a solid base plate under the patient's head, which is fastened to the treatment couch. Adjustable bite blocks are often used in conjunction with a Timo head-and-neck support to steady the head and neck region (Figure 16-8).

Due to the enhancement of the specialty with 3D conformal therapy and dose escalation, it is essential that precise tumor control occur and that side effects be minimized. The ability to provide tight target margins, standardize dose, and maintain daily treatment reproducibility is directly related to the precision of patient positioning and immobilization. Patient position has the following limitations that preclude exactness: variance among accelerators, simulators, and treatment planning coordinate systems; daily organ movement; organ movement during the treatment processes; patient movement during treatment; rotation of the skeleton; and treatment setup errors. Appropriate patient positioning and immobilization help to diminish errors and facilitate the delivery of precise radiation. Studies have concluded that immobilization systems assist in reducing the need for large target margins.[7–9] Even more precise immobilization devices will be needed in the future to allow for the higher doses of 3D conformal radiation therapy. The combination of CT simulation with radiation therapy in the same treatment room and on the same machine (tomotherapy) is also a future possibility.

The multidisciplinary team must make it a priority to provide safe, secure, and comfortable surroundings for patients undergoing arduous, prolonged treatment. Nurses are in a key position to coordinate this effort by ensuring that patients are provided with comprehensive informed consent about these procedures and are encouraged to ask questions in order to demystify fears of the unknown associated with radiation therapy and treatment protocols.

Treatment Techniques and Delivery: Advanced Topics in Radiation Oncology

Computed Tomography Based Simulation

Computerized tomography and simulation were heretofore considered separate pretreatment procedures. Recently, CT and simulation have been studied and are now considered a combined entity for radiation treatment planning. A CT simulator is a single diagnostic treatment-planning machine that combines both procedures in one unit and therefore minimizes the number of patient visits

for pretreatment planning. In addition, CT simulation has increased speed, efficiency, and accuracy of treatment planning and delivery. To accomplish this procedure, the patient is placed on the CT simulator table, and the tumor and normal structures are outlined on each CT slice. A computer performs a 3D transformation of the CT slices and creates a digitally reconstructed radiograph (DRR).[10] The DRR resembles a normal diagnostic film, however the images are digital and are manipulated to provide improved contrast and detail (Figure 16-9). Radiation oncologists draw blocks directly on the DRR to accurately differentiate the tumor from normal surrounding tissue. The mold room uses the DRR to construct blocks. The DRR and all CT slices and outlines are then digitized into the treatment-planning computer. A contemporary mode for retrieval and monitoring of DRRs is the local area network (LAN) that enables physicians to obtain DRR and port film images on their desktop computers to ensure clinical quality assurance.[11]

Contemporary treatment planning with computer-based simulation has begun to replace traditional simulators. Computer and technological advances are providing radiation oncology with the advantages of 3D conformal radiation therapy (3D CRT). In addition, CT and magnetic resonance imaging (MRI) provide 3D images of anatomy and tumor for more accurate treatment planning.[12] The virtual simulator is used to simulate the therapy machine and operates on a digital representation of the patient. Today, virtual simulation software is widely available for clinical treatment planning.[13] The process of virtual simulation differs from conventional simulation yet still accomplishes the development of a fully documented beam arrangement. The steps to achieve virtual simulation are detailed in Figure 16-10.[14] Patients are immobilized in hemibody foam torso casts and custom foam head support with thermal plastic facemasks. Patients are placed in the immobilization device and then registered electronically with the monitoring equipment on a CT scanner table. Head casts are secured to the CT table by use of a head holder. The body casts are also registered for daily alignment but with lasers. A coordinate system is used to localize objects and is tailored to the individual patient.

Once the CT scans have been completed, the structures to be treated, target volumes, and critical structures to avoid are identified. Structures are outlined on a computer display of the scans. These outlines delineate the parameters for creating 3D graphical displays and for performing volume, dose volume, and other geometric calculations. Drawing and defining these parameters is a time-consuming endeavor. Advances in computer algorithms for pattern recognition will likely replace the need for manual depictions.[13]

Virtual simulation is similar to physical simulation because it requires a machine that can imitate the motions of the actual treatment machine. The virtual simulator display has seven panels that provide a superset of the functions of both a conventional simulator and treatment machine. The unit control panel provides the same functions as the traditional simulator. The table can be oriented along three axes; the collimator or gantry can be

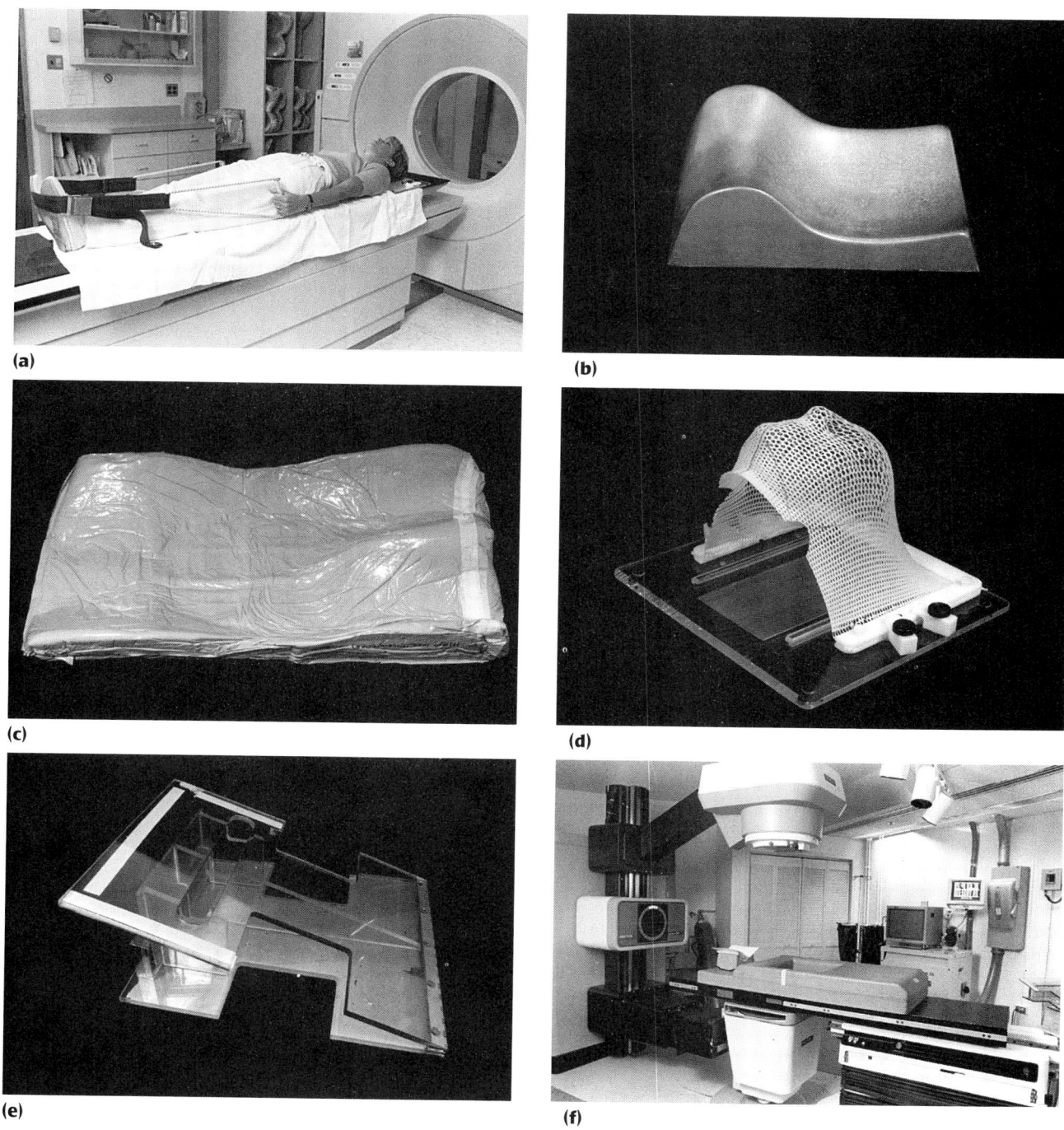

Figure 16-8 Positioning devices. **A.** Hand and foot strap to pull shoulders down and out of the radiation path when treating the base of the neck. **B.** Headrest for varying neck extension during treatment. **C.** The Alpha Cradle is an anatomically molded custom positioning device. **D.** Aquaplast is a head immobilization device of pre-cut thermoplastic sheets that are attached to a rigid frame. **E.** A breast board provides arms and breast support for improved treatment position. **F.** Belly board is a prone position support with a window cutout for the abdomen that minimizes the amount of intestine in the treatment field. (Photos courtesy of Fox Chase Cancer Center.)

rotated; and the jaws of the machine can be opened or closed by operating the corresponding control with a computer mouse. Documentation of conventional simulation consists of chart notes, simulation films, and skin marks. Virtual simulation documentation is related to these parameters and includes beam parameter settings and hard-copy block templates for the block fabrication room or multileaf collimator parameters. These are communicated over a computerized network that controls the multileaf collimator subsystem.[12]

Figure 16-9 A digitally reconstructed radiograph of the pelvis is used for radiation therapy planning and documentation of radiation treatment fields. (Photo courtesy of Fox Chase Cancer Center.)

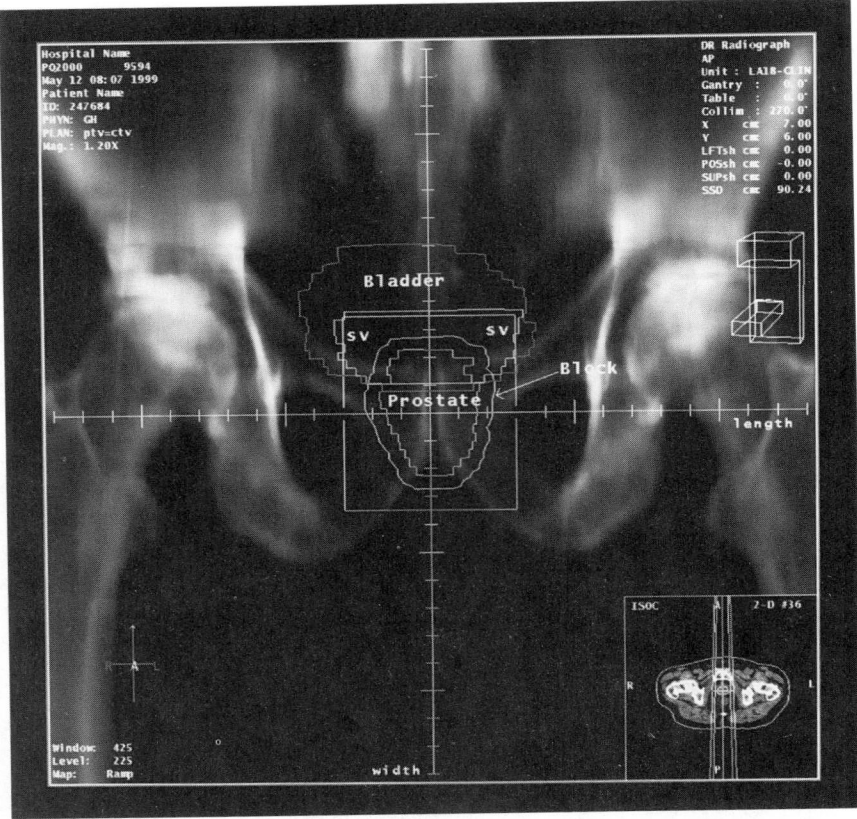

Virtual simulation provides the exact identification of structures that can be visualized on CT scans as well as conformation of beam outlines to target shapes with small margins from any direction. There are some precautions that need to be considered when using this advanced practice technique. Patient motion and internal organs are sometimes not visualized as clearly on virtual simulation as on fluoroscopic simulation. It is important to be aware of the potential for daily error due to the diminished visualization of structures. Virtual simulation often results in a CT study of greater than 100 scans, which is a large amount of data to review to form contours of structures. Virtual simulation is sometimes unable to provide a well-defined clinical target volume (CTV) for some tumor sites. If this occurs, it is necessary for radiation oncologists and dosimetrists to rely on the natural history of the patient's disease to identify the appropriate CTV.

The use of virtual simulation should be dovetailed with conventional simulation. Clinical diagnoses that require regional treatment such as breast or Hodgkin's disease may be best planned by conventional simulation. Conventional simulation is cost effective, uses minimal amount of data and personnel time, and should be considered the primary treatment-planning device within radiation oncology departments. Virtual simulation is integral for conformal treatment planning and for achieving complicated configurations. A dedicated CT simulator is usually considered only within a high-volume setting that can afford to support its use.[13]

Conformal Radiation Therapy: 3D Treatment Planning

Three-dimensional treatment planning and CRT delivers a radiation dose to a target with an improved margin for sparing normal tissue compared to standard two-dimensional treatment. Researchers worldwide developed 3D and conformal treatment methods.[12,15] The overall goal of the research and development of this treatment advance was to create a modality that would conform the radiation prescription to the target volumes and deliver lower doses to surrounding normal structures.[12] The most common clinical application of 3D CRT is for prostate cancer.[12] Table 16-4 describes the process of 3D treatment planning and CRT.

The process of 3D CRT is complicated and requires radiographic verification of the simulation procedure in some patients to confirm the accuracy of 3D plans. Block checks and a comparison of portal films with the DRR using bony landmarks is done. The dosimetrist provides dose calculations and treatment parameters recorded on the treatment record. Common tumor sites treated with 3D CRT include prostate, lung, head and neck, brain, and hepatobiliary tract. Clinical research in 3D CRT includes technical improvements with immobilization and dose delivery, reduction of dose to normal structures, and dose-escalation studies to increase dose to the target volume to improve local tumor control and survival.

Patient selection for 3D CRT must focus on individuals

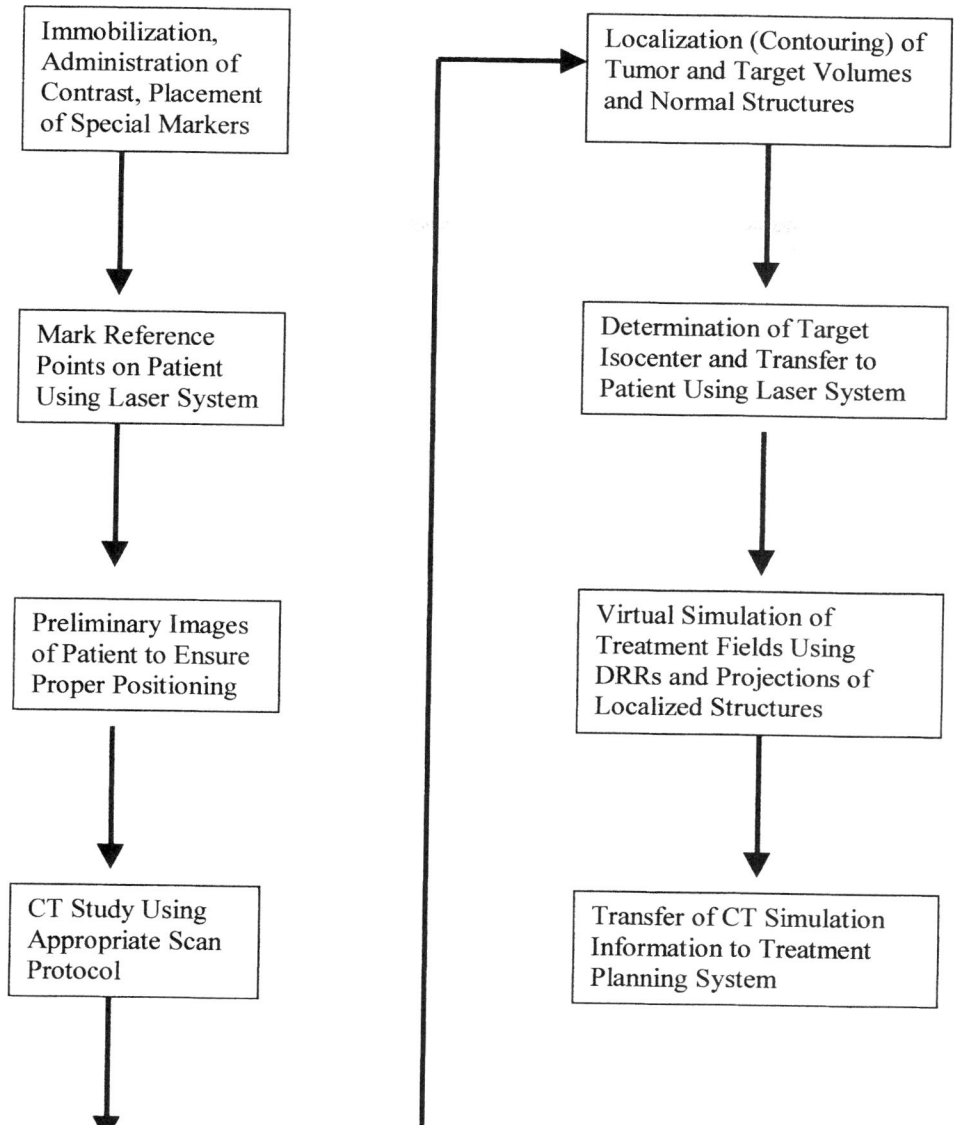

Figure 16-10
Computerized tomography simulation process. (Reprinted with permission from Hunt M: Localization and field design using a CT simulator, in Coia LR, Schultheiss TE, Hanks GE (eds): *A Practical Guide to CT Simulation.* Madison, WI, Advanced Medical Publishing, 1995, p. 37.[14])

who will benefit from this treatment delivery system. Patients with tumors surrounded by complicated anatomy, irregular-shaped tumors, or tumors near radiation-sensitive normal structures were identified to be such a population. Achieving dose escalation can be a challenge in certain sites with serial architecture (spinal cord and brain) due to the potential for complications. Some identified benefits of 3D CRT include improved local tumor control due to better coverage of target volume with a specific dose of radiation, less acute and late morbidity, establishment of dose-escalation studies, and improved survival. The efficiency of 3D CRT is improving, and more patients are being treated with the support of enhanced productivity statistics.

Three-dimensional treatment planning requires tremendous precision and accuracy. It is therefore essential that a quality assurance (QA) program include the entire multidisciplinary team, be thorough, and provide for monitoring and evaluation of all parameters of these advanced treatment modalities. The testing of hardware and software and methodical review of individual patient treatment plans must be included. The future directions of 3D physics and treatment planning will include the increased use of multimodality imaging to define the gross tumor volume (GTV) and CTV more precisely. Magnetic resonance imaging and angiography along with spectography, single photon emission computer tomography (SPECT), and positron emission tomography (PET) will be used to supplement CT data. Improved software for contouring normal structures and target volumes and virtual simulation will require less personnel time. Research will focus on the study of improved clinical outcomes as well as efficiency and cost-effectiveness in prospective clinical trials.[12]

Table 16-4 Process of 3D Treatment Planning and Conformal Radiation Therapy

- Clinical evaluation of patients, including tumor staging, functional status of uninvolved organs, and performance status

- CT simulation and placement of anatomical reference marks, and the creation of an immobilization device to assist with positioning

- Outline of target volumes (gross, clinical, and planning GTV, CTV, and PTV) and surrounding normal structures and transfer of this contour data to the 3D treatment planning system

- Virtual simulation with CT data for anatomical reconstruction and portal outline, dose planning, and beam selection for plan optimization including the generation of DRRs

- Portals are designed using the beam's eye view (BEV) and tool and beam arrangements using the room-eye view (REV), which is used to set the isocenter position and monitor beam arrangements

- Evaluations and rendering of the final plan once clinical precision is accomplished

- Review of final set of DRRs, and determination of cerrobend blocks or multileaf collimation settings

Data from Chao et al.[12]

Intensity-Modulated Radiation Therapy

Intensity-modulated radiation therapy (IMRT) is a new technology that can deliver a precise dose of radiation to the target and spare normal surrounding tissues. The beam intensity in IMRT varies across the treatment field and treats the tumor with a series of small beams of different strengths. These small beams are created by the use of a multileaf collimator or a dynamic multileaf collimator.[12] The tumor receives the dose from these beams using a crossfire technique, which creates a uniform dose, sparing the surrounding tissues. The difference between IMRT and 3D CRT is that 3D CRT uses radiation beams of uniform strength. The treatment planning software used for IMRT is based on inverse planning. The inverse planning algorithms start with the ideal distribution and find beam characteristics or profiles to produce the intended plan. This contrasts with conventional forward planning where a number of beams are directed from different directions. These conventional beams cannot treat a tumor surrounding a vital organ due to the inability to avoid dosing the normal tissue. The IMRT technology provides for separation of the tumor from adjacent structures and tissues.[12] It is considered the treatment planning system of the future and may replace 3D planning, however IMRT remains investigational and requires more clinical experience before its widespread application.[16]

Stereotactic Radiosurgery

Stereotactic radiosurgery is a 3D technique that delivers the entire desired dose in one fraction. Stereotactic principles guide radiosurgery and target intracranial lesions through the use of multiple beams. The concept of radiosurgery evolved in 1951 from Lars Leksell, a Swedish neurosurgeon. His work focused on the use of a specially designed isotope unit known as the gamma knife, which was responsible for the evolution of many radiosurgical procedures. Limited availability of the gamma knife made radiosurgery inaccessible until the mid-1980s,[16,17] when researchers began to adapt LINACs to administer radiosurgery. This made radiosurgery more available, as many radiation oncologists and neurosurgeons purchased hardware and software to upgrade their LINACs. Stereotactic techniques have expanded beyond the scope of neurosurgical procedures. During this last decade, stereotactic techniques have been applied to fractionated treatments, known as *stereotactic radiotherapy*, and applications outside of the brain.[17]

Radiosurgery techniques use a stereotactic frame fixed to the patient's skull to provide accurate landmarks for localization of intracranial targets (Figure 16-11). These targets are correlated with neuroimaging studies such as MRI, CT, and angiography. The purpose of the frame is to provide a basis for target identification within an x, y, and z coordinate system. This system is used to define the shape and extent of the target lesion.[12] Table 16-5 describes the unique features of stereotactic external-beam irradiation.[12]

Radiosurgery is indicated for distinct lesions, less than or equal to 4 cm, with the potential to respond to a single fraction of radiation. Ideal targets for radiosurgery are almost entirely spherical and small ($\leq$3 cm in maximum dimension). Irregular volumes can present the challenge of treating many isocenters to achieve conformation to the target volume. Primary and metastatic brain tumors are most commonly treated, however the greatest clinical experience has been treating arteriovenous malformations (AVMs).[12]

The two radiosurgery systems used are the gamma knife and the LINAC-based system. Both systems consist of a stereotactic frame, radiation delivery system, and computer hardware and treatment planning software. The radiosurgery system utilizes MRI or CT information to locate and determine target size and location, treatment planning needs, and type of radiation delivery. Although the systems vary, the clinical outcomes for treatment should be equal for similar patient groups. The cost of the gamma-knife system ranges from approximately $3.5–$4.2 million including new facility construction. The cobalt sources decay after 7 years and must be replaced at a significant cost. Use of the gamma knife is limited to radiosurgery. The unit contains cobalt distributed in 201 sources over a portion of a hemisphere so that circular beams from collimators may enter the skull through a large number of evenly distributed points. The gamma knife has a permanent 18,000-kg shield surrounding a hemispheric array of cobalt sources. Four interchangeable outer collimator helmets are used to vary the target volume. Individual collimators can be plugged in to conform the dose to the target shape. The target size is about 3–18 mm, with a 0.1-mm degree of accuracy.[12,18]

Figure 16-11 Stereotactic frame. **A.** Basic stereotactic system with angiographic localizer *(upper right)*, computerized tomographic localizer *(upper left)*, head ring with post and pins *(lower left)*, and a mount for positioning the patient onto the table *(lower right)*. **B.** Angiographic localizer. **C.** Computerized tomographic localizer. (Reprinted with permission from Khan, FM, Potish RA: *Treatment Planning in Radiation Oncology* Baltimore, Williams & Wilkins, 1998.[16])

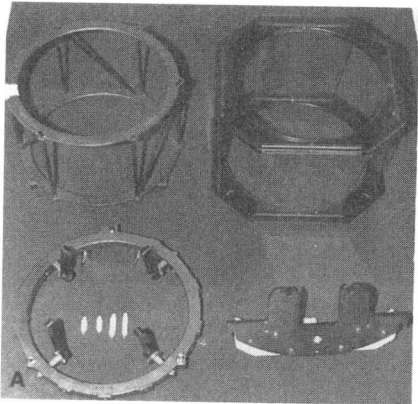
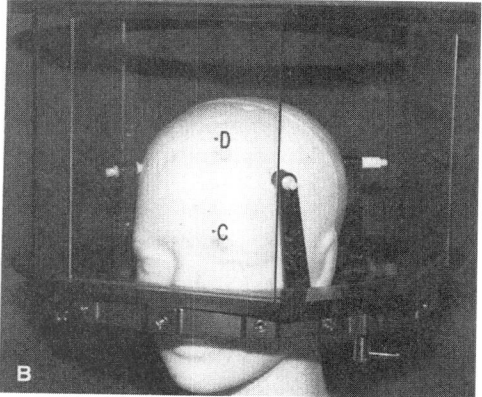
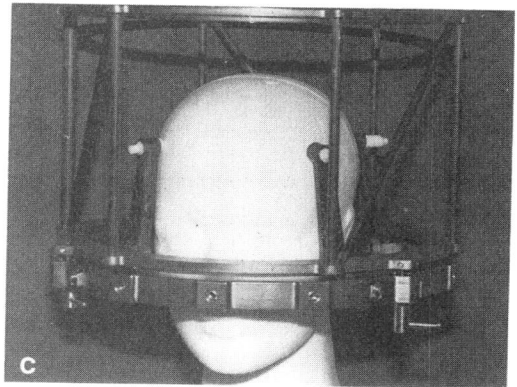

The LINAC can be adapted to administer stereotactic radiation at a much lower cost ($50,000–$300,000) than the gamma knife. Target sizes of the LINAC range from 10–50 mm with an accuracy of 0.1–1.0 mm. The LINAC administers radiosurgery in the following ways:

1. The gantry rotates through an arc for each of several stationary couch angles.
2. In dynamic stereotactic radiosurgery, the gantry and couch move simultaneously, and the beam of entry on the skull resembles a seam that provides an advantage so that beam entrance and exit doses do not overlap.

3. A rotating chair aligns and immobilizes the patient's head in a stationary radiation beam.

All techniques used to determine target volume depend on the location and type of lesion to be treated. A comparison of the accuracy of target localization, steepness of fall-off of radiation dose outside the target, and the ability to irradiate irregularly shaped targets has been made; they are comparable for both treatment systems.[18]

Approximately 6 months after radiosurgery, MRI is used to monitor the development of edema or potential radiation sequelae. The PET scan has recently emerged as a way to differentiate tumor from necrosis in previously irradiated patients.[12]

Table 16-5 Unique Features of Stereotactic External Beam Irradiation to the Brain

- Small volumes of 1–30 cm³ are treated.
- Single radiation fraction is commonly delivered.
- Target localization and treatment planning require expert and precise planning.
- High-dose gradients at field edges minimize dose deposition outside the target volume.
- Beams intersect at a common point within the skull; 3D distribution of beams minimizes the volume of normal tissue receiving moderate or high doses of radiation.

Data from Chao et al.[12]

Brachytherapy

Brachytherapy or implant therapy has been used clinically for more than 100 years. *Brachy,* from Greek meaning "short distance," is the term used to describe radiation treatment where the radiation source is in direct contact with the tumor. With brachytherapy, dose distribution is dependent on the inverse square law because the source is usually directly within the tumor volume. It is therefore crucial that the placement of the radiation sources be exact. Brachytherapy procedures can be done with either temporary or permanent implants. Temporary implants usually have long half-lives and higher energies than permanent implants. These radiation sources can be manufactured in several forms, such as needles, seeds, and ribbons (Figure 16-12). Temporary radiation sources are inserted into catheters that are surgically placed in the tumor. A few days postoperatively, the patient is brought to the radiation department for simulation. Wires with nonradioactive metal seeds are then threaded into these catheters. Films are taken and the image of the seed placement is digitized into a brachytherapy treatment-planning computer. Once the treatment plan is complete and the optimal dose rate is selected, the radioactive sources can be inserted. The implantation occurs in the patient's room. The duration is usually 1–3 days. Most temporary implants are loaded interstitially.[19]

Implantation techniques may be characterized in terms of the type of surgical approach within the target volume (interstitial, intracavitary, transluminal, or mold techniques), the means of controlling the dose delivered (temporary or permanent implants), and the dose rate (low, medium, or high). *Interstitial brachytherapy* is the surgical implantation of small radioactive sources directly into target tissues. Permanent interstitial implants remain placed forever. The initial source strength is chosen so that the prescribed dose is fully delivered when the implanted radioactivity has decayed to a negligible level. *Interstitial low-dose rate* (LDR) *brachythrapy* is commonly used to treat cancer of the oral cavity, oropharynx, prostate, and sarcoma. Intracavitary insertion consists of positioning applicators with radioactive sources into a body cavity close to the target tissue. The most commonly used intracavitary treatment technique is insertion of a tandem and colpostat for cervical cancer. Intracavitary implants are temporary; they are inserted in the patient for a specified time (usually 24–168 hours after source insertion for LDR therapy). *Transluminal brachytherapy* is the insertion of a line source into a body lumen to treat its surface and adjacent tissues. *Plesiocurie* or mold therapy is a surface-dose application, which consists of an applicator containing a variety of radioactive sources designed to deliver a uniform dose distribution to the skin or mucosal surface.[12]

The International Commission on Radiation Units and Measurements (ICRU) determines dose rates of implants.[20] Low-dose rate implants deliver doses at a rate of 40–200 cGy/hr (0.4–2.0 Gy/hr), requiring treatment times of 24–144 hours. High-dose rate (HDR) brachytherapy delivers dose rates in excess of 0.2 Gy/min (12 Gy/hr). Modern HDR remote afterloaders contain sources capable of delivering dose rates of 0.12Gy/sec (430 Gy/hr) at 1 cm distance, resulting in brief treatment times. A shielded vault and remote afterloading device are essential components of a HDR brachytherapy facility. Low-dose rate implant patients are confined to the hospital during treatment to manage the potential radiation safety hazard of the implant. High-dose rate brachytherapy is performed as an outpatient procedure. The ultra-low-dose rate range is not recognized by the ICRU report, however it is important in the implementation of treatment with permanent iodine 125 (I 125) and palladium 103 (Pd 103) seed implants. Clinical application and usefulness of radionuclides depend on physical properties such as half-life, radiation output per unit activity, specific activity, and photon energy. In the past, radium was the primary isotope used in brachytherapy. Due to its long half-life and high-energy output, radium has been replaced with cesium (Cs), gold (Au), and iridium (Ir). These isotopes have shorter half-lives than radium and can be shielded more easily due to low energies.[12]

Traditional implant systems known as Manchester, Quimby, and Paris were developed before computer-assisted dosimetry for implant therapy. These classic systems continue to guide the radiation oncologist in arranging and positioning sources for target volumes identified intraoperatively by palpation and direct visualization. Additionally, these systems continue to assist as the basis for dose prescription independent of the use of computer-

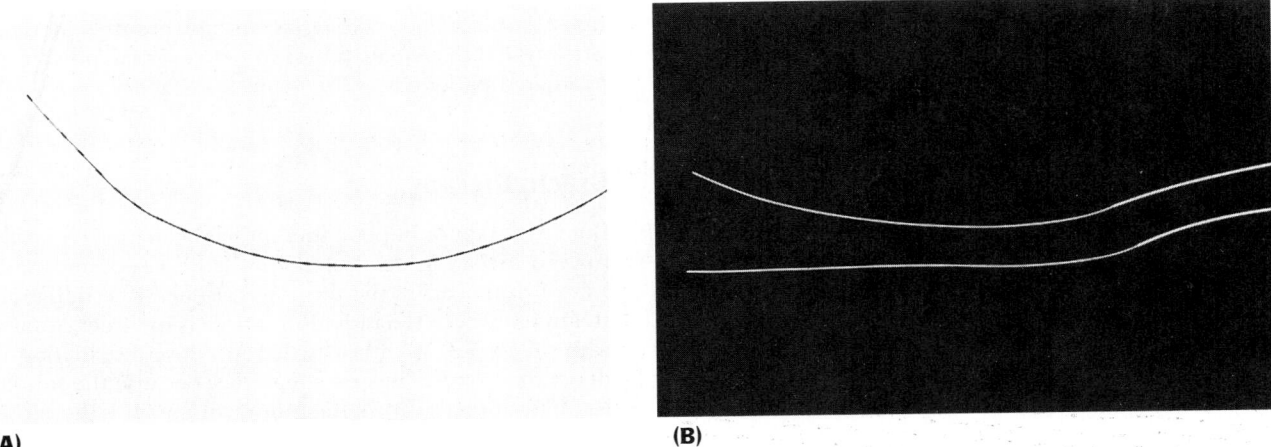

(A)　　　　　　　　　　　　　　　　　**(B)**

Figure 16-12 Brachytherapy sources. **A.** Iridium ribbon. **B.** Loading catheter for iridium seeds. (Photo courtesy of Fox Chase Cancer Center.)

assisted planning. Classic systems are useful for pre-planning of interstitial implants and for manually verifying postimplant computer plans.[12]

By using remote afterloading devices, radiation exposure can be diminished for hospital personnel and particularly for nursing staff who are primarily responsible for source loading and the care of implant patients. This delivery system consists of a pneumatically or motor-driven source transport system that robotically transfers radioactive material between a shielded safe and each treatment applicator. High-dose rate and LDR are the two types of remote afterloading that can be used. The most common LDR source is 137 Cs, which has a dose rate of about 1 cGy/min. The most common HDR source is 192 Ir, with a dose rate of 100 cGy/min.[4,12]

Pretreatment brachytherapy procedures are similar in remote afterloading brachytherapy. The treatment plan is developed by the physicists and approved by the radiation oncologists, then the patient is escorted and set up in the treatment room. The LDR or HDR source is connected to the end of a cable inside the afterloading unit. This unit has data from the planning computer. The cable is directed out of the unit into one of the patient's catheters. Several catheters can be connected to the unit. Each catheter is irradiated, one at a time, until the designated dose is achieved. The motor that drives the source out of the treatment unit is connected electronically to the treatment room door. If the need arises for cessation of treatment, opening the door will cause the source to draw back into the unit by an interlocking system. This safety device lessens the danger of personnel exposure. This interlock is the safety advantage integral to the use of this delivery system compared to manual afterloading.[21]

Low-dose rate remote afterloading is commonly used for intracavitary treatment of uterine cancer. All LDR procedures are done in the patient's room. The interlock is connected to the patients' door so that nurses can give care and family members can visit without risk. The most common applications of HDR brachytherapy include sarcomas and tumors of the vaginal apex, esophagus, lung, and floor of the mouth. Most HDR treatments are performed on an outpatient basis. This is a tremendous advantage of afterloading brachytherapy.[22,23]

Unsealed Radionuclide Therapy

Unsealed radionuclide therapy is used for the treatment of benign or malignant thyroid disease, hematological disease, malignant bone disease, and benign or malignant disease within a body cavity. Table 16-6 lists the currently approved nonsealed radionuclide sources. Strict guidelines exist for the use of these sources in women, hence verification of a nonpregnant and nonbreast-feeding condition must be established prior to the initiation of therapy. A negative B human chorionic gonadotropin test within 48 hours before therapy, documented hysterectomy or tubal ligation, a postmenopausal state with no menstrual bleeding for 2 years, or premenarche are sufficient clinical indicators to proceed with treatment. Breast-feeding must be stopped for 1 or 2 weeks prior to administration of an unsealed radioactive source.[12]

Specific Nuclear Regulatory Commission (NRC) guidelines must be followed for determining inpatient or outpatient dose, which is dependent on the total body burden of the radioisotope. Nurses must consistently but safely render care to patients receiving unsealed radioisotope therapy. It is essential that nurses reduce their exposure to emitted radiation by using the principles of time, distance, and shielding. Institutional policy and procedure must be in place to manage the total program and process as well as the possibility of emergency spills. Institutions administering both teletherapy and brachytherapy must have pre-established standards of nursing practice to ensure effective patient management as well as radiation safety. These nursing actions must focus on individual patient needs and provide detailed practice guidelines for both routine and emergency requirements. Table 16-7 provides an overview of Nursing Practice Standards from a national comprehensive cancer center (Fox Chase Cancer Center, Philadelphia, PA). These standards provide details of clinical actions for both routine and emergent situations.

Institutions administering unsealed radioactive sources must have strict quality assurance (QA) policies and procedures in place. These programs should be guided by the NRC and focus on the protection of patients, the public, and medical personnel from the potential hazards of unnecessary exposure. Table 16-8 lists the compo-

Table 16-6   Currently Approved Nonsealed Radionuclide Sources

Agent	Use
Sodium iodine (I 131)	Cure of hyperthyroidism; cure and palliation of thyroid carcinoma
Sodium phosphate (P 32)	Treatment of myeloproliferative disorders such as polycythemia vera and thrombocytosis
Colloidal chromic phosphate (P 32)	Intracavitary therapy for malignant ascites, malignant pleural effusion, and brain cysts
Strontium chloride (Sr 89)	Palliation of painful bony metastasis
Rhenium (Re 186)	Experimental. Investigated for use in treating radiation synovectomy, cystic craniopharyngioma, cystic astrocytoma, medullary thyroid carcinoma, bone metastasis. Intraperitoneal use for metastatic ovarian carcinoma.

Data from Chao et al.[12]

Table 16-7   Standards of Nursing Practice

Care of the patient receiving external beam radiation

1. Educate the patient with regard to goal of therapy and treatment experience, including simulation, setup, tattoos, blocks, and casts.
2. Be aware of patient's treatment field and teach patient symptom management of the associated general and site-specific reactions to therapy. Site-specific reactions may include diarrhea, nausea and vomiting, dysuria, dysphagia, esophagitis, mucositis, xerostomia, hair loss, and skin reactions.
3. Encourage rest periods as needed during the course of therapy to combat the anticipated side effect of fatigue.
4. Provide nutrition counseling to minimize weight loss. Encourage patient's consumption of appropriate diet for side effect management (e.g., high protein, high calorie, low residue, or soft).
5. Use skin-care products (i.e., soaps, creams, lotions, gels, etc.) only at the recommendation of the Radiation Oncology staff.
6. Initiate referral to Home Health Services if patient symptoms require continued follow-up and assessment in the home.

Care of patient receiving brachytherapy

1. Provide preimplant teaching to the patients and their families to promote basic knowledge and understanding of the goals of therapy and the treatment experience.
2. Observe principles of time, distance, and shielding while caring for the implant patient. Perform patient care from behind lead shields placed at the bedside.
3. Wear radiation film badge or direct reading dosimeter to record radiation exposure when in proximity of the implant patient.
4. Pregnant nurses are not to care for implant patients while they are loaded with radioactive sources.
5. Body fluids are *not* radioactive and may be disposed of according to routine institutional policy.
   Exception: Patients receiving systemic radioactive iodine will have contaminated body secretions. Patients' linens must remain in room in linen bag. Patient should be served meals with disposable utensils and paper products. Trash bin will also remain in room until radiation safety officer verifies it is no longer contaminated. Everything should remain in the patient's room until cleared by a Radiation Safety Officer.
6. Check radioactive sources at the beginning and end of each shift and document the status of the implant. Applicators should have caps on, and interstitial needles and catheters should be counted and observed for dislodgment.
7. If implant becomes dislodged, the nurse will retrieve the radioactive source using the provided long forceps and place it in source holder in the room. Notify the Radiation Oncologist immediately. There is 24-hour on-call coverage.
8. Know correct course of action if patient has a medical emergency.
9. Inform patient and visitors of hospital policy regarding visitation while patient has radioactive material in place. Children under 18 and pregnant women are prohibited from visiting. Any questions should be referred to the Radiation Safety Officer.

Reproduced with permission of Fox Chase Cancer Center, Department of Nursing, Philadelphia, PA

Table 16-8   Components of a QA Program for Administration of Unsealed Radioactive Sources

- Different foundations of the same isotope must be recognized when ordering them. For example, chromic P 32 is used for pleural or peritoneal instillation and sodium P 32 is used intravenously for polycythemia vera.
- The appropriate activity of isotope must be available on the date of administration, so the timing of the delivery and the availability must be considered.
- Safe handling is essential and the packaging must appropriately protect the shipment on receipt.
- Radioisotope activity must be determined with a dose calibrator that has been tested for linearity, constancy, and accuracy.
- Administration of an activity of a radiopharmaceutical that differs from the prescribed activity by more than 20% (either smaller or larger) is a misadministration. If the difference is between 10% and 20%, it is a recordable event. Compliance with Nuclear Regulatory Commission policy is mandatory.
- Prior to radioisotope administration, the following must occur: signed and dated informed consent and advanced directive, prescribed activity correct within 10%, and patient identification using two methods.

Data from Chao et al.[12]

nents of a QA program for administration of unsealed radioactive sources.[12]

Multimodality Fusion

The ability to correlate 3D images from various common imaging modalities (CT, MRI) has become a valuable tool in the practice of radiation oncology. Specialized computer software enables multimodality fusion and provides clinicians with the ability to identify structures in one imaging modality and then spatially register the structures in a different modality. The most frequently used 3D imaging modalities for treatment planning in radiation therapy are CT and MRI. Computerized tomography imaging is fast, cost-effective, and provides high resolution between structures. Magnetic resonance imaging is more costly, although it provides superior soft-tissue resolution compared to CT. Other less commonly used 3D treatment planning procedures include SPECT, PET, and ultrasound.

All of the 3D imaging techniques can be fused to any other technique. This is possible because 3D image data is stored in units known as voxels. A voxel is represented on a computer screen by a gray-scale level that represents a level characteristic to its imaging modality. The volume and size of the voxels are not equal when comparing two different imaging modalities. To equate two image sets of different size, the fusion software has to scale the lower resolution study to the same size voxel as the other study. This is done by interpolating between the voxels of the lower resolution study to create the same size voxel as the higher resolution image set. The images are packaged into equal volumes, and the minimum necessary to spatially register the studies is three unique points. These points have to represent the same point in space in each of the image sets. More points would increase the accuracy of the fusion. Scaling the images to the same resolution also allows them to be viewed together at any reference plane.[24,25]

Mathematical algorithms are often used in image fu-

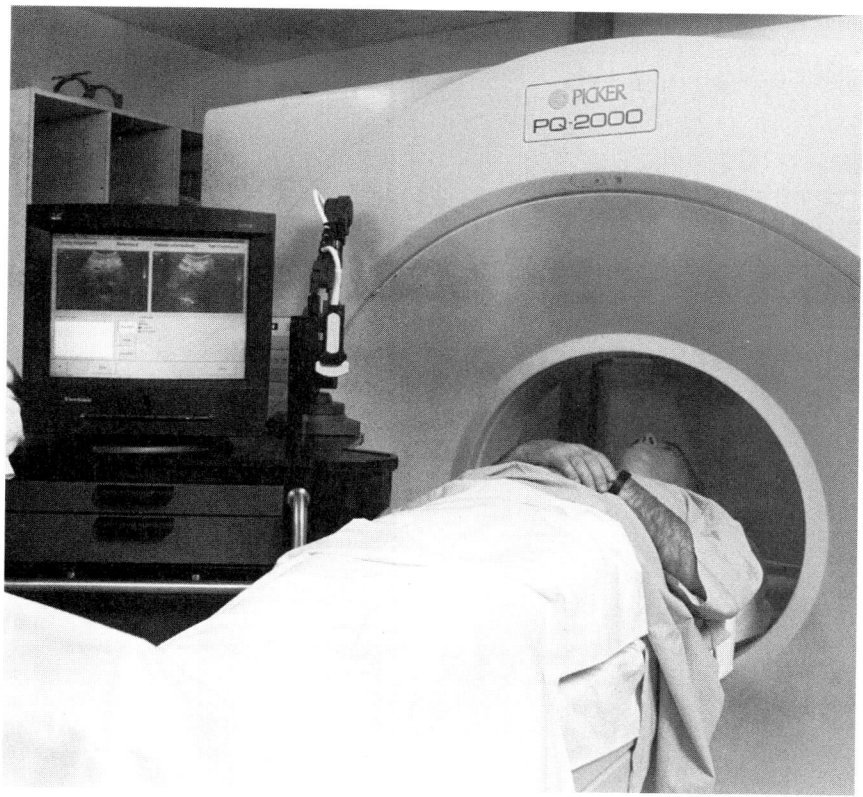

Figure 16-13 B-mode acquisition and targeting ultrasound localizing system. (Photo courtesy of Fox Chase Cancer Center.)

sion software. This registration technique works by trying to minimize the error between selected points in each study that are supposed to represent the same point in space in each study. Other sources of error in image fusion can be attributed to the accuracy of the imaging technique itself. The spatial accuracy of imaging modalities varies. Computed tomography has a superior spatial accuracy with an error of only a few millimeters over 30 cm. Spatial accuracy in MRI is not as good and can have errors up to 3–4 mm over 20 cm. Variation in patient positioning and patient motion during each of the imaging sessions can also be a great source of error. These potential errors require that the image fusion concentrate on the area of interest. The clinical application of multimodality image fusion will continue to be refined as imaging techniques and computer support evolves. This radiation planning technique has the potential to provide patients with the most exact treatment plan, which will enhance efficacy and minimize side effect profiles. The potential of this technique is still under study, but it appears to be promising.

B-Mode Acquisition and Targeting System

The B-mode acquisition and targeting (BAT) system (NOMOS Corporation, Sewickley, PA) is a patented ultrasound positioning system used for the delivery of radiation treatment to the prostate gland (Figure 16-13). This system provides a noninvasive way to deliver more precise

radiation therapy. Ultimately, it will offer the potential of improved cancer control by facilitating the safe delivery of higher radiation doses. The BAT technology combines an ultrasound probe and a 3D positioning tool to pinpoint target organs rapidly at the time of each radiation treatment session. This dramatically reduces the need to target an extra margin of tissue around the tumor site. These extra margins have traditionally been used to compensate for errors in localization of the radiation beam. As such, BAT results in a significant reduction in the amount of healthy tissue exposed to radiation. The BAT stereotactic localization device is essentially equivalent to CT scanning localization, accurate, simple to use, and adds no significant time to overall treatment.

The Food and Drug Administration (FDA) recently approved BAT. It is the only FDA-approved device of its kind on the market today. Preliminary feasibility trials occurred in 1999 at the Fox Chase Cancer Center in Philadelphia and at the Cleveland Clinic. These are the first two institutions in the world to use the BAT technology. To date, BAT has been exclusively used for prostate cancer. BAT is considered appropriate for any organ that can be visualized by ultrasound. Possible cancer sites for radiation treatment using BAT include the breast, liver, bladder, kidney, pancreas, and uterus. The ability of BAT to reduce treatment margins may allow for more successful, higher dose treatments while decreasing the risk of complications associated with either standard or escalated doses of radiation therapy. According to Gerald Hanks, MD, Chairman of Fox Chase Cancer Center Department of Radiation Oncology, the development of this ultrasound-based localization system holds great promise as a significant advancement in the treatment of solid tumors.[26]

Conclusion

The specialty of radiation oncology is a technological and clinical blend of skill and knowledge. This unique practice incorporates the talent and skills of a diverse team of professionals. Integral to the function of this complex environment is the professional oncology nurse. It is incumbent on these nurses to study, learn, and apply the scientific basis of radiation oncology practice to clinical situations. Patients treated with radiation are subject to rigorous procedures, prolonged treatment courses, and unfamiliar environments, all of which are compounded by the fear of a cancer diagnosis. Numerous questions and anxieties must be addressed. Nurses must creatively combine scientific and clinical knowledge into a pragmatic framework for patient management.

Radiation oncology continues to refine known treatment techniques and modalities and investigate new technology. Research studies focus on the enhancement of treatment planning techniques in order to provide patients with the most refined modalities. Although advanced treatment planning has become popular, few institutions have been able to implement it fully due to expense, additional staffing, and the need for sophisticated equipment. Economic restraint continues to plague institutions and hinder the installation of state-of-the-art equipment to deliver cutting-edge technology. By the time smaller, independent, less endowed radiation centers install a new technology it becomes obsolete. Therefore, it is not the pace of discovery and application of new treatment techniques that is problematic, but rather the frequent inability of institutions to keep pace economically. As such, radiation oncology professionals must advocate for the specialty so that scientific sophistication and clinical application are promoted and invoked in a timely, effective manner.

References

1. Rice AM: An introduction to radiotherapy. *Nurs Stand* 12: 49–54, 1997
2. Bucholtz JD: Comforting children during radiotherapy. *Oncol Nurs Forum* 21:987–994, 1994
3. Khan FM: *The Physics of Radiation Therapy.* Baltimore, Williams & Wilkins, 1994
4. Gazda MJ, Coia LR: Radiation treatment planning and techniques in cancer management: A multidisciplinary approach, in Pazdur R, Coia LR, Hosians WJ, Wagman LD (eds): *Medical, Surgical and Radiation Oncology* (ed 3). New York, PRR Inc., 1999, pp 649–660
5. Bentel GC: *Radiation Therapy Planning.* New York, McGraw-Hill, 1996
6. Reinstein LE: Patient positioning and immobilization, in Khan FM, Potish RA (eds): *Treatment Planning Radiation Oncology.* Baltimore, Williams & Wilkins, 1998, pp 55–88
7. Rosenthal SA, Roche M, Goldsmith BJ, et al: Immobilization improves the reproducibility of patient positioning during 6 field conformal radiation therapy for prostate carcinoma. *Int J Radiat Oncol Biol Phys* 27:921–926, 1993
8. Soffen EM, Hanks GE, Hwang CC, et al: Conformal static field therapy for low volume, low grade prostate cancer with rigid immobilization. *Int J Radiat Oncol Biol Phys* 20:141–146, 1991
9. Verhey LJ: Immobilizing and positioning patients for radiotherapy. *Semin Radiat Oncol* 5:100–114, 1995
10. Hunt M: Localization and field design using a CT simulator, in Coia LR, Schultheiss TE, Hanks GE (eds): *A Practical Guide to CT Simulation.* Madison, WI, Advanced Medical Publishing, 1995, pp 23–38
11. Das IJ, McGee KP, Desobry GE: The digitally reconstructed radiograph, in Coia LR, Schultheiss TE, Hanks GE (eds): *A Practical Guide to CT Simulation.* Madison, WI, Advanced Medical Publishing, 1995, pp 39–50
12. Chao KSC, Perez CA, Brady LW: *Radiation Oncology: Management Decisions.* Philadelphia, Lippincott-Raven, 1999
13. Sherouse GW: Radiotherapy simulation, in Khan FM, Potish RA (eds): *Treatment Planning in Radiation Oncology.* Baltimore, Williams & Wilkins, 1998, pp 39–53
14. Hunt M: Localization and field design using a CT simulator, in Coia LR, Schultheiss TE, Hanks GE (eds): *A Practical Guide to CT Simulation.* Madison, WI, Advanced Medical Publishing, 1995, pp 25–38
15. Sterling TD, Knowlton KC, Weinkham JJ, et al: Dynamic display of radiotherapy plans using computer-produced films. *Radiology* 107:689–691, 1973
16. Khan FM, Potish RA: *Treatment Planning in Radiation Oncology.* Baltimore, Williams & Wilkins, 1998
17. Bova FJ, Meeks SL, Friedman WA: LINAC radiosurgery: System requirements, procedures and testing, in Khan FM, Potish RA (eds): *Treatment Planning in Radiation Oncology.* Baltimore, Williams & Wilkins, 1998
18. Schwartz M: Stereotactic radiosurgery: Comparing different technologies. *CMAJ* 158:625–628, 1998
19. Brenner DJ: Radiation biology in brachytherapy. *J Surg Oncol* 65:66–70, 1997
20. International Commission on Radiation Units and Measurements: *Dose and volume specification for reporting intracavitary therapy in gynecology,* Report No. 38. Bethesda, MD, ICRU, 1985
21. Orton CG, Ezell GA: Physics and dosimetry of high-dose-rate brachytherapy, in Perez CA, Brady LW (eds): *Principles and Practice of Radiation Oncology* (ed 3). Philadelphia, Lippincott-Raven, 1998, pp 469–485
22. Erickson B, Gillin MT: Interstitial implantation of gynecologic malignancies. *J Surg Oncol* 66:285–295, 1997
23. Gaspar LE: Brachytherapy in lung cancer. *J Surg Oncol* 67: 60–70, 1998
24. Quarantelli M, Alfano B, Larobina M, et al: Frequency and coding for simultaneous display of multi-modality images. *J Nucl Med* 40:442–447, 1999
25. McNeeley SW: Image fusion theory and demonstration. *Proceedings Radiation Oncology Conference,* Fox Chase Cancer Center, Philadelphia, PA 1998 p 206
26. Hanks G: *Fox Chase Cancer Center Local newsletter,* 25, 1999

CHAPTER 17

Radiation Therapy: Toxicities and Management

Karen E. Maher, RN, MS, ANP, AOCN

Introduction

Approximately 60% of oncology patients will receive radiation therapy during the course of their treatment. Irradiation may be administered at multiple points in the treatment continuum, as neoadjuvant therapy, preoperative and postoperative therapy, and adjunctive treatment. Palliative irradiation may occur at multiple times depending on disease course and patient response. Combined-modality therapy of chemotherapy and/or surgery and/or radiation therapy is commonly used in the treatment of cancer. The additive effects of combining these treatments with radiation generally result in more acute and prolonged toxicities. Performance status and comorbid conditions contribute to patient tolerance of irradiation and may predispose the patient to a more difficult course of therapy. This chapter reviews the radiobiologic rationale for radiation toxicities, site specific acute and late toxicities, and nursing assessment and management.

Radiobiology

Cellular response to radiation injury is directly related to the degree of mitotic activity. Actively replicating cells have four stages and one resting phase in their life cycle:

G_1 The gap between the end of mitosis and the start of DNA synthesis
S   DNA synthesis
G_2 The gap between DNA synthesis and mitosis
M   Mitosis
G_0 Resting phase

The cell is most sensitive to radiation during mitosis and the G_2 phase, with the greatest radioresistance occurring in the DNA synthesis phase.[1] (See Chapter 15.)

The term *radiosensitivity* refers to the response of tumor cells to radiation in terms of degree and speed of response. Poorly differentiated immature cells, rapidly proliferating cells, or cells with a high mitotic potential are more radiosensitive.

Another term frequently used is *radiocurability*. This refers to local or regional eradication of tumor cells by radiation, and means that the tumor-to-normal-tissue relations are such that curative doses of radiation can be applied without excessive damage to normal tissues. Examples of radiocurable tumors are carcinomas of the cervix, larynx, breast, and prostate.

The terms radiosensitivity and radiocurability are not interchangeable. For example, non-Hodgkin's lymphoma is very radiosensitive but may not be radiocurable. All tissues have a degree of radiosensitivity, but it is the effect on normal tissue surrounding the tumor that largely determines the maximum radiation dose and resulting toxicities.[2]

The goal of radiation therapy is to destroy cancer cells while maintaining the integrity of normal tissue. This is defined as the *therapeutic ratio* (Figure 17-1).[2] Providing radiation doses within the therapeutic ratio allows for tumor eradication or reduction and minimal residual injury to surrounding normal tissues and structures. However, because ionizing radiation does not differentiate between normal cells and cancer cells, it damages both. Malignant and normal cells differ little in their overall response to ionizing radiation. Achieving the therapeutic ratio requires a delicate balance between desired treatment outcome and toxicities.

Normal cells and cancer cells undergo some degree of repair to sublethal damage between doses of radiation.

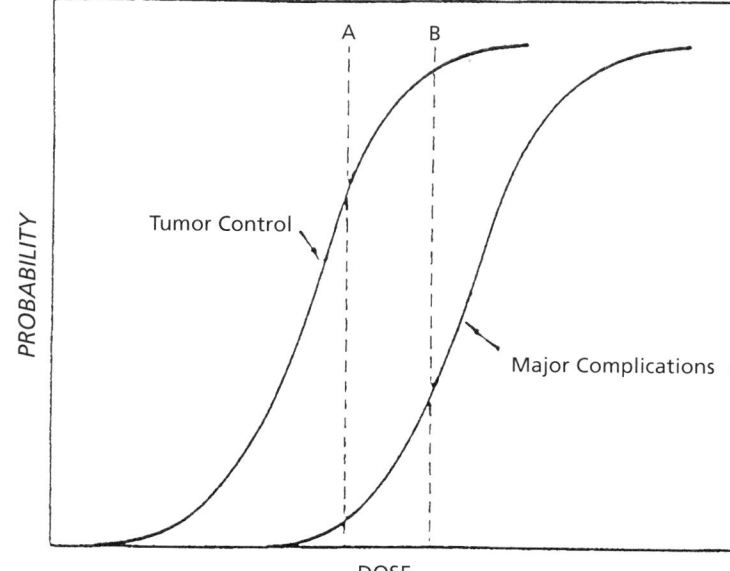

**Figure 17-1
Therapeutic Ratio.**
Sigmoid curves of tumor control and complications. (A) Dose for tumor control with minimum complications. (B) Maximum tumor dose with significant complications. (Reprinted with permission from Hellman, S: Principles of cancer management: radiation therapy, in DeVita VT, Hellman S, Rosenberg SA (eds): *Cancer: Principles and Practice of Oncology* (ed 5). Philadelphia: Lippincott-Raven, 1997, p. 320.[2])

A single dose of ionizing radiation will have a greater effect on cells than the same dose divided into several fractions. If the goal of radiation is maximum tumor cell kill while sparing normal tissue, dividing the radiation into equal doses or fractions is crucial to achieving the therapeutic ratio. Radiation is most commonly administered in a daily fraction, however *hyperfractionation* (two or more fractions per day separated by 4–6 hours) can be used in some patients. Fractionation is designed to take advantage of the "Four Rs" of Radiobiology:

1. *Repair:* The ability of cells to recover from sublethal radiation injury. Repair usually occurs within 24 hours but may occur in as little as 4 hours in some tissues. Normal cells repeatedly repair between daily doses. By contrast, tumor cells may initially repair, but as radiation continues their ability to repair decreases, thus increasing the radiation damage to tumor cells.

2. *Redistribution:* Fractionated radiation doses disrupt the cellular life cycle, causing mitotic delays in the tumor cell cycle. This theoretically enhances the effects of each succeeding radiation dose because more tumor cells are likely to be in mitosis at the same time, thus increasing the cell kill. Tumor cells may be more subject to redistribution, due in part to their erratic growth and development.

3. *Repopulation* (regeneration): Irradiated normal cells are able to complete their cell cycle and undergo successful mitoses between radiation doses. Tumor cells are more likely to die after radiation injury because of the abnormal features that result from growth and mitosis. Generally, tumor cell division stays ahead of cell death or loss, which contrasts with mature normal cell growth and division that matches cell loss.

4. *Reoxygenation:* It is believed that well-oxygenated cells do not allow reversal and repair of the chemical changes produced by radiation. The reoxygenation process involves radioresistant hypoxic tumor cells becoming radiosensitive aerated or oxygenated cells between radiation doses. In large tumors with necrotic central components, the effect of radiation is to continuously destroy the outer layers (like peeling an onion) to allow the central core to be exposed to capillary oxygenation and thus become more radiosensitive. This theory assumes there is adequate microcirculation of the tumor mass. It has been stated that reoxygenation may be the most important advantage of fractionation.[2]

In summary, fractionation of the total radiation dose spares normal tissue because repair of sublethal damage allows repopulation between doses. The redistribution and reoxygenation that occur between the daily fractions increase the radiosensitivity of the tumor cells to improve overall treatment outcome. The goal is to kill tumor cells and allow normal cells to regrow and repopulate surrounding tissue.[2]

Tissue and Organ Response to Radiation

Normal tissue response to ionizing radiation depends on the total dose, fractionation schedule (daily dose and overall length of treatment), and volume treated (Figure 17-2).[3] This concept, which will be repeated throughout the chapter, is integral to understanding the pathophysiology and occurrence of acute and late radiation-associated toxicities.[3] All cells and structures that lie within the path of the ionizing radiation beam are vulnerable. Tissue and organ systems within the body are composed of multiple cellular components that have differing radiation-tolerance parameters. Normal tissue and organ tolerance determines the limit of radiation that can be safely administered to a specific target area in the body. There is abundant literature documenting tolerance doses of tissues and structures within reasonably precise

Figure 17-2 Basic Factors Affecting Normal Tissue Response to Radiation. (Adapted with permission from Chao KS, Perez CA, Brady LW: Fundamentals of patient management, in Chao DS, Perez CA, Brady LW (eds): *Radiation Oncology Management Decisions.* Philadelphia, Lippincott-Raven, 1999, pp 1-13.[3])

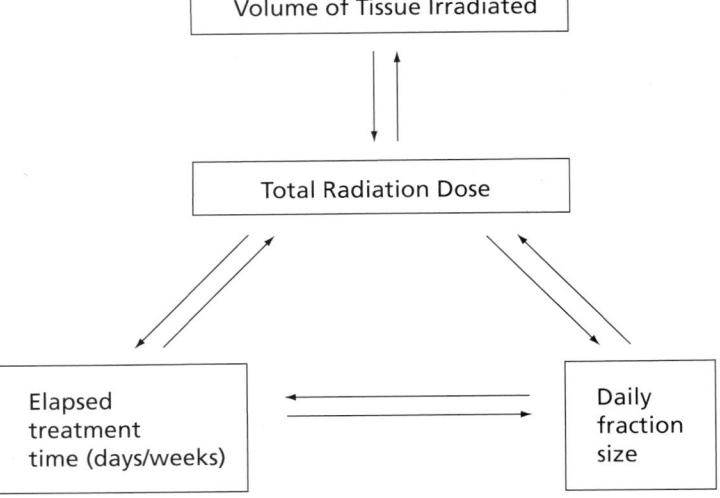

limits. Table 17-1 illustrates the cellular replacement times for certain body systems.[4,5] Information on tolerance doses has been revised in recent years because of advances in combined-modality therapy. When chemotherapy and radiation are used concurrently, acute and late reactions in various tissues generally occur at much lower doses than when radiation is used alone. In addition, combined-modality therapy can produce acute and late radiation injuries that are not commonly seen with either modality alone. Therefore, patients treated with combined-modality therapy are at risk for multiple toxicities that can be classified as acute, subacute, and late effects (Table 17-2).

Acute Effects

Acute effects of radiation occur primarily in rapidly renewing tissues.[2] Because the response of rapidly renewing tissues depends on the balance between cell birth and cell death, acute tissue reaction is affected by the time allowed for repopulation and is therefore dependent on field size, daily radiation dose, and overall length of treatment (number of treatments). The concept of fractionation of radiation therapy is *crucial* to allowing normal cell repopulation (recall the Four R's of Radiobiology). Uninterrupted treatment would quickly overwhelm the body's ability to repair normal tissues and therefore would

Table 17-1 Selected Cellular Systems in Normal Tissue and Approximate Turnover/Replacement Time

System	Turnover/Replacement Time*
Integumentary	
Epidermis	30 days
Basal cells	Nadir: 21 days
	Re-epithelialization: 28–31 days
Endothelial cells	Unknown
Blood	
RBC's	120 days
Granulocytes	6–10 hr in blood, 2–3 days in tissue
Lymphocytes	100–300 + days
Platelets	5–10 days
Respiratory tract	
Tracheal epithelium	50 days
GI tract	
Oral mucosa	10–14 days
Stomach	3–9 days
Small intestine	1.5 days
Colon	10 days
Skin	20 days
GU tract	
Urinary bladder	50 days
Testis	20 days
Lung alveolar cells	10–30 days
Eye	
Cornea	7 days

*Turnover/replacement time is the time required for replacement of number of cells equal to that in the whole population of the system. Data from Coia, Moylan[4] and Archambieu, Pezner.[5]

Table 17-2 Phases of Radiation Effect: Acute, Subacute, Late

Acute Effect Phase
- Evidence of radiation effect is seen in hours to days.
- Proliferating cells are more radiosensitive than quiescent cells.
- Brisk reactions heal completely, but significant residual damage may be present.
- Tissues most at risk:

Bladder	Ovary, testis
Bone marrow	Salivary gland
Colon	Skin
Esophagus	Small bowel
Lymph nodes	Stomach
Oral mucosa	Vagina

Subacute Effect Phase
- Evidence of damage of clinical significance is seen in weeks to a few months after completing radiation.
- Tissues most at risk:

Brain	Liver
Heart	Lung
Kidney	Spinal cord

Late Effect Phase
- If given sufficient doses of radiation, all tissues can manifest late effects.
- Radiation causes injury to vasculoconnective tissue and parenchymal cells.
- Occurs in tissues with low cell turnover
- Dependent on fractionation, treatment volume, total radiation dose
- Tissues most at risk:

Bile ducts	Lymph tissue
Bone	Pancreas (endocrine)
Brain	Pituitary
Breast	Thyroid
Cartilage	

cause unacceptable toxicities. As a result, treatment schedules are generally 5 days per week, with 2 consecutive days of break or rest. Occasionally, treatment breaks are necessary to allow healing of normal tissue. Acute toxicities vary with each patient, are site-specific and generally short-term, and resolve after completion of treatment. The time to complete resolution of acute toxicities depends on the specific tissues treated and the degree of reaction to the radiation.

Subacute Effects

Subacute effects are those toxicities that are clinically evident within weeks to a few months after completing radiation. Pneumonitis is a subacute clinical syndrome that may occur after chest irradiation. (Pneumonitis is described in detail later in the chapter.)

Late Effects

Late effects are due to the dose-limiting factors in radiation.[2] The extent and degree of late effects are dependent on the size of the daily fraction and the total radiation dose, total treatment time, size of the treatment field, type of radiation (photons vs. electrons), and concurrent chemotherapy. The mechanism of late radiation injury is not definitively known.

Assessment and Management of Skin Reactions, Fatigue, and Myelosuppression

Role of the Radiation Therapy Nurse

The role of the radiation therapy (RT) nurse has only recently been more clearly defined, in contrast to the medical oncology nurse who has had an established role in the administration of chemotherapy and management of symptoms.[6] With increasingly aggressive cancer treatment regimens, the patient is at risk for multiple toxicities and the RT nurse must be prepared to assess and intervene as indicated. New and innovative strategies for teaching about and managing toxicities necessitate a dialogue among all professionals involved in the patient's treatment to produce optimum outcomes. Radiation therapy nurses are responsible for teaching, assessing, and managing toxicities, and helping patients through a course of irradiation. Radiation therapy can engender many fears for patients, their family, and friends. Misinformation is common, and patient's friends and family may reinforce concerns due to erroneous assumptions and lack of accurate information. It is essential that the RT nurses and physicians educate both the patient and family before beginning a course of treatment.

Hinds et al evaluated the functions and methods preferred by patients for receiving information related to radiation therapy.[7] Findings concluded that information allowed patients to be active participants in their care, reduced anxiety, and helped patients feel prepared for the treatments. Poroch demonstrated that radiation therapy patients who received structured teaching interventions, including sensory and procedural information, were significantly less anxious and more satisfied during the course of their treatment than the cohort control group that received standard information used in the radiation therapy department.[8] Patient education should include an overview of the treatment plan, myths and misconceptions, information on the actual treatments (including sensory information), the simulation process, expected outcome (cure, control, or palliation), specific side effects of treatment, and symptom management.[9]

The experience of cancer and its treatment generate high levels of distress and difficulty in coping. Even though cancer treatment is stressful, cessation of treatment is also associated with emotional stress due to uncertainty about tumor recurrence.[10] The staff in radiation oncology departments form brief, intense relationships with patients and their families. Each individual staff member and radiation program deals with the ending of a course of therapy in a different way. While patients are always pleased to be finishing treatment, it is important to acknowledge the ending of this portion of their cancer therapy. Often radiation therapy is the last treatment modality, after surgery and chemotherapy, and patients are indeed "finished" with treatment at the completion of the radiation course. This can be an uncertain time with patients experiencing multiple concerns regarding time to resolution of treatment-related toxicities, monitoring for cancer recurrence, and perhaps most difficult—resuming a "normal" life. Cancer counseling or other supportive care can be extremely helpful at this point in the treatment continuum.

In general, the management of toxicities related to radiation therapy is similar to measures used for managing chemotherapy-related side effects. It may not always be clear whether the chemotherapy or radiation is causing the specific toxicity. It is important that medical and radiation oncology nurses collaborate in planning management of side effects. While the side effects of radiation are site specific, most patients are at risk for some degree of skin reaction, fatigue, and occasionally myelosuppression.

Skin Reaction

Early radiation machines used much lower and less penetrating energies, thus most of the radiation dose was superficial. The degree of skin erythema was frequently used as an indication of overall radiation dose. Therefore, when the patient's skin became severely erythematous or desquamated, the radiation course ended. Modern megavoltage radiation equipment, such as the linear accelerator, have been called "skin-sparing" treatment machines. Despite advanced technology in the science and delivery of radiation, the radiation beam still must first pass through the skin to reach the targeted tissue or organ. Fortunately, the dreaded and frequently severe skin reactions previously associated with radiation therapy are rarely seen with the modern treatment techniques and equipment now in common use.

Typical skin response to radiation depends on numerous radiation- and patient-related factors. Radiation factors affecting skin reaction include the beam type and energy, daily treatment dose, tissue equivalent (bolus) material on the skin surface during treatment, accelerated dose fractionation, and location and size of the treatment fields. The field location and beam arrangement (single vs. opposed vs. multibeam) defines the skin surface(s) at risk. Patient factors affecting skin reaction include skin folds in the treatment fields, nutritional status, individual radiosensitivity, and comorbid conditions such as ataxia-telangiectasias and autoimmune illness (Table 17-3).[11]

Skin response to radiation is dependent on dose and reflects changes in the cellular components of the epidermis, dermis, and vasculature.[12] The epidermis and dermis are continuously renewing their cellular populations so

Table 17-3 Typical Factors Influencing Skin Response to Radiation

Radiation-related:
- Total dose and total time
- Daily fraction size
- Type of radiation beam (photons vs. electrons)
- Use of tissue equivalent bolus material
- Size of treatment field

Patient-related:
- Anatomic location of treatment field(s)
- Characteristics of skin in treatment field(s)
- Proximity of tumor to skin surface
- Concomitant chemotherapy
- Comorbid conditions
- Nutritional status

Inflammatory response:
- Histamine and serotonin released
- Local microcirculation increases tissue perfusion
- Infiltration by leukocytes

Acute changes
- May occur within 2–3 weeks after start or completion of treatment
- Usually repairable
- Types:
  Erythema/epilation
  Dry desquamation
  Moist desquamation

Chronic changes
- May occur several months to years after completion of treatment
- May be permanent
- Types:
  Tissue necrosis or ulceration
  Fibrosis
  Edema
  Hyperpigmentation

Adapted with permission from Strunk B, Maher KE: Collaborative nurse management of multifactorial moist desquamation in a patient undergoing radiotherapy. *J Enterost Ther Nurs* 20:152–157, 1993.[11]

that cell production equals cell loss. Acute skin effect is a reflection of the inability of cells in the epidermis and dermis to keep up with the accelerated loss caused by the radiation.

Acute skin effects

Acute skin reactions vary in intensity and duration depending on the factors mentioned earlier. The single most important factor is the location of radiation field. For example, a woman undergoing breast irradiation is more at risk for an acute skin reaction due to the curved, tangential radiation fields that result in a higher dose to the skin surface and skin folds. Compare this to a man receiving four-field radiation to the pelvis (small, relatively flat surfaces) for prostate cancer. In this situation, a skin reaction is rarely seen.

The degree of skin reaction can be visually assessed and may progress in a stepwise fashion from erythema to dry desquamation to moist desquamation.[13] The stages of potential acute skin reactions are outlined in Table 17-4.[13] It is important to understand that not all patients experience each stage of skin reaction and that some patients have several stages occurring simultaneously. Most patients demonstrate some degree of skin dryness, itching, and erythema. Erythema can progress to include dermal edema and discomfort. Dry desquamation of the skin can occur as erythema resolves. Moist desquamation of skin in the treatment field involves the epilation of the epidermis and exposure of the dermis. Patients with moist desquamation have pain and may need treatment suspended to allow for healing. *Burn* is not an appropriate term to describe a skin reaction to radiation, as it implies that too much radiation was administered or that an error was made in the treatment prescription.[14] Most radiation oncology nurses and staff avoid use of the word *burn*;

however, this is how patients commonly describe their skin reactions. Generally, acute skin symptoms begin about 3 weeks (2700–3000 cGy) into a course of treatment and are confined to the treatment field. Acute skin reactions heal completely and do not predict for late skin manifestations.

Concurrent chemotherapy and irradiation can result in more severe and prolonged acute skin reactions. The degree of skin effect is dependent on the specific chemotherapeutic agents used and the site of radiation. For example, patients receiving concurrent chemotherapy and radiation for cancers of the oropharynx, hypopharynx, or nasopharynx (skin of neck and face), or of the anus and vulva (perianal/perineal skin) are at risk for enhanced skin reaction due to multiple skin folds and extensive mucosa in the radiation fields. An erythematous skin recall reaction may occur in patients who have undergone irradiation and then are given anthracyclines (e.g., doxorubicin) in close proximity to completion of radiation. There are no systematic methods available to confirm skin recall, the doses of chemotherapy or radiation required, or the time interval involved.[5]

Late skin effects

The late changes to skin produced by radiation can be functionally limiting if neuropathy, arthropathy, contraction, and necrosis are produced. Management of late skin effects is directed at relieving symptoms, promoting healing, and surgical intervention as indicated. The late effects of radiation on the skin are dose dependent. The time interval to development of clinically evident skin changes is a result of the response of the cellular components in the epidermis, dermis, and microvasculature. The evolution of skin effects reflects a continuous remodeling of these cellular populations.[5]

Table 17-4 Acute Effects of Radiation on Skin

Tissue Response	Onset/Duration	Clinical Presentation	Physiological Rationale
Erythema Phase I (transient)	Within hours to days of first treatment Resolves after several days but will recur if treatment continues	Faint, often unnoticed redness	Thought to be a vascular response to extracapillary cell injury
Phase II (erythema proper)	Following 2–3 wk of standard fractionated radiation therapy Resolves 20–30 days following last treatment	Redness that outlines treatment field Intensifies as treatment continues	Intensity greater with higher radiation doses and larger treatment fields (greater amount of vasculature)
		Increased skin temperature	Increased blood flow through dermis from vasodilation
		Edema	Capillary vasodilation with endothelial swelling and increased capillary permeability. Histamine and serotonin are released and microcirculation increases tissue perfusion allowing infiltration of the area by leukocytes.
Pruritus	Occurs most commonly when exposure exceeds 20–28 Gy	Itching	Thinning of the epidermis with decreased sebaceous and sweat gland function results in dehydration of the stratum corneum, the water-retaining skin layer.
Hyperpigmentation	Following 2–3 wk of standard fractionated radiation therapy Usually resolves 3 mo to 1 yr following completion of treatment, but may be chronic	Tanned appearance	Cornified basal cells carry more melanin into superficial layers of the epidermis and radiation stimulates tyrosinase to convert tyrosine to melanin. Increased melanocyte activity causes cells to become darker. Darker-skinned people may have more hyperpigmentation because they traditionally have more melanin.
Dry desquamation	Following 3–4 wk of standard fractionated radiation therapy Resolves 1–2 wk after completion of treatment	Dryness, flaking, and peeling often accompanied by itching	Each dose of radiation destroys a fixed percentage of basal cells. Surviving basal cells become cornified and are shed at an increased rate. Noncycling basal cells are stimulated and cell cycle time is shortened.
Moist desquamation	Following 40 Gy or with trauma/excess friction Recovery usually 2–4 wk after completion of treatment	Brilliant erythema Sloughing skin Exposed dermis Serous exudate oozing from surface	Destruction of epithelium. All basal cells have been destroyed and no new cells are yet formed.
		Pain	Nerve endings in the dermis are exposed.
Skin regrowth following moist desquamation	Dependent on severity Usually complete 2–3 mo following completion of treatment	Small areas of epithelium develop. New skin is smooth, pink, thin, and dryer	Epithelial cells migrate via proliferation from outside the treatment field and through peripheral migration.
		Gradual thickening of skin over time, but skin does not regain former thickness	Migration occurs best over moist healthy tissue. Fewer sweat and sebaceous glands result in chronic dryness.

Reprinted with permission from Goodman M, Hilderley LJ, Purl S: Integumentary and mucous membrane alterations, in Groenwald SL, Frogge MH, Goodman M, Yarbro CH (eds): *Cancer Nursing: Principles and Practice* (ed 4). Sudbury, MA, Jones and Bartlett, 1997, pp 772–773.[13]

A time period of varying length occurs in which the skin appears "normal" during radiation treatment. Then, within a period of time that may be measured in years, skin changes such as hyperpigmentation, scaling, atrophy, telangiectasias, subcutaneous fibrosis, and necrosis may develop and progress. Radiation dose schedules that produce late skin reactions are similar to those that produce acute skin reactions. However late effects on skin are more severe following schedules that include daily fractions of 250–300 cGy or higher. Most patients are treated using daily fractions of 180–200 cGy, thus markedly reducing the risk of late skin effects.[5] Potential late skin effects are outlined in Table 17-5.[13]

Skin care assessment and management

A major role of RT nurses is assessment of skin reactions, teaching skin care, and managing skin breakdown if it occurs.[14] There are many preventive and interventional skin care regimens in use, however there is a paucity of scientific data to support most practice interventions. It has long been believed that skin in the treatment field should have no product (such as topical emollients) applied prior to daily treatment. There is a common belief that the product applied to the skin acts as a bolus and will enhance skin reaction. Burch et al investigated what occurs on the skin surface when deodorants, powders, and creams are applied in the treatment area prior to radiation treatments.[15] The study was conducted using a phantom chamber to measure surface doses of radiation after various products were applied. Results included essentially no difference in surface dose. The limitation of the study is that it was conducted using a phantom and not human subjects.[15] Another study randomized 99 patients receiving radiation therapy to the breast or chest wall to one of three washing policies:

Group 1: No washing of skin in the treatment field

Group 2: Washing with water alone

Group 3: Washing with soap and water

The study concluded that there was little difference between washing with water alone and washing with soap and water.[16] Overall, skin reactions were less if the patients washed. Patients were also prescribed a topical cream for skin reactions, but whether the creams were beneficial was not tested, therefore no recommendations on their use can be made.[16]

At this time, the optimum skin care regimen remains unclear. The goals of skin care management are to enhance patient comfort, promote healing, and prevent infection if skin breakdown occurs.[12] Some general guidelines are suggested including gentle care of the skin in the treatment field, sun protection with sun-block products (SPF ≥ 15), and moist wound-healing principles for management of moist desquamation.[11,14] Because of the lack of definitive data regarding the efficacy of skin care products and regimens, most skin care guidelines are institution specific and based on habit and anecdotal experience. Most radiation oncology nurses and physicians have developed skin care protocols. Table 17-6 lists suggested skin care guidelines.

Fatigue

Fatigue during radiation is subjective, almost universal, and affected by multiple factors such as the extent of disease, age, concurrent chemotherapy, weight loss, pain, anemia, and length of radiation treatment. The specific etiology of radiation-related fatigue is unclear. Frequently, patients have undergone a surgical procedure(s) and received chemotherapy prior to radiation therapy. Thus, many patients come to the radiation experience familiar with fatigue and its impact on their life.

Although most cancer patients report that fatigue is a major obstacle to maintaining normal daily activities and quality of life, it is seldom assessed and treated in clinical practice.[17] Fatigue is best measured by patient self-report. Patients describe their fatigue in many ways including tiredness, weakness, exhaustion, lack of energy, malaise, impaired ability to concentrate, and overall impaired ability to complete activities of daily living.[18] It follows that such a potentially dramatic influence on physical and mental functioning may adversely affect quality of life.

Patients and families should be taught that fatigue is an expected effect of treatment and may be increased when receiving combined-modality therapy.[19] The degree of fatigue-related symptoms increases over the course of radiation treatment.[20,21] During a course of fractionated radiation therapy, fatigue is often cumulative and may peak after a period of weeks. Occasionally, fatigue persists for a prolonged period after the completion of radiation therapy.[17] An early study by King et al examined 96 subjects weekly during radiation therapy, and then monthly for 3 months after completing treatment.[22] The patients were receiving radiation for cancers of the chest, head and neck, prostate, bladder, and for gynecologic tumors. Overall, from 65%–93% of patients reported fatigue that gradually increased and was continuous by the last 2 weeks of treatment, and that persisted for several months postradiation. Fatigue symptoms tend to persist after other treatment-related side effects have resolved. It is important to observe for symptoms of clinical depression, especially in the patient experiencing prolonged fatigue.

Graydon et al evaluated the four strategies patients use to manage fatigue while undergoing chemotherapy or radiation therapy.[23] They are (1) reducing or stopping activity, (2) increasing activity (physical/social), (3) distraction, and (4) doing something different. Another study of 76 women undergoing radiation therapy for breast cancer reported that the strategies of sitting and sleeping were consistently the most frequently reported and believed to be somewhat effective.[24] What may make managing fatigue even more difficult is that it is a subjective experience. Patients can generally cope with other side effects such as nausea, vomiting, diarrhea, and skin

Table 17-5   Late Effects of Radiation on Skin and Connective Tissue

Tissue Response	Onset/Duration	Clinical Presentation	Physiological Rationale
Photosensitivity	Begins during treatment and is lifelong	Enhanced erythema over skin exposed to UV radiation from sun and tanning beds/booths	Destruction of melanocytes in the irradiated dermis and slower melanin production following irradiation reduce the skin's ability to protect itself from UV rays.
Pigmentation changes Hyperpigmentation	Refer to Table 17-4		
Hypopigmentation	May begin anytime following resolution of hyperpigmentation Permanent	Lack of skin color	Radiation doses necessary to eradicate cancer may permanently destroy melanocytes, which results in the skin's inability to form pigment.
Atrophy	Following epidermal regrowth Permanent	Thin and fragile epidermis	Newly formed epidermis is thinner. The epidermis thickens over time, but never attains its preirradiation thickness.
Fibrosis	Usually begins 4–6 mo following completion of treatment May worsen over time	Dense, hard, uneven skin texture If extensive, may cause considerable induration	Fibroblasts, responsible for producing collagen, demonstrate uneven cellular division resulting in faulty collagen remodeling. Fibrotic tissue results, giving the skin an uneven texture.
Telangiectasia	Occurs up to 8 yr following radiation therapy Permanent	Purple-red, spiderlike appearance of blood vessels in skin	Dose and fraction size–dependent. Basement membrane thickening results in a decreased permeability of material through capillary walls. With capillary occlusion, there are fewer functioning small vessels and a decreased capacity for capillary regeneration. This results in increased pressure of blood flow through remaining undamaged superficial structures.
Ulceration and necrosis	Rare May occur up to 20 yr following treatment Usually occurs as a result of inflammation and trauma to previously irradiated tissue	Painful ulcers with red, raised edges and a shaggy, necrotic base Usually shows little or no tendency to epithelialize or contract Despite local treatment, ulcers tend to deepen and become more painful	Although the mechanism is not clear, late ulceration and necrosis occur as a result of connective tissue damage. Electron microscopic studies suggest that permanent damage to fibroblasts and their precursor cells prevents stem cell replication, angiogenesis, and wound contraction. Occasionally, sustained vascular occlusion and tissue ischemia may be responsible for ulceration and necrosis.

Reprinted with permission from Goodman M, Hilderley LJ, Purl S: Integumentary and mucous membrane alterations, in Groenwald SL, Frogge MH, Goodman M, Yarbro CH (eds): *Cancer Nursing: Principles and Practice* (ed 4). Sudbury, MA, Jones and Bartlett, 1997, p 775.[13]

reactions, perhaps because there are concrete and effective interventions. Fatigue, on the other hand, does not lend itself to such concrete techniques.

Acknowledging fatigue as a "legitimate" toxicity of radiation therapy may be as important as suggestions for management. Educating patients and family members also includes helping them choose the most appropriate interventions to fight fatigue. Finding a balance of activity and energy conservation may be helpful for the chronic fatigue experienced with both chemotherapy and radia-

Table 17-6 Suggested Skin Care Guidelines for Patients During Radiation Therapy*

What to expect:

- When you are receiving radiation therapy, it is recommended that you pay special attention to your skin in the area being treated. Skin in the treated area will be more sensitive and can be more easily injured than usual.
- Skin in the treated area may become itchy, dry, red, and sore. Rarely, the skin blisters and peels. Your physician, nurse, and radiation therapist will be monitoring the skin. Ask questions if you have any symptoms or concerns.
- Most important: handle skin in the treated area *gently.*
- Do not remove temporary skin marks; tattoos are permanent and will not be affected.
- You will lose hair only in the immediate treated area.
- Wash skin in the treated area with warm, *not* hot, water.
- Wash—*never* scrub—the skin with care with a mild moisturizing soap (e.g., Dove, Tone) and pat dry.
- Avoid heating pads and ice packs on the treated area.
- Avoid using preshave lotions and hair removal products in the treated area.
- If possible, do not shave the treated area. If shaving is necessary, use an electric razor.
- Wear loose, soft clothing over the treated area.
- Do not expose the treated area to the sun. If sun exposure is unavoidable, use sunblock having SPF 15 or more.
- Avoid using tape on the treated area.
- Moisturizing the skin can be helpful. Talk with your nurse, radiation therapist, or physician; a list of recommended products may be available.

*Techniques for skin care management are institution specific and not necessarily based on established data as to the optimum regimen.

tion therapy.[19] Physical activity must be individualized and usually includes light exercise such as walking and gardening. Exercise has been shown to increase concentration and overall ability to think clearly, which allows patients to participate more fully in their care and daily activities. Other strategies to treat fatigue include modification of the patient's drug regimen, correction of metabolic abnormalities, and pharmacologic treatments for anemia (e.g., epoetin alfa), depression, or insomnia. Specific pharmacologic approaches include psychostimulant drugs and corticosteroids. Supportive therapies may also be helpful such as cognitive therapies, sleep hygiene strategies, and nutritional support.[17] (See Chapter 32 for a detailed discussion of fatigue.)

Myelosuppression

The bone marrow is an important dose-limiting cell-renewal tissue for chemotherapy, wide-field irradiation, and autologous bone marrow transplantation.[25] The bone marrow is so highly radiosensitive that injury to the bone marrow is produced by any dose of radiation. Following each dose of radiation, peripheral blood cells progressively decrease in number due to the destruction of both

mature and precursor cells. Lymphocytes are the most sensitive cells; hence lymphopenia develops early in the course of radiation therapy. Figure 17-3 illustrates the relative radiosensitivity of hematopoietic cell lines throughout their life cycle.[26] The radiation dose, site, and tissue volume all affect the acute response of the bone marrow to therapy. When small radiation fields comprising only 10%-15% of the bone marrow are radiated, the unexposed bone marrow responds by increasing its population of progenitor cells to meet the demands for hematopoiesis. Thus, acute myelosuppression is usually not seen unless large areas containing a substantial portion of marrow are within the radiation fields.[25] Approximately 40% of active bone marrow is in the pelvis, with the remaining 60% of active marrow distributed as illustrated in Figure 17-4.[27]

The acute effects of concurrent chemotherapy and radiation on the bone marrow are complex. Any treatment regimen combining chemotherapy and radiation therapy must take into account potential increased dose-limiting marrow suppression.[25] Growth factors supporting development of all hematologic cell lines are seldom needed when radiation is used as a single modality. However, in combined-modality therapy, growth factors are commonly part of treatment regimens due to the increased risk of pancytopenia.

Patients most at risk for cytopenia are those receiving concurrent chemo-radiation, total body irradiation, extended-field (whole-abdomen) radiation, and splenic radiation. Most radiation fields are designed to limit the amount of bone marrow exposed to radiation. However, it may be necessary to irradiate marrow producing areas in high-risk patients, such as those who have been heavily pretreated (chemotherapy and/or radiation) and those with bony metastases that require radiation therapy for pain management. The frequency of monitoring blood counts varies by individual radiation oncology practice.

The chronic or late effects of radiation on the bone marrow include increased hematopoietic activity in unexposed marrow segments, followed by extension of functioning marrow into previously quiescent areas such as the femora and humeri. Bone marrow regeneration is variable in each individual and generally lags behind the peripheral blood counts. Marrow recovery can occur over extended periods, with total recovery in 12–24 months, but this depends on the volume of marrow irradiated.[25] Generally, patients are not at greater risk for infection during the chronic recovery phase.

Acute Radiation Toxicities and Management: Site Specific

Acute toxicities or side effects are expected during a course of radiation therapy. Radiation toxicities directly correlate with the specific normal tissues and structures

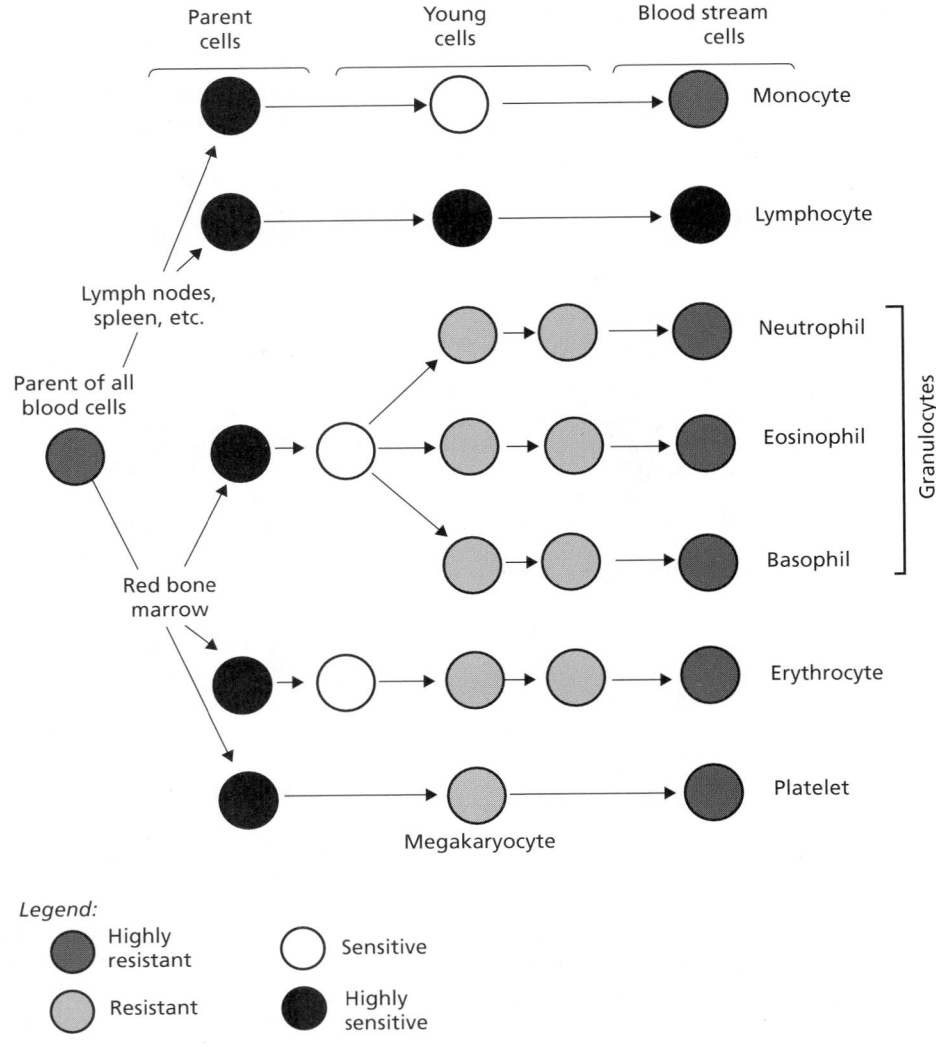

Figure 17-3 Radiosensitivity of hematopoietic blood cells. Note that lymphocytes remain highly sensitive to radiation throughout their life cycle. (Reprinted with permission from Casarett GW: *Radiation Histopathology* (vol. 1). Boca Raton: CRC Press, 1980.[26])

Parent cells | Young cells | Blood stream cells

Monocyte

Lymphocyte

Lymph nodes, spleen, etc.

Parent of all blood cells

Neutrophil

Eosinophil

Granulocytes

Basophil

Red bone marrow

Erythrocyte

Platelet

Megakaryocyte

Legend:

Highly resistant

Resistant

Sensitive

Highly sensitive

within the path of the radiation beam. Table 17-7 is a representative list of site specific acute toxicities. The goal of radiation is to maintain the therapeutic ratio to achieve maximum tumor cell kill with minimal toxicity to normal tissues and structures.

Because the radiation beam must pass through the skin, all patients are at some level of risk for an acute skin reaction. Also, as previously described, fatigue is an almost universal reaction to radiation therapy. When assessing patients, the nurse should be aware of potential skin reactions, fatigue, and myelosuppression, in addition to site specific effects. The following section addresses potential site specific acute radiation-related toxicities and management. The list of toxicities is representative and reflects policies and practices currently in the literature and at various institutions. It should be stressed that alternative methods for managing toxicities exist that are also appropriate. Acute toxicities are dependent on the site treated, daily dose, radiation energy used and size of the treatment field (the radiation therapy mantra).

Brain

Used in treatment for primary brain tumors or metastases, head and brain irradiation can result in the following toxicities.

Alopecia and scalp erythema

Because of the high mitotic rate of hair follicles of the scalp, hair loss will occur when the head is irradiated. Alopecia starts approximately 2–3 weeks (~2500–3000 cGy) into treatment. The extent of alopecia is dependent on the size of the field. If the whole brain is treated (i.e., diffuse or multiple metastases) total hair loss will result. Partial brain irradiation (i.e., primary brain tumor) results in alopecia that conforms to the edges of the treatment field(s). Hair almost always regrows with scalp doses of 5000–6000 cGy or less, and permanent hair loss usually occurs with doses of 6000 cGy or more.[28] Regrowth of hair may take from 3–6 months after completion of radia-

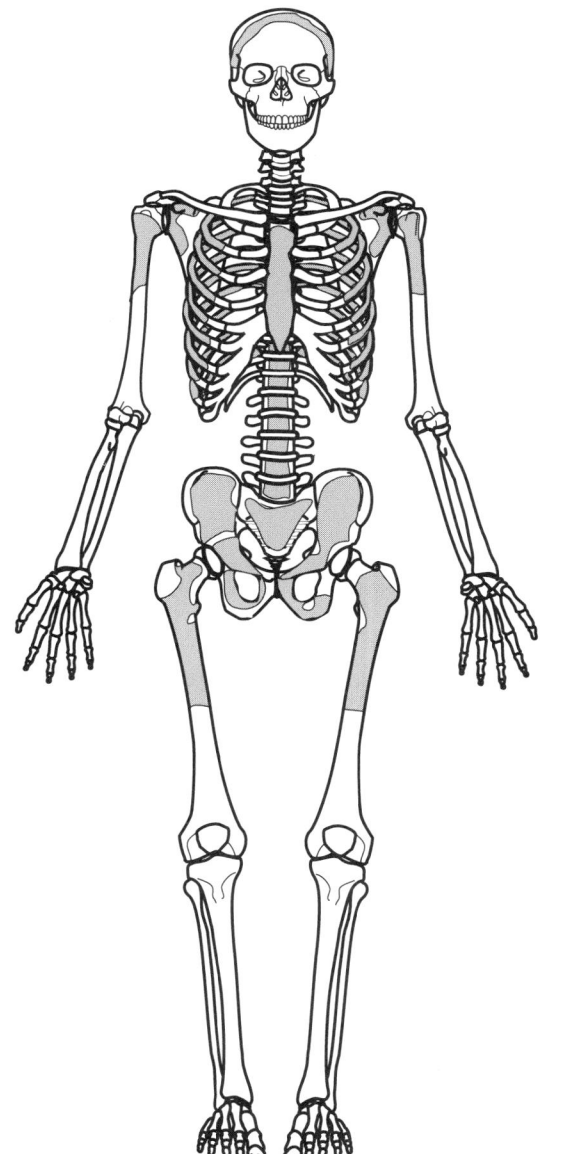

Figure 17-4 Bone Marrow Distribution. Bone marrow distribution in adult humans as determined by autopsy findings; active regions are shaded.

Table 17-7 Site Specific Acute Toxicities of Radiation Therapy*

CNS (primary brain tumors, brain metastasis)
  Brain
    Scalp, forehead erythema
    Alopecia
    External auditory canal irritation
    Transient increased cerebral edema
    Nausea/vomiting (rare)
  Spinal cord
    Lhermitte's syndrome (subacute)

Head and Neck (nasopharynx, oro/hypopharynx, larynx)
  Skin erythema
  Oral mucositis
  Esophagitis→dysphagia→odynophagia
  Xerostomia
  Dysgeusia, ageusia→anorexia

Breast
  Skin erythema that may progress to moist desquamation

Chest/Lung (lung, esophageal, gastric cancers)
  Skin erythema (anterior and posterior fields)
  Esophagitis→dysphagia/odynophagia
  Dysgeusia→anorexia
  Gastric reflux symptoms
  Pneumonitis (subacute)

Abdomen/Pelvis (GI, GU, gynecologic cancers)
  Nausea/vomiting (radiation site–dependent)
  Diarrhea
  Cystitis symptoms
  Mucositis of perianal region
  Vaginal dryness

*Acute toxicities are dependent on site treated (what normal structures are in the field), daily dose, radiation energy used, and volume treated (size of the field).

tion, and may be a different color and/or texture. Alopecia secondary to irradiation of the head is inevitable and there are no proven preventive strategies. Alopecia causes a major change in self-image and is a visible reminder of the cancer experience.

Management. Scalp irritation and erythema can be managed with gentle care to the scalp and hair. The hair should be washed with a mild shampoo. Irritants such as hair dyes, hot curlers and irons, and hair dryers that can further irritate the scalp should be avoided. Patients should be encouraged to consider hair coverings (e.g., wig, turban, scarves) prior to hair loss because it is much easier to match hair style and color before total alopecia occurs. The scalp tends to be sensitive after radiation-induced hair loss, especially with accompanying scalp erythema and irritation. Some patients cannot tolerate anything on the head.

Inform patients that there is significant body heat loss from the head and that, without the insulation of hair, they might feel cold, especially during sleep. During the day, the head and scalp should be protected from the sun with hats and sun-block products. Psychological interventions, such as support groups or patient-to-patient assistance, may help the patient cope with the effects of alopecia on self-image.

Ear and external auditory canal

If the ear is in the treatment field, the pinna and external auditory canal may become irritated, sore, and pruritic. Symptoms generally resolve within 1–2 weeks after completion of therapy.

Management. Instruct the patient to protect the ear from sun and cold exposure. For discomfort in the external auditory canal, ear drops with hydrocortisone can be prescribed.

Cerebral edema

Increased intracranial pressure (ICP), secondary to cerebral edema, is often present at diagnosis. Radiation-induced ICP occurs, though the mechanism is not well understood.[29] The incidence of ICP increases with the size of the initial fraction(s); for example, fractions of 200 cGy or more per day commonly result in ICP. Symptoms include exacerbation of the patients' presenting neurologic symptoms such as headache, nausea and vomiting, muscle or extremity weakness, seizures, and mental status changes.

Management. Patients with known brain tumors or metastasis are usually taking corticosteroids, and titrating the dose will often alleviate symptoms of ICP. The patient who is not taking corticosteroids and will begin brain radiation, especially whole-brain treatment, needs to be closely monitored. Cerebral edema can develop quickly. The steroid most commonly used to prevent cerebral edema is dexamethasone due to its rapid onset of activity and biologic half-life of 36–54 hours. The dose of dexamethasone varies, but a frequently used regimen is 12–16 mg per day (4 mg every 6–8 hours). Instruct patients not to abruptly discontinue the corticosteroid because of hypothalamic-pituitary axis (HPA) suppression which can result in adrenal insufficiency. Symptoms of adrenal insufficiency include fatigue, nausea, vomiting, diarrhea, and weight loss.

Patients and families should be educated regarding the multiple side effects of steroids, such as gastrointestinal (GI) effects (reflux, nausea), candidiasis (especially in the oral cavity), hyperglycemia in diabetics, psychologic changes such as mood swings, insomnia, and myopathy (especially proximal leg weakness). Antacid therapy (i.e., H2 blocker or acid-pump inhibitor) is recommended for prophylaxis of GI symptoms. Other steroid-induced toxicities are managed with medications such as lorazepam and temazepam for relaxation or sleep, systemic antifungals for candidiasis, and titration of oral antidiabetic agents or insulin for hyperglycemia.

Steroids relieve ICP symptoms relatively quickly, however most patients do not feel well while taking them and want to stop steroid therapy as soon as possible. Timing of a steroid taper is variable, but generally decreasing the dose by half every 4–7 days will not cause exacerbation of symptoms. If symptoms recur, instruct the patient to return to the previous steroid dose. Try not to begin a steroid taper on Friday (half-life of dexamethasone = 36–54 hours), because neurologic symptoms may recur on the weekend when radiation oncology staff are not as readily available.

Nausea and vomiting

Nausea and vomiting caused by brain irradiation is rare, short-lived, and can be well-controlled with antiemetics. Symptoms also may be secondary to cerebral edema, and increasing the corticosteroid dose may relieve symptoms.

Management. Antiemetic regimens include: Selective 5-HT3 receptor antagonists:

- Ondansetron 8 mg PO 1–2 hours prior to radiation and every 8 hours PRN

- Granisetron 2 mg PO 1 hour prior to dailey radiation

- Dolasetron mesylate 100 mg PO 1 hour prior to radiation

Phenothiazines:

- Prochlorperazine 5–10 mg PO 1 hour prior to radiation and every 4–6 hours PRN

- Prochlorperazine spansules 15 mg PO or suppositories 25 mg PR given approximately 1–2 hours prior to radiation

- Triethylperazine 10 mg PO 1 hour prior to radiation and every 8 hours PRN

Somnolence syndrome (subacute)

Symptoms of the somnolence syndrome include excessive sleepiness and fatigue, accompanied by anorexia and occasional mild headache. The somnolence syndrome is well recognized and occurs more frequently in children than in adults. The cause of the somnolence is unclear but believed to be related to transient demyelination secondary to radiation effect on oligodendrocytes.[30] Symptoms of somnolence occur 4–12 weeks after radiation is complete and can last for 2–8 weeks.

Management. Management is directed at supportive care as the syndrome runs its course. Supportive measures include maintaining nutrition (especially in children who may sleep a greater portion of 24 hours) and prevention of problems related to prolonged immobilization, such as venous thrombosis and skin breakdown.

Head and Neck

Used in treatment for cancers of the nasopharynx, oropharynx, hypopharynx, and larynx, head and neck irradiation can result in multiple toxicities. Assessment and management of toxicities related to irradiation for head and neck cancers is a major challenge for oncology nurses. There are numerous structures and systems in the head and neck region that result in multiple and often severe acute and late toxicities. Patients with head and neck cancer tend to have poor nutritional status, abuse tobacco and alcohol, and have functional deficits (i.e., speech, swallowing, chewing, airway compromise). Persons with head and neck cancer need advocacy and support from all members of the cancer care team to maintain compliance with the radiation schedule, as well as to manage the toxicities and needed self-care regimens. Suspension of radiation treatment may be needed to allow for healing of affected tissues.

Oral mucositis (stomatitis)

The epithelial cells of the mucous membrane lining the oral cavity are highly radiosensitive.[28] The reaction of the oral mucosa can range from erythema to painful ulcerated areas. A pseudomembrane can form and then slough off, leaving a painful, friable surface.[31] Areas of the buccal mucosa and buccal sulcus that are adjacent to metal tooth fillings are at greater risk for increased reaction due to radiation scatter from the metal filling. Mucositis will be enhanced and prolonged in patients who have preexisting poor oral or dental hygiene, continue to smoke, use chewing tobacco, consume alcohol, and have poorly fitting dentures. Combined-modality therapy with chemotherapeutic agents such as 5-fluorouracil will enhance mucositis of the oropharynx. The onset of oral mucositis is seen approximately 2–3 weeks after the start of treatment. Symptoms generally start as generalized oral discomfort and progress (depending on radiation dose) to pain such that eating, swallowing, and speaking are extremely painful, if not impossible.

Assessment for oral mucositis involves frequent inspection of the oral cavity. Evaluation schedules are patient specific, however weekly inspection is adequate early in the course of treatment (first 2–3 weeks), and then as symptoms indicate. A mouth care regimen should focus on hygiene, dental prophylaxis, and comfort.

Management. Management strategies include avoiding products that will further dry the mucous membranes, such as mouthwashes with alcohol and any glycerin-based product. Instruct the patient to gently brush teeth and tongue frequently with a soft toothbrush. Ideally, the patient should perform oral care four times daily and, if tolerated, continue flossing teeth. Mouth rinses with an isotonic saline solution (swish and spit) help loosen debris and cleanse the oral cavity. A common saline solution mixture is 1 teaspoon of salt and/or 1 teaspoon baking soda in a quart of water. This solution is mild and rarely causes increased discomfort. Patients should be encouraged to swish and spit the solution as often as possible, ideally every 1–2 waking hours. Topical anesthetics such as a 1:1:1 mixture of liquid antacid, diphenhydramine hydrochloride, and viscous lidocaine are helpful. Instruct patients to swish and swallow/spit 5–10 mL of the topical anesthetic 20 minutes prior to eating and drinking.

There are many commercially prepared topical anesthetics available. Systemic analgesics are often needed and are most convenient in the liquid form if odynophagia is present. Other recommendations include using dentures only when eating and a soft to liquid diet of bland foods at room temperature. Oral mucositis can dramatically decrease appetite and diminish caloric intake, which may necessitate nutritional supplements and

intravenous hydration. (See section below on esophagitis for further discussion of nursing management.)

Oral candidiasis

Candidiasis is an infection of the oral mucosa with a yeastlike fungi, most commonly *Candida albicans.* In patients undergoing head and neck irradiation candidiasis is common due to destruction of the protective oral mucosal barrier, resulting in an overgrowth of candida. The infection is characterized by white patches and clusters in the mouth. Assessment of the entire oral cavity includes the tongue, roof of mouth, and buccal sulci. A culture can be sent for microbiologic confirmation; however, the diagnosis is usually made on the basis of clinical findings.

Management. Antifungal medication is prescribed. There are various preparations of antifungal drugs, including swish and swallow, troches, and systemic oral agents. It is important to remember that most head and neck patients have concurrent xerostomia (see below) and, therefore, troches will be generally ineffective because they will not dissolve. A swish-and-swallow preparation demands a compliant patient, as it must be done 4–5 times daily. Daily oral administration of an oral medication such as fluconazole or ketoconazole may be more appropriate for these patients. Often, esophagitis and mucositis diminish somewhat when candidiasis is resolved. Head and neck patients endure multiple toxicities and candidiasis is one of many. Reassure the patient that this infection is fairly easily treated with medication.

Oral herpes

Oral herpetic lesions may occur with or without candidiasis. Herpes lesions appear as vesicles on the oral mucosa. Diagnosis is made by clinical assessment, culture, and microbiologic confirmation.

Management. Treatment with oral antiviral medications such as acyclovir or famciclovir are generally effective.

Xerostomia

The major salivary glands (parotid, submandibular, and sublingual) are highly radiosensitive. Together, the salivary glands produce more than 1 liter of saliva per day. Typically, about 60%–65% of the total salivary volume is produced by the parotid glands, 20%–30% by the submandibular glands, and 2%–5% by the sublingual glands. The parotid glands are composed of serous cells and produce watery and albuminous secretions. The submaxillary and sublingual glands, composed of mixed serous cells and mucous acini, have thicker secretions. Saliva plays an important role in mastication, digestion, swallowing, and speech. More than 99% of saliva is water. Saliva also contains inorganic ions, lipids, amino acids, proteins, and traces of hormone-like substances. The proteins, including the salivary enzymes, are derived from the serum or synthesized within the parotid glands. The secretory function of the salivary glands is controlled by the autonomic nervous system and may be stimulated by the sensation of taste, smell, or chewing, and by psychological factors and stimulation, such as esophageal and gastric irritations, from other organs.[32] Saliva provides lubrication for oral tissues and protection from bacterial infections. Saliva also inhibits enamel decalcification and provides an important excretory route for blood-borne urea, uric acid, and ammonia.

The serous cells of the salivary glands are more radiosensitive and the mucous cells more radioresistant. A 50% or more reduction in salivary flow has been detected after the first week of fractionated radiation therapy to the head and neck area. Salivary flow continues to decline and may become barely measurable by the end of a 6 to 8 week course of treatment. Because the parotid glands (serous, watery secretions) are more affected by the radiation, the remaining saliva becomes thick and ropy.[32] Generally, patients notice the onset of dry mouth within the first 2 weeks of radiation.

Management. Some strategies for managing oral dryness include increasing oral fluids (most patients find water most helpful, but relief is of short duration), sugarless candy or gum, and sugarless lemon-flavored drinks.[31,33] A dietary consult is helpful to assist patients with meal planning. Saliva substitutes and chemical salivary gland stimulants are available. The so-called artificial saliva products are helpful for some patients but only afford short-term relief of dryness. Pilocarpine hydrochloride is a cholinergic stimulant that acts on postganglionic cells innervating smooth muscles and exocrine glands (i.e., sweat and salivary glands).[32] Several studies have demonstrated that pilocarpine given orally can reduce the symptoms of postirradiation xerostomia in patients who have some residual salivary function.[34-37] The most common regimen consists of pilocarpine 5 mg qid and can be increased to 10 mg qid as indicated. Side effects include sweating (usually within 30 minutes of administration), and other cholinergic effects that are relatively mild with the 5-mg dose regimen. Some data suggest that pilocarpine given concurrently and 3 months postirradiation may decrease overall postirradiation xerostomia.[38]

Esophagitis and pharyngitis

The pharynx and esophagus are usually in the treatment fields for head and neck irradiation. The resulting mucositis causes dysphagia and odynophagia that can be so severe that patients may be unable to take food and fluids or swallow oral secretions. Symptoms usually start approximately 2 weeks into a course of therapy. If the patient is receiving concurrent chemotherapy, symptoms may occur sooner and be more severe. As with oral mucositis, patients who continue to smoke and use alcohol are more at risk for acute and prolonged symptoms.

Management. Nursing management and interventions are similar to those for oral mucositis. Esophagitis/pharyngitis is a potentially serious toxicity if patients are unable to maintain nutrition and hydration. Patients should be weighed once or twice weekly and carefully assessed as to oral intake. Enteral feeding and IV hydration are needed in many patients and should be discussed prior to initiating irradiation. When prescribing medication for the patient with odynophagia, liquids or crushable tablets should be considered. Patients quickly determine what they can swallow, and intake usually centers on soft to liquid foods. Consultation and collaboration with a dietitian helps the patient maintain a high nutritional status.

Taste changes (dysgeusia, ageusia)

Taste buds (receptors) are primarily located on the tongue, soft palate, glossopalatine arch, and posterior wall of the pharynx. Taste sensation includes sweet, sour, salty, and bitter. Because the taste buds are extremely radiosensitive, symptoms are noted early in the course of treatment, often during weeks 1 and 2.[31] Patients typically describe a decrease in taste (hypogeusia) and altered taste (dysgeusia). In some patients this will progress to loss of all taste (ageusia).

Taste is integrally bound to appetite and when one cannot taste food it may result in progressive anorexia and weight loss. Patients may describe a sensation of the food creating a "tasteless ball of goo" in their mouth. Add to this the symptoms of xerostomia and mucositis/esophagitis, and eating can become an ordeal.

Management. Encourage oral care prior to meals to help clear residual tastes and refresh the mouth for meals.[31] Enhancing the palatability of foods is discussed in Chapter 33, and applies to patients undergoing radiation. The loss of "salt" perception can be particularly problematic for some patients if they add significant quantities of salt to their food. In such a case, a dietary consult can be very helpful.

Laryngitis

If the larynx is in the radiation treatment field(s), patients will experience laryngitis due to edema of the vocal cords.[28] Symptoms include hoarseness that can be mild to so severe that speech is almost impossible.

Management. Patients should be instructed to avoid straining to speak; however, this is difficult to accomplish. Elderly patients or those who live alone may be anxious that they will not be able to communicate their needs should they be in an emergent situation. Speech therapists can be consulted for assistive devices such as those that amplify the voice.

Instruct patients to avoid tobacco and alcohol. It is important to remember that compliance with abstinence from tobacco and alcohol can be difficult, if not impossible, for this group of patients who often have many years of dependency and use. Management of laryngitis is similar to esophagitis, focusing on nutrition, hydration, lubrication, and pain relief.

Dental caries

Dental caries technically are not an acute toxicity of head and neck irradiation, but preventive management for this during treatment is mandatory. All teeth are at risk, not just those in the path of the radiation beam. Due to the shift in the pH of the mouth toward a highly acid oral environment, a markedly cariogenic flora develops. The teeth rapidly demineralize and enamel defects appear, especially on the cervical and incisal/occlusal surfaces. The resulting dental demineralization almost always leads to radiation-induced caries.[39]

Preventive management. Dentulous patients must have a dental evaluation prior to starting radiation. Questionable teeth are extracted, ideally at least 14 days prior to the initiation of irradiation. Most often, dental prophylaxis consists of daily fluoride solution or gel applied to a mold (tray) and placed on upper and lower teeth, then held in place for several minutes. A home care fluoride regimen is essential but may not be possible to maintain if severe mucositis is present. This argues for even greater compliance with the oral care regimen until fluoride prophylaxis can be resumed.

Breast

Used in treatment for breast carcinoma, breast irradiation can result in several toxicities. This discussion focuses on the effects of breast irradiation after breast-preserving surgery.

Skin reactions

Skin reaction is the primary acute side effect of breast irradiation. Due to the tangential angle of the beam, the skin dose is enhanced. Skin in the treatment fields demonstrate erythema and hyperpigmentation. Changes are usually clinically evident at approximately 3000 cGy with standard fractions of 180–200 cGy daily.[40] Skin reactions can progress to severe erythema and moist desquamation, especially in the inframammary crease and axilla. Women who are at most risk for developing moist desquamation are those with large pendulous breasts, and women who have recently completed or are receiving concurrent chemotherapy.

Management. See Assessment and Management of Skin Reactions, above. The patient may also experience transient discomfort in the breast and axilla during radiation. It is unclear as to the etiology, however surgical changes and possibly transient radiation-related edema may be the cause. Such symptoms usually respond to nonsteroidal anti-inflammatory drugs such as ibuprofen or naproxyn.

Esophagitis

Esophagitis may occur if the supraclavicular fossa is included in the treatment field. Symptoms are usually mild and limited in duration.

Management. See Management under Esophagitis and pharyngitis in Head and Neck.

Chest and Lung

Used in treatment for lung, esophageal, gastric cancers, Hodgkin's disease, and non-Hodgkin's chest lymphoma, chest and lung irradiation results in the following toxicities.

Esophagitis and pharyngitis

Most radiation treatment fields for treatment of lung, esophageal, and gastric cancers, and some lymphomas include the mediastinum and thus affect the esophagus and hypopharynx. The radiation causes inflammation and denudation of the surface of the epithelium of the pharynx and esophagus. The resulting mucositis causes dysphagia and odynophagia that may become severe. Patients often describe the feeling of a "lump" in the throat and a feeling of obstruction when swallowing. Symptoms start 2–3 weeks after initiation of radiation, or sooner if the patient is receiving concurrent chemotherapy.[41] The treatment fields are usually angled (versus initial direct anterior-posterior fields) approximately two-thirds of the way into treatment, thus minimizing some of the dose to the pharynx and esophagus so symptoms lessen. Depending on the length (top to bottom) of the field and the site of esophageal or gastric cancer (e.g., tumor at the gastroesophageal junction), patients may experience gastric reflux that can exacerbate esophagitis symptoms.

Management. Management is similar to that described under Esophagitis and pharyngitis in the Head and Neck section. Dietary modifications are helpful and include a soft to liquid diet and nutritional supplements. Antacid therapy can be started for patients experiencing reflux symptoms. Close monitoring is essential as oral intake can decrease with fluid imbalance and weight loss occurring rapidly. Patients presenting with upper gastrointestinal and lung cancers frequently have impaired nutritional status and a history of tobacco and alcohol abuse, which can challenge optimum patient management.

Taste changes

It is unclear why patients receiving radiation to the chest experience taste changes. The cause is likely multifactorial, including prior or concurrent chemotherapy, fatigue, and medications such as opioids. Taste changes may lead to anorexia and, when combined with the previously described toxicities, can cause a cascade of effects including increased fatigue, weight loss, weakness, and delayed healing of acute side effects.

Management. Consultation with the oncology dietitian is helpful to define ways to maintain optimum nutritional status.

Pneumonitis (subacute)

Pneumonitis is not an infectious process, and *pneumonopathy* might be a more appropriate term. Pneumonitis is caused by a decrease in surfactant produced by the alveolar type-II pneumocytes, and endothelial cell and vessel permeability that negatively impacts perfusion.[28] Symptoms occur 1–3 months after completion of radiation and can be seen within days after administration of certain chemotherapeutic agents, such as bleomycin, chlorambucil, the nitrosureas, cyclophosphamide, methotrexate, and procarbazine. Symptomatic pneumonitis occurs in approximately 5%–15% of patients irradiated for mediastinal lymphoma or lung cancer, and approximately 1% of women treated for breast cancer.[42]

The severity of pneumonitis is dependent on the degree of pulmonary involvement, which is related to the amount of lung in the treatment fields. Symptoms include low-grade fever and nonspecific respiratory symptoms such as congestion, nonproductive cough, and a feeling of fullness in the chest. If symptoms progress, the patient may experience dyspnea, pleuritic chest pain, and increasing cough that may result in small amounts of sputum with hemoptysis. On examination, altered breath sounds are usually absent, and evidence of consolidation is sometimes found in the region corresponding to pneumonitis. Pleural friction rub or pleural fluid may be detected. Generally, the symptomatic phase of pneumonitis is relatively short in duration, and symptoms resolve completely.

Diagnosis of pneumonitis is made clinically with radiologic studies and symptom review. A chest x-ray (CXR) may reveal a diffuse infiltrate and possibly functional lung volume loss corresponding to the radiation field. Computerized tomography (CT) scans are more sensitive in evaluating lung density. Ventilation/perfusion scans are also used for diagnosis. Pulmonary function tests (PFT) will not demonstrate an abnormality until 4–8 weeks after completion of irradiation. A decrease in diffusion capacity is generally the most outstanding parameter on PFTs.[42]

Management. Treatment of the acute symptoms of pneumonitis includes absolute bed rest to conserve respiratory effort, bronchial dilators, oxygen therapy, and glucocorticoids. Treatment measures do not shorten the duration of pneumonitis; instead treatment aims to palliate symptoms. Pneumonitis can be severe with symptoms including fever and acute cor pulmonale that can lead to death. After the acute phase of pneumonitis, symptoms slowly improve, as damaged lung tissue regenerates.[42]

Nursing assessment includes evaluation of symptoms, and monitoring of oxygenation status and the patient's ability to complete activities of daily living. Acute cor pulmonale results primarily from disorders of the lungs and pulmonary vessels that cause hypertrophy or failure of the right ventricle. The occurrence of cor pulmonale is uncommon, but symptoms can be severe and debilitating. Signs of cor pulmonale relate to right-sided heart failure such as abdominal pain and bloating, peripheral edema especially of the lower extremities, weight gain, jugular venous distention, hepatomegaly, and hepatojugular reflex. Some nonspecific symptoms of cor pulmonale include tachycardia, pallor/cyanosis, fatigue, exercise intolerance, and weakness. Interventions for mild to moderate cor pulmonale secondary to radiation-induced pneumonitis include oxygen therapy, diuretics, and digoxin.

Abdomen and Pelvis

Used in treatment for gastrointestinal, genitourinary, and gynecologic cancers, abdomen and pelvis irradiation can result in the following toxicities.

Nausea and vomiting

Radiation therapy is a localized treatment, hence nausea and vomiting will not occur unless radiation fields include the whole abdomen, extended pelvic fields, epigastric region, paraaortic area, and in rare cases the chemoreceptor trigger zone (CTZ) in the cerebral cortex.[43] Symptoms of nausea and vomiting directly related to irradiation are fairly predictable and will occur 1–3 hours after the daily treatment. Nausea and vomiting are influenced by multiple other factors including medications (e.g., opioids, antibiotics), chemotherapeutic agents, constipation, pain, and metabolic alterations such as hypercalcemia.

Management. Patients who are at risk for nausea and vomiting should be premedicated with antiemetics approximately 1 hour prior to daily treatment, depending on medication and route of administration. The goal is to prevent an initial emetic episode. Around-the-clock administration of antiemetics may be necessary if symptoms warrant. It is difficult to definitively recommend whether patients should receive daily radiation treatment with an empty or full stomach. Generally, patients feel better and have less nausea if they eat small frequent meals or snacks, including prior to daily radiation. See Nausea and vomiting under Brain for a brief discussion of antiemetics commonly used in radiation therapy.

Diarrhea and proctitis

The size of the abdominal/pelvic radiation field generally determines the risk for diarrhea and proctitis. Diarrhea is a result of denuding of the intestinal mucosa, leading to decreased absorptive capacity and increased motility and peristalsis.[44] The small bowel is much more radiosensitive than the colon or rectum, and the extent of the small bowel's involvement greatly influences the severity of the symptoms. A patient undergoing whole-abdomen radiation is most at risk to experience watery diarrhea and cramping, while the patient with a relatively small pelvic field (e.g., radiation for prostate cancer) will most likely have frequent soft bowel movements rather than pronounced diarrhea.

Proctitis can be accompanied by tenesmus. Proctitis occurs most frequently in patients receiving radiation for rectal, anal, and prostate cancers due to the location of the inferior border of the treatment fields. Symptoms are compounded if concurrent chemotherapy is administered.

Management. Patients should be instructed regarding a low-residue diet and the use of antidiarrheals. A low-residue diet guideline is helpful to assist in teaching and for patient reference. Ethnic and geographic food patterns should be considered to support compliance.[43] An oncology dietitian consultation can be invaluable. It is helpful to advise the patient to have antidiarrheal medication (e.g., loperamide or diphenoxylate/atropine) on hand in case diarrhea occurs unexpectedly.

Proctitis symptoms can be treated with conservative management including sitz baths and anti-inflammatory agents such as pramoxine hydrochloride 1% and/or hydrocortisone acetate 1% (cream or foam). Gastro-intestinal-specific antispasmodics may decrease tenesmus symptoms. Diarrhea and frequent stools can result in painful irritation of the perianal region secondary to frequent cleansing. Helpful interventions include gently cleansing the perianal region (after each bowel movement) with warm water using a squirt bottle, pat dry, and then apply a barrier cream and using pre-moistened towelettes.

Assessment should start with the patient's definition of diarrhea and specific stool characteristics and frequency. Of most concern are frequent, watery stools that have the potential for inducing electrolyte imbalance and dehydration. Patients most at risk for dehydration due to diarrhea or vomiting include children, the elderly, debilitated individuals, and those receiving concurrent chemotherapy (e.g., 5-fluorouracil, cisplatin). It is essential to monitor weight frequently (daily if necessary), check orthostatic blood pressure, and assess skin and mucosal turgor. Some patients may require intravenous hydration and a break from radiation treatment.

Cystitis

Acute cystitis symptoms include dysuria, nocturia, hesitancy, urgency, and urinary frequency. The intensity and duration of symptoms are dependent on the volume of bladder in the radiation treatment field. As the radiation dose escalates, patients may experience tenesmus and bladder spasms that potentiate existing symptoms. Hematuria is uncommon. Symptoms of acute bladder irritation frequently occur 3–5 weeks after the initiation of radia-

tion therapy and usually subside 2–8 weeks after completion of treatment. Symptoms of cystitis subside with mucosal healing, pharmacologic intervention, and if needed a break from radiation treatment.[45]

Management. Pretreatment assessment of bladder function includes documentation of patterns of urinary elimination, such as symptoms of urgency, frequency, dysuria, and nocturia. A past history of urinary tract infections and medications used for treatment should be noted, as well as the presence of urinary diversions.[46]

Inflamed mucosal and ulceration of the bladder increase the potential for infection. Initial treatment consists of ruling out infection and antibiotic therapy if indicated. Infection often exacerbates bladder spasm and complicates delivery of radiation treatment. Antispasmodics help relieve dysuria and provide relief from bladder spasms. Optimal comfort is obtained if both infection and bladder spasm are treated simultaneously. Phenazopyridine hydrochloride is frequently used to treat dysuria symptoms. When taken orally, the majority of the drug enters the urine unchanged, where it acts as a topical analgesic within the bladder. When taking the drug, the patient's urine will be colored orange-red.

Symptoms such as mild urinary frequency are due to a modest reduction in bladder capacity. To increase storage capacity, antispasmodic medications such as oxybutynin chloride and flavoxate hydrochloride relax the bladder smooth muscle by inhibiting the muscarinic effects of acetylcholine. Side effects of antispasmodic therapy include hypertension, palpitation, arrhythmia, and stimulation of the central nervous system. Anticholinergic drugs should be used cautiously in those with cardiovascular diseases and hyperthyroidism and avoided in patients with bladder outlet obstructive symptoms. Relaxation of bladder smooth muscle can also be produced by blocking the alpha-1 adenoreceptors in the bladder with medications such as terazosin, or alpha-IA blocker such as tamsulosin which can decrease bladder outlet obstruction without affecting contractility. Use terazosin (alpha-1 blockers) cautiously in patients on antihypertensive medication.[45]

Instruct patients to maintain an adequate intake of fluids to promote frequent voiding and to decrease the potential for infection by diluting the bacterial population. Recommended fluid intake is 1–2 L/day. If voided urine is clear to light yellow in color, hydration is probably adequate. In addition, teaching patients to avoid foods that irritate the bladder mucosa may help to delay the onset of cystitis and decrease symptoms. These foods include coffee, tea, alcohol, spices, and tobacco products.[46] Encourage patients to report any signs of bladder irritation, such as dysuria, frequency, urgency with decreased urine volume, and any signs of hematuria or excessive mucus shreds in the urine. The nurse should also be aware of the baseline hemoglobin and hematocrit values as well as any coagulation studies. Hematuria usually causes minimal blood loss and rarely an anemia, but early documentation will assist in assessment of future problems. Acute cystitis symptoms cause discomfort and pain, and may significantly disrupt the patient's life. Reassure the patient that symptoms subside gradually over 2–8 weeks after completion of radiation.

Vaginal dryness

The most immediate response to irradiation of the vagina is loss of most or all of the vaginal epithelium, especially in areas in proximity to brachytherapy sources. This acute reaction results in vaginitis, with thinning and inflammation of the mucosa causing dryness, pruritus, and possibly a mucoid discharge.[47] Dyspareunia is common.

Patients report itching and discomfort, especially at the vaginal introitus that begins at variable points in the course of treatment. Onset of symptoms is usually early and more pronounced in women who have estrogen depletion.

Management.   Vaginal lubricants such as Astroglide® are advised to decrease dyspareunia. Acute radiation reactions such as erythema, moist desquamation, and confluent mucositis will resolve within 2–3 months after completion of irradiation. (See Chapter 37 for more on sexuality issues.)

Extremity

Used in treatment for sarcoma and bony metastasis, radiation to the extremities, due to minimal surrounding structures, generally results in few acute toxicities. Some fields for radiation of an extremity, such as the hip or femur, include surrounding pelvic structures, so the patient will be at risk for diarrhea due to bowel sensitivity. (See management of Diarrhea/proctitis under section on Abdomen and Pelvis Section, above.)

Eye

Used in treatment of intraocular malignancies, lymphoma and leukemia, CNS and head and neck cancers, and thyroid eye disease (benign pathology), eye irradiation can result in conjunctival edema and tearing.

Conjunctival edema and tearing

The eyelid, conjunctiva, cornea, sclera, and often the lacrimal gland are irradiated in treatment of ocular malignancies. Inflammatory response to radiation can occur within 24 hours following radiation, and the conjunctiva and other periocular tissues can develop edema secondary to diffuse infiltration by neutrophils. The conjunctiva will become erythematous, with periorbital edema occasionally developing within the first 24 hours after treatment. Other acute symptoms include transient eyelid erythema or edema, mild conjunctivitis, and loss of lashes. Patients may experience burning of the eye(s), sensation

of a foreign body, diminished vision, and excessive tearing.[48] Depending on the size of the radiation field, there may be alopecia of the eyebrow(s).

Management.   Ocular lubrication with an artificial tears solution or ointment, patching, and antibiotic drops as indicated is helpful. Toxicity-related symptoms peak within 10–20 days, resolve within 2–4 weeks, and heal completely within 8 weeks.[48]

Late Effects of Radiation: Site Specific

Since the earliest application of radiation in treating cancer, providers have been concerned about the late effects of radiation therapy on normal tissues and organs. The inability to precisely predict manifestations of late normal-tissue injury dictates the importance of vigilant patient follow-up. Late effects are usually progressive and can manifest months to years after completion of radiation therapy. Radiation-related second malignancies are a risk for some patients following successful radiation treatment.[49]

Radiation tissue tolerance, measured in degrees of minimal to maximum, can be a valuable guide for estimating long-term effects. The clinical applicability of tolerance doses has changed as a result of utilization of new agents such as biologic response modifiers, chemotherapeutic drugs, new modalities (hyperthermia, high dose rate brachytherapy, and radiosurgery), and these modalities' concurrent and subsequent use with traditional irradiation, chemotherapy, and surgery.[49]

Tissue and organ tolerance is determined by the radiosensitivity of relevant stem cell subpopulations, which may not always be proliferating or dividing. Within the radiation field(s), the most radiosensitive vital cell population determines whether there is organ tolerance or organ failure. Thus, the functional capacity of cells is often distinct from their regenerative capacity, permitting organ function to be preserved in the face of injury and allowing for recovery or repair from the radiation insult.[50] See Table 17-8 for radiation tolerance doses and complication end points, which are commonly referred to as late effects.[51]

All normal tissues do not follow the same behavior pattern in response to radiation. Late reactions occur in tissues that normally have low cell-cycle turnover or regeneration, such as the endothelium and connective tissues.[49] In such tissues, the radiation produces little change in the function of mature, differentiated cells, and therefore there is no early evidence of tissue malfunction until those mature cells gradually die due to normal wear and tear or additional trauma. When the tissue attempts to replace the lost cells by cellular division, the radiation damage inflicted on the tissues months or years earlier becomes manifest, as the cells are unable to produce viable new cells. In contrast, tissues in which the cells are normally being replaced every few hours or days (e.g.,

Table 17-8   Site Specific Late Effects of Radiation Therapy*

CNS
  Brain
    Focal/diffuse necrosis
    Leukoencephalopathy
    Pituitary/hypothalamic dysfunction
    Cognitive dysfunction
  Spinal cord
    Myelopathy/necrosis

Head and Neck
  Mucosa
    Paleness, thinning, telangiectasias
  Salivary gland
    Xerostomia
  Teeth/mandible
    Caries
    Temporomandibular joint fibrosis
    Osteoradionecrosis
  Thyroid
    Hypo-/hyperthyroid
    Thyroid cartilage necrosis
    Laryngeal edema
  Eye
    Cataracts
    Skin changes, loss of lashes
    Dry eye, corneal ulceration
    Visual loss/blindness

Chest
  Lung
    Pneumonitis (subacute)
    Pulmonary fibrosis
  Heart
    Cardiomyopathy
    Pericarditis
    Coronary artery disease
  Breast
    Skin tanning, fibrosis, telangiectasias
    Breast fibrosis, contraction, edema
    Increased risk of pathologic rib fracture
    Pneumonitis (subacute)
    Pulmonary fibrosis
    Pericarditis
    Arm edema if axilla supraclavicular lymph node treated

Bone
  Necrosis of femoral head

Gastrointestinal
  Esophagus
    Dysmotility
    Dysphagia/odynophagia
    Esophageal stricture
  Stomach
    Dyspepsia/gastritis
    Contracture
  Small/large bowel
    Mucosal injury
    Decreased motility, malabsorption
    Obstruction
  Rectum
    Proctitis
    Fistula
  Liver
    Radiation hepatitis
    Hepatic failure

Genitourinary
  Kidney
    Anemia
    Chronic radiation nephritis
    Hypertension
  Bladder
    Mucosal injury: hematuria
    Fistula
    Fibrosis
  Prostate
    Impotence
  Penis
    Mucosal changes
    Urethral stricture
  Vagina
    Thinning/atrophy/dry mucosa
    Narrowing, shortening, fibrosis

Reproductive
  Ovaries/testis
    Sterility

Hematopoietic
  Fibrosis
  Aplasia

Carcinogenesis
  Meningioma, nerve sheath glioma
  Sarcoma: bone/soft tissue
  Leukemias: acute myelogenous leukemia

*Because the tolerance levels of all tissues are known, the overall risk of radiation related late effects is very low. The percentage of risk varies by site, with bowel damage risk approximately 3%–5%, and upper extremity arm edema with lymph node radiation approximately 10%–15%.

skin and mucosa) quickly recognize that cell replacement is being impaired, even as treatment proceeds. These cells immediately activate compensatory mechanisms to speed up the rate of cell proliferation to counteract the accelerated rate of cell loss. Molecular biology, gene expression and cytokine cascade identification are key factors in the mechanisms responsible for late effects. Intercellular communication through autocrine, paracrine, and endocrine pathways via cytokine networks is the new pathophysiologic paradigm to explain the cellular process of late radiation effects.[52]

A model to aid understanding the clinical outcome of late effects of radiation, described by Marks, characterizes an organ as being composed of multiple functioning subunits (FSU) that operate in one of two ways, either as a parallel system or as a series system.[53] In a *parallel system*, organ function is generally maintained if damage occurs because the remaining FSUs operate independently from the damaged region, assuming there is adequate function in the remainder of the organ. Hence, part of an organ can be sacrificed or damaged beyond repair and the organ will still function adequately. The lung, liver, and kidney are highly sensitive to relatively low doses of radiation, but damage to part of these organs does not render them incapable of function. In a *series system*, damage to one portion of an organ may render the entire organ or system dysfunctional because the system must work in sequence. Examples include the gastrointestinal tract and neural tissues. This series system concept can encompass organ-to-organ interactions. Damage produced in one organ can have serious consequences in another organ, such as renal failure leading to overall multisystem failure and death.[53]

The impact of late radiation effects is now recognized as an important area of study, especially as it relates to quality of life. The dose-limiting organs in the treatment field define the amount of radiation prescribed. The risk of late effects related to radiation confirms the importance of accuracy in daily fraction dose, total radiation dose, volume treated, and patient comorbidities. The optimum dose-response curves to avoid late effects remain difficult to define despite extensive documentation of radiation injures in the literature. The accuracy of commonly used scales for quantification of acute and especially late reactions is important.[52]

In 1992, one group developed a grading scale for late effects of normal tissues (LENT). The goal was to create a simple, widely applicable, reproducible, and accurate scale—in ascending order of severity—of the complications of radiation treatment. The descriptors were divided into four major categories: subjective, objective, management, and analytic (SOMA). Each SOMA scale is site specific to more precisely define outcomes.[49] By monitoring different elements in the SOMA scales, it is hoped that the components of damage in individual organs may be differentiated, perhaps allowing more appropriate medical intervention to manage and alleviate symptoms.

By diligently measuring and reporting the outcomes of radiation treatment, one day we should be able to provide toxicity-free survival as well as achieve disease-free survival or local tumor control.[50]

The morbidity and the burden of specific late effects and toxicities may be perceived quite differently by patients and health care providers. This is especially true if the late effects and toxicities are protracted, irreversible, uncontrollable, painful, or socially disabling.[48] It is important to remember that the overall risk of late effects is small (but never zero) and that it varies by site treated. The risk of morbidity and mortality associated with no treatment for a primary or metastatic cancer is almost always greater than the risk of late effects. Ultimately, it is the patient and family who must decide how to weigh the risks and benefits of treatment.

Selected late effects on organ systems are discussed below. See Table 17-8 for a more inclusive list of site-specific late effects.

Central Nervous System

Brain necrosis

The onset of symptoms of brain necrosis can be as early as 6 months following radiation treatment, but the peak time of presentation of symptoms is 1–2 years after completion of radiation. Brain necrosis is typically not diffuse; instead, it is focal. Symptoms of brain necrosis include manifestations of increased intracranial pressure (ICP) such as headache, somnolence, intellectual and cognitive deficits, decrease in short- and long-term memory, seizures, and focal neurological deficits corresponding to the part of the brain irradiated. Magnetic resonance imaging (MRI) is the most sensitive tool available for diagnosing brain necrosis. Pathologic tissue confirmation may be necessary to differentiate necrosis from recurrent tumor.[50,54] Radiation-induced brain necrosis is usually progressive and fatal.

Management. If appropriate, surgical debulking of necrosis and use of corticosteroids can offer transient symptom relief.

Leukoencephalopathy

Leukoencephalopathy occurs almost exclusively after chemotherapy but can occur after brain irradiation, with or without chemotherapy.[50,54] It is characterized by multiple, noninflammatory necrotic foci in the white matter of brain tissue, with demyelination and reactive astrocytosis. Symptoms of leukoencephalopathy include lethargy, seizures, spasticity, paresis, and ataxia. Magnetic resonance imaging can be helpful in diagnosis. Leukoencephalopathy is generally irreversible.

Management. Treatment is limited to supportive measures, such as symptom management of seizures, and physical and occupational therapy consultations for assistance with motor dysfunction.

Cognitive and emotional dysfunction

The incidence and extent of radiation-related cognitive and emotional dysfunction is difficult to determine due to multiple variables, including underlying disease (primary tumor, leukemia), specific brain site, increased ICP, and effects of therapies including surgery and chemotherapy. Cognitive and emotional deficits following brain radiation are well documented in children, but the contribution by radiation alone is unclear because patients often receive systemic and intrathecal chemotherapy.[50,54]

Management. Neuropsychiatric consultation can be valuable for behavioral and pharmacologic management of specific dysfunctions.

Pituitary and hypothalamic dysfunction

Radiation damage can affect the hypothalamic-pituitary axis and cause permanent dysfunctions. Clinical syndromes include hypothyroidism, Addison's disease, diabetes insipidus, and decreased sexual hormone levels.[28] Growth hormone is commonly affected in children and must be monitored and replaced as needed.

Management.   Each specific syndrome is treated with replacement hormonal therapies and surveillance of hormone levels.

Spinal cord

Myelopathies are uncommon, but not rare, complications of cancer treatment. Because the multiple signs and symptoms of radiation myelopathy can occur in differing combinations at different rates of progression, it is not possible to make the diagnosis of radiation myelopathy based on symptoms alone. The initial signs are subtle and may not be noticed by patients. Symptoms include sensory deficits (unilateral or bilateral), that often manifest as diminished temperature sensation, leg weakness, clumsiness, and diminished proprioception. Objective signs and symptoms include changes in gait (often foot drop), spasticity, weakness, hemiparesis, Brown-Séquard syndrome, and possibly incontinence. Hyperreflexia and Babinski signs are often found on neurological examination. Pain may accompany symptoms. The patient may be asymptomatic until some trauma initiates a progressive neurological deficit. No specific combination of signs or symptoms can distinguish radiation myelopathy from myelopathies of many other etiologies.[54]

Management.   Management of radiation-induced spinal cord myelopathy has been primarily limited to administration of corticosteroids, with limited success. Response to corticosteroid therapy is transient with some improvement in symptoms and is likely due to a decrease in spinal cord edema. The prognosis in radiation myelopathy depends primarily on the degree to which the originally treated lesion transects the spinal cord and the anatomical level of the lesion. Complete transection of the cord is a sign of poor prognosis. Generally lesions at higher anatomical levels have a poorer prognosis than lesions at lower levels. The actuarial mortality from radiation-induced spinal cord myelopathy is 55% at 18 months for cervical lesions, and 25% at 18 months for thoracic lesions. Younger patients have a better prognosis than older patients.[54]

Head and Neck

There is the potential for multiple disabling late effects following head and neck irradiation. If the patient has also undergone surgical resection, there can be structural dysfunction in addition to the effects of irradiation. Persons with head and neck cancer usually require extensive rehabilitation to manage alterations related to speech, swallowing, eating, and respiratory function.

Xerostomia and dental caries

Xerostomia persists for months to years and almost always will be present to some degree. The extent of symptoms is dependent on the volume of salivary gland tissue irradiated, the total radiation dose, and individual patient response. As a consequence, patients may experience impaired ability to swallow, chew, talk, and wear dentures comfortably. Most patients permanently change the nature of their diet to some degree.

Radiation-induced dental effects are indirectly produced by salivary changes that occur when the parotid glands are included in the treatment portals, and rarely by direct effect of radiation on the teeth. Alteration of the normal oral microfloral balance to a more cariogenic one occurs as a result of changes in the salivary contents and a lowered oral pH. (See Xerostomia under Head and Neck section, above, for a more detailed outline of salivary composition.)

Dental decay and varying degrees of dental disintegration after irradiation typically develops along the gum line.[32] Thus, patients are at high risk for dental caries, periodontal disease, stomatitis, dysphagia, and altered taste.[31] Because of changes in the oral microflora secondary to xerostomia, candidiasis and other oral infections are more common. Long-term xerostomia and dental caries can be disabling and can significantly affect quality of life.

Management.   Management is as discussed in Xerostomia under Head and Neck section, above. The most important aspect of xerostomia management is compliance with life-long dental surveillance and prophylaxis.

Osteoradionecrosis

Osteoradionecrosis is a serious complication secondary to the effects of xerostomia and radiation to the maxilla and mandible. *Osteoradionecrosis* is characterized as a hypocellular and hypovascular dissolution of bone. Osteocytes and the supporting vasculature may be irreversibly injured by radiation. Osteoradionecrosis is progressive, can lead to intolerable pain or fracture, and may necessitate surgical resection. Patients most at risk are dentulous and require dental extractions after completing radiation therapy. Cooper and Fu believe that it is neither necessary nor advisable to extract all teeth before treatment as a preventive measure[32]; however, teeth of questionable viability should be extracted prior to initiating radiation therapy (see Dental caries under Head and Neck section, above). Nonirritating, well-fitting dentures do not appear to increase the incidence of osteoradionecrosis. Patients remain at risk for development of osteoradionecrosis for years following radiation therapy.

Most cases of osteoradionecrosis develop in the mandible. Osteoradionecrosis initially manifests as a nondescript erythematous change of the overlying mucosa, which then ulcerates to reveal the necrotic bone below. Necrotic bone has a dull appearance, unlike the pearly color of healthy periosteum.[32]

Management. Prevention of osteoradionecrosis includes meticulous oral and periodontal hygiene, with fluoride prophylaxis and frequent dental evaluation. Oral care must be maintained indefinitely because of impaired potential for healing in response to physical irritation, chemical agents, and microbial organisms.[32] Attempts should be made to replace or increase salivary flow (see Head and Neck section). Foods and beverages containing sucrose should be avoided. If caries develop, removal and restoration are advised immediately. Patients are at more risk for developing oral *Candida albicans* due to xerostomia, and prompt treatment helps maintain oral integrity. Optimum nutritional status is important for bone maintenance and healing. Head and neck patients are commonly at increased risk of nutritional compromise due to poor nutritional status at diagnosis and alterations in chewing and swallowing induced by surgery and radiation.

Treatment of osteoradionecrosis includes antibiotic therapy to help control acute pain, swelling, and suppuration. Surgical resection of osteoradionecrotic lesions is an option. One study demonstrated that 6 of 22 patients had lesions resected, with 3 patients demonstrating postsurgical recurrence. The preventive and therapeutic use of antibiotics and hyperbaric oxygen has been reported to be effective in some cases, but reproducible long-term benefit is equivocal.[32]

Hypothyroidism

Hypothyroidism is the most common clinical consequence of irradiation to the thyroid in patients who have received therapeutic doses to the neck area.[55] Patients should be monitored with periodic serum thyroid-stimulating hormone (TSH) and free-throxin 4 (FT4) screening.

Management. Hypothyroidism can be effectively treated with thyroid replacement.

Lung

Pulmonary fibrosis

Pulmonary fibrosis can develop insidiously in a previously irradiated lung field. There is debate as to whether one always has an acute phase of fibrosis, which may not be symptomatic but can be viewed radiographically. The degree of fibrosis stabilizes after 1–2 years. Radiation-induced lung injury is characterized by progressive fibrosis of the alveolar septa, which become thickened by bundles of elastic fibers. The alveoli subsequently collapse and are then obliterated by connective tissue. The hilum

or mediastinum may become retracted with a densely contracted lung segment, resulting in compensatory hyperinflation of adjacent or contralateral lung tissue.[42] These changes can lead to the appearance (usually within 1–2 years after radiation) of lung scarring on CXR that corresponds to the shape of the radiation portal; CT scan may provide more definitive imaging for diagnosis. Pulmonary function tests may suggest reduced tidal volume; however, PFTs do not demonstrate significant changes when small volumes of lung are irradiated, due to functional compensation by adjacent lung regions. Thus, PFTs are not the most accurate measurement of radiation-induced lung injury. Diffusion capacity may be the best measure of total lung function because this test is least likely to be affected by compensatory changes in unirradiated portions of the lung.[42]

Most patients with radiation-induced pulmonary fibrosis are asymptomatic. The clinical symptoms are directly related to the amount of lung parenchyma involved and the patients' preexisting pulmonary reserves. Symptoms are generally minimal if fibrosis is limited to less than 50% of one lung. If the volume of one irradiated lung increases above 50%, patients will likely become symptomatic to some degree. Symptoms include dyspnea on exertion, reduced exercise tolerance, orthopnea, cyanosis, and finger clubbing. In some instances, chronic respiratory failure can occur and may result in cor pulmonale and subsequent right heart failure.[42]

Management. Management of radiation-induced pulmonary fibrosis consists of supportive care, such as oxygen therapy and pulmonary rehabilitation exercises to manage respiratory symptoms.

Heart

Pericarditis

Pericarditis is a result of fibrosis in the parietal pericardium that may progress to constriction of the heart.

Management. If signs of heart failure occur, treatment is focused on increasing cardiac output to maintain system perfusion. Excessive pericardial fluid may accumulate rapidly to produce cardiac tamponade, which must be relieved by pericardiocentesis or pericardiectomy. Pericardial disease may develop several months to years after radiation therapy. Patients may exhibit symptoms of acute pericarditis or have a chronic pericardial effusion.[56]

Cardiomyopathy

The myocardium is involved less frequently than the pericardium. The myocardium can develop patches of diffuse fibrosis affecting the anterior wall of the left ventricle and, less frequently, the anterior wall of the right ventricle.[56]

Patients present with severe signs and symptoms of pericardial disease, with constriction and severe heart failure. The cardiomyopathy becomes evident when symptoms do not improve with pericardiectomy. Left ventricular ejection function (LVEF) studies can be used for monitoring during chemotherapy and radiation. Doses of radiation and anthracyclines normally considered safe may precipitate severe cardiomyopathy when both agents are used simultaneously or sequentially.[56]

Management. If signs of heart failure occur, treatment is focused on increasing cardiac output to maintain system perfusion.

Breast

The total radiation dose to the whole breast for management of microscopic residual disease is 4500–5000 cGy. In this dose range the incidence of late effects is very low. Higher doses to the whole breast ($\geq$6000–6500 cGy) are associated with atrophy, fibrosis, retraction, and telangiectasias that predispose the patient to a poor cosmetic outcome. Rarely, late effects occur that limit function, such as breast tissue contraction, necrosis, or neuropathy. Moist desquamation of the skin during radiation is not predictive of late effects.

Management. Management is directed at relieving symptoms; surgical intervention occurs as appropriate.[5] Surgical revision of a contracted painful breast can be difficult due to the risk of poor healing after definitive radiation doses to the breast and surrounding tissues. It must be emphasized that late effects as described, with a poor cosmetic outcome, are extremely rare today with the radiation doses used and modern high-energy equipment.

Abdomen and Pelvis

Small and large bowel injury

The radiation tolerance of the small and large bowel is a major dose-limiting factor in the treatment of many cancers of the abdomen and pelvis. Late radiation-related injury to the bowel is caused by fibrosis and ischemia. Symptoms include fecal frequency/urgency, bleeding, pain, fistula formation, and intractable diarrhea. Due to anatomically smaller lumen size, obstruction is more common in the small bowel than in the large bowel or rectum. The most important factors contributing to the extent of bowel injury include radiation dose (the rectum may be more tolerant than the remainder of the bowel), prior abdominal surgery, history of pelvic inflammatory disease, and concurrent chemotherapy. Some studies suggest that a history of hypertension or diabetes mellitus may be associated with a greater risk of late intestinal injury. The likelihood of severe late complications to the bowel is low, approximately 5% or less, with current treatment approaches and radiation doses.[57]

Management. Chronic radiation injury to the small and large intestine can be managed by a low-residue diet, stool softeners, and use of loperamide or diphenoxylate with atropine. If reduced rectal sphincter compliance is a problem, fiber laxatives can be used to provide form, consistency, and softening of the stool. For diarrhea caused by small bowel injury, several studies have suggested the use of cholestyramine. This presumably helps by reducing the level of intraluminal bile salts. Proctitis can be managed by a course of pentosan polysulfate, which may improve mucosal integrity. Severe injury that results in ulceration and bleeding can be controlled by endoscopic laser treatment or suction cautery. Partial small bowel obstruction may be managed by bowel rest and decompression followed by dietary modification. Surgery may be necessary to relieve more extensive bowel obstruction. However controversy exists as to the extent of surgical resection necessary—whether all adhesions within the bowel should be lysed versus limiting the resection to the area(s) acutely involved. Generally, it can be said that an aggressive surgical approach to resection will potentially have a better impact on the quality of life of the patient. Prior to surgery, consultation with the radiation oncologist is important to delineate the exact radiation dose given and the extent of the treatment field.[57]

Genitourinary System

Bladder

Most late radiation-induced complications of the bladder are related to contracture, bleeding, symptomatic cystitis, and rarely fistulas. Incontinence is not common, but if found is likely related to the additive effect of radiation and prior surgical manipulations of the bladder neck and urethra. The degree of late radiation-related symptoms is dependent on the amount of bladder included in the radiation treatment fields. Irradiation fields for prostate cancer include much less bladder volume than the treatment fields for bladder cancer.

Management. Treatment for late effects on the bladder is individualized and may include drug therapy to reduce cystitis symptoms (e.g., pentosan polysulfate) or surgical intervention for bleeding or to manage fistulas (e.g., vesicovaginal fistula).

Vagina

Chronic effects, occurring 12 months or more after completion of radiation, include thinning and atrophy of the vaginal epithelium and development of telangiectasias. Patients may experience a decrease in size of the vaginal vault due to narrowing, shortening (made more pronounced after radical hysterectomy), paravaginal fibrosis, loss of elasticity, adhesions, and marked decrease in vaginal lubrication. All these manifestations often result in dyspareunia. Brachytherapy results in more pronounced acute symptoms and can contribute to late effects.[47]

Management. Management begins with preradiation teaching so patients are aware of what to expect after radiation. If the patient is not sexually active, dilators can be used to maintain vaginal patency. Women should be instructed about the importance of keeping the vagina patent and minimizing fibrosis in order to facilitate future physical examinations essential for tumor surveillance. Problems with sexual adjustment after radiation therapy can be significant. Women may have depressive symptoms, fear of injury from intercourse, fear of recurrent cancer, poor communication with sex partner, feeling of being less feminine and desirable, and separation and loss of sex partner.[47] The nurse often is the most accessible and comfortable person with whom the patient can discuss this physically and emotionally complex topic.

Reproductive System

Ovary

The probability of sterility and endocrine insufficiency is related to radiation dose, fraction size, and patient age. Definitive external pelvic irradiation of doses exceeding 2400 cGy will produce permanent ovarian ablation in the adult female. If the woman is postmenopausal, there are few consequences. However, for the premenopausal woman, symptoms will be similar to those of menopause including: hot flashes, atrophic vulvitis, vaginitis with pruritus and dyspareunia, alterations in body fat distribution, changes in the breasts, accelerated bone demineralization, potential premature cardiovascular disease, and unpredictable effects on libido. The severity of these effects varies among individuals, based on body habitus and levels of estrogen production, both adrenal and peripheral.[47]

Management. Management of estrogen deficit produced by damage to the ovaries is dependent on the specific cancer. Estrogen replacement in women with breast cancer is controversial and seldom advised. For women with gynecological cancers, estrogen and progesterone replacement has a role. Women are advised to discuss the issue with their oncologists. Nontraditional medicine may be helpful in providing relief of menopausal symptoms with the use of natural and herbal preparations. Women with breast cancer are generally advised to avoid all estrogens, including phytoestrogens, until more is known regarding the pathophysiology of these substances and the specific malignancy.

The premenopausal woman who requires radiation therapy that will include the ovaries may have concerns regarding conservation of potential reproductive capability. Preventing ovarian ablation is an achievable goal in patients treated with radiation. A thorough discussion of the available alternatives should occur prior to selection of a definitive plan for treatment. Strategies for conserv-

ing reproductive capability include utilization of reproductive technology such as in vitro fertilization and transplantation of one or both ovaries to sites remote from the radiation fields. If the patient is receiving high-dose chemotherapy, ovarian ablation may occur despite efforts to remove them from path of the radiation beam.[47]

Testis

The testis is highly radiosensitive, and a small dose of 200–1000 cGy or fractionated dose of 100–200 cGy of radiation will cause permanent sterility. Young men who require radiation that may affect the testes should be referred for sperm analysis and sperm banking as appropriate. Testicular shields can be used but they will not prevent internal radiation scatter; therefore, the testes will receive some radiation dose.[58]

The severity of the impairment in spermatogenesis and length of recovery depend on the radiation dose to the testis. In the typical patient receiving irradiation for a classic seminoma, the remaining testis receives a dose in the range of 30–180 cGy. An even greater dose is delivered to the contralateral testis if the hemiscrotum is irradiated. Radiation doses of this magnitude usually produce temporary oligospermia or azoospermia followed by recovery 18–24 months later.[58]

Management. A patient may become fertile during the recovery phase, and should be counseled regarding this possibility. Mutations induced in germinal stem cells may produce abnormal spermatozoa. Fortunately, the potentially abnormal spermatozoa arising from these mutated stem cells tend to have poor fertilization potential. The occurrence of the mutations depends on the radiation dose delivered. No genetic abnormalities from ionizing radiation have been demonstrated in humans, which perhaps reflects the body's ability to repair such damage.[58] Patients are advised to practice birth control during and after irradiation. The length of time to practice birth control is not entirely clear, but generally 24 months are recommended to allow for recovery of normal spermatogenesis.

Sexual dysfunction

A comprehensive discussion of sexuality and interventions is beyond the scope of this chapter and the reader is referred to Chapter 37. However, it is important to recognize that sexual dysfunction in both men and women can occur after radiation therapy for various malignancies, especially gynecological and genitourinary cancers. Radiation therapy can cause significant sexual disruption. It is incumbent on oncology nurses to recognize that sexual dysfunction is a problem which may be of great concern to the patient and partner and therefore affect quality of life. Patients and their partners rarely verbalize issues or concerns about sexual dysfunction. Obtaining a sexual history prior to initiating treatment may allow for implementation of preventive measures that can lessen dysfunction. The direct effects of irradiation on normal tissue may progress over a number of years; thus, sexual dysfunction may be progressive and require life-long rehabilitation and interventions.[47]

Secondary Malignancies

In the retrospective evaluation of radiation-induced secondary malignancies, an important factor to remember is that many patients in the studies were originally treated in the 1950s and 1960s, with some being treated as far back as 1925. Thus, patients were treated with techniques and doses different from the more refined radiation therapy currently in use.[59] Some of the criteria for defining second cancer include:

- Secondary tumors must have a different histological appearance from primary tumors.

- Both the primary and secondary tumor must be malignant.

- Both must be anatomically separate and the second tumor cannot be a metastasis from the primary tumor.

- Secondary tumors must produce their own metastases.[59]

With increasing longevity, many patients may develop second cancers anywhere from 6 months to 20 years or more after completion of treatment for the primary cancer. Considering the difficulty of classifying and identifying secondary cancers induced by radiation, their incidence may be higher than current studies indicate. It is important to implement careful follow-up and surveillance for recent patients to determine whether changes in therapeutic technique and radiation doses have affected the incidence of second cancers.[59]

Most solid tumors (e.g., sarcoma) do not occur until 10 years or more after radiation exposure, and for some cancer sites (e.g., breast and bladder) excess risks emerge only 15 years or more after irradiation. Radiation-induced sarcomas of bone and soft tissue are the most frequent secondary malignant neoplasms in irradiated tissues. Sarcomas have a high tendency to recur locally, metastasize, and become one of the most fatal complications of radiation therapy.[59] Most of the knowledge about radiation effects in humans has come from epidemiological studies of atom bomb survivors in Japan, occupationally irradiated workers, patients exposed to large amounts of diagnostic radiation, and patients treated with radiation for malignant and nonmalignant diseases. Studies in the atom bomb survivors and in women treated for benign gynecological disorders have shown that the excess relative risk per gray tends to be fairly stable for at least 30 years following radiation. At present, it is not known whether the relative risk remains elevated throughout life or if the risk for different solid tumors versus leukemia or lymphomatous cancers varies. The risk of leukemia attributable to irradiation is observed within a few years from radiation exposure, with a peak after 5–9 years and a gradual decline thereafter. Continuous exposures, given at low-dose rates, are less leukemogenic than a single radiation dose. Age at exposure may be the greatest determinant of risk for radiation-induced cancer, especially in those patients irradiated as children and adolescents.[60]

Knowledge of the risk factors for second malignancy has made it possible to identify patient groups at high risk of developing second cancers due to treatments they received in the past. An example is the increased risk of breast cancer in women treated as youngsters with mantle irradiation for Hodgkin's disease. Previously irradiated patients should be closely monitored and screened as appropriate. Preventive strategies, such as smoking cessation, may substantially reduce risk of developing a treatment-related cancer.

The issue of treatment-induced second cancers must always be viewed in relation to the dramatic improvement in survival rates for various malignancies. The carcinogenic effects of therapeutic irradiation deserve more investigation. Issues to be clarified include the shape of the radiation dose-response curve in the higher dose range, the duration of radiation-induced cancer risk, the effects of dose fractionation, age at radiation exposure, the interaction of radiation therapy with environmental carcinogens, and genetic susceptibility. Because the mechanisms underlying the carcinogenic effects of radiation are still poorly understood, research should also focus on the identification of specific gene alterations associated with the development of radiation-induced cancer.[60]

The risk associated with cancer treatment should be weighed carefully against the consequences of not using such treatments. Changes in therapies to reduce the risk of late complications and second malignancies should be made only in the context of carefully designed clinical trials that evaluate whether the overall efficacy of treatment is maintained. In addition, for many new cancer treatments the long-term risk of second malignancies is not known.[60]

Conclusion

Cancer treatment with radiation therapy can be rigorous, with multiple acute toxicities and the risk of late effects. However, due to advances in technology (e.g., conformal therapy, stereotactic radiosurgery, and high-dose brachytherapy), treatment is associated with fewer side effects and optimum outcomes. While a toxicity-free course of radiation probably is not realistic, oncology nurses are skilled at managing side effects and supporting patients through a course of therapy. Balancing treatment outcomes, especially when palliation is the goal, with quality of life remains a priority. Oncology nurses are integral in caring for cancer patients and their families at each point on the treatment continuum.

References

1. Hall E: *Radiobiology for the Radiologist*. New York, Lippincott-Raven, 1994
2. Hellman S: Principles of cancer management: Radiation therapy, in DeVita VT, Hellman S, Rosenberg SA (eds): *Cancer: Principles and Practice of Oncology* (ed 5). Philadelphia, Lippincott-Raven, 1997, pp 307–332
3. Chao KS, Perez CA, Brady LW: Fundamentals of patient management, in Chao DS, Perez CA, Brady LW (eds): *Radiation Oncology Management Decisions*. Philadelphia, Lippincott-Raven, 1999, pp 1–13
4. Coia LR, Moylan DJ: *Introduction to Clinical Radiation Oncology* (ed 3). Madison, WI, Medical Physics Publishing, 1994
5. Archambieu JO, Pezner R: Pathophysiology of irradiated skin and breast. *Int J Radiat Oncol Biol Phys* 31:1171–1185, 1995
6. Wengstrom Y: Assessing nursing problems of importance for the development of nursing care in a radiation therapy department. *Cancer Nurs* 21:50–53, 1998
7. Hinds C, Streater A, Mood C: Functions and preferred methods of receiving information related to radiotherapy. *Cancer Nurs* 18:374–384, 1995
8. Poroch D: The effect of preparatory patient education on the anxiety and satisfaction of cancer patients receiving radiation therapy. *Cancer Nurs* 18:206–214, 1995
9. Dunne-Daly CF: Nursing care and adverse reactions of external radiation therapy: A self-learning module. *Cancer Nurs* 17:236–256, 1994
10. Christman NJ: Uncertainty and adjustment during radiotherapy. *Nurs Res* 39:17–20, 1990
11. Strunk B, Maher KE: Collaborative nurse management of multifactorial moist desquamation in a patient undergoing radiotherapy. *J Enterost Ther Nurs* 20:152–157, 1993
12. Sitton E: Managing side effects of skin changes and fatigue, in Dow KH, Bucholtz JD, Iwamoto RR, et al (eds): *Nursing Care in Radiation Oncology* (ed 2). Philadelphia, Saunders, 1997, pp 79–100
13. Goodman M, Hilderley LJ, Purl S: Integumentary and mucous membrane alterations, in Groenwald SL, Frogge MH, Goodman M, Yarbro CH (eds): *Cancer Nursing: Principles and Practice* (ed 4). Sudbury, MA, Jones and Bartlett, 1997, pp 768–822
14. Dunne-Daly CF: Skin and wound care in radiation oncology. *Cancer Nurs* 18:144–162, 1995
15. Burch SE, Parker SA, Vann AM, et al: Measurement of 6-MV x-ray surface dose when topical agents are applied prior to external beam irradiation. *Int J Radiat Oncol Biol Phys* 38:447–451, 1997
16. Campbell IR, Illingworth MH: Can patients wash during radiotherapy to the breast or chest wall? A randomized controlled trial. *Clin Oncol* 4:78–82, 1992
17. Portenoy RK, Itri LM: Cancer-related fatigue: Guidelines for evaluation and management. *Oncologist* 4:1–10, 1999
18. Piper BF: The Groopman article reviewed. *Oncol* 12:345–346, 1996
19. Clark PM, Lacasse C: Cancer-related fatigue: Clinical practice issues. *Clin J Oncol Nurs* 2:45–54, 1998
20. Greenberg DB, Sawicka J, Eisenthal S, et al: Fatigue syndrome due to localized radiation. *J Pain Sympt Manage* 7:38–45, 1992
21. Munro AJ, Potter S: A quantitative approach to the distress caused by symptoms in patients treated with radical radiotherapy. *Br J Cancer* 74:640–647, 1996
22. King KB, Nail LM, Kraemer K, et al: Patients' descriptions of the experience of receiving radiation therapy. *Oncol Nurs Forum* 12:55–61, 1985
23. Graydon JE, Bubela N, Irvine D, et al: Fatigue-reducing strategies used by patients receiving treatment for cancer. *Cancer Nurs* 18:23–28, 1995
24. Irvine DM, Vincent L, Graydon JE, et al: Fatigue in women with breast cancer receiving radiation therapy. *Cancer Nurs* 21:127–135, 1998
25. Mauch P, Constine L, Greenberger J, et al: Hematopoietic stem cell compartment: Acute and late effects of radiation therapy and chemotherapy. *Int J Radiat Oncol Biol Phys* 31:1319–1339, 1995
26. Casarett GW: *Radiation Histopathology* (vol. 1). Boca Raton, FL, CRC Press 1980
27. Hashimoto M: The distribution of active marrow in the bones of the normal adult. *Kyushu J Med Sci* 11:103–111, 1960
28. Bruner DW, Bucholtz JD, Iwamoto R, Strohl R (eds): *Manual for Radiation Oncology Nursing Practice and Education*. Pittsburgh, Oncology Nursing Press, 1998
29. Wara WM, Bauman GS, Sneed PK, et al: Brain, brain stem and cerebellum, in Perez CA, Brady LW (eds): *Principles and Practice of Radiation Oncology* (ed 3). Philadelphia, Lippincott, 1997, pp 777–828
30. Kun LE: The brain and spinal cord, in Cox JD (ed): *Moss' Radiation Oncology: Rationale, Technique, Results* (ed 7). St. Louis, Mosby, 1994, pp 737–742
31. Iwamoto RR: Cancers of the head and neck, in Dow KH, Bucholtz JD, Iwamoto RR, et al (eds): *Nursing Care in Radiation Oncology* (ed 2). Philadelphia, Saunders, 1997, pp 239–260
32. Cooper JS, Fu K: Late effects of radiation therapy in the head and neck region. *Int J Radiat Oncol Biol Phys* 31:1141–1164, 1995
33. Iwamoto RR: Radiation therapy, in Otto SE (ed): *Oncology Nursing* (ed 3). St. Louis, Mosby, 1997, pp 503–529
34. Mandel ID, Katz R, Zengo A, et al: The effects of pharmacologic agent on salivary secretion and composition in man. 1. Pilocarpine, atropine and anticholinesterases. *J Oral Ther Pharmacol* 4:192–199, 1968
35. Greenspan E, Daniels TE: Effectiveness of pilocarpine in postradiation xerostomia. *Cancer* 59:1123–1125, 1987
36. LeVeque FG, Montgomery F, Potter D, et al: A multi-center randomized, double-blind, placebo-controlled, dose-titration study of oral pilocarpine for treatment of radiation-induced xerostomia in head and neck cancer patients. *J Clin Oncol* 11:1124–1131, 1993
37. Johnson JT, Ferretti GA, Nethery WJ, et al: Oral pilocarpine for post irradiation xerostomia in patients with head and neck cancer. *N Engl J Med* 329:390–395, 1993
38. Zimmerman R, Mark R, Tran L, et al: Concomitant pilocarpine during head and neck irradiation is associated with decreased posttreatment xerostomia. *Int J Radiat Oncol Biol Phys* 37:571–575, 1997
39. Rothstein JP: *Oral Care of Cancer Patients* (ed 7). Tampa, Florida Division, American Cancer Society, 1998
40. Mazanec SR: Breast cancer, in Dow KH, Bucholtz JD, Iwamoto RR, et al (eds): *Nursing Care in Radiation Oncology* (ed 2). Philadelphia, Saunders, 1997, pp 101–135

41. Knopp JM: Lung cancer, in Dow KH, Bucholtz JD, Iwamoto RR, et al (eds): *Nursing Care in Radiation Oncology* (ed 2). Philadelphia, Saunders, 1997, pp 293–315

42. McDonald S, Rubin P, Phillips TL, et al: Injury to the lung from cancer therapy: Clinical syndromes, measurable endpoints, and potential scoring systems. *Int J Radiat Oncol Biol Phys* 31:1187–1204, 1995

43. Hilderley LJ: Radiotherapy, in Groenwald S, Frogge MH, Goodman M, Yarbro CH (eds): *Cancer Nursing: Principles and Practice* (ed 4). Sudbury, MA, Jones and Bartlett, 1997, pp 247–282

44. Stevens KR: Stomach and small intestine, in Cox JD (ed): *Moss' Radiation Oncology: Rationale, Technique, Results* (ed 7). St. Louis, Mosby, 1994, pp 428–439

45. Maher KE: Male genitourinary cancers, in Dow KH, Bucholtz JD, Iwamoto RR, et al (eds): *Nursing Care in Radiation Oncology* (ed 2). Philadelphia, Saunders, 1997, pp 184–221

46. McCarthy CP: Altered patterns of elimination, in Dow KH, Hilderley LH (eds): *Nursing Care in Radiation Oncology*. Philadelphia, Saunders, 1992, pp 126–148

47. Grigsby PW, Russell A, Bruner D, et al: Late injury of cancer therapy on the female reproductive tract. *Int J Radiat Oncol Biol Phys* 31:1281–1300, 1995

48. Gordon KB, Char DH: Late effects of radiation on the eye and ocular adnexa. *Int J Radiat Oncol Biol Phys* 31:1123–1140, 1995

49. Rubin R, Constine LS, Fajardo D. et al: RTOG late effects working group-overview: Late effects of normal tissues (LENT) scoring system. *Int J Radiat Oncol Biol Phys* 31:1041–1042, 1995

50. Rubin P, Constine LS, Williams JP: Late effects of cancer treatment: Radiation and drug toxicity, in Perez CA, Brady LW (eds): *Principles and Practice of Radiation Oncology* (ed 3). Philadelphia, Lippincott, 1997, pp 155–211

51. Rubin P: The law and order of radiation sensitivity, absolute vs. relative, in Vaeth JM, Meyer JL (eds): *Radiation Tolerance of Normal Tissues: Frontiers of Radiation Therapy and Oncology*, Basel, Switzerland, Karger, 1989, pp 7–40

52. Pavy JJ, Denekamp J, Letschert J, et al: EORTC late effects working group-late effects toxicity scoring: The SOMA scale. *Int J Radiat Oncol Biol Phys* 31:1043–1048, 1995

53. Marks LB: The impact of organ structure on radiation response. *Int J Radiat Oncol Biol Phys* 34:1165–1171, 1996

54. Schultheiss TE, Kun LE, Ang KK, et al: Radiation response of the central nervous system. *Int J Radiat Oncol Biol Phys* 31:1093–1112, 1995

55. Hancock SL, McDougall IR: Thyroid abnormalities after therapeutic external radiation. *Int J Radiat Oncol Biol Phys* 31:1165–1170, 1995

56. Stewart JR, Fajardo LF, Gillette LM, et al: Radiation injury to the heart. *Int J Radiat Oncol Biol Phys* 31:1205–1211, 1995

57. Coia LR, Myerson RJ: Late effects of radiation therapy on the gastrointestinal tract. *Int J Radiat Oncol Biol Phys* 31: 1213–1236, 1995

58. Hussey DH: The testicle, in Cox JD (ed): *Moss' Radiation Oncology: Rationale, Technique, Results* (ed 7). St. Louis, Mosby, 1994, pp 559–586

59. Haas R: Evaluating the risks of radiation-induced secondary cancers. *Radiat Ther* 4:104–112, 1996

60. Flora E, van Leeuwen A: Second cancers, in DeVita VT, Hellman S, Rosenberg SA (eds): *Cancer: Principles and Practice of Oncology* (ed 5). Philadelphia, Lippincott-Raven, 1997, pp 2273–2296

CHAPTER 18

Chemotherapy: Principles of Therapy

Peter V. Tortorice, PharmD, BCOP

Historical Perspective

The term *chemotherapy* was first coined to describe the use of chemicals or drugs to treat microbial diseases and later neoplastic diseases.[1] In the 1940s, nitrogen mustard, the first cytotoxic drug, was introduced for cancer chemotherapy. Nitrogen mustard—a derivative of mustard gas, which was used as a chemical deterrent in the two world wars—was developed as an antineoplastic agent after it was learned that soldiers exposed to this drug developed reversible leukopenia. Soon after the introduction of nitrogen mustard, methotrexate, cyclophosphamide, and fluorouracil were made available for treatment of advanced cancers. Two significant developments occurred in the 1960s and late 1970s that opened the door for modern-day cancer chemotherapy: (1) the introduction of platinum-coordinated complexes as cytotoxic therapy, and (2) the introduction of combination chemotherapy to improve response rates and survival without significantly affecting toxicity.

The screening, synthesis, and clinical testing of new compounds or analogues of currently active agents continued through the 1970s and 1980s. Among the most useful agents discovered during this period were the semisynthetic podophyllotoxin etoposide and paclitaxel, a natural product isolated from the Western yew tree. The development of the anthracycline analogue doxorubicin also had a significant impact on the treatment of breast cancer and sarcomas. The biologic response modifiers were first recognized as having antineoplastic activity in the 1980s. The search for new agents to treat cancer continues into the twenty-first century.

Strategies being emphasized for drug development in the new decade include drugs with novel mechanisms of action, monoclonal antibodies directed against specific cellular targets, drugs that modulate or reverse drug resistance, and drugs used for supportive care of the cancer patient. Supportive therapies that have made administering and managing chemotherapy easier and safer include simple and effective antiemetic therapy and hematopoietic growth factors.

Historically, the goals of early chemotherapy were primarily limited to palliation of symptoms. An increase in available agents and more experience with cytotoxic chemotherapy produced significant tumor regression and improved control of cancer. The development and acceptance of combination chemotherapy greatly improved the outcome of otherwise incurable neoplastic diseases. This approach to cancer treatment incorporated the theoretical point that targeting multiple biochemical processes would have a greater overall effect on tumor regression and remission. The goals of chemotherapy then shifted to a curative approach for those cancers in which complete responses to chemotherapy were seen. Cancers for which cures and increased survival have been accomplished using chemotherapy alone or in combination with other modalities such as surgery and radiation therapy are listed in Table 18-1. Although chemotherapy

Table 18-1 Chemotherapy-Sensitive Tumors

Relative Chemosensitivity and Expected Survival Outcome	Type of Cancer
Highly sensitive: Normal survival, possible cure	Acute leukemia in children Hodgkin's disease Diffuse large-cell lymphoma Burkitt's lymphoma Testicular carcinoma Embryonal carcinoma Ewing's sarcoma Wilms' tumor Skin cancer
Moderately sensitive: Increase in survival	Ovarian carcinoma Breast carcinoma Endometrial carcinoma Acute leukemia in adults Small cell lung cancer Prostate cancer Stomach cancer Cervical cancer Neuroblastoma
Minimally sensitive: Some increase in survival	Head and neck cancers Gastrointestinal cancers Endocrine gland tumors Malignant melanoma Osteogenic sarcoma Soft tissue sarcoma
Marginally sensitive: No documented increase in survival	Bladder cancer Esophageal cancer Non–small cell lung cancer Pancreatic carcinoma Hepatocellular carcinoma

has produced cures in a subset of patients with cancers such as acute leukemia, Hodgkin's disease, and testicular tumors, significant cure rates for the most common cancers such as breast cancer, lung cancer, and colon cancer have not been achieved.

The use of drugs to control or eradicate cancer has developed into the specialization of medical oncology. The treatment of individuals with cancer is one of the most rapidly expanding and dynamic fields in medicine and demands continuous reevaluation and reappraisal of new and established therapies. To continue to develop and improve cancer treatment, more patients need to participate in controlled clinical trials. It is estimated that fewer than 10% of eligible patients actively being treated for cancer are enrolled in clinical trials. The clinician is a key figure in encouraging cooperation not only from the patient and his or her family but also from the health care community, including providers and sponsors (third-party payers). Increased survival and, more important, the maintenance or improvement of quality of life for patients with cancer can be achieved with the appropriate use of chemotherapy.

Cancer Chemotherapy Drug Development

Drug discovery and the eventual development of cancer treatment compounds involve numerous strategies. The most successful methods seek to combine current knowledge of the biology of cancer and the pharmacologic properties of potentially therapeutic compounds. Synthesis and testing of analogues of compounds with known antineoplastic activity is one of the approaches that has had some success. Synthesis of chemically or mechanistically similar compounds having different pharmacokinetic or toxic properties has yielded clinically useful new agents. An example of this approach may be found with the introduction of the new camptothecins: topotecan and irinotecan. Both agents are effective topoisomerase I inhibitors but lack the unpredictable urotoxicity seen with earlier camptothecin derivatives. Another approach to developing new antineoplastic agents is further identifying the proposed mechanism of action for previously identified active compounds. The elucidation of the specific effects of paclitaxel on tubulin formation and the identification of etoposide as a topoisomerase inhibitor are examples of this approach to drug development.

The oncology research community is composed of national and local study groups, university-based research programs, and pharmaceutical manufacturers. The National Cancer Institute (NCI) assists in coordinating the massive efforts of researchers and clinicians in screening and developing drugs for use in cancer treatment. A significant amount of research and development, primarily by pharmaceutical manufacturers, is conducted outside the NCI.

The drug approval process in the United States is rigorous and comprehensive. New compounds undergo extensive testing in animals and then in humans before being submitted to the FDA for approval and becoming commercially available. Because of the unique and potentially life-threatening toxicities associated with antineoplastic drugs, this approval process may become both lengthy and expensive. The average time and cost to bring a drug to market may range from 10 to 12 years and from $40 to $80 million.

Preclinical Evaluation

The NCI coordinates the screening of more than 10,000 compounds each year in an effort to find new and potentially useful drugs for treating cancer. Less than 1% of screened compounds proceed to clinical trials. Compounds with known or suspected antineoplastic activity are screened by a number of methods, including transplantable rodent tumor models. Positive compounds are further evaluated against a panel of human tumor cell lines grown in defined media.[2] Cell lines in use include lung, ovarian, and renal cell cancer; malignant melanoma; brain tumors; and leukemias. Because of the interest in the impact drug resistance may have on chemotherapy effectiveness, a multidrug resistant (MDR) variant of a human breast cancer and murine leukemia cell lines are also available for testing.[3]

Compounds having demonstrated significant antineoplastic activity then undergo preclinical toxicology studies. The purpose of these studies is to determine a safe starting dose for use in humans. The lethal dose in 10% of animals tested (LD_{10}) is then used to calculate a starting dose for clinical trials. Although mice are the primary toxicology test animal, the dose determined for clinical trials is first tested in dogs to avoid excessive risk to humans. Body surface area (BSA) is the preferred reference point used for making interspecies dose comparisons.

Clinical Trials

Following the initial development and pharmaceutical preparation in the preclinical phase, new compounds must be tested in humans to evaluate their activity and toxicity in treating cancers. Table 18-2 briefly describes the phases of clinical trials conducted in the United States and lists the purpose and goals of each phase of testing. Although healthy volunteers are usually recruited for phase I testing, because of the potential for significant toxicity with antineoplastic drugs, patients with advanced cancer are enrolled in these trials. These patients may also benefit from the new therapies. The ideal patients for phase II testing are previously untreated; however, most tend to be patients who have shown little or no response to previous chemotherapy. Usually, response rates of higher than 20% indicate the agent may have therapeutic usefulness and warrants further clinical testing. Traditionally, response rates, duration of response, survival, and toxicity are measured; however, quality of

Table 18-2 Different Phases of Clinical Trials Conducted in the United States

Phase	Purpose	Comment
I	Determines maximum tolerated dose and describes pharmacology and pharmacokinetics in humans	Dosing starts at 10% of the LD_{10} in mice. Determine safe dose and schedule for phase II
II	Determines drug activity in specific tumors	Also determines administration schedule, toxicity, supportive care
III	New drug or drug combinations are compared against the standard therapy	Objective criteria: Response rate, duration of response, survival, toxicity, and quality of life
IV	Role of drug in adjuvant/curative setting	Determines other uses, doses, schedules, and combination regimens

life has also become a focus of clinical trials. At the conclusion of phase III testing, it should be known whether the new treatment is better than the standard therapy in terms of response, survival, toxicity, and what impact it has on the patient's quality of life. Phase IV studies generally involve the use of drugs in combination with other therapies where cure is the goal of treatment.

Scientific Basis of Chemotherapy

Researchers have only recently begun to identify what is thought to be the primary pharmacologic activity of many antineoplastic agents. The actual mechanism or combination of mechanisms responsible for killing tumor cells remains elusive. This disparity is partly a function of the lack of a clear understanding of how cancer cells originate, grow, and regress. The next section addresses tumor cell biology and how chemotherapeutic drugs may selectively exert their cytotoxicity.

The Cell Cycle

Much of what is known regarding the effects of cytotoxic chemotherapy relies on understanding the cell cycle. The cycle is made of five phases: G_1, S, G_2, M, and G_0. The phases describe periods of time for different cellular processes that ultimately result in a cell's reproduction or death (Figure 18-1). In any population, only some cells are actively proliferating. The *growth fraction* is the portion of cells actively cycling compared to the entire population. Following mitosis, a cell can do any one of the following: leave the cycle, differentiate, and eventually die; enter a resting state (G_0) and reenter the cycle at some later time (stem cells); or enter the G_1 phase and continue to cycle. Synthesis of RNA and proteins occurs predominantly in the G_1 phase. Synthesis, or *S phase*, is when DNA is being replicated and is a relatively short period compared with the overall time a cell is cycling. The G_2 *phase* is typically brief, occurring after DNA synthesis and just before cell division. Mitosis, or cell division, ensues during the *M phase*, resulting in two identical daughter cells. The time from mitosis to mitosis is described as the *cycling time*. Cells that have left the cycle to enter G_0 are considered to be in a *resting* or *dormant phase*. These cells can actively synthesize RNA and proteins and differentiate; however, they are typically resistant to the cytotoxic effects of chemotherapy.

Tumor Cell Kinetics

Tumor cells may be distinguished from cells of normal tissues by their loss of controlled cell division, lack of

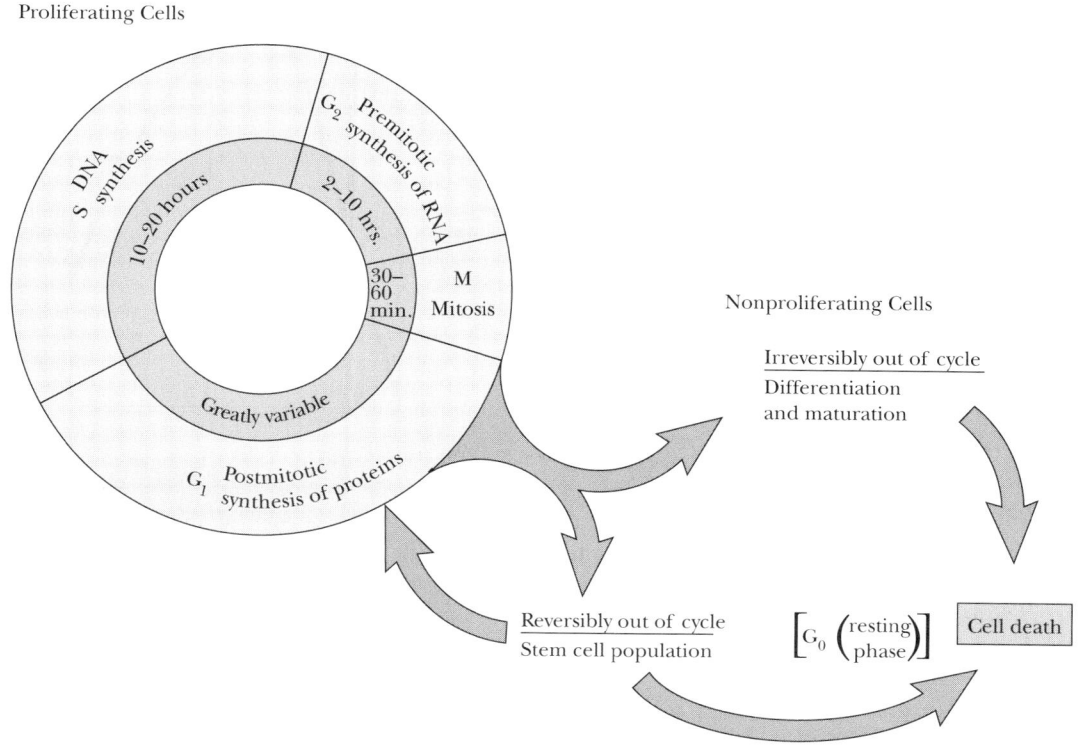

Figure 18-1 Diagrammatic representation of the life of a cell, emphasizing the relationships between the cell cycle and proliferating and nonproliferating cells.

differentiation, and ability to invade surrounding tissues and establish new growth at distant sites in the body. Theoretically, most antineoplastic agents utilize the rapid proliferation rate of tumor cells as a target for their cytotoxic effects. This is also the mechanism of many of the toxicities seen in cells of normal tissues because they are also going through the cell cycle and dividing, but at a much slower rate. A kinetic model has been developed to explain the selective effects of antineoplastic drugs on both normal and tumor cells.[4] The model states that (1) tumor growth is often exponential, (2) doubling times vary widely between tumors, and (3) chemotherapy-sensitive tumors tend to grow faster than slow-growing tumors that are less responsive to chemotherapy.

Doubling time of both malignant and normal tissues is widely variable. The factors that affect doubling time are cell cycle time, growth fraction, and cell loss by either cell death (apoptosis) or differentiation or metastasis. Cells with a rapid cycling time and a tumor with a large growth fraction should be the most responsive to cytotoxic therapy.[5] Although tumor cells may exhibit rapid cycling, the rate is not higher than what is seen with normal renewal tissues such as the bone marrow and gastrointestinal mucosa. Therefore, uncontrolled proliferation is not the sole distinguishing trait of tumor cells. Loss of homeostatic mechanisms, such as contact inhibition and cell differentiation and maturation, leads to an increased proliferative rate, which exceeds cell death. This leads to the accumulation of tumor cells.

The Effects of Chemotherapy on Tumor Cells

Cell kill hypothesis

The cell kill hypothesis is a basic principle often used to describe the effects of cancer chemotherapy on normal and tumor cells. The hypothesis describes a first-order kinetic process that predicts the number of cells killed based on the dose of chemotherapy given. This applies only to cells that are actively proliferating and assumes that treatment sensitivity does not change and that growth rate is constant. A model of this concept was originally described by Skipper et al in the early 1960s using a leukemia L 1210 tumor in mice.[6] The model is based on a log-kill relationship for dose of chemotherapy and a constant proportion of cells killed per treatment. If a given drug at a given dose produces a 1-log kill (or a 90%) reduction, then a tumor of 1×10^5 will be decreased to 1×10^4. A treatment with a 3-log kill is necessary to produce a tumor reduction of 99.9%. Essentially, no treatment can completely reduce the number of tumor cells to zero; therefore, the net effect on viable tumor cells is surviving cells plus regrowth before the next treatment. Because of these limitations, Skipper's model is not applicable to most human tumors. Malignancies that do follow this model include Burkitt's lymphoma and germ cell tumors. The cell kill hypothesis is still used today in determining tumor cell growth inhibition of newly derived anticancer compounds.

Gompertzian curve

The effect of antineoplastic drugs on human tumors cannot be fully explained by the cell kill model because not all tumor cells are in a proliferative state. A Gompertzian growth curve (Figure 18-2) probably best describes the growth of human tumors and the responses observed with the administration of antineoplastic drugs.[3,7] Tumor growth fraction and proliferative rate are not constant but instead decrease with time as a tumor goes from a small, undetectable clump of cells to a large mass. The doubling time of a tumor increases as the mass increases in size. Eventually, the tumor reaches a growth plateau phase where further increase in size becomes minimal because of the slower doubling time.

The Gompertzian curve also is useful in describing the observed tumor response to chemotherapy.[8] If cytotoxic chemotherapy is given in the growth phase of the tumor, the portion of cells actively proliferating (growth fraction) is large; therefore, a high percentage of cells will be susceptible to the effects of the drugs. However, in a more advanced stage of the disease, when growth has reached a plateau, fewer cells will be dividing and thereby will be less susceptible to chemotherapy.

When surgery or radiation therapy has been used to

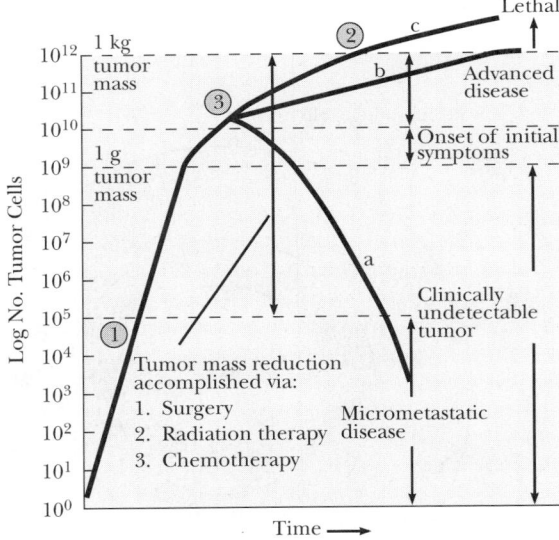

Figure 18-2 Gompertzian tumor growth curve: relationship of tumor mass, diagnosis, symptoms, and potential treatment regimens. Growth phases and chemotherapy response: (1) log phase (high growth fraction, short doubling time); (2) plateau phase (low growth fraction, longer doubling time); (3) initiation of chemotherapy treatments: (a) tumor cells responsive to drugs; (b) tumor exhibits initial response to treatment but develops resistance (secondary or somatic resistance); (c) tumor unresponsive to drug regimen (primary resistance). (Used with permission from Buick RN: Cellular basis of chemotherapy, in Dorr RT, Von Hoff DD (eds): *Cancer Chemotherapy Handbook* (ed 2). Norwalk, CT, Appleton & Lange, 1994, pp 3–14.[7])

reduce the tumor mass, chemotherapy may be useful in eradicating remaining residual and micrometastatic disease.[9] However, because metastatic cells are often the result of numerous prior divisions, the possibility that either primary or secondary drug resistance has developed is significant.

Mechanisms and sites of action of chemotherapy

Chemotherapeutic drugs induce their cytotoxicity on tumor cells and normal tissue by one or more mechanisms. Figure 18-3 illustrates the potential sites and proposed mechanisms of action for many of the drugs currently available for cancer chemotherapy. Central to the diagram is the genetic machinery, considered to be the focus for most effective cytotoxic drugs.

Chemotherapy Drug Selection and Factors Affecting Response to Chemotherapy

There is wide variability in both therapeutic response and unacceptable toxicity observed in patients receiving chemotherapy. This variability may be explained by differences in factors involving the patient with cancer, the chemotherapy being given, and the type of tumor being treated.

Patient factors include toxicity response, organ dysfunction, previous treatment, and age. The occurrence and severity of toxicity are widely variable between patients and often necessitate chemotherapy dose reduction or treatment delay. Preexisting organ dysfunction such as renal or hepatic insufficiency may also require dose or schedule alteration. Patients who have received previous chemotherapy may not be candidates to receive the same drug again or, likewise, a drug with similar toxicity. Patients who have received more than the recommended maximum lifetime dose of the anthracycline drugs (doxorubicin, daunorubicin, idarubicin) should not receive any more of these agents, as they greatly increase the patients' risk for developing severe cardiomyopathy. Drugs that are neurotoxic should be avoided in patients with preexisting neurologic defects. Previous bone marrow transplant or the use of severely marrow-toxic drugs may preclude the future use of full doses of myelosuppressive drugs. All these factors may have an adverse effect on a patient's antineoplastic response and the overall potential to cure or control the cancer.

Antineoplastic activity, pharmacokinetics, dose, and schedule are important drug factors that can influence chemotherapy response and toxicity. The relative cytotoxicity of any antineoplastic drug is dependent on the origin of the tumor and the presence of intrinsic drug resistance. Intrinsic resistance is probably a type of generic defense mechanism present in cells of certain histologic type. Pharmacokinetic factors determine the ability of chemo-therapeutic drugs to reach their cellular targets. Changes in these factors, such as decreased metabolic activation or increased drug clearance from the body, may decrease antitumor response. Similarly, alterations in protein binding of certain drugs, such as etoposide or teniposide, may enhance clinical toxicity. Poorly lipophilic drugs administered systemically are ineffective for tumors found in lipophilic tissues such as the central nervous system. Administration of drugs such as methotrexate or cytarabine directly into the intrathecal space will circumvent this obstacle. The ability to deliver the optimal dose of chemotherapy for a specific cancer is often limited by the patient's individualized maximum tolerated dose. The clinical use of hematopoietic growth factors such as granulocyte colony stimulating factor (G-CSF) and granulocyte-macrophage colony-stimulating factor (GM-CSF) has allowed the dose of myelotoxic drugs to be escalated in an attempt to improve response.

Tumor factors such as tumor growth and size significantly influence the response to chemotherapy. Larger tumors have small growth fractions and are therefore less responsive to the cytotoxic effects of antineoplastic drugs. The ability of chemotherapy to reach large solid tumors may be hindered by inadequate blood flow. Chemotherapy response is also influenced by tumor cell histology. Table 18-1 differentiates tumor types by their sensitivity to chemotherapy and what outcomes may be expected in patients successfully treated with chemotherapy. Selectivity of certain types of malignancies for specific chemotherapeutic agents is also seen. Fluorouracil is most active in cancers of endodermal tissue such as gastrointestinal and breast neoplasms. Epithelial tumors such as squamous cell cancers are especially sensitive to the cytotoxic effects of bleomycin.

Suboptimal Response to Chemotherapy and Strategies to Overcome Treatment Failure

Theoretical Basis for Chemotherapy Resistance

The failure of chemotherapy to control tumor growth and induce a remission is one of the most important problems facing the oncology clinician today. Several theories and models have been developed to explain this phenomenon. The previously described cell kill model served as an early attempt to explain neoplastic cell growth and lack of response to cytotoxic chemotherapy. According to the model, increasing the dose of a cytotoxic drug or adding other drugs results in an increase in cell kill. Therefore, the theory suggests, failure of chemotherapy to eradicate a tumor is the result of inadequate dose intensity or the presence of biochemically resistant tumor cells. Although this theory is applicable to tumor regression, clinical data do not necessarily support it.[8]

Another possible explanation for treatment failures

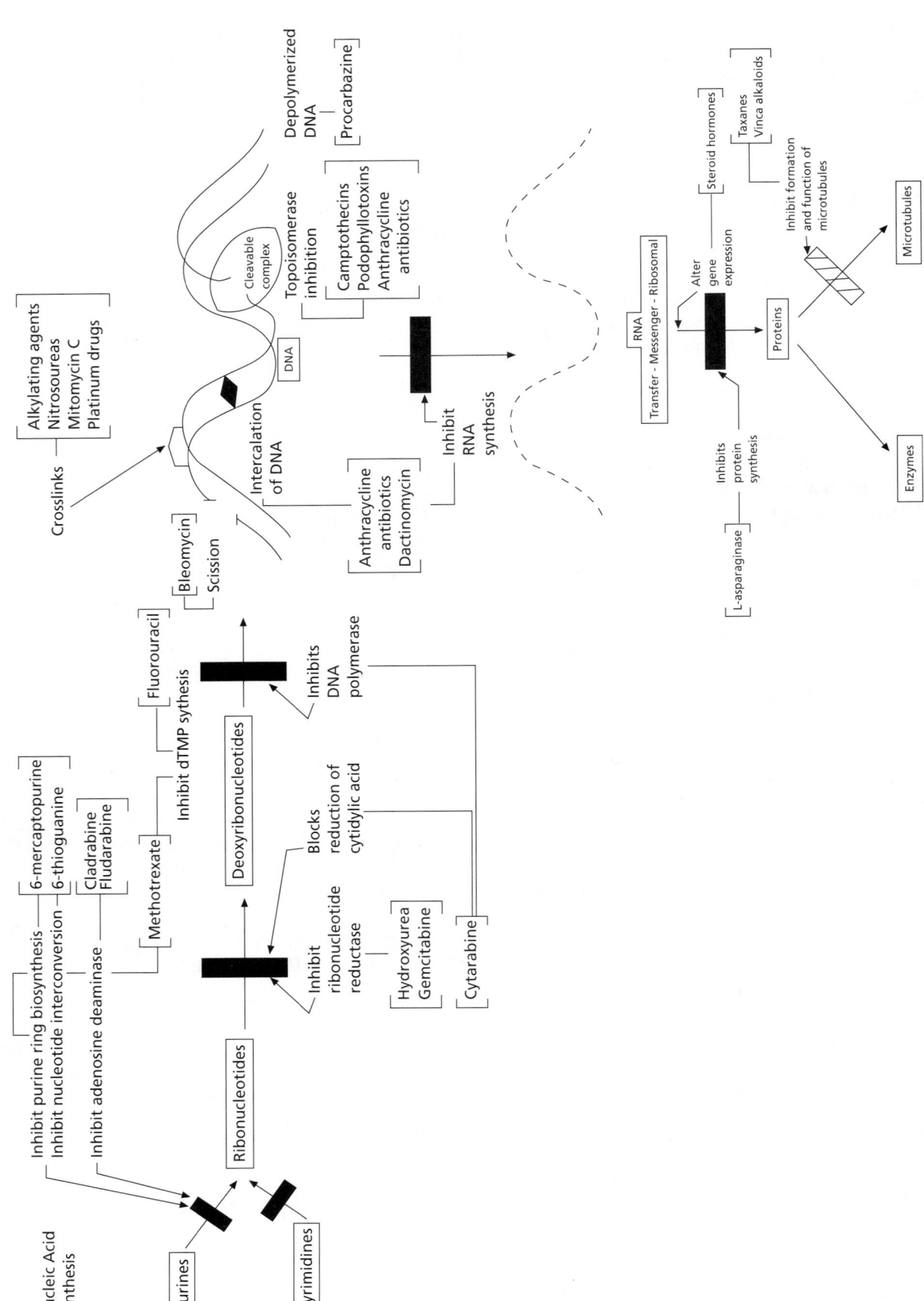

Figure 18-3 Mechanisms of action of chemotherapeutic agents.

is the stem cell concept. Stem cells continually produce progeny that go on to become mature cells but themselves do not differentiate. Stem cells constitute a small portion of the total population of cells. Therefore, eradicating the stem cell population would theoretically eliminate the source of malignant cells and induce tumor regression. However, this must be accomplished without greatly increasing the rate of genetic mutation and producing other biochemically resistant stem cell lines.

Currently, the most popular explanation for chemotherapy treatment failures is the development of drug resistance. The genetic instability of tumor cells with high mitotic rates is possibly responsible for the emergence of resistant clones within a population of tumor cells. A quantitative explanation of this process was first described by Goldie and Coldman in 1979.[10] Treatment failure could be explained by the existence of drug-resistant cells that resulted from random genetic mutations occurring before or during cytotoxic chemotherapy. The best chance for curing cancer would be to apply effective drugs early to reduce the total number of cancer cells while preventing resistant cells from developing, thus supporting the established concepts of combination chemotherapy.

Tumors that recur following effective initial treatment often present a treatment dilemma. Disease that recurs within 6 months usually is considered resistant to initial chemotherapy, and an alternative drug regimen is used. However, recurrence more than 6 months after treatment may be successfully treated with the same or a similar chemotherapy regimen. This phenomenon may be explained by either the reversion of resistant cells to drug-sensitive cells, or the predominance of initially sensitive cells in the relapsed tumor.[8] Although the Goldie and Coldman model presents an important concept of quantitative drug resistance, the assumptions are not always applicable to human tumors. Continued diligence in exploring the mechanisms behind chemotherapy treatment failure is a goal of modern chemotherapy.

Cytotoxic Drug Resistance

Although patient and drug factors play an important role in response to chemotherapy, genetic instability of the tumor cell and emergence of resistance are currently considered the most significant determinants of response.[11] Although much work is focusing on changing the biology or genetic composition of tumor cells, strategies for overcoming resistance need to be developed and implemented.

Cytotoxic drug resistance may be expressed as a temporary or permanent insensitivity to one or more antineoplastic drugs. Temporary or relative resistance is usually a function of the drug's inability to reach the target cells. Reasons why this could happen include poor blood supply, anatomic sanctuary sites such as the testes and central nervous system, or altered pharmacokinetic parameters. As yet undefined host defense mechanisms may also have

a negative impact on treatment success. In some conditions, temporary resistance may be reversed by altering drug delivery, dose, or scheduling of drug administration.

Permanent or phenotypic drug resistance is an inheritable type of resistance mechanism, which may result from a genetic mutation or preexisting trait.[12] This form of resistance may be present prior to treatment (*primary resistance*) or may develop after exposure to antineoplastic drugs (*secondary resistance*). Cytotoxic drug resistance may develop from genetic changes such as point mutations or gene amplification. *Point mutations* usually occur in a single cell and are independent of drug concentration. *Gene amplification* is influenced by drug concentration and occurs with repeated exposure over an extended period of time. Expression of the *MDR*-1 gene is associated with the development of the MDR phenotype.[13]

Biological basis of phenotypic drug resistance

Phenotypic drug resistance is believed to arise from spontaneous genetic mutations that regularly occur in a population of tumor cells.[12] Their model was based on Luria and Delbruck's observations of the development of acquired resistance in bacteria.[14] A mutational origin appears responsible for the development of antibiotic resistance in bacterial cells, which is analogous to cytotoxic drug resistance observed in tumor cells. Antibiotics or cytotoxic drugs selectively kill sensitive cells and leave behind phenotypically resistant cells that reproduce and expand the volume of resistant tumor cells. This process has been demonstrated in mouse lymphoma cells that exhibited resistance to folic acid antagonist after exposure to methotrexate.[15]

The development of drug resistance is dependent on the spontaneous mutation rate of tumor cells, the timing of a significant mutation relative to the tumor's growth, and overall tumor burden. All biological systems have an inherent probability of undergoing genetic variation from random changes. These random changes may result in minor effects, no effect, or a mutation that alters the cell's characteristics and sensitivity to cytotoxic drugs. Neoplastic cells are genetically unstable and exhibit a high rate of mutation. If mutations occur early in the growth of a population of tumor cells, a high fraction of resistant cells would result. A mutation occurring later would produce only a small fraction of resistant clones. If no resistant cells develop prior to treatment, then a cure would be probable with the appropriate chemotherapy. Cytotoxic therapy directed at minimal tumor burden has a much greater likelihood of being successful.

The Goldie and Coldman model provides a strong argument for the use of adjuvant and combination chemotherapy.[10] Adjuvant chemotherapy is used in an attempt to eradicate undetectable or micrometastatic tumor cells. If the probability of cure decreases as the number of tumor cells or the mutation rate increases, then eliminating all possible tumor cells or clones should induce a cure or a complete response. The model also supports the use of combination chemotherapy with non-cross-resistant drugs to potentially eliminate subpopulations of resistant tumor cells. The likelihood of a cell being resistant to two or more antineoplastic drugs simultaneously is less than that of being resistant to single agents when used alone.

Mechanisms of drug resistance

Tumor cells exposed to antineoplastic drugs sometimes develop mechanisms to protect themselves against the drug's cytotoxic effect. Table 18-3 lists possible mechanisms of resistance and the drugs most often affected.[7,16] Resistance may result from alterations in cytotoxic drug metabolism, alterations in cytotoxic targets, biochemical cofactor presence or absence, ability of cells to repair DNA lesions, or decreased intracellular drug concentrations. The most significant discovery explaining cytotoxic drug resistance is the P-glycoprotein (P-gp) efflux pump associated with overexpression of the *MDR*-1 gene.[13]

Types of multidrug resistance

Tumor cells that exhibit resistance to a group of drugs that are structurally dissimilar have unrelated cytotoxic mechanisms, or both are expressing a MDR. Resistance usually develops intrinsically or is acquired following exposure to a particular drug in the group.[13] Multidrug resistance may occur as a result of overexpression of P-gp membrane efflux pump, enhancements of the glutathione detoxification pathway, or alterations in topoisomerase enzyme systems. The identification and further investigation of this type of resistance and strategies to prevent MDR will have broad clinical implications for the use of chemotherapy as a form of cancer treatment.

P-glycoprotein-associated MDR phenotype.   The classic form of MDR is associated with overexpression of *MDR*-1 gene, which encodes for an energy-dependent cell membrane efflux pump, P-gp. This phenomenon was first described in tumor cells selected for resistance to dactinomycin that also exhibited resistance to vinca alkaloids, daunorubicin, and mitomycin.[13] Figure 18-4 is a model of P-gp structure.[17] The pump naturally functions to transport toxic molecules from inside the cell to the external environment and P-gp is found in low concentra-

Table 18-3 Possible Mechanisms of Cytotoxic Drug Resistance

Site or Type of Resistance	Mechanism of Resistance	Drugs Involved
Drug metabolism	Reduced drug activation	Cytarabine Fluorouracil 6-Mercaptopurine Methotrexate
	Increased drug deactivation	Alkylating agents Cytarabine Doxorubicin
Cytotoxic targets	Increased enzyme levels	Fluorouracil Methotrexate
	Alteration in enzyme-substrate binding	Doxorubicin Etoposide Fluorouracil 6-Mercaptopurine Methotrexate
Biochemical modification	Use of alternative (salvage) pathways	Cytarabine Fluorouracil 6-Mercaptopurine Methotrexate
	Decreased cofactor concentrations (reduced folate pool)	Fluorouracil
DNA repair systems	Increased DNA repair	Alkylating agents Cisplatin Mitomycin
Intracellular drug concentration	Decreased cellular uptake	Mechlorethamine Methotrexate
	Increased efflux (P-glycoprotein mediated)	Anthracycline antibiotics Etoposide Paclitaxel Vinca alkaloids

Data from Buick[7]; Yarbro.[16]

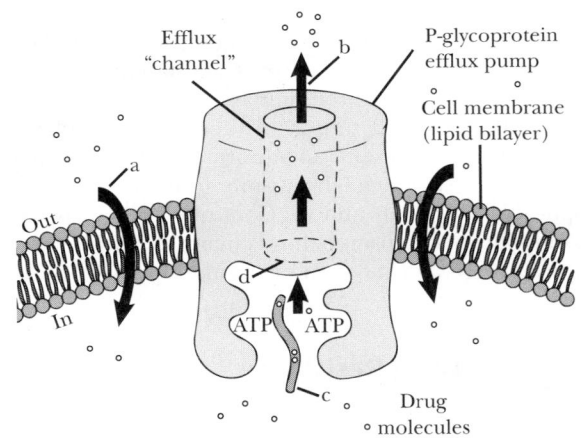

Figure 18-4 Model of P-glycoprotein as an energy-dependent (ATP) drug efflux pump.
Key: (a = drug influx; b = drug efflux via P-glycoprotein "channel"; c = possible carrier protein-assisted efflux; d = possible site for binding of pump inhibitors.)
In this model, drugs enter the cell by diffusing across the lipid bilayer (a), drugs bind directly to P-glycoprotein and are transported out of cell (b), drugs bind to a carrier protein and are transported out of cell (c), and efflux may be inhibited by the binding of chemosensitizers (d). (Adapted with permission from Dalton WS: Overcoming the multidrug-resistant phenotype, in DeVita VT, Hellman S, Rosenberg SA [eds]: *Cancer: Principles and Practice of Oncology* (ed 4). J.B. Lippincott Co., 1993, pp 2655–2666.)[17]

tions in normal tissues, including the renal tubules, colon, small intestine, bile canaliculi, and vascular epithelia of the brain and spinal cord.[18-20] Cytotoxic drugs that have entered the cell probably bind to a carrier protein before reaching their cellular targets and are transported out of the cell via the pump.[17] The actual process of drug binding and extruding from the cell is unknown. The list of drugs exhibiting P-gp-associated cross-resistance include several natural products and an antimetabolite (Table 18-4).

Levels of P-gp have been found in many human tumors, including acute and chronic leukemias, ovarian cancer, multiple myeloma, breast cancer, soft-tissue sarcomas, renal cell carcinoma, and small cell lung cancer.[21-24] The presence of P-gp has typically been associated with prior cytotoxic therapy, intrinsically resistant tumors, and inferior treatment outcomes. The detection of the *MDR*-1 gene product from cells of tumors typically resistant to chemotherapy, such as colon, kidney, liver, and pancreas, further supports the importance of P-gp in chemotherapy failure.[24] The presence of *MDR*-1 phenotype and overexpression of P-gp has been found to be a predictor of poor prognosis and shortened survival in patients with acute leukemias, multiple myeloma, and malignant lymphomas.[25,26] The development of immunohistochemical assays and monoclonal antibodies to identify tumor cells expressing P-gp will provide a greater understanding of the approaches needed to overcome these types of drug resistance.[27] Likewise, elucidating the structure and function of P-gp will contribute to the strategies to overcome this type of resistance.

Strategies for reversing P-gp-associated MDR. Approaches to overcoming MDR are receiving much attention. Strategies being investigated include the use of high-dose chemotherapy to increase intracellular cytotoxic drug concentrations, the use of non-cross-resistant drug regimens to prevent the emergence of resistant clones, and the use of modulators to inhibit or reverse the effects of specialized resistance mechanisms such as

P-gp-associated drug efflux. Several pharmaceutical agents currently available for treatment of nonmalignant conditions have been identified in vitro as modulators of P-gp-associated MDR, including calcium channel blockers, calmodulin inhibitors (phenothiazines), cyclosporine, and steroid hormones.[28] The two most widely investigated modulators are verapamil and cyclosporine. These drugs are believed to act directly by binding to special sites on the P-gp molecule and inhibiting the efflux of cytotoxic drugs. The specific binding sites and mechanism of interaction are not known; however, the outcome is decreased efflux and higher intracellular concentrations of the antineoplastic drug.[29] Responses were most often observed in patients with hematologic malignancies and some solid tumors such as breast cancer.

Of the compounds identified as MDR modulators or chemosensitizers, only two, verapamil and cyclosporine, have received significant attention in both clinical trials and clinical practice. High-dose verapamil was given to patients with multiple myeloma receiving VAD chemotherapy (vincristine, doxorubicin, and dexamethasone).[30] The patients who expressed the *MDR*-1 gene showed a response when the modulator was added to the regimen. However, cardiotoxicity of the regimen, which was considered to be primarily the result of high-dose verapamil, has prevented the combination from being routinely used for reversing MDR. A trial using lower oral doses of verapamil with VAD chemotherapy showed no improvement in response or outcome compared to patient who received VAD without verapamil.[31]

Several trials have demonstrated that cyclosporine is an effective agent for reversing MDR in myeloma and acute myelocytic leukemia and for eliminating malignant cells that were positive for the presence of P-gp.[32,33] Because cyclosporine is an inhibitor of metabolic enzymes and has been documented to reduce the clearance of many chemotherapy drugs,[34,35] prolonged elimination of these chemotherapy drugs, *not* reversal or inhibition of the efflux pump, may be a contributing factor in the positive outcome of the studies. Cyclosporine use is also plagued by numerous and significant toxicities including renal insufficiency, hyperbilirubinemia, and neurotoxicity.

Before the use of modulators to reverse MDR is incorporated into clinical practice, other agents need to be developed that are more effective MDR-reversing agents and have no or minimal toxicity. These newer agents should also demonstrate a lack of interference in the activity or pharmacokinetics of the chemotherapeutic drug being used to treat the malignancy. Dex-verapamil is a stereoisomer of verapamil but lacks the cardiac toxicity associated with verapamil. When given along with EPOCH (etoposide, prednisone, vincristine, cyclophosphamide, doxorubicin) chemotherapy to patients with drug-resistant non-Hodgkin's lymphoma, responses were seen in 12% of patients.[36] The compound PSC-833, a nonimmunologic derivative of cyclosporine that lacks nephrotoxicity, has been tested in patients with multiple

Table 18-4 Chemotherapeutic Drugs Exhibiting Cross-Resistance in P-Glycoprotein-Associated Multidrug Resistance

Dactinomycin
Daunorubicin
Doxorubicin
Etoposide
Mitomycin
Mitoxantrone
Paclitaxel
Trimetrexate
Vinblastine
Vincristine

Data from Dalton.[17]

myeloma receiving VAD (vincristine, adriamycin, dexamethasone) chemotherapy.[37] The results of this phase I trial did not demonstrate a response in patients receiving the combination. The current data on resistance modulators suggests that only patients enrolled in clinical trials should receive these compounds. Other approaches to modulation of P-gp-associated MDR involve the inhibition of protein kinases, which are enzymes that control the phosphorylation of P-gp and thereby regulate its function.[38] Therapies aimed at suppressing MDR-1 gene expression may also be considered as alternative approaches to modulating resistance. Yet another strategy focuses on sequencing non-cross-resistant chemotherapy regimens to prevent the survival of resistant clones.[39]

Laboratory and clinical research is ongoing to identify compounds that may be used to reverse or prevent MDR. Ideal compounds should be potent inhibitors of MDR and easy to administer. Moreover, they should not negatively interfere with the pharmacology or pharmacokinetics of the chemotherapeutic regimen and should have minimal toxicity of their own. Modulators also should be evaluated for their effect on P-gp efflux pumps in normal tissues, such as the brain and gastrointestinal tract, because inhibition of cytotoxic drug removal could result in new or more severe toxicities in these cells.

Other forms of MDR associated with increased drug efflux. Multidrug resistance-associated protein (MRP) has been identified as a type of MDR not associated with overexpression of P-gp.[40] The natural substrates in cells of MRP include glutathione and leukotriene C4.[41] Expression of the MRP gene confers resistance to doxorubicin, vincristine, etoposide, and colchicine.[42] Elevated levels of MRP may have prognostic importance in patients with acute or chronic leukemias.[43] More recently, another carrier protein has been discovered termed lung cancer resistance-associated protein (LRP).[44] The LRP gene overexpression was associated with a poor prognosis and reduced overall survival in patients with advanced ovarian cancer.[45] Identifying and developing strategies or drugs to overcome these types of resistance are in the early phases of testing. Because glutathione is a natural substrate for MRP, depletion of glutathione may provide a mechanism for modulating this form of resistance.[41]

Other mechanisms of MDR. Another type of MDR has been described in cells cross-resistant to topoisomerase poisons such as etoposide, doxorubicin, daunorubicin, and topotecan. Although most of the drugs associated with this type of MDR are also associated with P-gp-mediated MDR, the pattern of resistance is different and cells retain sensitivity to vinca alkaloids.[46] Resistance may be conferred by the tumor cell's ability to decrease the activity of or change the binding properties of topoisomerase enzymes. Tumor cells that have developed resistance to one type of topoisomerase II poisons such as intercalators (e.g., doxorubicin) may not be resistant to an alternative type such as epipodophyllotoxins (e.g., etoposide). Therefore, resistance may be overcome by utilizing different types of topoisomerase II poisons.

Multidrug resistance may also be demonstrated in cells with increased detoxifying systems, such as glutathione S-transferase (GST) enzymes, and elevated glutathione levels.[47] These enzymes catalyze conjugation of electrophilic hydrophobic compounds, such as alkylating agents and their metabolites, with glutathione, which facilitates elimination from the tumor cell. Alkylating agents, their metabolites, and platinum compounds are among the most frequent substrates of these enzymes.[48] Strategies being investigated for reversing this type of resistance include administering inhibitors of GST and glutathione synthesis such as buthionine sulfoximine (BSO).[49] Further research is needed to determine the effects of BSO on chemotherapy response rates and duration before this modulator can be used in clinical practice.

Drug-gene interactions and chemotherapy resistance

DNA is the genetic blueprint found in all living cells and is composed of two complementary strands of nucleic acid base pairs. Genes are composed of sections of the double-stranded DNA that encode for specific proteins needed to carry out cellular growth, development, and reproduction. The majority of antineoplastic drugs exert their cytotoxicity by interfering with the replication, transcription, or repair of DNA. However, the direct mechanism or pathway that antineoplastic drugs use to induce cell death is largely unknown. There is much interest in exploring and describing the interactions these drugs have with genes and how cell death is induced.

Cells that are undergoing replication enter the cell cycle and progress through the four phases of the cycle resulting in the formation of two identical daughter cells. Checkpoints along the cycle are in place to ensure that DNA is undamaged before the cell is allowed to enter the S phase. The regulator protein that provides a checkpoint for cells with undamaged DNA is p53.[50] When cells with damaged DNA enter the cell cycle, those with normal p53 gene will be prevented from entering S phase and instead will undergo apoptosis or programmed cell death. However, cells with mutated p53 gene, also known as the tumor-suppressor gene, are often unable to undergo apoptosis and instead go on to replicate mutated cells.[51] This mutation is known to occur in most human tumors and may be an important determinant in the chemosensitivity of tumor cells to DNA-damaging drugs. Nonmutated or wild-type p53 is known to repress the MDR gene, and loss of normal p53 results in decreased chemosensitivity to MDR-sensitive antineoplastic drugs.[52]

Loss or mutations in p53 have been found in a number of solid tumors and chronic lymphocytic leukemia. Patients with advanced breast cancer who exhibited a poor response to doxorubicin chemotherapy and were more likely to relapse also were more likely to have p53 gene mutations.[53] Poor response to cisplatin chemotherapy and shorter disease-free survival was found in 60% of patients with ovarian cancer who had inactivation of p53 gene.[54] Other solid tumors with abnormal *p53* expression that have reduced response to chemotherapy and radiation therapy include non–small cell lung cancer, gastric cancer, and colorectal cancers.[55,56] Status of *p53* was the strongest prognostic factor for survival in a multivariate analysis conducted in patients with B-cell chronic lymphocytic leukemia.[57]

The proteins BCL-2 and BAX are members of a large family of related proteins that control a cell's decision to enter apoptosis. The ratio of these proteins appears to be the critical determinant of whether or not a cell undergoes apoptosis. The BCL-2 proteins block apoptosis, and elevated levels are associated with resistance to vincristine, methotrexate, fluorouracil, hydroxyurea, and cisplatin.[58] The BAX protein, however, urges the cell to enter apoptosis and is associated with increased chemosensitivity to paclitaxel, vincristine, and doxorubicin.[59] The BCL-2 protein can also block apoptosis even in the presence of tumors with high levels of *p53* expression, which is known to promote apoptosis. Most of the research on ways to enhance chemosensitivity related to BCL-2 and BAX is being conducted in vitro. The sequencing of chemotherapy drugs to increase the phosphorylation of BCL-2 has been suggested as a way of optimizing apoptosis in tumor cells.[60]

Chemotherapy as a Treatment for Cancer

Primary and Adjuvant Chemotherapy

Chemotherapy given with curative intent may be either primary therapy or adjuvant therapy. Chemotherapy is considered primary treatment for patients with cancers for which no effective alternative treatment is available or if the alternative treatment is less than optimal. *Induction* is a common term used to describe chemotherapy given to patients with leukemia or other advanced disease that is highly sensitive to drugs. *Neoadjuvant chemotherapy* describes chemotherapy given prior to alternative treatments in patients who present with primarily local disease.[61] This approach has had some success in preserving organ structure and function in cancers of the lung and larynx.[62,63] However, there is some concern that neoadjuvant treatment may delay the execution of definitive local therapy such as surgery or radiation therapy. Chemotherapy given concurrently instead of sequentially with radiation therapy is becoming a popular approach, especially for cancers of the head and neck.

Adjuvant chemotherapy is a well-established and routine part of treatment for cancers of the breast and bowel. Systemic therapy is usually given following surgical resection of the primary tumor with the intent of improving the potential for cure. Although effective chemotherapy would theoretically eradicate clinically undetected and micrometastatic disease, the overall effect on tumor recurrence has been less than dramatic.

Therapeutic Strategies

Combination chemotherapy

Administering a combination of clinically effective anticancer drugs is the standard chemotherapeutic approach for most malignancies. Although individually the drugs are biochemically and clinically active, they are rarely used alone as single agents. Combination chemotherapy was first applied with success in the treatment of leukemias and lymphomas and is now employed routinely for most other malignancies. The objectives of combination chemotherapy are achieving maximal tumor cell kill without excessive toxicity, providing cytotoxic drugs that are active against potentially resistant heterogeneous tumor populations, and avoiding selection of resistant cell lines. Table 18-5 delineates the principles by which antineoplastic drugs are usually chosen for combination regimens. When overlapping toxicities are unavoidable, as is often the case with bone marrow–suppressive drugs, administration of less than full doses or longer intervals between treatments may be necessary. Recovery time for normal tissues is typically used to determine the retreatment or cycle time. The time for the bone marrow to reach its nadir (lowest counts) and recover differs depending on the drugs administered. Nadir and recovery periods are critical for determining the length of a treatment cycle. Therefore, chemotherapy cycles for drugs with significant myelosuppression are approximately 3 to 4 weeks. The duration of treatment is usually based on the response rate or a number determined from clinical trials.

Dose intensity. Delivering a sufficient amount of drug over a specified period of time is of great importance in curing drug-sensitive malignancies. However, many situations often prevent the proper dose from being delivered, such as the necessity for a dose reduction or a delay in treatment because of unacceptable toxicity. Dose reductions as small as 20% do not affect clinical response rates for most drug-sensitive tumors; however, loss of cure is likely. Decreasing the dose or adjusting the schedule of treatment may explain the failure of chemotherapy to cure drug-sensitive tumors.

The concept of dose intensity has been developed to assist the researcher and clinician in evaluating the impact these changes in doses have on treatment outcomes.[64] Dose intensity is expressed as the amount of drug delivered per unit of time, or simply $mg/m^2/week$.

Table 18-5 Principles for Selection of Antineoplastic Drugs for Combination Chemotherapy Regimens

1. Choose drugs with single agent activity. Drugs producing complete responses are preferred.
2. Avoid drugs with overlapping toxicities.
3. Administer drugs at their optimal dose and schedule as previously determined by clinical trials.
4. Give chemotherapy at regular intervals (cycles) and minimize the time between cycles.

The effect of a new regimen on treatment outcome can be expressed as the relative dose intensity (RDI), which is calculated by dividing the dose intensity of a test regimen by that of a standard regimen. This calculation can be done for a single drug or for an average of all drugs in a combination regimen.[65] The impact of dose reductions or treatment delays is best evaluated when dose intensity is based on actual or received doses instead of intended or protocol doses.

The dose intensity has been applied to a number of diseases to improve response rates. Increasing the dose has improved outcomes in lymphomas and advanced tumors of the ovary, breast, and colon.[66,67] High-dose chemotherapy regimens with hematopoietic support are quickly becoming an acceptable treatment alternative for refractory lymphomas, breast cancer, childhood sarcomas, and neuroblastomas.

Chemoprotective agents

Antineoplastic drugs are among the most toxic drugs administered to humans. Some toxicities such as nausea, vomiting, mucositis, alopecia, and fatigue, are not life-threatening. Bone marrow suppression is both common and potentially life-threatening; however, it is dose dependent and can be managed by reducing doses, delaying therapy, or administering hematopoietic growth factors. Several drugs are known to induce life-threatening and permanent cellular injury. Chemoprotective and rescue agents have been developed and are under investigation for use in preventing or reversing drug-induced toxicity for some anticancer agents including cisplatin, doxorubicin, ifosfamide, and methotrexate. Availability of these compounds has permitted expanded clinical development and use of the anticancer drugs whose toxicity they ameliorate. Table 18-6 lists currently available chemoprotective and rescue agents, along with their clinical indications, proposed mechanisms of action, and toxicities.[68–70]

High-dose chemotherapy with peripheral blood stem cell transplant

High-dose chemotherapy with autologous rescue is being used more frequently in cancers that respond to increasing doses of marrow-ablative therapy such as leukemias, lymphomas, breast cancer, and ovarian cancer. This form of therapy, once available only at select treatment centers, is now being offered at most major medical centers and many large community hospitals. Reasons for the expansion of this form of cancer treatment include the curative potential, more experience with administering and managing these therapies, and advancements in supportive care for patients. The introduction of the hematopoietic growth factors (HGFs) such as G-CSF and GM-CSF has been among the major advancements in supportive care measures. Their availability has allowed for harvesting of hematopoietic stem cells from peripheral blood—in most situations avoiding costly and painful bone marrow harvesting. Peripheral blood stem cells (PBSCs) are committed progenitor cells existing in peripheral blood that have the capacity to restore hematopoiesis.[71]

Before receiving marrow-ablative chemotherapy, patients are given HGFs with or without chemotherapy, typically cyclophosphamide, to mobilize stem cells into the peripheral blood from the bone marrow.[72] Patients then undergo leukopheresis to remove mobilized stem cells from the peripheral blood.[73] Leukopheresis may be performed two to six times to collect an adequate number of cells ($8–10 \times 10^8$ peripheral blood mononuclear cells / kg). Following high-dose chemotherapy, radiation therapy, or both, which is intended to eradicate the cancer cells and by consequence the bone marrow stem cells, the patient's PBSCs are reinfused. As with other forms of hematopoietic cell transplantation, infused stem cells migrate to the bone marrow and engraft. Compared with patients receiving only autologous bone marrow, patients who receive PBSCs either alone or with bone marrow transplantation typically have fewer days of neutropenia and thrombocytopenia. Major disadvantages of PBSC transplantation include nausea, vomiting, and hypertension associated with infusion of the large amounts of the cryopreservative dimethyl sulfoxide (DMSO) and the large volume of PBSCs. Another concern is the potential to reinfuse mobilized tumor cells as well as hematopoietic stem cells. The significance of this contamination for relapse rates is yet to be determined.[74] The use of monoclonal antibodies to manufacture a product devoid of tumor cells is currently under investigation.

Table 18-6 Drugs Used as Chemoprotective and Rescue Agents for Cancer Chemotherapy

Chemoprotective Drug	Anticancer Drug	Mechanism of Action	Target Organ	Side Effects
Amifostine (Ethyol)	Cisplatin	Reduces DNA damage	Kidney	Hypotension, vomiting
Dexrazoxane (Zinacard)	Doxorubicin	Inhibits free radical formation	Heart	Myelosuppression, nausea and vomiting
Leucovorin (folinic acid)	Methotrexate	Circumvents enzyme inhibition	Bone marrow GI Kidney	Hypersensitivity, rash
Mesna (Mesnex)	Ifosfamide Cyclophosphamide	Binds toxic metabolites in bladder	Kidney Bladder	Nausea, vomiting, hypersensitivity

Data from Dorr,[68] Product Information: Etyol,[69] Seifert.[70]

Chemotherapy as a radiation sensitizer

The concomitant use of chemotherapy and radiation therapy has received significant attention in the literature.[75,76] The primary goal of this type of combined-modality treatment is to increase the effectiveness of the radiation and improve local-regional control of disease. A number of theoretical considerations may explain the improved results seen when chemotherapy and radiation are given concomitantly for specific tumors. The modalities affect different tumor cell subpopulations; therefore, their combined use may better eradicate cells resistant to the other modality. Tumor cell regrowth following radiation therapy is slowed by the addition of chemotherapy, and cells undergoing growth are more vulnerable to the cytotoxic effects of chemotherapy. The cytoreductive effects of chemotherapy improve tumor oxygen supply, resulting in an increased susceptibility to radiation effects. In addition, direct interaction of the combined modalities, as yet undefined, may explain the improved response seen especially at a local-regional level. A *positive interaction* is defined as enhanced radiation effects in tumor cells and less observed toxicity.[76] Significant improvement in quality of life may be achieved by using combined-modality regimens to preserve organs affected by cancer such as the larynx, anal canal, bladder, and esophagus.[77]

Chemotherapy and radiation therapy with fluorouracil has demonstrated improved overall survival for individuals with cancers of the head and neck, rectum, pancreas, and lung.[75] Cisplatin has also been investigated as a radiation enhancer, with the greatest activity seen in tumors sensitive to cisplatin.[78] Cisplatin combined with other antineoplastic drugs such as paclitaxel, fluorouracil, or etoposide for radiation enhancement have also been studied.[79,80] The results of clinical trials combining cisplatin and radiation, with or without fluorouracil, for head and neck cancer have shown improved disease-free survival over radiation alone.[81]

Modulation of fluorouracil by leucovorin

Leucovorin, or folinic acid, has been developed primarily as an antidote for antifolate therapy. Another emerging role of leucovorin is in the modulation of the cytotoxicity of fluorouracil. Although fluorouracil is the most active antineoplastic drug in cancers of the gastrointestinal tract, its ability to control progression of these cancers is modest. Therefore, investigators have sought to enhance fluorouracil's efficacy in an attempt to better control and potentially cure these cancers. In the presence of increased folate pools, the active form of fluorouracil binds more tightly to the target enzyme.[82]

The interaction of leucovorin and fluorouracil has been studied in more than 650 patients, with significantly improved response rates being seen with the combination compared with fluorouracil alone.[83] Although the optimal dose and schedule of leucovorin have not been determined, a prolonged or 5-day intermittent dosing schedule is preferred. The results of current trials suggest that a maximal benefit of combined therapy is seen in patients with less advanced disease.[83,84] Other drugs that have been tested as biochemical modulators of fluorouracil include methotrexate, N-(phosphonacetyl)-L-aspartate (PALA), and alfa-interferon.

Chronopharmacology and cancer chemotherapy

Chronopharmacology is described as the temporal variation in the handling of drugs by the body.[85] This new and emerging science examines the variance of chemical and physical processes of a biological system with respect to time. The antineoplastic and toxic effects of several anticancer drugs exhibit variable and predictable daily or circadian rhythms in murine and human trials.[86] Both normal and tumor cells exhibit circadian cytokinetic rhythms; however, generally these rhythms are asynchronic. By exploiting these differences in chronobiology, the timing of cancer chemotherapy may be able to maximize therapeutic activity and minimize toxicity.

Clinical trials have focused on minimizing the toxic effects of antineoplastic drugs; however, some information is available on improved efficacy with chronochemotherapy dosing regimens.[86,87] Floxuridine given by continuous hepatic artery infusion produced less toxicity with increasing dose intensity when the majority of the daily dose was given in the evening hours (3 P.M. to 9 P.M.).[88] The catabolism of fluorouracil follows a circadian variation that may be exploited to allow maximum dose delivery during a period of decreased catabolic activity.[89] Patients with metastatic colorectal cancer received cisplatin along with a continuous infusion of fluorouracil and leucovorin given as either a flat infusion or on a circadian-modified schedule.[90] In the circadian-modified schedule, stomatitis, hand and foot syndrome, and neutropenia were significantly reduced, whereas dose intensity and antitumor response were significantly increased. No differences were seen in survival; however, this approach deserves further study in cancers more responsive to chemotherapy. Several studies suggest that the ideal timing for doxorubicin is the early morning and for cisplatin late afternoon or early evening.[86] Other drugs that have been investigated for chronochemotherapy variability include cytarabine and methotrexate.

New Targets for Anticancer Therapy

The majority of cancer chemotherapy has been limited to drugs that are cytotoxic to the reproductive cycle and functions of tumor cells. Interest has grown in targeting other mechanisms of tumor growth, invasion, and metastasis. By targeting tumor cells with these types of therapy, toxicity to normal tissues should be less. Table 18-7 is a list of selected agents under development and their proposed anticancer targets.

Table 18-7 Drugs and New Targets for Anticancer Therapy under Development

Therapeutic Target	Drug in Development
Angiogenesis inhibitors	Angiostatin
	Endostatin
	Interferon alfa
	Interleukin-12
	Suramin
	Thalidomide
Matrix metalloproteinase inhibitors	Marimastat
	AG 3340
	CGS-72023A
Cycline-dependent kinase inhibitors	Flavopiridol
	Staurosporine
	UCN-01
Signal transduction inhibitors	Bryostatin
	Staurosporine
	Tamoxifen
	Thalidomide

Angiogenesis inhibitors

Tumors need an adequate blood supply to provide cells with nutrients and oxygen to grow and develop. Angiogenesis, the formation of new blood vessels, occurs as a tumor grows and displaces cells farther away from the primary blood source. If angiogenesis does not occur, then tumor growth is usually limited to a small clump of nonproliferative cells that are usually incapable of metastasizing.[91] Disease progression and prognosis have been shown to be dependent on microvessel density of breast, lung, and prostate tumors.[92] In order for primary tumors to metastasize they must have adequate access to vasculature so they can travel to distant sites and invade target organs.

There are several growth factors and oncogenes known to stimulate angiogenesis. Among the most potent mitogens for endothelial cells are vascular endothelial growth factor (VEGF) and basic fibroblast growth factor (bFGF).[93,94] Inhibition of these factors is being investigated as a potential therapeutic modality for controlling the growth of tumors and inhibiting the development of metastatic disease.[95] Agents that block mitogenic signals or that bind to mitogens are under investigation for their ability to limit tumor growth to a small clump of cells that are only a few millimeters in diameter. Among the most popular compounds that have demonstrated significant antiangiogenic activity are angiostatin, endostatin, interleukin 12, suramin, and thalidomide.[96,97] Alfa-interferon has been reported clinically to produce regression of pulmonary capillary hemangiomatosis in a child.[98]

Matrix metalloproteinase inhibition

Matrix metalloproteinase (MMP) inhibitors are being investigated for their ability not only to inhibit angiogenesis but also to inhibit invasion of tumor cells in target organs and tissues.[99] Representing a group of sixteen extracellular enzymes, MMPs are activated in normal processes including tissue growth, wound repair, and reproduction. Endogenous MMP inhibitors include alpha$_2$-macroglobulin and tissue inhibitor of metalloproteinases 1, 2, 3, and 4.[100] An imbalance in the amounts of MMPs and MMP inhibitors is what allows the degradation of extracellular matrix and permits tumor cells to grow and metastasize.[101] Therefore, inhibiting these enzymes might shift the balance away from activation of MMPs. Among the compounds being studied for oral use include marimastat, AG3340 (Agouron Pharmaceuticals, Inc., La Jolla, California), and CGS-72023A (Novartis Pharmaceutical Corporation, East Hanover, New Jersey).

Other novel targets

Cycline-dependent kinase (CDK) inhibitors are currently being investigated in preclinical and phase I and II trials for their role in stalling or blocking progression of the reproductive cell cycle. Responsible for regulating key checkpoints in the cell cycle, CDKs prevent cells with damaged DNA from replicating. By inhibiting the phosphorylation or activation of CDKs, cells with unreplicated or damaged DNA will go on to replicate and produce nonviable cells or cell death.[102] Agents currently in clinical trials include staurosporine and its derivative UCN-01, and flavopiridol. Intracellular signaling pathways regulate cell growth, differentiation, and death. Mutations within these pathways may lead to oncogene stimulation and other factors that promote tumor growth and metastasis. These signals are usually initiated with the activation of a transmembrane receptor by a second messenger. Inhibiting these receptors may have a negative effect on tumor growth and progression. Drugs that have signal transduction inhibition include suramin, tamoxifen, and thalidomide.

Pharmacology of Chemotherapeutic Drugs

Pharmacokinetics of Antineoplastic Drugs

Principles of pharmacokinetics

Pharmacokinetics is the study of the movement of drugs in the body. Several parameters have been used to describe the pharmacokinetics of drugs.[103] The *half-life* of a drug is the time required for the serum concentration of the drug to decrease by one-half. The drug's half-life determines the time required to reach steady-state concentrations in the serum and the appropriate dosing interval. The concept of steady-state serum concentration is less useful in chemotherapy compared to antibiotic or antiepileptic drug therapy because most antineoplastics are administered as single doses. However, knowing the half-life of a drug may be useful when evaluating the interval necessary for most of the drug to be removed from the body. This time period is equal to three half-lives of the drug. *Clearance* is the most important pharmacokinetic parameter because it determines the steady-state concentration and is independent of half-life. Clearance is determined by blood flow to an organ, usually the kidney or liver, and the organ's efficacy in extracting the drug from the blood. If a drug is cleared from the body by more than one organ, then the total clearance is a sum of the individual clearance of each extracting organ. Clearance may be altered by changes in blood flow to an organ, by enzyme function, and by protein binding. Cyclophosphamide is highly dependent on metabolizing enzymes for activation and inactivation. Therefore, induction or inhibition of enzymes may cause a more rapid or slower clearance of the drug. Changes in protein binding caused by either hypoalbuminemia or interactions with other drugs may alter the removal of highly protein-bound drugs such as etoposide or teniposide. The volume of distribution (V_D) relates the amount of drug in the body to the serum concentration. This parameter is usually different among individuals and is a function of the drug's protein-binding capabilities and its ability to distribute to extravascular compartments (tissue binding). Half-life is dependent on clearance and V_D; therefore, variability in half-life may be the result of changes in clearance, V_D, or both. Variability in these parameters may help explain the differences in response and toxicity seen among patients treated with similar doses and schedules of chemotherapy.

The basic principles of clinical pharmacokinetics may be divided into four major areas: absorption, distribution, metabolism, and excretion.

Absorption. Absorption from the gastrointestinal tract should be sufficient to ensure adequate bioavailability of the drug. Because the bioavailability of most anticancer drugs is poor and unpredictable, they are usually given parenterally to ensure accurate dosing and optimal systemic exposure. Drugs administered orally for cancer treatment include alkylating agents (cyclophosphamide, chlorambucil, and melphalan), etoposide, lomustine, methotrexate, and procarbazine. Although oral absorption is less than optimal for some of these drugs, the amount that reaches systemic circulation and, more important, the tumor is sufficient to produce a response.

Distribution. Distribution of drugs in the body is determined primarily by their ability to penetrate different tissues and their affinity for binding to plasma proteins. Drugs that are highly lipophilic tend to be more readily taken up by lipophilic tissues such as bone marrow, fat, and the central nervous system. Nitrosoureas such as carmustine and lomustine are useful for brain and hematopoietic malignancies because they readily penetrate these tissues. Decreased levels of plasma proteins, especially albumin, often occur in patients with cancer. This may be the result of nutritional deficiencies or decreased hepatic synthesis of albumin. The cytotoxic activity of

Table 18-8 Chemotherapy Drugs That Depend on Hepatic Metabolism for Activation and Clearance from the Body

Chemotherapy Drug	Activation	Clearance
Anthracycline antibiotics	X	X
Capecitabine	X	X
Cyclophosphamide	X	X
Dacarbazine	X	X
Hexamethylmelamine		X
Ifosfamide	X	
Nitrosoureas		X
Carmustine		
Lomustine		
Procarbazine	X	

highly protein-bound chemotherapy drugs such as etoposide and teniposide may be enhanced in these patients because a greater percentage of the drug is unbound. An increase in the unbound fraction can also occur if two highly bound drugs are administered concurrently. Methotrexate abnormally distributes in ascites and pleural effusions, delaying clearance and enhancing hematologic and mucosal toxicity.[104]

Metabolism. The metabolic activation and inactivation or catabolism of drugs is carried out primarily by the liver. Some of these enzymatic processes are also performed in normal and tumor cells. Several chemotherapy drugs require activation intracellularly or systemically before they are able to exert their cytotoxic effect (Table 18-8). Antimetabolites such as fluorouracil and cytarabine are phosphorylated to active nucleotides in tumor cells. Cisplatin undergoes a chemical aquation with water molecules intracellularly, which generates a positively charged species that, in turn, forms adducts with DNA molecules.[105] Cyclophosphamide and ifosfamide are transformed by hepatic microsomal enzymes into active alkylating species.[106] Some chemotherapeutic drugs are metabolized to inactive compounds, which are then excreted by the body (see Table 18-8). The rate of metabolic conversion may be affected by a number of factors, including hepatic dysfunction (either drug-induced or tumor-induced) or genetic differences in drug metabolism. Changes in liver function or metabolic enzymes may result in decreased cytotoxic activity, increased treatment-related toxicity, or both. Table 18-9 lists drugs known to

Table 18-9 Drugs Known to Enhance or Inhibit Hepatic Microsomal Metabolism

Enhance	Inhibit
Cyclophosphamide	Cimetidine
Phenobarbital	Alfa-interferon
Phenytoin	Ketoconazole
Rifampin	Verapamil

alter microsomal enzymes and potentially affect antineoplastic drug disposition.

Elimination. The kidneys are responsible for the majority of the elimination of drugs and drug metabolites from the body. A number of anticancer drugs are highly dependent on renal function for their elimination. Significant decreases in renal function can decrease the clearance of these compounds from the body and cause excessive toxicity (Table 18-10). Cisplatin and methotrexate are both eliminated primarily by the kidney and are nephrotoxic themselves; therefore, decreased renal function may produce enhanced toxicity and a further decline in renal function. The biliary tract is the primary route of elimination for vinca alkaloids, and urinary excretion is minimal.

Pharmacokinetic principles applied to chemotherapeutic drugs

Chemotherapeutic drugs must reach their target site in order to exert their antineoplastic activity. Often their targets are intracellular structures and molecules such as DNA, enzymes, and microtubules. Adequate blood supply to tumor cells is necessary for optimal delivery of chemotherapy to the drugs' site of action. Then, once at the tumor cell, the drug must be transported intracellularly via passive, facilitated, or active transport mechanisms.[104] Transport mechanisms may either facilitate drug entry into the cell or hasten its removal. As mentioned previously, efflux from the cell is a major limitation of antineoplastic drug efficacy. Systemic drug exposure is also an important parameter in ensuring the optimal cytotoxic response and minimal toxicity. The area under the serum concentration-time curve (AUC) is a measure of systemic drug exposure. Because the AUC is dependent on drug administration and elimination, changes in these parameters may greatly affect the systemic exposure. Patients with a more rapid drug clearance may need larger doses than those with a slower clearance. Therefore, methods of dose prediction based on target AUCs and a measure of drug elimination may provide a more optimal treatment intensity.

Pharmacokinetic parameters should be routinely applied in clinical practice to assist in delivering the optimal dose with the least risk of serious toxicity. Interpatient variability should always be considered when evaluating therapeutic or toxic response to therapy.

Table 18-10 Chemotherapeutic Agents Cleared by Kidneys That Have Increased Toxicity in Renal Insufficiency

Drugs Requiring Dose Modification	
Bleomycin	Cyclophosphamide
Carboplatin	Etoposide
Cisplatin	Methotrexate
	Streptozocin

Drug Interactions in the Patient Receiving Chemotherapy

A drug interaction occurs when the effects of one drug, therapeutic or toxic, are modified by the presence of another. Interactions may result in a beneficial effect such as improving therapeutic response or preventing or reducing toxicity. However, the majority produce undesirable outcomes such as a suboptimal therapeutic response or enhanced adverse effects. Tables 18-11 [68,107-115] and 18-12 [68,116,117] list numerous clinically significant drug interactions in patients receiving cancer chemotherapy.

Clinically significant drug interactions may be described as having a direct, indirect, or additive effect on the chemotherapy treatment. Direct interactions involve changes in the pharmacokinetics of the primary drug such as oral absorption, distribution, metabolism, and excretion. Drugs may also interact by indirectly altering the eliminating function of the organs of the body. Drug-induced renal or hepatic dysfunction may cause chemotherapy drugs to be eliminated more slowly, thereby increasing the potential for and severity of adverse reactions. Chemotherapeutic and other drugs occasionally share similar toxicities such as myelosuppression and gastrointestinal disturbances.

Not all drug interactions result in clinically significant therapeutic or toxic outcomes. Most interactions occur only under specific pharmacologic and physiologic situations; therefore, drug interactions should be judged by their overall effect on therapeutic response and patient care. The potential for serious interaction increases with the number of drugs a patient receives. Because most patients with cancer receive chemotherapy drugs, supportive care drugs, and conceivably pain management drugs, the potential for drug interactions is relatively high. Many patients with advanced disease have significant organ dysfunction, are elderly, or have concomitant illness, all of which contribute to the potential for harmful drug interactions.

Antineoplastic Drugs

Cancer chemotherapeutic drugs have traditionally been classified by their mechanism of action, chemical structure, or biological source. Grouping antineoplastic drugs into categories is done primarily for convenience. Although drugs within a class share some characteristics, there are often major differences in their indications, toxicities, and pharmaceutical properties. Figure 18-3 illustrates the proposed mechanisms and sites of action for most chemotherapeutic drugs. (See Chapter 20 for detailed descriptions of chemotherapy-induced toxicity and management of side effects, and Chapter 19, Appendix 19-B.)

Alkylating and alkylating-like agents

Classic alkylators. Alkylating agents were among the first drugs used to treat malignancies in humans, and they continue to play a major role in chemotherapy. This

Table 18-11   Selected Clinically Significant Drug Interactions in Patients Receiving Cancer Chemotherapy

Chemotherapy Drug	Interacting Drug	Pharmacokinetic/Pharmacodynamic Effect[a]	Management of Interaction
Asparaginase	Methotrexate	↓ toxicity[b]	Give methotrexate 3–24 hours prior
Bleomycin	Cisplatin	↓ renal elimination, ↑ pulmonary toxicity	Monitor renal function in patients previously treated with cisplatin
	Oxygen	↑ risk of acute pulmonary inflammation	Avoid inspired oxygen above 25%
Busulfan	Phenytoin[c]	↑ metabolic clearance, ↓ bone marrow cytotoxicity	Begin phenytoin therapy briefly before busulfan
Carmustine	Phenytoin	↓ phenytoin blood level, ↓ antiseizure effect	Monitor phenytoin level and adjust dose
Cisplatin	Anticonvulsant drugs (carbamazepine, phenytoin, valproic acid)	↓ oral absorption of anticonvulsant drug, ↓ blood levels	Monitor levels and increase dose as needed
	Sodium thiosulfate Mesna	Chemical incompatibility, ↓ cytotoxic and toxic effects Sodium thiosulfate may be used as an antidote for cisplatin toxicity	Do not administer in same infusion device
Cyclophosphamide	Allopurinol	↓ renal elimination of alkylating metabolite, ↑ toxicity	Monitor bone marrow and urologic toxicity
	Succinylcholine	↓ metabolic clearance of succinylcholine, Prolonged neuromuscular block	Use neuromuscular blocking drugs cautiously
Corticosteroids (dexamethasone, hydrocortisone, methylprednisolone)	Aminoglutethimide Mitotane	↑ metabolic clearance, ↓ therapeutic effect	Adjust corticosteroid dose to avoid adrenal crisis
Etoposide	Phenobarbital Phenytoin	↑ metabolic clearance, ↓ cytotoxicity	Avoid coadministration
	Highly protein-bound drugs	↓ protein binding, ↑ myelotoxicity	Avoid coadministration
Fluorouracil	Alfa interferon	↓ metabolic clearance, ↑ cytotoxicity	Monitor for severe gastrointestinal toxicity
	Metronidazole	↓ metabolic clearance, ↑ toxicity	Coadminister with caution
Ifosfamide	Antifungals (ketoconazole, itraconazole)	↓ clearance, ↑ toxicity	Avoid coadministration
	Phenobarbital	↑ metabolic activation, ↑ toxicity	Monitor bone marrow suppression and neurotoxicity
Alfa interferon	Theophylline	↓ metabolic clearance	Monitor theophylline blood levels
Interleukin-2	Corticosteroids	Block antitumor effect, ↓ tumor response rate	Use corticosteroids only for IL-2 toxicity management
Levamisole	Alcohol	Blocked metabolic clearance of alcohol, Disulfiram-like reaction (flushing, headache, nausea, vomiting, hypotension)	Avoid coadministration
Mercaptopurine	Allopurinol	↓ metabolic clearance, ↑ serum levels, prolonged bone marrow suppression	Decrease dose of mercaptopurine by 75%
	Cotrimoxazole (trimethoprim, sulfamethoxazole)	↑ oral absorption, ↓ metabolic activation	Monitor bone marrow suppression

(continued)

Table 18-11 Selected Clinically Significant Drug Interactions in Patients Receiving Cancer Chemotherapy (continued)

Chemotherapy Drug	Interacting Drug	Pharmacokinetic/Pharmacodynamic Effect[a]	Management of Interaction
Methotrexate	Cotrimoxazole	↓ renal clearance, additive antifolate activity, ↑ bone marrow toxicity	Monitor methotrexate levels and toxicity
	NSAIDs, salicylates	↓ renal clearance, ↓ protein binding, ↑ bone marrow and gastrointestinal toxicity	Monitor methotrexate levels and toxicity (*fatal* outcomes reported in cases of oral methotrexate and NSAID use)
	Probenecid Penicillin G	↓ renal clearance, ↑ toxic effects	Monitor methotrexate levels and toxicity
Paclitaxel	Cisplatin	↓ total body clearance, ↑ myelotoxicity	Give paclitaxel before cisplatin
Procarbazine	Ethanol	Blocks metabolism of alcohol, disulfiram-like reaction	Avoid coadministration
	Sympathomimetic drugs (ephedrine, epinephrine) Tricyclic antidepressant drugs (amitriptyline, imipramine)	MAO inhibition,[d] hypertensive crisis, tremor, excitation	Most interactions are not clinically important
Tamoxifen	Aminoglutethimide	↑ metabolic clearance	Avoid concurrent use
Teniposide	Highly protein-bound drugs[e]	↓ protein binding, ↑ in free (active) drug blood level	Avoid coadministration
Vinblastine	Phenytoin	↓ phenytoin blood level	Monitor phenytoin level and adjust dose as needed
Vincristine	Asparaginase	↑ risk of peripheral neurotoxicity	Give vincristine first

a. Refers to chemotherapy drug unless otherwise specified.

b. Result of methotrexate-induced block of protein synthesis.

c. For seizure prophylaxis for patients receiving high-dose busulfan for bone marrow transplant therapy.

d. Monoamine oxidase inhibition decreases the metabolism of sympathomimetic drugs, neurotransmitters released by tricyclic antidepressants, and endogenous amines.

e. Specifically sodium salicylate, sulfonamide drugs, and tolbutamide.

Data from Dorr,[68] Hansten,[107] Balis,[108] Finley,[109] Loadman,[110] Ignoffo,[111] Evans,[112] Thyss,[113] Ellison,[114] Fitzsimmons.[115]

group consists of a wide array of cytotoxic drugs that possess single-agent tumoricidal activity as well as a significant role in combination chemotherapy. Alkylating agents contribute electrophilic, alkyl groups (R-CH$_2$-CH$_2$) to attack electron-rich, nucleophilic sites on biological macromolecules such as DNA. The most common site of DNA alkylation is the N-7 position of guanine, with adducts at other positions on other bases being less frequent.[118] These DNA adducts may produce a variety of lesions, including strand breaks, nucleotide base deletions, and ring openings. Cytotoxicity and mutagenicity of alkylating agents usually result from these DNA adducts as well as interference with replication and transcription.[119,120] Many of the DNA lesions may be restored by repair enzymes; however, if the repair is only partial, additional DNA damage may result. Alkylators are non–cell cycle phase specific and are most active in the resting phase (G$_0$). Most alkylating agents are considered mutagens and potentially carcinogenic; therefore, the health care professional should be especially careful to avoid exposure when working with these compounds.

Mechlorethamine (nitrogen mustard) was the first alkylating agent introduced for cancer therapy. The drug spontaneously undergoes molecular rearrangement in aqueous solution to form a reactive species with two chloroethyl groups available for formation of cross-links of DNA strands.[118] Nitrogen mustard has a very short half-life and is usually undetectable in the blood within a few minutes of administration. It is a severe vesicant that must be handled with caution to prevent exposure of the clinician and to prevent extravasation during administration. Dose-limiting toxicities are myelosuppression, which may be severe, and rapid-onset nausea and vomiting. The major therapeutic role of mechlorethamine is in the MOPP (mechlorethamine, vincristine, procarbazine, prednisone) chemotherapy regimen for Hodgkin's disease. Other uses include topical application for mycosis fungoides or skin cancer, and intracavitary instillation for malignant pleural or pericardial effusions.

Melphalan, busulfan, and chlorambucil are usually given orally. Melphalan and busulfan are currently available as injectable products for specific indications. Mel-

Table 18-12 Chemotherapy Drug Interactions with Warfarin

Chemotherapy Drug	Possible Mechanism of Interaction	Effect on Prothrombin Time
Aminoglutethimide	↑ metabolic clearance	Shortens
Levamisole	Unknown	Prolongs
Mercaptopurine	Antagonize anticoagulant effect	Shortens
Mitotane	↑ metabolic clearance	Shortens
Tamoxifen	Unknown; enzyme inhibition and/or protein-binding displacement	Prolongs

Data from Dorr,[68] Hall,[116] Tenni.[117]

phalan was developed as a targeted agent for selective uptake in tumors actively using phenylalanine and tyrosine, such as melanin-producing malignant cells. The drug is transported into cells via two amino acid transport systems, a highly active L-amino acid system and a second, less active, amino acid system.[121] Absorption from the gastrointestinal tract is variable and is slowed when the drug is taken with food; therefore, it should be taken on an empty stomach. Melphalan may be given parenterally when the oral route is not appropriate; however, a 50% dose reduction should be considered in patients with a significant decrease in renal function. Chlorambucil is completely absorbed from the gastrointestinal tract. It has a predictable myelotoxicity profile and is well established in the treatment of chronic lymphocytic leukemia. Busulfan is a bifunctional alkylating agent with two reactive groups on opposite ends of the molecule, which form DNA adducts resulting in cross-linked strands.[118] In addition to its use in chronic myelogenous leukemia (CML), busulfan is also used in high-dose chemotherapy conditioning regimens and allogeneic or autologous bone marrow transplantation.

Cyclophosphamide and ifosfamide undergo a multistep activation process in vivo involving both hepatic microsomal and cellular enzyme systems to generate reactive chemical species. The two active metabolites of cyclophosphamide responsible for the majority of the drug's cytotoxicity are phosphoramide mustard and acrolein.[122] Acrolein is also primarily responsible for inducing hemorrhagic cystitis in approximately 10% of patients. This complication may be avoided by ensuring the patient is adequately hydrated and encouraging frequent urination within 24 hours of cyclophosphamide administration. Ifosfamide administration is associated with a much higher incidence of urotoxicity than cyclophosphamide. This is the result of an altered pharmacokinetic profile, which generates more urotoxic metabolite precursors than are found with cyclophosphamide.[123] Cystitis can be prevented by the coadministration of mesna, a compound that inactivates urotoxic metabolites in the bladder. Because cyclophosphamide and ifosfamide rely on both the kidneys and the liver for elimination, their toxicity may be prolonged in patients with compromised renal or hepatic failure.

Thiotepa is a polyfunctional alkylating agent that induces multiple types of DNA damage, including interstrand cross-links. Thiotepa may be administered by various routes: intravenous for breast cancer, intravesical for superficial bladder cancer, intrapleural for malignant pleural effusions, and intraperitoneal for refractory ovarian cancer. Thiotepa has some unique skin toxicities, including an acute erythroderma and dry desquamation of the palms and soles, and chronic darkening or bronzing of the skin when used in high-dose regimens.

Nitrosoureas decompose in aqueous solutions to form two reactive intermediates, a chloroethyldiazohydroxide and an isocyanate group.[124] The chloroethyldiazohydroxide form undergoes further decomposition to yield chloroethyl carbonium ions, which form adducts with DNA and induce interstrand cross-links. Isocyanate groups react with amine groups and produce carbamoylation reactions and thereby deplete glutathione and inhibit DNA repair. The interaction of chloroethyl carbonium ions with DNA is most likely the major cytotoxic effect. Nitrosoureas are distinct from other alkylators in that they are highly lipid soluble and readily cross the blood-brain barrier, lending themselves highly active in intracranial tumors. Other uses include Hodgkin's and non-Hodgkin's lymphoma and malignant melanoma.

Platinum-containing compounds. Drugs in this category constitute a highly active category of antineoplastic agents widely used for cancer treatment. Platinum compounds undergo an aquation reaction that enables them to react with macromolecules with strong binding sites such as DNA.[125] Cisplatin-induced DNA adducts and formation of intrastrand DNA cross-links correlate well with the drug's cytotoxicity and antitumor activity.[126,127] Although cisplatin and other platinum analogues behave similarly to alkylators, their cytotoxicity is probably the result of a combination of mechanisms of action, including inhibition of DNA and protein synthesis, alteration in cell membrane transport, and suppression of mitochondrial function.

Cisplatin and carboplatin are both highly dependent on renal elimination as their primary route of excretion. Cisplatin is removed from the blood in both its free and protein-bound forms following a triphasic elimination model. In the first two phases, primarily the unbound or free form of cisplatin is eliminated. Since 90% of the drug is excreted by the kidneys, adequate renal function is important in preventing drug accumulation and excessive toxicity. Patients who previously received cisplatin may be at increased risk for toxicity with carboplatin and should be evaluated for decreased renal function. Cisplatin given intraperitoneally produces peak levels that are as much as 21 times higher than peak plasma levels using similar doses.[128] Sodium thiosulfate may be administered systemically to decrease severe toxicities experienced with intraperitoneally administered cisplatin. Carboplatin elimination follows a triphasic pattern similar to that of cisplatin.[129] A formula derived by Calvert et al utilizing a patient's glomerular filtration rate and a desired systemic exposure (AUC) is widely used to calculate an individualized dose of carboplatin[130] (see Chapter 19). A measured or estimated creatinine clearance is commonly used for glomerular filtration rate and a target AUC is chosen based on prior and concurrent myelotoxic chemotherapy exposure.

Although both platinum analogues possess similar antitumor activity, there are significant differences in their dosing, administration, and side effect profiles. The dose-limiting toxicity of cisplatin is nephrotoxicity. Acute renal failure may occur within 24 hours of drug administration. Patients most at risk are those who receive inadequate hydration. Nephrotoxicity may usually be avoided by adequately hydrating the patient and administering diuretics such as furosemide, mannitol, or both. Carboplatin, although dependent on good renal function for elimination, is not necessarily nephrotoxic and rarely requires concomitant hydration and diuresis. Nausea and vomiting are common in patients receiving either platinum compound. However, emesis is often more severe and prolonged with cisplatin. Combination antiemetic regimens are usually necessary to prevent and treat this side effect, which is often most feared by the patient. Dose-limiting myelosuppression is much more of an issue with carboplatin than with cisplatin. Neurotoxicity and ototoxicity are more commonly associated with cisplatin.

Other alkylating-like drugs.

Other drugs with alkylating-like activity include dacarbazine, temozolomide, procarbazine, and altretamine (hexamethylmelamine). These drugs, like most other alkylating agents, are dependent on metabolic activation for the formation of reactive species. Dacarbazine functions primarily as an alkylating agent but may also act as an antimetabolite by inhibiting purine nucleoside incorporation into DNA.[131,132]

Dacarbazine does not appear to be cell cycle–phase specific and kills cells in all phases of the cycle. The drug is extremely sensitive to light and will undergo spontaneous decomposition to both active and inactive compounds. The most significant adverse events are nausea and vomiting, which may decrease with repeated courses. Other toxicities include a flulike syndrome, myelosuppression, and photosensitivity. Dacarbazine is also associated with hepatic venoocclusive disease characterized by fever and acute hepatic necrosis.[133] Temozolomide is a new monofunctional alkylating agent similar to dacarbazine. The drug requires dealkylation to produce an unstable intermediate that rapidly decomposes to release methyldiazonium.[134] Temozolomide is administered orally and has significant activity in patients with malignant gliomas (glioblastoma multiforme, anaplastic astrocytoma) and in advanced metastatic malignant melanoma.[135,136]

Procarbazine is administered orally and is a major therapeutic agent in the treatment of Hodgkin's disease and brain tumors. Two significant drug interactions are possible in patients taking procarbazine.[137] The first is the drug's ability to inhibit the enzyme monoamine oxidase, which is responsible for metabolism of amines. Inhibition of vasoactive amine metabolism may lead to hypertensive crisis, severe headache, sweating, and coma. Patients should avoid eating foods high in tyramine such as wine, ripe cheese, chocolate, and liver to prevent this drug interaction. The second interaction is seen when patients on procarbazine consume alcohol. They experience a disulfiram reaction, which is characterized by nausea, vomiting, palpitations, and sweating. Hexamethylmelamine is an orally administered agent whose mechanism of action is uncertain but probably of an alkylating type.

Antitumor antibiotics

Anthracycline antibiotics. The antitumor antibiotics constitute a large and diverse group of antineoplastic drugs originally derived from natural sources. Anthracyclines are a group of highly colored compounds known as *rhodomycins,* with both antineoplastic and antimicrobial activity. Anthracyclines (daunorubicin, doxorubicin, and idarubicin) and the chemically related anthracenediones (mitoxantrone) have multiple mechanisms of cytotoxicity, including intercalation, covalent DNA binding, free radical formation, and topoisomerase II enzyme inhibition. The two mechanisms now thought responsible for the majority of the cytotoxicity are free radical formation and inhibition of topoisomerase II enzyme. Anthracyclines can also interfere with the DNA unwinding process catalyzed by the nuclear enzyme topoisomerase II.[138,139] A "cleavable complex" is produced by inhibiting the enzyme's re-ligation function, thereby creating double-strand breaks in the DNA structure. Anthracyclines generate oxygen radicals by at least two mechanisms. The quinone structure common to all anthracyclines can donate an electron to an oxygen molecule and generate a superoxide. The superoxide is converted to hydrogen peroxide by superoxide dismutase and finally to a hydroxyl radical. Hydroxyl radical, the most reactive compound known, rapidly attacks DNA and cell membrane lipids.[140] An iron-anthracycline complex may also produce hydroxyl radical from hydrogen peroxide. Most normal tissues and tumor cells possess enzymes capable of detoxifying hydrogen peroxide. Both catalase and glutathione peroxidase convert hydrogen peroxide to water. Heart muscle cells lack the enzyme catalase, and anthracycline compounds destroy glutathione peroxidase.[141] This leaves cardiac tissue unable to detoxify hydrogen peroxide, which may then give rise to a reactive hydroxyl radical. There is now substantial evidence that the drug-iron complex plays an important role in the cytotoxicity of anthracyclines. Hydroxyl radical formation in cardiac tissue may be significantly decreased by the use of an edetate analogue dexrazoxane, that effectively chelates iron.

Anthracyclines are metabolized to both active and inactive compounds by the liver. The major metabolites of most anthracyclines are their alcohols, such as doxorubinicinol, which have antitumor activity but not as significant as do the parent compounds. The anthracycline dose should be reduced in patients with hepatic dysfunction, especially if the bilirubin is elevated. Dose adjustment is not necessary in renal failure because renal clearance of anthracyclines is minimal.

Cardiac toxicity of anthracyclines may manifest as acute changes in ECG and arrhythmias, which is more significant in patients with preexisting heart disease. However, the more common and often therapy-limiting cardiotoxicity is the development of cardiomyopathy leading to congestive heart failure.[140] Up to 10% of patients receiving a cumulative dose of doxorubicin greater than 550 mg/m[2] will develop this toxicity. Cardiac function is usually monitored with serial measurements of left ventricular function and ECG. Potential strategies to prevent or lessen cardiotoxicity include prolonged infusions of doxorubicin and cardioprotectant drugs such as dexrazoxane (Zinecard).

Mitoxantrone may be associated with less nausea, vomiting, and alopecia. Cardiac toxicity in patients treated with mitoxantrone appears to be less than that seen with doxorubicin.[142] However, there may be no difference in the incidence of cardiomyopathy at doses equipotent to doxorubicin. Daunorubicin, doxorubicin, and idarubicin are vesicants and can induce a severe extravasation injury characterized by pain, erythema, and tissue necrosis. Mitoxantrone is considered an irritant, and extravasation injury is much less common. Other toxicities of anthracyclines include mucositis, nausea, vomiting, and alopecia.

Liposomal encapsulation of doxorubicin and daunorubicin have provided two new anticancer agents with therapeutic and toxicity profiles different from the free form of these drugs. The mechanism of action is believed to be unchanged; however, the liposomal formulation changes the pharmacokinetics, allowing for a longer half-life and increased uptake by tumor cells.[143] Liposomal daunorubicin and liposomal doxorubicin are currently established treatments for Kaposi sarcoma in patients with acquired immunodeficiency syndrome (AIDS). There are also significant data suggesting activity in breast cancer. Less alopecia, nausea, vomiting, and neurotoxicity is seen with these agents compared with their nonliposomal or free drug formulations. Cardiac toxicity appears to be less dose-limiting with the liposomal encapsulated drugs. Doses greater than 1000 mg/m[2] have been given without significant changes in left ventricular function. An infusion reaction consisting of back pain, chest tightness, and flushing has been seen in approximately 7% of patients receiving their first dose of liposomal doxorubicin.[144] This rarely requires discontinuing treatment and is usually managed with administration of diphenhydramine and restarting the infusion at a slower rate. Palmar-plantar skin eruptions with swelling, pain, erythema, and desquamation of skin have also been seen in some patients receiving liposomal doxorubicin.

Other antitumor antibiotics. Bleomycin is a polypeptide composed of many low-molecular-weight proteins, isolated from the fungus *Streptomyces verticullus*. A drug-iron-oxygen complex binds to DNA by intercalation and generates oxygen radicals, which attack the nucleotide bases.[145] This results in single- and double-strand DNA breaks. Tumor cells are most sensitive to bleomycin in the premitotic, or G_2, phase, or in the mitotic phase of the cell cycle. Bleomycin has been used to synchronize cells into the G_2 and S phases so that other antineoplastic agents that act in those phases may have an increased cell kill potential. Bleomycin is also useful in combination chemotherapy regimens because of its lack of significant myelosuppressive effects.

Bleomycin is highly dependent on renal clearance for elimination from the body. Significant renal failure necessitates decreasing the dose by 50%–75% of full dose. Renal function of patients previously treated with renal toxic drugs or those who are currently receiving cisplatin should be monitored closely. Pulmonary toxicity of bleomycin may initially present as cough, dyspnea, and pleuritic chest pain. Patients at higher risk for developing bleomycin-related pulmonary fibrosis include older patients ($\geq$70 years), those with preexisting pulmonary disease, and those who have received mediastinal radiation therapy. Although a cumulative dose greater than 450 units is associated with a higher incidence of fibrosis, clinically significant pulmonary toxicity has been documented at lower doses.

Dactinomycin (actinomycin D) also binds to DNA by intercalation and induces single-strand breaks similar to those seen with doxorubicin.[146] The drug is currently limited to use in pediatric tumors and gestational trophoblastic neoplasms. Dactinomycin is not metabolized to a significant amount but instead is excreted unchanged in the urine and bile.

Mitomycin C is activated to an alkylating agent and its cytotoxicity is the result of cross-links with DNA, leading to inhibition of DNA synthesis and cell death. The drug is preferentially activated in hypoxic tissues such as the environment common to solid tumors.[147] Metabolism of mitomycin by the liver is poorly defined, and renal clearance plays only a minor role in total elimination. Mitomycin degrades at pHs lower than 6; therefore, when the drug is used intravesicularly for bladder cancer, a pH higher than 6 should be maintained in the bladder to ensure potency. A delayed and cumulative myelosuppression is seen with mitomycin. However, the development of a hemolytic-uremic syndrome resulting in renal failure, which is rarely reversible, is of more concern.

Antimetabolites

Antifolates. Antimetabolites used in cancer chemotherapy are structural analogues of nucleotide bases, which are the building blocks of DNA and RNA. The antineoplastic effect of this group of drugs is related to their ability to inhibit nucleic acid synthesis or to falsely be incorporated into the DNA double helix. Antifolate drugs methotrexate and trimetrexate inhibit the enzyme dihydrofolate reductase (DHFR), which catalyzes the reduction of dihydrofolate (folic acid) to tetrohydrofolate (folinic acid). Reduced folates act as 1-carbon donors necessary for the synthesis of purine and pyrimidine bases. Inhibition of DHFR by methotrexate depletes the intracellular reduced folate pool, thereby blocking de novo synthesis of nucleotide bases. These compounds also inhibit other folate-dependent enzymes such as thymidylate synthase, which catalyzes uracil to thymidine. Cytotoxicity is the result of an arrest of folate-dependent enzymatic reactions, including DNA, RNA, and protein synthesis.[148]

Rapidly proliferating cells in S phase are most susceptible to methotrexate-induced depletion of reduced folates. Therefore, longer exposure of tumor cells to methotrexate will allow more cells to enter the DNA synthesis phase of the cell cycle and result in enhanced cell kill. Most cells can function with relatively small amounts of DHFR to maintain sufficient reduced folate pools. Therefore, a high intracellular concentration of antifolate drugs should be maintained to ensure complete enzyme inhibition. This may be accomplished by administering large amounts of methotrexate such as those seen in treatment for malignant lymphomas and sarcomas. The ability to administer such high doses is possible only with the timely administration of leucovorin (folinic acid). Leucovorin circumvents methotrexate-induced enzyme blockade and "rescues" normal cells by providing them with the reduced folates they need for nucleic acid and protein synthesis.[149]

Methotrexate is one of the most extensively studied antineoplastic drugs for its pharmacokinetics, in part because there is a simple and readily available assay to measure the blood concentration of methotrexate. This assay is frequently used to monitor for potential toxicity when administering moderate to high doses of methotrexate. The drug is well absorbed orally at moderate to low doses. Elimination occurs primarily through renal excretion via glomerular filtration and active secretion in the proximal tubule.[150] As previously mentioned, excretion is highly dependent on adequate renal function and may be inhibited by a number of compounds. Doses should be reduced in patients with decreased renal function, and blood levels should be monitored following each dose. Patients with blood levels greater than 0.5 μM at 48 hours postdose are at increased risk for severe myelosuppression and mucositis.[151] Leucovorin therapy should be continued in these patients until methotrexate blood levels are below 0.05 μM. Dose reductions vary and should be proportionate with reductions in creatinine clearance. Patients with a creatinine clearance of 10-50 mL/minute should receive 30%–50% of the original dose, and those with creatinine clearance less than 10 mL/minute only 15% of original dose.[150] The pharmacokinetics of methotrexate are altered by distribution into third-space fluid collections such as ascitic accumulation in the peritoneal cavity. Elimination is prolonged and toxicity is increased because of the slow redistribution of the drug from the peritoneum back into the blood.[104]

Methotrexate-associated toxicities, besides myelosuppression and mucositis, include nephrotoxicity, hepatotoxicity, and pulmonary fibrosis. Hepatotoxicity may result from high-dose therapy and result in acute and reversible elevations in liver function enzymes. Methotrexate is useful as treatment or prophylaxis for meningeal leukemia; however, the drug poorly distributes into the cerebrospinal fluid (CSF). Therefore, methotrexate may be injected directly into the CSF by lumbar puncture or intraventricular device (Ommaya reservoir). Toxicities seen with intrathecal administration include severe headache, nuchal rigidity, vomiting, and fever; in severe cases, a demyelinating encephalopathy may develop.

Pyrimidine analogues. The fluoropyrimidine 5-fluorouracil (5-FU) undergoes extensive metabolism intracellularly to an active metabolite fluorodeoxyuridine monophosphate (FdUMP). FdUMP covalently binds with thymidylate synthase (TS) and inhibits the enzyme's ability to synthesize deoxythymidine triphosphate (dTTP), a precursor of DNA synthesis. Other metabolic pathways are conversion of 5-FU to fluorouradine triphosphate (FUTP), which may be incorporated into RNA, and conversion of FdUMP to the triphosphate form, which may be incorporated into DNA. Cytotoxicity of 5-FU by these metabolic pathways results in depletion of dTTP or false incorporation of other metabolites into DNA and RNA.[152,153] The administration of 5-FU and leucovorin concurrently enhances this reaction and increases the cytotoxic effect of 5-FU (see above Modulation of fluorouracil by leucovorin, under Therapeutic Strategies).

Rapidly cleared by the liver, 5-FU has a plasma half-life of 6–20 minutes. There may be considerable variation in half-life time among patients. The enzyme dihydropyrimidine dehydrogenase metabolizes 5-FU to dihydrofluorouracil in the liver and other tissues. Patients who are deficient in this enzyme experience greatly increased 5-FU levels and resultant toxicity.[154] When 5-FU or floxuridine is administered directly into the hepatic artery or portal vein, hepatic metastases are directly exposed to the drug with minimal systemic exposure because of the drug's significant first-pass clearance.

The major dose-limiting toxicity of 5-FU is dependent on the schedule of administration. Myelosuppression is more prominent when the drug is given by rapid bolus injection, whereas mucositis and gastrointestinal toxicity are more common with prolonged infusions over 4 to 5 days. Cholestatic jaundice and biliary sclerosis are complications of intrahepatic adminstration of fluoropyrimidines. Therapy with 5-FU has sometimes caused chest pain, elevation in cardiac enzymes, and ECG changes similar to those seen with myocardial ischemia. This syndrome may be associated with 5-FU-induced coronary vasospasm.[155]

Orally administered fluoropyrimidines have been avoided because of the erratic bioavailability seen with these drugs. However, recently three new approaches to orally administering fluoropyrimidines have been developed. Capecitabine is now FDA approved for the treatment of patients with metastatic breast cancer for which anthracyclines or paclitaxel are indicated. Capecitabine is a prodrug which undergoes numerous metabolic steps in both the liver and tissues to ultimately become fluorouracil.[156] The cytotoxic metabolite is more concentrated in tumor cells than normal cells because of the higher concentrations of thymidine phosphorylase, the enzyme responsible for the final conversion to fluorouracil. The major dose-limiting side effects include diarrhea, hand-and-foot syndrome, and stomatitis. Capecitabine is also active in colorectal cancer. Two other fluoropyrimidine compounds are under investigation for use in colorectal cancer. UFT is a combination of the fluorouracil prodrug ftorafur and uracil that is given in a 1-to-4 molar ratio by the oral route. The combination drugs produce higher tumor-to-serum fluorouracil ratios than ftorafur alone.[157] The pharmacokinetics of fluorouracil are significantly altered by the coadministration of 5-ethynyluracil, a potent inhibitor of dihydropyrimidine dehydrogenase that is responsible for the inactivation of fluorouracil.[158] The combination is being investigated for the orally administered treatment of colorectal cancer.

Cytarabine was originally isolated from the sponge *Cryptothethya crypta*. The parent drug is phosphorylated to ara-CTP, which competes with the normal substrate deoxycytidine triphosphate (dCTP) to inhibit DNA polymerase-alpha.[159] DNA polymerases are critical enzymes in the synthesis and repair of DNA. The metabolite ara-CTP may also incorporate into DNA and interfere with chain polymerization and repair of damaged DNA strands. As seen with other antimetabolites, tumor cells and normal tissues are most sensitive to cytarabine in the S phase of the cell cycle.

Cytarabine is rapidly converted to the inactive metabolite ara-U by the enzyme cytidine deaminase, which is present in many tissues, including the gastrointestinal epithelium and liver. The half-life is 7–20 minutes, with more than 70% of the dose appearing in the urine as ara-U. Cytarabine is usually administered by continuous infusion following a bolus dose. This regimen is used to maintain cytotoxic levels despite the drug's rapid inactivation and to maximally expose all cycling cells to the cytotoxic effects during the S phase of the cell cycle. Cytarabine may be used alone or in addition to methotrexate for meningeal leukemia; however, direct intrathecal administration is necessary to obtain sufficient drug concentrations in the CSF. Only small amounts of cytarabine are needed intrathecally because deamination is minimal in the CSF. Toxicity of cytarabine includes myelosuppression and gastrointestinal epithelial injury. When high-dose cytarabine is used for refractory acute myelogenous leukemia (AML), 20% of patients may experience a cerebral and cerebellar dysfunction. This syndrome is more often seen in individuals older than 50 and is characterized by slurred speech, ataxia, confusion, and coma.[160] High-dose cytarabine is also associated with conjunctivitis, which can usually be prevented by giving the patient steroid ophthalmic drops.

Gemcitabine is a pyrimidine analogue of deoxycytidine that is converted intracellularly to its diphosphate and triphosphate metabolites. Gemcitabine diphosphate is an inhibitor of ribonucleotide reductase and thereby inhibits de novo nucleotide synthesis.[161] Gemcitabine triphosphate inhibits DNA synthesis by competing with the physiologic substrate, deoxycytidine triphosphate, for DNA polymerase and incorporation into DNA. The reduction of intracellular deoxycytidine triphosphate induced by gemcitabine diphosphate enhances the incorporation of gemcitabine triphosphate into DNA, a mechanism referred to as "self-potentiation." Therefore, the half-life of gemcitabine is prolonged because of this phenomenon. Infusions should be limited to 30 minutes. Longer infusions are associated with a higher degree of myelotoxicity. Other important adverse effects include elevated liver transaminase enzymes, nausea and vomiting, and skin rash with or without pruritus.[162]

Purine analogues.   Thiopurines 6-mercaptopurine (6-MP) and 6-thioguanine (6-TG) are converted to their respective monophosphates, which inhibit purine synthesis and cause an accumulation of nucleic acid precursors. These precursors in turn facilitate the conversion of 6-MP and 6-TG to their active nucleotide forms. The triphosphate nucleotides of these drugs incorporate into DNA and induce strand breaks, which are correlated with cytotoxicity. Methotrexate, an inhibitor of de novo purine biosynthesis, is synergistic with the 6-thiopurines by blocking purine synthesis and enhancing thiopurine activation. The cytotoxicity of fludarabine and cladribine (2-chlorodeoxyadenosine) is associated with their ability to inhibit DNA polymerase and other enzymes utilized in the synthesis of DNA and RNA.[163,164]

Plant derivatives

Antineoplastic drugs derived from plant sources represent a large and diverse group of chemotherapeutic drugs. Many of the drugs in this group (plant alkaloids, paclitaxel) are naturally occurring alkaloids that were isolated from plant material. Others are the result of synthetic and semisynthetic processes used to manufacture analogues of compounds originally extracted from plants. Examples include etoposide, docetaxel, and topotecan. The discovery of new plant-derived compounds with antitumor activity is ongoing and will continue to provide important and novel agents for the treatment of cancer.

Vinca alkaloids.   Natural alkaloids present in small quantities in the periwinkle plant play a major role in cancer chemotherapy. Although the drugs in this group are dramatically similar in chemical structure, their antitumor activity and toxicity differ greatly. Vincristine has a broad spectrum of activity, including leukemia, lymphoma, breast cancer, lung cancer, and multiple myeloma, while vinblastine is used primarily in germ cell tumors and advanced Hodgkin's disease. Vinblastine is myelotoxic and neurotoxic; vincristine is also neurotoxic but has amazingly minimal myelotoxicity. Vinorelbine is the newest vinca alkaloid to become available in the

United States. It is active in breast cancer and non-small cell lung cancer and is both myelotoxic and neurotoxic. Vindesine is widely available in Europe but currently not available in the United States except in clinical trials.

Vinca alkaloids belong to a group of compounds now known as the *tubulin interactive agents.* They exert their cytotoxic effects primarily by interfering with normal microtubule formation and function, which is critical for the mitosis phase of the cell cycle and ultimately cell division. Microtubules have other important cellular functions that are affected by the vinca alkaloids, including maintenance of cell shape and intracellular transport. Vinca alkaloids bind to specific sites on tubulin, preventing formation of tubulin dimers and inhibiting the formation of microtubule structures. Although mitotic arrest is the primary mechanism of cell death, vinca alkaloids may have a cytolytic effect on resting cells in G_0 phase and other cells in G_1 or S phase.[165] Cells are sensitive to low concentrations of vincristine, and duration of exposure is critical in cytotoxic effect.

Despite the wide range of clinical uses of the vinca alkaloids, there is surprisingly little information available to describe their pharmacologic and pharmacokinetic profiles. This may be primarily the result of lack of a sensitive drug assay for quantitating the low concentration found in patients receiving vincas. Vincristine is highly bound to serum proteins, blood cells, and especially platelets. Vincristine is metabolized primarily by the liver and concentrates in the bile. Seventy percent of a dose is excreted in the feces, and approximately 10% is excreted in the urine.[166] Dose modification should be considered in patients with hepatic dysfunction, particularly patients with biliary obstructions. Vinblastine and vinorelbine have similar pharmacokinetic profiles, with excretion occurring primarily through the biliary tract. All the vinca alkaloids have a prolonged terminal elimination phase half-life of 1–4 days.

Vinca alkaloids are known for their peripheral neurotoxicity, which is frequently a cumulative dose-limiting toxicity. Peripheral neurotoxicity initially presents as sensory impairment (stocking-and-glove distribution) and paresthesias. Patients may later develop neuritic pain and motor dysfunction. Loss of deep tendon reflexes, foot and wrist drop, ataxia, and paralysis may occur with continued vinca alkaloid therapy. The only effective management is discontinuation of therapy. Accidental intrathecal administration of vincristine induces an ascending paralysis resulting in death. Constipation and abdominal pain are frequent complaints of older patients while on vincristine. Myelosuppression is also a dose-limiting toxicity of vinblastine and vinorelbine, but not vincristine. The vinca alkaloids are vesicants, and extravasation should be avoided.

Taxanes. The taxanes have emerged as an extremely important group of antitumor compounds with activity in a wide range of cancers. Taxanes are complex chemical structures that are difficult to synthesize in the laboratory, and extraction and isolation from plant material was the only source for paclitaxel until the early 1990s, when a semisynthetic process using a taxane precursor was developed. Because of the drug's poor water solubility, the injectable formulation must contain 50% polyoxyethylated castor oil (Cremophor EL) vehicle to maintain aqueous solubility. This creates problems with administration as Cremophor EL can leach hepatotoxic plasticizer from PVC plastic infusion devices and is also associated with severe hypersensitivity reactions.

Extracted and isolated from the bark of the Pacific yew tree *Taxus brevifolia*, paclitaxel has demonstrated antitumor activity in preclinical studies in a broad range of tumor models.[167] Paclitaxel and docetaxel preferentially bind to microtubules over tubulin dimers, and inhibit microtubule disassembly, which is necessary for normal functioning of microtubule structures.[168] Cells exposed to paclitaxel display many arrays of disorganized microtubules during all phases of the cell cycle.[169] Although taxanes have these distinct antimicrotubule effects on cells, the actual mechanism of cell death is unclear. The mechanism of action and cytotoxic effect of docetaxel are similar to those of paclitaxel.[170]

Hepatic metabolism and biliary excretion probably constitute the major routes of elimination for paclitaxel and docetaxel.[171,172] Urinary excretion accounts for less than 5% of total body clearance of the drug. Paclitaxel clearance is reduced by as much as 30% when given following cisplatin.[173] This interaction results in increased peak plasma concentrations of paclitaxel and more severe myelotoxicity than is seen with the reverse administration schedule. For routine use of paclitaxel with cisplatin or carboplatin, the paclitaxel should be given first, followed by cisplatin or carboplatin. The taxanes also exhibit a high degree of protein binding (90%–95%). Among the most significant toxicities associated with taxanes are myelosuppression, neurotoxicity, hypersensitivity, total body alopecia, and transient myalgias and arthralgias. Nail separation may occur especially when paclitaxel is given as a weekly 1-hour infusion. Hypersensitivity reactions were seen in 10% of patients receiving paclitaxel during early clinical trials.[174] Hypersensitivity reactions usually occur within the first 10 minutes of the initial infusion and may be characterized by hypotension, bronchospasm, dyspnea, abdominal and leg pain, and severe facial flushing. Major hypersensitivity reactions may be prevented in most patients by the preinfusion administration of a corticosteroid (dexamethasone), an antihistamine (diphenhydramine), and an H_2-blocking drug (cimetidine or ranitidine). Paclitaxel may be safely given parenterally with infusions lasting 24, 3, or 1 hours. The 3-hour infusion rate has been associated with less neutropenia than the 24-hour infusion.

The toxicity profile of docetaxel is different from that of paclitaxel.[175] The incidence of hypersensitivity reactions is lower with docetaxel, with severe reactions experienced in fewer than 1% of patients treated. Skin reactions, including pruritus, macular or papular lesions, erythema, and desquamation, are seen in 50%–70% of patients treated with docetaxel. Nail changes, consisting of an orange discoloration and thickening of the nails, were also observed in many patients in clinical trials. A more significant complication is fluid retention and weight gain, which can occur in 6% of patients. Characteristics of this side effect include peripheral edema, generalized edema, pleural effusion, and cardiac tamponade. A 5-day regimen of corticosteroid is useful in preventing and lessening the fluid retention, and is also useful for prevention of hypersensitivity reactions.

Epipodophyllotoxins. Podophyllotoxin, an extract of the mandrake plant, is an antimitotic drug that binds to tubulin and inhibits microtubulin formation. This compound was not further developed as an antitumor agent because of its unacceptable toxicity in humans. Etoposide and teniposide are glycosidic derivatives of podophyllotoxin that possess significant activity in many human tumors such as germ cell tumors and lung cancer, with a more predictable and mild toxicity profile. Initially, these drugs were thought to work as antimicrotubule agents similar to podophyllotoxin and vinca alkaloids. However, these agents produced no effect on microtubule assembly.[176] Cell cycle studies demonstrated epipodophyllotoxins induced arrest of cells in late S or early G phase instead of the expected M-phase arrest common with antimitotic drugs. Along with the observation of drug-induced DNA strand breaks, scientists have suggested the primary cytotoxic mechanism of these compounds is inhibition of topoisomerase II.[177] Epipodophyllotoxins stabilize the enzyme-DNA formation, thereby inhibiting the reunion of the two DNA strands originally cleaved by the enzyme. Additionally, the synergy of the etoposides with antimetabolite drugs may be the result of inhibition of nucleoside transport into the cell.

Etoposide and teniposide are highly protein-bound (94% and 99%, respectively) to the albumin. Drugs that interfere with the protein binding of teniposide may induce greater toxicity in patients receiving both drugs (see Drug Interactions in the Patients Receiving Chemotherapy, above). Renal clearance is the major route of elimination for etoposide, with approximately 40%–60% of the drug excreted unchanged in the urine. Biliary excretion and hepatic metabolism are responsible for elimination to a lesser extent.[178] Teniposide is more extensively metabolized, with only 5%–20% excreted unchanged in the urine. The cytotoxic effects of etoposide exhibit a schedule dependency in the treatment of extensive small-cell lung cancer.[179] Etoposide is available as an oral formulation, which has a bioavailability of approximately 50%.

The toxicities of both agents are similar, with myelosuppression, hypersensitivity, and infusion-related blood pressure changes being the most significant. Both agents are also poorly water-soluble, necessitating the addition of Tween 80 or Cremophor EL and other excipients to maintain the drugs in aqueous solution. The manufacturer of teniposide recommends avoiding the use of PVC plastic infusion devices to prevent exposing the patient to potentially hepatotoxic plasticizers leached from the plastic by the Cremophor vehicle.

Camptothecin derivatives. Camptothecin sodium was originally tested in the early 1970s as an antitumor compound. Despite the drug's significant activity in both preclinical and clinical trials, it was abandoned because of unpredictable and often severe hemorrhagic cystitis. Later interest in this group of drugs was renewed with the introduction of semisynthetic analogues of camptothecin. Topotecan and irinotecan have undergone extensive clinical evaluation and were recently approved by the FDA as single-agent therapy for refractory ovarian cancer and relapsed colon cancer, respectively. Their proposed mechanism of action is inhibition of topoisomerase I, an enzyme responsible for maintaining the three-dimensional structure of DNA. Topoisomerase inhibitors bind with the DNA-enzyme complex, thereby inducing DNA strand breaks and cell death.[180]

Camptothecins appear to exist in two species in aqueous solutions: a closed lactone ring, which possesses cytotoxic activity, and an open carboxylate form, which does not. The conversion is pH dependent, with the open form predominating in an alkaline environment and the closed, or active, form predominating in an acidic solution. Much of the unpredictable urotoxicity seen in early trials of camptothecin sodium may be explained by the lack of knowledge of the pH-dependent conversion and the shift of the equilibrium toward the active species in the acidic environment of the bladder. Irinotecan is a prodrug and must be converted to its active form via carboxylesterase in the body.[181] Myelosuppression is the major dose-limiting toxicity of topotecan, while diarrhea is the primary dose-limiting toxicity for irinotecan when administered on a once-weekly schedule. To effectively manage the diarrhea associated with irinotecan, patients should be instructed to start a high-dose loperamide regimen (2 mg of loperamide every 2 hours) until they are diarrhea-free for 12 hours.

Miscellaneous agents

L-asparaginase induces a rapid and complete depletion from the blood of the amino acid L-asparagine. This biochemical process is cytotoxic to tumor cells highly dependent on exogenous sources of the amino acid. The major cytotoxic effect is the inhibition of protein synthesis, with a secondary effect of inhibition of nucleic acid synthesis also observed in sensitive cells. L-asparaginase is considered cell cycle–phase nonspecific, despite the drug's ability to block cells in G_1 and S phases of the cell cycle. The drug's only antineoplastic use is as part of the induction and consolidation therapy for acute lymphocytic leukemia in both children and adults. L-asparaginase is extracted from *Escherichia coli* bacteria and is associated with a high incidence of anaphylaxis. Patients who develop severe hypersensitivity reactions to the bacterial source product may receive pegaspargase, which is chemically altered to be less immunogenic. Other toxicities seen with L-asparaginase include hyperglycemia, hypoprothrombinemia, and neurotoxicity.

Hydroxyurea is a DNA-selective antimetabolite that

inhibits ribonucleotide reductase and has minimal inhibitory effect on RNA and protein synthesis. Its major indication is in rapidly controlling blood counts in acute leukemia and other myeloproliferative diseases such as polycythemia vera and essential thrombocytosis. Allopurinol should be used in conjuction with hydroxyurea to prevent tumor lysis syndrome.

Estramustine is a unique compound made up of a molecule of estradiol phosphate combined with nitrogen mustard. Originally believed to have alkylating properties, the drug's mechanism of action is now thought to be related to antimicrotubule activity.[182]

Hormonal Therapy

Hormonal manipulations were among the first treatments used to control cancer. Initially they had limited potential to induce significant response in sensitive tumors; currently, however, they are critical components in the treatment for many different neoplasms. Table 18-13 lists the commonly used hormonal agents and their primary indications. Steroids and steroid analogues constitute the majority of drugs used for hormonal therapy. Their mechanism of action is incompletely understood but probably involves the inhibition of steroid-specific receptors located on the surface of cells. Blocking these receptors prevents the cell from receiving normal hormonal growth stimulation, thereby decreasing the growth fraction of the tumor.

Antiestrogens

Tamoxifen is a frequently used anticancer drug in the treatment of breast cancer. It is used in both the adjuvant setting and for treatment of metastatic disease in primarily estrogen receptor–positive tumors. Tamoxifen's primary mechanism of action is blocking estrogen stimulation of breast cancer cells.[183] This is achieved by the drug's ability to inhibit both the translocation and nuclear binding of the estrogen receptor. Tamoxifen is an estrogen antagonist (blocker) in breast tissue and an estrogen agonist (stimulator) on the endometrium, bone, and lipids. The most prominent toxicity is hot flashes, which affect approximately half of the women who use it.[184] Other side effects include a slight increased incidence of thromboembolic events and a potential to cause endometrial cancer. In a large randomized trial comparing tamoxifen and placebo in the prevention of breast cancer in women, it was found that women at risk were 50% less likely to develop a breast malignancy if they were taking tamoxifen 20 mg daily.[185] Another antiestrogen drug toremifene is thought to be a more pure antiestrogen. A trial comparing tamoxifen and toremifene indicated both were equally effective in treating metastatic breast cancer.[186] However, toremifene appears to be less carcinogenic at least in preclinical models.[187] Megestrol has also been used to treat metastatic breast cancer but more recently is primarily used for the treatment of anorexia-cachexia related to cancer.[188]

Table 18-13 Commonly Used Hormonal Agents and Primary Indications

Pharmacologic Class	Drug Name(s)	Primary Indication(s)
Corticosteroids	Dexamethasone Hydrocortisone Methylprednisolone Prednisone	Leukemias Hodgkin's disease Malignant lymphomas Breast cancer Multiple myeloma
Androgens	Fluoxymesterone Testosterone	Breast cancer
Estrogens	Conjugated estrogens Diethylstilbesterol Estradiol	Prostate cancer Breast cancer
Antiestrogens		
Progestins	Medroxyprogesterone Megesterol	Endometrial cancer Breast cancer
Estrogen-receptor antagonists	Tamoxifen (Nolvadex) Toremifene (Fareston)	Breast cancer
Aromatase inhibitors	Mitotane Anastrozole (Arimidex) Letrozole (Femara)	Adrenal cancer Breast cancer Breast cancer
LH-RH analogues	Goserelin (Zoladex) Leuprolide (Lupron)	Prostate cancer Breast cancer
Antiandrogens	Flutamide (Eulexin) Nilutamide (Nilandron) Bicalutamide (Casodex)	Prostate cancer

Aromatase inhibitors

Aromatase inhibitors suppress postmenopausal estrogen synthesis by inhibiting the peripheral conversion of androgens to estrogens. These agents have been primarily developed for the treatment of hormonally sensitive breast cancer. Ovarian production of estrogen is unaffected, therefore, these agents are only useful in postmenopausal women or oophorectomized premenopausal women. Aminoglutethamide was the first agent available but is now rarely used because of poor tolerance and need to replace corticosteroids along with the drug. Newer agents include anastrozole and letrozole. Both of these drugs are potent aromatase inhibitors and equally effective to aminoglutethamide, however, they only minimally effect the synthesis of corticosteroids, aldosterone, or thyroid hormone.

Gonadotropin-releasing hormone analogues

Luteinizing hormone releasing hormone (LH-RH) agonists are synthetic analogues of the naturally occurring hormone. Initially, these drugs induce an increase in testosterone levels secondary to their stimulation of LH release. However, with continued use, the pituitary gland becomes desensitized, resulting in a dramatic decrease in the production of estrogens and androgens. Leuprolide and goserelin are both available as slow-release depot injections that are given at monthly or every 4-month intervals. Castration levels of testosterone are achieved within 3–4 weeks with leuprolide[189] and within 1 month with goserelin.[190]

Antiandrogens

Antiandrogens are used in men with hormone-responsive metastatic prostate cancer, either as initial therapy or in combination with a gonadotropin-releasing hormone analogue. Their mechanism of action is binding to the androgen receptor and blocking the effects of dihydrotestosterone on prostate cancer cells.[191] Flutamide was the first antiandrogen available and the most frequent adverse events include diarrhea, gynecomastia, and occasionally hepatotoxicity. Other newer antiandrogens are nilutamide and bicalutamide. Both of these agents have equivalent activity to flutamide, however, they are usually better tolerated because of less diarrhea and a more simplified administration schedule.

Differentiation Agents

Retinoids

Retinoids, a class of compounds structurally related to vitamin A (retinol), have been found to influence proliferation and differentiation of normal and tumor cells.[192] The two compounds most studied for their effect on controlling or preventing tumor growth are 13-*cis* retinoic acid (isotretinoin) and all-trans retinoic acid (tretinoin). Isotretinoin is currently marketed as the anti-acne product Accutane, however, it is under extensive evaluation, often in combination with alfa-interferon, for the prevention of new and recurrent squamous cell tumors.[193] Isotretinoin reverses oral leukoplakia, a premalignant state of the oral cavity in heavy tobacco smokers.[194] Other potential uses for isotretinoin include myelodysplastic syndromes and acute and chronic leukemias.[195–197] Tretinoin (Vesanoid) has recently been approved for use in induction and maintenance regimens for acute promyelocytic leukemia. Toxicity of these compounds is similar to the pharmacologic effects of hypervitaminosis A, which include dry lips and mucous membranes, skin fragility, brittle nails, photosensitivity, and conjunctivitis.[198] Other side effects are headache, nausea and vomiting, transaminase and triglyceride elevations, arthralgia, and bone pain. Tretinoin is also associated with a severe leukocytosis, which may induce fevers, respiratory distress, pulmonary and pericardial effusions, and hypotension.[199] All retinoids are teratogens and therefore should never be given to pregnant female patients.

Other differentiation agents

Vitamin D_3 has demonstrated in vitro activity in decreasing growth of leukemia, breast, colon, and prostate cancer cell lines. Butyrate and phenylacetate are compounds known to induce differentiation in erythroleukemia, malignant gliomas, and prostate cancer. Amifostine, a cytoprotectant, is also known to promote multilineage hematopoiesis in patients with myelodysplastic syndrome.[200] Amifostine was usually given as an infusions of $200 \ mg/m^2$ three times weekly, and side effects consisted of hypotension and nausea and vomiting.

Conclusion

Drug therapy for the control and cure of cancer has come a long way from early experimentation with mustard gas derivatives. Currently, a multitude of drugs with a variety of treatment schedules are among the oncologist's armamentarium. Research efforts must continue to focus on improving the oncology patient's life by evaluating new drugs and therapies, as well as reevaluating old ones. Biological therapies are also being actively investigated for their ability to control tumor growth and generation. The development of gene-therapy approaches may hold the key to more effective and better-tolerated treatment for cancer. New knowledge of this type is expanding exponentially as technology enhances our ability to peer into the genetic workings of the tumor cell. Future directions for research in oncology should include combining chemotherapy and biological therapy, gene therapy, or all of these to achieve optimal patient outcomes.

References

1. Kennedy BJ: Evolution of chemotherapy. *CA Cancer J Clin* 41:261–263, 1991 (editorial)
2. Shoemaker RH, Wolpert-DeFilippes MK, Kern DH, et al: Application of a human tumor colony-forming assay to new drug screening. *Cancer Res* 45:2145–2153, 1985
3. DeVita VT: Principles of cancer management: Chemotherapy, in DeVita VT, Hellman S, Rosenberg SA (eds): *Cancer: Principles and Practice of Oncology* (ed 5). Philadelphia, Lippincott, 1997, pp 333–347
4. DeVita VT: Cell kinetics and chemotherapy of cancer. *Cancer Chemother Rep* 2:22–23, 1971
5. Charbit A, Malaise EP, Tubiana M: Relation between the pathological nature and the growth rate of human tumors. *Eur J Cancer* 7:307–315, 1971
6. Skipper HE, Schabel FM, Wilcox WS: Experimental evaluation of potential anticancer agents XII: On the criteria and kinetics associated with "curability" of experimental leukemia. *Cancer Chemother Rep* 35:1–111, 1964
7. Buick RN: Cellular basis of chemotherapy, in Dorr RT, Von Hoff DD (eds): *Cancer Chemotherapy Handbook* (ed 2). Norwalk, CT, Appleton & Lange, 1994, pp 3–14
8. Norton L: The Norton-Simon hypothesis, in Perry MC (ed): *Chemotherapy Source Book* (ed 2). Baltimore, Williams & Wilkins, 1996, pp 43–61
9. Norton L, Day R: Potential innovations in scheduling in cancer chemotherapy, in DeVita VT, Hellman S, Rosenberg SA (eds): *Important Advances in Oncology*. Philadelphia, Lippincott, 1991, pp 57–73
10. Goldie JH, Coldman AJ: A mathematic model for relating the drug sensitivity of tumors to their spontaneous mutation rate. *Cancer Treat Rep* 63:1727–1733, 1979
11. Skipper HE, Simpson-Herren L: Relationship between tumor cell heterogeneity and responsiveness to chemotherapy, in DeVita VT, Hellman S, Rosenberg SA (eds): *Important Advances in Oncology*. Philadelphia, Lippincott, 1985, pp 63–77
12. Goldie JH, Coldman AJ: The genetic origin of drug resistance in neoplasms: Implications for systemic therapy. *Cancer Res* 44:3643–3653, 1984
13. Shustik C, Dalton W, Gros P: P-glycoprotein-mediated multidrug resistance in tumor cells: Biochemistry, clinical relevance, and modulation. *Mol Aspects Med* 16:1–78, 1995
14. Luria SE, Delbruck M: Mutations of bacteria from virus sensitivity to virus resistance. *Genetics* 28:491–511, 1943
15. Law LW: Origin of the resistance of leukemic cells to folic acid antagonists. *Nature* 169:628–629, 1952
16. Yarbro JW: The scientific basis of cancer chemotherapy, in Perry MC (ed): *Chemotherapy Source Book* (ed 2). Baltimore, Williams & Wilkins, 1996, pp 3–18
17. Dalton WS: Overcoming the multidrug-resistant phenotype, in DeVita VT, Hellman S, Rosenberg SA (eds): *Cancer: Principles and Practice of Oncology* (ed 4). Philadelphia, Lippincott, 1993, pp 2655–2666
18. Gill DR, Hyde SC, Higgins CF, et al: Separation of drug transport and chloride channel functions of the human multidrug resistance P-glycoprotein. *Cell* 71:23–32, 1992
19. Cordon-Carlo C, O'Brien JP, Boccia J, et al: Expression of the multidrug resistance gene product (p-glycoprotein) in human normal and tumor tissues. *J Histochem Cytochem* 38:1277–1287, 1990
20. Sugawara I, Hamada H, Tsuruo T, et al: Specialized localization of P-glycoprotein recognized by MRK 16 monoclonal antibody in endothelial cells of the brain and the spinal cord. *Jpn J Cancer Res* 81:727–730, 1990
21. Marie J, Zittoun R, Sikic B: Multidrug resistance (*MDR-1*) gene expression in adult acute leukemias: Correlations with treatment and in vitro drug sensitivity. *Blood* 78:586–592, 1991
22. Bell DR, Gerlach JH, Kartner N, et al: Detection of P-glycoprotein in ovarian cancer: A molecular marker associated with multidrug resistance. *J Clin Oncol* 3:311–315, 1985
23. Schneider J, Bak M, Efferth TH, et al: P-glycoprotein expression in treated and untreated breast cancer. *Br J Cancer* 60:815–818, 1989
24. Goldstein LJ, Galski H, Fojo A, et al: Expression of a multidrug resistance in human cancers. *J Natl Cancer Inst* 81:116–176, 1989
25. Dan S, Esumi M, Sawada U, et al: Expression of a multidrug-resistance gene in human malignant lymphoma and related disorders. *Leuk Res* 15:1139–1143, 1991
26. Epstein J, Xiao HQ, Oba BK: P-glycoprotein expression in plasma-cell myeloma is associated with resistance to VAD. *Blood* 74:913–917, 1989
27. Beck WT, Grogan TM, Willman CL, et al: Methods to detect P-glycoprotein-associated multidrug resistance in patients' tumors: Finding of consensus recommendations. *Cancer Res* 56: 3010–3020, 1996
28. Ford JM, Hait WN: Pharmacology of drugs that alter multidrug resistance in cancer. *Pharmacol Rev* 42:155–199, 1990
29. Murren JR, DeVita VT: Another look at multidrug resistance. *PPO Updates* 9:1–12, 1995
30. Salmon SE, Dalton WS, Grogan TM, et al: Multidrug-resistant myeloma: Laboratory and clinical effects of verapamil as a chemosensitizer. *Blood* 78:44–50, 1991
31. Dalton WS, Crowley JJ, Salmon, et al: A phase III randomized study of oral verapamil as a chemosensitizer to reverse drug resistance in patients with refractory myeloma: A SWOG study. *Cancer* 75:815–820, 1995
32. Marie JP, Bastie JN, Coloma F, et al: Cyclosporin A as a modifier agent in the salvage treatment of acute leukemia (AL). *Leukemia* 7:821–824, 1993
33. List AF, Spier C, Greer J, et al: Phase I/II trial of cyclosporin as a chemotherapy-resistance modifier in acute leukemia. *J Clin Oncol* 11:1652–1658, 1993
34. Lum BL, Fisher GA, Brophy NA, et al: Clinical trials of modulation of multidrug resistance: Pharmacokinetic and pharmacodynamic considerations. *Cancer* 72:3502–3514, 1993
35. Erlichman C, Moore M, Thiessen JJ, et al: Phase I pharmacokinetic study of cyclosporin A combined with doxorubicin. *Cancer Res* 53:4837–4842, 1993
36. Wilson WH, Bates SE, Fojo A, et al: Controlled trial of dexverapamil, a modulator of multidrug resistance in lymphas refractory to EPOCH chemotherapy. *J Clin Oncol* 13:1995–2004, 1995
37. Sonneveld P, Marie JP, Huesman C, et al: Reversal of multidrug resistance by SDZ PSC 833, with VAD (vincristine, doxorubicin, dexamethasone) in refractory multiple myeloma. A phase I study. *Leukemia* 10: 1741–1750, 1996
38. Fan D, Regenass U, Bettran P, et al: Protein kinase C inhibitor staurosporin derivative CGP 41251 reverses MDR in murine and human cancer cell lines. *Anticancer Drugs* 5:29, 1994–1996, (suppl 1)
39. Bonadonna G, Zambetti M, Valagussa P: Sequential or alternating doxorubicin and CMF regimens in breast cancer with more than three positive nodes: Ten-year results. *JAMA* 273:542–547, 1995
40. Cole SPC, Sparks KE, Fraser K, et al: Pharmacological

characterization of multidrug resistant MRP-transfected human cells. *Cancer Res* 54:5902–5910, 1994

41. Zaman GJ, Lankelma J, van Tellingen O, et al: Role of glutathione in the export of compounds from cells by the multidrug resistance-associated protein. *Proc Natl Acad Sci USA* 92:7690, 1995 (Abstr)

42. Grant CE, Valdimarsson G, Hipfner DR, et al: Overexpression of multidrug resistance-associated protein (MRP) increases to natural product drugs. *Cancer Res* 54:357–361, 1994

43. Burger H, Booter K, Zaman GJR, et al: Expression of the multidrug resistance-associated protein (MRP) in acute and chronic leukemias *Leukemia* 8:990–997, 1994

44. Scheffer GL, Wijngaard PLJ, Flens MJ, et al: The drug resistance related protein LRP is a major vault protein. *Nature Med* 1:578–582, 1995

45. Izquierdo MA, van der Zee AGJ, Vermorken JB, et al: Drug resistance-associated marker LRP for prediciton of response to chemotherapy and prognosis in advanced ovarian carcinoma. *J Natl Can Inst* 87:1230–1237, 1995

46. Glisson BS: Multidrug resistance mediated through alterations in topoisomerase II. *Cancer Bull* 41:37–39, 1989

47. Mannervik B, Danielson UH: Glutathione transferases: Structure and catalytic activity. *Crit Rev Biochem* 23:283–337, 1988

48. Lazo JS, Basu A: Metallothionein expression and transient resistance to electrophilic antineoplastic drugs. *Cancer Biol* 2:267–271, 1991

49. Ozols RF, O'Dwyer PJ, Hamilton TC, et al: The role of glutathione in drug resistance. *Cancer Treat Rev* 17:45–50, 1990 (suppl A)

50. Symonds H, Krall L, Remington L, et al: p53 dependent apoptosis suppresses tumor growth and progression in vivo. *Cell* 73:703–711, 1994

51. Waldman T, Lengauer C, Kinzler K, et al: Uncoupling of S phase and mitosis induced by anticancer agents in cells lacking p21. *Nature* 381:713–716, 1996

52. Thottassery JV, Zambetta GP, Arimori K, et al: p53 dependent regulation of MDR1 gene expression causes selective resistance to chemotherapeutic agents. *Proc Natl Acad Sci USA* 94:11037, 1997 (Abstr)

53. Aas T, Borresen AL, Geisler S, et al: Specific p53 mutations are associated with de novo resistance to doxorubicin in breast cancer patients. *Nature Med* 2:811–814, 1996

54. Righetti SC, Della TG, Pilotti S, et al: A comparative study p53 gene mutations, protein accumulation, and response to cisplatin-based chemotherapy in advanced ovarian carcinoma. *Cancer Res* 56:689–693, 1996

55. Rusch V, Klimstra V, Venkatramen E, et al: Aberrant p53 expression predicts clinical resistance to cisplatin based chemotherapy in locally advanced non-small cell lung cancer. *Cancer Res* 55:5038–5042, 1992

56. Hamada M, Fujiwara T, Hizuta A, et al: The p53 gene is a potent determinant of chemosensitivity and radiosensitivity in gastric and colorectal cancers. *J Cancer Res Clin Oncol* 122:360–365, 1996

57. Dohner H, Fischer K, Bentz M, et al: p53 gene deletion predicts for poor survival and non-response to therapy with purine anologs in chronic B-cell leukemia. *Blood* 85:1580–1589, 1995

58. Simonian PL, Grillot DA, Nunez G: bcl-2 and bcl-XL can differentially block chemotherapy associated cell death. *Blood* 90:1208–1216, 1997

59. Strobel T, Swanson L, Korsmeyer S, et al: BAX enhances paclitaxel-induced apoptosis through a p53 independent pathway. *Proc Natl Acad Sci USA* 93:14094, 1996 (Abstract)

60. Lictra E, Todd MB, Dipaola RS: Vinblastine or paclitaxel enhance mitoxantrone antitumor activity in a sequence dependent manner in association with BCL-2 phosphorylation. *Proc Am Soc Clin Oncol* 17:247, 1998 (Abstr)

61. Frei A III, Clark JR, Miller D: The concept of neoadjuvant chemotherapy, in Salmon SE (ed): *Adjuvant Therapy of Cancer V.* Orlando, FL, Grune & Stratton, 1987, pp 67–72

62. Jacobs C, Pinto H: Adjuvant and neoadjuvant treatment of head and neck cancers: The next chapter. *Semin Oncol* 22:540–552, 1995

63. Friedland DM, Comis RL: Perioperative therapy of non-small cell lung cancer: A review of adjuvant and neoadjuvant approaches. *Semin Oncol* 22:571–581, 1995

64. Hryniuk WM: The importance of dose intensity in the outcome of chemotherapy, in DeVita VT, Hellman S, Rosenberg SA (eds): *Important Advances in Oncology 1988.* Philadelphia, Lippincott, 1988, pp 121–142

65. Hryniuk WM: Average relative dose intensity and the impact on design of clinical trials. *Semin Oncol* 14:65–74, 1987

66. Hryniuk WM, Levine MN: Analysis of dose intensity for adjuvant chemotherapy trials in stage II breast cancer. *J Clin Oncol* 4:1162–1170, 1986

67. Bonadonna G, Valagussa R: Dose-response effect of adjuvant chemotherapy in breast cancer. *N Engl J Med* 304:10–15, 1981

68. Dorr RT, Von Hoff DD (eds): *Cancer Chemotherapy Handbook* (ed 2). Norwalk, CT, Appleton & Lange, 1994

69. Product information: Etyol. Palo Alto, CA, Alza Pharmaceuticals, 1986

70. Seifert CF, Nesser ME, Thompson DF: Dexrazoxane in the prevention of doxorubicin-induced cardiotoxicity. *Ann Pharmacother* 28:1063–1072, 1994

71. Rice A, Reiffers J: Peripheral blood stem cells contain pluripotent stem cells. *Int J Cell Cloning* 10:101, 1992 (suppl 1)

72. Bregni M, Sierna S, Magni M, et al: Circulating hemopoietic progenitors mobilized by cancer chemotherapy and by rhGM-CSF in the treatment of high-grade non-Hodgkin's lymphoma. *Leukemia* 5:123–127, 1991 (suppl 1)

73. Kessinger A: Autologous transplantation with peripheral blood stem cells: A review of clinical results. *J Clin Apheresis* 5:97–102, 1990

74. Brugger W, Bross KJ, Blatt M, et al: Mobilization of tumor cells and hematopoietic progenitor cells into peripheral blood of patients with solid tumors. *Blood* 83:636–640, 1994

75. Vokes EE, Weichselbaum RR: Concomitant chemoradiotherapy: Rational and clinical experience in patients with solid tumors. *J Clin Oncol* 8:911–934, 1990

76. Rotman M, Rosenthal CJ: *Concomitant Continuous Infusion Chemotherapy and Radiation.* New York, Springer-Verlag, 1991

77. Wolf GT, Hong WK, Gross-Fischer S, et al: Induction chemotherapy plus radiation compared with surgery plus radiation in patients with advanced laryngeal cancer: The Department of Veterans Affairs Laryngeal Cancer Study Group. *N Engl J Med* 324:1685–1690, 1991

78. Begg AC, Van der Kolk PJ, Dewit L, et al: Radiosensitization by cisplatin of R1F1 tumor cells in vitro. *Int J Radiat Biol* 50:871–884, 1986

79. Kallman RF, Rapachhietta D, Zaghloul MS: Schedule-dependent therapeutic gain from the combination of fractionated irradiation plus c-DDP and 5-FU or plus C-DDP and cyclophosphamide in C3H/Km mouse model systems. *Int J Radiat Oncol Biol Phys* 20:227–232, 1991

80. Pfeffer MR, Teicher BA, Holden SA, et al: The interaction of cisplatin plus etoposide with radiation ± hyperthermia. *Int J Radiat Oncol Biol Phys* 19:1439–1447, 1990

81. Merlano M, Rosso R, Benasso M, et al: Alternating chemotherapy and radiotherapy vs radiotherapy in advanced inoperable SCC-HN: A cooperative randomized trial. *Proc Am Soc Clin Oncol* 10:198, 1991 (abstr)

82. Santi DV, McHenry CS, Sommer H: Interaction of thymidylate synthetase with 5-fluorouridylate. *Biochemistry* 13:471–480, 1974

83. Piedbois P, Buyse M, Rustum Y, et al: Modulation of fluorouracil by leucovorin in advanced colorectal cancer: Evidence in terms of response rate. *J Clin Oncol* 10:896–903, 1992

84. Gerstner J, O'Connell MJ, Wieand HS, et al: A prospectively randomized clinical trial comparing 5FU combined with either high or low dose leucovorin for the treatment of advanced colorectal cancer. *Proc Am Soc Clin Oncol* 10:134, 1991 (abstr)

85. Reinberg A, Smolensky MH: Circadian changes of drug disposition in man. *Clin Pharmacokinet* 7:401–420, 1982

86. Bjarnason GA, Hrushesky WJM: Circadian cancer chemotherapy: Clinical trials. *J Infus Chemother* 2:79–88, 1992

87. Caussanel JP, Levi F, Brienza S, et al: Phase I trial of 5-day continuous venous infusion of oxaliplatin at circadian rhythm-modulated rate compared with constant rate. *J Natl Cancer Inst* 82:1046–1050, 1990

88. Hrushesky W, von Roemelling R, Lanning R, Rabatini J: Circadian-shaped infusions of floxuridine for progressive metastatic renal cell carcinoma. *J Clin Oncol* 8:1504–1509, 1990

89. Harris BE, Song R, Song S, et al: Circadian variation of 5-fluorouracil catabolism in isolated perfused rat liver. *Cancer Res* 49:6610–6614, 1989

90. Levi FZ, DiPalma M: Improved therapeutic index through ambulatory circadian rhythmic delivery of high dose 3 drug chemotherapy in a randomized phase III multicenter trial. *Proc Am Soc Clin Oncol* 13:197, 1994 (Abstr)

91. Folkman J: What is the evidence that tumors are angiogenesis-dependent? *J Natl Cancer Inst* 82:4–6, 1990

92. Weidner N, Folkman J: Tumor vascularity as a prognostic factor in cancer. *Prin Pract Oncol Update* 11:1–5, 1997

93. Folkman J: Tumor angiogensis and tissue factor. *Nature Med* 2:167–168, 1996

94. Pepper MS, Ferrara N, Orci L, et al: Potent synergism between vascular endothelial growth factor and basic fibroblast growth factor in the induction of angiogenesis in vitro. *Biochem Biophys Res Commun* 189:824–831, 1992

95. Folkman J: Tumor angiogensis: Therapeutic implications. *N Eng J Med* 285:1182–1186, 1971

96. Masiero L, Figg WD, Kohn EC: Review of the clinical experience with CAI, thalidomide, TNP-470 and interleukin-12. *Angiogensis* 1:23–28, 1997

97. Boehm T, Folkman J, Browder T, et al: Antiangiogenic therapy of experimental cancer does not induce acquired drug resistance. *Nature* 390: 404–407, 1997

98. White CW, Sondheimer HM, Crouch EC, et al: Treatment of pulmonary hemangiomatosis with recombinant interferon alfa-2a. *N Eng J Med* 320:1197–1200, 1989

99. Chamber AF, Matrisian LM: Changing views of the role of matrix metalloproteinases in metastasis. *J Natl Cancer Inst* 89:1260–1264, 1997

100. Guedez L, Lim MS, Stetler-Stevenson WG: The role of metalloproteinases and their inhibitors in hematological disorders. *Crit Rev Oncog* 7: 205–225, 1996

101. Brown PD: Matrix metalloproteinase inhibitors in the treatment of cancer. *Med Oncol* 14:1–10, 1997

102. Poon RYC, Jiang W, Toyoshima H, et al: Cyclin-dependent kinases are inactivated by a combination of p21 and Thr-14/Tyr-15 phosphorylation after UV-induced DNA damage. *J Biol Chem* 271:13283–13291, 1996

103. Baur LA: Individualization of drug therapy: Clinical pharmacokinetics and pharmacodynamics, in DiPiro JT, Talbert RL, Hayes PE, et al (eds): *Pharmacotherapy* (ed 2). Norwalk, CT, Appleton & Lange, 1993, pp 15–31

104. Ratain MJ: Pharmacology of cancer chemotherapy, in DeVita VT, Hellman S, Rosenberg SA (eds): *Cancer: Principles and Practice of Oncology* (ed 5). Philadelphia, Lippincott-Raven, 1997, pp 375–385

105. Lippard SJ: New chemistry of an old molecule: cis(Pt NH$_3$)$_2$ Cl$_2$). *Science* 218:1075–1082, 1982

106. Moore MJ: Clinical pharmacokinetics of cyclophosphamide. *Clin Pharmacokinet* 20:194–208, 1991

107. Hansten PD, Horn JR (eds): *Drug Interactions and Updates.* Vancouver, WA, Applied Therapeutics, 1995

108. Balis FM: Pharmacokinetic drug interactions of commonly used anticancer drugs. *Clin Pharmacokinet* 11:223–235, 1986

109. Finley RS: Drug interactions in the oncology patient. *Semin Oncol Nurs* 8:95–101, 1992

110. Loadman PM, Bibby MC: Pharmacokinetic drug interactions with anticancer drugs. *Clin Pharmacokinet* 26:486–500, 1994

111. Ignoffo RJ: Drug interactions with antineoplastic agents. *Highlights on Antineoplastic Drugs* 7:2–7, 1989

112. Evans WE, Christensen ML: *Drug Interactions with Methotrexate.* Wayne, NJ, Lederle Laboratories, 1985

113. Thyss A, Milano G, Kubar J, et al: Clinical and pharmacokinetic evidence of a life-threatening interaction between methotrexate and ketoprofen. *Lancet* 1:256–258, 1986

114. Ellison NM, Servi RJ: Acute renal failure and death following sequential intermediate-dose methotrexate and 5-FU: A possible adverse effect due to concomitant indomethacin administration. *Cancer Treat Reports* 69:342–343, 1985

115. Fitzsimmons WE, Ghalie R, Kaizer H: The effect of hepatic enzyme inducers on busulfan neurotoxicity and myelotoxicity. *Cancer Chemother Pharmacol* 27:27–32, 1990

116. Hall G, Lind MJ, Huang M, et al: Intravenous infusions of ifosfamide/mesna and perturbation of warfarin anticoagulant control. *Postgrad Med J* 66:860–861, 1990

117. Tenni P, Lalich DL, Byrne MJ : Life-threatening interaction between tamoxifen and warfarin. *Br Med J* 298:93, 1989

118. Bubley GJ, Ogata GK, Dupuis NP, et al: Detection of sequence-specific antitumor alkylating agent DNA damage from cells treated in culture and from a patient. *Cancer Res* 54:6325–6329, 1994

119. Hanawalt PC, Cooper PK, Ganesan AK, et al: DNA repair in bacteria and mammalian cells. *Annu Rev Biochem* 48: 783–836, 1979

120. Bohr VA, Phillips DH, Hanawalt PC: Heterogeneous DNA damage and repair in the mammalian genome. *Cancer Res* 47:6426–6436, 1987

121. Begleiter A, Lam H-YP, Grover J, et al: Evidence for active transport of melphalan by two amino acid carriers in L5178Y lymphoblasts in vitro. *Cancer Res* 39:353–359, 1979

122. Hilton J: Role of aldehyde dehydrogenase in cyclophosphamide-resistant L 1210 leukemia. *Cancer Res* 44:5156–5160, 1984

123. Colvin M: The comparative pharmacology of cyclophosphamide and ifosfamide. *Semin Oncol* 9:2–7, 1982 (suppl 1)

124. Montgomery JA: Chemistry and structure: Activity studies of the nitrosoureas. *Cancer Treat Reports* 60:651–664, 1976

125. Pascoe JM, Roberts JJ: Interaction between mammalian

cell DNA and inorganic platinum compounds: I. DNA interstrand cross-linking and cytotoxic properties of platinum (II) compounds. *Biochem Pharmacol* 23:1345–1357, 1974

126. Fichtinger-Schepman AMJ, van der Veer JL, den Hartog JHJ, et al: Adducts of the antitumor drug cis-diamminedichloroplatinum (II) with DNA: Formation, identification and quantitation. *Biochemistry* 24:707, 1985

127. Bloommaert FA, van Kijk-Knijenburg HCM, Dijt FJ, et al: Formation of DNA adducts by the anticancer drug carboplatin: Different nucleotide sequence preferences in vitro and in cells. *Biochemistry* 34: 8474, 1995

128. Howell SB, Pfeifle CE, Wung WE, et al: Intraperitoneal cis-diamminedechloroplatin with synthetic thiosulfate protection. *Cancer Res* 43:1426–1431, 1983

129. Oguri S, Sakakibara T, Mase H, et al: Clinical pharmacokinetics of carboplatin. *J Clin Pharmacol* 28:208–215, 1988

130. Calvert AH, Newell DR, Gumbrell LA, et al: Carboplatin dosage prospect of evaluation of a simple formula based on renal function. *J Clin Oncol* 7:1748–1756, 1989

131. Montgomery JA: Experimental studies at Southern Research Institute with DTIC (NSC-45388). *Cancer Treat Reports* 60:125–134, 1976

132. Hayward IP, Parson PG: Epigenetic effects of the methylating agent 5-(3-methyl-1-triazeno) imidazole-4-carboxamide in human melanoma cells. *Aust J Exp Biol Med Sci* 62: 597–606, 1984

133. Sutherland CM, Krementz ET: Hepatic toxicity of DTIC. *Cancer Treat Reports* 65:321–322, 1981

134. Plowman J, Waud WR, Koutsoukous AD, Rubinstein LV, et al: Preclinical antitumor activity of temozolomide in mice: Efficacy against human brain tumor zenografts and synergism with 1,3-bis(2-chloroethyl)-1-nitrosourea *Cancer Res* 54:3793–3795, 1994

135. O'Reilly SM, Newlands ES, Glaser MG, et al: Temozolomide: A new oral cytotoxic chemotherapeutic agent with promising activitiy against primary brain tumors. *Eur J Cancer* 29A: 940–942, 1993

136. Brock CS, Newlands ES, Wedge SR, et al: Phase I trial of temozolomide using an extended continuous oral schedule. *Cancer Res* 58:4367–4367, 1998

137. Holt GA (ed): *Food and Drug Interactions: A Health Care Professional's Guide.* Chicago, Precept Press, 1992

138. Zhang H, D'Arpe P, Liu LF: A model for tumor cell killing by topoisomerase poisons. *Cancer Cells* 2:23–27, 1990

139. Zwelling LA: Topoisomerase II as a target of antileukemia drugs: A review of controversial areas. *Hematol Pathol* 3: 101–112, 1989

140. Myers CE: Anthracyclines, in Chabner B (ed): *Pharmacologic Principles of Cancer Treatment.* Philadelphia, Saunders, 1982, pp 416–434.

141. Allen A: The cardiotoxicity of chemotherapeutic drugs. *Semin Oncol* 19:529–542, 1992

142. Fisher GR, Patterson LH: Lack of involvement of reactive oxygen in the cytotoxicity of mitoxantrone, CI941 and ametantrone in MCF-7 cells: Comparison with doxorubicin. *Cancer Chemother Pharmacol* 30:451–458, 1992

143. Forssen EA, Coulter DM, Proffitt RT: Selective in vivo localization of daunorubicin small unilamellar vesicles in solid tumors. *Cancer Res* 56:2066–2075, 1996

144. Product information: Doxil. Menlo Park, CA, Sequus Pharmaceuticals, 1995

145. Kozarich JW, Worth L, Frank BL, et al: Sequence-specific isotope effects on the cleavage of DNA by bleomycin. *Science* 245:1396–1399, 1989

146. Ross WE, Bradley MO: DNA double-strand breaks in mammalian cells after exposure to intercalating agents. *Biochim Biophys Acta* 654:129–134, 1981

147. Anton DL, Friedman PA: Actinomycin. *Cancer Growth Prog* 10:131–132, 1989

148. Allegra CJ, Grem JL: Antimetabolites, in DeVita VT, Hellman S, Rosenberg SA (eds): *Cancer: Principles and Practice of Oncology* (ed 5). Philadelphia, Lippincott, 1997, pp 432–452

149. Pinedo HM, Zaharko DS, Bull JM, et al: The reversal of methotrexate cytotoxicity to mouse bone marrow cells by leucovorin and nucleosides. *Cancer Res* 36:4418–4424, 1976

150. Evans WE, Crom WR, Yalowich J: Methotrexate, in Evans WE, Schentag JJ, Juskow J (eds): *Applied Pharmacokinetics: Principles of Therapeutic Drug Monitoring* (ed 2). Spokane, WA, Applied Therapeutics, 1986, pp 1009–1056

151. Stoller RG, Hande KR, Jacobs SA, et al: Use of plasma pharmacokinetics to predict and prevent methotrexate toxicity. *N Engl J Med* 297:630–634, 1977

152. Heidelberger C, Chandhari NK, Dannenberg P, et al: Fluorinated pyrimidines: A new class of tumor inhibitory compounds. *Nature* 179:663–666, 1957

153. Mandel HG: Incorporation of 5-fluorouracil into RNA and its molecular consequences. *Prog Mol Subcell Biol* 1:82–135, 1969

154. Diasio RB, Schuetz JD, Wallace HJ, et al: Dihydrofluorouracil, a fluorouracil catabolite with antitumor activity in murine and human cells. *Cancer Res* 45:4900–4903, 1985

155. Burger AJ, Mannino S: 5-fluorouracil-induced coronary vasospasm. *Am Heart J* 114:433–436, 1987

156. Budman DR, Meropol NJ, Reigner B, et al: Preliminary studies of a novel oral fluoropyrimidine carbamate: Capecitabine. *J Clin Oncol* 16:1795–1802, 1998

157. Fuji S, Ikenaka K, Fukushima M, et al: Effect of uracil and its derivatives on antitumor activity of 5-fluorouracil and 1-(2-tetrahydrofuryl)-5-fluorouracil. *Jpn J Cancer Res* 69: 763–768, 1979

158. Baccanari DP, Davis ST, Knick V, et al: 5-ethynyluraci (766C85): A potent modulator of the pharmacokinetics and antitumor efficacy of 5-fluorouracil. *Proc Natl Acad Sci USA* 90:11064, 1993 (abstr)

159. Fram RJ, Egan EM, Kufe DW: Accumulation of leukemic cell DNA strand breaks with Adrimycin and cytosine arabinoside. *Leuk Res* 7:243–249, 1983

160. Baker WJ, Royer GL, Weiss RB: Cytarabine and neurologic toxicity. *J Clin Oncol* 9:679–693, 1991

161. Baker CH, Banzon J, Bollinger JM, et al: 2'-deoxy-2'methylenecytidine and 2'-dexoy-2', 2'-difluorocytidine 5'-diphosphate: Potent mechansim-based inhibitors of ribonucleotide reductase. *J Med Chem* 34:1879–1884, 1991

162. Hue YF, Reitz J: Gemcitabine: A cytidine analogue active against solid tumors. *Am J Health-Syst Pharm* 54:162–170, 1997

163. Tseng W-C, Derse D, Cheng Y-C, et al: In vitro biological activity of 9-beta-D-arabinofuranosyl-2-fluoroadenine and the biochemical actions of its triphosphate on DNA polymerase and ribonucleotide reductase from HeLa cells. *Mol Pharmacol* 21:474–477, 1982

164. Seto S, Carrera CJ, Kubota M, et al: Mechanism of deoxyadenosine and 2-chlorodoxyadenosine toxicity to nondividing human lymphocytes. *J Clin Invest* 75:377–383, 1985

165. Madoc-Jones H, Mauro F: Interphase action of vinblastine and vincristine: Differences in their lethal action through the mitotic cycle of cultured mammalian cells. *J Cell Physiol* 72:185–196, 1968

166. Nelson RL: The comparative clinical pharmacology and pharmacokinetics of vindisine, vincristine, and vinblastine in human patients with cancer. *Med Pediatr Oncol* 10: 115–127, 1982

167. Wani MC, Taylor HL, Wall ME, et al: Plant antitumor agents: IV. The isolation and structure of taxol, a novel antileukemic and antitumor agent from *Taxus brevifolia*. *J Am Chem Soc* 93:2325–2327, 1971

168. Schiff PB, Fant J, Horowitz SB: Promotion of microtubule assembly in vitro by taxol. *Nature* 22:665–667, 1979

169. Rowinsky EK, Donehower RC, Jones RJ, et al: Microtubule changes and cytotoxicity in leukemic cell lines treated with taxol. *Cancer Res* 48:4093–4100, 1988

170. Bissery MC, Guenard D, Gueritte-Voegelein F, et al: Experimental antitumor activity of taxotere (RP 56976, NSC 628503), a taxol analogue. *Cancer Res* 51:4845–4852, 1991

171. Rowisnky EK, Burke PJ, Karp JE, et al: Phase I clinical and pharmacokinetic study of taxol. *Cancer Res* 49:4640–4647, 1989

172. Extra JM, Rousseau F, Bruno R, et al: Phase I and pharmacokinetic study of taxotere (NSC 628503) given as a short intravenous infusion. *Cancer Res* 53:1037–1042, 1993

173. Citardi M, Rowinsky EK, Schaefer KL, et al: Sequence-dependent cytotoxicity between cisplatin and the antimicrotubule agents taxol and vincristine. *Proc Am Assoc Cancer Res* 31:2431, 1990 (Abstract)

174. Weiss RB, Donehower RC, Wiernik PH, et al: Hypersensitivity reactions from taxol. *J Clin Oncol* 8:1263–1268, 1990

175. Chevallier B, Fumoleau P, Kerbrat P, et al: Docetaxel is a major cytotoxic drug for the treatment of advanced breast cancer. *J Clin Oncol* 13:314–322, 1995

176. Loike D, Horwitz SB: Effects of podophyllotoxin and VP-6 on microtubule assembly in vitro and nucleotide transport in HeLa cells. *Biochemistry* 15:5435–5442, 1976

177. Yang L, Rowe RC, Liu LF: Identification of DNA topoisomerase II as an intracellular target of antitumor epipodophyllotoxins in Simian virus 40-infected monkey cells. *Cancer Res* 45:5872–5876, 1985

178. Creaven PJ: The clinical pharmacology of VM-26 and VP-16-213: A brief overview. *Cancer Chemother Pharmacol* 7: 133–140, 1982

179. Slevin ML, Clark PL, Joel SP, et al: A randomized trial to evaluate the effects of schedule on the activity of etoposide in small-cell lung cancer. *J Clin Oncol* 7:1333–1340, 1989

180. Jones SF, Burris HA: Topoisomerase I Inhibitors: Topotecan and irinotecan. *Cancer Pract* 4:51–53, 1996

181. Rothenberg ML, Kuhn JG, Burris HA, et al: Phase I and pharmacokinetic trial of weekly CPT-11. *J Clin Oncol* 11: 2194–2204, 1993

182. Stearns ME, Tew KD: Antimicrotubule effects of estramustine, an antiprostatic tumor drug. *Cancer Res* 45:3891–3897, 1985

183. Jaiyesimi IA, Buzdar AU, Decker DA, et al: Use of tamoxifen for breast cancer: Twenty-eight years later. *J Clin Oncol* 13: 513–529, 1995

184. Love RR, Cameron L, Connell B: Symptoms associated with tamoxifen treatment in postmenopausal women. *Arch Intern Med* 151:1842–1847, 1991

185. Fisher B, Costantino JP, Wickerham DL, et al: Tamoxifen for prevention of breast cancer: Report of the National Surgical Adjuvant Breast and Bowel Project P-1 study. *J Natl Cancer Inst* 90:1371–1388, 1998

186. Hayes DF, Vanzyl JA, Hacking A, et al: Randomized comparison of tamoxifen and two separate doses of toremifene in postmenopausal patients with metastatic breast cancer. *J Clin Oncol* 13:2556–2566, 1995

187. Styles JA, Davies A, Lim CK, et al: Genotoxicity of tamoxifen, tamoxifen epoxide and toremifene in human lymphoblastoid cells containing human cytochrome P450. *Carcinogenesis* 15:5–9, 1994

188. Loprinzi CL, Ellison NM, Schaid DJ, et al: Controlled trial of megestrol acetate for treatment of cancer anorexia and cachexia. *J Natl Cancer Inst* 82:1127–1132, 1990

189. Plosker GL, Brogden RN: Leuproelin: A review of its pharmacology and therapeutic use in prostate cancer, endometriosis and other sex-hormone-related disorders. *Drugs* 48: 930–952, 1994

190. Clayton RN, Bailey LC, Cottam J, et al: A radioimmunoassay for GnRH agonist analogue in serum of patients with prostate cancer treated with goserelin. *Endocrinology* 22: 453–462, 1985

191. Brogden RN, Chrisp P: Flutamide: A review of its pharmacodynamic, pharmacokinetic properties and therapeutic use in advanced prostatic cancer. *Drugs Aging* 1:104–118, 1991

192. Sporn MB, Roberts AB: Interactions of retinoids and transforming growth factor-beta in regulation of cell differentiation and proliferation. *Mol Endocrinol* 5:3–7, 1991

193. Lippman S, Parkinson D, Itri L, et al: 13-*cis*-Retinoic acid and interferon alpha-2a: Effective combination therapy for advanced squamous cell carcinoma of the skin. *J Natl Cancer Inst* 84:235–241, 1992

194. Hong WK, Endicott J, Itri LM, et al: 13-cis-retinoic acid in the treatment of oral leukoplakia. *N Eng J Med* 315: 1501–1505, 1986

195. Clark R, Ismail S, Jacobs A, et al: A randomized trial of 13-*cis*-Retinoic acid with or without cytosine arabinoside in patients with myelodysplastic syndrome. *Br J Haematol* 66: 77–83, 1987

196. Fontana J, Rogers J, Durham J: The role of 13-*cis*-Retinoic acid in the remission induction of a patient with acute promyelocytic leukemia. *Cancer* 57:209–217, 1986

197. Kramer Z, Boros L, Wiernik P, et al: 13-*cis*-Retinoic acid in the treatment of elderly patients with acute myeloid leukemia. *Cancer* 67:1484–1486, 1991

198. Kamm J, Ashenfelter K, Ehmann C: Preclinical and clinical toxicology of selected retinoids, in Sporn M, Roberts A, Goodman D (eds): *The Retinoids*. Orlando, FL, Academic Press, 1984, pp 287–326

199. Warrell RR: All-trans-Retinoic acid, in *American Society of Clinical Oncology Educational Book, 28th Annual Meeting, San Diego, California, May 17-19, 1992*, pp 107–112

200. List AF, Brasfield F, Heaton R, et al: Stimulation of hematopoiesis by amifostine in patients with myelodysplastic syndrome. *Blood* 90:3364–3369, 1997

CHAPTER 19

Chemotherapy: Principles of Administration

Michelle Goodman, RN, MS

Chemotherapy Administration

Chemotherapy is administered in a variety of care settings. The majority of cancer patients receive systemic chemotherapy in an ambulatory care setting that may be adjacent to a university hospital, or in a 23-hour unit designed to care for patients requiring lengthy infusions. Others may receive their chemotherapy in a freestanding clinic or in their homes. Few individuals actually require hospitalization for chemotherapy despite the fact that treatment regimens are currently more aggressive and dose-intensive in nature. Hospital admission is generally reserved for patients who require intensive monitoring or are acutely ill. Even bone marrow transplant and peripheral blood stem cell transplant programs are moving to the outpatient setting.[1]

The shift to outpatient ambulatory care services has grown out of the need for more efficient and economical health care delivery systems as hospitals cope with increases in managed care and capitation. Managed care is rapidly replacing fee-for-service in all aspects of the health care delivery system.[2] Oncology nurses are challenged with the increased responsibility of coordinating quality patient care with limited resources and support. Through team building and working with other disciplines, the nurse effectively assesses and develops a plan of care that ensures continuity regardless of the care setting. The real challenge lies in finding ways to promote self-care in an aging population with limited personal and social resources. This chapter deals with both basic and advanced principles of chemotherapy administration. It focuses on clinical practice, methods of drug delivery, and vascular access devices (VADs).

Professional Qualifications

Educational guidelines for nurses administering chemotherapy are almost universally implemented in a variety of practice settings.[3,4] Both the Intravenous Nurses' Society and the Oncology Nursing Society have published position statements regarding the administration of antineoplastic agents and the educational preparation of the nurse.[5,6]

Basic qualifications for nurses administering antineoplastic agents include:

- Current licensure as a registered nurse

- Certification in CPR

- Intravenous therapy skills

- Educational preparation and demonstrated knowledge in all areas related to antineoplastic drugs, including pharmacology, drug preparation, drug disposition, metabolism, elimination, and various drug interactions

- Demonstrated knowledge of prevention of medication errors and the skill of drug administration

- Ongoing acquisition of updated information and verification of continuing knowledge and skills

- Policies and procedures that govern specific actions (Table 19-1)

Formal instruction in chemotherapy administration techniques and certification programs are essential to ensure quality patient care as well as to achieve and maintain high safety standards.[7,8] Chemotherapy certification also provides proof of formalized training and skill demonstration, which is extremely important from a professional liability perspective. Antineoplastic agents have serious, even life-threatening side effects, and it is in the best interests of the patient, nurse, and institution that educational preparation be obtained and documented. Additionally, clinically oriented policies and procedures that are part of ongoing quality improvement help to provide a firm practical and legal foundation for this aspect of oncology nursing practice.

Handling Cytotoxic Drugs

Exposure to cytotoxic drugs is known to be potentially hazardous to one's health.[9–11] Direct exposure to cytotoxic agents can occur during admixture, administration, or handling, and involves inhalation, ingestion, or absorption.[12,13] The drugs are known to be mutagenic, teratogenic, and carcinogenic. Additionally, exposure has been reported to result in rashes, skin discolorations, scarring, blurred vision, and dizziness. Guidelines containing recommendations to prevent cytotoxic drug exposure of personnel and the environment have been established by the Occupational Safety and Health Administration (OSHA), Oncology Nursing Society, and American Society of Hospital Pharmacists. Detailed drug handling guidelines are outlined in Table 19-2.

Table 19-1 Institutional Policies and Procedures for Chemotherapy Administration

- Staff education for chemotherapy and other specialty procedures (i.e., vascular access devices [VADs], Ommaya reservoirs)
- Chemotherapy administration (all routes)
- Mechanisms for prevention and reporting of drug and dosing errors
- Vesicant management
- Allergic reactions
- Safe drug handling and disposal
- Patient and family education
- Management of VADs
- Documentation methods (extravasation record)
- Coordination of home care
- Outcome standards
- Oncology quality-improvement process

Table 19-2   Cytotoxic Drug Handling Guidelines

Preparation

- Verify current drug order with patient profile.
- Verify drug dose.
- Don a disposable gown that is lint-free, low- or nonpermeable, long-sleeved, cuffed, and solid-fronted.
- Don a pair of powder-free, thick, surgical-quality latex gloves, ensuring that the cuffs of the gloves overlap the cuffs of the gown.
- Admix all cytotoxic drugs in a class II biological safety cabinet (vertical air flow) that meets national standards and is inspected appropriately.
- Use a disposable, plastic-backed liner for the preparation area and appropriate equipment such as Luer-Lok syringes.
- Clean the cabinet daily with 70% alcohol, and decontaminate it weekly or if spills occur.
- Use aseptic technique.
- Take care to avoid drug dispersement by venting vials, handling ampules carefully, avoiding overfilling of containers, and adding diluents slowly.
- Attach and prime IV tubing before adding the cytotoxic drug to the IV solution.
- Wipe all syringes and containers, and label them appropriately, including a warning label indicating that the contents are cytotoxic.
- When dispensing vincristine, affix a label that indicates that the drug is lethal if injected intrathecally.
- Do not clip or recap needles; discard all sharps in an appropriately labeled, puncture-proof container.
- Discard protective clothing and used materials in a separate trash bag labeled "cytotoxic."
- Wash hands.
- Verify with pharmacist that the drug order is identical to the drug prepared and that the dose is customary and reasonable.

Administration

- Receive appropriately labeled cytotoxic drugs in clean, dry syringes or bags of IV fluids inside zipper-seal plastic bags. Inspect bags before opening to ensure no spillage in the bag.
- Wash hands. If dripping or splashing can occur, don a disposable gown that is lint-free, low- or nonpermeable, long-sleeved, cuffed, and solid-fronted.
- Don a pair of powder-free, thick, surgical-quality latex gloves, ensuring that the cuffs of the gloves overlap the cuffs of the gown, if a gown is being worn.
- Place a plastic-backed absorbent pad over the work area to absorb any drips.
- Use intravenous administration sets and syringes with Luer-Lok fittings.
- If the administration set is not attached to the intravenous fluids and primed by the pharmacist, it should be attached and primed

with caution to prevent exposure of the drug to the environment. It may be primed into a gauze pad inside a zipper-seal bag, or it may be piggybacked to plain fluids and primed by retrograde flow ("back-primed").

- Secure all connections and Y-sites with tape.
- Keep a gauze pad at hand to wipe droplets off Y-sites or connecting points.
- Do not expel air from syringes. If air is in a syringe, hold it in such a way that the air is up near the plunger and simply stop pushing on the plunger when all of the drug is injected.
- Do not use intravenous bottles with venting tubes.
- Monitor administration sets and connection sites for leakage.
- Do not clip or recap needles. Discard the needle-syringe unit into a convenient and appropriately labeled, puncture-proof container.
- Discard all gauze, tubing, bags, bottles, etc., in appropriately labeled bags, and seal. Remove gown and gloves and discard in a similar manner.
- Wash hands.

General Handling and Disposal

- Dispose of all sharps, containers, and cytotoxic waste according to appropriate state and federal guidelines (usually, incineration or burial in a hazardous waste landfill).
- Contain all grossly contaminated linen of treated patients within 48 hours in labeled double bags, and wash twice (same procedure as for infectious wastes).
- Obtain spill kits, and place them in the admixture and administration areas.
- Clean up spills using available kits and disposable towels or sponges. For large spills, double gloving is recommended.
- If direct exposure occurs, immediately rinse the area with running water. For eye exposure, rinse with an eye wash solution or sterile saline.
- Report all episodes of exposure to employee health or the equivalent resource.

Personnel

- Identify all personnel who handle cytotoxic drugs.
- Educate and train personnel in proper drug handling.
- Establish a mechanism to monitor cytotoxic drug handling practices, from receipt through disposal.
- Provide ready access to information regarding cytotoxic drugs.
- Address pregnancy and medical surveillance issues.
- Monitor all spills and occurrences of direct exposure through a quality-improvement program.
- Develop patient education materials as needed, particularly for use in the home.

Data from Oncology Nursing Society.[3] American Society of Hospital Pharmacists,[9] American Society of Hospital Pharmacists.[10] Occupational Safety and Health Administration.[13]

Personnel policies regarding pregnancy are quite varied, despite OSHA's suggestion that appropriate protective practices should reduce any potential reproductive hazards.[13] While OSHA recommends that employees be informed of potential risks and, if necessary, reassigned to other duties, it is not uncommon to find institutional policies that prohibit pregnant or lactating women from working with cytotoxic drugs, particularly in drug preparation. These precautionary measures are undertaken to protect the mother and developing fetus from the potential effects of drug exposure and the institution from potential liability. Another personnel issue is medical surveillance, which usually includes a preemployment health assessment, a baseline CBC, and thorough documentation of any risk factors in the health history.[14] More extensive testing is becoming less common, for there are no data to support a cause-and-effect relationship between precautionary cytotoxic drug handling and abnormal physical or laboratory findings.

Patient education regarding cytotoxic drug handling is important so that patients and family members understand why gloves and gowns are being worn and do not feel alienated by the practice. Education is a crucial element if chemotherapy is being provided in the home setting, as family members need to be instructed in drug containment practices. The health care professional should provide the patient with written instructions specifying that gloves be worn when working with the medications, used materials be placed in the provided containers, care be taken to avoid direct exposure, spills be cleaned up with the spill kit provided, and direct external exposure be managed with copious flushing and washing.[15] Despite proof that exposure to cytotoxic drugs can be harmful, a large percentage of health professionals continue to disregard personal protective measures.[16,17] There appears to be a perception that low-level exposure is not harmful, as no absolute scientific quantification of exposure has been defined. However, it is important to realize that stiff financial penalties against the institution can be incurred if OSHA ascertains noncompliance with established guidelines. The minimum standards to be met include (1) knowledge of the latest scientific information, (2) established policies and procedures, and (3) ongoing monitoring to ensure compliance and continuous quality improvement.

Patient and Family Education

Educating patients and their family members about cancer is usually initiated by the physician, who explains the diagnosis of cancer, treatment options, their risks and benefits, alternatives, and prognosis. Nurses are responsible for giving the patient and family specific information about treatment side effects and measures to recognize and minimize their consequences. Teaching self-care measures is critically important given the often limited resources and support services available. Self-care guides such as those detailed by Yarbro et al are ideal because

they can be photocopied, individualized, and given to the patient to reinforce teaching.[18] Identifying problems or side effects a patient might experience due to the chemotherapy as a whole rather than addressing each drug separately is most efficient, due to the wide range of side effects encountered. Some basic steps to follow when planning and implementing patient education are included in Table 19-3.

The patient and nurse should both be relaxed, with time to discuss the treatment and its side effects. Asking the patient if there are any questions helps to address concerns immediately and establishes an open exchange of information. Anxiety during the presentation is unavoidable, but the nurse should observe the patient's facial expressions and body language to help measure the information's impact on the patient; it is sometimes necessary to allow time for the facts to be assimilated. More complex instruction is required when a patient is entering a research protocol, as this involves a written informed consent, usually several pages in length, that is read to the patient or reviewed in great detail.

Follow-up includes assessment of the patient's understanding of the information imparted and determination that the desired outcome has been achieved. Observation of the patient and questioning regarding actions and activities are usually sufficient to ensure comprehension. Documentation in the patient record includes a detailed note or a checklist-type form[19–23] (see Chapter 20).

Professional Issues

The delivery of chemotherapy, as well as the education of the patient and family, is primarily the responsibility of the registered professional nurse. The nurse must be properly educated in the pharmacology of the drugs, including distribution and elimination patterns, the proper techniques of drug preparation and administration, and especially drug interactions. Appendix A and Appendix B describe the dosing, metabolism, preparation, administration precautions, and special considerations regarding the administration of the more common oral and intravenous antineoplastic agents.

Because the administration of chemotherapy is primarily the nurse's responsibility, the nurse must be skilled in venipuncture, accessing, and management of numerous types of VADs and drug administration systems. The nurse is also responsible for the prevention, early detection, and management of acute reactions associated with chemotherapy, including hypersensitivity, anaphylaxis, hypotension, extravasation, and nausea and vomiting. Through instructions, both oral and written, the nurse prepares the patient to manage the anticipated side effects of chemotherapy and to report symptoms early to the health care team so that more serious toxic reactions can be avoided.

One of the primary responsibilities of the nurse in the delivery of chemotherapy is to ensure that the correct dose of the appropriate drug is given to the appropriate

Table 19-3 Chemotherapy Patient Education Guidelines

Preparation

- Accompany the physician when the treatment plan is explained to the patient and family to better reinforce what they have been told.

- Identify learning needs and specific written instructions for prevention and management of side effects.

- Emphasize the importance of self-care strategies and provide the patient and family with self-care guidelines that are clearly written at an eighth-grade level of understanding.

- Determine whether audiovisuals are appropriate teaching aids. Test equipment and establish a time for patient/family to view.

- Review policies, procedures, and documentation forms.

Planning

- Know the basics about the patient to be taught and the goal of the treatment plan. Review the chart. It is especially important to know if the patient speaks and reads English, if that is the language being used.

- If possible, separate the teaching session from the actual drug administration procedure.

- Encourage the patient to have a family member present during instruction sessions.

- Assemble all teaching materials including calendar, prescriptions, drug information sheets, and other teaching materials before you begin, to avoid interruptions.

Presentation

- Introduce self and purpose.

- Determine if the patient has any specific questions or concerns to address before proceeding.

- Discuss the treatment process (i.e., starting intravenous infusion, administering drugs, length of time, immediate events, expected follow-up, monitoring side effects, and home care). Describe any sensations the patient might have during the infusion/injection (e.g., coolness, perirectal burning, light-headedness, nasal stuffiness).

- Describe the potential side effects and interventions in order to minimize their consequences. Include specific information about what to look for, what's normal, how to take a temperature, where to buy a wig, which mouth care regimen to use, and other appropriate recommendations. Provide written information regarding when to call the physician or nurse.

- Avoid overloading the patient with information about rare or unusual risks of chemotherapy. Give written information regarding this aspect of his or her treatment and elaborate where appropriate.

- Ensure that informed consent (written or verbal) has been obtained.

- Maintain a responsive atmosphere that is open to questioning.

- Give written instructions regarding activity, diet, hygiene, medications, and other self-care behaviors for the patient to follow for the next few days or weeks.

Follow-Up

- Document the encounter and the patient's response. (See Patient Teaching and Documentation Tool, Chapter 20.)

- Question the patient to assess his or her understanding of the information imparted.

- When possible, observe the patient to determine if his or her actions indicate an understanding of the information (e.g., hydration, mouth care, medications).

- It is optimal to contact the patient within 24 hours of drug administration to determine if there are any questions or problems to be resolved, especially if the patient and nurse are no longer together in the same setting (i.e., hospital or home).

---

individual. Despite the fact that safeguards are in place, serious errors in drug dosing do occur.[24,25] Such tragic events are regrettable but not so remarkable when one considers the number of chemotherapy doses given and the number of patients treated. Significant drug errors occur at a rate of less than 1%.[26]

As practitioners, it is important to consider the potential origins and the settings in which drug errors are likely to occur. Combinations of complicated regimens of potentially lethal drugs are currently being given in high doses in a variety of settings, not just the research institutions where procedures intended to guard against drug errors are usually in place. Consequently, even though the caregiver may recognize a cumulative dose as higher than the usual dose they may still fail to question the order. In addition, institutions are being pressured to dramatically scale back. As resources diminish and individuals are required to do more with less, the risk of error increases. Nurses are being required to be more efficient and to deliver the same quality of care with fewer support services. In some settings, in an effort to reduce expenditures, highly trained and experienced nurse practitioners are being replaced by individuals who are less experienced, less knowledgeable, and therefore less qualified, which increases the possibility of error.

In an effort to reduce the risk for drug error, the following safeguards should be instituted wherever chemotherapy is admixed and administered.

1. Only the most senior physician directly responsible for the care of the patient and most familiar with the drug regimen and dosing schedule should sign the chemotherapy orders.

2. The drug name should be written clearly and in full. Abbreviations are to be avoided, especially where drugs with similar sounding names are concerned (e.g., cisplatin and carboplatin, taxol and taxotere, mitomycin and mitoxantrone, vinblastine and vinorelbine, 5-FUdR and 5-FU).

3. When the drug order is written (usually in triplicate), the drug name, dose in mg/m^2, dose to be given, the total daily dose, and number of days that dose is given is indicated on the order sheet.

4. Cumulative dose for the course of treatment is not written on the order sheet in order to avoid that dose being given each day by mistake.

5. A carbon copy or a copy of the original order written by the physician is sent to the pharmacy for drug preparation. It is most important that the drug order not be transcribed or rewritten before it reaches the pharmacy.

6. Once the order reaches the pharmacy the order is checked by the pharmacist against previous orders for that patient. If the drug or dose varies from the previous order, the order should be verified. If the patient is on a research protocol, the pharmacy staff should have a copy of the protocol to verify the order.

7. The person writing the order for the drug should avoid the use of extraneous ".0" because "100.0" may be misread as "1000." Probability of error could be further reduced by spelling out the amount as "one hundred," which will rarely, if ever, be read as "one thousand."

8. In most settings, computer-generated labels are used. Ideally, the computer should be programmed *not* to print the label if the dose/cumulative dose are out of the ordinary and customary range. To override the computer and print the label would then require verification and authorization.

9. Drugs should be dispensed on trays or in plastic zipper-lock bags large enough to hold all the drugs to be given to one patient. Drugs intended for one patient may be confused with another patient's order if they are not isolated in a bag or on a tray.

10. Once the pharmacist signs off on the drug, verifying that it is the right dose of the right drug for the right patient, the complete order is given to the nurse. The nurse then checks the drugs against the original written order to again confirm the accuracy of the order prior to treating the patient.

11. If at all possible, the person preparing the drug should not be the same person double-checking the order to make certain that what was ordered was prepared. If a nurse is working alone in a clinic, the physician should be available to double-check the drugs prior to administration.

12. Everyone responsible for drug preparation and administration (pharmacist, pharmacy technicians, and nurses) needs to be properly trained in the specialty of chemotherapy drug preparation.

13. If the patient is receiving chemotherapy at home, the nurse must have proof of certification by an approved chemotherapy administration program to administer chemotherapy.

14. Policies and procedures for preventing and reporting drug errors are reviewed regularly according to institutional policy and procedure.

15. Policies and procedures for drug preparation and administration should be reviewed by committee on a yearly basis.

16. Everyone responsible for chemotherapy drug preparation and administration should be empowered with the ability to question the order. If there is any question related to the drug, dose, route, or schedule, the individual must clarify the order and be encouraged to do so.

17. Any protocol involving unusual dosing patterns or dose-intensive regimens should be reviewed carefully by all. No one should be expected to prepare or administer a drug with a dose-intensive schedule without the opportunity to review the protocol at least 24 hours in advance, especially if the study involves an investigational agent.

It is not uncommon in a busy outpatient clinic for a nurse to have no prior knowledge that a patient is beginning a new chemotherapy protocol before the patient appears in the clinic ready to be treated. This is not optimal because the nurse has no time to review the protocol and to prepare the patient's learning packet. Errors can be made whenever drugs are given in a hurried and unprepared manner. Communication between the physician, pharmacist, and nurse is critical to providing a safe level of care.

It is further recommended that all licensed registered nurses should have malpractice insurance, regardless of their practice setting but especially if their practice involves intravenous therapy.[27] To infiltrate a vesicant chemotherapeutic agent is not an act of negligence or malpractice. The issue is how much fluid infiltrated the tissues, over what length of time, the nurse's specific actions, and the completeness of the documentation and follow-up. At issue will also be the nurse's level of preparation and skill in intravenous drug administration and whether or not certification has been received to administer certain drugs, specifically vesicant chemotherapy. General certification in oncology nursing does not qualify the nurse to administer chemotherapy. Specific guidelines for certification and training to safely administer chemotherapy have been suggested by the Oncology Nursing Society Cancer Chemotherapy Guidelines.[3] Critical to these guidelines is the supervised training and experience of administering vesicant agents.

Specific policies and procedures that reflect standards of practice for intravenous drug administration should be readily available, reviewed frequently, and updated as necessary. If the nurse does not have knowledge of a specific procedure or does not follow it, he or she is not practicing according to the hospital's policy, and his or her actions are therefore indefensible in court. If the supervisor failed to inform the nurse of the policy and procedure, the supervisor (physician, nurse manager, hospital administration) may also be found at fault.

When a drug error occurs or an extravasation of a vesicant is suspected or certain, the nurse must document the event as thoroughly as possible to verify exactly what actions were taken to ensure optimal patient care. When the event involves infiltration of a vesicant agent, an extravasation record (Figure 19-1) is useful to prompt the nurse to document the event as thoroughly as possible. When called on to testify in a legal case, one cannot be

Patient _____ Date infiltration occurred _____

Drug _____ Dilution mg/mL _____ vesicant _____ irritant _____

Amount of drug infiltrated: < 1 mL_____ 1–3 mL_____ 3–5 mL_____ 5 mL_____ > 10 mL_____

Method of drug administration:

_____ Two-syringe technique IV push

_____ Side-arm with IV freely running

_____ Continuous infusion: rate _____ ml/hour

peristaltic pump _____ yes _____ no

_____ VAD: _____ port _____ tunneled catheter

type of needle _____

_____ Other _____

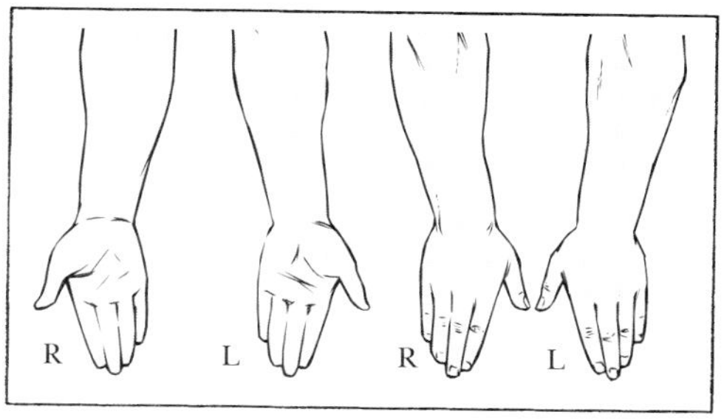

Description of site:

Size _____ Color _____ Texture _____
(Indicate location on diagram)

right arm   left arm
(attach photograph)

Process Documentation: Describe the events that occurred during the drug administration

S: (Patient's Symptoms) _____

_____

_____

O: (Clinical Symptoms) _____

_____

_____

A: (Assessment) _____ suspected extravasation _____ definite extravasation _____

_____

P: (Plan of care) Initial actions: _____

_____

Physician notified: _____ Instructions: _____

_____

Follow-up Instructions: _____

_____

Additional Comments: _____

Consultations: _____ Plastic Surgery _____ Physical Therapy _____ Other _____

Date of referral: _____ Follow-up _____

Return appointment: _____ Written instructions for site care reviewed with patient _____

(RN Signature _____)

Follow-up visit #1 (date _____) Describe site and care instructions (attach photo): _____

_____

Follow-up visit #2 (date _____) Describe site and care instructions (attach photo): _____

_____

Follow-up visit #3 (date _____) Describe site and care instructions: (attach photo): _____

Figure 19-1 Extravasation record. (Reprinted with permission from Goodman M, Rush Cancer Institute, Chicago.)

expected to recall events that occurred 5 years ago. If the nurse does not document the actions taken and what the patient reported at the time, it is as if nothing was done and what the patient currently says is true, no matter what the nurse did or what the patient reported initially. It is important to document, if possible, the amount of fluid infiltrated and the size of the involved area. The site should be drawn on the extravasation record to identify the location, and a color photograph should be attached to the extravasation record to compare to serial photographs to be taken on a weekly basis until the degree of damage can be determined. The format of an extravasation record should identify what the patient reported (subjective data), what the nurse observed (objective data), what the nurse did in detail (action), and the immediate plan of care, including instructions for the patient and follow-up site care (plan). The nurse must document that the physician was notified and that instructions for care were explained and given to the patient, including future plans for care such as a return appointment for evaluation and possible referral to a plastic surgeon and physical therapist.

Another issue that needs to be addressed is the patient's risk for extravasation. Often, patients are offered a VAD because of the nature of their treatment or their poor venous access and then refuse the device. This should be documented in the medical record. Ten years ago, before access devices were so readily available, it may have been acceptable to stick a patient three and four times with an angiocath or a scalp vein needle to secure an adequate, but likely suboptimal, venous access. Today, VADs are not only available but in many settings are the logical solution for any patient who requires chemotherapy for an indefinite period of time.

Chemotherapy is never (with rare exception) an emergency treatment in which a delay of 2 or 3 days to place an access device would be detrimental to the patient's condition. On the other hand, an extravasation is associated with extreme morbidity, and an access device is inevitable under these circumstances. It is in the best interest of the patient that the nurse refuse to attempt another venipuncture rather than forging ahead with even more risk of extravasation. Unfortunately, the pressure to complete the task at hand and the fact that refusing to try one more time might mean the drug will be wasted often leads to poor judgment. As nurses, we need to give each other permission to make the appropriate choice and provide the support needed once that choice is made.

Routes of Drug Administration

Dose Calculation

The dose of drug to be administered is generally based on the individual's body surface area, usually expressed in milligrams per square meter or milligrams per kilogram. The patient's body surface area is usually determined by a height and weight nomogram. There is controversy regarding the accuracy and safety of this method because some patients may have been heavily pretreated and therefore unable to tolerate higher doses of drugs or dose-intensive regimens. In addition, many patients are clinically obese, which is defined as weighing 30% or more over ideal body weight. Empiric decreases in the doses of anticancer agents given to obese patients based on ideal body weight are not supported by available data.[28] Georgiadis et al found no significant association between obesity and toxicity measured primarily as white blood cell nadir.[29] Bear in mind that inappropriate dose reduction may compromise efficacy, which is particularly meaningful when the intent of treatment is cure. However, in situations where a dose reduction is necessary and the patient's weight is significantly greater than their ideal, a simple method of calculating their dose is to take the average of the ideal and actual weight. If an ideal weight table is not available, start with 100 pounds for 5 feet and add 5 pounds for each additional inch. So, someone who is 5'5" would ideally weigh 125 pounds. That weight, plus their actual weight divided by two, would give the weight on which to calculate dose per square meter.

Attempts are often made to individualize the dose of a drug so that optimal therapeutic response is achieved without toxic effects. However, the outcome is generally less than ideal, and patients, especially the elderly, are frequently underdosed because of the potential for severe toxicity. It is often proposed that individual doses be calculated based on a person's physiological age rather than their chronological age. One example of this approach involves the application of the Calvert formula for carboplatin dosing.[30] The Calvert formula makes it possible to individualize the carboplatin dose in order to obtain a maximally effective dose with tolerable side effects.

Carboplatin is excreted by the kidneys, in particular glomerular filtration with little excretion or reabsorption by the renal tubules. Therefore, pretreatment assessment of renal function or glomerular filtration rate (GFR) can be used to individualize carboplatin dose in adults. The GFR is essentially equivalent to the creatinine clearance, which can be estimated from the patient's age, serum creatinine, and weight. Another factor in the Calvert formula involves the area under the curve (AUC), or target drug concentration for carboplatin. The AUC dosing correlates more closely with drug toxicity than do doses based on body surface area.[31] In the presence of impaired renal function, the delayed clearance of carboplatin would result in prolonged drug exposure (increased AUC); in patients with high renal clearance decreased AUC could result in subtherapeutic dosing. Because AUC or carboplatin exposure, rather than toxicity, is the measurement, it is not influenced by concurrent myelosuppressive therapy or supportive treatment. The following formula is applicable in single-agent, combination therapy, or high-dose studies:

Carboplatin dose (mg) = Target AUC × (GFR + 25)

where AUC = area under the curve;

GFR = glomerular filtration rate.

The AUC ranges from 4–11 and is selected for appropriate clinical situations. For example, if the patient has had prior treatment or is receiving carboplatin in combination with another myelosuppressive agent, an AUC of 4–5 might be selected. If the patient is receiving carboplatin alone and has not been previously treated with ablative chemotherapy, an AUC of 7–11 might be selected.

Pretreatment Considerations

Table 19-4 includes specific tasks involved in antineoplastic drug administration that are applicable in all practice settings. Of special note would be any procedure that would address patient safety such as anaphylaxis or extravasation. All emergency equipment should be available and in good working order. Standing orders for emergency care should be readily available as well as appropriate personnel in the event that an emergency situation should arise. In the current practice environment, it is not uncommon for one or two nurses to be the sole providers of care in an ambulatory care setting with a clinic full of patients who have seen the physician and are receiving their medicines or waiting to begin their treatment. The physicians often see their patients and leave to do rounds in the hospital or to go to another freestanding oncology facility. Standards of practice dictate that a physician be physically available where chemotherapy is administered. This applies to all settings where drugs of an experimental nature are given, but in fact reactions and emergency situations can arise when more commonly used drugs like etoposide are given. The first consideration is the safety of the patient, and the policies and procedures governing the setting in which chemotherapy is given should specifically indicate that a physician should be present physically, not just available by phone.

There are other specific factors to be considered for individual drugs (e.g., test dosing prior to administering bleomycin). While not a common practice, it is still considered appropriate to administer a test dose of bleomycin prior to administering the full dose because the first dose of bleomycin has been known to cause rare but severe allergic reactions, especially in patients with lymphoma.[31] Test dosing involves giving 0.5–1.0 unit of bleomycin intravenously, intramuscularly, or subcutaneously prior to the first dose of the drug. It is preferable to test dose 24 hours prior to administration, but it is commonly done 1 or 2 hours before the full dose, followed by close observation. Diphenhydramine 50 mg and acetaminophen 1000 mg may be given with the bleomycin and again 4 hours later. The hypersensitivity reactions including hypotension, rash, facial flushing, and bronchospasm can progress to anaphylaxis, but in general most patients experience only a relatively high fever, chills, and a flulike syndrome. These symptoms are usually preventable if the patient is given the diphenhydramine and acetaminophen and remembers to take it again 4 hours later.

Another issue involves prevention of hypersensitivity reactions (HSR) with paclitaxel or docetaxel. When paclitaxel is given, patients must remember to begin taking dexamethasone 20 mg by mouth 13 and 7 hours prior to dosing with taxol. In addition, patients are given diphenhydramine 50 mg IV and a histamine blocker (ranitidine 20 mg or cimetidine 300 mg) 30 minutes prior to paclitaxil. Most reactions, if they are going to occur with paclitaxil, occur within the first three courses and are thought to be due to Cremophor EL, the formulation vehicle.

In the case of etoposide, the primary reaction is hypotension. Severe hypotension can occur if the drug is infused in less than 45 minutes. Etoposide is formulated in benzyl alcohol and Tween 80. Caution should be taken when giving etoposide for the first and second time. The infusion is started slowly at a 60-minute rate, and all nursing personnel are informed that the patient is receiving the drug for the first or second time. The patient is instructed to report any light-headedness, dizziness, rash, or difficulty breathing. Bronchospasm with severe wheezing can occur and responds to antihistamines and glucocorticosteroids. It is advisable, especially if the individual is atopic or has a prior history of reaction to paclitaxel or cisplatin, to have diphenhydramine 50 mg available if needed. If the patient is receiving both paclitaxel and etoposide, special pretreatment and monitoring for hypersensitivity reactions may be needed.[32] Inhaled bronchodilators, epinephrine and diphenhydramine 50 mg, should be readily available in the treatment area.

Docetaxel is a drug similar to paclitaxel but is associated with less risk of HSR and initially, in phase 1 studies, was given without premedication. Currently, most patients are given dexamethasone 8 mg twice a day for 5 days beginning 1 day prior to docetaxel. This precaution appears to delay the onset and decrease the severity of fluid retention characterized by peripheral edema, pleural effusions, and ascites.

The last pretreatment consideration involves the sequencing of various drugs to either enhance cytotoxicity or minimize toxicity to normal tissues. For example, the administration of slightly higher doses of intravenous methotrexate 1 hour prior to 5-fluorouracil (5-FU), with leucovorin rescue 24 hours later, appears to enhance the cell kill effect of both the methotrexate and 5-FU. Similarly, the sequence of cisplatin before paclitaxel induces more profound neutropenia than the alternate sequence. The incidence of neutropenia is believed to be due to the lower paclitaxel clearance rates when cisplatin precedes paclitaxel.[33] In addition the cytotoxic effects of paclitaxel preceding platinol were additive, whereas the reverse sequence resulted in pronounced antagonism.[34] A study by Clark et al demonstrated that administering paclitaxel before carboplatin resulted in significantly greater cytotoxicity than when administering the drugs in the reverse sequence.[35] The toxicity profile was not

Table 19-4 Chemotherapy Administration Guidelines

Professional Preparation

- Maintain appropriate knowledge and skills regarding chemotherapy drug protocols and administration procedures.
- Review applicable policies and procedures.
- Review drug protocol and research guidelines.

Patient Preparation

- Verify patient identity (arm band, driver's license, verbalization of name).
- Ensure appropriate patient education.
- Confirm that appropriate laboratory tests have been completed and are within normal limits.
- Measure and record baseline vital signs.
- Verify patient's allergy history.
- Assess venous access status (i.e., need for VAD).
- Initiate pretreatment therapies, if ordered (e.g., hydration, test dosing).

Drug Preparation

- Verify drug order (including body surface area and dosage calculations).
- Obtain prepared drug, and double-check label for the correct drug, dose, route, and patient. If admixing, follow appropriate guidelines for cytotoxic drug admixture.
- Ensure rapid access to extravasation kit and medications necessary if allergic reaction occurs (parenteral diphenhydramine hydrochloride, epinephrine, and hydrocortisone should be immediately available).
- Obtain necessary supplies and equipment for safe drug administration.
- Wash hands, and don gloves and appropriate protective clothing.

Venipuncture Guidelines

- Establish work area with plastic-backed pad.
- Organize materials, needle box, syringes, flush, IV start materials, and IV fluids.
- Select needle size and type according to setting, patient's veins, and treatment to be administered.
- Determine appropriate site for venous access, avoiding:
  - limbs with recent (i.e., 30 min) venipunctures
  - limbs with axillary node dissections, extensive radiation therapy, or obstructive process
  - antecubital fossa (for peripheral sticks)
  - ecchymotic or sclerosed areas
  - bony prominences and joints
- Ensure adequate lighting and visualization of area to be accessed.
- Remove jewelry near access site.
- Select a large vein if administering drugs known to be irritating (mechlorethamine, BCNU, streptozotocin, paclitaxel, docetaxel, vinorelbine).
- Administer vesicants only at sites designated by established policies and procedures, specifically in areas with underlying subcutaneous tissue. Areas to be avoided when administering vesicants include veins over joints, bony prominences, neurovascular bundles, tendons, and areas of existing soft-tissue damage.
- For peripheral sites, begin at the most distal areas.
- Utilize an appropriate sterile technique for access.
- Achieve a "clean" venipuncture and determine patency. The needle should not puncture through the back of the vein and then be resettled within the vein. There should be a brisk, immediate blood return and no swelling at the needle site.
- Secure needle with tape, but ensure visualization of the site.
- Flush needle with sterile NS or D5W to clear the line and establish patency. Observe the site at this time to ensure that swelling is not occurring at the needle site.
- Use Luer-Lok fittings for intravenous (IV) sets and syringes; use sterile gauze or alcohol pad for priming IV sets.

Drug Administration Guidelines

- Check patient's condition periodically during drug administration, and explain actions being taken, when appropriate.
- Monitor the status of the venous access site periodically during the process.
- If administering a vesicant, observe the site continuously throughout the injection.
- Administer antiemetics (if not already given).
- Ensure drug containment at all times. Wipe any droplets at the connector or Y-site with a gauze pad.
- Administer chemotherapy drugs as ordered, using slow, steady pressure.
- Check for a blood return every few ml and before and after each drug.
- Flush between each drug with sterile NS or D5W to avoid drug admixture and potential precipitation.
- When administering short-term drips or infusions, establish the infusion, taping all connections securely, and set the appropriate flow rate.
- Generally, place long-term infusions on an infusion pump.
- Flush after last drug with sterile NS or D5W.
- If appropriate, discontinue the IV needle. For peripheral sites, hold pressure manually over the site for a few minutes, then apply small, sterile dressing.
- Do not clip or recap needles.

Postadministration Guidelines

- Discard all materials (needles, syringes, bags, tubing, gown, gloves, etc.) appropriately.
- Assess patient's status and provide for follow-up:
  - *Inpatient:* Call button within reach; fluids available, etc.
  - *Outpatient:* Transportation ready; return appointment and prescriptions obtained; telephone number of physician or nurse available
  - *Home care:* Caregiver available; telephone number of nurse-on-call available
- Document all actions (flow sheets or specialized forms are recommended). (See Chapter 20.)

VAD = vascular access device; NS = normal saline; BCNU = carmustine; D5W = 5% dextrose in water.

affected by sequence of drug administration. Therefore, to achieve the greatest efficacy with no increase in toxicity the paclitaxel is routinely administered prior to carboplatin.

Another example of the importance of sequencing in chemotherapy administration involves the administration of doxorubicin and paclitaxel. A moderate to severe mucositis can occur when paclitaxel is given prior to doxorubicin but not when it is given in the reverse sequence. The paclitaxel-related mucosal damage concomitant with neutropenia has been thought to contribute to the development of typhlitis, which can be life-threatening. Pharmacokinetic data indicate that when paclitaxel is given immediately prior to doxorubicin, there is a 31.6% average decrease in the clearance of doxorubicin, which contributes greatly to profound neutropenia.[36] Based on this, the sequence of doxorubicin followed by paclitaxel is recommended.

Chemotherapy was designed as a systemic treatment for cancer, having the ability to travel throughout the body via the bloodstream and to damage or kill dividing cells. It is now possible to direct drugs systemically as well as to almost every anatomical region in the body—to specific organs, inside body cavities, and to body spaces. Intravenous chemotherapy remains the most common route of drug delivery, but other systemic routes include oral, intramuscular, and subcutaneous. Regional drug delivery utilizes the following routes: topical, intraarterial, intraperitoneal, intrapleural, intravesical, intrathecal, and intraventricular. It is even possible to use these techniques to administer the drugs directly into the center of a tumor (intratumoral).

Topical

Cutaneous malignant lesions can be treated in a variety of ways, including the topical application of antineoplastic agents. This is most commonly done for cutaneous T-cell lymphoma, basal cell carcinoma, Kaposi's sarcoma, and squamous cell carcinoma. The agents used include nitrogen mustard for cutaneous T-cell lymphoma and fluorouracil for basal and squamous cell carcinomas.[37] The topical agent is usually applied once or twice daily until the lesions progress to the necrosis phase, which may take 1–3 weeks. The affected area is not washed vigorously during the treatment period. The expected result of topical antineoplastic administration is local sloughing of the affected area and eventual regranulation of normal tissue, so it is normal for the treated area to become red and tender, then to form a lesion that becomes necrotic, followed by superficial sloughing of the dead tissue and regrowth of healthy skin. It is unusual for the patient to experience any systemic side effects of the drugs unless the majority of the skin is being treated; incidences of mild, delayed side effects such as nausea have been reported.

Special nursing considerations for these patients include

- Patient education, with special consideration of body image issues

- Application of the drug using cotton swabs or non-metal applicators

- Close attention to application only in the prescribed (affected) area

- Careful avoidance of the eyes, nose, mouth, or other areas close to mucous membranes

- Utilization of safe drug-handling practices (e.g., gloves and strict attention to drug containment)

- When using nitrogen mustard, having sodium thiosulfate available (to neutralize the nitrogen mustard) and applying it to areas of the skin that may be inadvertently exposed (after removal of the drug)

- Application of dressings, if prescribed

- Observation for untoward sequelae (e.g., severe burning or rashes, which may require discontinuation of therapy or subsequent dose reduction)

- Monitoring disease response

Oral

A variety of antineoplastic agents are administered orally to treat numerous types of cancer (Appendix A).[38] The oral route is convenient, economical, noninvasive, and often less toxic. Most oral drugs are well absorbed as long as the gastrointestinal tract is functioning normally.

The nursing responsibilities for oral drug administration include safe handling (gloves are considered acceptable if physical contact with the tablet or capsule is required) and monitoring for drug absorption and compliance with the prescribed therapy. If the patient experiences emesis immediately after drug ingestion and the pills or capsules cannot be visualized, the drug is usually not repeated. Several oral antineoplastic agents are also available in parenteral forms, providing an option for patients intolerant of or noncompliant with oral regimens. Other recommendations include the following:

- Prescribe one "course" at a time, to avoid inadvertent overdosing that could be life threatening.

- Instruct the patient to take the medication on an empty stomach with water to enhance absorption, unless the drug is tolerated better with food, as is the case with prednisone, cyclophosphamide, and tamoxifen.

- Familiarize the patient with both generic and brand names of the drug, to avoid confusion or double dosing (many physicians prefer to prescribe brand name antineoplastic agents to avoid the possibility of the generics not being bioequivalent).

- Instruct the patient to maintain a record of drugs being taken.

- Obtain a list of any drugs currently being taken by the patient to ensure compatibility.

- Advise the patient to avoid taking any over-the-counter drugs without first checking with the physician or nurse.

- Question the patient at each visit regarding the medication (i.e., how much was taken, whether any doses were omitted, and why).

It is important that the patient comply with the treatment regimen to maximize the goal of therapy (i.e., remission or cure). Oral agents give the patient control over drug administration, and noncompliance is not common. However, tamoxifen can cause hot flashes and mood swings, cyclophosphamide and etoposide can cause emesis, and levamisole can cause neurotoxicity. A patient might decide to omit a dose in order to feel better temporarily. The patient needs to understand the importance of dosing and scheduling and how critical it is that the prescribed regimen be followed exactly. With therapy such as leucovorin following methotrexate, noncompliance could be fatal. It is common for patients receiving oral antineoplastic agents to be given a calendar with the doses indicated and space to record each dose. The nurse checks the previous treatment calendar and questions the patient about any omitted doses during each encounter. The regimen can often be modified to enhance the patient's tolerance of the side effects (e.g., administering an antiemetic to minimize nausea or changing the time of dose administration).

Intramuscular and Subcutaneous

Utilization of intramuscular or subcutaneous antineoplastic drug delivery was uncommon in the past, as only a few drugs were indicated by this route. The development of the biological agents (e.g., interferon, colony-stimulating factors) has increased the number of drugs given intramuscularly or subcutaneously. These convenient and quick routes are handled according to standard injection methods. Because some of the drugs can sting or burn, intramuscular injections are usually given into large muscles, with the Z-track method being optional. Subcutaneous injections of small volumes (up to 3 mL) are in the usual sites and should be rotated if given daily. Many drug manufacturers have distributed videos, charts, or posters that clearly outline the steps to follow for patients self-administering subcutaneous medications. One drug that is administered subcutaneously in a rather unique way is goserelin acetate (Zoladex), a hormonal agent used in the treatment of breast cancer and prostate cancer. It is actually a dry drug pellet that is implanted in the soft tissue of the abdomen, where it gradually is absorbed over 1–3 months. A local anesthetic such as Emla Cream (ASTRA, Inc., Westborough, MA) or a lidocaine injection or ice is usually used to minimize discomfort, as the needle is large (16-gauge).

Intravenous

The intravenous route of drug delivery is the most common and most reliable method of drug delivery. Detailed nursing actions concerning intravenous drug administration are included in Table 19-4 and Appendix 19B. Selection of a VAD, an angiocath, or a butterfly needle will be determined by the type of therapy the patient is to receive and the condition of the patient's veins. For most patients, a 21-gauge needle is adequate for extended infusions for hydration and for 3- and 4-hour infusions of chemotherapy. If an IV needs to stay in for more than 1 hour, it is best to place an angiocath that will be less likely to infiltrate and will be less traumatic to the veins. If the patient is to receive only an injection of chemotherapy and intravenous antiemetics without hydration, a 23- or 21-gauge butterfly needle is preferred because it is easy to insert into small veins and is less traumatic because it is not left in for an extended period of time. The problem with small butterfly needles (25-gauge) is that the blood return is often lost because the needle is so small. When giving a vesicant, it is always better to have blood return throughout the injection, so a smaller-gauge needle is not preferable in that situation. Unfortunately, patients often have such small veins that the smaller needles are needed. In this situation, choosing an angiocath which is thin-walled with an over-the-needle cannula, permits a large internal diameter once the stylet is removed without overly traumatizing the vein. Choosing the appropriate device is important but taking the time to find the most appropriate vein is even more important. Staying focused on finding the vein can be difficult considering the numerous distractions that exist in a busy ambulatory care center. The initial and careful assessment of both arms (if appropriate) is critical to vein selection. Too often the nurse fails to assess the veins properly, fails to distend the veins sufficiently prior to attempting venipuncture, and fails to apply adequate traction on the vein to prevent the vein from rolling. If a vein is not obvious, it is advisable to apply moist heat to the arms for 5–10 minutes and have the patient drink warm liquids prior to attempting venipuncture. If the patient is known to have small, hard-to-find veins, the patient should drink four to six glasses of fluid the morning of treatment, dress warmly, and practice vein distention by squeezing a handball for 10 minutes prior to the nurse attempting venipuncture. If the nurse has difficulty accessing an appropriate vein after one or two attempts, she should seek the assistance of a colleague. If a patient repeatedly requires more than three sticks and the plan is to have chemotherapy indefinitely, or at least for an extended period of time, a VAD is appropriate. The longer the patient has the device, the longer he or she benefits from having it placed. Even if a person has adequate veins, if he or she has metastatic disease and will require an access device at some point, it is appropriate to propose it early on in the course of treatment.

When selecting a vein, the general rule is to start distally and gradually proceed proximally. Another rule might be to select the best vein, provided that vein is not the antecubital vein. Some nurses might prefer the antecubital area for venous access because it contains large veins to facilitate rapid drug delivery. However, this area should be avoided, especially if the patient is receiving a vesicant agent. Placing a needle in the antecubital area restricts patient mobility and increases the risk of dislodgment. Any extravasation that occurs is difficult to detect because the area is dense and a lot of fluid can infiltrate before it is detected.

Another issue involves the order in which chemotherapeutic agents are given. Except where sequencing is important pharmacologically, the order of drug delivery is probably not critical. However, when administering a vesicant agent, it is wiser to administer the antiemetic and any antianxiolytic agent after the vesicant. No agent, except perhaps nitrogen mustard, causes emesis in the first hour, so giving the vesicant before the antiemetic is sound practice. It is important that the patient be alert and able to communicate how they are feeling throughout the injection of the vesicant. Reasons to give the vesicant before any other agent are (1) the venous integrity is greatest earlier in the procedure; (2) the nurse's assessment skills and the patient's level of awareness and sensitivity are most acute at the initiation of the infusion; (3) the possibility that the vein will be irritated by other drugs (e.g. decadron) or by movement is eliminated. The idea that if the vein takes the nonvesicants without any problem then the vesicant will infuse without difficulty is faulty reasoning. The risk of infiltration of any IV increases over time. Often, other drugs can cause venous irritation and even spasm that can result in a loss of blood return, a major assessment criteria for safe administration of chemotherapy.

Another factor in the intravenous administration of chemotherapy is the pain associated with the needle stick. Patients seldom become accustomed to the discomfort and often grow to dread the event more as time goes on. The pain of venipuncture can be dealt with in a number of ways; first-needle phobia is a major reason for insertion of a VAD. However, while the placement of an access device does diminish the discomfort of a needle stick, it by no means eliminates it. Ethyl chloride spray has been used to numb the site prior to needle stick, but it does not work well. Ice has been used over ports to ease the discomfort, but again patients will still feel the needle stick. There is one approach to pain prevention with a needle stick that works remarkably well and is especially indicated for anyone with a needle phobia and with children. Emla Cream or Disc is a mixture of lidocaine 2.5% and prilocaine 2.5%. A dollop of cream is placed over the vein, port, or selected site for injection approximately 1–4 hours prior to treatment. An occlusive dressing (provided with the 5-g tubes) is applied over the Emla Cream without spreading out the cream. The Emla Disc is often preferred as there is no need for an additional dressing since the Emla is self-contained within the disc. If the Emla Cream is used, the dressing is removed and the site is cleansed thoroughly prior to the needle insertion.

Having patients turn their heads away or close their eyes guarantees elimination of the psychological component of fear of needle sticks, although it does not totally eliminate the anticipation of the pain—until the patient sees how well the approach works to prevent pain and discomfort. Patients who in the past have experienced severe anxiety and pain with venipuncture claim they feel nothing when the needle goes in, not even pressure, especially when the Emla is in place for at least 2 hours. One word of caution—Emla should not be used in patients who are also receiving a vesicant agent peripherally because they may not be able to feel the pain if the vesicant should infiltrate. Using Emla Cream means that the nurse needs to take a little time to help the patient select the vein that will be used at the next treatment, and the nurse must try to access a vein in that area. In patients with few veins, it is a good idea to select two sites to prepare with the Emla Cream. Patients should be cautioned that it is not always possible to access a vein in a previously selected site. When it does work out, however, the patient is extremely appreciative. For the nurse, it is especially rewarding to be able to eliminate what is surely the most dreaded aspect of the patient's treatment. Even patients with ports become devoted users of Emla Cream.

Vesicant Extravasation Issues

Several of the most commonly administered chemotherapy drugs are vesicants, meaning that they cause tissue necrosis if they infiltrate or extravasate out of the blood vessel and into the soft tissue. While a few nonantineoplastic drugs are vesicants (e.g., levophed and dilantin), the number of antineoplastic vesicants is significant; they are listed in Table 19-5 along with the agents known

Table 19-5 Antineoplastic Vesicants and Irritants

Vesicants

Dactinomycin (Cosmegen)
Daunorubicin (Cerubidine)
Doxorubicin (Adriamycin)
Estramustin (Emcyt)
Idarubicin (Idamycin)
Mitomycin C (Mutamycin)
Nitrogen mustard (Mustargen)
Teniposide (Vumon)
Vinblastine (Velban)
Vincristine (Oncovin)

Irritants

Carmustine (BiCNU)
Dacarbazine (DTIC)
Etoposide (VP-16)
Liposomal doxorubicin (Doxil)
Mithramycin (Plicamycin)
Mitoxantrone (Novantrone)
Paclitaxel (Taxol)
Streptozocin (Zanosar)
Docetaxel (Taxotere)
Vinorelbine (Navelbine)

to be irritating to the vein during drug administration. It is critical that the nurse administering chemotherapy be aware of the drugs that are vesicants and use safety measures to try to prevent extravasation.

When infiltration of a vesicant occurs, underlying tissue is damaged. The damage can be severe enough to result in physical deformity or a functional deficit, such as loss of joint mobility, loss of vascularity, or loss of tendon function. If a sufficient amount of an irritant infiltrates, it too can cause significant damage beyond discoloration and pain. The following guidelines are suggested to minimize the risk of extravasation.

1. Be aware of certain patients at increased risk for extravasation:
   a. Patients unable to communicate to the nurse about the pain of extravasation
   b. Elderly, debilitated, or confused patients with diabetes or general vascular disease
   c. Any patient with fragile veins
2. Generally, avoid infusing vesicants over joints, bony prominences, tendons, neurovascular bundles, or the antecubital fossa.
3. Never give vesicants intramuscularly or subcutaneously.
4. Avoid giving vesicant drugs in areas where venous or lymphatic circulation is poor (e.g., operative side for a mastectomy patient, patient with superior vena cava syndrome) or in sites that have been previously irradiated.
5. Make sure the peripheral IV site is adequate and less than 24 hours old. A brisk blood return and easy flow of fluids are to be determined before administering vesicants in any IV needle or catheter (peripheral or central).
6. Visualize the needle or catheter insertion site, and observe the site continuously. (Never leave the patient unattended when administering a vesicant peripherally.)
7. When giving more than one chemotherapy agent, give the vesicant agent first.
8. Give vesicants in a steady, even flow, checking frequently (every 1–2 mL) for a blood return. When checking for a blood return, do so gently to avoid excessive pressure in the vein.
9. If a vesicant is ordered as an *infusion,* it is given through a central line only and checked every 1–2 hours in health care facilities and every 2–4 hours when the patient is receiving vesicant infusions in the home.
10. An extravasation kit containing all materials necessary to manage an extravasation should be available wherever vesicant agents are administered. Include in the kit a copy of the extravasation policy and procedure.

Despite these precautions, vesicant extravasation does occur, although the incidence is low among experienced oncology nurses in cancer specialty settings (0.1%) and somewhat higher in general hospital settings (2%–5%).[39]

Detection of a vesicant extravasation in its earliest stage is most likely to result in the least possible soft-tissue damage. The nurse should be aware of the following symptoms that could indicate extravasation; it is also important to note that an extravasation can occur without any symptoms.

- Swelling (most common)
- Stinging, burning, or pain at the injection site (not *always* present)
- Redness (not often seen initially)
- Lack of blood return (if this is *only* symptom, the IV should be reevaluated; if still no blood return, consider other options); lack of a blood return alone is not always indicative of an extravasation; extravasation can occur even if a blood return is present

If an extravasation is suspected, the infusion must be stopped immediately and the needle site inspected.

Chemotherapy drug extravasation is a known complication of cancer treatment. The occurrence of extravasation of vesicant chemotherapeutic agents is probably underreported, but according to the literature the incidence ranges from 0.5%–5.0% of patients receiving peripheral intravenous chemotherapeutic agents[40,41] and 6.4% of patients ($n = 300$) receiving vesicant chemotherapy via implanted vascular access ports.[42]

The most benign, inconsequential local reaction to chemotherapy is venous flare (see Color Plate 1 [Figure 19-2]). This reaction occurs most commonly in patients receiving doxorubicin and is characterized by a localized erythema, venous streaking, and pruritus along the injected vein. This localized allergic reaction is distinguishable from an extravasation by the absence of pain or swelling and the presence of a blood return. Once this important distinction is made, it is safe to continue injecting the agent. Flushing the vein with saline and slowing the injection rate appear to ease the symptoms, which dissipate without treatment within 20–30 minutes of the injection.

Another local tissue reaction characterized by pain, venous irritation, and chemical phlebitis can occur with certain nonvesicant chemotherapy agents. These agents are called *irritants* and are listed in Table 19-5. While any drug given in concentrated form in sufficient amount can cause tissue damage if infiltrated, these agents are not associated with ulceration if infiltrated. Irritants cause intravascular irritation often accompanied by pain (described as achiness or as tightness) only during the infusion and may, as is the case with carmustine, be a function of the diluent.

Vinorelbine can cause venous irritation. Infusing 250 mL of fluid and injecting the drug over 6–10 minutes followed by a 250-mL infusion of saline or dextrose in water will minimize discomfort when infusing vinorelbine into a peripheral vein. When administering vinorelbine into a central line the flush is probably not important but it is generally done as a precaution. Liposomal doxorubicin is an irritant that is given as an infusion over

30–60 minutes. If infiltrated, there may be redness and edema but no ulceration. A cold compress is appropriate to ease discomfort. With some irritants like dacarbazine or streptozocin, increasing the dilution, applying a cold pack, or slowing the drip rate will ease the pain associated with infusion.

The most devastating skin reactions caused by chemotherapy occur when a vesicant agent is infiltrated, causing an extravasation injury. The degree of injury to local tissues is related to the vesicant properties of the drug infiltrated, the concentration of the drug, and the amount of the drug infiltrated. For example, in the animal model 0.2 mL of doxorubicin at a concentration of 2 mg/mL produces a 1-cm diameter lesion taking 7–8 weeks to heal.[40]

By definition, an *extravasation* is the infiltration of a vesicant chemotherapeutic agent. A *vesicant* is a drug that, if infiltrated, is capable of causing pain, ulceration, necrosis, and sloughing of damaged tissue. While all vesicants are capable of causing significant ulceration and morbidity due to pain, tissue necrosis, and potential loss of function of the affected area, this rarely occurs when these drugs are given by professional nurses who are trained in the proper techniques of chemotherapy drug administration. Although infiltration of vesicant agents can occur even when these drugs are given by properly trained individuals, the sequelae are usually inconsequential and the wound usually heals spontaneously over time.

To infiltrate a vesicant agent is traumatic for patient and nurse, but it is not an act of negligence. In many situations, the patient is elderly with small frail veins, or obese with deep and difficult-to-access veins. In such cases, the occurrence of an extravasation is more a function of venous integrity than the administration technique. Patients should be thoroughly informed regarding the vesicant potential of the drugs they are receiving and the importance of reporting any pain, burning, or stinging during the injection.

To ensure the best outcome possible in the event of an extravasation, the nurse must be able to recognize that an infiltration has occurred and act appropriately. When vesicant agents are administered by nurses and physicians who are not trained in the skills of chemotherapy administration, the subtle early signs and symptoms of an extravasation may go unnoticed, resulting in extensive tissue damage and possible loss of function, even amputation (see Color Plates 2 and 3 [Figures 19-3 and 19-4]).

Prevention and assessment

Because there are no universally effective, optimal means of treating vesicant extravasation, the best approach is prevention. The Cancer Chemotherapy Guidelines and Recommendations for the Management of Vesicant Extravasation[3] is an excellent resource for nurses and physicians to implement preventive care and for the design of appropriate policies and procedures in individual practice settings. The official position of the Oncology Nursing Society is that all personnel who administer chemotherapy should receive training in chemotherapy drug administration and management of toxicities, including drug extravasation. Institutionally approved guidelines for extravasation management should be readily available, reviewed, and revised regularly as appropriate. The physician's guidelines or institutional protocol for the management of a presumed or proven extravasation should be readily available wherever vesicant drugs are administered and instituted immediately in the event of an extravasation. The procedure for documenting and reporting an actual or suspected extravasation should be clearly defined.

The signs and symptoms of an extravasation may be very obvious or extremely subtle. The one obvious sign of drug infiltration is a bleb formation at the injection site that is readily apparent in a superficial vein, or swelling that occurs in more deeply accessed veins. In the absence of pain, swelling, or diffuse induration, an extravasation may go unnoticed, especially when the vein lies deep within an obese limb. In this situation, a large amount of drug can infiltrate, especially if the drug is injected slowly.

Pain can be an early or late symptom depending on the patient's ability to report this sensation. If a patient is elderly and confused or heavily sedated, symptoms may go unreported. Any antiemetics, sedatives, or analgesics that may affect the patient's ability to readily report any change in sensation at the injection site should be withheld until after the vesicant has been safely administered. The report of any change in sensation such as pain, stinging, or burning at the injection site warrants further investigation to ensure an intact vein. The vesicant injection is stopped immediately and the vein is aspirated to ensure a blood return. In the absence of any swelling, pain, or evidence of infiltration, the injection of the vesicant may continue following a copious (30–40 mL) saline flush. If the patient again complains of discomfort despite the presence of a blood return and absence of swelling, the site should be flushed with saline once more and the IV discontinued. Drug administration is resumed at another appropriate site despite the absence of any evidence of extravasation. Mitomycin has been associated with subtle extravasation; therefore, in the presence of any discomfort, the nurse is cautioned to immediately stop the injection, flush copiously with saline, and restart the IV despite the absence of any objective signs of extravasation.

A blood return should be assessed every 1–2 mL of drug administration. The presence of a blood return is valuable to determine venous access but does not always ensure an intact vein. A blood return can be obtained in the presence of an extravasation as the needle may extend partially through the vein, allowing for a subtle leakage of the vesicant into the subcutaneous tissues. In this situation, the blood return will be weak instead of full and brisk. On the other hand, the absence of a blood return in no way confirms an extravasation. The needle bevel or cannula tip, on aspiration, may become positioned against the vein wall, preventing appropriate and obvious blood return. In this situation, the clinician may choose to restart the IV or rely on other measures of assessing venous integrity. Often, the patient does not have numerous venous access sites from which to choose. While one would always want to spare the patient another needle stick, it is often better to restart the IV elsewhere, especially when, after flushing with saline, there remains any doubt of an intact vein.

Rarely, if ever, is the administration of chemotherapy an emergency situation, meaning that if the nurse determines that the patient has no optimal means of safely receiving the vesicant agent, then the nurse should confer with the physician regarding placement of a VAD, after which the drug may be administered. In the current milieu of cancer treatment and with the variety of short- and long-term VADs available, the nurse should not feel compelled to administer vesicant agents in less than optimally safe circumstances. These devices have become a common method of drug delivery and, depending on the patient's individual treatment plan, may be recommended prior to beginning chemotherapy.

While generally considered a reliable and safe means of drug delivery, implanted ports and, less commonly, tunneled catheters do sometimes result in extravasations of vesicant agents. In the case of implanted ports, the cause of drug extravasation is usually a misplaced or displaced needle. In this situation, the drug extravasates into the port pocket or area surrounding the port. Another mechanism for drug extravasation from ports involves retrograde subcutaneous leakage from percutaneously inserted catheters obstructed by a fibrin sheath.[43,44] Extravasation may also occur into the subcutaneous tunnel, either from thrombosis and backtracking or from a damaged or fractured central venous catheter. Extravasation may also occur into the intrathoracic cavity as a complication of catheter placement.

Prior to injecting or infusing a vesicant into a tunneled central venous catheter or a nontunneled centrally or peripherally placed central venous catheter (e.g., peripherally inserted central catheter [PICC]), examine the exit site for leaks and the insertion site for evidence of swelling or venous thrombosis. Catheter displacement may be evidenced by the appearance of the cuff extruding from the exit site or of the obviously more white segment of catheter at the exit site, indicating that the catheter has been pulled or slipped out of place. Observe the insertion site (usually the ipsilateral supraclavicular area) for evidence of swelling during fluid bolus. Any evidence of swelling or subjective complaints by the patient of pain or discomfort during fluid bolus warrants investigation.

The presence of a blood return from an implanted port or a tunneled catheter usually confirms catheter tip placement. However, it is not uncommon for a catheter to be properly placed without evidence of catheter damage and still have an absent or intermittent blood return. The catheter or port remains safe to use, provided it flushes easily without subjective complaints. If, however, the patient complains of discomfort with fluid injection or if the flow demonstrates resistance, becomes sluggish, or does not flow freely with gravity, it is possible that the catheter tip is somehow intermittently obstructed, the

catheter has drifted or migrated into a smaller ancillary vein, or it has otherwise become bent or coiled, preventing backflow of blood (Figures 19-5 and 19-6). It is important in these situations to determine catheter placement by radiological means. The injection of fluid or chemotherapy should be withheld pending physician examination.

When giving vesicant agents through a port, whether by simple injection or long-term infusion, it is important to use a 90-degree bent huber-point needle rather than a straight needle. Straight needles can easily become dislodged because there is no way to stabilize them regardless of how brief the injection time. Patients are instructed to report any pain, burning, tightness, stinging, or discomfort over the chest area during the injection or infusion. When injecting a vesicant, the blood return is assessed before the injection and at the conclusion of the injection. During the short-term or long-term infusion of a vesicant, assessment of blood return is variable depending on the status of the patient. In some situations where the patient is confused or uncooperative, it is reasonable to question whether it is safe to use a port for long-term vesicant infusions because these needles can become dislodged even under the best conditions.

It is difficult to determine how frequently a catheter should be aspirated during the infusion of a vesicant in the hospitalized individual to determine the presence or absence of a blood return. If the catheter or port never

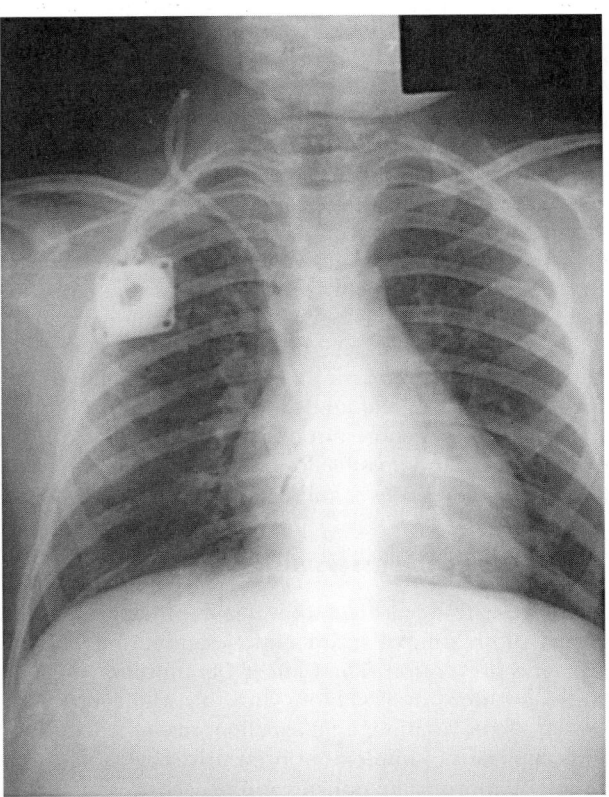

Figure 19-5 Catheter bent causing resistance during infusion and lack of blood return.

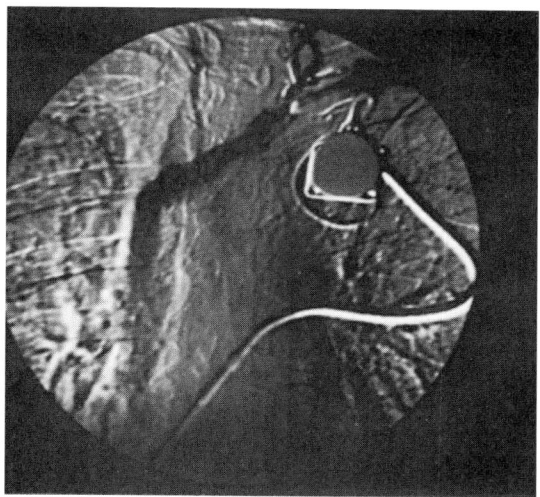

Figure 19-6 Catheter coiled around port as demonstrated by digital subtraction venogram.

had a blood return prior to instituting the vesicant infusion, then assessment of the site every hour as would be done with any intravenous infusion seems appropriate. If a blood return is known to exist, then assessment of blood return will vary from institution to institution, but assessment at the beginning of each shift seems appropriate, with hourly visual examination of the infusion/insertion site. More frequent catheter aspiration such as at the beginning and end of each shift or every 4 hours would appear excessive and could significantly increase risk for infection.

The ideal catheter for infusion of vesicant agents in the outpatient/home environment is the tunneled externally based catheter or PICC line. In some situations where a port is already in place, this device can safely be employed for vesicant infusions provided the patient is capable of regularly assessing the site for proper needle placement.

Management

If a frank extravasation has occurred, it will usually be obvious to patient and nurse at the time it occurs. In some situations, however, the actual symptoms are delayed for 24–48 hours. The patient may report a redness over the injection site that is warm to the touch. Most often, these delayed symptoms indicate that only a small amount of drug actually infiltrated. Color Plate 4 (Figure 19-7) depicts a doxorubicin extravasation 12 days after drug administration. There was no pain with movement of the area, which healed spontaneously without local treatment. Color Plate 5 (Figure 19-8) demonstrates erythema and edema at the injection site one week after doxorubicin administration. At the time of administration, blood return was lost and the patient complained of slight pain at the site. The drug was stopped. After flushing with saline, slight swelling was noted over the area. Ice was applied. This area progressed to blister for-

mation in 3 weeks, with clear demarcation of the damaged area (see Color Plate 6 [Figure 19-9]), which was surgically excised (see Color Plate 7 [Figure 19-10]).

When there is cause to believe that an extravasation of a vesicant agent has occurred during drug administration, prompt nursing action will, in general, minimize tissue damage. The nurse is responsible for ensuring that all antidotes and diluents are readily available and accessible. The following outlines appropriate steps to be taken if an extravasation is suspected.

1. Stop the administration of the chemotherapeutic agent. If injecting through the side arm of a free-flowing IV, stop the fluid flow immediately; failure to do so further disperses the infiltrated drug into the tissues.
2. Disconnect the intravenous tubing or syringe and attach an empty 10-mL syringe. Attempt to aspirate any residual drug in the tubing and at the site. Stabilize the extremity and tape the syringe in place.
3. If unable to aspirate any blood or residual drug from the tubing, remove the needle. Gentle apply a sterile 2 × 2 gauze pad over the needle entrance site.
4. Prepare the antidote according to institutional policy and procedure (Table 19-6).[45–47]
5. Replace syringe with antidote-filled syringe and inject the antidote.
6. If the needle has been removed, inject the antidote subcutaneously into the extravasation site using a single injection of a 25-gauge needle.
7. Remove the needle.
8. Avoid applying direct manual pressure to the site.
9. Photograph the extravasation site prior to applying a loose sterile dressing.
10. Apply a warm compress in the event of a plant alkyloid extravasation 15 minutes or more four times daily for 24 hours.
11. Apply ice for 15 minutes or more every 3–4 hours for 24–48 hours as tolerated in the event of an anthracycline extravasation.
12. Notify the attending physician that an extravasation has occurred or is suspected.
13. Instruct the patient on local care, systemic analgesics, and plan for follow-up.
    a. Elevate the extremity for 48 hours.
    b. After the first 48 hours, the patient should be encouraged to use the extremity normally. Failure to do so may result in stiffness, neuropathy, and causalgia.[46]
    c. Arrange for a return appointment once or twice weekly depending on the amount of drug suspected to have extravasated and the patient's individual concerns.
    d. Photograph the site weekly as appropriate. Document degree of erythema, induration, pain, and whether there is evidence of ulceration or necrosis.
    e. If pain persists beyond 7–10 days, confer with physician regarding a plastic surgery consultation, especially if there is evidence of ulcer demarcation.

Table 19-6 Management of Selected Vesicant Extravasations

Chemotherapeutic Agent	Mechanism of Tissue Damage and Clinical Course	Pharmacological Antidote	Local Management	Comments
Doxorubicin (Adriamycin)	Binds to nucleic acids leading to prolonged tissue damage Drug is steadily released from dead or dying cells, thereby causing damage to neighboring cells	None	Apply ice for 15 min q3–4h as tolerated × 24–48 hr Elevate the extremity for 48 hr Resume normal activities after 48 hr Physical therapy may be appropriate to prevent stiffness and neuralgia Topical (1–2 mL) dimethylsulfoxide (99%) applied to the site q6h may be beneficial	Less extensive (1–2 mL/2 mg/mL) extravasations tend to heal spontaneously More extensive (>3 mL) extravasations follow an indolent course, usually causing ulceration, eschar formation, and pain Surgical intervention with skin grafting may be required
Daunorubicin (Cerubidine, daunomycin)	Binds to nucleic acids leading to prolonged tissue damage (See doxorubicin) Severe pain may be noted during infusion of the drug Cellulitis may occur without extravasation	None	Ice or local cooling has not been beneficial, but may be used to increase comfort Heat increases ulceration Surgical excision is usually needed to remove necrotic tissue and locally entrapped drug Little information is currently available. Extravasations may be managed like doxorubicin extravasation	Topical DMSO 99% may help to minimize ulceration
Idarubicin (epirubicin, Idamycin)	Both drugs have vesicant properties similar to doxorubicin	None	Little information is currently available. Extravasations may be managed like doxorubicin extravasation	
Mechlorethamine (nitrogen mustard, Mustargen)	Drug rapidly fixes to tissues, causing immediate tissue damage Drug is probably not recycled locally Immediate, often intense pain is noted if extravasated Thrombophlebitis of the injected vein is common Perivenous hyperpigmentation may occur following a single injection	Isotonic sodium thiosulfate Mix 4 mL 10% sodium thiosulfate with 6 mL sterile H_2O or 1.6 mL 25% sodium thiosulfate with 8.4 mL sterile H_2O Yield 10 mL 1/6 molar solution sodium thiosulfate	Inject 1–4 mL 1/6 molar solution of sodium thiosulfate through existing IV line or subcutaneously if IV has been removed Inject 1 mL for each mg extravasated Topical cooling may promote comfort but does not appear to minimize ulceration	Sodium thiosulfate neutralizes nitrogen mustard Initiate local treatment immediately Ensure availability of sodium thiosulfate and sterile water for injection in extravasation kit prior to initiating injection of nitrogen mustard
Vincristine (Oncovin) Vinblastine (Velban) Teniposide (Vumon)	These agents do not bind to DNA, but inhibit mitosis. Tissue damage tends to follow a more indolent course	Hyaluronidase (Wydase) (refrigerate) Mix 150 U/mL hyaluronidase with 1 mL of sodium chloride	Inject 1.4 mL through existing IV line or subcutaneously if IV has been removed Administer 1 mL for each mL extravasated	Both hyaluronidase and heat act to enhance the systemic absorption from subcutaneous spaces

Table 19-6 Management of Selected Vesicant Extravasations (continued)

Chemotherapeutic Agent	Mechanism of Tissue Damage and Clinical Course	Pharmacological Antidote	Local Management	Comments
Vindesine (Eldisine)	Pain, localized swelling, and erythema typically occur if these drugs are extravasated		Apply warm compress 15 min four times a day × 48 hr	Local cooling, vitamin A cream, and hydrocortisone injection significantly increase vinca alkaloid skin ulcers
				Symptoms of vindesine extravasation may be delayed. Ulceration and delayed healing (6 mo) have been noted
Vinorelbine (Navelbine)		None		Vinorelbine may be associated with an intense aching along the injected vein 12–24 hr after the injection, persisting for 3–4 days. Systemic analgesics may be necessary.
				To reduce incidence of phlebitis administer vinorelbine over 6–10 min into the side-port or a free-flowing IV most distant from the patient.
Etoposide (VePesid)	Blister formation may occur within a week of extravasation and gradually resolve without frank ulceration	None		
	If ulceration does occur, healing is often prolonged, taking 5–6 mo			
Mitomycin C (Mutamycin)	Frank and obvious mitomycin C extravasation is associated with intense pain gradually resulting in painful ulceration, necrosis, and eschar formation	None	DMSO may provide some benefit in the treatment of mitomycin C extravasation, but further research is needed	Mitomycin C may cause dermal ulceration at sites distant from injection site
	Surgical debridement is usually necessary where significant extravasation has occurred		Protect from sunlight	Glucocorticoids appear to offer no therapeutic benefit in the treatment of immediate or delayed mitomycin C extravasations, and may even worsen ulceration
	Delayed skin ulceration may appear at a previous injection site			Neither heating nor cooling has proved therapeutic
	Extravasation may occur without any evidence of pain or swelling at the site with delay of ulceration occurring weeks to months later			
Dactinomycin (Actinomycin D, Cosmegen)	Dactinomycin is a potent intercalating agent that causes intense pain and ulceration if extravasated	None	Ice may be applied to the site to increase comfort Elevate area for 48 hr Resume normal activities after 48 hr Consult plastic surgeon if pain persists for >7–10 days	Neither topical cooling nor DMSO is effective local treatment for extravasation of dactinomycin Heat may significantly enhance tissue damage

DMSO = dimethyl sulfoxide.

    f. Consider physical therapy consultation to encourage normal use of the extremity during healing.

14. Complete extravasation documentation record (see Figure 19-1), paying special attention to subjective complaints and objective observations of the details immediately surrounding the extravasation event.

Paclitaxel and docetaxel are similar antineoplastic agents that are considered to be moderate irritants with the potential to cause ulceration if large amounts of the drug infiltrate. These drugs are routinely infused via peripheral veins, some with the assistance of an infusion pump. In most health care settings, vesicants are not administered with the force of a peristaltic infusion pump into a peripheral vein. In the case of these drugs, it is important to use caution in the manner in which they are given. There is evidence clinically that both paclitaxel and docetaxel cause a moderate degree of tissue damage when infiltrated, and most clinicians consider them to be irritants. Once infiltrated, the amount of tissue damage appears to be related to the amount and concentration of the drug infiltrated.[47] The injection of hyaluronidase (300 units) into the area of infiltration has been recommended.[3] Currently the application of heat to the site of infiltration of either paclitaxel or docetaxel is not recommended. Color Plate 8 (Figure 19-11) depicts a docetaxel infiltration. At four weeks, the area is peeling and somewhat tender. No ulceration occurred. The clear line of demarcation is the outline of the warm cloth that appeared to aggravate more than help the condition.[48]

Extravasation from a central venous catheter (tunneled, nontunneled, implanted port, or PICC line) may be substantial before detected because infusions are not monitored constantly and the vesicant may be more diluted than when given by intravenous injection. Therefore, pain at the site may not be noted early. Dressings over the port site may mask swelling. Because infusions tend to be given slowly, a considerable amount of drug can extravasate without obvious evidence of leakage. In the case of an implanted port, the cause is usually needle dislodgment from the port septum, where the needle is found lying in the subcutaneous tissue. The degree of tissue damage will depend on the concentration of the drug and the amount infiltrated. In some cases, there may be no tissue breakdown; in others, wide excision including mastectomy may be required for the wound to heal.

If an extravasation is suspected from a central venous catheter, the infusion is immediately stopped and the physician is notified. An attempt should be made to estimate the amount of drug extravasated. It may be possible to aspirate residual drug from the site. An antidote can be administered if available. Otherwise, the needle should be removed. Efforts to manually express fluid from the site should be avoided. Instead, a sterile dressing should be applied over the needle entrance site and changed frequently. Ice or warm packs should be applied per institutional policy and procedure. Appropriate documentation (extravasation documentation record) should be completed, and plans for careful follow-up and additional consultation with a surgeon may be appropriate.

Intraarterial

Intraarterial drug administration, a drug delivery practice that gained popularity in the early 1980s, involves cannulation of the artery that provides a tumor's blood supply and subsequent administration of the drug directly through the arterial catheter to the tumor bed.[49] This practice increases the concentration of the drug to known areas of tumor and decreases the systemic drug concentration and thus the side effects. The primary use of this route is the hepatic artery for the management of potential or actual metastasis of colon cancer to the liver. It has also been used for hepatocellular carcinoma. The antineoplastic drugs used include fluorouracil, floxuridine, doxorubicin, and mitomycin C, among others.

The most common method of intraarterial drug delivery involves placement of a silastic catheter into the main artery supplying the tumor. This catheter is then attached either to an implanted port or a pump (i.e., Medtronics or Infusaid pump). The Infusaid pump (Infusaid, Inc., Norwood, MA) and the Synchromed Infusion System (Medtronics, Inc., Minneapolis, MN) are examples of subcutaneously implanted pumps. The catheter is inserted into the appropriate artery and then attached to the pump located in a surgically created subcutaneous pocket, usually in the lower abdomen or upper chest. The pump chamber is accessed via a noncoring needle and filled with either chemotherapy or heparinized sterile saline. The flow rates are dependent on pump design and are either preset prior to implantation or adjustable via an external electronic wand that communicates with the internal pump. Obviously, care and maintenance of these devices by the nurse requires a formalized educational program and ongoing monitoring of pump functioning.

The implantable pump offers the patient the greatest level of freedom when receiving intraarterial chemotherapy, and the pump has lower complication rates than external methods. One potential disadvantage is the cost. The pump plus the implantation can be extremely costly, and insurance companies under managed care may not agree to pay. When compared to intermittent hospitalization, an ambulatory pump is usually deemed to be cost-effective if therapy is anticipated for a minimum of 3–6 months or longer. In fact, long-term therapy with an external pump can eventually cost more due to the cost of disposable supplies.

Nursing considerations involve monitoring for drug side effects and potential pump complications, such as infection, occlusion, extravasation, and malfunction. Some unique nursing actions are necessary when dealing with implantable pumps, such as not aspirating the center septum, monitoring or establishing pump flow rate, and detecting malfunctions. The oncology nurse is referred to the manufacturers' instructions and guidelines regarding the management of these advanced nursing responsibilities.

Intraperitoneal

Regional delivery of chemotherapy into the peritoneal space has been found to be a safe and effective treatment for locally recurrent ovarian and colon cancers. The antineoplastic agents used include cisplatin, carboplatin, etoposide, doxorubicin, and cytarabine, among others.

The semipermeable nature of the peritoneal space allows high concentrations of the drugs to be achieved at the tumor sites throughout but with lower concentrations entering the bloodstream. The procedure causes local side effects due to the large volume of fluid filling the space, and the drugs cause systemic side effects that are mild or delayed when compared to intravenous administration of the same drugs. It is possible with some of the drugs to minimize the systemic side effects by simultaneously infusing an agent intravenously to counteract drug side effects through the venous system. This is most commonly achieved during the intraperitoneal instillation of cisplatin by infusing intravenous sodium thiosulfate, which appears to decrease the renal toxicities of the cisplatin.[50]

There are three methods of accessing the peritoneal space: (1) intermittent placement of temporary indwelling catheters; (2) placement of a Tenckhoff external catheter; and (3) placement of an implantable peritoneal port.[51,52] Intermittent placement might be used if the therapy is planned for a short time, such as for symptom relief or palliation. Tenckhoff catheters or ports are placed when several months of therapy are planned, especially when the treatment goal is cure of minimal or microscopic residual disease. Tenckhoff catheters have the advantage of rapid flow rate (10–15 minutes for 2 L) and allow for catheter manipulation to dislodge fibrin deposits, if necessary. Because they are external, Tenckhoff catheters require care and maintenance by the patient and may result in an increased incidence of infection or leakage around the catheter. The implanted port is internal and requires no care when not accessed and so has a potentially lower rate of infection. Disadvantages include a slower flow rate (30–45 minutes for 2 L), a needle stick required for access, and a surgical procedure necessary for removal.

Nursing considerations include patient education, assessing the catheter or port patency, establishing access, administering systemic therapies as ordered, instilling the infusate, monitoring patient response to the procedure, draining the infusate (if ordered), side effect management, and documentation as outlined in Table 19-7.

Side effects of the drugs used for intraperitoneal chemotherapy are variable and depend on the agents being administered. Regardless of the drugs administered, complications specific to the intraperitoneal route include respiratory distress, abdominal pain, discomfort, and diarrhea, which are due to increased intraabdominal pressure. Appropriate interventions to manage these problems include elevation of the head of the bed, instructing the patient to roll from side to side to distribute the infusate, and administering analgesics. Mechanical difficulties can occur and include inflow or outflow occlusions caused by fibrin sheath formation over the catheter, other outflow occlusions, and catheter migration. Other complications include infection, chemical irritation of the peritoneal space, electrolyte imbalances, and with an implantable port drug extravasation.

In general, intraperitoneal chemotherapy is well tolerated by patients and provides a safe, effective treatment for the management of peritoneal disease, particularly ovarian carcinoma. Patients are frequently able to maintain a normal lifestyle, for this route is successfully utilized in inpatient, ambulatory, and home care settings, with fewer side effects than traditional intravenous therapy.

Intrapleural

Care of the patient with a pleural effusion traditionally involves insertion of chest tubes, drainage of the fluid, and sclerosis of the pleural space to prevent recurrence of the effusion. When the effusion is caused by malignant cells, the preferred treatment is sclerosis with an antineoplastic agent such as nitrogen mustard or bleomycin.[53] This is accomplished in the usual sterile manner by injecting the drug directly into the chest tube and clamping it for a specified time (e.g., 24 hours). The procedure can be repeated daily for several days if necessary. Nursing management of intrapleural chemotherapy includes patient education, safe drug handling, and side effect management. Nitrogen mustard is well known for its emetogenic properties, and treatment with adequate antiemetics is necessary. Also, severe pleural pain can accompany intrapleural nitrogen mustard, and a strong narcotic such as morphine sulfate is frequently ordered as a premedication and for 24–48 hours afterward. Use of a patient-controlled anesthesia (PCA) pump is ideal for patient control of the analgesic agent to ensure adequate pain control. Bleomycin does not cause pain but instead may cause mild nausea or fever and chills, similar to its intravenous side effect profile. In general, nursing care focuses on emesis control, pain control, respiratory status, chest tube security, and other comfort measures, depending on the drug used.

The process just described is a standard procedure that has been moderately successful for many years. The quest for newer and better forms of sclerosing therapy has led to a variety of alternatives that appear equal to or better than traditional therapy. These include:

- Use of other agents, including methylprednisolone,[49] doxorubicin hydrochloride–containing poly (L-lactic acid) microspheres (ADR-MS),[54] and cisplatin plus cytarabine[55] (all agents being used investigationally)

- Insertion of small-bore percutaneously placed catheters or implantable ports with drainage and subse-

Table 19-7 Nursing Considerations in Intraperitoneal Drug Administration

Patient Education

- Instruct the patient in the care of the catheter or port prior to its insertion.

- Immediately prior to initiating therapy, explain the drug administration process, side effects of the drugs, side effects of the route, and measures to manage/minimize the side effects.

- Teach the patient and/or family how to care for the catheter at home, if appropriate.

Pretreatment and Site Access

- Verify the drug order and normal serum electrolyte levels.

- Insert a urinary catheter to straight drainage, if ordered, and initiate intake and output measurements.

- Ensure that intravenous therapy is proceeding as ordered. (IP cisplatin infusions usually include prehydration for 12–24 hr with IV fluids containing potassium and magnesium supplements. A few moments before initiating the IP cisplatin, IV sodium thiosulfate is begun to neutralize the systemic cisplatin and to prevent renal toxicities and severe nausea and vomiting.)

- Gather appropriate supplies and materials, and wash hands.

- Assess the area around the catheter or port for redness, edema, warmth, or tenderness.

- Organize materials, don gloves (and gown if desired).

- Access external catheter directly after a thorough povidone-iodine scrub of the external hub using aseptic technique, *or*

- Access implanted port using aseptic technique and a large-gauge, noncoring, 90-degree needle of appropriate length (usually 1–1.5 in.); anesthetize the skin surface prior to access, if desired, with 2% xylocaine, Emla Cream, or ice.

- Flush the catheter with 10–20 mL of nonbacteriostatic sterile saline; catheter should flush easily.

- Administer antiemetics, if ordered.

Drug Administration

- Initiate IV sodium thiosulfate, if ordered.

- Position patient comfortably in a semi-Fowler's position (elevate head of bed).

- Open the clamp on the tubing, and infuse the warmed IP chemotherapy at the prescribed rate (usually over 30 min to several hours).

- Stop infusion immediately if severe pain is experienced and check for catheter migration (usually with x-ray verification).

- Slow the rate of infusion if the patient experiences shortness of breath or discomfort.

- Administer analgesics as prescribed, if necessary.

- Apply blankets if patient feels chilled.

- Close the clamp on the tubing when the infusion is complete, and encourage repositioning from side to side every 15 min during the dwell time (usually 2–4 hr).

- Monitor patient's comfort levels and observe for shortness of breath, abdominal discomfort, or diarrhea.

- After the prescribed dwell time, open the clamp to the drainage bag and allow the solution to drain. If flow is sluggish, check tubing for kinks, help patient roll from side to side, have patient use the Valsalva maneuver, apply manual pressure to the abdomen, or irrigate the catheter with normal saline.

- Recognize that the volume of drained fluid may be less than that infused, and reassure patient that the fluid will be reabsorbed and metabolized.

- Clamp tubing on drainage bag after fluid has drained (usually 30 min to 2 hr), and send specimen, properly labeled as cytotoxic, to cytology or dispose of in proper hazardous waste container.

Postadministration Care

- Flush catheter or port with nonbacteriostatic sterile saline; if using a port, follow with heparinized saline.

- Secure site using standard technique (i.e., cap and secure catheter or remove needle from port, and cover site with a small dressing, if necessary).

- Establish IV fluids as prescribed, or discontinue IV needle.

- Assess patient's status; ensure ability to perform self-care, if appropriate.

- Document procedure in medical record.

IP = intraperitoneal; IV = intravenous.

---

quent sclerosing instead of large-bore closed-tube thoracostomy[56,57] (see Chapter 30)

- Implantation of pleuroperitoneal shunts[58]

The most noteworthy of these advances is small-bore catheter placement, which is easily accomplished with only mild discomfort and without the major trauma of regular chest tube insertion. Also, for recurrent pleural effusion, thoracentesis can be performed repeatedly via an implantable port, with the catheter portion in the pleural space and the portal on the lower rib cage. Acceptance and clinical utilization of these techniques are variable, and the oncology nurse is encouraged to be aware of the specific procedures used and the established policies describing the nurse's role in administering intrapleural chemotherapy.

Intravesical

Direct instillation of chemotherapy into the bladder has proved to be an extremely effective and simple method of controlling superficial bladder cancer and carcinoma in situ. Agents such as thiotepa, doxorubicin, mitomycin C, and bacillus Calmette-Guérin (BCG) have all been shown to be effective, especially BCG. Instillation is usually weekly for 4–12 weeks and involves insertion of a urinary catheter, instillation of the drug (usually in 50–60 mL of sterile solution), and retention of the drug for 1–2 hours (with frequent movement to disperse the drug throughout the bladder) prior to unclamping the catheter or voiding. Some physicians prefer to have the urinary catheter remain clamped and in place for the dwell time. In this case, the fluid that drains from the catheter when it is unclamped should be contained and disposed of properly (i.e., sealed, then labeled as cytotoxic waste). If the physician prefers to withdraw the catheter after drug instillation and instructs the patient to void in 1–2 hours, the patient should flush the toilet twice after voiding. Local side effects such as bladder irritation or, with mitomycin C, dermatitis of the external genitalia can be experienced. A unique side effect of BCG is a "creepy-crawly" feeling sometimes referred to as "BCG-osis."[59,60] Patients report feeling as if their skin is creeping or little things are crawling on them. Administration of a mild sedative can be considered if this side effect occurs.

While initial studies of intravesical chemotherapy demonstrated an apparent decreased incidence of recurrent bladder tumors, this finding has not been corroborated by long-term studies. Therefore, it appears that the role of intravesical chemotherapy will be as a single postoperative instillation rather than as long-term maintenance therapy.[61]

Nursing considerations for patients receiving intravesical chemotherapy include patient education (stressing hand washing and personal hygiene), drug administration, side effect monitoring, and safe drug handling. For most oncology nurses, it is unusual to have experience with this method of drug delivery, as it is commonly performed in urologists' offices as part of a postoperative office visit.

Intrathecal or Intraventricular

Cancer cells can cross the blood-brain barrier and appear in the cerebrospinal fluid (CSF), resulting in central nervous system involvement of the malignancy. This phenomenon is seen most commonly in leukemia (meningeal leukemia) and to a lesser extent in other malignancies, such as breast cancer, lymphoma, and rhabdomyosarcoma (meningeal carcinomatosis). Unfortunately, available antineoplastic agents are unable to enter the CSF in sufficient concentrations to kill the cancer cells effectively, so chemotherapy is injected directly into the CSF as prophylaxis or to manage existing disease. The antineoplastic drugs used include methotrexate, cytarabine, thiotepa, and interferon. When prepared for use by this route, the preservative-free drug is always admixed under strictly sterile conditions with a preservative-free diluent such as sodium chloride USP (unpreserved) or Ringer's injection USP (unpreserved). Methotrexate is available in an unpreserved lyophilized form for intrathecal use. Cytarabine is supplied with a diluent that contains benzyl alcohol and should be replaced with an appropriate unpreserved diluent (sodium chloride or Ringer's solution).

The two primary methods of instillation are intrathecal and intraventricular. The intrathecal route is achieved by performing a standard lumbar puncture, using established techniques to ascertain placement, and injecting 10–12 mL of drug, followed by withdrawal of the needle. This procedure usually is performed by a physician or a nurse practitioner on a daily to weekly basis, depending on the protocol being followed. This method is quick and easy to perform but is disadvantageous because the drug may reach only epidural or subdural spaces. Even when it reaches the subarachnoid space, therapeutic levels of the drug usually are not achieved in the ventricles. For this reason, many physicians prefer intraventricular drug administration.

Central instillation of the drug into the ventricle can be achieved via an Ommaya reservoir (Figure 19-12), which is surgically implanted through the cranium. A skin flap is created, and the Ommaya reservoir is placed underneath the skin, with the catheter extending from the reservoir to the ventricle. Once the surgical site has healed, the only visible evidence of the device is a small bump on the head. Placement of this reservoir obviously involves greater risk than performance of a lumbar puncture, but it provides permanent intraventricular access for those patients in whom repeated translumbar puncture is impractical. Ommaya reservoirs are usually accessed by

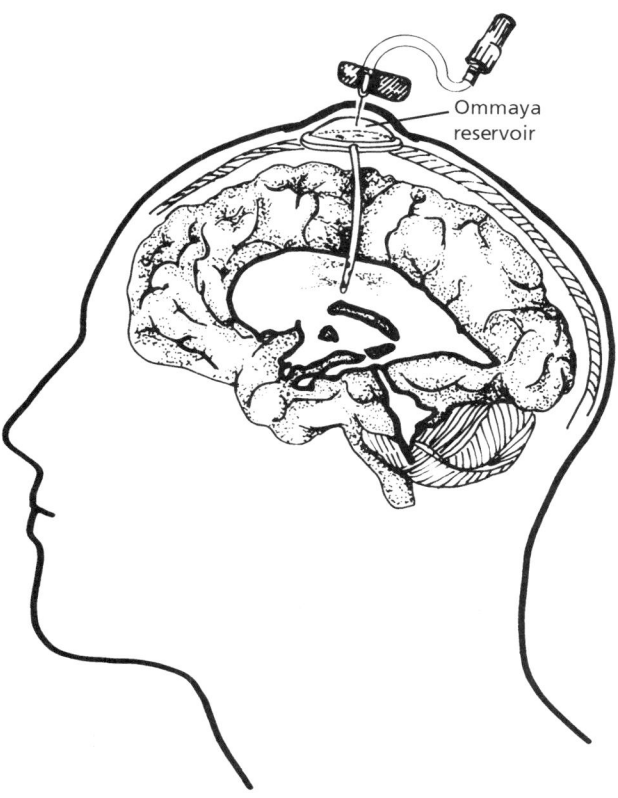

Figure 19-12 Ommaya reservoir placement.

specially trained nurses. The patient is typically in a supine position but can be sitting if that is more comfortable. The site is assessed for tenderness, redness, or warmth. The area above the Ommaya reservoir is prepared in a sterile manner with betadine in a standard circular motion, using three swabs (shaving a small area is desirable). Access is achieved using a small-gauge, noncoring needle (Table 19-8). Cerebrospinal fluid, in a volume equal to the amount of drug to be injected, is gently aspirated and if necessary can be sent for cytology or laboratory studies.

The drug is administered slowly, and resistance should not be felt. The reservoir volume is approximately 1.5–2.0

Table 19-8 Intraventricular Chemotherapy: Use of the Ommaya Reservoir

Description: The Ommaya reservoir has a catheter that rests in the lateral ventricle. The general uses of the reservoir include:
1. Sample CSF
2. Monitor CSF pressure
3. Administer analgesics into the CSF
4. Administer antibiotics into the CSF
5. Administer chemotherapy into the CSF

Equipment: Accessing the Ommaya reservoir is a sterile procedure; assemble all equipment before you begin:

Sterile gloves
Betadine swabs #3
Alcohol wipes #3
Shave/prep kit (optional)
25-gauge Butterfly needle with attached tubing
Premixed drugs (preservative-free)
Equipment for specimen collection: 3-mL syringes, collection tubes, requisitions
Small dressing or adhesive strip

Procedure:
NOTE: Shave area if needed prior to establishing a sterile field.
1. Assemble equipment; prepare a sterile field.
2. Position patient in a semirecumbent position. Support head with pillow.
3. Examine reservoir for any signs of infection. Palpate disc to locate center.
4. Cleanse area over disc in a circular motion with Betadine swabs (x3).
5. Repeat using alcohol.
6. Using a sterile procedure puncture the disc perpendicularly with the needle. Normally, CSF is clear and colorless as it rises into the tubing. Aspirate slightly to collect 2–3 mL of CSF. Set aside to flush the reservoir after drug instillation. Aspirating the CSF from the reservoir is not contraindicated but should be done gently as it may cause the reservoir catheter to become obstructed. If this occurs, flush to clear and continue collection.
7. Obtain CSF specimens for cytology/microbiology with separate syringes and set aside.
8. Attach syringe of medicine and inject drug slowly over 5–10 minutes. The fluid being injected should be amply diluted to prevent irritation to the meninges (e.g., methotrexate is usually mixed in 12 mL of preservative-free solvent).
9. Follow medicine with 2–3 mL of CSF flush.
10. Remove needle, and apply a small dressing.

---

mL, and the needle usually is flushed with a small volume of nonbacteriostatic saline to clear the drug from the needle prior to its removal. After needle withdrawal, it is common to gently "pump" the reservoir to aid in adequate drug dispersement. The patient frequently will hear a slight whooshing or squishing sound when the reservoir is depressed and then refills. No heparinization or intermittent flushing is necessary, as CSF flows freely through the device. Patients are instructed to rest in a supine position for approximately 30 minutes following the procedure.

Regardless of the specific delivery method, nursing considerations include patient education, assessment of the access site, administration (or assistance with administration) of the drug, safe drug handling, and side effect management. Even though intravenous drugs do not cross the blood-brain barrier in sufficient concentration to treat meningeal disease, the intraventricular drugs are capable of entering the systemic bloodstream. Side effects of the drugs, such as nausea, stomatitis, and mild myelosuppression, are to be anticipated. Special care should be taken with methotrexate, particularly if it is given with another drug such as cytarabine or in conjunction with radiation therapy. Leucovorin may be given orally to prevent unnecessarily severe systemic toxicities. The expected side effects related to intraventricular drug administration include headache, nausea, vomiting, ataxia, blurred vision, and transient paresthesias. The most serious complication for which to observe is infection, which is manifested by tenderness, redness, drainage, warmth or fever, stiff neck, and headache (with or without vomiting). Acute chemical arachnoiditis characterized by headache, back pain, vomiting, fever, and nuchal rigidity has been reported. This reaction appears to be more common in the elderly and in the presence of reduced cerebral glucose and protein metabolism accompanied by altered blood-brain barrier permeability.[62]

Vascular Access Devices

The development of central venous catheters (CVCs) and other types of long-term VADs has enhanced the lives of oncology patients but added a new series of concerns and challenges for their caregivers. Device selection, patient selection, use, maintenance, complication management, and product development continue to be refined by practice and research. Use of VADs is not restricted to the cancer population, and the oncology nurse often serves as an expert resource to other users of the devices.

There are many different kinds of catheters, needles, and implantable ports used for cancer chemotherapy delivery. Some of the major VAD types and features are outlined in Table 19-9. The nurse has an important role in assessing the patient's vascular access needs and selecting or recommending placement of the proper device. Intermittent peripheral venous access is preferred for patients with good veins who are on limited intermittent

Table 19-9 Overview of Available Vascular Access Devices

Type	Description	Longevity	Comments
Peripheral needle Scalp vein Butterfly	• Stainless steel • Single lumen • 27- to 19-gauge	Minutes to days	• Excellent for short-term access, especially outpatient • Increased risk of infiltration with long-term use
Peripheral catheter Intima	• Catheter over needle • Teflon or polyurethane • Single and double lumen • 26- to 14-gauge	Hours to days	• Excellent for multiday infusional therapy • Provides greater patient mobility as less likely to infiltrate
Nontunneled central venous catheter	• Polyurethane or silicone catheter • Single, double, and triple lumen	Hours to months	• Excellent for emergency need for CVC • Can augment existing VAD for acute care needs or longer-term use • Inserted by physician at bedside or in procedure room
Peripherally inserted central catheters (PICCs)	• Silicone elastomer or other polymers • Single and double lumen • 24- to 16-gauge	Weeks to months	• Excellent for continuous infusion over several weeks or months • Can be inserted at bedside by specially trained nurse • Quick, easy central access without surgical procedure • Requires external site care and routine flushing
Tunneled central venous catheter	• Silicone catheter with Dacron cuff • Single, double, and triple lumen • 4.2–19.2 Fr; 40- to 90-cm length • Groshong has slit valve, requiring less flushing	Months to years	• Excellent for long-term, continuous, or intermittent therapy • Preferred for long-term TPN administration • Preferred by many for vesicant infusional therapy • Requires external site care and routine flushing
Implantable port	• Titanium, stainless steel, silastic, or plastic portal attached to catheter • Single and double lumen • Access with noncoring needle • Low profile ports available	Months to years	• Excellent for long-term, intermittent infusional therapy • No site care required when not in use so excellent for patients unable to perform site care • Surgical procedure required for removal
Peripheral port	• Titanium portal attached to silastic catheter • Single lumen • Access with noncoring 22-gauge needle	Months to years	• Ideal for intermittent access, particularly for those patients with active lifestyles or body image concerns • No external site care when not in use • Not ideal for blood draw due to small volume

CVC = central venous catheter; VAD = venous access device; TPN = total parenteral nutrition.

therapies not involving vesicant infusions. Even multiday infusional therapy can easily be administered through peripheral veins when vascular integrity is good. A VAD should be considered in patients with poor veins, requiring multi-infusional therapy (e.g., the patient with acute leukemia receiving chemotherapy, blood products, antibiotics, and total parenteral nutrition [TPN]), long-term therapy, or continuous infusion of vesicants.

As with other aspects of chemotherapy administration, education of both the nurse and the patient and family is essential when dealing with VADs. The oncology nurse should be knowledgeable in all aspects of VAD care: selection, placement, postinsertion care, accessing, flushing, site care, troubleshooting, repairing, and removing. There is no universal standard of care for these devices. There is a need for randomized prospective clinical trials to help define the standards of care for VADs. The nurse is urged to be familiar with the particular brands of devices, the manufacturers' recommendations, existing clinical practice trends, and the established policies and procedures of the employing institution.[63,64] Patient and family education is critical, as many devices have self-care aspects that must be considered when selecting the VAD. Any patient having an external device must be able to flush, clean, and care for the device. Consideration should be given to the patient's ability to understand instructions, physical ability to manipulate the catheter, financial ability to purchase supplies, access to a clean area in the home, willingness to perform self-care activities, and compliance in reporting problems. Many excellent booklets and videotapes have been developed by VAD manufacturers and also by hospitals and health care agencies, but their usefulness depends on the nurse's assessment of the patient's ability to understand and comply with the actions described.[65]

General Management

The selection, care, and maintenance of the long-term devices vary with the type of VAD and will be addressed separately for nontunneled CVCs, tunneled central venous catheters (TCVCs), and implantable ports. Many of the major complications are handled in similar ways, so the management of complications will be addressed together for all the devices, immediately following the discussion of general management. Most CVCs will be inserted so the catheter tip ends in the superior vena cava, but for those patients in whom this is not possible, a femoral approach with the catheter tip in the inferior vena cava may be an option.

Nontunneled central venous catheters

Short-term use of a nontunneled CVC, such as a standard subclavian line, is common practice in urgent situations. When an immediate need for a central line arises, it commonly is placed by a physician at the bedside, in the intensive care unit, or in the emergency room. For oncology patients, it is primarily intended to provide immediate access until the emergency can be resolved, or in some practices silastic catheters may be used for months with low infection rates.[66] These devices are also used in oncology patients whose need for multi-infusional therapy exceeds the capabilities of an existing tunneled CVC or implantable port. A multilumen subclavian catheter might be placed in a patient with acute leukemia who is on chemotherapy, hydration, antibiotics, TPN, blood products, and other medications or in a patient on a complex investigational drug protocol. The triple-lumen central catheter can augment the long-term device during the hospitalization and be removed prior to discharge or left in place for outpatient care. The oncology patient may have a CVC in place for apheresis or dialysis. These catheters are usually dedicated to those procedures and care is directed by those departments.

For long-term use, the gap that exists between the trauma of subclavian lines and the investment in a long-term tunneled catheter or port has been narrowed with the use of PICCs.[67] From the patient's viewpoint, the PICC is the least expensive and most easily inserted long-term

CVC, but it requires self-care capabilities and often a caregiver because it is located at the antecubital fossa and self-care has to be one-handed. These small-gauge, thin-walled catheters are inserted at the antecubital fossa into the basilic or cephalic vein (Figure 19-13). The procedure is performed by a physician or a specially trained nurse at the patient's bedside. The catheter can be advanced into the superior vena cava, in which case x-ray verification of placement is required. A few state boards of nursing consider the placement of a CVC to be outside the role of a professional nurse, so it is important for the nurse to verify that placement of a PICC is within the scope of nursing as defined by the state. Some states allow PICC insertion by a nurse if it is considered a long-line catheter and is only advanced into the axillary or subclavian veins, in which case x-ray verification of placement is not necessarily required but is preferred, especially for vesicant administration. Formal training in the intricacies of PICC insertion is required as the insertion techniques vary greatly among the specific devices and success is usually technique-dependent and due to repeated practice.[66-68]

Peripherally inserted central catheters are ideal for short-term access (1 week to several months) in patients with adequate antecubital veins, self-care capabilities, and the need for a wide variety of intravenous therapies, including antibiotics, chemotherapy, TPN, and analgesics. The thin, flexible nature of the catheter does not lend itself well to blood withdrawal, but it is not contraindicated and may be successfully achieved with gentle application of

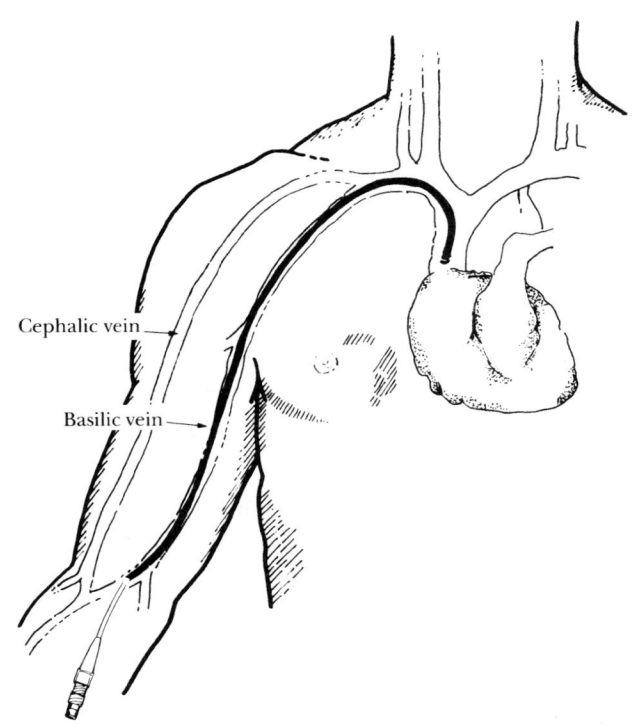

Figure 19-13 Placement of peripherally inserted central catheter (PICC).

pressure via the syringe used for blood withdrawal. The complication rate is similar to that for other VADs in terms of infection, clotting, and malfunction.[69] Some studies suggest a higher rate of phlebitis, which may be technique-dependent or caused by powdered gloves. Meticulous attention to sterile technique during insertion and rinsing the powder off the gloves prior to handling the PICC seem to decrease these complications. An overview of PICC features is given in Table 19-10.[68]

Tunneled central venous catheters

The TCVC provides safe and reliable long-term access (months to years) with a low incidence of infection, suitable for almost all hematology/oncology patients and many others as well. Tunneled CVCs continue to be well accepted and have been modified by the various manufacturers who now market similar devices. The unique features of the TCVC (Figure 19-14) include a Dacron cuff around which granulation tissue forms, actually helping to hold the catheter in place. The 4- to 10-inch tunnel through which the catheter is channeled serves to prevent the easy passage of bacteria from the skin into the vein. Also, the cuff is thought to help stop bacteria traveling along the subcutaneous portion of the catheter. A second cuff (VitaCuff; Vitaphore, San Carlos, CA) impregnated with silver ions can be attached to any catheter to help decrease the infection rate. The catheter material is usually radiopaque silicone to aid insertion and subsequent placement verification. The external portion of the TCVC has a Luer-Lok hub (to allow direct access with an intravenous infusion set) or placement of an as-needed heparin-lock adapter (to allow access via a needle or needleless system). Single-, double-, and triple-lumen TCVCs are available in various gauges and lengths (Figure 19-15). Areas of development include newer materials and antibiotic bonded catheters.[70]

One unique variation of a TCVC is the Groshong catheter (Figure 19-16), which features a closed-end radiopaque tip. Flow through the catheter is achieved via a

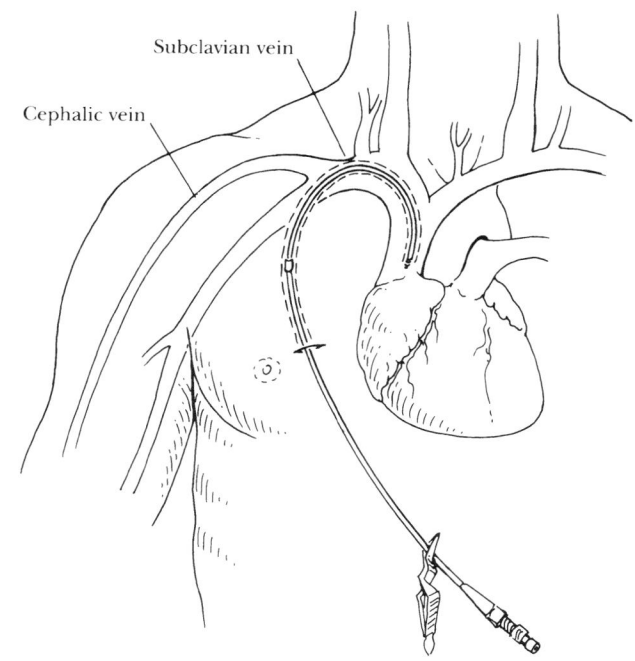

Figure 19-14 Tunneled central venous catheter placement.

patented slit valve, which opens out into the bloodstream when fluid is infusing into the catheter, opens inward into the catheter lumen when blood is being withdrawn from the catheter, and remains closed when no pressure is being applied. Groshong catheter technology has been applied to the other VADs, and Groshong ports and PICCs are available, as well as the tunneled and nontunneled CVCs. This design prevents the need for regular heparinization of the catheter, which usually is flushed with sterile normal saline (NS) once a week when not in use, making it advantageous in those patients for whom heparin is contraindicated.

Patient selection is a key issue with the TCVC because

Table 19-10 Peripherally Inserted Central Catheter (PICC) Overview

Catheter Features

- Multiple manufacturers and insertion techniques are available.
- Composed of silicone elastomer or other polymers.
- Available in single- and dual-lumen styles.
- Sizes range from 16–24 gauge and 20–60 cm in length.
- Insertion kits with introducers are available from some manufacturers.
- Cost effective compared to all other VADs.

Placement

- Successful placement is highly technique dependent; requires formal training.

- A sterile procedure at bedside; performed by registered nurse or physician.
- Requires adequate antecubital veins and x-ray verification.

Use

- Excellent for central access for 1 week to several months.
- Blood withdrawal can be difficult; may be dependent on catheter gauge.
- Requires regular flushing/heparinization.
- Requires sterile dressing.
- Easily removed by registered nurse at bedside.
- Over time, multiple insertions can cause venous scarring and decrease the ability to reuse the site.

VAD = vascular access device.

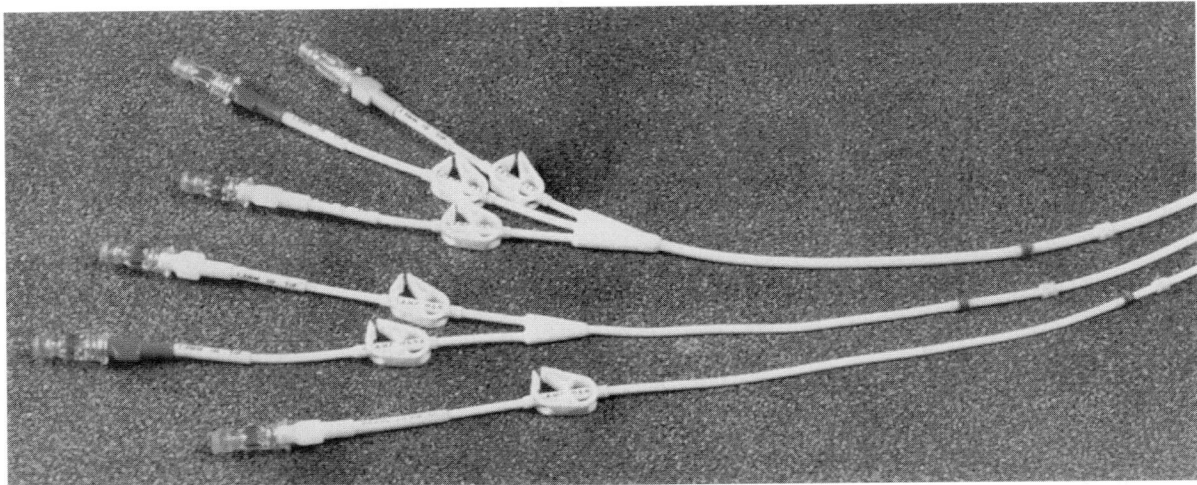

Figure 19-15   Hickman catheters—single, double, and triple lumen. (Courtesy of Bard Access Systems, Salt Lake City, UT.)

it requires regular care and maintenance. The patient or significant other must be willing and physically able to clean the exit site, flush the catheter, change the cap, and assess and report complications. The patient must be able to afford the equipment (needles, syringes, heparin or saline, and dressing materials) and must have access to a clean area in the home in which to perform self-care. Body image and patient lifestyle can be issues because of the catheter exit through the chest wall, which can be distressing or embarrassing to some patients, particularly adolescents. Also, whereas swimming in chlorinated pools is allowed by some practitioners, swimming in ponds, rivers, or the ocean usually is not recommended.

There are several major advantages of the TCVC, including its elimination of needle sticks for those people who have a needle phobia, and the ease with which it is removed when no longer needed for care. It also allows for a great deal of flexibility in terms of use, being a preferred device for long-term TPN, vesicant infusion therapy, and continuous infusions. It also is the only long-term device that offers a triple-access option. Finally, it is less expensive in terms of both the device and the

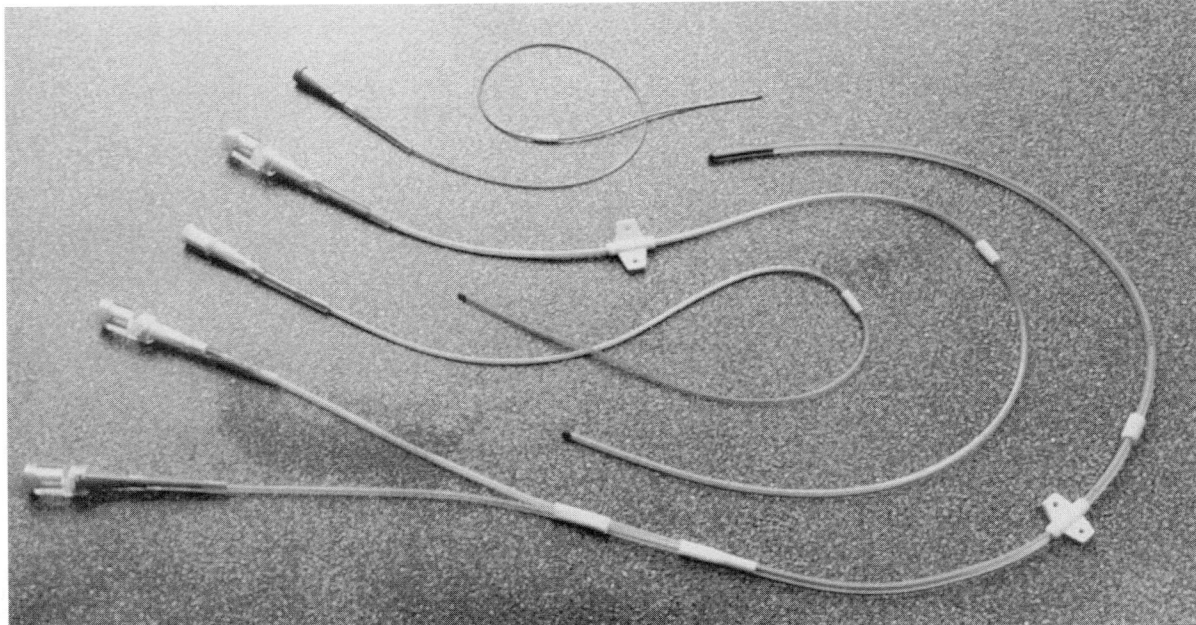

Figure 19-16   Various Groshong catheters. From top to bottom, pediatric, central venous catheter (CVC), tunneled central venous catheter (TCVC), dual-lumen TCVC. (Courtesy of Bard Access Systems, Salt Lake City, UT.)

insertion costs than an implantable port; however, there is some debate as to the long-term cost effectiveness, because supplies are needed for care and their cost depends on the regimen of care and frequency and type of flushing. An overview of TCVC features is given in Table 19-11.

Despite the common use of TCVCs for more than two decades, there is little standardization of their insertion and care. Insertion is not without risks, and complications include pneumothorax and arterial puncture.[71] Various techniques are used for placement, and experienced oncology nurses are beginning to work with physicians and patients prior to insertion to help select a site that is convenient when considering clothing and body contours. Adequate instruction of the patient and family both before and after placement is critical to a successful experience with a TCVC.

When developing policies and procedures governing the use of TCVCs, it is recommended that the following aspects of care be included:

- Requires sterile site care with dressings until the formation of granulation tissue and verification of normal absolute neutrophil counts, at which time site care involves bathing the chest wall and securing the catheter with tape to prevent dislodgment

- When not in use, requires daily, every other day, or even weekly flushing with 3–5 mL of heparinized saline (10 U/mL)

- Allows blood withdrawal for all laboratory tests (except coagulation studies), which can be achieved via vacutainer technique, if desired; vacutainer technique is preferred because it minimizes the risk of accidental needle sticks

- Whenever blood has been aspirated into the catheter, it is flushed with 20 mL of saline prior to heparin-locking or resuming an infusion

- Must avoid intraluminal mixing of potentially incompatible drugs, which can be achieved by flushing with plain fluid between each drug

- Must avoid scissors, sharp objects, and needles longer than 1 inch

- Access is either direct or via as-needed heparin-lock adapter cap; all connections must use Luer-Lok

- Continuous infusions should be directly connected to the catheter hub

Perhaps one reason there is so much variation in technique across treatment settings and facilities is because it may not really matter which type of dressing is used or how often and with what the catheter is flushed. Several small studies regarding dressings have suggested equivocal results. One study showed a slight increased risk of infection with transparent vs. gauze dressings, while the other showed no statistically significant difference between transparent, gauze, or no dressing.[72,73] Similarly,

Table 19-11 Tunneled Central Venous Catheter Overview

Catheter Features
- Multiple manufacturers.
- Composed of silicone or polyurethane with Dacron cuff.
- Available as single-, double-, and triple-lumen catheters.
- Sizes range from 4.2–19.2 Fr and 40–90 cm in length.
- Inner diameter ranges from 0.7–1.6 mm, with a priming volume of 0.3–2.5 mL.
- Insertion kits with introducers are available from all manufacturers.
- Cost-effective, especially with percutaneous insertion (eliminates operating room cost).

Placement
- Technique-dependent; training or observation of the technique is strongly encouraged.
- A sterile procedure, performed by physician, usually in operating room, although some can be inserted percutaneously at the bedside or in a radiology suite.
- Exit site on the nondominant side should be preselected by the nurse, with the patient erect and clothed to prevent placement at an inappropriate site (e.g., under the breast).
- Groshong catheters require a reverse tunneling technique and cannot be trimmed at the proximal end.
- Can be placed through numerous veins, including the jugular, cephalic, and subclavian veins for catheter tip placement in superior vena cava. Occasionally inguinal approach for tip placement in inferior vena cava is necessary.
- Frequently placed under fluoroscopy; x-ray verification of placement is required.
- Suture should be placed at exit site to retain proper catheter placement until granulation occurs around the cuff (usually within 2 wk), and then the suture should be removed.

Use
- Excellent for long-term access for several months to years.
- Preferred for TPN, vesicants, and continuous infusions.
- Requires regular flushing/heparinization (daily to weekly).
- Groshong requires weekly flushing with sterile NS when not in use.
- Requires exit site care.
- Blood withdrawal is easy; can use vacutainer technique.
- Usually removed by physician.

Differences with nontunneled CVCs
- Do not have Dacron cuffs.
- Insertion may take place at bedside or in procedure room.
- Nylon sutures remain in place for duration of catheter life.
- May be used for days to months.
- Easily removed by nurse or physician at bedside.

TPN = total parenteral nutrition; CVC = central venous catheter.

Kelley et al analyzed existing data regarding flushing regimens, conducted a 3-year study, and concluded that weekly flushing with heparin 100 units/mL was safe and effective for 86.5% of study participants.[74] Another group, routinely flushing with sterile saline weekly in pediatric patients, reported that the most striking finding of the study was that most infections occurred during the summer months, when children might be expected to be outside playing and swimming and are perhaps at high risk for infection.[75] Interpretation of these findings and resolution of some of these issues will continue to require assessment, documentation, and reporting of research study results.

One unique care issue related to TCVCs is fracture, puncture, or cutting of the external portion of the catheter. Puncture can be prevented by not using scissors or sharp objects near the catheter and limiting needles used for access to 1 inch in length or by using needleless systems. It is also advisable to avoid clamping the catheter continuously or, if a clamp is used, padding and rotating the clamp site. As long as at least 2 inches of undamaged catheter exits the skin, it can be repaired using a repair kit available from the manufacturer. Most repair kits are designed only for a specific catheter, especially the double- and triple-lumen repair kits when the break is in the main portion of the catheter. Emergency repairs to a single-lumen can be conducted via the following steps:

1. Clamp catheter close to chest wall.
2. Clean catheter with alcohol at the most distal undamaged point.
3. Using sterile scissors, cut the catheter.
4. Remove the inner metal stylus from a 14 - or 16-gauge peripheral IV catheter, and insert the IV catheter into the TCVC until the cut edge touches the hub.
5. Secure with tape or suture.
6. Attach heparin-lock adapter cap, unclamp, and gently flush catheter; heparinize or use in the normal manner.
7. Obtain a repair kit as soon as possible for permanent repair.

One major advantage of the TCVC is the ease with which it is removed by the physician when no longer needed or desired by the patient. Prior to withdrawal of the catheter, some catheter manufacturers suggest a short surgical incision, under local anesthesia, to mechanically release the Dacron cuff from the subcutaneous tissue. If the cuff is not removed with the catheter, it may become infected later. Catheter removal is achieved by cleaning the exit site and manually pulling on the catheter until it loosens in the tunnel. Pressure is then applied manually over the entrance site into the vein and maintained for several minutes after catheter removal. Steady, slow pressure is applied while pulling on the catheter until the entire catheter is removed and inspected to ensure that it is intact, because breakage or splintering can occur. A small dressing is applied to the exit site, if necessary.

Implantable ports

The implantable port has proved to be a unique development in vascular access devices because when it is not in use, it requires almost no care or maintenance (Figures 19-17 and 19-18). A *port* is a hollow housing of stainless steel, titanium, or plastic that contains a compressed latex septum over a portal chamber connected via a small tube to a silicone or polyurethane catheter that is inserted into a blood vessel. It is placed subcutaneously and accessed percutaneously using a special noncoring needle. The needle has an offset bevel, which prevents coring the septum and allows 1000–3600 punctures per port, depending on manufacturer and needle size. The plastic and titanium ports are advantageous because they cause little if any disturbance on x-ray film during imaging procedures. Ports are available with (1) the catheter permanently attached to the portal housing, in which case the surgeon adjusts the length by trimming the distal portion of the catheter prior to insertion; or (2) the catheter separate from the portal housing, in which case the surgeon trims the proximal end prior to attaching and securing it to the portal during the implantation procedure. They are available in single and double designs, with the double port having two distinct portal chambers to allow simultaneous administration of separate solutions. Most ports are accessed through the top. A portal design that provides access via the side, allowing the needle to be positioned parallel to the skin, is available but is not commonly used by practitioners today. An overview of port features is given in Table 19-12.

Port routes. There are five major types of ports: venous, arterial, peritoneal, intrapleural, and epidural. The unique portal design allows access to more than just the vascular system. While the portal housings are all essentially the same, the catheters are designed, located, and cared for differently. The arterial and epidural ports have specially designed catheters with very small lumens, as

Figure 19-17 Schematic drawing of an implantable port.

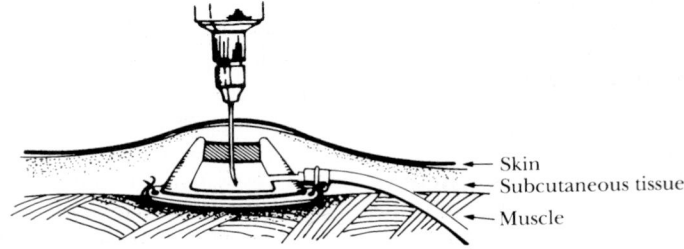

Skin
Subcutaneous tissue
Muscle

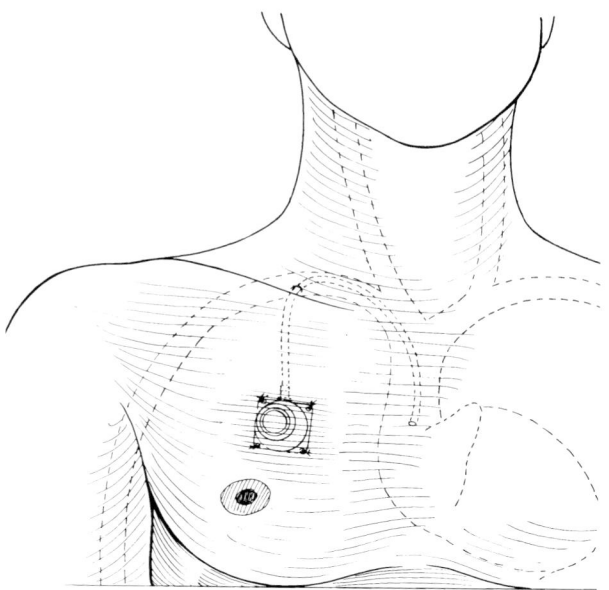

Figure 19-18 Venous port placement.

the flow rate through these devices is often as low as 2–3 mL per day. At the opposite end of the spectrum is the peritoneal catheter, which has a large lumen and multiple fluid outlet holes in the catheter to allow rapid infusion of fluids. The venous ports have varying-sized lumens and flow rates. Usually, venous ports are placed in the upper chest area. Arterial ports can be placed in any of the sites. Peritoneal ports are consistently placed on the lower rib cage, but could be on the lower abdomen. Epidural ports could be at either of the lower positions. Unfortunately, there is no standardized placement of the different types of ports, which creates major problems for the nurse unfamiliar with a new patient. It is imperative that the type of device and its purpose be determined prior to access of the port. Though not common, it is important to remember that ports can be located in other areas of the body. Most patients are given an identifying wallet card and information regarding their ports. If that information is unavailable and the patient is unsure of the device type, then the health care professional must seek the operative note in the hospital chart to confirm device type and catheter route.

Nursing issues related to arterial, peritoneal, epidural, and intrapleural ports are summarized in Table 19-13 and are discussed in some detail in the previous portion of this chapter dealing with routes of drug administration.

Port usage. The routine care of the venous port when not being used is to flush it once every 3–4 months with sterile heparinized saline (usually 5 mL of 100 U/mL solution). It is an ideal choice for patients who are unable or unwilling to care properly for an external device, receiving intermittent therapies, concerned about body image, or physically active (especially if swimming in unchlorinated bodies of water). Its major disadvantage is

Table 19-12 Port Overview

Port Features

- Available in standard size or low profile
- Composed of stainless steel, titanium, or plastic, with catheter of silicone or polyurethane.
- Available with preattached or attachable catheters in single and double designs.
- Can be accessed with a noncoring needle, usually through the top; side-access model is available.
- Types include venous, arterial, peritoneal, intrapleural, and epidural.
- Venous variations include central and peripheral insertion techniques.
- Insertion kits with introducers are available from all manufacturers.
- Expensive, both in terms of port cost and implantation procedure.
- Possibly the least expensive of all VADs for routine care and maintenance.

Placement

- Technique-dependent; training or observation of the technique is required.
- A sterile procedure, performed by surgeon in operating room.
- Exit site on the nondominant side should be preselected by the nurse, with the patient erect and clothed to prevent placement at an inappropriate site (e.g., under the breast, in the breast, or under the arm).
- Groshong port catheters cannot be trimmed at the proximal end.
- Frequently placed with fluoroscopy; x-ray verification of placement required.
- Suture line should not be over the top of the port.
- Port should be accessed with an infusion set and a dressing applied prior to leaving the operating room if it is to be used immediately; some practitioners prefer to wait 14 days prior to use to allow postoperative edema to resolve and wound to heal.

Use

- Can remain in place and functional for many years.
- Ideal for intermittent therapies.
- Must be accessed using noncoring needle.
- Ice or a local anesthetic such as Emla Disc can be used to decrease discomfort prior to accessing.
- When not in use, must be flushed every 4–6 weeks (usually with 3–5 mL of sterile 100 U/mL heparinized saline).
- For continuous access, site care is provided and needle is changed per established policy (usually every 7 days or prn).
- Blood withdrawal is easy; can use vacutainer technique.
- Removal requires surgical procedure.

VAD = vascular access device.

that it requires a needle to pass through the skin and into the port for usage. The procedure of accessing the port could introduce infective organisms, cause a hematoma in a thrombocytopenic patient, cause anxiety in a patient with a needle phobia, or result in extravasation

Table 19-13 Unique Types of Implantable Ports

Arterial

- Used to administer continuous or intermittent intra-arterial chemotherapy.
- Catheter is placed into an artery, and port is usually placed on the lower rib cage.
- Accessed and managed in the usual manner, except heparinization procedure may be different, with increased frequency (i.e., weekly) or higher concentrations of heparin (100–1000 U/mL).
- Catheter has a small lumen and seems to form clots more easily than venous catheters; hence the need for at least weekly flushing.

Peritoneal

- Used to administer intermittent intraperitoneal chemotherapy for ovarian or colon cancer.
- Catheter is placed in the peritoneal space, and port is usually placed on the lower rib cage but can be in the lower abdominal area.
- Accessed and managed in the usual sterile manner, except 19-gauge noncoring needles are used to facilitate large-volume infusions; the portal is flushed after use with sterile saline, and heparinization usually is not required.
- Catheter has a very large lumen with several ridges or cuffs to secure placement and multiple exit holes in the distal portion for rapid fluid infusion.

Epidural

- Used to administer intrathecal or epidural medications, including chemotherapy and analgesics.
- Catheter is placed into the intrathecal or epidural space and tunneled through a long subcutaneous passage from the spinal area to the side of the abdomen, where the port is placed on the lower rib cage or the abdominal area. The portal is designed with a 60-μm screen filter to remove particulate matter.
- Accessed using special 24-gauge noncoring needles, *always* with meticulous sterile technique, including sterile gloves, prep drape, and procedure tray.
- **Never to be flushed with heparin.**
- Preservative-free chemotherapy or morphine is instilled or infused into the port.
- After usage, 1–2 mL of sterile, preservative-free saline may be used to flush the line.
- Catheter has a small lumen (0.5-mm inner diameter), which is suitable for this type of drug delivery.

Intrapleural

- Used to drain pleural effusions periodically in patients who are unresponsive to sclerosing.
- Accessed with noncoring needle only.
- Patient's position is changed frequently during "tap."
- Flushed with 3 mL of saline.

of fluid around the port if performed incorrectly or if the needle subsequently becomes dislodged. There is also a remote possibility that the device could extrude through the skin.

Nursing management of ports involves assessing the site, accessing the device, infusing or withdrawing fluids, and flushing. The nurse should help select the portal site prior to implantation. With the patient erect and clothed, the nondominant side should be examined for a convenient location. Ideally, the port can be located over a rib in an area easy for the patient to visualize for care but not visible when clothed. Consideration should be given to clothing, brassiere straps, lifestyle (e.g., frequent holding of a telephone receiver between the head and shoulder), and physical activities (e.g., swimming). Thin patients may need low-profile ports; obese patients may need large ports. Also, in obese patients or large-breasted women, placement of the port near the sternum provides better needle stability and ease of access. Care should be taken to avoid placement of the port under the arm, under the breast, in the breast, or in the soft tissue of the abdomen (for nonvenous ports). The preferred site and an alternate should be marked on the skin as a reference for the surgeon. It is also helpful if the surgeon offsets the port pocket so that the suture line is 1–2 inches away from the top of the port.

Port access usually is achieved under sterile or aseptic technique after a betadine scrub using noncoring needles that can be either straight or bent at a 90-degree angle. The needle penetrates the septum and is advanced until it touches the bottom of the portal chamber. The most popular access needles are actually infusion sets consisting of needle, tubing, Luer-Lok hub, and containing a Y-site and a clamp. These infusion sets allow great flexibility and multiple access sites and can be left in place for up to 7 days. For long-term access, a sterile dressing (usually transparent) is placed over the site and assessed on a daily basis. Redness, rash, or blistering of the skin around the port could be indicative of an allergic reaction to the tape or dressing, and is resolved by using an alternative type of tape, dressing, or skin-disinfecting agent.

There are several other aspects of port accessing that are especially important to the patient. The area is tender and edematous for a week or so after implantation, causing manipulation of the device to be uncomfortable or even painful. Some practitioners prefer to wait until the site has healed and the edema is gone before using the port. When immediate use is indicated, the port should be accessed and dressed securely in the operating room. For routine use once the site is healed, the needle stick usually is not a concern to most patients and causes little discomfort. Occasionally, a patient will have a needle phobia or experience pain during insertion. Effective options to increase patient comfort include application of a small ice pack to the area for a few minutes or application of a topical anesthetic agent to numb the area before accessing. Most patients prefer to have the site anesthetized prior to access with application of a topical anesthetic such as ethyl chloride or Emla Cream.

All types of medications and fluids can be administered through venous ports, but some problems have been noted with TPN, which can cause drug crystals or sludge to build up inside the portal housing and occlude the device. As with TCVCs, blood withdrawal can be accomplished for all laboratory studies except those involving coagulation, and the vacutainer technique can be used. There is a concern when administering continuous-infusion vesicants because the needle could become dislodged from the septum and remain under the skin, causing a port pocket extravasation. For this reason, vesicant infusions are monitored frequently (every 1–2 hours), and some practitioners prefer that PICCs or TCVCs be placed instead of ports if it is known in advance that this type of therapy may be necessary.

As with other VADs, the nurse must know and assess for the signs and symptoms of complications with utilization of the device. The port should have a brisk blood return, easy flow of fluids, and there should be no edema, redness, or pain in the surrounding tissues. If any problems are noted, measures should be taken to resolve them; if necessary, verification of the patency of the port should be ascertained using x-ray film, venogram, or contrast study (cathetergram).

Peripheral implantable port. A variation of the venous port that combines the properties of a PICC and a port is the peripherally inserted port.[76] The P.A.S.-Port (Peripheral Access System, Pharmacia Deltec, Inc., Minneapolis, MN) allows the peripheral insertion of a port near the antecubital fossa. Insertion and proper placement are achieved using an electronic device that enables insertion at the bedside or in the physician's office. The P.A.S.-Port is about half the size of a regular port and allows patients to experience the advantages of port placement (unobtrusive, long-term access, intermittent use) without having to expose the chest area to achieve access. Access is achieved through a short (½-inch) noncoring needle or infusion set. In all other aspects except placement, it is managed like other implantable venous ports.

Complication Management

Occlusions, infections, and other complications can occur with all of the long-term VADs.

The incidence and type of complication depend on the device, insertion technique, care regimen, and to a great extent on physiological factors inherent in the introduction of a long-term catheter into the venous system.[77–80]

Intraluminal catheter occlusion

The complete inability to withdraw blood or infuse fluid in a VAD is most commonly the result of a blood clot within the catheter. It can also be caused by incompatible drugs or lipids that have crystallized or precipitated and have obstructed the catheter. The nurse is instrumental in assessing the catheter and its most recent usage to determine which of these causes are most likely to have occurred. Blood clots can build up over time (i.e., sluggish catheter) but can also appear suddenly. Drug precipitates tend to be more directly related to a recent infusion

and are seen more often with TPN and lipids.[81] Measures to prevent either occurrence include the following:[71,82–84]

- Maintain positive pressure within the catheter and vigorously flush the catheter provided there is no resistance. If there is intermittent resistance it may mean that the catheter is being pinched off at the level of the clavicle and first rib. Vigorously flushing in this situation can cause an aneurysm in the catheter.

- Advise patient to avoid excessive manipulation (i.e., pinching or bending) of external catheters.

- Vigorously flush with at least 20 mL of sterile NS after any blood has gotten into the catheter. This helps to prevent sludge build-up within the port.

- Document each patient's VAD experience, and adjust concentration, volume, and frequency of heparinized flush, as needed.

- Question patient and family regarding actual catheter maintenance activities to assess compliance with recommended care and usage.

- Flush between each drug with at least 10 mL of plain IV fluid to avoid incompatible drug admixture.

- Vigorously flush catheter every 8–12 hours when administering TPN or lipids.

- Do not administer IV fluid or TPN containing visible precipitates (which is more likely to occur if the solution is more than 24 hours old).

In the case of ports, the inability to infuse or aspirate is typically due to the needles being improperly placed in the septum rather than the portal. Advancing the needle into the portal usually will solve the problem. Also, if the patient has a low-profile port, the septum is not very deep and a 1-inch Huber-point needle will result in a portion of the needle tip being occluded in the septum. When the patient has a low profile port, a ¾-inch 22 Huber point needle will clear the septum and function properly.

Management of an occluded catheter when a blood clot is suspected involves the instillation of alteplase, a tissue plasminogen activator (tPA). Alteplase is prepared as a 2 mg/2 mL syringe and is instilled into the occluded catheter and allowed to dwell for 2 hours. After 2 hours, the nurse attempts to withdraw blood from the catheter. Aspiration of several milliliters of blood ensures removal of the drug and residual clot. The catheter is then irrigated with several milliliters of 0.9% sodium chloride. Urokinase, which currently is not available, has in the past been almost universally successful in clearing a clotted catheter. In the event urokinase is available for use, the procedure for using it follows. A dose of urokinase 5000 units in 1–3 mL is instilled using a 3-mL or larger syringe and a gentle to-and-fro motion. The catheter is then clamped for 30 minutes or longer, after which an attempt is made to aspirate the catheter contents. If successful, the catheter is flushed and used; if unsuccessful the procedure is repeated.[85] Certain drug precipitates can be cleared using 0.1 hydrochloric acid for some crystals or ethanol 70% for lipid deposits.[86–89] The process is similar to that used for urokinase, with the gentle instillation of 0.2–1.0 mL of drug. After a dwell time of 30–60 minutes, an attempt is made to aspirate the catheter contents. If TPN is not involved and a specific drug is known or suspected, a pharmacist should be consulted about possible agents that might dissolve the precipitate and enable it to be aspirated from the catheter. Figure 19-19 describes a possible decision-making matrix to consider when dealing with a completely occluded catheter.

Extraluminal catheter occlusion

Catheter sluggishness or partial occlusion can be due to two extraluminal phenomena: fibrin sheath formation and thrombosis. The catheter position can also affect flow, so a partial occlusion, in the absence of pain or discomfort, should first be managed by instructing the patient to change positions, raise the arms, deep breathe, and/or cough (Figure 19-20). Each of these might release the open lumen of the catheter from the vein wall and allow easy flushing and blood withdrawal. If a withdrawal occlusion exists (flushes easily but backflow is sluggish or nonexistent), fibrin sheath formation or thrombosis should be considered. Fibrin sheaths can form at the catheter insertion site and float, like a sleeve, around the outside of the catheter. If the sheath extends beyond the lumen, it can cause withdrawal occlusions. Lysis of the sheath may be achieved by instilling alteplase 2 mg/2 mL prefilled syringe or (if available) urokinase 5000–10,000 units into the catheter with an extended dwell time of 1–24 hours.[83]

Venous thrombosis can be caused by a variety of factors, including endothelial injury, hypercoagulability, multiple catheters, catheter stiffness (i.e., polyvinyl chloride), catheter size (i.e., larger bore), and catheter placement (i.e., left side or in a smaller vein). The incidence of catheter thrombosis with clinical symptoms appears to be as high as 10%. Actual incidence in the absence of clinical symptoms could be as high as 50%.[90] Signs and symptoms are related to impaired blood flow and include edema of the neck, face, shoulder, or arm; prominent superficial veins; neck pain; tingling of the neck, shoulder, or arm; and skin color or temperature changes. A variety of radiographic studies can be used to diagnose and define the extent of the thrombosis accurately.

Management of venous thrombosis usually involves anticoagulants or thrombolytic agents. Several authors report success with the continuous infusion, centrally and/or peripherally, of urokinase for 4–24 hours.[91] It is recommended that all lumens of a multilumenal device be treated. The serum fibrinogen level should be maintained at 80–100 mg/dL by titration of the urokinase.[91] The success of this treatment may be related to a short period of symptoms prior to the infusion. Prophylactic administration of low-dose warfarin (1 mg/day) appears to prevent or decrease the incidence of thrombus formation.[68,92]

Infection

Long-term central venous catheters are designed to minimize the risk of infection compared to regular venous catheters, but infection still occurs in 2.7%–60% of devices.[77,79] This wide range is probably dependent on the techniques used to insert and care for the VADs as well as the diagnoses and physical conditions of the patients involved. Infections can occur locally (on the skin), in the catheter tunnel/port pocket, or systemically. Infections are more common in patients with neutropenia (<500 granulocytes/mm^3), those with multilumen catheters, and those receiving TPN or chemotherapy. A study by Howell et al indicated that neutropenia was the only independent risk factor for catheter-related infections.[79]

Local infections at the catheter exit site or over the skin around the port needle insertion site usually are due to organisms on the skin such as *Staphylococcus aureus* and *Staphylococcus epidermidis*. Symptoms can include redness, warmth, discomfort, and exudate. Management includes culture of the area, increased frequency of dressing changes with meticulous site care, and administration of appropriate oral or intravenous antibiotics.[77,85] The needle should be removed from an implantable port if a skin infection occurs over the port, and it should not be reaccessed until the infection clears.

Infections in the catheter tunnel or port pocket usually involve a variety of different organisms and are manifested by redness, edema, tenderness or discomfort, exudate, skin warmth, and/or fever. After cultures have been taken, including aspiration of any port pocket exudate, appropriate intravenous antibiotic therapy is initiated. If the causative organism is identified and appropriate anti-infective therapy fails to resolve the infection, consideration should be given to removal of the device.

Systemic infections can be thrombus related or caused by intraluminal catheter colonization with a wide variety of infective organisms. Signs and symptoms include fever and chills. Blood cultures are taken through each lumen of the device as well as peripherally and can be positive either in the device only or via both routes. Administration of appropriate antibacterial or antifungal therapy is initiated, and blood cultures are repeated. Failure to resolve the infection is cause to consider removal of the device.

Preventing infection is a primary concern when caring for all types of VADs. Attention should be focused on the techniques used in routine maintenance, and care should be taken to employ measures to decrease the risk of infection such as decreasing the catheter manipulations and aseptic handling of the hubs. The VitaCuff is impregnated with silver ions and can be attached to any catheter before insertion to provide an antimicrobial barrier within the catheter tunnel. It has been reported to decrease the incidence of catheter infections.[93] Another preventive measure successful in decreasing catheter infection rates is the "locking" of the device with a heparinized vancomycin solution (instead of only heparinized

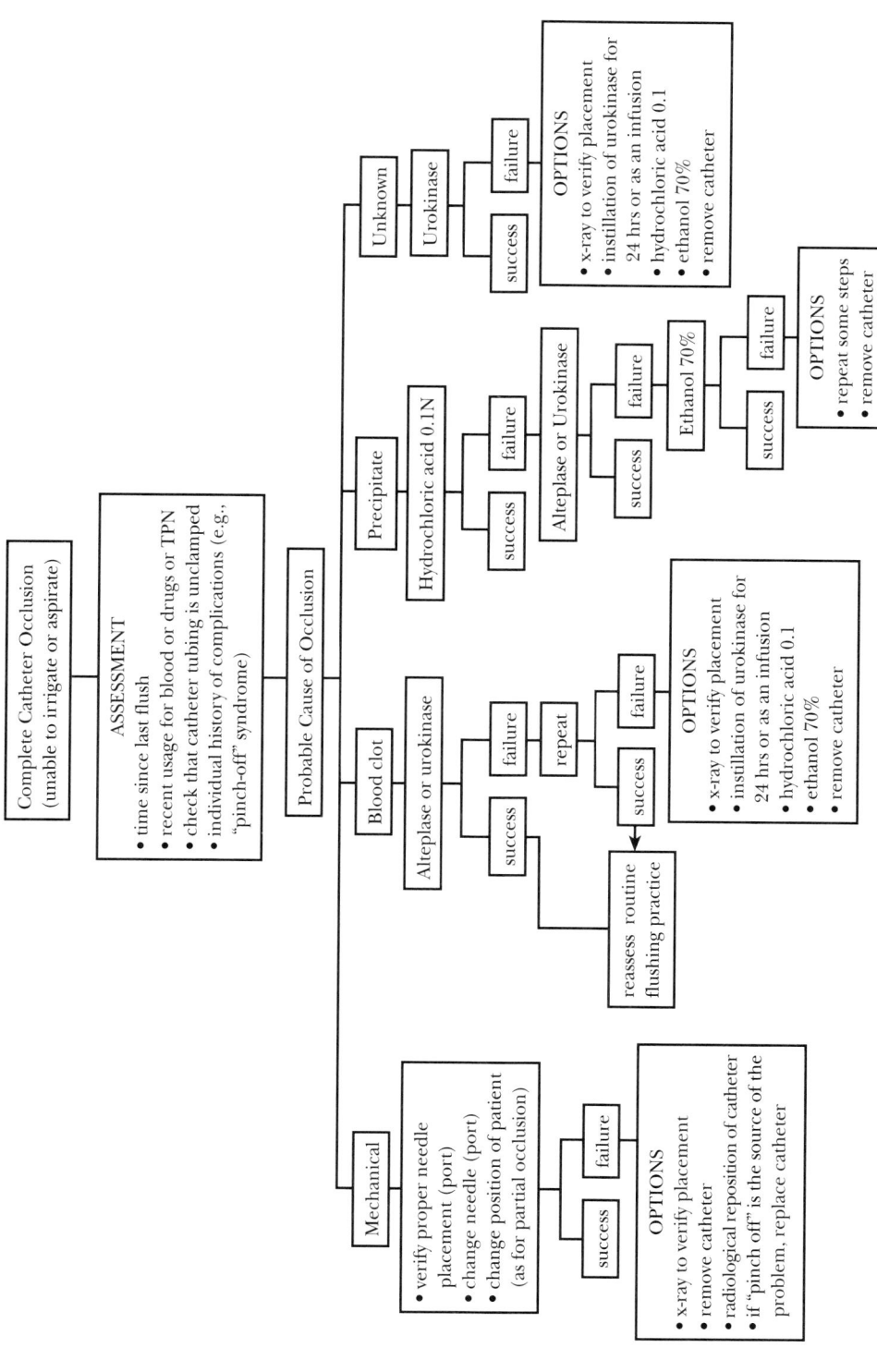

Figure 19-19 Managing complete catheter occlusion. (TPN = total parenteral nutrition.)

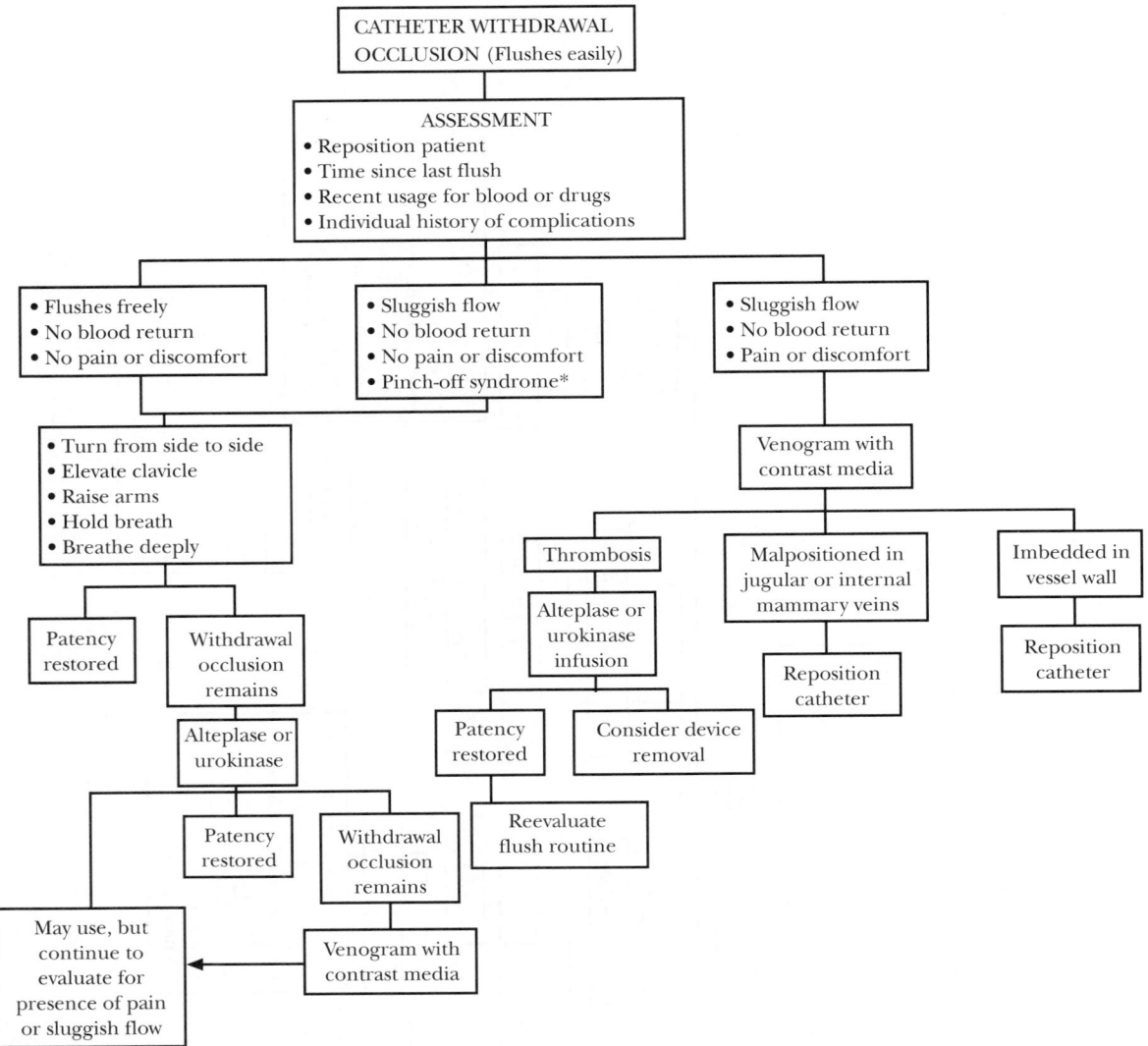

CATHETER WITHDRAWAL
OCCLUSION (Flushes easily)

ASSESSMENT
• Reposition patient
• Time since last flush
• Recent usage for blood or drugs
• Individual history of complications

• Flushes freely
• No blood return
• No pain or discomfort

• Sluggish flow
• No blood return
• No pain or discomfort
• Pinch-off syndrome*

• Sluggish flow
• No blood return
• Pain or discomfort

• Turn from side to side
• Elevate clavicle
• Raise arms
• Hold breath
• Breathe deeply

Venogram with
contrast media

Patency restored

Withdrawal occlusion remains

Thrombosis

Malpositioned in jugular or internal mammary veins

Imbedded in vessel wall

Alteplase or urokinase

Alteplase or urokinase infusion

Reposition catheter

Reposition catheter

Patency restored

Withdrawal occlusion remains

Patency restored

Consider device removal

May use, but continue to evaluate for presence of pain or sluggish flow

Venogram with contrast media

Reevaluate flush routine

*Severe degree of pinch-off syndrome may require catheter removal.

Figure 19-20 Managing catheter withdrawal occlusion.

saline).[94] No toxicities or complications have been noted, and no patients have experienced bacteremia due to intraluminal colonization of vancomycin-susceptible organisms, although infection due to other organisms has occurred. Another approach has been to investigate the use of antibiotic-bonded catheters and the possible impact of these catheters on infection rates.[70]

Other complications

Occlusions and device malfunctions can occur for a variety of other reasons, and careful assessment of the device when occlusion occurs should always include consideration of malpositioning or breakage. Catheters can be kinked, compressed by tumor, compressed between the rib and clavicle ("pinch-off sign"), malpositioned due to patient manipulation ("twiddler's syndrome"), malpositioned for other reasons, severed, punctured, split, or separated. The port access needle can be embedded in the septum; be inaccurately placed into the side of the port or catheter, instead of the portal housing; or become dislodged from the port and remain under the skin.

Thrombus formation can result in a retrograde flow of blood or fluid along the catheter tract, with subsequent extravasation into the subcutaneous tissues. Infusion of drugs into a severed, punctured, or separated catheter can also result in extravasation. Prevention of vesicant extravasation is discussed elsewhere in this chapter, but it is prudent to reiterate that all VADs should be patent and functioning appropriately before initiating vesicant therapy. Extravasation of vesicants into the chest wall or thorax can result in severe deformity, loss of function, or death.

All of the vascular access devices are popular, and manufacturers are continually developing new designs with innovative features every year. Oncology nurses frequently review these new devices and are called on to evaluate their effectiveness. Cost containment is a growing concern, and the best price usually can be achieved if all of the devices selected come from a limited number of vendors, thus consolidating buying power.

Reporting Defects

The Safe Medical Devices Act of 1995 requires health care facilities and manufacturers to report device-related events that did cause or could have caused serious injury or death. The MEDWatch system through the Food and Drug Administration (FDA) makes the reporting process simple and confidential. Forms can be obtained by calling 1-800-FDA-1088.[95]

Conclusion

Cancer chemotherapy administration is a rapidly evolving area of oncology nursing practice that offers exciting opportunities for both beginning and seasoned oncology nurses. The level of responsibility for monitoring patients receiving chemotherapy and managing many aspects of their care continues to increase. Expanded outpatient and home care settings, where the majority of chemotherapy is given, offer opportunities for triage assessment and nursing intervention at an increasingly autonomous level. The technical explosions in drug delivery systems are a constant informational challenge, as is maintaining the personal and rewarding relationships with patients for whom these advanced technologies are utilized.

Health care will continue to move toward more and more ambulatory and home care, with hospitals becoming virtually intensive care buildings. Reimbursement, lobbying, litigation, and legislation will continue to be issues of concern in the twenty-first century. The oncology nurse has a vital role in establishing effective policies and procedures by serving on institutional practice or policy committees. An oncology clinical practice committee with responsibility for reviewing and recommending procedures can also serve to evaluate new technologies. Methods for assuring competency also are being developed and documented.[96] Patient care evaluation and quality improvement are key responsibilities recognized by the Joint Commission on the Accreditation of Healthcare Organizations, which initiated clinical indicators for oncology to more closely monitor quality in the health care setting.

References

1. Herrmann RP, Leather M, Leather HL, et al: Clinical care for patients receiving autologous hematopoietic stem cell transplantation in the home setting. *Oncol Nurs Forum* 25: 1427–1432, 1998
2. Baird S: The impact of changing health care delivery on oncology practice. *Oncol Nurs Forum* 2:1–13, 1995
3. Oncology Nursing Society: *ONS Cancer Chemotherapy Guidelines and Recommendations for Practice*. Pittsburgh, Oncology Nursing Society Press, 1999
4. Alabama Board of Nursing: *Alabama Board of Nursing Administrative Code*. Montgomery, AL, Alabama Board of Nursing, 1990
5. Rutherford C: Position Paper—Administration of antineoplastic agents. *J Intraven Nurs* 15:8–9, 1992
6. Oncology Nursing Society: *Position Statement—Preparations of the professional registered nurse who administers and cares for the individual receiving chemotherapy*. Pittsburgh, Oncology Nursing Society Press, 1991
7. Krohner KM, Spitak AF: Cancer nursing education in the community hospital: Principles and practice. *Oncol Nurs Forum* 19:783–786, 1992
8. Creaton EM, Leonard ED, Day AL: A hospital-based chemotherapy education and training program. *Cancer Nurs* 14:79–90, 1991
9. American Society of Hospital Pharmacists: ASHP technical assistance bulletin on handling cytotoxic and hazardous drugs. *Am J Hosp Pharm* 47:1033–1049, 1990
10. American Society of Hospital Pharmacists: *Safe Handling of Cytotoxic and Hazardous Drugs Study Guide*. Bethesda, MD, American Society of Hospital Pharmacists, 1990
11. U.S. Department of Health and Human Services, Public Health Service, National Institutes of Health: *Recommendations for the Safe Handling of Cytotoxic Drugs*. NIH Publication No. 92-2621, 1996
12. McDiarmid MA, Gurley HT, Arrington D: Pharmaceuticals as hospital hazards: Managing the risks. *J Occup Med* 33: 155–158, 1991
13. Occupational Safety and Health Administration: *Work Practice Guidelines for Personnel Dealing with Cytotoxic (Antineoplastic) Drugs* (OSHA Instruction CPL 2-2.20B). Washington, DC, US Department of Labor Publication, 1995
14. Parillo VL: Documentation forms for monitoring occupational surveillance of health care workers who handle cytotoxic drugs. *Oncol Nurs Forum* 21:115–118, 1994
15. Blecke C: Home chemotherapy safety procedures. *Oncol Nurs Forum* 16:719–724, 1989
16. Valanis B, McNeil V, Driscoll K: Staff members' compliance with their facility's antineoplastic drug handling policy. *Oncol Nurs Forum* 18:571–576, 1991
17. Stajich GV, Barnett CW, Turner SV, et al: Protective measures used by oncologic office nurses handling parenteral antineoplastic agents. *Oncol Nurs Forum* 13:47–49, 1986
18. Yarbro CH, Frogge MH, and Goodman M (eds): *Cancer Symptom Management* (ed 2). Sudbury, MA, Jones and Bartlett, 1999
19. Spath ML, Rimkus CF, Saenz DA: A chemotherapy and infusion therapy flow sheet for outpatient oncology settings. *Oncol Nurs Forum* 25:129–132, 1998
20. Cushman KE: A tool for documenting chemotherapy administration quickly and completely. *Oncol Nurs Forum* 18: 599–600, 1991
21. Moore JM, Knobf MT: A nursing flow sheet for documentation of ambulatory oncology. *Oncol Nurs Forum* 18:933–939, 1991
22. Coker M, Lampert A: Teaching checklist for home infusion therapy. *Oncol Nurs Forum* 17:923–926, 1990
23. Pickett RR: Outpatient oncology chemotherapy documentation tool. *Oncol Nurs Forum* 19:515–517, 1992

24. Attilio R: Caring enough to understand: The road to oncology medication error prevention. *Hosp Pharm* 31:17–26, 1996

25. Phillips D, Christenfeld N, Glynn I: Increase in US medication error deaths between 1983 and 1993. *Lancet* 351:643–644, 1998

26. Rogers BB: Preventing and detecting cancer chemotherapy drug errors. *Oncol Nurs Updates* 6:1–12, 1999

27. Masoorlis S: Infusion therapy lawsuits: An occupational hazard. *J Intraven Nurs* 18:88–91, 1995

28. Baker K, Grochow LB, Donehower R: Should anticancer drug doses be adjusted in the obese patient? *J Natl Cancer Inst* 87:333–335, 1995

29. Georgiadis MS, Steinberg SM, Hankins LA, et al: Obesity and therapy-related toxicity in patients treated for small cell lung cancer. *J Natl Cancer Inst* 87:361–366, 1995

30. Calvert AH, Newell DR, Gumbrell LA, et al: Carboplatin dosage: Prospective evaluation of a simple formula based on renal function. *J Clin Oncol* 7:1748–1756, 1989

31. Riggs CE: Anti-tumor antibiotics and related compounds, in Perry MC (ed): *The Chemotherapy Source Book*. Baltimore, MD, Williams & Wilkins, 1992, pp 318–358

32. Friedland D, Gorman G, Treat T: Hypersensitivity reaction from taxol and etoposide. *J Natl Cancer Inst* 85:2036, 1993

33. Rowinsky EK, Gilbert MR, McGuire WP, et al: Serious hypersensitivity reactions related to its Cremophor EL formulation vehicle. *J Clin Oncol* 9:1692–1703, 1991

34. Van Hoefer U, Harstrick A, Wilke H, et al: Schedule dependent antagonism of paclitaxel and cisplatin in human gastric and ovarian carcinoma cell lines in vitro. *Eur J Cancer* 31A:92–97, 1995

35. Clark JW, Santos-Moore AS, Choy H: Sequencing of taxol and carboplatinum therapy. *Proc Am Assoc Cancer Res* 36:298, 1995 (abstr 1772)

36. Holmes FA, Newman RA, Madden T, et al: Schedule dependent pharmacokinetics (pk) in a phase I trial of taxol and doxorubicin as initial therapy for metastatic breast cancer. NCI Publication, A489, NCI-EORTC, 1–27 1994

37. Gilyon K, Kuzel T: Cutaneous T-cell lymphoma. *Oncol Nurs Forum* 18:901–908, 1991

38. Martin V, Walker FE, Goodman M: Delivery of cancer chemotherapy, in Stromborg MF, McCorkle R, Grant M (eds): *Cancer Nursing: A Comprehensive Textbook*. Philadelphia, Saunders, 1996, pp 397–399

39. Rudolph R, Larson DL: Etiology and treatment of chemotherapeutic agent extravasation injuries: A review. *J Clin Oncol* 5:1116–1126, 1987

40. Laughlin RA, Landeen JM, Habal MB: The management of inadvertent subcutaneous adriamycin infiltration. *Am J Surg* 137:408–412, 1979

41. Ignoffo RJ, Friedman MA: Therapy of local toxicities caused by extravasation of cancer chemotherapeutic drugs. *Cancer Treat Rev* 7:17–27, 1980

42. Brothers TE, Niederhuber JE, Roberts JA, Ensminger WD: Experience with subcutaneous infusion ports in three hundred patients. *Surg Gynecol Obstet* 66:295–301, 1988

43. Gemlo BT, Rayner AA, Swanson RJ, et al: Extravasation: A serious complication of the split-sheath introducer technique for venous access. *Arch Surg* 123:490–492, 1988

44. Mayo DJ, Pearson DC: Chemotherapy extravasation: A consequence of fibrin sheath formation around venous access devices. *Oncol Nurs Forum* 22:675–680, 1995

45. Bertelli G, Gozza GB, Vidili S, et al: Topical DMSO dimethylsulfoxide for the prevention of soft tissue injury after extravasation of vesicant cytotoxic drugs: Prospective clinical study. *J Clin Oncol* 13:2851–2855, 1996

46. Rudolph R, Larson DL: Etiology and treatment of chemotherapeutic agent extravasation injuries: A review. *J Clin Oncol* 5:1116–1126, 1987

47. Ajani J, Dodd LG, Daugherty K, et al: Taxol induced soft-tissue injury secondary to extravasation: Characterized by histopathology and clinical course. *J Natl Cancer Inst* 86:51–53, 1994

48. Goodman M: Taxol and Taxotere infiltrations: Special considerations in management. *Oncol Nurs Forum* 23:87, 1996

49. Bartal AH, Gazitt Y, Zidan G, et al: Clinical and flow cytometry characteristics of malignant pleural effusion in patients after intracavitary administration of methyl-prednisolone acetate. *Cancer* 67:3136–3140, 1991

50. Howell SB, Pfeifle CL, Wung WE, et al: Intraperitoneal cisplatin with systemic thiosulfate protection. *Ann Intern Med* 97:845–851, 1982

51. Zook-Enck D: Intraperitoneal therapy via the Tenckhoff catheter. *J Intraven Nurs* 13:375–382, 1990

52. Malloy J: Administering intraperitoneal chemotherapy: A new approach. *Nursing* 1:58–62, 1991

53. Moores D: Malignant pleural effusions. *Semin Oncol* 18:59–61, 1991 (suppl 2)

54. Ike O, Shimizu Y, Hitomi S, et al: Treatment of malignant pleural effusions with doxorubicin hydrochloride containing poly (L-lactic acid) microspheres. *Chest* 99:911–915, 1991

55. Rusch VW, Figlin R, Godwin D, et al: Intrapleural cisplatin and cytarabine in the management of pleural effusions: A Lung Cancer Study Group trial. *J Clin Oncol* 9:313–319, 1991

56. Parker LA, Charnock GC, Delany DJ: Small-bore catheter drainage and sclerotherapy for malignant pleural effusions. *Cancer* 64:1218–1221, 1989

57. Walsh FW, Alberts WM, Soloman DA, et al: Malignant pleural effusions: Pleurodesis using a small-bore percutaneous catheter. *South Med J* 92:963–965, 1989

58. Tsang V, Fernando HC, Goldstraw P: Pleuroperitoneal shunt for recurrent malignant pleural effusion. *Thorax* 45:369–372, 1990

59. Herr HW, Badalament RA, Amato DA, et al: Superficial bladder cancer treated with bacillus Calmette-Guerin: A multivariate analysis of factors affecting tumor progression. *J Urol* 141:22–29, 1989

60. Brosman SA, Lamm DL: The preparation, handling and use of intravesical bacillus Calmette-Guerin for the management of stage Ta, T1, carcinoma in situ and transitional cell cancer. *J Urol* 144:313–315, 1990

61. Lamm DL, Riggs DR, Traynelis CI: Apparent failure of current intravesical chemotherapy prophylaxis to influence the long-term course of superficial transitional cell carcinoma of the bladder. *J Urol* 153:1444–1450, 1995

62. Phillips PC: Methotrexate neurotoxicity, in Rottenberg DA (ed): *Neurologic Complications of Cancer Treatment*. Boston, Butterworth-Heinemann, 1991, pp 155–123

63. Oncology Nursing Society: *Access Device Guidelines: Recommendations for Nursing Education and Practice*. Pittsburgh, Oncology Nursing Society, 1996, pp 2–86

64. ACS Nursing Subcommittee: *Venous Access Devices Standards of Care*. Salt Lake City, American Cancer Society, 1990, p 8

65. Lucas AB: A critical review of venous access devices: The nursing perspective, in Hubbard SM, Greene PE, Knobf MT (eds): *Current Issues in Cancer Nursing Practice*. Philadelphia, Lippincott, 1991, pp 1–10

66. Raad I, Davis S, Becker M, et al: Low infection rate and long durability of nontunneled silastic catheters. *Arch Intern Med* 153:1791–1796, 1993

67. Alexander HR, Lucas A: New technologies in long-term venous access and peripherally inserted central venous catheters, in Alexander HR (ed): *Vascular Access in the Cancer Patient: Devices, Insertion Techniques, Maintenance, and Prevention of Complications.* Philadelphia, Lippincott, 1995, pp 130–146

68. Ryder M: Peripherally inserted central venous catheters. *Nurs Clin North Am* 28:937–971, 1994

69. Alexander HR: Infectious complications associated with long-term vascular access devices: Etiology, diagnosis, treatment, and prophylaxis, in Alexander HR (ed): *Vascular Access in the Cancer Patient: Devices, Insertion Techniques, Maintenance, and Prevention of Complications.* Philadelphia, Lippincott, 1995, pp 112–128

70. Maki DG, Wheeler SJ, Stoltz SM, et al: Clinical trial of a novel antiseptic-coated central venous catheter. *American Society of Microbiology,* p.327. 1991 (abstr)

71. Lucas A: Routine maintenance and care of long-term vascular access devices, in Alexander HR (ed): *Vascular Access in the Cancer Patient: Devices, Insertion Techniques, Maintenance, and Prevention of Complications.* Philadelphia, Lippincott, pp 148–164, 1995

72. Hoffman KK, Weber DJ, Samsa GP, et al: Transparent polyurethane film as an intravenous catheter dressing: A meta-analysis of the infection rates. *JAMA* 267:2072–2076, 1992

73. Hutchinson SK, Waskerwitz M, Martin K, et al: Non-occlusive, clean permanent right atrial dressing change procedures compared with occlusive, sterile permanent right atrial catheter dressing change procedures in children with cancer. *J Pediatr Oncol Nurs* 7:71, 1990

74. Kelly C, Dumenko L, McGregor SE, et al: A change in flushing protocols of central venous catheters. *Oncol Nurs Forum* 19:599–605, 1992

75. Wiernikowski JT, Elder-Thornley D, Dawson S, et al: Bacterial colonization of tunnelled right atrial catheters in pediatric oncology: A comparison of sterile saline and bacteriostatic saline flush solutions. *Am J Pediatr Hematol Oncol* 13:137–140, 1991

76. Winters V, Peters B, Coila S, et al: A trial with a new peripheral implanted vascular access device. *Oncol Nurs Forum* 17:891–896, 1990

77. Groeger S, Lucas A, Thaler H, et al: Infectious morbidity associated with long-term use of vascular access devices in patients with cancer. *Ann Intern Med* 153:1167–1174, 1993

78. Danzig L, Shat L, Collins K, et al: Bloodstream infections associated with a needleless system in patients receiving home infusion therapy. *JAMA* 23:1862–1864, 1995

79. Howell P, Walters P, Donowitz G, et al: Risk factors for infection of adult patients with cancer who have tunneled central venous access devices. *Cancer* 75:1367–1375, 1995

80. Keung Y, Watkins D, Chen S, et al: Comparative study of infectious complications of different types of chronic vascular access devices. *Cancer* 73:2832–2837, 1994

81. Kupensky D: Use of hydrochloric acid to restore patency in an occluded implantable port. *J Intraven Nurs* 18:198–201, 1995

82. Breaux CW, Duke D, Georgeson KE, et al: Calcium phosphate crystal occlusion of central venous catheters used for total parenteral nutrition in infants and children: Prevention and treatment. *J Pediatr Surg* 22:829–832, 1987

83. Wickham R, Purl S, Welker D: Long-term central venous catheters: Issues for care. *Semin Oncol Nurs* 8:133–147, 1992

84. Wickham R, Purl S, McHale M: Long-term central venous catheters, in Kitt S, Selfridge-Thomas J, Proehl J, Kaiser J (eds): *Emergency Nursing. A Physiologic and Clinical Perspective.* Philadelphia, Saunders, 1995, pp 640–664

85. Holcombe BJ, Forloines-Lynn S, Garmhausen LW: Restoring patency of long-term central venous access devices. *J Intraven Nurs* 15:36–41, 1992

86. Duffy LF, Kerzner B, Gevus V, et al: Treatment of central venous catheter occlusions with hydrochloric acid. *J Pediatr* 114:1002–1104, 1989

87. Pennington CR, Pithie AD: Ethanol lock in the management of catheter occlusion. *J Parenter Enteral Nutr* 11:507–508, 1987

88. Thompson B, Veal D: Pharmacologic treatment of pediatric catheter occlusion. *Hosp Pharm* 27:137–141, 1992

89. Shulman RJ, Reed T, Pitre D, et al: Use of hydrochloric acid to clear obstructed central venous catheters. *J Parenter Enteral Nutr* 12:509–510, 1988

90. Gray WJ, Bell WR: Fibrinolytic agents in the treatment of thrombotic disorders. *Semin Oncol* 17:228–237, 1990

91. Fraschini G, Jadeja J, Lawson M, et al: Local infusion of urokinase for the lysis of thrombosis associated with permanent central venous catheters in cancer patients. *J Clin Oncol* 5:672–678, 1990

92. Bern MM, Lokich JL, Wallach SR, et al: Very low doses of warfarin can prevent thrombosis in central venous catheters: A randomized perspective trial. *Ann Intern Med* 112:423–428, 1990

93. Flowers RH, Schwenzer KJ, Kopel RF, et al: Efficacy of an attachable subcutaneous cuff for the prevention of intravascular catheter-related sepsis. *JAMA* 261:878–883, 1989

94. Schwartz C, Hendrickson KJ, Roghmann K, et al: Prevention of bacteremia attributed to luminal colonization of tunneled central venous catheters with vancomycin-susceptible organisms. *J Clin Oncol* 8:1591–1597, 1990

95. Dessler DA: Introducing MEDWatch, a new approach to reporting medication and device adverse effects and product problems. *JAMA* 269:2765–2768, 1995

96. Dool J, Rodehaver CB, Fulton JS: Central venous access devices, issues for staff education and clinical competence. *Nurs Clin North Am* 28:973–984, 1993

97. Chabner B, Longo D (eds): *Cancer Chemotherapy and Biotherapy: Principles and Practice* (ed 2). Philadelphia, Lippincott-Raven, 1996, pp 600–824

98. Barton-Burke M (ed): *Cancer Chemotherapy: A Nursing Process Approach.* Sudbury, MA, Jones and Bartlett, 1996, pp 187–495

99. Dorr R, VanHoff DD (eds): *Cancer Chemotherapy Handbook* (ed 2). Norwalk, CT, Appleton and Lange, 1993, pp 112–935

100. Fischer DS, Knobf MT, Durivage HJ (eds): *Cancer Chemotherapy Handbook* (ed 4). St. Louis, Mosby, 1993, pp 58–215

Appendix 19A Oral Antineoplastic Agents

Drug and Disease Indications	Dose and Schedule	Side Effects: Acute or Delayed	Pharmacokinetics	Comments
Altretamine (Hexamethyl-melamine hexalene) Ovarian cancer	*Cap:* 50 mg and 100 mg clear *Dose:* 240–320 mg/m²/day	*Nadir:* 21–28 days Acute liver toxicity is dose-limiting; nausea and vomiting are dose-related Mild BMS (Bone Marrow Suppression) Abdominal cramping Diarrhea Peripheral neuropathies Agitation, confusion	Variable absorption Rapid metabolism Urine excretion 90% in 72 hr	• Pyridoxine 50 mg/day may decrease neuropathy. • Take with food, prophylactic antiemetics. • May worsen vincristine-related peripheral neuropathy.
Busulfan (Myleran) Leukemia	*Tab:* 2 mg white *Dose:* 4–12 mg/day for several weeks	*Nadir:* 10–30 days delayed marrow recovery Potentially teratogenic Pulmonary fibrosis with long-term use Dermatologic hyperpigmentation Gynecomastia Amenorrhea	Well absorbed Extensive hepatic metabolism to inactive compounds Renal excretion	• Bone marrow recovery may be delayed; therefore caution is advised with long-term use. Hydration and allopurinol may be indicated to prevent hyperuricemia. Total cumulative dose: 600 mg. • Long-term daily administration is not recommended due to the risk of second malignancies with chronic alkylating agents.
Capecitabine (Xeloda) Metastatic breast cancer	*Tab:* 150 mg light peach, 500 mg peach 2500 mg/m²/day × 14 days q 21 days swallow with water only; take with food	Mild BMS Dose-limiting toxicity is diarrhea Hand-foot syndrome, dermatitis, fatigue, anorexia, nausea, stomatitis	Metabolized to 5-FU; excreted in urine	• Administer in two oral doses, 12 hours apart, 30 minutes after a meal • Monitor coagulation profile in patients also taking coumarin
Chlorambucil (Leukeran) Leukemia Hodgkin's disease	*Tab:* 2 mg white *Dose:* 4–8 mg/m²/day × 3–6 wk 16 mg/m²/wk q 4 wk	*Nadir:* 7–10 days Severe BMS Slight nausea and vomiting Occasional dermatitis Abnormal liver function Pulmonary fibrosis with prolonged use Second malignancy Sterility	Hepatic metabolism to active compound Renal excretion of 50% of unchanged drug	• Good oral absorption. • Concomitant barbiturate administration may enhance toxicity. Marrow suppression may be prolonged.
Cyclophosphamide (Cytoxan) Breast cancer Multiple myeloma Small cell lung cancer Malignant lymphomas Leukemias	*Tab:* 25–50 mg *Dose:* 1–5 mg/kg/day 60–120 mg/m² Adjust dose in presence of renal dysfunction	*Nadir:* 7–14 days Bone marrow suppression (BMS) Anorexia, nausea, and vomiting Alopecia Hemorrhagic cystitis with gross or microscopic hematuria Amenorrhea Sterility	Activated in the liver Oral absorption in 1 hr 30% of drug excreted unchanged in urine	• Vigorous hydration (3 L/day). • Encourage frequent voiding to prevent hemorrhagic cystitis (a sterile inflammation of the urinary bladder). If patient complains of burning on urination or bladder incontinence, urinalysis may reveal occult blood. Control by withdrawal of the drug and hydration. • May take pills in divided doses early in the day and with meals or all at one time. Better tolerated with cold foods. • Barbiturates and other inducers of hepatic microsomal enzymes may enhance toxicity, e.g., cimetidine. Allopurinol may enhance BMS.
Hydroxyurea (Hydrea) Chronic myelocytic leukemia Melanoma Head and neck cancer	*Cap:* 500 mg *Dose:* 80 mg/kg/day every third day 750–1000 mg/m²/day × 5 Decrease dose in presence of renal dysfunction Store in tight container in a cool environment	*Nadir:* 13–17 days Acute nausea and vomiting Chronic and severe anemia Neurological seizures and hallucinations Dermatitis Dysuria Azotemia	Well absorbed Hepatic metabolism Renal excretion of 80% of compound in 12 hr Crosses into CSF	• Concomitant radiation and/or 5-fluorouracil (5-FU) may enhance neurotoxicity. • Dysuria and renal impairment may occur. • Consider pretreatment with allopurinol.
Lomustine (CCNU) Brain cancer Lymphomas	*Cap:* 100 mg green/green, 40 mg green/white, 10 mg white *Dose:* 100–130 mg/m² q 6–8 wk	*Nadir:* 28–42 days Severe cumulative BMS Nausea and vomiting 4–6 hr after dosing Anorexia Alopecia Stomatitis Hepatotoxicity	Absorbed rapidly (<60 min) Hepatic metabolism Renal excretion of 50% in 24 hr and 75% in 96 hr Crosses into CSF	• Dispense one dose at a time to prevent accidental overdose. • Take on an empty stomach just before bedtime. • Pretreat with aggressive antiemetics. • Protect pills from heat and humidity.

Appendix 19A Oral Antineoplastic Agents (continued)

Drug and Disease Indications	Dose and Schedule	Side Effects: Acute or Delayed	Pharmacokinetics	Comments

L-phenylanine mustard (melphalan, Alkeran)
   Multiple myeloma
   Ovarian cancer
	Tab: 2 mg white
	Dose: 0.1–0.15 mg/kg/day × 2–3 wk
	Reduce dose with hepatic or renal impairment
		Nadir: 10–18 days
		Nausea and vomiting usually mild
		Dermatitis
		Pulmonary fibrosis
		Long-term therapy can result in acute leukemia
			Hepatic metabolism
			Renal excretion 20%–35% (10% unchanged)
			20%–50% excreted in feces within 6 days
				• Protect pills from sunlight.
				• Take on an empty stomach.
				• BMS may be cumulative in older patients.
				• Leukemogenic.

6-Mercaptopurine (6-MP) Leukemia	*Tab:* 50 mg off-white *Dose:* 80–100 mg/m²/day Titrate dose based on blood counts Reduce dose in presence of hepatic or renal dysfunction	*Nadir:* 10–14 days Nausea, vomiting Mucositis Diarrhea Drug fever Intrahepatic cholestasis Pulmonary toxicity with prolonged use	Incomplete oral absorption Hepatic inactivation Renal excretion 10% unchanged in 24 hr	• Protect pills from light. • Administer as single dose on an empty stomach. • Increased toxicity with allopurinol (reduce dose by one-third to one-fourth of the original dose). • Administer with caution to patients on sodium warfarin (Coumadin). • Monitor liver function tests.

Methotrexate
   Squamous cell carcinoma
   Lung cancer
	Tab: 2.5 mg yellow
	Dose: 2.5–10 mg/day PO or 15–30 mg/day PO × 5 days q 1–3 wk
		Nadir: 7–10 days
		Nausea and anorexia can occur; stomatitis and ulcerations can occur and are dose-limiting.
			Serum half-life is 2–4 hr
			Excreted by the kidneys
				• Dose is reduced with renal impairment; dosing on an empty stomach may enhance bioavailability. Excretion may be impaired in patients with simultaneous administration or weak acids such as salicylates or vitamin C; oral dosing is generally well tolerated.
				• Avoid administration of methotrexate with ketoprotein or probenecid because toxicity of methotrexate may be enhanced.

Procarbazine (Matulane) Hodgkin's disease	*Cap:* 50 mg *Dose:* 100 mg/m²/day × 14 days q 4 wk; reduce dose in presence of hepatic or renal dysfunction	*Nadir:* 4 wk BMS, nausea, vomiting, and diarrhea gradually subside; flulike syndrome, paresthesias, neuropathies, dizziness, and ataxia	Well absorbed from the gastrointestinal tract Metabolized in the liver with a biological half-life of about 1 hr 70% of the drug is eliminated by 24 hr in the urine; 5% appears as unchanged drug	• Drug and food interactions can occur. • Central nervous system (CNS) depression can occur with concomitant administration of procarbazine and CNS depressants. • Hypertensive crisis can occur when procarbazine is administered with certain antidepressants (tricyclics and monoamine oxidase inhibitors) and tyramine-rich foods. • Severe nausea and vomiting can occur if taken with ethanol, mixed drinks, and beer.
Temozolomide (Temodar) Astrocytoma	*Cap:* 5 mg green, 20 mg brown, 100 mg blue, 250 mg black *Dose:* 150 mg/m²/day × 5 days q mo Dose escalation based on nadir counts	*Nadir:* Platelets by day 26, neutrophils by day 28 BMS is dose-limiting toxicity Nausea, vomiting, fatigue, and headache can be severe in 10% of cases	Rapidly absorbed with a mean elimination half-life of 1.8 hr Eliminated via the kidneys	• Take on an empty stomach at night with glass of water. • Capsules should not be opened or chewed.
6-Thioguanine Leukemia	*Tab:* 40 mg green/yellow *Dose:* 80–100 mg/m² Reduce dose if stomatitis occurs	*Nadir:* 7–28 days Stomatitis Diarrhea Hepatotoxicity	Variable, incomplete absorption Hepatic metabolism Renal excretion	• Administer on an empty stomach. • Does not require dose reduction when used in conjunction with allopurinol.

VP-16 (etoposide, VePesid)
   Lung cancer
   Testicular cancer
	Cap: 50 mg pink
	Dose: 2 × the IV dose or 100–200 mg/m²/day 3–5 × days q 3–4 wk
		Nadir: 7–14 days (white blood cell count)
		Nausea and vomiting: 9–16 days (platelets)
		Alopecia
		BMS is dose limiting
			Renal and hepatic metabolism
			Incomplete and variable absorption
				• Nausea is mild though can be more severe with oral route than with IV route.

Adapted and revised from Goodman M: Delivery of cancer chemotherapy, in Baird S, McCorkle R, Grant M (eds): *Cancer Nursing: A Comprehensive Textbook.* Philadelphia, Saunders, 1991, p 311.

Appendix 19B Intravenous Antineoplastic Agents

Dosage and Efficacy	Mechanism of Action and Metabolism	Administration Precautions	Side Effects
BLEOMYCIN (Blenoxane)			
Dosage: • May be given IM, SQ, IV, intratumoral, intra-arterial. • 10–20 U/m² once or twice a week • Intrapleural/pericardial sclerosing dose: 50–60 U/m² in 50–100 mL NS or D5W; not to exceed 40 U/m² in geriatric population *Efficacy:* • Cervical cancer • Head and neck cancer • Penis, skin, and testicular cancer • Hodgkin's and non-Hodgkin's lymphoma • Kaposi's sarcoma	*Mechanism of action:* • Cell-cycle phase specific for G₂ and M phase. Binds to DNA. • Inhibits cell progression out of G₂, resulting in cellular synchronization for subsequent drug therapy. *Metabolism:* • t½ = 20 min • Renal elimination	*Administration precautions:* • Administer with caution to patients with significant pulmonary or renal disease. Prior cisplatin therapy may reduce bleomycin clearance, increasing plasma half-life and toxicity. • Test dose: Bleomycin is associated with HSR and a test dose of 2 U IV in 50 mL D5W over 15 min followed by observation. Observe for anaphylactic reaction for 1–2 hours posttest dose. • Lymphoma patients are more at risk for HSR and should be tested for the first two doses.	*Side effects:* • Lifetime cumulative dose is 400 U. • 25% dose reduction for creatinine clearance of 30–50 mL/min • 50% dose reduction for creatinine clearance of 20–30 mL/min • Fever occurs in approximately 50% of patients. Premedicate with acetamino-phen 1 g and diphenhydramine 50 mg. (Repeat 6 hr later.) • Dermatological reactions such as hyperpigmentation, hyperkeratosis, and erythema on palms and fingers; urticaria, rash, mucositis, and alopecia • Anorexia and mild nausea • Interstitial pneumonitis and pulmonary fibrosis occur more commonly in patients who also have mediastinal radiation, are elderly, and receive higher cumulative doses.
CARBOPLATIN (Paraplatin)			
Dosage: • IV: 360 mg/m² q 4 wk • Higher doses are given in pretransplant protocols and intraperitoneally or intraarterially. • Dose calculations are most therapeutically based on the desired serum concentration (AUC), renal status, and whether or not the patient has been previously treated with chemotherapy (Calvert Method). • Note that doses calculated according to the Calvert formula are total mg, not mg/m² (see text).	*Mechanism of action:* • Maximal cytotoxicity occurs when cells are in the S-phase although cell kill by intrastrand DNA cross-linkage occurs throughout G₁, S, and G₂ phases of the cell cycle. *Metabolism:* • t½ = 2.5 hr • 60% eliminated unchanged in the urine • Major routes of elimination are glomerular filtration and tubular secretion.	*Administration precautions:* • Available as lyophilized (powdered) form to distinguish it from cisplatin, which is only available in aqueous solution. • Usually administered over 15–30 min in 500 mL of NS or D5W, without further hydration. • May also be administered as a continuous 24-hr or longer infusion. • Forms a precipitate when in contact with aluminum, causing loss of antitumor potency. • Injection site irritation and erythema can occur with infiltration but no ulceration or necrosis. • Physically compatible with ondansetron.	*Side effects:* • DLT: myelosuppression, particularly thrombocytopenia. Nadir occurs at 2–3 wk. • Nausea and vomiting are mild and rarely last beyond 24 hours. • Ototoxicity and neurotoxicity (paresthesias) are uncommon. • Alopecia, mucositis, and abnormal liver functions have been reported. • Nephrotoxicity occurs but is less common than with cisplatin.

Efficacy:
- Ovarian carcinoma
- Testicular cancer
- Head and neck cancer
- Cervical cancer
- Lung cancer

CARMUSTINE (BiCNU)

Dosage:
- IV: 150–200 mg/m² q 6 wk
- Higher doses have been used in pretransplant protocols.

Efficacy:
- Brain tumors
- Multiple myeloma
- Hodgkin's disease
- Non-Hodgkin's lymphoma
- Melanoma

Mechanism of action:
- Inhibits enzymatic reactions involved in DNA synthesis
- Inhibits DNA repair
- Acts predominantly during late G and early S phase
- Readily crosses the blood-brain barrier

Metabolism:
- Metabolized by the liver
- 80% eliminated via the kidneys
- t½ = 15–20 min

Administration precautions:
- Soluble in water and absolute alcohol.
- Protect from light.
- Administer in 100–500 mL D5W or NS as a 1- to 2-hr infusion.
- Infusion may burn as it goes in and should be monitored closely.
- Heat provides symptomatic relief.
- Slowing the infusion rate also eases vein discomfort.
- Hypotension can occur if the infusion is given rapidly.
- Facial flushing and dizziness occur infrequently.
- Compatible with ondansetron.
- Incompatible with polyvinylchloride infusion bags and with sodium bicarbonate.
- Avoid contact with skin; a brown stain may result.

Side effects:
- DLT: Leukopenia and thrombocytopenia occur 3–5 wk after treatment, recovery at 8 wk.
- Myelosuppression may be cumulative.
- Nausea and vomiting are common and require aggressive antiemetic therapy.
- Pulmonary fibrosis has been reported and generally presents as a dry cough and dyspnea.
- Alopecia is common.
- Elevation of LFTs and azotemia can occur with higher doses. Cimetidine has been shown to potentiate carmustine toxicity.

CISPLATIN (Platinol) AQUEOUS SOLUTION

Dosage:
- IV: 20–40 mg/m² day × 3–5 days q 3–4 wk
- 20–120 mg/m² single dose q 3–4 wk
- IP: 100–270 mg/m² in 2 L of warmed NS. Infuse via gravity over 10 min. Allow 4-hr dwell time.

Efficacy:
- Bladder

Mechanism of action:
- Binds to DNA affecting DNA replication
- Forms DNA protein cross-links
- Interacts with cellular glutathione

Metabolism:
- 90% bound to plasma proteins
- 20%–45% eliminated unchanged via kidney
- t½ = 60–90 hr

Administration precautions:
- Dose reductions: 25% dose reduction for patients with creatinine clearance of 30–50 mL/min and a 50% dose reduction for patients with creatinine clearance <30 mL/min
- Administer after appropriate hydration (1–2 L with mannitol).
- Maintain urinary output (125 mL/hr). Mixing

Side effects:
- Concomitant administration of probenecid enhances cisplatin renal toxicity.
- Monitor patient for HSR: tachycardia, wheezing, hypotension, and facial edema.
- Acute and delayed nausea and vomiting are preventable with aggressive antiemetics including 5 HT3 receptor antagonists, dexamethasone, and metoclopramide.

(continued)

Appendix 19B Intravenous Antineoplastic Agents (continued)

Dosage and Efficacy	Mechanism of Action and Metabolism	Administration Precautions	Side Effects
• Ovarian • Testicular carcinoma • Non–small cell lung cancer • Head and neck cancer	• 10% eliminated in bile	• cisplatin in 0.9% NaCl maintains drug stability. • Cisplatin may react with aluminum resulting in loss of cisplatin potency. • Physically compatible with ondansetron. • Sodium thiosulfate and mesna directly inactivate cisplatin. • Administer with caution in patients receiving other potentially nephrotoxic drugs (aminoglycosides).	• High frequency hearing loss may occur in up to 30% of patients. • Tinnitis, vestibular dysfunction, and ototoxicity occur infrequently and are preventable with adequate hydration and mannitol diuresis. • Peripheral neuropathy including numbness, tingling, and sensory loss occurs in arms and legs with long-term administration. • Hypomagnesemia is seen with high dose (> 200 mg/m^2) and is preventable with oral and IV supplements. • Hemolytic anemia is seen with higher doses and responds to recombinant erythropoietin.

CYCLOPHOSPHAMIDE (Cytoxan)

Dosage and Efficacy	Mechanism of Action and Metabolism	Administration Precautions	Side Effects
Dosage: • PO: 50–200 mg/m^2 PO each day × 14 days q 28 days • IV: 500 mg–1.5 g/m^2 IV q 3 wk or 60 mg/kg IV × 2 days prior to BMT *Efficacy:* • Breast • Ovary • Leukemias • Lymphomas • Multiple myeloma • Lung cancer	*Mechanism of action:* • Activated by hepatic microsomal enzymes; prevents cell division by cross-linking DNA strands • Non–cell-cycle phase specific *Metabolism:* • t½ = 3–10 hr • Metabolized in the liver • Excreted in the kidney (15% unchanged) • 33% of drug is excreted unchanged in the stool	*Administration precautions:* • When doses >1000 mg are given, patients should receive hydration of 500–1000 mL NS. • Administer IV dose slowly to prevent nasal congestion, headache, and dizziness. • Encourage fluid intake of 3 L/day while taking cyclophosphamide. • When taking oral doses, encourage patient to take all pills before 5 P.M. to minimize bladder contact with toxic metabolites. • Phenytoin and chloral hydrate may enhance the conversion of cyclophosphamide to toxic metabolites, thereby increasing toxicity.	*Side effects:* • Hemorrhagic cystitis occurs rarely with conventional doses. • Hydration and mesna are indicated with high-dose and pretransplant therapy. • SIADH can occur with high-dose cyclophosphamide. • Nausea and vomiting are preventable with aggressive antiemetic therapy. • Alopecia is common. Metallic taste occurs during injection and when taken orally. Encourage the patient to chew gum, peppermint, or lemon candy. • Myelosuppression (leukopenia) is dose-limiting. • Amenorrhea and reversible oligospermia occur and are dose dependent. • Cyclophosphamide 1 mg/mL is compatible with doxorubicin, cisplatin, mesna, and other drugs. • Blurring of vision has been reported. • Cardiac toxicity can occur with high-dose therapy, especially if given with radiation to the chest area.

CYTARABINE (Cytosar; ARA-C, Cytosine Arabinoside)

Dosage:
- IV: 5–10 day CI (continuous infusion) of 100–200 mg/m²

  or
- Intrathecal: 5–70 mg/m² 1–3×/week

  or
- Subcutaneous: 1 mg/kg 1–2×/week or 100 mg bid × 5 days q 28 days

Efficacy:
- Acute leukemia
- Myeloid leukemia
- Acute nonlymphocytic leukemia
- Meningeal leukemia

Mechanism of action:
- Inhibits DNA polymerase causing DNA chain elongation and arrest
- Cell-cycle phase specific for the S phase
- Antimetabolite

Metabolism:
- Metabolized in the liver
- At 24 hr, 90% of the drug is eliminated in the urine
- $t\frac{1}{2}$ = 2–3 hr

Administration precautions:
- Given IV push or IV infusion over 30 min
- 5- to 10-day continuous infusions may be optimal for antitumor cytotoxicity because of the S-phase specificity.
- For intrathecal use, mix drug with lactated Ringer's solution or NS without preservatives.
- Rotate sites for SQ injections.

Side effects:
- Myelosuppression is the DLT. Nadir at 5–7 days, recovery in 2–3 wk.
- Anemia is common.
- Nausea, vomiting, anorexia, metallic taste, stomatitis, and diarrhea are reported.
- Minimal alopecia
- Skin erythema can occur. Arthralgias and myalgias occur.
- After intrathecal use, patients may experience nausea, vomiting, fever, and headache.
- Ocular toxicity: excessive tearing, photophobia, and blurred vision.
- High-dose therapy can lead to CNS toxicity: lethargy, confusion, ataxia.
- Cytarabine may decrease the cellular uptake of methotrexate.
- Compatible with vincristine, prednisolone, sodium phosphate, and ondansetron.
- Physical changes are noted with methotrexate and 5-FU and heparin.
- Compatible with vancomycin for 4–8 hr.

DACARBAZINE (DTIC)

Dosage:
- 375 mg/m² q 3–4 wk

  or
- 150–250 mg/m²/qd × 5 days q 3–4 wk

  or
- 850 mg/m² on day 1 q 3–4 wk

Efficacy:
- Malignant melanoma
- Soft-tissue sarcomas
- Hodgkin's disease

Mechanism of action:
- Causes cross-linkage and breaks in DNA strands.
- Inhibits RNA and DNA synthesis.
- Cell-cycle phase nonspecific, but has more activity in late G_2.

Metabolism:
- Activated by liver microsomes
- Excreted renally
- $t\frac{1}{2}$ = 35 min

Administration precautions:
- Reconstitute with D5W or saline
- Solution can be painful and should be administered slowly in 250–500 mL of solution over 30–60 min. Moist heat along the vein eases pain.
- Stable for 8 hr at room temperature, 72 hr if refrigerated.
- Drug should be protected from light.
- May turn to a pinkish color if exposed to light.
- HSR can occur; hypotension occurs with high-dose therapy.

Side effects:
- DLT: moderate degree of myelosuppression.
- Nadir occurs at 21–25 days.
- Anemia can occur.
- Severe nausea and vomiting can occur.
- Aggressive pretreatment with antiemetic therapy is needed. Nausea and vomiting lessen by day 3–4 of treatment.
- Hepatotoxic; monitor liver functions
- Flulike syndrome may occur with fever, myalgia, and malaise at about 7 days, lasting 1–3 wk.
- Photosensitivity can occur; protect skin from sunlight.

(continued)

Appendix 19B Intravenous Antineoplastic Agents (continued)

Dosage and Efficacy	Mechanism of Action and Metabolism	Administration Precautions	Side Effects

DACTINOMYCIN (Actinomycin D; ACT-D, Cosmegen)

Dosage and Efficacy	Mechanism of Action and Metabolism	Administration Precautions	Side Effects

Dosage:
• 10–15 μ/kg/day × 5 days q 3–4 wk
  or
• 2.4 mg/m² in divided doses over 1 wk
  or
• 2 mg/m² IV q 3–4 wk
 	
Efficacy:
• Wilms' tumor
• Embryonal rhabdomyosarcoma
• Choriocarcinoma
• Malignant melanoma
• Hodgkin's and non-Hodgkin's lymphoma
	Mechanisms of action:
	• Binds between purine-pyrimidine base pairs in DNA.
	• Inhibits the synthesis of DNA-dependent RNA and messenger RNA.
	• Action is cell-cycle nonspecific but is more active during G₁ and in cells that are cycling.
	
	Metabolism:
	Excreted unchanged in bile and urine
		Administration precautions:
		• Reconstitute with preservative-free sterile water for injection. Preserved diluent may cause precipitation. Use drug as soon as possible.
		• Monitor liver functions; dose reductions may be necessary.
		• Use extreme caution during administration.
		• Dactinomycin is a severe vesicant.
		• Dactinomycin is compatible with ondansetron.
		• When calculating dose, double-check the order since the drug is ordered both as μg/kg and mg/m².
			Side effects:
			• DLT: myelosuppression occurs within 7–10 days of dosing.
			• Nadir may be delayed, occurring at 3 wk.
			• Due to its immunosuppressive effects, avoid administering dactinomycin to patients who have an active viral infection.
			• Nausea and vomiting can be severe. Aggressive pretreatment with antiemetics is appropriate.
			• Mucositis and diarrhea can be severe; institute preventive oral hygiene regimen.
			• Alopecia occurs commonly.
			• Erythema, hyperpigmentation, and an acnelike rash occur commonly.
			• Dactinomycin can cause a radiation recall reaction.
			• Hepatic venoocclusive toxicity manifested as elevated SGOT and bilirubin can occur.

DAUNORUBICIN (daunomycin, Cerubidine)

Dosage and Efficacy	Mechanism of Action and Metabolism	Administration Precautions	Side Effects
Dosage: • 30–60 mg/m² daily × 3–5 days q 3–4 wk *Efficacy:* • ALL • AML • Acute monocytic leukemia • Acute nonlymphocytic leukemia	*Mechanism of action:* • Intercalates DNA, thereby blocking DNA, RNA and protein synthesis. It is an anthracycline antitumor antibiotic. *Metabolism:* • Metabolized in the liver • About 40% of the drug is eliminated via the bile • 20%–25% is eliminated via the urine • t½ = 20–25 hr	*Administration precautions:* • 20-mg vial is reconstituted with 4 mL of sterile water = 5 mg/mL. • QS to 15–20 mL of NS • Stable for 24 hr at room temperature and 48 hr under refrigeration. • Incompatible with heparin, 5-FU, and dexamethasone • Compatible with ondansetron • CAUTION: Because the solution is red, as is doxorubicin and with a similar sounding name, the vial should be double-checked against the order. • Urine will be pink to red for 12–24 hr after administration.	*Side effects:* • DLT: myelosuppression. • WBC nadir occurs at 7–14 days; recovery at 3 wk. Thrombocytopenia and anemia occur. • Stomatitis occurs, but is mild. • Diarrhea occurs infrequently. • Nausea and vomiting occur 1–5 hr after dosing but is prevented with aggressive antiemetic therapy. • Alopecia is abrupt and involves all body hair. • Hyperpigmentation of the nails occurs. Urticaria and a generalized rash have been reported. • Monitor liver functions. If elevated LFTs are noted, dose reduction is indicated.

- Daunorubicin is a severe vesicant. Extreme caution should be used in administration of this drug.
- Administer via the side arm of a freely running IV or by the two-syringe technique.
- Cardiac toxicity can occur. Dose is limited to 500–600 mg/m².
- Manifestation of CHF is characterized by dyspnea on exertion, fatigue, and arrhythmias.

DOCETAXEL (Taxotere)

Dosage:
- 80–100 mg/m² q 3 wk as a 1-hour infusion

Efficacy:
- Ovarian cancer
- Breast cancer
- Non-small cell lung cancer

Mechanism of action:
- Antimicrotubule agent—a mitotic spindle poison. Enhances microtubule assembly and inhibits the depolymerization of tubulin. This process leads to increased bundles of microtubules in the cell. The cell is then unable to divide.

Metabolism:
- Metabolized in the liver, excreted in the feces, and minimally excreted in the urine.
- t½ = 11 hr

Administration precautions:
- Docetaxel solution contains 2 mg (40 mg/mL) of docetaxel in polysorbate/tween 80. Refrigerated vial sits at room temperature for 5 min. Once mixed with solvent the solution contains 10 mg/mL. The appropriate amount of docetaxel is mixed with D5W in a concentration <1 mg/mL. Once diluted, docetaxel is stable for 8 hr at room temperature.
- Avoid infiltration: The drug is an irritant, but can cause tissue damage depending on the concentration.
- Hyaluronidase SQ injections (maximum volume of 3 mL) have been recommended for treatment of infiltration. Apply cold to the site, not heat.
- Monitor liver functions carefully; dose adjustments are appropriate if LFTs are elevated 2.5× normal.

Side effects:
- The DLT for docetaxel is neutropenia and thrombocytopenia.
- All patients receive dexamethasone 8 mg PO bid × 5 days starting 1 day prior to docetaxel.
- Diphenhydramine 50 mg is also given 30 min prior to prevent hypersensitivity reactions.
- If mild HSR occurs with flushing, skin reactions, or pruritus, the infusion rate is slowed with observation. If the patient experiences rash, flushing, mild dyspnea, or chest discomfort, the infusion is stopped and the patient is treated with IV diphenhydramine and dexamethasone. The infusion may be resumed after symptoms abate.
- If severe symptoms such as generalized urticaria, angioedema, or hypotension occur, the infusion is stopped and the patient is treated with antihistamine, steroid, and if necessary epinephrine or bronchodilators. The patient may still receive the docetaxel depending on the severity of the response. If the patient reacts a second time the patient probably should not receive the drug again.
- Nausea and vomiting are minimal.
- Alopecia occurs within 3 wk of the first treatment.
- Nail separation may occur.
- Drug-associated fluid retention or edema including pleural effusions, ascites, and peripheral edema occur and may be managed with a diuretic, which may or may not be helpful.

(continued)

Appendix 19B Intravenous Antineoplastic Agents (continued)

Dosage and Efficacy	Mechanism of Action and Metabolism	Administration Precautions	Side Effects
	DOXORUBICIN (Adriamycin, Rubex)		
Dosage: • 60–75 mg/m² as bolus or as a continuous infusion over 3–4 days q 3–4 wk. Higher doses are used in dose-intensive regimens. • Doxorubicin may also be given intraarterially, intrapleurally, and by bladder instillation. *Efficacy:* • Acute nonlymphocytic leukemia • Acute lymphocytic leukemia • Wilms' tumor • Neuroblastoma • Soft-tissue sarcoma • Breast cancer • Hepatocellular carcinoma • Ovarian carcinoma	*Mechanism of action:* • Binds directly to DNA base pairs and inhibits DNA, RNA, and protein synthesis. Antitumor antibiotic. Cell-cycle specific for the S-phase. *Metabolism:* • Extensively metabolized by the liver • 40%–50% of the drug is eliminated in the bile. • 5% is eliminated in the urine. • t½ = 18–30 hr	*Administration precautions:* • Available in liquid and lyophilized form. • Reconstitute with sterile water for injection, D5W, NS to form a solution of 2 mg/mL. • Stable for 35 days at room temperature. • Incompatible with heparin, dexamethasone, 5-FU, furosemide, aminophylline. • Compatible with cyclophosphamide, cisplatin, dacarbazine, droperidol, vinblastine, vincristine, and ondansetron. • Doxorubicin turns the urine a reddish orange for 8–10 hr after administration. • Since doxorubicin is metabolized and eliminated by the liver, liver function tests are monitored frequently. Elevation in bilirubin to 1.2–3 mg/dL warrants a 50% dose reduction; bilirubin of 3 mg/dL calls for a 75% dose reduction. • Administer with extreme caution. Doxorubicin is a severe vesicant. It will cause tissue damage, ulceration, and necrosis if infiltrated. Inject through the side arm of a freely running and well-established IV or by using the two-syringe technique. • CAUTION: It has a similar name and color to daunorubicin. Check the drug order against the vial to ensure the right dose of the right drug.	*Side effects:* • DLT: Myelosuppression, especially leukopenia. Nadir occurs at 10–14 days. Recovery is swift at 3 wk. • Cardiac toxicity can occur. Dose is limited to 450–550 mg/m². Doxorubicin causes damage to the myocyte of the heart, causing various degrees of damage, but manifests as CHF as the heart begins to function less efficiently as a pump. • MUGA scans are done periodically to monitor left ventricular function. Early symptoms of CHF include tachycardia, dyspnea on exertion, arrhythmias, and EKG changes. • Alopecia occurs predictably and is dose dependent. Doses greater than 50 mg are associated with moderate to severe loss. Doses of 90–100 mg cause hair loss in 2.5 wk. • Stomatitis is dose-limiting and can be more severe with continuous infusions. Continuous infusions are only given through central lines, never through peripheral lines. • Nail bed changes occur and include hyperpigmentation especially in blacks and in individuals of Mediterranean descent.
	DOXORUBICIN HYDROCHLORIDE LIPOSOME INJECTION (Doxil)		
Dosage: • 20 mg/m² over 30 min q 3 wk *Efficacy:* • AIDS • Kaposi's sarcoma	*Mechanism of action:* • Anti-tumor antibiotic binds directly to DNA • Inhibits DNA and RNA synthesis • Drug is encapsulated in stealth liposomes to prolong circulation time *Metabolism:* • Slower clearance from body than doxorubicin • t½ = 55 hr	*Administration precautions:* • Dilute in 250 mL 5% dextrose USP. • Drug is an irritant.	*Side effects:* • Acute infusion reaction may occur with flushing, shortness of breath, facial swelling, headache, chills, back pain, chest and throat tightness, and/or hypotension. Stop infusion. Restart if symptoms abate. • Hand-foot syndrome may require dose reduction. • Stomatitis may occur. • BMS is dose limiting. • Cardiac toxicity may occur. • Less incidence of alopecia compared to doxorubicin.

ETOPOSIDE (VePesid, VP-16)

Dosage:
- 50–100 mg/m² IV qd × 5 (testicular cancer) q 3–4 wk
- 75–200 mg/m² IV qd × 3 (small cell lung cancer) q 3–4 wk. Oral dose is twice the intravenous dose.
- 400 mg/m²/day × 3 days prior to bone marrow transplant.

Efficacy:
- Small cell lung cancer
- Testicular cancer

Mechanism of action:
- Inhibits DNA synthesis in S and G₂. Causes single-strand breaks in DNA.
- Cell-cycle phase specific for S and G₂ phase.

Metabolism:
- Extensively protein bound. Metabolized in the liver. Excreted in the bile and urine
- t½ = 8–14 hr

Administration precautions:
- Following dilution in NS or 5% dextrose, the drug is stable for 72–96 hr at room temperature. At room temperature, stability is dependent on concentration:
  .6 mg/mL = 24 hr
  1 mg/mL = 4 hr
  2 mg/mL = 2 hr
- Etoposide is administered slowly over at least 30–45 min.
- Hypotension can occur, monitor patients for drug sensitivity.

Side effects:
- DLT: Leukopenia, dose-related. Nadir occurs 7–14 days, recovery by day 21.
- Nausea and vomiting are uncommon. Anorexia occurs, especially with oral dosing.
- Alopecia occurs more commonly with IV dosing. Radiation recall and pruritus can occur.
- HSR reactions are rare.

5-FLUOROURACIL (5-FU, Adrucil)

Dosage:
- Doses vary: 300–600 mg/m² IV × 5 days q 3–4 wk
- 450–600 mg/m² IV weekly
- 800–1200 mg/m² continuous infusion × 14–21 days to toxicity

Efficacy:
- Cancer of the breast, colon, rectum, pancreas, stomach, head and neck

Mechanism of action:
- Inhibits the formation of thymidine, which is necessary for DNA synthesis. Causes abnormal RNA synthesis. Acts synergistically with methotrexate.
- Cell-cycle phase specific for the S-phase.

Metabolism:
- Poorly absorbed by mouth. After IV administration, the drug is metabolized to active metabolites.
- Approximately 45% of the drug is metabolized by the liver.
- 15% is eliminated unchanged in the urine.
- t½ = 10–20 min

Administration precautions:
- May be given a variety of ways: IV as a continuous infusion, IV push, arterial infusion, intracavitary, or intraperitoneally.
- Store at room temperature and protect from light.
- Incompatible with daunorubicin, doxorubicin, idarubicin, cisplatin, cytarabine, and diazepam.
- Compatible with vincristine, methotrexate, potassium chloride, and magnesium sulfate.

Side effects:
- Myelosuppression may be dose-limiting, but less common with continuous infusion.
- Mucositis is most common DLT with continuous infusions. Symptoms of erythema, soreness, and ulceration may begin within 5–8 days of therapy. Sucking on ice chips as tolerated may decrease oral stomatitis. Diarrhea can be severe, even life threatening, especially when 5-FU is given in higher doses with leucovorin.
- Nausea, vomiting, and anorexia occur less frequently, but are more common when 5-FU is given simultaneously with radiation to the abdomen.
- Skin and nail bed changes occur, especially with continuous infusion. Partial nail loss can occur as well as banding. Palmar-plantar erythrodysesthesias can be severe, necessitating dose reduction and treatment delays. Hyperpigmentation and photosensitivity are common. Patients are cautioned to protect themselves from the sun. Excessive lacrimation due to tear duct stenosis and blurred vision occur in about 25% of patients.

(continued)

Appendix 19B Intravenous Antineoplastic Agents (continued)

Dosage and Efficacy	Mechanism of Action and Metabolism	Administration Precautions	Side Effects
			• Headache, cerebellar ataxia, nystagmus, and confusion occur with higher doses.
			• Administering 5-FU based on the patient's circadian rhythm may lessen toxicity in general.
			• Alopecia is dose dependent.
			• Ataxia occurs in elderly patients. Other CNS changes include headache, drowsiness, and blurred vision.

FLOXURIDINE (FUDR, 5-FUDR)

Dosage and Efficacy	Mechanism of Action and Metabolism	Administration Precautions	Side Effects
Dosage: • 0.1–0.6 mg/kg/day by intrahepatic infusion. Therapy is continued to toxicity, usually 7–14 days. • Circadian infusion protocols have been used. • Intravenous doses range from 0.5–1.0 mg/kg/day for up to 2 weeks by continuous infusion. *Efficacy:* • Adenocarcinoma metastatic to the liver	*Mechanism of action:* • Antimetabolite, similar to 5-FU, interrupts DNA synthesis causing cell death. Cell-cycle phase specific for the S-phase. *Metabolism:* • Metabolized to 5-FU when given IV. • 70%–90% of the drug is metabolized by the liver, and metabolites are excreted by the kidneys and lungs. When given, intrahepatic FUDR has a much higher first pass extraction rate compared to 5-FU and therefore the cytotoxic effect is more localized to the liver. • t½ = 0.3–3.6 hr	*Administration precautions:* • Caution should be exercised as both 5-FU and floxuridine (also called 5-FUDR) are supplied in 500-mg vials and the doses of each are dramatically different. With such similar names it is important to note that mistaking 500 mg of FUDR for 500 mg of 5-FU could be lethal. • FUDR 500-mg vial of lyophilized powder is reconstituted with sterile water. • Generally given via an intraarterial infusion pump • Heparin is added to the FUDR to prevent clotting of the catheter due to the slow infusion rate.	*Side effects:* • When given as an intraarterial infusion an H2 antihistamine such as ranitidine may be recommended (150 mg bid) to prevent peptic ulcer disease. • The intraarterial route is usually associated with less systemic toxicity. • Bone marrow suppression is more common with IV bolus injections. • Nausea, vomiting, and anorexia are common. Abdominal cramps with severe diarrhea are indications to interrupt therapy. Mucositis does not occur often and if it occurs is an indication to interrupt the treatment and to reduce the dose. • Skin changes can occur and include edema, dermatitis, rashes, and pruritus as well as hyperpigmentation. • Alopecia can occur but is usually mild.

GEMCITABINE (Gemzar)

Dosage and Efficacy	Mechanism of Action and Metabolism	Administration Precautions	Side Effects
Dosage: • 800–1000 mg/m² weekly × 3 weeks q 4 wk *Efficacy:* • Pancreas cancer • Non-small cell lung cancer	*Mechanism of action:* • Antimetabolite • Inhibits DNA synthesis • Cell-cycle specific for the S-phase *Metabolism:* • Eliminated by kidneys	*Administration precautions:* • Reconstitute with sodium chloride to a solution containing 10 mg/mL. • Dilute in 100–1000 mL of saline and infuse over 30 min to 3 hr.	*Side effects:* • Myleosuppression, especially thrombocytopenia, can be dose-limiting. • Flulike syndrome with fever, mild nausea, and vomiting can occur. Fever generally occurs within 8 hr of dosing. Acetaminophen generally relieves symptoms.

- Breast cancer

- t½ = 20 min

- Rash may occur within 2–3 days of the infusion. Topical steroids may be helpful.
- Peripheral edema may occur.

IDARUBICIN (Idamycin)

Mechanism of action:
- Cell-cycle phase specific for S-phase
- Analog of daunorubicin
- Inhibits RNA synthesis

Metabolism:
- Excreted primarily in the bile and urine
- 25% of the drug is eliminated over approximately 5 days
- t½ = 13–26 hr
- Metabolized in the liver to active form

Dosage:
- 12 mg/m²/day for 3 days
- Doses vary
- Generally given in combination with other drugs

Efficacy:
- Acute nonlymphocytic leukemia

Administration precautions:
- Reconstituted with NS.
- Protect from light.
- Caution is used during administration because drug is a vesicant.

- Incompatible with 5-FU, etoposide, dexamethasone, heparin, hydrocortisone, methotrexate, and vincristine.

Side effects:
- DLT: Leukopenia and thrombocytopenia are expected.
- Urine can be pink to red for 48 hr after administration.
- Nausea can be mild to moderate and preventable with standard antiemetic.
- Diarrhea and mucositis can occur.
- Alopecia occurs gradually.
- Cumulative cardiomyopathy and CHF can occur with large cumulative doses.

IFOSFAMIDE (Ifex)

Mechanism of action:
- Ifosfamide is an alkylating agent. It is a prodrug and requires activation in the liver by microsomal enzymes.

Metabolism:
- Metabolized by the liver to inactive metabolites.
- 15%–56% of the drug is excreted unchanged in the urine.
- t½ = 7–15 hr
- Drug elimination may be hindered by renal dysfunction.

Dosage:
- IV: 1.0–1.2 g/m²/day over a 5-day period q 3–4 wk. Higher doses of 2.5–3.7 g/m²/day over a 2- to 3-day period.
- Mesna at a dose of 20% of the ifosfamide dose is given just prior to the ifosfamide and q 4 h for 2 more doses. Mesna may be given IV or PO.

Efficacy:
- Testicular cancer
- Soft-tissue sarcoma
- Hodgkin's and non-Hodgkin's lymphoma
- Acute leukemias
- Ewing's sarcoma
- Osteosarcoma

Administration precautions:
- Ifosfamide is administered over at least 30 min with aggressive hydration to reduce the incidence of hemorrhagic cystitis.
- The uroprotectant mesna is also given either as a continuous infusion or in divided doses q 4 h × 3 doses.
- Ifosfamide and mesna are compatible and can be infused concurrently when high-dose ifosfamide is given.

Side effects:
- Myelosuppression is the DLT.
- WBC nadir usually occurs 7–10 days posttreatment.
- Urinary tract toxicity is the dose-limiting toxicity and is manifested as hemorrhagic cystitis. Patients may complain of dysuria and frequency 2–3 days after the infusion. Encourage oral intake of 2–3 L per day prior to and after dosing. Encourage patients to empty their bladders every 2–3 hr.
- Nausea and vomiting are common with higher doses. Symptoms are preventable with serotonin antagonist therapy.
- Avoid sedation with neurotoxic drugs that can exacerbate the lethargy and confusion that can occur due to the accumulation of chloracetylaldehyde, a metabolite with neurotoxic properties.
- Alopecia is more common with higher doses and occurs usually within 3 wk of therapy.

(continued)

Appendix 19B Intravenous Antineoplastic Agents (continued)

Dosage and Efficacy	Mechanism of Action and Metabolism	Administration Precautions	Side Effects
	IRINOTECAN (Camptosar, CPT-11)		
Dosage: • 125–150 mg/m² IV over 90 min weekly × 4 wk q 6 wk *Efficacy:* • Adenocarcinoma • Colon/rectal cancer	*Mechanism of action:* • Topoisomerase I inhibitor • Blocks DNA and RNA synthesis in dividing cells *Metabolism:* • Metabolized to its active form in liver • 20% drug excreted in urine • 30% excreted in bile • t½ = 6–10 hr	*Administration precautions:* • Dilute in 5% dextrose: stable for 24 hr at room temperature. • Drug is an irritant.	*Side effects:* • Dose-limiting toxicities are diarrhea and myelosuppression. • Loperamide is administered for diarrhea. • Flushing and diaphoresis may occur during infusion. • Moderate to severe nausea and vomiting may occur.
	L-ASPARAGINASE (Elspar) Erwinia Asparaginase		
Dosage: • Used in combination with other drugs, active in ALL 200 IU/day for 28 days, 1000 IU/kg × 10 days 　　　　or • 20,000 IU/m²/wk *Efficacy:* • ALL	*Mechanism of action:* • Inhibits protein synthesis *Metabolism:* • Biphasic elimination • t½ = 4–9 hr and 1.4–1.8 days • Binds to vascular binding sites • May be eliminated by the liver	*Administration precautions:* • Dilute in nonpreserved sterile saline or water. • Use within 8 hr. • Refrigerate before and after reconstitution. • Do not infuse through a filter. • IV slow push over 30 min, or IM. • Do not use if solution is cloudy. • Skin test with 2 IU intradermal at least 1 hr prior to dosing. • Administer subsequent doses with caution despite negative skin test.	*Side effects:* • Anaphylactic reactions can occur in 20%–35% of patients. • Monitor closely with appropriate support. • IM use is associated with delayed allergic response. • If HSR occurs, the Erwinia preparation may be used with prophylactic premedication. • Urticarial eruptions are common. • Incidence of reactions increases with each subsequent dosing. • Slight anemia can occur; leukopenia is rare. • Malaise, anorexia, nausea, and vomiting occur frequently. • Hepatic toxicity is uncommon. • Lethargy, somnolence, disorientation, and loss of recent memory occur with higher doses.
	MECHLORETHAMINE HYDROCHLORIDE (nitrogen mustard, Mustargen)		
Dosage: • IV: 6 mg/m² on days 1 and 8 • Topically: 10 mg/60 mL ointment *Efficacy:* • Hodgkin's disease	*Mechanism of action:* • Alkylating agent results in abnormal base pairing causing DNA miscoding, cross-linking of DNA, and strand breakage. • Cell-cycle nonspecific	*Administration precautions:* • Once reconstituted with sterile water or NS the drug should be used within 60 min because of its instability. • Nitrogen mustard should be administered by IV push via a freely running IV line.	*Side effects:* • Myelosuppression is the DLT. • Leukopenia occurs 8–14 days following treatment. Severe thrombocytopenia may occur.

Efficacy:
- CML
- Lymphosarcoma

Metabolism:
- Rapidly deactivated in the blood
- t½ = 15 min

Administration precautions:
- Administering nitrogen mustard via direct IV push technique can cause venous thrombosis and pain.
- Nitrogen mustard is a severe vesicant and must be given with extreme caution.
- Assess for a blood return every 1 mL of injection.
- If extravasation occurs, inject a solution of sodium thiosulfate (1/6 molar) into the area to neutralize the drug.
- For 1 mg of nitrogen mustard infiltrated, inject 2 mL of the 10% thiosulfate solution.
- Preparation: 4 mL sodium thiosulfate injection (10%) diluted with 6 mL of sterile water for injection.

Side effects:
- Severe nausea and vomiting within 1 hr of IV administration. Patients should be premedicated with aggressive antiemetic therapy.
- Alopecia is common. A metallic taste is common during the injection and can be masked by encouraging the patient to chew gum or bite on a lemon rind.
- Amenorrhea and impaired spermatogenesis occurs and is dose dependent.

MELPHALAN (Alkeran, L-PAM, L-Phenylalanine Mustard)

Mechanism of action:
- Alkylating agent; cycle specific
- Forms DNA cross-links

Metabolism:
- 80%–90% of the drug is bound to plasma proteins
- 10%–15% of the drug is eliminated unchanged in the urine
- t½ = 1.5–4.0 hr

Dosage:
- IV: 16 mg/m² q 3 wk × 4 doses then q 4 wk
- PO: 2 mg/kg/day × 5 days q 4–6 wk
- BMT: 50–60 mg/m² IV

Efficacy:
- Multiple myeloma
- Epithelial carcinoma of the ovary
- BMT

Administration precautions:
- Reconstitute with 10 mL of supplied diluent for a concentration = 5 mg/mL.
- Dilute in NS to a concentration of 0.45 mg/mL and use within 60 min.
- Do not refrigerate reconstituted product.
- When taken orally, peak plasma levels are reached within 2 hr. The drug is poorly absorbed when taken with food.

Side effects:
- Myelosuppression is the DLT.
- GI: mild anorexia, nausea and vomiting when taken orally. Nausea and vomiting can be severe with higher IV doses. Mucositis, diarrhea, and oral ulceration occur infrequently. Leukopenia and thrombocytopenia peak at 2–3 wk and may be cumulative with a prolonged recovery period of 6 or more wk.
- Pruritus, dermatitis, and rash may occur. Alopecia is not common with oral dosing.
- Amenorrhea and oligospermia are common.
- Second malignancies (leukemias) have been reported.

METHOTREXATE (MTX, Mexate, amethopterin)

Mechanism of action:
- MTX tightly binds to dihydrofolate reductase thereby blocking the reduction of dihydrofolate to tetrahydrofolic acid, the active form of folic acid. This process effectively arrests DNA, RNA, and protein synthesis.
- Antimetabolite
- Cell-cycle specific for the S-phase of the cell cycle

Dosage:
- 15–30 mg/day × 5 days or 20–30 mg/m² twice weekly
- Single doses of 1.5–20 g/m² with leucovorin rescue
- Intrathecal dosing 10–15 mg in 7–15 mL of preservative-free saline

Efficacy:
- Trophoblastic neoplasms

Administration precautions:
- Lower doses (<100 mg) are usually given IVP without leucovorin rescue.
- When given with 5-FU for breast cancer, the MTX dose is followed in 1 hr by the 5-FU. The drugs are synergistic when given this way.
- Leucovorin rescue is needed because the dose of MTX is generally >100 mg.

Side effects:
- Myelosuppression is the DLT. Leukopenia is dose-dependent and is more likely to occur with prolonged exposure.
- Nausea and vomiting are common with higher doses. Diarrhea can be dose limiting. Stomatitis is more common with higher doses and more lengthy infusions.
- Skin erythema, hyperpigmentation, photosensitivity, rash, folliculitis, and pruritus

(continued)

Appendix 19B Intravenous Antineoplastic Agents (continued)

Dosage and Efficacy	Mechanism of Action and Metabolism	Administration Precautions	Side Effects
• Acute leukemias • Meningeal leukemias • Carcinoma of the breast • Osteogenic sarcoma • Burkitt's lymphoma	*Metabolism:* • MTX is distributed freely in water, which means that it will circulate in third space fluid, increasing the toxicity of the drug since it is not being metabolized. Patients with effusions or ascites should be monitored carefully to avoid severe toxicity. • MTX is highly protein bound and should not be given with acids that may compete for binding (elimination) sites, which would increase the AUC of the MTX, resulting in extreme toxicity. • 90% of MTX is eliminated from the kidneys in the urine as unchanged drug. • BUN and creatinine levels should be monitored regularly. If there is evidence of renal impairment lower doses should be given with leucovorin rescue.	• Preservative-free MTX used for intrathecal injection should be prepared just prior to use. • Protect infusions from light.	may occur. MTX can cause enhanced radiation side effects if given simultaneously. • Renal dysfunction is dose-related and more common in patients who are dehydrated. When given in higher doses, the patient's urine pH must be >7 to prevent precipitation of the MTX in the renal tubules, with subsequent renal damage. Administer bicarb as directed. The BUN and creatinine are monitored prior to high-dose therapy. • Neurological dysfunction can occur with intrathecal administration, especially if cranial radiation has also been given. • Photophobia, excessive lacrimation, and conjunctivitis have been noted.

MITOMYCIN (Mutamycin, mitomycin C)

Dosage and Efficacy	Mechanism of Action and Metabolism	Administration Precautions	Side Effects
Dosage: • 20 mg/m² as a single dose repeated q 6–8 wk • For bladder instillation: 20–40 mg is mixed with 20–40 mL of water or saline and is given q 1–2 wk *Efficacy:* • Adenocarcinoma of the stomach, pancreas • Cancer of the bladder, breast	*Mechanism of action:* • Antitumor antibiotic • Active during the G₁ and S-phase of the cell cycle • Disrupts DNA synthesis secondary to alkylation *Metabolism:* • Mitomycin is inactivated by microsomal enzymes in the liver and is metabolized in the spleen and kidneys. • 10%–30% of the drug is eliminated unchanged in the urine • $t\frac{1}{2}$ = 0.5–1.0 hr	*Administration precautions:* • Reconstitute in sterile water: 10 mL in 5 mg vial = 0.5 mg/mL. Use within 3 hr. • Mitomycin is a severe vesicant. Administer with caution. • Give IV push through the side arm of a freely running IV to minimize venous irritation. Assess for a blood return every 1 mL of drug. Discontinue the injection immediately if the patient complains of pain or burning. • Mitomycin can cause tissue damage without evidence of drug infiltration. • Skin ulceration may occur at sites distant from the site of drug administration.	*Side effects:* • Myelosuppression is the DLT. • Leukopenia and thrombocytopenia occur late at 4–5 wk with recovery at 7–8 wk. Both are cumulative. • Anemia and hemolytic–uremic syndrome have been reported. • Nausea and vomiting are mild. • Alopecia is mild, photosensitivity, skin rash, and pruritus are uncommon. • Venoocclusive disease of the liver with abdominal pain, hepatomegaly, and liver failure occur in patients receiving mitomycin and BMT. • Pulmonary fibrosis has been reported.

MITOXANTRONE (Novantrone)

Dosage and Efficacy	Mechanism of Action and Metabolism	Administration Precautions	Side Effects
Dosage: • 10–12 mg/m²/day × 5 days for induction of acute nonlymphocytic leukemia; 12 mg/m² q 3–4 wk	*Mechanism of action:* • Antitumor antibiotic • Intercalates into DNA; disrupts cell division	*Administration precautions:* • Dark blue solution in vials • Dilute in at least 50 mL D5W or NS. • Stable for 7 days at room temperature.	*Side effects:* • Leukopenia is the DLT. • Nausea and vomiting are mild and preventable. Alopecia is common. Diarrhea and stomatitis may occur.

Efficacy:
- Acute monocytic leukemia
- AML
- Acute promyelocytic leukemia
- Breast cancer
- Primary hepatocellular carcinoma

Metabolism:
- Metabolized in the liver and excreted in the bile and urine
- t½ = 24–37 hr

- Administer IV over at least 5 min as an infusion.

- Cumulative cardiomyopathy can occur. Monitoring the left ventricular ejection fraction is indicated, especially in patients who are at risk for heart disease or who have received doxorubicin in the past.
- Blue discoloration of the sclera may occur. The urine may remain blue-green for 48 hr following treatment.

PACLITAXEL (Taxol)

Dosage:
- 200–250 mg/m² q 3 wk or in heavily pretreated patients
- 135–170 mg/m² q 3 wk or weekly in divided doses

Efficacy:
- Ovarian carcinoma
- Breast cancer
- Non-small cell lung cancer

Mechanism of action:
- Promotes assembly of microtubules and stabilizes them, thereby blocking mitosis.
- Paclitaxel also prevents transition of the cell from G_0 phase to S phase by blocking cellular response to growth factors.

Metabolism:
- The majority of paclitaxel is protein bound.
- Elimination is primarily hepatic; minimal renal excretion
- t½ = 1.3–8.0 hr

Administration precautions:
- Formulated in 50% polyoxyethylated castor oil (Cremophor EL) and 50% dehydrated alcohol.
- Administer only in glass bottles or non-PVC containers (polyolefin containers using polyethylene-lined nitroglycerin tubing sets).
- Cremophor-containing solutions will leach the plasticizer DEHP from PVC containers. DEHP can cause liver toxicity.
- Inline filtration is needed (.02 μm) due to the natural origins of the drug.
- Administration rate varies from 1–3 hr to 24–96 hr. In general, the longer the infusion, the more likely the patient will experience myelosuppression that is dose limiting.
- Hypersensitivity reactions can occur with paclitaxel infusion and are thought to be related to the Cremophor EL. Patients are premedicated with dexamethasone 20 mg at 13 and 7 hr prior to treatment; with diphenhydramine 50 mg IV 30 min prior, and with an H_2 blocker (cimetidine 300 mg or pepcid 20 mg) 30 min prior.
- When administering paclitaxel with doxorubicin, the doxorubicin is given first; likewise when paclitaxel is given with cisplatin or carboplatin, the paclitaxel is given first to avoid disruption in the elimination of the platinum compound and enhanced toxicity.
- Synergistic with herceptin.

Side effects:
- HSRs occur infrequently with proper premedication. Most HSRs occur within the first or second dosing. Symptoms include dyspnea, urticaria, flushing, and hypotension.
- DLT is myelosuppression.
- Leukopenic nadir occurs 7–10 days after dosing, with recovery at 15 days. Anemia and thrombocytopenia occur less frequently.
- Peripheral neuropathy occurs more commonly in patients who are also receiving cisplatin. Hyperesthesias and burning pain in the feet may also occur. Myalgias and arthralgias occur usually 3–4 days after dosing.
- Alopecia is complete at 3 wk.
- Mucositis occurs more commonly with prolonged infusions. Nausea and vomiting are mild. Diarrhea occurs infrequently. Paclitaxel is an irritant but can cause blistering and skin breakdown if large amounts of more concentrated drug are infiltrated.

(continued)

Appendix 19B Intravenous Antineoplastic Agents (continued)

Dosage and Efficacy	Mechanism of Action and Metabolism	Administration Precautions	Side Effects
	TENIPOSIDE (Vumon, VM-26)		
Dosage: • 100 mg/m² 1–2 times weekly and 20–60 mg/m² × 5 days or 90 mg/m²/day × 5 days for lung cancer *Efficacy:* • Relapsed or refractory acute lymphoblastic leukemia • Small-cell lung cancer	*Mechanism of action:* • Plant alkaloid, topoisomerase II inhibitor • Phase specific, acts in late S phase and early G₂ phase *Metabolism:* • Bound to plasma protein; metabolized in the liver with less than 10% of the unchanged drug in feces • Eliminated in the urine • t½ = 20 hr	*Administration precautions:* • Dosage is diluted in sodium chloride and is physically stable for approximately 24 hr at room temperature in glass containers. Drug may precipitate in plastic containers. • Administer over at least a 45-min period to avoid severe hypotension. • Avoid extravasation. • Local phlebitis may occur. • HSRs occur and include blood pressure changes, bronchospasm, tachycardia, urticaria, facial flushing, diaphoresis, periorbital edema, vomiting, and/or fever.	*Side effects:* • Leukopenia is the DLT occurring at 10–14 days. • Nausea and vomiting are rare. • Alopecia occurs gradually; skin rash is rare. • With high-dose therapy, severe skin rashes can occur. • Hemolytic anemia with renal failure has occurred. • HSR may be related to the Cremophor EL vehicle. • Secondary malignancies occur infrequently. • Hyperbilirubinemia, SGOT, and SGPT elevations can occur.
	THIOTEPA (Thioplex)		
Dosage: • 12–16 mg/m² q 1–4 wk • 900 mg/m² (transplant dose) • 30–60 mg q wk × 4 wk for intravesicular use • 1.0–10 mg/m² 1–2 times per wk for intrathecal use *Efficacy:* • Breast cancer • Ovarian cancer • Superficial bladder cancer • Lymphoma • Hodgkin's disease	*Mechanism of action:* • An alkylating agent similar to nitrogen mustard *Metabolism:* • Variably absorbed through the bladder mucosa following intravesical injection • Metabolized in the liver • t½ = 2–3 hr	*Administration precautions:* • 15-mg vial is reconstituted with 1.5 mL of sterile water and further diluted with saline for intrathecal use (preservative free). • Intravenous and intravesical solutions may be diluted with saline, D5W, or lactated Ringer's solution and are chemically stable for at least 5 days in the refrigerator and 24 hr at room temperature. • Intravesical instillation involves placement of a catheter in the bladder and instillation of the drug with retention of the liquid for up to 2 hr. The patient is repositioned q 15 min to maximize exposure to the tissues of the bladder. • Intrathecal doses are mixed in up to 20 mL of Ringer's lactate to maximize CNS distribution. • Intravenous administration may be given IVP or as an infusion. Thiotepa is not a vesicant.	*Side effects:* • Myelosuppression is the DLT and may be cumulative. • Leukopenia occurs 7–10 days postinjection. • Thrombocytopenia may be delayed. • Nausea and vomiting are not common in nontransplant doses. • Stomatitis may be severe in transplant doses. • Abdominal pain, hematuria, dysuria, frequency, and urgency occur with intravesical instillation. • Second malignancies have been reported.

TOPOTECAN (Hycamtin)

Dosage:
- 1.3–1.6 mg/m² IV infusion over 30 min, 2 hr, or 24 hr

  or
- 1.5–2.0 mg/m²/day as a 30-min infusion × 5 days

Efficacy:
- Small cell lung cancer
- Ovarian cancer
- Esophageal cancer

Mechanism of action:
- Topoisomerase I inhibitor causes single strand breaks in DNA, causing the cell to die during DNA replication

Metabolism:
- Up to 48% of the drug is eliminated unchanged in the urine
- t½ = 3 hr

Administration precautions:
- 5-mg vial is reconstituted with 2 mL of sterile water and diluted in D5W.
- Stable for up to 48 hr at room temperature.
- Given intravenously as an infusion.

Side effects:
- Leukopenia is the DLT, and the nadir occurs at day 10–12 with recovery at 3 wk.
- Thrombocytopenia and anemia occur but are not usually dose limiting.
- Mild to moderate nausea and vomiting may occur. Diarrhea has been reported to occur during or shortly after the infusion.
- Fever and mild flulike symptoms are reported.
- Alopecia and skin rash may occur.
- Elevated LFTs are common.
- Headache, dizziness, lightheadedness, and peripheral neuropathy have been reported.

VINBLASTINE (Velban)

Dosage:
- 6–10 mg/m² q 2–4 wk; 1.7–2.0 mg/m²/day weekly as a continuous infusion or over a period of 96 hr

Efficacy:
- Hodgkin's disease
- Non-Hodgkin's lymphoma
- Testicular cancer
- Kaposi's sarcoma
- Breast cancer
- Melanoma
- Cancers of the kidney, bladder, and cervix
- Head and neck cancers
- Lung cancer
- Ovarian cancer

Mechanism of action:
- Cell-cycle phase specific for the M phase
- A plant alkaloid that binds to tubulin causing inhibition of the microtubule assembly, which inhibits mitotic spindle formation.

Metabolism:
- Metabolized by the liver
- Less than 1% is eliminated unchanged in the urine
- t½ = 20 hr

Administration precautions:
- Reconstituted with 10 mL of bacteriostatic NS to yield a concentration of 1 mg/mL.
- Dose may be further diluted with D5W or NS for continuous infusion.
- Continuous infusions may only be given through central lines because vinblastine is a severe vesicant if infiltrated.
- Store in the refrigerator. Stable for 14 days at room temperature and for 30 days under refrigeration.

Side effects:
- Leukopenia is the DLT.
- Thrombocytopenia and anemia are less common.
- Nausea and vomiting, anorexia, diarrhea, and mucositis are rare.
- Peripheral neuropathy, constipation, paralytic ileus, and urinary retention may occur.
- Alopecia occurs with higher doses.
- Rash and photosensitivity may occur.
- Infiltration may cause ulceration depending on the amount of drug extravasated.
- Treatment with hyaluronidase and heat may minimize ulceration.
- Incompatible with heparin and furosemide.
- Compatible in solution with doxorubicin, metoclopramide, dacarbazine, and bleomycin.

(continued)

Appendix 19B Intravenous Antineoplastic Agents (continued)

Dosage and Efficacy	Mechanism of Action and Metabolism	Administration Precautions	Side Effects
	VINCRISTINE (Oncovin)		
Dosage: • 0.5–1.4 mg/m² q 1–4 wk • Continuous infusion regimens of 0.5 mg/day to 0.5 mg/m²/day × 4 days may be used. *Efficacy:* • Acute leukemia • Hodgkin's disease • Non-Hodgkin's lymphoma • Rhabdomyosarcoma • Neuroblastoma • Wilms' tumor • Ewing's sarcoma • Melanoma • Multiple myeloma • Breast cancer • Lung cancer	*Mechanism of action:* • Plant alkaloid • Binds to tubulin, causing inhibition of microtubule assembly, which inhibits mitotic spindle formation • M phase specific. *Metabolism:* • Metabolized by the liver. • 40%–70% excreted in the bile. • t½ = 70–100 hr	*Administration precautions:* • Store in the refrigerator. • Stable for at least 30 days at room temperature. • Doses for continuous infusion are further diluted with NS or D5W. • Compatible with doxorubicin, bleomycin, cytarabine, fluorouracil, methotrexate, and metoclopramide. • Vincristine is a vesicant that should be given with caution and through a central line when given as a continuous infusion. • Hyaluronidase plus heat to disperse the antidote are indicated if the drug should infiltrate. • Greater than 2 mg total dose is usually contraindicated due to the toxicity of the drug. • Vincristine is lethal if given intrathecally and should be labeled as such when dispensed by the pharmacist. • Administer with caution in patients with obvious liver dysfunction.	*Side effects:* • Myelosuppression is mild. Nausea, vomiting, anorexia, and diarrhea are rare. • Constipation and abdominal pain may occur due to the neurological toxicity of the drug. • Prophylactic stool softeners and laxatives may be indicated in patients at high risk for constipation. • Alopecia is minimal. Paresthesias, ataxia, hoarseness, myalgias, headache, and seizures may occur. • Severe pain in the jaw may occur.
	VINORELBINE TARTRATE (Navelbine)		
Dosage: • PO: 40-mg capsule for oral use • IV: 30–40 mg/m² weekly *Efficacy:* • Breast cancer • Ovarian cancer • Head and neck cancer • Esophageal cancer • Non-small cell lung cancer • Lung cancer • Germ cell cancers	*Mechanism of action:* • Cell-cycle specific • Produces cell blockade in G₂ and M phase • Blocks polymerization of microtubules • Impairs mitotic spindle *Metabolism:* • Hepatic elimination • Binds to plasma proteins • Nonrenal elimination	*Administration precautions:* • Venous irritation occurs in about 25% of patients. Symptoms include erythema and pain at the site, vein discoloration and tenderness along the vein. • Administer drug over 6–10 min through the side arm of a freely running IV. Inject through the port farthest from the IV site. • Follow injection with 75–125 mL of IV fluid to flush the line (peripheral IV sites only). • Local tissue damage/necrosis, phlebitis may occur if the drug infiltrates. • Dose reduction may be appropriate for	*Side effects:* • DLT: Noncumulative neutropenia • Alopecia/hair thinning after several treatments • Anorexia • Asthenia • Peripheral neuropathy • Constipation occurs in about ⅓ of patients and increases after several treatments. • Fatigue can be cumulative. • Arthralgias and myalgias • Rash (rare)

- Hodgkin's disease

patients with impaired liver function: If bilirubin is >2.1, the dose of vinorelbine is reduced 50%–75% (i.e., 15–7.5 mg/m^2).
- Pain at the tumor site can occur during administration.
- Vinorelbine is compatible with metoclopramide, ondansetron, chlorpromazine, promethazine, and dexamethasone.
- Vinorelbine is incompatible with 5-FU, thiotepa, furosemide, amphotericin, ampicillin, piperacillin, aminophylline, and sodium bicarbonate.

- Typhlitis with abdominal pain and fever occur 3–4 days after treatment in heavily pretreated patients.
- Jaw pain is rare.

ALL = acute lymphocytic leukemia; AML = acute myelogenous leukemia; AUC = area under the curve; BMT = bone marrow transplant; CHF = congestive heart failure; CI = continuous infusion; D5W = 5% dextrose in water; DLT = dose-limiting toxicity; 5-FU = fluorouracil; 5HT3 = serotonin receptor; GI = gastrointestinal; HSR = hypersensitivity reaction; IM = intramuscular; IP = intraperitoneal; IT = intrathecal; IV = intravenous; IVP = intravenous push; IU = International unit; LFT = liver function test; MUGA = ejection fraction; NS = normal saline; PVC = polyvinyl chloride; QS = quantity sufficient; SIADH = syndrome of inappropriate antidiuretic hormone; SGOT = serum glutamic oxaloacetic transaminase; SGPT = serum glutamic pyruvic transaminase; SQ = subcutaneous; t½ = half-life.

CHAPTER 20

Chemotherapy: Toxicity Management

Dawn Camp-Sorrell, RN, MSN, FNP, AOCN

Introduction

Chemotherapy is administered based on a dose-response relationship (i.e., the more drug administered, the more cancer cells killed). The more cancer cells killed, more normal cell are also killed, subsequently, in acute and chronic toxicity, it affects the quality of life. Characteristically, chemotherapeutic agents have a narrow therapeutic index, with anticipated acute toxicities expressed in rapidly dividing normal tissues, such as the bone marrow, the gastrointestinal tract, the gonads, and the hair follicles. Acute and long-term toxicities from chemotherapy may also be a function of the drug's effect on specific cells of a given organ. The incidence and severity of toxicities are related to the drug's dosage, administration schedule, specific mechanism of action, as well as concomitant illness and specific measures used to prevent or minimize toxicities. Chemotherapeutic agents cause side effects that can appear immediately or after a few days (acute), within a few weeks (intermediate), or months to years after chemotherapy administration (long-term).[1]

Because virtually every organ is affected by chemotherapy, the toxicities of the drug will commonly determine the maximum amount of drug that can be administered safely. Side effects such as stomatitis, alopecia, myelosuppression, nausea, vomiting, anorexia, and diarrhea are common, depending on the agent administered. These are expected side effects that can be managed effectively and generally do not warrant reducing the dose or discontinuing the drug. *Toxic effects* refer to life-threatening, often dose-limiting effects characteristic of high dosages. Cumulative and irreversible damage to certain vital organs, such as the heart, limits the total dosage of chemotherapy.[1]

Providing nursing care to the patient receiving chemotherapy presents many challenges. Interventions focus on preventing or minimizing side effects caused by the chemotherapeutic agent. The key is to assess accurately the patient's status and to complete a health history to detect risk factors before initiating therapy that provides baseline data. After the patient begins treatment, it is important to assess any changes from the baseline and to evaluate the effectiveness of the interventions implemented.

Pretreatment Evaluation: Risk Analysis

Individuals with an overall weak physical condition and poor nutritional status are not likely to tolerate a vigorous treatment course.[2] Patients previously treated with multiple chemotherapy agents, radiation, or biotherapy may lack marrow reserve, placing them at a higher risk for infection, bleeding, or anemia. The inability or unwillingness of an individual to perform self-care may increase the severity of a side effect and also delay the seeking of appropriate care from health care professionals.

Preexisting disorders such as hepatic or renal dysfunc-

tion can alter the absorption, distribution, metabolism, and excretion of chemotherapy, causing abnormal accumulations of the drug and its metabolites.[3] Hypovolemia due to nausea and vomiting, diarrhea, inadequate dietary intake, third spacing (the shift of fluid from the vascular space to the interstitial space), or hypoalbuminemia may increase the risk of acute renal failure.[4] Thus, the patient could be placed at a higher risk for organ toxicities.

Because the incidence of cancer increases with age, nurses must be aware of possible additional risks for the elderly. Age-related changes in physical stature, body composition, kidneys, liver, and other organs influence the pharmacokinetic and pharmacodynamic properties of drug therapy, possibly prolonging the agent's half-life.[4] Many elderly people, especially those over age 85, are physically frail secondary to chronic and debilitating illness or poor nutrition or as a result of aging. Chronic illnesses such as arthritis, heart disease, diabetes, glaucoma, high blood pressure, cognitive deficits, and hearing and vision loss are common in the elderly.[3] These conditions may interfere with an individual's ability to perform basic activities of daily living and, consequently, elderly patients may be unable to perform preventive measures to minimize side effects.

Gradual but substantial changes occur in body composition with age. The percentage of body fat increases, with a corresponding decrease in muscle mass and percentage of body water. Decreases occur in cardiac output, kidney function, hepatic blood flow, the ability to conjugate drugs, and the effectiveness of the immune system.[2,3] Cardiovascular changes occur including thickening of blood vessel walls, atherosclerotic plaque formation, and loss of elastin fibers, which can lead to cardiac hypertrophy, diastolic dysfunction, and myocardial ischemia.[5] With advancing age, the kidneys atrophy, bringing subsequent decrease in renal function. Vasoconstriction of the renal vasculature decreases renal blood flow, glomerular filtration rate, and the ability to concentrate and dilute urine, resulting in a decreased creatinine clearance.[4] Bone marrow reserves decrease, and the ability to replicate myeloid and erythroid progenitor cells decreases. In addition, the functional ability of peripheral mononuclear cells is impaired.[5,6]

Historically, elderly patients (age >60) with cancer have not been treated as aggressively as their younger counterparts because it was speculated that the elderly would not be able to tolerate the stresses imposed by chemotherapy. This trend is changing, however, and many elderly patients now receive aggressive treatment for their cancer.[5–12] Numerous studies have looked at the consequences of treating older patients with chemotherapy. Although the study results are often variable and contradictory, the degree of tolerance to chemotherapy has depended on the type of malignancy and dose intensity.

In general, for many solid tumors, elderly patients tolerate chemotherapy, used either for adjuvant or palliation therapy, as well as young patients.[9] Cisplatin in moderate doses (60–100 mg/m^2) has been found to be safe in patients 80 years or older.[12] Geriatric patients with a systemic malignancy such as lymphoma or acute leukemia usually develop more treatment-related toxicity than younger patients. However, geriatric patients can achieve complete response from chemotherapy if they survive the intensive initial therapy.[11]

While it is critical to be knowledgeable regarding the potential problems the elderly may encounter as a consequence of physiologic aging, age alone has not been shown to be a significant factor in the incidence and severity of toxicity to chemotherapy.[9–12] Chronic illness that often accompanies longevity is a better predictor for tolerance than age alone. The one exception has been hematologic toxicity, probably related to decreased marrow reserve or renal function. Health care professionals, therefore, should monitor hematologic values closely to minimize potential ill effects. Patients older than 70 years with normal renal and hepatic function and without serious medical conditions have been found to tolerate chemotherapy as well as individuals in younger populations.[10–12]

Quality of Life and Chemotherapy Toxicity

Treatment considerations include the patient's quality of life, the impact chemotherapy will have on the patient's quality of life, and the patient's physical and mental well-being.[13] Complications or side effects from chemotherapy are weighed against its potential antineoplastic benefits. If tumor control or palliation is the goal, the side effects are weighed against such benefits of chemotherapy as pain control and prolonged survival time.

In the past, cancer treatment was evaluated by tumor response and survival rates rather than by functional ability or quality of life.[14] Quality of life is difficult to measure. It should be based on the physical, psychological, social, and spiritual characteristics of what gives life value to the individual.[15] Quality of life is recognized as an acceptable end point in clinical trials, which have been influenced by viewing cancer as a chronic condition instead of as an acute event. Groups of cancer survivors have indicated to the health care community that quality of life is as important to the patient as the overall therapeutic effect.[16]

Physical symptoms (i.e., nausea, pain, rashes, stomatitis, etc.) can result in significant distress that has a marked impact on the patient's quality of life.[17] It is important to realize that the patient's perception of cancer and chemotherapy treatment will influence how the individual reacts and ultimately adapts.[16] Side effects can impair a patient's abilities to function at work or at home, maintain sexual relationships, and engage in social activities. The degree of self-reported symptoms relates to the individual's perceived quality of life, such as when an increase in symptoms correlates with a decrease in quality of life.[16] Feelings of helplessness are heightened because patients are dependent on health care professionals to deliver their treatment. Anxiety can develop at key decision points, such as diagnosis, beginning of treatment, while awaiting test results, when the treatment plan is altered, or when the chemotherapy treatment plan has been successfully completed.[15] Chemotherapy-related changes in physical appearance are often described as a distressing aspect of cancer treatment. Weight changes and alopecia commonly occur and can be especially devastating because they are physical manifestations of having cancer.[15]

In an effort to minimize acute and chronic toxicities, chemoprotectant agents are being developed to improve the patient's quality of life.[18] Agents can be given prior to the chemotherapy agent to decrease the incidence of the expected toxicity, such as amifostine to minimize nephrotoxicity. Other agents, such as growth factors, are given concurrently with the chemotherapy and are directed at modulating the acute phase of the wound-healing response and decreasing inflammatory cascades. Rescue agents, such as leucovorin, are given after methotrexate to help minimize acute reactions.[18,19]

To help the patient cope with potential side effects, the nurse should foster a trusting relationship with the patient so that communication is open and sufficient information can be provided to help the patient retain control over his or her care. An important aspect of establishing a partnership with the patient and family in the pretreatment phase is knowing what concerns about the treatment need to be explored and what information needs to be provided. Such information helps patients formulate questions about available options when making difficult decisions about their care. When participating actively, the patient's feelings of control are enhanced, resulting in an improved functional status, sense of well-being, and performance of effective self-care.[20] Nurses must focus on developing practical interventions to reduce the psychological distress of treatment and to provide needed information, thereby increasing the patient's quality of life.

Self-Care

There is undeniable evidence that cost factors are dictating the administration of health care. Institutional, state, and federal regulatory bodies have assumed increasing jurisdiction over how and where patients will be treated. Diagnostic-related groups (DRGs) and prospective payment, cost-control measures by other insurers, as well as increased out-of-pocket medical expenses for consumers have combined to create a shift from hospital-based care to outpatient and home-care settings.[20] The change from inpatient to outpatient administration of chemotherapy shifts the responsibility for managing the treatment of side effects from health care providers to patients and their families. To facilitate self-care, nurses must understand the nature, incidence, and relative severity of each side effect, and be aware of effective self-care activities for reducing the severity of side effects.

With increasing severity of a side effect, patients become more immobilized and may delay initiating self-care behaviors for several days. Therefore, follow-up by the nurse must be initiated at least 1–3 days after chemotherapy to assess the patient and to determine whether side effects are being managed adequately. Patient education is essential to ensure that the patient and family understand what self-care measures need to be taken for the side effects experienced.[20]

One of the key goals of nursing care is to minimize toxicity, therefore the patient and caregiver must be instructed how to initiate self-care activities. *Self-care* is any activity initiated by patient, family, or friends to alleviate or minimize a side effect.[21] Self-care activities are initiated before treatment and are used throughout the treatment phase to manage or minimize side effects. In situations where patients are unable or unwilling to participate, efforts must be made to include family members or visiting nurses to ensure compliance. Without compliance, the side effects can be severe and may lead to further complications, which may result in hospitalization and death. Side effects that seem to be the most distressing to patients include fatigue, nausea, vomiting, alopecia, anorexia, and mouth sores.[15] Nurses must continue to develop effective strategies to assist patients in minimizing these side effects. Documenting strategies that have been successful, including those suggested by the patient, can serve as a useful resource for future patient instruction.

Patient Education and Follow-Up

Although teaching may be initiated while the patient is still hospitalized, most teaching regarding chemotherapy takes place in the outpatient setting and is provided by the nurse who will administer the drugs. The intent of teaching is more than to give information: it provides support and knowledge to empower the patient to manage self-care effectively.[20,21] Teaching patients about their treatment reduces fear, increases self-confidence, improves compliance, and enhances their participation in self-care.[20]

One approach to identifying the informational needs of the patients and family members is to focus on the various phases of cancer care: diagnosis, treatment, rehabilitation, survivorship, and recurrent disease. Goals of chemotherapy teaching include:

1. Helping the patient adjust to the treatment
2. Explaining how the treatment will affect the cancer
3. Imparting the sequence of administration
4. Recognizing and controlling side effects
5. Encouraging self-care behaviors that minimize side effects

6. Listing side effects that should be reported to the health care professional

All information offered to the patient is documented in the patient's record (Figure 20-1) for future reference as well as to comply with professional regulations. It is important to reinforce teachings periodically, as retention without reinforcement is short-lived.

In the outpatient setting, the nurse frequently screens phone calls and triages the patient to assist in evaluating symptomatology and initiating the appropriate treatment measures. The nurse must gather sufficient data to determine whether the patient needs medical intervention and, if so, whether the patient will be cared for most appropriately in the outpatient setting or in the hospital. Figure 20-2 is a telephone triage flowchart listing basic steps that might be appropriate in managing patient problems over the phone. Obviously, the nurse needs to be highly knowledgeable about the patient's history, the last chemotherapy treatment, and whether this complaint is related to the treatment, the disease, or is unrelated.

Objective and subjective data must be gathered methodically in order to formulate an opinion about the patient's account. After consulting with the physician, the nurse once again speaks to the patient, either to gather more information or to relay instructions to the patient or family regarding care. Examples of specific phone-triage flowcharts are included in the discussion of various chemotherapy side effects later in the chapter.

Chemotherapy Toxicities

Grading of Toxicities

Standardization of assessment and documentation of side effects are crucial in evaluating the therapeutic use of chemotherapy. Specific therapies can be assessed by comparing their benefits with toxicity occurrence. To assess toxicity, the following information should be considered as it relates to chemotherapy administration:

- Which toxicities occurred
- Toxicity severity
- Time of onset
- Duration of effect
- Interventions used to minimize the effect

In the recognition and evaluation of toxicities, one must discriminate between an expected and a toxic reaction from chemotherapy and distinguish these from complications related to the cancer. For example, if a patient with lymphoma presents to the clinic with a complaint of paresthesias, numbness, and tingling, the patient must be evaluated for possible spinal cord compression from tumor progression and for peripheral toxicity from vincristine administration.

CHEMOTHERAPY TEACHING CHECKLIST

Assessment Summary:

_____

_____

_____

_____

_____

_____

Patient
name: _____
Primary
nurse: _____

Drugs: _____

_____

LEARNING NEED	TEACHING INITIATED (DATE & INITIALS)	KNOWLEDGE CONFIRMED (DATE & INITIALS)	COMMENTS
1. Patient education booklets/drug cards			
2. Viewed chemotherapy video Other:			
3. Common side effects and treatment			
a. Nausea and vomiting—antiemetics			
b. Stomatitis—mouth care			
c. Alopecia—wigs/scarves			
d. Decreased white blood cells—infection precaution			
e. Decreased red blood cells—fatigue			
f. Decreased platelets—bleeding precaution			
g. Skin and nail bed changes			
h. Loss of appetite—nutrition			
i. Diarrhea—medication/diet			
j. Constipation—diet/medication			
k. Flulike symptoms			
l. Urine discoloration			
m. Hemorrhagic cystitis			
n. Premedications (chemoprotectants, steroids, etc)			
o. Other			
4. Specific teaching			
a. Subcutaneous injections			
b. Maintaining adequate nutrition			
c. Precautions to report during drug administration:			
(1) Stinging, burning pain			
(2) Flushing of face			
(3) Metallic taste			
(4) Feeling of numbness			
(5) Itching at site (or generalized itching)			
(6) Allergic reactions			

Figure 20-1 Chemotherapy teaching checklist

(continued)

LEARNING NEED	TEACHING INITIATED (DATE & INITIALS)	KNOWLEDGE CONFIRMED (DATE & INITIALS)	COMMENTS

d. Reproductive changes
  *Dyspareunia
  *Menopausal symptoms
  *Vaginal discomfort			

e. Activity			
f. Interaction with other drugs/food			
g. Vascular access device			
h. Perineal burning (Decadron)			
i. Peripheral edema			
5. Symptoms to report to physician:			
a. Bleeding			
b. Prolonged nausea or vomiting			
c. Fever/chills			
d. Stomatitis			
e. Diarrhea/constipation			
f. Numbness or tingling of extremities			
g. Difficulty breathing or shortness of breath			
h. Other			
6. Prescriptions given to patient with Instructions: □ Antiemetics _____ □ Wig □ Blood counts □ Other			
7. Schedule/calendar of drug treatment			
8. Instructions to obtain blood counts			
9. Follow-up or referral to community resources			

Comments: _____

_____

_____

_____

Patient signature: _____

RN signature: _____

Figure 20-1   Chemotherapy teaching checklist (continued)

Using specific parameters and operational definitions to define the degree of a given toxicity ensures consistency in documenting observed reactions (Table 20-1). Toxicity grading scales have been developed by the World Health Organization and various cooperative study groups to provide consistency in reporting. Adequate assessment and documentation of the side effect experienced, the patient's overall response to the regimen, and subsequent quality of life can be essential for evaluating the impact of treatment. Decisions regarding the need for appropriate adjustments in the treatment plan can be determined on the basis of sound, objective data documented by the nurse.[15,22]

Specific guidelines need to be taught and given in written form to the patient and caregiver to ensure that they report any type of toxicity. Misinterpretation of a patient's report can negatively affect changes made in the treatment protocol. Nurses will continue to be chal-

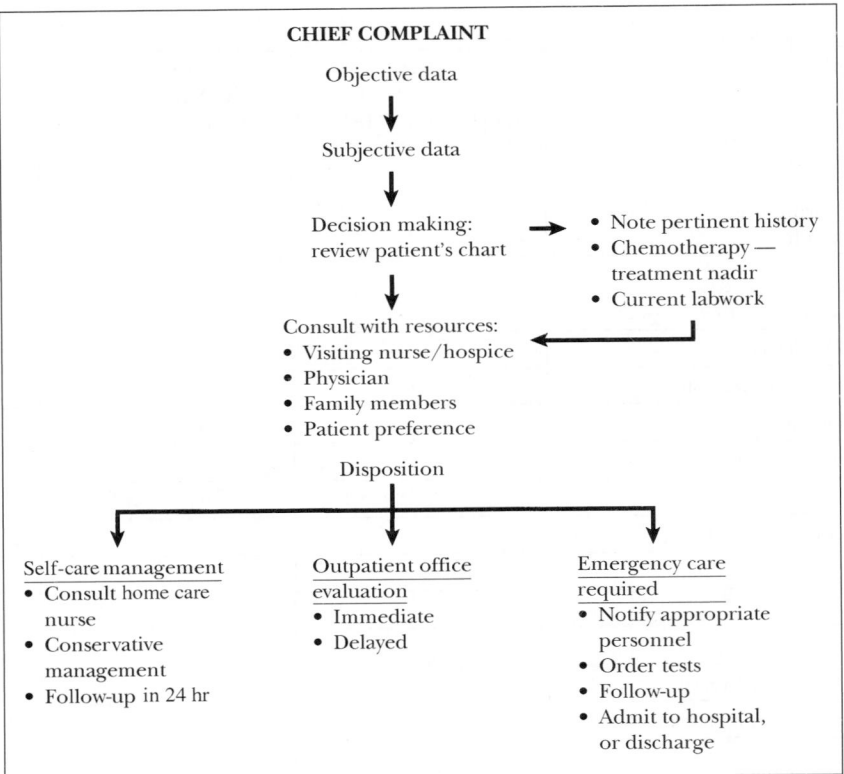

Figure 20-2 Telephone triage flowchart

lenged to design effective assessment and documentation systems that ensure accurate patient observation and reporting of toxicities, especially in the home setting.

Systemic Toxicities

Bone marrow suppression

Myelosuppression is the most common dose-limiting side effect of chemotherapy and can also be the most lethal.[23] All hematopoietic cells divide rapidly, regardless of their developmental stage, and are therefore vulnerable to chemotherapy. Proliferating progenitor cells that produce the mature granulocytes, erythrocytes, and thrombocytes in the peripheral circulation are commonly destroyed. As immature cells in the marrow and preexisting mature cells are destroyed, the nadir becomes apparent, usually 7–14 days after chemotherapy. At the same time, cells in the bone marrow are maturing and are ready to be released into the peripheral blood. Within a short period of time (3–4 weeks), the nadir will resolve.[24] However, when high doses are administered, the stem cell population may fail to repopulate quickly enough, resulting in a prolonged nadir period.

The majority of chemotherapy drugs cause some degree of myelosuppression.[23] Agents most active against cells that are cycling or those active during a specific phase of the cell cycle can produce rapid cytopenia. Because alkylating agents and nitrosoureas affect cycling cells and noncycling cells, these drugs are more likely to destroy the marrow stem cells. Antimetabolites, vinca alkaloids, and antitumor antibiotics are most damaging to cells that are in a specific phase of the cell cycle; thus, myelosuppression is less severe with these agents.[23] However, dose intensification and drug combinations can produce severe and prolonged neutropenia. For many drugs, myelosuppression can be the dose-limiting toxicity, especially for newer agents such as paclitaxel, docetaxel, vinorelbine, and gemcitabine.[25-33] Paclitaxel can cause neutropenia, with the severity dependent on the administration schedule, dose, extent of previous treatment, and pharmacological exposure to the drug. Although preliminary data reveal that 3-hour infusion induces less neutropenia, the neutropenic effect is not cumulative, and permanent toxicity does not occur to the bone marrow. Gemcitibine can cause myelosuppression, especially thrombocytopenia. The hematologic toxicity has been found to be cumulative with the maximum tolerated dose of 1500 mg/m²/week over a 30-minute infusion. Docetaxel results in an early short-lasting type of neutropenia at a dose of 100 mg/m² or greater when infused over 1 hour every 3 weeks. The nadir usually occurs at day 8 and resolves in 1 to 2 weeks, which has not been found to be a cumulative effect.

Risk factors such as tumor cells in the bone marrow, prior treatment with chemotherapy or radiation, and a high negative nitrogen balance will compromise the marrow and increase the degree and duration of cytopenia.[23] It has been recognized that an increased risk of infection

Table 20-1   Grading Toxicities from Chemotherapeutic Agents

Toxicity	Grade ≥ 1	Grade 1	Grade 2	Grade 3	Grade 4
HEMATOLOGIC					
WBC (1000/mm³)	≥4.0	3.0–3.9	2.0–2.9	1.0–1.9	<1.0
Granulocytes (1000/mm³)	≥2.0	1.5–1.9	1.0–1.4	0.5–0.9	<0.5
Platelets (1000/mm³)	≥100	75–99	50–74	25–49	<25
Hemoglobin (g/100 mL)	≥11	9.5–10.9	8.0–9.4	6.5–7.9	<6.5
Hemorrhage	None	Slight, no transfusion	Mild, 1–2 transfusions/ episode	Gross, 3–4 transfusions/ episode	Massive, >4 transfusions/ episode
Infection/fever	None	Temp: <38°C No antibiotics	Temp: 38°–40°C Broad-spectrum antibiotics	Temp: >40°C Antifungal coverage	Signs of sepsis: reevaluate medication
GASTROINTESTINAL					
Nausea/vomiting	None	Slight nausea, 1 episode of vomiting Maintains intake	Occasional nausea, 2–5 episodes of vomiting Maintains intake	Frequent nausea, 6–10 episodes of vomiting Intake decreased	Constant nausea, >10 episodes of vomiting No intake
Diarrhea	None	2–3 stools	4–6 stools Moderate cramps	7–9 stools Severe cramps	>10 stools; needs rehydration
Constipation	None	Dry, hard passage of painful stool Stool softener	No stool >2 days Laxatives	No stool >4 days Rule out obstruction or cause	—
Stomatitis	None	Painless ulcers, erythema, or mild soreness	Painful erythema, edema, or ulcers, but can eat	Painful erythema, edema, ulcers, cannot eat	Requires parenteral or enteral support
Esophagitis/dysphagia	None	Painless ulcers, erythema, mild soreness, or dysphagia	Painful erythema, edema, ulcers, or moderate dysphagia, but can eat without narcotics	Cannot eat solids, or requires narcotics to eat	As above or complete obstruction or perforation
Taste	Normal	Slightly altered taste, metallic taste	Markedly altered taste	—	—
DERMATOLOGIC					
Skin	None	Scattered macular or papular eruption or erythema; asymptomatic	Scattered macular or papular eruption, or erythema with pruritus or other associated symptoms	Generalized symtomatic macular, papular, or vesicular eruption	Exofoliative dermatitis or ulcerating dermatitis
Local	None	Pain	Pain and swelling with inflammation or phlebitis	Ulceration	Plastic surgery indicated
OTHER					
Myalgia/arthralgia	None	Mild	Decrease in ability to move	Disabled	—

occurs among individuals suffering from protein-calorie malnutrition, causing lymphopenia, diminished levels of the complement system, and a decrease of certain immunoglobulins. In addition, myelotoxicity caused by chemotherapy and radiation therapy is enhanced by protein deprivation resulting from cancer cachexia. Younger patients are less likely to demonstrate severe cytopenia due to chemotherapy because their marrow is more cellular and has a decreased percentage of fat.

Differences in the lengths and kinetics of the life cycles of particular blood cells account for the frequency of neutropenia, thrombocytopenia, and anemia. Maturation of cells in the bone marrow takes 8 to 10 days, with variation in the life span for each cell type.

Red blood cells (RBCs) have a life span of 120 days. Chemotherapy-induced anemia occurs rarely because the bone marrow begins to recover before the number of circulating RBCs decreases significantly. Although low hemoglobin and hematocrit levels will not prevent administration of chemotherapy, low levels affect how the patient feels and functions. Anemia is manifested by pallor, hypotension, headaches, irritability, and fatigue (see Chapter 32). Tachycardia and tachypnea may be present due to the hypoxic effects on the heart. Secondary problems include skin or mucous membrane breakdown arising from decreased tissue oxygenation, and cardiopulmonary stress. The incapacitating symptoms of anemia have a profound impact on quality of life.[17,34] Anemia can usually be corrected with RBC transfusion.

Anemia of chronic disease is associated with erythroid hypoplasia of the bone marrow.[35] This results in a slight decrease in reticulocytosis, hypoferremia, and a decrease in serum erythropoietin. Actions of certain chemotherapeutic agents such as cisplatin may inhibit the maturation of the erythroid lineage cells in the bone marrow.[36]

Erythropoietin can be administered in an attempt to correct anemia induced by chemotherapy. Erythropoietin is a growth factor for erythroid progenitor cells that promotes proliferation and maintains their survival.[37] The usual dose is 150 U/kg subcutaneously three times a week until the target hematocrit is reached. Weekly erythropoietin administration at a dose of 400 U/kg has been found to be as effective compared to three weekly injections.[37] The target range, which is monitored weekly, is 36%–40%.[34] Once the patient reaches the target range, a maintenance dose is administered. Although a response from erythropoietin may take 2 to 8 weeks, the maintenance dose is the dose the patient was receiving when the target hematocrit was reached. Only 50%–60% of anemic cancer patients respond to epoetin alfa, and it may require up to 12 weeks of treatment to determine if the patient is benefiting from the drug; by monitoring for an increase in hemoglobin level and in reticulocyte count.[34]

Patients with iron deficiency require iron supplementation because adequate iron stores are necessary to support erythropoiesis. The most common side effect from erythropoietin is hypertension, therefore the patient's blood pressure should be monitored frequently.[35]

The life span of platelets is 7 to 10 days. Thrombocytopenia usually occurs 8–14 days after chemotherapy and in most cases concomitantly with neutropenia. Chemotherapy may be suspended if the count drops below 100,000/mm³. Thrombocytopenia is a potential or actual dose-limiting toxicity of gemcitabine, carboplatin, dacarbazine, 5-FU, lomustine, mitomycin-C, thiotepa, and trimetrexate. A cumulative and delayed onset of thrombocytopenia has been observed with carmustine, fludarabine, lomustine, mitomycin-C, streptozocin, and thiotepa. When platelets are less than 50,000 cells/mm³, a moderate risk of bleeding exists. As the platelets continue to decrease below 10,000 cells/mm³, a severe risk exists for fatal gastrointestinal, central nervous system, and respiratory tract hemorrhage. Manifestations of thrombocytopenia are easy bruising; bleeding from gums, nose, or other orifices; and petechiae on the upper and lower extremities, pressure points, elbows, and palate (Figure 20-3).[23] Transfusion of platelets is a common therapeutic intervention for platelet count below 10,000–20,000 cells/mm³, although it is often dependent on the patient's symptoms.[38]

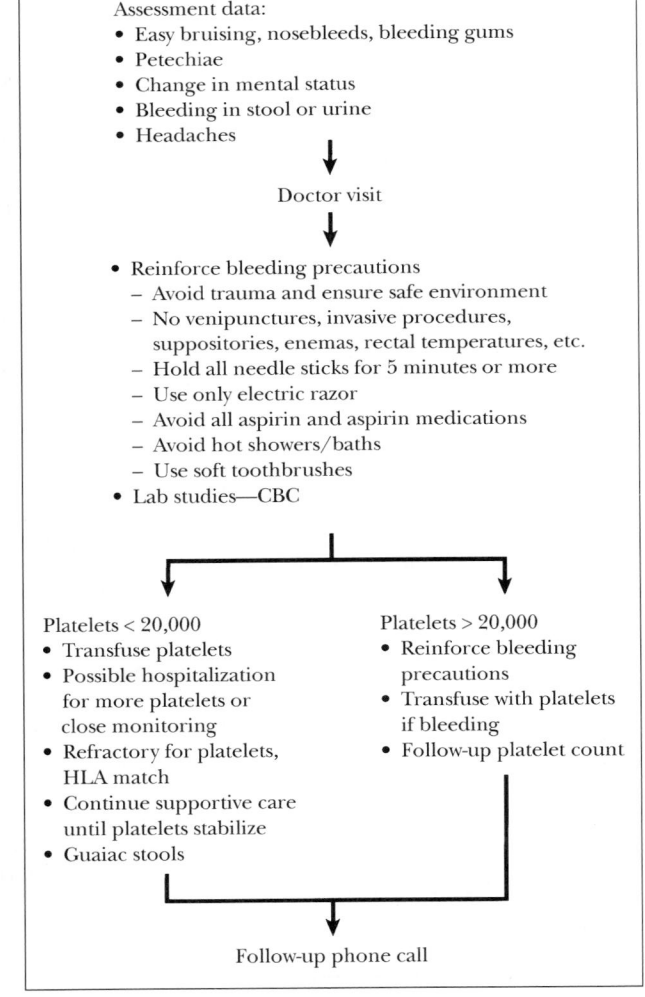

Figure 20-3 Thrombocytopenia telephone triage flowchart.

In an attempt to minimize the occurrence of chemotherapy-induced thrombocytopenia, interleukin 11 (IL-11) has been approved as a growth factor for megakaryocytes in nonmyeloid malignancies and in nonmyeloablative chemotherapy regimens. Interleukin 11 causes proliferation of hematopoietic stem cells and megakaryocyte progenitors and also induces megakaryocytic maturation.[39] Interestingly, IL-11 causes this effect independently of thrombopoietin. The dose is 50 µg/kg administered daily subcutaneously until the platelet count is greater than 50,000 cells/mm³.[40] Interleukin 11 is discontinued 2 days prior to the next chemotherapy treatment. Side effects from IL-11 are thought to occur secondary to an increase in intravascular fluid from renal sodium retention and plasma volume expansion including dyspnea, edema, and an increase in pleural effusion formation.[39,40] Subsequently, patients with a history of congestive heart failure or coronary heart disease are usually not candidates for IL-11.

The life span of the granulocyte is 6–8 hours after release from the marrow. Neutropenia typically develops 8–12 days after chemotherapy, with recovery in 3–4 weeks. Chemotherapy is usually withheld if the patient's white blood cell (WBC) count is between 1000 and 3000/mm³ or if the absolute neutrophil count (ANC) is below 1500/mm³. Neutropenia generally is defined as an ANC below 1500 cells/mm³. In normal individuals, neutrophils, including both the segmented and slightly less mature band forms, are found in concentrations ranging from 1830–7250 cells/mm³. Profound neutropenia (grade 4) usually is defined as an ANC less than 500 cells/mm³.[23]

It is important to note that neutropenia can occur when total WBC count is within a normal range (4000–10,000/mm³). Consequently, quantitating the ANC is essential to achieving a correct assessment of neutrophil status. An ANC is calculated by multiplying the total WBC count by the differential proportion of combined band and segmented neutrophils in a blood sample.

WBC (segmented neutrophils + band neutrophils)
= ANC

Thus, in a patient with a WBC count of 4000 cells/mm³, a differential of 34% segmented neutrophils plus 3% band neutrophils yields an ANC of

4000 cells/mm³ × .37 = 1480 cells/mm³.

Monocyte count should also be monitored because an increase in monocytes precedes and predicts resolution of neutropenia.[23]

Since the prime function of neutrophils is phagocytosis, neutropenia eliminates one of the body's prime defenses against bacterial infection. Infections, due to invasion and overgrowth of pathogenic microbes, increase in frequency and severity as ANC decreases. In addition, risk for severe infections increases when the nadir persists for more than 7–10 days.[41]

Signs of an infection may not be apparent with the inhibition of phagocytic cells. The only response may be fever and at times this may not be present. It is estimated that 80% of the infections that occur arise from endogenous microbial flora of the gastrointestinal or respiratory tract.[24,41,42] When the neutrophil count is less than 500 cells/mm³, approximately 20% or more of febrile episodes will have an associated bacteremia caused principally by aerobic gram-negative bacilli (*Escherichia coli, Klebsiella pneumoniae, Pseudomonas aeruginosa*) and gram-positive cocci (coagulase-negative staphylococci, streptococci species, and *Staphylococcus aureus*).[41,42]

Chemotherapy-induced damage to the alimentary canal and respiratory tract mucosa facilitates the entry of infecting organisms; therefore, pneumonia and sinusitis are commonly seen. The nurse must assess for inflammation at the sites most commonly infected, including the periodontium, pharynx, lower esophagus, lung, perineum, anus, skin, and venous access exit sites. Prevention, early detection, good hand-washing technique, and prompt management of infections in patients with neutropenia are essential if sepsis and septic shock are to be avoided (Figure 20-4).[43]

Once appropriate cultures are obtained, broad-spectrum antibiotics are used to treat chemotherapy-induced infections: (1) until cultures indicate eradication of the causative organism, (2) for a minimum of 7 days, or (3) until the neutrophil count is greater than 500/mm³.[42] Extended-spectrum cephalosporins (ceftazidime) and the carbapenems (imipenem) are agents most often used for empiric monotherapy. Combination therapy with anti-

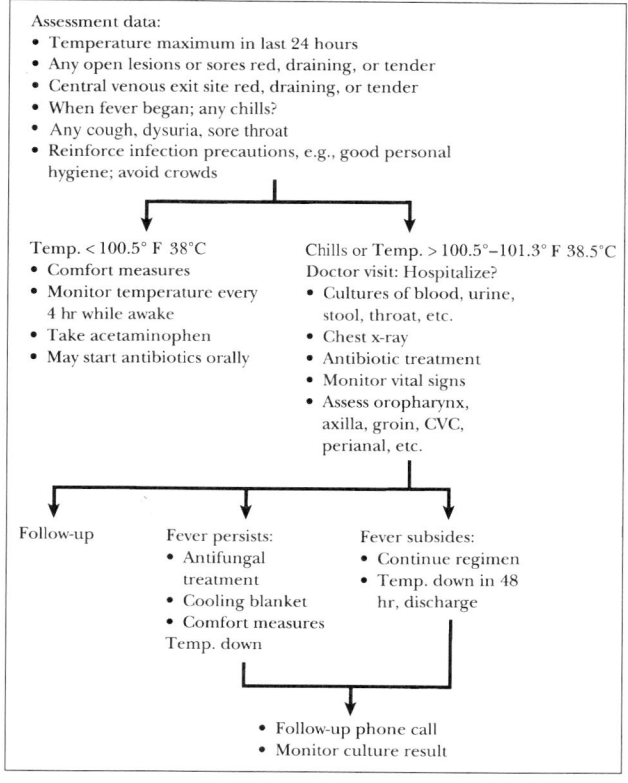

Figure 20-4   Fever telephone triage flowchart.

pseudomonal third-generation cephalosporins and aminoglycosides or penicillin is generally used.[24] Other combinations include a β-lactam (penicillin) with an aminoglycoside or another β-lactam.[41,42,44] With the increased predominance of gram-positive organisms in febrile neutropenic patients, the use of vancomycin with an antipseudomonal β-lactam agent has been beneficial. Although effective, such combinations should not be used routinely because of potential emergence of vancomycin-resistant organisms. Empiric use of vancomycin is recommended in patients known to be colonized with methicillin-resistant organisms, in patients with a venous access device infection, and in patients on quinolone prophylaxis with severe mucositis who are at risk for a streptococcal infection or positive blood cultures prior to susceptibility information.[41]

Until recently, all febrile neutropenic patients were treated with hospital-based parenteral antibiotics. Risk assessment is now used to determine the need for hospitalization and the route of antibiotic therapy.[41,44] Neutropenia induced by solid tumor treatment is usually less than 10 days in duration, whereas neutropenia associated with hematologic malignancies often lasts 15 to 20 days. High-risk patients include those with hematologic malignancies and bone marrow transplant recipients with prolonged neutropenia. These patients need to be hospitalized and given broad-spectrum parenteral therapy until resolution of fever and neutropenia and until cultures indicate eradication of causative organisms. Moderate-risk patients include those with a comorbidity such as hypertension or renal failure; they need to be stabilized in the hospital and discharged early with parenteral or oral antibiotics. Low-risk patients can be given outpatient therapy with either oral ciprofloxacin or ciprofloxacin plus amoxicillin.[41]

Fever persisting for more than 3 days without identification of an infected site or organism suggests (1) a nonbacterial cause, (2) resistance to the antibiotic, (3) emergence of a second bacterial infection, (4) inadequate antibiotic serum and tissue levels, (5) drug fever, or (6) infection at avascular sites (abscess).[44] At this point, antifungal therapy is started. Antiviral drugs are usually not recommended unless mucosal lesions or viral disease is suspected. Risk for recurrent fever and infection are significant for neutropenic patients or those with poor marrow recovery such as in disease-related bone marrow dysfunction.[24]

Protective isolation has no effect on the host's endogenous flora and no impact on organisms transmitted by water or food. It is not surprising that when careful hand washing and handling of food and other supplies are conducted, the addition of protective isolation offers no benefit in decreasing infections in neutropenic patients. Thus, hand washing is the best preventive method for minimizing infection in the neutropenic patient.[43]

Among all the problems identified with myelosuppression, infection is the most serious and is associated with significant morbidity and mortality.[41] For this reason, much attention has been focused on the therapeutic application of recombinant colony-stimulating factors (CSFs) to augment neutrophil counts. Hematopoietic growth factors are a family of glycoprotein hormones that act as natural regulators of hematopoiesis to promote the proliferation and differentiation of hematopoietic progenitor cells along multiple pathways.[45,46] While hematopoietic stimulants have not changed the decline rate of granulocytes, they have shortened the duration of neutropenia, thereby dramatically reducing the morbidity and mortality from infections. The discovery of CSFs offers hope that the myelosuppression associated with chemotherapy can be ameliorated and that full dosages of chemotherapy can be used in cancer therapy.

The American Society of Clinical Oncologists has developed clinical practice guidelines for appropriate use of CSFs.[45] After reviewing available literature, the following guidelines were developed to assist the practitioner in use of CSFs:

1. CSFs are appropriate to initiate if subsequent chemotherapy regimens are delayed from prolonged neutropenia and if dose reduction is not possible.
2. CSFs are appropriate in febrile neutropenia in conjunction with antibiotics only in clinical deterioration such as multiorgan failure.
3. CSFs are appropriate when febrile neutropenia is expected in >40% of patients such as results from high-dose chemotherapy.
4. CSFs are appropriate with autologous bone marrow transplants, to shorten neutropenia and infectious complications.
5. CSFs are effective in mobilizing peripheral blood progenitor cells for transplantation.

Inconclusive data exist on the use of CSFs with other conditions, especially febrile neutropenia. Although growth factors have made a tremendous impact on decreasing duration of neutropenia thereby decreasing the incidence of infections, reduced efficacy occurs with multiple courses and with bone marrow depletion. Another limitation is that there are specific lineage growth factors affecting only a segment of one tissue compartment.[18] Studies continue to find the most effective growth factor. Experimental data have suggested that the pineal hormone melatonin may counteract chemotherapy-induced myelosuppression. Studies have shown melatonin to inhibit the production of free radicals that mediate chemotherapy-induced toxicity.[47]

Although clinical experience is limited, granulocyte CSFs may have a potential role in treating fungal infections. Colony-stimulating factors have been shown to enhance activity of phagocytic cells against *Candida* species.[48]

Gastrointestinal tract

Chemotherapy-induced gastrointestinal toxicity can be the most devastating experience for the patient. Although numerous pharmacological interventions have been developed to minimize these toxicities, the occurrence can lead to delay of treatment, fluid and electrolyte imbalances, weight loss, and malnutrition.

Diarrhea.   Chemotherapy-induced diarrhea occurs due to a combination of factors, including an imbalance between absorption and secretion in the small bowel.[49,50] Diarrhea is an increase in stool volume and liquidity, resulting in three or more bowel movements per day. Chemotherapy produces acute damage to the intestinal mucosa that is characterized by necrosis of the cells that line the intestinal crypt, resulting in extensive bowel wall inflammation. Without crypt cells, replacement of cells in the intestinal villi is hampered, resulting in a decreased absorptive surface. Because of the intestinal inflammation, factors such as prostaglandins and cytokines are secreted that further stimulate the secretion of intestinal fluids and electrolytes from crypt cells.[51]

The degree and duration of diarrhea depends on the agent, dose, nadir, and frequency of chemotherapy administration. Incidence and severity of diarrhea have increased with newer chemotherapy agents, adjunct therapies, and aggressive treatment approaches.[49] Alterations in mucosal integrity, coupled with the destruction of brush-border enzymes essential for carbohydrate and protein digestion, produce moderate to severe diarrhea immediately following chemotherapy and up to 14 days after chemotherapy. With 5-FU and leucovorin therapy, patients may experience abdominal cramps and rectal urgency, which can evolve into nocturnal diarrhea or fecal incontinence leading to lethargy, weakness, orthostatic hypotension, and fluid and electrolyte imbalance. Without adequate management, prolonged diarrhea will cause dehydration, nutritional malabsorption, and circulatory collapse.

Although 5-FU is the most common drug to cause diarrhea, other agents include methotrexate, docetaxel, actinomycin D, doxorubicin, trimetrexate, and irinotecan. Combination chemotherapy and multimodal treatment can result in severe diarrhea. Antiemetics such as metoclopramide and prokinetic agents can cause diarrhea by increasing bowel transit time.[52]

Thorough evaluation to determine the cause of the diarrhea provides a firm foundation for planning interventions. Management may be limited to dietary measures, such as a low-residue, high-caloric, protein diet or pharmacological measures. Stool cultures need to be obtained initially to rule out an infectious process so that appropriate therapy can be implemented. *Clostridium difficile* has been reported in patients receiving chemotherapy who have had prior antibiotic exposure. Antidiarrheal agents should never be given to counteract diarrhea resulting from an infection, as these agents slow the passage of stool through the intestines, prolonging the mucosal exposure to the organism's toxins. Usually when the diarrhea is a result of an organism, it will resolve in a few days with the use of vancomycin or metronidazole.[53]

Pharmacological intervention for diarrhea is varied. Anticholinergic drugs such as atropine sulfate and scopolamine reduce gastric secretions and decrease intestinal peristalsis. Opiate therapy binds to receptors on the smooth muscle of bowel, slowing down the intestinal motility and increasing fluid absorption. Loperamide is a long-acting opioid agonist without central opioid activity. Although the recommendation is a maximum of 16 mg in 24 hours, an increase of the loperamide dose must be used to control irinotecan-induced diarrhea. Current recommendations are 4 mg initially followed by 2 mg every 4 hours until the diarrhea stops.[33] Octreotide acetate, a synthetic analog of the hormone octapeptide, inhibits the release of gut hormones, including serotonin and gastrin, from the gastrointestinal tract. It affects the gastrointestinal tract by prolonging intestinal transit time, increasing intestinal water and electrolyte transport, and decreasing mesenteric blood flow. Octreotide acetate is indicated for patients who have excessive diarrhea as a result of gastrointestinal resections or when other pharmacological treatments have proved ineffective in managing chemotherapy-induced diarrhea.[51,53] Other pharmacologic agents are under investigation for diarrhea including clonidine, calcium channel blockers, nonsteroidal anti-inflammatory drugs, and leukotriene-synthesis inhibitors.[52]

Chemotherapy usually is administered despite the occurrence of diarrhea. However, diarrhea can be severe enough to be a dose-limiting toxicity of some chemotherapeutic agents such as irinotecan or combination therapy, specifically 5-FU and leucovorin. The nurse must carefully monitor the patient's status to provide appropriate therapy, such as antidiarrheal medications, fluid and electrolyte replacements, and perirectal care to prevent further complications (Figure 20-5).

Constipation.   Constipation is defined as infrequent, excessively hard and dry bowel movements resulting from a decrease in rectal filling or emptying.[54] Risk factors that contribute to constipation include narcotic analgesics, a decrease in physical activity, a low-fiber diet, a decrease in fluid intake, and bed rest. Other medications such as anticholinergics, calcium channel blockers, iron, calcium, and anticonvulsants decrease stool frequency. Vincristine, vinblastine, and vinorelbine are the most common chemotherapy agents to cause constipation, as a result of autonomic nerve dysfunction manifested as colicky abdominal pain and ileus. Rectal emptying is specifically diminished because nonfunctional afferent and efferent pathways from the sacral cord are interrupted. Symptoms occur 3–7 days after drug administration and may be accompanied by evidence of peripheral nerve dysfunction.[55]

Patients are instructed to be aware of bowel movements. If a bowel movement does not occur every other day, a laxative must be taken. If there are no results, the physician should be asked for further instructions. Laxative therapy or prophylactic stool softener is recommended prior to the administration of drugs known to contribute to constipation, especially if the patient has a history of or is at risk for constipation. The patient should be encouraged to increase the amount of high-fiber foods

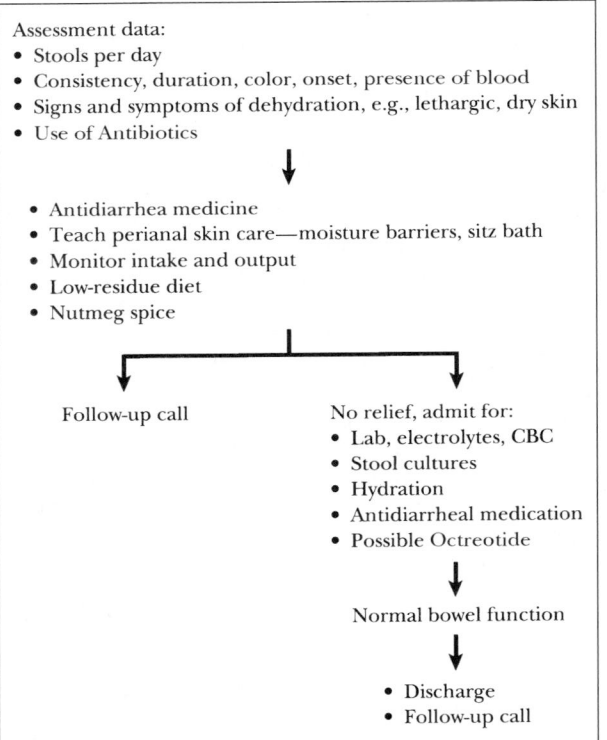

Figure 20-5 Diarrhea telephone triage flowchart

ent vagal motor nuclei; and histamine in the VC and the vestibular apparatus. Chemotherapy damages the enterochromaffin cells of the duodenal mucosa causing serotonin release that binds to vagal afferent receptors. These afferent receptors send impulses to the emetic center.[56]

Vestibular-cerebellar afferent pathway areas transmit impulses to the cerebellum and then to the VC, which is experienced as motion sickness. When rapid motion change occurs, the receptors of the labyrinth in the inner ear are stimulated, which is associated with nausea.[56] Obstruction, irritation, inflammation, or delayed gastric emptying may stimulate the gastrointestinal tract through vagal visceral afferent pathways.[55] Conditioned and anticipatory responses are controlled by the cerebral cortex and limbic system, which can be stimulated by sights, sounds, or odors that the patient associates with chemotherapy, thereby making the patient nauseated.[56]

Although nausea, retching, and vomiting commonly occur together, they are considered separate conditions.[58] *Nausea* is described as a subjective conscious recognition of the desire to vomit and is manifested by an unpleasant wavelike sensation in the epigastric area, at the back of the throat, or throughout the abdomen. Nausea is mediated by the autonomic nervous system and accompanied by symptoms such as tachycardia, perspiration, light-headedness, dizziness, pallor, excess salivation, and weakness.

Retching is a rhythmic and spasmodic movement, in-

in the daily diet as well as to increase fluid intake. The patient also should be encouraged to increase physical activity, if that is tolerated. It should be stressed to the patient never to wait more than 3 days for a bowel movement before calling the physician, since a complication such as impaction or ileus can arise (Figure 20-6).

Nausea and vomiting. During the past decade, the management of chemotherapy-related nausea and vomiting has vastly improved. Understanding the pathophysiology of the symptoms, the efficacy and limitations of pharmacological interventions, and the use of nonpharmacological techniques is essential in minimizing nausea and vomiting. Emesis is a complicated process that requires coordination by the vomiting center (VC) in the lateral reticular formation of the medulla (Figure 20-7). The VC lies close to the respiratory center on the floor of the fourth ventricle and is directly activated by the visceral and vagal afferent pathways from the gastrointestinal tract, chemoreceptor trigger zone (CTZ), vestibular apparatus, and the cerebral cortex. When the VC is stimulated, emesis is induced via impulses to the salivation and respiratory centers and to the pharyngeal, gastrointestinal, and abdominal muscles.[56]

The VC is rich in neurotransmitter receptors sensitive to chemical toxins in the blood and cerebrospinal fluid.[57] The major receptors are dopamine, serotonin (5-HT), and muscarinic cholinergic in the CTZ; muscarinic and dopamine in the VC, vestibular apparatus, and the effer-

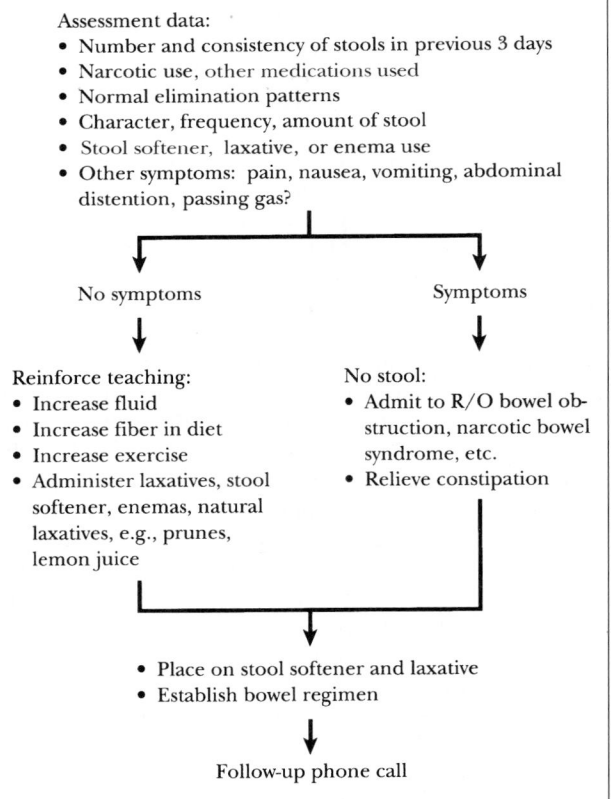

Figure 20-6 Constipation telephone triage flowchart

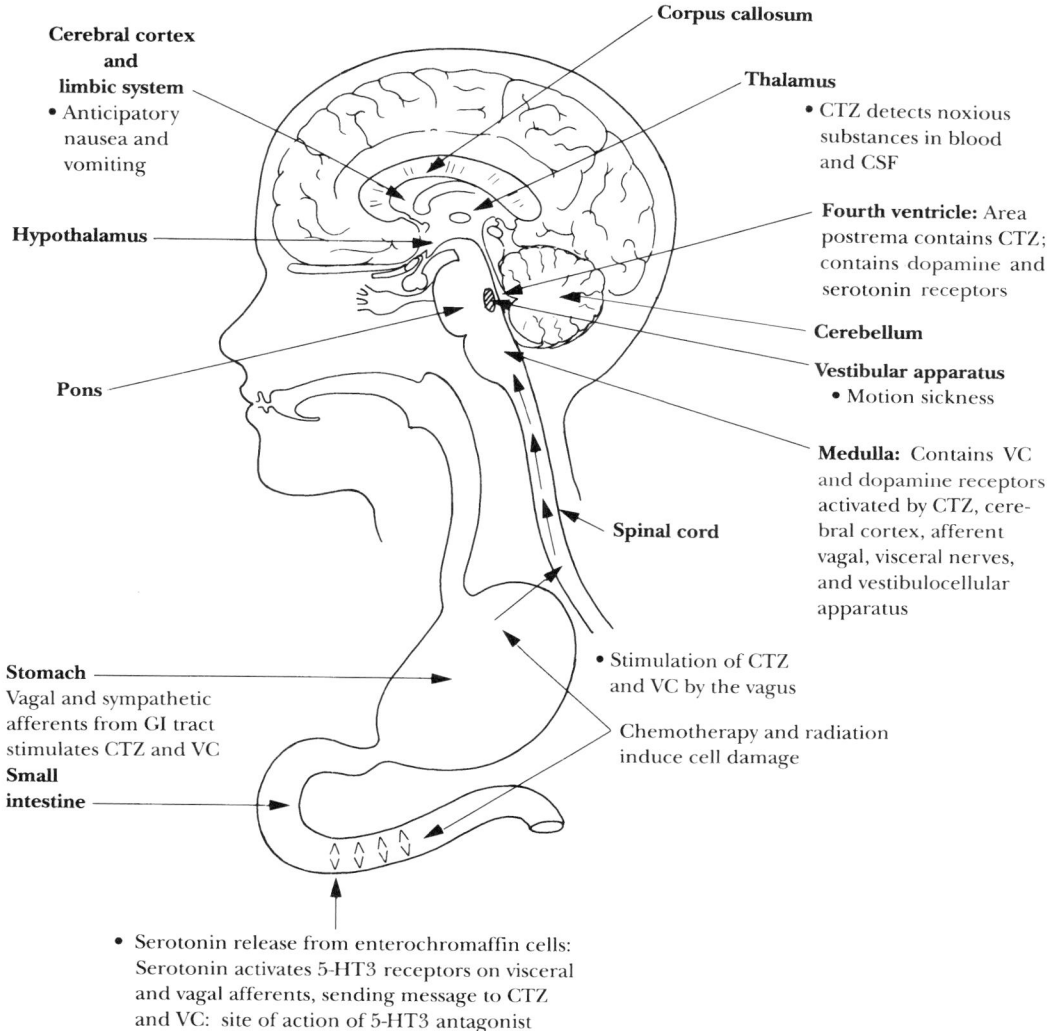

Figure 20-7 Pathways of nausea and vomiting

volving the diaphragm and abdominal muscles, controlled by the respiratory center in the brain stem near the VC. Negative intrathoracic pressure and positive abdominal pressure result in unproductive retching. When the negative pressure becomes positive, vomiting occurs. *Vomiting* is a somatic process performed by the respiratory muscles causing the forceful oral expulsion of gastric, duodenal, or jejunal contents through the mouth.[58]

Nausea and vomiting can be classified as acute, delayed, and anticipatory. *Acute nausea and vomiting* occur from a few minutes to 1–2 hours after treatment, resolving within 24 hours. The pattern is determined by the emetogenicity of the chemotherapy and pretreatment with an antiemetic agent. *Delayed nausea and vomiting* persist or develop 24 hours after chemotherapy, perhaps due to the ongoing effect that the metabolites of chemotherapy continue to exert on the CNS or gastrointestinal tract. Although cisplatin is thought to be the culprit, cyclophos-

phamide, doxorubicin, and ifosfamide can cause delayed nausea. If nausea was controlled within the first 24 hours after therapy, delayed patterns are less likely to occur. However, despite effective antiemetic regimens, patients still experience a significant amount of delayed nausea and vomiting.[14] *Anticipatory nausea and vomiting* occur in 25% of patients as a result of classic operant conditioning from stimuli associated with chemotherapy, usually 12 hours prior to administration. Such conditioned responses are experienced after a few sessions of chemotherapy and occur most commonly when efforts to control emesis are unsuccessful. Lorazepam has been found to relieve anticipatory effects as well as delayed nausea.[59]

It is possible to predict the degree and severity of nausea and vomiting as well as the onset and duration (Table 20-2). Mechlorethamine, for example, induces emesis within 30 minutes of intravenous administration,

Table 20-2 Emetogenic Potential of Chemotherapeutic Agents

Incidence	Level	Agent	Onset (hours)	Duration (hours)
Very high (>90%)	5	Cisplatin (>50 mg/m²)	1–6	24–48 +
		Dacarbazine	1–3	1–12
		Mechlorethamine	0.5–2	8–24
		Melphalan—high dose	0.3–6	6–12
		Streptozocin	1–6	12–24
		Cytarabine—high dose (> l g/m²)	1–4	12–48
High (60%–90%)	4	Carmustine (>100 mg/m²)	2–4	4–24
		Cyclophosphamide (>600 mg/m²)	4–12	12–24
		Procarbazine	24–27	variable
		Etoposide—high dose	4–6	24 +
		Semustine	1–5	12–24
		Lomustine	4–6	12–24
		Dactinomycin	2–5	24
		Plicamycin	1–6	12–24
		Methotrexate—high dose	1–12	24–72
		Actinomycin-D	1–12	24–48
		Cytarabine (500 mg/m²)	1–12	24–48
		Epirubicin/Idarubin	6–12	24 +
Moderate (30%–60%)	3	Doxorubicin (>50–75 mg/m²)	4–6	6 +
		Mitoxantrone	4–6	6 +
		5-Fluorouracil	3–6	24 +
		Mitomycin C	1–4	48–72
		Carboplatin	4–6	12–24
		Daunorubicin (<50 mg/m²)	2–6	24
		L-Asparaginase	1–4	2–12
		Topotecan	6–12	24–72
		Ifosfamide (<1.5 g/m²)	3–6	24–72
		Irinotecan	6–12	24 +
		Epirubicin	—	—
		Idarubicin	—	—
Low (10%–30%)	2	Bleomycin	3–6	—
		Cytarabine (<20 mg/m²)	6–12	3–12
		Etoposide	3–8	—
		Melphalan	6–12	—
		6-Mercaptopurine	4–8	—
		Methotrexate (<100 mg/m²)	4–12	3–12
		Vinblastine	4–8	—
		Hydroxyurea	—	—
		Teniposide	—	—
		Gemcitabine	—	—
		Vinorelbine	—	—
		Fludarabine	—	—
		Hydroxyurea	—	—
		Topotecan	—	—
		Capecitabine	—	—
		Gemcitabine	—	—
		Trimetrexate	—	—
Very low (<10%)	1	Vincristine	4–8	—
		Chlorambucil	48–72	—
		Busulfan	—	—
		Thioguanine	—	—
		Hormones	—	—
		Paclitaxel	4–8	—
		Docetaxel	—	—
		Thiotepa	—	—

whereas other highly emetic agents cause emesis at least 1 hour after infusion. With moderately to highly emetic drugs, emesis develops within 6 hours of administration. Drugs with low emetic potential usually cause emesis 12–48 hours after administration. Variability in occurrence and onset suggests that each drug may cause emesis via different mechanisms or by stimulating different pathways.[57,60] Rate and route of chemotherapy administration also affect emetic onset, intensity, and duration. For example, rapid infusion of cytarabine is more often associated with an earlier onset of severe emesis than is slower infusion.

An emesis model has been devised to illustrate the mechanisms involved in acute and delayed nausea and vomiting. According to this model, emesis results from various mechanisms within separate phases. Phase I is considered to be serotonin sensitive and in this phase serotonin inhibitors are most beneficial. Phase II is the prokinetic sensitive phase, which may persist for several days. Drugs that enhance gastric emptying are beneficial during this phase such as metoclopramide. Phase III is considered to be the steroid-sensitive phase in which steroids can minimize nausea and vomiting. This model also provides the rationale for using different antiemetics at different times to effectively control nausea and vomiting.[56]

Management begins with obtaining an in-depth emetic history and developing a preventive action plan with antiemetics (Table 20-3). Characteristics that affect the occurrence of nausea and vomiting include susceptibility to motion sickness, poor previous emetic control, fatigue, poor social functioning, and being young. Individuals with a heavy alcohol intake seem to have a decreased occurrence of nausea and vomiting.[57,61]

Successful antiemetic regimens interrupt the stimulation of the VC. Combination regimens must be individualized and developed according to the emetic potential of the chemotherapy regimen, expected duration of the nausea and vomiting, and current pattern of symptoms. Numerous combinations are being investigated extensively to eliminate the stimulation of the VC. These regimens use drugs with proven single-agent antiemetic activity, optimum doses, routes, and minimum overlapping toxicities (Figure 20-8).[62] For example, combinations of dopamine antagonists with steroids have been found to provide complete control of nausea and vomiting in up to 100% of patients undergoing high-dose cisplatin-based regimens. The combination of ondansetron and dexamethasone have been found more efficacious than ondansetron alone in controlling emesis.[63]

With the addition of the serotonin inhibitors, the management of chemotherapy-induced nausea and vomiting has improved. After extensive review of studies using serotonin inhibitors, several findings were supported: (1) no greater efficacy is found among ondansetron, granisetron, dolasetron, or tropisetron; (2) efficacy appears more pronounced for cisplatin-containing regimens; (3) less efficacy is found for delayed nausea and vomiting; (4) dexamethasone increases efficacy; (5) efficacy seems to diminish over repeated days or repeated chemotherapy cycles.[63,64]

Further classification has been proposed to determine the emetogenicity of combination chemotherapy (see Table 20-2).[60] Initially, the most emetogenic agent in the combination is identified. Other agents are then assessed for emetogenic potential with these considerations: (1) level 1 agents do not significantly contribute to the overall emetogenicity of the combination; (2) one or more level 2 agents increase the emetogenicity of the combination by one level greater than the most emetogenetic agents; and (3) the emetogenicity of the combination is increased by one level per agent when a level 3 or 4 agent is added to the regimen.[60]

Behavioral interventions such as progressive muscle relaxation, hypnosis, and systematic desensitization can be taught to the patient to help interrupt the association of nausea and vomiting with chemotherapy. The nurse can try to minimize in the environment any aversive sounds or smells that could stimulate the VC. Distraction with audiotapes, radio, or television programs should be provided in the treatment area to help minimize nausea. Each of these techniques has been found effective in decreasing the frequency and duration of vomiting as well as in decreasing anxiety.[65]

It is important to teach the patient about the potential side effects of antiemetic therapy, such as drowsiness and diarrhea. If the patient is returning home after an emetogenic chemotherapy treatment, ensure that someone can provide transportation and care in the immediate hours following therapy. Phone follow-up 24–48 hours after treatment is essential to ensure that appropriate antiemetic management is being followed (Figure 20-9).

Mucositis.   *Mucositis* is a general term that describes the inflammatory response of mucosal epithelial cells to the cytotoxic effects of chemotherapy. Painful ulceration, hemorrhage, and secondary infection may develop when mucositis is not detected early or continues untreated. Because all mucous membrane–covered surfaces exhibit similar patterns of growth, replacement, and function, any mucous membrane within the gastrointestinal tract from the mouth to rectum or vagina can be adversely affected by chemotherapy.

The epithelial cells lining the gastrointestinal mucosa renew rapidly, which enables them to replace cells lost when food is chewed, swallowed, digested, and eliminated from the body. Mucositis results when these mucosal cells are damaged by chemotherapy and are unable to adequately repair and replace normal cell loss.[66] Manifestations of gastrointestinal toxicity include mucositis in the oral cavity (stomatitis), esophagus (esophagitis), in the intestines as diarrhea (enteritis), and in the vagina (vaginitis).

Stomatitis.   Chemotherapy-induced oral complications can be acute or chronic. Acute reactions include mucosal inflammation and ulceration, infection, and mucosal bleeding. Although chronic complications can

Table 20-3 Antiemetic Therapy

Classification	Drugs	Availability/Dose	Schedule	Duration	Half-Life	Comments
Benzodiazepines *Mechanism of action* CNS depressant; interferes with afferent nerves from cerebral cortex; sedative *Common side effects* Sedation, amnesia, confusion	Lorazepam Diazepam	Tablet: 1–3 mg PO or sublingual IV: 0.5–2.5 mg Tablet: 2–4 mg IV: 2–10 mg	q3–4h q4–6h	4–8 hr 4–8 hr	10–15 hr 30–40 hr	Reduces anticipatory nausea and vomiting. May aggravate CNS effects of ifosfamide. Use with caution in patients with hepatic and renal dysfunction.
Butyrophenones *Mechanism of action* Dopamine antagonist in the CTZ, esophagus, and stomach *Common side effects* Sedation, hypotension, tachycardia, EPS	Droperidol Haloperidol	IM: 2.5–10 mg IV: 0.5–2.5 mg Tablet: 3–5 mg IM: 1–5 mg IV: 1–3 mg	q3–4h q4h q2–6h	2–4 hr 2–6 hr	10 hr 12–18 hr	Diphenhydramine 25–50 mg PO or IV will prevent EPS. EPS more common in young patients. May have additive effects. Use caution in patients with cardiac disorders.
Cannabinoids *Mechanism of action* Suppresses pathways to VC (speculated) *Common side effects* Sedation, dizziness, dysphoria, dry mouth, disorientation, impaired concentration, orthostatic hypotension, tachycardia	Dronabinol	Tablet: 5–10 mg	q4h	4–6 hr		May be difficult to obtain in outpatient setting. Elderly patients generally do not tolerate side effects. Generally used for second-line antiemetic therapy.
Phenothiazines *Mechanism of action* Blocks dopamine receptor in the CTZ; inhibits VC by blocking autonomic afferent impulses via vagus nerve *Common side effects* Sedation, orthostatic hypotension, EPS, dizziness, drowsiness	Prochlorperazine Promethazine Thiethylperazine Chlorpromazine Perphenazine Trimethobenzamide	Tablet: 5–25 mg Sustained release: 10–30 mg PO IM/IV: 20–40 mg Rectal: 25 mg q4h Tablet: 12.5–25 mg IM/IV: 10–25 mg Rectal: 25 mg Tablet: 10 mg IM: 10 mg Rectal: 10 mg Tablet: 25–50 mg IM/IV: 25–50 mg Rectal: 25–100 mg Tablet: 4 mg IM/IV: 5 mg Capsule: 250 mg Rectal: 200 mg IM: 200 mg	q4–6h q10–12h q3–4h q4–6h q4–6h q4–6h q4–6h q4–6h q6–8h q6–8h q6–8h	3–4 hr 10–12 hr 3–4 hr 3–4 hr 3–4 hr 3–4 hr 6–8 hr 6–8 hr 3–4 hr 3–4 hr 3–4 hr 3–4 hr 3–4 hr		Administer IV dose over 15–30 min. EPS more common in person <30 years. Side effects can be cumulative in the elderly. Do not exceed 5 mg/min with IV dose. Dystonia can occur with chlorpromazine, especially with IV dosing. Chlorpromazine generally second-line antiemetic therapy. Diphenhydramine can prevent EPS and dystonia. Sustained-release form of Prochlorperazine (currently not available) can prevent delayed nausea and vomiting.
Substituted Benzamide *Mechanism of action* Dopamine antagonist; accelerates gastric emptying and small-bowel transit; CTZ *Common side effects* Sedation, diarrhea, anxiety, EPS, fatigue, headache	Metoclopramide	Tablet: 5–10 mg IV: 1–3 mg/kg	q2–3h × 3–5 doses	2–3 hr	4–6 hr	EPS more common in young patients. Administer over 15 min to prevent intense anxiety. Use with caution in patients with renal dysfunction.

Table 20-3 Antiemetic Therapy (continued)

Classification	Drugs	Availability/Dose	Schedule	Duration	Half-Life	Comments
5-HT agonists *Mechanism of action* Increases gastric emptying *Common side effects* Diarrhea, headache, abdominal pain, flatulence	Cisapride	Tablet: 10 mg	before meals and at bedtime			Usually well tolerated.
Steroids *Mechanism of action* Antiprostaglandin synthesis activity? *Common side effects:* Insomnia, euphoria, anxiety, hypertension, edema, facial flushing	Dexamethasone	Tablet: 2–4 mg IV: 10–20 mg IV: 125–250 mg	q4–6 h q3h		2–3 hr	Rapid infusion causes perineal itching. Taper dose to prevent insomnia, anxiety, and euphoria. Acne may occur.
Antihistamines *Mechanism of action* Histamine H1; receptor antagonist *Common side effects* Sedation, hypotension	Diphenhydramine	Tablet: 25–50 mg IM/IV: 12.5–50 mg	q3–4h		5–8 hr	Prevents acute dystonic reactions. Use with caution in patients with hepatic dysfunction.
Serotonin Inhibitors *Mechanism of action* Serotonin receptor; (5-HT3) antagonist *Common side effects* Hypotension, headache, constipation, sedation minimal	Ondansetron	IV: 16–32 mg/24 hr 0.15–0.18 mg/kg PO: 4-mg and 8-mg tablets Sublingual: investigational	q12h q8h	8 hr	3–4 hr	Transient elevations of LFTs may occur with cisplatin and ondansetron administration.
	Granisetron	IV: 10 µg/kg	30 min prior to chemo	12 hr	8–10 hr	Single dose of granisetron may be sufficient for a 12-hr time period. Classification not recommended for delayed or anticipatory nausea/vomiting.
	Dolasetron	IV: 1.8 mg/kg PO: 100 mg		12hr	8–10 hr	
	Tropisetron	IV: 5 mg PO: 5 mg everyday × 5 days	30 min prior to chemo			
Anticholinergic *Common side effects* Dry mouth, sedation, blurred vision, restlessness	Scopolamine	Patch: 0.5 mg/24 hr every 3 days		72 hr		May irritate skin. May be difficult to obtain.

VC = vomiting center; CTZ = chemoreceptor trigger zone; EPS = extrapyramidal symptoms; LFTs = liver function tests

occur from chemotherapy, these changes are usually a result of radiation-induced changes to healthy tissue and include xerostomia, taste alterations, trismus, and soft-tissue and bone necrosis.

The risk of developing stomatitis is not the same for all patients, nor is it equal in similar drug regimens. Diagnosis and aggressiveness of the chemotherapy regimen are predictors of oral complications. Breast cancer patients can have as low as 12% risk compared with 70%

in leukemia patients.[67] The frequency of oral problems is two to three times higher in patients with hematologic malignancies than with solid tumors. Stomatitis occurs more commonly in younger than in older patients. The higher mitotic index of the oral mucosa and higher incidence of hematologic malignancies in the younger patient population may explain the age-related risk factor.[67]

Preexisting oral disease (dental caries, partially erupted third molars) as well as poor oral hygiene and

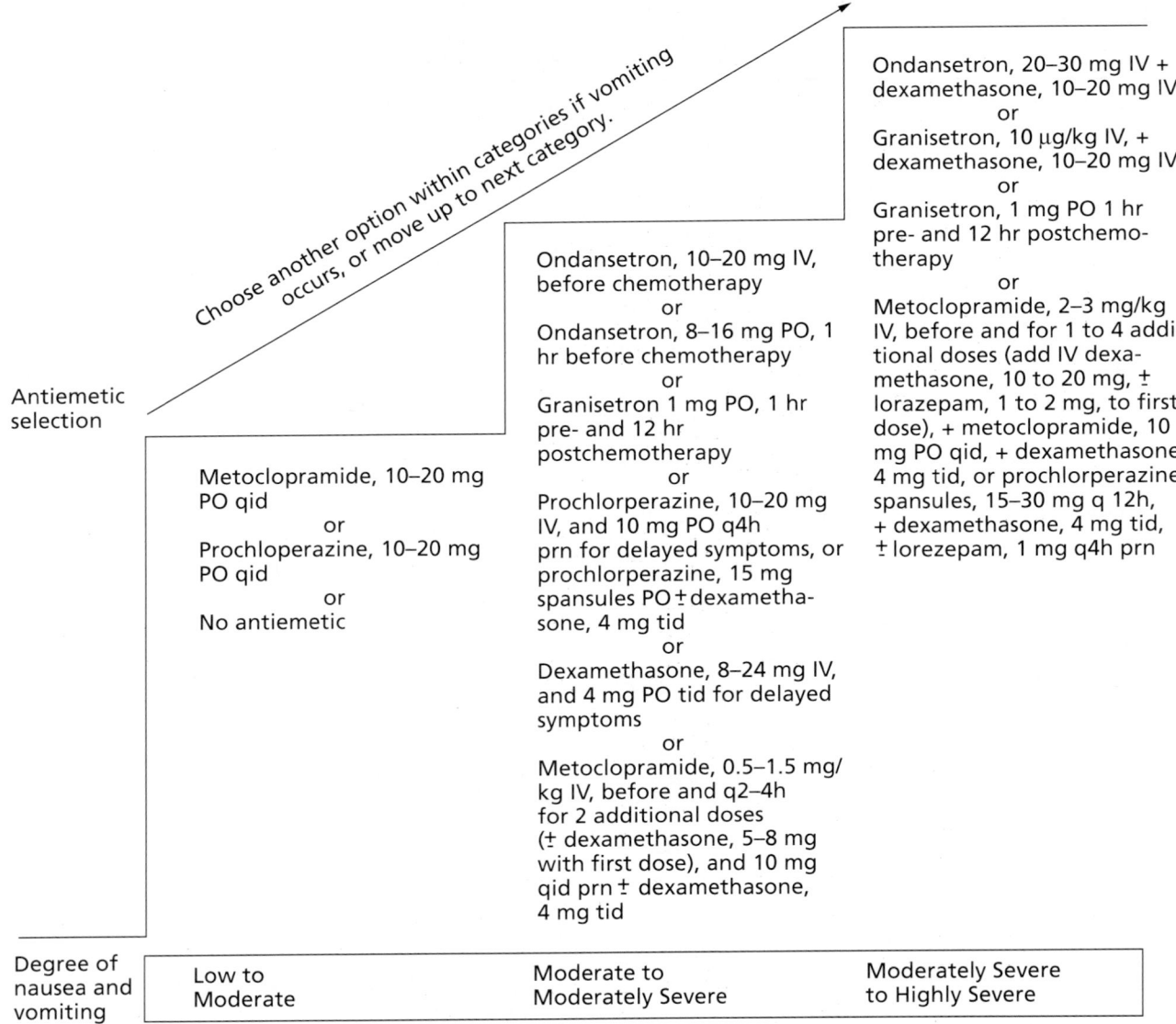

Choose another option within categories if vomiting occurs, or move up to next category.

Antiemetic selection

Metoclopramide, 10–20 mg PO qid
or
Prochloperazine, 10–20 mg PO qid
or
No antiemetic

Ondansetron, 10–20 mg IV, before chemotherapy
or
Ondansetron, 8–16 mg PO, 1 hr before chemotherapy
or
Granisetron 1 mg PO, 1 hr pre- and 12 hr postchemotherapy
or
Prochlorperazine, 10–20 mg IV, and 10 mg PO q4h prn for delayed symptoms, or prochlorperazine, 15 mg spansules PO ± dexamethasone, 4 mg tid
or
Dexamethasone, 8–24 mg IV, and 4 mg PO tid for delayed symptoms
or
Metoclopramide, 0.5–1.5 mg/kg IV, before and q2–4h for 2 additional doses (± dexamethasone, 5–8 mg with first dose), and 10 mg qid prn ± dexamethasone, 4 mg tid

Ondansetron, 20–30 mg IV + dexamethasone, 10–20 mg IV
or
Granisetron, 10 µg/kg IV, + dexamethasone, 10–20 mg IV
or
Granisetron, 1 mg PO 1 hr pre- and 12 hr postchemotherapy
or
Metoclopramide, 2–3 mg/kg IV, before and for 1 to 4 additional doses (add IV dexamethasone, 10 to 20 mg, ± lorazepam, 1 to 2 mg, to first dose), + metoclopramide, 10 mg PO qid, + dexamethasone, 4 mg tid, or prochlorperazine spansules, 15–30 mg q 12h, + dexamethasone, 4 mg tid, ± lorezepam, 1 mg q4h prn

Degree of nausea and vomiting

Low to Moderate	Moderate to Moderately Severe	Moderately Severe to Highly Severe

(Change within categories if side effects or vomiting occur; move up if nausea and vomiting are not controlled.) Always make sure that patients receiveing moderately severe and greater emetogenic chemotherapy receive antiemetics for delayed nausea and vomiting, try ondansetron, 8 mg PO, if other antiemetics are ineffective.

Figure 20-8   Antiemetic selection for chemotherapy (Reprinted with permission from Wickham R: Nausea and vomiting, in Yarbro CH, Frogge MH, Goodman M (eds): *Cancer Symptom Management* (ed 2). Sudbury, MA, Jones and Bartlett, 1999.)[62]

local irritants (ill-fitting dental prostheses, tobacco, alcohol) will predispose chemotherapy patients to an increased risk of oral complications. Periodontitis, a common oral disease, causes a tenfold increase in bacterial and fungal organisms in the oral cavity. Depletion of protein stores and malnutrition increase the risk of infection by altering the integrity of the epithelial barrier and depressing the immune system.[68]

The majority of chemotherapy agents can cause some degree of stomatitis. Those agents most associated with stomatitis are the antimetabolites and antitumor antibiotics, in particular bleomycin, doxorubicin, daunorubicin, docetaxel, 5-FU, methotrexate, and high-dose therapy with busulfan, etoposide, melphalan, and thiotepa. Less commonly associated drugs include cytarabine, paclitaxel, vinblastine, gemcitabine, and vincristine. *Trans*-retinoic acid can cause cracked and inflamed lips.[69] Mucositis is observed more often with 5-FU when combined with other mucositis-producing drugs, such as methotrexate and doxorubicin, and when 5-FU is given concurrently with leucovorin.

Although stomatitis is dose-related and is more common with higher doses, those who develop stomatitis with one cycle of therapy will almost assuredly develop recurrence in subsequent courses unless the drugs or doses are changed.[68] This is especially the case when the body

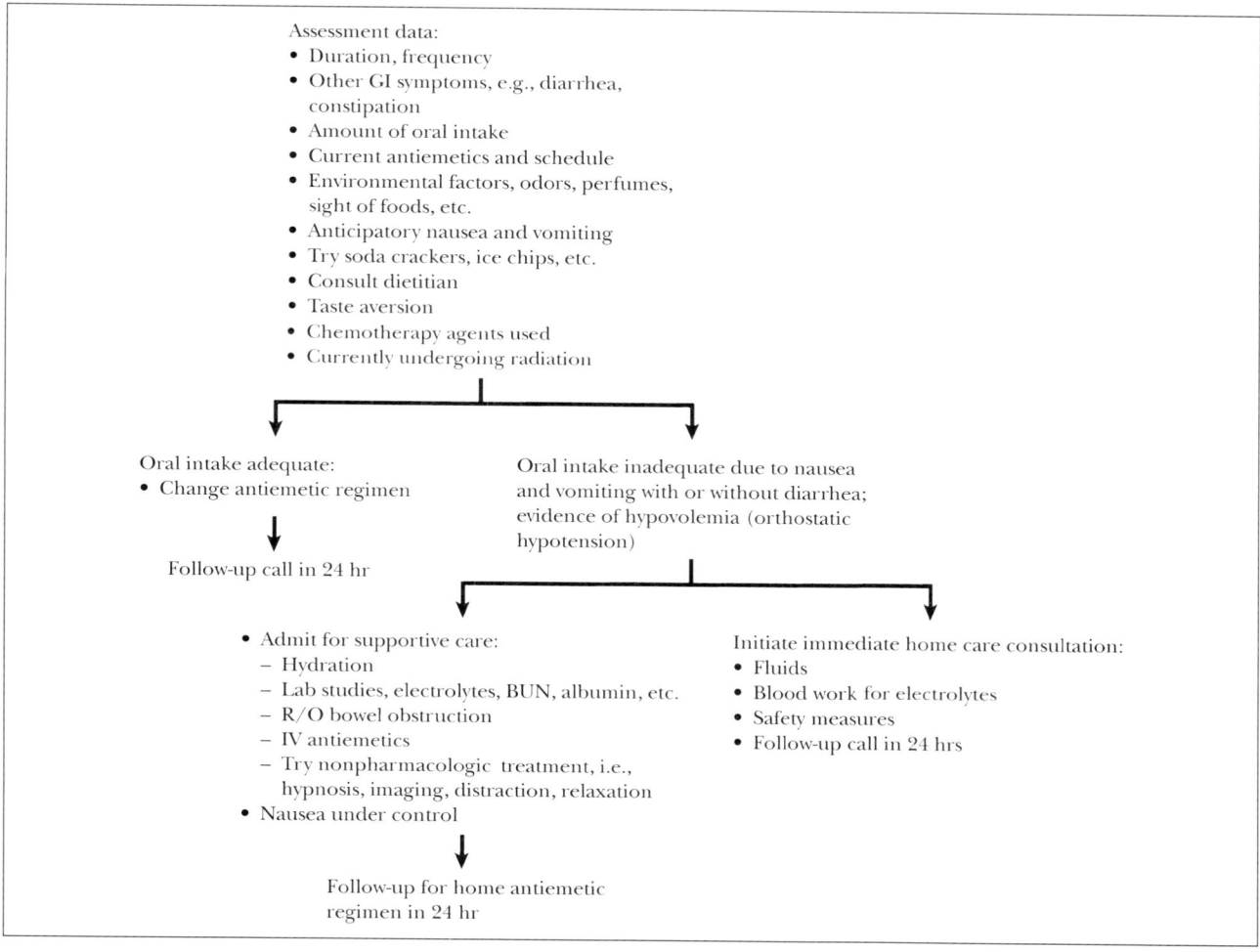

Assessment data:
• Duration, frequency
• Other GI symptoms, e.g., diarrhea, constipation
• Amount of oral intake
• Current antiemetics and schedule
• Environmental factors, odors, perfumes, sight of foods, etc.
• Anticipatory nausea and vomiting
• Try soda crackers, ice chips, etc.
• Consult dietitian
• Taste aversion
• Chemotherapy agents used
• Currently undergoing radiation

Oral intake adequate:
• Change antiemetic regimen

Follow-up call in 24 hr

Oral intake inadequate due to nausea and vomiting with or without diarrhea; evidence of hypovolemia (orthostatic hypotension)

• Admit for supportive care:
  – Hydration
  – Lab studies, electrolytes, BUN, albumin, etc.
  – R/O bowel obstruction
  – IV antiemetics
  – Try nonpharmacologic treatment, i.e., hypnosis, imaging, distraction, relaxation
• Nausea under control

Follow-up for home antiemetic regimen in 24 hr

Initiate immediate home care consultation:
• Fluids
• Blood work for electrolytes
• Safety measures
• Follow-up call in 24 hrs

Figure 20-9 Nausea and vomiting telephone triage flowchart

is unable to adequately eliminate a stomatotoxic drug. For example, in the presence of renal dysfunction or liver dysfunction, excretion of methotrexate and doxorubicin, respectively, may be compromised.

Direct stomatotoxicity results from the cytotoxic action of drugs on the cells of the oral basal epithelium, causing a decrease in the rate of cell renewal. The sequela are a thinned atrophic mucosa and initiation of an inflammatory response (stomatitis). Most often affected are the nonkeratinized mucosal areas, including the buccal and labial mucosa, tongue, soft palate, and floor of the mouth. Rarely are the gingiva or hard palate involved.[67]

Histologic changes can occur within 5–7 days of initial drug exposure. Dry mucosa, tongue, or lips; burning sensation in the oral cavity; and increased salivation result. Visible signs of inflammation and oral ulceration can be observed 7–10 days following therapy. Changes in the oral cavity correlate with the timing of myelosuppression, as leukocytes and the oral mucosal cells have similar cell renewal rates. Without complications and further insult from repeated drug administration, stomatitis is self-limiting and gradually reverses itself within 2–3

weeks as the granulocyte count returns to normal, often preceding bone marrow recovery by 2–3 days. Improvement in the status of the oral mucosa can therefore be predictive of a WBC count recovery.[66]

A baseline assessment of the oral cavity should be done prior to the initiation of treatment. Dental prophylaxis, restoration, and repair should be completed before treatment begins. Once treatment is initiated, an oral assessment should be repeated at regular intervals; outpatients should be instructed on self-assessment.[68] Nursing management of stomatitis will depend on its severity, which is often described as mild, moderate, or severe (see Table 20-1).

Research has substantiated that oral complications can be reduced or eliminated by meticulous oral assessment with interventions before, during, and between courses of chemotherapy.[68] Table 20-4 describes various oral cleansing agents and devices, different means of lubricating and coating the oral cavity, and basic solutions and measures to manage oral discomfort. Developing a plan of care that the patient finds acceptable may be more beneficial than employing complicated regimens.

Table 20-4 Prevention and Management of Perioral Complications of Cancer Treatment

Plan/Agent	Schedule	Action	Comments
BASIC ORAL CLEANSING			
Cleansing Mouth Rinses			
Normal saline	4×/day	Mechanical plaque control; removes and washes away loose debris	Nonirritating; no unpleasant taste
		Physical; moistens and soothes oral mucosa	Mixture preparation: 1 teaspoon salt in 1 quart warm water; use sterile saline if granulocytopenic or mouth ulcers present
Sodium bicarbonate solution	4×/day	Mechanical plaque control; loosens hardened crusts and debris	Decreases odor; unpleasant taste reported
		Mucosolvent Reduces acidity	Mixture preparation: 1 tsp baking soda in 8 oz water for thick paste of sodium bicarbonate; water applied to gingival sulcus for use in mechanical plaque debridement
Hydrogen peroxide	4×/day	Mechanical plaque control; loosens hardened crusts and debris	
Antimicrobial Mouth Rinses			
Peridex	15 mL rinse 3×/day; do *not* swallow	Broad-spectrum antimicrobial agent used to suppress oral microflora and prevent dental plaque formation	Efficacy for the prophylaxis of therapy-induced mucositis is controversial
		Decreases bacterial cloud in mouth	Most common local side effect from long-term use is staining of teeth and tongue. No systemic toxicity has been reported.
		Prevents oral candidal infections	
Chlorhexidine	15-mL swish, gargle, and spit q8h	Antibacterial and antifungal action; used for high-risk patients	Augments protective effect of fluoride
			May cause brown discoloration of teeth
			Mixture preparation: dilute 3% hydrogen peroxide to ¼ strength. *Note:* Mix just prior to usage to maintain oxidizing effect; refrigerated solution may also provide local anesthetic effect
MAINTENANCE OF ORAL MOISTURE			
Oral Care			
Orabalance®	Use after rinsing mouth and after brushing	Relief of dry mouth	A nondrying moisturizing gel; may be applied around the teeth and along gum line
Saliva substitutes			
Moi-Stir®	As needed	Mouth-moistening salivary supplement	Available in oral swabsticks and spray
Xerolube®	As needed	Mouth moisturizer; caries inhibition	Includes fluoride as an added benefit
Sialogogues			
Salagen®	5 mg 3×/day	Stimulates saliva production from functioning salivary glands	Investigational use for patients with radiation-induced xerostomia
			Contraindicated in patients with uncontrolled asthma or narrow-angle glaucoma; use caution with cardiovascular disease.

Table 20-4   Prevention and Management of Perioral Complications of Cancer Treatment (continued)

Plan/Agent	Schedule	Action	Comments
RELIEF OF PAIN AND INFLAMMATION			
Coating Agents			
Orabase®	As needed	Topical anesthetic for localized areas of pain	Quick onset of action (30 sec), but short duration of action (5–15 min) Does not change consistency after application
Hurricane®	As needed	Topical anesthetic	Available as spray, liquid, or gel Onset of action, 30 sec; duration 15 min No systemic absorption
Oratect-gel®	As needed, no more than 4×/day	Topical anesthetic	Gel dries in about 30–60 sec to form a protective film Maximum protection lasts about 2 hr Film dissipates gradually over 6 hr Do not try to mechanically remove Mild, transient stinging when applied
Zilactin®	Dry lesions; apply 4×/day	Provides a protective coating and leads to pain relief	Forms protective film over oral ulcers that can last 5 hr Gel forms an opaque white film inside the mouth and a transparent film extraorally when dried Mild, transient burning sensation with application of gel
Topical Anesthetic Rinses			
Xylocaine viscous 2% solution	15 mL swish and swallow q3h, as needed	Topical anesthetic for generalized areas of pain	Onset of action is 5 min Duration of action is approximately 20 min Systemically absorbed Watch for CNS and cardiac toxicity Swish and swallow for brief pain relief (e.g., before meals)
Dyclonine hydrochloride 0.5% or 1% solution	15 ml swish and spit, as needed	Topical anesthetic for generalized areas of pain	Minimally absorbed Decreasing potential for CNS and cardiac toxicity
Combination mixtures (e.g., viscous xylocaine 2%, Benadryl® elixir 12.5 mg/mL, Maalox®)	4×/day	Topical anesthetic for generalized areas of pain	Benadryl may exacerbate xerostomia
Ulcerease®	15-mL swish	Anesthetic mouth rinse	Contains no alcohol Use full strength May apply directly to ulcers with cotton swab after rinsing
Sucralfate suspension	1 g/15 mL swish; 15 mL 4×/day	Binds to ulcerated tissue protecting it from further insult and may promote healing	No anesthetic action Suspension may aggravate nausea
Vitamin E	1 mL topically to oral lesions 2×/day	Promotes healing of mouth ulcers and controls pain	Anecdotal and research-based studies conclude vitamin E may help speed healing of chemotherapy-induced stomatitis
Systemic Analgesics			
Nonsteroidal anti-inflammatory agents (e.g., Trilisate®)	Depends on agent used Doses vary	Mild to moderate pain	Longer duration of action than aspirin No effect on platelets Minimal GI side effects
Narcotic agents (e.g., morphine)	Depends on agent used Dose varies	Moderate to severe pain	

Because reinforcement promotes compliance, nurses should continually review with the patient the individual plan for oral care and assess its continued acceptability. Generally, the recommendation is that routine oral care be performed at least after meals and at bedtime, and that the frequency be increased as the severity of stomatitis increases.[68]

Mouth rinses enhance removal of loosened debris and should be nonirritating and nondehydrating. Several solutions for rinsing have been studied and include normal saline, chlorhexidine, benzydamine, sodium bicarbonate, and hydrogen peroxide, as well as several combinations of these. Normal saline may be the least damaging; sodium bicarbonate is effective as a cleansing agent, but some patients complain of the bad taste and a too concentrated solution can change the oral cavity pH; hydrogen peroxide breaks down new tissues and should be avoided when fresh granulation surfaces are visible in the mouth; chlorhexidine and benzydamine cleanse the oral cavity, yet poor taste yields poor compliance. To date, the optimum cleansing agent for stomatitis has not been determined.[66,68]

The oral cavity is susceptible indirectly to infection because of chemotherapy-induced neutropenia. Chemotherapy weakens host defenses by changing the oral flora to become primarily gram-negative and reducing salivary and mucous gland function.[66] An overgrowth of normal oral microorganisms results in invasion of both endogenous and exogenous pathological organisms capable of producing oral infections. Mucosal disruption becomes an important portal of entry and compromises the integrity of the oral mucosa as the first line of defense. Pathogenic organisms can further contaminate the lungs and gastrointestinal tract, disseminating infection systematically.

Bacterial, fungal, and viral infections are all common in the myelosuppressed patient. Organisms such as *Streptococcus* species, *Candida* species, and herpes simplex virus (HSV) are the major oral infectious pathogens. Each infection has certain clinical features, such as the white or "cottage cheese" appearance of *Candida albicans* or the painful vesicular lesions or herpes simplex, that assist in identifying the pathogen. The proper identification of the pathogen requires a culture, and management will depend on the identified pathogen.[66]

The most frequent cause of oral infection is fungal. *C. albicans* is the predominating organism and pseudomembranous candidiasis (oral thrush) the most common clinical manifestation. Oral *Candida* infections are traditionally treated with topical antifungal agents such as nystatin oral rinses or clotrimazole troches.[66] The nystatin liquid must be swished in the mouth for 5 minutes and then spit out or swallowed, 4 times daily. The troche, given five times a day, must be sucked in the mouth until dissolved, approximately 30 minutes. Long-term use of oral troches should be avoided as they contain large quantities of sugar that may result in dental caries. If xerostomia is present, the troche will take longer to dissolve. Patients should be instructed to cleanse the mouth before administering the agent and not to eat or drink for at least 30 minutes after application. This will permit drug contact with the mucosal surfaces to exert an antifungal effect. Denture wearers should be instructed to soak their appliance overnight with 100 mL nystatin suspension. The plastic in dentures can act as a reservoir to reinfect the treated mucosa.

Alternatives for oropharyngeal candidiasis refractory to topical treatment are the systemic oral antifungal agents, ketoconazole 200 mg daily or fluconazole 100 mg daily. Absorption of ketoconazole is dependent on gastric acidity; therefore, patients are instructed to avoid the use of antacids and other medications that alter gastric pH within 2 hours of taking ketoconazole. A course of low-dose intravenous amphotericin B is indicated for nonresponsive infection and in severe esophageal and disseminated candidal infections.[66]

Herpes simplex virus is the most common viral pathogen affecting the oral cavity. Vesicle fluid should be obtained for a culture to confirm the presence of HSV. When no vesicles are present, the base of the lesion should be swabbed using a viral culture swab. Swabs used for nasopharyngeal cultures (calcium alginate swabs) inactivate the virus and should not be used. Reactivation of latent HSV is the cause of the majority of HSV infections.

Immunocompromised patients who are seropositive are at risk. For patients with limited tissue involvement, acyclovir ointment can be applied topically every 3–6 hours while awake. Patients should be instructed to use gloves or cotton swabs when applying ointment, as autoinoculation with the virus can occur. Extensive tissue involvement for disseminated herpes requires systemic acyclovir therapy, either orally or parenterally. Acyclovir prophylaxis may be used to prevent infection in selected high-risk populations such as bone marrow transplant.[66]

Bacterial infections may affect the gingiva, the mucosa, or the teeth. Bacterial culture isolate and positive blood cultures confirm the diagnosis, however clinical features (pain, fever, oral lesions) may be present without positive blood cultures. Parenteral antibiotic therapy based on the causative organisms is the treatment of choice.

Oral pain is the major clinical problem associated with stomatitis. Pain results due to sloughing of the superficial epithelium, inflammation of the oral mucosa, and ulceration, making it difficult for the patient to practice adequate oral hygiene, eat properly, and communicate. Minimizing the pain can be accomplished with topical anesthetics and systemic analgesics (see Table 20-4).

Oral bleeding and hemorrhage are indirect stomatotoxic sequela from chemotherapy-induced thrombocytopenia. Bleeding results when the oral mucosa is traumatized or because of underlying periodontal disease and may occur anywhere in the mouth. The lips, tongue, and gingiva are the most common sites. For patients with a platelet count less than $20,000/mm^3$, less vigorous oral hygiene regimens should be used to clean the oral cavity. Management of bleeding with topical coagulants (thrombin-soaked gauze) and pressure is often helpful.

Although the treatment of stomatitis remains palliative and symptom-oriented, studies are ongoing to evaluate prophylactic measures to alleviate this side effect. Clinical trials with CSFs administered to patients undergoing chemotherapy have incidentally reported a decrease in the occurrence and severity of stomatitis along with restoration of neutrophil counts and function.[70]

Lisofylline, an anti-inflammatory agent, has been found to suppress the production of the inflammatory cytokines thought to cause mucositis during chemotherapy.[18] Initial testing in bone marrow transplant patients indicated a decrease in treatment-related infections and mucositis and an increase rate of bone marrow engraftment. The drug was given intravenously over 10 minutes every 6 hours during the conditioning regimen and continued until day 21 after transplant.

A keratinocyte growth factor that enhances the growth of keratinocytes, or epithelium cells, is currently being studied in the prevention of chemotherapy-induced mucositis.[18] This naturally occurring cytokine produced by the subepithelial fibroblasts within the skin and intestinal wall has been shown to increase growth of the epithelium in animals.

Taste alterations.

Patients receiving chemotherapy may be susceptible to taste alterations. There can be actual or perceived changes in taste. The drugs cause direct injury to taste cells composing the taste buds, resulting in taste changes that vary widely and are highly individualized. Commonly induced changes include lowered threshold for bitter taste, increased threshold for sweet taste, and complaints of metallic taste. Chemotherapy drugs frequently associated with taste alterations are cyclophosphamide, dacarbazine, doxorubicin, 5-FU, levamisole, methotrexate, nitrogen mustard, cisplatin, and vincristine.

Some agents like doxorubicin and methotrexate may alter taste acuity, while others like cyclophosphamide and vincristine can be tasted while injected. Chemotherapy-induced taste alterations can further be influenced by poor oral hygiene, infection of the oral cavity, dentures, and unpleasant odors.[68]

Unless patients are specifically questioned, taste alterations are seldom reported spontaneously. When questioned, patients may report their taste changes as reasons for their loss of appetite or decreased weight. Nursing interventions are aimed at teaching patients self-care measures to maintain optimal nutrition. Eating hints should be customized in accordance with each patient's change in taste appreciation.

Esophagitis.

Histologically, the mucosal lining of the esophagus is the same as the oral cavity. The esophagus is lined with stratified squamous epithelial cells. Destruction and inadequate replacement of these epithelial cells caused by chemotherapy agents will result in an inflammatory response called *esophagitis*. Similar to stomatitis, esophagitis can progress to ulceration, hemorrhage, and secondary infection and cause pain sufficient to make eating very difficult.[55] Treatment may be discontinued

temporarily to allow recovery of these cells, which parallels recovery of the WBC count.

The most common early symptoms of esophagitis include dysphagia (difficulty swallowing), odynophagia (painful swallowing), and epigastric pain. Esophageal pain that worsens and becomes continuous and substernal indicates progressive esophagitis. Any patient who develops oral mucositis following chemotherapy is at risk for spread to the esophageal mucosal tissue. Prior or concurrent radiation may augment the severity and extent of mucosal injury. Some drugs such as dactinomycin and doxorubicin potentiate radiation injury to the esophagus, while others including 5-FU, hydroxyurea, procarbazine, and vinblastine produce an additive toxic effect with radiation.[55]

Although management of esophagitis varies greatly, all management is directed at symptom relief and supportive care (Table 20-5). Interventions are initiated to minimize irritation and promote comfort. This is best accomplished through dietary manipulation, topical anesthesia, and systemic analgesia when needed.

If nutritional status becomes compromised, patients may benefit from commercially prepared supplements. A nutritionist may be helpful in determining which products would best meet the individual needs of the patient. Some patients may require a feeding tube, usually a gastrostomy, if esophagitis is severe. Occasionally, a tube will be placed prior to initiating treatment if nutritional problems are anticipated. Local anesthetics are often used every 3–4 hours as needed and prior to meals to help alleviate the pain associated with esophagitis (see Table 20-4). If topical anesthetic preparations do not relieve the discomfort, narcotic analgesics may be needed. Tablets may need to be crushed and given in food, considering narcotic elixirs often contain alcohol, which can further irritate the mucosa.

Superimposed *Candida* infections may also present significant problems for patients with cancer.[55] Symptoms of *Candida* infection are often difficult to distinguish from treatment-induced esophagitis and may include dysphagia and pain. Prompt and appropriate medical treatment is necessary in order to prevent a systemic spread. Esophageal candidiasis is most commonly treated using ketoconazole, fluconazole, or nystatin oral suspension.[66]

Integument.

The effects of chemotherapy on the skin and mucous membranes can be profound. The oncology nurse is commonly faced with the challenge of deciding how to minimize and manage these side effects.

Hyperpigmentation.

Numerous chemotherapeutic agents are associated with hyperpigmentation (discoloration) of the skin, nails, and mucous membranes. While the etiology of hyperpigmentation is poorly understood, it is possible that the drug or a metabolic by-product of the drug stimulates melanocytes to produce increased quantities of melanin.[71] It is unclear why some drugs

Table 20-5 Self-Care Guidelines for Esophagitis and Dysphagia

While receiving chemotherapy, you may begin to develop a sore throat or a feeling like food is getting stuck when you swallow. This usually begins gradually after about 2 weeks of treatment and may become more severe as treatment continues. It is *temporary* and will gradually begin to get better about 2 weeks after treatment is finished.

The following guidelines were designed to help you to be more comfortable during treatment and to make sure that you are eating and drinking enough liquids.

1. Tell your nurse or doctor if you have a sore throat or are having trouble swallowing.
2. Change your diet to include foods that are soft and moist. Using sauces and gravies is helpful.
3. Avoid foods that are spicy, salty, dry, or rough in texture.
4. Drink at least eight glasses of liquid each day. Fruit nectar is often very soothing. Avoid alcoholic beverages, citrus juices, and carbonated beverages—they will irritate your throat.
5. Avoid very hot foods.
6. Eat or drink cold foods such as ice cream, frozen juice bars, and gelatin. This may help to soothe the throat, especially before eating a meal.
7. Take small bites and chew foods well.
8. Use a straw to make swallowing easier.
9. Avoid using commercial mouthwashes because they often contain alcohol, which can irritate your throat.
10. Try not to smoke. It can be difficult to stop smoking during a stressful time, but your nurse or doctor can provide you with some helpful suggestions.
11. Placing a cool air humidifier with tap water in the room where you spend most of your time during the day and where you sleep at night may help to keep your mouth and throat from getting dry.
12. If your doctor prescribes medicine to help with the pain and discomfort, do not be afraid to take it. Taking this medicine will make you more comfortable and help you to eat and drink.
13. Notify your nurse or doctor if taking pills becomes difficult. Some, but not all, pills can be crushed and taken in ice cream or applesauce.
14. Keep your mouth fresh and clean. Baking soda (1 tsp mixed in 1 qt of water) works well to rinse your mouth and gargle. This can be done every 2 hr.
15. If it becomes more difficult to eat, change your foods to include very soft, blended, and/or liquid foods. Your nurse or doctor may suggest liquid food supplements.
16. Tell your nurse or doctor if you notice any of the following:
    • Unable to drink fluids
    • Dizziness, extreme tiredness, or weakness
    • Chills or fever of 100.8°F (38.2°C) or higher
    • Urinating small amounts of dark urine

are associated with widespread hyperpigmentation and others cause darkening confined to a specific area such as the tongue, nails, or mucous membranes. Hyperpigmentation occurs more commonly in dark-skinned individuals.

Busulfan can cause hyperpigmentation involving the neck, upper trunk, nipples, and abdomen, which is frequently associated with busulfan-induced pulmonary fibrosis. Hyperpigmentation caused by cyclophosphamide may be diffuse or confined to the palms, soles, nails, or

gums. Skin contact with carmustine or nitrogen mustard can result in a contact dermatitis followed by postinflammatory hyperpigmentation.[71] After several infusions, irinotecan can cause hyperpigmentation that fades after the drug regimen is stopped.[33]

5-Fluorouracil can cause hyperpigmentation, especially in those patients who receive high-dose weekly infusions with or without leucovorin. Hyperpigmentation occurs most readily in sun-exposed areas.[72] Serpiginous hyperpigmented streaks overlying veins used repeatedly for 5-FU infusions occur without any clinical evidence of cutaneous inflammation, phlebitis, or sclerosis (Figure 20-10).

Bleomycin may cause hyperpigmentation over the veins into which the drug is administered. However, bleomycin is more commonly associated with hyperpigmentation over pressure points or with linear streaks occurring in areas of intense scratching, presumably due to localized vasodilation that results in an increased bleomycin concentration in the skin (Figure 20-11).[73]

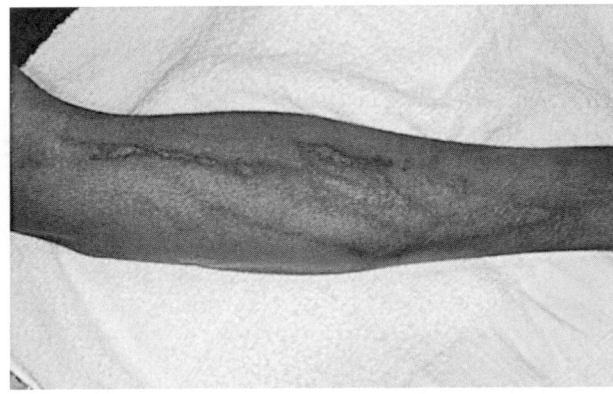

Figure 20-10 Serpiginous hyperpigmentation following 5-fluorouracil infusion

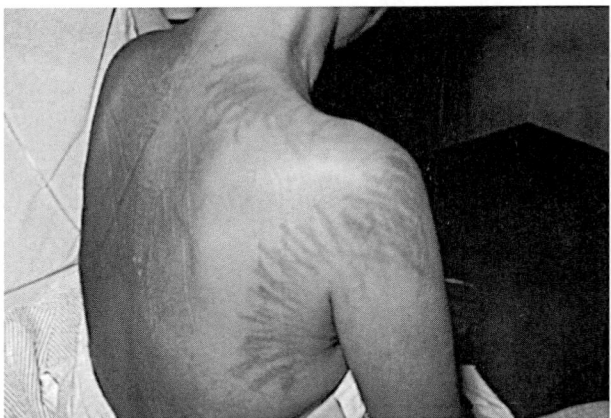

Figure 20-11 Flagellate streaks of hyperpigmentation in an Asian woman occurring in areas of intense scratching following intracavitary (intrapleural) bleomycin

Doxorubicin, busulfan, cyclophosphamide, 5-FU, and etoposide have been associated with hyperpigmentation of the oral mucosa and tongue, especially in blacks. Doxorubicin and 5-FU also may cause skin darkening over the interphalangeal and metacarpophalangeal joints. The mechanism of this effect is not known, but phalangeal darkening decreases once therapy is terminated.[71]

Hypersensitivity. Cutaneous hypersensitivity reactions (HSRs) to chemotherapy occur infrequently and tend not to be dose-related. Cutaneous manifestations of immediate HSRs (type I reactions) generally present as urticaria, angioedema, or anaphylaxis. L-asparaginase, for example, is a polypeptide of bacterial origin that causes HSR in 10%–20% of patients receiving the drug. Acute urticaria is the most frequent manifestation of L-asparaginase HSR, with 10% of these patients progressing to life-threatening anaphylaxis.[71]

Paclitaxel can cause hypotension, rash, dyspnea, and bronchospasm within 10 minutes of initiating the drug, suggesting a nonimmunologic anaphylactoid reaction.[25] The cause of this HSR is believed to be to due the drug vehicle, Cremophor EL (polyoxyethylated castor oil). Measures to minimize HSR with paclitaxel include prolonging drug infusion time (6–24 hours) and using a three-drug prophylactic regimen consisting of an antihistamine, corticosteroid, and H_2 receptor antagonist. Despite these precautions, approximately 2% of patients will experience HSRs after receiving paclitaxel.[25]

Docetaxel is associated with HSR, most notably skin rash, anaphylaxis, and fluid retention. Pretreatment with 8 mg of dexamethasone twice daily starting 1 day prior to dosing and continuing for a total of 5 days has minimized these reactions.[26]

Parenteral cisplatin, carboplatin, and nitrogen mustard can cause a type I HSR in approximately 5% of patients.[71] The manifestations of this reaction include anxiety, pruritus, cough, dyspnea, angioedema, bronchospasm, rash, urticaria, and hypotension. These symptoms are usually relieved by prompt administration of antihistamines.

Teniposide and parenteral etoposide can cause HSR with the initial dosing, manifesting as dyspnea, wheezing, hypotension, urticaria, pruritus, angioedema, facial flushing, and rash. The incidence is higher with teniposide as it is admixed with Cremophor EL (polyoxyethylated castor oil). Decreasing the infusion rate and premedicating with an antihistamine and a steroid generally permits further drug administration.[71]

Other drugs that can produce rash, urticaria, pruritus, or angioedema include procarbazine, cytarabine, levamisole, topotecan, trimetrexate, anthracycline antibiotics, melphalan, and methotrexate. Trans-retinoic acid causes dry skin with mild exfoliation similar to a rash associated with pruritus.[69]

A common side effect of aminoglutethimide is a morbilliform maculopapular rash sometimes associated with fever. The pruritic rash usually disappears and does not necessitate cessation of therapy. Rarely, it can progress and cause desquamation. Hydrocortisone may be given in higher than usual doses for the first 2 weeks of therapy in an attempt to decrease severity of the skin rash.

Dactinomycin folliculitis presents as diffuse erythematous papules over the face and trunk, resembling acne, and appearing approximately 5 days after therapy. The rash resolves in 3–5 days. Folliculitis has also been reported following high-dose methotrexate.[71]

Erythema multiforme has been infrequently associated with chemotherapeutic agents. Patients receiving high-dose combination chemotherapy are more at risk for erythema multiforme. This reaction is characterized by target lesions over the extremities, often involving the mucous membranes. Busulfan, etoposide, procarbazine, hydroxyurea, bleomycin, methotrexate, and cytarabine have been associated with such lesions, which occasionally develop into generalized blistering.[74]

Acral erythema. An intensely painful erythema, scaling and epidermal sloughing from the palms and soles followed by desquamation and reepithelialization of the skin has been reported with continuous infusions of 5-FU, doxorubicin, paclitaxel, high-dose cytarabine, and floxuridine. The condition, also called *palmar-plantar erythrodysesthesia,* may represent a direct toxic effect on the epidermis and dermal vasculature or an accumulation of the chemotherapeutic agent in eccrine structures, causing erythema of the palms and soles where there are a high concentration of eccrine glands.[74,75] Chemotherapy is usually suspended until symptoms subside and is then resumed at a lower dose. However, the symptoms may recur and may necessitate cessation of therapy.

Pruritus. An allergic dermatitis may result from chemotherapy causing localized and generalized pruritus. Pruritus can be overwhelming and distressing to the individual, as it commonly interferes with rest and sleep and can result in skin breakdown and infection.

Assessment requires a thorough evaluation of the possible cause of the itching and any factors that might aggravate the condition. If pruritus is chemotherapy induced, the condition generally resolves when the drug is stopped or gradually dissipates following antihistamine therapy.

Nursing management focuses on skin care and comfort. Medicated baths, anesthetic creams, and emollient creams may be soothing. Soaps made especially for sensitive skin should be used when skin cleansing is required. The patient is encouraged to use alternate cutaneous stimulation methods to relieve the urge to scratch. These include massage, pressure, or rubbing the area with a soft cloth. Distractions such as music, imagery, or relaxation may ease the itch sensation. Perfumes, cosmetics, starch-based powders, and deodorants should be avoided.[72,74]

Environmental factors include keeping the room humidity at 30%–40% and the room temperature cool. Cotton clothing and sheets should be washed in hypoallergenic soaps. Medications such as antihistamines or corticosteroids may be used to minimize itching.

Photosensitivity. Photosensitivity is an enhanced skin response to ultraviolet (UV) rays. This enhanced response may present like a sunburn with erythema, edema, blisters, hyperpigmentation, and desquamation or peeling.[71] Rarely, photoallergy, similar to contact dermatitis, with immediate wheal and flare reactions or delayed reactions occur. Photosensitivity has been reported following skin exposure to UV light following administration of 5-FU, dacarbazine, trans-retinoic acid, vinblastine, and high-dose methotrexate. In general, the exposed area becomes erythematous within a few hours and gradually subsides. Dacarbazine, however, has been associated with pruritus and erythematous eruptions on the face, neck, and dorsal surfaces of both hands after sun exposure occurred within 1–2 hours following drug administration.[71]

Nurses must educate patients on the dangers of UV exposure. Verbal and written instructions concerning ways to reduce the risk of developing a photosensitivity reaction are given to the patient. Sun exposure, particularly between the hours of 10 A.M. and 3 P.M., and tanning booths should be avoided. Protective clothing and a hat should be worn even on cloudy days.

Most important, nurses provide instructions regarding the proper use of sunscreen based on the individual's skin type. Sunscreens contain a sun protection factor (SPF) that defines the ratio of the time it takes to develop erythema with and without the sunscreen applied. For example, an individual who can only be in direct sunlight for 30 minutes without erythema may, by applying a sunscreen with an SPF of 8, remain outside for 240 minutes (30 × 8) without burning. The higher the SPF number, the more complete the sun protection. Products with an SPF higher than 15 are recommended for protection following chemotherapy. Sunblocks with an SPF of 25 or more are available and recommended for children and fair-skinned individuals. In general, the greater the SPF, the greater the chance of skin irritation. Some sunscreens are water-resistant, but in general they should be applied frequently and directly to the skin. To maximize its effectiveness, sunscreen should be applied at least 15–30 minutes before sun exposure and as often as indicated by activities in which the individual is engaged.

Alopecia. Alopecia is the most noticeable cutaneous side effect of chemotherapy and often one of the most distressing.[76] Although, certainly not a life-threatening event, loss of hair has a profound social and psychological impact on individuals and their acceptance of treatment. Some may even refuse potentially curative therapy for fear of this effect.

Chemotherapy agents affect actively growing (anagen) hairs. Because anagen hair is the most rapidly proliferating cell population in the human body, alopecia is a common toxicity. Extent of hair loss can range from thinning of scalp hair to total body hair loss.[71] Chemotherapy causes the hair shaft to be fragile or defective and thereby subject to breakage with minimal trauma.

Higher doses of chemotherapy or more potent epilators cause complete mitotic arrest, resulting in atrophy of the root and loss of the hair root bulb. Hair falls out spontaneously or is lost easily when combed or washed. Drugs of less intensity temporarily inhibit or slow cellular activity, causing bulb deformity and narrowing of the hair shaft. When hair growth resumes, narrow, weakened hair shafts are prone to breakage at the point of constriction. The hair root however, remains intact and active, leaving a thinning pattern of hair loss.

With an average 85% of scalp hair follicles in the anagen phase at any given time, the most common location for hair loss is the scalp. The majority of other body hair follicles (eyebrows, axilla, pubic area) are in the less active catagen and telogen phases and therefore are not initially affected. However, with multiple exposures from long-term therapy these hairs may also be lost as the hairs enter the anagen phase.[71]

Unlike natural hair loss, chemotherapy-induced alopecia occurs rapidly and usually starts 2–3 weeks following a dose of chemotherapy. Hair loss is usually asymptomatic; however, some patients have described intense scalp discomfort 1–2 days prior to and during hair shedding.

Chemotherapy-induced alopecia is temporary and reversible. After discontinuation of the drugs, regrowth is visible in 4–6 weeks, but complete regrowth may take 1–2 years. As hair grows back, alterations in hair pigmentation (lighter or darker), hair texture (finer or coarser), and hair type (straight or curly) may be evident.[71]

The severity and duration of chemotherapy-induced alopecia are related to the type of drug, combination of drugs, dose of drug, method of administration, and pharmacokinetics. Hair loss can be described as minimal (less than 25%), moderate (25%–50%), or severe (>50%) loss of heat or body warmth from head as well as sun exposure, which indicates the need for head covering. Chemotherapy agents most frequently associated with moderate to severe hair loss include trimetrexate, cyclophosphamide, doxorubicin, dactinomycin, daunorubicin, etoposide, idarubicin, ifosfamide, irinotecan, mechlorethamine, paclitaxel, topotecan, and vincristine. Mild hair loss is associated with bleomycin, carmustine, epirubicin, 5-FU, methotrexate, melphalan, mitomycin, mitoxantrone, teniposide, and vinorelbine.

Bolus intravenous administration of chemotherapy results in immediate peak serum levels with subsequent exposure and damage of sensitive growing hairs, resulting in hair loss. Infusions over several hours or longer are associated with greater likelihood of alopecia. The risk of alopecia appears to be decreased with low-dose continuous infusion. This may be related to the fact that high peak serum levels are necessary to cause hair loss.[77]

A patient-related factor that may influence the degree of scalp hair loss is the variability of scalp hair growth among individuals. Individuals who have relatively few hairs in the anagen phase will be less sensitive to the effects of chemotherapy. Another factor to consider is the condition of the patient's hair before treatment. Damaged hair (tinted, permed) may potentiate the risk for alopecia.

Until the early 1990s, scalp hypothermia was the technique used to prevent or minimize hair loss. However, because there was risk of scalp micrometastasis, these techniques are no longer recommended.[78] Therefore, more emphasis needs to be placed on the psychological support of the patient experiencing hair loss from chemotherapy and use of creative measures to preserve self-image.[79]

It is essential that the patient and family be informed of the timing, extent, and duration of hair loss at the onset of therapy. While these factors are not always known, many times they are; for instance, when high-dose doxorubicin and cyclophosphamide are used, hair loss is nearly complete by 3 weeks. Patients should be encouraged to discuss their feelings regarding hair loss.[79] It is often helpful for patients to prepare for alopecia by procuring a scalp prosthesis (wig or hairpiece) before it becomes necessary. This often reduces the anxiety associated with the uncertain timing of hair loss and makes it easier for a stylist to match color and style. Patients should be encouraged to question their insurance carriers regarding coverage for "cranial therapeutic prosthesis" for treatment-induced alopecia. Some insurance companies will reimburse with a physician's prescription or letter.

Certain measures can be used to minimize or delay hair loss and scalp irritation. Some clinicians advise patients to cut long hair short in anticipation of hair loss. Short hair may make hair loss less noticeable, make remaining hair appear thicker, and possibly decrease the weight on the hair shaft.[79] Once hair loss is significant, the patient may be advised to shave the remaining scalp hairs. This practice allows the hair to grow in at the same length, often permitting the patient to go without a wig sooner. In addition, shaving the head rids the patient of the problem of continuous shedding of hair. Measures to minimize hair loss include use of mild protein-based shampoos with conditioners, avoidance of daily shampooing, allowing hair to dry naturally, and grooming hair with a wide-toothed comb. Hair care practices such as blow-drying, perming, or coloring hair are controversial and areas for further nursing research. Claims have been made that these practices cause the hair to become brittle and fall out earlier during chemotherapy.

Nails. Changes in the fingernails and toenails are commonly seen during chemotherapy.[80] Pigmentation is seen most commonly and occurs with more regularity and intensity in blacks than in whites. The pigment generally is deposited at the base of the nail, causing transverse dark bands that correlate with the times the drug was administered. This reaction occurs most commonly with paclitaxel, docetaxel, doxorubicin, and cyclophosphamide but has been reported with melphalan, 5-FU, daunomycin, idarubicin, and bleomycin. If continuous infusion therapy of these drugs is given, the nails darken evenly.

Beau lines (transverse white lines or grooves in the nail) indicate a reduction or cessation of nail growth in response to chemotherapy. A partial separation of the nail plate (onycholysis) can be seen with 5-FU, doxorubicin, paclitaxel, docetaxel, and bleomycin.[71]

Vaginitis. Potentially, any drug known to cause oral mucositis may be associated with painful irritation and inflammation of the vagina. Because the vagina is near the vulva, women may experience both vulvar and vaginal irritation (vulvovaginitis). Symptoms may occur 3–5 days after chemotherapy is given and resolve 7–10 days later. The nurse should inquire as to whether the patient is experiencing any discomfort because such information probably will not be volunteered. Symptoms include vaginal discharge, itching, odor, pain, soreness, bleeding, or dyspareunia. The vulvar and vaginal membranes should be inspected for signs of impaired integrity such as erythema, swelling, or ulceration.

Nursing interventions are directed toward measures to decrease inflammation of mucous membranes, to increase comfort, and to minimize complications. Comfort can be provided with cold compresses or cool sitz baths for relief of pruritus, and warm compresses for severe inflammation. Patients are instructed to wear cotton underpants and to avoid pantyhose and tight-fitting clothes. Analgesics may be needed for severe discomfort or pain. Exposure to physical and chemical irritants (tampons, genital deodorant sprays, deodorant-containing vaginal pads) should be avoided.

Cultures should be obtained if an infection is suspected such as *Candida vaginitis*. Medical treatment is based on etiology and includes topical and systemic medications. The treatment of choice for *Candida vaginitis* is miconazole nitrate or clotrimazole cream or suppositories. When vaginal creams are prescribed, patients should be taught not to use tampons, which will absorb the medication. If a suppository is ordered, the patient should be instructed where it is to be inserted. The importance of completing the course of therapy should be stressed as recurrence is common if therapy is stopped early. *Trichomonas vaginitis* is treated systemically with metronidazole, and the partner is recommended for therapy as well.

Prevention of chemotherapy-induced vaginitis includes educating the patient regarding good personal hygiene and sexual activity. The nurse's goal is to help the patient maintain a healthy vagina, thereby reducing the potential for secondary vaginal infections. The perineum should be cleansed following each urination and bowel movement with mild soap and water and then pat or air dried. Soap and water remove most odors from noninfectious causes, but persistent genital odor should be investigated. Routine douching is not recommended.

The patient is instructed to use a water-based lubricant during vaginal intercourse to avoid mucosal irritation. Condoms should be used to prevent transmission of organisms through nonintact mucosa. Vaginal intercourse should be avoided in the presence of mucosal ulcerations and while neutrophil and platelet counts are low. Alternative methods of sexual activity should be suggested.

Organ Toxicities

Certain chemotherapy drugs may cause direct damage to specific cells of a given organ or cause indirect damage by the effects of cellular breakdown by-products. In general, organ toxicities are predictable based on the cumulative dose, the presence of concomitant organ dysfunction, the age of the patient, and the manner in which the drug is given. Of interest is the fact that the toxicity profile may be changing as a result of the more widespread use of dose-intensive regimens, multimodality treatment, chemoprotectants, and CSFs. These approaches to managing the disease are likely to result in more organ toxicities as myelosuppression becomes less prominent. Each of the major organ toxicities are discussed. Tables 20–6 through 20–11 provide a review of major toxicities in terms of risk factors, signs of toxicity, preventive measures, grading, and management.

Cardiotoxicity

Cardiotoxicity is described as an acute or chronic process. The acute form consists of transient electrocardiogram (ECG) changes that occur in approximately 10% of patients receiving chemotherapy. Acute effects are immediate in onset and resolve quickly without serious complications. These effects are not dose related and are not an indication to stop the drug. Less than 5% of patients develop chronic cardiotoxicity from a cumulative drug effect that requires immediate discontinuation of the drug.[81,82] Chronic effects occur weeks or months after administration, involving nonreversible cardiomyopathy, presenting as a classic biventricular congestive heart failure (CHF) with a characteristic low-voltage QRS complex. Signs and symptoms are classical for CHF, including complaints of a nonproductive cough, dyspnea, and pedal edema. Generally, it is poorly responsive to diuretics or digitalis, becoming progressively worse, with a 60% mortality.

Anthracyclines are known to cause cardiotoxicity by directly damaging the cardiac myocyte cells. The incidence of cardiotoxicity is 2%–3% after cumulative doses are administered.[81] Total cumulative dosages have been established at 550 mg/m^2 for doxorubicin, 400 mg/m^2 for epirubicin, and 600 mg/m^2 for daunomycin, with a decrease in dose to 450 mg/m^2 if mediastinal radiation has been administered.[81,83]

The mechanism of action occurs in the presence of oxygen, where the anthracyclines form a bond or union with iron or copper. These complexes inhibit lipid peroxidation, allowing a free oxygen radical to damage the myocyte directly. This results in a loss of myocardial fibrils, mitochondrial changes, and cellular destruction. As a result, the myocyte has limited contractility, leading to

hypertrophy of the cardiac muscle, which increases the demand for oxygen.[81,82]

In an attempt to decrease cardiotoxicity occurrence, altering the dose scheduling of doxorubicin to frequent lower doses has resulted in reduction of cardiotoxicity without compromise of antitumor effects.[81] The use of liposome doxorubicin has demonstrated a reduction of cardiotoxicity.[84] Chemoprotectants are being evaluated to protect the cardiac tissue by blocking damage to the myocyte. In animal studies calcium antagonists, catechin, and combination of selenium and amifostine have been found to reduce anthracycline-induced cardiotoxicity.[81,85,86]

Dexrazoxane (Zinecard) is currently approved for patients with metastatic breast cancer who have received cumulative doses of 300 mg/m^2 and are continuing treatment with doxorubicin (not for initial treatment). Patients have been able to tolerate greater cumulative doses of doxorubicin with a decreased risk of cardiac events. The agent is administered 30 minutes prior to doxorubicin, calculated on a 10:1 ratio. Thus, with a 50-mg dose of doxorubicin, 500 mg of dexrazoxane would be administered.[87] This compound has permitted doses of doxorubicin up to 700 mg/m^2 to be administered without cardiotoxicity occurring. It appears to interfere with the intracellular process responsible for anthracycline-induced cardiomyopathy.[87]

In an attempt to reduce further the cardiotoxicity from the anthracyclines, analogs that have greater antitumor activity and may have reduced cardiotoxicity have been developed. Epirubicin, idarubicin, esorubicin, and aclarubicin appear to be similar to doxorubicin, but the cardiotoxicity is significantly less. Although mitoxantrone has been associated with rare cardiac events, it is considered to be less cardiotoxic.[81]

Acute pericarditis has been reported with high-dose cyclophosphamide therapy (90–270 mg/kg) used in the bone marrow transplant (BMT) population, with subsequent pericardial effusion and cardiac tamponade.[82] Cyclophosphamide damages the myocytes in a manner similar to anthracyclines, where swelling and decreased contractility lead to less effective pumping of the heart. Hemorrhagic myocardial necrosis has been reported, with leakage of blood through capillaries. Transient complete heart block requiring temporary pacemaker support has been reported. Toxicity ranges from minor, transient ECG changes and asymptomatic elevation of cardiac enzymes to fatal myopericarditis and myocardial necrosis.[82]

Myocardial ischemia has been reported with 5-FU infusion in patients with or without preexisting heart disease. Coronary vasospasm with resulting angina pectoris, myocardial infarction, S-T segment elevations, and ventricular ectopy has been described. The pathophysiology is unclear, although a direct cardiomyopathic effect from the release of vasoactive substances in the presence of 5-FU has been suggested.[88] It has been speculated that angina is a coronary artery spasm of the Prinzmetal type that responds to nitrates. Cessation of therapy does not appear to be absolutely necessary, as patients who have such a syndrome can be pretreated with calcium antagonists known to prevent coronary artery spasm.

Asymptomatic bradycardia has been reported in about 30% of patients with ovarian cancer who have received paclitaxel.[82] Other cardiac disturbances that have been reported in 5% of patients include atrioventricular conduction blocks, left bundle branch blocks, ventricular tachycardia, and symptoms of cardiac ischemia. Most paclitaxel-related cardiac disturbances were not associated with clinical symptoms and were noted incidentally during continuous cardiac monitoring. Paclitaxel infusion is not discontinued unless associated with progressive atrioventricular conduction disturbances. The mechanism is unclear; however, it is speculated to be the result of the administration vehicle Cremophor EL (polyoxyethylated castor oil), which causes activation of selected cardiac-histamine receptors. Stimulation of these receptors in the cardiac tissue increases myocardial oxygen demand and produces coronary vasoconstriction. Although cardiac disturbances are usually benign, a case report documents the occurrence of myocardial ischemia during paclitaxel administration that resulted in death.[89]

Cardiac function should be evaluated throughout therapy for patients at high risk for cardiotoxicity or those who will be receiving high dosages of paclitaxel, an anthracycline, cyclophosphamide, or Herceptin . Methods to evaluate cardiac function include noninvasive monitoring with ECG, echocardiography, and radionuclide cardiography. An ejection fraction less than 45% or a decrease of 5% or more from the resting value is considered abnormal. Further doses of cardiotoxic chemotherapy are not recommended.[82] Although an endomyocardial biopsy can reveal damage to the myocyte prior to clinical detection, the procedure is costly and technically difficult and requires considerable expertise. Recently, the serum concentrations of cardiospecific proteins that are released from damaged myocyte have been evaluated in rats.[90] Cardiac troponin T levels were found to be useful in detecting early cardiac injury induced by anthracyclines.

The lifelong cardiotoxic effects of conventional anthracycline therapy highlight the need for monitoring cardiac dysfunction. Radionuclide cardiography and echocardiograms are the noninvasive methods most commonly used, despite their insensitivity for detecting early signs of cardotoxicitiy.[81] Considering the occurrence of late-onset cardiac dysfunction, long-term follow-up is recommended, with noninvasive testing based on the patient's risk factors and cardiac symptoms. Low-risk patients have been defined as those receiving less than 200 mg/m² of an anthracycline and no mediastinal radiation or exhibiting no cardiac abnormality. High-risk patients are considered to have received more than 500 mg/m² of an anthracycline, to have received mediastinal radiation, or to have abnormal cardiac function. Long-term follow-up recommendations include a minimum of one echocardiogram yearly and a cardiac scan every 5 years if the patient remains asymptomatic.

Accurate documentation and monitoring of total cumulative dosages are essential. Cardiac assessment is imperative to evaluate for a third heart sound or gallop, which could indicate cardiac insufficiency. Cardiac monitoring may be necessary for administering high dosages of chemotherapy, such as with cyclophosphamide. Once the patient develops chronic cardiotoxicity, nursing interventions include teaching the patient about energy conservation, managing fluid retention, and minimizing sodium in the diet. Supportive care with digitalis, angiotensin-converting enzyme (ACE) inhibitors to enhance the cardiac output, and diuretics to manage fluid should also be instituted. Eventually, the patient may need supplemental oxygen and vasodilator medications to relieve dyspnea. Heart transplantation has become an accepted procedure to treat end-stage heart disease from anthracycline cardiomyopathy.[91] The degree of cardiac injury determines the limitations on activities of daily living the individual will experience. Few are prepared for this debilitating effect, and nurses must initiate interventions that will assist the patient and family in coping. Patients are also taught the importance of close cardiac follow-up, once the treatment is complete, to monitor for late cardiac effects (Table 20-6).

Neurotoxicity

Chemotherapy-induced neurotoxicity can arise as a direct or an indirect damage to the CNS, peripheral nervous system, cranial nerves, or any combination of the three. The majority of patients experience temporary neurotoxicity; however, some will have permanent neurological deficits. Significant neurotoxicity usually requires suspending the treatment until the symptom resolves and reinstituting with a 50% dose reduction or discontinuing the drug.[92]

The central and peripheral nervous systems are protected against potentially neurotoxic effects by the blood-brain barrier and blood-nerve barriers. If intact, these barriers exclude most chemotherapeutic agents that are water soluble and also exclude relatively large molecules. Biopsies of damaged nerves from chemotherapy have demonstrated a mild decrease in the number of large diameter myelinated nerve fibers, and ultrastructural studies have shown scattered degenerating nerve fibers both in the axon and in the myelin sheaths. Severity of neurotoxicity is usually dose-related, with symptoms exhibited in a variable and unpredictable fashion.

The CNS is made up of collections of neurons, and their connections are organized into the brain and spinal cord areas. Damage to the CNS primarily involves the cerebellum, which produces altered reflexes, unsteady gait, ataxia, and confusion. The peripheral nervous system is basically a set of communication channels located outside the CNS, consisting of the cranial and spinal nerves. Damage to the peripheral nervous system produces paralysis or loss of movement and sensation to those areas affected by the particular nerve. The autonomic nervous system (ANS) includes those peripheral nerves that regulate functions occurring automatically in the

Table 20-6 Organ Toxicity of Chemotherapy Agents: Cardiotoxicity

Toxicity/ Symptoms	Grade	General Risk Factors	Chemotherapy Agent/Risk Factors	Mechanism of Damage	Protective/ Management Measures
×b Tachycardia • Dyspnea • Nonproductive cough • Neck vein distention • Gallop rhythm • Rales • Pedal edema • Cardiomegaly • Dull or sharp precordial pain, may radiate to neck and shoulder • Cardiac friction rub • ST-T wave changes • Supraventricular • Tachyarrhythmias • T-wave flattening	Cardiac Dysrhythmias 0 = None 1 = Asymptomatic, transient, requires no therapy 2 = Recurrent or persistent, requires no therapy 3 = Requires treatment 4 = Requires monitoring; hypotension, ventricular tachycardia, or fibrillation Cardiac Function 0 = None 1 = Asymptomatic decline of resting ejection by less than 20% of baseline 2 = Asymptomatic, decline of resting ejection fraction by more than 20% of baseline 3 = Mild CHF, responsive to therapy 4 = Severe or refractory CHF	• Age, geriatric and pediatric • Cumulative dose • Schedule of drug administration • History of cardiac disease (e.g., atherosclerosis, mitral valve prolapse, CHF, hypertension) • Use of combination drugs • Hepatic dysfunction • Prior mediastinum radiation • Prior anthracycline exposure	Anthracyclines • Doxorubicin (>550 mg/m^2) • Daunorubicin (>600 mg/m^2) • Dactinomycin • Doxorubicin-enhanced effect with: actinomycin, mitomycin, vincristine, melphalan, bleomycin cyclophosphamide • Mitoxantrone (>160 mg/m^2) • Cyclophosphamide, High-dose (>144 mg/kg × 4 days) • 5-Fluorouracil • Paclitaxel • Herceptin	Acute Changes: • Hypereosinophilia of myocytes Chronic Changes: • Loss of contractile elements • Mitochondrial changes • Myocyte damage • Hemorrhagic myocardial necrosis • Fibrin deposition in interstitium • Coronary spasm of the Prinzmetal type • Speculated to be related to Cremaphor EL (polyoxyethylated castor oil), the administration vehicle for Paclitaxel that causes activation of selected cardiac histamine receptors	• Limit cumulative dose of doxorubicin to <550 mg/m^2 • Administer doxorubicin at lower doses more frequently • ECG before treatment • Radionuclide cardiac scan • Administer dexrazoxane before anthracycline dose • Administer calcium channel blockers before anthracycline dose • Limit cumulative dose of daunorubicin to <600 mg/m^2 • Avoid alcohol, smoking, and cocaine use • Moderate exercise and low-fat, low-salt diet • Prevent thrombus with daily aspirin or warfarin • Herceptin is not given concurrent with doxorubicin

CHF = congestive heart failure

body, such as the cardiovascular, respiratory, and endocrine systems. Damage to the ANS causes ileus, impotence, or urinary retention.

Vincristine is well known for potential peripheral neuropathy characterized by myalgia and loss of the deep tendon reflex at the ankle, progressing to complete areflexia, distal symmetric sensory loss, motor weakness, foot drop, and muscle atrophy.[92] Autonomic neuropathy is characterized by ileus, constipation, impotence, urinary retention, or postural hypotension. The mechanism of damage is believed to involve disruption of the microtubule in the neural tissues, which thereby inhibits the mitotic spindle movements necessary for the mitosis

phase of cellular reproduction.[74] Vincristine doses greater than 2 mg increase the risk of neurotoxicity.

Neuropathy related to cisplatin is reversible, although cases of persistent progression after the discontinuation of the drug have been reported.[92] Cisplatin affects the large-diameter fibers of the neural tissues, resulting in sensory changes. The earliest sign of peripheral neuropathy is decreased vibratory sense, described as hand and feet paresthesia, with the classic stocking-glove distribution. Sensory loss occurs initially; without dose modification, loss of the Achilles reflex, muscle weakness, and loss of the deep tendon reflex occur. Symptoms of neuropathy are seen at cumulative doses of 300–500 mg/m^2. As the neuropathy progresses, position sense is impaired and a marked sensory ataxia develops. Peripheral neuropathy has been reported from combined paclitaxel and cisplatin. Sensory-motor neuropathy occurs 1–21 weeks after initiation of therapy. Neuropathy appears to be progressive with additional courses, and more pronounced with higher doses of paclitaxel (cumulative dose of ≥1500 mg/m^3).[93]

High-tone hearing loss is speculated to be related to the loss of hairs in the organ of Corti resulting from cisplatin. Rapid drug delivery, simultaneous administration of aminoglycosides, and dehydration seem to increase the potential for ototoxicity. The loss can be reversed with discontinuation of the drug; however, permanent damage has been reported, resulting in the need for a hearing aid.[92]

Neurotoxicity characterized by metabolic encephalopathy manifested as blurred vision, seizures, motor system dysfunction, urinary incontinence, cranial nerve dysfunction, subclinical electroencephalographic changes, or irreversible coma has been reported in 5%–30% of patients treated with ifosfamide.[94] Signs have occurred within 2 hours of bolus administration and up to 28 days after therapy. Within 48–72 hours of cessation of ifosfamide, most abnormalities spontaneously clear. Risk factors associated with neurotoxicity include duration of administration, hepatic insufficiency, previous cisplatin, presence of bulky disease, low serum albumin, and high serum creatinine.[94] Although the cause is not completely understood, the encephalopathy is thought to result from an accumulation of drug metabolites (chloracetaldehyde), thus causing direct CNS damage.

After several courses, high-dose methotrexate (>1 g/m^2) occasionally causes encephalopathy that usually is transient and reversible.[92] Intrathecal methotrexate may cause a chemical meningitis, with fever, headache, muscle rigidity, and cerebrospinal fluid leukocytosis. This is rare, but it occurs within hours of the intrathecal injection and resolves spontaneously.

5-Fluorouracil may cause an acute cerebellar dysfunction, which is usually more common in the elderly. It is characterized by rapid onset of gait ataxia, limb incoordination, dysarthria, nystagmus, and diplopia. Effects are reversible with drug withdrawal or dose reduction. Multifocal cerebral demyelination has been described to occur as the result of 5-FU and levamisole or leucovorin administration.[95] Symptoms that have been exhibited include acute confusion, ataxia, slurred speech, and restlessness. With steroid use and discontinuing chemotherapy, the patient's symptoms improve.

High-dose cytarabine can cause encephalopathy, leukoencephalopathy, and sometimes peripheral neuropathy with doses greater than 18 g/m^2. High doses increase the transport rate over the cell membranes, enhancing the intracellular drug concentrations and prolonging the cellular exposure to the drug's metabolites. CNS toxicity usually occurs 5–7 days after the start of therapy.[92] Ocular toxicity (conjunctivitis, photophobia, burning, and decreased acuity) and cerebellar and cerebral dysfunction

can also occur. Once the drug is stopped, the neurological symptoms may resolve partially or completely.

Arthralgia and myalgia have been reported to occur infrequently with docetaxel administration. If symptoms occur, they are usually experienced a few days after administration and lasting up to 4 days.[96] Severity of discomfort can be reduced by the use of prophylactic analgesics such as ibuprofen. Transient myalgia and arthralgia are common after paclitaxel.[97] Symptoms usually occur 2–3 days after treatment and resolve in approximately 6 days. The shoulder and paraspinal muscles seem to be the most common area of occurrence, however other muscle groups can be affected. Trans-retinoic acid commonly causes myalgia, arthralgia, and muscle weakness.[69]

One of the principal nonhematologic toxicities of paclitaxel is sensory neuropathy, which is experienced at doses 250 mg/m^2 or greater. Symptoms consist of numbness, tingling, or burning pain of the lower extremities. Perioral numbness has been reported that may be asymmetrical at onset and progress in a symmetrical pattern. Neurotoxicity is typically cumulative, with large-fiber modalities (vibration, proprioception) more frequently affected than loss of small-fiber modalities (pain and temperature).[93] Mild symptoms improve or resolve within several months after the discontinuation of paclitaxel. Amitriptyline has been found to be beneficial in relieving discomfort of the symptoms. Autonomic neuropathy has been reported with high doses of paclitaxel (250 mg/m^2 or greater) and is exhibited as paralytic ileus and orthostatic hypotension. Patients with diabetes mellitus experience this neuropathy more frequently.[93] Transient encephalopathy has been reported after paclitaxel infusion and is exhibited as confusion, word-finding difficulty, and behavioral changes. Symptoms appear 1 week after paclitaxel infusion and resolve spontaneously.[98]

Docetaxel administration can produce mild sensory neuropathy. At a cumulative dose of 600 mg/m^2, severe and disabling neuropathy can develop. Symptoms include paresthesia, numbness, loss of sensory qualities, and a decrease in deep tendon reflexes.[96]

Chemoprotectants have been evaluated in minimizing chemotherapy-induced neurotoxicity. Amifostine has been found to decrease cisplatin-induced neurotoxicity and may protect against ototoxicity.[18] Prosaposin, a neurotrophic factor, has been found to facilitate nerve regeneration in rats. Findings suggest the prevention of paclitaxel-induced neurotoxiciy.[99]

Astute neurological assessment is critical in patients receiving potentially neurotoxic agents. Baseline assessment should include sensory function, motor function, gait, range-of-motion, cranial nerves, and reflexes. Renal and hepatic functions should be monitored closely.[93] Chemotherapy agents such as ifosfamide and cytarabine will have increased neurotoxicity with renal dysfunction. Sedatives, antiemetics, and tranquilizers, which are CNS depressants, must be used with caution because their usage may increase toxicity. In addition other causes of these symptoms, such as electrolyte imbalances, metastasis, or other medical conditions, can cause similar effects. Neurotoxicity will affect patients by decreasing their mobility, ability for self-care, and ability to perform fine-motor skills such as writing and buttoning a shirt. An occupational therapist may need to be consulted to help the patient adapt to loss of motor skills. Patients must be taught the importance of reporting any change in status, such as numbness and tingling of the extremities. If neurological deficits become severe, safety measures must be initiated to protect the patient from harm (Table 20-7).

Pulmonary toxicity

Pulmonary toxicity is usually irreversible and progressive as a result of chemotherapy administration. The initial site of damage seems to be the endothelial cells, with an inflammatory-type reaction resulting in drug-induced pneumonitis. Another type of damage occurs as a result of an immunologic mechanism. Either the lung or the drug may act as the antigen in an allergic-type reaction.[100] Chronic exposure to chemotherapy causes an extensive alteration of the pulmonary parenchyma, with changes in the connective tissue, obliteration of alveoli, and dilatation of air spaces, known as *honeycombing*.[100] Continuous injury and repair result in restrictive lung disease, increased work of breathing, and a functionally reduced lung volume, leading to impaired gas exchange. Hypoxemia results because oxygen does not diffuse in the damaged areas while perfusion continues.

Pulmonary toxicity usually presents clinically as dyspnea, unproductive cough, bilateral basilar rales, and tachypnea. The chest x-ray may be within normal limits, but can show a pattern of diffuse interstitial markings. Arterial blood gases reveal hypoxia, with hypocapnia and respiratory alkalosis. The most sensitive pulmonary function test is the carbon-monoxide diffusion capacity, which becomes abnormal before clinical symptoms occur.[101] Other pulmonary function tests can show a restrictive pattern when pulmonary fibrosis has occurred. The best method to establish a pathological diagnosis is to obtain involved tissues by an open-lung biopsy or a fiberoptic bronchoscopy. Bacterial or fungal infections and metastasis can then be ruled out.

Bleomycin is known to cause pulmonary toxicity. The incidence is 5% for a total cumulative dose of 450 units and 15% for higher dosages. Bleomycin is concentrated preferentially in the lung and is inactivated by a hydrolase enzyme. This enzyme is relatively deficient in lung tissue as compared with other tissues, such as the liver. These findings may explain the relative sensitivity of bleomycin to lung tissue, causing (1) early endothelial cell damage, (2) decrease in type I pneumocytes, with subsequent proliferation, and (3) migration of type II pneumocytes into alveolar spaces, inducing interstitial changes.[102] Following destruction of type I cells, repair is characterized by hyperplasia and dysplasia of the type II pneumocytes. Fibroblast proliferation, with subsequent pulmonary fibrosis, is probably the basis for irreversible changes induced by bleomycin.[102]

Cytarabine exerts a direct toxic effect on the pneumocytes and capillary endothelial cells to diminish the integrity of cell membranes and increase capillary permeability. A capillary leak syndrome, involving primarily the lung, occurs 2–21 days after the first dose, resulting in pulmonary edema and respiratory failure, with features of adult respiratory disease (ARD). It appears to be related to high doses and continuous administration.[100]

Mitomycin C damage to the lung presents as diffuse alveolar damage with capillary leak and pulmonary edema. Incidence ranges from 3%–36%, occurring 6–12 months after therapy; however, occurrence may be after a brief exposure. If dyspnea occurs with a normal chest radiograph, it may be necessary to discontinue mitomycin from the treatment plan.[100]

Cyclophosphamide causes pulmonary toxicity in less than 1% of patients and is associated with high doses (120 mg/kg/day for 4 days). Histological findings include endothelial swelling, pneumocyte dysplasia, edema, fibrosis, and fibroblast proliferation. The result of damage is alveolar hemorrhage and fibrin deposition.[100]

Carmustine inhibits lung glutathione disulfide reductase, which mediates the resultant cellular injury. Damage occurs after a long latency period, averaging 3 years, but may occur after only 6 weeks of therapy. High-dose carmustine has an incidence of 20%–30% when a cumulative dose of 1500 mg/m² is given. An insidious cough with dyspnea or sudden respiratory failure occurs. It has been suggested that this reaction may be more common when cyclophosphamide is given simultaneously.[103] Glucocorticoid administration has improved symptoms; however, mortality still occurs in a small percentage of patients.

Methotrexate can also produce an acute or a chronic process related to endothelial injury.[104] Diffuse alveolar damage is characterized by the disappearance of type I pneumocytes, hyaline membrane formation, and the presence of inflammatory cells in the alveoli and interstitium. The incidence is less than 1%, with an acute onset of pulmonary edema producing ARD or more gradual systemic toxicity (such as fever, chills), and malaise being present before the appearance of pulmonary symptoms. Radiographic features may be unique, with pleural effusion occurring alone or in conjunction with pulmonary infiltrates, peripheral consolidations, or chronic eosinophilic pneumonia.

An uncommon side effect of docetaxel is fluid retention. The incidence is related to the cumulative dose, which can be disabling, worsening with higher doses. Fluid retention is exhibited peripherally, as abdominal ascites, as a pleural effusion, or as a combination of the two. The fluid retention is reversible and can be controlled with diuretics.[26]

Trans-retinoic acid can cause a syndrome of high fever, respiratory distress, pulmonary infiltrates, and pericardial or pleural effusion that occurs 2 days to 3 weeks after initiating treatment. Retinoic acid syndrome can be reversed with the administration of corticosteroids.[69] Irinotecan can cause dyspnea on exertion and pneumonitis with pulmo-

Table 20-7   Organ Toxicity of Chemotherapy Agents: Neurotoxicity

Toxicity/Symptoms	Grade	General Risk Factors	Chemotherapy Agent/Risk Factors/ Symptoms	Mechanism of Damage	Protective/ Management Measures
Cerebellar • Unsteady gait • Nystagmus • Ataxia • Dizziness • Seizures • Hemiparesis • Confusion • Coma Autonomic • Ileus • Constipation • Impotence • Urinary retention • Postural hypotension Peripheral/Cranial • Facial palsies • Diplopia • Paresthesia of hands and feet • Muscle atrophy • Foot drop • Loss of deep tendon reflexes • Areflexia • Sensory loss • Sensory perception loss • Hoarseness	Neurocerebellar 0 = None 1 = Slight incoordination dysdiadokinesis 2 = Intention tremor dysmetria, slurred speech 3 = Locomotor ataxia 4 = Cerebellar necrosis Neurocortical 0 = None 1 = Mild somnolence or agitation 2 = Moderate somnolence or agitation 3 = Severe somnolence or agitation, confusion, disorientation, hallucination, aphasia 4 = Coma, seizures, psychosis Neurosensory 0 = None 1 = Mild paresthesias, loss of deep tendon reflexes 2 = Mild or moderate objective sensory loss, moderate paresthesias 3 = Severe objective loss, or paresthesias that interfere with function Neuromotor 0 = None 1 = Subjective weakness 2 = Mild objective weakness 3 = Objective weakness with impairment of function 4 = Paralysis	• Dosage • Cranial radiation • Intrathecal administration • Age • CNS depressants (i.e., antiemetics, tranquilizers, and sedatives) • History of diabetes, chronic alcohol abuse	Ifosfamide • High doses • Cerebellar and cranial dysfunction Vincristine • Dose related >2 mg/m^2 of unit dose • Hepatic dysfunction • Autonomic, peripheral dysfunction Cisplatin • Dose-related • Renal dysfunction • Dehydration • Autonomic, peripheral dysfunction • Concurrent treatment with vincristine or etoposide Methotrexate • High dose (>1 g/m^2) • Cerebellar dysfunction • Concurrent cranial radiation therapy • Intrathecal dose • Increases effect with cytarabine, daunorubicin, salicylates, sulfonamides, vinblastine, vincristine Cytarabine • High doses (>2 g/m^2) • Cerebellar and peripheral effects 5-Fluorouracil • Cerebellar dysfunction • Dose and schedule related Taxanes • Peripheral neuropathies • Myalgias/arthralgia	• Accumulation of drug metabolite (chloracetaldehyde) with direct CNS effect • Disrupts microtubules in the neural tissues • Damages large fibers, resulting in sensory change • Damage/loss of inner hair cells in the organ of Corti • Demyelination of nerve fibers	• Place on bowel regimen • Oral diazepam 5 mg every 6 hr at the time of treatment, to manage muscle spasms • Eliminate furosemide • Avoid concurrent administration of aminoglycosides • Audiometric testing for high risk • Ethyol (amifostine) • Withhold therapy for severe toxicity, i.e., muscle weakness or pain • Neurologic recovery, start drug at 50% dose reduction • Monitor neurologic signs and symptoms • Monitor electrolytes • Institute safety measures • Administer amifostine with cisplatin

nary infiltrates.[33] Busulfan can cause pulmonary fibrosis when a dose of more than 500 mg is given.[100]

Gemcitabine can cause mild self-limiting dyspnea to fatal pulmonary toxicity. The symptoms exhibited include tachypnea, marked hypoxemia and interstitial infiltrates on chest x-ray consistent with pulmonary edema. Administration of corticosteroids and diuretics seem to reverse the toxicity.[105]

Because lung damage is usually irreversible and progressive, it is imperative to detect evidence of pulmonary toxicity as early as possible. The causative agent may be discontinued or dose-reduced to prevent further damage to lung tissue. High concentrations of inspired oxygen are toxic to the lungs, and the simultaneous administration of various chemotherapy drugs may induce lung damage.[101] Nurses need to be aware of this phenomenon and must monitor the patient's oxygen saturation and breath sounds closely for early signs and symptoms of pulmonary toxicity.

When oxygen saturation is compromised due to restrictive lung damage, the patient experiences dyspnea on exertion or at rest. As a result, the patient must expend increased effort to perform simple activities of daily living. Nursing care is centered on teaching the patient to prioritize daily activities and to use breathing techniques such as pursed lips to lessen the effects of dyspnea. Supplemental oxygen therapy may be necessary to relieve the dyspnea. The family and patient must be taught how to administer the oxygen and what safety precautions to institute for oxygen therapy. Steroids are usually administered to lessen the pulmonary symptoms. Single-lung transplantation may be an option for drug-induced pulmonary toxicity.[106] To prevent further complications, the nurse must also teach the patient how to mobilize secretions by maintaining an adequate fluid intake and performing effective cough and deep-breathing techniques (Table 20-8).

Hepatotoxicity

Chemotherapy agents can cause a variety of hepatotoxic reactions. The initial site of damage seems to be the parenchymal cells. Obstruction to hepatic blood flow results in fatty changes, hepatocellular necrosis, cholestasis, hepatitis, and venoocclusive disease (VOD). Hepatotoxicity usually is diagnosed initially by transient elevations of the hepatic enzymes during treatment, which can progress to hepatomegaly, jaundice, and abdominal pain. Unless extensive fibrosis or necrosis has occurred, hepatotoxicity is reversible.[107]

Liver toxicity induced by high-dose methotrexate is transient and usually does not result in chronic liver disease. Elevation of hepatic enzyme levels is common, rising with successive courses and tending to be higher in patients treated on a daily schedule than those treated on intermittent schedules. Chronic inflammatory infiltrates in the portal tracts, focal liver cell necrosis, fibrosis, and cirrhosis may occur. However, all abnormalities usually resolve within 1 month following cessation of methotrexate therapy.[108]

High-dose cytarabine may induce intrahepatic cholestasis, possibly as a result of injury to the hepatocyte transport system. Changes are reversible; therefore, they do not appear to limit cytarabine use.[107] 5-Fluorouracil with combination levamisole has resulted in increase in alkaline phosphatase, transaminase, and bilirubin. These changes resolve with the discontinuation of therapy; medical intervention is not needed.[109] Gemcitabine, irinotecan, trimetrexate, and antitumor antibiotics can cause a transient increase of hepatic enzymes that resolve after discontinuing the drug.[27,33,107]

Fluorodeoxyuridine, usually administered as a continuous arterial dose, can cause chemical hepatitis, with increases in transaminases, alkaline phosphatase, and serum bilirubin levels. Stricture of intrahepatic or extrahepatic bile ducts can also occur. Toxicity appears to be both time and dose dependent. Liver function usually normalizes when the drug is discontinued. However, the development of biliary sclerosis is irreversible.[107]

Hepatocellular disease occurs with the administration of 6-mercaptopurine in daily doses exceeding 2 mg/kg. Histological pattern includes features of intrahepatic cholestasis and parenchymal cell necrosis. Moderate elevations occur in transaminases, alkaline phosphatase, and serum bilirubin, with episodes of jaundice occurring 30 days after initiation of therapy.[107]

Few guidelines exist for the use of drugs when hepatic dysfunction is present. Known hepatotoxic drugs must be avoided when liver function test results are abnormal. Impaired liver function delays excretion and results in increased accumulation in the plasma and tissues, especially for drugs such as doxorubicin, daunorubicin, paclitaxel, docetaxel, vincristine, and vinblastine, which are excreted primarily by the liver into the bile. It has been recommended to reduce or not to administer these agents if the serum bilirubin is between 1.5 and 3 mg/dL. If the SGOT is between 60 and 180 international units, the drug should be reduced by 50%.[107]

Hepatic toxicity is uncommon, but it can be a serious consequence of chemotherapy administration, ranging from transient enzyme elevations to permanent cirrhosis. Because there are many disease- and treatment-related factors that can be hepatotoxic, it is difficult to attribute hepatic toxicity definitively to specific agents. During chemotherapy administration, the nurse monitors liver function tests closely, as enzymatic changes may be the first clinical evidence of hepatotoxicity. Third spacing (the shift of fluid from the vascular space to the interstitial space) can occur as a result of hepatotoxicity. Signs of fluid shift are decreased blood pressure, increased pulse rate, low central venous pressure, decreased urine output, increased specific gravity, low levels of serum albumin, and hemoconcentration. Albumin is administered to replace the plasma protein and assist with absorption of the fluid. Fluid restriction minimizes third spacing, which enhances renal blood flow, decreases systemic congestion, and improves patient comfort. Other supportive care measures include diuretics, decreased protein intake, lactulose, and emotional support (Table 20-9).

Table 20-8   Organ Toxicity of Chemotherapy Agents: Pulmonary Toxicity

Toxicity/ Symptoms	Grade	General Risk Factors	Chemotherapy Agent/Risk Factors	Mechanism of Damage	Protective/ Management Measures
• Low-grade fever • Nonproductive cough • Dyspnea • Tachycardia • Diffuse basilar crackles • Wheezing • Pleural rub • Fatigue • Malaise • Chest pain • Night sweats • Tachypnea • Cyanosis • Edema	Dyspnea 0 = None 1 = Asymptomatic with abnormal PFTs 2 = Dyspnea on exertion 3 = Dyspnea at normal activity 4 = Dyspnea at rest Pulmonary Fibrosis 0 = Normal 1 = Radiographic changes, no symptoms 2 = N/A 3 = Changes with symptoms Pulmonary Edema 0–2 = None 3 = Radiographic changes and diuretics required 4 = Requires intubation Pneumonitis (noninfectious) 0 = Normal 1 = Radiographic change, symptoms do not require steroids 2 = Steroids required 3 = Oxygen required 4 = Requires assisted ventilation Pleural Effusion 0 = None 1–4 = Present ARDs 0 = None 1 = Mild 2 = Moderate 3 = Severe 4 = Life threatening	• Age • Preexisting lung disease, e.g., COPD, TB • History of smoking • Cumulative dose • Long-term therapy • Mediastinal radiation • High inspired concentration of oxygen • Renal insufficiency	Bleomycin • Synergistic with vincristine • Cumulative dose >450 mg/m^2 • Oxygen exposure >50% Mitomycin • History of cyclophosphamide and/ or methotrexate administration • Oxygen concentrations >50% Carmustine • Dose related (>1500 mg/m^2) • Concurrent administration with cyclophosphamide Busulfan Cyclophosphamide: • High dose >120 mg/kg/day × 4 days Methotrexate Cytarabine • High doses (5 g/m^2) Gemcitabine	• Initial injury to capillary endothelium cells • Necrosis of type I epithelial cells • Hypertrophy of type II alveolar pneumocytes • Pulmonary fibrosis • Hypersensitivity reaction or immune complex related • Damage similar to bleomycin • Increased effect with VM-26, vincristine • Inhibition of glutathione reductase in alveolar macrophages • Hyperplasia and dysplasia of the type II pneumocytes • Alveolar hemorrhage and fibrin deposition • Increased effect with cisplatin, VM-26, vincristine • Capillary leak syndrome, pulmonary edema • Interstitial pneumonitis • Capillary leak syndrome • Capillary endothelial damage • See cytarabine	• Assess for risk factors • Obtain baseline pulmonary function tests • Monitor cumulative dose • Limit cumulative dose • Limit oxygen to keep arterial PO$_2$ >60 mm Hg • Discontinue drug if dyspnea occurs • Assess for pulmonary symptoms • Administer steroids and oxygen • Monitor activities to minimize energy • Stop or reduce dose of drug • Fluid restriction • Administer diuretics • Follow-up with PFTs

PFT = pulmonary function test; COPD = chronic obstructive pulmonary disorder; TB = tuberculosis.

Table 20-9 Organ Toxicity of Chemotherapy Agents: Hepatotoxicity

Toxicity/ Symptoms	Grade	General Risk Factors	Chemotherapy Agent	Mechanism of Damage	Protective/ Management Measures
• Elevated bilirubin, LDH, SGOT, alkaline phosphatase, SGPT • Chemical hepatitis • Jaundice • Ascites • Decreased albumin • Cirrhosis • Hepatomegaly • Right upper quadrant pain • Fatigue • Anorexia • Nausea • Decreased clotting factor synthesis • Hyperpigmentation of skin	Bilirubin 0–1 = Normal 2 = <1.5 3 = 1.5–3.0 4 = >3.0 SGOT/SGPT 0 = Normal 1 = <2.5 2 = 2.6–5.0 3 = 5.1–20 4 = >20 Alkaline Phosphatase 0 = Normal 1 = 2.5 2 = 2.6–5.0 3 = 5.1–20 4 = >20 Liver Clinical 0–2 = No change 3 = Precoma 4 = Hepatic coma	• Prior liver damage, e.g., hepatitis • Dose • Diabetes mellitus • Tumor involvement • Irradiation of liver • Alcoholism • Liver infections • Concurrent administration of hepatotoxic drugs, e.g., phenothiazines • Age • Hepatic dysfunction • Total bilirubin >2 mg/100 mL • Obesity	• Methotrexate • 6-Mercaptopurine • Cytarabine • Fluorodoxyuridine • Nitrosoureas • Etoposide, high dose • Cisplatin, high dose • L-Asparaginase • Amsacrine • Cyclophosphamide, high dose • Doxorubicin • Vincristine • Vinblastine • Docetaxel • Irinotecan • Gemcitabine • Trimetrexate	Direct Toxic Effects • Parenchymal cell damage • Intrahepatic cholestasis • Hepatic fibrosis • Fatty changes	• Reduce dose in presence of liver dysfunction for drugs metabolized in liver, e.g., vinca alkaloids or doxorubicin • Avoid alcohol intake • Monitor liver function tests • If bilirubin >1.5 mg, reduce dose by 50% • If bilirubin >3.0 mg, reduce dose by 75% • Avoid hepatotoxic drugs

Hemorrhagic cystitis

Hemorrhagic cystitis is a bladder toxicity resulting from cyclophosphamide and ifosfamide therapy. Hemorrhagic cystitis ranges from microscopic hematuria to frank bleeding, necessitating invasive local intervention with instillation of sclerosing agents. Symptoms range from transient irritative urination, dysuria, and suprapubic pain to life-threatening hemorrhage. Transient cystitis has an early onset and short duration due to the direct effect of the deposition of acrolein, a by-product of metabolism, on the urothelium.[110]

After oral or intravenous administration, cyclophosphamide is metabolized by hepatic microsomal enzymes to hydroxycyclophosphamide and later by target cells to phosphamide mustard (active) and acrolein (urinary metabolite). The binding of acrolein to the bladder mucosa results in inflammation and ulceration. Approximately 10% of people receiving cyclophosphamide experience microscopic hematuria.[111] Early diagnosis is accomplished by urine dipstick or visual observation of red-tinged urine. If necessary, a confirmed diagnosis can be accomplished by cystoscopy, which shows discrete bleeding capillaries or diffuse mucosal ulceration, hemorrhage, and necrosis.[112]

When hemorrhagic cystitis develops, drug therapy probably should be discontinued. In many patients, discontinuation will lead to amelioration of the symptoms without sequelae; however, microhematuria can continue long after discontinuing cyclophosphamide. When therapy is not stopped, up to 55% of patients have persistent symptoms. Extensive chronic bleeding and mucosal inflammation can produce long-term cystitis, irreversible bladder fibrosis, bladder contraction, and an increased risk for bladder cancer.[112] In high doses, Mesna has been successful in protecting the bladder from the harmful effects of acrolein.[112]

Ifosfamide has a slower rate of metabolic activation into acrolein, allowing larger dosages to be administered as compared to cyclophosphamide. Mesna, a uroprotectant, contains a sulfhydryl group believed to bind acrolein within the urinary collecting system and detoxifies ifosfamide. Mesna is administered before ifosfamide and then intermittently up to 24 hours afterward to protect the bladder. Mesna can be administered intravenously, orally, or subcutaneously.[110]

Gemcitabine can cause microscopic hematuria and proteinuria, especially with repeated cycles. In clinical trials, the occurrence was not found to be correlated with a cumulative dose or with treatment duration.[27] In rare instances, irinotecan caused hematuria.[33]

Protection of the bladder from either drug focuses on hyperhydration, frequent voiding, and diuresis. If cystitis occurs, the treatment includes bladder irrigation through a three-way Foley catheter to clear developing clots. The various solutions that cause a protein precipitate to form over the bleeding surfaces include saline, potassium aluminum sulfate, silver nitrate, and formalin. Vasopressins such as amino caproic acid may be administered intravenously or orally to decrease clotting. Cystoscopy may be necessary to cauterize bleeders, if the bladder irrigations were ineffective in controlling the bleeding. As a last resort, a cystectomy may be necessary.[112]

During administration of chemotherapy agents, the nurse should monitor the urine for blood, through dipsticking or observation. Strict intake and output measures are imperative to ensure minimal contact of acrolein with the bladder mucosa. The patient must be taught to maintain adequate hydration and to void frequently. If feasible, cyclophosphamide should be administered early in the day so the patient can drink fluids and void frequently without interruption of sleep. Insertion of a Foley catheter may be necessary when high doses of cyclophosphamide are administered, to ensure that the agent is being cleared from the bladder continuously (Table 20-10).

Nephrotoxicity

Nephrotoxicity is a dose-limiting side effect of some chemotherapeutic agents. Serious fluid and electrolyte imbalances that can progress to renal failure are the result of the direct and indirect effects of these agents on the kidney. Many chemotherapy agents are both metabolized and excreted by the kidneys; others are merely excreted as metabolites or as unchanged drugs. The manner in which chemotherapy damages the kidney varies from direct renal cell damage to an obstructive nephropathy resulting from precipitate formation. Renal failure, acid/base disorders, or electrolyte abnormalities may also occur as a result of tumor lysis syndrome or uric acid nephropathy.[113] When renal clearance of a specific drug with linear pharmacokinetics is 35%–40% and the patient has moderate-to-severe renal function, a significant increase of the drug in the area under the plasma concentration curve (AUC) can occur.[114] For patients with preexisting renal disease or who exhibit early signs of renal toxicity, the dosage may need to be reduced or the agent eliminated from the treatment plan.

Cisplatin can cause mild-to-severe nephrotoxicity, with specific damage to the proximal and distal tubules. Platinum metal chelates in the renal tubules cause direct damage to the proximal tubular cells, damaging the tubular basement membranes, and can cause focal tubular necrosis.[114] Acute damage can occur within 3–21 hours after cisplatin administration, as evidenced by renal enzyme changes when precautions are not taken. Renal dysfunction can persist for several years following cisplatin administration and may be irreversible.[113] Damage is characterized by degeneration of renal tubular epithelium, thickening of tubular basement membrane, and mild interstitial fibrosis. To avoid toxicity, patients should receive vigorous saline hydration of 1–2 liters as well as diuresis during therapy.

The use of mannitol in facilitating and inducing diuresis is a means of ensuring adequate urine flow. Mannitol possibly prevents immediate binding of cisplatin onto the renal tubules. Loop diuretics such as furosemide must be used with caution, as an increase in cisplatin toxicity has been reported. Frequent determinations of renal function should be obtained, and if the creatinine clearance falls to less than 50 mg/mL, the drug should be withheld until renal function improves. Daily magnesium supplementation may be indicated during cisplatin ther-

Table 20-10   Organ Toxicity of Chemotherapy Agents: Hemorrhagic Cystitis

Toxicity/ Symptoms	Grade	General Risk Factors	Chemotherapy Agent/Risk Factors	Mechanism of Damage	Protective/ Management Measures
• Gross hematuria • Dysuria, urgency • Suprapubic pain	0 = None 1 = Micro only 2 = Gross, no clots 3 = Gross, with clots 4 = Requires transfusion	• Dose-related • Pelvic radiation	Cyclophosphamide • High dose (>2.5 g) Ifosfamide • Single high dose vs multiple dose Gemcitabine Irinotecan	• Drug metabolite acrolein damages bladder mucosa Synergistic Effect • Cisplatin • VM-26 • Vincristine	• Vigorous hydration • Frequent emptying of bladder, especially at night • Monitor urine for blood • 3-way Foley irrigation with saline, alum, or formaldehyde • Administer amino caproic acid IV or PO • Mesna given in a dose of 20%–30% of ifosfamide q4h × 3

apy, and electrolyte levels should be monitored frequently.[113]

Amifostine, recently approved by the FDA, is an organic thiophosphate used to reduce the cumulative renal toxicity associated with repeated administration of cisplatin in patients with advanced ovarian or non–small cell lung cancer. Amifostine's ability to protect normal tissue without compromising tumor cell kill is attributed to the higher capillary alkaline phosphatase activity, higher pH, and better vascular bed of normal tissue as compared to cancer tissue. Other benefits seen with amifostine administration include (1) reduced occurrence of hypomagnesemia, (2) protected effect of the kidneys from nephrotoxic antibiotics, and (3) reduced cumulative nephrotoxicity associated with cisplatin.[115,116]

Amifostine is dephosphorylated at the tissue site by alkaline phosphatase to form free thiol. Within the cell, thiol neutralizes reactive components of cisplatin before damage occurs to the DNA and RNA of the normal cell. Thiol acts as a potent scavenger of oxygen-free radicals and superoxide anions. This phenomenon is important because free radicals can damage cell membranes, DNA, and other vital cell components.[115,116]

Amifostine 740 mg/m^2 or 910 mg/m^2 is administered to the patient over 5–15 minutes intravenously after the patient has been adequately hydrated with 1 liter of fluid. Fifteen minutes after the amifostine, cisplatin is administered. The most common side effect has been transient systolic hypotension; therefore, it is recommended that amifostine be administered with the patient in a supine position. The blood pressure is monitored every 5 minutes throughout the infusion and 5 minutes after the infusion. If the blood pressure drops below threshold from the baseline, the infusion is interrupted. The infusion can be restarted if the blood pressure returns to threshold within 5 minutes and if the patient is asymptomatic. If the blood pressure does not return to threshold, the infusion is discontinued and the next dose is reduced to 740 mg/m^2.[115]

Transient systolic hypotension is short term and reversible. It is treated with fluid administration and by placing the patient in the Trendelenburg position. Increased nausea and vomiting have occurred, which may be a potentiating effect with cisplatin. Antiemetics must be given prior to amifostine administration and continued with cisplatin. Other side effects that have been observed include flushing, feeling of warmth or coldness, chills, syncope, somnolence, hiccups, and sneezing.[116]

Another compound being studied in an attempt to minimize cisplatin-induced nephrotoxicity is silibinin. This compound is a flavonoid extracted from *Sylibum marianum* that has both antioxidant, anti-inflammatory, and RNA and protein synthesis stimulating properties. In studies with rats, silibinin prevented cisplatin-induced nephrotoxicity.[117] Selenium has been successful in reducing nephrotoxicity as well as bone marrow suppression in patients receiving cisplatin-based chemotherapy.[118]

Standard doses of methotrexate are not associated with renal toxicity unless the patient has preexisting renal dysfunction. High doses (>1 g/m^2) can cause an obstructive nephropathy from precipitation of methotrexate or its metabolites in the renal tubules. Risk factors associated with drug-induced nephrotoxicity include (1) low urine pH, (2) dehydration, (3) low methotrexate clearance, (4) decreased urine output, and (5) concurrent intrathecal treatment.[119] In general, urinary alkalization to maintain a urine pH greater than 7 with simultaneous administration of sodium bicarbonate or diamox prevents precipitate formation, permitting high-dose therapy.

Streptozocin in doses over 1.5 g/m^2 is associated with renal dysfunction in more than 65% of patients. Characteristically, streptozocin causes a tubulointerstitial nephritis and tubular atrophy due to direct damage of the tubules. This toxicity is manifested by hypokalemia, proteinuria, increased blood urea nitrogen (BUN), and increased creatinine levels.[113] Renal function tests and creatinine clearance tests should be obtained before beginning streptozocin therapy. Patients who develop an elevation of serum creatinine, even if it subsequently returns to normal, are cautioned against receiving further streptozocin, as severe toxicity may occur.

Lomustine and carmustine can cause a delayed renal failure months or years following therapy. Azotemia and proteinuria are manifested, followed by progressive renal failure, often requiring dialysis. It appears that the incidence of renal failure increases dramatically after a total dose of 1500 mg/m^2.[113]

Mitomycin C has been associated with a syndrome of renal failure and microangiopathic hemolytic anemia. This toxicity occurs in approximately 20% of patients who have received a cumulative dose of 100 mg or more after approximately 6 months of therapy and is characterized by an abrupt onset of microangiopathic hemolytic anemia, thrombocytopenia, azotemia, proteinuria, and hematuria. It is generally reversible.[113]

Nurses play a vital role in preventing nephrotoxicity. Preventive management includes aggressive hydration with hypertonic saline, diuresis, urinary alkalinization, and careful monitoring of urine output. Renal function tests, especially creatinine clearance, should be monitored before and after administering nephrotoxic drugs. Patients that must receive other nephrotoxic drugs, such as aminoglycosides or contrast dye, should be monitored closely for early signs and symptoms of toxicity. Assessment of renal function should continue throughout treatment and periodically after the completion of therapy (Table 20-11).

Conclusion

Advances in cancer therapy are made by continual investigations, evaluation of treatment results, and their incorporation into the practice of oncology. Because of the amount of time spent directly with the patient receiving chemotherapy, the nurse is often the health care provider

Table 20-11 Organ Toxicity of Chemotherapy Agents: Nephrotoxicity

Toxicity/ Symptoms	Grade	General Risk Factors	Chemotherapy Agent/Risk Factors	Mechanism of Damage	Protective/ Preventive Measures	General Management
• Increased BUN, creatinine • Oliguria • Azotemia • Proteinuria • Decreased creatinine clearance • Hyperuricemia • Hypomagnesemia • Hypocalcemia	Creatinine 0 = WNL 1 = <1.5 2 = 1.5–3.0 3 = 3.1–6.0 4 = >6.0 Proteinuria 0 = No change 1 = 1+ or <3 g/L 2 = 2–3+ or 3–10 g/L 3 = 4+ or >10 g/L 4 = Nephrotic syndrome Hematuria 0 = None 1 = Micro 2 = Gross, no clots 3 = Gross, with clots 4 = Requires transfusion BUN mg% 0 = WNL <20 1 = 21–30 2 = 31–50 3 = >50	• Age • Dose of agent • Preexisting disease of kidneys, renal insufficiency • Nutritional status • Duration of cancer therapy • Concurrent: —Aminoglycoside therapy —Amphotericin-B • Renal damage • Dehydration • Large tumor mass • Ileal conduits • Contrast dye • History of sodium-retaining states (e.g., cirrhosis, CHF, nephrosis) • K and Mg depletion	Nitrosoureas • Cumulative dose of 1200 mg/m^2 for carmustine and lomustine Mitomycin C • Increased effect with vincristine and VM-26 Anthracyclines • High dose (1.5 g/m^2/wk) Streptozocin • Dose (>1.5 g/m^2/wk) Cisplatin • Multiple doses (>50 mg/m^2) • High dose • Increased effect with cyclophosphamide Methotrexate • High dose (>1 g/m^2) • Enhanced effect with cisplatin	• Direct cell damage in glomerulus • Chronic interstitial nephritis • Tubular atrophy • Direct cell damage in glomerulus • Microangiopathic hemolytic anemia • Tubular atrophy • Diffuse tubulointerstitial nephritis • Tubulointerstitial nephritis • Tubular atrophy • Direct cell damage in tubules • Necrosis of proximal and distal renal tubules • Precipitation of metabolites in the acid environment of the urine • Obstructive nephropathy	These following four measures apply to all drugs • Monitor renal function tests • Saline diuresis • Hydrate patient (3000 mL/day) • Decrease uric acid production with allopurinol • Stop drug if creatinine does not return to baseline • Diuresis with mannitol • Administer amifostine 15 min before administration • Maintain alkalinization of urine pH >7 • Administer leucovorin • Administer bicarbonate • Avoid vitamin C Acids (ASA, vitamin C) compete for drug elimination sites, which increases serum concentration of methotrexate	• Substitute analogue drug • Reduce dose for creatinine clearance (normal 125 mL/min) 30–60 mL/min: Cisplatin, 50% Methotrexate, 50% Mitomycin, 75% Nitrosoureas, hold dose 10–30 mL/min Cisplatin, hold dose Mitomycin, 75% <10 mL/min Cyclophosphamide, 50% Mitomycin, 50% Avoid nephrotoxic drugs and contrast dye

Note: Pharmacokinetics of the following drugs suggest dose reduction when the patient has renal impairment:
fludarabine
carboplatin (increased thrombocytopenia with renal dysfunction)
ifosfamide (increased CNS toxicity)
melphalan IV

pentostatin (increased serious toxicity)
etoposide (increased bone marrow toxicity)
topotecan (increased neutropenia)
bleomycin (increased pulmonary toxicity)
dacarbazine
hydroxyurea (increased bone marrow toxicity)

best able to recognize subtle changes in the patient's status that could be indicative of pending complications from chemotherapy. Nursing responsibilities are multifaceted and include patient education, ongoing physical assessments, identification of risk factors, and prompt therapeutic interventions, with ongoing evaluation for modification.

Occurrence of side effects does not necessarily preclude withholding of chemotherapy but instead alerts nurses to the need for careful assessment, management, and evaluation. The nurse's assessment of a patient's response to treatment and assistance in preventing or managing side effects can make a difference in the patient's overall perceived quality of life. Once the treatment is complete, nurses can be instrumental in encouraging patients to have a yearly comprehensive physical examinations to detect cancer recurrence and long-term effects of chemotherapy.

References

1. Lowenthal RM, Eaton K: Toxicity of chemotherapy. *Hematol Oncol Clin North Am* 10:967–990, 1996

2. Yanick R, Ries LA: Cancer in the older persons. *Cancer* 74: 1995–2003, 1994

3. Yanick R, Havlik RJ, Wesley MN, et al: Cancer and comorbidity in the elderly patient: A descriptive profile. *Ann Epidemiol* 6:399–412, 1996

4. Kintzel PE, Dorr RT: Anticancer drug renal toxicity and elimination: Dosing guidelines for altered renal function. *Cancer Treat Rev* 21:23–64, 1995

5. Vose JM: Cytokine use in the older patient. *Semin Oncol* 22: 6–8, 1995 (suppl 1)

6. Lipschitz DA: Age-related declines in hematopoietic reserve capacity. *Semin Oncol* 22:3–5, 1995 (suppl 1)

7. Boyle DM: Realities to guide novel and necessary nursing care in geriatric oncology. *Cancer Nurs* 17:125–136, 1994

8. Cohen HJ: Biology of aging as related to cancer. *Cancer* 74:2092–2100, 1994

9. Leslie WT: Chemotherapy in older cancer patients. *Oncology* 6:74–80, 1992

10. Gomez H, Mas L, Casanova L: Elderly patients with aggressive non-Hodgkin's lymphoma treated with CHOP chemotherapy plus granulocyte-macrophage colony stimulating factor: Identification of two age subgroups with differing hematologic toxicity. *J Clin Oncol* 16:2352–2358, 1998

11. Cascinu S, Del Ferro E, Catalano G: Toxicity and therapeutic response to chemotherapy in patients aged 70 years or older with advanced cancer. *Am J Clin Oncol* 19:371–374, 1996

12. Thyss A, Saudes L, Otto J, et al: Renal tolerance of cisplatin in patients more than 80 years old. *J Clin Oncol* 12: 2121–2125, 1994

13. Carlson RW: Quality of life issues in the treatment of metastatic breast cancer. *Oncology* 12:27–31, 1998 (suppl 4)

14. Morrow GR, Stern RM, Pierce HI, et al: Initial control of chemotherapy-induced nausea and vomiting in patient's quality of life. *Oncology* 12:32–37, 1998 (suppl 4)

15. Cella DR: Quality of life: Concepts and definition. *J Pain Symptom Manage* 9:186–192, 1993.

16. Youngblood M, Williams PD, Eyles H, et al: A comparison of two methods of assessing cancer therapy-related symptoms. *Cancer Nurs* 17:37–44, 1994

17. Demetri GD, Kris M, Wade J, et al: Quality of life benefit in chemotherapy patients treated with epoetin alfa is independent of disease response or tumor type: Results from a prospective community oncology study. *J Clin Oncol* 16: 3412–3425, 1998

18. Trotti A: Toxicity antagonists in cancer therapy. *Curr Opin Oncol* 91:569–578, 1997

19. Schuchter LM: Current role of protective agents in cancer treatment. *Oncology* 11:505–518, 1997

20. Whelan RJ, Mohide EA, Willan AR, et al: The supportive care needs of newly diagnosed cancer patients attending a regional cancer center. *Cancer* 80:1518–1524, 1997

21. Grahn G, Danielson M: Coping with the cancer experience. II. Evaluating an education and support programme for cancer patients and their significant others. *Eur J Cancer Care* 5:182–187, 1996

22. Yarbro CH: Nursing implications in the administration of cancer chemotherapy, in Perry MC (ed): The *Chemotherapy Source Book*. Baltimore, Williams & Wilkins, 1996, pp 1029–1039

23. Hoagland HC, Gastineau DA: Hematologic complications of cancer chemotherapy, in Perry MC (ed): *The Chemotherapy Source Book*. Baltimore, Williams & Wilkins, 1996, pp 559–570

24. Glauser M: Empiric therapy of bacterial infections in patients with severe neutropenia. *Diagn Microbiol Infect Dis* 31:467–472, 1998

25. Rowinsky EK, Eisenhauer EA, Chaudhry V, et al: Clinical toxicities encountered with paclitaxel (Taxol). *Semin Oncol* 20:1–15, 1993 (suppl 3)

26. Pronk LC, Stoter G, Verweij J: Docetaxel (taxotere): Single agent activity, development of combination treatment and reducing side effects. *Cancer Treat Rev* 21:463–478, 1995

27. Guchelaar HJ, Richel DJ, van Knapen A: Clinical, toxicological and pharmacological aspects of gemcitabine. *Cancer Treat Rev* 22:15–31, 1996

28. Michael M, Moore M: Clinical experience with gemcitabine in pancreatic carcinoma. *Oncology* 11:1615–1621, 1997

29. Hudis CA, Seidman AD, Crown JPA, et al: Phase II and pharmacologic study of docetaxel, an initial chemotherapy for metastatic breast cancer. *J Clin Oncol* 14:58–65, 1996

30. Hohneker J: A summary of vinorelbine (Navelbine) safety data from North American clinical trials. *Semin Oncol* 21: 42–47, 1994 (suppl 10)

31. Toso C, Lindley C: Vinorelbine: A novel vinca alkaloid. *Am J Health-Syst Pharm* 52:1287–1304, 1995

32. Rowinsky EK, Kaufman SH: Topotecan in combination chemotherapy. *Semin Oncol* 24:S20–S26, 1997 (suppl 20)

33. Wiseman LR, Markham A: Irinotecan: A review of its pharmacological properties and clinical efficacy in the management of advance colorectal cancer. *Drugs* 54:606–623, 1996

34. Ludwig H, Fritz E: Anemia of cancer patients: Patient selection and patient stratification for epoetin treatment. *Semin Oncol* 25:35–38, 1998 (suppl 7)

35. Krantz SB: Pathogenesis and treatment of anemia of chronic disease. *Am J Med Sci* 307:353–359, 1994

36. Vose JM, Armitage JO: Clinical applications of hematopoietic growth factors. *J Clin Oncol* 13:1023–1035, 1995

37. Tsukuda M, Yuyama S, Kohno H: Effectiveness of weekly subcutaneous recombinant human erythropoietin administration for chemotherapy induced-anemia. *Biotherapy* 11: 21–25, 1998

38. Goldberg GL, Gibbon DG, Smith HO, et al: Clinical impact of chemotherapy-induced thrombocytopenia in patients with gynecologic cancer. *J Clin Oncol* 12:2317–2320, 1994

39. Issacs C, Nicholas JR, Bailey FA, et al: Randomized placebo-controlled study of recombinant human interleukin 11 to prevent chemotherapy-induced thrombocytopenia in patients with breast cancer receiving dose-intensive cyclophosphamide and doxorubicin. *J Clin Oncol* 15:3368–3377, 1997

40. Tepler I, Elias L, Smith JW: A randomized placebo-controlled trial of recombinant human interleukin 11 in cancer patients with severe thrombocytopenia due to chemotherapy. *Blood* 87:3607–3614, 1996

41. Rolston KV: Expanding the options for risk-based therapy

in febrile neutropenia. *Diagn Microbial Infect Dis* 31:411–416, 1998

42. Giamarellou H: Empiric therapy for infections in the febrile, neutropenic, compromised host. *Med Clin North Am* 79:559–580, 1995

43. Verhoef J: Prevention of infections in the neutropenic patient. *Clin Infect Dis* 17:559–567, 1993 (suppl 2)

44. Hughes WT, Armstrong D, Bodey GP, et al: 1997 guidelines for the use of antimicrobial agents in neutropenic patients with unexplained fever. *Clin Infect Dis* 25:551–573, 1997

45. Miller L, Ozer H, Anderson JR, et al: American Society of Oncology recommendations for the use of hematopoietic colony-stimulating factors: Evidence-based, clinical practice guidelines. *J Clin Oncol* 12:2471–2508, 1994

46. Maher DW, Lieschke GJ, Green M, et al: Filgrastim in patients with chemotherapy-induced febrile neutropenia: A double-blind, placebo-controlled trial. *Ann Intern Med* 121:492–501, 1994

47. Lissoni P, Tancini G, Barni S, et al: Treatment of cancer chemotherapy–induced toxicity with the pineal hormone melatonin. *Support Care Cancer* 5:126–129, 1997

48. Rodriguez-Adrian LJ, Grazziutti ML, Rex JH, Anaissis EJ: The potential role of cytokine therapy for fungal infections in patients with cancer: Is recovery from neutropenia all that is needed? *Clin Infect Dis* 26:1270–1278, 1998

49. Engelking C, Rutledge D, Ippoliti C, et al: Cancer related diarrhea: A neglected cause of cancer-related symptom distress. *Oncol Nurs Forum* 25:859–860, 1998

50. Hogan CM: The nurse's role in diarrhea management. *Oncol Nurs Forum* 25:879–886, 1998

51. Cascinu S: Drug therapy in diarrheal diseases in oncology/hematology patients. *Crit Rev Oncol Hematol* 18:37–50, 1995

52. Wadler S, Benson AB, Engelking C, et al: Recommended guidelines for the treatment of chemotherapy-induced diarrhea. *J Clin Oncol* 16:3169–3178, 1998

53. Ippoliti C: Antidiarrheal agents for the management of treatment-related diarrhea in cancer patients. *Am J Health-Syst Pharm* 55:1573–1580, 1998

54. Vickery G: Basics of constipation. *Gastroenterol Nurs* 20:125–128, 1997

55. Maule WF: Gastrointestinal toxicity of chemotherapeutic agents, in Perry MC (ed): *The Chemotherapy Source Book.* Baltimore, Williams & Wilkins, 1996, pp 697–707

56. Andrews PRL, Davis CJ: The physiology of emesis induced by anticancer therapy, in Reynolds DJM, Andrews PRL, Davis CJ (eds): *Serotonin and the Scientific Basis of AntiEmetic Therapy.* Philadelphia. Oxford Clinical Communications, 1995, pp 25–49

57. Osoba D, Zee B, Pater J, et al: Determinants of post chemotherapy nausea and vomiting in patients with cancer. *J Clin Oncol* 15:116–123, 1997

58. Rhodes VA: Criteria for assessment of nausea, vomiting, and retching. *Oncol Nurs Forum* 24:13–19, 1997 (suppl)

59. Malik IA, Khan WA, Qazilbash M: Clinical efficacy of lorazepam in prophylaxis of anticipatory, acute, and delayed nausea and vomiting induced by high doses of cisplatin. *Am J Clin Oncol* 18:170–175, 1995

60. Hesketh PJ, Kris MG, Grunberg SM, et al: Proposal for classifying the acute emetogenicity of cancer chemotherapy. *J Clin Oncol* 15:103–109, 1997

61. Goodman M: Risk factors and antiemetic management of chemotherapy induced nausea and vomiting. *Oncol Nurs Forum* 24:20–32, 1997 (suppl)

62. Wickham R: Nausea and vomiting, in Yarbro CH, Frogge

MH, Goodman M (eds): *Cancer Symptom Management* (ed 2). Sudbury, MA, Jones and Bartlett, 1999, pp 228–263

63. Roila F, Ballatori E, Tonato M, Del Favero A: 5-HT3 receptor antagonists: Differences and similarities. *Eur J Cancer* 13:1364–1370, 1997

64. Hesketh P, Navari R, Grate T, et al: Double-blind, randomized comparison of the antiemetic efficacy of intravenous dolasetron mesylate and intravenous ondansetron in prevention of acute cisplatin induced emesis in patients with cancer. *J Clin Oncol* 14:2242–2249, 1996

65. King CR: Nonpharmacologic management of chemotherapy induced nausea and vomiting. *Oncol Nurs Forum* 24:41–48, 1997 (suppl)

66. Symonds RP: Treatment-induced mucositis: An old problem with new remedies. *Br J Cancer* 77:1689–1695, 1998

67. Raybould TP, Ferretti GA: Oral care of the cancer patients in Macdonald JS, Haller DG, Mayer RJ (eds): *Manual of Oncologic Therapeutics.* Philadelphia, Lippincott, 1995, pp 456–466

68. Larson PJ, Miaskowski C, MacPhail L, et al: The PRO-SELF mouth aware program: An effective approach for reducing chemotherapy-induced mucositis. *Cancer Nurs* 21:263–268, 1998

69. Levien TL, Baker DE: Reviews of tramadol and tretinoin. *Hosp Pharm* 31:54–73, 1996

70. Chi KH, Chen SY, Chan VK, et al: Effect of granulocyte-macrophage colony stimulating factor (GM-CSF) on oral mucositis in head and neck patients after cisplatin, 5FU leucovorin chemotherapy. *Proc Am Soc of Clin Oncol* 13:428, 1994 (abstr 1469)

71. Hood A: Dermatologic toxicity, in Perry MC (ed): *The Chemotherapy Source Book.* Baltimore, Williams & Wilkins, 1996, pp 595–606

72. Gallagher J: Management of cutaneous symptoms. *Semin Oncol Nurs* 11:239–247, 1995

73. Rest EB, Horn TD: Dermatology, in Armitage JO, Antman KH (eds): *High Dose Cancer Therapy (ed 2).* Baltimore, Williams & Wilkins, 1995, pp 578–608

74. Armstrong T, Rust D, Kohtz JR: Neurological, pulmonary, and cutaneous toxicities of high dose chemotherapy. *Oncol Nurs Forum* 24:23–33, 1997 (suppl)

75. de Argila D, Dominguez JD, Iglesias L: Taxol-induced acral erythema. *Dermatology* 192: 377–378, 1996

76. Freedman TG: Social and cultural dimensions of hair loss in women treated for breast cancer. *Cancer Nurs* 17:334–331, 1994.

77. Pickard-Holly S: The symptom experience of alopecia. *Semin Oncol Nurs* 11:235–238, 1995

78. Camp-Sorrell D: Scalp hypothermia devices: Current status. *ONS News* 6:1,5, 1991.

79. Anderson MS, Johnson J: Restoration of body image and self-esteem for women after cancer treatment: A rehabilitative strategy. *Cancer Pract* 2:345–349, 1994

80. Borecky DJ, Stephenson JJ, Keeling JH, et al: Idarubicin-induced pigmentary changes of the nails. *Cutis* 59:203–204, 1997

81. Shan K, Lincoff AM, Young JB: Anthracycline-induced cardiotoxicity. *Ann Intern Med* 125:47–58, 1996

82. Ewer MS, Benjamin RS: Cardiotoxicity of chemotherapeutic drugs, in Perry MC (ed): *The Chemotherapy Source Book.* Baltimore, Williams & Wilkins, 1996, pp 649–663

83. Berchem GJ, Ries F, Hanfelt J, et al: Epirubicin cardiotoxicity: A study comparing low with high-dose-intensity weekly schedules. *Support Care Cancer* 4:308–312, 1996

84. Muggia FM: Clinical efficacy and prospects for use of pegylated liposomal doxorubicin in the treatment of ovarian and breast cancers. *Drugs* 54:22–29, 1997(suppl 4)

85. Kozluca O, Olcay E, Surucu S, et al: Prevention of doxorubicin induced cardiotoxicity by catechin. *Cancer Lett* 99: 1–6, 1996

86. Dobric S, Dragojevic-Simic V, Bokonjic D, et al: The efficacy of selenium, WR-2721, and their combination in the prevention of adriamycin-induced cardiotoxicity in rats. *J Environ Pathol Toxicol Oncol* 17:291–299, 1998

87. Bates M, Lieu D, Zagari M, et al: A pharmacoeconomic evaluation of the use of dexrazoxane in preventing anthracycline-induced cardiotoxicity in patients with stage IIIB or IV metastatic breast cancer. *Clin Ther* 19:167–184, 1997

88. Weidmann B, Teipel A, Niederie N: The syndrome of 5-fluorouracil cardiotoxicity: An elusive cardiopathy. *Cancer* 73: 2001–2002, 1994

89. Soe MS, Berkman A, Mardelli, J: Case report: Paclitaxel-induced myocardial ischemia. *Med J* 45:41–43, 1996

90. Herman EH, Lipshultz SE, Rifai N, et al: Use of cardiac troponin T levels as an indicator of doxorubicin-induced cardiotoxicity. *Cancer Res* 58:195–197, 1998

91. Deng MC, Kececioglu D, Weyand M, et al: Successful long-term course after heart transplantation for anthracycline cardiomyopathy in a young boy despite neurological complications. *Thorac Cardiovasc Surg* 42:122–124, 1994

92. MacDonald DR: Neurotoxicity of chemotherapeutic agents, in Perry MC (ed): *The Chemotherapy Source Book.* Baltimore, Williams & Wilkins, 1996, pp 745–765

93. Berger T, Malayeri R, Doppelbauer A: Neurological monitoring of neurotoxicity induced by paclitaxel/cisplatin chemotherapy. *Eur J Cancer* 33: 1393–1399, 1997

94. Cain JW, Bender CM: Ifosfamide-induced neurotoxicity: Associated symptoms and nursing implications. *Oncol Nurs Forum* 22:659–666, 1995

95. Fassas ABT, Gattani AM, Morgello S: Cerebral demyelination with 5-fluorouracil and levamisole. *Cancer Invest* 12: 379–383, 1994

96. Hilkens PHE, Verweij J, Stoter G, et al: Peripheral neurotoxicity induced by docetaxel. *Am Acad Neurol* 46:104–111, 1996

97. Kunitoh H, Saijo N, Furuse K, et al: Neuromuscular toxicities of paclitaxel 210 mg/m² by 3-hour infusion. *Br J Cancer* 77:1686–1688, 1998

98. Perry JR, Warner E: Transient encephalopathy after paclitaxel (Taxol) infusion. *Neurology* 46:1596–1599, 1996

99. Campana WM, Eskeland N, Calcutt NA, et al: Prosaptide prevents paclitaxel neurotoxicity. *Neurotoxicology* 19: 237–244, 1998

100. Koh DW, Castro M: Pulmonary toxicity of chemotherapy drugs, in Perry MC (ed): *The Chemotherapy Source Book.* Baltimore, Williams & Wilkins, 1996, pp 665–695

101. Chap L, Shpiner R, Levine M, et al: Pulmonary toxicity of high-dose chemotherapy for breast cancer: A non-invasive approach to diagnosis and treatment. *Bone Marrow Transplant* 20:1063–1067, 1997

102. Sleijfer S, van der Mark TW, Koops S, Mulder NH: Decrease in pulmonary function during bleomycin-containing combination chemotherapy for testicular cancer: Not only a bleomycin effect. *Br J Cancer* 71:120–123, 1995

103. Kalaycioglu M, Kavuru M, Tuason L, Bolwell B: Empiric prednisone therapy for pulmonary toxic reaction after high-dose chemotherapy containing carmustine (BCNU). *Chest* 107:482–487, 1995

104. Cannon GW: Methotrexate pulmonary toxicity. *Rheum Dis Clin North Am* 23:917–937, 1997

105. Pavlakis N, Bell DR, Millward MJ, Levi JA: Fatal pulmonary toxicity resulting from treatment with gemcitabine. *Cancer* 80:286–291, 1997

106. Santamauro JT, Stover DE, Jules-Elysee K, et al: Lung transplantation for chemotherapy-induced pulmonary fibrosis. *Chest* 105:310–312, 1994

107. King PD, Perry MC: Hepatotoxicity of chemotherapeutic agents, in Perry MC: *The Chemotherapy Source Book.* Baltimore, Williams & Wilkins, 1996, pp 709–726

108. West SG: Methotrexate hepatotoxicity. *Rheum Dis Clin North Am* 23:883–915, 1997

109. Moertel CG, Fleming TR, Macdonald JS, et al: Hepatic toxicity associated with fluorouracil plus levamisole adjuvant toxicity. *J Clin Oncol* 11:2386–2390, 1993

110. Markman M, Kennedy A, Webster K, et al: Continuous subcutaneous administration of mesna to prevent ifosfamide-induced hemorrhagic cystitis. *Semin Oncol* 23: 97–98, 1996 (suppl 6)

111. Grochow LB: Covalent DNA-binding drugs, in Perry MC (ed): *The Chemotherapy Source Book.* Philadelphia, Williams & Wilkins, 1996, pp 295–316

112. West NJ: Prevention and treatment of hemorrhagic cystitis. *Pharmacotherapy* 17:696–706, 1997

113. Patterson WP, Reams GP: Renal and electrolyte abnormalities due to chemotherapy, in Perry MC (ed): *The Chemotherapy Source Book.* Philadelphia, Williams & Wilkins, 1996, pp 727–744

114. Choudhury D, Ahmed Z: Drug-induced nephrotoxicity. *Med Clin North Am* 81:705–717, 1997

115. Viele CS, Holmes BC: Amifostine: Drug profile and nursing implications of the first pancytoprotectant. *Oncol Nurs Forum* 25:515–523, 1998

116. Alberts DS, Bleyer WA: Future development of amifostine in treatment. *Semin Oncol* 23:90–99, 1996 (suppl 8)

117. Gaedeke J, Fels LM, Bokemeyer C, et al: Cisplatin nephrotoxicity and protection by silibinin. *Nephrol Dial Transplant* 11:55–62, 1996

118. Hu YJ, Chen Y, Zhang YQ, et al: The protective role of selenium on the toxicity of cisplatin-contained chemotherapy regimen in cancer patients. *Biol Trace Elem Res* 56: 331–341, 1997

119. Relling MV, Fairclough D, Ayers D, et al: Patient characteristics associated with high-risk methotrexate concentrations and toxicity. *J Clin Oncol* 12:1667–1672, 1994

CHAPTER 21

Principles of Bone Marrow and Hematopoietic Cell Transplantation

Marie Bakitas Whedon, MS, ARNP, FAAN
Mary Roach, MS, RN, AOCN

Introduction

Bone marrow transplantation (BMT) is now all but an historical term given the significant changes in conceptualization and terminology used to describe a treatment originally designed to cure disorders of the hematopoietic system. Rarely is "bone marrow" tissue actually transplanted to repair the diseased or dysfunctional hematopoietic system of persons with malignant and nonmalignant diseases. Rather, advances in technology have allowed an apheresis process, similar to donating a unit of blood, to become the major method of acquiring or "harvesting" hematopoietic "seeds"—the pluripotential stem cells. These cells, acquired from a healthy related or unrelated volunteer donor or the patient, are used in a variety of ways to aid in the cure or control of disease.

This chapter describes historical developments that have led to the current treatment traditionally known as BMT. Advances in science have caused broadened treatment indications and the development of practice and treatment standards. The health care economic environment has also influenced current and likely future directions in transplantation. The chapter concludes with a discussion of financial and reimbursement trends that have resulted in changes in care such as the movement of transplantation to the outpatient clinic and home. The transplant procedure is described in Chapter 22, and Chapter 23 discusses the acute and long-term effects of transplantation and nursing care.

The ABCs of Bone Marrow Transplantation

For clarity and consistency, a brief discussion of transplant terminology is important. Bone marrow was the human material previously used for transplantation, hence the acronym BMT. The term *autologous* resulted in the acronym ABMT and was used when an individual served as his or her own source of marrow. Discovery of the presence of hematopoietic stem cells in peripheral circulation, similar to those harvested from the bone marrow, led to the nomenclature *peripheral blood stem cell* (PBSC). However, due to the lack of worldwide scientific agreement on a single terminology, regional differences in language complicate the plethora of labels and acronyms referring to similar treatments formerly known as BMT. Common terms include peripheral blood stem cell transplantation (PBSCT), blood cell transplantation (BCT), and high-dose therapy with stem cell "rescue." More recently the broad term hematopoietic cell transplantation (HCT) has gained acceptance.[1]

This confusing transplant terminology presents challenges to professionals and also to patients and families who are trying to comprehend the type of treatment they are to receive and the goals of treatment. Use of the word *transplant* itself has led to confusion. For instance, in *traditional* BMT, healthy bone marrow was removed from a donor (allogeneic) and given to a patient with a bone marrow disease (such as the marrow malignancy leukemia, or a marrow defect like aplastic anemia) to replace the defective organ. This particular situation was truly a *transplant*.

However, when a tissue-compatible healthy donor was not available, control of the disease was sometimes possible by removal of the person's own bone marrow (autologous). Autologous marrow was purged of malignant cells with agents like chemotherapy or biological response modifiers and returned to the patient. In this case, the intent was again to replace the diseased hematopoietic organ with a presumably healthier one,[2] yet autologous marrow was not really *transplanted* but rather reinfused.

Concurrent with the development of autologous marrow removal and reinfusion technology was the advent of high-dose or dose-intensive chemotherapy regimens to cure previously incurable cancers like neuroblastoma.[3] The term *rescue* was used to indicate how this new procedure prevented treatment-related, lethal hematopoietic complications such as irreversible bone marrow destruction, immunosuppression, and fatal sepsis. Autologous marrow rescue or support procedures signaled a new era in the field of transplantation for patients with both hematologic and solid tumors. Today, patients with incurable cancers can safely receive potentially curative doses of chemotherapy and radiation therapy, while sparing their marrow from destruction.[4]

Finally, the source of hematopoietic stem cells has evolved from being marrow-derived (BMT) to being obtained primarily by pheresis from peripheral circulation (PBSCT). Most procedures known as BMTs are neither bone marrow cells nor transplants. In fact, stem cells from healthy donors are more frequently obtained from peripheral blood rather than from the bone marrow of the donor's iliac crest.[5,6] For the remaining discussion, the terms *transplantation* and HCT will be used regardless of whether stem cells are obtained from marrow or peripheral blood and administered for replacement. The terms *rescue* or *support* will be used rather than transplant when referring to the enhancement of a normal hematopoietic system following high-dose therapy.

Historical Developments

The notion of using bone marrow to treat patients with blood disorders dates back to the late nineteenth century, with the first reports of bone marrow extract given by mouth to patients with anemia. Over the next 50 years, there were sporadic attempts to use bone marrow orally, intramuscularly, and intravenously to treat anemias and leukemias.[7] Figure 21-1 offers a timeline of developments in transplantation.

After World War II and detonation of the first nuclear bombs, interest in ameliorating the effects of radiation increased. In 1951, Jacobson et al observed that lethally

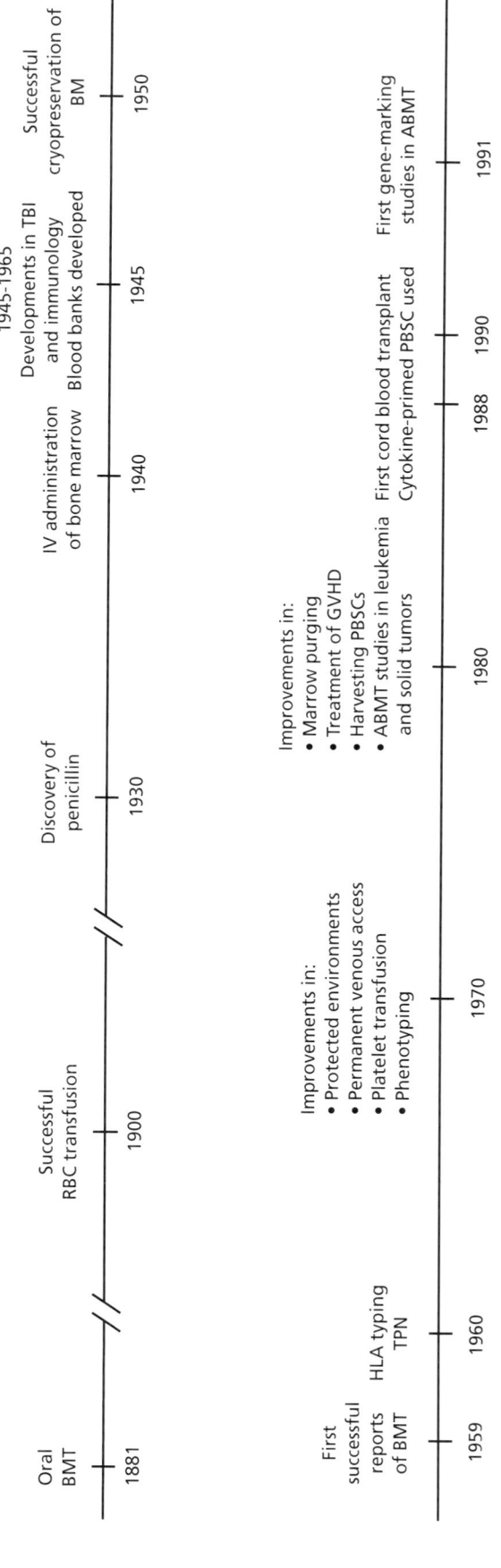

Figure 21-1   Time line to transplantation. (BMT = bone marrow transplant; RBC = red blood cell; IV = intravenous; TBI = total body irradiation; BM = bone marrow; HLA = human leukocyte antigen; TPN = total parenteral nutrition; GVHD = graft-vs-host disease; PBSC = peripheral blood stem cells; ABMT = autologous bone marrow transplantation)

irradiated mice could survive if given an intraperitoneal injection of cells from the spleen.[8] Further studies that same year demonstrated the same result with an infusion of intravenous bone marrow from the animal's twin,[9] confirming that the recovery of marrow function was a result of the colonization of the transplanted marrow cells.[7] Despite marrow recovery, death ensued due to severe diarrhea, weight loss, and skin lesions.[10] This was called *secondary disease,* now known to have been graft-versus-host disease (GVHD).[7]

Based on this experience with animals, patients with leukemia were given high doses of radiation to treat their leukemia and infused with healthy donor marrow in an attempt to cure them. In 1957, Thomas et al reported a successful human BMT and transient engraftment.[11] However, these early attempts at BMT were done without knowledge of tissue typing or GVHD and were disappointing. After initial enthusiasm, attempts at human transplantation were largely abandoned.

Still, animal—primarily canine—research continued and led to early understanding of the genetics of the histocompatibility system and development of immunosuppressive drugs to treat GVHD.[12] Understanding histocompatibility was crucial to success in transplantation. This knowledge led to human leukocyte antigen (HLA) typing that allowed selection of appropriate donors and reduction in the incidence of GVHD resulting from poorly matched transplants.[7] In 1963, the first BMT in a patient with leukemia with engraftment and survival for more than 1 year was reported.[13]

The modern era of transplantation is generally agreed to date from the late 1960s and early 1970s. Advances in supportive care including antibiotics, platelet collection and transfusion, and isolation techniques led to improved outcomes in transplant.[12] The Hickman catheter was developed to facilitate frequent and prolonged venous access.[14] Patients with aplastic anemia and leukemia were treated and cured with cyclophosphamide, with or without total body irradiation, and BMT.[12]

The subsequent two decades have seen major changes in the field of transplantation. The use of stem cell sources other than bone marrow has dramatically changed the way transplants are performed. The ability to cryopreserve peripherally derived stem cells, their ability to reconstitute the hematopoietic system, and data that supports the effectiveness of dose-intense chemotherapy in solid tumors have contributed to the increase in the use of autologous stem cell rescue.[3,15] Peripheral blood stem cells are also now being used in allogeneic transplants.[6,16] This allows for the collection of donor stem cells without an operative procedure and the concomitant risk of anesthesia. Umbilical cord blood, rich in stem cells, is now also being used as a stem cell source in transplant.[17–19]

The use of colony-stimulating factors (CSF) like granulocyte- and granulocyte-macrophage colony-stimulating factors (G-CSF and GM-CSF) to facilitate collection of hematopoietic cells and to shorten the period of myelosuppression following transplant has had a significant effect on the safety, cost, and numbers of transplants performed.[20,21] Research has led to the investigation of many different CSFs (stem cell factor, interleukin-3, megakaryocyte growth and development factor) that may improve mobilization and collection of stem cells. Ex vivo expansion to grow stem cell colonies may decrease the number of stem cell collections required, increase the number of mature post-progenitor cells thereby reducing the duration of myelosuppression following high-dose chemotherapy, and generate populations of specific cells (dendritic cells) that may be of use as adoptive immunotherapy after transplant.[22]

Major research issues concerning allogeneic transplant include improving conditioning regimens to reduce relapse rates from malignant disease, improving GVHD prevention and treatment, and improving prevention and treatment of infectious complications. With improvements in management of GVHD, which is a greater risk in unrelated donor transplant, the use of unrelated donors for allogeneic transplant has dramatically increased.[23,24]

Another area of active investigation is gene therapy. Much of the early work in developing gene therapy protocols was done using the hematopoietic stem cell.[25] In gene therapy, the HSC is removed and its cellular DNA is manipulated in one of several ways. Reinfusion of the altered stem cell serves as a vehicle to deliver normal human genes or gene products.[25] In 1990, the first approved gene therapy was administered to a young girl with severe combined immunodeficiency disease.[26] Gene therapy techniques have been used for cell tracking, to map the destination of tumor-infiltrating lymphocytes, and to assess the contribution of malignant cells in autologous stem cell products to relapse. Other studies have focused on transfecting bone marrow cells with drug-resistance genes to confer on them protection from high-dose chemotherapy.[27,28]

Changes in the financing of health care in the United States has also affected transplantation. Pressure to contain costs has contributed to the shift of portions of transplantation care to the outpatient and home setting with the attendant need to educate patients and caregivers.[29,30]

Types of Transplantation

Different types of HCT are described in terms of the hematopoietic stem cell source: an identical twin (syngeneic), a donor (allogeneic), or the person's own (autologous). For each donor type, the stem cell source can be marrow or peripheral blood. Figure 21-2 compares relative numbers of allogeneic and autologous transplants worldwide since 1970.[31] Umbilical cord blood is another potential stem cell source.

Syngeneic

A syngeneic donor is an identical twin of the recipient. They share identical genes and thus are a perfect HLA

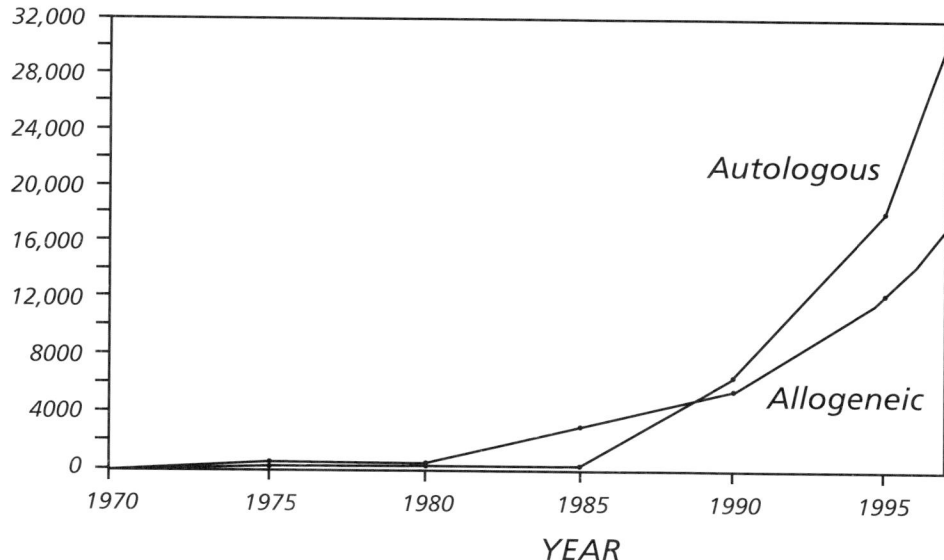

Figure 21-2 Annual number of transplants. (Reprinted with permission from Rizzo DJ: New summary slides show current trends in BMT. *ABMTR Newsletter* 5:4, 1998.[31])

match. Sharing identical tissue types avoids the development and complications of GVHD. However, the risk of relapse is greater in patients transplanted for leukemia because of the lack of the graft-versus-leukemia (GVL) effect.[32] Graft-versus-leukemia (described more fully later) is a reaction that occurs when the donor graft recognizes residual recipient leukemia cells as foreign and destroys them.

Allogeneic

Allogeneic transplant involves the removal of stem cells from a donor which are then infused into the person with the disease. Allogeneic BMTs were originally done for bone marrow failure (aplastic anemia) or malignancy (leukemia). Allogeneic donors can be related or unrelated to the recipient. Because complications are reduced, the closer the HLA match between donor and recipient the better; an identical HLA match is best. The genes encoding the HLA are inherited, so the patient's family members (usually the siblings) are typed to determine their HLA antigen profile and how closely their type matches that of the patient. HLA typing involves taking a blood sample to test for these antigens on the surface of the blood lymphocytes.

A related donor is preferred because the HLA system characterizes major histocompatibility antigens, but minor antigens also exist that are not yet identifiable. A relative has a greater chance than an unrelated donor to share these minor antigens, thus the ideal donor is an HLA-identical relative.[33] However, given the small average family size in the United States, an individual has only a 35% chance of having an HLA-matched sibling.[34] A partially matched sibling or other family member can also serve as a donor, depending on the degree and character of the match.[35]

If the patient does not have a suitable family donor, a search for an unrelated donor can be undertaken. The National Marrow Donor Program (NMDP), a donor registry developed in 1986, allows patients without a related donor to find an HLA-matched or partially matched unrelated donor. Four and one-half million people have been registered as potential unrelated donors worldwide.[36] Although morbidity and mortality are generally greater in unrelated donor transplants than in matched related transplants (largely due to GVHD), the number of these transplants is increasing[35,37] (Figure 21-3).[31] Because HLA type is linked to ethnic origin and minorities are underrepresented in transplant registries, a major goal of the NMDP is to evaluate HLA type in more members of ethnic minorities.[36]

The source of allogeneic stem cells, regardless of the donor, has historically been bone marrow. With the successful use of PBSCs in autologous transplant, the use of PBSCs in allogeneic transplant is being investigated.[5,6] Advantages with the use of PBSCs in allogeneic transplants include:

1. Shorter duration of myelosuppression, resulting in a decrease in transfusions, bacterial and fungal infections, and the use of antibiotics.
2. No increase in incidence of acute GVHD when compared to allogeneic bone marrow as a stem cell source.
3. Less donor morbidity when bone marrow harvest is not required.

Concerns about the use of PBSCs involve the lack of data on long-term outcomes and the risk of using CSFs to mobilize stem cells in donors.[5,6]

Autologous

When the stem cell donor is the patient, the transplant is termed *autologous*. Autologous stem cells, collected and

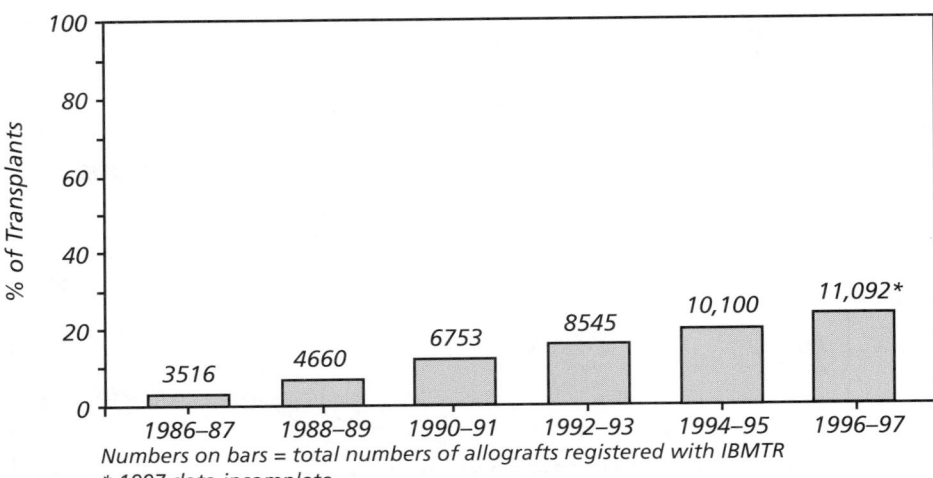

Figure 21-3 Percent of allogeneic transplants from unrelated donors. (IBMTR = International Bone Marrow Transplant Registry.) (Reprinted with permission from Rizzo DJ: New summary slides show current trends in BMT. *ABMTR Newsletter* 5:4, 1998.[31])

cryopreserved, are used as a rescue following dose-intensive chemotherapy, with or without radiation therapy, that would otherwise be lethal to the hematopoietic system. Early autologous transplants used harvested bone marrow from the patient. But as mentioned previously, in the early 1980s, it was found that stem cells also circulated in the peripheral blood, albeit in small numbers. The ability of PBSCs to restore hematopoeisis just as well as bone marrow–derived stem cells, caused this to become the major technique used.[15,24]

Peripheral blood stem cells have several advantages over bone marrow. First, general anesthesia, which is generally used for marrow harvest, is avoided. Second, cell collection is performed as an outpatient procedure. Third, more rapid hematologic engraftment occurs after PBSCs are infused than occurs with marrow infusion.[38] Chemotherapy and/or CSFs are used to increase the number of stem cells in the peripheral blood and reduce the number of phereses needed to collect an adequate number of stem cells.

Determining the number of stem cells needed to reliably reconstitute bone marrow function has been an active area of research. A number of techniques have been used. Cells with the CD34 antigen include committed hematopoeitic progenitor cells as well as pluripotent stem cells.[39] Many transplant centers now use the number of CD34+ cells present to determine adequate colonies available to reconstitute hematopoiesis. Studies have shown that infusion of $\geq 5 \times 10^6$ CD34+ cells/kilogram reduces the time to platelet and neutrophil recovery.[40,41]

Umbilical Cord Blood

The presence of hematopoietic stem cells in umbilical cord blood was first reported in 1974.[42] Cord blood was first proposed as a possible stem cell source for transplant in the 1980s.[43] Now umbilical cord blood is used as a stem cell source for for both related and unrelated donor transplants.

Cord blood represents a stem cell source that is abundant, correlated with lower infectious disease and tumor contamination risk, and associated with less GVHD.[44] Disadvantages to the use of cord blood is that the stem cell numbers may not be sufficient to restore hematopoiesis in adults. Furthermore, though the incidence of acute GVHD with cord blood appears no higher than with other stem cell sources, the incidence of chronic GVHD is unknown.[44,45]

Most cord blood transplants to date have been done in children. There is some evidence that lower numbers of mononuclear cells in cord blood are needed to restore marrow function as opposed to bone marrow–derived stem cells.[46] The *ex vivo* expansion and cryopreservation of cord blood stem cells are also being explored in view of their use in adults.[17]

Umbilical cord blood has the possibility of greatly increasing the pool of donors for unrelated transplants as well as increasing minority representation in donor registries.[45] Already, public cord blood banks exist in New York, Milan, and Dusseldorf, and more are being created worldwide. Several private, commercial cord blood banks have also been developed for autologous and related cord blood storage.[19]

The National Heart, Lung, and Blood Institute is sponsoring a clinical trial to address some of the unanswered clinical questions regarding cord blood transplant. The goal is to collect HLA type, infectious disease information, and cryopreserve 15,000 units of cord blood to be used for transplant in malignant and nonmalignant diseases under one protocol in order to define basic safety and efficacy questions of cord blood transplant.[47]

Transplantation Indications and Outcomes

Original indications for transplant were aplastic anemia or leukemias that were treated with syngeneic or allogeneic BMT. These diseases and acquired hematologic disorders are still treated with transplantation, but the indications for transplant have grown significantly over the last two decades. Figure 21-4 shows a comparison of allogeneic and autologous transplants for different diseases performed in 1997.[31] Other indications for allogeneic transplantation include nonmalignant inherited diseases such as immunodeficiency disorders, sickle cell disease, storage diseases, thalassemia, and Fanconi's anemia. Under investigation is treatment of some congenital disorders while the fetus is still in utero.

Most transplants are autologous and performed to treat a variety of solid tumors, primarily breast cancer.[4,24,38,48] Researchers are also investigating the role of autologous transplant in autoimmune disorders.[24,49] Important considerations in determining the role of transplantation for specific patients are prognostic factors for that individual's disease, the timing of transplant in the disease course, and consideration of the patient's risk factors for transplant. The National Comprehensive Cancer Network (NCCN) has a special panel to determine how BMT fits into practice guidelines for all types of cancers.[50] Table 21-1 presents malignant and nonmalignant diseases treated with transplantation.[16]

Hematologic Malignancies

Leukemias continue to be the most frequent diagnosis treated with allogeneic transplant.[24,51] Bone marrow transplant is the only potentially curative therapy for patients with acute myelogenous leukemia (AML) who fail induction therapy. About a third of patients who relapse and then attain a second complete remission can be cured with BMT. These outcomes are superior to those achieved without transplant.[34] The best outcomes for allogeneic transplant are achieved in first complete remission; however, it is unclear if this is superior to initial chemotherapy followed by transplant in the case of relapse.[52] Compared

to allogeneic transplant, autologous transplant results in a higher relapse rate but lower treatment-associated mortality. Allogeneic transplant appears to have an advantage over autologous transplant in first remission for individuals with high-risk disease; results are comparable for allogeneic and autologous transplant in second remission.[34,36]

Acute lymphocytic leukemia (ALL) is the most common childhood leukemia. Allogeneic transplant is indicated in second remission and in first remission for children with poor prognostic features.[53,54] In adults, the indications are similar to those in children: Bone marrow transplant remains the most effective therapy following initial relapse and is generally recommended for adults with high-risk disease (Philadelphia chromosome positive).[34,55] Autologous transplant is used in ALL for older patients and for those lacking a suitable donor, but relapse rates are much higher than with allogeneic transplant.[55]

Allogeneic bone marrow transplant is the only curative therapy for chronic myelogenous leukemia (CML).[56] Patients transplanted in the early chronic phase within 1 year of diagnosis have the best outcome. Transplantation in later stages of CML (accelerated and blast phase) are associated with worse outcomes. Autologous transplant for CML, although not curative, may be associated with longer survival than conventional chemotherapy.[57]

The use of transplantation in chronic lymphocytic leukemia (CLL) is relatively new. Because it is largely a disease of older adults and often has an indolent course, conservative therapy has been the traditional approach. However, with a decrease in the morbidity and mortality of transplant and the development of new drugs with activity in CLL, transplantation is being increasingly considered.[58] Autologous and allogeneic transplants for CLL in younger patients are being evaluated.[59-61]

Patients with relapsed or resistant intermediate- and high-grade non-Hodgkin's lymphoma and relapsed Hodgkin's disease are candidates for transplantation. Patients whose tumors remain sensitive to chemotherapy

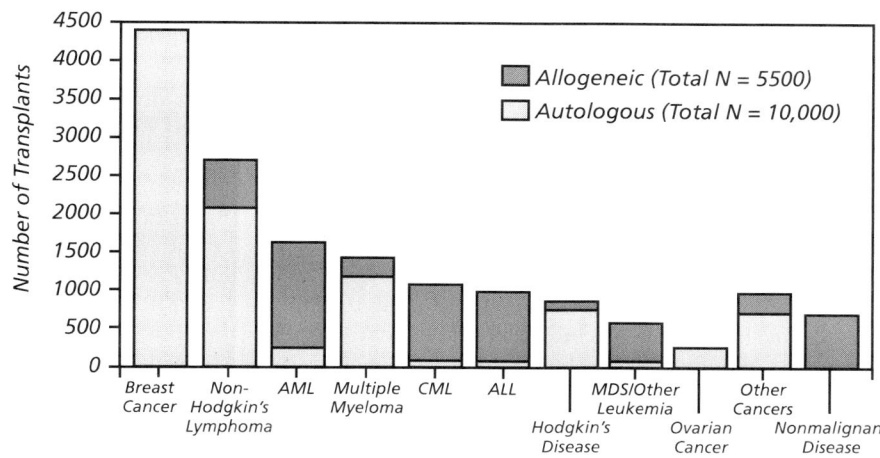

Figure 21-4 Indications for blood and marrow transplantation in North America, 1997. (AML = acute myelogenous leukemia; CML = chronic myelogenous leukemia; ALL = acute lymphocytic leukemia; MDS = myelodysplastic syndrome.) (Reprinted with permission from Rizzo DJ: New summary slides show current trends in BMT. *ABMTR Newsletter* 5:4, 1998.[31])

Table 21-1 Diseases Treated with Transplantation

Malignant Diseases	Nonmalignant Diseases
Hematologic malignancies	Hematologic disorders
Acute lymphocytic leukemia	Severe aplastic anemia
Acute myelogenous leukemia	Diamond-Blackfan anemia
Chronic lymphocytic leukemia	Fanconi's anemia
Chronic myelogenous leukemia	Sickle cell anemia
Myelodysplastic syndrome	Beta thalassemia major
Monosomy 7 syndrome	Chédiak-Hagashi syndrome
Non-Hodgkin's lymphoma	Chronic granulomatous disease
Hodgkin's lymphoma	Congenital neutropenia
Multiple myeloma	Reticular dysgenesis
Solid tumors	Congenital immunodeficiencies
Neuroblastoma	Severe combined immunodeficiency (SCID)
Brain tumor	Wiskott-Aldrich syndrome
Testicular germ cell tumors	Functional T-cell deficiency
Breast cancer	Mucopolysaccharidoses
Lung cancer	Hurler's disease
Ovarian cancer	Hunter's disease
Melanoma	Sanfilippo syndrome
Glioma	Morquio syndrome
Sarcoma	Lipidoses
Other solid tumors	Adrenoleukodystrophy
	Methachromatic leukodystrophy
	Gaucher disease
	Miscellaneous
	Osteopetrosis
	Langerhan cell histiocytosis
	Lesch-Nylan syndrome
	Glycogen storage diseases

and are treated with high-dose chemotherapy and stem cell rescue have a 40%–60% chance of 5-year disease-free survival.[36,62] Low-grade lymphoma, like CLL, is often a slowly progressive disease and has been managed conservatively in the past. There is some evidence that autologous transplant may prolong disease-free survival as compared with standard chemotherapy; allogeneic transplant is also being evaluated.[63]

Myelodysplastic syndrome (MDS) and myeloproliferative disorders represent a variety of clonal hematopoietic diseases.[64,65] Allogeneic transplant is the only curative therapy available for myelodysplasia but is usually reserved for patients under age 55 with excess blasts or complex cytogenetic abnormalities.[65] Autologous transplant for MDS is also under investigation.[64] Allogeneic transplantation is an option for myeloproliferative disorders, primarily agnogenic myeloid metaplasia (myelofibrosis), and essential thrombocytopenia and polycythemia vera unresponsive to conventional therapy.

Transplantation is being increasingly used to treat multiple myeloma, a disease incurable with standard chemotherapy. Allogeneic transplant is curative for some patients with advanced myeloma.[66] However, this approach has a relatively high treatment-related mortality and is generally reserved for younger patients. Results of a randomized trial comparing high-dose chemotherapy and autologous transplant to conventional chemotherapy in myeloma demonstrated that high-dose therapy significantly improves disease-free and overall survival.[67]

Solid Tumors

One of the major changes in the field of transplantation over the last decade has been the increase in the use of high-dose chemotherapy (HDC) and autologous stem cell rescue to treat solid tumors, especially breast cancer.[68] The concept of dose-response underlies this therapy. In animal models, doubling the chemotherapy dose increases tumor cell kill by tenfold or more.[68] High doses of alkylating agents are also known to overcome some tumor cell drug resistance. However, myelosuppression is the dose-limiting toxicity of most chemotherapy drugs, especially alkylating agents. These high doses of chemotherapy (conditioning therapy) can be delivered if marrow function is "rescued" by infusion of stem cells collected prior to HDC.

In solid tumors, HDC and stem cell rescue can be effective if three conditions are met: (1) the tumor is sensitive to standard-dose chemotherapy; (2) there is a dose-response effect in the tumor type treated; and (3) myelosuppression is the dose-limiting toxicity of the conditioning therapy.[2–4] A number of solid tumors meet these criteria and HDC is under investigation in their treatment.

The first trials of HDC for breast cancer were conducted in the early 1980s in women with refractory metastatic disease. Although HDC yielded a higher complete response rate, survival was not improved.[4,68] The introduction of "induction" chemotherapy prior to HDC and rescue reduced tumor burden in women with newly diagnosed metastatic disease. Although more complete remissions resulted from this approach, the majority of patients continued to relapse. The best outcomes occurred in women who achieved a complete remission with induction therapy prior to transplantation. Studies using this apppproach demonstrated 20%–30% disease-free survival at 3 years.[69]

Prospective, randomized trials are needed to define effectiveness of HDC and rescue in metastatic breast cancer. One randomized study of 90 women with newly diagnosed breast cancer reported improved response rate, response duration, and overall survival with HDC and autologous stem cell rescue.[70] Another single-institution, randomized study reported greater disease-free survival in patients with metastatic breast cancer treated with HDC and stem cell support.[71] Data from the largest randomized trial of HDC and stem cell rescue in chemotherapy-sensitive metastatic disease (184 evaluable patients) showed no difference in overall survival and no difference in time to disease progression.[72] A smaller randomized study (61 patients) of women with chemotherapy-sensitive metastatic breast cancer also showed no difference in progression-free or overall survival between HDC and stem cell rescue and standard dose chemotherapy.[73] Further follow-up is needed to clarify the role of HDC in metastatic breast cancer.

Although randomized trials are needed to define the role of HDC in breast cancer, enrollment in these trials has been difficult. Many women (and some professionals) have believed that more intensive therapy improves the chance for cure and are unwilling to be randomized to the standard-dose arm. The conflicting results obtained in the metastatic breast cancer trials highlight the critical need for new approaches to be evaluated by clinical research before broad application outside of clinical studies.

Given the initially encouraging outcomes in metastatic breast cancer, this approach was extended to women with high-risk (node positive) locally advanced breast cancer. Preliminary results from the randomized, multicenter trial comparing HDC to conventional dose chemotherapy in women with more than ten positive nodes at diagnosis showed no difference in overall survival, though there were fewer relapses in the HDC arm.[74] Two other studies evaluating HDC and stem cell rescue in high-risk breast cancer showed conflicting results. A large randomized Scandinavian study showed no overall benefit to HDC, while a smaller South African study showed fewer relapses and lower mortality in the HDC arm.[75,76] Another trial is evaluating HDC in women with four to nine positive nodes. Novel investigations of biotherapy combined with HDC/rescue for breast cancer are also under way.[77]

Other solid tumors are being treated with HDC and autologous stem cell support. Ovarian cancer exhibits chemotherapy sensitivity and responds to dose intensity. The majority of patients with germ cell tumors are cured with conventional dose chemotherapy. Transplantation is an option with superior outcomes over salvage chemotherapy in some patients who relapse following first-line chemotherapy.[78] Clinical trials are ongoing to establish the role of HDC in this disease.[79,80] High-dose chemotherapy has also been used in brain tumors. It is more successful in chemosensitive tumors, but phase III trials have yet to be done to evaluate the response and survival impact in selected tumor subtypes.[81] Other solid tumors that have been treated with HDC include neuroblastoma, malignant melanoma, and small-cell lung cancer.

Nonmalignant Diseases

A variety of congenital and acquired nonmalignant diseases are treated with allogeneic transplantation. Most transplants for these indications are done in children.[53] In adults, aplastic anemia is the most common nonmalignant disease treated with BMT.

Current Investigations/Future Applications

Research is ongoing in all diseases treated with transplantation, particularly to define ways to improve out-comes. Some methods being investigated include purging methods in autologous transplant, improved conditioning regimens to prevent relapse in malignant diseases, better prevention and treatment of GVHD and infections during transplant, CD34+ cell selection and ex vivo expansion, and the incorporation of research in gene therapy into transplantation.[24]

In addition, new indications for transplantation are also being explored. Transplantation is a novel approach in some incurable nonmalignant diseases such as sickle cell anemia, inborn errors of metabolism, and autoimmune disorders. The latter resulted because patients transplanted for hematologic malignancies who had preexisting autoimmune diseases sometimes experienced a remission of their autoimmune disorder.[82,83] The mechanisms responsible for this response are not clear, but clinical trials examining the feasibility of allogeneic and autologous transplant for severe, life-threatening autoimmune diseases (e.g., rheumatoid arthritis) are being designed.[83–85]

Outcomes

Cure

In the best of all possible worlds the transplant recipient survives the procedure and is cured of his or her disease. In an increasing number of diseases, this is the case. Transplantation is known to be curative in several malignant and nonmalignant disorders. Reductions in treatment-associated mortality have helped to make this possible. Astute nursing care is one factor that can prevent deaths due to treatment complications. Other factors influencing the mortality rate include type and stage of disease at time of transplant, type of transplant (allogeneic vs. autologous), degree of HLA match of donor in allogeneic transplant, age of patient, and experience of the transplant center. Overall, allogeneic transplant has a higher transplant-related mortality risk (about 20%–30%) than autologous transplant. The autologous transplant-related mortality is under 5% at most centers.[24] Table 21-2 lists the estimated 5-year disease-free survival of various diseases following transplantation.

Even when cured of their original disease, survivors can have disabilities following transplant. (Acute and long-term complications are described in detail in Chapter 23.) Long-term complications that can have the greatest impact on the quality of survival include chronic GVHD (allogeneic), continued immune dysfunction resulting in infections (especially from chronic GVHD), pulmonary complications from conditioning therapy, reproductive effects, effects on sexual functioning, thyroid dysfunction, and the development of cataracts. In pediatric patients, there may be adverse effects on growth and development and learning difficulties in school.[86] The long-term sequelae of autologous transplant are generally less given the absence of GVHD and the avoidance, in

Table 21-2   Estimated 5-year Disease-Free Survival (DFS) Following Transplantation

Disease	Stage	5-yr DFS Allogeneic	5-yr DFS Autologous
AML	1st CR	45–70%	35–45%
AML	2nd CR	20–45%	15–40%
ALL	1st CR	45–60%	30–60%
ALL	2nd CR	20–40%	15–40%
MDS	Combined	20–45%	ND
CML	Chronic	60–75%	50%
CML	Accelerated	30–45%	25%
CML	Blast crisis	10–20%	
NHL	1st relapse, 2nd CR	30–50%	45–60%
HD	1st relapse, 2nd CR	10–30%	40–60%
MM	Combined	30–50%	30%
CLL		20–55%	ND
Breast cancer	Stage IV	ND	15–30%
Breast cancer	Stage III	ND	55%
Breast cancer	Stage II	ND	70%
Germ cell	Recurrent	ND	15–20%
Brain tumors		ND	13%

ALL = acute lymphocytic leukemia; AML = acute myelogenous leukemia; CLL = chronic lymphocytic leukemia; CML = chronic myelogenous leukemia; CR = complete remission; HD = Hodgkin's disease; MDS = myelodysplastic syndrome; MM = multiple myeloma; ND = no data; NHL = non-Hodgkin's lymphoma.

most conditioning regimens, of the use of total body irradiation.

However, allogeneic and autologous transplant share some potential long-term effects including the risk of cognitive effects and second malignancies. Several studies have demonstrated cognitive deficits prior to transplant in some patients and impairment of cognitive functioning during transplant hospitalization.[87] Clinically, patients report difficulty with memory and concentration following transplant. Clearly, more study is needed in this area to delineate the effect of intensive therapy on cognitive functioning.

Secondary malignancies following treatment with chemotherapy and radiation are another potential consequence of transplantation.[88] Lymphoproliferative disorders, solid tumors, leukemia, and myelodsyplastic syndrome have all been reported after transplantation. The incidence of solid tumors in one analysis was 6.7% at 15 years after transplantation.[88] For hematologic malignancies, estimated incidence ranged from 4%–18% in 1254 patients following autologous transplantation.[86]

Causes are thought to be multifactorial, including conditioning chemotherapy and radiation, immunosupression, Epstein-Barr virus infection, and GVHD. Transplant patients should be evaluated for the development of secondary malignancies as an integral part of their preventive health care.

Relapse

Relapse of disease following transplant remains a major problem hindering the success of this procedure. Reasons for relapse depend on the stage of disease at transplant and differ between autologous and allogeneic transplants. In general, the later the transplant is performed in the course of a disease, the worse the outcome. Patients with leukemia who receive transplants during relapse have worse outcomes than those who receive transplants during remission. In solid tumors, patients with a minimal tumor burden at time of transplant fare better than those with more disease.

In allogeneic transplant, relapse results from inadequate conditioning therapy that fails to eradicate the cancer. The absence of a sufficient GVL effect may also play a role in relapse. For example, syngeneic transplants for leukemia have higher relapse rates than allogeneic transplants likely due to a lack of a GVL effect.

Relapse following allogeneic transplant is very difficult for patients and families because this is often the only hope for curing their disease. However, other possibilities are developing. Second transplants have been performed for relapsed disease, though the risk of complications is high. Taking advantage of the GVL effect in patients with CML, infusion of donor mononuclear cells can induce a complete remission in the majority of patients with less toxicity than a second transplant.[89] Withdrawal of immunosuppression in order to trigger GVL is another option in treating relapsed leukemias after allogeneic transplant. Still, there is a risk of significant GVHD.[90]

In autologous transplant, the failure of HDC to eradicate the tumor (inherent disease resistance) and acquired drug resistance are factors related to relapse. Further autologous transplant lacks the benefit of the GVL effect. It is usually not possible to determine if relapse resulted from insufficient tumor chemosensitivity or a developed drug resistance.[91] Some transplant protocols are now incorporating strategies to overcome drug resistance. Promising posttransplant immunotherapy strategies to reduce disease relapse include the use of cytokines and interleukins (IL-2, IL-12, interferon), ex vivo activated cellular immunotherapy, immunomodulating agents such as cyclosporine and thalidomide, and monoclonal and bispecific antibodies.[92] Tumor contamination of autologous stem cell product is also a known contributor to relapse. Attempts to purge stems cells of malignant cells continue to be investigated. After HDC, second transplant is an option in selected patients, especially those who experience an extended disease-free interval after treatment.

Hematopoietic and Immunologic Concepts of Transplantation

The hematopoietic system and normal immunology are described in Chapters 3 and 31. Major concepts related to transplantation are reviewed here.

Normal Hematopoiesis and Peripheral Blood Stem Cells

The bone marrow contains a supply of all blood cells from the earliest pluripotential stem cell to mature fully functional red, white, and megakaryocytic blood cells (Figure 21-5). Although only about 5% of marrow cells are pluripotential stem cells, this amount is capable of dividing and differentiating (under the influence of various cytokines) into all lines of mature blood cells. Hence, an ongoing, lifetime supply of blood cells necessary to support life is readily available. It is this principle that has enabled stem cell transplantation and reconstitution of hematopoiesis into a recipient devoid of hematopoietic cells.[39,93–95] Similarly, removal of an adequate number of pluripotential stem cells from a patient that can then be reinfused following lethal doses of chemotherapy and radiation therapy allows the person to survive.[40,41]

Blood cells express certain antigens (referred to as cell differentiation or cluster designation antigens, or CD followed by a number) at different stages of maturation.[93] These antigenic markers provide a useful label for identifying cells of interest. Hematopoietic cells that express (are positive for) the CD34 antigen are called CD34+ (positive). These are the cells of greatest interest in transplantation. This early cell is present at 10–100 times greater frequency in the bone marrow than in the peripheral blood. Moreover, the ability to identify it, increase its numbers, and separate it from other cells in the circulation allows it to be obtained for transplantation using only minimally invasive harvesting techniques as compared to traditional bone marrow harvesting.[39,93,94]

In addition to the hematopoietic stem cells, the marrow microenvironment must be intact for homing and reconstitution of hematopoiesis to occur. Both the "seed" and the "soil" are important aspects of normal recovery. It is truly remarkable that both marrow and peripherally derived stem cells, after infusion, can locate their place in the bone marrow.[95] Destruction of marrow architecture by treatment (e.g., radiation) or disease can interfere with resuming normal hematopoiesis following stem cell infusion.

Hematopoietic Stem Cells: Mobilization/Priming

Hematopoietic stem cells have receptors on their cell walls for various cytokine growth factors. These growth factors, which are made endogenously or their commer-cially available counterparts, which are made through recombinant DNA processes, stimulate pluripotential stem cells to differentiate and mature. These products are administered in transplantation and cause the body to overproduce pluripotential stem cells beyond the body's required needs and induce cell differentiation and maturation. Within 2 days of administration of hematopoietic growth factors (HGFs), the number of HSCs increases.[96] The administration of HGFs takes place right before pheresis so that more cells are available to be collected from the circulation. This process is referred to as *mobilization*. *Priming*, a related process also resulting from HGF infusion, stimulates the cells to move toward maturity, so once infused (or in the case of autologous transplant reinfused) nearly mature, functionally active cells are readily available to protect the body from foreign invaders.[93]

Administration of chemotherapy, usually cyclophosphamide, is another method to mobilize stem cells. Following the marrow suppressive effects of chemotherapy, the body responds (within 2 days) with a rebound stem cell production. Physicians take advantage of this normal body response to raise the number of circulating stem cells available for collection. Sometimes HGFs and chemotherapy are used in combination to mobilize stem cells. Mobilization reduces the number of phereses needed to collect adequate cells to reconstitute hematopoiesis. The primed cells reduce the period of immunosuppression. Mobilization and priming have improved transplantation by making the collection procedure more efficient and the recovery period quicker and safer for the patient.[20–22]

Recombinant Hematopoietic Growth Factors

Hematopoietic growth factors used for mobilization include stem cell factor, IL-3, G-CSF, and GM-CSF alone or in combination. Collection of peripheral blood progenitor stem cells has been shown to (1) increase the yield of mononuclear cells expressing the CD34 antigen (e.g., CD34+ cells) and other committed progenitor cells collected during pheresis, and (2) hasten the hematopoietic recovery of the recipient.[20] Hastened recovery of neutrophils and platelets in mobilized cells versus steady-state peripheral stem cells or bone marrow is likely due to the maturational effect of the cytokines on the progenitors. Cytokine-induced maturational effects on some of the early progenitors decrease the normal lag time of cell maturation after infusion. The clinical significance of using cytokine-mobilized PBSCs is a decreased length of time of the patient's nadir (lowest point of blood counts following chemotherapy), which reduces complications of infection and bleeding.[20]

Expansion of Stem Cells

Another technique to obtain cells needed for transplantation or rescue is known as *stem cell expansion*. In this case, a select number of CD34+ cells are collected, and in vitro

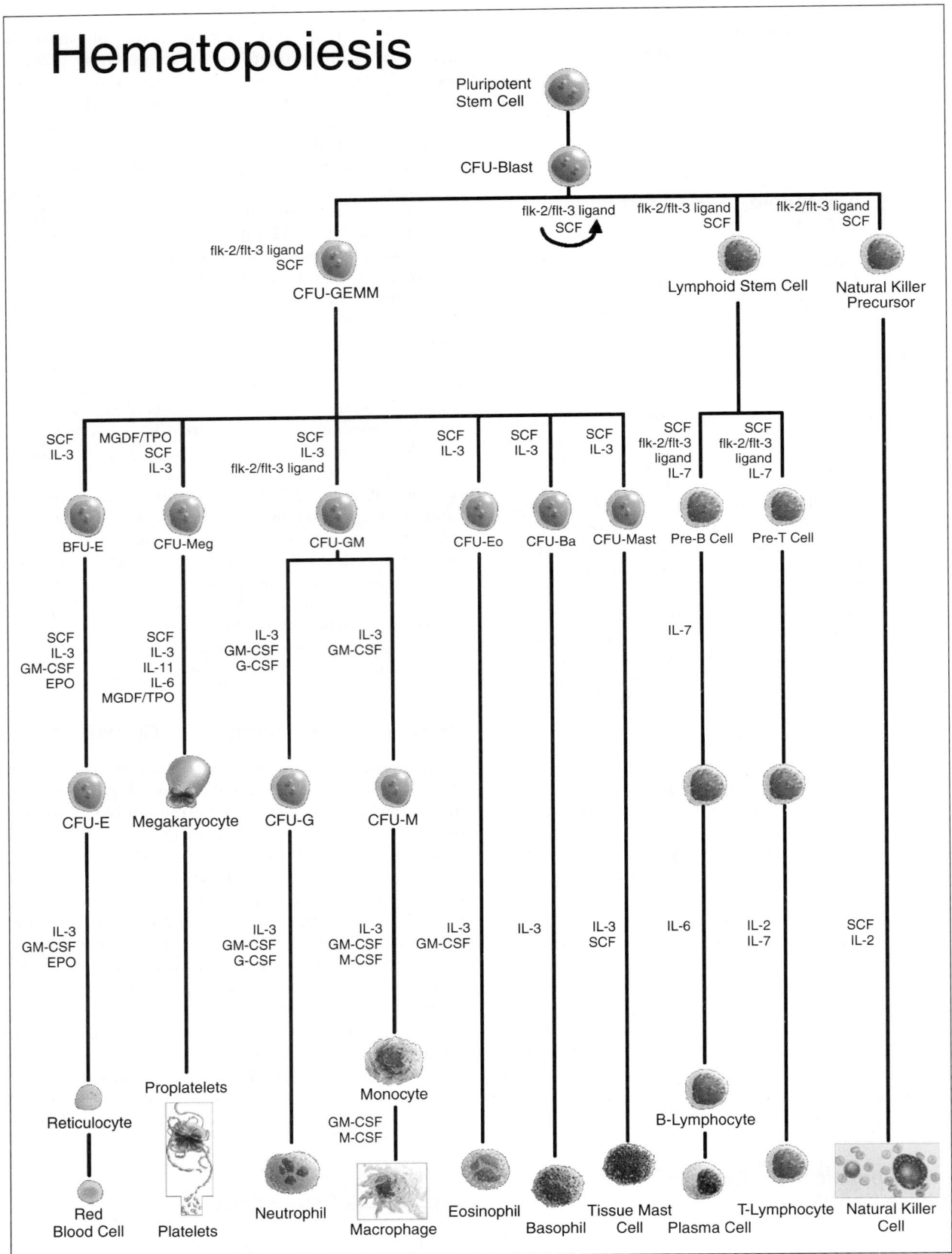

Figure 21-5   Hematopoietic tree. (Reprinted with permission from Amgen, Inc., Thousand Oaks, CA)

a cytokine "soup" is added (Figure 21-6). In appropriate culture medium the cells multiply, making it possible to expand the few collected cells to a number of cells capable of replacing the adult hematopoietic system.[94,96]

Purging

A concern of collection of HSCs from either marrow or circulation is the inability to assure that only nonmalignant normal cells will be collected.[36] This is of particular concern when harvesting cells from a person with a hematopoietic malignancy such as leukemia. However, it is also possible to harvest malignant cells metastatic to the bone in solid tumors, even if the patient has undetectable disease. A variety of techniques have been developed to attempt to eradicate these cells from the harvested product. Physical, chemical, and immunological methods are used to destroy or eliminate malignant cells, although it is unclear whether these methods are successful or reduce relapse of disease.[36]

Human Leukocyte Antigen

Blood-forming cells, like other human tissue, possess inherited characteristics (antigens) on their cell wall. Like a fingerprint, these antigens are unique to the individual from whom they are derived.[97] Also, just like the inherited characteristics of hair color or height, the HLA-6 antigen code on chromosome 6 (also known as the major histocompatibility complex [MHC]) is a result of a set of genes derived from each parent. Stem cells possess three classes of HLAs. Most important to transplantation are the A, B, and C genes on the class I region, and the D gene (broken down into three subtypes, DR, DP, DQ) on the class II region. Class I molecules are found on all nucleated cells of the body, and class II molecules are located primarily on immune cells such as lymphocytes and macrophages.[97] The most important function of these molecules is to present peptides to the immunological T cells so that body cells may be recognized as self.[97]

Determining compatibility between the patient and a donor is essential to the success of an allogeneic transplant. Serological, cellular, and molecular methods are used to test for compatibility between the HLA type of the donor and the recipient. Complications of HLA incompatibility can be life-threatening and include GVHD and rejection.

In the case of allogeneic transplantation, it is generally the immunocompetent donor graft that, after infusion into the immunoincompetent host, recognizes the host as "foreign." This results in an acute and chronic form of GVHD. The development of GVHD is the greatest predictor of outcome in allogeneic transplantation. (Prevention, clinical consequences, and treatment of GVHD are discussed in detail in Chapter 23.)

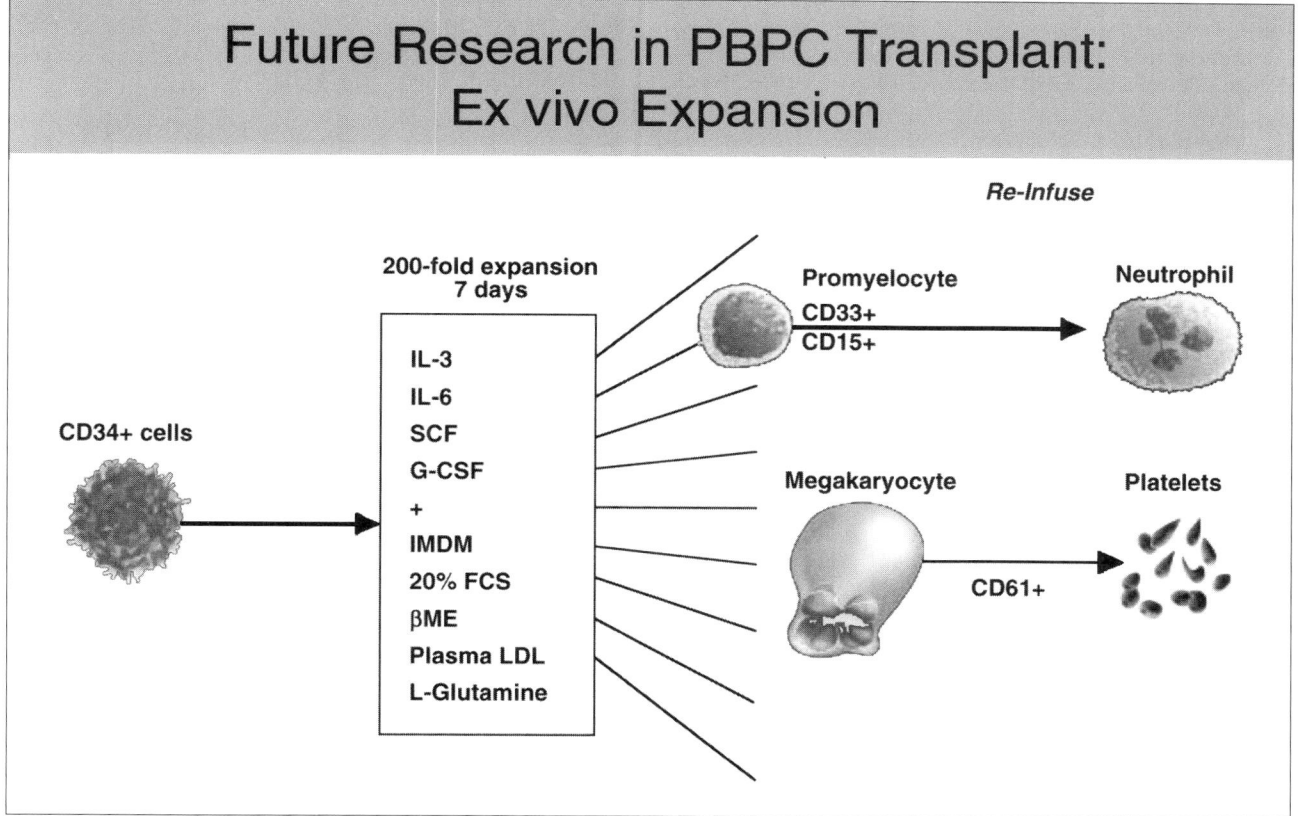

Figure 21-6   Stem cell expansion. (Reprinted with permission from Amgen, Inc., Thousand Oaks, CA)

Identification of an HLA-compatible donor is a necessary first step in allogeneic transplantation. An identical twin is the most compatible donor for transplantation, as the HLA type is also identical. The next step is to look within the recipient's immediate family. There is an approximately 25% chance of a person having an HLA match within their immediate family, as illustrated in Figure 21-7.[97] Lacking an acceptable match within the family, a search for a phenotypically compatible match from a volunteer donor registry (e.g., NMDP) is sought. A sample of the recipient's blood is HLA-typed and matched by computer (NMDP search software is called Search Tracking and Registry [STAR]) against the HLA types of volunteer donors from the registry. From receipt of a request for a report of potential donors, it takes approximately 24 hours for the report to be produced and sent to the requesting physician. If an acceptable match is found, the transplant may proceed. However, if a six antigen match is not found, less compatible but acceptable matches may be identified. In such cases, the recipient may be referred to a specialized center that performs mismatched unrelated transplants. Specialized centers are used because physiologic consequences of transplanting mismatched stem cells can result in significant acute side effects that require the management of a team specialized in these complications.

Prophylaxis and Treatment of Graft-versus-Host Disease

The better the compatibility between donor and recipient, the lower the incidence and severity of GVHD.[97]

Methods used to offset this serious complication include prophylaxis and treatment with immunosuppressive agents and T-cell depletion of the donor stem cell product.

Immunosuppression

Immunosuppressive medications like cyclosporine, methotrexate, and steroids are commonly used to prevent or treat GVHD. Immunosuppressives blunt the reaction of the newly developed donor immune system and keep it from identifying the host or patient as foreign. Immunosuppressive drugs may need to be taken for months to years following an allogeneic transplant. Although patients experience side effects like frequent colds and susceptibility to infection, they avoid or minimize the more harmful complications of GVHD.[12]

T-cell depletion

Under normal immunologic conditions, T cells play a major role in recognition of self from nonself proteins. In the case of allogeneic transplantion, active donor T cells within the stem cell graft have this same capability. As a result, donor T cells may recognize the recipient tissues as foreign, initiating a GVHD reaction. To avoid or lessen this serious consequence, several methods have been attempted to deplete the donor product of T cells, including physical, immunological, and pharmacological techniques. Regardless of technique, the desired outcome is reduction or elimination of T cells capable of initiating life-threatening GVHD.

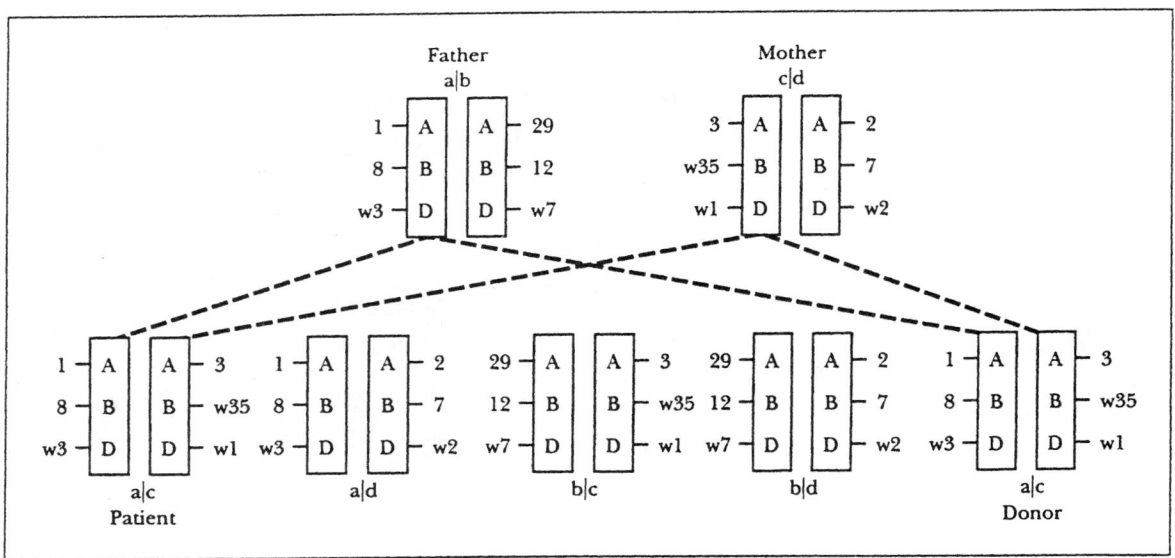

Figure 21-7 Diagram of possible combinations of human leukocyte antigen (HLA) region of chromosome-6 inherited by offspring from parents. The recipient and donor have inherited the same two haplotypes and are genotypically HLA identical.

Graft-versus-Leukemia Effect

The donor marrow, in addition to causing the complication of GVHD, can also exert a beneficial effect against the malignancy. The immunocompetent donor cells can recognize the patient's malignant cells as foreign and eliminate them. This effect was originally identified in leukemia patients and was termed GVL. It was observed that relapses were noted much less often in patients with GVHD than in patients who did not have this complication. Furthermore, syngeneic or autologous transplants lacking GVHD were noted to have higher relapse rates not only in leukemia but in other disease types.[32]

ABO Mismatch

Occasionally, a recipient may receive a HCT from a donor who possesses a different ABO blood type. Effective removal of red blood cells from the stem cell product has enabled successful transplantation in this case. After transplantation, the recipient will have the donor ABO blood type.

Standards for Transplantation

The unprecedented growth of transplant programs outside of established, academic centers in the late 1980s and 1990s raised many questions about the quality of care being provided.[98,99] In response to this concern, the Foundation for the Accreditation of Hematopoietic Cell Therapy (FAHCT) was formed in 1996, and Standards for Hematopoietic Progenitor Cell Collection, Processing, and Transplantation were published.[100] FAHCT standards were developed from and based on work of the Regulatory Affairs Committee of the International Society for Hematotherapy and Graft Engineering (ISHAGE) and a subcommittee of the Clinical Affairs Committee of the American Society of Blood and Marrow Transplantation (ASBMT). In order to be considered for accreditation, a program must perform at least ten transplants of each type during the year prior to which accreditation is being requested. Therefore, a program seeking accreditation for both autologous and allogeneic transplantation must perform ten procedures of each type. This mimimum requirement is consistent with earlier standards from the American Society of Hematology/American Society of Clinical Oncology[101] and the American Society for Blood and Marrow Transplantation,[102] following International Bone Marrow Transplant Registry (IBMTR) findings of higher treatment-related mortality and treatment failure in programs performing five or fewer transplants per year.[103]

Although FAHCT standards deal primarily with the medical and laboratory practices of transplantation, standards for nurses are also addressed and include the following major points:

- Nurses and nurse supervisors should be formally trained and experienced in the management of patients receiving hematopoietic progenitor cell transplants.

- Training should include hematology/oncology patient care, administration of high-dose therapy and growth factors, managment of infectious complications associated with compromised host defense mechanisms, administration of blood components, and an appropriate degree of intensive medical/pediatric nursing care.[100]

Transplant nursing standards have come from a variety of sources.[104–106] Within the Oncology Nursing Society (ONS), a special interest group (SIG) comprised solely of nurses with an interest in caring for patients undergoing transplant and rescue procedures exists and has proposed educational and practice standards for the field.[104] Annually, the ONS/BMT SIG also publishes a directory of HCT programs that includes contact information and other program information to assist nurses in networking on clinical and administrative issues.[105] Similar organizations exist for transplant nurses in Canada and Europe (the European Bone Marrow Transplant [EBMT] group).

International and interdisciplinary collaboration and networking has assisted in defining standards for specialized education of nurses and quantifying appropriate nursing staff ratios to care for these patients.[98] Standards have been especially helpful in guiding programs under development to identify appropriate nursing care practice and educational requirements. Program standards for ratios or categories of personnel are less well described, specifically for outpatient programs.

The complexity and specialization of transplant care within and across many different health care settings has given rise to multiple nursing roles within the field.[99,106–108] Transplant nursing coordinators and case managers are nurses who have specialized knowledge about patient evaluation, eligibility, and advocacy. Nurses in these roles assist patients to obtain appropriate testing, education, and insurance eligibility prior to the procedure.[99] Following transplant, these same nurses maintain contact with patients to guide them through the postprocedure adaptation and continued medical follow-up phase.

A variety of nursing roles have become integral to the continuum of HCT care. Changes in medical staffing and education have led to the incorporation of the nurse practitioner role as vital to the care of patients during the acute-care phase of transplantation. A handbook of care practices has helped to define the scope of practice for nurse practioners interested in the high-intensity care required by these patients.[108] Community and home-care nurses also provide increasing amounts of specialized care, requiring in-depth HCT knowledge about issues formerly in the domain of the inpatient nurse.[106,107]

National Marrow Donor Program

Prior to 1986, allogeneic transplant candidates lacking an HLA-matched relative either did not receive a transplant or were forced to independently canvas the world in search of a donor.[97] In July 1986, the U.S. Congress passed legislation creating a central registry of volunteers willing to donate marrow. The contract awarded to the NMDP created a registry that harnessed and regulated a national network of transplant, donor, and collection centers that work together to serve patients in need. As of January 1998, more than 3 million donors were listed and more than 7000 unrelated transplants had been facilitated by the center.[23]

International Bone Marrow Transplant Registry

Since the development of BMT, thousands of procedures have been performed by hundreds of programs worldwide for many different diseases. Despite this, few programs treat a large enough volume of patients to determine overall procedure efficacy. The IBMTR formed in 1970, the Autologous Bone Marrow Transplant Registry (ABMTR) formed in 1990, and the European Bone Marrow Transplant (EBMT) group are three international organizations studying and developing a scientific evidence base for the transplant procedure.[24,85,98] These groups maintain databases of procedures performed and their outcomes from a large percentage of transplant programs. For example, the IBMTR database includes information on about 40% of all allogeneic transplants done between 1970 and 1994.

Collaborating clinical treatment centers regularly and voluntarily report standardized information to these central agencies about the types of transplants performed, aspects of the process, and outcomes of the procedures. The growth of the database of autologous and hematopoietic procedures has been captured by the ABMTR to which 160 centers contribute data, summarizing about 50% of the autotransplants done between 1989 and 1994.[98] Updates of this data can be viewed on the IBMTR Web site (see Table 21-4). The pooled data are regularly analyzed and shared through a variety of peer-reviewed mechanisms (journal articles, newsletters, Web sites, scientific slides, and presentations) to inform the scientific and lay communities about state-of-the-art care and promising trends in the procedure.[31]

Contemporary Issues and Future Directions

Financial/Reimbursement Issues

Transplantation has achieved distinction within and outside of the oncology community as much for its financial controversies as its scientific discoveries. Reasons for this include the following:

- It is a costly, widely used procedure that lacks clear efficacy in some diseases.
- Insurance denials have generated high publicity court cases of patients suing for insurance coverage.
- HCT programs were perceived to be high-profit centers, which led to exponential growth of programs.[109]
- Provision of an unprecedented level of high-intensity care in outpatient clinics and at home in order to decrease the economic burden.[110]

Whether the outcomes of these financial trends are considered positive or negative likely depends on one's perspective whether patient, provider, or payer.[111]

Costs of a transplant procedure range from $50,000–$100,000, depending on the type, complexity, and institutional charging structure.[111] Lengthy hospital stays in high-tech environments, extensive use of high-cost pharmaceuticals, and stem cell acquisition and processing procedures account for much of the costs. In the early days, HCT procedures were done at a limited number of well-established academic centers. Public fundraisers, research dollars, and fee-for-service insurances covered the procedure costs.[112] Once the promise of cure in previously incurable solid tumors spread throughout the medical and lay community (particularly in breast cancer), a chain of events was set into motion that has greatly influenced many areas of modern health care.[113–115] One of the most significant changes in HCT was the financial impetus (rather than an evidence-based initiative) for shifting high-tech care to the outpatient environment.

Simultaneously, the growth of capitated and managed care plans has affected the financial concerns and issues of HCT. These plans employ "gatekeepers" who may create barriers for eligible patients to receive this treatment. It is estimated that between 1990 and the beginning of the twenty-first century, the outpatient cancer market will far surpass inpatient oncology reimbursements. Outpatient reimbursements are expected to grow from $85 billion to $290 billion per year.[110] Outpatient transplant procedures account for a significant portion of this care. A percentage of the rising costs results from the volume of procedures that can be performed outside the confines of the previously limited specialized inpatient isolation environments.[114–116] The good news is that at lower costs per procedure, more eligible patients might be able to receive this treatment. It is likely that each outpatient procedure costs insurers less than when performed in the inpatient environment. Unaccounted are the costs of care that have simply been shifted to unpaid at-home family caregivers and the out-of-pocket costs for services that were previously covered (e.g., some medications, home care, etc.).

Not all scientific advances have increased HCT costs. For instance, Pajeau et al report a cost savings when mobilized PBSC were used as compared with marrow because of faster immune recovery, decreased hospitalization, and lower pharmacy costs.[117] Other efficiencies have been gained by consolidating all HCT services into a single team of staff and location of care.[111] It is unclear how these scientific and economic, health care forces will interact to shape the future of transplantation.

Outpatient and Home Care Issues

Several variations on traditional inpatient care have evolved for pediatric marrow transplantation,[118] patients receiving allogeneic PBSCTs,[117] and adults undergoing HCT.[119] Patient evaluation and immunosuppressive therapies were the first interventions to be regularly performed outside of the inpatient setting. Chemotherapy and severe neutropenia are now being managed by a combination of outpatient nurses, homecare nurses, and family or other caregivers. Additionally, most acute symptoms are being managed in the clinic and in the home. Positive patient outcomes from decreased isolation of confined environments include improved quality of life for patients without apparent increased morbidity or mortality.[113,114,116,120] Additional information about outpatient transplant options and models of care are summarized in Table 21-3. (See also Chapter 22.)

Web Sites

The Internet contains a vast amount of information for patients and professionals regarding transplantation. Due to the lack of regulation on the Internet, nurses should explore patient on-line support groups or "chat rooms" before recommending them to patients. However, a few on-line resources and support groups are well established and provide appreciated connections for patients who may feel isolated when separated from the treatment center. The *Blood and Marrow Transplant Newsletter*, a quarterly paper version of an on-line site, is produced by BMT survivor Susan Stewart. (Obtain by writing or calling: Blood & Marrow Transplant Newsletter, 2900 Skokie Valley Road, Highland Park, IL 60035; phone: 847-433-3313, toll-free: 1-888-597-7674; fax: 847-433-4599.) Created in 1994 under the name BMT Newsletter, with the cooperation of HCT medical and nursing professional volunteer writers and reviewers, it was one of the first comprehesive sources of information about the procedure for patients. This resource is a mainstay of HCT patient education. A listing of helpful Web sites is included in Table 21-4.

Table 21-3 Models of Blood Cell Transplant (BCT) Care

Type	Description
Traditional BCT	Outpatient pretransplant evaluation, central catheter placement, apheresis, mobilization, cryopreservation Inpatient administration for dose-intensive chemotherapy/irradiation through supportive care and hematopoietic recovery Outpatient care until stabilized engraftment, with subsequent return to referring physician
Early-discharge BCT	Outpatient pretransplant evaluation, central catheter placement, apheresis, mobilization, cryopreservation Inpatient dose-intensive chemotherapy/irradiation Outpatient supportive care during hematopoietic recovery, and stabilized engraftment with subsequent return to referring physician Inpatient admission per institutional protocol
Outpatient BCT	Outpatient pretransplant evaluation, central catheter placement, apheresis, mobilization, cryopreservation Outpatient dose-intensive chemotherapy/irradiation, outpatient supportive care during hematopoietic recovery, and stabilized engraftment with subsequent return to referring physician Inpatient admission per institutional protocol

Reprinted with permission from Bedell MK, Mroz WT: The bone marrow and blood stem cell transplant marketplace, in Whedon MB, Wujcik D (eds): *Marrow and Blood Stem Cell Transplantation: Principles, Practice and Nursing Insights* (ed 2). Sudbury, MA, Jones and Bartlett, 1997, pp 459–473[112]

Table 21-4 Web Sites Containing Transplant Information

International Bone Marrow Transplant Registry
http://www.ibmtr.org
Provides scientific information to professionals on the state of the science of autologous and allogeneic HCT

National Marrow Donor Program
http://www.marrow.org
www.bmtinfo.org
Provides information about becoming a marrow donor or searching for an unrelated marrow donor

Blood and Marrow Transplant Newsletter
http://www.bmtnews.org
Provides access to the electronic newsletter and other publications in addition to HCT news items, a patient-survivor link service, and an attorney referral service regarding insurance reimbursement difficulties

BMT-Talk
http://www.ai.mit.edu/people/laurel/Bmttalk/bmt-talk.html
Home page for the mailing list BMT-Talk that hosts communications between more than 200 HCT patients and survivors

BMT Resource NetMarks
http://www.uokhsc.edu/sections/hemaonco/bmtmark.htm
A directory of HCT-related information on the Internet

National BMT Link
http://comnet.org/nbmtlink
Connects HCT patients with survivors who can provide psychosocial support

Conclusion

Since the earliest days of transplantation, nurses have been on the forefront contributing to the art and science of patient care and research. Many scientific advances have led to a redesign of how care is provided. Nurses have provided the leadership and clinical expertise to ensure that patients and their families experience appropriate and safe levels of service. As the future creates challenges in all aspects of health care, many of the lessons from transplant science (e.g., immunology, genetics) to economics (e.g., centers of excellence, high-tech outpatient care) will continue to guide the fields of oncology and oncology nursing.

References

1. Thomas ED, Forman SJ, Blume KG (eds): *Hematopoietic Cell Transplantation* (ed 2). Malden, MA, Blackwell Science, 1999

2. Whedon MB, Damianos F: Nursing care issues in patients undergoing autologous bone marrow transplantation. *Oncology* 7:78–92, 1993

3. Wingard JR: Bone marrow to blood stem cells: Past, present, future in, Whedon MB, Wujcik D (eds): *Marrow and Blood Stem Cell Transplantation: Principles, Practice and Nursing Insights* (ed 2). Sudbury, MA, Jones and Bartlett, 1997, pp 3–24

4. Peters WP, Ross M, Vredenburgh JJ, et al: High-dose chemotherapy and autologous bone marrow support as consolidation after standard-dose adjuvant therapy for high-risk primary breast cancer. *J Clin Oncol* 11:1132–1143, 1993

5. Goldman JM: Peripheral blood stem cells for allografting. *Blood* 85:1413–1416, 1995.

6. Wagner ND, Quinones VW: Allogeneic peripheral blood stem cell transplantation: Clinical overview and nursing implications. *Oncol Nurs Forum* 25:1049–1055, 1998

7. Santos GW: Historical background, in Atkinson K (ed): *Clinical Bone Marrow Transplantation*. Cambridge, Cambridge University Press, 1994, pp 1–9

8. Jacobson LO, Simmons EL, Marks EK, et al: Recovery from radiation injury. *Science* 113:510–511, 1951

9. Lorenz E, Uphoff DE, Reid, TR, et al: Modification of acute irradiation injury in mice and guinea pigs by bone marrow injection. *Radiology* 58:863–877, 1951

10. Cohen JA, Vos O, Van Bekkum DW: The present status of radiation protection by chemical and biological agents in mammals, in de Hevesy GC, Forssberg AG, Abbott JD (eds): *Advances in Radiology*. Edinburgh, Oliver and Boyd, 1957, pp 134–144

11. Thomas ED, Lochte HL Jr, Lu WC, et al: Intravenous infusion of bone marrow in patients receiving radiation and chemotherapy. *N Engl J Med* 257:491–496, 1957

12. Thomas ED, Storb R: The development of the scientific foundation of hematopoietic cell transplantation based on animal and human studies, in Thomas ED, Forman SJ, Blume KG (eds): *Hematopoietic Cell Transplantation* (ed 2). Malden, MA, Blackwell Science Inc, 1999, pp 1–11

13. Mathé G, Amiel JL, Schwarzenberg L, et al: Hematopoietic chimera in man after allogeneic (homologous) bone marrow transplantation. *Br Med J* 2:1633–1635, 1963

14. Hickman RO, Buckner CD, Clift RA: A modified right atrial catheter for access to the venous system in marrow transplant recipients. *Surg Gynecol Obstet* 148:871–875, 1979

15. Kessinger A: Reestablishing hematopoiesis after dose-intensive therapy with peripheral stem cells, in Armitage JO, Antman K (eds): *High-Dose Cancer Therapy*. Baltimore, Williams & Wilkins, 1992, pp 182–194

16. O'Connell SA, Schmit-Pokorny K: Blood and marrow stem cell transplantation: Indications, procedure, process, in, Whedon MB, Wujcik D (eds). *Marrow and Blood Stem Cell Transplantation: Principles, Practice and Nursing Insights* (ed 2) Sudbury, MA, Jones and Bartlett, 1997, 66–99

17. Almici C, Carlo-Stella C, Wagner JE, et al: Clonogenic capacity and *ex vivo* expansion potential of umbilical cord blood progenitor cells are not impaired by cryopreservation. *Bone Marrow Transplant* 19:1079–1084, 1997

18. Davison DB: Bone marrow, peripheral blood stem cell, and umbilical cord blood procurement, in Shapiro TW, Davison DB, Rust DM (eds): *A Clinical Guide to Stem Cell and Bone Marrow Transplantation*. Sudbury, MA: Jones and Bartlett, 1997, pp 113–124

19. Fisher CA, McGrath MB, Cannon ME: Related and autologous cord blood banking, in Broxmeyer HE (ed): *Cellular Characteristics of Cord Blood and Cord Blood Transplantation*. Bethesda MD, AABB Press, 1998, pp 199–216

20. Chao NJ, Schriber JR, Grimes K, et al: Granulocyte colony-stimulating factor "mobilized" peripheral blood progenitor cells accelerate granulocyte and platelet recovery after high-dose chemotherapy. *Blood* 81:2031–2035, 1993

21. Schmitz N, Linch DC, Dreger P, et al: Randomized trial of filgrastim-mobilised blood progenitor cell transplantation versus autologous bone-marrow transplantation in lymphoma patients. *Lancet* 347:353–357, 1996

22. Kanz L, Brugger WL: Mobilization and ex vivo manipulation of peripheral blood progenitor cells for support of high-dose cancer therapy, in Thomas ED, Blume SJ, Forman SJ (eds): *Hematopoietic Cell Transplantation* (ed 2). Malden, MA, Blackwell Science, 1999, pp 455–468

23. Bishop MR: Bone marrow transplantation from unrelated donors. *ASCO Education Book*, American Society of Clinical Oncology, Alexandria, VA, spring: 88–92, 1998

24. Horowitz MM: Uses and growth of hematopoeitic cell transplantion, in Thomas ED, Blume SJ, Forman SJ (eds): *Hematopoietic Cell Transplantation* (ed 2). Malden, MA, Blackwell Science, 1999, pp 12–18

25. Keating A, Leslie K: Gene therapy and bone marrow transplantation, in Atkinson K (ed): *Clinical Bone Marrow Transplantation*. Cambridge, Cambridge University Press, 1994, pp 715–724

26. Blaese RM: The ADA human gene therapy clinical protocol. *Hum Gene Ther* 1:327–362, 1990

27. Banerjee D, Shao S, Li H, et al: Gene therapy utilizing drug resistance gene: A review. *Stem Cells* 12:378–385, 1994

28. Zhang W, Fang X: Gene therapy strategies for cancer. *Expert Opin Invest Drugs* 4:487–514, 1995

29. Buchsel PC, Kapustay PM: Models of ambulatory care for blood cell and bone marrow transplantation, in Whedon MB, Wujcik D (eds): *Marrow and Blood Stem Cell Transplantation: Principles, Practice and Nursing Insights* (ed 2). Sudbury, MA, Jones & Bartlett, 1997, pp 525–561

30. Kelley CH, McBride LH, Randolph SR, et al: *Home Care Management of the Blood Cell Transplant Patient* (ed 3). Sudbury MA, Jones and Bartlett, 1998

31. Rizzo DJ: New summary slides show current trends in BMT. *ABMTR Newsletter* 5:4, 1998

32. Fefer A: Graft-versus-tumor responses, in Thomas ED,

Blume SJ, Forman SJ (eds): *Hematopoietic Cell Transplantation* (ed 2). Malden, MA, Blackwell Science, 1999, pp 316–326

33. Goulmy F: Human minor histocompatibility antigens: New concepts for marrow transplantation and adoptive immunotherapy. *Immunol Rev* 157:125–140, 1997

34. Appelbaum FR: The use of bone marrow and peripheral blood stem cell transplantation in the treatment of cancer. *CA Cancer J Clin* 46:142–164, 1996

35. Beatty PG: Marrow transplantation using volunteer unrelated donors in a comparison of mismatched family donor transplants: A Seattle perspective. *Bone Marrow Transplant* 14:S39–41, 1994 (suppl 4)

36. Atkinson K: *The BMT Data Book*. Cambridge, Cambridge University Press, 1998

37. Gordon-Smith EC: A consensus statement on unrelated donor bone marrow transplantation from the consensus panel chaired by EC Gordon-Smith. *Bone Marrow Transplant* 19: 959–962, 1997

38. Crilley P, Goldstein LJ: Peripheral blood stem cell transplant in breast cancer. *Semin Oncol* 22:238–249, 1995

39. Wujcik D: Hematopoiesis, in Whedon MB, Wujcik D (eds): *Blood and Marrow Stem Cell Tranplantation: Principles, Practice, and Nursing Insights* (ed 2). Sudbury, MA, Jones and Bartlett, 1997, pp 25–42

40. Kiss JE, Rybka WB, Winkelstein A, et al: Relationship of CD34 + cell dose to early and late hematopoiesis following autologous peripheral blood stem cell transplantation. *Bone Marrow Transplant* 19:303–310, 1997

41. Sola C, Maroto P, Salazar R, et al: High-dose chemotherapy (HDC) and peripheral blood stem cell (PBSC) autologous transplantation: Influence of the number of infused CD34 + cells in hematopoetic recovery and support measures required. *Proc Am Soc Clin Oncol* 15:538, 1996 (abstr)

42. Kundtzon S: *In vitro* growth of granulocytic colonies from circulating cells in human cord blood. *Blood* 43:357–361, 1974

43. Broxmeyer HE, Kurtzberg J, Gluckman E: Human umbilical cord blood as a potential source of transplantable hematopoietic stem/progenitor cells. *Proc Natl Acad Sci USA* 86: 3828–3832, 1989

44. Weber-Nordt, RM Schott E, Finke J, et al: Umbilical cord blood: An alternative to the transplantation of bone marrow stem cells. *Cancer Treat Rev* 22:381–391, 1996

45. Wagner JE: Allogeneic umbilical cord blood transplantation. *Cancer Treat Res* 77:187–216, 1997

46. Laporte J-P, Gorin, N-C, Rubinstein P, et al: Transplantation from an unrelated donor in an adult with chronic myelogenous leukemia. *N Engl J Med* 335:167–170, 1996

47. Broxmeyer HE, Smith FO: Cord blood stem cell transplantation, in Thomas ED, Blume SJ, Forman SJ (eds): *Hematopoietic Cell Transplantation* (ed 2). Malden, MA, Blackwell Science, 1999, pp 431–443

48. Rosti G, Phillip T, Chauvin F, et al: European group for blood and marrow transplantation (EBMT) registry in solid tumors: 13 years of experience. *Bone Marrow Transplant* 19:S86, 1997 (suppl 1)

49. Snowden JA, Biggs JC, Brooks PM: Autologous blood stem cell transplantation for autoimmune diseases. *Lancet* 348: 1112–1113, 1996

50. Vaughan WP, Silver SM, Beatty PG et al: Incorporating bone marrow transplantation into NCCN guidelines. *Oncology* 12:390–392, 1998

51. Gratwohl A, Passweg J, Baldomero H, et al: Special report: Blood and marrow transplantation activity in Europe 1996. *Bone Marrow Transplant* 22:227–240, 1998

52. Stockerl-Goldstein KE, Blume KG: Allogeneic hematopoietic cell transplantation for adult patients with acute myeloid leukemia, in Thomas ED, Blume SJ, Forman SJ (eds): *Hematopoietic Cell Transplantation* (ed 2). Malden, MA, Blackwell Science, 1999, pp 823–834

53. Dini G, Cornish JM, Gadner H: Bone marrow transplant indications for childhood leukemias: Achieveing a consensus. The EBMT Pediatric Diseases Working Party. *Bone Marrow Transplant* 18:4–7, 1996 (suppl 2)

54. Abramovitz LZ, Senner AM: Pediatric bone marrow transplantation update. *Oncol Nurs Forum* 22:107–115, 1995

55. Gale RP, Butturini A, Horowitz M: HLA-identical sibling bone marrow transplantation for acute lymphoblastic leukemia, in Atkinson K (ed): *Clinical Bone Marrow Transplantation*. Cambridge, Cambridge University Press, 1994, pp 191–196

56. Passweg JR, Rowlings PA, Horowitz MM: Related donor bone marrow transplantation for chronic myelogenous leukemia. *Hematol Oncol Clin North Am* 12: 81–92, 1998

57. Bhatia R, Forman SJ: Autologous transplant for the treatment of chronic myelogenous leukemia. *Hematol Oncol Clin North Am* 12:151–172, 1998

58. Hays K, McCartney S: Nursing care of the patient with chronic lymphocytic leukemia. *Semin Oncol* 25:75–79, 1998

59. Khouri IF, Keating MJ, Vriesendrop HM, et al: Autologous and allogeneic bone marrow transplantation for chronic lymphocytic leukemia: Preliminary results. *J Clin Oncol* 12: 748–758, 1994

60. Rabinowe SN, Soiffer RJ, Gribben JG, et al: Autologus and allogeneic bone marrow transplantation for poor prognosis patients with B-cell chronic lymphocytic leukemia. *Blood* 83:1366–1376, 1993

61. Flinn IW, Vogelsang G: Bone marrow transplantation for chronic lymphocytic leukemia. *Semin Oncol* 25:60–64, 1998

62. Philip T, Guglielmi C, Hagenbeek A, et al: Autologous bone marrow transplantation as compared with salvage chemotherapy in relapses of chemotherapy-sensitive non-Hodgkin's lymphoma. *N Engl J Med* 333:1540–1545, 1995

63. Horning SJ: High-dose therapy and transplantation for low-grade lymphoma. *Hematol Oncol Clin North Am* 11:919–935, 1997

64. Greenberg P: NCCN practice guidelines for the myelodysplastic syndromes. *Oncology* 12:53, 1998

65. Anderson JE: Allogeneic hematopoietic cell transplantation for myelodysplatic and myeloproliferative disorders, in Thomas ED, Blume SJ, Forman SJ (eds): *Hematopoietic Cell Transplantation* (ed 2). Malden, MA, Blackwell Science, 1999, pp 872–886

66. Bensinger WI, Buckner CD, Gahrton G: Allogeneic stem cell transplant for multiple myeloma. *Hematol Oncol Clin North Am* 11:147–157, 1997

67. Attal M, Harousseau JL: Standard therapy versus autologous transplantation in multiple myeloma. *Hematol Oncol Clin North Am* 11:133–146, 1997

68. Peters WP, Baynes RD: Autologous hematopoietic cell transplantation for breast cancer, in Thomas ED, Blume SJ, Forman SJ (eds): *Hematopoietic Cell Transplantation* (ed 2). Malden, MA, Blackwell Science, 1999, pp 1029–1042

69. Ljungman P, Björkstrand B, Fornander T, et al: High-dose chemotherapy with autologous stem cell support in patients with responding stage IV breast cancer. *Bone Marrow Transplant* 22:445–448, 1998

70. Bezwoda WR, Seymour L, Dansey RD: High-dose chemotherapy with hematopoietic rescue as primary treatment for metastatic breast cancer: A randomized trial. *J Clin Oncol* 13:2483–2489, 1995

71. Peters WP, Jones RB, Vredenburgh J, et al: A large, prospective, randomized trial of high-dose combination alkylating agent (CPB) with autologous cellular support (ABMS) as consolidation for patients with metastatic breast cancer achieving complete remission after intensive doxorubicin-based induction therapy (AFM). *Proc Am Soc Clin Oncol* 15: 121, 1996 (abstr 149)

72. Stadtmauer EA, O'Neill A, Goldstein LJ, et al: Phase III randomized trial of high-dose chemotherapy (HDC) and stem cell support (SCT) shows no difference in overall survival or severe toxicity compared to maintenance chemotherapy with cyclophosphamide, methotrexate and 5-fluorouracil (CMF) for women with metastatic breast cancer who are responding to conventional induction chemotherapy: The 'Philadelphia' Intergroup Study (PBT-1). *Proc Am Soc Clin Oncol* 18:1a, 1999 (abstr 1)

73. Lotz J-P, Curé H, Janvier M, et al: High-dose chemotherapy (HD-CT) with hematopoietic stem cells transplantation (HSCT) for mestastatic breast cancer (MBC): Results of the French Protocol PEGASE 04. *Proc Am Soc Clin Oncol* 18:43a, 1999 (abstr 161)

74. Peters W, Rosner G, Vredenburgh J, et al: A Prospective, randomized comparison of two doses of combination alkyating agents (AA) as consoldiation after CAF in high-risk primary breast cancer involving ten or more axillary lymph nodes (LN): Preliminary results of CALGB 9082/SWOG 9114/NCIC MA-13. *Proc Am Soc Clin Oncol* 18:1a, 1999 (abstr 2)

75. The Scandinavian Breast Cancer Study Group 9401: Results from a randomized adjuvant breast cancer study with high dose chemotherapy with CTC· supported by autologous bone marrow stem cells versus dose escalated and tailored FEC therapy. *Proc Am Soc Clin Oncol* 18:2a, 1999 (abstr 3)

76. Schmitz N, Sextro M, Pfistner B, et al: High-dose therapy (HDT) followed by hematopoietic stem cell transplantation (HSCT) for relapsed chemosensitive Hodgkin's disease (HD): Final results of a randomized GHSG and EBMT trial (HD-R1). *Proc Am Soc Clin Oncol* 18:2a, 1999 (abstr 4)

77. Foelber R: Autologous stem cell transplant plus interleukin-2 for breast cancer: Review and nursing management. *Oncol Nurs Forum* 25:563–568, 1998

78. Nichols CR: Hematopoietic cell transplantation in germ cell tumors, in Thomas ED, Blume SJ, Forman SJ (eds): *Hematopoietic Cell Transplantation* (ed 2). Malden, MA, Blackwell Science, 1999, pp 1049–1057

79. Fennelly D: The role of high-dose chemotherapy in the management of advanced ovarian cancer. *Curr Opin Oncol* 8:415–425, 1996

80. Fennelly DW, Aghajanian C, Shapiro F, et al: Dose escalation of paclitaxel with high-dose carboplatin using peripheral blood progenitor cell support in patients with advanced ovarian cancer. *Semin Oncol* 24:S2–26–S2–30, 1997

81. Prados MD, Berger MS, Wilson CB: Primary central nervous system tumors: Advances in knowledge and treatment. *CA Cancer J Clin* 48:331–360, 1998.

82. Burt RK: BMT for severe autoimmune diseases: An idea whose time has come. *Oncology* 11:1001–1017, 1997

83. Marmont AM: Stem cell transplantation for severe autoimmune disorders, with special reference to rheumatic diseases. *J Rheumatol* 48:13–18, 1997 (suppl)

84. Nash RA, McSweeney PA, Storb R, et al: Development of a protocol for allogeneic marrow transplantation for severe systemic sclerosis: Paradigm for autoimmune disease. *J Rheumatol* 48:72–78, 1997 (suppl)

85. Tyndall A, Gratwohl A: Special report. Blood and marrow stem cell transplants in auto-immune disease: A consensus report written on behalf of the European League against Rheumatism (EULAR) and the European Group for Blood and Marrow Transplantation (EBMT). *Bone Marrow Transplant* 19: 643–645, 1997

86. Deeg HJ: Delayed complications after hematopoietic cell transplantation, in Thomas ED, Blume SJ, Forman SJ (eds): *Hematopoietic Cell Transplantation* (ed 2). Malden, MA, Blackwell Science, 1999, pp 776–788

87. Ahles TA, Tope DM, Furstenberg C, et al: Psychologic and neuropsychologic impact of autologous bone marrow transplantation. *J Clin Oncol* 14:1457–1462, 1996

88. Curtis RE, Rowlings PA, Deeg HJ, et al: Solid cancers after bone marrow transplantation. *N Engl J Med* 336: 897–904, 1997

89. Porter DL, Antin JH: Infusion of donor peripheral blood mononuclear cells to treat relapse after transplantation for chronic myelogenous leukemia. *Hematol Oncol Clin North Am* 12:123–149, 1998

90. Kolb HJ: Management of relapse after hematopoietic cell transplantation, in Thomas ED, Blume SJ, Forman SJ (eds): *Hematopoietic Cell Transplantation* (ed 2). Malden, MA, Blackwell Science, 1999, pp 929–936

91. Doroshow JH: Pharmacological basis for high-dose chemotherapy, in Thomas ED, Blume SJ, Forman SJ (eds): *Hematopoietic Cell Transplantation* (ed 2). Malden, MA, Blackwell Science, 1999, pp 103–122

92. Negrin RS: Prevention and therapy of relapse after autologous hematopoietic cell transplantation, in Thomas ED, Blume SJ, Forman SJ (eds): *Hematopoietic Cell Transplantation* (ed 2). Malden, MA, Blackwell Science, 1999, pp 1123–1134

93. Sutherland CW: The hematology and immunology of peripheral stem cell transplantation, in Buchsel P (ed): *Advanced Concepts in Peripheral Stem Cell Transplantation*. Pittsburgh, Oncology Education Services, 1997, pp 8–16

94. DeMeyer E: Advanced concepts in peripheral stem cell transplantation, in Buchsel P (ed): *Advanced Concepts in Peripheral Stem Cell Transplantation*. Pittsburgh, Oncology Education Services, 1997, pp 17–22

95. O'Mara A, Whedon M: Nursing assessment: Hematologic system, in Lewis S, Heitkemper M (ed): *Medical-Surgical Nursing: Assessment and Management of Clinical Problems*. St. Louis, Mosby, 1999, pp 719–736

96. Ezzone S (ed): *Peripheral Blood Stem Cell Transplantation: Recommendations for Nursing Education and Practice*. Pittsburgh, Oncology Nursing Press, 1997

97. Hegland J: Transplant immunology: HLA and issues of stem cell donation, in Whedon MB, Wujcik D (eds): *Marrow and Blood Stem Cell Transplantation: Principles, Practice and Nursing Insights* (ed 2). Sudbury, MA, Jones and Bartlett, 1997, pp 43–65

98. Ezzone S, Fliedner M: Transplant networks and standards of care: International perspectives, in Whedon MB, Wujcik D (eds). *Marrow and Blood Stem Cell Transplantation: Principles, Practice and Nursing Insights* (ed 2). Sudbury, MA, Jones and Bartlett, 1997, pp 474–496

99. Whedon MB, Fliedner M: Nursing issues in hematopoeitic cell transplantation, in Thomas ED, Forman SJ, Blume KG (eds): *Hematopoietic Cell Transplantation* (ed 2). Malden, MA, Blackwell Science, 1999, pp 381–385

100. Foundation for the Accreditation of Hematopoietic Cell Therapy (FAHCT): *Standards for Hematopoietic Progenitor Cell Collection, Processing and Transplantation*. First Edition-North America, Omaha, NE, September 1996

101. American Society of Hematology/American Society of Clinical Oncologists: Recommended criteria for the performance of bone marrow transplantation. *Blood* 75:1209, 1990

102. Phillips G, Armitage J, Bearman S, et al: American Society for Blood and Marrow Transplantation guidelines for clinical centers. *Biol Blood Marrow Transplant* 1:54–55, 1995.

103. Bortin MM, Horowitz MM, Rimm AA: Progress report from the International Bone Marrow Transplant Registry. *Bone Marrow Transplant* 10:113–122, 1992

104. Ezzone S, Camp-Sorrell D (eds): *Manual for Bone Marrow Transplant Nursing.* Pittsburgh, Oncology Nursing Press, 1994

105. Oncology Nursing Society: *Bone Marrow Transplant Nursing Resource Directory.* Pittsburgh, Oncology Nursing Press, 1998

106. Brighton S, Whedon MB: Implications of bone marrow transplantation for nursing, in McMillan S, Holley S (eds): *Instructor's Resource Manual for the ONS Core Curriculum.* Philadelphia, Saunders, 1995, pp 213–221

107. Roach M, Whedon MB: Bone marrow transplantation, in Fink R, Gates R (eds): *Oncology Nursing Secrets.* Boston, Henlay & Belfus, 1997, pp 62–72

108. Shapiro TW, Davison DB, Rust DM: *A Clinical Guide to Stem Cell and Bone Marrow Transplantation.* Sudbury, MA, Jones and Bartlett, 1997

109. Engelking C: Peripheral blood stem cell therapy for breast cancer: Arguing the case. *Innov Breast Cancer Care* 3:51, 67, 1998

110. Guidelines, Protocols Described for Outpatient BMT Program. *Oncol News* 7:25, 1998

111. Giles K, Vaughn WP: A model of care for bone marrow transplantation patients: Update 1998. *Oncol Issues* 14: 21–25, 1999

112. Bedell MK, Mroz WT: The bone marrow and blood stem cell transplant marketplace, in Whedon MB, Wujcik D (eds): *Marrow and Blood Stem Cell Transplantation: Principles, Practice and Nursing Insights* (ed 2). Sudbury, MA, Jones and Bartlett, 1997, pp 459–473

113. Peters WP, Kurtzberg J, Rosner G, et al: Comparative effects of G-CSF and GM-CSF on priming peripheral blood progenitor cells for use with autologous bone marrow after high-dose chemotherapy. *Blood* 81:1709–1719, 1993

114. Lawrence CC, Gilbert CJ, Peters WP: Evaluation of symptom distress in a bone marrow transplant outpatient environment. *Ann Pharmacother* 30:941–945, 1996

115. Health Insurance: *Coverage of Autologous Bone Marrow Transplantation for Breast Cancer.* Washington D.C. Government Accounting Office/HEHS-96-83, 1996

116. Meisenberg BR, Miller WE, McMillan R, et al: Outpatient high-dose chemotherapy with autologous stem-cell rescue for hematologic and nonhematologic malignnacies. *J Clin Oncol* 15:11–17, 1997

117. Pajeau TS, Wateers TM, Bennett CL, et al: Economic analysis of allogeneic blood stem cell versus allogeneic bone marrow transplantation for hematologic malignancies. *Proc Am Soc Clin Oncol* 16:419a, 1997 (abstr 1499)

118. Fidler P, Hibbs C: Bone marrow transplant today—Home tomorrow: Ambulatory care issues in pediatric marrow transplantion. *J Pediatr Oncol Nurs* 14:228–238, 1997

119. Herrmann RP, Leather M, Leather HL, et al: Clinical care for patients receiving autologous hematopoietic stem cell transplantation in the home setting. *Oncol Nurs Forum* 25: 1427–1432, 1998

120. Frappier B, Schmit-Pokorny K: Using a classroom setting to provide patient education on high dose therapy and stem cell transplantation. *Oncol Nurs Forum* 24:341, 1997

CHAPTER 22

Techniques of Hematopoietic Cell Transplantation

Debra Wujcik, RN, MSN, AOCN

Kathy Price, RN, OCN®

Introduction

Bone marrow transplantation (BMT) has been a treatment for patients with hematologic malignancies since the mid-1900s. The original procedure required harvesting pluripotent stem cells (PPSCs) from the bone marrow of a human leukocyte antigen (HLA)–matched donor. The patient received preparative therapy that included high-dose myeloablative chemotherapy and total body irradiation (TBI). The harvested cells were then reinfused into the patient. Intense supportive care was required for 4–6 weeks until the donor cells migrated to the bone marrow and began to produce new hematopoietic cells. This is the process for allogeneic BMT.

High-dose chemotherapy for the treatment of solid tumors produced improved response rates, but the dose-limiting toxicity was myelosuppression. Patients needed a rescue of stem cells to recover hematopoietic function. Harvesting the patient's own stem cells, freezing them, and reinfusing them after conditioning therapy expanded the use of BMT to autologous BMT.

The discovery that PPSCs circulated in the peripheral blood stream led to new techniques to collect, preserve, and reinfuse cells. Collection of cells through apheresis was easier and less costly than bone marrow harvest. There is controversy as to whether PPSCs and the peripheral blood progenitor cells (PBPCs) are equivalent in terms of durability of hematopoietic reconstitution. However, transplantation with cells obtained from peripheral circulation now represents approximately 75% of the autologous transplants performed for solid tumors.[1]

The terminology for transplantation is confusing and ever changing. Despite attempts to achieve consensus, there is not universal acceptance. Key terms for understanding the literature are listed in Table 22-1. For the purposes of this chapter, the general term for transplantation is hematopoietic cell transplantation (HCT). Bone marrow transplantation designates transplant with hematopoietic cells obtained from the bone marrow. Blood cell transplantation (BCT) refers to transplant with cells from the peripheral circulation, and umbilical cord transplantation (UCBT) refers to transplant with cells from the umbilical cord.

There are an estimated 30,000–40,000 HCTs per year,

with an expected growth rate of 10%–20% per year.[2] A number of variables contribute to the growth: increased efficacy of HCT with increased use in more disease sites, better understanding of optimal timing for HCT, increased donor availability, improved conditioning strategies, and improved supportive care. Techniques for HCT differ according to the source of cells and type of transplant. The techniques for HCT must meet standards set by the Foundation for Accreditation of Hematopoietic Cell Therapy (FAHCT) (Table 22-2).[3]

This chapter reviews the techniques of HCT throughout the process. Procedures to obtain cells for transplant, cell processing and storage, preparative regimens, and reinfusion of cells are discussed. Nursing indications for patient education, assessment, and management of complications are presented.

Patient Evaluation

The first step in patient evaluation for HCT is determining whether the patient is a candidate for transplantation and which type of transplant is most appropriate. The disease, stage of disease, performance status of the patient, availability of an appropriate protocol, and donor availability are considered. The type of transplant the patient will receive is decided early in the process because insurance preauthorization, timing, and scheduling are influenced by this information.[4]

Physical Evaluation

The clinical evaluation occurs simultaneously with an insurance preauthorization process. There is documented improved response to transplantation when there is low tumor burden and if the disease is chemotherapy sensitive. Also, the earlier the stage of disease at the time of transplant, the better the survival. The clinical evaluation includes determining if any organ dysfunction secondary to disease or prior therapy is present. Specifically, the lungs and heart are evaluated. Other screening tests include viral studies to rule out HIV or hepatitis, among others (Table 22-3).[5,6]

Psychosocial Evaluation

The psychosocial evaluation begins with education of the patient and family about the rationale, risks, and benefits of HCT. Discussion should include acute and long-term effects. The assessment of patient and family understanding of the informed consent provides the nurse with a basis for further counseling. The coping strategies of the patient and family are identified. Problems such as drug, alcohol, or tobacco addictions are addressed.[7] Sources of support and available resources are identified. A plan is developed for managing life activities during the trans-

Table 22-1 Terminology of Hematopoietic Cell Transplantation

Source of hematopoietic cells	Procedure
Bone marrow	Bone marrow harvest
Peripheral circulation	Apheresis
Umbilical cord blood	Delivery room collection

Type of transplant	Donor of cells
Allogeneic	HLA-matched related donor
	HLA-matched unrelated donor
Autologous	Patient
Syngeneic	HLA-identical twin

Table 22-2 Standards for Hematopoietic Cell Transplantation

PERSONNEL

Director	Licensed and board certified; 1 year specific clinical training or 2 years as attending for patients undergoing transplantation
Other physicians	Trained under the Director with demonstrated competency in the management of myelosuppressed patients
Surgeon	Skilled in catheter placement
Consultants	Consultants available who are board certified in pulmonary, gastroenterology, nephrology, infectious disease, cardiology, psychiatry, and radiation oncology
Nurses	Formally trained and experienced in care of transplantation patients; skills in administration of chemotherapy and blood components and management of infections
Technologist	Trained for handling of stem cells

CELL COLLECTION FACILITY REQUIREMENTS

Facility medical director	Director shall have 1 year's experience in the collection procedure with 10 collection procedures of each type
Personnel	Adequate numbers of trained personnel
Laboratory	Accredited laboratory to perform all required tests
Facility	Transfusion facility or blood bank providing 24-hour blood component support including irradiated blood components
Collection procedures	Standard operating manual describing all procedures

CELL PROCESSING

Laboratory director	Requires relevant doctoral degree with training and experience for the scope of activities
Processing procedures	Standard operating manual for all procedures; methods for processing shall be validated to result in acceptable hematopoietic progenitor cell viability and recovery
Records	Detailed worksheets maintained for all procedures; objectives and acceptable end points for each procedure are specified; director or designee reviews every record

Data from Foundation for the Accreditation of Hematopoietic Cell Therapy.[3]

plant period such as child care, transportation, employment, and who will stay with the patient during HCT.

Financial Evaluation

The insurance evaluation must occur early in the evaluation process due to the expense ($75,000–$150,000) and the frequent investigational nature of HCT.[8] An insurance counselor or transplant coordinator works closely with the transplant team to keep them advised of potential reimbursement obstacles. Preauthorization of insurance coverage is usually required. Sometimes during this process, it is learned that the patient must go to a different transplant center where the insurance company has an existing contract. Successful preauthorization is dependent on the case manager's knowledge of the patient's history and the transplant process, as well as experience in negotiations with the insurers.[9,10] It is common for institutions to negotiate with the insurer to provide all care for a set or capitated fee.

In general, insurers provide coverage for allogeneic and autologous BMT for patients with acute leukemia in remission, resistant non-Hodgkin's lymphoma, advanced Hodgkin's disease, recurrent neuroblastoma, and medulloblastoma. Autologous transplant for patients with solid tumors continues to increase in use but remains controversial.[11] Often, patients without insurance coverage must raise their own funds and have a certain amount raised before the transplant.

Some patients with breast cancer have to sue insurers to obtain coverage for autologous HCT. Several payers such as Blue Cross and Blue Shield (BC/BS) have agreed to support patients enrolled in clinical trials until the results are known.[12] Recent reports of several large randomized studies still do not provide conclusive evidence that high-dose therapy followed by stem cell rescue for high-risk or metastatic breast cancer patients improves survival.[13–15]

Education

Beginning with the initial period of evaluation and continuing throughout the process of HCT, the patient and family require extensive education (Table 22-4). It is useful to provide written and oral instructions and allow sufficient time for patients and family members to synthesize information and ask questions.[16] Use of critical pathways may allow the teaching to be presented in a

Table 22-3   Baseline Evaluation for Patients Undergoing Hematopoietic Cell Transplantation

Test	Comment
Complete blood count, including differential and reticulocyte	Establish baseline
Complete blood chemistry profile, urinalysis	Establish baseline; ensure renal and liver function
Prothrombin time, partial thromboplastin time	Establish baseline; ensure coagulation ability
Thyroid function tests	Establish baseline for comparison after total body irradiation
Chest x-ray (PA-Lat)	Establish baseline pulmonary status
Cardiac ejection fraction by (resting) MUGA scan, 12-lead ECG	Establish baseline cardiac function for comparison during and after conditioning therapy
Pulmonary function tests (including DLCO)	Establish baseline pulmonary function
Type and screen	Confirm patient blood typing
Herpes simplex virus serology, Epstein Barr virus serology, *Varicella zoster* serology	Establish previous viral exposure and risk of reactivation of infection
Human immunodeficiency virus antibody, human T-cell leukemia virus 1 antibody	Rule out eligibility for transplantation
Toxoplasma serology (IgG)	Establish previous toxoplasma exposure and risk of reactivation of infection

PA-Lat = posterior, anterior, and lateral; MUGA = multigated angiogram; ECG = electrocardiogram; DLCO = diffusion of lung with carbon dioxide.

consistent, sequential manner with reinforcement at the appropriate time.[9,17]

Cells for Transplantation

The process of obtaining stem cells for HCT differs according to the type of transplant. With BMT, the cells are obtained through a bone marrow harvest. In BCT, the pluripotent stem cells and progenitor cells are collected from the peripheral blood. Each procedure has unique steps for donor preparation, the actual procedure, and for managing complications.

Bone Marrow Harvest

The cells harvested from the bone marrow are PPSCs. These are cells that have the capacity for both myeloid and lymphoid (multilineage) differentiation, proliferation, and self-renewal.[18,19] The exact number of PPSCs needed to repopulate a marrow destroyed by chemotherapy and radiation has not been determined. However, 5% of the 1×10^6 or 1×10^7 nucleated cells found in adult human marrow contain sufficient PPSCs for transplant.[20] It is generally agreed that the minimum threshold below which acceptable hematopoietic reconstitution may not occur is $15–20 \times 10^4$ colony forming units–granulocyte macrophages (CFU-GM)/kg or $1–2 \times 10^6$ CD34$^+$ cells/kg of body weight.[21,22]

The cells needed for successful engraftment after high-dose chemotherapy and irradiation are difficult to isolate. The CD34 antigen is an antigen expressed on the surface of early progenitor cells. The CD34 antigen does not appear on the PPSC but is present on the committed progenitors. Currently, the CD34 assay is the best technique available to identify the cells that have proved to be correlated with successful engraftment.[23–25]

Procedure

The bone marrow harvest is usually done in the operating room with the patient anesthetized. Multiple aspirations are obtained from each posterior iliac crest to obtain the necessary volume of PPSCs. Marrow may be aspirated from the anterior iliac crests and the sternum if the cell yield from the posterior iliac crests is not adequate. The marrow is placed in a heparinized tissue culture medium, filtered for removal of fat and bone particles, then sent to the laboratory for processing and cryopreservation. The procedure usually takes 1–2 hours.[4]

Postoperatively, pressure dressings are applied to the puncture sites. The nurse assesses the patient for bleeding, pain, and fluid balance. Because 400–600 mL of whole blood are aspirated during the harvest, the patient may receive an autologous unit of blood that was collected before the procedure. The complication rate for bone marrow harvest is low, and the patient is usually discharged following recovery the same day or the next day.[4] The donor may experience pain at the collection sites, which is controlled by mild analgesics. The donor's body will replace the cells that were removed within a few weeks.

A double or triple lumen silicone catheter is placed centrally to use for reinfusion of bone marrow cells, ad-

Table 22-4 Topics for Education of Hematopoietic Cell Transplantation Patients

Phase	Bone Marrow Transplant	Both	Blood Cell Transplant
Evaluation		Overview	
		Tests	
		Laboratory specimens	
		Local housing	
Catheter		Placement	
		Catheter care	
		Complications	
Procurement of cells	Harvest procedure		Mobilization
	Complications		Pheresis
			Complications
Conditioning	Specific drugs +/−		Specific drugs
	total body irradiation		Irradiation rare
Reinfusion		Preparation	
		Procedure	
		Complications	
Supportive care		Antibiotics	
		Hematopoietic growth factors	
		Blood products	
		Total parenteral nutrition	
Discharge		Criteria for discharge	
		Continued care at home	

ministration of conditioning chemotherapy and hydration, and supportive therapy such as antibiotics and transfusions of blood products. The catheter is placed at the time of harvest or at the first day of conditioning therapy unless the patient has a preexisting catheter from prior therapy. Catheter care includes insertion site care, dressing changes, and flushing procedures. The patient is instructed on the signs and symptoms of infection and management of complications such as occlusion or accidental puncture of the catheter.

Harvest for allogeneic bone marrow transplant

The replacement marrow for allogeneic BMT is obtained from a related or unrelated HLA-matched donor. Prior to harvest, several issues need to be addressed for the normal donor. Donor preparation includes education and medical evaluation. The standard physical evaluation of the donor includes a complete medical history and physical examination, psychosocial evaluation, EKG, chest x-ray, and laboratory evaluation. Laboratory evaluation includes CBC with differential, serum tests for major organ function (renal and hepatic), hepatitis screen (A, B, C), HIV, CMV, HSV, ABO and Rh, and histocompatible tissue typing.[4] The infectious disease screening is performed within 30 days prior to the collection.[3]

To maintain maximum viability, cells harvested from a donor are given as soon as possible. The timing of allogeneic marrow harvest is carefully coordinated with the transplant team. Because cells are processed and delivered to the recipient within hours of collection, cryopreservation is unnecessary.

A thorough description of the harvesting procedure and the potential impact that the harvest may have on the donor and the relationship with the recipient should be discussed with the donor. Unrelated donors should also receive counseling prior to donation. The donor should not feel pressured into donating. To preserve confidentiality and avoid contact between a potential donor and the patient or the patient's family, the identity of an unrelated donor remains unknown to both the patient and the transplanting center.[4]

There are many limitations to allogeneic BMT. The biggest drawback is the availability of an appropriate marrow donor. Only one in four persons needing a BMT has a related match. The National Marrow Donor Program provides a pool of nearly 2 million potential donors but the registry is hindered by the numbers of donors from different races. The best opportunity to find a match is within one's own race and the largest race in the registry is white. The frequency of specific HLA types differs among racial and ethnic groups. Most HLA pairs occur in all ethnic groups, but a few are limited to a single ethnic group. The frequency of an HLA pair can also vary within the ethnic group, depending on the geographic location of the population.[26]

Histocompatibility is another limitation of allogeneic BMT. The greater the histoincompatibility between patient and donor, the greater the risk of graft failure, graft rejection, and graft-versus-host disease (GVHD).[26] If there is a major ABO incompatibility between the donor and recipient, the bone marrow will be depleted of red cells or plasma.[4]

Harvest for autologous bone marrow transplant

The process of obtaining bone marrow for autologous BMT is the same as for allogeneic BMT, but the volume harvested may be greater if there is a need for purging or other manipulation to remove tumor cells. The bone marrow is harvested when the patient is in remission and recovered from other treatment. The cells are then processed and frozen until needed.

Blood Cell Apheresis

Another option for transplant is the use of stem cells obtained from the peripheral circulation. Some PPSCs circulate in the peripheral blood in small numbers, and committed progenitors circulate in greater numbers.[27] *Progenitors* are cells that have limited ability to divide and are irreversibly committed to one or more lines of differentiation.[28] The colony-forming unit–granulocyte, erythrocyte, macrophage, megakaryocyte (CFU-GEMM) and colony-forming unit–lymphocyte (CFU-L) are committed stem cells. Although they are irreversibly committed to the separate lineages, they remain capable of differentiating to one of several cell lines.[18] (See Figure 21-5 in the previous chapter, which illustrates the hematopoietic cascade.)

The PBPCs represent 1%–10% of the marrow progenitors. Once it was proved that these cells could be reinfused into animals (mice, dogs, and baboons) and restore hematopoiesis, the process was applied to humans.[29] The first transplant using cells obtained from peripheral blood was reported in 1985, with several more the following year.[30]

This process has historically been referred to as peripheral blood stem cell transplant (PBSCT) or peripheral blood progenitor cell transplant (PBPCT). The process involves obtaining and infusing an unspecified number of true PPSCs with or without committed progenitor and precursor cells.[19,31] The current terminology for this process is *blood cell transplant* (BCT). Blood cell transplant is considered to be more precise and so is preferred to other terms to differentiate the PPSC obtained from the bone marrow for allogeneic and autologous BMT from the combined PPSC and committed progenitors obtained from the peripheral blood for BCT.[19]

There are advantages to using peripheral PPSCs and progenitor cells obtained from peripheral blood. Neutrophils and platelets recover more rapidly when progenitor cells are used.[32,33] This is because the committed progenitors collected for BCT are further along the differentiation pathway than are the PPSCs harvested from the bone marrow. Also, no anesthesia is required for BCT so there is less risk of complications and fewer medical contraindications than with bone marrow harvest. Patients who cannot have bone marrow harvested due to contraindications to anesthesia, marrow involvement, or prior radiation therapy to large areas of bone marrow may be able to undergo BCT. Disadvantages to using PBSCs include the cost of multiple aphereses and purging procedures, the requirement for mobilization, and the necessity for vascular access.[34]

As with BMT, there are several types of BCT. A patient may use their own cells (autologous), cells obtained from an identical twin (syngeneic), or cells obtained from a matched related or unrelated donor (allogeneic).[35–37] The procedure for collection of the PBSCs and progenitors is the same for each type of BCT.

Blood cell transplant mobilization

Purpose. The purpose of mobilization for BCT is to release an increased number of PPSCs and progenitor cells into the peripheral blood stream. The number of progenitor cells in the blood stream in the steady state is only 1%–10% of the marrow progenitors.[33] In order to collect enough stem cells from the blood, stem cells must be mobilized or moved from the bone marrow to the blood.[38,39] The number of PPSCs and progenitors can be increased up to 100- to 500-fold through the use of hematopoietic growth factors (HGFs), chemotherapy, or both.[33,40] Without mobilization, 10–14 apheresis procedures are required to obtain the required number of cells needed for BCT.[22,28] There is disagreement regarding the optimal number of cells needed for successful engraftment. However, there is agreement that the minimal number of cells required for BCT is 5–7 $\times$ 10^8 mononuclear cells/kg or $\geq$ 1–5 $\times$ 10^6 CD34$^+$ cells/kg.[41] Engraftment of both granulocytes and platelets is significantly influenced by the number of CD34$^+$ cells per kg infused, and some suggest that doses of 15 $\times$ 10^6 CD34$^+$ cells/kg shorten hematopoietic recovery and may improve quality of life.[42,43] With appropriate mobilization, this usually requires 1–3 apheresis procedures. However, the optimal process for mobilization is not yet defined.

Chemotherapy mobilization. Chemotherapy is used for mobilization either alone or in combination with HGFs. Chemotherapy alone causes an increase in the number of circulating progenitor cells in the peripheral blood. However, the results using chemotherapy are variable and less predictable than with HGFs. Rebound leukocytosis occurs after single-agent chemotherapy with high-dose cyclophosphamide or with multiple drug regimens using etoposide, cyclophosphamide, and cisplatin.[40] Cyclophosphamide is the most commonly reported chemotherapeutic agent for mobilization.[44] Dosages vary between 2–4 grams administered intravenously as an inpatient or outpatient regimen. Blood counts are monitored daily or every other day to track the recovery of the absolute neutrophil count (ANC). Collection begins when the ANC is between 1000 cells/mm^3 to 5000 cells/mm^3. It is important not to use drugs that induce thrombocytopenia at the time of maximum progenitor output or to use drugs that are damaging to progenitor cells such as carmustine or melphalan.[28]

Chemotherapy alone for mobilization is useful for tumor reduction in patients with residual malignancy[37], but there are disadvantages as well. Fever and pancytopenia that occur as side effects of the drugs can interfere with the schedule for apheresis. In addition, because the rebound leukocytosis occurs 10–14 days after chemotherapy, it is often difficult to plan ahead for collection of cells.[44,45]

The use of chemotherapy and HGFs together usually leads to the collection of more cells than either method alone.[38] The efficiency of the collection is influenced by individual and technical factors. The patient's pretreatment with chemotherapy or radiation therapy may cause bone marrow damage, making it difficult to mobilize a sufficient number of progenitors. Some data indicates that the patient's age and sex negatively influence the yield of progenitors, with female patients and older patients (>55 years) having lower yields.[40]

Hematopoietic growth factor mobilization. The administration of HGFs alone can result in the collection of adequate numbers of stem cells. Hematopoietic growth factors stimulate enhanced proliferation and maturation of neutrophils and provide a much more controlled response for mobilization. Granulocyte-macrophage colony-stimulating factor or granulocyte colony-stimulating factor (G-CSF) are the agents most commonly used for mobilization.[37] Granulocyte colony-stimulating factor is indicated for mobilization at 10 μg/kg/day given subcutaneously for 4–6 days. Patients or a family member are taught self-administration. Collection of hematopoietic cells begins on day 4 or day 5 of growth factor administration.[46,47] Daily injections continue until collection is completed. The type of growth factor used results in different mobilization, with G-CSF producing a greater yield of stem cells than patients receiving GM-CSF.[48]

Patient and caregiver education regarding administration and side effects of HGF/chemotherapy mobilization is important. Hematopoietic growth factors can produce adverse reactions including nausea, diarrhea, rash, fever, malaise, pleural effusion, increased clotting of the catheter, vomiting, bone pain, headache, chills, dyspnea, and edema.[49] Bone pain is the most predominant symptom and can be treated effectively with acetaminophen. Local irritation may occur at the injection site. Patients must be instructed to report this symptom immediately to prevent any skin breakdown and possible infection. Patients mobilized with chemotherapy need instruction regarding monitoring their temperature and reporting a temperature greater than 100.4°F (40.2°C), chills, or any change in their clinical condition.[38]

Combinations. Newer agents being evaluated for mobilization include stem cell factor, erythropoietin (EPO), PIXY 321 (a fusion molecule made from a combination of GM-CSF and interleukin-3 [IL-3]), and IL-3 used alone or in sequence with GM-CSF and G-CSF.[21,37] None of these agents given alone is better than G-CSF, but they can be effectively combined with G-CSF or GM-CSF. Attempts are currently being made to amplify the number of stem cells ex vivo with stem cell factor, IL-1, IL-3, IL-6, gamma interferon, and EPO.[50,51] This process allows for the collection of a small amount of cells that are grown and expanded in the laboratory until the desired number of cells is produced.[52]

Hematopoietic growth factor mobilized PBSCs are being used more frequently as an alternative to marrow collection in the allogeneic transplantation setting.[35,36] Reports increasingly show that PBSCs alone are equal or even superior to bone marrow with regard to the speed of engraftment and the ability of PBSCs to provide long-term hematopoietic reconstitution.[53] The safety considerations for normal PBSC donors have not been fully addressed. Short- and long-term effects of HGF mobilization and collection in normal donors is currently under investigation and not yet well defined. Further data are needed to answer the many questions regarding the safety of this practice.[35–37,53]

Blood cell transplant apheresis

A single apheresis can obtain the desired number of cells if there is no malignancy in the bone marrow, if the patient received minor pretreatment with chemotherapy, and if appropriate mobilization is used.[45] Although usually two or three procedures are needed, strategies are being investigated to decrease the number to one.[54] Two benefits of a single apheresis approach would be the decreased volume withdrawn from the patient and the decreased dimethylsulfate (DMSO) reinfused into the patient.[22]

Patient preparation

The preparation of the patient for apheresis includes extensive education, placement of the central venous catheter (CVC), and beginning specific medications. Teaching at this time includes catheter care, process of apheresis, mobilization, and potential complications.[16]

Catheter placement. The patient undergoing BCT requires a catheter that is stiffer than the traditional CVC used for BMT due to the need for high volume and pressure during apheresis (i.e., about 60–70 mL/min vs. 30 mL/min). Subclavian silicone catheters placed centrally and used in BMT are not stiff enough to withstand the rapid withdrawal of blood. A more rigid catheter used for dialysis was frequently used for BCT apheresis in the past. This catheter was replaced by another after apheresis for extended use during BCT. The PermCath (Quinton, Boothel, WA) is a double-lumen catheter suitable for use during apheresis, conditioning chemotherapy, and supportive care. More choices are now available including The Pheres-Flow (Horizan Medical Products, Inc., Manchester, GA) triple-lumen catheter. This catheter is intended for long-term access and is able to withstand the pressures and flow rates required during apheresis, with the added benefit of a third port.

The catheter is inserted in an outpatient setting, usually at the beginning or during the period of mobilization, and used throughout BCT. Normal donors for allogeneic transplantation may have large-gauge peripheral catheters placed in bilateral antecubital veins. If peripheral access is not achievable, a temporary CVC can be placed prior to collection and removed immediately following completion of the collection.

Medications. The mobilization process is initiated at the appropriate time. If an HGF is being used, the patient must learn subcutaneous administration. It is usually administered daily for 5–6 days, with the collection of cells beginning on day 4 or 5. If chemotherapy is used for mobilization, the drugs are given and the patient returns home. Blood counts are monitored daily or every other day and apheresis begins when the desired WBC is achieved.[4] To prevent platelet clumping during apheresis, ibuprofen 200 mg is given daily starting several days before apheresis begins. At the same time, calcium carbonate (Oscal-D) 500 mg orally three times daily is prescribed to minimize hypocalcemia during apheresis.

Procedure

Equipment. Blood cell separators have been used since the 1980s for various clinical indications such as plasma apheresis and leukapheresis. Cells can be harvested by automated continuous- or discontinuous-flow blood cell separators.[48] The Fenwal CS 3000 (Fenwal Laboratories, Deerfield, IL), Cobe Spectra (Cobe Laboratories, Lakewood, CO), and the Haemonetics V-50 or M30 (Haemonetics Corp., Braintree, MA) are the most commonly used machines.[4,48] Third-generation machines are now in use.[40,55] These include the CS 3000 Plus, a totally computerized continuous-flow device, the Fresenius AS 104, AS.TEC 204 (Fresenius, Bad Homburg, Germany), and the Excel (Dideco, Mirandola, Italy), which are semiautomated continuous-flow separators. These machines operate with cyclic phases of separation, spillover, concentration, and collection. The Cobe Spectra, also a semiautomated continuous-flow separator, operates with a computer program using centrifugation.

Collection. Collection of cells begins once the WBC count is adequate. When chemotherapy is used for mobilization, the WBC must be greater than 10,000 cells/mm³, and clear evidence of rising counts must be present prior to collection of cells. If growth factor is used to stimulate neutrophil production, a count of greater than 20,000 cells/mm³ indicates that the patient is ready to be apheresed. Baseline blood specimens including RBC, platelet, and calcium are drawn. Next, the patient is connected to the machine using the CVC. About 7–15 liters of blood are processed through the machine in a 2–4 hour period. The mononuclear cell layer is drawn off of the blood and the rest is returned to the patient. Chilling can occur due to the large volume of blood leaving the body, then cooling to room temperature before being returned to the patient. However, the patient is generally comfortable during the procedure and can watch television or use other diversional activities.

Large-volume leukapheresis. Cells are collected daily on an outpatient basis until the desired amount is obtained, which usually requires 2–4 days. Large-volume leukapheresis (LVL) is becoming the standard procedure. The modernization of leukapheresis equipment makes possible the processing of large volumes of blood at one time.[54] Large-volume leukapheresis processes at least three blood volumes (15–35 liters) during a single apheresis over approximately 3–5 hours. The large blood volumes are achieved on the Cobe machines by increasing the blood flow rate. This would normally increase the consumption of anticoagulant used to prevent clotting, resulting in citrate reactions. If the flow rate is changed by increasing the inlet to anticoagulant ratio, then the anticoagulant ratio to the patient is not increased. When using this method, anticoagulant needs to be added directly to the product by 5%–10%, depending on the patient's platelet count. For platelet counts >200,000 mm³, 10% anticoagulant is added to product to prevent clumping. (L Sanders, A Thomas, personal communication, March, 1999).

Complications

There are several potential procedure complications that can be avoided or minimized by early intervention.[16] A large volume of the anticoagulant, sodium citrate, is used to keep the blood from clotting.[40] The citrate binds to ionized serum calcium causing hypocalcemia. This causes the patient to experience tingling in the extremities and around the mouth. Nurses routinely give calcium carbonate (TUMS) (SmithKline Beecham) at the beginning of apheresis and as needed throughout the procedure. Intravenous calcium gluconate may be needed if the hypocalcemia becomes severe. Hypovolemia may also be problematic, especially for patients with a history of cardiac problems. The patient may complain of light-headedness, chilling, dizziness, shaking, and experience dysrhythmia. Thrombocytopenia is problematic with some types of equipment because platelets are destroyed by the process. Because platelet counts may drop by 50% during the apheresis procedure, the patient should have an adequate platelet count (>100,000/mm³) before the procedure.[49] Occasionally, the blood flow rate through the CVC may be altered or decreased. Usually a position change by the patient quickly remedies the problem.

Human Cord Blood

Another alternative for obtaining bone marrow stem cells is using placental or umbilical cord blood. Since 1988, there have been an estimated 500 related or unrelated donor umbilical cord blood transplants, and large-scale collection and storage of UCB stem cells is currently under way.[56,57] Cells are collected immediately after delivery of the placenta.

Advantages of using UCB include immediate availability, absence of donor risk, absence of donor attrition, and low risk of transmissible infectious disease such as cytomegalovirus and Epstein Barr virus. A decreased risk of GVHD is considered an advantage because the fetal cells are not competent immunologically. Umbilical cord blood may allow expansion of available donor pools in targeted ethnic and racial minorities currently underrepresented in all marrow donor registries.[57,58] Disadvantages of using UCB include the lowered risk of GVHD in patients with hematologic malignancy. The lowered risk may cause a potentially higher risk of relapse as there is no graft-versus-leukemia effect. Other disadvantages include an increased risk of genetic disorder transmission and insufficient numbers of cells for engraftment for larger recipients.

FAHCT standards require a personal and family history of the biological mother (and father if available) to be obtained and documented prior to or within 48 hours of UCB collection. Infectious disease testing of the maternal donor is required no more than 30 days prior to or within 48 hours of UCB collection. Cord blood is not accepted for unrelated transplant if there is a history of a genetic disorder in the immediate family that may affect the recipient.[3]

The outcomes from UCB transplants are being evaluated. There is one report of 143 UCB transplants from 45 centers. The 1-year survival rate of 78 recipients from related donors was 63%; and in 65 patients receiving unrelated UCB transplants, 1-year survival was 29%.[59] Many issues need to be resolved, including optimal methods for harvesting, processing, storing, ethical and regulatory issues, minimum number of cells needed for engraftment in larger recipients, risk of chronic and acute GVHD with mismatched donors, the malignancy relapse rate, the potential for gene therapy, ex vivo expansion, and immunologic reconstitution following transplant.[58]

Cell Processing and Storage

Cell Identification

The cells obtained from the bone marrow, peripheral blood, or umbilical cord are processed and cryopreserved in the same way. The American Association of Blood Banking (AABB) and FAHCT have strict standards for processing and storage of the cells.[3,60] Processing begins with the identification of the cells needed for engraftment. Previously, the CFU-GM assay was used to identify the adequate dose. This technique requires 14 days, which is problematic when trying to determine if additional cells should be collected. More recently, the CFU-GM assay has been replaced by CD34 assay. In most studies, there is a correlation between CD34+ cells and CFU-GM. The CD34+ assay is an easier, standardized method that provides a real number of circulating progenitor cells, not a number predicted after growth in culture.[61,62] At present, CD34+ selection is the most reproducible and standardizable technique available. However, most agree that further development of techniques to identify the number and type of cells essential for engraftment is needed.[28,63]

Processing

After collection, the stem cells are processed by weighing and calculating the concentration of cells per milliliter. For concentrations exceeding 2×10^8 nucleated cells/mL, additional plasma may be collected and added to adjust the volume to the optimal freezing concentration of 2×10^8 nucleated cells/mL. The product is tested for tumor or other outside contamination, total CD34+ count, mononuclear cell counts, and viability of the cells.[4] FAHCT describes the product as "minimally manipulated" cells since they have not been exposed to any ex vivo procedures that selectively remove, enrich, or expand the cell populations.[3]

Quality management of collected cells is strictly defined and monitored through the American Association of Blood Banks and FAHCT (see Table 22-2). The laboratory must document the testing of the components, laboratory control procedures, and the sterility and accuracy of all supplies and reagents. Equipment is kept clean and calibrated. Component identification and labeling is done in a manner to prevent mislabeling of components.

Tumor Contamination

One of the main reasons for using blood rather than bone marrow–derived cells for autologous transplantation was to avoid tumor contamination from bone marrow.

Minimal residual disease is especially important for patients with hematologic malignancy. The outcome after either autologous BMT or BCT in patients with acute myelogenous leukemia is similar. Therefore, the shortened nadir period produced by BCT may be the only advantage of one procedure over the other. Gene-marking experiments have clearly indicated that relapses can originate from tumor cells contaminating the cryopreserved cells.[52] The development of sensitive methods for the detection of tumor cells indicates that contamination of peripheral blood with malignant cells is common.[64]

Cell sorting

CD34 assays are useful to separate the malignant cells in a positive selection process. CD34 antigens are not present in breast tumors, neuroblastoma, lymphoma, and multiple myeloma cells.[65] Therefore, PPSCs and progenitor cell isolates should be free from tumor contamination. That is, in theory, selecting only CD34+ cells should produce a product that is free from malignant cells for those diseases.[52,66]

Mobilized peripheral CD34+ progenitors can be highly purified with good recovery and can result in complete and sustained engraftment.[52] Methods currently in use include magnetic activated cell sorting of the product and continuous flow technology for cell enrichment. One method, Ceprate™, stem cell concentration kit (Cell Pro, Inc., Bothell, WA) was recently approved by the Food and Drug Administration (FDA) for both bone marrow stem cell and PBPC processing.

Purging techniques

Purging of autologous bone marrow and peripheral blood cells is another strategy to decrease the risk of tumor contamination. Purging is done after harvest or apheresis and before cryopreservation. A number of procedures are used to remove the malignant cells, all of which have potential to harm the PPSCs and progenitor cells.[67,68] This manipulation often results in delayed or failed engraftment.

Several different approaches are used for purging. Pharmacologic methods use chemotherapeutic agents such as 4-hydroperoxycyclophosphamide (4HC) or mafosfamide. Immunologic methods use monoclonal antibodies (MoAbs) and toxins. A MoAb must specifically target the malignant cell and have no effect on hematologic stem cells in order to effectively purge the tissue. If the targeted antigen is present at high concentration on the cell surface, there is increased cell killing. Because the MoAbs are not toxic themselves, they are combined with other agents or toxins. Physical methods are used to mark the malignant cells, then separate them from the isolate.[65] To date, there are no randomized trials to identify the best purging methods.

Manipulation of hematopoietic progenitor cells includes ex vivo expansion, gene manipulation, and T-cell depletion. *Ex vivo expansion* involves the expansion in culture of one or more populations of cells. There are reports that selected CD34$^+$ cells grown for 7–14 days in liquid culture systems with various combinations of HGFs, such as stem cell factor, IL-3 or IL-6 with G-CSF or GM-CSF, and EPO, produce an increase in numbers of CFU-GM. The long-term durability of these cells is not proven.[1] Umbilical cord blood cells have also been expanded in culture using PIXY 321, flt-3 ligand, and EPO. To date, these expanded populations of cells have not been reinfused into humans.[58]

Gene manipulation involves the insertion of one or more genes into one or more populations of cells. An example of this is the insertion of multidrug resistance gene (MDR-1) into PBPCs in order to confer resistance to drugs such as paclitaxel. Following engraftment of modified PBPCs, the patient can tolerate repeated exposure to high-dose paclitaxel.[69,70]

Marrow stem cells usually contain 10%–15% mature T lymphocytes. Patients who receive these T lymphocytes and have no posttransplant immunosuppression experience 80%–100% incidence of grade 2–4 acute GVHD.[71] Depletion of the T lymphocytes greatly decreases this risk and can be accomplished through a variety of laboratory techniques. Clinical trials continue to evaluate the most effective procedures.

Freezing of cells

Cells for autologous transplant or umbilical cord cells being harvested and stored for later use are frozen. Cryopreservation is necessary to prevent stem cell damage and assure viability of the stem cells. Cells are frozen and stored at temperatures below 32°F (0°C). Dimethylsulfate is added so that cells will not lyse when thawed. Freezing of the cells begins at -1°C (33.8°F)/minute down to -40°C (-40°F), and -2°C (28.4°F)/minute from -40°C (-40°F) to -80°C (-112°F). The cells are stored in liquid nitrogen between -100°C (-148°F) and -196°C (-321°F).[72] Freezers for component storage must have an alarm system that signals a change in temperature. The alarm system must be monitored 24 hours per day. Newer techniques for cryopreservation using a methanol bath and nonprogrammed freezer are being developed. This process is simpler and less costly, enabling use in almost any institution.[73]

Conditioning Therapy

Conditioning therapy is the regimen used to prepare the patient to receive the transplanted stem cells. The goal of the preparative regimen varies depending on the type of transplant and the disease indication.[74–76] The goal for allogeneic transplantation is to eradicate remaining disease, ablate the marrow to make room for donor marrow, and suppress the immune system to prevent GVHD. In autologous transplantation, immunosuppression is not needed as the patient is the source of cells. However, antitumor and ablative effects are still needed.

Total Body Irradiation

Total body irradiation is used for immunosuppression and tumor eradication. Advantage of this systemic treatment include (1) no sanctuary sites of tumor, (2) even distribution of the dosage, (3) no detoxification or excretion needed after administration, and (4) the dose can be tailored for the patient's specific needs (i.e., boosted or shielded).[77] Total body irradiation was originally given as a single fraction of 10 Gy. This dose produced idiopathic interstitial pneumonitis in more than 70% of patients. The dose is now fractionated and given at 1.5–2.0 Gy twice daily for 3 days for a total dose of up to 12 Gy.[78]

The procedure for TBI takes 20–30 minutes per fraction. The patient usually is placed in a side-lying position and changes to the opposite side midway through the procedure. Toxicities of TBI are both acute and delayed and can be more severe depending on the chemotherapeutic agents administered (Table 22-5).[79]

Chemotherapy

Total body irradiation and high-dose cyclophosphamide have been tested alone as preparative regimens for allogeneic BMT, but the results were not sufficient. The combination provided an excellent response in hematologic malignancies and became the gold standard in the 1970s and 1980s.[2] Busulfan was tested to replace TBI and was found to be effective, though there are different toxici-

Table 22-5 Toxicities of Total Body Irradiation

Toxicities	Onset	Duration
Acute		
Nausea	Immediate	48 hr
Severe vomiting	3–5 days	3–5 days
Diarrhea	3–5 days	3–5 days
Fever	Immediate	24 hr
Skin erythema	Immediate	3–4 days
Severe skin changes	4–10 days	Variable
Oral mucositis	4–10 days	Variable
Parotitis	24 hours	24–48 hr
Delayed		
Interstitial pulmonary pneumonitis	2 mo	
Gonadal dysfunction	Variable	
Cataracts	10 yr	
Second malignancy	10 yr	

ties.[74] Cyclophosphamide and busulfan are most often used in allogeneic BMT centers without TBI capability. The regimens for preparation for autologous transplant vary according to the underlying disease. The agents are selected for maximum effect against specific malignancies (Table 22-6).[74–76] The dosages that constitute high-dose therapy are those that increase systemic exposure threefold as compared to a standard dose.[74]

Reinfusion

Reinfusion of the bone marrow stem cells or PBPCs should occur 24 hours after high-dose chemotherapy in order to prevent damage to the reinfused stem cells by residual chemotherapy. The exception to this guideline is for thiotepa, which requires 48 hours for protection of the transplanted cells.

Blood cell transplant reinfusion

If PBPCs are collected in more than one apheresis, the volume to be transplanted is contained in more than one bag. On the day of transplantation, day 0, the cells are transported in the frozen state to the patient's bedside. The primary container is sealed and aseptic. A secondary container is provided to prevent leakage. The outer shipping container is thermally insulated at whatever level is needed to maintain the frozen state until reaching the bedside. A basket of supplies needed during reinfusion should be available at bedside. After patient identification is verified per patient armband, the cells are thawed quickly in a warm water bath 98.6–104°F (37–40°C). Rapid warming prevents small ice crystals from forming by recrystallization. Cells are fragile and should not be manipulated prior to infusion. To preserve viability of cells, they are infused immediately, within 10–20 minutes of thawing per bag. A second bag of cells should not be thawed until the previous bag is completely infused.

A connector is inserted to break the vacuum and provide a needle puncture site. Using a 60-mL syringe, the cells are withdrawn from the collection bag. The cells are administered through a tunneled CVC by IV push via a separate line infusing preservative-free normal saline. The saline should help to minimize blood cell clumping. There should not be any filters on the IV line. The bag is emptied and rinsed with 10–20 mL of preservative-free saline. The process is repeated until each bag is infused. Depending on the volume of the DMSO, the patient may receive 1–3 bags, wait several hours, then resume. Dimethylsulfate is 10% of the volume of each bag. The maximum DMSO per day the patient should receive is 1 mL/kg; DMSO causes the patient to have an immediate garlic taste. Because DMSO is excreted by the lungs, the same odor is obvious in the immediate area of the patient's room. Some patients report a lessened taste if they suck on hard candies during and after the infusion. Nausea can be associated with reinfusion. It is temporary and usually not disturbing. Still, patients are premedicated with an antiemetic. Shortness of breath or complaints of chest tightness are associated with both the cells passing through the lungs and the temperature of the cells. Reducing the rate of infusion should alleviate these symptoms.

Bone marrow transplant reinfusion

Allogeneic hematopoietic cells are infused through the CVC much like any blood product would be given. The cells arrive at the bedside within hours of collection. Ideally, there is minimal manipulation of these life-giving cells. Patient identity is verified using the patient armband. The patient is premedicated to lessen the side effects most commonly associated with the infusion. Premedications may include a prophylactic antiemetic such as lorazepam. Diphenhydramine chloride, meperidine hydrochloride, hydrocortisone, acetaminophen, and methylprednisolone may be given as prophylaxis for transfusion-related hemolytic reactions. Furosemide and mannitol are given to prevent fluid overload. The patient is usually hydrated prior to, during, and following the infusion. Strict intake and output should be monitored to prevent fluid overload. Vital signs are monitored as per blood transfusion standards. Cells are infused using an infusion pump. It is important to avoid any filters on the IV tubing. The infusion bags should be gently agitated periodically to prevent fat cells from clumping in the product.

Inpatient Issues

A number of factors have influenced the transition of transplant care from inpatient to outpatient settings: technological advances, improved symptom management, cost containment initiatives, and patient advocacy.[80] Patients receiving allogeneic transplants generally receive the conditioning treatment and immediate posttrans-

Table 22.6 Common Chemotherapeutic Agents Used in Hematopoietic Cell Transplantation

Diseases	Conditioning Regimen	Acronym
Hematologic, general	Busulfan/cyclophosphamide	BU/CY
	Busulfan/cyclophosphamide/total body irradiation	BU/CY/TBI
	Busulfan/melphalan	BU/MEL
	Cyclophosphamide/total body irradiation	CY/TBI
	Cytarabine/total body irradiation	Ara-C/TBI
Hematologic, acute leukemia	Cyclophosphamide/etoposide/total body irradiation	CY/VP/TBI
	Cyclophosphamide/cytarabine/total body irradiation	TCC
	Etoposide/total body irradiation	VP/TBI
Non-Hodgkin's Lymphoma	Carmustine/etoposide/cytarabine/cyclophosphamide	BEAC
Hodgkin's and non-Hodgkin's lymphoma	Carmustine/etoposide/cytarabine/melphalan	BEAM
	Cyclophosphamide/carmustine/etoposide	CBV, BCV
Hodgkin's, non-Hodgkin's lymphoma, multiple myeloma	Busulfan/cyclophosphamide/etoposide	BU/CY/VP
Multiple myeloma	Melphalan/total body irradiation	Mel/TBI
Breast	Mitoxantrone/etoposide/thiotepa	MVT
Breast, solid tumors	Cyclophosphamide/carmustine/cisplatin	CBP
	Cyclophosphamide/thiotepa/carboplatin	STAMP-5, CCT
	Cyclophosphamide/thiotepa/cisplatin	CTP
Breast, solid tumors, testicular	Cyclophosphamide/etoposide/cisplatin	CVP, CPE
Solid tumors	Ifosfamide/carboplatin/etoposide	ICE

plant care in the hospital. Use of HGFs has decreased the length of the nadir, allowing for earlier discharge. In addition, many institutions have outpatient facilities (hotel accommodations) available 7 days per week to allow for daily assessments and treatments while providing for social/family needs.

Outpatient Issues

Blood cell transplant developments that support outpatient care have greatly influenced the move to outpatient care. These include decreased number of aphereses, greater number and applications of HGFs, intravenous antibiotics and antiemetics[81], increased numbers of BCT procedures, standardization of care, and increased numbers of community centers.[80] The cost-effectiveness of BCT is difficult to evaluate. A cost-effectiveness analysis that measures the value (years of life saved) over cost of medical interventions is frequently used to support continued use of BCT.[8]

Advances in BMT include improved management of GVHD, increased long-term disease-free survival, increased availability of donors through the National Marrow Donor Program, and more diseases being treated with BMT. Also, more alternative care models and strate-

gies are being utilized. These provide safe, quality, cost-effective care to reduce or eliminate the need for hospitalization.[80] Ruiz-Arguelles et al recently reported using noncryopreserved cells to successfully transplant patients in an outpatient setting using a 1-day conditioning regimen of high-dose melphalan in patients with hematologic malignancy.[82]

Successful outpatient models have modified chemotherapy regimens to decrease side effects such as mucositis and hemorrhagic cystitis. Drug combinations that have been shown to be successfully used for outpatient transplantation, are melphalan, carmustine/triethylenethiophosphormide (thiotepa), cyclophosphamide/mesna/thiotepa, and busulfan. Duke's program is the most successful program to date. Women with breast cancer receiving autologous BMT are hospitalized for chemotherapy, then discharged to a nearby hotel. The women are seen daily in the outpatient clinic and 67% are readmitted for a short period (<5 days).[81] Others have also used a hotel to support outpatient care.[83] Patients in the Duke program received empiric ceftazidime every 8 hours during the period of neutropenia. Two doses were administered in the outpatient clinic and the night dose was administered at the hotel by a visiting nurse. This model adjusted the level of care provided in the clinic according to the length of time after transplant. During the first 2 weeks posttransplant, patients received physician assessments one to two times per day. More stable patients were seen by the physician two to three times per week.

Autologous BCT in the home was reported by Hermann et al.[84] Twenty-five adults with multiple myeloma, non-Hodgkin's lymphoma, or Hodgkin's disease received all care at home except for the infusion of blood stem cells. Participation in the program required the availability of a caregiver. A clinical nurse specialist made visits to the home twice a day and reported to the physician and evening nursing staff on the BMT patient unit. Sixty percent of patients required admission to the hospital for a median of 5 days for management of complications, which is comparable to other outpatient models. Patients participating in the program expressed high satisfaction with the care received at home.

Outpatient TBI is also being evaluated. Sixty-eight pediatric patients received outpatient TBI in preparation for transplantation.[85] To control the nausea and vomiting usually associated with TBI, the patients receive an oral 5HT-3 antagonist every 8 hours. Due to the efficacy of this classification of antiemetics, the nausea and vomiting was well-controlled with only one patient requiring intravenous hydration and one patient requiring hospitalization for intractable diarrhea and dehydration.

The clinic/home care option for transplant is not available for all patients. Patient selection requires assessment of medical condition, functional status, family support, and psychosocial history.[38] Geographical distance from the center is considered if there is no adequate housing nearby. Both the patient and caregiver must be able to understand the treatment and demonstrate ability to fully cooperate with all required treatments. Studies comparing the cost and safety implications for patients receiving HCT in various settings are ongoing. Meisenberg compared the cost and safety data for ninety-four patients receiving autologous BCT in three settings: inpatient, partial outpatient, and total outpatient.[86] The average length of stay was 17.3, 8.2, and 2.7 days, respectively. The mean procedure costs were $39,700, $36,200, and $29,400, respectively. There was no difference in toxicity or overall response. As efforts continue to reduce the cost of HCT, it will be interesting to see if the patients who have available caregivers providing a significant amount of care will receive direct benefit through premium discounts or reimbursement for care provided.

Conclusion

The nurse caring for patients undergoing HCT will continue to be challenged by the rapid progress and changes in the field. The technical developments for the mobilization, collection, processing, and reinfusion of hematopoietic cells require professionals who are committed to continual study. Participation in ongoing research will produce conditioning regimens modified for outpatient administration and more effective medications for symptom management. As HCT care continues to be delivered outside of the standard inpatient unit, the nurse must collaborate more closely with family caregivers and community health professionals.

References

1. Boiron JM, Reiffers J, Lowenthal RM: Blood cell transplantation: Past, present and future. *Hematol Cell Ther* 38:399–407, 1996
2. Horowitz MM: Uses and growth of hematopoietic cell transplantation, in Thomas ED, Blume KG, Forman SJ (eds): *Hematopoietic Cell Transplantation* (ed 2). Boston, Blackwell Science, 1999, pp 12–18
3. Foundation for the Accreditation of Hematopoietic Cell Therapy: *Standards for Hematopoietic Progenitor Cell Collection, Processing and Transplantation.* Omaha, NE, FAHCT 1996, pp 1–58
4. O'Connell SA, Schmit-Pokorney K: Blood and marrow stem cell transplantation: Indications, procedures, process, in Whedon MB, Wujcik D (eds): *Blood and Marrow Stem Cell Transplantation: Principles, Practice, Nursing Insights* (ed 2). Sudbury, MA, Jones and Bartlett, 1997, pp 66–99
5. Jassak PF, Riley MB: Autologous stem cell transplant. *Cancer Pract* 2:141–145, 1994
6. Wujcik D, Downs S: Bone marrow transplantation. *Crit Care Nurs Clin North Am* 4:149–166, 1992
7. Blume KG, Amylon MD: The evaluation and counseling of candidates for hematopoietic cell transplantation, in Thomas ED, Blume KG, Forman SJ (eds): *Hematopoietic Cell Transplantation* (ed 2). Malden, MA, Blackwell Science, 1999, pp 371–380
8. Yee GC: Peripheral blood progenitor cell transplantation: Economic issues. *Pharmacotherapy* 18:9–16, 1998
9. King CR: Peripheral stem cell transplantation: Past, present, and future, in Buchsel PC, Whedon MB (eds): *Bone Marrow Transplantation: Administrative and Clinical Issues.* Sudbury, MA, Jones and Bartlett, 1995, pp 187–211
10. Buchsell PC, Kapustay PM: Peripheral stem cell transplantation, in Hubbard SM, Goodman M, Knobf MT (eds): *Oncology Nursing.* Philadelphia, Lippincott, 1995, pp 1–14
11. Wodinsky HB, Dillman RO, MacDonald SA: Assessing peripheral blood stem cell transplant technology. *J Oncol Manage* 3:22–27, 1994
12. Mahaney FXJ: Bone marrow transplant for breast cancer: Some insurers pay, some insurer's don't. *J Natl Cancer Inst* 86:420–421, 1994
13. Peters WP, Rosner G, Vredenburgh J, et al: A prospective, randomized comparison of two doses of combination alkylating agents (AA) as consolidation after CAF in high-risk primary breast cancer involving ten or more axillary lymph nodes (LN): Preliminary results of CALGB 9082/SWOG 9114/NCIC MA-13. *Proc Am Soc Clin Oncol* 18:1a 1999 (abstr A2)
14. Bezwoda WR: Randomized, controlled trial of high dose chemotherapy (HD-CNVp) vs. standard dose (CAF) chemotherapy for high risk, surgically treated, primary breast cancer. *Proc Am Soc Clin Oncol* 18:2a 1999 (abstr A4)
15. Stadtmauer EA: Phase III randomized trial of high-dose chemotherapy (HDC) and stem cell support (SCT) shows no difference in overall survival or severe toxicity compared to maintenance chemotherapy with cyclophosphamide, methotrexate and 5-fluorouracil (CMF) for women with

metastatic breast cancer who are responding to conventional induction chemotherapy: The Philadelphia intergroup study (PBT-01). *Proc Am Soc Clin Oncol* 18:1a, 1999 (abstr A1)

16. Walker FE, Roethke SK, Sandman V, et al: Guiding patients and their families through peripheral stem cell transplantation with the help of a teaching booklet. *Oncol Nurs Forum* 21:585–591, 1994

17. Burns JM, Tierney K, Long GD, et al: Critical pathways for administering high-dose chemotherapy followed by peripheral blood stem cell rescue in the outpatient setting. *Semin Oncol Nurs* 22:1219–1224, 1995

18. Wujcik D: Hematopoietic growth factors, in Rieger PT (ed): *Biotherapy: A Comprehensive Overview.* Sudbury, MA, Jones and Bartlett, 1995, pp 113–133

19. Coiffier B, Philip T, Burnett AK, et al: Consensus conference on intensive chemotherapy plus hematopoietic stem cell transplantation in malignancies, Lyon, June 4-6, 1993. [Review]. *Ann Oncol* 5:19–23, 1994

20. Spangrude GJ: Biological and clinical aspects of hematopoietic stem cells. [Review]. *Annu Rev Med* 45:93–104, 1994

21. To LB, Haylock DN, Simmons PJ, et al: The biology and clinical uses of blood stem cells. *Blood* 89:2233–2258, 1997

22. Korbling M, Juttner C, Henon P, et al: Blood versus bone marrow transplants, in Gale RP, Juttner C, Henon P (eds): *Blood Stem Cell Transplants.* New York, Cambridge University Press, 1994, pp 87–98

23. Bensinger W: Isolating stem and progenitor cells, in Gale RP, Juttner CA, Henon P (eds): *Blood Stem Cell Transplants.* New York, Cambridge University Press, 1994, pp 32–42

24. Hogge DE, Sutherland HJ, Lansdrop PM, et al: The elusive peripheral blood hemopoietic stem cell. *Semin Hematol* 30: 82–91, 1993

25. Shpall EJ, Warkentin PI, Jones RB: Guidelines for the procurement and manipulation of stem cells for transplantation, in Thomas ED, Blume KG, Forman SJ (eds): *Hematopoietic Cell Transplantation* (ed 2). Malden, MA, Blackwell Science, 1999, pp 417–430

26. Hegland J: Transplant immunology: HLA and issues of stem cell donation, in Whedon MB, Wujcik D (eds): *Blood and Marrow Stem Cell Transplantion* (ed 2). Sudbury, MA, Jones and Bartlett, 1997, pp 43–65

27. Eaves CJ, Eaves AC: Stem and progenitor cells in the blood, in Gale RP, Juttner CA, Henon P (eds): *Blood Stem Cell Transplants.* New York, Cambridge University Press, 1994, pp 20–31

28. Juttner CA, Henon P, Gale RP: Blood stem cell transplants: Current state, future directions, in Gale RP, Juttner CA, Henon P (eds): *Blood Stem Cell Transplant.* New York, Cambridge University Press, 1994, pp 167–180

29. Thomas ED, Storb R: The development of the scientific foundation of hematopoietic cell transplantation based on animal and human studies, in Thomas ED, Blume KG, Forman SJ (eds): *Hematopoietic Cell Transplantation* (ed 2). Malden, MA, Blackwell Science, 1999, pp 1–11

30. Korbling M, Fliedner TM: History of blood stem cell transplants in Gale RP, Juttner CA, Henon P (eds): *Blood Stem Cell Transplants.* New York, Cambridge University Press, 1994, pp 9–19

31. Craig JL, Turner ML, Parker AC: Peripheral blood stem cell transplantation. *Blood Rev* 6:59–67, 1992

32. Sheridan W, Juttner CA, Szer J, et al: Granulocyte-colony-stimulating factor (G-CSF) in peripheral blood stem cell (PBSC) and bone marrow (BM) transplantation. *Blood* 76: 565, 1990

33. Sacher RA: Bone marrow and stem cell transplantation—Where are we going? *Semin Hematol* 30:130–133, 1993

34. Champlin RE: Peripheral blood progenitor cells: A replacement for marrow transplantation? *Semin Oncol* 2:15–21, 1996

35. Anderlini P, Korbling M, Dale D, et al: Allogeneic blood stem cell transplantation: Considerations for donors. *Blood* 90:903–908, 1997

36. Arcese W, Aversa F, Bandini G, et al: Clinical use of allogeneic hematopoietic stem cells from sources other than bone marrow. *Haematologica* 83:159–182, 1998

37. Kapustay PM: Blood cell transplantation: Concepts and concerns. *Semin Oncol Nurs* 13:151–163, 1997

38. D'Andrea B, Belliveau D, Birmingham J, et al: High-dose chemotherapy followed by stem cell transplant: The clinic/home care experience. *J Care Manage* 3:46–84, 1997

39. Poloquin CM: Overview of bone marrow and peripheral blood stem cell transplantation. *Clin J Oncol Nurs* 1:11–17, 1997

40. To LB: Mobilizing and collecting blood stem cells, in Gale RP, Juttner CA, Henon P (eds): *Blood Stem Cell Transplants.* New York, Cambridge University Press, 1994, pp 56–74

41. Bender JG, To LB, Williams S, et al: Defining a therapeutic dose of peripheral blood stem cells. [Review]. *J Hematother* 1:329–341, 1992

42. Ketterer N, Salles G, Raba M, et al: High CD34(+) cell counts decrease hematologic toxicity of autologous peripheral blood progenitor cell transplantation. *Blood* 91: 3148–3155, 1998

43. Perez-Simon JA, Caballero M, Corral MJ, et al: Minimal number of circulating CD34+ cells to ensure successful leukapheresis and engraftment in autologous peripheral blood progenitor cell transplantation. *Transfusion* 38: 385–391, 1998

44. To LB, Shepperd KM, Haylock DN: Single high doses of cyclophosphamide enable the collection of high numbers of hemopoietic stem cells from the peripheral blood. *Exp Hematol* 18:442–447, 1990

45. Korbling M, Fliedner TM, Holle R, et al: Autologous blood stem cell (ABSCT) versus purged bone marrow transplantation (pABMT) in standard risk AML: Influence of source and cell composition of the autograft on hemopoietic reconstitution and disease-free survival. *Bone Marrow Transplant* 7:343–349, 1991

46. Sheridan WP, Begley CG, Juttner CA: Effect of peripheral-blood progenitor cells mobilized by filgrastim (G-CSF) on platelet recovery after high-dose chemotherapy. *Lancet* 339: 640–644, 1992

47. Henon P, Becker M: Cytokine enhancement of peripheral blood stem cells. *Stem Cells* 11:65–71, 1993

48. Moog R, Muller N: Technical aspects and performance in collecting peripheral blood progenitor cells. *Ann Hematol* 77:143–147, 1998

49. Wagner ND, Quinones VW: Allogeneic peripheral blood stem cell transplantation: Clinical overview and nursing implications. *Oncol Nurs Forum* 25:1049–1055, 1998

50. Brugger W, Mocklin W, Heimfeld S, et al: Ex vivo expansion of enriched peripheral blood CD34+ progenitor cells by stem cell factor, interleukin-1 beta (IL-1beta), IL-6, IL-3, interferon-gamma, and erythropoietin. *Blood* 81:2579–2584, 1993

51. Purdy MH, Hogan CJ, Hami L, et al: Large volume ex vivo expansion of CD34-positive hematopoietic progenitor cells for transplantation. *J Hematother* 4:515–525, 1995

52. Handgretinger R, Lang P, Schumm M, et al: Isolation and transplantation of autologous peripheral CD34+ progeni-

tor cells highly purified by magnetic-activated cell sorting. *Bone Marrow Transplant* 21:987–993, 1998

53. Watanabe T, Takaue Y, Kawano Y: Peripheral blood stem cell transplantation: An update. *J Med Invest* 44:25–31, 1997

54. Jones HM, Jones SA, Watts MJ, et al: Development of a simplified single-apheresis approach for peripheral-blood progenitor-cell transplantation in previously treated patients with lymphoma. *J Clin Oncol* 12:1693–1702, 1994

55. Valbonesi M: Hemopoietic stem cells: Technical and methodological considerations. [Review]. *Stem Cells* 11:58–63, 1993

56. Cairo MS, Wagner JE: Placental and/or umbilical cord blood: An alternative source of hematopoietic stem cells for transplantation. *Blood* 90:4665–4678, 1997

57. Kline RM, Bertolone SJ: Umbilical cord blood transplantation: providing a donor for everyone needing a bone marrow transplant? *South Med J* 91:821–828, 1998

58. Koller MR, Manchel I, Maher RJ, et al: Clinical-scale human umbilical cord blood cell expansion in a novel automated perfusion culture system. *Bone Marrow Transplant* 21:653–663, 1998

59. Gluckman R, Rocha V, Boyer-Chammard A, et al: Outcome of cord-blood transplantation from related and unrelated donors. Eurocord Transplant Group and the European Blood and Marrow Transplantation Group. *N Engl J Med* 337:373–381, 1997

60. Bone marrow and peripheral blood progenitor cells, in Klein HG (ed): *16th Edition Standards for Blood Banks and Transfusion Services* (ed 16). Bethesda, MD, American Association for Blood Banks, 1994, pp 47–51

61. Di Nicola M, Siena S, Bregni M, et al: Quantization of CD34 + peripheral blood hematopoietic progenitors for autografting in cancer patients. *Int J Artif Organs* 16:80–82, 1993

62. Demirer T, Buckner CD, Bensinger WI: Optimization of peripheral blood stem cell mobilization. *Stem Cells* 14:106–116, 1996

63. Bender JG, Unverzagt K, Walker DE, et al: Phenotypic analysis and characterization of CD34 + cells from normal human bone marrow, cord blood, peripheral blood, and mobilized peripheral blood from patients undergoing autologous stem cell transplantation. *Clin Immunol Immunopathol* 70:10–18, 1994

64. Brenner MK, Rill DR: Gene-marking to improve the outcome of autologous bone marrow transplantation. *Lancet* 3:33–36, 1993

65. Shpall EJ, Jones RB, Bearman SI, et al: Transplantation of enriched CD34-positive autologous marrow into breast cancer patients following high-dose chemotherapy: Influence of CD34-positive peripheral-blood progenitors and growth factors on engraftment. *J Clin Oncol* 12:28–36, 1994

66. Berenson R: Human stem cell transplantation. *Leuk Lymphoma* 11:137–139, 1993

67. Freedman AS, Nadler LM: Developments in purging in autotransplantation. *Hematol Oncol Clin North Am* 7:687–715, 1993

68. Gulati SC, Duensing S: Evaluating the benefit of purging in stem cell transplantation. [Review]. *Cancer Invest* 12:447–449, 1994

69. Korbling M, Champlin R: Peripheral blood progenitor cell transplantation: A replacement for marrow auto- or allografts. *Stem Cells* 14:185–195, 1996

70. Hanania EG, Fu S, Zu Z, et al: Chemotherapy resistance to taxol in clonogenic progenitor cells following transduction of CD34 selected marrow and peripheral blood cells with a retrovirus that contains the MDR-1 chemotherapy resistance gene. *Gene Ther* 2:285–294, 1995

71. Kernan NA: T-cell depletion for the prevention of graft versus host disease, in Thomas ED, Blume KG, Forman SJ (eds): *Hematopoietic Cell Transplantation* (ed 2). Malden, MA, Blackwell Science, 1999, pp 186–196

72. Meagher RC, Herzig RH: Techniques of harvesting and cryopreservation of stem cells. *Hematol Oncol Clin North Am* 7:501–533, 1993

73. Hernandez-Navarro F, Ojeda E, Arrieta R, et al: Hematopoietic cell transplantation using plasma and DMSO without HES, with non-programmed freezing by immersion in a methanol bath: Results in 213 cases. *Bone Marrow Transplant* 21:511–517, 1998

74. Doroshow JH: Pharmacological basis for high-dose chemotherapy, in Thomas ED, Blume KG, Forman SJ (eds): *Hematopoietic Cell Transplantation* (ed 2). Malden, MA, Blackwell Science, 1999, pp 103–122

75. Dix SP, Yee GC: Pharmacologic and biologic agents, in Whedon MB, Wujcik D (eds): *Blood and Marrow Stem Cell Transplantation: Principles, Practice, and Nursing Insights* (ed 2). Sudbury, MA, Jones and Bartlett, 1997, pp 100–150

76. Conditioning regimens and management of common toxicities, in Shapiro TW, Davison DB, Rust DM (eds): *Stem Cell and Bone Marrow Transplantation*, Sudbury, MA, Jones and Bartlett, 1997, pp 39–80

77. Shank B: Radiotherapeutic principles of hematopoietic cell transplantation, in Thomas ED, Blume KG, Forman SJ (eds): *Hematopoietic Cell Transplantation* (ed 2). Boston, Blackwell Science, 1999, pp 151–167

78. Lin H, Dryzmala RE: Total body and hemibody irradiation, in Perez CA, Bracy LW (eds): *Principles and Practice of Radiation Oncology*. Philadelphia, Lippincott-Raven, 1997, pp 333–342

79. Dudjak L: Alternatives in dose fractionization and treatment volume, in Dow KH, Hilderly LJ (eds): *Nursing Care in Radiation Therapy*. Philadelphia, Saunders, 1992, pp 285–294

80. Buchsel PC, Kapustay PM: Models of ambulatory care for blood cell and bone marrow transplantation, in Wheden MB, Wujcik D (eds): *Blood and Marrow Stem Cell Transplantation: Principles, Practice, and Nursing Insights* (ed 2). Sudbury, MA, Jones and Bartlett, 1997, pp 525–561

81. Peters WP, Ross M, Vredenburgh JJ, et al: The use of intensive clinic support to permit outpatient autologous bone marrow transplantation for breast cancer. *Semin Oncol* 21:25–31, 1994

82. Ruiz-Arguelles GJ, Ruiz-Arguelles A, Perez-Romano B, et al: Non-cryopreserved peripheral blood stem cell autotransplants for hematological malignancies can be performed entirely on an outpatient basis. *Am J Hematol* 58:161–164, 1998

83. McGuire TR, Tarantolo MD, Reed E: Peripheral blood progenitor cells: Enabling outpatient transplantation. *Pharmacotherapy* 18:17S–23S, 1998

84. Herrmann RP, Leather M, Leather HL, et al: Clinical care for patients receiving autologous hematopoietic stem cell transplantation in the home setting. *Oncol Nurs Forum* 25:1427–1432, 1998

85. Applegate GL, Mittal BB, Kletzel M, et al: Outpatient total body irradiation prior to bone marrow transplantation in pediatric patients: A feasibility analysis. *Bone Marrow Transplant* 21:651–652, 1998

86. Meisenberg BR, Ferran K, Hollenbach K, et al: Reduced charges and costs associated with outpatient autologous stem cell transplantation. *Bone Marrow Transplant* 21:927–932, 1998

CHAPTER 23

Complications of Hematopoietic Cell Transplantation

Susan A. O'Connell MSN, RN, OCN®

INTRODUCTION

Marrow and blood stem cell transplantation, also known as hematopoietic cell transplantation, is a widely used therapeutic modality in the field of cancer care that offers a long-term, disease-free survival in more than 50% of some patients with previously fatal diseases. *Transplantation* is defined as the transfer of living tissues or organs from one part of the body to another or from one individual to another. There are three major types of marrow and blood stem cell transplantation: autologous, allogeneic, and syngeneic. Their names indicate the source of the marrow or blood cells that are transplanted or infused into the recipient.

Both acute and chronic complications can occur in all three types of transplantation. There are specific complications, however, that occur only in allogeneic transplantation; these are discussed in detail in this chapter. This therapy challenges clinicians to manage the associated complications and psychosocial issues. Complications are generally the result of (1) the conditioning regimens (chemotherapy and radiation), (2) graft-versus-host disease, or (3) problems associated with the original disease, and (4) the adverse effects of the medications. Figure 23-1 illustrates the sequence of major complications occurring during the first year following hematopoietic cell transplantation. Acute complications of hematopoietic cell transplantation generally occur during the first 100 days, whereas chronic complications tend to occur after day 100. This chapter reviews both acute and chronic complications of marrow and blood cell transplantation as well as important supportive management and psychosocial issues encountered by patients, families, and donors.

Acute Complications

Acute Graft-Versus-Host Disease

Graft-versus-host disease (GVHD) remains a major complication of allogeneic bone marrow transplant (BMT), with an overall incidence occurring in 25%–70% of patients despite GVHD prophylaxis.[1] The primary organs affected by GVHD are the skin, gastrointestinal tract, and liver. Graft-versus-host disease is an immunologic disease and occurs in an acute and chronic form. It is thought to be a graft-host response in which the grafted donor T-lymphocytes recognize disparate non–human leukocyte antigen (HLA) host cell antigens and initiate cytotoxic injury directed against host (patient) tissue.

Acute GVHD occurs during the first 100 days posttransplant, with the median day of onset being day 17.[2] Acute GVHD occurs in 15%–80% of patients undergoing allogeneic BMT.[3] High-risk factors for the development of acute GVHD include unrelated donor and HLA-mismatched donor, sex mismatching, donor parity, older age, and the type of GVHD prophylaxis that was used. Table 23-1 shows the influences of these factors on the incidence of GVHD.[4]

Clinical features of acute GVHD usually begin with a macropapular rash that may be pruritic or painful, red in color, and initially involves the palm and soles. As the rash progresses, the cheeks, neck, and trunk are affected, often with papule formation. A hyperacute, or severe, form of GVHD includes fever, influenza-like symptoms, generalized erythroderma, and desquamation developing 7–14 days after transplant. A skin biopsy is performed to confirm the diagnosis.

Symptoms of intestinal GVHD include profuse diar-

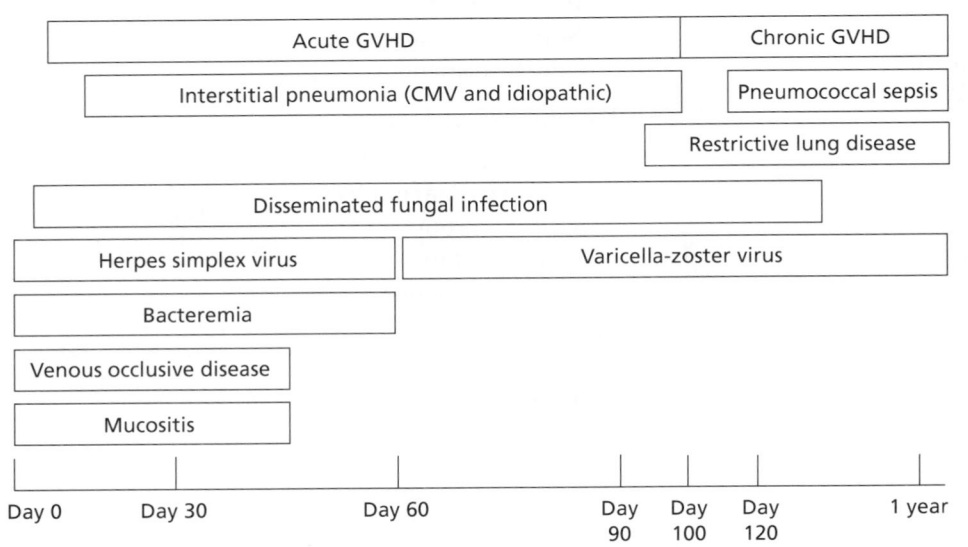

Figure 23-1 Sequence of major complications occurring during the first year following hematopoietic cell transplantation (GVHD = graft-versus-host disease; CMV = cytomegalovirus.)

Table 23-1 Influences on Incidence of Graft-Versus-Host Disease (GVHD)

Degree of Significance	Less GVHD	More GVHD
More significant		
Donor-recipient relationship	Identical twins	Mismatched relative
	Self (autologous)	Unrelated donor
	Matched sibling	
Type of prophylaxis	T-cell depletion	None
	MTX + CSP combined	MTX alone
		CSP alone
Donor-recipient sex match	Male to male	Parous female to male
	Male to female	
	Nulliparous female to male	
Less significant		
Age of recipient and donor	Younger	Older
BMT conditioning regimen	Less intensive	More intensive
Post-BMT viral infection (particularly cytomegalovirus)	No	Yes

MTX = methotrexate; CSP = cyclosporine; BMT = bone marrow transplant.

Reprinted with permission from Treleaven J, Wiernik P (eds): *Color Atlas and Text of Bone Marrow Transplantation.* London, Mosby-Wolfe, 1995, p 144.[4]

rhea (several liters per day), gastrointestinal bleeding, crampy abdominal pain, and ileus. Some patients present with anorexia and dyspepsia and may not have lower tract involvement. Gastrointestinal endoscopy and biopsy are necessary to confirm the diagnosis. Liver GVHD usually presents with elevated liver enzymes, liver tenderness, hepatomegaly, and eventually jaundice. A biopsy of the liver is usually not required if the patient already has documented GVHD of the skin or gut but is useful in some cases. Thrombocytopenia, anemia, capillary leak syndrome, hemolysis, and ocular symptoms have been reported in patients with acute GVHD.[5]

Tables 23-2 and 23-3 present a commonly used system for the staging and grading of acute GVHD. In general, grade I acute GVHD has a favorable prognosis and does not require treatment. Grade II GVHD is a moderately severe disease that usually results in multiorgan involvement and requires therapy. A recent modification of grade II disease includes symptoms of nausea, anorexia, food intolerance, or vomiting confirmed to be enteric GVHD on upper intestinal biopsy.[6] Grade III disease is severe, multiorgan GVHD, and grade IV disease is life-threatening or fatal acute GVHD. The overall grade of acute GVHD predicts the clinical course. There is usually a lower survival probability in those with higher grades (III and IV) of GVHD.

Several methods are used to prevent the incidence and decrease the severity of acute GVHD. Because histocompatibility is a key determinant of the kinetics of GVHD, molecular characterization of class I and II antigens can be a powerful asset in the selection of the best available family or unrelated donor.[7] Matching seronegative marrow recipients with seronegative donors also appears to reduce the risk of both cytomegalovirus (CMV) infection and GVHD.[8] Laminar airflow (LAF) protective isolation with gut decontamination has been shown to decrease the incidence of acute GVHD and improve survival in transplant patients with aplastic anemia prepared with cyclophosphamide (CY) alone.

Prophylaxis

Single-agent immunosuppression (e.g., procarbazine, cyclosporine, methotrexate, FK-506 [tacrolimus]), and combination immunosuppresive agents (e.g., methotrexate, cyclosporine, steroids, FK-506,) all show a reduction in the incidence and severity of acute GVHD.[7] Studies evaluating antibody prophylaxis using intravenous immu-

Table 23-2 Staging of Acute Graft-Versus-Host Disease

Stage	Skin	Liver	Gut
1 (mild)	Maculopapular rash <25% body	Bilirubin 2–3 mg/dL	Diarrhea 500–1000 mL/day or persistent nausea
2 (moderate)	Maculopapular rash 25–50% body	Bilirubin 3–6 mg/dL	Diarrhea 1000–1500 mL/day
3 (severe)	Generalized erythroderma	Bilirubin 6–15 mg/dL	Diarrhea >1500 mL/day
4 (life-threatening)	Desquamation and bullae	Bilirubin >15 mg/dL	Pain +/− ileus

Data from Sullivan[5]; Weisdorf et al.[6]

Table 23-3 Grading of Acute Graft-Versus-Host Disease

| Grade | Stage | | | |
	Skin	Liver	Gut	Functional Impairment
0	0	0	0	0
I	1–2	0	0	0
II	1–3	1	1	1
III	2–3	2–3	2–3	2
IV	2–4	2–4	2–4	3

Data from Sullivan.[7]

noglobulin, antihuman thymocyte globulin (ATG), and anti-T-cell monoclonal antibodies against the interleukin-2 (IL-2) receptor agents show beneficial results in the prevention or severity of GVHD.[7] Antibody inhibition of interleukin-1 (IL-1) and tumor necrosis factor (TNF) in murine models showed a reduction of GVHD and mortality, however human trials failed to show a reduction in the incidence of acute GVHD.[9] Similarly, an anti-CD5-immunotoxin conjugate did not appear to be of benefit in clinical trials to prevent GVHD.[10] Depletion of T cells in the marrow showed significant reductions in the incidence and severity of acute GVHD, but results to date are offset by an increase in the rate of graft failure and recurrent leukemia.[11] New immunosuppressive agents being investigated as single agents or in combinations to prevent GVHD include trimetrexate, fludarabine, rapamycin (sirolimus), and ultraviolet radiation.[7] Agents to prevent T-cell activation or proliferation or to promote donor-specific anergy via blockage of B7 family costimulation are moving toward clinical trials.[12]

Treatment

Cytotoxic agents and glucocorticoids are used to treat diagnostically confirmed acute GVHD. Treatment is mandated for grade II–IV acute GVHD and consists of continuing the original immunosuppressive prophylaxis (cyclosporine [CSP] or FK-506) and adding methylprednisolone (MP).[13] Most centers use a steroid taper schedule based on patient response rather than a fixed dose schedule.[13]

Patients in whom initial therapy for GVHD failed may receive a variety of salvage regimens including OKT3 monoclonal antibody, mitogenic anti-CD3, antibody specific for the IL-2 receptor, therapies to downregulate IL-1 with IL-1 receptor or IL-1 receptor antagonist, ATG ultraviolet radiation, FK-506 and mycophenolate mofetil (MMF).[7] In addition, the dose of prednisone is increased.

Gut rest, hyperalimentation, pain control, and antibiotic prophylaxis are routine elements of supportive care for patients with GVHD. Oral agents may be used to improve nausea, oral intake, and diarrhea. Antiviral prophylaxis may be especially important in preventing inter-

stitial pneumonia in patients with refractory GVHD. New antifungal agents, such as liposomal amphotericin, may be useful in preventing and treating serious mycotic infections.

Outcome is predicted by the overall grade of acute GVHD and response to treatment. Mortality in patients with grade II–IV acute GVHD is lowest in those who achieve a complete response to initial treatment for GVHD.[14] Factors associated with a decrease in survival include HLA-nonidentical marrow donors, liver abnormalities in addition to GVHD, early time of onset, and type of treatment for GVHD.[7]

Nursing management of patients experiencing acute GVHD is complex and requires expert skills and knowledge. Important nursing interventions include:

- Careful assessment to identify early clinical manifestations and to distinguish GVHD from other complications
- Identification of high-risk patients and knowing the period when acute GVHD is most likely to occur
- Providing appropriate skin care for patient comfort and prevention of infection
- Monitoring of fluid balance including intake and output, daily weights, serum electrolytes
- Providing adequate nutritional support including monitoring of caloric intake, consulting with the nutritional support team, and administration of nutritional supplementation
- Preventing complications associated with gastrointestinal bleeding by monitoring stools, hemoglobin and hematocrit, and administration of blood product therapy
- Pain management for individuals experiencing abdominal pain from liver or gut involvement with acute GVHD
- Prevention and treatment of infections
- Monitoring and administration of medications used to prevent or treat acute GVHD, including patient education of the medication program and side effects.

Infection

Infections contribute significantly to morbidity and mortality in patients undergoing marrow and blood cell transplantation. The high-dose chemotherapy and radiation therapy used as the preparative conditioning regimen prior to transplantation results in prolonged severe neutropenia, placing these patients at high risk for developing bacterial, viral, and fungal infections. The degree and severity of neutropenia is directly related to the risk of infection. Other factors that would place the transplant patient at higher risk of developing an infection include type of transplant (allogeneic or autologous), history of infections, placement of central venous catheters, and damaged oral or gastrointestinal mucosa.[15] Patients undergoing allogeneic transplantation have an increased risk of infection because of the need for immunosuppression following marrow or blood stem cell transplant to prevent GVHD. Many centers prophylactically treat patients with antibiotics, although this practice is changing due to the concern of the development of antibiotic resistance. Hematopoietic growth factors have been found to reduce the duration and severity of neutropenia following marrow and blood stem cell transplant.[16]

During the first 3 months posttransplant, recipients are at high risk for developing bacterial, fungal (candida and aspergillus), herpes simplex virus, *Pneumocystis carinii*, and cytomegalovirus infections. Common sites of infection are the oral cavity, gastrointestinal mucosa, skin, and catheter sites. Bacterial infections are the most common type of infection following high-dose therapy, with 15%–25% of patients developing bacteremia. When a patient develops neutropenic fever, empiric antibiotics are initiated. These antibiotics usually involve a combination of an aminoglycoside, penicillin, and possibly vancomycin.[17] Acyclovir is commonly administered prophylactically to prevent reactivation of the herpes simplex virus and to treat some other types of herpes infections. Ganciclovir prophylaxis has been found to be effective in suppressing CMV infection and disease.[18] Detecting fungal infections is extremely difficult. Supportive care includes antifungal medications such as amphotericin B and rooms with HEPA filters or laminar airflow (LAF) rooms.

Early detection of infections is an important nursing consideration in the management of the marrow and blood stem cell transplant patient. Nurses should assess patients every 4 hours for infections. This assessment should include monitoring vital signs, assessing catheter sites and the oral mucosa, auscultating lung sounds, evaluating mental status, and monitoring laboratory values.

Gastrointestinal Complications

The incidence of intestinal complications remains high (up to 90%) in the patient undergoing marrow and blood cell transplant. However, the severity of these complications has decreased because of the development of more effective strategies to prevent and treat these disorders. Common causes of gastrointestinal complications include the conditioning regimen, GVHD, medications, and infections.

Nausea, vomiting, and anorexia are problems that most patients experience following the conditioning regimen (high-dose chemotherapy and radiation therapy). Inability to eat is currently a major reason for prolonged hospitalization and parenteral nutrition. Mucositis, which is also caused from the conditioning regimen, can produce swelling, pain, and in severe cases sloughing of the oropharyngeal epithelium, and may be worsened by superinfection and methotrexate therapy.[19] Oral mucositis reaches a peak 10–14 days following transplant and can lead to nausea and anorexia.[19] Mucositis pain can be effectively treated with

opioids but can lead to gastric stasis, intestinal ileus, anorexia, and vomiting.[20] After a period of 10–15 days, persistent gastrointestinal problems are usually caused by acute GVHD, infections, or medications.[21]

Acute GVHD may cause early gastrointestinal manifestations including anorexia, nausea, vomiting, abdominal pain, and diarrhea. Endoscopic biopsy is often needed to confirm the diagnosis of acute GVHD and rule out an infectious process.

Medications that may produce gastrointestinal complications include oral nonabsorbable antibiotics (nystatin), cyclosporine, trimethoprim-sulfamethoxazole, intravenous amphotericin, and high-dose opioids; they are frequent causes of nausea and occasionally protracted vomiting. Oral magnesium and nonabsorbable antibiotics can cause mild diarrhea.[22]

Infections of the gastrointestinal system may also cause anorexia, vomiting, and diarrhea. Common infections of the gastrointestinal system include CMV, fungal esophagitis, bacterial esophagitis, aspergillus, toxoplasma, or viruses.[21] Diarrhea associated with infections and acute GVHD is seen as early as day 7 in mismatched BMT patients.[23]

Hepatic Complications

Venoocclusive disease (VOD) is a result of combination chemotherapy, or chemotherapy plus irradiation therapy causing cellular damage to the liver. Venoocclusive disease is a disease of the small blood vessels in the liver and is characterized by an occlusion in the venous outflow tract of the liver. It develops in 10%–60% of patients during the first few weeks after transplant. The onset of VOD is usually before day 30 following transplantation. It varies in severity from mild, reversible disease to severe disease associated with multiorgan failure. Symptoms that determine the clinical diagnosis include jaundice, fluid retention, and hepatomegaly. Additional symptoms are liver tenderness, increased bilirubin, edema, and ascites.[24] Laboratory studies, ultrasound, computerized tomography (CT) scans, and liver biopsy are methods used to diagnose VOD. There is no definitive method to prevent or treat VOD. Approximately 70% of patients recover from VOD with supportive care only.[24] The overall goal of treatment is to support the patient and manage symptoms until VOD has run its course and the regenerative capabilities of the liver have had a chance to repair the damage from the disease. The management of VOD symptoms includes maintaining fluid and electrolyte balance, minimizing adverse effects of ascites, adjusting drugs to reflect impaired hepatic and renal function, avoiding compounding encephalopathy with drugs that alter mental status, and monitoring and treating coagulopathy. The overall goals of these efforts are to improve the impaired flow of blood through the liver and kidneys, redistribute body fluids appropriately, assist the body's compensatory efforts, and counter inappropriate compensatory actions that the body institutes.[25]

Other causes of liver injury following transplantation include infections (viral, fungal, and bacterial), GVHD, drugs, and total parenteral nutrition (TPN).[21]

Nursing care of the patient with hepatic complications includes:

- Identifying patients at high risk for developing liver complications

- Assessment of skin color, fluid balance, liver enlargement, or tenderness

- Monitoring bilirubin and other liver function tests

- Patient education regarding liver biopsy and other diagnostic tests

- Management of fluid balance

- Pain management

- Administration of medications used for treatment of hepatic complications such as thrombolytic therapy or antibiotic therapy.

Neurological Complications

Neurological and neuromuscular complications occur in up to 70% of marrow recipients as a result of the conditioning regimen, immunosuppressive drugs, and infection.[26] The peak time of onset is from pretransplant to 21 days after transplantation.[22] Neuropathy and somnolence occur pretransplant, while confusion or disorientation peak in the second week posttransplant.[27] Leukoencephalopathy occurs in 7% of marrow transplant recipients who have had prior cranial irradiation and intrathecal methotrexate.[28]

Nurses are often the first to recognize early neurological complications in the marrow and blood stem cell transplant patient. Routine neurological assessment should be performed in these patients to permit early recognition and treatment in an effort to prevent or limit neurological morbidity.

Hematologic Complications

Hematologic dysfunction is a major complication of marrow and blood cell transplantation. Patients undergoing high-dose chemotherapy and radiation therapy experience pancytopenia and immune dysfunction due to the ablation of hematopoiesis. Neutropenia may last for 2 or 3 weeks following transplant.[29] Nursing care of the neutropenic patient includes the prevention, early detection, and prompt management of infections. A comprehensive physical assessment including monitoring vital signs, with special attention to the oral mucosa, catheter sites, lungs, and rectal area, is required for the marrow and blood cell transplant patient who is neutropenic. The administration of hematopoietic growth factors, monitoring laboratory values, and patient education on neutropenic precautions are important nursing interventions.

Anemia and thrombocytopenia are expected events following marrow or blood stem transplantation. Multiple transfusions of red blood cells and platelets are required, especially during the first 30 days after transplant. Most transplant centers suggest maintaining the hemoglobin above 8.0 g/dL and platelet count above 20,000 mm³. It is recommended that red cells and platelets be depleted of leukocytes to prevent alloimmunization.[30] This can be accomplished through the use of a filter. Either random or single donor platelets can be used. If patients become refractory to platelet transfusion, HLA-matched unrelated or family donor platelets can be used. The use of CMV antibody–negative blood components in CMV antibody–negative patients has been suggested.[30] The risk of developing CMV infection is approximately 40% in CMV-negative patients who receive unscreened blood products. To prevent transfusion-associated GVHD, blood components are irradiated, which interferes with the ability of the lymphocytes to proliferate. Nurses must have a thorough understanding of the unique transfusion requirements of the marrow and blood stem cell transplant patient in order to closely monitor patient symptomatology and intervene accordingly.

Failure to engraft is another hematologic complication that can occur following blood or marrow cell transplantation. Following the myeloblative conditioning regimen, the blood cells are destroyed and hematopoiesis, or the process of blood cell formation, does not occur. The two general mechanisms of a failure of engraftment are (1) failure of donor cells to establish residence in the host, and (2) active rejection of transplanted donor cells by the host (recipient).[31] In sibling donor allogeneic transplant, the incidence of graft failure is 1–2%. After allogeneic transplantation, as many as 10% of patients will not engraft or, after initial engraftment, will experience a period of poor graft function.[32] The use of T-cell-depleted marrow as a donor source and the use of non-HLA identical donors is associated with an incidence of graft rejection as high as 15%. If graft failure occurs, treatment may include the administration of hematopoietic growth factors and a second marrow infusion or further cytoreduction with chemotherapy and radiation followed by second marrow or blood cell transplantation.[33]

Pulmonary Complications

Pulmonary complications following marrow or blood cell transplantation are a major cause of morbidity and mortality, affecting between 40% and 60% of patients.[34] Pulmonary complications include pneumothorax, pulmonary edema, pulmonary hemorrhage, and pulmonary infections including bacterial, viral, and fungal infections.

Pneumothorax may be associated with pretransplant placement of a central line. Spontaneous pneumothorax may also occur in the acute phase of transplant. Predisposing factors for pneumothorax include high-dose steroids, total body irradiation (TBI), and poor nutrition with recent weight loss.

Pulmonary edema can be seen in the first few days

following marrow or blood cell transplant and is due to fluid overload. Previous exposure to anthracyclines and the use of cyclophosphamide and TBI during conditioning can exacerbate this complication.

Pulmonary hemorrhage is usually associated with infection and thrombocytopenia. More rarely, acute hemorrhagic pulmonary edema can occur and is more common among HLA-matched unrelated transplant patients receiving high doses of cyclosporine. Pulmonary hemorrhage has a high mortality rate. Transient hypoxia may occur at the time of marrow infusion due to small particles of bone and fat in the marrow.

Bacterial respiratory infections occur in 20%–50% of individuals during the acute neutropenic phase following blood or marrow cell transplant. Between 8% and 25% of patients develop interstitial pneumonitis 30–100 days after transplant.[31] In half of the cases, CMV infection is the responsible organism. The remaining cases are due to other unidentifiable agents that are termed *idiopathic.* The incidence of pulmonary respiratory infections has decreased due to the routine use of prophylactic antimicrobial agents. Diffuse idiopathic pulmonary injury has an incidence of 7%–15% and a mortality that exceeds 60%.[35] The risk factors for idiopathic pneumonia include the type of chemotherapy in the preparative regimen, preexisting pulmonary abnormality, older age, TBI in the preparative regimen, methotrexate to prevent GVHD, and severe GVHD. Occasionally, patients respond to steroid treatment, but most do not. The mortality of marrow transplant patients with pneumonitis who require intubation and mechanical ventilation is greater than 90%.[36] Bronchoalveolar lavage has become the gold standard for diagnosing pneumonitis following marrow transplant; open lung biopsy is rarely used.

The herpes virus and CMV account for the majority of posttransplant viral respiratory infections. Herpes simplex pneumonitis occurs mainly in the first few weeks after transplant.[36] Other respiratory viruses that have been implicated in episodes of posttransplant pneumonitis include respiratory syncytial virus (RSV), the parainfluenza viruses, and adenovirus.

Respiratory fungal infections are mainly due to *Aspergillus* species, *Candida* species, and occasionally *Cryptococcus neoformans.* During the first 3 weeks posttransplant, the risk of developing *Aspergillus* infection has been estimated at 1% per day, with the risk increasing to 4.3% per day after day 22.

Pneumocystis carinii pneumonia (PCP) is an opportunistic organism that occurs in immunocompromised patients with defective T-cell function. The peak time for posttransplant development of PCP is between 30 and 100 days, and the organism is implicated in up to 4% of cases of infectious pneumonitis.

Cardiac Complications

Cardiac dysfunction can occur in the marrow or blood cell transplant patient who has received high-dose cyclo-

phosphamide. Cyclophosphamide is associated with a 5%–10% incidence of detectable hemorrhagic cardiomyopathy when used at transplant doses. The clinical picture consists of congestive heart failure, pericardial effusion, loss of electrocardiogram (ECG) voltage, and cardiomegaly developing in the first 10 days posttransplant. Minor ECG changes, such as ST-T wave segment changes, supraventricular arrhythmias, or pericarditis without hemodynamically significant effusion develop in the majority of patients receiving cyclophosphamide-containing regimens. The dose of cyclophosphamide is a major factor in the development of cardiac toxicity. The contribution of prior anthracycline therapy, mediastinal radiation therapy, or TBI to the development of cardiac toxicity is unclear. Baseline multiple gated aquisition (MUGA) scans are performed to measure left ventricular ejection fraction (LVEF) prior to transplant. Patients whose LVEF is less than 50% are excluded from transplantation at some centers. Most centers conduct daily ECGs prior to and during the administration of cyclophosphamide. Carmustine (BCNU) is another chemotherapeutic agent that is used in some transplant preparative regimens and has been reported to be associated with cardiac toxicity.[37]

Treatment of cardiac complications consists of symptomatic pharmacological support and fluid management. Pericardiocentesis or placement of a pericardial window may be necessary for hemodynamically significant pericardial effusions.[38] Routine nursing care should include identifying high-risk patients, managing fluids, and monitoring cardiac behavior as needed.

Oral Complications

Complications of the oral cavity develop in almost all patients undergoing blood or marrow cell transplantation. Oral complications are the direct or indirect result of the toxicities from the conditioning regimen. Herpes simplex virus and *Candida albicans* account for most oral infections, although their incidence has been dramatically reduced by the institution of prophylactic agents. Early intervention for oral complications may result in the institution of prompt treatment and prolonged survival.

Mucositis, often severe and extremely painful, develops in more than 75% of bone marrow transplant recipients, and its prevention, unfortunately, remains unsatisfactory.[39] Mucositis management can be challenging for the clinician and patient. Management is centered on supportive care approaches. Appropriate management is based on the severity of tissue damage and symptoms, prevention and treatment of infection, nutritional support, and proper assessment to determine the need for analgesics and opioids.[40]

Nurses are responsible for assessing the oral cavity frequently, educating patients regarding the rationale for the oral hygiene program, monitoring the compliance of the oral care protocol, and evaluating the effectiveness of the interventions. (See Chapter 20 for a detailed discussion on oral care protocols.) Many centers have teams including dentists and dental hygienists that focus on the prevention and treatment of oral complications.

Renal Complications

Renal failure related to chemotherapy, antibiotic therapy, cyclosporine, and FK-506 given prior to transplant is a frequent occurrence in the early posttransplantation period.[41] Renal impairment also occurs as a result of organ system dysfunction. The transplant nurse needs to monitor the fluid balance (weight, input, output, assessment of fluid status on physical examination), blood pressure, laboratory values, mental status, and medications to prevent acute renal failure, or to promote recovery following a diagnosis of acute renal failure. Medical management of the transplant patient in acute renal failure includes the administration of diuretics or volume replacement, correcting electrolyte imbalances, reducing further nephrotoxins, and managing infections. Hemodialysis or continuous renal replacement therapy (CRRT) may be required to help correct acute renal failure.[42]

Late Complications

The number of marrow and blood cell recipients is increasing rapidly. Most patients are able to live a relatively normal productive life. Some, however, develop delayed or long-term complications that compromise quality of life. Some delayed complications are transplant related (e.g., GVHD, immunodeficiency); others are due to the intensity of the preparative regimen (e.g., infertility, cataracts). Other delayed complications are related to the underlying disease (e.g., recurrence of disease), and many are multifactorial in etiology (e.g., secondary malignancies, chronic pulmonary disease).[43]

Chronic Graft-Versus-Host Disease

Chronic GVHD is the most common delayed complication, occurring in as many as 40%–60% of allogeneic transplant recipients.[44] It may develop from 2 months to 2 years after allogeneic transplant.[45] Risk factors include HLA disparity, prior acute GVHD, and increasing patient age. Some controversial risk factors include the use of blood stem cells versus marrow, the infusion of donor lymphocytes, unirradiated buffy coat or marrow reinfusions, and splenectomy. A reduction in chronic GVHD with prolonged cyclosporine prophylaxis or random red-cell transfusions given shortly before transplant has been shown.[5]

Chronic GVHD can affect the skin, liver, eyes, oral cavity, lungs, intestine, nerves, muscles, vagina, kidneys, and marrow function. Limited chronic GVHD includes localized skin involvement and hepatic dysfunction due to chronic GVHD. Extensive chronic GVHD involves either generalized skin involvement and localized skin involve-

ment or hepatic dysfunction due to chronic GVHD, plus liver histology or involvement of the eye, minor salivary glands, oral mucosa, or any other target organ.

Morbidity and mortality are highest in patients with a progressive onset of chronic GVHD directly following acute GVHD, intermediate in those with a quiescent onset following resolution of acute GVHD, and lowest in patients with a de novo onset. Death is usually due to infection. Figure 23-2 identifies possible GVHD complications.

Methods to prevent chronic GVHD have been studied and include modification of thymic function, T-cell depletion, the administration of intravenous immunoglobulin or immunosuppressive drugs, and prolonged immunosuppression.[5] These methods have proved to be either unsuccessful or controversial.

Medical management of chronic GVHD includes a combination of corticosteroids and immunosuppressive drugs (cyclosporine, FK-506). Azathioprine (AZT) may be added as secondary treatment. Thalidomide, clofazimine, psoralen-UV-A (PUVA), extracorporeal photopheresis, and low-dose total lymphoid irradiation are currently being studied in patients with steroid-refractory chronic GVHD.[5]

Antimicrobial prophylaxis is an important aspect of the treatment of patients with chronic GVHD. The relationships between immunodeficiency, GVHD-associated immunosuppression, and infection are complex interactions that are of critical importance in the management of these patients. Other supportive measures include replacement intravenous immunoglobulin, use of artificial tears, avoidance of sun exposure, physical therapy, and psychosocial support.[31]

Nursing care of the patient with chronic GVHD is complex and requires expert skills, knowledge, and creativity. Daily assessments, identifying high-risk patients, skin and wound care, pain management, monitoring lab values (e.g., Hgb, Hct, liver function tests), prevention and treatment of infection, administration of medications (e.g., intravenous immunoglobulin, immunosuppresive drugs, corticosteroids), and providing psychosocial support are all important components of nursing care of the patient with chronic GVHD.

Late Infectious Complications

Late infections occur in the blood and marrow transplant patient, especially in patients with chronic GVHD. Despite improvement in hematopoietic function, there are still marked abnormalities in the patient's immunologic defense. The major risk factors for infection in the postengraftment period (days 30–100) include the rate and extent of recovery of the host's new immune system, the presence of GVHD and its effects on immune recovery and mucosal barriers, and the use of immunosuppressive agents for the treatment of GVHD.[46]

The time of greatest immune deficiency after transplant is between the loss of native immunity and passively transferred donor immunity and the development of new

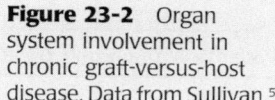

Figure 23-2 Organ system involvement in chronic graft-versus-host disease. Data from Sullivan.[5]

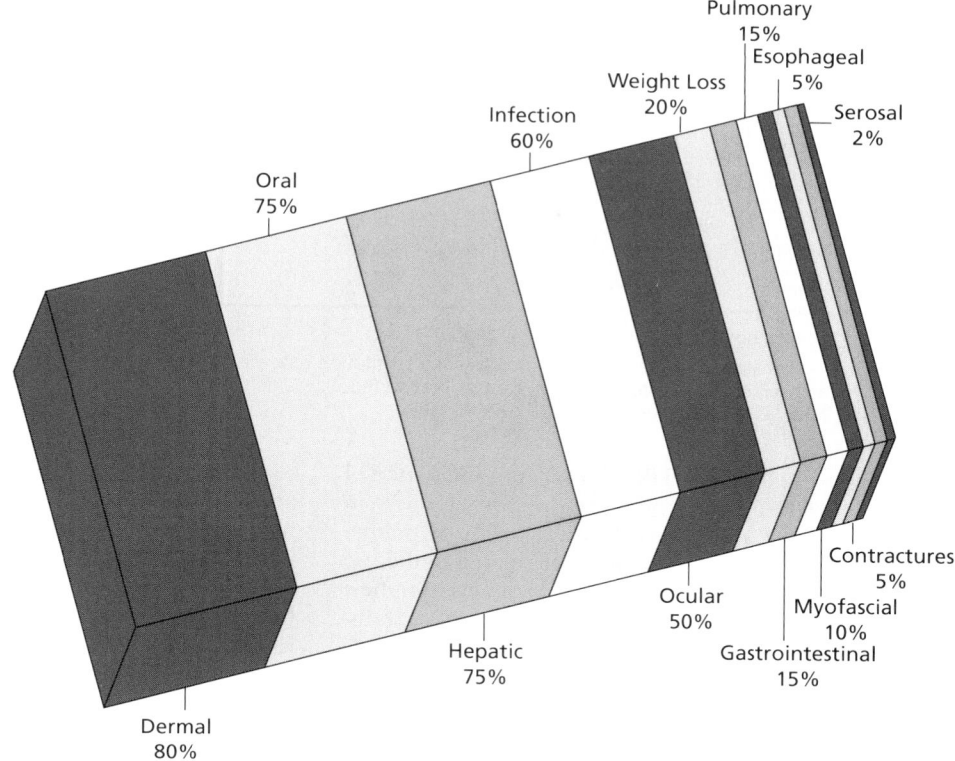

transplanted donor-related immune function. This occurs from days 50–100 after transplantation and corresponds to the time of greatest risk for infection during the postengraftment period. Recovery of immune function may be further delayed by the presence of GVHD. Because of the effect of chronic GVHD on immune function and the fact that the process of chronic GVHD damages epithelial cells in the skin, liver, and mucous membranes, GVHD is a major risk factor for infection during this phase of transplantation.[47]

Infections that occur secondary to defects in cell-mediated immunity predominate during this phase of transplantation. In patients with damaged anatomic barriers as a result of acute GVHD, bacterial and fungal infections may also occur. The single most significant pathogen in the postengraftment period is CMV.

The late phase of bone marrow transplantation occurs approximately 100 days after transplantation. This also represents the time at which chronic GVHD becomes evident. The major predispositions to infection are the effect of GVHD on target organs and the delay in recovery of the immune system that GVHD produces. In the absence of chronic GVHD, infection is unusual. The defects in immune function, which usually resolve by 1 year after transplantation, are persistent in the presence of chronic GVHD.

The infections that occur during the late posttransplantation period are commonly localized to the skin, upper respiratory tract, and lungs. Viral infections, primarily those due to VZV, are responsible for more than

40% of infections during this period. Bacterial infections, particularly those involving the lungs and upper respiratory tract, account for more than 33% of infections, while fungal infections are implicated in the remaining 20% of episodes.[48]

Medical management of late infectious complications includes prevention and prompt treatment of common infections found in the postengraftment and late posttransplantation phase and treatment of chronic GVHD. Nursing care of the patient during the postengraftment and late posttransplantation phase includes frequent assessment for signs of infection, identification of patients at high risk for infection, administration of antibiotics and intravenous immunoglobulin, and patient education regarding infection prevention.

In order to regenerate the immune system after transplantation, it is important to revaccinate the patient who is 1 year or more out from transplant.[31] Table 23-4 illustrates the timing of immunization following transplant.[51]

Ophthalmologic Complications

Cataracts are a common complication, occurring more often in women than men, and the incidence increases with age. Radiation therapy, chemotherapy, and glucocorticoids are thought to enhance cataract formation. In patients conditioned with TBI, cataracts develop approximately 1 year after transplant.[49] When patients are given single-dose TBI, the incidence of cataracts is 80% at 5–6

Table 23-4   Timing of Immunization Following Bone Marrow Transplant

Vaccine	Patients Without Chronic GVHD	Patients With Chronic GVHD
Diphtheria-tetanus toxoid	3–6 mo	3–6 mo
Oral poliovirus (Sabin)	Not recommended	Not recommended
Inactivated poliovirus (Salk)	6–12 mo	Not indicated if on IV immunoglobulin
Measles-mumps-rubella	1–2 yr	Not recommended
Varicella	2 yr	Not recommended

GVHD = graft-versus-host disease

Reprinted from Parkman R, Weinberg KI: Immunological reconstitution following hematopoietic stem cell transplantation, in Thomas ED, Blume KG, Forman SJ (eds): *Hematopoietic Cell Transplantation* (ed 2). Malden, MA, Blackwell Science, Inc., 1999, p 709. Reprinted by permission of Blackwell Science, Inc.[49]

years. When fractionated TBI is given, the incidence of cataracts is 30%–50%.[51] The incidence of cataracts in patients who have not been exposed to TBI or cranial irradiation is 20% and is thought to be related to the use of steroids.[51] Overall, the incidence of cataracts is highest in patients who received cranial irradiation prior to transplant. Although eye shielding might prevent cataracts, there is some reluctance to do so due to the relapse of leukemia observed in the ocular bulb. The treatment of choice is lens extraction and implantation of an artificial lens.

Other ophthalmic complications of marrow or blood cell recipients are generally related to immunosuppresive therapy, chronic GVHD, and associated infections. Graft-versus-host disease and infections may also cause scar formation. Long-term antibiotics and artificial tears can prevent some infections and scarring. Sicca syndrome, or dry-eye syndrome, has been observed in patients with chronic GVHD and some patients without chronic GVHD. A Schirmer's test is used to determine ocular lubrication. A reading of less than 10 confirms ocular sicca. Artificial tears can alleviate discomfort, however further treatment is sometimes required. Treatment is usually ligation of the canaliculi that normally drain the lacrimal fluid. Nursing management of the patient with potential or actual ophthalmic complications should include identifying high-risk patients and educating these patients regarding regular ophthalmologic follow-up.

Urologic Complications

Cystitis with microscopic or macroscopic hematuria occurs in 10%–15% of patients following marrow or blood stem cell transplant.[52] The cyclophosphamide metabolite acrolein causes inflammation of the bladder mucosa, which can be particularly severe in patients conditioned with a combination of cyclophosphamide plus busulfan.[53] In most patients, cystitis is an acute problem. Some patients, however, develop protracted hematuria and scarring of the bladder wall and present with a chronic problem of urinary frequency. Medical treatment consists of bladder irrigation, cystoscopic fulguration, and in

some severe cases cystectomy with construction of an artificial bladder from a bowel loop. Antispasmodic treatment may be helpful for patients with severe scarring. Viruses (e.g., CMV) may also be responsible for hematuria.

Patients receiving immunosuppressive therapy for GVHD, particularly women with vaginal GVHD, are at risk for recurrent urinary tract infections. Treatment is antibiotic therapy.

Late renal failure following transplant was once thought to be an infrequent problem. Renal insufficiency has been found, however, in 20%–25% of patients by 2 years after BMT, particularly in patients treated aggressively with nephrotoxic chemotherapy (e.g., platinum-based agents). Some patients have also shown features of hemolytic-uremic syndrome. Once nephropathy develops, control of hypertension is the mainstay of therapy.

Nurses need to assess for urologic complications and educate patients to report immediately urinary frequency, dysuria, hematuria, and abdominal pain so that prompt diagnosis and treatment can be initiated. Monitoring renal function tests and hemoglobin and hematocrit values are important nursing considerations.

Oral/Dental Complications

The incidence of chronic oral GVHD is approximately 80%, affecting the oral and pharyngeal mucosa. An oral sicca syndrome related to conditioning therapy or chronic GVHD may result in poor oral hygiene with recurrent infection and periodontitis. Dental decay may occur because of the altered consistency and reduced volume of saliva, so there is a lack of cleansing by saliva. Patients also experience pain in the oral cavity and may be hesitant to brush their teeth or perform good oral hygiene. Treatment includes meticulous oral hygiene, fluoride treatment, artificial saliva, and other supportive care measures.

Nursing management includes the teaching of comfort measures such as the use of topical medications to alleviate pain, burning, and soreness. Soft, bland diets are recommended. Artificial saliva and sugarless gums, hard candy, and mints can stimulate saliva production and alter taste. Vigorous oral hygiene measures including brushing teeth at least three times a day using a soft toothbrush, application of topical fluoride as ordered, flossing, and mouth rinses should be encouraged. Many centers have dentists and oral hygienists who specialize in dental complications and can be consulted for this late complication.

Pulmonary Complications

Chronic pulmonary complications affect at least 15%–20% of patients after blood and marrow cell transplant.[54] These complications include late interstitial pneumonitis, restrictive pulmonary changes, obstructive pulmonary disease, and progressive bronchiolitis obliterans.

Late interstitial pneumonitis occurs almost exclusively in patients with chronic GVHD.[54] They may fail to respond to bronchodilators but get better with immunosuppressive therapy. Most of these patients have clinical symptoms and pathological findings of GVHD, and treatment with immunosuppressive agents is usually required. Some patients show signs of interstitial fibrosis. Infectious organisms may be the cause of late interstitial pneumonitis in some patients. Late occurrences of CMV infections, including pneumonitis, is observed in 10%–15% of patients 1 year or later after transplant.[55] Treatment involves the administration of ganciclovir.

Restrictive pulmonary changes may occur and are not correlated with the type of conditioning regimen or with chronic GVHD and generally do not produce severe symptoms. They are, however, associated with an increase in long-term mortality. At 3 months posttransplantation, pulmonary function tests (PFT) frequently show a decline in total lung capacity and diffusing capacity. One-third of patients have restrictive defects (<80% of predicted values) at that time.[56] Routine evaluation of lung capacity is warranted. Aggressive bronchial hygiene and prophylaxis and prompt treatment of infections with antibiotic therapy might be useful in reducing severe infectious complications and in slowing disease progression.

Obstructive pulmonary disease is found in approximately 25% of patients by 3 months posttransplantation.[55] This number may not be significantly different from pretransplant findings as many patients have abnormal PFT values before transplant. The pathogenesis of obstructive pulmonary disease after blood or marrow stem cell transplantation is not fully understood. These obstructive changes might represent sequelae to extensive restrictive changes in the small airways or, as in obstructive bronchiolitis, may be related to small-airway destruction. Recurrent aspirations secondary to esophageal abnormalities (e.g., associated with GVHD) or purulent sinus secretions contribute to airway inflammation and the development of obstructive lung disease. Patients with chronic GVHD may also have low IgG and IgA levels, which may further contribute to infections. Obstructive pulmonary disease generally does not respond to bronchodilator treatment,

and only 30%–40% of patients improve on immunosuppressive therapy, with glucocorticoids given alone or in combination with cyclosporine.

Progressive bronchiolitis obliterans affects approximately 10% of all patients with active chronic GVHD.[57] It occurs as early as 3 months and as late as 2 years after blood or marrow stem cell transplant. The clinical course of bronchiolitis varies from mild, with slow deterioration, to diffuse necrotizing fatal bronchiolitis of the small airways. Generally, the disease does not respond well to conventional therapy of chronic GVHD with glucocorticoids. Combination therapy with glucocorticoids and cyclosporine is indicated. Azathioprine is sometimes added if pulmonary function continues to deteriorate.[57]

Late pulmonary complications require nurses to educate patients about their pathogenesis and the subtle signs and symptoms that they should report. Nursing care should include evaluating routine vital signs and pulmonary assessment, including observation for dyspnea or cough. Nurses should be aware of the patient's baseline PFTs and monitor results of routine follow-up studies.

Cardiac Complications

Delayed cardiac complications following marrow or blood cell transplantation may occur, however, the incidence is low. Table 23-5 lists risk factors for cardiac complications after BMT. Pretransplantation evaluation of ejection fraction has not been a reliable tool in predicting cardiac complications. It has been suggested that cardiac toxicity can be avoided if cyclophosphamide is administered as a dose per square meter rather than per kilogram.[58]

Anecdotal reports indicate that late cardiomyopathy due to BMT can be treated successfully by orthotopic cardiac transplantation.[59] Some cases of myocardial infarction have occurred at various time intervals after BMT but a cause-effect relationship has not been proved.[60]

Nurses should perform cardiac assessment routinely on the patient at risk for cardiac complications. Patient education should include signs and symptoms of cardiac

Table 23-5 Potential Risks for Cardiac Complications following Hematopoietic Stem Cell Transplantation

- Prior anthracycline therapy
- Mediastinal radiation therapy
- Total body irradiation
- Pretransplant ejection fraction <50%
- Prior carmustine (BCNU) therapy
- Prior high-dose cyclophosphamide
- Sepsis
- History of mitral valve disease
- Diagnosis of Hurler's syndrome or thalassemia

problems that require prompt reporting to the transplant team.

Endocrine Dysfunction

Endocrine dysfunction is not usually a life-threatening complication following marrow or blood cell transplantation. It can, however, affect the patient's quality of life in terms of functional ability. Cytotoxic therapy and in particular radiation therapy damage the endocrine glands. The intensive therapy given prior to transplantation and the conditioning regimen used in the preparation for transplant are expected to cause endocrine insufficiency.

Thyroid dysfunction is noted in a significant proportion of patients following transplant. There is a 30%–60% incidence of detecting elevated thyroid stimulating hormone at 5 years, with 5%–25% of pediatric transplant patients developing clinical symptoms of thyroid deficiency.[63] One study showed the incidence of thyroid dysfunction was 57% at 3 months and 29% at 14 months, suggesting that some spontaneous recovery has occurred.[61] The incidence is higher in children than in adults. The risk is higher in those receiving single-dose irradiation rather than fractionated irradiation and in those receiving pretransplant cranial irradiation. Yearly thyroid assessment in both adult and pediatric patients at risk is recommended. Thyroid replacement therapy is usually indicated for patients with hypothyroidism.

Growth disorders in children have been found to be multifactorial in origin. Busulfan conditioning regimens are much less frequently associated with growth disturbance. Recent data have shown that select patients have a good response to early initiation of growth hormone replacement.[62] Sexual development is also adversely affected in children. Approximately 60% of prepubertal boys undergoing TBI have delayed puberty, and 65% of prepubertal girls have delayed development with associated primary ovarian failure.[31]

Avascular Necrosis of the Bone

Avascular necrosis of the bone is a direct result of bone softening associated with glucocorticoid therapy given for management of GVHD. It may occur after a long delay or even after short courses of high-dose therapy.[63] It occurs in approximately 4%–8% of patients as early as 2 months and as late as 10 years after transplantation.[31] It affects the weight-bearing bones in particular. Patients may present with complaints of pain and limited range of motion. Treatment includes joint replacement, particularly in weight-bearing joints such as the hip, pain management, physical therapy, and sometimes antimicrobial therapy. Nurses need to monitor patients for bone pain, particularly in the weight-bearing joints, joint contractures, and limited range of motion if they have a history of steroid therapy following transplant.

Secondary Malignancies

As the number of patients surviving hematopoietic cell transplantation is increasing, secondary malignancies have been recognized as a complication. These secondary malignancies are composed of lymphoproliferative disorders, hematopoietic disorders, and solid tumors.[64]

Posttransplantation lymphoproliferative disorders (PTLDs) occur within months of transplantation. Factors associated with increased risk of PTLD include T-cell depleted marrow, HLA mismatch donor, use of ATG, and an underlying diagnosis of primary immunodeficiency. Complete responses to secondary malignancies have been achieved with interferon alfa and intravenous immunoglobulin.[65] Another effective treatment is monoclonal antibody directed at B-cell antigens CD21 and CD24. Preliminary data suggest that cellular therapy (i.e., donor leukocyte infusions, gene-marked Epstein-Barr virus [EBV]–specific T lymphocytes, thymidine kinase [TK]-transduced cells) can be effective in the treatment of PTLD.[66]

Solid tumors occur after allogeneic, syngeneic, and autologous marrow and blood stem cell transplantation. These tumors arise in the host cells and occur several years following transplant. A recent study of 2150 patients undergoing either allotransplantation or autotransplantation noted that 15 patients developed a solid tumor for a cumulative probability of 5.6% at 13 years.[65] Total body irradiation used in the conditioning regimen was the major risk factor. An analysis of 20,000 patients who underwent transplant in Seattle or were reported to the International Bone Marrow Transplant Registry indicates a risk of solid tumors of 2.2% at 10 years and 6.7% at 15 years after transplantation.[67] Common tumor types included head and neck cancer, squamous cell carcinomas, and melanomas of the skin, liver, brain, thyroid, bone, and connective tissue. Dose of TBI and risk of malignancy were positively correlated. Squamous cell carcinoma of the buccal cavity was strongly linked with male gender and chronic GVHD. The overall risk was highest in young patients who received transplants for acute leukemia and declined with increasing age at time of transplant. The etiology of solid tumor development following blood and marrow stem cell transplantation is multifactorial. Prevention of chronic GVHD and omission of irradiation when possible are important prophylactic measures.

The development of myelodysplastic syndrome (MDS) and leukemia after high-dose chemotherapy and autologous transplantation has been widely reported in recent years. Govindarajan et al noted that the University of Minneapolis estimated the probability of MDS in patients who received transplants for Hodgkin's disease or non-Hodgkin's lymphoma at 13.5% at 6 years.[68] Significant risk factors were the use of peripheral blood rather than marrow stem cells and age over 35 years at time of transplant. The extent of therapy given before transplant is a major factor contributing to the development of MDS or leukemia.

Treatment of posttransplantation MDS includes chemotherapy that is usually not well tolerated and allogeneic, blood and marrow stem cell transplantation. Transplantation is potentially curative, but the success rates are 10%–15%.[69]

Nursing measures for patients at high risk for developing secondary malignancies include close monitoring and reporting of suspicious signs and symptoms. Patients require education about warning signs and symptoms of cancer, routine cancer screening, and measures to prevent cancer development.

Neurological Complications

Delayed neurological complications can occur months or years after hematopoietic cell transplantation. Intrathecal chemotherapy, cranial irradiation, infections, systemic chemotherapy, chronic GVHD, and recurrent disease contribute to these complications. Several clearly documented cases of peripheral neuropathy with reduced nerve conduction velocity related to chronic GVHD have been reported.[70] Children are especially vulnerable to late neurological complications, with an incidence of approximately 7%.[70] Adults with prior central nervous system disease are also at risk.

Leukoencephalopathy, a severe syndrome where white matter of the brain is damaged, is related to extensive intrathecal administration of methotrexate alone or in combination with cranial irradiation and the use of TBI. It has been observed predominantly in pediatric patients, however, it has occurred infrequently in recent years due to a more judicious use of intrathecal therapy, brain shielding when appropriate, or omission of cranial irradiation whenever possible.

Infections of the CNS (e.g., *Toxoplasma gondii*) have occurred 6–8 months after hematopoietic transplantation.[71] Patients with chronic GVHD are particularly prone to develop septicemia and meningitis caused by encapsulated organisms. It is recommended that patients with chronic GVHD who receive immunosuppressive therapy also be given prophylactic antibiotics.[72]

Patients with neurological complications may have impaired memory, shortened attention span, and defects in verbal fluency. Children, particularly those who also received cranial irradiation, are likely to score lower than control subjects in visual-motor, processing tasks, and various IQ tests.[73]

Medical management is symptom management, supportive care, prevention and treatment of infections, and referral for neurological evaluation. Nurses are often the first to detect subtle neurological changes. CNS assessments are part of routine follow-up care. Prompt reporting of changes in neurological assessment is key to a positive outcome for adverse CNS effects.

Graft Rejection

Graft rejection or graft failure is a result of genetic disparity between the donor and recipient. Two forms of graft rejection are observed. *Primary rejection* is the absence of any sign of hematological function of the graft. *Late rejection* is defined as graft loss after initial graft function. At the present time, it is not clear whether the pathogenesis of late graft failure is the same as that for primary nonengraftment. Primary nonengraftment appears to result from a host-mediated graft rejection. Late graft failures have not necessarily been associated with an abrupt host-type lymphocytosis; rather, grafts fail with a steady decline in the absolute neutrophil count. The risk of graft failure with HLA-genotypically identical transplants is approximately 2%; with HLA-haploidentical transplants donors the risk is 3%–15%; with one disparity in the donor, the risk of rejection is 5%; with two or three disparities, the risk of rejection is 15%.[74] Several factors associated with an increased risk for graft rejection other than HLA mismatch include transfusion-induced alloimmunization of the recipient against the donor before transplant, patient diagnosis of acute myelogenous leukemia, conditioning regimen, pre- and posttransplant immunosuppressive regimen, depletion of T cells in the donor marrow, and transplantation of a lower marrow cell dose.[74]

In certain patients, recovery of autologous myeloid cells can occur, especially if the patient is treated with hematopoietic growth factors. If unsuccessful, patients with primary or late graft rejection can sometimes be rescued with a second transplant.[32]

Nurses play a key role in providing psychosocial support to the patient and family at the time of graft failure. Many patients are devastated when learning of this serious complication and have few treatment options left. Issues regarding second transplant or other treatment options, symptom management, and do-not-resuscitate (DNR) orders emerge. The nurse's role as patient advocate in ensuring that the patient has the information necessary to make informed decisions is critical.

Relapse

Although hematopoietic cell transplantation has proved successful for many diseases, relapse remains a major problem. Relapse in the patient with leukemia is infrequent before day 100 unless the patient has shown persistence of marrow tumor cells at days 7–21 after transplant.[75] In the case of chronic myelogenous leukemia (CML), cytogenetic evidence of relapse may predate morphological evidence by many months. There are a variety of tests that can help detect relapse of disease (i.e., cytogenetics, restriction fragment length polymorphism analysis, Y chromosome DNA detection).[76] When relapse occurs, it generally indicates that disease is still present in the host cells and that the conditioning regimen was not adequate to completely eradicate the tumor cells found in the marrow or other organs.

Treatment options include second transplant, standard or low-dose chemotherapy and irradiation, experimental trials (e.g., new agents, monoclonal antibodies, irradiation alone or in combination with chemotherapy), supportive care, or hospice care. Relapse of disease is a devastating event for patients and their families as the disease is usually no longer considered curable. Most patients are not able to undergo second transplant, have exhausted their treatment options, and are physically, emotionally, and financially drained.

Nurses play an important role in supporting patients and their families at the time of relapse. The transplant nurse works with the transplant team to provide information to the patient about their treatment options and to support their informed decisions. If the patient chooses palliative or hospice care, the transplant nurse can facilitate a smooth transition to these services so that the patient and family do not feel abandoned by the transplant team.

Supportive Management

Nutritional Support

The benefits of maintaining nutritional intake during marrow or blood cell transplant are well established. Developments in the use of hematopoietic growth factors have reduced the period of neutropenia and therefore have reduced the requirement to use parenteral nutrition for all patients throughout the course of transplant. The resolution of mucositis and the ability of transplant recipients to resume oral intake frequently coincide with the appearance of circulating neutrophils.[77]

While nutritional support remains an essential aspect of supportive care, the range of options is now varied. Nutritional support recommendations are currently based on the nutritional status of the individual patient, and total parenteral nutrition is no longer indicated for all patients undergoing blood or marrow stem cell transplant. Guidelines for the prescription of total parenteral nutrition vary from center to center.

Pain Management

Individuals undergoing marrow or blood cell transplantation may experience pain at various stages of the transplant process. Table 23-6 outlines sources of pain in the transplant patient according to the phase of transplant.

When a marrow or blood stem cell transplant patient reports pain, analgesic medications are often considered as a first line of treatment. It is important for the transplant nurse to consider nonpharmacological modalities as part of the treatment plan as well. Marrow and blood cell transplant patients with mucositis treated with optimal opioid and other analgesic methods experience only 50%–60% reductions in pain.[78]

Nurses and other members of the transplant team need to assess frequently for pain, identify its cause, implement pain management strategies (pharmacological and/or nonpharmacological) and evaluate the effective-

Table 23-6 Sources of Pain in the Marrow and Blood Stem Cell Transplant Patient

Pretransplant phase
Blood stem cell mobilization
Marrow harvest
Placement of central venous access device
Diagnostic procedures (marrow biopsy, lumbar puncture)
Disease-related pain

In-hospital, peritransplant period
Mucositis
Conditioning regimen-related cutaneous burns
Neuropathic-type pain associated with immunosuppressive drugs
Liver distention associated with VOD or infection
Bone pain associated with growth factors
Gastritis
Rectal pain/hemorrhoids
Painful urination from hemorrhagic cystitis
Diagnostic procedures
Disease-related pain

Postengraftment period
Graft-versus-host disease
Bone pain associated with steroid tapering
Herpes zoster infection
Diagnostic procedures (marrow biopsy, lumbar puncture)
Peripheral neuropathies from conditioning regimen
Gut pain from CMV
Disease-related pain

VOD = venous occlusive disease; CMV = cytomegalovirus.

ness of the pain management plan. Many centers have pain consult services that can work with the transplant team in the management of pain in the marrow and blood cell transplant patient.

Psychosocial Issues

Fertility and Sexuality

As the number of long-term survivors undergoing hematopoietic cell transplant increases, the issues of fertility and normal sexual function are becoming increasingly important problems. One of the major complications following high-dose chemoradiotherapy is infertility. This is a frequent concern of young patients about to undergo hematopoietic cell transplantation. The prospect of infertility post-transplant is as upsetting as the diagnosis of cancer itself. Disappointment over the prospect of infertility is not limited to patients who have never had children but extends to some individuals who already have children and would like to expand their family. Nurses can advise patients that it is sometimes possible to conceive a child after transplant. Men are sometimes able to cryopreserve sperm for future use and women are able to cryopreserve eggs for implantation following transplantation. While these steps are not guaranteed to result in a successful pregnancy, it may comfort patients to know that it is possible. It is also important for the patient to understand that although the technology is available, the procedure is expensive and there is not always sufficient time to collect sperm or eggs before proceeding to blood or marrow transplant. Often, previous chemotherapy or radiation therapy has reduced the quality and quantity of viable sperm necessary for storage.

Impairment of ovarian function following radiation therapy depends on the dose of radiation and the patient's age. Patients who are young and receive TBI can, on rare occasions, recover ovarian function and fertility. For most patients, however, infertility is a long-term problem.

The majority of men who have undergone TBI are azoospermic and have elevated follicle-stimulating hormone levels. Total body irradiation has less effect on testosterone levels, with some patients having normal luteinizing hormone levels and normal levels of testosterone. Some patients, however, experience hypogonadism that requires replacement therapy with transdermal testosterone patches or intramuscular injections. The effect of these therapies on sexual satisfaction is an important one.

Although women are usually informed that they will be infertile posttransplant, many are not warned that they may have premature menopause. For some women, this is a serious quality-of-life issue. When menopause occurs, it can shock and anger the unprepared patient. It is important to inform patients that they may become menopausal and to assure them that steps can be taken to overcome some of the consequences of premature menopause, such as osteoporosis. Women who hope to become pregnant after transplant, with the help of assisted reproduction techniques, should be assured that premature menopause will not eliminate this option.

Many transplant survivors experience significant, long-term changes in sexuality following treatment. Problems including lack of libido, inability to perform, and pain are reported both by persons with normal and abnormal hormone levels posttransplant. Little research has been done on the issue of sexuality posttransplant. What has been done suggests that women experience difficulty with sexuality posttransplant more frequently than do men.[79] It also appears that women who begin hormone replacement therapy within a year after their transplant experience fewer difficulties with sexuality than those who do not.[79]

Changes in sexuality can seriously stress a relationship, particularly if the survivor's partner believes that the problem is purely psychological rather than physical. While fatigue and psychological trauma do indeed affect sexuality, it is important that patients and their partners know that physical changes occur following transplant that may affect the survivor's sexuality as well. Patients should be advised that they may need to develop new approaches to intimacy after transplant to enable both partners to have a satisfying sexual relationship. Patients should be encouraged to report sexual difficulties and be provided with referrals to experts who may be able to help resolve some of the problems.

Cognitive Functioning

One complication that is often overlooked in the transplant population is the change in cognitive ability that may be experienced both short-term and long-term. It is widely known that learning difficulties are experienced by children following hematopoietic cell transplantation. Little information is available on cognitive changes experienced by some adult survivors of hematopoietic cell transplantation.

Some problems that have been identified by patients include memory difficulties, poor concentration, stuttering, difficulty in spelling, inability to perform jobs that were previously mastered, and difficulty learning new tasks. Many patients compensate by changing the way they manage information; for example, making lists, writing down all appointments, taking notes, and so on. For others, the solution is not so simple, and their problem may interfere with their ability to perform a job or learn a new skill.

Nurses should advise patients that changes in cognitive abilities may occur. If problems with cognitive functioning occur, the patient will know that the problem is not unique. Education of family members about possible cognitive changes is important so that they understand that the patient's new forgetfulness is not simply laziness but a consequence of the treatment.

Support Groups

While it is impossible to predict what a patient's quality of life will be following blood or marrow stem cell transplantation, it is sometimes useful for patients to hear about survivors or to speak to them directly. Sharing the results of one quality-of-life study in which 74% of the 125 patients reported that their quality of life was as good or better than it was pretransplant may alleviate the fear many patients experience.[80] Offering patients and their families the opportunity to talk to a survivor of blood or marrow transplantation can, for some, be quite encouraging. Hearing from a survivor who has gone through the transplant process can often provide hope to the patient and family. Many centers have support groups for patients and family members. Sometimes patient support groups are held separately from family support groups so the unique issues of each group can be addressed. Often, social workers, transplant nurses, psychologists, and other members of the transplant team are intimately involved in facilitating the groups.

Quality of Life

Quality-of-life studies in patients following hematopoietic cell transplant have steadily increased in the past few years. The high interest in this area parallels the growing number of patients who are long-time survivors and the major studies specific to quality of life in the hematopoietic cell transplantation population.[89–90] Table 23-7 summarizes the findings from eight of these studies.[82]

Through these studies we are beginning to learn how blood and marrow stem cell transplantation affects various aspects of patients' lives. Quality-of-life studies in this population are still limited and suffer from small samples, retrospective designs, and populations of mixed medical diagnoses.

Nurses caring for transplant survivors can provide patient support and teaching regarding sexual functioning. Referrals for psychological counseling, infertility programs, vocational counseling, financial counseling, rehabilitation programs, and support groups should be considered early in the transplant process.

Impact on Donor

Both allogeneic and syngeneic blood and marrow transplantation requires collection of marrow or stem cells from a healthy individual. The donor may or may not be related to the recipient. Issues surrounding the act of

Table 23-7 Summary of Major Quality-of-Life Studies

Author(s)	Population Studied	Major Findings
Chao et al[83]	58 HCT patients, followed for 1 year after transplant	Increase in global QOL from 90 days to 1 year; 63% employed full-time by 1 year; 53% maintained stable weight by 1 year; 34% reported frequent colds at day 90 and at 1 year; 72% good sleep patterns by 1 year; 98% appearance back to normal by 1 year; 64% sexually satisfied at 90 days and 180 days
Andrykowski et al[84]	28 adult HCT patients studied pretransplant and at 1 year posttransplant	Decrease in sexual relationships, blurred vision, increase in vigor, trend toward improved functional status; physical and psychosocial status improved for some and declined for others; males and older patients had greatest decline
McQuellon et al[85]	24 breast cancer patients, autologous transplant, compared pretransplant and at day 100	Improved overall physical functioning by day 100; 33% had depressive symptoms pretransplant; at day 100, 25% had concerns related to job or work, 42% finance, 51% general physical health, 26% general frame of mind, 34% appearance, 37% health or life insurance, 33% personal or intimate physical relations, 38% planning for the future
McQuellon et al[86]	86 allogeneic and autologous patients followed pretransplant through first year	24% depressed when admitted for transplant; 20% continued to be distressed at 1 year; physical status improved at time of discharge and day 100; psychological distress continued below baseline level and did not rise above baseline until 1 year; overall QOL decreased from before hospitalization to discharge and then improved at 100 days and 1 year; some deficits (e.g., fatigue) continued and remained at 1 year; majority of patients' QOL and psychological distress did not improve at 1 year; even after 1 year, 20%–25% of patients had persistent concerns
Whedon et al[87]	29 autologous patients measured 1–6 years after transplant	Global QOL was high; distress over visual changes and reproductive concerns and family stress; major concerns over sexual functioning and fertility changes; 66% returned to work; sense of purpose and maintaining hope reported
Grant et al[88]	450 long-term survivors	Moderate QOL scores that increased from 1 year to 5 years or more after BMT; fear of recurrence decreased as time since transplant increased; fatigue was a considerable problem during first year and showed little improvement across time
Bush et al[80]	125 long-term survivors	79% reported QOL to be same or better than before BMT; 80% rated current weight and QOL as good to excellent; survivors after 10 years had moderate emotional and sexual dysfunction, fatigue, eye problems, sleep disturbance, general pain and cognitive dysfunction, although severity of distress associated with these complications was low; 74% employed, 7% disabled, 5% seeking employment; long-term survivors had good mood and low psychological distress scores compared to other cancer populations; concerns about illness were mild and included a lack of social support as time after transplant increased
Molassiotis et al[89]	91 long-term survivors of allogeneic or autologous transplant compared to 73 patients receiving maintenance chemotherapy	Most transplant survivors reported good to excellent QOL; 20% had not returned to full-time employment even at 40 months' posttransplant; borderline anxiety and depression found in both groups; physical well-being better in autologous group than allogeneic group; more sexual dysfunction reported in transplant group; social support high in transplant group

marrow or blood stem cell donation revolve around the physical and psychological outcome of the transplant and the motivational factors underlying the marrow donation. The donation of marrow or blood stem cells requires a high level of commitment and some degree of health risk on the part of the donor. Limited studies have been conducted on such donor issues. Most of what we have learned about the physical and psychological sequelae of marrow donation comes from a comprehensive study of several hundred adult unrelated marrow donors recruited from 1987 to 1991 through the National Marrow Donor Program (NMDP). Results showed that a sizable minority of donors experienced their donation as stressful and inconvenient, with 12% admitting to some degree of worry about their own health.[90] Donors were, however, generally quite positive about their donation. At 1 year after donation, 87% of the donors stated that they believed their donation experience was "very worthwhile," while 91% indicated that they would be willing to donate again in the future. Some evidence suggest that donors with longer marrow collection times and those who experienced lower-back pain or difficulty walking following the donation viewed their experience as more stressful and experienced less positive psychosocial outcomes.

Unrelated blood and marrow stem cell transplantation is reliant on the recruitment and maintenance of a large and suitable pool of volunteer marrow donors. Consequently, it is important to understand what motivates donors. Switzer et al identified six distinct types of donor motives: exchange-related, idealized helping, normative, positive feeling, empathy-related, and past experience–based.[91] Donor motives predicted donor reactions to donation. Donors reporting exchange motives or simple helping motives experienced greater predonation ambivalence and more negative postdonation reactions. Donors who reported empathy and positive feeling motives evidenced less predonation ambivalence and more positive postdonation reactions.

Suggestions that the donor may experience "survivor guilt" following the death of the recipient can be found in the literature. It has also been suggested that the donor may experience guilt and self-blame should their marrow fail to engraft or should GVHD contribute to the death of the recipient. The lack of research in this area makes it difficult to formulate any firm conclusions in this area. One study showed that the death of the recipient produced feelings of guilt and responsibility in a few instances.[90] Grief, however, was universally experienced by unrelated donors in learning of the recipient's death and was often surprisingly intense considering that they were strangers. One would expect more negative reactions and profound grief in donors with a prior relationship to the recipient. We do not have any studies that have looked at that population.

Nurses working with donors need to assist in the evaluation of the motivational factors underlying their desire to donate. The relationship between the donor and recipient should also be explored. Physical and psychological follow-up is warranted in caring for the donor.

Conclusion

Marrow and blood stem cell transplantation is a complex process and requires expert nursing care. Patients experiencing acute and chronic complications as well as psychosocial difficulties rely on the skilled, compassionate nurse to help guide them through this process. Being equipped with knowledge about the various complications that may occur and their management is essential in facilitating the smooth transition of the patient to the successful survivor.

References

1. Woo SB, Lee SJ, Schubert MM: Graft-vs.-host disease. *Crit Rev Oral Biol Med.* 8:201–216, 1997
2. Bortin MM, Horowitz MM, Rimm AA: Increasing utilization of allogeneic bone marrow transplantation. *Ann Intern Med* 116:505–512, 1992
3. Kanfer E: The diagnosis and management of early complications, in Treleaven J, Barrett J (eds): *Bone Marrow Transplantation in Practice.* New York, Churchill Livingstone, 1992, pp 315–327
4. Treleaven J, Weirnitz P (eds): *Color Atlas and Text of Bone Marrow Transplantation.* London, Mosby-Wolfe, 1995, p 144
5. Sullivan KM: Graft-versus-host disease, in Forman SJ, Blume KG, Thomas ED (eds): *Bone Marrow Transplantation.* Malden, MA, Blackwell Science, 1994, pp 339–362
6. Weisdorf DJ, Snover DC, Haake R, et al: Acute upper gastrointestinal graft-versus-host disease: Clinical significance and response to immunosuppressive therapy. *Blood* 76:624–629, 1990
7. Sullivan K: Graft-versus-host disease, in Thomas ED, Blume K, Forman S (eds): *Hematopoietic Cell Transplantation* (ed 2). Malden, MA, Blackwell Science, 1999, pp 515–536
8. Weisdorf D, Hakke R, Blazar B, et al: Risk factors for acute graft-versus-host disease in histocompatible donor bone marrow transplantation. *Transplantation* 51:1197–1203, 1991
9. McCarthy PL, Abhyankar S, Neben S, et al: Inhibition of intereukin-1 by an interleukin-1 receptor antagonist prevents graft-versus-host disease. *Blood* 78: 1915–1918, 1991
10. Weisdorf D, Filipovich A, McGlave P, et al: Combination graft-versus-host disease prophylaxis using immunotoxin (anti-CD5-RTA) plus methotrexate and cyclosporine or prednisone after unrelated donor marrow transplantation. *Bone Marrow Transplant* 12:531–536, 1993
11. Marmount AM, Horowitz MM, Gale RP, et al: T-cell depletion of HLA-identical transplants in leukemia. *Blood* 78: 2120–2130, 1991
12. Gribben JG, Guinan EC, Boussiotis VA, et al: Complete blockade of B7 family-mediated costimulation is necessary to induce human alloantigen-specific anergy: A method to ameliorate graft-versus-host disease and extend the donor pool. *Blood* 87:4887–4893, 1996
13. Ruuru T, Niederwieser D, Gratwohl A, et al: A survey of the prophylaxis and treatment of acute GVHD in Europe: A report of the European Group for Blood and Marrow Transplantation (EBMT). Chronic Leukaemia Working Party of the EBMT. *Bone Marrow Transplant* 19:759–764, 1997
14. Martin PJ, Schoch G, Fisher L, et al: A retrospective analysis

of therapy for acute graft-versus-host disease: Initial treatment. *Blood* 76:1464–1472, 1990

15. O'Connell S, Schmit-Pokorny K: Blood and marrow stem cell transplantation: Indications, procedure, process, in Whedon MB, Wujcik D (eds): *Blood and Marrow Stem Cell Transplantation: Principles, Practice, and Nursing Insights* (ed 2). Sudbury, MA, Jones and Bartlett, 1997, pp 66–99

16. Johnston E, Crawford J: Hematopoietic growth factors in the reduction of chemotherapeutic toxicity. *Semin Oncol* 25:552–561, 1998

17. Reed E: Infectious complications during autotransplantation. *Hematol Oncol Clin North Am* 7:717–735, 1993

18. Goodrich J, Bowden R, Fisher L, et al: Ganciclovir prophylaxis to prevent cytomegalovirus disease after allogeneic marrow transplant. *Ann Intern Med* 118:173–178, 1993

19. Schubert MM, Williams BI, Lloid ME, et al: Clinical assessment scale for the rating of oral mucosal changes following bone marrow transplantation. *Cancer* 69:2469–2477, 1992

20. Shuhart MC, McDonald GB: Gastrointestinal and hepatic complications, in Forman SJ, Blume KG, Thomas ED (eds): *Bone Marrow Transplantation*. Malden, MA, Blackwell Science, 1994, pp 454–481

21. Strasser S, McDonald G: Gastrointestinal and hepatic complications, in Thomas ED, Blume K, Forman S (eds): *Hematopoietic Cell Transplantation* (ed 2). Malden, MA, Blackwell Science, 1999, pp 627–658

22. Buchsel PC: Bone marrow transplantation, in Groenwald SL, Frogge MH, Goodman M, Yarbro CH (eds): *Cancer Nursing: Principles and Practice* (ed 4). Sudbury, MA, Jones and Bartlett, 1997, pp 459–506

23. Hill HH, Chapman RC, Kornell JA, et al: Self-administration of morphine in bone marrow transplant patients with reduced drug requirement. *Pain* 40:121–129, 1990

24. McDonald G: Venoocclusive disease of the liver following marrow transplantation. *Marrow Transplant Rev* 3(4):49–54, 1993

25. Baglin TP, Harper P, Marcus RE: Venocclusive disease of the liver complicating ABMT successfully treated with recombinant tissue plasminogen activator. *Bone Marrow Transplant* 5:439–441, 1990

26. Openshaw D, Slatkin N: Neurological complications, in Thomas ED, Blume KG, Forman SJ (eds): *Hematopoietic Cell Transplantation* (ed 2). Malden, MA, Blackwell Science, 1999, pp 659–673

27. Meyers CA, Weitzner M, Byrne K, et al: Evaluation of the neurobehavioral functioning of patients before, during, and after bone marrow transplantation. *J Clin Oncol* 12:820–826, 1994

28. Furlong T: Neurologic complications of immunosuppressive cancer therapy. *Oncol Nurs Forum* 20:1337–1352, 1993

29. Hiemenz JW, Greene JN: Special considerations for the patient undergoing allogeneic or autologous bone marrow transplantation. *Hematol Oncol Clin North Am* 9:961–1002, 1993

30. McCullough J: Principles of transfusion support before and after hematopoietic cell transplantation, in Thomas ED, Blume KG, Forman SJ (eds): *Hematopoietic Cell Transplantation* (ed 2). Malden, MA, Blackwell Science, 1999, pp 685–703

31. Smith B: Stem cell transplantation, in DeVita VT, Hellman S, Rosenberg SA (eds): *Cancer: Principles and Practice of Oncology* (ed 5). Philadelphia, Lippincott-Raven, 1997, pp 2621–2639

32. Nemunaitis J, Singer JW, Buckner CD, et al: Use of recombinant human granulocyte-macrophage colony-stimulating factor in graft failure after bone marrow transplantation. *Blood* 76:245–253, 1990

33. Wagner J, Storb R: Allogeneic transplantation for aplastic anemia, in Thomas ED, Blume KG, Forman S (eds): *Hematopoietic Cell Transplantation* (ed 2). Malden, MA, Blackwell Science, 1999, pp 791–806

34. Height S, Sheilds M: Problems following bone marrow transplantation, in Treleaven J, Wiernik P (eds): *Color Atlas and Text of Bone Marrow Transplantation*. London, Mosby-Wolfe, 1995, pp 169–180

35. Crawford S: Critical care and respiratory failure, in Thomas ED, Blume K, Forman S (eds): *Hematopoietic Cell Transplantation* (ed 2). Malden, MA, Blackwell Science, 1999, pp 515–536

36. Chan CK, Hyland RH, Hutcheon MA: Pulmonary complications following bone marrow transplantation. *Clin Chest Med* 111:323–332, 1990

37. Kupari M, Violin L, Suokas A, et al: Cardiac involvement in bone marrow transplantation; electrocardiographic changes, arrhythmias, heart failure and autopsy findings. *Bone Marrow Transplant* 5:91–98, 1990

38. Peterson FB, Bearman SI: Preparative regimens and their toxicity, in Forman SJ, Blume KG, Thomas ED (eds): *Bone Marrow Transplantation*. Malden, MA, Blackwell Science, 1994, pp 96–113

39. Eisen D, Essel J, Broun ER: Oral cavity complications of bone marrow transplantation. *Semin Cutaneous Med Surg* 16:265–272, 1997

40. Schubert M, Peterson D, Lloid M: Oral complications, in Thomas ED, Blume K, Forman S (eds): *Hematopoietic Cell Transplantation* (ed 2). Malden, MA, Blackwell Science, 1999, pp 751–763

41. Zager RA: Acute renal failure in the setting of bone marrow transplantation. *Kidney Int* 46:1443–1458, 1994

42. King C, Hoffar N, Murray M: Acute renal failure in bone marrow transplantation. *Oncol Nurs Forum* 19:1327–1335, 1992

43. Corcoran-Buchsel P: Long-term complications of allogeneic bone marrow transplantation: Nursing implications. *Oncol Nurs Forum* 13:61–70, 1986

44. Deeg HJ: Delayed complications after hematopoietic cell transplantation, in Thomas ED, Blume K, Forman S (eds): *Hematopoietic Cell Transplantation* (ed 2). Malden, MA, Blackwell Science, 1999, pp 776–788

45. Armitage JO: Bone marrow transplantation. *N Engl J Med* 330:827, 1994

46. Sable CA, Donowitz GR: Infections in bone marrow transplant recipients. *Clin Infect Dis* 18:273–284, 1994

47. Randolph S, Leum E, Buchsel PC: Long-term complications of BMT, in Buchsel PC, Whedon MB (eds): *Bone Marrow Transplantation: Administrative and Clinical Strategies*. Sudbury, MA, Jones and Bartlett, 1995, pp 323–350

48. Saral R: Candida and aspergillus infections in immunocompromised patients: An overview. *Rev Infect Dis* 13:487–492, 1991

49. Parkman R, Weinberg KI: Immunological reconstitution following hematopoietic stem cell transplantations, in Thomas ED, Blume KG, Forman SJ (eds): *Hematopoietic Cell Transplantation* (ed 2). Malden, MA, Blackwell Science, 1999, pp 704–711

50. Benyunes MC, Sullivan KM, Deeg HJ, et al: Cataracts after bone marrow transplantation: Long-term follow-up of adults treated with fractionated total body irradiation. *Int J Radiat Oncol Biol Phys* 32:661–670, 1995

51. Belkacemi Y, Ozsahin M, Pene F, et al: Cataractogenesis after total body irradiation. *Int J Radiat Oncol Biol Phys* 35:53–60, 1996

52. Yang DD, Hurd DD, Case LD, et al: Hemorrhagic cystitis in bone marrow transplantation. *Urology* 44:322–328, 1994

53. Stella F, Battistelli S, Marcheggiani F, et al: Urothelial cell changes due to busulfan and cyclophosphamide treatment in bone marrow transplantation. *Acta Cytol* 34:885–890, 1990

54. Kantrow SP, Hackman RC, Boeckh M, et al: Idiopathic pneumonia syndrome: Changing spectrum of lung injury after marrow transplantation. *Transplantation* 63:1079–1086, 1997

55. Boeckh M, Riddell SR, Cunningham T, et al: Increased risk of late CMV infection and disease in allogeneic marrow transplant recipients after ganciclovir prophylaxis is due to a lack of CMV-specific T-cell responses. *Blood* 88:302a, 1996, (abstr)

56. Crawford SW, Pepe M, Lin D, et al: Abnormalities of pulmonary function tests after marrow transplantation predict nonrelapse mortality. *Am J Respir Crit Care Med* 152:690–695, 1995

57. Deeg HJ, Socie G, Schoch G, et al: Malignancies after marrow transplantation for aplastic anemia and Fanconi anemia: A joint Seattle and Paris analysis of results in 700 patients. *Blood* 87:386–392, 1996

58. Braverman AC, Antin JH, Plappert MT, et al: Cyclophosphamide cardiotoxicity in bone marrow transplantation: A prospective evaluation of new dosing regimens. *J Clin Oncol* 9:1215–1223, 1991

59. Ramrakha PS, Marks DI, O'Brien SG, et al: Orthotopic cardiac transplantation for dilatated cardiomyopathy after allogeneic bone marrow transplantation. *Clin Transplant* 8:23–26, 1994

60. Hochster H, Wasserheit C, Speyer J: Cardiotoxicity and cardioprotection during chemotherapy. *Curr Opin Oncol* 7:304–309, 1995 (review)

61. Toubert ME, Socie G, Gluckman E, et al: Short and long-term follow-up of thyroid dysfunction after allogeneic bone marrow transplantation without the use of preparative total body irradiation. *Br J Haematol* 98:453–457, 1997

62. Huma Z, Boulad F, Black P, et al: Growth in children after bone marrow transplantation for acute leukemia. *Blood* 86:819–824, 1995

63. Fink JC, Leisenring WM, Sullivan KM, et al: Avascular necrosis following bone marrow transplantation: A case control study. *Bone* 22:67–71, 1998

64. Deeg HJ, Socie G: Malignancies after hematopoietic stem cell transplantation: Many questions, some answers. *Blood* 55:233–239, 1998

65. Bhatia S, Ramsay NK, Steinbuch M, et al: Malignant neoplasms following bone marrow transplantation. *Blood* 87:3633–3639, 1996

66. Heslop HE, Ng CY, Li C, et al: Long-term restoration of immunity against Epstein-Barr virus infection by adoptive transfer of gene-modified virus-specific T lymphocytes. *Nat Med* 2:551–555, 1996

67. Curtis RE, Rowlings PA, Deeg HJ, et al: Solid cancers after bone marrow transplantation. *N Engl J Med* 336:897–904, 1997

68. Govindarajan R, Jagannath S, Flick JT, et al: Preceding standard therapy is the likely cause of MDS after autotransplants for multiple myeloma. *Br J Haematol* 85:349–353, 1996

69. Anderson JE, Gooley TA, Schoch G, et al: Stem cell transplantation for secondary acute myeloid leukemia: Evaluation of transplantation as initial therapy or following induction chemotherapy. *Blood* 89:2578–2585, 1997

70. Greenspan A, Deeg HJ, Cottler-Fox M, et al: Incapacitating peripheral neuropathy as a manifestation of chronic graft-versus-host disease. *Bone Marrow Transplant* 5:349–352, 1990

71. Slavin MA, Meyers JD, Remington JS, et al: Toxoplasma gondii infection in marrow transplant recipients: A 20 year experience. *Bone Marrow Transplant* 13:549–557, 1994

72. Sullivan KM, Wade JC, Bowden RA: Management of the immunocompromised host, in Schrier SL, McArthur JR (eds): *Hematology*. St. Louis, American Society of Hematology, 1993, pp 163–174

73. Chou RH, Wong GB, Kramer JH, et al: Toxicities of total-body irradiation for pediatric bone marrow transplantation. *Int J Radiat Oncol Biol Phys* 34:843–851, 1996

74. Anasetti C: Hematopoietic cell transplantation from HLA partially matched related donors, in Thomas ED, Blume K, Forman S (eds): *Hematopoietic Cell Transplantation* (ed 2). Malden, MA, Blackwell Science, 1999, pp 515–536

75. Sale G, Shulman H, Hackman R: Pathology of hematopoietic cell transplantation, in Thomas ED, Blume K, Forman S (eds): *Hematopoietic Cell Transplantation* (ed 2). Malden, MA, Blackwell Science, 1999, pp 515–536

76. Radich J, Appelbaum F, Bryant E, et al: PCR detection of the bcr-abl fusion transcript after bone marrow transplant for chronic myeloid leukemia predicts subsequent relapse: A multivariate model of 356 patients. *Blood* 85:2632–2638, 1995

77. Weisdorf S, Schwarzenberg SJ: Nutritional support of hematopoietic stem cell recipients, in Thomas ED, Blume K, Forman S (eds): *Hematopoietic Cell Transplantation* (ed 2). Malden, MA, Blackwell Science, 1999, pp 515–536

78. Syrjala KL, Donaldson GW, Davis MW, et al: Relaxation and imagery and cognitive-behavioral training reduce pain during cancer treatment: A controlled clinical trial. *Pain* 63:189–198, 1995

79. Syrjala K, Abrams K: Ask the doctor. *Blood Marrow Transplant News* 8:1–11, 1997

80. Bush N, Haberman M, Donaldson G, et al: Quality of life of adult long-term survivors of bone marrow transplantation. *Soc Sci Med* 40:479–490, 1995

81. Whedon M, Ferrell BR: Quality of life in adult bone marrow transplant patients: Beyond the first year. *Semin Oncol Nurs* 10:42–57, 1994

82. Grant M: Assessment of quality of life following hematopoietic cell transplantation, in Thomas ED, Blume K, Forman S (eds): *Hematopoietic Cell Transplantation* (ed 2). Malden, MA, Blackwell Science, 1999, pp 407–413

83. Chao NJ, Tierney K, Bloom JR, et al: Dynamic assessment of quality of life after autologous bone marrow transplantation. *Blood* 80:825–830, 1992

84. Andrykowski MA, Brady MJ, Greiner CB, et al: 'Returning to normal' following bone marrow transplantation: Outcomes, expectations and informed consent. *Bone Marrow Transplant* 15:573–581, 1995

85. McQuellon RP, Craven B, Russell GB, et al: Quality of life in breast cancer patients before and after autologous bone marrow transplantation. *Bone Marrow Transplant* 18:579–584, 1996

86. McQuellon RP, Russell GB, Rambo TD: Quality of life and psychological distress of bone marrow transplant recipients: The "time trajectory" to recovery over the first year. *Bone Marrow Transplant* 21:477–486, 1998

87. Whedon M, Stearns D, Mills LE: Quality of life of long-term adult survivors of autologous bone marrow transplantation. *Oncol Nurs Forum* 10:1527–1535, 1995

88. Grant M, Ferrell B, Rivera L, et al: Cross-sectional study on quality of life in 450 adults surviving from 1 to 15 years post HCT. (in press).

89. Molassiotis A, van den Akker OB, Milligan DW, et al: Quality of life in long-term survivors of marrow transplantation:

Comparison with a matched group receiving maintenance chemotherapy. *Bone Marrow Transplant* 17:249–258, 1996

90. Butterworth VA, Simmons RG, Bartsch G, et al: Psychosocial effects of unrelated bone marrow donation: Experiences of the National Marrow Donor Program. *Blood* 81:1947–1959, 1993

91. Switzer GE, Simmons RG, Dew MA: Helping unrelated stranger: Physical and psychological reactions to the bone marrow donation process among anonymous donors. *J Appl Soc Psychol* 26:469–490, 1996

CHAPTER 24

Biotherapy

Linda A. Battiato, RN, MSN, OCN®
Vera S. Wheeler, RN, MN, OCN®

Introduction

Biological agents have started to gain acceptance as standard therapy in oncology care. They are used for primary or supportive care in solid tumors and hematological malignancies and in the bone marrow transplant setting. Use of biological agents is found across the continuum of cancer care including diagnosis, adjuvant therapy, treatment of metastatic disease, and even cancer prevention. While many advances have been made, biotherapy continues to mature with further development of scientific knowledge and biotechnology and broader clinical experience with current cytokines, monoclonal antibodies, and other biological agents.

This chapter describes the major current applications of biotherapy and those being investigated in clinical trials. Major toxicities commonly experienced by patients receiving these therapies are also addressed.

Foundation Concepts for Biotherapy

Immune Defense against Malignancy: An Overview

Immune surveillance

Immune surveillance is a theory that was first proposed in the 1950s to explain the role of the immune system in defending against neoplastic cells. Tumor cells express abnormal tumor antigens on their surfaces that can be recognized and subsequently destroyed by immune cells. The immune system is believed to destroy many circulating malignant cells before they can become established sites of tumor. Although the response of immune defense cells to specific tumors has been demonstrated, the theory fails to explain why some cancers elude immune detection and response. Abbas et al suggest that immunosurveillance may be most effective in a subset of virally caused cancers.[1]

Tumor escape mechanisms

Several mechanisms of immune evasion have been proposed to explain how tumors escape immune system detection. These mechanisms include down-regulation of major histocompatibility class I expression, lack of co-stimulatory signals needed for antigen presentation, or tumor secretion of immunosuppressive products. Tumors may also escape immune system detection because they are weakly immunogenic. An immunogenic tumor is made of cells that express one or more antigens that could be recognized by the immune system. A tumor-bearing host may be immunologically tolerant to tumor antigens because of inappropriate antigen presentation to the immune system or because of neonatal exposure to such antigens. Induction of suppressor T cells may also inhibit the immune response to cancer.[2]

Effector mechanisms of immune function

Defense against foreign antigens, either exogenous microbes or endogenous altered or virally transformed cells, is accomplished through components of the immune response. Effector or cell-killing mechanisms are initiated through a complicated recognition system of self/nonself surface molecules known as the major histocompatibility complex (MHC). The primary defense against transformed cells is cell-mediated immunity carried out by T lymphocytes and aided by B cells and humoral immunity. Stimulated by the presence of an antigen, the macrophage activates a T-helper (T_H) cell. The activated T_H cell, along with cytokines, initiates a B-cell response and the generation of antibody, an increase in cytotoxic T8 cells, activation of natural killer (NK) cells, and the stimulation of hematopoietic stem cells. (For a complete review of the immune system defense against malignancy and the specific cells adapted to cancer therapy as biologic agents, see Chapter 3.)

Cytokines

Cytokines are glycoprotein products of immune cells, such as lymphocytes and macrophages, that coordinate and initiate effector defense functions. Cytokines include the interleukins, interferons, colony-stimulating factors, and tumor necrosis factor. Some of the interleukins have a primary role in hematopoiesis, while others are more active in the immune system and some have overlapping properties. Cytokines are not cytotoxic agents themselves, with the exception of tumor necrosis factor-alpha (TNF-α) and lymphotoxin (TNF-β). The primary host defense cytokines include interleukins 1, 2, 4, 6, and 12; interferons α, β, γ; TNF-α; TNF-β; and transforming growth factor beta (TGF-β).

Cytokines generally share certain properties:

- They mediate and regulate immune defense functions of the body by providing communication and coordination among a variety of diverse immune cells; they have been called the "hormones" of the immune system.

- They have brief half-lives and usually function over short distances.

- They are produced by many different cell types and also act on diverse cell targets both within the immune system and in other organ targets such as the liver.

- Their actions are overlapping, redundant, and sometimes contradictory. They can influence the stimulation of other cytokines to produce synergistic effects as in a cytokine network or to antagonize the actions of other cytokines.

- They bind to surface receptors of target cells and act as regulators of cell growth or as mediators of defense functions.[1,3]

The cytokine network is an overlapping, interactive communication pattern within the immune system. The secretion of one cytokine (or the administration of a recombinant form) can initiate a large release of secondary cytokines. Figure 24-1 illustrates one aspect of this network. When a bolus of high-dose interleukin 2 (IL-2) is administered, it potentially stimulates three cell types: NK, macrophage, and cytotoxic T lymphocyte (CTL) cells. These cells secrete a variety of cytokines responsible for flulike symptoms and potential tumor cell killing. Other administered cytokines will engage in their own unique interactions within the cytokine network.

Origins of Biotherapy

Coley's toxins

William Coley, a New York surgeon, observed in 1893 that a patient with metastatic sarcoma had a complete remission of his cancer after two episodes of erysipelas, a streptococcal infection. Coley continued to explore the relationship of acute infection and tumor regression by injecting live and later killed bacterial extracts into patients' tumors. These extracts, known as Coley's toxins, were administered in a highly variable manner but are believed to have contained *Streptococcus pyogenes* with *Serratia marcescens* and *Bacillus prodigiosus*. Patients received these injections for weeks, months, or even up to a year. They reacted with fever, chills, and other systemic effects that Coley believed were an essential part of the treatment. Although approximately one-fourth of Coley's patients had a complete regression of their tumor, interest in these toxins waned with the onset of radiation therapy and chemotherapy.[3,4] It is now believed that the active ingredient in these toxins was endotoxin, a component

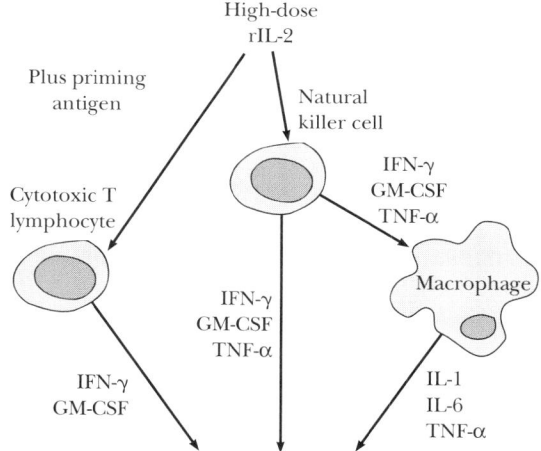

Figure 24-1 High-dose rIL-2 cytokine cascade: rIL-2 given parenterally can result in a massive release of cytokines and symptoms of inflammation from the activation of peripheral blood mononuclear cells and their pyrogenic cytokines.[3] (GM-CSF = granulocyte-macrophage colony stimulating factor; IFN = interferon; IL-1 = interleukin 1; IL-6 = interleukin 6; TNF-α = tumor necrosis factor-alpha)

in bacterial cell walls that generated TNF and other cytokines in the patient.

BCG and modern immunotherapy

In the 1960s and 1970s, nonspecific immunopotentiators such as bacillus Calmette-Guérin (BCG) were being tested in clinical trials. BCG was originally developed as a vaccine for tuberculosis. The use of BCG as adjuvant therapy after chemotherapy demonstrated increased survival of children with acute lymphoblastic leukemia and sparked interest in immunotherapy as a cancer treatment.[5] However, many subsequent clinical studies showed little difference in the cancer recurrence rates using BCG, *Corynebacterium parvum,* and other immunopotentiators. Interest in immunotherapy again faded.

Biological response modifiers

Advances in molecular biology and computerization, and the advent of genetic engineering in the early 1980s provided a large number of new substances from the mammalian genome that were capable of modulating immune functions. Oldham describes biological response modifiers (BRMs) as a "medicine cabinet" of new biologicals that may directly or indirectly have antitumor activity.[5] Unlike previous immunotherapeutic agents, these were homogenous, pure substances that were capable of more specific effects in the immune system. Biological response modifiers are defined as "agents or approaches that will modify the relationship between tumor and host by modifying the host's biological response to tumor cells, with resultant therapeutic benefit."[6,p3] These agents can be classified as: (1) agents that restore, augment, or modulate host-antitumor immune mechanisms; (2) cells or cellular products that have direct antitumor effects such as TNF; and (3) biological agents that have other biological, antitumor effects; for example, interfering with the metastatic ability of tumor or differentiating agents.[7] Today, BRMs are more broadly defined and encompass a greater number of substances than those used in the earlier field of immunotherapy, even though the terms are sometimes used interchangeably. *Biotherapy,* or *biological therapy,* have become the more prevalent terms. *Biother-*

apy is defined as the use of agents derived from biological sources or that affect biological responses.[8] It now describes agents that are biological in origin that may not have antitumor effects but have other biological effects such as affecting hematopoiesis.[9]

Recombinant DNA Technology

Recombinant DNA, or the combining of genes from different sources to produce an organism with new qualities, is an important basic principle to biotherapy. (Table 24-1 defines terms used in biotechnology.) This advance in molecular biology has enabled the current generation of biological agents to be available for use in cancer therapy. When the process of recombinant DNA was discovered in the 1970s, there was much controversy over how this new technology might be used or misused. However, recombinant DNA technology produces proteins that have created a new class of drugs called *biopharmaceuticals.* Table 24-2 identifies major classifications of biopharmaceuticals presently available or in clinical trials.

The process of recombinant DNA starts with the isolation of a specific segment of one strand of DNA (Figure 24-2). This segment, a sequence of base pairs responsible for the manufacture of a particular protein, is cut from the DNA strand using a specific restriction enzyme. The remaining "sticky ends" enable the fragment to be joined to DNA in the plasmid by the binding of complementary base pairs, thymine to adenine and guanine to cytosine. The splice in the DNA strand is completed by another enzyme, and the plasmid is inserted into a bacterial cell and cultured to produce the desired protein.[10]

This process, called *polymerase chain reaction* (PCR), is used to create copies of a specific segment of DNA without vectors and bacteria. Short-stranded DNA fragments, known as *primers,* correspond to the short segment of DNA to be amplified. The DNA and primers are separated by heating and by the addition of DNA polymerase that generates new additions to the strands, doubling the number of DNA fragments. These cycles are repeated within minutes and can generate millions of copies of the DNA fragments.[10]

The future of biotherapy is influenced by new develop-

Table 24-1   Common Terms for Biotechnology

Biopharmaceuticals: Proteins, usually the product of recombinant DNA technology, that are used as drugs (e.g., interferon, human growth hormone).

Gene: A unit of DNA that forms a discrete part of a chromosome of an organism.

Genetic engineering: The formation of new combinations of genes that are placed into an organism in which these genes do not occur naturally.

Polymerase chain reaction (PCR): A method of gene amplication that does not require use of bacterial vectors.

Plasmid: An autonomously replicating, circular molecule of DNA. It is used as a vector for the introduction of a gene.

Restriction enzymes: Enzymes that act like "molecular scissors," cutting strands of DNA at specific cleavage sites to make specific DNA fragments.

Recombinant DNA: A genome containing genes from different sources that have been combined by genetic engineering methods.

Vector: A carrier for the DNA in genetic engineering. Typical vectors are plasmids and viruses.

Table 24-2 Major Classifications of Biopharmaceuticals

Category	Examples
1. Enzymes and enzyme regulators	Alteplase; tissue plasminogen activator or TPA (Activase)
	Ceredase-glucocerebrosidase for Gaucher disease (Cerezyme)
2. Hormones and hormonelike growth factors	Human insulin (Humulin)
	Erythropoietin (Procrit)
	Platelet-derived growth factor (PDGF)
3. Cytokines	Alfa-interferon (Intron A)
	Aldesleukin, interleukin-2 (Proleukin)
	Filgrastim (Neupogen)
4. Vaccines	Hepatitis B vaccine (Recombivax)

many separate subclasses of interferon into one molecule. Future generations of biological products continue to develop with ongoing technological and theoretical advances.

ments in biotechnology. The first generation of biotechnology produced recombinant versions of immune cell proteins such as alfa-interferon and interleukin 2. These were pure, homogenous, contaminant-free products used in clinical trials to modulate or initiate antitumor responses. A second generation of biotechnological products has been evaluated. They are genes for the naturally occurring proteins that have been combined to make hybrid products.[11] The aim is to eliminate troublesome side effects and increase the effectiveness of the agents. These agents are called *fusion proteins*. Examples of these agents include PIXY 321, which combines granulocyte-macrophage colony-stimulating factor (GM-CSF) and IL-3, and DAB-IL-2, an immunotoxin. Consensus interferon is another example of combining active portions of

Hematopoietic Growth Factors

One of the most successful applications for biotherapy has been hematopoietic growth factors (HGFs). Unlike other applications in which cytokines are administered as primary anticancer therapy, HGFs are used as supportive therapy to myelosuppressive chemotherapy or bone marrow transplantation (BMT). Chemotherapy administration is associated with many side effects including neutropenia, anemia, and thrombocytopenia. All of these "cytopenias" can adversely affect the patient and clinical outcomes by causing dose-reductions and interruptions of treatment schedules, life-threatening sequelae, troublesome symptoms, and impaired quality of life.

Hematopoiesis

Hematopoiesis, the process of blood cell formation, takes place in the bone marrow. From one originating stem cell, the bone marrow is capable of producing ten distinct cells that function in body defense (neutrophil, eosinophil, basophil, mast cell, monocyte/macrophage, B and

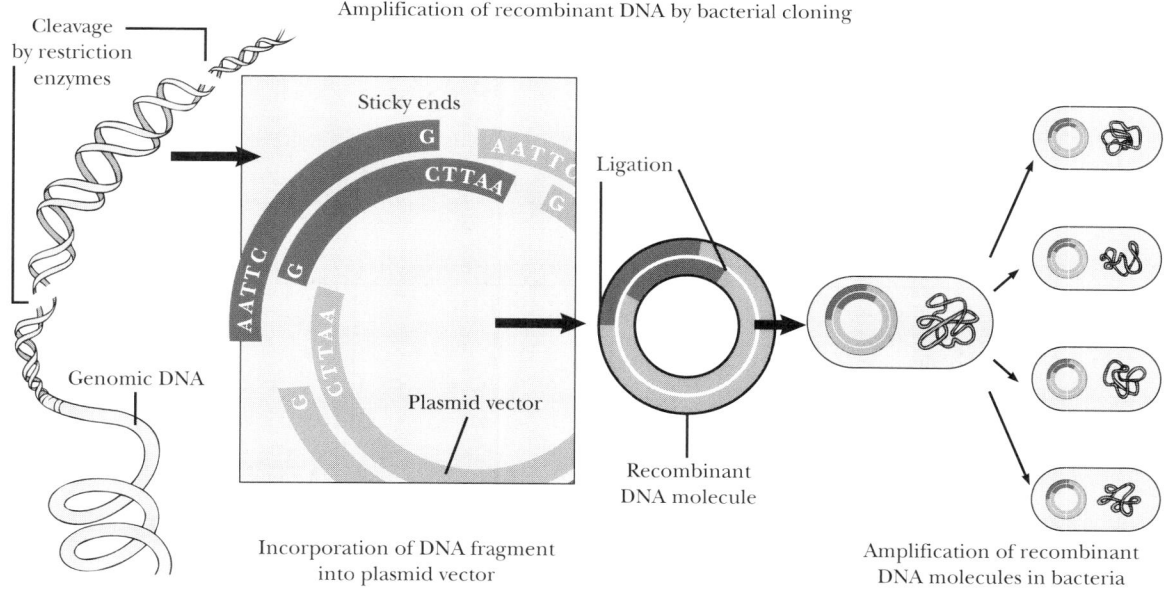

Figure 24-2 Amplification of recombinant DNA by bacterial cloning. In the example shown, the DNA segment to be amplified is separated by cleavage with a restriction enzyme that produces "sticky ends." The restriction enzyme cuts each strand as well as the plasmid DNA at a single site, generating "sticky ends" on the plasmid that are complementary to the ends of the DNA fragments. The cut ends of the DNA fragments and the plasmid form smooth joints with ligase enzyme. The new molecule is carried into bacteria that replicate the plasmid as they grow in culture. (Data from Rosenthal.[10])

T lymphocyte, natural killer cell), oxygen-carrying capability (erythrocyte), and clotting (platelet). As shown in Figure 24-3, these mature cells develop from cell lineages that gradually produce a more differentiated, specialized cell in the bone marrow under the influence of growth factors. Hematopoietic growth factors are cytokines, hormones, colony-stimulating factors, and other molecules that influence the development of bone marrow–derived cells to their mature form. These growth factors are usually synthesized by stromal cells in the bone marrow or rarely by nonhematopoietic cells (e.g., the synthesis of erythropoietin by kidney and liver cells). (See Chapter 3 for additional information on hematopoiesis.)

Recombinant Growth Factors

Recombinant DNA technology has allowed production of the naturally occurring growth factors for clinical use. Some HGFs are *lineage specific,* that is, they stimulate only one blood cell line (e.g., granulocyte colony-stimulating factor [G-CSF] and erythropoietin [EPO]). Other HGFs stimulate more than one hematopoietic lineage and are considered multilineage.[12] Table 24-3 lists the HGFs that are FDA-approved for clinical use. With the exception of GM-CSF, the approved HGFs have mostly single-lineage effects. While effects on more than one hematopoietic lineage are clearly seen in laboratory and preclinical mod-

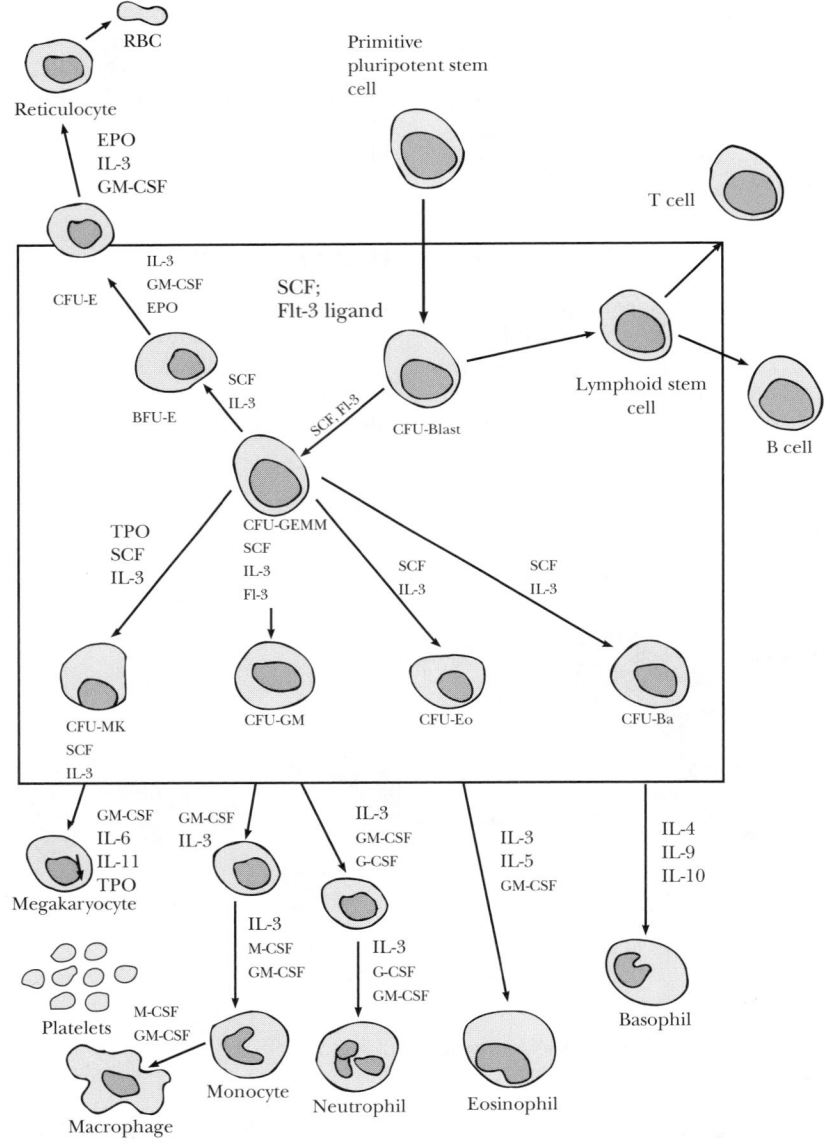

Figure 24-3   The Hematopoietic Cascade. (CFU = colony-forming unit; BFU = burst-forming unit; GEMM = granulocyte/ erythrocyte/monocyte/megakaryocyte; GM = granulocyte-monocyte; MK = megakaryocyte; Eo = eosinophil; Ba = basophil; SCF = stem cell factor; TPO = thrombopoietin; Flt = Flt-3 ligand.

Table 24-3 FDA-Approved Hematopoietic Growth Factors

Agent	Generic Name	Trade Name	Indications	Dose	Route
G-CSF	Filgrastim	Neupogen (Amgen, Inc., Thousand Oaks, CA)	Decrease neutropenia after chemotherapy in nonmyeloid malignancies, after induction/consolidation chemotherapy for AML and in BMT PBPC mobilization	Chemotherapy: 5 µg/kg/day, administer 24 hr after chemotherapy, for up to 2 wk until ANC nadir >10,000/mm³ BMT: 10 µg/kg/day, then titrate per counts	SC, IV
GM-CSF	Sargramostim	Leukine (Immunex Corp, Seattle, WA)	Accelerate bone marrow recovery after BMT, in allogeneic BMT with delayed or failed engraftment, after induction therapy in AML, PBPC mobilization	250 µg/m²/day until ANC >1500/mm³ × 3 days	SC, IV
Erythropoietin alfa	Epoietin alfa	Procrit (Ortho Biotech, Inc., Raritan, NJ); Epogen (Amgen, Inc., Thousand Oaks, CA)	Treatment of anemia in patients with chronic renal failure, cancer patients on chemotherapy, HIV+ patients receiving AZT, surgical patients	For chemotherapy, recommended starting dose 150 units/kg, 3×/wk × 8–12 wk; adjust to maintain desired hematocrit	SC, IV
Interleukin-11	Oprelvekin	Neumega (Genetics Institute, Cambridge, MA)	Prevent thrombocytopenia and reduce need for patient transfusions following myelosuppressive chemotherapy	Adults: 50 µg/kg/day until post-nadir patient count is >50,000/mm³ (max 21 days)	SC

AML = acute myelogenous leukemia; BMT = bone marrow transplantation; PBPC = peripheral blood progenitor cell; ANC = absolute neutrophil count; AZT = zidovudine.

els, the multilineage HGFs have not had a clinically significant impact on reducing pancytopenias. Some cytokines such as IL-1, IL-6, and GM-CSF have pleiotropic actions and have been evaluated for use as HGFs, antitumor agents, and for other diverse applications. The major cell lineages and related HGFs, along with the status of these growth factors as biopharmaceutical agents for clinical use, are discussed in the next section.

Hematopoietic Progenitor Cells and Hematopoietic Growth Factors

Multipotential precursor cells

The hematopoietic stem cell (HSC), also called a totipotent stem cell, is a self-renewing, originating cell that divides asynchronously. In other words, one daughter cell replaces the parent stem cell and the other becomes a hematopoietic progenitor cell (HPC), losing its capacity for self-renewal. The HSC is also a rare cell, believed to be 1 cell per 100,000 nucleated marrow cells, and usually resides in a noncycling or G_0 state. It is unclear what stimulates an HSC to enter the cell cycle as it is not believed to be responsive to any of the known growth factors.[13]

Hematopoietic progenitor cells are multipotential precursor cells, also referred to as stem cells, that are responsive to growth factors. They are cells capable of repopulating the marrow after myelosuppressive therapy

and maintaining hematopoiesis. These pluripotent cells have CD34-positive surface markers.[14]

Stem cell factor. One of the major HGFs that influences multipotential precursor cells (or colony-forming unit [CFU] blasts) to develop into myeloid or lymphoid lineages is stem cell factor (SCF). Stem cell factor is also known as steel factor or kit ligand, names derived from its discovery in Steel mutant mice and as the ligand for c-*kit* proto-oncogene. Stem cell factor stimulates undifferentiated multipotential progenitor cells and committed cell lineage precursors (e.g., CFU-granulocyte erythrocyte monocyte megakaryocyte [CFU-GEMM]) to further develop into mature cells (see Figure 24-3). When administered alone, SCF has demonstrated little colony-stimulating activity. However, in combination with other HGFs such as G-CSF, GM-CSF, IL-3, or EPO, it increases the number and size of cell colonies, suggesting that it influences early progenitor activity.[15]

Stem cell factor has been studied in clinical trials for preventing chemotherapy-induced myelosuppression and for peripheral blood progenitor cell (PBPC) mobilization. Phase I clinical trials of recombinant methionyl human SCF were completed in patients with advanced lung and breast cancer. The most frequent side effects were injection site reactions and mild to severe symptoms of hypersensitivity reactions, with urticaria, dyspnea, and throat tightness. These symptoms were believed to result from mast cell stimulation. Patients were given H_1-receptor antagonist medication with future SCF doses.[16,17]

Clinical trial results suggest that SCF may be most clinically useful combined with G-CSF for PBPC mobilization.[17] Clinical trials have shown improved mobilization of PBPC by combining SCF with G-CSF. In phase III trials in patients with breast cancer and patients with lymphoma, fewer apheresis procedures were required to collect adequate numbers of PBPCs after mobilization with a combination of SCF/G-CSF compared to G-CSF alone. When used in lower doses and with antihistamine premedication, SCF has been well tolerated.[18,19]

Flt-3 ligand. Flt-3 ligand is an early-acting growth factor that stimulates the proliferation of hematopoietic stem cells and primitive progenitor cells in combination with other growth factors. Although it has its own unique features, Flt-3 ligand is similar in some respects to kit ligand (SCF). Flt-3 ligand has activity on stem cells and appears to act as a critical early regulator of myelopoiesis/erythropoiesis and lymphopoiesis.[20] Flt-3 ligand has been shown to synergistically enhance G-CSF mobilization of hematopoietic stem and progenitor cells in mice.[21] Flt-3 ligand in combination with G-CSF may be useful in mobilizing PBPCs in humans. Because Flt-3 does not affect mast cells, administration of this agent would be expected to produce fewer allergic reactions than SCF. Early clinical trials of Flt-3 ligand are under way in humans. In addition to its hematopoietic effects, Flt-3 ligand may have other immune-mediated antitumor effects.[20]

Interleukin-3. This cytokine is also known as IL-3 or multi-CSF. Its major role is to promote growth and differentiation of multipotential committed progenitor cells such as CFU-GEMM for the myeloid cell lineages and the lymphoid progenitor cells.[22] Interleukin-3 has been tested in clinical trials to evaluate its potential to reverse myelosuppressive effects after chemotherapy and autologous stem cell transplantation and for its ability to restore hematopoiesis in patients with aplastic anemia and myelodysplastic syndrome.[23–25] Interleukin-3 has also been studied after autologous stem cell transplantation.[17] Modest increases in neutrophils, eosinophils, reticulocytes, and platelets were noted in these studies but at doses that resulted in moderate to severe toxicity. Interleukin-3 has been given sequentially with GM-CSF to mobilize peripheral blood progenitor cells, but toxicity prevented the administration of effective doses of IL-3. Lack of efficacy and significant toxicity have discouraged further investigation of this cytokine.[17]

PIXY 321. PIXY 321 is a synthetic molecule, combining IL-3 and GM-CSF, made by genetic-engineering techniques. The coding regions of these cytokines are combined to make a product ten times more potent a stimulator of erythroid burst-forming unit (BFU-E) and CFU-GEMM than either substance alone.[15] PIXY 321 has been studied for its ability to ameliorate chemotherapy-induced myelosuppression and for PBPC mobilization. Phase I studies demonstrated the safety of this agent.[26] Phase III randomized studies of PIXY 321 after chemo-

therapy and autologous BMT have shown no benefit over GM-CSF alone.[27,28]

Neutrophil and monocyte/macrophage cell lineages

The monocyte/macrophage and neutrophil lineages (see Figure 24-3) develop from the common multipotential progenitor cell, the CFU-GEMM, into the CFU-GM under the influence of SCF and IL-3. The CFU-GM differentiates into a monocyte with stimulation of IL-3, GM-CSF, and M-CSF. The latter CSFs may influence development of the macrophage from the monocyte.

The CFU-GM can also differentiate into the neutrophil under the influence of IL-3, GM-CSF, and G-CSF. Granulocyte colony-stimulating factor acts on committed granulocyte precursors to increase the number of progeny. Although G-CSF is considered to be a lineage-specific HGF, it also has been found to have some effect on multipotential precursor cells.[22]

Granulocyte colony-stimulating factor. Granulocyte colony-stimulating factor is a single-lineage CSF that is the prime growth factor in the late development of neutrophils, stimulating their proliferation and activation. It increases the mature cells' infection-fighting capability.

Filgrastim (Neupogen) is a recombinant form of G-CSF that was first approved by the FDA for use in decreasing neutropenia related to chemotherapy in patients with nonmyeloid malignancies. Granulocyte colony-stimulating factor has been shown to decrease the duration of neutropenia, the number of episodes of neutropenic fever, and the number of hospital days in patients receiving chemotherapy.[29] Colony-stimulating factors such as G-CSF are sometimes used in clinical practice to treat established febrile or afebrile neutropenia; however, this approach is not supported in the literature.[30]

Granulocyte colony-stimulating factor is approved for use after induction or consolidation chemotherapy for acute myeloid leukemia. Concerned that CSF use would stimulate leukemic blast proliferation, practitioners were initially reluctant to use them in patients with myeloid malignancies. Use of G-CSF has not been associated with enhancement of leukemic growth, nor has it negatively impacted remission rate or survival in adults with acute myelogenous leukemia (AML).[30] Granulocyte colony-stimulating factor is also indicated to reduce the duration of neutropenia in patients receiving BMT and for the mobilization of PBPCs; it is approved for congenital, cyclic, or idiopathic neutropenia. The most frequent side effect of G-CSF is bone pain. Transient liver function alterations have also been observed.[30]

Granulocyte-macrophage colony-stimulating factor. Granulocyte-macrophage colony-stimulating factor is a multilineage growth factor that stimulates the proliferation and differentiation of hematopoietic progenitors of neutrophil, eosinophil, and monocyte colonies and also has effects on maturing monocytes and macrophages. In addition to its vital role in hematopoiesis, GM-CSF has diverse biologic effects on the immune system. It enhances several functional activities of mature effector cells involved in antigen presentation and cell-mediated immunity, including neutrophils, monocytes, macrophages, and dendritic cells.[31]

Sargramostim (Leukine) is a recombinant form of GM-CSF that is approved by the FDA for use in accelerating bone marrow recovery after autologous BMT, in allogeneic BMT with failed or delayed engraftment, and after induction therapy in acute myeloid leukemia. It is also indicated to mobilize progenitor cells for PBPC transplantation or autologous BMT.[31]

While the approved indications for GM-CSF are based on its myeloproliferative effects, potential clinical applications are being evaluated based on its ability to enhance immune function. Granulocyte-macrophage colony-stimulating factor may be useful as prophylaxis or as adjunctive treatment of bacterial or fungal infections in cancer patients receiving myelosuppressive chemotherapy and patients with advanced HIV infections. Patients who are HIV positive and have received GM-CSF in clinical trials have shown a significant increase in CD4 counts and a decreased viral load.[31]

Side effects of sargramostim include fever, lethargy, myalgia, bone pain, anorexia, injection site redness, and rash. It is sometimes associated with a "first dose reaction," characterized by flushing, tachycardia, hypotension, dyspnea, nausea, and vomiting.[32]

Macrophage colony-stimulating factor. Macrophage colony-stimulating factor is a lineage-specific CSF that stimulates the differentiation and maturation of promonocytes into monocytes and macrophages. It also acts on mature cells to enhance their phagocytosis of bacteria, fungi, and potential tumor cells.

Clinical trials of E. coli–derived recombinant M-CSF as an antitumor agent have shown limited clinical benefit.[33] Macrophage colony-stimulating factor has been studied as an antifungal agent in a small uncontrolled trial in patients undergoing BMT. A benefit from M-CSF was suggested for patients with candidal infections, but not for aspergillus. Randomized clinical trial data are needed to further define the potential of M-CSF as an antifungal agent.[34]

Erythrocyte lineage

The red blood cell (RBC) or erythrocyte is the mature cell of a specialized cell lineage that starts with the CFU-GEMM (see Figure 24-3). The first committed progenitor cell for this lineage is the BFU-E. Initially, these cells are stimulated by SCF, IL-3, and GM-CSF, and they develop EPO receptors making them responsive to EPO. They evolve into erythroid colony-forming units (CFU-E) and to the reticulocyte in the presence of the hormone EPO. As the cells mature to erythrocytes, they lose their surface receptors to EPO.[35]

Erythropoietin. Erythropoietin is a hormone normally synthesized by peritubular cells in the kidney and secondarily by hepatocytes. Its production and plasma levels are closely regulated by many factors, including tissue oxygenation. Erythropoietin production is increased by hypoxia and decreased by inflammatory cytokines such as IL-1, IFN-γ, and TNF.

Two identical recombinant products of epoetin alfa or EPO are available for use—Epogen (Amgen, Thousand Oaks, CA) and Procrit (Ortho Biotech, Raritan, NJ). Both products are approved for all indications, but each pharmaceutical company has restricted marketing rights for certain indications. The recombinant forms of EPO are approved for anemia associated with chronic renal failure for patients on dialysis, anemia associated with cancer chemotherapy, anemia related to zidovudine (AZT) therapy in HIV-infected patients, and anemia in surgical patients to reduce the need for allogeneic transfusion.

In cancer patients receiving chemotherapy, clinical trials have documented the efficacy of EPO in increasing hemoglobin levels and reducing transfusion use.[36] Studies of patients with cancer have consistently shown that EPO improves quality of life.[37–39] Myelodysplastic syndrome (MDS) responds poorly to EPO, but an increased response rate has been observed with EPO in combination with G-CSF.[40] Erythropoietin may have a role in mobilizing erythroid progenitor cells and other precursor cells in the setting of high-dose chemotherapy with bone marrow or PBPC support.[41]

For treatment of anemia after chemotherapy, the FDA-approved schedule of EPO is three times per week. Recent clinical trial data has shown that once-weekly dosing is similar to three-times weekly dosing in increasing hemoglobin and quality of life.[42] Because of the length of time required for erythropoiesis, a clinically significant increase in hematocrit can occur as late as 6–8 weeks after treatment. Erythropoietin is generally well-tolerated in oncology patients. Subcutaneous administration of EPO may cause burning at the injection site, and IV administration may cause transient flushing.[43]

Platelet cell lineage

The platelet cell is another highly specialized cell of the bone marrow that develops from the multipotential myeloid progenitor cell (see Figure 24-3). The first committed cell is CFU-megakaryocyte (CFU-MK). It is stimulated by SCF, IL-3, and thrombopoietin. The CFU-MK becomes more differentiated under the influence of several additional growth factors including GM-CSF, IL-6, and IL-11 as the megakaryocyte cell fragments into platelets.

Several growth factors have been evaluated for their ability to stimulate platelet production following chemotherapy. Many agents believed to have potential (IL-1, IL-3, IL-6, SCF, and PIXY 321) have been found to be either ineffective or too toxic, and clinical trials evaluating them as thrombopoietic agents have been abandoned for the most part.[17] Recombinant IL-11 and thrombopoietin have shown the most promise for use as thrombopoietic agents. Interleukin-11 is the only FDA-approved thrombopoietic growth factor, and thrombopoietin is in clinical trials.

Interleukin-11. Interleukin-11 is produced by fibroblasts, endothelial cells, adipocytes, and monocytes. It regulates platelet development by acting on primitive stem cells and early and late megakaryocyte progenitors. Interleukin-11 also synergizes with other early-acting hematopoietic growth factors to promote megakaryocyte colony formation. Interleukin-11 stimulates megakaryocyte maturation, ultimately increasing platelet production.[44,45]

Interleukin-11 has demonstrated efficacy in reducing the need for platelet transfusions in patients undergoing chemotherapy in a phase II randomized clinical trial. In this trial, patients who had experienced thrombocytopenia in previous chemotherapy cycles were randomized to receive IL-11 or placebo with their next cycle of chemotherapy. Patients treated with IL-11 were significantly more likely to avoid the requirement for platelet transfusion versus those in the placebo group.[46] A phase II study of patients with metastatic breast cancer receiving chemotherapy showed a trend toward decreased transfusion use in the IL-11 group. For all of those patients that required platelet transfusions, the mean number of platelet transfusions required was significantly less in patients receiving IL-11.[47]

The recombinant form of IL-11, oprelvekin (Neumega), is indicated for prevention of severe thrombocytopenia and reduction of the need for platelet transfusions following myelosuppressive chemotherapy.[48] In clinical trials, the most common adverse events associated with oprelvekin included peripheral edema, dyspnea, tachycardia, and conjunctival redness. Most adverse events were mild to moderate in severity, associated with fluid retention, and reversible after discontinuation of dosing.[49] Ongoing clinical trials are evaluating the use of rIL-11 in MDS, BMT, and leukemia as well as for the prevention of stomatitis.[48]

Thrombopoietin. Described as the primary regulator of platelet production, this growth factor regulates all stages of platelet production by promoting proliferation of megakaryocyte progenitors and megakaryocyte maturation. Thrombopoietin (TPO) is made primarily in the liver and kidney. It has several names—MGDF, TPO, c-*mpl* ligand—as it was characterized independently by five groups of researchers. However, it is believed to be the same molecule.[50]

Two forms of recombinant human thrombopoietin have been studied in clinical trials. The full-length glycosylated molecule is referred to as recombinant human thrombopoietin (rhTPO) (Genentech, Inc., San Francisco, CA). A truncated form of the molecule covalently bound to polyethylene glycol is referred to as pegylated recombinant human megakaryocyte growth and development factor (PEG-rHuMGDF) (Amgen). Both of these agents have undergone investigation in several clinical settings. Clinical studies with PEG-rHuMGDF have been halted due to the development of neutralizing antibodies that were associated with thrombocytopenia. No neutralizing antibodies have been seen with rhTPO, and trials with rhTPO are ongoing.[51,52]

Early clinical trials of TPO have shown that this cytokine has the ability to attenuate thrombocytopenia and enhance platelet recovery after moderately myelosuppressive chemotherapy. Initial results of trials of TPO in combination with G-CSF for the mobilization of PBPCs are encouraging. A single dose of rhTPO has been associated with a dose-dependent rise in circulating platelet counts and a potent PBPC mobilization effect. Thrombopoietin is being evaluated for its ability to enhance platelet recovery after bone marrow transplant and chemotherapy in patients with AML and for increasing the apheresis yield of platelets in normal donors and cancer patients. In general, TPO has been safe and well-tolerated, although thrombotic episodes have been reported in patients receiving PEG-rHuMGDF.[51,52]

Interleukin-1. Interleukin-1 is a pleiotropic cytokine with broad hematopoietic and immunostimulatory effects. There are two forms of IL-1, IL-1α and IL-1β. In hematopoiesis, IL-1 induces the production of several growth factors, including GM-CSF, G-CSF, and IL-6, and it synergizes with CSFs in the proliferation of hematopoietic progenitor cells.[53] Although IL-1 has some multilineage effects, as a growth factor it has shown the most potential as a platelet-stimulating factor. Platelet-stimulating effects of IL-1 may be related to secondary stimulation of IL-6. Recombinant IL-1α has shown definite activity in increasing platelet counts after high-dose chemotherapy regimens containing carboplatin but not without significant side effects, including dose-limiting hypotension.[54] Usefulness of IL-1 appears limited by its severe toxicities.[55] (See under Anticancer Cytokine Therapy for a further description of IL-1).

Interleukin-6. Interleukin-6 is a cytokine with many actions within the immune system and in hematopoiesis. It is believed to have a role in thrombopoiesis as a cofactor in stimulating the CFU-MK progenitor cell. It is synergistic to other growth factors such as IL-1 and IL-3 in increasing the number of CFU-MK colonies. Interleukin-6 also promotes differentiation and maturation of megakaryocytes.[56]

The ability of IL-6 to accelerate platelet recovery has been studied in several clinical trials. Because of unacceptable toxicities (headache, fever, myalgia, and stimulation of acute-phase reactants) and only modest thrombopoietic effects, it does not appear that IL-6 will be a clinically useful agent.[17]

Anticancer Cytokine Therapy

Interferon

Interferon (IFN) was the first cytokine to be explored as an anticancer biological agent. It has been extensively studied, both in natural and recombinant forms, in a variety of doses and schedules. The early enthusiasm for interferon as a "magic bullet for cancer" did not become a reality, but now interferons are being used as part of biological therapy in low- and high-dose regimens and in combination with other cytokines and chemotherapy regimens.[57]

Interferon was discovered in 1957 with the observation that cells infected with a virus produced a substance that prevented further viral infection to nearby cells.[58] In the 1970s and 1980s, the anticancer qualities of IFN led to clinical trials using a natural product extracted from leukocytes and later recombinant varieties when they became available. Table 24-4 describes IFNs presently approved by the FDA for clinical use.

Types

There are three major types of IFN in the body: α, β, and γ. Interferon-α and -β are type-I IFN and are located on chromosome 9. While IFN-β has only one form, there are more than 24 subtypes of IFN-α. Interferon-α is primarily made by virally stimulated leukocytes; IFN-β is made by activated fibroblasts. Interferon-γ is the only type-II IFN, and its gene is located on chromosome 12. It is made by antigen-activated T cells and NK cells as part of an immune response. All three of these IFNs have recombinant forms and are approved for use in cancer and other diseases. Currently IFN-α is the only type of IFN with approved indications in oncology.

There is also a second-generation type of interferon called consensus IFN (CIFN) (rIFN-con-1, Infergen). Consensus IFN, a type-I interferon that does not occur in nature, was bioengineered by combining the amino acid sequences of the first eight known subtypes of IFN-α.[59] Toxicities are similar to those experienced with IFN-α. Consensus IFN is approved for use in chronic hepatitis C. Consensus IFN is being evaluated in clinical trials in various malignancies. A polyethylene-glycol-modified IFN (PEG intron) has been developed and is in early clinical trials. This agent has a longer half-life than the naturally occurring protein and requires less frequent administration.[60]

Another new class of IFN has also been identified. Interferon-τ, or trophoblast IFN, is a new class of IFN that has a structure similar to IFN-α. The major function of trophoblast IFN is to signal receptors in the endometrium to maintain an appropriate environment for the embryo. Preliminary laboratory studies suggest that trophoblast IFN may have antiviral and antineoplastic activity.[58,61]

Biological activity

The interferons have multiple activities that vary significantly among the interferon types. Activities of the interferons include antiviral activity, direct antiproliferative activity, immunomodulation, inhibition of angiogenesis, regulation of differentiation, oncogene suppression, and enhancement of cell-surface antigen expression. Interferons α and β exert direct antitumor activity. They slow the growth and proliferation of tumor cells by pro-

Table 24-4   Types of Interferons: A Comparison of Characteristics

Type/Subtype	Primary Function	Cell Source	Commercial Product	FDA-Approved Uses
Type I				
INF-α	Antiviral; antiproliferative	Leukocytes; host cells infected by virus	Leukocyte IFN IFN Alfa 2A Roferon (Roche)	• Chronic hepatitis C • Chronic myelogenous leukemia • HCL • AIDS-related Kaposi sarcoma
			IFN Alfa 2B Intron A (Schering)	• HCL; AIDS-related Kaposi sarcoma • Chronic hepatitis B • Adjuvant therapy for follicular lymphoma with anthracycline-containing chemotherapy • Condyloma acuminata • Adjuvant melanoma
			Infergen (Amgen)	• Chronic hepatitis C
IFN-β	Antiviral; antiproliferative	Fibroblast; endothelial cells	Interferon Beta 1b Betaseron (Berlex/Chiron Labs)	• Relapsing, remitting multiple sclerosis
			Interferon Beta 1a Avonex (Biogen)	
Type II				
IFN-γ	Immunomodulatory	Activated T cells; NK cells	IFN Gamma 1b Actimmune (Genetech)	• Chronic granulomatous disease

longing the cell cycle. The chief function of IFN-γ is immunomodulation. It induces class-II MHC receptor molecules, activates macrophages, and increases the cytotoxicity of T cells and NK cells. Interferon-γ also induces other cytokines such as IL-2 and TNF-α.[61-64]

Side effects

Side effects of IFN depend on the IFN type, dose level, and schedule. The higher the dose, the more severe the side effects. Table 24-5 lists typical side effects of IFN. Patients receiving IFN-α experience the worst flulike symptoms on the first dose. Flulike symptoms typically develop 2–4 hours after IFN administration and last for approximately 8 hours. With continued administration, patients develop tachyphylaxis or the lessening of intensity and disappearance of symptoms. However, if the IFN is stopped and restarted, the acute symptoms recur. Patients receiving IFN-γ do not experience tachyphylaxis to acute symptoms. Fatigue is the primary dose-limiting toxicity of IFN therapy.[61,64]

Clinical application of alfa-interferon

Interferon-α was first approved for use in hairy cell leukemia (HCL). However, other more active drugs have generally replaced its use in HCL. It is also approved for use in a high-dose regimen for AIDS-related Kaposi's sarcoma and CML. Interferon-α is approved for use in follicular lymphoma when used in combination with an anthracycline-containing regimen. The addition of IFN-α to a doxorubicin-containing regimen for patients with advanced-stage follicular lymphoma increased the progression-free survival and overall survival compared to chemotherapy alone.[65] Interferon-α is also approved for use in various forms of hepatitis and for condyloma acuminata.

Interferon-α is indicated for use as an adjuvant for surgical patients with malignant melanoma who are at high risk for systemic recurrence because of the thickness of the primary lesion or local lymph node involvement.

Table 24-5 Common Toxicities Related to Interferon Administration

Acute:

Fever, chills, rigor
Malaise
Myalgia
Headache
Nausea, vomiting, diarrhea

Chronic:

Anorexia
Weight loss
Fatigue
Mental slowing
Confusion
Neutropenia, thrombocytopenia
Increased liver enzymes

In a pivotal randomized clinical trial, IFN-α was associated with a 42% improvement in 5-year relapse-free survival rate and an improvement in overall survival in the adjuvant setting.[66] A subsequent follow-up trial demonstrated an improvement in relapse-free survival, but no statistically significant difference in overall survival.[67] The adjuvant melanoma regimen involves a 4-week induction phase of IFN at 20 MIU/m² IV 5 days/week, followed by a 48-week maintenance phase of IFN at 10 MIU/m² SC 3 days/week. Side effects with this regimen may be substantial. Nursing management involves assessment of side effects, which may require nursing support or dose modifications.[68]

Interferon-α has shown activity in renal cell carcinoma, multiple myeloma, cutaneous T-cell lymphoma, and squamous and basal cell cancer of the skin. Interferon-α has been used in many clinical trials in combination with other biological agents and chemotherapy.

Interleukins

Interleukins are cytokines that act primarily between lymphocytes. The word *interleukin* literally means "between white cells." However, since their discovery, ILs have been found to have broader activity, interacting with other immune cells and body organs that have a role in the inflammatory immune response.

Interleukins are referred to by several names, as they were discovered by a variety of researchers and given functional names to describe their identified action. To minimize confusion, the International Congress of Immunology designates interleukins by number as soon as the interleukin gene is described. To date, eighteen have been identified, and the search for new interleukins continues.[69] Interleukin-2 is the only interleukin approved by the FDA as an anticancer agent.

Unlike other forms of cancer therapy such as chemotherapy, interleukins are not directly cytotoxic to tumor cells. Rather, they act as messengers to initiate, coordinate, and sometimes amplify potent immune defense activities. As such, they require a functional, intact immune system to achieve their therapeutic effects.

Immunosuppressive agents such as corticosteroids can block the therapeutic actions of interleukins and other cytokines when they are used as anticancer therapy. This has implications for health care professionals when selecting medications for the management of symptoms commonly associated with cytokine therapy.

The following section highlights IL-2 and its clinical use and discusses other interleukins that have been evaluated for use as antitumor agents.

Interleukin-2

Biologic effects. First identified as a T-cell growth factor, IL-2 is a lymphokine that causes immune activation and release of other cytokines. Interleukin-2 has no direct antitumor activity but stimulates the activation of immune cells capable of targeting and killing cancer cells. Produced by activated T lymphocytes, IL-2 increases and stimulates the following immune system cells: cytotoxic lymphoid cells, NK and lymphokine-activated killer (LAK) cells, B cells, complement factors, and monocytes and macrophages. Interleukin-2 also stimulates the production of other cytokines such as IFN-γ, TNF, and GM-CSF. Interleukin-2 facilitates the migration of immunologically active cells to the tumor site. Dose-dependent immunomodulatory and antitumor activity of IL-2 in animal models led to the development of high-dose IL-2 regimens for clinical investigation.[70,71]

Clinical application.   Recombinant IL-2 (rIL-2), also known as aldesleukin (Proleukin), was first approved for the treatment of metastatic renal cell cancer (RCC) and has subsequently been approved for metastatic melanoma. Initial approval for rIL-2 in RCC was based on a multicenter study of 255 patients in which 14% of participants responded to the therapy. For those patients who responded, the remission was durable and averaged 20.3 months.[72] A 1996 update of the long-term response data from these patients indicated a 15% overall response rate and a median response duration for all objective responders of 54 months, with a range of 3 months to 8.9 years.[73]

High-dose rIL-2 received approval for use in malignant melanoma based on a retrospective analysis of 266 patients treated in all trials of high-dose bolus rIL-2 conducted between 1985 and 1993. The median response duration in this analysis was 6.5 months, with 60% of responders remaining progression-free at 5 years.[74]

In initial clinical studies, IL-2 was given by IV bolus infusion at doses of 600,000 to 720,000 IU/kg every 8 hours as tolerated.[75] The regulatory approved dose of rIL-2 for RCC and melanoma is 600,000 IU/kg every 8 hours by a 15-minute infusion for 5 days (maximum of 14 doses per cycle as tolerated). Following 9 days of rest, the schedule is repeated. Patients are retreated depending on results of tumor evaluation 4 weeks after completion of a course of therapy and prior to starting another treatment course.

Side effects.   The side effects of IL-2 are described in Table 24-6. It is important to note that the side effects of IL-2 are dose dependent. High-dose bolus rIL-2 is associated with severe dose-limiting multisystem side effects. Lower doses of rIL-2 are associated with many of the same side effects, but they are generally less severe. Interleukin-2 induces proinflammatory cytokines such as IL-1, TNF-α, and IFN-γ. These and other substances such as nitric oxide play a major role in rIL-2 toxicity.[76] Many IL-2 side effects are due to a dose-related capillary leak syndrome and are reversible when therapy is stopped.[77]

Patients must be carefully screened prior to beginning IL-2 treatment to ensure adequate renal, hepatic, neurologic, cardiac, and pulmonary function. Treatment-related mortality with high-dose bolus IL-2 has decreased significantly as clinicians have had more experience with this agent and have learned to select appropriate patients.

The multiorgan toxicity of this regimen has limited its use to patients with excellent organ function and performance status who are being treated by experienced clinicians in an intensive-care setting.[76,78]

Alternate IL-2 regimens.   In an attempt to minimize toxicity, clinical trials have examined various doses, routes, and schedules of rIL-2 in metastatic RCC. Numerous publications in the literature describe the use of rIL-2 outside of the approved regimen. Lower dose intravenous (bolus or continuous infusion) regimens have generally resulted in decreased toxicities and have allowed patients to be treated in conventional hospital settings. Subcutaneous rIL-2 regimens have safely been given in the outpatient setting. These regimens are also associated with fewer side effects than high-dose bolus therapy. Transient inflammation and local induration at injection sites occurs in most patients receiving subcutaneous rIL-2. Fever, chills, fatigue, and nausea are the most common side effects seen with subcutaneous rIL-2.[79-81]

Alternate regimens of rIL-2 alone or in combination with IFN have successfully reduced acute toxicities and expense associated with inpatient regimens while maintaining comparable response rates. Patients with poorer functional status such as the elderly and those with concomitant systemic disease are more likely to tolerate the lower dose regimens. Recent data suggests, however, that the duration of response may be less with low-dose regimens.[73,78,80,82] It has been suggested that until long-term follow-up of low-dose rIL-2 regimens documents durable responses and survival, high-dose rIL-2 is the therapy of choice for patients with metastatic RCC who are able to tolerate this therapy.[73,78,80,82] In metastatic melanoma, high-dose rIL-2 has been associated with superior overall response rates that are more durable and of higher quality than those obtained with lower doses of rIL-2 or alternative administration schedules or routes.[76]

IL-2: Other directions.   Toxicity-reduction strategies such as administering IL-2 with agents that block the effects of IL-1 and TNF are being evaluated to ameliorate severe high-dose IL-2 toxicities.[76] The role of IL-2 as adjuvant treatment for patients with high-risk stage III RCC is being studied in a large randomized clinical trial. Studies are also investigating the potential use of IL-2 in HIV infection[83] and as a vaccine adjuvant in cancer and infectious disease. Low-dose or ultra-low-dose long-term pulse therapy with IL-2 has been studied as a means to provide longer-lasting immune stimulation.[84]

Hematologic malignancies and BMT are emerging areas for rIL-2 trials, though the role of rIL-2 in these settings is uncertain.[85] Interleukin-2 has been evaluated as consolidative immunotherapy after BMT or stem cell transplant at the time of minimal residual disease with the intent of reducing relapse rates.[86] Positive preliminary results have encouraged development of phase III trials. Interleukin-2 has been given after autologous BMT with the intent of augmenting the graft versus tumor effect to improve relapse rates.[87] It also has been studied in

Table 24-6 Side Effects of Interleukin-2

System	Manifestation	Comment	Management Guidelines
General—flulike	Fever, malaise, chills/rigors Myalgias/arthralgias Headache Fatigue	Fever occurs within 2–8 hours of drug administration; most severe after initial doses Chills/rigors occur 2–8 hours after IV administration and within 30–60 minutes after SC administration	Premedicate with acetaminophen and/ or NSAIDs Narcotics (i.e., meperidine or dilaudid) may be given to control chills
Gastrointestinal	Nausea, vomiting, diarrhea, anorexia, taste changes, stomatitis	Mild to moderate and dose-dependent Resolve rapidly after treatment is discontinued	Antiemetics Avoid concomitant use of corticosteroids (may reduce effectiveness of therapy) Antidiarrheal agents Dietary modifications
Dermatologic	Pruritic, macular erythematous rash that can progress to dry desquamation Injection-site nodules and induration with SC administration Peeling skin on palms and soles	Dermatologic reactions can be mild to moderate or severe Skin nodules from SC injections usually disappear within a few months after treatment is discontinued	Antipruritics Water-based moisturizers Emollient lotions Avoid drying soaps, excessive heat Rotation of injection sites
Neurologic	Confusion, hallucination, agitation, cognitive changes, depression, sleep disturbances	Dose-related; may be dose-limiting with high-dose May be seen after a few doses; reversible	Establish safety measures; discontinuation of agent may be necessary Antidepressants as appropriate Sedative; antianxiety medication
Cardiovascular/ Pulmonary	Hypotension, tachycardia, arrhythmias, fluid retention, edema, weight gain, dyspnea	Partially related to capillary leak syndrome—increased capillary permeability causes fluid to leak from vascular bed into tissues	Assess heart/lung sounds, vital signs, weight Use of diuretics discouraged with high-dose IL-2 (may result in depletion of intravascular volume and hypotension) Vasopressors and judicious use of fluids for high-dose IL-2 Diuretics may be used at completion of high dose therapy
Renal	Increased creatinine, BUN; oliguria, azotemia	Related to decreased renal perfusion associated with decrease in intravascular volume and peripheral vascular dilatation Concomitant use of NSAIDS may contribute further to renal toxicity	Monitor lab values, I & O Renal dose vasopressors may be needed to maintain kidney perfusion
Hepatic	Elevated SGOT, SGPT, LDH, alkaline phosphatase, bilirubin Jaundice	Dose-related Reversible	Monitor lab values Assess for jaundice, hepatomegaly
Hematologic	Thrombocytopenia, anemia leukopenia, eosinophilia Impaired neutrophil function with decreased chemotaxis	Generally mild	Monitor CBC Administer prophylactic antibiotics for patients with central lines receiving high-dose IL-2 Assess for infection, bleeding, fatigue, SOB Support with blood products

NSAIDs = nonsteroidal anti-inflammatories; I & O = intake and output; SOB = shortness of breath.

patients with AML with relapsed and refractory disease and in second remission with encouraging results.[88]

Interleukin-1

Interleukin-1 is one of the oldest known cytokines having broad, pleiotropic effects on the body. Interleukin-1 is identified as the prototypic proinflammatory cytokine and is a primary coordinator of the body's inflammatory response to microbial invasion. It is described as having a major role in a variety of inflammatory and autoimmune diseases and is responsible for the harmful host effects of acute sepsis. In host defense, IL-1 stimulates both T and B lymphocytes and is a cofactor in the activation of

NK cells. It also stimulates secondary cytokine production of IL-2, IL-3, CSFs, IL-6, and TNF. These actions frequently manifest in the side effects experienced by patients receiving recombinant IL-1 (rIL-1) or cytokines that induce endogenous IL-1 production. Interleukin-1-induced septic shock appears to be mediated by the ability of IL-1 to increase plasma concentrations of molecules such as platelet-activating factor, prostaglandins, and nitric oxide, which are potent vasodilators.[89]

Several clinical studies have explored the potential side effects, dose-limiting toxicities, and antitumor potential of IL-1α and IL-1β. Both forms of IL-1 have been associated with symptoms typical of acute sepsis including fever, rigors, nausea, and dose-limiting hypotension sometimes requiring vasopressor support. No significant antitumor responses have been reported with IL-1.[90–92]

Another member of the IL-1 family is the IL-1 receptor agonist (IL-1RA). By blocking the binding of IL-1 to its cell-surface receptors, IL-1RA inhibits IL-1 activity.[89] It has been identified as having a possible role in decreasing IL-1-induced side effects associated with IL-2 administration, but success with this approach has been limited.[76]

Interleukin-4

Interleukin-4 is primarily a growth factor for B cells and a cofactor for T-cell development. It is capable of stimulating the growth and activation of mast cells and eosinophils. Truitt et al reviewed more than ten phase I/II studies of recombinant IL-4 (rIL-4), starting in 1988, to evaluate the toxicity and potential efficacy of this agent. Common side effects seen with rIL-4 include flulike symptoms, fluid retention, and significant nasal congestion, headache, and malaise. None of the studies reported significant response in patients receiving rIL-4, likely further limiting study of single-agent rIL-4 as an anticancer agent.[93,94]

Interleukin-6

Interleukin-6, like IL-1, has pleiotropic or wide-ranging actions to promote host defense. The primary sources of IL-6 are the monocyte/macrophage and activated T-helper cells. Interleukin-6 also inhibits tumor growth and is a cofactor in thrombopoiesis and B-cell differentiation.[62] First identified as IFN-α2 due to its similarity to α- and β-interferons and its antiviral activity, IL-6 is also known as a hybridoma growth factor in the production of monoclonal antibodies and the growth of myeloma.[93] Like IL-1, IL-6 is a pyrogenic cytokine capable of inducing fever. Administration of IL-6 has been associated with fever, headache, fatigue, myalgia, reversible anemia, and induction of acute-phase proteins. Clinical trials with recombinant IL-6 (rIL-6) have failed to show significant antitumor effect, likely limiting its clinical usefulness.[93]

Interleukin-12

Interleukin-12 is a multifunctional cytokine that promotes cell-mediated immunity through its effects on T and NK cells. Interleukin-12 facilitates type-1 helper T-lymphocyte responses, enhances the lytic activity of NK cells, augments the specific CTL responses, and induces the secretion of IFN-γ. Preclinical models of IL-12 have demonstrated significant antitumor activity. Interleukin-12 has also been shown to play an important role in the promotion of the host resistance to infection by bacterial, fungal, and protozoan pathogens.[95–97]

Recombinant IL-12 (rIL-12) has been studied in phase I and II clinical trials. Early studies of IV bolus rIL-12 were complicated by severe toxicities and treatment-related deaths, thus clinical development was temporarily halted.[98] Subsequent studies found that administering a test dose of rIL-12 prior to initiating daily intravenous dosing is necessary to attenuate the severe toxicity. Recombinant IL-12 has been given safely as an IV bolus with the use of a test dose and in subcutaneous regimens. Common side effects seen with rIL-12 include fever, chills, fatigue, stomatitis, liver function test abnormalities, and transient leukopenia.[76,99]

Clinical trials using rIL-12 in RCC have shown limited response, and trials in other malignancies including melanoma are ongoing.[76] Interleukin-12 is also being evaluated after transplantation, in the HIV setting and as a vaccine adjuvant. Recombinant IL-12 may have potential in combination with other cytokines such as IL-2 and as an antiviral agent for the treatment of hepatitis B and hepatitis C virus.[97]

Combination Therapy

In an attempt to improve and optimize response in certain malignancies, various combinations of cytokines and chemotherapeutic agents have been evaluated. The important variables of agent, dose, route, sequencing of agents, and duration of treatment are only a few that may influence significantly the therapeutic outcome for the patient. Many combinations of cytokines have been evaluated such as rIL-2 and rIL-4, rIL-2 and rTNF-α; the most widely studied combination is rIL-2 and IFN-α. A clinical advantage from the addition of IFN-α to rIL-2 has not been demonstrated in RCC and melanoma.[100] An ongoing randomized phase III trial in the Cytokine Working Group is comparing the efficacy of high-dose bolus rIL-2 with an outpatient subcutaneous regimen of rIL-2 and IFN-α in metastatic RCC.

Biochemotherapy

This form of combination therapy involves combining a cytokine or group of cytokines with chemotherapy. This therapy attempts to preserve the immune function stimulated by the cytokines along with tumoricidal effects of chemotherapy and improve response rates of either treatment modality alone. Synergy between chemotherapeutic and biological agents and the lack of cross-resistance provides a sound basis for the development of biochemotherapy regimens.[101] Numerous studies have evaluated rIL-2 or IFN-α in combination with various chemotherapy agents in several malignancies.

Biochemotherapy has been most actively studied in metastatic melanoma. Encouraging results have been seen with studies that combine cisplatin-based chemotherapy with high-dose IL-2 alone or with lower doses of IL-2 and IFN. Combined results from a variety of regimens show a response rate of approximately 50%, with a median survival of 11–12 months. These regimens have been administered either in a sequential or concurrent fashion. Most biochemotherapy regimens require inpatient admission and are associated with significant side effects including severe myelosuppression, nausea and vomiting, and moderately severe hypotension as well as constitutional symptoms. Outpatient biochemotherapy regimens have also been developed. It is uncertain how these regimens compare to chemotherapy alone or inpatient biochemotherapy regimens. Despite some promising results, biochemotherapy remains investigational. More phase III trial data (including survival rates and durability of responses) comparing biochemotherapy with chemotherapy or immunotherapy alone are needed to clearly establish a role for biochemotherapy in the treatment of metastatic melanoma.[76]

Tumor Necrosis Factors

Tumor necrosis factors are a group of glycoproteins produced by immune cells in response to a pathogen. They are the active substances first seen in Coley's toxins. Cachectin, or TNF-α, is produced primarily by macrophages, NK cells, and T cells. These cells elicit a variety of immune response actions including increased catabolism, enhanced phagocytosis, and tumor destruction.[62]

Lymphotoxin, or TNF-β, is also a cytokine produced by T cells in response to antigen. It is a cytotoxin that when released is capable of killing any nearby cells. The cell killing of TNF-β is enhanced by IFN-γ.[62] Tumor necrosis factor is one of the few cytokines that has direct, tumoricidal capability. Although the exact method of cell killing is yet unknown, TNF is capable of damaging tumor blood vessels, leading to necrosis and loss of nutrients and oxygen.[102]

The recombinant form of TNF-α (rTNF-α) was evaluated in phase I clinical trials in 1987. Toxicities included severe constitutional symptoms and hypotension, resembling symptoms of septic shock.[103] While rTNF-α was shown to be effective in preclinical trials, in murine tumors, the maximum tolerated dose (MTD) of TNF-α in clinical studies was substantially less than the effective dose in murine tumors.[104]

Subsequent clinical trials have focused on using rTNF-α in a regional infusion as a way to limit systemic toxicity yet increase the dose to tumors to obtain local control and make limb-sparing surgery possible.[105] Patients with melanoma and sarcoma whose tumors are confined to a limb have received rTNF via isolated limb perfusions with melphalan or with melphalan and IFN-γ. Significant and sometimes dramatic necrosis of melanoma or sarcoma tumors has been seen with this treatment, which has produced response rates up to 90%.[106–108] Side effects have included fever and chills, skin rash, limb swelling, and hypotension in the immediate postoperative period. Systemic toxicities are a result of the leak of perfusate from the extremity to the systemic circulation.[106–108] Tumor necrosis factor is approved in Europe for isolated limb perfusion of locally advanced grade 2–3 soft-tissue sarcomas in extremities.[108] Tumor necrosis factor has also been administered with melphalan via isolated hepatic perfusion for unresectable cancers confined to the liver, with significant regression of bulky hepatic cancers seen in the majority of patients.[109]

Activated Cell Therapy (Adoptive Immunotherapy)

The discovery and development of recombinant cytokines such as IL-2 have facilitated the development of activated cell therapy. These activated cells are immune cells that are removed from the patient and placed in culture with rIL-2, which greatly increases their numbers and enhances their cytolytic capacity. The cells are then administered to the patient as adoptive immunotherapy. Activated cells are capable of targeting cancer cells without killing normal cells.

There are two types of activated cells: LAK cells and tumor-infiltrating lymphocytes (TIL). Lymphokine-activated killer cells are primarily made up of NK cells activated on exposure to high levels of IL-2. They are nonspecific killer cells that can lyse tumor cells without major histocompatibility complex (MHC) recognition and specificity.[110]

Lymphokine-Activated Killer Cells

Therapy with LAK begins with the administration of high-dose rIL-2 to stimulate cell production. These cells are then removed by a series of plasmaphereses and are cultured in rIL-2 for several days. They are returned to the patient along with additional rIL-2 doses as tolerated.

The side effects of the therapy are caused by the rIL-2 administered with the cells and include fever, chills, hypotension, oliguria, weight gain, mental status changes, and pruritus. Only pulmonary congestion and dyspnea are attributable to LAK cells themselves.

One of the first patients with melanoma to be given IL-2/LAK therapy had a durable complete remission. However, long-term evaluation of IL-2/LAK therapy has shown that only 5%–10% of patients with melanoma or RCC have responded to therapy. The addition of LAK cells has not demonstrated an advantage in response rates over patients receiving high-dose rIL-2 alone.[111]

Tumor-Infiltrating Lymphocytes

Tumor-infiltrating lymphocytes are a second type of activated cell used in cell transfer therapy. They are derived from tumor sites and are cytotoxic to autologous (patient's own) but not allogeneic (others of the same type) tumors. They are also 50–100 times more potent than LAK. Though the TIL cell population may vary according to the type of cancer, in melanoma approximately 60% are CD4/CD8 cells, and NK cell numbers are low. They also differ from LAK as they travel to tumor sites, recognizing MHC and tumor antigens.[112]

Therapy with TIL begins with isolation of these cells from fresh resected tumor that is enzymatically digested into single cell suspensions. Tumor cells and TIL are then cultured in a medium containing antibiotics and rIL-2. Within 2 weeks, tumor cells disappear; over 30 days, the number of TIL rapidly increases and is allowed to grow to a size predicted from preclinical studies to be therapeutically effective. The cells are then removed from culture, washed, and prepared for reinfusion. They are administered intravenously in saline in divided doses depending on the total numbers of cells. High-dose rIL-2 is also administered as tolerated to keep the cells active.[113]

The toxicity of TIL therapy reflects the same side effects of high-dose rIL-2. Side effects directly related to TIL infusions are pulmonary symptoms such as dyspnea, pulmonary congestion, and hypoxia.

Rosenberg et al reported the 5-year National Institutes of Health (NIH) experience with TIL therapy in malignant melanoma: 86 patients were treated with TIL and rIL-2 with or without cyclophosphamide.[114] The objective response rate was 34%, with more patients responding to TIL derived from subcutaneous metastatic tumor deposits than to TIL derived from lymph nodes. No significant difference was reported for patients who also received cyclophamide. Some patients responded to TIL who had previously failed to respond to high-dose rIL-2 alone; however, only one complete response and no durable responses occurred in this group. Considering that IL-2 plus TIL therapy is not sufficiently superior to IL-2 alone and that this regimen is costly and time and labor intensive, clinical usefulness of this treatment modality appears limited.[76]

As cancer therapy moves to a molecular-based level, a new generation of more effective TIL may be created. Early gene-therapy trials used TIL transduced with genes for cytokines such as TNF and IL-2 that were designed to deliver high concentrations of TNF to tumor sites with decreased systemic effects.[115] Tumor-infiltrating lymphocytes have been instrumental in the identification of melanoma-associated antigens (MAA), which have a role in cancer vaccine therapy. They also have shown an ability to recognize MAA and have subsequently been used to clone the genes that encoded the MAA that they recognized. The availability of the gene sequences of MAA has provided new opportunities for developing immunization strategies involving the delivery of the desired gene product to the patient in the form of a recombinant virus.[76]

Monoclonal Antibodies

Antibodies are proteins made by the immune system, each in response to a specific antigen. Monoclonal antibodies (MAb) are artificially produced antibodies that are the product of a single clone of cells sensitized to a specific antigenic protein present on the surface of a target tumor. Monoclonal antibody therapy, also known as *serotherapy* or *passive immunotherapy*, was one of the first forms of modern biotherapy to use a highly specific cytotoxic agent directed against cancer cells while sparing normal tissue.

Manufacture of Antibodies and the Hybridoma Technique

In the 1970s, the hybridoma technique enabled researchers to create highly specific antibodies in large quantities, which made it possible to develop MAbs into a potential cancer therapy. However, it also introduced one of this therapy's biggest problems—the use of foreign immunogenic protein.

As shown in Figure 24-4, the hybridoma process begins by immunizing a mouse with a selected antigen. B cells within the spleen of the mouse soon produce immunoglobulin directed against the injected antigen. The mouse spleen cells are then fused in polyethylene glycol with immortal B cells—myeloma cells—that are capable of continued antibody production in cell culture. Thus, B spleen cells with the desired genetic antibody information are combined with cells having continued antibody production potential. These hybrid daughter cells are separated using a medium that eliminates all nonhybrid cells; clones that produce the desired antibody against the immunizing antigen are then selected. Finally, the selected cell clones are stored or cultured for mass production.[116–118]

This classic method of MAb production has been modified through the use of genetic engineering techniques. Recombinant DNA allows MAb structure to be reshaped to include portions made from human protein or to delete undesired sections of the antibody structure.[119] Newer methods of MAb production include the use of transgenic animals or the genetic engineering of a mouse to produce human instead of mouse antibodies. Some biotechnology companies are evaluating the use of bacteria such as *E. coli* as antibody factories to mass-produce a specific antibody.[120]

Structure

Monoclonal antibodies are made of two heavy and two light polypeptide chains that are linked by disulfide bonds to form a Y (Figure 24-5). The site where the antibody binds with the specific antigen is called the variable region (Fab) because it varies greatly from one antibody to another. The stem of the Y links the antibody to other cells that participate in the immune response. This area is called the constant region (Fc) of the molecule because it is constant within all classes of antibodies.[121]

The first generation of MAbs were made from murine proteins. The repetitive use of antibodies containing foreign protein is strongly immunogenic in immunocompetent patients. It is estimated that 50% of patients develop human antimouse antibody (HAMA) on the first exposure, and up to 90% of patients who receive three or more MAb doses develop HAMA.[120] Human antimouse antibody can bind to the MAb, increasing its clearance from the body and potentially leading to increased toxicity.

In an attempt to decrease the incidence of HAMA, changes in the structure of MAbs have been made to

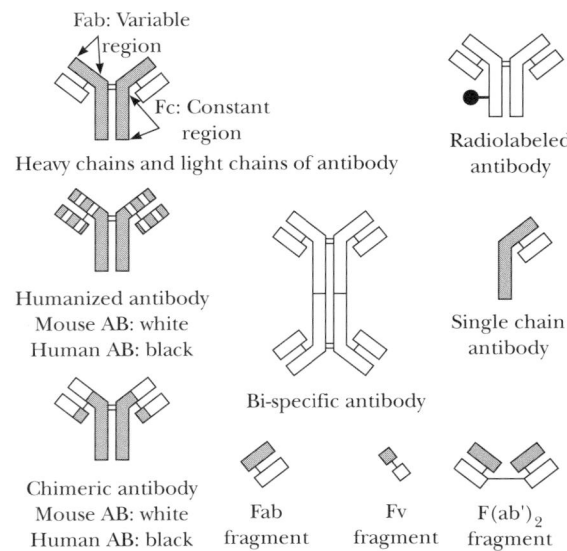

Figure 24-5 Antibody anatomy: variations on the structure of murine, human, and chimeric antibodies.

include more human protein, which is less immunogenic. Figure 24-5 shows some of the major modifications of MAb. Chimera antibodies combine the mouse Fab or variable portion with a humanized constant region or Fc. These MAbs have a longer circulating half-life and are less immunogenic than murine antibodies, which allows for repeated dosing.[119] The human Fc portion of a chimeric MAb improves its ability to mediate complement-dependent cytotoxicity (CDC) and antibody-dependent cell-mediated cytotoxicity (ADCC), which makes it more potent than the parent murine MAb. Another MAb design is predominately human protein and is called *humanized antibody*. Short segments of murine antibody have been inserted in the variable end on a human antibody structure.

Another approach to antibody design has been to decrease the size of the antibody and use the antibody fragments. These fragments—Fab, F(ab')$_2$, or Fv—lack a constant Fc region and thus cannot attach to host cells. They are less immunogenic and are able to penetrate tissues more than an intact antibody but are rapidly cleared from the circulation. Antibody fragments are also used as vehicles for toxins or radioisotopes.[122]

Mechanism of action

The first generation of MAb was used in its native, unconjugated form and functioned like human immunoglobulin. This form of unaltered antibody is dependent on host immune mechanisms for cell killing because the antibody itself is not a cytotoxic agent. Some of these immune mechanisms include activation of the complement cascade on the surface of tumor cells, which can result in cell killing through enzymes; enabling phago-

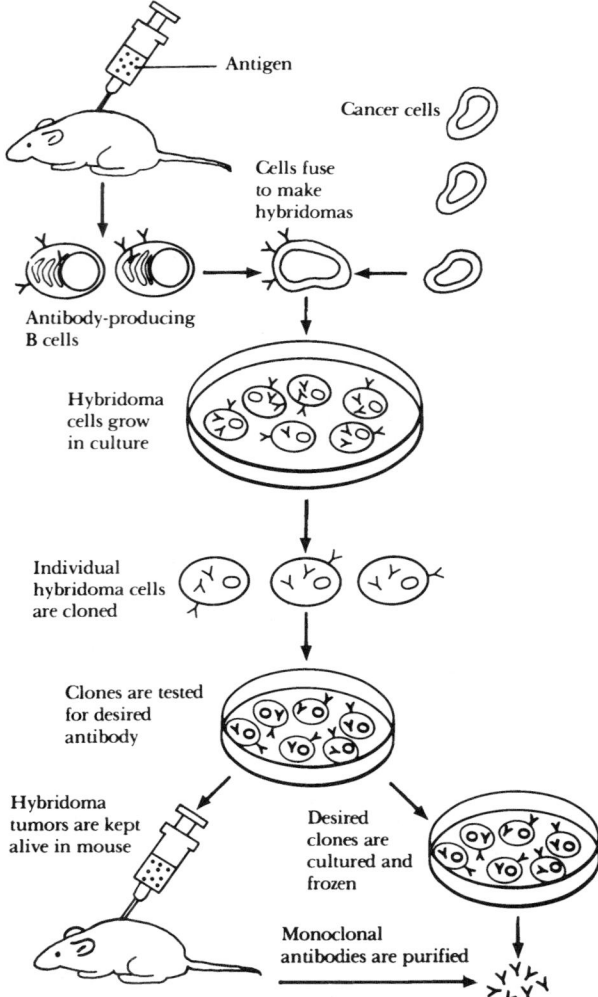

Figure 24-4 A diagram of the hybridoma technology for manufacturing monoclonal antibodies. Reprinted from Schindler LW: Understanding the Immune System. NIH Publication No. 88-529. Bethesda, MD, US Department of Health and Human Services, 1988.[116]

cytic cells to attach to and ingest tumor cells; and enhancing NK cell tumor destruction by ADCC.[121]

Antigen identification

The specificity of MAbs is dependent on identifying antigenic proteins on the surface of tumors that are not present on normal tissues. Monoclonal antibodies have been developed and directed toward many tumor-associated antigens. Some of the categories of MAb antigen targets include oncofetal antigens (carcinoembryonic antigen; CEA), differentiation antigens, tissue-specific antigens (prostate-specific antigen; PSA), growth factors (epidermal growth factor), and oncogene products (c-erbB2). Anti-idiotypic antibodies can also be used as surrogate antigens. An *idiotype* is the specific binding region of an antibody. Anti-idiotype MAbs are directed to the antigen-binding sites of antitumor antibodies and mimic the original tumor antigen.[117,121,123]

Monoclonal Antibodies in Cancer Therapy

Monoclonal antibodies have three essential roles in cancer therapy:

1. Diagnostic and screening functions; radioisotope-labeled MAbs are capable of identifying sites of tumor in the patient that may not be detectable by other methods.
2. Purging autologous bone marrow of malignant cells ex vivo.
3. Cancer therapy capable of killing tumor cells with high specificity.

Cancer therapy with MAbs has made great strides in the 1990s and is the focus of the following discussion.

Unconjugated monoclonal antibodies

Unconjugated MAbs are the simplest of the MAb therapies. As noted earlier, these were the first generation of MAb to be studied. In this approach, the MAb itself mediates cell death through various immune mechanisms. Selecting the proper target antigen has been essential to the development of MAb therapy. Hematologic malignancies have been extensively studied as ideal tumor models for MAb therapy because they express a variety of well-defined cell-surface antigens.[124] The first MAb approved for therapeutic use in oncology, rituximab (Rituxan), is an unconjugated MAb directed against the CD20 antigen. The second MAb approved for therapeutic use is trastuzumab (Herceptin), the anti-Her-2 MAb. (These MAbs are discussed in detail later under Approved Therapeutic Monoclonal Antibodies.)

An extensively studied unconjugated MAb is the CAMPATH-1 MAb, which is targeted against CD52, an antigen expressed by both B and T cells as well as monocytes and granulocytes. The humanized version, CAMPATH-1H, has shown efficacy in refractory chronic lymphocytic leukemia (CLL), with response rates from 42%–80%, and pivotal trials are underway to secure approval for its use in this malignancy. CAMPATH-1H is associated with significant toxicity including infusion-related reactions and grade IV neutropenia, thrombocytopenia, and lymphopenia. CD10 and CD25 have been studied as antigen targets for the therapy of acute lymphocytic leukemia (ALL). CD10 is also known as the CALLA, or the common ALL antigen, which is expressed by a large proportion of ALL cells. Trials have also used unconjugated MAb to treat patients with cutaneous T-cell lymphoma and AML with limited success.[124]

Monoclonal antibodies have also been extensively studied in various solid tumors, but generally the results have been less encouraging than in hematologic malignancies. Monoclonal antibody 17-1A is an antibody targeted toward a surface antigen in gastrointestinal cancers that has been widely studied in colorectal cancer.[121,124]

Antibody conjugates

Because of the limited efficacy seen with unconjugated MAb in early trials, another strategy was developed to use the ability of MAb to bind specifically to a target, spare normal tissues, and deliver a cell poison to the tumor cell. These carrier or conjugated MAbs are capable of cell killing and do not require the host's immune competence. Conjugated MAbs have three major divisions: immunotoxins, antibody drug conjugates, and radioimmunoconjugates.

Immunotoxins. An immunotoxin (IT) is a molecule formed when an MAb or fragment is conjugated to a plant or bacterial cell toxin. Ricin is the most commonly used plant toxin; however, some studies have tried saporin or gelonin. These are potent cell poisons, only minute amounts of which need to be incorporated into a cell to inhibit protein synthesis and cause cell death. Pseudomonas exotoxin (PE) and diphtheria toxin are the two most frequently used bacterial toxins.

First-generation ITs used a toxin chemically coupled to an unaltered MAb. These bonds were sometimes unstable and could separate in vivo.[125] Unexpected toxicity occasionally occurred. One example was the MAb OVB3 coupled to PE, or OVB3-PE. When this agent was tested in phase I studies in patients with ovarian cancer, unexpected severe neurotoxicity occurred due to cross-reactivity and binding of the MAb to neural tissue.[125] Efforts were then directed at decreasing toxicity and increasing efficacy.

Second-generation ITs use recombinant DNA technology to reshape both the MAb carrier and toxin, splicing desired genes and removing sites of binding from the toxin to decrease toxicity. Monoclonal antibody fragments can be combined with altered PE to decrease binding to hepatocytes, which has resulted in hepatic necrosis.

Most ITs have shown little activity in clinical trials and have been associated with significant toxicities such as dose-limiting vascular leak syndrome. Frequent development of HAMA or antitoxin responses have also occurred, which prohibited retreatment of patients. Of all MAb-based therapies, ITs may be farthest from clinical use as they are not as easy to use as other MAb therapies and do not have the low side effect profile of the unconjugated MAbs.[124]

Antibody-drug conjugates. Monoclonal antibodies have been linked to chemotherapeutic agents with the goal of increasing drug concentration at the tumor site. However, difficulty getting sufficient concentrations of drug at the site of bulky, often necrotic, and poorly vascularized tumors has been a limiting factor.

Radioimmunoconjugates. Monoclonal antibodies or MAb fragments have been used as carriers of radiation to tumor sites. Radiation has the advantage of killing tumor cells without requiring cell uptake. The most frequently used radionuclides are beta emitters such as iodide I 131 (I^{131}) and yttrium Y 90 (Y^{90}). They have a relatively short half-life and are capable of transmitting energy a distance of several cell diameters.[119] Several radioimmunoconjugates (RIC) have been under investigation. Trials of RIC in non-Hodgkin's lymphoma have reported response rates from 20%–30% with I^{131} conjugates that target a number of antigens including HLA-DR, CD20, CD21, and CD22. Even higher responses have been seen in studies in non-Hodgkin's lymphoma that used myeloablative doses of RIC with stem cell support. It has been suggested that RICs may become part of myeloablative combination chemotherapy regimens and may augment or replace total body irradiation. Initial studies have also shown promising results with RIC in the treatment of leukemias.[124]

Problems with RICs include potential liver damage due to radiation effects during MAb clearance, stability of the conjugated MAb, and the ability of the MAb to reach its target.[118,119] The infusion of RIC can be associated with acute systemic side effects such as fever, chills, rash, and nausea, and may also stimulate HAMA response in about 15%–25% of patients. Radioimmunoconjugates are also associated with a significant degree of myelosuppression that may be affected by prior radiation therapy and chemotherapy. Radioimmunoconjugates require an on-site radiopharmacy and dosimetry calculations, both of which may limit application of RICs to a small number of centers.[124]

Problems in Monoclonal Antibody Therapy

In addition to the problems with HAMA previously noted, other problems encountered in MAb therapy center on the characteristics of the tumor target. Unbound circulating antigen from the tumor can bind MAbs and prevent them from reaching their target. Also, tumors modulate or change surface antigens, making it difficult for the MAb to link to the target. Often, tumors are bulky, hypoxic, and poorly vascularized, making it difficult for circu-

lating MAbs to gain access. For these reasons, MAbs can have low uptake rates, particularly in solid tumors.[126]

Side Effects of Monoclonal Antibody Therapy

The side effect profile of MAbs depends on the agent used and whether the MAb is conjugated and the nature of the conjugate. Because some or all of the MAb consists of foreign proteins, acute infusion-related allergic reactions are common. Reactions can be mild to moderate and include fevers, chills, rigors, nausea and vomiting, fatigue, headache, rhinitis, and pruritus. More severe hypersensitivity reactions may include urticaria, pruritus, dyspnea, hypotension, bronchospasm, and rarely anaphylaxis. Symptoms usually begin within 30 minutes to 2 hours after the start of the first infusion and are usually limited to the duration of the infusion. This constellation of symptoms, which has been referred to as an *infusion-related symptom complex,* is more commonly seen with the agent rituximab, than with the humanized MAb, trastuzumab, because it is chimeric and contains a murine region. The use of chimeric MAbs has not eliminated infusion-related toxicities, but with chimeric MAbs infusion-related toxicities decrease substantially with second and subsequent doses.[124,127]

Another potential reaction to MAb therapy is serum sickness. This may occur 2–4 weeks after therapy and results from circulating immune complexes. It is characterized by urticaria, pruritus, malaise and other flulike symptoms, arthralgia, and generalized adenopathy.[128]

Approved Therapeutic Monoclonal Antibodies

Rituximab

Rituximab (Rituxan) is a chimeric murine/human MAb directed against the CD20 antigen found on the surface of B lymphocytes. It consists of variable regions from the heavy and light chains of the murine anti-CD20 antibody (IDEC 2B8) grafted onto a human IgG1 constant backbone (Figure 24-6). Studies have shown that the human Fc regions enhanced the ability of the chimeric C2B8 antibody to initiate complement-mediated lysis and ADCC. The CD20 cell-surface antigen is expressed by more than 90% of B-cell lymphomas and chronic lymphocytic leukemias. The CD20 antigen is suited for targeted therapy because it is not found on precursor B cells or stem cells. Furthermore, the CD20 antigen does not circulate in the bloodstream and does not impede tumor-cell targeting. Because CD20–anti-CD20 antigen-antibody complexes are not internalized by the cell, the cell surface-bound antibody persists for a longer time, allowing optimal interaction between the antibody and host immune effector cells or complement. Rituximab is thought to cause cell lysis through the induc-

Figure 24-6 Chimeric Rituximab-engineered antibody. The human Fc domain and kappa constant regions may contribute to the infrequency of host-antibody response. (Reprinted with permission from Genetech, Inc. San Francisco, CA and IDEC.)

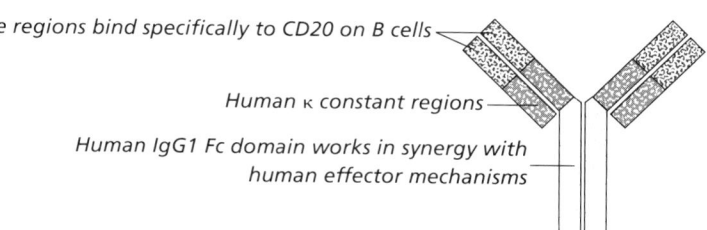

Murine variable regions bind specifically to CD20 on B cells

Human κ constant regions

Human IgG1 Fc domain works in synergy with human effector mechanisms

tion of ADCC and CDC (Figure 24-7). It also has been shown to trigger apoptosis (programmed cell death).[124,127]

Clinical trials.   Treatment with rituximab resulted in an overall 48% response rate in a pivotal multicenter phase II study in patients with relapsed or refractory low-grade or follicular CD20-positive B-cell non-Hodgkin's lymphoma. Side effects were mild to moderate and were mostly infusion related. An infusion-related symptom complex consisting of fever, chills and rigors, nausea, asthenia, and headache occurred in a majority of patients during the first infusion. These reactions occurred within 30 minutes to 2 hours after the start of the first infusion and decreased in incidence with subsequent infusions. Other events seen less frequently include neutropenia, leukopenia, thrombocytopenia, hypotension, bronchospasm, angioedema, and recurrences of preexisting cardiac conditions.[129]

Clinical use.   Rituximab is indicated for the treatment of patients with relapsed or refractory low-grade or follicular CD20-positive B-cell non-Hodgkin's lymphoma. It is administered by intravenous infusion once weekly for four doses. Current studies are looking at ways to improve response rates by combining rituximab with chemotherapy such as CHOP (cyclophosphamide, doxorubicin, vincristine, prednisone) or other biologic agents such as interferon. A study combining rituximab with CHOP in intermediate-grade non-Hodgkin's lymphoma resulted in an overall response rate of 97% and showed that these two modalities could be safely administered together. Rituximab also is being evaluated as adjuvant therapy for patients with intermediate-grade non-Hodgkin's lymphoma and in other B-cell malignancies such as CLL and multiple myeloma. Trials evaluating the use of rituximab after bone marrow or stem cell transplantation are underway.[124,129,130]

Trastuzumab

Trastuzumab (Herceptin) is a MAb directed against the human epidermal growth factor receptor (HER2/neu) (also known as c-erbB2) proto-oncogene. Overexpression of HER2 is found in 25%–30% of human breast cancers. In clinical studies, HER2 protein overexpression and HER2 gene amplification have been associated with a higher frequency of tumor recurrence and a decreased overall survival time.[131,132]

Because of its role in the pathogenesis of breast cancer, strategies to interfere with the function of the HER2 receptor protein have been evaluated. Trastuzumab is a recombinant DNA-derived humanized MAb that binds to the extracellular domain of the HER2 protein, inhibiting signal transduction and cell proliferation. Trastuzumab has been shown to inhibit the proliferation of human tumor cells that overexpress HER2, both in vitro and in animals. Trastuzumab enhances antibody cellular cytotoxicity.[133]

Clinical trials.   In two phase II clinical trials, the anti-HER2/neu MAb, trastuzumab, showed significant activity both as a single agent and in combination with traditional cytotoxic chemotherapy in the treatment of HER2/neu overexpressing metastatic breast cancer. The beneficial treatment effects were limited to patients with the highest level of HER2 protein overexpression. Overall, trastuzumab was generally well-tolerated in both studies. Mild infusion-associated symptoms such as chills and fever were reported by about 40% of patients and primarily occurred with the first infusion. An increased risk of cardiac dysfunction was observed in patients who received trastuzumab in combination with anthracyclines and cyclophosphamide. Anemia, leukopenia, diarrhea, and an increased incidence of infection were rarely seen with trastuzumab.[134,135]

Figure 24-7 Rituximab mechanism of action. Rituximab binds CD20, which is present on normal and malignant pre-B mature B cells; may induce antibody-dependent cell-mediated cytotoxicity (ADCC) and complement-dependent cytotoxicity; and triggers apoptosis.

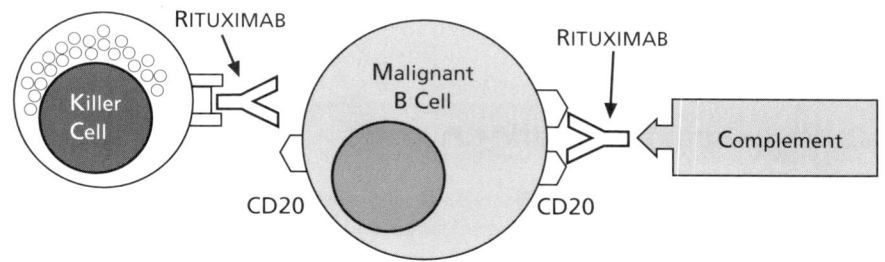

Clinical use. Trastuzumab is indicated as a single agent for the treatment of patients with metastatic breast cancer whose tumors overexpress the HER2 protein and who have received one or more chemotherapy regimens for metastatic disease. Trastuzumab combined with paclitaxel is indicated for patients with metastatic breast cancer who have not received chemotherapy for metastatic disease and whose tumors overexpress the HER2 protein. Trastuzumab is administered by intravenous infusion. Because of the increased incidence of cardiac dysfunction in patients treated with trastumuzab, patients should undergo a thorough cardiac assessment prior to treatment and frequent monitoring for deteriorating cardiac function. Extreme caution should be used in treating patients with preexisting cardiac dysfunction.[133]

Fusion Proteins

As noted earlier, an immunotoxin is an MAb conjugated to a toxin. A fusion protein made of a growth factor or cytokine linked to a toxin is called a *recombinant toxin,* a *chimeric toxin,* or oncotoxin. Sometimes, however, the term *immunotoxin* is loosely applied to all of these molecules.[136] Several fusion proteins have been evaluated as anticancer therapy, and $DAB_{389}IL-2$ is the first to be approved as a therapeutic cancer agent.

$DAB_{389}IL-2$

$DAB_{389}IL-2$ is a diphtheria toxin fused to IL-2. This fusion protein binds to cells containing IL-2 receptors and causes a series of reactions that inhibit protein synthesis, ultimately resulting in cell death. The human IL-2 receptor exists in three forms, and its expression has been reported to occur in patients with cutaneous T-cell lymphoma (CTCL), CLL, Hodgkin's, and non-Hodgkin's lymphoma. CD25 is one of the IL-2 receptor subunit components.[137,138]

In a phase III randomized trial of patients with CTCL, 30% of heavily pretreated refractory patients had objective responses to $DAB_{389}IL-2$. In addition, treatment with $DAB_{389}IL-2$ improved quality of life in the responding patients.[139] $DAB_{389}IL-2$ (denileukin-difitox; Ontak) is approved for treatment of persistent or recurrent CTCL in patients whose malignant cells express the CD25 component of the IL-2 receptor. Side effects of $DAB_{389}IL-2$ include acute hypersensitivity-type reactions, vascular leak syndrome, flulike symptoms, nausea, vomiting, and diarrhea.[137–139]

Other Immunomodulating Agents

An *immunomodulating agent* can be broadly defined as a substance that stimulates host defense mechanisms or indirectly augments aspects of immunity that are benefi-cial in cancer therapy. *Immunostimulants* are often nonspecific agents that target key immune cells such as the monocyte/macrophage, provoking secondary responses involving increased cytokines, cytotoxic cell activation, and increased immunoglobulins.

Nonspecific immunostimulation is based on the theory that the host's responsiveness to a tumor can be increased through overall stimulation of host-defense mechanisms using nontumor-related antigenic agents such as microorganisms.[140] In localized therapy, the tumor may be an "innocent bystander" but killed in the reaction to the provoking agent. This concept has been pursued in numerous clinical studies since the 1970s, with occasional positive outcomes.[4] These results underscore the need to better understand the complexities of the host-tumor relationship in order to apply this theory to clinical practice.

Some immunomodulating agents, such as cancer vaccines, provide active specific immunotherapy directed to a specific tumor target. Immunomodulator agents also include those that target specific aspects of host defense to stimulate cell differentiation (e.g., thymic hormones acting on T-cell differentiation); chemical substances that act as nonspecific immunostimulants (e.g., levamisole); vitamin preparations such as retinoids; and even chemotherapeutic agents such as cyclophosphamide that may decrease suppressor T-cell function or stimulate immune cells after initial immunosuppression.[140]

Nonspecific immunomodulating agents require that the host be capable of developing an immune response. Permanent damage to the immune system or persistent immunosuppression will interfere with the agent's effectiveness. In addition, the patient's tumor burden should be low. Large, bulky tumors are believed to significantly suppress host-defense mechanisms. Therefore, immunomodulators are frequently used as adjunctive therapy with surgery or chemotherapy to reduce the patient's tumor burden.[140,141]

The following sections briefly describe immunomodulating agents that are approved for cancer therapy or for clinical trials.

BCG (Bacillus Calmette-Guérin)

This nonspecific immunostimulant was originally derived from attentuated *Mycobacterium bovis* isolated in 1920. There are various BCG strains available which vary according to the number of organisms per unit of dose administered. BCG has been administered intradermally, subcutaneously, by scarification, or via intracavitary infusion. It produces localized side effects of swelling, pain, inflammation, and ulceration of the injection site, as well as systemic flulike symptoms of fever, chills, malaise, and arthralgia. Patients can have hypersensitivity reactions to BCG preparations if they have had previous exposure to BCG or a positive purified protein derivative (PPD). A small number of patients receiving BCG may develop a disseminated BCG infection.[140,142,143]

Special precautions are used with the patient receiving BCG, particularly intralesional therapy.[142] They include:

- Assessing the patient's potential for a hypersensitivity reaction to BCG before and during therapy. Patients with prior exposure to this agent will have a more rapid response that can be severe and can lead to anaphylaxis. Changes in the BCG dosage may be required.

- Premedicating patients with acetaminophen and diphenhydramine, which may decrease the severity of systemic flulike symptoms.

- Monitoring patients for prolonged flulike symptoms and organ dysfunction (liver, kidney, and pulmonary abnormalities) that suggest potential BCG infection.

- Observing universal precautions. All BCG syringes and other materials that have come in contact with BCG should be disposed of as hazardous waste to prevent environmental contamination. Consult the health agency's epidemiology official for other BCG safety guidelines.

BCG (Thera Cys, Tice BCG) is FDA-approved as a bladder instillation for intravesical treatment of carcinoma in situ of the bladder. Patients receive repeated 2-hour bladder instillations of BCG weekly for 6 weeks as an induction therapy followed by maintenance therapy (given at varying intervals depending on product and physician preference) for 12–24 months. The side effects of intravesical BCG therapy include hematuria and dysuria from the inflammatory mucosal reaction to BCG, fever, and rarely disseminated BCG infection. A long-term outcome of BCG bladder instillations can be a contracted bladder. BCG has also been studied as an intralesional injection for superficial metastatic malignant melanoma lesions. Approximately 60% of immunocompetent patients with melanoma receiving intralesional therapy achieved complete control of superficial lesions. Long-term survival occurred in approximately one-fourth of responding patients.[142]

Retinoids

Retinoids are a group of small-molecule hormones that are natural derivatives of retinol or vitamin A. They include all-*trans*-retinoic acid (ATRA, or tretinoin), 13-*cis*-retinoic acid (13-*cis*-RA, or isotretinoin), and 9-*cis*-retinoic acid (9-*cis*-RA, or alitretinoin).

Retinoids are essential in the physiologic processes of vision, fertility, and embryonal growth. In cancer, retinoids act as immunomodulators by inducing cellular differentiation and suppressing proliferation.[144,145] Cancers that may be responsive to retinoids include leukemias, melanoma, neuroblastoma, and various epithelial cancers.

Retinol is absorbed from the gastrointestinal tract and is bound in the circulation to retinol-binding plasma proteins in minute amounts. Intracellularly, retinol is oxidized to form 13-*cis*-RA, 9-*cis*-RA, or other compounds. They target receptors in the nucleus capable of binding retinol as well as steroids, estrogen, and thyroid. Here, they interact with DNA to affect cellular growth and functions. For example, retinol can suppress the synthesis of stromelysin by tumor cells, a compound that allows tumors to metastasize by degrading stromal tissue.

Clinically, dramatic effects have been seen using retinoids in acute promyelocytic leukemia (APL). Tretinoin acts on APL cells to increase their differentiation into mature granulocyte cells and induce clinical remission.[145,146] Tretinoin (Vesanoid) is approved for the induction of remission in patients with APL. Trials have shown that in appropriate combinations with chemotherapy, incorporation of tretinoin into induction regimens doubles the disease event–free survival in APL. Used alone, tretinoin can induce a remission in the majority of newly diagnosed patients, but the remission often is not durable. Tretinoin may have a role as maintenance therapy in APL.[147]

A serious side effect of retinol therapy in APL is retinoic acid syndrome.[144,148] Patients receiving retinoids can exhibit fever, respiratory distress, interstitial pulmonary infiltrates, pleural effusions, and weight gain. Retinoic acid syndrome can be fatal if not promptly recognized and treated, usually with high-dose corticosteroids. It occurs in approximately 25% of patients and can appear within 2–21 days of onset of therapy. Symptoms do not abate or reverse when the drug is discontinued.[148]

Isotretinoin (Accutane) is an actively studied retinoid in oncology. The combination of 13-*cis* RA plus IFN-α improved response rates in RCC compared to IFN-α alone. Responses have also been achieved with this combination in advanced squamous cell carcinoma of the skin and cervix. Common retinoid side effects include headache, mucocutaneous dryness, alteration in liver enzymes, and elevation of triglycerides.[149,150] In addition, isotretinoin and all known oral retinoids are teratogenic. Isotretinoin and other retinoids have shown activity in chemoprevention trials.[151–153]

Alitretinoin is a naturally occurring retinoid that activates all known retinoid receptor subtypes.[144] It is FDA approved as Panretin gel, which is indicated for the topical treatment of cutaneous lesions in patients with HIV-related Kaposi sarcoma.

Cancer Vaccines

While it once appeared that cancer vaccine research had been largely abandoned, it has recently experienced a resurgence and is once again an active area of research with definite clinical potential. An increased understanding of older vaccine technologies along with newer advances in biotechnology and gene therapy have been responsible for renewed interest in cancer vaccine therapy.[154] It is difficult to stay abreast of this constantly changing and developing field.

Cancer vaccine therapy is classified as a type of active specific immunotherapy. The term *vaccine* is commonly associated with the practice of administering microbes or derivatives of microbes to prevent infectious diseases. Use of vaccines in other areas led to the hope that immunizing against tumors could lead to immune responses potent enough to affect the growth of established cancers.[155] In cancer, vaccine therapy involves administering antigens (constructed or derived from natural sources) to patients to stimulate their own immune system to recognize and destroy the tumor. The cellular arm of the immune response (responsible for cell-mediated immunity), in particular the CD8+ cytotoxic T-cell (CTL) arm, has been identified as being best able to recognize tumor cells as foreign and lead to their destruction.[156] Vaccine therapy requires that the patient be immunocompetent and not have a large tumor burden.[157]

Antigen presentation is required for the development of an effective antitumor CTL response.[158] The initial aim of any vaccine is to present the antigen to the immune system in a way that will activate or enhance a cell-mediated antitumor response that exists but failed to reject the malignancy.[159] After the antigen is taken up and digested by antigen-presenting cells (APC), the antigen is bound to glycoproteins encoded by the MHC and presented on the surface of the APC, along with costimulatory molecules (such as molecules of the B7 family).[160] Tumor vaccines may work to increase antigen presentation to immune cells or increase costimulatory signals to induce an immune response or a combination of both.[161]

Tumor Antigens

A prerequisite for tumor vaccination is the identification of tumor antigens recognized by T cells that will be used to construct a vaccine. The ideal antigen(s) should be able to stimulate a clinically effective immune response, and they must be expressed in vivo by the tumor being treated. Unfortunately, the ideal antigen does not exist.[162] Three main categories of antigens have been identified. *Unique tumor-* or *patient-specific antigens* are only expressed in the tumor from which they were identified and are unique to a certain patient. *Shared tumor-specific antigens* are expressed in many tumor types with a common histology but not in normal tissue. *Tissue-specific differentiation antigens* are expressed by the normal tissue from which the tumor arose. Other antigen sources include mutated oncogenes (i.e., K-*ras*, HER2/neu), viral-transforming proteins, embryonic proteins, and mutated tumor-suppressor proteins.[155,163] A critical question in vaccine development is whether effective tumor immunity can be induced by immunization to a single antigen, or whether responses to multiple antigens on cancer cells are needed for cells to be destroyed.[162]

Vaccine Approaches

Intact tumor cells

The easiest way to make a cancer vaccine is to use intact, inactivated tumor cells as an antigen source. These vaccines may be either autologous or allogeneic.[154]

Autologous vaccines. Among the earliest vaccines, autologous vaccines are derived by isolating proteins or peptides from a patient's tumor cells. These tumor cells are obtained from surgery or biopsy, then irradiated or somehow killed or attenuated before being reinfused to the patient. Autologous vaccines have many limitations including cost and time required to generate specific vaccines for each individual patient.[155,164]

Heat-shock protein (HSP) vaccines are a recently developed type of autologous vaccine. Made by cells in response to heating or other stress, HSPs serve as carriers for peptides, some of which may have been derived from tumor proteins. They are autologous because they must be extracted from a given tumor and provide immunologic protection against only that tumor.[155]

Allogeneic vaccines. Allogeneic tumor vaccines are developed by establishing tissue-culture lines from metastatic tumors of several patients, growing them in large batches, mixing the various cell lines, and inactivating them, usually by radiation.[154] Allogeneic vaccines have more usefulness in a large population because they can be made from cell lines selected to provide multiple tumor-associated antigens and a broad range of HLA expression. Allogeneic cells have been found to be more immunogenic than autologous cells. One example of an allogeneic vaccine is a polyvalent antigen-enriched whole-cell melanoma vaccine (PMCV) or CancerVax. This is a live-cell preparation of several melanoma cell lines combined with BCG as an adjuvant. A polyvalent-shed antigen vaccine that is prepared from four melanoma cells lines has been developed and is being studied in melanoma.[158,164]

A related allogeneic strategy involves the preparation of crude extracts of tumor cells prepared from allogeneic cells. An example is the melanoma lysate vaccine, melacine, which was developed from two melanoma cell lines and is administered to patients with the adjuvant, DETOX. Another immunization strategy involves the infection of allogeneic tumor cells with viruses such as the vaccinia virus to create oncolysates that are made of both viral and tumor antigens. The viral antigens act as an immunologic adjuvant that enhances immune responses to the tumor antigens. Two examples of this type of vaccine are the vaccinia melanoma oncolysate (VMO) vaccine and a vaccinia melanoma cell lysate (VMCL) vaccine.[155,165]

Purified extracts

Investigators have found chemical components on the surface of cancer cells and have been able to prepare vaccines consisting of purified or synthesized preparations of these components called *gangliosides*. Gangliosides are present on the surface of many melanoma cells and are important immunogenic antigens in melanoma patients. An actively studied ganglioside, GM2, is found in the cell membrane of virtually all melanoma cells and is a normal component of other tissues. For use in a vaccine, GM2 is extracted from animal sources and then extensively purified. A polyvalent ganglioside vaccine that may be able to overcome the problem of antigenic heterogeneity and potentially induce a more potent immune response not possible with single ganglioside vaccines is currently in development.[166] Another approach to ganglioside vaccination under investigation is the administration of anti-idiotype antibodies that mimic the ganglioside.[167]

Peptides

Intracellular proteins have been discovered that can be expressed on the cell surface in the form of small peptides. These proteins undergo intracellular processing and are broken down into units that are carried to the cell surface and bound to the MHC. These peptides can be characterized, synthesized, and used as vaccines. An example of peptide vaccines are those derived from a series of melanoma-associated proteins encoded by the Melanoma AntiGEn(MAGE) family of proteins. The MAGE proteins were first found in melanoma cells but also have been identified in some lung, gastrointestinal, and breast cancers. Another set of peptides found on the surface of most melanoma cells is made from proteins involved in the synthesis of melanin. These tissue-specific differentiation protein antigens are found on normal melanocytes in the skin and the choroid of the eye and include tyrosinase, gp100, and MART-1.[154]

Dendritic cell vaccines

Dendritic cells (DCs) are the most effective APCs. Consequently, DC-based vaccines are an active area of clinical investigation and represent a direct and efficient method of improving antigen presentation. Dendritic cell-based vaccine therapy involves generating DCs from cancer patients, loading the DCs with antigen, and reinfusing them into the patient.[156] It is possible to obtain both CD34+ hematopoietic stem cells and functional DCs from the same leukapheresis collection to peripheral blood stem cell transplantation (PBSCT) and immunization purposes, respectively.[168] Because Flt-3 ligand mobilization has been found to augment DC in the blood, this could eliminate the need to culture peripheral blood mononuclear cells to generate DCs.[156]

Tumor Vaccine Adjuvants

The development of adjuvants to boost the immune response to an antigen is critical to the development of effective vaccines. Multiple approaches to augment vaccine immunogenicity have been used and several are under investigation. A bacterial preparation such as BCG is frequently used as a nonspecific immunostimulant. DETOX (Ribi Immunochemicals Hamilton, Montana) is an adjuvant composed of portions of *Salmonella minnesota* and *Mycobacterium phlei* combined with the tumor vaccine. In other studies, viral proteins, called *viral oncolysates*, are added to tumor cell preparations to stimulate the immune system. Other adjuvants include alum, or QS21, or slow-release vehicles such as liposomes. Other approaches include adding the antigen to strongly immunogenic molecules such as keyhole limpet hemocyanin (KLH).[154,162]

Several cytokines have been shown to augment antigen presentation during vaccine therapy and have been investigated as vaccine adjuvants. Cytokine gene-transduced cellular vaccines can avoid systemic toxicity associated with cytokines and have been shown to have enhanced immunologic activity. Granulocyte-macrophage colony-stimulating factor is the most potent cytokine gene used to modify tumor immunogenicity. Phase I studies with GM-CSF gene-transduced autologous vaccines have shown safety, and phase II trials are planned. Interferon-γ, IL-7, IL-2, IL-4, IL-12, and TNF-α gene-transduced tumor vaccines have also been evaluated and have been generally well-tolerated. Administration of liposomal cytokine preparations with vaccine also have improved immune response with less toxicity.[169]

Gene Therapy and Vaccine Development

The application of gene-transfer technologies has led to the development of cytokine gene-transduced tumor vaccines that have been shown to have enhanced immunologic activity. The use of GM-CSF-activated tumor peptide-pulsed DC is supported by basic research on cytokine gene therapy applied to cancer immunotherapy.[169] Most current studies use retroviral vectors to add the desired cytokine gene to the tumor cell DNA. Innovations in gene therapy have also led to the development of recombinant and synthetic antigens. Scientists now have the ability to clone the genes encoding the tumor antigens recognized by tumor cells. Tumor-associated antigens can be made synthetically or by recombinant DNA technology.[155] Antigens made by synthetic, or recombinant DNA technology can be altered to facilitate immune recognition.

Viral and bacterial vaccine vectors have been identified as ways to deliver antigens. *Listeria monocytogenes* is a vaccine carrier that naturally infects APC and may deliver immunogens to the antigen-processing and presentation pathways. Also, the bacterium itself acts as a danger signal for the immune system because it stimulates the innate immune response producing cytokines and mediators that enhance antigen presentation.[170]

Clinical Use of Cancer Vaccines

Although many clinical trials have been carried out in patients with metastatic disease, cancer vaccine therapy may be most useful in the management of cancer patients after surgery, in patients with minimal residual disease, and in patients expected to have tumor recurrence. The amount of an immune response needed to prevent tumor implantation is less than what is required to slow the growth of an established tumor.[170]

In contrast to chemotherapy, which exerts direct cytotoxic effects on tumor cells and causes prompt cell kill, vaccines act more indirectly, and frequently immune response take 4–8 weeks to develop following initial immunization.[164] Table 24-7 illustrates the differences between antitumor responses induced by chemotherapy and cancer vaccines. Studies of cancer vaccines are usually long-term and require years to demonstrate survival difference. In vaccine trials, development of an antibody response or strong delayed-type hypersensitivity (DTH) reaction was strongly correlated with an improved clinical outcome.[162]

Because they possess a degree of inherent immunogenicity, the most common targets for tumor vaccine strategies have been melanoma and, to a lesser degree, RCC. Melanomas are good candidates for vaccine therapy because they express well-characterized antigens. Also, because they often metastasize to superficial sites, tumors can be removed easily so that cells can be extracted for vaccine preparation.[158,162] Several vaccines for melanoma are in advanced stages of clinical trials (Table 24-8).

Other less immunogenic tumors have also been identified as targets for vaccine therapy. With certain chemical manipulations and strategies to enhance immunogenicity, they also can be recognized by the immune system. In colorectal cancer, vaccines are being studied that immunize against carcinoembryonic antigen (CEA).[171] Several prostate cancer vaccines are in development.[172] Breast cancer vaccine development has focused on induction of T-cell responses to HER2/neu.[173] Idiotype-specific tumor proteins are being studied as vaccines in patients with low-grade follicular lymphoma and multiple myeloma. Vaccines against the HIV virus are in development.

Vaccine Administration and Nursing Management

Most vaccines are either given by the intradermal (ID) or subcutaneous routes. The ID route is more painful, and sometimes vaccines must be administered in several injections. Prophylactic analgesia with a topical anesthetic such as Emla cream has been reported to be effective in eliminating the discomfort associated with multiple ID injections. The most proximal portion of the leg or arm is preferable for ID injections.[174]

Nursing assessment after vaccine administration involves measurement of induration, erythema, or edema at vaccine sites and identification of systemic symptoms. Most vaccines studied in clinical trials thus far have been associated with little toxicity. Side effects with some vaccines have been related to the adjuvant. Local injection site reactions are the most common side effect. Local response can include swelling, erythema and tenderness, or pruritus that can last from 1–7 days. An acute reaction in the first 15 minutes suggests an antibody-mediated hypersensitivity allergic reaction that is different from the expected cellular immune response. Patients can become sensitized to proteins in the vaccine preparation and can develop a local hypersensitivity reaction.[174]

Part of the nursing role with vaccine therapy may include measuring and photographing vaccine sites and assisting with punch biopsies of vaccine sites. Delayed-type hypersensitivity skin testing is often done in patients receiving cancer vaccine therapy to evaluate the presence of an antitumor immune response. Nurses are often involved in the application and interpretation of DTH skin tests.[174]

Future of Vaccine Therapy

Although randomized trials have not yet shown significant improvements in the survival of patients receiving vaccine therapy, clinical data with melanoma vaccines are encouraging. Therapeutic cancer vaccines may offer an attractive alternative to traditional therapies because their minimal toxicities may allow patients to maintain a better quality of life. Future studies will focus on ways to improve the immune response to vaccine therapy and improve vaccine specificity and potency. Discoveries of new antigens will enhance vaccine development. New innovations to improve vaccine therapy are developing at a rapid pace. As basic research in cytokine gene therapy continues to

Table 24-7 Contrasts Between Antitumor Responses Induced by Chemotherapy and Active Immunotherapy With Cancer Vaccines

	Chemotherapy	Active Immunotherapy
Mechanism of response	Direct: Drug is toxic to cancer cells	Indirect: Cytotoxic T cells and antibodies activated to kill tumor
Intermediate steps	Rapid: Drug quickly metabolizes to active state	Slow: 8–12 weeks to maximum activation of immune response
Clinical response	Rapid: 2–4 weeks	Slow: 3–6 months
Duration of response	Short: Weeks to months	Long: Most responses last months to years
Side effects	Substantial: Severe toxicity may occur	Few: Usually mild side effects

Reprinted with permission from Chan A, Morton D: Active immunotherapy with allogeneic tumor cell vaccines: Present status. *Semin Oncol* 26:612, 1998.[164]

Table 24-8 Examples of Melanoma Vaccines in Advanced Stages of Clinical Trials

Vaccines	Description	Comment
Cancer Vax (Polyvalent whole-cell melanoma vaccine; adjuvant—BCG)	Allogeneic; developed from 3 melanoma cell lines that include 11 tumor-associated antigens and 8 melanoma-associated antigens	Phase III trials ongoing • Cancer Vax vs. IFN-α for adjuvant melanoma • Cancer Vax and BCG vs. placebo and BCG in stage IV melanoma
Polyvalent shed antigen	Allogeneic; prepared from 4 melanoma cell lines	Small phase III pilot trial showed efficacy over placebo; other trials ongoing
Melacine (adjuvant—Detox)	Allogeneic; developed from 2 melanoma cell lines	Trial in stage IV melanoma showed no difference between melacine and low-dose cyclophosphamide vs. 4-drug chemotherapy regimen, but less toxicity improved quality of life Ongoing studies of melacine and IFN-α vs. IFN-α in stage III and IV melanoma
GMK (GM2 ganglioside conjugated to KLH with adjuvant QS-21)	Purified extract ganglioside vaccine targeted against GM2 melanoma antigen	Phase III multicenter, intergroup randomized trial to compare GMK melanoma vaccine vs. IFN for adjuvant mellanoma treatment ongoing

Data from Conforti et al,[158] Bystryn,[162] Chan and Morton,[164] Mitchell,[165] Livingston.[166]

be applied to cancer vaccine therapy, even more advances are likely to be made in this field. Further results of clinical trials using immunostimulatory gene transfer and genetically modified tumor vaccines are anxiously awaited and will tell us more about the future of cancer vaccine therapy.

Nursing Management of the Patient Receiving Biotherapy

Biotherapy, like chemotherapy, has a distinctive constellation of common side effects. Patients frequently experience fever and chills, headache, malaise, and arthralgia. Some patients experience injection site redness, induration, and pain. A few patients may develop generalized swelling, rash, weight gain, hypotension, and occasionally respiratory changes.

Not all biological agents have the same profile of toxicities. High-dose cytokines, particularly high-dose rIL-2, can result in a broad spectrum of toxicities affecting nearly all organ systems. In contrast, CSFs, particularly G-CSF (filgrastim), are well-tolerated. One possible explanation for this variability is that a few cytokines, particularly IL-1, IL-2, and IL-6, like native interleukins, are capable of initiating broad, inflammatory activities throughout the body, either directly or when mediated through secondary cytokines. Other agents have a narrow range of activity.

Effects of Dose and Schedule

Biological agents differ from chemotherapy in the dose level required to achieve therapeutic effects. Often, the best results from chemotherapy are obtained from high-

dose, intensive regimens given at the maximum tolerated dose (MTD). Biological agents, on the other hand, may stimulate the desired biological activity at a dose level far less than the MTD. This dose is called the optimal biological dose (OBD).[175] Thus, the evaluation of a new biological agent is more complex than evaluation of a new drug. Different symptoms predominate with variations in the method of administration (subcutaneous versus parenteral), dose level, and schedule. For example, lower dose subcutaneous rIL-2 administration is associated with less severe toxicities than high-dose bolus rIL-2.

Preparation, Administration, and Safe Handling of Biological Agents

Biological agents such as recombinant growth factors are reconstituted predominantly by nurses and patients. Patients commonly self-inject these agents. Biopharmaceuticals must be handled differently than drugs. *Biopharmaceuticals* are protein-based agents that often require refrigerated storage. Patients who travel should be cautioned that these products cannot tolerate the extremes in temperature commonly found in car trunks and airplane baggage holds. When the lyophilized product is reconstituted, the vial should not be shaken or the diluent directed into the dried powder. Excessive foaming that can denature the protein may occur. Finally, some biopharmaceuticals are not compatible with all plastic syringes and intravenous tubing. The package insert can provide valuable information on storage and compatibility of a particular product. Many pharmaceutical companies offer toll-free numbers to answer questions and supply additional information regarding their products.

At present, there are no known safety hazards associated with exposure to cytokines, MAbs, or cell therapies. However, the use of simple barriers is recommended to prevent inadvertent exposure to immunogenic substances. For products containing BCG, it is recommended that barriers be used with special disposal to prevent environmental contamination with *Mycobacterium*. The Oncology Nursing Society has published a monograph on biotherapy that provides more specific instructions on safe handling.[176]

Side Effects and Key Nursing Strategies

Flulike syndrome

Flulike syndrome (FLS) is a constellation of nonspecific symptoms that typically occurs when one develops an influenza infection. The major symptoms include chills and possible rigors, moderate to high fever 100–104°F (37.8–40°C), myalgias, arthralgias, and malaise. These symptoms may be associated with one or more related symptoms such as headache, anorexia, nausea, vomiting, diarrhea, sinusitis, and hyperalgesia. Fever patterns of some of the biological agents are shown in Table 24–9.[177]

Body temperature is controlled by preoptic anterior hypothalamic brain centers in a feedback mechanism with peripheral sensors (Figure 24-8). According to the set-point theory of temperature control, the hypothalamic centers "sense" deviations from a set temperature range of 97.5 to 99.5°F (36.4–37.3°C) and regulate thermal balance with heat-producing vasoconstriction and shivering or with heat loss actions such as vasodilation and sweating.[178,179] Pyrogenic pathogens, toxins, or drugs stimulate the release of endogenous pyrogenic cytokines such as IL-1, TNF, and IL-6 that act on thermal brain centers via prostaglandin release to create an upward reset of the body's temperature set point. Feedback mechanisms now read the body temperature as cold and initiate heat-producing actions such as involuntary muscular contractions or rigors. The hypothalamic temperature set point can be returned to normal when blood levels of endogenous pyrogen at the brain centers fall or are blocked by antipyretics such as aspirin.[179] The excess heat is then released through diaphoresis.

Shivering or rigors requires a large energy expenditure and increased oxygen consumption three- to fivefold greater than normal.[178] This involuntary, vigorous exer-

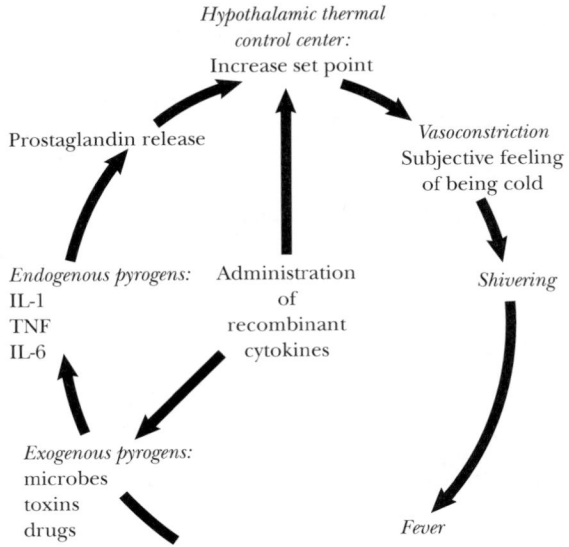

Figure 24-8 Pathogenesis of cytokine-related fever.

cise may put a strain on both the cardiovascular system and the large muscle groups of the body. Therefore, it is important to control rigors as soon as they occur to prevent undue cardiovascular stress.

Flulike syndrome is most frequently a side effect of cytokine therapy, although not all cytokines produce the full spectrum of symptoms or at the same intensity. *Tachyphylaxis,* or the development of tolerance to a symptom with repeated frequent doses, commonly occurs with IFN therapy. The FLS symptoms are most severe with the first doses and then lessen and disappear. The FLS symptoms return only when the therapy is stopped and restarted.

Monoclonal antibody therapy has its own FLS pattern of symptoms. Some MAbs do not cause fever at all; others create a biphasic fever pattern, with fever occurring at the onset of administration and then several hours after completion. Arthralgias, possibly due to circulating immune complexes, rather than myalgias may accompany the fever.[180]

Colony-stimulating factors such as G-CSF and EPO generally do not cause fever; GM-CSF is an exception. Fever may accompany GM-CSF administration, probably through stimulation of endogenous pyrogen release from monocytes and macrophages.

Nursing management. Guidelines for the nursing management of FLS in a patient receiving biological therapy are as follows:

- *Evaluate the risk for FLS symptoms:* Cytokine therapy, monoclonal antibody infusions, and the first dose of interferons are the highest risk.

- *Premedicate* the patient 1 hour prior to the first dose: Common medications are acetaminophen and indomethacin (optional).

Table 24-9 Fever Patterns

Agent	Onset (hr)	Peak (hr)	Duration (hr)
Interferon	2–4	6	4–8
IL-2 (bolus)	2–4	6	4–8
IL-2 (continuous)	Elevated throughout after infusion		
Monoclonal antibodies	0.5–1.0	2	8–12

Adapted with permission from Haeuber D: The flu-like syndrome. In Rieger PT (ed): *Biotherapy: A Comprehensive Overview.* Sudbury, MA, Jones and Bartlett, 1995, pp 243–258.[177]

- *Keep the patient warm:* Use warm blankets at the first sign of a chill.

- *For rigors:* Administer meperidine 25–50 mg parenterally, as appropriate to the patient-care setting.

- *For arthralgia, myalgia, or headache:* Continue the use of acetaminophen and indomethacin as appropriate.

- *For uncontrolled, high fevers:* Use cooling blanket or tepid bath.

- *Consider other sources of fever:* Infection may be a complication of cytokine therapy, particularly if the patient is receiving high-dose IL-2. If fever persists and is accompanied by hypotension, consider the following possible sources of infection: pulmonary, urinary tract, IV site, or central venous catheter, existing wound or skin lesion, or septicemia from unknown sources.

Fatigue

Fatigue is a symptom commonly experienced by cancer patients and especially those receiving radiation therapy and chemotherapy. It is also a common side effect of many types of biotherapy and is severe enough in certain high-dose, long-term cytokine regimens to be a dose-limiting factor. Fatigue is of special concern for patients who are receiving adjuvant therapy with IFN for melanoma as their total treatment lasts for 1 year.

Fatigue's subjective nature can make definition challenging. Aistairs defines fatigue as subjective feelings of generalized weariness, weakness, exhaustion, and lack of energy resulting from prolonged stress that is directly or indirectly attributable to the disease process.[181] Winningham describes fatigue as a subjective feeling of tiredness that is multidimensional and multisensory.[182] She distinguishes *acute fatigue*—that which is protective and disappears after a short rest—from *chronic fatigue*, which is not relieved by rest and is constant and debilitating. All of these definitions help define the experience of biotherapy-related fatigue: A chronic fatigue characterized by generalized weariness, weakness, exhaustion, and feelings of tiredness. It can be accompanied by other symptoms such as fever, myalgia, and headache. Fatigue from biotherapy is a symptom that can disrupt physical, psychological, and spiritual well-being.[183]

Interferon. When IFN-α was first investigated in phase I/II clinical trials, the impact of severe fatigue on a patient's functional status was recognized for the first time. Quesada et al note that daily schedules of IFN at doses of 20 MIU or more can result in profound toxicity including fatigue.[184] Davis describes the patient experience of fatigue while receiving escalating doses of IFN-α as fatigue increasing over time and positively related to the dose level.[185] Patients reported feeling tired all the time. They had increased leg weakness and needed to lie down. Maintenance of nutrition and fluid balance became a problem as patients were too tired to make the

effort to eat or even lift food to their mouths. Donnelly describes the fatigue associated with adjuvant IFN therapy in melanoma and notes that in addition to the fatigue associated with the FLS, patients experienced a mental fatigue accompanied by cognitive deficits, such as mental slowing, moderated depression, persistent somnolence, and severe headache.[68]

Interleukin. Fatigue is a common side effect with nearly all interleukins such as IL-1, IL-2, IL-4, and IL-6, particularly in long-term outpatient regimens. When interleukins are combined with IFN, fatigue appears to be additive.

Monoclonal antibodies, colony-stimulating factors. Fatigue is not a common side effect of either MAbs or CSFs.

Nursing management. The following are nursing guidelines for the care of patients experiencing biotherapy-related fatigue.

- *Assessment:* Evaluate the patient self-report of fatigue for perception of amount of fatigue, peak severity, patterns of activity and sleep, impact on self-care activities, and nutritional balance.

- *Patient education:* Teach patient and family the relationship of fatigue to therapy, methods of saving energy, and value of activity despite fatigue.

- *Maintain activity:* Plan with patient how to maintain activity and prevent prolonged bedrest. Patients receiving IFN who maintained activity despite fatigue were observed to have improved functioning.[185]

Cardiovascular and respiratory changes

Cardiovascular changes are associated most frequently with high-dose IL-2, and usually occur in association with the capillary leak syndrome (CLS). These changes include supraventricular arrhythmias such as atrial fibrillation and supraventricular tachycardia, symptoms of ischemia, and decreased cardiac contractility.[186] These symptoms occur in approximately 10% of patients undergoing treatment. Myocarditis and myocardial infarction have also occurred, possibly in patients who may have had underlying coronary artery disease.

Cytokines such as rIL-1, rIL-2, and TNF typically cause hypotension, decrease in central venous pressure, and oliguria necessitating fluid administration. Monoclonal antibody therapy with Herceptin has resulted in signs and symptoms of cardiac dysfunction such as dyspnea, increased cough, paroxysmal nocturnal dyspnea, peripheral edema, S3 gallop, or reduced ejection fraction. The probability of cardiac dysfunction in patients treated with trastuzumab was highest in patients who received trastuzumab concurrently with anthracyclines.[133]

Cardiovascular changes associated with rIL-11 therapy include peripheral edema, dyspnea, and tachycardia. These events are associated with fluid retention that is mainly due to volume expansion caused by renal sodium retention, not a capillary leak syndrome. Less commonly, arrhythmias (atrial fibrillation and flutter) and palpitations have occurred in patients following treatment with rIL-11.[48]

Respiratory changes may arise from various sources. Hypersensitivity reactions may cause wheezing and bronchospasm. Respiratory changes may occur in high-dose IL-2 therapy, with pulmonary edema, dyspnea, shortness of breath, and hypoxia. The administration of activated cell therapy can worsen these symptoms.[186]

Nursing management

- *Monitor:* Assess the patient's cardiovascular and respiratory status at frequent intervals during high-dose IL-2 therapy. Evaluate left ventricular function in all patients prior to and during treatment with trastuzumab. Assess for cardiovascular changes in patients receiving rIL-11, and monitor electrolytes closely if diuretics are prescribed.[48]

- *Patient education:* Teach patient to report chest pain, edema, palpitations, or changes in respiration that occur during therapy.

Capillary leak syndrome

The capillary or vascular leak syndrome is an important side effect that is unique to biological agents, most frequently described in patients receiving high-dose rIL-2. It is the extravasation of fluids and albumin into body tissues, associated with a decreased peripheral vascular resistance, hypotension, and intravascular volume.[186] Compensatory mechanisms of oliguria, increased creatinine levels, tachycardia, and weight gain also occur as fluids are administered to maintain the blood pressure. Major organ dysfunction such as mental status changes, nausea and diarrhea, and pulmonary edema occur with a rapid weight gain, sometimes up to 10% of pretreatment body weight.

Capillary leak syndrome can occur rapidly or increase gradually over hours. Although it is a toxicity most frequently associated with high-dose IL-2 therapy, it has been reported in varying degrees with other cytokines and high-dose GM-CSF. It rarely occurs with MAb therapy, but it occurs commonly with immunotoxin therapy. It has not been described with IFNs and nonspecific immunomodulators.

Nursing management

- *Monitor:* Assess regularly the patient's blood pressure, pulse, respiratory status, urine output, and body weight during therapy. Have the patient remove all restrictive jewelry, particularly rings, before treatment begins.

- *For hypotension and oliguria:* Administer fluid boluses per physician order with caution. Low-dose vasopressors may be administered to increase urine output.

Intensive care monitoring may be required if patient does not respond to above measures.

- *Patient education:* Instruct patient to stand gradually and allow blood pressure to adjust to the upright position. Request that patient report symptoms of dizziness.

Dermatologic changes

The skin is not generally considered a primary immune organ; however, it often exemplifies what is happening in the person's immune system. Administration of biological agents can stimulate immunoreactive cells such as Langerhans cells in the skin that function like macrophages and, along with activated T cells, release cytokines and vasoactive substances contributing to the redness, swelling, and itching seen in patients receiving cytokine therapy.[187]

Allergic reactions, particularly to a foreign protein such as MAb, can occur. These symptoms include acute development of an erythematous rash on the face and upper body, swelling, hives, and pruritus.

Interleukin-2 therapy, particularly high-dose IL-2, can create similar reactions but over a longer period of time. Erythema starting on the face and upper body progresses to severe dryness and flaking; pruritus can be intense. In severe cases, skin erosions and the sloughing of the palms, soles, and nails can occur, with gradual healing after therapy ends.[77,81] Hair thinning may occur, but alopecia is rare. Patients with preexisting psoriasis can experience a worsening of their disease with IL-2 therapy, possibly due to T-cell activation.

When cytokines such as IL-2 and GM-CSF are given subcutaneously, inflammatory reactions at the injection site often occur. Swelling and pain resolve within days, but a firm nodule may remain at the site for months.[81] As described earlier, vaccine therapy may be associated with local cutaneous reactions.

Nursing management. Interventions that may aid healing, decrease discomfort, and prevent infectious complications are as follows:

- *Apply hypoallergenic emollient lotions and creams* on the skin frequently. Instruct patient to use bath oil and hypoallergenic soaps for bathing.

- *For pruritus:* For severe itching, administer antipruritic medications such as hydroxyzine HCL, or diphenhydramine. Use lorazepam with severe itching as needed. Use colloidal oatmeal baths (Aveeno).

- *For subcutaneous site inflammation:* Rotate sites and do not reuse until firmness resolves. Use local anesthetics and possibly cooling for inflammation.

Gastrointestinal symptoms

Anorexia, nausea, vomiting, and diarrhea can occur primarily with cytokine therapy, but also with MAb therapy in association with flulike symptoms. It can be sporadic and may not require medication.

The most severe nausea, vomiting, and diarrhea occur with IL-2 therapy, particularly high-dose regimens. In a few patients, it was a dose-limiting factor to treatment. Rosenberg et al reported that approximately one-third of patients receiving high-dose IL-2 regimens experienced nausea, vomiting, and diarrhea at grade 3 or 4 toxicity.[75] Biochemotherapy regimens are associated with significant nausea and vomiting, often requiring aggressive antiemetic therapy with 5HT3 antagonists.[76]

There are few studies exploring the cause of gastrointestinal problems with IL-2 therapy. The most likely possibility is the vascular leak syndrome or the leakage of fluid and albumin into the gastrointestinal tract. Diarrhea can be severe, with loss of fluid and electrolytes. Colon perforation and gastrointestinal bleeding have also been reported, particularly in early studies with IL-2.[186]

Nursing management.   The interventions for nausea, vomiting, and diarrhea previously used with chemotherapy may be applicable for use in IL-2 therapy. One exception is that steroids should not be used as an antiemetic because of their effects on immune function. The following interventions may be useful in managing IL-2-related gastrointestinal symptoms:

- *Evaluate:* Know the potential that the type of therapy has for moderate to severe nausea, vomiting, or diarrhea.

- *For nausea and vomiting:* Medicate patients either with antiemetics on an as-needed basis, or administer on a regular schedule, depending on severity of symptoms.

- *For diarrhea:* Use antidiarrheal medications as needed, starting with the least potent. Observe patient for symptoms of bowel stasis, distention, and signs of an acute abdomen.

- *Monitor:* Assess patients for symptoms of fluid and electrolyte imbalance.

Neurological effects

Patients receiving IFN-α or IL-2 can experience simple memory changes, increased anxiety, nightmares, and other sleep disturbances. One symptom frequently encountered but poorly described is the loss of concentration or an inability to pay attention.[188] More severe symptoms of disorientation, somnolence, and even coma can occur. These symptoms are reversible with supportive care. However, unless therapy is stopped when early signs of neurotoxicity appear, symptoms may worsen and persist for days to weeks before improving.[189]

Neurological changes are infrequent in cytokine therapy and are rare in MAb or other biological therapy. Although rare, neurotoxicity can be severe, particularly in high-dose IFN-α or rIL-2 therapy. When these cytokines are combined, the incidence of neurotoxicity is significantly higher than with IL-2 or IFN-α alone.

Rosenberg et al reported that in 283 patients receiving high-dose IL-2, 14% experienced disorientation, 5% somnolence, and 2% coma.[75] Marincola et al reviewed 189 patients who received varying dose combinations of IFN-α and high-dose IL-2.[189] They found a greater incidence of neurotoxicity than previously reported for either agent alone.

Nursing management.   The following are interventions to be used with patients receiving high-dose IL or IFN-α therapy:

- *Assessment:* Assess patient prior to start of therapy for baseline neurologic functioning. Elderly patients are at increased risk. High-dose IL-2 is usually omitted rather than delayed for severe neurotoxicity, so the nurses assessment of neurologic changes is crucial to patient management.

- *Patient education:* Teach patient and family members early signs of mental status changes that should be reported to the health team.

- *Monitor:* Protect patient from harm and observe frequently when mental status changes occur.

- *Decrease stress:* Reduce environmental demands that increase attentional fatigue.[189]

Anaphylactic reactions

Type I hypersensitivity reactions (anaphylaxis) are rarely seen with the administration of biological agents. However, anaphylaxis is always a concern when administering agents that are designed to stimulate or potentiate immune function.

Anaphylaxis results from the stimulation of mast or basophil cells when IgE antigen complexes bind to surface receptors. This results in the release of mediators such as histamine, leukotrienes, and prostaglandins.[190] Within minutes, the patient develops symptoms of redness, swelling, urticaria, nervousness, angioedema, respiratory distress, abdominal cramping, and hypotension.

Anaphylactoid reactions have most commonly occurred with MAb therapy. Most of these reactions occurred with MAb in their early development and in administration to patients with lymphoma or leukemia, or when MAbs were administered by rapid infusion.[118]

Nursing management

- *Review emergency procedures:* Have essential drugs, steroids, epinephrine, and antihistamines available when administering MAb or other biological agents to patients with a history of hypersensitivity reactions.

- *Patient education:* Instruct patient and family about the symptoms of hypersensitivity. Request that they call their physician if symptoms occur or seek immediate medical assistance if symptoms develop rapidly.

Monoclonal Antibody Infusion–Related Symptom Complex

This constellation of symptoms is unique to patients receiving MAb therapy. See Table 24-10 for general management guidelines.

Biotherapy and Quality of Life

The subjective symptoms frequently experienced by patients receiving biotherapy offer great opportunities for nurse researchers to better define the symptom experience and interventions to decrease the burden experienced by the patient. Fever and chills; arthralgia and myalgia; fatigue; nonspecific neurological changes, particularly in the elderly; nausea and vomiting with cytokines; and pruritus are typical symptoms for which significant improvements in understanding and intervention might occur. These symptoms can significantly affect quality of life (QOL) and present excellent opportunities for QOL research. Nurses may also be involved in outcome studies to determine the impact of biologic therapy on QOL when compared to more conventional therapy. While side effects of some biologic agents can negatively affect QOL, many supportive care and therapeutic agents can actually improve QOL.

Economic and Reimbursement Considerations

In this age of managed care and cost containment, most medical treatments are under close scrutiny to determine

---

Table 24-10 General Guidelines for Monoclonal Antibody Administration and Infusion-Related Symptom Complex

- Monitor vital signs per protocol
- Consider premedication with acetaminophen and diphenhydramine
- Decrease subsequent infusion rates according to manufacturer's guidelines if initial dose well-tolerated
- Medicate with acetaminophen, diphenhydramine for fever, chills; may need to slow infusion
- Medicate with antiemetics for nausea and vomiting
- Stop infusion for mild to moderate hypersensitivity reactions (hives, rash, pruritus, fever), notify physician, treat reaction; may be able to resume infusion when symptoms subside
- Stop infusion for severe hypersensitivity reaction (hypotension, bronchospasm, angioedema); resume infusion at 50% rate reduction when symptoms subside
- Keep emergency medications and O_2 available for severe hypersensitivity reactions

---

their clinical benefit and cost-benefit ratios. This may be particularly true with biological therapy, which can be associated with considerable costs. Economic considerations have led to the incorporation of pharmacoeconomic analysis into clinical trials and the development of clinical practice guidelines.[9,191] For example, the American Society of Clinical Oncology has developed guidelines for the appropriate use of CSFs. Part of their recommendations are based on a cost analysis of the incidence level at which the estimated additional cost of G-CSF equaled the estimated cost savings from avoided hospitalization.[192] Clinical trials are evaluating alternate doses and schedules of G-CSF to maximize efficacy and minimize cost. Future trials will evaluate the cost effectiveness of platelet growth factors compared with platelet transfusion.[193] Identifying patients most likely to respond to EPO can avoid the cost of treating patients who will not respond.[194] Defining response criteria for all types of biological therapy will help reduce costly interventions and facilitate selection of patients most likely to benefit.[191]

While not traditionally in the nurse's realm, the changing health care environment requires nurses to be involved in and have a heightened awareness of insurance and reimbursement issues. Nurses can advocate for patients receiving biological therapy by assessing their insurance status (e.g., do they have private insurance, an HMO, Medicare or Medicaid, or are they uninsured?). Knowledge of insurance requirements to obtain prescriptions at a given pharmacy is necessary if patients are self-administering subcutaneous biological agents (e.g., IFN, hematopoietic growth factors) at home. Knowledge of a patient's home-care coverage is helpful if using home-care support for injection teaching and supplies or to administer biological agents. Medicare guidelines restricting home self-injection of most biological agents impact nurses who must coordinate alternate arrangements for treatment. Nurses may be involved in making referrals to or collaborating with social workers or insurance specialists for reimbursement issues. Most pharmaceutical companies have patient assistance programs and reimbursement specialists that may be helpful for patients and health care professionals. Nurses may have a role in educating insurance companies and providing them with data to support treatment decisions for a given therapy and in helping patients to advocate for themselves.[195,196]

The Future of Biotherapy

From mid-1980 to the late 1990s, there has been tremendous growth in the field of biotherapy. The approval by the FDA of several growth factors and IL-2 began to establish biotherapy as a qualified cancer therapy. Numerous studies of cytokines, activated cells, and hematopoietic growth factors have been published, and vaccine therapy has experienced a rebirth. New indications have emerged for existing biological agents such as IL-2 and IFN. The approval of MAbs and a platelet growth factor has brought even more biological agents into clinical practice.

The new millennium, however, will likely bring yet-unknown changes to the field of biotherapy. Research and development support and reimbursement money will become increasingly scarce. Biotherapy may indirectly benefit as it may force prioritization and refocusing on biological agents that are practical, economically feasible, and the best possibilities for improving the treatment of cancer. Finally, the incorporation of gene-transfer technology into biotherapy provides promising new avenues that may bring effective treatment, a cure, or even the prevention of cancer.

References

1. Abbas AK, Lichtman AH, Pober JS: *Cellular and Molecular Immunology.* Philadelphia, Saunders, 1991
2. Shu S, Plautz E, Krauss JC et al: Tumor immunology. *JAMA* 278:1972–1981, 1997
3. Balkwill FR: *Cytokines in Cancer Therapy.* Oxford, Oxford University Press, 1989
4. Oettgen HF, Old LJ: The history of cancer, in DeVita V, Hellman S, Rosenberg SA (eds): *Biologic Therapy of Cancer.* Philadelphia, Saunders, 1991, pp 104–110
5. Oldham RK: Cancer biotherapy: General principles, in Oldham RK (ed): *Principles of Cancer Biotherapy* (ed 2). New York, Marcel Dekker, 1991, pp 1–22
6. Mihich E, Fefer A (eds): *National Cancer Institute Monograph, 63.* NIH publication No. 83-2606. Bethesda, MD, National Institutes of Health, 1983
7. Clark J, Longo D: Biological response modifiers. *Mediguide Oncol* 6:1–4, 1986
8. Rieger PT: *Biotherapy, A Comprehensive Overview.* Sudbury, MA, Jones and Bartlett, 1995
9. Rieger PT: The use of biotherapy in patients with cancer, in *Anemia and Fatigue in Cancer Patients: Nursing Care Management. A Nursing Symposium.* Newtown, PA, Associates in Medical Marketing, 1997, pp 26–35
10. Rosenthal N: Tools of the trade—Recombinant DNA. *N Engl J Med* 331:315–317, 1994
11. Richards B: New ways for biotechnology to detect and treat old and new diseases. *Biotechnol Educ* 3:2–8, 1992
12. Pitler L: Hematopoietic growth factors in clinical practice. *Semin Oncol Nurs* 12:115–129, 1996
13. Ratajczak MZ, Gewirtz AM: The biology of hematopoietic stem cells. *Semin Oncol* 22:210–217, 1995
14. Golde DW: The stem cell. *Sci Am* 261:86–93, 1991
15. Bernstein SH, Kufe DW: Future of basic/clinical hematopoiesis research in the era of hematopoietic growth factor availability. *Semin Oncol* 19:441–448, 1992
16. Sheridan WP, McNiece I: Stem cell factor, in Armitage JO, Antman KH (eds): *High-Dose Cancer Therapy* (ed 2). Baltimore, Williams & Wilkins, 1995, pp 429–444
17. Maslak P, Nimer SD: The efficacy of IL-3, SCF, IL-6, and IL-11 in treating thrombocytopenia. *Semin Hematol* 35: 253–260, 1998
18. Schpall EJ, Wheeler CA, Turner SA, et al: A randomized phase III study of PBPC mobilization by stem cell factor (stemgen) and filgrastim in patients with high risk breast cancer. *Blood* 90:591a, 1997 (abstr 2627) (suppl)
19. Stiff P, Gingrich S, Luger RA, et al: Improved PBPC collection using Stemgen/rm (stem cell factor, SCF) and Filgrastim (G-CSF) compared with G-CSF alone in heavily pretreated lymphoma and Hodgkin's Disease patients. *Blood* 90:591a, 1997 (abstr 2628) (suppl)
20. Lyman SD, Jacobsen SEW: C-kit ligand and flt-3 ligand: Stem/progenitor cell factors with overlapping yet distinct activities. *Blood* 91:1101–1134, 1998
21. Yoshikazu S, Shimazaki C, Ashihara E, et al: Synergistic effect of flt-3 ligand on the granulocyte colony-stimulating factor–induced mobilization of hematopoietic stem cells and progenitor cells into blood in mice. *Blood* 89: 3186–3191, 1997
22. Guillaume T, Symann M: Interleukin 3: General biology, preclinical and clinical studies, in Armitage JO, Antman KH (eds): *High-Dose Cancer Therapy* (ed 2). Baltimore, Williams & Wilkins, 1995, pp 372–401
23. Kurzrock R, Talpaz M, Estrov Z, et al: Phase I study of recombinant human interleukin 3 in patients with bone marrow failure. *J Clin Oncol* 9:1241–1250, 1991
24. Lindemann A, Ganser A, Hermann F, et al: Biologic effects of recombinant human interleukin 3 in vivo. *J Clin Oncol* 9:2120–2127, 1991
25. Postmus PE, Gietema JA, Damsma O, et al: Effects of recombinant human interleukin 3 in patients with relapsed small cell lung cancer treated with chemotherapy: A dose-finding study. *J Clin Oncol* 10:1131–1140, 1992
26. Vadhan-Raj S, Papadopoulos NE, Burgess MA, et al: Effects of PIXY 321, a granulocyte-macrophage colony stimulating factor/interleukin-3 fusion protein, on chemotherapy-induced multilineage myelosuppression in patients with sarcoma. *J Clin Oncol* 12:715–724, 1994
27. O'Shaughnessy JA, Tolcher A, Riseberg D, et al: Prospective randomized trial of 5-fluorouracil, leucovorin, doxorubicin, and cyclophosphamide chemotherapy in combination with the interleukin-3/granulocyte-macrophage colony-stimulating factor (GM-CSF) fusion protein (PIXY 321) versus GM-CSF in patients with advanced breast cancer. *Blood* 87:2205–2211, 1996
28. Vose J: Granulocyte-macrophage colony stimulating factor interleukin-3 fusion protein versus granulocyte-colony stimulating factor after autologous bone marrow transplant for non-Hodgkins lymphoma: Results of a randomized double-blind trial. *J Clin Oncol* 15:1617–1623, 1997
29. Crawford J, Ozer H, Stoller R, et al: Reduction by granulocyte colony-stimulating factor of fever and neutropenia induced by chemotherapy in patients with non-small cell lung cancer. *N Engl J Med* 325:164–179, 1991
30. Johnston EM, Crawford J. Hematopoietic growth factors in the reduction of chemotherapeutic toxicity. *Semin Oncol* 25:552–561, 1998
31. Armitage JO: Emerging applications of recombinant human granulocyte-macrophage colony stimulating factor. *Blood* 92:4491–4508, 1998
32. Lieschke GJ, Burgess AW: Granulocyte colony-stimulating factor and granulocyte-macrophage colony-stimulating factor, part I. *N Engl J Med* 327:28–35, 1992
33. Griffin JD: Hematopoietic growth factors, in DeVita V, Hellman S, Rosenberg SA (eds): *Cancer Principles and Practice of Oncology* (ed 5). Philadelphia, Lippincott-Raven, 1997, pp 2639–2657
34. Neumanitis J: Use of macrophage colony stimulating factor in the treatment of fungal infections. *Clin Infect Dis* 26: 1279–1281, 1998

35. Spivak JL: Cancer-related anemia: Its causes and characteristics. *Semin Oncol* 21:3–8, 1994 (suppl 3)

36. Thatcher N: Management of chemotherapy-induced anemia in solid tumors. *Semin Oncol* 25:23–26, 1998 (suppl 7)

37. Demetri GD, Kris M, Wade J, et al: Quality-of-life benefit in chemotherapy patients treated with epoetin alfa I independent of disease response or tumor type: Results from a prospective community oncology study. *J Clin Oncol* 16:3412–3425, 1998

38. Glaspy J, Bukowski R, Steinberg D, et al: Impact of therapy with epoetin alfa on clinical outcomes in patients with nonmyeloid malignancies during cancer chemotherapy in community oncology practice. *J Clin Oncol* 15:1218–1234, 1997

39. Leitgeb C, Pecherstorfer M, Fritz E, et al: Quality of life in chronic anemia of cancer during treatment with recombinant human erythropoietin. *Cancer* 73:2535–2542, 1994

40. Casadevall N: Update on the role of Epoetin Alfa in hematologic malignancies and myelodysplastic syndromes. *Semin Oncol* 25:12–18, 1998 (suppl 7)

41. Henry DH: Epoetin Alfa and high-dose chemotherapy. *Semin Oncol* 25:54–57, 1998 (suppl 7)

42. Gabrilove JL, Einhorn LH, Livingston RB, et al: Once-weekly dosing of Epoetin Alfa is similar to three-times-weekly dosing in increasing hemoglobin and quality of life. *Proc Am Soc Clin Oncol* 18:574a, 1999 (abstr 2216)

43. Jilani SM, Glaspy JA: Impact of epoetin alfa in chemotherapy-associated anemia. *Semin Oncol* 25:571–576, 1998

44. Du X, William DA: Interleukin-11: A multifunctional growth factor derived from the hematopoietic microenvironment. *Blood* 83:2023–2030, 1994

45. Du X, William DA: Interleukin-11: Review of molecular, cell biology and clinical use. *Blood* 89:3897–3908, 1997

46. Tepler I, Elias L, Smith JW, et al: A randomized, placebo-controlled trial of recombinant human IL-11 in cancer patients with severe thrombocytopenia due to chemotherapy. *Blood* 87:3607–3614, 1996

47. Isaacs C, Robert NH, Bailey FA, et al: A randomized, placebo-controlled study of recombinant human interleukin-11 to prevent chemotherapy-induced thrombocytopenia in patients with breast cancer receiving dose-intensive cyclophosphamide and doxorubicin. *J Clin Oncol* 15:3368–3377, 1997

48. Rust DM, Wood LS, Battiato L: Oprelvekin: An alternative treatment for thrombocytopenia. *Clin J Oncol Nursing* 3:57–62, 1999

49. Smith JW, Beach S, Loewy JA, et al: Integrated analysis of two placebo-controlled studies of Neumega (rhIL-11) to prevent severe chemotherapy-induced thrombocytopenia. *Proc Am Soc Clin Oncol* 16:11a, 1997 (abstr 388)

50. Kauchansky K. Thrombopoietin: The primary regulator of platelet production. *Blood* 86:419–431, 1995

51. Vadhan-Raj S: Recombinant human thrombopoietin: Clinical experience and in vivo biology. *Semin Hematol* 35:261–268, 1998

52. Prow D, Vadhan-Raj S: Thrombopoietin: Biology and potential clinical applications. *Oncology* 12:1597–1608, 1998

53. Fibbe WE, Rillemze R: The role of interleukin-1 in hematopoiesis. *Acta Haematol* 86:148–154, 1991

54. Vadhan-Raj S, Kudella AP, Garrison L, et al: Effects of interleukin 1 alpha on carboplatin-induced thrombocytopenia in patients with recurrent ovarian cancer. *J Clin Oncol* 12:707–714, 1994

55. Weber JS, Gordon MS: Platelet-stimulating factors, in DeVita VT, Hellman S, Rosenberg SA (eds): *Biologic Therapy of Cancer* (ed 2). Philadelphia: Lippincott, 1995, pp 183–189

56. Weber J: Interleukin 6: Multi-functional cytokine. *Biol Ther Cancer Updates* 3:1–9, 1993

57. Jenks S: After the early hype, interferons spark interest. *J Natl Cancer Inst* 85:773–775, 1993

58. Johnson HM, Bazer FW, Fuller W, et al: How interferons fight disease. *Sci Am* 264:68–75, 1994

59. Glaspy JA, Souza L, Scates S, et al: Treatment of hairy cell leukemia with granulocyte colony-stimulating factor and recombinant consensus interferon or recombinant interferon-alpha-2b. *J Immunother* 11:198–208, 1992

60. Bukowski R, Ernstoff M, Gore M, et al: Phase I study of polyethylene glycol (PEG) interferon alpha-2B (PEG INTRON) in patients with solid tumors. *Proc Am Soc Clin Oncol* 18:446a, 1999 (abstr 1719)

61. Stadler R: Interferons in dermatology: Present day standard. *Dermatol Clin* 16:377–392, 1992

62. Tizard IR: *Immunology, An Introduction* (ed 3). Fort Worth, Texas, Saunders, 1992

63. Rosenberg SA: Principles of cancer management: Biologic therapy, in DeVita VT, Hellman S, Rosenberg SA (eds): *Cancer: Principles and Practice of Oncology* (ed 5). Philadelphia, Lippincott-Raven, 1997, pp 349–373

64. Ballow M, Nelson R: Immunopharmacology: Immunomodulation and immunotherapy. *JAMA* 278:2008–2017, 1997

65. Sodal-Ceigny P, Lepage E, Brousse N: Doxorubicin-containing regimens with or without Interferon Alfa-2b for advanced follicular lymphomas: Final analysis of survival and toxicity in the Groupe d'Etude des Lymphomes Folliculaires 86 Trial. *J Clin Oncol* 16:2332–2338, 1998

66. Kirkwood JM, Strawderman MH, Ernstoff MS. Interferon-Alfa-2b adjuvant therapy of high-risk resected cutaneous melanoma: The Eastern Cooperative Oncology Group Trial EST 1684. *J Clin Oncol* 14:7–17, 1996

67. Kirkwood JM, Ibrahim J, Sondak V, et al: Preliminary analysis of the E1690/S911/C9190 Intergroup Postoperative adjuvant trial of high- and low-dose IFNalfa2b (HDI and LDI) in high-risk primary or lymph node metastatic melanoma. *Proc Am Soc Clin Oncol* 18:2072, 1999 (abstr 2072)

68. Donnelly S: Patient management strategies for Interferon Alfa-2b as adjuvant therapy of high-risk melanoma. *Oncol Nurs Forum* 25:921–927, 1998

69. Dinarello CA: IL-18: A TH1-inducing, proinflammatory cytokine and new member of the IL-1 family. *J Allergy Clin Immunol* 103:11–24, 1999

70. Rubin JT: Interleukin-2: Its biology and clinical application in patients with cancer. *Cancer Invest* 11:460–472, 1993

71. Sharp E. The interleukins, in Rieger PT (ed): *Biotherapy: A Comprehensive Overview,* Sudbury, MA, Jones and Bartlett, 1995, pp 93–111

72. Fisher RI: Introduction: Interleukin-2—Advances in clinical research and treatment. *Semin Oncol* 20:1–2, 1993 (suppl 9)

73. Fisher RI, Rosenberg SA, Sznol M, et al: High-dose aldesleukin in renal cell carcinoma: Long term survival update. *Cancer J Sci Am* 3:S70–S77, 1997 (suppl 1)

74. Atkins MB, Lotze M, Wiernik P, et al: High dose IL-2 therapy alone results in long term durable complete responses in patients with metastatic melanoma. *Proc Am Soc Clin Oncol* 16:494, 1997 (abstr 1780)

75. Rosenberg SA, Yang JC, Topalian SL, et al: Treatment of 283 consecutive patients with metastatic melanoma or renal cell cancer using high-dose bolus interleukin 2. *JAMA* 271:907–913, 1994

76. Atkins MB: Immunotherapy and experimental approaches for metastatic melanoma. *Hematol Oncol Clin North Am* 12: 877–902, 1998

77. Parkinson DR, Sznol M: High-dose interleukin-2 in the therapy of metastatic renal cell carcinoma. *Semin Oncol* 22: 61–66, 1995

78. Rosenberg SA: Keynote Address: Perspectives on the use of interleukin-2 in cancer treatment. *Cancer J Sci Am* 3: S2–S6, 1997 (suppl 1)

79. Gold PJ, Thompson JA, Markowitz DR, et al: Metastatic renal cell carcinoma: Long term survival after therapy with high-dose continuous-infusion interleukin-2. *Cancer J Sci Am* 3:S85–S91, 1997 (suppl 1)

80. Yang JC, Rosenberg SA: An ongoing prospective randomized comparison of interleukin-2 regimens for the treatment of metastatic renal cell cancer. *Cancer J Sci Am* 3: S79–S84, 1997 (suppl 1)

81. Sleijfer DT, Janssen RAJ, Buter J, et al: Phase II study of subcutaneous interleukin-2 in unselected patients with advanced renal cell cancer on an outpatient basis. *J Clin Oncol* 10:1119–1123, 1992

82. Dutcher JP, Atkins M, Fisher R. Interleukin-2-based therapy for metastatic renal cell cancer: The Cytokine Working Group Experience, 1989–1997. *Cancer J Sci Am* 3:S73–S78, 1997 (suppl 1)

83. Levy Y, Capitant C, Houhou S, et al: Immunological efficacy of IL-2 therapy in HIV patients: Results of a randomised trial comparing subcutaneous PEG, continuous IV IL-2 with antiretroviral therapy. *Blood* 92:169a, 1998 (abstr 681)

84. Lissoni P: Effects of low-dose recombinant interleukin-2 in human malignancies. *Cancer J Sci Am* 3:S115–S120, 1997

85. Fefer A: Interleukin-2 in the treatment of hematologic malignancies. *Cancer J Sci Am* 3:S35–S36, 1997 (suppl 1) (editorial)

86. Fefer A, Robinson N, Benyunes MC, et al: Interleukin-2 therapy after bone marrow or stem cell transplantation for hematologic malignances. *Cancer J Sci Am* 3:S48–S53, 1997 (suppl 1)

87. Mazumder A: Experimental evidence of interleukin-2 activity in bone marrow transplantation. *Cancer J Sci Am* 3: S37–S42, 1997 (suppl 1)

88. Meloni G, Vignett M, Pogliani E, et al: Interleukin-2 therapy in relapsed acute myelogenous leukemia. *Cancer J Sci Am* 3:S43–S47, 1997 (suppl 1)

89. Dinarello CA, Wolff S: The role of interleukin 1 in disease. *N Engl J Med* 328:106–113, 1993

90. Smith JW, Urba WJ, Curti BD, et al: The toxic and hematologic effects of interleukin-1 alpha administered in a phase I trial to patients with advanced malignancies. *J Clin Oncol* 10:1141–1152, 1992

91. Crown J, Jakubowski A, Kemeny N, et al: A phase I trial of recombinant human interleukin-1B alone and in combination with myelosuppressive doses of 5-fluorouracil in patients with gastrointestinal cancer. *Blood* 78:1420–1427, 1991

92. Dinarello CA: Interleukin-1. *Cytokine Growth Factor Rev* 8: 253–265, 1997

93. Truitt RL, Borden EC, Keever CA: Role of IL-4, IL-6, and IL-12 in cancer therapy, in DeVita VT, Hellman S, Rosenberg SA (eds): *Biologic Therapy of Cancer* (ed 2). Philadelphia, Lippincott, 1995, pp 279–293

94. Wheeler V: Interleukins: The search for an anticancer therapy. *Semin Oncol Nurs* 12:106–114, 1996

95. Hiscox S, Jiang WG: Interleukin-12, an emerging antitumour cytokine. *In Vivo* 11:125–132, 1997

96. Fujiwara H, Hamaoka T: Antitumor and antimetastatic effects of interleukin 12. *Cancer Chemother Pharmacol* 38: S22–S26, 1996 (suppl)

97. Carreno V, Quiroga JA: Biological properties of interleukin-12 and its therapeutic use in persistent hepatitis B virus and hepatitis C virus infection. *J Viral Hep* 2:83–86, 1997 (suppl 4)

98. Atkins MB, Robertson MJ, Gordon M, et al: Phase I evaluation of intravenous recombinant human interleukin-12 in patients with advanced malignancies. *Clin Cancer Res* 3:409, 417, 1997

99. Motzer RJ, Rakhit A, Schwartz LH, et al. Phase I trial of subcutaneous recombinant human interleukin-12 in patients with advanced renal cell carcinoma. *Clin Cancer Res* 4:1183–1191, 1998

100. Atkins MB, Sparano J, Fisher RI, et al: Randomized phase II trial of high-dose interleukin-2 either alone or in combination with interferon alpha-2b in advanced renal cell cancer. *J Clin Oncol* 11:661–670, 1993

101. Legha SS, Ring S, Eton O, et al: Development of a biochemotherapy regimen with concurrent administration of cisplatin, vinblastine, dacarbazine, interferon alfa, and interleukin-2 for patients with metastatic melanoma. *J Clin Oncol* 16:1752–1759, 1998

102. Old LJ: Tumor necrosis factor. *Sci Am* 258:59–75, 1988

103. Feinberg B, Kurzrock M, Talpaz M, et al: A phase I trial of intravenously-administered recombinant tumor necrosis factor-alpha in cancer patients. *J Clin Oncol* 6:1328–1334, 1988

104. Fraker DL, Alexander HR: The use of tumor necrosis factor in isolated limb perfusions for melanoma and sarcoma. *Princ Pract Oncol Upd* 7:1–10, 1993

105. Sleijfer S, Mulder NH. Tumour necrosis factor: The decline and fall of a biological agent and its resurrection. *Clin Oncol* 6:127–132, 1994

106. Gutman M, Inbar M, Lev-Shlush D, et al: High dose tumor necrosis factor-alpha and melphalan administered via isolated limb perfusion for advanced limb soft tissue sarcoma results in a >90% response rate and limb preservation. *Cancer* 79:1129–1136, 1997

107. Fraker DL, Alexander R, Andrich M, et al: Treatment of patients with melanoma of the extremity using hyperthermic isolated limb perfusion with melphalan, tumor necrosis factor, and interferon gamma: Results of a tumor necrosis factor dose-escalation study. *J Clin Oncol* 14: 479–489, 1996

108. Eggermont AMM, Schraffordt Koops H, Slausner JM, et al: Limb salvage by isolated limb perfusion with TNF and melphalan in patients with locally advanced soft tissue sarcomas: Outcome of 270 ILPs in 246 patients. *Proc Am Soc Clin Oncol* 18:535a, 1999 (abstr 2067)

109. Alexander RH, Bartlett D, Libutti SK, et al: Isolated hepatic perfusion with tumor necrosis factor and melphalan for unresectable cancers confined to the liver. *J Clin Oncol* 16: 1479–1489, 1998

110. Rosenberg SA: Adoptive immunotherapy for cancer, in Paul WE (ed): *Immunology, Recognition and Response*. New York, Freeman, 1990, pp 109–121

111. Sznol M, Parkinson DR: Clinical applications of IL-2. *Oncology* 8:61–66, 1994

112. Platsoucas CD, Freedman RS: Tumor-infiltrating lymphocytes in gene therapy. *Cancer Bull* 45:118–124, 1993

113. Topalian SL, Solomon D, Avis FP, et al: Immunotherapy of patients with advanced cancer using tumor-infiltrating lymphocytes and recombinant interleukin-2: A pilot study. *J Clin Oncol* 6:839–853, 1988

114. Rosenberg SA, Yannelli JR, Yang JC, et al: Treatment of patients with autologous tumor-infiltrating lymphocytes and interleukin 2. *J Natl Cancer Inst* 86:1159–1164, 1994

115. Rosenberg SA: Gene therapy for cancer. *JAMA* 268: 2416–2419, 1992

116. Schindler LW: *Understanding the Immune System.* NIH Publication No. 88-529. Bethesda, MD, U.S. Department of Health and Human Services, 1988

117. Goldenberg DM: Recent advances in cancer detection and therapy with radiolabeled antibodies. *Mediguide Oncol* 10: 1–10, 1990

118. DiJulio JE, Liles TM: Monoclonal antibodies, in Rieger PT (ed): *Biotherapy, A Comprehensive Overview.* Boston, Jones and Bartlett, 1995, pp 135–160

119. Lobuglio AF, Saleh MN: Monoclonal antibodies, in Niederheber JE (ed): *Current Therapy in Oncology.* New York, Decker, 1993, pp 41–49

120. Gibbs WW: Try, try again. *Sci Am* 263:101–103, 1993

121. Bacquiran DC, Dantis L, McKerrow J. Monoclonal antibodies: Innovations in diagnosis and therapy. *Semin Oncol Nurs* 12:130–141, 1996

122. Pai LH, Pastan I: Immunotoxins and recombinant toxins, in DeVita V, Hellman S, Rosenberg SA (eds): *Biologic Therapy of Cancer* (ed 2). Philadelphia, Lippincott, 1995, pp 521–533

123. Schlom J: Monoclonal antibodies in cancer therapy: Basic principles, in DeVita VT, Hellman S, Rosenberg SA (eds): *Biologic Therapy of Cancer* (ed 2). Philadelphia, Lippincott, 1995, pp 507–521

124. Multani PS, Grossbard ML: Monoclonal antibody-based therapies for hematologic malignancies. *J Clin Oncol* 16: 3691–3710, 1998

125. Pai LH, Pastan I: Immunotoxins and recombinant toxins for cancer treatment, in DeVita VT, Hellman S, Rosenberg SA (eds): *Important Advances in Oncology.* Philadelphia, Lippincott, 1994, pp 3–19

126. Goldenberg DM: Challenges to the therapy of cancer with monoclonal antibodies. *J Natl Cancer Inst* 83:78–79, 1991

127. Press O: Prospects for the management of non-Hodgkin's lymphomas with monoclonal antibodies and immunoconjugates. *Cancer J Sci Am* 4:S19–S26, 1998 (suppl 2)

128. Dillman JB: Toxicity of monoclonal antibodies in the treatment of cancer. *Semin Oncol Nurs* 4:107–111, 1988

129. McLaughlin P, Grillo-Lopez AJ, Link BK, et al: Rituximab chimeric anti-CD20 monoclonal antibody therapy for relapsed indolent lymphoma: Half of patients respond to a four-dose treatment plan. *J Clin Oncol* 16:2825–2833, 1998

130. McLaughlin P, White CA, Grillo-Lopez AJ, et al: Clinical status and optimal use of Rituximab for B-cell lymphomas. *Oncology* 12:1763–1770, 1998

131. Slamonn DJ, Clark GM, Wong SG, et al: Human breast cancer: Correlation of relapse and survival with amplification of the HER-2/neu oncogene. *Science* 235:177–182, 1987

132. Slamon DJ, Godolphin W, Jones LA, et al: Studies of the HER-2/neu proto-oncogene in human breast and ovarian cancer. *Science* 244:707–712, 1989

133. Herceptin. Trastuzumab anti-HER2 monoclonal antibody. Complete prescribing information (product monograph). San Francisco, Genentech, 1998

134. Cobleigh MA, Vogel CL, Tripathy NJ, et al: Efficacy and safety of Herceptin (humanized anti-HER-2 antibody) as a single agent in 222 women with HER-2 overexpression who relapsed following chemotherapy for metastatic breast cancer. *Proc Am Soc Clin Oncol* 16:97a, 1998 (abstr 376)

135. Slamon D, Leyland-Jones B, Shak S, et al: Addition of Herceptin (humanized anti-HER-2 antibody) to first line chemotherapy for HER-2 overexpressing metastatic breast cancer (HER-2/MBC). *Proc Am Soc Clin Oncol* 16:98a, 1998 (abstr 377)

136. Pai LH, Paston I: Immunotoxin therapy, in DeVita VT, Hellman S, Rosenberg SA (eds): *Cancer: Principles and Practice of Oncology* (ed 5). Philadelphia, Lippincott-Raven, 1997, pp 3045–3057

137. Nichols J, Foss F, Kuzel RM, et al: Interleukin-2 fusion protein: An investigational therapy for interleukin-2 receptor expressing malignancies. *Eur J Cancer* 33:S34–36, 1997 (suppl)

138. Duvic M, Cather J, Maize J, et al: DAB389IL-2 fusion toxin produces clinical responses in tumor stage cutaneous T cell lymphoma. *Am J Hematol* 58:87–70, 1998

139. Saleh MN, LeMaistre CF, Kuzel TM, et al: Antitumor activity of DAB 389IL-2 fusion toxin in mycosis fungoides. *J Am Acad Dermatol* 39:63–73, 1998

140. Hersh EM, Taylor CW: Immunotherapy by active immunization: Use of nonspecific stimulants and immunomodulators, in DeVita V, Hellman S, Rosenberg SA (eds): *Biologic Therapy of Cancer.* Philadelphia, Lippincott, 1991, pp 613–626

141. Spreafico F: The use of levamisole in cancer patients. *Drugs* 19:105–116, 1980

142. Morton DL, Hunt KK, Bauer RL, et al: Immunotherapy by active immunization of the host using nonspecific agents—Clinical applications using intralesional therapy. In DeVita V, Hellman S, Rosenberg SA (eds): *Biologic Therapy of Cancer.* Philadelphia, Lippincott, 1991, pp 627–642

143. Herr H: Instillation therapy for bladder cancer, in DeVita V, Hellman S, Rosenberg SA (eds): *Biologic Therapy of Cancer.* Philadelphia, Lippincott, 1991, pp 643–650

144. Parkinson DR, Smith MA, Cheson BD, et al: Trans-retinoic acid and related differentiation agents. *Semin Oncol* 19: 734–741, 1992

145. Warrell RP: Applications for retinoids in cancer therapy. *Semin Hematol* 31:1–13, 1994 (suppl 5)

146. Miller WH, Dmitrovsky E: Retinoic acid and its rearranged receptor in the treatment of acute promyelocytic leukemia, in DeVita V, Hellman S, Rosenberg SA (eds): *Important Advances in Oncology 1993.* Philadelphia, Lippincott, 1993, pp 81–93

147. Slack JL: Recent advances in the biology and treatment of acute promyelocytic leukemia, in Michael C. Perry (ed): *American Society of Clinical Oncology Educational Book.* Alexandria, VA, ASCO, 1998, pp 54–65

148. Gillis JC, Goa KL: Tretinoin. *Drugs* 50:897–923, 1995

149. Moore DM, Kalvakolano DV, Lippman SM, et al: Retinoic acid and interferon in human cancer: Mechanisms and clinical studies. *Semin Hematol* 31:31–37, 1994 (suppl 5)

150. Lippman SM, Lotan R, Schleuniger U: Retinoid-interferon therapy of solid tumors. *Int J Cancer* 70:481–483, 1997

151. Levine N: Role of retinoids in skin cancer treatment and prevention. *J Am Acad Dermatol* 39:S62–S66, 1998 (suppl)

152. Singh DK, Lipmann SM: Cancer chemoprevention. Part 1: Retinoids and carotenoids and other classic antioxidants. *Oncology* 12:1643–1657, 1998

153. DiGiovanna JJ: Retinoid chemoprevention in the high-risk patient. *J Am Acad Dermatol* 39:S82–S85, 1998 (suppl)

154. Berd D: Cancer vaccines: Reborn or just recycled? *Semin Oncol* 25:605–610, 1998

155. Restifio NP, Sznol M: Cancer vaccines, in DeVita VT, Hellman S, Rosenberg SA (eds): *Cancer: Principles and Practice of Oncology* (ed 5). Philadelphia, Lippincott-Raven, 1997, pp 3023–3043

156. Gilboa E, Nair SK, Lyerly KH: Immunotherapy of cancer with dendritic-cell-based vaccines. *Cancer Immunol Immunother* 46:82–87, 1998

157. Ruddon RW: *Cancer Biology* (ed 3). New York, Oxford University Press, 1995

158. Conforti AM, Ollila DW, Kelley MC, et al: Update on active specific immunotherapy with melanoma vaccines. *J Surg Oncol* 66:55–64, 1997

159. Kang N, Truman H, Sanders R, et al: Melanoma antigens and targets for vaccination. *Br J Hematol* 58:282–286, 1997

160. Maxwell-Armstrong CA, Durrant LG, Scholefield JH: Colorectal cancer vaccines. *Br J Surg* 85:149–154, 1998

161. Hallin P, Adams VR: Cancer Vaccines (Part 1 of 2). *J Am Pharm Assoc* NS31:588–589, 1997

162. Bystryn JC: Vaccines for melanoma: Design strategies and clinical results. *Dermatol Clin* 16:269–275, 1998

163. Pardoll DM. Cancer vaccines. *Nat Med Vaccine Suppl* 5:525–531, 1998

164. Chan A, Morton D: Active immunotherapy with allogeneic tumor cell vaccines: Present status. *Semin Oncol* 25:611–622, 1998

165. Mitchell M: Perspectives on allogeneic melanoma lysates in active specific immunotherapy. *Semin Oncol* 25:623–635, 1998

166. Livingston P: Ganglioside vaccines with emphasis on GM2. *Semin Oncol* 25:636–645, 1998

167. Foon K, Goutam S, Hutchins L, et al: Antibody responses in melanoma patients immunized with an anti-idiotype antibody mimicking disialoganglioside GD21. *Clin Cancer Res* 4:1117–1124, 1998

168. Choi D, Perrin M, Hoffmann S, et al: Dendritic cell-based vaccines in the setting of peripheral blood stem cell transplantation: CD34pos cell-depleted mobilized peripheral blood can serve as a potent source of dendritic cells. *Clin Cancer Res* 4:2709–2716, 1998

169. Simons JW, Mikhak B: Ex vivo gene therapy using cytokine-transduced tumor vaccines: Molecular and clinical pharmacology. *Semin Oncol* 25:661–676, 1998

170. Paglia P, Guzman CA: Keeping the immune system alerted against cancer. *Cancer Immunol Immunother* 46:88–92, 1998

171. Zbar AP, Lemoine NR, Wadhwa M, et al: Biological therapy: Approaches in colorectal cancer. Strategies to enhance carcinoembryonic antigen (CEA) as an immunogenic target. *Br J Cancer* 77:683–693, 1998

172. Hwang LC, Fein S, Levitsy H, et al: Prostate cancer vaccines: Current status. *Semin Oncol* 26:192–201, 1999

173. Disis ML, Cheever M: Her-2/neu oncogenic protein: Issues in vaccine development. *Crit Rev Immunol* 18:37–45, 1998

174. Weber CE: Cytokine-modified tumor vaccines: An antitumor strategy revisited in the age of molecular medicine. *Cancer Nurs* 21:167–177, 1998

175. Rieger PT: Dosing and scheduling biological response modifiers, in Rieger PT (ed): *Biotherapy: A Comprehensive Overview.* Boston, Jones and Bartlett, 1995, pp 43–66

176. Conrad KJ, Horrell CJ (eds): *Biotherapy: Recommendations for Nursing Course Content and Clinical Practicum.* Pittsburgh, Oncology Nursing Press, 1995

177. Haeuber D: The flu-like syndrome, in Rieger PT (ed): *Biotherapy: A Comprehensive Overview.* Sudbury, MA, Jones and Bartlett, 1995, pp 243–258

178. Holtzclaw BJ: Shivering, a clinical nursing problem. *Nurs Clin North Am* 25:977–986, 1990

179. Dinarello CA, Cannon JG, Wolff S: New concepts on the pathogenesis of fever. *Rev Infect Dis* 10:168–189, 1988

180. Haeuber D: Recent advances in the management of biotherapy-related side effects: Flu-like syndrome. *Oncol Nurs Forum* 16:35–40, 1989 (suppl)

181. Aistairs J: Fatigue in the cancer patient: A conceptual approach to a clinical problem. *Oncol Nurs Forum* 14:25–30, 1987

182. Winningham ML: Fatigue, in Groenwald SL, Frogge MH, Goodman M, Yarbro CH (eds): *Cancer Symptom Management.* Sudbury, MA, Jones and Bartlett, 1996, pp 42–58

183. Skalla KA, Rieger PT: Fatigue, in Rieger PT (ed): *Biotherapy: A Comprehensive Overview.* Sudbury, MA, Jones and Bartlett, 1995, pp 221–242

184. Quesada JR, Talpaz M, Rios A, et al: Clinical toxicity of interferons in cancer patients: A review. *J Clin Oncol* 4:234–243, 1986

185. Davis C: Interferon-induced fatigue. *Oncol Nurs Bull* 1:4–5, 1987

186. Siegel JP, Puri RK: Interleukin-2 toxicity. *J Clin Oncol* 9:694–704, 1991

187. Dummer R, Miller K, Eilles C: The skin: An immunoreactive target organ during interleukin 2 administration? *Dermatologica* 183:95–99, 1991

188. Forman AD: Neurologic complications of cytokine therapy. *Oncology* 8:105–110, 1994

189. Marincola FM, White DE, Wise AP, et al: Combination therapy with interferon alfa-2a and interleukin-2 for the treatment of metastatic cancer. *J Clin Oncol* 13:110–112, 1995

190. Fox GW, Ream MA: Hypersensitivity reactions, in Yasko JM, Dudjak LA (eds): *Biological Response Modifier Therapy: Symptom Management.* Emeryville, CA, Park Row Publishers, 1990, pp 187–196

191. Szucs TD: The growing importance of cost-effectiveness in oncologic practice. *Curr Opin Oncol* 10:279–283, 1998

192. Ozer H, Miller L, Schiffer CA, et al: American Society of Clinical Oncology update of recommendations for the use of hematopoietic colony-stimulating factors: Evidence-based, clinical practice guidelines. *J Clin Oncol* 14:1957–1960, 1996

193. Rubenstein EB: Evaluating cost-effectiveness in outpatient management of medical complications in cancer patients. *Curr Opin Oncol* 10:297–301, 1998

194. Ludwig H, Fritz E: Anemia of cancer patients: Patient selection and patient stratification for epoetin treatment. *Semin Oncol* 25:33–38, 1998 (suppl 3)

195. Ritter B, Rohloff C: Administration of biochemotherapy in melanoma. *Biotherapy: Consider Oncol Nurses* 3:1–7, 1998

196. Houston D: Supportive therapies for chemotherapy patients. *Cancer Nurs* 20:409–413, 1997

CHAPTER 25

Gene Therapy

Dale Halsey Lea, RN, MPH

Introduction

The diagnosis, management, and treatment of human disease are being revolutionized by the genetic discoveries emerging from the Human Genome Project.[1] Gene therapy, under development since the 1960s, is moving forward at a rapid pace. Transferring corrected or altered genes into a person's cells has the potential to cure or improve a vast majority of health conditions that have thus far been resistant to treatment. Although gene therapy is thought by many to constitute the next major medical advance, the promise of the new technology also provokes concern at individual and societal levels. Ethical issues include the potential to manipulate egg and sperm to improve future genetics, the possibility of enhancing "desirable" characteristics, and the potential for discrimination against those who are identified as having "undesirable" genetic conditions and predispositions. Scientists, health care providers, and the public are debating ethical issues as the full potential of gene therapy and related technologies become available.[2–5]

Nurses, who provide care to patients throughout the health care system, must become knowledgeable about advances in gene therapy and its applications. Oncology nurses will increasingly be called on to participate in clinical trials, assist individuals and families in decision-making about gene therapy, and collaborate with other health care professionals to maintain continuity and coordination of care of individuals receiving gene therapy. As part of their responsibility to promote the health and welfare of individuals, families, and communities, oncology nurses participate in the development of social policies for safety, financial, and ethical issues related to gene therapy. Oncology nurses have opportunities to make valuable contributions to research regarding the impact of gene therapy treatments on the individual, family, and community. Perhaps most importantly, oncology nurses will need to develop knowledge and skills to assist those patients participating in gene therapy to successfully translate and integrate newly gained genetic information into their daily lives.[6–8]

This chapter provides an overview of gene therapy. The history, goals, and principles, and regulation of and current approaches to gene therapy are discussed. Current clinical applications of gene therapy as well as social and ethical considerations are described. The chapter outlines new directions for oncology nursing practice including assessing social, cultural, and family understanding of and responses to new genetic interventions, and in assuring continuity and coordination of patient and family care across the various health care settings.

Genetic Disorders

Only a small percentage of the human population (15%) has a rare genetic condition.[9] Genetic influences affect much larger populations by playing a part in the development of more common health conditions that occur later in life.[1] Health conditions including cancer, heart disease, Alzheimer disease, depression, and diabetes all have a genetic component. Heart and circulatory diseases alone, under genetic influence, affect some 2 million individuals; cancer affects 1 million more.[3,9]

Genes are made up of a chemical code (DNA) particular to each gene. One hundred thousand genes reside in each individual's human genome. The code differs in sequence from gene to gene and directs the composition and production of proteins that in turn make up living tissue and regulate all of the body's functions. Genetic disorders arise when an error in the complex, multistep process of replication and cell division occurs. The error may be slight—perhaps just one unit of the code is misspelled, repeated, or deleted—but its corresponding protein will be similarly improperly put together. When the protein is essential enough, the error may lead to a sequence of events that can lead to disability or even death.[3,10] Gene therapy interventions are being developed to treat three types of genetically caused conditions. These are single gene, multifactorial, and acquired genetic conditions.[11–13]

There are more than 10,000 genetic conditions that are caused by a single altered gene. These are called *Mendelian genetic disorders* and include such conditions as cystic fibrosis, hemophilia, sickle cell anemia, and Huntington disease.[4,14] Some forms of hereditary breast and colon cancer as well as other cancers are also caused by a single gene alteration. These and other single gene disorders are inherited in families in either an autosomal dominant, recessive, or X-linked manner. Individually, these conditions are rare, but together they represent an important cause of disease and disability.[9] Conditions caused by a combination of genetic and environmental influences are called *multifactorial genetic disorders*. These conditions, more complex and less well-defined than the single gene disorders, include heart disease, high blood pressure, cancer, and mental illness. Current research efforts are providing a better understanding of the genetic susceptibility to these and other multifactorial genetic conditions. *Acquired genetic conditions* are those that occur as a result of a viral infection such as hepatitis or acquired immunodeficiency syndrome. In these conditions, the disorder is caused by the new genetic information the virus carries into the host.[11–13]

Genetic disorders altogether account for up to 40% of pediatric and 50% of adult hospital admissions. The extent and nature of treatment, hospitalization, and long-term care contribute to increasing expense for patients, families, and the health care system. Gene therapy and other gene-based therapeutic interventions have the potential to offer alternative and possibly less invasive and less expensive ways of treating genetic-related health conditions.

History of Gene Therapy

The current concept of gene therapy is based on the premise that definitive treatment for genetic disorders should be possible by treatment directed to the site of the defect itself—the gene mutation—rather than to the secondary effects and symptoms of the mutant gene. Newer approaches to gene therapy unite pharmacotherapeutics with genetic principles and include the use of DNA to treat disease.[3,4] Gene therapy represents a comprehensive range of therapeutic interventions. Although gene therapy is often thought to be a new therapeutic concept, the idea that genes can be used to treat human disease can be traced back several decades. The term *gene therapy* is derived from the phrase *genetic engineering*. At the Sixth International Congress of Genetics held in 1932, *genetic engineering* was defined as the application of genetic principles to animal and plant breeding to distinguish it from the perception of eugenics.[15,16] Gene therapy as a therapeutic intervention has since evolved within the context of pharmacologic and surgical traditions. Screening and dietary treatment of phenylketonuria (PKU) to prevent severe mental retardation and other conventional therapeutic approaches such as liver transplantation can be viewed as gene therapy interventions because they were founded on an understanding of genetics and biochemistry. Genetic conditions involving hormone or clotting deficiencies can now be treated by genetically corrected replacement therapies. These interventions have led to impressive improvements in health outcomes.[9,17]

New applications of gene therapy are based on advances in our understanding of the human genome during the past 40 years. Table 25-1 outlines some of the important historical events leading to the possibility of gene therapy. Genetic correction of human disease has encountered numerous conceptual, technical, and ethical problems, many of which became apparent in the early 1980s after the reports of studies on the use of cloned human beta-globulin genes to treat patients with thalassemia.[18] Since those trials, research using model systems has helped to establish more firmly gene mutations as appropriate targets to treat some genetic disorders. Retroviral-mediated gene transfer is now the principal procedure used. Interest in conducting further research toward human gene therapy has increased and has led to the discovery of basic genetic concepts in bacteria and bacteriophages, recombinant DNA technology, and gene transfer techniques, and the application of these concepts to the treatment of human disease. The emerging field of gene therapy combines the ability to treat human disease with externally administered substances that have specific actions and the ability to alter tissue permanently. Gene therapy, as it is evolving, represents an entirely new branch of medicine that has the potential to revolutionize the way human disease is treated.[2–4]

Principles and Goals of Gene Therapy

Gene Therapy Defined

Gene therapy seeks to provide therapeutic benefit to a patient by introducing normal genes into the patient's cell nuclei to repair, enhance, replace, or compensate for an altered gene.[2,3,19] Gene therapy strategies under investigation include inserting a new functioning gene into the cells of a patient to correct a genetic abnormality or birth defect, thereby providing a new function for a cell. Gene therapy offers the potential for treatment of many genetic disorders as well as cancer, infectious diseases, and autoimmune disorders through the genetic modification of cells in the human body.

Current gene therapy initiatives are aimed at somatic cells, the nonreproductive cells of the body (e.g., skin, muscle, bone, and liver). This type of gene therapy, called *somatic gene therapy*, can correct inherited genetic disorders and is limited to only one generation. Gene therapy aimed at altering sperm and ova (reproductive cells) is called *germ-line gene therapy*. In the United States, only somatic gene therapy has been approved for use in clinical trials. Germ-line gene therapy has been limited to animal studies and is not presently considered to be ethically acceptable in the treatment of humans. The ethical issues raised by the prospect of germ-line gene therapy are multiple. The introduction of an altered gene into a fertilized egg, for example, carries the potential risk of introducing a new gene mutation that would be present in an individual at birth and could then be passed on to future generations.[6,13,20]

Enhancement gene therapy and eugenics are two other possible uses of gene therapy. The principle behind *enhancement gene therapy* is the placement of genes in an embryo or offspring that would improve a societally desir-

Table 25-1   Gene Therapy: Historical Development

Year	Discovery
1944	Hereditary material is determined to be DNA (deoxyribonucleic acid)
1953	Discovery of DNA structure
1961	Discovery of the genetic code
1973	Establishment of a technique for recombining different genes in living cells
1976	Discovery of first cancer gene
1977	Recombinant DNA techniques used to make human growth hormone
1978	Cloning of gene for human insulin leads to the development of humulin (1982) for treatment
1983	Development of polymerase chain reaction (PCR) technique
1985	Identification of first genetic marker for cystic fibrosis
1986	Identification of tumor-suppressor genes
1990	Initiation of the Human Genome Project
1990	Initiation of first human gene therapy trial

Data from Culver[3]; Rimoin et al.[9]

able trait such as decreased weight or increased height. Gene therapy used for *eugenic purposes* involves the introduction of specific genetic traits into a population to develop "desirable" human attributes such as intelligence. These two applications of gene therapy, like germline gene therapy, are not considered by most to be ethically acceptable.[20–22]

Gene Identification and Characterization

The normal function of the gene of interest and the characterization of the protein that it makes must be completely understood before a plan for gene correction can be made. Several mechanisms can cause an altered gene to produce a defective protein or result in abnormal regulation of gene expression. There may be, for example, an alteration in a gene that is critical for cell survival. Depending on where in the gene the actual defect has occurred, the resulting defective protein is either nonfunctional or poorly expressed. Adenosine deaminase (ADA) deficiency is an example of this type of gene defect, in which damage to the ADA gene results in T-lymphocyte death and severe combined immunodeficiency. An abnormality in a regulatory gene is another mechanism that can cause problems. Certain genes are responsible for the control of the production of a specific gene product. When these genes are defective, functional gene products are not produced in adequate quantities. The gene defect present in thalassemia is an example of this type of gene abnormality.[3]

A therapeutic intervention using gene therapy is considered when the gene function and regulation are known and the variations in gene expression among populations have been discovered. At present, the best candidates for gene therapy are those disorders that involve relatively simple "housekeeping" genes. These genes are not involved with regulation of gene expression and are not critical to the development and differentiation of the abnormal cell lines.[3]

Gene Transfer Methods

The most pressing technological hurdle facing gene therapy researchers is the discovery of efficient methods to transfer genes into human cells.[2,23] Successful gene therapy requires efficient gene delivery and continuous corrective activity of the transferred gene in the patient.[24] Gene transfer methods currently under investigation include recombinant virus vectors, chemical, physical, and fusion methods, and receptor-mediated endocytosis. Each of these techniques has demonstrated advantages and disadvantages, and each may someday find successful clinical application.[2,3]

Assuring that the transferred gene is integrated into the DNA of the target cell is as important as finding the proper transfer method. Stable integration of the corrected gene, for example, is critical when introducing

modifications into cells that have not yet reached maturity or are rapidly dividing. These cells produce future cell populations; maintaining gene correction as the cells divide and reproduce helps to provide long-term benefit to patients. In contrast, gene insertion into nondividing and terminally differentiated tissues such as liver or skeletal muscle may not require integration as a feature of the gene transfer method.[3]

Gene transfer in vitro and in vivo

Two general approaches—in vitro and in vivo—have been used to transfer a corrected or altered gene.[2,6,8,13,25] The in vitro approach is used most widely in clinical trials because it has the advantage of eliminating the possibility of gene transfer into germ line tissues. The technique is also often more efficient than in vivo transfer.

The in vitro approach requires that the defective cells or cells of interest be removed from the patient first. The corrected or marker gene is then inserted into the cells, and the altered cells are returned to the individual. Cells most commonly used for this approach include lymphocytes, skin fibroblasts, and tumor and bone marrow cells.[6,13,17] These cells are readily accessible, amenable to manipulation, and able to survive for long periods of time following reinfusion. The in vitro method has not been successful with nondividing cells such as kidney, liver, or brain because they cannot be grown in sufficient numbers for efficient stable gene transfer and are difficult to reimplant.

In vivo gene transfer to achieve gene therapy has been developed on the basis of direct delivery of therapeutic genes to target body cells. In vivo is more promising for its potential to directly affect disease sites with minimal risk to the individual. In vivo approaches to gene therapy are currently being used in clinical trials for cystic fibrosis (CF), muscular dystrophy, melanoma, and heart, lung, and metabolic conditions.[2,3,26] Another in vivo approach that has not yet been used but is under development is a method whereby the altered gene could be directly injected into the bloodstream.[2]

Both in vitro and in vivo gene transfer methods require a carrier, or vector, to transfer the augmented or functional genes into the target cells. The two major vector systems currently used for gene transfer are viral and nonviral.

Vectors for Gene Transfer

Effective gene therapy of inherited and acquired genetic disorders requires success in four main areas: (1) efficient delivery of the gene to the target tissue; (2) sustaining long-term gene expression; (3) ensuring that the gene transfer will not harm the patient in any way; and (4) transferring the corrected gene to nondividing cells. An additional but equally important goal is to develop a cost-effective means to manufacture the vector.[2,3,5,26] A variety of vector systems to achieve the goal of gene transfer have been developed and evaluated: viral vectors such as retrovirus, adenovirus, adeno-associated virus, and herpes virus vectors. Several nonviral vectors including liposomes, molecular conjugates, and other particulate vectors also have been created for gene transfer. Viral methods of gene transfer are referred to as *viral transduction*, whereas nonviral methods are called *physical transfection* of the therapeutic gene. Each vector has met with some success in delivering the therapeutic gene to the target tissue; each has distinct problems and disadvantages as a vector.[6-8, 16]

Viral Vectors

Most current gene therapy uses viral vectors to deliver the therapeutic gene to the target tissue. All viruses used have been disabled of any pathogenic effects by removing the genes required for replication of the virus and replacing them with therapeutic genes and selection markers (Figure 25-1).[27] The use of viruses is a potentially powerful technique because many have evolved the specific mechanisms to deliver DNA to cells. Humans, however, have an immune system designed to defend against viruses, and attempts to transfer genes in viral vectors have been complicated by host responses.[2,5]

Retroviral vectors

A retrovirus is composed of RNA that can insert itself readily into dividing cells. Retroviruses are considered the most promising gene transfer vehicle. Approximately 60% of the approved gene therapy clinical protocols use retroviral vectors.[2] These RNA viruses are able to carry out efficient gene transfer into many types of cells and can integrate into the host cell genes with stability. The therapeutic gene carried into the cell by the retrovirus will be inherited by all future generations of the cell and will provide the possibility of long-term gene expression (Figure 25-2).[3] Most retroviral vectors appear to have minimal risk because they have evolved into relatively nonpathogenic parasites. The murine leukemia virus (MuLV) in particular has traditionally been used as a vector of choice for clinical gene therapy protocols, and a variety of packaging methods to enclose the vector genome within the viral particles have been developed. The chosen vector has all of the viral genes removed, is replication defective, and can accommodate up to 8 kilobases (units of 1000 bases in a DNA sequence) of therapeutic DNA.[2,13]

Retroviruses, although advantageous in many ways, pose several challenges. First, retroviral vectors integrate into host cells randomly. Consequently, it is not possible to predict into which of the 46 chromosomes the altered gene will insert itself. The lack of specificity for the host cells works against direct delivery of the vector to the body. Of equal concern is the fact that the random insertion of the retrovirus will disrupt normal genes essential for proper cell function and lead to harmful physiologic effects that favor cancer development. Those retroviruses receiving the most study fail to transfer the therapeutic genes into nondividing cells. Current retrovirus vectors are useful only when the membrane surrounding the cell nucleus of the host cell dissolves, and this event occurs only during cell division.[2,3,23]

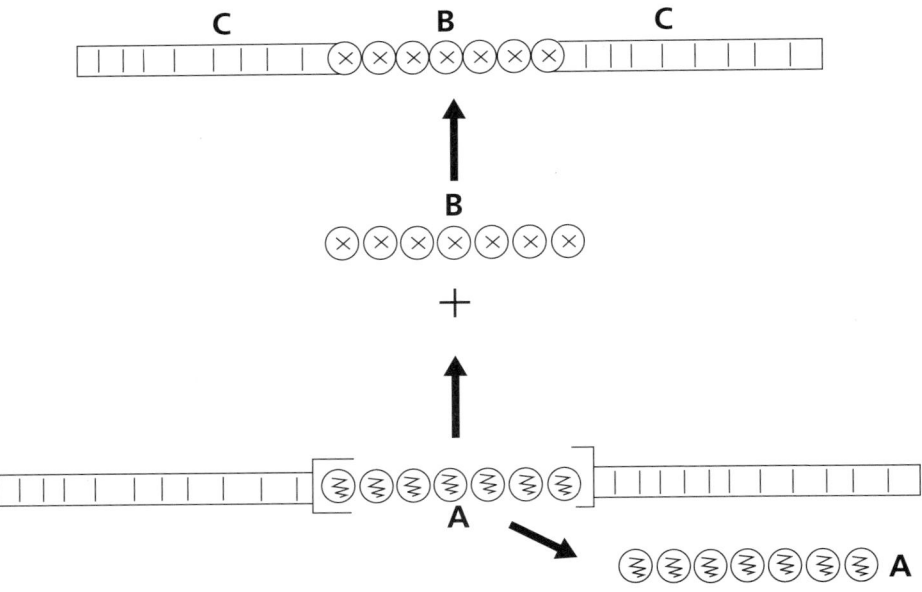

Figure 25-1 Viral vector with therapeutic gene. Preparation of viral vectors by removal of the disease-producing viral gene (**A**) and replacement with the therapeutic gene (**B**). Viral genes necessary for invasion of the cell (**C**) are maintained.

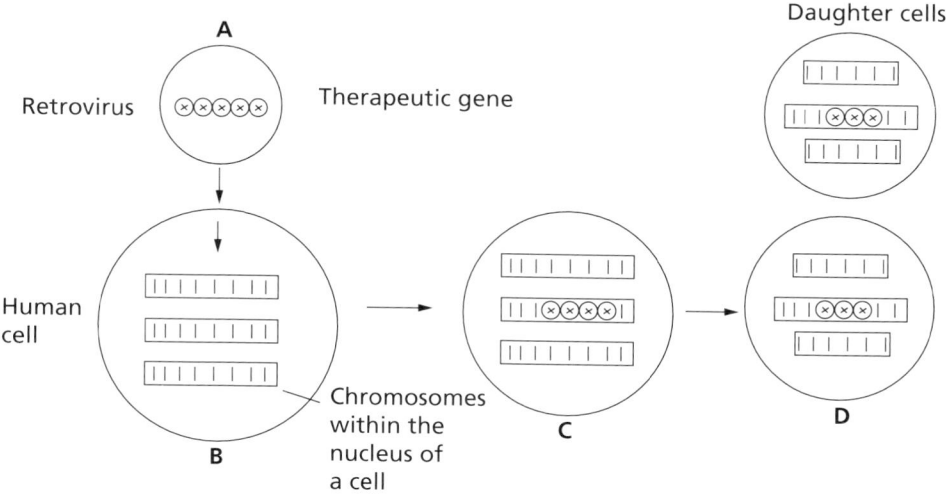

Figure 25-2   Retroviral delivery of a therapeutic gene. **A.** A retrovirus with the therapeutic gene invades the cell. **B.** Reverse transcriptase makes a DNA copy of the retroviral RNA. The viral DNA and the therapeutic gene are part of the nucleus and are incorporated into one of the 46 human chromosomes. **C.** The therapeutic effect remains if the cell replicates, providing daughter cells with a copy of the therapeutic gene **D.**

Lentiviral vectors

Lentiviruses, which belong to the retrovirus family, are now being used in gene therapy because they can infect both dividing and nondividing cells. Human immunodeficiency virus (HIV) is the most well-known lentivirus used for gene transfer in vivo. When lentivirus vectors have been injected into rodent brain, liver, muscle, or eye cells, the viruses have produced sustained therapeutic gene expression over 6 months—the longest time tested thus far. To date, lentiviral vectors have not produced a cellular immune response at the site of the injection, nor have they generated any potent antibody response.[24,28,29]

Researchers are making progress in confronting the shortcomings of retroviruses as gene delivery vehicles. To increase the specificity and enable retroviruses to direct themselves to particular cells in the body, researchers are finding ways to alter the viral envelope (the outermost surface). Retroviruses will deposit their therapeutic genes into a cell only if proteins projecting from the surface find a specific match or receptor on the cell. A retrovirus needs to bind its viral proteins to the cell's receptors in order to fuse its envelope with the cell membrane and release the therapeutic gene into the cell's interior. Investigators are finding ways to replace or modify natural envelope proteins or to add new proteins or protein parts to existing envelopes. These additions make retroviruses more selective about the cells they invade.[2]

Adenoviral Vectors

Adenoviruses are a family of viruses that cause benign respiratory tract infections in humans. They also have the capacity to infect both dividing and nondividing cells,

making them useful for gene therapy. Adenoviruses are large and can hold large segments of therapeutic DNA. They can be produced in large amounts in culture. They have been the vectors of choice for many protocols designed to treat the pulmonary complications of cystic fibrosis as well as for a variety of clinical protocols to treat cancer. In contrast to the retrovirus, which contains RNA, adenoviruses contain DNA and thus do not integrate into host DNA but instead replicate themselves outside of the nucleus of the host cell. Because of this limited integration, expression of the therapeutic gene is short-lived and regular reapplication of gene therapy using adenovirus vectors is necessary (Figure 25-3).[3,11,12]

The potential usefulness of adenoviral vectors stems from the fact that they do not require actively dividing cells to introduce their therapeutic gene. Adenoviruses, however, are a common cause of upper respiratory tract infections in humans. For the purpose of gene therapy, unfortunately, most of the human population may experience an active immune response to antibodies from a previous infection, which could reduce the effectiveness of gene therapy. Another potential concern with using adenoviral vectors is that the integrated gene may not lead to uniform correction of the gene defect because it may not remain active in the host cell. Other viral vectors that may potentially enhance the delivery of therapeutic genes are therefore being explored.[6,8,13]

Newer adenoviral vectors

The adeno-associated virus (AAV) is one of the newer viral vectors under investigation; it is a simple, nonpathogenic virus composed of a single strand of DNA. In order to replicate, AAV needs additional genes. A helper virus,

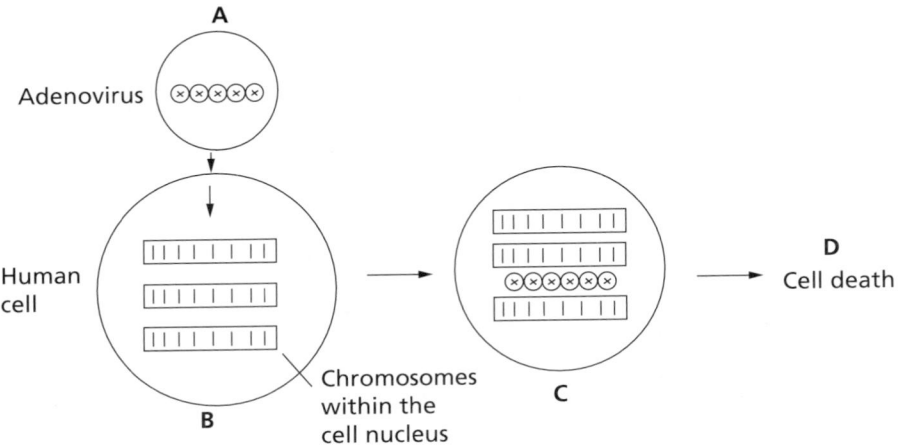

Figure 25-3   Adenoviral delivery of a therapeutic gene. **A.** An adenovirus with therapeutic gene invades the cell. **B.** The viral DNA and the therapeutic gene are part of the nucleus but are not incorporated into a chromosome. **C.** The therapeutic effect is lost when the cell dies **D**.

usually adenovirus or herpes simplex virus, serves the purpose. The AAV virus can infect a variety of types of cells, and although it appears to integrate in a nonspecific manner, it has been shown to integrate preferentially into chromosome 19. Preparation of the AAV is labor intensive, however, and the potential for an immune response remains since 80% of the adult population has antibodies to AAV. Still, AAV shows promise as a potential vector for in vivo gene therapy.[2]

Other viruses that are being considered and developed for use as vectors for gene therapy are the herpes simplex virus, which infects cells of the nervous system, and vaccinia-virus. These viral vector systems produce a transient response, and many people have an immunity to components of the virus from being infected previously.[2,5]

Nonviral Vectors

Nonviral vector delivery systems for gene transfer may, in time, have more therapeutic potential than viral methods because of ease of manufacturing and safety issues. To enhance integration into the human genome, nonviral methods rely on transfer of therapeutic genes into human cells by chemical methods such as precipitation with calcium phosphate and encapsulation of therapeutic genes into liposomes or molecular conjugates (complexes of lipids and DNA). Physical methods being explored and developed include direct microinjection of DNA into cells by particle acceleration. The efficiency of this process appears to be low, but intramuscular injection of "naked" DNA has been used successfully to establish cellular and humoral responses, suggesting that simple intramuscular administration of DNA could be used to create gene vaccines.[2,21]

Nonviral gene delivery systems may provide a means for achieving short-term expression of therapeutic gene

products in certain tissues with a high degree of safety. Studies to date suggest that nonviral delivery systems have toxicities and safety profiles similar to conventional drugs and other biological products. There have been no reports of significant toxicity to naked DNA in animal or human studies to date. Several organs appear to be particularly acceptable targets for nonviral gene therapy: lung, liver, and endothelial tissue. Other targets include tissues that are accessible to direct interstitial injection such as muscle, skin, and tumor masses.[13]

One of the greatest challenges for gene therapy is the development of safe and cost-effective therapeutic gene delivery systems that can be used along with conventional pharmaceutical and biological products. Current viral and nonviral vectors do not yet provide a completely satisfactory means of being propagated in proliferating cells. To increase the possibilities of success, the minichromosome, an artificial chromosome formed by reducing an existing chromosome, is under investigation. Using a method called telomere-mediated fragmentation, chromosomes are reduced to a size that can serve as a natural human vector for therapeutic genes.[30] Nonviral gene therapy methods offer the potential for therapeutic interventions that may be acceptable to physicians and patients and offer safety and efficiency similar to conventional therapeutic modalities.[31]

Clinical Protocols for Gene Therapy

The Severe Combined Immunodeficiency Disease Protocol

Although attempts at human gene therapy began in the 1960s, 1990 was an important landmark in the evolution of gene therapy. The first approved clinical protocol for gene therapy was initiated in 1990. Two girls with adenosine deaminase (ADA) deficiency, a rare genetic condition that produces severe immunodeficiency in children, were injected with white blood cells carrying a therapeutic gene. The clinical protocol called for inserting the ADA gene into T lymphocytes. Adenosine deaminase is an enzyme needed for normal immune system functioning. It prevents the build-up of deoxyadenosine, a metabolic product that becomes toxic to immune cells, especially lymphocytes, when present in high concentrations. ADA deficiency accounts for 25% of cases of severe combined immunodeficiency disease (SCID).[32] The clinical protocol for treating ADA deficiency had two major influences on gene therapy. It demonstrated the safety of retroviral gene transfer, and it showed that patients could benefit from gene therapy.[2,8,22,23] Examples of other single gene disorders for which gene therapy is being investigated are listed in Table 25-2.

Gene Therapy Regulation

More than 300 clinical protocols have been approved throughout the world and more than 3000 patients have been treated with therapeutic genes since the initiation of the SCID protocol.[2] Guidelines for clinical gene therapy protocols have been established by the National Institutes of Health (NIH) in the document, "Points to Consider in the Design and Submission of Human Somatic Cell Gene Therapy Protocols." The guidelines require that proposals for human gene therapy go through several levels of review. Each proposed protocol must first be reviewed by local bioethics and biosafety committees and must be in accord with the standards of conventional research. The Human Gene Therapy Research Subcommittee and the Recombinant DNA Advisory Committee (RAC) then review the protocol. These two committees serve in an advisory capacity to the Director of the NIH who approves all gene transfer and gene therapy proposals.[33] The Food and Drug Administration (FDA) addresses the scientific methodology and preclinical safety testing and also has created a set of guidelines for the initiation

of gene therapy. The FDA's guidelines are separate from the Human Genome Research Subcommittee and RAC guidelines and address the characteristics, production, and certification of the biological substances being used for gene transfer.[13,34,35]

At the time this chapter was written (February 1999), 280 clinical protocols were approved in the United States. The majority of these (69.8%) are for the treatment of cancer. Genetic diseases such as cystic fibrosis and other single gene disorders make up approximately 14.5% of clinical gene therapy protocols. Clinical gene therapy trials for the treatment of AIDS (10.9%) and for conditions such as peripheral artery disease, rheumatoid arthritis, and coronary artery disease (4.8%) also are being carried out. The majority of these approved protocols are phase I clinical trials. Updated information about the current number and type of clinical protocol is available through the online Web site of the Office of Recombinant DNA Activities.[36]

Cancer Gene Therapy

Treatment of cancer using gene therapy is aimed at the inhibition of oncogene function and restoration of tumor suppressor function.[13,16] Proto-oncogenes are normal cellular genes that are essential for cellular growth and development. Oncogenes stimulate neoplastic growth and are activated by proto-oncogenes that encode a growth factor or another protein and disturb normal cell development and regulation. Antioncogenes are those genes that block the action of growth-inducing proteins. These genes are also called tumor-suppressor genes to denote their ability to block the action of oncogenes. When functioning normally, tumor-suppressor genes and proto-oncogenes work together to enable the body to perform vital functions such as replacing dead cells and repairing defective ones.[10,16,21]

Two types of gene transfer are used in clinical cancer gene therapy trials: gene marking and gene therapy. Gene marking involves labeling cells for future identification. A gene that has been genetically marked is introduced

Table 25-2   Examples of Approved Single-Gene Clinical Gene Therapy Trials

Inherited Genetic Condition	Target Tissue	Vector	Gene/Gene Product
Cystic fibrosis	Respiratory tract	Adenovirus, adeno-associated virus, liposomes	CFTR
Familial hypercholesterolemia	Hepatocytes	Retrovirus	LDL receptor
Severe immunodeficiency due to ADA deficiency	Lymphocytes	Retrovirus	ADA
Alpha-1 antitrypsin deficiency	Respiratory tract	Liposomes	Alpha-1 antitrypsin
Gaucher's disease	Lymphocytes	Retrovirus	Glulocerebrocidase
Hunter's syndrome	Lymphocytes	Retrovirus	Iduronate-sulfatase

CFTR = cystic fibrosis transmembrane conductance regulator; LDL = low density lipoprotein; ADA = adenosine deaminase.
Data from Anderson[2]; Wheeler.[8]

into cells most commonly using a retrovirus as a vector for the desired gene. The approach is being used to determine the source of relapse in individuals undergoing autologous bone marrow transplantation.[13,37] Gene therapy studies involve modification of the content or expression of altered genes in somatic cells by transferring the functional or enhanced genes. Gene therapy interventions currently under investigation include suicide genes, antisense oligonucleotides, and insertion of therapeutic genes into progenitor cells.[10,13,17]

Gene-marking protocols

The first clinical gene-marking protocol took place in 1989. The study's purpose was to evaluate the effectiveness of immunotherapy for treatment of malignant melanoma using the neomycin resistance (Neo r) gene in tumor-infiltrating lymphocytes (TIL). The studies involved "marking" TIL with a neomycin resistance gene. The goals of the study were to: (1) demonstrate the safety of transferring an exogenous gene into a patient, and (2) show that the genes could be later detected and that the fate of TIL cells over time could be followed. Gene marking was the first method used for improving outcomes of blood cell transplantation and remains one of the major areas of concentration for gene transfer in the treatment of cancer. Use of this technique is providing a way to analyze more accurately the efficiency of different purging techniques.[2,8,38-40]

TIL gene-marking protocol for melanoma. Tumor-infiltrating lymphocytes are cytotoxic cells present in metastatic deposits of melanoma. The gene-marking protocol used in the TIL protocol involves removal of TIL from each patient, insertion of a marker gene into TIL using a retroviral vector, and reinfusion of the marked cells into each patient in conjunction with interleukin-2. Blood samples were periodically obtained from participating patients and from tumors to determine how many marked TILs were present in both, and to determine a correlation between the presence of TILs and clinical response. Researchers found that TILs could be detected in the bloodstream and in tumors after several months, and that the participating patients did not experience any adverse effects. Important clinical information gained from this study included confirming the safety of the procedure and proof that marked cells could be isolated from patients and reinfused.[39]

Gene-marking studies for leukemia and neuroblastoma Gene-marking studies also are being used with patients who have leukemia and neuroblastoma. In these clinical trials, marked genes are reinfused to study bone marrow reconstitution and the problem of relapse in autologous bone marrow transplantation. Studies of children with acute myelogenous leukemia who relapse after autologous bone marrow transplant are addressing the reason for relapse. Does the relapse occur as a result of the presence of residual cancer genes in the transplanted bone marrow that were not destroyed by purging tech-

niques, or as a result of continued residual disease in the patient that is not being effectively eradicated by chemotherapy?[28,37] In these protocols, a portion of harvested bone marrow cells is exposed to a retroviral vector with a marker gene—Neo r. The marked cells, along with unmarked bone marrow cells, are purged of malignant cells, and reinfused into the patient. If leukemia cells in relapsed patients are found to have originated in the marked stem cells, this suggests that stronger purging techniques could be used. If the relapsed leukemia cells are unmarked, indicating that they arose from cells not destroyed by therapy, then more strenuous conditioning protocols would be indicated.[8,38,39]

Gene-marking studies for stem cell transplantation and hematopoietic reconstitution. More recent gene-marking studies have been combined with other therapeutic effects of stem cell transplantation to address issues for future recipients of bone marrow or stem cell transplantation. A study initiated in 1994 is examining long-term hematopoietic reconstitution. In this study, a retroviral vector is used to mark stem cells. Participating patients are followed with peripheral blood testing every 6 months for 5 years to determine the extent to which these cells contribute to long-term hematopoietic reconstitution.[41] Other marking studies involve the investigation of hematopoietic reconstitution in adult patients undergoing bone marrow and blood cell transplant for lymphoma or metastatic breast cancer. The purpose of these studies is to learn whether stem cells should be used in place of or in addition to bone marrow cells, and to determine the number of stem cells required for successful engraftment.[42]

Cord blood and gene marking. In a recent gene-marking study, researchers reported results of cord blood transplantation. Cord blood collected at birth has been demonstrated to be effective for hematopoietic reconstitution with limited graft-versus-host disease (GVHD). The current study was designed to address questions regarding the ability to transfer the expression of new genetic material into myeloid progenitor cells from cord blood using an adeno-associated vector.[43] Cord blood was effectively transferred without preincubation of the cells with growth factors. The results of this study are promising and this area is becoming an important focus of research for engraftment in adults.[44]

Gene therapy protocols

A number of protocols are investigating the transfer of genes that can correct an error (gene alteration) or add a new function (gene addition). These clinical protocols include addition of a function to deliver a drug directly to a tumor or to modify the effects of chemotherapy, a "suicide gene" approach, and enhancing antigenicity. Such studies are founded on earlier gene marker studies that showed that a new gene could be safely inserted into patients and followed over time.

Tumor necrosis factor clinical protocols. In one of the first gene therapy protocols, researchers added a gene for tumor necrosis factor (TNF) to a vector containing TILs aimed at sites of malignant melanoma. The purpose of the study was to improve TIL immunotherapy by adding a gene to the TILs to increase their therapeutic effect.[40] Tumor necrosis factor is known as a powerful anticancer agent but has not been shown to be an effective cancer treatment when used in humans because of the highly toxic side effects when used in large doses. To avoid toxicity and increase tumoricidal activity, TILs were isolated from melanoma patients, and the TNF gene inserted into TIL. This allowed the TIL to move into tumor deposits to deliver a high dose of TNF to the tumor only, avoiding toxic side effects. Preliminary studies show that it is possible to insert a new gene into lymphocytes, reinsert the altered genes with a new function into a patient's cells, and achieve successful treatment without harm to the patient.[45,46]

Multidrug resistance gene clinical protocols. The multidrug resistance (MDR-1) clinical gene therapy trials for breast cancer are another example of gene addition therapy. P-glycoprotein is a product of the MDR-1 gene, and its function is to move drugs continuously out of a cell.[3] Researchers hypothesized that introducing MDR-1 into bone marrow progenitor cells would modify the effects of high-dose chemotherapy and prevent dose-limiting myelosuppression.[47–49] In these clinical protocols, patients with advanced breast cancer were treated initially with standard chemotherapy protocols to induce remission. Bone marrow progenitor cells were removed from the patient and cultured with a retrovirus carrying the genetic material for the MDR-1 gene. The retrovirus was used to transfer the MDR-1 gene into a portion of the patient's bone marrow cells. The MDR-1 gene confers resistance to the toxic effects of chemotherapy on the progenitor bone marrow cells and their offspring by pumping the chemotherapy out of the cells before the drugs are able to destroy the cell. It is hoped that MDR-1-marked cells will contribute to the rebuilding of the bone marrow following intense chemotherapy, an option not currently available due to the sensitivity of newly engrafted cells to chemotherapeutic agents.[50,51]

"Suicide" gene therapy protocols. These clinical trials involve transfer of a gene that produces an enzyme whose activity converts a nontoxic prodrug to its toxic form—a "suicide gene." The gene transfer is targeted to tumor cells to make them susceptible to an agent that does not cause harm to normal cells but kills malignant cells. The suicide gene is toxic to dividing cells only, thus sparing the normal cells and nondividing tumor cells. At present, replication-defective retroviral vectors are used because of their ability to transfer genes solely to actively dividing cells. The HSV-TK gene therapy protocol is an example of the use of a suicide gene; HSV-TK protocols use the herpes simplex virus thymidine kinase. Any cell that incorporates the *HSV-TK* gene becomes sensitive to the antiviral drug ganciclovir and can be destroyed on exposure. Retroviral vectors transfer genes to actively dividing cells, and therefore, this type of gene therapy is well suited for the treatment of brain tumors, as only the malignant cells are dividing and replicating. When a patient is treated with ganciclovir, the tumor cells are killed.

The National Cancer Institute (NCI) has conducted a clinical gene therapy trial in patients with brain tumors using intratumoral gene transfer with HSV-TK plus intravenous ganciclovir.[52] All patients received an injection of HSV-TK-producer cells directly into the tumor under magnetic resonance imaging guidance. Those patients with surgically accessible tumors had a craniotomy 7 days after the infusion, and the lining of the tumor cavity was infused with HSV-TK-producer cells. Ganciclovir also was given intravenously for 2 weeks beginning on the fifth postoperative day. Ganciclovir was given intravenously for 14 days to patients with inoperable brain tumors beginning 7 days after the HSV-TK injection. Initial results of these trials have shown promise, and use of this gene therapy method continues to be studied in patients with melanoma, brain, ovarian, and breast cancers.[53–55]

The Genetic Therapy Inc./Novartis Company (Gaithersburg, Maryland) is carrying out a similar trial targeting glioblastoma multiforma, a malignant brain tumor. The goal of the trial is the insertion of a gene capable of directing cell killing into a malignant tumor while protecting normal brain cells. This trial is one of the only phase III trials currently under way. The retroviral vector being injected into the tumor mass contains the *NEO-R* gene as a selective marker and *HSV-TK*. The only dividing cells in the area of a growing brain tumor are tumor cells and blood vessel cells. Because the retroviral vector only transduces the actively dividing cells, only tumor and blood vessel cells are affected. When ganciclovir is given to the patient, only the cells expressing the *HSV-TK* gene will take up the drug and incorporate it into their DNA synthesis and be killed. At present, forty centers in North America and Europe are involved, and an estimated 250 patients are enrolled.[56]

Nonviral Gene Therapy

Liposomes. A growing number of gene therapy protocols are investigating the use of nonviral methods to transfer therapeutic genes. Liposomes are nontoxic lipids that are being used as gene transfer vectors for the treatment of certain cancers. Liposome vectors contain DNA within a lipid structure that can be directly delivered to the cell as the liposome fuses with the cell membrane. This gene therapy method is being investigated with the *p53* tumor-suppressor gene in the treatment of patients with melanoma. The *p53* gene is a tumor-suppressor gene whose role is essential in helping to regulate cell proliferation and differentiation. The *p53* gene is inactivated in patients with the Li-Fraumeni familial cancer syndrome. In clinical gene therapy trials with patients who have Li-Fraumeni syndrome, the *p53* gene is inserted into cells after having been incorporated into a liposome, thus restoring to normal cells their ability to inhibit tumor activity.[46,57]

Antisense oligonucleotides. New genetic therapies for cancer treatment are being developed that specifically target DNA and RNA. Use of specific segments of DNA—antisense oligonucleotides—is one example of this new methodology. Antisense oligonucleotides are nucleic-binding agents. They are short strands of nucleotides that predictably combine with other nucleotides. This property allows for design of a treatment drug that can recognize a unique site on a specific gene. Antisense oligonucleotide segments are short strands of nucleic binding agents that contain a DNA sequence capable of binding with an RNA message. This property allows them to be targeted to specific errors in gene expression including that of a single base-pair mutation. Oligonucleotides can be inserted into cells to interfere with the translation of RNA into an oncogene protein. When transferred into patients, they prevent the oncogene's RNA message from being translated into a functional oncogene protein. One clinical trial under way is examining the use of oligonucleotide gene therapy in patients with acute myelogenous leukemia. In this study, antisense oligonucleotides are being used to destroy cancer cells in ex vivo blood cell purging. The specific oligonucleotide is targeted to an RNA segment that carries the *p53* gene to block overexpression. Another trial is investigating the use of antisense oligonucleotides to eliminate cancer cells during ex vivo blood cell purging as a treatment for patients with chronic myelogenous leukemia. A messenger RNA, transcribed from the *MYB* gene, is used to restore normal regulation and proliferation of blood cells. Therapies are still being perfected using antisense oligonucleotides Successful outcomes resulting from these gene therapies suggest that they may one day become common treatments for health conditions that now have no effective treatment, or for patients who experience relapse.[16,38]

Other nonviral gene therapies under investigation. DNA complexes that contain lipid, protein, peptide, or polymeric carriers as well as ligands capable of binding to cell-surface receptors on target cells are being used to deliver therapeutic genes to somatic tissue. This type of gene transfer method is currently under investigation to transfer genes to the lung, liver, endothelium, epithelium, and tumor cells. These gene therapy products are referred to as *gene drugs*. Methods to deliver gene drugs include aerosol spray, injection, and the *gene gun*, a needle-free injection device.[32,38]

Gene delivery using the aerosol method is being investigated as a therapeutic intervention for patients who have cystic fibrosis (CF), an autosomal recessive inherited condition that affects 1 in 2500 individuals and leads to airway obstruction and digestive problems caused by thick and sticky mucous. There are currently sixteen clinical gene therapy trials under way for the treatment of CF.[2,58] The findings from this research may lead to gene therapy treatment for other pulmonary complications, wound healing, and cardiac muscle damage from chemotoxicity.[38]

Studies of nonviral gene therapy methods are laying the groundwork for new gene treatments of both acute and chronic disease, and for the possibility of altering the dose and frequency of therapeutic gene administration in response to the patient's changing clinical needs. HER-2, for example, a protein located in cell surfaces, when overexpressed causes cancers to become more aggressive. The *HER-2* oncogene is overexpressed in 20%–30% of breast cancers, and these tumors seem to be more aggressive and somewhat more resistant to chemotherapy than those not overexpressing the oncogene. Clinical trials involving the use of gene therapy to deliver an antibody against the HER-2 protein have led to the creation of a genetically engineered drug that hones in on the HER-2 and blocks proliferation and thus decreases tumor growth.[59-62]

The safety profile for this class of drugs may be comparable to conventional drugs and biological products. To date, there are no reports of significant adverse effects when DNA is directly injected into muscle and other tissue, nor has there been any evidence of antinuclear antibodies in human subjects participating in clinical trials using direct delivery of "naked" DNA, or protein-DNA complexes.[63]

Gene therapy vaccines. A number of phase II trials are being carried out to investigate gene therapy vaccines against cancer. One of the trials currently under way is for head and neck squamous cell carcinoma and another for metastatic malignant melanoma. In these trials, an HLA gene (B27) that the tumor does not produce is injected directly into the tumor mass. Expression of this foreign antigen is expected to stimulate the patient's immune system to react against the cancer. Data collected to date on treated patients indicate that their immune systems, in addition to responding to B27, responded to other antigens on tumor cells, thereby producing an immune attack on nontransduced tumor cells. No evidence of toxicity in any of the 200 patients treated was reported over a 2-year period.[2,64]

Ethical, Social, and Legal Issues

No discussion of gene therapy would be complete without giving consideration to ethical issues. Ethical ramifications associated with gene therapies have been a societal concern since the first half of the twentieth century, during the eugenics movement, and as a result of the atrocities committed during World War II. The Nuremberg Code and the Declaration of Helsinki have since provided guidelines relating to research design, informed consent, and research reporting for researchers.[21,65-67] As gene therapy has evolved over the past 25 years, professional and public scrutiny has focused on the ethical implications of the technology. Organized religions have taken an active part in discussions on the ethical implications of human gene therapy. Churches and religious leaders have made valuable contributions to ethical dialogues by maintaining active communication with scientists, particularly those on regulatory committees and involved with the scientific literature. The continuing dialogue among theologians, ethicists, and scientists has helped to shape and implement regulatory processes for gene therapy designed to safeguard against misuse.[6,68,69]

The guidelines, "Points to Consider," were developed in 1988 by the NIH to solidify ethical concerns and to assist investigators and reviewers of human gene therapy proposals in addressing difficult issues.[6,34,35] The points, revised in 1990, provide a foundation for current and future clinical genome research. Information from the document was condensed to form six sets of ethical guidelines:

1. Concern for the clinical benefit of all persons receiving gene therapy
2. Assurance of informed consent
3. Fair selection of persons for gene therapy research protocols
4. Attention to the need for biosafety protocols
5. Public involvement in genetic research policy
6. Attention to long-term consequences of genetic research.

These considerations provide an ethical framework for researchers and health care professionals to address the multitude of questions that are evolving as recombinant techniques and gene therapy become more common.[22,35]

Assessing Clinical Benefits

Consideration of the assessment of clinical benefits in "Points to Consider" focuses on the researcher's responsibility to ensure that the risk to the participant for any gene therapy protocol is outweighed by the benefit of the treatment. To meet this consideration, researchers need to have adequate knowledge of the treatment to determine whether the participant will benefit more from the gene therapy trial than from any alternative treatment for the condition. NIH Director Harold Varums convened a panel in 1995 to assess the NIH investment in gene therapy research.[70] The panel concluded that gene therapy had been oversold to the public, and that gene therapy publicity is already causing some patients to forego conventional therapeutic interventions. Panel members emphasized the importance of research aimed at developing a better understanding of the underlying mechanisms that contribute to genetic disease. This kind of research, conducted to support ethical and scientifically sound development and application of gene therapy trials, will better meet the needs of the patients participating in the trials.[70]

Participant Selection and Informed Consent

The "Points to Consider" document also notes that potential research subjects should choose freely to participate in gene therapy. The choice of the participants must be equitable and candidates for gene therapy research need to be chosen fairly from among multiple populations. Those who are considered to be vulnerable populations such as prisoners should not serve as subjects.[22,34,71] Participant selection also involves compassionate or "emergency" use of gene therapy. A request was made to the NIH RAC Committee in 1993 for compassionate use of a gene therapy protocol, for example, for a patient with limited life expectancy. The request, although finally granted, generated many questions regarding emergency access to gene therapy and fairness of selection to other participants. If one patient is granted permission, how does a researcher decide about other applicants? How does the researcher maintain the integrity of the research data if emergency-use patients, who do not meet the clinical trial research criteria, are accepted into the protocol? These and other concerns about subject selection are presented to the RAC Committee and underscore some of the inherent issues in regulation of any new and as yet unproven therapy.[6,72]

Clinical research always involves an informed consent process to ensure that subjects participating in the research are doing so freely and voluntarily and with full information about the risks and benefits.[73–75] This precedent does not require that protocols be completely risk-free or that the benefits be unequivocally established before clinical trials are proposed. Rather, the premise of informed consent is that risks are honestly described, and the patient considering the research ultimately decides the value of the potential benefits and the possible risks. When minors are involved as participants in gene therapy clinical trials, the "Points to Consider" document emphasizes the need for informed assent by the minor in addition to obtaining parental permission.[76] The informed consent process for gene therapy protocols should also include discussion of plans for follow-up with primary care providers, social workers, geneticists, and psychologists in addition to the clinical investigators. Including these professionals in a follow-up plan ensures that participants will receive support in all areas of health care including reproduction and psychological development, normal processes that may be influenced by participation in gene therapy.[33]

The issue of informed consent becomes more problematic when germ-line therapy is considered. Germ-line gene therapy would alter the genes of future generations, and possibly create unknown long-term consequences. Germ-line gene therapy also raises the ethical concern that future unborn generations would not be able to give informed consent before gene therapy makes deliberate changes to their genetic code. For this and other ethical reasons, germ-line therapy is currently prohibited.[2,22,77]

Safety Issues

Short- and long-term side effects and toxicities associated with new gene therapy interventions also are of concern.

Program needs for implementing human clinical gene therapy trials include the importance of staff expertise, training of professional support staff, and patient and family counseling. These are deemed essential to assure the safety and successful implementation of gene therapy research.[78]

Patient safety

To date, no severe toxicity directly related to gene-altered cells has been reported.[2] This does not mean that patients undergoing gene therapy do not experience any side effects. As with any research drug protocol, during administration, patients need to be observed and evaluated for an allergic reaction to the foreign protein. Common side effects reported thus far include fever, chills, headache, fatigue, myalgias, nausea, and vomiting. Less common side effects reported include anorexia, diarrhea, and central nervous system effects such as extremity weakness, anemia, and leukopenia.[22] Table 25-3 summarizes reported side effects observed with some of the more common vectors. Concern that the disabled retrovirus may be able to restore its replication capacity through mutation, or that it may activate cancer genes has been expressed. No evidence of these side effects has been reported.[2,13,22]

Researchers cannot at this time predict the long-term risks to patients undergoing gene therapy or to their children. Some adverse effects may not become apparent for years. Vigilant follow-up care is needed to identify, diagnose, and prevent side effects. Long-term follow-up care may not be built into gene therapy protocols. Nurses caring for individuals who have undergone gene therapy must therefore be aware of this potential gap and develop a plan for following and monitoring patients.[6,12,24,31]

Public safety

The safety of those working with this new method of drug delivery is a second important concern. Safety involves protecting providers, families, and the public from the possibility of infectious transmission of recombinant genes with viral vectors. To date, infectious spread of recombinant viruses has not been observed, and the risk of this complication is considered to be remote. Not all gene therapy protocols use retroviral vectors and those that do may not all use them in the same way. Implementing universal precautions in consultation with nursing and hospital infection control officers is one safety measure that has been put in place for clinical trials using viral vectors, as these precautions are considered sufficient to prevent transmission of known pathogens such as hepatitis and HIV.[6,8,33]

Equal Access to Gene Therapy and Confidentiality of Genetic Information

As more is learned about the safety and efficacy of gene therapies to treat cancer, additional ethical issues will arise concerning the cost, availability, and allocation of these therapies. The average estimated cost for developing a new agent for gene therapy is $125 million.[2,13,79] What are the ethical implications of treatments developed for individuals with end-stage disease versus research directed toward prevention and cause of disease? Additionally, as with any costly treatment, will only a select few be able to afford access to gene therapy? Only selected medical centers can provide gene therapies, which could translate to additional patient expense for travel and lodging. Insurance companies do not pay for lodging and travel to centers for treatment. Patients could spend large amounts of out-of-pocket money just to get and stay there unless this is covered by research money. The potential for an ever-widening disparity in health and quality-of-life between individuals becomes a greater possibility than before.[13]

The potential for gene therapy as a viable intervention raises several other ethical concerns. Genetic testing and gene therapies reveal information about individuals and family members. This information has the potential to label currently healthy individuals as "at risk." As genetic testing and therapeutics become more common, personal and family genetic information may inadvertently become public. The Americans with Disabilities Act of 1990 offers protection against genetic discrimination in the workplace, but many questions remain about the possibilities for genetic discrimination by insurance companies and employers. Confidentiality, although viewed as the foundation of the patient-provider relationship, needs to be enforced in all areas of genetic testing and research. In a recent study by Geller et al, more than 32% of physicians reported that they would automatically provide genetic test results to a patient's insurance company without obtaining authorization from the patient.[80] These researchers document the pressing need to educate all primary care providers about the nature of genetic information and the risks associated with disclosure of such information to third parties.[80]

Table 25-3 Adverse Effects Reported in World-Wide Clinical Trials for Cancer Gene Therapy

Vector	Adverse Effect
Retrovirus	Erythema and induration, pruritus and pain, fever, elevation of LFTs, peritumor edema, abdominal pain, diarrhea, nausea, increased local edema, seizures abducens, paresis, confusion, intratumoral hemorrhage, mild exacerbation of graft-versus-host disease
Adenovirus	Fever, abnormal liver function, fatigue, pulmonary infiltrate, transient lung function abnormalities
Liposome	Injection pain, transient pneumothorax
Plasmid	Fever

LFTs = liver function tests.
Data from Lea[7]; Anderson[2,12]; Cuaron and Gallucci.[38]

Emerging Ethical Issues in Gene Therapy

The RAC, which advises the NIH Director on gene therapy, is currently engaged in discussions about fetal gene therapy. Two serious and life-threatening genetic disorders—ADA deficiency and alpha-thalassemia—are under consideration for fetal gene therapy. Current issues being debated include whether it is better to treat a disease for which backup therapies exist, as they do for ADA deficiency, or to go forward with gene treatment for alpha-thalassemia, a blood disorder that is often fatal to fetuses. At this stage, participants in the discussions agree that more data are needed about the safety and efficacy of fetal gene therapy as well as information on the possible alteration of fetuses' germ-line cells.[81]

The first gene therapy policy conference organized by the RAC in 1997 focused on another critical issue in gene therapy: the possibility that genetic engineering may be used for nondisease conditions—for enhancement or "cosmetic" purposes. The RAC's concern is that enhancement engineering is being considered already and that, without vigilance on the part of the RAC and FDA, could bypass these regulatory processes. A U.S. biotechnology company, for example, recently developed the technology for transferring genes into hair follicles to stimulate hair growth. The clinical objective is to reverse hair loss that occurs as a result of chemotherapy.[2,82] The indication stated when applying to the FDA for approval and product licensing is "chemotherapy-induced alopecia." Once a product such as this is licensed for any indication, however, it can be prescribed for other uses if the clinician feels it is clinically justified. One result could be millions of balding men being prescribed gene therapy for hair loss. The members of the conference concluded that the FDA should include a risk-benefit analysis that takes into account the possibility of "off label" use for cosmetic reasons when considering gene therapy products. This is one of the ways in which society may use genetic therapies for enhancement purposes.[2]

Information to educate the public about gene therapy and related social and ethical issues is available. Documents such as "Gene Therapy for Human Patients: Information for the General Public," from the NIH are essential to continuing public discussion and debate regarding the safe and ethical use of gene therapy.[83] Table 25-4 lists on-line resources regarding gene therapy and the Human Genome Project.

Practice Implications for Oncology Nurses

The evolution of genetics and its important role in health and disease are leading to continuous changes in nursing practice. To meet the changing clinical and educational needs of individuals, families, and communities, oncology nurses and the entire nursing community need to be knowledgeable and fluent in handling new genetic con-

Table 25-4 Internet Resources for Gene Therapy

- *http://www.ncgr.org*—National Center for Genome Resources
- *http://www.nci.nih.gov*—National Cancer Institute
- *http://www.nhgri.nih.gov*—National Human Genome Research Institute
- *http://www.ncbi.nlm.nih.gov/*—National Center for Biotechnology Information
- *http://www.alessexcellence.org/ae/aepc/NIH/index.html*—Understanding gene testing
- *http://rex.nci.nih.gov/INFO_CANCER/Cancer_facts/Section7/FS7_10.html*—Immunotherapy and Gene Therapy of Cancer
- *http://rex.nci.nih.gov/INFO_CANCER/Cancer_facts/Section7/FS7_18.html*—Questions and Answers About Gene Therapy

cepts and information.[84,85] Oncology nurses caring for individuals who are participating in gene therapy trials will be involved in providing direct care, educating individuals and the public, and advocating for fair and equitable use and for the confidentiality and privacy of genetic information. Roles for oncology nurses providing genetic-related health care in these areas are outlined in Table 25-5. Two emerging roles for oncology nurses are provider of genetic services and clinical investigator in nursing genetic research.[13,86–88]

Provider of Genetic Services

The identification of cancer susceptibility genes and gene therapy developments are expanding the role for oncology nurses as genetics service providers. Oncology nurses now have the opportunity to participate in counseling individuals and families with increased risk of cancer by identifying risk factors and genes associated with cancer predisposition. Although these services are not uniformly available, many centers, clinics, and community practices are increasing their activities in this area.[13,87,88]

Genetics services include identifying individuals and families in need of further genetic evaluation and testing, referring to more specialized genetics professionals, and participating in the genetic counseling process. These services are a critical component of cancer risk assessment and treatment. Oncology nurses, by virtue of their specialized training and knowledge in cancer and their sensitivity to the influence of family and cultural beliefs on health care decisions, can incorporate components of the genetic counseling process into the care of individuals receiving gene therapy and their families.[7,83,84] (The reader is referred elsewhere[7,87,88] for a more detailed discussion of genetic counseling and nursing participation in this service.)

Nursing Research

Gene therapy, as a clinical treatment for cancer, is in its early stages. Many issues regarding response to gene

Table 25-5 Nursing Responsibilities in Caring for Patients and Families Undergoing Gene Therapy

Direct Caregiver

- Provides anticipatory guidance
- Assures informed decision-making/consent
- Develops treatment and management plans
- Administers gene therapy
- Observes patients for expected and unexpected side effects of treatment, including psychosocial and emotional response
- Participates in developing long-term follow-up plans
- Assures coordination and collaboration of care with all health care providers involved in patient/family care before, during, and after gene therapy

Educator

- Serves as an information source to patients, families, and the public
- Provides relevant, accurate, and understandable information to patients, both in written and verbal format
- Assures that patient/family questions will be answered at all times

Advocate

- Assures privacy and confidentiality of genetic information
- Protects against discrimination
- Advocates for fair and equitable use of gene therapies for all populations
- Promotes public understanding of somatic gene therapy

Genetics Services Provider

- Gathers relevant family history information
- Identifies individuals and families in need of further genetic education and counseling
- Assesses psychosocial, ethnocultural, and educational background
- Provides psychosocial support in follow-up to genetic counseling

Research Investigator

- Participates in or conducts clinical research trials in gene therapy
- Serves as a preceptor to other nurses
- Develops research protocols that will address patient/family response and adaptation to genetic information, including gene therapy

Reprinted with permission from Lea DH: Gene therapy: Current and future implications for oncology nursing practice. *Semin Oncol Nurs* 13:115–122, 1997.[13]

therapy remain for patients undergoing gene therapy. The oncology nurse needs to consider the following issues:

- The long-term physical and psychosocial ramifications of gene therapy.

- How individuals and families adapt to new genetic information and therapies.

- How cultural and family backgrounds may influence individual's decision making.

- Identification of educational materials and methods that are best suited for providing information about gene therapy.

- Preparation of primary care practitioners, especially nurses, to care for individuals and families throughout life following gene therapy.

Oncology nurses as direct caregivers, educators, and advocates can have an instrumental role in initiating and participating in nursing research to help address these issues.[13,89,90] Oncology nurses can also play a leading role in developing longitudinal research efforts focusing on the continuum of identifying individual responses and adaptation to genetic cancer risk, testing, treatment, and posttreatment. Nurses can identify fluctuations in the coping process and recognize optimal times for psychosocial interventions and support. Other areas for oncology nursing research include determining effective means for tailoring information to differing educational and cultural backgrounds, and developing nursing management approaches to family concerns with regard to gene therapy.[88]

Conclusion

Oncology nurses practicing in all settings will be challenged as they care for individuals before, during, and after gene therapy interventions. They can meet these challenges through preparation to support and facilitate patient's decision making and their adaptation to genetic interventions, to face ethical and social issues, and to promote and advocate for safe and fair use of this new technology. Oncology nurses can best prepare themselves for these tasks by becoming knowledgeable about all aspects of gene therapy and, as with any new clinical situation, by examining their views and values and their role in the effective delivery of genetic health care.

References

1. Guyer M, Collins FS: The Human Genome Project and the future of medicine. *Am J Dis Child* 8:20–26, 1993
2. Anderson WF: Human gene therapy. *Nature* 392:25–30, 1998 (suppl)
3. Culver KW: *Gene Therapy: A Handbook for Physicians*. New York, Leibert, 1994
4. Lyon J: *Altered Fates and the Retooling of Human Life*. New York, Norton, 1995
5. Verma IM, Somia N: Gene therapy: Promises, problems and prospects. *Nature* 389:239–242, 1997
6. Jenkins J, Wheeler V, Albright L: Gene therapy for cancer. *Cancer Nurs* 17:447–456, 1994

7. Lea DH, Jenkins J, Francomano C: *Genetics in Clinical Practice: New Directions for Nursing and Health Care.* Sudbury, MA, Jones and Bartlett, 1998

8. Wheeler VS: Gene therapy: Current strategies and future applications. *Oncol Nurs Forum* 22:20–26, 1995 (suppl)

9. Rimoin DL, Connor JM, Pyeritz RE (ed): *Emery and Rimoin's Principles and Practice of Medical Genetics* (ed 3). New York, Churchill Livingstone, 1996

10. Thompson MW, McInnes RR, Willard HF (eds): *Thompson and Thompson: Genetics in Medicine.* Philadelphia, Saunders, 1991

11. Anderson WF: Gene therapy for genetic diseases. *Hum Gene Ther* 5:282–282, 1994a

12. Anderson WF: Gene therapy. *Sci Am* 9:124–128, 1995

13. Lea DH: Gene therapy: Current and future implications for oncology nursing practice. *Semin Oncol Nurs* 13:115–122, 1997

14. McKusick VA: *Mendelian Inheritance in Man: Catalogs of Autosomal Dominant, Autosomal Recessive and X-linked Phenotypes* (ed 11). Baltimore, MD, The Johns Hopkins University, 1994

15. Lederberg J: The genetics of human nature. *Social Res* 40:375–406, 1973

16. Wolf JA, Lederberg J: An early history of gene transfer and gene therapy. *Hum Gene Ther* 5:469–480, 1994

17. Mastrangelo MJ, Berd D, Nathan FE, et al: Gene therapy for human cancer: An essay for clinicians. *Semin Oncol* 3:4–21, 1996

18. Friedman T: Progress toward human gene therapy. *Science* 244:1275–1280, 1989

19. Rosenecker J, Schmalix WA, Schindlehauer D, et al: Towards gene therapy of cystic fibrosis. *Eur J Med Res* 8:149–156, 1998

20. Anderson WF: Human gene therapy. *Science* 256:808–813, 1992

21. Robinson KD, Abernathy E, Conrad KJ: Gene therapy of cancer. *Semin Oncol Nurse* 12:142–151, 1996

22. Sommers MS, Shackmann J: Designer genes and critical care nursing: The future is now. *Heart Lung* 24: 228–238, 1995

23. Jenks SN, Blaese MR: Still blazing a path of his own. *J Natl Cancer Inst* 90:1188–1191, 1998

24. Kafri T, Blomer U, Peterson DA, et al: Sustained expression of genes delivered directly into liver and muscle by lentiviral vectors. *Nature Genet* 17:314–317, 1997

25. Pickler RH, Munroe CL: Gene therapy for inherited disorders. *J Pediatr Nurs* 10:40–47, 1995

26. Bilbao G, Feng M, Rancourt C, et al: Adenoviral/retroviral vector chimeras: A novel strategy to achieve high-efficiency stable transduction in vivo. *FASEB J* 11:624–634, 1997

27. Schneirle BS, Groner B: Retroviral targeted delivery. *Gene Ther* 3:1069–1073, 1996

28. Naldini L, Blomer P, Gallay D, et al: In vivo gene delivery and stable transduction of non-dividing cells by a lentiviral vector. *Science* 272:263–267, 1996

29. Friedman T: Overcoming the obstacles to gene therapy. *Sci Am* 276:80–86, 1997

30. Calos M: The potential of extrachromosomal replicating vectors for gene therapy. *Trends Genet* 12:463–466, 1996

31. Ledley FD: After gene therapy: Issues in long-term clinical follow-up and care. *Adv Genet* 32:1–16, 1995

32. Morsy MA, Kohnosuka M, Clemens P, Casky T: Progress towards gene therapy. *JAMA* 270:2338–2345, 1993

33. Ledley FD: Clinical considerations in the design of protocols for somatic gene therapy. *Hum Gene Ther* 2:77–83, 1991

34. Jeungst E: The NIH "Points to consider" and the limits of human gene therapy. *Hum Gene Ther* 1:425–433, 1990

35. National Institutes of Health: Points to consider in human somatic cell therapy. *Hum Gene Ther* 2:251–256, 1991

36. ORDA Report: Documents—Recombinant DNA in *Office of Recombinant DNA Activities.* Available at http://www.nih.gov/od/orda/protocol.pdf

37. Brenner M, Rill DR, Moen RC, et al: Gene-marking to trace origin of relapse after autologous bone marrow transplant. *Lancet* 341:85–87, 1993

38. Cuaron LJ, Gallucci B: Gene therapy and blood cell transplantation. *Semin Oncol Nurs* 13:200–207, 1997

39. Platsoucas CD, Freedman RS: Tumor-infiltrating lymphocytes in gene therapy. *Cancer Bull* 45:118–124, 1993

40. Rosenberg SA, Aebersold PM, Cornetta K, et al: Gene transfer into humans: Immunotherapy of patients with advanced melanoma using tumor-infiltrating lymphocytes modified by retroviral gene transduction. *N Engl J Med* 323a:570–578, 1990 (suppl)

41. Schuening F, Miller D, Totok-Storb B, et al: Study on contribution of genetically marked peripheral blood repopulating cells to hematopoeitic reconstitution after transplantation. *Hum Gene Ther* 5:1523–1534, 1994

42. Douer D, Levine A, Anderson WF, et al: High-dose chemotherapy and autologous bone marrow plus peripheral blood stem cell transplantation for patients with lymphoma or metastatic breast cancer: Use of marker genes to investigate hematopoietic reconstitution in adults. *Hum Gene Ther* 7:669–684, 1996

43. Broxmeyer HE, Cooper S, Etienne-Julan M, et al: Cord blood transplantation and the potential for gene therapy: Gene transduction using a recombinant adeno-associated viral vector. *Ann NY Acad Sci* 770:105–115, 1995

44. Almici C, Carlo-Stella C, Wagner J, et al: Umbilical cord blood as a source of hematopoietic stem cells: From research to clinical application. *Haematologica* 80:473–479, 1995

45. Rosenberg SA: Gene therapy for cancer. *JAMA* 268:2418–2419, 1992a

46. Freeman FM, Zwiebel JA: Gene therapy of cancer. *Clin Invest* 6:676–688, 1993

47. Biedler JL: Genetic aspects of multidrug resistance. *Cancer* 70:1799–1809, 1992 (suppl)

48. Deisseroth AB: Current trends and future directions in the genetic therapy of human neoplastic disease. *Cancer* 72:2069–2074

49. Deisseroth AB, Kavanagh JJ, Hanania EG, et al: Gene therapy: Chemoprotection, immunoenhancement and modification of tumor cells. *Cancer Bull* 45:139–145, 1993

50. Culver KW, Blaese RM: Gene therapy for cancer. *Trends Genet* 5:174–178, 1994

51. O'Shaughnessy JA: Clinical protocol: Retroviral mediated transfer of the human multi-drug resistance gene (MDR-1) into hematopoeitic stem cells during autologous transplantation after intensive chemotherapy for metastatic breast cancer. *Hum Gene Ther* 5:981–991, 1994

52. Jenks S: Dramatic new strategies for brain tumors emerge. *J Natl Cancer Inst* 85:662–663, 1993a

53. Oldfield EH, Ram Z, Culver KW, et al: Gene therapy for the treatment of brain tumors using intra-tumoral transduction with the thymadine kinase gene and intravenous ganciclovir. *Hum Gene Ther* 4:39–69, 1993

54. Culver KW: Clinical applications of gene therapy for cancer. *Clin Chem* 4:510–512, 1994.

55. Vile R, Russel SJ: Gene transfer technologies for the gene therapy of cancer. *Gene Ther* 1:(2)88–98, 1994

56. Ram Z, Culver KW, Oshiro EM, et al: Therapy of malignant brain tumors by intratumoral implantation of retroviral vector-producing cells. *Nature Med* 3:1354–1361, 1997

57. Yarbro JW: Oncogenes and cancer suppressor genes. *Semin Oncol Nurs* 8:30–39, 1992

58. Davies JL, Geddes DM, Alton EWFW: Prospects for gene therapy for cystic fibrosis. *Mol Med Today* 4:292–299, 1998

59. Holzman D: her-2/NEU gene bumped into the limelight. *J Natl Cancer Inst* 88:147–148, 1996

60. Hortobagyi GN: Treatment of breast cancer. *N Engl J Med* 339:974–984, 1998

61. Slamon DJ, Clark GM, Wong SG, et al: Human breast cancer: Correlation of relapse and survival with amplification of the HER-2/neu oncogene. *Science* 235:177–182, 1987

62. Slamon D, Leyland-Jones B, Shak S, et al: Addition of herceptin (humanized anti-HER2 antibody) to first line chemotherapy for HER2 over-expressing metastatic breast cancer markedly increases anticancer activity: A randomized, multinational controlled phase III trial. *Proc Am Soc Clin Oncol* 17:98a, 1998 (abstr)

63. Ledley F: Nonviral gene therapy: The promise of genes as pharmaceutical products. *Hum Gene Ther* 6:1129–1144, 1995

64. Nabel G, Gordon D, Bishop DK, et al: Immune response in human melanoma after transfer of an allogenic class I major histocompatibility complex gene with DNA-liposome complexes. *Proc Natl Acad Sci USA* 93(26):15388–15393, 1996

65. Areen J: The greatest rewards and the heaviest penalties. *Hum Gene Ther* 3:277–278, 1992

66. Harrison L: Issues related to the protection of human research participants. *J Neurosci Nurs* 25:187–193, 1993

67. Howell JD: The history of eugenics and the future of gene therapy. *J Clin Ethics* 2:274–278, 1991

68. Gustafson JM: A Christian perspective on genetic engineering. *Hum Gene Ther* 5:747–754, 1994

69. Nelson JR: The role of religions in the analysis of ethical issues of human gene therapy. *Hum Gene Ther* 1:143–148, 1990

70. Orkin SH, Motulsky AG: *Report and Recommendations of the Panel to Assess the NIH Investment in Research on Gene Therapy.* Available at http://www.nih.gov/od/orda/panelrep.htm

71. Subcommittee on Human Gene Therapy, Recombinant DNA Advisory Committee, National Institutes of Health. Points to consider in the design and submission of protocols for the transfer of recombinant DNA into the genome of human subjects. *Hum Gene Ther* 1:93–103, 1990

72. Capron A, Leventhal B, Post L: Requests for compassionate use of gene therapy: Memorandum from the subcommittee to the RAC, January 13, 1993. *Hum Gene Ther* 4:199–200, 1993

73. Surgeon General: U.S. Public Health Service Investigation involving human subjects, including clinical research: Requirements for review to insure the rights and welfare of individuals. *Public Policy Order No. 129*, 1966

74. Code of Federal Regulations: Title 45, Part 46: *Protection of Human Subjects* (revised March 8, 1983). 1980

75. Faden R, Beauchamp T: *A History and Theory of Informed Consent.* New York: Oxford University Press, 1986

76. Koalata G: Ethicists wary over new gene technique's consequences. *New York Times*, Nov 22: B9, 1994

77. Fletcher JC, Richter G: Human fetal gene therapy: Moral and ethical questions. *Hum Gene Ther* 7:1605–1614, 1996

78. McGarrity GJ: Resource needs for institutional programs in human gene therapy. *Hum Gene Ther* 3:279–284, 1992

79. Mayer D: Biotherapy: Recent advances and nursing implications. *Nurs Clin North Am* 25:291–309, 1990

80. Geller G, Tambor ES, Chase GA, et al: Physicians' attitudes toward disclosure of genetic information to third parties. *J Law Med Eth* 21:238–240, 1993

81. Jenks S: Researchers seek guidance on "preproposal" for *in utero* gene therapy. *J Natl Cancer Inst* 90:1507, 1998

82. Li L, Hoffman RM: The feasibility of targeted selective gene therapy of the hair follicle. *Nature Med* 1:705–706, 1995

83. McGarrity GJ, Walters L: Gene therapy for human patients: Information for the general public. *NIH Pub No 90-2885.* 1–13, April 1990

84. Hayflick SJ, Eiff PM: Role of primary care providers in delivery of genetic services. *Community Genetics* 1:18–22, 1998

85. Piste C: Molecular medicine and information-based targeted healthcare. *Nature Biotech* 16:19–21, 1998 (suppl)

86. Andrews LB, Fullarton JE, Holtzman NA, Motulsky AG: *Assessing Genetic Risks: Implications for Health and Social Policy.* Washington, National Academy Press, 1994

87. Loescher LJ: Genetics in cancer prediction, screening and counseling: Genetics in cancer prediction and screening (Part I). *Oncol Nurs Forum* 22:10–15, 1995 (suppl)

88. Loescher LJ: Genetics in cancer prediction, screening, and counseling: The nurse's role in genetic counseling (Part II). *Oncol Nurs Forum* 22:16–19, 1995 (suppl)

89. Cogliano-Shutta NA: Pediatric Phase I clinical trials: Ethical issues and nursing considerations. *Oncol Nurs Forum* 13:29–32, 1986

90. Jassak PF, Ryan MP: Ethical issues in clinical research. *Semin Oncol Nurs* 5:102–108, 1989

CHAPTER 26

Late Effects of Cancer Treatment

Ida Marie (Ki) Moore, RN, DNS, FAAN
Wendy Hobbie, RN, MSN, CRNP

Scope of the Problem

Long-term disease-free survival from pediatric and adult cancers continues to improve. For white adults, 5-year survival for all cancer sites was 50% in 1974–1976, 52% in 1980–1982, and 60% in 1986–1993. Survival rates for blacks have also increased, but are 10%–15% lower than those of whites for the most common cancers except lung cancer. For children, improvements in long-term disease-free survival have been even more dramatic. Five-year relative survival for all cancer sites in children under the age of 15 years was 56% in 1974–1976, 65% in 1980–1982, and 72% in 1986–1993.[1] It is estimated that there will be 180,000–220,000 childhood cancer survivors in 2000, and that by 2010, 1 in every 250 young adults between the ages of 15 and 45 years will be a survivor of childhood cancer.[2,3]

Biological cure refers to a patient who has no evidence of disease, has the same life expectancy as a person who never had cancer, and ultimately dies of unrelated causes.[4] Because of the aggressive nature of cancer treatment, cure is not without consequences. The consequences or late effects of cancer result from the physiological effects of particular treatments or from the interactions among treatment, the individual, and the disease. In contrast to the acute side effects of chemotherapy and radiation that are due to death of proliferative cells in tissues with relatively rapid renewal, late biological toxicity is believed to progress over time and by different mechanisms.

Most patients appear clinically healthy shortly after the completion of cancer therapy, but they may have subclinical tissue damage that may be detected by sensitive screening tests. Individuals with subclinical tissue damage can function well and be asymptomatic if compensatory mechanisms are adequate. Late effects, or the late expression of tissue damage, occur when physiological stress or developmental changes overwhelm compensatory mechanisms.[5] Late effects can appear months to years after treatment and can be mild to severe to life-threatening. Their impact depends on the age and developmental state of the patient. Younger individuals may be more resilient than older adults to the acute side effects of treatment, but children are often at greater risk than adults for late effects.

A great unknown is what will happen to individuals who received intensive treatment in their youth as they age. Although we may not be able to detect any obvious side effects soon after the completion of treatment, the effect of even subtle tissue damage on the process of aging is unknown. For adults, the cumulative effects of treatment toxicity combined with hereditary predisposition to particular health problems and exposure to damaging agents such as alcohol, cigarette smoke, or pollutants on organ systems are unknown. This chapter summarizes what is currently known about long-term tissue injury and the development of secondary cancers following cancer treatment. Assessment and management of late effects are also discussed. Finally, as more is learned about the pathophysiological mechanisms responsible for late effects, strategies for protecting healthy tissues can be developed and tested; this information regarding causes of late effects is included whenever possible.

Central Nervous System

Neuropsychological, neuroanatomical, and neurophysiological changes can occur as a result of central nervous system (CNS) treatment. These late effects have been observed in survivors of acute lymphoblastic leukemia (ALL) and brain tumors, and following bone marrow transplant.

Neuropsychological Late Effects

Declines in general intellectual abilities (intelligence quotient, IQ) and academic achievement, as well as deficits in visual-motor integration, attention, memory, visual-motor skills, and verbal fluency are the most frequently reported neuropsychological late effects of CNS treatment.[6–25] Nonverbal skills are especially vulnerable to the deleterious effects of CNS treatment, and deficits in these areas may be among the first to appear.

Neuropsychological late effects progress over time and become observable as cognitive abilities begin to lag behind age and developmental expectations. Age at time of CNS treatment is an important consideration because of the vulnerability of the developing brain to the damaging effects of radiation and chemotherapy. Children with ALL who receive cranial radiation before age 5 are at greatest risk for cognitive deficits, and 85% of children with brain tumors who receive radiation therapy before age 3 experience significant cognitive impairments, such as a decline in full-scale IQ of 15–25 or more points.[5,18,26–31]

The type of CNS treatment that has been most closely associated with neuropsychological deficits is cranial radiation alone or in combination with intrathecal (IT) chemotherapy. Children and adults treated for brain tumors with relatively high doses of cranial radiation consistently demonstrate deficits in intellectual abilities, memory, reasoning, visuospatial abilities, and mathematical skills.[6–18,26–31] There is a relationship between the radiation dose and the severity of late effects. Survivors of brain tumors often have the most serious cognitive deficits, while children who receive lower cranial radiation doses as part of bone marrow conditioning regimens experience mild to no observable impairments.[27–36] In addition to age and radiation dose, girls may be more severely affected than boys in terms of general cognitive performance such as IQ scores.[37] Balsom et al found that the protective effect of preirradiation IT methotrexate was most significant in girls less than 5 years of age at the time of CNS treatment.[38]

There is less information about the effects of IT chemotherapy alone or in combination with moderate to high-dose systemic chemotherapy on long-term cognitive and academic abilities. Findings from several studies suggest that IT chemotherapy combined with systemic methotrexate (1 g/m²) for treatment of ALL is associated with neurological toxicity comparable to that of cranial radiation.[25,39,40] High-dose carmustine (BCNU), cytosine, arabinoside, fludarabine, and spiromustine have been associated with acute and chronic neurotoxicities.[41]

Neuroanatomical Changes

Computerized tomography (CT) and magnetic resonance imaging (MRI) have been used to evaluate structural changes after CNS treatment. Atrophy, leukoencephalopathy, and white matter changes or calcifications have been found in more than 50% of children with ALL who received either systemic medium to high-dose methotrexate (2 g/m²) or systemic and IT methotrexate plus cranial radiation. A greater percentage of abnormal scans occurred in children who received radiation.[42,43]

Diffuse brain atrophy, as measured by the size of the CNS compartments, has also been documented in children who had either completed or were receiving ALL treatment. The highest incidence of brain atrophy (71% overall) occurred during the administration of IT chemotherapy, suggesting that CNS damage begins during treatment.[44] In addition to atrophy, perfusion defects have been identified in children with ALL whose treatment regimens included either IT and intravenous methotrexate or cranial radiation.[45]

Mechanisms of Injury

There are several possible mechanisms by which radiation and chemotherapy damage nonmalignant CNS tissue. Radiation injury to endothelial cells in small and medium-sized cerebral vessels causes deposition of calcium and mineralized debris. The result is some degree of occlusion, depending on the lumen size of the vessel. Dystrophic calcification of surrounding neural tissue also occurs.[42,43,47] Vascular endothelial damage can also perturb the normally tight junctions of the blood-brain barrier, allowing greater concentrations of systemic chemotherapy to penetrate the CNS.

Radiation and methotrexate damage oligodendroglia, the myelin-producing cells in the CNS. Occlusive changes in vessels and decreased perfusion cause necrosis of glial cells and neurons.[43,48] Decreased white matter glucose metabolism (detected by [¹⁸F] fluorodeoxyglucose positron emission tomography) in children with ALL treated with cranial radiation and IT chemotherapy suggests that the predominant and direct neurotoxic effect of radiation is injury to white matter.[49] Methotrexate also causes myelin damage. Methotrexate blocks the synthesis of tetrahydrofolate by inhibition of the enzyme dihydrofolate reductase. Tetrahydrofolate is required as an intermediate carrier of one-carbon groups necessary for the synthesis of many biological macromolecules such as myelin

proteins and lipids.[50,51] Injury to gray matter structures can also occur but is thought to be less common than vascular or white matter damage. Vascular endothelial damage and decreased perfusion may contribute to gray matter damage.[43,47,48] A decrease in white matter glucose metabolism may also reduce or interfere with neuronal functions such as synaptic connectivity.[49]

Vision and Hearing

Visual defects and hearing loss also can occur following CNS treatment. Enucleation, which may be necessary in the treatment of ocular tumors such as retinoblastoma, is the most disabling visual deficit. Cataracts have been associated with cranial irradiation (2–16 Gray [Gy]) and long-term corticosteroid therapy. Cataracts are due to radiation damage to the germinative zone of lens epithelial cell DNA as well as direct cytoplasmic effects such as disruption of membrane channels.[52]

Retinopathy can also occur following radiation to the eye, orbit, nasal cavity, paranasal sinus, or nasopharyngeal area.[53,54] The mean time to onset of symptoms in one study was 2.8 years after treatment, and the earliest symptom was usually diminished vision.[53] The risk of radiation retinopathy increased with doses in the 45–55 Gy range. However, chemotherapy and concurrent chronic illness, such as diabetes mellitus, may increase the risk.[53] Radiation retinopathy is primarily due to vascular changes such as thickened arteriolar walls, lumenal narrowing and occlusion, and ischemia.[52] A dose-per-fraction effect may be important for children who receive radiation therapy as conservative therapy for retinoblastoma. In one study, hypofractionation was found to increase the risk of subsequent retinopathy.[54]

The pathogenesis of radiation retinopathy involves obstruction of small vessels with resulting ischemia, edema, and neovascularization of the optic disk.[54] Conjunctivitis, telangiectasis, corneal ulceration, optic neuropathy, and atrophy or stenosis of the lacrimal system can also occur but at radiation doses between 30 and 75 Gy.[52]

Chemotherapy can cause ocular effects that may or may not be reversible. Conjunctivitis, keratitis, retinal hemorrhage, retinopathy, optic neuritis, and blurred vision are the more commonly reported ocular toxicities of systemic chemotherapy.[52,55] Less is written about the mechanisms of ocular toxicity following chemotherapy, however one study suggests direct vascular injury.[56]

Visual defects can be assessed by visual examination, slit-lamp examination, ultrasound, fluorescein angiogram, or MRI.[52] Visual evoked potentials may be helpful in monitoring changes in sensory visual pathway or visual pathway damage in young children who can not communicate visual symptoms or cooperate with more standard vision assessment methods.[57]

Hearing loss, especially in the high-tone range, is most closely associated with cisplatin.[58–60] A study of children with brain tumors treated with dose-intensive induction chemotherapy suggests that carboplatin-based high-dose therapy also results in significant ototoxicity.[61] Treatment regimens that combine cranial radiation and cisplatin-based chemotherapy increase the risk for sensorineural hearing loss.[62,63] Concurrent ifosfamide therapy also can exacerbate cisplatin-induced hearing loss. Patients who receive ifosfamide in combination with cisplatin are more likely to require amplification than those who receive cisplatin in combination with other drugs such as methotrexate and doxorubicin.[64]

One of the most consistently reported risk factors for cisplatin-based ototoxicity is drug dose. A cumulative dose of more than 600 mg/m^2 greatly increases the risk for persistent hearing loss in adults and children.[58–60] High cumulative doses of cisplatin can also impair renal function. Children with malignant brain tumors who were treated with eight drugs (including cisplatin) in one day and who developed severe renal insufficiency were at greatest risk for significant hearing loss.[65] Iris and skin pigmentation may also affect cisplatin-induced ototoxicity. In a study of 19 children who had audiological assessments before and after cisplatin therapy for various solid tumors, a weak association between iris pigmentation and decreased auditory threshold was found. Children with brown or black eyes had greater hearing loss than did those with blue or hazel eyes, suggesting that pigmentation influences host susceptibility to cisplatin ototoxicity.[66] History of noise exposure has also been found to be a risk factor for adults.[59]

Periodic audiometric evaluations can be used to monitor for ototoxicity that is manifested as a deterioration of pure-tone thresholds. Acoustic reflex threshold measures may also be useful for detecting early sensorineural hearing loss. This method may be particularly useful in young children.[67]

Damage to the hair cells of the cochlea is the most common mechanism of ototoxicity following cisplatin.[66] Postirradiation hyperemia may increase the sensitivity of the cochlea to cisplatin damage.[64] Recurrent otitis media, a common problem in children receiving chemotherapy, as well as the use of antibiotics that are ototoxic, also can contribute to hearing loss. Little is known about effective methods for protecting the auditory system from the damaging effects of chemotherapy and radiation. However, two studies report an otoprotective effect of sodium thiosulfate (SDS). In these studies, high doses of SDS were administered to patients with malignant brain tumors after recovery of blood-brain barrier disruption. Sodium thiosulfate is thought to bind and inactivate DNA alkylating agents such as cisplatin and carboplatin. In both studies, hearing loss was decreased in patients treated with SDS.[68,69]

Immune System

Immunosuppression is one of the most serious acute toxic effects of chemotherapy and radiation. Some aspects of immune function can remain impaired for years after treatment. For example, high-dose chemotherapy fol-

lowed by bone marrow transplantation has been found to induce a profound and prolonged impairment of hematopoiesis. Diminished stem cell self-renewal and low levels of erythroid and megakaryocyte progenitors have also been reported.[70] Radiation in conjunction with multiagent chemotherapy can result in more frequent and more severe immune system impairment.[71,72]

The clinical significance of these long-term alterations in immune function is not well understood. There is no evidence that patients with persistent immunologic abnormalities are at greater risk for infections. One group of patients at increased risk of infection are those who have undergone splenectomy. Overwhelming bacterial infections, primarily pneumococcal, are a major concern to these individuals because of the protective role of the spleen against encapsulated organisms. Persistent immune defects have not been linked to the occurrence of second malignancies. This may change, however, as survival time increases for larger numbers of patients.

Cardiovascular System

Anthracyclines, such as daunorubicin and doxorubicin, have improved survival in patients with acute leukemias, lymphomas, pediatric solid tumors, and other cancers. One of the most serious late effects of these drugs is cardiac toxicity, which typically presents as cardiomyopathy, with clinical signs of congestive heart failure.[73] Pathophysiological changes associated with cardiomyopathy include decreased contractility and stroke volume, increased left ventricular afterload, and increased end systolic wall stress. Recent evidence indicates that structural damage to the heart can exist prior to the onset of symptoms.[74,75] In a study of cardiac function in long-term survivors of malignant bone tumors, 18 of 31 patients (58%) had cardiac abnormalities 2.3–14.1 years after treatment with doxorubicin, however 12 of the 18 patients (67%) were asymptomatic.[75]

The risk and severity of cardiotoxicity is related to cumulative dose,[76–78] schedule of administration (continuous versus intermittent), and presence of other factors such as mediastinal irradiation. Cumulative doses of 550 mg/m^2 have been associated with cardiac toxicity in adults; similar abnormalities can occur after lower doses in children. Lipshultz et al found that 57% of children with acute leukemia treated with doxorubicin developed abnormalities of left ventricular afterload or contractility.[77] The cumulative dose of doxorubicin was the most significant predictor of abnormal cardiac function. However, cardiac toxicity has been observed in children treated with anthracycline doses (90–270 mg/m^2), suggesting that there may be no completely safe drug dose.[78]

Individuals who received radiation therapy to a field that includes the heart, such as mediastinal radiation for Hodgkin's disease or other lymphomas, also are at risk for cardiotoxicity. Delayed radiation injury to the heart can be manifested as pericardial disease, myocardial disease, or coronary heart disease.[79–81] An acceleration of coronary artery disease that results in angina and myocardial infarction may occur in some patients. Patients with pericardial damage secondary to mediastinal irradiation may have overt symptoms and abnormalities that are visible on x-ray examination. Pericardial damage may be self-limiting, but life-threatening pericardial effusions with tamponade can occur.[81] Some evidence suggests that use of current radiation blocking techniques that protect some portions of the ventricles from irradiation result in more modest and less frequent cardiac toxicity.[82] In general, peripheral vascular disease is a rare cardiovascular late effect. However, approximately 50% of patients with germ cell tumors of the testes treated with cisplatin, vinblastine, and bleomycin report having Raynaud's phenomenon.[80] A case of episodic complete heart block after high-dose cyclophosphamide and thiotepa has also been reported.[83]

Mechanisms of Injury and Cardioprotection

The mechanisms of cardiac damage following anthracyclines include inhibited expression of genes encoding for cardiac muscle protein, binding to membranes rich in cardiolipin, and the formation of free radicals.[84] The heart is particularly sensitive to free radical–induced damage because of low levels of free radical scavengers. Drugs that prevent the formation of superhydroxide radicals are being investigated for efficacy in preventing doxorubicin-induced cardiotoxicity. Results to date from animal and human studies are encouraging.[84–86]

Rats treated with doxorubicin were injected with an antibody that binds specifically to myosin in injured cells. The investigators reported a strong positive correlation between the intensity of antibody binding and loss of contractile function.[87] The value of indium–111-antimyosin scintigraphy in early detection of myocardial damage in children treated with doxorubicin was pilot-tested in a group of eight patients. Results suggest that this method may be suitable to detect early myocardial damage after a cumulative doxorubicin dose of 150 mg/m^2 and may be useful in identifying children who are at increased risk for developing late cardiac sequelae.[88]

Cardiac damage following radiation primarily involves the endothelial cells of the myocardial capillaries. The injury causes swelling, microvascular thrombosis, or rupture. The result is obstruction or destruction of the myocardial microvasculature. In contrast to the effects of anthracyclines, direct damage of myocytes has not been observed in humans.[81] While pharmacologic cardioprotection has not been reported, the use of current radiation techniques that shield the heart may afford similar protection.[82]

Pulmonary System

Pneumonitis and pulmonary fibrosis are the major biological late effects of treatment to the pulmonary system.

These problems can be caused by chemotherapy, radiation therapy, and recurrent respiratory infections in immunosuppressed patients.[89–91] Alkylating agents (primarily busulfan) and the nitrosourea agents (e.g., lomustine and carmustine) have been associated with the development of pulmonary fibrosis. In one study, 30% of long-term survivors of Hodgkin's disease experienced respiratory symptoms and associated reductions in lung function.[91] The mechanisms of bleomycin injury include formation of free radicals and lipid peroxidation of phospholipid membranes. Subsequently, interstitial edema and damage to type 1 pneumocytes occurs.[89] Late lung injury is characterized by progressive fibrosis and collapse of alveoli.[89]

Pulmonary fibrosis is the most common type of chronic lung damage following radiation therapy. Obstructive lung disease also can occur. Pulmonary damage is more likely when higher radiation doses are used and when larger lung volumes are irradiated. For example, only 13% of children with immunodeficiency disorders who received total body irradiation prior to bone marrow transplant developed chronic interstitial lung disease.[92] Radiation therapy also can potentiate the long-term toxicity induced by other agents such as bleomycin and nitrosoureas. The late phase of fibrosis is characterized by loss of capillaries and type I pneumocytes and increased deposition of collagen.[90] Evidence suggests that activation of cells, such as the macrophage, that produce cytokines and growth factors is an important mechanism of radiation-induced lung injury. For example, in vitro studies demonstrate increased synthesis of tumor necrosis factor-alpha (TNF-α) and fibroblastic growth factors.[90]

Acute pulmonary toxicity is mediated by cellular activation of genes that result in production of cytokines such as interleukin-1 (IL-1), transforming growth factor-beta, and TNF-α. These cytokines are also thought to contribute to late tissue injury. Future prevention strategies for pulmonary late effects may use gene therapy. For example, overexpression of a transgene for a free radical scavenger (manganese superoxide dismutase) that was delivered to the lungs of mice prior to radiation resulted in increased survival and decreased alveolitis and fibrosis.[93]

Gastrointestinal System

Radiation and radiation-enhancing chemotherapeutic agents can have long-term effects on the gastrointestinal tract and the liver. Late effects of radiation on the esophagus result primarily from damage to the esophageal wall, although mucosal ulcerations may also persist.[94] The major significant late effect of gastric irradiation is ulceration due to destruction of mucosal cells of the gastric mucosa. Although rare, vascular abnormalities and altered digestive system activity can result in malabsorption.

Moderate to severe intestinal injury following pelvic radiation usually appears within 2–5 years after irradiation. Late radiation injury to the small and large intestine can result in increased frequency of bowel actions and greater stool weight; decreased bile acid, vitamin B_{12}, and fat absorption; more rapid gastric emptying and small bowel transit; as well as bleeding, pain, fistula formation, and obstruction.[95,96] Histologic changes due to radiation injury include atypical epithelial cells, intestinal wall fibrosis, serosal thickening, and vascular sclerosis.[97] The technique and field of radiation impact the probability of late gastrointestinal injury. For example, conformal radiation therapy allows for a higher tumor dose while irradiating a smaller volume of normal tissue. Therefore, the incidence and severity of injury to normal gastrointestinal tissues should be less.[98] Although chemotherapy can augment acute gastrointestinal radiation toxicity, the effect of chemotherapy on late toxicity is not well established.

Late effects in the liver are more common and include hepatic fibrosis, cirrhosis, and portal hypertension. Radiation therapy in combination with radiation-enhancing agents, such as actinomycin D and possibly vincristine, can result in hepatic fibrosis. Portal hypertension can occur if the fibrosis is severe. Hepatic arterial infusion chemotherapy for management of liver metastases can result in significant hepatotoxicity. In a recent study, 30 women with metastatic breast carcinoma to the liver underwent systemic chemotherapy alone or in combination with 3–5 cycles of hepatic arterial infusion chemotherapy. Morphological changes in the liver that were attributed to the toxic effects of treatment were identified in 27 women. These included fatty changes, severe cirrhotic changes, and localized atrophy.[99] Chemotherapy-induced hepatic injury is usually due to the breakdown of drugs into free radicals that impair cell function and result in cell death.[99]

The administration of blood products as part of the supportive care of myelosuppressed patients can cause chronic hepatitis. Hepatitis C, transmitted by blood transfusions or by lifestyle practices, is now the most common chronic blood-borne infection in the United States and has become an important cause of late gastrointestinal toxicities.[100,101] Patients can be screened for hepatitis C infection by serological tests for anti-HCV antibody.

Renal System

Nephritis and cystitis are the major long-term renal toxicities that result from cancer treatment. Damage to the nephrons and bladder has been documented in patients treated with cyclophosphamide, ifosfamide, and cisplatin.[102] The hemorrhagic cystitis that can occur following cyclophosphamide therapy may persist, and the risk is increased by concurrent pelvic radiation. Acrolein, a metabolite of cyclophosphamide, is thought to be responsible for hemorrhagic cystitis. Mesna, a sulfhydryl compound, binds to acrolein within the urinary tract, and

thereby decreases the incidence of renal toxicity with cyclophosphamide and ifosfamide.[103] Pharmacological strategies that may be effective in protecting the kidney from chemotherapy-related injury include calcium chloride, N-acetylcysteine, and amifostine.[103–106]

Children with unilateral nephrectomy who receive ifosfamide may develop Fanconi's syndrome. Renal phosphate and amino acid loss, renal tubular acidosis, and dehydration can occur and result in metabolic bone disease, growth failure, and decompensated renal tubular insufficiency.[106] Radiation also can damage the kidneys. Radiation doses of 20 Gy or less may minimize the risk of renal toxicity, whereas concurrent administration of radiation-enhancing drugs increases the risk. Clinical manifestations of nephritis include proteinuria, hypertension, anemia, and progressive renal failure, although early detection and intervention may prevent irreversible damage. The compensatory hypertrophy of the remaining kidney following nephrectomy for renal tumors such as Wilms' tumor has not been associated with any biological consequences. However, urinary tract infections or trauma to the remaining kidney obviously can be a serious problem. Children with bilateral Wilms' tumor are at risk for renal failure, and in these patients kidney parenchymal–sparing procedures offer the potential advantage of decreasing the risk of end-stage renal failure.[107]

Endocrine System

Cancer treatment can adversely affect a number of endocrine functions, including metabolism, growth, secondary sexual development, and reproduction. These late effects result from damage to the target organ (i.e., thyroid, ovary, and testis), and the hypothalamic pituitary axis. Table 26-1 summarizes the major endocrine sequelae, related risk factors, and recommendations for evaluation.

Thyroid

Direct damage to the thyroid gland causes primary hypothyroidism, with a decreased production of thyroxine (T_4) and triiodothyronine (T_3). These hormones have biological effects on oxygen consumption, the central and peripheral nervous systems, skeletal and cardiac muscle, carbohydrate and cholesterol metabolism, and growth and development.[108] Primary hypothyroidism can be compensated when there is only partial organ damage and some function is preserved. The compensated state is maintained by an increased production of thyrotropin-releasing factor (TRF) and thyroid-stimulating hormone (TSH) from the hypothalamus and pituitary. This chronic overstimulation is of concern because it is believed to

Table 26-1   Endocrine Late Effects, Risk Factors, and Evaluation Methods

Organ	Chemotherapy	Radiation	Risk Population	Evaluation
Thyroid	None known	>2000 cGy or >750 cGy TBI = overt or compensated hypothyroidism Graves' disease	Young children Tumors of head and neck Brain tumors Leukemia with cranial radiation BMT Lymphomas (HD, NHL)	T_4, free T_4, TSH, T_3
Ovaries	MOPP/COPP Cyclophosphamide Ifosfamide Busulfan BCNU/CCNU (age and dose dependent)	400–1000 cGy (age dependent)	>40 yr Abdominal and pelvic tumors HD Spinal radiation	LH, FSH, estradiol drawn on days 5–8 of menstrual cycle
Testes	MOPP/COPP Cyclophosphamide Ifosfamide Busulfan BCNU/CCNU	<400 cGy = azoospermia, possible recovery >600 cGy = permanent azoospermia > 2400 cGy = Leydig cell damage, decreased testosterone	HD and NHL Pelvic tumors Testicular tumors Leukemia with testicular infiltrates	LH, FSH, testosterone, semen analysis
Hypothalamic-pituitary axis	None currently identified	>2400 cGy = hypothalamic dysfunction >4000 cGy = pituitary dysfunction	Leukemia with CNS radiation CNS tumors Head and neck tumors	Growth charts (sitting and standing height) Somatomedin-C LH, FSH, estradiol, testosterone, prolactin T_4, TSH, free T_4, T_3 Bone age Cortisol levels Growth hormone (even in adults at risk)

increase the risk of malignant transformation in previously damaged cells.[109,110] Overt or compensated primary hypothyroidism has been documented in 4%–80% of patients who received radiation to the neck for Hodgkin's disease, other lymphomas, and carcinomas.[111–113] Damage to the thyroid gland usually occurs after radiation doses of more than 20 Gy in multiple fractions. In general, the incidence and severity of thyroid dysfunction appear to increase with higher radiation doses and may be due to damage to thyroid follicular cells, thyroid vasculature, or connective tissue. There are no chemotherapeutic agents that have been associated with long-term thyroid damage. The importance of age at time of irradiation has been difficult to assess. Although hypothyroidism usually develops 3–4 years after treatment, it can occur as late as 7–14 years later.[113,114]

When the hypothalamic pituitary axis is in the field of radiation to the nasopharynx of the CNS, secondary hypothyroidism can occur. Decreased levels of TRF, TSH, T_3, and T_4 have been reported in patients who received at least 55 Gy of external beam radiation for nasopharyngeal, paranasal sinus, or brain tumors that did not involve the hypothalamus or pituitary.[115,116] These studies found no difference in the development of secondary hypothyroidism between children and adults although most subjects were adults. As with primary thyroid dysfunction, secondary hypothyroidism may not develop until years after the completion of therapy. Hyperthyroidism has also been reported after radiation to the mantle region. The incidence is low and the mechanism is unclear.[115]

Growth

Growth hormone deficiency resulting in short stature is one of the most common long-term endocrine consequences of radiation to the CNS in children.[116] Growth impairment with deficient growth hormone release and decreased linear growth rate has been found in 50%–100% of children with brain tumors who received 24 Gy or more of cranial or craniospinal radiation.[116–119] Children with ALL who received radiation for CNS prophylaxis have demonstrated a similar pattern of growth disturbances.[120,121] Pituitary dysfunction requires radiation doses of at least 40 Gy, but damage to the hypothalamus occurs with lower doses.[122] Although the belief has been that growth disturbances as a result of hypothalamic damage require doses of at least 24 Gy,[121,122] Starceski et al observed a 25% decline in height percentile in children treated with 24 Gy and a 14% decline in children treated with 18 Gy.[123] In both groups, growth velocity decreased significantly over 3 years following treatment and did not recover. Clayton and Shalet also found that dose of whole-brain radiation (27–47.5 Gy) and time from irradiation were significant predictors of growth hormone deficiency.[124] The overall incidence of growth hormone deficiency (74%) 5 years after treatment was comparable across radiation doses; however, children who received 30 Gy or more of radiation developed growth hormone deficiency earlier. The fewer the number of fractionations for a given radiation dose, the greater the risk of long-term sequelae. Children treated with cranial radiation before age 5 are believed to be more susceptible to growth deficits, which may become most apparent during periods of rapid growth.[125] Growth retardation may be more pronounced in children who receive cranial and spinal irradiation because of spinal shortening.[119]

Chemotherapy in combination with cranial radiation may increase the risk for growth failure. In a study of 38 prepubertal children who survived medulloblastoma, those who received chemotherapy plus radiation had significantly poorer growth over a 4-year period than those who received only radiation.[126]

There has been controversy regarding the use of growth hormone in children treated for malignancies. The concern stems from the potential side effects of growth hormone including the development of leukemia. Another related concern is that growth hormone may stimulate cancer cell growth and result in a relapse or recurrence of the primary disease. However, recent studies indicate that the incidence of relapse or recurrence is not higher in children who receive growth hormone when compared to untreated controls.[127,128]

Another area of research is the use of growth hormone in adults who have growth hormone deficiency. Aside from increasing linear growth, growth hormone is important in defining body composition, bone mineral density, muscle strength, exercise performance, cardiovascular system, metabolism, and immune function.[129,130] Studies have documented that growth hormone–deficient adults are at increased risk for osteoporitic fractures, heart disease, decreased lean body mass, and muscle strength. Therefore, it is important that at-risk adults are evaluated for growth hormone deficiency and are referred to an endocrinologist for evaluation and consideration for hormone replacement.[129,130]

Secondary Sexual Development and Reproduction

Chemotherapy, specifically alkylating agents (e.g., cyclophosphamide, mechlorethamine, busulfan, and procarbazine), can cause permanent damage to the gonads. Primary ovarian failure, with amenorrhea, decreased estradiol, and elevated gonadotropins (luteinizing hormone [LH] and follicle-stimulating hormone [FSH]), has been reported in women who received these agents for Hodgkin's disease, breast cancer, and ovarian germ cell tumors.[131,132] In younger patients, ovarian damage is manifested as failure to develop secondary sexual characteristics or as arrested pubertal development.[133]

Damage to the germinal epithelium of the testis with decreased or absent spermatogonia can occur in males treated with alkylating agents. Leydig cell damage is unusual; thus, testosterone production and pubertal development are often not affected. Testicular damage with azoospermia is most frequent in males with Hodgkin's disease who received MOPP (mechlorethamine, vincristine, procarbazine, and prednisone) but also has been observed in males with ALL or rhabdomyosarcoma treated with cyclophosphamide and cytosine arabinoside.[134,135] Impaired testicular function has also been documented in men who received higher dose cisplatin and etoposide for germ cell cancer.[136]

Age at time of treatment, gender, total drug dose, and the use of combinations of alkylating agents are important risk factors for gonadal failure. The quiescence of the prepubertal gonad provides some protection, whereas the incidence of gonadal damage increases with age and stage in pubertal development. The testis appears to be more sensitive than the ovary to the damaging effects of therapy. Rivkees and Crawford reported that the incidence of gonadal dysfunction increased from 0% in prepubertal girls and 14% in prepubertal boys to 71% in sexually mature women and 95% in mature men.[134] Byrne et al found that the fertility of men treated with alkylating agents was half that of the fertility of control subjects, whereas the fertility of women was unimpaired.[137]

The risk of gonadal failure also increases with greater total doses of alkylating agents and the use of more than one drug, such as in MOPP therapy. Cumulative cyclophosphamide dose is an important risk factor for recovery of spermatogenesis. Radiation is another cause of gonadal dysfunction. Pathological changes in women who receive radiation to the ovaries include reduced numbers of oocytes, inhibited follicle development, atrophic ovaries, and strong fibrohyalinization.[138,139] Older women are at greater risk for ovarian failure following radiation. Ovarian function may be preserved in girls who receive 8 Gy; however, ovarian failure has been reported in 100% of women older than 40 years of age treated with 400 cGy.[139]

The testis is extremely sensitive to the damaging effects of radiation. The threshold dose required to damage the germinal epithelium is as low as 3–4 Gy, while the Leydig cells are more resistant, with permanent damage occurring following doses at 20 Gy.[140] Scatter to the ovaries and testes as a result of abdominal or craniospinal irradiation also can result in long-term damage.[136,140,141] In a large retrospective cohort study of 2283 survivors of childhood cancer, Byrne et al found that radiation therapy directed below the diaphragm depressed fertility in men and women by approximately 25%, and combined therapy involving infradiaphragmatic radiation and alkylating agents reduced fertility to almost 50% of that in the control subjects.[137] Testicular damage and ovarian failure occur infrequently after treatment for leukemia with regimens that do not include alkylating agents or cytosine arabinoside, and there does not appear to be an increased frequency of adverse pregnancy outcome (spontaneous abortions and stillbirths) compared with the general population.[142] In addition to the damaging effects of chemotherapy and radiation therapy on stem cells, retroperitoneal lymph node dissection can contribute to ejaculatory dysfunction.[135]

Radiation to the cranium or nasopharynx can damage the hypothalamic pituitary axis, causing secondary gonadal failure. Subnormal levels of LH, FSH, and prolactin-inhibiting factor (PIF) have been found in males and females treated for head and neck tumors with 4–78 Gy of radiation.[143] In addition to the effects of low LH and FSH levels on ovarian and testicular function, the decrease in PIF and resultant increase in prolactin caused irregular menses, anovulatory periods, low testosterone, reduced libido, and impotence.[144] In children, cranial radiation is thought to disrupt CNS mechanisms influencing puberty. The result is early puberty, and the most profound disturbance occurs in children irradiated at a young age.[145]

Sexual Dysfunction

Other than gonadal failure, a number of treatment-related factors may impair sexual functioning. Sexual issues are complex and include physiological and psychological components. These effects are more often noted in adult survivors of cancer but will become apparent in childhood survivors as they enter adulthood. The most common problems include decreased libido, erectile dysfunction, and dyspareunia. Cancer-related therapies that often lead to the development of sexual dysfunction include radiation to the pelvis and surgical changes and removal of gonads, which can result in decreased hormonal production, fibrosis of tissue, decreased blood flow, and nerve damage. Researchers have reported sexual dysfunction in approximately 50% of women who survive breast cancer.[146] These findings are similar to those noted in survivors of gynecological cancer.[147,148] Seventy percent of men who have had radical prostatectomies report erectile dysfunction.[149,150]

Lack of physical energy or syndromes resulting in chronic pain and psychological concerns also compound the complex issues of sexual dysfunction.[146] Questions regarding sexual functioning and satisfaction should be incorporated into routine follow-up visits so that a treatment plan can be developed.

Treatment programs are influenced by many factors including the initial diagnosis, type of treatment, available intervention, and willingness of the survivor. For example, some women who are diagnosed with breast cancer cannot receive estrogen replacement. However, less risky alternatives (estrin vaginal ring and water-based lubricants) to combat some of the menopausal symptoms are becoming available.[151,152] Interventions for erectile dysfunction have poor acceptance in general. Penile injections, vacuum devices, and intraurethral medications have low satisfaction and high dropout rates.[153–155] Sildenafil has a high acceptance rate among patients; however, many cancer survivors will not achieve an adequate erection with this medication alone.[153–155] Although treatment programs may be difficult to develop due to the multifaceted aspects of sexual dysfunction, the health care provider's approach to this subject matter may greatly increase patient awareness and compliance with intervention programs.

Offspring

There has long been concern regarding the effects of cancer therapy on the offspring of survivors. The effects of antineoplastic therapy on a fetus in the first and second trimester can be devastating.[156] However, the potential mutagenic effects of cancer therapy on offspring years after the completion of treatment has been less well understood due to the small numbers of offspring. The largest study to date involved 5847 offspring of 14,652 survivors of childhood cancer. These researchers found no increased risk of nonhereditary cancers among offspring. There was also no increased risk of birth defects.[157] In opposition to a previous report that wives of men treated for Hodgkin's disease appeared to have an increased incidence of spontaneous abortions,[158] more recent data do not support these results.[159] Li et al noted that women who were treated with flank irradiation for Wilms' tumor had small but otherwise healthy infants.[160] The most recent studies have been very encouraging to survivors and their families. However, survivors interested in having children should obtain their treatment records and be evaluated by a reproductive endocrinologist and geneticist in order to make an informed decision.

Musculoskeletal System

The treatment most frequently associated with late effects in the musculoskeletal system and related tissues is radiation. Cosmetic and functional alterations of the bone, soft tissue, and teeth are frequently reported in children who have been treated with radiation. Factors that can dramatically affect the degree of disfigurement include age at diagnosis, total dose and volume of tissue irradiated, and fraction size.[161] Children treated before age 6 or those undergoing rapid growth during puberty are at highest risk for musculoskeletal changes secondary to radiation.

Uneven irradiation to the vertebrae, soft tissue, and muscles (e.g., radiation to one side of the body) for the treatment of intraabdominal tumors frequently results in scoliosis, kyphosis, or both. Although more recent protocols have been modified to minimize these problems, skeletal abnormalities may occur in some children and tend to become more apparent during periods of rapid growth such as the adolescent growth spurt. In a study of 31 children successfully treated for Wilms' tumor with surgery, chemotherapy, and radiation, ten children developed an orthopedic abnormality requiring intervention or a scoliotic curve greater than 20 degrees.[162] Other factors associated with the occurrence of significant late orthopedic problems were higher radiation dose (mean dose of 28.9 Gy) and larger irradiated field (150 cm²).

Spinal shortening, another radiation-related effect, is caused by damage to the growth centers in the vertebral bodies.[163] Children who receive spinal radiation frequently do not achieve their full height potential; those who receive craniospinal irradiation are at great risk for growth retardation because of central (hypothalamic-pituitary), as well as direct (skeletal), effects.[161]

The late effects on long bones include functional limitations, shortening of the extremity, osteonecrosis, increased susceptibility to fractures, and poor healing. Avascular necrosis and osteoporosis are also noted following radiation and prolonged use of corticosteroids.[164]

Surgical procedures such as amputation or limb disarticulation have obvious immediate and lasting cosmetic, as well as physical and psychological consequences. Physical problems that may arise following these procedures include but are not limited to recurrent infections, the need for surgical revisions of internal prosthesis, and poorly fitting external prosthetics.[165] The decision regarding amputation versus limb salvage has been controversial for years. Advocates of limb salvage focus on the survivor's desire to maintain their limb while advocates of amputation focus on the quality-of-life issues and high functioning of amputees. This issue is not likely to be resolved easily because prognosis is not affected by the procedure used at time of diagnosis.[166,167]

Altered growth of facial bones following maxillofacial or orbital irradiation or surgery causes facial asymmetry. This is a difficult problem that frequently occurs in children treated for tumors such as rhabdomyosarcoma. Maxillofacial irradiation also can cause a number of dental problems such as foreshortening and blunting of the roots, incomplete calcification, delayed or arrested tooth development, caries, and loosening.[168] Recently, dental problems in patients who were treated with chemotherapy have been reported and include abnormal occlusion, hypoplasia, enamel opacities, and radiological abnormalities.[168]

Men and women who receive chemotherapeutic agents that impair gonadal function may lose bone mineral density. In a study of 29 men previously treated for Hodgkin's disease, a significant reduction in forearm cortical bone mineral content and in lumbar spine bone mineral density was identified.[169]

Late radiation damage to muscle can occur, especially following treatment of soft tissue sarcomas of the extremities. Mechanisms of injury that have been identified primarily from animal studies include a direct effect on myocytes resulting in cell death; vascular damage with ischemia; atrophy and fibrosis; and inflammation with a preferential increase in type III collagen.[170] Muscle damage can progress over time; the risk increases with larger radiation doses and decreases with dose fractionation.

The skin and breast tissue may also be impacted by radiation. Radiation most profoundly affects the breast bud. The result is uneven development of breast tissue.[171,172] Permanent alopecia can occur following higher doses of radiation (>40 Gy) such as is used in treatment of brain tumors.[173] Other skin and related changes include contractures noted following infiltrations and edema secondary to disrupted lymphatic flow.[173] Lymphedema is noted in 10%–15% of women postmastectomy.[174] The incidence is greater following high-dose radiation therapy or a history of one or more infections.[175] A variety of interventions for lymphedema, such as sequential pneumatic compression sleeve and manual massage, are available but results have been variable.[175]

Fatigue

Fatigue is a complex phenomenon that is reportedly experienced by 78%–96% of individuals with cancer.[176] The exact mechanism by which fatigue occurs remains unknown. Several theories have been proposed as models to explain and evaluate fatigue. These include stress response,[177] neurophysiological factors,[178] reduced skeletal muscle protein stores,[179] and a multifaceted model that incorporates biochemical, physiologic, and behavioral aspects.[180] Application of these theories to individuals who have completed treatment is not clear. However, several studies have documented fatigue in survivors years following the completion of treatment. Whedon et al documented fatigue in survivors of bone marrow transplantation 1–18 years after treatment.[181] Fatigue plays a significant role in a survivor's perception of quality of life posttreatment.[181] Ferrell et al noted that in 687 survivors, fatigue was one of the most negative items affecting quality of life.[182] Seventy-five percent of women treated with radiation and 61% of women treated with chemotherapy for breast cancer complained of decreased stamina 2–10 years after treatment.[183] Information about fatigue among childhood cancer survivors is minimal. Currently available literature predominantly describes fatigue in children with cognitive deficits following whole-brain radiation.[184,185] Anecdotally, some children experience fatigue many years following radiation treatment to the CNS, chest, and total body. Fatigue is most likely an underappreciated problem reported in children.

Although the etiology of fatigue in the surviving population is poorly understood, it is imperative that the prevalence of this problem be explored. Questions regarding the symptom of fatigue should be incorporated into the annual evaluation. Physiological causes for fatigue should be ruled out when possible, and strategies for decreasing fatigue, such as adequate nutrition and hydration; modified activity and rest patterns; stress management; and cognitive therapies should be used.[176]

Second Malignant Neoplasms

It has been clearly established that adults and children who have received chemotherapy, radiation therapy, or both for a primary malignancy are at increased risk for the development of a second malignant neoplasm. For example, in patients with Hodgkin's disease, there is a 77-fold increased risk of the development of leukemia within 4 years of initial treatment.[186] For children, the overall risk is estimated to be at least ten times greater than the cancer incidence among age-matched children.[187] Among a cohort of 981 children who were followed from 4.3 to 26.5 years after completion of ALL therapy, the estimated cumulative risk of second malignant neoplasms within 20 years was 2.9%, and the corresponding risk for cases with radiation therapy was 8.1%, compared with 0.3% for those who received only chemotherapy.[188]

Malignant transformation of normal cells is due to nonlethal damage to the DNA that is not repaired. Alkylating agents and ionizing radiation are the treatments most closely linked to a second malignant neoplasm. In addition to the type and dose of treatment received, the risk of the development of a second cancer depends on several predisposing factors. Some tumors have a common underlying etiologic factor. For example, patients with bladder cancer are at greater risk for the development of lung cancer because both tumors are associated with smoking.[189] Genetic susceptibility is a second factor.[187] Children with the genetic form of retinoblastoma (which is usually bilateral) have a much higher incidence of sarcomas (as a second malignant neoplasm) than those with the nongenetic form of the disease.[190]

Following Chemotherapy

Acute nonlymphocytic leukemia (ANL) following treatment with alkylating agents is the most common chemotherapy-related second malignant neoplasm. The disease usually is preceded by a period of prolonged pancytopenia and can occur as early as 1.3 years following the initiation of chemotherapy for the primary malignancy. The incidence of treatment-related ANL peaks at 5 years and plateaus at 10 years following treatment.[191]

Acute nonlymphocytic leukemia following Hodgkin's disease has been studied intensively in large cohorts of patients.[191-194] The overall cumulative risk has been reported to be 3.3% at 15 years postdiagnosis but varies from 0.6% in patients who received only radiation therapy

to 17% in those treated with combination chemotherapy.[191,195] The treatment regimen with the greatest leukemogenic potential is MOPP, presumably due to the mechlorethamine and procarbazine.[189,193-195] A dose-response relationship between alkylating agents and the occurrence of a second malignant neoplasm has been reported.[195] The addition of radiation to the MOPP regimen does not appear to significantly increase the risk of ANL,[195] whereas the recent use of ABVD (doxorubicin, bleomycin, vinblastine, and dacarbazine) and a regimen involving procarbazine, melphalan, and vinblastine have not been found to carry an increased risk of acute leukemia, which is attributed to lower total dose of alkylating agents.[191,195] The risk of ANL in children previously treated for Hodgkin's disease has been associated with disease relapse, treatment with alkylating agents and radiation, and splenectomy.[196,197]

In patients with multiple myeloma, the risk of the development of ANL is unusually high—more than 200 times that of the incidence in the general population. The drug most closely associated with ANL is melphalan, although multiple myeloma may also be associated with an increased risk of ANL that is unrelated to treatment.[198]

Although the incidence is not as great as with Hodgkin's disease or multiple myeloma, treatment-related acute leukemia has occurred in patients with non-Hodgkin's lymphoma,[199] breast cancer,[200] lung cancer,[201] ovarian cancer,[202] and in survivors of childhood cancer.[203-205] Alkylating agents, primarily cyclophosphamide and melphalan, have been linked to the occurrence of ANL. Acute nonlymphocytic leukemia was two to three times more likely to develop in women who received melphalan for the treatment of ovarian cancer than in those who received cyclophosphamide, which suggests that, of the two drugs, melphalan has the greater leukemogenic potential.[206] There is also concern among some cancer researchers that etoposide may increase the risk for ANL.[201] Intercalating topoisomerase II inhibitors (doxorubicin, dactinomycin), when combined with alkylating agents and radiation, may cause secondary AML. A review of 3696 patients treated for cancer at St. Jude Children's Research Hospital, Memphis, Tennessee, between 1980 and 1992 revealed 36 cases of secondary AML. Chromosomal abnormalities (11q23 and/or 21q22) were identified with alkylating agents and intercalating agents. Four cases with the chromosomal abnormalities had not received epipodophyllotoxin treatment.[205]

Following Radiation

Sarcomas of the bone and soft tissue are the most common second malignant neoplasm after radiation therapy. Although the latency period can be as short as 5 months, it ranges from 10–20 years following radiation.[207] The incidence has been found to peak at 15–20 years after the initial diagnosis.[167,190] Malignant transformation can occur in doses ranging from 10–80 Gy. The relative risk increases from 8% following doses of 10–20 Gy to 40%

following doses of 60 Gy.[207] It has been postulated that the decreased risk following doses of 80 Gy is due to the phenomenon of cell killing rather than nonlethal cell damage.

In a large study of 9170 survivors of childhood cancer, 48 cases of bone cancer occurred as opposed to the 0.4 expected (relative risk 133).[207] The risk was highest among children treated for retinoblastoma (relative risk 999) and Ewing's sarcoma (relative risk 649) but also was increased significantly in patients treated for rhabdomyosarcoma, Wilms' tumor, and Hodgkin's disease. Of the patients with sarcoma, 84% had received radiation, and 83% of the subsequent tumors occurred within the field of radiation.

Acute nonlymphocytic leukemia following radiation therapy is uncommon but has been reported in childhood cancer[195] and non-Hodgkin's lymphoma.[193] Women with breast cancer treated with postoperative radiation also have a slightly increased risk of ANL.[200] In addition to sarcomas and leukemia, a variety of other solid tumors have been linked to treatment with radiation. A slightly excessive number of tumors of the bladder, rectum, uterus, bone, and connective tissue has been reported in women who received radiation for gynecologic cancer.[208,209] Brain tumors can occur after cranial irradiation for CNS prophylaxis in childhood ALL.[188,210,211] Twenty-four second malignant CNS neoplasms were found in a cohort study of 9720 children treated for ALL.[210] This represented a 22-fold excess of CNS tumors. All CNS tumors developed in children treated with cranial radiation; the risk was greatest in children who were age 5 or younger at the time of diagnosis.

In a study of survivors of Hodgkin's disease, a 17% cumulative risk of second cancers was noted 20 years posttreatment. The most common tumors were lung and breast cancer, with 77% occurring in or adjoining the field of radiation.[212] In another study of childhood survivors of Hodgkin's disease, breast cancer was the most common solid tumor. Individuals at highest risk were those girls who received mantle radiation between the ages of 10 and 16 years and those receiving higher doses (>30 Gy).[213] With the recently observed risk for breast cancer following radiation, routine evaluation has become controversial in young women (<30 years of age). Currently, mammography is thought to be the best available technique for breast cancer screening. However, with younger women there is concern about the accuracy of mammography in dense breast tissue. Some clinicians are recommending baseline mammography 5–10 years after radiation or the age of 30. Others have recommended possible chemoprevention with tamoxifen and retinoids for those in the highest risk categories.[213–215] However, there is consensus that women who receive radiation to the breast (especially those treated between the ages of 10 and 16 years and who receive higher radiation doses) need close monitoring. Aggressive evaluation of any breast mass and examination of the contralateral breast (due to the increase risk of synchronous bilateral disease) is imperative.[216–218]

Early Detection and Prevention, Health Maintenance and Promotion

"Comprehensive care of cancer survivors demands maximum efforts to prevent, minimize, and effectively treat long-term medical sequelae through the survivorship trajectory."[219,p890]

Early detection and prevention of late toxicities is a relatively new area of investigation. If early indicators of late tissue damage are identified, interventions designed to diminish the severity and overall impact of the toxicity can be developed and tested. Knowledge of the mechanisms responsible for delayed tissue damage following radiation and chemotherapy is increasing and provides the basis for interventions designed to inhibit specific pathways or scavenge toxic by-products. In addition, understanding the etiology of posttreatment effects will assist in the development of treatment modifications that will decrease late effects for future generations but not compromise disease control and overall survival rates.

Researchers in pediatric oncology have led the way in developing comprehensive care clinics that meet the unique needs of childhood cancer survivors. Since the early 1980s, Meadows and Hobbie have focused on the role of the health care team in posttreatment management of survivors.[218] Since that time, more than ninety institutions that care for children with cancer have developed programs to meet the needs of cancer survivors. The most recent trend in program development is that of young adult follow-up programs for childhood cancer survivors.[220] These programs attempt to bridge the gap between pediatric and adult health care systems. All of these follow-up programs have a foundation in education, health promotion, and maintenance. The focus is on modifiable risk factors in an at-risk population that will attenuate late effects in at-risk organs.

In an effort to provide organization for follow-up care and universal guidelines, cooperative organizations that initiate and coordinate multicenter clinical trials have formed specific subcommittees to develop standard criteria for monitoring late injury to normal tissue. The SOMA scales (subjective, objective, management, and analytical evaluation of injury) are intended to address the need for sensitive and uniform criteria for monitoring late reactions.[221]

Survivors of cancer require lifelong follow-up care to maximize the opportunity to provide education about previous treatment, potential and actual late effects, and lifestyle choices that may modify the expression of late effects. The health care team should focus on modifiable risk factors such as smoking, drinking, dietary habits, and exercise.[219]

Follow-up programs for adult cancer survivors are rare. At completion of treatment, the individual with cancer returns to a primary care provider with episodic visits to the oncologist to rule out disease recurrence. Insurance issues, institutional resistance, and financial constraints are often cited as common causes for lack of follow-up programs.

Strategies for Prevention

Strategies for preventing late effects are emerging. Drugs that bind or metabolize intracellular mediators of cell injury are under development and testing. For example, drugs such as dexrazone bind intracellular iron and inhibit the formation of free radicals responsible for anthracycline-induced cardiac toxicity.[73] An adrenocorticotropic hormone [ACTH (4-9)] analog, Org 2766, has been found to minimize cisplatin neuropathy in men treated for testicular cancer. Preliminary evidence suggests that Org 2766, a neuropeptide, does not protect against the neurotoxic effects of cisplatin but ameliorates the neuropathy by enhancing endogenous nerve repair mechanisms.[222]

Conclusion

This chapter has provided a comprehensive review of the biological late effects that can be caused by curative cancer therapy. Long-term surveillance for these toxic effects is a recent and challenging area for oncology nurses and physicians. A long-range perspective is essential because the latency period for some late toxicities is many years after completion of treatment and the consequences of permanent tissue damage across the lifespan are unknown.

General recommendations for long-term follow-up include an annual physical examination with a complete blood cell count and urinalysis. Evaluation of specific toxicity to organ systems and second malignancies depends on the initial diagnosis, type and amount of treatment received, and host risk factors. For some late toxicities, surveillance guidelines have been standardized. The Cardiology Committee of the Children's Cancer Study Group recently published guidelines for cardiac monitoring of children during and after anthracycline therapy.[223] Recommendations for late cardiac follow-up include (1) an electrocardiogram (ECG) and echocardiogram every 2–3 years, and (2) a radionuclide angiocardiogram and 24-hour continuous taped ECG every 6 years posttherapy. These recommendations may change as more sensitive methods of detecting subclinical organ damage become available, but they still serve as a model for establishing long-term evaluation guidelines for all late toxicities. However, a careful balance between monitoring and the creation of needless anxiety that could hinder the patient's overall rehabilitation and emotional adjustment must be achieved. Tempering information regarding late effects with modifiable risk factors, wellness, and health promotion offers the best opportunity for early identification of late effects and maximizes survivor compliance and sense of well being.

References

1. Landis SH, Murray T, Bolden S, et al: Cancer statistics, 1998. *CA Cancer J Clin* 48:6–29, 1998
2. Bleyer A: The impact of childhood cancer on the United States and the world. *CA Cancer J Clin* 40:355–367, 1990
3. Hammond D: Historical overview of childhood cancer. Plenary Session: Workshop on Quality of Life in Children's Cancer: Implications for Practice and Research. Atlanta, GA, January 1995
4. van Eys J: Living beyond cure: Transcending survival. *Am J Pediatr Hematol Oncol* 9:114–118, 1987
5. Schwartz CL: Late effects of treatment in long-term survivors of cancer. *Cancer Treat Rev* 21:355–366, 1995
6. Anderson V, Smibert E, Ekert H, et al: Intellectual, educational, and behavioural sequelae after cranial irradiation and chemotherapy. *Arch Dis Child* 70:476–485, 1994
7. Butler RW, Hill JM, Steinherz PG, et al: Neuropsychologic effects of cranial irradiation, intrathecal methotrexate, and systemic methotrexate in childhood cancer. *J Clin Oncol* 12:2621–2629, 1994
8. Cousens P, Waters B, Said J, et al: Cognitive effects of cranial irradiation in leukaemia: A survey and meta-analysis. *J Child Psychol Psychiatry* 29:839–852, 1988
9. Dowell RE, Copeland DR, Francis DJ, et al: Absence of synergistic effects of CNS treatments on neuropsychologic test performance among children. *J Clin Oncol* 9:1029–1036, 1991
10. Giralt J, Ortega JJ, Olive T, et al: Long-term neuropsychologic sequelae of childhood leukemia: Comparison of two CNS prophylactic regimens. *Int J Radiat Oncol Biol Phys* 24:49–53, 1992
11. Halberg FE, Kramer JH, Moore IM, et al: Prophylactic cranial irradiation dose effects of late cognitive function in children treated for acute lymphoblastic leukemia. *Int J Radiat Oncol Biol Phys* 22:13–16, 1991
12. Hongwei Q, Jianjun F, Yonghong Z, et al: Intelligence function in children with acute lymphoblastic leukemia after treatment. *Chin Med Sci J* 8:91–94, 1992
13. Jankovic M, Brouwers P, Valsecchi MG, et al: Association of 1800 cGy cranial irradiation with intellectual function in children with acute lymphoblastic leukaemia. *Lancet* 344:224–227, 1994
14. Kato M, Azuma E, Ido M, et al: Ten-year survey of the intellectual deficits in children with acute lymphoblastic leukemia receiving chemoimmunotherapy. *Med Pediatr Oncol* 2:435–440, 1993
15. Kleinman SN, Waber DP: Prose memory strategies of children treated for leukemia: A story grammar analysis of the Anna Thompson passage. *Neuropsychology* 8:464–470, 1994
16. MacLean WE, Noll RB, Stehbens JA, et al: Neuropsychological effects of cranial irradiation in young children with acute lymphoblastic leukemia 9 months after diagnosis. *Arch Neurol* 52:156–160, 1995
17. Rodgers J, Britton PG, Morris RG, et al: Memory after treatment for acute lymphoblastic leukaemia. *Arch Dis Child* 67:266–268, 1992
18. Smibert E, Anderson V, Godber T, et al: Risk factors for intellectual and educational sequelae of cranial irradiation in childhood acute lymphoblastic leukaemia. *Br J Cancer* 73:825–830, 1996
19. Waber DP, Bernstein JH, Kammerer BL, et al: Neuropsychological diagnostic profiles of children who received

CNS treatment for acute lymphoblastic leukemia: The systemic approach to assessment. *Dev Neuropsychol* 8:1–28, 1992

20. Waber DP, Tarbell NJ, Kahn CM, et al: The relationship of sex and treatment modality to neuropsychological outcome in childhood acute lymphoblastic leukemia. *J Clin Oncol* 10:810–817, 1992

21. Williams KS, Ochs J, Williams MJ, et al: Parental report of everyday cognitive abilities among children treated for acute lymphoblastic leukemia. *J Pediatr Psychol* 16:13–26, 1991

22. Brown RR, Sawyer MB, Antoniou G, et al: A 3 year follow-up of the intellectual and academic functioning of children receiving central nervous system prophylactic chemotherapy for leukemia. *J Dev Behav Pediatr* 17:392–398, 1996

23. Copeland DR, Moore BD, Francis DJ, et al: Neuropsychologic effects of chemotherapy on children with cancer—a longitudinal study. *J Clin Oncol* 14:2826–2835, 1996

24. Mulhern RK, Fairclough D, Ochs J: A prospective comparison of neuropsychologic performance of children surviving leukemia who received 18-Gy, 24-Gy, or no cranial irradiation. *J Clin Oncol* 9:1348–1356, 1991

25. Ochs J, Mulhern R, Fairclough D, et al: Comparison of neuropsychologic functioning and clinical indicators of neurotoxicity in long-term survivors of childhood leukemia given cranial radiation of parenteral methotrexate: A prospective study. *J Clin Oncol* 9:145–151, 1991

26. Christie D, Leiper AD, Chessells JM, et al: Intellectual performance after presymptomatic cranial radiotherapy for leukaemia: Effects of age and sex. *Arch Dis Child* 73:136–140, 1995

27. Mulhern RK, Hancock J, Fairclough D, et al: Neuropsychological status of children treated for brain tumors: A critical review and integrative analysis. *Med Pediatr Oncol* 20:181–191, 1992

28. Glauser TA, Packer RJ: Cognitive deficits in long-term survivors of childhood brain tumors. *Childs Nerv Syst* 7:2–12, 1991

29. Sue E, Kalifa C, Brauner R, et al: Brain tumors under the age of three: The price of survival. *Acta Neurochir (Wien)* 106:93–98, 1990

30. Hoppe-Firsch E, Renier D, Lellouch-Tubiana A, et al: Medulloblastoma in childhood: Progressive intellectual deterioration. *Childs Nerv Syst* 6:60–65, 1990

31. Radcliffe J, Bunin GR, Sutton LN, et al: Cognitive deficits in long-term survivors of childhood medulloblastoma and other noncortical tumors: Age-dependent effects of whole brain radiation. *Int J Dev Neurosci* 12:327–334, 1994

32. Kramer JH, Crowe AB, Larson DA, et al: Neuropsychological sequelae of medulloblastoma in adults. *Int J Radiat Oncol Biol Phys* 38:21–26, 1997

33. Archibald YM, Lunn D, Ruttan LA, et al: Cognitive functioning in long-term survivors of high-grade glioma. *J Neurosurg* 80:247–253, 1994

34. Kramer JH, Crittenden MR, Halberg FE, et al: A prospective study of cognitive functioning following low-dose cranial radiation for bone marrow transplantation. *Pediatrics* 90:447–450, 1992

35. Parth P, Kennedy RS, Lane NE, et al: Motor and cognitive testing of bone marrow transplant patients after chemoradiotherapy. *Percept Mot Skills* 68:1227–1241, 1989

36. McGuire T, Sanders JE, Hill D, et al: Neuropsychological function in children given total body irradiation for marrow transplantation. *Exp Hematol* 1:19:578, 1991 (abstr)

37. Brown RT, Madan-Swain A: Cognitive, neuropsychological, and academic sequelae in children with leukemia. *J Learn Disabil* 26:74–90, 1993

38. Balsom WR, Bleyer WA, Robinson LL, et al: Intellectual function in long-term survivors of childhood acute lymphoblastic leukemia: Protective effect of pre-irradiation methotrexate. A Children's Cancer Study Group Study. *Med Pediatr Oncol* 19:486–492, 1991

39. Kaufmann PM, Moore IM, Espy KA, et al: Attention and learning strategies following triple intrathecal chemotherapy for childhood leukemia. Abstract prepared for the *International Neuropsychological Society* and *Australian Society for the Study of Brain Impairment 2nd Pacific Rim Conference*, Cairns, Queensland, Australia, July 5–8, 1995

40. Andrews-Espy K, Moore IM, Kaufmann PM, et al: Neuropsychological declines in survivors of childhood ALL. *J Pediatr Psychol* (2000, in press)

41. Hussain M, Wozniak AJ, Edelstein MB: Neurotoxicity of antineoplastic agents. *Crit Rev Oncol Hematol* 14:61–75, 1993

42. Hertzberg H, Huk WJ, Ueberall MA, et al: CNS late effects after all therapy in childhood. Part I: Neuroradiological findings in long-term survivors of childhood ALL—An evaluation of the interferences between morphology and neuropsychological performance. *Med Pediatr Oncol* 28:387–400, 1997

43. Kingma A, Mooyaart EL, Kamps WA, et al: Magnetic resonance imaging of the brain and neuropsychological evaluation in children treated for acute lymphoblastic leukemia at a young age. *Am J Pediatr Hematol Oncol* 15:231–238, 1993

44. Prassopoulos P, Cavouras D, Golfinopoulos S, et al: Quantitative assessment of cerebral atrophy during and after treatment in children with acute lymphoblastic leukemia. *Invest Radiol* 31:749–754, 1996

45. Harila-Saari AH, Ahonen KA, Vainionpää LK, et al: Brain perfusion after treatment of childhood acute lymphoblastic leukemia. *J Nucl Med* 38:82–88, 1997

46. Chen CY, Zimmerman RA, Faro S, et al: Childhood leukemia: Central nervous abnormalities during and after treatment. *Am J Neuroradiol* 17:295–310, 1996

47. Hazuka MB, Kinzie JJ, Davis KA, et al. Treatment-related central nervous system toxicity: MR imaging evaluation with CT and clinical correlation. *Magn Reson Imaging* 7:669–676, 1989

48. Ueberall MA, Wenzel D, Hertzberg H, et al. CNS late effects after ALL therapy in childhood. Part II: Conventional EEG recordings in asymptomatic long-term survivors of childhood ALL—An evaluation of the interferences between neurophysiology, neurology, psychology, and CNS morphology. *Med Pediatr Oncol* 29:121–131, 1997

49. Phillips PC, Moeller JR, Sidtis JJ, et al: Abnormal cerebral glucose metabolism in long-term survivors of childhood acute lymphocytic leukemia. *Ann Neurol* 29:263–271, 1991

50. Asato R, Akiyama Y, Ito M, et al: Nuclear magnetic resonance abnormalities of the cerebral white matter in children with acute lymphoblastic leukemia and malignant lymphoma during and after central nervous system prophylactic treatment with intrathecal methotrexate. *Cancer* 70:1997–2004, 1992

51. Surtees R, Clelland J, Hann I, et al: Demyelination and single-carbon transfer pathway metabolites during the treatment of acute lymphoblastic leukemia: CSF studies. *J Clin Oncol* 16:1505–1511, 1998

52. Gordon KB, Char DH, Sagerman RH, et al: Late effects of radiation on the eye and ocular adnexa. *Int J Radiat Oncol Biol Phys* 31:1123–1139, 1995

53. Parsons JT, Bova FJ, Fitzgerald CR, et al: Radiation retinopathy after external-beam irradiation: Analysis of time-dose factors. *Int J Radiat Oncol Biol Phys* 30:765–773, 1994

54. Coucke PA, Schmid C, Balmer A, et al: Hypofractionation in retinoblastoma: An increased risk of retinopathy. *Radiother Oncol* 28:157–161, 1993

55. Al-Tweigeri T, Nabholtz JM, Mackey JR, et al: Ocular toxicity and cancer chemotherapy. *Cancer* 78:1359–1373, 1996

56. Defer G, Fauchon F, Schaison M, et al: Visual toxicity following intra-arterial chemotherapy with hydroxyethyl-CNU in patients with malignant gliomas. *Neuroradiology* 33:432–437, 1991

57. Taylor MJ, McCulloch DL: Visual evoked potentials in infants and children. *J Clin Neurophysiol* 3:357–372, 1992

58. Bokemeyer C, Berger CC, Kuczyk MA, et al: Evaluation of long-term toxicity after chemotherapy for testicular cancer. *J Clin Oncol* 14:2923–2932, 1996

59. Bokemeyer C, Berger CC, Hartmann JT, et al: Analysis of risk factors for cisplatin-induced ototoxicity in patients with testicular cancer. *Br J Cancer* 77:1355–1362, 1998

60. Skinner R, Pearson ADJ, Amineddine HA, et al: Ototoxicity of cisplatinum in children and adolescents. *Br J Cancer* 61:927–931, 1990

61. Freilich RJ, Kraus DH, Budnick AS, et al: Hearing loss in children with brain tumors treated with cisplatin and carboplatin-based high-dose chemotherapy with autologous bone marrow rescue. *Med Pediatr Oncol* 26:95–100, 1996

62. Walkwe DA, Pillov J, Waters KD, et al: Enhanced cisplatin ototoxicity in children with brain tumors who have received simultaneous or prior cranial irradiation. *Med Pediatr Oncol* 17:48–52, 1989

63. Miettinen S, Laurikainen E, Johansson R, et al: Radiotherapy enhanced ototoxicity of cisplatin in children. *Acta Otolaryngol (Stockh)* 529:90–94, 1997

64. Meyer WH, Ayers D, McHaney VA, et al: Ifosfamide and exacerbation of cisplatin-induced hearing loss. *Lancet* 341:754–755, 1993

65. Ilveskoski I, Saarinen UM, Wiklund T, et al: Ototoxicity in children with malignant brain tumors treated with the "8 in 1" chemotherapy protocol. *Med Pediatr Oncol* 27:26–31, 1996

66. Todd NW, Alvarado CS, Brewer DB, et al: Cisplatin in children: Hearing loss correlates with iris and skin pigmentation. *J Laryngol Otol* 109:926–929, 1995

67. Park KR: The utility of acoustic reflex thresholds and other conventional audiologic tests for monitoring cisplatin ototoxicity in the pediatric population. *Ear Hear* 17:107–115, 1996

68. Neuwelt EA, Brummett RE, Doolittle ND, et al: First evidence of otoprotection against carboplatin-induced hearing loss with a two-compartment system in patients with central nervous system malignancy using sodium thiosulfate. *J Pharmacol Exp Ther* 286:77–84, 1998

69. Madasu R, Ruckenstein MJ, Leake F, et al: Ototoxic effects of supradose cisplatin with sodium thiosulfate neutralization in patients with head and neck cancer. *Arch Otolaryngol Head Neck Surg* 123:978–981, 1997

70. Domenech J, Linassier C, Gihana E, et al: Prolonged impairment of hematopoiesis after high-dose therapy followed by autologous bone marrow transplantation. *Blood* 85:3320–3327, 1995

71. Van Rijswijk RF, Sybesma JPH, Kater L: A prospective study of the changes in the immune status before, during and after multiple agent chemotherapy for Hodgkin's disease. *Cancer* 51:637–644, 1983

72. Mauch P, Constine L, Greenberger J, et al: Hematopoietic stem cell compartment: Acute and late effects of radiation therapy and chemotherapy. *Int J Radiat Oncology Biol Phys* 31:1319–1339, 1995

73. Hershko C, Link G, Tzahor M, et al: The role of iron and iron chelators in anthracycline cardiotoxicity. *Leuk Lymphoma* 11:207–214, 1993

74. Sorensen K, Levitt G, Sebag-Montefiore D, et al: Cardiac function in Wilms' tumor survivors. *J Clin Oncol* 13:1546–1556, 1995

75. Postma A, Bink-Boelkens MTE, Beaufort-Krol GCM, et al: Late cardiotoxicity after treatment for a malignant bone tumor. *Med Pediatr Oncol* 26:230–237, 1996

76. Steinherz LJ, Steinherz P, Tan G, et al: Cardiac toxicity 4–20 years after completing anthracycline therapy. *Proc Am Soc Clin Oncol* 8:296, 1989 (abstr)

77. Lipshultz SE, Colan SD, Gelber RD, et al: Late cardiac effects of doxorubicin therapy for acute lymphoblastic leukemia in childhood. *N Engl J Med* 324:808–815, 1991

78. Sorensen K, Levitt G, Bull C, et al: Anthracycline dose in childhood acute lymphoblastic leukemia: Issues of early survival versus late cardiotoxicity. *J Clin Oncol* 15:61–68, 1997

79. Stewart JR, Fajardo LF, Gillette SM, et al: Radiation injury to the heart. *Int J Radiat Oncol Biol Phys* 31:1205–1211, 1995

80. Benoff LJ, Schweitzer P: Radiation therapy-induced cardiac injury. *Am Heart J* 129:1193–1196, 1995

81. Stewart JR, Fajardo LF, Gillette SM, et al: Radiation injury to the heart. *Int J Radiat Oncol Biol Phys* 31:1205–1211, 1995

82. Constine LS, Schwartz RG, Savage DE, et al: Cardiac function, perfusion, and morbidity in irradiated long-term survivors of Hodgkin's disease. *Int J Radiat Oncol Biol Phys* 39:897–906, 1997

83. Ramireddy K, Kane KM, Adhar GC: Acquired episodic complete heart block after high-dose chemotherapy with cyclophosphamide and thiotepa. *Am Heart J* 127:701–704, 1994

84. Seifert CF, Nesser ME, Thompson DF: Dexrazoxane in the prevention of doxorubicin-induced cardiotoxicity. *Ann Pharmacother* 28:1063–1072, 1994

85. Basser RL, Green MD: Strategies for prevention of anthracycline cardiotoxicity. *Cancer Treat Rev* 19:57–77, 1993

86. Hochster H, Wasserheit C, Speyer J, et al: Cardiotoxicity and cardioprotection during chemotherapy. *Curr Opin Oncol* 7:304–309, 1995

87. Khaw BA, Gold HK, Yasuda T, et al: Scintigraphic quantification of myocardial necrosis in patients after intravenous injection of myosin-specific antibody. *Circulation* 74:501–508, 1986

88. Kremer LCM, Tiel-van Buul MMC, Ubbink MC, et al: Indium-111-antimyosin scintigraphy in the early detection of heart damage after anthracycline therapy in children. *J Clin Oncol* 17:1208–1211, 1999

89. McDonald S, Rubin P, Phillips TL, et al: Injury to the lung from cancer therapy: Clinical syndromes, measurable endpoints, and potential scoring systems. *Int J Radiat Oncol Biol Phys* 31:1187–1203, 1995

90. Morgan GW, Breit SN: Radiation and the lung: A reevaluation of the mechanisms mediating pulmonary injury. *Int J Radiat Oncol Biol Phys* 31:361–369, 1995

91. Lund MB, Kongerud J, Nome O, et al: Lung function impairment in long-term survivors of Hodgkin's disease. *Ann Oncol* 6:495–501, 1995

92. Chou RH, Wong GB, Kramer JH, et al: Toxicities of total-body irradiation for pediatric bone marrow transplantation. *Int J Radiat Oncol Biol Phys* 34:843–851, 1996

93. Epperly M, Bray J, Kraeger S, et al: Prevention of late effects of irradiation lung damage by manganese superoxide dismutase gene therapy. *Gene Ther* 5:196–208, 1998

94. Coia LR, Myerson RJ, Tepper JE: Late effects of radiation therapy on the gastrointestinal tract. *Int J Radiat Oncol Biol Phys* 31:1213–1236, 1995

95. Yeoh E, Horowitz M, Russo A, et al: Effect of pelvic irradiation on gastrointestinal function: A prospective longitudinal study. *Am J Med* 95:397–406, 1993

96. Yeoh E, Horowitz M, Russo A, et al: A retrospective study of the effects of pelvic irradiation for carcinoma of the cervix on gastrointestinal function. *Int J Radiat Oncol Biol Phys* 26:229–237, 1993

97. Saclarides TJ: Radiation injuries of the gastrointestinal tract. *Surg Clin North Am* 77:261–267, 1997

98. Schultheiss TE, Hanks GE, Hunt MA, et al: Incidence of and factors related to late complications in conformal and conventional radiation treatment of cancer of the prostate. *Int J Radiat Oncol Biol Phys* 32:643–649, 1995

99. Shirkhoda A, Baird S: Morphologic changes of the liver following chemotherapy for metastatic breast carcinoma: CT findings. *Abdom Imaging* 19:39–42, 1994

100. Alter MJ, Mast EE, Moyer LA, et al: Hepatitis C. *Infect Dis Clin North Am* 12:13–25, 1998

101. Hubbard P: Hepatitis C. *Hepatology* 2:17–18, 23–26, 29–31, 1998

102. Efros MD, Ahmed T, Coombe N, et al: Urologic complications of high-dose chemotherapy and bone marrow transplantation. *Urology* 43:355–360, 1994

103. Sheikh-Hamad D, Timmins K, Jalali Z: Cisplatin-induced renal toxicity: Possible reversal by N-Acetylcysteine treatment. *J Am Soc Nephrol* 8:1640–1645, 1997

104. Foster-Nora JA, Siden R: Amifostine for protection from antineoplastic drug toxicity. *Am J Health Syst Pharm* 54:787–800, 1997

105. Capizzi RL, Oster W: Protection of normal tissue from the cytotoxic effects of chemotherapy and radiation by amifostine: Clinical experiences. *Eur J Cancer* 31A:S8–S13, 1995

106. Rossi R, Kleinebrand A, Gödde A, et al: Increased risk of ifosfamide-induced renal Fanconi's syndrome after unilateral nephrectomy. *Lancet* 341:755, 1993

107. Ritchey M, Green DM, Thomas P, et al: Renal failure in Wilm's tumor patients: A report from the national Wilms' tumor study group. *Med Pediatr Oncol* 26:75–80, 1996

108. Ganong WF: The thyroid gland, in Ganong WF (ed): *Review of Medical Physiology*. Palo Alto, CA, Appleton & Lange, 1987, pp 262–275

109. Morgan GW, Freeman AP, McLean RG, et al: Late cardiac, thyroid and pulmonary sequelae of mantle radiotherapy for Hodgkin's disease. *Radiat Oncol Biol Phys* 11:11, 1985

110. Moroff SV, Fluks JZ: Thyroid cancer following radiotherapy for Hodgkin's disease: A case report and review of the literature. *Med Pediatr Oncol* 14:216–220, 1986

111. Smith RE, Adler RA, Clark P, et al: Thyroid function after mantle radiation in Hodgkin's disease. *JAMA* 245:46–49, 1981

112. Mortilmer RH, Hill GE, Galligan JP, et al: Hypothyroidism and Graves' disease after mantle irradiation: A follow-up study. *Aust N Z J Med* 16:347–351, 1986

113. Josensuu H, Viikari J: Thyroid function after postoperative radiation therapy in patients with breast cancer. *Acta Radiol Oncol* 25:167–170, 1986

114. Constine LS, Rubin P, Woolf PD: Hyperprolactinemia and hypothyroidism following cytotoxic therapy for central nervous system malignancies. *J Clin Oncol* 5:1841–1851, 1987

115. Samaan NA, Vieto R, Scholtz PN, et al: Hypothalamic, pituitary and thyroid dysfunction after radiotherapy to the head and neck. *Int J Radiat Oncol Biol Phys* 8:1857–1867, 1982

116. Sklar CA, Constine LS: Chronic neuroendocrinological sequelae of radiation therapy. *Int J Radiat Oncol Biol Phys* 31:1113–1121, 1995

117. Davies HA, Didcock E, Didi M, et al: Disproportionate short stature after cranial irradiation and combination chemotherapy for leukemia. *Arch Dis Child* 70:472–475, 1994

118. Kao GD, Willi SM, Goldwein J: The sequellae of chemoradiation therapy for head and neck cancer in children: Managing impaired growth, development, and other side effects. *Med Pediatr Oncol* 21:60–66, 1993

119. Braumer R, Rappaport R, Prevot C, et al: A prospective study of growth hormone deficiency in children given cranial irradiation, and its relation to statural growth. *J Clin Endocrinol Metab* 68:346–351, 1989

120. Hakami N, Mohammad A, Meyer J: Growth and growth hormone of children with acute lymphoblastic leukemia following central nervous system prophylaxis with and without cranial irradiation. *Am J Pediatr Hematol Oncol* 2:311–316, 1985

121. Robison LL, Nesbit ME, Sather HN, et al: Height of children successfully treated for acute lymphoblastic leukemia: A report from the late effects study committee of Children's Cancer Study Group. *Med Pediatr Oncol* 13:13–21, 1985

122. Cicognani A, Cacciari E, Veechi V, et al: Differential effects of 18- and 24-Gy cranial irradiation on growth rate and growth hormone release in children with prolonged survival after acute lymphoblastic leukemia. *Am J Dis Child* 141:550–552, 1986

123. Starceski PJ, Lee PA, Blatt J, et al: Comparable effects of 1800- and 2400-rad cranial irradiation on height and weight in children treated for acute lymphoblastic leukemia. *Am J Dis Child* 141:550–552, 1987

124. Clayton PE, Shalet SM: Dose dependency of time of onset on radiation-induced growth hormone deficiency. *J Pediatr* 118:226–227, 1991

125. Brauner R, Czernichow P, Rappaport R: Greater susceptibility to hypothalamopituitary irradiation in younger children with acute lymphoblastic leukemia. *J Pediatr* 108:3332, 1986

126. Olshan JS, Gubernick J, Packer RJ, et al: The effects of adjuvant chemotherapy on growth in children with medulloblastoma. *Cancer* 70:2013–2017, 1992

127. Moshang T, Rundle AM, Graves DA, et al: Brain tumor recurrence in children treated with growth hormone: The National Cooperative Growth Study experience. *J Pediatr* 128:S4–7, 1996 (suppl)

128. Shalet SM, Brennan BD: Growth and growth hormone treatment for childhood leukemia. *Hormone Research* 50:1–10, 1998

129. Carroll PV, Emanuel CR, Thorner M, et al: Growth hormone deficiency in adulthood and the effects of growth hormone replacement: A review. *J Clin Endocrinol Metab* 83:382–395, 1998

130. Chipman JJ, Attanasio AF, Birkett MA, et al: The safety profile of Growth Hormone replacement therapy in adults. *Clin Endocrinol (Oxf)* 46:473–481, 1997

131. Jordan VC, Fritz NF, Tormey DC: Endocrine effects of adjuvant chemotherapy and long-term tamoxifen adminis-

tration on node-positive patients with breast cancer. *Cancer Res* 47:624–630, 1987

132. Gershenson DM: Menstrual and reproductive function after treatment with combination chemotherapy for malignant ovarian germ cell tumors. *J Clin Oncol* 6:270–275, 1988

133. Torano AE, Halperin EC, Leventhal BG: The ovary, in Schwartz CL, Hobbie WL, Constine LS, Ruccione KS (eds): *Survivors of Childhood Cancer: Assessment and Management.* Philadelphia, Mosby, 1994, pp 213–224

134. Rivkees SA, Crawford JD: The relationship of gonadal activity and chemotherapy-induced gonadal damage. *JAMA* 259:2123–2125, 1988

135. Heyn R, Raney RB, Hays DM, et al: Late effects of therapy in patients with paratesticular rhabdomyosarcoma. *J Clin Oncol* 10:614–623, 1992

136. Petersen PM, Hansen SW, Giwercman A, et al: Dose-dependent impairment of testicular function in patients treated with cisplatin-based chemotherapy for germ cell cancer. *Ann Oncol* 5:355–358, 1994

137. Byrne J, Mulvihill JJ, Myers MH, et al: Effects of treatment on fertility in long-term survivors of childhood or adolescent cancer. *N Engl J Med* 317:1315–1321, 1987

138. Nicosia S, Matus-Ridley M, Meadows AT: Gonadal effects of cancer therapy in girls. *Cancer* 55:2364–2372, 1985

139. Fischer B, Bheung A: Delayed effect of radiation therapy with or without chemotherapy on ovarian function in women with Hodgkin's disease. *Acta Radiol Oncol* 23:43–48, 1984

140. Shalet SM, Horner A, Ahmed SR, et al: Leydig cell damage and testicular function combination chemotherapy in childhood for acute lymphoblastic leukemia. *Med Pediatr Oncol* 13:65–68, 1985

141. Hamre MR, Robison LL, Nesbit ME, et al: Effects of radiation on ovarian function in long-term survivors of childhood acute lymphoblastic leukemia: A report from the Children's Cancer Study Group. *J Clin Oncol* 5:1759–1765, 1987

142. Green DM, Hall B, Zevon M: Pregnancy outcome after treatment for acute lymphoblastic leukemia during childhood or adolescence. *Cancer* 64:2335–2339, 1989

143. Saman N, Vieto R, Schultz B, et al: Hypothalamic, pituitary and thyroid dysfunction after radiotherapy to the head and neck. *Int J Radiat Oncol Biol Phys* 8:1857–1867, 1982

144. Buvat J, LeMarie A, Burat-Herbaut M, et al: Hyperprolactinemia and sexual function in men. *Horm Res* 22:196–203, 1984

145. Ogilvy-Stuart AL, Clayton PE, Shalet SM: Cranial irradiation and early puberty. *J Clin Endocrinol Metab* 78:1282–1286, 1994

146. Schover LR, Montague DK, Lakin MM: Sexual problems, in DeVita VT, Hellman S, Rosenberg SA (eds): *Cancer: Principles and Practice of Oncology* (ed 5). Philadephia, Lippincott-Raven, 1997, pp 2857–2872

147. Ganz PA, Rowland JH, Desmond K, et al: Life after breast cancer: Understanding women's health related quality of life and sexual functioning. *J Clin Oncol* 16:501–514, 1998

148. Andersen BL: Quality of life for women with gynecologic cancer. *Curr Opin Obstet Gynecol* 7:69–76, 1995

149. Fossa SD, Woehre H, Kurth KH, et al: Influence of urologic morbidity on quality of life in patients with prostate cancer. *Eur Urol* 31:3–8, 1997

150. Robinson JW, Dufour MS, Fung TS: Erectile functioning of men treated for prostate carcinoma. *Cancer* 79:538–544, 1997

151. Ayton RA, Darling GM, Murkies AL, et al: A comparative

study of safety and efficacy of continuous low dose oestradiol release from a vaginal ring compared with conjugated equine oestrogen vaginal cream in the treatment of postmenopausal urogenital atrophy. *Br J Obstet Gynaecol* 103:351–358, 1996

152. Baker VL: Alternatives to oral estrogen replacement: Transdermal patches, percutaneous gels, vaginal creams and rings, implants and other methods of delivery. *Obstet Gynecol Clin North Am* 21:271–297, 1994

153. Hanash KA: Comparative results of goal oriented therapy for erectile dysfunction. *Br J Urol* 157:2135–2138, 1997

154. Dewire DM, Todd E, Meyers P: Patient satisfaction with current impotence therapy. *Wis Med J* 94:542–544, 1995

155. Jarow JP, Nana-Sinkam P, Sabbagh M, et al: Outcome analysis of goal directed therapy for impotence. *J Urol* 155:1609–1612, 1996

156. Mirkes PE: Cyclosphosphamide teratogenesis: A review. *Teratogenesis Carcinog Mutagen* 5:75, 1985

157. Sankila R, Olsen J, Anderson H, et al: Risk of cancer among offspring of childhood cancer surivivors *N Engl J Med* 338:1339–1344, 1998

158. Holmes GE, Holmes FF: Pregnancy outcome of patients treated for Hodgkin's Disease. *Cancer* 257:216, 1978

159. Aisner J, Seirnick PH, Pearl P: Pregnancy outcome in patients treated for Hodgkin's Disease. *J Clin Oncol* 41:1317, 1993

160. Li F, Gimbrere K, Gelber RD, et al: Outcome of pregnancy in therapy on the gastrointestinal tract. *Int J Radiat Oncol Biol Phys* 31:1213–1236, 1995

161. Silber JH, Littman PS, Meadows AT: Stature loss following skeletal irradiation for childhood cancer. *J Clin Oncol* 8:304–312, 1990

162. Rate WR, Bulter MS, Robertson WW, et al: Late orthopedic effects in children with Wilms' tumor treated with abdominal irradiation. *Med Pediatr Oncol* 19:265–268, 1991

163. Shalet SM, Gibson B, Swindell R, et al: Effect of spinal irradiation on growth. *Arch Dis Child* 62:461–464, 1987

164. Felix C, Blatt J, Goodman MA, Medina J: Avascular necrosis of bone following combination chemotherapy for acute lymphocytic leukemia. *Med Pediatr Oncol* 13:269, 1985

165. Mosher RB, McCarthy BJ: Late effects in survivors of bone tumors. *J Pediatr Oncol Nurs* 15:72–84, 1998

166. Marcove RC, Sheth DS, Healey J, et al: Limb sparing surgery for extremity sarcoma. *Cancer Invest* 12:497–504, 1994

167. Greenberg DB, Goorin A, Gebhardt MC, et al: Quality of life in osteogenic survivors. *Oncology* 8:19–25, 1994

168. Maguire A, Craft AW, Evans RGB, et al: The long-term effects of treatment on the dental conditions of children surviving malignant disease. *Cancer* 60:2570–2575, 1987

169. Holmes SJ, Whitehouse RW, Clark ST, et al: Reduced bone mineral density in men following chemotherapy for Hodgkin's disease. *Br J Cancer* 70:371–375, 1994

170. Gillette EL, Mahler PA, Powers BE, et al: Late radiation injury to muscle and peripheral nerves. *Int J Radiat Oncol Biol Phys* 31:1309–1318, 1995

171. Furst CJ, Lundell M, Ahlback SO, et al: Breast hypoplasia following irradiation of the female breast in infancy and early childhood. *Acta Oncol* 28:519–523, 1989

172. Rosenfield NS, Haller JO, Berdon WE: Failure of development of the growing breast after radiation therapy. *Pediatr Radiol* 19:124–127, 1989

173. Marcus RB, McGrath B, O'Conner K, et al: Long term effects on the musculoskeletal and integumentary systems and the breast, in Schwartz CL, Hobbie WL, Constine LS, Ruccione KS (eds): *Survivors of Childhood Cancer: Assessment*

and Management. Philadelphia, Mosby-Yearbook, 1994, pp 263–292

174. Ragnarsson KT: Principles of cancer rehabilitation medicine, in Holland JF, Bast RC, Morton DL, et al (eds): *Cancer Medicine.* Baltimore, Williams & Wilkins, 1997, pp 1382–1383

175. Segerstrom K, Bjerle P, et al: Factors that influence the incidence of brachial edema after treatment of breast cancer. *Scand J Plast Reconstr Surg Hand Surg* 26:223–227, 1992

176. Miakowski C, Portenoy RK: Update on the assessment & management of cancer-related fatigue. Principles & Practice of Supportive Oncology Updates 1:1–10, 1998

177. Aistars J: Fatigue in the cancer patient: A conceptual approach to a clinical problem. *Oncol Nurs Forum* 14:25–30, 1987

178. Funk SG, Tornquist EM, Champagne MT, et al: *Key Aspects of Comfort Management of Pain, Fatigue and Nausea.* New York, Springer, 1989

179. St. Pierre BA, Kaspar CE, Lindsey AM: Fatigue mechanisms in patients with cancer: Effects of tumor necrosis factor and exercise on skeletal muscle. *Oncol Nurs Forum* 19:419–425, 1992

180. Piper BF, Lindsey AM, Dodd MJ: Fatigue mechanisms in cancer patients: Developing nursing theory. *Oncol Nurs Forum* 14:17–23, 1987

181. Whedon M, Stearns D, Mills LE: Quality of life of long term adult survivors of autologous bone marrow transplantation. *Oncol Nurs Forum* 22:1527–1535, 1995

182. Ferrell BR, Grant M, Dean GE, et al: Bone tired: The experience of fatigue and its impact on quality of life. *Oncol Nurs Forum* 23:1539–1547, 1996

183. Berglund G, Bolund C, Fornander T, et al: Late effects of adjuvant chemotherapy and postoperative radiotherapy on quality of life among breast cancer patients. *Eur J Cancer* 27:1075–1081, 1991

184. Radclifte J, Packer RJ, Atkins TE, et al: Three and four year cognitive outcomes in children with noncortical brain tumors treated with whole brain radiotherapy. *Ann Neurol* 32:551–554, 1992

185. Brouwers P: Neuropsychological abilities of long term survivors of childhood leukemia, in Aaronsen NK, Beckmann J (eds): *The Quality of Life of Cancer Patients.* New York, Raven Press, 1987, pp 153–165

186. Roller AC, Pembrook L, Plese L, et al: One-in-five Hodgkin's patients still at risk after 15 years. *Oncol Nurs Update* 2:13, 1987

187. Meadows AT: Second malignant neoplasms in childhood cancer survivors. *J Assoc Pediatr Oncol Nurs* 6:7–11, 1989

188. Nygaard R, Garwicz S, Haldorsen T, et al: Second malignant neoplasms in patients treated for childhood leukemia. *Acta Paediatr Scand* 80:1220–1228, 1991

189. Fraser MC, Tucker MA: Second malignancies following cancer therapy. *Semin Oncol Nurs* 5:43–55, 1989

190. Tucker MA, D'Angio GI, Boice JD, et al: Bone sarcomas linked to radiotherapy and chemotherapy in children. *N Engl J Med* 317:588–593, 1987

191. Tucker MH, Coleman CN, Cox RS, et al: Risk of second cancers after treatment for Hodgkin's disease. *N Engl J Med* 318:76–81, 1988

192. Valagussa P, Santoro A, Fossati-Bellani F, et al: Second acute leukemia and other malignancies following treatment for Hodgkin's disease. *J Clin Oncol* 4:830–837, 1986

193. Coleman M, Easton DF, Horwich A, et al: Second malignancies and Hodgkin's disease: The Royal Marsden Hospital experience. *Radiother Oncol* 11:229–238, 1988

194. Blayney DW, Longo DL, Yound RC, et al: Decreasing risk of leukemia with prolonged follow-up after chemotherapy and radiation for Hodgkin's disease. *N Engl J Med* 316:710–714, 1987

195. Meadows AT: Second malignant neoplasms. *Clin Oncol* 4:217–261, 1985

196. Pui CH, Hancock ML, Raimondi SC, et al: Myeloid neoplasia in children treated for solid tumors. *Lancet* 336:417–421, 1990

197. Meadows AT, Obringer AC, Marrero O, et al: Second malignant neoplasms following childhood Hodgkin's disease: Treatment and splenectomy as risk factors. *Med Pediatr Oncol* 17:477–484, 1989

198. Green MH: Epidemiologic studies of chemotherapy related acute leukemia, in Castellani A (ed): *Epidemiology and Quantitation of Environmental Risk in Humans from Radiation and Other Agents.* New York, Plenum, 1985, pp 499–514

199. Pedersen-Bjergaard J, Ersboll J, Sorensen HM, et al: Risk of acute nonlymphocytic leukemia and preleukemia in patients treated with cyclophosphamide for non-Hodgkin's lymphomas. *Ann Intern Med* 103:195–200, 1985

200. Fisher B, Rockete H, Fisher ER, et al: Leukemia in breast cancer patients following adjuvant chemotherapy or postoperative radiation: The NSABP experience. *J Clin Oncol* 3:1640–1658, 1985

201. Ratain MJ, Kaminer LS, Bitran JD, et al: Acute nonlymphocytic leukemia following etoposide and cisplatin combination chemotherapy for advanced non-small cell carcinoma of the lung. *Blood* 70:1412–1417, 1987

202. Kaldor JM, Day NE, Pettersson F, et al: Leukemia following chemotherapy for ovarian cancer. *N Engl J Med* 322:1–6, 1990

203. Tucker MA, Meadows AT, Boice JD Jr, et al: Leukemia after therapy with alkylating agents for childhood cancer. *J Natl Cancer Inst* 78:459–464, 1987

204. Moss TS, Stauss LC, Das L, et al: Secondary leukemia following successful treatment of Wilm's tumor. *Am J Pediatr Hematol Oncol* 11:158–161, 1989

205. Sandoval C, Pui CH, Bowman LC, et al: Secondary acute myeloid leukemia in children previously treated with alkylating agents, intercalating topoisomerase II inhibitors, and irradiation. *J Clin Oncol* 11:1039–1045, 1993

206. Greene MH, Harris EL, Gershenson DM, et al: Melphalan may be a more potent leukemogen than cyclophosphamide. *Ann Intern Med* 105:360–367, 1986

207. Tucker MA, D'Angio GJ, Boice JD, et al: Bone sarcomas linked to radiotherapy and chemotherapy in children. *N Engl J Med* 317:588–593, 1987

208. Boice JD Jr, Blettner M, Kleinerman RA, et al: Radiation dose and second cancer risk in patients treated for cancer of the cervix. *Radiat Res* 116:3–55, 1988

209. Storm HH: Secondary primary cancer after treatment for cervical cancer: Late effects of radiotherapy. *Cancer* 61:679–688, 1988

210. Rimm IJ, Li FC, Tabell NJ: Brain tumors after cranial irradiation for childhood acute lymphoblastic leukemia: A 13 year experience from the Dana Farber Cancer Institute and The Children's Hospital. *Cancer* 59:1506–1508, 1987

211. Neglia JP, Meadows AT, Robison LL, et al: Second neoplasms after acute lymphoblastic leukemia in childhood. *N Engl J Med* 325:1330–1336, 1991

212. Nyandoto P, Muhonen T, Joensuu H: Second cancers among long term survivors from Hodgkin's disease. *Int J Radiat Biol Phys* 42:373–378, 1998

213. Bhatia S, Robison LL, Oberlin O, et al: Breast cancer and

other second neoplasms after childhood Hodgkin's disease. *N Engl J Med* 334:745–751, 1996

214. O'Brien PC, Barton MB, Fisher R: Breast cancer following treatment for Hodgkin's disease: The need for screening in a young population. *Australas Radiol (Sydney)* 39:271–276, 1995

215. Dershaw DD, Yahalom J, Petick JA: Breast carcinoma in women previously treated for Hodgkin's disease: Mammographic evaluation. *Radiology* 184:421–423, 1992

216. Colvett KT: Bilateral breast carcinoma after radiation therapy for Hodgkin's disease. *South Med J* 88:239–242, 1995

217. Peters MH, Sonpal IM, Batra MK: Breast cancer in women following mantle irradiation for Hodgkin's disease. *Am Surg* 61:763–766, 1995

218. Meadows AT, Hobbie WL: Medical consequences of cure. *Cancer* 58:524, 1986

219. Harpham WS: Long term survivors, in Berger A (ed): *Principles and Practice of Supportive Oncology.* Philadelphia, Lippincott-Raven, 1998, p 890

220. Oeffinger KC, Eshelman DA, Tomlinson GE, Buchanan GR: Programs for adult survivors of childhood cancer. *J Clin Oncol* 16:2864–2867, 1998

221. Pavy JJ, Denekamp J, Letschert J, et al: Late effects of toxicity scoring: The SOMA scale. *Int J Radiat Oncol Biol Phys* 31:1043–1047, 1995

222. van Gerven JMA, Hovestadt A, Moll JW: The effects of an ACTH (4-9) analogue on development of cisplatin neuropathy in testicular cancer: A randomized trial. *J Neurol* 241:432–435, 1994

223. Steinherz LS, Graham T, Hurwitz R, et al: Guidelines for cardiac monitoring of children during and after anthracycline therapy: Reports of the Cardiology Committee of the Children's Cancer Study Group. *Pediatrics* 89:942–949, 1992

CHAPTER 27

Alternative and Complementary Therapies in Cancer Management

Terri Ades, CS, RN, MS, AOCN
Connie Henke Yarbro, RN, MS, FAAN

Introduction

Scope of the Issue

Each year more than 1 million Americans are diagnosed as having cancer, and more than half of these are cured with scientific conventional therapies. Likewise, each year thousands of cancer patients and many others who fear they might develop cancer devote countless hours and invest billions of dollars in the use of alternative cancer therapies that are outside the realm of mainstream, conventional medicine. Often, these treatments offer individuals a chance to participate in their own care, reflecting the naturalistic approaches so popular with the public today. Others will use these methods as complementary techniques to help control symptoms of their disease or side effects from proven cancer therapy.[1,2] In 1997, 42% of Americans used some form of alternative therapy, and approximately 39 million people sought advice or treatment from an alternative medical practitioner.[3]

Whether labeled "unconventional," "unsound," "unproven," "unorthodox," or "questionable," alternative treatments range from those that are both fraudulent and dangerous to health to those that are harmless and expensive. Patients spend an estimated $13 billion each year on alternative medicine.[4–6] According to Eisenberg and colleagues[3] estimated expenditures for professional services in alternative medicine increased 45%, excluding inflation between 1990 and 1997, and were conservatively estimated at $22.6 billion in 1990 and $32.7 billion in 1997, with at least $12.2 billion paid out-of-pocket in 1997. Total 1997 expenditures relating to alternative therapies were estimated at $27 billion.[7]

Because the field of alternative and complementary therapies has become more widespread and popular, Congress mandated the establishment of the Office of Alternative Medicine (OAM) in 1992 at the National Institutes of Health (NIH); in 1998 it became the National Center for Complementary and Alternative Medicine (NCCAM). The NCCAM supports clinical research centers in conducting research on complementary and alternative medicine therapies and studies, to examine the efficacy, safety, and validity of these therapies. Medical schools have established departments and courses on alternative medicine.[8] More health insurers are expanding coverage to include alternative health care. Communication via the Internet has provided the public with the latest information and sources of many alternative therapies, though the reliability of much of this information remains questionable.

Definitions

Today, "alternative" is the popular lexicon for unconventional, unproven, or questionable therapies. The American Cancer Society (ACS) defines *alternative therapies* as unproven or disproven methods that are used in the place of mainstream, or conventional treatment, whereas *complementary therapies* are supportive therapies that are used to complement standard conventional therapy.[9] This definition is based on the use of the method rather than what the method is. The use of the phrase "alternative and complementary" provides an opportunity to make a distinction between the two—those that could be helpful (complementary) with conventional treatment and those replacing conventional, mainstream treatment (alternative), which may be harmful. The acronym CAM, or complementary and alternative medicine, is used indiscriminately, implying that complementary and alternative therapies are the same, thus further confusing the public. A newer phrase adds even more confusion; *integrative therapy* is defined as the combined offering of conventional therapy and CAM.

Oncology nurses are involved with complementary therapies that have been scientifically evaluated and proved to be helpful adjuncts in the care of patients with cancer (e.g., relaxation techniques, biofeedback, music therapy). In some situations, complementary methods can be used inappropriately as alternative therapies; for example, if they are touted as a cure for disease an individual may delay seeking conventional treatment.

Alternative methods of cancer management include diagnostic tests or therapeutic methods that have not shown efficacy in animal tumor models or in scientific clinical trials but that are promoted for general use in cancer prevention, diagnosis, or treatment. Such methods may not be safe for the consumer, because they have not met the requirements of the U.S. Food, Drug, and Cosmetic Act.

Prevalence

The use of alternative and complementary therapies is widespread. A review of published data identified twenty-six surveys of cancer patients in thirteen countries, including five surveys from the United States.[10] The average prevalence of use of complementary/alternative medicine across all studies was 31%. The most commonly used therapies included dietary approaches, hypnotherapy, imagery/visualization, megavitamins, spiritual healing, and herbs. Other studies confirm these findings.[11–13]

Studies of use of complementary and alternative therapies by the general public in the United States reported prevalence rates of 33%–50%.[14–16] However, a recent study reported that the use of unconventional therapies was substantially lower than previously reported.[17] Druss and Rosenheck reported that 6.5% of the U.S. population visited practitioners for both unconventional and conventional therapies but that only 1.8% used conventional services exclusively.[17]

Prevalence rates from all alternative and complementary studies in the United States and internationally range from less than 10% to more than 50%. This broad span might be explained by the various, inconsistent definitions of what constitutes alternative and complementary therapies. Often, studies neglect to include their definition of alternative and complementary therapies. As a result, a study may use the term CAM when referring to complementary therapies only.

Studies also report information about the types of therapies used. A large study of adults in the United States conducted in 1991 showed that relaxation techniques (13%), chiropractic (10%), and massage (7%) were most commonly used. Herbal remedies were reported used by only 3% of the respondents.[16] A similar study of the general public in 1997, however, identified the most common alternative and complementary therapies to be herbal remedies, used by 17% of the respondents, chiropractic used by 16% of those surveyed, massage therapy (14%), and vitamin therapy (13%).[15]

In 1994, the Food Supplement Act was passed, which allowed herbal medicines and other food supplements to be sold over-the-counter without review by the Food and Drug Administration (FDA); this likely explains the increased use of herbal remedies from 3% in 1991 to 17% in 1997. It is estimated that sales of dietary supplements have doubled since passage of the 1994 law. Expanding insurance coverage of chiropractic care during that time period may account for the increase in its use.

Who Seeks Alternative and Complementary Cancer Treatments and Why

The typical person who seeks alternative and complementary therapies tends to be white, female, better educated, of higher socioeconomic status, and younger than those who do not seek its use.[10,18–21]

A recent study of 1305 individuals with a variety of illnesses found that most of these alternative medicine users appeared to find these health care alternatives more consistent with their values, beliefs, and philosophies toward health and life.[7] Users approach their health in what might be described as a holistic manner. They are more likely to have had some type of transformational experience that has changed their world view in some significant way. They are also more likely to report poorer health status than nonusers. This group did not use alternatives because they were dissatisfied with conventional medicine. Though the study did not include individuals with cancer, it did include people with chronic illnesses such as diabetes, digestive problems, anxiety, depression, addictive problems, headaches, muscle strains, and chronic pain. The author's definition of alternative medicine included therapies that are used as complementary.

Using an alternative method of therapy may provide an individual with a greater sense of self-control. The desire for control may stem from an individual feeling like a passive recipient of treatments rather than a partner in treatment decision making. With alternative therapies, patients feel that they are contributing to their health,

thus gaining confidence and a greater sense of well-being.[22–24]

Burstein et al analyzed the use of alternative medicine by 480 women with newly diagnosed early-stage breast cancer.[25] Twenty-eight percent of the women began use after surgery, but 10.6% had used alternative medicine before their breast cancer diagnosis. Of particular importance is the finding that those who began alternative medicine after surgery had greater psychosocial distress and worse quality of life. These results contrast significantly with the commonly held view that the seeker of alternative therapies is psychologically strong, self-assertive, and well-adjusted.[26]

Most patients learn about unconventional treatments by word of mouth, through the mass media (e.g., books, newspapers, television, radio, Internet), from advocacy groups, and at health food stores. Although many patients using alternative therapies continue with standard conventional treatment, most such patients did not inform their doctor that they were taking an alternative treatment.[27]

Historical Perspectives

For thousands of years, individuals in need have turned to people offering what might help ease their medical problems. Popular folk remedies for the treatment of cancer have been available for centuries. Only in recent times has the scientific method, in conjunction with organized medicine and government, been able to provide a measure of confidence that a treatment is safe and effective.

Legislation

Before the Food and Drug Act of 1906, thousands of unproven treatments were promoted to the American public. Often, the treatments were not harmful in and of themselves. However, as an anonymous physician noted in a letter to the *National Quarterly Review* in 1861, "Quackery kills a larger number annually than the disease it pretends to cure."[28,29]

In 1906, President Theodore Roosevelt signed into law the Pure Food and Drug Act, which forbade including misleading or false statements on the labels of remedies. However, Janssen reported that in 1910, in a crucial test of the new law, the U.S. Supreme Court ruled that the law involved only truthful labeling of ingredients used in drugs, not the false therapeutic claims on the drug label.[29] Justice Oliver Wendell Holmes, Jr., concluded that individuals could not be prosecuted for what he termed "mistaken praise" of their treatments, even though the claims were false.

Noting the dangers of permitting unsafe and ineffective drugs on the market, President Taft implored Congress, in 1911, to pass tougher legislation:

There are none so credulous as sufferers from disease. The need is urgent for legislation which will prevent the raising of false hopes of speedy cures of serious ailment by misstatements of facts as to the worthless mixtures on which the sick will rely while their disease progresses unchecked.[30]

In 1912, Congress passed the Sherley Amendment, which made it a crime to make false or fraudulent claims regarding the therapeutic efficacy of a drug. However, the impact of this legislation was somewhat limited, in that it was still necessary to prove that the promoter of the product intended to defraud the public. Mistaken claims could still be made, and patients could continue to be defrauded. In 1938, Congress eliminated this difficulty by passing legislation requiring scientific proof of safety before a drug could be marketed.

The Food and Drug Act of 1962

In 1962, Congress clarified some of the language of the previous legislation and further added that drugs must demonstrate efficacy in addition to safety before they can be marketed. Thus, the process was created by which a substance became approved for prescription use by the FDA.

The Food and Drug Commissioner noted that the Food and Drug Act of 1962 means that the freedom to choose an ineffective drug was properly surrendered in exchange for the freedom from danger to each person's health and well-being from the sale and use of worthless drugs.[31] Likewise, those in government have decided over the years that only individuals certified by experts may practice medicine and are qualified to help patients who would choose to seek their assistance. Though the Food and Drug Act of 1962 frequently has been challenged by those who promote unconventional methods, the Act was upheld by a decision of the U.S. Supreme Court in 1973.

Dietary Supplement and Health Education Act of 1994

Unlike prescribed or over-the-counter medicines made by pharmaceutical companies, there is no government regulation of herbs and other "food supplements," except that marketers are not able to make direct claims for prevention or cure. They can make general function, wellness, and nutritional support statements on package labels that imply health benefits, even though such benefits may not be well established by properly designed scientific studies. Based on the Dietary Supplement and Health Education Act of 1994, herbal products are not reviewed or regulated by the FDA, unless it appears that a product is causing death or serious toxicities. Before 1994, the FDA studied many herbal ingredients and eliminated them from legal sale. Today, however, products containing those same ingredients are available but without FDA approval. The FDA can only stop production of a product when it proves that the product is dangerous

to the health of Americans. Manufacturers are not required to show that their products are safe or effective.

Other government controls that apply to the sale of nutritional supplements and herbal remedies include the U.S. Postal Service, which controls products marketed through the mail. On several occasions, the Postal Service has challenged products shipped through the mail system that make unproven claims of cure for cancer and other diseases. The Federal Trade Commission regulates the advertising of food, cosmetics, nonprescription products, and some other health-related goods and services that are sold across state lines.

Individual states also have regulatory powers through licensing laws. State boards can regulate medical and dental practices. A few states have new laws regulating alternative and complementary therapies and their use by physicians. Despite these many safeguards, the public still has limited protection against the marketing of products that often promise much and produce little if any benefit. Some products marketed in health food stores have recently been removed from shelves only after serious harm and even death from the products were reported.[32]

Past Unproven Methods

Questionable approaches to cancer treatment have existed for centuries, but a popular new alternative seems to develop and thrive almost every decade. Examples of unorthodox approaches, arranged according to their eras of popularity, are identified in Table 27-1. From the nineteenth century "holistic" or "natural" movement to the early and mid-1900s so-called drug approach, then back to the holistic, natural, or diet-oriented regimens of today, many of the popular alternative therapies parallel the most promising developments in scientific clinical trials.[33,34] For example, during the 1960s and 1970s, when chemotherapeutic agents were being developed as an effective treatment for cancer, spurious compounds (e.g., Krebiozen and laetrile) were being promoted to cancer patients. In the 1980s, the cancer clinical trials of immunotherapy and biologics corresponded with the unproven use of immunoaugmentative therapy and other compounds that are purported to boost the immune system.

Popular Alternative and Complementary Methods of Today

Alternative methods of cancer treatment are primarily related to lifestyle and, as such, cannot be regulated by the FDA. Many of the unproven methods place responsibility for a healthy lifestyle on the patient and, have an aura of respectability in relation to conventional scientific medicine, that is concerned with diet, environmental carcinogens, lifestyle, and relation between emotions and physiological responses.[35]

Table 27-1 Popular Alternative Treatments in the United States

1800–1850
Thompsonianism: Emetics and hot baths

1850–1900
Homeopathy: Use of highly distilled or diluted inorganic and organic substances

1890s
Naturopathy: Diets, massages, colonic irrigation
Early osteopathy and chiropractic: Spinal manipulation

1900s
Tablet, ointment, and tonic cancer cures

1920s
"Energy" cancer cures: Cosmic energy, radio waves, light therapy, psychic diagnoses and treatments

1940s
Koch's glyoxylide

1950s
Hoxsey's cancer treatment

1960s
Krebiozen

1970s
Laetrile

1980s–1990s
Metabolic therapies: Diets, megavitamins, minerals, enzymes, colonic irrigation, nutritional supplements, macrobiotic diets
Pharmacologic and biologic therrapies: Antineoplastons, DMSO, Greek cancer cure, live-cell therapy, Cancell, herbal remedies, oxymedicine, immunoaugmentative therapy, shark cartilage
Electronic devices
Behavioral and psychological: Mental imagery, spiritual healing, mind healing, therapeutic touch

DMSO = dimethyl sulfoxide

In a study of contemporary unorthodox cancer treatments, Cassileth et al reported that 13% of 304 patients being treated at the University of Pennsylvania Cancer Center had turned to practitioners of alternative methods at one time or another.[22] An additional 365 patients who received alternative treatments were identified by contacting questionable practitioners and clinics. The total sample of 669 patients was interviewed. Among all patients who had turned to alternative therapy, the most commonly used remedies were, in descending order, metabolic therapy, diet therapies, megavitamins, mental imagery, spiritual or faith healing, and immune boosting therapy. The first three involved some form of nutritional therapy and were selected twice as frequently as the other regimens. This finding is supported by Read et al who found a high rate of vitamin, mineral, or herbal supplementation in a group of 32 patients with cancer.[36]

Thus, nutritional therapy represents a major type of alternative cancer treatment. In part, this may reflect public perceptions of the relationship between nutrition and health; in part it may reflect the fact that the FDA cannot regulate foods and vitamins in the same way it regulates drugs. In addition, other pharmacologic and biologic approaches and herbal approaches have gained popularity.[2] The following discussion reviews the more common alternative and complementary therapies and is categorized using the Center for Complementary and Alternative Medicine nomenclature: diet and nutrition, pharmacologic and biologic approaches, mind-body techniques, herbal remedies, alternative medical systems, manual healing methods, and bioelectromagnetics.

Diet and Nutrition

Dietary alternative cancer treatments often extend current scientific knowledge of the protective and risk-reducing effects of vegetables, fruits, fiber, and avoidance of dietary fat to the idea that foods or food supplements can cure cancer. Typically, proponents refer to these as "noninvasive and nontoxic" approaches to cancer treatment.

There are many different types of metabolic regimens for the prevention of cancer and for cancer treatment. These include restricted diets or fasting, specific dietary modification, macrobiotic diets, enzyme therapy, cellular therapy, megavitamins, detoxification with colonic irrigations, and the development of an appropriate mental attitude.[37] Metabolic therapy is based on the concept that cancer results from impaired metabolism that causes a build-up of toxins in the body. Some believe that detoxification and manipulation of diet can remove these toxins, reestablish metabolic balance, and strengthen the immune system to accomplish cure.[33,37]

Gerson regimen

The Gerson treatment for cancer, developed by German physician Dr. Max Gerson in the 1920s, is the original "metabolic" therapy. It proposes that constipation or inadequate elimination of wastes from the body interferes with metabolism and healing.[38] According to Gerson, cure can be achieved through manipulation of diet and *detoxification*, or purging the body of so-called toxins. There are many adaptations of Dr. Gerson's original program, but all have a consistent approach, which includes (1) avoidance of exposure to carcinogens, (2) positive mental outlook, and (3) eliminating wastes from the body. The daily schedule for the first 3–4 weeks includes thirteen glasses of raw vegetable and fruit juices a day, 5 coffee enemas 4 hours apart, castor oil and castor oil enema every other day, and supplemental vitamins, minerals, and enzymes. Salt, water, coffee, berries, nuts, fish, meat, and dairy products are forbidden.[38,39] Other components that have been added to the regimen are oral and rectal hydrogen peroxide; rectal ozone gas treatments; "live-cell" therapy; intravenous glucose, insulin, and potassium; laetrile, and vaccines.[2]

Several reports have noted that promotional brochures from the Gerson Institute claim to cure 90% of patients with early cancer and 50% of patients with advanced cancer; however, these claims are not supported by data or statistics.[2,38] What has been reported is that repeated enemas and purgatives are more likely to lead to metabolic imbalance than to correct it, and that coffee enemas have resulted in patient deaths.[40–42]

Macrobiotic diets

Over the years, a variety of diet therapies have been purported to be useful in the treatment of cancer. Today, the macrobiotic diet is probably the most popular, both in attempting to cure cancer and to prevent cancer. This diet has its origin in Zen mysticism, which proposes two antagonistic and complementary forces, yin and yang, that govern all things in the universe. Each food is classified as yin or yang, whereas each tumor is classified as being caused by an imbalance of either yin or yang. The diet is matched to the tumor to restore the balance between yin and yang, resulting in a cure or prevention, as the case may be. In addition to diet, balance is also achieved through cooking techniques and attitude toward life.[43]

The original version of the diet, developed by George Ohsawa (1893–1966), involved ten different macrobiotic diets. In the 1970s, Michio Kushi recommended a more standard macrobiotic diet that was less restrictive.[44] This diet consisted of 50%–60% whole cereal grains, 20%–25% vegetables, 5%–10% soups, 5%–10% beans and sea vegetables, occasional fish and fruits, and liquids sparingly. Foods that are not allowed because they are excessively yin or yang include: meat, animal fat, poultry, eggs, dairy products, bananas, citrus fruits, potatoes, tomatoes, spinach, coffee, sugar, and vitamin supplements. The macrobiotic diet uses only plant proteins and is high in bulk and low in fat. Soy is an important component of the diet.

Macrobiotic therapy can result in malnutrition and a deficiency in protein and vitamins. With adequate planning, vegetarian diets can be nutritionally sound, but for the cancer patient who may be immunosuppressed, a macrobiotic diet could be harmful. There is no evidence that the macrobiotic diet is beneficial in patients who have been diagnosed with cancer.[45] However, specific nutrients such as soy are being investigated for their potential anticancer properties. The NCCAM recently funded a pilot study of the cancer-preventive effects of the macrobiotic diet.

Megavitamins

The use of supplemental vitamins contrasts ironically with alternative medicine's emphasis on "natural" foods and therapies. Whereas certain cancers have been associated with low intake of some vitamins (e.g., lung cancer and vitamin A), there is no clear-cut evidence that large doses of vitamins prevent cancer.

Antioxidant nutrients in fruits and vegetables appear to protect the body against the oxygen-induced damage to tissues that constantly occurs as a result of normal metabolism. Because such damage is associated with increased cancer risk, these nutrients are believed to protect against cancer.[46] Antioxidants include vitamins C and E, selenium, and carotenoids. Studies suggest that people who eat more fruits and vegetables containing these antioxidants have a lower risk for cancer.[47] Clinical studies of antioxidant supplements, however, have not demonstrated a reduction in cancer risk.[48,49]

In 1968, Nobel Laureate Linus Pauling claimed that massive doses of vitamin C could cure cancer. Widespread interest among cancer patients prompted a series of NCI-sponsored clinical trials of vitamin C. The studies documented no consistent benefit from vitamin C in patients with advanced cancer.[50–52] There are theoretical reasons that ascorbic acid, acting as an antioxidant, might reduce the incidence of some cancers, and studies of the role of vitamin C in cancer continue.[53] However, megadoses of vitamin C can cause severe kidney damage.[54]

Pharmacologic and Biologic Approaches

Pharmacologic and biologic therapies are highly controversial. The more popular treatments in this category include antineoplastons, shark cartilage, and the immunoaugmentative therapies.

Antineoplaston therapy

Antineoplastons, developed by Stanislaw R. Burzynski, are only available in his clinic in Houston, Texas. Burzynski originally isolated the antineoplastons from the blood and then the urine of individuals without cancer; subsequently they were synthesized in the laboratory. He claims that antineoplastons are natural peptides and amino acid derivatives that cause cancer cells to change to normal cells and inhibit the growth of malignant cells.

Burzynski has numerous publications on antineoplastons in which he claims their effectiveness; however, many of these publications are duplications, published overseas and in non-peer-reviewed journals. Laboratory analysis by a respected scientist concluded that antineoplastons did not normalize cancer cells.[55] Still, some scientists believe that the compounds may show evidence of activity.[2,56]

Because of encouraging clinical evidence, a small clinical trial was initiated, but the study failed to accrue patients. The Burzynski Institute in Houston, Texas, continues research under a treatment investigational new drug (IND), but early data have been criticized as uninterpretable.[57]

Immunoaugmentative therapy

Immunoaugmentative therapy (IAT) for cancer was developed by the late Dr. Lawrence Burton (doctor of zoology) and given at his clinic in the Bahamas. This therapy is based on the theory that stimulation of the immune system will enable the body's normal defenses to destroy tumor cells.[2,34,58,59]

Immunoaugmentative therapy regimens are based on the determination of the individual's daily or twice-daily blood levels of tumor antibody, tumor complement, blocking protein factor, and deblocking protein factor. Based on these results, Burton determined dosages for daily injections of tumor complement obtained from patients with cancer, and tumor antibody and deblocking protein factor, which are obtained from the serum of persons without cancer.

Controlled clinical trials of IAT have not been done. An NCI analysis of the IAT materials revealed that the materials were dilute solutions of blood plasma, with no biologic activity and none of the components that were suggested.[60] Scientific documentation of this therapy is lacking.[2,33,59,61]

Safety concerns have arisen over the years. Unopened vials of treatment materials examined by NCI were found to be unsterile and contaminated with various bacteria;[62] skin abscesses at the injection site of IAT materials have been reported;[63] and in 1985 antibodies to hepatitis B and acquired immunodeficiency syndrome (AIDS) were found in the IAT serum.[60] Numerous attempts have been made to design a scientific clinical trial to evaluate IAT, but agreement could not be reached on the design of the trial.[2] Immunoaugmentative therapy has declined in popularity but remains an alternative approach to the treatment of cancer.

Cancell

Cancell, also known as Entelev, Jim's Juice, Croinic Acid, and Sheridan's Formula, popular in Florida and the midwestern United States, is a mixture of synthetic chemicals created for their electrical properties. James Sheridan, a chemist, developed the formula as a result of what he describes as a dream and inspiration from God. The active ingredients include inositol, nitric acid, sodium sulfite, potassium hydroxide, sulfuric acid, and catechol. Proponents claim that the formula reacts with the body electrically and lowers the voltage of the cell structure.[64] Because cancer cells are weak, they convert directly to waste material in the presence of low voltage. The body then eliminates the waste material. The cancer cells are replaced with normal cells, and the cancer no longer exists.

Additional recommendations include daily bromelain (pineapple enzyme); glutathione before each meal for patients with liver involvement, AIDS, or herpes virus; and butylated hydroxytoluene (BHT) every night for patients with AIDS, herpes, or Epstein-Barr virus. Promotional literature notes that vitamins will interfere with function of Cancell, and that it cannot be used with any other cancer therapy.[64] Although the FDA obtained a permanent injunction prohibiting the distribution of Cancell in interstate commerce,[65] Cancell continues to be distributed as "a gift" to anyone who requests it.

Dimethyl sulfoxide

This agent has been used as an industrial chemical solvent and as a preservative for culture cells. It is rapidly absorbed through the intact skin. Dimethyl sulfoxide (DMSO) 50% solution, is approved by FDA for bladder instillations. The industrial form has been used alone or in combination with laetrile and other forms of "metabolic" therapy, with claims that it will restore the cancer cell to a normal cell. A review of the literature revealed no evidence that DMSO results in objective benefit in the treatment of cancer patients.[66]

Cell therapy

Cell therapy, also referred to as live-cell therapy, fresh-cell therapy, or cellular therapy, is the injection of cells from animal embryos or fetuses. The type of cells given supposedly matches the diseased tissue or organ in the patient. Proponents claim that the live cells contain active agents (not identified) that stimulate the immune system and repair and regenerate the host cells.[2,67] Cellular therapy is promoted for a variety of indications (e.g., menstrual disorders, premature aging, sterility, neoplastic conditions in early and advanced states).[68]

Live-cell therapy was developed by Dr. Paul Niehans of Switzerland. Currently, Dr. Wolfram Kuhnau, an associate of Dr. Niehans, heads the live-cell therapy program in Tijuana, Mexico. In a review of the literature, no scientific evidence was found that live-cell therapy was effective in the treatment of cancer. Serious side effects (brucellosis, encephalomyelitis, anaphylactic shock) have resulted from live-cell therapy.[67]

Oxymedicine

Oxygen treatments (hydrogen peroxide, ozone gas, antioxidant enzymes) have gained popularity among the promoters of alternative cancer regimens. Hydrogen peroxide is administered by various routes: oral, rectal, intravenous, and vaginal. It is used as a part of the cancer cure offered in a hospital in Tijuana, Mexico, where patients receive dilute infusions of 35% food-grade hydrogen peroxide during their stay at the clinic.[2] Promoters claim that it stimulates immunity, oxidizes toxins, and kills bacteria and viruses.[2] Ozone gas can be administered by rectal infusion, intramuscularly, or in blood transfusion. Ozone enemas are a part of the Gerson regimen in Tijuana. Published information on ozone therapy in the treatment of cancer is minimal. Oxidizing agents such as hydrogen peroxide and ozone can be harmful, causing oxygen emboli and death.[69-71]

Shark cartilage

Interest in shark cartilage as a treatment for cancer was generated in 1992 by William Lane's book, *Sharks Don't Get Cancer*, and by media coverage of the use of shark cartilage in patients in Cuba. Proponents claim that shark cartilage is a protein that inhibits angiogenesis. The molecules of the active ingredients in the shark cartilage sold in health food stores are too large to be absorbed, and the ingested product decomposes into inert ingredients.[1] Despite this, many Americans are taking shark cartilage. Attempts were made by the NIH Office of Alternative Medicine to investigate the effectiveness of shark cartilage; however, the shark cartilage received was contaminated.[1] A recent phase I–II clinical trial found no clinical benefit of shark cartilage.[72] The declining success of shark cartilage as a cancer treatment has led to its promotion for other diseases.

Mind-Body Techniques

Mind-body techniques are popular complementary methods used by cancer patients.[18,19] Good documentation exists for the effectiveness of meditation, biofeedback, and yoga in stress reduction and the control of specific physiologic responses.[73,74]

Some proponents, however, claim that mind-body techniques can prevent or cure cancer. Studies suggesting that social support and prayer influence the course of cancer are widely publicized. One of the early studies, reported in *Lancet* in 1989, suggested that women with breast cancer who attended a weekly support group had twice the survival of women who did not attend a support group.[75] Results of this study have not been replicated.

Bernie Siegel, a popular proponent of the causal link between mind and cancer, places responsibility on the individual by emphasizing a positive attitude toward survival.[76] He believes that medical treatment is only as effective as the patient's unconscious mind allows. Positive reinforcement and stress reduction can allow healing to take place. However, evaluation of Siegel's work with "exceptional cancer patients" (ECaP), those encouraged to maintain positive attitudes and to assume responsibility for their own health, versus non-ECaP patients, those receiving no encouragement, revealed no difference in length of survival when both groups received standard treatment for their breast cancer.[77]

Many people find empowerment and comfort through various aspects of spiritual or faith healing. Cassileth and Brown found that 71 of their 378 patients were attracted to this method of therapy, which involved use of prayer, "laying on of hands," incantation, or other ways of obtaining divine intervention to rid themselves of the disease.[33] On the other hand, many patients resort to commercialized faith healers who defraud people of their money by claiming they can cure cancer. Other healers espouse self-love as a way to improve health.[78]

The belief that individuals can use mind-body work to prevent or cure cancer is attractive because it places control over the course of illness with the patient. However, the idea that patients can influence the course of their disease through mind-body techniques is not substantiated and can create feelings of inadequacy and guilt when the disease does not respond to the patient's best mental efforts.[79] Holland notes that some methods that require patients to accept the idea that emotions contributed to their cancer may render patients vulnerable to guilt and depression.[80]

Herbal Remedies

Herbs have been used to treat cancer for thousands of years. Plant products are the source of many effective cancer chemotherapeutic agents. The Natural Products Board of the NCI has tested more than 53,000 natural products in the past 10 years. Approximately one-third of all new cancer therapies come from a natural source.[96]

Two alkaloids isolated from the *Vinca rosea* plant are used in chemotherapy regimens against a variety of cancers. Vincristine sulfate and vinblastine sulfate are chemotherapy agents isolated from the herb periwinkle. Even though periwinkle has been most effective in cancer treatment, it is extremely toxic. The components, chemicals, or alkaloids of plants are tested in clinical trials to determine safety and efficacy, not the plant itself. Other cancer therapies from natural sources include paclitaxel, cytosine arabinoside, camptothecin, and zidovudine (azidothymidine; AZT).

Herbals, or whole plants, are not examined for safety and efficacy by the FDA, and they can be harmful. Still, the public equates marketing terms as "natural" or "environmentally friendly" with safety and often chooses these products over drugs for cancer treatment. This thinking has led health professionals and the public to believe that herbs are at worst harmless and at best beneficial.[81] Reliable resources describing their use and safety are lacking.[24,27]

Some form of herbal medicine is found in most parts of the world and across all cultures. Herbal remedies such as essiac tea, pau d'arco tea (taheebo), iscador, and chaparral tea are popular alternative cancer therapies.[1,27]

Essiac is one of the most popular herbals in North America. Discovered by a native Canadian healer, essiac was popularized by a Canadian nurse, Rene Caisse. Essiac, which is Caisse spelled backwards, is made up of four herbs: burdock, Indian rhubarb, sorrel, and slippery elm. When studied by the NCI, no anticancer effect was found. Essiac is illegal in Canada,[82] but it is available in health food stores in the United States.

Pau d'arco tea is an old Inca Indian herbal used for many illnesses, including cancer. The remedy is made from the bark of an evergreen tree in South America. Its active ingredient, lapachol, has been isolated and has demonstrated anticancer activity. The dose needed for activity, however, is too toxic for humans.[81,83]

Iscador, a derivative of mistletoe, is popular in Europe where it is available in clinics as a cancer treatment. Studies have examined its effectiveness as a cancer treatment, but definitive data have not been reported.[82] In Canada the herbal was removed from market because of controversy around its efficacy and safety. High doses cause liver hemorrhage, anemia, and thymus degeneration in experimental animals.[83,84]

Chaparral tea, promoted as a cancer treatment, can cause liver damage and liver failure. In 1992 the FDA issued a warning about this toxic effect.[85]

Alternative Medical Systems

The more popular healing systems, based on concepts of human physiology, are traditional Chinese medicine and ayurvedic medicine. Traditional Chinese medicine explains the body in terms of the body's relationship with the environment and cosmos. Chi, the life force said to run through all of nature, flows in the body through vertical energy channels known as meridians. The twelve meridians, which correspond to the twelve main rivers of ancient China, are believed to be dotted with acupoints. Each acupoint corresponds to a specific body organ or system, so that putting a needle into the acupoint or pressing the acupoint can reduce the life-force imbalance that is causing the problem in a specific organ.

Qi Gong and tai chi are therapeutic tools used along with acupuncture and acupressure to strengthen and balance chi. Herbal remedies are also used for most ailments, including cancer.[86]

India's Ayurvedic medicine was popularized by best-selling author Deepak Chopra.[87] The term *ayurveda* comes from the word *ayur* meaning life and *veda* meaning knowledge. The ayurveda healing technique is based on the classification of people into one of three body types. Specific remedies for disease and treatments for health promotion are available for each body type. The system has a mind-body component and uses such techniques as yoga and meditation to keep consciousness in balance. It also emphasizes detoxification and cleansing of all body orifices.

Manual Healing Methods

Manual healing includes touch and manipulation techniques. Hands-on massage is a useful complementary therapy for some patients with cancer for stress reduction.

One of the more popular manual healing methods for patients with cancer, therapeutic touch ("T touch"), involves no direct touch. Instead, healers move their hands a few inches above the patient's body and sweep away "blockages" to the patient's energy field. One study showed that experienced therapeutic touch practitioners were not able to detect energy fields.[88] Therapeutic touch is taught in North American nursing schools and widely practiced by nurses in the United States and other countries.[89] The value of chiropractic treatment for low back pain was supported in an NIH consensus statement. Its value continues to be disputed among mainstream physicians.[90]

Bioelectromagnetics

Bioelectromagnetics is the study of interactions between living organisms and their electromagnetic fields. These therapies use the low-frequency of the electromagnetic spectrum to produce magnetic fields that are thought to penetrate the body and heal damaged tissues, including those damaged by cancer.[91] Years ago, based on the belief that magnets placed at the foot of a patient's bed would pull out the cancer, magnets were sold for cancer cures. Today, simple magnets are sold to reduce pain. They can be purchased as arm, leg, or body bands, or as shoe inserts. The sale of these products stems from anecdotal reports and data from preliminary studies demonstrating magnet-induced pain relief for post-polio pain and pain occurring from localized muscle and bone injuries.[92,93]

Practitioners of Alternative Methods

Strategies Used by Promoters

Promoters of alternative cancer methods devote much money to public relations and media presentations that use scientific words or phrases in a misleading and deceptive manner while retaining a strong emotional impact. Omitted from such presentations is the fact that the remedy has never been objectively tested and found to be valid; they do not acknowledge that any patients have failed to benefit from the regimen. Instead, promoters rely heavily on testimonials and anecdotes that do not separate fact from fiction, coincidence, or the natural history of the disease. They also claim that a conspiracy exists within organized medicine or the government to keep "cures" from the American public so the "establishment" does not lose the money and business generated from cancer patients.

As with all advertising, the strategies used by the promoters of alternative treatment methods have become very sophisticated. Their claims are attuned to the times: (1) at a time when nutrition and mental attitude are being emphasized by the public, this reasonable interest is being exploited for personal profit; (2) at a time when society is emphasizing risk reduction, prevention of cancer is represented by advocates of alternative methods as achievable with their remedies; (3) there has been a tendency to combine many alternative methods to make objective evaluation difficult; and (4) a rising distrust of health professionals is being exploited. It is paradoxical that highly motivated and better-educated individuals are more likely to turn to questionable methods because of the promise that "you control your disease."[22,23]

Safety and Efficacy

Any claim for a new method of cancer management in the United States must meet certain scientific standards and be capable of confirmation before it receives approval by the federal government for interstate distribution. Most alternative approaches for the treatment of cancer lack scientifically interpretable and reproducible data.[2]

In 1992 the NIH were congressionally mandated to establish the NIH Office of Alternative Medicine.[94] Its stated purpose is to investigate unconventional medical practices. Currently, fourteen CAM Research Centers are supported by the NIH. The funded center to study alternative medicine and cancer is the Center for Alternative Medicine Research in Cancer at the University of Texas Health Science Center in Houston.[95] In October 1998, Congress elevated the Office to the NIH Center for Complementary and Alterative Medicine, with $50 million appropriated for its support.

Hawkins and Friedman, from the NCI Cancer Therapy Evaluation Program, Division of Cancer Treatment, note that the pivotal question for the NCI in trying to improve cancer therapy is whether the treatment in question is effective, regardless of the source.[96] Thus, the best way for the NCI to resolve the controversies surrounding unconventional treatment approaches is to identify potential approaches for further evaluation by advising investigators in the preparation of best-case series and the conduct of pilot clinical trials.

The federal and state governments participate in the regulation of alternative treatment methods. The FDA has regulatory authority over the manufacturing and marketing of food, drugs, devices, and cosmetics so safety and efficacy are ensured. The FDA regulations do not apply to treatment regimens or practices but only to specific substances used in treatment (e.g., laetrile, antineoplastons, IAT). The Federal Trade Commission (FTC) monitors the advertising of foods and over-the-counter drugs and prohibits false or deceptive advertising. The U.S. Postal Service has authority to monitor for false advertising of mail-order products. State laws regulate commerce within states (intrastate). For example, it is legal to manufacture and prescribe treatments that are not approved by the FDA, but only in the state in which the manufacture of the treatment takes place (e.g., Cancell in Michigan; antineoplastons in Texas). It is illegal to transport unapproved drugs across state lines; however, such transport continues via underground networks. Some states have enacted laws that exempt alternative treatments from state regulation. For example, Oklahoma and Florida enacted provisions to legalize the use of IAT, although they later repealed the laws.

In addition to scientific investigation and legislative regulation, education plays a major role in the control of alternative cancer treatment. Private and government organizations provide information to health professionals and the public. The ACS maintains an extensive database of information and through their Web site and toll-free phone service provides reliable information to the public about various types of alternative therapies. Through their call center, the ACS can also identify the types of therapies that are of greatest interest to the public. Other private organizations involved with the control of alternative methods are the American Society of Clinical Oncology, the American Medical Association, and the National Council Against Health Fraud (NCAHF). The NCI also receives inquiries through their Cancer Information Service. Table 27-2 identifies reliable sources of information on alternative cancer remedies.

A note of caution is needed, as there are currently no government standards on the quality of herbal products sold in the United States. Herbals may be sold to manufacturers as whole plants or plant parts, cut pieces or finely ground particles. The purity and concentration of a product is questionable. Assays are needed to identify the purity and concentration of the herbal. Manufacturers have little incentive to do assays because there is no pressure for quality control. Adulteration, substitution, and contamination have been reported. Analysis of 54 ginseng products revealed that 45% contained no ginseng at all.[85] Some dietary herbals have been found to contain senna (a potent laxative) and ephedra (ephedrine found in some herbals sold as energy boosters). Table 27-3 identifies herbals with serious side effects.

Role of Nurses/Nursing Interventions

Advances in science and technology over the past 30 years have resulted in major challenges for health care professionals providing care to patients with cancer. It has become a major challenge to maintain knowledge of the numerous drug combinations, biological therapies, and treatment protocols for the different types of cancer. Along with this progress has come the continued development of alternative cancer treatments and combinations of these treatment regimens. Nurses provide support,

Table 27-2 Sources of Information on Alternative Therapies

Cancer-specific information

American Cancer Society
1-800-ACS-2345
http://www.cancer.org

University of Texas Center for Alternative Medicine Research in Cancer
http://www.sph.uth.tmc.edu/utcam/default.htm

NIH Center for Complementary and Alternative Medicine
http://altmed.od.nih.gov/

CancerGuide by Steve Dunn: http://cancerguide.org

Alternative methods information

Quackwatch
http://www.quackwatch.com

National Council for Reliable Information
http://www.ncahf.org

Herb and food supplement information

American Botanical Council
http://www.herbalgram.org

US Pharmacopoeia Consumer Information
http://www.usp.org

Table 27-3   Herbals With Serious Side Effects

Aloe—can cause potassium loss over time. Should not be used with digitalis or prescription diuretics.

Cascara—can cause potassium loss over time. Should not be used with digitalis or prescription diuretics.

Chaparral—can cause liver damage; contraindicated in anyone with a history of liver disease.

Chaste Tree Berry—may activate the pituitary resulting in early onset of menstruation after delivery. May interfere with dopamine-receptor antagonists.

Chomper—has been found to be contaminated with digitalis.

Comfrey—linked to the development of liver damage and cancer when taken orally.

Echinacea—contraindicated in patients with autoimmune diseases due to its immunosuppressive effects with use after 6-8 weeks.

Feverfew—may interact with anticoagulants to increase bleeding.

Ginger—inhibits platelet aggregation which can result in prolonged bleeding.

Gingko—selective agonist of platelet aggregation which can result in prolonged bleeding time.

Ginseng—over-use can cause headache, insomnia, and palpitation. Use with caution in patients with hypertension.

Jin Bu Huan—can cause hepatitis and slow heart rate.

Hawthorn—high doses cause CNS depression and hypotension. May interact with blood pressure and heart medications.

Kava—high doses can cause muscle weakness. Potentiates alcohol and other CNS depressants.

Licorice—high doses can cause pseudoaldosteronism resulting in hypertension, water retention, and potassium loss. Contraindicated in patients with liver disorders, hypokalemia, or who are taking cardiac glycosides.

Ma Huang (contains ephedra)—can cause hypertension and CNS stimulation. Can cause hyperglycemia.

Pau D'Arco—active ingredients shown to be toxic in humans. Has anticoagulant effects.

Senna—can cause potassium loss over time. Should not be used with digitalis or prescription diuretics.

St. John's Wort—contraindicated with prescription anti-depressants. May act as a MAO inhibitor.

Data from Cassileth,[66] Beckwith.[97]

care, and comfort for patients within a health care system with rapidly changing and complex scientific treatment modalities. How is it possible to sort through the confusing array of facts and choices available? How can we identify therapies proven scientifically from those therapies that have not been evaluated?

Some nurses are vulnerable to the appealing simplicity of "holistic" medicine. The movement away from high technology is evident in several articles in which nurses discussed the use of reflexology, aromatherapy, massage, herbalism, and dietary practice.[98–100] Reflexology on the feet is supposed to correspond to specific organs and to balance the body's energy. The NCAHF newsletter considers it "fringe nursing" and notes that nurses undermine their credibility by promoting such therapies.[101] Several state boards of nursing award continuing education credits for nonscientific seminars on such topics as crystal healing, fire walking, reflexology, therapeutic touch, applied kinesiology, and aromatherapy.[102,103]

Behavioral methods (mental imagery, biofeedback, and even humor, which some clinicians and patients are using more systematically) are of major interest to nurses and are supportive elements of the care for patients with cancer. How does a nurse sort through the beneficial or detrimental aspects of these methods? With nutritional interventions, such as vitamin supplements, patients feel that they are doing something for themselves. How can nurses help them develop a plan of self-care, and when does that cross over into promoting ineffective cancer remedies?

Two recent articles highlight the problem that nurses face. Spiegel et al reported that psychosocial intervention significantly increased survival in patients with metastatic breast cancer.[104] A larger randomized study is needed to verify their results. A second study, by Cassileth et al, further confounds the situation by providing convincing evidence that for patients with extensive cancer, there is no difference in survival between patients who received a particular unconventional treatment regimen versus conventional therapy.[21] They noted that quality of life was better among conventionally treated patients. This finding is supported by Burstein et al who reported greater psychosocial distress and worse quality of life in women with early stage breast cancer who used alternative medicine for the first time.[25] Deprived of our conventional wisdom regarding unconventional treatments, how are we to respond to patients who say, "Why not? It can't hurt, and it might help!"

The responsible position requires that nurses deal realistically with the complexities and limitations of modern cancer care as well as the subtlety and seductiveness of the alternative cancer treatment industry. Four specific steps will assist in this difficult task: (1) identification of alternative therapies, (2) assessment of communication channels and patient motivation, (3) maintenance of positive communication channels, and (4) maintenance of patient participation in their health care.

Identification of Alternative and Complementary Therapies

The health professional must be informed both of the most frequently encountered alternative methods and of the particular aims of a given individual's therapy. The health professional should be able to explain the risks of alternative methods, such as toxicity or, in instances where the alternative method is being used as a sole form of therapy, the risk of further progression of disease. For individuals using an alternative method in combination with standard therapy, it is still important to know the

Table 27-4 Questions Patients Should Ask Their Health Care Provider When Considering Complementary and Alternative Therapies

- What benefits can be expected from this therapy?
- What are the risks associated with this therapy?
- Do the known benefits outweigh the risks?
- What side effects can be expected?
- Will the therapy interfere with conventional treatment?
- Will the therapy be covered by health insurance?

Reprinted from CANCERNET (database online). Q and A About Complementary and Alternative Medicine in Cancer Treatment. Bethesda MD: NCI; 1999. Accessed 11/16/99. Available at http://cancernet.nci.nih.gov/cgi-bin/srchcgi.exe?DBID=pdq&TYPE=search&SFMT=pdq_statement/1/0/0&ZUI=600914.[105]

side effects for which to look. A drug analysis may prove valuable for any substances the patient has been given by an unproven methods clinic. The risks of adverse effects can be increased when drugs are mixed with unorthodox substances, and the patient must be informed that all risks may not be known. Table 27-4 provides a list of questions patients should ask their health care provider when considering complementary and alternative therapies.[105] Table 27-5 lists some of the useful complementary approaches that may help patients feel better and improve their quality of life.

Assessment of Communication Channels and Patient Motivation

Communication patterns between the patient and family must be evaluated. The family may become preoccupied

Table 27-5 Helpful Complementary Approaches

Aromatherapy

Art therapy

Biofeedback

Herbals
    ginger tea for nausea or heartburn
    camomile tea for indigestion
    valerian tea for sleep problems

Massage therapy

Meditation

Music therapy

Physical activity

Prayer, spiritual practices

Support groups

T'ai chi

Yoga

Well-balanced diet

with seeking different therapies as a means of coping with stress. Such a situation may be intense enough to cause the family to exclude the patient from the decision-making process. Thus, the patient is separated from the family's communication system and from the psychological and physical support that is so important. In this case, the family must be made aware of the impact their actions may have on the patient. A social worker, chaplain, or patient-family support group might facilitate more effective communication within the family.

Maintenance of Positive Communication Channels

It is important for the physician and health care professional to discuss alternative methods of cancer management with patients, as patients are likely to hear about a variety of methods. By initiating such a discussion, the health care professional helps keep communication channels open for further inquiry by the patient and family. The increase in centers that are now providing integrative and complementary therapy has created an environment in which questions are openly addressed during the patient's visit. However, many patients are still not comfortable discussing their interest in complementary and alternative methods. Table 27-6 identifies some potential questions to ask in order to assess a patient's possible interest or motivation for seeking alternative methods of cancer therapy. These questions provide an opportunity

Table 27-6 Questions That May Be Helpful in Assessing a Patient's Possible Interest in Seeking Alternative Cancer Remedies

- Do you feel like an active participant in your health care?
  If not: How would you like to play a more active role?
- Are you having difficulty accepting your diagnosis?
- Do you feel a sense of helplessness and hopelessness?
- Do you feel depressed?
- Do you feel anxious?
- What type of diet do you follow?
- Do you take supplemental vitamins?
  If so: What kind?
- Do you frequent health food stores?
- Have you received any information regarding alternative methods of cancer treatment?
  If so:
  - Are you considering using this therapy?
  - What benefits do you perceive you will derive from this therapy?
  - Is your family encouraging you to pursue this therapy?
  - Would you like us to review the information?

to discover unmet needs of the patient and family, assess their understanding of the therapies they have been receiving, assess their potential interest in unproven methods, and provide reinforcement to the patient and family that discussion of alternative treatment methods will not cause rejection or impair their communication with the health care team. A nonjudgmental attitude facilitates the assessment of the motivations of patient and family in wanting to try an unproven method. In turn, the patient and family likely will be more receptive to the information provided by a health care professional who offers no negative response or moral judgment.

Maintenance of Patient Participation in Their Health Care

Many patients turn to alternative cancer remedies because they do not feel like an active participant in their care and have lost hope that conventional therapy will work. It is important for patients and family to participate in health care. Patient education can increase patient satisfaction, increase patient knowledge, and enhance self-care. For example, information on diet and nutrition provided in a positive context will help the patient feel a part of the therapeutic effort and may prevent the use of questionable dietary therapies. In the event of advancing illness or when conventional treatment modalities have been exhausted, hope and a sense of participation can sometimes be generated if we offer the patient participation in a clinical trial of investigative therapy.

If the patient pursues alternative methods, health care professionals should communicate that they will continue to provide care and would like to be kept informed of the treatments the patient is going to pursue. The patient should be urged to continue standard medical care.

Conclusion

The health professionals caring for patients with cancer must be kept informed of alternative and complementary methods. The terms questionable, unconventional, quackery, alternative, and complementary suggest that the substance or method is being promoted even though it has not been proven effective. Therapies must be tested to determine their safety and efficacy. The present system relies on the scientific method to determine what therapies will be on the market, and improvements are continually being made in methods of evaluation. In this way, the health care consumer is protected from unsafe therapies. As nurses, we have the responsibility to stay informed in order to help patients make educated health care choices. The challenge for health care professionals is to remain nonbiased and to accept the patient's choice of treatment.

References

1. Cassileth BR, Chapman CC: Alternative and complementary cancer therapies. *Cancer* 77:1026–1033, 1996
2. Office of Technology Assessment: *Unconventional Cancer Treatments.* OTA-H-405. Washington, DC, U.S. Government Printing Office, 1990
3. Eisenberg DM, Davis RB, Ettner SL, et al: Trends in alternative medicine use in the United States, 1990–1997: results of a follow-up national survey. *JAMA* 280:1569–1575, 1998
4. Ernst E, Resch KL, Mills S, et al: Complementary medicine—a definition. *Br J Gen Pract* 45:506, 1995
5. Cassileth BR: This study "medicalizes" self-help activities by labeling them unconventional. Invited comment on Eisenberg DM, Kessler RC, Foster C, et al: Unconventional medicine in the US. *N Engl J Med* 328:246–252, 1993
6. Cassileth BR, Lusk EJ, Strouse TB, Bodenheimer BJ: Contemporary unorthodox treatments in cancer medicine: A study of patients, treatments and practitioners. *Ann Intern Med* 101:105–112, 1984
7. Astin J: Why patients use alternative medicine. *JAMA* 19:1548–1553, 1998
8. Auer T: Training in alternatives: The next revolution in medicine. *Alt Ther Health Med* 1:16–17, 1995
9. American Cancer Society: *Operational Statement on Complementary and Alternative Methods of Cancer Management.* Atlanta, GA, American Cancer Society, 1999
10. Ernst E, Cassileth BR: The prevalence of complementary/alternative medicine in cancer: A systematic review. *Cancer* 83:777–782, 1998
11. Miller M, Boyer MJ, Butow PN, et al: The use of unproven methods of treatment by cancer patients: Frequency, expectations, and cost. *Support Care Cancer* 6:337–347, 1998
12. Crocetti E, Crotti N, Feltin A, et al: The use of complementary therapies by breast cancer patients attending conventional treatment. *Eur J Cancer* 34:324–328, 1998
13. Fernandex CV, Stutzer CA, MacWilliam L, et al: Alternative and complementary therapy use in pediatric oncology patients in British Columbia: Prevalence and reasons for use and nonuse. *J Clin Oncol* 16:1279–1286, 1998
14. Elder NC, Gillcrist A, Minz R: Use of alternative health care by family practice patients. *Arch Fam Med* 6:181–184, 1997
15. The Landmark Report. Nov, 1997. Available at: http://www.landmarkhealthcare.com. Accessed 12/28/98
16. Eisenberg DM, Kessler RC, Foster C, et al: Unconventional medicine in the US. *N Engl J Med* 328:246–252, 1993
17. Druss BG, Rosenheck RA: Association between use of unconventional therapies and conventional medical services. *JAMA* 282:651–656, 1999
18. Lerner IJ, Kennedy BJ: The prevalence of questionable methods of cancer treatment in the United States. *CA Cancer J Clin* 42:181–191, 1992
19. Cassileth BR: Unorthodox cancer medicine. *Cancer Invest* 4:591–598, 1986
20. Downer SM, Cody MM, McCluskey P, et al: Pursuit and practice of complementary therapies by cancer patients receiving conventional treatment. *BMJ* 309:86–89, 1994
21. Cassileth BR, Lusk EJ, Guerry D, et al: Survival and quality of life among patients receiving unproven as compared with conventional cancer therapy. *N Engl J Med* 324:1180–1185, 1991

22. Cassileth BR, Lusk E, Strouse T, et al: Contemporary unorthodox treatments in cancer medicine. *Ann Intern Med* 101: 105–112, 1984

23. Hiratzka S: Knowledge and attitudes of persons with cancer toward use of unproven treatment methods. *Oncol Nurs Forum* 12:36–41, 1985

24. Montbriand MJ: Freedom of choice: An issue concerning alternative therapies chosen by patients with cancer. *Oncol Nurs Forum* 20:1195–1201, 1993

25. Burstein HJ, Gelber S, Guadagnoli E, et al: Use of alternative medicine by women with early-stage breast cancer. *N Engl J Med* 340:1733–1739, 1999

26. Holland JC: Use of alternative medicine—A marker for distress? (editorial) *N Engl J Med* 340:1758–1759, 1999

27. Montbriand MJ: An overview of alternate therapies chosen by patients with cancer. *Oncol Nurs Forum* 21:1547–1554, 1994

28. Janssen WF: The cancer "cures": A challenge to rational therapeutics. *Analytical Chem* 50:197A–202A, 1978

29. Janssen WF: Cancer quackery—The past and the present. *Semin Oncol* 6:526–536, 1979

30. Message from President Taft. *Congressional Record* (21 June 1911), 62nd Cong., 1st sess., 2380

31. Kennedy D: Commissioner decision on status. *Fed Register* 42:39806–39967, 1977

32. American Cancer Society: Regulatory and safety issues for drugs, nutritional supplements, and herbs. Available at: http://www.cancer.org/alt_therapy/index.html. Accessed on 11/23/99

33. Cassileth B, Brown H: Unorthodox cancer medicine. *CA Cancer J Clin* 38:176–186, 1988

34. Curt GA: Unsound methods of cancer treatment. *PPO Updates* 4:1–10, 1990

35. Cassileth BR: Historical trends and patient characteristics, in Barrett S, Cassileth BR (eds): *Dubious Cancer Treatment.* Tampa, FL, American Cancer Society, Florida Division, 1991, pp 27–34

36. Read MH, St. Jeor S, Seymour K, et al: Supplementation practices of a group of patients with cancer. *J Am Diet Assoc* 90:278–279, 1990

37. Miller NJ, Howard-Ruben J: Unproven methods of cancer management. Part I: Background and historical perspectives. *Oncol Nurs Forum* 10:46–52, 1983

38. American Cancer Society: Unproven methods of cancer management: Gerson Method. *CA Cancer J Clin* 40:252–256, 1990

39. Gerson M: The cure of advanced cancer by diet therapy: A summary of 30 years of clinical experimentation. *Physiol Chem Phys* 10:449–464, 1978

40. Eisele JE, Reay DT: Deaths related to coffee enemas. *JAMA* 244:1608–1609, 1980

41. Istre GR, Kreiss K, Hopkins RS, et al: An outbreak of amebiasis spread by colonic irrigation at a chiropractic clinic. *N Engl J Med* 307:339–342, 1982

42. Markman M: Medical complications of "alternative" cancer therapy. *N Engl J Med* 312:1640–1641, 1985 (letter)

43. Ohsawa G: *Cancer and the Philosophy of the Far East.* Binghamton, NY, Swan House Publishing, 1971

44. Kushi M: *Macrobiotic Approach to Cancer.* Wayne, NJ, Avery Publishing, 1982

45. American Cancer Society: Unproven methods of cancer management: Macrobiotic diets for the treatment of cancer. *CA Cancer J Clin* 39:248–251, 1989

46. Willet WC. Micronutrients and cancer risk. *Am J Clin Nutr* 59:1162s–1165s, 1994 (suppl 5)

47. Steinmetz KA, Potter JD: Vegetables, fruits, and cancer. II. Mechanisms. *Cancer Causes Control* 2:427–442, 1991

48. Block G: Vitamin C and cancer prevention: The epidemiologic evidence. *Am J Clin Nutr* 53:270s–282s, 1991 (suppl 1)

49. Byers T, Perry G: Dietary carotenes, vitamin C and vitamin E as protective antioxidants in human cancers. *Annu Rev Nutr* 12:139–159, 1992

50. Creagan ET, Moertel CG, O'Fallon JR, et al: Failure of high-dose vitamin C to benefit patients with advanced cancer. *N Engl J Med* 301:687–690, 1979

51. Moertel CG, Fleming TR, Creagan ET, et al: High-dose vitamin C versus placebo in the treatment of patients with advanced cancer who have had no prior chemotherapy. *N Engl J Med* 312:137–141, 1985

52. Tschetter L, Creagan ET, O'Fallon JR, et al: A community-based study of vitamin C (ascorbic acid) therapy in patients with advanced cancer. *Proc Am Soc Clin Oncol* 2:92, 1983 (abstr)

53. Marwick C: Cancer institute takes a look at ascorbic acid. *JAMA* 264:1926, 1990

54. Swartz RD, Wesley JR, Sommermeyer MG, et al: Hyperoxaluria and renal insufficiency due to ascorbic acid administration during total parenteral nutrition. *Ann Intern Med* 100: 530–531, 1984

55. Green S: "Antineoplastons": An unproved cancer therapy. *JAMA* 267:2924–2928, 1992

56. NCI plans trials of Burzynski's "Antineoplaston"; JAMA Report says no antitumor activity in tests. *Cancer Letter* 18: 1–4, 1992

57. Experts say interpretable results unlikely in Burzynski's antineoplastons studies. *Cancer Letter* 24:1–16, 1998

58. Zavertnik JJ: Immuno-augmentative therapy, in Barrett S, Cassileth BR (eds): *Dubious Cancer Treatment.* Tampa, FL, American Cancer Society, Florida Division, 1990, pp 63–72

59. American Cancer Society: Questionable methods of cancer management: Immuno-augmentative therapy (IAT). *CA Cancer J Clin* 41:357–364, 1991

60. Curt GA, Katterhagen G, Mahaney FX: Immunoaugmentative therapy: A primer on the perils of unproved treatments: *JAMA* 255:505–507, 1986

61. Easy cures for cancer still find support. *JAMA* 246:714–716, 1981

62. Curt GA: Warning on immunoaugmentative therapy. *N Engl J Med* 311:859, 1984

63. Centers for Disease Control: Cutaneous nocardiosis in cancer receiving immunotherapy injections—Bahamas. *Morb Mortal Wkly Rep* 33:471–477, 1984

64. Sopack E, Howell MI: *Important Information About Cancell* (promotional literature). November 1988

65. *U.S. vs. James V. Sheridan and Edward J. Sopack.* Complaint for permanent injunction filed in the U.S. District Court of the Eastern District of Michigan, February 21, 1989

66. Cassileth BR: *The Alternative Medicine Handbook.* New York, Norton, 1998

67. American Cancer Society: Unproven methods of cancer management: Fresh-cell therapy. *CA Cancer J Clin* 41: 126–128, 1991

68. Alvarez G: Live-cell therapy at the Manner Clinic. *Manner and Metabolic Research Foundation Newsletter* 1:2–3, 1992

69. Sleigh JW, Linter SPK: Hazards of hydrogen peroxide. *Br Med J* 291:1706, 1985

70. Bassan NM, Dudai M, Shaley O: Near-fatal systemic oxygen embolism due to wound irrigation with hydrogen peroxide. *Postgrad Med J* 58:448–451, 1982

71. American Cancer Society: Questionable methods of cancer management: Hydrogen peroxide and other "hyperoxygenation" therapies. *CA Cancer J Clin* 43:47–55, 1993

72. Miller DR, Anderson GT, Stark JJ, et al: Phase I/II trial of the safety and efficacy of shark cartilage in the treatment of advanced cancer. *J Clin Oncol* 16:3649–3655, 1998

73. NIH Technology assessment panel on integration of behavioral and relaxation approaches into the treatment of chronic pain and insomnia, *JAMA* 276:313–318, 1996

74. Sundar S, Agrawal SK, Singh VP, et al: Role of yoga in management of essential hypertension. *Acta Cardiol* 39: 203–208, 1984

75. Spiegal D, Bloom JR, Kraemer H, Gottheil E: Effect of psychosocial treatment on survival of patients with metastatic breast cancer. *Lancet* 2:888–891, 1989

76. Siegel B: *Love, Medicine & Miracles.* New York, Harper & Row, 1986

77. Gellert GA, Maxwell RM, Siegel BS: Survival of breast cancer patients receiving adjunctive psychosocial support therapy: A 10-year follow-up study. *J Clin Oncol* 11:66–69, 1993

78. Irish AC: Maintaining health in persons with HIV infection. *Semin Oncol Nurs* 5:302–307, 1989

79. Cassileth BR: The social implications of mind-body cancer research. *Cancer Invest* 7:361–364, 1989

80. Holland JC: Why patients seek unproven cancer remedies: A psychological perspective. *CA Cancer J Clin* 32:10–14, 1982

81. Montbriand MJ: Past and present herbs used to treat cancer: Medicine, magic, or poison? *Oncol Nurs Forum* 26: 49–60, 1999

82. Workshop on Alternative Medicine: *Alternative medicine: Expanding medical horizons. A Report to the National Institutes of Health on alternative medical systems and practices in the US.* Washington, DC, US Government Printing Office, 1992

83. Bisset NG: *Herbal Drugs and Phytopharmaceuticals: A Handbook for Practice on a Scientific Basis.* Boca Raton, FL, CRC Press, 1994

84. Tyler VE: *The Honest Herbal* (ed 3). Binghamton, NY, Pharmaceutical Products, 1993

85. Gordon DW, Rosenthal G, Hart J, et al: Chaparral ingestion: The broadening spectrum of liver injury caused by herbal medications. *JAMA* 273:489–490, 1995

86. Tyler VE: *Herbs of Choice: The Therapeutic Use of Phytochemedicinals.* New York, Pharmaceutical Products Press, 1994

87. Chopra D: *Ageless Body, Timeless Mind.* New York: Harmony Books, 1993

88. Rosa L, Rosa E, Sarner L, et al: A close look at Therapeutic Touch. *JAMA* 279:1005–1010, 1998

89. Scheiber B: Therapeutic Touch: Evaluating the "Growing Body of Evidence" Claim. *The Scientific Review of Alternative Medicine* 1:13–15, 1997

90. Shekelle PG: What role for chiropractic in healthy care? *N Engl J Med* 339:1074–1075, 1998

91. Burton Goldberg Group: *Alternative Medicine: The Definitve Guide.* Puyallup, WA: Future Publishing, 1993, p 571

92. Vallbona C, Hazlewood CF, Jurida G: Response of pain to static magnetic fields in post polio patients: A double-blind study. *Arch Phys Med Rehabil* 78:1200–1203, 1997

93. Pujol J, Pascual-Leone A, Dolz C, et al: The effect of repetitive magnetic stimulation on localized musculoskeletal pain. *Neuroreport* 9:1745–1748, 1998

94. Senate Appropriations Report. *Unconventional medical practices,* 1992, page 141

95. Senate gives NIH director authority to permit research by unconventional MDs. *Cancer Letter* 18:3–4, 1992

96. Hawkins MJ, Friedman MA: Commentary: National Cancer Institute's evaluation of unconventional cancer treatments. *J Natl Cancer Inst* 84:1699–1702, 1992

97. Beckwith J: Idaho Drug Information Center, Pharmacist's Letter and Prescriber's Letter. *Herbal Medicine.* Document #131033, Stockton CA, 1998

98. Passant H: A holistic approach in the ward. *Nurs Times* 86: 26–28, 1990

99. Evans M: Reflex zone therapy for mothers. *Nurs Times* 86: 29–31, 1990

100. Smith M: Healing through touch. *Nurs Times* 86:31–32, 1990

101. National Council Against Health Fraud: Fringe nursing. *National Council Against Health Fraud Newsletter* 13:4, 1990

102. National Council Against Health Fraud: Registered nurses get CE credit for crystal healing coursework. *National Council Against Health Fraud Newsletter* 13:3, 1990

103. National Council Against Health Fraud: Colorado RN confronts pseudoscience in nurses continuing education. *National Council Against Health Fraud Newsletter* 15:3, 1992

104. Spiegel D, Bloom JR, Kraemer HC, et al. Effect of psychosocial treatment on survival of patients with metastatic breast cancer. *Lancet* 2:888–890, 1989

105. CANCERNET (database online). Q and A About Complementary and Alternative Medicine in Cancer Treatment. Bethesda, MD: NCI; 1999. Accessed 11/16/99. Available at http://cancernet.nci.nih.gov/cgi-bin/srchcgi.exe?DBID =pdq&TYPE=search&SFMT=pdq_statement/1/0/0& ZUI=600914

Symptom Management

CHAPTER 28

Assessment of Cancer Pain

Katherine A. Yeager, MS, RN
Deborah B. McGuire, PhD, RN, FAAN
Vivian R. Sheidler, MS, RN

Introduction and Background

Pain is one of the most prevalent symptoms faced by patients with cancer. Fear of unrelieved pain is rightly a concern for both patients and their families, because despite the availability of information and technology that can relieve most cancer pain, it often remains under-treated.[1] The purpose of this chapter is to describe the causes and manifestations of cancer pain, the scope of the cancer pain problem, and key components of assessment. In Chapter 29, management of cancer pain is discussed.

Definitions of Pain

Historically, pain has not been easy to define. During the seventeenth century, pain was viewed as a signal of bodily injury, with scant attention paid to its nonphysical aspects. In the twentieth century, researchers formulated concepts of pain that recognized and included not only the physical "alarm" aspect but other neurological activities, cultural factors, individual personality, and experiential variables.

The International Association for the Study of Pain (IASP) developed a definition of pain acceptable to both clinicians and researchers: "Pain is an unpleasant sensory and emotional experience associated with actual or potential tissue damage, or described in terms of such damage."[2,p.250] This definition accounted for both sensory and emotional aspects of pain as well as for pain of pathophysiological and psychological origin. It incorporated the essential elements of subjectivity and individual uniqueness in the pain experience.

In addition to this definition of pain, the IASP published a list of pain terms, with their definitions (e.g., allodynia and causalgia), which it viewed as a "minimum standard vocabulary for members of different disciplines who work in the field of pain."[2] In 1986 the IASP published additional pain terms with definitions, descriptions of chronic pain syndromes, and a classification and coding schema for these different syndromes.[3] A more recent publication lists a full taxonomy of chronic pain,[4] which includes many different types of cancer-related pain. It is important to note, however, that controversy exists about the appropriateness of applying the IASP definition of pain to individuals who cannot report pain (e.g., infants), because the definition implies that verbal self-report is necessary for pain to be present.[5]

It is commonly accepted that chronic pain and acute pain are distinctly different phenomena. Bonica defined acute pain as "a complex constellation of unpleasant sensory, perceptual, and emotional experiences and certain associated autonomic, psychologic, emotional, and behavioral responses."[6,p.19] IASP defined it as "Pain of recent onset and probably limited duration," which usually has "an identifiable temporal and causal relationship to injury or disease."[7,p.2] Chronic pain generally continues past the time of injury and may not have an identifiable etiology or any overt behavioral signs or physiological changes. Bonica noted that acute pain may recur periodically when an individual has recurrent acute pathophysiological processes, such as those commonly seen in persons with cancer.[6] Thus, cancer pain can be chronic in the case of progressive disease, or acute, depending on the status of the disease.

Theories and Mechanisms of Pain

Closely related to definitions of pain are theories of pain. Various theories have been proposed over the years and, as with definitions of pain, many began with one or two simple anatomical or clinical aspects of pain and then expanded to include a multitude of anatomical, neural, physiological, clinical, and psychological variables. Until the midtwentieth century, several traditional but opposing theories of pain were prominent. Since then, additional theories have been developed in attempts to explain the phenomenon of pain in a more comprehensive fashion.[8] Most notable of these is the *gate control theory of pain*, proposed by Melzack and Wall in 1965[9] and revisited not long ago.[10] It is now abundantly clear that pain has a sensory component as well as a reactive (emotional) component. Novy et al described these newer theories as being comprehensive rather than restrictive because they incorporated multiple aspects of pain.[8] Much research is being conducted to elucidate the specific processes and phenomena responsible for producing the sensory and emotional puzzle called pain. While it is not possible to describe these efforts in any detail in this chapter, a brief overview of general mechanisms of pain is provided next.

When considered strictly in terms of the pathophysiological and biochemical processes that cause it, pain experienced by patients with cancer is no different than pain experienced by other individuals. Etiological, clinical, and psychosocial characteristics of both tumor- and treatment-related cancer pain, however, distinguish it from other types of pain. These differences are elaborated on later in the chapter; in this section the basic mechanisms of pain in general are considered.

The perception of and response to pain are due to four distinct processes that operate simultaneously and are required for pain to occur (Table 28-1).[11] The first of these processes, *transduction*, begins when a noxious (painful or tissue-damaging) stimulus affects a peripheral sensory nerve ending, depolarizing it and setting off electrical activity that initiates the phenomenon of pain perception. *Transmission*, the next process, consists of the series of subsequent neural events that carry the electrical impulses throughout the nervous system, from peripheral to central. *Modulation*, the third process, is a neural activity that controls pain transmission neurons originating in the periphery and/or the central nervous system (CNS). The fourth process, *perception*, is less an actual physiological/anatomic process than it is the vague sub-

Table 28-1 Mechanisms of Pain

Process	Anatomic and Physiological Components	Description
Transduction	• Peripheral nerve fibers • Chemical substances	Noxious stimulus depolarizes peripheral nerve and sets off electrical activity
Transmission	• Afferent nerve fibers • Dorsal horn of spinal cord • Spinothalamic pathways • Thalamus and cortex	Neural events that occur subsequent to transduction and carry electrical impulses throughout the nervous system, from peripheral to central
Modulation	• Periaqueductal gray • Descending neurons • Dorsal horn of spinal cord • Opiate receptors • Opioid peptides • Neurotransmitters	A central neural activity that controls transmission of pain impulses and contributes to variability of pain
Perception	• Transmission system • Modulation system • Cortical processes	Neural activities involved in transmission and modulation result in a subjective correlate of pain that encompasses complex behavioral, psychological, and emotional factors

Data from Fields.[11]

jective correlate of pain (how it feels) that encompasses complex behavioral, psychological, and emotional factors that are little understood. (The reader interested in more detail is referred to Fields,[11] Wilkie,[12] and Wall and Melzack.[13]) Figure 28-1 shows schematically where transmission and modulation occur.

Cancer Pain as a Multidimensional Phenomenon

The notion of sensory and reactive aspects of pain—developed and nurtured through the gate control theory of pain—has been used by researchers to develop a multidimensional conceptual framework for cancer pain. Ahles et al hypothesized five dimensions: (1) *physiologic* (organic etiology of pain), (2) *sensory* (intensity, location, quality), (3) *affective* (depression, anxiety), (4) *cognitive* (manner in which pain influences an individual's thought processes, how the individual views her- or himself, or the meaning of pain), and (5) *behavioral* (pain-related behaviors such as medication intake and activity level).[14] In a study of 40 patients with cancer who had tumor-related pain, Ahles et al confirmed this framework. One of the conclusions that Ahles et al reached was that treatment for cancer pain could consist of specific therapeutic modalities targeted to each of the five dimensions.[14]

McGuire adapted Ahles's conceptual framework to conduct a descriptive study of 40 cancer patients with pain and 40 without pain and found support for the five dimensions of the model.[15] Individuals with cancer pain used a number of cognitive and behavioral coping strategies that they reported as moderately effective at reducing and controlling their pain.[16] Last, results suggested that there was a sixth important area—the *sociocultural dimension*[17]—which includes demographic, social, and cultural characteristics that are related to the experience of pain. The six dimensions are complex, interrelated, and contribute to the individual's perception of and response to pain.[17] Reviews of research literature indicate substantial support for this conceptualization of pain, both for cancer pain and other types of pain.[17,18] Further discussion of each dimension follows.

Physiological dimension

Ahles et al originally described the physiological dimension as consisting of the organic etiology of pain.[14] This definition was based on earlier work by researchers at Memorial Sloan-Kettering Cancer Center in New York who described three types of pain observed in patients with cancer, each with a different etiology: (1) pain associated with direct tumor involvement, (2) pain associated with cancer therapy, and (3) pain unrelated to either the tumor or its treatment.[19] Sources of pain associated with cancer treatment are many, ranging from initial diagnostic procedures causing acute, short-term pain, to standard therapeutic modalities (surgery, radiation therapy, chemotherapy) causing acute, short-term and/or chronic long-term pain. An example of acute, short-term pain is that associated with mucositis in patients receiving bone marrow transplantation.[20,21] Additional work is aimed at describing more fully treatment-related pain syndromes in specific populations, such as marrow transplant pa-

Transmission

Modulation

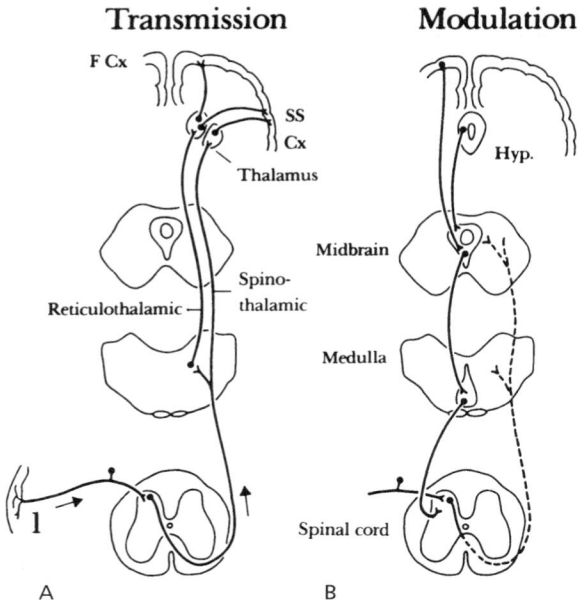

Figure 28-1 Pain transmission and modulation. **A.** Transmission system for nociceptive messages. Noxious stimuli activate the sensitive peripheral ending of the primary afferent nociceptor by the process of transduction (*l*). The message is then transmitted over the peripheral nerve to the spinal cord, where it synapses with cells of origin of the two major ascending pain pathways, the spinothalamic and spinoreticulothalamic. The message is relayed in the thalamus to both the frontal (*F Cx*) and the somatosensory cortex (*SS Cx*). **B.** Pain modulation network. Inputs from frontal cortex and hypothalamus (*Hyp.*) activate cells in the midbrain, which control spinal pain transmission cells via cells in the medulla. (Reprinted with permission from Fields HL: *Pain.* New York: McGraw-Hill, 1987.[11])

tients.[22] The third type of pain described by Foley was pain unrelated to either cancer or its treatment.[19] She estimated that it accounted for 3%–10% of the pain seen in cancer patients. Individuals with cancer pain are just as likely as the average individual to have pain from migraine headache, osteoarthritis, or degenerative disk disease. The presence of such pain, however, is important, and should be carefully assessed to be sure that it is *not* cancer related.

The work of these researchers has led to a greater understanding of the epidemiology and pathophysiology of cancer pain, including three specific pain syndromes that occur in patients with cancer and are usually caused by tumor.[23] These syndromes of somatic, visceral, and neuropathic pain are characterized by pain of different qualities, located in different anatomical parts of the body, and caused by different mechanisms. Distinctions between somatic and visceral pain, and neuropathic pain, lie not only in the mechanisms causing the pain but also in responses to treatment. Characteristics of these pain syndromes are shown in Table 28-2. Although these three syndromes are usually associated with tumor-related pain,

they may apply to treatment-related pain as well.[24,25] It is important to note that many cancer patients with pain will have one or more of these three syndromes simultaneously,[26] and that each syndrome responds differently to therapeutic modalities.[27] These three syndromes are described in detail by Caraceni,[28] who also discusses pain due to treatment and draws clinical correlations to the various types of cancer pain.

A recently described new type of cancer pain is *breakthrough* or *incident pain*,[29] defined as episodes of pain that "interrupt a tolerable background pain," which is usually chronic cancer-related pain. Petzke et al reported data demonstrating that breakthrough (they called it transitory) pain can be somatic, visceral, and/or neuropathic in origin.[30]

Related to etiology of pain are two other characteristics. *Duration* of pain refers to whether pain is acute or chronic. The second characteristic related to etiology of pain is the *pattern* that pain displays. Cancer pain is often described as continuous or constant, but it is also intermittent, brief, or transient, as evidenced by breakthrough pain, pain on movement, and other clinical manifestations of pain. Additionally, patients with cancer may have pain that lasts 1 hour or more to the entire day,[31] and many experience two or more patterns of pain simultaneously.

Sensory dimension

The sensory dimension of cancer-related pain relates to where the pain is located and what it feels like. Three specific components of this dimension are location, intensity, and quality.

Location.　This first component of pain is important. Many patients with cancer have been reported to have pain at two or more locations.[31–33] The number of separate locations of pain has clear implications for the sensory dimension, for the entire pain experience, and for assessment and management.

Intensity.　Intensity of pain, or how strong it feels, is the second important component of the sensory dimension. Intensity is a perceived, and therefore a subjective, phenomenon with variation due to an individual's sensation threshold (defined by Twycross[34] as the least stimulus at which a person perceives a sensation). Individual threshold may be affected by a variety of factors, such as physical comfort, mood, medications, and social environment, thus causing perceived intensity of pain to increase or decrease. Intensity is the most commonly assessed aspect of pain and is characterized by words such as *none, mild, moderate, severe, intolerable, excruciating, bad,* and *intense.* Recent data suggest, however, that intensity of cancer pain may be less for many patients than the intensity of common pains such as headache, stomachache, or toothache.[35] However, patients did report that when their cancer pain was at its worst, it was severe and often inadequately controlled.

Table 28-2   Cancer Pain Syndromes

Type of Pain	Physiological Structures	Mechanism of Pain	Characteristics of Pain	Examples of Acute Pain	Sources of Chronic Pain
Somatic pain	Cutaneous: Skin and subcutaneous tissues Deep somatic: Bone, muscle, blood vessels, connective tissues	Activation of nociceptors	Localization of cutaneous pain: Well localized Localization of deep somatic pain: Less well defined Common descriptions: Constant, achy	Postoperative incisional pain Pain at the insertion sites of tubes and drains Bone of hip fractures Skeletal muscle	Bony metastases Degenerative or osteoarthritis Rheumatoid arthritis Compression fractures from osteoporosis Back pain Peripheral vascular disease Chronic stasis ulcers
Visceral pain	Organs and linings of body cavities	Activation of nociceptors	Localization: Poorly localized, diffuse, deep Common descriptions: Cramping, splitting	Chest and abdominal tubes and drains Bladder distention or spasms Intestinal distention Pericarditis Constipation	Organ metastases Spastic bowel Inflammatory bowel disease Hiatal hernia Chronic hepatitis
Neuropathic pain	Nerve fibers Spinal cord Central nervous system	Nonnociceptive Injury to the nervous system structures	Localization: Poorly localized Common descriptions: Shooting, hot-burning, fiery, electric shocklike, sharp, painfully numb	Phantom limb pain Postmastectomy pain Nerve compression	Diabetic neuropathy Herpes zoster–related pain Cancer-related nerve injury Chronic phantom limb pain Trigeminal neuralgia Central poststroke pain Postmastectomy syndrome

Quality.   The third component of the sensory dimension is the quality of pain, which refers to how it actually feels. Melzack and Torgerson were among the first to systematically study words that people used to describe pain.[36] They composed a list of 102 words from the clinical literature on pain and organized them into classes that described sensory, affective, and evaluative properties of pain. Words placed in the sensory category referred to temporal, spatial, pressure, and thermal. Examples of these sensory words are *pulsing, radiating, penetrating,* and *burning,* respectively. Some studies have revealed that patients with cancer pain use certain words more commonly than others to describe sensory aspects of their pain.[37–40] Words commonly used by patients in these studies included *sharp, tender, aching, throbbing, sore, stabbing, heavy, shooting,* and *gnawing.*

Affective dimension

The affective dimension consists of depression, anxiety, or other psychological factors or personality traits associated with pain.[14] In 1988 Dalton and Feuerstein reviewed literature relating to biobehavioral factors of pain as well as affective, behavioral, and cognitive responses to pain.[41] Although their review included both anecdotal and research reports relevant to the affective dimension of pain, it was clear that little research existed. A previous edition of this chapter identified 21 studies related to the affective dimension of cancer pain[42] and, in tabular format, indicated what psychological parameters were measured and what their relationships were to pain. Research and review articles[17,18,40–43] also support the importance of the affective dimension in cancer pain, especially as related to mood changes and other transient affective states.

It is evident that parameters relevant to the affective dimension of pain range from specific personality traits (e.g., neuroticism) to affective disorders (e.g., depression) to general concepts such as psychological well-being and mood. Taking into account the strong and weak points of studies in this area, it is possible to conclude that (1) specific personality factors probably are not related to the experience of cancer pain; (2) there is little evidence that affective disorders such as depression and anxiety are *strongly* related to pain; and (3) much more research is needed on relationships among these psychological parameters and the experience of cancer pain.

Cognitive dimension

The cognitive dimension of cancer pain, as conceived by Ahles et al,[14] encompassed the manner in which the pain influences a person's thought processes or the manner in which the person views her- or himself. In their study, Ahles et al found support for this dimension by assessing the meaning of each patient's pain. Almost two-thirds believed their pain was an indicator of progressive disease, and these individuals had significantly elevated anxiety and depression scores.

Spiegel and Bloom found that in patients with metastatic breast cancer, the belief that pain indicated worsening disease was significantly correlated with reports of more pain, more anxiety, and more depression.[44] Similarly, McGuire found that 40% of patients with tumor-related pain considered pain an indicator of disease progression.[15] Barkwell reported that cancer patients with pain ascribed words like *challenge, punishment,* and *enemy* to their pain. She found that patients who viewed pain as a challenge reported less pain and had lower depression and higher coping scores than those who viewed pain as punishment or as an enemy. Ferrell and Dean emphasized the importance of helping cancer patients determine the meaning of their pain so that they could better cope with it.[46]

In another aspect of the cognitive dimension, researchers have examined the effects of opioid analgesics on the cognitive function of patients with pain. They found that cognitive deficits occurred as opioids were first prescribed or when doses were adjusted upward, but that these deficits were transient, with functioning returning to baseline when drug doses were stabilized for approximately 2 weeks.[47,48] Thus, level and quality of cognition in relation to pharmacologic therapy appear to be part of the cognitive dimension of pain, as these may influence the ability of individuals to report pain.

Finally, several researchers have examined cognitive strategies used by patients with cancer to cope with pain. Such strategies clearly fall within the cognitive dimension of pain because they result from cognitive processes. Specific strategies include various forms of distraction (e.g., reading, watching television), use of coping self-statements, reinterpretation of painful sensations, selective inattention, withdrawal, suppression of pain, and trying to accept pain.[16,47,49,50]

Behavioral dimension

The behavioral dimension of pain includes a variety of observable behaviors related to pain. Until recently, there was little research supporting this dimension of the cancer pain experience. Ahles et al focused on level of activity and intake of analgesics as manifestations of this dimension in their study.[14] They found that cancer patients with pain spent significantly less time walking or standing than those who did not have pain. Furthermore, 77% of the patients with pain reported that people in their immediate environment could tell when they were in pain because of their facial expressions, changes in mood or activity, or verbal complaints.

Communication of pain to others, however, remains problematic in some patient populations. For example,

Francke and Theeuwen learned that patients who had undergone breast cancer surgery did not readily report their pain and expressed concern about "annoying" the staff.[51] A variety of behaviors have been described that indicate the presence, and possibly even the severity, of cancer pain. Keefe et al conducted a study of the behavioral manifestations of pain in patients with head and neck cancer who were undergoing treatment for their disease.[52] Guarded movements and grimacing were found to be the major behavioral indicators of pain, with grimacing correlating significantly with patients' reports of pain intensity. In addition, the amount of time patients spent walking or standing tended to decrease over the treatment period, and time spent reclining increased. As treatment progressed, the number of simple daily activities that caused pain increased significantly.

Another component of the behavioral dimension of pain consists of simple strategies or activities that patients engage in to control pain. Several studies have examined these activities. In a survey of 351 hospitalized patients, some of whom had cancer, researchers noted that the most commonly cited ($\geq$33%) pain reduction methods involved medications, rest or lying down, heat, and distraction.[53] Several studies found that cancer patients used an array of nonanalgesic, behaviorally oriented pain control methods, including heat, distraction, position change, massage, nonnarcotic drugs, exercise, pressure/manipulation, immobilization, guarding, and analgesics.[49,50,54,55]

Sociocultural dimension

The sociocultural dimension of cancer pain consists of a variety of demographic, ethnic, cultural, spiritual, and related factors that influence a person's perception of and response to pain. Historically, few researchers have examined relationships among these factors and cancer pain, but research activity in these areas is increasing as health care providers recognize the important influences of demographic and cultural characteristics on responses to pain and its treatment.

Sociocultural variables studied in patients with cancer pain have included sex, race, age, and cultural background. In a study of cancer inpatients, McGuire noted that females and nonwhites had significantly lower scores on the McGill Pain Questionnaire than males or whites.[56] In a subsequent study of inpatients and outpatients, blacks and older patients had less pain and depression.[15] A study by Greenwald indicated that despite few differences between ethnic identity and pain report, the ways in which people described affective aspects of pain using the McGill Pain Questionnaire varied across ethnic groups.[57] He concluded that specific ethnic identities conditioned the individual expression of pain, even though assimilation into the American population had occurred.

McMillan found that cancer patients with pain who were over age 55 years reported less pain intensity than those who were younger.[58] On the other hand, another study found that the pain intensity of patients who were over 65 years of age was similar to that of those under 65.[59] More recently, age has been related to doses of opioids in patients with cancer. Vigano et al. reported that while elderly patients reported similar pain intensity to younger patients, they required significantly lower doses of opioids.[60]

Cleeland et al, using the Brief Pain Inventory (BPI), reported in their landmark study that female patients with metastatic cancer were significantly more likely to experience inadequate management of their pain, manifested by less and shorter pain relief, and more pain-related functional impairment.[61] These results suggest that gender may be linked, in as yet unclear ways, to efficacy of pain management in patients with cancer.

As noted earlier, the research literature supporting the sociocultural dimension of cancer is just beginning to emerge. Fink and Gates reviewed relationships among culture, pain, and cancer, and clearly demonstrated that in both noncancer and cancer populations that demographic and cultural factors are important in patients' perceptions of and responses to pain.[62]

One additional component in this dimension that influences cancer pain assessment and management is the patient's family. A significant amount of literature has accumulated that addresses areas such as differences in perceptions of pain between patient and family caregivers,[63] influences of the family on pain management[64] including drug prescriptions,[65] and relationships between knowledge of pain and pain reporting.[66] Clearly, family caregivers, particularly in the home setting, play a major role in assessing and managing pain.[67] This role is just beginning to be explored by clinicians and researchers.

Implications of the multidimensional model

The multidimensional conceptualization of cancer pain has been described as consisting of six interrelated dimensions,[17] a proposition that is confirmed by research findings. Glajchen et al studied 191 outpatients with cancer and found that pain disrupted their mood, activities, and enjoyment of life.[68] They demonstrated relationships among pain intensity, family communication related to pain, and patients' educational level. These investigators concluded that psychological factors (affective and behavioral dimensions), demographics (sociocultural dimension), and medical factors (physiological, sensory, and behavioral dimensions) could interfere with assessment and management of cancer pain. In another study, Lancee et al tested a model for determinants of distress in cancer patients in 1309 individuals with cancer.[69] Among their most striking findings was that pain (and other symptoms) had a direct effect on distress (affective dimension), and that pain was the single most significant factor related to distress. Additionally, pain exerted an indirect effect on distress through its effects on functional impairment (behavioral dimension) and cancer-related fears (cognitive dimension). Williamson and Schulz demonstrated in 268 younger (aged 30–64 years) and older (65–90 years) patients with cancer that the effects of

pain on depression (affective dimension) are mediated by functional disability (behavioral dimension).[70] This impairment was more distressing to the younger patients than to the older ones. These investigators also noted that patients' overall levels of depression were below those considered at risk for clinical depression.

The multidimensional conceptualization of cancer pain, as initially defined by Ahles et al,[14] expanded by McGuire,[17] and supported by the research of many investigators, provides a relevant conceptual approach to pain assessment and management. Various parameters within the dimensions of pain (e.g., duration and pattern in the physiological; intensity and quality in the sensory; mood changes in the affective; effects of pain on functioning in the behavioral) are important for nurses to assess. Similarly, various parameters within the dimensions of pain can be targeted for specific interventions that affect the organic etiology causing pain, transmission of pain, or patients' responses to pain (see Chapter 29). As examples, a painful bony metastatic lesion (physiological dimension) can be treated with radiation therapy; pain intensity (sensory dimension) can be ameliorated using analgesics; and responses to pain (cognitive dimension) can be altered using distraction strategies.

Scope of the Cancer Pain Problem

Pain in the patient with cancer has long been recognized as a challenging clinical problem. The Oncology Nursing Society's (ONS) recent position paper on cancer pain management[1] emphasized the fact that cancer pain often is managed inadequately, despite nearly a decade of work attempting to alleviate this problem. A comprehensive understanding of the scope of the cancer pain problem, and why it is still not adequately managed, requires knowledge of its prevalence, significance, and the professional issues involved in its management.

Prevalence

The incidence of cancer pain for all cancer diagnoses during all stages of the disease has been difficult to quantify. Most studies report prevalence data rather than incidence data. Problems affecting the accuracy of prevalence data include (1) lack of systematic data collection and pain measurement techniques, (2) lack of documentation regarding the extent of patients' disease, (3) lack of identification of pain's etiology, and (4) inclusion of multiple cancer diagnoses as a single group.[71] Despite these problems, however, researchers have examined the prevalence of cancer pain in a number of studies.[72] Prevalence of pain by clinical setting, regardless of cancer diagnosis, indicates that patients in hospice and specialty units report a higher prevalence of pain than patients in other settings. This observation can be understood by recognizing that patients with advanced, metastatic disease are often referred to these settings for terminal care. Likewise, patients with advanced disease report more severe pain than those who are in the early stages of their illness.[72-75]

The severity of cancer pain, as opposed to the presence of pain, has been used as a means of reporting not only prevalence of pain but also its characteristics. Several studies revealed that patients with cancer-related pain described it as ranging from mild or moderate to severe to excruciating.[72] Most patients, however, reported pain in the mild to moderate rather than in the severe range.[35] Examination of pain prevalence data by cancer diagnosis shows the likelihood of pain becoming a significant problem with the progression of disease, particularly in common solid tumors such as lung and breast cancer. Several cancers, notably pancreatic and primary bone, exhibit relatively high prevalence rates of pain across all stages of disease.[76,77] Literature related to pain from cancer treatment (i.e., peripheral blood stem cell and bone marrow transplantation, postmastectomy) has identified unique concerns and treatment challenges.[77-79]

Taken together, the published studies on the prevalence of cancer pain indicate several important things. First, knowledge of cancer pain comes primarily from prevalence studies, as there are few published reports on the incidence of cancer pain. Second, pain clearly is more prevalent in those patients with advanced stages of disease and those being treated in hospice or specialty units. Third, certain common malignancies are more often associated with cancer pain, and it is these malignancies in which pain is better studied and understood. Finally, much of the available data are derived from patients with tumor- and/or treatment-related pain, rendering accurate rates for any specific type of pain difficult to ascertain.

Because of the complicated nature of cancer pain, with its different etiologies,[25] varied presentations,[26] multiple dimensions,[17] and variety of treatments, and the previously mentioned difficulties with studying the incidence and prevalence of the problem, we can speculate that the true prevalence of pain is much greater than existing reports indicate.

Significance

Although cancer pain clearly is a multidimensional phenomenon, the impact on patients who have it, or on their families and friends, is only beginning to be understood. Cancer pain is a significant problem for a variety of reasons. It is already well known that individuals with cancer-related pain exhibit a variety of pain-related behaviors[55] and experience many physical and psychosocial problems.[14,15,38,74,80,81] Additionally, recent years have witnessed an explosion of clinical research, sociocultural, political, regulatory/legal, health policy, and professional activities that have increased knowledge about pain and have influenced in both positive and negative ways how pain is managed. These developments encompass quality of life,

family and home care issues, ethical concerns related to use of advanced technologies, financial costs associated with cancer pain, managed care, regulatory influences on use of controlled substances, legal impediments to adequate management of pain, health policy initiatives in pain, increased emphasis on cancer pain by national and international agencies, and increased federal and private research funding opportunities. The brief discussion that follows provides a cursory overview of these developments and demonstrates the far-reaching significance of the cancer pain problem.

Quality of life is a construct that has been examined in people with cancer pain as a domain of concern[40,82] as well as a potential outcome variable in treatment. Research has included a quality-of-life tool in the clinical arena to evaluate pharmacological interventions with respect to their impact on pain intensity as well as on the total person.[83] Additional research has documented the scope and extent of pain's influence on quality of life. For example, Strang and Qvarner demonstrated in 84 patients with cancer-related pain that there was not only significant physical suffering but also negative influences on daily functional activities and concentration.[84] Ferrell and colleagues validated a conceptual model of quality of life in patients with cancer pain that included four domains: physical well-being and symptoms, social concerns, psychological well-being, and spiritual well-being.[85] Research focused on this model has demonstrated quite clearly that quality of life is significantly affected by cancer pain, and that its assessment is important in evaluating both patients' responses to pain interventions and their overall status.[86]

The impact of pain on family caregivers, particularly in the home environment, is an area that has been studied in some depth. A study of 85 family caregivers of patients with cancer pain[87] revealed that pain caused a significant burden for families. Descriptions of pain centered on four themes: anatomical descriptions of pain, hidden pain (patient hides it), family fear and suffering, and overwhelming or unendurable pain. Families' experience of pain included three themes: helplessness, coping by denial of their own feelings (i.e., pretending to "be strong"), and a wish for the patient's death (a "welcome relief" from the suffering).

A second part of this same study[88] documented that family members played a major caregiving role in managing their loved one's pain. With respect to pharmacological interventions, they decided what medications to give and when, monitored them around the clock, kept records, dealt with fears of addiction, and assumed total responsibility for pain medications. In the realm of nonpharmacological interventions, they provided a number of physical interventions (e.g., positioning and/or mobility, massage, application of cold and heat) as well as cognitive interventions (e.g., being there, touch, talk). This research also revealed the questions and concerns family caregivers had about pain and its management, including their advice to professional caregivers (i.e., be there, offer hope, explain, be honest, listen, educate, give enough medicine) and their own personal perspectives (the future, understanding why, death, and fears about medications and handling pain at home).

Data from this same study, conducted in a community hospital, a national cancer center, and a home-based community hospice, were examined in relation to caregiver burden and family factors influencing pain management.[89] Areas of burden included physical dimensions, psychological responses, and interference with normal activities. Families of patients cared for in all three sites rated patients' pain and distress as severe, but caregivers in the home hospice setting reported lower burden, better mood, less distress, and more feelings of being supported in their attempts to care for their loved one.

Research suggests that patients and their family caregivers do not always agree on the presence and severity of pain and other symptoms.[90] A study of 170 caregivers of cancer patients who died in 1994 found that caregivers reported effective pain relief in only 46% of the patients.[65] No differences were observed in degree of pain or effectiveness of pain interventions when comparing rural, urban, or suburban locations or different care settings. Another study of 78 patient-caregiver dyads found that when dyads were noncongruent in assessment of patients' pain, caregivers experienced higher caregiver strain.[64] These issues document the significant impact pain has on the family system of cancer patients and provide many directions for nursing practice.

Ethical concerns related to the use of high technology in medicine[91] are important issues, particularly with respect to costs, access, social justice, informed consent, and autonomy. In the management of cancer pain, the potential for violations of accepted principles of biomedical ethics (autonomy, beneficence, nonmaleficence, and justice) has been clearly explicated.[92] Examples include decision making by health caregivers who as experts feel they can make decisions for patients, lack of respect for patients' values, inadequate concern for the vulnerability of people in pain, conflicts of interest when caregivers have ownership in companies manufacturing or distributing high-technology equipment, selection of therapies that may not provide the best benefits for patients, implementation of therapies that increase risk of harm, denial of access to needed therapy because of reimbursement issues, and use of inappropriate interventions to increase reimbursement. Whedon and Ferrell provided an excellent discussion of considerations in using high-technology management in cancer patients with pain.[93] They emphasized the appropriate use of such technology, delineating the need for specific guidelines in clinical practice and for use of pain management principles in deciding on, selecting, and implementing various advanced technologies.

The costs associated with caring for patients with cancer-related pain have been explored empirically. Data from admissions records over a 12-month period in a national cancer center revealed that 26% of 5772 patients studied had at least one hospital admission for inadequately controlled pain, and that 54% of admissions for uncontrolled pain occurred within 2 weeks of the patient's most recent discharge.[94] The 255 readmissions for uncontrolled pain observed in this study were estimated to cost approximately $5 million over a 1-year period. The investigators suggested that predischarge education related to pain management and potential barriers to effective pain management in the home and/or community needs careful exploration. Because reimbursement for unplanned readmissions for pain control may be limited, tremendous costs to both patients and health care facilities may result. Because nurses influence both the cost and the effectiveness of care for patients with cancer-related pain, assessing the cost effectiveness of different approaches of pain management is an important part of the nurse's role in the changing health care environment.[95]

A different perspective on costs is provided by a landmark legal case that involved the inadequate management of pain in a terminally ill cancer patient admitted to a nursing home in North Carolina.[96] In this case, opioid analgesics were withheld from the patient by the nurse because of concerns about addiction, and other medications were substituted. The family of the patient proved that failure of the nurse and her employer to fulfill their obligations and responsibilities resulted in increased pain and suffering and in "emotional and mental anguish." This "inhuman treatment" resulted initially in a $15 million jury award for compensatory and punitive damages. Although the award was later set aside and a confidential settlement figure agreed on,[97] the case underscored the importance of ethical and professional obligations to relieve pain and suffering and of individualized plans of care for patients with pain.

Problems of inadequate medical coverage and uneven reimbursement policies for health care including prescription drugs, medical equipment, and professional services, affect pain management for cancer patients, particularly the elderly, poor, and minorities. Access to opioid analgesics is limited by some state-controlled substance regulations and by some mail-order pharmacy policies.[98,99] Ferrell and Griffith presented an in-depth analysis of cost issues related to pain management, specifically costs associated with oral medications, parenteral and spinal analgesics, personnel, surgical and anesthetic procedures, radiation therapy, unrelieved pain at home, nondrug interventions, and morbidity.[100] They also discussed cost savings by various care settings, costs to justify services, reimbursement biases, conflict of interest, and indirect costs to patients and families.

In the world of managed care, many blame the changing health care delivery systems (including managed care organizations) for creating roadblocks to effective pain treatments. Some argue that a broad range of social and political issues create roadblocks, including organized medicine's failure to meet the needs of people in pain.[101] The Oncology Nursing Society recognizes that the cost-reduction emphasis in health care restructuring threatens the delivery of quality cancer care and calls on nurses to make decisions guided by quality rather than cost alone when caring for patients in pain.[102] Opportunities have been identified for improvement in response to managed care, including curbing the practice of providing excess care, giving greater emphasis on palliation and supportive care, allowing for flexible provider roles, relocating research dollars to reward innovations and reduce duplication, and providing more community education.[103]

Regulatory and legal developments also have come to the forefront in the cancer pain issue. Because fear of regulatory scrutiny has been identified as a barrier in cancer pain management, state and national laws and regulations are also problematic.[104-106] Pain management advocates throughout the United States have helped to defeat legislation that potentially limits patient access to opioids. For example, state-run multiple-prescription programs, which are intended to decrease substance abuse fraud and drug abuse, result in rapid decreases in the number of appropriate prescriptions written for controlled substances. Several states are considering repealing their triplicate prescription laws.[107] Other positive efforts in the legislative arena include the passage of intractable pain treatment laws, pain summit meetings, and, more recently, the establishment of state pain commissions.[108]

This brief review has highlighted several areas that demonstrate the far-reaching significance of the cancer pain problem. In addition, health policy initiatives and professional organizational efforts to reduce pain and improve its management are another recent and critically important development.[108,109] Such initiatives have occurred both within the United States and internationally. Increased funding opportunities for basic and applied research on pain are more available than in past years, with some agencies specifically targeting pain.[18,110]

Finally, another area of enormous significance to the cancer pain problem is the extensive evidence suggesting that cancer pain is poorly managed worldwide by health professionals from a number of disciplines. Nurses in particular suffer from a lack of research-based knowledge about the prevalence of pain, the impact it has on patients and others, and effective ways of managing it. The next section explores a number of professional issues that influence management of pain.

Professional Issues

Organizational efforts

Organizations and agencies involved with cancer treatment and pain management have directed their efforts toward improving pain management. The most recent ONS position paper[1] highlighted the fact that control of cancer pain is largely inadequate. Further, the paper pointed out that individuals with cancer pain have the right to have pain recognized as a problem and dealt with expediently. Similarly, the World Health Organization (WHO) has designated the relief of cancer pain as one of the goals of its cancer control program.[111] Addi-

tionally, the NIH consensus statement[112] recommended using multiple treatment modalities to help control cancer pain. At a national level, the American Pain Society (APS) published revised performance improvement standards on pain management[113] as well as publishing the fourth edition of its principles for using analgesics to treat acute and cancer pain.[114] The American Society of Clinical Oncology (ASCO) issued a formal statement on the rights of patients to receive adequate pain management and published an educational curriculum for oncologists and oncologists in training.[115] The Agency for Health Care Policy and Research (AHCPR) has clinical practice guidelines for the management of cancer-related pain.[116] Finally, the International Association for the Study of Pain (IASP) published a pain curriculum for use in basic nursing education,[117] predicated on the notion that because nurses have frequent contact with patients receiving care in many settings, they need comprehensive knowledge about pain. The position papers, guidelines, recommendations, and curricula from these various groups have developed in part because of the compelling evidence documented over at least two decades that unrelieved cancer pain is a significant clinical problem.

Obstacles to successful management

A number of obstacles to pain management can be attributed to health care professionals, patients and family, and the health care system (Table 28-3). Inaccurate knowledge about pharmacological principles represents a major problem area, as documented by many studies. Questionnaires administered to nurses, physicians, and students, as well as reviews of patients' records, indicate that in those individuals with cancer pain, there are problems such as prolonged dosing intervals (i.e., not commensurate with the duration of action of the drug), lack of knowledge about equal analgesic doses, misconceptions about morphine's effectiveness as an oral analgesic, and use of doses too low to provide relief of pain.[61,118-123] In a recent landmark case, the Oregon Board of Medical Examiners took action against a physician for undertreat-

Table 28-3 Obstacles to Successful Pain Management

- Lack of understanding about pain
- Expectation that pain should be present
- Relief of pain not viewed as a goal of treatment
- Inadequate or nonexistent assessment
- Undertreatment with analgesics
- Inadequate knowledge of analgesics and other drugs
- Fears of addiction, sedation, and respiratory depression
- Inadequate knowledge of other interventions for pain
- Perceptual differences between patients and health care providers
- Legal impediments

ment of pain. The physician was required to go through an educational program and work with another physician in his field to assess his practice and make improvements.[124]

Issues surrounding addiction and potential toxicities of potent opioids also have been cited as reasons for suboptimal pain control.[125–129] Although some evidence strongly suggests that addiction is not a problem for individuals who require opioids,[130] nurses, physicians, and medical students fear iatrogenically induced addiction and certainly overestimate its risk when opioids are prescribed.[131–133]

Ferrell et al reviewed 14 pharmacology or medical-surgical nursing textbooks published since 1985 and found that only 1 out of 14 defined opioid addiction correctly and described accurately the likelihood of addiction developing with legitimate opioid use.[134] This finding underscores the principal reason why there is so much confusion about addiction.

A more fundamental problem that nurses have demonstrated is a deficiency in the assessment of pain. A lack of basic assessment skills, failure to acknowledge and document the existence of pain, and inaccurate or nonexistent documentation when the problem is known to exist prohibit patients from receiving reasonable pain control.[32,135–137] Although there is strong evidence suggesting that systematic pain assessment and documentation can improve pain management,[138] these very basic nursing actions are not performed consistently.

Several other problems have been identified as obstacles to successful management of pain.[101] Patients' reluctance to report pain to their health care providers and concerns about analgesics are major problems.[139] Perceptual differences between patients and professionals about severity of existing pain have been documented by several investigators.[128,138,140] And last, the role of government agencies, such as the Drug Enforcement Agency, and existing legal statutes have contributed to inadequate prescribing by physicians because of fear of regulatory scrutiny.[105,141,142]

Improvements in management

Nurses and physicians have acknowledged their educational deficiencies related to cancer pain and its management.[127,143,144] The need for structured educational content in basic health professions' educational programs has been encouraged.[112,117,145–152] In nursing, Spross et al delineated positions involving not only basic and graduate nursing school education but also continuing education.[152] ASCO recommends education about cancer pain management for all fellowship training programs,[115] and as noted earlier the IASP[117] has recommendations on pain curriculum in basic nursing education.

Initial efforts at improving pain management consisted of integrating both patients and caregivers into quality assurance efforts[153,154] and using a multidisciplinary team to get current pain knowledge into practice.[155] More recently, clinicians have reported a variety of creative programs in clinical and institutional settings that have improved pain management outcomes.[156–159] A structure common to several of these programs is teams or clinical partners who participate jointly in the educational activities, thus supporting the interdisciplinary nature of cancer pain practice.

In addition to such institutional programs, improvement of pain management can be accomplished through formal performance improvement programs.[154,160–162] The APS quality improvement guidelines for acute and cancer pain are applicable to both inpatient and outpatient settings.[113] Major programmatic efforts, such as the state cancer pain initiatives and the WHO Cancer Control Program, have made the cancer pain problem much more visible, leading to heightened efforts to improve the care of patients with cancer pain.

Delivery of pain management services

The delivery of pain management services is a controversial issue.[163] Individual practitioners who take care of oncology patients should possess basic skills in assessment and management. Recognizing the significant educational needs mentioned earlier, some practitioners may feel more comfortable in referring a patient to a "specialist" for pain management, if one is available. A specialist may be an anesthesiologist, a medical or radiation oncologist, a neurologist, a neurosurgeon, a nurse, a pharmacist, a psychologist, a psychiatrist, or a social worker. Instead of an individual specialist, there may be a multidisciplinary pain team that can provide services.[164] When a referral is made to a specialist or to a pain team, several questions must be answered:

1. What is the level of responsibility of the consultant for the individual patient?
2. What role does the primary provider have after the consultation?
3. Does the patient incur significant additional costs by receiving care from a specialist or a multidisciplinary team?
4. If there are several options for a patient's pain management plan, how are decisions made, and who helps the patient and family with those decisions?

Gonzales et al reported that in 64% of 276 patients referred for a pain consultation, the outcome of the evaluation (which usually required further diagnostic tests and analgesic changes) led to identifying the etiology of the pain problem.[165] Metastatic disease was the most common cause of the pain. In addition, 22% of the patients received treatment for their pain problem with radiation, surgery, or chemotherapy. Walsh described a palliative care service that saw approximately 400 patients per year.[166] This consultant and management service was part of a hematology/medical oncology department and was involved in research activities as well as providing full clinical services. Bascom described an interdisciplinary team that provided comfort care for any seriously ill patients with comfort care needs, not just the traditional hospice patients. This team provided a broader focus of care and cared for patients referred for consultation which would not have been served under a traditional model of palliative care.[167] When clinical settings had a formal service, only 40% of the nurses associated with the group spent more than 50% of the day in pain-related activities, indicating that most were involved in activities other than pain management. Although these multidisciplinary approaches to managing cancer-related pain may be optimal, utilization of resources, costs, and outcomes in today's health care climate needs careful consideration.

Issues surrounding continuity of care have also affected pain management for the patient with cancer. Patients may be seen by a number of different physicians in different settings, but no one is willing to take the responsibility for managing the patient's pain. Often, poor communication across different settings (i.e., hospital and community care setting) compound this problem.[168]

Principles of Assessment and Management

Effective clinical assessment and management of cancer pain rest on recognition and use of a number of critical principles. First is the importance of the nursing role in assessment and management.[169] The ONS position paper[152] delineated the nurse's role as (1) describing pain, (2) identifying aggravating and relieving factors, (3) determining the meaning of pain, (4) determining its cause, (5) determining individuals' definitions of optimal pain relief, (6) deriving nursing diagnoses, (7) assisting in selecting interventions, and (8) evaluating efficacy of interventions. Although nurses certainly contribute to the goals of the physician establishing and treating the cause of pain, the nurses' emphasis is on the individual as a whole person, and on his or her response to pain. Thus, the nurses' focus is on individual definitions of optimal pain relief, psychosocial and physical problems amenable to nursing interventions, and evaluation of the overall response to treatment. Nurses are also interested in how pain affects an individual's significant others and support systems. It is also important to recognize that in today's health care environment, the continuum of care spans inpatient and outpatient facilities, private offices, long-term care facilities, and the home setting. Thus, pain care occurs in multiple settings and, as indicated earlier, includes both chronic and acute pain.

In addition to the critical importance of the nurse's role, there are other principles of assessment and management that are implicit in successful nursing management of cancer pain. These principles consist of use of an interdisciplinary approach in delivery of pain management services, a well-conceived scope of practice for nurses, thorough assessment and documentation, incorporation of guidelines and standards into clinical practice and evaluation of outcomes, and approaches to managing pain in special populations of individuals. Each of these areas is explored in the following sections.

Interdisciplinary Approach

The multidimensional conceptualization of cancer pain requires the involvement of multiple health care disciplines in assessment and management.[116] Treatment approaches, delineated in Chapter 29, consist of chemotherapy, radiation therapy, surgery, anesthetic techniques, pharmacological agents, cognitive/behavioral methods, physical techniques, and many more. Clearly, there is no one best way to treat cancer pain and no one best discipline or person prepared for managing cancer pain. Thus, input is required from specific health care professionals, including nurses, pharmacists, social workers, occupational therapists, physical therapists, psychologists, and physicians from many specialties and subspecialties (e.g., internal medicine, anesthesiology, surgery, radiation oncology, psychiatry).

Nursing's Scope of Practice and Responsibilities

Nurses are an integral part of the interdisciplinary team approach to managing cancer pain. Because of their prolonged contact with cancer patients in a variety of settings, and their relationships with these individuals and their families, oncology nurses are best prepared to assume a leadership role in the assessment and management of cancer pain. Assumption of such a role is consistent with the ONS's mission of improving the care of persons with cancer.[1] The ONS position paper[152] delineated a scope of practice for nurses with different levels of expertise (e.g., nurses and oncology clinical nurse specialists). These levels of expertise were made operational with specific knowledge and skills associated with each level. With the publication of the new scope and standards of oncology nursing practice,[170] the idea of levels of expertise can be easily translated into the general oncology nursing practice and advanced oncology nursing practice described in this publication. At the generalist level, the nurse needs a cancer pain–specific knowledge base that enables appropriate assessment, development of a care plan based on the nursing process, evaluation of the plan, and consultation with others when needed. At the advanced level, the nurse (an individual with a master's degree) should have substantially more theoretical knowledge and clinical expertise in cancer pain that allows assessment, diagnosis, analysis of complex problems, and the use of relevant research and theory to problem-solve.

It is clear that assumption of a leadership role in effective management of cancer patients' pain is a nursing responsibility. The scope of nursing practice delineated in the original ONS position paper on pain[152] as well as the new paper on cancer pain management[1] provide the foundation for all positions relevant to nurses' roles and responsibilities in caring for persons with cancer-related pain.

Assessment and Documentation

Literature documenting nurses' problems with assessing cancer pain has been discussed previously, including the relationship between pain assessment and barriers to adequate pain management. This section presents the rationale for and basic principles of assessment, assessment parameters, tools for assessing pain, documentation of pain assessment, and strategies for incorporating assessment into institutional practice including evaluation of outcomes.

Rationale and basic principles

Systematic nursing assessment of pain is important for several reasons. First, it establishes a baseline from which to plan and begin interventions. Second, it assists in the selection of interventions. Third, it makes evaluation of the interventions possible. Assessment of pain is a critical process that aids in the clinical management of pain and, indeed, goes hand-in-hand with successful management. Current clinical guidelines and other sources identify assessment as key to managing pain.[114–116]

The timing of assessments is critical as well. Any cancer patient with pain who enters any health care setting should have an initial or baseline assessment. After the initiation of interventions, continuous or ongoing assessment is necessary for evaluation and revision of treatment plans. This approach to assessment is modeled on the nursing process. Collection of pain assessment data should be systematic and organized, as is the collection of general nursing data.

In addition, there are some "pitfalls" in assessment of pain. They include (1) the belief that patients with pain will demonstrate changes in vital signs or display overt behavioral manifestations of pain; (2) the belief that all pain should have a documented organic cause; (3) the belief that all pain in cancer patients is due to tumor rather than to "normal" pain such as migraine headache or arthritis; and (4) being overwhelmed with clinical responsibilities and thus becoming insensitive to patients' pain and their related needs. Awareness and avoidance of these "pitfalls" should help nurses perform good pain assessments.

Assessment parameters

The multidimensional conceptualization of pain described previously provides guidance in assessing pain.[17] The range of assessment parameters is quite wide and represents each of the multiple dimensions of cancer pain.[17] Key clinical parameters that require assessment in each dimension are highlighted in Table 28-4. Basic techniques for assessing pain, including the extremely important pain history, are discussed in other sources.[169,171,172]

Assessment tools

There is extensive literature on instruments to measure clinical pain, but a lengthy discussion is impossible

---

Table 28-4   Assessment Parameters Using the Multidimensional Conceptualization of Cancer Pain

Physiological	Sensory	Affective
• Onset	• Location	• Distress
• Associated factors	• Intensity	• Anxiety
• Duration	• Quality	• Depression
• Type of pain (acute or chronic)	• Pattern	• Mental state
• Syndrome		• Perception of suffering
• Anatomy		• Irritability/agitation
• Physiology		• Pain relief

Cognitive	Behavioral	Sociocultural
• Meaning of pain	• Activities of daily living	• Ethnocultural/background
• Thought processes	• Behaviors (pain-related, preventive, or controlling)	• Family/social life
• Coping strategies	• Use of medications	• Work/home responsibilities
• Knowledge	• Sleep/rest patterns	• Environment
• Attitudes/beliefs	• Fatigue and other symptoms	• Familial attitudes/beliefs/behaviors
• Previous treatments		• Personal attitudes/beliefs
• Influencing factors (positive and negative)		• Communication with others
• Level of cognition and/or impairment		• Interpersonal relationships

here. The reader is referred to several recent publications in which this literature is reviewed and discussed, both in relation to pain in general and cancer pain in particular.[171-173] The section below presents a general discussion about types of tools, their appropriate uses, and considerations in selecting tools in an effort to help readers select the best tool for a given situation.

Pain assessment tools can be classified by the number of dimensions of pain they assess.[173] Unidimensional tools focus on one dimension of the pain experience, such as the sensory dimension, and within that dimension may focus on a specific parameter, such as pain intensity. Ten-centimeter visual analog scales (VAS) (anchors of no pain and worst possible pain) or verbal descriptor scales (VDS) (words such as *none, mild, moderate,* and *severe*) measuring pain intensity are examples of commonly used unidimensional tools. Although most VASs and VDSs are of the paper-and-pencil variety, there are some different formats. For example, a format consisting of a 5×20 cm plastic device with a sliding marker moving within a groove that measures 10 cm was tested and found to be reliable and valid at assessing pain intensity in cancer patients.[174] Pain relief can also be measured with VASs and VDSs simply by changing anchor and descriptor words. As another example, a numeric rating scale version of the VDS was demonstrated to be reliable and valid when verbally administered in a 0–10 format without visual cues.[175] Although these scales have documented reliability and validity in measuring cancer-related pain,[173] they measure only one parameter of one dimension of pain and thus are limited in their representation of the total pain experience. However, because pain intensity is such a salient aspect of pain, these scales are an excellent means to evaluate the success of specific interventions for pain.[176] It is important, however, to note that patients' reports of cancer pain intensity may vary in relation to their reported intensity of other types of pain,[35] with implications for interpretation as well as patient teaching. Indeed, the APS quality improvement guidelines[113] recommended regular use of pain intensity and relief scales, as did the AHCPR guidelines for both cancer pain and acute pain management.[116,177] Other unidimensional tools consist of body diagrams to assess location of pain and rating scales to assess behavioral indicators of pain[173] (see Table 28-4).

Multidimensional tools focus on two or more dimensions of the pain experience (see Table 28-4). The McGill Pain Questionnaire (MPQ)[178] is perhaps the most well-known example. The MPQ was originally developed to measure multidimensional aspects of pain in many diseases but has been shown to be reliable and valid in a number of different populations of patients with cancer.[173] Another comprehensive multidimensional (sensory, affective, cognitive, behavioral, sociocultural) tool is the Brief Pain Inventory (BPI), developed initially for assessing pain in general but used fairly extensively for cancer pain.[163,173] Recent research suggests that the BPI is a good tool for use in low-income blacks.[179-181] There are also several multidimensional tools that are short and

easy to administer. For example, Melzack developed the short-form version of the MPQ[182] to assess sensory (including intensity and quality) and affective dimensions of pain; the BPI also exists in a short version.[113] Additional multidimensional methods for assessing pain have been developed to assist nurses in making both baseline and ongoing assessments, taking the form of comprehensive questionnaires and flow sheets.[138,171,172] Use of diaries to record pain at home is becoming more common, as is an emphasis on assessing functional status as it relates to pain.[172,183] Finally, clinicians and researchers have recently begun to recognize the importance of interactions between pain and other symptoms such as fatigue, sleep, and psychological distress.[184-187] Some symptoms, such as pain, fatigue, emotional distress, and sleep alterations, appear to be associated with one another in patients with cancer-related pain.[184,187] Recent studies indicate that patients with cancer often suffer not only from pain but from numerous other symptoms. The most commonly observed symptoms are fatigue, weakness, lack of energy, worrying or feeling sad, and feeling drowsy or having difficulty sleeping.[185,186] These clinical observations have resulted in attempts to construct new multidimensional tools to assess common cancer-related symptoms simultaneously, including pain. The Memorial Symptom Assessment Scale (MSAS), for example, is designed to collect information about the prevalence, characteristics, and distress of 32 common symptoms, including pain.[188] The MSAS has good preliminary evidence of reliability and validity, and may be useful to nurses wishing to perform a comprehensive symptom assessment.

The choice of tools for assessing pain depends on several considerations.[169] Of foremost concern are the dimensions of pain that are most relevant in a given situation. For example, the behavioral dimension assumes primary importance in an adult patient with cancer experiencing acute confusion or cognitive failure,[189,190] whereas the sensory and affective dimensions may predominate in an alert and oriented postoperative patient. The tool selected should be able to assess the relevant parameters of the dimension(s) of interest. The purpose of the assessment (i.e., baseline versus ongoing) is a second major consideration. In general, baseline assessments will require a more detailed and comprehensive tool, while ongoing assessments can use brief, simple tools.

Another consideration relates to the pain interventions being used. Effects of treatments aimed at the physiological and sensory dimensions (e.g., analgesics) should be evaluated by assessing parameters such as location, intensity, and quality. Treatments aimed at the cognitive, affective, and behavioral dimensions (e.g., distraction and relaxation) should be evaluated using tools assessing parameters of those dimensions (see Table 28-4). Still another important area relates to specific patient and setting factors, such as age, cognitive abilities, type of pain, level of acuity, physical function, literacy and language issues, personal preference, and type of clinical setting (inpatient, outpatient, home, hospice). Some of these patient-related factors may influence whether the tools selected are subjective (patient self-report) or objective (observational) in nature.

Finally, issues related to time, feasibility, and relevance to the clinical setting are a major consideration. Important considerations include the amount of time required to complete tools, format and amount of writing, overlap with existing documentation, relevance of parameters to setting and to clinicians, personal comfort and preference, and lines of responsibility and accountability.

Problem identification and documentation

The outcome of a thorough baseline assessment of the patient with cancer-related pain should be identification of problems that structure the design and implementation of the management plan. McCaffery and Beebe cited 18 nursing diagnoses that the nurse should consider as part of the assessment process: anxiety, constipation, ineffective individual coping, diversional activity deficit, fatigue, fear, knowledge deficit (specify), impaired physical mobility, powerlessness, feeding self-care deficit, bathing/hygiene self-care deficit, dressing/grooming self-care deficit, toileting self-care deficit, sexual dysfunction, sleep pattern disturbance, social isolation, spiritual distress (distress of the human spirit), and altered thought processes.[191] Carpenito's text on nursing diagnoses includes such relevant diagnoses as activity intolerance, anxiety, constipation, family coping, fatigue, and fear, among many others.[192] The inclusion of *all* relevant clinical problems and nursing diagnoses will emphasize the need for multiple disciplines being involved in using multiple interventions for pain.

Of critical importance is the need for nurses to document their assessment in a manner appropriate for their clinical settings. The APS quality improvement standards[130] recommended the documentation of pain intensity and pain relief on standard patient records, such as the vital sign sheet or patient flow sheet. Similarly, the AHCPR guidelines on cancer pain management[116] suggested incorporation of assessment data into routine institutional records. The use of standardized pain assessment and documentation appears to have a positive impact on pain intensity and to facilitate management of pain.[138,161,193,194]

Incorporation into Practice and Evaluation of Outcomes

Successful management of cancer pain will ultimately depend on the extent to which systematic processes, tools, documentation procedures, and lines of formal accountability and responsibility for pain management are incorporated into institutional settings. The ONS position paper on cancer pain management,[1] as mentioned previously, places the coordination of pain management squarely on the oncology nurse. Several creative programs for helping oncology nurses assume this role were noted

earlier.[157–160] The AHCPR cancer pain guidelines[116] provide a useful framework for incorporating sound pain assessment and management principles into clinical practice. Similarly, the use of components of the APS performance improvement standards,[113] such as assessment of patient satisfaction with pain management, can give clues to approaches that are working or that need improvement.[195] Strong institutionally supported programs for incorporating pain management into ongoing quality improvement mechanisms, such as the one described by Bookbinder et al,[161] have been successful in decreasing pain problems. Implementation of any effort to positively affect pain management must of necessity include evaluation of outcomes.[196,197] Recent work by a variety of authors has addressed mechanisms for assessing outcomes, both subjective patient reports and objective measures, and has emphasized the importance of continually evaluating outcomes in order to assure adequate pain management.[198–200]

Special Populations

Because cancer is a group of diseases that affects individuals across the life span, the pain associated with it likewise occurs in groups of varying age, background, and clinical characteristics. Several populations—the elderly, individuals with substance abuse history, individuals with diverse sociocultural backgrounds, and the terminally ill—require special consideration in the areas of pain assessment and management.

The elderly

The elderly population in the United States (individuals aged 65 and older) more than doubled between 1950 and 1980 (from 12.3 million to 25.5 million), and one projection for the year 2030 is that the elderly population will increase to 64.3 million people.[201] As this population increases in number, one would expect to see a corresponding increase in the incidence of cancer and cancer-related deaths. Current American Cancer Society statistics indicate that for the five leading cancer sites, 51% of cancer deaths are in individuals between ages 55 and 74, and 37% are in individuals aged 75 or older.[202]

The problem of cancer pain in elderly patients with cancer has been grossly neglected,[203–205] and prevalence surveys of pain are lacking. Ferrell reviewed 11 geriatric medicine textbooks and found only 2 with chapters on pain in the elderly, with negligible content about cancer-related pain.[206]

A misconception that lay individuals have about pain among the elderly is that pain is a normal sequela of aging. As a result of this belief, elderly patients may not report pain as a problem since it is considered "normal." In one study of "younger" elderly versus "older" elderly, there was a trend for the older elderly to report pain less often.[207] Similarly, if health care professionals are told about pain by elderly patients, they may dismiss the complaint as insignificant since pain becomes a manifestation of the aging process. While it may be true that people develop more chronic diseases as they age,[208] the experience of pain does not need to be an expectation.

The normal process of aging creates unique problems in the management of cancer pain, especially as related to assessment. Ferrell et al found that 71% of patients in a long-term care facility had pain and an average of five chronic medical conditions.[209] With the prevalence of more chronic diseases, there potentially will exist multiple causes of the same complaint. The elderly experience greater alterations in the musculoskeletal system and are more vulnerable to acute and soft-tissue pain.[210] Chronic problems such as arthritis, degenerative disk disease, osteoporosis, and peripheral neuropathy may confuse the pain problem for individuals who also have cancer-related pain.

Another unique problem is that the elderly may experience significant sensory and cognitive impairment.[191,204,210–212] The symptoms associated with these potential impairments alert the health care professional to be especially astute in obtaining a careful, detailed pain history.[191,204,210] The risk of historical inadequacies through the underreporting of symptoms, memory deficits, and concomitant depression-related symptomatology may lead to an inaccurate pain diagnosis and inappropriate treatment. A very important piece of assessment data to obtain in the elderly is any change from baseline behaviors, usual routines, and social interactions. A gradual loss of physical health, changes in family structure, limited economic resources, and a loss of social status can greatly influence a patient's quality of life and, therefore, the problem of pain.[191,213,214]

Still another major unique problem is the issue of the sensitivity of elderly patients to both perception of pain and sensitivity to pharmacological interventions. The literature about perceptual sensitivity reveals contradictions. Bayer et al reviewed symptoms of acute myocardial infarction in elderly patients and found that chest pain was reported less frequently than other symptoms, especially by patients over 85 years old.[215] They proposed several explanations to account for this finding: higher pain threshold, autonomic dysfunction, or cortical failure from neurological disease. In a review of the relationship between age and experimentally induced pain, Harkins et al found no major age differences in pain sensitivity but noted that interindividual changes in pain sensitivity may have accounted for some differences.[213] Similarly, Bressler et al found no statistically significant differences in reports of pain intensity in cancer outpatients under versus over 60 years of age.[38]

The final issue relevant to pain in the elderly follows naturally from the issues already discussed. If assessment of cancer pain in the elderly is complicated by the possibility of multiple causative factors, sensory and cognitive impairment, differences in sensitivity, and pain relief because of normal physiological aging, does this population of patients receive adequate analgesic management? A study of 13,625 patients in nursing homes found that

4003 of these patients reported daily pain.[216] Only 26% of the patients received morphine, and 26% of the patients who reported daily pain received no analgesia. Independent predictors of failing to receive analgesic agents were minority race, low cognitive performance, and the number of other medications being administered. Several reports indicate that the elderly have fewer opioids prescribed for them than younger patients.[204,205,217,218] Portenoy et al raised a very important issue in this regard: If the elderly perceive pain less often, indicating a lower prevalence of pain, then less frequent prescribing of analgesics is appropriate.[203] If, however, the elderly experience pain similar to the younger population of patients and choose not to report the pain, or respond more slowly to painful stimuli, indicating a higher prevalence of pain, then underprescribing creates needless suffering. As in other areas related to cancer pain, more well-controlled, epidemiological studies of the prevalence of pain in the elderly are needed to help delineate the scope of the problem in this vulnerable population and to assist in answering questions about appropriate management.

In summary, the problem of cancer pain in the elderly population is an important one. As individuals enter the later stages of life, the risk of developing cancer increases, and thus the risk of cancer pain increases. Specific attention to the unique physiological, pharmacological, psychological, and sociological issues for these individuals is crucial for appropriate, successful management of cancer pain.

Substance abuse history

The national problem of drug abuse creates challenges for health care professionals when pain and substance abuse occur simultaneously. Comptom identified specific management strategies in dealing with patients with active addiction.[219] The first step in treating a patient with a current or past history of addiction is for the clinician to acknowledge his or her personal biases and make a conscious effort to put those biases aside. General guidelines for these patients include openly discussing the patient's addiction and encouraging the patient to express fears of how this may affect treatment, accept and act on the patient's report of pain with appropriate assessment and treatment, develop a treatment plan and if feasible give the patient a written copy, consult an addiction specialist and a pain specialist if available, begin with nondrug or nonopioid analgesia but if pain relief is inadequate use opioids, and assess the patient's motivation for drug treatment and have referral references available. For patients in the inpatient setting, consider using intravenous patient-controlled analgesia to give the patient more control and reduce potential confrontations with the staff. For patients in the outpatient setting, if opioid analgesics are required, select long-acting formulations such as transdermal fentanyl or controlled-release morphine.

With all patients having any previous or current substance abuse history, it is important that an adversarial relationship not begin or escalate between patient and staff. As with any other patient, the substance abuse patient's report of pain should not be questioned or doubted.[191] Appropriate medications should not be withheld as a form of punishment,[191] and pain relief should not become a bargaining tool.[220] Communication among all members of the health team, including the patient, about how pain will be managed should be instituted early in the course of contact with the patient. Sometimes a contract may be useful for establishing realistic goals between the health care provider and the patient. Regularly scheduled meetings to review the goals of care may avoid unnecessary conflict. In order to provide a consistent approach to management, several authors recommend having only one physician assume responsibility for writing all opioid orders and, likewise, one nurse assume responsibility for coordinating nursing care.[220-222] The assistance of professionals experienced in substance abuse, analgesic management, and cognitive-behavioral approaches to pain may be helpful in developing a successful plan of care.

Individuals with a substance abuse history may require much higher doses of opioids for pain because of tolerance.[221] When a patient reports increasing pain that requires higher doses of opioids, the clinician should focus on the changing pain pattern as the reason for the need for more opioids and *not* on "drug seeking behavior." Twycross recommended changing a patient from parenteral analgesics to oral or rectal routes so that the association between street drugs and pain relief is not present.[34] Regardless of any history of substance abuse, the patient is entitled to receive reasonable, adequate care for a concomitant cancer pain problem. Obstacles to achieving this goal need to be discussed, examined, and resolved to ensure pain relief.

Culturally diverse populations

Nurses' assessment and management of individuals with cancer pain can be influenced by a number of factors, ranging from attitudes, beliefs, and personal history of pain to stereotypical notions about how people of specific ethnocultural backgrounds respond to pain.[72] As the racial and cultural diversity of the United States increases, more and more nurses find themselves caring for patients of ethnocultural backgrounds different from their own. The notion of "cultural competence" has come to the forefront of clinical practice and is exceedingly important in relation to pain assessment and management.[223] In this section, approaches for dealing with culturally diverse patient populations are discussed.

According to Donnelly and Sutterley, the American health care system's philosophies have their roots in white, middle-class values and beliefs.[224] That is, in the American system of health care, provision frequently is not made for acknowledging the individual's ethnocultural perspective, let alone understanding or using it in planning health care interventions. There is a tendency

on the part of nurses and other health care providers to become ethnocentric—that is, to believe that their own health practices are superior to those of others.[225] Because nurses espouse the notion of holistic care tailored to individuals' unique and specific needs, the idea of not only accepting but incorporating cultural diversity into plans for care is essential to achieving truly holistic care.

Different ethnic groups express pain and suffering differently.[62,226] The nurse's interpretation of individuals' behaviors and verbalizations related to pain should be based on knowledge of how the patients' culture views responses to pain.[62,225] Respect for cultures other than one's own and for the fact that people have specific beliefs and behaviors that emanate from their cultural background is known as *cultural sensitivity.*

Although providing nursing care for people who are culturally diverse can be extremely challenging, the nurse's commitment to delivering total care and supporting an individual's integrity and dignity can be exemplified by learning as much as possible about the individual's ethnocultural background and its influences on health and illness beliefs and behaviors.[227] Several authors have made recommendations that should be useful to nurses caring for individuals of culturally diverse backgrounds. Fong discussed the importance of developing rapport as the foundation of successful nursing interventions.[225] She urged the use of good manners, maintaining a broad and open attitude, and maintaining flexibility. Kagawa-Singer highlighted the importance of developing good communication with patients and their family, followed by facilitation of their integrating the disease process and its treatment into their lives.[227] A key principle is the use of negotiation to achieve feasible treatment plans and to enlist the patient's and family's participation in reaching treatment goals. These recommendations are generically useful and include identification and achievement of mutual goals, compromise and integration of different health care practices into the care plan, identification and discussion of nursing interventions with patient and family, stressing the importance of health education, use of vital teaching materials if language is a problem, and seeking additional information and assistance from cultural organizations and resources when necessary.

Although little has been written specifically on dealing with cancer pain in individuals of different cultural backgrounds, Fink and Gates provided an excellent review.[62] They discuss variables related to culture and pain, for example, the meaning of pain, gender, age, living and working environments, social class, religion, language, and level of assimilation and acculturation. Finally, in patients who are culturally different from their caregivers, as well as in those who are similar, the area of spirituality is important. This construct is beginning to receive more attention, particularly as it relates to cultural differences, the nursing process, chronic illness, and dying.[228] Of special note are Jacik's work on the spiritual care of the dying adult[229] and Johnston Taylor and Ersek's work on the ethical and spiritual dimensions of cancer pain management.[230]

Palliative and terminal care

Twycross wrote in 1987 that "the aim of terminal care is to help the patient, despite the cancer and increasing physical limitations, to go on having a good quality of life until he dies."[231,p.173] Wanzer et al described the physician's responsibility toward dying individuals, emphasizing the "art of deliberately creating a medical environment that allows a peaceful death."[232,p.846] The parallel for nursing is obvious—the nurse must practice the art of creating a nursing environment that allows a peaceful death.

In recent years, this approach has evolved into the multidisciplinary specialty of palliative care. Philosophical, organizational, and practical aspects of providing palliative care to terminally ill individuals with cancer pain have been described for inpatient and home hospice settings,[229,233-237] the home care setting,[34,238] extended care facilities,[239] and general inpatient and cancer settings.[166,240-242] Several key aspects of caring for these individuals exist, regardless of setting, and need to be considered by nurses who are involved in palliative care.

The focus of terminal care is on relief of pain and other symptoms and on psychological support of both the patient and the family. Teamwork is requisite to the success of these efforts. Death often is accompanied by great fear, a normal human response that is part of the survival instinct.[230] In the care of terminal illness, not only are the dying afraid of death, but the living are as well. Withdrawal from those who are dying is a common reaction, yet remaining with the individual is one of the most important aspects of terminal care. Jacik wrote: "Human presence is a priceless source of comfort to dying persons."[229,p.267] For those dying with pain, the knowledge that health care providers and others are not only present but continually focusing on relieving the pain serves as a great comfort.

Related to continual efforts at relieving pain are the issues of assessment and treatment, particularly when pain worsens or new pain appears. The goal of minimizing pain and increasing comfort in the terminally ill individual must not obstruct the normal response to complaints of pain or restrict the range of interventions that might be considered or attempted. There is no reason why terminally ill people with worsening or new symptoms of pain should be evaluated, diagnosed, and treated any differently than nonterminally ill individuals with cancer pain. For example, the development of new and painful metastatic lesions of the bone in a home hospice patient should not preclude use of radiation therapy if appropriate, even if it means that the patient must be moved. The goal is increased comfort, and all possible means to achieve it should be considered.

A flexible and adjustable care plan to meet the patient's changing needs as the disease progresses is essential.[232] Research indicates that pain and other symptoms during the last 4 weeks of life assume tremendous variability.[243] Tailoring of palliative care to meet these diverse needs involves the use of multiple interventions, including pharmacological therapies, and the expertise to use these interventions properly. Often there is inadequate knowledge of pharmacokinetics, neurology, and medical oncology.[244] Similarly, underutilization of opioids and adjuvant drugs can erode patients' confidence in the medical system and bring their dying into sharper focus. The WHO guidelines for cancer pain relief have been applied successfully to terminal cancer patients with pain.[245] Nonpharmacological, noninvasive interventions for pain are also appropriate in the terminal cancer patient.

Recent research has indicated the importance of addressing family factors that influence pain management, as well as the burdens with which home caregivers must deal with.[87-89] As with all areas of health care, the cost aspects of palliative cancer care are being closely scrutinized.[246] Hospice care is often viewed as less expensive, but data does not support this. The analysis of this issue is difficult because some of the savings may be related to home care where cost shifting occurs. Family members may be paying out-of-pocket costs and providing labor and losing wages due to time out of work.[246] These activities, the ongoing need for assessment of pain, coordination of pain management, and support of the family members are well within the scope of practice for oncology nurses engaged in palliative care.

The current issues of suicidal ideation or actual suicide in persons with progressive cancer accompanied by severe pain has been followed closely by those working in palliative care.[247-250] Foley reviewed the issues surrounding patients' requests for physician-assisted suicide as an option in the face of uncontrolled pain and multiple other adverse symptoms.[251] She commented that physicians are not adequately trained to care for dying patients and, furthermore, are deterred from appropriate terminal care by economic considerations. She urged improved physician-patient communication, patient-centered care, better judgments about when to withhold or withdraw care, and familiarity with concepts of palliative care as ways to reduce physician-assisted suicide and euthanasia. Breitbart described specific factors that may make patients more likely to engage in suicidal ideation: pain and suffering, advanced disease with poor prognosis, depression and hopelessness, delirium, loss of control, preexisting psychopathology, prior family or personal history of suicide, and exhaustion or fatigue.[252]

Coyle has addressed the role of nursing in relation to current debates about euthanasia and physician-assisted suicide in patients with terminal cancer.[253] She emphasized the need for nurses to understand the issues surrounding these debates, including specific definitions, ethical principles underlying positions for or against euthanasia, and the positions of professional and global health organizations. She indicated that nurses also needed to understand the factors just cited that may make patients more vulnerable to considering suicide as an option, and to use all resources at their disposal to derive appropriate and individualized management plans for such individuals. Also useful when dealing with pain management and the dying are the discussions presented by

Hammes and Cain.[254,255] Through the use of case studies, they review the ethics of pain management in regards to respecting patient wishes and present some excellent case studies in an effort to strengthen clinical judgment in difficult cases.

Conclusion

When caring for special populations with cancer pain, a number of basic principles and special considerations need to be employed by nurses. Foremost is the need for an interdisciplinary approach. Exceedingly important as well, however, are a thorough understanding of the scope of nursing practice; accurate assessment and diagnosis; appropriate attention to developmental, clinical, and cultural issues; and knowledge about palliative care. Awareness and use of the information just presented will help nurses to identify and assess cancer pain and to plan, implement, coordinate, and evaluate its interdisciplinary management.[1] Specific approaches to the management of cancer pain are presented in the next chapter.

References

1. Oncology Nursing Society: Cancer pain management. *Oncol Nurs Forum* 25:817–818, 1998
2. International Association for the Study of Pain Subcommittee on Taxonomy: Pain terms: A list with definitions and usage. *Pain* 6:249–252, 1979
3. International Association for the Study of Pain: Pain terms: A current list with definitions and notes on usage. *Pain* 3: S216–S221, 1986 (suppl)
4. Task Force on Taxonomy: *Classification of Chronic Pain: Descriptions of Chronic Pain Syndromes and Definitions of Terms* (ed 2). Seattle, International Association for the Study of Pain Press, 1994
5. Rollin BE: Some conceptual and ethical concerns about current views of pain. *Pain Forum* 8:78–83, 1999
6. Bonica JJ: Definitions and taxonomy of pain, in Bonica JJ (ed): *The Management of Pain*, vol 1 (ed 2). Philadelphia, Lea & Febiger, 1990, pp 18–27
7. International Association for the Study of Pain Task Force on Acute Pain. *Management of Acute Pain: A Practical Guide.* Seattle, International Association for the Study of Pain Press, 1992
8. Novy DM, Nelson DV, Francis DJ, et al: Perspectives of chronic pain: An evaluative comparison of restrictive and comprehensive models. *Psychol Bull* 118:238–247, 1995
9. Melzack R, Wall PD: Pain mechanisms: A new theory. *Science* 150:971–979, 1965
10. Melzack R: Pain: Past, present, and future. *Can J Exp Psychol* 47:615–629, 1993
11. Fields HL: *Pain.* New York, McGraw-Hill, 1987
12. Wilkie DJ: Neural mechanisms of pain: A foundation for cancer pain assessment and management, in McGuire DB, Yarbro CH, Ferrell BR (eds): *Cancer Pain Management* (ed 2). Sudbury, MA, Jones and Bartlett, 1995, pp 61–87
13. Wall PD, Melzack R: *Textbook of Pain* (ed 3). New York, Churchill Livingstone, 1994
14. Ahles TA, Blanchard EB, Ruckdeschel JC: The multidimensional nature of cancer-related pain. *Pain* 17:277–288, 1983
15. McGuire DB: Cancer-related pain: A multidimensional approach. *Dissert Abstr Int* 48(03), Sec B:705, 1987
16. McGuire DB: Coping strategies used by cancer patients with pain. *Oncol Nurs Forum* 14:123, 1987 (abstr)
17. McGuire DB: The multiple dimensions of cancer pain: A framework for assessment and management, in McGuire DB, Yarbro CH, Ferrell BR (eds): *Cancer Pain Management* (ed 2). Sudbury, MA, Jones and Bartlett, 1995, pp 1–17
18. NINR Priority Expert Panel on Symptom Management: Acute Pain: *Symptom Management: Acute Pain*, vol 6. NIH publication No. 94-2421. Bethesda, MD, National Institute of Nursing Research, U.S. Department of Health and Human Services, U.S. Public Health Service, National Institutes of Health, 1994
19. Foley KN: Pain syndromes in patients with cancer, in Bonica JJ, Ventafridda V (eds): *Advances in Pain Research and Therapy*, vol 2. New York, Raven Press, 1979, pp 59–75
20. Gaston-Johansson F, Franco T, Zimmerman L: Pain and psychological distress in patients undergoing autologous bone marrow transplantation. *Oncol Nurs Forum* 19:41–48, 1992
21. McGuire DB, Altomonte V, Peterson DE, et al: Patterns of mucositis and pain in patients receiving preparative chemotherapy and bone marrow transplantation. *Oncol Nurs Forum* 20:1493–1502, 1993
22. Yeager KA, McGuire DB, De Loney V: Profiles of pain in bone marrow/stem cell transplant and leukemia patients. *Oncol Nurs Forum* 26:358, 1999 (abstr)
23. Portenoy RK: Cancer pain: Epidemiology and syndromes. *Cancer* 63:2298–2307, 1989
24. Payne R: Cancer pain: Anatomy, physiology, and pharmacology. *Cancer* 63:2266–2274, 1989
25. Kelly JB, Payne R: Pain syndromes in the cancer patient. *Neurol Clin* 9:937–953, 1991
26. Banning A, Sjogren P, Henriksen H: Pain causes in 200 patients referred to a multidisciplinary cancer pain clinic. *Pain* 45:45–48, 1991
27. Samuelsson H, Hedner T: Pain characterization in cancer patients and the analgetic response to epidural morphine. *Pain* 46:3–8, 1991
28. Caraceni A: Clinicopathologic correlates of common cancer pain syndromes. *Hematol Oncol Clin North Am* 10:57–78, 1996
29. Portenoy RK, Payne D, Jacobsen P: Breakthrough pain: Characteristics and impact in patients with cancer pain. *Pain* 81:129–134, 1999
30. Petzke F, Radbruch L, Zech D, et al: Temporal presentation of chronic cancer pain: Transitory pains on admission to a multidisciplinary pain clinic. *J Pain Symptom Manage* 17: 391–401, 1999
31. Arathuzik D: Pain experience for metastatic breast cancer patients. *Cancer Nurs* 14:41–48, 1991
32. Donovan MI, Dillon P: Incidence and characteristics of pain in a sample of hospitalized cancer patients. *Cancer Nurs* 10:85–92, 1987
33. Twycross RG, Fairfield S: Pain in far-advanced cancer. *Pain* 14:303–310, 1982
34. Twycross R: *Pain Relief in Advanced Cancer.* Edinburgh, Churchill Livingstone, 1994
35. Berry DL, Wilkie DJ, Huang H, et al: Cancer pain and

common pain: A comparison of patient-reported intensities. *Oncol Nurs Forum* 26:721–726, 1999

36. Melzack R, Torgerson WS: On the language of pain. *Anesthesiology* 34:50–59, 1971

37. Dubuisson D, Melzack R: Classification of clinical pain descriptions by multiple group discriminant analysis. *Exp Neurol* 51:480–487, 1976

38. Bressler LR, Hange PA, McGuire DB: Characterization of the pain experience in a sample of cancer outpatients. *Oncol Nurs Forum* 13:51–55, 1986

39. Zimmerman L, Duncan K, Pozehl B, et al: Pain descriptors used by patients with cancer. *Oncol Nurs Forum* 14:67–71, 1987

40. Padilla GV, Ferrell B, Grant MM, et al: Defining the content domain of quality of life for cancer patients with pain. *Cancer Nurs* 13:108–115, 1990

41. Dalton JA, Feuerstein M: Biobehavioral factors in cancer pain. *Pain* 33:137–147, 1988

42. McGuire DB, Sheidler VR: Pain, in Groenwald SL, Frogge MH, Goodman M, Yarbro CH (eds): *Cancer Nursing: Principles and Practice* (ed 2). Sudbury, MA, Jones and Bartlett, 1990, pp 385–441

43. Spiegel D, Sands S, Koopman C: Pain and depression in patients with cancer. *Cancer* 74:2570–2578, 1994

44. Spiegel D, Bloom J: Pain in metastatic breast cancer. *Cancer* 52:341–345, 1983

45. Barkwell DP: Ascribed meaning: A critical factor in coping and pain attenuation in patients with cancer-related pain. *J Palliat Care* 7:5–14, 1991

46. Ferrell BR, Dean G: The meaning of cancer pain. *Semin Oncol Nurs* 11:17–22, 1995

47. Bruera E, Macmillan K, Hanson J, et al: The cognitive effects of the administration of narcotic analgesics in patients with cancer pain. *Pain* 39:13–16, 1989

48. Sjogren P, Banning A: Pain, sedation and reaction time during long-term treatment of cancer patients with oral and epidural opioids. *Pain* 39:5–11, 1989

49. Wilkie DJ, Keefe FJ: Coping strategies of patients with lung cancer-related pain. *Clin J Pain* 7:292–299, 1991

50. Arathuzik D: The appraisal of pain and coping in cancer patients. *West J Nurs Res* 13:714–731, 1991

51. Francke AL, Theeuwen I: Inhibition in expressing pain: A qualitative study among Dutch breast cancer patients. *Cancer Nurs* 17:193–199, 1994

52. Keefe FJ, Brantley A, Manuel G, et al: Behavioral assessment of head and neck cancer pain. *Pain* 23:327–336, 1985

53. Donovan MI: Nursing assessment of cancer pain. *Semin Oncol Nurs* 1:109–115, 1985

54. Barbour LA, McGuire DB, Kirchhoff KT: Non-analgesic methods of pain control used by cancer outpatients. *Oncol Nurs Forum* 13:56–60, 1986

55. Wilkie D, Lovejoy N, Dodd M, et al: Cancer pain control behaviors: Description and correlation with pain intensity. *Oncol Nurs Forum* 15:723–731, 1988

56. McGuire DB: Assessment of pain in cancer inpatients using the McGill Pain Questionnaire. *Oncol Nurs Forum* 11:32–37, 1984

57. Greenwald HP: Interethnic differences in pain perception. *Pain* 44:157–163, 1991

58. McMillan S: The relationship between age and intensity of cancer-related symptoms. *Oncol Nurs Forum* 16:237–241, 1989

59. Ferrell BA, Ferrell BR: The experience of pain and quality of life in elderly patients. *Gerontology* 28:76A, 1988 (suppl)

60. Vigano A, Bruera E, Suarez-Almazor ME: Age, pain intensity, and opioid dose in patients with advanced cancer. *Cancer* 83:1244–1250, 1998

61. Cleeland CS, Gonin R, Hatfield AK, et al: Pain and its treatment in outpatients with metastatic cancer. *N Engl J Med* 330:592–596, 1994

62. Fink RS, Gates R: Cultural diversity and cancer pain, in McGuire DB, Yarbro CH, Ferrell BR (eds): *Cancer Pain Management* (ed 2). Sudbury, MA, Jones and Bartlett, 1995, pp 19–39

63. Yeager KA, Miaskowski C, Dibble SL, et al: Differences in pain knowledge and perception of the pain experience between outpatients with cancer and their family caregivers. *Oncol Nurs Forum* 22:1235–1241, 1995

64. Miaskowski C, Zimmer EF, Barrett KM, et al: Differences in patients' and family caregivers' perceptions of the pain experience influence patient and caregiver outcomes. *Pain* 72:217–226, 1997

65. Bucher JA, Trostle GB, Moore M: Family reports of cancer pain, pain relief, and prescription access. *Cancer Pract* 7: 71–77, 1999

66. Elliott VA, Elliott TE, Murray DM, et al: Patients and family members: The role of knowledge and attitudes in cancer pain. *J Pain Symptom Manage* 12:209–220, 1996

67. Ferrell BR: Patient and family caregiver perspectives. *Oncology* 13(suppl 2) 5:15–19, 1999

68. Glajchen M, Fitzmartin RD, Blum D, Swanton R: Psychosocial barriers to cancer pain relief. *Cancer Pract* 3:76–82, 1995

69. Lancee WJ, Vachon MLS, Ghadirian P, et al: The impact of pain and impaired role performance on distress in persons with cancer. *Can J Psychiatry* 39:617–622, 1994

70. Williamson GM, Schulz R: Activity restriction mediates the association between pain and depressed affect: A study of younger and older adult cancer patients. *Psychol Aging* 10: 369–378, 1995

71. Coyle N, Foley K: Prevalence and profile of pain syndromes in cancer patients, in McGuire DB, Yarbro CH (eds): *Cancer Pain Management*. Philadelphia, Saunders, 1987, pp 21–46

72. McGuire DB, Sheidler VR: Pain, in Groenwald SL, Frogge MH, Goodman M, Yarbro CH (eds): *Cancer Nursing: Principles and Practice* (ed 4). Sudbury, MA, Jones and Bartlett, 1997, pp 529–584

73. Grond S, Zech D, Diefenbach C, et al: Assessment of pain: A prospective evaluation in 2266 cancer patients referred to a pain service. *Pain* 64:107–114, 1996

74. Cleeland CS: The impact of pain on the patient with cancer. *Cancer* 54:2635–2641, 1984

75. Twycross R, Harcourt J, Bergl S: A survey of pain in patients with advanced cancer. *J Pain Symptom Manage* 12:273–282, 1996

76. Miaskowski C, Dibble SL: The problem of pain in outpatients with breast cancer. *Oncol Nurs Forum* 22:791–797, 1995

77. Stevens PE, Dibble SL, Miaskowski C: Prevalence, characteristics, and impact of postmastectomy pain syndrome: An investigation of women's experiences. *Pain* 61:61–68, 1995

78. Pederson C, Paran L: Pain and distress in adult and children undergoing peripheral blood stem cell or bone marrow transplant. *Oncol Nurs Forum* 26:575–582, 1999

79. Nielsen B, Miaskowski C, Dibble SL: Pain with mammography: Fact or fiction? *Oncol Nurs Forum* 20:639–642, 1993

80. Ferrell BR, Schneider C: Experience and management of cancer pain at home. *Cancer Nurs* 11:84–90, 1988

81. Norvell K, Zimmerman L: Psychological variables, and cancer pain. *Oncol Nurs Forum* 16:160, 1989 (suppl)

82. Ferrell BR, Wisdom C, Wenzl C: Quality of life as an outcome variable in the management of cancer pain. *Cancer* 63:2321–2327, 1989

83. Ferrell B, Wisdom C, Wenzl C, et al: Effects of controlled release morphine on QOL for cancer pain. *Oncol Nurs Forum* 16:521–526, 1989

84. Strang P, Qvarner H: Cancer-related pain and its influence on quality of life. *Anticancer Res* 10:109–112, 1990

85. Ferrell BR, Grant M, Padilla G, et al: The experience of pain and perceptions of quality of life: Validation of a conceptual model. *Hosp J* 7:9–24, 1991

86. Ferrell BR: The quality of lives: 1,525 voices of cancer. *Oncol Nurs Forum* 23:907–916, 1996

87. Ferrell BR, Rhiner M, Cohen MZ, et al: Pain as a metaphor for illness: Part I. Impact of cancer pain on family caregivers. *Oncol Nurs Forum* 18:1303–1309, 1991

88. Ferrell BR, Cohen MZ, Rhiner M, et al: Pain as a metaphor for illness: Part II. Family caregivers' management of pain. *Oncol Nurs Forum* 18:1315–1321, 1991

89. Ferrell BR, Ferrell BA, Rhiner M, et al: Family factors influencing cancer pain management. *Postgrad Med J* 67: S64–S69, 1991 (suppl)

90. Kurtz ME, Kurtz JC, Given CC, et al: Concordance of cancer patient and caregiver symptom reports. *Cancer Pract* 4: 185–190, 1996

91. Ishay R: High technology in medicine: Ethical aspects. *Isr J Med Sci* 25:274–278, 1989

92. Ferrell BR, Rhiner M: High-tech comfort: Ethical issues in cancer pain management for the 1990s. *J Clin Ethics* 2: 108–112, 1991

93. Whedon M, Ferrell BR: Professional and ethical considerations in the use of high-tech pain management. *Oncol Nurs Forum* 18:1135–1143, 1991

94. Ropchan R, Ferrell BR, Grant M, et al: Pain management as a nursing administration concern. *Oncol Nurs Forum* 19: 317, 1992 (abstr)

95. Bruner DW: Cost-effectiveness and palliative care. *Semin Oncol Nurs* 14:164–167, 1998

96. Angarola RT, Donato BJ: Inappropriate pain management results in high jury award. *J Pain Symptom Manage* 6:407, 1991

97. Cushing M: The legal side: Pain management on trial. *Am J Nurs* 92:21–22, 1992

98. Angarola RT, Joranson DE: Healthcare reimbursement policies: Do they block acute and cancer pain management? *APS Bull* 4:7–9, 1994

99. Joranson DE: Are health-care reimbursement policies a barrier to acute and cancer pain management? *J Pain Symptom Manage* 9:244–253, 1994

100. Ferrell BR, Griffith H: Cost issues related to pain management: Reports from the cancer pain panel of the Agency for Health Care Policy and Research. *J Pain Symptom Manage* 9:221–234, 1994

101. Steig RL, Lippe P, Shepard TA: Roadblocks to effective pain treatment. *Med Clin North Am* 83:809–821, 1999

102. Oncology Nursing Society: Position Paper on Quality Cancer Care. *Oncol Nurs Forum* 24:951–953, 1997

103. Simmons WJ, Goforth L: The impact of managed care on cancer care: Review and recommendations. *Cancer Pract* 5: 111–118, 1997

104. Angarola RT, Wray SD: Legal impediments to cancer pain treatment, in Hill CS, Fields WS (eds): *Advances in Pain Research and Therapy,* vol 11. New York, Raven Press, 1989, pp 213–231

105. Portenoy RK: The effect of drug regulation on the management of cancer pain. *NY State Med J* 91:13S–18S, 1991

106. Joranson DE, Gilson AM: Regulatory barriers to pain management. *Semin Oncol Nurs* 14:158–163, 1998

107. Angarola RT, Bormel FG: Proposed legislative changes and access to pain medications. *APS Bull* 6:8–9, 1996

108. Joranson DE: State pain commissions: New vehicle for progress? *APS Bull* 6:7–9, 1996

109. Spross JA: Cancer pain relief: An international perspective. *Oncol Nurs Forum* 19:5–11, 1992 (suppl)

110. National Institute of Nursing Research: Symptom Management: Acute Pain RFA: NR-94-003. *NIH Guide* 23, 1994

111. World Health Organization: *Cancer Pain Relief* (ed 2). Geneva, World Health Organization, 1996

112. National Institutes of Health: The integrated approach to the management of pain. *NIH Consensus Development Conference Statement* 6, 1986

113. Anonymous: American Pain Society Quality of Care Committee: Quality improvement guidelines for the treatment of acute pain and cancer pain. *JAMA* 274:1874–1880, 1995

114. American Pain Society: *Principles of Analgesic Use in the Treatment of Acute Pain and Cancer Pain* (ed 4). Skokie, IL, APS, 1998

115. Ad Hoc Committee on Cancer Pain of the American Society of Clinical Oncology: Cancer pain assessment and treatment curriculum guidelines. *J Clin Oncol* 10:1976–1982, 1992

116. Jacox A, Carr DB, Payne R, et al: *Management of Cancer Pain: Clinical Practice Guideline No. 9.* AHCPR publication No. 94-0592. Rockville, MD, Agency for Health Care Policy and Research, U.S. Department of Health and Human Services, Public Health Service, 1994

117. Ad hoc Committee: Pain curriculum for basic nursing education. *IASP Newsletter* Sept/Oct:4–6, 1993

118. Sheidler VR, McGuire DB, Grossman SA, et al: Analgesic decision-making skills of nurses. *Oncol Nurs Forum* 19: 1531–1534, 1992

119. Schauer PK, Wetterman TL, Schauer AR: Physicians' attitudes and knowledge about the management of cancer-related pain. *Conn Med* 52:705–707, 1988

120. McCaffery M, Ferrell BR: Nurses' knowledge about cancer pain: A survey of five countries. *J Pain Symptom Manage* 10: 356–369, 1995

121. Hill CS: The barriers to adequate pain management with opioid analgesics. *Semin Oncol* 20:1–5, 1993

122. Wallace KG, Reed BA, Pasero C, et al: Staff nurses perceptions of barriers to effective pain management. *J Pain Symptom Manage* 10:204–213, 1995

123. Ferrell BR, McCaffery M: Nurses' knowledge about equianalgesia and opioid dosing. *Cancer Nurs* 20:201–212, 1997

124. Barnett EH: Case marks big shift in pain policy. *The Oregonian,* September 2, 1999

125. Marks R, Sachar E: Undertreatment of medical inpatients with narcotic analgesics. *Ann Intern Med* 78:173–181, 1973

126. Hauck SL: Pain: Problem for the person with cancer. *Cancer Nurs* 9:66–76, 1986

127. Myers JS: Cancer pain: Assessment of nurses' knowledge and attitudes. *Oncol Nurs Forum* 12:62–66, 1985

128. Weis OF, Sriwatanakul K, Alloza JL, et al: Attitudes of patients, housestaff, and nurses toward post-operative analgesic care. *Anesth Analg* 62:70–74, 1983

129. Elliott TE, Elliott BA: Physician attitudes and beliefs about use of morphine for cancer pain. *J Pain Symptom Manage* 7:141–148, 1992

130. Porter J, Jick H: Addiction rare in patients treated with narcotics. *N Engl J Med* 302:123, 1980

131. Weissman DE, Dahl JL: Attitudes about cancer pain: A survey of Wisconsin's first-year medical students. *J Pain Symptom Manage* 5:345–349, 1990

132. Edgar L, Hamilton J: A survey examining nurses' knowledge of pain control. *J Pain Symptom Manage* 7:18–26, 1992

133. McCaffery M, Ferrell BR, O'Neil-Page E, et al: Nurses' knowledge of opioid analgesic drugs and psychological dependence. *Cancer Nurs* 13:21–27, 1990

134. Ferrell BR, McCaffery M, Rhiner M: Pain addiction: An urgent need for change in nursing education. *J Pain Symptom Manage* 7:117–124, 1992

135. Camp LD: Comparison of medical, surgical and oncology patients' descriptions of pain and nurses' documentation of pain assessments. *J Adv Nurs* 12:593–598, 1987

136. Dalton JA: Nurses' perceptions of their pain assessment skills, pain management practices, and attitudes toward pain. *Oncol Nurs Forum* 16:225–231, 1989

137. Paice JA, Mahon SM, Faut-Callahan M: Factors associated with adequate pain control in hospitalized patients diagnosed with cancer. *Cancer Nurs* 14:298–305, 1991

138. Faries JE, Mills DS, Goldsmith KW, et al: Systematic pain records and their impact on pain control: A pilot study. *Cancer Nurs* 14:306–313, 1991

139. Ward SE, Goldberg N, Miller-McCauley V, et al: Patient-related barriers to management of cancer pain. *Pain* 52: 319–324, 1993

140. Grossman SA, Sheidler VR, Swedeen K, et al: Correlation of patient and caregiver ratings of cancer pain. *J Pain Symptom Manage* 6:53–57, 1991

141. Weissman DE, Joranson DE, Hopwood MB: Wisconsin physicians' knowledge and attitudes about opioid analgesic regulations. *Wis Med J* 90:671–675, 1991

142. Hill CS: Pain management in a drug-oriented society. *Cancer* 63:2382–2386, 1989

143. Pritchard AP: Management of pain and nursing attitudes. *Cancer Nurs* 11:203–209, 1988

144. Von Roenn JH, Cleeland CS, Gonin R, et al: Physician attitudes and practice in cancer pain management: A survey from the Eastern Cooperative Oncology Group. *Ann Intern Med* 119:121–126, 1993

145. Pilowsky I: An outline curriculum on pain for medical school. *Pain* 33:1–2, 1988

146. Ferrell BR, McGuire DB, Donovan MI: Knowledge and beliefs regarding pain in a sample of nursing faculty. *J Prof Nurs* 9:79–88, 1993

147. Wisconsin Cancer Pain Initiative Nursing Education Committee: *Competency Guidelines for Cancer Pain Management in Nursing Education and Practice.* Madison, WI, Wisconsin Cancer Pain Initiative, 1995

148. Zahn ML: Pain management instruction in nursing curricula. *J Nurs Educ* 34:262–267, 1995

149. Weissman DE: Cancer pain education for physicians in practice: Establishing a new paradigm. *J Pain Symptom Manage* 12:1–8, 1996

150. Dalton JA, Blau W: Changing the practice of pain management. *Pain Forum* 5:266–272, 1996

151. Breitbart W: The practice of pain management—change from within or from without. *Pain Forum* 5:275–278, 1996

152. Spross JA, McGuire DB, Schmitt R: Oncology Nursing Society position paper on cancer pain. *Oncol Nurs Forum* 17: 595–614, 751–760, 825, 944–955, 1990

153. Max MB: Improving outcomes of analgesic treatment: Is education enough? *Ann Intern Med* 113:885–889, 1990

154. Miaskowski C, Donovan M: Implementation of the American Pain Society Quality Assurance Standards for Relief of Acute Pain and Cancer Pain in oncology nursing practice. *Oncol Nurs Forum* 19:411–415, 1992

155. Weissman DE, Abram SE, Haddox AD, et al: Educational role of cancer pain rounds. *J Cancer Educ* 4:113–116, 1989

156. Weissman DE, Dahl JL: Update on the cancer pain role model education program. *J Pain Symptom Manage* 10: 292–297, 1995

157. Ferrell BR, Dean GE, Grant M, et al: An institutional commitment to pain management. *J Clin Oncol* 13:2158–2165, 1995

158. Ferrell BR, Grant M, Ritchey KL, et al: The pain resource nurse training program: A unique approach to pain management. *J Pain Symptom Manage* 8:545–556, 1993

159. McMenamin E, McCorkle E, Barg F, et al: Implementing a multidisciplinary cancer pain education program. *Cancer Pract* 3:303–309, 1995

160. Ward SE, Gordon D: Application of the American Pain Society quality assurance standards. *Pain* 56:299–306, 1994

161. Bookbinder M, Kiss M, Coyle N, et al: Improving pain management practices, in McGuire DB, Yarbro CH, Ferrell BR (eds): *Cancer Pain Management* (ed 2). Sudbury, MA, Jones and Bartlett, 1995, pp 321–361

162. Ferrell B, Whedon M, Rollins B: Pain and quality assessment/improvement. *J Nurs Care Qual* 9:69–85, 1995

163. Portenoy RK, Coyle N: Controversies in the long-term management of analgesic therapy in patients with advanced cancer. *J Pain Symptom Manage* 5:307–319, 1991

164. Williams A, Kedziera P, Osterlund H, et al: Models of healthcare delivery in cancer pain management. *Oncol Nurs Forum* 19:20–26, 1992 (suppl)

165. Gonzales GR, Elliott KJ, Portenoy RK, et al: The impact of a comprehensive evaluation in the management of cancer pain. *Pain* 47:141–144, 1991

166. Walsh TD: Continuing care in a medical center: The Cleveland Clinic Foundation Palliative Care Service. *J Pain Symptom Manage* 5:273–278, 1990

167. Bascom PB: A hospital-based comfort care team: Consultation for seriously ill and dying patients. *Am J Hosp Palliat Care* 14:57–60, 1997

168. Redmond K: Organizational barriers in opioid use. *Support Care Cancer* 5:451–456, 1997

169. McGuire DB: Comprehensive and multidimensional assessment and measurement of pain. *J Pain Symptom Manage* 7: 312–319, 1992

170. American Nurses Association and Oncology Nursing Society: *Statement on the Scope and Standards of Oncology Nursing Practice.* Washington, DC, 1996

171. McCaffery M, Pasero C: *Pain: Clinical Manual* (ed 2). St. Louis, Mosby, 1999

172. Vallerand AH: Measurement issues in the comprehensive assessment of cancer pain. *Semin Oncol Nurs* 13:16–24, 1997

173. McGuire DB: Measuring pain, in Frank-Stromborg M, Olsen S (eds): *Instruments for Clinical Nursing Research* (ed 2). Sudbury, MA, Jones and Bartlett, 1997, pp 528–564

174. Grossman SA, Sheidler VR, McGuire DB, et al: A comparison of the Hopkins Pain Rating Instrument with standard visual analogue and verbal descriptor scales in patients with cancer pain. *J Pain Symptom Manage* 7:196–203, 1992

175. Paice JA, Cohen FL: Validity of a verbally administered numeric rating scale to measure cancer pain intensity. *Cancer Nurs* 20:88–93, 1997

176. Collins SL, Moore RA, McQuay HJ: The visual analogue

pain intensity scale: What is moderate pain in millimetres? *Pain* 72:95–97, 1997

177. Acute Pain Management Guideline Panel: Acute Pain Management: Operative or Medical Procedures and Trauma. Clinical Practice Guideline. AHCPR publication No. 92-0032. Rockville, MD, Agency for Health Care Policy and Research, Public Health Service, U.S. Department of Health and Human Services, 1992

178. Melzack R: The McGill Pain Questionnaire: Major properties and scoring methods. *Pain* 1:277–299, 1975

179. McGuire DB, Strickland OL: Assessment of cancer-related pain in low-income African Americans: Reliability, validity, and clinical utility of the Brief Pain Inventory and three pain intensity scales. *Proc 8th World Congress on Pain.* Seattle, WA, International Association for the Study of Pain, 1996, p 174.

180. Uki J, Mendoza T, Cleeland CS, et al.: A brief cancer pain assessment tool in Japanese: The utility of the Japanese Brief Pain Inventory—BPI-J. *J Pain Symptom Manage* 16: 364–373, 1998

181. Saxena A, Mendoza T, Cleeland CS: The assessment of cancer pain in north India: The validation of the Hindi Brief Pain Inventory—BPI-H. *J Pain Symptom Manage* 17: 27–41, 1999

182. Melzack R: The short-form McGill Pain Questionnaire. *Pain* 30:191–197, 1987

183. de Wit R, van Dam F, Hanneman M, et al: Evaluation of the use of a pain diary in chronic cancer pain patients at home. *Pain* 79:89–99, 1999

184. McGuire DB, Grimm PM, Baxendale-Cox L, et al: *Pain, fatigue, and sleep alterations in cancer: A multidimensional perspective.* Proc 12th Annual Meeting of the American Pain Society. Glenview, IL, American Pain Society, 1994, p. A-12 (abstr)

185. Portenoy RK, Thaler HT, Kornblith AB, et al: Symptom prevalence, characteristics and distress in a cancer population. *Qual Life Res* 3:183–189, 1994

186. Donnelly S, Walsh D: The symptoms of advanced cancer. *Semin Oncol* 22:67–72, 1995

187. Miaskowski C, Lee K: Pain, fatigue, and sleep disturbance in oncology outpatients receiving radiation therapy for bone metastases: A pilot study. *J Pain Symptom Manage* 17: 320–322, 1999

188. Portenoy RK, Thaler HT, Kornblith AB, et al: The Memorial Symptom Assessment Scale: An instrument for the evaluation of symptom prevalence, characteristics and distress. *Eur J Cancer* 30A:1326–1336, 1994

189. Stiefel F, Fainsinger R, Bruera E: Acute confusional states in patients with advanced cancer. *J Pain Symptom Manage* 7:94–98, 1992

190. Bruera E, Fainsinger RL, Miller MJ, et al: The assessment of pain intensity in patients with cognitive failure: A preliminary report. *J Pain Symptom Manage* 7:267–270, 1992

191. McCaffery M, Beebe A: *Pain: Clinical Manual for Nursing Practice.* St. Louis, Mosby, 1989

192. Carpenito LJ: *Nursing Diagnosis: Application to Clinical Practice* (ed 4). Philadelphia, Lippincott, 1992, pp 211–248

193. Jadlos MA, Kelman GB, Marra K, et al: A pain management documentation tool. *Oncol Nurs Forum* 23:1451–1454, 1996

194. Kravitz RL, Delafield JP, Hays RD, et al: Bedside charting of pain levels in hospitalized patients with cancer: A randomized controlled trial. *J Pain Symptom Manage* 11:81–87, 1996

195. Miaskowski C, Nichols R, Brody R, et al: Assessment of patient satisfaction utilizing the American Pain Society's Quality Assurance Standards on acute and cancer-related pain. *J Pain Symptom Manage* 9:5–11, 1994

196. Grant M, Ferrell BR, Rivera LM, et al: Unscheduled readmissions for uncontrolled symptoms: A health care challenge for nurses. *Nurs Clin North Am* 30:673–682, 1995

197. Dalton JA: Outcomes that provide evidence of change in cancer pain management. *Nurs Clin North Am* 30:683–695, 1995

198. de Wit R, van Dam F, Vielvoye-Kerkmeer A, et al: The treatment of chronic cancer pain in a cancer hospital in the Netherlands. *J Pain Symptom Manage* 17:333–350, 1999

199. de Wit R, van Dam F, Abu-Saad HH, et al: Empirical comparison of commonly used measures to evaluate pain treatment in cancer patients with chronic pain. *J Clin Oncol* 17: 1280–1287, 1999

200. Calvin A, Becker H, Biering P, et al: Measuring patient opinion of pain management. *J Pain Symptom Manage* 17: 17–26, 1999

201. Gilford DM (ed): *The Aging Population in the Twenty-First Century: Statistics for Health Policy.* Washington, DC, National Academy Press, 1988

202. Parker SL, Tong T, Bolden S, et al: Cancer statistics, 1996. *CA Cancer J Clin* 46:5–27, 1996

203. Portenoy RK: Optimal pain control in elderly cancer patients. *Geriatrics* 42:33–44, 1987

204. Ferrell BA, Ferrell BR: Assessment of chronic pain in the elderly. *Geriatr Med Today* 8:123–134, 1989

205. Harkins SW: Geriatric pain: Pain perceptions in the old. *Clin Geriatr Med* 12:434–459, 1996

206. Ferrell BA: Pain in the elderly, in Watt-Watson JH, Donovan MI (eds): *Pain Management: Nursing Perspective.* St. Louis, Mosby, 1992, pp 349–369

207. Thomas MR, Roy R: Age and pain: A comparative study of the "younger and older" elderly. *Pain Manage* 1: 174–179, 1988

208. Office of Technology Assessment: *Technology and Aging in America.* Publication No. OTA-BA-264. Washington, DC, Office of Technology Assessment, 1985

209. Ferrell BA, Ferrell BR, Osterweil D: Pain in the nursing home. *J Am Geriatr Soc* 38:409–414, 1990

210. Newton PA: Chronic pain, in Cassel KY, Walsh JR (eds): *Geriatric Medicine,* vol 2. *Fundamentals of Geriatric Care.* New York, Springer-Verlag, 1984, pp 236–274

211. Lamy PP: Pain management, drugs, and the elderly. *J Am Health Care Assoc* 10:32–36, 1984

212. Ferrell BA, Ferrell BR, Rivera L: Pain in cognitively impaired nursing home patients. *J Pain Symptom Manage* 10: 591–598, 1995

213. Harkins SW, Kwentus J, Price DD: Pain in the elderly, in Bendetti C, Chapman CR, Morrica G (eds): *Advances in Pain Research and Therapy,* vol 7. New York, Raven Press, 1984, pp 103–121

214. Ferrell BR, Grant MM, Riner M, et al: Home care: Maintaining quality of life for patient and family. *Oncology* 6: 136–140, 1992 (suppl)

215. Bayer AJ, Chadha JS, Farag RR, et al: Changing presentations of myocardial infarction with increasing old age. *J Am Geriatr Soc* 34:263–266, 1986

216. Bernabei R, Gambassi G, Lapane K, et al: Management of pain in elderly patients with cancer. *JAMA* 279:1877–1882, 1998

217. Faherty BS, Grier MR: Analgesic medication for elderly people post-surgery. *Nurs Res* 33:369–372, 1984

218. Portenoy RK, Kanner RM: Patterns of analgesic prescrip-

tion and consumption in a university-affiliated community hospital. *Arch Intern Med* 145:439–441, 1985

219. Compton P: Substance abuse, in McCaffery M, Pasero C (eds): *Pain: Clinical Manual* (ed 2). St. Louis: Mosby, 1999, pp 428–466

220. McCaffery M, Vourakis C: Assessment and relief of pain in chemically dependent patients. *Orthop Nurs* 11:13–27, 1992

221. Coyle N, Foley KM: Alteration in comfort: Pain, in Baird SB, McCorkle R, Grant M (eds): *Cancer Nursing: A Comprehensive Textbook.* Philadelphia, Saunders, 1991, pp 782–805

222. Hoffman M, Provatas A, Lyver A, et al: Pain management in the opioid-addicted patient with cancer. *Cancer* 68: 121–122, 1991

223. Lavizzo-Mourey R, Macknzie E: Cultural competence: Essential measurements of quality for managed care organizations. *Ann Intern Med* 124:919–921, 1996

224. Donnelly GF, Sutterley DC: From the editors (editorial). *Top Clin Nurs* 7: v, 1985 (entire issue on cultural diversity and nursing practice)

225. Fong CM: Ethnicity and nursing practice. *Top Clin Nurs* 7: 1–10, 1985

226. Douglas MK: Cultural diversity in the response to pain, in Puntillo KA (ed): *Pain in the Critically Ill: Assessment and Management.* Gaithersburg, VA, Aspen, 1991, pp 65–76

227. Kagawa-Singer M: Ethnic perspectives of cancer nursing: Hispanics and Japanese-Americans. *Oncol Nurs Forum* 14: 59–65, 1987

228. Carson VB (ed): *Spiritual Dimensions of Nursing Practice.* Philadelphia, Saunders, 1989

229. Jacik M: Spiritual care of the dying adult, in Carson VB (ed): *Spiritual Dimensions of Nursing Practice.* Philadelphia, Saunders, 1989, pp 254–288

230. Johnston Taylor E, Ersek M: Ethical and spiritual dimensions of cancer pain management, in McGuire DB, Yarbro CH, Ferrell BR (eds): *Cancer Pain Management* (ed 2). Sudbury MA, Jones and Bartlett, 1995, pp 41–60

231. Twycross RD: Terminal care: Organization and technical aspects, in Swerdlow M, Ventafridda V (eds): *Cancer Pain.* Lancaster, England, MTP Press, 1987, pp 173–184

232. Wanzer SH, Federman DD, Adelstein SJ, et al: The physician's responsibility toward hopelessly ill patients. *N Engl J Med* 320:844–849, 1989

233. Burchman SL: Hospice care of the cancer pain patient, in Abram SE (ed): *Cancer Pain.* Boston, Kluwer, 1989, pp 153–169

234. Kane RL, Bernstein L, Wales J, et al: Hospice effectiveness in controlling pain. *JAMA* 253:2683–2686, 1985

235. Austin C, Cody OP, Eyres PJ, et al: Hospice home care pain management: Four critical variables. *Cancer Nurs* 9:38–65, 1986

236. Fainsinger R, Miller MJ, Bruera E: Symptom control during the last week of life on a palliative care unit. *J Palliat Care* 7:5–11, 1991

237. Pickett M, Cooley ME, Gordon DB: Pallative care: past, present and future. *Semin Oncol Nurs* 14:86–94, 1998

238. Ventafridda V, Ripamonti C, DeConno F, et al: Symptom prevalence and control during cancer patients' last days of life. *J Palliat Care* 6:7–11, 1990

239. Degner LF, Fujii SH, Levitt M: Implementing a program to control chronic pain of malignant disease for patients in an extended care facility. *Cancer Nurs* 5:263–268, 1982

240. Bruera E, MacMillan K, Hanson J, et al: Palliative care in a cancer center: Results in 1984 versus 1987. *J Pain Symptom Manage* 5:1–5, 1990

241. Miller RD, Walsh TD: Psychosocial aspects of palliative care in advanced cancer. *J Pain Symptom Manage* 6:24–29, 1991

242. Chan H, Woodruff RK: Palliative care in a general teaching hospital: Assessment of needs. *Med J Aust* 155:597–599, 1991

243. Coyle N, Adelhardt J, Foley KM, et al: Character of terminal illness in the advanced cancer patient: Pain and other symptoms during the last four weeks of life. *J Pain Symptom Manage* 5:83–93, 1990

244. Mount B: Challenges in palliative care (keynote address). *Am J Hosp Care* 2:22–29, 1985

245. Grond S, Zech D, Schug SA, et al: Validation of World Health Organization Guidelines for cancer pain relief during the last days and hours of life. *J Pain Symptom Manage* 6:411–422, 1991

246. Bailes JS: Cost aspects of palliative cancer care. *Semin Oncol* 22:64–66, 1995

247. Foley K: Competent care for the dying instead of physician-assisted suicide. *N Engl J Med* 336:54–58, 1997

248. Emanuel E: Pain and symptom control: Patients' rights and physicians' responsibilities. *Hematol Oncol Clin North Am* 10:41–56, 1996

249. Goldstein F: Inadequate pain management: A suicidogen. *J Clin Pharmacol* 37:1–3, 1997

250. Bretscher ME, Creagan ET: Understanding suffering: What palliative medicine teaches us. *Mayo Clin Proc* 72:785–787

251. Foley KM: Pain, physician-assisted suicide, and euthanasia. *Pain Forum* 4:163–178, 1995

252. Breitbart W: Cancer pain and suicide, in Foley KM, Bonica JJ, Ventafridda V (eds): *Advances in Pain Research and Therapy.* New York, Raven Press, 1990, pp 399–412

253. Coyle N: The euthanasia and physician-assisted suicide debate: Issues for nursing. *Oncol Nurs Forum* 19:41–46, 1992 (suppl)

254. Hammes BJ, Cain JM: The ethics of pain management for cancer patients: Case studies and analysis. *J Pain Symptom Manage* 9:166–170, 1994

255. Cain JM, Hammes BJ: Ethics and pain management: Respecting patients' wishes. *J Pain Symptom Manage* 9: 160–165, 1994

CHAPTER 29

Management of Cancer Pain

Rosemary C. Polomano, PhD, RN, FAAN
Deborah B. McGuire, PhD, RN, FAAN
Vivian R. Sheidler, MS, RN

Introduction

New developments in the understanding of pain and its effects on human responses have led to advances in the utilization of pharmacotherapy, nonpharmacological approaches, and invasive interventional techniques that target the physiological and psychosocial aspects of the pain experience. The multidimensional aspects of pain associated with cancer often require a combination of these modalities in order to achieve maximum pain-relieving benefits. Pain management, while it is still evolving as a specialty in health care, is now based on proven scientific principles and evidenced-based information. Research into the basis for pain and its specific mechanisms has guided the implementation of a wide variety of therapies that now offer patients with cancer-related pain better pain control and improved physical and emotional well-being. The content presented in this chapter will enable nurses to identify effective pharmacotherapy and nonpharmacologic interventions so that these may be implemented to prevent the worsening of pain and to alleviate suffering.

Specialized Pain Care

Growing numbers of health care professionals (e.g., advanced practice nurses, medical oncologists, internal medicine physicians, anesthesiologists, clinical pharmacists) have sought specialization in pain care. The integration of multidisciplinary services (pain management teams, hospice, palliative care and supportive care teams, and pain clinics and centers) into the health care system has had a significant impact on the education of health professionals and the delivery of pain care. Such multidisciplinary groups have generated databases that have been useful in understanding the incidence of pain syndromes and referral patterns for the treatment of complex pain problems requiring more attention.[1–3]

Nurses and other health care professionals need to be aware of inpatient, outpatient, and home care resources that are available to them and their patients, both through their institutions and health systems and referral agencies. In addition, many health systems,[4] professional organizations,[5–11] government agencies,[12,13] and international organizations[14] have published evidence- and consensus-based guidelines to define "best practices" for the management of acute and chronic cancer pain. These documents offer a compilation of assessment and treatment clinical care guidelines in the form of protocols, algorithms, and outcome-based criteria; information on pharmacotherapy and other interventions; citations from the literature; and educational resources that are available to both clinicians and patients in order to promote optimal pain practices.

End-of-Life Issues

End-of-life issues are now being addressed by professionals who provide palliative and supportive care services in hospitals, at home, in long-term care facilities, and in free-standing institutions. However, many believe that these services should be rendered much sooner, and that patients should be able to make informed decisions about their care before they become too sick to determine what level of care is needed.[15] Changes in patterns for health care reimbursement, active cancer treatment at the end of life, and the reluctance of health professionals to refer patients for end-of-life care clearly emphasize the importance of more aggressive pain care earlier in the course of the disease. Constraints imposed by managed care organizations on end-of-life services reinforce the need for clinicians who care for patients in all phases of their illness to be educated and trained in pain management.[16]

There is a growing body of evidence-based information to address palliative care for specific populations such as the elderly. Older patients with cancer present with more complex clinical problems and pain. Cancer pain is often accompanied by long-term pain from nonmalignant diseases. In order to manage this pain effectively, health professionals must be aware of the physiological changes associated with aging that may complicate treatment with drug therapy. Still more important is the ability to apply this information when designing analgesic regimens for elders at the end of life. Elders represent a vulnerable population of patients who may not be afforded aggressive, specialized pain care. Cleary and Carbone documented that elders were less likely to receive interventional therapy for pain and expert pain care despite the fact that they experienced a higher incidence of symptoms at the end of life.[17] Investigators who are part of the SUPPORT (Study to Understand the Prognosis and Preferences for Outcomes and Risks of Treatment) Project have documented that, more often than not, older persons who are seriously ill die in the hospital with significant pain and distressing symptoms.[18]

Interventions

Interventions and techniques for managing cancer pain can be categorized into three major approaches (Figure 29-1). The first approach, treat the underlying pathology, uses treatments aimed at targeting the underlying pathophysiological mechanisms for pain with antineoplastic therapies or surgical interventions. The primary goal of these treatments is to control, reduce, or eradicate the tumor. The second category, change perception or sensation of pain, utilizes pharmacological and interventional techniques to either diminish or interrupt painful sensory input from the periphery or alter pain perception and sensations at the level of the sensory cortex in the brain. The third category, diminish emotional or reactive component, implements cognitive or behavioral strategies as a means to alter the central processing of pain. The goal of this last approach is to positively affect the contextual aspects of pain by alleviating or reducing emotional distress or negative reactions to pain. A wide variety

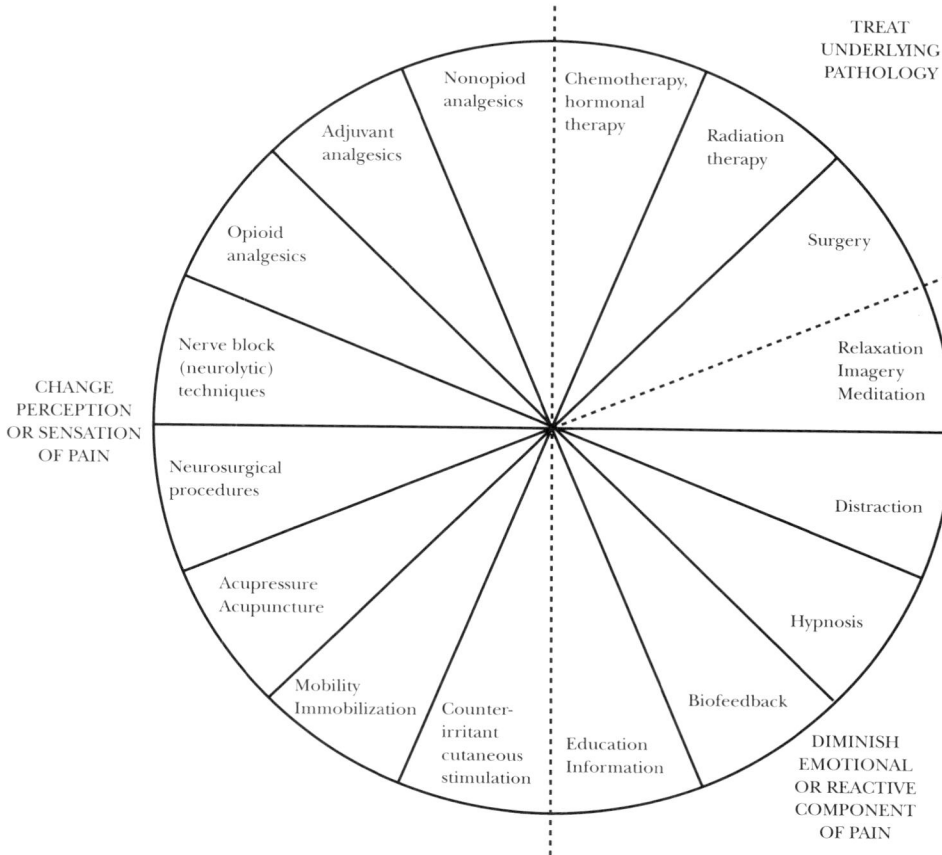

Figure 29-1 Three major approaches to interventions for cancer pain.

of nonpharmacological techniques can be used to achieve this outcome. More often than not, any combination of these three major approaches will be applied simultaneously to achieve the greatest impact on relieving pain.

Because pain management has evolved as a specialty among multiple groups of health care professionals, interdisciplinary efforts typically afford the greatest benefits in treating cancer-related pain. Multi-treatment modalities have become the mainstay to manage chronic cancer pain; therefore, the following sections address specific interventions within each of the three major treatment categories. Successful plans of care for managing pain demand advanced knowledge of the physiology and pathophysiology of pain, underlying principles of pain control, and indications and mechanisms of action for pharmacotherapy, nonpharmacological strategies, and interventional techniques. Moreover, nurses must collaborate with physicians and other health professionals to assess pain, design optimal analgesic therapy, and evaluate responses to pain treatments.

Treatment of Underlying Pathology

Typically, the three major cancer treatment modalities—chemotherapy, radiation therapy, and surgery—are em-

ployed as curative and adjunctive therapies; however, they can also be effective in the control and palliation of cancer pain. The primary intent of palliation is to reduce symptoms and improve quality of life. Hormonal therapy, another treatment modality, is similar to chemotherapy in that hormonal agents can also be administered for the purpose of arresting cancers and relieving symptoms. Whether treatments are given to control or palliate advanced cancer, the assessment of pain and pain relief are paramount in monitoring the success of therapy (see Chapter 28 for more on pain assessment). New complaints of pain during therapy should raise suspicion of tumor progression, not simply growing tolerance to drug therapy.[19] A multitude of pain interventions can now be used across the continuum of care. These interventions have specific indications for alleviating cancer pain and are reviewed in several comprehensive pain texts.[20–22]

Chemotherapy

Only recently has pain relief been measured as outcome criterion for evaluating responses to chemotherapy. Because concerns with quality of life are now emphasized with palliative chemotherapy,[23,24] clinicians are encouraged to incorporate assessments of pain and its relief into clinical care practices. Pain intensity, perceptions of pain relief, quality and character of the pain, analgesic requirements, and functional level are all critical end points that can be used to evaluate responses to palliative therapy. The toxicities of any therapeutic modality must be weighed against the benefits of relieving pain and distressing symptoms from advanced cancer. Comprehensive staging systems for evaluating cancer pain, such as one described by Bruera et al,[25] provide a systematic way to measure pain as an indicator of the efficacy of cancer treatment protocols with chemotherapy and other treatments.

Hormonal therapy has an important role in the palliation of painful symptoms. While this form of therapy has relatively few side effects, hormonal manipulation is only an option for patients with certain types of cancer such as cancers of the breast and prostate. Specific hormones can reduce the size of the tumor or slow its growth, typically in painful locations such as the bone and soft tissues.[26] The time course for improvement is more gradual with hormonal therapy compared to other treatments, sometimes taking 3–6 weeks before improvements in pain can be observed.[27] It provides palliation with fewer side effects and may afford significant relief of pain, sometimes even for prolonged periods of time. Investigators have reported favorable responses in painful bony metastases from breast and prostate cancers using a variety of therapies, including estrogen, androgen, progestin, aminoglutethimide, and corticosteroids. The benefits of chemotherapy and steroids have also been investigated for the palliation of hormone-resistant prostate cancer. In a randomized-controlled trial with end points of pain control and quality of life, the addition of mitoxantrone to prednisone therapy prolonged the duration of palliation compared to prednisone therapy alone.[28]

Radiation Therapy

Alleviation of pain and improvements in symptoms and quality of life have been the major objectives for palliative radiation therapy. About 70% of patients with bony metastases will derive a significant benefit from external radiation therapy, but much depends on the type of tumor, histology, location, and extent of the cancer.[29] Unfortunately, there is no way of knowing who will benefit from radiation for palliation of symptoms; however, characteristics of pain prior to treatment may be important predictors. Rutten et al found that the presence of radiating pain and the pain intensity before therapy are predictors of responses to treatment.[30] Scott stresses the importance of assessing quality of life during palliative radiation therapy and provides a variety of measurement tools that incorporate measures for pain.[31]

The use of external beam radiation has had a long-standing role in the management of painful bone metastases, most often for cancers of the breast, lung, and prostate.[32,33] In addition, it is standard treatment for relieving pain from epidural cord compression, and it

may be helpful in treating pain from headaches and increased intracranial pressure due to brain metastases.[34] Radiation therapy may also be useful for alleviating pain resulting from nerve root infiltration, pelvic and abdominal metastases from colorectal or cervical carcinomas, and local symptoms from lung and head and neck cancers.[27]

The onset and duration of pain relief are influenced by several factors, such as the radiation energy source, dose per fraction, total dose, length of treatment, and certainly the type of cancer and the location.[27] The optimal dose and fractionation of palliative radiation for bony metastases remains controversial. Gaze et al studied the effects of two fractionation schedules and found that a single treatment with 10 Gy was just as effective as 22.5 Gy in five fractionated doses.[35] The cost of palliative radiation therapy for metastatic bone disease is a concern. A preliminary evaluation of radiation therapy and chronic opioid therapy showed that brief courses of radiation therapy were significantly better in reducing pain and more cost-effective.[36]

New evidence is available to document the efficacy of radiopharmaceutical agents in relieving pain caused by bone metastases. Strontium-89, a beta-emitter radionuclide, has been shown to decrease bone pain and decrease analgesic requirements in patients with prostate and breast cancer.[37–41] Patients receive the drug intravenously as outpatients no less than every 3 months. The agent, a calcium analog, is localized in the bone in sites of increased osteogenesis from primary bone tumors or metastatic spread. Pain relief can be anticipated 7–21 days following treatment, with maximum effects within 6 weeks. The duration of relief can last up to 6 months.[42] Toxicities include myelosuppression and a temporary painful flare in the location of the pain within a few days after administration. For the first week following administration, patients need to be advised about (1) using a toilet instead of a urinal, (2) double flushing of the toilet after use, (3) cleaning excreta off of the toilet and flushing it down the toilet, (4) washing hands after using or cleaning the toilet, and (5) immediately laundering clothes separately should they be soiled with blood or urine.[42] Samarium sm 153 lexidronam is another radiopharmaceutical that is also indicated for the relief of pain associated with osteoblastic lesions of the bone.[42]

Surgery

Surgical intervention as a palliative measure is generally performed to prevent or treat complications or oncological emergencies such as obstruction or compression of vital organs or the spinal cord. Palliative surgery can help resolve these serious and often life-threatening complications. In addition, surgical intervention can alleviate tumor burden in order to maximize responses to other modalities such as radiation therapy or chemotherapy. Studies have shown that surgical palliation for pancreatic cancer, gastric and esophageal cancers, and pleural meso-thelioma has improved quality of life, disease symptoms, and morbidity.[43–45] There are little data, however, to demonstrate the long-term outcomes for pain control with these procedures.

Surgical ablation of endocrine glands may indirectly affect tumor growth that is dependent on the production of certain hormones (e.g., hypophysectomy or bilateral oophorectomy for advanced breast cancer, and orchiectomy for advanced prostate cancer), thus alleviating pain. Orthopedic procedures are performed to prevent or stabilize fractures of the long bones, spine, and pelvis.

There are data to document the success of palliative surgical procedures in relieving pain. Harrington described the various innovations in surgical interventions for bony structures invaded by tumors and summarized the favorable outcomes, including pain relief by location and type of procedure.[46] For example, 82% of patients with compromised neurological function from vertebral metastases improved by at least one functional grade following decompression and stabilization.

Other surgical palliative techniques for pain include procedures to implant devices for localization of chemotherapy perfusions or to insert radioactive isotopes. Table 29-1 outlines painful conditions from advanced cancer and the types of palliative procedures that can be performed to relieve pain.[47]

Technological advancements allow for less invasive techniques for tumor ablation and relief of pain. Interventional radiologists insert percutaneous transhepatic biliary drains to relieve hepatic congestion and pain associated with biliary obstruction. Embolization and chemo-embolization alleviate pain from organ enlargement or tumor encroachment. Gastroenterologists perform endoscopic placement of stents to relieve pressure, and drains to alleviate congestion. Photodynamic therapy can be used to reduce tumors in certain areas. (For specific information on these techniques for pain control, consult these sources.[48,49]) A variety of neurosurgical procedures can be performed to interrupt the transmission of pain by disrupting pain pathways; these are discussed in the next section.

The treatment modalities previously described offer one approach to relieving cancer pain—treatment of the underlying pathology. Nursing responsibilities in caring for patients are fairly standard and quite similar to those when the same methods are used as first-line, curative therapies.

Table 29-1 Examples of Palliative Surgical Procedures

Site and Clinical Condition	Type of Tumor	Palliative Surgical Procedures
Soft tissue/skin metastasis	Breast carcinoma Ulcerating or fungating lesions	Surgical excision Simple mastectomy
	Melanoma	Local excision
Abdominal Intestinal obstruction	Colorectal and ovarian carcinoma, peritoneal carcinomatosis	Colectomy (resection and anastomosis) Colostomy Gastrointestinal bypass Placement of gastric or intestinal tube for decompression
	Pancreatic carcinoma	Choleduocojejunosotomy
Serious ascites	Colon, breast and ovarian carcinomas	Peritoneovenous shunt
Acute urinary tract obstruction	Upper tract: Flank and retroperitoneal tumor Pelvic tract: Cancer of cervix, prostrate, rectum	Nephrostomy Cutaneous ureterostomy, cystotomy
Rectovessical fistula Rectovaginal fistula	Rectal and cervical carcinoma	Colostomy Colostomy
Malignant lesions of the skeleton Lesions of the extremities	Sarcomas, epithelial tumors, metastatic visceral tumors	Reductive surgery (amputation) Disarticulation
Pathological fractures Extremities	Metastases from lung, breast, prostate, renal, thyroid carcinomas Primary advanced bone and soft-tissue tumors	Intramedullary fixation Prosthetic or replacement reconstruction Amputation
Vertebra	Same as above	Spine stabilization
Neuraxial nervous system involvement Spinal cord compression	Metastases from lung, breast, prostate, renal, thyroid carcinomas Lymphomas, sarcomas	Decompression laminectomy

Data from Lillemoe[43]; Harrington[46]; Azzarelli, et al.[47]

Change in Perception/Sensation of Pain

The second major approach to treating cancer pain, changing the perception and sensation of pain, requires knowledge and skills regarding pharmacotherapy and invasive and noninvasive interventional techniques. Figure 29-1 represents a number of interventions that can be used to modify noxious sensory input in the periphery and at the level of the spinal cord and brain.

Pharmacologic Therapy

Pharmacologic therapy with several classes of drugs (e.g., nonopioids, opioids, and adjuvant agents) is generally considered the mainstay for treating cancer pain and is employed for a wide variety of painful conditions. Nurses have a major responsibility to be familiar with all of the pharmacological options for pain, including indications for their use, drug classifications, mechanisms of action, routes of administration, usual starting doses, adverse effects and interventions to manage them, and important outcome measures for monitoring their effectiveness.

Drug therapy with opioid and nonopioid adjuvant medications remains the primary method to control cancer-related pain. Regardless of the point at which a patient with cancer experiences pain, pharmacological interventions should be considered. (For a comprehensive overview of pharmacological agents used in the management of cancer pain, consult these references.[50-54])

It is critical to understand the classifications of analgesics, pharmacological properties, mechanisms of action, adverse effects, and associated terminology for analgesic medications that are outlined in Table 29-2.[51,55,56] These terms are especially important as they relate to the administration of opioid analgesics. Confusion exists among health professionals regarding the meaning of *tolerance, physical dependence,* and *addiction.* Unfortunately, widespread misconceptions about these conditions have negatively influenced prescribing patterns for opioid analgesics.

Nonopioids

Although the class of nonopioid analgesics varies in its chemical structure and classification, it is often grouped into distinct categories: para-aminophenol derivatives (e.g., acetaminophen [Tylenol]), salycylic acid derivatives (e.g., aspirin and choline magnesium trisalicylate [Trilisate]), and a variety of subclasses of other nonsteroidal anti-inflammatory drugs (NSAIDs).[57] All of these drugs possess antipyretic and analgesic properties and exert their analgesic effects in the periphery. Para-aminophenol derivatives such as acetaminophen have no anti-inflammatory properties. In addition, nonopioid drugs do not produce physical dependence, tolerance, or addiction, and they have a maximum ceiling effect for their analgesic potential. Acetaminophen and choline magnesium trisalicylate have no antiplatelet properties, while the NSAIDs and aspirin do affect platelet function and coagulation. This potential hematological effect is caused by irreversible acetylation of platelet cyclooxygenase, which inhibits platelet aggregation.[57]

The mechanism of action for these drugs has been well described. The NSAIDs inhibit cyclooxygenase in peripheral tissues, which prevents arachidonic acid from converting to prostaglandin.[57] This action alters transduction in the nociceptors, or pain receptors, of primary afferents. Prostaglandins are associated with pain that results from injury or inflammation, and they can sensitize pain receptors to mechanical and chemical stimulation. There is a new generation of NSAIDs called cyclooxygenase-2 or Cox-2 inhibitors. Agents that are currently on the market include celecoxib (Celebrex) and rofecoxib (Vioxx). Work is currently under way to establish their efficacy in the treatment of cancer-related pain syndromes.[58]

Table 29-2 Common Terminology Associated with Analgesics

Efficacy	Degree of analgesic provided by a given dose of an analgesic administered under a particular set of conditions
Dose response	Increase in dose accompanied by increase in effectiveness
Relative analgesic potency	Ratio of doses of two drugs
Relative analgesic potential	Relationship between efficacy and adverse effects
Half-life	Time it takes a drug to fall to half its original concentration in the blood
Opiate receptors	Specific recognition sites on which opioids produce their actions
Tolerance	A pharmacological phenomenon that develops when a given dose of a drug produces a decreased effect or when larger doses must be given to obtain the effects observed from the original dose
Physical dependence	An altered physiological state produced by the repeated administration of a drug and that necessitates the continued administration of the drug to prevent the appearance of withdrawal
Addiction	A behavioral pattern of drug use characterized by overwhelming involvement with its use; also known as *psychological dependence*

Data from McCaffery and Beebe[51]; Pasternak[55]; Reisine and Pasternak.[56]

Nonopioids are indicated for cancer pain that is considered mild to moderate in intensity. Non-cancer-related pain, such as that caused by arthritis, primary dysmenorrhea, muscle sprains, orthopedic injuries, and dental pain, is commonly managed with nonopioids. The NSAIDs can be useful for metastatic bone pain; pain from mechanical compression of tendons, muscles, pleura, and peritoneum; soft tissue pain; and nonobstructive visceral pain.[57]

Some studies evaluating the effects of NSAIDs for cancer pain indicate that the drugs are efficacious in providing pain relief.[59–61] These investigations document their effectiveness as adjuncts to opioid analgesics for bony metastases or as single agents for the initial treatment of mild pain. For the most part, investigators caution that nonopioid agents have limited benefits for patients with advanced cancer because of low maximal efficacy.[11,62]

The combination of nonopioids and opioids administered simultaneously may enhance analgesia. Earlier studies of patients with cancer demonstrated the beneficial effect of aspirin and morphine over morphine alone.[63] Another nonopioid, ibuprofen, was the drug of choice in two studies, the first involving two different doses of methadone[64] and the second involving a variety of scheduled opioids.[65] Both studies showed increased analgesic efficacy with the ibuprofen/opioid combination compared to an opioid alone. Eisenberg et al conducted a meta-analysis of 25 studies using 16 NSAIDs in 1545 patients.[66] Contrary to prior findings, the addition of NSAIDs to single or multiple doses of weak opioids offered no improvements in analgesic effects. They also cautioned that there was a lack of evidence to support the practice of using NSAIDs for patients experiencing pain from bony metastases. This is an important point, because many sources such as clinical practice guidelines advocate the use of NSAIDs in treating pain caused by metastatic disease in the bones.

Major toxicities from NSAIDs include gastrointestinal effects such as nausea, vomiting, epigastric pain, hemorrhagic ulcers, bleeding, diarrhea, and constipation.[67,68] The loss of the cytoprotective effect of prostaglandin on the gastrointestinal epithelium causes the occurrence of gastrointestinal side effects.[69] The elderly are at significantly increased risk for developing hemorrhagic ulcer disease, especially with higher doses.[70,71] Other potential toxicities include renal dysfunction, sodium and water retention, skin rashes, headaches, and cognitive dysfunction. While there is limited information comparing the efficacy and side effect profiles among NSAIDs, Brooks and Day have compiled data to guide clinicians in selecting one agent over another.[72]

Recent guidelines published by the American Geriatrics Society outline pain management strategies for elders.[8] The panel of expert geriatric clinicians and researchers stressed several important points about the use of both NSAIDs and acetaminophen in older patients. First, high-dose long-term NSAIDs should not be administered because of gastrointestinal and renal toxicities. If used chronically, doses should be prescribed on an as-needed basis rather than daily or around the clock. Second, short-acting NSAIDs instead of long-acting agents are recommended. Third, daily doses of acetaminophen should not exceed 4000 mg. Patients who are elderly must be frequently reminded about these precautions as they may use over-the-counter preparations without notifying their health professionals.

The selection of a nonopioid for an individual patient is often based on the prescriber's preference and experience with particular agents. To date, there is little evidence to indicate advantages of any one agent over another. Table 29-3 lists the commonly used agents and usual dosages. Formulations that are available in tablet, suspension, and suppository and that can be administered less frequently may simplify drug-dosing schedules. Table 29-4 highlights important considerations for the use of nonopioids.

The benefits of nonopioids for patients with severe pain who require higher than usual doses of opioids have

Table 29-3 Nonopioids Commonly Used in Analgesic Treatments of Cancer Pain

Name	Half-Life	Dosing Interval	Starting Dose (mg/day)	Maximum Dose (mg/day)
Acetaminophen	2–3 h	q4h	2000	4000
Acetylsalicylic acid	2–3 h	q4h	2000	6000
Choline magnesium trisalicylate	9–17 h	q12h	2000	4000
Diclofenac	1–2 h	q8–12h	75–100	200
Diflunisal	8–12 h	q8–12h after loading dose	500–1000	1500
Ibuprofen	3–4 h	q4–6h	1600	3200
Indomethacin	4–5 h	q8–12h	50–75	150–200
Ketorolac	4–9 h	q6h after loading dose	60–120	150
Naproxen	10–20 h	q6–8h	750	1250

Data from American Geriatrics Society Panel on Chronic Pain in Older Persons[8]; Jacox et al[12]; United States Pharmacopeial Convention, Inc.[42]; and Insel.[57]

not been established. Nonopioids can be considered either alone or in conjunction with an opioid when pain is mild. In summary, nonopioids are useful in the management of cancer-related pain. Optimal use of this group of drugs requires a careful medical and analgesic history, especially for patients with complex health problems.[73]

Steroids

Steroids are essential for reducing swelling, inflammation, and compression, resulting from the direct or indirect effects of tumor growth, that may lead to permanent nerve damage. Walsh suggested that steroids can be effective for problems such as bone metastases, lymphedema, compression from solid tumors, and brachial and lumbosacral plexopathies.[74] Emergent steroid therapy is warranted for impending spinal cord compression and the severe pain that accompanies tumor encroachment on spinal nerves.[75] In the end-of-life phase of illness, steroids can act as an appetite stimulant[76] and antiemetic.[77]

The pain-relieving qualities of steroids when used as adjuvant analgesics with opioids have been observed clinically and have been reported in the literature. Bruera et al compared methylprednisolone 32 mg/day with placebo in a 14-day randomized double-blind study to evaluate pain relief and other associated symptoms.[78] Pain improved significantly with the methylprednisolone as opposed to the placebo. The researchers found improvements in appetite (77%) and daily activity (68%) and decreases in depression (71%) and analgesic consumption (57%). Dexamethasone has been shown to reduce pain and fatigue and increase activity levels for patients with advanced lung cancer.[79]

Some adverse effects caused by steroids, particularly an increase in appetite and elevation of mood, may be desirable for some patients, especially those with advanced disease. However, other toxicities, such as proximal myopathy, steroid-induced hyperglycemia, and cushingoid side effects, need to be considered seriously if steroids are used early in the disease course to treat pain. It is generally recommended that steroids be reserved for those patients with advanced disease or for short-term use.[53]

Opioids

Opioid analgesics comprise a class of analgesics that act centrally by interfering with pain perception in the brain. They are classified into three major categories:

1. *Morphine-like opioid agonists.* Opioid agonists comprise the subclass of opioids that are most useful for managing cancer pain. These agents bind with mu and kappa opioid receptors. The mu receptor is an important opioid receptor as it is responsible for supraspinal analgesia, respiratory depression, euphoria, and physical dependence. In contrast, the kappa receptor affects spinal analgesia, miosis, and sedation. Commonly used opioids classified as morphine agonists include codeine, fentanyl, hydrocodone, hydromorphone, levorphanol, meperidine, morphine, methadone, and oxycodone.
2. *Opioid antagonists.* These agents exert no agonistic effects on opioid receptor activity; therefore, they possess no analgesic properties. Naloxone (Narcan) is a pure opioid antagonist.
3. *Opioid agonist-antagonists.* Drugs in this category include partial agonists and mixed agonist-antagonists. Mixed agonist-antagonists (e.g., butorphanol and nalbuphine) act competitively at different receptor sites, and the partial agonists, which include buprenorphine, act at only one receptor site (mu).[56] It is generally accepted by cancer pain experts that opioid agonist-antagonist drugs have very limited usefulness in cancer pain management because of their propensity to induce opioid withdrawal and cause severe CNS side effects. As a result, these drugs are not discussed in this chapter.

There is certain critical information that nurses, physicians, and pharmacists must know before opioids are prescribed, dispensed, or administered to patients with cancer-related pain. Mechanism of action, purpose and

Table 29-4 Considerations in the Use of Nonopioid Analgesics

Problem	Suggested Nonopioids
Need for strong anti-inflammatory activity	All drugs except acetaminophen
Need for parenteral route	Ketorolac
Risk of thrombocytopenia or other hematological disorder	Acetaminophen, choline magnesium trisalicylate
Impaired renal function	Acetaminophen, diflunisal, sulindac
Altered gastrointestinal function	Acetaminophen, choline magnesium trisalicylate, salsalate
Compliance	Diflunisal, naproxen, piroxicam, choline magnesium trisalicylate
Risk of significant adverse side effects	Avoid indomethacin, phenylbutazone, oxyphenbutazone
Need for chronic use	Avoid mefanamic acid, maclofenamate
Cost	Aspirin, acetaminophen

Table 29-5 Dose Equivalents for Opioid Analgesics in Opioid-Naive Adults and Children ≥50 kg body weight[a]

Drug	Approximate Equianalgesic Dose		Usual Starting Dose for Moderate to Severe Pain	
	Oral	Parenteral	Oral	Parenteral
OPIOID AGONIST[b]				
Morphine[c]	30 mg q3–4h (repeat around-the-clock dosing)	10 mg q3–4h	30 mg q3–4h	10 mg q3–4h
	60 mg q3–4h (single dose or intermittent dosing)			
Morphine, controlled-release[c,d] (MS Contin, Oramorph)	90–120 mg q12h	N/A	90–120 mg q12h	N/A
Hydromorphone[c] (Dilaudid)	7.5 mg q3–4h	1.5 mg q3–4h	6 mg q3–4h	1.5 mg q3–4h
Levorphanol (Levo-Dromoran)	4 mg q6–8h	2 mg q6–8h	4 mg q6–8h	2 mg q6–8h
Meperidine (Demerol)	300 mg q2–3h	100 mg q3h	N/R	100 mg q3h
Methadone (Dolophine, others)	20 mg q6–8h	10 mg q6–8h	20 mg q6–8h	10 mg q6–8h
Oxymorphone[c] (Numorphan)	N/A	1 mg q3–4h	N/A	1 mg q3–4h
COMBINATION OPIOID/NSAID PREPARATIONS[e]				
Codeine[f] (with aspirin or acetaminophen)	180–200 mg q3–4h	130 mg q3–4h	60 mg q3–4h	60 mg q2h (IM/SQ)
Hydrocodone (in Lorcet, Lortab, Vicodin, others)	30 mg q3–4h	N/A	10 mg q3–4h	N/A
Oxycodone (Roxicodone, also in Percocet, Percodan, Tylox, others)	30 mg q3–4h	N/A	10 mg q3–4h	N/A

q = every; N/A = not available; N/R = not recommended; NSAID = nonsteroidal anti-inflammatory drug; IM = intramuscular; SQ = subcutaneous.

[a]*Caution:* Recommended doses do not apply for adult patients with body weight less than 50 kg.

[b]*Caution:* Recommended doses do not apply to patients with renal or hepatic insufficiency or other conditions affecting drug metabolism and kinetics.

[c]*Caution:* For morphine, hydromorphone, and oxymorphone, rectal administration is an alternate route for patients unable to take oral medications. Equianalgesic doses may differ from oral and parenteral doses because of pharmacokinetic differences.

[d]Transdermal fentanyl (Duragesic) is an alternative option. Transdermal fentanyl dosage is not calculated as equianalgesic to a single morphine dose. See the package insert for dosing calculations. Doses above 25 μg/h should not be used in opioid-naive patients.

[e]*Caution:* Doses of aspirin and acetaminophen in combination opioid/NSAID preparations must also be adjusted to the patient's body weight. Aspirin is contraindicated in children in the presence of fever or other viral disease because of its association with Reye's syndrome.

[f]*Caution:* Codeine doses above 65 mg often are not appropriate because of diminishing incremental analgesia with increasing doses but continually increasing nausea, constipation, and other side effects.

Note: Published tables vary in the suggested doses that are equianalgesic to morphine. Clinical response is the criterion that must be applied for each patient; titration to clinical responses is necessary. Because there is not complete cross-tolerance among these drugs, it is usually necessary to use a lower than equianalgesic dose when changing drugs and to retitrate to response.

Reprinted from Jacox A, Carr DB, Payne R, et al: *Management of Cancer Pain: Adults' Quick Reference Guide No. 9.* AHCPR Publication No. 94-0593. Rockville, MD, Agency for Health Care Policy and Research, U.S. Department of Health and Human Services, Public Health Service, 1994.[12]

category, common starting dose, equivalence to other analgesics, duration of effect, half-life of the drug, available routes, and adverse effects that are common and unique to certain agents must be known. Ferrante describes the principles of opioid therapy, pharmacodynamic properties, and physiological considerations for both oral and parental opioids.[80] Table 29-5 contains information about the relative potencies of commonly used analgesics for moderate to severe pain.

All opioid analgesics share common effects as a result of their action. Central nervous system, respiratory, cardiovascular, gastrointestinal, genitourinary, and dermato-

logical effects of these drugs are outlined in Table 29-6. The four most common side effects, however, are sedation, respiratory depression, nausea and vomiting, and constipation.[56] Sedation, a common problem, is addressed in the section that follows on psychostimulants.

Respiratory depression rarely occurs if opioids are given based on rational use and commonly accepted principles. If it does occur, it can be treated easily and successfully with naloxone or with nalmefene, which has a longer duration of action than naloxone. The amount of naloxone a patient receives should be titrated to changes in respiratory rate. Rapid bolus injections of naloxone

Table 29-6 Common Side Effects of Opioid Analgesics

System	Side Effect
Central nervous	Sedation, drowsiness, mental clouding, euphoria, analgesia, nausea, vomiting, ↓ physical activity, lethargy, mood changes
Respiratory	↓ Respiratory rate, ↓ ventilatory minute volume, ↓ tidal exchange, ↓ P_{O_2}, ↑ P_{CO_2}
Cardiovascular	Hypotension from peripheral vasodilation or histamine release
Gastrointestinal	*Stomach:* ↓ motility; *small intestine:* ↓ propulsive contractions, delayed digestion from ↓ biliary and pancreatic secretions; *large intestine:* ↓ or absent propulsive peristaltic waves, causing delay in passage of contents; *biliary tract:* ↑ pressure from morphinelike drugs, causing epigastric distress to biliary colic
Genitourinary	↑ Tone and amplitude of ureter contractions, ↑ tone of bladder muscles→urgency, ↑ tone of vesical sphincter
Dermatological	Vasodilation of cutaneous blood vessels→ ↑ warmth and flushing of skin on face, neck, and upper thorax, sweating, pruritus

↑ = increased; ↓ = decreased; → = leading to
Data from Reisine and Pasternak.[56]

should be avoided in opioid-tolerant patients to avoid precipitating acute physiological withdrawal that can cause nausea, vomiting, agitation, diaphoresis and intense pain, and lead to life-threatening seizures. Respiratory depression is a concern when patients who have been maintained on opioid agonist drugs receive an interventional anesthetic procedure that may totally eliminate their pain. The stimulus of pain on respiratory function is eliminated, which places the patient at risk for respiratory depression.

The chemoreceptor trigger zone (CTZ) in the brain is sensitive to chemical stimuli such as opioids. Similar to the effect of chemotherapy-related nausea and vomiting, the CTZ and the vomiting center can be stimulated to produce nausea and vomiting. In a retrospective review of 260 patients receiving opioids, Campora et al found that of patients who received morphine ($n = 71$), 18.3% had moderate to severe nausea and 28% had vomiting.[81]

If a patient experiences opioid-related nausea and vomiting, there are many options available. Portenoy and Coyle[82] recommended the following:

1. Treat aggressively on initial presentation.
2. Use antiemetics that act at the CTZ, such as prochlorperazine and thiethylperazine.
3. Use metoclopramide if gastroparesis is a possible etiology of the nausea and vomiting.
4. Use an antivertigo drug such as cyclizine or scopolamine if symptoms worsen with movement.
5. Consider drug combinations.

6. Maximize dose response, especially if symptoms partially improve.
7. Prescribe antiemetics on an around-the-clock basis for 1–2 weeks.

Constipation is a significant clinical problem for patients taking chronic opioid therapy. The gut rarely accommodates or becomes tolerant to the effects of opioid analgesics; therefore, measures to prevent constipation must always accompany opioid administration. If measures to prevent and aggressively treat constipation are not instituted, patients can experience serious problems such as a bowel obstruction. The problem may be compounded by change in eating patterns, decreased fluid intake, inactivity, intraabdominal metastases, or concurrent administration of other drugs that cause constipation (e.g., vinca alkaloid antineoplastic agents, tricyclic antidepressants). Dietary measures include encouraging patients to increase their fluid intake and dietary fiber consumption. The patients or a family member should keep a record of when the patient has had a bowel movement.

The use of laxative preparations generally is necessary when patients must take opioids. Table 29-7 lists six categories of laxatives, their mechanisms of action, and commonly available preparations. Patients frequently require laxatives from more than one category, such as a stimulant laxative and a detergent laxative. It is also important to keep in mind that stool softeners alone have little effect on opioid-induced constipation. Additionally, there is little evidence to support a strong correlation between opioid dose and the need for a laxative. In the clinical setting, however, an increase in the dose of opioids often necessitates an increased need for laxatives. More detailed guidelines regarding the assessment and management of constipation are available.[83,84]

Oral naloxone has recently been investigated as an agent to reverse opioid-induced constipation. Because of its poor bioavailability, higher doses than would be administered by the parenteral route are necessary. It is suggested that 4 mg daily to a maximum of 12 mg is within a safe dosing range and that dosing intervals be no closer than every 6 hours.[85]

Properties inherent in opioids complicate a patient's therapy if health care professionals are not aware of the correct terminology and its implications for clinical practice. Table 29-2 includes definitions of *tolerance, physical dependence,* and *addiction. Tolerance* is a gradual resistance that requires that doses of specific analgesics be adjusted to accommodate the pharmacological phenomenon. *Physical dependence* is an issue when patients no longer require opioids for pain control and they must be tapered slowly off of them. It is also an issue if a patient inadvertently receives an agonist-antagonist drug, causing acute withdrawal, or if naloxone is required to slowly reverse opioid-induced respiratory depression. The problem of addiction was addressed earlier in this chapter, but to reiterate, *addiction* is not a problem for patients who require opioids for justifiable medical indications such as disease-related pain.

Table 29-7 Laxatives for Opiate-Induced Constipation

Category	Action	Common Preparations
Bulk	Increases size, weight, and frequency of stool; requires high fluid intake	Metamucil, Maltsupex Psyllium
Saline	Draws water into intestinal lumen and distends bowel; changes stool consistency	Milk of magnesia, magnesium citrate
Stimulant	Increases motor activity by direct action on the bowel	Bisacodyl, senna, Ex-Lax, Cascara
Lubricant	Reduces friction and coats the stool	Mineral oil
Osmotic	Increases volume in colon; promotes water retention	Lactulose, sorbitol
Detergent	Reduces surface tension	Docusate; available in combination with stimulant laxatives

Responsiveness to opioids may be a function of the mechanism for the pain. There has been considerable controversy over the last few years regarding the use of opioids for neuropathic pain. Historically, neuropathic pain was thought to be less responsive to opioid analgesics. Portenoy et al suggested that patients may, in fact, just require higher doses of opioids to relieve neuropathic pain and that opioids should not be excluded as a viable option for patients who have pain resulting from nerve injury.[86] Cherny et al evaluated opioid responsiveness to single doses of morphine or heroin among 168 patients with neuropathic pain and/or nociceptive pain.[87] Those with a definite or possible/probable component of neuropathic pain had significantly less pain relief compared to subjects with nociceptive pain. Patients with head and neck cancer who were experiencing neuropathic pain required greater escalations in their opioid doses compared to other pain syndromes.[88]

In addition to pain mechanisms, other factors such as age influence requirements for opioid analgesics. While older patients have been noted to have the same pain intensity levels as younger adults, elderly patients may require lower amounts of opioid analgesics to achieve a comparable effect.[89]

Specific drug selection. In some circumstances, the selection of an opioid or other analgesic may be arbitrary or based on the prescriber's experience. The World Health Organization (WHO) Analgesic Ladder and Guidelines for cancer pain relief have been utilized widely, both in the United States and internationally. When this stepwise model based on pain severity is used appropriately, there are major benefits and substantial evidence to support guidelines for analgesic prescribing.[90] More important, the oral route of administration for opioids is the most convenient and is preferred to other routes.[12]

Some investigators have attempted to describe physician-prescribing patterns for the treatment of cancer pain. Cherny et al conducted a survey to determine strategies used by physicians in selecting opioid analgesics and routes of administration for inpatients with cancer pain.[91] There were 182 changes in opioid regimens or doses for 80 of the 100 patients evaluated. The frequency of changes before discharge or death were attributed to the following: 31.4% for convenience and adequate pain relief, 25% to diminish side effects, 19.3% to reduce invasiveness of the therapy, and 17.7% to improve pain control and decrease opioid toxicity.

Various patient-related factors contribute to the selection of a specific opioid. These factors include pain intensity, patient age, concomitant medical illnesses, and specific drug characteristics. Opioid administration guidelines are described in Table 29-8.[52] The sections that follow outline specific analgesic drugs and considerations for the clinical management of cancer pain.

Morphine. Morphine remains the standard by which equianalgesic comparisons are established. In addition, morphine remains the most frequently used opioid analgesic for moderate to severe cancer pain in the United States as well as in many foreign countries.[92–94] It is available for oral, parental, rectal, and neuraxial (intraspinal, epidural, or subarachnoid) administration. Controlled-release or long-acting morphine permits 8- to 12-hour (MS Contin, Oramorph) or 24-hour (Kadian) dosing schedules as opposed to 3- to 4-hour dosing. Depending on the manufacturer, controlled- or sustained-released preparations come in multiple dosing strengths (15-, 30-, 60-, 100-, and 200-mg) to allow flexibility in dosing schedules. Patients taking MS Contin every 12 hours with supplemental short-acting opioids reported significantly better compliance with prescribed amounts of opioids and improvements in quality of life compared to a schedule that included short-acting opioids alone.[95] Numerous studies, both controlled and uncontrolled, have demonstrated the efficacy and safety of controlled-released morphine.[95–97]

Even though morphine is considered an effective oral analgesic agent, it is much less potent when taken orally than administered parenterally. Parenteral (IV, IM) to oral potency ratios vary from 1:6 for single oral doses to 1:3 for chronic dosing schedules.[12] A possible explanation for this discrepancy from single to chronic oral dosing might be related to the by-products of morphine metabolism—morphine-3- and morphine-6-glucuronide. The accumulation of these metabolites with repeated dosing

---

Table 29-8   Guidelines for the Use of Opioids in Chronic Cancer Pain

1. Consider the role of this treatment in a multimodal approach.
2. Drug selection
   a. Consider pain intensity, age, whether major organ failure is present (especially renal, hepatic, or respiratory), and presence of coexisting disease.
   b. Consider pharmacological issues (e.g., accumulation of metabolites and effects of concurrent drugs and possible interactions).
   c. Consider individual differences (note prior treatment outcomes) and patient preference.
   d. Be aware of available routes of administration (e.g., oral, intravenous, subcutaneous) and formulation (e.g., controlled release or immediate release).
   e. Be aware of cost differences.
3. Route selection
   a. Use least invasive route possible.
   b. Consider patient compliance and convenience.
4. Dosing and dose tritration
   a. Consider previous dosing requirement and relative analgesic potencies when initiating therapy.
   b. Start with low dose and increase until adequate analgesia is achieved or dose-limiting side effects are encountered.
   c. Consider dosing schedule (e.g., around-the-clock or as needed).
   d. Consider "rescue" doses for breakthrough pain.
   e. Recognize that tolerance is rarely the "driving force" for dose escalation; consider disease progression or psychological factors when increasing dose requirements occur.
5. Trials of alternative opioids: Given individual differences in the response to various opioids, consider a trial of another opioid following treatment failure; be aware of incomplete cross tolerance.
6. Treatment of side effects
   a. Be aware of the prevalence and impact of opioid side effects.
   b. Consider a preventive approach in the management of constipation.
7. Monitoring
   a. Monitor pain intensity and pain relief on an ongoing basis.
   b. Make necessary modifications to treatment plan.
   c. Be aware of potential for withdrawal if considering cessation of opioid therapy and need for tapering schedule.

Reprinted with permission from Coyle N, Cherny N, Portenoy RK: Pharmacologic management of cancer pain, in McGuire DB, Yarbro CH, Ferrell BR (eds): *Cancer Pain Management* (ed 2). Sudbury, MA, Jones and Bartlett, 1995, pp 131–158.[52]

---

may not only be responsible for analgesia, but they also are attributed to the development of adverse side effects, especially in patients with altered renal function due to morphine.[98-100]

Fentanyl.   Fentanyl is available as a parenteral agent and in transdermal and transmucosal delivery systems. Further information regarding fentanyl's use in the management of cancer pain is provided in later sections.

Hydromorphone.   Hydromorphone (Dilaudid) can be administered orally, rectally, and parenterally and is a useful alternative to morphine, particularly for the elderly, as there are no known toxic metabolites that may accumulate with repeated dosing.[56]

Methadone and levorphanol.   Both of these opioid analgesics have a prolonged plasma half-life (see Table 29-5) that does not correspond to the average duration of analgesia. When patients are initially placed on fixed schedules of these drugs, they are at risk of developing prolonged sedation and respiratory depression as the drug level in their plasma rises. Both are available in oral and parenteral preparations.

While methadone, a synthetic opioid agent, is a second choice agent, it possesses several desirable characteristics such as excellent oral and rectal absorption, no active metabolites, high potency at a low cost, potentially longer intervals between administration, and incomplete

cross-tolerance with mu opioid agonist agents.[101] Standard equianalgesic conversion tables may be unreliable, necessitating individualized determinations for methadone doses.[101] Because dosing schedules for methadone can vary, it is generally recommended that initial therapy begin with longer dosing intervals of 6–8 hours, until responses to analgesia and the effects of its long plasma half-life can be evaluated. Methadone is one of the choice opioids for patients who are allergic to morphine because its chemical structure is so different.[53] Methadone is not recommended for elderly patients due to its long plasma half-life and the possibility of drug accumulation.

Levorphanol is another synthetic potent mu opioid receptor agonist, but it also binds to kappa receptors that may be responsible for central nervous system side effects such as delirium and hallucinations.[102] Because levorphanol may be infrequently prescribed, it may be difficult to obtain from retail pharmacy chains. Similar to methadone, its extended serum half-life (>12 hours) makes it less desirable for the elderly.

Oxycodone.   Historically, oxycodone has been used in relatively low doses (e.g., 10 mg q4h), either alone or in combination with aspirin or acetaminophen. Glare and Walsh demonstrated the efficacy of high-dose oxycodone (e.g., 360 mg/day) for patients with cancer pain.[103] Current thinking is that oxycodone does not have an upper limit or a ceiling effect, and it does not possess active toxic metabolites. Oxycodone is now available as a controlled-release preparation (OxyContin) in 10-, 20-, 40-, 80-mg tablets for every 12-hour dosing. Multiple dosing strengths permit flexible schedules with low- and high-dose regimens.[104]

Opioids not recommended for cancer pain. Meperidine (Demerol) is not recommended for the treatment of chronic cancer pain.[13] Even though its use has declined considerably, some clinicians are not aware of its poor oral efficacy and risk for producing serious toxic side effects such as agitation, tremors, myoclonus, and seizures. Additionally, it has poor oral efficacy.[56,105]

Proproxyphene, the active opioid in Darvocet, is structurally similar to methadone, but it is a very weak opioid with few advantages in the treatment of chronic pain. Its short analgesic duration and longer plasma half-life with accumulation of a toxic metabolite possesses several risks when administered to elders.[8]

Other agents

Tramadol is a new centrally acting binary analgesic that binds weakly to mu opioid receptors.[106] It has opioid agonists and monaminergic agonist actions. It can be considered a weak opioid similar to codeine. The normal dose range is 50–100 mg every 4–6 hours, and side effects include dizziness, nausea, sedation, dry mouth, and diaphoresis. To date, there have been limited studies with patients who have cancer.[107]

Adjuvant analgesics

Adjuvant analgesics are defined as those medications that enhance the action of pain-modulating systems. In general, adjuvant analgesics are indicated primarily for uses other than pain management. According to Breitbart, psychotropic drugs such as antidepressants, anticonvulsants, and psychostimulants play an important role at each step of the WHO Analgesic Ladder, especially in the treatment of neuropathic pain.[108] He provides an excellent overview of considerations in selecting these agents for pain control and offers guidelines for their use in clinical practice. Although there are several different classes of adjuvant analgesics, only the most common agents are discussed below.

Tricyclic antidepressants. Tricyclic antidepressants have demonstrated significant benefits for the management of neuropathic pain. These drugs act by inhibiting the uptake of neurotransmitters (norepinephrine and serotonin) into nerve terminals.[109] This subclass of antidepressants has demonstrated efficacy in the treatment of many chronic nonmalignant neuropathic pain syndromes, such as postherpetic neuralgia and diabetic neuropathy.[110–112] For the treatment of cancer pain, these agents have been effective in relieving pain due to infiltration of nerves or from treatment-related injury such as postmastectomy pain syndrome.[113,114] Tricyclic antidepressants help to reduce continuous dysesthetic and

burning sensations and the cutaneous hypersensitivity associated with nerve injury. Although selective serotinin reuptake inhibitors (SSRIs; e.g., fluoxetine, paroxetine, sertraline) have not been proven to exert analgesic effects, treatment with any of these agents can substantially improve the depression that accompanies chronic pain. Interactions do occur with concomitant administration of tricyclic antidepressants and SSRIs, therefore, nurses should consult the drug information literature for recommended dosing modifications and approaches for monitoring adverse effects.

A partial list of tricyclic antidepressants is provided in Table 29-9, along with dose ranges for maximal benefits and a side effect profile rating.[109] Payne recommends that a low starting dose of 10 mg be administered at bedtime, especially for elderly patients.[53] The dose can be increased to 25 mg in 3 days, then escalated by 25 mg every 3–7 days as tolerated. It is often necessary to reach daily doses of 75–150 mg before significant pain-relieving effects are observed. Tricyclic antidepressants are contraindicated for patients with cardiac conduction abnormalities. Slower and lower incremental increases may be necessary for elderly patients.

The major adverse effects from tricyclic antidepressants are anticholinergic effects such as dry mouth, constipation, postural hypotension and urinary retention, and sedation. These can be troublesome, especially if a patient is already receiving opioid analgesics that cause similar problems.

Anticonvulsants. The site and mechanism of action for anticonvulsants for cancer-related pain are not well understood. Similar to tricyclic antidepressants, anticonvulsants are used to treat neuropathic pain. For the most part, they have become standard therapy for the treatment of trigeminal neuralgia, diabetic neuropathy, and herpes zoster–related pain.[115] Agents such as carbamazepine (Tegretol), gabapentin (Neurontin), phenytoin (Dilantin), valproate, and clonazepam (Klonopin) are particularly effective for neuropathic pain syndromes associated with shooting, electric shock–like, or lancinating sensations.[109]

Anticonvulsant drugs may be beneficial for the treatment of direct peripheral nerve injuries such as herpes zoster–related pain or centrally mediated pain from nerve damage. Recent studies have documented the efficacy of gabapentin for the treatment of neuropathic pain.[116,117] McCaffery provides anecdotal evidence that gabapentin is effective for lancinating pain.[118]

Gabapentin has significant advantages over the other agents because of its relatively low toxicity. Unlike carbamazepine and clonazepam, gabapentin is less sedating. In addition, gabapentin does not produce the hematological effects that are often a concern with carbamazepine and phenytoin. While somnolence, dizziness, ataxia, fatigue, and cognitive dysfunction have been linked to gabapentin, many of these adverse effects can be prevented with slow dose escalations. An initial dose of 100 mg twice daily can be administered, with dose increases of 100

Table 29-9 Properties of Common Tricyclic Antidepressants Used as Analgesics for Neuropathic Pain

Drugs	Relative Anticholinergic Effects	Relative Sedative Effects	Usual Starting Dose	Usual Daily Therapeutic Dosing Range	Half-Life (hr)	Comments
Tertiary amine agents Amitriptyline	++++	++++	10–25 mg at hs	50–150 mg	30–45	Lower initial doses and gradual titration for elders. Risk for orthostatic hypotension moderate to high. Increased risk for constipation.
Doxepin	++	+++	10–25 mg at hs	50–150 mg	8–25	
Secondary amine agents Desipramine	+	+	25 mg at hs	100–150 mg	12–25	Lower toxicity profile. Recommended for elderly patients
Nortriptyline	++	++	25 mg at hs	100–150 mg	18–45	

Data from United States Pharmacopeial Convention, Inc[42]; Coyle, et al[52]; Lipman.[109]

mg/day every 3–5 days, as tolerated, to achieve a thrice daily dosing schedule. Typically, patients will require at least 900–1200 mg per day; however, higher daily doses of 3600 mg have been suggested to maximize pain control.[119] Table 29-10 lists common doses and toxicities of five common anticonvulsants.

NMDA receptor antagonist. Data from animal models suggest that NMDA (N-methyl-D-aspartate) receptor activity plays an important role in many chronic pain states. While the function of these receptors is not altogether understood, there is compelling evidence from animal models that activation of NMDA receptors in the spinal cord as a result of nerve damage or inflammation contributes to increased pain.[120] The NMDA receptors may also be responsible, in part, for tolerance that develops to opiate analgesics.[121] Both dextromethorphan (DM) and, to a lesser extent, ketamine are NMDA antagonists. The effectiveness of dextromethorphan in humans has not been well studied alone or in combination with other analgesics. Mercadante et al added DM to therapy with NSAIDS and morphine and found that no significant benefits were derived by the addition of DM.[122]

Ketamine, a parenteral anesthetic, has potent analgesic properties at lower doses. It also seems to exert its greatest effect on neuropathic pain syndromes. Mercadante reviews its efficacy and synergistic actions with opioid analgesics.[123] Low-dose intravenous ketamine in doses of 0.1–1.5 mg/kg per hour have shown promising effects in relieving chronic neuropathic pain.[124] Intravenous ketamine is expensive and inconvenient to administer. As a result, investigators continue to study the effects of this preparation with patients experiencing severe chronic cancer pain. Long-term subcutaneous continuous infusions of ketamine are an alternative to intravenous administration.[125] Clark et al reported their experience with the successful management of cancer pain with oral ketamine.[126]

Psychostimulants. Psychostimulants are useful in counteracting the sedation that accompanies opioid analgesics. If the sedation is present without any other CNS problems, such as delirium or confusion, and if pain occurs when the opioid dose is lowered, a psychostimulant may be indicated. In addition, these agents can potentiate opioid analgesia and allow more rapid escalations of opioid doses to treat complex pain syndromes.

Typically, amphetamines (e.g., dextroamphetamine) or the drug methylphenidate are used to counteract opioid-induced sedation. Amphetamines are more powerful CNS stimulants than methylphenidate; however, both decrease the central depression caused by sedating drugs. It is believed that this effect is possible through stimulation of the cortex and reticular activating system.[127] The recommended starting dose for methylphenidate is 10 mg; recommended starting dose for dextroamphetamine is 2.5 mg. The initial dose is given in the morning, and if the morning dose is well tolerated an early afternoon dose may be administered to counteract midday sedation. Doses can be titrated to response, with an expected benefit within 2 days.[128] Methylphenidate is particularly effective at treating opioid-induced sedation.[129]

The more desirable side effects are increased alert-

Table 29-10   Anticonvulsants for Pain Management

Drug	Dose	Indications	Adverse Effects
Carbamazepine	100–200 mg PO bid Increase every other day to 800 mg/day in divided doses.	Useful for paroxysmal and lancinating, shooting, electric shock–like pains	Sedation, drowsiness, diplopia, ataxia, hematological toxicity
Clonazepam	0.5–1.5 mg/day PO Maximum 3–4 mg/day in divided doses.	Same as above Useful for preexisting anxiety	Sedation, ataxia, behavioral disturbances, mood or mental changes
Gabapentin	300–900 mg tid (900–2400 mg) PO Initial dose 100 mg tid, then increase by 100 mg/day as tolerated. May titrate up to 3600 mg/day. For elders, increase slowly: 100 mg/day q3–5 days.	Same as above	Sedation, ataxia, dizziness, difficulty concentrating, visual abnormalities
Phenytoin	300–500 mg/day PO	Same as above	Sedation, drowsiness, ataxia, diplopia, nausea, skin rash, or hypertrichosis
Valproic acid	15–60 mg/kg/day PO in divided doses	Same as above	Behavioral, mood, or mental changes; hepatotoxicity, visual disturbances, coagulopathy or thrombocytopenia, bleeding

Data from Jacox et al[12]; Payne[53]; Rowbathum et al.[119]

ness, increased ability to concentrate, mood elevation, euphoria, and an increase in motor and speech activity. Unpleasant side effects include confusion, agitation, dysphoria, apprehension, and fatigue.[127]

The use of psychostimulants has become an acceptable practice based on data from earlier studies of patients with cancer. A controlled clinical trial comparing methylphenidate (15 mg/day) to placebo demonstrated superior effects of methylphenidate in increasing analgesia while decreasing sedation.[130] Subsequently, Bruera et al found that 91% of patients reported improvement in somnolence 48 hours after treatment.[131] They also noted that patients became tolerant to methylphenidate with an initial dose of 15 mg/day and a mean maximal daily dose of 42 mg ± 6 mg after 39 ± 20 days. In a double-blind, placebo-controlled trial with methylphenidate, Wilwerding et al reported an improvement in opioid-induced drowsiness and an increase in nighttime sleep.[129]

Phenothiazines/antihistamines.   According to Dundee and Moore, the myth that promethazine potentiates analgesia with promethazine originated from "observations after its [promethazine's] use with large doses of pethidine [meperidine] or other analgesics, and erroneously attributing reductions in barbiturate dosage and side effects during anesthesia to the promethazine."[132,p.96] Even though promethazine was purported to have antianalgesic properties almost 30 years ago, the potentiation myth is still widely believed today. Similarly, Keats et al, found that promethazine did not increase analgesic efficacy, meperidine-induced respiratory depression, or prevent meperidine-induced nausea and vomiting, but that it did increase the sedative effects of meperidine.[133] Meth-

otrimeprazine (Levoprome) is the only phenothiazine that has demonstrated analgesic properties.[7]

Haloperidol (Haldol) has not been found to possess any opioid-sparing effects.[134] However, this agent can be used to treat opioid-induced acute confusional states (hallucinations, agitation from delirium).[135]

Hydroxyzine (Vistaril) does have mild analgesic, antiemetic, sedating, and antihistamine effects, but its analgesic benefits have only been demonstrated with intramuscular injection. Oral hydroxyzine is a useful adjunct for nausea and anxiety.[7]

Bisphosphonates

These powerful inhibitors of bone resorption are used for treating disorders such as Paget's disease and hypercalcemia of malignancy. There are data to support the usefulness of these agents for relieving bone pain and improving outcomes for patients with metastatic bone involvement. Ernst et al found a statistically significant decrease in pain scores and an increase in activity level with clodronate 600 mg when compared with placebo in 24 patients with metastatic bone pain.[136] When clodronate 300 mg was given intravenously for 10 days to men with metastatic prostate cancer, there was a reported notable improvement in bone pain.[137]

Pamidronate also has significant benefits in relieving pain from bony metastases that do not respond to NSAIDS and steroids. A double-blind, placebo-controlled trial with pamidronate 90 mg administered as a 4-hour infusion for nine cycles to patients with multiple myeloma showed that patients who received the drug had a significant decrease in bone pain.[138] While the cost of therapy and the time necessary to administer the infusion are important to consider with its use, economic considerations must be weighed against more costly alternatives such as surgery or radiation.[139]

Routes of opioid administration

A variety of routes of opioid administration are available. Individualized plans of care should be developed in collaboration with the patient and physician. Six routes of opioid administration are briefly described below: (1) oral (which may also include sublingual and transmucosal, although they are infrequently used), (2) transdermal, (3) rectal, (4) topical, (5) parenteral (which includes intramuscular, subcutaneous, and intravenous) delivered by intermittent bolus or infusion, and (6) intraspinal or neuraxial (which includes epidural, subarachnoid, and intraventricular) by intermittent bolus or continuous infusion via external or implanted pumps.

Oral. The oral route is preferred over all other routes because it is an effective, comparatively inexpensive, convenient, and safe way to administer opioids. Oral dosing schedules should be used for as long as possible. If patients have a functional gastrointestinal system and can swallow the required number of tablets or amount of oral solution to achieve adequate pain control, then the oral route is the most appropriate route of administration.

Switching patients from the oral route to an alternate route should be considered if high doses of oral opioids are ineffective or if toxicities occur that cannot be successfully managed. For example, severe nausea and vomiting that cannot be controlled with aggressive antiemetic therapy may be one reason to convert patients to another route of administration. Difficulty swallowing, mechanical obstruction of the gastrointestinal tract, and inability to ingest large amounts of oral medication may necessitate the use of other dosing formulations. High doses of oral opioids are often necessary, but as long as effective pain relief can be achieved, high doses are not a reason to switch patients to alternate routes of administration.

The scheduling of oral medications should be on a fixed-interval basis, except in a few circumstances when it may be necessary to use a variable dosing schedule. These include (1) initial dose titration with methadone and levorphanol; (2) concomitant therapies, such as radiation and chemotherapy that may relieve pain, thus reducing the need for scheduled opioid analgesics; (3) simultaneous scheduling with around-the-clock administration to provide for incident or breakthrough pain (this also applies to continuous infusions); and (4) pain that is intermittent.

Sublingual. Opioids such as morphine or oxycodone can be administered by the sublingual route using concentrated oral solution preparations. For patients who are unable to take oral medication, this route can be used intermittently for short-term management of breakthrough pain or on a regular schedule in the last few days or weeks of life. It is important, however, to recognize that sublingual administration may yield fluctuating serum concentrations with erratic pain control; thus, vigilant assessment is necessary.

Transmucosal. The transmucosal route of administration is now possible with a new delivery system for oral transmucosal fentanyl citrate (OTFC). Farrar et al conducted a randomized, double-blind, placebo-controlled trial to evaluate the safety and efficacy of transmucosal fentanyl citrate in the treatment of breakthrough pain in cancer patients.[140] The preparation was effective in relieving pain within 15 minutes, and patients receiving the transmucosal fentanyl used fewer "rescue" doses with other opioids. Readers are advised to consult information from the manufacturer regarding dosing guidelines and equinanalgesic conversions to other opioids.

Transdermal. The transdermal fentanyl system (Duragesic) is currently the only commercially available opioid preparation in the form of a patch, with dosing strengths of 25-, 50-, 75-, and 100-μg. Fentanyl, which is 75–100 times more potent than morphine, is delivered through the skin in a constant-release delivery system. Approximately 92% of the drug is absorbed into the systemic circulation by 72 hours,[42] requiring applications of the patch every 3 days. While the preparation has been shown to produce effects on pain relief, sleep, and symptoms comparable to controlled-released oral morphine, greater patient satisfaction has been reported with the transdermal system.[141] Its use, however, is reserved for patients with steady-state pain who cannot ingest oral medication. Significant delays in achieving analgesia can be encountered if this system is used for patients with rapidly escalating pain. Rescue or supplemental opioid medication is generally needed to control incident or breakthrough pain. Patterns for the use of supplemental medication must be assessed. The patch dose should be raised if there is an increased need for additional supplemental medication 48 hours following the application. Some patients may require patch changes every 48 hours, but this should only be considered when an increase in the dose has been tried.

Calis et al provide an excellent review of the pharmacology, efficacy, and clinical issues related to transdermal fentanyl.[142] Although randomized, well-controlled clinical trials using transdermal fentanyl are lacking, many open-labeled studies indicate that this delivery system provides effective pain relief.[143,144] Data on equianalgesic conversions to oral morphine have been published.[145] The toxicities from transdermal fentanyl are similar to those from other opioid agonist analgesics.

There are several unique features of the transdermal delivery system that have important clinical implications. First, after removing the patch, release of the drug from the skin depot will continue for several hours. This is important if patients experience significant sedation or respiratory depression, because simply removing the patch does not eliminate the risk of further problems from drug toxicity. Therefore, continued monitoring for side effects is necessary. Second, variability in body temperature of 3°C can increase the serum concentrations by 25%. Finally, variability in skin thickness can significantly affect serum concentrations. Thin skin can produce 1.5 times and broken skin 5 times the normal serum value. Thus, an individual with thick skin may absorb less of the drug.[146] Payne presented important clinical guidelines for using transdermal fentanyl, including the following: (1) follow similar principles for chronic opioid use; (2) use in patients with stable baseline pain and minimal incident pain; (3) provide liberal rescue analgesia, especially during the first 24 hours; (4) use rescue doses to calculate dose increases; (5) rotate skin sites; (6) clarify patient and family expectations; and (7) allow several weeks for therapeutic trial.[147] Patients must be advised to avoid local heat (e.g., heating pads, moist heat, prolonged hot showers, electric blankets) on or around the area where the patch is applied as heat may accelerate drug absorption.

Using a research-based approach, Wakefield et al identified the need for nursing education to ensure the appropriate use of more expensive drug delivery systems.[148] It is critical that nurses understand the pharmacodynamics of the transdermal fentanyl system, proper placement of the patch on the upper torso of the body, and more importantly practice implications should side effects occur. Advantages and disadvantages of transdermal fentanyl are highlighted in Table 29-11.

Rectal.   With the advent of the transdermal fentanyl system and innovations in infusional delivery devices, there is no longer as much need for rectal administration of opioids. There may be circumstances, however, when the rectal route is an acceptable alternative. Patients who are unable to take oral medication in the last few days of life may benefit from rectal opioids. Rectal preparations are commercially available for nonopioids (e.g., acetaminophen, aspirin, indomethacin) and opioids (e.g., morphine, hydromorphone, oxymorphone). Many of these opioid agonist products do not allow for flexible titration because of low-potency dosing strengths. For example, hydromorphone comes in a 3-mg suppository, so patients who require high doses of hydromorphone would potentially need more suppositories per dose. Similarly, even though morphine is available in 10-, 20-, and 30-mg strengths, the same problem exists for patients who require high doses. Today, many pharmacies can compound higher dose strengths and even prepare medications for rectal use that are not available from pharmaceutical manufacturers.

Controlled trials using the rectal route of administration in opioid-tolerant patients are lacking. However, one recent well-controlled randomized trial comparing a solution of morphine, 10 mg, administered orally versus rectally in opioid-naive patients showed significant differences in pain intensity, with reduction in pain relief taking 10 minutes for the rectal route versus 60 minutes for the oral route.[149] Bioavailability of rectally administered morphine is quite variable. Administration of oral controlled-release morphine (MS Contin) by the rectal route has been studied, but it is not a route approved by the U.S. Food and Drug Administration (FDA). Cole and Hanning described the advantages and disadvantages of the rectal route of opioid administration, which are summarized in Table 29-12.[150]

Topical.   Topical agents are generally effective in reducing inflammation and the cutaneous hypersensitivity that accompanies neuralgias and neuropathic pain. Capsaicin, manufactured from hot peppers, is a safe and effective analgesic agent, offering a wide range of uses for the treatment of arthritis pain, herpes zoster–related pain, diabetic neuropathy, and postmastectomy pain.[151] When applied regularly to the skin of painful areas, capsaicin depletes the nerve terminals of substance P, a peptide responsible for the transmission of pain. The first few applications are often associated with increased pain, but over time (typically a few days), some patients will experience a decrease in pain and hypersensitivity of the skin. The addition of a topical anesthetic when using capsaicin and initiating therapy with the lower concentration of the cream or lotion may improve compliance with initial therapy. Capsaicin is available in nonprescription strengths of 0.025% (Zostrix Cream, Capzacin-P Cream, and Capsin Lotion) and 0.075% (Zostrix-HP Cream, Capsin Lotion). Patients are advised to wash their hands thoroughly after use and to avoid touching the affected area after applying the preparation.

EMLA cream (eutectic mixture of local anesthetics; specifically, prilocaine and lidocaine) is another topical agent that reduces the cutaneous hypersensitivity associated with neuropathic pain. Once applied, it is necessary to cover the area with an occlusive dressing such as a

Table 29-11   Advantages and Disavantages of the Transdermal Fentanyl System

Advantages	Disadvantages
FENTANYL TO ORAL	
• Convenient	• More expensive
• Continuous delivery	• Slower onset
• Long duration	• Slower titration
	• Difficult to reverse side effects immediately
FENTANYL TO IV/SQ	
• Less invasive	• Slower onset
• No needles or pumps	• Slower titration
• Less expensive	• Difficult to reverse side effects immediately
• Easy for caregiver	• More experience with pump-delivery systems
• Requires less technical nursing time	

Data from Calis et al[142]; Payne.[147]

Table 29-12 Advantages and Disadvantages of Rectal Opioid Administration

Advantages	Disadvantages
• Absorption is not delayed by alterations in GI tract, such as vomiting	• Wide variation in systemic availability
• Useful if patients have difficulty swallowing, are unconscious, or NPO	• Delayed or limited absorption due to small surface area
• Drug can be removed if an adverse drug reaction develops	• Defecation or constipation may impair absorption
• Digestive enzymes do not affect drug breakdown	• Rectal-wall enzymes or microorganisms may degrade drug
• No unpleasant taste	• Invasive
• Significant first-pass effect from the liver may be avoided	• Self-medication may be difficult or impossible
• Easier to learn than sophisticated pump technology	
• Low cost	

GI = gastrointestinal; NPO = nothing by mouth.
Data from Cole and Hanning.[150]

transparent (TegaDerm, or plastic wrap) or nonabsorbable covering. While the efficacy of topical NSAIDs has not been established, there are various preparations (e.g., ketoprofen gel) that are compounded for individual client use.

Parenteral. Intramuscular injections of opioid medication may be used to treat acute pain, such as postoperative pain, however, intramuscular injections are painful and should only be used for short-term pain control. Intermittent subcutaneous injections can be administered to control both acute and chronic cancer-related pain, if peripheral or central venous access is not possible. If prolonged analgesic administration is required, intermittent injections should not be used and other routes that do not produce pain on administration should be considered.

Intravenous bolus is a common alternative to intramuscular or subcutaneous injections; however, scheduled bolus injections produce significant peak-and-trough effects with fluctuating levels of pain relief. If doses need to be given every 2 hours or less, then continuous parenteral infusion may be more appropriate. Continuous parenteral infusions are indicated for gastrointestinal problems such as uncontrollable vomiting or obstruction, the inability to ingest oral analgesics, inadequate pain relief or unacceptable toxicities from oral or intermittent bolus injections, and the impracticality of frequent, repeated injections.[152]

The safety and efficacy of continuous intravenous infusions have been demonstrated.[152-155] Continuous infusions provide the patient with steady blood levels of the opioid and can avoid the potential side effects and return of pain associated with intermittent dosing. Guidelines for initiating and managing continuous infusions have been based on clinical experience rather than on controlled studies.[154,155] These guidelines are useful for initiating infusions and determining parameters for titrating doses. A summary of the management of continuous infusional therapy appears in Table 29-13.

Continuous subcutaneous. Continuous subcutaneous opioid infusions provide an acceptable alternative to intravenous administration in circumstances when long-term intravenous access is not available or is limited. Ambulatory, computerized infusion devices have facilitated the use of subcutaneous infusions at home. Because subcutaneous infusions are relatively easy to initiate, patients can be switched over to a subcutaneous infusion in the home providing that necessary resources (drug-delivery system, skilled home care professionals) are in place.

Morphine and hydromorphone[156,157] and metha-

Table 29-13 Suggestions for the Management of Continuous Intravenous Infusion of Opioid Analgesics

1. All infusions should be administered with a flow-calibrated infusion pump.
2. Convert the patient's current opioid drugs to an equal analgesic parenteral dose of the drug that will be used for the infusion.
3. If the drug to be used for the infusion is the same one the patient is currently receiving, divide the parenteral dose by 24 to determine the hourly infusion rate.
4. If the drug to be used for the infusion is a different drug, use only half of the parenteral dose, and then divide by 24 to determine the hourly infusion rate.
5. Administer a loading dose at the beginning of the infusion and with each increase in the infusion rate. The amount of the loading dose depends on the patient's current opioid requirements.
6. Titrate the infusion until the patient reports pain relief or unacceptable side effects. Titration may occur the following ways:
   a. Increase the infusion rate by 10%–20% every few hours if the patient is receiving close monitoring.
   b. Administer additional doses of a short-acting opioid (preferably the same drug as the infusion) q1–2h prn. Give 25%–50% of the hourly dose for prn dosing. Increase the infusion rate q12–24h by the amount equal to the total number of milligrams during the preceding period divided by the number of hours in that period. Use this method if the patient is not receiving dose monitoring.

Data from Portenoy RK.[154]

done[158] have been the most commonly used opioids for subcutaneous administration; however, recent evidence shows that continuous subcutaneous infusions of fentanyl are also safe and effective.[159] A small-gauge butterfly needle (25 or 27) or commercially available needle system (e.g., Sub-Q-Set) is inserted into the subcutaneous tissue below the clavicle bone of the anterior chest or in the abdomen. Frequency of needle site changes is quite variable depending on the volume of drug per hour, the volume and number of demand or bolus doses, and the drug. Reports have ranged from every 6 hours to every 21 days.[160] Macmillan et al studied 45 patients receiving subcutaneous infusions and found that the average duration of a needle remaining in place without toxicities was 7.3 days ± 5.2 (range 1–29).

Continuous subcutaneous infusions of opioids are indicated for patients who (1) are unable to take oral medication due to nausea, vomiting, or a mechanical obstruction in the gastrointestinal tract; (2) are unable to use alternative routes because doses may be too high; (3) have limited or no venous access; and (4) are unable to maintain control with oral administration. Problems associated with subcutaneous continuous infusions have included local skin irritation, leakage, swelling, and discomfort at the needle site. Teflon catheters appear to last longer than metal needles.[161] Bruera et al reported that patients preferred this system for analgesic administration because they achieved better pain control and increased mobility and found it easy to administer.[162] Moulin et al used a randomized, double-blind crossover design to compare subcutaneous and intravenous hydromorphone infusions.[163] They concluded that there were no significant differences between the two routes with regard to pain intensity, pain relief, mood, and sedation. In fact, they strongly recommended abandoning the intravenous route for management. In another prospective trial, Lang et al compared intermittent oral or subcutaneous with continuous subcutaneous administration and found statistically significant improvements in pain relief and fewer toxicities for the subcutaneous route.[164]

An important clinical issue for subcutaneous infusions is the volume and concentration of the drug infused. Differences in volume and concentration and how these affect pain relief have been studied. Morphine and hydromorphone can be reconstituted to make concentrations as high as 60 mg/mL and 100 mg/mL, respectively.[42] Bruera et al demonstrated that with a mean hydromorphone concentration of 30 ± 15 mg/mL, hydromorphone can be safely given in concentrations higher than those commercially available.[165] The volume per 24 hours without the addition of substances like hyaluronidase has been reported at 24–48 mL/day.[155,162] An earlier study by Bruera et al reported on the successful use of hyaluronidase with a dextrose/saline solution to deliver subcutaneous hydration and opioid analgesics.[166] The rate of infusion was 20–100 mL/hour.

Patient-controlled analgesia. Advances in computerized software for infusion devices have made patient-controlled analgesia (PCA) a common and acceptable method for delivering opioid analgesia through parenteral (IV and SQ) routes. Intravenous PCA for postoperative pain has become the mainstay for intravenous administration of opioids. Use of PCA for chronic cancer-related pain has also evolved into an effective approach for parenteral drug delivery. Patient-controlled analgesia (PCA) is designed to allow patients to self-administer analgesics within a preset interval that is programmed into the infusion device. Regimens for acute pain such as postoperative pain include a self-administered or demand dose, but a continuous background infusion or basal rate of an opioid analgesic (e.g., morphine, fentanyl, hydromorphone, and less often meperidine) may be added. Demand-dosing schedules usually include small doses of the opioid with short *lock-out intervals* (5–15 minutes), the time allowed between doses. Patients can access self-administered doses frequently to control short-term pain. In doing so, peaks and troughs for serum levels that are often associated with conventional as needed (PRN) parenteral administration are avoided. On the other hand, PCA regimens for the management of chronic cancer pain almost always include a basal rate that is supposed to deliver the bulk of the analgesic therapy. Higher demand doses at less frequent intervals are used to supplement the basal rate. This practice is intended to prevent the patient from working too hard to maintain adequate analgesia. In general, the benefits of PCA include better overall pain control, more prompt administration of opioids to control predictable or unpredictable bouts of pain, increased onset of analgesic action, and greater patient satisfaction.

Patient-controlled analgesia has also been successfully used in adolescents and adults to treat severe mucositis pain from the preparative regimen for bone marrow transplantation.[167] Bruera et al reported similar efficacy and toxicity with subcutaneous PCA and subcutaneous continuous infusions in 22 patients.[168] Each PCA bolus dose was equivalent to 4 hours of the infusion. Kerr et al reported that patients had improvement in pain control using PCA with subcutaneous and intravenous opioid infusions.[169] Maximum hourly doses for the opioids in the study were hydromorphone 60 mg, morphine 80 mg, and meperidine 50 mg. While morphine and hydromorphone remain the most frequently administered opioids for PCA, methadone can also be safely administered by this route.[170]

Sophisticated computer software technology for infusion devices as well as demonstrated efficacy and safety have contributed to more frequent use of PCA infusion devices by both inpatients and outpatients. While its use with inpatients is rarely disputed, the appropriateness of PCA for control of chronic cancer-related pain at home has been debated. Ferrell et al identified appropriate indications for the use of PCA: (1) administration of oral medication is not possible; (2) the patient may benefit from increased self-control; and (3) severe breakthrough pain needs to be controlled.[171] They also cautioned that PCA was *not* appropriate with increased sedation or confusion; if oral therapy was not maximized; in potential conflict of interest if the prescriber and owners of the equipment or supplier were the same; when convenience was assumed; and if home health care nurses were inadequately trained.

Intermittent subcutaneous. When it is not possible to administer continuous subcutaneous infusions due to economic considerations, availability of home health resources, or patient acceptance, short-term intermittent subcutaneous injections are possible.[172] A subcutaneous needle system can be placed in a fashion similar to that for continuous infusions. The same needle and administration set are used for multiple scheduled injections throughout the day. This approach can also be used on an intermittent, as-needed basis for breakthrough pain in patients who are using transdermal fentanyl and are unable to take medications orally.

Intraspinal (neuraxial). The identification of opiate receptors in the brain and spinal cord and the results of early animal work involving spinal opioids have provided the bases for use of intraspinal or neuraxial (epidural and intrathecal [subarachnoid]) opioid administration for cancer pain. Epidural therapy is delivered into the epidural space, an area outside the dura over the subarachnoid space. The epidural space consists of fat, veins, and some arteries. The subarachnoid space, below the dura, is where cerebral spinal fluid circulates. The route of delivery into the subarachnoid space is termed *intrathecal administration*. The potency of opioids is approximately 10 times greater when injected into the subarachnoid space by intrathecal administration compared to the epidural route.

In an early study, Arner and Arner evaluated a hierarchy of responses to epidural analgesia with different pain problems.[173] From best response to least response, these are (1) somatic continuous pain, (2) visceral continuous pain, (3) somatic intermittent pain, (4) visceral intermittent pain, (5) neuropathic pain, either intermittent or continuous, and (6) cutaneous pain.

Morphine and fentanyl have been the most common agents used for intraspinal opioid administration; however, hydromorphone has also been used. The combination of opioids and anesthetic agents such as bupivacaine or ropivacaine is often used, especially in patients who have not been treated successfully with opioids alone.[174,175] Anesthetic agents, which act in part by reducing cell membrane permeability to sodium ions, act directly on the nerve roots. Although there are added risks of motor, sensory, and sympathetic complications, the use of anesthetic agents can provide patients with effective pain relief. Nonopioids such as clonidine, an alpha-adrenergic agonist, have also been studied and are more effective than placebo for patients with neuropathic pain.[176]

Criteria for determining the appropriateness of a patient for intraspinal opioids have been established by several investigators and clinicians.[177–179] These include:

- Opioid-responsive pain, but unacceptable toxicities from systemic opioids

- Pain below the midcervical dermatome
- Neuroablative or anesthetic procedures unsuccessful or not indicated
- Life expectancy of more than 3 months
- Satisfactory home and family support
- Successful response to trial of opioids or anesthetic agent through temporary catheter

Penn and Paice suggest that responses to trials of intraspinal therapy be based on a decrease in systemic opioids, the degree of pain relief, and improvements in activity level.[180]

Administration of intraspinal analgesics can be accomplished through a percutaneous externalized catheter, tunneled implantable externalized catheter (DuPen, Davol Inc., Cranston, RI), implantable reservoir or a port for injection (either as a bolus injection or continuous infusion [Port-a-Cath, SIMS Delta, Inc., St. Paul MN]) and totally implantable drug-delivery systems (SynchroMed Infusion System, Medtronic, Inc., Minneapolis, MN.) Factors that determine which type of system should be used include life expectancy, route of administration (epidural vs. intrathecal), clinician expertise, opioid and anesthetic requirements, home care support, and economic considerations. Externalized catheters and implantable ports are generally used for epidural therapy and require an infusion device for drug delivery. Totally implantable drug-delivery systems are more costly and typically used when life expectancy is believed to be greater than 3 months. Advantages and disadvantages of intraspinal drug delivery systems are highlighted in Table 29-14.[12]

Paice et al conducted a multicenter survey of physicians to examine use of intraspinal opioids for both cancer- and noncancer-related pain.[181] They concluded that there was little agreement as to the critical outcomes that should be measured to evaluate the success of therapy. Numerous reports have documented the outcomes of intraspinal therapy. Complications and rate of occurrence have been attributed to the type of technology or catheter, placement of the catheter (epidural vs. intrathecal), and duration of therapy. Complications include catheter-related problems, such as dislodgement, obstruction or occlusion, breakage, or leakage from the catheter. Externalized epidural catheters are more vulnerable to kinking and tearing. Overall, the incidence of catheter-related problems, 10%–40%, was similar to those reported by others. Of interest, patients with neuropathic pain tended to require higher doses at 6 months of therapy.

Drug-induced toxicities such as urinary retention, pruritus, nausea, vomiting, and respiratory depression can occur with intraspinal therapy. Respiratory depression rarely occurs with patients who are tolerant to opioids; however, intrathecal therapy tends to pose the greatest risk.[182] Motor impairment is more pronounced with the use of a local anesthetic such as bupivacaine that acts on both sensory and motor nerves. Ropivacaine, which is selective for just sensory nerves, tends to produce fewer motor problems.[183] This agent may be a better op-

Table 29-14 Advantages and Disadvantages of Intraspinal Drug Administration

System	Advantages	Disadvantages
Percutaneous temporary catheter	Used extensively both intraoperatively and postoperatively. Useful when prognosis is limited (<1 month).	Mechanical problems include catheter dislodgement, kinking, or migration.
Permanent silicone rubber epidural	Catheter implantation is a minor procedure. Dislodgement and infection less common than with temporary catheters. Can deliver bolus injections, continuous infusions, or PCA (with or without continuous delivery).	
Subcutaneous implanted injection port	Increased stability, less risk of dislodgement. Can deliver bolus injections or continuous infusions (with or without PCA).	Implantation more invasive than external catheters. Approved only for epidural catheter in U.S. Potential for infection increases with frequent injections.
Subcutaneous reservoir	Potential for reduced infection in comparison to external system.	Difficult to access, and fibrosis may occur after repeated injection.
Implanted pumps (continuous and programmable)	Potential for decreased risk of infection.	Need for more extensive operative procedure. Need for specialized, costly equipment with programmable systems.

PCA = patient-controlled analgesia.

Reprinted from Jacox A, Carr DB, Payne R, et al: *Management of Cancer Pain; Adults' Quick Reference Guide No. 9.* AHCPR Publication No. 94-0593. Rockville, MD, Agency for Health Care Policy and Research, U.S. Department of Health and Human Services, Public Health Service, 1994, p 14.

tion for patients who are elderly or already weak and debilitated. Another important concern is the risk of infection, which is possible with all types of delivery systems but is greater with externalized infusion systems. DuPen et al reported a 5.4% incidence of infection (1 per 1702 catheter-days).[184] Most reported infections were exit site or superficial epidural track infections. Catheters were removed only if a patient had a positive culture or if an infection was present in the epidural space.

Recently, intraspinal clonidine has been administered for the treatment of neuropathic pain. Clonidine, an alpha$_2$-agonist, is believed to interfere with norepinephrine and epinephrine at the level of the spinal cord. These neurotransmitters are thought to be implicated in the transmission of pain from nerve injury. Eisenach et al,[176] in a study of 85 patients with severe cancer pain taking large doses of opioid, compared epidural clonidine at a dose of 30 μg per hour to placebo over 14 days. The group receiving the clonidine experienced a decrease in blood pressure and heart rate, and those with a component of neuropathic pain had a decrease in pain. Hypotension, defined as a serious side effect, was evident only in patients in the clonidine group and in one member of the placebo group. While guidelines for monitoring patients receiving epidural clonidine vary, frequent monitoring of the blood pressure and heart rate is most critical in the first 12–24 hours after initiating therapy and when dose escalations are made. The nurse should collaborate with the prescribing physician to determine specific monitoring parameters.

The care of patients who are receiving intraspinal therapy at home requires coordination between the physician or team responsible for maintaining therapy and home health agency professionals. The basic knowledge and competency levels that are required to take care of patients receiving intraspinal opioids have been determined.[185,186] Nurses must possess an understanding of the anatomy and physiology of the spinal cord, pharmacological properties of drugs used in neuraxial therapy, potential complications of therapy, and care of external catheters and the exit site. The nurse must also be familiar with the operational features of external infusion devices and implantable infusion systems. Guidelines for patient monitoring, drug administration, and protocols involving potential complications and emergency situations must be defined in the plan of care.

Prior to initiating intraspinal therapy, the patient and family are informed about the expectations for the therapy, possible complications, the need for diagnostic tests, the costs involved, possible expected outcomes, alternative forms of therapy, and options for home care. Next, the patient and family must be prepared for the placement procedure. Olsson et al[186] and Paice[187] have formulated plans of care for patients receiving intraspinal opioids that include nursing diagnoses, patient outcomes, and nursing interventions. Nursing diagnoses include (1) potential alteration in respiratory function; (2) potential alteration in comfort related to pruritus, nausea, vomiting, pain on injection, and inadequate pain relief; (3) potential alteration in elimination (urinary); (4) knowledge deficit regarding epidural analgesia; and (5) potential infection at the catheter site. After careful assessment, a decision about inserting a permanent catheter or an implantable infusion system is made.

Externalized catheters (Arrow International Inc., Reading, PA. Dupen catheter) and implantable ports (e.g., Arrow Port-a-Cath) that are accessed require local skin care at the exit site. Admittedly, there are no universally acceptable protocols for cleansing and dressing the site; however, many agree that there is a possibility that caustic agents such as iodine and acetone can migrate into the epidural space. Paice et al recently conducted a study to evaluate potential hazards of using providine-iodine to cleanse the catheter exit site.[188] Cleansing with commercially available pledgets rather than iodine swabs or gauze pads was associated with the least amount of contamination into the catheter.

Plans for home care focus on optimizing the patient's regimen before discharge. Because hospital length of stay may be limited, dose titration often must resume at home. Plans for follow-up, outpatient management, and coordination of home care activities are essential. It is critical to ensure that any home health or home infusion agency to which the patient is referred is familiar with prescribed protocols for catheter care and patient monitoring. The agency should have experience in the home management of intraspinal therapy and be able to identify problems and promptly respond to them. The availability of agency resources must be determined, especially to safeguard against a disruption in therapy should problems with the catheter or infusion device occur. Implantable SynchroMed Infusion Systems require a portable computer for programming and interrogating the internal device. Should a patient experience side effects, it is critical that the agency be able to immediately access and use the computer or be able to promptly transport the patient to a facility where a computer is available.

Technology-Supported Pain Care

Concerns about the appropriateness of some of the routes of administration described above, such as PCA and home use of neuraxial opioids, reflect the broader dilemma facing technology-supported pain care. The Oncology Nursing Society developed a resolution to address the appropriateness of technology in pain management including use of neuraxial (intraspinal, epidural, and subarachnoid) routes, intravenous administration, and subcutaneous infusions.[189] This document delineated the appropriate implications for technology-supported pain care and stressed the significant financial, physical, and psychological burdens that are placed on the patient and family when such therapy is used. While no one would argue that all patients are unequivocally entitled to receive pain relief, the process of selecting the methods to provide such relief and allocating resources remains an issue for debate. Ferrell and Rhiner used a biomedical ethical perspective in approaching this problem.[190] Ethical principles and decision-making are relevant to the determinations of who should receive technology-supported pain therapies. Whedon and Ferrell provided a case-study analysis of patient situations to illustrate the importance of appropriate patient selection, the need for a thorough assessment to determine the efficacy of the treatment, informed consent issues, financial implications, burden placed on the family, conflict of interest, and complications or morbidity.[191] Indiscriminate use of these therapies without clear indications can lead to undue emotional stress for patient and family, disruptions in the home environment, financial worries, and inappropriate use of health care resources.

Nurses are seldom able to make the final decision about whether a patient should receive technology-supported pain care, but they are in a position to identify appropriate indications and weigh the benefits against the risks and costs of therapy. Nurses can also assume a lead role in establishing standards for the use of pain technology, as there is evidence to suggest that clinicians are generally inconsistent in how they implement such therapies.[191]

Drug Therapy for the Elderly

Treatment of pain in the elderly requires knowledge of their specialized needs due to the physiological and lifestyle changes that occur with aging. The application of information regarding the pharmacodynamics of analgesics is critical in selecting agents that have a low side effect profile. Table 29-15 outlines the important considerations for use of analgesics in the elderly.[8,109,192]

Nerve Blocks and Neuroablative Procedures

Temporary nerve blocks and permanent neurolytic blocks or neuroablation are procedures used to modulate neural responses to noxious stimuli in cancer-related pain. The injection of a local anesthetic into a nerve, nerve root, or epidural space prevents the generation and conduction of nerve impulses. Temporary or nondestructive nerve blocks serve two functions: (1) this technique is used for the treatment of intractable pain such as neuropathic pain caused by invasion or compression of intraspinal nerve roots; and (2) it is helpful as a prognostic/diagnostic technique to differentiate visceral pain from somatic pain, demonstrate neural pathways for selected pain conditions, and determine who might benefit from a more permanent block or neuroablative procedures.[193] While adequate relief of pain may be achieved, it is short-term because the effects of the local anesthetic generally wear off in 6–8 hours.

Neurolytic or destructive nerve blocks provide more prolonged pain relief than nondestructive nerve blocks and can minimize the need for systemic medication, thus reducing drug-related toxicities. There are several factors that must be considered before a neurolytic procedure is performed.[194] First, neurolytic blocks are most useful in treating pain that is well-defined or localized. Second, pain relief in response to a temporary block with a local anesthetic may be evaluated; however, short-term blocks do not always predict responses to neurolytic techniques. Third, the patient and family must understand the long-term neurological consequences (bowel and bladder dys-

Table 29-15 Special Considerations for Pain Assessment and Pain Management in the Elderly

Age-Related Changes	Specific Interventions for the Elderly
Mental status ↓ Mental acuity Short-term memory deficits ↓ Information processing ↑ Susceptibility to sedating effects of analgesics Organic brain syndrome	• Use caution with psychoactive agents. • Select opioid agents with ↓ sedating effects (e.g., hydrocodone, oxycodone, hydromorphone). • Select adjuvant agents with ↓ sedating effects (e.g., gabapentin and desipramine). • Initiate therapy with one-half the usual starting dose for adults. • Institute safety precautions. • Use appropriate age-specific pain measures for the elderly and cognitively impaired.
Vision and hearing ↓ Visual acuity ↓ Hearing	• Use pain assessment measures and teaching materials that are easy to read. • Modify the environment (e.g., proper lighting, reduce noise and external stimuli). • Speak clearly and maintain eye contact. • Use medication labels that can be read easily. • Ensure proper functioning of hearing aids. • Avoid drugs that are contraindicated with glaucoma (e.g., agents with anticholinergic effects).
Musculoskeletal Degenerative joint disease Osteoporosis Joint stiffness ↓ Mobility	• Begin with nonopioid agents. • Do not exceed daily recommended doses for acetaminophen of >4000 mg/day. • Use NSAIDs appropriately for mechanisms of pain that involve inflammation. • Discontinue therapy with NSAIDs if analgesia is not effective. • Encourage exercise and physical therapy programs. • Institute treatment with methods of cutaneous stimulation. • Administer effective supplemental analgesia for provoked pain associated with activity.
Pulmonary ↓ Pulmonary reserves COPD Emphysema	• Use caution with opioid and other analgesic agents that cause sedation. • Initiate opioid therapy with one-half the usual starting dose for adults, especially for opioid-naive patients. • Remember that the risk of respiratory depression from opioids is minimized if doses are escalated safely. • Respiratory depression from opioids is rarely a problem for patients who are opioid-dependent and tolerant to their effects.
Cardiovascular Reduced blood volume ↓ Cardiac output and reserve ↓ Circulation Conduction abnormalities	• Drug absorption, distribution, and excretion may be altered by cardiovascular changes associated with aging. • Administer NSAIDs cautiously to patients with congestive heart failure due to a reduction in prostaglandins that are necessary to maintain renal perfusion; this increases the risk for fluid retention and peripheral edema. • Avoid tricyclic antidepressants if patients have cardiac conduction defects.
Gastrointestinal Changes in salivary flow and dentition ↓ Fluid intake Dehydration ↓ Gastric emptying	• Avoid NSAIDs in patients with a history of peptic ulcer disease. • Avoid NSAIDs in patients concurrently taking anticoagulants (e.g., warfarin). • Use caution with tricyclics with ↑ anticholinergic effects (amitriptyline). • Use opioids cautiously in patients who are dehydrated, as they may be more susceptible to opioid-related side effects.
Renal ↓ Renal filtration and renal clearance Renal insufficiency	• Obtain baseline BUN, creatinine, and creatinine clearance prior to initiating therapy with NSAIDs, and monitor renal function closely for long-term NSAID use. • Consider lower doses of NSAIDs to reduce the risk of renal toxicity with long-term use. • Administer short-acting NSAIDs on a prn rather than RTC basis. • Avoid opioids with toxic active metabolites that are excreted by the kidney (meperidine, proproxyphene). • Use caution with morphine due to morphine-3- and morphine-6-glucuronide, which may accumulate with impaired renal function
Genitourinary Benign prostatic hypertrophy in men Urinary incontinence, stress incontinence in women	• Patients who are opioid-naive are most at risk for urinary retention. • Use caution with anticholinergic agents (e.g., amitriptyline) that may cause urinary retention. • Instruct patients taking opioids or tricyclic antidepressants to report changes in urination, and be aware of signs of urinary tract infections.

↓ = decreased; ↑ = increased; NSAID = nonsteroidal anti-inflammatory drug; COPD = chronic obstructive pulmonary disease; BUN = blood urea nitrogen.

Data from American Geriatrics Society Panel on Chronic Pain in Older Persons[8]; Hofmann et al[17]; Lipman[109]; Dellasega and Keiser.[192]

function, motor impairment, sensory alterations) in the area affected by the block. A nerve block with local anesthetic will give the patient some sense of how it feels to experience altered sensations over the affected site. Fourth, the patient's length of survival is taken into account. Because neurolysis of nerves may not be permanent and some regeneration can be expected within weeks to months, neurolytic procedures are generally reserved for patients with a limited life expectancy.

Unfortunately neurolytic agents cannot discriminate between pain fibers, A-delta and C-fibers, and other fibers (e.g., motor). Therefore, both sensory and motor impairment can result from neurolytic procedures. Celiac plexus and superior hypogastric neurolytic blocks are recommended for patients with intraabdominal metastases and pelvic pain.[195] Lillemoe et al,[196] in an evaluation of the effect of chemical splanchnicectomy (destruction of the splanchic nerves) with alcohol on pain in patients with unresectable pancreatic carcinoma, demonstrated significant reductions in pain compared to injections with saline. Neurolysis of the brachial plexus may be useful for upper extremity pain, but because the brachial plexus has a high number of motor nerves, weakness of limb or loss of function can result.[197] Chemical nerve destruction in the lumbosacral area can lead to bowel and bladder impairment and lower extremity weakness.

Alcohol and phenol are the two most common agents used for chemical neurolysis. Alcohol is administered directly into the nerve, nerve root, or plexus. Injections can be painful, but this is transient and pain can be effectively managed with additional pain medication. The alcohol can be absorbed, and depending on the concentration and volume, patients may experience the short-term systemic effects of alcohol intoxication. It may be necessary to implement patient safety measures and close observation should this occur. Phenol has a higher affinity than alcohol for vasculature, therefore, the injury to blood vessels may account for neurological damage.[198] Regardless of the agent used, patients may experience heightened pain 12–24 hours following the procedure. A flexible schedule with short-acting analgesics should be used to treat transient exacerbations of pain. Twenty-four to 48 hours following the procedure and regularly thereafter for 1–2 weeks, the patient should be assessed for a decrease in pain and a reduction in analgesics.

Destructive neurosurgical procedures most often are used when standard pharmacological and nonpharmacological strategies are no longer effective. Patients are carefully selected for these procedures due to the potential motor and sensory impairment. Several neurosurgical techniques can be performed. The indications and implications for preprocedure and postprocedure care are outlined by Tasker:[199]

- *Peripheral neurectomy:* Destroys sensory modalities (from peripheral nerve; not recommended for pain in extremities)

- *Rhizotomy:* Eliminates all sensation entering dorsal spinal cord; preserves motor function; indicated for involvement of a limited number of dermatones; percutaneous procedure is an option for debilitated patients

- *Cordotomy:* Involves interruption of ascending pain and temperature fibers in anterolateral spinal cord; preserves major sensory function; good for unilateral pain

- *Myelotomy:* Interrupts pain and temperature fibers as they cross before reaching opposite spinothalamic tract; used for bilateral pain

The nursing responsibilities for patients undergoing anesthetic and neurodestructive procedures include (1) knowledge about the purpose of the procedure and how it is performed; (2) potential complications based on type of block, agent, and location; and (3) potential benefit of the procedure. An efficient way of obtaining some of this information is to participate in the explanation of the procedure to the patient and to talk with the anesthesiologist or neurosurgeon. Because this requisite information is based on the patient's individual pain problem, standard reference materials may provide incomplete information. The Core Curriculum for Neuroscience Nursing[200] is a useful resource for nurses caring for patients undergoing neurodestructive procedures.

Diminishing the Emotional and Reactive Components of Pain

This approach to managing pain is an area in which nurses can discuss cognitive, behavioral, informational, and other strategies; prepare patients for these therapies; and mobilize the necessary resources to implement them. Interventions included in this approach do not generally affect the underlying pathology or alter the perception or sensation of pain, but rather help in a variety of ways to decrease patients' emotional responses to pain, enabling them to deal with it more positively and proactively.

Because both nurses and physicians may have little information about nonpsychiatric, nonpharmacologic interventions, individuals with cancer often have greater awareness of these approaches than health care providers.[201] Such techniques can be helpful in reducing pain and should be encouraged as part of a comprehensive pain management effort. Indeed, clinical practice guidelines[12] and nursing specialty organizations[202] urge a combination of therapeutic approaches.

Aside from being underutilized, the efficacy of these interventions is only beginning to be systematically tested with rigorous research designs in the clinical environment. Although there are methodologic and logistical difficulties inherent in conducting nonpharmacological intervention studies with cancer patients,[203,204] the usefulness of nonpharmacologic strategies needs evaluation, particularly in terms of how they should be used in conjunction with pharmacologic approaches to therapy.

The role of these techniques is clearly that of an adjuvant to standard pharmacological therapy.[205] Drugs are used to treat the somatic (physiological and sensory) dimensions of pain, while nondrug methods are aimed at treating the affective, cognitive, behavioral, and sociocultural dimensions of pain. The benefits of many of the techniques are that they may increase the patient's sense of personal control, reduce feelings of helplessness, provide opportunities to become actively involved in care, reduce stress and anxiety, elevate mood, raise pain threshold, and thereby reduce pain.

Spross and Burke published an excellent and comprehensive summary of the use of nonpharmacologic noninvasive interventions for patients with cancer pain.[206] They used the multidimensional conceptualization of pain presented earlier in this text (see Chapter 28) to describe numerous strategies available for managing pain, review research and anecdotal evidence for the efficacy of the strategies, and discuss the knowledge and skills nurses needed to implement them in clinical settings. They grouped noninvasive measures into the categories of interpersonal/spiritual, cognitive, behavioral, physical, and environmental. Each technique they describe was included because it met one or more of the following criteria: easy to learn, easy to use in the clinical setting, not completely discussed in other resources readily available to nurses, important or efficacious in relieving cancer pain, potentially effective for relieving pain despite little scientific support, or documented efficacy in patients with noncancer pain.

McCaffery and Pasero addressed nonpharmacologic pain interventions.[205] They noted that although sufficient research still did not exist to document the efficacy of these techniques, a number of them were easily and quickly implemented, specifically cutaneous stimulation, distraction, and relaxation. They recommend that these techniques be incorporated into the care plan where appropriate and when patients are willing.

Many of the treatment strategies aimed at diminishing the emotional and reactive components of pain are classified as cognitive, behavioral, or cognitive *and* behavioral techniques. *Cognitive methods* are those that attempt directly to modify thought processes in order to attenuate or relieve pain; they can be applied to thoughts, images, and attitudes. Examples include information, distraction, imagery, calming self-statements, identification of detrimental responses to pain, and informational or educational programs about pain and its management. *Behavioral methods* are those that modify physiological reactions to pain or behavioral manifestations of pain. Examples include relaxation, meditation, music therapy, and various desensitization strategies. Sometimes cognitive and behavioral techniques are used together, such as relaxation and guided imagery.

Another category of nonpharmacologic interventions are those that diminish the emotional and reactive components of pain by providing cutaneous stimulation; examples include applications of heat, cold, massage, and vibration. Although these methods technically fall within the major treatment approach of changing perception or sensation of pain, they are included here because they are traditional nursing interventions that also involve use of specific behaviors to ameliorate pain.

Finally, a separate category of behavioral interventions that change perception or sensation of pain and also diminish affective reactions is based on mobility/mobilization and immobilization in order to improve functional status. Most of these interventions are simple and can be initiated when ongoing assessment of pain suggests a need for them.

In each of the following sections, selected interventions are discussed briefly. Additional information, including research evidence supporting their efficacy in cancer pain and details on implementing them, can be found in Spross and Burke[205] and McCaffery and Pasero.[206] Our discussion is limited only to those techniques that are clearly within the scope of nursing practice and can be used without significant additional training. Table 29-16 provides additional information about these techniques.

Cutaneous Stimulation

This group of methods is thought to help relieve pain by physiologically altering the transmission of nociceptive stimuli; these methods are based on the gate-control theory of pain and additional basic and clinical research findings related to mechanisms of pain.[207] Heat can be applied with hot packs, a heating pad, a hot water bottle, or a shower or bath. Cold can be applied with cold packs, cold cloths, ice, gel packs, or cold water. Massage is administered via fingers or hands and can be accompanied by a variety of topical local anesthetic agents such as capsaicin, EMLA, or lidocaine.[205] Vibration can be administered with a variety of stimulators including transcutaneous electrical nerve stimulators in some cases. Some of these methods are used frequently at home by patients with pain, and combinations are common. The research testing these methods is still somewhat sparse. One experimental study suggested that massage was an effective short-term intervention in male cancer patients with pain.[208] Another study indicated that 30 minutes of massage therapy reduced cancer patients' anxiety and pain perception, and enhanced their feelings of relaxation.[209] Some patients taking opiates do derive benefit from transcutaneous electrical nerve stimulation (TENS).[208] Rhiner et al reported in a study of cancer pain that heat and massage/vibration were the most common methods selected by elderly cancer patients.[210] Kingdon et al present brief clinically oriented guidelines for using some of these techniques.[211]

Immobilization/Mobilization and Functional Status

Even when good pharmacological therapy has been instituted, some individuals may still experience pain on

Table 29-16 Selected Nonpharmacological Interventions for Pain

Technique	Examples	Advantages	Disadvantages
Cutaneous stimulation	Superficial heating or cooling, vibration, massage	Many methods; makes pain tolerable; reduces pain, patients are receptive; can apply stimulation at site of pain or other sites; can provide distraction	Not for therapeutic or curative purposes; can damage tissue if applied incorrectly
Immobilization/mobilization	Splinting, bracing, walking, exercise, rest	Decreases pain, improves range of motion, conserves energy, improves functional status, promotes relaxation	Discomfort on physical exertion; decrease in functional status
Distraction	*Internal:* Mental images, counting, singing silently; *external:* music, reading, television, conversation	Decreased pain intensity, increased pain tolerance; more acceptable pain sensation; greater sense of control; improved mood	Not helpful for vigilant patients; may have no effect on pain intensity; may be hard to enact; may not 'look like' they are in pain resulting in doubt about pain and/or failure to medicate after distraction; awareness of pain and fatigue may increase; irritability
Relaxation	Slow breathing, progressive muscle relaxation, relaxing mental imagery, repetitive activity or thought	Reduces anxiety, may reduce pain; promotes sleep; decreases fatigue and skeletal muscle tension; increases confidence in ability to handle pain	Can be time-consuming; difficult to teach, practice, and use effectively; is an adjunct method that does not directly relieve pain; often difficult to distinguish between relaxation and imagery
Comprehensive models	Cognitive/behavioral interventions, psychoeducational approaches	Address multiple dimensions of pain; individualized; include patient and family; problem-focused; requires interdisciplinary team	May be difficult to assemble an appropriate interdisciplinary team depending on setting and resources; can be complex and time-consuming

Data from McCaffery and Pasero.[205]

movement. Methods such as complete or partial immobilization of the body or parts of the body and positioning of specific body parts may be quite helpful.[212,213] In other circumstances, mild exercise such as joint range of motion and stretching may help decrease pain. Finally, rest or lying down may help in some instances, perhaps partly because of the relaxation that occurs. Pain assessment tools that address patients' functional status, such as the Brief Pain Inventory,[12,214] can be helpful in determining the impact of pain on daily activities or sleeping and provide rationale for implementing some of these interventions in order to improve functional status.

Although existing research is primarily descriptive,[213,215] it does suggest benefit from these methods. One study examined the use of a therapeutic bed and found it effective in promoting comfort in selected cancer patients.[216] Additional information on these techniques and more can be found in Kingdon et al,[211] Spross and Burke,[206] and McCaffery and Wolff.[212]

Distraction

Distraction is usually defined as a method of diverting one's attention away from sensations or feelings related to pain. Distraction can be significantly helpful in reducing pain. A classic example is the focusing exercises (accompanied by relaxation techniques) taught in childbirth education classes. There are many individual distraction techniques and strategies; examples include conversation, verbalization to self or others, deep thinking, visualization and imagery, mind-body separation, routines/rituals, breathing exercises, counting, reading, and watching television. Additional distraction strategies used by patients with cancer-related pain are music,[217,218] and humor.[210,219–221] Many professional caregivers do not realize the broad scope and variety of distraction strategies, nor the fact that some strategies may work for one individual and not for another. A careful appraisal of patients' preferences and willingness to try such techniques is an important part of the care plan.

Descriptive studies of both inpatients and outpatients with cancer-related pain[213,215,222–224] revealed that distraction strategies such as reading and television helped to reduce pain to some degree. In one of these studies,[223] patients with cancer pain employed a variety of cognitive and behavioral coping techniques (ignoring pain, reinterpreting the sensation, increasing physical activity, etc.) and rated them as moderately effective at reducing pain. More recently, Rhiner et al reported that 50% of patients in their study of cancer pain selected distraction strategies for pain relief.[210] So again, although the scientific evidence is not strong, it is sufficient for caregivers to consider incorporation of such distraction strategies into the pain management plan.

Relaxation and Guided Imagery

Relaxation training helps produce physiological and mental relaxation. The two most common methods are *progressive muscle relaxation*, which is the systematic tensing/relaxing of sixteen muscle groups, and *self-relaxation*, which is the passive, quiet, and still use of autogenic phrases such as "my arms are warm and heavy." Training usually occurs in six to ten sessions with a therapist. Audiotapes can be used at home afterward, and individuals are encouraged to practice and use their new skills. *Guided imagery*, in which an individual visualizes pleasant places or things, is frequently used in conjunction with relaxation.

Though the literature on these techniques in the patient population with cancer is scanty, it was recently reviewed and discussed in depth by Wallace.[225] Of eight studies testing relaxation and imagery for cancer pain, only three[226–228] demonstrated significantly decreased pain intensity. Other studies showed only slight improvement,[229] no difference,[230,231] or worse pain.[232] Effects of relaxation and imagery on the affective dimension of pain, or other components such as perceptions of control over pain or functional status, were equivocal. One additional study not discussed by Wallace[225] was that of Syrjala et al,[233] which demonstrated that transplant patients with acute oral pain from mucositis who received a relaxation and imagery intervention experienced less pain than those who did not. Overall, however, the effectiveness of this group of interventions stills needs careful investigation, particularly when used with opioid analgesics.

Comprehensive Cognitive/Behavioral/ Educational Methods

Several individuals have proposed comprehensive cognitive, behavioral, and educational approaches for cancer pain. These approaches are based on cognitive and social learning models in which pain can be described in terms of objective qualities (e.g., location and intensity) and psychological significance. In one model, therapists provide short-term therapeutic interventions that are adaptable to the individual.[234] More recently, Loscalzo wrote that comprehensive psychological approaches are time-limited, problem-focused, practical, and aimed at both patient and family.[235] The major focus of this framework is to understand how an individual patient's view of the world influences his interpretation and behavior, and to use this information to develop comprehensive psychobehavioral approaches. Strictly speaking, this approach is usually implemented by providers such as psychiatric social workers or psychologists,[235,236] but many elements

are germane to nursing practice. Indeed, there is mounting evidence that nurses have developed effective cognitive/behavioral/educational approaches to symptom management and that, more importantly, collaborative interdisciplinary teams of health care providers have developed management approaches that improve patient outcomes.[237–239]

In summary, the evidence available suggests that many of the nonpharmacological techniques described may be useful in alleviating cancer pain, but clearly much more systematic research is needed to document their efficacy, whether used alone in selected pain situations or as part of a comprehensive treatment plan. Most of these techniques are familiar to nurses and can be used in a variety of settings. Specific references can assist nurses with the information needed to use the techniques effectively.[205,206,240] Many of these techniques require patient and family education and a willingness to try them as adjuncts to pharmacological therapy. Integrated with the use of such techniques, however, should be the nurse as coach, a professional education counseling model that complements patient teaching.[241] The nurse as coach focuses on facilitating the cognitive emotional processing of the patient and enhances self-care skills and cognitive control, areas particularly important in pain management.

Education and Information

Accurate and appropriate education and information for patients with cancer-related pain and their caregivers are an essential aspect of comprehensive pain management. Patients' knowledge about and attitudes toward cancer pain can positively or negatively affect its management.[242] The importance of education was highlighted in the Agency for Health Care Policy and Research (AHCPR) guidelines on cancer pain, which explicitly stated, "Because of the many misconceptions regarding pain and its treatment, education about the ability to control pain effectively and correction of myths about the use of opioids should be included as part of the treatment plan."[12,p.83] These guidelines include a patient guide specifically designed to help patients learn why pain control is important and how to work most effectively with their health care providers.

Barriers, challenges, and solutions to the problem of pain education for patients, families, and nurses have been discussed in depth by Grant and Rivera[243] and by McCaffery and Pasero.[205] Both provide a comprehensive list of resources for pain that include professional and volunteer organizations, publications, and information on patient service programs. The latter reference also provides a number of Web sites with useful information for patients, their families, and professional health care providers. With the explosion of Internet technology and patients' use of it, nurses and other health care providers need to be aware of these many resources.

Although an in-depth discussion of patient and family

education is beyond the scope of this chapter, two key areas must be emphasized. First is the need to select appropriate content for pain education. Much of this content is based on the AHCPR guidelines,[12] the Wisconsin Cancer Pain Initiative,[244] and work by individual investigators.[245] Table 29-17 displays key areas of content for teaching patients and their families and other caregivers. Second is the importance of incorporating sound teaching principles into the plan. Table 29-18 delineates specific guidelines for providing education to patients and families.[12,226,243] Recent research testing pain education programs for cancer pain indicates that patients, families, and health care providers can all benefit from systematically implemented comprehensive programs.[246,247] Additionally, a variety of patient education and documentation tools have been developed to help nurses with pain management.[248,249] Pain education is clearly an essential role for nurses caring for patients with cancer-related pain, as it helps patients and families cope with pain, and improves quality of life.

Conclusion

The multidimensional aspects of cancer pain have been presented in order to heighten nurses' awareness of the physiological mechanisms and psychosocial aspects of pain, including cognitive, behavioral, and sociocultural issues. The unique and complex nature of pain requires

Table 29-17 Content Outline for Pain Education

Importance of treating cancer pain

Causes of cancer pain

Assessing and reporting pain

Available treatment/choosing the right treatments

Beliefs and attitudes about pain treatments/barriers
  Nonopioids
  Opioids
  Other

Side effects of pain medicine

How to take pain medicine
  Routes
  Timing

Nonmedicine pain treatments
  Self-administered cognitive, behavioral, and physical methods
  Radiation therapy
  Neurological therapy
  Surgical therapy

Participation of friends and family in pain treatment

General symptom control

Having a plan and communicating with health care professionals

Data from Jacox et al[12]; Weissman and Dahl[244]; Rhiner and Coluzzi.[245]

Table 29-18 Teaching Principles for Pain Education

- Use only accurate up-to-date information that is predominantly researched-based.
- Assess patient and family's educational needs, cultural background, and prior experiences, and provide content accordingly (individualize).
- Provide both oral and written information that has appropriate literacy levels.
- Involve family members or other caregivers.
- Establish mutually agreeable goals with patient and family or other caregivers.
- Keep teaching sessions brief and take breaks as needed.
- Provide most important material first, based on needs assessment.
- Use a variety of teaching strategies that encourage active, participative learning.
- Use materials that are clear, concise, and have illustrations, if possible.
- Use large print for elderly.
- Consider the patient's physical comfort and select an appropriate environment.
- Tailor teaching to patient's setting (e.g., home or community-based).
- Work closely with other professional health care providers (e.g., home health nurse, physician) to implement teaching plan.

Data from Jacox et al[12]; Ferrell et al[226]; Grant and Rivera[243]; Weissman and Dahl.[244]

specialized care that is best rendered by interdisciplinary collaboration. Combinations of pharmacological, non-pharmacological, and interventional techniques are becoming the mainstays for cancer pain management. Knowledge of all of these strategies is required for nurses so that they can help develop comprehensive plans of care. Earlier interventions with aggressive treatment of pain and palliative care services will provide more assurance that pain and suffering can be alleviated at the end-of-life phase of illness.

Future changes in the health care system will make it necessary for nurses to use research-based data and published clinical care guidelines to define "best practices" that yield maximum benefits for pain relief. Nurses will need to closely examine their practices as they are asked to do more with fewer health care resources. Employers, managed care, and third party health care payers will hold nurses accountable for their practice; therefore, it will be imperative to monitor nursing care through patient-oriented outcomes. As advances in pain therapy expand, greater demands will be placed on nurses to acquire the higher levels of knowledge necessary to care for patients with cancer-related pain. The greatest challenge will be to integrate this knowledge to its fullest, to continue to investigate innovative ways to treat pain, and to impart this knowledge to patients and other health professionals.

References

1. Banning A, Sjogren P, Henriksen H: Pain causes in 200 patients referred to a multidisciplinary cancer pain clinic. *Pain* 45:45–48, 1991

2. Kiar M: The therapy of cancer pain and its integration into a comprehensive supportive care strategy. *Ann Oncol* 8:S15–S19, 1997 (suppl 3)

3. Janjan NA, Payne R, Gillis T, et al: Presenting symptoms in patients referred to a multidisciplinary clinic for bone metastases. *J Pain Symptom Manage* 16:171–178, 1998

4. Wisconsin Cancer Pain Initiative Nursing Education Committee: *Competency Guidelines for Cancer Pain Management in Nursing Education and Practice.* Madison, WI, Wisconsin Cancer Pain Initiative, 1995

5. Spross JA, McGuire DB, Schmitt R: Oncology Nursing Society position paper on cancer pain. *Oncol Nurs Forum* 17: 595–614, 751–760, 825, 944–955, 1990

6. Ad Hoc Committee on Cancer Pain of the American Society of Clinical Oncology: Cancer pain assessment and treatment curriculum guidelines. *J Clin Oncol* 10:1976–1982, 1992

7. American Pain Society: *Principles of Analgesic Use in the Treatment of Acute Pain and Cancer Pain* (ed 4). Skokie, IL, APS Press, 1999

8. American Geriatrics Society Panel on Chronic Pain in Older Persons: The management of chronic pain in older persons. *J Am Geriatr Soc* 46:635–651, 1998

9. Ad Hoc Committee on Cancer Pain of the American Society of Clinical Oncology: Cancer pain assessment and treatment curriculum guidelines. *J Clin Oncol* 10:1976–1982, 1992

10. Practice guidelines for cancer pain management. A report by the American Society for Anesthesiologists Task Force on Pain Management, Cancer Pain Section. *Anesthesiology* 84:1243–1257, 1996

11. Acute Pain Management Guideline Panel: *Acute Pain Management: Operative or Medical Procedures and Trauma: Clinical Practice Guidelines.* AHCPR publication No. 92-0032. Rockville, MD: Agency for Health Care Policy and Research, Public Health Service, U.S. Department of Health and Human Services, 1992

12. Jacox A, Carr DB, Payne R, et al: *Management of Cancer Pain: Adults' Quick Reference Guide No. 9.* AHCPR Publication No. 94-0593. Rockville, MD, Agency for Health Care Policy and Research, U.S. Department of Health and Human Services, Public Health Service, 1994

13. World Health Organization: *Cancer Pain Relief* (ed 2). Geneva, WHO, 1996

14. Portenoy RK: Report from the International Association for the Study of Pain Task Force on cancer pain. *J Pain Symptom Manage* 12:93–96, 1996

15. Pickett M, Cooley ME, Gordon DB: Palliative care: Past, present, and the future. *Semin Oncol Nurs* 14:86–94, 1998

16. Randal J: Hospice services feel the pinch of managed care. *J Natl Cancer Inst* 88:860–862, 1996

17. Cleary JF, Carbone PP: Palliative medicine in the elderly. *Cancer* 80:1335–1347, 1997

18. Lynn J, Teno JM, Phillipps RS, et al: Perceptions by family members of the dying experience of older and seriously ill patients. SUPPORT Investigators. Study to understand prognosis and preference for outcomes and risks of treatment. *Ann Intern Med* 126:97–106, 1997

19. Collins E, Poulain P, Gauvain-Piquard A, et al: Is disease progression the major factor in morphine "tolerance" in cancer pain treatment? *Pain* 55:319–326, 1993

20. Patt RB: *Cancer Pain.* Philadelphia, Lippincott, 1993

21. McGuire DB: The multiple dimensions of cancer pain: A framework for assessment and management, in McGuire DB, Yarbro CH, Ferrell BR (eds): *Cancer Pain Management* (ed 2). Sudbury, MA, Jones and Bartlett, 1995, pp 1–17

22. Berger AM, Portenoy RK, Weissman DE (eds): *Supportive Oncology Care.* Philadelphia, Lippincott-Raven, 1998

23. Payne SA: A study of quality of life in cancer patients receiving palliative chemotherapy. *Soc Sci Med* 35:1505–1509, 1992

24. Ellison NM: Palliative chemotherapy. *Am J Hosp Palliat Care* 15:93–103, 1998

25. Bruera E, Schoeller T, Wenk R, et al: A prospective multicenter assessment of the Edmonton Staging System for Cancer Pain. *J Pain Symptom Manage* 10:348–355, 1995

26. Kurman MR: Systemic therapy (chemotherapy) in the palliative treatment of cancer pain, in Patt RB: *Cancer Pain.* Philadelphia, Lippincott, 1993, pp 251–274

27. Janjan NA, Weissman DA: Primary cancer treatment: Antineoplastic, in Berger AM, Portenoy RK, Weissman DE (eds): *Supportive Oncology Care.* Philadelphia, Lippincott-Raven, 1998, pp 43–59

28. Tannock IF, Osoba D, Stocker MR, et al: Chemotherapy with mitoxantrone plus prednisone or prednisone alone for symptomatic hormone-resistant prostate cancer: A Canadian randomized trial with palliative endpoints. *J Clin Oncol* 14:1756–1764, 1996

29. Arcangeli G, Micheli A, Arcangeli G, et al: The responsiveness of bony metastases to radiotherapy: The effect of site, histology and radiation dose on pain relief. *Radiat Oncol* 14:95–101, 1989

30. Rutten EH, Crul BJ, van der Toorn PP, et al: Pain characteristics help predict the analgesic efficacy of radiotherapy for the treatment of cancer pain. *Pain* 69:131–135, 1997

31. Scott CB: Issues in quality of life assessment during cancer therapy. *Semin Radiat Oncol* 8:5–9, 1998 (suppl 4)

32. Needham PR, Hoskin PJ: Radiotherapy for painful bone metastases. *Palliat Med* 8:95–104, 1994

33. Hoskin PJ: Radiotherapy for bone pain. *Pain* 63:137–139, 1995

34. Ashby M: The role of radiotherapy in palliative care. *J Pain Symptom Manage* 6:380–388, 1991

35. Gaze MN, Kelly CG, Kerr GR, et al: Pain relief and quality of life for bone metastases: A randomized trial of two fractionation schedules. *Radiat Oncol* 45:109–116, 1997

36. Macklis RM, Cornelli H, Lasher J: Brief courses of palliative radiotherapy for metastatic bone pain: A pilot cost-minimization comparison with narcotic analgesics. *Am J Clin Oncol* 21:617–622, 1998

37. Porter AT: Use of strontium-89 in metastatic cancer: US and UK experience. *Oncology* 8:25–29, 1994 (suppl)

38. Robinson RG, Preston DF, Baxter KG, et al: Clinical experience with strontium-89 in prostatic and breast cancer patients. *Semin Oncol* 20:44–48, 1993 (suppl 2)

39. Kan MK: Palliation of bone pain in patients with metastatic cancer using strontium-89 (Metastron). *Cancer Nurs* 18: 286–291, 1995

40. Baumrucker S: Palliation of painful bone metastasis: Strontium-89. *Am J Hospice Palliat Care* 15:113–115, 1998

41. Bucholtz J: *Patient Information, Strontium-89.* Baltimore, The Johns Hopkins Oncology Center Division of Radiation Oncology, 1993

42. United States Pharmacopeial Convention, Inc.: *USP DI Drug Information for the Health Care Professional* (ed 19). Englewood, CO, Micromedex, 1999

43. Lillemoe KD: Palliative surgery for pancreatic cancer. *Surg Clin North Am* 7:199–216, 1998

44. Branicki J, Law SY, Fok M, et al: Quality of life in patients with cancer of the esophagus and gastric cardia: A case for palliative resection. *Arch Surg* 133:316–322, 1998

45. Soysal O, Karaoglanoglu N, Demiracan S, et al: Pleurectomy/decortication for palliation in malignant pleural mesothelioma: Results of surgery: *Eur J Cardiothoracic Sur* 11: 210–213, 1997

46. Harrington KD: Orthopaedic surgical management of skeletal complications of malignancy. *Cancer* 80:1614–1627, 1997 (suppl 8)

47. Azzarelli A, Crispino S: Palliative surgery in cancer pain treatment, in Swerdlow M, Ventafridda V (eds): *Cancer Pain.* Lancaster, England, MTI Press, 1987, pp 97–103

48. Polomano RC, Soulen M, McDaniel C: Sedation and analgesia with interventional radiology for oncology patients. *Crit Care Nurs Clin North Am* 9:335–353, 1997

49. Kochman ML, Soulen M, Polomano RC: Palliative endoscopy and interventional radiology, in Berger A, Portenoy RK, Weissman DE (eds): *Principles and Practice of Supportive Oncology.* Philadelphia: Lippincott-Raven, 1998, pp 651–666

50. Twycross R: *Pain Relief in Advanced Cancer.* Edinburgh, Churchill Livingstone, 1994

51. McCaffery M, Beebe A: *Pain: Clinical Manual for Nursing Practice.* St. Louis, Mosby, 1989

52. Coyle N, Cherny N, Portenoy RK: Pharmacologic management of cancer pain, in McGuire DB, Yarbro CH, Ferrell BR (eds): *Cancer Pain Management* (ed 2). Sudbury, MA, Jones and Bartlett, 1995, pp 131–158

53. Payne R: Pharmacological management of pain, in Berger A, Portenoy RK, Weissman DE (eds): *Principles and Practice of Supportive Oncology.* Philadelphia: Lippincott-Raven, 1998, pp 61–75

54. Levy MH: Pharmacological treatment of cancer pain. *N Engl J Med,* 335:1124–1132, 1996

55. Pasternak GW: Biochemistry and pharmacology of multiple mu opioid receptors, in Foley KM, Inturrisi CE (eds): *Advances in Pain Research and Therapy,* vol 8. New York, Raven, 1986, pp 337–344

56. Reisine T, Pasternak G: Opioid analgesics and antagonists, in Hardman JG, Gilman AG, Limbard LE, et al (eds): *Goodman and Gilman's The Pharmacological Basis of Therapeutics* (ed 9). New York, McGraw-Hill, 1996, pp 521–556

57. Insel PA: Analgesic-antipyretic and antiinflammatory agents: Drugs employed in the treatment of gout, in Hardman JG, Gilman AG, Limbard LE, et al (eds): *Goodman and Gilman's The Pharmacological Basis of Therapeutics* (ed 9). New York, McGraw-Hill, 1996, pp 617–657

58. Lipsky PE: Specific Cox-2 inhibitors in arthritis, oncology, and beyond: Where is the science headed? *J Rheumatol* 26: 25–30, 1999 (suppl 56)

59. Turnbull R, Hills LJ: Naproxen versus aspirin as analgesics in advanced malignant disease. *J Palliat Care* 1:25–28,1986

60. Levick S, Jacobs C, Loukas DF: Naproxen sodium in treatment of bone pain due to metastatic cancer. *Pain* 35: 253–258, 1988

61. Ventafridda V, De Conno F, Panerai AE, et al: Nonsteroidal anti-inflammatory drugs as the first step in cancer pain therapy: Double blind, within-patient study comparing nine drugs. *J Int Med Res* 18:21–29, 1990

62. Cherny NI, Portenoy RK: The management of cancer pain. *CA Cancer J Clin* 44:263–303, 1994

63. Houde RW, Wallenstein SL, Rogers A: Clinical pharmacology of analgesics: A method of assaying analgesic effect. *Clin Pharmacol Ther* 1:163–174, 1960

64. Ferrer-Brechner T, Ganz P: Combination therapy with ibuprofen and methadone for chronic cancer pain. *Am J Med* 77:78–83, 1984

65. Weingart WA, Sorkness CA, Earhart RH: Analgesia with oral narcotics and added ibuprofen in cancer patients. *Clin Pharm* 4:53–58, 1985

66. Eisenberg E, Berley CS, Carr DB, et al: Efficacy and safety of nonsteroidal inflammatory drugs for cancer pain: A meta-analysis. *J Clin Oncol* 12:2756–2765, 1994

67. Henry D, Lim LL-Y, Rodriquiz LAG, et al: Variability in risk of gastrointestinal complications with individual nonsteroidal anti-inflammatory drugs: Results of a collaborative meta-analysis. *Br J Med* 312:1563–1566, 1996

68. Allison MC, Howatson AG, Torrance CJ, et al: Gastrointestinal damage associated with the use of nonsteroidal antiinflammatory drugs. *N Engl J Med* 327:749–754, 1992

69. Griffin MR, Piper JM, Daughterty JR, et al: Nonsteroidal anti-inflammatory drug use and increased risk for peptic ulcer disease in elderly persons. *Ann Intern Med* 114: 257–263, 1991

70. Shorr RI, Ray WA, Daugherty JR, et al: Concurrent use of nonsteroidal anti-inflammatory drugs and oral anticoagulants places elderly persons at high risk for hemorrhagic peptic ulcer disease. *Arch Intern Med* 153:1665–1670, 1993

71. Tamblyn R, Berkson L, Dauphinee WD, et al: Unnecessary prescribing of NSAIDs and the management of NSAID-related gastropathy in medical practice. *Ann Intern Med* 127:429–438, 1997

72. Brooks PM, Day RO: Nonsteroidal anti-inflammatory drugs—Differences and similarities. *N Engl J Med* 324: 1716–1724, 1991

73. Ruoff G: Management of pain in patients with multiple health problems: A guide for practicing physicians. *Am J Med* 105:53S–60S, 1998

74. Walsh TD: Adjuvant analgesic therapy in cancer pain, in Foley KM, Bonica JJ, Ventafridda V (eds): *Advances in Pain Research and Therapy,* vol 16. New York, Raven, 1990, pp 155–169

75. Loblaw DA, Laperriere NJ: Emergency treatment of malignant extradural spinal cord compression: An evidenced-based guideline. *J Clin Oncol* 16:1613–1624, 1998

76. Bruera E: Clinical management of anorexia and cachexia in patients with advanced cancer. *Oncology* 49:35–42, 1992 (suppl 2)

77. Vigano A, Watanabe S, Bruera E: Anorexia and cachexia in advanced cancer patients. *Cancer Surv* 21:99–115, 1994

78. Bruera E, Roca E, Cedaro L, et al: Action of oral methylprednisolone in terminal cancer patients: A prospective randomized double blind study. *Cancer Treat Rep* 69: 751–754, 1985

79. Robertson CL, Marques CB, Gralla RJ, et al: Documenting the rapidity of pain relief and palliation of other lung cancer symptoms with the use of dexamethasone. *Proc Am Soc Clin Oncol* 16:A280, 1997 (abstr)

80. Ferrante FM: Principles of opioid pharmacotherapy: Practical implications of basic mechanisms. *J Pain Symptom Manage* 11:265–273, 1996

81. Campora E, Merlini L, Pace M, et al: The incidence of

narcotic-induced emesis. *J Pain Symptom Manage* 6: 428–430, 1991

82. Portenoy RK, Coyle N: Controversies in the long-term management of analgesic therapy in patients with advanced cancer. *J Pain Symptom Manage* 5:307–319, 1991

83. Bruera E, Suarez-Almazor M, Velasco A, et al: The assessment of constipation in terminally ill cancer patients admitted to a palliative care unit: A retrospective review. *J Pain Symptom Manage* 9:515–519, 1994

84. McMillan SC, Williams FA: Validity and reliability of the Constipation Assessment Scale. *Cancer Nurs* 12:183–188, 1989

85. Culpepper-Morgan JA, Inturrisi CE, Portenoy RK, et al: Treatment of opioid-induced constipation with oral naloxone. *Clin Pharmacol Ther* 52:90–95, 1992

86. Portenoy RK, Foley KM, Inturrisi CE: The nature of opioid responsiveness and its implications for neuropathic pain: New hypotheses derived from studies of opioid infusions. *Pain* 43:273–286, 1991

87. Cherny NI, Thaler HT, Friedlander-Klar H, et al: Opioid responsiveness of cancer pain syndromes caused by neuropathic or nociceptive mechanisms: A combined analysis of controlled, single-dose studies. *Neurology* 44:857–861, 1994

88. Mercadante S: Opioid responsiveness in patients with advanced head and neck cancer. *Support Care Cancer* 6: 482–485, 1998

89. Vigano A, Bruera E, Suarez-Almazor ME: Age, pain intensity, and opioid dose in patients with advanced cancer. *Cancer* 83:1244–1250, 1998

90. Zech DF, Grond S, Lynch J, et al: Validation of World Health Organization Guidelines for cancer pain relief: A 10-year prospective study. *Pain* 63:65–76, 1995

91. Cherny NJ, Chang V, Frager G, et al: Opioid pharmacotherapy in the management of cancer pain: A survey of strategies used by pain physicians for the selection of analgesic drugs and routes of administration. *Cancer* 76:1283–1293, 1995

92. Tsuneto S, Havashi A, Miyazaki M, et al: Clinical survey of controlled release morphine for cancer pain relief in a Japanese hospice. *Postgrad Med J* 67:79–81, 1991 (suppl)

93. Vijayaram S, Ramamani PV, Chandrashekhar NS, et al: Continuing care for cancer pain relief with oral morphine solution: One year experience in a regional cancer center. *Cancer* 66:1590–1595, 1990

94. Ferrell BR, Wisdom C, Wenzl C: Quality of life as an outcome variable in the management of cancer pain. *Cancer* 63:2321–2327, 1989

95. Brescia FJ, Walsh M, Savarese JJ, et al: A study of controlled-release oral morphine (MS Contin) in an advanced cancer hospital. *J Pain Symptom Manage* 2:193–198, 1987

96. Khojasteh A, Evans W, Reynolds RD, et al: Controlled-release oral morphine sulfate in the treatment of cancer pain with pharmacokinetic correlation. *J Clin Oncol* 5: 956–961, 1987

97. Thirwell MP, Sloan PA, Maroun JA, et al: Pharmacokinetics and clinical efficacy of oral morphine solution and controlled-release morphine tablets in cancer patients. *Cancer* 63:2275–2283, 1989

98. Portenoy RK, Thaler HT, Inturrisi CE, et al: The metabolite morphine-6-glucuronide contributes to the analgesia produced by morphine infusion in patients with pain and normal renal function. *Clin Pharmacol Ther* 51:422–431, 1992

99. Portenoy RK, Foley KM, Stulman J, et al: Plasma morphine

and morphine-6-glucuronide during chronic morphine therapy for cancer pain: Plasma profiles, steady state concentrations, and the consequences of renal failure. *Pain* 47:13–19, 1991

100. Faura CC, Moore RA, Horga JF, et al: Morphine and morphine-6-glucuronide plasma concentrations and effect in cancer pain. *J Pain Symptom Manage* 11:95–102, 1996

101. Ripamonti C, Zecca E, Bruera E: An update on the clinical use of methadone for cancer pain. *Pain* 70:109–115, 1997

102. Tive L, Ginsberg K, Pick CG, et al: κ3 receptors and levorphanol analgesia. *Neuropharmacology* 9:851–856, 1992

103. Glare PA, Walsh TD: Dose-ranging study of oxycodone for chronic pain in advanced cancer. *J Clin Oncol* 11:973–978, 1993

104. Grandy RP, Reder RF, Fitzmartin RO, et al: Steady-state pharmacokinetic comparison of controlled-release oxycodone tablets vs oxycodone oral liquid. *J Clin Pharmacol* 34: 1015, 1994

105. Kaiko RF, Foley KM, Grabinski PY, et al: Central nervous system excitatory effects of meperidine in cancer patients. *Ann Neurol* 13:180–185, 1983

106. Dayer P, Collart L, Desmeules J: The pharmacology of tramadol. *Drugs* 47:3–7, 1994 (suppl 1)

107. Wilder-Smith CH, Schimke J, Osterwalder B, et al: Oral tramadol, a mu-opioid agonist and monamine reuptake blocker, and morphine for strong cancer-related pain. *Ann Oncol* 5:141–146, 1994

108. Breitbart W: Psychotropic adjuvant analgesics for pain in cancer and AIDS. *Psychol Oncol* 7:333–345, 1998

109. Lipman AG: Analgesic drugs for neuropathic and sympathetically maintained pain. *Clin Geriatr Med* 12:501–515, 1996

110. Max MB, Lynch SA, Muir J, et al: Effects of desipiramine, amitriptyline, and fluoxetine on pain in diabetic neuropathy. *N Engl J Med* 326:1250–1256, 1992

111. Watson CPN, Chipman M, Reed K, et al: Amitriptyline versus maprotiline in postherpetic neuralgia: A randomized, double-blind crossover trial. *Pain* 48:29–36, 1992

112. Max MB: Thirteen consecutive well-designed randomized trials show that antidepressants reduce pain in diabetic neuropathy and postherpetic neuralgia. *Pain Forum* 4: 248–253, 1995

113. Martin LA, Hagan NA: Neuropathic pain in cancer patients: Mechanisms, syndromes, and clinical controversies. *J Pain Symptom Manage* 14:99–117, 1997

114. Eija K, Tasmuth T, Pertti J: Amitriptyline effectively relieves neuropathic pain following treatment of breast cancer. *Pain* 64:293–302, 1995

115. McQuay H, Carroll D, Jadad AK, et al: Anticonvulsant drugs for management of pain: A systematic review. *Br Med J* 311:1047–1052, 1995

116. Beydoun A, Uthman BM, Sackellares JC: Gabapentin: Pharmacokinetics, efficacy, and safety. *Clin Neuropharmacol* 18: 469–481, 1995

117. Rosner H, Rubin L, Kestenbaum A: Gabapentin adjunctive therapy in neuropathic states. *Clin J Pain* 12:56–58, 1996

118. McCaffery M: Gabapentin for lancinating pain. *Am J Nurs* 98:12, 1998

119. Rowbotham M, Harden N, Stacey B, et al: Gabapentin for the treatment of postherpetic neuralgia: A randomized controlled trial. *JAMA* 280:1837–1842, 1998

120. Tal M, Bennett GJ: Dextrophan relieves neuropathic heat-evoked hyperalgesia in the rat. *Neurosci Lett* 151:107–110, 1993

121. Vaccarino AL: Tolerance to morphine analgesia basic issues to consider. *Pain Forum* 8:25–28, 1999

122. Mercadante S, Casuccio A, Genovese G: Ineffectiveness of dextromethorphan in cancer pain. *J Pain Symptom Manage* 16:317–322, 1998

123. Mercadante S: Ketamine in cancer pain: An update. *Palliat Med* 10:225–230, 1996

124. Backjona M, Arndt G, Gombar KA, et al: Response of neuropathic pain syndromes to ketamine: A preliminary study. *Pain* 56:51–57, 1994

125. Mercandante S, Lodi F, Sapio M, et al: Long-term ketamine subcutaneous infusions in neuropathic cancer pain. *J Pain Symptom Manage* 10:564–568, 1995

126. Clark JL, Kalan GK: Effective treatment of severe cancer pain of the head using low-dose ketamine in an opioid-tolerant patient. *J Pain Symptom Manage* 10:310–314, 1995

127. Hoffman BB, Lefkowitz RJ: Catecholamines and sympathomimetic drugs, in Gilman AG, Rall TW, Nies AS, et al (eds): *Goodman and Gilman's The Pharmacological Basis of Therapeutics* (ed 8). New York, Pergamon, 1990, pp 187–220

128. Bruera E, Watanabe S: Psychostimulants as adjuvant analgesics. *J Pain Symptom Manage* 9:412–415, 1994

129. Wilwerding MB, Loprinzi CL, Mailliard JA, et al: A randomized, crossover evaluation of methylphenidate in cancer patients receiving strong narcotics. *Support Care Cancer* 3:135–138, 1995

130. Bruera E, Chadwick S, Brenneis C, et al: Methylphenidate associated with narcotics for the treatment of cancer pain. *Cancer Treat Rep* 71:67–70, 1987

131. Bruera E, Brenneis C, Patterson AH, et al: Use of methylphenidate as an adjuvant to narcotic analgesics in patients with advanced cancer. *J Pain Symptom Manage* 4:3–6, 1989

132. Dundee JW, Moore J: The myth of phenothiazine potentiation. *Anaesthesiol* 16:95–96, 1961

133. Keats AS, Telford J, Kurosu Y: "Potentiation" of meperidine by promethazine. *Anesthesiology* 22:34–41, 1961

134. Hanks GW, Thomas PJ, Trueman T, et al: The myth of haloperidol potentiation. *Lancet* 2:523–524, 1983

135. Stiefel F, Fainsinger R, Bruera E: Acute confusional states in patients with advanced cancer. *J Pain Symptom Manage* 7:94–98, 1992

136. Ernst DS, MacDonald N, Paterson AHG, et al: A double-blind, crossover trial of intravenous clodronate in metastatic bone pain. *J Pain Symptom Manage* 7:4–11, 1992

137. Adami S, Mian M: Clodronate therapy of metastatic bone disease in patients with prostatic carcinoma. *Recent Result Cancer Res* 116:67–72, 1989

138. Berenson JR, Lichtenstein A, Porter L, et al: Efficacy of pamidronate in reducing skeletal events in patients with advanced multiple myeloma. *N Engl J Med* 334:488–493, 1996

139. Strong KM, McPherson ML: Pamidronate. *Am J Hos Palliat Care* 15:54–55, 1998

140. Farrar JT, Cleary J, Rauck R, et al: Oral transmucosal fentanyl citrate: Randomized, double-blind, placebo-controlled trial for treatment of breakthrough pain in cancer patients. *J Natl Cancer Inst* 90:611–616, 1998

141. Payne R, Mathias SD, Pasta DJ, et al: Quality of life and cancer pain: Satisfaction and side effects with transdermal fentanyl versus oral morphine. *J Clin Oncol* 16:1588–1593, 1998

142. Calis KA, Kohler DR, Corso DM: Transdermally administered fentanyl for pain management. *Clin Pharm* 11:22–36, 1992

143. Maves TJ, Barcellos WA: Management of cancer pain with transdermal fentanyl: Phase IV trial, University of Iowa. *J Pain Symptom Manage* 7:S58–S62, 1991

144. Levy MH, Rosen SM, Kedziera P: Transdermal fentanyl: Seeding trial in patients with chronic cancer pain. *J Pain Symptom Manage* 7:S48–S50, 1992

145. Hanks GW, Fallon MT: Transdermal fentanyl in cancer pain: Conversion from oral morphine. *J Pain Symptom Manage* 10:87, 1995

146. Gupta SK, Southam M, Gale R, et al: System functionality and physiochemical model of fentanyl transdermal system. *J Pain Symptom Manage* 7:S17–S26, 1992

147. Payne R: Transdermal fentanyl: Suggested recommendations for clinical use. *J Pain Symptom Manage* 7:S40–S44, 1992

148. Wakefield B, Johnson JA, Kron-Chalupa J, et al: A research-based guideline for appropriate use of transdermal fentanyl. *Oncol Nurs Forum* 29:1505–1513, 1998

149. De Conno F, Ripamonti C, Saita L, et al: Role of rectal route in treating cancer pain: A randomized crossover clinical trial of oral versus rectal morphine administration in opioid-naive cancer patients with pain. *J Clin Oncol* 13:1004–1008, 1995

150. Cole L, Hanning CD: Review of the rectal use of opioids. *J Pain Symptom Manage* 5:118–126, 1990

151. Hautkappe M, Roizen MF, Toledano A, et al: Review of the effectiveness of capsaisan for painful cutaneous disorder and neural dysfunction. *Clin J Pain* 14:97–106, 1998

152. Portenoy RK, Moulin DE, Rogers A, et al: IV infusions of opioids for cancer pain: Clinical review and guidelines for use. *Cancer Treat Rep* 70:575–582, 1986

153. Ferris FD, Kerr IG, DeAngelis C, et al: Inpatient narcotic infusions for patients with cancer pain. *J Palliat Care* 6:51–59, 1990

154. Portenoy RK: Continuous infusion of opioid drugs. *Med Clin North Am* 71:233–241, 1987

155. Coyle N, Mauskop A, Maggard J, et al: Continuous infusions of opiates in cancer patients with pain. *Oncol Nurs Forum* 13:53–57, 1986

156. Coyle N, Cherny NI, Portenoy RK: Subcutaneous infusions at home. *Oncology* 8:21–27, 1994

157. Coyle N, Adelhardt J: Cancer patients and subcutaneous infusions. *Am J Nurs* 96:61, 1996

158. Poniatowski BC: Continuous subcutaneous infusions for pain. *J Intraven Nurs* 14:30–35, 1991

159. Watanabe S, Pereira J, Hanson J, et al: Fentanyl by continuous infusion for the management of cancer pain: A retrospective study. *J Pain Symptom Manage* 16:323–326, 1998

160. Sheidler VR: New methods in analgesic delivery, in McGuire DB, Yarbro CH (eds): *Cancer Pain Management.* Philadelphia, Saunders, 1987, pp 203–222

161. Macmillan K, Bruera E, Kuehn N, et al: A prospective comparison study between a butterfly needle and a teflon cannula for subcutaneous narcotic administration. *J Pain Symptom Manage* 9:82–84, 1994

162. Bruera E, Brenneis C, Michaud M, et al: Patient-controlled subcutaneous hydromorphone versus continuous subcutaneous infusion for the treatment of cancer pain. *J Natl Cancer Inst* 80:1152–1154, 1988

163. Moulin DE, Kreeft JH, Murray-Parsons N, et al: Comparison of continuous subcutaneous and intravenous hydromorphone for management of cancer pain. *Lancet* 337:465–468, 1991

164. Lang AH, Abbrederis K, Dzien A, et al: Treatment of severe cancer pain by continuous infusion of subcutaneous opioids. *Recent Results Cancer Res* 121:51–57, 1991

165. Bruera E, MacEachern T, MacMillan K, et al: Local tolerance to subcutaneous infusions of high concentrations of hydromorphone: A prospective study. *J Pain Symptom Manage* 8:201–204, 1993

166. Bruera E, Legris MA, Kuehn N, et al: Hypodermoclysis for the administration of fluids and narcotic analgesics in patients with advanced cancer. *J Natl Cancer Inst* 81: 1108–1109, 1989

167. Mackie AM, Coda BC, Hill HH: Adolescents use patient-controlled analgesia effectively for relief from prolonged oropharyngeal mucositis pain. *Pain* 46:265–269, 1991

168. Bruera E, Brenneis C, Michaud M, et al: Patient-controlled subcutaneous hydromorphone versus continuous subcutaneous infusion for the treatment of cancer pain. *J Natl Cancer Inst* 80:1152–1154, 1988

169. Kerr IG, Sone M, DeAngelis C, et al: Continuous narcotic infusion with patient controlled analgesia for chronic cancer pain in outpatients. *Ann Intern Med* 108:554–557, 1988

170. Fitzgibbon DR, Ready LB: Intravenous high-dose methadone administered by patient controlled analgesia and continuous infusion for the treatment of cancer pain refractory to high-dose morphine. *Pain* 72:259–261, 1997

171. Ferrell BR, Nash CC, Warfield C: The role of patient-controlled analgesia in the management of cancer pain. *J Pain Symptom Manage* 7:149–154, 1992

172. Crane RA: Intermittent subcutaneous infusion of opioids in hospice home care: An effective, economical, manageable option. *Am J Hosp Care* 11:8–12, 1994

173. Arner S, Arner B: Differential effects of epidural morphine in the treatment of cancer-related pain. *Acta Anaesthesiol Scand* 29:32–36, 1985

174. DuPen SL, Kharasch ED, Williams A, et al: Chronic epidural bupivacaine-opioid infusion in intractable cancer pain. *Pain* 49:293–300, 1992

175. Nitescu P, Appelgren L, Linder LE, et al: Epidural versus intrathecal morphine bupivacaine: Assessments of consecutive treatments in advanced cancer patients. *J Pain Symptom Manage* 5:18–26, 1990

176. Eisenach JC, DuPen S, Dubois M, et al: Epidural clonidine analgesia for intractable cancer pain. *Pain* 61:391–399, 1995

177. Paice JA, Magolan JM: Intraspinal drug delivery. *Nurs Clin North Am* 26:477–498, 1991

178. Onofrio BM, Yaksh TL: Long-term pain relief produced by intrathecal morphine infusion in 53 patients. *J Neurosurg* 72:200–209, 1990

179. Paice JA, Williams AR: Intraspinal drugs for pain, in McGuire DB, Yarbro CH, Ferrell BR (eds): *Cancer Pain Management* (ed 2). Sudbury, MA, Jones and Bartlett, 1995, pp 131–158

180. Penn RD, Paice JA: Chronic intrathecal morphine for intractable pain. *J Neurosurg* 67:182–186, 1987

181. Paice JA, Penn RD, Shott S: Intraspinal morphine for chronic pain: A retrospective, multicenter study. *J Pain Symptom Manage* 11:71–80, 1996

182. Krames ES: Intrathecal infusional therapies for intractable pain: Patient management guidelines. *J Pain Symptom Manage* 8:36–46, 1993

183. Scott DA, Emanuelsson BM, Mooney PH, et al: Pharmacokinetics and efficacy of long-term epidural ropivacaine infusion for postoperative analgesia. *Anesth Analg* 85: 1322–1330, 1997

184. DuPen SL, Peterson DG, Williams A, et al: Infection during chronic epidural catherization: Diagnosis and treatment. *Anesthesiology* 73:905–909, 1990

185. American Association of Nurse Anesthetists Position Statement: Provision of pain relief by medication administered via continuous epidural, intrathecal, intrapleural, peripheral nerve catheters, or other pain relief devices, American Association of Nurse Anesthetists, Park Ridge, IL, June 1990

186. Olsson GL, Leddo CC, Wild L: Nursing management of patients receiving epidural narcotics. *Heart Lung* 18: 130–138, 1989

187. Paice JA: Intrathecal morphine infusion for intractable cancer pain: A new use for implanted pumps. *Oncol Nurs Forum* 13:33–39, 1986

188. Paice JA, DuPen A, Schwertz D: Catheter port cleansing techniques and entry of povidone-iodine into the epidural space. *Oncol Nurs Forum* 26:603–605, 1999

189. Oncology Nursing Society: Resolution: Use of technology in pain management. Pittsburgh, 1991 Congress Oncology Nursing Society

190. Ferrell BR, Rhiner M: High-tech comfort: Ethical issues in cancer pain management for the 1990s. *J Clin Ethics* 2: 108–112, 1991

191. Ferrell BR, Rhiner M: Use of technology in the management of cancer pain. *J Pharm Care Pain Symptom Control* 2: 17–35, 1994

192. Dellasega C, Keiser CL: Pharmacologic approaches to chronic pain in the older adult. *Nurse Pract* 22:20–24, 1997

193. Hogan OH, Abram SE: Neural blockade for diagnosis and prognosis. *Anesthesiology* 86:216–241, 1997

194. Coles PG, Thompson GE: The role of neurolytic blocks in the treatment of cancer pain. *Int Anesthesiol Clin* 29:93–104, 1991

195. Patt RB, Reddy SK, Black RG: Neural blockade for abdominopelvic pain of oncologic origin. *Int Anesthesiol Clin* 36: 87–104, 1998

196. Lillemoe KD, Cameron JL, Kaufman HS, et al: Chemical splanchnietomy in patients with nonresectable pancreatic cancer: A prospective randomized trial. *Ann Surg* 217: 456–457, 1993

197. Patt RB: Peripheral neurolysis and the management of cancer pain, in Patt RB: *Cancer Pain*. Philadelphia, Lippincott, 1993, pp 359–376

198. Rosen SM: Procedure control of cancer pain. *Semin Oncol* 21:740–747, 1994

199. Tasker RR: Neurosurgical and neuroaugmentation intervention, in Patt RB: *Cancer Pain*. Philadelphia, Lippincott, 1993, pp 471–500

200. Amidei CS: Pain and pain syndromes, in Cammermeyer M, Appeldorn C (eds): *Core Curriculum for Neuroscience Nursing* (ed 3). Chicago, American Association of Neuroscience Nurses, 1990

201. Peteet J, Tay V, Cohen G, et al: Pain characteristics and treatment in an outpatient cancer population. *Cancer* 57: 1259–1265, 1986

202. Oncology Nursing Society: Cancer pain management. *Oncol Nurs Forum* 25:817–818, 1998

203. Mock V, Hill MN, Dienemann JA, et al: Challenges to behavioral research in oncology. *Cancer Pract* 4:267–273, 1996

204. McGuire DB, DeLoney VG, Yeager KA, et al: Maintaining study validity in a changing clinical environment. *Nurs Res* (in press)

205. McCaffery M, Pasero C: *Pain: Clinical Manual* (ed 2). St. Louis, Mosby, 1999

206. Spross JA, Burke MW: Nonpharmacological management of cancer pain, in McGuire DB, Yarbro CH, Ferrell BR

(eds): *Cancer Pain Management* (ed 2). Sudbury, MA, Jones and Bartlett, 1995, pp 159–205

207. Wilkie DJ: Neural mechanisms of pain: A foundation for cancer pain assessment and management, in McGuire DB, Yarbro CH, Ferrell BR (eds): *Cancer Pain Management* (ed 2). Sudbury, MA, Jones and Bartlett, 1995, pp 61–87

208. Weinrich SP, Weinrich MC: The effect of massage on pain in cancer patients. *Appl Nurs Res* 3:140–145, 1990

209. Ferrell-Torry AT, Glick OJ: The use of therapeutic massage as a nursing intervention to modify anxiety and the perception of cancer pain. *Cancer Nurs* 16:93–101, 1993

210. Rhiner M, Ferrell BR, Ferrell BA et al: A structured non-drug intervention program for cancer pain. *Cancer Pract* 1:137–143, 1993

211. Kingdon RT, Stanley KJ, Kizior RJ: *Handbook for Pain Management.* Philadelphia, Saunders, 1998

212. McCaffery M, Wolff M: Pain relief using cutaneous modalities, positioning, and movement, in Turk DC, Feldman CS (eds): *Noninvasive Approaches to Pain Management in the Terminally Ill.* New York, Haworth Press, 1992, pp 121–153

213. Wilkie DJ, Keefe FJ: Coping strategies of patients with lung cancer-related pain. *Clin J Pain* 7:292–299, 1991

214. McGuire DB: Measuring pain, in Frank-Stromborg M, Olsen S (eds): *Instruments for Clinical Health-care Research* (ed. 2). Philadelphia, Saunders, 1997, pp 528–564

215. Barbour LA, McGuire DB, Kirchhoff KT, et al: Non-analgesic methods of pain control used by cancer outpatients. *Oncol Nurs Forum* 13:56–60, 1986

216. Walsh M Sr, Brescia FJ: Clinitron therapy and pain management in advanced cancer patients. *J Pain Symptom Manage* 5:46–50, 1990

217. Beck S: The therapeutic use of music for cancer-related pain. *Oncol Nurs Forum* 18:1327–1337, 1991

218. Zimmerman L, Pozehl B, Duncan K, et al: Effects of music in patients who had chronic cancer pain. *West J Nurs Res* 11:298–309, 1989

219. Ditlow F: The missing element in health care: Humor as a form of creativity. *J Holistic Nurs* 11:66–79, 1993

220. Fritz DJ: Noninvasive pain control methods used by cancer outpatients. *Proc. Oncol Nurs Soc*, 1988, p 108 (abstr 27)

221. Nevo O, Keinan G, Teshimovsky-Arditl M: Humor and pain tolerance, *Humor* 6:71–88, 1993

222. Arathuzik D: The appraisal of pain and coping in cancer patients. *West J Nurs Res* 13:714–731, 1991

223. McGuire DB: Coping strategies used by cancer patients with pain. *Oncol Nurs Forum* 14:123, 1987

224. Wilkie DJ, Lovejoy N, Dodd M, et al: Cancer pain control behaviors: Description and correlation with pain intensity. *Oncol Nurs Forum* 15:723–731, 1988

225. Wallace KG: Analysis of recent literature concerning relaxation and imagery interventions for cancer pain. *Cancer Nurs* 20:79–87, 1997

226. Ferrell BR, Ferrell BA, Ahn C, et al: Pain management for elderly patients with cancer at home. *Cancer* 74:2139–2146, 1994 (suppl)

227. Graffam S, Johnson A: A comparison of two relaxation strategies for the relief of pain and its distress. *J Pain Symptom Manage* 2:229–231, 1987

228. Sloman R: Relaxation and the relief of cancer pain. *Nurs Clin N Am* 30:697–709, 1995

229. Fleming U: Relaxation therapy for far-advanced cancer. *Practitioner* 229:471–475, 1985

230. Arathuzik D: Effects of cognitive-behavioral strategies on pain in cancer patients. *Cancer Nurs* 17:207–214, 1995

231. Dalton JA: Education for pain management: A pilot study. *Patient Ed Couns* 9:155–165, 1987

232. Dalton JA, Toomey T, Workman MR: Pain relief for cancer patients. *Cancer Nurs* 11:322–328, 1988

233. Syrjala KL, Donaldson GW, Davis MW, et al: Relaxation and imagery and cognitive-behavioral training reduce pain during cancer treatment: A controlled clinical trial. *Pain* 63:189–198, 1995

234. Fishman B, Loscalzo M: Cognitive behavioral interventions in management of cancer pain: Principles and applications. *Med Clin North Am* 71:271–287, 1987

235. Loscalzo M: Psychological approaches to the management of pain in patients with advanced cancer. *Hematol Oncol Clin North Am* 10:139–155, 1996

236. Roth-Roemer S, Abrams JR, Syrjala KL: Nonpharmacologic approaches to adult cancer pain management. *APS Bull* 6: 1–4, 9, 1996

237. Dalton JA, Blau W, Lindley C, et al: Changing acute pain management to improve patient outcomes: An educational approach. *J Pain Symptom Manage* 17:277–287, 1999

238. Donovan MI, Evers K, Jacobs P, et al: When there is no benchmark: Designing a primary care-based chronic pain management program from the scientific basis up. *J Pain Symptom Manage* 18:38–48, 1999

239. Miaskowski C, Crews J, Ready LB, et al: Anesthesia-based pain services improve the quality of postoperative pain management. *Pain* 80:23–29, 1999

240. Watt-Watson J, Donovan MI: *Pain Management: Nursing Perspective.* St. Louis, Mosby-Year Book, 1992

241. Lewis FM, Zahlis EH: The nurse as coach: A conceptual framework for clinical practice. *Oncol Nurs Forum* 24: 1695–1702, 1997

242. Riddell A, Fitch MI: Patients' knowledge of and attitudes toward the management of cancer pain. *Oncol Nurs Forum* 24:1775–1784, 1997

243. Grant MM, Rivera LM: Pain education for nurses, patients, and families, in McGuire DB, Yarbro CH, Ferrell BR (eds): *Cancer Pain Management* (ed 2). Sudbury, MA, Jones and Bartlett, 1995, pp 289–319

244. Weissman DE, Dahl JL: Update on the Cancer Pain Role Model Education Program. *J Pain Symptom Manage* 10: 292–297, 1995

245. Rhiner M, Coluzzi PH: Family issues influencing management of cancer pain, in McGuire DB, Yarbro CH, Ferrell BR (eds): *Cancer Pain Management* (ed 2). Sudbury, MA, Jones and Bartlett, 1995, pp 207–230

246. De Wit R, van Dam F, Sandbelt L, et al: A pain education program for chronic pain patients: Follow-up results from a randomized clinical trial. *Pain* 73:55–69, 1997

247. Elliott TE, Murray DM, Oken MM, et al: The Minnesota Cancer Pain Project: Designs, methods, and education strategies. *J Cancer Ed* 10:102–112, 1995

248. Jadlos MA, Kelman GB, Marra K, et al: A pain management documentation tool. *Oncol Nurs Forum* 23:1451–1454, 1996

249. Wholihan D: A patient-education tool for patient-controlled analgesia. *Oncol Nurs Forum* 24:1801–1804, 1997

CHAPTER 30

Infection

Jan M. Ellerhorst-Ryan, RN, MSN, CS

Scope of the Problem

Infection in patients with cancer is a problem of great concern to health care providers. The types of infections presenting the greatest problems for cancer patients have changed over the years as a result of emerging resistant and opportunistic organisms. Effective antibiotic therapy has decreased mortality among cancer patients, but more aggressive cancer treatments, such as bone marrow transplant and intensive chemotherapy, have also created physiological and immunological challenges that are yet to be resolved.

Incidence

Infectious complications account for 70%–75% of deaths in patients with acute leukemia and are associated with up to 50% of deaths in those with solid tumors.[1] To understand why individuals with cancer are susceptible to infection requires an appreciation of normal host defenses and the mechanisms by which they are impaired by cancer and cancer therapy.

Etiology and Risk Factors

Infectious processes may be the result of the underlying malignancy, intensive treatment modalities, prolonged hospitalization, or a combination of these factors. The term *immunocompromised host* refers to a person who has one or more defects in natural defense mechanisms significant enough to predispose to severe, sometimes life-threatening infection.[2] Examples of defective protective mechanisms and factors contributing to infection in people with cancer are listed in Table 30-1.[3]

Physiological Alterations

Normal Anatomy, Physiology, and Scientific Principles

Integumentary, mucosal, and chemical barriers

Intact skin constitutes the most important physical barrier against invasion by both exogenous and endogenous organisms. The skin is made up of cornified layers of epithelial cells that cover the body and protect tissues against dehydration and invasion by harmful bacteria. When a break in the skin occurs, environmental microbes and those that normally inhabit hair follicles and sebaceous glands may enter the body and cause infection.

A second major defense against infection is the mucociliary activity found in the mucous membranes. The cilia of the epithelial cells that line the respiratory tract beat rhythmically to propel mucus and entrapped foreign par-

Table 30-1   Altered Protective Mechanisms Associated with Cancer and Cancer Treatment

Protective Mechanism	Defect
Skin, mucous membrane	Disrupted integrity due to cytotoxic agents, radiation, surgery, tumor invasion, vascular access catheters/devices, malnutrition
Normal flora	Alterations in endogenous microbes due to antibiotic use, hospitalization
Normal drainage mechanisms	Disrupted drainage due to central nervous system involvement, obstruction by tumor
Neutrophils	Decreased number due to cytotoxic agents, radiation, bone marrow involvement by tumor; disrupted phagocytic function due to corticosteroid therapy
Cellular immunity	Impaired response due to Hodgkin's disease, corticosteroid therapy, cytotoxic agents, malnutrition
Humoral immunity	Impaired response due to chronic lymphocytic leukemia, multiple myeloma, cytotoxic agents

ticles toward the nose and throat. In the gastrointestinal tract, the cilia propel bacteria and waste products to be removed in the feces. Microorganisms constitute up to 60% of the weight of the stool; therefore, an intact gastrointestinal mucous membrane is essential to prevention of infection.

A variety of other mechanisms serve to protect the body from microbial invasion. Resident microbial flora prevent pathogenic colonization by competing for surface-binding sites and nutrients and by producing metabolic products that are toxic to other organisms.[4] Acid pH inhibits or prevents bacterial growth on the skin and in the stomach, bladder, and vagina. Microbicidal elements found in prostatic fluid and in tears also provide a protective effect.

Leukocytes

Leukocytes, particularly polymorphonuclear neutrophils (PMNs), represent a significant defense against infection. Polymorphonuclear neutrophils, which are also referred to as *polys* or *segmented neutrophils (segs)*, are short-lived white blood cells (WBCs) that respond quickly to bacterial invasion. They are the most numerous of the leukocytes, constituting 55%–70% of circulating WBCs. The primary function of PMNs is the destruction and elimination of microorganisms through phagocytosis, the process of engulfing and ingesting foreign matter. In addition, PMNs secrete chemotactants, chemical substances that alert the body to the presence of an invader. Chemotactants stimulate increased production of PMNs and macrophages and direct them to the site of invasion. Without sufficient numbers of PMNs, the body's ability to mount an inflammatory response is compromised.

Monocytes and macrophages

Monocytes and macrophages constitute what was previously referred to as the reticuloendothelial system. Monocytes are released from the bone marrow before they complete the maturation process; thus, they are initially only capable of limited phagocytosis. After migrating into the tissues, full maturation occurs and the cells are then referred to as *macrophages*. Under normal conditions, more than 95% of these cells are mature tissue macrophages, while less than 2% are circulating monocytes.[5]

Macrophages can survive from several months to several years. They are highly phagocytic and play important roles in the inflammatory, cellular, and humoral responses. Following initial contact with a foreign protein, macrophages process and present antigens to lymphocytes, which in turn stimulate the immune response and cytokine production. Monocytes also produce specific components required for the complement cascade.[6]

Lymphocytes

Lymphocytes, the cells responsible for cellular and humoral immunity, provide long-term protection against a variety of microorganisms. They usually constitute 25%–30% of the total WBC count. *B lymphocytes,* responsible for humoral immunity, produce antibodies that neutralize, destroy, or facilitate phagocytosis of foreign proteins. *T lymphocytes,* providers of cellular immunity, initiate a variety of activities that directly or indirectly result in elimination of microorganisms or other foreign substances. T-helper cells are the most numerous of T-lymphocyte subsets, normally constituting more than 75% of total T-lymphocyte counts. T-helper cells serve as the principal regulators of immune function through secretion of protein mediators (*cytokines*) that act on other cells involved in the immune and inflammatory responses.[7] Cytokines produced by T-helper cells include interleukin-2 through interleukin-6, gamma-interferon, and granulocyte-macrophage colony-stimulating factor (GM-CSF). (See Chapter 3 for a more detailed discussion of the immune response.)

Cytokines

Cytokines are small protein hormones synthesized by a variety of leukocytes. Cytokines produced by mononuclear phagocytes (monocytes, macrophages, PMNs, and eosinophils) are referred to as *monokines,* whereas cytokines secreted by T and B lymphocytes are called *lymphokines.*

Cytokines initiate and regulate a number of inflammatory and immune responses. They include interferons, interleukins, growth factors, and colony-stimulating factors. (See Chapters 3 and 24 for specific information about cytokines and cytokine activity.)

Pathophysiology

Alterations in nonspecific defenses

Disruptions in protective barriers. Skin and mucous membrane integrity is frequently impaired by cancer and cancer therapy. Primary and metastatic tumor growth invades healthy tissue and disrupts normal circulation, resulting in ulceration, perforation or fistula formation, and necrosis. Chemotherapy and radiation may further alter the integrity of skin and mucosal surfaces, particularly in the gastrointestinal tract.

Diagnostic and treatment strategies typically involve a variety of invasive procedures, including surgery, venipuncture, peripheral intravenous infusions, bone marrow biopsies and aspirations, vascular access catheters, "fingersticks," and bronchoscopy. Infection rates associated with diagnostic and therapeutic interventions are high, depending on the type of tumor or treatment.

Host defenses are further compromised by neurological consequences of primary or metastatic disease involving the central nervous system (CNS). Examples include aspiration pneumonia due to impaired cough and gag reflex and urinary tract infections associated with inability to empty the bladder.

Changes in normal flora. Undisturbed, endogenous microbial flora exist as a carefully balanced synergistic microenvironment within the host. Alterations in normal flora predispose individuals with cancer to serious opportunistic or nosocomial infection.

More than 80% of infections developing in individuals with cancer arise from endogenous organisms, with many acquired during hospitalization.[8-10] Institutional sources of potential infection include personnel, food, air, water, equipment, and procedures. The most significant factor contributing to preventable transmission of infectious agents during hospitalization is poor hand washing by health care personnel.[11] Antibiotics, used both for treatment and prophylaxis, commonly alter normal flora, allowing overgrowth of pathogenic organisms and emergence of resistance.[1]

Obstruction. Obstruction, usually associated with solid tumors or lymphoma, may contribute to risk of infection by interfering with normal clearing and drainage mechanisms. Sites most often involved include the pulmonary system, biliary tree, gastrointestinal system, and urinary tract.

Neutropenia

There is a direct relationship between the number of circulating PMNs and incidence of infection. Individuals whose neutrophil count is less than 1000 cells/mm³ are considered to be neutropenic and at increased risk of infection (Figure 30-1). When the neutrophil count is less than 500 cells/mm³, risk of infection is significant. As the length of therapy and the duration and severity of neutropenia increase, so does the incidence of sepsis.[2,8,9]

Because of the short life span of circulating PMNs, their absolute number must be determined on a daily basis for neutropenic individuals. The absolute neutrophil count (ANC) is calculated using data from the total WBC and the differential, which specifies the percentage of WBCs by cell type. The differential also notes the presence of abnormal or premature WBCs. The ANC is determined by multiplying the percentage of PMNs and bands by the total number of WBCs. For example, a patient may have the following hematologic profile:

Total WBC = 2100 cells/mm³
Differential: = 28% PMNs
18% bands
42% lymphocytes
1% eosinophils
1% basophils
10% monocytes

To calculate the ANC, use the following formula:

$$ANC = total\ WBC\ (\%PMNs + \%bands)$$
$$= 2100(28\% + 18\%)$$
$$= 966$$

The individual in this example is considered neutropenic because the ANC is less than 1000. The total WBC count may be approximately the same from one day to the next, but the percentage of PMNs and bands may vary significantly. The WBC count alone will not always provide enough information to determine the presence of neutropenia.

Implanted vascular access devices.   Surgically placed central venous catheters and ports provide long-term access for blood sampling and infusion therapy. These devices, however, are not without risk of complications, the most common being infection and thrombosis. Three

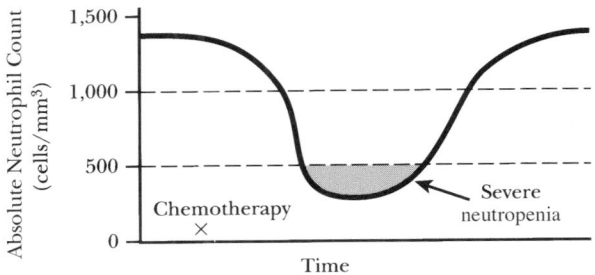

Figure 30-1 Chemotherapy cycle. Days of risk for infection vary according to type of chemotherapy agent administered and individual response to treatment. The fall in the neutrophil count may begin a few days after chemotherapy or may be delayed for more than a week. Severe neutropenia occurs when absolute neutrophil counts are less than 500, and may persist for several days, a week, or sometimes longer.

different types of infection are associated with vascular access catheters and devices: exit site infections, tunnel-track infection, and catheter-related bacteremias.

The incidence of catheter-related bacteremia is influenced by specific therapy, degree of catheter use, patient population, catheter insertion technique, and care and maintenance procedures. However, neutropenia remains the primary risk factor for infection in vascular access catheters.[12]

Thrombus and fibrin-sleeve formation have also been associated with catheter-related infection.[13] Thrombotic complications have been observed more frequently in patients with triple-lumen catheters than in those with double-lumen catheters and in patients with catheter tips placed above the T3 level.[14] Urokinase is used in combination with antibiotic therapy to improve treatment outcome for catheter-related infections. It is thought that urokinase enhances antimicrobial therapy by removing sites of bacterial and fungal colonization in the lumen of the catheter.[15]

Immunosuppression

Infection.   Although infection is commonly viewed as a result of compromised immunity, certain infections actually contribute to impairment of immune function. Depression of lymphocyte function in vitro has been associated with a variety of viral infections, including cytomegalovirus (CMV), herpes simplex virus (HSV), and Epstein-Barr virus (EBV).[8,16]

Acquired immunodeficiency syndrome.   Acquired immunodeficiency syndrome (AIDS) is characterized by loss of T-helper cells, resulting in progressive loss of immunocompetence, development of opportunistic infections and chronic wasting, impairment of the CNS, and emergence of unusual malignancies. The virus that causes AIDS, human immunodeficiency virus (HIV), has been isolated in blood, saliva, tears, urine, cerebrospinal fluid, semen, vaginal secretions, and breast milk. However, only blood, semen, and vaginal secretions are proven vectors. While breast-feeding has contributed to mother-to-child transmission, most infants are infected in utero or during labor and delivery.[17]

Common opportunistic infections associated with AIDS include CMV, HSV, herpes zoster, *Candida albicans*, *Cryptococcus*, *Pneumocystis carinii*, *Toxoplasma gondii*, *Cryptosporidium*, *Mycobacterium avium* complex (MAC), and tuberculosis.

Infection with HIV is not synonymous with AIDS. AIDS is part of a continuum of illnesses related to infection with HIV. Many persons with primary HIV infection are asymptomatic even though they demonstrate seropositivity for antibodies to HIV. Others may have symptoms that can develop 2–6 weeks after primary infection, including lymphadenopathy, fever, rigors, arthralgia, rash, abdominal cramping, and diarrhea. These symptoms are often accompanied by mild immunologic deficiencies, including lymphopenia and diminished T-cell response to mitogen.[18]

Tumor-associated abnormalities

The types of infections that occur in persons diagnosed with cancer are somewhat predictable. Abnormal cell-mediated immunity in Hodgkin's disease and acute leukemia is associated with increased incidence of infection by intracellular pathogens, including herpes viruses, *Cryptococcus neoformans*, *Brucella* species, *Mycobacterium tuberculosis*, *Listeria monocytogenes*, *Salmonella* species, and *T. gondii*.[1,11] Other malignancies such as advanced lung cancer and intracranial tumors are associated with a decreased sensitivity and an impaired ability to respond to a challenging antigen.

The spleen has two major roles in infection management. The spleen serves as a mechanical filter, removing bacteria from the bloodstream, and it also participates in antibody production.[1,4,19] Asplenic individuals have decreased levels of the complement factor properdin, which impairs opsonization and increases susceptibility to infection. The risk of overwhelming sepsis and death in persons with asplenia, especially those with Hodgkin's disease, is at least 50 times greater than in the normal population.[19] It has been noted, however, that individuals with Hodgkin's disease in complete remission have a 2.30% cumulative risk of overwhelming postsplenectomy infection, whereas the rate of infection increases to 15.25% for those in whom relapse has occurred.[20]

Febrile episodes occur most frequently in individuals with lymphoma and leukemia.[21] Although fever may be caused by the underlying cancer, 55%–70% of fevers result from infection, especially during periods of neutropenia.[22] Lymphomas, hypernephromas, and hepatomas may cause fever unrelated to infection. In addition, tumor masses that cause local obstruction or compromise blood supply to normal tissue can predispose tissue to necrosis, local infection, and fever. Fever caused by an underlying cancer cannot be distinguished, on the basis of duration or the degree of temperature elevation, from fever caused by infection. Excluding febrile episodes related to the administration of blood products and chemotherapeutic agents, which resolve spontaneously, fevers in the individual with cancer warrant thorough and prompt evaluation to rule out infection as the cause.

Nutrition

Cancer can affect nutritional status in several ways. The tumor can interfere with the functional capacity of gastrointestinal structures or organs and may cause inlet or outlet obstruction. Chronic obstruction can compromise the blood supply to surrounding tissue, especially if vascular impairment is severe or prolonged. The resulting necrosis and ulceration will predispose the affected areas to hemorrhage and infection.

Cachexia is a complex metabolic syndrome characterized by significant involuntary weight loss. The exact mechanisms responsible for cachexia are not completely understood, but it is believed that faulty metabolism of nutrients is a major factor. Nutritional research suggests that the failure of certain cachectic cancer patients to increase lean body mass despite adequate nutritional support results from the tumor effects on the host's metabolism.[23]

There is substantial evidence to support the existence of a relationship between malnutrition and a variety of immune deficiencies. Cell-mediated immunity is most often affected, with decreased lymphocyte numbers and diminished response to antigen. Phagocytosis, leukocyte chemotaxis, and the complement system are also impaired.[24,25] Immune defects related to nutritional deficiencies can be corrected by oral supplementation or parenteral nutritional support.

Cancer therapy

Surgery.   Surgery is commonly employed in diagnosis, staging, and treatment of individuals diagnosed with cancer. Various factors can increase the incidence of infectious postoperative complications, including the duration of preoperative hospitalization, extent of surgery, length of the procedure, presence and degree of hemorrhage and tissue ischemia, nutritional status of the patient, prior chemotherapy or corticosteroid administration, and, most importantly, presence of infection or wound contamination during surgery. Preoperative prophylactic antibiotics may be given to provide protection during the perioperative risk period. The choice of antibiotic is based on the operative site, potential pathogens, presence of prior infection, or heavy colonization with particular microorganisms.[26]

The surgical wound is the most common site of infection during the postoperative period. Wound infections range in severity from minor inflammatory responses to major potentially life-threatening infections. Distinctive patterns of microorganisms are usually seen in different hospital environments. Each institution's infection-control team monitors patterns, trends, and incidence of specific microorganisms resulting in infection. Special concern must be directed toward the detection of resistant organisms, which can develop with astonishing rapidity within the hospital environment, causing significant morbidity. A greater risk of sepsis accompanies certain surgical procedures. Surgical instrumentation of the genitourinary and gastrointestinal tracts is associated with higher incidence of morbidity and mortality.

Radiation therapy and chemotherapy.   Radiation therapy and chemotherapy interfere with essential metabolic functions of the cell and can cause inflammation and ulceration of normal tissues, predisposing the host to infection. Doses of chemotherapy and radiation that can be safely administered are determined by toxicity to normal tissues. Fractionation of radiation doses and administration of chemotherapy in intermittent cycles have been effective in enhancing therapeutic benefit while limiting toxicity.

The major risks associated with therapeutic radiation and cytotoxic chemotherapy relate to the induction of neutropenia and immunosuppression. Chemotherapy can induce immunological defects that lead to bacterial, fungal, parasitic, or viral infection. Not all chemotherapeutic agents, however, produce immunologic compromise. The potential toxicities and side effects of each agent should be reviewed and incorporated into the patient's plan of care and assessment. (See Chapter 20 for specific information concerning management of chemotherapy toxicity.)

During radiation therapy, leukocytes are the first blood cells to decrease, followed by platelets and erythrocytes. Blood counts are routinely monitored during radiation, especially if the treatment field is large or includes significant areas of bone marrow. Intensive radiation therapy results in a substantial reduction in cellular immune function that may persist for more than 1 year following treatment.[16]

Depending on the total dose and type of radiation, skin and mucous membrane integrity may be impaired, thereby predisposing to infection. Radiation reactions include epilation, erythema, dry and moist desquamation, mucositis, and necrosis. (See Chapter 17 for a discussion of nursing care for the patient receiving radiation therapy.)

Risk assessment for the febrile neutropenic person with cancer

Severity of neutropenia is well documented to be the single most important predictor of infection in the neutropenic individual. However, clinical investigations have revealed several other factors that contribute to overall risk of infection. These factors are summarized in Table 30-2.[8] Further studies will determine the safety of managing low-risk febrile neutropenic patients in the outpatient or home setting and/or with less aggressive antimicrobial therapies.[27]

Clinical Manifestations

Bacterial Infections

Changing patterns in bacterial infections are primarily the result of improvements in antibiotic therapy. During the 1950s and 1960s, *Staphylococcus aureus* was the most commonly identified organism in immunocompromised persons. Development of beta-lactamase-resistant penicillins provided highly effective therapy against *S. aureus* and led to the subsequent emergence of gram-negative organisms as the predominant pathogen. Empirical use of combination antibiotic therapy, incorporating third-generation cephalosporins, has greatly reduced the number of documented gram-negative infections. However, a recent resurgence of gram-positive infections is believed to be the result of increased use of central venous access catheters and the prevalence of methicillin-resistant strains of *Staphylococcus*.[8,9,28] In addition, an increase in the number of multidrug resistant gram-negative organisms has been noted in many institutions, due in part to excessive antibiotic use.

Gram-negative organisms

Despite current shifts in the patterns of infection, the primary cause of infection in neutropenic patients continues to be gram-negative organisms, especially *Escherichia coli*, *Klebsiella pneumoniae*, and *Pseudomonas aeruginosa*.[2,8,28,29] The most significant consequence of gram-

Table 30-2   Estimating Risk for Complications in Patients with Febrile Neutropenia

Factor	Low Risk	High Risk
Anticipated duration of neutropenia	Short (≤7 days)	Longer than 7 days
Type of cancer treatment	Solid tumor Maintenance therapy for leukemia	Leukemia induction Bone marrow transplant
Comorbid conditions	None	Systemic hypotension Altered mental status New neurologic changes Respiratory failure Dehydration Abdominal pain Hemorrhage Cardiac compromise/arrhythmia Vascular access catheter tunnel infection or extensive cellulitis Acute renal or liver failure
Other	Fever of undetermined origin	Bacteremia, pneumonia, or other serious infection Age Inpatient status

Adapted with permission from Freifeld AG, Pizzo PA, Walsh TJ: Infections in the cancer patient, in DeVita VT, Hellman S, Rosenberg SA (eds): Cancer: Principles and Practice of Oncology (ed 5). Philadelphia, Lippincott-Raven, 1997, pp 2659–2702.[8]

negative infection is the potential for endotoxic or systemic shock. Endotoxins are lipopolysaccharide protein complexes found on the outer membrane of gram-negative organisms. The release of endotoxin by these organisms initiates a cascade of events that, unless interrupted, will rapidly lead to death for the neutropenic patient. The actions of endotoxins include release of endogenous pyrogens, resulting in a febrile response; alteration of the vascular endothelium, causing formation of microthrombi; activation of the complement, coagulation, and fibrinolytic systems; and release of bradykinin, histamine, and serotonin, producing vasodilation and increased capillary permeability.[30] Without early detection and prompt initiation of treatment, endotoxic shock leads to hypotension, tissue ischemia, multisystem failure, and death. (See Chapter 40 for more on septic shock.)

Gram-positive organisms

S. aureus (coagulase positive) and *Staphylococcus epidermidis* (coagulase negative) are responsible for most gram-positive infections occurring during periods of neutropenia and are usually associated with skin or vascular access infections. Other emerging gram-positive pathogens for neutropenic patients include enterococcus and diphtheroids. Individuals who are asplenic or have impaired humoral response have a higher incidence of *S. pneumoniae* infections.[9,29]

Although less common, infection with gram-positive organisms may result in shock produced by secretion of noxious proteins called *exotoxins*. The most well known exotoxin, produced by *S. aureus*, is associated with toxic shock syndrome and characterized by high fever, rash, vomiting, diarrhea, myalgia, and hypotension.[31]

Treatment

Empirical antibiotic therapy is treatment initiated before infecting organisms have been identified. To date, a standardized regimen for treatment of bacterial infections in individuals with neutropenia has not been defined. Selection of antibiotic agents must be individualized to consider the probable cause of infection and likely site of origin, as well as institutional patterns of infection and antibiotic resistance. In general, the empirical antibiotic regimen should cover a broad spectrum of pathogens without significant risk for emergence of resistant organisms or drug-related toxicity. Common combination therapies include a cephalosporin or extended-spectrum penicillin and an aminoglycoside. Third-generation cephalosporins (e.g., ceftazadime) and carbapenems (e.g., imipenem), which have a broad range of activity and high bactericidal levels, may be effective when used as single agents.[32-34] Vancomycin may be added if gram-positive organisms are involved or suspected.

Mycobacterial Infections

Although mycobacterial infections are uncommon in individuals with cancer, they tend to be associated with defects in cellular immunity. Latent infections with *M. tuberculosis* may be reactivated, particularly in persons with carcinoma of the head, neck, and lung.[8,9] *Mycobacterium arium* complex, common in individuals with AIDS, has also been observed in those with hairy cell leukemia and in individuals undergoing intensive chemotherapy for non-Hodgkin's lymphoma.[2]

Treatment

While isoniazid is the treatment of choice for tuberculosis, it is not effective therapy for MAC. Combination therapy has been more successful in treating MAC, including amikacin, rifampin, ciprofloxacin, ethambutol, clofazamine, and clarithromycin.[35]

Fungal Infections

In humans, fungi can exist in harmony with other endogenous flora in a carefully balanced synergistic microenvironment. Alterations in this environment, such as disrupted integumentary and mucosal barriers, treatment-induced neutropenia, immunosuppression, and alterations in normal flora can lead to invasive fungal infection. Fungal infections have become an increasingly important cause of morbidity and mortality in individuals with cancer, particularly hematologic and lymphoreticular neoplasms.

Factors predisposing to fungal infection include severe prolonged neutropenia, implanted vascular access catheters, administration of parenteral nutrition or corticosteroids, extended use of broad-spectrum antibiotics, and damage to oropharyngeal or gastrointestinal mucosa due to disease or treatment. Immunosuppressed individuals who develop new or progressive pulmonary infiltrates while receiving broad-spectrum antibiotics present a major challenge for differential diagnosis. The possibility of fungal infection must be considered.

Candida

Candida is the most common cause of invasive fungal infection. The presence of *Candida* in the sputum, mouth, or throat cannot be definitively correlated with infection because *Candida* can reside harmlessly in the healthy host. However, the immunosuppressed person is at risk when neutropenia occurs or when cellular immunity is impaired. Broad-spectrum antibiotics alter the function of normal bacterial flora and therefore are associated with increased risk of fungal overgrowth and infection.

Dermatologic infections with *Candida* occur most frequently in skin folds, such as the groin, perineum and perianal areas, and under the breasts. Oral candidiasis (thrush) is a common yeast infection that can disseminate throughout the gastrointestinal tract. Disseminated candidiasis often involves the lungs, kidneys, bones, joints, and CNS.

Aspergillus

Aspergillus is another common fungus that causes serious infections in individuals with cancer, particularly those who are neutropenic and/or are receiving immunosuppressive therapy. The fungus enters the host through the upper airway and typically causes pneumonia or sinus infection. Extrapulmonary sites of infection include CNS, liver, kidney, skin, and heart valves. Nosocomial transmission of *Aspergillus* has occurred in hospitals where spores contained in construction materials were disseminated through the ventilation system.

Aspergillosis is characterized by blood vessel invasion, which can lead to thrombosis and infarction of pulmonary arteries and veins. Blood cultures are rarely positive, even in disseminated aspergillosis. The infection is difficult to diagnose, often necessitating aggressive treatment before the diagnosis is confirmed. Without prompt and aggressive therapy with amphotericin, *Aspergillus* pneumonia is almost always fatal in neutropenic patients.

Cryptococcus

Cryptococcus neoformans, a yeast found in soil and in pigeon excreta, is generally acquired by inhalation. The infection appears most often in individuals with advanced Hodgkin's disease and other lymphomas. It commonly occurs as an insidious meningoencephalitis. Headache, low-grade fever, vomiting, and diplopia are typical symptoms. Cerebrospinal fluid examination is often unremarkable, with only 50%–60% having detectable organism by India ink preparation. Diagnosis is usually made by documenting cryptococcal antigen in the serum or cerebrospinal fluid.[9,29]

Intrathecal administration of antifungal agents may be required for individuals whose cerebrospinal fluid does not clear with IV therapy. As with other fungi, cryptococcal infection can also occur in the lungs and disseminate to visceral organs.

Histoplasma

Histoplasmosis generally occurs as a pulmonary infection, usually in individuals with lymphoreticular neoplasms. The infection commonly disseminates, causing adenopathy and hepatosplenomegaly, which may be confused with the underlying neoplasm. Disseminated histoplasmosis can occur in individuals whose cancer is in remission, as well as in those with active disease; therefore, histological examination of biopsy material for *Histoplasma* is necessary if this organism is suspected as a cause of infection.

Phycomycetes

The phycomycetes (*Mucor, Rhizopus,* and *Absidia*) are opportunistic fungi widespread in dust and air. The lungs, nasal sinuses, and gastrointestinal tract are the three major sites of infection. After the fungi are inhaled into the lungs, the disease may disseminate to other body sites. Person-to-person transmission is rare.

Coccidioides

Coccidioides is found in the soil of the southwestern United States and typically enters the body by inhalation. The organism is rapidly phagocytized in individuals who have a competent immune system and may cause no symptoms. Immunocompromised individuals, however, are susceptible to the development of serious pulmonary infection.[36]

Treatment

Two major problems in treatment of fungal infections are the difficulty associated with culturing organisms from infected tissues and the limited number of effective agents available to manage severe fungal infections.

Amphotericin B is the drug of choice for treatment of systemic fungal infections. However, it is associated with significant side effects and toxicities, including fever, chills, rigors, nausea, vomiting, hypotension, bronchospasm, and occasionally seizures. Premedication with acetaminophen, antihistamines, or low-dose IV hydrocortisone generally reduces the reactions associated with the drug. Intravenous meperidine (1 mg/kg) can be used to ameliorate fever and chills that frequently accompany the initial administration of amphotericin.[37]

The major toxicity of amphotericin is nephrotoxicity. With continued administration, elevated levels of creatinine and blood urea nitrogen can occur. Electrolyte imbalances, particularly hypokalemia, are common and warrant careful monitoring of fluid and treatment.

The antifungal agent fluconazole is well absorbed and is able to penetrate into cerebrospinal fluid, the eye, and peritoneal fluid. It is available in oral and parenteral form. Fluconazole is most often used to treat cryptococcal meningitis and oropharyngeal, esophageal, and systemic *Candida* infections. Fluconazole is also indicated for *Candida* prophylaxis in patients undergoing bone marrow transplant. Side effects include exfoliative skin disorders (blistering, peeling, etc.), hepatotoxicity, and, less frequently, gastrointestinal disturbances and headaches.[37]

Ketoconazole, another oral antifungal agent, is used to treat disseminated and pulmonary coccidioidomycosis, candidiasis, and histoplasmosis. It is ineffective in treatment of fungal meningitis because of poor penetration into the cerebrospinal fluid. The most common side effects are nausea, vomiting, and diarrhea. Rare instances of hepatotoxicity have been reported. High-dose ketoconazole therapy has been shown to suppress corticosteroid secretion, resulting in menstrual irregularities and decreased male libido.[37]

The oral agent itraconazole may be used in the treatment of aspergillosis in persons who are intolerant of or resistant to amphotericin. It may also be prescribed for treatment of histoplasmosis. Itraconazole should be taken with food to increase absorption. Patients with achlorhydria may require dosage elevations to compensate for decreased drug absorption.[37]

Clotrimazole and nystatin are indicated in the treatment and prophylaxis of oropharyngeal candidiasis. Lozenges should dissolve slowly in the mouth and should not be chewed or swallowed. Nystatin suspension should be held in the mouth or swished through the mouth as long as possible, then swallowed. Both drugs are poorly absorbed from the gastrointestinal tract and therefore are not used to treat systemic mycosis.[37]

Flucytosine (5-FC) is another antifungal agent used for treatment of *Candida* and *Cryptococcus* infections. The major limitation to its use is the rapid onset of drug resistance. Flucytosine is well absorbed orally, with side effects that include nausea, vomiting, diarrhea, myelosuppression, skin rash, and hepatotoxicity.[37] Flucytosine is commonly used in combination with amphotericin.

Viral Infections

Viruses, the smallest known infectious microorganisms, are visible only with the aid of an electron microscope. Viruses have no intrinsic energy system and consist only of a deoxyribonucleic acid (DNA) or ribonucleic acid (RNA) nucleus surrounded by a protein coat. Viruses are replicated by host cell mechanisms after invasion by a single virus. The primary virus invades the cell and initiates the formation of similar viruses by the host cell. Common viruses cause measles, mumps, rubella, respiratory infections, colds, and bronchitis. Most viral infections in granulocytopenic patients are caused by herpes viruses and herpes simplex virus (HSV), varicella zoster virus (VZV), and CMV.

Herpes simplex

Herpes simplex virus can cause serious infection in persons with cancer, from either primary exposure to or reactivation of a latent virus. Major sites of infection are the oropharynx, esophagus, eyes, skin, urogenital tract, and perianal area. In rare cases of HSV dissemination, pulmonary, CNS, and hepatic involvement may be seen.

Individuals with impaired cell-mediated immunity are at increased risk for recurrent HSV infections resulting in extensive mucocutaneous ulceration. Progression of the ulcers occurs as the virus, unimpeded by T-cell response, spreads across the squamous epithelium.[38] Lesions in the immunocompromised host tend to be more invasive, slower to heal, and associated with prolonged viral shedding.[39]

Varicella zoster

Primary infection with VZV ("chickenpox") can cause serious vesicular eruption in individuals with cancer, especially children, and results in a mortality rate of up to 18%.[40] Following primary infection, reactivation ("shingles") can occur because the virus remains dor-

mant in the spinal ganglia. Incidence of reactivation approaches 30% in those with Hodgkin's disease or following bone marrow transplant (BMT).[41,42] Radiation therapy can also increase the risk of developing VZV infection. Usually, dermatomes involved with VZV lesions have previously been encompassed in a radiation field.

Diagnosis of zoster is based on a history of chickenpox, characteristic dermatomal distribution of vesicular lesions, and positive culture results. Because skin lesions (vesicles) can become confluent, meticulous skin care is required to prevent secondary bacterial infection.

The major complication of VZV infection is visceral dissemination, resulting in pneumonitis, hepatitis, and meningoencephalitis. However, even in the immunocompromised patient, disseminated VZV is rarely fatal.[40] The risk of visceral dissemination is increased in individuals receiving chemotherapy during the time of infection, especially if lymphopenia occurs (<500 lymphocytes/mm³). Disseminated VZV is frequently complicated by secondary bacterial infections.

Varicella is highly contagious, and the risk of spread to other seronegative immunocompromised individuals is substantial, especially in adults with Hodgkin's disease and children with leukemia. Because of the severity of VZV infection in persons with cancer, infected individuals have been treated with varicella zoster-immune globulin (VZIG). When administered within 72 hours of exposure to VZV, VZIG generally modifies the infection to a subclinical or mild form. Management of individuals with cancer who are seronegative and who have been exposed to VZV includes interruption of cancer therapy and administration of VZIG. Whenever possible, cancer treatment should not be reinstituted until the end of the incubation period, approximately 21 days. When clinical evidence of VZV infection occurs in individuals with cancer, immunosuppressive agents should be withheld until all skin lesions have dried and scabbed.

Cytomegalovirus

Cytomegalovirus infection is usually a result of viral reactivation, particularly in association with immunosuppression. It is a common cause of interstitial pneumonitis in individuals with impaired cellular immunity or following BMT. Cytomegalovirus pneumonia characteristically occurs within 3 months of transplant and is often fatal.[29,39]

Cytomegalovirus retinitis is the most common opportunistic ocular infection noted in immunocompromised persons, especially those with AIDS. Direct viral invasion of retinal cells results in tissue damage, necrosis, and high risk of retinal detachment. Less commonly, CMV will infect the gastrointestinal tract, resulting in esophagitis, gastritis, or enteritis.

Hepatitis virus

Hepatitis in individuals with cancer can occur as a primary infection with one of the hepatitis viruses (A, B [HBV], or C [HCV]) or as a secondary infection with other viruses. HBV and HCV are the major causative organisms in transfusion-related hepatitis.

Viral hepatitis occurs as an acute or chronic infection. Asymptomatic carriers may exhibit mild hepatic dysfunction. Although transfusions of blood products constitute the primary route of transmission, nonparenteral transmission occurs through sexual intercourse and contact with contaminated saliva, urine, and feces. Risk of infection to health care providers is high and warrants strict adherence to universal precautions outlined by the Centers for Disease Control, (CDC). See Table 30-3.[43] The CDC guidelines have been incorporated into the rules regarding occupational exposure to blood-borne pathogens released by the Occupational Safety and Health Administration (OSHA).[44]

Treatment

Acyclovir is an antiviral agent preferentially taken up by cells infected with HSV and VZV. Treatment with acyclovir decreases viral shedding from infected cells, accelerates healing of lesions, and decreases pain and itching. Acyclovir offers significant prophylaxis against recurrent infection for immunocompromised individuals, especially those who have had allogeneic BMT. It is available in parenteral, oral, and topical forms; however, it is not well absorbed from the gastrointestinal tract.

Table 30-3 Universal Precautions for Prevention of Transmission of Human Immunodeficiency Virus, Hepatitis B Virus, and Other Blood-Borne Pathogens

1. Never recap, bend, break, or clip needles.
2. Place needles and sharps promptly in an approved puncture-resistant container designated for needle disposal.
3. Use approved disposal containers in all areas.
4. Do not overfill containers.
5. Close container securely when three-quarters full.
6. Bag closed containers in red bags.
7. Protect open wounds from coming in contact with potentially infected materials.
8. Be sure to cover properly any broken skin surfaces.
9. Gloves are necessary when:
   a. drawing blood
   b. handling specimens that have obvious blood in them
   c. starting intravenous infusions (IVs)
   d. cleaning blood spills
   e. performing cardiopulmonary resuscitation (CPR)
   f. suctioning (especially a new tracheostomy)
   g. changing dressings
10. Wear mask, gloves, and protective eyewear when:
    a. blood splattering may occur
    b. inserting or maintaining arterial lines
    c. doing oral care
    d. doing emergency procedures
    e. doing invasive procedures
    f. doing hemodialysis or hemapheresis
    g. doing peritoneal dialysis
11. Change gloves between patients.
12. Wash hands thoroughly before leaving the patient's room.

Data from Centers for Disease Control.[43]

Side effects are minimal and consist primarily of nausea, vomiting, diarrhea, and anorexia. Phlebitis is common with intravenous administration. Acute renal failure may occur if acyclovir is given by rapid injection, especially in patients with other risk factors for renal insufficiency.[37]

Valacyclovir is a prodrug form of acyclovir used to treat HSV and VZV. It is rapidly absorbed in the gastrointestinal tract and converted to its active form. Most commonly reported side effects are headache and nausea.[37]

Famcyclovir is indicated in the treatment of herpes zoster and has been found to decrease the duration of postherpetic neuralgia by approximately 50%. Therapy is most effective when initiated within 48 hours of the onset of rash. Famcyclovir is well absorbed from the upper intestine. There have been no reports of serious side effects; however, adults with impaired renal function may require dosage adjustment.[37]

Vidarabine is an intravenous antiviral agent primarily used as second-line therapy for VZV and HSV infections. Due to poor solubility, the drug commonly requires 1.5–2.0 liters of fluid volume for administration. Toxicities include bone marrow suppression, gastrointestinal disturbances, and neurological effects such as tremor, confusion, alterations in mentation and behavior, and ataxia.[45]

Ganciclovir is used in treatment of CMV infection. It is a virostatic agent and therefore does not eliminate existing CMV but suppresses viral replication. Ganciclovir is currently available in parenteral and oral forms and as an intraocular implant for individuals with CMV retinitis who are intolerant of other forms of the drug. The most significant toxicities of ganciclovir are neutropenia and thrombocytopenia.[37]

Foscarnet is another virostatic agent that suppresses CMV replication. It also may be prescribed for acyclovir-resistant HSV infection. Oral absorption is poor; intravenous administration is required to achieve therapeutic serum levels. Primary side effects include anemia, nephrotoxicity, and hypocalcemia. Less common effects are CNS disturbances, including paresthesia, irritability, tremor, and headache.[37]

Cytomegalovirus hyperimmune globulin may be given in combination with either ganciclovir or foscarnet for immunocompromised patients with CMV pneumonitis.[39]

Protozoa and Parasites

Protozoal infections are associated with defects in cell-mediated immunity. These organisms are ubiquitous, causing few problems, if any, in individuals who are immunocompetent. In the immunocompromised host, however, protozoal infections are often difficult to treat and quickly become life-threatening.

Pneumocystis carinii

Pneumocystis carinii is most often classified as a protozoan based on its appearance, growth characteristics, and susceptibility to antiprotozoal agents. However, molecular and genetic analysis suggests that it is more closely related to fungi.[46] *P. carinii* causes infection in malnourished infants, children with primary immunodeficiency disorders, persons with AIDS, and those with cancer undergoing immunosuppressive therapy.

Clinical manifestations of *P. carinii* pneumonia (PCP) include fever, nonproductive cough, tachypnea with intercostal retraction, and potentially life-threatening respiratory compromise. Rales are often absent. Chest radiographs reveal diffuse interstitial infiltrates, although some cases may present with unremarkable findings. Pulse oxymetry or arterial blood gases typically demonstrate hypoxia. Fiberoptic bronchoscopy with bronchioalveolar lavage may be required to confirm the diagnosis.

Toxoplasma

T. gondii is an obligate intracellular parasite found in soil, cat excreta, and undercooked meats. It can remain encapsulated in host tissues, with reactivation of latent organisms causing infection. Persons at greatest risk include those with AIDS and those receiving immunosuppressive therapy for hematological malignancies or prevention of organ transplant rejection. Involvement of the CNS occurs in more than 50% of infected individuals who typically present with focal seizures, mental status changes, and localized headaches. However, in immunocompromised individuals the infection may be disseminated at the time of diagnosis.[29,47,48]

Cryptosporidium

Although a common cause of enteritis in individuals with AIDS, cryptosporidiosis has only occasionally been observed in other immunocompromised patients. Routes of transmission include person-to-person, animal-to-person, and environmental, particularly via contaminated water. When severe immune deficiencies are present, cryptosporidiosis results in voluminous watery diarrhea and secondary malnutrition, dehydration, and electrolyte imbalance.

Treatment

Untreated PCP is fatal. The treatment of choice for *P. carinii* is trimethoprim-sulfamethoxazole. Side effects include rash, nausea, vomiting, hepatotoxicity, and myelosuppression.

In individuals with known history of sulfonamide sensitivity, dapsone-trimethoprim, clindamycin plus primaquine, or atovaquone may be prescribed. Gastrointestinal absorption of atovaquone is low and variable. Absorption is significantly improved when the drug is administered with a high-fat meal. Atovaquone is usually well tolerated, with fever and skin rash the most common side effects. Side effects of dapsone may be more problematic, including hemolytic anemia, hypersensitivity reactions, blood dyscrasias, hepatic toxicity, and peripheral neuropathy. The most significant complication associated with clinda-

mycin is the development of antibiotic-associated pseudo-membranous colitis, also know as *Clostridium difficile* colitis. The condition is characterized by severe abdominal cramping and severe watery, sometimes bloody, diarrhea.[37]

Pentamidine is effective in treating PCP unresponsive to trimethoprim-sulfamethoxazole. Side effects, however, are troublesome, including azotemia, hypocalcemia, and hepatotoxicity. Rapid intravenous infusion may result in a precipitous fall in blood pressure. Severe, prolonged hypoglycemia, sometimes resulting in insulin-dependent diabetes, has also been reported, usually associated with higher doses, longer duration of therapy, and retreatment within 3 months.[37]

Trimetrexate may be given intravenously to treat moderate to severe PCP in patients who are intolerant of or resistant to other less aggressive therapy. Leucovorin must be concurrently administered to prevent potentially life-threatening bone marrow depression or gastrointestinal ulceration.[37]

Prophylactic treatment of patients at high-risk for PCP is most often accomplished with trimethoprim-sulfamethoxazole. Alternative agents include aerosolized pentamidine, dapsone, pyrimethamine plus sulfamethoxazole or clindamycin, and atovaquone.[47]

Treatment with pyrimethamine plus sulfamethoxazole has been effective against *T. gondii* in immunocompromised patients. Clindamycin can be substituted in patients with known allergies to sulfonamides.[47,48]

To date, there is no known treatment for cryptosporidiosis other than supportive therapy with antidiarrheal agents and replacement of fluid and electrolytes.[49]

Therapeutic Approaches and Nursing Care

Prevention

Because most cancer care is delivered in the outpatient or home setting, nursing care focuses on prevention of infection, measures to optimize the person's health status, and aggressive therapeutic interventions when infection occurs. The individual with cancer and his or her family need to be well informed about protective self-care measures and symptoms of infection to report to the health care team. When an infection develops, prompt initiation of medical and nursing interventions is imperative to prevent life-threatening complications. Nursing care strategies for patients at risk for infection, including assessment parameters, interventions, and instructions for patients and caregivers, are summarized in Table 30-4.[49]

Reducing environmental pathogens

The single most important intervention to prevent infection is meticulous hand washing by every person who enters the room or comes in contact with the individual at

Table 30-4   Nursing Care of Patient at Risk for Infection

Problem	Assessment	Nursing Intervention	Patient/Significant Other Teaching
Potential for systemic infection	a. *Patient history:* factors that compromise immune function (e.g., cancer treatment, steroid use, nutritional status, chronic infections, HIV+) b. Absolute neutrophil count c. Vital signs d. Comprehensive physical assessment e. Response to antimicrobial, colony-stimulating factor therapy	a. Strict hand-washing measures b. Appropriate protective measures (e.g., private room, protective isolation, dietary restrictions) c. Adequate fluid/dietary intake d. Adequate periods of rest e. Aseptic technique for invasive procedures, dressing changes, etc.	a. Importance of hand washing b. Rationale for protective measures c. Importance of optimizing health status (e.g., diet, rest, personal hygiene) d. Signs/symptoms of infection to report to health care team e. Ability to read thermometer
Potential/actual disruption of skin integrity	a. *Patient history:* recent trauma to skin or conditions that predispose to disrupted skin integrity b. *Physical assessment:* special attention to skin folds, wound sites, lesions suspicious for primary, recurrent malignancy c. Characteristics of open areas (e.g., size, depth, discharge)	a. Meticulous personal hygiene, particularly to high-risk areas b. Electric razors, dressing supplies less likely to traumatize skin c. Moisturizing lotions, mild soaps to prevent drying, chapping, cracking of skin d. Adequate fluid, dietary intake e. Caution when moving bedfast patient f. Activity consistent with health status g. Special mattress to minimize pressure areas h. Cultures of suspicious areas i. Aseptic technique for dressing changes j. Referral to home care agency for postdischarge follow-up	a. Self-care information regarding maintenance of skin integrity (e.g., avoiding exposure to sun, use of skin care products) b. Rationale for precautions c. Signs/symptoms to report to health care team d. Proper techniques for wound care, dressing changes
Potential/actual pulmonary infection	a. *Patient history:* dysphagia, diminished gag reflex, tobacco use, asbestos exposure, COPD, HIV+, radiation therapy to chest, pulmonary toxicity due to chemotherapy b. *Physical assessment:* Respiratory rate, effort, use of accessory muscles; chest auscultation c. Recent changes in pulmonary status (cough, sputum)	a. Cough/deep breathing exercises b. Activity appropriate for health status c. Adequate hydration d. Staff/visitors with respiratory infection restricted e. TB testing f. Review of x-ray, lab test results g. Sputum specimen for culture h. Aseptic technique when suctioning i. Supplemental O_2	a. Proper performance of cough/deep breathing exercises b. Strategies for smoking cessation c. Signs/symptoms to be reported to health care team d. Home safety precautions when using O_2 e. Information about community resources
Potential/actual disruption of oral mucosa	a. *Patient history:* chemotherapy, radiation therapy to head/neck, HIV+, tobacco/alcohol use, periodontal disease, hydration/nutritional status b. *Physical assessment of oral cavity:* color, moisture, lesions, ulcerations, amount and character of saliva c. Patient's routine for oral hygiene, presence of oral pain	a. Oral hygiene plan—toothbrush, toothpaste, dental floss; cotton swab or Toothettes® if pain, bleeding preclude use of toothbrush b. Normal saline, ¼ str. hydrogen peroxide, or sodium bicarbonate mouth rinses c. Adequate fluid intake d. Topical or systemic analgesia for oral or esophageal pain e. Water-soluble lubricant	a. Dietary modifications to reduce trauma to oral mucosa (avoiding spicy foods, temperature extremes, high acid content) b. Consistent, thorough oral assessment and hygiene c. Avoidance of tobacco, alcohol d. Signs/symptoms to be reported to health care team e. Use of dentures for meals only if oral mucous membrane integrity disrupted
Potential/actual disruption of rectal mucosa	a. *Patient history:* diet, sexual practices, medications, chemotherapy, HIV+, change in bowel habits	a. Dietary modifications to reduce rectal trauma (increase fiber for constipation; low residue for diarrhea)	a. Factors that increase risk of infection and strategies to reduce risk; dietary modification, alternative sexual practices, etc.

Table 30-4 Nursing Care of Patient at Risk for Infection (continued)

Problem	Assessment	Nursing Intervention	Patient/Significant Other Teaching
Potential/actual disruption of rectal mucosa *(cont.)*	b. *Physical assessment of rectal area:* erythema, ulceration, hemorrhoids, bleeding c. Character, frequency of bowel movements	b. Avoid invasive procedures (e.g., rectal temperatures, suppositories, enemas) c. Hygiene plan to prevent/minimize anorectal excoriation, promote comfort (e.g., sitz baths, cotton balls or soft wipes instead of toilet tissue) d. Stool softeners or antidiarrheal agents	b. Signs/symptoms to be reported to health care team
Potential/actual genitourinary (GU) infection	a. *Patient history:* benign prostatic hypertrophy, HIV +, bladder-toxic chemotherapy; symptoms of GU infection (dysuria, urinary frequency, urgency, hematuria, pruritis, vaginal/penile discharge) b. *Physical assessment of genitalia:* lesions, ulcerations, discharge c. Characteristics of urine—color, turbidity, odor	a. Adequate hydration b. Urine specimen (straight catheterization or clean catch) for culture and routine analysis c. Culture genital discharge, lesions d. Avoid indwelling urinary catheters e. Antispasmodic; analgesic agents as indicated	a. Rationale, importance of adequate hydration b. Signs/symptoms to be reported to health care team

Adapted with permission from Ellerhorst-Ryan JM: Nursing care plan for the immunocompromised patients, in Workman ML, Ellerhorst-Ryan JM, Koertge VH (eds.): *Nursing Care of the Immunocompromised Patient.* Philadelphia, Saunders, 1993.[49]

risk for infection. Neutropenic patients are advised of their risk and are encouraged to remind staff, family, and visitors about hand-washing precautions.

When hospitalized, the patient is given a private room. Nursing assignments include consideration for whether a staff member has had a recent immunization or transmissible infection. Ideally, staff members caring for a patient with an active infection are not also assigned to a neutropenic patient. However, this precaution is probably unnecessary if thorough and meticulous hand washing is consistently performed. Visitors are also screened for recent immunization or transmissible infection.

When the ANC is less than 1000/mm3, live plants, cut flowers, and fresh fruit should not be brought into the patient's room. During times when granulocytes are adequate, bacterial content can be decreased by adding 1 teaspoon of chlorine bleach to each quart of water used in flower vases. Water in pitchers, denture cups, and nebulizers is changed at least once a day.

The consumption of noncarbonated bottled water may place neutropenic individuals at risk for infection. Although current data is limited, studies have found *Stenotrophomonas* and *Pseudomonas* species present in noncarbonated bottled water. Carbonated products, on the other hand, did not yield bacteria on culture, probably because of low pH which prevents bacterial survival. Bottled water is often viewed as a healthy alternative to tap water. Until safety is demonstrated, drinking only carbonated forms of bottled water may be advisable until sufficient granulocyte recovery is present.[50]

During neutropenic episodes, invasive procedures are kept to a minimum, with adherence to strict aseptic tech-

nique when they are performed. Indwelling urinary catheters are also avoided whenever possible. If any type of catheter placement is necessary, the smallest lumen size available is selected and the duration of use is kept as brief as possible. Communicating with laboratory staff to coordinate blood sampling can prevent unnecessary venipuncture.

Optimizing health status

Adequate nutritional intake during periods of increased risk requires a high-calorie, high-protein diet. If severe neutropenia is anticipated, a low-bacteria cooked-food diet may be prescribed to minimize pathogenic colonization of the gut. A low-bacteria diet excludes fresh fruit, raw vegetables, fresh eggs, cold cuts, and many dairy products.[51]

Fluid intake is monitored to ensure adequate hydration, especially during periods of nausea, vomiting, and diarrhea, and when therapy includes agents with bladder and renal toxicity. Supplemental intravenous fluid administration may be needed periodically.

Activities are organized to allow for periods of rest. Certain individuals may become frustrated or discouraged by their lack of stamina or endurance. Assisting them with realistic goal setting and planning may enable them to accomplish desired tasks without further compromising their health status.

Strategies to maintain skin and mucous membrane integrity are implemented. Meticulous personal hygiene is imperative, with strict attention to skin folds, including the axillae, perineum, groin, buttocks, and under the breasts. Mild soap and a water-soluble lubricant can help prevent drying of the skin. Shaving with an electric razor will reduce the occurrence of accidental cuts. Fingernails and toenails should be kept short; toenails that are difficult to trim should be brought to the attention of a podiatrist.

The optimal plan for oral hygiene includes use of a soft to medium toothbrush, toothpaste, and dental floss. However, periods of thrombocytopenia and oral stomatitis may require substitution of sponge toothbrushes and normal saline. Oral care is performed after meals, at bedtime, and as indicated while the patient is awake. A number of proven strategies for prevention and treatment of stomatitis are available (see Chapter 20).[52] To be maximally effective, the chosen protocol must be performed consistently and on a regular basis.

Enemas, rectal temperatures, and suppositories are likely to traumatize fragile rectal mucosa and are avoided as much as possible in the high-risk patient. Prophylactic stool softeners are often recommended, particularly if hemorrhoids are present.

Activity consistent with current health status is encouraged to maintain optimal circulatory and pulmonary function. The patient is instructed and assisted in performing coughing and deep breathing exercises.

Although impaired cellular immunity and neutropenia are the primary causes of immunosuppression in individuals with cancer, humoral immunity can also be affected by either disease or treatment. Impaired humoral immunity compromises the efficacy of immunization, especially if chemotherapy is administered at the same time. Persons with cancer, especially those with acute leukemia, should receive pneumococcal and other vaccines only while in remission, since antibody response is limited during chemotherapy.

Management

Early detection

Despite strict adherence to protective measures, prolonged or severe neutropenia will allow rapid progression of a localized infection to potentially life-threatening sepsis. When the inflammatory response is diminished or absent, classic signs and symptoms of infection—fever, erythema, edema, pain, and purulence—may not be present, making early identification difficult.

During neutropenic periods, patients need nurses with diligent physical assessment skills, including the ability to listen carefully to information provided by the patient and significant others and to identify subtle clues indicative of infection. The most reliable indicator of infection is a low-grade fever. A temperature elevation of 1 degree that persists for 24 hours may be the only early evidence of infection.

Respiratory system. The high incidence of pneumonia in immunocompromised patients mandates thorough assessment of the respiratory system. During hospitalization, chest auscultation is performed every 2–4 hours, depending on extent of risk, and with each nursing visit when at home. Neutropenic individuals may experience only slight temperature elevation and mild dyspnea if pneumonia is present. Assessment findings for upper respiratory infection range from pain, swelling, erythema, and discharge in nonneutropenic individuals to vague discomfort and possibly mild erythema in neutropenic individuals.

Oropharynx. The oral mucosa is often traumatized by chemotherapeutic agents, especially the antimetabolites and antibiotics. Local infections can occur if inflamed or injured mucosal surfaces become colonized with bacteria, predisposing to systemic infection. Teeth and gums in poor condition can become a source of sepsis during periods of granulocytopenia. Stomatitis can compromise nutritional status and fluid intake; when severe, it can necessitate interruption of chemotherapy.

The oral cavity is regularly inspected for white plaques, gingival edema, erythema, bleeding, and ulceration. Complaints of oral pain and dysphagia should be followed up with bacterial, fungal, and viral cultures.

Gastrointestinal system. Disruption of intestinal mucosa by anticancer therapy facilitates bacterial invasion and increases the potential for sepsis. If a granulocytopenic patient receiving broad-spectrum antibiotics complains of dysphagia and retrosternal burning, *Candida* or HSV esophagitis must be considered. Gastritis, enteritis, and colitis typically present with nausea, vomiting, diarrhea, and abdominal pain or tenderness. Hepatitis results in fatigue, anorexia, early satiety, and clay-colored stools. The perirectal area should be routinely inspected for signs of inflammation, infection, hemorrhoids, and fissures. Complaints of perineal itching, tenderness, constipation, or pain with defecation can indicate early stages of perirectal cellulitis.

Central nervous system. Subtle changes in neurological function may signify either the onset of an infection or progression of malignancy. The development of any neurological abnormality warrants immediate attention.

Infections of the CNS present with a variety of symptoms, depending on the type and extent of infection. Typical complaints include headache, fever, visual impairment, personality changes, focal neurological signs, nuchal rigidity, altered mental status, and seizures.

Urinary tract. Urinary tract infections (UTIs) are common, especially in those cancer patients who have fever and neutropenia. Classic symptoms of UTI are typically absent in neutropenic patients. Observation of the clinical characteristics of the urine, specifically if cloudy and foul-smelling, is usually more helpful. *Candida* infection can result in erythema and pruritus in the perineal area.

Skin. Skin integrity should be regularly assessed, with special attention given to known areas of disruption at increased risk of breakdown.

Cardiovascular system. Symptoms of cardiovascular infection are generally nonspecific: fever, chills, malaise, and night sweats. Indications of possible cardiac infection include new or changing murmurs, thromboemboli, unexplained heart failure, and arrhythmias.

Nursing care during episodes of infection

Infection in the neutropenic patient is always considered a potentially life-threatening emergency. Fatality rates in untreated individuals during the first 48 hours of infection can exceed 50%.[10]

Cultures are obtained from all potential sites of infection, including urine, sputum, wound, stool, and blood. If vascular access catheters are present, culture specimens are obtained both from peripheral veins and through the catheter.

After culture specimens have been obtained, empirical broad-spectrum antibiotic therapy is promptly initiated and the patient's response closely observed. Monitoring for efficacy of antimicrobial treatment includes assessing vital signs every 2–4 hours; reviewing reports of chest x-rays and laboratory data, including arterial blood gases, blood counts, chemistry profiles, culture results, and serum antibiotic levels; and observing for signs of septic shock. If little or no improvement is apparent following 3–5 days of antibiotic treatment, cultures are repeated and the physician consulted about modifying the prescribed antimicrobial regimen.

Other supportive nursing care strategies include restoring circulatory fluid volume by administering intravenous fluids, blood or blood products, and vasopressors; and maintaining adequate oxygenation through the use of supplemental oxygen and, if necessary, mechanical ventilation. Additional measures are taken to promote optimal nutritional status by monitoring dietary intake, consulting with the dietitian, and conferring with the physician if enteral or parenteral nutrition is indicated.

Treatment of infection

Persons with cancer who are not immunocompromised or neutropenic can be treated with appropriate antibiotic therapy for the specific infectious agent identified. Cultures are performed before the initiation of therapy and antibiotics are changed, if necessary, when the results of sensitivity testing are known. However, empirical treatment with a broad-spectrum antibiotic is initiated if a serious infection develops rapidly.

Patients who have fever during periods of neutropenia will have a thorough physical examination, chest radiograph, and appropriate laboratory studies. After cultures of all potential sources of infection have been obtained, empirical broad-spectrum antibiotic therapy is initiated.

Neutropenic patients may not manifest clinical evidence of infection because neutropenia prevents the mounting of an inflammatory response. Progression to systemic infection and septic shock is usually rapid. There-fore, individuals with neutropenia must be evaluated at frequent intervals for signs and symptoms of infection. Common sites of infection identified in patients with neutropenia and fever are listed in Table 30-5.

Empirical antibiotics. Empirical antibiotic therapy in the patient with fever and neutropenia reduces the number of infections that could become severe enough to be demonstrated by microbiological culture or clinical documentation. The decreasing incidence of septic shock in this high-risk population suggests that prompt aggressive antibiotic therapy is effective in reducing the serious morbidity associated with gram-negative sepsis. The particular empirical antibiotic regimen selected must be broad, achieve high bactericidal levels, and be as nontoxic and simple to administer as possible.[8] Drug levels may be monitored periodically while the patient is receiving nephrotoxic antibiotics, and dosage adjustments made when indicated to maintain safe therapeutic levels.

Isolation precautions and protected environments. Persons with cancer receiving intensive therapeutic regimens are significantly more susceptible to infection than those receiving less intensive therapy. These severely immunocompromised persons are often placed on "protective" regimens intended to reduce the risk of infection. One such regimen, routine protective isolation, does not appear to reduce the risk of infection any more than consistent and frequent hand washing during patient care. Routine protective isolation fails to reduce the risk of infection from endogenous microorganisms or from colonization by contaminated hands of health care personnel.[53]

Efforts to exclude all microorganisms through use of patient isolator units (usually laminar air flow rooms), nonabsorbable prophylactic antibiotics, and sterilization of the patient's food and water may prevent or delay the onset of some infections. Therefore, these procedures have been recommended by some investigators for immunocompromised patients who have a predictable period of significant risk; for example, following bone marrow transplant or high-dose chemotherapy.[54,55]

Laminar air flow rooms are protected environments developed to shield the compromised host from exoge-

Table 30-5 Common Sites of Infection in Neutropenic Patients

Mouth and pharynx

Respiratory tract

Skin and soft tissue

Intravenous and vascular access catheters

Perineal area

Urinary tract

Gastrointestinal tract

nous and endogenous sources of infection. In this sophisticated isolation system, air is circulated through high-efficiency particulate air filters capable of removing from the air particles that are larger than 0.3 μm with a greater than 99.7% efficiency. The unidirectional (laminar) air flow significantly reduces air turbulence, which decreases the potential for microbial contamination in the consistently clean, protected environment. Semiportable units with horizontal air flow can be installed in regular hospital rooms.

To create an environment as free of microorganisms as possible, patients undergo cutaneous and gastrointestinal decontamination with oral nonabsorbable antibiotics before entry into the room. All objects brought into the room are sterilized by steam or gas, and food is semisterile. Anyone who has physical contact with the patient wears gloves, mask, and gown.

The disadvantages of laminar air flow rooms are that the protective environment is elaborate, cumbersome, and expensive. In addition, the patient may experience depression due to social isolation and possibly psychotic episodes because of sensory deprivation. Although laminar air flow rooms reduce incidence of infection and improve short-term survival, they have not affected long-term survival.

Granulocyte replacement.

Initial attempts at granulocyte replacement were in the form of granulocyte transfusions. However, limited efficacy, high cost, and serious complications, including development of lymphotoxic antibodies, made the procedure impractical.

Granulocyte colony-stimulating factor (G-CSF) and granulocyte-macrophage colony stimulating factor (GM-CSF) are hormonelike glycoproteins that promote the proliferation and maturation of phagocytes. Studies have shown that the duration of granulocytopenia following chemotherapy administration is markedly decreased when G-CSF or GM-CSF is used. In addition, mean recovery time for neutrophils following BMT is significantly shorter with the addition of CSFs.

Approach to the patient with gram-negative sepsis

Shock develops in approximately 27%–46% of patients with gram-negative bacteremia,[56] resulting in inadequate tissue perfusion and circulatory collapse. Mortality approaches 80% unless vigorous treatment is begun promptly. The clinical syndrome is a result of a number of interrelated factors that include the direct effect of bacterial endotoxin on the cardiovascular system, activation of the coagulation and complement cascade systems, nutritional status of the patient, and the nature of the underlying disease. Signs and symptoms depend on the stage of shock, the causative organism, and the age of the patient. The first sign of impending shock in the immunocompromised host may be limited to a low-grade fever, shaking chills, and mild hypotension. Early recognition of sepsis and aggressive intervention are essential if irreversible damage to vital organs and subsequent death

are to be averted (see Chapter 40 for more on septic shock).

Approach to the HIV-infected patient with cancer

Nursing care of persons with AIDS, with or without malignancy, presents a unique challenge. These individuals are at increased risk for opportunistic infection not only because of HIV-related impairment of cellular immunity but also because of neutropenia secondary to cancer treatment and antimicrobial therapy (e.g., ganciclovir). Most opportunistic infections are the consequence of T-helper cell depletion and are caused by mycobacterial, viral, fungal, and protozoal organisms. Antimicrobial therapy is sometimes continued indefinitely to prevent recurrent symptoms of infection. Side effects of therapy and progression of AIDS typically result in anorexia, nausea and vomiting, diarrhea, and malabsorption, which further compromise immune function.

Continuity of Care

Education about risk of infection begins at the time of diagnosis. The patient and family are instructed about the impact of cancer and cancer treatment on the inflammatory and immune responses. They are also taught about blood counts, anticipated time until the nadir is reached, and self-care activities to minimize risk of infection. Information provided about prescribed dietary restrictions to prevent pathogenic colonization of the gut also includes the importance of thoroughly cleaning kitchen equipment, such as blenders and food processors, between uses.

The patient and caregiver must understand the necessity of communicating to the health care team any deviations from normal health status. Instructions include specific signs and symptoms of infection that are to be reported promptly. Temperatures are to be checked at least daily and at the same time of day. If the patient or caregiver is visually impaired or has difficulty reading a glass thermometer, a digital thermometer should be obtained.

If antibiotic therapy will be administered at home, patients and family members are informed of potential side effects, particularly those that are to be reported promptly to the health care team. Instructions include the dosing interval, dietary considerations that affect drug absorption, and the importance of compliance with the prescribed antibiotic therapy. If G-CSF/GM-CSF therapy is initiated, preparation and administration techniques are observed until safe and accurate performance of procedures has been adequately demonstrated. Referral to a home health agency should always be considered for an individual who is at risk for infection, especially if caregiver support is inadequate, if home environmental concerns are present (e.g., no indoor plumbing, possible insect or rodent infestation), or if reinforcement of instruction is indicated.

Conclusion

Individuals with cancer are especially prone to developing infections as a result of impaired host defense mechanisms. Compromised immunity may be due to infection, nutritional deficiencies, tumor-associated factors, and cancer treatment. Most infections in this population are opportunistic and involve gram-negative and gram-positive microorganisms, although viruses, fungi, and protozoa are also involved in the spectrum of causative agents.

Infection in the immunocompromised person with cancer can quickly progress to life-threatening sepsis. Diligent nursing care directed toward prevention, early detection, and aggressive treatment is of primary importance for patient survival during high-risk periods.

References

1. Zembower T: Epidemiology of infectious complications in cancer patients, in Noskin GA (ed): *Management of Infectious Complications in Cancer Patients*. Boston, Kluwer Academic, 1998, pp 33–75

2. Schimpff SC: Infections in the cancer patient: Diagnosis, prevention, and treatment, in Mandell GL, Bennett JE, Dolin R (eds): *Principles and Practice of Infectious Diseases* (ed 4). New York, Churchill Livingstone, 1995, pp 2666–2675

3. Schwartsmann G, Dekker AW, Verhoef J: Complications of cytotoxic therapy, in Peckham M, Pinedo HM, Veronisi U (eds): *Oxford Textbook of Oncology*. New York, Oxford University Press, 1995, pp 2307–2327

4. DePauw BE, Donnelly JP, Fullberg B: Host impairments in patients with neoplastic disease, in Noskin GA (ed): *Management of Infectious Complications in Cancer Patients*. Boston, Kluwer Academic, 1998, pp 1–32

5. Locksley RM, Wilson CB: Cell mediated immunity and its role in host defense, in Mandell GL, Bennett JE, Dolin R (eds): *Principles and Practice of Infectious Diseases* (ed 4). New York, Churchill Livingstone, 1995, pp 102–149

6. Weinberg JB: Mononuclear phagocytes, in Lee GR, Foerster J, Lukens J, et al (eds): *Wintrobe's Clinical Hematology* (ed 10). Baltimore, Williams & Wilkins 1999, pp 377–414

7. Andre-Schwartz J, Schwartz R: Structure and function of the immune system, in Hoffman R, Benz EJ, Shatil SJ, et al (eds): *Hematology: Basic Principles and Practice* (ed 2). New York, Churchill Livingstone, 1995, pp 86–102

8. Freifeld AG, Pizzo PA, Walsh TJ: Infections in the cancer patient, in DeVita VT, Hellman S, Rosenberg SA (eds): *Cancer: Principles and Practice of Oncology* (ed 5). Philadelphia, Lippincott-Raven, 1997, pp 2659–2702

9. Rolston K, Bodey GP: Infections in patients with cancer, in Holland JF, Bast RC, Morton DL, et al (eds): *Cancer Medicine*, (ed 4). Baltimore, Williams & Wilkins, 1997, pp 3303–3333

10. Zimmer SH, Klatersky J: Infectious considerations in cancer, in Calabrisi P, Schein PS (eds): *Medical Oncology* (ed 2). New York, McGraw-Hill, 1993, pp 1073–1100

11. Varivarian D, Bodey GP: Infections associated with malignancy, in Gorbach SL, Bartlett JG, Blacklow NR (eds): *Infectious Diseases* (ed 2). Philadelphia, Saunders, 1998, pp 1222–1227

12. Howell PB, Walters PE, Donowitz GR, et al: Risk factors for infection of adult patients with cancer who have tunnelled central venous catheters. *Cancer* 75:1367–1375, 1995

13. Raad II, Luna M, Khalil SA, et al: The relationship between the thrombotic and infectious complications of central venous catheters. *JAMA* 271:1014–1016, 1994

14. Eastridge BJ, Lefor AT: Complications of indwelling venous access devices in cancer patients. *J Clin Oncol* 13:233–238, 1995

15. Jones GR, Konsler GK, Dunaway RP, et al: Prospective analysis of urokinase in the treatment of catheter sepsis in pediatric hematology-oncology patients. *J Pediatr Surg* 28:350–355, 1993

16. Sloas M, Rubin M, Walsh TJ, et al: Clinical approach to infections in the compromised host, in Hoffman R, Benz EJ, Shatil SJ, et al (eds): *Hematology: Basic Principles and Practice* (ed 2). New York, Churchill Livingstone, 1995, pp 1414–1472

17. Rogers MF, Lindegren ML: Epidemiology of pediatric HIV infection, in Wormser GP (ed): *AIDS and Other Manifestations of HIV Infection*. Philadelphia, Lippincott-Raven, 1998, pp 19–25

18. Siciliano RF: Immunodeficiency in HIV-1 infection, in Wormser GP (ed): *AIDS and Other Manifestations of HIV Infection*. Philadelphia, Lippincott-Raven, 1998, pp 257–278

19. Lynch AM, Kapila R: Overwheming postsplenectomy infection. *Infect Dis Clin North Am* 10:693–705, 1996

20. Baccarani M, Fiacchini M, Galiene P: Meningitis and septicemia in adults splenectomized for Hodgkin's disease. *Scand J Haematol* 36:492–498, 1986

21. Cleary JF: Fever and sweats, in Berger A, Portenoy RK, Weissman DE (eds): *Principles and Practice of Supportive Oncology*. Philadelphia, Lippincott-Raven, 1998, pp 119–131

22. Klatersky J: Febrile neutropenia. *Support Care Cancer* 1: 233–239, 1993

23. Blackburn G, Apovian CM, Bothe A: Nutritional factors in cancer, in Calabrisi P, Schein PS (eds): *Medical Oncology* (ed 2). New York, McGraw-Hill, 1993, pp 1149–1172

24. Chandra RK: Basic immunology and its application to nutritional problems, in Forse RA (ed): *Diet, Nutrition, and Immunity*. Boca Raton, FL, CRC Press, 1994, pp 1–8

25. Youkeles LH, Rosen MJ: Epidemiology of sepsis in the immunocompromised host, in Fein AM, Abraham EM, Balk RA, et al (eds): *Sepsis and Multiorgan Failure*. Baltimore, Williams & Wilkins, 1997, pp 35–42

26. Sawyer RG, Pruett TL: Wound infections. *Surg Clin North Am* 74:519–536, 1994

27. Rolston KVI, Rubenstein EB, Freifeld A: Early empiric antibiotic therapy for febrile neutropenia patients at low risk. *Infect Dis Clin North Am* 10:223–237, 1996

28. Meunier F: Infections in patients with acute leukemia and lymphoma, in Mandell GL, Bennett JE, Dolin R (eds): *Principles and Practice of Infectious Diseases* (ed 4). New York, Churchill Livingstone, 1995, pp 2674–2686

29. Noskin GA, Phair JP, Murphy RL: Diagnosis and management of infection in the immunocompromised host, in Shulman ST, Phair JP, Peterson LR, Warren JR (eds): *Biologic and Clinical Basis of Infectious Diseases* (ed 5). Philadelphia, Saunders, 1997, pp 361–381

30. Warren JR: Sepsis, in Shulman ST, Phair JP, Peterson LR, Warren JR (eds): *Biologic and Clinical Basis of Infectious Diseases* (ed 5). Philadelphia, Saunders, 1997, pp 475–489

31. Shulman ST: Staphylococci, staphyococcal disease, and toxic shock syndrome, in Shulman ST, Phair JP, Peterson LR, Warren JR (eds): *Biologic and Clinical Basis of Infectious Diseases* (ed 5). Philadelphia, Saunders, 1997, pp 505–514

32. Bow EJ, Loewen R, Vaughn D: Reduced requirement for antibiotic therapy targeting gram-negative organisms in febrile, neutropenic patients with cancer who are receiving antibacterial chemoprophylaxis with oral quinolones. *Clin Infect Dis* 20:907–912, 1995

33. Freifeld AG, Walsh T, Marshall D: Monotherapy for fever and neutropenia in cancer patients: A randomized comparison of ceftazidime versus imipenem. *J Clin Oncol* 13:165–176, 1995

34. DePauw BE, Raemaekers JMM, Schattenberg T, et al: Empirical and subsequent use of antibacterial agents in the febrile neutropenic patient. *J Intern Med* 242:69–77, 1997 (suppl 740)

35. Eccles E, Ptak J: Mycobacterium avium complex infection in AIDS: Clinical features, treatment and prevention. *J Assoc Nurses AIDS Care* 6:37–47, 1995

36. Phair JP: Fungal infections of the respiratory tract, in Shulman ST, Phair JP, Peterson LR, Warren JR (eds): *Biologic and Clinical Basis of Infectious Diseases* (ed 5). Philadelphia, Saunders, 1997, pp 176–191

37. United States Pharmacopeial Convention, Inc.: *Drug Information for the Health Care Professional* (ed 18). Rockville, MD, USPC, 1998

38. Katz BE: Viral infections, infectious mononucleosis and chronic fatigue syndrome, in Shulman ST, Phair JP, Peterson LR, Warren JR (eds): *Biologic and Clinical Basis of Infectious Diseases* (ed 5). Philadelphia, Saunders, 1997, pp 98–109

39. Snoeck R, DeClercq E: Herpesvirus infections in immunocompromised patients, in Klatersky J (ed): *Infectious Complications of Cancer.* Norwell MA, Kluwer Academic, 1995, pp 149–171

40. Whitley RJ: Varicella-zoster virus, in Mandell GL, Bennett JE, Dolin R (eds): *Principles and Practice of Infectious Diseases* (ed 4). New York, Churchill Livingstone, 1995, pp 1345–1351

41. Finberg RW: Infection in the patient with neoplastic disease, in MacDonald JS, Haller DG, Mayer RJ (eds): *Manual of Oncologic Therapeutics* (ed 3). Philadelphia, Lippincott, 1995, pp 415–429

42. Rosenberg SA: Hodgkin's disease, in Calabrisi P, Schein PS (eds): *Medical Oncology* (ed 2). New York, McGraw-Hill, 1993, pp 401–415

43. Centers for Disease Control: Universal precautions for prevention of transmission of human immunodeficiency virus, hepatitis B virus and other blood-borne pathogens. *MMWR Morb Mortal Wkly Rep* 37:377–387, 1988

44. Occupational Safety and Health Administration, United States Department of Labor: Occupational exposure to bloodborne pathogens. *Fed Register* 56:64175–64182, 1992

45. Hayden FG: Antiviral agents, in Mandell GL, Bennett JE, Dolin R (eds): *Principles and Practice of Infectious Diseases* (ed 4). New York, Churchill Livingstone, 1995, pp 441–450

46. Walzer PD: *Pneumocystis carinii*, in Mandell GL, Bennett JE, Dolin R (eds): *Principles and Practice of Infectious Diseases* (ed 4). New York, Churchill Livingstone, 1995, pp 2475–2487

47. Beaman MH, McCabe RE, Wong S, et al: *Toxoplasma gondii*, in Mandell GL, Bennett JE, Dolin R (eds): *Principles and Practice of Infectious Diseases* (ed 4). New York, Churchill Livingstone, 1995, pp 2455–2475

48. Zinner SH: New and unusual infection in neutropenic patients, in Klatersky J (ed): *Infectious Complications of Cancer.* Norwell, MA, Kluwer Academic, 1995, pp 173–184

49. Ellerhorst-Ryan JM: Nursing care plan for immunocompromised patients, in Workman ML, Ellerhorst-Ryan JM, Koertge VH (eds): *Nursing Care of the Immunocompromised Patient.* Philadelphia, Saunders, 1993

50. Wilkinson FH: Bottled water as a source of multi-resistant *Stenotrophomonas* and *Pseudomonas* species for neutropenic patients. *Euro Cancer Care* 7:12–14, 1998

51. Carter LW: Bacterial translocation: Nursing implications in the care of patients with neutropenia. *Oncol Nurs Forum* 21:857–865, 1994

52. Wilkes JD: Prevention and treatment of oral mucositis following cancer chemotherapy. *Semin Oncol* 25:538–551, 1998

53. Lynch P, Jackson MM, Cummings JM, et al: Rethinking the role of isolation practices in the prevention of nosocomial infections. *Ann Intern Med* 107:243–245, 1987

54. Poe SS, Larson E, McGuire D, et al: A national survey of infection prevention practices on bone marrow transplant units. *Oncol Nurs Forum* 21:1687–1694, 1994

55. Lynch LS: Infection in cancer patients, in Haskell CM (ed): *Cancer Treatment* (ed 4). Philadelphia, Saunders, 1995, pp 206–216

56. Rangel-Fraust MS, Wenzel RP: Epidemiology and natural history of bacterial sepsis, in Fein AM, Abraham EM, Balk RA, et al (eds): *Sepsis and Multiorgan Failure.* Baltimore, Williams & Wilkins, 1997, pp 27–34

CHAPTER 31

Bleeding

Barbara Holmes Gobel, RN, MS

Scope of the Problem

Bleeding represents one of the most complex clinical challenges in the supportive care of the patient with cancer. The numerous and unique complications of each cancer, combined with the often toxic effects of various cancer treatments, create a difficult problem in the diagnosis and management of bleeding. There are no specific incidence rates for this complication, as bleeding can occur with any cancer. However, bleeding does occur more frequently in individuals with hematologic cancers compared with those having solid tumors. Hematologic cancers affect the bone marrow, usually resulting in thrombocytopenia or platelets with altered function. Appropriate supportive measures are vital to the total care of an individual with bleeding.

Multiple hemostatic abnormalities may be involved in cancer-associated bleeding. Considerable differences exist in the presentation, proper management, and implications of these clinical problems. Minor bleeding may be the initial symptom that leads to the diagnosis of cancer. More severe bleeding may indicate the onset of a progressive or terminal phase of the cancer. Because the morbidity and mortality of many bleeding problems are significant, prevention of the problem is clearly the best management plan. Rapid recognition, assessment, and knowledgeable treatment of the bleeding complications of cancer will significantly improve the patient's quality of life and potential for survival.

The cornerstone of treatment for cancer-associated bleeding is blood component therapy. An important adjunct to blood component therapy, particularly in terms of preventing bleeding, is the use of the recombinant colony-stimulating factors that are capable of stimulating the proliferation and maturation of bone marrow cells. They are in part responsible for improving the results of chemotherapy dose-intensification protocols, which may increase the survival of many patients with cancer. In addition to blood component therapy and recombinant colony-stimulating factors, numerous medications are used with bleeding problems.

This chapter includes a review of the process of hematopoiesis, followed by a discussion of coagulation and fibrinolysis. Pathophysiology of bleeding covers both platelet abnormalities and the problems associated with hypocoagulation. Clinical manifestations of bleeding and the causes of bleeding are reviewed. Care of the individual with cancer who is experiencing bleeding, including both nursing and medical support, is reviewed. Finally, blood component therapy and its use in cancer therapy is discussed.

Physiology of Bleeding

Hematopoiesis

Hematopoiesis is the process by which blood cells are formed. During fetal development, the blood-forming organs include the spleen, liver, and bone marrow. The bone marrow is the primary site of hematopoiesis at the time of birth. During childhood, hematopoiesis takes place in the ribs, skull, spleen, pelvis, liver, sternum, vertebrae, and the proximal epiphyses of the long bones; all but the liver are involved in adult hematopoiesis.[1] Bone marrow provides a specialized environment in which hematopoietic progenitor cells proliferate and become committed to differentiate.[2] Within the marrow, various elements—including the structural or stromal elements (fibroblasts, endothelial cells, fat cells) and the accessory cells (macrophages and lymphocytes) of the marrow—interact either to enhance or inhibit hematopoiesis.

All of the blood cell lines derive from a pluripotent stem cell, or common progenitor cell, that is capable of extensive, possibly lifelong self-renewal and can differentiate to all cell lineages.[3] The stem cell is not normally in an active cycle. When the cell must undergo division, following injury or after marrow depletion, for example, a daughter cell leaves the stem cell pool and passes through a series of divisions and maturational changes, culminating in the formation of the mature blood cells found in circulating blood. The processes of proliferation, differentiation, and maturation are mediated by various humoral factors, predominantly by an expanding set of hematopoietic growth factors, or colony-stimulating factors (CSFs). See Figure 31-1 for an outline of blood cell development and the factors that mediate this process.

Early on in blood cell development, the progeny of the pluripotent stem cell forms a population of multipotent progenitor cells that are uncommitted to any cell line and have a limited self-renewing capacity. The colony-forming unit CFU-GEMM is an example of the multipotent stem cell for granulocytes, erythroid, monocyte, and megakaryocyte lines and can develop into any one of these lines. The lymphoid cell line follows a separate course of differentiation and maturation.[4]

As cells continue to differentiate, they become committed to specific cell lines. At this level, progenitor cells are called *unipotent* or *bipotent*, describing their ability to follow one or two cell lines, respectively. These cells include CFU-GM (granulocyte, monocyte, and macrophage), CFU-EO (eosinophil), burst-forming unit-erythroid (BFU-E) and CFU-E (erythroid), and CFU-Mega (megakaryocyte) and are committed stem cells.[1,4] Committed stem cells become increasingly differentiated and morphologically recognizable as belonging to a specific cell line. Ultimately, the cell undergoes further division and becomes a mature component of the circulating blood.

Colony-stimulating factors

Colony-stimulating factors are a set of hormone-like glycoproteins or cytokines that mediate hematopoiesis for all blood cell lines; they govern the production of blood at every level of cell development, including the pluripotent stem cells.[5] Some CSFs appear to have an effect on more than one blood cell line. Interleukin-3 (IL-3), also called multi-CSF, is a growth factor for a variety

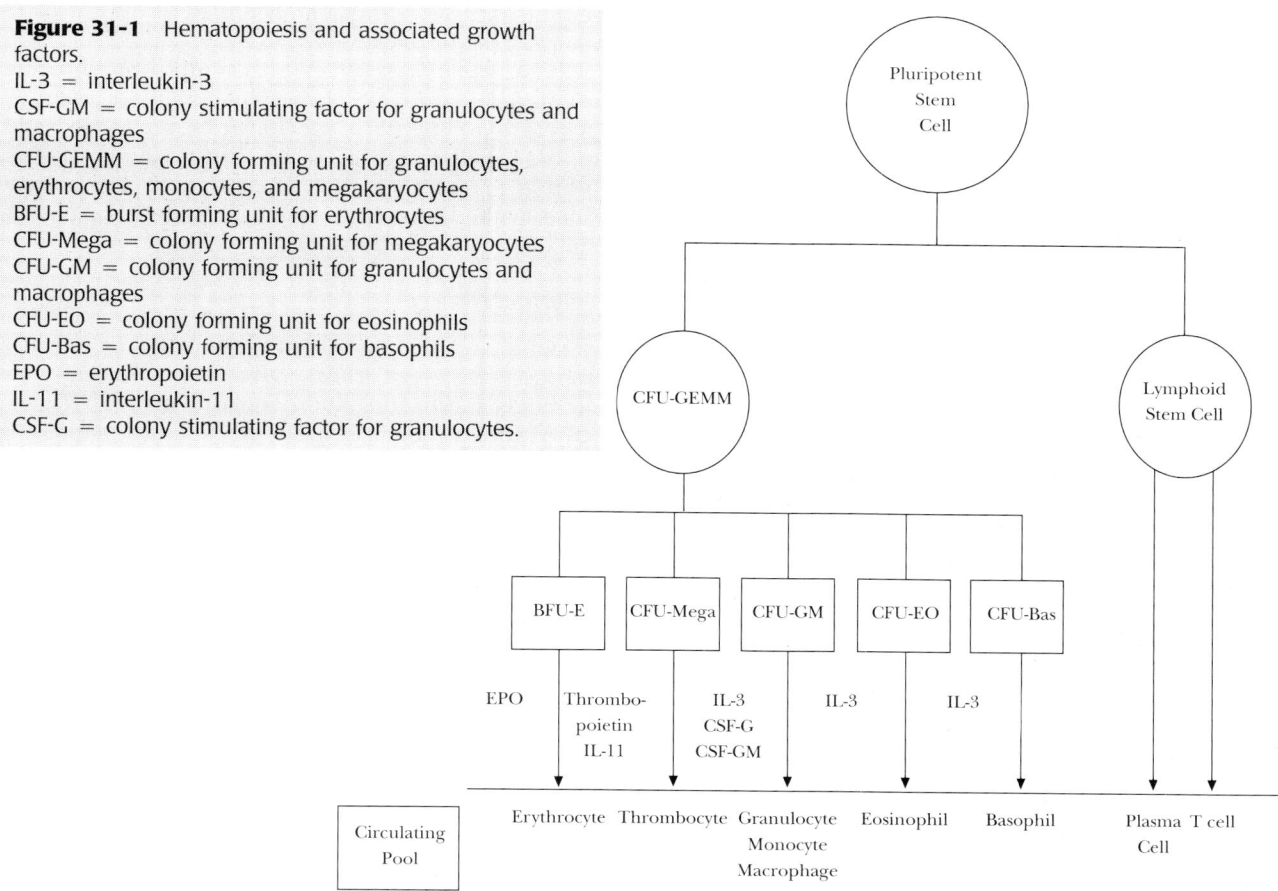

Figure 31-1 Hematopoiesis and associated growth factors.
IL-3 = interleukin-3
CSF-GM = colony stimulating factor for granulocytes and macrophages
CFU-GEMM = colony forming unit for granulocytes, erythrocytes, monocytes, and megakaryocytes
BFU-E = burst forming unit for erythrocytes
CFU-Mega = colony forming unit for megakaryocytes
CFU-GM = colony forming unit for granulocytes and macrophages
CFU-EO = colony forming unit for eosinophils
CFU-Bas = colony forming unit for basophils
EPO = erythropoietin
IL-11 = interleukin-11
CSF-G = colony stimulating factor for granulocytes.

of progenitor cells as is granulocyte-macrophage colony-stimulating factor (GM-CSF) (see Figure 31-1). These CSFs stimulate the growth of multipotential hematopoietic progenitor cells and cells already committed to myeloid, erythroid, or megakaryocytic lines.[4] Other CSFs stimulate production of cells along single blood cell lines. Granulocyte-CSF (G-CSF) macrophage-CSF, and erythropoietin (EPO) stimulate the growth of predominantly granulocytes, monocytes, and red blood cells, respectively.[6] It is hypothesized that an overlap of the effects of one factor on another probably occurs and that CSFs are not truly lineage specific.[7] Colony-stimulating factors appear to act on specific cells because of receptors that reside on the target cell membrane. The different distribution of these specific receptors may help to explain why they are responsive to some CSFs and not others.

Hemostasis

Hemostasis is the process by which the fluid component of blood becomes a solid clot. This process is initiated by vascular or tissue injury and culminates in the formation of a firm mechanical barrier, or a clot (made up of platelets and fibrin). The sequence of events after injury includes local constriction, platelet adherence to structures in the vessel wall, aggregation of platelets to

form a hemostatic plug, and coagulation or solid-clot formation.

When blood vessel injury occurs, vasoconstriction initially provides minimal control of bleeding. Within seconds, platelets are attracted to and adhere to the underlying layer of collagen of the exposed subendothelial tissue.[8] Platelets then release a number of components, including calcium, serotonin, proteolytic enzymes, cationic proteins, thromboxane A, and nucleotide adenosine diphosphate (ADP)[8]; ADP causes platelets to swell and become "sticky," thus increasing their adherence to one another. Increasing levels of ADP lead to clot contraction, degranulation, and ultimately fusion of the platelets. The end result of ADP-mediated platelet accumulation is the formation of a large platelet aggregate, or a hemostatic plug. Activated platelets also provide an anionic phospholipid surface for the clotting reactions that lead to thrombin generation, an essential precursor to fibrin. This mass of platelets fills the gap in the vessel wall and arrests bleeding, usually within 5 minutes. This primary hemostatic mechanism produces only a temporary cessation of bleeding.

Coagulation

Coagulation may be considered a mechanism for rapid replacement of an unstable platelet plug with a stable fibrin clot. A series of interdependent, enzyme-mediated reactions activate fibrin; the fibrin clot is the final product of hemostasis. When these enzymes or coagulation factors are stimulated, they become active in a sequential manner, not in numerical order (Table 31-1). This process is often referred to as the *coagulation cascade*. Multiple inhibitors and control mechanisms keep these reactions localized to the site of the injury. Figure 31-2 shows the mechanism of normal blood coagulation.

The coagulation cascade is initiated when procoagulant substances, the most significant of which is tissue factor (TF), are released during blood vessel injury. *Tissue factor* is a transmembrane glycoprotein present on the surface of many cell types that is not normally in contact with the circulation but is exposed to blood after vascular damage; it also plays a significant role in inflammation.[9] On activation TF binds with coagulation factors that then trigger both the intrinsic and the extrinsic pathways of coagulation. The intrinsic pathway of coagulation is known as the *contact activation pathway*. It is activated by trauma or infection that causes inflammatory proteins to be released into the circulation. The extrinsic pathway of coagulation is activated by tissue injury. These two pathways collaborate at various stages and together are known as the *common pathway of coagulation*.

The activation of prothrombin is an intermediary step in the activation of thrombin. Prothrombin is converted to thrombin, the most powerful of the coagulation enzymes. Thrombin then acts on fibrinogen to form fibrin.[10] The fibrin clot is soluble until it becomes polymerized by factor XIIIa (fibrin stabilizing factor), which converts it into a stable, or insoluble, clot. Hemostasis is complete when the fibrin network alone is able to resist the hydrostatic pressure in the vessel.

Fibrin formation is an essential component of hemostasis, inflammation, and tissue repair, but it is a temporary reaction. The fibrin clot must be remodeled and removed to restore normal tissue structure and function, as well as to restore normal blood flow. This is accomplished by the fibrinolytic system that controls the enzymatic degradation of fibrin.

Fibrinolysis

Fibrinolysis, or clot breakdown, is initiated by enzymes known as *plasminogen activators*, that are present in most body fluids and normal and neoplastic tissues[11] (Figure 31-3). Plasminogen, an inactive precursor of plasmin, is activated to plasmin in the presence of thrombin. Plasmin is responsible for the lysis of fibrin clots. The breakdown of fibrinogen and fibrin results in polypeptides called *fibrin degradation products* (FDPs) or *fibrin split products* (FSPs). These FDPs are powerful anticoagulant substances that have a destructive effect on fibrin in the platelet plug. When these products are increased in the circulation there is a predisposition to bleeding.[12]

Pathophysiology of Bleeding

Bleeding in the patient with cancer is primarily due to alterations in hemostatic mechanisms that can be attributed to either platelet abnormalities or coagulation abnormalities. Abnormalities of platelet production, function, survival, and metabolism frequently occur in individuals with cancer and may be due to a variety of causes. Generally, mechanical or humoral effects of the tumor itself or abnormalities in the host induced by the tumor or treatment of the tumor cause these platelet abnormalities. Coagulation problems may be related both to hypocoagulation and hypercoagulation. Bleeding in the patient with cancer may also result from structural alterations such as blood vessel damage by infection or treatment-related damage.

Platelet Abnormalities

Thrombocytopenia

Thrombocytopenia, a reduction in the number of circulating platelets, is the most frequent platelet abnormality associated with cancer. Thrombocytopenia may be caused by a decrease in platelet production, a change in platelet distribution (e.g., sequestration of platelets in the spleen), platelet destruction, vascular dilution, drug therapies (see Treatment Effects under Clinical Manifestations), or disseminated intravascular coagulation (DIC, see Chapter 39).[13–17]

Platelet production. The most common cause of thrombocytopenia in patients with cancer is a disorder involving decreased megakaryocytopoiesis (i.e., platelet

Table 31-1 Normal Coagulation Factors

Factor	Factor Name	Normal Range
I	Fibrinogen	142–366 mg/dL
II	Prothrombin	80%–120%
III	Tissue factor, tissue thromboplastin (extrinsic prothrombin activator)	80%–120%
IV	Calcium	8.5–10.5 mg/dL
V	Proaccelerin, accelerator globulin	50%–150%
VI	Not assigned	
VII	Proconvertin, serum prothrombin conversion accelerator (SPCA)	60%–140%
VIII	Antihemophilic globulin (AHG), antihemophilic factor (AHF)	60%–150%
IX	Plasma thromboplastin component (PTC), Christmas factor	60%–150%
X	Stuart-Prower factor	60%–150%
XI	Plasma thromboplastin antecedent (PTA)	60%–135%
XII	Hageman factor	50%–150%
XIII	Fibrin stabilizing factor (FSF)	Present

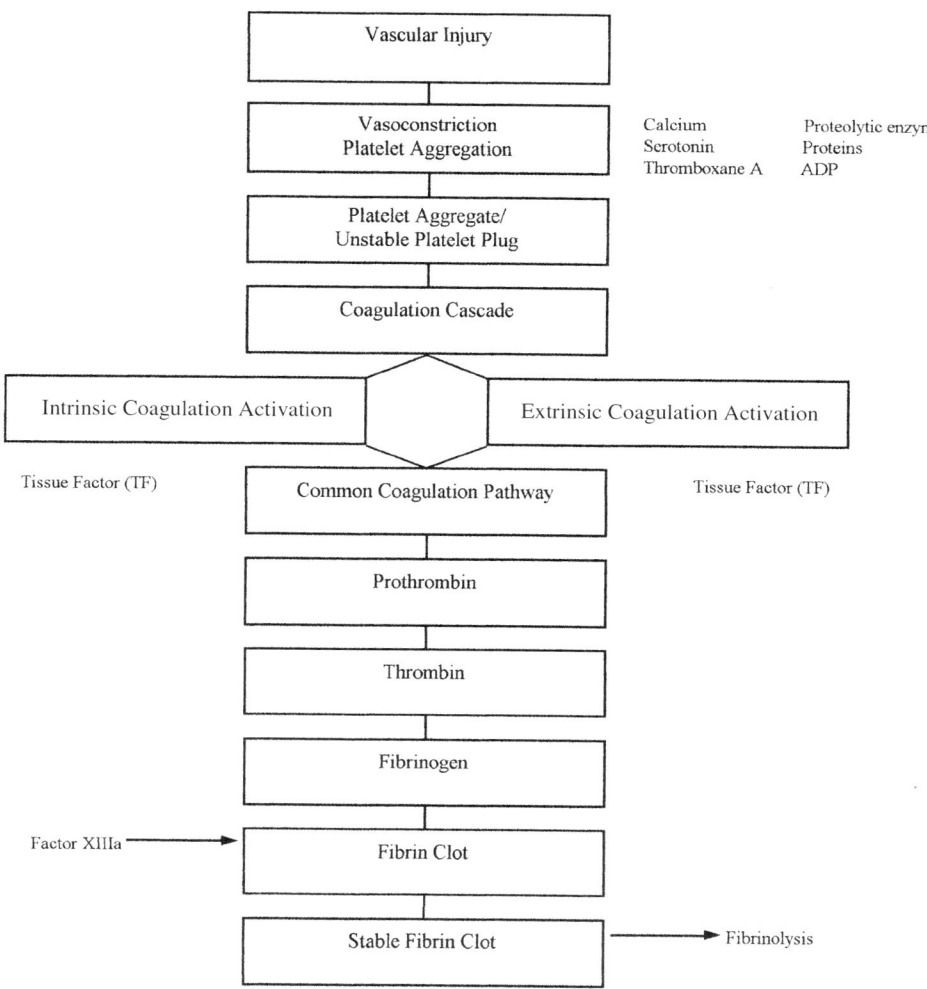

Figure 31-2 Mechanism of normal blood coagulation.

production in the bone marrow). This decreased production of platelets may be due to tumor invasion of the bone marrow or to acute or delayed effects of chemotherapy or radiation therapy. When tumor invasion is the cause of the decrease in platelet production, the resulting thrombocytopenia is generally a part of the total picture of pancytopenia. A low platelet count is directly proportional to the degree of bone marrow infiltration by tumor cells.

Platelet distribution. Thrombocytopenia due to an abnormal distribution of platelets can occur in cancer patients with hypersplenism. An enlarged spleen may sequester up to 90% of the platelet population, making them unavailable to the circulation. Tumor metastasis to the spleen, particularly due to lung, breast, colon, prostate, and stomach cancers and lymphomas, are known to cause hypersplenism and subsequent platelet sequestration. Thrombocytopenia can also be due to congestive splenomegaly related to splenic vein obstruction in pancreatic cancer.[18] The thrombocytopenia related to hypersplenism is generally mild (platelet count of

40,000–100,000 cells/mm^3). The absence of a palpable spleen rules out this type of thrombocytopenic disorder.

Platelet destruction. Thrombocytopenia can also be due to an immune-mediated thrombocytopenia, or idiopathic thrombocytopenia purpura (ITP). The rapid destruction of platelets in ITP is due to an autoimmune process in which antibodies are formed against the individual's own platelets. This condition results in normal or increased numbers of megakaryocytes (immature platelets) in the bone marrow and decreased numbers of circulating platelets in the general circulation. Signs and symptoms of ITP include petechiae, purpura, ecchymosis, thrombocytopenia, and bleeding (gingival, urinary, gastrointestinal, and occasionally cerebral).[19] ITP occurs most frequently in individuals with lymphoproliferative disorders such as chronic lymphocytic leukemia (CLL), acute lymphocytic leukemia (ALL), and non-Hodgkin's lymphoma.[16,20] It is rarely associated with solid tumors.[21]

Platelet dilution. Multiple blood transfusions may aggravate thrombocytopenia. Blood can be stored up to 21

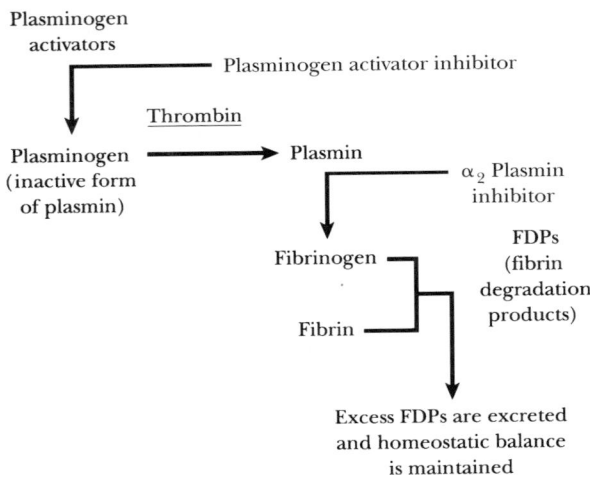

Figure 31-3 Fibrinolysis.

days with minimal decrease in red cell survival. However, the platelets in the stored blood lose effectiveness after 24 hours of storage. This dilutional effect is in direct proportion to the amount of blood transfused.[13,22]

Thrombocythemia/thrombocytosis

Thrombocythemia and thrombocytosis are a result of overproduction of platelets. Thrombocythemia, also known as *essential* or *primary thrombocythemia*, is characterized by an abnormal expansion of the megakaryocytic progenitor cell portion of the marrow. It is one of a group of related chronic myeloproliferative disorders that includes polycythemia vera, chronic myelogenous leukemia (CML), agnogenic myeloid metaplasia, and idiopathic myelofibrosis.[13,21,23] Thrombocytosis, also known as *secondary* or *reactive thrombocytosis*, occurs in approximately 30%–40% of patients with cancer. Thrombocytosis is seen in lung, breast, kidney, ovarian, pancreatic, and gastrointestinal carcinomas, and in Hodgkin's disease, splenectomized patients, and in individuals with widespread cancer.[24]

The major complications related to an increased platelet count are bleeding and thrombosis. The most common sites of bleeding and potential hemorrhage associated with these conditions are the mucosa and the gastrointestinal tract. Bleeding can also occur in other sites such as the skin and the genitourinary tract.[25] Thrombosis may result in symptoms associated with venous thrombosis, pulmonary embolism, transient cerebral ischemia, myocardial infarction, and angina, or portal mesenteric vein occlusion.[21]

Altered platelet function

At times, patients with cancer may bleed despite normal platelet counts and coagulation factors. Alterations in platelet function may be responsible for this type of bleeding. A variety of hematologic diseases are associated with abnormal platelet function. Hemostatic abnormali-

ties associated with abnormal platelet function include multiple myeloma, Waldenström's macroglobulinemia, acute myelogenous leukemia, chronic myelogenous leukemia (CML), and ALL in children.[26,27] The major abnormality noted in these diseases is a decrease in the procoagulant activity of the platelets, which is a measure of platelet factor III. Also noted in these diseases are platelets that are larger or smaller than normal, abnormally shaped platelets, and a variation in the number of storage pool granules. In multiple myeloma, the qualitative defect in platelet function can occur as a result of the M protein coating the platelet and interfering with platelet aggregation.[28] Abnormal platelet function has also been described in patients with thrombocytosis associated with the myeloproliferative disorders; this may help to explain the increased incidence of hemorrhage in patients with an increased platelet concentration.

Hypocoagulation

The most significant factor leading to a state of hypocoagulation is liver disease. Liver disease may result from infection, chemotherapy, tumor invasion, or surgical resection. Regardless of etiology, liver disease has been reported to cause prolonged bleeding time, reduced platelet aggregation, and procoagulant activity.[29] Liver disease interferes with the synthesis of plasma coagulation factors I, II, V, VII, IX, and X. In addition to the decreased production of these factors, liver disease may also interfere with their functioning. Decreased liver function contributes to diminished liver clearance of FDPs and activated clotting factors, which further inhibits the coagulation mechanism.

A deficiency of vitamin K may also cause a hypocoagulation syndrome. This may be seen in patients with cancer who lack vitamin K in their diet, with biliary obstruction, malabsorptive states, intestinal sterilization due to antibiotic administration, and impaired clotting factor synthesis due to liver disease.[30] A deficiency of vitamin K results in a greatly reduced chemical activation of vitamin K–dependent proteins: factors II, VII, IX, and X; the result is a state of decreased hemostasis.

Individuals who undergo extensive surgical procedures and receive large amounts of frozen plasma may demonstrate a prolonged prothrombin time and a prolonged partial thromboplastin time. These individuals are prone to postsurgical bleeding. Frozen plasma has deficient levels of factors V and VIII, which can also lead to a state of decreased hemostasis.

Isolated factor deficiencies are also related to cancer. Acquired von Willebrand's disease has been demonstrated to occur in solid tumors, hematologic cancers, myeloproliferative disorders, macroglobulinemia, and lymphoproliferative disorders. A small number of patients with malignant B-cell disease and Wilms' tumor have been reported to develop acquired von Willebrand's disease.[31] Patients with this syndrome demonstrate bruising, mucosal bleeding, and gastrointestinal hemorrhage. Coagulation studies shows a prolonged bleeding time and diminished or absent factor VIII procoagulant activity,

(VIII:c), von Willebrand's factor antigen (vWF:Ag), and ristocetin cofactor activity.[29]

Conditions related to hypocoagulation are less common than the other types of hemostatic alterations discussed in this chapter. Although any type of coagulation abnormality can lead to bleeding, hypocoagulation disorders less frequently cause serious bleeding when they do occur. Hemorrhages tend to develop in the deeper areas of the body, such as the subcutaneous or intramuscular tissues. Bleeding into the joints, especially of the distal extremities, may occur in hypocoagulation disorders.

Clinical Manifestations

The platelet count is considered to be the single most significant factor for predicting bleeding in the patient with cancer. Gaydos et al first reported an association between a low platelet count and an increased risk of bleeding in 1962.[32] Regardless of the cause, the risk of spontaneous hemorrhage is considered to be greater than 50% when the platelet count is less than 20,000 cells/mm[3]. Manifestations of a low platelet count may include easy bruising, petechiae, ecchymosis, melana, hematuria, and bleeding from the gums, nose, mouth, or other orifices.

Tumor Effects

Tumor-related bleeding in cancer can occur through different mechanisms. Tumor invasion in the bone marrow, due either to solid tumors or hematologic malignancies, can cause bleeding. Tumor-related bleeding may also be due to tumor extension into surrounding structures or blood vessels. Tumor-related bleeding may also be manifested as DIC.

Tumor invasion

Tumor invasion into the bone marrow can be caused by primary tumor in hematologic diseases that are intrinsic to the marrow or by metastatic spread of tumor to the marrow from cancers of various organs. This type of tumor invasion is called *myelophthisis*. Tumor invasion that causes bleeding is common in Hodgkins's and non-Hodgkin's lymphoma, leukemia, malignant melanoma, and neuroblastoma. Bleeding related to tumor invasion is also common in carcinoma of the lung, breast, prostate, thyroid, kidney, and adrenal glands.[33] Tumor invasion can result in anemia, thrombocytopenia, granulocytopenia, and neutropenia. The decrease in production of normal marrow elements is thought to be a response to the physiologic "crowding out" of normal cells, competition for cell nutrients, and the invading cells' metabolic end products, which are toxic to normal cells.

Tumor extension

Tumor extension may occur in surrounding structures or blood vessels. Bleeding is a common presenting symptom of cancer, generally occurring as a result of tumor and local invasion. Blood loss and the resulting iron-deficiency anemia are frequently the initial signs of lung, gynecologic, genitourinary, or colorectal carcinomas.[34–37] Clinically, the individual may present with symptoms ranging from minor incidents of bleeding to gross blood loss.

Frequently, the most dramatic cause of bleeding in the patient with cancer is the invasion, erosion, and subsequent rupture of blood vessels. Any tumor involvement of vascular tissue or any tumor lying in close proximity to major vessels is seen as a risk for bleeding. Cancers of the large bronchi or lung may erode into the bronchial artery or branches of the pulmonary artery. Hemoptysis from tumor erosion into pulmonary blood vessels may appear as streaks of blood or gross blood loss. Head and neck tumors may also be associated with serious bleeding. Invasive cancers, particularly at the base of the tongue, can erode branches of the external carotid artery. Massive vaginal bleeding due to pelvic tumor masses that invade major pelvic vessels is commonly seen in patients with cervical cancer and occasionally in patients with endometrial or ovarian cancer.

More gradual bleeding involving smaller circulatory structures is usually less obvious and therefore more difficult to diagnose. Melena due to colorectal carcinoma or the microscopic bleeding of macroglobulinemia can persist undetected until manifested by iron deficiency anemia. A continual loss of 6–8 mL of blood per day will eventually precipitate classic iron deficiency because the compensatory need for cell production exceeds the iron-producing capacity of the normal adult diet.

The most definitive test for iron deficiency anemia is a bone marrow biopsy, which demonstrates absent stainable iron stores.[38] On examination, the red blood cells are small (microcytic) and irregularly shaped, with decreased amounts of hemoglobin (hypochromic). The serum ferritin level is decreased, which reflects a depletion in total body iron stores. The serum iron assay is often low but may be normal, and the iron-binding capacity is increased. The reticulocyte count is usually normal.[39,40]

The homeostatic mechanisms in the body provide such remarkable compensatory adaptation that iron deficiency anemia may be quite serious before the person actually develops significant symptoms. It is important to remember, therefore, that the onset of symptoms may reflect the rate of the progression of the anemia better than does the severity. Fatigue, weakness, irritability, dyspnea, and tachycardia are typical clinical symptoms experienced by individuals with anemia.

Treatment Effects

Chemotherapy effects

Bleeding in cancer may be related to chemotherapy, radiation therapy, surgery, or medication effects. Chemotherapy is the cancer treatment most often associated with hematologic toxicity, including thrombocytopenia.

The effects of chemotherapy are due in large part to the particular drugs used, dosages, schedules, routes of administration, previous cancer treatments, and any concomitant therapies. Chemotherapy-induced thrombocytopenia is usually caused by the destruction of the proliferating cells of the platelet line. As these cells are destroyed, the circulatory platelets are cleared at the end of their life span, and the nadir of a patient's blood cell count occurs. Considering that the average life span of a platelet is only 7 days, this accounts in part for the high incidence of thrombocytopenia related to chemotherapy.

Chemotherapy drugs act at specific points in the cell cycle and, on that basis, are classified as *cell-cycle phase specific* (CCS) drugs or *cell-cycle phase nonspecific* (CCNS) drugs. Cell-cycle phase specific drugs such as cytarabine or methotrexate have their impact on proliferating cells and do not destroy cells in the resting phase of the cell cycle. These agents have an early nadir and recovery occurs relatively rapidly (7–14 days). Cell-cycle phase nonspecific drugs such as carmustine and busulfan destroy cells in the resting phase of the cell cycle, damaging nonproliferating stem cells. These drugs have a delayed nadir (4–5 weeks) and delayed recovery (6 weeks).[41] Table 31-2 provides a list of chemotherapy agents associated with moderate to severe thrombocytopenia.

Radiation therapy effects

Radiation therapy can also cause hematologic toxicity, particularly when large areas of bone marrow are treated. The most significant factor that determines the risk of bone marrow depression related to radiation therapy is the volume of productive bone marrow in the radiation field. This risk factor is even more important than the therapeutic dose or the fractionation schedule.[42] Radiation-induced hematologic toxicity is usually caused by damage to the nonproliferating stem cells or to the cells in the resting phase of the cell cycle. Megakaryocytes are affected 1–2 weeks after exposure to the radiation, and take about 2–6 weeks for recovery. Radiation therapy is local treatment, except for total nodal or total body irradiation, and does not usually cause the nadirs in blood count seen with chemotherapy. The localized nature of this treatment generally allows the untreated marrow to compensate for the damage to the treated marrow.

Surgical effects

Surgical causes of bleeding in cancer may occur in an attempt to manage the cancer itself. For example, there is potential for a carotid artery rupture after a radical neck dissection for the treatment of head and neck cancer. Carotid artery rupture occurs more frequently when the patient has received prior radiation therapy. Prophylactic arterial ligation may be performed to minimize the risk of a carotid hemorrhage. The patient who undergoes a ligation of the external carotid arteries runs the risk of a stroke. Small transient bleeding usually occurs before any vessel rupture. Careful observation can assist in predicting and controlling such a complication.

Medication effects

Numerous drugs are known to affect platelet number and function. At times, some of these drugs are administered deliberately for their antithrombotic effect (e.g., heparin), with diminished platelet number or function being the therapeutic goal. However, this is an undesired side effect for many of the drugs administered to patients with cancer.

Thrombocytopenia is the most common of the drug-induced blood dyscrasias, as any drug can cause unexpected thrombocytopenia.[43] Drug-induced thrombocytopenia may be caused by immune-mediated suppression or destruction of platelets, a decreased production of platelets, or a nonimmune direct effect on circulating platelets (as occurs with the use of heparin).[43] Quinine and quinidine are drugs known to cause drug-induced immune thrombocytopenia.[17] When patients have been sensitized to the use of these drugs, the platelet count drops rapidly, with bleeding occurring within hours or days of ingestion. Many drugs can cause a decreased production of platelets including thiazide diuretics as well as furosemide, antimetabolites, antimitotic agents, antitumor antibiotics, benzene and benzene derivatives, ionizing radiation, nitrogen mustard, estrogens, and alcohol. Chronic alcohol use results in a decreased platelet production as well as reduced platelet survival, which can lead to an increased incidence of bleeding.[44] Heparin is the most common cause of drug-induced thrombocytopenia; this may be due to either a direct aggregating effect of heparin, leading to reversible platelet clumping in which complications are unlikely, or to heparin-induced thrombocytopenia (HIT). The latter is more serious and can lead to bleeding. In HIT, heparin binds to platelet membranes, which results in platelet clumping and a decrease in the peripheral platelet count. Low-molecular-weight heparins are associated less often with HIT.[43]

Many drugs are known to affect platelet aggregation, as demonstrated by a prolonged bleeding time. Still, only aspirin has been shown to cause a significant increased risk of bleeding. Aspirin works primarily by inactivating platelet cyclooxygenase. Inactivation of cyclooxygenase decreases platelet aggregation, prevents release of vasoactive substances, and prolongs the bleeding time.[45] This platelet aggregation abnormality is so characteristic that abnormal platelet aggregation patterns of any etiology are often designated as *aspirin-like*.[27] The bleeding time can be prolonged for up to 4 days after a single dose of aspirin, until normal platelet turnover results in a significant number of new platelets with normal function. The mechanism of action of nonsteroidal anti-inflammatory drugs appears to be similar to that of aspirin inhibition of platelet cyclooxygenase; these drugs have only a temporary effect, causing inhibition only as long as the active drug is present in the circulation.

Table 31-2 Chemotherapeutic Agents Associated with Significant Thrombocytopenia

Chemotherapeutic Agent	Degree of Suppression	Nadir (days)	Recovery (days)	Comments
Busulfan	Moderate	21–28	42–56	Cell-cycle phase nonspecific (CCNS), cumulative toxicity
Carmustine	Marked	28–42	35–42	CCNS, cumulative
Chlorambucil	Moderate	21–28	42–56	CCNS, cumulative
Cladribine	Moderate	14	60	CCS Cell-cycle phase specific
Cyclophosphamide	Moderate (dose-related—100 mg/m²)	7–14	21	CCNS, cumulative
Cytarabine	Marked	10	21	CCS
Dacarbazine	Marked (dose-related—200 mg/m² IV daily × 5 days)	10–14	21–28	CCNS
Dactinomycin	Marked	14	21–28	CCNS
Daunorubicin hydrochloride	Marked	10	21–28	CCNS
Docetaxel	Moderate to marked	8	14	CCS
Doxorubicin	Moderate to marked (dose-related)	10–14	21	CCNS
Epirubicin hydrochloride	Moderate	10–14	21	CCNS
5-Fluorouracil	Moderate (dose-related—12–15 mg/kg)	9–21	21	CCS
Gemcitabine	Moderate			CCS
Hycamptin	Moderate	10–12	15–21	CCS
Hydroxyurea	Moderate	7	14	
Idarubicin	Moderate	10–15	25	CCNS
Lomustine	Marked	21–28	42	CCNS, cumulative
Mechlorethamine	Moderate	10–14	21–28	CCNS, cumulative
Methotrexate	Moderate (dose-related—100 mg/m²)	10	14	CCS
Mitomycin C	Marked	21–28	42–56	CCNS, cumulative
Paclitaxel	Marked	8–15	21	CCS
L-phenylalanine	Moderate	14–21	21–28	CCNS, cumulative
Plicamycin	Moderate	14	21	CCNS
Procarbazine	Moderate	14	21–28	
Streptozocin	Moderate			CCNS, cumulative
6-Thioguanine	Moderate to marked	14–28	28–35	CCS
Triethylenephosphoramide	Moderate	14–21	40–50	CCNS
Vinblastine	Moderate to marked	10	21	CCS
Vinorelbine	Mild to moderate	14	21	CCS

The mechanism by which antibiotics cause prolonged bleeding times is not entirely clear. It is thought that high-dose β-lactam penicillins inhibit platelet function by binding to platelet membrane components, which are necessary for platelet adhesiveness interactions.[46] The frequency of clinically significant hemorrhage due solely to the effect of antibiotics on platelet function is rare, but the risk of bleeding may be increased in patients with coexisting hemostatic defects such as thrombocytopenia or vitamin-K deficiency.[27] The cephalosporins may cause a similar pattern of platelet dysfunction (as well as affecting the abdominal flora), decreased vitamin K absorption, and affect coagulation.[12] Psychotropic drugs, such as tricyclic antidepressants and phenothiazines, may cause impaired platelet aggregation with resultant prolonged bleeding times. However, this effect has not been found to be associated with an increased risk of bleeding.[27]

Infection-Related Effects

Localized infections, including viral and bacterial infections, that occur at sites of blood vessels may cause cavitational or local ulcerations that, in turn, may cause bleeding. Systemic infections, particularly gram-negative bacteremias, can stimulate DIC, which can result in life-threatening bleeding and thrombosis.

Miscellaneous Effects

The production of high viscosity proteins in multiple myeloma and Waldenström's macroglobulinemia can cause bleeding. Although rare, this overproduction of abnormal proteins has been identified in 4% of individuals with immunoglobulin G (IgG) myeloma and in 5%–10% of individuals with immunoglobulin A (IgA) myeloma.[47] In multiple myeloma, this overproduction of proteins (immunoglobulins) increases the viscosity of the blood, resulting in poor circulatory movement with increased risk for clotting and bleeding.[48] A clinical triad of symptoms occur with this hyperviscosity syndrome, including bleeding, visual changes, and neurologic deficits.[48]

Thrombocytopenia associated with multiple myeloma is usually associated with chemotherapy or radiation therapy. Thrombocytopenia may also be seen when the myeloma expands within the marrow compartment, further contributing to the risk of bleeding. Moreover, a qualitative defect in platelet function can occur, as the M protein (myeloma protein or malignant protein of myeloma) coating the platelet interferes with its function.[49]

Assessment for Bleeding

Assessment for bleeding in the patient with cancer begins with a thorough history and physical examination. The assessment may be comprehensive, as when interviewing a person suspected of having cancer, or cursory, as when caring for an individual with acute blood loss due to cancer. A number of laboratory screening tests provide information about the risk of bleeding, measure actual blood loss, and help to determine the pathophysiology of the bleeding. Diagnostic tests may also be ordered to evaluate internal hemorrhage, including magnetic resonance imaging and angiography (MRI/MRA) scans, computerized tomography (CT) scans, plain film radiographs, and ultrasound. The information gathered in the assessment of bleeding is critical in preparing an appropriate plan of care.

Patient/Family History

The patient/family history is a vital component of a complete assessment. Because bleeding is a common problem in many malignancies, we must remain alert to findings that suggest bleeding disorders. Key aspects of a comprehensive history for the individual at risk for bleeding include:

- **Bleeding tendencies**, including easy bruising, excessive nosebleeds, gingival bleeding, presence of petechiae, change in color of stools or urine, stomach discomfort, vision problems, and painful joints

- **Signs or symptoms of anemia**, which may signify undetected long-term bleeding

- **Medications**, including chemotherapy or any over-the-counter medications that might interfere with the coagulation mechanism or that might uncover an important symptom for which the person is taking medication

- **Acute bacterial or viral infections** that may increase the risk of disseminated intravascular coagulation

- **General performance status** that helps to identify the effects of the disease or the presence of complications

- **Transfusion history**, including blood components required and the response to therapy (may provide information regarding potential risk of alloimmunization to prior blood products)

- **Nutritional status**, to identify vitamin K or vitamin C deficiency or generalized malnutrition that will affect the person's hematologic system

- **Immunologic disorders**, such as ITP that increase the risk of bleeding

- **Family history** of any bleeding abnormalities

Physical Examination

Physical examination of the patient with actual or potential bleeding requires a thorough head-to-toe approach. Diagnostic signs can be subtle, including skin petechiae noticed while bathing the patient, traces of blood as the patient brushes his or her teeth, and oozing from venipuncture sites or sites of injections. Such observations can lead to early diagnosis of bleeding problems and might prevent an incident of spontaneous hemorrhage.

The major problem associated with active bleeding is hemorrhage. Although bleeding can occur from any part of the body, common sites of hemorrhage include the gums, nose, brain, bladder, and the gastrointestinal tract. An examination of all body systems is done on a routine basis for any patient known to have a bleeding disorder (Table 31-3).

Screening Tests

Several screening tests provide information about hemostatic function, more specifically about the phases of hemostasis and fibrinolysis. The hematologic alterations leading to bleeding are complex, and test results vary depending on the degree of the original coagulation dysfunction and the cascading effect of related hemostatic mechanisms. Some of the most common screening tests of hemostatic functions are discussed next. A listing of tests of hemostasis is found in Table 31-4.

Platelet count

The platelet count is the best indicator of potential risk of bleeding in a patient with cancer. Normal platelet counts are considered to be 150,000–400,000 cells/mm³; platelet counts below 100,000 cells/mm³ are considered indicative of thrombocytopenia. Spontaneous hemorrhage generally is not a concern until the platelet count drops below 15,000 cells/mm³. Thrombocytosis occurs when the count rises above 400,000 cells/mm³.

Bleeding time

This test measures the time it takes for a small skin incision to stop bleeding. The results depend on the platelet number and function and the ability of the capillary wall to vasoconstrict. A normal bleeding time varies from 1–9 minutes. The bleeding time is prolonged when platelets are lacking or with a severe factor deficiency. Examples of disease states in which a prolonged bleeding time may be found include thrombocytopenia, von Willebrand's disease, infiltration of the marrow by tumor, and consumption of platelets in DIC. A prolonged bleeding time is also found with drugs that affect platelet function such as aspirin.

Whole-blood retraction test

This test, which measures the speed and extent of blood clot retraction in a test-tube, is done to determine the degree of platelet adequacy. A normal clot shrinks to half its normal size in 1–2 hours, disappearing completely in 24 hours. With thrombocytopenia or abnormally functioning platelets, clot retraction is slower and the clot stays soft and watery.

Bone marrow aspirate

In most cases, the definitive test to determine the etiology of thrombocytopenia is the bone marrow aspirate. If the platelet count is low, the bone marrow aspirate will demonstrate few megakaryocytes because of underproduction of cells. This may occur when there is crowding of the marrow by disease. The bone marrow aspirate

---

Table 31-3 Physical Examination of the Patient with Actual or Potential Bleeding

Central nervous system
Mental status changes including confusion, lethargy, restlessness, changes in cognition, alteration in level of consciousness, obtundation, seizures or coma; changes in neurologic signs including: widening pulse pressure, pupil size and reactivity, motor strength and coordination, speech and paralysis, and complaints of headache (all may indicate intracranial hemorrhage or impaired tissue perfusion)

Eyes[a] and ears
Visual disturbances including diplopia, blurred vision, and partial field loss; increased injection on the sclera, periorbital edema, subconjunctival hemorrhage (homogeneous red color that is sharply outlined on the sclera), headache, eye or ear pain

Nose, mouth and throat
Petechiae on nasal/oral mucosa, ulcerations, gingival or mucous membrane bleeding, epistaxis

Cardiovascular
Changes in vital signs, color and temperature of all extremities, peripheral pulses (all may demonstrate changes in peripheral perfusion); tachycardia, hypotension; observe for angina

Pulmonary
Respiratory rate and depth: dyspnea, tachypnea, and shortness of breath (may indicate an inability to compensate for blood loss); crackles, wheezes, stridor, dyspnea, tachypnea, orthopnea, hemoptysis (usually bright red in color and frothier than hematemesis), and cyanosis (all possible signs of bleeding in the lungs)

Abdominal
Pain (close attention to location); right upper quadrant pain and abdominal distention may be indicative of hepatomegaly; left flank or shoulder pain may be indicative of splenomegaly; vague abdominal pain may be indicative of retroperitoneal bleeding: palpable spleen, blood around rectum, tarry stools, frank or occult blood in stools, hematemesis; observe for bleeding hemorrhoids (may respond to local measures)

Genitourinary system
Blood in the urine (measure for frequency and size of clots), dysuria, burning, frequency and pain on urination (all are associated with hematuria); character and amount of menses; decreased urine output (if urine drops below 30 mL/hr it may be due to acute tubular necrosis secondary to thrombi, bleeding, or hypovolemia and associated shock)

Musculoskeletal system
Warm, tender, swollen joints with diminished mobility for active and passive range of motion (may indicate bleeding into the joints)

Integumentary system[b]
Bruising, petechiae, purpura, ecchymoses, hematomas, acrocyanosis (irregularly shaped cyanotic patches on the periphery of the arms and legs associated with bleeding due to DIC); pallor and jaundice (indicative of anemia and liver dysfunction), oozing from venipuncture sites or injections, biopsy sites, central lines, catheters, or nasogastric tubes

---

DIC = disseminated intravascular coagulation.

[a] Bleeding in the optic fundus could lead to permanent visual impairment.

[b] Assess entire skin surface, including intertriginous areas.

Table 31-4 Tests of Hemostasis

Test	Measures	Normal Value
PLATELET FUNCTION		
Platelet count	Number of circulating platelets	150,000–400,000/mm³
Bleeding time	Platelet plug formation; response of small vessels	1–9 min
Clot retraction	Ability of platelets to support retraction of a clot	50% retraction within 1 hr; compare with normal value
Bone marrow biopsy	Etiology of thrombocytopenia	Megakaryocytes present
COAGULATION		
Partial thromboplastin time (aPTT)	Diminished or absent coagulation factors	Varies; compare with normal control (usually 30–40 sec)
Prothrombin time (PT)	Diminished or absent coagulation factors	Varies; compare with normal control (approximately 70%–130%)
Thrombin time	Fibrinogen concentration; structure of fibrinogen; presence of inhibitors	Varies: compare with normal value (approximately 200–400 mg/dL)
Specific factor assays	Concentration of functional factor in plasma	50%–150% activity in pooled normal plasma
FIBRINOLYSIS		
Fibrin degradation product (FDP) assay	Presence of FDP in serum	10 µg/mL

will demonstrate adequate to increased levels of megakaryocytes if the platelets are being destroyed in the peripheral blood by the immune system. This may occur with diseases such as ITP or as a result of marrow toxic therapy.

Partial thromboplastin time (activated)

A normal activated partial thromboplastin time (aPTT) is approximately 30–40 seconds. The aPTT screens for coagulation deficiencies in the intrinsic and common pathways of coagulation. A prolonged aPTT is evidenced when any clotting factor, except for factors VII or XIII, exists in inadequate quantities. A prolonged aPTT may be seen with consumptive coagulopathy, liver disease, biliary obstruction, and with circulating anticoagulants such as heparin. There is a risk of spontaneous hemorrhage if the aPTT is greater than 100.[50]

Prothrombin time

The prothrombin time (PT) screens for coagulation deficiencies along the extrinsic or common pathways of coagulation. The PT is prolonged when clotting factors I, II, V, VII, or X are deficient. Prolonged PT values are seen in liver disease (hepatitis and tumor involvement), in obstructive biliary disease (e.g., bile duct obstruction secondary to tumor), and with coumarin ingestion.[51]

Taken together, the aPTT and the PT can give a fair indication of the nature of the clotting defect. If both the aPTT and the PT are normal and the patient is bleeding, the vessels or platelets are probably defective. Likewise, if either the aPTT or the PTT is prolonged and the patient is bleeding, the defect is likely in the clotting mechanism.

International normalized ratio

The effects of anticoagulation therapy are often measured by the international normalized ratio (INR). The normal INR is less than 2.0. An INR greater than 2.0 is considered anticoagulated (e.g., for the treatment of deep vein thrombosis or pulmonary edema).

Fibrin degradation products test

The measurement of FDPs provides an indication of the activity of the fibrinolytic system. Agglutination is demonstrated if the patient's blood contains degradation fragments. Levels of FDP greater than 10 µg/mL indicate increased fibrinolysis, as seen in DIC and primary fibrinolytic disorders.

Therapeutic Approaches and Nursing Care

Prevention of Bleeding

General measures

Bleeding precautions are instituted for any patients at risk for bleeding, to maintain their physical safety.

These measures are taught to both patient and family so they are aware of the potential risks of bleeding. Table 31-5 is a care plan for a patient experiencing thrombocytopenia or bleeding. Environmental safety is critical in patients at risk for bleeding; bumps or falls can be dangerous and even fatal.

Diligent measures to maintain skin integrity are instituted. Personal hygiene is essential for maintaining skin integrity. The use of a good emollient lotion helps to minimize dryness and potential breaks of the skin. In addition, paper tape or similar tapes should be used rather than adhesive tape to avoid trauma to the skin.

All unnecessary procedures are avoided in the patient at risk for bleeding, including intramuscular or subcutaneous injections, rectal temperatures or suppositories, and indwelling catheters. If the patient requires parenteral administration of medications, the intravenous route is used whenever possible. Intramuscular and subcutaneous injections place the patient at risk for the development of hematomas, which can become sites of infection when granulocytopenia is present. If injections are unavoidable, the smallest possible gauge needle is used. Pressure to the injection site is applied for several minutes, followed by the application of a pressure bandage to avoid a hematoma. Cold compresses may be used to assist in vasoconstriction. Similar care is taken at venipuncture sites.

The mouth and gums are easily damaged when the platelet count is low, and they become an excellent potential source of bleeding and infection. A systematic mouth care regimen should be instituted to minimize this problem. A lubricant to the lips, gums, and tongue will help avoid dryness and cracking. Soft-bristled toothbrushes help avoid trauma to sensitive gums. When the platelet count drops below 20,000–30,000 cells/mm³ or if the gums and mouth are bleeding, bristled toothbrushes should be avoided and mouth swabs or Toothettes used. Most commercial mouthwashes are avoided as they contain a high alcohol content that is irritating and drying to the gums and mouth. When the gums and mouth are

Table 31-5   Care Plan for the Patient Experiencing Thrombocytopenia/Bleeding

Patient Problem	Expected Outcomes	Nursing Interventions

Potential for bleeding related to thrombocytopenia	The patient will be free of bleeding.
	
	The patient/significant other will be able to state signs/symptoms indicative of bleeding.
	
	The patient/significant other will be able to demonstrate knowledge of their understanding of bleeding precautions.
		1. Monitor platelet count and other coagulation tests and report abnormal values.
		2. Assess vital signs q4h or as indicated.
		3. Hold myelosuppressive agents as indicated.
		4. Test all excreta for occult blood and report positive results.
		5. Assess patient for any signs/symptoms of bleeding (see Table 31-3).
		6. Maintain and reinforce bleeding precautions when the patient's platelet count is ≤20,000/mm³ or the patient is bleeding.
		  a. Use an emollient lotion on patient's skin.
		  b. Use only electric razor.
		  c. Use soft toothbrush or moistened cloth.
		  d. Use only alcohol-free mouthwash.
		  e. Avoid use of dental floss and toothpicks.
		  f. Avoid venipuncture, invasive procedures, rectal thermometers or suppositories.
		  g. Apply pressure to puncture sites for at least 5 min.
		  h. Avoid forceful coughing, sneezing, or nose blowing.
		  i. Avoid constipation; may require stool softeners.
		  j. Avoid cutting toenails and fingernails.
		  k. During menses, monitor pad count.
		  l. Avoid aspirin or any medications that may cause/aggravate thrombocytopenia.
		  m. Avoid tight-fitting or constrictive clothing.
		7. Administer recombinant thrombopoietin (rHIL-11) as indicated.
		8. Administer platelet transfusion if ordered.
		  a. Premedicate client as indicated.
		  b. Use leukocyte reduction filter on platelet transfusion as indicated.
		  c. Use HLA-matched platelets, if refractory to platelets.
		  d. Monitor, document, and notify physician if any allergic reaction (fever, chills, rash, hives, skin flushing).
		  e. Obtain posttransfusion platelet count.

irritated, dentures should not be replaced, particularly if they fit poorly. Patients requiring oxygen via nasal cannula or endotracheal tube are assessed for irritation to the mucosa. A lubricant may need to be applied to the nares to minimize drying and cracking.

Prevention of forceful coughing, sneezing, nose blowing, or vomiting can be critical in a patient at risk for bleeding. Cough medication, especially containing codeine or hydrocodone, may help to minimize bleeding related to coughing. Teaching the patient to gently clean the nares with tissue or a cotton swab dipped in saline may minimize bleeding related to nose blowing. Antiemetics minimize the potential of nausea and vomiting as well as keeping gastric juices from irritating the esophagus.

Bowel strain caused by constipation can initiate rectal bleeding. Prescription stool softeners may be necessary to avoid constipation. Instruction regarding proper diet and exercise to avoid constipation are also appropriate.

Colony-stimulating factors

The use of recombinant colony-stimulating growth factors to accelerate hematologic recovery following ablative chemotherapy or radiation therapy continues to be an area of intensive investigation. Studies in both animals and humans have clearly shown that the administration of growth factors can reduce the hematopoietic toxicities that follow exposure to chemotherapy and radiation therapy. Use of CSFs, specifically G-CSF and GM-CSF, has been found to shorten the duration of neutropenia, thus reducing morbidity and mortality associated with infection.[52,53]

Recombinant human interleukin-11 (rhIL-11). An exciting adjunct therapy for the treatment of bone marrow suppression associated with severe thrombocytopenia is the use of rhIL-11. Several different cytokines or growth factors have been evaluated for stimulation of megakaryocyte proliferation and maturation in patients undergoing chemotherapy,[54–60] but to date only rhIL-11 has demonstrated significant clinical efficacy in a randomized placebo-controlled trial.[61] This study included patients with a variety of cancer diagnoses who were receiving different chemotherapy regimens and who had already received platelet transfusions for severe thrombocytopenia resulting from the chemotherapy. Patients who received rhIL-11 in a dose of 5 μg/kg tolerated it well, and it significantly reduced the requirement for platelet transfusions compared to the group receiving placebo. Most adverse events in the study were mild to moderate in severity and were reversible after discontinuation of the drug. Adverse effects included edema, dyspnea, headache, palpitations, and atrial arrhythmia.[61] Another more recent study involving rhIL-11 demonstrated effective reduction of chemotherapy-associated thrombocytopenia in patients with breast cancer receiving dose-intensive chemotherapy.[62] This study is of particular interest because it demonstrated that the reduction of treatment-associated thrombocytopenia and the need for platelet transfusions in patients who receive dose-intensive chemotherapy may allow for chemotherapy to be administered at the intended doses as planned.[62]

Erythropoietin. The hematopoietic growth factor that regulates the proliferation, differentiation, and viability of erythrocyte progenitor cells and mature erythrocytes is known as EPO. Erythropoietin or epoietin alfa has been shown to be an effective treatment for anemia associated with cancer and chemotherapy-associated anemia in some patients. As it naturally occurs, EPO is produced in the kidney in response to hypoxia or decreased oxygen-carrying capacity of the blood. Cloning of the erythropoietin gene was accomplished in 1985,[63,64] which allowed for large-scale production using recombinant DNA technology.

Several studies have demonstrated that EPO administration is well tolerated and effective in the management of anemias associated with cancer and cancer chemotherapy. These findings also indicate that the administration of EPO increases the hemoglobin concentration and reduces red cell transfusion requirements in patients with cancer who receive chemotherapy and are anemic.[65–68] Of interest, EPO appears to have a beneficial effect on patient reported functional capacity, including energy level and quality of life, in patients with cancer who receive chemotherapy, independent of tumor response.[68–71] Improvement in functional status can be attributed to an increase in hemoglobin level, which supports the need to aggressively manage anemia in this patient population.[71] The response rate to EPO is about 50%–60% for patients with hematologic malignancies or solid tumors; response rates are poor in patients with myelodysplastic syndromes.[72,73] The use of EPO is being studied in some novel clinical applications such as a supportive strategy prior to high-dose chemotherapy and as a synergistic enhancer of blood progenitor cell mobilization in combination with G-CSF.[74,75]

Radiation and chemotherapy protectors

Another approach to preferentially protecting normal tissues from the toxicities of chemotherapy and radiation therapy is the administration of cytoprotectant agents before the cancer treatment. Some of these agents have been used for many years, including leucovorin (prevents myelosuppression and mucositis associated with high-dose methotrexate) and mesna (prevents hemorrhagic cystitis associated with cyclophosphamide and ifosfamide). One of the most promising of the newer cytoprotectant agents is amifostine (Ethyol). Amifostine is a naturally occurring thiol that protects cell damage by scavenging free radicals.[76] Amifostine has been demonstrated through randomized clinical trials to reduce the incidence and severity of cisplatin-induced renal toxicity for advanced ovarian and non–small cell lung cancers.[77–80] In addition to amifostine's approved indication, data suggest that it substantially reduces the severity of treatment-associated thrombocytopenia.[81,82] Data also demonstrate, the reduction of treatment-associated neutropenia, neurotoxicities, musculoskeletal toxicities, cardiotoxicity, and mutagenicity with the use of amifostine.[82–84]

Amifostine is given as an intravenous solution over 15 minutes prior to chemotherapy.[85] The established effective dose is 740–910 mg/m² prior to chemotherapy.[86] Amifostine is generally well tolerated, with transient side effects including nausea and vomiting, hypotension, hiccups, sneezing, a metallic taste in the mouth during the infusion, a flushed feeling, somnolence, and in rare cases hypocalcemia.[80,87,88] Pretreatment with newer antiemetics, such as odansetron or granisetron, can generally alleviate the problem of nausea and vomiting. Because of the hypotensive effects of amifostine, the patient is usually treated in a supine position with blood pressure monitoring every 5 minutes.[89] Clinical sequelae of amifostine-related hypotension are extremely rare.[76]

Management of Bleeding

General measures

If acute bleeding occurs, direct measures to stop the bleeding are instituted immediately. Direct, steady pressure is applied at the site of bleeding. Mechanical pressure such as insertion of an occlusion balloon catheter into the bronchus or the use of nasal packing during epistaxis can be used if the site of bleeding is not directly exposed. Iced saline gastric lavages or enemas may help to control gastrointestinal bleeding. Hypovolemic shock is to be avoided in situations of acute hemorrhage. Control of life-threatening hemorrhage is generally achieved with a combination of packed red cells with crystalloids or albumin as opposed to whole blood (see Blood Component Therapy, below).

Minor vascular bleeding due to capillary destruction is best controlled by treating the underlying malignancy. If iron deficiency anemia has occurred, oral or parenteral iron supplements are indicated. Oral iron supplements are often recommended because they are safe and usually correct the anemia within 6 weeks, but therapy generally continues for 4–6 months to adequately replace the iron stores.[39,40] Parenteral iron supplements may be given if the patient is not able to tolerate oral therapy or has a malabsorption problem. Iron dextran, generally given intravenously, requires a test dose because it is associated with a small risk of anaphylaxis.[39]

Physical and emotional rest are essential when the patient is bleeding. Rest helps to decrease pulse rate and blood pressure, allowing for clot formation. A state of active bleeding is frightening and anxiety-producing for the patient and family. A calm approach and reassurance are essential when managing an individual who is actively bleeding. Sedation can also be used to decrease anxiety and the metabolic rate.

Thrombocytopenia

Although thrombocytopenia may be the immediate cause of bleeding in individuals with platelet disorders, therapy must address the underlying cause of the decreased platelet level. When decreased platelet production is the result of tumor infiltration of marrow, the best therapy is treatment of the tumor itself. The hematologic complications will remain or worsen as long as marrow involvement persists. Platelet transfusions are often given to maintain a safe level of circulating thrombocytes until tumor regression occurs and marrow function returns. If platelet production has been depressed by chemotherapy or radiation therapy, in addition to platelet support the dosage or administration schedule of the treatment can be altered to maintain safe levels of platelet production.[90]

Platelet distribution.   Thrombocytopenia related to platelet sequestration due to an enlarged spleen is treated most effectively by aggressive tumor therapy. Chemotherapy and radiation therapy are usually most effective for this condition. Sequestration of platelets is at times reversible with epinephrine, which causes a release of trapped platelets from an enlarged spleen. Transient control of platelet sequestration has also been achieved with corticosteroid therapy. Steroids have a capillary-stabilizing effect that is important in minimizing the bleeding potential of thrombocytopenia. Splenectomy may be considered if other methods fail to control the sequestration of platelets.

Platelet destruction.   Individuals who are found to have asymptomatic ITP may be followed closely with no treatment. Individuals who experience severe thrombocytopenia are generally treated with prednisone therapy (1 mg/kg body weight).[91] This low-dose prednisone therapy may need to be maintained to keep the platelet count greater than 50,000 cells/mm³. If the platelet count drops during tapering of the prednisone, a high dose of the drug may be required.[92]

Platelet transfusions are seldom indicated for patients with ITP because the survival time of transfused platelets is shortened. Platelet transfusions may be used for controlling severe hemorrhage.[91] Intravenous immunoglobulin therapy plays an important role in managing acute bleeding. The efficacy of platelets has been found to be improved immediately after an infusion of intravenous immunoglobulin. The recommended dose of immunoglobulin is 1 g/kg/day for 2 days.[93]

Splenectomy for the management of ITP was used for many years before glucocorticoids were introduced. The decision to undergo splenectomy for the treatment of ITP is determined by the course and severity of the disease. Splenectomy may be done early on in the course of severe thrombocytopenia that is unresponsive to prednisone, or it may be done after several months if disease remission cannot be attained.[91] If patients fail prednisone therapy or lack a response to splenectomy, other treatments include splenic radiation or partial splenic embolization, vincristine, vinblastine, bleomycin, danazol, colchicine, anti-D antibody, and alfa-interferon.[94–99]

Drug-induced platelet abnormalities must be assessed carefully in context of the patient's total clinical profile. Aspirin has been demonstrated to cause an increased risk of bleeding. Because of this risk, the patient with cancer should avoid taking aspirin or any compounds containing aspirin. A prolonged bleeding time due to aspirin may be corrected by infusion of desmopressin (DDAVP).[100] The clinical risk for bleeding associated with nonsteroidal anti-inflammatory drugs is much less than the risk associated with aspirin ingestion. However, they should be used cautiously in patients with preexisting thrombocytopenia. The potential for beta-lactam-induced bleeding generally does not prohibit patients from being treated with appropriate antibiotic coverage; these patients need to be monitored closely for any signs or symptoms of bleeding. Platelet transfusions may be used during periods of thrombocytopenia to avoid hemorrhage as well as during periods of acute bleeding.

Hypocoagulation

Effective tumor therapy is the best means to control abnormalities related to hypocoagulation. Plasma and plasma derivative therapy may be used discriminately in specific clinical situations. Specific replacement of diminished factors is difficult because of the complex nature of these abnormalities. Generally, the treatment of specific inhibitors of coagulation factors depends on the severity of the abnormality.[101]

Liver disease associated with bleeding and clotting can be treated with infusion of fresh-frozen plasma or prothrombin complex concentrate (contains prothrombin and factors VII, IX, and X) when rapid correction of abnormalities is required. Prothrombin complex may also be given when attempting to shorten a prolonged prothrombin time, as before a needle biopsy of the liver. Albumin can be used as a volume expander in cases of active bleeding. Albumin is safer than plasma because it carries no risk of hepatitis transmission. It may, however, precipitate congestive heart failure in patients with compromised cardiovascular function. When albumin is used as a volume expander, the patient's cardiac and renal status must be monitored closely. Desmopressin may be infused when the patient with liver disease has a prolonged bleeding time, with mild to moderate amounts of bleeding.[27,100]

Generally, subcutaneous vitamin K (menaphthone, AquaMEPHYTON) is administered to correct the protein defects when this vitamin is deficient, as demonstrated by a prolonged prothrombin and bleeding time.[102] The patient is also instructed on dietary sources of vitamin K if absorption of the vitamin is not a problem. The major sources of dietary vitamin K are liver (92 g/100 g), broccoli (175 mg/100 g), and spinach (415 g/100 g).[103] Prothrombin complex concentrates or fresh-frozen plasma can be used in situations of vitamin-K deficiency with concomitant severe bleeding.[101]

Isolated factor deficiencies are best treated with specific plasma components if they can be identified. Patients with acquired von Willebrand's disease are generally treated when they experience bleeding or when they require an invasive procedure. The severity of the bleeding dictates the type and amount of therapy used. Treatment for bleeding due to this syndrome includes fresh-frozen plasma, cryoprecipitate, packed red cells and platelet concentrates, along with high-dose corticosteroids, factor VIII concentrates, DDAVP infusions, epsilon-aminocaproic acid (amicar), intravenous gammaglobulin, and extracorporeal immunoabsorption.[104,105]

Blood Component Therapy

In recent years, various professional societies and governmental organizations, including the American Society of Anesthesiologists and the College of American Pathologists, have developed "guidelines" and "practice parameters" for the use of blood component therapy. These guidelines have been prompted by the recognition that even though blood component administration has clearly accepted benefits, it still has significant complications, including transfusion reactions, transmittal of bacterial or parasitic diseases, immunosuppression, and high cost.[106,107]

Red blood cell therapy

In any patient, the clinical concern for the adverse physiologic effects of anemia is usually the basis for considering red blood cell replacement. Generally, the decision to transfuse is based on an overall clinical picture, including any underlying cardiac or pulmonary conditions or any concurrent conditions that might impair the patient's tolerance of anemia.[108] Among the causes of anemia frequently seen in patients with cancer, the two most common are decreased red cell production secondary to myelosuppressive therapy and the primary disease process.

Most practice guidelines agree that red blood cell transfusion is rarely indicated when the hemoglobin concentration is greater than 10 g/dL.[106,107] To date, no controlled studies have been done to determine the hemoglobin concentration at which red blood cell transfusions improve clinical outcomes. Physiologic signs of anemia (pallor, fatigue, rapid pulse, hyperventilation, and shortness of breath) should be relieved when the hemoglobin is raised to 10 or 11 g/100 mL.[22] The transfusion of 1 unit of red blood cells increases the hematocrit by 3% or the hemoglobin concentration by 1 g/dL in a 70-kg nonbleeding patient.

Packed erythrocytes usually are the therapy of choice. The advantage of packed red blood cells is that they provide more than 70% of the hematocrit of whole blood with only one-third of the plasma. This prevents unnecessary volume, electrolyte load, and anticoagulants that may otherwise be transfused.

Leukocytes in red blood cell transfusions can cause reactions if the recipient has antileukocyte antibodies, which can develop from previous transfusions or pregnancies. These antigenic reactions occur much more frequently in the oncology patient population (8.7%) compared with other patient groups.[109] Transfusion of packed red cells in these patients can cause fever and chills, and the patient can eventually become alloimmunized, or refractory to transfusions. This condition is demonstrated when transfusion of a unit of red cells fails to achieve the expected increase in the hemoglobin level. The use of leukocyte-reduced blood component therapy is indicated for these patients. Leukocyte reduction of blood products may be obtained by the use of bedside leukocyte reduction filters or the use of prestorage leukocyte reduction filtering in the laboratory. Currently, most leukocyte-reduced blood component therapy is done with bedside filters. However, there is a shift in the industry to provide blood that has already been leukocyte-reduced in the laboratory.

Red blood cells can be stored up to 5 weeks at 1–6°C in CPDA-1 anticoagulant or for 6 weeks if stored as an additive system unit.[106] The units may also be frozen for prolonged storage. Red blood cell units may be saline washed to remove almost all of the plasma.

Platelet therapy

The use of platelet transfusions has proved to have tremendous therapeutic value in controlling and preventing hemorrhage in patients undergoing chemotherapy for leukemia and other cancers.[110,111] Traditionally, attempts have been made to maintain the patient's platelet count above 20,000 cells/mm³ to minimize the potential for spontaneous bleeding.[112–114] More recent experience indicates that platelet counts in the range of 10,000–20,000 cells/mm³ can be monitored safely without use of prophylactic transfusions.[115–118] The debate about when to prophylactically transfuse platelets arises from concerns about transfusion-associated risks and the cost of transfusion.[106,107,119] In addition to the actual platelet count, patient-related information—such as the type of leukemia; presence of fever, infection, or DIC; administration of drugs that interfere with platelet function; and whether the patient requires any invasive procedures—should be taken into account when determining the appropriateness of transfusion therapy.[111,120,121] It is generally accepted that platelets are not transfused due to thrombocytopenia associated with increased platelet destruction, such as occurs in ITP. Platelet transfusions in these conditions are rarely indicated and usually ineffective.

Platelets can be obtained from differential centrifugation of donated whole blood or from platelet pheresis of single donors. A donor can be pheresed frequently (up to every other day) if the donor's platelets provide the patient with good platelet count increases. One unit of platelets is routinely obtained from 500 mL of fresh whole blood (Table 31-6). Platelets are stored at room temperature, and with gentle agitation for up to 5 days. Contaminating microorganisms may reach unacceptably high titers beyond 5 days.

Theoretically, 1 unit of platelets should increase the recipient's platelet count by 10,000 cells/mm³. However, the effectiveness of platelet transfusions is variable and depends on several factors. Failure to achieve adequate increases in the circulating platelet count may be due to fever, infection, hypersplenism, DIC, previous administration of amphotericin B, prolonged storage, and human leukocyte antigen (HLA) antibody grade.[120,122]

Fever and infection enhance the consumption of platelets and can increase the occurrence of hemorrhage. Patients with fever or sepsis may require more frequent platelet transfusions to maintain adequate platelet counts. Patients with fever can be premedicated with antipyretics prior to platelet transfusion in an attempt to minimize platelet destruction; premedication may also consist of corticosteroids and antihistamines. Demerol may be given if the patient is having shaking chills.

Patients with hypersplenism who are receiving platelet transfusions will have a reduced recovery of circulating platelets that is generally proportionate to the size of their spleen. If platelets are transfused while the patient is actively bleeding, increased increments will not be detected by blood counts. The effectiveness of platelet transfusions in this case is determined by clinical improvement and control of the bleeding. Amphotericin B can also decrease the recovery and survival of transfused platelets. It has been found in a prospective study that if amphotericin B is given 2 hours before or after the platelet transfusion, a decrease in platelet survival is not demonstrated.[123]

The preparation and storage of platelets are also important factors in determining the quality of the platelet transfusion. To be most effective, platelets must be fresh and metabolically active. Maximum effectiveness remains for up to 6 hours after platelets are obtained. Storage longer than 24 hours at 22°C causes significant loss of platelet function due to release of ADP and alterations in platelet membrane permeability.

Alloimmunization. Platelet survival is greatly decreased when alloimmunization to the platelet transfusion develops. Alloimmunization results when repeated transfusions of random-donor platelets fail to provide a therapeutic increment in the platelet count and may even cause a decrease in the platelet count posttransfusion.[124] The patient is then considered to be refractory to platelet transfusions. In most cases, alloimmunization is due to formation of antibodies to human leukocyte antigen (HLA) on the platelet cell surface and from contamination of white cells in the platelet concentrate.[125–127] Patients that are refractory to random-donor platelets may

Table 31-6 Platelet Transfusion Therapy

Specific Component	Content and Volume	General Indications	Complications	Nursing Considerations
Random donor (RD) • Fresh—best • Frozen and cryopreserved (limited application because of poor recovery)	• Multiple donors (4+) approximately 200 mL • Plasma, WBCs, few RBCs	• Bleeding and bleeding prophylaxis • Prophylactic for platelet count of 10,000–20,000/mm³	• Exposure of patients to multiple tissue antigens, which initiates antigen-antibody formation, leading to refractoriness • Hepatitis (increased risk with pooled products) • Allergic reactions may be seen more often if leukocyte reduction filter is not used	• Gently agitate bag occasionally to prevent platelet clumping. • Rapid infusion (per patient tolerance). • Tubing should include a 170–220-μm in-line blood filter. • A leukocyte reduction blood filter may be required. • Less expensive than single donor or HLA-matched platelet concentrates. • May require UVB irradiation if patient is severely immunosuppressed.
Single donor (SD) • Fresh (maximum effectiveness up to 6 hr)	• One donor • 1 unit ∝ 300 mL • Plasma, WBCs, RBCs • Number of platelets in a SD unit equals approximately the number of platelets in 5 RD units	• Bleeding and bleeding prophylaxis • Severe febrile reactions associated with random donor platelets • Often used once a patient is refractory to random donor platelets • Patients who require long-term platelet therapy • Minimizes the transmission of viral disease	• Refractoriness to platelets may occur over time	• Rapid infusion (generally 30 min+). • Tubing as above. • Leukocyte reduction blood filter may be required.
Human-leukocyte antigen (HLA) matched concentrate	• One donor compatible at the HLA complex • 1 unit ∝ 300 mL • Plasma, WBCs, RBCs	• When patients become refractory to RD and SD platelets • Minimizes transmission of viral disease	• Minimal	• HLA-matched platelets minimize patient exposure to multiple tissue antigens (HLA complex found on all blood cells—acts as a genetic monogram). • Rapid infusion (30 min+). • Tubing as above. Generally see more effective increases in the platelet count than with RD or SD.

∝ = approximately.

respond either to HLA-matched platelets or single-donor platelet transfusions, as they significantly reduce the number of platelet and leukocyte antibodies to which the recipient is exposed.[128] Elimination of antigen-presenting cells from platelet concentrates may be done with the use of leukocyte-reduction filters or by treating the platelet concentrate with ultraviolet light (UVB).[128–132] (See Transfusion Complications, for more information regarding irradiation of blood products.)

Febrile nonhemolytic transfusion reactions can occur in platelet and red blood cell transfusions but are more common in platelet transfusions.[133] It has been demonstrated that unfiltered platelet concentrates accumulate high levels of cytokines, which can produce the signs and symptoms of a febrile transfusion reaction.[133] This reaction causes allergic symptoms including hives, chills, fever, and skin flush, all of which may result in a poor increment related to the platelet transfusion. These reactions can be avoided by leukocyte depletion from the platelet concentrate during preparation or the use of a bedside leukocyte-reduction filter.[120] Premedicating the patient with acetaminophen prior to platelet transfusion decreases the frequency and severity of platelet transfusion reactions.[134]

The use of intravenous γ-globulin (IV IgG) is generally reserved for treating bleeding in patients with immune disorders such as ITP. The use of IV IgG does, however, continue to be investigated for the support of individuals refractory to all types of available transfusions. Some investigators have found that high-dose IV IgG (400 mg/kg/day for 5 days) improves the response to platelet concentrates in platelet-refractory patients.[135,136] This therapy is expensive but may be justified in the refractory patient with uncontrolled bleeding.

Plasma therapy

Fresh frozen plasma, the most frequently used of the plasma products, contains all of the labile clotting factors and the plasma proteins. Plasma proteins such as albumin and cryoprecipitate can be isolated and removed from plasma. The most common use of plasma and plasma components in cancer is with coagulation disorders. Plasma component therapy is also administered for shock, severe bleeding, bleeding associated with infections, and management of acute DIC. Plasma can be used to treat deficiencies of factors II, V, VIII, X, XI, and XIII.[137]

The amount and frequency of transfusions depends on several factors including the severity of the deficiency, specific factor deficiency, and the severity of bleeding. Another important dosing consideration in plasma therapy is the metabolic half-life of plasma and plasma derivatives. Replacement therapy is given in doses high enough to compensate for the decrease in plasma level as it is metabolized.[101] The metabolic half-life varies for each of the factors. Plasma and plasma factors usually are infused rapidly so the maximum plasma level is reached before metabolic changes or degradation occurs. Table 31-7 explains commonly used plasma components.

Transfusion Complications

There are many risks associated with blood component therapy, including transfusion reactions and transmission of diseases. While most reactions occur shortly after the transfusion, some reactions can occur several days to weeks after the transfusion. The acute reactions include acute hemolytic transfusion reactions (AHTR), febrile reactions, bacterial contamination of blood resulting in sepsis, and allergic reactions. Delayed transfusion reactions include the development of graft-versus-host disease (GVHD) and the transmission of diseases, particularly viral diseases. Table 31-8 lists transfusion reactions, and Table 31-9 explains the nursing management of transfusion reactions.

Immediate blood transfusion reactions

Immediate blood transfusion reactions may be due to an immune response to the blood component, as occurs with AHTR. The most severe type of AHTR is caused by the transfusion of ABO-incompatible blood. The most common cause of this reaction is clerical error involving basic misidentification of the patient.[108,138] Other immediate complications may be related to the method of administration (circulatory overload with respiratory distress, air embolism, or hypothermia), the age of the blood product, citrate toxicity, hypocalcemia, or hyperkalemia. Bacterial contamination of blood, which can result from bacteria entering blood bags during component preparation or from improperly cleansed skin at venipuncture sites, can cause fatal septic transfusion reactions.[139–141] Treatment of this reaction includes fluid infusion along with blood product and respiratory support. Broad-spectrum antibiotics are used until the results of blood cultures are available.[108]

Other immediate blood transfusion reactions include febrile reactions and allergic reactions. A febrile reaction is generally diagnosed in an individual with a temperature increase of more than 1°F that occurs during or shortly after transfusion without another identified cause. Shaking chills often accompany the fever. Reactions are seen most frequently in recipients of multiple transfusions, such as patients with cancer and multiparous women. Treatment consists of acetaminophen for the fever, meperidine for severe rigors, and steroids for dyspnea. Premedication with acetaminophen and steroids is used for patients who have a history of febrile reactions. Febrile reactions can generally be prevented by the use of bedside leukocyte-reduction filters or the use of prestorage leukocyte-reduced blood, because most febrile reactions are due to antileukocyte antibodies in the recipient that are directed against the donor blood. The removal of 2 or 3 log 10 of leukocytes can prevent most febrile reactions.[108] Bedside filters require no special processing of the blood.

Allergic reactions account for about 1% of transfusion reactions.[108] Allergic reactions may be mild, manifested by clinical signs and symptoms such as hives, urticaria, and cutaneous erythema. Allergic reactions may be severe,

Table 31-7 Commonly Used Plasma Components

Component	Content Volume and Route	Shelf Life	Indications	Complications	Nursing Considerations
Normal human plasma (fresh or frozen)	Plasma; all plasma proteins and clotting factors; 200 mL, IV route	1 yr frozen; 6 hr thawed	Severe blood loss; clotting factor deficiency (II, V, VII, X, XI, and XIII); plasma volume expander without increasing the hematocrit	Volume overload; hepatitis and other viruses; allergic reactions; hypernatremia, hypocalcemia	Requires ABO compatibility. Average adult dose is 3–5 units (12–15 mL/kg) given as rapidly as possible, generally over less than 30 min (depending on the patient's cardiovascular status); smaller doses may need to be given at periodic intervals; administer fresh-frozen plasma immediately after thawing to minimize deterioration of factors V and VIII; infusion should be slowed or stopped if patient demonstrates signs of citrate toxicity.
Normal human serum albumin	Aqueous fraction of pooled plasma 5%: 250 mL and 500 mL; 25%: 25 mL and 50 mL, IV route	3–5 yr	Rapid volume expansion	No hepatitis risk	Monitor cardiac and renal function closely; congestive heart failure may be precipitated by compromised function; each unit must be used immediately after opening as albumin does not contain preservatives; rate of administration of 5% solution should not be >2–4 mL/min; rate of administration of 25% solution should not be >1 mL/min.
Cryoprecipitate	Fibrinogen, factors VIII (100 units) and XIII, von Willebrand factor, fibronectin; 10–20 mL, IV route	1 yr frozen; 6 hr thawed	Severe von Willebrand's disease; hypofibrino-genemia (DIC); fibronectin may have a role in wound healing	Hepatitis and other viruses	Best to be ABO-compatible; should be kept at room temperature until infused; administer within 30 min; infusion of cryoprecipitate will increase circulating plasma fibrinogen to pre-bleeding levels; a "fibrin sealant" can be made by adding bovine thrombin to cryoprecipitate; it may stop bleeding when applied topically.
Fibrinogen	Fibrinogen; 10 mL, IV route	1 yr frozen	Clotting disorders; hemophilia A or B		Monitor cardiac and renal function closely; administer rapidly; 1 unit should raise level 10 units.
Purified AHF concentrate	Factor VIII (lyophilized); IV route	Per pharmacy label	Severe von Willebrand's disease; hemophilia A	High hepatitis risk (C)	Rate of administration is 2 mL/min, can be up to 10 mL/min; if patient's pulse increases significantly, rate of administration should be decreased.
Immune globulin	Immunoglobulin from large pools of human plasma, IV and IM route	Per pharmacy label	Bleeding disorders, hypogamma-globulinemia, ITP		May be given to clients who are refractory to a variety of platelet transfusions (random donor, single donor, HLA-matched platelets).
Antithrombin III (AT-III) concentrates	Antithrombin III (lyophilized)	Per pharmacy label	Antithrombin III deficiency		
Recombinant factor VIII	Factor VIII, IV route	Per pharmacy label	Hemophilia, especially for those patients who have never been exposed to blood products or have no evidence of transfusion-transmitted viruses		
Heat-treated lyophilized prothrombin complex concentrates (PCC)	Prothrombin factors VII, IX, X; IV route	Per pharmacy label	Bleeding disorders; hemophilia B; factor VIII inhibitor	High hepatitis risk (C); thrombosis; no HIV with currently available products	Monitor patient for signs/symptoms of thrombosis (no lab test measures PCC effectiveness).

DIC = disseminated intravascular coagulation; ITP = immune thrombocytopenic purpura; HLA = human leukocyte antigen.

Adapted and reprinted from Gobel BH: Plasma and plasma derivatives therapy for coagulation disorders. *Semin Oncol Nurs* 6:129–135, 1992.[101]

Table 31-8 Transfusion Reactions

Immediate

Acute hemolytic transfusion reaction (e.g., ABO incompatibility)
Bacterial contamination—shock, sepsis
Circulatory overload
Air embolism
Citrate toxicity
Hypocalcemia
Hyperkalemia
Hypothermia
Iron overload
Respiratory distress
Febrile reactions (temperature rise over 1°F), chills
Allergy—urticaria, anaphylaxis
Bacterial contamination

Delayed

Delayed hemolytic transfusion reaction
Graft-vs-host disease
Infection–hepatitis (A, B, or C), rotovirus, cytomegalovirus, human immunodeficiency virus, human T-cell lymphotrophic virus type 1, parasites, malaria, babesiosis
Alloimmunization
Bacterial contamination

manifested by bronchospasm, laryngeal edema, and anaphylaxis. A mild allergic reaction is treated with diphenhydramine or another antihistamine; prevention includes premedication with diphenhydramine. Washing the cells with saline helps to prevent allergic reactions. This process of washing the unit of blood rids the unit of plasma, suspending the cells in saline. If the patient has a severe allergic reaction, the patient will be treated as anyone with an anaphylactic reaction.

Delayed blood transfusion reactions

A serious delayed transfusion reaction in patients who are severely immunosuppressed is GVHD. Patients who are at risk for developing this complication include bone marrow transplant recipients, peripheral blood stem cell recipients, patients undergoing combination treatment for Hodgkin's and non-Hodgkin's lymphoma, and leukemia patients undergoing induction chemotherapy. This complication can occur following the transfusion of blood products containing viable lymphocytes. The donor-competent T lymphocyte immunologically attacks the immunocompromised host tissue after transfusion. Graft-versus-host disease is generally manifested in the skin, liver, and gastrointestinal tract and can be fatal.[142] Posttransfusion GVHD is fatal almost 90% of the time due to the development of bone marrow hypoplasia or aplasia.[143] To prevent posttransfusion GVHD, it is generally recommended that all blood products given to the severely immunocompromised patient be irradiated with at least 2500 cGy.[144] Irradiation of blood is done to inhibit proliferation of lymphocytes without impairment of platelets, red blood cells, or granulocytes. There is additional cost associated with irradiation of blood components. Currently, the cost of an irradiator and the radiation

source is approximately $50,000. Because of the additional cost, it is generally recommended that irradiated blood products only be used for specific indications.[143]

Transmission of diseases through blood products, particularly viral diseases, is a major concern of the public. Transmission of viral disease by blood has been steadily decreasing over the years.[137,145] The risk of HIV infection from 1 unit of volunteer donor blood is extremely small (1:450,000 to 1:660,000).[146] Other diseases of concern include rotovirus, hepatitis virus (particularly A, B, and C), human T-cell lymphotrophic virus (HTLV), parvovirus B19, malaria, babesiosis, and cytomegalovirus (CMV).[147–149] Immunocompromised patients are most susceptible to severe infections caused by parvovirus B19, malaria, babesiosis, and CMV.

Cytomegalovirus infection is one of the leading causes of death in bone marrow transplant recipients.[137] The CMV infection is caused by remaining leukocytes in the transfused blood. The use of CMV-seronegative blood products is currently the standard of care for severely immunosuppressed patients or for bone marrow transplant recipients who are seronegative and have seronegative bone marrow donors.[150,151] The demand for CMV-negative blood products may exceed the supply at many blood centers and in areas where CMV-negative blood cannot be found (e.g., Washington, D.C.), as the number of transplants has increased. Studies have shown that leukocyte-reduced blood products may significantly reduce the risk of CMV transmission.[151] Thus, if CMV-seronegative blood is not available when needed, a physician may order the use of a leukocyte-reduction filter with the blood product or substitute a prestorage leukocyte-reduced filtered unit or a frozen deglycerolized unit of blood (a more traditional method of leukocyte depletion).

Home Transfusion Therapy for the Cancer Patient

The home health care (HHC) industry has grown tremendously during the past decade. Services that are now provided in the home include complex intravenous therapy, including blood transfusion therapy. Services provided in the home are motivated by many changes in the health care environment and third-party reimbursement policies. Reimbursement agencies often prefer HHC services that cost substantially less than hospitalization but perhaps more than services rendered in the hospital outpatient setting.[152,153]

Blood transfusions administered in the home are usually provided by a HHC agency that contracts with a hospital transfusion service or an independent blood provider. Some hospitals have their own HHC programs that include blood transfusion as one of the available services. Limited information is available regarding out-of-hospital blood transfusion practices, as well as transfusion administration in the home. The American Association of Blood Banks (AABB) has provided some written instructions

Table 31-9 Nursing Management of Selected Transfusion Reactions

Type	Signs/Symptoms	Nursing Actions
Acute hemolytic transfusion reaction • ABO incompatibility	Fever, chills, hypotension, increased pulse rate, nausea/vomiting, flushing, low back pain, decreased urine output, hematuria, dyspnea, bleeding, anaphylaxis, shock	1. Stop transfusion. 2. Maintain patent IV line with normal saline. 3. Verify client and the blood unit with another nurse (the majority of reported fatalities with an acute hemolytic transfusion reaction involve human error). 4. Place in supine position. 5. Maintain open airway; provide CPR if necessary. 6. Obtain vital signs and record. 7. Notify physician. 8. Monitor intake and output. 9. Administer fluids and medications per physician order. 10. Vital signs per institutional guidelines. 11. Obtain blood and urine specimens. 12. Notify blood bank and return remainder of blood to blood bank. 13. Document event. 14. Admit patient to hospital if outpatient.
Febrile nonhemolytic transfusion reaction (FNHTRS) • Antileukocyte antibodies in the recipient directed against the donor blood	Fever (>1°F) ± chills, headache, hypotension, increased pulse rate, dyspnea, chest pain, nausea/vomiting	1. Stop transfusion. 2. Maintain patent IV line with normal saline. 3. Obtain and monitor vital signs and record. 4. Notify physician. 5. Assist in ruling out infection. 6. Administer medications and fluids per physician order: acetaminophen for fever, meperidine for chills and rigors, antihistamine for dyspnea. 7. Continue transfusion if symptoms are not severe. 8. Notify blood bank. 9. Document event. 10. For clients who are known to have FNHTRS or for clients who are at high risk for FNHTRS (multiply transfused clients) acetaminophen and antihistamines/steroids may be given before the transfusion to minimize or eliminate the transfusion reaction. The use of a leukocyte reduction filter may be indicated.
Allergic (usually mild) reaction • Recipient antibodies against immunoglobulin components or other soluble proteins in the plasma	Hives, urticaria, cutaneous erythema; may develop severe allergic or even fatal anaphylaxis	1. Obtain and monitor vital signs and record. 2. Slow or stop transfusion rate, depending on symptoms. 3. Measures to correct shock, maintain renal circulation, and to correct the bleeding depending on symptoms. 4. Notify physician. 5. Administer medications per physician order: antihistamines if reaction is mild. 6. Notify blood bank. 7. Document event.
Bacterial contamination • Cold-growing organisms	Fever, chills; may result in endotoxin shock	1. Stop transfusion. 2. Maintain patent IV line. 3. Measures to correct shock and to maintain renal circulation. 4. Obtain vital signs and record. 5. Notify physician. 6. Notify blood bank and return remainder of blood to blood bank. 7. Obtain blood and urine cultures of the client and the unit of blood. 8. Administer antibiotics per physician order. 9. Document event. 10. Admit client to hospital if outpatient.
Delayed hemolytic reaction • Development of alloantibodies to transfused blood	Delayed (7–10 days to weeks) decreased hemoglobin, low-grade fever, jaundice (increase in bilirubin and LDH)	Notify blood bank.

regarding out-of-hospital blood transfusions for blood providers.[154]

There are a number of advantages to home transfusion therapy for the cancer patient, including the potential for decreased cost, convenience for the patient and family, the ability to be treated in a familiar environment, and no risk of nosocomial infection.[155,156] It has been estimated that home infusion therapy services can reduce patient care costs by 30%–50% from inpatient costs.[157] Blood transfusion in the home has the potential disadvantage of increased risk of harm due to distance from emergency medical services. As such, the transfusionist may have a limited ability to manage adverse events.

Measures to improve safety of home transfusions must be carefully considered. Agencies or institutions that provide home transfusion therapy should establish appropriate selection criteria for inclusion in a home transfusion therapy program. Table 31-10 lists recommendations for selection criteria and safety considerations for a home transfusion program. These recommendations are based on the out-of-hospital transfusion guidelines of the Transfusion Practices Committee of the AABB.[154] Compliance with AABB standards is required by all AABB-accredited institutions.[158] These standards are widely regarded as the criteria that will help to ensure safe transfusion.[156] Another possible safety consideration is using only leukocyte-reduced blood components. Routinely using filtered blood may help to reduce the febrile nonhemolytic reaction rate.

Blood administration considerations

Once the patient has been accepted as a candidate for home transfusion therapy, a number of appointments are made and documents are established. Appointments are made with the patient for type and crossmatch samples and for the actual transfusion. The type and cross-match sample must be drawn within 48 hours of the actual transfusion. Once an informed consent is signed by the patient, a means of identification is placed on the patient. A unique patient identification number is required by AABB standard I1.000 and J1.000.[158] This unique identification number should be used for both identification of patients' samples for compatibility testing and at the time of transfusion. It is recommended that a commercial wristband system that uses preprinted numbers be used to increase patient safety. Documentation records include physician's written orders for the blood transfusion, a signed informed consent, laboratory results, nursing progress notes, and a blood transfusion flow record.

Nurses who administer blood in the home setting take on a great deal of responsibility. Institutional policies and procedures must be adhered to closely in order to maximize patient safety. Standard A2.200 of the AABB requires that each blood provider keep a manual detailing all procedures performed.[158] The home blood transfusion protocol outlined in Table 31-11 covers general administration considerations. Another AABB standard to follow in home transfusions is a protocol to identify, diagnose, and manage suspected transfusion reactions.

Once the transfusion is complete, the nurse discontinues the blood bag yet maintains a patent intravenous line. The nurse remains with the patient for at least 30–60 minutes after the transfusion to observe the patient and to monitor vital signs. If the patient is stable after this time, the intravenous line can be discontinued. All transfusion supplies are collected in a biohazard bag for disposal. Documentation of the entire blood transfusion process must be detailed and complete. Follow-up of the transfused patient should be done within 24 hours.

Table 31-10 Recommendations for Selection Criteria and Safety Considerations for a Home Blood Transfusion Program

Inclusion criteria

Cooperative patient

Stable cardiopulmonary status of the patient

Physical limitations that make transportation difficult

Absence of reactions to the most recent blood transfusion

A diagnosis supporting the need for blood transfusion therapy

Patients who do not have an acute need for blood, or who do not require more than 2 units in a 24-hour period

Safety considerations

A telephone available for medical needs or the need to call an ambulance

Presence of a responsible adult in the home during and after the blood transfusion

Conclusion

Bleeding associated with cancer represents a complex clinical challenge to the nurse. Bleeding can occur as a result of the cancer itself or as a complication of the treatment of the cancer. Bleeding can be occult and chronic, or it can be acute and life-threatening. Nurses who work with patients who have cancer must be prepared to meet the complex needs of these patients. Early detection of the signs and symptoms of bleeding allows for prompt diagnosis and treatment of the bleeding, thus preventing further complications. Management of bleeding is often as complex as the bleeding process itself. A variety of medications may be used to prevent and treat bleeding disorders. The cornerstone therapy in the prevention and management of bleeding is blood transfusion therapy. An important adjunct to blood transfusion therapy in preventing and treating a bleeding problem is the use of recombinant colony-stimulating factors. Exciting research continues in this area to identify as yet unknown CSFs that may benefit the patient with bleeding.

Table 31-11 Home Transfusion Protocol

Nursing Actions	Rationale

1. Gather supplies:
  • IV pole and pump (if required)
  • Blood filter (if required)
  • Saline
  • Appropriate blood tubing
  • Leukocyte reduction blood filters per institutional policies and procedures
  • Needles, syringes, appropriate for type of vascular access device to be used
  • Transfusion flow sheet
  • Emergency drug kit (including epinephrine 1:10,000 and 1:1000 and diphenhydramine hydrochloride 50 mg), extra saline bag
  • Transfusion reaction protocol
  • Emergency plan to transport patient (physician's phone #, hospital, and ambulance phone number)
	Most electromechanical pumps can safely administer RBC transfusions. Combining other solutions (including glucose) with RBCs can cause agglutination or hemolysis of the RBCs. All blood components require an in-line blood filter of 170 μm, at minimum. Some centers require all blood component therapy to be transfused through leukocyte reduction blood filters or similar device.

2. a. Check the physician's order to confirm the product type, dose, and rate of infusion.	All blood components must be administered with a physician's written order.
b. Review client medical history/allergies, etc.	Some medical conditions (e.g., congestive heart failure) may make it necessary to modify usual administration practices (i.e., administer blood over the longest, most appropriate length of time).

c. Obtain blood component from blood bank, on departure to client's home.
    • Check unit for client's full name, client's identification number, unique identifying numbers of the unit, the ABO and Rh type of the donor(s) and client, expiration date. Cross-check with blood bank employee and sign off.
    • Secure client's record and interpretation of compatibility test to the blood container.
    • Examine unit for unusual color, clots, or excessive air.
	The primary cause of acute fatal transfusion reactions is major ABO incompatibility related to clerical errors.
	
	Abnormalities may be an indication of contamination and/or improper collection or storage techniques.
	RBCs cannot be returned to storage if the temperature exceeds 10°C.

3. Transport the blood at a temperature between 1°C and 10°C (cool but not frozen).
  • Best achieved by transporting RBCs in an insulated container with wet ice.
  • Transport platelets at room temperature (between 20°C and 24°C); *do not* transport with wet ice.
  • Blood components are not to be placed in the client's refrigerator at home.
	Platelets have best biologic activity if stored at room temperature.
	
	Temperatures in home refrigerators are not regulated.

4. Confirm client identity:
  • Verbally against the client record.
  • Confirm client identification using the medical bracelet or other identification means and identify RBC compatibility on the tag attached to the unit and on all forms.
	As above.

5. Initiate blood component therapy:
  • Explain procedure to client/family.
  • Review with client and caregiver the signs/symptoms of adverse reactions; provide them with emergency phone numbers.
  • Premedicate client as ordered.
  • Establish baseline vital signs/record.
  • Start RBC transfusion slowly.
  • Vital signs per home transfusion flow sheet
  • Observe for transfusion reaction.
  • Adjust flow rate per order.
  • Infuse RBCs within 4 hr.
  • Observe and monitor vital signs 30 min after completion.
	Transfusion reactions may be immediate or delayed.
	
	May be required to alleviate allergic reactions.
	
	Symptoms of a transfusion reaction (especially RBCs) are usually evident during infusion of first 50 mL of blood.
	
	Minimize the risk of bacterial contamination.

6. Documentation:
  • Client identification procedure
  • General condition of client and vital signs throughout procedure
  • Record medication on flowsheet, etc.
  • Record time of arrival/departure.
	All to be part of the legal record.

REFERENCES

1. Haeuber D, Spross JA: Bone marrow, in Gross J, Johnson BL (eds): *Handbook of Oncology Nursing* (ed 2). Sudbury, MA, Jones and Bartlett, 1994, pp 373–399

2. Anderson KC: Hematologic complications and blood product support, in Holland JF, Bast RC, Morton DL, et al (eds): *Cancer Medicine* (ed 4). Baltimore, Williams & Wilkins, 1997, pp 3155–3177

3. John WJ, Patchell RA, Foon KA: Paraneoplastic syndromes, in DeVita VT, Hellman S, Rosenberg SA (eds): *Cancer: Principles and Practice of Oncology* (ed 5). Philadelphia, Lippincott-Raven, 1997, pp 2367–2422

4. Quesenberry PJ: Hematopoietic stem cells, progenitor cells, and cytokines, in Beutler E, Lichtman MA, Coller BS, Kipps TJ (eds): *Williams Hematology* (ed 5). New York, McGraw-Hill, 1995, pp 211–228

5. Reiger PT, Haeuber D: A new approach to managing chemotherapy-related anemia: Nursing implications of epoetin alfa. *Oncol Nurs Forum* 22:71–81, 1995

6. Griffin JD: Bone marrow dysfunction in the cancer patient: Hematopoietic growth factors, in DeVita VT, Hellman S, Rosenberg SA (eds): *Cancer: Principles and Practice of Oncology* (ed 5). Philadelphia, Lippincott-Raven, 1997, pp 2639–2657

7. Grosh WW, Quesenberry PJ: Recombinant human hematopoietic growth factors in the treatment of cytopenias. *Clin Immunol Immunopathol* 62:525–538, 1992

8. Jobe MI: Mechanisms of coagulation and fibrinolysis, in Lotspeich-Steininger CA, Stein-Martin EA, Koepke JA (eds): *Clinical Hematology: Principles, Procedures, Correlations.* Philadelphia, Lippincott, 1992, pp 579–598

9. Jesty J, Nemerson Y: The pathways of coagulation, in Beutler E, Lichtman MA, Coller BS, Kipps TJ (eds): *Williams Hematology* (ed 5). New York, McGraw-Hill, 1995, pp 1227–1238

10. Bick RL, Strauss JF, Frenkel EP: Thrombosis and hemorrhage in oncology patients. *Hematol Oncol Clin North Am* 10:875–907, 1996

11. Francis CW, Marder VJ: Mechanisms of fibrinolysis, in Beutler E, Lichtman MA, Coller BS, Kipps TJ (eds): *Williams Hematology* (ed 5). New York, McGraw-Hill, 1995, pp 1252–1260

12. Pruett J: Bleeding, in Groenwald SL, Frogge MH, Goodman M, Yarbro CH (eds): *Cancer Symptom Management.* Sudbury, MA, Jones and Bartlett, 1996, pp 269–288

13. Bick RL: Platelet function defects associated with hemorrhage or thrombosis. *Med Clin North Am* 78:577–607, 1994

14. Kirchner JT: Acute and chronic immune thrombocytopenic purpura. *Postgrad Med* 92:112–126, 1992

15. Lapka DMV, Wild LD, Barbour LA: Heparin-induced thrombocytopenia and thrombosis: A case study and clinical overview. *Oncol Nurs Forum* 21:871–876, 1994

16. Rutherford CJ, Frenkel EP: Thrombocytopenia: Issues in diagnosis and therapy. *Med Clin North Am* 78:555–575, 1994

17. Casini A: Quinine-induced pancytopenia and coagulopathy. *Ann Intern Med* 120:90–91, 1994

18. Rosen PJ: Bleeding problems in the cancer patient. *Hematol Oncol Clin North Am* 6:1315–1328, 1992

19. Shuey KM: Platelet-associated bleeding disorders. *Semin Oncol Nurs* 12:15–27, 1996

20. Kiefel V, Santoso S, Mueller-Eckhardt C: Serological, bio-chemical, and molecular aspects of platelet autoantigens. *Semin Hematol* 29:26–33, 1992

21. Schwartz CL, Cohen HJ: Myeloproliferative and myelodysplastic syndromes, in Pizzo PA, Poplack DG (eds): *Principles and Practice of Pediatric Oncology* (ed 2). Philadelphia, Lippincott, 1993, pp 519–536

22. Beutler E, Masouredis SP: Preservation and clinical use of erythrocytes and whole blood, in Beutler E, Lichtman MA, Coller BS, Kipps TJ (eds): *Williams Hematology* (ed 5). New York, McGraw-Hill, 1995, pp 1622–1635

23. Shafer AI: Essential (primary) thrombocythemia, in Beutler E, Lichtman MA, Coller BS, Kipps TJ (eds): *Williams Hematology* (ed 5). New York, McGraw-Hill, 1995, pp 1622–1635

24. Eichinger S, Bauer KA: Coagulopathic complications, in Holland JF, Bast RC, Morton DL, et al (eds): *Cancer Medicine* (ed 4). Baltimore, Williams & Wilkins, 1997, pp 3179–3190

25. Ravdi ML, Stocco F, Rossi C, et al: Thrombosis and hemorrhage in thrombocytosis: Evaluation of a large cohort of patients (357 cases). *J Med* 22:213–217, 1991

26. Gobel BH: Bleeding disorders, in Groenwald SL, Frogge MH, Goodman M, Yarbro CH (eds): *Cancer Nursing: Principles and Practice* (ed 4). Sudbury, MA, Jones and Bartlett, 1997, pp 604–639

27. Shattil SJ, Bennett JS: Acquired qualitative platelet disorders due to diseases, drugs, and foods, in Beutler E, Lichtman MA, Coller BS, Kipps TJ (eds): *Williams Hematology* (ed 5). New York, McGraw-Hill, 1995, pp 1386–1400

28. Sheridan CA: Multiple myeloma. *Semin Oncol Nurs* 12:59–69, 1996

29. Gralnick A, Ginsberg D: Von Willebrand's disease, in Beutler E, Lichtman MA, Coller BS, Kipps TJ (eds): *Williams Hematology* (ed 5). New York, McGraw-Hill, 1995, pp 1458–1480

30. Green D: Disorders of vitamin K-dependent coagulation factors, in Beutler E, Lichtman MA, Coller BS, Kipps TJ (eds): *Williams Hematology* (ed 5). New York, McGraw-Hill, 1995, pp 1481–1485

31. Murakawa M, Okamura T, Tsutsumi K, et al: Acquired von Willebrand's disease in association with essential thrombocythemia: Regression following treatment. *Acta Haematol* 87:83–90, 1992

32. Gaydos LA, Frierich EJ, Mantel N: The quantitative relation between platelet count and hemorrhage in patients with acute leukemia. *N Engl J Med* 266:905–909, 1962

33. Weber MS: Thrombocytopenia. *Am J Nurs* 94:46–52, 1994

34. Glover J, Miaskowski C: Small cell lung cancer: Pathophysiologic mechanisms and nursing implications. *Oncol Nurs Forum* 21:87–95, 1994

35. Walczak JR, Klemm PR, Guarnieri C: Gynecologic cancers, in Groenwald SL, Frogge MH, Goodman M, Yarbro CH (eds): *Cancer Nursing: Principles and Practice* (ed 4). Sudbury, MA, Jones and Bartlett, 1997, pp 1145–1198

36. Lind J, Hagan L: Bladder and kidney cancer, in Groenwald SL, Frogge MH, Goodman M, Yarbro CH (eds): *Cancer Nursing: Principles and Practice* (ed 4). Sudbury, MA, Jones and Bartlett, 1997, pp 889–915

37. Hoebler L: Colon and rectal cancer, in Groenwald SL, Frogge MH, Goodman M, Yarbro CH (eds): *Cancer Nursing: Principles and Practice* (ed 4). Sudbury, MA, Jones and Bartlett, 1997, pp 1036–1054

38. Erickson JM: Anemia. *Semin Oncol Nurs* 12:2–14, 1996

39. Massey AC: Microcytic anemias: Differential diagnosis and management of iron deficiency anemia. *Med Clin North Am* 76:549–566, 1992

40. Fairbanks VF, Beutler E: Iron deficiency, in Beutler E, Lichtman MA, Coller BS, Kipps TJ (eds): *Williams Hematology* (ed 5). New York, McGraw-Hill, 1995, pp 490–511

41. Fischer DS, Knobf MT, Durivage HJ (eds): *The Cancer Chemotherapy Handbook* (ed 4). St. Louis, Mosby, 1993

42. Hilderley LJ: Radiotherapy, in Groenwald SL, Frogge MH, Goodman M, Yarbro CH (eds): *Cancer Nursing: Principles and Practice* (ed 4). Sudbury, MA, Jones and Bartlett, 1997, pp 247–282

43. Peterson CW: Drug-induced blood disorders, in Young LY, Koda-Kimble MA (eds): *Applied Therapeutics: The Clinical Use of Drugs* (ed 6). Vancouver, Applied Therapeutics, Inc., 1995, pp 89-1–89-16

44. Peltz S: Severe thrombocytopenia secondary to alcohol use. *Postgrad Med* 89:75–85, 1991

45. Welty TE: Cerebrovascular disorders, in Young LY, Koda-Kimble MA (eds): *Applied Therapeutics: The Clinical Use of Drugs* (ed 6). Vancouver, Applied Therapeutics, Inc., 1995, pp 53-1–53-18

46. Manson SD, Elson S: Alterations in body defenses, in Shekelton ME, Litwak K (eds): *Critical Care Nursing of the Surgical Patient*. Philadelphia, Saunders, 1991, pp 850–868

47. Patterson WP, Caldwell CW, Doll DC: Hyperviscosity syndromes and coagulopathies. *Semin Oncol* 17:210–216, 1990

48. Hussein M: Multiple myeloma: An overview of diagnosis and management. *Clev Clin J Med* 61:285–298, 1994

49. Kyle RA: Diagnostic criteria of multiple myeloma. *Hematol Oncol Clin North Am* 6:347–358, 1992

50. McFarland MB, Gant MM: *Nursing Implications of Laboratory Tests* (ed 3). Albany, NY, Delmar Publishing, 1994, pp 64–91

51. Kee JL: *Handbook of Laboratory and Diagnostic Tests with Nursing Implications* (ed 2). Norwalk, CT, Appleton & Lange, 1994, pp 203–204

52. Dierdorf R, Krueter U, Jones TC: Use of granulocyte-macrophage colony stimulating factor in treatment of prolonged haematopoietic dysfunction after chemotherapy alone or chemotherapy plus bone marrow transplantation. *Med Oncol* 14:91–98, 1997

53. Morstyn G, Foote M, Perkins D, et al: The clinical utility of granulocyte colony-stimulating factor: Early achievements and future promise. (Review) *Stem Cells* 1:213–220, 1994

54. Collins C, Livingston RB, Ellis G, et al: Effect of PIXY321 on hematologic recovery after high-dose cyclophosphamide (CTX), etoposide (VP-16) and cisplatin (CDDP) (CEP) in women with breast carcinoma. *Blood* 82:366, 1993 (suppl 1, abstr)

55. Williams DE, Farese A, MacVitte TJ: PIXY321, but not GM-CSF plus IL-3 promotes hematopoietic reconstitution following lethal irradiation. *Blood* 82:366, 1993 (suppl 1, abstr)

56. Demetri GD, Bukowski RM, Samuels B, et al: Stimulation of thrombopoiesis by recombinant human interleukin-6 (IL-6) pre and post-chemotherapy in previously untreated sarcoma patients with normal hematopoiesis. *Blood* 82:367, 1993 (suppl 1, abstr)

57. Crawford J, Figlin R, Chang A, et al: Phase I/II trial of recombinant human interleukin-6 (IL-6) and granulocyte colony stimulating factor (rhG-CSF) following ifosphamide, carboplatin and etoposide (ICE) chemotherapy in patients with advanced non-small cell lung carcinoma (NSCLC). *Blood* 82:367, 1993 (suppl 1, abstr)

58. Veldhuis GJ, Willemse PHB, Sleijfer DT, et al: Toxicity and efficacy of escalating dosages of recombinant human interleukin-6 after chemotherapy in patients with breast cancer or non-small cell lung cancer. *J Clin Oncol* 13: 2585–2593, 1995

59. Schulz G, Krumwieh D, Oster W: Adjuvant therapy with recombinant interleukin-3 and granulocyte-macrophage colony-stimulating factor. *Pharmacol Ther* 52:85–94, 1991

60. Tepler I, Elias L, Smith JW, et al: A randomized placebo-controlled trial of recombinant human interleukin-11 in cancer patients with severe thrombocytopenia due to chemotherapy. *Blood* 87:3607–3614, 1996

61. Weich NS, Neben TY, Donaldson D, et al: Effects of interleukin-11 on megakaryocytes. *Blood* 88:60a, 1996 (suppl 1, abstr)

62. Isaacs C, Robert NJ, Bailey FA, et al: Randomized placebo-controlled study of recombinant human interleukin-11 to prevent chemotherapy-induced thrombocytopenia in patients with breast cancer receiving dose-intensive cyclophosphamide and doxorubicin. *J Clin Oncol* 15:3368–3377, 1997

63. Erslev AJ: Erythropoietin. *N Engl J Med* 324:1339–1344, 1991

64. Erickson N, Quesenberry PJ: Regulation of erythropoiesis. *Med Clin North Am* 76:745–755, 1992

65. Case DC Jr, Bukowski RM, Carey RW, et al: Recombinant human erythropoietin therapy for anemic cancer patients on combination chemotherapy. *J Natl Cancer Inst* 85: 801–806, 1993

66. Henry DH: Recombinant human erythropoietin for the treatment of anemia in patients with advanced cancer. *Semin Hematol* 30:12–26, 1993 (suppl 6)

67. Thatcher N: Management of chemotherapy-induced anemia in solid tumors. *Semin Oncol* 25:23–26, 1998

68. Pawlicki M, Jassem J, Bosze P, et al: A multicenter study of recombinant human erythropoietin (epoetin alpha) in the management of anemia in cancer patients receiving chemotherapy. *AntiCancer Drugs* 8:949–957, 1997

69. Demetri GD, Kris M, Wade J: Quality-of-life benefit in chemotherapy patients treated with epoetin alfa is independent of disease response or tumor type: Results from a prospective community oncology study. *J Clin Oncol* 16: 3412–3425, 1998

70. Jilani SM, Glaspy JA: Impact of epoetin alfa in chemotherapy-associated anemia. *Semin Oncol* 25:571–576, 1998

71. Glaspy J, Bukowski R, Steinberg D, et al: Impact of therapy with epoietin alfa on clinical outcomes in patients with nonmyeloid malignancies during cancer chemotherapy in community oncology practice. *J Clin Oncol* 15:1218–1234, 1997

72. Ludwig H, Fritz E: Anemia of cancer patients: Patient selection and patient stratification for epoetin treatment. *Semin Oncol* 25:35–38, 1998 (suppl 7)

73. Hellstrom-Lindberg E: Efficacy of erythropoietin in the myelodysplastic syndromes: A meta-analysis of 205 patients from 17 studies. *Br J Haematol* 89:67–71, 1995

74. Henry DH: Epoietin Alfa and high-dose chemotherapy. *Semin Oncol* 25:54–57, 1998 (suppl 7)

75. Henry DH: Hematological toxicities associated with dose-intensive chemotherapy, the role for and use of recombinant growth factors. *Ann Oncol* 8:S7–S10, 1997 (suppl 3)

76. Schuchter LM, Meropol N, Glick JH: Radiation and chemotherapy protectors, in DeVita VT, Hellman S, Rosenberg SA (eds): *Cancer: Principles and Practice of Oncology* (ed 5). Philadelphia, Lippincott-Raven, 1997, pp 3087–3092

77. Kemp G, Rose P, Lurain J, et al: Amifostine pretreatment for protection against cyclophosphamide-induced and cis-platin-induced toxicities: Results of a randomized control trial in patients with advanced ovarian cancer. *J Clin Oncol* 14:2101–2112, 1996

78. McGuire WP, Hoskins WJ, Brady MF, et al: Assessment of

dose-intensive therapy in suboptimally debulked ovarian cancer: A Gynecologic Oncology Group study. *J Clin Oncol* 13:1589–1599, 1995

79. Alberts DS, Green S, Hannigan EV, et al: Improved therapeutic index of carboplatin plus cyclophosphamide versus cisplatin plus cyclophosphamide: Final report by the Southwest Oncology Group of a phase III randomized trial in stages III and IV ovarian cancer. *J Clin Oncol* 10:706–717, 1992

80. Schuchter LM, Glick J: The current status of WR-2721 (amifostine): A chemotherapy and radiation protector. *Biol Ther Cancer* 3:1–7, 1993

81. Budd GT, Ganapathy R, Adelstein DJ, et al: Randomized trial of carboplatin plus amifostine versus carboplatin alone in patients with advanced solid tumors. *Cancer* 80:1134–1140, 1997

82. Alberts DS, Bleyer WA: Future development of amifostine in cancer treatment. *Semin Oncol* 23:90–99, 1996 (suppl 8)

83. Capizzi R: Amifostine: The preclinical basis for broad-spectrum selective cytoprotection of normal tissues from cytotoxic therapies. *Semin Oncol* 23:2–17, 1996 (suppl 8)

84. List AF, Brasfield F, Heaton R, et al: Stimulation of hematopoiesis by amifostine in patients with myelodysplastic syndrome. *Blood* 90:3364–3369, 1997

85. *Physician's Desk Reference* (ed 53). Ethyol. Montvale, NJ, Medical Economics Company, 1999, pp 513–515

86. Schuchter LM: Guidelines for the administration of amifostine. *Semin Oncol* 23:40–43, 1996 (suppl 8)

87. Foster-Nora JA, Siden R: Amifostine for protection from antineoplastic drug toxicity. *Am J Health Syst Pharm* 54:787–800, 1997

88. Spencer CM, Goa KL: Amifostine: A review of its pharmacodynamic and pharmacokinetic properties and therapeutic potential as a radioprotector and cytotoxic chemo-protector. *Drugs* 50:1001–1031, 1995

89. Lindeman K: Administration of the cytoprotectant amifostine. *Clin J Oncol Nurs* 2:101–104, 1998

90. Camp-Sorrell D: Chemotherapy: Toxicity management, in Groenwald SL, Frogge MH, Goodman M, Yarbro CH (eds): *Cancer Nursing: Principles and Practice* (ed 4). Sudbury, MA, Jones and Bartlett, 1997, pp 385–425

91. George JN, El-Harake MA, Raskob G: Chronic idiopathic thrombocytopenic purpura. *N Engl J Med* 331:1207–1211, 1994

92. Tardio DJ, McFarland JA, Gonzalez MF: Immune thrombocytopenia purpura: Current concepts. *J Gen Intern Med* 8:60–63, 1993

93. Blanchette VS, Kirby MA, Turner C: Role of intravenous immunoglobulin G in autoimmune hematologic disorders. *Semin Hematol* 29:72–82, 1992 (suppl 2)

94. Kirchner JT: Acute and chronic immune thrombocytopenic purpura. *Postgrad Med* 92:112–126, 1992

95. Calverly BC, Jones FW, Kelton JG: Splenic radiation for corticosteroid-resistant immune thrombocytopenia. *Ann Intern Med* 116:977–981, 1994

96. Naouri A, Feghati B, Chabal J, et al: Results of splenectomy for idiopathic thrombocytopenic purpura. *Acta Haematol* 89:200–203, 1993

97. Figueroa M, Gehlsen J, Hammond D, et al: Combination chemotherapy in refractory immune thrombocytopenic purpura. *N Engl J Med* 328:1226–1235, 1993

98. Miyazaki M, Itoh H, Kaiho T, et al: Partial splenic embolization for the treatment of chronic idiopathic thrombocytopenic purpura. *Am J Roentgenol* 163:123–126, 1994

99. Najean Y, Dufour V, Rain JD, et al: The site of platelet destruction in thrombocytopenic purpura as a predictive

100. index of the efficacy of splenectomy. *Br J Haematol* 79:271–276, 1991

100. Lethagen S, Rugarn P: The effect of DDAVP and placebo on platelet function and prolonged bleeding time induced by oral acetyl salicylic acid intake in healthy volunteers. *Thromb Haemost* 67:185–196, 1992

101. Gobel BH: Plasma and plasma derivatives therapy for coagulation disorders. *Semin Oncol Nurs* 6:129–135, 1990

102. Shetty HGM, Backhouse G, Bentley DP, et al: Effective reversal of warfarin-induced excessive anticoagulation with low-dose vitamin K. *Thromb Haemost* 67:13–19, 1992

103. Green D: Disorders of vitamin K-dependent coagulation factors, in Beutler E, Lichtman MA, Coller BS, Kipps TJ (eds): *Williams Hematology* (ed 5). New York, McGraw-Hill, 1995, pp 1481–1485

104. Jakaway JL: Acquired von Willebrand's disease. *Hematol Oncol Clin North Am* 6:1409–1417, 1992

105. Eikenboom JCJ, VanderMeer FJM, Briet E: Acquired von Willebrand's disease due to excessive fibrinolysis. *Br J Hematol* 81:618–624, 1992

106. Simon RL, Alverson DC, AuBuchon J, et al: Practice parameters for the use of red blood cell transfusions. *Arch Pathol Lab Med* 122:130–138, 1998

107. Stehling LC, Doherty DO, Faust RJ, et al: Practice guidelines for blood component therapy. A report by the American Society of Anesthesiologists Task Force on Blood Component Therapy. *Anesthesiology* 84:732–747, 1996

108. Synder EL, Mechanic SA: Bone marrow dysfunction in the cancer patient, in DeVita VT, Hellman S, Rosenberg SA (eds): *Cancer: Principles and Practice of Oncology* (ed 5). Philadelphia, Lippincott-Raven, 1997, pp 2607–2620

109. Mohandas K, Aledort L: Transfusion requirements, risks, and costs for patients with malignancy. *Transfusion* 35:427–430, 1995

110. Heyman MR, Schiffer CA: Platelet transfusion to patients receiving chemotherapy, in Rossi EC, Simon RL, Moss GS, Gould SA (eds): *Principles of Transfusion Medicine* (ed 2). Baltimore, Williams & Wilkins, 1996, pp 263–273

111. Slichter SJ: Principles of platelet transfusion therapy, in Hoffman R, Benz EJ Jr, Shattil SJ, et al (eds): *Hematology: Basic Principles and Practice* (ed 2). New York, Churchill Livingston, 1995, pp 1987–2006

112. Beutler R: Platelet transfusions: The 20,000/µL trigger. *Blood* 81:1411–1413, 1993

113. Pisciotto PT, Benson K, Hume H, et al: Prophylactic versus therapeutic platelet transfusion practices in hematology and/or oncology patients. *Transfusion* 35:498–502, 1995

114. Higby DJ, Cohen E, Holland JF, et al: The prophylactic treatment of thrombocytopenic leukemic patients with platelets: A double blind study. *Transfusion* 14:440–446, 1974

115. Rebulla P, Finazzi F, Marangone F, et al: The threshold for prophylactic platelet transfusions in adults with acute myeloid leukemia. *N Engl J Med* 337:1870–1875, 1997

116. Heckman KD, Weiner GJ, Davis CS, et al: Randomized study of prophylactic platelet transfusion threshold during induction therapy for adult acute leukemia: 10,000/µL versus 20,000/µL. *J Clin Oncol* 15:1143–1149, 1997

117. Lawrence JB, Yomtovian R, Hammons T, et al: Lowering the prophylactic platelet transfusion (ProPltTx) trigger: A prospective analysis. *Transfusion* 34 (suppl 53S, abstr) 1994

118. Wandt H, Frank M, Schneider C, et al: The 10,000/µL trigger compared to 20,000/µL for prophylactic platelet transfusion in AML: A prospective comparative multicenter study. *Blood* 88:443a, 1996 (suppl 1, abstr)

119. DeChristopher PJ, Anderson RR: Risks of transfusion and

organ and tissue transplantation: Practical concerns that drive practical policies. *Am J Clin Pathol* 107:S2–S11, 1997 (suppl 1)

120. Hussein MA, Hoeltge GA: Platelet transfusion therapy for medical and surgical patients. *Cleve Clin J Med* 63:245–250, 1996

121. Bishop AF, Matthews JP, McGarth K, et al: Factors influencing 20-hour increments after platelet transfusion. *Transfusion* 31:392–396, 1991

122. Norol F, Kuentz M, Cordonnier C, et al: Influence of clinical status on the efficiency of stored platelet transfusion. *Br J Haematol* 86:125–129, 1994

123. Hussein MA, Zuccaro K, Long T: Amphotericin-B does not adversely affect platelet recovery or survival when spaced by two hours from the platelet transfusion. *Blood* 86:899a, 1995 (abstr)

124. Walter-Coleman S: Transfusion therapy for patients critically ill with cancer. *AACN Clin Issues Crit Care Nurs* 7:37–45, 1996

125. Petranyi GG, Reti M, Harsanyi V, et al: Immunologic consequences of blood transfusion and their clinical manifestations. *Int Arch Allergy Immunol* 114:303–315, 1997

126. Meryman HT, Mincheff MS: Mechanism of alloimmunisation to HLA antigens, in Hogman CF (ed): *Leukocyte Depletion of Blood Components*. Amsterdam, VU University Press, 1994, pp 5–10

127. Murphy S: Preservation and clinical use of platelets, in Beutler E, Lichtman MA, Coller BS, Kipps TJ (eds): *Williams Hematology* (ed 5). New York, McGraw-Hill, 1995, pp 1361–1363

128. Lunban NLC, DePalma L: Use and administration of blood and components, in Chernow B (ed): *Essentials of Critical Care Pharmacology* (ed 2). Baltimore, Williams & Wilkins, 1994, pp 224–234

129. Saarinen UM, Koskimies S, Myllyla G: Systematic use of leukocyte-free blood components to prevent alloimmunisation and platelet refractoriness in multitransfused children with cancer. *Vox Sang* 65:286–292, 1993

130. Higgins VL: Leukocyte-reduced blood components: Patient benefits and practical applications. *Oncol Nurs Forum* 23:659–667, 1996

131. Anderson KC, Goodnough LT, Sayers M, et al: Variation in blood component irradiation practice: Implications for prevention of transfusion-associated graft-versus-host disease. *Blood* 77:2096–2102, 1991

132. Pamphilon DH, Blendell EL: Ultraviolet-B irradiation of platelet concentrates: A strategy to reduce transfusion recipient allosensitization. *Semin Hematol* 29:18–29, 1992

133. Aye MT, Palmer DS, Giulivi A: Effect of filtration of platelet concentrates on the accumulation of cytokines and platelet release factors during storage. *Transfusion* 35:117–124, 1995

134. Sharma S, Zuccaro K, Andresen S, et al: Premedication for platelet transfusion. A prospective study on four commonly used regimens. *Blood* 86:354a, 1995 (abstr)

135. Berkman SA, Lee ML, Gale RP: Clinical uses of intravenous immunoglobulins. *Ann Intern Med* 27:245–247, 1990

136. Kickler T, Brain HT, Piantadosi S, et al: A randomized placebo-controlled trial of intravenous gammaglobulin in alloimmunized thrombocytopenic patients. *Blood* 75:313–319, 1990

137. Menitove JE, Gill JG, Montgomery RR: Preparation and clinical use of plasma and plasma preparations, in Beutler E, Lichtman MA, Coller BS, Kipps TJ (eds): *Williams Hematology* (ed 5). New York, McGraw-Hill, 1995, pp 1649–1663

138. Linden JV, Paul B, Dressler KP: A report of 104 transfusion errors in New York State. *Transfusion* 32:601–603, 1992

139. Goldman M, Blajchman MA: Blood product associated bacterial sepsis. *Transfus Med Rev* 5:73–79, 1991

140. Ness P: Bacterial transmission by transfusion, in Rossi EC, Simon TL, Moss GS, Gould SA (eds): *Principles of Transfusion Medicine* (ed 2). Baltimore, Williams & Wilkins, 1996, pp 739–758

141. Wagner SJ, Friedman LI, Dodd RY: Transfusion-associated bacterial sepsis. *Clin Microbiol Rev* 7:290–297, 1994

142. Buschel PC: Allogeneic bone marrow transplantation, in Groenwald SL, Frogge MH, Goodman M, Yarbro CH (eds): *Cancer Nursing Principles and Practice* (ed 4). Sudbury, MA, Jones and Bartlett, 1997, pp 459–506

143. Wallerstein RO, Deisseroth AB: Bone marrow dysfunction in the cancer patient: Use of blood and blood products, in DeVita VT, Hellman S, Rosenberg SA (eds): *Cancer: Principles and Practice of Oncology* (ed 4). Philadelphia, Lippincott, 1993, pp 2262–2275

144. Moroff G, Luban NLC: Prevention of transfusion associated graft vs host disease. *Transfusion* 32:102–109, 1992

145. Dodd RY: The risk of transfusion transmitted disease. *N Engl J Med* 327:419–425, 1992

146. Lackritz EM, Satten GA, Aberle-Grasse J, et al: Estimated risk of transmission of the human immunodeficiency virus by screened blood in the United States. *N Engl J Med* 333:1721–1728, 1995

147. Luban NLC: Human parvovirus: Implications for transfusion medicine. *Transfusion* 34:821–827, 1994

148. Popovsky MA: Transfusion-transmitted babesiosis. *Transfusion* 31:296–301, 1991

149. Schreiber GB, Busch MP, Kleinman SH, et al: The risk of tranfusion-transmitted viral infections. *N Engl J Med* 334:1685–1690, 1996

150. Bowden RA, Schlicter SJ, Sayers MH, et al: Use of leukocyte-depleted platelets and cytomegalovirus seronegative red blood cells for prevention of primary cytomegalovirus infection after marrow transplant. *Blood* 78:248–250, 1991

151. Bowden RA, Schlicter SJ, Sayers MH, et al: A comparison of filtered leukocyte-reduced and cytomegalovirus (CMV) seronegative blood products for the prevention of transfusion-associated CMV infection after marrow transplant. *Blood* 85:3598–3603, 1995

152. Benson K, Balducci L, Milo KM, et al: Patient's attitudes regarding out-of-hospital blood transfusions. *Transfusion* 36:140–143, 1996

153. Douglas L: Out-of-hospital transfusions: Home transfusion therapy programs, in Fridey JL, Kasprisin C, Issitt LA (eds): *Out-of-Hospital Transfusion Therapy*. Bethesda, MD, American Association of Blood Banks, 1994, pp 43–57

154. Fridley JL, Kasprisin C, Issitt LA (eds): *Out-of-Hospital Transfusion Therapy*. Bethesda, MD, American Association of Blood Banks, 1994

155. McAbee RR, Grupp K, Horn B: Home intravenous therapy: Part 1. Issues. *Home Health Care Serv Q* 12:59–107, 1991

156. Benson K, Popovsky MA, Hines D: Nationwide survey of home transfusion practices. *Transfusion* 38:90–96, 1998

157. Home infusion therapy fact sheet. *J Nurs Adm* 22:8, 1992

158. Klein HG (ed): *Standards for Blood Banks and Transfusion Services* (ed 17). Bethesda, MD, American Association of Blood Banks, 1996

CHAPTER 32

Fatigue

Roxanne W. McDaniel, PhD, RN
Verna A. Rhodes, EdS, RN, FAAN

Scope of the Problem

Fatigue is a symptom we all experience at some point in our lives. For healthy individuals, it occurs as a result of physical exertion, stress, or lack of sleep. For individuals with cancer, fatigue is one of the most common and distressing problems, but its cause is not clearly understood.[1,2] The fatigue individuals with cancer experience may result from the disease itself, treatment modalities, psychological factors, or decreased functional capacity. Unfortunately, it is not limited to the period of active disease and treatment, and may last for years after treatment is completed when the individual is considered to be in remission.[3,4]

Definitions

Fatigue has an impact on all aspects of life.[5] Because it is a multifaceted problem, no general definition has been proposed that applies to every situation. Fatigue is a consequential side effect of cancer therapy that has received limited attention until recently. Still, this subjective symptom impacts all dimensions of an individual's quality of life; it can even hamper one's capacity for self-care. Both fatigue and quality of life are self-perceived states that necessitate thorough assessment approaches. Fatigue has been variously characterized as tiredness, weariness, exhaustion, lack of energy, incapacitation, decreased stamina, inability to sustain exertion, generalized lassitude, sleepiness, confusion, inadequate concentration, and a sense of inadequacy.[6–10] Descriptors frequently used by individuals with cancer include "pooped"; "worn out"; "no get-up-and-go"; "no pep"; "no interest"; "no energy"; "listless"; and having a strong desire to stop, rest, lie down, or sleep. Although individuals with cancer may describe feelings of weakness, they have differentiated fatigue from weakness and tiredness.[9] Early definitions of fatigue were derived from psychology, pathology, and physiology. More recently, fatigue has been defined by its cause, such as cancer-related fatigue.

Since the mid-1980s, nurse researchers have contributed greatly to the definition and study of fatigue. Nail and King describe fatigue as a human response to cancer and to the treatment for cancer.[11] Irvine et al describe fatigue as a subjective, self-recognized phenomena that is experienced as weariness, tiredness, or lack of energy and which varies in frequency and duration.[12] The North American Nursing Diagnosis Association defines fatigue as "an overwhelming sense of exhaustion and decreased capacity for physical and mental work regardless of adequate sleep."[13,p332] Piper defines fatigue as "a universal feeling of tiredness that is expected to occur normally at certain times of the day (because of circadian rhythmicity) or after certain types of activity or exertion."[14,p279] Hart, Freel, and Milde describe generalized fatigue as being a subjective self-evaluation of unpleasant sensations, such as decreasing physical and mental abilities, and decreased participation in activities.[15] According to Varicchio, fatigue can be emotionally or physiologically engendered, and may be a warning sign.[16] Several common themes can be identified from these definitions.

Fatigue also has been defined as either acute or chronic in nature. Acute fatigue serves as a protective mechanism to prevent harmful exhaustion. It is considered to be "normal" tiredness from physical or mental exertion.[8] Acute fatigue is generally localized and usually has an identifiable source with rapid onset and short duration. It does not adversely or permanently affect the ability to participate in the activities of daily living. Chronic fatigue, on the other hand, serves no useful purpose. It is often associated with a physical or psychological problem.[17] The onset is slow and insidious, and it has a constant and recurrent nature.[8]

Cimprich identified attentional fatigue that occurs in serious illness.[18] *Attentional fatigue* is a decrease in mental acuity and the physical discomfort an individual experiences when trying to focus attention or concentrate on an activity. For example, when concentrating on listening, a person may try to block out distractions such as unwanted noise or thoughts. Directing attention also helps in planning and organizing daily or weekly activities. Cimprich believes that prolonged demands on attention can lead to attentional fatigue and related impairments in key areas of functioning.[18] Systemic fatigue may influence attentional fatigue, and individuals with cancer are at particular risk for developing attentional fatigue due in part to the systemic nature of the disease, metabolic changes in their bodies, treatment effects, and the overwhelming amounts of information given to them regarding their disease.

Incidence

Fatigue is experienced daily by most people, but in a severe form it ultimately leads to a decreased ability to function. For healthy individuals, fatigue may be relieved by rest. Fatigue can have a protective role or it may be pathological in nature. It is one of the most common and distressing symptoms associated with the diagnosis and treatment of cancer.[19,20] Individuals with cancer were the first to identify fatigue as a cancer-related symptom.[21] Cancer fatigue is not generally relieved by rest. It is estimated that 72%–99% of individuals with cancer complain of fatigue during the course of their disease and treatment.[22,23] In individuals who are receiving chemotherapy, the reports of fatigue have ranged from 60% to almost 100%.[12,20,22] In a study by Vogelzang et al, of 419 patients with cancer, more than 78% experienced fatigue throughout the course of their disease and treatment, and 32% experienced it on a daily basis.[20] Cancer fatigue has been associated with surgery,[18] the use of interleukin-2, tumor necrosis factor, and colony-stimulating factor,[24–26] radiation therapy[27,28] and chemotherapy,[29,30] and concurrent illness.[31] The fatigue associated with cancer and its treatment interferes with normal activities of daily living and may negatively impact quality of life.

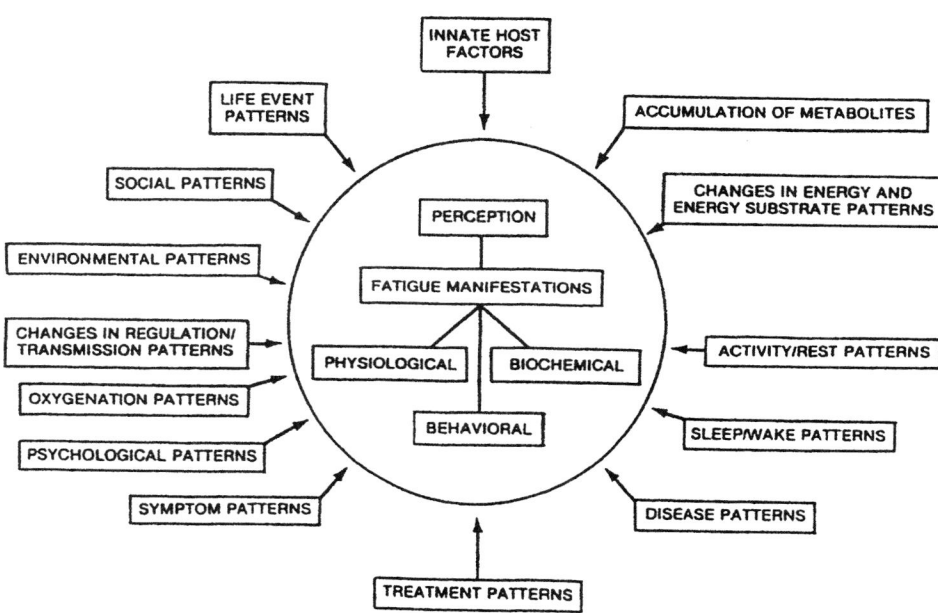

Figure 32-1 Piper's Integrated Fatigue Model. (Reprinted with permission from Winningham, Nail, Burke, et al: Fatigue and the cancer experience: The state of the knowledge. *Oncol Nurs Forum* 21:23–36, 1994.[8])

Etiology and Risk Factors

Although the exact cause of fatigue is unknown, it is considered to be a complex feedback system of regulated physiologic, psychological, and situational factors.[31] Various models and frameworks have been proposed to explain the mechanisms underlying fatigue. Two models that are frequently cited in relation to cancer fatigue are Piper's Integrated Fatigue Model (IFM) (Figure 32-1)[8] and Winningham's Psychobiologic-Entropy Model (Figure 32-2).[32] Piper's IFM considers fatigue in relation to physical, psychological, and treatment factors, as well as symptom patterns. Winningham's model considers fatigue as an energy deficit that leads to decreased activity

and secondary fatigue, causing decreased functional status.

Several physiologic factors have been associated with fatigue in individuals with cancer. They include anemia,[19,33,34] chronic pain,[35] infection, fever, surgery,[36] and inadequate nutrition related to gastrointestinal disturbances such as nausea, vomiting, and retching. Dehydration and electrolyte imbalances, acid-base imbalances, pain, hypoxia, neurologic toxicities, effects of drug therapies, cardiac abnormalities, dizziness, fever, constipation, and hormonal changes are other physiologic factors associated with cancer fatigue. Cancer fatigue is also related to radiation therapy, chemotherapy, biologic response modifiers, and multimodal therapy.

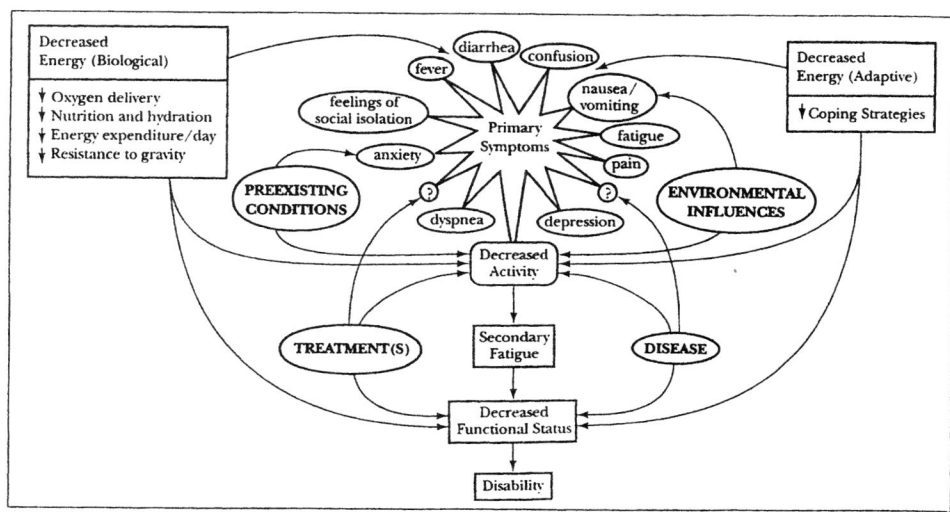

Figure 32-2 Winningham's Psychobiologic-Entropy Model of Functioning. (Copyright 1995, 1998 by Maryl L. Winningham. All rights reserved. Used by express written consent of author.)

Anemia

Anemia is a common complication of cancer and has been related to nutritional deficiencies, hemorrhage, hemolysis, hemodilution, infection, paraneoplastic syndromes, and sequelae of intensive treatment. Although chronic anemia associated with cancer is seldom life-threatening, it causes quality-of-life problems for individuals with cancer and is often exacerbated by intensive chemotherapy or combined modalities such as chemotherapy plus radiation therapy. The relationship between anemia and fatigue was demonstrated in a study by Cella who found that patients with hemoglobin levels greater than 12 g/dL reported significantly less fatigue and fewer nonfatigue anemia symptoms than patients with hemoglobin levels less than 12 g/dL.[19] Anemia is one of the most frequent disease- or treatment-related causes of fatigue. There are multiple causes of cancer-related anemia, including blood loss, iron or vitamin deficiency, myelosuppression caused by treatments, hemolysis, or tumor involvement of the marrow.

Severe myelosuppression can occur as the result of chemotherapy and radiation therapy to the bone marrow, particularly in the pelvis or spine. The increasing doses of chemotherapy and more intense courses of chemotherapy and radiation have made stem-cell depletion more common. Iron-deficiency anemia occurs most often in individuals with cancer when chronic blood loss is common, such as those with genitourinary and gastrointestinal cancers and cancers of the head and neck.

Pain

Pain associated with cancer can interfere with the activities of daily living. Many studies report decreased functional capacity, diminished strength, and decreased endurance. Pain has been associated with psychological effects that contribute to fatigue, such as personal distress, depression, and increased anxiety, fear, and somatic preoccupation. One study found that pain and fatigue, mobility, and difficulties in sleeping were among the problems that patients with colorectal and gastric cancer were most concerned about following surgery.[37] Hickok et al found in a retrospective study of 50 patients receiving radiation therapy for histologically diagnosed lung cancer, that 40 had pain.[38] Fatigue developed in 39 of the patients but closely followed development of pain in only 11 patients. Pain was independently associated with lack of energy in a study of 187 patients with metastatic and locally advanced cancer.[35] Fatigue and pain were found to be frequent and problematic side effects for women who were receiving treatment for breast cancer.[39]

Surgery

Fatigue is a frequent sequela of surgery. It is thought to be caused by injury to tissue and the surgical stress response, with subsequent increased demands on organ function, and by the effects of anesthesia and analgesics given before and after surgery. Changes in organ function may result from endocrine and metabolic changes due to the trauma of surgery.[40] Salmon and Hall have proposed that postoperative fatigue is the result of physiologic, psychological, and cultural factors that serve to maintain homeostasis while retaining the capacity to respond to new stressors.[41] This response is supported by cultural belief in the necessity of convalescence.[41] Fatigue following surgery has been found to last up to 6 months or longer. In a study of 60 patients with colorectal cancer, those who had conventional surgery had greater fatigue than those who had laparoscopic surgery.[37] A time-series study of women who had surgery for breast cancer found that fatigue and pain were the most frequently reported symptoms at 6 weeks, 3 months, and 6 months following surgery.[42] Advances in surgical techniques, such as laparoscopic surgery, may decrease the fatigue experienced by individuals with cancer. In a study of 60 patients with colorectal cancer, postoperative fatigue and analgesic requirements were lower after laparoscopic colorectal surgery than after conventional surgery.[36] Attentional fatigue has also been identified following surgery. In a study of women with breast cancer, Cimprich found that being older and having more extensive surgery increased the likelihood of attentional fatigue.[43]

Inadequate nutrition related to gastrointestinal disturbances such as nausea, vomiting, and retching has been well documented in the literature. However, fatigue can be the cause of decreased nutritional intake as well, which leads to a cycle of decreased nutrition and increased fatigue.

Psychological factors

Several psychological factors have been associated with fatigue in individuals with cancer, including anxiety, depression,[27,44-46] anticipatory nausea and vomiting, and pain. Anxiety and depression in individuals with cancer are frequently related to the stress associated with the diagnosis and treatment of cancer. Those patients with cancer at greatest risk for depression have inadequate pain control, preexisting mood disorders, advanced disease, or are in poor physical condition.[47] A higher incidence of anxiety and depression in individuals with cancer has been correlated with treatment-related fatigue. However, Hickok et al found fatigue in 39 of the 50 patients (78%) with lung cancer, but only 12% had depression.[38]

Situational factors associated with fatigue include sleep disturbances, decreased activity, immobility, and polypharmacy for concomitant health problems. Frequently, individuals who are experiencing fatigue are encouraged to get more rest. This decreased activity leads to muscle wasting and lowers functional capacity and endurance. Foltz et al found that more than 50% of the patients who had received at least one cycle of chemotherapy as inpatients reported having fatigue and sleeping difficulties following their hospitalization.[48] Another study compared 61 women who had received chemotherapy for breast cancer to 59 women with no history of cancer. Those who had received chemotherapy had more severe fatigue that was correlated with poorer quality of sleep.[49]

Radiation therapy

Fatigue associated with radiation therapy may be caused by anemia, an accumulation of cell-destruction end products, or increased energy requirements to repair damaged epithelial tissue. Radiation therapy has known and predictable side effects depending on the site of radiation treatment. For example, individuals who receive radiation to the bronchus experience cough and difficulty swallowing, while those who receive radiation for gynecologic cancer experience diarrhea, urinary frequency, and urinary burning.[50] The incidence of fatigue in individuals receiving radiation therapy has been well documented.[27,28]

Fatigue is the most commonly reported systemic side effect of radiation therapy. It has been reported to occur in 65%–78% of individuals receiving radiation therapy[38] and has been related to length of treatment, pain, depression, and weight loss. Radiation therapy has a cumulative effect, and many individuals report worsening symptoms later in their treatment. A study of cancer patients receiving radiation therapy found that just after radiation therapy, fatigue either increased or remained stable while depression decreased.[46] At 9 months, fatigue had decreased, whereas levels of depression remained stable. Vogelzang et al conducted a survey of 419 cancer patients who had received chemotherapy, radiation therapy, or both, and found that 78% experienced fatigue during the course of their disease and treatment.[20] Thirty-two percent of these patients experienced daily fatigue; in addition 32% reported that fatigue significantly affected their daily routine. Most of these patients considered fatigue a symptom that had to be endured; half of these patients did not discuss treatment options for fatigue with their oncologists.

The cumulative effect of radiation therapy was demonstrated in a study of 76 patients with breast cancer who were receiving external radiation therapy and were followed from the start of treatment to 6 months posttreatment.[27] Fatigue significantly increased over the course of treatment and was highest at the last week of treatment. Three months after treatment, fatigue returned to pretreatment levels. Fatigue in this study was not found to be influenced by age, stage of disease, time since surgery, weight, or length of time since diagnosis. It was significantly related to symptom distress, psychologic distress, and self-reported fatigue-relief strategies. In a study of patients who had completed radiation treatment for prostate or breast cancer, Walker et al found that fatigue was the most frequently reported continuing side effect.[51]

Chemotherapy

Fatigue is frequently reported by individuals during the course of their chemotherapy. Chemotherapy-related fatigue may be associated with anemia or with an accumulation of cell-destruction end products. The side effects associated with chemotherapy vary according to the type and dose of chemotherapy, but fatigue is the side effect most frequently reported.[3,24,30,39] The chemotherapy agents that are more likely to cause anemia are thiotepa, mechlorethamine hydrochloride, cactinomycin, cytarabine, cyclophosphamide, cladribine, cisplatin, carboplatin, busulfan, and aldesleukin.[52] Persistent fatigue has often been reported as a long-term side effect of adjuvant chemotherapy.

The impact of fatigue associated with chemotherapy has been demonstrated in numerous studies. Patterns of fatigue, activity, and rest were examined in a study of 72 women receiving adjuvant chemotherapy for breast cancer.[53] The Piper Fatigue Scale was used to measure fatigue at 48 hours after treatment and at treatment cycle midpoints. Wrist actigraphs which provide continuous monitoring of activity and motion were used to measure activity and rest cycles for 96 hours during each treatment and for 72 hours at each treatment-cycle midpoint. Fatigue scores were significantly different over time, and they were higher at treatment and lower at cycle midpoints. Activity levels were also significantly different over time and reflected the fatigue pattern. In a study of 307 women receiving treatment for breast cancer, fatigue was the most common and problematic side effect.[39]

A qualitative study of 127 adult patients was conducted to explore the experience of fatigue from the perspective of patients undergoing chemotherapy. Eight major categories of fatigue were identified, along with the dimensions and properties of fatigue. The descriptions provided by these patients demonstrate the subjective nature of the phenomenon as well as the impact of fatigue on their lives.[54] Another qualitative study of cancer patients receiving chemotherapy examined patients' perceptions of fatigue and tiredness and the nature, pattern, and causes of fatigue in relation to cancer and its treatment. Data were collected during two interviews at the beginning and end of a cycle of chemotherapy and with a diary. Fatigue at some point during the chemotherapy cycle was reported by almost 90% of the patients. Fatigue was most frequently associated with type of cancer, chemotherapy regimen, and changes in sleep patterns.[55]

Several studies have reported fatigue as a long-term side effect of chemotherapy. In a study of 21 women with breast cancer, fatigue was among the most frequently described problems immediately after completing chemotherapy and 6 months later. Most patients had not expected to experience chemotherapy-related problems 6 months after treatment. Fatigue interfered with the daily lives of these women.[3] The long-term effects of chemotherapy were examined in a study of 86 women who had completed adjuvant cytotoxic and/or hormonal therapy for early-stage breast cancer between 2 and 5 years prior.[56] The Functional Living Index—Cancer, the Symptom Distress Scale, the Medical Outcomes Study Short Form 36 were used to collect data. Overall, the women reported a high level of quality of life. Fatigue was the most frequently reported symptom (31.4%), followed by insomnia (23.3%), and local numbness at the surgical site (22.1%).

The characteristics of fatigue were examined in a comparison study of 61 women who had completed chemotherapy for breast cancer an average of more than 15 months prior and 59 women with no history of cancer.[49] The women who had received chemotherapy reported more severe fatigue and worse quality of life because of fatigue. Their fatigue was significantly related to other symptoms including poorer sleep quality and more menopausal symptoms. A study of 109 women who had completed treatment for stage I to stage III breast cancer within the previous 1 to 6 years had similar findings. Low to moderate fatigue was found to persist. When other variables were taken into account, fatigue was found to be significantly related to treatment with chemotherapy.[57]

These studies demonstrate the prevalence and severity of fatigue in individuals receiving chemotherapy for cancer. Fatigue is not only the most prevalent side effect, it interferes with activities of daily living and has a negative impact on quality of life. The persistent fatigue that has been demonstrated following chemotherapy needs to be further investigated.

Biologic response modifiers

Biologic response modifiers have the potential to improve both quality and quantity of life for many individuals. However, their effectiveness is often limited by side effects. One of the most common side effects associated with biologic response modifiers is fatigue.[58-61] The fatigue caused by biologic response modifiers may be due to neuromuscular fatigue,[59] changes in sleep patterns,[62] or immune-mediated endocrine disease that occurs during alfa-interferon therapy.[60]

The prevalence of fatigue in individuals receiving this therapy has been demonstrated in several studies. In a study of 92 patients with multiple myeloma who were receiving alfa-interferon, neutropenia and fatigue were the most common adverse effects.[63] A study by Johnston evaluated the efficacy and toxicity of combination biochemotherapy compared to chemotherapy alone in 65 patients with metastatic melanoma.[64] Patients treated with combination chemotherapy had significantly higher fatigue than those treated with chemotherapy alone (26% vs. 13%), and response rates were not improved with combination therapy. The dose-limiting effects of interferon were shown in a study of 13 patients with metastatic melanoma. Seven of the patients required 50% dose reduction because of fatigue and other side effects.[65]

The fatigue and other side effects associated with biologic response modifiers have led to decreased dosages and termination of treatment in some cases. Because fatigue is one of the dose-limiting side effects associated with biologic response modifiers, the positive results found by Karp with low-dose interleukin-2 are particularly encouraging.[66] This also highlights the need for more studies of low-dose biotherapy.

Physiologic Alterations

Pathophysiology

Fatigue is frequently classified as either central or peripheral. According to the central-peripheral model of fatigue, the central and peripheral mechanisms may operate alone or together to produce fatigue.[67] *Central fatigue* originates in the central nervous system and refers to impairments or efforts in the central processing of stimuli that originate in working muscles. Causes of central fatigue may include impaired spinal cord transmission, inhibition of voluntary effort, or nerve cell malfunction. Another cause of central fatigue may be increased 5-hydroxytryptamine. According to Davis, there is increasing evidence that increased brain serotonin (5-HT) can lead to central fatigue, thereby causing a deterioration in performance.[68] *Peripheral fatigue* refers to muscle exhaustion during exertion and occurs because of impairments in the peripheral nerves and contracting muscles.[69] Sites and mechanisms of peripheral fatigue that have been examined include neuromuscular junction, altered muscle metabolites, and peripheral changes in muscle function.[70] The fatigue experienced by individuals with cancer may be due to the central and peripheral release of cytokines and lymphokines by white blood cells,[59] which lead to loss of muscle protein. Much of the research on cytokines and lymphokines has been done on animals and individuals with chronic fatigue. Interleukin-1 (IL-1) and other cytokines are associated with muscle loss, decreased activity, and slower recovery time following activity. Increased levels of cytokines have been found in individuals with chronic fatigue syndrome,[71] and there is evidence that some cytokines are involved in sleep regulation.[72]

Theories of Causation

Several hypotheses have been developed to explain the possible physiologic causes of cancer fatigue. The causes of fatigue in individuals with cancer may be related to the primary tumor and metastasis to one or more systems. For example, cardiac or pulmonary function may be compromised as a result of a tumor, or severe anemia may lead to decreased oxygenation. Cancers that affect the endocrine glands may cause fatigue due to metabolic changes.[73] In addition, the malignant process is thought to cause changes in protein turnover and abnormalities in glucose and lipid metabolism that cause physiologic changes in tumor-free muscle tissue in individuals with cancer, which can result in fatigue.[74,75] The secretion of cytokines by monocytes and inflammatory cells stimulated in response to the cancer cells may also cause cancer-related fatigue due to loss of muscle.[73] Concomitant health problems such as chronic obstructive pulmonary disease may contribute to or exacerbate cancer fatigue.

Clearly, cancer fatigue is a complex problem that is impacted by the malignancy, tumor metastasis, psychological factors, and treatment effects.

Clinical Manifestations

The manifestations of fatigue can be either subjective or objective. Subjective signs are those that only the individual can evaluate, while objective signs can be assessed by another. According to Piper et al, subjective manifestations are the individual's perception of the occurrence and distress caused by the fatigue.[8] This may include the emotional or psychological and physical feelings of fatigue, the perception of interference with daily living activities, and the amount of distress caused by the fatigue. Objective manifestations may include weight loss, decreased energy, apathy, anemia, weakness, lack of motivation, decreased attention, excessive sleepiness, or changes in sleep patterns.

Assessment of Fatigue

Fatigue must be assessed in relation to the individual's expectations, daily patterns of living, state of health/ health deviations, environmental conditions, and prescribed diagnostic, therapeutic, and rehabilitative measures. The occurrence and distress of tiredness, weakness, lack of energy, and decreased concentration must be assessed as different entities. Fatigue is frequently associated with physical functioning or the ability to perform certain tasks. Although the Karnofsky Performance Status, an instrument useful for determining equivalent baseline performance between individuals or among groups, has often been used in cancer clinical trials, it inadequately portrays the complexities of fatigue.[76] Another instrument frequently used in clinical practice to rate fatigue is the Common Toxicity Criteria (CTC). Fatigue is rated on the CTC on a Likert-type scale from 0 to 4. The absence of fatigue is 0; fatigue that is above baseline, but does not alter normal activities is rated 1; moderate fatigue or fatigue causing difficulty in performing some activities is rated 2; severe fatigue or the loss of ability to perform some activities is rated 3; and fatigue that is disabling or causes a person to become bedridden is rated 4.

These measures of fatigue are used by practitioners to evaluate an individual's level of fatigue. However, it is more important to assess the individual's perception of fatigue as fatigue is often a subjective symptom. In a study of 2252 patients with cancer of the prostate, there were significant differences in patient and physician assessment of several domains including fatigue.[77] Physicians underestimated all patient symptoms. The differences in patient and nurse assessment of symptoms were also demonstrated in a study of hospice patients' perceptions of their symptom experiences and those of the hospice nurse assessing them.[78] Patients and nurses both completed the Adapted Symptom Distress Scale (ASDS-2) Form 2 on patient admission, and at 2 and 4 weeks after admission. In this study hospice nurses overestimated their patients' symptom experiences, including fatigue. Another study investigated the agreement between family caregivers' reports and cancer patients' reports of symptoms. Although the rate of agreement between patient and caregiver was highest for fatigue, the overall accuracy of caregiver reports was approximately 71%.[79] These studies highlight the importance of having patients assess their own fatigue.

Several instruments have been used to assess an individual's level of fatigue. These include single-item self-report scales, comprehensive instruments that include measures of fatigue or fatigue subscales, and multiple-item fatigue instruments. The most commonly used single-item scales are visual analog scales and Likert-type scales that ask individuals to rate the presence or severity of fatigue. The Rhoten Fatigue Scale, an example of a visual analog type of scale, rates fatigue from 0 "not tired, peppy" to 10 "total exhaustion."[80] It can be completed in a minimal amount of time and can be used by either the individual or the health care provider. Some comprehensive instruments that include measures of fatigue are the ASDS-2, a 31-item Likert-type instrument with 13 subscales[9]; the RAND Health Survey, a 36-item self-rating scale with 8 subscales[81]; and the Sickness Impact Profile, a 136-item instrument with 12 subscales.[82] Some of the more frequently used multiple-item fatigue instruments include the Revised Piper Fatigue Scale,[83] a 22-item Likert-type scale, with 4 subscales and 4 short answer questions; and the Fatigue Symptom Checklist, a 30-item self-report instrument with 3 subscales.[84]

The choice of which instrument to use to assess fatigue depends on the individual population and purpose of the assessment. Single-item scales are easy to administer and time-efficient in clinical practice. The multiple-item fatigue instruments generally have demonstrated greater reliability and validity, but may be too time consuming and taxing to use in daily clinical practice. The comprehensive instruments generally have similar advantages and disadvantages to the multiple-item fatigue instruments but are able to assess multiple symptoms. The subscales of the comprehensive instruments have demonstrated reliability and validity and can be used separately to assess individual symptoms, thereby decreasing the number of items to assess a symptom such as fatigue.

Cognitive, mental, affective, and temporal effects have also been identified as components of fatigue. Cimprich examined loss of concentration and decrease in memory or alertness. Assessment tools used previously to evaluate attention and concentration focused on global impairments such as psychiatric disturbances but were not always able to detect subtle impairments.[18] Clinical assessment for loss of concentration should begin with the initial contact and continue over time. Areas to be assessed include level of alertness, attention span, ability to focus and concentrate on an intended activity, and subjective perception of loss of concentration in daily life.

Two common tools currently used to detect cognitive or mental dysfunction include the Mini–Mental State Exam (MMSE) and the Cognitive Capacity Screening Examination (CCSE). The MMSE is a simple questionnaire that assesses orientation, registration, attention and calculation, recall, and language.[85] It is scored between 0 (worst possible score) and 30 (perfect score). Normal values are often considered to be 24 or higher in individuals who have command of the English language and have at least an eighth grade education. The CCSE is a 30-item instrument developed to assess cognitive impairment in nonpsychiatric patients.[86]

The temporal component of fatigue is linked to an individual's 24-hour circadian pattern. The temporal component considers what time of day individuals might have more energy and looks for patterns of fatigue. Assessment of the temporal component examination is important in differentiating between acute and chronic fatigue and in determining appropriate interventions. The affective dimension of fatigue includes distress, irritability, impatience, and lack of motivation. These represent the emotional meanings that fatigue may have, and raise the question of depression and how it relates to fatigue.

History and Physical Examination

Assessment of fatigue should include a careful history describing the pattern of fatigue and identifying the factors that contribute to its development. The initial assessment should include the pattern, onset, duration, and intensity of fatigue. Factors that increase or alleviate fatigue should also be explored. The history should include concurrent health problems, current medications, and associated treatment side effects. Patterns of sleep and rest and the effects of fatigue on activities of daily living and lifestyle are important areas to assess. Fatigue assessment should also include nutritional intake, change in appetite and weight, and psychological factors. A complete physical examination helps differentiate between physical weakness and fatigue; it should include diagnostic and laboratory tests for anemia and other physiologic causes of fatigue.

The importance of comprehensive assessment of fatigue was demonstrated in a qualitative study by Glaus et al that explored themes of fatigue in individuals with cancer and compared fatigue/tiredness in 20 patients with cancer and in 20 healthy individuals.[87] In unstructured interviews to discover the experiences and descriptions of fatigue, three categories emerged in both groups. Fifty-nine percent of patients with cancer and 55% of healthy individuals provided themes that were classified as physical, including decreased physical performance, weakness, and unusual need for rest or sleep. Themes classified as affective, including decreased motivation, no energy, anxiety, and sadness, were identified by 29% of patients with cancer and 21% of healthy individuals. More

healthy individuals (24%) identified themes in the cognitive category than did patients with cancer (12%). Both groups identified physical themes as being most frequent, but patients with cancer described the fatigue as unusual tiredness while healthy individuals described it as normal tiredness.

A thorough assessment is necessary to provide information about both the physical and psychological factors producing fatigue in the individual with cancer. Assessment of basic conditioning factors, including personal and sociocultural factors, patterns of living, health state, and developmental state, provides the foundation for interventions and helps patients develop self-care behaviors and coping strategies to manage the effects of fatigue on lifestyle.[21,88] A comprehensive assessment of the patient's health care situation must include the perspectives of physician and patient. For an example of an initial assessment form that includes data based on the patient's perspective, see Figure 32-3. These data, the pathophysiology of the present and past medical diagnoses, clinical manifestations, usual treatment, and nursing management, are essential for the development of an appropriate patient-centered plan of care.

Therapeutic Approaches and Nursing Care

A variety of therapeutic approaches is required to assist the patient who is experiencing fatigue. Assisting the patient with cancer-related fatigue to maintain quality of life is the desired outcome of nursing care. Nursing interventions must meet both the psychological and physical needs of the patient and consider the causes of fatigue. Cancer-related fatigue may be caused by anemia, inadequate nutrition, infection, anxiety or depression, changes in rest and sleep patterns, or decreased mobility. Interventions for fatigue discussed in this section include preparatory information to aid in management, and self-care activities including conservation of energy, exercise, rest and sleep, treatment of anemia, and motivational strategies.

Management of Fatigue

Individuals with cancer have attempted to alleviate their fatigue by adopting various self-care behaviors. Orem defines self-care as the activities that individuals initiate and perform on their own behalf to maintain life, health, and well being.[88] Self-care includes not only self-responsibility, independence, interdependence, and attendance to mind, body, and spirit but prophylactic measures, self-determination regarding therapy, and the decision to seek and secure appropriate health care assistance. Individuals learning to live with the effects of their pathologic conditions and medical care measures frequently have to develop a new repertoire of skills and knowledge. As

Personal and Sociocultural

Age: <u>36</u>
Gender: <u>Female</u>
Family: <u>Married (2nd marriage); 2 daughters, 15 and 8 years, and an 8-month-old son (older daughter from first marriage); mother and father deceased, 1 sister, 2 brothers; husband is self-employed carpenter</u>

Educational Level: <u>College Graduate</u>
Occupation: <u>Teacher (Elementary)</u>
Religion: <u>Church of God (attends regularly)</u>
Sociocultural Orientation: <u>White, middle class, raised in a rural Midwest community</u>
Relevant Life Experiences: <u>Both parents died with cancer at an early age (before patient turned 28)</u>
Social Roles: <u>Wife, mother, sister, breadwinner</u>

Patterns of Living

Living Environmental and Family System: <u>Lives with husband and children 100 miles from treatment center</u>

Health Habits (Self-Care Practices): <u>Considers herself to have good personal hygiene: teeth in good repair; sees dentist regularly; overweight; doesn't exercise; inconsistent with BSE: has not enrolled in cancer-screening program; sees doctor for yearly Pap smear; obtains a suntan every summer—occasionally sunburns; Tylenol for headaches; daily multiple vitamins; birth control pills for 13 years; and again after birth of 8-month-old son</u>

- Activity Patterns
  Usual/Routine: Household, church/community/school (children and employment)
  Preferred/Selected: Maintain employment; selected church and family activities

- Sleep/Rest Patterns
  Usual: 6–7 hours/weeknight
  Preferred: 8 hours/night

Nutritional Patterns:

Number of meals/snacks per day: <u>3 meals (light breakfast, large evening meal) and 2 snacks, A.M. and P.M.</u>
Food likes and dislikes: <u>Prefers starches, desserts; limited meat, dairy products (except ice cream), fresh fruits or vegetables</u>

Preferred Learning Style: <u>Is an avid reader; feels comfortable in groups but prefers reading and one-to-one demonstrations</u>

Health State and Health Care Systems

Present Health State: <u>Recently diagnosed with breast cancer; sought medical help after she discovered a breast lump while taking a shower; had (L) mastectomy with reconstruction; preparing to take adjuvant chemotherapy. Regular menstrual cycle since age 12 years. Questions the amount of time treatment will take from her many activities.</u>

Previous Health Concerns and Self-Care Actions: <u>3 normal pregnancies—only hospitalizations were for childbirth</u>

Perception of Health Care: <u>Views system as helpful—patient wants to be an informed customer and involved in decision-making</u>

Developmental State: <u>Early adult transitions</u>

Self-Management System for Care—Physical, Emotional, Spiritual: <u>Acknowledges some fear of cancer due to experience with parents. Lack of preventive health care due to fear of cancer experience with parents; looks to close friends for emotional support; feels she has strong spiritual faith; considers minister a close friend.</u>

Rationale

Assessment of factors affecting patient's perspective of health situations

Experiences influencing the seeking and securing of appropriate medical assistance and management of health state

Factors to be considered when assisting this patient. Modifying self-concept, self-image, and learning to live with the effects of pathologic conditions, e.g., fatigue and medical care measures.

Considerations for maintaining a balance of activity and rest. Regularly evaluate the severity of fatigue, and the individual's perception of what limitations are acceptable.

Data helpful to develop a nutritional dietary plan for potential energy requirements of health

A guide regarding the type of patient education

Provides information on coping strategies

An index of patient's life experiences and possible effects on perceptions of present health state

Figure 32-3   Patient assessment form.

health-related limitations in self-care are encountered, the goal of nursing is to teach strategies that will allow the individual to continue self-care. Patient education is dependent on an accurate assessment of the individual's basic conditioning factors, self-care abilities and capabilities, and therapeutic self-care demands.

Initial and ongoing assessments reveal information essential for effective education. Goals for education based on the assessment and deficits should be established with the individual and family. Ongoing assessments must be sensitive to comments from the individual or family that may indicate fatigue or decreased energy; remarks revealing any other limiting factors must also be considered. Following diagnosis and prior to treatment, individuals with cancer are often bewildered and overwhelmed by the quantity of general information about the treatment and its potential side effects that is thrust on them. In fact, many have indicated uncertainty as to what to really expect.[89] Often, health care professionals provide only procedural information about specific events that will happen and recommend actions that the individual should take as part of self-management.[90]

Preparatory sensory information

Preparatory sensory information incorporates sensory, procedural, and temporal information that reflects the experience of an event from the patient's point of view. Information that clearly describes what patients can expect before, during, and after treatment is crucial for effective patient education.[7] Information conveyed in a positive, nonthreatening manner and given before the treatment allows the patient to formulate a more effective mental image about the pending experience. An accurate mental image also decreases ambiguity about the event, activates innate coping strategies, and permits effective cognitive management of the fatigue experience. The goals and behaviors of patients with cancer are largely determined by their perceptions of the illness. Therefore, it is important to understand an individual's perception and its potential influence on actual experience and self-care/coping behaviors. For example, symptoms such as fatigue and weakness require that individuals modify their behavior to maintain normal self-care function and allow them to continue with valued activities. In addition, the individual's expectations about an experience and the actual experience have been shown to be related.[10] Studies have demonstrated that preparation for stressful happenings can reduce symptom experience (occurrence and distress) and facilitate adaptation.[7,91–93] Rhodes et al found a statistically significant relationship ($P = .015$) between patients' expectations of symptom experience and the symptom distress they experienced. Often, fatigue is referred to as a side effect that may convey a sense of secondary importance to the disease process and treatment.[54] Yet, fatigue is often a chief concern of individuals receiving chemotherapy.[21,30,54] The preparation individuals receive may yield unrealistic expectations for their experience, as the dimensions of cancer-related fatigue are unlike anything they have previously experienced.[54]

Information about fatigue, including neutral descriptions of specific sensations to be experienced and realistic expectations, helps the patient cope and develop self-care behaviors more easily. For example, if an individual is starting a treatment regimen whose participants have experienced little or no fatigue, then it is appropriate to give this factual information to prepare the patient. The amount of factual information provided will depend on what individuals want to know and what they need to know to safely live with their treatment and its side effects. For example, if a treatment regimen consists of combination antineoplastic agents, it is not important for the individual to know the drugs most likely to cause neutropenia, hence fatigue, but it is important for the patient to know when this potential side effect might occur and how to manage it.

Self-Care Activities

The nursing management of fatigue may best be addressed by instruction for self-care activities. This includes teaching about energy conservation, relaxation techniques, diversional activities, medication information, dietary modifications, and emotional support. A general teaching guide about fatigue for patients has been developed to assist nurses in designing and implementing individualized teaching (Table 32-1). In a study evaluating the strategies patients use to cope with fatigue during chemotherapy, patients identified 31 different self-care actions to relieve their fatigue.[30] These actions provided partial relief 53.7% of the time, nearly complete relief 25.5% of the time, and complete relief only 11.5% of the time. Most self-care activities such as resting, napping, and modifying activity were chosen because they seemed sensible; less than 7% of self-care was based on the advice of others. Similar to Dodd's studies, these findings indicate that the self-care activities attempted for fatigue are only partially effective against this severe treatment side effect.[90,94,95] Individualized educational strategies are considered to be the most effective preventive interventions; however, definitive research is needed.

Conservation of energy

The conservation of energy in the patient experiencing cancer-related fatigue can be accomplished by rescheduling activities to allow for rest periods or to decrease the amount of time that energy is needed.[96] An individual may develop an activity plan that enlists others to perform activities that are deemed less important, allowing the patient to conserve energy for activities that are deemed more important.[31] Other activities may need to be abandoned or completed in a different manner. The environment may also need modification to decrease energy demands.

Employers, family, and friends must be made aware of the likelihood of this unseen symptom and be willing to develop flexible strategies to help the patient manage fatigue, such as decreasing nonessential activities, enlisting the aid of others, and allowing a flexible work schedule. Table 32-2 provides a patient guide with strategies to manage fatigue.

Exercise

With the increased emphasis on cancer-related fatigue in recent years, more studies have examined the causes of fatigue and requisite interventions and self-care behaviors to manage fatigue in adults with cancer. Winningham was one of the first researchers to look at exercise and

Table 32-1 Teaching Guide About Fatigue

Self-Care Behaviors/Interventions	Expected Patient Outcome
Nursing Diagnosis: Lack of understanding of fatigue and possible causes and effects.	
• Assess and differentiate potential causes of patient's feelings of fatigue, tiredness, weakness.	Patient and significant others understand the causes of fatigue and the difference between fatigue, tiredness, and weakness. The patient and participants also understand the purpose of antineoplastic therapies and are better prepared.
• Fatigue (related to cancer): subjective experience; intensity, duration and distress vary; not completely relieved with rest or sleep; multidimensional and multicausal.	
• Tiredness: subjective experience; relieved with rest or sleep.	
• Weakness: subjective and objective; lack of physical strength of a given anatomical part or a generalized feeling of insufficient strength.	
• Explain that fatigue is multicausal: Therapeutic interventions of physiologic/biochemical changes Psychosocial, economic stress factors Imbalance of rest and activity (decreased activity) Insufficient sleep Inadequate nutrition	Patient will verbalize descriptions of fatigue and its sensations.
• Explain the purpose of antineoplastic therapy (e.g., chemotherapy, radiation therapy, biological response therapy [to destroy cancer cells]).	An understanding of fatigue patterns based on kind of therapy.
• Discuss possible patterns of fatigue occurrence; provide possible patterns (e.g., nadir 10–14 days postchemotherapy).	
• Provide preparatory information (procedural, temporal, and sensory for specific therapy and diagnosis, if known).	
• Appraise the existence of fatigue; measure fatigue occurrence and fatigue distress separately on a scale from 1 to 10.	Uses a numerical visual analog scale to measure the occurrence and distress of fatigue.
• Suggest recording level of fatigue at multiple points in time.	
• Encourage patients to discuss fatigue with family and health care providers; cumulative effect of radiation therapy and energy changes may be gradual.	
• Assess usual activity level and threshold.	
• Check laboratory reports and appraise effects.	
Nursing Diagnosis: Insufficient knowledge to institute appropriate self-care actions to manage fatigue.	
• Decrease nonessential activities; increase dependence on others for home management (meal preparation, cleaning, grocery shopping), transportation; avoid unscheduled extra demands; plan, prioritize, pace, and modify activities.	Patient and participants develop helpful strategies to manage fatigue by utilizing family and friends for essential activities.
• Suggest a journal, log, or diary of activities, feelings, and an evaluation of self-care actions.	Patient will use a journal of self-care actions.
• Teach diversional techniques, relaxation procedures, and distraction/diversion.	Diversional activity and relaxation techniques will be incorporated in daily life.
• Provide information concerning counseling or support groups.	
• Maintain a list of names and phone numbers of individuals volunteering assistance.	
• Limit energy expenditure.	

fatigue.[32] Exercise as an intervention to manage fatigue in women with breast cancer has been examined by Mock et al.[97,98] A study of women receiving chemotherapy for breast cancer compared women who participated in a structured walking program and attended support group meetings to women who received conventional supportive care. Women in the intervention group had significantly less fatigue than women in the conventional care group.[97] Another study of 46 women receiving radiation therapy for breast cancer found that a self-paced walking exercise decreased fatigue during treatment.[98] Suh and Lee had similar findings when they investigated the effects of a walking exercise on fatigue in 34 women receiv-

ing adjuvant chemotherapy for breast cancer.[99] Fatigue scores were considerably lower for women in the walking group.

Graydon et al conducted two interviews with women receiving either chemotherapy or radiation therapy for cancer to determine their level of fatigue and the effectiveness of the strategies used to relieve fatigue.[100] Patients were significantly more fatigued at the second interview, the midpoint of any chemotherapy cycle or the end of a 5- or 6-week course of radiation therapy. However, those with more effective fatigue-relieving strategies were less fatigued, relatively speaking, at that time. Sleep and exercise were the most effective strategies used to relieve

Table 32-2 Strategies to Manage Fatigue: A Patient Guide

Energy Conservation

- Limit energy expenditure.
- Determine the amount of activity you can do comfortably; preserve normality (e.g., going to work, maintaining a routine).
- Plan/schedule and rearrange activities and work (e.g., schedule therapy at most convenient hour or prior to weekend or days off work).
- Plan a variety of new/enjoyable activities to avoid the performance of a routine. Reserve energy for fun activities.
- Develop some meaningful goals, both short-term and long-term.
- Decrease nonessential activities.
- Increase dependence on others for home management (e.g., cleaning, shopping, meal preparation), transportation, and care.
- Avoid energy-consuming activities.
- Consider energy-saving techniques of daily living (e.g., avoid toweling—use a terry cloth robe; sit rather than stand for chores and other pertinent activities; use assistive devices).
- Invite family members' energy-saving ideas and aids:
    Wear school clothes 2 days to reduce laundry.
    Eliminate homemade desserts and eat prepared desserts.

Rest, Sleep, and Exercise

- Space periodic rest periods with activity/exercise during the day. Rest before becoming too tired! Try to keep ahead of the game!
- Avoid the use of stimulants, including caffeine.
- Avoid alcohol.
- Use relaxation techniques (e.g., progressive muscle relaxation, guided imagery).
- Follow an individualized plan of exercise with intermittent rest periods during the day.
- Participate in nonstrenuous exercise (e.g., walking may help to relieve fatigue).
- Participate in yoga, stretching exercises.
- Establish a regular bedtime.
- Take a warm bath.
- Sip warm milk or herbal teas.
- Listen to soothing music.
- Have a back massage.
- Read a relaxing book.
- Establish a quiet environment.

Motivation

- Encourage verbalization of thoughts and feelings regarding what makes life meaningful.
- Emphasize the positive aspects of life (e.g., the quality of our days, not the number of days makes life worthwhile). Uncertainty exists except for the present moment.
- Encourage participation and control in their treatment plan.
- Provide reminders that although illness is not desired, *everyone* can choose the way they wish to respond.
- Utilize appropriate humor (e.g., cartoons, videos, enjoyable people).
- Encourage communication with friends and loved ones.
- Encourage environmental change (e.g., indoor/outdoor).
- Encourage storytelling (e.g., life's accomplishments/events).

fatigue. Another study reported that exercise and rest were the most commonly used strategies to manage fatigue in 219 cancer survivors.[101] Of interest, patients with breast cancer reported greater benefits from exercise than those with non-Hodgkin's lymphoma. The findings from these studies indicate that exercise is an effective intervention for fatigue. Friendenreich and Courneya conducted a comprehensive review of the literature on exercise and rehabilitation of patients with cancer.[102] The nine studies available were all of patients with breast cancer. Based on a qualitative review, Friendenreich and Courneya concluded that exercise improved physiologic and psychological well-being; however, these findings should only be considered preliminary because of methodological problems in the studies. The findings from this analysis of published literature supports the need for more research to identify the optimal level of exercise for managing cancer-related fatigue, and the need for studies to determine which individuals will benefit most from exercise to reduce fatigue.

Exercise programs must be tailored to the individual based on age, gender, condition, and concurrent major health problems. For example, if a patient has other health problems such as cardiovascular disease or gross obesity (50% over ideal body weight), rhythmic walking activity should be modified. It is important to assess what the patient has previously been doing and what they currently are able to do comfortably. Patients who have been accustomed to an active exercise program may need to be cautioned about the intensity, frequency, and type of activity that may be appropriate. Additional studies on the effectiveness of specific exercise interventions for cancer-related fatigue are needed.

Rest and sleep

Rest and sleep are often the most recommended interventions for individuals with cancer who are experiencing fatigue. Rest may include napping, taking it easy, or removing oneself from areas of high activity and noise. Rest and napping were among the most frequently cited self-care strategies in the study by Richardson and Ream[30] but were less effective in relieving fatigue than going to bed early. Fatigue, the second most common symptom in a study of individuals who had received chemotherapy, was most often managed by increasing time spent resting and sleeping. For some individuals, rest and sleep can relieve or reduce fatigue. In caring for the individual with fatigue, it is important to schedule medications, treatments, and other activities around periods of rest and sleep. Corticosteroids are frequently used in antineoplastic drug regimens and in antiemetic drug protocols. While there are several adverse neurologic effects from glucocorticoids, sleep disruption, insomnia, restlessness, and increased motor activity are the most offensive to the patient combating cancer-related fatigue. An inability to concentrate or to maintain attention is extremely distressful and may lead to increased uncertainty, anxiety, and depression.[52] Other symptoms that may increase fatigue or interfere with rest and sleep must be assessed. A balance of activity and rest, neither too little nor too much, is essential to avoid increased perceptions of fatigue. A journal or diary of self-care activities and outcomes can be an extremely useful aid for reassessment, planning, and instruction.[48,103,104] In fact, this tool often fosters patient introspection that may direct a change in their self-care activities. The nurse may detect patterns of cause and effect that will help in guiding the patient's care. Figure 32-4 is an example of a self-care journal for fatigue.

Treatment of anemia

Cancer-related fatigue that is caused by anemia may be due to myelosuppression resulting from treatment,

hemolysis, blood loss, tumor involvement, or iron or vitamin deficiency.[6] Treatment of cancer-related fatigue caused by anemia improves the quality of life of these individuals. Red blood cell transfusions have been the usual treatment for severe anemia, with the goal of raising hemoglobin levels. However, due to the risks associated with transfusion, individuals with mild to moderate anemia have generally not been treated. For many of these individuals and those with more severe anemia, the use of recombinant human erythropoietin (epoetin alfa) has been effective in increasing hemoglobin concentration and hematocrit, and in significantly reducing transfusion requirements in patients with chemotherapy-induced anemia.[105] Erythropoietin has been effective in preventing and treating anemia in 50%–60% of the patients who receive it.[106,107] Studies have shown that treatment with erythropoietin is associated with a significant increase in energy level, functional status, and overall enhanced quality of life.[106,108,109] The treatment of cancer-related anemia with blood transfusion or erythropoietin is costly. Meadowcroft et al found that blood transfusions were less costly than erythropoietin in managing anemia in breast cancer patients, but there were no standard guidelines for transfusion.[110] Other studies have examined the financial costs of transfusions and the costs to the patient in terms of risk.[111,112] The findings highlight the need for careful assessment and monitoring of patients receiving transfusions or erythropoietin. Further studies that look at all of the cost-benefits of these treatments for anemia are needed.

Motivational strategies

Limited information is available regarding the relationship of motivation, hope, and uncertainty to fatigue. However, some similarities have been recognized between depression and fatigue. While health care providers and researchers have been aware of the psychosocial aspects of an individual's care and have recognized the interaction between physical and psychosocial rehabilitation, few have studied the mobilizing factors in cancer care. Hope has been defined as a multidimensional force composed of feelings, thoughts, and experiences that act as motivators, moving people toward a desired goal.[113] Because hope is a motivational force that maintains energy, it is essential in inspiring a patient's pursuit of health and self-care, but it also may effect strategies designed to manage fatigue. Motivational strategies to raise levels of hope can be designed to mobilize the human spirit and empower the individual to take self-improving action. Some motivational strategies are included in Table 32-2.

Conclusion

Fatigue is a major debilitating symptom for individuals with cancer, affecting activities of daily living, impacting treatment choices, and decreasing quality of life. Among the many symptoms associated with cancer and its treat-

INSTRUCTIONS

Please keep daily records in this journal, beginning on the day of your outpatient visit. Carry the journal and a pencil with you at all times so that you can record activities and results as they occur. The more detailed your journal is, the more valuable it will be in assessing your progress. In addition, your careful records will assist us in planning your care and in serving other patients. Your help is greatly appreciated.

The directions below will help you determine what information to put in each column of the journal. In addition, please refer to the sample entries on the next page.

Date, time	Record the date and time of each entry.
How I felt before self-care activity	Record entries as often as desired and on awakening, at noon, midafternoon or early evening, and before going to bed at night.
Self-care activity	Record the names of the medications taken and describe any action you took to improve how you were feeling.
Result	Describe how you felt an hour after completing the self-care activity; you may use the following code: 1 = I felt better 2 = no change 3 = I felt worse

Self-Care Journal Sample

Sample journal entries are shown below. Remember that details are important; if in doubt, include it.

Date/Time	How I Felt Before Self-Care Activity	Self-Care Activity	Result
6/18/99 7 AM	Awakened by alarm, tired, no energy. Hungry	Showered. Dried with terry cloth robe. Ate wheat toast & jam, boiled egg, orange juice & coffee	2
8:15	Need to rest after dressing	Sat in recliner on patio listening to birds	1
8:50	Lack of stamina	Husband drove to work	2
10:30	Weary from decision making	Walked in courtyard for 10 minutes.	1
12:00	Looking forward to seeing friends	Enjoyed lunch with two friends	1
3:00	Less able to concentrate	Called neighbor for ride home from work	2
5:30	Frustrated with childrens' lack of understanding about tiredness	Explained tiredness using marbles to represent mother's energy; removed ½ marbles to show energy needed to fight disease.	1
7:30	Tired, but more able to cope	Reading, while husband takes children to mall.	1

Figure 32-4 Self-care journal for fatigue. (Copyright 2000 by Verna A. Rhodes and Roxanne W. McDaniel. All rights reserved. Used with consent of the authors.)

ment, fatigue is one of the most prevalent symptoms, yet the least understood. Fatigue is the most frequently occurring side effect in individuals receiving chemotherapy and is a major dose-limiting side effect associated with biologic response modifiers. The fatigue individuals with cancer experience is not limited to the time of actual disease but may be a continuing problem even after treatment and during remission.

Several theories and models have been proposed to explain the cancer-related fatigue. However, to date there is no conclusive evidence to support any of these theories. The increased research on cancer-related fatigue has provided information about relationships between type of cancer, treatment modality, and development of fatigue. Other factors that may influence fatigue such as anxiety, depression, and pain have also been investigated. A major limitation of these studies is a lack of consistent measurement. Several studies report the severity and incidence of fatigue from the perspective of health care providers, individuals with cancer, and caregivers. Because fatigue is a subjective symptom, assessment must be based on the individual's perception.

Interventions to prevent or alleviate fatigue have been studied primarily in women with breast cancer. These studies provide support for the efficacy of exercise in this population. However, there has been limited research on exercise interventions in other populations. Qualitative studies have documented the incidence of fatigue and self-care activities used to manage fatigue. Other interventions to decrease fatigue such as resting, rearranging schedules to manage activities, and eliminating nonessential activities have been suggested. Education has been suggested as a strategy to provide information about symptoms associated with the diagnosis and treatment of fatigue and strategies to alleviate it. Providing preparatory sensory information has been effective in reducing side effects associated with medical procedures and has decreased symptom distress. However, limited research has examined the effectiveness of this approach in helping individuals manage fatigue. Further research is needed to identify self-care activities and to test interventions that are effective in managing fatigue.

References

1. Ashbury F, Findlay H: Patients' experiences with cancer in Canada. *Proc Annu Meet Am Soc Clin Oncol* 16:A201, 1997 (abstr)

2. Buckingham R, Fitt J, Sitzia J: Patients' experiences of chemotherapy: Side-effects of carboplatin in the treatment of carcinoma of the ovary. *Eur J Cancer Care* 6:59–71, 1997

3. Beisecker A, Cook MR, Ashworth J, et al: Side effects of adjuvant chemotherapy: Perceptions of node-negative breast cancer patients. *Psychol Oncol* 6:85–93, 1997

4. Dow KH, Ferrell BR, Leigh S, et al: An evaluation of the quality of life among long-term survivors of breast cancer. *Breast Cancer Res Treat* 39:261–273, 1996

5. Ferrell BR, Grant M, Dean GE, et al: "Bone tired": The experience of fatigue and its impact on quality of life. *Oncol Nurs Forum* 23:1539–1547, 1996

6. Aistars J: Fatigue in the cancer patient: A conceptual approach to a clinical problem. *Oncol Nurs Forum* 14:25–30, 1987

7. McDaniel RW, Rhodes VA: Development of a preparatory sensory information videotape for women receiving chemotherapy for breast cancer. *Cancer Nurs* 21:143–148, 1998

8. Winningham ML, Nail LM, Burke MB, et al: Fatigue and the cancer experience: The state of the knowledge. *Oncol Nurs Forum* 21:23–36, 1994

9. Rhodes VA, Watson PM, Johnson MH, et al: Patterns of nausea, vomiting, and distress in patients receiving antineoplastic drug protocols. *Oncol Nurs Forum* 14:35–44, 1987

10. Rhodes VA, Watson PM, McDaniel RW, et al: Expectation and occurrence of postchemotherapy side effects. *Cancer Pract* 3:247–253, 1995

11. Nail LM, King KB: Fatigue. *Semin Oncol Nurs* 3:257–262, 1987

12. Irvine DM, Vincent L, Graydon JE, et al: The prevalence and correlates of fatigue in patients receiving chemotherapy and radiotherapy. *Cancer Nurs* 17:367–378, 1994

13. Johnson M, Maas M: *Nursing Outcomes Classification (NOC)*. St. Louis, Mosby, 1997

14. Piper B: Fatigue, in Carrieri-Kohlman V, Lindsey AM, West CM (eds): *Pathophysiological Phenomena in Nursing: Human Responses to Illness* (ed 2). Philadelphia, Saunders, 1993, pp 279–302

15. Hart LK, Freel MI, Milde FK: Fatigue. *Nurs Clin North Am* 25:967–976, 1990

16. Varicchio C: Selecting a tool for measuring fatigue. *Oncol Nurs Forum* 12:122–127, 1985

17. Glaus A: Assessment of fatigue in cancer and non-cancer patients and in healthy individuals. *Support Care Cancer* 1:305–315, 1993

18. Cimprich B: Attentional fatigue following breast cancer surgery. *Res Nurs Health* 15:199–207, 1992

19. Cella D: The Functional Assessment of Cancer Therapy-Anemia (FACT-A) Scale: A new tool for the assessment of outcomes in cancer anemia and fatigue. *Semin Hematol* 34:13–19, 1997 (suppl 2)

20. Vogelzang NJ, Breitbart W, Cella D, et al: Patient, caregiver, and oncologist perceptions of cancer-related fatigue: Results of a tripart assessment survey. The Fatigue Coalition. *Semin Hematol* 34:4–12, 1997 (suppl 2)

21. Rhodes VA, Watson PM, Hanson B: Patients descriptions of the influence of tiredness and weakness on self-care abilities. *Cancer Nurs* 11:186–194, 1988

22. Blesch KS, Paice JA, Wickham R, et al: Correlates of fatigue in people with breast or lung cancer. *Oncol Nurs Forum* 18:81–87, 1991

23. Skalla K, Lacasse C: Patient education for fatigue. *Oncol Nurs Forum* 19:1537–1539, 1992

24. Dean GE, Spears L, Ferrell BR, et al: Fatigue in patients with cancer receiving interferon alpha. *Cancer Pract* 3:164–172, 1995

25. Piper BF, Rieger PT, Brophy L, et al: Recent advances in the management of biotherapy related side effects: Fatigue. *Oncol Nurs Forum* 16:27–34, 1989

26. Robinson KD, Posner JD: Patterns of self-care needs and interventions related to biologic response modifier therapy: Fatigue as a model. *Semin Oncol Nurs* 8:17–22, 1992

27. Irvine DM, Vincent L, Graydon JE, et al: Fatigue in women with breast cancer receiving radiation therapy. *Cancer Nurs* 21:127–135, 1998

28. Munro AJ, Potter S: A quantitative approach to the distress caused by symptoms in patients treated with radical radiotherapy. *Br J Cancer* 74:640–647, 1996

29. Mast ME: Correlates of fatigue in survivors of breast cancer. *Cancer Nurs* 21:136–142, 1998

30. Richardson A, Ream EK: Self-care behaviours initiated by chemotherapy patients in response to fatigue. *Int J Nurs Stud* 34:35–43, 1997

31. Nail L, Winningham M: Fatigue and weakness in cancer patients: The symptom experience. *Semin Oncol Nurs* 11:272–278, 1995

32. Winningham ML: The role of exercise in cancer therapy, in Eisinger M, Watson RW (eds): *Exercise and Disease*. Boca Raton, FL, CRC Press, 1992, pp 63–70

33. Cella D: Factors influencing quality of life in cancer patients: Anemia and fatigue. *Semin Oncol* 25:43–46, 1998 (suppl 7)

34. Koeller JM: Clinical guidelines for the treatment of cancer-related anemia. *Pharmacotherapy* 18:156–169, 1998

35. Hwang SS, Chang VT, Corpion C, et al: A preliminary study of clinical predictors for lack of energy in patients (pts) with advanced cancer. *Proc Annu Meet Am Soc Clin Oncol* 16: A241, 1997 (abstr)

36. Schwenk W, Bohm B, Muller JM: Postoperative fatigue after laparoscopic or conventional colorectal resections: A prospective randomized trial. *Surg Endosc* 12:1131–1136, 1998

37. Forsberg C, Bjorvell H, Cedermark B: Well-being and its relation to coping ability in patients with colo-rectal and gastric cancer before and after surgery. *Scand J Caring Sci* 10:35–44, 1996

38. Hickok JT, Morrow GR, McDonald S, et al: Frequency and correlates of fatigue in lung cancer patients receiving radiation therapy: Implications for management. *J Pain Symptom Manage* 11:370–377, 1996

39. Longman AJ, Braden CJ, Mishel MH: Pattern of association over time of side-effects burden, self-help, and self-care in women with breast cancer *Oncol Nurs Forum* 24:1555–1560, 1997

40. Kehlet H: Multimodal approach to control postoperative pathophysiology and rehabilitation. *Br J Anaesth* 78:606–617, 1997

41. Salmon P, Hall GM: A theory of postoperative fatigue. *J R Soc Med* 90:661–664, 1997

42. Wyatt GK, Friedman LL: Physical and psychosocial outcomes of midlife and older women following surgery and adjuvant therapy for breast cancer. *Oncol Nurs Forum* 25:761–768, 1998

43. Cimprich B: Age and extent of surgery affect attention in women treated for breast cancer. *Res Nurs Health* 21:229–238, 1998

44. Dimeo F, Stieglitz RD, Novelli-Fischer U, et al: Correlation between physical performance and fatigue in cancer patients. *Ann Oncol* 8:1251–1255, 1997

45. Longman AJ, Braden CJ, Mishel MH: Side effects burden

in women with breast cancer. *Cancer Pract* 4:274–280, 1996

46. Visser MR, Smets EM: Fatigue, depression and quality of life in cancer patients: How are they related? *Support Care Cancer* 6:101–108, 1998

47. Breitbart W: Identifying patients at risk for, and treatment of major psychiatric complications of cancer. *Support Care Cancer* 3:45–60, 1995

48. Foltz AT, Gaines G, Gullatte M: Recalled side effects and self-care actions of patients receiving inpatient chemotherapy. *Oncol Nurs Forum* 23:679–683, 1996

49. Broeckel JA, Jacobsen PB, Horton J, et al: Characteristics and correlates of fatigue after adjuvant chemotherapy for breast cancer. *J Clin Oncol* 16:1689–1696, 1998

50. Fieler VK: Side effects and quality of life in patients receiving high-dose rate brachytherapy. *Oncol Nurs Forum* 24:545–553, 1997

51. Walker BL, Nail LM, Larsen L, et al: Concerns, affect, and cognitive disruption following completion of radiation treatment for localized breast or prostate cancer. *Oncol Nurs Forum* 23:1181–1187, 1996

52. McEvoy GK (ed): American Hospital Formulary Service Drug Information. Bethesda, MD, American Society of Health-System Pharmacists, 1998

53. Berger AM: Patterns of fatigue and activity and rest during adjuvant breast cancer chemotherapy. *Oncol Nurs Forum* 25:51–62, 1998

54. Messias DK, Yeager KA, Dibble SL, et al: Patients' perspectives of fatigue while undergoing chemotherapy. *Oncol Nurs Forum* 24:43–48, 1997

55. Richardson A, Ream E: The experience of fatigue and other symptoms in patients receiving chemotherapy. *Eur J Cancer Care* 5:24–30, 1996 (suppl)

56. Lindley C, Vasa S, Sawyer WT, et al: Quality of life and preferences for treatment following systemic adjuvant therapy for early-stage breast cancer. *J Clin Oncol* 16:1380–1387, 1998

57. Mast ME: Survivors of breast cancer: Illness uncertainty, positive reappraisal, and emotional distress. *Oncol Nurs Forum* 25:555–562, 1998

58. Borden EC, Parkinson D: A perspective on the clinical effectiveness and tolerance of interferon-alpha. *Semin Oncol* 25:3–8, 1998 (suppl 1)

59. Dalakas MC, Mock V, Hawkins MJ: Fatigue: Definitions, mechanisms, and paradigms for study. *Semin Oncol* 25:48–53, 1998 (suppl 1)

60. Jones TH, Wadler S, Hupart KH: Endocrine-mediated mechanisms of fatigue during treatment with interferon-alpha. *Semin Oncol* 25:54–63, 1998 (suppl 1)

61. Weiss K: Safety profile of interferon-alpha therapy. *Semin Oncol* 25:9–13, 1998 (suppl 1)

62. Spath-Schwalbe E, Hansen K, Schmidt F, et al: Acute effects of recombinant human interleukin-6 on endocrine and central nervous sleep functions in healthy men. *J Clin Endocrinol Metab* 83:1573–1579, 1998

63. Blade J, San Miguel JF, Escudero ML, et al: Maintenance treatment with interferon alpha-2b in multiple myeloma: A prospective randomized study from PETHEMA (Program for the Study and Treatment of Hematological Malignancies, Spanish Society of Hematology). *Leukemia* 12:1144–1148, 1998

64. Johnston SR, Constenla DO, Moore J, et al: Randomized phase II trial of BCDT [carmustine (BCNU), cisplatin, dacarbazine (DTIC) and tamoxifen] with or without interferon alpha (IFN-alpha) and interleukin (IL-2) in patients with metastatic melanoma. *Br J Cancer* 77:1280–1286, 1998

65. Rosenthal MA, Oratz R: Phase II clinical trial of recombinant alpha 2b interferon and 13 cis retinoic acid in patients with metastatic melanoma. *Am J Clin Oncol* 21:352–354, 1998

66. Karp SE: Low-dose intravenous bolus interleukin-2 with interferon-alpha therapy for metastatic melanoma and renal cell carcinoma. *J Immunother* 21:56–61, 1998

67. Maclaren DPM, Gibson H, Parry-Billings M, et al: A review of metabolic and physiological factors in fatigue. *Exerc Sport Sci Rev* 17:29–66, 1989

68. Davis JM: Central and peripheral factors in fatigue. *J Sports Sci* 13:549, 1995

69. Porth CM: *Pathophysiology: Concepts of Altered States.* Philadelphia, Lippincott, 1998

70. Holder-Powell HM, Jones DA: Fatigue and muscular activity: A review. *Physiotherapy* 76:672–676, 1990

71. Gupta S, Aggarwal S, See D, Starr A: Cytokine production by adherent and non-adherent mononuclear cells in chronic fatigue syndrome. *J Psychiatr Res* 31:149–156, 1997

72. Vgontzas AN, Papanicolaou DA, Bixler EO, et al: Elevation of plasma cytokines in disorders of excessive daytime sleepiness: Role of sleep disturbance and obesity. *J Clin Endocrinol Metab* 82:1313–1316, 1997

73. Morant R: Asthenia in cancer patients—A double edged inflammatory response against the tumor? *J Palliat Care* 7:22–24, 1991

74. Mulligan K, Bloch AS: Energy expenditure and protein metabolism in human immunodeficiency virus infection and cancer cachexia. *Semin Oncol* 25:82–91, 1998 (suppl 6)

75. Theologides A: Anorexins asthenins and cachectins in cancer. *Am J Med* 81:296–298, 1986

76. Karnofsky DA, Burchenal JH: The clinical evaluation of chemotherapeutic agents in cancer, in MacLeod CM (ed): *Evaluation of Chemotherapeutic Agents.* New York, Columbia University Press, 1949, pp 191–205

77. Litwin MS, Lubeck DP, Henning JM, et al: Differences in urologist and patient assessments of health related quality of life in men with prostate cancer: Results of the CaPSURE database. *J Urol* 159:1988–1992, 1998

78. Rhodes VA, McDaniel RW, Matthews C: Comparison of hospice nurses and patients perceptions of symptom experience. *Cancer Nurs* 21:312–319, 1998

79. Kurtz ME, Kurtz JC, Given CC, et al: Concordance of cancer patient and caregiver symptom reports. *Cancer Pract* 4:185–190, 1996

80. Rhoten D: Fatigue and the postsurgical patient, in Norris CM (ed): *Concept Clarification in Nursing.* Rockville, MD, Aspen Systems Corporation, 1982, pp 277–300

81. Hays RD, Sherbourne CD, Mazel RM: The RAND 36 items health survey 1.0. *Health Econ* 2:217–227, 1993

82. Bergner M, Bobbitt R, Pollard W, et al: The Sickness Impact Profile: Validation of a health status measure. *Med Care* 14:57–67, 1976

83. Piper BF, Dibble SL, Dodd MJ, et al: The revised Piper Fatigue Scale: Psychometric evaluation in women with breast cancer. *Oncol Nurs Forum* 25:677–684, 1998

84. Yoshitake H: Relations between the symptoms and the feeling of fatigue. *Ergonomics* 45:422–432, 1969

85. Folstein M, Folstein S, McHugh P: Mini-Mental State Examination: A practical guide for grading the cognitive state of patients for clinicians. *J Psychiatr Res* 12:189–198, 1975

86. Jacobs JW, Bernard MR, Delgado A, et al: Screening for organic mental syndromes in the medically ill. *Ann Intern Med* 86:40–46, 1977

87. Glaus A, Crow R, Hammond S: A qualitative study to ex-

plore the concept of fatigue/tiredness in cancer patients and healthy individuals. *Support Care Cancer* 4:82–96, 1996

88. Orem DE: *Nursing Concepts of Practice* (ed 5). St. Louis, Mosby Year Book, 1995

89. Rhodes VA, McDaniel RW, Hanson B, et al: Sensory perceptions of patients on selected antineoplastic protocols. *Cancer Nurs* 17:45–51, 1994

90. Dodd MJ: Patterns of self care in cancer patients receiving radiation therapy. *Oncol Nurs Forum* 11:23–27, 1984

91. Moore SM: Effects of interventions to promote recovery in coronary artery bypass surgical patients. *J Cardiol Nurs* 12:59–70, 1997

92. Gammon J, Mulholland CW: Effect of preparatory information prior to elective total hip replacement on psychological coping outcomes. *J Adv Nurs* 24:303–308, 1996

93. Johnson JE: Coping with radiation therapy: Optimism and the effect of preparatory interventions. *Res Nurs Health* 19: 3–12, 1996

94. Dodd M: Assessing patients' self-care for side-effects of cancer chemotherapy. *Cancer Nurs* 5:447–451, 1982

95. Dodd M: Patterns of self-care in patients with breast cancer. *Western J Nurs Res* 10:7–24

96. Mock V: Breast cancer and fatigue: Issues for the workplace. *AAOHN J* 46:425–431, 1998

97. Mock V, Barton Burke M, Sheehan P, et al: A nursing rehabilitation program for women with breast cancer receiving adjuvant chemotherapy. *Oncol Nurs Forum* 21: 899–907, 1994

98. Mock V, Dow KH, Meares CJ, et al: Effects of exercise on fatigue, physical functioning, and emotional distress during radiation therapy for breast cancer. *Oncol Nurs Forum* 24:991–1000, 1997

99. Suh E, Lee EO: The effects of rhythmic walking exercise on physical strength, fatigue, and functional status of breast cancer patients in adjuvant chemotherapy. *Oncol Nurs Forum* 25:331, 1998

100. Graydon JE, Bubela N, Irvine D, et al: Fatigue-reducing strategies used by patients receiving treatment for cancer. *Cancer Nurs* 18:23–28, 1995

101. Schwartz AL: Patterns of exercise and fatigue in physically active cancer survivors. *Oncol Nurs Forum* 25:485–491, 1998

102. Friendenreich CM, Courneya KS: Exercise as rehabilitation for cancer patients. *Clin J Sport Med* 6:237–244, 1996

103. Nail LM, Jones LS, Greene D, et al: Use and perceived efficacy of self-care activities in patients receiving chemotherapy. *Oncol Nurs Forum* 18:883–887, 1991

104. Richardson A, Ream E, Wilson-Barnett J: Fatigue in patients receiving chemotherapy: Patterns of change. *Cancer Nurs* 21:17–30, 1998

105. Adamson JW, Ludwig H: Predicting the hematopoietic response to recombinant human erythropoietin (Epoetin alfa) in the treatment of the anemia of cancer. *Oncology* 56:46–53, 1999

106. Ludwig H, Fritz E: Anemia of cancer patients: Patient selection and patient stratification for epoetin treatment. *Semin Oncol* 25:35–38, 1998 (suppl 7)

107. Beguin Y: Prediction of response to optimize outcome of treatment with erythropoietin. *Semin Oncol* 25:27–34, 1998 (suppl 7)

108. Glaspy J: The impact of epoetin alfa on quality of life during cancer chemotherapy: A fresh look at an old problem. *Semin Hematol* 34:20–26, 1997 (suppl 2)

109. Henry D: Haematological toxicities associated with dose-intensive chemotherapy, the role for and use of recombinant growth factors. *Ann Oncol* 8:S7–S10, 1997 (suppl 3)

110. Meadowcroft AM, Gilbert CJ, Maravich-May D, et al: Cost of managing anemia with and without prophylactic epoetin alfa therapy in breast cancer patients receiving combination chemotherapy. *Am J Health System Pharm* 55:1898–1902, 1998

111. Mohandas K, Aledort L: Transfusion requirements, risks, and costs for patients with malignancy. *Transfusion* 35: 427–430, 1995

112. Ortega A, Dranitsaris G, Puodziunas A: A clinical and economic evaluation of red blood cell transfusions in patients receiving cancer chemotherapy. *Int J Tech Assess Health Care* 14:788–798, 1998

113. Dufault K, Martocchio G. Hope: Its spheres and dimensions. *Nurs Clin North Am* 20:379–391, 1985

CHAPTER 33

Nutritional Disturbances

Ann T. Foltz, RN, DNS

Scope of the Problem

Nutritional disturbances in individuals with cancer occur along a continuum of nutritional adequacy, and range from optimal nutrition to malnutrition. Malnutrition is manifested as both undernutrition and overnutrition. Optimal nutrient intake provides adequate energy and protection from disease. When intake of nutrients is less than adequate or more than required, nutritional stores are reduced below normal or increased above normal, respectively. Nutritional lesions of varying magnitudes result, depending on the type and extent of the deficiency or excess.[1]

In the United States, recognition of the relationship between cancer and nutrition began in the 1930s[2] and became the subject of systematic research in the 1970s.[3] The research studies were of two main categories. One category, the relationship of nutrient intake to the development of cancer, has been discussed elsewhere in this text (see Chapter 3). The second category, cancer-induced nutritional problems and their management, is considered in this chapter.

Undernutrition is the most common nutritional problem in both pediatric and adult cancer populations with cancer.[4-9] However, the evidence that both undernutrition and overnutrition negatively affect morbidity, survival, and quality of life[6-12] emphasizes the need for oncology nurses to evaluate the nutritional status of all individuals under their care.

Definitions

The two opposite end points of malnutrition in individuals with cancer are obesity and cancer cachexia. *Obesity* is frequently defined as weighing 120% or more of ideal body weight, but this definition can be misleading. While obesity is identified with surplus fat, weight above the normal range can occur with increased muscle mass or fluid retention. For this reason, evaluation of body composition should be made when weight tables are used to diagnose obesity.

Terms used to describe nonmalignant nutritional deficiencies, and occasionally malignant starvation, are *kwashiorkor* (protein malnutrition with an adequate caloric intake) and *marasmus* (simple starvation with protein-calorie malnutrition). *Cachexia,* a general term meaning ill health, can occur in nonneoplastic diseases, such as sepsis, cardiac failure, and starvation. Although some investigators suggest using the term *anorexia-cachexia cancer syndrome* (ACCS) to refer to the disorder in populations with cancer,[5] this distinction is rarely made. Cancer cachexia is characterized by anorexia, weight loss, skeletal muscle atrophy, and asthenia (loss of strength).[5,7] Other symptoms of cancer cachexia are early satiety, edema, anemia,[7] reduced attention span, organ dysfunction,[13] metabolic abnormalities,[3,13,14] and susceptibility to other diseases.[3,14,15]

Cancer-associated cachexia can be differentiated into primary and secondary types.[15] *Primary cachexia* results from tumor-produced metabolic abnormalities or host responses. Successful treatment of primary cachexia relies on effective cancer treatment. When cure or significant control is not possible, palliation of cachexia may be possible for some interval of time. *Secondary cachexia* results from mechanical effects of the tumor or treatment. Secondary cachexia can be treated with a variety of approaches and is often more amenable to intervention than the primary form. *Repletion* describes the reestablishment of adequate nutritional status and normal body composition.

Other terms are commonly used to describe conditions that result from cancer or its treatment. These include *hypogeusia* (decreased taste sensitivity), *dysgeusia* (perverted taste perception), *odynophagia* or *dysphagia* (painful swallowing), *hyposmia* (diminished ability to smell), and *inanition* (progressive deterioration with muscle wasting and energy loss).

Incidence

Neither the incidence nor the prevalence of malnutrition is accurately documented in patients with cancer. From 40%–80% of patients with cancer develop some degree of malnutrition during their illness.[8,16,17] The absence of more accurate statistics arises from several factors. One problem is that nutritional status is rarely assessed when cancer is diagnosed, especially in the obese. Because assessment of nutritional status frequently is delayed, the opportunity to find more easily treated, minimal nutrient deficiencies in early stages is often lost. In addition, there is no consensus on what indicators of nutritional status should be used. Although weight is universally accepted as part of nutritional assessment, there is little agreement on what other parameters must be included. Recommendations vary from a careful clinical examination[18] to the use of an array of laboratory tests.[3,4,7,19,20] There is also no agreement on how malnutrition should be graded. In clinical trials, study groups have developed toxicity scales for weight change and anorexia; however, these scales are better suited to determine side effect profiles rather than malnutrition levels.

Overnutrition is most commonly documented in breast cancer. The incidence of obesity among women recently diagnosed with breast cancer ranges from 24%–38%.[11,12,21] In addition, from 40%–70% of women with breast cancer receiving adjuvant chemotherapy gain weight, and some become obese.[11,21,22] Concern about weight changes arises not only from cardiac or quality-of-life issues, but also because of findings that women with breast cancer who are obese have poorer survival than women who are not.[10–12,21,23] Overnutrition can exist in other cancers as well. In a survey of the weight and nutritional status of 99 consecutive cancer patients admitted for treatment, Colletti et al found that 4% were underweight and 43% were overweight.[24] Whether increased weight has negative consequences in types of cancer other than breast cancer is not clear.

Risk Factors

Individuals who are nourished adequately at the time of the cancer diagnosis have fewer problems with both the cancer and its treatment. The body's response to the tumor and the tumor-initiated metabolic changes are primary sources for malnutrition.[7,15,16,25–28] In addition, treatment imposes a burden by requiring repair of treatment-induced damage and by reducing the ability of the body to absorb nutrients.

The risk factors for overnutrition among cancer patients are less well understood than the risks for undernutrition. There is some suggestion that treatment, especially chemotherapy, alters either the appetite-controlling hormones or the psychological restraints on nutritional intake.[23,29,30]

External and internal factors

External factors include the environmental and political climate surrounding an individual. This climate encompasses the overall health of the country's economy, which has an impact on transportation, access to food shopping, availability of different nutrients, adequacy of housing and food preparation facilities, and availability of programs that offer food assistance. These environmental factors influence the individual, who possesses cultural and attitudinal concepts about nutrition and eating behaviors. Internal factors that influence a person's tendency to develop nutritional deficiencies include age, body image, past history of food fads or eating disorders, social support, educational level, alcohol or tobacco intake, and the presence of comorbid diseases. The effect of these factors on nutrition among individuals with cancer is an area of fairly recent exploration.[31,32] Much more research in this area is needed before individuals at risk can be reliably identified.

Cancer-related factors

The type of cancer affects the probability of malnutrition. Individuals with breast cancer or leukemia are at low risk.[3,4] From 20%–30% of patients with non-Hodgkin's lymphoma have significant weight loss; unfavorable histologies are correlated with higher weight loss.[4] Individuals with cancers of the aerodigestive (upper respiratory and digestive) and gastrointestinal tracts are at special risk for undernutrition from mechanical obstruction and physiological dysfunction due to local tumor compression.[3,6,33–35] Host responses to the cancer and the cancer itself cause changes in metabolism and energy needs and may explain why those with advanced disease are more likely to have nutritional problems.[25–28,36]

Treatment-related factors

All cancer therapies can cause nutritional deficiency. The magnitude of the treatment-related risk depends on the area of treatment, type of treatment, number of therapeutic modalities used, dosages of therapy used, and length of treatment.

Surgery. The effects of surgery on an individual's nutritional status depend on the extent of the procedure as well as the site of operation. Complications associated with surgery also are related to the nutritional status of the individual prior to the operation. Malnourished individuals have higher incidences of morbidity and mortality than do those who are adequately nourished.[8,13,34,35] This is of particular relevance to individuals with cancers of the aerodigestive or gastrointestinal tract. These patients may come to surgery with nutritional deficits because of cancer-related disruption of intake or absorption. In addition, they often have had multiple tests requiring restricted diets.

Surgery itself alters function. Major aerodigestive resections may produce hyposmia, dysgeusia, or impaired swallowing, resulting in reduced intake. Rearranged anatomy, common with gastric and esophageal resections, can create multiple lesions affecting nutrition. Patients with abdominal and pelvic incisions experience an ileus after surgery, complicating the ability to take adequate nutrition postoperatively.[37] Resections of large segments of the bowel can lead to malabsorption of fat, inadequate caloric intake, vitamin B_{12} deficiency, anemia, and fluid-electrolyte imbalance.[3,38] These problems can become chronic, resulting in reliance on enteral or parenteral feedings.

For individuals with other cancer sites, nutritional problems resulting from surgery are often limited to the immediate perioperative period. Interruption of oral intake is usually minimal. Use of antibiotics in the perioperative period, although disruptive to digestive processes that utilize intestinal bacteria, can be offset by intake of acidophilus-containing products. Surgical procedures create the same response to injury as does surgery for nonmalignant diseases. This stress is added to the psychological stress of dealing with a cancer diagnosis. Catecholamine, glucocorticoid, and glucagon outputs are increased, resulting in increased energy needs, loss of nitrogen, and water and sodium retention. Surgery can increase energy requirements by 28 kcal/kg/day or 1.5 times normal dietary requirements.[39] For this reason, surgical candidates must be assessed carefully prior to treatment so that any nutritional deficiencies can be addressed proactively.

Radiation. Radiation therapy can alter nutritional status by both systemic and local effects. The extent of the alteration varies with the area of the body being treated and the duration of treatment. Radiation alters function in the treatment area and poses particular problems for patients with aerodigestive or gastrointestinal cancers. Acute effects are transient and include anorexia, diarrhea, bleeding, nausea, vomiting, weight loss, mucositis, esophagitis, gastritis, xerostomia, and changes in taste. Local desquamation reactions can temporarily increase energy needs.[40] Some of these changes, especially xerostomia, can become chronic.

Indirect effects of radiation can also influence nutritional status. Fatigue and appetite changes commonly occur among individuals receiving radiation therapy. These symptoms can alter the person's desire and ability to procure, prepare, and ingest food.[41] Delayed effects of radiation, such as intestinal strictures, fibrosis or obstruction, fistulas, and hepatic or pulmonary fibrosis, cause mechanical problems in gut function and oxygenation. These in turn interrupt the person's ability to absorb, process, and ingest food and may necessitate long-term management.[42,43]

Chemotherapy. Chemotherapy causes a number of direct and indirect effects on nutrition. Direct effects include alteration of the intestinal absorptive surface, excitation of the chemoreceptor trigger zone and true vomiting center, and interference with specific metabolic and enzymatic reactions. The majority of chemotherapeutic agents, because of the damage they cause to frequently reproducing cells, alter the length and surface area of intestinal villi. Subsequent reduced ability of the gut to absorb nutrients and water can induce diarrhea and malabsorption.

Direct excitation of the centers for nausea and vomiting occurs to varying degrees with the majority of chemotherapy drugs.[44,45] The variability is dependent on the drug, dosage, and individual response. In addition to these nonspecific changes in nutritional intake, some drugs cause specific nutritional problems. For example, cisplatin can cause magnesium wasting, which may require replacement therapy.

Indirect effects of chemotherapy on nutrition include interference with nutrient intake related to anorexia, fatigue, constipation, taste changes, and food aversions. The number and magnitude of these various effects depend on the drugs chosen, their dosages, and the frequency and duration of drug administration. Although these side effects clearly alter nutrient intake during treatment, their significance to overall nutritional status has not been adequately studied.[46]

Biotherapy/immunotherapy. The effects of biotherapy on nutritional status are both direct and indirect. Agents like the interferons and interleukins cause anorexia, malaise, mucositis, nausea, and vomiting. Biotherapy-induced fevers produce a direct increase in energy and fluid needs. Indirect influences, such as fatigue and flulike symptoms, can make food procurement and preparation difficult.[47,48] The magnitude and duration of these side effects are variable and may decrease over time. Their clinical effect on nutritional status is not well documented.[49–51]

Normal Nutritional Physiology

There are several models that depict the complex relationships influencing nutrition; those used in much of the cancer literature are specific to the disease state.[3,52,53]

An alternative approach, use of a model of normal nutrient intake, demonstrates the effect of a variety of diseases on nutrition. This can be especially helpful for persons with comorbid diseases, which are common in the older cancer population. One such universal model suggests that nutritional status is a function of an energy exchange system made up of four compartments: the reference compartment, set point, controller, and body storage.[54]

The *reference compartment* is the repository of the standards governing nutrient intake. The standards have physiological (e.g., growth factors, insulin, glucose, thyroxine, smell/taste transmitters), psychological (e.g., body image, self-esteem, meaning/sight/smell of food), and cultural (e.g., acceptable foods, eating patterns, social importance of food) determinants. These standards are monitored by the *set point*. The standards are maintained by the *controller*, largely through balancing energy intake and expenditure. Energy is obtained through the ingestion, digestion, and metabolism of macronutrients (carbohydrates, protein, lipids, and water) and micronutrients (minerals and vitamins). The controller requires an intact gastrointestinal tract, including proper secretory and motility function, to work properly.

The result of the controller activity is the *body storage*, or body composition. The components of the body compartment include fat, protein (skeletal muscle, viscera, plasma, bone, cartilage, collagen), glycogen, minerals, and water (intracellular and extracellular). The percentage of each of the components varies with genetics, gender, and age. The body storage provides feedback to the set point regarding its status via physiological, psychological, and cultural perceptions (serum glucose, conditioned responses, perceived images, etc.). Under stress, feedback may be directed to the reference compartment, with the possibility that standard levels will be changed. The interplay among the compartments, in the setting of an adequate nutrient intake, results in sufficient body storage for energy needs and protection from illness.

Pathophysiology

Cancer, host response, and cancer treatment alter normal physiology. The alterations that affect nutritional status occur in the reference compartment, set point, and controller. These changes result in modified body storage, with the potential for development of obesity or cachexia.

Cancer-Induced Changes in the Reference Compartment

Changes in appetite

There is some evidence that loss of appetite is related to circulating factors produced by the cancer and the host.[5,7,55–59] These factors may be produced peripherally but have a central effect on the reference standards for appetite. Cytokines, including tumor necrosis factor (TNF), gamma interferon, and interleukins-1 and -2, have been proposed as one class of circulating anorectic agents.[55,58] There is also support for an effect of serotonin and bombesin on appetite suppression, especially among individuals with carcinoid or lung cancers.[3] Animal studies support the importance of serotonin and ammonia as anorectics in cancer; studies in humans have been limited.[57] Increased circulating lipids and lactic acid caused by tumor metabolism can also decrease appetite.[3]

Loss of appetite may be precipitated by cancer-induced psychological distress as well. Depression, anxiety, or situational factors (isolation, hospital food) may negatively influence food intake. Cancer-induced pain and pain medication can also reduce intake.

Increased appetite has been reported among women with breast cancer. Investigators suggest that increased as well as decreased appetite may occur as a function of psychological distress.[29,53] Many well women regularly limit their food intake. Following a breast cancer diagnosis, these women may lose their restraint, eat more, and gain weight. Additional study in this area is needed.

Changes in taste and smell

Altered taste and smell sensors, with loss of taste and olfactory cues, change the normal references that are part of appetite and intake. Changes may be caused by direct tumor invasion; cancer-induced deficiencies of zinc, copper, nickel, vitamin A, and niacin; or cancer-associated circulating factors. Circulating factors are hypothesized sources of taste changes occurring early in the disease process.

Physiological increases in the recognition thresholds for sweet, sour, and salt and decreases in the recognition levels for bitter are common. These threshold changes can lead to meat and other food aversions. Psychological factors may also contribute to food aversions. The hedonistic component of eating can be negatively influenced by alterations in taste or smell, leading to a reduced interest in eating and loss of appetite.

Changes in electrolyte balance

Alterations in micronutrient availability occur in paraneoplastic syndromes. Cancer can cause hypercalcemia and hypocalcemia, hyponatremia, hyperphosphatemia and hypophosphatemia. At least some of these abnormalities are caused by tumor-produced hormones and can be life-threatening. They also cause altered mental status as well as taste changes, with associated problems in intake and adherence to treatment regimens.

Cancer-Induced Changes in the Controller

Changes in energy expenditure

Patients with cancer can have increased energy needs initiated by cancer-induced sepsis, fistulas, or lesions. These energy demands can produce malnutrition in some patients, but they are not responsible for cachexia. Although early research suggested that cachexia results from tumor-driven increases in energy expenditure, data are far from consistent. Cancer patients have exhibited increased, decreased, and normal resting energy rates. Proposed mechanisms for those patients who do have increased energy expenditure include heightened cytokine activity, especially tumor necrosis factor and interleukin-6, increased use of futile metabolic cycles, and inappropriate energy production in response to decreased intake.[57–61] Although there is some support for each of the mechanisms in some patients, none are universally found in cachexic patients. Regardless, increased energy expenditure may be a problem for a subset of patients with cancer, but it does not explain cancer cachexia in all cases.

Changes in nutrient metabolism

Cancer is associated with abnormalities in carbohydrate, protein, and lipid metabolism. Changes in carbohydrate metabolism include increased Cori cycle activity, altered peripheral utilization of glucose, increased glucose turnover, and glucose intolerance.[25–28] Glucose intolerance has been linked to insulin resistance, delayed glucose clearance, reduced glucose uptake in skeletal muscles, and an inability to produce glycogen in muscle. Unlike diabetics, individuals with cancer have normal plasma insulin levels. It is not known whether cancer patients also have normal insulin secretion. The origin of the glucose intolerance is unknown, but researchers have suggested that some cases may be the result of cytokines produced by the host in response to the tumor.[58] Indirect effects of cancer that alter glucose metabolism include reduced activity and infection.

Increased hepatic glucose production has been reported in both undernourished and normal-weight patients with cancer.[25,58,59] The elevated glucose level is one of the features that differentiates cancer starvation/cachexia from normal starvation responses. In normal starvation, hepatic glucose production falls; this does not occur in cancer cachexia. The lack of a normal response to a decreased intake may be related to the reliance of cancer on glucose or it may be the product of a cancer-associated abnormal growth hormone.[57,58]

Individuals with cancer may develop altered protein metabolism. Some studies indicate that the tumor preferentially takes up nitrogen-containing materials.[3] Glutamine, an abundant amino acid required for DNA synthesis, may be one of the substances taken up by cancers to the detriment of the host. In addition to the shunting of needed proteins to the cancer, there can be increased muscle breakdown and hepatic protein activity.[5,28,62] Despite the increased hepatic activity, protein synthesis does not match protein catabolism. The net result is increased whole-body protein turnover. However, not all researchers find increased protein turnover, especially among cancer patients who are maintaining their weight.[63]

Abnormal lipid metabolism noted in cancer includes increased lipid mobilization and turnover, elevated triglyceride levels, decreased lipogenesis, altered glycerol transport, and decreased lipoprotein lipase activity.[3,5] To some degree, the alteration in fat metabolism may be related to insulin resistance, with preferential oxidation of fat rather than carbohydrates.

Changes in the gastrointestinal tract

Controller function is heavily dependent on an intact gastrointestinal system. Cancer can produce direct negative effects on the digestive system. Cancers of the aerodigestive structures can cause primary reduction in food and nutrient intake associated with the following:

- Difficulty chewing or swallowing
- Partial or complete obstruction
- Dysmotility
- Inactivation of bile salts, pancreatic enzymes
- Blind loop syndrome
- Fistulas
- Interference associated with pain (ulceration, nerve compression, etc.)
- Bowel wall, mesenteric infiltration
- Protein-losing enteropathy

The type and magnitude of the nutritional deficit depend on the tumor site and size. Nongastrointestinal cancers can cause alterations in nutritional status by interfering with food intake or increasing energy demand. Examples of these types of direct and indirect interference with intake include pain, dyspnea, blockages of mesenteric or peritoneal lymphatics, paraneoplastic syndromes that alter fluid or mineral balance, and altered cognitive function. Ulcerated lesions, both external and internal, increase nutrient need.

Changes in body storage

The degree of body storage alteration varies along the continuum of malnutrition. With small changes in nutrient intake or absorption, there may be no obvious change in body composition. In patients with weight gain, the compartment in which the change occurred should be determined. The most commonly affected compartments are the extracellular fluid and adipose tissue compartments. The most striking change in body composition is seen in cachexia. The total body fat and skeletal muscle components can drop as much as 85% and 75%, respectively.[55] Reduction in intracellular water and mineral supplies also occurs, although not to the same degree. Feedback signals from the body storage compartment are

deranged, reflecting the effect of cytokine activity and metabolic dysfunction. The altered feedback perpetuates the nutritional deficiencies.

Treatment-Induced Changes in the Reference Compartment

Changes in appetite

Just as cancer causes changes in appetite, so can therapy. Depressed appetite can be caused by biotherapeutic agents, notably tumor necrosis factor, interferon, and the interleukins.[47] Psychological responses to having and being treated for cancer with any modality can alter mood and change appetite. Medications prescribed for treatment also affect mood and appetite. Some of the drugs produce increased, rather than decreased, appetite or nutrient intake. Corticosteroids, prescribed in both pediatric and adult populations, can increase appetite.

Surgical anesthesia, chemotherapy, and radiation produce indirect effects on appetite through the induction of nausea, vomiting, and food aversions. Anticipatory nausea and vomiting become conditioned responses to chemotherapy. The clinical significance of these changes is unclear, because some patients alter choice of foods and eating patterns but not their total intake when faced with these symptoms.[50,51,64]

Taste changes can follow head and neck surgery, radiation, and chemotherapy. These changes may be temporary and are sometimes related to zinc deficiency. However, radiation and surgical alterations in gustatory and olfactory structures can be permanent. This may result in an alteration of the normal references for food acceptability or in a general reduction in intake over time.

Treatment-Induced Changes in the Controller

Changes in energy expenditure

Treatment can affect energy needs both directly and indirectly. Some biotherapeutic agents elicit shaking chills and fever, which increase energy demands. Increased energy needs from fever and infection can also accompany bone marrow suppression. Moreover, antifungal agents administered to immunocompromised patients cause fever and chill responses. Nutritional needs increase as the body responds to repair damage induced by surgery, radiation, or chemotherapy. Energy requirements are related to the type and magnitude of the treatment.

Changes in the gastrointestinal tract

Surgical resection removes or bypasses areas of the aerodigestive or gastrointestinal tract, causing a number of nutritional lesions. Chemotherapy and radiation cause direct injury to the intestinal villi, reducing the absorptive surface. Secondary candidiasis throughout the gastrointestinal tract can occur following antibiotic therapy associated with any treatment. These are major threats to the proper absorption of both macronutrients and micronutrients. Side effects of treatment include anorexia, nausea, vomiting, lactose intolerance, diarrhea, and constipation, all of which can create obstacles to normal gut function and intake. In addition, chronic changes can occur. Total bowel resection, bone marrow transplant–induced graft-versus-host disease, and radiation enteritis can lead to long-term patient dependence on parenteral nutritional support.

Clinical Manifestations

The most common clinical manifestation identified with cancer is cancer cachexia, which is characterized by skeletal muscle wasting, weight loss, and reduced function. The patient may complain of loss of appetite, inability to eat, or early satiety. However, because the nutrient deficiencies occur along a continuum, nutritional deficits can exist without these cardinal or extreme signs and symptoms. This is especially true of obese individuals, in whom weight loss can be overlooked. Fluid changes, such as edema or effusions, can mask protein and fat loss. The fact that nutritional disturbances can be subtle and are frequently nonspecific makes the need for assessment that much more important.

Screening, Assessment, and Grading

The goal of screening in nutrition is to identify those persons who are likely to have or to develop nutritional problems associated with their cancer. Nutritional screening is a far newer entity than nutritional assessment and is still developing standardized approaches. Nutritional assessment, a more precise and diagnostic procedure, consists of four elements: anthropometrics, laboratory findings, clinical examination, and dietary evaluation. Although nurses play an integral part in accurate nutritional assessment, registered dietitians and nutritionists are more frequently responsible for the nutritional assessment. Nurses often conduct screening for and early detection tests of nutritional deficits or excesses. Therefore, this discussion concentrates on screening and anthropometrics. For more detailed information on assessment, the reader is referred to other sources.[3,65,66]

Nutritional Screening

The need to assess nutritional status quickly and efficiently has led to the development of a number of screening instruments. The Patient-Generated Subjective Global Assessment (PG-SGA) is currently endorsed by the American Dietetics Association for oncology patients and has been used by oncology nurses in a variety of settings. The PG-SGA was modified by Otterly from the Subjective Global Assessment of Nutritional Status (SGA), an instrument with proven sensitivity and specificity.[65,67–69] Both the SGA and PG-SGA evaluate weight change, dietary intake changes, gastrointestinal symptoms lasting more than 2 weeks, and activity levels. The PG-SGA includes cancer-specific symptoms and a refinement of the activity-level estimation. The patient is able to complete a portion of the assessment, thus decreasing clinician time in data collection. The clinician, taking into consideration the diagnosis, stage of cancer, estimated treatment- and tumor-associated metabolic demand, and findings from a focused physical examination, determines a rating of well-nourished, moderately (or suspected) malnourished, or severely malnourished.

There are also a number of formulas that integrate several objective measures into assessment of nutritional risk (Table 33-1). These include the Nutritional Index (NI),[70] the Prognostic Nutritional Index (PNI),[71] the Hospital Prognostic Index (HPI),[72] and the Nutrition Risk Index (NRI).[73] These indices are especially helpful in identifying which individuals undergoing head and neck or gastrointestinal surgery might benefit from nutritional intervention prior to and following surgery. The HPI and NRI utilize measures that are commonly used and readily available.

Nutritional Assessment

Anthropometrics

Anthropometrics, the measurement of the weight, size, and proportions of the body, commonly include height, weight, and skin-fold thickness. Serial weight measurement is perhaps the single most important indicator of nutritional status for the clinician, although its importance is often underemphasized. It is also the anthropometric measure most often provided by nursing staff. Standard weight measurement is inexpensive, quick, and practical.

Weight should not be considered as a sole determinant of nutritional status, however, as weight alone does not reveal body composition. Weight among individuals with cancer may reflect tumor mass or fluid retention while masking loss of lean body mass. For example, children with abdominal masses are at risk for being considered at normal weight for height, despite loss of lean body mass.[4,9] Adults with ascites are at similar risk. There have been attempts to improve body composition determination through a variety of measures: ultrasound, computerized tomography, magnetic resonance imaging, dual-photon and dual-energy radiographic absorptiometry, neutron activation, total body potassium, total body

Table 33-1 Nutritional Assessment Formulas

Nutritional Formula	Formula	Key to Formula
Nutritional index (NI)	$1.9579 - 0.0017 \times (IgM \times prealbumin) - (0.0075 \times complement\ factor\ C3) - (0.0066 \times fibrinogen) + (0.033 \times cholesterol) - (0.1858 \times vitamin\ A–binding\ protein) + (0.6636 \times thyroxine-binding\ globulin)$	IgM, complement, fibrinogen, cholesterol, vitamin A–binding protein, and thyroxine are measured in mg/dL
Prognostic nutritional index (PNI)	$158 - (16.6 \times albumin) - (0.78 \times triceps\ skin\ fold) - (0.2 \times transferrin) - (5.8 \times delayed\ hypersensitivity\ reaction)$	Albumin is measured in g; triceps skin fold in mL; transferrin in mg/dL; delayed hypersensitivity as 0 (nonreactive), 1 (<5 mm reactivity), or 2 (≥5 mm reactivity)
Hospital prognostic index (HPI)	$(0.91 \times albumin) - (1.00 \times delayed\ hypersensitivity) - (1.44 \times sepsis\ rating) + (0.98 \times diagnosis\ rating) - 1.09$	Albumin is measured in g; delayed hypersensitivity as 1 (positive to 1 or more antigen) or 2 (nonreactive); sepsis as 1 (present) or 2 (absent); diagnosis as 1 (cancer present) or 2 (cancer not present)
Nutrition risk index (NRI)	$(15.19 \times albumin) + (0.417 \times \%\ usual\ body\ weight)$	Albumin is measured in g; % usual body weight is actual weight/usual weight $\times$ 100

water, and bioelectrical impedance. These techniques vary in their invasiveness, availability, and expense. At this point the primary use of these types of measures is in nutritional research, not routine assessment.[3,19] For the most part, clinical body composition estimates rely on weight measures coupled with additional anthropometrics, such as height or skin folds.

Weight combined with height measurement is an indirect indicator of body composition. It can be used to screen for both undernutrition and overnutrition. The Metropolitan Life Insurance Company Height-Weight Table has frequently been used as such a screening device. Because of possible inaccuracy, stemming from clinician estimation rather than calculation of frame size and reliance on data from white, insured persons aged 25–59 as the basis of the table, there are concerns in using the Metropolitan table. Although Metropolitan standards have been shown equivalent to nonwhite U.S. populations, there have been few comparisons with black women and the majority of Asian Pacific populations.[74] Moreover, there continues to be considerable controversy over what should be considered the normal range of age-related weight increases.[75] Thus, the Metropolitan tables should be used in conjunction with other measures to determine nutritional status and with an understanding of their limitations.

Weight and height can also be used to calculate the body mass index (BMI). The BMI is considered a more accurate estimation of total body fat than the Metropolitan weight tables. The BMI has limited utility in individuals with increased lean muscle mass or with large frames. It is also more relevant for determining obesity than for assessing undernutrition. The formula for BMI calculation is:

Weight in kilograms/height in meters squared

OR

Weight in pounds/height in inches squared x 704.5

BMI ranges:

<18.5	=	Underweight
18.5–24.9	=	Normal weight
25.0–29.9	=	Overweight
>30.0	=	Obese

The result of the BMI calculation can be compared to the BMI ranges above or plotted on a nomogram. It has been suggested that the acceptable BMI should increase with age to reflect the normal aging process, but standards for such increases have not been universally accepted.

Another important function of the anthropometric measures of height and weight is their use in calculating an individual's caloric needs. Resting metabolic rate nomograms have been developed for this purpose. Formulas are also commonly used. Caloric prescriptions for individuals with cancer are frequently based on the Harris-Benedict (HB) equation:

For women: 655 + (9.6 × weight in kg) + (1.7 × height in cm) − (4.7 × age in years)

For men: 66 + (1.37 × weight in kg) + (5 × height in cm) − (6.8 × age in years)

or the ideal weight formula (Table 33-2). These equations indicate the number of calories expended while the individual is at rest, or the *resting energy expenditure* (REE). This number is corrected for the level of required energy and varies according to activity, treatment, and morbid condition (Table 33-3). Kondsup et al advise factoring for activity level, stress, and desired weight gain.[76] However, there have been few estimates of energy required by individuals with cancer and those that are available suggest that determining the appropriate caloric need is difficult. Ulander et al found that although 66% of patients with colon cancer expended less than their esti-

Table 33-2 Ideal Weight Formula

For women:
- Ideal weight calculation: Add 100 pounds for first 60 inches, 5 pounds for each inch over 60 inches; divide by 2.2 to obtain ideal weight in kilograms
- Multiply ideal kilogram calculation by 24 hours and by 0.9 calories/kg = resting needs

For men:
- Ideal weight calculation: Add 106 pounds for first 60 inches, add 6 pounds for each inch over 60 inches; divide by 2.2 to obtain ideal weight in kilograms
- Multiply ideal kilogram calculation by 24 and by 1.0 calories/kg = resting needs

For children:
- For children under the age of 12, energy needs are often set at 1000 calories plus 100 calories for each year of age

mated basal energy postoperatively, they also lost weight, indicating that providing adequate nutrition based on HB estimates did not translate into weight maintenance.[37] Ringold-Smith et al reported that the HB equation overestimated the energy requirements before bone marrow transplant and underestimated needs after transplant. Thus, careful choice of correction factors is needed.[77]

Despite the overall importance, practicality, and clinical relevance of weight and height measures in nutritional assessment, the reliability of both measures is questionable when calibration checks of scales and uniform measuring methods are not practiced. Scales should be calibrated regularly. Self-calibrating scales also should be tested periodically. Using patient-reported weight and height should be discouraged. Training in accurate measurement and monitoring for quality assurance could improve the assessment process.

Additional anthropometrics used in nutritional assessment include skin-fold thickness and body-part circumferences to assess fat and muscle compartments. The assumptions underlying the use of skin-fold measures in this way is under debate, as is the number and specific skin-fold measures that should be included in assessment. In addition, reliability of measurement is dependent on training and quality control. For these reasons, skin-fold

Table 33-3 Correction Factors for Caloric Needs Above Resting Energy Expenditure

Patient Situation	Energy Correction Factor
On bed rest	1.2
Out of bed	1.3
Fever	1.0 + 0.13/°C
Surgery	1.0–1.2
Sepsis	1.4–1.8

measures are usually performed by a dietitian or nutritionist.

Laboratory Tests

Table 33-4 lists the laboratory tests commonly used to evaluate nutritional status.[3,20,65,66] It is important to remember that these tests are nonspecific for malnutrition. Example test results include low blood count, decreased lymphocyte count, and delayed hypersensitivity testing, all of which can be affected by both cancer and cancer treatment. In addition, the tests are often not sensitive to nutritional deficiencies. For example, severe nutritional deficiencies may exist before albumin levels fall. Serum albumin is a poor marker for screening or early detection but an excellent indicator of prognosis.[78] Another consideration is cost. Some of the more sensitive measures, like prealbumin or retinol-binding protein, are expensive and inadequately covered by insurance.[20]

Physical Examination

Physical examination is limited in its ability to distinguish between the effects of cancer and those of nutritional deficiency. The fact that physical changes such as glossitis, muscle wasting, or diarrhea exist in many patients with cancer secondary to their disease or treatment does not minimize their usefulness as indicators of problems in energy intake, absorption, or need. Physical examination may also identify other cancer-related changes, such as fevers, fistulas, or external lesions that influence the intake or expenditure of energy.[15]

Dietary Information

Dietary intake information is used to identify existing and potential nutritional excesses and deficits. In a full diet history, information that reflects both diet and general health is included. General questions alert the nurse to the need for more in-depth study of dietary intakes. Dietary information is obtained using a number of approaches: 24-hour recall surveys, food frequency measures, diet diaries, calorie counts, or monthly purchase records. The last method is rarely used in clinical practice. Any of the types of food-intake recordings provide information about energy, nutrient, vitamin, and mineral intakes. Obtaining this information requires variable amounts of time for data entry into nutrient analysis programs. The need for this depth of assessment will depend on the setting. Full dietary assessments are usually conducted by dietitians or nutritionists. However, the nurse should be alert to nursing assessment items of weight change, recent changes in intake, symptoms that influence eating or food preparation, and indications that alternative or complementary nutritional products are in use. Table 33-5 lists the strengths and weaknesses of the various diet history measures.

Table 33-4 Selected Laboratory Tests Used in Nutritional Assessment

Test	Comments
Complete blood count	Identifies macrocytosis (sign of possible folate or B_{12} deficiency) and anemia (may identify iron-deficiency anemia)
Tests of immune function	
Total lymphocyte count	A nonspecific measure of immune function; an indirect indicator of nutritional status. Levels below 1200 cubic centimeters suggest nutritional deficiency and increased morbidity and mortality in cancer patients.
Delayed hypersensitivity	This testing is based on the relationship between malnutrition and immune deficiency. Anergic responses are related to increased infection and mortality rates.
Iron studies	
Transferrin	Can be used to identify iron and is an indicator of protein status.
Protein studies	These measures indicate the state of protein catabolism, anabolism, and distribution.
Albumin	Albumin is not sensitive to minimal protein deficits and may be both insensitive and nonspecific to malnutrition in situations where major trauma exists. Low albumin levels are associated with increased surgical morbidity and mortality, with longer hospital and intensive care stays. Because the half-life of albumin is 18–20 days, it is not useful for detecting rapid changes in nutritional status.
Transferrin	Transferrin represents visceral protein stores to a greater extent than total protein or albumin measures. It has a half-life of 8–10 days and may be more useful in monitoring changes in nutritional status. Levels of transferrin are increased with iron deficiency and decreased with age, fluid overload, and antibiotic therapy. Total iron-binding capacity can be used to derive transferrin levels when transferrin testing is not available.
Prealbumin	Prealbumin is a transport protein for thyroxine- and retinol-binding protein. The serum half-life is 2–3 days and has potential advantages in monitoring changes in nutritional status. It has been used to measure the effectiveness of parenteral nutrition.
Creatinine height index (CHI)	Urinary creatinine excretion is a measure of muscle metabolism and lean body mass (protein stores). Holding weight constant, actual creatinine excretion is compared to ideal creatinine excretion rate. The CHI is more sensitive to malnutrition than the height-weight standards, especially among persons with edema or obesity. However, its measurement requires stable dietary intake and normal renal function.
Nitrogen	Measures of nitrogen balance can be obtained by collecting 24-hour protein intake history and urinary urea nitrogen and using the formula: Nitrogen balance = nitrogen intake − nitrogen output Where nitrogen intake = protein intake in g/24 hr (6.25 g protein/g nitrogen), and nitrogen output = urinary urea nitrogen + 4 g nitrogen

Functional Assessment

Assessment of the ability to perform the activities of daily living, especially in the areas of food procurement and preparation, are part of a thorough nutritional assessment. Performance level assessments also have for two decades been used to determine the relationship of nutrition to function.[79] The use of more specific measures, such as muscle strength, have for two decades been suggested as sensitive indicators of both positive and negative changes in food intake.[80] However, the use of such measures remains uncommon except in research situations.

Nutrition-Related Symptom Assessment

Assessment of symptoms that interfere with intake is part of an oncological nutritional assessment. These symptoms include anorexia, nausea, vomiting, diarrhea, constipation, mouth sores, dry mouth, pain when eating or swallowing, other pain, taste change, fatigue, difficulty in swallowing, indigestion, early satiety, cramping, and bloat-

ing. Linear analogue self-assessment, Likert scales, or narrative grading scales are useful in identifying the severity of the problem and the effectiveness of intervention[7,37,81] (Figure 33-1).

Therapeutic Approaches and Nursing Care

Because malnutrition is associated with increased morbidity and mortality rates,[81–85] intervention to prevent or minimize nutritional problems is a worthy goal. Research in this area is ongoing and explores nutritional manipulation in cancer prevention, as an adjunct to standard cancer therapy and as a mode of therapy. In addition, there are continuing studies of interventions that minimize the threats of treatment to the host's nutritional status.[84,86–88] Optimal nutrition planning utilizes a nutritional team with expertise in cancer-associated malnutrition.[7] When that is not available, a general nutritional support team

Table 33-5   Comparison of Dietary Intake Assessments

Assessment Method	Strengths	Weaknesses
Diet history	In-depth picture of dietary patterns and influencing factors (socio-economic, cultural, personal, religious)	Time-consuming
24-Hour recall	Usually accurate recall of previous 24 hours; interview time short	Accuracy depends on patient's memory, ability to estimate portions, willingness to report all foods and beverages consumed; 24-hour period sampled may not be representative
Diet diary	Representative of actual intake; description of intake patterns may suggest interventions	Accuracy depends on patient's memory, ability to estimate portions, willingness to report all foods and beverages consumed; can be tedious
Calorie count	Accurate report of nutrient values taken during hospitalization	Accuracy depends on skill of recorder; patient's visitors may ingest part; hospital food choices may not reflect normal diet patterns

may be of assistance. Development of a nutritional care plan may require the collaboration of nurses, physicians, dietitians, pharmacists, speech therapists, and social workers. The patient and family or significant others are an integral part of the effort. Without their participation in goal setting and method choice, it is unlikely that any intervention will be successful.

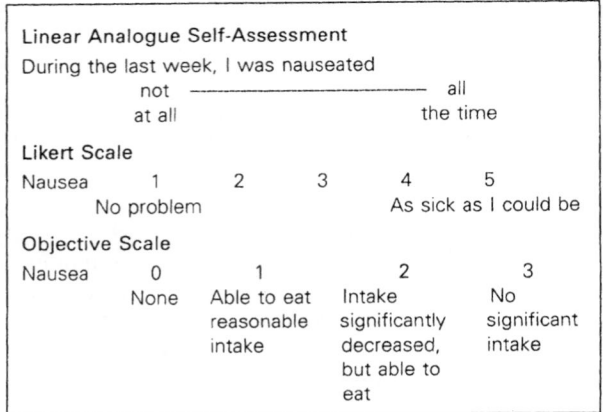

Figure 33-1   Examples of nutritionally linked symptom measurement

Intervention must also be based on realistic goals and ethical considerations. Goals may target specific or general dietary components to influence morbidity, mortality, appetite, function, or well-being. For patients in whom response to treatment is expected or for whom morbidity will be reduced, intervention is a sound practice. Goal setting within an ethical context can be more difficult for individuals with progressing disease, anorexia, and weight loss. Often, family members concentrate on reversing the patient's lack of appetite and weight loss. This can put undue stress on the patient and the family relationship. Interventions with minimal chances of success also interfere with progress toward closure, can be costly, and often are associated with their own morbidity. Allowing dehydration, which is often seen by family members as lack of care, has been found to be ethically and legally acceptable.[88] However, if eating is a major source of comfort or quality of life, then the use of interventions that improve appetite and alter the metabolic abnormalities should be considered.

Nutritional Interventions

The nutritional assessment, described previously and performed by members of the nutritional team, provides the basis for the nutritional prescription and development of intervention strategies. The possible prescriptions range from oral supplementation or deletion of specific nutrients to institution of total parenteral nutrition. Strategies include verbal counseling to alter intake or manage symptoms, prescription of medications to minimize side effects, or identification of resources to facilitate treatment with oral supplements, tube-administered enteral, or total parenteral nutrition. The level of intervention and accompanying strategy are dictated by the patient's baseline nutritional state, disease status, risks for malnutrition from treatment, anticipated response to therapy, and resources. Algorithms for individuals at normal weight and those who are undernourished are provided in Figures 33-2 and 33-3.

Nutritional Prescription

Alteration in specific dietary components

The development of some nutrient deficiencies is common across diseases. For example, low serum iron and potassium are not unusual in a number of chronic diseases. In patients with cancer, these deficits arise from a combination of chemotherapy-related effects on bone marrow, anemia of chronic disease, medications for comorbid conditions, and antibiotic use. Other deficiencies that are more specific to cancer include hypomagnesemia related to platinum chemotherapy; hyponatremia and hypercalcemia, resulting from paraneoplastic syndromes; and zinc deficiency accompanying head and neck cancers. Intervention with parenteral fluids or supplements

Figure 33-2 Nutritional support algorithm for individuals well nourished at baseline. (GI = gastrointestinal tract; PHA = peripheral hyperalimentation; TPN = total parenteral nutrition)

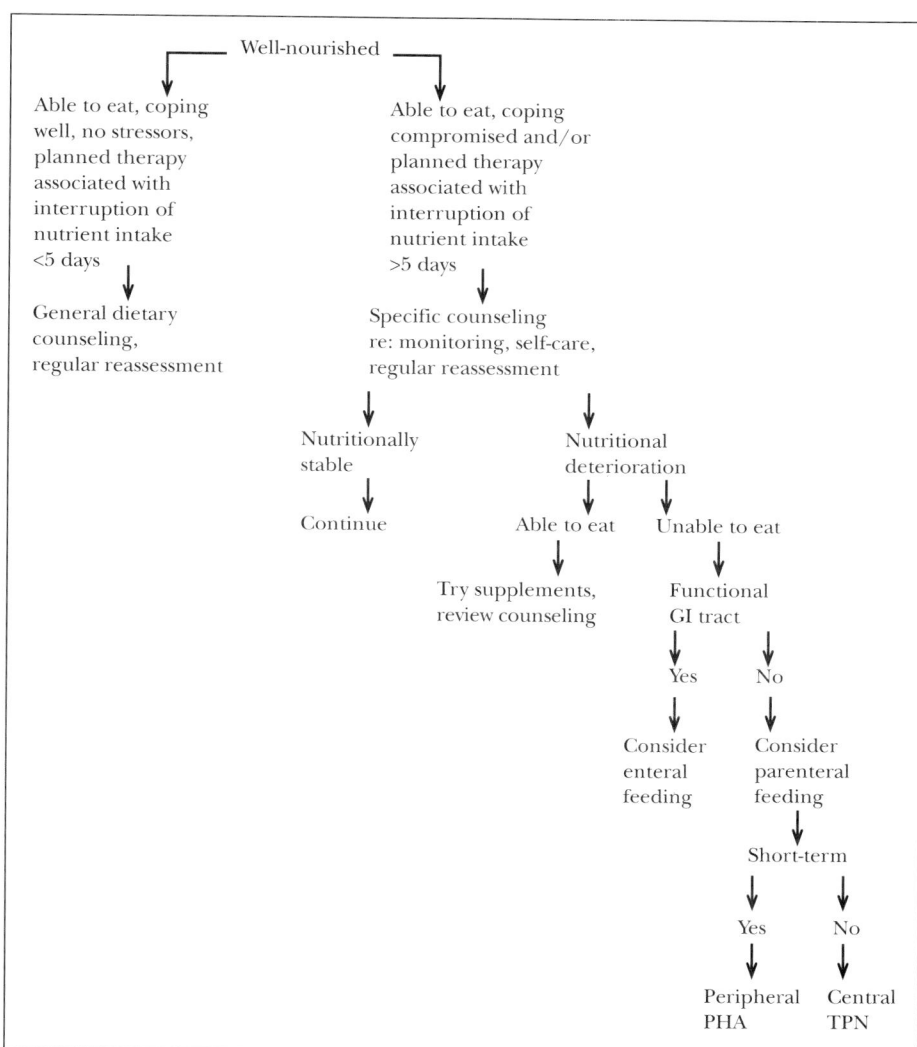

may be required for some patients; in others, oral mineral supplementation is used to control these problems. Educating the patient about foods that are good sources of the deficient mineral may also be helpful.

In addition to reversing known deficiencies, supplemental nutrients are given to minimize the side effects and maximize the therapeutic effect of standard treatment. Studies indicate that diets augmented with arginine improve cell-mediated immunity. Arginine in combination with omega-3 fatty acids improves healing and reduces complication rates among patients recovering from cancer surgery.[89,90,91] Glutamine supplementation acts as a chemotherapy sensitizer and protector for normal cells.[90,92,93] The increased use of these approaches depends on additional study to verify effectiveness, target population, dosages, and scheduling.

Reduction of specific macronutrients has also been the target of nutritional intervention. Dietary fat intake has become a target for specific treatment, especially among patients with breast cancer.[11,23,94–97] Clinical trials indicate that verbal counseling results in significantly decreased fat intake within 3 months among patients with breast cancer.[95–97] The altered intake pattern is sustained past the period of counseling. Several of the trials have found documented increased survival among participants.[10,23,94] Reduction of fat in combination with other diet manipulations are also being tested. Garritson et al found that a high-fiber, low-fat diet with added omega-3 fatty acids increased levels of helper T-cells and decreased numbers of suppressor T-cells among individuals with breast cancer.[94] A similar research effort found that patients with pancreatic and prostate cancers who ate a low-fat, high-fiber, and lower-calorie diet in addition to standard therapy had improved survival times.[97]

In a case study, fat intake was prescribed as salvage therapy.[98] Two children with advanced malignant astrocytoma who had exhausted other treatment measures were placed on a high-fat diet. The diet produced ketogenesis and reduced tumor uptake of glucose. The disease was stabilized in both children and one demonstrated im-

Figure 33-3 Nutritional support algorithm for individuals undernourished at baseline. (GI = gastrointestinal tract; PHA = peripheral hyperalimentation; TPN = total parenteral nutrition)

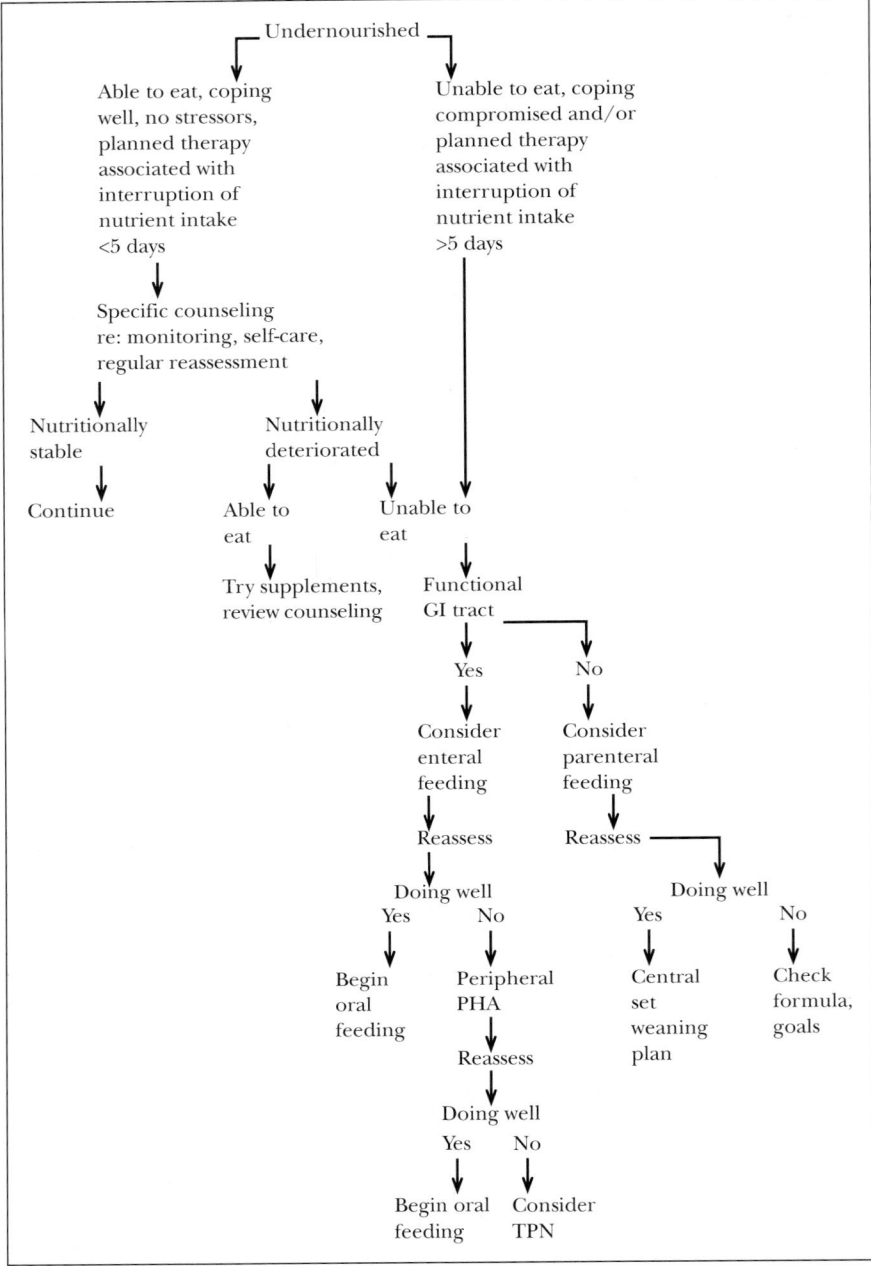

proved cognitive function. This trial utilized what is known about the dependency of the nervous system on glucose and the alteration of carbohydrate metabolism in cancer.

Alteration in general intake

A more traditional nutritional goal has been the improvement of the patient's overall intake to aid general nutritional status, minimize treatment side effects, and maximize treatment delivery. Increases in nutrient intake can significantly reduce the morbidity and mortality of severely malnourished patients in certain settings. However, the complex interaction of nutrition, cancer, and host can alter the usual response to increased intake. Investigators report that increased caloric intake may neither reverse weight loss nor improve survival.[23,50,64,84,94] Because of this complexity, specialized nutritional augmentation is not recommended for individuals who are adequately nourished, are not anticipated to be unable to eat for 10–14 days, or who have uncontrolled disease.[40,99] These criteria may provide direction for health care pro-

parenteral feeding.[40,73,99] The largest group of cancer patients receiving home parenteral nutrition are those with severe enteritis following curative radiation treatment.[119]

Other uses of aggressive nutritional support are controversial, in part because of problems of design or methodology in the extant research. Many of the studies have small sample sizes. The studies frequently have different nutritional outcomes, differing patient populations, and different feeding formulas. They also reveal that, although subsets of patients benefit from nutritional repletion, aggressive nutritional intervention does not alter morbidity or mortality for the majority of individuals with cancer. In addition, the risks associated with the various treatments must also be considered. The problems and common solutions associated with enteral and parenteral nutritional interventions are listed in Tables 33-7 and 33-8. The role of aggressive nutritional intervention in cancer treatment continues to require study. As the nutritional abnormali-

Table 33-7 Common Enteral Feeding Problems and Solutions

Problem	Solution
Diarrhea	Give formula at room temperature; use lactose-free formula; add fiber; add antidiarrheal medicine; reduce rate of feeding; reduce volume or use continuous feeding schedule; reduce strength of formula; review other potential sources (medications, treatment)
Regurgitation	Check tube placement; check residuals and withhold feedings if more than 100–200 mL; keep in Fowler's position; use small bore tube; place tube distally (jejunum, duodenum); consider drugs to increase motility
Nausea	Check tube placement; reduce rate; reduce anxiety; change formula; review other potential sources (infection, medications, treatment)
Distention	Use low-fat or hydrolyzed formula; encourage activity; review other potential sources (obstruction, constipation, organomegaly)
Dehydration	Increase water intake to ensure adequate amounts (usually 1 mL/kcal); control (diarrhea, nausea); watch for glucosuria
Fluid overload	Reduce water intake
Constipation	Increase water; increase fiber; increase activity
Local irritation	Clean area around tube; apply skin-protecting agents; monitor for otitis media if using nasal tubes
Mouth dryness	Frequent mouth rinsing; use xerostomia products; sugarless gum or mints if medically allowed
Tube obstruction	Use room temperature feedings; irrigate with water; use pump with high-density formulas (>1.5 kcal/mL) or small-bore tubes; use liquid medicines rather than crushing pills whenever possible
Metabolic imbalance	Monitor carbon dioxide levels; reduce carbohydrate in formula; monitor glucose; monitor potassium and supplement if needed

Table 33-8 Parenteral Feeding Considerations

General Indications: Presence of protein-calorie malnutrition; nonfunctioning gastrointestinal tract; unable to begin enteral feedings for 7 or more days; high-output fistulas; in combination with enteral feedings for some bowel resections; severe radiation enteritis with or without malignant disease; temporary malabsorption secondary to aggressive therapy (e.g., bone marrow transplant); obstructed bowel but otherwise acceptable quality of life

COMMON PARENTERAL FEEDING PROBLEMS AND SOLUTIONS

Problem	Solutions
Pneumo-hemothorax	Put patient in Trendelenburg position for line placement; check x-ray postprocedure
Embolism	Follow flushing regimen; avoid use of small diameter syringes when flushing; avoid exposure to free air
Obstruction	Flush per protocol; check for flow per protocol; treat with antiembolics per institutional protocol
Dislodgment	Assess for patency; be alert to patient complaints of pain or swelling in area of catheter insertion
Metabolic abnormalities	Monitor levels of glucose, ammonia, phosphate, liver enzymes, magnesium, potassium, hemoglobin/hematocrit
Infection	Perform careful site care and evaluation; monitor temperature, glucose levels, glucosuria
Trace element deficiency	Monitor vitamin and trace element
Bleeding	Monitor vitamin K administration

ties created by cancer are better understood, more appropriate interventions will be developed.[3,40,90,97]

Complementary, Alternative, and Questionable Nutritional Interventions

Selected traditional cancer centers are engaging in rigorous study of complementary and alternative medicine (CAM). This recent interest arises from at least two factors. One factor is the finding that from 49%–76% of individuals with cancer combine conventional and alternative or complementary therapies.[120–122] Nutritional approaches are the most commonly used complementary treatments. Secondly, there is increasing research evidence of effectiveness in some of the products used in CAM. These elements make it essential for nurses to understand both the benefits and disadvantages of CAM.

A number of therapeutic approaches rely heavily on nutritional components and have questionable or potentially harmful effects; these are listed in Table 33-9. As well, a number of readily available herbs and chemical supplements of unknown efficacy are advertised as helpful in improving health (Table 33-10). (See Chapter 27 for more detailed information on CAM). Knowledge about these products is constantly changing. It is essential for the nurse to remember several important details in gen-

Table 33-9 Questionable Dietary Treatments for Cancer

Diet/Additive	Proposed Activity	Comments/Side Effects
Antineoplastin/Burzynski therapy (peptide preparation originally derived from blood and urine)	Peptides are cytotoxic to cancer cells	FDA clinical trial showed no efficacy.
Cancell (nitric acid, sodium sulfate, sulfuric acid, potassium hydroxide)	Combination of ingredients alters electrical charges, creating lower voltage in cells. Cancer cells are susceptible to change and are converted to waste material.	Clinical trials showed no efficacy.
Gerson diet (daily coffee enemas, vegetarian diet, no sugar or salt, organic food purchased from Gerson Clinic)	Cleanses body of cancer toxins; reverses liver damage caused by toxins	Food requires extensive processing; expensive; enemas may cause perforated colon, enzyme imbalances
Macrobiotic diet (50%–60% calories from whole grains, 25%–30% from vegetables, 10%–25% from beans, seaweed, soy products); some rely heavily on rice with mineral and vitamins, including Laetrile; lifestyle changes (clothing choice, family involvement)	Cleanses body; "starves" cancer cells	Although properly constructed macrobiotic diets are adequate, many practitioners do not provide sufficient balanced nutrients. Protein, calorie, iron, vitamin B_{12}, and vitamin D deficiencies can occur.
Nieper Diet (restricted flour, red meat, sugar, coffee, tea; emphasizes eggs, whole grain products, B_{17} [Laetrile], carrot juice, high-doses of vitamins A, E, C, D, zinc, magnesium, calcium)	Cleanses body; "starves" cancer cells	Oral Laetrile associated with cyanide poisoning; high-dose vitamins associated with decreased immune function, liver damage, and renal toxicity

Data from American Cancer Society[123]; Cassileth.[124]

eral counseling about the use of herbs or chemical supplements:

- Preparations that may be useful in prevention of disease do not always have a salutary effect when the disease exists (e.g., saw palmetto reduces prostate size, possibly through phytoestrogenic action and may alter the effectiveness of hormonal drug treatment in prostate cancer).

- Preparations may be adulterated or contaminated with dangerous materials (e.g., lead and plant fillers containing digitalis or phytoestrogens have been found in some products).

- The complex interaction of nutrients, host, cancer, and cancer treatment, herbs and supplements can alter the metabolism of drugs, cancer, and the host in unknown ways (e.g., antioxidant supplements may alter the effectiveness of radiation or antimetabolite chemotherapy).

- There are positive effects from some supplements, and identifying accurate information can be difficult. (e.g., Internet sites abound; information from those selling products should be questioned).

Conclusion

Nutrition influences carcinogenesis itself as well as the quantity and quality of life once the disease exists. The nurse's ability to take full advantage of nutritional interventions is hampered by insufficient understanding of the pathophysiology of the tumor-host relationship. Without this knowledge, it is difficult to match a specific intervention with a specific nutritional problem.

This lack of knowledge emphasizes the importance of nursing care. Nurses are in the best position to detect undernutrition and overnutrition among individuals with cancer throughout the disease course. The nurse attends to basic nutritional information during the diagnostic process: height, weight, recent weight change, eating problems, unhealthy and healthful food choices, social situations that interfere with food procurement, and psychological responses that alter intake. Given this base, the nurse can work with other care providers to prioritize and define nutritional care. The nurse continues the assessment function throughout the patient's treatment and follow-up. Nutritional intervention can be devised in the overall context of the clinical situation and in accordance with the patient's beliefs and desires.

Although the scientific information is still far from complete, early nutritional intervention—when the tumor burden is relatively small—has the best chance to alter patient outcomes. This is particularly true for those undergoing surgery. Appropriate nutritional intervention reduces morbidity, length of hospital stay, and possibly mortality in these patients. For some patients the need for nutritional support will continue for a period following hospitalization. Understanding the limitations of nutritional interventions is important for both nurses

Table 33-10 Herbal, Vitamin, and Mineral Supplementation Associated with Alternative/Complementary Treatments for Cancer[130-132]

Herb, Vitamin, Mineral	Proposed Activity	Clinical Trial Results	Comments/Side Effects
Angelica	↑ Red blood cells, immune system	None available	May have estrogenic effect, ↑ sun sensitivity
Astragalus	↑ Interferon, T-cell count, stem cells; reduces side effects	Used in China; no clinical trial data available in U.S.	May cause diarrhea, bloating
Buckthorn	Cytotoxic action	None available	Strong laxative
Burdock, Turkey rhubarb, sorrel, slippery elm (essiac)	Cytotoxic combination	NCI-led animal studies negative; case studies describe minimal, possibly psychological, positive effects; drug company submitting trial to NCI	Contamination of burdock with belladonna in past; no other side effects reported
Cascara sagrada	Toxic to herpes simplex	Antileukemic activity in animals; no trials conducted in humans	Increases intestinal musculature contractility; diarrhea
Cat's claw	↑ Immune function; scavenge free radicals; one component alkaloid treats leukemia	NCI testing finds insufficient activity for cytotoxic testing; trials ongoing in Europe	May inhibit platelet aggregation; Often adulterated
Echinacea	Stimulates tumor necrosis factor, macrophage function; ↑ immune system function, ↑ healing; antibacterial action	Single study indicated that echinacea, combined with standard treatment, increase survival time in colon cancer	Often adulterated; not recommended for long-term use in individuals with HIV
Garlic	Chopped garlic transforms to allicin, an antibiotic antiprotozoan	Epidemiologic study suggests ↓ garlic intake associated with ↑ gastric cancer among Chinese	May interfere with clotting; cause gastric irritation
Ginseng	↑ Interferon production, antiherpetic; cytotoxic in animal trials; may ↑ survival in gastric cancer	Used in China; no clinical trial data available in U.S.	Commonly adulterated; may contain phytoandrogens
Gotu kola	Contains flavinoids; ↑ healing	None available	Sedative effect; interferes with diabetic drugs
Kombucha (Manchurian, Kargasok) tea	Fermentation product of yeasts and bacteria thought to be cytotoxic	No support for action	Contains alcohol, acetates, acetic acid, lactate; can leach lead from storage containers; has caused life-threatening acidosis in humans
Milk thistle (silymarin)	Protects liver cells from damage; antioxidant	Animal studies indicate a protective effect against skin cancers and chemotherapy-induced liver damage; reduces effect of tumor-promoting agents; no human trials conducted to date	
Mistletoe (Iscador)	Contains cytotoxic plant products; used in Europe	Associated with ↑ survival times in 10/11 studies; studies in Europe complicated because of preparation safety problems; may soon be studied in U.S.	Mistletoe can absorb harmful products from host plants; mistletoe berries are poisonous
Naturin[129]	↑ Helper T-cells, natural killer cell activity; ↓ radiation and chemotherapy cell injury	Still in trials for effectiveness, dosage[127]	
PC-SPES[128]	Herbal combination with estrogenic activity; used in treatment of prostate cancer	Clinical testing indicates significant estrogenic effect	Has similar side effects as other estrogens (breast tenderness, ↓ libido, venous thrombosis); may interfere with standard treatments for prostate cancer
Pycnogenol	Antioxidant; ↑ natural killer cell cytotoxicity	Uncontrolled studies performed in France; U.S. animal trials find natural killer enhancement; no human trials available	Side effects include allergic reactions, diarrhea; may interfere with oxidative action of radiation therapy; preparations vary in strength

Table 33-10   Herbal, Vitamin, and Mineral Supplementation Associated with Alternative/Complementary Treatments for Cancer[130–132] (continued)

Herb, Vitamin, Mineral	Proposed Activity	Clinical Trial Results	Comments/Side Effects
Rosemary	Antioxidant; inhibits cancer development; ↓ gastric upset; antibacterial action	None found	Large amounts cause intestinal cramping and irritation
Saw palmetto	↓ prostate size (benign disease)	Used in Europe; FDA banned labeling for prostate enlargement in U.S.	May interfere with prescription drugs, including those for prostatic hypertrophy and prostate cancer
Tea (green or black)[129]	Antioxidant activity may prevent cancer	Intake associated with ↑ survival time in Japanese breast cancer patients (stage I/II only)	Contains caffeine
Tumeric	Antioxidant (curcumin) may prevent cancer; decreases urinary mutagens in smokers	None available	Can cause stomach upset
White willow	Contains a salicylate (salicin); may mimic aspirin-like effects in prevention of esophageal, gastric, and colorectal cancers	None available	Side effects same as with all salicylates (gastric upset, tinnitus, rash, etc.)
DHEA	↑ Immune function; ↓ viral load (AIDS)		May have estrogenic effect
Vitamin A, retinoids, vitamin D	↑ Immune function, healing	Clinical trial results inconsistent	Long-term, high doses associated with liver damage, soft tissue calcification
Vitamin B₆ (pyridoxine)	↑ Immune function, healing	None available	Limb numbness, paresthesias
Niacin	↑ Immune function, healing; detoxifies system	None available	Doses above 3 g can cause liver damage, peptic ulcer, cardiac dysrhythmias and infarct, arthritis, skin rashes, flushing, diarrhea, nausea
Vitamin C	Antioxidant; ↑ differentiation, repair	No support for action	Kidney stones, rebound scurvy
Zinc	Adequate zinc levels promote healing; ↓ morbidity	Relationship to adequate zinc and survival reported in head/neck cancer patients	>60 mg/day associated with altered copper metabolism, reduced antioxidant function and immune response

NCI = National Cancer Institute; HIV = human immunodeficiency virus; PC-SPES = 8-herb dietary supplement; FDA = U.S. Food and Drug Administration; DHEA = dehydroepiandrosterone; AIDS = acquired immunodeficiency syndrome.
Data from Cassileth[124]; Shew et al[128]; Nakachi et al[129]; Tyler[130]; Farnsworth[131]; DiPaola et al.[132]

and patients. Assisting patients to make the best decisions for themselves may reduce frustration and use of questionable methods.

Nurses also should be attuned to newer approaches in the use of nutrition as therapy. Determining what part nutritional interventions will play in the cancer armamentarium needs additional study. Further, nurses have an obligation to continue research into the self-care actions routinely prescribed in dealing with nutritional disturbances. Many of the actions commonly suggested are based on anecdotal evidence alone. Much more study is needed before a nurse can accurately predict which self-care actions will be effective for a given patient. With the base of nursing research added to that of other disciplines, oncology nurses can positively influence the incidence and prevalence of nutritional deficiencies in cancer.

References

1. Chandra R: Nutrition and immunity: Lessons from the past and new insights into the future. *Am J Clin Nutr* 53: 1087–1101, 1991
2. Warren S: The immediate causes of death in cancer. *Am J Med Sci* 184:610–615, 1932
3. Shils ME: Nutrition and diet in cancer management, in Olson J, Shike ME (eds): *Modern Nutrition in Health and Disease* (ed 8). Philadelphia, Lea and Febiger, 1994, pp 1319–1342

4. Edelstein S: Nutritional assessment in cancer cachexia. *Pediatr Nurs* 17:237–240, 1991

5. Nelson K, Walsh D, Sheehan F: The cancer anorexia-cachexia syndrome. *J Clin Oncol* 12:213–225, 1994

6. McCarter MD, Gentilini OD, Gomez ME, Daly JM: Perioperative oral support with immunonutrients in cancer patients. *Journal of Parenteral & Enteral Nutrition* 22:206–211, 1998

7. Ottery FD: Cancer cachexia. *Cancer Pract* 2:123–131, 1994

8. The Veteran's Affairs Total Parenteral Nutrition Cooperative Study Group: Perioperative total parenteral nutrition in surgical patients. *N Engl J Med* 325:525–532, 1991

9. Andrassy RJ, Chwals WJ: Nutritional support of the pediatric oncology patient. *Nutrition* 14:124–129, 1998

10. de Lorgeril M, Salen P, Martin JL, et al: Mediterranean dietary patterns in a randomized trial: Prolonged survival and possible reduced cancer rate. *Arch Intern Med* 158:1181–1187, 1998

11. Goodwin PJ, Boyd NF: Body size and breast cancer prognosis. *Breast Cancer Res Treat* 16:205–214, 1990

12. Bastarrachea J, Hortobagyi GN, Smith TL, et al: Obesity as an adverse prognostic factor for patients receiving adjuvant chemotherapy for breast cancer. *Ann Intern Med* 119:18–25, 1993

13. Heys S, Park G, Forlick P, et al: Nutrition and malignant disease: Implications for surgical practice. *Br J Surg* 79:614–623, 1992

14. Langstein H, Norton J: Mechanisms of cancer cachexia. *Hematol Oncol Clin North Am* 5:103–120, 1991

15. Ottery FD: Supportive nutrition to prevent cachexia and improve quality of life. *Semin Oncol* 22:98–111, 1995

16. Coates K, Morgan S, Barollucci A, et al: Hospitalized malnutrition: A reevaluation 12 years later. *J Am Diet Assoc* 93:27–33, 1993

17. Tchekmedyian NS, Zahyra D, Halpert CR, et al: Assessment and maintenance of nutrition in older cancer patients. *Oncology* 6:105–111, 1992 (suppl 2)

18. Baker J, Detsky A, Wesson D, et al: Nutritional assessment: A comparison of clinical judgement and objective measures. *N Engl J Med* 306:969–972, 1982

19. Lipkin E, Bell S: Assessment of nutritional status. *Clin Lab Med* 13:329–352, 1993

20. Charney P: Nutrition assessment in the 1990s: Where are we now? *Nutr Clin Pract* 10:131–139, 1995

21. Senie RT, Rosen PP, Rhodes P, et al: Obesity at diagnosis of breast carcinoma influences duration of disease-free survival. *Arch Intern Med* 116:26–33, 1992

22. Levine E, Raczynski J, Carpenter J: Weight gain with breast cancer adjuvant treatment. *Cancer* 67:1954–1959, 1991

23. Holm L, Nordevang E, Hjalmer M, et al: Treatment failure and dietary habits in women with breast cancer. *J Natl Cancer Inst* 85:32–36, 1993

24. Colletti R, Copeland K, Devlin J, et al: Effect of obesity on plasma insulin-like growth factor in cancer patients. *Int J Obes* 15:523–527, 1991

25. Tayek JA: Review of cancer cachexia and abnormal glucose metabolism in humans with cancer. *J Am Coll Nutr* 11:445–456, 1992

26. Heber D, Tchekmedyian NS: Pathology of cancer. *Oncology* 49:28–31, 1992

27. Moldawer L, Rogy M, Lowry S: The role of cytokines in cancer cachexia. *J Parenter Enter Nutr* 16:43S–49S, 1992

28. Heber D, Byerly L, Tchekmedyian NS: Hormonal and metabolic abnormalities in the malnourished cancer patient. *J Parenter Enter Nutr* 16:60S–64S, 1992

29. Grindel CG: Weight gain in breast cancer patients receiving adjuvant chemotherapy as a function of restraint and disinhibition. *Oncol Nurs Forum* 17:23–27, 1990

30. Foltz AT: Weight gain among Stage II breast cancer patients: A study of five factors. *Oncol Nurs Forum* 12:21–26, 1985

31. Larson PJ, Lindsey AM, Dodd MJ, et al: Influence of age on problems experienced by patients with lung cancer undergoing radiation therapy. *Oncol Nurs Forum* 20:473–480, 1993

32. Waltman N, Bergstrom N, Armstrong N, et al: Nutritional status, pressure sores, and mortality in elderly patients with cancer. *Oncol Nurs Forum* 18:405–410, 1991

33. Staal-van den Brekel A, Schols A, ten Velde G, et al: Analysis of the energy balance in lung cancer patients. *Cancer Res* 54:6430–6433, 1994

34. Daly JM, Redmond HP, Lieberman M, et al: Nutritional support of patients with cancer of the gastrointestinal tract. *Surg Clin North Am* 71:523–536, 1991

35. Guo CB, Ma DQ, Zhang W: Applicability of the general nutritional status score to patients with oral and maxillofacial malignancies. *Int J Oral Maxillofac Surg* 23:167–169, 1994

36. Tchekmedyian NS, Zahyra D, Halpert CR, et al: Clinical aspects of nutrition in advanced cancer. *Oncology* 49:3–7, 1992

37. Ulander K, Jeppsson B, Grahn G: Postoperative energy intake in patients after colorectal cancer surgery. *Scand J Caring Sci* 12:131–138, 1998

38. Deutsch J: Normal digestive physiology and the evaluation of function. *Semin Oncol* 25:4–11, 1998

39. Williamson J: Physiologic stress: Trauma, sepsis, burns, and surgery, in Mahon L, Arliln M (eds): *Krause's Food, Nutrition and Diet Therapy* (ed 4). Philadelphia, Saunders, 1992, pp 503–504

40. Rivadeneira D, Evoy D, Fahey T, et al: Nutritional support of the cancer patient. *CA Cancer J Clin* 48:69–80, 1998

41. Winningham ML, Nail LM, Barton-Burke M, et al: Fatigue and the cancer experience: The state of the knowledge. *Oncol Nurs Forum* 21:23–26, 1994

42. Zimmermann F, Geinitz H, Feldmann H: Therapy and prophylaxis of acute and late radiation induced sequelae of the esophagus. *Strahlenther Onkol* 174:78–81, 1998 (suppl 3)

43. Donner C: Pathophysiology and therapy of chronic radiation-induced injury to the colon. *Dig Dis* 16:253–261, 1998

44. Jenns K: The importance of nausea. *Cancer Nurs* 17:488–493, 1994

45. Hesketh P, Kris M, Grunberg S, et al: Proposal for classifying the acute emetogenicity of cancer chemotherapy. *J Clin Oncol* 15:103–109, 1997

46. Bond S, Ham A, Wolton S, et al: Energy intake and basal metabolic rate during maintenance chemotherapy. *Arch Dis Child* 67:1318–1319, 1992

47. Wujcik D: An odyssey into biologic therapy. *Oncol Nurs Forum* 20:879–887, 1993

48. Samlowski WE, Wieble G, McMurry M, et al: Effects of total parenteral nutrition (TPN) during high dose interluekin 2 therapy for metastatic cancer. *J Immunother* 21:65–74, 1998

49. Hawthorn J: *Understanding and Management of Nausea and Vomiting.* Cambridge, MA, Blackwell Science, 1995

50. Ovesen L, Hannibal J, Allingstrup L: Dietary intake in patients with small cell lung cancer. *Eur J Clin Nutr* 46:435–437, 1992

51. Mattes RD, Curran WJ Jr, Alavi J, et al: Clinical implications of learned food aversions in patients with cancer treated with chemotherapy or radiation therapy. *Cancer* 70: 192–200, 1992

52. Grant M, Padilla GV, Rhiner M: Patterns of anorexia in cancer patients, in *Maintaining Nutritional Status in Persons with Cancer* (Pub No.71–25M-3332–03PE). Alanta, American Cancer Society, 1991, pp 12–27

53. Goodwin P, Esplen MJ, Butler K, et al: Multidisciplinary weight management in locoregional breast cancer. *Breast Cancer Res Treat* 48:53–64, 1998

54. Cioffi L: General theory of critical periods and the development of obesity, in Smogyi J (ed): *Nutritional, Psychological and Social Aspects of Obesity*. Basel, Karger, 1968, pp 17–28

55. Fearnon KCH: The mechanisms and treatment of weight loss in cancer. *Proc Nutr Soc* 51:251–256, 1992

56. Goodwin WJ, Byers PM: Nutritional management of the head and neck cancer patient. *Med Clin North Am* 77: 597–610, 1993

57. Meguid M, Muscaritoli M, Beverly J, et al: The early cancer anorexia paradigm: Changes in plasma free tryptophan and feeding indexes. *J Parenter Enter Nutr* 16:56S–59S, 1992

58. McNamara MJ, Alexander AR, Norton JA: Cytokines and their role in the pathophysiology of cancer cachexia. *J Parenter Enter Nutr* 16:50S–55S, 1992

59. Tchekmedyian NS, Heber D: Cancer and AIDS cachexia: Mechanisms and approaches to therapy. *Oncology* 7:55–59, 1993 (suppl)

60. Lowry S: Cancer cachexia revisited: Old problems and new perspectives. *Eur J Cancer* 27:1–3, 1991

61. Theologides A: Anorexins, asthenins, and cachectins in cancer. *Am J Med* 81:696–698, 1991

62. Istafan N, Wan J, Bistrian B: Nutrition and tumor promotion. *J Parenter Enter Nutr* 16:76S–82S, 1991

63. Mulligan K, Bloch A: Energy expenditure and protein metabolism in human immunodeficiency virus infection and cancer cachexia. *Semin Oncol* 25:82–91, 1998 (2 suppl 6)

64. Sarna L, Lindsey AM, Dean H, et al: Nutrient intake, weight change, symptom distress, and functional status over time in adults with lung cancer. *Oncol Nurs Forum* 20:481–489, 1993

65. McMahon K, Decker G, Ottery F: Integrating proactive nutritional assessment in clinical practices to prevent complications and cost. *Semin Oncol* 25:20–27, 1998 (2 suppl 6)

66. Gilbride J, Castro J: Malnutrition in the hospital, in Simko M, Cowell C, Gilbride J (eds): *Nutritional Assessment* (ed 2). Gaithersburg, MD, Aspen, 1995, pp 25–40

67. Detsky AS, McLaughlin JR, Baker JP, et al: What is subjective global assessment of nutritional status? *J Parenter Enter Nutr* 11:8–13, 1987

68. Ottery FD: Definition of standardized nutritional assessment and interventional pathways in oncology. *Nutrition* 12:S15–S19, 1996

69. Bowers JM, Dols CL: Subjective global assessment in HIV-infected patients. *J Assoc Nurs AIDS Care* 7:83–89, 1996

70. Buzby GP, Mullen JL, Matthews DC, et al: Prognostic nutritional index in gastrointestinal surgery. *Am J Surg* 139: 160–167, 1980

71. Whitney E, Cataldo C, Rolfes S: *Understanding Normal and Clinical Nutrition* (ed 3). St. Paul, MN, West Publishing, 1991

72. Harvey K, Moldwater L, Bistrian B, et al: Biological measure for the formulation of a hospital prognostic index. *Am J Clin Nutr* 34:2012–2015, 1981

73. Schlag P, Decker-Baumann C: Strategies and needs for nutritional support in cancer surgery. *Recent Results Cancer Res* 121:233–252, 1991

74. Robinett-Weiss N, Hixson M, Kier B, et al: The Metropolitan height-weight tables. *J Am Diet Assoc* 84:1480–1481, 1984

75. Willett W, Stampfer J, VanItallie T: New weight guidelines for Americans: Justified or injudicious. *Am J Clin Nutr* 53: 1102–1103, 1991

76. Kondsup J, Bak L, Hansen B, et al: Outcome from nutritional support using hospital food. *Nutrition* 14:319–321, 1998

77. Ringold-Smith K, William R, Horowitz E, et al: Determination of energy expenditure in the bone marrow transplant patient. *Nutr Clin Prac* 13:215–218, 1998

78. Vanek V: Use of serum albumin as a prognostic or nutritional marker. *Nutr Clin Prac* 13:110–112, 1998

79. Lindsey AM, Larson PJ, Dodd MJ, et al: Comorbidity, nutritional intake, social support, weight and functional status over time in older cancer patients receiving radiotherapy. *Cancer Nurs* 17:113–124, 1994

80. Klidgjian A, Archer T, Foster K, et al: Detection of dangerous malnutrition. *J Parenter Enter Nutr* 6:119–121, 1982

81. Nail LM, Jones L, Lauver D, et al: Use and perceived adequacy of self-care activities in patients receiving chemotherapy. *Oncol Nurs Forum* 18:883–887, 1991

82. Skolin I, Alexsson K, Ghannad P, et al: Nutrient intake and weight development in children during chemotherapy for malignant disease. *Oral Oncol* 33:364–368, 1997

83. Van Eys J: Benefits of nutritional intervention on nutritional status, quality of life, and survival. *Int J Cancer* 11: 66–68, 1998 (suppl)

84. Lundholm K, Hyltander A, Sandstrom R: Nutritional support in cancer treatment. *Curr Opin Oncol* 3:621–627, 1991

85. Goodman M, Kolonel L, Wilkens L, et al: Dietary factors in lung cancer diagnosis. *Eur J Cancer* 28:495–501, 1992

86. Filston H: What's new in pediatric surgery. *Pediatrics* 96: 748–757, 1995

87. Cady B: Basic principles in surgical oncology. *Arch Surg* 132:338–346, 1997

88. Taylor MA: Benefits of dehydration in terminally ill patients. *Geriatr Nurs* 16:271–272, 1995

89. Feyer P, Zimmermann JS, Titlbach OJ, et al: Radiotherapy-induced emesis: An overview. *Strahlenther Onkol* 174:56–61, 1998 (suppl 3)

90. Chuntrasakul C, Siltharm S, Sarasombath S: Metabolic and immune effects of dietary arginine, glutamine, and omega 3 fatty acids supplementation in immunized patients. *J Med Assoc Thai* 81:334–343, 1998

91. Imoberdorf R: Immuno-nutrition. *Support Care Cancer* 5: 381–386, 1997

92. Zeigler TR, Bye RL, Persinger RL, et al: Effects of glutamine supplementation on circulating lymphocytes after bone marrow transplantation. *Am J Med Sci* 31:4–10, 1998

93. Klimberg VS, Pappas A, Nwokedi E, et al: Effect of supplemental glutamine on methotrexate concentration in tumors. *Arch Surg* 127:1317–1320, 1992

94. Garritson BK, Niklein A, Peters GN, et al: Effect of major dietary modification on the immune system in patients with breast cancer. *Cancer Pract* 3:329–342, 1995

95. White E, Shattuck A, Dristal A, et al: Maintenance of a low-fat diet: Follow-up of the Women's Health Trial. *Cancer Epidemiol Biomarkers Prev* 1:315–323, 1992

96. de Waard F, Ramlan R, Mulders Y, et al: A feasibility study on weight reduction in obese postmenopausal breast cancer patients. *Eur J Cancer Prev* 2:233–238, 1993

97. Carter J, Saxe G, Newbold V, et al: Hypothesis: Dietary management may improve survival from nutritionally

linked cancers based on analysis of representative cases. *J Am Coll Nutr* 12:209–226, 1993

98. Nebeling C, Miraldi F, Shurin S, et al: Effects of a ketogenic diet on tumor metabolism and nutritional status in pediatric oncology patients. *J Am Coll Nutr* 14:202–208, 1995

99. Klein S, Koretz RL: Nutrition support in patients with cancer: What do the data really show? *Nutr Clin Pract* 9:91–100, 1994

100. Smith M, Holcombe J, Stullenbarger E: A meta-analysis of intervention effectiveness for symptom management in oncology nursing research. *Oncol Nurs Forum* 21:1201–1209, 1994

101. Foltz A, Gullatte M, Gaines G: Post-hospitalization self-care actions among medical oncology patients. *Oncol Nurs Forum* 23:679–683, 1996

102. Ottery FD, Walsh D, Strawford A: Pharmacological management of anorexia/cachexia. *Semin Oncol* 25:35–44, 1998

103. Loprinzi CL: Management of cancer anorexia/cachexia. *Support Care Cancer* 3:120–123, 1995

104. Kardinal CL, Loprinzi CL, Scaid DJ, et al: A controlled trial of cyproheptadine in cancer patients with anorexia and/or cachexia. *Cancer* 65:2657–2662, 1990

105. Bruera E, Roca E, Cedaro L, et al: Action of oral methylprednisolone in terminal cancer patients. *Cancer Treat Rep* 69:751–754, 1992

106. Tchekmedyian NS, Hickman M, Siau J, et al: Megestrol acetate in cancer anorexia and weight loss. *Cancer* 69:1268–1274, 1992

107. Breura E, Macmillan K, Kuehn N, et al: A controlled trial of Megestrol acetate on appetite, caloric intake, nutritional status, and other symptoms in patients with advanced cancer. *Cancer* 66:1279–1282, 1990

108. Kornblith AB, Hollis D, Zuckerman E, et al: Effect of Megestrol acetate on quality of life in a dose-response trial in women with advanced breast cancer. *J Clin Oncol* 11:2081–2089, 1993

109. Loprinzi CL, Michalek JC, Scaid DJ, et al: Phase III evaluation of four doses of Megestrol acetate as therapy for patients with cancer anorexia and/or cachexia. *J Clin Oncol* 11:762–767, 1993

110. Plasse TF, Gortner RW, Krasnow SH, et al: Recent clinical experience with dronabinol. *Pharmacol Biochem Behav* 40:695–700, 1991

111. Nelson KA, Walsh TD, Deeter P, et al: A phase II study of delta-9–tetrahydrocannabinol for appetite stimulation in cancer-associated anorexia. *J Palliat Care* 10:14–18, 1994

112. Pearlstone D, Wolf R, Berman R, et al: Effect of systemic insulin on protein kinetics in postoperative cancer patients. *Ann Surg Oncol* 1:321–332, 1994

113. Cerosimo E, Pisters PW, Pesola G, et al: The effect of graded doses of insulin on peripheral glucose uptake and lactate release in cancer cachexia. *Surgery* 109:459–467, 1991

114. Kosty MP, Fleishman SB, Herndon JE, et al: Cisplatin, vinblastine and hydrazine sulfate in advanced non-small cell lung cancer. *Proc Am Soc Clin Oncol* 11:294, 1992 (abstr)

115. Goldberg R, Loprinzi C, Mailliard J, et al: A randomized placebo-controlled evaluation of pentoxifylline in patients with cancer anorexia and cachexia. *Proc Am Soc Clin Oncol* 13:459, 1994 (abstr)

116. Haslett PA: Anticytokine approaches to the treatment of anorexia and cachexia. *Semin Oncol* 25:53–57, 1998 (suppl 6)

117. Muurahainen N, Mulligan K: Clinical trials in human immunodeficiency virus wasting. *Semin Oncol* 25:104–111, 1998 (suppl 6)

118. Daly JM, Weintraub FN, Shou J, et al: Enteral nutrition during multimodal therapy in upper gastrointestinal cancer patients. *Ann Surg* 221:327–338, 1995

119. Howard L: Home parenteral nutrition in patients with a cancer diagnosis. *J Parenter Enter Nutr* 16:93S–99S, 1992

120. Montbriand MJ: An overview of alternate therapies chosen by patients with cancer. *Oncol Nurs Forum* 21:1547–1554, 1994

121. Montbriand MJ: Abandoning biomedicine for alternative therapies: Oncology patients' stories. *Cancer Nurs* 21:36–45, 1998

122. Ernst E, Cassileth BR: The prevalence of complementary/alternative medicine in cancer. *Cancer* 83:777–785, 1998

123. American Cancer Society: *Nutritional Therapies: Questionable Methods of Cancer Management* (Publ. no. 93–2M–N0315). Atlanta, American Cancer Society, 1993

124. Cassileth BR: *The Alternative Medicine Handbook.* New York, Norton, 1998

125. Oguchi J, Shikama N, Sasaki S. et al. Mucosa-adhesive water-soluble polymer film for treatment of acute radiation-induced oral mucositis. *Int J Radiat Oncol Biol Phys* 40:1033–1037, 1998

126. Foltz AT: Nutritional disturbances, in Groenwald SL, Frogge MH, Goodman M, Yarbo CH (eds): *Cancer Nursing: Principles and Practice* (ed 4). Sudbury, MA, Jones and Bartlett, 1997, pp 655–683

127. Spaulding-Albright N: A review of some herbal and related products commonly used in cancer patients. *J Am Diet Assoc* 97:S208–215, 1997 (10 suppl)

128. Shen RN, Lu L, Jia XQ, et al: Naturin. *In Vivo* 10:201–209, 1996

129. Nakachi K, Suemasu K, Suga K, et al: Influence of drinking green tea on breast cancer malignancy among Japanese patients. *Jpn J Cancer Res* 89:254–261, 1998

130. Tyler VE: *Herbs of Choice.* Binghamton, NY, Haworth Press, 1993

131. Farnsworth NR: Relative safety of herbal medicines. *J Am Botan Council Herb Res Found HerbalGram* 29:36A–G, 1993

132. DiPaola RS, Zhang H, Lambert GH, et al: Clinical and biologic activity of an estrogenic herbal combination in prostate cancer. *N Engl J Med* 339:839–841, 1998

CHAPTER 34

Hypercalcemia

Rita S. Wickham, RN, PhD, AOCN

Scope of the Problem

Definition

Hypercalcemia is the most common metabolic complication of malignancy and can be life-threatening for some patients. Hypercalcemia is diagnosed when the serum calcium exceeds 11.0 mg/dL (or is greater than 5.5 mEq/L, or 2.74 mmol/L; or is greater than 1.35 mmol/L of *ionized* calcium). However, this definition is simplistic and does not capture the severity of hypercalcemia, which can be symptomatic with relatively small increases in serum calcium levels. Other factors, such as the rapidity of development, renal function, age, relative physical health, concomitant medications, and previous episodes of hypercalcemia, are also important.[1] Hypercalcemia occurs because of a breakdown of normal calcium homeostasis and almost always develops in patients whose cancer is advanced; prognosis is limited (approximately 2–6 months).[2] Nevertheless, prompt recognition and treatment usually enhances quality of life, and antiresorptive therapies may increase duration of survival for some individuals.

Incidence

It is estimated that 10%–40% of cancer patients experience hypercalcemia as a relatively late complication of malignancy, but incidence varies widely by tumor type (Table 34-1).[1–10] Because they occur frequently, breast cancer (with multiple bone metastases) and lung cancer account for 22%–60% of all cases.[2] While hypercalcemia is frequent among patients with uncommon malignancies, it is rare in some common malignancies, such as colorectal and prostate cancer, and virtually never occurs in patients who have primary bone tumors. An iatrogenic cause of transient hypercalcemia in some women with breast cancer is tumor flare, which occurs with the initiation of hormone therapy.[1] It has been proposed that the incidence of hypercalcemia may actually be decreasing because of the widespread use of bisphosphonates.[11]

Etiology and Risk Factors

More than 90% of patients who develop hypercalcemia have primary hyperparathyroidism or malignant disease. Other causes of hypercalcemia are infrequent and include drug effects, congenital problems, thyroid or renal dysfunction, and immobilization (Table 34-2).[2,12–14]

Hyperparathyroidism is the most frequent etiology of hypercalcemia, but patients with this condition usually are not acutely symptomatic because hypercalcemia develops over a long period of time, and homeostatic mechanisms can come into play. Thus, patients with primary hyperparathyroidism are commonly ambulatory, and hypercalcemia is typically diagnosed by routine laboratory tests.[2] On the other hand, hypercalcemia due to cancer is usually steadily and rapidly progressive, so homeostatic mechanisms are overwhelmed. Cancer-induced hypercalcemia most often rapidly leads to symptoms, even with relatively low serum calcium levels, which necessitates hospitalization, prompt diagnosis, and treatment. Most patients have obvious widespread metastases when hypercalcemia is diagnosed but may or may not have bone metastases, depending on the primary pathogenic mechanisms involved.

Table 34-1 Incidence of Hypercalcemia in Particular Malignancies

Malignancy	Reported Incidence	References
Lung		1,5,10
Squamous cell	35%	
Other	11%	
Breast	17–40%	2,10
Hematologic		4,9,10
Adult T-cell lymphoma/leukemia	50%	
Multiple myeloma	20–40%	
Lymphoma	<10%	
Genitourinary	12%	10
Head and neck (squamous)	2.5–25% (varies by site)	3,10
Renal cell	6%	1
Unknown primary	7%	1
Liver (primary)	3%	1,10
Other: cholangiocarcinoma, clear cell carcinoma of the ovary, pancreatic islet cell, vipoma	1%	2,6
Prostate, uterine, colorectal, primary bone, parathyroid, chronic lymphocytic leukemia, chronic myelogenous leukemia, acute leukemia, small cell lung cancer	<1%	2,7–10

Table 34-2 Etiologies of Hypercalcemia

Relative Frequency	Comments
FREQUENT	
Primary hyperparathyroidism	• Develops over a long period, usually asymptomatic
	• Parathyroid adenomas cause >80% of cases
Malignancy	• More likely to occur rapidly, leading to neurological, cardiovascular, gastrointestinal, and fluid volume deficit symptoms
	• May be accompanied by other symptoms of advanced cancer
RARE	
Dietary (or Drug)	
Vitamin D intoxication	• Chronic ingestion of >50,000 IU/day or excessive ingestion of foods high in vitamin D
Vitamin A intoxication	• Chronic ingestion of >50,000 units/day
Milk-alkali syndrome	• Associated with chronic use of milk and antacids; leads to mild metabolic alkalosis and renal calcium reabsorption
Drugs	
Lithium	• Alters "set point" for PTH secretion, causing mild hypercalcemia
Thiazide diuretics	
Tamoxifen, estrogens, antiestrogens	• Increases bone resorption
Theophylline toxicity	• May increase effect of PTH
Endocrine disorders	• No specific information available regarding mechanisms
Hyperthyroidism	
Pheocromocytoma	
Adrenal insufficiency (Addison's disease)	
Thyrotoxicosis	
Granulomatous diseases	
Sarcoidosis	• Increased 1-alpha-hydroxylase activity leading to elevated serum 1,25-dihydroxyvitamin D
Histoplasmosis	
Tuberculosis	
Coccidioidomycosis	
Other	
Familial hypocalciuric hypercalcemia	• Autosomal dominant inherited condition
Diuretic phase of acute renal failure	• Increased renal calcium reabsorption
Acute and chronic renal failure	• Increased resorption of calcium from bone
Paget's disease	• Increased renal calcium reabsorption
Immobilization	• Increased resorption of calcium from bone

PTH = parathyroid hormone.

Hypercalcemia of Malignancy: Physiologic Alterations

The fundamental cause of hypercalcemia is that more calcium is resorbed from bone than is deposited in bone, which is usually coupled with secondary impaired renal excretion of excessive serum calcium.[5,11,12,15] Tumors, or normal tissues surrounding them, produce and secrete one or several hormone-like polypeptides (cytokines) or other regulatory factors, which subsequently act systemically or locally to impair normal calcium homeostasis. The pathophysiology of hypercalcemia differs somewhat depending on the underlying malignancy, but these mechanisms result in only subtle differences in organ effects that do not generally require different treatments. Therefore, it is probably most useful to bear in mind that

there are no absolute divisions in types of malignancy-induced hypercalcemia, and pathogenic processes most likely occur along a continuum rather than being discrete etiologic groups.[15]

One of two mechanisms is usually the primary cause of hypercalcemia: humoral hypercalcemia of malignancy (HHM) or local osteolytic hypercalcemia (LOH). Humoral hypercalcemia occurs most frequently and is estimated to cause nearly 80% of hypercalcemia cases, whereas LOH causes 20%–30% of cases.[10,14] The broad classifications of HHM and LOH are not totally inclusive for all malignancies, and particular tumors may elaborate other cytokines or hormones that have effects on organ systems involved in calcium homeostasis. For instance, hematologic malignancies may produce 1,25-dihydroxyvitamin D, which causes increased calcium resorption from bone, increased absorption of dietary calcium from the gut, and possibly impaired glomerular filtration of calcium.[9] In addition, immobilization because of poorly controlled pain or other symptoms, or renal failure may worsen hypercalcemia.

Humoral Hypercalcemia of Malignancy

Patients with HHM, who may or may not have bone metastases, have tumors that elaborate and secrete humoral factors (hormones and cytokines) that act systemically or locally to induce excessive calcium resorption from bone and resultant hypercalcemia.[5] The most important hormone is parathyroid hormone–related peptide (PTHrP), which is detectable in the serum of about 80% of hypercalcemic patients who have solid tumors.[16,17] Both parathyroid hormone (PTH) and PTHrP probably evolved from the same ancestral gene, and while the gene for PTHrP is more complex than that for PTH, both gene products share similar structure and biologic function.[10,15,18] That is, the release of either is associated with increased osteoclast bone resorption, reduced bone formation, and increased tubular resorption of calcium. Parathyroid hormone and PTHrP are both normally expressed in fetal and adult tissues, but serum PTHrP levels are undetectable in healthy adults. Parathyroid hormone–related peptide has multiple roles in the differentiation and physiologic functioning of normal tissues, including cartilage and bone, skin, breast, pancreatic islets, kidney, mammary epithelium, placenta, smooth muscle function, and in immune functions.[17,19]

Parathyroid hormone–related peptide does have some distinct roles, such as the establishment of bone metastases in breast cancer and an autocrine function in the growth of some tumors.[16,20] It is elaborated by some malignant tumors that are not accompanied by extensive bone metastases, including squamous cell carcinomas of the lung, head, and neck; breast malignancies; and adenocarcinomas of the kidney, lung, pancreas, or ovary.[15] Ectopic PTHrP does not respond to normal negative feedback loops, and serum calcium levels rise to dangerous levels.

Tumor-produced PTHrP probably does not account for all of the clinical features of HHM, and effects on the bone, kidney, and intestine of patients with cancer may be influenced by other tumor-produced factors, such as interleukins, tumor growth factor (TGF), tumor necrosis factor (TNF), and epidermal growth factor (EGF).[21,22] High production of any of these factors can directly increase osteoclastic bone resorption, and they can also potentiate the effects of PTHrP on osteoclast activity and calcium homeostasis.[15] Furthermore, PTHrP-induced renal tubular calcium resorption occurs in many patients with solid tumors, and in some patients with multiple myeloma and breast cancer, in whom circulating PTHrP is usually not an important factor. In these patients, volume depletion impairs glomerular filtration and leads to increased sodium and calcium resorption in the proximal convoluted tubules. However, increased renal tubular calcium resorption persists even after dehydration is corrected.[15]

Local Osteolytic Hypercalcemia

In patients who have breast cancer or multiple myeloma, hypercalcemia usually occurs late in the disease and almost never develops unless the patient has extensive osteolytic bone metastases.[2,9] However, tumor cells do not resorb bone but produce local cytokines or other regulatory factors that induce local bone absorption, osteolysis, and hypercalcemia.[15] Increased levels of osteoclast-regulating factors are found adjacent to and within skeletal metastases, and induce osteoclasts to migrate to the tumor site and become active. This leads to uncoupling of bone formation and destruction of bone.[23–25] Local production of PTHrP by tumor cells is probably the most important mechanism of LOH, as breast cancer patients with LOH have been shown to have increased PTHrP near tumor cells in bone, but no increases occur in the primary tumor, soft tissue metastases, or plasma.[26] This finding is consistent with the "seed and soil" theory. That is, bone provides a fertile environment for tumor cell growth, which is enhanced by PTHrP production in this microenvironment. Similarly, multiple myeloma almost always causes destructive osteolytic bone lesions throughout the skeleton, leading to diffuse osteopenia. Bone destruction is the consequence of myeloma-produced mediators, such as IL-6, IL-1β, and TNF-α, and lymphotoxin.[9]

Normal Anatomy and Physiology: Scientific Principles

Normal Calcium Homeostasis

The body's total calcium content is approximately 1 kg, of which 99% is bound in bones and teeth. Only the remaining 1% of calcium, which is found in the serum, is of interest. Forty-five to 50% of serum calcium is ionized (Ca^{2+}), which is the biologically active form. Forty percent is bound to protein, primarily albumin, and a small amount is bound to globulin.[12–14] The remaining 10%–15% is complexed with bicarbonate, citrate, or phosphate. Normal serum calcium levels reflect ionized and bound forms (unless ionized calcium is specifically measured), and are maintained in a constant narrow range. The ranges vary slightly by gender, and for men are approximately 9.0–10.3 mg/dL (or 4.5–5.2 mEq/L, or 2.25–2.57 mmol/L), and for women 8.9–10.2 mg/dL (or 4.4–5.1 mEq/L, or 2.22–2.54 mmol/L).[27]

Only ionized Ca^{2+} is physiologically active and filtered in the kidney. Ca^{2+} has multiple effects on parathyroid function; the kidney and other organs and tissues; and in modulating enzyme function, intracellular and extracellular signaling, bone functioning, clotting factors, and adhesion molecules.[12,28] Among its most important activities, Ca^{2+} regulates many intracellular and extracellular functions, particularly the electrical potential of cells and thus neuromuscular conductivity and transmission.

Despite the fact that calcium levels fluctuate each day with dietary calcium consumption and bone remodeling, serum calcium remains within a remarkably narrow range because of the actions of several calciotropic hormones (parathyroid hormone, 1,23-dihydroxyvitamin D, and calcitonin) on target organ systems (bone, gastrointestinal tract, and kidney). For instance, 200–400 mg of calcium is released and is taken up by bone each day during bone remodeling. Under normal circumstances, calcium fluxes across bone surfaces not involved in remodeling are greater than those involved in remodeling.[4] Bone surface cells not actively involved in bone remodeling communicate with deeper osteocytes, which can rapidly interact to regulate calcium transport from the extraosseous extracellular fluid to the serum. This system has the potential capacity to move large volumes of calcium from bone to serum, which occurs under the influence of parathyroid hormone.

Each day, approximately 900 mg of calcium is consumed in the diet, and the influence of 1,25-dihydroxyvitamin D causes about 350 mg to be absorbed from the gastrointestinal tract. Of this, 150 mg is released into intestinal secretions, so the net absorption of dietary calcium is 200 mg. The excess is excreted by the kidney and maintains serum calcium balance.[12]

Calciotropic hormones

Parathyroid hormone, 1,25-dihydroxyvitamin D, and calcitonin are the primary hormones regulated by calcium concentrations in the extracellular fluid, particularly by effects on bone.[4,29] The first two serve to increase the serum calcium level, while calcitonin will decrease it over the short run. Other hormones (e.g., thyroxin, glucocorticoids, estrogens) also influence bone cell function.

Parathyroid hormone. Parathyroid hormone is a single-chain polypeptide secreted by the chief cells of the parathyroid gland in response to low serum calcium levels. The secretion of PTH may also be influenced by other factors, such as prostaglandins, adrenergic agonists, magnesium, and vitamin D metabolites, which can recruit and attract osteoclasts to bone surfaces and lead to subsequent bone resorption. Parathyroid hormone acts predominantly on bone and kidney. In bone, it increases the size and volume of the ruffled border of osteoclasts, which leads to increased bone resorption, and inhibits osteoblasts. The net effect is an increase in calcium release from bone.[4,29] Parathyroid hormone also has a powerful action on the kidney to resorb calcium in the distal convoluted tubule, and promotes the synthesis of 1,25-dihydroxyvitamin D in the proximal tubules of the kidney. This, in turn, increases calcium absorption in the gut.

1,25-dihydroxyvitamin D. 1,25-dihydroxyvitamin D is synthesized by the body via conversion of precursors in the skin by ultraviolet light (sunlight), which are further acted on by the liver and ultimately by the kidney.[4,29] Final hydroxylation occurs in the kidney and may be stimulated by PTH or low extracellular phosphate levels; other hormones (e.g., calcitonin, estrogen, growth hormone, prolactin) may also have some influence. Conversely, when the serum calcium or phosphate is high, synthesis is inhibited. The major effect of 1,25-dihydroxyvitamin D is to provide sufficient amounts of calcium and phosphate for bone mineralization. In the face of low serum calcium levels or during periods of increased physiologic need, 1,25-dihydroxyvitamin D acts primarily on the gut to promote absorption of dietary calcium.

1,25-dihydroxyvitamin D has powerful stimulatory effects on bone resorption and enhances the differentiation of osteoclast precursors into osteoclasts; it also influences both the resorption of bone and the mineralization of the matrix, along with calcium and phosphate resorption from bone.[4,12,29] In addition, it stimulates calcium and phosphate absorption in the gut.

Calcitonin. Calcitonin is synthesized by the parafollicular (C) cells of the thyroid and acts to lower serum calcium levels and, secondarily, to control the movements of other ions (e.g., phosphate, magnesium, sodium). The synthesis of calcitonin is regulated by extracellular calcium, food intake, and some gastric hormones (gastrin, glucagon, secretin, and cholecystokinin-pancreozymin).[4,29] The prime target organs are calcitonin receptors in the bone (osteoclasts) and the kidney.

Calcitonin does not play a major role in day-to-day serum calcium homeostasis but does enhance the body's ability to deal with rapid changes in serum calcium load or depletion. Thus, calcitonin is released in response to a rapid increase in serum calcium, such as would occur after the ingestion of a high calcium-containing meal. As extracellular calcium is lowered, calcitonin release is inhibited.[4] Calcitonin also acts to decrease serum calcium by exerting a direct effect on osteoclast differentiation, maturation, number, mobility, and cellular function.[29] Under the influence of calcitonin, osteoclasts rapidly lose their ruffled border and move away from the resorptive surface, so calcium is not transported from bone to the extracellular fluid. In the kidney, calcitonin receptors are found in the ascending limb of the loop of Henle, the proximal end of the distal convoluted tubule, and the cortical segment of the collection tubule. When calcitonin binds to these receptors, tubular resorption is reduced and, consequently, calcium, sodium, potassium, chloride, phosphate, and water are excreted.

Other factors. Other factors, including other hormones and cytokines, are known to play some role in calcium balance. For instance, thyroid hormone stimulates osteoclasts and thus bone resorption; glucocorticoids exert complex effects on bone metabolism, and prolonged use may inhibit bone matrix synthesis; and estrogens have complex and interactive effects with calcitonin, PTH, and vitamin D. Estrogen receptors have been identified on the osteoblasts and osteoclasts of humans and animals.[30] When estrogen is administered over a long period, the net effects are a decreased rate of bone turnover, osteoclast inhibition, and bone stabilization.[29]

Several cytokines interact synergistically and antagonistically with each other or with other hormones to exert important effects on bone-cell function, metabolism, and bone turnover.[29] Cytokines involved mainly in bone formation include insulin-like growth factors 1 and 2 and bone morphogenetic proteins. Those that primarily cause bone resorption include IL-6 and colony-stimulating factors. Those that both form and resorb bone include TGF-β, platelet-derived growth factors, and IL-1. Prostaglandins may also influence local bone-cell activity.

Bone

Living bone is specialized connective tissue consisting of bone cells and hydroxyapatite, an organic matrix composed mainly of calcium and phosphate and strengthened by crystalline salts.[31] Bone cells include osteoclasts and osteoblasts, as well as bone-lining cells and osteocytes, which arise from osteoblasts. The functions of osteoblasts and osteoclasts are controlled by hormones and local factors, including weight bearing. Both types of bone cells are intimately involved in remodeling bone (each elaborates and secretes substances that induce the formation and activity of the other) and in releasing and depositing calcium into bone.[4,31]

Osteoclasts arise from pluripotent hematopoietic bone marrow stem cells, specifically the monocyte cell line.[23,24,31] As such, osteoclasts share a common initial differentiation pathway with macrophages, but their differentiation is influenced by the sequential expression of different sets of genes, cytokines, and growth factors. Osteoclasts are morphologically, cytochemically, and immunophenotypically similar to other cells in the mononuclear-phagocytic system. They are rich in enzymes that degrade bone matrix, and can release local factors that contribute to resorption of bone. Osteoclasts play a major role in bone remodeling and are the *only* cells that can resorb bone; they can increase bone resorption to fulfill calcium requirements of body homeostasis when necessary.[24]

Osteoblasts arise from local mesenchymal osteoprogenitors (preosteoblasts) found near bone-forming surfaces. The primary role of these cells is to synthesize the mineralized bony matrix; they also can mature to become flattened bone-lining cells that cover bone surfaces or migrate into bone to become osteocytes maintaining the bone matrix.[31,32] Osteoblasts and preosteoblasts, but not osteoclasts, have receptors for PTH, PTHrP, and 1,25-dihydroxy-vitamin D.[23] Osteoblasts produce several factors (e.g., granulocyte-macrophage colony-stimulating factor [GM-CSF], granulocyte colony-stimulating factor [G-CSF], and macrophage colony-stimulating factor [M-CSF], IL-1, IL-6, TNF) that have subsequent effects on osteoclast differentiation and function.[30,31]

After skeletal maturation, remodeling occurs in which a fraction of bone is removed and replaced each year without changing the size or shape of the bone. Bone remodeling, which occurs on the bone surfaces and within bone, is integral to maintaining the structural integrity and tensile strength of bone and to serum calcium regulation.[4,31] At any one time, only about 10% of the skeleton is undergoing active remodeling.[25] Bone remodeling continues throughout life and is *coupled;* that is, resorption at a particular site exactly equals bone formation at that site. Sometime after the fifth decade of life, bone remodeling becomes uncoupled, and bone formation does not keep pace with resorption. Thus, skeletal mass decreases, skeletal strength is reduced, and the risk for fractures increases.[31]

The functions of remodeling are to replace bone matrix that has developed defects from normal use, to prevent the propagation of fatigue cracks that can progress to fractures, and to play a role in mineral homeostasis.[29] It is not known how the body determines and controls the sites of remodeling, but weight bearing is an important factor and osteocytes may act as mechanosensors with bone.[24] The minimal intensity and type of mechanical forces (load) necessary to maintain normal bone density have not been identified, but empirical and clinical evidence suggest that markedly decreased loading has negative effects on bone strength and mass. For instance, prolonged immobilization of a limb or skeletal traction causes bone resorption to exceed bone formation. Even vigorous activity after such restriction can delay regained bone density for many months in children, and bone density may never reach previous levels in older people.[29]

Normal Bone Remodeling

The cycle of bone remodeling lasts approximately 3 months in adult bone, and has three phases: activation, resorption, and reversal.[25] This process maintains bone mass and equilibrates the balance between resorption and formation (Figure 34-1).

Activation

The activation phase initiates remodeling and corresponds to osteoclast differentiation in response to soluble factors released by osteoblasts.[30] Activation is not random but occurs at sites where remodeling and restructuring are necessary; osteoclasts are also found at active bone resorption sites in pathologic conditions characterized by extensive osteolysis.[4] Mononuclear preosteoclasts that have proliferated in the bone marrow are attracted to bone sites where resorption of bone will occur.[24] Resident bone cells, genes, and growth factors induce mononuclear precursors to fuse into multinucleated osteoclasts. Local osteoblasts and bone marrow stromal cells affect PTH, PTHrP, and prostaglandins to stimulate the formation of osteoclasts and resorptive activity. Genes that may be important for osteoclast formation and activity include the proto-oncogenes *FOS, MYC,* and *SRC.*[30]

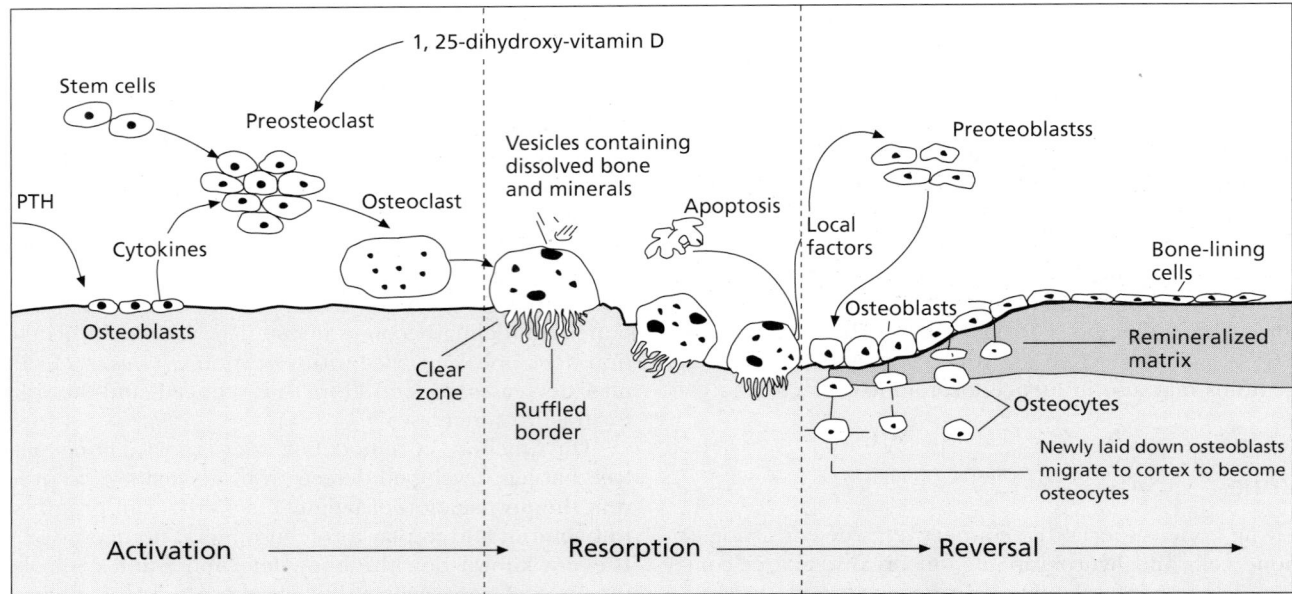

Figure 34-1 Bone remodeling involves coordinated processes of osteoblasts and osteoclasts that maintain bone mass. Activation commences as the parathyroid gland secretes parathyroid hormone (PTH), signaling osteoblasts to secrete cytokines. These cytokines, along with calcitriol, cause preosteoclasts to fuse into multinucleated osteoclasts. During resorption, osteoclasts are firmly attached to bone surfaces by the clear zone. The clear zone encloses an acidic environment, in which the ruffled border dissolves the bone matrix. The dissolved bone and minerals are resorbed via endocytosis into vesicles, transported through the cell cytoplasm, and released from the opposite cell membrane into the serum. At the end of resorption, osteoclasts release local factors to induce preosteoblast formation and then undergo apoptosis. During reversal, osteoblasts secrete new bone matrix and some osteoblasts migrate to the cortex to become osteocytes. The remaining osteoblasts become bone-lining cells.

Growth factors that have been identified near bone and are known to play some role in the formation of osteoclasts include M-CSF, and cytokines (IL-1, IL-6, IL-11), leukemia inhibitory factor, and TNF.[4] Calcitriol is also essential for the formation of osteoclasts and the differentiation of osteoclast precursors.

Resorption

The second phase of bone remodeling, resorption, lasts approximately 15–30 days.[4,30] During this time, osteoclasts resting directly on the bone surface have two specialized plasma membranes: a ruffled border and a clear zone. The ruffled border is the bone-resorbing organ, and the clear zone surrounding it attaches the osteoclast to the underlying bone by means of integrins.[23,24,30] The highly infolded ruffled border is a specialized lysosomal membrane that forms by rapid fusion of acidic intracellular vesicles and secretes proteolytic enzymes, such as lysosomal cysteine proteinases and matrix metalloproteinases, which can dissolve hydroxyapatite crystals. In vitro studies using rat cells showed that osteoclasts are tightly sealed to the bone surface during resorption to isolate the resorption area from the extracellular fluid. Dissolved bone mineral is endocytosed in vesicles through the ruffled border membrane, transported through the osteoclast, and emptied from a secretory area in the opposite cell membrane into the serum.[33–35] Osteoclasts are probably removed by apoptosis, or programmed cell death, after they fulfill their resorptive task.[24]

Reversal

In the reversal phase of bone remodeling, osteoclasts from the old matrix release local factors that stimulate undifferentiated mesenchymal cells, or *preosteoblasts*, to start filling the resorption cavity. These precursor cells assume the appearance of osteoblasts and secrete a specialized extracellular matrix, which subsequently mineralizes.[29] Approximate 10%–20% of the osteoblasts become embedded in the mineralized matrix and become osteocytes; the remainder become flattened and elongated to cover the bone surface.[25,32]

The Role of the Kidney

The kidney is the major regulator of serum calcium levels and, as mentioned previously, under normal circumstances excretes the excess dietary calcium that has been absorbed in the gut (approximately 200 mg/day). Renal excretion can increase to approximate 600 mg per day when necessary to maintain a normal serum calcium.[36] However, severe hypercalcemia overwhelms the kidneys' ability to concentrate urine and excrete high amounts of calcium liberated from the bone. This effect is exacerbated in HHM, in which a tumor elaborates and secretes PTHrP into the serum. The PTHrP causes the kidney to resorb calcium despite the presence of hypercalcemia. Furthermore, high concentrations of calcium in the urine impede sodium and water reabsorption, which results in excessive urine formation (polyuria).[27] If uncorrected, fluid volume is lost and dehydration results. This sets up a vicious circle, because renal blood flow decreases in the face of dehydration and fluid volume deficit; glomerular filtration decreases; and sodium and calcium are resorbed in the proximal tubules, which worsens hypercalcemia.

The Role of the Gastrointestinal Tract

With the exception of rare tumors that produce 1,25-dihydroxyvitamin D, the gastrointestinal tract does not play a role in HHM. This is because 1,25-dihydroxyvitamin D is produced only when serum calcium is low and is inhibited by high serum calcium levels.

Clinical Manifestations of Hypercalcemia

Individuals who develop hypercalcemia exhibit a constellation of unpleasant, nonspecific signs and symptoms that may be misinterpreted as manifestations of terminal cancer, or as side effects of chemotherapy, radiation therapy, or other medications (e.g., opioids). There is great variability in how patients present: Some are asymptomatic, and few have all the symptoms. Predominant signs and symptoms reflect calcium's roles on neuromuscular (CNS and peripheral), gastrointestinal, renal, and cardiovascular functioning (Table 34-3).[4,12,37] In general, elevated calcium levels exert a depressive effect on neuromuscular excitability.

There is little relationship between symptoms and serum calcium levels. However, patients with serum calcium levels of greater than 14 mg/dL usually have symptoms; those who rapidly develop hypercalcemia are likely to have severe symptoms; and older or debilitated individuals are more likely than young people to experience neuromuscular signs and symptoms.[1,27]

Neuromuscular Signs and Symptoms

Neurologic effects of hypercalcemia occur in the central nervous system (CNS) and in the periphery. The CNS effects are more obvious, and peripheral effects are more likely to be attributed to advanced cancer. Effects in the CNS begin with impaired concentration and perhaps mild confusion or disturbing nightmares.[4] Progressive confusion, lethargy, other CNS symptoms, and ultimately coma occur if hypercalcemia is uncorrected and serum calcium rises to greater than 15 mg/dL. Conversely, when hypercalcemia is adequately treated, severe CNS effects may resolve more slowly than serum calcium normalizes.

Table 34-3 Manifestations of Hypercalcemia Associated with Cancer

Organ System	Signs and Symptoms
Neurological **Central nervous system**	Altered cognition Confusion Apathy Drowsiness or lethargy **Late:** Obtundation, coma
Peripheral neuromuscular	Muscle weakness Hypotonia Decreased respiratory muscle capacity Decreased or absent deep tendon reflexes
Renal	Polyuria Polydipsia Dehydration (dry mucous membranes, orthostatic hypotension, etc.) Occasional nephrocalcinosis
Cardiovascular	Prolonged P-R interval Widened QRS Shortened QT, ST intervals Bradycardia (with rapid increases) **Late:** Widened T waves, broadened T wave, heart block, ventricular arrhythmias, asystole Enhanced sensitivity to digitalis Hypertension (if intravascular volume is maintained)
Gastrointestinal	Increased gastric acid secretion Anorexia Nausea and vomiting Constipation Acute pancreatitis (rare) **Late:** Obstipation

(The clinical picture of hypercalcemia varies in patients with hyperparathyroidism, who are more likely to experience anxiety, memory difficulties, and restlessness.[12]) Peripheral effects occur because elevated serum calcium depresses neuromuscular excitability in smooth and striated muscle, and results in weakness, hypotonic muscles, and absent deep-tendon reflexes.[27]

Gastrointestinal Signs and Symptoms

The dampening effect of increased serum calcium on neuromuscular excitability also occurs in the autonomic nervous system. Gastrointestinal motility slows and gastric acid secretion increases, which may intensify nausea, vomiting, and anorexia.[27] Constipation is aggravated by dehydration and may progress to obstipation, which in turn worsens nausea and anorexia.

Renal Manifestations

Hypercalcemia reduces the kidney's ability to concentrate urine, possibly because antidiuretic hormone (ADH) is inhibited.[27] Polyuria results in dehydration and reduced extracellular volume, which in turn leads to decreased renal perfusion and decreased GFR. In the face of decreased GFR and dehydration, more sodium and calcium are resorbed in the proximal tubules.[4] Signs of dehydration are evident and may include thirst, dry mucosa, decreased or absent perspiration, poor skin turgor, and concentrated urine (late).

Cardiovascular Manifestations

High levels of serum calcium increase cardiac contractility and irritability, and slow cardiac conduction.[27] Electrocardiogram changes may include a prolonged P-R interval, a widened QRS, or a shortened Q-T interval. T-waves appear wide secondary to the increased Q-T interval. As in other organ systems, symptoms worsen as serum calcium increases. Bradycardia is unusual but may occur when the serum calcium increases rapidly.[38] Bradyarrhythmias can progress to bundle branch block and, at 18 mg/dL, atrioventricular block may occur and can progress to complete heart block or asystole.[27] Calcium and digitalis have a synergistic effect on the heart, and digoxin excretion in the urine will be impaired during hypercalcemia.[4]

Assessment and Grading

While there is no standard grading toxicity criteria for hypercalcemia, several authors concur on levels of severity based on a range of normal serum calcium values of 8.5–10.5 mg/dL.[27,39] Hypercalcemia may be graded mild (<12 mg/dL), moderate (12–14 mg/dL), severe (14–16 mg/dL), or life-threatening (>16 mg/dL). These values assume a normal serum albumin and must be adjusted if this is not the case (see Diagnostic studies below). Grading, in conjunction with clinical symptoms, is useful in diagnostic and treatment decisions.

Diagnostic Work-up for Hypercalcemia

The diagnostic work-up for hypercalcemia includes a history, physical examination, and laboratory tests, and is important because 20%–25% of patients with cancer may experience hypercalcemia from other causes. These include primary hyperparathyroidism (4%); hormone manipulation with tamoxifen, estrogens, androgens, or progestins for breast cancer (2%); vitamin D intoxication (2%); or other idiopathic causes (16%).[2] Confirming hypercalcemia thus depends on confirming a syndrome, and single symptoms are insufficient to diagnose the problem.

Patient and family history

The patient or family history is important to identifying hypercalcemia and confirming a cancer-related

cause. The patient, or family members if the patient is confused or obtunded, provides important information that guides further diagnostic tests as well as medical treatment and nursing care. Most patients who present with hypercalcemia have a known diagnosis of malignant disease and have obvious signs of advancing disease. If the primary diagnosis is not immediately known, the patient's gender, general appearance, and duration and pattern of symptoms may provide some clues regarding the underlying cause. For example, the incidence of primary hyperparathyroidism is greatest in elderly women who have symptoms of mild hypercalcemia for longer than 6 months, whereas hypercalcemia related to malignancy has a rapid onset of symptoms.[15] The nurse should gather information regarding the patient's chief complaints, the presenting symptoms over time, the cancer diagnosis (if confirmed), known metastases, current antineoplastic therapy (especially estrogen or antiestrogen therapy), medication and dietary supplement history, and concomitant health problems (Table 34-4).[1,15] It is also important to do a pain assessment, particularly when the patient has known bone metastases, because poorly relieved pain can interfere with physical activity and mobility.

Physical examination

The physical examination is not specific for hypercalcemia per se, because of the previously discussed nonspecificity of signs and symptoms in multiple systems. When hypercalcemia is suspected, a broad-based assessment focuses on the patient's neurological assessment (level of consciousness, presence of confusion), muscular assessment (muscle weakness, flaccidity, absent deep-tendon reflexes), gastrointestinal assessment (nausea, abdominal distention, diminished bowel sounds, palpable feces in the colon), fluid volume status (obvious signs of dehydration), and cardiovascular assessment (irregular or slow heart rate). In addition, the nurse assesses the patient's performance status and physical appearance, because many patients have advanced disease. Thus, they may appear to be weak or fatigued and have muscle wasting and obvious weight loss.

Diagnostic studies

In most instances, the history and physical examination support a clear diagnosis of cancer-related hypercalcemia. In these individuals, the serum calcium confirms the diagnosis. However, it is not unusual for patients with advanced cancer to experience anorexia and cachexia, which result in low serum protein levels. Under normal circumstances, ionized calcium and calcium bound to albumin are at approximate equilibrium. However, when a patient has less serum albumin to bind with calcium, a greater portion of the total serum calcium portion *must* be ionized. One formula used to adjust serum calcium is based on a normal serum albumin value of less than 4.0 g/dL and can be adjusted for serum calcium values expressed as mg/dL, mEq/L, or mmol/L calcium (Table

Table 34-4 Focused History for Suspected Hypercalcemia

Focus	Comments
Chief complaint/reason for seeking care	Most commonly neurological/mental status symptoms, but may be other symptom(s) of advanced cancer, GI symptom, pain, polyuria, etc.
Symptom(s)	
Onset/duration	Recent onset or long-standing symptoms?
Progression	Rapid or slow worsening of symptoms?
Severity	Patient's rating
Associated symptoms	If patient does not volunteer, ask about frequent urination, thirst, constipation (ask if they are taking an opioid analgesic), weakness, fatigue.
Effects on important ADLs, QOL	Altered ambulation, nightmares
Diagnosis of cancer confirmed?	Is this a malignancy in which hypercalcemia occurs?
Known bone metastases?	Breast cancer and multiple myeloma are frequently associated with hypercalcemia.
Previous episodes of hypercalcemia	Associated with increased risk for occurrence.
Current therapy for cancer	
Chemotherapy	Can therapy be the cause of some of the symptoms?
New estrogen or antiestrogen	Has bone pain increased with new hormone (may indicate tumor flare)?
Medications	Ask about over-the-counter medications in addition to prescription drugs.
Megavitamins	Do CV assessment; report bradycardia or irregular HR to MD; hold digoxin until after consulting with MD.
Thiazide diuretic	
Lithium	
Digitalis	
Other	Ask about:
	Activity level, especially bedrest
	Whether pain, nausea/vomiting, or other unrelieved symptoms interfere with activity
	Current/usual appetite and diet
	Weight loss in last 6 months; calculate percent weight loss (>10% may indicate protein/calorie malnutrition).

GI = gastrointestinal; ADL = activities of daily living; QOL = quality of life; CV = cardiovascular; HR = heart rate; MD = physician.

34-5).[1,13,15] The results are considered to be rough estimates of total serum calcium but are easily calculated and clinically useful.

In rare instances, a patient with cancer will have primary hyperparathyroidism. If this is suspected, the immunoradiometric assay (IRMA) for PTH may be done. This test can confirm a malignant cause of hypercalcemia if PTH is suppressed, whereas it will be elevated in primary hyperparathyroidism.[15]

Therapeutic Approaches and Nursing Care

Treatment decisions are based on the severity of hypercalcemia, the necessity of hospitalization for treatment, and whether a decision not to treat hypercalcemia is appropriate if all definitive treatment options have been exhausted.[5] Most patients will be treated, and those who have moderate or greater hypercalcemia are hospitalized for treatment and close monitoring. A summary of proposed treatment options is included in Table 34-6.[13,27,39]

There is no consensus regarding the treatment of patients with mild hypercalcemia whose symptoms may go unnoticed or are thought to be caused by other problems.[40] These individuals may be managed with oral fluids and antiresorptive therapy in ambulatory settings. In cases of moderate hypercalcemia, severity of symptoms guides the choice and speed of therapy. Thus, moderately hypercalcemic patients who have serious manifestations (e.g., altered mental status, ECG changes, nausea and vomiting, polyuria) are treated in the same manner as those with more severe hypercalcemia. Severe and life-threatening hypercalcemia (>15 mg/dL) are always considered medical emergencies, and patients require immediate antiresorptive therapy in addition to saline, no matter how symptomatic they may be.[13,39] Initial treatment may include the use of the most rapid osteoclast inhibitor, calcitonin, in conjunction with the bisphosphonate pamidronate.

Goals of Therapy

The medical goals of hypercalcemia management are: (1) to correct dehydration; (2) to increase renal excretion of calcium with vigorous saline diuresis; (3) to inhibit calcium resorption from bone with antiresorptive agents; and (4) to treat the underlying malignancy, if possible. No matter how mild or severe hypercalcemia is, dehydration with oral or intravenous saline-containing fluids is always

Table 34-5 Formulas for Adjusting Serum Calcium for Low Serum Albumin

Calcium in mg/dL =
(base albumin concentration [4.0 mg/dL] − measured serum albumin concentration [g/dL]) × 0.8 mg/dL + reported serum calcium

Example: The patient's reported serum calcium is 11.8 mg/dL, and serum albumin is 2.5 g/dL.

(4.0 g/dL − 2.5 g/dL) = 1.5 g/dL × 0.8 = 1.2
11.8 + 1.2 = 13 mg/dL (corrected serum calcium)

Calcium in mEq/L =
(base albumin concentration [4.0 mg/dL] − measured serum albumin concentration [g/dL]) × 0.4 mg/dL + reported serum calcium

Example: The patient's reported serum calcium is 5.9 mEq/L, and serum albumin is 2.5 g/dL.

(4.0 g/dL − 2.5 g/dL) = 1.5 g/dL × 0.4 = 0.6
5.9 + 0.6 = 6.5 mEq/L (corrected serum calcium)

Calcium in mmol/L
(base albumin concentration [4.0 mg/dL] − measured serum albumin concentration [g/dL]) × 0.2 mg/dL + reported serum calcium

Example: The patient's reported serum calcium is 2.95 mmol/L, and serum albumin is 2.5 g/dL.

(4.0 g/dL − 2.5 g/dL) = 1.5 g/dL × 0.2 = 0.3
2.95 + 0.3 = 3.25 mmol/L (corrected serum calcium)

the essential first step to restore fluid balance and subsequently increase urinary calcium excretion.

Saline diuresis

Rehydration with intravenous 0.9% normal saline is critical to restore intracellular, extracellular, and vascular volumes, thus increasing GFR, calcium filtration, and excretion. The rate of normal saline administration is based on patient parameters, such as severity of hypercalcemia, severity of dehydration, and cardiovascular tolerance for volume expansion.[39] If tolerated, the patient may receive 100–250 mL (or more) of normal saline per hour for 24–48 hours to correct dehydration. The administration of 4–5 liters of normal saline over 24 hours results in modest decreases in serum calcium (perhaps 1–2 mEq/L), but this effect is temporary and is only equivalent to the degree that dehydration increased serum calcium.[12,40]

Saline diuresis may be contraindicated in patients experiencing renal failure or congestive heart failure. Such patients must be treated cautiously, and a loop diuretic, most commonly furosemide, must be added *only* after fluid balance has been restored.[12] However, furosemide can increase dehydration and electrolyte imbalance (particularly potassium) and is not be recommended, unless fluid overload is a major concern.

Pharmacologic interventions

The effect of normal saline diuresis is temporary, so definitive therapy including an antiresorptive drug to correct hypercalcemia is necessary (Table 34-7). According to recent reviews, the agent of choice to treat cancer-related hypercalcemia includes a bisphosphonate, particularly for all patients whose corrected serum calcium is greater than 13 mg/dL (or 3.0 mmol/L).[15,27,40] Furthermore, according to Body et al, no other agents, except for corticosteroids (which are not antiresorptive) in hematologic malignancies and calcitonin on the first day or two of treatment, are indicated to treat hypercalcemia.[40] Therefore, other antiresorptive agents that have been used to treat hypercalcemia, including plicamycin and gallium nitrate, will be briefly discussed. In rare instances, dialysis may also be indicated for severely hypercalcemic patients.

Bisphosphonates

Bisphosphonates, particularly pamidronate, are the most effective and least toxic agents used to treat hypercalcemia and thus have become the treatment of choice. Etidronate—the first bisphosphonate—became commercially useful in the 1930s as a water-softening agent in dish detergents, soaps, and toothpastes.[41] Bisphosphonates prevent precipitation of calcium phosphate in such products and have similar functions in bone. They are structural analogs of pyrophosphate, a component of crystalline bone, and are selectively taken up in bone undergoing active remodeling. Bisphosphonates have a high affinity for hydroxyapatite, bind rapidly to form stable compounds that resist lysis, and remain bound in bone for more than 1 year. In addition, they alter the structure, function, and viability of osteoclasts.[1,27,39]

Three generations of bisphosphonates have been developed, with each subsequent class having greater antiresorbing potencies. Etidronate, a first-generation agent, has a relative potency of one; while the second-generation agents clodronate and pamidronate have potencies of 10 and 100, respectively; and a third-generation agent alendronate has a potency of 1000.[42] Furthermore, even more powerful agents have been developed and are currently being studied. Etidronate and pamidronate are commercially available in the United States for the treatment of hypercalcemia, and clodronate is available in Europe. New, more potent bisphosphonates including zoledronate are being evaluated for their place in treating hypercalcemia.

Bisphosphonates are highly effective in decreasing hypercalcemia, lead to relatively durable normalization of serum calcium values, and have fewer adverse effects when compared to other antiresorptive agents. Approximately 60%–75% of intravenous doses accumulate in bone, and the remainder is excreted by the kidneys.[43] No oral bisphosphonates are available because they are poorly absorbed by this route, and the large doses necessary to effect a therapeutic response also cause gastrointestinal toxicities such as esophageal irritation.[1,40] Few studies have been well designed to compare the effectiveness of different bisphosphonates. In one study of patients who received pamidronate, clodronate, or etidronate,

Table 34-6 Therapy Options Based on Severity of Hypercalcemia

Grade/Level	Serum Calcium	Treatment Options
Normal	8.5–10.5 mg/dL 4.25–5.25 mEq/L 2.2–2.65 mmol/L	
Mild	<12 mg/dL <6 mEq/L >2.65–3.0 mmol/L	• Rehydrate with oral fluids or IV 3–4 L of normal saline over 24 h and observe • Manage associated symptoms. • Antineoplastic therapy for primary cancer. • If symptomatic, treat as for moderate to severe hypercalcemia.
Moderate	12–14 mg/dL 6–7 mEq/L 3.0–3.5 mmol/L	• Rehydrate with IV normal saline (3–4 L in first 24 h) to induce diuresis. • Add furosemide 20–40 mg q12h, *only* after dehydration corrected, if indicated (e.g., CHF, peripheral edema related to low albumin). • Pamidronate 60–90 mg IV over 2–24 h. • Antineoplastic therapy for underlying cancer.
Severe	14–16 mg/dL 7–8 mEq/L 3.5–4.0 mmol/L	• Rehydrate with IV normal saline (4–6 L in first 24 h) to induce diuresis. • Add furosemide 20–40 mg q12h, after dehydration corrected, if indicated (as above). • Pamidronate 90 mg IV over 2–24 h. • Antineoplastic therapy for underlying cancer.
Life-threatening	>16 mg/dL >8 mEq/L >4.0 mmol/L	• Rehydrate with IV normal saline (4–6 L in first 24 h) to induce diuresis. • Add furosemide 20–40 mg q12h, after dehydration corrected, if indicated (as above). • Salmon calcitonin 4 IU/kg SQ q12h; increase dose to 8 IU/kg SQ q6h if no response within 6 h. • Pamidronate 90 mg IV over 2–24 h (or plicamycin 25 μg/kg IV over 15–30 min). • Antineoplastic therapy for underlying cancer.

80%, 40%, and 33%, respectively, experienced normocalcemia. In addition, normocalcemia persisted three times longer in patients who received pamidronate.[37] However, patients who received clodronate were treated with a suboptimal dose.

Pamidronate. There is widespread consensus that pamidronate (Aredia) is the current drug of choice to treat hypercalcemia.[1,15,27,40,43] Pamidronate is more effective than etidronate, has no severe adverse effects or organ toxicities, and is comparatively convenient to administer. Thus, the need to use agents such as plicamycin or gallium nitrate has essentially disappeared. There is a dose-related response to pamidronate, in that only 30% of patients who received 30 mg experienced normocalcemia, while response rates of patients who received 60 mg and 90 mg were 61% and 100%, respectively.[44] Other studies confirm that 90 mg is effective in more than 95% of patients.[15,45] Unlike etidronate, pamidronate can be safely administered to patients with impaired renal function and is administered as an intravenous infusion over a relatively short period (2, 4, or up to 24 hours). The onset of action of is 24–48 hours, calcium nadirs at 5–6 days, and normal calcium is maintained for an average of 28 days.[27,46,47] Calcitonin, in addition to pamidronate, may be administered to patients experiencing severe or life-threatening hypercalcemia in order to achieve a more rapid reduction of serum calcium.

The adverse effects of pamidronate are few and mild. They include mild fever (elevations of 1–2°C), flulike syndrome with malaise, and an infusion site reaction characterized by mild erythema and discomfort.[44,48]

Etidronate. Etidronate (Didronel) was the initial bisphosphonate used to treat hypercalcemia, but is the least potent agent in the class and is no longer used for this purpose.[37] This agent is administered as an intravenous infusion over at least 2 hours for 3 days. Less than 50% of treated patients will experience normocalcemia, and it persists for a shorter period than with bisphosphonates. Furthermore, when used over extended periods, etidronate not only inhibits bone resorption but bone remineralization as well and can cause osteomalacia.[48]

Calcitonin

Calcitonin has the most rapid onset of action and lowers serum calcium by decreasing renal tubular resorption of calcium and, secondarily, by blocking osteoclast resorption.[12,14,27,37] Calcitonin is useful for initial treatment but only results in modest decreases in the calcium level and rapidly loses its effectiveness. Tachyphylaxis de-

Table 34-7 Antiresorptive and Other Agents to Treat Hypercalcemia

Agent	Mechanism of Action	Administration Considerations	Adverse Reactions	Comments
Bisphosphonates Pamidronate (Aredia)	Bind to hydroxyapatite; inhibit number and action of osteoclasts	60–90 mg IV over 2–24 h	Transient fever Flulike syndrome Site reaction	• Aredia is the agent of choice to treat hypercalcemia, because of high effectiveness and low toxicity
Etidronate (Didronel)	As above	7.5 mg/kg IV over ≥2 h × 3 days	Taste disturbances	• Least effective bisphosphonate • Prolonged use impairs bone remineralization
Calcitonin-salmon (Calcimar)	Inhibits osteoclast action; decreases renal reabsorption of calcium	4 IU/kg SQ q12h Increase to 8 IU/kg q6h prn	Allergic reactions	• Most rapid onset of action • Administer intradermal test dose • Wheal or mild erythema contraindicate further use • Tachyphylaxis occurs in 2–7 days
Plicamycin (Mithracin)	Causes death of osteoclasts by DNA intercalation Inhibits renal tubular reabsorption of calcium	25 μg/kg IV over 4–6 h	Nephrotoxicity Hepatotoxicity Increased prothrombin time Nausea and vomiting Thrombocytopenia	• Rapid onset of action • Dose may be repeated in 24–48 h if no decrease in calcium • More toxic than bisphosphonates • Contraindications: renal insufficiency, thrombocytopenia, hepatic failure • Not recommended
Gallium nitrate (Ganite)	Stabilizes bone crystals Inhibits osteoclasts	100–200 mg/m² over 24 h for up to 5 days	Nephrotoxicity (noncumulative) Nausea and vomiting	• Patient must be hospitalized for treatment • Not recommended
Corticosteroids Hydrocortisone	Inhibit lymphoid tissue growth	100–300 mg IV or PO over 3–5 days	Hyperglycemia Fluid retention	• Not used except for steroid-sensitive tumors (multiple myeloma, lymphoma) • May enhance effect of calcitonin
Prednisone	Inhibit down regulation of steroid receptors Increase urinary excretion of calcium	40–100 mg/day		• Slow acting, not specific; never used routinely or alone • Adverse effects preclude long-term use

velops in 2–7 days. Occasionally, a corticosteroid is administered with calcitonin to enhance and prolong its effect.[13,14] Calcitonin may be combined with pamidronate if the patient's serum calcium is greater than 13 mg/dL (3.3 mmol/L).[14]

Salmon calcitonin (Calcimar), which is more potent than human or porcine calcitonin, is used and may decrease serum calcium by as much as 2–3 mg/dL within 1–2 days. However, it can cause allergic reactions, so an intradermal test dose should be given.[37] If a wheal forms or mild erythema occurs at the site, further treatment with calcitonin is contraindicated. Other toxicity includes nausea, flushing, and abdominal cramps.

The usual initial dose of calcitonin is 4 IU/kg subcutaneously every 12 hours. Most patients will start to respond within 2–4 hours, so the serum calcium should be rechecked 5–6 hours after the first dose. If there has been no response, intravenous hydration with normal saline (plus furosemide, as indicated) will continue, and the dose of calcitonin may be increased to 8 IU/kg every 6 hours.

Other agents

Plicamycin. Plicamycin (Mithracin) was developed as an antineoplastic agent that was noted to cause hypocalcemia, and thus it became the first-line agent for hypercalcemia.[12,14] Plicamycin intercalates DNA in osteoclasts, causing cell death, and also inhibits renal tubular resorption of calcium.[37] It has a rapid onset of action and begins to lower calcium within 12 hours. However, only 30%–50% of patients achieve normocalcemia, which typically persists for only 7–10 days, when rebound hypercalcemia may occur.[27]

Plicamycin is an irritant, and infiltration may lead to local tissue reactions. The usual dose is 25 μg/kg administered as an intravenous infusion over 4–6 hours. The dose may be repeated in 24–48 hours if serum calcium does not decrease, and it is not unusual for the patient to require multiple doses to control hypercalcemia.[27,37] Plicamycin is more toxic than bisphosphonates, which poses a problem in patients who may already have received a great deal of chemotherapy. This drug can cause cumulative nephrotoxicity, hepatotoxicity, nausea and vomiting, thrombocytopenia, and an increased prothrombin time.[14,27]

Gallium nitrate. Gallium nitrate is a highly effective agent that normalizes calcium in almost all hypercalcemic patients. It is more efficacious than calcitonin, plicamycin, and etidronate.[49] Gallium localizes to sites of bone resorption and binds to hydroxyapatite—which stabilizes bone crystals and produces hydroxyapatite more resistant to osteoclast-mediated absorption—and also inhibits osteoclasts.[37] The serum calcium starts to decrease within 24–48 hours; normocalcemia occurs in 4–7 days and lasts for approximately 1 week.

Gallium nitrate is not generally used because of expense, inconvenience, and toxicities.[1] Patients must be hospitalized for several days to receive this agent, which is administered by continuous intravenous infusion with adequate intravenous hydration. The recommended dose is 100–200 mg/m² over 24 hours for up to 5 days.[37] Gallium can exacerbate renal insufficiency or lead to reversible, noncumulative nephrotoxicity in other patients. This is preventable by maintaining the patient's urine output at 2 liters per day. Other minor adverse effects include nausea and vomiting and constipation (may be related to hypercalcemia).

Corticosteroids

Corticosteroids do not play a major role in managing hypercalcemia but are occasionally useful in treating hypercalcemia associated with steroid-sensitive malignancies, such as multiple myeloma and lymphomas. They are also occasionally used as adjuncts with calcitonin to prevent attenuation of its effect.[1] Corticosteroids may be administered orally or parentally and act to inhibit 1,25-dihydroxy-vitamin D-mediated absorption of calcium from the gut.[27] Corticosteroids induce a slow response over 1–2 weeks.

Dialysis

Peritoneal or hemodialysis are rarely used to treat hypercalcemia. An indication for dialysis is the severely hypercalcemic patient who has a treatable malignancy but is experiencing renal insufficiency.[14,27] Dialysis can reduce serum calcium by 3–12 mg/dL in 24–48 hours. However, large amounts of phosphate are lost as well, which aggravates hypercalcemia. Thus, phosphate is typically added to the next dialysate or to the diet.

Prevention

Until recently, there were no preventive measures for hypercalcemia. However, pamidronate has been approved by the U.S. Food and Drug Administration for patients who have osteolytic bone metastases and who are not hypercalcemic, and thus is recommended postdischarge to maintain normal serum calcium levels.[15] This is based on data that confirms pamidronate can decrease skeletal complications, including hypercalcemia, pathologic fractures, bone pain, and the need for radiation therapy or surgery.[40,42] In addition, patients experience recalcification of lytic metastases and fewer new lytic metastases to bone, which enhances their quality of life. Such benefits occur in patients with breast cancer, multiple myeloma, and bony metastases from other diseases. Pamidronate 60–90 mg administered intravenously over 2 hours every 3–4 weeks is effective to preventively treat hypercalcemia and bone metastases.[43] Preventive management is advantageous and less costly because patients are treated in outpatient settings and avoid complications that require hospitalization.[42,48]

Other General Measures and Nursing Care

When caring for patients at risk for or actually experiencing hypercalcemia, nurses focus not only on administering medically ordered therapies but also on managing associated symptoms, maintaining patient safety, and minimizing risk for recurrence, which includes patient/family education. In addition, when patients no longer respond to anticancer or hypercalcemic therapies, the nurse focuses on the emotional and physical care of the patient at the end-stage of disease.

During the initial treatment phase of moderate to life-threatening hypercalcemia, patients are receiving large volumes of intravenous normal saline to induce rehydration and urinary calcium excretion. It is important to assess and manage fluid balance and potential electrolyte imbalance that may occur during vigorous diuresis, including marked decreases in sodium, potassium, phosphate, and magnesium. Laboratory results of these electrolytes should be assessed daily or more often if necessary.[27] Vital signs and symptoms of fluid overload should also be monitored at least every 4 hours during hydration and drug treatment. Cardiovascular status should be assessed, and the patient may require cardiac monitoring. If there is any question about the patient's cardiac status, the nurse should hold a dose of digoxin until after consultation with the patient's physician.[4,27] Likewise, if the patient has been taking tamoxifen or another hormone for breast cancer, the nurse should discuss administration with the physician.

Safety is another major concern for patients who have altered thinking, confusion, sleepiness, and muscle weakness. A major goal is to protect patients from falls and injury, particularly if they are voiding frequently and get up to use the bathroom or commode. In addition, the family or care providers may misconstrue lethargy as depression, which might be assumed to be a normal emotional response to the diagnosis.[27] Performing a Mini-Mental Status examination can help to differentiate confusion and lethargy from depression.

The nurse also focuses on increasing patient activity and ambulation, particularly in patients who are bedridden, because exercise and weight-bearing are critical to maintaining bone mass; inactivity leads to lost bone mass. This may mean controlling other symptoms that are interfering with the patient's ability or willingness to be active. For instance, it is not unusual for hypercalcemic patients to have painful bone metastases, or nausea and vomiting, either of which may limit activity.

Continuity of Care

Unless prophylactic treatment for hypercalcemia or treatment for the underlying malignancy is planned, the patient is likely to become hypercalcemic again. It is therefore not only useful to teach the patient and their family the most common signs and symptoms of hypercalcemia, but also to explore with them the pattern of symptoms they experienced. Helping them to strategize about actions to decrease their risk for hypercalcemia and advice on when to seek medical attention can then be personalized. Teaching should include instructions to maintain fluid intake at 3–4 liters per day (and telephoning their nurse or physician if they are unable to), along with liberal salt intake (unless there is a medical contraindication). Pain control and management of nausea and vomiting and other symptoms are important. The goal to maintain or increase mobility must be addressed within the context of performance status, pain and other symptom control, and nutritional status. Most patients can be encouraged to eat whatever tastes good, and calcium does not need to be withheld from the diet; it will not be absorbed from the gut if the patient is hypercalcemic.[15]

Conclusion

Hypercalcemia occurs as a relatively late complication of advanced cancer in a significant number of individuals. It negatively affects patients' quality of life and may ultimately lead to their death. It is important that nurses know which patients are at risk and the signs and symptoms of hypercalcemia. While the currently recommended "best" therapy for hypercalcemia, pamidronate, may not prolong survival, it represents a major advance because it can be used prophylactically and be administered over a relatively short time in an outpatient setting. Many patients will thus be prevented from experiencing common unpleasant and distressing signs and symptoms of hypercalcemia. Managing hypercalcemia is a reasonable palliative care goal that enhances most patients' quality of life.

References

1. Harvey HA: The management of hypercalcemia of malignancy. *Support Care Cancer* 3:123–129, 1995
2. Raue F: Epidemiological aspects of hypercalcemia of malignancy, in Raue W (ed): *Recent Results in Cancer Research.* Berlin, Springer-Verlag, 1994, pp 99–106
3. Muggia FM: Overview of cancer-related hypercalcemia: Epidemiology and etiology. *Semin Oncol* 17:3–9, 1990 (suppl 5)
4. Mosekilde L, Eriksen EF, Charles P: Hypercalcemia of malignancy: Pathophysiology, diagnosis and treatment. *Crit Rev Oncol Hematol* 11:1–27, 1991
5. Warrell RP: Etiology and current management of cancer-related hypercalcemia. *Oncology* 6:37–43, 1992
6. Orloff JJ, Stewart AF: Disorders of serum minerals caused by cancer, in Coe FL, Favus MJ (eds): *Disorders of Bone and Mineral Metabolism.* New York, Raven, 1992, pp 539–561
7. Mao C, Carter P, Schaefer P, et al: Malignant islet cell tumor associated with hypercalcemia. *Surgery* 117:37–40, 1995
8. Brown EM, Harris HW, Vassilev PM, et al: The biology of the extracellular Ca^{2+}-sensing receptor, in Bilezikian JP, Raisz LG, Rodan GA (eds): *Principles of Bone Biology.* New York, Academic, 1996, pp 243–262
9. Roodman GD: Mechanisms of bone lesions in multiple myeloma and lymphoma. *Cancer* 80:1557–1563, 1997
10. Heys SD, Smith IC, Eremin O: Hypercalcemia in patients with cancer: Aetiology and treatment. *Eur J Surg Oncol* 24: 139–142, 1998
11. Mundy GR: Mechanisms of bone metastasis. *Cancer* 80: 1546–1556, 1997
12. Bleyer A, Goldfarb S: Calcium metabolism, in Szerlip HM, Goldfarb S (eds): *Workshops in Fluid and Electrolyte Disorders.* New York, Churchill Livingstone, 1993, pp 165–191
13. Kaye TB: Hypercalcemia: How to pinpoint the cause and customize treatment. *Postgrad Med* 97:153–155, 159–160, 1993
14. Kovacs CS, MacDonald SM, Chik CL, et al: Hypercalcemia of malignancy in the palliative care patient: A treatment strategy. *J Pain Symptom Manage* 10:224–232, 1995
15. Mundy GR, Guise TA: Hypercalcemia of malignancy. *Am J Med* 103:134–145, 1997
16. Guise TA, Yin JJ, Taylor SD, et al: Evidence for a causal role of parathyroid hormone-related protein in the pathogenesis of human breast cancer-mediated osteolysis. *J Clin Invest* 98: 1544–1549, 1996
17. Rankin W, Grill V, Martin TJ: Parathyroid hormone-related protein and hypercalcemia. *Cancer* 80:1564–1571, 1997
18. Blind E: Humoral hypercalcemia of malignancy: Role of parathyroid hormone-related protein, in Raue F (ed): *Hypercalcemia of Malignancy.* New York, Springer-Verlag, 1994, pp 20–41
19. Philbrick WM, Wysolmerski JJ, Galbraith S, et al: Defining the roles of parathyroid hormone-related protein in normal physiology. *Physiol Rev* 71:127–173, 1996
20. Mundy GR, Guise TA: Role of parathyroid hormone-related peptide in hypercalcemia of malignancy and osteolytic bone disease. *Endocr Rel Cancer* 5:15–26, 1998

21. Pfeilschifter J: Cytokines as mediators of hypercalcemia of malignancy, in Raue F (ed): *Hypercalcemia of Malignancy*. New York, Springer-Verlag, 1994, pp 1–19

22. De La Mata J, Uy HL, Guise TA, et al: Interleukin-6 enhances hypercalcemia and bone resorption mediated by parathyroid hormone-related in vivo. *J Clin Invest* 95:2846–2852, 1995

23. Athanasou NA: Cellular biology of bone-resorbing cells. *J Bone Joint Surg* 78-A:1096–1113, 1996

24. Vaananen K: Osteoblast function: Biology and mechanisms, in Bilezikian JP, Raisz LG, Rodan GA (eds): *Principles of Bone Biology*. New York, Academic, 1996, pp 103–113

25. Kanis JA, McCloskey EV: Bone turnover and biochemical markers in malignancy. *Cancer* 80:1538–1545, 1997

26. Powell GJ, Southby J, Danks JA, et al: Localization of parathyroid hormone-related protein in breast cancer metastasis: Increased incidence in bone compared with other sites. *Cancer Res* 51:3059–3061, 1991

27. National Cancer Institute: *PDQ Physician Statement: Hypercalcemia*. Updated 09/1998. Available at: http://www.oncolink.edu/pdq_html/5/engl/504462.more.html. Accessed March 28, 1999

28. Brown EM, Vickery AL: Weekly clinicopathological exercises: Case 32-1996: A 44-year-old woman with a long history of intermittent hypercalcemia, a new neck mass, and hypercalcemic crisis. *N Engl J Med* 335:1213–1220, 1996

29. Buckwalter JA, Glimcher MJ, Cooper RR, et al: Bone biology. Part II: Formation, form, modeling, and regulation of cell function. *J Bone Joint Surg* 77-A:1276–1289, 1995

30. de Vernejoul MC: Dynamics of bone remodelling: Biochemical and pathophysiological basis. *Eur J Clin Chem Biochem* 34:729–734, 1996

31. Marks SC, Hermey DC: The structure and development of bone, in Bilezikian JP, Raisz LG, Rodan GA (eds): *Principles of Bone Biology*. New York, Academic, 1996, pp 3–14

32. Aubin JE, Liu F: The osteoblast lineage, in Bilezikian JP, Raisz LG, Rodan GA (eds): *Principles of Bone Biology*. New York, Academic, 1996, pp 51–67

33. Nesbitt SA, Horton MA: Trafficking of matrix collagens through bone-resorbing osteoclasts. *Science* 276:266–269, 1997

34. Mostov K, Werb Z: Journey across the osteoclast. *Science* 276:219–220, 1997

35. Salo J, Lehenkari P, Mulari M, et al: Removal of osteoclast bone resorption products by transcytosis. *Science* 276:270–273, 1997

36. Mundy GR: General concepts of calcium homeostasis, in Mundy GR (ed): *Calcium Homeostasis: Hypercalcemia and Hypocalcemia*. New York, Oxford University Press, 1990, pp 1–16

37. Watters J, Gerrard G, Dodwell D: The management of malignant hypercalcaemia. *Drugs* 52:837–848, 1996

38. Badertscher E, Warnica JW, Ernst DS: Acute hypercalcemia and severe bradycardia in a patient with breast cancer. *Can Med Assoc J* 148:1506–1508, 1993

39. Bilezikian JP: Management of acute hypercalcemia. *N Engl J Med* 326:1196–1203, 1992

40. Body JJ, Bartl R, Burckhardt P, et al: Current use of bisphosphonates in oncology. *J Clin Oncol* 16:3890–3899, 1998

41. Marwick C: Study of bisphosphonates lead to new view of bone remodeling, therapy for skeletal malignancy. *JAMA* 278:803–804, 1997

42. Bloomfield DJ: Should bisphosphonates be part of the standard therapy of patients with multiple myeloma or bone metastases from other cancers? An evidence-based review. *J Clin Oncol* 16:1218–1225, 1998

43. Hortobagyi GN, Theriault RL, Lipton A, et al: Long-term prevention of skeletal complications of metastatic breast cancer with pamidronate. *J Clin Oncol* 16:2038–2044, 1998

44. Nussbaum SR, Younger J, VandePol CJ, et al: Single-dose intravenous therapy with pamidronate for the treatment of hypercalcemia of malignancy: Comparison of 30-, 60-, and 90-mg dosages. *Am J Med* 95:297–304, 1993

45. Thurlimann B: *Bisphosphonates in Clinical Oncology: The Development of Pamidronate*. New York, Springer, 1998, pp 33–51

46. Wimalawansa SJ: Optimal frequency of administration of pamidronate in patients with hypercalcaemia of malignancy. *Clin Endocrinol* 41:591–595, 1994

47. Purohit OP, Radstone CR, Anthony C, et al: Randomised double-blind comparison of intravenous pamidronate and clodronate in the hypercalcaemia of malignancy. *Br J Cancer* 72:1289–1293, 1995

48. Fulfaro F, Casuccio A, Ticozzi C, et al: The role of bisphosphonates in the treatment of painful metastatic bone disease: A review of phase III trials. *Pain* 78:157–169, 1998

49. Patel S, Lyons AR, Hosing DJ: Drugs used in the treatment of metabolic bone disease. *Drugs* 46:594–617, 1993

CHAPTER 35

Paraneoplastic Syndromes

Irene Stewart Haapoja, RN, MS

Introduction

Paraneoplastic syndromes (PNSs) can be described as the "remote" or indirect effects of cancer. These rare diseases result from the secretion of substances, usually proteins, by the primary tumor or its metastases. These substances, also known as *mediators*, include hormones, growth factors, cytokines, antibodies, and other immune products, which indirectly result in a multitude of disorders of the endocrine, neurologic, hematologic, immunologic, cutaneous, musculoskeletal, renal, and gastrointestinal systems (Figure 35-1). It is important for oncology nurses to understand these syndromes in order to recognize them as potential early warning signs of a malignancy, as a complication of malignancy, or as an indication of recurrent disease. Early detection and prompt effective treatment may minimize the morbidity associated with these syndromes and their potential impact on quality of life.

It is estimated that a PNS will exist at the time of diagnosis in 10%–15% of all patients with cancer, and that up to 50% of cancer patients may encounter a tumor-specific PNS over the course of their disease. If the more generalized PNSs—anorexia-cachexia, tumor fever, and anemia of chronic disease—are included, then almost all patients with cancer will experience at least one paraneoplastic manifestation.[1,2] While PNSs can occur with any malignancy, they most frequently occur with lung cancer, specifically small cell lung carcinoma. The true incidence of PNSs is difficult to determine because they occur infrequently, they are associated with both benign and malignant disease, they are difficult to define in specific terms, and the diagnosis is often made by exclusion. Some general concepts exist concerning these syndromes:[1]

- They may precede a diagnosis of malignancy or may occur concurrently; however, most appear in the later stages of the disease course.

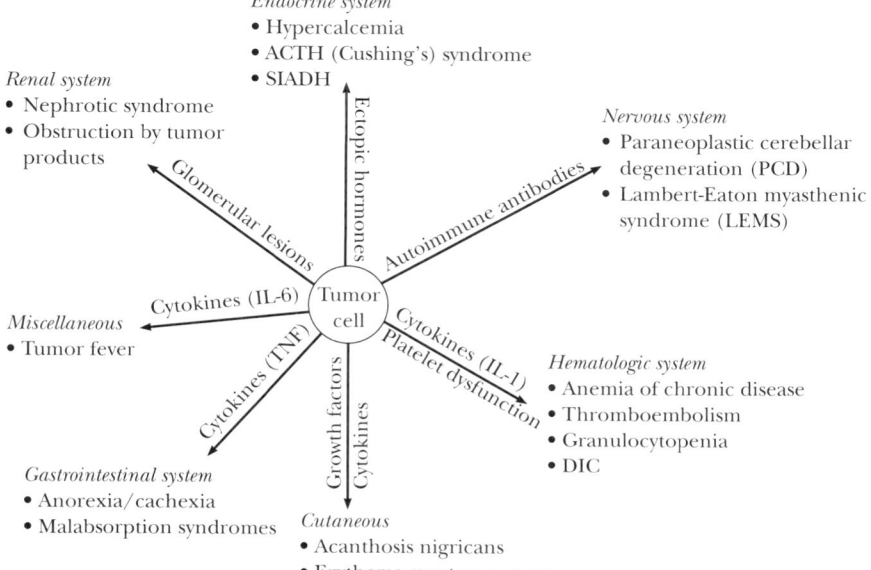

Figure 35-1 Paraneoplastic syndromes: Ectopic tumor effects. (ACTH = adrenocorticotropic hormone; SIADH = syndrome of antidiuretic hormone secretion; DIC = disseminated intravascular coagulation.)

Renal system
- Nephrotic syndrome
- Obstruction by tumor products

Miscellaneous
- Tumor fever

Gastrointestinal system
- Anorexia/cachexia
- Malabsorption syndromes

Endocrine system
- Hypercalcemia
- ACTH (Cushing's) syndrome
- SIADH

Nervous system
- Paraneoplastic cerebellar degeneration (PCD)
- Lambert-Eaton myasthenic syndrome (LEMS)

Hematologic system
- Anemia of chronic disease
- Thromboembolism
- Granulocytopenia
- DIC

Cutaneous
- Acanthosis nigricans
- Erythema gyratum repens

Tumor cell

Glomerular lesions · Cytokines (IL-6) · Ectopic hormones · Autoimmune antibodies · Cytokines (IL-1) · Platelet dysfunction · Cytokines (TNF) · Growth factors · Cytokines

- They rarely occur with childhood malignancies with the exception of Wilms' tumor and neuroblastoma.

- The existence of a PNS frequently predicts a poor prognosis with regard to the malignancy; however, the severity of the PNS may not necessarily correlate with the extent of malignant disease.

- A PNS may be useful as a monitoring tool to evaluate response of the malignancy to treatment and as an indication of recurrent disease.

- The primary treatment of a PNS is treatment of the underlying malignancy. Response of the PNS to therapy frequently correlates with tumor response, especially in the case of the endocrine- or hormone-related PNSs. Unfortunately, the individual may be left with permanent deficits caused by the PNS even when the malignancy has been successfully eradicated, as is often seen with the neurologic PNSs.

It is important to understand that many of these PNSs are extremely rare; in some instances only a few cases exist in the literature. Despite their rarity, PNSs are now being viewed as mechanisms for providing a greater understanding of tumor biology.[2] The "bystander effect" describes the pathogenic mechanism by which tumor cells must rely on normal tissue to produce PNSs. The "bystanders" are either normal cells that are mistaken for tumor cells by the patient's autoimmune response, as in the case of the neurologic PNSs, or are the normal systems recruited through tumor secretion of hormone, cytokine, or endocrine mediators to produce the endocrine, hematologic, and cutaneous PNSs.[3] A review of the major PNSs affecting each body system is presented next.

ENDOCRINE PARANEOPLASTIC SYNDROMES

Scope of the Problem

The endocrine PNSs are the most frequently occurring PNSs and the most well defined in terms of their etiology, clinical presentation, and disease course. These syndromes result from ectopic (tumor) synthesis of naturally occurring hormones or hormone precursors.[4] Definitive diagnosis depends on evidence that the tumor is synthesizing and secreting clinically significant amounts of the hormone, that the syndrome improves with successful treatment of the malignancy, and that it returns with recurrence of the malignancy. Confirmation that tumor tissue is synthesizing and secreting hormone can be done by in vitro testing; however, this extensive testing is not usually clinically useful and is rarely performed.[5]

Tumor cells have been shown to have the ability to produce almost every known hormone and hormone-releasing factor, resulting in the potential existence of multiple endocrine PNSs (Table 35-1).[6] The most common and well-known endocrine PNSs are hypercalcemia, paraneoplastic adrenocorticotropic hormone (pACTH) syndrome, and syndrome of inappropriate antidiuretic hormone (SIADH).

Definitions

Each endocrine PNS arises from tumor secretion of substances resulting in excessive amounts of circulating hormones that interrupt normal homeostatic mechanisms. *Paraneoplastic* or *humoral hypercalcemia* is defined as an elevated serum calcium level caused by tumor secretion of parathyroid hormone-related protein (PTHrP) and is usually distinguished from hypercalcemia arising from bony metastases. The normal range of serum calcium in adults is 8.5–10.5 mg/dL; hypercalcemia exists if the level exceeds 11.0 mg/dL.

Paraneoplastic ACTH syndrome is the development of pituitary-independent Cushing's disease caused by the secretion of ACTH by malignant cells and must be distinguished from pituitary-dependent Cushing's disease produced by a pituitary neoplasm or hyperplasia.[6]

Syndrome of inappropriate antidiuretic hormone secretion was initially described by Schwartz et al in 1957 as the secretion of antidiuretic hormone (ADH) by the pituitary in response to a thoracic tumor.[7] In 1963 Amatruda et al demonstrated that tumor production of ADH, not the pituitary, resulted in SIADH.[8] Today, SIADH is described as tumor production of ADH or arginine vasopressin (AVP), resulting in a syndrome of hyponatremia, urine inappropriately higher in osmolality than the plasma, and high urinary sodium concentrations despite serum hyponatremia.[4] This syndrome is more commonly referred to as SIAD, or syndrome of inappropriate diuresis, to reflect that vasopressin may not be the only agent to effect sodium excretion.[9]

Incidence

Hypercalcemia is the most common metabolic complication of malignancy, occurring in approximately 10% of patients with cancer, of which 10%–15% do not have metastatic bone disease. The malignancies most often associated with hypercalcemia are squamous cell carcinomas of the lung (15%), head and neck, and esophagus, followed by breast, uterine, cervical, lymphoma, multiple myeloma, and renal cell carcinomas.[4,6]

Although pACTH syndrome occurs rarely, it is considered the second most frequent PNS. Bronchogenic carcinoma accounts for 60%–70% of the cases of pACTH syndrome. Small cell lung carcinoma represents the majority of these cases; approximately 5% of small cell lung cancer patients will develop the syndrome during the course of their disease. Adenocarcinoma of the lung is

Table 35-1 Endocrine Paraneoplastic Syndromes

Syndrome	Hormone	Associated Malignancy	Clinical Presentation	Comments
Hypercalcemia	Parathyroid hormone-related protein (PTHrP)	*Solid Tumors:* Squamous cell • Lung cancer • Head and neck • Esophagus • Cervix • Breast • Ovarian • Bladder	• Confusion • Weakness • Lethargy	
	Osteoclast activating factors 1,25 hydroxyvitamin D	*Hematologic:* Multiple myeloma Acute leukemia Lymphoma		
Paraneoplastic ACTH (Cushing's) syndrome	Adrenocorticotropic hormone (ACTH)	Small cell lung carcinoma (6%) Carcinoid Pancreatic Medullary thyroid Pheochromocytoma	• Hypokalemia • Muscle weakness/ atrophy • Weight loss • Hypertension	
Syndrome of inappropriate antidiuresis	Arginine vasopressin (AVP) Atrial natriuretic hormone (ANP)	Small cell lung carcinoma (80%) Pancreatic Thymus Breast	• Water intoxication • Hyponatremia	
Paraneoplastic growth hormone–releasing hormone syndrome (acromegaly)	Growth hormone–releasing hormone (GHRH)	Bronchial carcinoid Pancreatic carcinoma	• Acromegaly	Rapid onset
Paraneoplastic osteomalacia	1,25 hydroxyvitamin D	"Strange tumors in strange places" Soft tissue, bone tumors • Hemangioma • Angiosarcoma • Osteoblastoma	• Skeletal pain • Muscle weakness	Occurs in young adults
Paraneoplastic secretion of human chorionic gonadotropin	Human chorionic gonadotropin (HCG)	Ovarian Testicular Large cell lung cancer Gastric Breast Melanoma	Usually asymptomatic • Dysfunctional bleeding • Gynecomastia	
Hypoglycemia	Insulin-like growth factors	Mesothelioma Fibrosarcoma Neurofibrosarcoma Hepatoma	• Diaphoresis • Confusion— may progress to stupor/coma	Many patients asymptomatic unless fasting
Paraneoplastic erythrocytosis	Erythropoietin	Uterine fibroma Cerebellar hemangioblastoma Hepatocellular carcinoma	• ↑ RBCs • ↑ Hgb/Hct • ↑ Red blood cell mass	Remission achieved by surgical resection of tumor

RBC = red blood cell; Hgb = hemoglobin; Hct = hematocrit.

less often associated (5%). Other malignancies associated with pACTH syndrome include pancreatic carcinoma, carcinoid tumors, hepatocellular carcinoma, pheochromocytoma, colon carcinoma, and medullary thyroid cancer. Adrenocorticotropic hormone–secreting bronchial carcinoid tumors represent a subset of patients with a more aggressive variant of carcinoid. These tumors have a higher incidence of local and lymphatic spread but, contradictorily, are often cured with surgical resection.[10] Paraneoplastic ACTH syndrome occurs more often than the benign form of Cushing's disease.[11]

Syndrome of inappropriate antidiuretic hormone secretion is primarily associated with small cell lung cancer, which accounts for about 80% of cases. Most of these patients may have some aspects of SIADH without clinical evidence of the syndrome. Only about 9%–14% percent of patients with small cell lung cancer have full-blown SIADH.[6] Other cancers associated with SIADH include non-small cell lung cancer, carcinoid tumors, squamous cell cancer of the head and neck; carcinomas of the prostate, esophagus, pancreas, and colon; thymoma; and Hodgkin's and non-Hodgkin's lymphomas. Central nervous system metastases, such as meningeal carcinomatosis, have also been associated with SIADH. The incidence of SIADH with cancers other than small cell lung cancer is extremely limited; these cancers may actually have a small cell component to their histology.[4]

Etiology and Risk Factors

The etiology of paraneoplastic hypercalcemia involves tumor secretion of bone-resorbing cytokines, prostaglandins, transforming growth factors, 1,25-dihydroxyvitamin D, and PTHrP. Of these substances, PTHrP is the primary factor in the development of paraneoplastic hypercalcemia. Although this etiology has been distinguished from bone-related hypercalcemia in the past, there appears to be a paraneoplastic component to the development of hypercalcemia in patients with bone metastases. Many patients with bone metastases never develop hypercalcemia because their homeostatic mechanisms are able to compensate for the excess calcium. No relationship has been found between the incidence of hypercalcemia and the extent of bony disease.[12]

The etiology of pACTH syndrome is ectopic secretion of ACTH by neoplastic cells, resulting in an excess of ACTH in the body. This leads to bilateral adrenal hyperplasia and the symptoms of Cushing's disease. Adrenocorticotropic hormone syndrome has been widely reported, with more than 75% of the cases associated with tumors located in the chest and mediastinum.[6] The prognosis of the patient diagnosed with pACTH syndrome is poor because ACTH may function as a growth factor for neoplastic cells, particularly small cell lung cancer tissue. In addition, excessive cortisol levels suppress immune function, leading to an increased risk of infection. The median survival of small cell lung cancer patients with pACTH averages 3–7 months.[13] Patients with pACTH syndrome are especially at risk for developing fungal infections.[14] They also are at risk for gastrointestinal ulceration and bleeding due to high cortisol levels.[15]

The etiology of SIADH as a PNS is related to ectopic production of vasopressin by malignant cells. The severity of SIADH usually correlates with the extent of malignant disease. Although structurally identical, ectopic AVP is not subject to normal physiologic controls.[16] Small cell carcinoma of the lung accounts for 80% of the malignancies associated with SIADH. Cyclophosphamide and vincristine, drugs frequently used in the treatment of small cell lung cancer, have also been associated with the development of SIADH. Cyclophosphamide's direct effect on the renal tubule, combined with the vigorous hydration used to prevent hemorrhagic cystitis, can result in SIADH. In this instance, SIADH represents a secondary paraneoplastic syndrome.[4] Other factors contributing to the multifactorial etiology of SIADH in the patient with small cell lung cancer include smoking (nicotine), stress, pain, nausea, and the use of morphine, all of which can increase AVP production.[16]

Pathophysiology

The pathophysiology of the endocrine PNSs is related to the effect of ectopic hormone production on the normal hormonal physiologic pathways affecting the release and inhibition of various hormones.

Normal calcium homeostasis is maintained by the interactions of multiple factors that affect bone resorption and osteolysis. Prostaglandins (PGE_1, PGE_2), parathyroid hormone (PTH), osteoclast-activating factor, and thyroxine (T_4) stimulate bone resorption and osteolysis. Calcitonin and estrogen inhibit these mechanisms. Paraneoplastic or humoral hypercalcemia in solid tumors is most often caused by tumor secretion of PTHrP, which is structurally similar to PTH and is present in small amounts in normal tissue. The PTHrP binds to PTH receptors and mimics the effect of PTH, inducing bone resorption and phosphaturia.[17,18] In addition to inducing hypercalcemia, PTHrP may act as a growth factor for malignant cells.

Hypercalcemia associated with multiple myeloma and lymphomas results from local bone destruction rather than from the effects of PTHrP. These tumors secrete osteoclast-activating factors that stimulate osteoclasts to resorb bone. Osteoclast-activating factors are made from one or several cytokines, such as interleukin-1-β, released from malignant plasma cells.[11] Another cytokine, tumor necrosis factor (TNF)-β, is secreted by multiple myeloma cells and stimulates bone resorption. Lymphoma, small cell lung cancer, and malignant melanoma cells may produce active metabolites of vitamin D, which stimulate calcium absorption from the gut.[4]

Paraneoplastic ACTH syndrome is related to tumor secretion of ACTH, which stimulates the adrenal cortex to increase glucocorticoid production, resulting in excessive amounts of corticosteroids and leading to the development of Cushing's disease. The ACTH is actually part of a precursor molecule, which contains melanocyte-stimulating hormone (MSH) and immunologic forms of beta-endorphin. Due to the increased levels of MSH, patients with pACTH syndrome may manifest marked hyperpigmentation. This precursor molecule contains many biologically inactive products; therefore, even though up to one-third of small cell lung cancer patients have increased serum ACTH levels, only 1%–2% develop Cushing's syndrome.[11]

The body's fluid and sodium balance are impacted by SIADH. Normally, the body maintains fluid volume and concentration within a very narrow range regulated by the effect of the neurohypophyseal peptide AVP on the kidney. When AVP is present, the collecting duct is permeable to water, resulting in water reabsorption and concentrated urine. Suppression of AVP leads to urine dilution. Malignant secretion of AVP overrides the normal negative feedback mechanism that suppresses AVP release when serum osmolality, blood volume, and sodium levels are homeostatic. The excess AVP stimulation leads to a scenario of water intoxication from an expanded extracellular volume, serum hypoosmolality, hyponatremia, and hypertonic urine.[11]

Clinical Manifestations

In many patients, the gradual onset of hypercalcemia is asymptomatic and found only during routine electrolyte measurement. A rapid increase in calcium occurs with highly proliferative tumors, causing accelerated bone resorption that overwhelms the kidney's ability to excrete the excess calcium. The acute symptoms of hypercalcemia ensue and include polyuria, polydipsia, nausea, vomiting, anorexia, constipation, lethargy, weakness, and dehydration. Nausea, vomiting, and polyuria can exacerbate the dehydration, which then decreases the glomerular filtration rate and can worsen the hypercalcemia. Occasional complaints are headaches, irritability, anxiety, and insomnia. Confusion, disorientation, hallucinations, and coma are late signs of progressively elevated serum calcium.[19] Obviously, these symptoms can arise from a multitude of oncologic complications and therapies, making it difficult to detect the onset of hypercalcemia without frequent laboratory evaluation.

Excess calcium ions adversely affect cardiac muscle contractility, cell membrane permeability, and the conduction of electrical impulses through the heart. The resulting cardiovascular effects include heart block, bradycardia, ventricular arrhythmias, and asystole.[19] Cushing's disease is a disorder of excess ACTH. Patients with pACTH syndrome are most likely to exhibit hypokalemia, metabolic alkalosis, glucose intolerance, hypertension, proximal muscle weakness, and peripheral edema.[5,15] The classic features of Cushing's disease, including the fat distribution changes such as buffalo hump and moon face, plethora, and cutaneous hyperpigmentation, may be absent because these patients do not survive long enough to develop these characteristics.

Water intoxication accounts for the signs and symptoms seen with SIADH, although most patients are asymptomatic. Edema is rare because the retained water is distributed into cells and not interstitially. When the serum sodium level has fallen to 115–120 mEq/liter (normal range = 137–145 mEq/liter), symptoms may include nausea, weakness, anorexia, fatigue, and muscle cramps. These vague, nonspecific complaints can be easily attributed to the cancer and often are not identified as early signs of hyponatremia. The symptomatology that a pa-

tient exhibits is dependent on both the severity of the hyponatremia and the rate at which it developed.[16]

As the hyponatremia worsens, symptoms may progress to include altered mental status, confusion, lethargy, combativeness, or psychotic behavior. When the hyponatremia is extremely severe (100–110 mEq/liter), seizures, coma, and death may occur.[4]

Assessment

Diagnostic Studies

Diagnosis of hypercalcemia is based on combining the clinical picture with an elevated calcium level. The normal range for serum calcium is 8.5–10.5 g/dL. Hypercalcemia is defined as a serum calcium level greater than 11.0 mg/dL. Measurement of ionized calcium levels is preferred to total serum calcium because it does not include protein-bound calcium and is considered more accurate.

Diagnosis of pACTH syndrome is made primarily by lab testing. Plasma cortisol and 24-hour urinary free-cortisol levels may be obtained. With ectopic ACTH, cortisol levels may be 140 times the normal level.[19] The simplest test to do is a dexamethasone suppression test. The patient receives 2 mg of dexamethasone every 6 hours for 48 hours, or a single 8 mg dose at midnight before obtaining a cortisol level at 8 A.M. the following morning. If the plasma cortisol levels do not suppress, the test is positive.[17] Petrosal sinus sampling may be used to differentiate between a primary pituitary Cushing's disease and ectopic ACTH. Catheters are inserted into the petrosal sinuses, which are the veins that drain the pituitary and are located between the jugular vein and the cavernous sinus. Simultaneous ACTH levels are obtained from the petrosal sinus and from a peripheral vein in the forearm. If ACTH levels are higher in the sinus than in the forearm, this finding suggests a pituitary adenoma. If the levels are similar, an ectopic source of ACTH is suspected. A more recent development in the diagnosis of pACTH is the discovery that most neuroendocrine malignancies express somatostatin and octreotide receptors.[20] These receptors are absent from pituitary adenomas, and pituitary Cushing's disease does not respond to somatostatin analogs. In some instances, ACTH-producing malignancies are difficult to detect, especially in the case of bronchial carcinoid tumors. A diagnostic study that has been successful in locating these tumors is the 111 indium-DTPA (diethylenetriamine pentaacetic acid)-labeled octreotide scan. This scan is able to discover and localize somatastatin receptive tumors by their uptake of octreotide in 80% of patients.[20]

Most cases of SIADH are diagnosed inadvertently when hyponatremia is found through routine serum chemistry studies. The diagnosis of SIADH requires the presence of hyponatremia in addition to plasma hypoosmolality and inappropriately concentrated urine. Plasma osmolality must be less than 280 mOsm/kg, and concurrent urinalysis must show increased levels of sodium (> 20 mEq/liter). Serum chemistries frequently show a low blood urea nitrogen (BUN), creatinine, albumin, and uric acid as a result of the increased extracellular fluid volume. Measurement of serum AVP levels is possible by radioimmunoassay but is rarely done. The levels may be normal or elevated.[15] Other conditions that cause hyponatremia must be ruled out, such as dehydration, fluid retention, or abnormal renal, adrenal, or thyroid function.

Therapeutic Approaches and Nursing Care

Treatment of hypercalcemia involves vigorous hydration and the use of drug therapy. Intravenous pamidronate sodium has proved to be the most effective and least toxic therapy for hypercalcemia associated with solid tumors.[15]

Nursing care involves being able to recognize the subtle signs of early hypercalcemia and taking appropriate action (see Chapter 34 for more on hypercalcemia).

Treatment of pACTH syndrome is primarily focused on treatment of the malignancy. Measures directed at controlling cortisol production and enhancing quality of life include:

- Aminoglutethimide: Can be effective in lowering cortisol levels due to its ability to block hormone production from the adrenal gland. Glucocorticoid replacement may be necessary (dexamethasone).

- Metyrapone: Inhibits enzymes needed to produce cortisol; 500–750 mg qid has a rapid onset and long duration of action.[21]

- Ketoconazole: An imidazole derivative that impairs corticosteroid production. Doses range from 400–1200 mg/day; it is most commonly used because of its rapid onset and minimal toxicities, but corticosteroid supplementation may be necessary due to profound adrenal suppression.[22]

- Mitotane: An oral adrenal cytotoxic agent with slow onset of action.

- Bilateral adrenalectomy: Used rarely in cases when the Cushing's syndrome is resistant to medical intervention or the patient has an indolent tumor and a longer life expectancy.

- Octreotide, as well as being useful as a diagnostic tool, also has a therapeutic effect through its ability to suppress ectopic ACTH secretion. It has been used successfully in the treatment of ACTH-secreting bronchial carcinoid tumors through continuous subcutaneous infusion.[20,23]

The prognosis for patients with pACTH is poor. The response rates to combination chemotherapy are usually very low. The presence of Cushing's syndrome at the time of diagnosis is considered an adverse prognostic factor, worse than if it develops later at the time of recurrence. Patients with pACTH syndrome usually die of pneumonia or opportunistic fungal infections instead of progressive disease.[6] Achieving control of the Cushing's syndrome through normalization of the cortisol level prior to initiating chemotherapy may reduce the potential for infection.

The treatment of SIADH, as with all PNSs, is directed at the underlying malignancy. However, stabilization of the patient and correction of the hyponatremia are essential. The severity of the hyponatremia and water intoxication determines the treatment of the SIADH. Nursing management of patient experiencing SIADH focuses on thorough neurologic assessment and monitoring fluid balance. (See Chapter 43 for more on SIADH.)

NEUROLOGIC PARANEOPLASTIC SYNDROMES

Scope of the Problem

Neurologic PNSs are uncommon, occurring in less than 1% of patients with cancer, yet they account for some of the most interesting and frustrating of the syndromes.[24] As opposed to most of the other PNSs, the neurologic syndromes do not always correlate with the status of the underlying malignancy, as nervous tissue is unable to repair certain types of damage. In some cases, the malignancy may resolve and the patient is left to cope with the permanent neurologic damage.[4]

Most neurologic disorders in patients with cancer are attributable to the effects of metastatic disease or treatment. However, the existence of paraneoplastic syndromes has been well established in some cases, such as thymoma and myasthenia gravis. It is important to note that these neurologic PNSs can also have a benign etiology. The possibility of cancer occurring simultaneously depends on the type of PNS; for example, two-thirds of patients with Lambert-Eaton myasthenic syndrome (LEMS) have or will develop lung cancer, whereas malignancy is much less commonly associated with sensorimotor peripheral neuropathy. In general, the faster the onset of the neurologic syndrome, the higher the odds that it is malignant in origin. Any segment of the nervous system, including the brain, spinal cord, and peripheral nervous system, may be affected by a PNS. In some cases, more than one area may be affected at the same time.[25]

Unlike the endocrine PNSs, in which the tumor secretes excessive amounts of a naturally occurring hormone, the neurologic PNSs are thought to occur from an autoimmune reaction to the tumor. Antibodies secreted by the immune system, in response to antigens shared by the tumor and nervous tissue, may attack nerve cells such as Purkinje cells, resulting in the neurologic syndrome. This theory, which has evolved in the last 20 years, has increased the interest of the scientific community in PNSs. Identification of autoantibodies causing PNS may lead to new diagnostic tests and the possibility of earlier diagnosis and treatment of both the malignancy and the PNS.[25] Unfortunately, except for LEMS, no direct evidence exists supporting the role of autoantibodies in the advent of the neurologic PNSs. Further investigation is needed to determine if autoantibodies are capable of direct neuronal damage, if they act in conjunction with the immune system, or are a sign of autoimmunity but are not specifically responsible for clinical disease.[26] The presence of autoimmune antibodies, indicating a significant antitumor immune response by the patient, has been associated with the spontaneous regression of small cell lung carcinoma.[27] A study of patients with small cell lung cancer having low titers of anti-Hu antibodies, but without evidence of any PNS, determined that these patients experienced better responses to treatment and improved survival.[28]

The neurologic PNSs can be categorized by the portion of the nervous system that is affected: Purkinje cell degeneration (paraneoplastic cerebellar degeneration), dorsal root ganglion degeneration (subacute sensory neuropathy), neuromuscular transmission failure (LEMS and myasthenia gravis), and general damage to the central and peripheral nervous system (paraneoplastic encephalomyelitis).[29] Two of the major neurologic PNSs, paraneoplastic cerebellar degeneration (PCD) and LEMS, are discussed in greater detail.

Definitions

Subacute cerebellar degeneration is a group of paraneoplastic neurologic disorders known to be caused by antineuronal antibodies that are characterized by progressive ataxia and severe vision changes. A number of antibodies have been identified in relation to PCD: anti-Yo, anti-Hu, anti-Ri, Hodgkin's, and PCD/LEMS. In more than 50% of patients, the onset of PCD usually predates diagnosis of the cancer by several months. Occasionally, the malignancy is not detected for years and is discovered only on autopsy.[30]

Lambert-Eaton myasthenic syndrome is a paraneoplastic antibody-mediated autoimmune disorder, characterized by weakness and easy fatigability of muscles, that primarily affects patients with small cell lung carcinoma.[31]

Incidence

Paraneoplastic cerebellar degeneration is a rare disorder, with fewer than 300 cases having been reported in the literature. In some instances a PNS may go undetected and therefore unreported due to the subtle nature of the symptoms. This is not the case with PCD, where symptoms are severe and easily identifiable. The malignancy most often associated with PCD is ovarian cancer. Other cancers in which PCD may occur include small cell lung cancer, Hodgkin's lymphoma, and to a lesser extent breast cancer. The autoantibody involved may differ depending on the malignancy (Table 35-2).

Lambert-Eaton myasthenic syndrome occurs in approximately 6% of patients with small cell lung cancer and has been incidentally reported in patients with breast, gastric, prostate, bladder, ovarian, and rectal cancers. An average of 40% of LEMS cases do not have a malignant etiology but result from a variety of autoimmune diseases, including rheumatoid arthritis, scleroderma, and multiple sclerosis.[31]

Etiology and Risk Factors

Both paraneoplastic neurologic syndromes result from the patient's immune system producing antibodies that mistake normal nerve cells for tumor cell antigens. The paraneoplastic cerebellar degeneration disorders arise from the presence of anti-Purkinje cell antibodies associated with specific neoplasms. The similarity between tumor cell antigens and onconeural antigens expressed by cerebellar Purkinje cells causes the immune system to mistakenly attack the Purkinje cells, with severe neurologic consequences.[30]

As a PNS, LEMS may be the result of autoantibodies attacking the neuromuscular structures involved in muscle nerve contraction. Small cell lung carcinoma is thought to originate from neuroectodermal tissue; therefore, tumor cells may express neural antigens containing voltage-gated calcium channels (VGCCs) on their cell surface. The immune response to the presence of malignant cells produces immunoglobulin G (IgG) antibodies against these tumor antigens. These IgG antibodies mistakenly attack VGCCs in normal nerve tissue, leading to the development of LEMS.[31]

Pathophysiology

Paraneoplastic cerebellar degeneration is a result of the loss or dysfunction of cerebellar Purkinje cells. The cerebellum is the area of the brain that assists in the coordination of movement. It processes sensory information to coordinate the activity of descending motor pathways. Coordinated gait, balance, head and eye movements, and muscle tone are the result of optimum cerebellar functioning. If cerebellar function is impaired, any or all of the following may occur: ataxia (staggered gait), intention tremors, loss of balance, loss of reflexes, or dysarthria (slow slurred speech). The cerebellum is only involved in the coordination of motor function; dysfunction does not produce sensory deficits.[32] However, sensory input from afferent fibers elicits action potentials in Purkinje cells, causing neuron discharge and transfer of electrical impulses to the cerebellar tissue.

Table 35-2 Autoantibody-Associated Paraneoplastic Cerebellar Degeneration Syndromes

Antibody	Malignancy	Syndrome	Clinical Features	Comments
Anti-Yo	• Ovarian carcinoma • Breast carcinoma	Paraneoplastic cerebellar degeneration (PCD)	• Occurs only in women • Occurs prior to malignant diagnosis in majority of patients • Localized tumor • Symptoms include severe dysarthria, oscillopsia, and diplopia	• Treatment with steroids or plasmapheresis is rarely effective • PCD remains unchanged even if malignancy is cured • 100 patients reported
Anti-Hu	• Small cell lung cancer (SCLC) • Prostate carcinoma • Adenocarcinoma of lung • Sarcoma	Paraneoplastic encephalomyelitis sensory neuropathy (PEM/SN)	• 60% of women • Occurs prior to malignant diagnosis • Sensory neuropathy may involve all 4 extremities	• 10% of SCLC patients have the Anti-Hu antibody but do not develop the syndrome • Death usually occurs from autonomic nervous system failure, not progressive disease • Treatment with steroids or plasmapheresis is rarely effective • Presence of the antibody indicates an indolent disease course
Anti-Ri	Not associated with a particular malignancy seen in lung, breast cancer	Paraneoplastic opsoclonus-myoclonus (POM)	• Involuntary eye movement in all directions • Truncal ataxia	• Clinical course is pattern of improvement and exacerbations independent of course of malignancy • Extremely rare (< 20 patients studied)
Hodgkin's	• Hodgkin's lymphoma	PCD	• Male to female ratio is 6:1 • Younger age (20–40 years) • Diagnosis usually made at time of malignant diagnosis • Signs and symptoms similar to Anti-Yo PCD	• Only PCD syndrome in which remission occurs in conjunction with response of lymphoma to treatment
PCD/LEMS (antibody negative)	• SCLC	PCD combined with Lambert-Eaton myasthenic syndrome (LEMS)	• Subacute onset of PCD • Lower extremity weakness • Occurs prior to malignant diagnosis • In some patients PCD is predominant; in others LEMS is predominant	• LEMS component may respond to plasmapheresis, steroids, or successful antineoplastic treatment; however, PCD component is usually unresponsive to therapy • More common than other PCD syndromes except Anti-Yo (30 patients reported)

Antineural Antibodies

The belief that PCD is an autoimmune disorder is based on the idea that the patient's immune response to the tumor produces antibodies that unfortunately recognize Purkinje cells as being similar to tumor cells, thereby attacking and destroying or disabling them.[30]

Several antibodies have been identified related to the development of PCD. These polyclonal IgG antibodies have been measured in the serum and cerebrospinal fluid (CSF) of patients with PCD. Not all patients with PCD have had antibodies present in their serum and CSF; however, the syndrome has been clinically identical to that in patients with antibodies. The presence of antibodies appears to have a positive prognostic significance, as it is associated with a more indolent tumor course.

Western blot analysis allowed the antibodies to be first identified in the early 1980s. Initially designated *anti-*

Purkinje cell antibody, the first antibody identified has since been labeled *anti-Yo* (after the first two letters of the last name of the patient studied). Subsequent antibodies identified are *anti-Hu, anti-Ri, Hodgkin's*, and *PCD/LEMS*. How these autoantibodies are currently described is subject to controversy. Generic nomenclature based on immunohistochemistry alone utilizes terms such as anti-Purkinje cell antibody (APCA), antineuronal nuclear antibody type-1 (ANNA-1), and antineuronal nuclear antibody type-2 (ANNA-2). Antibody- and antigen-specific nomenclature utilizes a combination of immunohistochemistry and western blot analysis (anti-Yo, anti-Hu, etc.).[33] In 1994, an international symposium concluded that the two terminologies were not interchangeable and that detection of anti-Yo or anti-Hu antibodies in a patient's serum or CSF was more specifically related to the presence of an underlying malignancy.[34] Each antibody is associated with different malignancies, and PCD has since been categorized according to the autoantibody involved (see Table 35-2).

The pathophysiology involved in LEMS is a specific abnormality at the cholinergic presynaptic junction. In normal neural function, nerve impulses are transmitted from one cell to another via electrical or chemical synapses. The structures involved with the transmission of a nerve impulse across a chemical synapse include the presynaptic neuron, a neurotransmitter substance, the synaptic cleft, and the postsynaptic cell. These structures are known as the *neuromuscular junction* (NMJ), which facilitates chemical impulses between motor neurons and skeletal muscle fibers. A nerve impulse or action potential is conducted from the motor neuron to the presynaptic neuron. Depolarization of the neuron plasma membrane opens calcium channels. Calcium influx stimulates the synaptic vesicles to fuse with the plasma membrane and release acetylcholine (ACh) into the synaptic cleft. The synaptic vesicles are located in zones in the presynaptic nerve terminal that contain rows of large intramembrane particles. These particles are VGCCs that regulate ACh release. Acetylcholine is a neurotransmitter that crosses the synaptic cleft and combines with an ACh receptor protein (AChR) on the postsynaptic muscle cell. This AChR complex increases conductance of Na^+ and K^+ currents, allowing depolarization of the postsynaptic muscle end plate. This end plate potential (EPP) triggers the action potential that results in muscle contraction.[31,32]

In LEMS, the presence of tumor cells stimulates an autoimmune response that produces IgG antibodies against calcium channels expressed by both the cancer and the neuromuscular junction. The IgG autoantibodies block the VGCCs in the presynaptic nerve terminal, resulting in insufficient ACh release into the synaptic cleft and therefore very low-amplitude muscle action potentials.[35]

Clinical Manifestations

The onset of PCD usually occurs prior to the diagnosis of cancer. Neurologic signs and symptoms that are usually

bilateral, symmetrical, and progressive characterize the cerebellar dysfunction. The initial symptoms are a slight difficulty in walking that rapidly progresses to severe ataxia. This deterioration may occur over days or weeks, with the movements of the arms, legs, and trunk becoming progressively uncoordinated. The patient may experience dysarthria, nystagmus, and oscillopsia, a subjective sensation that objects in the visual field are oscillating. Assistance may be needed to walk and sit, and eventually all activities of daily living are compromised. Communication may be difficult due to the dysarthria and the fact that most patients are unable to write due to hand tremors. Reading and watching television are challenging if not impossible due to the oscillopsia.[30]

Patients with PCD frequently have other mild neurologic deficits. These include sensorineural hearing loss, dysphagia, diplopia, and peripheral neuropathy. Signs of mild dementia may occur, but this is difficult to assess due to the impaired ability to communicate. Vertigo is frequently present.[36]

Eventually, the symptoms of PCD peak in their severity and stabilize. Unfortunately, even if the underlying malignancy is successfully treated, the neurologic symptoms rarely improve. However, there is a wide variety in the degree of severity of PCD. Some patients may experience only mild ataxia and impairment of writing and speaking abilities. A few patients may experience an improvement in neurologic symptoms as their tumor responds to therapy.[30]

Muscle weakness and easy fatigability characterize LEMS, with the muscle groups of the pelvic girdle and thighs primarily affected, the arms and shoulders to a lesser extent. Patients with LEMS complain of difficulty in climbing stairs, rising from a chair or toilet, walking, or running. Additional symptoms may include double- or blurred vision, dysarthria, dysphagia, ptosis, parasthesias, and muscle pain.[4] The weakness associated with LEMS tends to amplify toward the end of the day. It may temporarily improve with voluntary effort from the patient. The autonomic nervous system may also be affected in LEMS due to antibody attack on smooth muscle, resulting in complaints of constipation, urinary retention, abnormal sweating, postural hypotension, and dry mouth.[31]

Assessment

Diagnostic Studies

Routine neurologic diagnostic studies include magnetic resonance imaging (MRI), computerized tomography (CT) scan of the brain, and lumbar puncture. Patients with PCD initially may have a normal MRI or CT brain scan. As the cerebellar failure progresses over a few months, these scans may exhibit diffuse cerebellar atrophy and a dilated fourth ventricle.[36] A positron emission tomography (PET) scan may show abnormal metabolism of the cerebral hemispheres. Initial analysis of CSF obtained via lumbar puncture may show elevated protein levels, an increased IgG, and increased lymphocytes. However, after the neurologic symptoms have plateaued, the CSF frequently reverts to normal.[19]

The diagnosis of LEMS rests in part on distinguishing it from another neurologic disorder—myasthenia gravis (MG). Lambert-Eaton myasthenic syndrome is similar to MG but with some distinctions. In LEMS, in contrast to MG, muscle strength improves with exercise. The drug edrophonium (Tensilon), while very effective for the treatment of MG, has little effect in LEMS. The serum of MG patients contains ACh receptor antibodies that are not present in the serum of patients with LEMS.

Electromyography is used to assess compound muscle action potentials. Repeated nerve stimulation will cause an increase in muscle action potential, resulting in a temporary increase in muscle strength in LEMS. Patients with MG will experience a progressive decrease in muscle response.

Therapeutic Approaches and Nursing Care

Rarely does PCD respond to treatment. The treatments that have been attempted include corticosteroids such as prednisone and dexamethasone. More recently, plasmapheresis has been used in an effort to remove the autoantibodies and antigen-antibody complexes, much as it is used to treat other autoimmune disorders. It has not proved to be successful. This may be due to the fact that the Purkinje cells may have been attacked and quickly destroyed early in the course of the syndrome, long before the diagnosis of PCD was made and treatment initiated. The drug clonazepam has been used to treat the ataxia associated with PCD; doses range from 0.5–1.5 mg daily.[30]

The most challenging issues for nurses caring for patients with PCD is helping them accept that the neurologic symptoms may be permanent despite possible cure or improvement of their cancer. For most patients and families the symptoms occur very rapidly, with little chance to adapt to the deterioration in abilities and the increasing dependence on others. Nursing interventions are directed toward maximizing the patient's cognitive, visual, motor, and communication abilities.[16] Rehabilitation, psychological support, and counseling are essential to helping the patient and family adapt to changing roles and needs. With the advent of the Internet, a variety of Web sites have been developed as resources for the patient and family coping with a neurologic PNS. The International Paraneoplastic Association (http://paraneoplastic.hypermart.net/), founded in 1998, provides information, research links, support for caregivers, and coping and rehabilitation resources.

Treatment of LEMS, as with the previous PNSs, is based on treatment of the underlying malignancy. Frequently, the symptoms associated with LEMS improve with tumor response. If the neurologic symptoms do not improve, a variety of medications and plasmapheresis may be implemented. The drugs used to treat LEMS are pharmacologic agents that promote ACh release from the nerve terminal such as 3,4-diaminopyridine and guanidine. Guanidine is effective but has significant side effects such as seizures. 3,4-Diaminopyridine is the treatment of choice. It affects K^+ channels, thereby increasing the amount of ACh released into the synaptic cleft. Steroids, immune suppression, gamma globulin, and plasmapheresis have been utilized in the treatment of LEMS with mixed success. Plasmapheresis alone is associated with short-term clinical improvement. Weekly plasmapheresis, in combination with prednisone and azathioprine, has produced the most sustained clinical benefit.[37,38]

Patients with a neurologic disorder such as LEMS require a great deal of emotional support. The initial phases of the illness can be frightening, as LEMS patients must learn to deal with a diagnosis of cancer as well as a potentially disabling neurologic disease. The needs of the LEMS patient include ongoing assessment of neurologic status and comprehensive patient education regarding measures to cope with the chronic muscle weakness and fatigue.[39] Figure 35-2 depicts partial amputations of the fingertips and loss of the nails due to paraneoplastic sensory neuropathy, discussed in the case study (Table 35-3).

HEMATOLOGIC PARANEOPLASTIC SYNDROMES

Scope of the Problem

Hematologic abnormalities are frequent problems for oncology patients and often are associated with tumor infiltration of the bone marrow or the effect of antineoplastic therapy. However, the most common hematologic problem is anemia of chronic disease or malignancy. Tumor secretion of cytokines, colony-stimulating factors, and factors that affect coagulation can produce a variety of hematologic disorders, including anemia, granulocytopenia, eosinophilia, thrombocytosis, thromboembolism, nonbacterial thrombotic endocarditis, thrombocytopenia, and coagulopathies such as disseminated intravascular coagulation (DIC). Blood coagulation abnormalities have been reported in more than 90% of patients with cancer.[40] Anemia of malignancy and thromboembolism will be discussed in more detail.

Definitions

Anemia in the patient with cancer may be due to the effects of chemotherapy or radiation, bleeding, bone marrow invasion by tumor, or a primary hematologic disorder. Anemia as a remote effect of neoplastic disease is much

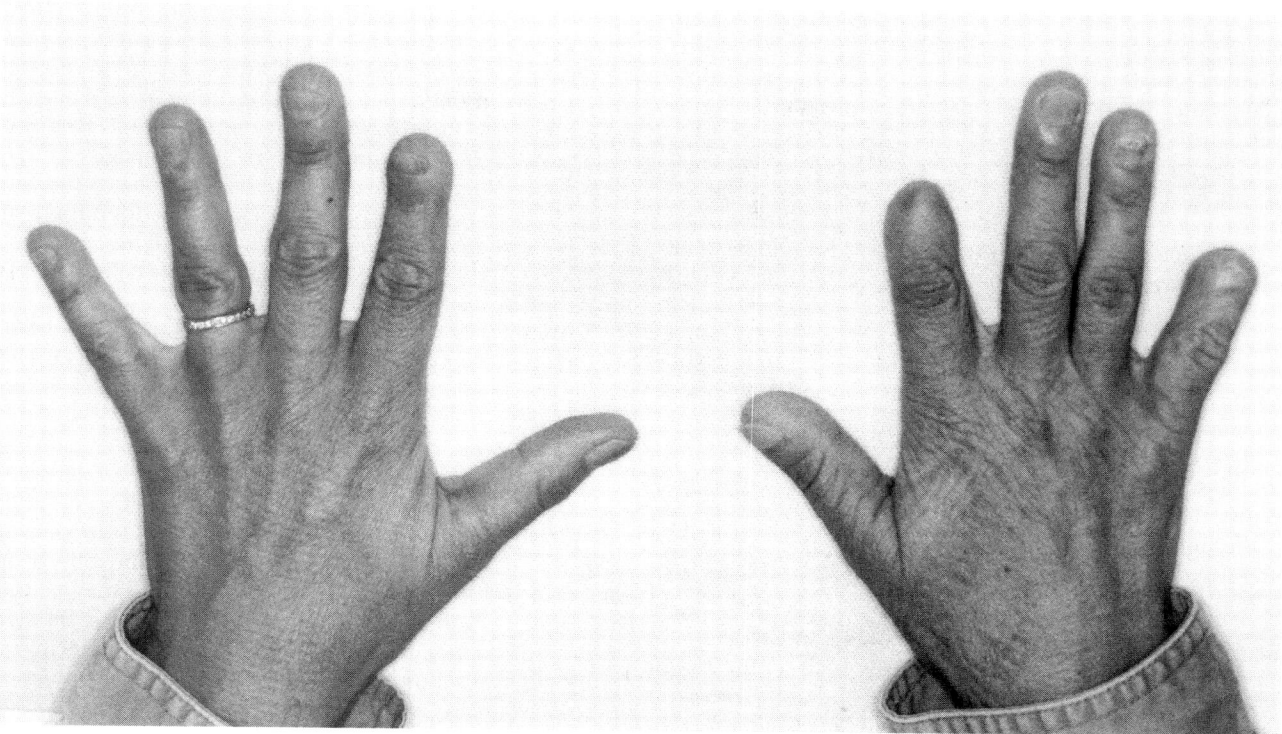

Figure 35-2 Hands of patient from a case study in Table 35-3, showing partial amputations of tips of fingers and lack of nails due to paraneoplastic sensory neuropathy.

Table 35-3 Case Study

Subject: Neurological paraneoplastic syndrome associated with large cell lymphoma

Summary: A 38-year-old woman presenting with a profound ascending sensory neuropathy was subsequently diagnosed with a large cell lymphoma of the lung. She later developed an autonomic neuropathy manifested by orthostatic hypotension and gastroparesis. She received 6 cycles of standard CHOP chemotherapy followed by radiation therapy for residual lung disease. She remains in complete remission three years following treatment.

Clinical symptoms: Initial complaints included fatigue, numbness and tingling of the arms and legs, right-sided facial numbness, difficulty ambulating, and dizziness when standing. Physical exam revealed severe orthostatic hypotension, the absence of fingernails, and sores on fingertips from patient biting. She also developed ulcerations of her lower extremities from trying to do housework.

Clinical course and treatment: The orthostatic hypotension has been successfully managed with fludrocortisone (Florinef), prednisone, and somatostatin (Sandostatin). She underwent three courses of plasmapheresis, which provided marked improvement of the fatigue but no change in the sensory neuropathy. However, in the past 2 years the sensory neuropathy has slightly improved. She currently ambulates with a wide-based gait using a single-prong cane. Following chemotherapy she developed osteomyelitis resulting in the partial amputation of several fingers (see Figure 35-2).

CHOP = cyclophosphamide, doxorubicin, vincristine, prednisone.

less common and is caused by tumor product impairment of bone marrow function and red cell metabolism.[4] When the cause of anemia in a patient with cancer cannot be determined, the diagnosis of "anemia of chronic disease or chronic malignancy" is often made. This syndrome is characterized by a normocytic/normochromic anemia that is not associated with a particular malignancy.[4]

Patients with cancer have a higher risk of thromboembolism (TE) or clot formation due to the hypercoagulable state induced by the malignancy. Paraneoplastic TE was first identified in 1865 by Trousseau, who noted an increased incidence of migratory venous thrombosis in patients with cancer. The definition of Trousseau's syndrome has been expanded over the years to reflect a better understanding of the effect of cancer cells on vasculature and the coagulation pathways. Trousseau's syndrome now describes a variety of thromboembolic disorders affecting both veins and arteries, including specific types of peripheral vascular disease and ischemic heart disease.[41]

Incidence

The incidence of anemia of malignancy is difficult if not impossible to determine because of the inability to separate treatment-related effects from a possible paraneoplastic etiology. Many oncology patients will experience some degree of anemia during their disease course, primarily related to treatment effects. Anemia of chronic malignancy is a diagnosis most commonly applied to patients with advanced disease.

The incidence of TE in patients with cancer has been estimated to be between 1% and 11%. The thromboemboli are frequently found at the time of autopsy. The malignancies primarily associated with TE include small cell lung cancer and non-small cell lung cancer, and colon, pancreas, and—to a lesser extent—breast, prostate, ovarian, and bladder carcinomas. The type of cancer most often implicated is mucin-secreting adenocarcinoma of the gastrointestinal tract. The incidence of TE appears to rise during chemotherapy and hormonal therapy, possibly related to the thrombogenic effect of antineoplastic agents and hormones. The exact mechanism is unknown but may involve a reduction in antithrombin fibrin and fibrinolytic activity.[42,43]

Etiology and Risk Factors

The etiology of anemia of malignancy is multifactorial. It involves the tumor secretion of cytokines, such as interleukin-1 (IL-1), affecting red cell metabolism; other factors include protein-calorie malnutrition, bone marrow failure, and chronic hemorrhage. Protein-calorie malnutrition will produce insufficiencies in iron and folic acid, and general hypoproteinemia. Heavily treated patients who have received multiple courses of chemotherapy and radiation are susceptible to bone marrow failure, which may be manifested by deficiencies in a single cell line such as red cells or platelets but more commonly presents as pancytopenia. Chronic microscopic bleeding usually results from the presence of primary or metastatic disease of the gastrointestinal tract, genitourinary system, or upper and lower respiratory tract.[44]

The etiology of TE is the ability of tumor cells to affect systemic activation of coagulation and cause platelet dysfunction. Thromboembolic disease that is refractory to anticoagulation therapy is often indicative of underlying cancer. Several prospective studies have confirmed a relationship between recurrent, episodic idiopathic deep vein thrombosis (DVT) and the subsequent development of malignancy.[45,46] Idiopathic DVT (no identifiable risk factors) is associated with an estimated 10%–20% risk of malignancy. A significant proportion of these tumors are very small, present at an early stage, and are therefore potentially curable.[45]

Pathophysiology

The multiple factors involved in the advent of anemia of malignancy include tumor secretion of cytokines that affect red cell metabolism and function. Interleukin-1 has the ability to interfere in the transfer process of iron molecules from the reticuloendothelial system to red cell precursors in the bone marrow, resulting in an iron-rich bone marrow but iron-deficient erythrocytes.[44] Another function of IL-1 is stimulation of macrophages in the spleen, causing a decrease in red cell life span. A protein called *anemia-inducing substance* has been identified in the plasma of patients with advanced malignancies that reduces the osmotic resistance of red blood cells, increasing their susceptibility to destruction.[47]

Tumor cells may remotely precipitate paraneoplastic TE by any one of three mechanisms: activation of the coagulation pathway, damage to the endothelial lining of blood vessels, or platelet activation.[41] (A review of the coagulation pathway and the association between clotting and cancer is discussed in Chapter 31.) Cancer cells are known to play a role in activation of the extrinsic clotting pathway. They may induce the cleavage of fibrinogen to fibrin and activate clotting factors such as factor VII or factor X, initiating the clotting cascade. This may be the combined result of direct and indirect effects of cancer cells. Stimulation of the patient's immune system by tumor cell antigens may activate monocyte-macrophages. These monocyte-macrophages, in turn, activate the clotting pathway through the expression of tissue factors. One theory describes the interaction of tumor cells, platelets, and inflammatory cells, causing the formation of a *fibrin gel*, a product essential to tumor growth and the development of metastases.[40]

Patients with cancer experience a variety of platelet disorders such as thrombocytopenia and platelet dysfunction. The exact mechanism by which tumor cells affect these disorders is unclear. One theory involves the production of thrombin.[41] Malignant cells may indirectly inflict damage to vascular endothelium via their activation of platelets. Platelets facilitate tumor cell adhesion to blood vessel walls through two mechanisms: the secretion of substances that promote further endothelial damage and the stimulation of increased platelet aggregation. This ability to affect platelet function is integral to the tumor's ability to invade, implant, and promote angiogenesis.[45]

Clinical Manifestations

Anemia of malignancy is characterized by a low hemoglobin around 10 g/dL, and may be as low as 7.0–8.0 g/dL, which may or may not be symptomatic. Patients may complain of fatigue, dyspnea on exertion, reduced mental acuity, anorexia, and headaches. Physical signs include pallor, postural hypotension, edema, and splenomegaly. Paraneoplastic TE is characterized by venous or arterial thrombosis that may be recurrent and migratory, frequently occurring in veins in which DVTs are uncommon. Signs and symptoms are consistent with the presence of a DVT, including pain and edema of the extremity.

Assessment

Diagnostic Studies

Anemia of malignancy is primarily a diagnosis of exclusion based on laboratory results, combined with the clinical picture. It is characterized by a low serum iron and low iron-binding capacity. Other laboratory tests include hemoglobin, hematocrit, reticulocyte count, and serum ferritin. Bone marrow biopsy and aspirate may be performed. Trousseau's syndrome is diagnosed on the basis of the clinical presentation, combined with ultrasound or radiographic confirmation of a thrombosis. Doppler ultrasound is most commonly performed.

Therapeutic Approaches and Nursing Care

Anemia of malignancy is usually managed through the use of transfusions whenever the patient becomes symptomatic or the hemoglobin falls below 8.0 g/dL. Growth factors are employed conservatively due to the need for repeated injections and high cost. Iron, vitamin therapy, and steroids may be used but are generally not effective. Migratory TE is difficult to treat successfully. Anticoagulation therapy including heparin, warfarin, or Lovenox is often instituted. Acute episodes of TE are managed with intravenous continuous-infusion heparin. Long-term management with warfarin therapy following the acute episode is usually unsuccessful. The advent of low-molecular-weight subcutaneous heparin has shown potential for the prevention of recurrent clot formation.

RENAL PARANEOPLASTIC SYNDROMES

Scope of the Problem

Most renal complications of malignancy are related to the effects of tumor infiltration on the kidneys, renal vein thrombosis, amyloidosis, urethral or ureteral obstruction, and complications of treatment, specifically chemotherapy. The only true renal PNSs are nephrotic syndrome produced by glomerular lesions and obstruction of the glomerulus by tumor products.[4] *Obstruction by tumor products* refers to the secretion of substances by malignant cells causing renal dysfunction. These are rare disorders such as mucoprotein secretion by

pancreatic carcinoma cells, resulting in intrarenal obstruction; and lysozyme secretion associated with acute leukemia, resulting in renal potassium wasting and hypocalcemia. Nephrotic syndrome will be discussed in more detail.

Definitions

The presence of paraneoplastic lesions in the renal glomerulus leads to a disease known as *nephrotic syndrome*, which is defined as impaired renal function resulting in massive proteinuria. Nephrotic syndrome fits the definition of a PNS in that it may precede the diagnosis of malignancy; a reduction in tumor burden by surgery or antineoplastic therapy is associated with a decrease in proteinuria; and increased proteinuria corresponds with tumor recurrence.[2]

Incidence

The incidence of nephrotic syndrome as a PNS is difficult to determine. A review of 101 patients with nephrotic syndrome of unknown origin by Lee et al in 1966 revealed 11 patients with evidence of malignancy.[48] Hodgkin's lymphoma is the primary malignancy associated with nephrotic syndrome. To a lesser degree, it is associated with non-Hodgkin's lymphomas such as Burkitt's lymphoma. Paraneoplastic nephrotic syndrome has also been reported in patients with lung, breast, colon, and prostate carcinomas as well as carcinoid tumors. Nephrotic syndrome precedes a diagnosis of cancer by up to several months and possibly years in approximately 45% of cases; it follows a malignant diagnosis in 15%–20% of cases. The remaining 30%–40% of cases are diagnosed concurrently.[49]

Etiology and Risk Factors

Nephrotic syndrome is most commonly known as a benign disorder, either resulting from a primary glomerular disease or occurring secondary to infection, drugs, or systemic diseases such as diabetes mellitus, systemic lupus erythematous, or rheumatoid arthritis.[50] The etiology of paraneoplastic nephrotic syndrome is the presence of glomerular lesions, with the type of lesion varying with the malignancy involved. In patients with carcinoma and nephrotic syndrome, the etiology may involve products of the immune system, specifically antigen-antibody complexes, that become trapped within the glomerulus and impair glomerular function. The presence of nephrotic syndrome is considered a poor prognostic factor; however, death usually results from tumor progression and not from renal failure. Median survival following the diagnosis of nephrotic syndrome averages 12 months, and approximately 3 months from a malignant diagnosis.[51] However, successful eradication of the malignancy is associated with remission of the nephrotic syndrome.

Pathophysiology

The glomerulus is the portion of the renal nephron, or functional unit of the kidney, responsible for the ultrafiltration of plasma and eventual urine formation. *Ultrafiltration* refers to the removal of plasma proteins and the passive flow of protein-free fluid from the glomerular capillaries into Bowman's space and the renal tubules.[32] The basement membrane of the glomerular capillaries is the main filtration barrier to plasma proteins and the location of most glomerular lesions. The glomerular lesions associated with the presence of a malignancy vary with the type of malignancy involved. The renal lesion present in 80% of patients with Hodgkin's lymphoma is known as *lipoid nephrosis*. Lipoid nephrosis is characterized by the presence of nephrotic syndrome and minimal glomerular changes on histologic examination, and is also called *minimal change disease*.[52] Lipoid nephrosis may be linked to deficiencies in T-cell function, which are frequently seen in lymphomas. Membranous glomerulopathy and membranoproliferative glomerulonephritis represent the types of glomerular lesions seen in 20% of Hodgkin's lymphoma patients.[53]

Carcinomas are most often associated (80%–90%) with membranous glomerulonephritis, a type of glomerular lesion containing deposits of IgG and complement. Antigen-antibody complexes may become trapped in the glomerulus, resulting in lesions that adversely affect renal function. These types of complexes have been isolated from the kidneys of patients with lung and colon carcinomas and nephrotic syndrome. An example is the discovery of tumor-directed antibody and carcinoembryonic antigen present in the glomeruli of a patient with gastric carcinoma.[54]

The leakage of plasma proteins into the urine leads to the development of hypoalbuminemia, which in turn causes peripheral edema from the decrease in plasma oncotic pressure. The low plasma oncotic pressure instigates a series of homeostatic mechanisms, such as increased vasopressin secretion, in an effort to restore the plasma volume. The subsequent sodium and water retention further aggravate the peripheral edema, leading to anasarca. Another effect of insufficient plasma oncotic pressure is increased hepatic lipoprotein synthesis, resulting in hyperlipidemia—specifically, elevated cholesterol and low-density lipoprotein levels.[50]

Clinical Manifestations

The clinical manifestations of nephrotic syndrome may precede a malignant diagnosis by 2–18 months. The cardinal sign of nephrotic syndrome is massive proteinuria, accompanied by hypoalbuminemia, hyperlipidemia, and edema. Signs and symptoms include brown, foamy urine and facial and peripheral edema, which may progress to anasarca or edema of all body tissues. The combined water and electrolyte retention may cause mild to moderate hypertension.

Assessment and Grading

Diagnostic Studies

As with many PNSs, paraneoplastic nephrotic syndrome is a diagnosis of exclusion. Renal vein thrombosis, amyloidosis, and drug-related or benign disease etiologies must be ruled out. Nephrotic syndrome is diagnosed primarily by percutaneous renal biopsy, combined with the clinical picture. On renal biopsy, minimal change disease is manifested by hyalinization of the glomeruli and narrowing or obliteration of the capillary walls, but completely normal capillary basement membranes without evidence of immune deposits.[52] Renal biopsy results from patients with membranous glomerulonephritis related to carcinoma show fine holes in the glomerular basement membrane and focal capillary irregularities caused by granular deposits of IgG and possibly complement.[49]

Renal ultrasound may be utilized to eliminate renal vein thrombosis or hydronephrosis as an etiology for the nephrotic syndrome. Findings usually reveal enlarged, occasionally asymmetric kidneys and increased echogenicity consistent with parenchymal disease.

Laboratory studies include urinalysis, 24-hour urine collection, and serum chemistry profile. Urinalysis shows moderate heme, 2^+–4^+ protein, and 2^+ granular casts. A 24-hour urine examination may contain protein levels of 3800–7000 mg. The chemistry profile may reveal an elevated creatinine, BUN, and cholesterol, with a decreased albumin.

Gallium scan may be performed and will show uptake by the kidneys. It can be utilized as a screening tool for patients with idiopathic nephrotic syndrome to screen for occult lymphoma.[55]

Therapeutic Approaches and Nursing Care

The primary treatment of paraneoplastic nephrotic syndrome is focused on the underlying malignancy. The development of acute renal failure is a concern but rarely occurs. Resolution of the nephrotic syndrome is fairly rapid following tumor response to therapy. Sherman et al report two cases of nephrotic syndrome associated with Hodgkin's lymphoma, characterized by anasarca, hypertension, hypoalbuminemia, and massive proteinuria.[56] In both cases, the patients received mantle radiation to the neck, axillae, supraclavicular areas, and mediastinum. Within 1 week of the radiation, spontaneous diuresis occurred, the hypoalbuminemia resolved, and a significant decrease in the proteinuria was noted.

Another case of nephrotic syndrome associated with adenocarcinoma of unknown primary etiology was reported by Robinson et al.[55] In this situation, the nephrotic syndrome preceded the malignant diagnosis by 1 year, and it waxed and waned with the malignancy. Recurrence of disease was heralded by symptoms of the nephrotic syndrome.

Management of the nephrotic syndrome itself includes the use of steroids and diuretics. The use of glucocorticoids is standard (i.e., prednisone 40–100 mg/day × 4 weeks followed by a reduced dose for an additional 4 weeks). A response to steroids is usually seen in 8–24 weeks. Side effects include muscle weakness, increased appetite, and the development of cushingoid symptoms. Loop diuretics are commonly used to relieve the edema. A high-protein diet may be recommended; however, most of the dietary protein will be excreted in the urine, and many cancer patients find this type of diet difficult to tolerate. Cytotoxic drugs such as cyclophosphamide and chlorambucil may be used but are usually reserved for patients who cannot tolerate steroids.[54]

MISCELLANEOUS PARANEOPLASTIC SYNDROMES

Cutaneous Paraneoplastic Syndromes

Malignant disease has always been associated with the development of a wide variety of cutaneous syndromes or dermatoses. In contrast to the previous PNSs, no one malignancy is predominantly associated with cutaneous PNSs in general, although some are pathognomonic for a certain malignancy. The etiology of most cutaneous PNSs is unknown. Possible theories include the secretion of transforming-growth factor alpha, resulting in abnormal stimulation of epidermal cells, peptide production by the tumor, or a type of autoimmune reaction involving dermal infiltration by neutrophils, lymphocytes, and eosinophils.[57,58]

Cutaneous PNSs are extremely rare; for example, only 50 reported cases of erythema gyratum repens exist[59] (Figure 35-3).[60] These syndromes range from extremely rare but frequently associated with malignancy, to those that are equally associated with benign and malignant disease, to those that are infrequently associated with malignancy. Diagnosis of a cutaneous PNS is made on the basis of physical examination and skin biopsy. The presence of the syndrome should lead to a search for a malignant cause, if not previously diagnosed, or for recurrent disease in the patient with a history of malignancy.[57] A true cutaneous PNS must meet two criteria:

(1) the appearance of the dermatosis must follow the development of the malignancy; and (2) the disease course of both the dermatosis and the malignancy must coincide.[58] The dermatoses considered to be true PNSs are described in Table 35-4.

The primary treatment of cutaneous PNS is treatment of the underlying malignancy. Topical and systemic corticosteroid therapy have been used with some success.[59] Other measures are strictly supportive, including nonsteroidal anti-inflammatory medications, lubricating lotions, and analgesics as needed. Nursing care depends on the severity of the syndrome and may involve the use of wet dressings and antihistamines to prevent scratching and secondary infection. Patient education and emotional support are essential as the patient must cope with the effects of the syndrome while waiting for the malignancy to respond to treatment.

Anorexia-Cachexia Syndrome

The predominant and most well known PNSs affecting the gastrointestinal system are anorexia and cachexia. Malabsorption syndromes are a rare phenomenon associated with histologic abnormalities of the small bowel, characterized by a flattening of the mucosa and villous atrophy. The malignancies related to malabsorption syndromes include colon, lung, prostate, and pancreatic carcinomas, and lymphomas.[4] *Anorexia* refers to a loss of appetite and subsequent reduction in food intake. *Cancer cachexia* is a syndrome defined as progressive loss of body fat and lean body mass associated with anorexia, early satiety, profound weakness, anemia, fatigue, impaired immune function, and poor performance status.[61,62] The incidence of anorexia and cachexia in the oncologic population is difficult to determine but is estimated to occur in 60%–70% of patients with advanced malignant disease. It is considered a major contributing factor in the cause of death in 50% of patients with advanced disease.[63]

Anorexia-cachexia does not result from the nutritional demands of the malignancy or reduced food intake, but from multiple metabolic and physiologic abnormalities. Anorexia-cachexia differs from other PNSs in that it is not associated with a specific malignancy but can occur with any cancer. A study conducted by the Eastern Cooperative Oncology Group (ECOG) determined that patients with breast carcinoma, sarcoma, non-lymphocytic leukemia, and favorable prognosis non-Hodgkin's lymphoma experienced the lowest incidence of weight loss (31%–40%); patients with less favorable prognosis non-Hodgkin's lymphoma, prostate, colon, and lung carcinomas were associated with a 48%–61% incidence of weight loss; and the highest incidence of weight loss was found in patients with gastric and pancreatic cancers (83%–87%).[62] Anorexia-cachexia is more commonly associated with end-stage disease but can occur any time during the disease process and is usually related to the amount of tumor burden. The timing of the syn-

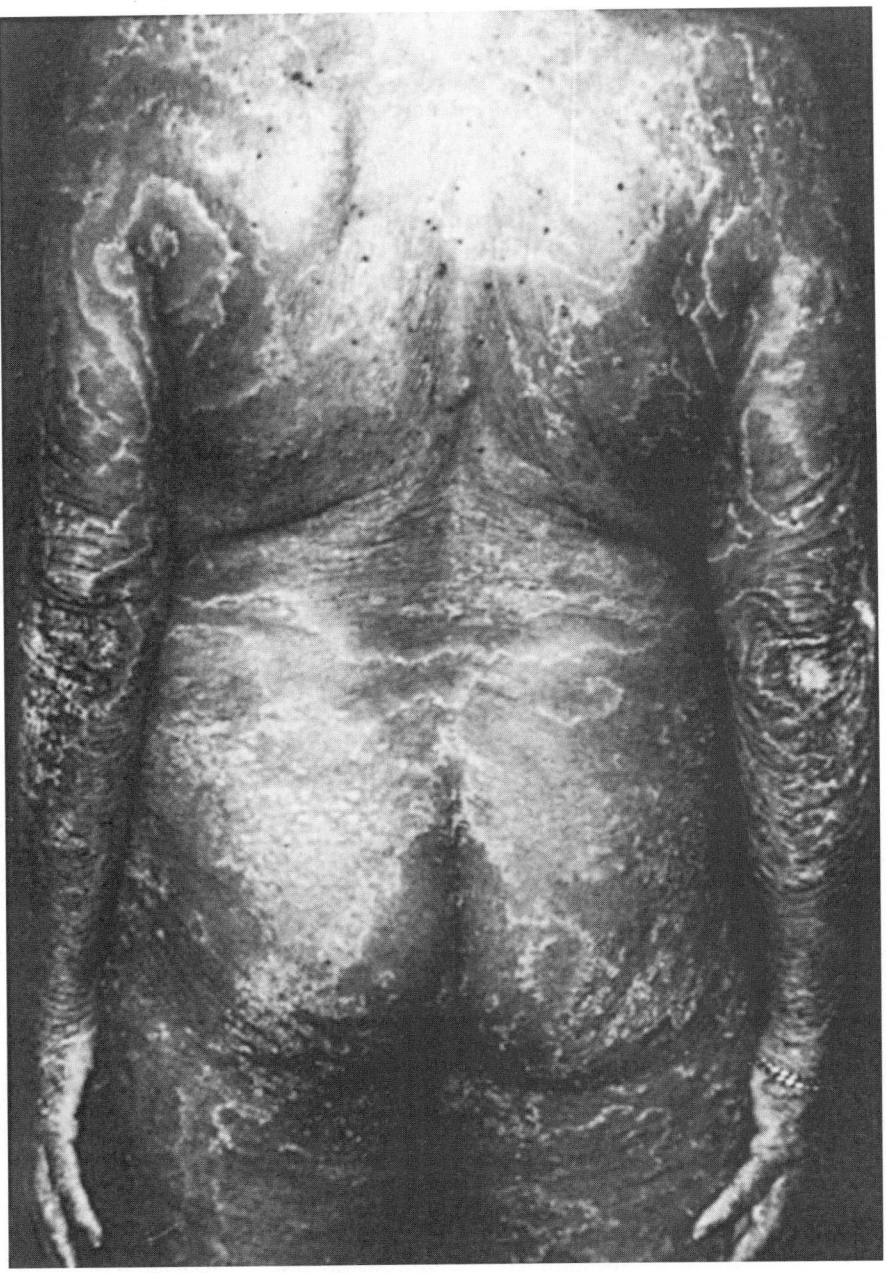

Figure 35-3 Patient with erythema gyratum repens showing classic "wood grain" pattern most pronounced in the intertriginous areas. (Photo reproduced with permission from Appell ML, Ward WQ, Tyring SK: Erythema gyratum repens—A cutaneous marker of malignancy. *Cancer* 62:548–550. Copyright © 1988 American Cancer Society. Reprinted by permission of Wiley-Liss, Inc., a subsidiary of John Wiley and Sons, Inc.)[60]

drome differs with the type of histology. Anorexia-cachexia is a dominant feature of lung cancer, occurring much earlier in the disease course than is seen in patients with breast cancer. The syndrome can severely impact a patient's ability to tolerate antineoplastic therapy and may potentiate adverse reactions.[63]

Several mediators including peptides, hormones, cytokines, and tumor-related factors play a role in the cancer cachexia syndrome. The anorexia associated with the syndrome may be related to the presence of appetite-suppressing neuropeptides. In normal appetite physiology, neuropeptide Y (NPY) is secreted by the hypothalamus and binds to the Y-5 receptor in the hypothalamus, lead-ing to appetite stimulation. Malignant cells may produce a peptide known as leptin that preferentially binds to the Y-5 receptor, inhibiting the effect of NPY, and producing satiety.[64] Hormones involved in the anorexia-cachexia syndrome include insulin, insulin-like growth factor, epinephrine, corticotropin, and human growth hormone. The body's normal response to decreased nutrient intake is conservation of glucose and protein stores through a reduction in glucose production, protein synthesis, and protein breakdown. With the anorexia-cachexia syndrome, this ability is impaired, and protein and fat breakdown occur at a higher rate, corresponding with the development of insulin resistance.[62,65]

Table 35-4 Paraneoplastic Cutaneous Syndromes

Disorder	Clinical Presentation	Associated Malignancy	Comments
Pigmented lesions			
• Acanthosis nigricans	• Velvety, brown, symmetrical lesions with hyperkeratosis that occur primarily in flexural areas—axilla, posterior neck, perineum, umbilicus	• 90% of cases associated with malignancy • 60% gastric carcinoma • 5% lung carcinoma	• Usually associated with advanced disease
• Sign of Leser-Trelat	• Multiple seborrheic (wart-like) lesions	• Adenocarcinomas • Non-Hodgkin's lymphoma • GI malignancies—43%	• Rapid development signals malignancy • Pruritic
• Sweet's syndrome (acute, febrile neutrophilic dermatosis)	• Painful erythematous plaques covering arms, head, and neck	• 10%–15% of cases associated with a malignancy, usually hematologic, leukemias (AML), myeloma • GU, GI, breast—less common	
• Bazex's syndrome	• Scaly, pruritic psoriasiform rash affecting nails, nose, ears, elbows, knees, fingers, and toes	• Squamous cell carcinomas of head and neck, esophagus, lung • Vulvar, esophageal, and uterine carcinomas	• Males primarily affected • Females less common • 100% association with malignancy
Erythemas			
• Erythema gyratum repens (*repens* is latin for "to crawl or creep")	• Expanding, scaly, concentric bands (gyri) with a "wood grain" pattern	• 32% lung carcinoma • Breast • Esophagus • Uterine	• Pruritic • Moves rapidly across skin surface—about 1 cm per day • 2:1 male to female ratio • 100% association with malignancy • Tumor resection results in complete resolution within 6 weeks
• Glucagonoma syndrome (necrolytic migratory erythema)	• Erythematous patches • Stomatitis	• Islet cell tumors of pancreas	• Tumor resection results in clearance of the eruption within 48 hours
• Flushing	• Intermittent episodes of facial flushing	• Carcinoid • Medullary thyroid carcinoma	
Endocrine/metabolic lesions			
• Porphyria cutanea tarda	• *Early:* Photosensitive subepidermal vesicles, fragile skin, hyperpigmentation • *Late:* Alopecia, scarring, sclerodermoid changes	• Liver carcinoma	• Often painful, pruritic
• Systemic nodular panniculitis	• Fever, erythematous SQ nodules, fat necrosis of bone marrow, lungs, and other organs; abdominal pain	• Pancreatic adenocarcinoma	• Occurs rarely; also associated with benign pancreatic disease
Miscellaneous			
• Pruritus	• Generalized itching with areas of excoriation from scratching • Chronic, intensive itching of nostrils associated with advanced brain tumors	• Hodgkin's and T-cell lymphomas • Polycythemia vera • CNS malignancies	• 25% of Hodgkin's lymphoma patients experience generalized itching • May be presenting symptom of malignancies
• Hypertrichosis lanuginosa (malignant down)	• Fine, silky hair occurring primarily on forehead and ears	• Lung, colon carcinomas, also bladder, uterine	• Rapid onset • 90% association with malignancy
• Hypertrophic pulmonary osteoarthropathy (HPO)	• Painful, symmetric arthropathy involving fingers, wrists, elbows, and knees caused by periostitis	• Intrathoracic malignancies primarily lung carcinomas (88%) • Histologies most common are large cell and adenocarcinoma of the lung	• Associated with clubbing of fingers and toes • May resemble rheumatoid arthritis • Usually precedes diagnosis of malignancy

GI = gastrointestinal; AML = acute myelogenous leukemia; GU = genitourinary; SQ = subcutaneous; CNS = central nervous system.

The major cytokine involved in the anorexia-cachexia syndrome is tumor necrosis factor-alpha (TNF-α), also known as cachectin. Interleukin-1β, IL-6, and gamma interferon may also play roles. The effect of TNF is alteration of metabolic controls, affecting the mechanisms that regulate hunger, satiety, taste, and metabolism—specifically, lipid metabolism.[4] Tumor necrosis factor is a protein secreted by monocytes and macrophages that was initially named *cachectin* after its discovery in parasite-infected rabbits who developed anorexia and tissue wasting. Giving recombinant TNF to laboratory animals produces anorexia and weight loss but is dependent on the method of administration. Intermittent bolus administration allowed the animals to become tolerant to the effects of the TNF and subsequently begin eating and gaining weight. Continuous-infusion TNF produced more profound anorexia, weight loss, loss of muscle mass, and eventually death.[63]

Tumor-related factors that contribute to the anorexia-cachexia syndrome include an acidic peptide known as *proteoglycan*, which has been isolated in the urine of patients with cancer who have experienced significant weight loss. Animal studies have demonstrated proteoglycan's ability to mobilize free-fatty acids and amino acids, suggesting that its role is to provide nutrients for tumor growth. Eicosapentaenoic acid is an antagonist to the effect of proteoglycan and may eventually play a role in the treatment of anorexia-cachexia.[62,66]

Nursing assessment of the cancer patient's nutritional status, including appetite, weight, and weight loss, is critical in allowing early diagnosis and intervention. (See Chapter 33 for nutritional and pharmacologic interventions.)

Tumor Fever

Tumor fever is a PNS primarily associated with lymphomas, and less often with leukemias, myelodysplastic syndromes, renal cell carcinoma, hepatoma, osteogenic sarcoma, and metastatic liver disease. Although less common in solid tumors, tumor fever has been documented as a sign of metastatic disease in patients with breast and nasopharyngeal carcinomas, and is frequently associated with the presence of other paraneoplastic syndromes.[67,68] Tumor fever is produced by tumor secretion of one or multiple pyrogenic cytokines, specifically IL-1α, IL-1β, interferon-α, TNF-α, TNF-β, and IL-6, that act directly on the hypothalamus, causing the release of prostaglandin E_2, which increases the body's temperature set-point. Leukemia and lymphoma cell lines are capable of intrinsic production of these cytokines, whereas solid tumors may promote cytokine release from "bystander" endothelial cells or monocytes.[69]

The majority of patients with tumor fever do not follow a specific pattern. Fever patterns occur most commonly with lymphomas, specifically Hodgkin's lymphoma. In Hodgkin's lymphoma the presence of fever at the time of diagnosis is considered a poor prognostic indicator. A particular tumor fever known as Pel Ebstein fever also occurs in Hodgkin's lymphoma, with a pattern of a 3- to 10-day period of fever alternating with afebrile periods.[70]

The primary therapy for tumor fever is treatment of the underlying malignancy. Chemotherapy often leads to defervescence of the fever as the tumor burden is reduced. However, because of the malaise that chronic fever may produce, symptomatic relief is important. Medications that may provide temporary relief are primarily nonsteroidal anti-inflammatory drugs (NSAIDs), specifically naproxen, indomethacin, or diclofenac, all of which have been shown to be equally effective in controlling tumor fever. Failure of one NSAID does not preclude the use of a second drug. These drugs are so effective at controlling tumor fever that they have been used to distinguish between fever due to infection and that caused by malignancy. They have also been used as a diagnostic tool in patients with cancer who have fever of unknown origin (FUO). The mechanism by which NSAIDs affect tumor fever is unknown but may involve their ability to block prostaglandin E_2 synthesis.[69,71]

Ocular Paraneoplastic Syndromes

The ocular paraneoplastic syndromes are extremely rare disorders that have been documented in both adults and children. The two syndromes that have been most clearly defined are opsoclonus and cancer-associated retinopathy. Opsoclonus is an involuntary eye-movement disorder in which the eye moves primarily horizontally with frequent vertical and rotating jerks. These movements continue despite closing the eyes or sleeping.[72] In children, opsoclonus has been associated with neuroblastoma and is usually the presenting symptom leading to diagnosis of the malignancy. Opsoclonus in adults, 70% of which occurs in patients with small cell lung cancer or breast carcinoma, usually presents in patients over 40 years of age, accompanied by tremors and gait disturbances.[26] It has been linked to the presence of cerebellar degeneration and may have a similar autoimmune pathophysiology. Anti-Hu and anti-Purkinje cell antibodies have been found in the serum of patients with opsoclonus and may produce the syndrome by attacking cerebellar cells.[73] Oral steroids and intravenous immunoglobulin have been used with variable success.[74]

Cancer-associated retinopathy (CAR) is a paraneoplastic syndrome primarily associated with small cell lung cancer but also has been documented in patients with non-small cell lung cancer, and cervical, breast, and endometrial carcinomas. The discovery of antiretinal antibodies, known as anti-CAR antibodies, suggests an abnormal autoimmune response. Patients experience unilateral or bilateral visual loss related to retinal degeneration, occasionally leading to blindness. Initial symptoms include blurred vision and abnormal color perception. Visual disturbances such as sparkles, shimmering, or distortions are common. Vision may deteriorate rapidly, or over several years, and may occur prior to or concurrently with diagnosis of the malignancy. Physical examination usually demonstrates abnormalities in the retinal vasculature and a significant decrease in the number of retinal ganglion cells. Oral steroids again may be beneficial.[26,75]

Conclusion

The PNSs represent a fascinating group of diseases that may affect the endocrine, neurologic, hematologic, renal, gastrointestinal, and cutaneous systems. These syndromes range in incidence from extremely rare, such as the paraneoplastic cerebellar disorders and cutaneous syndromes, to quite prevalent, such as anorexia-cachexia and anemia of chronic disease. Nursing management of these syndromes can be quite challenging, ranging from the ability to detect the subtle neurologic changes of SIADH, to the support and rehabilitation of the patient with LEMS. As we gain a greater understanding of the substances that tumor cells secrete, the mechanisms involved, and their effect on normal tissue, we may be able to provide better treatments for PNSs, prevent their occurrence, and impact the diagnosis and management of cancer itself.

References

1. Eckhardt SL: Paraneoplastic syndromes. *Cancer Surv* 21:197–209, 1994
2. Nathanson L, Hall TC: Introduction: Paraneoplastic syndromes. *Semin Oncol* 24:265–268, 1997
3. Hall TC: Paraneoplastic syndromes: Mechanisms. *Semin Oncol* 24:269–276, 1997
4. John WJ, Foon KA, Patchell RA: Paraneoplastic syndromes, in Devita VT, Hellman S, Rosenberg SA (eds): *Cancer: Principles and Practice of Oncology* (ed 5). Philadelphia, Lippincott-Raven, 1997, pp 2397–2422
5. Anderson KM: Paraneoplastic syndromes, in Bone R (ed): *Quick Reference to Internal Medicine*. New York, Igaku-Shoin Medical Publishers Inc., 1993, pp 1061–1065
6. Block JB: Paraneoplastic syndromes, in Haskell CM, Berek JS (eds): *Cancer Treatment* (ed 4). Philadelphia, Saunders, 1995, pp 245–264
7. Schwartz WB, Bennett W, Curelop S, et al: A syndrome of renal sodium loss and hyponatremia probably resulting from inappropriate secretion of antidiuretic hormone. *Am J Med* 23:529–534, 1957
8. Amatruda TT, Mulrow PJ, Gallagher JC, et al: Carcinoma of the lung with inappropriate antidiuresis: Demonstration of an antidiuretic-hormone-like activity in tumor extract. *N Engl J Med* 269:544–550, 1963
9. Moses AM, Scheinman SJ: Ectopic secretion of neurohypophyseal peptides in patients with malignancy. *Endocrinol Metab Clin North Am* 20:489–506, 1991
10. Shrager JB, Wright CD, Wain JC, et al: Bronchopulmonary carcinoid tumors associated with Cushing's syndrome: A more aggressive variant of typical carcinoid. *J Thorac Cardiovasc Surg* 114:367–375, 1997
11. Becker KL, Silva OL: Paraneoplastic endocrine syndromes, in Becker KL (ed): *Principles and Practice of Endocrinology and Metabolism* (ed 2). Philadelphia, Lippincott, 1995, pp 1842–1852
12. Ralston SH: Pathogenesis and management of cancer-associated hypercalcemia. *Cancer Surv* 21:179–196, 1994
13. Marchioli CC, Graziano SL: Paraneoplastic syndromes associated with small cell lung cancer. *Chest Surg Clin North Am* 7:65–80, 1997
14. Pierce ST: Paraendocrine syndromes. *Curr Opin Oncol* 5:639–645, 1993
15. Shepard FA, Laskey J, Evans WK, et al: Cushing's syndrome associated with ectopic corticotropin production and small cell lung cancer. *J Clin Oncol* 10:21–27, 1992
16. Zumsteg MM, Casperson DS: Paraneoplastic syndromes in metastatic disease. *Semin Oncol Nurs* 14:220–229, 1998
17. Odell WD: Endocrine/metabolic syndromes of cancer. *Semin Oncol* 24:299–317, 1997
18. Kaplan M: Hypercalcemia of malignancy: A review of advances in pathophysiology. *Oncol Nurs Forum* 21:1039–1046, 1994
19. Midthun DE, Jett JR: Clinical presentation of lung cancer, in Pass HI, Mitchell JB, Johnson DH, Turrisi AT (eds): *Lung Cancer: Principles and Practice*. Philadelphia, Lippincott-Raven, 1996, pp 421–435
20. von Werder K, Muller OA, Stalla GK: Somatostatin analogs in corticotropin production. *Metabolism* 45:129–131, 1996
21. Comi RJ, Gorden P: Long-term medical treatment of ectopic ACTH syndrome. *South Med J* 91:1014–1018, 1998
22. Winquist EW, Laskey J, Crump M, et al: Ketoconazole in the management of paraneoplastic Cushing's syndrome secondary to ectopic adrenocorticotropin production. *J Clin Oncol* 13:157–164, 1995
23. Van den Bruel A, Bex M, Van Dorpe J, et al: Occult ectopic ACTH secretion due to recurrent lung carcinoid: Long-term control of hypercortisolism by continous subcutaneous infusion of octreotide. *Clin Endocrinol* 49:541–546, 1998
24. Dalmau JO, Posner JB: Paraneoplastic syndromes affecting the nervous system. *Semin Oncol* 24:318–328, 1997
25. Posner JB, Furneaux HM: Paraneoplastic syndromes, in Waksman BH (ed): *Immunologic Mechanisms in Neurologic and Psychiatric Disease*. New York, Raven, 1990, pp 187–219
26. Dropcho EJ: Neurologic paraneoplastic syndromes. *J Neurosci* 153:264–278, 1998
27. Darnell RB, DeAngelis LM: Regression of small cell lung carcinoma in patients with paraneoplastic neuronal antibodies. *Lancet* 341:21–22, 1993
28. Graus F, Dalmau J, Rene R, et al: Anti-Hu antibodies in patients with small cell lung cancer: Association with complete response to therapy and improved survival. *J Clin Oncol* 15:2866–2872, 1997
29. Posner JB, Dalmau J: Paraneoplastic syndromes. *Curr Opin Immunol* 9:723–729, 1997
30. Posner JB: Paraneoplastic cerebellar degeneration. *Principles and Practice of Oncology Updates* 5:1–13, 1991
31. Lang B, Newsom-Davis J: Immunopathology of the Lambert-Eaton myasthenic syndrome. *Springer Semin Immunopathol* 17:3–15, 1995
32. Berne RM, Levy MN: *Principles of Physiology*. St. Louis, Mosby, 1994, p 134
33. Nath U, Grant R: Neurological paraneoplastic syndromes. *J Clin Path* 50:975–980, 1997
34. Moll JWB, Antoine JC, Brashear HR, et al: Guidelines for

the detection of paraneoplastic antineuronal-specific anti-bodies: Report from the workshop to the fourth meeting of the International Society of Neuroimmunology on Para-neoplastic Neurological Disease, 22–23 October 1994, Rot-terdam, the Netherlands. *Neurology* 45:1937–1941, 1995

35. Lennon VA, Kryzer TJ, Griesmann GE, et al: Calcium-chan-nel antibodies in the Lambert-Eaton syndrome and other paraneoplastic syndromes. *N Engl J Med* 332:1467–1474, 1995

36. Posner JB: Paraneoplastic syndromes. *Neurol Clin* 9:919–936, 1991

37. Newsom-Davis J, Murray N: Plasma exchange and immuno-suppressive drug treatment in the Lambert-Eaton myas-thenic syndrome. *Neurology* 34:480–485, 1984

38. Dau PC, Denys EH: Plasmapheresis and immunosuppressive drug therapy in the Lambert-Eaton syndrome. *Ann Neurol* 11:570–575, 1982

39. Struthers CS: Lambert-Eaton myasthenic syndrome in small cell lung cancer: Nursing implications. *Oncol Nurs Forum* 21: 677–683, 1994

40. Rickles FR, Edwards RL: Activation of blood coagulation in cancer: Trousseau's syndrome revisited. *Blood* 62:14–31, 1983

41. Naschitz JE, Yeshurun D, Lev LM: Thromboembolism in cancer. *Cancer* 71:1384–1390, 1993

42. Levine MN, Gent M, Hirsh J, et al: The thrombogenic effect of anticancer drug therapy in women with stage II breast cancer. *N Engl J Med* 318:404–407, 1988

43. Bick RL, Strauss JF, Frenkel EP: Thrombosis and hemor-rhage in oncology patients. *Hematol Oncol Clin North Am* 10: 875–907, 1996

44. Turner AR: Haematological aspects of palliative medicine, in Doyle D, Hanks GWC, MacDonald N (eds): *Oxford Textbook of Palliative Medicine*. New York, Oxford University Press, 1994, pp 486–491

45. Silverstein RL, Nachman RL: Cancer and clotting: Trous-seau's warning. *N Engl J Med* 327:1163–1164, 1992

46. Prandoni P, Lensing AWA, Buller HR, et al: Deep-vein throm-bosis and the incidence of subsequent symptomatic cancer. *N Engl J Med* 327:1128–1133, 1992

47. Honda K, Ishiko O, Tatsuta I, et al: Anemia inducing sub-stance from plasma of patients with advanced malignant neoplasms. *Cancer Res* 55:3623–3639, 1995

48. Lee JC, Yamaguchi H, Hopper J Jr: The association of cancer and the nephrotic syndrome. *Ann Intern Med* 64:41–51, 1966

49. Becker BN, Goldin G, Santos R, et al: Carcinoid tumor and the nephrotic syndrome: A novel association between neoplasia and glomerular disease. *South Med J* 89:240–242, 1996

50. Glassock RJ, Brenner BM: The major glomerulopathies, in Isselbacher KJ, Braunwald E, Wilson JD, et al (eds): *Har-rison's Principles of Internal Medicine*. New York, McGraw-Hill, 1994, pp 1295–1306

51. Eagen JW, Lewis EJ: Glomerulopathies of neoplasia. *Kidney Int* 11:297–306, 1977

52. Sherman RL, Susin M, Weksler ME, et al: Lipoid nephrosis in Hodgkin's disease. *Am J Med* 52:699–706, 1972

53. Gagliano RG, Costanzi JJ, Beathard GA, et al: The nephrotic syndrome associated with neoplasia: An unusual para-neoplastic syndrome. *Am J Med* 60:1026–1031, 1976

54. Juweid M, Kim CK, Heyman S: Nephrotic syndrome as an unusual paraneoplastic syndrome of Hodgkin's disease

demonstrated on Gallium-67 scan. *Clin Nucl Med* 19: 224–227, 1994

55. Robinson WL, Mitas JA, Haerr RW, et al: Remission and exacerbation of tumor-related nephrotic syndrome with treatment of the neoplasm. *Cancer* 54:1082–1084, 1984

56. Sherman RL, Susin M, Weksler ME, et al: Lipoid nephrosis in Hodgkin's disease. *Am J Med* 52:699–706, 1972

57. Cohen PR: Cutaneous paraneoplastic syndromes. *Am Fam Physician* 50:1273–1282, 1994

58. McLean DI, Haynes HA: Cutaneous manifestations of inter-nal malignant disease, in Fitzpatrick T (ed): *Fitzpatrick Derma-tology and General Medicine* (ed 4). New York, McGraw-Hill, 1993, pp 2229–2248

59. Boyd AS, Neldner KH, Menter A: Erythema gyratum repens: A paraneoplastic eruption. *J Am Acad Dermatol* 26:757–762, 1992

60. Appell ML, Ward WQ, Tyring SK: Erythema gyratum re-pens—a cutaneous marker of malignancy. *Cancer* 62: 548–550, 1988

61. Cotran RS, Kumar V, Robbins SL: *Robbins Pathologic Basis of Disease* (ed 5). Philadelphia, Saunders, 1994, pp 52–73

62. Puccio M, Nathanson L: The cancer cachexia syndrome. *Semin Oncol* 24:277–287, 1997

63. Alexander HR, Norton JA: Pathophysiology of cancer cachexia, in Doyle D, Hanks GWC, MacDonald N (eds): *Oxford Textbook of Palliative Medicine*. New York, Oxford Uni-versity Press, 1994, pp 316–329

64. Gerald C, Walker MW, Criscione L, et al: A receptor subtype involved in neuropeptide-Y-induced food intake. *Nature* 382: 168–171, 1996

65. Vigano A, Watanabe S, Bruera E: Anorexia and cachexia in advanced cancer patients. *Cancer Surv* 21:99–115, 1994

66. Beck SA, Smith KL, Tisdale MJ: Anti-cachetic and anti-tumor effect of eicosapentaenoic acid and its effect on protein turnover. *Cancer Res* 51:6089–6093, 1991

67. Drenth JP, de Kleijn EH, de Mulder PH, et al: Metastatic breast cancer presenting as fever, rash, and arthritis. *Cancer* 75:1608–1611, 1995

68. Liaw CC, Chen JS, Wang CH, et al: Tumor fever in patients with nasopharyngeal carcinoma: Clinical experience of 67 patients. *Am J Clin Oncol* 21:422–425, 1998

69. Dinarello CA, Bunn PA: Fever. *Semin Oncol* 24:288–298, 1997

70. Morant R, Hans-Jorg S: The management of infections in palliative care, in Doyle D, Hanks GWC, MacDonald N (eds): *Oxford Textbook of Palliative Medicine*. New York, Oxford Uni-versity Press, 1994, pp 378–384

71. Tsavaris N, Zinelis A, Karabelis A, et al: A randomized trial of the effect of three non-steroidal antiinflammatory agents in ameliorating cancer-induced fever. *J Intern Med* 228: 451–455, 1990

72. Amin AR, Jakobiec FA, Dreyer EB: Ocular syndromes associ-ated with systemic malignancy. *Int Ophthalmol Clin* 37: 281–302, 1997

73. Hersh B, Dalmau J, Dangond F, et al: Paraneoplastic opsoclo-nus-myoclonus associated with anti-Hu antibody. *Neurology* 44:1754–1755, 1994

74. Pless M, Ronthal MB: Treatment of opsoclonus-myoclonus with high-dose intravenous immunoglobin. *Neurology* 46: 583–584, 1996

75. Wiggs JL: Ocular syndromes associated with systemic ma-lignancy, in Albert DM, Jakobiec FA (eds): *Principles and Practices of Ophthalmology: Clinical Practice*. Philadelphia, Saunders, 1994, pp 3350–3355

CHAPTER 36

Malignant Effusions and Edemas

Claire Works, RN, MS, ARNP
Mary B. Maxwell, RN, PhD

Introduction

Fluid derangements are common in individuals with cancer. Abnormal leakage from blood into tissues (edema) or cavities (effusions) occurs with many kinds of malignancy. Usually associated with advanced disease but sometimes occurring as the presenting symptom, effusions and edema interfere with normal body function at the site where they develop and add new problems to those manifestations already present as a result of the underlying cancer and its treatment. Although all cancers can metastasize to any of the body's serous cavities, *malignant effusions* occur most commonly in the pleural space of the lung (pleural effusion), the peritoneal cavity in the abdomen (ascites), or the space surrounding the heart (pericardial effusion). The brain is a frequent site for *malignant edema*. This chapter discusses normal fluid regulation in relation to fluid derangements seen in patients with cancer and compares and contrasts the various effusions. The pathophysiology, clinical manifestations, assessment, and interventions for the six most common fluid retention sites are presented.

Normal Fluid Regulation

The distribution pattern of body water is termed *fluid spacing*. *First spacing* describes a normal distribution of fluid in both the extracellular and intracellular compartments. *Second spacing* refers to an excess accumulation of interstitial fluid (edema), while *third spacing* is fluid retention in areas that usually have no fluid or a minimum of fluid (effusion). Edema or effusion represents a disturbance in the normal distribution of extracellular fluid.

Extracellular fluids are separated into interstitial and intravascular compartments by the semipermeable mem-

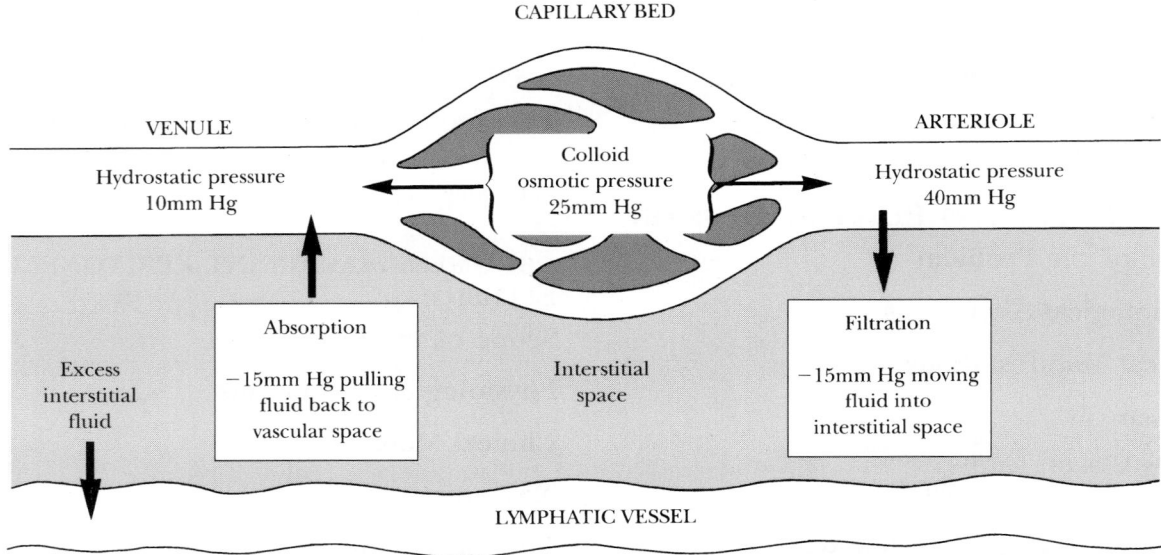

CAPILLARY BED

VENULE — Hydrostatic pressure 10mm Hg

Colloid osmotic pressure 25mm Hg

ARTERIOLE — Hydrostatic pressure 40mm Hg

Absorption
−15mm Hg pulling fluid back to vascular space

Excess interstitial fluid

Interstitial space

Filtration
−15mm Hg moving fluid into interstitial space

LYMPHATIC VESSEL

Figure 36-1 As described by Starling's law, the colloid osmotic pressure, hydrostatic pressure, capillary permeability, diffusion, and filtration pressure are all factors influencing fluid movement across the capillary membrane from the blood to the interstitial space.

branes surrounding capillaries and cells. These membranes serve as the points where exchange takes place between each cell and its respective fluid environment (the interstitial fluid), and between the interstitial fluid and the plasma within the circulatory system. Various pressures, as described by Starling's law, influence fluid movement across the capillary membranes (Figure 36-1). More fluid moves out of the intravascular into the interstitial compartment than returns via the capillary membrane. The lymphatic capillaries take up the excess interstitial fluid and return it to the bloodstream via the lymphatic and thoracic ducts. Lymphatic drainage is particularly important for the removal of proteins that leak into the interstitial spaces, thereby keeping the interstitial osmotic pressure low. Edema results from any augmentation of the forces influencing movement of fluids from the intravascular compartment into the interstitial compartment.

Fluid Disturbances in Cancer

Effects of Cancer and Cancer Treatment

Cancer, either a primary tumor or a metastatic lesion, can affect fluid pressure dynamics in several negative ways: by direct extension of the tumor, by seeding of body cavities with malignant cells, by lymphatic or venous obstruction, and by causing severe hypoproteinemia (Table 36-1). The four fluid retention states discussed in this chapter are directly due to cancer. Also, cancer treatments can affect or be altered by effusions/edemas. For instance, methotrexate given at routine doses can cause excessive myelosuppression in a patient who is experiencing third spacing. As a result of the syndrome of inappropriate antidiuretic hormone (SIADH), a severe fluid imbalance, termed *water intoxication,* can occur. It usually develops in patients with lung cancer or in patients receiving antineoplastic agents or analgesics (cyclophosphamide, vincristine, morphine).

General Considerations: Similarities and Differences

Incidence

Much of the data on incidence of effusion and edema are from autopsy reports in earlier years, when postmortem examinations were routinely carried out. Because autopsies are currently performed for only 10% of cancer deaths, the actual incidence of metastasis and malignant fluid retention is less clear today.[1] It is surmised that the incidence of these later complications is on the rise because longer survival after diagnosis is occurring as a result of improved treatments for primary disease.[2] While pericardial effusion is usually seen only in end-stage disease, in contrast, pleural effusion, ascites, and cerebral edema may be the first indication of cancer.

Table 36-1   Causes of Malignant Edema (According to Underlying Physiological Mechanism)

HYDROSTATIC PRESSURE ABNORMALITIES

Increased Capillary Fluid Pressure
  Increased venous pressure
    Vein obstruction
      Tumor
      Thrombophlebitis
    Increased total volume with decreased cardiac output
    Fluid overload
  Sodium and water retention, increased aldosterone from:
    Decreased renal blood flow
      Renal failure
    Increased aldosterone
      Corticosteroid therapy
    Inability to metabolize aldosterone
      Liver metastasis

ONCOTIC PRESSURE ABNORMALITIES

Decreased Capillary Oncotic Pressure
  Loss of serum protein
    Anemia
    Bleeding
  Decreased protein intake
    Malnutrition
  Decreased albumin production
    Liver metastasis

Increased Interstitial Oncotic Pressure
  Increased capillary permeability to protein
    Inflammatory reactions
      Seeding of cavity surfaces with tumor cells
      Infection
  Obstructed lymphatics: decreased removal of tissue fluid and protein
    Malignant disease
    Surgical removal of lymph nodes

Rapid versus slow accumulation

Cavities and tissues can accommodate surprisingly large volumes of fluids if the abnormal liquid accumulates slowly over time. However, a rapid increase in volume, even a small amount, tends to overwhelm compensatory mechanisms, and life-threatening symptoms can occur. Malignant effusions and edemas usually begin slowly but then increase and expand exponentially.

Assessment

Many more malignant pleural effusions than pericardial effusions are symptomatic. Thus, pericardial effusions are more difficult to diagnose. Often the individual's history and physical examination point to the likely etiology of the effusion/edema. The most helpful diagnostic tools for pleural effusion are the chest x-ray and examination of the pleural fluid, while the echocardiogram is the most important tool in pericardial effusions. The physical examination helps determine the diagnosis of ascites. Brain lesions causing cerebral edema are usually diagnosed with computerized tomography (CT).

Transudates versus exudates

Fluid accumulation at an effusion site can be classified as either a transudate or an exudate. Classification has diagnostic implications and can be a distinguishing characteristic between a malignant or a nonmalignant cause. A *transudate* is a low-protein fluid that has leaked from blood vessels due to mechanical factors, as in cirrhosis, congestive heart failure, or nephrotic syndrome. In contrast, an *exudate* is protein-rich fluid that has leaked from blood vessels with increased permeability. Most malignant effusions are exudates, caused by irritation of the serous membrane by sloughed cancer cells or solid tumor implants. The malignant exudate contains cells or cellular debris released by the resulting inflammation. Transudates and exudates can be distinguished by fluid protein to serum protein ratios, and by fluid lactate dehydrogenase (LDH) to serum LDH ratios.[2]

Treatment

For effusions, systemic treatment is usually employed first if the underlying cancer is responsive to chemotherapy. Otherwise, local therapy for malignant effusions is similar: drain the fluid, attempt to obliterate the third space, and prevent reaccumulation. No single clearly superior approach for local control of any of the effusions has been demonstrated by randomized clinical trial. A variety of treatment techniques have been advocated.

Cerebral edema is treated quite differently, with steroids, surgery, and radiation therapy. The main goals of treatment for malignant effusions and edemas are similar (Table 36-2). Specific therapy depends on the site where the fluid has accumulated and the individual patient and tumor-related factors (Table 36-3).[3]

Nursing Care

Although most patients will develop edemas or effusions when their cancer is advanced, ongoing **assessment** of each patient for signs or symptoms of fluid retention is crucial so that interventions can be instituted early. When fluid accumulation occurs, the patient and family will need **emotional support** to counteract the stress and fears associated with advancing disease, cosmetic appearance

Table 36-2 Goals of Treatment for Malignant Effusions or Edemas

Short-term Goals
  Determine underlying cause
  Relieve discomfort
  Prevent fluid reaccumulation

Long-term Goals
  Prevent complications
  Prolong survival
  Enhance quality of life

Table 36-3 Factors Influencing Treatment Choices for Malignant Effusions/Edemas

PATIENT-RELATED FACTORS

Severity of symptoms
Performance status
Concomitant medical problems
Motivation

TUMOR-RELATED FACTORS

Location and extent of tumor
Responsiveness to chemotherapy or radiation
Natural history of tumor: type, histology, aggressiveness
Concurrent therapies

changes, and the necessity for further medical intervention. With the treatment of effusions, the nurse will probably assist with potentially painful diagnostic and sclerosing procedures. Important nursing interventions include minimizing discomfort, providing reassurance, and **monitoring** the patient during and after these procedures for untoward reactions. **Patient education** will prepare the patient and family for tests and procedures and teach them to recognize and report side effects or complications. Assessment is important in early detection of fluid derangements. Keeping records of fluid intake and output, evaluating the rate of fluid reaccumulation after cavity drainage, and monitoring electrolytes and proteins are essential. **Skin care** of the affected area is necessary with ascites. **Pain evaluation and control** are often in order because the abnormal fluid accumulation can put pressure on nerve endings in surrounding structures. **Medications** (steroids, diuretics) may need to be administered and assessment for iatrogenic complications completed. If life-threatening cardiac tamponade or brain herniation occurs, **emergency care** is needed. Using the elements emphasized here, a complete plan of care for actual and potential problems specific to the fluid retention state should be developed for each patient. Additional detailed nursing care plans are available for selected aspects of fluid retention management (Table 36-4).[4-11]

LUNG: MALIGNANT PLEURAL EFFUSION

Scope of the Problem

Although it is usually stated that approximately half of all newly diagnosed pleural effusions in adults are malignant, there are no recent reports on the incidence of pleural effusion.[12] Table 36-5 shows the tumor types associated with malignant pleural effusion and the incidence for each type.

Fifty percent of all patients with cancer will develop pleural effusion at some time during their disease.[13] It may be the first sign of malignancy. Pleural effusion later

Table 36-4 Nursing Care Plans for Patients with Malignant Effusions or Edemas

Effusion or Edema Type	Plans	Reference
Pleural effusion	Nursing management during chest tube insertion and pleural sclerosing	Rossetti[4]
	Thoracostomy management in the home (patient education)	Hewitt and Jansen[5]
Pericardial effusion	Nursing plan of care for patients experiencing cardiac tamponade	Joiner and Kolodychuk[6]
	Nursing care plan for patients with pericardial window surgery for cardiac tamponade	Wojciechowicz[7]
	Nursing interventions for common complications of medical treatment for pericardial effusion	Mangan[8]
Peritoneal effusion	Patient care standards for patients with peritoneovenous shunt	Kehoe[9]
Lymphedema	Nursing interventions for patients with lymphedema	Getz[10]
	Guidelines for the care of the patient with altered tissue perfusion (lymphedema)	Kennelly and Yurkovic[11]

in the disease progression is an ominous sign, but it does not necessarily mean the beginning of the terminal stage. Lung and breast cancer account for approximately 75% of malignant pleural effusions.[14,15] A median survival time of 14 months for breast cancer patients with effusions has been reported, compared with 6 months for patients with lung and other tumors, and 16 months for patients with mesothelioma.[15] Most patients (90%) will have effusions of more than 500 mL, and approximately one-third will present with bilateral pleural effusions.[16]

Physiological Alterations

Pleural fluid is a filtrate from the parietal pleura. It is formed and removed more slowly than formerly believed, with 100–200 mL being produced each 24 hours and then removed by the parietal pleural stomata.[14] The space between the parietal and visceral pleura contains a small amount of fluid (5–15 mL) that acts as a lubricant, allowing the two surfaces to move without friction. The

Table 36-5 Incidence of Pleural Effusion Related to Tumor Type

Tumor Type	Incidence (%)
Lung cancer	35
Breast cancer	23
Adenocarcinoma, unknown primary	12
Leukemia/lymphoma	10
Reproductive tract	6
Gastrointestinal tract	5
Genitourinary tract	3
Primary unknown	3
Others	5

Adapted with permission from Olopade OI, Ultmann JE: Malignant Effusions. *CA: Cancer J Clin* 41:166–179, 1991.[2]

parietal pleura contains nerve endings for pain, but the visceral pleura does not. In the presence of a massive effusion process, the interpleural space may contain as much as 1500 mL of fluid (Figure 36-2).

There are five ways that fluid equilibrium in the pleural space can be disturbed by cancer, either directly by origination in the pleura or indirectly via metastatic spread:

1. Most commonly, implantation with cancer cells on the pleural surface leads to increased capillary permeability and leakage from the intravascular to the interstitial compartment. This occurs with pleural effusions in patients with solid tumors such as lung cancer.
2. Obstruction of pleural or pulmonary lymphatic channels by malignant processes can prevent resorption of fluid. This is seen in pleural effusions related to lymphomas or breast cancer.
3. The pulmonary veins can be obstructed by tumor, leading to increased capillary hydrostatic pressure in the visceral pleura. This is another mechanism seen in lung cancer.
4. The pleural space colloid osmotic pressure may be increased by necrotic malignant cells being shed into the pleural space. This leads to a reduced absorption of fluid by the visceral pleural capillaries. It may be seen with lung and breast cancers.
5. The thoracic duct may be perforated, producing a chylous pleural effusion. This sometimes occurs with lymphoma.[2,14]

In addition, tumor-related pathologies that can cause pleural effusion include superior vena cava syndrome (SVCS) endobronchial obstruction with atelectasis, postobstructive pneumonitis, and pericardial constriction.

Clinical Manifestations

The extent of alteration of respiratory function depends on the amount and rate of pleural fluid accumulation as well as the patient's underlying pulmonary status. The

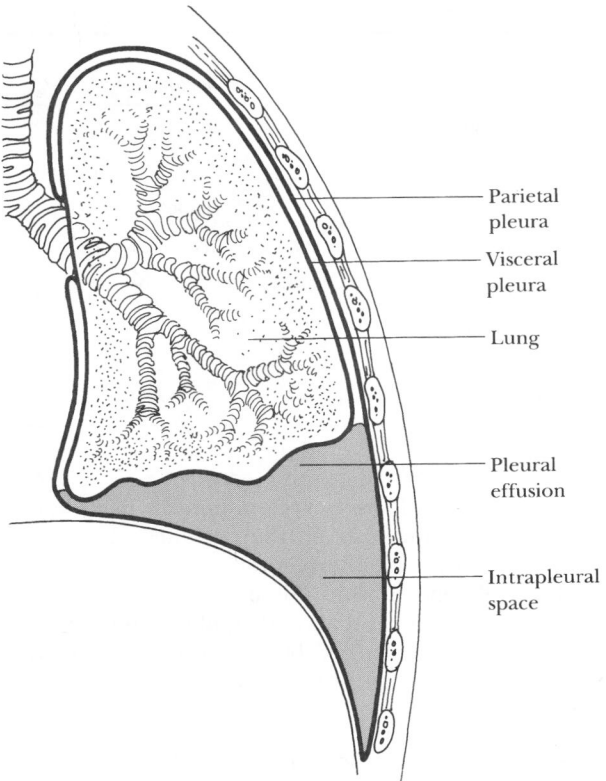

Figure 36-2 In the lung, fluid is constantly being filtered across the intrapleural space from the parietal pleural surface and reabsorbed through the visceral pleura. When obstruction by malignant processes prevents reabsorption, fluid accumulates in the intrapleural space and pleural effusion results.

Parietal pleura

Visceral pleura

Lung

Pleural effusion

Intrapleural space

Table 36-6 Assessment of the Patient with Suspected Pleural Effusion
SUBJECTIVE INDICATORS
Dyspnea
Orthopnea
Dry, nonproductive cough
Chest pain, chest heaviness
OBJECTIVE INDICATORS
Labored breathing
Tachypnea
Dullness to percussion
Restricted chest wall expansion
Impaired transmission of breath sounds
LABORATORY INDICATORS
Fluid visualized on chest x-ray
Positive pleural fluid cytology

fluid accumulation restricts lung expansion, reduces lung volume, alters the ventilation and perfusion capacity, and results in abnormal gas exchange and hypoxia. Malignant pleural effusion may develop slowly over a period of several months. Pleural effusions due to noncancer causes usually have a more abrupt onset.

When pleural effusion develops in the patient with advanced cancer, it is often difficult to sort out the respiratory effects of the pleural fluid accumulation as opposed to shortness of breath due to thoracic muscle weakness and general debilitation. Breathing difficulties may also be aggravated by the side effects of chemotherapeutic agents (bleomycin and methotrexate) or prior lung irradiation.

Common presenting symptoms and signs are distressing to most patients (Table 36-6). Patients experience dyspnea, cough, and chest pain. The dyspnea progresses to orthopnea as the effusion worsens. The symptoms are related to compression of the lung from the increasing fluid accumulation.[17] The degree of subjective symptoms produced by a pleural effusion is dependent on the amount of fluid involved and on the rapidity with which it has accumulated.[18] Although the majority of cancer patients with pleural effusions are symptomatic, 23% are not, with the effusion being found incidentally.[14]

Assessment

Radiographic Examination

Chest x-rays are important in visualizing free fluid in the pleural cavity and relating accumulation to other structures. Most pleural effusions begin in the subpulmonic area between the lung and the diaphragm and appear as an elevated diaphragm on the affected side. The fluid casts an opaque shadow that has the same density as the heart. The larger the effusion, the more opaque it will appear. A pleural effusion will not be detected on a posterior-anterior chest film unless it contains at least 200–300 mL of fluid. A small effusion shows haziness at the base of the lung and obliterates the costophrenic angle. A lateral decubitus x-ray film is the best way to identify a small effusion, because gravity will cause the fluid to shift to a position along the dependent lateral rib cage where it is easier to visualize.[19]

Clues to the type of cancer causing the pleural effusion may be seen on x-ray. Mediastinum shift away from the effusion points to a disseminated nonthoracic tumor, such as breast or ovary. If the mediastinum is shifted toward the effusion, carcinoma of the lung, with some degree of bronchial obstruction, is probably involved. Mesothelioma or fixed central nodal metastasis is indicated if no mediastinal shift is seen.[12] If there is suspicion of pleural mesothelioma, ultrasound or CT can be useful.[2]

Pleural Fluid Examination

Any new pleural effusion must be aspirated to confirm the presence of malignant cells and to rule out nonmalignant causes. Pleural fluid cytological analysis yields a definitive diagnosis in approximately 70% of patients with malignant pleural effusion.[15] Thoracoscopy with direct pleural biopsy leads to a diagnosis 100% of the time. If possible, the pleural fluid should be removed at the same time as the diagnostic thoracentesis, providing immediate relief for the distressing symptoms of large (1000–1500 mL) effusions.[2] Fluid should be removed slowly to avoid re-expansion pulmonary edema.

It is important to determine whether the fluid is an exudate or a transudate. Because malignant effusion is almost always an exudate, a transudative fluid would indicate a nonmalignant cause. The aspirated fluid is sent for cultures, gram and acid-fast stains, cell counts, and chemistry studies. Characteristics of the fluid that are helpful diagnostically are appearance (straw-colored, bloody, turbid, or milky) and levels of glucose amylase, protein, LDH, and lymphocytes.[2] The majority of malignant pleural effusions are grossly bloody.[20]

Therapeutic Approaches and Nursing Care

How the malignant pleural effusion is treated depends on the type of tumor and previous therapy (Figure 36-3). Small, asymptomatic effusions caused by lymphomas, testicular carcinomas, leukemia, breast cancer, small cell lung cancer, and ovarian cancer are first treated with systemic chemotherapy or hormonal therapy. Unless the patient has been aggressively treated in the past and the tumor has become resistant to certain drugs, these types of tumors will usually respond and the effusion will disappear.[20] Patients with chemotherapy-resistant tumors (melanoma, non-small cell lung cancer) will require alternative treatment approaches. If the underlying disease is unresponsive to therapy and the patient is symptomatic, palliative measures should be implemented.

Removal of Fluid

Relief of symptoms is a short-term treatment goal that is usually achieved when the pleural fluid is mechanically drained. However, the fluid tends to reaccumulate when it is not possible to control the underlying cancer. Long-range treatment goals are directed toward the obliteration of the pleural space so that pleural fluid cannot reaccumulate.

Thoracentesis. In a thoracentesis the pleural fluid is removed by needle aspiration through the chest wall. The patient is placed in an upright sitting position, with arms and shoulders raised. This elevates and separates the ribs to make needle insertion easier. After the thoracentesis is completed and the pleural fluid has been drained, the patient is assessed for complications such as pneumothorax, pain, hypotension, or pulmonary edema. Patient education and support as well as medication and local anesthesia are important measures to prevent anxiety and discomfort during any of these therapeutic procedures.[16]

Although thoracentesis alone is effective for diagnosis,

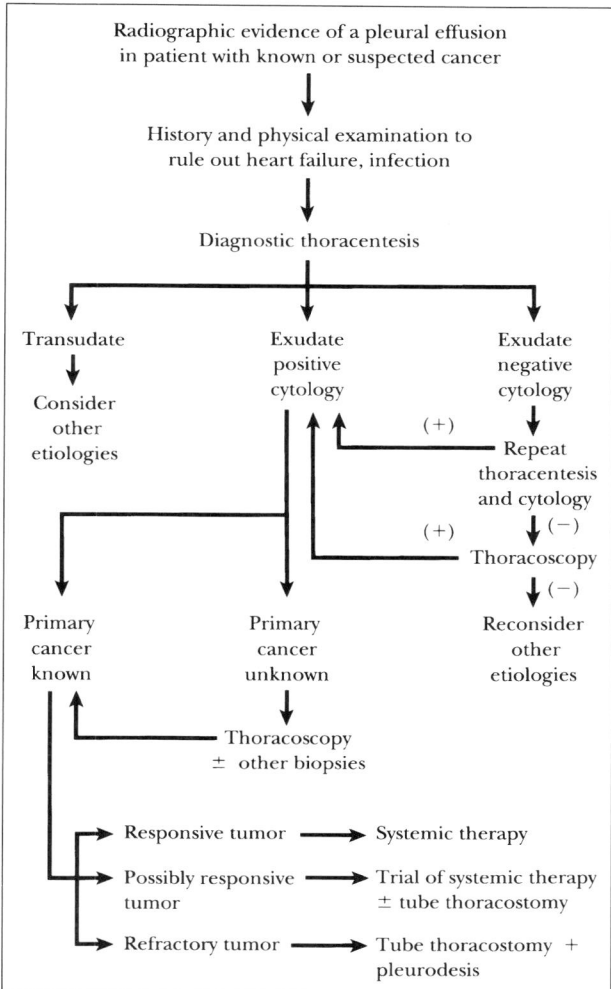

Figure 36-3 Algorithm for diagnosis and management of malignant pleural effusion. (Reprinted with permission from Ruckdeschel, JC: Management of malignant pleural effusion: An overview. *Semin Oncol* 15:24–28, 1988 (suppl)[21]

palliation, or relief of acute respiratory distress, it is of little value for treating recurrent malignant effusions because the fluid usually reaccumulates quickly. In one study of 94 patients, the average reaccumulation time was 4 days and there was a 97% chance of recurrence within a month of the thoracentesis.[2] The risks of repeated thoracentesis include hypoalbuminemia, electrolyte imbalance, pneumothorax, fluid loculation, and infection.

Thoracentesis via an implanted port and intrapleural catheter is an alternative approach that can be advantageous for the patient whose cancer is refractory to treatment and thus will likely experience repeated pleural fluid reaccumulation. Pleural fluid removal via an implanted port and interpleural catheter can be completed by the nurse in the ambulatory or home setting (Figure 36-4). Using the implanted port reduces the risk of pneumothorax and infection that can occur with repeated traditional percutaneous aspiration approaches. In addi-

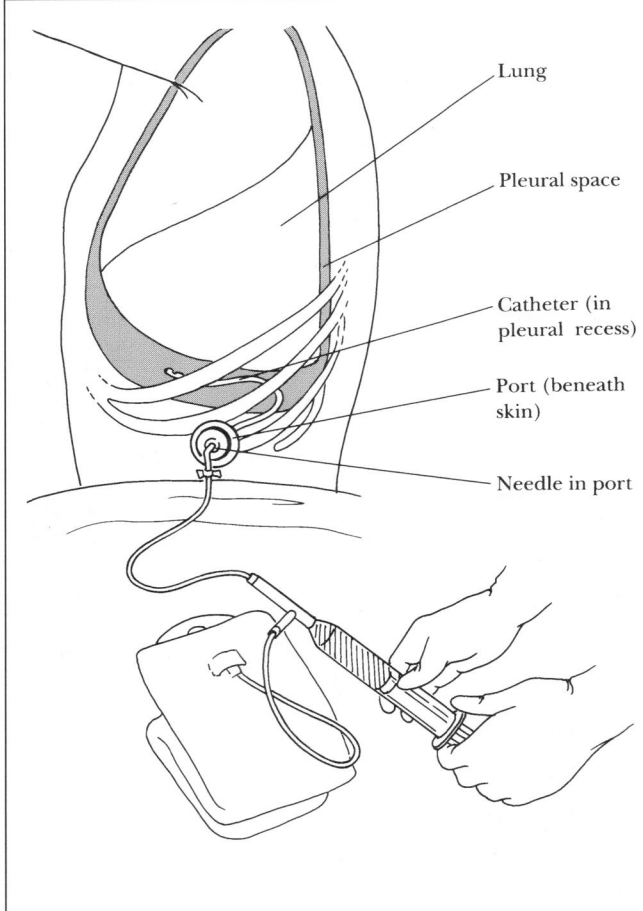

Lung

Pleural space

Catheter (in pleural recess)

Port (beneath skin)

Needle in port

Assemble equipment:
1. Thoracentesis tray
2. Size 19g 90° Huber point needle with tubing and clamps
3. Heparin-saline solution (100 μ/ml 3 ml)
4. Betadine swabs
5. Sterile gloves (2 pairs)

Procedure:
1. Place patient in a comfortable position on side.
2. Open thoracentesis tray.
3. Place sterile Huber needle on sterile tray.
4. Don sterile gloves.
5. Connect 60-ml syringe to 2-way connector.
6. Connect one end of 2-way connector to the drainage bag and one end to sterile Huber needle (see illustration).
7. Prep site over port using sterile technique.
8. Change gloves.
9. Clamp Huber needle tubing.
10. Access port.
11. Tape needle securely.
12. Unclamp Huber needle tubing.
13. Draw back on plunger (fluid should be yellowish).
14. Fill syringe. Push on plunger to empty syringe into drainage bag. Repeat procedure until desired amount is obtained.
15. If the tube seems plugged, clamp the catheter, disconnect at 2-way valve and clear mucous plug.
16. If drainage seems to slow down or stop, have patient change position.
17. When tap is complete (1500 ml or so), clamp catheter. Disconnect drainage tube and flush with 3–5 cc of heparinized saline.
18. Withdraw needle from port.
19. Apply Band-Aid™.

Do not attempt to access port with thoracentesis needle. Must use Huber point needle. Procedure can be repeated as necessary.

Figure 36-4 Thoracentesis via an implanted port. (Procedure compliments of Michelle Goodman, RN, MS, Rush Presbyterian St. Luke's Medical Center.)

tion, there can be significant reduction of health care resources consumed because nurses can evacuate the fluid accumulation before the symptoms of effusion become disabling. There is also a reduced need for repeat radiological examinations. Because a Huber point needle is used to access the implanted port, the patient experiences less pain than occurs with the large-gauge thoracentesis needle or a thoracostomy tube. Ease of performing the thoracentesis procedure, along with reduced pain and anxiety, significantly improves the patient's experience.

Indwelling catheter. Another option for management of recurrent pleural effusion is placement of a Tenckhoff catheter. This is an externally draining catheter that is positioned in the pleural space. Tenckhoff catheters are placed in the operating room under local anesthesia. The patient or home care nurse empties the accumulated fluid as needed. These catheters function reliably and have been well-tolerated by patients.[22]

Thoracostomy tube. A thoracostomy tube may be inserted via video-guided thoracoscopy to facilitate fluid drainage and then left in place to assess the degree of fluid reaccumulation. However, chest tube drainage alone is only partially effective. Measures to prevent fluid reaccumulation are also needed. Nursing assessments while a thoracostomy tube is in place include observing for pneumothorax, pain, hypotension, and pulmonary edema as well as care of the closed-chest drainage system.[17] Care is taken to ensure that the chest tube remains patent since exudate fluid tends to clot. Thoracostomy tubes can also be used to instill sclerosing agents into the pleural space.

Obliteration of the Pleural Space

If the pleural space can be obliterated, then the reaccumulation of pleural fluid may be prevented. Obliteration is achieved by instilling a chemical agent that causes *pleurodesis;* that is, the visceral and parietal pleura become permanently adhered together. The chemical agent causes mesothelial fibrosis and the obliteration of small pleural blood vessels.[2]

Chemical agents. Over the years, many chemicals have been used as sclerosing agents to prevent pleural effusion recurrence. Chemical sclerosing does not prolong the patient's life but may enhance quality of life by relieving symptoms and reducing the time a patient spends in the hospital. Agents used for pleural instillation in the past (nitrogen mustard, quinacrine, 5-fluorouracil, talc) have had side effects, such as nausea and vomiting, hypotension, pain, and bone marrow depression.

Tetracycline was previously the agent of choice for intrapleural sclerotherapy, but it is no longer available.[17] Doxycycline (an analog of tetracycline) is currently under study as a sclerosing agent. Bleomycin and sterilized talc are the two agents commonly used for pleurodesis.[16,17]

The selected sclerosing agent is instilled into the pleural space via the thoracentesis needle or the thoracostomy tube. Because the overall objective is to expose as much of the pleura as possible to the chemical, most of the pleural fluid will have to be removed and the lung reexpanded before the agent is instilled. The patient will be asked to move around and change position frequently to help distribute the agent. Nursing management during chest tube insertion and pleural sclerosing includes patient education and reassurance, pain control, positioning, and the management of the chest tube drainage as well as maintaining the drainage system.[20,23] Chest tube insertion and pleural sclerosing can be difficult and painful procedures for patients, who may already be debilitated due to their underlying disease.

Biological agents may be utilized as sclerosing agents in the future. Interleukin-2, with or without lymphokine-activated killer cells, has shown promise.[17] Interferons have not produced impressive results. *Corynebacterium parvum* provides no increased efficacy compared to other agents, has significant toxicity, and requires multiple instillations.[17] Interest in using radioactive isotopes (gold, phosphorus) has subsided, as both isotopes are difficult to work with and less effective than other treatment approaches.[17]

New technology using small-bore needles may permit management of malignant pleural effusions on an outpatient basis. At one institution, 28 outpatients were treated using radiologically placed small-bore catheters connected to a plastic bag with a one-way valve system for gravity drainage. Drainage was followed by intrapleural instillation of bleomycin. With palliation results comparable to in-hospital methods, greater patient comfort and lower health care costs can result from new approaches in outpatient management of effusion.[24]

Surgical methods. If a pleural effusion remains uncontrolled after other approaches have been tried, surgery is another option. If a patient has a good life expectancy and a good performance status, pleural stripping is advocated. Success rates approach 90%, but there can be serious complications such as air leak, bleeding, pneumonia, and empyema.[2]

Pleurectomy (removal of most of the parietal pleura) has been reported to be effective in some cases. This procedure should be used only for a very narrowly defined group of patients.[17] Also, a pleuroperitoneal shunt has been developed for control of malignant effusion.

The shunt is inserted into the subcutaneous tissue (placement usually requires general anesthesia), and pleural fluid is diverted to the peritoneal cavity via manual compression of the shunt's main valve pump. The patient must be motivated, because he is required to conscientiously pump the valve intermittently (100 compressions five times a day) to prevent clogging. Shunt malfunction has plagued this procedure.[17]

Radiation. Although external beam radiation may be used as local treatment for mediastinal tumors (lymphoma and lung), hemithoracic radiation is not recommended as a first-line management of malignant pleural effusions due to the hazard of pulmonary fibrosis. Radiation is limited to treatment of the underlying disease, not the resultant effusion.

Which treatment is best? Despite decades of experience with palliation of malignant pleural effusion, there is an urgent need for controlled studies using larger numbers of patients. Few studies have addressed such important factors as improvement, quality of life, performance status, or exercise tolerance. In summary, some general guidelines for treatment can be advanced:

- Small, symptomless effusions often can be left alone.

- If the underlying cancer will probably respond to treatment, specific treatment of larger effusions should wait (as long as the patient's symptoms are tolerable).

- The patient's overall prognosis should be considered before embarking on an aggressive approach.

- If pleurodesis is the option selected, it should be performed early.

- If the effusion recurs or lung expansion is compromised due to pleural disease, pleuroperitoneal shunting may be attempted.[13]

HEART: MALIGNANT PERICARDIAL EFFUSION

Scope of the Problem

Autopsy series indicate that metastasis to the heart and pericardium occurs in up to 20% of patients.[2] Pericardial metastases are found at autopsy in 35% of patients with lung cancer and 25% of patients with breast cancer.[20] However, only 30% of affected patients are symptomatic. Because pericardial effusion is not easily detected by routine tests, it is often not discovered while the patient is alive. Pericardial effusion occurs most often with cancers of the lung and breast, leukemia, and lymphoma. Melanoma and sarcoma also can cause pericardial metastases. The majority (60%–75%) of all pericardial effusions occur in patients with lung and breast cancers.[20]

Pathophysiology

The pericardial sac or cavity that surrounds the heart is completely closed. Two layers make up the sac: a tough outer fibrous pericardium called the *parietal pericardium* and an inner layer of serous pericardium called the *visceral pericardium* (Figure 36-5).[8] Malignant pericardial effusion collects within this cavity. The cavity ordinarily contains less than 50 mL of fluid, which serves as a lubricant.

Pericardial metastasis results from lymphatic or hematogenous spread or from direct invasion by an adjacent primary tumor. Tumor implants may stud the pericardial surface or completely encase the pericardium. Pericarditis secondary to prior radiation therapy can cause severe pericardial thickening. The majority of pericardial effusions result from obstruction of lymphatic and venous drainage of the heart. This obstruction disturbs the intrapericardial pressure and results in fluid build-up. The effects of pericardial fluid accumulation are largely dependent on the rate of exudation, the physical compliance capacity of the pericardial cavity, ventricular function, myocardial size, and blood volume. If the fluid accumulation is gradual, as is usually the case with metastatic spread, the pericardium can stretch to accommodate up to 2 liters of fluid without symptoms.[17] However, rapid build-up of even 250 mL will result in obvious and severe symptoms.[20]

Clinical Manifestations

Pericardial effusions become symptomatic when the accumulated fluid burden creates enough pressure to impair ventricular filling in diastole. Systemic circulatory effects of decreased cardiac output and impaired venous return lead to generalized congestion. The body tries to compensate in several ways: (1) a tachycardia is created by adrenergic stimulation to offset decreased stroke volume; (2) systemic and pulmonary venous pressure increase in an attempt to increase venous return to the heart; and (3) the adrenergic stimulation increases the ejection fraction, leading to increased peripheral resistance that will support arterial blood pressure.[6]

Most persons with pericardial effusions are asymptomatic, so cardiac involvement may be overlooked. Symptoms are related to the rate at which the effusion accumulates. A small effusion (250 mL) that accumulates rapidly may be symptomatic, while a large volume (1000 mL) effusion with gradual onset may be asymptomatic.[20] The individual may have only nonspecific symptoms at first: dyspnea, cough, orthopnea, and chest pain.[17] Often, the patient is mistakenly treated for right heart failure; unfortunately, the administration of diuretics exacerbates the overall pericardial effusion problem.[17] The clinician should have a high index of suspicion for pericardial involvement whenever patients with cancer exhibit cardiovascular symptoms. If not diagnosed early, pericardial effusion can lead to a life-threatening emergency.

Signs and symptoms of a developing pericardial effusion are often insidious (Table 36-7). These findings can be subdivided into three categories of indicators (subjective, objective, laboratory).[6] Cardiac tamponade is an oncological emergency and is discussed in detail in Chapter 38.

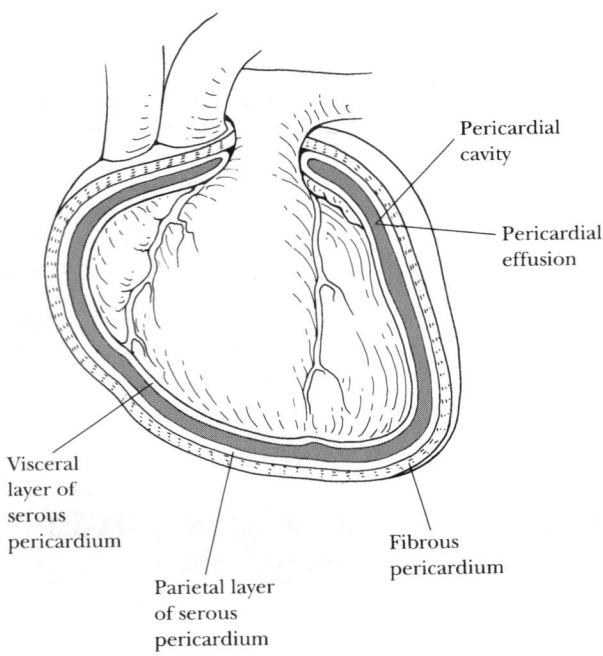

Figure 36-5 The pericardium is composed of two main compartments, the parietal pericardium and the visceral pericardium. Where the great vessels attach to the heart, these layers become continuous with each other to form the pericardial space. If venous or lymphatic drainage of the heart becomes obstructed by tumor-related processes, seepage of fluid through the visceral pericardium into the pericardial space leads to pericardial effusion. (Adapted from the *Oncology Nursing Forum* with permission from the Oncology Nursing Press. Mangan C: Malignant pericardial effusion: Pathophysiology and clinical correlates. *Oncol Nurs Forum* 19:1216, 1992.)[8]

Labels in figure: Pericardial cavity; Pericardial effusion; Fibrous pericardium; Parietal layer of serous pericardium; Visceral layer of serous pericardium

Assessment

Radiography

Echocardiography is the fastest, least invasive, and most precise method for visualization and quantification of malignant pericardial effusion. It also allows for evaluation of ventricular function. An upright anteroposterior (AP) x-ray view of the chest reveals cardiomegaly ("water bottle heart") but is not diagnostic. Bilateral pleural effusion, mediastinal widening, and hilar adenopathy can be observed. A small pericardial effusion may not be apparent on x-ray. Difficult-to-detect lesions may be better visualized by CT.

Table 36-7   Assessment of the Patient with Suspected Pericardial Effusion (Order of Frequency Encountered)

Signs and Symptoms

SUBJECTIVE INDICATORS

Dyspnea
Cough
Chest pain
Orthopnea
Weakness
Dysphagia
Syncope
Palpitations

OBJECTIVE INDICATORS

Pleural effusion
Tachycardia
Jugular venous distention
Hepatomegaly
Peripheral edema
Pulsus paradoxus
Hypotension
Distant heart sounds
Rales
Pericardial rub

LABORATORY INDICATORS

Echocardiographic fluid
Abnormal ECG
Abnormal chest x-ray
Positive pericardial fluid cytology
Positive pericardial biopsy

Electrocardiography

Electrocardiograph (ECG) changes with pericardial effusion include tachycardia, atrial and ventricular arrhythmia, low QRS voltage, and nonspecific ST- and T-wave changes. Electrical alternans can occur with large effusions.[17]

Pericardial Fluid Examination

Fluid withdrawn from the pericardial cavity by pericardiocentesis (needle aspiration using a subxiphoid approach) that has a bloody appearance is indicative of malignancy, especially with lung cancer.[8] Such fluid is always exudative. Cytological examination can reveal tumor cells, but false-negatives are possible. The ability to make the diagnosis based on cytology can be difficult, particularly with effusions due to lymphoma or mesothelioma.[17]

Therapeutic Approaches and Nursing Care

Various medical and surgical treatment options for pericardial effusion exist, but there are no prospective, ran-

domized trials comparing them.[16] Choice of treatment depends on the size of the effusion, the patient's symptoms, performance status, and prognosis.[17] If the individual is asymptomatic, it is usually expedient to simply watch and wait (Figure 36-6).

Removal of Fluid

Pericardiocentesis alone. Percutaneous pericardiocentesis (performed since 1840) guided by echocardiography is an important diagnostic tool and is useful for initial drainage of fluid from the pericardium. This leads to dramatic relief of symptoms with minimal risk.[20,25,26] The use of echocardiography has significantly reduced the major risks of the pericardiocentesis procedure, including myocardial or coronary artery laceration, pneumothorax, and abdominal organ trauma.[25] Pericardial drainage alone is not definitive treatment, most effusions reaccumulate a short time after the tap.[20] Nursing care during the pericardiocentesis includes explaining the procedure to the patient and attempting to reduce anxiety and discomfort; positioning the patient in a semi-Fowler's position; maintaining asepsis; and having available a good light source, a defibrillator, and emergency medications. The nurse must continuously monitor the patient and the ECG during the pericardiocentesis, and

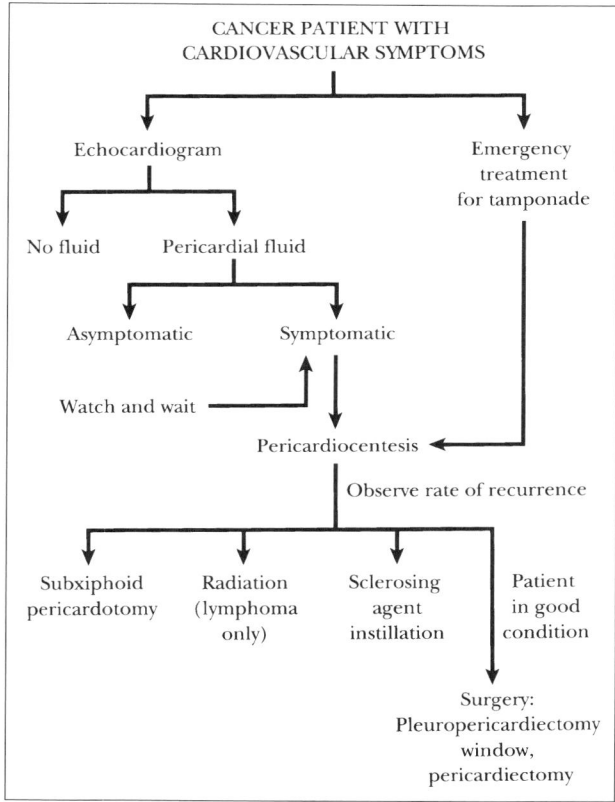

Figure 36-6   Algorithm for diagnosis and management of malignant pericardial effusion.

afterward monitor for complications. Emergency support measures such as intravenous fluids, oxygen, and drugs to increase cardiac output and blood pressure must be available.[6,8,27]

Subxiphoid pericardiotomy. Under local anesthesia using a subxiphoid approach, subxiphoid pericardiotomy (pericardial window) allows for a longer period of drainage and permits examination of the pericardial space as well as obtaining a pericardial biopsy. Complications are rare, and the recurrence rate is low.[25,28] Nursing care is the same as for pericardiocentesis.

Balloon pericardiotomy. After accessing the pericardial space by a conventional pericardiocentesis, a guide wire is threaded into the pericardium and a balloon-dilating catheter inflated to create a window. Fluid then drains into the pleural space. Balloon pericardiotomy can be performed under local anesthesia and in most cases allows for early hospital discharge.[26,29]

Pericardioperitoneal shunt. A Denver pleuroperitoneal shunt has been used successfully to drain the pericardial effusion into the peritoneal cavity. The procedure is performed under local anesthesia and the patients are discharged 2–4 days later. In comparison, the more traditional methods of pericardial drainage led to higher postoperative morbidity and mortality and a much longer hospital stay.[30] This newer approach will need further study but could result in improved clinical outcomes.

Obliteration of the Pericardial Space

Pericardiocentesis with sclerosing agent instillation. Various agents have been used to sclerose the pericardium. Sclerosing agents used in pericardial effusions include doxycycline, thiotepa, bleomycin, minocycline, 5-fluorouracil, cisplatin, and nitrogen mustard. Radioactive gold or chromic phosphate have also been tried but are not commonly used due to logistical problems.[17] Immunostimulating agents, such as interleukin-2, have been used but have not been shown to be more effective than conventional sclerosing agents.[17] The degree of response and toxicity varies with each agent.

Surgery. Surgical intervention, including pericardiopleural window via thoracotomy and pericardiectomy, is generally reserved for medically appropriate patients whose malignant effusion is unresponsive to other therapies or who have required repeated pericardiocentesis. General anesthesia and thoracotomy are required. Cardiac tamponade symptoms are usually present. A less invasive approach is the use of videothoracoscopic surgery for pericardiectomy. The videothoracoscopic approach is more complex and requires a surgeon with specialized experience. A thoracotomy or video-assisted thoracoscopic surgery is the treatment of choice for patients with both pericardial and pleural effusions.[31]

A nursing care plan for patients with a pericardial effusion undergoing pericardial window surgery includes preoperative measures to (1) maintain blood pressure and heart rate, (2) maintain urine output and mental status, (3) provide sufficient oxygen, and (4) decrease pain and anxiety. Nursing measures postoperatively include prevention of infection, atelectasis, pleural effusion, and pneumothorax, as well as ongoing assessment for cardiac arrhythmia due to surgical irritation or the presence of the pericardial catheter. Prevention of anxiety and pain and bleeding due to the catheter and maintaining free-flowing pericardial drainage are important.[32]

Recurrence following surgical intervention is rare. A reported experience with subxiphoid partial pericardiectomy, with or without a sclerosing agent, concluded that this procedure is a safe and effective treatment for malignant pericardial effusions. It was suggested that patients with symptomatic malignant pericardial effusions be treated first with subxiphoid partial pericardiectomy, thus reserving sclerosant instillation for those who have persistent drainage after surgery.[33]

Radiation. The use of external beam radiation is most effective in highly radiosensitive cancers, such as lymphomas and leukemias.[17,26] Response rates are generally greater than 50%.[26] Carcinoma of the lung and breast are also sufficiently radiosensitive for radiation to be considered in the treatment plan.

ABDOMEN: MALIGNANT PERITONEAL EFFUSION

Scope of the Problem

Malignant peritoneal effusion (ascites) is associated with ovarian, uterine, cervical, pancreatic, colorectal, and gastric carcinomas.[20,34] Gynecological tumors account for about 75% of malignant ascites in women, while only 10% have a gastrointestinal etiology. More than 50% of men with malignant ascites have a gastrointestinal tumor.[34] The appearance of ascites in patients with advanced disease is prognostically grim, and palliation is usually all that can be offered. Life expectancy is a few months.

Physiological Alterations

The peritoneal cavity is covered by a serous lining composed of the visceral peritoneum, which lines and supports the abdominal organs and the parietal peritoneum. The parietal peritoneum covers the abdominal and pelvic walls and the undersurface of the diaphragm (Figure 36-7). As with the other third spaces, a small amount of fluid lubricates the cavity. Normally, the volume of peritoneal fluid is regulated by the pressure gradient balances described previously, with lymphatic channels draining 80% of all lymphatic peritoneal fluid.[35] When the production of peritoneal fluid exceeds the ability of the lymphatic channels to drain the cavity (the thoracic duct may be dilated to five to ten times the normal size), ascites develops.

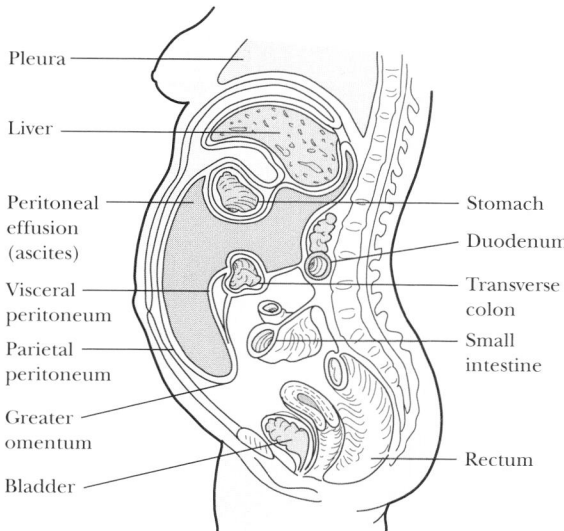

Figure 36-7 The peritoneal cavity is covered by the visceral peritoneum that lines and supports the abdominal organs, and the parietal peritoneum that covers the abdominal and pelvic walls and the undersurface of the diaphragm. If, due to malignant processes, the volume of fluid accumulating in the peritoneal space exceeds the capacity of lymphatic channels to drain the cavity, ascites develops.

Table 36-8 Assessment of the Patient with a Peritoneal Effusion

SUBJECTIVE INDICATORS
Indigestion and early satiety
Swollen ankles
Easily fatigued
Shortness of breath

OBJECTIVE INDICATORS
Weight gain
Distended abdomen
Fluid wave—"puddle sign"
Shifting dullness
Bulging flanks
Everted umbilicus
Stretched skin

LABORATORY INDICATORS
Abdominal flat plate
Ultrasound
Abdominal CT
Paracentesis

The most common cause of ascitic fluid build-up is tumor seeding the peritoneum, resulting in obstruction of the diaphragmatic and abdominal lymphatics. This occurs primarily with gynecological cancers. Excess intraperitoneal fluid production may also be a factor contributing to ascites. The tumor itself may elaborate humoral factors that cause increased capillary leakage of proteins and fluids into the peritoneum. In patients with diffuse liver metastasis and venous obstruction, hypoalbuminemia and low serum protein may play a part in the development of a transudative ascites.

Clinical Manifestations

The pressure of the ascitic fluid volume on nearby organs is uncomfortable and restrictive. Several liters of ascitic fluid can be accommodated in the abdomen. Some people report gaining 50–60 pounds of body weight as a result of excess fluid. This massive accumulation of fluid leads to negative body image changes, anorexia, early satiety, and difficulty in breathing and walking. Subjective, objective, and laboratory findings illustrate the typical profile of a person with ascites (Table 36-8). Most physical signs appear after 1 liter or more of fluid is present.

Assessment

Peritoneal effusion is diagnosed primarily by physical examination, with malignant characteristics confirmed by

paracentesis. An abdomen filled with more than 500 mL of fluid appears as a single curve from the xiphoid process to the pubis, with the umbilicus frequently everted. The following signs are characteristic of free fluid: bulging flanks, tympany at the top of the abdominal curve, elicitation of a fluid wave, and shifting dullness. A small effusion is hard to detect. The "puddle sign" is said to detect as little as 120 mL of free fluid in the abdominal cavity. To elicit the puddle sign, the patient lies prone for 5 minutes, then rises on elbows and knees. A stethoscope is applied to the most dependent part of the abdomen, and the clinician repeatedly flicks the near flank with a finger. As the stethoscope is moved across the abdomen away from the examiner, the sound becomes louder. Small volumes of fluid in the abdomen can also be detected by ultrasonic examination. Detecting ascites in obese patients is difficult, even when it is marked.

Therapeutic Approaches and Nursing Care

Many treatment approaches have been tried, but an optimal intervention has yet to be found.[34] No controlled trials comparing alternative therapies have been reported. It is difficult to carry out research in individuals whose longevity is limited to only a few months. An algorithm for the management of the patient with ascites includes the multiple factors influencing selection of treatment (Figure 36-8). Nursing care measures focus on maintaining fluid and electrolyte balance, comfort measures, and early recognition of complications.

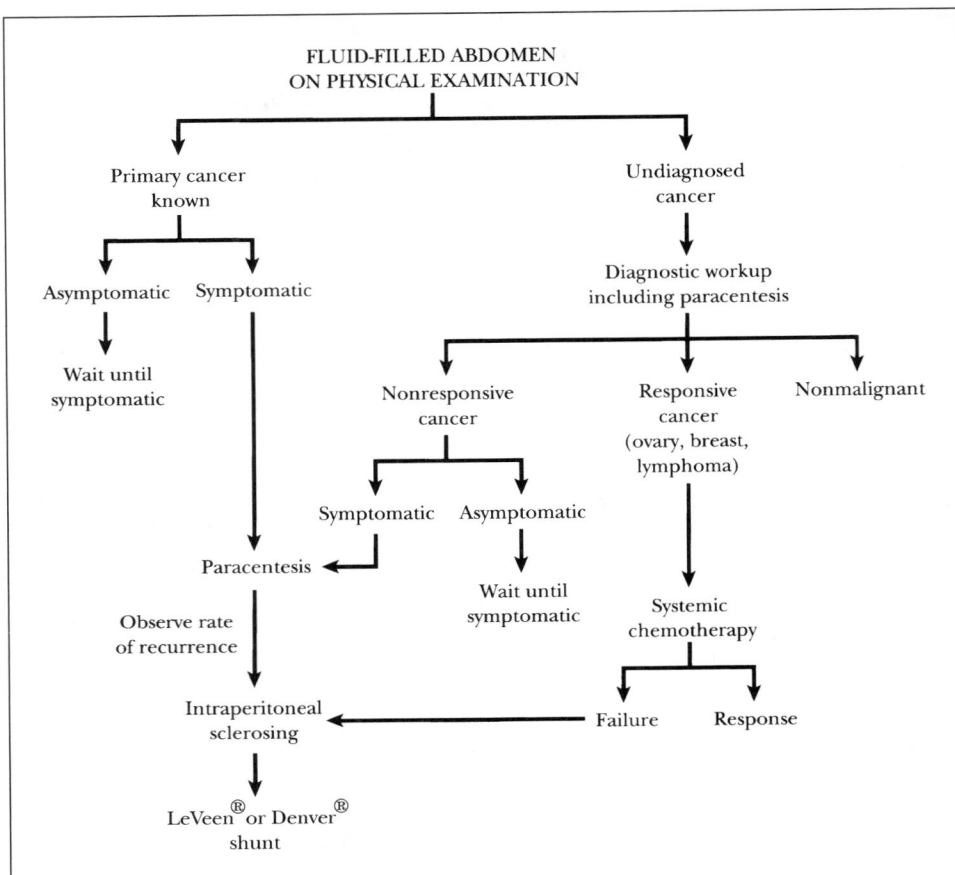

Figure 36-8 Algorithm for diagnosis and management of malignant peritoneal effusion.

Diet and Diuresis

Although diet and diuresis are important as therapy for individuals with ascites due to cirrhosis, sodium restriction and diuretics are usually ineffective in malignant ascites. Unless the underlying malignancy causing the ascites responds to antineoplastic therapy, the pathophysiology of ascites will remain unaltered and fluid accumulation will continue despite exogenous fluid restriction measures.

Removal of Fluid

Paracentesis. Aside from its usefulness as a diagnostic tool, fluid removal by paracentesis alone is of little therapeutic benefit. It is usually reserved until a large volume of fluid has accumulated and the patient is profoundly symptomatic because the fluid reaccumulates rapidly. Of particular note, removal of 2–3 liters of fluid and repeated paracentesis taps can lead to severe protein depletion, postural hypotension, and electrolyte abnormalities. Injury to the viscera and the introduction of infection can occur. Although caution is urged regarding rapidly removing large volumes of ascitic fluid, there has been recent anecdotal evidence that rapid decompression via paracentesis is not harmful with malignant ascites, probably because the mechanism of its production differs from that of cirrhotic ascites.[36] In addition, there has been a report of successful drainage of ascitic fluid with

a temporary catheter inserted with CT guidance.[37] With this method, fluid may be drained gradually and multiple paracenteses may be avoided.

Obliteration of the intraperitoneal space. In the past, intracavity therapy has consisted of instillation of a radioactive colloid suspension (no longer in favor) or a chemotherapeutic agent. The chemotherapy instillation is designed to provoke an inflammatory response leading to sclerosis of the peritoneal space linings. Although sclerosing therapy is effective in treating pleural effusions, it is less successful with ascites.[34] Modest responses to bleomycin instillation for palliation have been reported with no significant side effects. Doxorubicin, nitrogen mustard, and tetracycline instillations have been tried with small groups of individuals. Cisplatin has been administered intraperitoneally.

Access to the peritoneal cavity for drug administration is an important technical problem. The peritoneum can be entered on a temporary basis with various catheters, but repeated puncture of the abdominal wall and peritoneum is risky. Adhesions can occur, which increases the risk of bowel perforation and peritonitis. The Tenckhoff catheter is often used to provide repeated access to the peritoneum. It can remain in place indefinitely and allows peritoneal fluid sampling in addition to drug instillation. Unfortunately, the Tenckhoff catheter sometimes needs to be removed due to obstruction or infection.[34] Using a Groshong catheter for draining malignant ascites is an alternative to conventional paracentesis.[38] Use of the Groshong catheter prevents needle access and does not require surgical removal on completion of chemotherapy. Complex dressing changes like those required by the Tenckhoff catheter are unnecessary.

Recently, there has been some interest in the combination of debulking surgery with intraperitoneal hyperthermic chemotherapy administration. This approach has been used in patients with and without ascites. While it is too early to evaluate the effectiveness of this intervention, it is postulated to prolong survival and perhaps even prevent the development of malignant ascites.[39]

Peritoneovenous shunting. Shunt devices (LeVeen® and Denver®) can be used to recirculate ascitic fluid continuously to the intravascular space. One end of a catheter is implanted in the peritoneal cavity and a tube is channeled through subcutaneous tissue to the superior vena cava, where the other end is implanted. A pressure differential between the abdominal cavity and the thoracic vein enables fluid to ascend from the peritoneal cavity into the superior vena cava. Because neoplastic ascites tend to contain more particulate matter than other fluid types (usually an exudate), a Denver® shunt may be preferred as it has a subcutaneous pump that can be manually compressed to prevent clogging of the tubing.[20] Despite this potential advantage, a functional superiority of one over the other of these devices has not been documented in the literature, leaving the choice to the clinician's personal preference.[20]

Peritoneovenous shunting is no panacea. It is usually reserved for individuals in whom all other treatment options have failed. Median survival time after shunt placement is 2–4 months, so it is difficult to obtain objective evaluation criteria. When the shunt is functioning well, it provides good palliation. Complications can occur, with clotting occurring most frequently, but sometimes disseminated intravascular coagulation and pulmonary embolism develop. In some instances, postoperative complications might be predicted by a preoperative procedure designed to assess patient tolerance to the proposed permanent shunt. Termed *peritoneovenous autotransfusion*, this preoperative evaluation can be accomplished by using an external shunting system trial over 48 hours.[40]

Nursing care of the patient with a peritoneovenous shunt includes teaching the patient and family the purpose and care of the shunt, signs and symptoms of problems with the shunt, and recognition and prevention of infection, as well as alleviating anxiety. In addition, nursing care includes measures related to the peritoneal effusion and advanced cancer.

BRAIN: MALIGNANT CEREBRAL EDEMA

Scope of the Problem

Cerebral edema results from an increase in the fluid content of the brain. There are three major types of

cerebral edema: vasogenic edema (extracellular, the most common type), cytotoxic edema (intracellular, due to metabolic abnormalities), and interstitial edema (due to cerebrospinal fluid blockage). Malignant cerebral edema is usually the vasogenic type caused by increased permeability of the cerebral capillary endothelial cells. Many brain tumors obstruct the outflow of cerebrospinal fluid, resulting in interstitial edema.[41] Although the edema can be iatrogenic, caused by radiation therapy, surgery, or chemotherapy, most cerebral edema accompanies primary or metastatic brain tumors or carcinomatous meningitis.

Any cancer can metastasize to the brain; brain metastasis occurs in 25%–35% of all persons with cancer. The cancers that most commonly metastasize to the brain are lung, breast, melanoma, renal, and thyroid.[42]

Physiological Alterations

Mechanisms thought to play a role in the formation of malignant cerebral edema are (1) direct injury to the vascular endothelium by the expanding tumor, (2) dysplastic vascular structures within tumor lesions, (3) biochemically mediated alterations of capillary permeability (including the excretion of a permeability factor by tumor cells), and (4) a less stable blood-brain barrier.[43] Capillary permeability varies depending on histology and tumor size. Edema develops as water and ions passively diffuse into the brain's extracellular space to maintain isotonicity. The white matter of the brain is primarily affected (Figure 36-9). The progression of edema through brain tissue

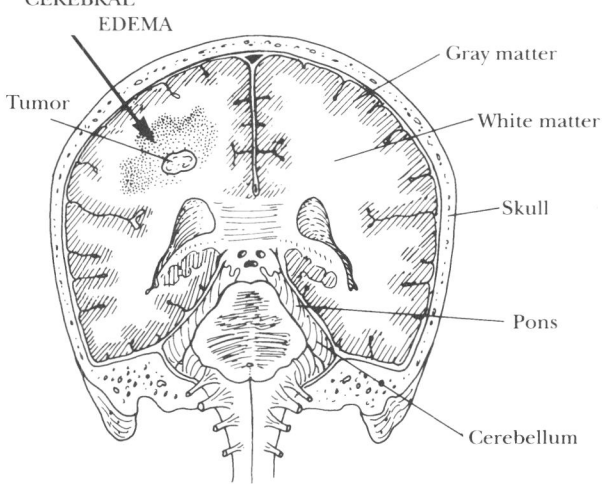

Figure 36-9 Vasogenic edema of the brain due to a primary tumor or metastatic lesion is characterized by increased permeability of brain capillary endothelial cells. The white matter of the brain is primarily affected. The progression of edema through the white matter of brain tissue occurs as bulk flow regulated by cerebral perfusion pressure.

occurs as bulk fluid flow regulated by cerebral perfusion pressure.

How cerebral edema leads to neurological dysfunction is not clear, but it is probably related to tissue ischemia and toxic inhibition of local neuron activity induced by metabolic abnormalities in the surrounding extravascular fluid. When the edema exceeds the limits of compensatory mechanisms, brain herniation can occur.

Clinical Manifestations

Neurological deficits in patients with brain tumors are due in equal measure to peritumoral edema and the tumor mass itself.[41] Initial symptoms of intracerebral tumors are headache, nausea and vomiting, personality changes, diminished cognition, and somnolence[41] (Table 36-9). Symptoms may be so subtle that they are only apparent to those who know the patient well. Family members may notice the patient's lack of persistence in tasks, undue irritability, emotional lability, inertia, faulty insight, forgetfulness, reduced range of mental activity, indifference to common social practices, and lack of initiative and spontaneity. These early symptoms are often incorrectly attributed to worry, anxiety, or depression. Patients themselves often complain only of being weak, tired, or dizzy. As time progresses, the symptoms become more pronounced.

About 20% of patients with intracerebral tumors present with seizures.[41] Headache, another common early symptom, is due to distortion and traction of pain-sensitive structures by the edema. Intermittent at first, headache usually is present in the morning and gradually increases in duration and frequency. Clinical signs may be observed that relate to specific parts of the brain, and these can be localized to the affected area by neurological assessment.[44]

Assessment

Neurological examination, CT scanning, and magnetic resonance imaging (MRI) are the primary studies used for diagnosing a brain tumor mass. Magnetic resonance imaging is best for visualizing cerebral edema.[44] Surgery, such as stereotactic biopsy, is required for a definitive tissue diagnosis. Other conditions (abscess, multiple sclerosis) can have a radiographic appearance similar to that of a tumor.[45]

Therapeutic Approaches and Nursing Care

Aggressive therapy is warranted to sustain or restore neurological function. Surgery, radiation therapy, and chemotherapy all have a role in treating brain tumors and, thus, in reducing cerebral edema. Steroids are also commonly used to reduce edema. In most patients, neurological symptoms improve with treatment. Some brain tumors are curable. In others, remissions may be lengthy or brief, depending on the tumor type.

Nursing management of patients with cerebral edema focuses on assessment, administration of medication, monitoring for side effects associated with these medications, the institution of safety and seizure precautions, and prevention of complications of immobility. Interventions may be targeted to the patient's specific neurological deficits.

Early detection of brain herniation is essential to preserve brain function. The nurse must be sensitive to changes in vital signs and be able to intervene rapidly. Hypertension exacerbates cerebral edema.[32] With advanced cerebral edema and the resultant increased intracranial pressure, changes in vital signs such as bounding radial pulse, elevated temperature, and respiratory impairment may be seen. Decreased level of consciousness, change in pupil size and reaction to light, and altered motor response, in addition to other vital sign changes, should alert the nurse to impending brain herniation, an oncologic emergency.[44]

Steroids, Anticonvulsants, and Osmotherapy

The single most important adjunctive treatment to combat the effects of vasogenic cerebral edema is the use of glucocorticoids (dexamethasone, prednisone). High doses of dexamethasone (30–60 mg in four to six divided

Table 36-9 Assessment of the Patient with Cerebral Edema

Signs and Symptoms

SUBJECTIVE INDICATORS

Headache
Weakness, focal
Mental disturbance
Seizures
Gait disorder
Visual disturbance
Language disturbance

OBJECTIVE INDICATORS

Hemiparesis
Impaired cognition
Sensory loss, unilateral
Papilledema
Ataxia
Aphasia

LABORATORY INDICATORS

Computerized tomography (CT) brain
Magnetic resonance imaging (MRI)

doses) are given.[45] When symptoms are controlled, the steroid dose is tapered until symptoms again become apparent. The dose is then adjusted until the symptoms subside.[41] Steroid withdrawal can result in headache, lethargy, postural dizziness, and nausea, which mirror symptoms associated with either adrenal suppression or progressive edema. Dexamethasone is the preferred agent because of its minimal sodium-retaining properties and relative potency.

Patients who have had seizures are placed on anticonvulsant therapy. Some clinicians prescribe prophylactic anticonvulsants when an intracerebral tumor is diagnosed.[41] Seizure control is very important, as seizures cause a transient increase in intracranial pressure.[46] Careful monitoring of anticonvulsant drug levels is necessary to maintain efficacy and prevent side effects.

Mannitol is an osmotherapy agent that can be used to reduce profound cerebral edema on a temporary basis. It creates an osmotic gradient that pulls fluid out of the brain and causes diuresis.[47] Mannitol should be tapered slowly, as abrupt withdrawal can cause rebound edema.[42]

Surgery

Surgery is the primary modality for the treatment of brain tumors. Surgical debulking is the most effective means of reducing intracranial pressure and preventing further edema formation.[41] Recent technological advances in surgical technique and imaging have made most brain tumors accessible to surgery. Multiple factors influence the decision regarding surgical excision of metastatic brain lesions, including the number of lesions and the extent of systemic disease.[48] If surgical resection is not possible, needle biopsy should be performed for tissue diagnosis. Treatment for brain tumors should be initiated only after definitive tissue diagnosis.[41] There may be a temporary increase in brain edema immediately postoperatively.

Radiation Therapy

Many unifocal primary brain tumors are potentially curable with radiation therapy. However, these tumors tend to infiltrate diffusely into surrounding tissue, necessitating a wide irradiation field.[41] The tolerance of normal tissue to radiation is dose-limiting. Because it is assumed that microscopic tumor is present in metastatic disease, the radiation port usually encompasses the whole brain. The optimum fractionation schedule and duration of therapy are the subject of clinical trials.[41,48] Radiation therapy causes an acute increase in brain edema, characterized by headache, nausea, vomiting, and worsened neurological symptoms. Long-term effects of radiation include cognitive dysfunction.[41] Interstitial brachytherapy (the implantation of seeds containing iodine 120 or iridium 192) can sometimes be used to achieve a high-dose "local" boost to the tumor while minimizing radiation exposure for normal brain tissue.

Chemotherapy

Several chemotherapeutic agents (carmustine, lomustine, procarbazine) are effective against primary brain tumors.[43] Obstacles to the use of chemotherapy include delivery of the agent across the blood-brain barrier and central nervous system toxicity. Regional drug delivery methods include intraarterial and intrathecal chemotherapy. Patients with edema due to carcinomatous meningitis are aggressively treated with intrathecal chemotherapy.

Conclusion

When fluid accumulates abnormally in the patient with cancer, the consequences can range from life-threatening to merely irksome. A variety of interventions can be employed, mostly for palliation, depending on the amount of fluid present and the site where it is retained. Aggressive medical and nursing care can alleviate discomfort and may prolong life, or at least maintain its quality. Without exception, these conditions are most effectively treated by controlling the underlying disease. The best hope for eliminating malignant effusions and edemas would be to discover a cure for cancer, or at least more effective therapies.

References

1. Hill RB, Anderson RE: The autopsy in oncology. *CA Cancer J Clin* 42:47–56, 1992
2. Olopade OI, Ultmann JE: Malignant effusions. *CA Cancer J Clin* 41:166–179, 1991
3. Gobel BH, Lawler PE: Malignant pleural effusions. *Oncol Nurs Forum* 12(4): 49–54, 1985
4. Rossetti AC: Nursing care of patients treated with intrapleural tetracycline for control of malignant pleural effusion. *Cancer Nurs* 8:103–109, 1985
5. Hewitt JB, Jansen WB: A management strategy for malignancy-induced pleural effusion: Long-term thoracostomy drainage: *Oncol Nurs Forum* 14:17–22, 1987
6. Joiner GA, Kolodychuk GR: Neoplastic cardiac tamponade. *Crit Care Nurs* 11:50–58, 1991
7. Wojciechowicz V: Peripheral window surgery for cardiac tamponade. *Crit Care Nurs* 5:28–33, 1985
8. Mangan CM: Malignant pericardial effusions: Pathophysiology and clinical correlates. *Oncol Nurs Forum* 19:1215–1221, 1992
9. Kehoe C: Malignant ascites: Etiology, diagnosis, and treatment. *Oncol Nurs Forum* 18:523–530, 1991
10. Getz DH: The primary, secondary, and tertiary nursing interventions of lymphedema. *Cancer Nurs* 8:177–184, 1985
11. Kennelly LF, Yurkovic CA: Altered tissue perfusion, peripheral, related to lymphedema, in McNally JC, Somerville ET, Miaskowski C (eds): *Guidelines for Oncology Nursing Practice.* Philadelphia, Saunders, 1991, pp 387–391
12. Moores DW: Malignant pleural effusion. *Semin Oncol* 18: 59–61, 1991 (suppl)

13. Miles DW, Kough RK: Diagnosis and management of malignant pleural effusion. *Cancer Treat Rev* 19:115–168, 1993

14. Lynch TJ: Management of malignant pleural effusions. *Chest* 103:385S–389S, 1993 (suppl)

15. Keller SM: Current and future therapy for malignant pleural effusion. *Chest* 103:63S–67S, 1993 (suppl)

16. Pass HI: Malignant pleural and pericardial effusions, in DeVita VT, Hellman S, Rosenberg SA (eds): *Cancer: Principles and Practices of Oncology* (ed 5). Philadelphia, Lippincott-Raven, 1997, pp 2586–2598

17. Robinson LA, Ruckdeschel JC: Management of pleural and pericardial effusions, in Berger A, Portenoy RK, Weissman DE (eds): *Principles and Practice of Supportive Oncology*. Philadelphia, Lippincott-Raven, 1998, pp 327–352

18. Davey SS, McCance KL, Budd MC: Alterations of pulmonary function, in McCance KL, Huether SE (eds): *Pathophysiology: The Biologic Basis for Disease in Adults and Children* (ed 2). St. Louis, Mosby, 1994, pp 1148–1190

19. Ferri FF: Procedures and interpretation of results, in Ferri FF (ed): *Practical Guide to the Care of the Medical Patient* (ed 4). St. Louis, Mosby, 1998, pp 801–830

20. Yarbro JW: Effusions, in Abeloff MD, Armitage JO, Lichter AS, et al (eds): *Clinical Oncology*. New York, Churchill Livingstone, 1995, pp 709–725

21. Ruckdeschel JC: Management of malignant pleural effusion: An overview. *Semin Oncol* 15:24–28, 1988 (suppl)

22. Robinson RD, Fullerton DA, Albert JD, et al: Use of pleural Tenckhoff catheter to palliate malignant pleural effusion. *Ann Thorac Surg* 57:286–288, 1994

23. Luketich JD, Kiss M, Hershey J, et al: Chest tube insertion: A prospective evaluation of pain management. *Clin J Pain* 14:152–154, 1998

24. Belani CP, Aisner J, Patz E, et al: Ambulatory sclerotherapy for malignant pleural effusion. *Proc Am Soc Clin Oncol* 14:524, 1995 (abstr)

25. Fiocco M, Krasna MJ: The management of malignant pleural and pericardial effusions. *Hematol Oncol Clin North Am* 11:253–265, 1997

26. Vaitkus PT, Hermann HC, LeWinter MM: Treatment of malignant pericardial effusion. *JAMA* 272:59–64, 1994

27. Okamoto H, Shinkai T, Yamakido M, et al: Cardiac tamponade caused by primary lung cancer and the management of pericardial effusion. *Cancer* 73:93–98, 1993

28. Latham RJ, Cohen DJ, Kuntz RE, et al: Pericardial effusion in patients with cancer: Outcome with contemporary management strategies. *Heart* 75:67–71, 1996

29. Keane D, Jackson J: Managing recurrent malignant pericardial effusions: Percutaneous balloon pericardiotomy may have a role. *BMJ* 305:729–730, 1992

30. Wang N, Feikes JR, Morensen T, et al: Pericardioperitoneal shunt: An alternative treatment for malignant pericardial effusion. *Ann Thorac Surg* 57:289–292, 1994

31. Girardi LN, Ginsberg RJ, Burt ME: Pericardiocentesis and intrapericardial sclerosis: Effective therapy for malignant pericardial effusions. *Ann Thorac Surg* 64:1422–1428, 1997

32. Dragonette P: Malignant Pericardial effusion and cardiac tamponade, in Chernecky CC, Berger BJ (eds): *Advanced and Critical Care Oncology Nursing*. Philadelphia, Saunders, 1998, pp 425–443

33. Chan A, Rischin D, Clark CP, et al: Subxiphoid partial pericardiectomy with or without sclerosant instillation in the treatment of symptomatic pericardial effusions in patients with malignancy. *Cancer* 68:1021–1025, 1991

34. Marincola FM, Schwartzentruber DJ: Malignant ascites, in DeVita VT, Hellman S, Rosenberg SA (eds): *Cancer: Principles and Practices of Oncology* (ed 5). Philadelphia, Lippincott-Raven, 1997, pp 2586–2598

35. Zehner LC, Hoogstraten B: Malignant effusions and their management. *Semin Oncol Nurs* 1:259–268, 1985

36. Ratliff CR, Hutchinson M, Conner C: Rapid paracentesis of large volumes of ascitic fluid. *Oncol Nurs Forum* 18:1461, 1991

37. Mercadante S, La Rosa S, Nicolosi G, et al: Temporary drainage of symptomatic malignant ascites by a catheter inserted under computed tomography. *J Pain Symptom Manage* 15:374–378, 1998

38. Hrozencik SP, Ness EA: Intraperitoneal chemotherapy via the Groshong catheter in the patient with gynecologic cancer. *Oncol Nurs Forum* 18:1245, 1991

39. Loggie BW, Perini M, Fleming RA, et al: Treatment and prevention of malignant ascites associated with disseminated intraperitoneal malignancies by aggressive combined-modality therapy. *Am Surg* 63:137–143, 1997

40. Kehoe C: Malignant ascites: Etiology, diagnosis, and treatment. *Oncol Nurs Forum* 18:523–530, 1991

41. Levin VA, Leibel SA, Gutin PH: Neoplasms of the central nervous system, in DeVita VT, Hellman S, Rosenberg SA (eds): *Cancer: Principles and Practice of Oncology* (ed 5). Philadelphia, Lippincott-Raven, 1997, pp 2022–2082

42. Ferri FF: Neurology, in Ferri FF (ed): *Practical Guide to the Care of the Medical Patient* (ed 4). St. Louis, Mosby, 1998, pp 672–709

43. Ito U, Reulen HJ, Tomita H, et al: A computed tomography study on formation, propagation, and resolution of edema fluid in metastatic brain tumors, in Long D (ed): *Advances in Neurology*, vol 52. New York, Raven, 1990, pp 342–357

44. Saba MT, Magolan JM: Understanding cerebral edema: Implications for oncology nurses. *Oncol Nurs Forum* 18:499–505, 1991

45. Hochberg F, Pruitt A: Neoplastic diseases of the central nervous system, in Isselbacher KJ, Braunwald E, Wilson JD, et al (eds): *Harrison's Principles of Internal Medicine* (ed 13). New York: McGraw-Hill, 1994, pp 2256–2269

46. Gelb DJ, Chimowitz MI: Stroke, in Gelb DJ (ed): *Introduction to Clinical Neurology*. Boston, Butterworth-Heinemann, 1995, pp 103–122

47. Poole RM, Gelb DJ: Acute mental status changes, in Gelb DJ (ed): *Introduction to Clinical Neurology*. Boston, Butterworth-Heinemann, 1995, pp 253–268

48. Loeffler JS, Patchell RA, Sawaya R: Metastatic brain cancer, in DeVita VT, Hellman S, Rosenberg SA (eds): *Cancer: Principles and Practice of Oncology* (ed 5). Philadelphia, Lippincott-Raven, 1997, pp 2523–2536

CHAPTER 37

Sexual and Reproductive Dysfunction

Linda U. Krebs, RN, PhD, AOCN

Scope of the Problem

Although increasingly recognized as consequences of cancer or cancer therapy, sexual and reproductive dysfunctions often have been dismissed as normal side effects about which the caregiver can do little or nothing. Indeed, these dysfunctions often have gone underdiagnosed, underrated, or both because of lack of concern, information, or knowledge on the part of the caregiver, or because of fear, lack of knowledge, or embarrassment on the part of the patient or family. Often, problems related to sexuality and reproduction are not addressed unless the patient is extremely assertive or presents to the health care provider in a crisis situation.[1]

Of all the complications associated with cancer, difficulties in the ability to feel comfortable with one's own sexuality and body image, to be sexually intimate, and to bear children have remained major concerns that affect all aspects of the patient's and family's lives. For some patients, sexual or reproductive dysfunctions may be temporary, with full recovery expected when therapy is completed. For many others, however, alterations in sexual or reproductive function are permanent, requiring adaptations in management of intimate relationships and lifelong plans to bear and raise children. Even short-term, temporary alterations can have long-term effects on the patient and family, influencing lifestyles and life choices.

Sexuality and reproductive ability are intrinsic components of every individual, involving all aspects of our being.[2] The sexuality and reproductive capacity of the individual with cancer may be affected by a variety of factors, including the biological process of cancer, the effects of treatment, additional health problems and medications, and the psychological and social issues, such as religious and cultural norms, surrounding the patient and family.[3] Physiological problems of infertility and sterility, changes in body appearance, and the inability to have intercourse are exacerbated by the psychological and psychosexual issues of alteration in body image, fear of abandonment, loss of self-esteem, alterations in sexual identity, and concerns about self. Without appropriate education, counseling, and support, it may be difficult for the patient and family to adapt to the alterations that cancer can produce.

Physiological Alterations

The pituitary and the hypothalamus regulate gonadal function. The pituitary is divided into two distinct parts—the anterior and posterior portions—and is attached to the hypothalamus by the pituitary or hypophysial stalk, through which runs a minute blood vessel system, the hypothalamic-hypophysial portal vessels.[4,5]

Hypothalamic-releasing or hypothalamic-inhibiting hormones are secreted within the hypothalamus and then spread via the portal vessel system to the anterior pitu-itary, where they act to influence glandular secretion. When produced in appropriate amounts, these hormones institute a feedback mechanism that shuts off hormonal secretion at the hypothalamus and pituitary level.[4,5]

In gonadal function, luteinizing hormone–releasing hormone (LHRH) or gonadotropin-releasing hormone (GnRH) is secreted by the hypothalamus and stimulates the anterior pituitary to produce luteinizing hormone (LH) and follicle-stimulating hormone (FSH). Luteinizing hormone and FSH stimulate the testis and ovary to produce the appropriate hormones. When blood levels of these hormones are adequate, the hormones exert a negative feedback on the pituitary, thus decreasing glandular secretion.[4,5]

Follicle-stimulating hormone and LH play major roles in the control of male sexual function. Luteinizing hormone acts on the interstitial Leydig cells to produce testosterone; FSH, in conjunction with testosterone, is responsible for the conversion of spermatogonia into spermatocytes. A reciprocal inhibition of hypothalamic/anterior pituitary secretion of gonadotropic hormones by testicular hormones keeps the level of hormones stable. In this system, the hypothalamus secretes GnRH, which causes the anterior pituitary to secrete LH. In turn, LH stimulates the Leydig cells to produce testosterone. The testosterone then negatively feeds back to the hypothalamus, inhibiting production of GnRH. Spermatogenesis is controlled in much the same manner, with FSH stimulating the Sertoli cells to convert spermatids into sperm. The Sertoli cells then secrete a hormone called *inhibin* that, through negative feedback, causes a decrease in FSH production, thus keeping spermatogenesis at a constant rate (Figure 37-1).[4,5]

The female hormonal system, like the male, consists of three levels of hormones: GnRH from the hypothalamus, LH and FSH from the anterior pituitary, and estrogen and progesterone from the ovary. In the nonpregnant female, monthly rhythmic changes in the rates of secretion of female hormones and responding changes in the sexual organs result in the female sexual (menstrual) cycle. As a result, a single mature ovum is released from an ovary, and the endometrium of the uterus is prepared for implantation. Follicle-stimulating hormone is responsible for growth of the ovarian follicle, which eventually will become the mature ovum. At the beginning of menstruation, FSH and LH increase, causing rapid cellular growth in about 20 follicles. Eventually, one follicle begins to outgrow the others, causing atresia of the remaining follicles. During follicle growth, estrogen is secreted, probably causing a positive feedback mechanism that results in a surge of LH. This surge of LH, which occurs two days before ovulation, is necessary for follicular growth and ovulation. Around the time of ovulation, the ruptured follicle, under the stimulation of LH, becomes the corpus luteum that secretes both estrogen and progesterone. After several days, the estrogen and progesterone create negative feedback to decrease secretion of FSH and LH. The

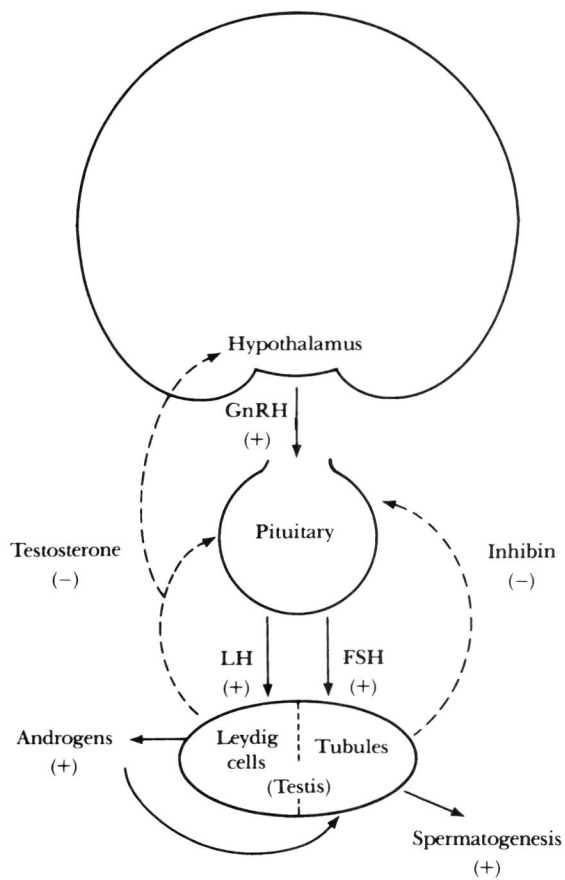

Figure 37-1 Normal testicular function. FSH = follicle-stimulating hormone; GnRH = gonadotropin-releasing hormone; LH = luteinizing hormone. (Data from Guyton and Hall[4]; Marieb.[5])

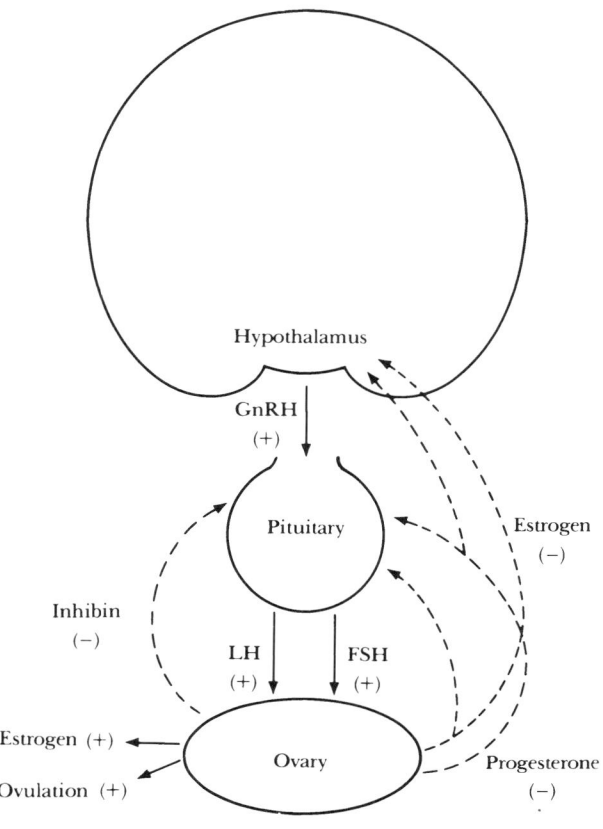

Figure 37-2 Normal ovarian function. FSH = follicle-stimulating hormone; GnRH = gonadotropin-releasing hormone; LH = luteinizing hormone. (Data from Guyton and Hall[4]; Marieb.[5])

corpus luteum, which also secretes inhibin, slowly degenerates, creating a loss of the feedback mechanism and an associated rise in secretion of FSH and LH, beginning a new ovarian cycle and leading to menstruation (Figure 37-2).[4,5]

Ovarian failure and germinal aplasia can occur as a result of disease, therapy, nutritional status, psychological factors, or any combination of these. Ovarian failure also is related to age; as women near menopause, ovarian failure is more likely. In ovarian failure, damage to ovarian follicles causes decreased levels of estrogens and progesterones, which results in increased levels of LH and FSH with no compensating feedback mechanism. In addition, inhibin may be produced and may react further to alter FSH production. Ovulation ceases, menstruation becomes erratic or ceases, and early menopause often results (Figure 37-3).[4,5] In the male, damage to the Leydig cells results in decreased testosterone production; LH and FSH will be elevated. Initially, Leydig cell activity may be sufficiently compensated to produce adequate amounts of testosterone, but continued damage results

in temporary, but more often permanent, sterility (Figure 37-4).[4,5]

Clinical Manifestations: Effect of Cancer Therapy on Gonadal Function

Surgery

Some surgical procedures for cancer of the gastrointestinal and genitourinary tracts cause sexual dysfunction through the removal of sexual organs, damage to nerves that enervate sexual organs, or alteration of normal function. In addition, surgery for cancers of the head and neck and the breast, and amputation alter body image and may affect sexual identity. Organ dysfunction, either through loss of or alteration in normal function, is most common in cancers of the colon, rectum, bladder and associated urinary structures, and male and female genital tracts. Even when organs are not removed, normal

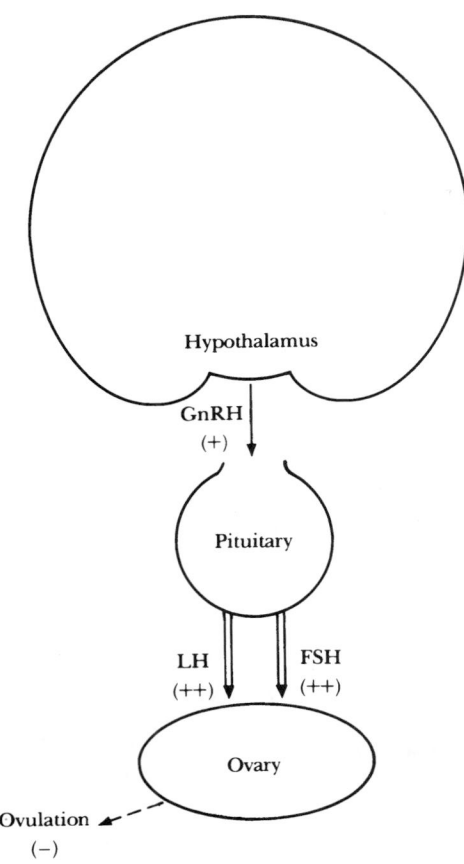

Figure 37-3 Ovarian failure. (FSH = follicle-stimulating hormone; GnRH = gonadotropin-releasing hormone; LH = luteinizing hormone.) (Data from Guyton and Hall[4]; Marieb.[5])

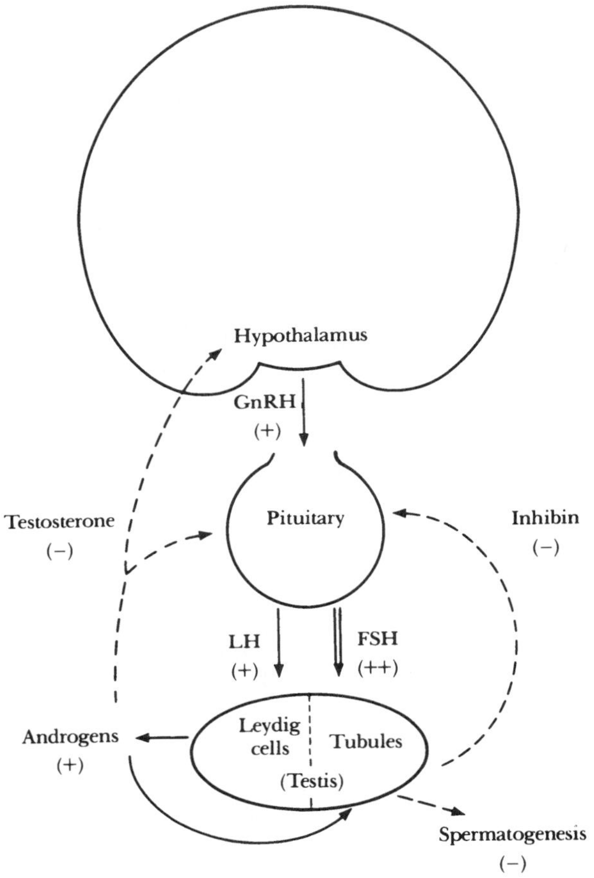

Figure 37-4 Germinal aplasia. (FSH = follicle-stimulating hormone; GnRH = gonadotropin-releasing hormone; LH = luteinizing hormone.) (Data from Guyton and Hall[4]; Marieb.[5])

function may be disrupted through removal of tumor tissue surrounding an organ, lymph node dissection, or associated physiological and psychological abnormalities related to the type of surgery required.

Cancer of the colon and rectum

Surgery for cancer of the colon and rectum may cause sexual dysfunction in both men and women. In general, sexual dysfunctions in women are more commonly related to psychosocial issues, whereas in men dysfunctions may be both physical and psychosocial. The most common surgery for colon cancer is some degree of colectomy, with or without a colostomy. While previously cancer of the rectum and anus often required an anterior or an abdominoperineal resection (APR), sphincter-preserving surgery without need for an ostomy is now the most common surgical procedure for rectal cancer.[6] Though this saves the sphincter, the surgery is associated with increased bowel frequency, a sense of urgency, fecal leakage, rectovaginal fistula and bladder, and erectile dysfunction in many patients.[7–9]

For those in whom an APR is necessary, sexual dysfunc-

tion may be related to the placement of the colostomy, to removal of or interference with sexual organ function, or some combination of the two. A colostomy can be associated with sexual dysfunction because of negative changes in the patient's body image and self-esteem, and the responses of family and friends. In an extensive review of quality-of-life literature for patients with and without a stoma, the majority of patients with a stoma had some type of sexual dysfunction. The most common complaints were erectile dysfunction and ejaculatory impotence in men and dyspareunia and orgasmic dysfunction in women. As a group, those with a stoma were less sexually active and experienced more generalized distress than those without a stoma. Of additional importance was the finding that all patients with colorectal cancer experienced some degree of sexual dysfunction and decreased quality of life, regardless of the type of therapy.[7]

For the woman with an APR, the ovaries or uterus may be removed at the time of surgery in addition to colostomy, thus causing dysfunction from primary inability to bear children or from alterations in normal hormonal patterns. In addition, women may have part of the vagina removed, or healing of the perineal wound may result in vaginal scarring that causes painful or incomplete vaginal intercourse. A decreased incidence of orgasm and vaginal lubrication, reduced libido, and dyspareunia have also been noted but are much less common.[10,11]

For the man who has an APR, sexual dysfunction is more severe, with 30%–60% of men experiencing decreased desire, 30%–75% having erectile dysfunction, and 65%–85% experiencing ejaculatory dysfunction.[11] Age appears to be a factor, with the older patient more likely to suffer complete or incomplete erectile impotence.[12] This is most likely due to damage to parasympathetic and sympathetic nerves that control both erection and ejaculation. In addition to erectile dysfunction, decreased amount and force of ejaculation or retrograde ejaculation may occur. This result, which may be temporary or permanent, adds to the trauma of surgery for the patient because the outcome is unpredictable. Sexual dysfunction defined by cessation of sexual relationship, absence of erection, absence of ejaculation, or inability to penetrate occurs in 15% of men who have a high anterior resection, whereas 54% of men with an APR experience some type of dysfunction.[13] For all patients, damage to nerves enervating the pelvic plexus appears to be the most common denominator in organic sexual dysfunction. If complete nerve-sparing procedures are undertaken successfully, erectile and ejaculatory functions are maintained and the majority of men are able to have sexual intercourse and achieve orgasm.[14]

Cancers of the genitourinary tract

Bladder cancer. The treatment of bladder cancer may alter sexual function in men and women. Repeated cystoscopy for local treatment of transitional cell cancer has been noted to cause pain with coitus for women, transient pain during erection and ejaculation in men, and temporary decrease in desire for both. Transurethral resection or partial cystectomy may result in mild pain or dyspareunia; however, normal sexual function should not be altered. For some patients, urinary incontinence may cause cessation of normal activities for fear of having an accident. In addition, body image and self-esteem may be altered due to the need to use incontinence pads or other protective materials.

Radical cystectomy results in sexual dysfunction for both men and women because of organ removal and damage to nerves. Erectile dysfunction has been noted to be more than 90% in men undergoing radical cystectomy.[15] Orgasm may be experienced but is usually less intense and without ejaculate.[11] Sexual interest and penile sensation are not altered.[16,17] For the woman who has radical cystectomy, the surgery usually includes removal of the bladder and urethra, the uterus, ovaries, fallopian tubes, and the anterior portion of the vagina. Although vaginal reconstruction typically is performed, the resulting vagina may be more narrow and shallow and provide less lubrication than before surgery, leading to difficulty with penetration. In addition, the removal of the ovaries, with associated estrogen loss, leads to dryness,

inelasticity of the vagina, dyspareunia, and menopausal symptoms. Vaginal dilation and the liberal use of lubrication may provide relief.[2,11,12]

For both sexes, urinary diversion is a necessity with radical cystectomy; this may result in alterations in self-esteem and body image and may lead to a decrease or cessation of all sexual activities, with women reporting decreased desire and feelings of decreased attractiveness.[15,18,19] In the past, the ileal conduit, which necessitated the continuous use of an ostomy appliance, was the most common method for urinary diversion. Today the surgical development of a Kock pouch, or continent reservoir, has become more widely employed, resulting in overall improved sexual adjustment due to decreased odor and leakage.[15,19] Most recently, the construction of a neobladder, made from the ileum and the large intestine, has allowed patients to maintain bladder function and normal voiding patterns.[20] While most commonly used in men, women also may benefit; however, women have a 70% chance of being hypercontinent, requiring self-catheterization.[21] In studies comparing the neobladder to the ileal conduit, improved quality of life and decreased alterations in sexual functioning were noted in both men and women who had bladder substitution.[18,19]

Penile cancer/cancer of the male urethra. Cancer of the penis and male urethra are rare. Primary treatment is total or partial penectomy. The degree of limitation primarily relates to the amount of tissue removed.[16] Partial penectomy does not result in loss of erectile, ejaculative, or orgasmic abilities, whereas erectile ability obviously is absent with total penectomy.[11,22] Desire remains, and stimulation of the remaining genital tissue can produce orgasm.[15,23] Ejaculation, through the perineal urethrostomy, should continue. New techniques to create a penis have been used after a total penectomy. A semirigid or inflatable prosthesis restores the ability to have intercourse and has been reported to increase erectile ability, libido, and frequency of intercourse.[23,24] Successful placement rates of 83% for malleable and mechanical prostheses and 67% for inflatable prostheses have been reported, with an overall mechanical failure rate of 7%.[25] Those treated with radiation therapy had significantly fewer concerns related to sexual dysfunction than those with partial or total penectomy who noted decreased interest, enjoyment, frequency, and ability.[26]

Testicular cancer. The treatment of testicular cancer includes an orchiectomy and typically retroperitoneal lymph node dissection and removal of a pelvic mass, usually followed by chemotherapy or radiation therapy. Unilateral orchiectomy will not result in infertility or sexual dysfunction, providing that the contralateral testis is normal and the individual is fertile at diagnosis. Infertility before any definitive therapy is well documented and may be related to hormonal imbalance or may result from subacute chronic illness.[27–29] If bilateral orchiectomy is performed, sterility and decreased libido, related to loss of testosterone, will result. Retroperitoneal lymph node dissection (RPLND) done for staging or as treatment may result in temporary or permanent loss of ejaculation, whereas potency and the ability to have an orgasm remain.[29-31] Whenever possible, nerve-sparing RPLND should be done as these procedures are associated with preservation of ejaculatory function and fertility.[15,29,32] In some individuals, retrograde ejaculation has been noted. Additionally, decreased libido and arousal, decreased pleasure and intensity of orgasm, and erectile dysfunction have been described.[15,33] In approximately one-fourth of those undergoing retroperitoneal surgery, complete absence of ejaculation also is experienced.[33] For most patients, discussions about sexuality before, during, and following treatment are crucial.[34] Prior to therapy, an important aspect of discussion should be information about sperm banking.

Prostate cancer.

Therapy for prostate cancer consists of various combinations of surgery, chemotherapy, radiation therapy, and hormonal manipulation, all of which have a potential to alter sexual function. Surgical treatment of prostate cancer includes prostatectomy or bilateral orchiectomy. Transurethral resection of the prostate generally does not cause impotence or erectile dysfunction; however, retrograde ejaculation occurs in approximately 90% of all patients. Transabdominal resection of the prostate results in retrograde ejaculation in 75%–80% of patients and may cause erectile dysfunction.

The perineal approach, or radical prostatectomy, may result in permanent damage to erectile function with concomitant loss of emission and ejaculation.[15,16,35] Alterations in desire, penile sensation, and the ability to reach orgasm should not occur.[32] Radical prostatectomy is associated with a statistically significant decrease in sexual function, including the ability to achieve and frequency of erections, when patients are compared to those treated solely with radiation therapy.[36]

Nerve-sparing or potency-sparing surgery was developed by Walsh in the 1980s and, according to Church,[37] probably has been the most significant surgical development in the treatment of prostate cancer. Prior to the development of this procedure, 2%–15% of patients experienced urinary incontinence, and 80%–90% experienced impotence. With current techniques, approximately 60%–70% of men will maintain potency,[38] although the exact percentage varies among individual reports and by whether the patient had a non-nerve-sparing, unilateral nerve-sparing, or bilateral nerve-sparing procedure.[39,40] Bilateral orchiectomy causes sexual dysfunction through gradual diminution of libido, impotence, gynecomastia, penile atrophy, and body image changes.[17,35] Testicular implants filled with saline may be of benefit in managing body image changes. Various methods, including the use of penile prostheses, suction or vacuum devices, intracorporeal injections of papaverine hydrochloride or prostaglandin E_1, or medications such as yohimbine hydrochloride, have been used to restore erectile potential. Indeed, those who used erectile aids after surgery had the best sexual outcomes when compared to those with or without nerve-sparing surgery

who did not use them.[41] Most recently, sildenafil citrate (Viagra) has been tried to manage erectile dysfunction in men who have had radical prostatectomy, with 80% of patients who had undergone a bilateral nerve-sparing procedure able to achieve erection and maintain vaginal intercouse for a mean of 6.92 minutes. All reported spousal satisfaction. None of the patients with unilateral or non-nerve-sparing procedures was able to attain an erection.[42]

Fear of failure may also play a role in erectile dysfunction. Because return of full erection potential may take as long as 2 years, it is suggested that the patient wait a minimum of 6 months after surgery to see if function will return.[43,44] With new techniques, sterility in individuals with retrograde ejaculation is not as frequent. Because of the ability to separate sperm from urine, artificial insemination of the mate may be possible.[32]

Gynecologic malignancies

Surgical management of gynecologic malignancies includes surgery of the vulva, vagina, uterus and uterine cervix, ovary, and fallopian tube, and pelvic exenteration. Although the majority of gynecologic surgeries are invisible assaults to femininity, sexual identity and sexual functioning are often permanently affected. It is imperative that sexual and reproductive counseling be provided to the patient and family before surgical intervention because most surgeries permanently alter fertility and may alter sexuality. Studies have shown that women treated for gynecologic malignancy are likely to experience alterations in sexuality and sexual functioning, including decreased desire, dyspareunia, recurrent vaginal infections, vaginal atrophy and dryness, decreased sense of feeling feminine, cessation of all sexual activities, and difficulties related to menopausal symptoms and infertility.[45-48]

Vulvar cancer.

Treatment for vulvar cancer will not alter fertility but may affect sexuality, with 21%–90% of women reporting cessation of all sexual activities following radical vulvectomy.[45] In general, good cosmetic results occur with treatment of early disease except for the simple vulvectomy, which removes the labia and subcutaneous tissue, with retention of the clitoris. Introital stenosis may result but may be easily managed through the use of lubrication and vaginal dilators. Whenever possible, conservative therapy should be employed in order to minimize cosmetic alterations, maintain body image, and minimize sexual dysfunction.

Radical vulvectomy frequently results in delayed wound healing, altered body image, abnormalities in sensory perception of the genital area, leg edema, decreased range of motion in lower extremities, altered orgasmic potential, and introital stenosis.[35,47,49,50] Evaluation of lymph nodes prior to radical surgery may allow for more limited surgeries with less compromise to sexuality.[51] In those who undergo radical pelvic surgery, generalized sexual dysfunction, including pain, anxiety, and decreased desire, is common, occurs earlier, and persists unless appropriately treated. In general, if cure is a possibility, women have been willing to live with sexual dysfunction and body image changes, provided adequate information and discussion about causes of dysfunction and alternative methods of sexual satisfaction are given.[52] All women need education on the effects of removal of tissue and on body image prior to surgery to promote self-esteem, function, and compliance with care.

Vaginal cancer.

Vaginal cancer is rare. Surgery for the majority of gynecological cancers results in some abnormality and need for reconstruction of the vagina. A shortened vagina can cause considerable sexual dysfunction because of decreased vaginal length and width, lack of lubrication, and pain on intercourse. Total vaginectomy without reconstruction precludes vaginal intercourse; however, there are multiple techniques for vaginal reconstruction. Reconstruction can be accomplished using the large or small bowel, the umbilicus, gracilis or rectus musculocutaneous flaps, or a pedicle graft from the greater omentum.[53–55] It has been noted that in 30%–70% of patients who do have reconstruction, there is a return of orgasmic sensations if they existed before surgery. Despite this finding, reconstruction should not be considered a panacea for sexual dysfunction, as some women complain that the new vagina is too large, too small, or has a persistent, annoying discharge.[55,56]

Cervical cancer and endometrial cancer.

Treatment for cervical intraepithelial neoplasia and carcinoma in situ includes conization, laser therapy, cryosurgery, loop electrosurgical excision (LEEP), or simple hysterectomy.[51,56] All but the last usually have no effect on fertility (conization may result in cervical stenosis or incompetence), nor should they cause any physiological sexual dysfunction. Simple hysterectomy precludes further childbearing but should not affect sexual functioning. Treatment for invasive disease is usually radical hysterectomy, with or without bilateral salpingo-oophorectomy. If oophorectomy is included, menopausal symptoms, with hot flashes and decreases in vaginal lubrication and elasticity, may severely alter sexual functioning.[35,51,56] Approximately 50% of patients treated for early-stage cervical cancer have a marked decrease in their sexual relationships and experience extreme fatigue, lack of energy, depressed mood, weight gain, and anxiety.[57]

In women with endometrial cancer, effects of treatment and uncertainty about the future increase sexual difficulties.[58] Of those satisfied with their current sexual functioning, the majority notes that return to normalcy occurred gradually over a prolonged period.

Although sexual feeling should not be altered after a radical hysterectomy, delayed bowel and bladder function may occur and necessitate discharge from the hospital with a urinary catheter. Long-term catheter placement may alter body image and affect sexuality. Intercourse can be accomplished through securing the catheter to the abdomen and making changes in coital position.[50,59] It also should be remembered that many women measure femininity by the ability to bear children. If this ability is removed, sexual dysfunctions may occur even in the absence of organic cause.

Ovarian cancer.

Initial treatment for ovarian cancer is surgery, usually consisting of a radical hysterectomy with bilateral salpingo-oophorectomy and omentectomy. Fertility is lost and the associated menopausal symptoms occur. In the young woman with ovarian teratoma or borderline malignant epithelial neoplasia, it is possible to maintain fertility if disease is confined to one ovary and is of low grade. Adequate staging is essential, and the patient must be willing to comply with all follow-up recommendations.[60–62] Treatment usually continues with combination chemotherapy, thus further compounding sexual and reproductive dysfunctions, including alterations in libido, frequency of intercourse, and desire for close physical contact.[45]

Pelvic exenteration

Although pelvic exenteration may be performed in the man or woman with advanced colorectal or bladder cancer, the most common indication for pelvic exenteration is a locally advanced gynecologic malignancy. An anterior pelvic exenteration preserves the rectum, whereas a posterior exenteration preserves the bladder. A total pelvic exenteration involves removing the vagina, uterus, ovaries, fallopian tubes, bladder, and rectum; in the man, the prostate, seminal vesicles, and vas deferens are removed.[51,56] In patients with total pelvic exenteration, a urinary conduit and colostomy are created and a neovagina may be constructed.[35,51,54] In the woman, reproductive and sexual dysfunctions are profound. Dysfunction related to removal of all pelvic organs with resulting ostomies is obvious. In addition, body image, sexual identity, and self-esteem are disturbed, and appropriate interventions and education need to be provided. In the woman with vaginal reconstruction, intercourse may be possible; however, the physiological and psychological ramifications of this surgery may result in inability and lack of desire to participate in sexual activities.[35,55]

Breast cancer

Although some surgeries may not be strictly related to sexual functioning, they may cause dysfunction as a result of the psychological issues related to the particular body part. The most likely assault to body image and sexual identity with resultant sexual dysfunction is surgical removal of all or part of the breast. Although fertility is not altered by mastectomy or lumpectomy, the inability or difficulty in breast-feeding should pregnancy be accomplished may be a major assault to the woman's femininity. In addition, removal or partial removal of a breast may result in sexual dysfunction because of fear of rejection, physical discomfort, anxiety about initiating sexual activities, feelings of being defective or different, or any combination of these factors.[45] In particular, Lewis et al noted that single women with children were more likely to be burdened by a breast cancer diagnosis than their married counterparts.[63]

Although it had been previously reported that the use of breast-preserving surgery (lumpectomy) caused significantly less alteration in body image, sexual desire, and frequency of intercourse,[56,64] recent studies have shown no difference between women receiving lumpectomy and radiation therapy and women undergoing mastectomy.[65–68] Having the ability to choose the type of therapy also did not play a role in overall sexual adjustment.[69] In general, breast reconstruction does not appear to influence overall sexual adjustment following mastectomy;[70] however, Neill et al reported decreased consequences of breast cancer in 11 women who did undergo reconstruction.[69] Whenever possible, surgical options, including breast reconstruction, should be made available to the woman with breast cancer.

Head and neck cancer

Although not generally considered an area responsible for sexual dysfunction, surgical treatment for cancers of the head and neck region are responsible for varying degrees of alteration in body image, leading to changes in sexuality and intimacy. Results of disease and treatment are readily apparent. Even with reconstructive surgery or the use of prostheses to ameliorate deformities, sexuality may be affected by the alterations in sensation, breathing, and voice; by the ability to use the mouth and tongue or similar abnormalities. Difficulty with arousal and orgasm and cessation of sexual activities also have been reported.[71] Presurgical counseling and long-term follow-up may be necessary for sexual rehabilitation.[59,69,72]

Radiation Therapy

Radiation therapy can cause sexual and reproductive dysfunction through primary organ failure (e.g., ovarian failure and testicular aplasia), alterations in organ function (e.g., decreased lubrication and impotence), and the temporary or permanent effects of therapy not associated with reproduction (e.g., diarrhea and fatigue). Permanent effects most commonly are related to total dose, location, length of treatment, age, and prior fertility status.[73] In the woman, fertility depends on follicular maturation and ovum release. Radiation therapy to the ovaries has its most direct effect on the intermediate follicles. If these follicles are damaged by radiation and insufficient small follicles remain, permanent sterility results. In the man, although the Leydig cell and mature sperm are relatively radioresistant, immature sperm and spermatogonia are extremely radiosensitive. Small doses of radiation will begin the process of infertility, which, depending on total dose, may be permanent.[74]

In women, temporary or permanent sterility is related to the dose of radiation, the volume of tissues radiated, the time period the ovaries are exposed to radiation, and age.[73,74] Because a woman has fewer oocytes as she nears menopause, radiation injury at that point in the life span is more likely to be permanent. A radiation dose of 600–1200 cGy is capable of inducing menopause; however, younger women appear to be more resistant to this effect and may not experience permanent sterility until a dose of greater than 2000 cGy. In women older than 40, a dose of 600 cGy often is associated with subsequent menopause and the associated menopausal symptoms of hot flashes, amenorrhea, dyspareunia, loss of libido, and vaginal atrophy.[73,75] For some women, the use of exogenous estrogens may alleviate these side effects.

Movement of the ovaries out of the radiation field (oophoropexy), with appropriate shielding, has helped maintain fertility even when relatively high doses of radiation have been given. Ovaries can be moved to the midline of the uterus or to the iliac crests. In young women or those desiring to maintain both reproductive capacity and hormonal function, ovarian transposition, with the ovaries moved to the upper abdomen, can be undertaken.[73] Successful pregnancies, without evidence of fetal congenital anomalies, have been reported following oophoropexy.[73,76,77]

In addition to sterility or transient infertility, radiation therapy can produce other sexual dysfunctions, which may be temporary or permanent. Decreases in sexual enjoyment, ability to attain orgasm, libido, and frequency of intercourse and sexual dreams, as well as vaginal stenosis or shortening, vaginal irritation, increased risk of infection, and decreased lubrication and sensation have been reported in women treated with radiation therapy. Painful intercourse and menstrual changes have also been reported.[78–81]

In men, temporary or permanent azoospermia also is a function of age, dose, tissue volume, and exposure time. When the testis is exposed to radiation, a reduction in sperm count begins within 6–8 weeks and continues for up to 1 year after completion of therapy. Doses of less than 500 cGy usually are associated with temporary sterility, whereas doses of greater than 500 cGy usually result in permanent sterility.[74] The return of normal spermatogenesis is related to total testicular dose, with a dose of less than 100 cGy taking 9–12 months for recovery, whereas 200–300 cGy may take 2–3 years and 400–600 cGy 5 years or more.[82]

Below-diaphragm irradiation for Hodgkin's disease has been associated with long-term elevation of FSH, with the majority of patients remaining azoospermic more than a decade following treatment.[83] In a follow-up of 60 long-term survivors of childhood acute lymphoblastic leukemia, Sklar et al found that 50% of men exposed to craniospinal and extended abdominal field radiation experienced decreased testicular volume, abnormal germ cell function, and elevated FSH levels.[84] Generally, shielding the testicle results in a mean dose of less than 44 cGy to the testicle. Thus, for those not requiring primary testicular irradiation, adequate testicular shielding may alleviate the sequelae of infertility.[85]

The majority of men treated by external beam for prostate cancer have temporary or permanent impotence. Impotence is believed to be caused by fibrosis of pelvic vasculature or radiation damage of pelvic nerves. In addition to impotence, patients experience decreased frequency of ejaculation and libido. Those who receive irradiation to the whole pelvis are likely to experience more severe side effects.[86] Interstitial therapy appears to decrease the incidence of impotence even in those with prior prostate surgery provided the patient received a bilateral nerve-sparing procedure. Newer radiation delivery methods, such as three-dimensional conformal radiation therapy, and use of smaller radiation therapy ports have decreased the incidence of impotence in patients with prostate cancer.[87–90] In addition to difficulty in gaining or maintaining an erection, a decreased libido, inability to ejaculate, inability to lubricate, inability to achieve orgasm or reduced intensity of orgasm, and decreased sexual pleasure are common findings in men who receive radiation to the pelvis.

Along with direct assaults to sexual and reproductive function by radiation therapy, the general side effects and accompanying psychological effects frequently can alter sexual function. Severe fatigue can limit all activity. Nausea, vomiting, and diarrhea can decrease energy, sexual desire, and feelings of desirability and can interfere with a sense of general well-being. Inflammation, pain, and limited range of motion may make sexual activities difficult or impossible. In addition to physical limitations, fear, depression, anxiety, stress, body image alterations, and lowered self-esteem may be additional burdens.[91] The appropriate use of energy-conserving strategies, medications, lubricants, dilators, prostheses, time, and counseling may alleviate side effects, promote a sense of well-being, and improve sexual function.

Chemotherapy

Chemotherapy-induced reproductive and sexual dysfunction is related to the type of drug, dose, length of treatment, age and sex of the individual receiving treatment, and length of time after therapy. In addition, the use of combination therapy, with multiple agents and drugs given to combat side effects of chemotherapy, also plays a role in infertility or sexual dysfunction.

Infertility and sterility after chemotherapy have been noted since the early 1970s, with reports of amenorrhea and azoospermia after single-agent or combination therapy.[92] Adult men are more likely to experience long-term side effects regardless of age, whereas women are more apt to have permanent cessation of menses as they near age 40.[93,94] The principal drugs that induce infertility are the alkylating agents, but others have been implicated, in particular, cytosine arabinoside, 5-fluorouracil, vinblastine, vincristine, cisplatin, and procarbazine. Combinations of these drugs appear to prolong infertility[95–99] (Table 37-1).

Men

Infertility occurs in men primarily through depletion of the germinal epithelium that lines the seminiferous

Table 37-1 Chemotherapeutic Agents Affecting Sexual or Reproductive Function

Agent	Complication
ALKYLATING AGENTS	
Altretamine	Amenorrhea, oligospermia, azoospermia, decreased libido, ovarian dysfunction, erectile dysfunction
Busulfan	
Chlorambucil	
Cisplatin	
Cyclophosphamide	
Ifosfamide	
Melphalan	
Nitrogen mustard	
ANTIMETABOLITES	
Cytosine arabinoside	As for alkylating agents
Fludarabine phosphate	
5-Fluorouracil	
Methotrexate	
ANTITUMOR ANTIBIOTICS	
Dactinomycin	As for alkylating agents
Daunorubicin	
Doxorubicin	
Plicamycin	
PLANT PRODUCTS	
Vinblastine	Decreased libido, ovarian dysfunction, erectile dysfunction
Vincristine	Retrograde ejaculation, erectile dysfunction
MISCELLANEOUS AGENTS	
Aminoglutethimide	Irregular menses, acne
Androgens	Masculinization (women)
Antiandrogens	Decreased libido, impotence
Antiestrogens	Gynecomastia, impotence
Corticosteroids	Transient impotence
Estrogens	Gynecomastia, acne
Goserelin acetate	Impotence
Interferons	Amenorrhea, pelvic pain
Procarbazine	As for alkylating agents
Progestins	Menstrual abnormalities, change in libido, masculinization (women)

Data from Schilsky and Erlichman[93]; Wilkes et al[95]; Langhorne[96]; Glasel[97]; Guy and Ingram[98]; Martin et al.[99]

tubules. On testicular biopsy, the interstitial Leydig cells appear normal, whereas the tubules are abnormal, contain Sertoli cells, and have depleted or absent germinal epithelium. Clinically, testicular volume decreases, oligospermia or azoospermia occurs, and infertility results.[100] Following drug-induced azoospermia, the process of spermatogenesis must start all over, as if the patient were going through puberty. Initially, the germ stem cell must repopulate the testicle, then spermatogenesis should occur. This process may take several years.[101]

Single-agent and combination chemotherapy have been reported to cause germinal aplasia, with alkylating agents the most extensively studied. Cumulative doses of greater than 400 mg/m² of cisplatin have been associated with irreversible damage to gonadal function.[102] Stoter et al evaluated 48 men with testicular cancer who had been treated with platinum, vinblastine, bleomycin (PVB) plus maintenance chemotherapy.[103] With a minimum follow-up of seven years, 40% of participants reported a negative alteration in sexual life, with 21% experiencing decreased sexual desire, 8% experiencing erectile dysfunction, and 15% experiencing ejaculatory dysfunction. Fertility may improve with time, however, and there are reports of slow recovery of spermatogenesis, culminating with the ability to father children, in patients who had initially been rendered azoospermic or oligospermic following combination chemotherapy for testicular cancer.[104–106]

Hormonal manipulation and treatment with estrogens are well known as a cause of sexual dysfunction. The majority of patients who receive androgen-ablative therapy experience a major reduction in interest in sexual intercourse and are unable to attain or maintain an erection.[107] In some instances, the addition of finasteride has been shown to maintain potency while also maintaining the androgen-abalative effect.[108] Gynecomastia and decreases in libido, sexual excitement, and the ability to achieve sexual fulfillment are significant problems.[95,98]

Additional side effects of chemotherapy include partial or total impotence, ejaculatory difficulties, and decreased desire, arousal, and orgasmic ability. Sexual dysfunction may be related to chemotherapy-induced angiopathy, particularly with drug regimens that contain cisplatin, vinblastine, and bleomycin sulfate.[109] Semen cryopreservation prior to initial therapy should be considered for all men interested in fathering a child.

Women

Women experience sexual and reproductive dysfunction from chemotherapy as a result of hormonal alterations or direct effects that cause ovarian fibrosis and follicle destruction. Previous sexual health may also play a role. Follicle-stimulating hormone and LH levels are elevated and estradiol is decreased, leading to amenorrhea, menopausal symptoms, dyspareunia, and vaginal atrophy and dryness.[95,100,110]

Like men, women experience reproductive dysfunction from both single-agent and combination chemother-apy; however, age appears to play a more significant role in infertility in women than in men, with women younger than 30 years able to tolerate much higher doses of chemotherapy without resultant permanent amenorrhea and premature menopause.[111,112] Amenorrhea has been noted in women with breast cancer treated with daily doses of cyclophosphamide and in women with Hodgkin's disease or breast cancer treated with combination chemotherapy, particularly when the regimen contains an alkylating agent.[95,111,113] Permanent amenorrhea may be evident by cessation of therapy but often occurs gradually over time.[112] In an analysis of nine studies, Chapman concluded that amenorrhea occurred more commonly in women older than 40 and that ovarian failure correlated most closely to that seen in women treated solely with cyclophosphamide.[101] Additionally, Chapman postulates that ovarian dysfunction occurs at all ages but is more reported and diagnosed in women closer to menopause.

It appears that any combination of drugs containing an alkylating agent is apt to cause infertility, and as women near menopause, permanent cessation of menses is more likely. When hormonal manipulation includes androgens, not only sexual and reproductive function but also body image and feelings of sexual identity are affected. Chemotherapy contributes significantly to sexual dysfunction not only through menopausal symptoms but also through increased risk of urinary tract infections and candidal infections, vaginal irritation, exacerbations of genital herpes and human papillomavirus, and alterations in desire and arousal due to decreases in circulating androgens. In addition, the use of hormonal therapies, such as tamoxifen and aminoglutethimide, have been associated with menopausal symptoms and decreased sexual desire.[95,110,114–116] Appropriate support and counseling should be provided.

Children

The effect of chemotherapy on gonadal function in children has been extensively studied.[117,118] Primary effects include delayed sexual maturation and alterations in reproductive potential. While the effects of chemotherapy are different in girls and boys, the primary effects appear to be age-related. Prepubescent boys seem to be minimally affected by chemotherapy and progress into and through puberty without major difficulty.[118] Young men treated during puberty, however, appear to be more likely to have gonadal dysfunction, with profound effects on both germ cell production and Leydig cell function, resulting in increases in FSH and LH and a decrease in testosterone levels.[80,101] It should be noted, however, that because the reserve supply of spermatogonia in young men is much smaller than in adults, chemotherapy has the potential to significantly alter spermatogenesis. This cannot be easily assessed until puberty.[101] The majority of girls treated with combination therapy appear to have normal ovarian function; however, long-term follow-up is needed to assess whether these individuals will experience premature menopause.[101,118]

Other issues

Drugs used to manage chemotherapy side effects can alter sexual function. Impotence, decreased sexual desire, decreased sense of sexual fulfillment, and decreased ability to achieve orgasm all have been associated with these agents (Table 37-2).[92,95,97,119]

Biological Response Modifiers

Although frequently used in the adjuvant setting and for treatment of earlier stage disease, biological response

Table 37-2 Cancer-Associated Drugs That Affect Sexual and Reproductive Function

Agent	Complication
ANTIDEPRESSANTS	
Amitriptyline	Impotence, altered libido
Clonazepam	
Imipramine	
Selective serotonin reuptake inhibitors (SSRIs)	
ANTIEMETICS/SEDATIVES/TRANQUILIZERS	
Chlorpromazine	Sedation, orgasm without ejaculation, impotence, decreased sexual interest, decreased intensity of orgasm, gynecomastia
Diazepam	
Lorazepam	
Metoclopramide	
Prochlorperazine	
Scopolamine	
ANTIHISTAMINES	
Diphenhydramine	Sedation, decreased sexual interest
NARCOTICS	
Codeine	Decreased libido, sedation, impaired potency
Fentanyl	
Hydromorphone	
Morphine	
STEROIDS	
See Table 37-1	
MISCELLANEOUS	
Cimetidine	Impotence
Dronabinol	Altered libido, sedation
Ketoconazole	Decreased libido

Data from Schilsky and Erlichman[93]; Wilkes et al[95]; Glasel.[97]

modifiers (BRMs) have not yet been studied sufficiently with regard to their sexual side effects. Rieger noted that most changes in sexuality are related to known BRM side effects, including fatigue, mucous membrane dryness, flulike symptoms, and body image changes.[120] Some information is available on the use of the interferons, in particular alfa-interferon, alone or in combination with other agents. Decreased libido, amenorrhea, pelvic pain, uterine bleeding, and erectile dysfunction have been reported with alfa-interferon, and animals exposed to all interferons have demonstrated an increased rate of spontaneous abortion.[95,121] Additionally, the retinoids have been associated with spontaneous abortion and fetal malformation.[122] In addition to drug-induced dysfunction, the usual side effects of fatigue and flulike symptoms affect interest in and comfort with sexual activities. No studies are available for the use of BRMs in human pregnancy and lactation; information often is extrapolated from animal data. Currently, the use of these agents in pregnancy and while lactating is contraindicated. Research on the subject of gonadal dysfunction related to BRMs is extremely important.

Stem Cell and Marrow Transplantation

As long-term survival from transplantation increases, issues related to sexuality and sexual dysfunction have become more evident. The late effects of bone marrow transplantation (BMT) include chronic fatigue, body image alterations, gonadal dysfunction, and infertility. Women experience decreased sexual desire and satisfaction, vaginal atrophy and decreased vaginal lubrication, and painful intercourse, as well as feelings of loss of femininity.[123] Men frequently experience premature ejaculation due to prolonged abstinence, while long-term consequences include decreased desire, body image alterations, and impotence or erectile difficulties.[124] The germ-free environment and long hospitalization required with transplantation can affect sexuality and intimacy due to lack of privacy and limited physical contact. Additionally, lack of energy and chronic fatigue impede normal activities in up to 50% of all patients who receive transplants.[125] The combination of high-dose chemotherapy and total body irradiation (TBI) exacerbates sexually-related side effects.[123]

Primary gonadal dysfunction has been described in all transplant patients, whether or not the patients received TBI. Recovery of gonadal function is rare in both men and women (<10%) and is related to age, and the use of TBI and combination versus single-agent chemotherapy.[123,126] Still, successful pregnancy has been reported following transplantation. Increasing age and the use of TBI seemed most integral to the inability to conceive or father a child.[127] Assisted reproduction techniques have been shown to benefit those desiring a child following transplant.[128]

Numerous authors have investigated quality of life in survivors of BMT.[129–132] Decreased energy and moderate to severe fatigue were experienced by more than 50% of BMT survivors up to ten years after transplant.[125,129,130] Other major concerns included infertility, inability to perform sexually, and alterations in sexual intimacy, pleasure, and the ability to achieve orgasm and an erection.[129,130] Sexual and reproductive implications of treatment should be discussed and counseling provided prior to, throughout, and following treatment.

Therapeutic Approaches and Nursing Care

Sexual Counseling

All patients should receive information about the possible side effects of disease and treatment on sexuality and reproduction. Potential side effects include alterations in physical function and libido, menopausal symptoms, problems with erection and ejaculation, and infertility. Patients deserve the opportunity to have their sexual problems thoughtfully identified, and good communication among all parties is essential.[133] Potential side effects and possible methods for management should be discussed with the patient (and partner if available) at diagnosis, throughout treatment, and during follow-up visits.

In order to effectively assess a patient for alterations in sexuality, the nurse must understand the patient's medical, psychiatric, and psychosexual status, evaluate present relationships, and provide recommendations and encouragement.[134] Nurses should include sexuality in their assessment of all patients and should provide hope, reassurance, and basic information.[12] Potential methods for assessment of sexual dysfunction include the use of the ALARM model and the model proposed by Auchincloss (Table 37-3).[56,134]

Once sexual functioning has been assessed, interventions are necessary to maintain optimal sexual functioning and to promote adaptation to the sexual and reproductive side effects of disease and treatment. Interventions should include the patient's partner whenever possible. The PLISSIT model is another method of intervention (Table 37-4). This model can help the majority of patients without the need for intensive therapy.[135] In order to maintain integrity and to improve quality of life,

Table 37-3 Evaluation of Sexual Dysfunction

ALARM Model	Auchincloss Model
A– Activity (sexual)	Evaluate sexual status:
L– Libido/desire	Present sexual function
	Past experiences
A– Arousal and orgasm	Relationships
R– Resolution/release	Evaluate medical, psychological,
M– Medical data	and cancer status

Data from Anderson and Lamb[56]; Auchincloss.[134]

Table 37-4 PLISSIT Model for Intervention

P – Permission

LI – Limited information

SS – Specific suggestions

IT – Intensive therapy

Data from Annon.[135]

it is essential that all patients receive counseling about sexual dysfunction, that open communication be encouraged, and that interventions be individualized and valued by the participants.

Nursing Assessment and Management

Not every nurse can be a sexual counselor; however, listening to concerns of patient and family, presenting factual information in a nonthreatening manner, managing noncomplex disease- and treatment-related symptoms, and providing appropriate referrals can be easily incorporated into routine care. Many health care providers rarely discuss issues related to sexual and reproductive concerns for a variety of personal and professional reasons. Primary reasons cited include personal discomfort, lack of training or knowledge, and fears of embarrassing themselves or their patients. Additional reasons include lack of time, concerns about the appropriateness of such discussions when dealing with a life-threatening illness, and the belief that these subjects are not part of the nurse's job description.[3,136,137]

Although not always accurately portrayed, sexuality is more than the act of intercourse. It includes intimacy, touching, a multitude of activities to show affection, and a variety of methods to communicate with others. Cancer and treatment may disrupt or permanently alter one's ability to maintain previous sexual patterns or may cause infertility; however, cancer cannot alter the fact that one is a sexual being. This information needs to be reiterated and reinforced to the patient and family.[3,136]

Assisting patients and families with sexual alterations is congruent with and integral to the nurse's role in providing holistic care. There are many simple, easy-to-follow methods; however, in order for nurses to provide assistance, they must understand their own sexual identity, what constitutes acceptable sexual patterns and practices, as well as the sociocultural, environmental, and other beliefs that may impact how the nurse interacts with others as sexual beings.[3,15,78,79,136–141]

Asking about the patient's sexual practices early in the clinical assessment legitimizes and normalizes the subject and gives patients permission to discuss sexual issues. Current practices, cultural and religious beliefs, and general intimacy issues should be incorporated in the discussion. Additionally, whenever possible and appropriate, the patient's partner should be included. Medical jargon and value-oriented terminology should be avoided, and questions and responses should acknowledge the subject and related concerns as being normal and important.[3,58,136–142]

Nurses must provide factual information about disease, treatment, and potential side effects. Discussing potential alterations in sexual functioning, including fertility issues, prior to or early in treatment and continuing these discussions well into the follow-up phase is essential. Information is needed to dispel myths, decrease anxiety, minimize embarrassment, provide a basis for alternative strategies, and open lines of communication between the patient and others.[3,136,137,139,141,142]

Managing the side effects of cancer and treatment is also integral to the nurse's role. Offering simple suggestions and appropriately managing side effects may be sufficient for most patients to continue or reinstitute sexual activities and enhance intimacy. In addition to management of such traditional symptoms as pain, nausea, vomiting, and bone marrow depression, nurses should provide information and strategies about the importance of communication and openness; the need for exercise, rest, and adequate nutrition; the use of contraception; setting the stage for sexual activities (candles, music, sexy clothing); experimentation with alternative methods of intimacy and the liberal and adequate use of lubricants, foreplay, and more comfortable positions. Energy conservation techniques and information on the timing of medications and methods to maintain cleanliness and personal hygiene are also important.[3,15,58,79,136–141]

Finally, knowing when to make referrals and recognizing appropriate community resources are essential. Areas of referral include hormonal therapies, vacuum devices or medications to manage erectile dysfunction, sperm banking and other fertility-preserving options, and reconstructive surgery and prostheses. Some patients will require psychosexual counseling; others will not. Individualization of education and counseling is important for each patient. It is crucial that the nurse (or others) not invent sexual concerns for those who do not have them; rather, the nurse anticipates, recognizes, advocates, and assists those who do.

Fertility Considerations and Procreative Alternatives

Fertility and pregnancy following cancer diagnosis are fraught with a multitude of concerns, particularly the ability to conceive, carry to term, and deliver a healthy newborn with no congenital abnormalities and no increased risk for future malignancies because of either parent's previous diagnosis and treatment for cancer. Radiation therapy and chemotherapy, alone or in combination, have the potential to induce infertility. Proved fertility is measured by pregnancy rates and even when fertility is preserved, conception may be delayed. Information about procreative alternatives, the potential for infertility, and issues related to genetic inheritance, mutagenicity, and timing of pregnancy must be thoroughly discussed with potential parents prior to their attempting conception.[143,144]

Mutagenicity

Mutagenicity is the ability to cause an abnormality in the genetic content of cells, resulting in cell death, alteration(s) in growth and replication, or no noticeable alteration in cell function. Possible germ cell mutations may not be evident for generations of offspring.[145]

Numerous researchers have investigated the offspring of individuals exposed to chemotherapy or radiation therapy as children, adolescents, or young adults as a method to adequately assess mutagenicity following therapy.[101,146–149] While several specific instances of fetal wasting or congenital malformations, such as an increase in first pregnancy miscarriages[146] and congenital cardiac abnormalities,[147,148] were identified, no statistical difference in congenital malformations, still births, or low birth weights was seen.[146–150] Additionally, chromosome analyses of offspring of parents treated for Hodgkin's disease were normal,[149] and no increased risk of genetic disease was identified in more than 4500 children of adult survivors of childhood cancer.[151] In all studies, it has been difficult to specifically implicate germ cell mutations as the cause of adverse outcomes of pregnancy. Follow-up over several generations of patients and their offspring will be needed before definitive answers are obtained.

Teratogenicity

Teratogenicity is the ability of a toxic compound to produce alterations in an exposed fetus. Both chemotherapy and radiation therapy are known to have teratogenic effects on the fetus, causing spontaneous abortion, fetal malformation, or fetal death, especially during the first trimester. Low-dose radiation has also been implicated in fetal malignancy.[152–154]

Radiation exposure during the first trimester represents the greatest risk to the fetus, with exposure of 100 cGy or more resulting in fetal death, microcephaly, eye anomalies, and intrauterine growth retardation. In the second or third trimester, fetal death is unlikely, but growth retardation, sterility, and cataracts are common findings.[154]

Chemotherapy, particularly when received during the first trimester, has been related to congenital abnormalities, with approximately 10% of fetuses experiencing some type of anomaly. In general, the alkylating agents and antimetabolites have been most often associated with fetal malformations. Chemotherapy during the second or third trimester may cause premature birth or low birth weights, but congenital abnormalities are not increased over the incidence with normal pregnancy.[152,155–157] The timing of chemotherapy is critical. Chemotherapy given prior to the fifth week of gestation is most likely to result in spontaneous abortion if severe damage to the blastocyst occurs. Between the fifth and twelfth week, structural damage is most common and congenital malformations occur.

After the twelfth week, fetal growth restriction is most common. Additionally, effects also are related to drug dose, length of exposure, frequency of administration, and type and number of drugs administered[156] (Table 37-5).

Reproductive Counseling

Discussions concerning fertility and reproduction issues need to be held prior to the onset of therapy and should continue well into posttreatment and follow-up. Current fertility status, desire for future childbearing, and contra-

Table 37-5 Teratogenetic Effects of Chemotherapy

Agent	Complication
ALKYLATING AGENTS	
Altretamine	Spontaneous abortions Skeletal malformations
Busulfan	Spontaneous abortions Skeletal malformations
Chlorambucil	Spontaneous abortions Skeletal malformations
Cyclophosphamide	Spontaneous abortions Skeletal malformations
Ifosfamide	Spontaneous abortions Skeletal malformations
Nitrogen mustard	Spontaneous abortions Skeletal malformations
Nitrosoureas	Spontaneous abortions Skeletal malformations
ANTIMETABOLITES	
Cytosine arabinoside	Spontaneous abortions Skeletal malformations
5-Fluorouracil	Spontaneous abortions Skeletal malformations
6-Mercaptopurine	Spontaneous abortions Skeletal malformations
Methotrexate	Spontaneous abortions Skeletal malformations
MISCELLANEOUS AGENTS	
Daunorubicin	Spontaneous abortions
Glucocorticoids	Spontaneous abortions
Hydroxyurea	Spontaneous abortions
Procarbazine	Atrial/septal defects
Retinoids	Spontaneous abortions, malformations
Thalidomide	Skeletal malformations
Vinblastine	Spontaneous abortions

Data from Wilkes et al[95]; Glasel[97]; Rieger[122]; Green et al[148]; Robinson and Krebs[152]; Barnicle.[155]

ception practices should be investigated during the initial assessment. Potential alterations should be openly discussed and referrals made as appropriate. Counseling for possible risks of mutagenicity, increased cancer risk, and unknown sequelae of treatment for progeny should be included.[144,158,159] Birth control methods need to be implemented to minimize the possibility of an unplanned pregnancy during therapy. In addition, methods to maintain fertility during therapy should be investigated.

For those receiving radiation therapy, appropriate shielding of the testes or ovaries or oophoropexy to position the ovaries outside the radiation field may be of benefit.[77,159,160] Birth control pills in women and GnRH analogs in men have been postulated to protect the germ cells from damage by chemotherapeutic agents. To date, no study has shown benefit in treating men with GnRH analogs, however some benefit has been shown in animal studies.[161] Studies in these areas continue.

Because it is often difficult to predict when an individual receiving chemotherapy is infertile, it is extremely important that methods to prevent pregnancy are discussed and appropriate drugs or devices provided. It has also been suggested that following cancer therapy an individual should wait a minimum of 2 years before attempting conception. This suggestion is made both to prevent pregnancy during the time recurrence is most likely and to allow for the recovery of spermatogenesis or ovarian function if it has been temporarily altered by therapy.[152,162] It should be noted, however, that this time frame may be too long for some women at risk for early menopause and that no benefit is known to be derived from a prolonged waiting time.[143,153]

Semen Cryopreservation and Sperm Recovery

Semen storage for use in artificial insemination has been available for many years. Although initially used to establish pregnancy in infertile couples, sperm banking has more recently been used to preserve procreation abilities in men undergoing cancer therapy. Unfortunately, the option to bank sperm will not be available to every man undergoing cancer therapy. Many men will be subfertile or infertile at the time of diagnosis, particularly those with testis cancer or Hodgkin's disease.[163,164] In addition, although newer techniques, such as mapping and fine-needle aspiration of the testis to recover sperm after treatment,[160] are being investigated, sperm banking is most effective when completed prior to initiation of therapy. Thus, anyone with rapidly progressing disease frequently cannot delay the start of therapy to complete the cryopreservation process. Still, cryopreservation of sperm has provided a viable option for improving fertility prospects in men with various forms of cancer,[112,163,165,166] and any semen sample that contains even one motile or viable sperm can be preserved.[160]

Even if artificial insemination is never completed, the knowledge that semen has been banked and is available when needed can provide a significant psychological boost for the male undergoing cancer therapy.[165,167] All aspects of the sperm-banking process, from initial visit through the completion of insemination, should be fully discussed with the patient so that informed decisions can be made.

For those who have maintained some degree of fertility but experience retrograde ejaculation, a trial of a sympathomimetic agent may prove beneficial. If this procedure is not helpful, sperm can be harvested from urine, washed, and used for insemination. For true ejaculation, a rectal probe that electrically stimulates the vas deferens, seminal vesicle, and prostate to initiate the ejaculatory reflex may be of benefit. In addition, some men will benefit from sperm aspiration from the vas deferens or epididymis, followed by *intracytoplasmic sperm injection* (ICSI) in which a single sperm is injected into a single egg. Scientists also are investigating the potential for restoration of spermatogenesis through transplantation of the male germ cell.[160]

In Vitro Fertilization/Embryo Transfer

In vitro fertilization (IVF)—used for male infertility due to low sperm counts or for female infertility due to severe endometriosis, immunological infertility, or absent or damaged fallopian tubes—has undergone remarkable technological advances, with more than 30,000 fertilization cycles undertaken each year.[168] In vitro fertilization requires ovarian stimulation followed by ova retrieval via ultrasound-guided needle aspiration of the preovulatory follicles. Laparoscopy also may be used. The retrieved oocytes are then incubated with sperm for 5–26 hours. Following incubation, the embryos are transferred to the uterus and released. Successful pregnancy rates are approximately 20%. Human embryo cryopreservation has been used for more than 15 years and is now considered to be a routine procedure. The process of retrieval is the same. For those who used both fresh and cryopreserved embryos, the successful pregnancy rate increased by 8%.[169] In addition, the use of ICSI has increased the rate of successful fertilization, thereby increasing the potential for a successful pregnancy.[160,164,166]

Now that cryopreservation of embryos is routine, researchers are investigating new techniques to cryopreserve oocytes that could later be autotransplanted into the infertile woman or isolated and allowed to mature in vitro. Concerns about the best method for implantation and the potential for reintroduction of malignant cells have impacted use, however thawed oocytes appear to be viable and the procedure promising. Currently, it appears that in vitro maturation followed by ICSI and IVF will be most beneficial.[170–172]

Pregnancy and Cancer

Although pregnancy complicated by a diagnosis of cancer is a rare event, it creates multiple problems for all con-

cerned. Uncertainty about the prognosis of mother and fetus, the rigors of treatment, and the long-term sequelae of cancer for patient, infant, and family compound events that normally are surrounded by a myriad of conflicting emotions. Only with comprehensive care by many health care and ancillary individuals can a positive outcome for mother, fetus, and family be anticipated.

Cancer is the second-leading cause of death during the reproductive years. It is estimated that cancer complicates about 1 in 1000 pregnancies and that approximately 1 in 118 women with cancer also have a concomitant pregnancy. The most commonly associated cancers are lymphoma, leukemia, malignant melanoma, and cancers of the breast, cervix, ovary, and colorectum—the cancers most common during the reproductive years.[173,174]

In general, most cancers do not adversely affect a pregnancy, nor does the pregnancy adversely affect the cancer outcome, although it is possible that the treatment necessary to manage the cancer may have an adverse effect on the pregnancy. Therapeutic abortion has not been shown to be of benefit in altering disease progression and should not be considered unless continued pregnancy will compromise treatment and thus prognosis. The wishes of the patient and family must be considered, with therapeutic options, including prognosis for mother and fetus, being fully explained.

It was previously believed that cancer associated with pregnancy was more aggressive and that the outcome for all patients was dismal. It is now recognized that delay in diagnoses may be a more likely cause of advanced disease at the time of diagnosis. Diagnosing cancer during a pregnancy is difficult, and signs and symptoms of the disease may be misconstrued or underestimated. Treatment options should be evaluated as though the patient were not pregnant and therapy instituted when appropriate.[152,162,173,175]

Medical Management of Commonly Associated Cancers

Breast cancer

Breast cancer is the cancer most commonly associated with pregnancy, occurring in 1 of every 3000 pregnancies.[162,176–178] Among all women with breast cancer who are still in their childbearing years, one in three will be pregnant at the time of diagnosis.[152,173]

Breast examination should be part of the initial prenatal visit. Although breast enlargement during pregnancy makes examination difficult, it is essential that all women have a thorough examination. If the woman does not practice breast self-examination (BSE), BSE education should be included. If a mass is felt, prompt evaluation is necessary. Although a mammogram is difficult to interpret because of density of the breast, it may be safely undertaken if appropriate fetal shielding is used.[179] Even if a mammogram shows negative results, a breast mass must be investigated until a definitive diagnosis is made.[176,180–184]

Treatment of breast cancer in the pregnant woman should be the same as in the nonpregnant woman. Initial diagnosis should be attempted by fine-needle aspiration, followed by open biopsy if a definitive diagnosis cannot be made.[176] Biopsy with the patient under local anesthesia has not been shown to cause fetal harm and should be performed without delay.[180,181,185] Once a definitive diagnosis is made, further therapy can be tailored to time of gestation, physician recommendations, and patient wishes. In general, modified mastectomy with lymph node sampling is the standard treatment for early disease. Depending on gestational age, adjuvant chemotherapy can often be delayed until after delivery. For the woman desiring breast-conserving surgery, lumpectomy with lymph node sampling may be done if she is close to term, but radiation therapy and chemotherapy will be delayed until delivery. For advanced disease, surgery and chemotherapy should be undertaken without delay. Therapeutic abortion may be suggested during the first trimester in order to prevent chemotherapy exposure to the fetus.[176,180,181,185–187] Chances for survival have been considered poor, with reports of 30%–57% survival rates.[183] However, when patients are matched stage for stage with nonpregnant control subjects, there appear to be no differences in survival rates.[183,188] Delay in diagnosis, often for more than 3 months may be the most important factor leading to decreased survival.

Pregnancy safety following cancer treatment has been extensively evaluated, particularly for women treated for breast cancer. There appears to be no decrease in survival for women who become pregnant following breast cancer treatment.[153,189–195] It even is possible that a further pregnancy may actually protect against recurrence. However, it may be that there are inherent differences between those able to conceive and those unable to conceive, thus altering the survival statistics for this population.[196,197] While increasing, the number of reported pregnancies remains small and thus most likely represents a select and nongeneralizable subset of women with breast cancer. For those desiring future pregnancies, a wait of from 1–5 years following cessation of all treatment, including adjuvant tamoxifen, is recommended.[176,177,194,197] Those who are known to be *BRCA1* positive should consider genetic counseling prior to attempting conception.[198]

Breast-feeding after breast cancer diagnosis also has been highly debated. For the woman who has received primary breast radiation, it has been suggested that breast-feeding occur only on the nonirradiated side, primarily because of the possible increase in mastitis associated with breast-feeding in the irradiated breast but also due to diminished or absent lactation.[177,178,193] Pregnancy subsequent to breast irradiation often results in breast asymmetry, with little enlargement of the irradiated breast and minimal to no lactation from the radiated side.[189]

Cancer of the cervix

The second most common cancer during pregnancy is cancer of the cervix, which occurs in 1 in 400 pregnancies.

Approximately 1 in every 100 women diagnosed with cervical cancer will be pregnant at the time of diagnosis. Carcinoma in situ is most commonly found, with invasive disease seen in only 2%–5% of all patients. Signs and symptoms of cervical cancer are similar to those found in the nonpregnant patient, with the majority of pregnant patients experiencing vaginal bleeding or discharge.[199] Diagnosis is most commonly made by Papanicolaou smear. If the smear is abnormal, colposcopy with appropriate biopsies should be undertaken. Cone biopsy is rarely indicated but may be used to confirm a diagnosis of microinvasion. However, it is not without risks and is associated with a 30% complication rate, including hemorrhage, premature delivery, and infection.[51,62,152,200] More recently, loop electrode excision has been proposed to minimize the potential complications of conization; however, loop excision does not appear to improve disease-free surgical margins and is associated with an increased incidence of cervical hemorrhage.[200] Laser vaporization may be of benefit but has not been tested in pregnancy. Of importance is the fact that it does not impact subsequent pregnancies as is common with conization.[201]

For carcinoma in situ, the pregnancy may be allowed to continue. Biopsy should be repeated every 6–8 weeks and, unless there is progression, definitive therapy delayed until after delivery. If frank invasion is found, treatment consistent with standard practice for nonpregnant women should not be delayed. During the first two trimesters, surgery or radiation therapy without therapeutic abortion is usually undertaken. Early stage disease (IA and IB) may be treated with radical hysterectomy and pelvic lymph node dissection, while in advanced disease, radiation therapy is the most common treatment. During the third trimester, fetal viability usually can be awaited and the baby can be delivered by cesarean section, after which the appropriate cancer therapy is given.[51,199,202–205]

Controversy exists over the safety of vaginal delivery. In reviewing the current literature, Nevin et al found that many believed vaginal delivery would disseminate the cancer or cause hemorrhage or infection[204]; thus, cesarean section was recommended. Others have suggested that vaginal delivery actually may be associated with an improved overall survival and should be allowed if possible. Recurrence in the episiotomy has been reported following vaginal delivery.[206] Careful follow-up for recurrence is essential. The definitive approach remains unclear.

Ovarian cancer

Ovarian masses are common during pregnancy, occurring once in every 81 pregnancies. In general, only 2%–5% of these are malignant, for an estimated 1:9000 to 1:25,000 case ratio. Most patients are asymptomatic, with an adnexal mass noted at the first prenatal visit.[152,207] There are a variety of ways to approach a pelvic mass during pregnancy, including the use of ultrasonography and magnetic resonance imaging.[207,208] In general, any mass that is unilateral, greater than 6 cm, solid, and lasts into the second trimester must be evaluated.[207,209]

If malignancy is diagnosed, treatment should proceed as in the nonpregnant woman. Early disease (stage IA) of low-grade histological findings can be managed by unilateral oophorectomy and biopsy of the other ovary. The pregnancy may be allowed to continue. For all other stages, standard therapy of radical hysterectomy, omentectomy, node biopsy, and peritoneal washings should be carried out. If the woman is near term, a cesarean section, followed by the appropriate therapy, may be performed. Unfortunately, 30%–50% of all women will be diagnosed with stage III or IV disease. Although recent management of stage III disease has resulted in improved survival, in general the prognosis for long-term survival is poor.[51,207,210] As in the treatment of all cancers, the wishes of the patient must be considered. It is not uncommon for a pregnant woman with advanced disease to delay treatment until the fetus is viable. Palliative treatment should be instituted at the earliest possible time.

Malignant melanoma

Malignant melanoma is one of the most rapidly increasing cancers. It occurs most often in a preexisting mole in fair-haired individuals with blue or green eyes and an inability to tan when exposed to the sun; the peak incidence is during the third and fourth decades. At least 35% of women diagnosed with melanoma will be in their childbearing years.[211,212]

Melanoma arising during pregnancy has been postulated to be associated with poor prognosis because it is hormonally influenced and thus exacerbated by pregnancy. At present this has yet to be definitely proved. What is known is that melanoma that occurs during pregnancy more often is found on the trunk, a site associated with a poor prognosis.[211] Also, these melanomas tend to be thicker, also synonymous with a poor prognosis.[213] In addition, all pigmented areas darken during pregnancy, making diagnosis of early changes more difficult. Biopsy and removal of questionable lesions are indicated. There appears to be no difference in survival between the pregnant and nonpregnant woman with melanoma.[211,214,215]

Treatment consists of wide excision with skin graft if necessary. Lymph node dissection remains controversial. Adjuvant therapy is being investigated, but no definite answers are available for the pregnant patient. The benefits of chemotherapy and BRMs remain unclear. However, while chemotherapy regimens can be safely administered during the second and third trimesters,[216] the adjuvant use of alfa-interferon should be delayed until postpartum due to increased fetal and maternal complications associated with high-dose regimens.[211] For individuals with advanced disease, therapeutic abortion followed by palliative chemotherapy is advised. For the individual with brain metastasis, surgery or radiation therapy with appropriate fetal shielding may be undertaken.

Malignant melanoma is known to metastasize to the placenta and fetus. The placenta should be carefully evaluated at delivery and the infant monitored for development of melanoma.[217-219] Further pregnancies should not be undertaken until at least 2 years after diagnosis and treatment.[220]

Lymphomas

Both non-Hodgkin's lymphoma (NHL) and Hodgkin's disease (HD) occur with pregnancy, although the incidence is rare, with HD occurring in 1 in 6000 pregnancies and NHL rarely associated.[221,222] Hodgkin's disease usually occurs as asymptomatic lymphadenopathy of the cervical, supraclavicular, or mediastinal regions. Disease confined to the neck or axilla usually can be treated with radiation therapy combined with fetal shielding. Because more extensive disease requires combination chemotherapy, a therapeutic abortion is suggested during the first half of pregnancy. During the last half of pregnancy, therapy will be defined by the stage of the pregnancy. If viability is imminent, therapy may be delayed or single-drug treatment instituted and delivery awaited. For rapidly progressing disease, combination chemotherapy should be instituted immediately.[221-223] Pregnancy does not appear to negatively impact the clinical course of HD.[224]

Fewer than 100 cases of NHL and pregnancy have been reported in the literature. In general, pregnant patients tend to be diagnosed later and have a poor prognosis with increased risk of relapse after remission.[225] Although NHL is known to metastasize to the placenta and fetus and thus requires careful observation at delivery, NHL has not developed in these infants.[226]

Leukemia

Leukemia occurs in 1 in 75,000 pregnancies. Diagnosis is often made on routine complete blood count. Treatment should be instituted immediately unless the fetus is viable or near viability. If the fetus is viable, delivery should not be delayed. If the fetus is near viability, leukapheresis may be utilized until delivery is possible. Combination chemotherapy has been administered safely in the second and third trimesters, with no increased incidence of neonatal birth defects.[227] Improved treatment and supportive care regimens have decreased the incidence of life-threatening complications and increased remission induction rates, thus initial survival of the pregnant woman and her fetus is common.[223] Therapeutic abortion is suggested in the first trimester to avoid fetal exposure to chemotherapy.[228,229]

Effects of Treatment and Malignancy on the Fetus

Surgery

Maternal surgery can be safely accomplished with minimal risk to the fetus.[51,207] Pelvic surgery is more easily accomplished during the second trimester. There is little risk to the fetus from short exposure to anesthetic agents after the first trimester. Adequate ventilation and prevention of hypotension are of prime importance. As long as competent surgeons and anesthesiologists with appropriate fetal monitoring equipment are available, no harm to the fetus should occur.[75,180,207]

Radiation

Radiation doses of greater than 250 cGy during pregnancy have been associated with fetal damage—for example, mental retardation, skin changes, and spontaneous abortions (depending on stage of gestation). Low doses of radiation associated with diagnostic x-ray studies (<0.5 cGy) are probably not harmful if adequate fetal shielding is provided.[179] Radiation to the pelvis should be avoided.[154,179,230] Long-term effects of low-dose radiation remain unknown, but the concerns of chromosomal aberrations and an increase in childhood cancer in children exposed in utero remain. Follow-up over many generations may be necessary to determine the exact effects.[51,231]

Chemotherapy

Chemotherapy has been administered prior to and concurrent with pregnancy. As previously noted, chemotherapy during the first trimester has been associated with fetal wastage, malformations, and low birth weights. Many studies indicate that the incidence of fetal malformations is low (<10%) and may be minimized or avoided with careful selection of agents. Latent effects are still unknown, and offspring need continuous evaluation. It is important to note that pharmacokinetics of chemotherapeutic agents may be altered by the normal physiological changes of pregnancy. Monitoring for unexpected toxicities or altered response patterns is of extreme importance. Additionally, evaluation of the fetus for toxicities from administration of drugs immediately prior to delivery is paramount. Both neonatal metabolism and drug excretion may be suboptimal, and the placenta, which is the normal mechanism for excretion, has been eliminated.[156,178,232]

Maternal-fetal spread

Only a few cancers spread from the mother to the fetus, with melanoma, NHL, and leukemia the most common. Because few series have been compiled, the exact incidence is unknown. Dildy et al reviewed cases of maternal malignancy metastatic to products of conception and reported on 53 cases.[233] The most common cancer was malignant melanoma. Metastasis to the placenta occurred in twelve patients and spread to the fetus in seven. The second most common were the hematological malignancies (leukemia and lymphoma), involving eight instances of placental spread and four cases of fetal spread. Breast and lung cancers were next; however, no cases of spread to the fetus have been reported. In most instances, there is spread to the placenta but no fetal involvement. Because of the rare incidence of metastatic involvement to the infant, evaluation of the placenta and fetus is essential in women with disseminated cancers.[178]

Nursing Management of the Pregnant Patient

Nursing management of the pregnant patient with a concomitant diagnosis of cancer can be extremely complicated. Interventions including psychosocial, educational, and ethical considerations must be developed and implemented. It has been suggested that pregnancy and cancer be treated as a high-risk event with all the associated needs.[173,178] Careful explanations of all aspects of care, with special emphasis on support of the patient and her family, need to be included. Normal activities of pregnancy may be delayed or prevented by disease or treatment, and fears of fetal demise, cancer therapy, and death may prevent resolution of ambivalence toward pregnancy and establishment of emotional affiliation to the growing child. Ethical considerations become apparent as plans for pregnancy are contrasted with needs for therapy. In some instances therapeutic abortion may be necessary for optimal treatment; in other instances therapy delays may be requested to provide for the safety of the fetus. Nonjudgmental care by health care personnel is essential during these difficult times.

Nursing care of the woman with cancer and her baby is extremely complex and of utmost importance. With a focus on educational interventions, psychological support, and coordination of care, the nurse has an important role in the final outcome. Treatment plans; coordination of follow-up; education about cancer, pregnancy, and treatment; and emotional support of the patient and significant others are integral components of the comprehensive care needed by the pregnant woman with cancer. Without these essential elements, it may not be possible to provide the necessary care for a positive or improved maternal and fetal outcome.

Conclusion

Sexual and reproductive dysfunction in patients with cancer occurs much more frequently than previously recognized. Almost every patient exposed to cancer or cancer treatment may experience some form of sexual dysfunction at some point during the illness. With cancer survival rates improving and with the understanding that sexual and reproductive function are important to all individuals, it is essential that sexuality and sexual function be assessed and evaluated prior to therapy and that appropriate interventions be implemented throughout treatment and the follow-up period.

References

1. Ganz PA: Current issues in cancer rehabilitation. *Cancer* 65:742–751, 1990
2. Anastasia PJ: Altered sexuality, in Carroll-Johnson RM, Gorman LM, Bush NJ (eds): *Psychosocial Nursing Care Along*

the Cancer Continuum. Pittsburgh, Oncology Nursing Press, 1998, pp 227–240

3. Nishimoto PW: Sexuality, in Gates RA, Fink RM (eds): *Oncology Nursing Secrets.* Philadelphia, Hanley & Belfus, 1997, pp 312–324

4, Guyton AC, Hall JE: *Human Physiology and Mechanism of Disease* (ed 6). Philadelphia, Saunders, 1997, pp 648–669

5. Marieb EN: *Human Anatomy and Physiology* (ed 5). Menlo Park, CA, Benjamin/Cummings, 1998, pp 1030–1077

6. Enker WE: Total mesorectal excision—The new golden standard of surgery for rectal cancer. *Ann Med* 29:127–133, 1997

7. Sprangers MAG, Taal BG, Aaronson NK, et al: Quality of life in colorectal cancer: Stoma vs. nonstoma patients. *Dis Colon Rectum* 38:361–369, 1995

8. Sugarbaker PH: Rectovaginal fistula following low circular stapled anastomosis in women with rectal cancer. *J Surg Oncol* 61:155–158, 1996

9. Sugihara K, Moriya Y, Akasu T, et al: Pelvic autonomic nerve preservation for patients with rectal carcinoma: Oncologic and functional outcome. *Cancer* 78:1871–1880, 1996

10. Dobkin KA, Broadwell DC: Nursing considerations for the patient undergoing colostomy surgery. *Semin Oncol Nurs* 2: 249–255, 1986

11. Andersen BL: How cancer affects sexual functioning. *Oncology* 4:81–88, 1990

12. Schrover LR: Sexual dysfunction, in Holland JC (ed): *Psychooncology.* New York, Oxford University Press, 1998, pp 494–499

13. Koukouras D, Spiliotis J, Scopa CD, et al: Radical consequence in the sexuality of male patients operated for colorectal carcinoma. *Eur J Surg Oncol* 17:285–288, 1991

14. Masui H, Ike H, Yamaguchi S, et al: Male sexual functioning after autonomic nerve-sparing operation for rectal cancer. *Dis Colon Rectum* 39:1140–1145, 1996

15. Ofman US: Preservation of function in genitourinary cancers: Psychosexual and psychosocial issues. *Cancer Invest* 13:125–131, 1995

16. Smith DB, Babaian RJ: The effects of treatment for cancer on male fertility and sexuality. *Cancer Nurs* 15:271–275, 1992

17. Ofman US: Psychosocial and sexual implications of genitourinary cancers. *Semin Oncol Nurs* 9:286–292, 1993

18. Bjerre BD, Johansen C, Steven K: Health-related quality of life after cystectomy: Bladder substitution compared with ileal conduit diversion. *Br J Urol* 75:200–205, 1995

19. Bjerre BD, Johansen C, Steven K: A questionnaire study of sexological problems following urinary diversion in the female patient. *Scan J Urol Nephrol* 31:155–160, 1997

20. Kelly LP, Miaskowski C: An overview of bladder cancer: Treatment and nursing interventions. *Oncol Nurs Forum* 23:459–468, 1996

21. Hautmann RE, Paiss T, de Petriconi R: The ileal neobladder in women: 9 years experience with 18 patients. *J Urol* 155:76–81, 1996

22. D'Ancona CA, Botega NJ, DeMoraes C, et al: Quality of life after partial penectomy for penile carcinoma. *Urology* 50:593–596, 1997

23. Dobkin PL, Bradley I: Assessment of sexual dysfunction in oncology patients: Review, critique, and suggestions. *J Psychosoc Oncol* 9:43–74, 1991

24. Tefilli MV, Dubocq F, Rajpurkar A, et al: Assessment of psychosexual adjustment after insertion of inflatable penile prosthesis. *Urology* 52:1106–1112, 1998

25. Nukui F, Okamoto S, Nagata M, et al: Complications and reimplantation of penile implants. *Int J Urol* 4:52–54, 1997

26. Opjordsmoen S, Waehre H, Aass N, et al: Sexuality in patients treated for penile cancer: Patients' experience and doctors' judgement. *Br J Urol* 73:554–560, 1994

27. Foster RS, McNulty A, Rubin LR, et al: The fertility of patients with clinical stage I testis cancer managed by nerve-sparing retroperitoneal lymph node dissection. *J Urol* 152: 1139–1143, 1994

28. Donohue JP, Foster RS, Rowland RG, et al: Nerve-sparing retroperitoneal lymphadenectomy with preservation of ejaculation. *J Urol* 144:287–292, 1990

29. Brock D, Fox S, Gosling G, et al: Testicular cancer. *Semin Oncol Nurs* 9:224–236, 1993

30. Lamb MA: Sexuality and sexual functioning, in McCorkle R, Grant M, Frank-Stromborg M, Baird SB (eds): *Cancer Nursing: A Comprehensive Textbook* (ed 2). Philadelphia, Saunders, 1996, pp 1105–1127

31. Arai Y, Kawakita M, Okada Y, et al: Sexuality and fertility in long-term survivors of testicular cancer. *J Clin Oncol* 15: 1444–1448, 1997

32. Ohl DA, Sonksen J: What are the chances of infertility and should sperm be banked? *Semin Urol Oncol* 14:36–44, 1996

33. Van Basten JP, Jonker-Pool G, van Driel MF, et al: Sexual functioning after multimodality treatment for disseminated nonseminomatous testicular germ cell tumor. *J Urol* 154:1411–1416

34. Aass N, Grunfeld B, Kaalhus O, et al: Pre- and post-treatment sexual life in testicular cancer patients: A descriptive investigation. *Br J Cancer* 67:1113–1117, 1993

35. Murphy GP, Morris LB, Lange D: *Informed Decisions.* New York, Viking, 1997

36. Yarbro CH, Ferrans CE: Quality of life of patients with prostate cancer treated with surgery or radiation therapy. *Oncol Nurs Forum* 25:685–693, 1998

37. Church PA: Prostate cancer, in Steele G, Cady B (eds): *General Surgical Oncology.* Philadelphia, Saunders, 1992, pp 275–285

38. Richie JP: Localized prostate cancer: Overview of surgical management. *Urology* 49:335–337, 1997(suppl 3A)

39. Talcott JA, Rieker P, Clark JA, et al: Patient-reported symptoms after primary therapy for early prostate cancer: Results of a prospective cohort study. *J Clin Oncol* 16:275–283, 1998

40. Geary ES, Dendinger TE, Freiha FS, et al: Nerve sparing radical prostatectomy: A different view. *J Urol* 154:145–149, 1995

41. Perez MA, Meyerowitz BE, Lieskovsky G, et al: Quality of life and sexuality following radical prostatectomy in patients with prostate cancer who do or do not use erectile aids. *Urology* 50:740–746, 1997

42. Zippe CD, Kedia AW, Kedia K, et al: Treatment of erectile dysfunction after radical prostatectomy with sildenafil citrate (Viagra). *Urology* 52:963–966, 1998

43. Einhorn C: Helping the prostate surgery patient face sexual dysfunction. *Innov Urol Nurs* 3:1, 9, 1992

44. Meredith CE: Treatment options for men with erectile dysfunction. *Innov Urol Nurs* 3:2–4, 8, 11, 1992

45. Thranov I, Klee M: Sexuality among gynecologic cancer patients: A cross-sectional study. *Gynecol Oncol* 52:14–19, 1994

46. Auchincloss SS: After treatment: Psychological issues in gynecologic cancer survivorship. *Cancer* 76:2117–2124, 1995 (suppl 10)

47. Steginga SK, Dunn J: Women's experiences following treat-

ment for gynecologic cancer. *Oncol Nurs Forum* 24: 1403–1408, 1997

48. Anderson BL: Stress and quality of life following cervical cancer. *Monogr J Natl Cancer Inst* 21:65–70, 1996

49. Weijmar Schultz WCM, Van de Weil HBM, Bouma J, et al: Psychosexuality after cancer of the vulva. *Cancer* 66: 402–407, 1990

50. Lamb MA: Psychosexual issues: The woman with gynecologic cancer. *Semin Oncol Nurs* 6:237–243, 1990

51. DiSaia PJ, Creasman WT: *Clinical Gynecologic Oncology* (ed 5). St. Louis, Mosby, 1997

52. Corney RH, Crowther ME, Howells A: Psychosexual dysfunction in women with gynaecological cancer following radical pelvic surgery. *Br J Obstet Gynaecol* 100:73–78, 1993

53. Chun JK, Behnam AB, Dottino P, et al: Use of the umbilicus in reconstruction of the vulva and vagina with a rectus abdominus musculocutaneous flap. *Ann Plastic Surg* 40: 659–663, 1998

54. Esrig D, Freeman JA, Stein JP, et al: New technique of reconstruction following anterior exenteration. *Urology* 49: 768–771, 1997

55. Louis-Sylvestre C, Haddad B, Paniel BJ: Creation of a sigmoid neovagina: Technique and results in 16 cases. *Eur J Obstet Gynecol Reprod Biol* 75:225–229, 1997

56. Andersen BL, Lamb M: Sexuality and cancer, in Murphy GP, Lawrence W, Lenhard RE (eds): *American Cancer Society Textbook of Clinical Oncology* (ed 2). Atlanta, American Cancer Society, 1995, pp 699–713

57. Cull A, Cowie VJ, Farquarson DIM, et al: Early stage cervical cancer: Psychosexual and sexual outcomes of treatment. *Br J Cancer* 68:1216–1220, 1993

58. Lamb MA, Sheldon TA: The sexual adaptation of women treated for endometrial cancer. *Cancer Pract* 2:103–113, 1994

59. Shell JA: Impact of cancer on sexuality, in Otto S (ed): *Oncology Nursing* (ed 3). St. Louis, Mosby Year Book, 1997, pp 737–760

60. Tserkezoglou AJ: Malignant ovarian neoplasms: The place of conservative therapy. *Ann N Y Acad Sci* 816:362–368, 1997.

61. Zanetta G, Chiari S, Rota S, et al: Conservative surgery for stage I ovarian carcinoma in women of childbearing age. *Br J Obstet Gynaecol* 104:1030–1035, 1997

62. De Stefano MS, Bertin-Matson K: Gynecologic cancers, in McCorkle R, Grant M, Frank-Stromborg M, Baird SB (eds): *Cancer Nursing: A Comprehensive Textbook* (ed 2). Philadelphia, Saunders, 1991, pp 698–728

63. Lewis FM, Zahlis EH, Sjands ME, et al: The functioning of single women with breast cancer and their school-aged children. *Cancer Pract* 4:15–24, 1996

64. Schain WS: The sexual and intimate consequences of breast cancer treatment. *CA Cancer J Clin* 38:154–161, 1988

65. Fallowfield LJ, Hall A: Psychosocial and sexual impact of diagnosis and treatment of breast cancer. *Br Med Bull* 47: 388–399, 1991

66. Schover LR: The impact of breast cancer on sexuality, body image and intimate relationships. *CA Cancer J Clin* 41:112–120, 1991

67. Omne-Ponten M, Holmberg L, Burns T, et al: Determinants of the psycho-social outcome after operation for breast cancer: Results of a prospective comparative interview study following mastectomy and breast conservation. *Eur J Cancer* 28A:1062–1067, 1992

68. Wilmoth MC, Townsend J: A comparison of the effects of lumpectomy versus mastectomy on sexual behaviors. *Cancer Pract* 3:279–285, 1995

69. Neill KM, Armstrong N, Burnett CB: Choosing reconstruction after mastectomy: A qualitative analysis. *Oncol Nurs Forum* 25:743–750, 1998

70. Fallowfield L: Offering choice of surgical treatment to women with breast cancer. *Patient Education & Counseling* 30:209–214, 1997

71. Monga U, Tan G, Ostermann HJ, et al: Sexuality in head and neck cancer patients. *Arch Phys Med Rehab* 78:298–304, 1997

72. Lamb MA: Effects of cancer on the sexuality and fertility of women. *Semin Oncol Nurs* 11:120–127, 1995

73. Granai CO, Amado PM, Goldstein AS, et al: The effects of cancer therapy on fertility. *Clin Adv Oncol Nurs* 3:1, 3, 7–9, 1991

74. Hilderley LJ: Radiotherapy, in Groenwald S, Frogge MH, Goodman M, Yarbro CH (eds): *Cancer Nursing: Principles and Practice* (ed 4). Sudbury, MA, Jones and Bartlett, 1997, pp 247–282

75. Stair J: Sexual dysfunction: Infertility, in McNally JC, Sommerville ET, Miaskowski C, Rostad M (eds): *Guidelines for Oncology Nursing Practice* (ed 2). Philadelphia, Saunders, 1991, pp 345–349

76. Haie-Meder C, Milka-Cabanne N, Michel G, et al: Radiotherapy after ovarian transposition: Ovarian function and fertility preservation. *Int J Radiat Oncol Biol Phys* 25:419–424, 1993

77. Morice P, Thiam-Ba R, Castaigne D, et al: Fertility results after ovarian transposition for pelvic malignancies treated by external irradiation or brachytherapy. *Hum Reprod* 13: 660–663, 1998

78. Smith DB: Sexuality, in Gross J, Johnson BL (eds): *Handbook of Oncology Nursing* (ed 2). Sudbury, MA, Jones and Bartlett, 1994, pp 557–571

79. Cartwright-Alcarese F: Addressing sexual dysfunction following radiation therapy for a gynecologic malignancy. *Oncol Nurs Forum* 22:1227–1232, 1995

80. Fieler VK: Side effects and quality of life in patients receiving high-dose rate brachytherapy. *Oncol Nurs Forum* 24: 545–553, 1997

81. Flay LD, Matthews JH: The effects of radiotherapy and surgery on the sexual function of women treated for cervical cancer. *Int J Radiat Oncol Biol Phys* 31:399–404, 1995

82. Rowly MJ, Leach DR, Warner GA, et al: Effects of graded doses of ionizing radiation on human testes. *Radiat Res* 59: 665–678, 1974

83. Shafford EA, Kingston JE, Malpas JS, et al: Testicular function following the treatment of Hodgkin's disease in childhood. *Br J Cancer* 68:1199–1204, 1993

84. Sklar CA, Robison LL, Nesbit ME, et al: Effects of radiation on testicular function in long-term survivors of childhood acute lymphoblastic leukemia: A report from the Children's Cancer Study Group. *J Clin Oncol* 8:1981–1987, 1990

85. Centola GM, Keller JW, Henzler M, et al: Effect of low-dose testicular irradiation on sperm count and fertility in patients with testicular seminoma. *J Androl* 15:608–613, 1994

86. Beard CJ, Lamb C, Buswell L, et al: Radiation-associated morbidity in patients undergoing small-field external beam irradiation for prostate cancer. *Int J Radiat Oncol Biol Phys* 41:257–262, 1998

87. Formenti SC, Lieskovsky G, Simoneau AR, et al: Impact of moderate dose of postoperative radiation on urinary continence and potency in men with prostate cancer

treated with nerve sparing prostatectomy. *J Urol* 155: 616–619, 1996

88. Sharkey J, Chovnick SD, Behar RJ, et al: Outpatient ultrasound-guided palladium 103 brachytherapy for localized adenocarcinoma of the prostate: A preliminary report of 434 patients. *Urology* 51:796–803, 1998

89. Zeitlin SI, Sherman J, Raboy A, et al: High dose combination radiotherapy for the treatment of localized prostate cancer. *J Urol* 160:91–95, 1998

90. Zelefsky MJ, Wallner KE, Ling CC, et al: Comparison of the 5-year outcome and morbidity of the three-dimensional conformal radiotherapy versus transperineal permanent iodine-125 implantation for early-stage prostate cancer. *J Clin Oncol* 17:517–522, 1999

91. Shell JA: Knowledge deficit related to radiation therapy, in McNally JC, Sommerville ET, Miaskowski C, Rostad M (eds): *Guidelines for Oncology Nursing Practice* (ed 2). Philadelphia, Saunders, 1991, pp 62–69

92. Longo DL, Fisher RI: Medical problems in long-term survivors of Hodgkin's disease. *Intern Med Spec* 4:165–171, 1983

93. Schilsky RL, Erlichman C: Late complications of chemotherapy: Infertility and carcinogenesis, in Chabner B (ed): *Pharmacologic Principles of Cancer Treatment.* Philadelphia, Saunders, 1982, pp 109–128

94. Chapman RM: Effect of cytotoxic therapy on sexuality and gonadal function. *Semin Oncol* 9:84–94, 1982

95. Wilkes GM, Ingwersen K, Burke MB: *1999 Oncology Nursing Drug Handbook.* Sudbury, MA, Jones and Bartlett, 1999

96. Langhorne M: Chemotherapy, in Otto S (ed): *Oncology Nursing* (ed 3). St. Louis, Mosby Year Book, 1997, pp 530–572

97. Glasel M: Effects on reproduction/sexual function, in Tenenbaum L (ed): *Cancer Chemotherapy and Biotherapy: A Reference Guide* (ed 2). Philadelphia, Saunders, 1994, pp 273–285

98. Guy JL, Ingram BA: Medical oncology: The agents, in McCorkle R, Grant M, Frank-Stromborg M, Baird SB (eds): *Cancer Nursing: A Comprehensive Textbook* (ed 2). Philadelphia, Saunders, 1996, pp 359–394

99. Martin V, Walker FE, Goodman M: Delivery of cancer chemotherapy, in McCorkle R, Grant M, Frank-Stromborg M, Baird SB (eds): *Cancer Nursing: A Comprehensive Textbook* (ed 2). Philadelphia, Saunders, 1996, pp 395–433

100. Schilsky RL, Lewis BJ, Sherins RJ, et al: Gonadal dysfunction in patients receiving chemotherapy for cancer. *Ann Intern Med* 93:109–114, 1980

101. Chapman RM: Gonadal toxicity and teratogenicity, in Perry MC (ed): *The Chemotherapy Sourcebook.* Baltimore, Williams & Wilkins, 1992, pp 710–753

102. Pont J, Albrecht W: Fertility after chemotherapy for testicular germ cell cancer. *Fertil Steril* 68:1–5, 1997

103. Stoter G, Koopman A, Vendrik CP, et al: Ten-year survival and late sequelae in testicular cancer patients treated with cisplatin, vinblastine and bleomycin. *J Clin Oncol* 7: 1099–1104, 1989

104. Lampe H, Horwich A, Norman A, et al: Fertility after chemotherapy for testicular germ cell cancers. *J Clin Oncol* 15:239–245, 1997

105. Peterson PM, Giwercman A, Skakkebaek NE, et al: Gonadal function in men with testicular cancer. *Semin Oncol* 25: 224–233, 1998

106. Stephenson WT, Poirier SM, Rubin L, et al: Evaluation of reproductive capacity in germ cell tumor patients following treatment with cisplatin, etoposide, and bleomycin. *J Clin Oncol* 13:2278–2280, 1995

107. Shrover L: Sexual rehabilitation after treatment for prostate cancer. *Cancer* 71:1024–1030, 1993 (suppl 3)

108. Brufsky A, Fontaine-Rothe P, Berlane K, et al: Finasteride and flutamide as potency-sparing androgen-ablative therapy for advanced adenocarcinoma of the prostate. *Urology* 49:913–920, 1997

109. Van Basten JP, Hoekstra HJ, van driel MF, et al: Sexual dysfunction in nonseminoma testicular cancer patients is related to chemotherapy-induced angiopathy. *J Clin Oncol* 15:2442–2448, 1997

110. Knopf MT: Natural menopause and ovarian toxicity associated with breast cancer therapy. *Oncol Nurs Forum* 25: 1519–1530, 1998

111. Chapman RM, Sutcliffe SB, Malpas JS: Cytotoxic-induced ovarian failure in women with Hodgkin's disease: II. Effects on sexual function. *JAMA* 242:1171–1181, 1979

112. Averette HE, Boike GM, Jarrell MA: Effects of chemotherapy on gonadal function and reproductive capacity. *CA Cancer J Clin* 40:199–209, 1990

113. Young-McCaughan S: Sexual functioning in women with breast cancer after treatment with adjuvant therapy. *Cancer Nurs* 19:308–319, 1996

114. Schover LR: Sexuality and body image in younger women with breast cancer. *Monogr Natl Cancer Inst* 16:177–182, 1994

115. Pansacreta JV, McCorkle R: Providing accurate information to women about tamoxifen therapy for breast cancer: Current indications, effects, and controversies. *Oncol Nurs Forum* 25:1577–1583, 1998

116. Sitzia J, Huggins L: Side effects of cyclophosphamide, methotrexate and 5FU (CMF) chemotherapy for breast cancer. *Cancer Pract* 6:13–21, 1998

117. Meadows AT: Follow-up and care of childhood cancer survivors. *Hosp Pract* 15:99–108, 1991

118. Levy MJ, Stillman RJ: Reproductive potential in survivors of childhood malignancy. *Pediatrician* 18:61–70, 1991

119. Wilson B: The effects of drugs on male sexual function and fertility. *Nurse Pract* 16:12–24, 1991

120. Rieger PT: Patient management, in Rieger PT (ed): *Biotherapy: A Comprehensive Overview.* Sudbury, MA, Jones and Bartlett, 1995, pp 195–219

121. Intron-A (package insert). Kenilworth, NJ, Schering Corporation, 1995

122. Rieger PT: *Clinical Handbook for Biotherapy.* Sudbury, MA, Jones and Bartlett, 1999

123. Buchsel PC, Leum EW, Randolph SR: Delayed complications of bone marrow transplantation: An update. *Oncol Nurs Forum* 23:1267–1291, 1996

124. Molassiotis A, van den Akker OB, Milligan DW, et al: Gonadal function and psychosexual adjustment in male long-term survivors of bone marrow transplantation. *Bone Marrow Transplant* 16:253–259, 1995

125. Belec RH: Quality of life: Perceptions of long-term survivors of bone marrow transplantation. *Oncol Nurs Forum* 19: 31–37, 1992

126. Singhal S, Powles R, Treleaven J, et al: Melphalan alone prior to allogeneic bone marrow transplantation from HLA-identical sibling donors for hematologic malignancies: Alloengraftment with potential preservation of fertility in women. *Bone Marrow Transplant* 18:1049–1055, 1996

127. Milliken S, Powles R, Parikh P: Successful pregnancy following bone marrow transplantation for leukaemia. *Bone Marrow Transplant* 5:135–137, 1990

128. Rio B, Letur-Konirsch H, Ajchenbaum-Cymbalista F, et al: Full-term pregnancy with embryos from donated oocytes

in a 36-year-old woman allografted for chronic myeloid leukemia. *Bone Marrow Transplant* 13:487–488, 1994

129. Whedon M, Stearns D, Mills LE: Quality of life of long-term adult survivors of autologous bone marrow transplantation. *Oncol Nurs Forum* 22:1527–1537, 1995

130. Haberman M, Bush N, Young K, et al: Quality of life of adult long-term survivors of bone marrow transplantation: A qualitative analysis of narrative data. *Oncol Nurs Forum* 20:1545–1553, 1993

131. Ferrell B, Grant M, Schmidt GM, et al: The meaning of quality of life for bone marrow transplant survivors: Part 1. The impact of bone marrow transplant on quality of life. *Cancer Nurs* 15:153–160, 1992

132. Ferrell B, Grant M, Schmidt GM, et al: The meaning of quality of life for bone marrow transplant survivors: Part 2. Improving quality of life for bone marrow transplant survivors. *Cancer Nurs* 15:247–253, 1992

133. Granai CO, Amado PM, Goldstein AS, et al: Female sexuality and cancer. *Clin Adv Oncol Nurs* 3:1–3, 7–9, 1990

134. Auchincloss S: Sexual dysfunction after cancer treatment. *J Psychosoc Oncol* 9:23–42, 1991

135. Annon JS: *The Behavioral Treatment of Sexual Problems.* Honolulu, Mercantile Printing, 1974, pp 43–47

136. Smith DB: Sexuality and the patient with cancer: What nurses need to know. *Oncol Patient Care* 4:1–3, 15, 1994

137. Shell JA: The psychosocial impact of ostomy surgery. *Progressions* 4:3–6, 8–11, 14, 15, 1992

138. Ofman US: Psychosexual aspects of sexuality in the patient with cancer. *Oncol Patient Care* 4:7, 8, 14, 15, 1994

139. Shell JA, Smith CK: Sexuality and the older person with cancer. *Oncol Nurs Forum* 21:553–558, 1994

140. Small EC: Psycho-sexual issues. *Obstet Gynecol Clin North Am* 21:773–780, 1994

141. Baron RH: Dispelling the myths of pregnancy-associated breast cancer. *Oncol Nurs Forum* 21:507–512, 1994

142. Hughes MK: Sexuality issues: Keeping your cool. *Oncol Nurs Forum* 23:1597–1600, 1996

143. Nicholson HS, Byrne J: Fertility and pregnancy after treatment for cancer during childhood or adolescence. *Cancer* 71:3392–3399, 1993 (suppl)

144. Klein CE: Fertility and the cancer survivor. *Coping* 9:48–49, 1995

145. Byrne J: Fertility and pregnancy after malignancy. *Semin Perinatol* 14:423–429, 1990

146. Hawkins MM: Is there evidence of therapy-related increases in germ cell mutation among childhood cancer survivors? *J Natl Cancer Inst* 83:1643–1650, 1991

147. Senturia YD, Peckham CS: Children fathered by men treated with chemotherapy for testicular cancer. *Eur J Cancer* 26:429–432, 1990

148. Green DM, Zevon MA, Lowrie G, et al: Congenital anomalies in children of patients who received chemotherapy for cancer in childhood and adolescence. *N Engl J Med* 325:141–146, 1991

149. Swerdlow AJ, Jacobs PA, Marks A, et al: Fertility, reproductive outcomes, and health of offspring of patients treated for Hodgkin's disease: An investigation including chromosome examinations. *Br J Cancer* 74:291–296, 1996

150. Hansen PV, Glavind K, Panduro J, et al: Paternity in patients with testicular germ cell cancer: Pretreatment and post-treatment findings. *Eur J Cancer* 27:1385–1389, 1991

151. Byrne J, Rasmussen SA, Steinhorn SC, et al: Genetic disease in offspring of long-term survivors of childhood and adolescent cancer. *Am J Hum Genet* 62:45–52, 1998

152. Robinson WA, Krebs LU: Oncologic disease, in Abrams R, Wexler P (eds): *Medical Care of the Pregnant Patient: Concepts and Management.* Boston, Little, Brown, 1983, pp 307–319

153. Reichman BS, Green KB: Breast cancer in young women: Effect of chemotherapy on ovarian function, fertility, and birth defects. *Monogr Natl Cancer Inst* 16:125–129, 1994

154. Mayr NA, Wen B, Saw CB: Radiation therapy during pregnancy. *Obstet Gynecol Clin North Am* 25:301–321, 1998

155. Barnicle MM: Chemotherapy and pregnancy. *Semin Oncol Nurs* 8:124–132, 1992

156. Buekers TE, Lallas TA: Chemotherapy in pregnancy. *Obstet Gynecol Clin North Am* 25:323–329, 1998

157. Zemlickis D, Lishner M, Degendorfer P, et al: Fetal outcome after in utero exposure to cancer chemotherapy. *Arch Intern Med* 152:573–576, 1992

158. Shahin MS, Puscheck E: Reproductive sequelae of cancer treatment. *Obstet Gynecol Clin North Am* 25:423–433, 1998

159. Rieker PP: How should a man with testicular cancer be counseled and what information is available to him? *Semin Urol Oncol* 14:17–23, 1996

160. Turek PJ, Lowther DN, Carroll PR: Fertility issues and their management in men with testis cancer. *Urol Clin North Am* 25:517–531, 1998

161. Kreuser ED, Klingmuller D, Thiel E: The role of LHRH-analogues in protecting gonadal functions during chemotherapy and irradiation. *Eur Urol* 23:157–164, 1993

162. Mott-Smith ME, Stolberg L: Sexual function and pregnancy, in Casciato DA, Lowitz BB (eds): *Manual of Clinical Oncology* (ed 3). Boston, Little, Brown, 1995, pp 575–582

163. Lass A, Akagbosu F, Abusheikha N, et al: A programme of semen cryopreservation for patients with malignant disease in a tertiary infertility centre: Lessons from 8 years' experience. *Human Reprod* 13:3256–3261, 1998

164. Petersen PM, Skakkebaek NE, Vistisen K, et al: Semen quality and reproductive hormones before orchiectomy in men with testicular cancer. *J Clin Oncol* 17:941–947, 1999

165. Sweet V, Servy EJ, Karow AM: Reproductive issues for men with cancer: Technology and nursing management. *Oncol Nurs Forum* 23:51–58, 1996

166. Naysmith TE, Blake DA, Harvey VJ, et al: Do men undergoing sterilizing cancer treatments have a fertile future? *Hum Reprod* 13:3250–3255, 1998

167. Koeppel KM: Sperm banking and patients with cancer: Issues concerning patients and healthcare professionals. *Cancer Nurs* 18:306–312, 1995

168. Meacham RB, Lipshultz LI: Assisted reproductive technologies for male factor infertility. *Curr Opin Obstet Gynecol* 3:656–661, 1991

169. Mandelbaum J, Belaisch-Allart J, Junca AM, et al: Cryopreservation in human assisted reproduction is now routine for embryos but remains a research procedure for oocytes. *Hum Reprod* 3:161–177, 1998 (suppl 13)

170. Abir R, Fisch B, Raz A, et al: Preservation of fertility in women undergoing chemotherapy: Current approach and future prospects. *J Assist Reprod Genet* 15:477–496, 1998

171. Donnez J, Bassil S: Indications for cryopreservation of ovarian tissue. *Hum Reprod Update* 4:248–259, 1998

172. Newton H: The cryopreservation of ovarian tissue as a strategy for preserving the fertility of cancer patients. *Hum Reprod Update* 4:237–247, 1998

173. Krebs LU: Pregnancy and cancer. *Semin Oncol Nurs* 1:35–41, 1985

174. Waalen J: Pregnancy poses tough questions for cancer treatment. *J Natl Cancer Inst* 83:900, 1991

175. Zemlickis D, Lishner M, Degendorfer P, et al: Maternal and

fetal outcome after invasive cervical cancer in pregnancy. *J Clin Oncol* 9:1956–1961, 1991

176. Sorosky JI, Scott-Connor CEH: Breast disease complicating pregnancy. *Obstet Gynecol Clin North Am* 25:253–263, 1998

177. Dow KH (ed): *Pocket Guide to Breast Cancer.* Sudbury, MA, Jones and Bartlett, 1999, pp 183–190

178. Krebs LU: Cancer and pregnancy, in Gates RA, Fink RM (eds): *Oncology Nursing Secrets.* Philadelphia, Hanley & Belfus, 1997, pp 400–405

179. Pelsang RE: Diagnostic imaging modalities during pregnancy. *Obstet Gynecol Clin North Am* 25:287–300, 1998

180. Fiorica JV: Special problems: Breast cancer and pregnancy. *Obstet Gynecol Clin North Am* 21:721–732, 1994

181. Petrek JA: Breast cancer during pregnancy. *Cancer* 74: 518–527, 1994 (suppl)

182. Zemlickis D, Lishner M, Degendorfer P, et al: Maternal and fetal outcome after breast cancer in pregnancy. *Am J Obstet Gynecol* 166:781–787, 1992

183. Shapiro CL, Mayer RJ: Breast cancer in pregnancy. *Adv Oncol* 8:25–29, 1992

184. Samuels TH, Liu FF, Yaffe M, et al: Gestational breast cancer. *Can Assoc Radiol J* 49:172–180, 1998

185. Hoover HC: Breast cancer during pregnancy and lactation. *Surg Clin North Am* 70:1151–1163, 1990

186. Barnavon Y, Wallack K: Management of the pregnant patient with carcinoma of the breast. *Surg Gynecol Obstet* 171: 347–352, 1990

187. Van der Vange N, van Dongen JA: Breast cancer and pregnancy. *Eur J Surg Oncol* 17:1–8, 1991

188. Petrek JA, Dukoff R, Rogato A: Prognosis of pregnancy-associated breast cancer. *Cancer* 67:869–872, 1990

189. Higgins S, Haffty BG: Pregnancy and lactation after breast-conserving therapy for early stage breast cancer. *Cancer* 73: 2175–2180, 1994

190. von Schoultz E, Johansson H, Wilking N, et al: Influence of prior and subsequent pregnancy on breast cancer prognosis. *J Clin Oncol* 13:430–434, 1995

191. Dow KH, Harris JR, Roy C: Pregnancy after breast-conserving surgery and radiation therapy for breast cancer. *Monogr Natl Cancer Inst* 16:131–137, 1994

192. Shivvers SA, Miller DS: Preinvasive and invasive breast and cervical cancer prior to or during pregnancy. *Clin Perinatol* 24:369–389, 1997

193. Surbone A, Petrek JA: Childbearing issues in breast carcinoma survivors. *Cancer* 79:1271–1278, 1997

194. Danforth DN: How subsequent pregnancy affects outcome in women with a prior breast cancer. *Oncology* 5:23–35, 1991

195. Collichio FA, Agnello R, Staltzer J: Pregnancy after breast cancer: From psychosocial issues through conception. *Oncology* 12:759–769, 1998

196. Sankila R, Heinavaara S, Hakulinen T: Survival of breast cancer patients after subsequent term pregnancy: "Healthy mother effect." *Am J Obstet Gynecol* 170:818–823, 1994

197. Petrek JA: Pregnancy safety after breast cancer. *Cancer* 74: 528–531, 1994

198. Johannsson O, Loman N, Borg A, et al: Pregnancy-associated breast cancer in BRCA1 and BRCA2 germline mutation carriers. *Lancet* 352:1359–1360, 1998

199. Roberts JA: Management of gynecologic tumors during pregnancy. *Clin Perinatol* 10:369–382, 1983

200. Connor JP: Noninvasive cervical cancer complicating pregnancy. *Obstet Gynecol Clin North Am* 25:331–342, 1998

201. Van Rooijen M, Persson E: Pregnancy outcome after laser

202. Sood AK, Sorosky JI: Invasive cervical cancer complicating pregnancy. *Obstet Gynecol Clin North Am* 25:343–352, 1998

203. Duggan B, Muderspach LI, Roman LD, et al: Cervical cancer in pregnancy: Reporting on planned delay in therapy. *Obstet Gynecol* 82:598–602, 1993

204. Nevin J, Soeters R, Dehaeek K, et al: Cervical carcinoma associated with pregnancy. *Obstet Gynecol Surv* 50:228–239, 1995

205. Sivanesaratnam V, Jayalakshmi P, Loo C: Surgical management of early invasive cancer of the cervix associated with pregnancy. *Gynecol Oncol* 48:68–75, 1993

206. Cliby WA, Dodson MK, Podratz KC: Cervical cancer complicated by pregnancy: Episiotomy site recurrences following vaginal delivery. *Obstet Gynecol* 84:179–183, 1994

207. Boulay R, Podczaski E: Ovarian cancer complicating pregnancy. *Obstet Gynecol Clin North Am* 25:385–399, 1998

208. Bromley B, Benacerraf B: Adnexal masses during pregnancy: Accuracy of sonographic diagnosis and outcome. *J Ultrasound Med* 16:447–452, 1997

209. Grendys EC Jr, Barnes WA: Ovarian cancer in pregnancy. *Surg Clin North Am* 75:1–14, 1995

210. King LA, Nevin PC, Williams PP, et al: Treatment of advanced epithelial ovarian cancer in pregnancy with cisplatin-based chemotherapy. *Gynecol Oncol* 41:78–80, 1991

211. Squatrito RC, Harlow SP: Melanoma complicating pregnancy. *Obstet Gynecol Clin North Am* 25:407–416, 1998

212. Teplitzky S, Sabates B, Yu K, et al: Melanoma during pregnancy: A case report and review of the literature. *J LA State Med Soc* 150:539–543, 1998

213. Travers RL, Sober AJ, Berwick M, et al: Increased thickness of pregnancy-associated melanoma. *Br J Dermatol* 132: 876–883, 1995

214. Slingluff CL, Reintgen DS, Vollmer RT, et al: Malignant melanoma arising during pregnancy: A study of 100 patients. *Ann Surg* 211:552–559, 1990

215. Wong JH, Sterns EE, Kopald KH, et al: Prognostic significance of pregnancy in stage I melanoma. *Arch Surg* 124: 1227–1231, 1989

216. Dipaola RS, Goodin S, Ratzell M, et al: Chemotherapy for metastatic melanoma during pregnancy. *Gynecol Oncol* 66: 526–530, 1997

217. Anderson JF, Kent S, Machin GA: Maternal malignant melanoma with placental metastasis: A case report with literature review. *Pediatr Pathol* 9:35–42, 1989

218. Brossard J, Abish S, Bernstein ML, et al: Maternal malignancy involving the products of conception: A report of malignant melanoma and medulloblastoma. *Am J Pediatr Hematol Oncol* 16:380–383, 1994

219. Ferreira CM, Maceira JM, Coelho JM: Melanoma and pregnancy with placental metastases. Report of a case. *Am J Dermatol* 20:403–407, 1998

220. Mackie RM, Bufalino R, Morabito A, et al: Lack of effect of pregnancy on outcome of melanoma. *Lancet* 337:653–655, 1991

221. Ward FT, Weiss RB: Lymphoma in pregnancy. *Adv Oncol* 8:18–22, 1992

222. Kennedy BJ: Hodgkin's disease. *CA Cancer J Clin* 43: 325–346, 1993

223. Peleg D, Ben-Ami M: Lymphoma and leukemia complicating pregnancy. *Obstet Gynecol Clin North Am* 25:365–383, 1998

224. Anselmo AP, Cavalieri E, Enrici RM, et al: Hodgkin's dis-

ease during pregnancy: Diagnostic and therapeutic management. *Fetal Diagn Test* 14:102–195, 1999

225. Gelb AB, van de Rijn M, Wamke RA, et al: Pregnancy-associated lymphomas: A clinicopathologic study. *Cancer* 78:304–310, 1996

226. Meguerian-Bedoyan Z, Lamant L, Hopfner C, et al: Anaplastic large cell lymphoma of maternal origin involving the placenta: Case report and literature survey. *Am J Surg Pathol* 21:1236–1241, 1997

227. Ramirez-Smiley M, Ingle B: Leukemia during pregnancy. *Oncol Nurs Forum* 22:1363–1368, 1995

228. Henderson ES: A selected overview, in Gunz FW, Henderson ES (eds): *Leukemia* (ed 4). Orlando, FL, Grune & Stratton, 1983, pp 785–798

229. Caligiuri MA: Leukemia in pregnancy. *Adv Oncol* 8:10–17, 1992

230. Cygler J, Ding GX, Kendal W, et al: Fetal dose for a patient undergoing mantle field irradiation for Hodgkin's disease. *Med Dosim* 22:135–137, 1997

231. Jankowski CB: Radiation and pregnancy: Putting the risks in proportion. *Am J Nurs* 86:260–265, 1986

232. Doll DC: Chemotherapy in pregnancy, in Perry MC (ed): *The Chemotherapy Sourcebook*. Baltimore, Williams & Wilkins, 1992, pp 703–709

233. Dildy GA, Moise KJ, Carpenter RJ, et al: Maternal malignancy metastatic to the products of conception: A review. *Obstet Gynecol Surv* 44:535–540, 1989

Oncologic Emergencies

CHAPTER 38

Cardiac Tamponade

Roberta Kaplow, RN, PhD, CCNS, CCRN

Scope of the Problem

Definitions

Cardiac tamponade results from an excess accumulation of fluid in the pericardial sac (pericardial effusion). The fluid collection causes an increase in pressure around the heart—hemodynamically significant compression of the heart—resulting in diminished flow of blood to the ventricles.[1,2] The net effect is a decrease in cardiac output and impaired cardiac function. Because the interference with filling of the ventricles and cardiac pumping can result in pulseless electrical activity, cardiovascular collapse, and death,[3] cardiac tamponade is a life-threatening complication of cancer. An individual may be considered to have a cardiac tamponade when the pericardial effusion has caused the described hemodynamic instability and compensatory mechanisms have failed.[4]

Incidence

The diagnosis of cardiac tamponade is often missed because many patients with pericardial effusions are asymptomatic.[4] However, the presence of a pericardial effusion has been reported on autopsy in up to 20% of individuals with a cancer diagnosis.[5,6] When signs and symptoms of a pericardial effusion do present, they are often attributed to the primary malignancy.[4] Patients with pericardial effusions are at risk for developing cardiac tamponade if left untreated.[7] Malignancies, the most common cause of cardiac tamponade, account for 16%–41% of the incidence of this complication.[1,3,7]

Etiology and Risk Factors

Several tumors are associated with the development of pericardial effusions including lung (40%), breast (23%), lymphoma (11%), and leukemia (5%).[5,8,9] Together, these tumors account for approximately 75% of pericardial effusions.[3,4] When these tumors metastasize to the pericardium or myocardium, obstruction of venous and lymphatic drainage occurs and an excess amount of pericardial fluid accumulates (pericardial effusion). Cardiac tamponade (hemodynamically significant compression of the heart by pericardial fluid)[2] can also result from constriction of the pericardium by tumor or postradiation pericarditis.[10]

Several cancers have been implicated in the development of cardiac tamponade. In addition to the four malignancies associated with the development of pericardial effusion, other malignancies include malignant melanoma, gastric, ovarian, kidney, pancreas, and head and neck cancers, and mesothelioma.[1,7] Cardiac tamponade usually occurs as a result of a tumor's metastasizing to the pericardium or from tumor invasion from adjoining tissue.[5] Individuals who have received greater than 4000 cGy of radiation therapy to the pericardium may also develop cardiac tamponade.[1]

While it cannot be prevented, nurses must be aware of cardiac tamponade as a potential complication of both the malignant process and the cancer treatment modalities. Often, clinical manifestations are vague or attributed to the underlying malignancy or other etiology. This poses a challenge for the nurse and other members of the health care team. Accurate and early detection of signs and symptoms and prompt treatment of cardiac tamponade are essential to minimize morbidity and mortality.[7]

Physiologic Alterations

Normal Anatomy and Physiology

The pericardium is a fibrous double-layered sac surrounding the heart. The functions of the pericardium include protection of the heart from friction, infection, and inflammation, stabilization of cardiac position against gravity, and support of the heart chambers.[4,10,11] A small amount of low protein fluid in the pericardium helps attain these goals. The normal amount of fluid in the pericardium is approximately 15–50 mL. The fluid is drained by the lymphatic system into the mediastinum.

Normally, intrapericardial pressure is lower than ventricular diastolic pressure and is equal to pleural pressure. This normal pressure gradient between the heart chambers and the pericardium allows the heart chambers to fill. Intrapericardial pressure normally ranges from 2–3 mm Hg during inspiration and 5–7 mm Hg during expiration.[1,4]

Pathophysiology

The amount of fluid surrounding the heart in an individual with pericardial effusion can range from approximately 50 mL to greater than one liter. This fluid may impair the ventricle's ability to fill during diastole.

The degree of pathophysiologic changes that occur depends on how quickly the excess fluid has accumulated. When accumulated gradually, the pericardium has time to compensate for the increased volume before a tamponade (decreased cardiac output) will occur. When fluid accumulates acutely, intrapericardial pressure rises to 20 mm Hg or higher. This increase in intrapericardial pressure accounts for the hemodynamic instability and impaired cardiac function associated with cardiac tamponade[1,4] (Figure 38-1).

The excess pericardial fluid compresses the heart and prevents it from filling adequately. Right ventricular filling is contingent upon a gradient between central venous pressure and right ventricular diastolic pressure. The increase in intrapericardial pressure that results from the excess fluid accumulation affects this gradient, and right

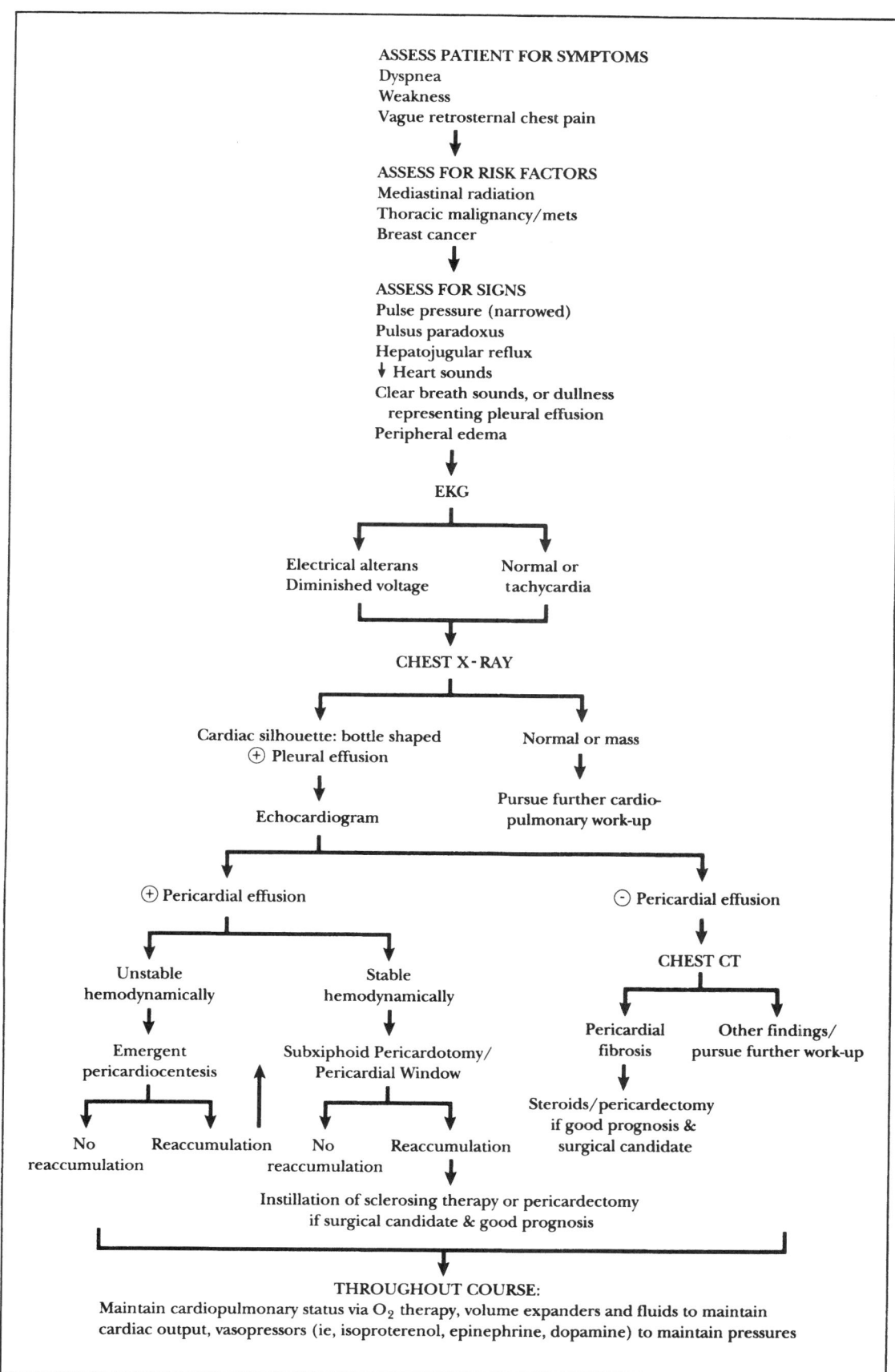

Figure 38-1 Clinical pathway for cardiac tamponade.

ventricular filling cannot be adequately sustained. Decreased right ventricular filling and compression of the right ventricle results in a decrease in blood leaving that chamber. Thus, the amount of blood entering, and subsequently leaving, the left side of the heart is decreased. The compression also causes an increase in intracardiac diastolic pressures on the right and left sides, and equalization of filling pressures in each of the heart chambers.[1,4]

Hence, the development of cardiac tamponade from a pericardial effusion is based on the compliance of the pericardium, rate of accumulation of fluid, and the amount of fluid that accumulates.[10] If the fluid accumulates slowly, the pericardium will expand to accommodate the excess fluid[1,10] and the body attempts to compensate.

Compensatory mechanisms include an increased production of endogenous catecholamines from the sympathetic nervous system. Catecholamine production results in an increase in heart rate (positive chronotropy), an increase in contractility (positive inotropy), and an increase in peripheral vasoconstriction of the arterial and venous beds. If the tamponade is severe, compensatory mechanisms include an increase in systemic vascular resistance—the amount of work the heart has to do to eject blood. If the fluid accumulates quickly, the pericardium will not stretch,[4] compensatory mechanisms cannot be activated, and hemodynamic instability ensues.

Clinical Manifestations

The signs and symptoms of cardiac tamponade are variable and depend on the rate and amount of pericardial fluid accumulation and the individual's baseline cardiac function.[1,4,11] A summary of the signs and symptoms appears in Table 38-1. If fluid accumulation occurs slowly, signs and symptoms may include fatigue, shortness of breath, neck vein distention, hepatomegaly, and abdominal distention.[10] As the amount of fluid increases, cardiovascular signs and symptoms become more prominent. One of the earliest is an elevation in central venous pressure. This is a result of the increase in intrapericardial pressure from the fluid accumulation and occurs in 50%–63% of individuals.[4] Elevation in central venous pressure may be indicated by neck vein distention. Ordinarily, when a person inspires, there is a decrease in intrathoracic pressure with a resultant increase in blood return to the heart and collapse of neck veins. When an individual has cardiac tamponade, blood cannot return to the heart and neck vein distention occurs.

Other signs and symptoms of increased fluid accumulation include the presence of distant heart sounds, decreased or absent apical pulse, and decreased cardiac output.[10] Distant or muffled heart sounds are the result of fluid surrounding and compressing the heart, thus creating a barrier between the heart and the examiner's stethoscope.[3]

If fluid accumulation is rapid, the body does not have time to develop compensatory mechanisms. The resultant clinical signs are an increase in ventricular diastolic and pulmonary venous pressures, and a decrease in stroke volume (the amount of blood ejected by the heart with each beat), cardiac output, and arterial blood pressure. These signs will be accompanied by tachypnea, dyspnea, and orthopnea.[3,10] Other signs the individual will present with include hypotension[4,7] and resting tachycardia.[4]

Table 38-1 Cardiac Tamponade: Clinical Presentation and Pathologic Response

Pathology	Clinical Presentation: Signs and Symptoms	Pathophysiology and Compensatory Mechanisms
Decrease in cardiac output	Increased resting heart rate	Increased heart rate decreases cardiac output
	Peripheral vasoconstriction causing cyanosis	Blood is shunted from the peripheral circulation to supply vital organs
	Decreased renal output	Decreased renal perfusion
	Narrowing pulse pressure	Systolic pressure falls as cardiac output decreases; arteries constrict to maintain perfusion
	Paradoxical pulse	With inspiration, the diaphragm compresses the pericardial sac. The left ventricle receives less blood and cardiac output is reduced causing a decreased systolic blood pressure on inspiration
	Anxiety, restlessness, confusion	Cerebral anoxia due to inadequate perfusion
	Symptoms of shock	Cardiac decompensation
Compression of heart and structures in chest	Dysphagia, cough, retrosternal chest pain	Fluid collection around heart compresses the trachea, esophagus, and adjacent nerves
Venous congestion	Peripheral edema, jugular venous distention	With decrease in ventricular filling, venous return is reduced causing vascular congestion
Distention and filling of pericardial sac	Dullness to percussion, weak heart sounds, chest fullness/discomfort	Fluid surrounding heart decreases heart sounds

As an early sign of cardiac tamponade, dyspnea can progress and occur at rest as cardiovascular impairment attenuates.[4] It is not uncommon for individuals to be able to speak only one word before becoming dyspneic.[3] The etiology of dyspnea is felt to be the decrease in cardiac output or the decrease in lung expansion by the pericardium. Cyanosis results from the decrease in venous return and venous hypertension. Tachypnea results from the decrease in cardiac output and resultant hypoxia. No adventitious sounds are audible with the disorder as there is no pulmonary congestion.

Individuals with cardiac tamponade often have a pulsus paradoxus, a decrease in systolic arterial blood pressure of greater than 10 mm Hg during inspiration. The etiology of pulsus paradoxus is felt to be due to impaired cardiac filling and should be suspected when a palpated pulse decreases in intensity or disappears upon inspiration and becomes stronger upon exhalation.[6] To measure the extent of a pulsus paradoxus, the blood pressure cuff should be inflated above the level of the individual's systolic pressure and deflated at a rate of 3 mm/second. The first systolic pressure reading heard only during exhalation should be noted. The sound disappears upon inspiration. The systolic pressure reading that is audible during both inspiration and exhalation is then noted. If the difference between the two systolic pressure sounds is greater than 10 mm Hg, the individual has a pulsus paradoxus.

As the cardiac tamponade increases, stroke volume continues to decrease, systemic vascular resistance increases, systolic blood pressure falls, diastolic blood pressure increases, and pulse pressure (the difference between systolic and diastolic blood pressure) narrows.

The "classic" signs of cardiac tamponade—elevated central venous pressure, hypotension, and distant heart sounds—are known as "Beck's triad."[2] However, while a significant percentage of individuals manifest one or two of the signs, all three signs only occur in advanced stages of tamponade.[4]

Individuals with cardiac tamponade may also present with mental status changes, including lethargy, restlessness, confusion, and decreased level of consciousness. These signs and symptoms result from the hemodynamic instability and decreased cardiac output and hypoxia. Individuals may also manifest hepatojugular reflux, an increase in jugular venous pressure of 1 cm or more.[5] To assess, the individual is placed in a supine position with the head of the bed elevated so that jugular venous palpations are discernible. Pressure is exerted for 30–60 seconds over the right upper quadrant of the abdomen. The test is positive if there is an elevation in the jugular venous pressure. The result is due to elevation of central venous pressure.

Prolonged periods of hypotension cause hypoperfusion to the kidneys. This can result in oliguria or anuria. Prolonged hypotension and decreased cardiac output may also result in decreased peripheral perfusion. This may be manifested by weakness, fatigue, dyspnea, chest pain, and cool, clammy extremities.

Other findings may include peripheral edema, anxiety, apprehension, and agitation, cough, hiccups, hoarseness, and dysphagia. The latter four symptoms are related to compression of the esophageal and tracheal nerves. Individuals may also develop chest pain or heaviness.[1,4]

Less common signs and symptoms include peripheral edema, low-grade fever, hepatomegaly, abdominal pain, and nausea. The latter two symptoms are felt to be due to hepatic and intestinal congestion.

Assessment

Physical Exam

As discussed previously, any of the aforementioned clinical manifestations may be noted, depending on the rate of accumulation of the fluid, the amount of fluid accumulated, and the baseline cardiac function of the individual (see Figure 38-1).

Diagnostic tests

Several tests and procedures aid in the diagnosis of cardiac tamponade. These include echocardiography, chest radiograph, computerized tomography (CT) scan, magnetic resonance imaging (MRI), pulmonary artery catheterization, electrocardiogram, fluoroscopy, serum laboratory tests, and pericardiocentesis with pericardial fluid evaluation.

Echocardiography. Echocardiography is the most sensitive and precise method for the diagnosis of cardiac tamponade since as little as 15 mL of fluid may be detected. During an echocardiogram, ultrasonic waves are produced via a probe. The waves create a picture of the heart and can depict heart functioning. An echocardiogram will reveal compression of the right ventricular free wall during early diastole and collapse of the right atrial and ventricular free walls during diastole in individuals with cardiac tamponade. Since the right side of the heart contains less myocardium than the left side, the pressure being exerted by the pericardial fluid can cause the right side to collapse. In addition to pericardial fluid, an echocardiogram will reveal a low ejection fraction and, possibly, a pericardial mass. Quantification of the pericardial fluid is also possible.[12]

When fluid separates the pericardium from myocardium, pericardial effusion is visualized as an "echo-free" clear space separating the moving cardiac walls from the immobile pericardium.[12] A two-dimensional echocardiography is useful for the detection of fluid as well as for selecting the appropriate site to perform a pericardiocentesis.

Echocardiography is also helpful in the assessment of hemodynamic effects of the tamponade. While echocardiography is helpful in diagnosing cardiac tamponade, it may become difficult to perform in a hemodynamically unstable individual as this procedure can be time-consuming.[7]

Radiograph. Chest radiograph is not a definitive diagnostic method for cardiac tamponade because fluid may not appear radiographically and the cardiac silhouette may appear normal. Radiograph films are abnormal in 90% of individuals but changes are considered nonspecific in 50% of the cases.[13] However, cardiac tamponade may be suspected if the chest radiograph reveals an enlarged heart, mediastinal widening, dilated cardiac silhouette, cardiomegaly, and pleural effusions. The cardiac silhouette may appear like a "water-bottle heart"[4] (Figure 38-2). However, the cardiac silhouette will appear enlarged only after at least 250 mL of pericardial fluid has accumulated.[10] Lung fields are usually clear in individuals with cardiac tamponade.[12] A confirmation of the diagnosis must be made with either echocardiography, ultrasound, MRI, or CT scan. Each of these can show fluid in the pericardium better than an ordinary radiographic study. It has been suggested that any individual with a cancer diagnosis who has change in the size and shape of the heart with clear lung fields on a radiographic study should be evaluated for the presence of pericardial effusion.[4]

Computerized tomography. A CT scan may indicate the presence of a cardiac tamponade, and it is useful for determining the pericardial thickness and presence of a pleural effusion or masses. As a diagnostic test, a CT scan has limited usefulness due to the blurring of the pericardial contents as a result of cardiac motion during the study.[4] A CT scan will provide no data regarding cardiac functioning in the presence of a tamponade.[3]

Magnetic resonance imaging. An MRI also has limited usefulness in the diagnosis of cardiac tamponade. While an MRI does afford the clinician a more defined view of the myocardium compared to CT, it offers no benefit over echocardiography.[4]

Pulmonary artery catheterization. Insertion of a pulmonary artery catheter will reveal equalization of right- and left-sided heart pressures and a decrease in cardiac output. Right atrial mean, right ventricular diastolic, and pulmonary artery wedge pressures equalize in individuals with cardiac tamponade.

The individual with cardiac tamponade will manifest other changes in the hemodynamic profile. Findings include decreased pulse pressure, tachycardia, increased systemic vascular resistance (the amount of work the heart has to do to eject blood), increased central venous pressure, increased left atrial pressure, increased pulmonary artery pressures, increased pulmonary artery occlusive pressure (wedge pressure), decreased blood pressure, and decreased cardiac output. As insertion of a pulmonary artery catheter is invasive and not without associated complications, it is rarely indicated since echocardiography is a reliable, noninvasive diagnostic method.[4]

Electrocardiography. Findings on electrocardiogram are nonspecific. Those findings consistent with the diagnosis of cardiac tamponade include tachycardia, atrial and ventricular dysrhythmias (e.g., atrial fibrillation and premature ventricular contractions), changes in shape and amplitude of the P wave, low-voltage QRS complexes and T waves and electrical alternans. The decrease in voltage of the complexes may be the result of the fluid in the pericardium compressing on the heart. ST segment elevation may be present in leads I, II, AVL, and AVF and may be depressed in lead AVR. The ST segment elevation and T wave changes may be due to inflammation. Electrical alternans is a change in the direction and amplitude of the QRS and T wave and is usually seen with every other beat. It may result from changes in cardiac position during depolarization.[4,10]

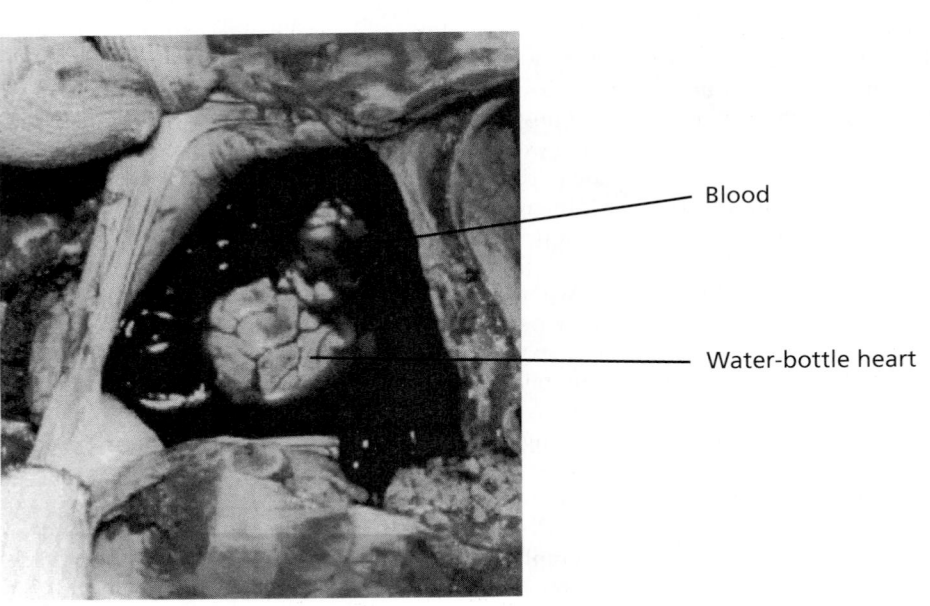

Figure 38-2 Water-bottle heart. Source: http://www.cyber-nurse.com/veetac/horrorctam.htm.

Blood

Water-bottle heart

Another sequela to cardiac tamponade is pulseless electrical activity. This will be manifested with the presence of electrical activity on electrocardiogram in the absence of a detectable pulse.

Fluoroscopy. This diagnostic procedure is rarely used for cardiac tamponade. Like echocardiography, it is a time-consuming test. Furthermore, cardiac enlargement cannot be distinguished from cardiac tamponade with this procedure.

Serum laboratory tests. Laboratory tests that may be obtained include hematocrit and arterial blood gas. While results of laboratory tests do not confirm the diagnosis of cardiac tamponade, they can support the findings of other diagnostic tests and guide management. Hematocrit levels may be unchanged or decreased in cardiac tamponade, depending on the etiology. Results of arterial blood gases may reveal an increase in pH and decrease in $PaCO_2$ (respiratory alkalosis).

Pericardial fluid evaluation. To determine if a pericardial effusion is malignant in nature, a pericardiocentesis may be performed in individuals with a large effusion (>1 cm of clear space seen on echocardiogram). The procedure is usually done under ultrasound, echocardiography, or fluoroscopy guidance in order to minimize the risk of complications such as cardiac puncture, ventricular tachycardia, or tension pneumothorax. The fluid is sent to the lab for cytology and lactic dehydrogenase (LDH) and total protein levels. Malignant effusions may appear bloody, serosanguinous, or serous.[5]

Therapeutic Approaches and Nursing Care

Prevention

A preventive measure for cardiac tamponade is successful treatment of the underlying malignancy. Treatment of the underlying cause may prevent reaccumulation of fluid. Long-term therapeutic interventions include instillation of a sclerosing agent, insertion of a pericardial window, or pericardiectomy.

Management

Several therapeutic approaches are available to treat pericardial effusions and subsequent cardiac tamponade. Factors that are considered in selecting an intervention include the individual's presenting symptoms, diagnosis, disease stage, prognosis, and physical condition.[3,14]

Individuals may require stabilization of their hemodynamic status prior to initiation of any other therapeutic intervention. Regardless of the therapeutic approach selected, the goals of therapy include enhancing cardiac function, pericardial fluid removal, prevention of reaccumulation, and minimizing complications.

Supportive Care

Prior to treatment for cardiac tamponade, individuals can be stabilized with oxygen to reduce cardiac workload and with aggressive fluid volume resuscitation and administration of inotropic agents to enhance cardiac output and prevent diastolic collapse.[2,7,12,13] Administration of intravenous fluids such as crystalloids, blood, or plasma will increase ventricular filling and cardiac output. Attainment of a systolic blood pressure of 90 mm Hg or higher will improve ventricular filling pressure. Titration of inotropic agents such as dopamine, norepinephrine, or dobutamine, which stimulate beta$_1$ receptors, may be employed to enhance contractility and cardiac output. Logically then, use of beta-blockers should be avoided. Agents that stimulate alpha-receptors, causing vasoconstriction, will increase the amount of work the heart must do to eject blood and decrease cardiac output. Conversely, use of arterial vasodilators such as nitroprusside will decrease the amount of work the heart must do to eject blood and may help increase blood pressure. Administration of diuretics will decrease circulating volume, thereby decreasing ventricular filling, and therefore should not be given. Use of positive-pressure ventilation should, ideally, be avoided as it is associated with an increase in intrathoracic pressure and subsequent decrease in cardiac output. Maintaining the individual on bedrest in semi-Fowler's position may be helpful as it further decreases cardiac workload.

Pericardiocentesis

A pericardiocentesis—removal of fluid from the pericardial sac—is the most common approach used for the management of cardiac tamponade. It relieves the increased end diastolic pressure and decreased ventricular filling. Improvement in clinical status is usually seen after as little as 25–50 mL of fluid are removed.

A pericardiocentesis can be performed at the bedside with cardiac monitoring available. The individual is placed in semi-Fowler's position, the site is cleansed with an antibacterial solution, and local anesthesia is injected into the site. The semi-Fowler's position is assumed so that most of the fluid will be in the most dependent position. A 16-gauge to 18-gauge intracardiac needle attached to a 30–50 mL syringe is inserted into the pericardial sac using a subxiphoid approach under ultrasound guidance or with electrocardiogram (ECG) monitoring. When using ECG monitoring, alligator clamps are attached to the hub of the needle and to a V-lead on the ECG machine. When the needle comes in contact with the pericardium, the QRS voltage will increase. If the needle comes in contact with the myocardium, the individual may develop ectopic beats (premature atrial or ventricular contractions) or ST segment elevation. Once in the pericardial sac, fluid is gradually aspirated with the syringe.

Once the pericardiocentesis is completed, a catheter

may be inserted into the site. The catheter may be left in place and effusion allowed to drain until the output is 50–100 mL in 24 hours.

Nursing care during the pericardiocentesis procedure is reviewed in Table 38-2. Several complications may occur during the procedure, including dysrhythmias, pneumothorax, laceration of the coronary arteries, laceration of the lung, myocardial puncture (right atrium or right ventricle), trauma to abdominal organs (especially the liver), infection, introduction of air into the heart, and hypotension. Nursing monitoring for signs and symptoms

---

Table 38-2 Pericardiocentesis: Nursing Care

Preprocedure

- Describe possible sensations that may be experienced by the patient during the procedure (initial stick of the small needle for administration of the local anesthetic, burning during administration of the local anesthetic, pressure sensation during insertion of the pericardiocentesis needle, and some pain if the needle touches the pericardium during the procedure [the pericardium, which has nerve endings, is not anesthetized by the local anesthesia])
- Procure all needed equipment
- Supportive therapy with oxygen, aggressive fluid resuscitation, and administration of vasoactive agents, as clinically indicated and prescribed
- Assess for signs and symptoms of cardiac tamponade and obtain baseline hemodynamic parameters
- Ensure that signed consent has been obtained
- Explain procedure to individual
- Ensure IV access
- Position supine with HOB elevated to 30 degrees, as tolerated and suggested by physician performing procedure
- Connect to cardiac monitor, ECG machine, noninvasive blood pressure monitoring device, and pulse oximeter
- Administer sedation/anxiolytics, as prescribed
- Connect alligator clamp to hub of intracardiac needle and to V-lead on ECG machine or cardiac monitor

During procedure

- Monitor cardiac rhythm, vital signs, and hemodynamic status
- Observe for complications related to procedure
- Monitor amount and characteristics of drainage being aspirated
- Administer sedation or anxiolytics as needed

Postprocedure

- Assess for complications
- Assess for improvement in hemodynamic status and resolution of other signs and symptoms of cardiac tamponade
- Assess amount and characteristics of drainage if catheter left in place
- Ascertain that pericardial fluid specimens are sent to the lab for analysis
- Document vital signs, medications administered, and response to the procedure according to institutional policy and procedure

---

of any of these complications is important. The incidence of these complications is decreased when the procedure is conducted under direct visualization or electrocardiographic guidance. In addition, there is a decreased risk of complications with larger amounts of fluid in the pericardial sac.[4] Given the decreased morbidity associated with direct visualization and guidance, unguided pericardiocentesis procedures are recommended in emergent situations only.[3]

Frequent monitoring of vital signs, hemodynamic status (i.e., central venous pressure), and for presence of dysrhythmias during and following the procedure is essential. If the individual is in the intensive care unit, monitoring for cardiac dysrhythmias and of pulmonary artery pressures (if the individual has a pulmonary catheter in place) are conducted.

Pericardiocentesis with Sclerosing

As many as 56% of patients will experience reaccumulation of pericardial fluid after a pericardiocentesis.[3,5] In an attempt to prevent reaccumulation of fluid, management of cardiac tamponade includes instillation of a sclerosing agent into the pericardial sac every one to two days via the pericardiocentesis catheter. This procedure is done once pericardial fluid output is reduced to 50–100 mL in 24 hours. Sclerosing agents include bleomycin, doxycycline, mitomycin C, cisplatin, fluorouracil, minocycline, or radioisotopes. Instillation of a sclerosing agent creates an inflammatory response of the pericardium. In one study, minocycline was reported to control pericardial effusions for more than 30 days in more than 90% of individuals.[15] The catheter remains in place until less than 25 mL/24 hours pericardial fluid is drained. The catheter is removed after two days due to the risk of infection.

Side effects of administration of sclerosing agents include pain, fever, and myelosuppression. Investigators of one clinical trial reported individuals' experiencing shorter hospitalizations and less retrosternal pain after receiving bleomycin as compared to doxycycline.[16]

Biologic response modifiers, such as interleukin 2, have been used to control the recurrence of pericardial effusions. Data suggest that approximately 67% of the cases can be controlled with these substances.[17] Radioisotopes such as gold and chromic phosphate have also been used to control pericardial effusions. Only partial effectiveness has been reported.[4]

Nursing care of individuals undergoing pericardiocentesis with sclerosing are similar to those described for individuals undergoing pericardiocentesis.

Pericardiotomy

A pericardiocentesis usually provides only temporary relief from signs and symptoms of cardiac tamponade until the underlying malignancy is treated. A pericardiotomy is an alternative method to prevent the reaccumulation of fluid. It involves incision of the pericardium and insertion of a balloon catheter into the pericardial sac.

The procedure can be performed at the bedside either percutaneously or using a subxiphoid approach under local anesthesia and is associated with minimal risks. A vertical incision is made below the xiphoid process and tissue displaced so that the pericardium can be visualized and incised. Once in place, the balloon is dilated to form a pericardial window, allowing pericardial fluid to drain. Nursing care of the individual undergoing a pericardiotomy is the same as the care of an individual undergoing a pericardiocentesis. A thoracotomy with pericardiotomy can also be performed under general anesthesia in the operating room.

Pleuropericardial Window

Another treatment approach, a pleuropericardial window, may be performed in the operating room under general anesthesia. The procedure entails removal of a piece of the pericardium, usually 4 cm. The purpose of a pericardial window is to drain the fluid from the pericardial sac if the effusion and tamponade are recurrent.[1] As this procedure is not well tolerated in a critically ill person, stabilization should first be accomplished. The procedure can also be performed using local anesthesia in 30–45 minutes.

A pleuropericardial window is usually performed on individuals refractory to other therapies. Preoperative nursing management for this individual includes patient education and supportive therapy. Postoperative prevention of complications is essential. Patency of the drainage catheter must also be maintained. Reported morbidities include infection, atelectasis, pleural effusion, pneumothorax, dysrhythmias, pain, and bleeding.

Pericardiectomy

A pericardiectomy is the excision of part to all of the pericardium. It involves a thoracotomy or median sternotomy. The pericardium is resected to facilitate drainage of fluid into the pleural space. The procedure is performed in the operating room under local or general anesthesia. General anesthesia is used for individuals with hemodynamic stability. The procedure is indicated for individuals with constrictive pericardial disease, which may occur in individuals with cancer with radiation pericarditis, for individuals with recurrent cardiac tamponade, and for individuals with long-term survival.[3] Complications associated with this procedure are laceration of the myocardium, bleeding, scarring, and infection. Cardiopulmonary bypass is usually required when a complete pericardiectomy is performed.[2]

Postprocedure nursing care associated with a pericardiectomy is similar to that for a pericardiocentesis. In addition, assessment for complications, including bleeding and hematoma formation, must be conducted. Neurovascular checks, hemodynamic monitoring including monitoring of urinary output, and assessment for reoccurrence of cardiac tamponade are also conducted.[3]

Chemotherapy and Radiotherapy

Administration of systemic chemotherapy and radiotherapy to the pericardium has been effectively used to control pericardial effusions.[4,14] It has been reported that up to 67% of individuals did not experience recurrence of the effusion following pericardiocentesis and administration of chemotherapy.[18] It has further been suggested that hormonal therapy may be effective in managing pericardial effusions in individuals with breast cancer. Administration of systemic chemotherapy is recommended in individuals with chemosensitive tumors such as lymphoma, leukemia, testicular cancer, and small cell lung carcinoma.

Use of external beam radiotherapy has also been reported in the management of pericardial effusions. Approximately 67% of individuals have had a positive result following administration of 1500–4000 cGy. A complication of this therapy is development of pericardial inflammation. Hence, radiotherapy is recommended for the individual with a radiosensitive tumor (such as lymphoma or leukemia) who has not received radiotherapy in the past and who is hemodynamically stable.[4]

Nursing care of individuals receiving systemic chemotherapy and radiotherapy for cardiac tamponade include providing patient education materials to facilitate the decision-making process regarding treatment options and specific information related to antineoplastic toxicities.

Continuity of Care

Management of an individual with cardiac tamponade poses several challenges for the nurse. It encompasses assessment and management of physiologic alterations, psychosocial support, and individual and family education.[7]

Assessment

Ongoing assessments must be performed to detect pericardial fluid accumulation. Evidence of any signs and symptoms of reaccumulation should be investigated immediately. Postprocedure wound assessments must also be performed. These assessments may be conducted in the home, the ambulatory setting, or the hospital.[3,14]

Physiologic Management

Nursing care associated with therapeutic approaches include ongoing assessment, monitoring of vital signs, respiratory and cardiovascular status, positioning, administration of supportive therapies, premedications, and ECG monitoring.[1,3] Following any therapeutic intervention, nursing management includes monitoring for signs and symptoms of any complications related to the procedure.

Psychosocial Support

Once fluid has accumulated and interventions are required, emotional support must be provided to combat the fear and anxiety associated with experiencing a life-threatening oncologic emergency.[1,3,19] The acute onset of the signs and symptoms as well as the need for admission to a critical care unit are additional sources of anxiety.

Providing an explanation of anticipated interventions and allowing the individual to verbalize concerns is essential. In addition to the reduction in psychosocial distress, support may result in a concomitant decrease in cardiac work load.

Patient and Family Education

Individuals and families must be educated about signs and symptoms of recurrence and actions to take in the event of recurrence. Early intervention is pivotal in trying to decrease complications and improving individual outcomes. Educational endeavors should also include information about the diagnostic and therapeutic interventions the individual will be experiencing.

Individuals and their families should also be aware of the prognosis associated with cardiac tamponade following treatment. Reportedly, individuals with cardiac tamponade may recover from the critical event with a good functional status. Length of survival depends on the malignant etiology and the extent of disease. A mean survival time of 3–18 months has been reported, depending on the underlying malignancy.[4]

Nursing Care

In addition to the nursing care delineated for the specific therapeutic interventions, several nursing diagnoses can be derived for the individual with a cardiac tamponade. A plan of care addressing the diagnoses appears in Table 38-3.

Table 38-3 Cardiac Tamponade: Nursing Care

Decreased cardiac output r/t decreased ventricular filling

Expected Outcome:	Individual's cardiac output will return to within normal limits.
Interventions:	Assess for signs and symptoms of decreased cardiac output:

  decreased blood pressure
  increased heart rate
  decreased level of consciousness
  cool, pale, and clammy skin
  decreased urine output (less than 0.5 mL/kg/hour)
  faint or absent peripheral pulses
  distant or muffled heart sounds
  weakness
  dizziness
  shortness of breath

Assess for signs and symptoms of cardiac tamponade.

Monitor vital signs and hemodynamic parameters (blood pressure, heart rate, respiratory rate, central venous pressure, pulmonary artery pressures) and sPO$_2$ hourly and prn.

Auscultate breath sounds q4h and prn.

Hourly I/O.

Assess cardiac rhythm and ECG tracings for electrical alternans, dysrhythmias, and for changes.

Administer aggressive fluid therapy and vasoactive agents, as prescribed.

Administer supplemental oxygen as prescribed.

Assist individual to assume a position of comfort.

Alteration in tissue perfusion r/t decreased cardiac output.

Expected Outcome:	Individual will attain and maintain normal tissue perfusion.
Interventions:	Assess for signs and symptoms of altered tissue perfusion:

  cool skin
  altered mental status
  increased capillary refill time

Monitor ABG results for acid-base imbalance.

Administer supplemental oxygen as prescribed.

Table 38-3   Cardiac Tamponade: Nursing Care (continued)

Impaired gas exchange r/t pericardial effusions (compensation by respiratory system for change in cardiac output could lead to impaired gas exchange).

Expected Outcome: Individual will maintain adequate gas exchange.

Interventions: Assess for signs and symptoms of impaired gas exchange:
  mental status changes
  tachypnea
  tachycardia or bradycardia
  dyspnea
  orthopnea
  use of accessory muscles
  presence of adventitious breath sounds
  activity tolerance
  SPO$_2$ levels

Monitor ABG results.

Administer supplemental oxygen, as prescribed.

Monitor vital signs hourly and prn.

Auscultate breath sounds q4h and prn.

Provide measures to minimize anxiety (e.g., anxiolytics, calm environment, relaxation techniques).

Assist to assume a position of comfort (e.g., semi-Fowler's).

Plan activities to allow for frequent rest periods.

Potential for infection r/t procedure and antineoplastic therapy.

Expected Outcome: Individual will not develop infection related to invasive procedures or antineoplastic therapy.

Interventions: Assess for signs and symptoms of infection:
  fever
  tachycardia
  tachypnea
  increased WBCs
  redness or discharge from catheter sites
  positive blood culture results

Maintain aseptic or sterile technique with all indwelling catheters according to institutional policy and procedure.

Administer antibiotic therapy as prescribed.

Perform sterile dressing changes to catheter sites according to institutional policy and procedure.

Anxiety r/t procedure, symptoms, and onset of critical illness compounding a cancer diagnosis and lack of information

Expected Outcome: Individual will verbalize a decrease in anxiety related to presence of symptoms and potential treatment modalities.

Interventions: Assess patient's degree of anxiety by observing behavioral manifestations and listening for verbal cues.

Encourage patient to verbalize feelings.

Explain all procedures and rationale for symptoms to individual and clarify misconceptions.

Allow time for individual and significant other to ask questions.

Anticipate that information may need to be reinforced.

Administer anxiolytics for treatment modalities, as prescribed.

Lack of knowledge r/t procedures and possible symptoms

Expected Outcomes: Individual will verbalize an increase in knowledge of symptoms and treatment modalities.

Individual will verbalize the signs and symptoms to report.

Interventions: Explain all procedures and rationale for symptoms to individual.

Allow time for individual and significant other to ask questions.

Assess individual understanding of information; reinforce as needed.

Provide written education information when preparing for discharge (e.g., signs and symptoms of reaccumulation of fluid and actions to take).

SPO$_2$ = PO$_2$ saturation

Conclusion

Cardiac tamponade is a life-threatening oncologic emergency that requires immediate management. Signs and symptoms of cardiac tamponade may occur slowly, over time, or acutely. Individuals require ongoing monitoring of their hemodynamic status to ensure the appropriate therapies are implemented. Despite the high level of acuity that the individual initially may present, prompt intervention and relief of the tamponade is usually associated with improved quality of life for a reasonable amount of time.[4]

Cardiac tamponade is not an uncommon oncologic emergency. It has been suggested that the incidence of cardiac tamponade due to malignancy may increase. This is attributed to the improvements in antineoplastic therapies and subsequent increase in survival time.[7]

No one therapeutic intervention is preferred in the management of cardiac tamponade. The decision is based on numerous factors, including the individual's disease type, prognosis, expected survival time, and clinical status.[4] Prompt and accurate nursing recognition and knowledge of the etiology, signs and symptoms, pathophysiology, and management of the problem are pivotal to decrease the morbidity and mortality associated with this oncologic emergency.

References

1. Uaje C, Kahsen K, Parish L: Oncology emergencies. *Crit Care Nurs Q* 18:26–34, 1996
2. Schwartz DE: Pericardial disease, in Parsons PE, Wiener-Kronish JP (eds): *Critical Care Secrets.* Philadelphia, Hanley & Belfus, 1992, pp 152–159
3. Beauchamp KA: Pericardial tamponade: An oncologic emergency. *Clin J Oncol Nurs* 2:85–95, 1998
4. Robinson LA, Ruckdeschel JC: Management of pleural and pericardial effusions, in Berger AM, Portenoy RL, Weissman DE (eds): *Principles and Practice of Supportive Oncology.* Philadelphia, Lippincott-Raven, 1998, pp 327–352
5. Maher EA, Shepherd FA, Dodd TJ: Pericardial sclerosis as the primary management of malignant pericardial effusion and cardiac tamponade. *J Thorac Cardiovasc Surg* 112:637–643, 1996
6. Pass HI: Malignant pleural and pericardial effusions, in DeVita VT, Hellman S, Rosenberg SA (eds): *Cancer: Principles and Practice of Oncology* (ed 5). Philadelphia, Lippincott, 1997, pp 2586–2598
7. Joiner GA, Kolodychuk GR: Neoplastic cardiac tamponade. *Crit Care Nurse* 11:50–58, 1991
8. Wilkes JD, Fidias P, Vaickus L, et al: Malignancy-related pericardial effusion: 127 cases from the Roswell Park Cancer Institute. *Cancer* 76:1377–1387, 1995
9. Laham RJ, Cohen DJ, Kuntz RE, et al: Pericardial effusion in patients with cancer: outcome with contemporary management strategies. *Heart* 75:67–71, 1996
10. Hambach C: Opening a window on pericardial effusion. *Nursing 98:*28:1–4, 1998
11. Miaskowski C: Oncologic emergencies, in Baird SB, McCorkle R, Grant CM (eds): *Cancer Nursing: A Comprehensive Textbook.* Philadelphia, Saunders, 1991, pp 885–893
12. Barbiere CC: Cardiac tamponade: diagnosis and emergency intervention. *Crit Care Nurse* 10:20–22, 1990
13. Saleh TG, Elfenbein GJ: Oncologic emergencies. *J Am Acad Physician Assist* 4:7–20, 1991
14. Lawler PE: Effusions, in Groenwald SL, Frogge MH, Goodman M, Yarbro CH (eds): *Cancer Symptom Management.* Sudbury, MA, Jones & Bartlett, 1996, pp 399–414
15. Lashevsky I, Ben Yosef R, Rinkevich D, et al: Intrapericardial minocycline sclerosis for malignant pericardial effusion. *Chest* 109:1452–1454, 1996
16. Liu G, Crump M, Goss PE, et al: Prospective comparison of the sclerosing agents doxycycline and bleomycin for the primary management of malignant pericardial effusion and cardiac tamponade. *J Clin Oncol* 14:3141–3147, 1996
17. Lissoni P, Barni S, Ardizzoia A: Intracavity administration of interleukin-2 as a palliative therapy for neoplastic effusions. *Tumori* 78:118–120, 1992
18. Vaitkus PT, Herrmann HC, LeWinter MM: Treatment of malignant pericardial effusion. *JAMA* 272:59–64, 1994
19. Maxwell MB: Malignant effusions and edema, in Groenwald SL, Frogge MH, Goodman M, Yarbro CH (eds): *Cancer Nursing. Principles and Practice* (ed 4). Sudbury, MA, Jones & Bartlett, 1997, pp 721–743

CHAPTER 39

Disseminated Intravascular Coagulation

Barbara Holmes Gobel, RN, MS

Scope of the Problem

Definitions

Disseminated intravascular coagulation (DIC) is the most common serious thrombotic state that occurs in individuals with cancer. DIC represents an inappropriate and exaggerated overstimulation of normal coagulation, in which thrombosis and then hemorrhage occurs. This seemingly paradoxical situation results in hypercoagulation, in which multiple small clots are formed in the microcirculation of many organs, and fibrinolysis, in which there is consumption of clots and clotting factors. Ultimately the body becomes unable to respond to vascular or tissue injury through stable clot formation, and hemorrhage occurs. The hemorrhage associated with DIC may be profound, but it is the intravascular coagulation that leads to irreversible morbidity and mortality in this population of patients.[1]

DIC can be chronic or acute in nature. If only a minor imbalance is present related to the intravascular coagulation, the syndrome may be chronic. Chronic DIC generally presents as localized thrombotic events, e.g., deep vein thrombosis. Acute DIC, which can be life-threatening, occurs when the intravascular coagulation becomes overwhelming to the body. Acute DIC is seen in certain defined clinical situations such as sepsis, acute leukemia, and tumor lysis. This chapter will deal with the acute form of DIC.

Incidence

Although DIC is considered to be a problem commonly associated with malignancy, its incidence is difficult to estimate as it varies depending on the type of associated neoplasm. Abnormal blood coagulation studies that demonstrate laboratory evidence of DIC are frequently reported in patients with disseminated solid malignancies (particularly the adenocarcinomas) and leukemia (particularly acute promyelocytic leukemia [APL]).[2-4] Overall, DIC is estimated to occur in 10% of all patients with cancer,[5] although it often remains undetected until severe hemorrhage occurs and frequently is only discovered at the time of autopsy.

Etiology and Risk Factors

DIC in the cancer population is always secondary to either the malignancy itself or to an underlying condition such as infection. Table 39-1 lists common causes of DIC in cancer. The most common cancers associated with acute DIC include acute leukemia and the mucin-producing adenocarcinomas. APL is the malignancy most commonly associated with DIC, which has been reported to occur in up to 85% of patients with APL.[6] DIC associated with APL can occur before and in conjunction with chemotherapy administration.[6] A procoagulant substance has

Table 39-1 Common Causes of DIC in Cancer

Neoplasms
- Solid tumors—lung, breast, ovary, stomach, pancreas, prostate, melanoma, gallbladder
- Leukemia—acute promyelocytic, acute myelogenous, chronic myelogenous, acute lymphoblastic

Infections
- Gram-negative bacteria—pseudomonas, salmonella, hemophilus, meningococcus, enterobacteriaceae
- Gram-positive bacteria—pneumococcus, staphylococcus, hemolytic streptococci
- Viremias—hepatitis, varicella, cytomegalovirus, human immunodeficiency virus
- Septic shock

Liver disease
- Obstructive jaundice
- Fulminant hepatic failure

Intravascular hemorrhage
- Acute hemolytic transfusion reaction
- Multiple transfusions of whole blood
- Minor hemolysis

Prosthetic devices
- Peritoneovenous shunts

been identified on the promyelocytic blast cells that is similar to thromboplastin. This substance is believed to be released from granulocytes on the promyelocytes, which subsequently initiates the clotting response.[7] It is important to note that with the use of new antileukemic drugs and the use of antifibrinolytic medications (to prevent bleeding), the mortality rate associated with APL has decreased significantly.[8] One of the antifibrinolytic agents that has shown great promise in the reduction of bleeding during treatment of APL is tranexamic acid.[9,10]

The solid tumors that are most commonly associated with DIC are the adenocarcinomas, including those of the lung, breast, stomach, pancreas, and prostate. Of these solid tumors, breast and prostate cancers are probably the most commonly seen DIC-related cancers. (The incidence of these cancers is significantly higher than the incidence of APL.) In addition to an unidentified procoagulant substance thought to be released from these cancers directly stimulating the coagulation system, tumors may also release necrotic tissue or tissue enzymes into the circulation thereby activating the coagulation mechanism.[11]

Infection and sepsis associated with cancer are the most common causes of acute DIC, and can be associated with a variety of bacterial, fungal, and viral infections. Sepsis, especially from gram-negative bacteria, is the most frequent cause of DIC.[12,13] It is believed that bacterial endotoxins released from gram-negative bacteremia activate one of the clotting factors (factor XII); this factor can initiate coagulation as well as stimulate fibrinolysis (the breakdown of clots), thus setting up DIC. Gram-positive organisms are thought to initiate coagulation by the same mechanism as endotoxins.[1] The triggering mechanism associated with viruses, including varicella, hepatitis, cytomegalovirus (CMV), or human immunodeficiency virus (HIV) is unclear.

Primary liver disease or liver metastasis can increase the risk of DIC. The liver replaces clotting factors and inhibitors as they are consumed.[13] The liver also clears activated coagulation factors and fibrinolytic degradation products from the systemic circulation. Hepatic failure then disrupts the normal balance of coagulation, which can lead to DIC.

Hemolytic transfusion reactions may be complicated by shock, renal failure, and DIC with severe bleeding.[13] These reactions are probably due to generalized endothelial injury caused by activated complement, cytokines, and neutrophil products.[14] DIC may also occur after massive transfusions, but its etiology is unknown.[13]

Prosthetic devices, such as a peritoneovenous shunt, are used to shunt ascitic fluid into the systemic circulation. Ascitic fluid contains collagen and other procoagulant substances. When these substances are shunted into the general circulation, DIC can be triggered.[15]

Physiologic Alterations

Pathophysiology

Although DIC is triggered by a number of defined clinical events such as infection or the malignancy itself, once initiated the pathophysiology is similar in all disorders. When one of these events occurs, the coagulation system is activated, thus activating thrombin and simultaneously activating the fibrinolytic system with the production of plasmin.[16] As discussed in Chapter 31 on "Bleeding Disorders," in which there is a thorough discussion of the physiology of coagulation, thrombin is the central proteolytic enzyme of blood coagulation. The presence of thrombin is also necessary for the breakdown of clots, or fibrinolysis.

Excess circulating thrombin cleaves fibrinogen, which leaves behind fibrin monomers that polymerize into fibrin clots in the circulation.[1] These excess clots trap platelets that lead to microvascular and macrovascular thrombosis with subsequent impaired organ perfusion and end-organ damage.[1,16,17] This entrapment of platelets also leads to a worsening of the thrombocytopenia, which is generally seen with acute DIC. As this process continues clotting factors are consumed, overwhelming their potential for production. At the same time, excess circulating thrombin assists in the conversion of plasminogen to plasmin, causing fibrinolysis, which in turn results in increased amounts of fibrin degradation products that have strong anticoagulant properties, leading to hemorrhage.[18] Excess plasmin can inactivate clotting factors, but it can also activate the complement and kinin systems. Activation of these systems can lead to increased vascular

permeability, hypotension, and shock. The clinical picture of acute DIC is a hemodynamically unstable patient who is experiencing a combination of extreme thrombosis and bleeding. Figure 39-1 depicts the process of DIC.

Clinical Manifestations

Signs and symptoms of acute DIC are variable and complex. Recognizing this syndrome in its early phase and treating it promptly are crucial to the prognosis of the affected patient. Unfortunately, DIC is often a fatal process as it frequently goes unrecognized until severe hemorrhage occurs. Some early specific signs of DIC that should forewarn of the problem of DIC include petechiae, purpura, hemorrhagic bullae, acral cyanosis, and at times frank gangrene.[17,19,20] Systemic signs and symptoms of DIC include fever, hypoxia, acidosis, hypotension, and proteinuria.[19,21] If severe, the patient will demonstrate a clinical picture of shock.

Bleeding is the most obvious sign of a hemorrhagic disorder and can occur from any orifice or opening on the surface of the skin. Patients may ooze blood from surgical, venipuncture, or wound sites. Overt hemorrhage involving multiple unrelated sites is not uncommon in the patient with acute DIC. Hemoptysis, intraperitoneal hemorrhage, and intracranial bleeding all pose life-threatening events for the patient with DIC.

Thrombus formation often occurs simultaneously with bleeding in DIC. Thrombi generally form in the

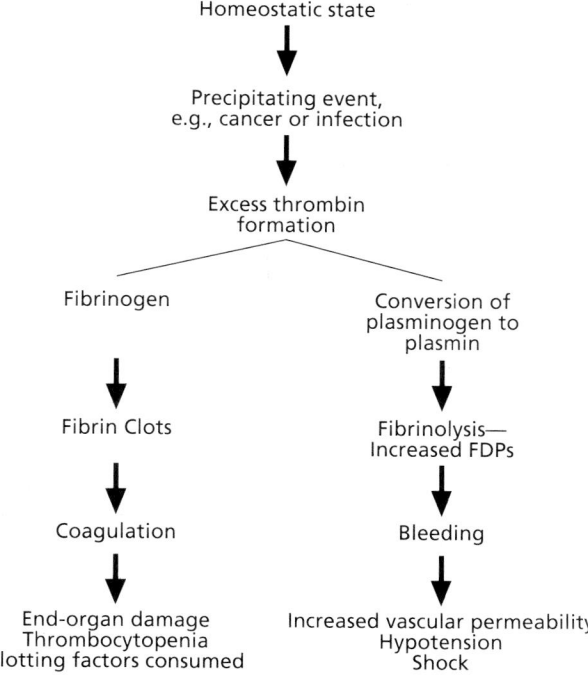

FIGURE 39-1 The process of DIC.

superficial and smaller veins, and may be clinically unde-tectable. Subtle signs and symptoms of thrombi include red, indurated tender areas found in multiple organ sites. When thrombosis occurs, the signs and symptoms may include focal ischemia, acral cyanosis, superficial gan-grene, altered sensorium, ulceration of the gastroin-testinal tract, and dyspnea (which can lead to acute respiratory distress syndrome). Widespread thrombosis (purpura fulminans—irregular hemorrhagic skin le-sions) and significant bleeding can occur simultane-ously.[22]

Assessment

There is no specific laboratory finding that is absolutely diagnostic of DIC. A battery of lab tests in conjunction with clinical evidence must be used to confirm the diagno-sis, as well as to monitor response to treatment. A number of clinical conditions will affect these tests, which makes their interpretation difficult. For example, multiple blood product transfusions will dilute clotting factors or platelets, and liver disease with portal hypertension can lead to thrombocytopenia and the activation of the fi-brinolytic system.

Traditionally, a "classic triad" of tests have been used to help support the diagnosis of DIC: the prothrombin time (PT), the platelet count, and the plasma fibrinogen level.[22,23] It has been found, however, that these findings are not as predictive of DIC as once was thought. The PT, while expected to be prolonged in DIC (because of a depletion of clotting factors), is normal in up to 50% of the patients diagnosed with DIC. This is because of interference of circulating activated clotting factors or fibrin degradation products (FDPs). The same has been found for the activated partial thromboplastin time (aPTT).[16,19] The platelet count is usually decreased in

DIC, but the mere presence of thrombocytopenia is nei-ther sensitive nor specific for DIC.[13] The fibrinogen con-centration does screen for clinically significant clotting factor deficiency, but this test too may be misleading due to circulating activated factors.[13,17] The presence of schistocytes—red cell fragments—in the blood smear is a frequent but nonspecific finding for acute DIC. (The presence of schistocytes supports the diagnosis of chronic DIC more significantly, as they are found in almost all such cases.)[23,24]

Newer, more sophisticated tests have become available for a more accurate laboratory diagnosis of DIC. Table 39-2 lists the laboratory tests used to support the diagnosis of DIC. One of these newer tests is the D-dimer assay. The D-dimer is a neoantigen formed as a result of plasmin digestion of fibrin. This test is specific for FDPs, which are increased in acute DIC.[24] Another test used to screen for excess FDPs is the FDP titer. FDP titers are found to be elevated in most patients with DIC.[1]

Other tests may be done to document accelerated coagulation and accelerated fibrinolysis, which may also help to support a diagnosis of DIC. A decreased level of antithrombin III (AT III) demonstrates accelerated coagulation, which is suggestive for DIC. Measuring the products of coagulation factor activation provides more information about the dynamics of DIC. The plasma level of fibrinopeptide A reflects the rate of fibrin formation, and levels of prothrombin activation peptide (F1 and F2) and thrombin–antithrombin complexes (TAT) are indicators of the rate of thrombin formation.[13,16]

In addition to FDP titers and the D-dimer assay tests to detect accelerated fibrinolysis in DIC, plasminogen and α2-antiplasmin levels may be drawn. The presence of lower or falling levels of plasminogen and α2-antiplasmin levels suggests hyperfibrinolysis.[16] These tests also help to support the diagnosis of DIC.

The above-mentioned screening tests—an elevated D-dimer assay, elevated FDP titer, a decreased AT III level,

Table 39-2 Laboratory Studies for DIC

Test	Result	Comments
D-dimer assay	Elevated	Neoantigen formed when plasmin digests fibrin Specific for increased FDPs
FDP titer	Elevated	Increased consumption of clots Specific for increased FDPs
Platelet count	Decreased	Frequent, but nonspecific finding in DIC
Peripheral smear	Schistocytes	Frequent, but nonspecific finding in DIC
Antithrombin III level	Decreased	Demonstrates accelerated coagulation
Fibrinopeptide A level	Elevated	Reflects the rate of fibrin formation, demonstrates accelerated coagulation
Prothrombin fragments (F1 & F2)	Elevated	Reflects the rate of thrombin formation, demonstrates accelerated coagulation
Thrombin-antithrombin (TAT) complexes	Elevated	Reflects the rate of thrombin formation, demonstrates accelerated coagulation
Plasminogen levels	Decreased	Suggests hyperfibrinolysis
α2-antiplasmin levels	Decreased	Suggests hyperfibrinolysis

a decreased fibrinopeptide A level, and the presence of schistocytes in the presence of a thrombocytopenic patient—would be considered to be positive laboratory diagnostic findings for DIC.[1,13,16]

Therapeutic Approaches and Nursing Care

Prevention

DIC related to cancer cannot necessarily be prevented as it often occurs as a result of the malignancy itself or treatment of the malignancy, e.g., chemotherapy or the administration of blood products. The potential for preventing DIC related to infection may result from aggressive management of the neutropenic patient. Early detection of the signs and symptoms of DIC allow for the best chance for prompt diagnosis and treatment, resulting in a better prognosis for the patient with DIC.

Prevention of further complications of DIC includes removal of any tight or restrictive clothing. If edema is present, it should be measured daily. Elastic support stockings may help minimize stasis and promote venous return. Other measures to decrease stasis and promote venous return include assisting the patient with leg lifts or elevating the legs to 15–20 degrees at intervals, and teaching the patient to wiggle his or her toes and perform ankle circles frequently while in bed. Compression to the knee vessels is minimized by avoiding placing anything under the knees while in bed (pillows, knee gatches), by avoiding crossing of the knees or legs, and by avoiding dangling the legs over the side of the bed.[11]

Management

Treatment of the underlying etiology is critical in the management of DIC.[16,21,22] Until the underlying stimulus of DIC is managed successfully, all other therapy will only provide an interval of symptomatic relief. Thus, the patient who is experiencing DIC related to sepsis must be treated aggressively with antibiotic therapy while being hemodynamically supported.

Early detection of the signs and symptoms of DIC may allow for prompt diagnosis and treatment. The major complications related to DIC include: (1) bleeding with the potential for hemorrhage resulting in hypoxia, acidosis, hypotension, proteinuria, and altered fluid balance, and (2) thrombus formation. Ongoing monitoring of the bleeding process is essential to minimize blood loss. See Table 39-3 for a review of the physical examination of the patient with actual or potential bleeding. Oxygen therapy is initiated immediately for the hypoxia and associated acidosis. Fluid replacement therapy must also be initiated promptly, as the patient can quickly become hypovolemic with significant bleeding. Fluid replacement therapy will also help manage the associated proteinuria

Table 39-3   Physical Examination of the Patient with Actual or Potential Bleeding

Integumentary system
- Bruising, petechiae, purpura, ecchymoses, acrocyanosis (irregularly shaped cyanotic patches on the periphery of arms and legs associated with bleeding due to DIC)
- Oozing from venipuncture sites or injections, biopsy sites, central lines, catheters, or nasogastric tubes
- Color and condition of gingival tissues

Eyes[a] and ears
- Visual disturbances, increased injection on the sclera, periorbital edema, subconjunctival hemorrhage (homogeneous red color that is sharply outlined on the sclera), headache, eye or ear pain

Nose, mouth, and throat
- Petechiae on nasal/oral mucosa, epistaxis, tenderness or bleeding from gums or oral mucosa

Cardiopulmonary system
- Crackles, wheezes, stridor, dyspnea, tachypnea, orthopnea, cyanosis, and hemoptysis (all possible signs of bleeding in the lungs), vital sign changes, decrease in color and temperature of all extremities, decreased peripheral pulses, tachycardia
- Observe for angina

Gastrointestinal system[b]
- Pain, bleeding, blood around rectum, tarry stools, frank or occult blood in stools, hemoptysis
- Observe for bleeding hemorrhoids (may respond to local measures)

Genitourinary system
- Bleeding, character, and amount of menses
- Monitor intake and output (if urine drops below 30 mL/hr it may be due to acute tubular necrosis secondary to thrombi, bleeding, or hypovolemia)

Musculoskeletal system
- Check for complaint of painful joints while performing active or passive range of motion, which may indicate bleeding into the joints

Central nervous system
- Mental status changes, including restlessness, confusion, lethargy, dizziness, obtundation, seizures, or coma (may indicate intracranial hemorrhage or impaired tissue perfusion)

[a]Bleeding in the optic fundus could lead to permanent visual impairment.

[b]Guaiac all excreta for blood.

and hypotension. Fluid replacement may include albumin, hydroxyethyl starch, plasma protein fraction, and intravenous (IV) solutions.[1,7] The administration of blood components such as red blood cells, platelets, and fresh frozen plasma may also double as replacement fluids. Caution must by used in treating the bleeding patient to avoid fluid overload and complications such as congestive heart failure.

Education is a necessary component of care when a patient is at risk for or is experiencing DIC. Patients and families are taught to report any bleeding or unusual symptoms. They are taught to save all excreta for the nurse to examine for blood. The patient and family will also need excellent psychosocial support should the patient develop this paradoxical situation of hemorrhage and thrombus formation.

Managing intravascular clotting

Much of the recent literature advocates that once treatment for the underlying stimulus of DIC is initiated, the intravascular clotting be treated next.[1,16,17] Although the bleeding associated with DIC is obvious and may be dramatic, it is the thrombotic process that has the greatest impact on morbidity and mortality in patients with DIC. Thus, an anticoagulant such as heparin may be initiated to stop the intravascular clotting process. Bick[1,3,19,21] has written extensively on the process of DIC and its management, and he recommends the use of subcutaneous (SQ) low-dose heparin initially. Effectiveness of low-dose heparin is generally seen within about 3 to 4 hours after initiation of therapy, first by correction of lab values and then by a cessation of clinically significant bleeding and thrombosis. Low-dose SQ heparin is generally considered to be safer than a higher dose of IV heparin, as it is associated with minimal chance of an increased risk of hemorrhage and the dose and route can be adjusted based on the patient's symptoms. Heparin use is contraindicated in patients with any signs of intracranial bleeding (e.g., cerebral vascular accident or headache), open wounds, or recent surgery. Antithrombin III is another anticoagulant that may be used for acute DIC.[16] Newer agents of potential benefit include recombinant hirudin, defibrotide, and gabexate.[25–28]

Blood component therapy

After attempts have been made at treating the underlying stimulus of DIC and managing the thrombotic state of the patient, blood component replacement therapy may be initiated. Most reports regarding blood component replacement therapy stress the importance of identifying the missing or lacking component and administering that specific component. There is, however, some controversy over its use in this setting. In addition to the problem of the lack of clinical trials in managing patients with DIC, another problem lies in the fact that certain blood components that may be deemed beneficial for the bleeding may be harmful for the process of coagulation. For example, fresh frozen plasma (FFP) is advocated by some authors for continued bleeding in a patient with DIC, as it provides a balanced substitution of coagulation factors.[13,29,30] Other authors cite concerns about the use of FFP in a patient with acute DIC because it contains fibrinogen, which can potentially create higher levels of FDPs that in turn can further impair hemostasis.[1,15,16] Cryoprecipitate (a concentrated source of fibrin and factor VIII) may be used to treat the severely bleeding patient who is hypofibrinogenemic, yet it too may create increased levels of FDPs.[29,31] Platelets may be given if the platelet count drops below 20,000 cells/mm³. A platelet count of 50,000 cells/mm³ in a bleeding patient may require platelet transfusion because of possible platelet dysfunction.[29] Washed packed red blood cells may also be given for the patient who is hemorrhaging. As mentioned before, volume expanders may include albumin, plasma protein fraction, and hydroxyethyl starch.[1]

Fibrinolytic inhibitors

In rare instances, fibrinolytic medications may be used in managing ongoing DIC. These medications may be used when the patient continues to bleed after being treated by the other three measures listed above: treating the underlying stimulus of DIC, treating the thrombotic process, and administering missing blood components. Two of these medications are epsilon-amino-caproic acid (EACA, Amicar) and tranexamic acid (retinoic acid). These medications are given only after the intravascular coagulation process and fibrin deposition have been alleviated, as they can lead to widespread fibrin deposition in the microcirculation and result in ischemic organ dysfunction.[17,22] Amicar is generally given by slow IV push every hour for 24 hours, or until bleeding stops. In addition to the problem of increased fibrin deposition, Amicar can cause ventricular arrhythmias, severe hypotension, and severe hypokalemia.[1] Retinoic acid is a newer agent with fewer undesirable effects.[20] It is being used more frequently in the management of APL, where there is a high risk of DIC. Addition of retinoic acid to the treatment plan of APL may result in less hemorrhage and transfusion requirements.[10]

Continuity of Care

The care of patients with acute DIC is complex and challenging. Most patients experiencing this syndrome will be managed primarily in the intensive care setting. The patient who is bleeding and intravascularly clotting at the same time will require aggressive hemodynamic support. The treatments used for the bleeding and clotting—anticoagulants, blood components, and possibly fibrinolytic inhibitors—have serious potential side effects that require intensive assessment and monitoring. However, because the process of DIC may occur over hours to days, patients at risk for DIC may be cared for in any setting. Nurses need to be aware of risk factors for the development of acute DIC related to cancer. With prompt recognition of a bleeding or clotting problem, there is the potential for prompt treatment of this potentially fatal syndrome.

Conclusion

Acute DIC related to cancer can be due to a number of causative factors, including the cancer itself or a process such as infection. The primary management of patients with acute DIC is to treat the underlying pathology creating the DIC condition. Patients may also be treated aggressively to maintain their hemodynamic status, as well as with a variety of medications and blood components.

Because DIC contributes greatly to morbidity and mortality in patients with cancer, nurses play a valuable role in the prompt recognition of its signs and symptoms. Early recognition of the signs and symptoms of bleeding or clotting can lead to prompt treatment of this challenging problem. It is hoped that future research will identify more clearly the most appropriate treatment for acute DIC.

References

1. Bick RL: Disseminated intravascular coagulation: objective clinical and laboratory diagnosis, treatment, and assessment of therapeutic response. *Semin Thromb Hemost* 22:69–88, 1996
2. Bick RL: Coagulation abnormalities in malignancy. *Semin Thromb Hemost* 18:353–372, 1992
3. Bick RL: Alterations of hemostasis in malignancy, in Bick RL, Bennett JM, Brynes RK (eds): *Hematology: Clinical and Laboratory Practice.* St. Louis, Mosby, 1993, pp 1583–1590
4. Murphy-Ende K: Disseminated intravascular coagulation, in Chernecky CC, Berger BJ (eds): *Advanced and Critical Care Oncology Nursing.* Philadelphia, Saunders, 1998, pp 119–139
5. Bavier AR: Coagulopathies, in Gross J, Johnson BL (eds): *Handbook of Oncology Nursing* (ed 2). Sudbury, MA, Jones and Bartlett, 1994, pp 729–794
6. Bunn RA, Ridgeway EC: Paraneoplastic syndromes, in DeVita VT, Hellman S, Rosenberg SA (eds): *Cancer: Principles and Practice of Oncology* (ed 4). Philadelphia, Lippincott, 1993, pp 2026–2071
7. Goodnough LT: Management of disseminated intravacular coagulation, in Rossi EC, Simon TL, Moss GS (eds): *Principles of Transfusion Medicine.* Baltimore, Williams and Wilkins, 1991, pp 373–382
8. Kurtz A: Disseminated intravascular coagulation with leukemia patients. *Cancer Nurs* 16:456–463, 1993
9. Seto AH, Dunlap DS: Tranexamic acid in oncology. *Ann Pharmacother* 30:868–870, 1996
10. Shpilberg O, Blumenthal R, Sofer O, et al: A controlled trial of tranexamic acid therapy for the reduction of bleeding during treatment of acute myeloid leukemia. *Leuk Lymphoma* 19:141–144, 1995
11. Gobel BH: Bleeding disorders, in Groenwald SL, Frogge MH, Goodman M, Yarbro CH (eds): *Cancer Nursing Principles and Practice* (ed 4). Sudbury, MA, Jones and Bartlett, 1997, pp 604–639
12. Bone RC: Modulators of coagulation. A critical appraisal of their role in sepsis. *Arch Intern Med* 152:1381–1389, 1992
13. Williams EC, Mosher DF: Disseminated intravascular coagulation, in DeVita VT, Hellman S, Rosenberg SA (eds): *Cancer*

Principles and Practice of Oncology (ed 5). Philadelphia, Lippincott-Raven, 1997, pp 1758–1769
14. Butler J, Parker D, Pillai R: Systemic release of neutrophil elastase and tumor necrosis factor alpha following ABO incompatible blood transfusion. *Br J Haematol* 78:525–526, 1991
15. Lankiewicz MW, Bell WB: Disseminated intravascular coagulation, in Bell WB (ed): *Hematologic and Oncologic Emergencies.* New York, Churchill Livingstone, 1993, pp 110–119
16. Staudinger T, Locker GJ, Frass M: Management of acquired coagulation disorders in emergency and intensive-care medicine. *Semin Thromb Hemost* 22:93–104, 1996
17. Bick RL: Disseminated intravascular coagulation: objective criteria for diagnosis and management. *Med Clin North Am* 78:541–543, 1994
18. Gobel BH: Disseminated intravascular coagulation. *Semin Oncol Nurs* 15:174–182, 1999
19. Bick RL, Baker WF: Disseminated intravascular coagulation syndromes. *Hematol Pathol* 6:1–24, 1992
20. Bick RL: Disseminated intravascular coagulation. *Hematol Oncol Clin North Am* 6:1259–1285, 1992
21. Bick RL: Disseminated intravascular coagulation, in Bick RL (ed): *Disorders of Thrombosis and Hemostasis: Clinical and Laboratory Practice.* Chicago, ASCP Press, 1992, 137–173
22. Marder JV, Martin SE, Coleman RW: Clinical aspects of consumptive thrombohemorrhagic disorders, in Coleman RW, Hirsh J, Marder JV, Salzman EW (eds): *Hemostasis and Thrombosis* (ed 3). Philadelphia, Lippincott, 1993, pp 665–693
23. Rutherford CJ, Frenkel EP: Thrombocytopenia: issues in diagnosis and therapy. *Med Clin North Am* 78:555–575, 1994
24. Bick RL, Baker W: Diagnostic efficiency of the D-dimer assay in DIC and related disorders. *Thromb Res* 65:785–790, 1992
25. Vinazzer HA: Antithrombin III in shock and disseminated intravascular coagulation. *Clin Appl Thromb Hemost* 1:62–65, 1995
26. Dickneite G, Czech J: Combination of antibiotic treatment with the thrombin inhibitor recombinant hirudin for the therapy of experimental *Klebsiella pneumoniae* sepsis. *Thromb Haemost* 71:772–778, 1994
27. Nowak G, Markwardt F: Hirudin in disseminated intravascular coagulation. *Haemostasis* 21 (Suppl 1): 142–148, 1991
28. Okamura T, Niho Y, Itoga T, et al: Treatment of disseminated intravascular coagulation and its prodromal stage with gabexate mesilate (FOY): a multi-center trial. *Acta Haematol* 90:120–124, 1993
29. Gilbert JA, Scalzi RP: Disseminated intravascular coagulation. *Emerg Med Clin North Am* 11:465–480, 1993
30. Kithchens CS: Disseminated intravascular coagulation, in Brain MC, Carbone PP, Kelton JG, Schiller JH (eds): *Current Therapy in Hematology-Oncology,* St. Louis, Mosby, 1995, pp 182–187
31. Menitove M, Gill JG, Montgomery RR: Preparation and clinical use of plasma and plasma fractions, in Beutler E, Lichtman MA, Coller BS, Kipps TJ (eds): *Williams Hemotology* (ed 5). New York, McGraw Hill, 1995, pp 1649–1663

CHAPTER 40

Septic Shock

Jennifer Petersen, RN, MS, OCN®

Scope of the Problem

Septic shock is characterized by hypotension, hypoxemia, organ dysfunction, and possibly even death. Following the invasion of bacteria, viruses, and/or fungi into the body, a battle between microbial factors and the host's immune and inflammatory response ensues. Early recognition and intervention frequently make the difference between living and dying in this oncologic emergency. Oncology nurses are in a pivotal position to optimize patient outcomes by understanding the risk factors, pathophysiology, clinical presentation, and therapeutic interventions of septic shock.

Definitions

Septic shock is not an all-or-nothing phenomenon. Rather, each phase represents a progressive stage of the same pathologic process. In 1991 the American College of Chest Physicians/Society of Critical Care Medicine (ACCP/SCCM) standardized definitions of the phases involved in septic shock: infection, bacteremia, systemic inflammatory response syndrome (SIRS), sepsis, severe sepsis, septic shock, and multiple organ dysfunction syndrome (MODS).[1]

According to Bone et al,[1] sepsis is a systemic inflammatory response to infection as evidenced by elevation of temperature, heart rate, and respiratory rate. The white blood count may be greater or less than normal. As symptoms progress, hypoperfusion, hypotension, and organ dysfunction occur, indicating severe sepsis. Septic shock is characterized by severe sepsis with hypoperfusion and hypotension that persist despite aggressive fluid challenge. Although MODS is potentially reversible, pathophysiologic abnormalities are so severe that homeostasis cannot be maintained without prompt and exact intervention.[2] The presence of MODS is an important prognostic indicator for septic shock; in fact, severe prolonged dysfunction of three or more organs correlates with a mortality rate of 90% or greater.[2]

Incidence

Advances in medical technology have produced novel methods of treatment and supportive care. These advances have increased the survival of the immunocompromised patient. An estimated 500,000 cases of sepsis occur annually in the United States.[3] Septicemia is the thirteenth leading cause of death.[3] Accordingly, septic shock remains the number one cause of death in medical and surgical intensive care units with mortality rates of approximately 40%–60%.[3,4] Although fungal, viral, and protozal infections can cause septic shock, the most common source continues to be bacterial, causing approximately 40%–60% of cases.[4] Gram-negative organisms have historically accounted for 50%–60% of septic shock cases, while gram-positive infections have been implicated in 5%–10% of cases.[3] The incidence of gram-positive sepsis is rising sharply due to increased use of intravascular devices and pneumonia, as well as the emergence of antibiotic-resistant organisms.[4] In an estimated 10%–30% of cases of septic shock, an initiating organism is never identified.[4]

Etiology and Risk Factors

The risk of developing septic shock mirrors the complexity of the oncology patient based on type, degree, and duration of immune deficiency. Immune function of individuals with cancer is threatened by numerous factors including the nature of their malignancy, antineoplastic therapy, as well as comorbid conditions (see Figure 40-1).[5] Understanding the normal host's defense is key to recognizing the risk factors of sepsis and septic shock in the oncology population. In general the individual is armed with nonspecific host defenses such as intact skin and mucous membranes, stomach acidity, flow of secretions, and proper nutrition.[6] These protective mechanisms are threatened, however, by cytotoxic drugs, radiation, surgery, invasive procedures, or the tumor itself.

Kumar[6] divides the host defenses that make up the immune system into four specific categories: (1) polymor-

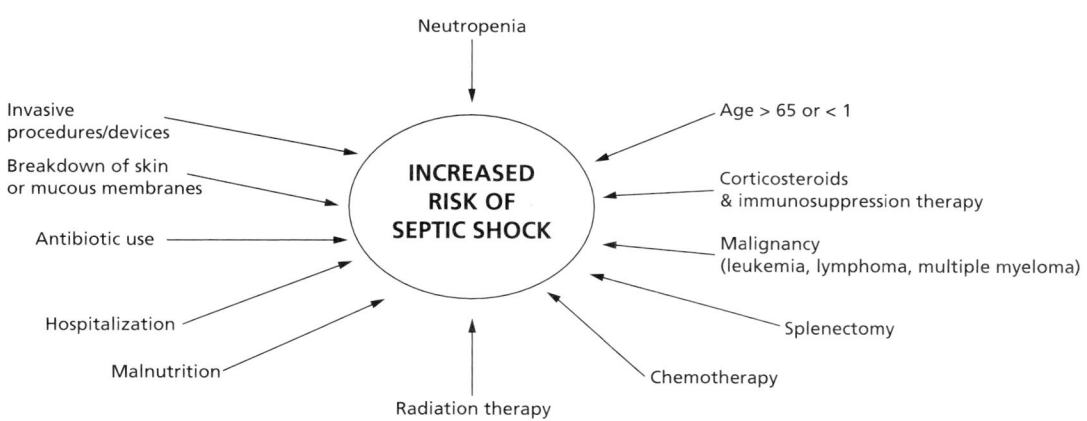

Figure 40-1   Risk factors for septic shock

phonuclear neutrophils(PMNs), (2) cell-mediated immunity, (3) humoral immunity, and (4) the complement cascade. In the first category of host defense, PMNs—otherwise known as granulocytes—phagocytoze and kill microbes. The most common defect in this host defense is called *granulocytopenia* which is a decrease in the number of PMNs. This is the single most important risk factor for sepsis in individuals with cancer.[7] Granulocytopenia occurs secondary to leukemia, bone marrow infiltration (or myelophthisis), total body irradiation, and cytotoxic chemotherapy. Individuals with a granulocyte count of less than $500/mm^3$ are at greatest risk of developing septic shock.

The second category of host defense is cell-mediated immunity, which serves to eliminate pathogens, malignant cells, and viruses by employing monocytes, macrophages, and T lymphocytes. Aberrant or ineffectual cell-mediated immunity is a result of lymphoma, HIV, and immunosuppressive/cytotoxic chemotherapy. The third type of host defense involves humoral immunity consisting of B lymphocytes that produce antibodies to foreign antigens. Antibodies tag microorganisms to be phagocytized. A humoral immunity defect occurs in patients with multiple myeloma, chronic lymphocytic leukemia, asplenism, and cytotoxic chemotherapy. The fourth category of immune function, the complement cascade, primarily induces inflammation and activation of phagocytic cells. Alterations in the complement cascade are observed in individuals with multiple myeloma. Chapter 3 provides a detailed review of the immune system.

Physiologic Alterations

Normal Physiology

If a microbial intruder such as bacteria, fungus, or a virus invades the body, it is recognized as foreign by white blood cells (WBCs). An adequate intact immune system promptly recruits neutrophils, macrophages, lymphocytes, and antibodies to the nidus of infection to prevent host colonization. At this point, microbes and their toxins are neutralized and eliminated via phagocytosis. If the virulence of the pathogen exceeds the capabilities of the host's defense, sepsis and possibly septic shock follow. As previously noted, an individual with cancer is particularly at risk due to multiple immune defects.

Pathophysiology

The pathophysiology of septic shock is a systemic biphasic process characterized by an initial pro-inflammatory response to ensure short-term survival and a longer compensatory anti-inflammatory response.[8,9] When checks and balances between these two normal protective phases fail, widespread systemic inflammation and shock may follow. If the invading organism overcomes local immune efforts, translocation into the bloodstream by the organism itself or by its cellular components occurs. For example, during bacterial proliferation or lysis, a structural component in the cell membrane of gram-negative microorganisms called "endotoxin" is released. Endotoxin is a potent trigger that ultimately causes the cellular and hemodynamic alterations seen in septic shock. According to Parrillo,[10] human and animal research have demonstrated that small doses of endotoxin injected into subjects produce fever, tachycardia, hypotension, decreased systemic vascular resistance, and myocardial depression. In addition, higher levels of endotoxemia generally correlate with an increased severity of septic shock.[10] Similarly, gram-positive organisms trigger septic shock via liberation of exotoxins, enterotoxins, peptidoglycans, and lipoteichoic acid.[4]

Bacterial toxins essentially serve as alarms to host immunity to prepare for an attack against the invading pathogen.[11] This counterattack by the host's immune system consists of the stimulation of macrophages, monocytes, neutrophils, and plasma cells that activates an outpouring of several endogenous cytokines and mediators (see Figure 40-2).[12,13] The primary pro-inflammatory cytokines are tumor necrosis factor (TNF), interleukin 1 (IL1), and interleukin 6 (IL6).[9] These cytokines promote the release of secondary mediators that function in a variety of ways to ultimately reduce injury, promote healing, and battle pathogenic organisms.[9] Ironically, without proper regulation, the same protective process may induce fatal systemic inflammation and septic shock. In the attempt to modulate the inflammatory response, several anti-inflammatory substances such as endogenous corticosteroids and catecholamines are released, which results in rebound immunosuppression.

Endogenous mediators and inflammatory cells have a profound effect on the vasculature, heart, and other organs.[10] The vascular endothelium is responsible for anticoagulation, vasoregulation, and the maintenance of oxygen delivery to tissues.[14] As a result of its large systemic surface area, endothelium is constantly exposed to toxins and inflammatory mediators that induce vascular abnormalities during septic shock.[14] Endotoxin, TNF, and IL1 promote tissue factor expression on endothelial cells, which activates coagulation via the extrinsic pathway.[4] As septic shock progresses, fibrinolysis, coagulopathies, and possibly even disseminated intravascular coagulation (DIC) may occur.[4,15]

In response to endotoxin, the endothelium releases endothelium-derived relaxing factor, or nitric oxide, which causes vasodilatation and decreased arterial and venous tone.[10,16] The primary compensatory role of nitric oxide is to sustain visceral blood flow; when produced in excess, however, nitric oxide is thought to be responsible for the myocardial depression as well as the pathologic hypotension observed as the hallmark of septic shock.[17] Other vascular abnormalities include venous pooling, decreased venous return, and maldistribution of blood volume.[4] In addition, increased microvascular permeability renders vessels porous to fluids and solutes, resulting in hypovolemia via capillary leak and third spacing.[4] Migration and adhesion of neutrophils, platelets, red blood

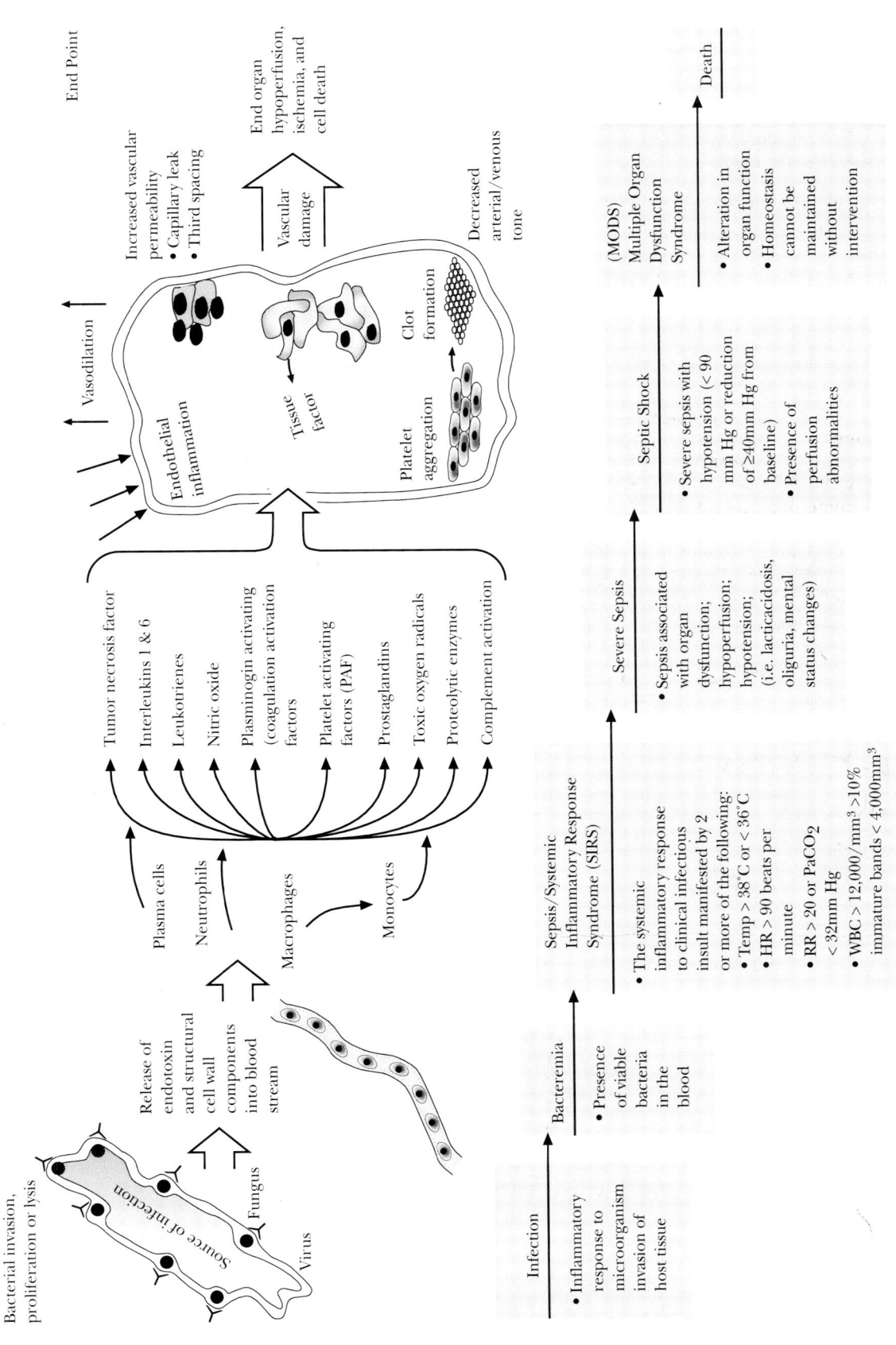

Figure 40-2   Pathophysiology of the septic shock cascade. Data from Bone et al[1]; Huddleston[12] Wheller, Bernar.[13]

cells (RBCs), and fibrin form sludging in the microvasculature. Obstruction of blood flow and inadequate nutrient exchange results in tissue hypoxia and metabolic abnormalities.[10]

Clinical Manifestations

Classic initial presentation of septic shock is manifested by fever, shaking chills, hypotension, tachycardia, tachypnea, and mental status changes. Such manifestations vary according to the stage of septic shock as well as the immunologic integrity of the individual with cancer. Frequently, signs and symptoms are subtle or absent. For example, a study by Le Gall et al[18] observed 1130 patients with severe sepsis and found 55% had fevers > 38° C, 15% were hypothermic (< 36° C), and 30% were normothermic. Attention to all clinical changes, therefore, is crucial for early recognition and treatment of the sepsis syndrome. The clinical picture of septic shock illustrates the effects of coagulopathy, hypotension, hypoperfusion, and ultimately tissue ischemia on virtually every organ system in the body (see Table 40-1).[19–22]

Mental status changes range from apprehension, agitation, withdrawal, confusion, obtundation, to coma.

Table 40-1 Clinical Manifestations of Organ Dysfunction in Septic Shock

Organ system	Severe Sepsis	Septic Shock
Central Nervous System	- Apprehension - Confusion - Disorientation - Agitation	- Obtundation - Coma
Cardiovascular	- Sinus tachycardia - Cardiac output normal to increased - BP < 90 mm Hg, or 40 mm Hg ↓ baseline - Systemic vascular resistance ↓	- Acrocyanosis - Tachycardia - Dysrhythmias - Hypotension - Cardiac output normal or high - Systemic vascular resistance ↑ or ↓
Pulmonary	- Tachypnea - Shallow breaths - Hypoxic on room air - Respiratory and metabolic acidosis - ↓ Breath sounds & crackles	- Shortness of breath (if not ventilated) - Refractory hypoxemia - Respiratory & metabolic acidosis - ↓ Breath sounds, crackles, and wheezes - Pulmonary edema - Acute respiratory distress syndrome
Renal	- ↓ Urine output - Increased osmolality	- Oliguria - Anuria - BUN ↑ - Creatinine ↑ - Acute renal failure
Hematology	- Leukopenia or leukocytosis - Thrombocytopenia - PT/PTT prolonged - Fibrinogen ↓ - Fibrin degradation products ↑	- Leukopenia or leukocytosis - Thrombocytopenia - Anemia - PT/PTT prolonged - Fibrinogen ↓ - Fibrin degradation products ↑
Metabolic & Electrolyte	- Temp > 38°C or < 36°C - Lactic acidosis - Hyperglycemia	- Temp > 38°C or < 36°C - Lactic acidosis - Hyperglycemia or hypoglycemia - ↓ Albumin - ↓ Potassium - ↓ Sodium - ↓ Calcium - ↓ Magnesium - ↓ Phosphate
Integument	- Dry, warm, and flushed skin	- Cold, pale, & clammy skin
Gastrointestinal	- Nausea and vomiting - ↓ GI motility	- ↓ GI motility - GI bleeding - ↑ Liver function tests - Jaundice

These changes arise from cerebral hypoxia, cerebral edema, and metabolic abnormalities.[21] Mentation changes often precede hypotension and temperature abnormalities in septic shock presentation.[4]

Cardiovascular manifestations of septic shock include increased heart rate and increased cardiac output (CO), decreased systemic vascular resistance (SVR), hypovolemia, hypotension, widened pulse pressure, arrhythmias, and decreased ejection fraction.[21] Interestingly, studies have postulated that coronary blood flow remains relatively adequate during septic shock and that, if myocardial dysfunction occurs, it is a result of circulating myocardial depressants.[10] These depressants have been identified as nitric oxide, tumor necrosis factor (TNF), and interleukin-1 (IL-1), and, when measured in high levels, denote a poor prognosis.[4] The skin and extremities are initially warm, dry, and flushed due to massive vasodilatation. Later in septic shock, the skin becomes cold, pale, and "clammy" as a result of maldistribution of blood flow.[21]

Dyspnea and tachypnea are always observed in septic shock. In many cases, pulmonary symptoms herald the onset of septic shock.[21] Due to hyperventilation, respiratory alkalosis soon follows.[22] Ventilation/perfusion inadequacy occurs because of increased capillary permeability and edema causing hypoxemia.[23] Refractory hypoxemia, pulmonary edema, adult respiratory distress syndrome (ARDS), respiratory acidosis, and ultimately respiratory failure will follow if the septic shock cascade is not blunted.[21] Urinary output ranges from a decreased urine output to anuria as septic shock progresses toward acute renal failure. Elevation in serum BUN and creatinine are observed.

Hematologic findings reveal leukocytosis due to increased neutrophil production and liberation of WBCs from the vessel wall into circulation (demargination) or leukopenia due to consumption, sequestration, or decrease in the number of WBCs from underlying malignancy.[22] Granulocytopenia in septic shock generally correlates with a poor prognosis.[21] Thrombocytopenia may result from decreased production, increased destruction, pooling, and sludging of platelets in the microvasculature. Prolonged PT/PTT, decreased fibrinogen, and elevated fibrin degradation products (FDP) may indicate DIC.[22] Clinical indicators of DIC include thrombosis, ischemia, and bleeding. Anemia is commonly seen as a result of hemodilution, hemorrhage, and shortened RBC survival.[21]

Alterations in glucose metabolism caused by sepsis initially present as hyperglycemia. Blood glucose levels rise sharply in response to release by the sympathetic nervous system of endogenous catecholamines, epinephrine, norepinephrine, glucocorticoids, as well as simultaneous gluconeogenesis.[24] Hypoglycemia may be seen in late prolonged septic shock, indicating hepatic failure and demise of compensatory mechanisms.[24] Elevated serum lactate levels reflect anaerobic metabolism in response to tissue hypoxia that can occur early in the process.[25] Also observed are lowered levels of albumin, sodium, potassium, calcium, and magnesium.[22]

The gastrointestinal (GI) tract is highly vascular and thus sensitive to ischemic conditions during septic shock.[26] Tissue hypoxia and bowel wall edema may result in decreased GI motility, nausea, vomiting, and ileus.[21] As a result of coagulopathies and tissue injury, GI bleeding and stress ulcers occur later in septic shock. Hyperbilirubinemia and transaminase elevation are observed in response to hepatocyte hypoperfusion. Considering the magnitude of functions performed by the liver (vascular, immune, metabolic, coagulation, detoxification, storage, and secretory), liver failure significantly affects all other organ systems' and impedes the body's attempt to regain homeostasis. Mortality rates with liver failure due to septic shock reach 90%–100%.[27]

Assessment

Patient History

When caring for an individual in septic shock, understanding past and present medical history helps identify risk factors and pinpoint the infectious source. Depending on the time and place of septic shock presentation, this information may come directly from the patient, a family member, or from the medical record. Information regarding current cancer treatment (chemotherapy, radiation, steroids or other immunosuppressive drugs, dosages and schedule) is important in determining the type, degree, and duration of immunosuppression. History of prior infections and antibiotic use may provide clues to the development of secondary infections or resistant organisms. Individuals who are older than 65, have indwelling catheters, and have poor nutritional status are at a significant risk for sepsis and possibly septic shock.

Physical Exam

The physical examination serves a dual purpose: (1) to assess the degree of organ dysfunction resulting from septic shock, and (2) to investigate the source of infection. Assessment of vital signs is performed with the first suspicion of a patient's being septic and is repeated as frequently as needed depending on the stage of shock. Ideally, monitoring of blood pressure (BP), pulse, and oxygen saturation should be continually performed and recorded using an electronic monitoring device if the patient is not in the intensive care setting. The assessment of vital signs as well as of weight gain or loss provides noninvasive feedback regarding the severity of shock as well as a measure of the benefits of therapeutic interventions. A thorough assessment should be performed since almost every organ system is affected during septic shock (see Table 40-1). The search for the focus of infection in an individual with cancer includes assessments of the mouth, pharynx, GI tract, respiratory tract, perianal region, urinary tract, skin, and catheter site.

Early hospital discharge, as well as the increasing complexity of cytotoxic treatment in the ambulatory setting, translates into many immunocompromised individuals caring for themselves at home. Initial assessment of sepsis and early septic shock is sometimes done via telephone triage by a practitioner in the outpatient setting. Figure 40-3 illustrates guidelines for a verbal assessment to examine risk factors, determine severity of condition, as well as identify the urgent need to seek medical evaluation.

Diagnostic Studies

Many diagnostic tests are available to evaluate severity of septic shock and to determine the source of infection. Blood cultures are drawn expeditiously from two separate sources (two venipuncture sites, or one venipuncture site and one central line) using 10% providone iodine or 1%–2% tincture of iodine allowed to dry as a skin preparation. Central line access and the culture bottles are cleansed with 70% alcohol.[28] Cultures of other body fluids such as urine, stool, sputum, or other exudate are collected as clinically relevant. Cultures should be repeated

every 24 hours if septic shock persists. Frequent monitoring of the complete blood count (CBC), electrolytes, lactic acid, arterial blood gases (ABGs), coagulation profiles, and liver functions provide information about the severity of septic shock, organ dysfunction, and response to therapeutic interventions.[29] To further evaluate organ function and to determine the infectious source, other tests such as echocardiograms, computerized tomography (CT) scans, ventilation/perfusion scan, and angiography may be performed[30] (see Table 40-2).

Therapeutic Approaches and Nursing Care

Prevention

Basic infection precautions should be instituted and consistently practiced across all settings in oncology care (see

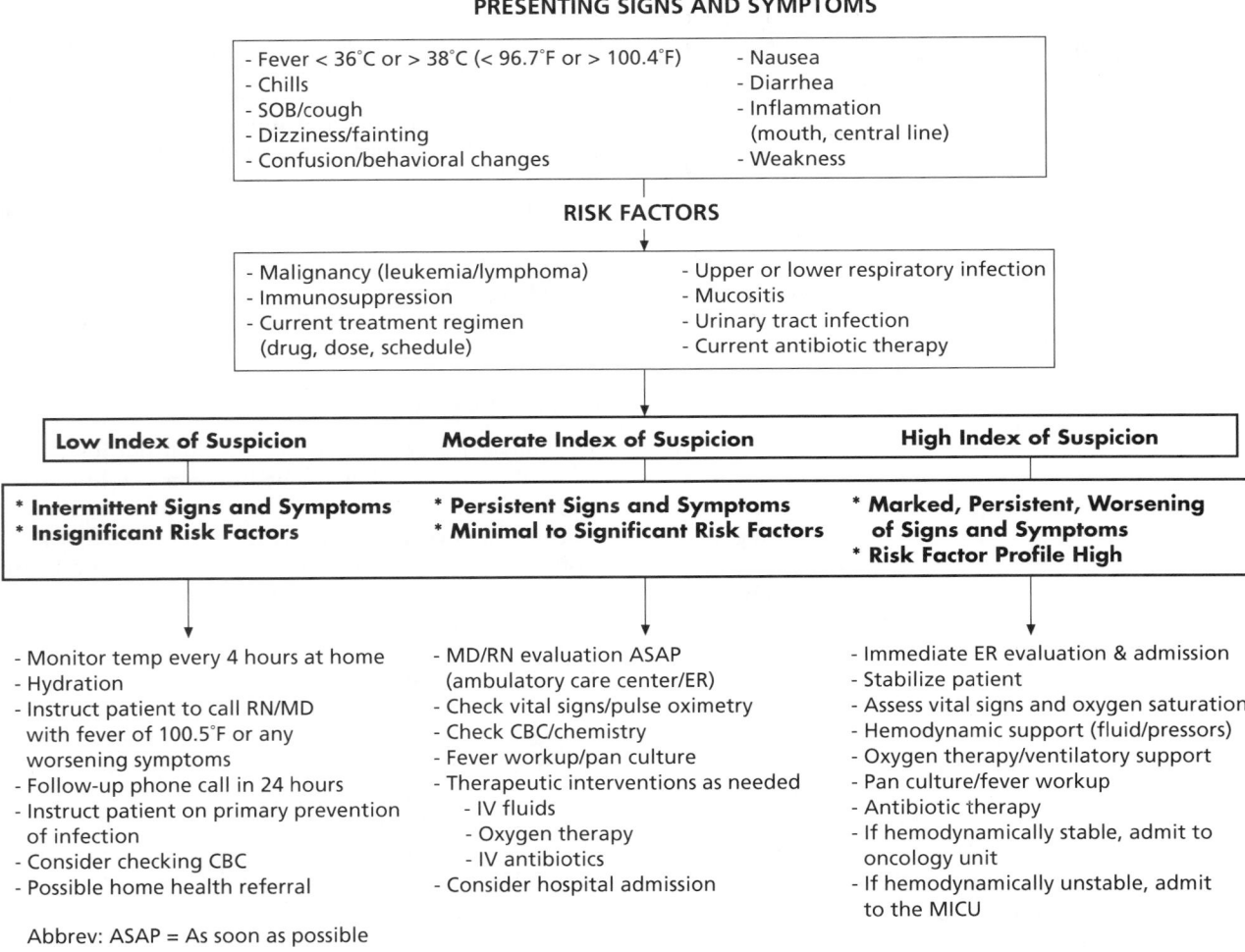

PRESENTING SIGNS AND SYMPTOMS

- Fever < 36°C or > 38°C (< 96.7°F or > 100.4°F)   - Nausea
- Chills   - Diarrhea
- SOB/cough   - Inflammation
- Dizziness/fainting   (mouth, central line)
- Confusion/behavioral changes   - Weakness

RISK FACTORS

- Malignancy (leukemia/lymphoma)   - Upper or lower respiratory infection
- Immunosuppression   - Mucositis
- Current treatment regimen   - Urinary tract infection
  (drug, dose, schedule)   - Current antibiotic therapy

Low Index of Suspicion	Moderate Index of Suspicion	High Index of Suspicion
* Intermittent Signs and Symptoms * Insignificant Risk Factors	* Persistent Signs and Symptoms * Minimal to Significant Risk Factors	* Marked, Persistent, Worsening of Signs and Symptoms * Risk Factor Profile High

- Monitor temp every 4 hours at home
- Hydration
- Instruct patient to call RN/MD with fever of 100.5°F or any worsening symptoms
- Follow-up phone call in 24 hours
- Instruct patient on primary prevention of infection
- Consider checking CBC
- Possible home health referral
	- MD/RN evaluation ASAP (ambulatory care center/ER)
	- Check vital signs/pulse oximetry
	- Check CBC/chemistry
	- Fever workup/pan culture
	- Therapeutic interventions as needed
	    - IV fluids
	    - Oxygen therapy
	    - IV antibiotics
	- Consider hospital admission
		- Immediate ER evaluation & admission
		- Stabilize patient
		- Assess vital signs and oxygen saturation
		- Hemodynamic support (fluid/pressors)
		- Oxygen therapy/ventilatory support
		- Pan culture/fever workup
		- Antibiotic therapy
		- If hemodynamically stable, admit to oncology unit
		- If hemodynamically unstable, admit to the MICU

Abbrev: ASAP = As soon as possible
        MICU = Medical intensive care unit

Figure 40-3 Telephone triage evaluation for suspected septic shock for patients in the home setting.

Table 40-2 Common Diagnostic Studies in Septic Shock Evaluation

Diagnostic Studies	Implications/Comments
Cultures of blood and body fluids (urine, sputum, drainage, stool)	Should be obtained expeditiously before starting antibiotics to properly identify pathogen Should be repeated every 24 hours if sepsis persists Results will show presence of a specific organism or no growth
Complete blood count	↑ WBCs in presence of infection or inflammation ↓ hemoglobin/hematocrit may reflect hemorrhage, hemodilution, or RBC destruction. ↓ platelet count may reflect decreased production, ↑ destruction, pooling or sludging; a ↓ platelet count may also signal early coagulopathies (DIC)
Chemistry (electrolytes and liver function tests)	↑ BUN, ↓ creatinine may reflect dehydration and/or renal hypoxia Initial ↑ in glucose due to the body's compensatory anti-inflammatory response and gluconeogenesis ↓ in glucose in prolonged shock as liver failure occurs Initially liver function test may remain normal but ↑ transaminase and bilirubin occur in prolonged septic shock
Serum lactate	↑ Levels are indicative of tissue hypoxia and anaerobic metabolism; helpful in evaluating metabolic acidosis
Prothrombin time/ partial thrombo-plastin time (PT/PTT)	Prolonged PT/PTT commonly occur during septic shock and may or may not indicate DIC ↓ PT may indicate hepatic failure
Pulse oximetry	↓ levels indicate decreased tissue perfusion and oxygenation; pulse oximetry should be monitored frequently Evaluates oxygenation efforts and respiratory status; if septic shock persists, more invasive monitoring of oxygenation is done via an arterial line in intensive care
Arterial blood gases (ABGs)	A ↓ percentage oxygen saturation indicates oxygenation of blood and decrease tissue perfusion ABGs indicate presence and degree of severity of respiratory and metabolic acidosis
Chest x-ray	Evaluates presence or progression of pulmonary edema, pneumonia, adult respiratory distress syndrome Posterior/anterior/lateral views are preferred but if only a portable x-ray is possible, films should be obtained with the patient in an upright position
Electrocardiogram	↑ heart rate in presence of fever, hypoxia, hypotension, hypermetabolism Dysrhthmias
Urinalysis	↑ in WBCs and bacteria may indicate infectious source ↑ RBCs/occult blood may be suggestive of bleeding due to coagulopathy
Antibiotic levels	The timing of blood level will depend on the chosen antibiotic These levels provide valuable information regarding appropriate posing based in renal function and drug clearance
Fibrinogen degradation products (FDPs)	↑ levels seen during fibrinolysis and DIC

Abbrev: BUN = Blood urea nitrogen
DIC = disseminated intravascular coagulation

Chapter 30). The key to preventing progression from infection to septic shock is early recognition and intervention. Physicians and nurses must have the knowledge, experience, and advanced clinical judgment to anticipate and manage the complications associated with septic shock. Also, patients should be informed of the importance of prompt reporting of signs and symptoms of infection. The sophisticated technology and advanced skills inherent in supportive ancillary disciplines such as pharmacy, respiratory care, and laboratory services as well as the services of subspecialists in infectious disease, pulmonology, and intensive care are essential.

The major therapeutic goals in septic shock management are threefold: (1) hemodynamic support, (2) treatment of the infection, and (3) oxygenation. The overall goal is to restore oxygen to tissues. These interventions are performed simultaneously as prompt treatment increases chances of survival.

Hemodynamic Support

Major fluid volume depletion exists in patients with septic shock due to decreased venous tone, vascular pooling, capillary leak, and third spacing of fluid. The hallmark of septic shock is profound hypotension. Reinstating adequate circulating volume raises blood pressure and enhances cardiac performance, systemic perfusion, and normalization of oxidative metabolism.[31]

Fluid resuscitation

It is not known whether crystalloid or colloid solutions are superior for fluid resuscitation. Crystalloids (normal saline, lactated Ringer's) are used most commonly during early stabilization of septic shock.[32] Fluids ideally should be given in predetermined boluses followed by end point assessments of BP, heart rate, and urine output.[32,33] Initially, a rapid infusion of 500–1000 mL rate should be administered and repeated until the systolic BP is at least 90 mm Hg.[16,33] If 2–3 liters fail to show rapid clinical benefit as evidenced by increased BP and urine output, visible jugular veins, and improved mentation, then intravascular monitoring (pulmonary artery catheter or central venous catheter) is indicated, if not already in place.[32,33] During persistent septic shock, 6–10 liters of crystalloids may be given within the first 24 hours.[32] Colloids (plasma protein fraction, albumin, geletans, and dextrans) are also used in fluid resuscitation for mobilization of extracellular volume into the intravascular space, or plasma expansion. Studies have failed to demonstrate superiority of one solution over the other; however, it has been postulated that crystalloids may be best in early shock and colloids best in late shock.[16,33,34]

Complications of fluid resuscitation include peripheral and pulmonary edema, and hemodilution. The clinical benefits of restoring hemoglobin levels via packed RBC transfusion vary on an individual basis. Transfusion will increase the volume and oxygen-carrying capacity of blood, which can be beneficial for underlying cardiac disease.[4,23,33] Raising the hemoglobin and hematocrit increases viscosity levels in the circulating volume, however, which reduces cardiac output, blood flow, and perfusion, most notably in the microvasculature.[35] The recommended range for hemoglobin is 10–12 g/dL and for hematocrit, from 30%–35%.[35]

Fluid resuscitation restores blood pressure in approximately 30%–40% of septic hypotensive patients.[36] When such efforts fail, vasopressor and inotropic drugs are added. Of note, there is a greater than 80% chance of death in individuals requiring pharmacological intervention.[23] Koscove[33] emphasizes the importance of maximum volume replacement before any vasoactive drugs are initiated to provide for adequate preload and maximal drug efficacy.

Vasopressors and inotropic support

Dopamine is employed as first-line therapy for its vasopressor and inotropic effects. A starting dose of 2 μg/kg/min (renal and splanic perfusion) is given and is titrated up to 25 μg/kg/min (vasoconstriction) until a systolic BP of 90 mm Hg is attained.[36] If dopamine alone is inadequate, norepinephrine (0.02 to > 0.40 μg/kg/min) is added for increased vasopressor support, or dobutamine (2–20 μg/kg/min) for increased inotropic support.[23,33,36] If the above measures fail to restore hemodynamic stability, epinephrine is given, which generally heralds a very poor prognosis.[23]

Treatment of Infection

Extensive investigation of agents to interrupt the septic shock cascade is ongoing; however, the current mainstay is prompt and appropriate initiation of antibiotics. Blood cultures provide critical information regarding offending pathogens and antibiotic sensitivity and therefore must be collected before any antimicrobial therapy is started. Until a definitive source of infection is identifed, empiric antibiotics are administered as soon as possible to kill or inhibit microorganism growth. The immunocompromised individual requires broad-spectrum antibiotic coverage against common gram-negative organisms (*Pseudomonas aeruginosa, Escherichia coli, Klebsiella*) and gram-positive organisms (*coagulase-negative staphlococci, S. aureus, streptococci, S. pneumoniae, Corynebacterium*).[37] One choice for treatment is double gram-negative coverage of a beta-lactam (e.g., cefipime 2 g IV q 8 hours) with an aminoglycoside (e.g., tobramycin sulfate 5 mg/kg IV q 24 hours). An equally effective treatment is single-agent therapy with a carbapenem (e.g., imipenum/cilastin sodium 500 mg q 6 hours) or a third-generation cephalosporin. These therapies are considered effective for initial coverage until culture and sensitivity results are available to refine antimicrobial therapy.[7,23,33,38] If infection of an indwelling catheter is suspected, adding vancomycin hydrochloride 1 g q 12 hours initially is generally acceptable; however, survival advantages have not been observed.[7]

Septic shock may progress rapidly as antibiotics lyse bacteria, which elevates endotoxin levels in the bloodstream, a phenomenon known as the *Jarisch-Herxheimer reaction*.[39] Initiating antibiotic therapy as soon as possible limits the numbers of circulating pathogens, which ultimately limits the amount of endotoxin liberated from the bacterial cell wall. Another means to limit endotoxin levels is avoiding, if possible, antibiotics known to promote endotoxin release such as aztreonam, cefotaxime sodium, ceftazidime, and the quinolones.[39]

Oxygen Therapy and Respiratory Support

As soon as septic shock is suspected, oxygen therapy should be initiated by nasal cannula and increased as needed based on oxygen saturation, arterial blood gases (ABGs), and lactate levels.[23] As interstitial and alveolar edema continue to worsen, ventilation/perfusion mismatch occurs, taxing the respiratory effort and increasing oxygen demands. Early intubation and mechanical ventilation is encouraged to increase oxygen delivery and decrease oxygen demand until septic shock can be reversed.[23]

Supportive care in the situation of septic shock also includes management of coagulopathies, electrolyte replacement, thermoregulation, and nutrition. Steroid use in treatment of septic shock remains controversial. Over the past decade researchers have agreed that steroid use does not improve survival and may increase morbidity and mortality.[40] However, a recent study demonstrated that low doses of hydrocortisone were beneficial in quickly reversing shock, thereby decreasing mortality.[41] Other research efforts directed at the modulation of endotoxin, cytokines, nitric oxide, and other pathway inhibitors are currently ongoing, but have thus far failed to improve outcomes in septic shock.

Conclusion

Septic shock remains an oncologic emergency of great significance. Although this topic continues to be widely studied, a "magic bullet" treatment does not yet exist. It is therefore imperative for oncology nurses to best employ the treatments available to us today. An understanding of the population at risk for developing a life-threatening infection along with early recognition and treatment are the best resources for improved patient outcomes.

References

1. Bone RC, Balk RA, Cerra FB, et al: Definition for sepsis and organ failure and guidelines for the use of innovative therapies in sepsis. *Chest* 101:1644–1655, 1992

2. Marshal JC: Criteria for the description of organ dysfunction in sepsis and SIRS, in Fein AM, Abraham EM, Balk RA, et al (eds): *Sepsis and MultiOrgan Failure*. Baltimore, Williams & Wilkins, 1997, pp 286–296

3. Rangel-Frausto MS, Wenzel RP: The epidemiology and natural history of bacterial sepsis, in Fein AM, Abraham EM, Balk RA, et al (eds): *Sepsis and Multiorgan Failure*. Baltimore, Williams & Wilkins, 1997, pp 27–34

4. Astiz ME, Rackow EC: Septic shock. *Lancet* 351:1501–1505, 1998

5. Youkeles LH, Roses MJ: The epidemiology of sepsis in the immunocompromised host, in Fein AM, Abraham EM, Balk RA, et al (eds): *Sepsis and Multiorgan Failure*. Baltimore, Williams & Wilkins, 1997, pp 35–42

6. Kumar A: Care of the immunocompromised patient in the intensive care unit, in Murray MJ, Coursin DB, Pearl RG, Prough DS, et al (eds): *Critical Care Medicine Perioperative Management*. Philadelphia, Lippincott-Raven, 1997, pp 669–690

7. Pizzo PA: Empirical therapy and prevention of infection in the immunocompromised host, in Mandell GL, Bennet JE, Dolin R (eds): *Principles and Practice of Infectious Diseases*. New York, Churchill Livingstone, 1995, pp 2686–2696

8. Deutschman CS: Care of the patient with sepsis or the systemic inflammatory response syndrome, in Murray MJ, Coursin DB, Pearl RG, Prough DS, et al (eds): *Critical Care Medicine Perioperative Management*. Philadelphia, Lippincott-Raven, 1997, pp 631–642

9. Bone RC: Systemic inflammatory response syndrome: a unifying concept of systemic inflammation, in Fein AM, Abraham EM, Balk RA, et al (eds): *Sepsis and Multiorgan Failure*. Baltimore, Williams & Wilkins, 1997, pp 3–10

10. Parrillo JE: Pathogenic mechanisms of septic shock. *N Engl J Med* 328:1471–1477, 1993

11. Opal SM, Yu RL: Antiendotoxin strategies for the prevention and treatment of septic shock—new approaches and future directions. *Drugs* 55:497–508, 1998

12. Huddleston Secor V: The systemic inflammatory response syndrome: role of inflammatory mediators in multiple organ dysfunction syndrome, in Huddleston Secor V (ed): *Multiple Organ Dysfunction and Failure: Pathophysiology and Clinical Implications* (ed 2). St Louis, Mosby-Year Book, 1996, pp 46–72

13. Wheeler AP, Bernard GR: Treating patients with severe sepsis. *N Engl J Med* 340:207–214, 1999

14. Huddleston Secor V: Multiple organ dysfunction syndrome: background, etiology, and sequence of events, in Huddleston Secor V (ed): *Multiple Organ Dysfunction and Failure: Pathophysiology and Clinical Implications* (ed 2). St. Louis, Mosby-Year Book, 1996, pp 1–18

15. Levi M, Van Der Poll T, Ten Cate H: The cytokine-mediated imbalance between coagulant and anticoagulant mechanisms in sepsis and endotoxaemia. *Eur J Clin Invest* 27:3–9, 1997

16. Ognibene FP: Pathogenesis and innovative treatment of septic shock. *Adv Intern Med* 42:313–338, 1997

17. Kilbourn R: The discovery of nitric oxide as the key mediator in septic shock. *Sepsis* 1:85–91, 1998

18. Le Gall J, Lemeshow S, Leleu G, et al: Customized probability models for early severe sepsis in adult intensive care patients. *JAMA* 273:644–650, 1995

19. Robbins EV: Maldistribution of circulating volume, in Huddleston Secor V (ed): *Multiple Organ Dysfunction and Failure: Pathophysiology and Clinical Implications* (ed 2). St. Louis, Mosby-Year Book, 1996, pp 107–134

20. Ellerhorst-Ryan J: Infection, in Groenwald SL, Frogge MH, Goodman M, Yarbro CH (eds): *Cancer Nursing: Principles and Practice* (ed 4). Sudbury, MA, Jones and Bartlett, 1997, pp 585–603

21. Rodrigues JC, Fein AM: Diagnostic approach and clinical manifestations of severe sepsis, in Fein AM, Abraham EM, Balk RA, et al (eds): *Sepsis and Multiorgan Failure*. Baltimore, Williams & Wilkins, 1997, pp 269–276

22. Huddleston Secor V: Multiple organ dysfunction syndrome: overview and conclusions, in Huddleston Secor V (ed): *Multiple Organ Dysfunction and Failure: Pathophysiology and Clinical Implications* (ed 2). St. Louis, Mosby-Year Book, 1996, pp 402–423

23. Wiessner WH, Casey LC, Zbilut JP: Treatment of sepsis and septic shock: a review. *Heart Lung.* 24:380–389, 1995

24. Kimbrell JD: Alterations in metabolism, in Huddleston Secor V (ed): *Multiple Organ Dysfunction and Failure: Pathophysiology and Clinical Implications* (ed 2). St. Louis, Mosby-Year Book, 1996, pp 148–163

25. Astiz ME, Rackow EC: Mechanism and classification of shock, in Fein AM, Abraham EM, Balk RA, et al (eds): *Sepsis and Multiorgan Failure*. Baltimore, Williams & Wilkins, 1997, pp 11–20

26. O'Neill PL: Gastrointestinal system: target organ and source of multiple organ dysfunction syndrome, in Huddleston Secor V (ed): *Multiple Organ Dysfunction and Failure: Pathophysiology and Clinical Implications* (ed 2). St. Louis, Mosby-Year Book, 1996, pp 215–236

27. Lohrman J: Hepatic dysfunction, hypermetabolism, and multiple organ dysfunction syndrome, in Huddleston Secor V (ed): *Multiple Organ Dysfunction and Failure: Pathophysiology and Clinical Implications* (ed 2). St. Louis, Mosby-Year Book, 1996, pp 196–214

28. O'Grady NP, Barie PS, Bartlett JG, et al: Practice guidelines for evaluating new fever in critically ill adults. *Clin Infect Dis* 26:1042–1059, 1998

29. Huddleston Secor V: The inflammatory/immune response: implications for the critically ill, in Huddleston Secor V (ed): *Multiple Organ Dysfunction and Failure: Pathophysiology and Clinical Implications* (ed 2). St. Louis, Mosby-Year Book, 1996, pp 19–45

30. Arons MM, Wheeler AP: Imaging in sepsis, in Fein AM, Abraham EM, Balk RA, et al (eds): *Sepsis and Multiorgan Failure*. Baltimore, Williams & Wilkins, 1997, pp 327–336

31. Zimmerman JL, Dellinger RP: A care map for severe sepsis, in Fein AM, Abraham EM, Balk RA, et al (eds): *Sepsis and*

Multiorgan Failure. Baltimore, Williams & Wilkins, 1997, pp 467–474

32. Astiz ME, Castro V, Rackow EC: Fluids and resuscitation in sepsis, in Fein AM, Abraham EM, Balk RA, et al (eds): *Sepsis and Multiorgan Failure.* Baltimore, Williams & Wilkins, 1997, pp 494–502

33. Koscove EM: Sepsis and septic shock, in Brillman JC, Quenzer RW (eds): *Infectious Disease in Emergency Medicine* (ed 2). Philadelphia, Lippincott-Raven 1998, pp 129–152

34. Krau SD: Selecting and managing fluid therapy. *Crit Care Nurs Clin North Am* 10:401–410, 1998

35. Von Rueden KT, Dunham CM: Evaluation and management of oxygen delivery and consumption in multiple organ dysfunction syndrome, in Huddleston Secor V (ed): *Multiple Organ Dysfunction and Failure: Pathophysiology and Clinical Implications* (ed 2). St. Louis, Mosby-Year Book, 1996, pp 384–401

36. Vincent JL: Pharmacologic management of shock: support of the cardiovascular system, in Fein AM, Abraham EM, Balk RA, et al (eds): *Sepsis and Multiorgan Failure.* Baltimore, Williams & Wilkins, 1997, pp 462–466

37. Cunha BA, Gill MV: Antimicrobial therapy in sepsis, in Fein AM, Abraham EM, Balk RA, et al (eds): *Sepsis and Multiorgan Failure.* Baltimore, Williams & Wilkins, 1997, pp 483–493

38. Freifeld AG, Walsh T, Marshall D: Monotherapy for fever and neutropenia in cancer patients: a randomized comparison of ceftazidime versus imipenem. *J Clin Oncol* 13:165–176, 1995

39. Casey LC: Antibiotics: more than just "bug" killers. *Crit Care Med* 25:1270–1274, 1997

40. Matot I, Sprung CL: Corticosteroids in septic shock: resurrection of last rites? *Crit Care Med* 26:627–630, 1998

41. Bollaert PE, Charpentier C, Levy B: Reversal of late septic shock with surpaphysiologic doses of hydrocortisone. *Crit Care Med* 26:245–251, 1998

CHAPTER 41

Spinal Cord Compression

Anne Marie Flaherty, RN, MSN, AOCN, CNSC

Scope of the Problem

Definition

Although rare, spinal cord compression is a devastating complication of progressive cancer. It is a malignant process that causes disruption in neurologic function when a tumor and its destructive effects on the vertebral column compress neural tissue and its blood supply.[1]

Incidence

While only about 5% of individuals with cancer have spinal cord compression on autopsy, the neurologic deterioration can render a person paralyzed if prompt medical attention is not instituted.[2] Approximately 18,000–20,000 cases are diagnosed annually, about twice that of traumatic spinal cord injuries.[3] The incidence of spinal cord compression may actually be increasing due to improved treatments and prolonged survival currently seen in various cancers. Its incidence is most closely associated with that of bone metastases and in particular vertebral metastases. Spinal cord compression is now referred to as a skeletal-related event or a consequence of bone metastasis. The most important prognostic factor is the

neurologic function prior to the initiation of treatment. In the classic study by Gilbert and colleagues, the majority of those who were ambulatory prior to treatment remained so after completion.[4]

In this chapter, the discussion is primarily related to metastatic epidural spinal cord compression and not primary spinal cord tumors. Oncology nurses are in the best position to identify those at risk to develop spinal cord compression and those with early stage spinal cord compression so that treatment is instituted prior to neurologic deterioration. The primary goal is to preserve and maintain the neurologic status of the individual.

Pathophysiology

Anatomy of the Spinal Cord

The spinal cord consists of ascending and descending nerve tracts that carry impulses to and from the brain and peripheral nerves. These impulses result in sensory information and motor ability.[5] The spinal cord is protected by three connective tissue membranes known as the leptomeninges: (1) pia mater, the innermost layer; (2) arachnoid, the middle layer; and (3) dura mater, the outermost layer. See Figure 41-1(A). The spinal cord is

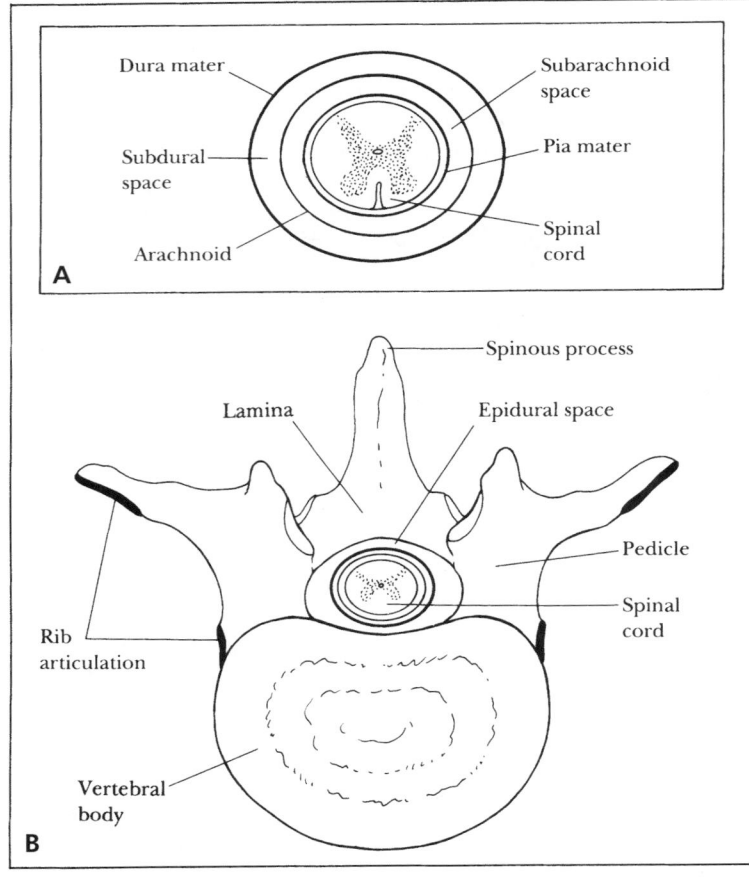

Figure 41-1 (A) The cross-section illustrates the leptomeninges or membranes surrounding the spinal cord and spaces between the membranes. (B) Cross-section of vertebra and spinal cord. The vertebra consists of the vertebral body, pedicles, laminae, and spinous process. The spinal cord spans the length of the vertebral column in the canal formed by the vertebrae.

surrounded by the vertebral column—a bony structure that consists of stacked vertebrae and provides flexibility and support.[6] Each vertebra consists of a vertebral body, two laminae, two pedicles, and a spinous process. See Figure 41-1(B). The spinal cord starts at the base of the brain and ends in the space between the first two lumbar vertebrae. The cauda equina refers to a group of lumbar and sacral nerve roots emerging from the end of the spinal cord. The spinal cord is larger in the cervical and lumbar regions and thus these vertebrae are also larger to accommodate the cord.

The spinal cord is arranged into distinct regions including the butterfly-shaped gray matter, which has anterior horns controlling motor function, lateral horns controlling autonomic functions, and the posterior horns related to sensation. The lateral and anterior spinal cord white matter includes corticospinal tracts and additional nerve tracts that control fine motor control and tone. The spinocerebellar tracts are associated with muscle stretch and tone sensation. The lateral spinothalamic tract carries pain fibers and the dorsal columns transmit fine touch and positional sense (Figure 41-2).[7]

Etiology

Spinal cord compression can arise from either primary tumors within the spinal cord and its protective layers or as a result of metastatic disease. Primary tumors of the spine that arise within the cord itself are called *intramedullary* and those that develop within the dural layers are called *extramedullary–intradural*. These tumors include malignancies such as ependymoma, astrocytoma, oligodendroglioma, and meningioma.[5]

Metastasis to the spine can be classified as intramedul-lary, leptomeningeal, and epidural. Intramedullary and leptomeningeal metastases are rare and arise from hematogenous spread via paravertebral and extradural plexi as well as growth along nerve roots from paravertebral tumors. Intramedullary metastases are most often associated with breast and lung cancer while leukemia and lymphoma are more likely to result in leptomeningeal carcinomatosis.[8,9] Epidural metastasis is the most common type of metastasis to the spine. It occurs because of the extension of a tumor from the vertebral column, the extension of a tumor through the intervertebral foramina, or direct tumor deposits in the epidural space. Figure 41-3 illustrates the various locations of spinal metastases. Eighty-five percent of cases of epidural metastasis involve the vertebral column, while 10%–15% of cases develop compression from paravertebral tumors that extend through the foramina. Direct epidural metastasis is rather uncommon.[9]

The skeleton is the third most frequent site of metastasis after the lung and liver, and the vertebral column is the most common site for skeletal metastasis.[10] The vertebral body rather than the pedicles or laminae is most often involved. The vertebral column is rich with growth factors, which are present in the bone marrow and help support malignant growth. Another factor encouraging metastatic growth in the vertebral column is its blood supply. The Batson plexus is a low-pressure, valveless venous system that drains thoracic, abdominal, and pelvic organs when thoracic and abdominal pressure is raised during coughing or straining. The proximity of the plexus may also explain why most spinal cord compression occurs anteriorly or anteriolaterally closest to the posterior portion of the vertebral body.[11] Epidural compression occurs when bony disease in the vertebra causes either extraosseous extension of tumor or destruction and col-

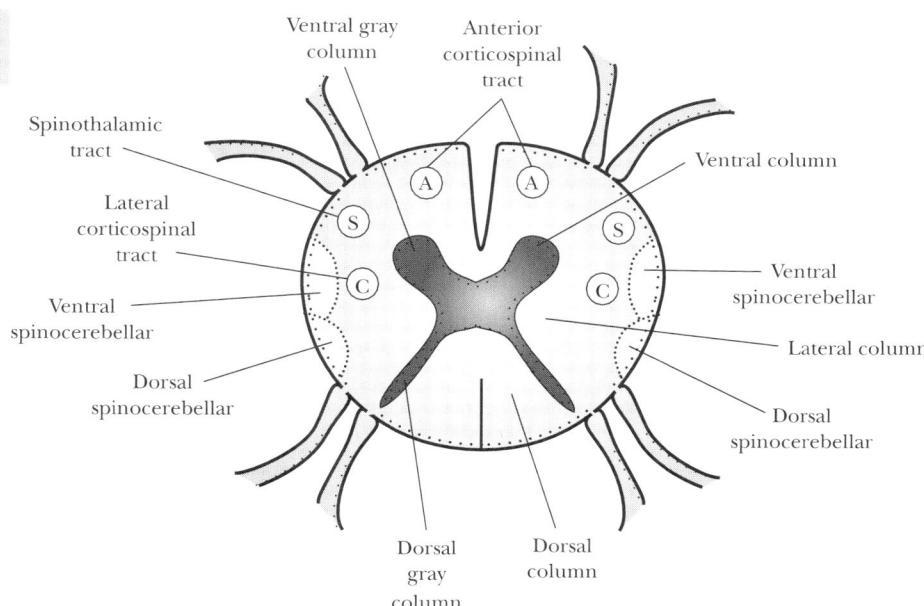

Figure 41-2 Cross-section of spinal cord and spinal tracts.

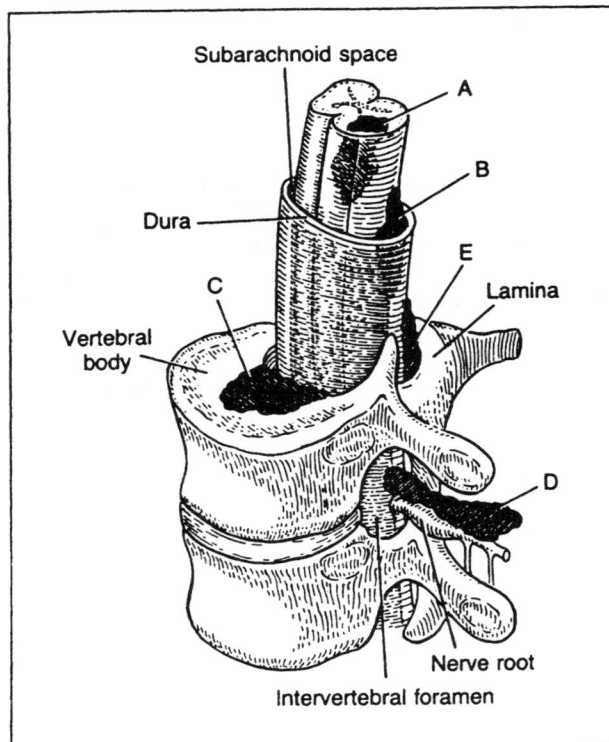

Figure 41-3 Locations of metastases to the spine. Intramedullary metastases are located within the spinal cord (A) Leptomeningeal metastases are in the subarachnoid space (B) and are extramedullary and intradural. Epidural metastases arise from the extension of metastases located in the adjacent vertebral column (C), in the paravertebral spaces through the intervertebral foramina (D), or rarely, in the epidural space itself (E). As these epidural metastases grow, they compress adjacent blood vessels, nerve roots, and spinal cord, resulting in local and referred pain, radiculopathy, and myelopathy. (Reprinted with permission from Byrne TN: Spinal cord compression from epidural metastasis. *N Engl J Med* 325:614–619, 1992. Copyright © 1992 Massachusetts Medical Society. All rights reserved.)[9]

Pathogenesis

Early in spinal cord compression there is compression of the epidural venous plexus, which causes ischemia and vasogenic cord edema.[13] This results in a conduction block and demyelination. There is new evidence that compressed neural tissue leads to a series of neurochemical changes caused by the release of seratonin, prostaglandin, and glutamide. These neurotoxic chemicals cause further tissue damage and neurologic changes.[3] Later in the course of spinal cord compression, parenchymal blood supply is disrupted, which causes further cord damage.

Site of Compression

The site of epidural metastasis and cord compression is related to the origin of the primary cancer and depends on the anatomic location of the tumor, vascular supply, and venous drainage. The thoracic spine is the most frequent site of epidural compression accounting for about 70% of cases.[2] This can be explained by the fact that the most frequent cancers associated with bone metastases—breast, lung, and prostate—most often cause thoracic compression. As well, there are more thoracic vertebrae than lumbosacral or cervical. Although lumbosacral metastases on autopsy are more common, they are asymptomatic and often go undetected.[14] About one-third of all patients with spinal cord compression will have multiple sites of metastases.[15]

Clinical Manifestations and Physical Assessment

It is not clear what specific pathophysiologic changes cause each of the clinical manifestations associated with spinal cord compression. These manifestations of cord compression depend upon the level of the lesion and compression but not necessarily upon which part of the cord—anterior, posterior, or lateral—is actually compressed.[13]

The symptoms of cord compression usually start as mild and noncontributory, but will become more pronounced. These symptoms most often follow a progressive pattern that the clinician must be aware of in order to diagnose cord compression early and preserve neurologic function (Table 41-1). The initial symptom is back pain that is accompanied or followed by motor weakness and decreased sensation. This weakness then progresses to motor and sensory loss, loss of proprioception, vibratory sense, and bowel and bladder dysfunction.[16]

Back Pain

Back pain is the presenting symptom in over 95% of individuals with spinal cord compression. Approximately one-third of individuals who present with back pain have

lapse of bony structures into the epidural space (see Figure 41-3).[9] While extraosseous extension of a tumor most often causes compression, if vertebral collapse and angulation of the spine are present, the prognosis is not as favorable.[12] Cancers associated with epidural compression via vertebral metastasis include cancers of the breast, lung, prostate, and kidney, and multiple myeloma and melanoma.

While vertebral metastasis is the most common mechanism for spinal cord compression, tumors can compress the cord by direct extension through the intervertebral foramina (see Figure 41-3).[9] Lymphomas and neuroblastoma travel through this space and compress the spine without invasion of the bony structures. Some tumors—e.g., colon, kidney, prostate, and head and neck—extend directly into the vertebral structures or epidural space without metastases.[13]

Table 41-1 Assessment of the Patient with Suspected Spinal Cord Compression

History

I. Risk factors (type of primary tumor, presence of bony metastases)

II. Medication profile, with review of potential side effects

III. Symptom analysis—back pain
  A. Distinguish other pain, if any, from pain due to bone metastases: has location, intensity, character changed?
  B. Perform systematic assessment
    1. Location (is pain localized, radicular, referred?) Compare with dermatome chart
    2. Does the pain radiate? To where?
    3. Onset of pain
    4. Character (is it constant or intermittent?)
    5. Quality (have patient describe—is it squeezing, bandlike?)
    6. Intensity (have patient rate on scale from 0–5, with 5 being the worst)
    7. Aggravating factors (lying down, coughing, sneezing, straining?)
    8. Alleviating factors (sitting up, medications?)

IV. Focused history
  A. Musculoskeletal: Has the patient noticed any weakness? Any heaviness or stiffness of the limbs? Any difficulty walking, gait disturbances? Falls? Lack of coordination? Paralysis? Onset/course?
  B. Sensory: any numbness or paresthesia? Where? Have patient describe it. Any changes in sensation to touch, temperature? Areas of no sensation? Any loss of position sense?
  C. Autonomic function:
    1. Assess usual patterns of elimination
    2. Any bladder difficulties (urgency, initiating voiding, retention, overflow, incontinence)? Onset?
    3. Any bowel difficulties (expelling fecal contents, constipation, absence of sensation or numbness in rectum, incontinence with loss of sphincter control? Onset?

Physical Exam

I. General observations: orientation to person, place, time; accuracy as a historian, presence of family members

II. Focused exam
  A. Percuss vertebrae along spinal cord. Note level of pain if any.
  B. Ask patient to do straight leg raising (SLR) if pain in back or on neck flexion—does this elicit pain?
  C. Evaluate urinary system; if retention, discuss with MD need for straight catheterization to evaluate postvoiding residual (residual of >150 mL considered retention)
  D. Evaluate rectal sphincter tone
  E. Evaluate motor strength
  F. Evaluate sensory function
  G. Evaluate reflexes: look for hyperactive deep tendon reflexes or absence of superficial reflexes

Reprinted with permission from Wilkes GM: Neurological disturbances, in Yarbro CH, Frogge MH, Goodman M (eds): *Cancer Symptom Management* (ed 2). Sudbury, MA, Jones and Bartlett 1999, p 353.[16]

75% blockage of the spinal cord despite a normal neurologic exam.[17] Central back pain is caused by vertebral collapse or stretching of the periosteum of the involved bony structure. The pain can be localized within one or two vertebrae of the compression. Almost half of the cases of epidural compression involve one vertebra while 25% involve multiple contiguous vertebrae; the remaining cases involve multiple separate vertebrae.[7] Back pain can also be radicular in nature, meaning the pain moves or radiates from one location to another. It is caused by the tumor irritating the nerve roots such that the pain follows the distribution of the nerve. Radicular pain with cervical and lumbosacral compression is usually unilateral while thoracic compression is usually associated with bilateral pain.[16] Radicular pain with thoracic compression is described as a constrictive-band-like pain while cervical and lumbosacral compression may cause pain that radiates to a limb. Radicular pain is more common in lumbar and cervical spinal cord compression.[15]

Back pain often heralds an impending cord compression and can be present a few days to months. The pain is similar to that associated with degenerative disease or herniated disc in that it can be elicited with movement, valsalva maneuver, cough, and straight leg raising or neck flexion. Back pain from cord compression differs from degenerative disease in that lying supine does not alleviate the pain. Lying down increases venous congestion and edema, which cause individuals to complain of being unable to sleep at night and to find comfort in a recliner or chair. Epidural compression can occur at any level in the spine, whereas degenerative changes are most often seen in the cervical and lumbar spine.[10] Sometimes it may be difficult to distinguish pain related to spinal cord compression, but suspicion should be raised when there is a change in the nature, intensity, or location of back pain.

On physical exam the clinician tries to elicit the back pain by percussing the vertebrae and having the patient perform leg raising or neck flexion. This will help identify the level of compression. The assessment also includes a description of the nature and character of the pain, its intensity, and alleviating as well as aggravating factors.

Motor Weakness and Motor Loss

In general, muscle weakness follows pain as cord compression progresses. Rarely is weakness, which is a prelude to loss of motor function, a presenting symptom of cord compression. About three-fourths of individuals are obviously paraparetic at the time of diagnosis and even more cases are identified during a neurologic exam. The weakness is usually described as a heaviness or stiffness and involves proximal muscles that are used to climb stairs or get out of a chair.[2]

About 95% of patients who have weakness have a greater than 75% blockage of the spinal cord.[4] On physical exam the strength of the extremities and gait are assessed in order to determine motor loss. This is important in identifying early neurologic deficits that represent a more urgent clinical condition. Ambulation at the time of diagnosis is critical because less than 25% of paralyzed patients will regain their ability to ambulate after treatment of spinal cord compression.[18]

Sensory Disturbances and Sensory Loss

Sensory changes are less common than motor weakness, but early complaints include numbness or paresthesia. The sensory loss ascends to the level of the compression as it progresses and can correspond to within two vertebral bodies of the site of the lesion. Clinicians should be aware that this is not always reliable since multiple lesions may be present and multiple dermatomes may be affected. In addition, many sensory and motor pathways cross and overlap so that identification of the level of the lesion can be extremely difficult.

As the compression progresses, sensory loss is accompanied by loss of proprioception, position sense, vibration, temperature sense, and deep pressure.[19] Loss of pain and temperature sensation below a specific dermatome indicates disruption of the spinal thalamic pathway in the lateral column of the spinal cord's white matter. Ataxia and loss of vibration accompany sensory loss and are associated with disruption in the posterior spinocerebellar pathways or posterior columns.[20] Deep tendon reflexes may be decreased at the level of the lesion and hyperactive below that level.[13]

Autonomic Dysfunction

Autonomic dysfunction includes an array of bowel and bladder disturbances that are due to disruption in lower motor neuron function.[16] This is a late sign of spinal cord compression and includes sphincter problems that result in bowel and bladder incontinence or retention.

The individual may experience difficulty initiating urinary flow. This may occur with retention, frequency, or incontinence. Urinary retention is defined as a postvoid residual of greater than 150 mL when one is catheterized after micturation.

Early bowel problems may be present when the individual complains of difficulty expelling stool and experiences loss of feeling. This may lead to constipation or incontinence. Poor sphincter tone is a late sign of autonomic dysfunction and is a poor prognostic sign.[13] Usually those individuals who have autonomic dysfunction are also nonambulatory and rarely regain the ability to ambulate (Table 41-2).

Diagnostic Evaluation

Plain Films and Bone Scans

Plain radiologic films of the painful area of the vertebral column will demonstrate vertebral body collapse, pedicle erosion, and osteolytic or osteoblastic lesions in more than 83% of cases of epidural metastasis.[21] The degree of vertebral destruction caused by metastatic disease as seen on plain films may be directly related to the incidence of spinal cord compression. For plain films to demonstrate osteolytic osseous destruction, greater than 50% of bone must be affected.[22] While bone scan is more sensitive than x-rays, it is often not as helpful as plain films in diagnosing areas of potential cord compression. Bone scans pinpoint the area of disease but do not identify the degree of bone destruction or epidural cord compression. Also, if there is widespread disease, many vertebral bodies may be positive and the level or degree of actual compression not identified.

Magnetic Resonance Imaging

Magnetic resonance imaging (MRI) has emerged as the safest and preferred tool for the diagnosis of spinal cord compression. It is noninvasive and provides a variety of images to help visualize different abnormalities in the

Table 41-2 Relationship of Pretreatment Neurologic Status to Ambulation after Treatment

Pretreatment Neurologic Status	Treatment	Posttreatment Neurologic Status
52% of patients ambulatory with minimal impairment	Dexamethasone 10 mg IV followed by 4 mg q6h	94% of patients ambulatory
39% of patients paraparetic and nonambulatory	Radiation 200–300 cGy every day for a total of 2000–3000 cGy	60% of patients ambulatory
9% of patients paraplegic		1% of patients ambulatory

Data from Maranzano, Latini.[28]

spinal cord and surrounding structures. While it is equal to a myelogram with computerized tomography (CT) scan diagnosis of cord compression due to extradural masses, MRI is far superior in diagnosis of paravertebral masses, intramedullary disease, and bone metastases.[23] An MRI is performed with and without gadolinium since paravertebral masses, leptomeningeal disease, and intramedullary tumors are better visualized with gadolinium.

Based on the bone scan, spine films, and clinical presentation, the site of compression can be generally identified. If only a specific area of the spine is examined by MRI, additional sites of compression may not be identified and go untreated. Approximately 10%–30% of patients with clinical symptoms of spinal cord compression have multiple lesions on MRI. The entire spine therefore should be imaged in order to identify additional areas that are not near the symptomatic lesion. A sagittal MRI survey of the entire spine can be obtained to identify sites of compression and then more detailed images can be obtained to further visualize the type and degree of compression.[24]

Individuals who suffer from claustrophobia may not be able to tolerate the MRI exam. In this case the patient may be referred to an "open" MRI facility. A sedative such as lorazepam may also be helpful. Persons who have a pacemaker or metal implantation near the area to be imaged are advised not to undergo an MRI.

Myelogram with Computerized Tomography

If an MRI is unable to be performed, myelography with CT scan is comparable in adequately diagnosing spinal cord compression. Contrast is injected via a lumbar puncture into the subarachnoid space, and flow is observed to identify any defects. If a complete block is observed, a cervical or cisternal puncture is required to determine the upper level of the block. Cerebrospinal fluid (CSF) withdrawn prior to the instillation of contrast is analyzed for malignant cells, cell count, glucose, and protein. Presence of malignant cells in the CSF confirms leptomeningeal carcinomatosis or tumor in the lining or meninges. This may be present along with spinal cord compression.

Myelography is not without risks. It is invasive and therefore requires proper coagulation as well as adequate renal function for the use of contrast. The MRI is preferred if available to the patient. The positron emission Tomography (PET) scan is not indicated in identifying spinal cord compression because, although it measures the metabolic activity of a tumor, it does not adequately define anatomic features or clearly demonstrate spinal cord compression.

There are algorithms that aid clinicians in promptly diagnosing spinal cord compression (Figure 41-4).[10,13] There are also differing opinions about how to treat symptomatic individuals regardless of the presence of actual spinal cord compression. In any case, it is important to identify all areas of disease, distinguish which areas may cause neurologic sequelae, and identify adequate treat-

ment ports for radiation. If this can be done more expeditiously and less expensively without many different types of imaging, some physicians feel that less is better. If the clinical condition demonstrates obvious signs of epidural compression, however, then emergent MRI with gadolinium is warranted. In addition, if other areas of early cord compression are not identified, they may go untreated and become symptomatic with neurological deterioration.[10]

Therapeutic Approaches

Medical Management

Epidural spinal cord compression is a life-threatening condition requiring immediate intervention so that the neurologic condition is at least preserved. Disease progression can cause rapid deterioration and paraplegia, quadriplegia, and even respiratory arrest if the cervical spine is involved. The major therapeutic approaches include steroids, radiation therapy, and surgery, including either laminectomy or vertebral body resection with stabilization. While controversy exists over which treatment or combination of treatments is the best approach, posttreatment neurologic status is most directly related to pretreatment neurologic status.[25,26] The goals of treatment include decompression of neural tissue, eradication of tumor cells, relief of pain, preservation of neurological function, and prevention of recurrence and progression.[2]

Steroids

The usual treatment for spinal cord compression, regardless of the type of cancer, is steroids combined with radiotherapy. Steroids are instituted prior to definitive treatment because they relieve pain and improve neurologic function by reducing spinal cord edema.[24] The traditional dosing for steroids is a bolus of dexamethasone 10 mg intravenously (IV) followed by 4 mg every 6 hours. One nonradomized study compared high-dose dexamethasone to a lower dose and found no difference in overall neurologic recovery.[27] Side effects, however, are more common with higher doses (100 mg) of steroids and should be reserved for those with significant neurologic symptoms or rapidly progressing symptoms.[9] The steroid therapy continues during the early phase of definitive treatment and may begin to be tapered if the individual's neurologic status is improving or stabilized. The taper continues unless symptoms worsen, and then doses should be increased and tapered again after restabilization. Tapering is a priority in order to avoid the long-term side effects of steroid therapy such as hyperglycemia, gastric ulceration, immunosuppression and opportunistic infections, psychosis, and proximal muscle weakness in an already immunologically compromised individual. Complications associated with steroid use are more common when serum albumin is low and the length of administration is longer than 3 weeks.[25]

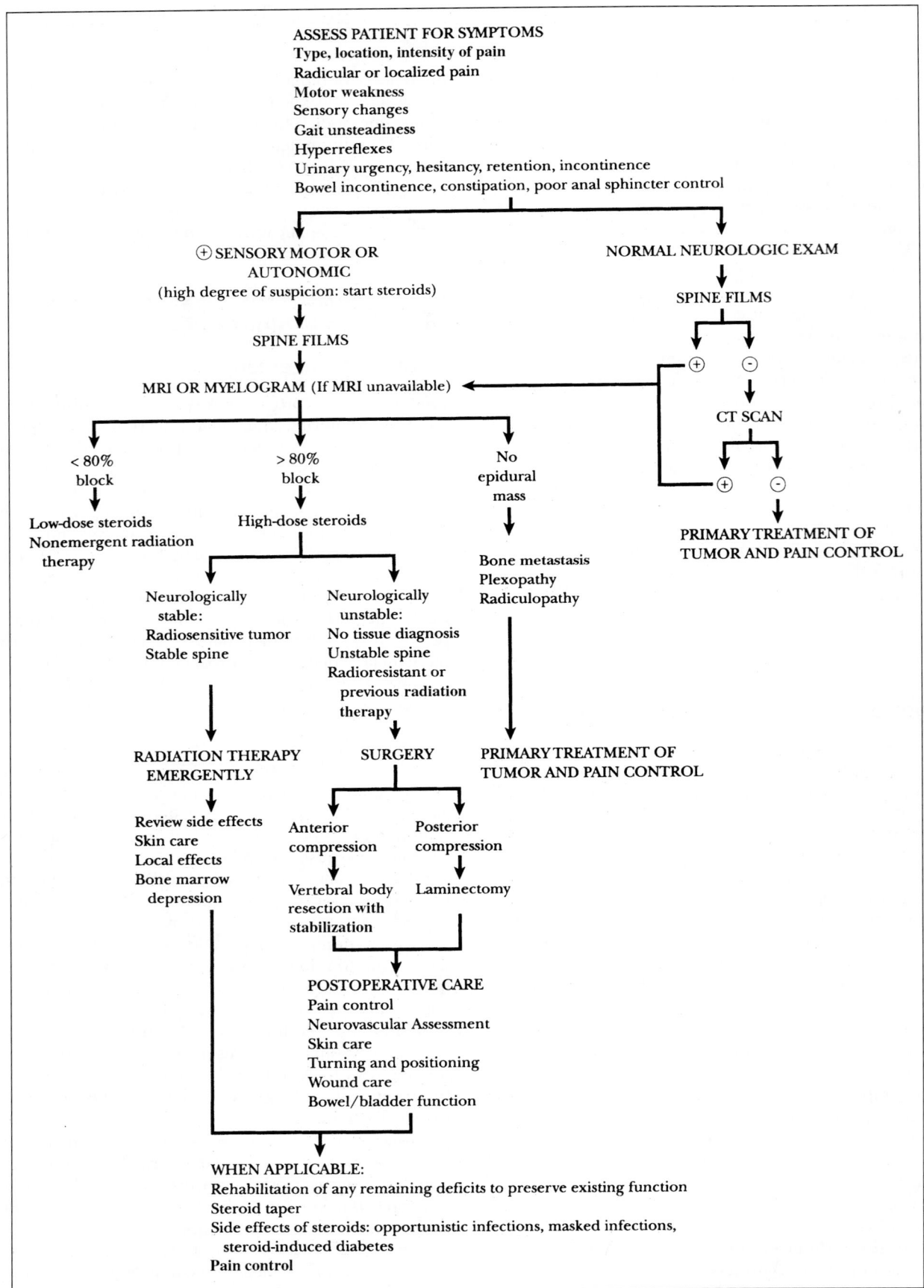

Figure 41-4 Clinical pathway for spinal cord compression.

Radiation

Radiation therapy is the standard treatment for spinal cord compression from epidural metastasis. The radiation port is identified by myelogram or MRI and extends one or two vertebrae above and below the level of the compression. This ensures that the metastatic disease is fully treated. The usual dosage range is 2000–4000 cGy given in 5–20 fractions over 2–4 weeks. The length of treatment is determined partly by histology, since most solid tumors respond at 3000 cGy delivered in 10 fractions. Neuroblastoma and lymphoma have favorable histologies and respond with 2000–3000 cGy while more radiation-resistant tumors such as melanoma require more than 3000 cGy.[28,29] Overall, breast and prostate cancer, myeloma, and lymphoma respond to radiation better than melanoma, sarcoma, and lung cancer.[26,28]

As demonstrated in Table 41-2, the degree of neurologic impairment prior to initiating treatment is predictive of recovery of ambulation posttreatment. Maranzano and associates[28] evaluated the effect of radiation and steroids on neurologic status in cord compression. The majority of individuals were ambulatory (52%) and 94% of these patients remained so. Paraparetic and paralyzed cases did not respond as well with only 60% and 11%, respectively, remaining ambulatory after treatment. Median survival time was longer for those who remained ambulatory, for females, and for those with favorable histologies such as myeloma and breast and prostate cancers.[26] Again, the major conclusion drawn from this study is the importance of early diagnosis.

Between 15%–25% of individuals with spinal cord compression will experience a local recurrence, the majority within a couple of vertebrae of the initial site of cord compression.[30] Additional radiation may or may not be an option due to the maximum amount the spinal cord can tolerate without injuring the healthy neural tissue. If excessive radiation is given, the cord may become damaged and result in further weakness, sensory changes, or autonomic dysfunction. One study reviewed cases of reirradiation for recurrent spinal metastasis and risk of radiation myelopathy, ability to walk, and survival. Results showed that reirradiation often preserves ambulation with the minimal risk of radiation myelopathy. Initial radiation doses averaged 3000 cGy while reirradiation doses averaged 5425 cGy; median survival was 4.7 months.[31]

The side effects of radiation are minimal and relate to where on the spinal column the radiation is directed. Radiation is generally well tolerated, but patients with preexisting bone metastasis and less-than-optimal bone marrow function may incur further suppression of marrow function due to radiation effects. Skin reactions are usually very mild and doses are delivered in such a fashion that surrounding tissue is minimally affected.

Surgical interventions

In the past, surgery was indicated for those with neurologic deficits that progressed during radiation and that presented acutely with rapid deterioration, with spinal instability, or with local recurrence after completion of radiation. The development of MRI, which provides detailed imaging of the tumor and neural structures, and new spine stabilization techniques have made surgery a more effective and earlier option.[32] Surgical decompression with laminectomy or vertebral body resection can promptly relieve spinal cord compression. Traditionally, laminectomy removed the lamina, spinous process, and posterior portion of the tumor. Complete resection was not possible since most epidural metastases are anterior to the spine in the posterior portion of the vertebral body. The primary goal was to decompress the spine by providing an alternate space for the tumor and to stabilize the spine using rods.

A newer surgical approach is to completely resect the tumor and reconstruct the spine so that stability is achieved.[33] In order to accomplish this, surgery may include multiple approaches. Because the majority of tumors are anterior, an anterior approach is most often required. The diseased vertebral body is resected and reconstructed with methylmethacrylate or other material, then the spine is further stabilized with either an anterior or posterior device that attaches to healthy adjoining vertebral bodies.[34] The spine can also be stabilized with bone grafting or fusion posteriorly. The anterior approach requires a thoracotomy for thoracic and some cervical vertebrae. For lumbar resection a retroperitoneal approach is used, while an anterior lateral approach is required for most cervical lesions.[35]

There are now various types of surgical procedures aimed at tumor resection and stabilization: posterior approach laminectomy for posterior tumors; anterior approach with resection and stabilization with a combination of methylmethacrylate, instrumentation or bone grafting, and either a "staged" or simultaneous anterior and posterior approach with anterior resection and posterior stabilization through instrumentation or posterior fusion and grafting.[32,33,35]

Surgery is usually followed by radiation therapy in order to achieve maximal results. Since radiation will interfere with bone grafting and healing it must be timed appropriately. Data based on animal studies suggest that the best time to initiate radiation is no sooner than 4 weeks postoperatively.[36] Wound and bone healing should be well established at that time.

The most promising results from these surgical techniques are relief of pain and spinal stability, which allows for full ambulation and neurologic recovery. No study has prospectively compared the various therapeutic modalities. The problem with most surgical studies is that the population is highly selective and more favorable conditions are treated in a more traditional approach. In one review, Siegal and Siegal analyzed data from various studies and found that decompression surgery with spine stabilization resulted in neurologic recovery in 63% of those who had a laminectomy and 73% of those who had a vertebral body resection.[37] This is compared to about 44% of those who have either radiation alone or laminectomy alone. In addition, pain was relieved in more than 85% of those who had the decompressive surgery with spine stabilization.[37]

Surgery, while it has many advantages, is not without risk. Surgical morbidity with resection and stabilization has been estimated as high as 48% and mortality about 6%.[33] Complications encountered postoperatively include infection, CSF leakage, progression of neurologic deficits, instrumentation or stabilization failure, and hemorrhage.[32]

Surgery must be carefully considered on an individual, case-by-case basis. Two important factors are the performance status of the individual prior to surgery and whether the benefit outweighs the risk. Surgery is indicated when tissue is needed for histologic diagnosis, especially if this is the only accessible area of disease. Extensive bone destruction, vertebral collapse, and spine instability (particularly when accompanied by intractable pain) may be best treated with a surgical approach. In addition, if the patient is currently receiving steroid and radiation therapy and experiences rapid neurologic deterioration, surgery may be warranted. Surgery should also be considered in those cases of solitary recurrence in the spinal cord. The desire to maintain and improve the quality of life for those with metastatic cancer motivates the use of this aggressive approach.

Chemotherapy

Chemotherapy may be a treatment option in extremely chemosensitive tumors such as Hodgkin's and non-Hodgkin's lymphoma, neuroblastoma, or germ cell tumors.[38,39] It may also be used as an adjuvant therapy to surgery and radiation, but is generally not the primary treatment in an acute situation. Hormone therapy is another option for those with prostate and breast cancer. Usually these patients have had the disease a long time and have been treated with hormone manipulation and may be resistant. The hormone-sensitive cases may benefit from a trial in addition to standard therapy for spinal cord compression. New hormone manipulation treatments for breast cancer such as aromatase inhibitors may be effective in tamoxifen/megestrol-resistant cancers.[40]

Another new therapy has emerged as a preventive treatment for spinal cord compression. Bisphosphonates are bone resorption inhibitors that have been used to treat hypercalcemia from malignancy.[41] Recent research has shown that bisphosphonates delay the onset and reduce the frequency of skeletal-related episodes (SREs) such as pathologic fracture, bone pain, and spinal cord compression. They have also reduced the need for palliative radiotherapy and orthopedic surgery.[42–44] While bisphosphonates have clearly improved the quality of life for those with metastatic breast cancer and myeloma, the results show them to be less effective for metastatic prostate cancer. It may be that prostatic bone metastases are less responsive to bisphosphonates because they are more osteoblastic than osteolytic in nature.

Pamidronate is the current recommended bisphosphonate, administered IV as a 90-mg dose in 250 mL of normal saline or dextrose over 2 hours every 3–4 weeks. Oral bisphosphonates such as alendronate are not as effective; but a current trial is investigating the use of zoledronate, a potent bisphosphonate, as a 5-minute monthly IV injection to see if a more convenient and less costly method will yield equal results. The side effects of pamidronate include flulike symptoms most often after the first few treatments, local reaction at the injection site, arthralgias, and myalgias. Overall, pamidronate is very well tolerated.

Symptom Management

The nursing care of the individual experiencing spinal cord compression is primarily concerned with early detection and symptom management. Clinical problems evolve from the rapidity of onset, level and degree of compression, presenting symptoms, as well as type and response to treatment. Assessment is crucial throughout this emergency for evaluation of neurologic status and preservation of maximal function. Assessment includes monitoring of sensory and motor function as well as of bowel and bladder function.

Pain

Table 41-3 lists the most frequent problems associated with epidural spinal cord compression and management goals with interventions to help direct care. Since more than 95% of patients with spinal cord compression have pain, knowledge of pain management is essential. Pain assessment is crucial to help identify intensity, location, factors that help and those that exacerbate pain, and other symptoms that accompany pain. Oncology nurses need extensive knowledge of the principles of analgesia, opioids, equianalgesia, cost analyses of various regimens, and nonpharmacologic approaches. In addition, adjunct agents such as nonsteroidal anti-inflammatory drugs (NSAIDs), anticonvulsants, and antidepressants may be helpful in pain management.

An "analgesic ladder" approach has been developed by the Cancer Pain Relief and Palliative Care Program of the World Health Organization.[45] This approach helps clinicians select agents based on the patient's severity of pain and provides a standard for pain management. Many large institutions have "pain teams" that act as consultants for individuals with unusual or refractory pain. NSAIDs are very useful in managing bone pain, but bleeding and renal problems may occur and individuals require close monitoring when these agents are used on a regular basis.

Recently, anticonvulsants and antidepressants have emerged as useful agents to treat neuropathic pain that occurs when peripheral nerves or their roots are compressed or infiltrated.[46] This type of pain typically does not easily respond to opioids and requires adjunct agents. Epidural cord compression may also cause spastic reactions below the level of the compression and require the use of benzodiazepines. Effective analgesia is established

Table 41-3 Symptom Management

Problems	Patient Goals	Interventions
Pain due to irritation and compression of nerve roots and neural tissue as evidenced by localized or radicular pain	Maximum comfort as reported on a pain scale during rest and activity by appropriately using various types of analgesics and nonpharmacologic interventions	• Analgesic regimen • Dexamethasone • NSAIDs • Opioids • Anticonvulsants/antidepressants • Complementary medicine: capsicum cream, hydrotherapy, massage
Immobility due to compression of neural tissue, motor neurons as evidenced by proximal muscle weakness that progresses to motor loss	Maintain optimum level of mobility, range of motion, and strength through an activity and exercise program	• Referral to physical therapy • Obtain equipment and devices to preserve alignment, enhance mobility, and stabilize spine • Assist home care agency in organizing environment to be conducive to mobility
Risk of injury related to sensory loss, which includes paresthesia, loss of temperature, position and vibratory senses, and light touch	Safety will be preserved at all times	• Assess degree of sensory changes: touch, temperature, paresthesia • Assess environment for physical, thermal, chemical hazards and organize environment to minimize hazards • Assist patient with ADLs as indicated
Bladder dysfunction due to disruption of lower motor neurons (autonomic function) as evidenced by incontinence, frequency, and/or retention	Maintain adequate urinary elimination with early identification and treatment of urinary tract infections	• Fluid intake greater than 2 quarts/day • Adequate intake of juices to maintain acidity, e.g., cranberry • Straight catheterization/indwelling catheter to maintain continence and empty bladder • Change indwelling catheter each week • Urinalysis/urine culture for pain, burning, foul smelling/cloudy urine, fever, increased WBC count • Prompt treatment of urinary tract infection with antibiotic sensitive to the organism identified • Daily perineal hygiene
Bowel disturbances due to opioid use and disruption of lower motor neurons (autonomic function) as evidenced by constipation, incontinence, and/or difficulty expelling stool	Maintain adequate bowel elimination and prevent ileus from constipation	• Establish bowel regimen including stool softner, i.e., docusate sodium intestinal lubricants, mineral oil, laxatives; senna products, magnesium-based products, i.e., milk of magnesia, magnesium citrate • Dietary recommendations include fresh fruits, vegetables, high-fiber cereals • Adequate fluid intake greater than 2 quarts/day • Provide periodic perineal hygiene

Data from Wilkes.[16]

early and adjusted as steroids and radiation relieve pain. A variety of agents and types of administration are available to provide comfort.

Complementary medicine offers a unique approach to pain management through therapies that enhance well-being and control symptoms. Warm baths and Jacuzzi as part of hydrotherapy promote muscle relaxation and overall relaxation. A professional massage can help relieve pain by working on specific muscle groups that are affected by the spinal cord compression. Capsicum cream contains a powerful pain-relieving chemical found in hot red peppers. This cream may help relieve the back pain associated with cord compression.[47]

Mobility

Quality of life is deeply affected by changes in one's ability to ambulate and function independently. It is crucial, therefore, that the oncology nurse identify any motor or sensory changes early before more profound loss is encountered. Preserving and maximizing function are a priority since many have rehabilitative potential after treatment is initiated.

If spine and vertebral instability is present at diagnosis, the patient should be fitted for a stabilization brace to provide support until surgery can be performed. This brace is worn whenever the patient is moved or gets out of bed and postoperatively until the stabilization materials or bone grafts heal and strengthen the structures surrounding the spine. If the patient undergoes a thoracotomy for anterior resection or a two-step procedure of anterior and posterior resection, postoperative care includes turning and positioning with special attention to preserving alignment and spine stabilization during recovery. Neurologic assessment is critical in the postoperative phase as well as pain control, wound care, and preliminary rehabilitation.[48]

Physical therapy is essential for patients who experience any motor weakness. If recovery is realistic, therapy is directed toward regaining full mobility and strength.

If there is permanent weakness or motor loss, the goals of therapy included maintaining existing function, strength, and range of motion. Assistive devices such as walkers, commodes, wheelchairs, and transfer boards may be required to maximize the patient's mobility. This equipment can be individualized to the patient's needs and physical environment.

Bowel and bladder dysfunction

Autonomic disturbances include bowel and bladder incontinence and retention. Weakness of sphincters can lead to incontinence while paralysis of muscles associated with emptying the bladder and rectum can lead to retention and constipation. Establishment of daily elimination regimens will help manage any bowel and bladder dysfunctions.

If a patient is dexterous with a good prognosis, intermittent self-catheterization is the most effective method for urinary continence. It provides control and continence, ease of mobility without external devices, and reduces the incidence of urinary tract infections. On the other hand, patients with advanced cancer would benefit from an indwelling urinary catheter.

Fluid intake, daily perineal hygiene, and catheter care with scheduled changes will reduce the incidence of urinary tract infections associated with indwelling catheters. Fluid intake should exceed 2 liters per day and contain liquids that maintain acidity, e.g., cranberry juice. Nurses must be vigilant about early diagnosis of urinary tract infections by watching for such symptoms as foul smelling or cloudy urine, elevated white count on complete blood count (CBC), and fever. Treatment with a fluoroquinolone or sulfa-based antibiotic will usually cover most common organisms associated with urinary infections.

Bowel control can be established with the appropriate use of diet, stool softeners, lubricants, and laxatives. In addition to maintaining fluid intake, dietary adjustments to help reduce constipation and establish a regular pattern include increasing fiber. For oncology patients, however, these are very difficult to accomplish due to anorexia and fatigue. A bowel regimen will reduce the incidence of constipation as well as establish continence. Stool seepage is less likely if the rectum is evacuated on a regular basis. If muscle tone and sphincter control are disrupted, medication can assist in developing regular bowel habits.

Many lubricants and laxatives are available. Compliance, degree of being palatable, ease of use, and individual preference are factors to consider when selecting laxatives and lubricants for each individual. The regimen usually consists of a stool softener and laxative. Lubricants, e.g., mineral oil, are essential if the patient has refractory constipation or impaction.

Laxatives are classified as saline, osmotic, or stimulant. Saline-type laxatives include magnesium citrate and magnesium hydroxide. Most common osmotic laxatives are lactulose and sorbitol. Senna products, bisacodyl (Dulcolax), and cascara are stimulant laxatives that are frequently prescribed.[49] A combination of these types of laxatives may be required to adequately establish regularity. Usually rectal suppositories and enemas are reserved for impaction and severe cases of constipation. In spinal cord compression, however, rectal suppositories may be needed to stimulate the intestinal nerve plexus in order to evacuate the rectum.[49]

Skin care

Skin care is essential during radiation therapy, particularly if the patient is receiving higher doses or treatment to a large port. The radiation oncology nurse should perform routine assessment so that skin problems are identified promptly. During radiation therapy, skin should not be washed with soap and topical creams and oils are avoided. Once radiation is completed, water-soluble lotion such as Aquafor may be applied. Usual skin reactions are redness and mild discomfort similar to a sunburn. While skin reactions from spine irradiation are rare, silver nitrate cream can be applied if an open area develops.

Conclusion

Spinal cord compression is one of the most common neurologic emergencies facing the individual with cancer. Prompt recognition and treatment preserve neurologic function and prevent permanent deficits, such as paraplegia and bowel and bladder incontinence or retention. Magnetic resonance imaging has emerged as the safest and most clinically useful diagnostic tool in spinal cord compression. Although radiation therapy has been the primary treatment, new surgical techniques are emerging as feasible options to restore ambulation and relieve pain. Nurses play a pivotal role in identifying those at risk and early cases of spinal cord compression.

References

1. Snell RS: *Neuroanatomy. A review.* Boston: Little, Brown, 1992
2. Byrne TN: Metastatic epidural spinal cord compression, in Black PH, Loeffler JS (eds): *Cancer of the Nervous System.* London, Blackwell Scientific, 1997, pp 664–673
3. Siegel, T: Spinal cord compression: from laboratory to clinic. *Eur J Cancer* 31A:1748–1753, 1995
4. Gilbert RW, Kim JH, Posner JB: Epidural spinal cord compression from metastatic tumor: diagnosis and treatment. *Ann Neurol* 3:40–51, 1978
5. Schaefer SL: Oncologic complications: spinal cord compression, in Otto SE (ed): *Oncology Nursing.* St. Louis, Mosby-Year Book, 1991, pp 468–526
6. Waxman SG, DeGroot J: *Correlative Neuroanatomy.* Norwalk, CT, Appleton & Lange, 1995
7. Michalski JM, Garcia DM: Spinal canal, in Perez CA, Brody LW (eds): *Radiation Oncology.* Philadelphia, Lippincott-Raven, 1997, pp 849–866

8. Byrne TN, Waxman SG: Spinal cord compression: diagnosis and principles of treatment. *Contemporary Neurology Series,* vol. 33. Philadelphia, F. A. Davis, 1990

9. Byrne TN: Spinal cord compression from epidural metastasis. *N Engl J Med* 325:614–619, 1992

10. Bridwell KH: Treatment of metastatic prostate cancer of the spine. *Urol Clin North Am* 18:153–159, 1991

11. Batson OV: The function of the vertebral veins and their role in the spread of metastasis. *Ann Surg* 112:138–149, 1940

12. Flynn DF, Shipley WU: Management of spinal cord compression secondary to metastatic prostate carcinoma. *Urol Clin North Am* 18:145–152, 1991

13. Deangelis LM, Posner JB: Neurologic complications, in Holland JF, Frei E, Bast RC, et al (eds): *Cancer Medicine* (ed 4). Baltimore, Williams & Wilkins, 1997, pp 3117–3150

14. Perrin RG, Janjan NA, Langford LA: Spinal axis metastasis, in Levin V (ed): *Cancer of the Nervous System.* London, Blackwell Scientific, 1997, pp 259–280

15. Helweg–Larsen S, Hansen SW, Sorenson PS: Second occurrence of symptomatic metastatic spinal cord compression and findings of multiple spinal epidural metastases. *Int J Radiat Oncol Biol Phys* 33:595–597, 1995

16. Wilkes GM: Neurological disturbances, in Yarbro CH, Frogge MH, Goodman M (eds): *Cancer Symptom Management,* (ed 2). Sudbury, MA, Jones and Bartlett, 1999, pp 344–381

17. Helweg–Larsen S, Sorenson PS: Symptoms and signs in metastatic spinal cord compression: a study of progression from first symptoms until diagnosis in 153 patients. *Eur J Cancer* 30A:396–399, 1994

18. Kim RY, Spencer SA, Meredith RF, et al: Extradural spinal cord compression: analysis of factors determining functional prognosis. *Radiology* 176:279–289, 1990

19. Schiff D, Batchelor T, Wen PY: Neurologic emergencies in cancer patients. *Neurol Clin* 16:449–483, 1998

20. Chipps EM, Clanin NJ, Campbell VG: *Neurologic Disorders.* St. Louis, Mosby, 1992

21. Held JL, Peahota A: Nursing care of the patients with spinal cord compression. *Oncol Nurs Forum* 20:1507–1516, 1993

22. Bucholtz JD: Central nervous systems metastases. *Semin Oncol Nurs* 14:61–72, 1998

23. Helweg–Larsen S, Wagner A, Kjaer L, et al: Comparison of myelography combined with post-myelographic spinal CT and MRI in suspected metastatic disease of the spinal canal. *J Neurooncol* 13:231–235, 1992

24. Fuller BG, Heiss J, Oedfield EH: Spinal cord compression, in DeVita VT, Hellman S, Rosenberg SA (eds): *Cancer Principles and Practice* (ed 5). Philadelphia, Lippincott-Raven, 1997, pp 2476–2485

25. Hoegler D: Radiotherapy for palliation of symptoms in incurable cancer. *Curr Probl Cancer* 3:135–183, 1997

26. Kim RY, Spencer SA, Meredith RF, et al: Extradural spinal cord compression: analysis of factors determining functional prognosis—prospective study. *Radiology* 176:279–282, 1990

27. Heimdal K, Herschberg H, Slettebo H, et al: High incidence of serious side effects of high dose dexamethasone treatment in patients with epidural spinal cord compression. *J Neurooncol* 12:141–146, 1992

28. Maranzano E, Latini P: Effectiveness of radiation therapy without surgery in metastatic spinal cord compression: final results from a prospective trial. *Int J Radiat Oncol Biol Phys* 32:959–967, 1995

29. Levov M, Dale J, Stein M, et al: The management of meta-static spinal cord compression: a radiotherapeutic success ceiling. *Int J Radiat Oncol Biol Phys* 27:231–236, 1993

30. Kaminski HJ, Dewon VG, Ruff RL: Second occurrence of spinal epidural metastases. *Neurology* 41:744–749, 1991

31. Schiff D, Shaw EG, Cascino TL: Outcome after spinal reirradiation for malignant epidural spinal compression. *Ann Neurol* 37:583–589, 1995

32. Cooper PR, Errico TJ, Mantin R, et al: A systemic approach to spinal reconstruction after anterior decompression for neoplastic disease of the thoracic and lumbar spine. *J Neurosurg* 32:1–8, 1993

33. Sundaressan N, Sachdew VP, Holland JF, et al: Surgical treatment of spinal cord compression from epidural metastasis. *J Clin Oncol* 13:2330–2335, 1995

34. Arbit E, Galicich JH: Vertebral body reconstruction with a modified Harrington rod distraction system for stabilization of the spine affected with metastatic disease. *J Neurosurg* 83: 617–620, 1995

35. Gokaslan ZL: Spine surgery for cancer. *Curr Opin Oncol* 8: 178–181, 1996

36. Bouchard JA, Koka A, Bensusan JS, et al: Effects of irradiation on posterior spinal fusions: a rabbit model. *Spine* 19: 1836–1841, 1994

37. Siegal T, Surgical management of malignant epidural tumors compressing the spinal cord, in Schmidek HH, Sweet WH (eds): *Operative Neurosurgical Techniques.* Philadelphia, Saunders, 1995, pp 1997–2025

38. Wong ET, Portlock CS, O'Brien JP, et al: Chemosensitive epidural spinal disease in non Hodgkin's lymphoma. *Neurology* 46:1543–1547, 1996

39. Cooper K, Bajorin D, Shapiro W, et al: Decompression of epidural metastases from germ cell tumors with chemotherapy. *J Neurooncol* 8:275–279, 1990

40. Harvey HA, Manni A: Clinical use of aromatase inhibitors in breast carcinoma, in Holland JF, Frei E, Bast RC, et al (eds): *Cancer Medicine* (ed 4). Baltimore, Williams & Wilkins, 1997, pp 1113–1124

41. Rogers MJ, Watts DJ, Russell RG: Overview of bisphospho-nates. *Cancer* 80:1652–1660, 1997

42. Hortobagyi GN, Theriault RL, Porter L, et al: Efficacy of pamidronate in reducing skeletal complications in patients with breast cancer and lytic bone metastases. *N Engl J Med* 335:1785–1791, 1996

43. Lipton A: Bisphosphonates and breast carcinoma. *Cancer* 80:1668–1673, 1997

44. Berenson J, Lichtenstein A, Porter L, et al: Long term pamidronate disodium therapy leads to a reduction in skeletal related episodes (SRE's) in stage III multiple myeloma patients and an improvement in survival in those on salvage therapy. *Blood* 86:442–447, 1995

45. World Health Organization: *Cancer Pain Relief* (ed 2), with a guide to opioid availability. Geneva: World Health Organization, 1996

46. Portenoy RK: Contemporary diagnosis and management of pain in oncologic and AIDS patients. Newtown, PA, Handbooks in Health Care Inc., 1997

47. Cassileth BR. Complementary and alternative therapies. Philadelphia, Lippincott, Williams & Wilkins, 1998

48. Dyck S: Surgical instrumentation as a palliative treatment for spinal cord compression. *Oncol Nurs Forum* 18:515–521, 1991

49. Curtiss CP: Constipation, in Yarbro CH, Frogge MH, Goodman M (eds): *Cancer Symptom Management.* Sudbury, MA, Jones & Bartlett, 1999, pp 512–521

CHAPTER 42

Superior Vena Cava Syndrome

Ellen Sitton, RN, MSN, OCN®

Scope of the Problem

Superior vena cava syndrome (SVCS) refers to signs and symptoms that occur when blood flow through the superior vena cava (SVC) is compromised. This results in venous congestion proximal to the occlusion and restricted cardiac output. Increased venous pressures occur in the head, neck, upper extremities, and upper thorax. Compression of the upper central venous return by a malignant tumor in the mediastinum is the most common cause of SVCS. Less common causes include obstruction by a benign process, tumor invasion, and thrombosis of the SVC. Manifestations of compromise of the SVC generally develop gradually but may occur quickly. SVCS is not considered an oncologic emergency in the absence of respiratory distress or cerebral edema.[1,2] The syndrome is rarely fatal in itself and the underlying disease process determines prognosis.[3] Treatment decisions are determined by diagnosis.

Incidence

SVCS is relatively uncommon and appears in only 3%–4% of individuals with cancer.[4] However, 78%–95% of SVCS presents in individuals with cancer.[2,5,6] Any primary or metastatic tumor in the mediastinum can obstruct the SVC.

The incidence of SVCS not directly related to cancer appears to be increasing.[4,6–9] As many as 15%–22% of SVCS may be caused by nonmalignant conditions including thrombus formation and compression.[6,10] Thrombus formation related to vascular access devices, central venous monitoring catheters, and cardiac pacemaker electrodes account for 3%–5% of SVCS.[3] Compression of the SVC can be caused by benign tumor, mediastinal fibrosis, histoplasmosis, and thoracic aortic aneurysm. SVCS recurs in approximately 10%–20% of cases especially with lymphoma.[3]

SVCS in the pediatric population is rare. Causes for 70% of pediatric SVCS include surgery for congenital heart disease, ventriculoatrial shunt for hydrocephalus, and central venous catheters.[6] The most common malignancies causing SVCS are non-Hodgkin's lymphoma, Hodgkin's disease, and acute lymphoblastic leukemia. In children the trachea and right main stem bronchus are easily compressed and have small diameters. Respiratory symptoms such as cough, dyspnea, air hunger, and wheezing caused by tracheal compression often predominate in children.[11]

Etiology and Risk Factors

When SVCS was first described in 1757, causes were generally reported as tuberculosis and syphilitic aortic aneurysms.[5] Currently, cancer is the predominate etiology. The most common types of cancer associated with SVCS are lung cancer (67%–80%), lymphoma involving the mediastinum (8%–14%), and metastatic breast cancer (less than 3%)[6,8,12,13] (see Table 42-1). The most common malignant etiology of SVCS is locally advanced bronchogenic carcinoma. Forty-two percent of SVCS due to lung cancer are caused by small cell and 26% by squamous cell lung cancer,[6,13,14] both of which tend to present more centrally than peripherally.[15] SVCS occurs in 3%–10% of all individuals with lung cancer.[16] However, small cell lung cancer has an associated incidence of SVCS of 9%–19%.[6,17] Individuals with right lung cancer are four times more likely to develop the syndrome than those with left lung cancer due to the location of the SVC nearer to the right lung.[4] SVCS occurs in approximately 3%–8% of cases of lymphoma.[10] High-grade lymphomas such as diffuse large cell and lymphoblastic lymphoma are more likely to cause SVCS than lower grade lymphomas.[4] SVCS is rarely caused by Hodgkin's lymphoma in spite of the high incidence of mediastinal involvement.

Pathophysiology

Normal Anatomy and Physiology

Structures in the mediastinum include the SVC, aorta, pulmonary artery, sternum, vertebrae, trachea, right bronchus, and perihilar and paratracheal lymph nodes. The SVC is located in the right anterior superior mediastinum. The junction of the right and left brachiocephalic veins is the beginning of the SVC, which is approximately 6–8 cm in length (see Figure 42-1). The SVC extends to the right atrium where it is anchored to the pericardial sac in a relatively fixed position. It is a thin-walled large blood vessel (1.5–2.0 cm in diameter) that carries venous blood from the head, neck, upper extremities, and upper thorax to the right atrium of the heart. Blood flow is at low pressure, a factor that may contribute to intraluminal thrombus formation.[12] One major vein, the azygos vein, empties into the SVC at the level of the right main stem bronchus carrying blood returned from the posterior torso (see Figure 42-2). Most structures in the mediastinum are relatively rigid except for the SVC, which can easily be compressed. Lymph nodes surround the SVC and can be a major factor in SVC obstruction when they are invaded by cancer (see Figure 42-3). A moderate increase in lymph node size can cause SVC compromise.

Partial or complete occlusion of the SVC results in

Table 42-1 Cancer Etiology of SVCS

Type of Cancer	Percentage
Lung cancer	67–80
Lymphoma	8–14
Metastatic breast cancer	< 3

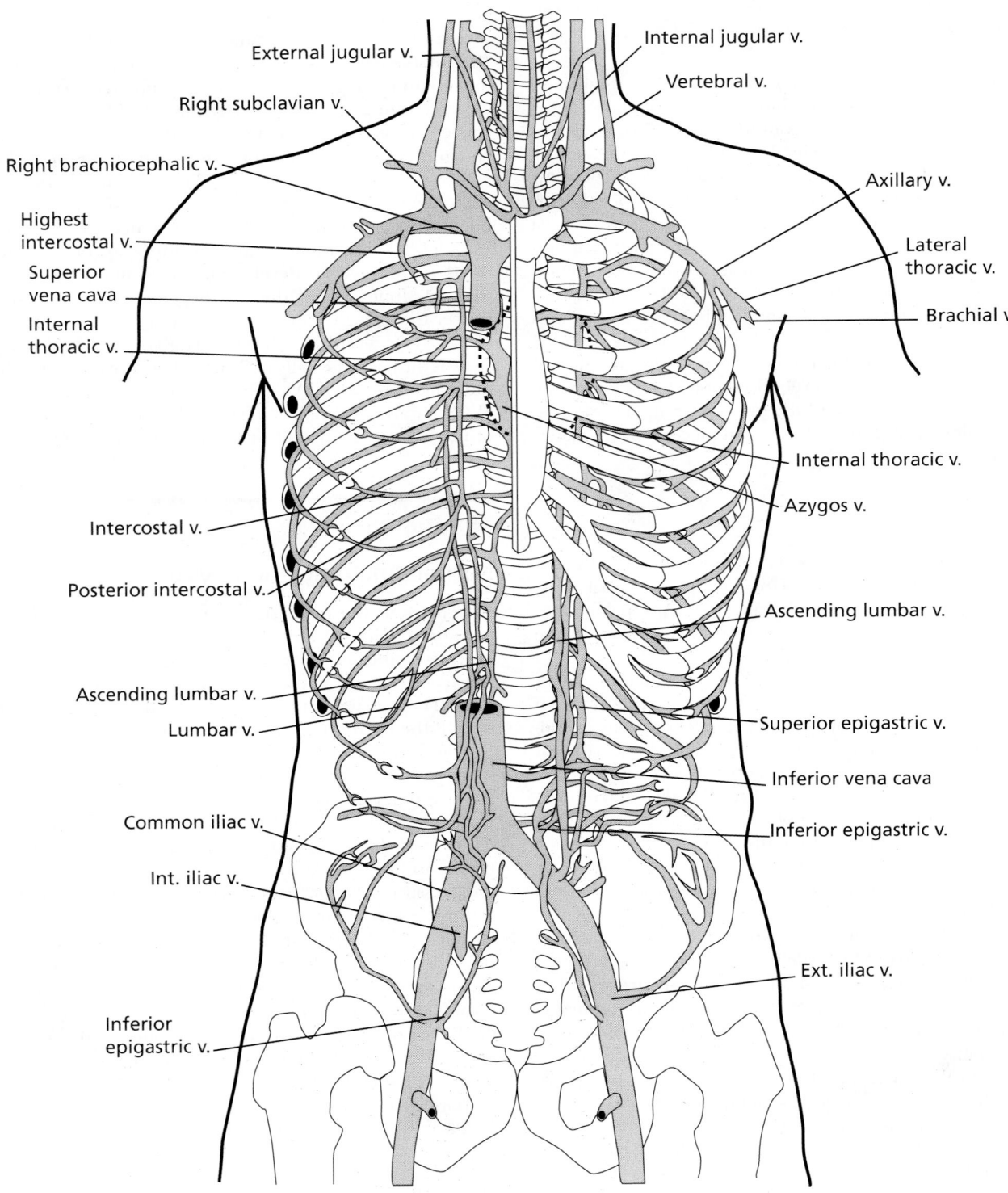

Figure 42-1   Anterior view of SVC and venous drainage.

increased venous pressure (venous hypertension) causing venous stasis and vein engorgement in the areas normally drained by the SVC. Blood from the upper body bypasses the SVC obstruction and is diverted into various venous collateral venous pathways in the area to return blood to the right atrium.[16] The specific pathways develop in direct relation to the location and extent of obstruction of the SVC. Collateral circulation is generally associated with

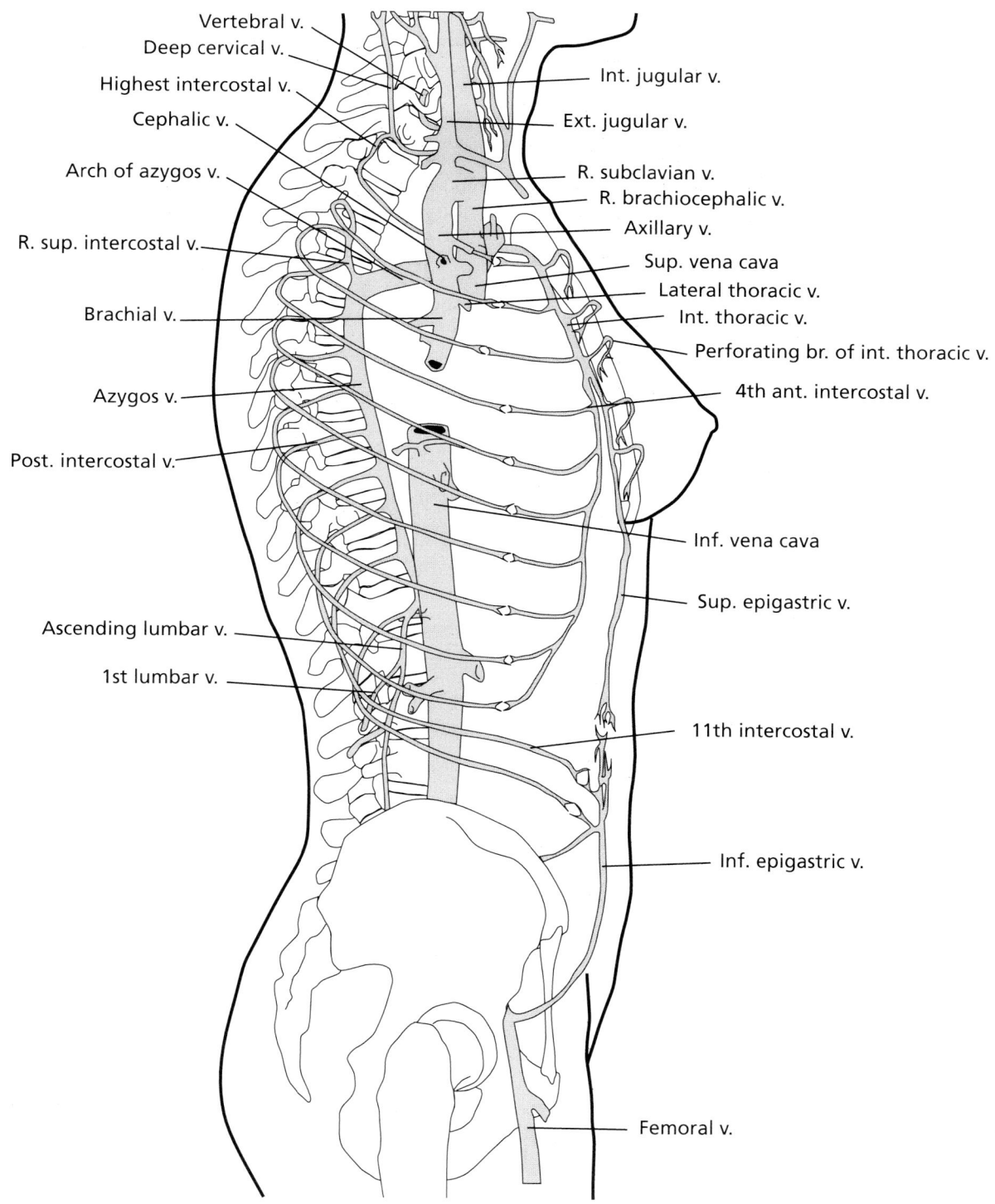

FIGURE 42-2 Lateral view of SVC and venous drainage.

four interconnected venous pathways: (1) azygos and hemiazygos, (2) internal mammary, (3) lateral thoracic and superficial thoracoabdominal, and (4) vertebral venous plexus.[16,18] The azygos pathway branches posteriorly from the SVC and is the most common venous collateral route. When the azygos vein is also obstructed as it enters the SVC, the other three routes develop to a higher degree. The azygos vein can also be compressed by lymph nodes invaded by cancer. SVCS that develops rapidly may preclude the development of collaterals.

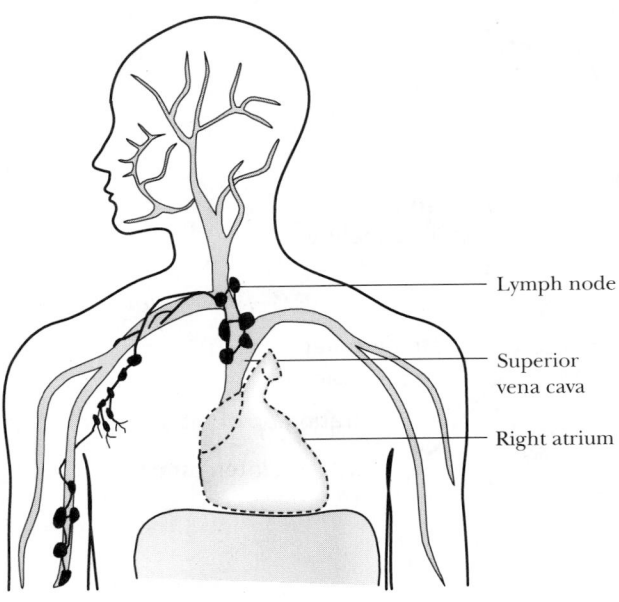

FIGURE 42-3 Lymph nodes near the SVC.

- Lymph node
- Superior vena cava
- Right atrium

The degree of obstruction of the SVC may vary dramatically. Stanford and Doty[9] used venographic patterns to classify individuals with SVCS into four categories based on the severity of obstruction and the extent of collateral venous circulation. In type I partial SVC obstruction (up to 90% stenosis) is observed and the azygos–right atrial pathway is not obstructed. Blood flow is in the normal direction. In type II, individuals have 90%–100% SVC obstruction with patency and normal direction of blood flow in the azygos–right atrial pathway. In type III, there is 90%–100% SVC obstruction with reversal of azygos blood flow. Type IV is complete obstruction of the SVC and one or more of the major vena cava tributaries including the azygos systems. With types III and IV there is blood flow into the inferior vena cava. The development of collateral circulation correlated with the extent of SVC obstruction and patency of the azygos system. In type I there is little or no collateral development, and in types II and IV there is moderate collateral development. Collateral circulation is most evident in category III individuals with complete or near complete SVC obstruction and reversal of azygos pathways. When collateral circulation is central rather than peripheral there is a higher incidence of cerebral and respiratory compromise. Types III and IV categories account for 85% of compromise symptoms.[9,19]

Pathophysiology

SVCS may be caused by external compression by primary or metastatic cancer, direct invasion by tumor, or thrombus formation within the vessel. All types of obstruction reduce venous blood return to the heart from the upper body, increase venous congestion, and decrease cardiac output. Increased venous pressures may cause pleural or pericardial effusion and edema of the face, neck, upper thorax, and upper extremities. Tumor invasion or compression of other structures such as the esophagus, trachea, or pericardium interferes with function of these organs.

Changes in blood composition, reduced blood flow, and damaged vein wall contribute to intraluminal thrombus formation.[20] Individuals with cancer often have hypercoagulability states that can contribute to thrombus formation.[12,16,20–22] When SVCS occurs as a result of tumor compression or invasion of the SVC, secondary intravascular venous thrombosis may increase the size of the obstruction.[9,16] Irritation of the vessel wall may be caused when drugs are infused through a catheter that is immobilized by a thrombus allowing chemical exposure of the vein to infused chemotherapeutic agents and other drugs.[21,23] Indwelling central vascular catheters may cause mechanical slowing of blood flow[22] and irritation and inflammation of the vessel wall, especially in the presence of infection.[3,15] Mechanical trauma of the vein wall during central line catheter placement can result in accumulated fibrin and aggregation of blood components that may cause the catheter to adhere to the vein wall and induce thrombus formation.[21]

Clinical Manifestations

Clinical manifestations of SVCS are related to the underlying disease processes and SVC obstruction-related venous hypertension of the upper body, decreased cardiac output, and venous collateral circulation.[16] Signs and symptoms of SVCS are progressive if the cause is not corrected. Initial signs and symptoms may be vague and barely noticeable or may develop rapidly. Early recognition and treatment of SVCS may prevent progression of life-threatening respiratory and cerebral complications. Figure 42-4 describes a clinical pathway for SVCS.

Assessment

Assessment of individuals at high risk for SVCS—such as those with lung cancer, mediastinal lymphoma, or long-term central venous catheter—is essential in both the inpatient and outpatient settings. The history and a physical examination will reveal the severity and duration of symptoms of the individual with SVCS. Clinical manifestations are related to the extent and location of obstruction and the development of collateral circulation.[24] Signs and symptoms often develop gradually and may be vague initially. Mild symptoms may disappear after the individual has been upright for several hours. Gradual, slow progression of obstruction causes slow onset of symptoms due to the development of collateral circulation that compensates for the obstruction.[25] Symptoms that manifest a rapid onset preclude the benefit of collateral pathways that develop over time. Intravascular thrombosis may be associated with rapid onset of symptoms. Approximately 20%–31% of individuals with SVCS have a history of less

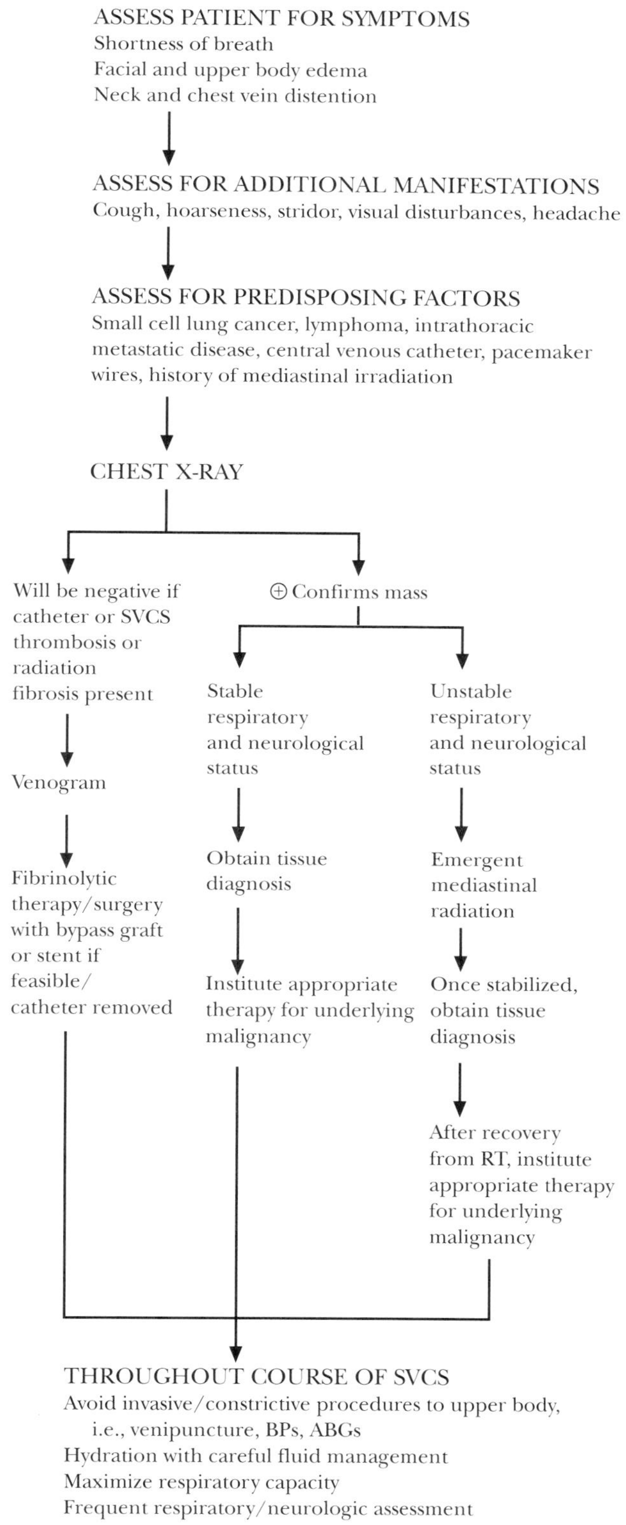

ASSESS PATIENT FOR SYMPTOMS
Shortness of breath
Facial and upper body edema
Neck and chest vein distention

↓

ASSESS FOR ADDITIONAL MANIFESTATIONS
Cough, hoarseness, stridor, visual disturbances, headache

↓

ASSESS FOR PREDISPOSING FACTORS
Small cell lung cancer, lymphoma, intrathoracic
metastatic disease, central venous catheter, pacemaker
wires, history of mediastinal irradiation

↓

CHEST X-RAY

Will be negative if
catheter or SVCS
thrombosis or
radiation
fibrosis present

↓

Venogram

↓

Fibrinolytic
therapy/surgery
with bypass graft
or stent if
feasible/
catheter removed

⊕ Confirms mass

Stable
respiratory
and neurological
status

↓

Obtain tissue
diagnosis

↓

Institute appropriate
therapy for underlying
malignancy

Unstable
respiratory
and neurological
status

↓

Emergent
mediastinal
radiation

↓

Once stabilized,
obtain tissue
diagnosis

↓

After recovery
from RT, institute
appropriate therapy
for underlying
malignancy

THROUGHOUT COURSE OF SVCS
Avoid invasive/constrictive procedures to upper body,
   i.e., venipuncture, BPs, ABGs
Hydration with careful fluid management
Maximize respiratory capacity
Frequent respiratory/neurologic assessment

FIGURE 42-4   Clinical pathway for SVCS.

than 2 weeks' duration of symptoms, 31%–35% of individuals present with symptoms that have been present 3–4 weeks, while 27% have symptoms for 5 weeks or longer.[6,13]

Patient history

Because 67%–80% of malignant causes of SVCS are related to lung cancer, individuals with a history of smoking or other risk factors for lung cancer may be at a relatively high risk for development of SVCS. Metastatic or primary cancer in the mediastinum is also a risk factor for SVCS. A rare risk factor is previous mediastinal irradiation.[26] Assess for the presence of a central catheter. Two placement factors correlate with an increased incidence of catheter-related thrombosis when they are both present: left-sided, long-term indwelling vascular access catheter and catheter tip in the upper half of the vena cava.[23] Two possible explanations for the increased thrombosis are (1) the left brachiocephalic vein forms a more marked angle with the vena cava and the wall of the vena cava may be injured at insertion, and (2) chronic microtrauma from a catheter tip that did not clear the angle may occur with each heartbeat and be further injured by infused drugs, especially chemotherapy. Signs and symptoms of SVCS may be more pronounced in individuals who have preexisting coronary artery disease, hypertension, or heart failure possibly due to increased strain on the cardiovascular system.[26]

Physical exam

Symptoms of SVCS are generally typical and include dyspnea, nonproductive cough, and sensation of fullness of the face, neck, upper trunk, and extremities[27,28] (see Table 42-2). Bending over, stooping, or lying flat may aggravate symptoms. Dyspnea is the most common symptom of SVCS in individuals with lung cancer and lymphoma.[12] Classic clinical findings are neck vein distention, chest wall vein distention, edema of the face and upper extremities, and periorbital edema. Dilated veins

Table 42-2   Early and Late Signs and Symptoms of SVCS

Early	Late
Respiratory System	
• Vague breathing changes (e.g., heaviness; shortness of breath on exertion)	• Stridor
	• Respiratory distress
	• Facial flushing
• Dyspnea	• Anxiety
• Tachypnea (> 30 per minute)	• Laryngeal changes (hoarseness, stridor due to edema or nerve compression)
• Orthopnea	
• Nonproductive cough	
• Hoarseness (secondary to paralysis of vocal cord) (laryngeal edema)	
• Fatigue	

(continues)

Table 42-2 Early and Late Signs and Symptoms of SVCS (continued)

Early	Late
Cardiovascular System	
• Neck vein distention	• Tachycardia
• Blood pressure higher in upper than lower extremities	• Decreased or absent peripheral pulses
• Facial swelling and conjunctival edema especially in the morning upon arising; may decrease as day progresses	• Congestive heart failure
	• Chest pain (due to pleural effusion)
• Nasal stuffiness, epistaxis	• Decreased blood pressure
• Feeling of fullness in ear	• Cyanosis
• Periobital edema	
• Redness and edema in conjunctiva	
• Fullness of face	
• Facial erythema	
• Swelling of neck, arms, and hands (tight collar, tight rings, tight watch)	
• Pitting edema of arms and hands	
• Visible collateral veins on the chest and/or breast; veins tortuous, prominent, and dilated	
• Cyanosis of upper torso (due to venous stasis)	
• Weight gain over 1–2 weeks	
Central Nervous System	
• Mild headache	• Severe headache
• Mood changes	• Irritability
• Anxiety	• Visual disturbances, blurred vision
• Lethargy	• Dizziness, syncope
• Lightheadedness especially on exertion	• Mental status changes: confusion, change in level of consciousness, stupor, coma
	• Seizures
	• Papilledema
	• Horner's (unilateral ptosis, unilateral constricted pupil, loss of sweating on same side forehead)
Gastrointestinal System	
• Nausea	• Dysphagia
	• Hemoptysis

over the trunk and upper extremities appear prominent and tortuous and are palpable. Physical assessment may also reveal plethora, facial flushing, cyanosis, dizziness, and tachypnea. Infrequently, the individual may experience hoarseness, chest pain, dysphagia, dizziness, and hemoptysis. Signs that rarely occur are Horner's syndrome (unilateral ptosis, constricted pupil, and ipsilateral loss of sweating from pressure on the cervical sympathetic nerves) and a paralyzed vocal cord causing hoarseness or stridor (due to cervical sympathetic nerve compromise of recurrent laryngeal nerve entrapment or involvement by lymph nodes). Laryngeal edema may cause stridor, cyanosis, hoarseness, and use of accessory muscles for breathing. Airway obstruction and cerebral edema are indications for immediate treatment. Headache, visual disturbances, anxiety, irritability, lethargy, papilledema, confusion, and change in level of consciousness may indicate venous congestion severe enough to cause increased intracranial pressure. Cerebral or airway compromise negatively affect survival.[9]

Individuals with catheter-related thrombosis may experience shoulder or retrosternal pain exacerbated by injection into the catheter.[23] Thrombosis rarely causes a complete obstruction of the SVC.[29]

Diagnostic studies

Because SVCS may be the presenting symptom of underlying pathology, determination of the etiology of SVCS is important prior to treatment. A significant number of cases are caused by nonmalignant etiologies. When cancer is present, accurate histologic diagnosis is necessary to plan appropriate anticancer treatment. A chest x-ray in an individual with SVCS will be positive in approximately 80%–85% of cases.[3,8] Findings often include superior mediastinal widening due to presence of tumor. Pleural effusion may be found due to venous hypertension and thoracic lymphatic obstruction.[16] Chest x-ray may be normal if the etiology is an indwelling catheter with an intravascular thrombus.[8]

In the individual not yet diagnosed the least invasive method to obtain a tissue diagnosis is used. Sputum cytology identifies the underlying cancer in 50% of cases and thoracentesis for pleural effusion will establish the diagnosis of cancer in approximately 70%.[8] Diagnostic tests including fiberoscopy, lymph node biopsy, mediastinoscopy, and thoracotomy in the presence of SVCS have not been found to result in serious complications related to the syndrome.[2] Biopsy of a mass or palpable lymph node may be performed. Bone marrow biopsy is indicated when bone marrow involvement is suspected. It reveals only about 25% of cancers.[8] Mediastinoscopy and thoracotomy are performed only when other procedures have failed to reveal a diagnosis and lung cancer is suspected. Both risk disruption of chest wall collateral pathways. Additional tests may include arterial blood gases, electrolytes, kidney function tests, complete blood count, and coagulation studies.

A computerized tomography (CT) scan provides detailed information related to mediastinal structures and the extent of disease involvement. Evaluation of critical structures such as the SVC, other vascular structures, lymph nodes, bronchi, and spinal cord provides information necessary for treatment planning. Recent advances in CT technology have expanded its role in investigating vascular pathology.[30] It is useful in determining the location and extent of thrombi, vascular compression and invasion, and pathways of venous circulation including collaterals. The CT is also used to localize a tumor for CT-guided biopsy and to determine radiation treatment fields. Magnetic resonance imaging (MRI) is currently being investigated as a noninvasive diagnostic tool to visualize vascular pathways as well as mediastinal structures.

Contrast venography can detect compromise in circulation and patterns of collateral development. It is especially useful when a surgical bypass procedure is considered. However, it is an invasive procedure that requires contrast material and similar information can be obtained from such studies as CT and MRI.

Therapeutic Approaches and Nursing Care

Management

The treatment of SVCS is based on the cause of the obstruction, severity of symptoms, prognosis, patient preferences, and goals of treatment (palliation or cure). Historically SVCS was treated as a medical emergency with immediate mediastinal irradiation. Radiation therapy without histologic diagnosis can interfere with subsequent diagnosis and treatment plan. Whenever possible, the treatment plan is determined after the diagnosis has been made. Nursing management includes measures to relieve symptoms of the SVCS and of treatment (see Table 42-3).

Thrombolysis

Catheter-related thrombosis threatens loss of the central line, interruption of treatment, and continued clot formation. SVCS related to thrombosis in the presence of a central venous access device (VAD) catheter is treated with infusion of a thrombolytic agent such as streptokinase, urokinase, or tissue plasminogen activator (t-PA) and heparin. The agent may be infused through the catheter or a different venipuncture site. Urokinase has been reported to be more effective than streptokinase and has demonstrated lower occurrence of bleeding, pyrogenic side effects, and allergic response.[6,31] Urokinase has a relatively short half-life and demonstrates faster lysis of clots than streptokinase. Thrombolysis with urokinase is discontinued at 48 hours or when the thrombus is no longer present, a local complication occurs, or fibrinogen level decreases below 100 mg/dL. Thrombolysis with streptokinase or urokinase in association with a central venous catheter is achieved in 73%–87%.[7,32] Delivering

the drug through a peripheral vein can prolong thrombolysis when it travels through collateral circulation in part bypassing the site of obstruction.[7] Delay in treatment for more than 5 days after the onset of symptoms has been associated with the failure of treatment to successfully treat the thrombus.[7]

Tissue plasminogen activator is also an effective thrombolytic therapy. It is administered as a bolus infusion and has several advantages over urokinase including less likelihood of hemorrhage, faster lysis of clot, and higher probability of success when administered more than 5 days after clot formation.[4,31] Febrile reactions are more common with t-PA.

Nursing care during thrombolytic or anticoagulation administration includes bleeding precautions. Assess for bleeding and monitor vital signs. Monitor for intracranial hemorrhage related to increased intracranial pressure secondary to venous hypertension. Effects of thrombolytic agents continue for several hours after infusion and monitoring for bleeding is continued. Heparin infusion is generally also administered followed by conversion to low-dose warfarin. Heparin and warfarin are not effective in clot lysis but may stop progression of the clot and prevent new thrombus formation. Coagulation studies are monitored with fibrinogen levels and partial thromboplastin times prior to thrombolytic therapy and every 6 hours during therapy.[10] Treatment decisions include whether to save the catheter or remove it. The central line may be salvaged with successful thrombolysis.[32] Thrombolytic agents are contraindicated in individuals with bleeding disorders, increased intracranial pressure, intracranial or intraspinal surgery, history of hemorrhagic stroke, and cerebral metastasis.[4,20]

External compression or tumor invasion of the SVC may cause intravascular thrombus formation. Because of ongoing venous stasis, anticoagulation with heparin or oral anticoagulants may be used to decrease the extent and prevent progression of thrombus formation.[5]

Chemotherapy

When the etiology of SVC is cancer, treatment is most often multidrug chemotherapy and/or radiation therapy. With the exception of very responsive tumors, time is required for either chemotherapy or radiation therapy to alleviate symptoms. However, collateral circulation may be sufficient to maintain patient status until treatment becomes effective. Insufficient collateral drainage may precipitate venous hypertension and cerebral or airway compromise.

Multidrug chemotherapy is especially effective in the treatment of SVCS caused by small cell lung cancer and non-Hodgkin's lymphoma. Symptom relief often occurs after the first week of treatment. Venous stasis may cause local drug concentration in the upper thorax. A long-term venous access catheter or femoral vein catheter may be necessary to administer chemotherapy.[4]

Chan and colleagues[17] found significant improvement in symptoms with treatment of SVCS in small cell lung

Table 42-3 SVCS Treatment Approaches: Management of Side Effects

Possible Side Effects of Treatment Approaches	Management of Side Effects
Thrombolytic and Anticoagulation Therapy • Hemorrhage related to anticoagulation or thrombolysis	• Bleeding precautions • Assess for bleeding (e.g., petechiae, bruising, epistaxis, gingival bleeding, hematuria, melena, mental status changes) • Monitor coagulation studies
Chemotherapy • Myelosuppression • Nausea • Vomiting • Stomatitis • Alopecia	• Avoid upper extremity IV access • Myelosuppression: assess for infection and bleeding; minimize risk of infection; bleeding precautions • Nausea and vomiting: antiemetics; nonpharmacologic interventions; small frequent meals; bland diet • Stomatitis: oral care; soft toothbrush; topical anesthetics; analgesics; avoid irritants; bland diet • Alopecia: assess perception of hair loss; provide resources for head coverings and support groups
Radiation Therapy • *Early*: esophagitis, cough, nausea, skin reaction, fatigue • *Late*: pneumonitis (depends on amount of lung treated), pulmonary fibrosis, esophageal sequelae (rare: stenosis, ulceration, fistula), cardiac changes (rare: pericardial effusion, constrictive pericarditis, cardiomyopathy), spinal cord myelopathy, brachial plexopathy	• Esophagitis: topical anesthetics such as viscous lidocaine; agents such as liquid antacids that coat mucosa; analgesics; avoid irritants; soft diet • Cough: antitussives possibly with codeine • Nausea: antiemetics; small frequent meals; bland diet • Skin reactions: topical moisturizing creams; protect from irritants • Fatigue: balance rest/activity; prioritize and pace activities; plan rest prn • Pneumonitis: bed rest; bronchodilators; corticosteroids
Stent Placement • Groin hematoma • Femoral-site deep vein thrombosis • Access-site cellulitis • Pleuritic chest pain • Stent migration • Stent fracture • Shoulder pain • Occlusion • Pulmonary embolism • SVC perforation	• Catheter access site: assess for bleeding; infection; pain • Occlusion: assess for recurrent SVCS • Pulmonary embolism: assess breathing; assess pain • SVC perforation: assess for bleeding
Vein Graft Surgery • Infection • Postoperative complications	• Nursing care for postoperative thoracotomy

cancer in 93% after chemotherapy and 94% after mediastinal irradiation. Several studies have demonstrated an advantage for combined chemotherapy and radiation therapy.[6,17] Initial multidrug chemotherapy to decrease tumor volume may allow smaller subsequent radiation fields to be used. Combined chemotherapy and radiation therapy is often used to treat non-Hodgkin's lymphoma. In individuals who have had previous mediastinal irradiation, chemotherapy is the treatment of choice. Chemotherapy regimens for small cell lung cancer often include drugs such as cyclophosphamide, doxorubicin, etoposide, cisplatin, and vindesine.[2]

Nursing care of the individual receiving chemotherapy depends upon the agents administered. Combined chemotherapy and radiation therapy results in a higher incidence of esophagitis and neutropenia.[3,33] Nursing management may be required for myelosuppression, nausea and vomiting, stomatitis, esophagitis, and alopecia. When chemotherapy is administered, arm veins in the involved extremities should not be used.[6] Venous stasis due to obstruction may result in local accumulation of the drug with poor absorption and irritation of the vessel wall. Because of the risk for extravasation and tissue damage, administering irritant or vesicant chemotherapy through lower extremity peripheral veins is not recommended. Placement of a long-term vascular access device into the inferior vena cava via the femoral vein is needed to safely administer chemotherapy.

Radiation therapy

Tumor type and extent, any history of previous irradiation in the area, and performance status determine the radiation dose prescribed. Radiation therapy for SVCS is often administered for 2–3 days as high-dose fractions of 4 Gy and subsequently as daily fractions of 1.8–2.0 Gy until the total prescribed dose is completed.[33] Higher initial daily doses are believed to result in more rapid decrease in symptoms than standard dose fractions.[13] Some investigators have found that symptom relief is not enhanced by the higher initial fractions and recommend standard fractionation throughout the treatment.[14] Radiation is generally 30–50 Gy administered over 2–5 weeks but may be as high as 60–70 Gy in 6–7 weeks. Lymphomas are more responsive to radiation and generally require less than other tumor types. Radiation fields for mediastinal treatment generally include mediastinal, hilar, and supraclavicular lymph nodes and any adjacent lung lesions.[33] Symptom relief generally occurs at 2 weeks from the start of radiation therapy with maximum relief at 3 weeks.[5] Good to excellent relief of SVCS symptoms occurs in about 70% of those with lung cancer and 95% with lymphoma.[33] No explanation has been found for the fact that SVCS in small cell lung cancer is a positive prognostic indicator with higher 5-year survival than small cell lung cancer without SVCS.[14]

Side effects of irradiation to the mediastinum depend upon the total dose, dose per fraction, volume of normal tissue included in the field, and whether chemotherapy is combined with radiation therapy. Side effects that occur during and for 1 month after radiation therapy are considered early side effects. Nursing management is often necessary for esophagitis, cough, nausea, skin reaction, and fatigue. Symptomatic treatment helps minimize these side effects. Late effects of radiation therapy to the mediastinum include pneumonitis, pulmonary fibrosis, esophageal ulceration or stenosis, cardiac changes, spinal cord myelopathy, and brachial plexopathy.

In SVCS caused by non–small cell lung carcinoma (NSCLC), radiation therapy is the treatment of choice.[6] Effective symptom relief is high; however, prognosis is poor. Radiation therapy is also the treatment of choice in individuals without a histologic diagnosis in whom rapid deterioration in mental status (increased intracranial pressure) or severe upper airway compression occurs (e.g., obstruction of the bronchus). In addition to SVCS, radiation therapy may be prescribed to treat other symptoms such as hemoptysis, cough, and bone pain.

Stent placement

Until recently, radiation therapy and chemotherapy have been considered the standard treatment for SVCS.

The intravascular placement of self-expanding stents to relieve SVC obstruction was first published in 1992 by Rocchini and colleagues.[34] Endovascular techniques may be used to revascularize the SVC after unsuccessful thrombolysis or in cases of tumor compression or invasion. Percutaneous placement of metallic intravascular stents has been used to successfully treat SVC obstruction in 68%–100% of cases.[35] The stent is generally placed by an interventional radiologist under local anesthesia. Immediate improvement in symptoms is reported in 22% of cases and an additional 70% experience improvement in 12 hours.[5] Resolution of peripheral edema generally occurs within 1 to 7 days.[35] Low-pressure venous blood flow may contribute to thrombus formation in the stented area. Heparin is generally administered during the procedure and may be converted to oral warfarin therapy for 3–6 months after stent placement to prevent thrombus formation. Anticoagulant therapy after stent placement is controversial. When a thrombus is present, thrombolysis may be performed before stent placement. This procedure decreases the size of the thrombus and the amount of potential embolic material. Recurrent SVC obstruction is observed in up to 45% of cases, possibly due to malignant invasion through the stented area, compression by tumor, intimal thickening, or thrombus formation.[35] Stent placement is contraindicated in cases of tumor invasion of the vessel.

Nursing management after stent placement includes care for potential complications such as groin hematoma or infection and femoral site deep vein thrombosis. Administer analgesics for pleuritic chest pain and shoulder pain after stent placement. Assess for signs of pulmonary embolism and bleeding due to SVC perforation. Complications include stent migration, fracture, and occlusion.

Surgery

Surgical bypass using a reconstructed saphenous vein graft to relieve obstruction of the SVC has been performed in individuals with benign SVCS but has been limited in the individual with cancer, especially in those with advanced disease. The newly constructed vein connects the brachiocephalic or left jugular vein with the right atrium and bypasses the obstructed SVC. This treatment is effective but involves radical surgery. When advanced disease is present in the chest, treatment is generally palliative.

Nursing care

The nurse evaluates the individual's and family's responses to interventions and treatment. Goals of nursing management include ongoing assessment of status, maintenance of adequate cardiopulmonary function, maximization of oxygenation and perfusion, and provision of comfort measures to relieve dyspnea and anxiety (see Table 42-4). Assessment of the cardiac, respiratory, and central nervous systems is important in the individual with SVCS. Baseline assessment includes vital signs,

Table 42-4 Nursing Diagnoses for SVCS

Problem	Expected Outcomes	Nursing Interventions
Decreased cardiac output related to decreased venous return	Maintain adequate oxygenation	Assess respiratory system (cyanosis, hoarseness, stridor, dyspnea, tachypnea, cough, rales/rhonchi)
Altered tissue perfusion related to venous congestion and venous hypertension	Maintain airway	Assess cardiac system (tachycardia, dysrhythmias, hypotension, reduced pulse quality)
Ineffective breathing pattern related to airway compression by tumor	Maintain optimal venous drainage	Monitor blood pressure on lower extremity
Activity intolerance related to reduced cardiac output	Maintain adequate hydration	Administer oxygen
	Reduce edema	Monitor oxygen saturation
	Reduce fatigue	Administer corticosteroids for laryngeal edema
		Position upright
		Monitor for dysphagia
		Administer diuretics and fluids
		Monitor fluid balance
		Remove rings and constrictive clothing
		Avoid venipuncture in upper extremities
		Avoid Valsalva maneuver, bending, stooping, lying flat, coughing
		Administer cough suppressants
		Administer analgesics for discomfort
		Minimize activity
Neurologic changes related to increased intracranial pressure	Prevent neurologic complications	Assess central nervous system (altered mental status, lethargy, headache, vomiting, visual changes)
		Administer corticosteroids for cerebral edema
		Position upright
Bleeding related to thrombolytic and anticoagulant treatment	Prevent bleeding	Assess for bleeding
	Reduce thrombus	Administer thrombolytics and anticoagulants
		Monitor coagulation studies
		Teach bleeding precautions
Anxiety related to respiratory distress	Relieve anxiety	Provide emotional support
		Assure relief of symptoms with successful treatment
		Maintain calm environment
		Teach relaxation techniques
		Administer anxiolytics, mild sedatives
Fatigue related to disease process, treatment, and reduced cardiac output	Minimize fatigue	Teach use of energy conservation techniques
	Perform activities of daily living	Prioritize activities
		Assist with activities of daily living
Altered body image related to edema	Reduce edema	Educate individual and family that edema will decrease with successful treatment
	Reassure that edema will resolve	
Knowledge deficit	Recognize early symptoms of SVCS	Educate individual and family to recognize signs and symptoms of recurrent SVCS
		Educate about treatment and side effect management

appearance, activity level, and mental status. Individuals who are at high risk for SVCS are monitored for early signs and symptoms of obstruction. In the individual diagnosed with lung cancer or mediastinal lymphoma, the nurse must be alert for signs and symptoms of SVCS.

Raising the head of the bed and administering oxygen may contribute to the relief of dyspnea and other symptoms related to reduced cardiac output and increased venous pressure. Minimizing activity level may also reduce dyspnea. Avoid peripheral upper extremity venipuncture and intravenous (IV) therapy. A femoral or central venous line with the tip past the obstruction may be necessary to administer drugs or chemotherapy.[24] Bronchial compression or laryngeal edema may create an emergency situation in which immediate treatment is needed. Changes in neurologic status may also indicate an emergency situation.

Steroids and diuretics are frequently prescribed, although their efficacy is not well documented. Corticosteroids are used to relieve laryngeal and cerebral edema.[10] Diuretics, low-sodium diet, and decreased activity contribute to reduced cardiac output. Efforts to reduce edema through diuretics and low salt intake must be done carefully to avoid an increased risk of thrombus formation with dehydration. Overhydration will exacerbate SVCS.

Venous access of the involved extremity in the individual with SVCS should be avoided whenever possible. Lower extremities can be used for venipuncture and blood pressure measurement. Remove rings and loosen constrictive clothing.

The Valsalva maneuver increases venous pressure and should be prevented by administration of medications such as stool softeners and cough suppressants when indicated. Symptoms of SVCS may cause fear and anxiety in the individual with this syndrome. Provide a calm and restful environment, provide support, and administer medications that reduce anxiety, discomfort, and other symptoms when necessary. Assure the individual that changes in physical appearance such as periorbital and facial edema (plethora) and fullness will decrease with successful treatment.

Continuity of Care

Rehabilitation after relieving the signs and symptoms of SVCS is rapid when the underlying disease is controlled. Routine follow-up for the diagnosis is generally adequate. With a growing emphasis on ambulatory care, there is an increased need for health care providers to prepare individuals and family members to perform self care at home. The nurse provides education related to symptom management at home and identification of symptoms that may indicate recurrent SVCS. When SVCS reappears, it may be related to progression of underlying disease.[25] Monitor for bleeding if anticoagulation therapy is administered. Monitor for side effects of therapy.

Conclusion

SVCS is a relatively rare complication; it can develop rapidly but generally develops gradually. While most SVCS is caused by an underlying malignancy, there are a significant number of cases related to nonmalignant causes. Treatment is based on the etiology. When the cause is unknown initially, every effort is made to establish the diagnosis prior to treatment. Early detection and treatment of SVCS can prevent progression to severe complications.

The overall prognosis and psychosocial factors are considered in the treatment plan. Individuals and families are taught measures to reduce and minimize manifestations of SVCS and side effects of treatment. After successful treatment they are educated to report signs and symptoms of recurrent SVCS. The nurse assists the individual with continued management of the underlying disease. The greatest impact on future trends of this complication rely on new and effective treatment of lung cancer and lymphoma, which are most frequently associated with SVCS.

References

1. Pinover WH, Coia LR: Palliative radiation therapy, in Berger AM, Portenoy RK, Weissman DE (eds): *Principles and Practice of Supportive Oncology.* Philadelphia, Lippincott-Raven, 1998, pp 603–626
2. Urban T, Lebeau B, Chastang C, et al: Superior vena cava syndrome in small-cell lung cancer. *Arch Intern Med* 153: 384–387, 1993
3. Kreamer K: Superior vena cava syndrome, in Johnson BL, Gross J (eds): *Handbook of Oncology Nursing* (ed 3). Sudbury, MA, Jones and Bartlett, 1998, pp 645–654
4. Mack KC: Superior vena cava syndrome, in Gates RA, Fink RM (eds): *Oncology Nursing Secrets.* Philadelphia, Hanley & Belfus, 1997, pp 356–362
5. Nicholson AA, Ettles DF, Arnold A: Treatment of malignant superior vena cava obstruction: metal stents or radiation therapy: *J Vasc Interv Radiol* 8:781–788, 1997
6. Yahalom J: Oncologic emergencies, in DeVita VT, Hellman S, Rosenberg SA (eds): *Cancer: Principles and Practice of Oncology* (ed 5). Philadelphia, Lippincott-Raven, 1997, pp 2469–2476
7. Gray BH, Olin JW, Graor RA, et al: Safety and efficacy of thrombolytic therapy for superior vena cava syndrome. *Chest* 99:54–59, 1991
8. O'Brien JF: The oncologic crisis Part 2: Cardiorespiratory and neurologic emergencies. *Emerg Med* 28:21–44, 1996
9. Stanford W, Doty DB: The role of venography and surgery in the management of patients with superior vena cava obstruction. *Ann Thorac Surg* 41:158–163, 1986
10. Kee ST, Kinoshita L, Razavi MK, et al: Superior vena cava syndrome: treatment with catheter-directed thrombolysis and endovascular stent placement. *Radiology* 206:187–193, 1998
11. Kelly KM, Lange B: Oncologic emergencies. *Pediatr Clin North Am* 44:809–830, 1997

12. Abner A: Approach to the patient who presents with superior vena cava obstruction. *Chest* 103:394s–397s, 1993

13. Armstrong BA, Perez CA, Simpson JR, et al: Role of irradiation in the management of superior vena cava syndrome. *Int J Radiat Oncol Biol Phys* 13:531–539, 1987

14. Wurschmidt F, Bunemann H, Heilmann HP: Small cell lung cancer with and without superior vena cava syndrome: A multivariate analysis of prognostic factors in 408 cases. *Int J Radiat Oncol Biol Phys* 33:77–82, 1995

15. Nally AT: Critical care of the patient with lung cancer. *AACN Clinical Issues* 7:79–94, 1996

16. Baker GL, Barnes HJ: Superior vena cava syndrome: etiology, diagnosis, and treatment. *Am J Crit Care* 1:54–64, 1992

17. Chan RH, Dar AR, Yu E, et al: Superior vena cava obstruction in small-cell lung cancer. *Int J Radiat Oncol Biol Phys* 38:513–520, 1997

18. Bashist B, Parisi A, Frager DH, et al: Abdominal CT findings when the superior vena cava, brachiocephalic vein, or subclavian vein is obstructed. *Am J Radiol* 167:1457–1463, 1996

19. Alimi YS, Gloviczki P, Vrtiska TJ, et al: Reconstruction of the superior vena cava: benefits of postoperative surveillance and secondary endovascular interventions. *J Vasc Surg* 27:287–301, 1998

20. Hadaway LC: Major thrombotic and nonthrombotic complications: loss of patency. *J Intrav Nurs* 21:S143–S160, 1998

21. Bagnall-Reeb H: Diagnosis of central venous access device occlusion. *J Intrav Nurs* 21:S115–S121, 1998

22. Shelton BK: Superior vena cava syndrome, in Ziegfeld CR, Lubejko BG, Shelton BK (eds): *Manual of Cancer Nursing*. Philadelphia, Lippincott, 1998, pp 401–409

23. Puel V, Caudry M, LeMetayer P, et al: Superior vena cava thrombosis related to catheter malposition in cancer chemotherapy given through implanted ports. *Cancer* 72:2248–2252, 1993

24. Camp-Sorrell D, Mayo DJ: Superior vena cava syndrome. *Clin J Oncol Nurs* 2:153–154, 1998

25. Stewart IE: Superior vena cava syndrome: an oncologic complication. *Semin Oncol Nurs* 12:122–317, 1996

26. Loney M: Superior vena cava syndrome, in Chernecky CC, Berger BJ (eds): *Advanced and Critical Care Oncology Nursing: Managing Primary Complications*. Philadelphia, Saunders, 1998, pp 603–621

27. Hunter JC: Structural emergencies, in Itano JK, Taoka KN (eds): *Core Curriculum for Oncology Nursing* (ed 3). Philadelphia, Saunders, 1998, pp 340–354

28. Shuey KM: Heart, lung, and endocrine complications of solid tumors. *Semin Oncol Nurs* 10:177–188, 1994

29. Mayo DJ, Pearson DC, Horne MK: Superior vena cava thrombosis associated with a central venous access device: a case report. *Clin J Oncol Nurs* 1:5–10, 1997

30. Naik KS, Chalmers AG: Pictorial review: the differential diagnosis of early inferior vena caval opacification on dynamic CT. *Clin Radiol* 52:504–509, 1997

31. Greenberg S, Kosinski R, Daniels J: Treatment of superior vena cava thrombosis with recombinant tissue type plasminogen activator. *Chest* 99:1298–1301, 1991

32. Seigel EL, Jew AC, Delcore R, et al: Thrombolytic therapy for catheter-related thrombosis. *Am J Surg* 166:716–719, 1993

33. Emami B, Graham MV: Lung, in Perez CA, Brady LW (eds): *Principles and Practice of Radiation Oncology* (ed 3). Philadelphia, Lippincott, 1998, pp 1181–1220

34. Rocchini AP, Meliones JN, Beekman RH, et al: Use of balloon expandable stents to treat experimental peripheral pulmonary artery and SVC stenoses: preliminary experience. *Pediatr Cardiol* 13:92–96, 1992

35. Hochrein J, Bashore TM, O'Laughlin MP, et al: Percutaneous stenting of superior vena cava syndrome: a case report and review of the literature. *Am J Med* 104:78–84, 1998

Syndrome of Inappropriate Antidiuretic Hormone

Irene Stewart Haapoja, RN, MS

Scope of the Problem

Paraneoplastic syndromes are diseases resulting from tumor secretion of substances that affect systems at a distance from the primary tumor or its metastases. Syndrome of inappropriate antidiuretic hormone (SIADH) is a paraneoplastic syndrome most often associated with lung carcinomas. The endocrine paraneoplastic syndromes, of which SIADH is the most common and well known, usually follow a chronic course corresponding to the status of the malignancy. However, SIADH can present emergently as a life-threatening oncologic complication.

Definitions

SIADH was first described by Schwartz and associates in 1957 as the secretion of antidiuretic hormone by the pituitary in response to a thoracic tumor.[1] Subsequent research determined that SIADH resulted from tumor, not pituitary, secretion of antidiuretic hormone (ADH).[2] SIADH is currently defined as tumor secretion of ADH or its biologically active form arginine vasopressin (AVP), causing a syndrome of hyponatremia, urine osmolality disproportionately higher than plasma osmolality, and elevated urinary sodium concentrations.

The acronym *SIAD*, or *syndrome of inappropriate diuresis*, has been used to describe SIADH, reflecting the possibility that ADH may not be the only hormone affecting sodium excretion.[3] In some patients with small cell lung cancer (SCLC), atrial natriuretic peptide (ANP), a hormone arising from cardiac atrial tissue, has been identified as the cause of hyponatremia.[4] In other patients, ectopic ADH and ANP secretion both contribute to the etiology of SIADH.

Incidence

SIADH is a rare emergency in the general oncology population, occurring in only 1%–2% of cancer patients.[5] It is primarily associated with SCLC, which is rare itself as it accounts for less than 25% of all lung cancers. Small cell lung cancer is associated with close to 80% of all cases of SIADH, with the majority being subclinical or nonsymptomatic. A diagnosis of SIADH is not considered a negative prognostic factor in SCLC, nor is it related to a patient's potential response to chemotherapy.[6] Approximately 9%–14% of SCLC patients with SIADH have clinical evidence of the syndrome with signs and symptoms ranging from vague nausea and weakness to life-threatening seizures and coma.[7]

Etiology and Risk Factors

SIADH is caused by the ectopic production of vasopressin by malignant cells. While structurally identical to normal ADH, ectopic ADH is not regulated. In some patients, ectopic secretion of ANP alone may be responsible for the development of hyponatremia; in others the syndrome may result from tumor secretion of both ADH and ANP.[8] In a series of 263 lung cancer patients, 21 of the 133 patients with SCLC were hyponatremic. Eleven of these patients had tumor cell lines assayed for the presence of ADH and ANP. Nine patients' tumors produced ANP, seven produced ADH, and five produced both ANP and ADH.[9] The more severe cases of hyponatremia are associated with ectopic ADH, rather than ANP, production.[8]

Nonmalignant causes of SIADH may also occur in the oncology population and include infectious diseases (pneumonia, tuberculosis, and empyema); pain, nausea, and emotional stress; drugs (vincristine, vinblastine, cyclophosphamide, morphine); and general anesthesia, all of which increase AVP production.[10,11] See Table 43-1.

Patients who are at risk for the development of SIADH are primarily those with lung carcinomas, especially SCLC. Other patients at risk include those with carcinomas of the pancreas, brain, head and neck (especially oral cavity, but less often larynx, nasopharynx, and esophagus), prostate, duodenum, and ovary. The syndrome has also been described in patients with mesothelioma,

---

Table 43-1   Nonmalignant Causes of SIADH[11]

Pulmonary
- Infection (tuberculosis, lung abscess, pneumonia, empyema)
- COPD

Central Nervous System
- Trauma (subdural hematoma, skull fracture, concussion, stroke, subarachnoid hemorrhage, cerebral vascular thrombosis)
- Intracranial space-occupying lesions (primary or metastatic tumors)
- Infection (encephalitis, meningitis)
- Guillain-Barré syndrome
- Vasculitis (lupus)
- Acute intermittent porphyria
- Pain and emotional stress

Drugs
- Chemotherapeutic agents (vincristine, vinblastine, cyclophosphamide, ifosfamide, cisplatin)
- Narcotics (morphine, barbiturates)
- General anesthesia
- Nicotine
- Chlorpropamide (Diabinese)
- Carbamazepine (Tegretol)
- Tricyclic antidepressants

Surgery
- Neck dissection
- Mitral stenosis correction

Hodgkin's and non-Hodgkin's lymphomas, thymoma, and acute myelogenous leukemia (AML).[12-20] The patients at highest risk are those with tumors of squamous cell or neuroendocrine histology. See Table 43-2.

Physiologic Alterations

Normal Physiology and Scientific Principles

Understanding how the body maintains its fluid balance is key to comprehending the impact of ectopic ADH production. Constant regulation of body water within a very narrow range is achieved by the presence of ADH or AVP and its effect on the kidney. Arginine vasopressin is produced by the hypothalamus and stored in the posterior pituitary, where it is released in response to changes in plasma osmolality or volume. Normally, plasma osmolality is maintained within a narrow range of 286–294 mOsm/kg. Conditions such as dehydration, positive-pressure breathing, and vasodilation result in an increase in plasma osmolality, which is detected by the osmoreceptors in the hypothalamus and pressoreceptors in the left atrium and carotid sinus. These receptors stimulate the release of AVP, which acts to conserve water and concentrate the urine by binding to the V_2 receptor on the cell surface of the renal collecting duct.[10] The resulting receptor–hormone complex activates adenylate cyclase, increases the concentration of cyclic adenosine monophosphate (AMP), and stimulates prostaglandin E production. The presence of cyclic AMP activates protein kinase A, causing the phosphorylation of unidentified proteins. These proteins stimulate exocytosis or the insertion of water channels into the cell membrane. The water channels allow the cell membrane to become permeable to water. In general, the number of water channels correlates with the plasma concentration of AVP.[21] Inhibition of AVP release causes the water channels to be reinternalized back into the cell.[10,21] See Figure 43-1.

Table 43-2 Malignancies Associated with SIADH[12-20]

Malignancy	Incidence of SIADH
Small cell lung cancer	11%–46%
Duodenal and pancreatic carcinoma	
Prostate carcinoma	Five cases reported
Lymphomas (Hodgkin's and non-Hodgkin's)	
Chronic lymphocytic leukemia	Two cases reported
Head and neck carcinomas	3%
Gynecological	
Ovarian carcinoma (neuroendocrine)	One case reported
Cervical (small cell)	Two cases reported
Ovarian teratoma (germ cell)	One case reported
Papillary serous carcinoma peritoneum	One case reported
Thymic neuroblastoma	Four cases reported

The presence of AVP increases the transfer of water from the duct to the renal capillaries. At the same time, it increases the permeability of the collecting duct to urea and increases sodium absorption in the ascending limb of the loop of Henle. The resulting increase in plasma volume and normalization of plasma osmolality provides the feedback loop that inhibits AVP release. Cold weather, recumbency, and negative-pressure breathing can also inhibit AVP release.

The release of AVP is also regulated by certain neurotransmitters and neuropeptides. Angiotensin II, histamine, and bradykinin all appear to stimulate the release of AVP. On the other hand, AVP release may be inhibited by the presence of prostaglandins, dopamine, serotonin, and substance P, as evidenced by the antidiuretic effects of pain, nausea and vomiting, and emotional stress. The exact relationships, however, are unclear.[10]

Pathophysiology

The ability of neoplastic cells to synthesize, store, and release AVP results in excessive amounts of AVP leading to a condition known as *water intoxication*. The presence of extreme amounts of AVP causes water to be conserved in the kidney and produces a concentrated urine (urine osmolality > 300 mmol/kg). The increase in free water in the extracellular fluid (ECF) leads to plasma hypoosmolality and dilutional serum hyponatremia. Sodium continues to be excreted from the kidney in parallel to the sodium intake. Intracellular edema occurs as the plasma water follows an osmotic gradient, moving extracellular to intracellular.[22] Cerebral edema eventually occurs and leads to a disruption of neural function and death.

Clinical Manifestations

Water intoxication accounts for the symptomatology of SIADH. Edema is rare since the excess water is distributed intracellularly and not interstitially. Moderate hyponatremia (serum sodium level of 115–120 mEq/L) may cause nausea, weakness, anorexia, fatigue, and muscle cramps. These vague, nonspecific complaints can easily be attributed to the primary malignancy and are often not identified as early signs of hyponatremia. The symptoms that a patient exhibits are dependent upon the severity of the hyponatremia and the rate it developed. Rapid onset hyponatremia (72 hours or less) is associated with the most severe symptomatology.

As hyponatremia worsens, symptoms progress to include changes in mental status, such as confusion, lethargy, combativeness, or psychotic behavior. These signs and symptoms result from brain cell edema. Severe hyponatremia (100–110 mEq/L) is associated with refractory seizures, coma, and death.[6]

PRINCIPAL CELL

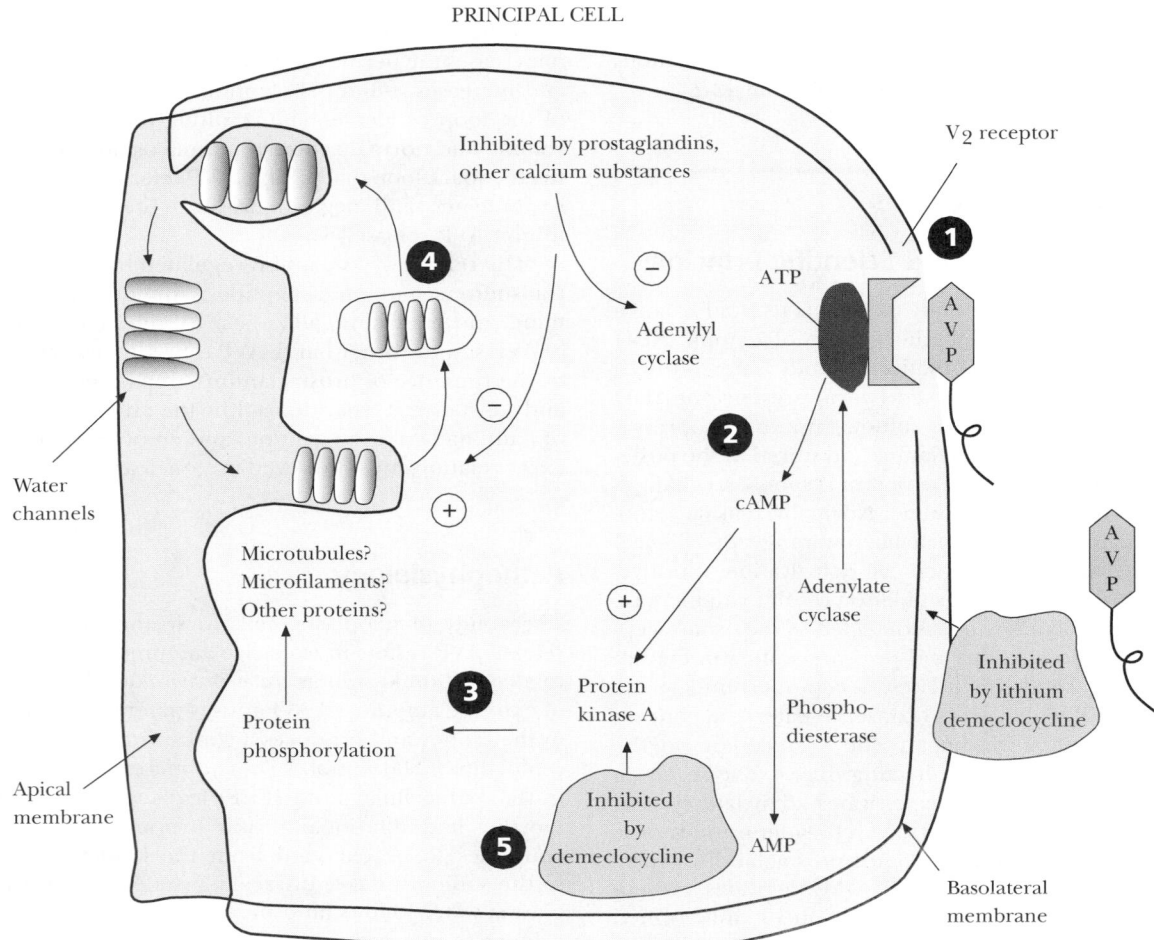

Figure 43-1 Action of AVP in the renal collecting duct. (1) AVP binds to the V_2 receptor on the principal cell. (2) The receptor-hormone complex activates a guanine nucleotide binding protein (GTP), which stimulates an enzyme, adenylate cyclase. This enzyme converts adenosine triphosphate (ATP) to cyclic 3′,5′-adenosine monophosphate (cAMP). AVP also stimulates prostaglandin E production, which acts as a feedback inhibitor of adenylate cyclase (3). The formation of cAMP initiates a chain of events: protein kinase A is activated causing the phosphorylation of unidentified proteins and microtubules. (4) The phosphorylated proteins cause the insertion of water channels into the apical membrane (exocytosis), allowing the membrane to become water permeable. When AVP is removed, the water channels are reinternalized into the cell (endocytosis), and the membrane becomes impermeable to water. (5) Demeclocycline inhibits adenylate cyclase stimulation by AVP and the stimulation of protein kinase A, preventing the formation of water channels. Data from Moses, Streeten[10]; Valtin, Schafer[21]

Assessment and Grading

Assessment of the patient with SIADH focuses on a skillful neurologic exam. Due to the nonspecificity and vagueness of the symptoms related to mild hyponatremia, SIADH may go undiagnosed until the hyponatremia becomes severe and cerebral edema produces neurologic changes. With regard to patients with SCLC, the presence of SIADH does not appear to negatively correlate with the stage of disease, response to chemotherapy, or survival.[6,8]

The diagnosis of SIADH is most frequently made concurrently with discovery of the malignancy. It may also occur with recurrence of malignancy. Most cases are inadvertently diagnosed when hyponatremia is found through routine serum chemistry studies. Ectopic SIADH is a diagnosis of exclusion. Other nonmalignant etiologies must be ruled out, such as infection, pneumothorax, or drug-related SIADH. The diagnosis of SIADH requires the presence of hyponatremia in addition to decreased plasma osmolality and inappropriately concentrated urine. See Table 43-3. Plasma osmolality must be less than 280 mOsm/kg and concurrent urinalysis must show increased levels of sodium (>20 mEq/L). Serum chemistries frequently show a low BUN, creatinine, albumin, and uric acid—a dilutional effect as a result of the increased

Table 43-3 Criteria for the Diagnosis of SIADH

- Serum osmolality (<275 mOsm/kg)
- Serum sodium (<130 mEq/L)
- Urine osmolality (urine osmolality > serum osmolality)
- Urinary sodium (>25 mEq/L)
- Euvolemia
- Decreased levels of BUN, uric acid, creatinine, and albumin
- Lack of edema
- Normal renal, adrenal, and thyroid function

extracellular fluid. Measurement of serum AVP levels is possible by radioimmunoassay but is rarely done. The AVP levels may be normal or elevated.[7]

A diagnostic study for SIADH that is rarely performed is the *water load test,* which is performed in the morning with the patient drinking 20 mL/kg of their body weight within 10–20 minutes. Urine output is collected every hour for 4–5 hours, while the patient remains supine. Between 65%–80% of the water load should be excreted within the 4–5 hour time period, with a corresponding urinary hypoosmolality. If less than 40% of the water load is excreted, the diagnosis points to SIADH. The water load test should not be performed if the serum sodium level is 125 mEq/L or lower due to the risk of potentiating water intoxication and causing renal insufficiency.[10]

Therapeutic Approaches and Nursing Care

The only potential cure for SIADH is successful treatment of the underlying malignancy. In the meantime, stabilization of the patient and correction of the hyponatremia is essential. The severity of the hyponatremia and water intoxication determine the treatment of SIADH. Fluid restriction to 800–1000 mL/day is the initial treatment of choice for mild hyponatremia (serum sodium between 125–134 mEq/L), and may be the only therapy necessary. Fluid restriction allows the plasma osmolality, and the sodium level, to gradually increase through eventual loss of free water.

Severe, symptomatic, acute hyponatremia (serum sodium concentration < 110–115 mEq/L) resulting from SIADH is an oncologic emergency requiring immediate attention. Hypertonic (3%) saline given intravenously at a rate of 0.1 mL/kg/minute over 24 hours should increase the serum sodium by 10 mmol/L per day.[7] Intravenous furosemide (1 mg/kg) is often used to expedite water loss. Such therapeutic endeavors are instituted only in carefully controlled situations, such as an intensive care setting. The patient must be monitored carefully and the serum sodium and electrolytes checked frequently, at least every 1–3 hours. Frequent neurologic assessments of the severely hyponatremic patient are essential. These

assessments should include an evaluation of mental status and level of conciousness. Restriction of oral fluids should also be instituted. The patient's fluid balance is monitored and the patient is weighed daily. The rate of correction of the serum sodium should be no faster than 0.5 mEq/L per hour, and the initial therapy discontinued once the patient becomes mildly hyponatremic (serum sodium 125–130 mEq/L) in an effort to avoid neurologic complications. Correcting the serum sodium too rapidly may cause brain damage from brain cell dehydration. It can also lead to an irreversible neurodegenerative disorder known as *central pontine myelinolysis* (CPM),[23] which results from osmotic injury to endothelial cells in the brain and a breakdown of the blood-brain barrier; primarily in the pons and thalamus. Severe edema develops causing demyelination of white matter that can be seen on computerized tomography (CT) or magnetic resonance imaging (MRI). Symptoms of CPM range from dysphagia to quadraparesis.[24]

Chronic mild to moderate hyponatremia may be managed with certain oral medications. Demeclocycline (600–1200 mg daily) is an antibiotic that is most frequently used to treat chronic SIADH. It stimulates diuresis by impairing the effect of AVP on the renal tubule. Demeclocycline allows a normal daily intake of water and other fluids. Superinfections, azotemia, and hematologic changes may occur. Some patients develop diabetes insipidus. The patient's renal function should be frequently monitored while taking demeclocycline. Acute renal failure has occurred in patients with liver cirrhosis who were being treated for SIADH with demeclocycline. Another drug occassionally used to treat SIADH is urea, which produces an osmotic diuresis and also allows normal fluid intake.[18]

A newer, more specific treatment for hyponatremia is the use of vasopressin (AVP) receptor antagonists. Currently, peptide and nonpeptide AVP antagonists are being evaluated for their use in the treatment of SIADH. These antagonists work by binding to the V_2 (vasopressin) receptors on the surface of renal cell collecting ducts, thereby blocking the effect of ectopic AVP. The difficulty in bringing peptide antagonists to the clinical setting is that they are not specific to V_2 receptors and with chronic use become less effective. They are only available in parenteral form. The nonpeptide AVP antagonists have proved more promising. They are specific to the V_2 receptors and can be given orally. These agents are currently in phase I trials.[25]

Outpatient oncology nurses, especially those caring for newly diagnosed lung cancer patients, should maintain a high index of suspicion for the development of SIADH. Obtaining a complete patient history, conducting a careful nursing assessment, and reviewing serum chemistries assist with early diagnosis. Figure 43-2 describes clinical symptoms and phone triage for SIADH. Patients and their family members are instructed regarding the early symptoms of hyponatremia (nausea, weakness, muscle cramps, confusion, lethargy) and are encouraged to report these symptoms promptly. Communication be-

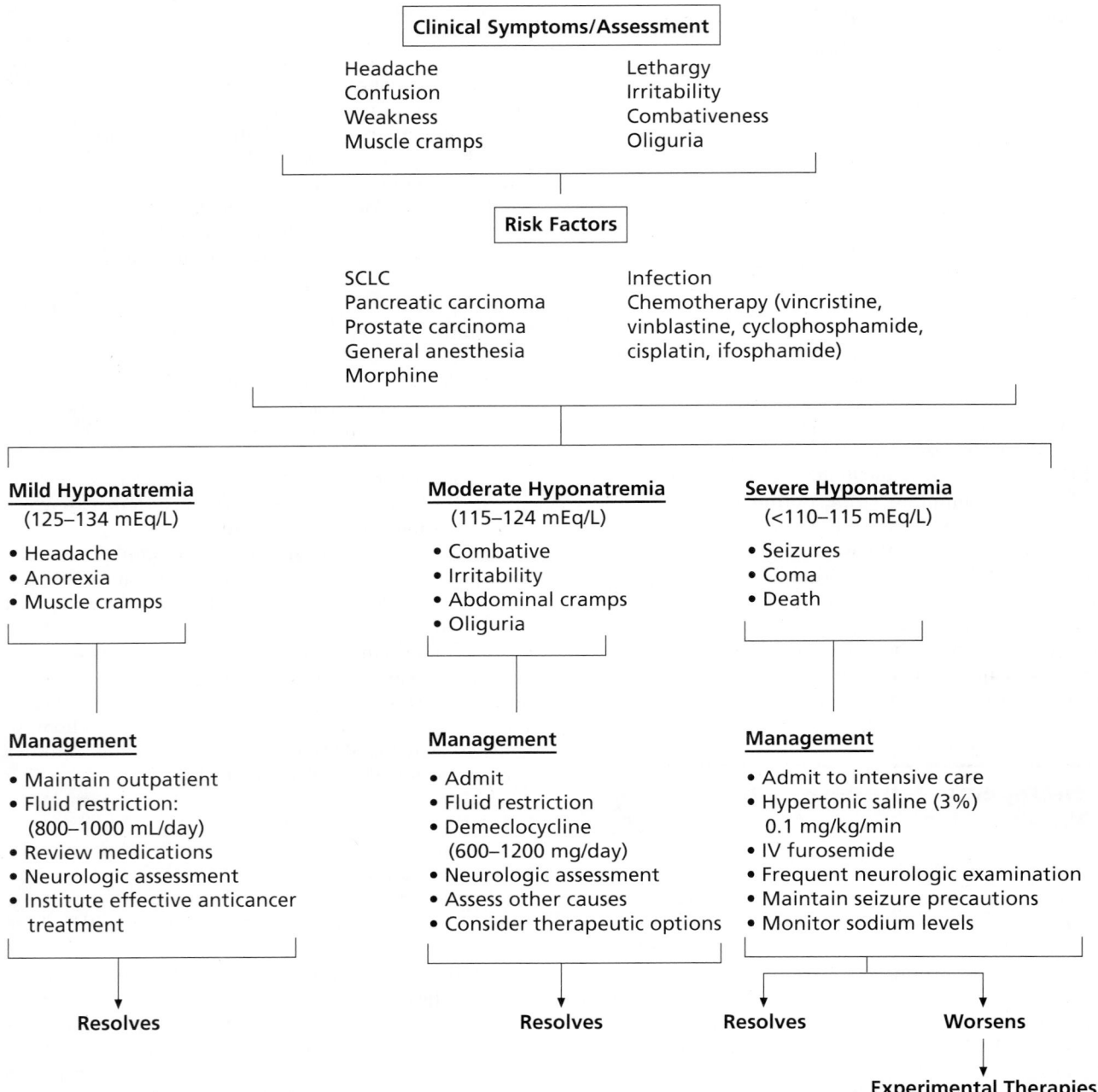

Figure 43-2 Phone triage: SIADH.

tween inpatient and outpatient nurses regarding the hospitalization course, current medications, and status at discharge is essential.

for oncology patients, especially the small cell lung cancer population, must have a high index of suspicion for the presence of SIADH. Early intervention can prevent serious complications resulting from hyponatremia.

Conclusion

SIADH is a paraneoplastic syndrome primarily associated with SCLC that most frequently follows a chronic course but can present as an oncologic emergency. Nurses caring

References

1. Schwartz WB, Bennett W, Curelop S, et al: A syndrome of renal sodium loss and hyponatremia probably resulting

from inappropriate secretion of antidiuretic hormone. *Am J Med* 23:529–534, 1957

2. Amatruda TT, Mulrow PJ, Gallagher JC, et al: Carcinoma of the lung with inappropriate antidiuresis. Demonstration of an antidiuretic-hormone-like activity in tumor extract. *N Engl J Med* 269:544–550, 1963

3. Moses AM, Scheinman SJ: Ectopic secretion of neurohypophyseal peptides in patients with malignancy. *Endocrinol Metab Clin North Am* 20:489–506, 1991

4. Shimizu K, Nakano S, Nakano Y, et al: Ectopic atrial natriuretic peptide production in small cell lung cancer with the syndrome of inappropriate antidiuretic hormone secretion. *Cancer* 68:2284–2288, 1991

5. Eckhardt SJ: Paraneoplastic syndromes. *Cancer Surv* 21:197–209, 1994

6. John WJ, Foon KA, Patchell RA: Paraneoplastic syndromes, in DeVita VT, Hellman S, Rosenberg SA (eds): *Cancer: Principles & Practice of Oncology* (ed 5). Philadelphia, Lippincott-Raven, 1997, pp 2397–2422

7. Block JB: Paraneoplastic syndromes, in Haskell CM, Berek JS (eds): *Cancer Treatment.* Philadelphia, Saunders, 1995, pp 245–264

8. Marchioli CC, Graziano SL: Paraneoplastic syndromes associated with small cell lung cancer. *Chest Surg Clin North Am* 7:65–80, 1997

9. Gross AJ, Steinberg SM, Reilly JG, et al: Atrial natriuretic factor and arginine vasopressin production in tumor cell lines from patients with lung cancer and their relationship to serum sodium. *Cancer Res* 53:67–74, 1993

10. Moses AM, Streeten DH: Disorders of the neurohypophysis, in Fauci AS, Braunwald E, Isselbacher KJ, et al (eds): *Harrison's Principles of Internal Medicine* (ed 14): 1997, pp 2003–2012

11. Mesko TW, Garcia O, Yee LD, et al: The syndrome of inappropriate secretion of antidiuretic hormone (SIADH) as a consequence of neck dissection. *J Laryngol Otol* 111:449–453, 1997

12. Ferlito A, Rinaldo A, DeVaney K: Sydrome of inappropriate antidiuretic hormone secretion associated with head and neck cancers: review of the literature. *Ann Otol Rhinol Laryngol* 106:878–883, 1997

13. Taskin M, Barker B, Calanog A, et al: Syndrome of inappropriate antidiuresis in ovarian serous carcinoma with neuroendocrine differentiation. *Gynecol Oncol* 62:400–404, 1996

14. Argani P, Erlandson RA, Rosai J: Thymic neuroblastoma in adults—report of three cases with special emphasis on its association with the syndrome of inappropriate secretion of antidiuretic hormone. *Anat Pathol* 108:537–543, 1997

15. Successful treatment of syndrome of inappropriate antidiuretic secretion (SIADH) in 2 patients with CNS involvement of chronic lymphocytic leukaemia. *Eur J Haematol* 58:207–208, 1997 (letter to the editor)

16. Lam SK, Cheung LP: Inappropriate ADH secretion due to immature ovarian teratoma. *Aust NZ J Obstet Gynaecol* 36:104–105, 1996

17. Ishibashi-Ueda H, Imakita M, Yutani C, et al: Small cell carcinoma of the uterine cervix with syndrome of inappropriate antidiuretic hormone secretion. *Mod Pathol* 9:397–400, 1996

18. Bunn PA, Ridgway EC: Paraneoplastic syndromes, in DeVita VT, Hellman S, Rosenberg SA (eds): *Cancer: Principles and Practice of Oncology* (ed 3). Philadelphia: Lippincott, 1996, pp 1896–1940

19. Gasparini M, Broderick GA, Narayan P: The syndrome of inappropriate antidiuretic hormone secretion on a patient with adenocarcinoma of the prostate. *J Urol* 150:978–980, 1993

20. Resnik E, Bender D: Syndrome of inappropriate antidiuretic hormone secretion in papillary serous surface carcinoma of the peritoneum. *J Surg Oncol* 61:63–65, 1996

21. Valtin H, Schafer JA: *Renal Function* (ed 3). Boston, Little, Brown, 1995

22. Hawthorne Maxson JL: Syndrome of inappropriate antidiuretic hormone secretion, in Chernecky C, Berger BJ (eds): *Advanced and Critical Care Oncology Nursing: Managing primary complications.* Philadelphia, W.B. Saunders, 1998, pp 622–636

23. Gross P, Reimann D, Neidel J, et al: The treatment of severe hyponatremia. *Kidney Int* 53:S-6–S-11, 1998 (suppl 64)

24. Norenberg MD, Leslie KO, Robertson AS: Association between rise in serum sodium and central pontine myelinolysis. *Ann Neurol* 11:128–135, 1982

25. Ishikawa S, Toshikazu S: Vasopressin receptor antagonists Therapeutic efficacy of vasopressin receptor antagonists. *Intern Med* 37(2):217–219, 1998

CHAPTER 44

Tumor Lysis Syndrome

Jean Lydon, RN, MS, AOCN

Scope of the Problem

Tumor lysis syndrome (TLS) is a metabolic complication of effective cancer therapy that occurs when large numbers of tumor cells are destroyed rapidly. Tumor cell destruction causes high levels of intracellular components—primarily potassium, phosphorus, and uric acid—to be released into the bloodstream. Metabolic abnormalities associated with TLS include hyperuricemia, hyperkalemia, hyperphosphatemia, and hypocalcemia. This syndrome can lead to life-threatening complications including cardiac arrhythmias, renal failure, and acute respiratory distress syndrome. Although the most frequent cause of TLS is the administration of systemic chemotherapy, any form of cancer therapy that causes rapid cell lysis and necrosis of a tumor mass can induce this syndrome.

The true incidence of TLS is not known. There have been several case reports of this syndrome, but very few studies done to determine its incidence in children and adults. The National Cancer Institute (NCI) conducted the initial review of the frequency of TLS in 37 patients with Burkitt's lymphoma. In this series, azotemia—defined as serum creatinine ≥ 1.6 mg/dL—occurred in 14 patients. In these azotemic patients, the incidence of posttreatment abnormalities were as follows: hyperuricemia in 21%, hyperphosphatemia in 100%, hypocalcemia in 100%, and hyperkalemia in 21%.[1] In two retrospective studies, laboratory evidence of metabolic changes associated with TLS occurred frequently (42%–70%), whereas life-threatening clinical TLS requiring specific additional interventions was infrequent (3%–6%).[2,3]

TLS occurs more frequently in patients with aggressive hematologic malignancies than in those with solid tumors. Hematologic malignancies commonly associated with TLS include Burkitt's lymphoma, acute lymphoblastic lymphoma, diffuse histiocytic lymphoma, acute lymphocytic leukemia, acute myelogenous leukemia, and chronic myelogenous leukemia in blast crisis.[2,4–6] The incidence of TLS in patients with more indolent hematologic malignancies such as chronic lymphocytic leukemia and prolymphocytic leukemia has increased in recent years, presumably due to more effective and intensive treatments and the use of new chemotherapeutic agents.[7] Although rare in patients with solid tumors, TLS has been reported in a variety of solid tumors including metastatic seminoma,[8] small cell lung cancer,[9,10] metastatic breast carcinoma,[11] metastatic medulloblastoma,[12] hepatoblastoma,[13] and Merkel cell carcinoma.[14]

Etiology and Risk Factors

Analysis of tumor, patient, and treatment characteristics can help identify those patients most likely to develop TLS (see Figure 44-1). TLS can occur with any malignancy in which there is a large tumor burden, a high growth fraction, and/or effective therapy, usually chemotherapy.[6,9,15] Additional risk factors for the development of TLS that are commonly seen in patients with large, bulky tumors include extensive lymph node involvement, enlarged spleen, multiple metastases, elevated levels of lactic dehydrogenase (LDH), white blood cell (WBC), and uric acid levels. Studies with ionizing radiation in both murine cell models and human malignancies utilizing flow cytometric techniques support the findings that TLS occurs more frequently in malignancies involving B cells and activated T cells.[16] Patients with pretreatment renal impairment as a result of dehydration, metabolic disturbances, or obstruction are at greater risk for TLS because they are less able to clear cellular breakdown products.[2,17] Lastly, patients with preexisting metabolic disturbances are at increased risk for TLS. Significant hyperphosphatemia, hyperuricemia, and/or hyperkalemia may exist prior to initiating cytotoxic therapy. For example, the lymphoblasts of leukemia patients contain four times more phosphate than do normal mature lymphoblasts. Thus, in patients with high levels of lymphoblasts, phosphate metabolism is increased, causing significant hyperphosphatemia before initiating treatment. Serum uric acid and uric acid excretion can be affected by the degree of elevation in the WBC count; the degree of enlargement of lymph nodes, spleen, and liver; dehydration; baseline renal insufficiency; acidic urine; and decreased urinary flow rate 24 hours prior to treatment.[8] In the patient with cancer, hyperkalemia may be present before initiating cytoxic therapy due to renal insufficiency, dehydration, adrenal insufficiency, acidosis, and/or medications. In summary, the addition of cytotoxic therapy in the patient with pretreatment hyperphosphatemia, hyperuricemia, and/or hyperkalemia increases the risk of TLS.[1,2,4,7,8]

Physiologic Alterations

The kidneys regulate fluid and electrolyte balance by filtering essential substances from the blood—selectively reabsorbing needed fluid and electrolytes and excreting those not needed into the urine. Normally, small and controlled amounts of potassium, phosphorus, and uric acid are present in the blood. In the intracellular fluid, potassium is the major cation and phosphorus is the major anion. When cells are destroyed, the DNA in the nucleus of the cell is released into the blood and the purines are converted in the liver to uric acid. Uric acid production requires cell catabolism but relies on the kidney for excretion. At normal rates of production and excretion, excesses of potassium, phosphorus, and uric acid do not occur.[18,19] When massive amounts of cells are destroyed, however, these substances are released into the blood, causing abnormally high levels of these minerals. There is an inverse relationship between phosphorus and calcium, whereby if one mineral increases, the other decreases in the same proportion. Thus when tumor cells lyse, which results in the release of large amounts of

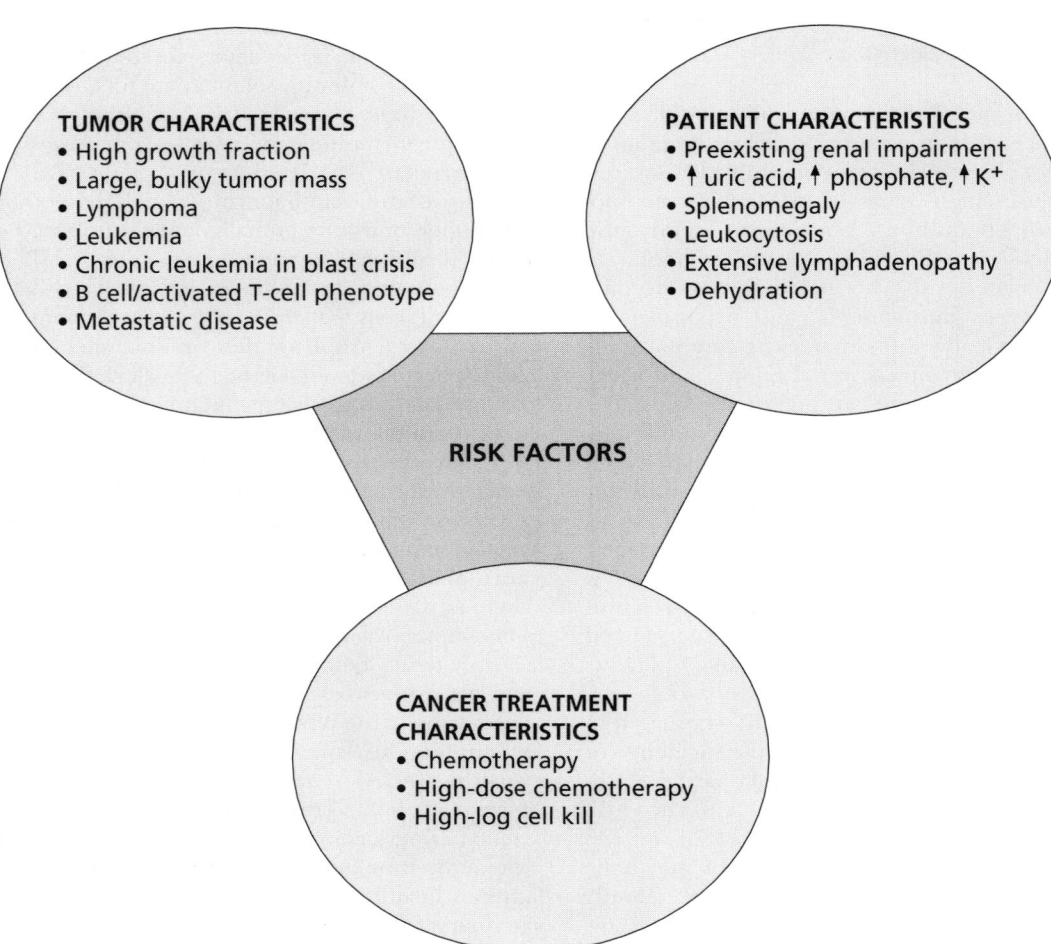

Figure 44-1 Risk factors for TLS comprise tumor, patient, and cancer treatment characteristics.

phosphorus into the blood, there is a proportional decrease in serum calcium resulting in hypocalcemia.[7,9]

Patients with massive tumor burdens have rapidly dividing cells that may be more sensitive to chemotherapeutic agents that are cytotoxic to dividing cells. Effective cancer therapy—usually chemotherapy—can initiate TLS by causing the cell membrane to rupture, releasing intracellular contents into the extracellular fluids and subsequently into the bloodstream. Tumor lysis syndrome usually occurs 6–72 hours following chemotherapy and lasts 5–7 days. It is during this posttherapy time that increased tumor cytolysis occurs.[1,20,21] Pathophysiologically, these events can lead to acute renal failure and cardiac conduction abnormalities.

The acute renal failure secondary to TLS is primarily due to hyperuricemia and hyperphosphatemia. Uric acid nephropathy is a complication that can occur secondary to hyperuricemia whereby uric acid crystals form in the collective ducts of the kidneys and ureters. These crystallizations lead to obstructive uropathy resulting in decreased glomerular filtration, increased hydrostatic pressure, obstructed urine flow, and eventually acute renal failure. Similarly, calcium phosphate salts secondary to hyperphosphatemia may precipitate in the renal tubules and cause renal failure. Although the kidneys normally can accommodate moderate elevations in uric acid and phosphorus by increasing excretion, continued tumor lysis overwhelms the body's homeostatic mechanisms, ultimately resulting in acute renal failure. Renal insufficiency in turn exacerbates the existing hyperkalemia and hypocalcemia.[18,19,22]

The cardiac conduction abnormalities related to TLS are due to hyperkalemia. Ninety-eight percent of the body's potassium (K+) is in the intracellular compartment. When cell lysis occurs, potassium is released from the intracellular compartment to the extracellular compartment and serum potassium levels increase. Hyperkalemia has a major depressant affect on cardiac function resulting in bradycardia, heart block, and cardiac standstill. Electrocardiogram changes reveal widening of the QRS complex, tall T waves, and flat or absent P waves. At serum concentrations of greater than 9 mEq K, conduction is so delayed that the heart becomes flaccid and if not recognized and treated immediately, cardiac arrest will result.[4,18,19,23]

Clinical Manifestations

The four major clinical manifestations of TLS are hyperuricemia, hyperkalemia, hyperphosphatemia, and hypocalcemia. These manifestations may occur individually, together, or in combination. The severity of these metabolic alterations is related to tumor burden and renal dysfunction, which determine the signs and symptoms observed in TLS.

The early manifestations of TLS include fatigue/lethargy, nausea, vomiting, anorexia, diarrhea, cloudiness of urine, flank pain, muscle weakness, and cramps. These initial symptoms can be vague, mild complaints easily attributed to a side effect of treatment. As the potassium level increases, elevations in blood pressure and heart rate may occur. A patient in the early phase of TLS may exhibit minimal renal symptoms. As the metabolic abnormalities increase, however, the patient will become more symptomatic and exhibit further TLS-related symptoms. Gastrointestinal symptoms will increase in severity and the patient may experience severe abdominal cramping and pain. Neuromuscular symptoms will also increase from mild paresthesias and muscle irritability to tetany and convulsions. Specific electrocardiogram changes are evident in the early and late phases of TLS. Prolongation of the QT interval and ST segment, and lowering and inversion of the T wave are early electrocardiogram (ECG) changes associated with TLS. Late TLS-associated ECG changes include tall T waves, shortened QT interval, widened QRS, loss of P wave, and sine wave. Initially the patient may exhibit an increase in blood pressure and heart rate, but as these metabolic disturbances continue, a decrease in blood pressure and heart rate occurs. Persistent hypocalcemia and hyperkalemia result in neurologic changes including memory loss, delirium, and hallucinations. Severe azotemia, which generally presents as increased serum urea and creatinine levels, and anuria due to progressive renal impairment are seen in the later phases of TLS. If TLS is unrecognized, untreated, or continues despite treatment, complete anuria, cardiac arrest, and death may occur.[4,7,22–24] In summary, the physical consequences of TLS affect all body organs and frequently result in severe systemic effects. Figure 44-2 provides an overview of early and late signs and symptoms of TLS by body systems.

Assessment and Grading

Knowledge of TLS as a potential complication of cytotoxic therapy in patients with rapidly proliferating tumors is essential. The diagnosis of TLS is primarily based on laboratory and clinical findings of four metabolic abnormalities: hyperuricemia, hyperkalemia, hyperphosphatemia, and hypocalcemia. An accurate assessment of the patient prior to initiating cytotoxic therapy is necessary to rule out pretreatment TLS and to establish baseline laboratory and clinical data. Initially, a complete history and physical is performed and risk factors for TLS are identified. In taking the patient history, information regarding weight, nutritional and hydration status, past and current medications, and history of chronic health problems or organ dysfunction is obtained. Assessment of risk factors is necessary for the prevention and management of TLS but can also assist the physician to determine the best setting for initiating cytotoxic therapy. Patients at high risk of developing TLS (e.g., high-grade lymphoma, acute leukemia, preexisting renal impairment, elevated LDH pretreatment) may require hospitalization for their treatment, whereas those patients at low risk (e.g., solid tumor, low-grade lymphoma, adequate renal function, normal pretreatment LDH) can be treated as an outpatient. Specific laboratory parameters evaluated prior to, during, and after treatment include serum potassium, phosphorus, calcium, uric acid, blood urea nitrogen (BUN), creatinine, LDH, complete blood count (CBC), and platelet count, and urinary pH and sediment. Assessment of the physical signs and symptoms of TLS related to gastrointestinal, neuromuscular, neurologic, cardiovascular, and renal function is critical to TLS management (see Figure 44-2). Renal function is closely monitored by analyzing serum electrolytes, BUN, and creatinine and urinary pH and sediment every 4–6 hours or more frequently if necessary. Cardiac function is evaluated by frequent vital signs, ECG, and if necessary a chest x-ray and multigated acquisition heart scan (MUGA) to assess for fluid overload and the heart's left ventricular ejection fraction (LVEF).

TLS has been broadly defined as the metabolic abnormalities that occur after rapid tumor cell destruction. However, a specific grading scale or guideline related to the degree or type of metabolic abnormality required to qualify for TLS is lacking. In reviewing the literature, two grading scales have been used to study patients with TLS. Razis and associates developed a grading scale for the evaluation of 41 patients with acute leukemia at high risk for TLS, which was divided into three grades (grade I, II, III) based on severity of metabolic parameters.[5] In Hande and Garrow's[2] retrospective analysis of 102 patients receiving chemotherapy for intermediate to high-grade non-Hodgkin's lymphoma, TLS was divided into either "laboratory tumor lysis syndrome" (LTLS) or "clinical tumor lysis syndrome" (CTLS). LTLS was defined as any two of the following metabolic changes occurring within four days of treatment: a 25% increase in serum phosphate, potassium, uric acid, or urea nitrogen concentrations or a 25% decline in the serum calcium concentration. CTLS was defined as LTLS plus one of the following: a serum potassium greater than 6 mEq/L, a creatinine level greater than 2.5 mg/dL, a calcium level less than 6 mg/dL, the development of a life-threatening arrhythmia, or sudden death.[2] Development of a

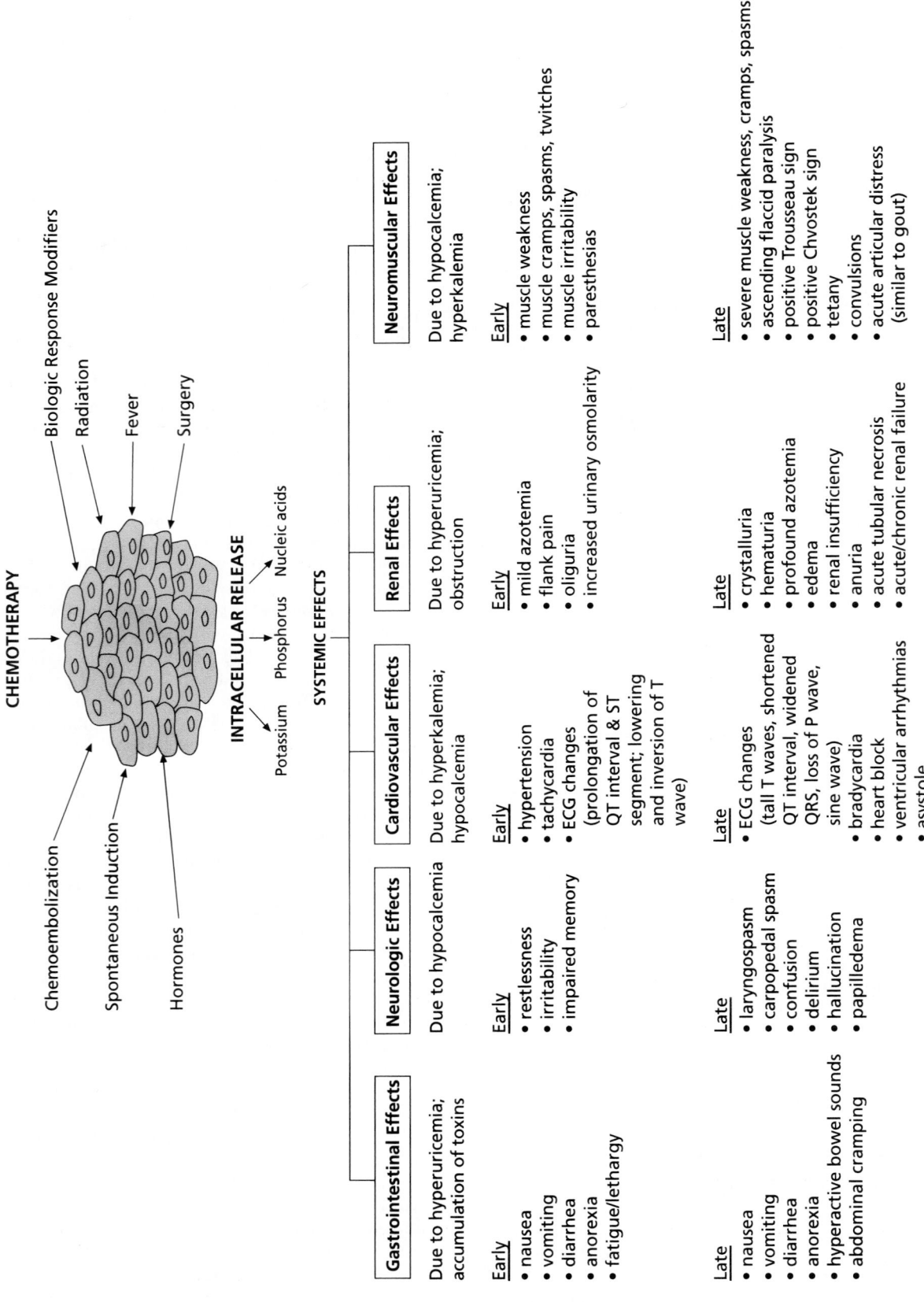

Figure 44-2 TLS results in multiple systemic effects occurring early and late in the disease and treatment.

standardized grading scale for TLS would increase our knowledge of the incidence, tumor types, risk factors, and morbidity and mortality rates associated with this syndrome. Furthermore, specific prevention and treatment programs based on the grade of TLS could be developed and evaluated.

Therapeutic Approaches

The primary goal of TLS management is prevention. Recognition of patients at risk for this syndrome allows preventive measures to be instituted prior to treatment, thereby decreasing the risk of severe electrolyte imbalances. The four key elements of TLS prevention and intervention are (1) aggressive hydration and diuresis, (2) allopurinol, (3) urinary alkalinization, and (4) early identification and correction of electrolyte imbalances.[1,17]

The most important mechanism for preventing uric acid nephropathy and acute renal failure is by aggressively hydrating a patient with at least 3 liters/m[2]/per day, and ensuring an adequate urinary output of 100–200 cc/hour. Diuretics (loop or osmotic) are often used to maintain this urinary flow rate and to prevent renal tubular damage. The use of diuretics is particularly important for elderly patients and those at risk for fluid overload. These measures improve glomerular filtration; enhance excretion of potassium, phosphate, and uric acid; and inhibit calcium reabsorption. It is important that aggressive hydration, with or without diuretics, begin 24–48 hours prior to treatment and continue for several days posttreatment.[1,4,6,17]

Allopurinol is the second key element of TLS prevention and intervention. Allopurinol inhibits the enzyme xanthine oxidase and prevents the formation of uric acid, which in turn prevents uric acid nephropathy. The standard dose of allopurinol is 300 mg per day given for several days before, during, and after cytotoxic therapy. However, for high-risk patients with normal renal function, a loading dose of 500 mg/m[2] followed by a daily dose of 200 mg/m[2] has been recommended.[1] The use of allopurinol must be closely monitored because of possible side effects such as fever, rash, eosinophilia, exfoliative dermatitis, and the infrequent occurrence of xanthine crystal nephropathy. Furthermore, it may be necessary to reduce the standard dose of allopurinol based on the creatinine clearance rate in patients with renal impairment. Allopurinol should be reduced or discontinued once hyperuricemia is controlled.[1,17]

The third key element of TLS prevention and intervention, alkalinization of the urine, is controversial. Urinary alkalinization increases the solubility of uric acid. Overly rigorous alkalinization can cause severe complications, however, most notably calcium phosphate precipitation in the renal tubules. This in turn can further decrease the calcium level and increase the symptoms of hypocalcemia. Therefore, urinary alkalinization measures to prevent renal complications secondary to TLS must be

individualized and used cautiously. Alkalinization of the urine can be achieved by adding 50–100 mEq of sodium bicarbonate to each liter of intravenous (IV) hydration and/or administering acetazolamide 250–500 mg IV daily.[25]

The last key element of TLS prevention and intervention is the early identification and treatment of life-threatening electrolyte imbalances. Early identification of TLS requires frequent laboratory assessment of electrolytes and renal function, as well as careful assessment of the signs and symptoms associated with each metabolic abnormality. Accurate phone triage is critical to the management of TLS on an outpatient basis (see Figure 44-3). Prompt recognition and treatment of these metabolic abnormalities often reduces the need for hospitalization by preventing the development of clinical TLS. However, if TLS metabolic abnormalities and/or clinical symptoms persist for 48–72 hours despite aggressive preventive and treatment measures, hospitalization is necessary.

Laboratory values and the patient's clinical condition can change dramatically over a few hours, necessitating more intensive monitoring and treatment. The patient would be admitted to the intensive care unit if the laboratory and/or clinical signs and symptoms of TLS continue to worsen despite preventive and treatment measures, or if the patient develops renal, respiratory, or cardiac failure. These patients often require aggressive hemodynamic monitoring and mechanical ventilation. Dialysis may be necessary if vigorous conservative measures are unsuccessful at normalizing electrolytes or establishing urinary flow.

Suggested criteria for dialysis therapy in TLS include patients who have the following serum blood levels: (1) potassium > 6 mEq/L, (2) phosphorus > 10 mg/dL, (3) uric acid > 10 mg/dL, or (4) creatinine > 10 mg/dL. Dialysis is also recommended for patients with fluid volume overload, renal insufficiency, symptomatic hypocalcemia, and for those patients unresponsive to other corrective treatment measures.[26] Hemodialysis, peritoneal dialysis (PD), and continuous hemofiltrations have been used in the treatment of both children and adults with TLS. Unfortunately, data comparing the various modalities are sparse and each type has specific advantages and disadvantages. Dialysis has been particularly successful in treating obstructive nephropathy, acute renal failure, and accompanying metabolic abnormalities associated with TLS.[27,28] While dialysis has generally been used in patients who have failed conventional management, Saccente and associates[29] studied the prospective use of continous veno-venous hemofiltration (CVVH) in high-risk patients. Similar to continuous arteriovenous hemofiltration (CAVH) that allows for the slow adjustment of fluid and solutes, CVVH eliminates the need for arterial access by adding a blood pump that provides the filtration pressure for the system. Saccente and colleagues concluded that the use of CVVH at the time of the chemotherapy treatment could potentially decrease the morbidity and mortality associated with induction chemotherapy in high-risk patients. The small sample size in this study

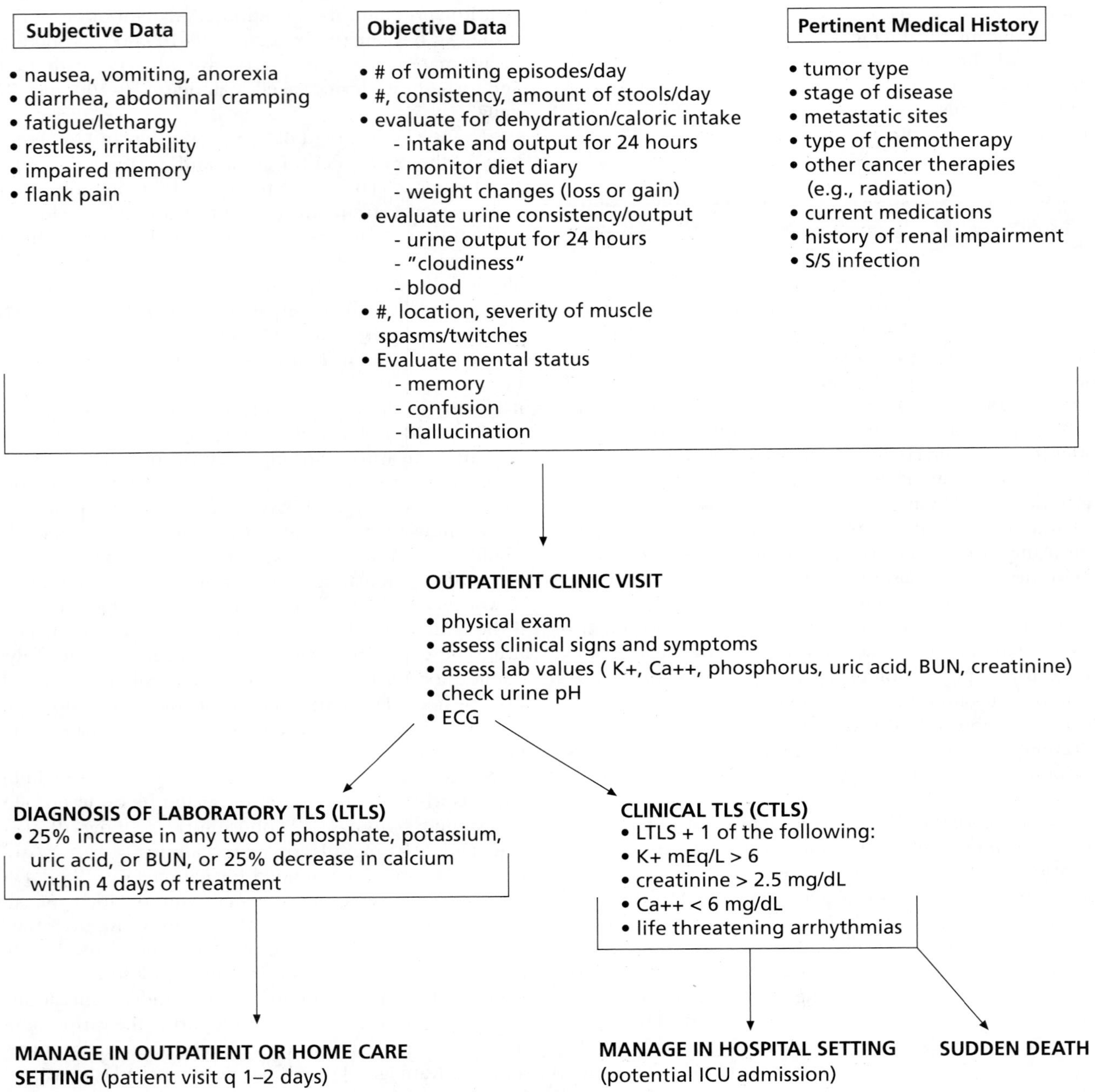

Subjective Data	Objective Data	Pertinent Medical History

• nausea, vomiting, anorexia
• diarrhea, abdominal cramping
• fatigue/lethargy
• restless, irritability
• impaired memory
• flank pain
	• # of vomiting episodes/day
	• #, consistency, amount of stools/day
	• evaluate for dehydration/caloric intake
	  - intake and output for 24 hours
	  - monitor diet diary
	  - weight changes (loss or gain)
	• evaluate urine consistency/output
	  - urine output for 24 hours
	  - "cloudiness"
	  - blood
	• #, location, severity of muscle
	  spasms/twitches
	• Evaluate mental status
	  - memory
	  - confusion
	  - hallucination
		• tumor type
		• stage of disease
		• metastatic sites
		• type of chemotherapy
		• other cancer therapies
		  (e.g., radiation)
		• current medications
		• history of renal impairment
		• S/S infection

OUTPATIENT CLINIC VISIT

• physical exam
• assess clinical signs and symptoms
• assess lab values (K+, Ca++, phosphorus, uric acid, BUN, creatinine)
• check urine pH
• ECG

DIAGNOSIS OF LABORATORY TLS (LTLS)
• 25% increase in any two of phosphate, potassium, uric acid, or BUN, or 25% decrease in calcium within 4 days of treatment

CLINICAL TLS (CTLS)
• LTLS + 1 of the following:
• K+ mEq/L > 6
• creatinine > 2.5 mg/dL
• Ca++ < 6 mg/dL
• life threatening arrhythmias

MANAGE IN OUTPATIENT OR HOME CARE SETTING (patient visit q 1–2 days)

MANAGE IN HOSPITAL SETTING (potential ICU admission)

SUDDEN DEATH

Figure 44-3 Phone triage assessment of TLS and patient disposition (S/S = signs and symptoms, ICU = intensive care unit)

prohibits generalization, but the results support further investigation of this technique in a larger number of patients.[29] Management and potential outcomes of TLS are presented in Figure 44-4.

Precise morbidity and mortality rates for patients who develop TLS are not known. In the TLS literature, some authors report resolution of TLS with treatment, while others report death despite appropriate treatment.[14,23] A classic study by Cohen and associates reported death in 6 of 37 patients with Burkitt's lymphoma, with only one death attributed to a TLS complication.[1] In the Hande and Garrow study of 102 patients with non-Hodgkin's lymphoma receiving chemotherapy, 42% of patients had LTLS and only 6% had CTLS. No deaths were reported in this study.[2] Retrospective and prospective studies, rather than case reports, are needed to define morbidity and mortality associated with TLS. It seems likely, however, that the occurrence and resolution of TLS depend not only on specific risk factors but on the early identification and initiation of preventive measures.

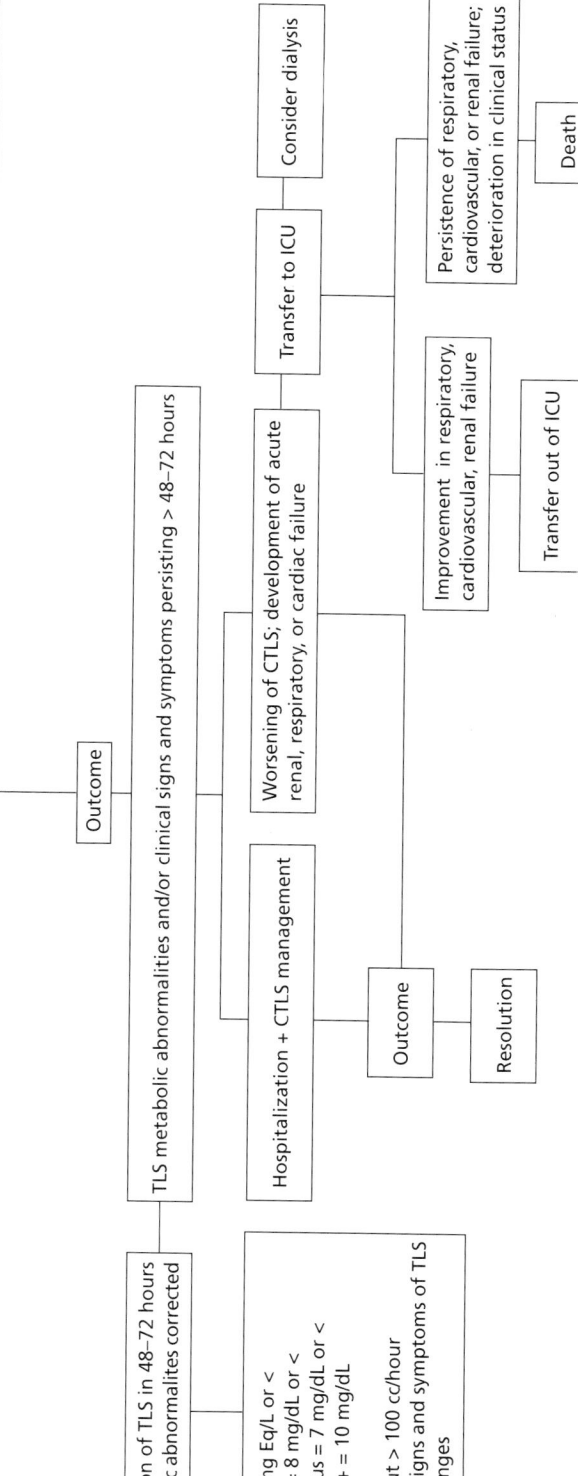

Management of Hyperuricemia

- increase or continue allopurinol until uric acid normal
- IV hydration > 3L/m²/day
- maintain urinary alkalinization (pH > 7) until uric acid normal
- administer acetazolamide 250–500 mg IV/day if volume load a problem or hyperuricemia refractory to above measures; initiate low-dose dopamine for oliguria or preexisting fluid retention

Management of Hypocalcemia

- monitor ECG
- institute seizure precautions
- administer 1–3 amps of 10% calcium gluconate IV over 3–5 minutes with ECG monitoring for severe changes
- administration of CA++ supplements is controversial

General Principles—Management

- withhold further antitumor therapy until TLS resolves
- assess clinical signs and symptoms
- monitor electrolytes and renal function q 6–12 hours for LTLS & q 4 hours for CTLS
- ensure hydration of > 3L/m²/day
- allopurinol (100–300 mg/m²/day)
- alkalinize urine (pH > 7)
- administer sodium bicarbonate (50 mEq/L) if pH < 7
- monitor urine pH 3–4 times/day for LTLS and q 4 hours for CTLS
- administer nonthiazide diuretic if u/o < 100 cc/hour
- monitor I & O
- weigh daily
- monitor ECG
- monitor arterial blood gas
- specific dietary restrictions

Management of Hyperkalemia

- assess clinical signs and symptoms
- monitor ECG
- administer kayexalate resin 15–30 g orally or rectally for K+ < 7 and no ECG change
- administer 1–3 amps of 10% calcium gluconate IVP over 3–5 minutes with ECG monitoring for K+ > 7 and ECG changes
- administer Na bicarbonate 50–150 mEq/L
- administer D10W with 10–15 units of regular insulin over 1 hour in patient who is oliguric
- restrict dietary K+

Management of Hyperphosphatemia

- administer phosphate binding antacids (amphogel 30 cc TID or neutraphos 2 tabs PO TID)
- eliminate other sources of phosphorus (diet, medications)
- administer hypertonic glucose & insulin infusion
- monitor calcium

Figure 44-4   Principles of management of TLS. (IVP = intravenous push, u/o = urinary output, F/O = intake and output)

Nursing Care

When caring for a patient at risk for TLS, the goal of nursing care is prevention and minimization of the syndrome. Prevention, early identification, and intervention of TLS require knowledge of risk factors, laboratory and clinical signs and symptoms of each metabolic abnormality, and treatment measures. Whether TLS is a potential problem for an individual or has already occurred, two major nursing responsibilities are education and assessment. Education of the patient and family of the risk factors, clinical manifestations, possible treatment measures, and of when to seek medical help is key to prevention of TLS. All patients at risk for TLS should receive both verbal and written information regarding the syndrome. Figure 44-5 provides a teaching tool for patients at risk for TLS. The importance of patient and family teaching regarding the complications of cancer therapy has become increasingly clear as the majority of cancer therapies are given on an outpatient basis and the complexities of cancer therapies has increased.

Another major responsibility of the nurse is the accurate and continual assessment of the patient before, during, and after cancer therapy. Baseline and ongoing assessment of laboratory parameters and clinical manifes-

PROBLEM: Tumor Lysis Syndrome (TLS) is a rare problem that can occur when tumor cells are "killed." As tumor cells break down, you can have problems getting these cells out of the body. Three problems can occur if TLS is not treated: 1) the kidneys will have trouble getting rid of water and waste products from your body; 2) the muscles and nerves in your body can become more excited and not work as well; 3) the heart can become weak and/or stop working. However, by learning about TLS and following your doctor or nurse's orders, you can prevent or lessen the symptoms of TLS.

SIGNS/SYMPTOMS: Tell your doctor or nurse if you have any of these symptoms:

- nausea, vomiting, diarrhea, loss of appetite
- very tired
- muscle cramps, weakness, spasms, or twitches
- pain in your side
- "cloudy " urine or blood in the urine

- swelling or weight gain
- numbess or tingling in your hands or feet
- shortness of breath or trouble with breathing
- swelling or pain in your joints

WAYS TO PREVENT TLS

- increase fluids – drink _____ per day
- take medicine (Allopurinol)

- check blood counts
- check weight every day

WAYS TO TREAT TLS

- stop cancer treatment for a short time
- check blood counts often
- IV fluids

- take medicines (Allopurinol, "water pills")
- keep track of fluid intake and urine output
- special diet

WHERE TO TREAT TLS: Treatment of "mild" TLS can be done in the office, clinic, or by having a home health nurse visit. Treatment of "severe" TLS is done in the hospital.

SCHEDULE:

MEDICINE(S): _____

_____

_____

BLOOD DRAW(S): _____

_____

_____

SPECIAL INSTRUCTIONS: _____

_____

_____

PHONE NUMBERS:

DOCTOR: _____   PHONE: _____

NURSE: _____   _____

OTHER: _____   _____

Figure 44-5 Tumor lysis syndrome patient care guide.

tations will detect subtle changes, thereby preventing serious and life-threatening complications of TLS. A thorough physical assessment is conducted prior to, during, and after cancer therapy to determine the effect of the metabolic abnormalities on many organ systems. The nurse will utilize certain diagnostic tests such as Chvostek's sign, Trousseau's sign, deep tendon reflexes, and ECG to assist in monitoring the clinical status of a patient with potential or actual TLS.

The medical management of TLS requires active participation of nurses in various health care settings. They are responsible primarily for the day-to-day management of the patient. Specific responsibilities include drawing of blood; administration of chemotherapy, hydration, electrolytes, diuretics, and blood products; and documentation of pertinent findings and interventions in the medical record. Since patients with potential or actual TLS often traverse different health care settings in the treatment of their disease, the nurse must serve as the liaison or coordinator to ensure continuity of care. It is the oncology nurse's responsibility to communicate all patient-related findings to physicians and other health care providers. The oncology nurse's role in the provision of emotional support to the patient and family cannot be understated. It is often difficult for patients and families to understand how such a severe and life-threatening complication can occur when the treatment is working so well against the disease.

Conclusion

Tumor lysis syndrome is an oncologic emergency that in many cases can be predicted, allowing for timely preventive and supportive treatment measures. The syndrome is a set of metabolic disturbances resulting from rapid cellular destruction due to effective antineoplastic therapy. With advances in cancer therapy, particularly newer and more complex therapies, the incidence of TLS may increase. Therefore, heightened awareness and knowledge of this potentially fatal complication is essential for prevention and management. As more patients receive treatment on an outpatient basis, education of patients and families and careful follow-up care is required. Although our knowledge of TLS risk factors, prevention measures, and management strategies has increased, further research is needed to identify the true incidence and associated morbidity and mortality of this syndrome. Oncology nurses' early recognition of TLS and prompt intervention may prevent this serious complication.

References

1. Cohen LF, Balow JE, Magrath IT, et al: Acute tumor lysis syndrome: a review of 37 patients with Burkitt's lymphoma. *Am J Med* 68:486–491, 1980

2. Hande KR, Garrow GC: Acute tumor lysis syndrome in patients with high-grade non-Hodgkin's lymphoma. *Am J Med* 94:133–139, 1993

3. Kedar A, Grow W, Neiberger RE: Clinical versus laboratory tumor lysis syndrome in children with acute leukemia. *Pediatr Hematol Oncol* 12:129–134, 1995

4. Jones DP, Mahmoud H, Chesney RW: Tumor lysis syndrome: pathogenesis and management. *Pediatr Nephrol* 9:206–212, 1995

5. Razis E, Arlin ZA, Ahmed T, et al: Incidence and treatment of tumor lysis syndrome in patients with acute leukemia. *ACTA Haematol* 91:171–174, 1994

6. Fleming DR, Doukas MA: Acute tumor lysis syndrome in hematologic malignancies. *Leuk Lymphoma* 8:315–318, 1992

7. McCroskey RD, Mosher DF, Spencer CD, et al: Acute tumor lysis syndrome and treatment response, in patients treated for refractory chronic lymphocytic leukemia with short course, high dose cytosine arabinoside, cisplatinum and etoposide. *Cancer* 66:246–250, 1990

8. Barton JC: Tumor lysis syndrome in non-hematopoietic neoplasms. *Cancer* 64:738–740, 1989

9. Hussein AM, Feun LG: Tumor lysis syndrome after induction chemotherapy in small cell lung carcinoma. *Am J Clin Oncol* 13:10–13, 1990

10. Kalemkerian GP, Darwish B, Vaterasian ML: Tumor lysis syndrome in small cell carcinoma and other solid tumors. *Am J Med* 103:363–367, 1977

11. Skalarin NT, Markham M: Spontaneous recurrent tumor lysis syndrome in breast cancer. *Am J Clin Oncol* 18:71–73, 1995

12. Tomlinson GC, Solberg LA Jr: Acute tumor lysis syndrome with metastatic medulloblastoma. *Cancer* 53:1783–1785, 1984

13. Lobe TE, Karkera MS, Custer MD, et al: Fatal refractory hyperkalemia due to tumor lysis, during primary resection for hepatoblastoma. *J Pediatr Surg* 25:249–250, 1990

14. Dirix LY, Prove A, Becquart D, et al: Tumor lysis syndrome in a patient with metastatic Merkel cell carcinoma. *Cancer* 67:2207–2210, 1991

15. Nomdedeu J, Martino R, Sureda A, et al: Acute tumor lysis syndrome complicating conditioning therapy for bone marrow transplantation in patients with chronic lymphocytic leukemia. *Bone Marrow Transplant* 13:659–660, 1994

16. Fleming DR, Henslee-Downey PJ, Coffey CW: Radiation induced acute tumor lysis syndrome in the bone marrow transplantation. *Bone Marrow Transplant* 8:235–236, 1991

17. Chasty RC, Liu-Yin JA: Acute tumor lysis syndrome. *Br J Hosp Med* 49:488–492, 1993

18. Ganding WF: *Review of Medical Physiology* (ed 17). Norwalk, CT, Appleton & Lange, 1995

19. Bullock J, Boyle J, Wang MP: *Physiology* (ed 3). Philadelphia, Williams & Wilkins, 1995

20. O'Brien JF: The oncologic crisis part 7: septic, hematologic and metabolic emergencies. *Emerg Med* 28:24–38, 1996

21. Simmons ED, Somberg KA: Acute tumor lysis syndrome after intrathecal methotrexate administration. *Cancer* 67:2062–2065, 1991

22. Polcheldy C: Hyperuricemia in leukemia and lymphoma. *N Y State J Med* 73:1085–1092, 1973

23. Drakos P, Bar-Ziv J, Catane R: Tumor lysis syndrome in non hematologic malignancies: report of a case and review of the literature. *Am J Clin Oncol* 17:502–505, 1994

24. Rohaly-Davis J, Johnston K: Hematologic emergencies in the intensive care unit. *Crit Care Nurs Q* 18:35–43, 1996

25. Ten Harkel ADJ, Kis-vanHolthe JE, Vanweel M, et al: Alkalin-

ization and the tumor lysis syndrome. *Med Pediatr Oncol* 31: 27–28, 1998

26. Robison J: Tumor lysis syndrome, in Chernecky C, Berger B (eds), *Advanced and Critical Care Oncology Nursing.* Philadelphia, Saunders, 1998, pp 637–654

27. Bishof NA, Welch TR, Strife F, et al: Continuous hemodiafiltration in children. *Pediatrics* 85:819–823, 1990

28. Heney D, Essex-Cater A, Brocklebank JT, et al: Continuous arteriovenous haemofiltration in the treatment of tumour lysis syndrome. *Pediatr Nephrol* 4:245–247, 1990

29. Saccente SL, Kohart EC, Berkow RL: Prevention of tumor lysis syndrome using continuous veno-venous hemofiltration. *Pediatr Nephrol* 9:569–573, 1995

The Care of Individuals with Cancer

CHAPTER 45

AIDS-Related Malignancies

James C. Pace, DSN, RN, MDiv, ANP-CS

Introduction

An Overview of HIV Disease

The history of the acquired immunodeficiency syndrome (AIDS) pandemic in the United States began in 1981 when the first description of what would soon be referred to as AIDS appeared in the Centers for Disease Control's *Morbidity and Mortality Weekly Report* of June 5, 1981. This report described the occurrence of a rare type of pneumonia in five young men from Los Angeles. From that moment on, similar cases across the United States and Europe began to paint images of people who shared a clinical picture of severe immunosuppression. Over the next few years, the human immunodeficiency virus (HIV) was identified and named. Much has been learned in two decades.

HIV and AIDS are not synonymous terms. The term *AIDS* is used to indicate only the most severe clinical conditions and diseases observed in the continuum of HIV infection. The natural history of HIV infection spans a range of conditions from an initial symptom-free period of ten years or more (with CD4+ T-cell counts > 500/mm³) to clinically apparent disease states (CD4+ T-cell counts > 200/mm³ and < 500/mm³) with constitutional symptoms (to include candidiasis [oral and/or genital], cervical dysplasia, herpes zoster, pelvic inflammatory disease, and peripheral neuropathy), to conditions characterized by severe immunodeficiency (CD4+ T-cell counts < 200/mm³), serious opportunistic infections, and malignancies.[1] Once advanced HIV disease occurs with CD4+ T-cell counts < 50/mm³, death becomes likely within one year.[1] The last decade of the twentieth century has led to many breakthroughs in the prevention, treatment, and understanding of HIV disease and AIDS; however, the discovery of a cure is hindered because HIV is able to change its genetic make-up rapidly, allowing for multiple mutations of the virus that are resistant to current treatment approaches.[1]

Malignancies and HIV Disease

Malignancies have long been associated with both congenital and acquired immunodeficiency disorders. For example, patients undergoing organ transplantation with subsequent receipt of immunosuppressive drugs developed Kaposi's sarcoma approximately two years from the time of transplant 400–500 times more frequently than expected.[2] Non-Hodgkin's lymphoma (NHL) occurs at an average of three years from time of transplant, and is seen 25–50 times more frequently than expected, while anogenital cancers occur approximately eight years from transplantation, with a frequency of 100 times greater than expected.[2] In early 1981, the AIDS was initially recognized from the outbreak of Kaposi's sarcoma along with another opportunistic infection, *Pneumocystis carinii* pneumonia (PCP), among young, previously healthy homosexual men.[3–5] The model of transplant-related cancers is remarkably similar to the cancers that have been described in association with HIV: Kaposi's sarcoma became an AIDS-defining condition at the onset of the epidemic, while NHL and cervical cancer became AIDS-defining in 1985 and 1993, respectively.[2] The presence of an AIDS defining condition indicates that the HIV infection has reached a level where it meets the Centers for Disease Control (CDC) criteria for AIDS. Additional malignancies associated with HIV/AIDS include anal cancer, Hodgkin's disease, seminoma, melanoma, oropharyngeal cancer, and multiple myeloma. At this writing, more than 640,000 cases of AIDS have been documented in the United States.[4] The most recent estimate of HIV prevalence indicates that between 650,000 and 900,000 Americans are living with HIV.[6] Statistical models suggest that at least 40,000 persons in the United States are being infected each year and roughly the same number die each year of HIV-related illness.[7] Because the number of persons infected each year was roughly the same as the number who died each year, prevalence since 1992 has been stable. Recently, however, because of the use of highly active antiretroviral therapies (HAART), more persons with HIV are living longer, and the prevalence of AIDS increased from 1995 to 1996.[8] The implication is that this population is living longer in an advanced state of immunodeficiency that allows for the occurrence of some form of cancer. Of those persons now living with AIDS, it is postulated that approximately 40% will experience an AIDS-related malignancy. Ongoing research is required to determine if the incidence and variety of cancers will continue to increase, as HIV infected patients live longer due to effective treatment. To date, no cure or vaccine has been discovered for HIV infection, and predictions are that AIDS will continue long into the twenty-first century.

KAPOSI'S SARCOMA

In 1872 the Hungarian physician Moriz Kaposi first described this disease as "multiple idiopathic pigmented hemangiosarcoma."[9] He described the condition as localized, nodular, brown-red tumors that appeared first on the soles and then the hands. He recognized the disease as rare, affecting men over age 40. He was aware of the multifocal nature of the disease, the occurrence of visceral involvement, and the vascular nature of the tumor (*classic* Kaposi's sarcoma).[9] In the 1950s and 1960s, *endemic* Kaposi's sarcoma (KS), a more aggressive form of the disease that occurred in younger individuals, was described in central Africa. During the 1970s, KS was reported among a new group of patients receiving immunosuppressive therapy for renal transplantation and other medical conditions.[10,11] Individuals infected with HIV, especially homosexual or bisexual men, are currently the group with the highest incidence of an aggressive form of KS known as *epidemic* or *AIDS-associated* KS.[5,12] Thus, variations in pattern, clinical manifestation, and course of KS has contributed to the creation of four separate classifications of KS: (1) classic, or non-HIV related KS, usually in men of Mediterranean descent; (2) endemic KS occurring in men, women, and children in certain areas of Africa; (3) KS associated with iatrogenic immunosuppression, sometimes referred to as *renal transplant* KS; and (4) epidemic, or HIV-related KS which occurs primarily in men who have sex with men (MSM).[13] The most notable characteristics that distinguish HIV-related KS from the other three classifications of KS are its fulminate, widely disseminated course and shorter survival.[13] Histopathologically, all four variations of KS are essentially the same.[13]

Epidemiology

Prior to the AIDS epidemic, KS was considered to be a rare disease with an annual incidence in the United States of 0.021–0.061 per 100,000 population.[14] Since the AIDS pandemic, more than 24,000 cases of AIDS-associated KS have been reported to the CDC. Throughout the course of HIV infection, KS has been reported in approximately 40% of homosexual/bisexual men, 11% of heterosexual men, and 2% of women.[15] The reasons for this predisposition in homosexual men is uncertain, although it has been historically postulated that there exists a sexually transmitted cofactor which might be spread via receptive anal sex. Consistent with this idea is that HIV-infected women who are diagnosed with KS are most likely to have acquired HIV by heterosexual contact with a bisexual male.[16] The incidence of AIDS-associated Kaposi's sarcoma has steadily decreased since the mid 1980s. To date, AIDS-associated KS is seen in approximately 14% of all cases of AIDS reported to the CDC.[17] This downward trend has been attributed to a number of explanations, several of which are widely disputed in current literature. Among reasons given for the decreased incidence of KS are the decline in use of unlabeled amyl nitrate, an inhalant recreational drug and a possible mutagen,[18] and changes in sexual practices such as decreased anal lingus, anal intercourse, and anal fisting that may increase the chance for developing Kaposi's sarcoma.[19] Primarily, however, the decrease in KS is attributed to the use of highly active antiretroviral therapy used to decrease viral loads (HIV RNA quantitation), to increase CD4+ T-cell counts, to offset future infections with opportunistic infections, and to improve the patient's prognosis in terms of life span.

While the incidence of KS as an AIDS defining illness has declined in recent years, the disease is now more common in patients with more severe underlying immunosuppression and history of prior AIDS-defining illnesses.[20] Despite this fact, the median survival appears to have improved over time.[20]

Etiology and Related Pathophysiology

Several risk factors are implicated in the development of KS. First, underlying immunosuppression exists. It is interesting to note that in the transplant recipient population, once immunosuppressant therapy is discontinued, there is a resultant spontaneous regression of KS in approximately 20%–30% of cases.[2] There is a relationship between HLA-DQI and the development of KS, as opposed to other AIDS-defining illnesses, thus a genetic predisposition may exist.[21] A third factor may relate directly to the HIV virus. When the *tat* gene of HIV is inserted into the fertilized ova of inbred mice, skin tumors develop that closely resemble KS in approximately 15% of the male offspring. It is believed that the *tat* gene serves as the malignant event, transforming a normal mesenchymal cell, presumably of vascular endothelial origin, into the malignant phenotype. It is also believed that the tat protein functions as a growth factor for KS.[22]

KS-associated Herpes Virus (KSHV)/Human Herpes Virus 8 (HHV-8)

Unique DNA sequences have been found in KS tissues that were absent in normal, uninvolved skin.[23] These DNA sequences were found to have similarity to two known herpes viruses—the Epstein-Barr virus (EBV) and the herpes virus saimiri, which causes fulminate lymphoma in New World monkeys. This virus, dubbed *KSHV (KS-associated herpes virus)*, and now termed *HHV-8 (human herpes virus type 8)*, is present in almost all cases of KS including classic Mediterranean KS, endemic KS from Africa, transplant-associated KS, and AIDS-associated KS.[24] HHV-8 has been found to have a very narrow spectrum of human illness, including KS and a newly described type of lymphoma termed *body cavity based lymphoma.*[25]

The Multicenter AIDS Cohort Study (MACS) provides further data that indicates HHV-8 may be etiologic in the pathogenesis of KS. MACS reported that in a study of 40 homosexual/bisexual men who developed KS, 80% were seropositive to HHV-8 prior to the development of KS. The median time between seroconversion to HHV-8 and the diagnosis of KS was 33 months with a range of 6–75 months. These 40 men were matched to 40 control homosexual/bisexual men who eventually developed AIDS based on an illness other than KS. Only 18% of those in the control group were seropositive for HHV-8 prior to the development of AIDS.[26] From this study, it can be deduced that HHV-8 is present in KS tissues from all forms of the disease and that infection by HHV-8 occurs prior to the development of KS. Studies are evaluating the role of therapy against HHV-8 and prevention/treatment of KS. It is postulated that HHV-8 is present within prostatic tissues and secretions, and perhaps in sperm as well. The virus is also present in the nasal secretions and bronchoalveolar lavage fluids of patients who have pulmonary KS.

Growth Factors and KS

HIV disease causes the infected mononuclear cell to synthesize a whole range of inflammatory cytokines and angiogenic factors to include interleukin 6 (IL-6), Oncostatin-M, tumor necrosing factor-alpha (TNFα), tumor growth factor-alpha (TGFα), and others.[27] These inflammatory cytokines actually function as growth factors for KS. The KS cell is also capable of synthesizing its own angiogenic and growth factors, including IL-6, vascular growth endothelial factor, basic fibroblast growth factor, transforming growth factor-beta, and others, which function in an autocrine fashion by up-regulating growth of the cells from which they came. These angiogenic factors and cytokines constitute the climate in which the KS cells live and grow, which ensures the continued growth of surrounding vessels and KS cells. Based on these findings, new treatment protocols are aimed at down-regulating these cytokines in order to retard growth and development of disease.

Thus, the complete pathogenesis of KS involves the following multiple steps:

- A genetic predisposition
- Relative immunodeficiency
- HHV-8 becoming activated leading to a chain of events that causes the transformation of a normal vascular endothelial cell to that of a malignant phenotype

- In the HIV/AIDS environment, the associated inflammatory cytokines and angiogenic factors released from HIV-infected cells increase the growth of transformed KS cells leading to eventual wide spread clinical disease

Prevention, Screening, and Early Detection

Comprehensive histories and full body assessments of the person with HIV should comprise the continuous screening for the possibility of malignancies. As the patient's immune system becomes further compromised, the health care provider must be alert to any signs and symptoms of KS. Examination of the upper body (head, neck, and arms), the oral cavity, and the lower body, (legs and feet) are the first steps in screening and detection. As of yet, there is no known way to prevent KS. Early detection, of course, leads to earlier treatment strategies and increased survival time. Since there is increasing evidence that KS is associated with an oncogenic virus that may be sexually transmitted, teaching safer sex strategies and related practices might contribute to decreased rates of transmission.

Clinical Manifestations

KS usually presents with the appearance of single or multiple pink, red, or violaceus macular papules or nodules that are nonblanching, painless, nonpruritic, and palpable.[28,29] In some persons, discrete patch-stage lesions appear and are often mistaken for bruises, purpura, or diffuse cutaneous hemorrhages.[13] These patches can form plaques that eventually coalesce and form nodular tumors. New, multifocal lesions can occur at any time and most frequently include the tip of the nose, eyelid, hard palate, posterior pharynx, glans penis, thigh, and sole of the foot (see Figure 45-1).[28,29] In rare circumstances, the skin over the tumor can break down causing bleeding, necrosis, and pain. Lymphatic involvement at the site(s) can lead to lymphatic obstruction resulting in lymphedema (severe in some circumstances) of the face, penis, scrotum, and lower extremities. These areas of edema are usually firm and nonpitting.[28]

Extracutaneous sites for AIDS-KS involve the mucous membranes, gastrointestinal (GI) tract, lung, liver, spleen, adrenal gland, pancreas, and testis.[30] The most commonly affected extracutaneous site is the GI tract, although this site is often clinically unapparent. Pulmonary KS may be present with related dyspnea, hemoptysis, or both, and may be difficult to distinguish clinically and radiologically from PCP.

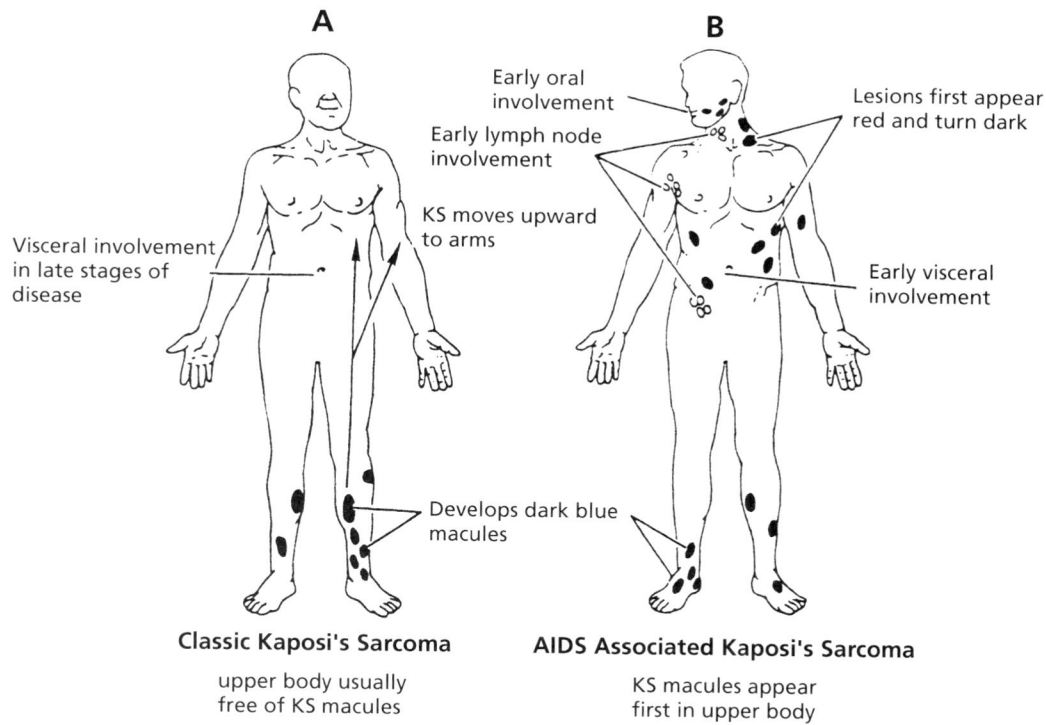

Figure 45-1 Classic and AIDS-associated Kaposi's sarcoma. A. Patients with classic KS (non-AIDS-related) demonstrate violet to dark blue bruises, spots, or macules on their lower legs. Gradually, the lesions enlarge into tumors and begin to form ulcers. KS lesions may, with time, spread upward to the trunk and arms. The movement of KS appears to follow the veins and involves the lymph system. In the late stages of the disease, visceral organs may become involved. B. For AIDS patients, initial lesions appear in greater number and are smaller than in classic KS. They first appear on the upper body (head and neck) and arms. The lesions first appear as pink or red oval bruises or macules that, with time, become dark blue and spread to the oral cavity and lower body, the legs, and feet. Visceral organs may be involved early on and the disease is aggressive. However, death is usually caused by opportunistic infection. (Reprinted with permission from Stine GJ: *AIDS Update 1998.* Englewood Cliffs, NJ, Prentice Hall, 1998, 127–158.)[29]

Assessment

A complete history and physical examination of the patient includes past history of drug use, sexual practices, ethnic ancestry (paying close attention to those born in the Caribbean, Mexico, Central America, or Africa), a close examination of the sclera, oral cavity (to include the hard palate, gum line, tongue, and tonsils), and skin (to include soles of the feet, legs, abdomen, arms, palms of the hands, neck, and face). Suspicious lesions, after careful examination by experienced health care providers, are biopsied before a diagnosis of KS can be established. Suspected KS involvement of other organs will lead to such diagnostic procedures as bronchoscopy and endoscopy of the upper and lower GI tract.

Diagnosis

In terms of diagnosis, KS lesions are readily recognized by most clinicians. In 1987, the CDC revised the definition of AIDS to include the presumptive diagnosis of KS based on characteristic gross appearance of any erythematous or violaceus plaquelike lesion on skin or mucous membrane.[31] However, the CDC urges clinicians to use caution with presumptive diagnoses and to make such decisions only when laboratory evidence supports the diagnosis of HIV infection. Definitive diagnosis is by punch biopsy of an accessible cutaneous lesion that can support a histologic diagnosis. Such definitive diagnoses are usually required before treatment with chemotherapy or radiation.

Prognostic Factors for Survival and Staging System of AIDS-Related KS

Several factors are associated with a poorer prognosis in AIDS-related KS:

- CD4 cell count $< 200/\text{mm}^3$
- History of AIDS prior to development of KS
- History of systemic "B" symptoms, such as fever, drenching night sweats, and/or weight loss[32]

Table 45-1 Staging for AIDS-Related Kaposi's Sarcoma

	Good Risk	Poor Risk
Tumor (*T*)	Confined to skin and/or lymph nodes and/or minimal oral disease (confined to palate)	Tumor associated edema or ulceration
		Extensive oral KS
		Gastrointestinal KS
		KS in visceral organs
Immune System (*I*)	CD4 cells > 200/mm³	CD4 cells < 200/mm³
Systemic Illness (*S*)	No history of opportunistic infection or thrush	History of opportunistic infection or thrush
	No systemic "B" symptoms*	Systemic "B" symptoms*
	Karnofsky performance status > 70%	Karnofsky performance status < 70%
		Other HIV-related illness

*Systemic "B" symptoms are unexplained fever, night sweats, >10% involuntary weight loss, or diarrhea persisting for more than two weeks.

Reprinted with permission from Krown SE, Metroka C, Wernz JC, et al: Kaposi's sarcoma in AIDS: a proposal for a uniform evaluation, response, and staging criteria. *J Clin Oncol* 7:1201–1207, 1989.[33]

The AIDS Clinical Trials Group (ACTG) has developed a staging system for AIDS-related KS termed *TIS* (see Table 45-1).[33] This acronym recognizes that factors related to the tumor (*T*), the immune system (*I*), and the presence of other associated illnesses (*S*) all are important in determining the state and prognosis of the patient's KS. This staging system's validity was confirmed in a study of 294 patients enrolled in eight ACTG sponsored trials.[34]

Therapeutic Approaches for AIDS-Related KS

AIDS-KS is a multicentric disease with wide dissemination at the outset despite the absence of visible lesions. The pace of the disease is variable—some patients progress extremely rapidly while others have disease states that remain quiet for years. Since there is no curative treatment at present, most clinicians find it reasonable to "watch and wait" in the initial phase of disease. The pace of the disease process is monitored and specific treatments are begun as necessary (see Table 45-2).[2]

Localized KS

Treatment for localized KS includes the use of cosmetics, surgical excision, cryotherapy, or laser therapy. In addition, local injections of vincristine (0.1 mg); vinblastine (0.1–0.2 mg) or interferon-α (1 million units) have all been used effectively in approximately 60%–90% of treated lesions.[2] Chemotherapeutic agents injected into the skin may be locally painful but are usually without systemic complications. Local radiotherapy has also been found useful. Local skin toxicities with "usual" doses of

radiotherapy are common due to the extreme sensitivity of normal skin fibroblasts.[35] Lower dose fractions of radiotherapy such as 150 cGy per day are often employed in AIDS-related KS with treatment periods limited to five to ten days. Following a week of rest, further radiation may be given if needed. In terms of edema and lymphedema, local radiation is helpful only with periorbital edema; it

Table 45-2 Treatment Guidelines in AIDS-Related Kaposi's Sarcoma

Extent of Disease	Treatment
Few, small lesions	No treatment, "watch and wait"
Few lesions, cosmetically or psychologically unacceptable	Cosmetic makeup
	Surgical excision
	Local treatments: Local injections: IFN-α, vinblastine, vincristine, liquid nitrogen cryotherapy, argon laser therapy, hCG
	Experimental: β-hCG, topical 9 cis-retinoic acid
Extensive mucocutaneous KS +/− asymptomatic visceral disease	Radiation therapy
Limited lymphedema	IFN-α plus antiretrovirals
	Experimental protocol
Rapidly progressive mucocutaneous KS	Systemic chemotherapy with single or multiple agents: ABV Doxil or DaunoXome Paclitaxel Experimental: 9 cis-retinoic acid; 9 AC topotecan; hCG
Symptomatic visceral disease	
Pulmonary KS	
Lymphedema	

Data from Levine.[2]

is less effective with lymphedema involving the upper or lower extremities.[2]

Extensive Disease

Biologic response modifiers.   Local treatment is not effective with extensive disease. For these patients with poor prognostic disease, approximately 40% will respond to interferon-α; with good prognostic factors, 60% of patients respond to interferon-α when combined with antiretroviral therapy.[36]

Antiretroviral drugs such as zidovudine (AZT), didanosine (ddI), and zalcitabine (ddC) have all shown therapeutic results when combined with interferon-α at subcutaneous doses of 10 million units or less given each day.[36] Higher doses of interferon are required if not combined with antiretrovirals (up to 36 million units/day).[36] The higher the dosage of interferon, the greater the complaints of such side effects as fatigue, fever, and systemic symptoms. While interferon is effective, complete response is usually not achieved. Nevertheless, the use of such therapy is correlated with prolonged survival rates in those who do respond to such therapy.

Chemotherapy for AIDS-Related KS

Since the use of chemotherapeutic drugs is associated with further immune compromise in most cases, the decision to treat with chemotherapy protocols requires thoughtful consideration. Indications for the use of chemotherapy include the following:

- Rapid progression of disease

- Presence of symptomatic visceral disease

- Presence of pulmonary KS

- Presence of significant lymphedema

Single agents such as vincristine, vinblastine, doxorubicin, bleomycin, and etoposide are usually quite effective.[37] ABV combination chemotherapy—adriamycin 20 mg/m[2], bleomycin 10 mg/m[2], and vincristine 2 mg given intravenously (IV) every two weeks—was shown to be more effective than single agent therapy with response rates as high as 80%.[38] Recent trials with liposomes embedded with chemotherapeutic agents have demonstrated greater tumor penetration with decreased systemic toxicities. Liposomal anthracyclines have been compared with ABV therapy with similar or somewhat better results. Doxil (liposomal doxorubicin) every two weeks[39] or DaunoXome (liposomal daunomycin) every two weeks[40] have been associated with partial remission rates of 43% and 25%, respectively. The toxicities of these agents include neutropenia and a syndrome of back pain, chest tightness, and flushing. These symptoms usually occur during infusion of the drug and tend to resolve upon subsequent slowing of the infusion and end with the infusion's completion. In addition, the use of paclitaxel in patients with relapsed AIDS-KS has been shown to be efficacious. Low doses of paclitaxel (100 mg/m[2]) IV every two weeks were licensed in 1997 for the treatment of relapsed KS and has demonstrated partial remissions with acceptable levels of toxicity (neutropenia and alopecia) in 57% of patients and complete remissions in 2% of patients studied.[41] In patients with advanced KS, paclitaxel in a regimen given over three hours every three weeks may be an important new therapy and is currently being studied.

Experimental Therapies for AIDS-Related KS

If HHV-8 is as instrumental in the pathogenesis of KS as is currently postulated, then agents that block HHV-8 will be an important potential treatment option. Several antiherpetic agents including acyclovir, foscarnet, ganciclovir, and cidofovir are being studied to evaluate their ability to prevent the development of KS. Results of these trials are eagerly anticipated.

Clinical trials are underway to determine if IL-4 and cis-retinoic acid (to down-regulate IL-6), tecogalen, and fumagillan (to down-regulate the angiogenic factors necessary for KS growth) block angiogenic and/or growth factors that may be associated with AIDS-related KS. Initial trials have been promising. Gill and associates[42] reported that the beta chain of human chorionic gonadotropin (hCG) is associated with decreased growth of KS lines in vitro and complete remission in 83% of KS lesions after intralesional therapy. The mechanism of response appears to be apoptotic death.

Nursing Care

Nursing care of the person with KS is first directed toward any potential knowledge deficit. The patient may not know what to look for or may believe simple nevi or bruises are indicative of KS long before the possibility for the actual occurrence of KS. For the patient who is diagnosed with KS, explaining treatment options and the availability of standard or investigational treatment, and ensuring that the patient understands any and all drugs and modalities (including radiotherapy and the use of immunotherapy) that may be used is essential for the patient to feel informed and in control. All patients need counseling regarding safer sex techniques and how to avoid exposure to other infections. Teaching about the need for adequate rest, good nutrition, and stress reduction rounds out the educational/counseling needs of the patient. Answering the questions of family members and significant others helps establish a supportive "team" that is ready to rally around the patient whenever needed.

As KS progresses, the obstructive and compressive nature of the tumor dictates the range of nursing care measures needed. Small, frequent, high-protein and high-calorie meals may be necessary to maintain the patient's weight. Anorexia, diarrhea, and weight loss may necessitate various teaching strategies, dietary modifications and supplements, and nursing protocols for symptom management. Good oral hygiene and meticulous skin care of the mouth, lips, and gums are warranted. Soft toothbrushes and toothettes can spare the mucosa abrasion and further damage that may have been caused by the disease process itself or the effects of radiation. Frequent monitoring of the patient's intake and output, and the presence of nausea, vomiting, diarrhea, and anorexia will help to assess the patient's hydration and the potential need for intravenous fluid replacements. Continuous assessment of the patient's level of pain and provision of comfort and pain relief measures is an essential aspect of care.

Cutaneous KS can lead to skin integrity breakdown if the lymphatic system is blocked due to tumor invasion. Such blockage can lead to chronic edema, ulceration, and constant weeping of the lesions themselves and the surrounding tissues. Nutritional irregularities, weight loss, and decreased mobility can lead to further tissue damage and breakdown. Meticulous skin inspection and care is essential. The skin must be kept clean and dry and free from possible contamination due to incontinence. The rectal area, the ankles, the elbows, and the heels of the feet should be continually assessed for their integrity and the potential for breakdown. Ointments, lamb's wool, and egg crate mattresses, are all a part of the nurse's armamentarium in the quest to maintain skin integrity.

Pulmonary KS, which can cause severe respiratory compromise and resultant distress, is an indicator of an extremely poor prognosis. Assessing the patient's respiratory status includes the evaluation of chest sounds, presence of cough, respiratory rate and volume, color of skin and nail beds, and assessment of temperature and related vital signs. Oxygen and other ventilatory needs in home or hospital requires education, planning, and assessing for the means of their proper functioning, upkeep, and service.

Decreased mobility and functional status require the assessment of support systems and prevention of their "burn-out" over time. Because of limitations in time, availability, and financial resources, persons with AIDS are often moved from care giver to care giver. When these supports can no longer provide the needed care and attention required by the patient, he or she is often forced to return to the homes of their elderly parent(s) or their parent's relatives for provision of care. This places multiple burdens on the care givers over time who may have various health care needs of their own. Securing help in the home, hospital, or long-term care facility may be necessary for those patients whose support systems are few or incapacitated over time.

Above all else, the nurse must always be aware of how this diagnosis is affecting the patient's self image. Body image disturbances are frequent when the lesions are visible on the face and extremities. Weight loss can give the appearance of being emaciated, wasted, or cachectic.

Patients may experience a range of distressed reactions from others, including close friends and family, and may become extremely depressed and withdrawn. The nurse who fosters an atmosphere of acceptance combined with accurate and adequate information can promote the ventilation of feelings, fears, and frustrations.

Utilizing all members of the interdisciplinary team helps in the discovery and planning of the patient's and family's full range of needs. Better health care outcomes in the long run are attained by making sure that the patient's legal needs are in order and by assessing the patient's and family's feelings regarding palliative or hospice care and resuscitative measures as early in the process as possible. Assessing the patient's spiritual/religious resources and potential areas of need ensures the incorporation of a holistic plan of nursing care.

Non-Hodgkin's (AIDS-Related) Lymphoma

Lymphoma is the second most common cancer in HIV (following KS) and the seventh most common cause of death for people with AIDS. A lymphoma is a neoplastic disorder (cancer) of the lymphoid tissue. The two most common types of lymphomas are non-Hodgkin's lymphomas (NHLs) and Hodgkin's disease. Burkitt's lymphoma is a rare variation of non-Hodgkin's lymphoma and is commonly reported in central Africa where its distribution appears to be determined by climatic factors, suggesting an insect vector and an infectious agent. Aggressive B-cell lymphoma (a non-Hodgkin's lymphoma) occurs in about 1%–5% of HIV-infected people and yet it makes up about 90%–95% of all lymphomas in people with HIV. The most common sites of non-Hodgkin's (AIDS-related) lymphomas are the brain, heart, or the anorectal area. In this section, AIDS-related lymphoma is understood to refer to a non-Hodgkin's lymphoma when found in persons who are infected with HIV/AIDS.

As early as 1982, physicians in San Francisco, Los Angeles, and New York noted that their homosexual patients were at increased risk for non-Hodgkin's lymphoma. These same physicians also began to notice links between NHL and the immunodeficiency disease state later termed AIDS. In 1987, the CDC included systemic high-grade, B-cell NHL in HIV-infected patients as a criterion for the diagnosis of AIDS.

Epidemiology

The incidence of NHL among persons with HIV/AIDS is much higher than in the general population. In a study involving hemophiliacs, there was a 29-fold increase in the risk of NHL among hemophiliacs with AIDS compared to hemophiliacs without HIV infection.[43] NHL is frequently the initial AIDS defining diagnosis. In a series of studies of persons with AIDS, NHL was the initial AIDS-defining illness in 3.5% of the cases in Europe[43] and 3.7% among persons with AIDS in studies conducted in the United States.[44,45] NHL may develop after another initial defining AIDS diagnosis such as recurrent pneumonia, wasting syndrome, esophageal candidiasis, or invasive cervical cancer. For example, one study reported that the rate of NHL among persons with AIDS was 2.4 per 100 patient-years.[45]

NHL occurs in all populations of persons with AIDS regardless of the way HIV was contracted. Some studies have revealed that there is a slightly higher incidence of NHL among men who have sex with men compared with other HIV patient populations.[45–47] Pederson and colleagues, however, found a slightly higher incidence of NHL among those with a history of injecting drugs rather than men who had sex with men.[44] It has also been postulated that white men and increasing age are also associated with the risk of developing AIDS-related NHL.[43–47] Lymphoma appears to be a late manifestation of HIV infection and occurs usually after fairly prolonged immunosuppression. NHL is the cause of death in approximately 16%–20% of HIV infected persons.[48]

Etiology and Related Pathophysiology

Lymphomas are cancers of the immune system and manifest in growth of lymph tissue cells with spread to other organs. Although AIDS-related NHL can originate as a malignancy of T cells, the vast majority begin as B lymphocyte malignant neoplasms. Such neoplasms are heterogeneous and they can range from being indolent to fulminant in their course.[49] It is well known that HIV infection induces chronic B-cell stimulation, proliferation, and activation. HIV also indirectly causes B-cell stimulation in response to the inflammatory cytokines IL-6 and IL-10, which are released from HIV-infected mononuclear cells, resulting in further B-cell stimulation.[50,51] This B-cell stimulation/proliferation leads to the polyclonal hypergammaglobulinemia that is so common in HIV infection as well as to the persistent generalized lymphadenopathy (PGL) that is also characteristic of HIV infection. In PGL, florid follicular (B-cell) hyperplasia is almost always seen. It has recently been demonstrated that the dendritic reticulum cells sequester HIV during the asymptomatic stages of infection and serve as sites from which uninfected CD4 cells, traveling through the node, are infected.[52]

It is also interesting to note that lymphocytes are the only cells that normally rearrange their DNA during the life span of the adult. Such DNA rearrangement allows the full range of antibody specificity that is required throughout the person's lifetime. In the milieu of chronic B-cell proliferation over a decade or more in the presence of HIV, it is not impossible to imagine genetic "errors" or "accidents" occurring over the course of normal DNA rearrangement. If even one piece of genetic information is translocated to a new site, there is the distinct possibility

of activation or dysregulation of an oncogene or tumor suppressor gene. This event allows a particular clone of B lymphocytes a growth advantage; the resultant development of a monoclonal B-cell lymphoma, caused by an earlier reactive B-cell response, would be exhibited.[53]

The brain is one of the most common sites of involvement; cerebral lymphoma accounted for 43% of all AIDS-related lymphomas.[45] In over 80% of AIDS-related NHL cases, the tumor is extranodal, making lymph-node-based tumors uncommon. Such extranodal disease is common to the GI tract, liver, orbit, gallbladder, jaw, rectum, earlobe, popliteal fossa, heart, lung, skin, pancreas, subcutaneous and soft tissue, epidural spaces, appendix, gingiva, parotid gland, paranasal sinuses, and the bone marrow.[54]

It is postulated that two herpes viruses, EBV and HHV-8, may play a role in the pathogenesis of AIDS-related NHL. In studies where pathologic tissue from patients with AIDS-related NHL was examined, Morgello[55] found EBV DNA in 50% of the cases; Levine and colleagues[54] found EBV DNA in 68% of AIDS-related NHL but only in 15% on non-HIV lymphomas. In the case of HHV-8, one particular type of lymphoma seems to be more common—namely, body-cavity-based lymphoma (BCBL), which exhibits itself as lymphomatous effusions involving pleura, pericardium, peritoneal cavity, and other sites without any evidence of solid tumor. In these cases, morphologic studies demonstrate a high proportion of BCBL cells containing HHV-8 DNA.[45,56–58] This disorder seems to be quite aggressive with median survival of only about 60 days.

Prevention, Screening, and Early Detection

There are no recommendations for primary prevention of NHL in HIV-infected persons. The key to improved outcome remains early detection. Teaching regarding the awareness and ability to identify early neurologic changes or unexplained abdominal pain as the prompt for obtaining imaging studies such as computerized tomography (CT) or magnetic resonance imaging (MRI) scans may detect the disease early in its course. Rapidly enlarging peripheral lymph nodes should be evaluated by tissue biopsy as soon as possible. Suspecting fevers of unknown origin and frequently assessing for any sudden elevation of the serum lactate dehydrogenase level are also ways to be cautiously suspicious for occult lymphoma.

Clinical Manifestations

Approximately 74% of persons with AIDS-related NHL present with nonspecific symptoms of weight loss, unexplained fever, and drenching night sweats.[54] It is also quite common to see elevations in the serum lactate dehydrogenase levels. Depending on where the tumor is located, associated signs and localized symptoms may also occur. NHL of the brain is associated with focal neurologic deficits such as hemiparesis, mental status changes, seizures, or headache.[45] GI tract lymphoma presents with abdominal pain, tenderness, weight loss, or GI bleeding.[59,60] Small bowel lymphoma may elicit the unusual manifestations of obstructive jaundice and small-bowel intussusception.[61,62]

Assessment

The patient will often present to the health care provider with complaints of fatigue, weight loss, fevers, and newly found, swollen, often tender, lymph nodes. On physical exam, the nurse may note the presence of enlarged cervical, axillary, and/or groin lymph nodes. Since such lymphadenopathy may already be present by virtue of the HIV infection, a careful history as to whether these areas have increased in size, number, and tenderness over time is important. The patient's current CD4+ T-cell count and viral load (and their current trends) can yield a measure of "risk" for lymphoma. The associated presence of fever or systemic complaints might suggest the possibility of lymphoma and may lead to biopsy and definitive diagnosis. Prior to the work-up required for staging, a careful history is taken to ascertain the presence or absence of "B" symptoms (fever, sweats, and weight loss of more than 10% of body weight). The physical exam is careful to note the size of the liver and spleen as well as the presence of abdominal tenderness. Laboratory data include complete blood count (CBC), differential cell and platelet count, sedimentation rate, serum chemistries, and liver function tests in order to screen for such conditions as hypercalcemia, hyperphosphatemia, and hyperuricemia. A chest x-ray and CT scan of the chest, abdomen, and pelvis are indicated to assess the extranodal involvement that is characteristic of HIV-related NHL. Bone marrow biopsy and lumbar puncture may be ordered by the clinician to assist with staging and the planning of therapy.

The prognosis for HIV-infected individuals with lymphoma is usually very poor. Lymphoma is a late-stage manifestation of HIV/AIDS, is usually accompanied by a low CD4+ T-cell count, and necessitates treatments (such as radiation and chemotherapy) that can themselves further weaken the immune system. Factors associated with decreased survival for persons with AIDS-related NHL include an elevated serum lactate dehydrogenase; stage III or IV disease; age over 35 years; poor performance status (Karnofsky scores less than 50%); CD4+ T-cell count less than 100/mm³; and a history of an AIDS-defining illness prior to the lymphoma.[63,64] The best prognosis is for the patient in whom the disease has not yet spread to the bone marrow and who has a CD4+ T-cell count over 200/mm³, a Karnofsky score over 70%, and no prior opportunistic infections. Median survival for those with even the best of prognoses is usually less than one year compared with four months for those with a poor prognosis.[63,64]

Diagnosis

As mentioned above, definitive diagnosis is arrived at with the pathologic examination of biopsy specimens or resected tissue or the cytologic examination of tissue fluid. Once lymphoma is diagnosed, a thorough staging evaluation is performed. Staging is done based on evaluations of the following parameters: CT scan of chest, abdomen, and pelvis; gallium-67 scan; lumbar puncture; bone marrow aspirate and biopsy; and culture to exclude other opportunistic infections in the presence of fever, night sweats, or weight loss. Such tests reveal the possibility for any of the following: lymphomatous masses, enlarged abdominal lymph nodes or extranodal masses, pleural effusions, lung nodules, axillary adenopathy, or interstitial lung disease.[65] Since many infections often present as "masses" or effusions, care must be taken to differentiate such infections from lymphoma. As mentioned previously, methods of obtaining specimens for definitive diagnosis include surgical biopsy or needle aspiration of tissue fluid. In the case of cerebral lymphoma, stereotactic biopsies reveal the cause of masses to the brain in a high percentage of cases.[66] Patients with neurologic symptoms should be evaluated as soon as possible with either CT or MRI scans of the brain; lumbar punctures should be performed if not contraindicated by such scanning. Because of the dangers posed with brain biopsies and the reluctance of many patients to undergo them, a two-week trial of empiric antitoxoplasmosis therapy is often attempted and actual biopsy of the brain reserved for those patients whose lesions do not exhibit a decrease in size with this therapy. Because toxoplasmosis is rare in those with negative toxoplasmosis serologies, brain biopsy should be performed in a timely fashion.[49] Several scanning devices have been developed in an effort to differentiate central nervous system (CNS) lymphoma from infection. Single positron emission computed tomography (SPECT) and positron emission tomography (PET) have shown a high degree of sensitivity and specificity for diagnosing cerebral malignant lesions in persons with AIDS.[67–70]

Therapeutic Approaches for Non-Hodgkin's Lymphoma

The treatment for AIDS-related lymphoma is difficult because of the underlying presence of immunosuppression, poor bone marrow reserve, and increased risk for opportunistic infections. In those patients who have CNS lymphoma, the treatment of choice is usually radiotherapy. Survival is poor with a mean length of only three months.[71] Multimodal therapy involving chemotherapy and radiotherapy is currently being studied in patients with primary CNS lymphoma.[45,72]

Systemic AIDS-related lymphoma is usually treated with chemotherapy, which in itself is problematic since it suppresses the immune system and may accelerate the course of HIV disease. Sparano and colleagues[73] found that patients with AIDS-related lymphoma who were treated with combination chemotherapy had a progressive decline in CD4 count, a twofold increase in the incidence of opportunistic infections, and short survival times. In response to these occurrences, Levine and colleagues[74] evaluated a low-dose chemotherapy regimen of methotrexate, bleomycin, doxorubicin, cyclophosphamide, vincristine, and dexamethosone (m-BACOD). The regimen was given over four months as opposed to the standard ten-month schedule. This low-dose regimen, given with intrathecal cytosine arabinoside to prevent CNS relapse, resulted in a complete remission rate of 51%. Responders usually survived a median of 18 months; the cause of death was usually an opportunistic infection.

In a recent study,[75] patients with AIDS-related lymphoma were stratified by prognostic category and then randomized to receive either low dose m-BACOD or a standard dose m-BACOD regimen given with granulocyte-macrophage colony-stimulating factor (GM-CSF) support. Results of this study (n = 198) reveal that complete remission rates were similar in the groups—median time to recurrence was greater than 190 weeks for those patients receiving the low-dose therapy and 106 weeks for patients receiving standard-dose chemotherapy. Median survival was 35 weeks in the low-dose group and 31 weeks in the standard-dose group. Thus, it appears that low-dose chemotherapy regimens are the treatment of choice for the majority of patients with AIDS-related lymphoma.

The administration of colony-stimulating factors (CSFs) such as G-CSF and GM-CSF is effective in reducing associated bacterial and fungal infections.[76] It is currently believed that antiretroviral therapy may enhance the clinical response of the patient to chemotherapy and that their combined efforts may exhibit antineoplastic effects. In studies[52,73,77] that compare regimens of combination chemotherapy with combination chemotherapy combined with antiretroviral drugs, preliminary results indicate that the combination of chemotherapy and antiretrovirals are associated with an increase in mucositis, anemia, and neurotoxicities. Protease inhibitors such as indinavir and saquinavir may alter the metabolism of such chemotherapeutic drugs (such as the CHOP regimen) leading to heretofore unexplained toxicities such as anemia and neurotoxicity.[52] Ongoing results of such trials are awaited with great interest.

Treatment for Relapsed or Refractory Disease

Few options exist for those patients who fail initial therapy. A response rate of about 20%–25% has been reported in patients with multiple relapses of AIDS-related lymphoma who were treated with mitoguazone.[52] Mitoguazone is not associated with bone marrow suppression and easily crosses the blood-brain barrier in levels that are potentially therapeutic; it is being studied as a first-line agent for those newly diagnosed with AIDS-related lymphoma. Other treatment modalities that have been used include (a) the infusional chemotherapy regimen of cyclophosphamide, doxorubicin, and etoposide,[78] (b) monoclonal antibodies conjugated to toxins such as B4-blocked ricin, (c) the use of IL-2, and (d) protocols that seek to determine if certain latent EBV proteins can be modulated in an attempt to render the tumor immunogenic and susceptible to the normal mechanisms of immune surveillance.[52]

Nursing Care

AIDS-related lymphoma is treated with radiation therapy, chemotherapy, or both. Teaching about the illness, management of side effects, how to avoid infections when neutropenic, care of the skin and mucous membranes, and the importance of adequate rest, nutrition, and sleep are all essential areas for the nurse to cover. In addition, some patients may be prone to tumor lysis syndrome if they are being treated for a bulky tumor. In the case of CNS lymphoma, the nurse must deal with safety issues related to the patient's potential for motor incoordination and cognitive deficits. As with KS, the patient's home environment must be assessed for the type and amount of support systems necessary for adequate and comprehensive care in the home setting. If these resources are not available or have been exhausted, transfer to a skilled nursing facility may be necessary. Providing emotional support to the patient and to the family and significant others is essential. Making decisions related to complex care management issues can oftentimes be challenging. The competence of the patient must be ascertained at each step of the treatment plan. Next of kin may step in and attempt to make decisions on the patient's behalf and may totally disregard those of the patient's long-term partner if there is not an authorized power of attorney in place. Exploring such legal and ethical issues as to "who is in charge" when the patient cannot make such decisions should be done early in the illness rather than waiting until it is too late.

If the mental deterioration is such that the patient becomes moribund or comatose, decisions related to placing the patient on life support (or the discontinuation of such therapy), starting intravenous or tube feedings, or the withdrawal of such support may surface. Once again, planning for the eventual likelihood of such circumstances with the patient and those close to the patient is best done early in the illness.

CERVICAL CANCER

Women represent the fastest rising population group at risk for HIV/AIDS in the United States.[79] Consistent with this statistic is the fact that cervical cancer became an AIDS-defining condition in 1993.[45]

Epidemiology

The true incidence of invasive cervical cancer in women with AIDS is unknown. In 1993, 1.3% of women with AIDS reported to the CDC had an initial AIDS diagnosis of invasive cervical cancer. This rate is thought to capture only a small portion of those women who actually have invasive cervical cancer.[45]

Etiology and Related Pathophysiology

Cervical intraepithelial neoplasia (CIN), also known as *cervical dysplasia*, is characterized by precursor lesions. In an HIV-positive woman, the progression of CIN to invasive cancer is a slow process, often taking several years. On average, CIN occurs in women ages 45–50.[45] When CIN is detected by Papanicolaou (Pap) smear in the early stages, treatment outcomes are favorable. However, in HIV-positive women, the occurrence of CIN has been noted to be more likely to rapidly progress, to be more advanced, to be more likely to occur between ages 16–48, to be less responsive to standard treatments, and to yield a poorer prognosis than in HIV-uninfected women.[80]

The CDC reports multiple risk factors for the development of CIN and cervical cancer in HIV-infected women. These risk factors include the following:

- Early age at first intercourse
- Multiple sex partners
- Sex with men who have sex with multiple partners
- Dietary deficiencies
- Cigarette smoking
- Use of oral contraceptives
- Immunosuppression
- Low socioeconomic status
- Lack of access to health care
- History of sexually transmitted diseases, especially human papillomavirus (HPV)
- Exposure to diethylstilbestrol in utero[81-83]

According to Klevens and associates,[84] there appears to be a greater incidence of AIDS-defining cervical cancer in women who are black, live in the South, are injecting drug users, and have a higher mean CD4 cell count than in women with other AIDS-defining illnesses.

There is a strong correlation between HPV, HIV, and cervical dysplasia. There are multiple types of HPV, including HPV 6 and HPV 11 that are associated with either viral condyloma or mild dysplastic changes (CIN I) and rarely progress to frank neoplasia. However, there are certain types of HPV—HPV 16, 18, 31, 33, 35, among others—that are often associated with the more advanced precursor lesions (CIN II and CIN III) and are found in most of the cases of invasive carcinoma. HPV types that are associated with high risk of cervical cancer produce viral proteins termed E6 or E7, which are crucial for malignant transformation. Studies have shown that HPV is detected in more than 95% of all cervical cancers.[45] As the CD4 cell count drops below 500/mm³, there also appears to be an increase in oncogenic HPV types as well as greater severity and prevalence of cervical dysplasia.[45] It is believed that approximately 50% of HIV infected women with CD4 cell counts less than 200/mm³ are infected with HPV 18.[85] Furthermore, it is now known that the HIV *tat* gene activates HPV.[2]

Pathogenesis and Staging

The early stage of cervical disease involves the microinvasion of the lesion into the basement membrane of the cervix. This microinvasion involves small fingerlike processes that extend into the stroma and if left undetected, measurable lesions that increase in size develop and extend into the endometrium and adjacent areas.[82] Cervical cancer is staged according to the standards of the International Federation of Gynecology and Obstetrics. The staging sequences range from 0–IV depending on the extent of tissue or organ involvement (see Chapter 50). CIN and carcinoma of the cervix have been conceptualized as a continuum progressing from mild dysplasia (grade I) to moderate dysplasia (grade II) to severe dysplasia and carcinoma in situ (grade III). A complete assessment involves a gynecologic oncologist and a radiation oncologist to determine the best individualized treatment plan possible.

Clinical Manifestations

There are no symptoms in the early stages of CIN. In such cases, CIN is usually discovered on Pap smears. The most common symptom of cervical cancer is vaginal bleeding, usually postcoital. Also present may be metorrhagia and a malodorous, blood-tinged vaginal discharge. With disease progression, there may be abdominal, pelvic, back, or leg pain; anorexia; weight loss; anemia as a result of vaginal bleeding; and edema of the leg(s) caused by the obstruction of lymph nodes. In advanced disease, there may be hematuria or rectal bleeding due to possible involvement of the bowel, bladder, or both.[86]

Assessment

In the history, the nurse should inquire about occurrence and duration of last normal menses. If the patient has a history of vaginal bleeding, the patient is asked about how current bleeding deviates from usual flow. A check to determine whether the woman is ovulating can be accomplished in part by asking about premenstrual symptoms, midcycle increase in mucus from the vagina, and biphasic temperatures. Questions related to abdominal pain, vaginal discharge, dysuria, birth control measures, sexual practices, use of oral contraceptives, recent trauma, potential family violence, past pregnancies, past medical history to include endocrine, and hematologic and gynecologic problems are essential. For women born between 1940 and 1974, the nurse should ask whether the patient's mother took diethylstilbestrol (DES) during pregnancy. On physical exam, the nurse should attempt to discover whether blood loss (if present) is significant by obtaining orthostatic blood pressure and pulse readings. The skin should be inspected for bruising, petechia, or purpura. A pelvic and speculum exam are performed checking for foreign bodies, infection, or organic pathology such as visible tumors. Diagnostic tests that may prove helpful include a urine or serum hCG, Pap smear with maturation index, saline vaginal wet prep, cervical culture for *Neisseria gonorrhoeae*, cervical culture for *Chlamydia trachomatis*, hemoglobin/hematocrit, or CBC.

Diagnosis

The Pap smear is the primary screening tool to ascertain the presence of abnormal cells, visible lesions, or both. Women with abnormal Pap smears are referred for colposcopic examinations and cervical biopsy to determine the presence of HPV and CIN.[82] In the case of the nonpregnant patient, an endocervical curettage is performed to obtain cervical cells. Conization is indicated if the lesion extends into the cervical canal and cannot be evaluated by colposcopy. Conization, or cone biopsy, is both a diagnostic and treatment method as it establishes the severity of CIN and removes a cone-shaped wedge of abnormal tissue. If invasive cervical cancer is found, the patient is usually anesthetized and the disease is staged to determine the spread of disease beyond the cervix.[82]

At the present time, many researchers are questioning the value of the routine Pap smear screening in the HIV-positive woman. It is a known fact that such Pap smears are also associated with false-negative readings in which a given Pap smear is considered normal while true CIN is confirmed by colposcopy and biopsy. Some investigators believe that all HIV-infected women should undergo baseline colposcopy with assessment of HPV status. Routine Pap screening would then be indicated for some patients while others whose baseline evaluation revealed any abnormal lesion or the presence of certain types of HPV would need to undergo serial colposcopy. Further study is needed before standards of care related to the optimal method for CIN screening in HIV-infected women can be established.

Prevention and the HIV-Positive Patient

Cervical cancer is preventable given adequate screening and early treatment of cervical dysplasia that can halt neoplastic progression. Current recommendations are that HIV-infected women have two Pap smears during the first year after diagnosis. Provided that both of these are negative, yearly Pap smears are then recommended. If a woman has a history of abnormal Pap smears before diagnosis with HIV, she should be referred for colposcopic examination with the appropriate treatment and follow-up.[86-88] There is some suspicion of an underdiagnosis of cervical cancer in women infected with HIV. Reasons for such underdiagnosis include fragmentation of care, limited access to such care (particularly in women of color), and the tendency to overlook gynecologic care and screening in the presence of more life-threatening care needs.[45,82,86] It goes without saying, therefore, that in women in whom CIN is diagnosed and in whom HIV status is unknown, HIV counseling and testing should be offered.

Therapeutic Approaches for Cervical Cancer

Approximately 40% of HIV infected women have abnormal Pap smears and/or colposcopic evidence of CIN (a precancerous lesion) when evaluated during routine gynecologic testing.[45] Low-grade CIN lesions (CIN I) are expected to regress spontaneously in seronegative women. High-grade CIN lesions—CIN II and III—eventually progress to invasive cervical cancer even in seronegative women. Well-established, definitive therapy for CIN II or III in such seronegative women includes the use of cryotherapy/cryosurgery, carbon dioxide (CO_2) laser therapy, cone biopsy or loop excision, and simple hysterectomy. Such therapies usually result in complete resolution of disease with eventual relapse in only 10%–15% of patients treated. In HIV-infected women with CIN I or II, such definitive therapy is associated with relapse in approximately 50% of patients after only one to two years.[88,89] In the HIV-infected population, optimal therapy for invasive cervical cancer is not yet known. Treatment may include single or combination strategies that include surgery, radiation, or chemotherapy. Chemotherapy often has limited effectiveness because cervical cancer responds poorly to chemotherapy. However, response rates of up to 70% have been reported with treatment that includes cisplatin, methotrexate, bleomycin, and doxorubicin.[82]

In most circumstances, when compared to seronegative counterparts, HIV-positive women with cervical cancer present with a higher grade of disease, a higher stage of disease, and early evidence of metastatic disease. In such cases, the relapse rate after definitive therapy is 100% with a median survival of less than one year.[90] In view of such relapse rates, there are several studies attempting to discover an agent that might prolong response. Such experimental approaches include the use of topical fluorouracil (5-FU) cream, oral difluoromethylornithine (DFMO), and HPV vaccines.[91] Also of note is the recent National Cancer Institute alert of February 22, 1999, urging physicians to begin treating metastatic cervical cancer with a combination of chemotherapy and radiation that will significantly reduce the death rate by 30%–50%. The implications of this government sponsored recommendation for the HIV-positive patient with metastatic cervical cancer awaits further study and guidelines.

Nursing Care

Women who have HIV have specific gynecologic needs that must be met in order to ensure them quality and comprehensive care. Some health care protocols require Pap smears every six months, others every year. Routine pelvic exams and explorations of the patient's sexual practices and habits acquaint the nurse with the specific and sometimes unique care needs of each patient. Continually assessing for such signs and symptoms as vaginal bleeding, dyspareunia, malodorous vaginal discharges, pelvic, back, or leg pain, and/or the presence of edema to the legs assures the patient that the nurse is not only interested in her full range of health care needs but is available to discuss potentially sensitive and embarrassing subject matters and questions.

Treatment of CIN and cervical carcinoma requires the nurse to educate the patient about the range of treatment modalities to include the possible side effects of radiation therapy and chemotherapy. Counseling the patient as to when to avoid sex, how to participate safely in sexual activities before and after therapies, and potential decisions regarding pregnancy and child birth foster an environment of trust, openness, and compassionate understanding.

Cervical cancer is considered to be a preventable cancer when adequate screening is provided and cervical dysplasia is treated. It is often the nurse who is at the forefront of making sure that all avenues are explored when it comes to comprehensive screening and detection and consistent health care over time.

Other Malignancies

In the past few years, several other cancers have been noted in persons with HIV. Lyter and colleagues[92,93] reported an increase in incidence of anal cancer, Hodgkin's disease, seminoma, melanoma, oropharyngeal cancer, and multiple myeloma in HIV-infected homosexual/bisexual men as compared to HIV-seronegative counterparts. Anal intraepithelial neoplasia (AIN) among HIV-positive men has increased substantially as persons with HIV and AIDS are living longer. Palefsky and colleagues[94] studied 348 HIV-positive men and 260 HIV-negative men over a four-year period. The risk for high-grade AIN was 19% among HIV-negative men, 30% among HIV-positive

men with a CD4 cell count greater than 500 mm³, and 52% among those with a CD4 cell count less than 200 mm³.[94] Routine screening for AIN by obtaining samples and smears through anoscopy should be considered in populations at risk.

Unlike non-Hodgkin's lymphoma, Hodgkin's disease (HD) is not an AIDS-defining illness. HD occurs with greater frequency, however, among HIV-infected individuals, is significantly more aggressive, and has not been successfully treated in the HIV-positive population. Frequent opportunistic infections and a depleted bone marrow reserve make it difficult to treat these individuals with chemotherapy regimens. Treatment measures, much like those used in NHL, have resulted in poor response rates and short survival times.

As persons with AIDS continue to live longer, it remains to be seen if the incidence and varieties of cancers will continue to increase. It may be difficult to determine if there is a direct relationship between these cancers and the HIV infection itself. Nevertheless, monitoring the HIV-infected population for cancer is important. If a malignancy is encountered in a patient that may be at risk for HIV/AIDS, exploration into HIV testing may indeed be warranted as an underlying immune deficiency will certainly influence future treatment plans.

The Double Trauma: AIDS *and* Malignancy

The stigma of AIDS involves a terrifying series of events and images: young people dying before their time, the relationship of sex and death, fear and homophobia, loss of insurance and career status, potential loss of disapproving family members and friends who find out that their child or loved one is a homosexual and/or drug user, discrimination and alienation/isolation, loss of self-control and functional status, loss of income and a new-found dependency on drug-assistance programs and AIDS-related programs and charities. The social meaning of AIDS intimately touches our ideas and feelings about religion, sexuality, social responsibility, individual privacy, health, promiscuity, and the prospect of living a "normal" lifespan. AIDS is a disease marked by a slow, progressive, and permanent course characterized by ever-increasing occurrences of a wide range of infections, drug side effects, eventual wasting, loss of independence, and eventual death. This is the worst case scenario of AIDS that lurks in the deepest recesses of the patient's consciousness at all times. There is no cure on the horizon.

When the diagnosis of a malignancy is added to that of AIDS, the addition of yet another "terminal" illness only reinforces the sense of living under a death sentence for those who strive to maintain a positive attitude, take care of themselves, and strictly adhere to complex medication regimens. There is the potential fear of utter vulnerability—having no resistance and no reserves to combat new infections currently held at bay. Issues related to additional expenses related to cancer treatments and their medical and nursing care needs only compound already strained financial reserves and plans for recovery or stabilization. One grieves for another aspect of the self that has been rendered sick and a yet deeper sense of helplessness is experienced as another domain of the medical establishment (the realm of oncology and hematology) must now become a part of the patient's culture. If the malignancy involves visible lesions, the HIV-infected individual encounters further issues related to body image and physical attractiveness.

The nurse can make an enormous difference in the care of the patient with AIDS who is diagnosed with a malignancy. The nurse who is comfortable with his or her own sense of sexuality and who keeps an open mind and heart can offer humane care to the person who is in need of human comfort and support. During the worst and best of times, the nurse can provide much-needed encouragement and a sense of worth and value to a patient population in need of hope, courage, and a sense of control.

Conclusion

HIV causes severe cellular immunodeficiency, which renders the infected individual vulnerable to opportunistic infections and neoplasms. The three most common cancers associated with AIDS are Kaposi's sarcoma, AIDS-related lymphoma, and cervical cancer in women. The nursing care for patients with these malignancies is oriented around screening and prevention, assessment, diagnosis, treatment, provision of supportive and emotional support, symptom management, discharge planning, home care, short-term hospital and outpatient care, sometimes skilled facility care, and, finally, terminal care and follow-up support to the family. The more compassionate, expert, and understanding the nursing care, the more humane and comfortable will be the health care experiences of the person with HIV/AIDS.

References

1. Flaskerud JH, Ungvarski PJ: Overview and update of HIV disease, in Ungvarski PJ, Flaskerud JH (eds): *HIV/AIDS: A Guide to Primary Care Management* (ed 4). Philadelphia, Saunders, 1999, pp 1–25

2. Levine A: AIDS-related malignancies. *Clin Care Options HIV* 2(3):1–10, 1996

3. Safai B, Schwartz JJ: Kaposi's sarcoma and the acquired immunodeficiency syndrome, in Devita VT, Hellman S, Rosenberg SA (eds): *AIDS: Etiology, Diagnosis, Treatment, and Prevention.* Philadelphia, Lippincott, 1992, pp 209–223

4. Centers for Disease Control and Prevention: Pneumocystis pneumonia—Los Angeles. *Morb Mortal Wkly Rep* 30:250, 1981

5. Centers for Disease Control and Prevention: Kaposi's sarcoma and Pneumocystis pneumonia among homosexual men—New York and California. *Morb Mortal Wkly Rep* 30: 305, 1981

6. Centers for Disease Control and Prevention: *HIV/AIDS Surveillance Report* 9(2):1–39. Atlanta, CDC, December 31, 1997

7. Centers for Disease Control and Prevention: HIV and AIDS trends: the changing landscape of the epidemic: a closer look. Atlanta, GA, Centers for Disease Control and Prevention, 1997

8. Centers for Disease Control and Prevention: Update: trends in AIDS incidence—United States, 1996. *Morb Mortal Wkly Rep* 46:861–866, 1997

9. Braun M: Classics in oncology: Idiopathic multiple pigmented sarcoma of the skin by Kaposi. *CA Cancer J Clin* 32: 340–347, 1982

10. Myers BD, Kessler E, Levi J, et al: Kaposi's sarcoma in kidney transplant recipients. *Arch Int Med* 133:307–311, 1974

11. Gange RW, Wilson JE: Kaposi's sarcoma and immunosuppressive therapy: an appraisal. *Clin Exp Dermatol* 3:135–146, 1978

12. Haverkos HW, Curran JW: The current outbreak of Kaposi's sarcoma and opportunistic infections. *CA Cancer J Clin* 32: 330–339, 1982

13. Friedman-Kien AE, Ostreicher R, Saltzman B: Clinical manifestations of classical, endemic, African, and epidemic AIDS-associated Kaposi's sarcoma, in Riedman-Kien AE (ed): *Color Atlas of AIDS*. Philadelphia, Saunders, 1989, pp 11–48

14. Rothman S: Remarks on sex, age, and racial distribution of Kaposi's sarcoma and on possible pathogenetic factors. *Acta Unio Int Contra Cancrum* 18:326–329, 1962

15. Beral V, Peterman TA, Berkelman RL, et al: KS among persons with AIDS. A sexually transmitted infection? *Lancet* 335:123–128, 1990

16. Lassoued K, Caluvel JP, Fegueux S, et al: AIDS associated Kaposi's sarcoma in female patients. *AIDS* 5:877–880, 1991

17. Centers for Disease Control: *HIV/AIDS Surveillance Report.* Atlanta, CDC, January 1990

18. Haverkos HW, Pinsky PF, Dortman DP, et al: Disease manifestation among homosexuals with acquired immunodeficiency syndrome: a possible role of nitrites in Kaposi's sarcoma. *Sex Transm Dis* 12:203, 1985

19. Kaldor JM, Tiondall B, Williamson P, et al: Factors associated with Kaposi's sarcoma in a cohort of homosexual and bisexual men. *J Acquir Immune Defic Syndr* 6:1145–1149, 1993

20. Miles SA, Wang H, Elashoff R, et al: Improved survival for patients with AIDS related Kaposi's sarcoma. *J Clin Oncol* 12:1910–1916, 1994

21. Mann DL, Murray C, O'Donnell M, et al: HLA antigen frequencies in HIV-1 related Kaposi's sarcoma. *J Acquir Immune Defic Syndr* 3:51–55, 1990

22. Vogel J, Hinrichs SH, Reynolds RK, et al: The HIV tat gene induces dermal lesions resembling Kaposi's sarcoma in transgenic mice. *Nature* 335:606–611, 1988

23. Chang Y, Cesarman E, Pessin MS, et al: Identification of herpesvirus-like DNA sequences in Kaposi's sarcoma. *Science* 266:1865–1869, 1994

24. Moore PS, Chang Y: Detection of herpesvirus-like DNA sequences in Kaposi's sarcoma in patients with and those without HIV infection. *N Engl J Med* 332:1186–1191, 1995

25. Cesarman E, Chang Y, Moore PS, et al: Kaposi's sarcoma-associated herpesvirus-like DNA sequences in AIDS-related body-cavity-based lymphomas. *N Engl J Med* 332:1186–1191, 1995

26. Gao SJ, Kingsley L, Hoover DR, et al: Seroconversion to

antibodies against Kaposi's sarcoma-associated herpesvirus-related latent nuclear antigens before the development of Kaposi's sarcoma. *N Engl J Med* 335:233–241, 1996

27. Ensoli B, Nakamura S, Salahuddin SZ, et al: AIDS-Kaposi's sarcoma derived cells express cytokines with autocrine and paracrine growth effects. *Science* 243:223–226, 1989

28. Heyer DM, Kahn JO, Volberding PA: HIV-related Kaposi's sarcoma, in Cohen PT, Sande MA, Volberding PA (eds): *The AIDS Knowledge Base*. Medical, 1990, pp 713.1–713.19

29. Stine GJ. *AIDS Update 1998*. Englewood Cliffs, NJ, 1998, pp 127–158

30. Safai B, Dias BM: Kaposi's sarcoma and cloacogenic carcinoma associated with AIDS, in Broder S, Merigan TC, Bolognesi D (eds): *Textbook of AIDS Medicine*. Baltimore, Williams and Wikins, 1994, pp 401–415

31. Centers for Disease Control: Revision of the CDC surveillance case definition for acquired immunodeficiency syndrome. *Morb Mortal Wkly Rep* 36(No. 1S):3S–15S, 1987

32. Chachoua A, Krigel R, Lafleur F, et al: Prognostic factors and staging classification of patients with epidemic Kaposi's sarcoma. *J Clin Oncol* 7:774–780, 1989

33. Krown SE, Metroka C, Wernz JC, et al: Kaposi's sarcoma in AIDS: a proposal for a uniform evaluation, response, and staging criteria. *J Clin Oncol* 7:1201–1207, 1989

34. Krown SE, Testa MA, Huang J. AIDS-related kaposi's sarcoma: prospective validation of the AIDS Clinical Trials Group Staging Classification. *J Clin Oncol* 75:3085–3092, 1997

35. Chak LY, Gill PS, Levine AM, et al: Radiation therapy for AIDS-related KS. *J Clin Oncol* 6:863–867, 1988

36. Mitsuyasu RT: Interferon alpha in the treatment of AIDS related KS. *Br J Haematol* 79:69–73, 1991

37. Lilenbaum RC, Ratner L: Systemic treatment of KS: current status and future directions. Editorial review. *AIDS* 8:141–151, 1994

38. Gill PS, Rarick MU, McCutchan JA, et al: A systemic treatment of AIDS-related KS: results of a randomized trial. *Am J Med* 90:427–433, 1991

39. Northfelt DWQ, Dezube B, Miller B, et al: Randomized comparative trial of doxil vs. adriamycin, bleomycin, and vincristine (ABV) in the treatment of severe AIDS related KS. *Blood* 86:382a, 1995

40. Gill PS, Wernz J, Scadden DT, et al: A randomized trial of liposomal daunorubicin (Daunoxome) versus adriamycine, bleomycin, and vincristine (ABV) in 232 patients with advanced AIDS related KS. *Proc Am Soc Clin Oncol* 14:291, 1995 (abstr)

41. Gill PS, Tulpule A, Reynld J, et al: Paclitaxel (Taxol) in the treatment of relapsed or refractory advanced AIDS-related Kaposi's sarcoma. *Proc Am Soc Clin Oncol* 15(854):306, 1996 (abstr)

42. Gill PS, Lunardi-Iskandar Y, Louis S, et al: The effect of preparation of human chorionic gonadotropin on AIDS-related KS. *N Engl J Med* 335:1261–1269, 1996

43. Ragni MV, Bele SH, Jaffee RA, et al: Acquired immunodeficiency syndrome-associated non-Hodgkin's lymphomas and other malignancies in patients with hemophilia. *Blood* 81:1889–1897, 1993

44. Pedersen C, Barton SE, Cjiesi A, et al: HIV related non-Hodgkin's lymphoma among European AIDS patients: AIDS in Europe Study Group. *Eur J Haematol* 55:245–250, 1995

45. Staats JA, Sheran M, Herr R: Adolescents and adults. Care management of AIDS-indicator diseases, in Ungvarski PJ,

Flaskerud JH (eds): *HIV/AIDS: A Guide to Primary Care Management* (ed 4). Philadelphia, Saunders, 1999, pp 194–254

46. Cote TR, Manns A, Hardy CR, et al: Epidemiology of brain lymphoma among people with or without acquired immunodeficiency syndrome: AIDS/Cancer Study Group. *J Natl Cancer Inst* 88:675–679, 1996

47. Serriano D, Salamina G, Francheschi S, et al: The epidemiology of AIDS-associated non-Hodgkin's lymphoma in the World Health Organization European Region. *Br J Cancer* 66:912–916, 1992

48. Peters BS, Beck EJ, Coleman DG, et al: Changing disease patterns in patients with AIDS in a referral centre in the United Kingdom: the changing face of AIDS. *Br Med J* 302:203–207, 1991

49. Kaplan LD, Northfelt DW: Malignancies associated with AIDS, in Sande MA, Volberding PA (eds): *The Medical Management of AIDS* (ed 5). Philadelphia, Saunders, 1997, pp 413–439

50. Emile D, Coumbaras J, Raphael M, et al: Interleukin-6 production in high-grade B lymphomas: correlation with the presence of malignant immunoblasts in acquired immunodeficiency syndrome and in human immunodeficiency seronegative patients. *Blood* 80:498–504, 1992

51. Masood R, Zhang Y, Bond MW, et al: Interleukin 10 is an autocrine growth factor for AIDS related B cell lymphoma. *Blood* 85:3423–3430, 1995

52. Levine A: Oncologic disorders and cytokines. *Clin Care Options for HIV* 4(2):1–19, 1998 (online)

53. Ballerini P, Gaidano G, Gon JZ, et al: Molecular pathogenesis of HIV associated lymphomas. *AIDS Res Hum Retroviruses* 8:731–735, 1992

54. Levine AM, Shibata D, Sullivan-Hurley J, et al: Epidemiological and biological study of acquired immunodeficiency syndrome-related lymphoma in the County of Los Angeles: preliminary results. *Cancer Res* 52:5482s–5484s, 1992 (suppl 19)

55. Morgello S: Epstein-Barr and human immunodeficiency viruses in acquired immunodeficiency syndrome-related primary central nervous system lymphoma. *Am J Pathol* 141:441–450, 1992

56. Carbone A, Gloghini A, Vaccher E, et al: Kaposi's sarcoma-associated herpesvirus DNA sequences in AIDS related and AIDS-unrelated lymphomatous effusions. *Br J Haematol* 94:533–543, 1996

57. Gessain A, Briere J, Angelin-Duclos C, et al: Human herpes virus 8 (Kaposi's sarcoma herpes virus) and malignant proliferations in France: a molecular study of 250 cases including two AIDS-associated body cavity lymphomas. *Leukemia* 11:266–272, 1997

58. Nador RG, Cesarman E, Chadburn A, et al: Primary effusion lymphoma: a distinct clinicopathologic entity associated with the Kaposi's sarcoma-associated herpes virus. *Blood* 88:645–656, 1996

59. Beck PL, Gill MJ, Sutherland LR: HIV-associated non-Hodgkin's lymphoma of the gastrointestinal tract. *Am J Gastroenterol* 91:2377–2381, 1996

60. Cappell MS, Botros N: Predominantly gastrointestinal symptoms and signs in 11 consecutive AIDS patients with gastrointestinal lymphoma. *Am J Gastroenterol* 89:545–549, 1994

61. Danin JD, McCarty M, Coker R: Case report: lymphoma causing small bowel intussusception in a patient with the acquired immune deficiency syndrome. *Clin Radiol* 46:350–351, 1992

62. Schoeppner HL, Wong DK, Bresalier RS: Primary small

bowel lymphoma manifested as obstructive jaundice in a patient with AIDS. *South Med J* 88:583–585, 1995

63. Levine AM, Sullivan-Halley J, Pike MD, et al: HIV related lymphoma: prognostic factors predictive of survival. *Cancer* 68:2466–2472, 1991

64. Straus D, Juang J, Testa M, et al: Prognostic factors in the treatment of HIV-associated non-Hodgkin's lymphoma: analysis of ACTG 142 (low dose vs. standard dose mBA-CODD + GM-CSF). *Blood* 86:604a, 1995

65. Sider L, Melany M. Thoracic AIDS-related lymphoma: CT appearance and CD4 counts. *AJR Am J Roentgenol* 160: 97–102, 1993 (suppl 4)

66. Iacoangeli M, Roselli R, Antinor A, et al: Experience with brain biopsy in acquired immune deficiency syndrome-related focal lesions of the central nervous system. *Br J Surg* 81:1508–1510, 1994

67. Hoffman JM, Waskin A, Schifter T, et al: FDG-PET in differentiating lymphoma from nonmalignant central nervous system lesions in patients with AIDS. *J Nucl Med* 34:567–575, 1993

68. Lorberboym M, Estok L, Machac J, et al: Rapid differential diagnosis of cerebral toxoplasmosis and primary central nervous system lymphoma by thallium-201 SPECT. *J Nucl Med* 37:1150–1154, 1996

69. O'Malley JP, Ziessman HA, Kuman PN, et al: Diagnosis of intracranial lymphoma in patients with AIDS: value of 201Tl single-photon emission computed tomography. *AJR Am J Roentgenol* 163:417–421, 1994

70. Pierce MA, Johnson MD, Maciunas RJ, et al: Evaluating contrast-enhancing brain lesions in patients with AIDS by using positron emission tomography. *Ann Int Med* 123: 594–598, 1995

71. Ling SM, Roach M, Larson DA, et al: Radiotherapy of primary central nervous system lymphoma in patients with and without human immunodeficiency virus: ten years of treatment experience at the University of California San Francisco. *Cancer* 73:2570–2582, 1994

72. Forsyth PA, Yahoalom J, DeAngelis LM: Combined-modality therapy in the treatment of primary central nervous system lymphoma in AIDS. *Neurology* 44:1473–1479, 1994

73. Sparano JA, Wiernik PH, Hu S, et al: Pilot trial of infusional cyclophsophamide, doxorubicin, and etoposide plus didanosine and filgrastim in patients with non-Hodgkin's lymphoma. *J Clin Oncol* 14:3026–3035, 1996

74. Levine AM, Tulpule A, Expina B, et al: Low dose methotrexate, bleomycin, doxorubicin, cyclophosphamide, vincristine, and dexamethasone with zalcitabine in patients with acquired immunodeficiency syndrome related lymphoma: effect on human immunodeficiency virus and serum interleukin-6 levels over time. *Cancer* 78:517–526, 1996

75. Kaplan L, Staus D, Testa M, et al: Randomized trial of standard dose mBACOD with GM-CSF vs. reduced dose mBA-COD for systemic HIV-related lymphoma. *Proc Am Soc Clin Oncol* 14:288, 1995 (abstr)

76. Newell M, Goldstein D, Milliken S, et al: Phase I/II trial of filgrastim (r-metHuG-CSF), CEOP chemotherapy and antiretroviral therapy in HIV-related non-Hodgkin's lymphoma. *Ann Oncol* 7:1029–1036, 1996

77. Levine AM, Tulpule A, Espina B, et al: Low dose m-BACOD with zalcitabine in patients with AIDS-related lymphoma: effect on HIV and serum interleukin-6 levels over time. *Cancer* 78:517–526, 1996

78. Sparano JA, Wiernik PH, Strack M, et al: Infusional cyclophosphamide, doxorubicine, and etoposide in HIV and HTLV-1 related non-Hodgkin's lymphoma: a highly active regimen. *Blood* 81:2810–2815, 1993

79. Centers for Disease Control: Characteristics of, and HIV infection among, women served by publicly funded HIV counseling and testing services: USA, 1989–1990. *Morb Mortal Wkly Rep* 40:195–203, 1991

80. Maimon M, Fruchter RG, Guy L, et al: Human immunodeficiency virus infections and invasive cervical carcinoma. *Cancer* 71:402–406, 1993

81. Centers for Disease Control: Risk for cervical disease in HIV infected women. *Morb Mortal Wkly Rep* 39:846–849, 1990

82. Peel KR: Premalignant and malignant disease of the cervix, in Whitefield CR (ed): *Dewhurst's Textbook of Obstetrics and Gynecology for Postgraduates* (ed 5). London, Blackwell Scientific, 1995, pp 717–737

83. Richart RM, Wright TC. Controversies in the management of low-grade cervical intraepithelial neoplasia. *Cancer* 71: 1413–1421, 1993 (suppl 4)

84. Klevens MR, Fleming PL, Mays MA, et al: Characteristics of women with AIDS and invasive cervical cancer. *Obstet Gynecol* 88:269–273, 1996

85. Vermund SH, Kelley KF, Kelin RS, et al: High risk of human papillomaviruses infection and cervical squamous intraepithelial lesions among women with symptomatic HIV infection. *Am J Obstetric Gynecol* 165:392–400, 1991

86. Hatch KD, FU YS: Cervical and vaginal cancer, in Berek JS, Adashi EY, Hillard PA (eds): *Novak's Gynecology* (ed 12). Baltimore, Williams and Wilkins, 1996, pp 1111–1122

87. Centers for Disease Control: USPHS/IDSA guidelines for the prevention of opportunistic infections in persons infected with human immunodeficiency virus. *Morb Mortal Wkly Rep* 46(RR-12):1–13, 1997

88. Denenberg R. Cervical cancer and women with HIV. GMHC: Treatment Issues 11(7/8):10–18, 1997

89. Maiman M, Fruchter RF, Serur E, et al: Recurrent cervical intraepithelial neoplasia in HIV seropositive women. *Obstet Gynecol* 82:170–174, 1993

90. Maiman M, Fruchter RG, Serur E, et al: HIV and cervical neoplasia. *Gynecol Oncol* 38:377–382, 1990

91. Levine A: Oncologic disorders and cytokines. *Clin Care Options for HIV* 4(2):1–19, 1998 (online)

92. Lyter DW, Bryant J, Thackeray R, et al: Incidence of human immunodeficiency virus related and nonrelated malignancies in a large cohort of homosexual men. *J Clin Oncol* 13: 2540–2546, 1995

93. Lyter DW, Kingsley LA, Rinaldo CR, et al: Malignancies in the Multicenter AIDS Cohort Study (MACS) 1984–1994. *Proc Am Soc Clin Oncol* 15:305, 1996 (abstr)

94. Palefsky JM. Anal human papillomavirus infection and anal cancer in HIV positive individuals: an emerging problem. *AIDS* 8:283–295, 1994

CHAPTER 46

Bone and Soft Tissue Sarcomas

Patricia A. Piasecki, RN, MS

Introduction

Bone and soft tissue malignancies are so uncommon that they are not listed among the five leading cancer sites. They occur in all age groups. Diagnosis and treatment of these lesions are complex. Key members of the health care team include the patient and family, the orthopedic surgeon, medical oncologist, radiologist, pathologist, radiation oncologist, thoracic surgeon, physical therapist, nurse, prosthetist, and social worker. Increased knowledge about bone and soft tissue sarcomas and a multidisciplinary approach have improved the results of treatment in recent years.

Epidemiology

The incidence of primary malignant bone and soft tissue tumors is remarkably low. These tumors constitute a small percentage of malignant tumors diagnosed in the United States.[1] The American Cancer Society estimates 2,500 new cases of bone cancer in 2000. Incidence is slightly higher for men. The estimated number of deaths in 2000 from bone cancer is 1400. In 2000, 8,100 new cases of soft tissue cancer are predicted. The estimated death toll from soft tissue tumors is 4600.[1]

Etiology

At present, relatively little is known regarding the cause of primary bone and soft tissue tumors. Consequently, prevention and detection of bone and soft tissue sarcomas remain difficult because few risk factors have been identified. Prior cancer therapy in the form of high-dose irradiation has been linked to the development of bone and soft tissue sarcoma. Chemicals such as vinyl chloride gas, arsenic, and dioxin or Agent Orange have been associated with the formation of soft tissue sarcomas. Exposure to alkylating agents such as melphalan, procarbazine, nitrosoureas, and chlorambucil predisposes patients to sarcomas. Immunosuppressed patients such as renal transplant recipients and persons with acquired immunodeficiency syndrome (AIDS) have a higher risk for soft tissue sarcomas. Neurofibromatosis patients have a 10% chance of one of their tumors transforming to a neurofibrosarcoma. Prolonged lymphedema following a mastectomy can lead to a lymphangiosarcoma.

Evidence of a familial tendency in bone cancer has been demonstrated by reports of siblings with osteosarcoma, Ewing's sarcoma, and chondrosarcoma. Bone and soft tissue sarcomas may be only part of a complex of different tumors that cluster in families. These findings suggest that common susceptibility may be the critical factor in predisposition to diverse forms of cancer.

Malignant bone neoplasms have been associated with a number of preexisting bone conditions. Paget's disease predisposes individuals primarily to osteosarcoma. The incidence of sarcomas in patients with symptoms of Paget's disease is under 10%. It has been proposed that the mechanisms responsible for the relationship are prolonged growth, an overstimulated metabolism, or both. The occurrence of bone tumors are also associated with hyperparathyroidism, chronic osteomyelitis, old bone infarct, osteochondromas, and enchondromas.

Molecular genetics are being studied in musculoskeletal tumors with the hope that genetic therapy will be a trend in the next decade. Osteosarcomas are noted to occur if both alleles at the *RB1* and *p53* are altered; these are tumor-suppressor genes.[2,3] Similar studies in chondrosarcoma cell lines are being performed. Neurofibrosarcoma patients have a loss of tumor-suppressor gene on chromosome 17p.[4] There is also ongoing research in this area.

Prevention, Screening, and Early Detection

Due to the relative low incidence of malignant bone and soft tissue sarcomas, there are no screening tests available for these tumors. For individuals with a family history of sarcoma or predisposing conditions such as neurofibromatosis or exposure to dioxin, annual physical exams are a prudent routine to adopt. Routine radiographic screenings are not advised. If bone pain or a mass is discovered it should be evaluated even if there is no predisposing condition.

Pathophysiology

Primary malignant bone and soft tissue tumors are derived from the cells that have a common ancestry, namely, the mesoderm or ectoderm. One group of bone and soft tissue tumors is produced by cells characterized by their ability to produce collagen. This group includes the osteogenic tumors arising from osteoblasts, the chondrogenic tumors arising from chondroblasts, and the fibrogenic tumors arising from fibroblasts. Another group originates in the bone marrow reticulum and includes round cell tumors such as Ewing's sarcoma and reticulum cell sarcoma. The third group arises in blood vessels of the bone and includes the angiosarcomas. Soft tissue sarcomas such as alveolar soft part sarcomas and epithelioid sarcomas have no known cellular origins.

Little can be said regarding the pathophysiology of bone and soft tissue tumors in general because of the individualized behavior demonstrated by the different types of tumors. Nearly every bone and soft tissue in the skeleton may be affected; however, individual tumors have a predilection for certain locations. Most often soft tissue sarcomas arise in the extremities but can involve head and neck and retroperitoneal areas. In addition, there are differences in cellular characteristics and in the progression of disease. In general, bone and soft tissue tumors tend to aggressively involve contiguous tissue and muscle and metastasize early to the lungs via the hematogenous route. Occasionally, soft tissue sarcomas can spread to regional lymph nodes.

Clinical Manifestations

Bone and soft tissue sarcomas can manifest with one or more of the following presentations:

1. Painful area on the musculoskeletal system
2. Pain at rest
3. Soft tissue or bony mass that may not be painful

Assessment

Patient and Family History

The evaluation of pain assumes a major focus in the interview. Obtaining information regarding the location, onset, duration, and quality of the pain assists in the differential diagnosis. It is important to rule out a traumatic injury to the area, which could result in a condition such as hematoma or myositis ossificans that can resemble tumors. More commonly, an injury merely brings a preexisting neoplasm to the attention of the individual. Bone tumor pain often has a gradual onset and may be present for a few months before the person seeks medical advice. An abrupt onset of pain does not necessarily rule out the presence of bone tumor because a pathological fracture may be the presenting symptom. Pain can be radicular. For example, a tumor of the hip can radiate pain via the obturator nerve and present with knee pain. Musculoskeletal tumor pain often is constant and worse at night. The severity of pain steadily increases as the tumor enlarges. Over-the-counter medications may not relieve the pain.

Soft tissue sarcomas present as painless masses unless they are impinging on nerves, blood vessels, or viscera. Other presenting symptoms such as a history of swelling need to be assessed during the patient interview. Attention is given to symptoms suggestive of pulmonary disease such as hemoptysis, chest pain, or cough. Family history of any cancer diagnosis and subsequent treatment, toxic substance exposure, and prior orthopedic conditions such as Paget's disease or neurofibromatosis should be noted.

To determine potential problems and needs, a psychosocial assessment should be incorporated into the initial interview. The individual may have a life-threatening tumor. The nature of family, peer, and love relationships and other support systems is explored. It often is helpful to identify the person in whom the patient most frequently confides as well as the person's usual coping strategies when confronting stress. To further delineate possible resources, the significance of personal relationships, work, and leisure activities is assessed. Inability to work is especially problematic if the patient is the policy holder of the medical insurance.

Physical Examination

The physical examination of the individual with a suspected bone or soft tissue lesion involves inspection and palpation of the affected area. Inspection may reveal a visible mass or swelling. Dilated surface veins may be evident. A firm, nontender, warm enlargement may be palpated over the affected portions, although malignant bone tumors are not always visible or palpable. Dimensions of the soft tissue mass should be noted. Evaluation for adenopathy and hepatomegaly also is performed. Limitations in motion of proximal joints are noted. Muscle atrophy can occur in a chronic setting and can be documented by measuring the affected and nonaffected limb. Analysis will most likely reveal an antalgic gait for a lower extremity tumor, as the patient will shorten the time spent on the affected limb. An assessment of neurovascular function of the affected limb is done.

Diagnostic Studies

Evaluation of the individual with symptoms suggestive of bone or soft tissue sarcoma necessitates the collaboration of the radiologist, orthopedic surgeon, and pathologist. Before any diagnostic conclusions are made, the person's clinical history is reviewed, as well as the radiological and histological features of the lesion.

Radiographs, although they frequently do not yield a specific diagnosis, provide the opportunity to view the location and the anatomy of the bony lesion, as well as the status of surrounding tissue. In general, radiographic changes can be appreciated only when the tumor is far advanced. Three basic patterns of tumor destruction that may be viewed radiographically are described as geographic, moth-eaten, or permeative. These patterns may be correlated with the pathological aggressiveness or quiescence of the tumor and may occur alone or in combination with one or both of the other patterns. The geographic pattern indicates that the tumor has a slow rate of growth. It is characterized by a large, well-defined hole in which the edge of completely destroyed bone interfaces with the edge of bone that is completely intact. The moth-eaten pattern indicates a moderately aggressive tumor. It is characterized by multiple holes that tend to coalesce. This pattern implies severe cortical destruction.

Finally, the permeative pattern indicates an aggressive tumor with a strong capacity for infiltration. It is characterized by multiple tiny holes in cortical bone. These holes diminish in size and number in the peripheral areas of the lesion. The moth-eaten pattern indicates that the tumor has breached the cortex and has extended longitudinally within the bone. Soft tissue sarcomas may have negative radiographs because radiographs best image bony tissue and poorly image the soft tissues.

Several other radiological methods may be used in the evaluation of primary malignant bone and soft tissue cancer. These include bone scans, arteriography, computerized tomography (CT), fluoroscopy, and magnetic resonance imaging (MRI). A bone scan is not helpful in distinguishing one bone condition from another but is useful in verifying the presence of abnormal bone when plain radiographs show normal findings. A bone scan helps to detect or exclude the presence of additional lesions in the skeleton. Likewise, arteriography is not diagnostic but aids in the planning of surgical, radiation, and perfusion chemotherapy treatments by outlining tumor margins and mapping arterial blood supply to the tumor. A CT provides an evaluation of the true bony extent of the disease. Fluoroscopy is used in the operating room to document the location in the bony lesion from which the biopsy specimen is taken.

The MRI is superior to a CT scan in demonstrating the tumor extent in marrow and soft tissue and in detecting recurrence in the presence of surgical clips and metallic prostheses. Magnetic resonance angiography can assist in surgical planning for vascularized graft harvest or evaluation of tumor bed.[5] Ultrasonography is useful in determining size and density of the soft tissue mass.

Biopsy is crucial for diagnosis. The biopsy should include the most representative section of the lesion as determined by the imaging. Biopsy tissue may be obtained by use of an open (incisional) or closed (needle) technique.

Open, or incisional, biopsy is the most common type of biopsy used for bone and soft tissue lesions. With the patient under general, regional, or local anesthesia, an incision is made over the tumor mass and a soft tissue sample is taken. Bone biopsies are more painful, weaken the bone, and need to be processed in the pathology department for a few days before diagnosis is made. Incisional biopsy yields a larger volume of tissue for examination but may cause larger hematoma, potentially spilling malignant cells.

The location and size of the incision are equally important to the surgeon and radiation oncologist. If resection of the tumor is performed, the site of the biopsy incision is removed en bloc with the tumor. The radiation oncologist includes the incision site in the field of treatment. Therefore, it is advisable for the orthopedic oncologist rather than the referring surgeon to perform the biopsy.

Frozen sections are done during incisional biopsy to ensure that representative material has been obtained.

In circumstances in which clinical and radiological findings are highly suggestive of a particular lesion such as chondrosarcoma, frozen sections are obtained with the intention of performing surgery while the patient is still anesthetized. For many bone tumors, however, it is advisable to await permanent paraffin sections.

Closed, or needle, biopsy is utilized on the basis that it is technically simple, involves minimal patient risk, is cost- and time-effective, may be repeated without any ill effects, and makes it possible to extract material from different depths of the tumor. This biopsy can be done by the surgeon under local anesthetic. In some centers radiologists perform CT-guided needle biopsies using intravenous (IV) sedation and local anesthetic. In addition, it is always possible to do incisional biopsy if the diagnosis remains unclear. Needle biopsy is approximately 80% accurate.[6] Needle biopsy is used for individuals with known metastatic disease and in deep lesions that would require large dissections.

In general, laboratory studies are not helpful in the diagnosis of musculoskeletal tumors. There are a few exceptions, which will be addressed in conjunction with the specific tumor type to which they apply. A CT of the chest and regional lymph nodes is done to determine the presence or absence of metastatic disease.

Prognostic Indicators

The prognosis for individuals with bone and soft tissue sarcoma is worse if the grade of the tumor is high, the location deep, and the tumor large. If there is distant metastasis to the lymph nodes, lungs, or other bones, the prognosis is also lowered. Nonresponsive tumors may be measured by serial positron emission tomography (PET) scanning before treatment, during treatment, and immediately prior to resection to identify the tumor's biological behavior.[7]

Classification and Staging

The classification of bone and soft tissue tumors currently is based on histological patterns, which in general correlate with the gross appearance, radiological features, and biological behavior of the tumor. Uncertainty with regard to the definition of terms used in pathological nomenclature and classification not only complicates the treatment of bone tumors but also impedes research efforts aimed at the development of staging classification for musculoskeletal tumors. Consequently, the American Joint Committee on Cancer has recommended that the *International Histological Classification of Tumors,* published by the World Health Organization, be used for specific definitions of histological typing.[8]

The World Health Organization scheme of classification (Table 46-1) is based on the type of differen-

Table 46-1   Histologic Typing of Primary Bone Tumors

Bone-forming tumors
  Benign
    Osteoma
    Osteoid osteoma and osteoblastoma
  Malignant
    Osteosarcoma
    Surface osteosarcoma
      Periosteal
      Periosteal or juxtacortical

Cartilage-forming tumors
  Benign
    Chondroma
    Osteochondroma (osteocartilaginous exostosis)
    Chondroblastoma (benign chondroblastoma; epiphyseal
      chondroblastoma)
    Chondromyxoid fibroma
  Malignant
    Chondrosarcoma
    Juxtacortical or periosteal chondrosarcoma
    Mesenchymal chondrosarcoma
    Clear cell chondrosarcoma
    Dedifferentiated chondrosarcoma

Giant cell tumor

Marrow tumors
  Ewing's sarcoma
  Neuroectodermal tumor of bone
  Bone lymphoma
  Myeloma

Vascular tumors
  Benign
    Hemangioma
    Lymphangioma
    Glomus tumor (glomangioma)
  Intermediate or indeterminate
    Hemangioendothelioma
    Hemangiopericytoma
  Malignant
    Angiosarcoma
    Malignant hemangiopericytoma

Other connective tissue tumors
  Benign
    Benign fibrous histiocytoma
    Lipoma
  Intermediate
    Desmoplastic fibroma
  Malignant
    Fibrosarcoma
    Liposarcoma
    Malignant mesenchymoma
    Undifferentiated sarcoma
    Malignant fibrous histiocytoma
    Leiomyosarcoma

Other malignant tumors
  Chordoma
  Adamantinoma

Other benign tumors
  Neurilemmoma (schwannoma, neurinoma)
  Neurofibroma

Tumor-like lesions
  "Brown tumor" of hyperparathyroidism

Data from Schajowicz.[9]

tiation shown by the tumor cells and the type of intracellular material they produce.[9] The main types of primary bone and soft tissue tumors are listed according to whether they are bone-forming, cartilage-forming, marrow-forming, vascular-forming, nerve-forming, or other connective tissue type.

The staging system for musculoskeletal sarcomas includes surgical grade, surgical site, presence of metastases including nodal involvement (Table 46-2).[8,10] Stage I includes low-grade lesions with low incidence of metastases, such as periosteal osteosarcoma. Stage II includes high-grade lesions with high incidence of metastases, such as classic osteosarcoma and angiosarcoma. The site is noted to be "A," which indicates an intracompartmental lesion, or "B," which indicates an extracompartmental lesion. Anatomic compartments have barriers to tumor extension. In bone these barriers are cortical bone and articular cartilage; in joints, articular cartilage and joint capsule; and in soft tissue, the major fascial septa and the tendinous origins and insertions of muscle. Lesions that involve the neurovascular bundle are extracompartmental. Stage III includes any site or grade lesion with metastases.[10]

Therapeutic Approaches and Nursing Care

The goals of treatment of primary malignant bone and soft tissue cancer include eradication of the tumor, avoidance of amputation when possible, and preservation of maximum function. The primary lesion is managed by surgery, radiotherapy, or chemotherapy, or a combination of these therapies. Treatment is highly individualized because an optimal treatment program has not been identified for each histological subtype.

Surgery

Surgical management of primary neoplasia of the bone is strongly influenced by the histopathological features, the anatomical site, and the physical size of the lesion. Clinical and radiographic data also are considered because they provide further information about the biological behavior of a given lesion.

Table 46-2 Anatomic Staging of Musculoskeletal Sarcomas

Rules for Classification

Clinical staging. Clinical staging includes physical examination, clinical laboratory tests, and biopsy of the sarcoma for microscopic diagnosis and grading.

Pathological staging. Pathological staging consists of the removal of the primary tumor, nodes, or suspected metastases.

Primary tumors (T)

Tx	Primary tumor cannot be assessed
T0	No evidence of primary tumor
T1	Tumor 5 cm or less in greatest dimension
T2	Tumor more than 5 cm in greatest dimension

Regional lymph nodes (N)

NX	Regional lymph nodes cannot be assessed
N0	No regional lymph node metastasis
N1	Regional lymph node metastasis

Distant metastasis (M)

MX	Presence of distant metastasis cannot be assessed
M0	No distant metastasis
M1	Distant metastasis

Tumor grade (G)

GX	Grade cannot be assessed
G1	Well differentiated
G2	Moderately well differentiated
G3–4	Poorly differentiated; undifferentiated

Stage grouping

Stage IA	G1	T1	N0	M0
Stage IB	G1	T2	N0	M0
Stage IIA	G2	T1	N0	M0
Stage IIB	G2	T2	N0	M0
Stage IIIA	G3–4	T1	N0	M0
Stage IIIB	G3–4	T2	N0	M0
Stage IVA	Any G	Any T	N1	M0
Stage IVB	Any G	Any T	Any N	M1

Data from American Joint Committee on Cancer.[8]

Twenty years ago, research indicated that no procedure short of ablation would control or eradicate aggressive forms of osteosarcoma, fibrosarcoma, and chondrosarcoma.[11] Historically, the amputation included the joint above the tumor. Tumors in inaccessible areas such as the pelvis, spine, or skull pose unique and difficult problems, with treatment frequently aimed at palliation.

In 1984 the National Institutes of Health held a conference to evaluate the efficacy of limb-sparing surgery. Experts reported their experiences with 2000 individuals diagnosed with sarcoma. The same disease-free survival rate was reported for individuals who underwent limb-sparing surgery as for those who underwent amputation.

The traditional contraindications for limb salvage are (1) inability to attain adequate surgical margin, (2) neurovascular bundle involved by tumor, (3) pathological fractures, and (4) age-group, that is, children younger than ten years, because of resultant limb length discrepancy. Recent chemotherapeutic responses have allowed

limb salvage in patients with osteosarcoma who sustain a pathological fracture. This group of patients had a slightly higher rate of local recurrence.[12]

Skeletally immature patients became candidates for limb salvage with the development of an expandable prosthesis in the early 1980s. The implantation of this prosthesis into the resected bone allows retention of the skeletally immature limb. Surgery is performed every 6–12 months to expand the prosthesis. Some patients need four expansions.[13] Complications include prosthetic loosening, mechanical failure of the implant, and flexion contracture. Rehabilitation of very young patients is difficult due to the rigors of the physical therapy.

Another option for skeletally immature patients with malignant neoplasm is the Van Nes rotationplasty. The procedure is utilized for distal femur lesions that otherwise would require an above-knee amputation. First, the bone and soft tissue of the thigh are resected while preserving the sciatic nerve. The proximal tibia is internally fixed to the proximal femur after rotating it 180°. The foot is backward. The foot is then used to fit a below-knee prosthesis.[14] The bone takes approximately three months to heal, and the prosthetic fitting ensues. Due to the unusual anatomy, prosthetic fitting and rehabilitation can be prolonged. The advantage of this surgery is that a larger portion of the limb is retained and, therefore, function is improved in terms of both energy and rigorous physical endeavors. The disadvantage of the surgery is the unusual limb appearance when the prosthesis is off. Complications include nonunion and infection.[15] It is another surgical option for young sarcoma patients.

A technique popularized by a Russian surgeon named Ilizarov is beginning to gain acceptance for pediatric tumor reconstruction. After the tumor is resected, bone transposition by distraction osteogenesis is accomplished by making cuts in the remaining proximal and distal bone segments (Figure 46-1). Utilizing an external fixator, these segments are gradually moved. In many months, the defect is closed. The biggest advantage is that the new bone is all from the patient. While infection, especially of pin sites, is a significant concern, it has not been a serious complication. The most problematic issue is the prolonged length the fixator needs to be retained, which is usually 12 months.[16]

Radical resection with reconstruction

In the preoperative period, it is necessary to discuss with the patient and family the postoperative management and rehabilitation of patients with radical resection and reconstruction. The patient, especially a younger one, should be aware that implant failure may occur and further surgery, including amputation, may be necessary. In one study only 67% of the metallic implants were functioning at ten years.[17]

Postoperative management in terms of levels of activity, mobilization, joint motion, weight bearing, the use of bracing devices, or external immobilization will vary according to the amount of bone and soft tissue resected,

cular function distal to the surgical site. Nerve injury may occur during the surgical procedure or postoperatively due to swelling, so the assessment provides the opportunity to observe for changes in sensation and motor function that occur. A splint may be ordered until the nerve recovers.

Blood loss and anemia can result from extensive tumor resection and reconstruction. These patients may be somewhat anemic preoperatively due to adjuvant treatments. Patients with malignancies cannot donate autologous blood but may elect to have their families and friends donate the 4–6 units of blood that may be necessary. Banked blood from the hospital is also available. A drainage tube is placed in the wound for 24–48 hours to prevent hematomas or seromas. Iron supplementation may be prescribed. The nurse monitors the patient's vital signs and laboratory values.[18]

Position restrictions are determined by the surgeon based on operative findings. Limb elevation, length of bedrest, and other restrictions are noted in the chart. Patients who undergo hip arthroplasty may return from surgery with an abductor pillow. For six weeks postoperatively, patients are restricted from flexing the hip over 90°, leg-crossing, or side-lying without a pillow between the legs. If these position restrictions are disregarded, a dislocation of the hip may occur, which is very painful and often shortens the leg. The patient will need to have the hip relocated under sedation or general anesthesia. Occasionally an open reduction is required. Following a dislocation, a hip spica cast or hip orthosis is applied for six weeks to allow the soft tissues to heal.

Postoperative pain occurs after these extensive procedures. Initially pain is managed with epidural catheter continuous infusions of narcotics or a patient-controlled analgesic pump. As pain decreases, milder narcotic tablets such as hydrocodone and nonsteroidal anti-inflammatory tablets are prescribed. Patients are discharged on these oral medications.

Wound necrosis can occur if large flaps are used to close the wound, especially if the surgical site was previously irradiated. Conservative treatments such as debridement and frequent dressing changes may be utilized. Plastic surgeons may be needed to employ a muscle flap (local or free) or split-thickness skin grafts to close the wound.

Postoperative infection remains a significant concern because adjuvant therapies such as chemotherapy may adversely affect patient immunity. Patients are given broad-spectrum antibiotics for 24 hours or longer after surgery and are taught lifelong prevention of implant infection, which could result from a hematogenous source. For example, an abscessed tooth could spill bacteria into the bloodstream and infect the implant. Written instructions are given to the patient (Table 46-3). Considerable bone damage can occur before detection of infection. Once infection is identified, treatment involves removal of the graft or implant, insertion of drains, immobilization, intravenous antibiotic therapy for six weeks, or antibiotic therapy for 6–12 months. Amputation of the

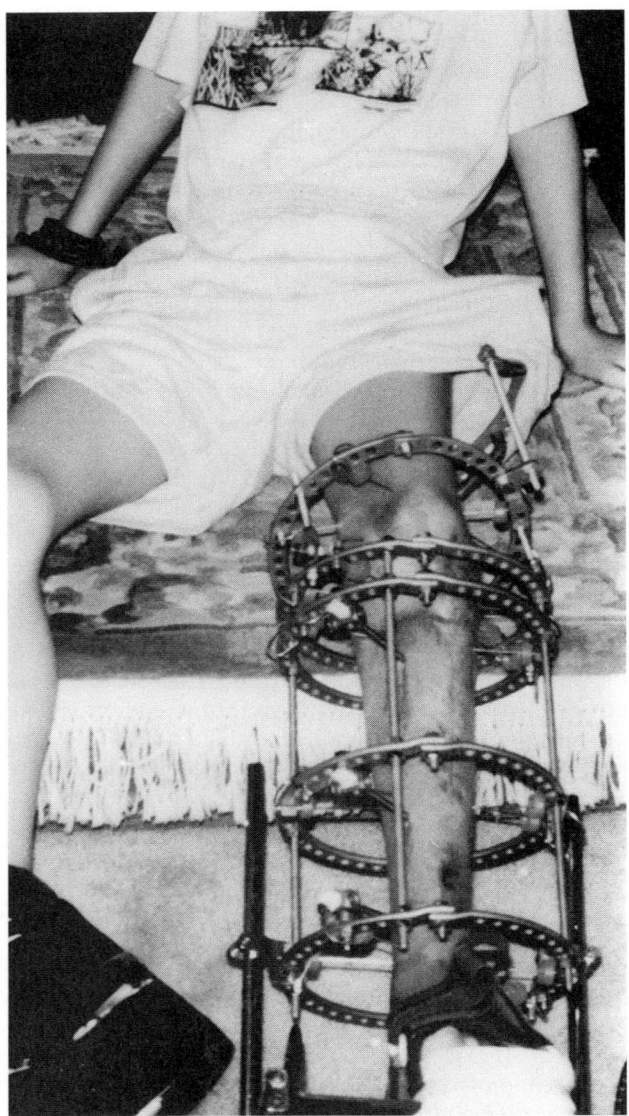

Figure 46-1   Photograph of a boy following a Ilizarov procedure.

and the location and stability of the implant or graft. When more extensive surgery is done, the actual function cannot be predicted as readily as when an amputation is planned. It is important to clarify this postoperatively.

Prevention of postoperative complications begins with preoperative teaching in conjunction with follow-up after surgery. The extensive nature of most resections requires longer exposure to anesthesia, necessitating attention to pulmonary hygiene. In the preoperative period the individual is familiarized with the pulmonary regimen. The patient is also instructed in isometric exercises and ankle pumps to prevent venous stasis. Malignancies, along with immobilization, increase the risk of deep vein thrombosis and pulmonary embolism.

The nurse conducts a baseline assessment of neurovas-

Table 46-3 Implant Infection Precautions

Source of Infection	What to Do
1. Invasive procedures: Surgery Proctoscopy Cystoscopy Endoscopy	Notify your doctor so antibiotics can be given to protect your implant.
2. Dental procedures: Cleaning Extraction Root canal Drilling	Notify your doctor or dentist prior to your appointment so antibiotics can be started before your exam.
3. Wound or abrasion that is red or pus-filled; fever, chills	Immediately see your doctor to determine if antibiotics are needed.
4. Infection in urinary tract, ears, throat, etc.	Immediately see your doctor to determine if antibiotics are needed.

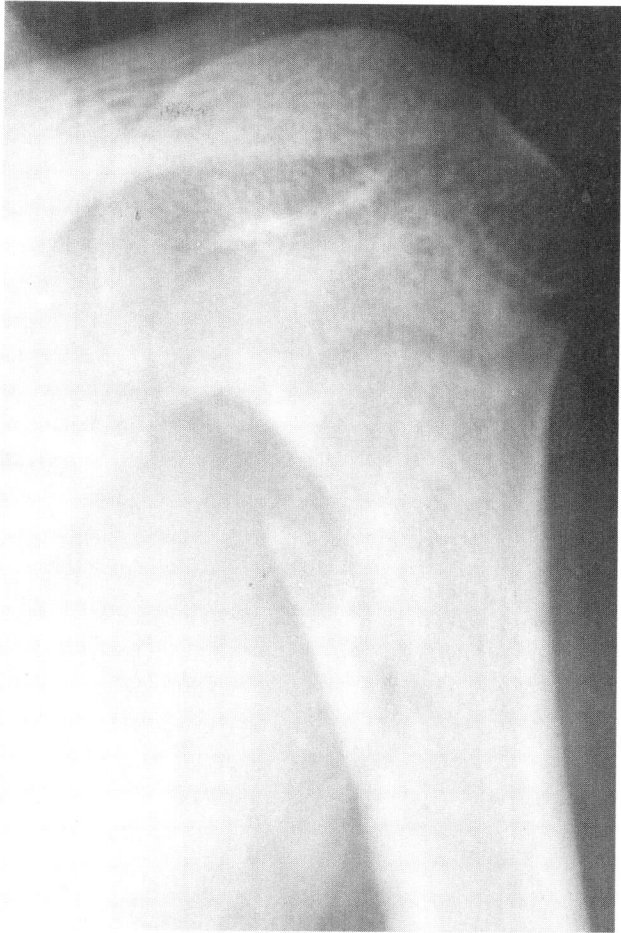

Figure 46-2 Radiograph of Ewing's sarcoma.

limb is a possibility if complications occur. The nurse must be vigilant in observing for signs of infection and in teaching patients about signs and symptoms to report.

Assessment for pneumonia, pulmonary embolism, and deep vein thrombosis is done during the postoperative period. Prophylactic anticoagulation with warfarin, low-molecular-weight heparin, sequential compressive embolic devices, and antiembolic stockings are often utilized for a few weeks.

Functional independence and a gradual adaptation to the changes in body image are the goals of rehabilitation. Resection often involves muscle tissue; therefore, physical therapy regimens often are used to improve and develop muscle tone. Assistive walking and brace devices may be needed if motor function is limited temporarily or permanently. For lower extremity resections, leg length discrepancies may necessitate gait retraining or may be managed simply through the use of shoe lifts. Finally, the importance of safety within the home environment cannot be overemphasized. The length of hospital stay ranges from four to seven days. Most patients who are discharged to their previous home environment are able to negotiate stairs. Lifelong activity restrictions, such as no jogging, heavy lifting, or racquet sports, may be imposed and thereafter alter the individual's career and recreation.

After wide resection, reconstruction to provide stability can be accomplished through the use of metal and synthetic materials; the use of bone autografts, which are those transplanted from one area to another in the same individual; or the use of bone allografts, which are those transferred between two genetically different members of the same species. The three most common methods of reconstruction after sarcoma resection are arthrodesis, arthroplasty with metallic or allograft implant, and intercalary allograft reconstruction (Figure 46-2 and Figure 46-3). Careful consideration should be given to type of reconstruction, particularly in view of the patient's functional needs.

Arthrodesis, or fusion, results in a stiff joint, which is a

handicap for the individual. This form of reconstruction, however, is sturdy and permits activities such as running and jumping. Revision surgery is less likely with this procedure. There are a variety of surgical techniques for arthrodesis that use metallic implants, allograft implants, or autograft bone. Complications include infection and nonunion. Patients who undergo segmental replacement have lower energy cost during gait than those with above-the-knee amputation, which could be a consideration in elderly patients who frequently have compromised cardiac status.

Arthroplasty with metallic or bone allograft implant or a combination of metal and allograft allows maintenance of joint function (Figure 46-4). The entire metallic prosthesis is cemented and allows the quickest recovery. The implant, however, is an artificial joint and will not tolerate percussive activities such as jogging and racquet sports or heavy lifting. Complications include infection, implant fracture, loosening of the implant, and nonunion. In any limb salvage surgery, muscle flaps and skin grafting may be necessary to assist in wound closure. In the tibia region, soft tissue reconstruction, in addition

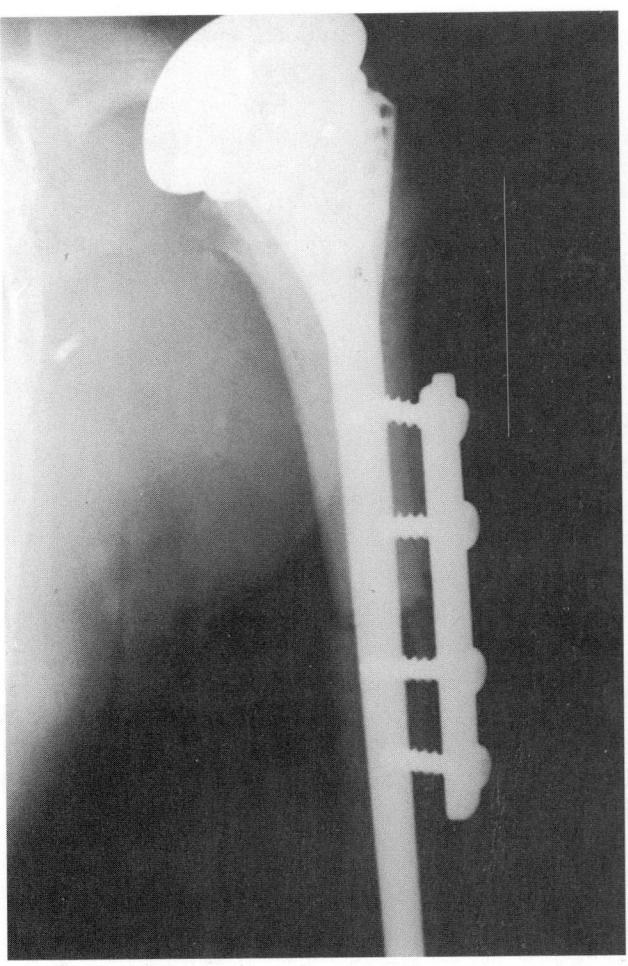

Figure 46-3 Resection of Ewing's sarcoma of the humerus with allograft reconstruction.

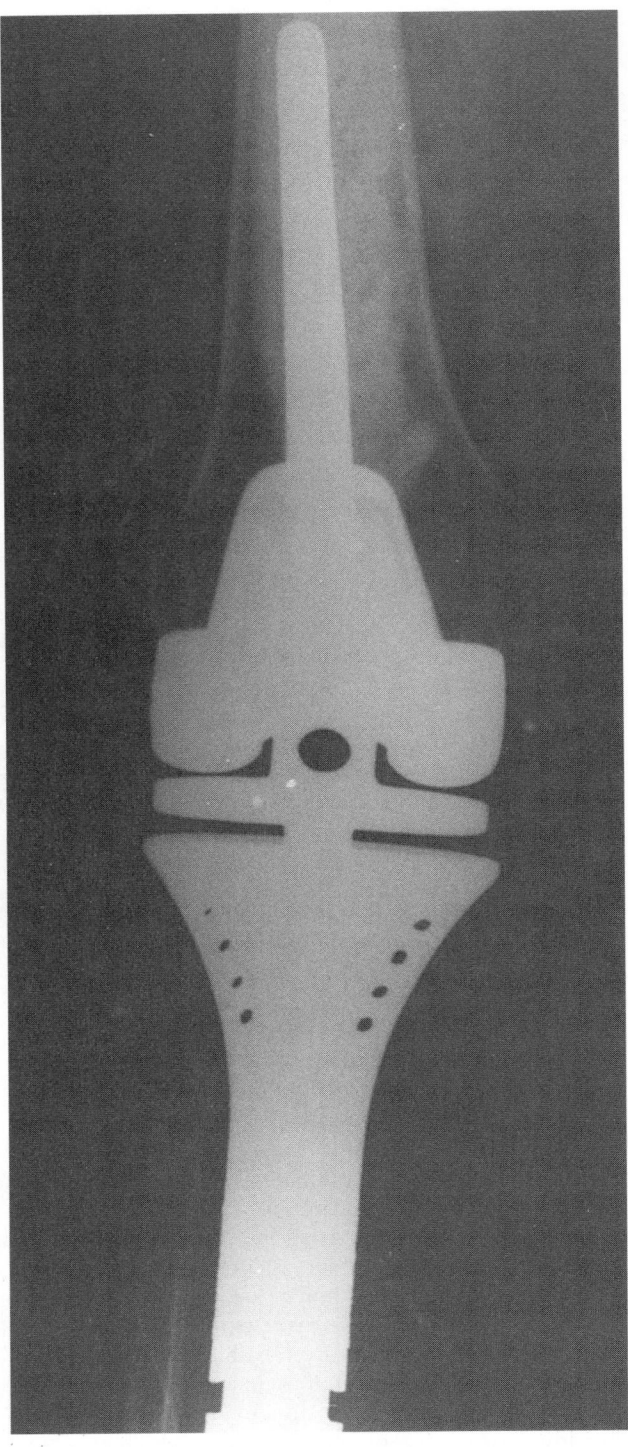

Figure 46-4 Malignant fibrous histiocytoma tibia and postresection with proximal tibia metallic arthroplasty.

to the bone reconstruction, may be needed. The most common local muscle flap used is the gastrocnemius muscle. It assists in eradicating dead space as well as providing coverage of the prosthesis. Frequently, skin grafts are used. The gastrocnemius muscle can also be used for knee extensor reconstruction.

Postoperatively, the patient is kept on bed rest for five days. The limb is monitored for wound necrosis, hematoma, pressure necrosis, and infection. The patient feels referred pain when the transposed muscle is touched. This is a normal sensation. The patient is discharged home in a windowed cast or a locked brace, and is allowed to walk for unlimited amounts of time at two weeks. Chemotherapy or radiation therapy is restarted at three weeks. Knee flexion exercises are started between six to eight weeks postoperatively in order to prevent an extensor lag.[19]

Free flaps are another coverage option. There have been studies to document use of the flaps with radiation and chemotherapy without increased complications.[20] In addition, it has been found that metallic proximal tibia implant patients have gait comparable to above knee prosthetics.[21]

Allografts

The use of allograft bone in tumor reconstruction has gained acceptance since the 1960s. In 1990, according to the American Association of Tissue Banks, an estimated 450,000 patients received transplants of bone, tendon, ligaments, and connective tissue. Among its advantages are that allograft tissue can be custom-sized in the surgical suite; there is no donor site morbidity or size limitation; and joint stability and function are improved by suturing allograft soft tissue attachments to host tissue, which is not possible with metallic implants. Allograft or cadaveric bone is procured in an operating room after consent is obtained from the next of kin. Often the donors have been involved in a motor vehicle accident or other fatal event. They may also donate heart, heart valves, lungs, liver, kidneys, corneas, and blood vessels. The donors are healthy and under 60 years of age. Thorough history and serological tests are performed to screen for viral or bacterial contamination. The chance of transplanting a human immune deficiency virus (HIV) allograft is calculated to be over one in a million.[22]

The bone is frozen, which diminishes its immune response. Bone allograft recipients do not require immuno-suppressive agents, which are often given to organ recipients. Freezing does inhibit cartilage viability, even when cryopreservation agents such as glycerol are applied to the articular surfaces. In a recent study by Enneking and Mindell, 16 retrieved cadaveric allografts were found to have no chondrocytes.[23] When a bone is needed by a surgeon, the medical director of the tissue bank selects an appropriately sized allograft utilizing recipient and allograft radiographs. Tissue typing is not performed. The tissue serves as a scaffold for the new host bone to grow into. The term *osteoconduction* describes this growth of capillaries and osteoprogenitor cells of the host into the allograft.

Osseous and osteochondral intercalary allografts provide a theoretically superior alternative to metallic implants because they provide joint mobility and are biological materials.

In an intercalary allograft, the allograft is placed between two segments of the host bone and actually heals to the host bone after being secured by metallic plates and screws. Research indicates successful results in the replacement of long bone tumors with fresh-frozen allografts.[24] Degenerative arthritis can occur in osteoarticular allografts but can be managed by nonsteroidal anti-inflammatory medications, another osteoarticular allograft, or composite implant.[25,26]

Long-term activity restrictions for individuals undergoing allografts are the same as for those receiving metallic implants. However, the individual needs to limit weight bearing and often must wear a cast or brace, sometimes for up to 6–12 months, until the allograft is healed to the host bone. Complications of this procedure include infection, allograft fracture, and nonunion. The incidence of infection is reported to be 5%.[27] Nonunion may require an autogenous iliac bone graft for one year following surgery. Chemotherapy retards allograft healing; postoperative chemotherapy was found to increase complications from 44%–51%.[24–28] The future of allograft reconstruction appears promising for individuals whose bone is destroyed by malignant tumors.

Metastatic sarcoma

The role of surgery in the management of disseminated disease has gained support in recent years. Sarcomas frequently metastasize to the lung before involving other sites. Twenty percent of patients with high-grade bone and soft tissue sarcomas have pulmonary lesions at the initial presentation. If untreated, most patients with pulmonary metastases will die within 18 months. A CT of the chest and chest x-ray are performed at the time of diagnosis and every three months to assess for extent of disease.[29] Individuals in whom lung metastases develop are good candidates for resection, provided the primary tumor is controlled, there is no indication of other visceral metastatic disease, and the pulmonary nodules are resectable. Wedge excision is the preferred procedure for lung lesions.[30] The nodule is adequately resected without compromising lung function. Patients generally recover rapidly after a thoracotomy or a sternotomy. If a thoracotomy is selected, two procedures are needed for those with bilateral pulmonary disease. The five-year actuarial survival rate is 50%.[31] The only factor predictive of survival after relapse is if the patient can be rendered surgically disease-free.

Radical resection without reconstruction

In soft tissue sarcomas and in bone sarcomas in expendable bones such as a fibula, clavicle, and sections of the pelvis, the resection is performed without any need for reconstruction. Nursing care is similar to that for patients with reconstruction. No lifelong infection concerns exist as no implants are placed.

Amputation

The psychological needs of the individual who undergoes amputation must be considered during preoperative preparation. It is reasonable to assume that the person facing an amputation has fears regarding death, disability, and deformity. In addition, the person may be concerned about the potential loss of social and economic self-sufficiency. These fears and concerns may lead to changes in self-esteem, which can be manifested by anxiety and depression. All these factors will affect the individual's readiness to learn and ability to participate in rehabilitation. Consequently, the plan of care includes interventions aimed at minimizing fear, decreasing anxiety, and promoting realistic optimism. The individual and family are encouraged to express their fears and doubts. Efforts are made to integrate their expectations with reality by providing accurate information from nursing and medical staff regarding the postoperative recovery period and future rehabilitation.

Following hemipelvectomy, the individual may harbor fears concerning sexual adequacy. A woman needs to be reassured that pregnancy and normal delivery are possible even after hemipelvectomy surgery. A decision concerning future pregnancies, however, may be influenced by the fact that the prosthesis cannot be worn during pregnancy. Impotence in a man following hemipelvectomy often is related to age. Loss of erectile capability is due primarily to a decrease in blood supply; however, pelvic nerve function may be compromised following hemipelvectomy. Most men recover potency over time. The younger the individual, the more rapid the recovery of potency.

To reduce anxiety it is sometimes helpful for the person undergoing surgery to meet preoperatively those individuals who will be involved in his or her postoperative care. Depending on the institution's program, this may include physical and occupational therapists, the prosthetist, the social worker, and the psychologist. Likewise, in some instances it may be helpful to arrange a preoperative visit from a person with an amputated limb who has mastered his prosthesis. Information regarding local organizations that train such volunteers can be obtained from the American Cancer Society. Care must be taken in assessing which individuals could benefit by interaction with these resources, however, as an overload of information may serve only to increase the person's anxiety and fear.

The nurse consults social service personnel to inform the patient and family about financial resources and rehabilitation programs available in the state. In general the available resources for individuals with cancer tend to be underutilized. Other support is available through groups such as the American Cancer Society and the American Handicapped Association.

It is important for the nurse to help establish realistic expectations regarding the patient's postamputation function. Many individuals who have lower extremity amputation can expect a return to full function and a relatively normal, active life through the use of a lower limb prosthesis and occasional walking aids. Amputees resume activities such as downhill skiing, swimming, basketball, and cycling with or without recreational prosthesis. It is estimated that 20,000 amputees participate in sporting activities, with more than 5000 participating in organized competition.[32] The person who has a hemicorporectomy is wheelchair-bound. Hemipelvectomy prostheses will approximate only soft tissue, and the use of a walker or crutches will be necessary for additional stability. Because of the significantly increased energy expenditure required, it may be necessary for the person with a more proximal amputation to spend more time in a wheelchair. Elderly patients or those with cardiac conditions may find prosthetic use tiring and may need to use at least a cane.

Ideally, the goal for the individual is independent function with the use of prostheses. In evaluating rehabilitation potential, the nurse considers other factors such as age, effects of adjuvant therapy, the existence of unrelated disease, and the patient's attitude. Prosthetic rehabilitation requires cooperation, coordination, and tremendous physical energy, and a comfortable prosthesis.[33] Lane and colleagues[34] have found that amputees who have received doxorubicin and bleomycin have greater resting heart rates, decreased walking velocity, and increased oxygen requirements. The longer the stump, the lower the energy cost. With this information, they have found patients with lightweight prosthetic devices and three-times-a-week supervised cardiovascular training increased their gait velocity and reduced net energy cost.[34]

Phantom limb phenomenon.   Preoperative teaching includes a discussion of phantom limb sensation and pain. It is a frightening experience for an individual with a recent amputation to feel sensation or pain, or both, in a limb that no longer exists. Consequently, the person who is not adequately prepared may neglect to report the occurrence of the phantom limb phenomenon and may harbor doubts about his sanity.

All individuals who have had an amputation can expect to feel some phantom limb sensation, whereas only some experience phantom limb pain. Phantom limb sensation is described as an awareness of the position or existence of the limb, and usually are experienced shortly after surgery. Itching, pressure, or tingling sensations may be described. Phantom limb pain usually occurs one to four weeks after surgery and is described as severe cramping, throbbing, or burning pain in various areas of the amputated limb. It may be triggered by fatigue, excitement, sickness, weather change, stress, and other stimuli. The incidence and severity of phantom limb pain are greater when the amputation site is more proximal. For many individuals, phantom limb pain resolves gradually in a few months. It is suggested that increased severity of phantom limb pain after a few months may be a symptom of locally recurrent cancer in a stump or it may be a sign of a neuroma.

Phantom limb pain is poorly understood but seems to depend on a combination of physical and emotional factors. The physical component relates to the surgical interruption of neural reflex pathways, with resultant transmission of abnormal patterns of nerve impulses. There is a correlation between the length of time a person experiences limb pain before surgery and the incidence and duration of phantom limb pain. Other factors that contribute to phantom pain include the maladaptive use of pain for secondary gain, the availability of support systems, and the ability to cope with loss.

A variety of measures are used to alleviate phantom limb pain. Simply applying heat to the stump or pressure with elastic bandages can be effective. Distraction and diversion techniques may decrease the person's awareness of the pain. Tranquilizers, local anesthesia, or muscle relaxants are occasionally effective in managing the pain. Recent studies show clonazepam or gabapentin to be useful drugs.[35] Psychotherapy and behavioral therapy also may be useful. Procedures that are available for intractable pain include hypnosis, nerve blocks, sympathectomy, cordotomy, acupuncture, biofeedback, and transcutaneous nerve stimulation. In rare cases revision of the stump with reamputation at a higher level may be done.

Amputation of the lower extremity.   Preoperative preparation of the individual facing a lower extremity amputation incorporates all the considerations routinely given to any person undergoing surgery. The individual who is to have a hemipelvectomy will need to know that a ureteral catheter will be inserted. A preoperative bowel cleansing will be given to decrease the content of the intestinal tract because of the slight chance that bowel would be penetrated intraoperatively.

General strengthening measures and mobility training should be initiated preoperatively by a physical therapist, if time and disease allow. Pull-ups provide preparation for walking with crutches.

The actual postoperative care varies according to whether the individual has had an immediate prosthetic fitting or a conventional delayed prosthetic fitting. Immediate postsurgical prosthetic fittings consist of a rigid dressing and cast applied to the stump at the time of surgery. A socket on the distal end of the cast is designed so that a pylon prosthetic unit may be attached to the cast (Figure 46-5). Restraining straps that go over the shoulder or attach to the waistband contribute to controlled pressure, improved stump shaping, and tissue support provided by the cast.

If a conventional delayed prosthesis fitting is planned, the patient will return from surgery with the stump covered with a dressing and an elastic bandage. To shrink and shape the stump, elastic bandages or elastic stump shrinkers are used until the first fitting (Figure 46-6). The individual is fitted with a temporary or intermediate prosthesis at approximately three to six weeks, when acute swelling has decreased. An intermediate prosthesis, however, lacks a cosmetic covering. Ambulation with weight bearing is encouraged as tolerated. Approximately three months after surgery, the individual is fitted with a permanent prosthesis, with or without immediate postsurgical fitting. Chemotherapy may change stump size and delay fitting of permanent prosthesis.

The relative advantages and disadvantages of immediate and delayed prosthesis fitting are summarized in Table 46-4. Postoperatively, the stump usually is elevated for 24 hours after surgery to prevent edema and promote venous return. To prevent hip contractures, the individual is assisted into the prone position three to four times a day for a minimum of 15 minutes and encouraged to assume that position for sleep. Exercises to maintain muscle tone and prevent edema, joint contractures, and muscle atrophy are initiated on the first postoperative day. Exercises include active range of motion, strengthening exercises for the upper extremities, and hyperextension of the stump.

Stump care involves frequent wrapping with elastic-bandages or stump shrinkers to facilitate stump shrinking or monitoring cast. Dangling transfer to a chair and crutch walking are encouraged on the first postoperative day. For the individual having a hemipelvectomy, mobilization also is possible on the second or third postoperative day. Length of stay ranges from two to five days depending on level of amputation. Below-knee amputees may have a two-day stay, while hip disarticulation patients may need five days.

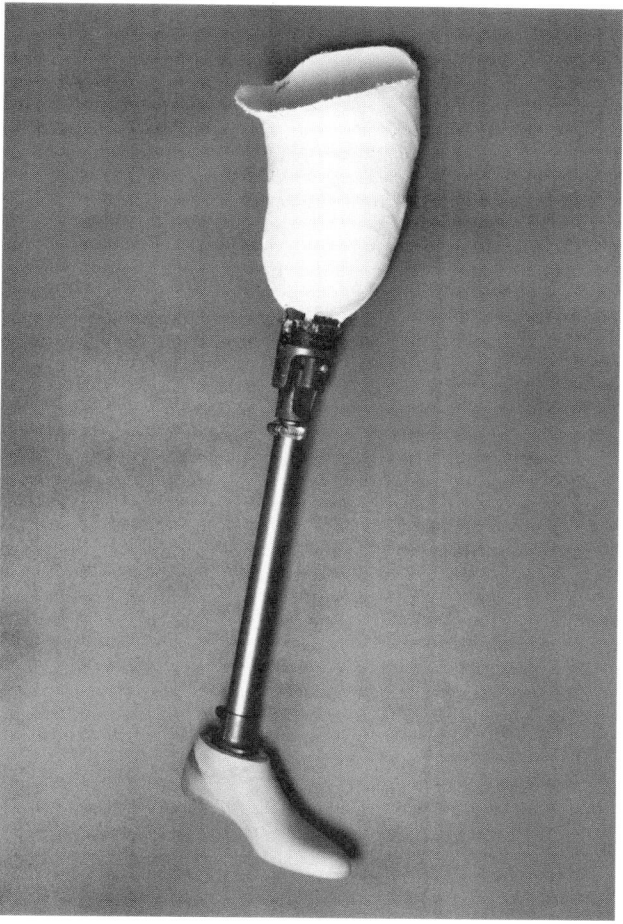

Figure 46-5 Immediate postsurgical prosthetic fitting with a pylon prosthetic unit attached to the cast.

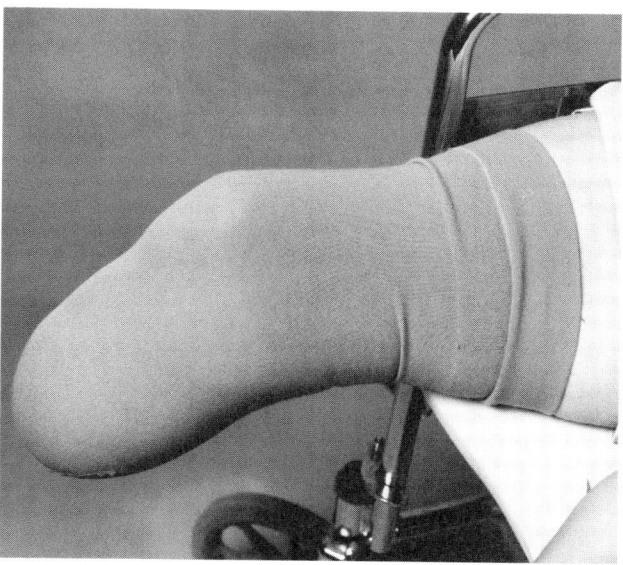

Figure 46-6 Elastic stump shrinker applied to shape stump.

Table 46-4 Relative Advantages and Disadvantages of Delayed Versus Immediate Prosthetic Fitting

	Delayed Fitting	Immediate Fitting
Advantages	Wound can be inspected for healing. Skin can be conditioned by Ace wraps and stump shrinkers.	Better emotional adjustment with immediate substitute limb. Motivation increased with early ambulation with limb. Decreased stump edema, pain, phantom limb pain, and contractures (caused by pressure of device).
Disadvantages	Edema delays shrinking and shaping of stump. Continuous rewrapping with elastic bandages is required. Attention must be given to prevention of contractures and other complications of immobility.	Wound cannot be visualized. Temporary prosthesis is heavy. Poor gait pattern can develop because of heavy prosthesis and discomfort in early ambulation period. Prosthetist must go to operating room to apply.

A sitting or bucket prosthesis may be needed for an individual with a hemipelvectomy because of the absence of an ischium on which to sit. Until the bucket prosthesis is fabricated, a pillow is placed under the surgical site for balance.

The nurse may make a referral to a home nurse, home physical therapist, and local rehabilitation programs involved with vocational rehabilitation. Most individuals with amputated limbs are capable of eventually returning to work with restrictions.

Teaching the individual how to care for the stump is an element of the rehabilitation program. The patient must perform daily stump hygiene with the use of a mild soap and water. The patient also should be instructed to avoid the use of skin creams, oils, and rubbing alcohol. Daily inspection for redness, blisters, or abrasions should be incorporated into the patient's routine. Stump socks or elastic wraps should fit properly and be changed daily. When the wound has healed, the individual can prevent edema by putting on the prosthesis immediately after arising and keeping it on all day. The individual with an immediate postsurgical prosthetic fitting also should be instructed regarding cast care and inspection for fit.

The individual is also taught how to put on and care for the prosthesis. The prosthesis socket is wiped out daily with a damp cloth. Care is taken to thoroughly dry the socket to prevent a source of skin irritation and prosthesis rust. The individual is taught the importance of never attempting to make mechanical adjustments to the prosthesis. Discomfort or difficulties necessitate a visit to the prosthetist.

The physician and prosthetist collaborate in planning the construction of the prosthetic device. The prosthetist is responsible for the construction and fit of the prosthesis and should be certified by the American Board for Certification of Prosthetists. Lower limb prostheses generally consist of a socket, suspension such as a waistband or suction or latex sleeve, knee joint, ankle joint, and foot (Figure 46-7). Many varieties of these components are available, which can be combined to meet the needs of each individual. For example, knee joints are available

that provide either mechanical or hydraulic assistance in controlling the swing phase of walking and provide increased stability during standing. Energy-storage prosthetic feet such as the Seattle foot are made with a flexible heel that releases the energy of foot fall at terminal stage

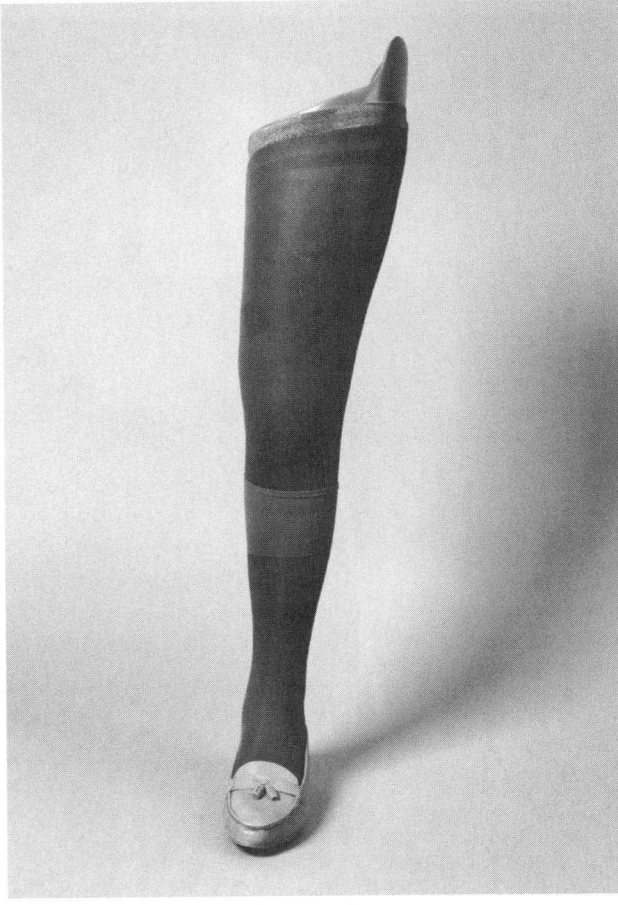

Figure 46-7 Lower limb prosthesis for an above-knee amputation.

to help initiate swing phase. These features, however, increase weight, cost, and maintenance. An above-knee prosthesis weighs approximately 3 kg and a below-knee prosthesis 1 kg. In designing the prosthesis, consideration is given to the person's age, ability, endurance, financial status, occupational goals, and motivation as well as comfort, fit, alignment, safety, ease of application, and appearance. The primary nurse can assess these factors and communicate them to the prosthetist.

After discharge, the individual with an amputation should be seen by the prosthetist every four to six weeks for the first year. The rehabilitation process is complete when the individual has attained an optimal level of independence and has successfully incorporated the prosthesis into his or her body image.

Amputation of the upper extremity.   Many of the considerations concerning preoperative, postoperative, and rehabilitative care discussed in the preceding section apply to individuals having an upper extremity amputation. There are, however, some significant differences.

Upper limb prostheses are far less satisfactory in both appearance and function than those created for lower extremities. The functional capabilities of the prosthesis for upper extremity amputation decrease as the level of amputation becomes more proximal. Power and motion are supplied in only a comparatively gross fashion. The most functional terminal (hand) device is a hook. The development of a substitute for the complex actions of the intricate muscles of the hand has thus far been impossible. Adequate cosmetic appearance can be obtained at the expense of function. Polyvinyl cosmetic gloves with realistic skin creases, veins, and hair are available. Skin tones are matched but the shade changes that occur in the normal hand as a result of position and season cannot be reproduced. In addition, the glove must be replaced frequently because ink, newsprint, and other stains are impossible to remove.

Conventional prostheses for the upper extremities consist of a hand terminal device, a harness to supply force from the proximal muscles, appropriate segments between them, including a socket for the stumps, and a cable system that provides motion at the terminal device and/or the elbow. Abduction of the scapula or flexion of the shoulder on the side of the prosthesis initiates movement. Flexion and extension of the wrist usually are omitted, although wrist units in flexed or extended positions are available. Pronation and supination are achieved by rotating the terminal device with the opposite hand. Likewise, opening and closing of the terminal device are accomplished through the use of the opposite hand.

Prostheses for interscapulothoracic amputations are fitted over the upper portion of the chest. Motion is severely limited because sources of power are unavailable. Some force can be initiated from the opposite shoulder and chest expansion. The primary function of the prosthesis, however, is cosmetic. Rejection of the upper ex-

tremity prosthetic devices occurs more often than with prostheses of the lower extremity because of a combination of poor function, low cosmetic value, and lack of motivation.

Upper extremity prosthetic research has been directed at the development of myoelectric limb substitution. In this system, electrical impulses from the contraction of extensor and flexor muscle in the stump are picked up by electrodes in the socket and are in turn amplified, switching on and off electrical motors in the prosthesis. An external battery pack may be worn to provide an additional electrical supply. Opening and closing of the terminal device, pronation and supination, and elbow flexion can be provided. The individual must be assessed first for the ability to elicit and control myoelectric signals. The advantages include an increase in control with less energy expenditure and improved physical appearance. The disadvantages include the cost of the device, electrical interference, or inadvertent contraction of the muscles when the user coughs or stretches.

The inadequacy of available upper limb prostheses can be disappointing for the person with an upper limb amputation. The nurse, in conjunction with the physician, provides information regarding the functional and cosmetic features of the upper extremity prostheses. It is important to discuss with the individual the negative social stigma attached to the hook, as well as its functional capabilities. Equal emphasis should be placed on the functional limitations and cosmetic value of the glove. Some individuals are willing to sacrifice function to obtain the best cosmetic replacement.

As with lower extremity amputations, immediate or delayed postsurgical prosthesis fitting is possible. When delayed fitting is planned, the individual will return from surgery with a soft dressing and elastic bandages covering the stump. Compression of the surgical area is to be avoided until healing takes place. Length of stay is one to two days.

As with the lower extremity amputation, independence and an adapted body image can be facilitated through psychological support, patient and family education, and appropriate referral to community resources. Rehabilitation goals emphasize using the remaining arm for activities of daily living. The patient should be evaluated preoperatively by an occupational therapist for information on one-handedness. Vocational rehabilitation assumes particular importance for the individual with an upper extremity amputation because the ensuing disability could prevent the resumption of previous employment.

Radiotherapy

The use of radiotherapy in the management of primary or metastatic malignant bone or soft tissue sarcoma depends on the radiosensitivity of the particular tumor type. Most bone tumors are relatively unresponsive to radiation. Consequently, radiation is reserved for palliation and may be used in conjunction with chemotherapy for inoperable tumors or in conjunction with surgery to reduce the tumor load of partially resectable tumors. Conventional radiation doses for palliative treatment of primary bone tumors often result in fibrosis and contractures that lead to amputation even if the tumor is controlled. Neutron beam therapy, however, which is produced by heavy particle accelerators, can deliver higher doses with fewer complications. At the Fermilab Neutron Therapy Facility in Batavia, Illinois, individuals were treated with neutron beam therapy for bone sarcoma in the axial skeleton or when surgery was refused for cosmetic or emotional reasons. The local control rate was 44%. Neutron beam irradiation may be an effective option for nonresectable sarcoma.[36]

In contrast, radiotherapy plays an integral role in the management of Ewing's sarcoma and soft tissue sarcomas. Complications of treatment include tendon contractures, edema of the involved extremity distal to the site of irradiation, cessation of growth of the extremity, and nonhealing fractures.

In soft tissue sarcomas, preoperative and postoperative radiation gave the same results, but preoperative radiation gave greater wound infections. Brachytherapy or loading catheters in surgical wounds may be used for the soft tissue sarcoma.

Regional hyperthermia is a technique of raising the temperature in a tumor to 42°C for approximately one hour. In a study of 40 patients with advanced sarcoma, regional hyperthermia along with ifosfamide plus etoposide was employed. There were 38 assessable patients, of whom only six had a complete response.[37] The treatment can be painful, with high systematic temperature and tachycardia occurring during the procedure. Complications include local infection, thrombosis, burns, and hematoma. Regional hyperthermia is not commonly utilized in the United States for sarcoma.

Chemotherapy and Immunotherapy

Since the addition of postoperative chemotherapy to the treatment of bone sarcomas in the early 1970s, survival rates have increased from 20% to more than 50%.[38] Currently chemotherapy is given preoperatively as well as postoperatively. The rationale for preoperative chemotherapy is to treat the micrometastasis, to decrease the primary tumor size, thereby increasing the likelihood of limb salvage surgery, and to assess the effectiveness of the chemotherapeutic agents for two to three months. The route of chemotherapy is either intravenous or intraarterial. The duration of treatment ranges from 6–12 months. Adjuvant chemotherapy for soft tissue sarcomas is considered experimental; it is discussed further in a later section.

Toxic effects are decreased by administering agents to counter the effects. Ifosfamide can cause hemorrhagic cystitis, but mesna, a sulfhydryl scavenger, can inactivate metabolites in urine and prevent this complication. It can also cause renal tubular defects and renal failure most commonly in children.[39] High-dose methotrexate can cause renal toxicities, but calcium leucovorin or citrovorum factor can ameliorate this toxicity. The systemic effects of chemotherapy such as neutropenia and thrombocytopenia may create wound complications.[40] Neutropenia may increase incidence of infection but not necessarily impede wound healing. Administration of granulocyte stimulators diminishes the severity of neutropenia, thereby enhancing the chemotherapeutic effect of a drug.

Classification of Certain Sarcomas

Osteosarcoma

Osteosarcoma is the most common osseous malignant bone tumor. Its incidence is greatest in individuals age 10 to 25 and it affects males twice as often as females. The incidence of osteosarcoma peaks again in older adults with Paget's disease. The increased incidence of osteosarcoma during adolescence has been correlated with skeletal growth patterns, which in turn may account for the greater overall occurrence in males.[9]

Osteosarcoma appears to arise from primitive bone-forming mesenchyma in the medullary cavity. Proliferating connective tissue generally gives rise to tumor osteoid and bone directly. The proliferating connective tissue also may form some tumor cartilage that undergoes rapid osseous transformation. Surface osteosarcoma includes periosteal and parosteal types.[41] Periosteal osteosarcoma, a variant of osteosarcoma, was originally described by Unni et al.[11] It occurs as a hard mass on the bone surface, especially the tibia and knee. The tumor is confined to the periosteum and cortex without a medullary component. Tumors are low to intermediate grade and usually nonmetastatic. Periosteal or juxtacortical osteosarcomas occur also on bony surfaces, especially the posterior femur and humerus. They are often low grade.

The histological pattern of osteosarcoma is so variable that no two specimens are exactly alike. Specimens have varying mixtures of malignant bone, malignant cartilage, and malignant stroma. Consequently, the tumor may be described as osteoblastic, chondroblastic, or fibroblastic, depending on which component is dominant. Whatever the pattern, the essential criteria for the diagnosis of osteosarcoma are the presence of frankly sarcomatous stroma and the formation of tumor osteoid and bone by malignant connective tissue.

The most frequent sites of osteosarcoma include the distal end of the femur, the proximal end of the tibia, and the proximal end of the humerus. Osteosarcomas may be discovered in the iliac bone, vertebral column, mandible, and in rare cases the scapula, clavicle, or bones in the hands and feet. Humeral and tibial lesions have a better prognosis.[42]

Metastatic spread occurs primarily to the lungs by the hematogenous route. Radiological evidence of pulmonary or bony metastases usually appears within 24 months of the definitive surgery. Late metastasis in one or more of the other bones occurs occasionally, often in the presence of pulmonary metastases.

Half of the individuals with osteosarcoma have an elevated serum alkaline phosphatase level. This level, which represents osteoblastic activity, tends to decline after removal of the tumor and to return to the initially high level in the presence of pulmonary metastasis. Those who present with markedly elevated levels have higher relapse rates.[43] In the normal growing child the levels are elevated. Other laboratory data do not appear to be significant in the diagnosis of osteosarcoma.

The classic radiological features of osteosarcoma include cortical bone destruction, extension of the tumor into soft tissue, and periosteal new bone formation that may appear in a perpendicular striated, or "sunburst," pattern. These findings can be diagnostic on plain radiographs.

The five-year survival rate for individuals treated with surgery alone or irradiation and surgery has been approximately 10%.[44] The high mortality rate is due principally to pulmonary metastasis, which is assumed to be present microscopically at the time of presentation. Reports evaluating adjuvant chemotherapy after surgery for osteosarcoma indicate a significant prolongation of the disease-free interval. Reports from the 1970s show that the five-year survival rate increased from 40% to 60% with the use of adjuvant chemotherapy using single agents. Current chemotherapy protocols have used doxorubicin, high-dose cyclophosphamide, or high-dose methotrexate with leucovorin rescue. Most agents are given on an outpatient basis either intravenously or intra-arterially. Bacci and colleagues[44] and Glasser and Lane[42] demonstrated an 87% disease-free state at two years to 77% at five years. When preoperative or primary chemotherapy is used, effectiveness is assessed at the time of tumor resection. This regimen allows an in vivo study of the tumor cells. During the 8–20 weeks of preoperative chemotherapy, physical examination of the tumor site is performed to assess for effectiveness of treatment by indices such as decreased pain and swelling. If there is 90% tumor necrosis, the high-dose methotrexate regimen is continued postoperatively for six months. The greater the necrosis, the greater the survival. If tumor necrosis is less, the chemotherapy is changed to ifosfamide and etoposide. The course is extended to 8–12 months.[45]

The improved results of chemotherapy have sparked interest in limb salvage resections. The chemotherapy can result in a decrease in the soft tissue component and ossification of the bony component. Surgery is planned after preoperative chemotherapy. The limb salvage criteria apply to these patients. Amputations are indicated for patients with large and invasive tumors. It is advisable to obtain a second opinion if an amputation is recommended. Local recurrence is as frequent in amputation surgery as in limb salvage surgeries (under 5%).[44] Resumption of chemotherapy after definitive surgery is delayed for one to two weeks.

Significant improvement of patient survival with metastatic disease was demonstrated in the 1980s. Of patients with osteosarcoma who had thoracotomies for metastases, 40% were free of disease more than two years after surgery.[30] No patients survived the development of pulmonary metastases unless they had surgical resection of gross disease. In these cases, chemotherapy is given after thoracotomy to eradicate microscopic disease.

Radiation is reserved for palliation or inoperable cases. Significant morbidity and mortality were reported when irradiation alone was used for treatment of the primary tumor.

Chondrosarcoma

Chondrosarcoma accounts for approximately 14% of malignant bone tumors. The incidence is greatest in individuals age 30 to 60 and among males.[9]

The occurrence of chondrosarcomas has been associated with syndromes of skeletal maldevelopment. Transformation of osteochondroma, multiple enchondromas, Ollier disease, or chondroplasia to chondrosarcoma has occurred. Chondrosarcoma arises from the cartilage and never has osteoid tissue.

There are both primary and secondary chondrosarcomas. The former includes central chondrosarcomas that arise in the medullary cavity. The latter includes those chondrosarcomas that arise from benign tumors.

The diagnosis of chondrosarcoma is based on cytological changes of the cartilage cells. A cartilage tumor is considered malignant in the presence of many cells with plump nuclei, that is, more than a few cells with two such nuclei or clumps of chromatin.

The most frequent sites of chondrosarcoma are the pelvic bone, long bones, scapula, and ribs. Less frequent sites are bones of the hand and foot, the nose, the maxilla, and the base of the skull.

Most chondrosarcomas do not tend to metastasize early but rather remain slow-growing and locally invasive. When advanced chondrosarcoma does become aggressive, it tends to metastasize via venous channels to the lungs and heart. Regional lymph nodes or other bones occasionally may be involved. Individuals with chondrosarcoma usually have a relatively long but unremarkable history. Medical advice often is sought for a slow-growing mass with intermittent dull, aching pain at the tumor site.

Radiographs of chondrosarcoma show a lobular pattern with or without calcification. If calcification is present, it usually is seen in a circular or semicircular pattern. Central chondrosarcomas in the long bones may show thickening of the cortex because of swelling of the shaft. The peripheral chondrosarcoma may demonstrate a vast, dense, blotchy appearance. Ragged, irregular, radiopaque streaks extending away from the central part of the lesion may be seen.

When the diagnosis of chondrosarcoma has been established, surgery is indicated. If the tumor is of central origin and has not extended through the cortex, wide resection and reconstruction are considered. Limb salvage surgery and amputation are options.

At present, chondrosarcoma remains nearly totally refractory to chemotherapeutic efforts inasmuch as chondrosarcomas usually have a poor blood supply. Consequently, drugs given IV do not reach the tumor in concentrations that are high enough to be effective. The benefit of chemotherapy as an adjuvant to surgery has not been established.

Radiotherapy, usually neutrons, has limited effectiveness and is reserved for palliation of advanced or inoperable chondrosarcomas.

Individuals with a diagnosis of chondrosarcoma have a considerably better prognosis than those with osteosarcoma. The overall survival rate of individuals treated with wide resection or amputation has been reported to be 50% at ten years.[9] In this series survival correlated well with the designated histological grade of the lesion.

Fibrosarcoma

Fibrosarcoma is rare, accounting for fewer than 7% of primary malignant bone tumors.[9] This type of neoplasm may occur at any age but is rare in children. There is no evident sex predominance.

Paget's disease may be a predisposing factor in the development of fibrosarcoma. In addition, the tumor may develop as a sequel to therapeutic irradiation or may develop at the site of an old bone infarct. Chronic osteomyelitis or fibrous dysplasia also may be a predisposing factor in the development of fibrosarcoma.

Fibrosarcoma is a malignant fibroblastic tumor that fails to develop tumor osteoid or bone in its local invasive growth site or in its metastatic foci. Periosteal new bone may be laid down as a direct extension of the tumor.

Like osteosarcoma, fibrosarcoma usually originates within the medullary cavity. It eventually penetrates the overlying cortex and extends into the periosteum and muscle. Occasionally a fibrosarcoma may arise periosteally and extend into the interior of contiguous bone.

Histological findings show that fibrosarcomas range from well differentiated to poorly differentiated. Rapidly growing tumors reflect cytological changes such as moderate anaplasia, cell irregularity, and many mitotic figures, and they tend to metastasize early. Less aggressive fibrosarcomas develop more slowly, taking longer to penetrate the cortex of the bone. Some fibrosarcomas are surprisingly indolent in their growth patterns and may show very little change over a period of years.

The femur and the tibia, the most common sites of occurrence, account for 50% of all fibrosarcomas. The neoplasm also may be observed in the humerus, radius, ulna, skull, and facial and pelvic bones. Metastasis occurs primarily to the lungs. Individuals with fibrosarcoma, like those with other primary bone tumors, usually have pain and swelling of the affected area.

When the diagnosis of fibrosarcoma has been estab-

lished, surgery is indicated. Limb and salvage amputations are options. Fibrosarcoma is considered to be radioresistant; consequently, the use of radiotherapy is reserved for inoperable tumors. Adjuvant chemotherapy programs after surgical treatment are being evaluated for reducing the incidence of microscopic residual metastatic disease.[9]

The prognosis for fibrosarcoma is guarded. The five- and ten-year survival rates after radical surgery have been reported at 28% and 21.8%, respectively.[9]

Ewing's Sarcoma

Ewing's sarcoma accounts for 6% of all malignant bone tumors.[9] Eighty percent of such tumors are diagnosed in individuals age 5 to 15, with more males affected than females. These patients are younger than any other patient affected by primary malignant bone tumors. The development of Ewing's sarcoma has not been strongly linked to any specific etiological factor.

Ewing's sarcoma is a primitive, multicentric tumor that appears to be derived from the mesenchymal connective tissue framework of bone marrow. The tumor usually arises in the marrow spaces in the shaft of long bones and rarely involves the epiphysis.

On microscopic examination, Ewing's sarcoma is characterized by the presence of uniform cells with indistinct borders. These cells are packed closely together and contain prominent round or ovoid nuclei and have finely divided chromatin.

No one site seems to predominate in the development of Ewing's sarcoma. The tumor commonly is situated in the pelvis and the diaphyseal or metadiaphyseal regions of long bones. Ewing's sarcomas metastasize early and most frequently involve the lungs. Bone marrow aspirate and biopsy is done at diagnosis. The lymph nodes and the skull are other frequent sites of metastasis. On autopsy, a considerable portion of skeleton is affected. It is unclear whether these bone lesions represent metastatic spread or independent development of disease in multiple sites. Metastasis may be present in nearly 20% of individuals at the time of diagnosis.

Many individuals have fever, anemia, high erythrocyte sedimentation rates, and sometimes leukocytosis at presentation. These symptoms can lead to an incorrect diagnosis of osteomyelitis. It has been observed that such findings result in a fulminating disease course that ends in death within a few months. Individuals who did not initially have such findings tended to survive longer. Wilkins and colleagues noted that normal lactic dehydrogenase, small distal primary lesion (< 8 cm), and the absence of metastasis were better prognostic factors for the patient with Ewing's sarcoma.[46]

Radiographs of Ewing's sarcoma show bone destruction that involves the shaft. Varying amounts of periosteal thickening may be present, with "onion" layers of laminated subperiosteal new bone. A large soft tissue mass frequently will be seen as well.

Initially treatment consisted of radiation with chemotherapy. Local recurrence rates of 21%–30% were theorized to have been caused by small foci of persistent tumor retained in each lesion.[46] Currently, integrated therapy with radiation and surgery in combination with chemotherapy is the treatment of choice for Ewing's sarcoma. Consequently, primary chemotherapy, as prophylactic therapy for micrometastases in bone and lung and to decrease tumor bulk in order to lessen the need for local therapy, is used as part of the initial treatment for all Ewing's patients. Using actinomycin, doxorubicin, vincristine, and cyclophosphamide, Wilkins and colleagues[46] reported an actuarial five-year disease-free survival rate of 40%–74%. Ifosfamide and etoposide are agents with a response rate approaching 50%.[47] Treatment usually takes place for 6–12 months and is often administered in an outpatient setting. Local treatment (surgery and/or radiation) begins approximately three months after the beginning of chemotherapy.

Ewing's tumor is extremely radiosensitive and capable of being cured locally with 50–60 Gy by means of shrinking fields. The National Cancer Institute reports a 3% incidence of radiation-induced sarcoma after combined chemotherapy and radiation in Ewing's patients.[48] In addition to this complication, growth plate injuries in skeletally immature patients, fibrosis of soft tissue, and joint contractures may occur.

Limb salvage and amputation are both options to be considered for local control of a Ewing's sarcoma. The goal is to eradicate the tumor and maintain function. Ideally, surgery only will be needed. If margins are close, surgery followed by radiotherapy improves the local control rate.[48]

Patients with metastases at the time of presentation are similarly treated, with a five-year survival rate of 30%. Ifosfamide is often utilized as a single agent for patients who have relapsed. There is ongoing research to evaluate its effectiveness as part of standard therapy for relapsed Ewing's sarcoma patients. Bone marrow transplants have also shown effectiveness.[49]

Soft Tissue Sarcomas

The histological subtypes of soft tissue sarcomas include malignant fibrous histiocytoma, liposarcoma, fibrosarcoma, synovial sarcoma, rhabdomyosarcoma, and leiomyosarcoma. They occur over 50% of the time in extremities; the remainder occur in the head and neck and retroperitoneum.

Soft tissue sarcomas invade surrounding tissue along the anatomic planes. They compress surrounding tissue and form a pseudocapsule, which contains tentacles of tumor. A marginal excision will never cure a soft tissue sarcoma. The local recurrence rate of this procedure is close to 100%.

Nodal metastases are common with a small amount of subtypes: synovial sarcomas (17%), epithelioid sarcoma (20%), and rhabdomyosarcoma (12%).[50] Lymph node involvement is a poor prognostic sign.

The more proximal lesions are usually larger since, in the retroperitoneum, buttock, or thigh, they can be disregarded until they are massive. A tumor that is superficial and smaller than 5 cm is felt to have a better prognosis.

Some histological subtypes such as rhabdomyosarcomas, synovial sarcomas, and malignant histiocytomas are considered poor prognosticators due to their high grade. However, any high-grade soft tissue sarcoma is ominous. Detectable pulmonary metastasis is more common in the high-grade soft tissue sarcomas. Typically, the first two years will reveal metastases and local recurrences. However, rhabdomyosarcomas in children are very sensitive to chemotherapy.

The five-year survival percentages of soft tissue sarcomas range from 30%–95% based on subtype and grade.[9] The range for extremity sarcomas is 90%–95%, for trunk sarcomas 50%–75%, and for retroperitoneal lesions 30%–50%. In each of the three locations, higher-grade sarcomas have a poorer survival rate.

It is not uncommon for the surgeon to surgically remove a mass and, after routine pathological examination, learn it is a malignant sarcoma. In this situation microscopic tumor is usually found at the surgical site. It is recommended that a reexcision of the tumor bed be performed immediately following the definitive diagnosis of sarcomas. Occasionally, the second surgical excision will reveal no evidence of microscopic tumor cells. It is vital to ensure that no cells are left behind in order to avoid a local recurrence.[51]

In the optimal situation, imaging (Figures 46-8, 46-9) is performed prior to biopsy of the tumor. If the tumor is small and superficial, a primary myectomy (en bloc resection of tumor) may be recommended. The patient is informed that no biopsy will be done prior to the resection. The advantage behind this surgical decision is to prevent cells from leaking during biopsy and also to avoid a second surgery. The disadvantage is that occasionally the final histology will reveal a benign diagnosis, which could have been removed in a less radical manner. In most cases an incisional biopsy is performed.

The timing of surgery is based on the need for radiation. If radiation is deemed unnecessary, as in a subcutaneous or intramuscular tumor with no impingement on neurovascular structure, a salvage or amputation surgery is performed. Larger tumors may be excised after pretreatment with radiation.

A wide excision is defined as more than 3 cm of normal tissue. This procedure controls local disease in 90% of persons. If the pathologist notes a lesser margin, radiation is given.

The advantage of postoperative radiation is that it allows for thorough histological grading and diagnosis. There is no delay in surgery. Wound healing is uncomplicated. At the time of surgery, the tumor margin can be outlined with a radiopaque clips. Currently, this radiation timing is utilized for sarcomas that are widely resected with or without a close margin. The dose is 60–65 Gy to the tumor bed with 45–50 Gy to all tissues disrupted during the procedure.

Preoperative radiation has the advantage of a small

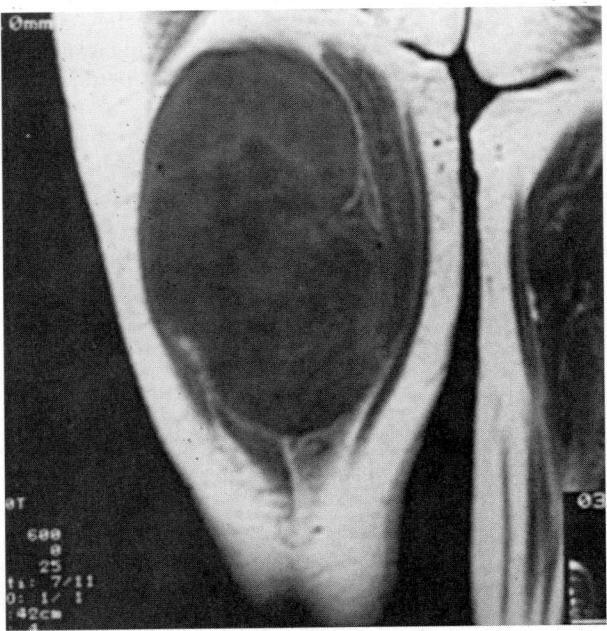 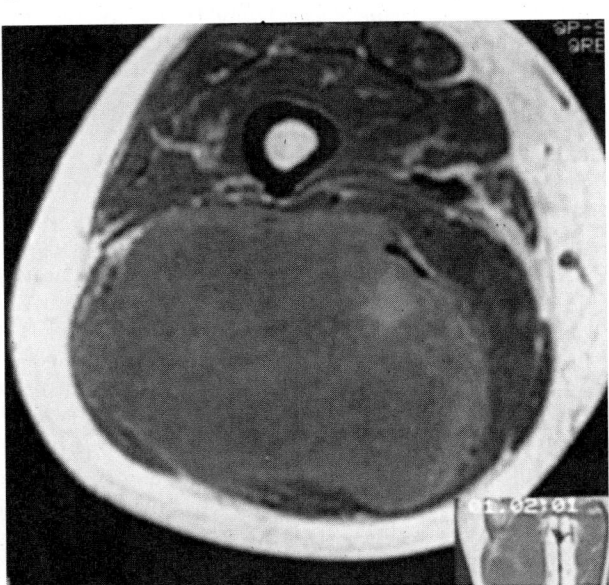

Figures 46-8, 46-9   MRI imaging of a 62-year-old female with an enlarging posterior thigh mass. Biopsy revealed a liposarcoma. Both axial (46-8) and coronal (46-9) views reveal the large mass, which was treated with preoperative irradiation and limb salvage surgery.

treatment area with fewer complications. It does require more preplanning with the surgeon and the radiation oncologist. The patient may be deemed to be a candidate for limb salvage surgery with preoperative irradiation if the tumor has regressed. A series of radiation administered preoperatively has a 24% wound complication rate, which is higher than postoperative radiation programs.[52] This may reflect patient selection with larger tumors. Surgery is delayed for three to six weeks following the cessation of radiation. If margins are close, additional radiation may be ordered. Another theoretical advantage of preoperative radiation is that the pseudocapsule surrounding the tumor becomes thicker and is easier and safer to remove.

In the 1980s a regimen of chemotherapy consisting of doxorubicin was given intraarterially, followed by 35 Gy of radiation. Local tumor control approached 90%, but the complication rate was very high at 35% and consisted of wound sloughs and fractures. Nevertheless, some centers continue to use this method.

Brachytherapy is a technique in which catheters are placed in the tumor bed during surgery and one to two days later loaded with radioactive sources such as iridium 192. This method is utilized with a large, deep tumor that is close to a neurovascular bundle. It is a technically tedious procedure. In a randomized prospective study, 117 patients who received brachytherapy were found to have decreased local recurrence compared with patients who received external beam.[53] The wound complication rate is 22%, which is significantly higher than in the external beam group. This treatment may be given in lower doses to minimize complications.

Patients with soft tissue sarcomas often achieve improved local control but frequently develop distant metastases. Initially, studies using chemotherapy, specifically doxorubicin, were solely for patients with metastatic soft tissue sarcoma. These patients had prolonged survival. However, cardiac toxicity is a concern.

Based on these results, trials were designed to examine the role of adjuvant chemotherapy in the management of soft tissue sarcoma. In the search to find better chemotherapy agents, multiagent trials for soft tissue sarcoma were initiated. Two studies showed improved disease-free survival but no improvement in overall survival utilizing doxorubicin and cyclophosphamide.[54,55] Recently, ifosfamide has been effective. The role of chemotherapy in the adjuvant setting for soft tissue sarcoma is still in its infancy. Further trials are needed to determine its utility. The use of cardioprotectants may permit safe dose escalation.

Metastatic Bone Tumors

Half of the 1 million cancers diagnosed in the United States each year metastasize to bone. The three mechanisms by which a tumor spreads from the primary site to bone are (1) direct extension to adjacent bones, (2) arterial embolization, and (3) direct venous spread through the pelvic and vertebral veins known as Batson's plexus. The common tumor locations are breast, lung, prostate, kidney, and thyroid. Other primary sites can metastasize but are less common. The mechanism for spread explains the affinity for bony metastasis to occur in the spine, pelvis, ribs, skull, and proximal long bones.

The patient commonly presents with skeletal pain that worsens with rest and a prior cancer history, and is greater than 40 years of age. An individual can experience a pathological fracture, in some reports up to 90%. Individuals with spinal metastasis may have radicular pain, paresthesias, heaviness of limbs, leg buckling, and episodes of dropping items.[56] Compression of the spinal cord, which needs immediate treatment to prevent progressive neurological injury, includes symptoms of pain, hyperreflexia, weakness of lower limbs, sensory loss, and loss of bowel and bladder control.[57] In addition, individuals can present with hypercalcemia due to extensive bone lysis. Tumor invading bone marrow can result in abnormal production of leukocytes, thrombocytes, and erythrocytes. Transfusions and antibiotic treatments or prophylaxis may be needed.

Diagnostic testing includes a biopsy if the individual has no known primary tumor. This biopsy is usually performed with a needle. A solitary lesion needs to be worked up as if it is a primary tumor, with local radiographic imaging such as a CT scan or MRI and a biopsy.[58] Other testing includes laboratory tests such as serum acid phosphatase, which may lead to the primary site. A technetium bone scan is utilized to determine which bones are involved. Plain radiographs of areas positive on bone scan as well as any painful sites are done. Half of trabecular bone is destroyed before plain radiographs reveal lesions. An MRI is useful for imaging spinal lesions as well as spinal cord compression.[59]

Chemotherapy for the primary site may result in pain reduction, decrease in the size of bony lesions, and stabilization of the number of lesions. Other treatments must be timed appropriately if myelosuppression occurs. Surgical wounds need one to two weeks to develop collagen synthesis before chemotherapy is reinstituted.

Radiation is most commonly given by the external beam route to the involved sites. The goal of this treatment is to relieve pain, improve bone strength, and improve neurological deficits. The most common dose is 30 Gy utilizing ten fractions. Pain relief usually occurs any time from 48 hours to eight weeks. Early pain relief can be attributed to release of chemical pain mediators and later pain cessation to tumor lysis. Systemic radiation for diffuse bony metastasis can be given with radioisotopes such as strontium 89.[60,61] Repeat visits to the radiation department are avoided by administering the medication as a single dose and often provide relief for 60% of those treated. Radiation may be utilized solely or combined with surgery.

Extremity lesions are managed by either arthroplasty or stabilization surgery. Pathological fractures preclude an individual's ability to walk, to maintain independence, and to experience pain relief. In addition, lesions greater than 2.5 cm in diameter that involve 50% of the cortex are at risk for fracture and need prophylactic stabilization.[62] Other researchers propose predicting the risk of pathological fracture by estimating load-bearing requirements.[63] It is recommended that impending fractures be stabilized to decrease surgical morbidity and decrease the hospitalization time. The range of surgical procedures include an intramedullary stabilizing device, internal fixation, and a prosthetic arthroplasty with or without an allograft. Bone cement or methylmethacrylate can be used to fill the cavity created by the tumor to further stabilize the implant. Rarely, an amputation may be done to relieve pain or to treat a nonhealing fracture. The surgical goal is to permit patients full weight bearing.

Spinal lesions require surgery if conservative treatment such as steroids, radiation, and bracing have failed, progressive neurological symptoms develop, and/or spinal instability is present. Bracing is rarely comfortable if the person has rib, pelvis, or other spine lesions. The procedure consists of debulking the tumor followed by stabilization using instrumentation such as Cotrel-Dubousset, Isola, or Moss. Vertebral body replacement may range from a Moss cage filled with methylmethacrylate, bone from patient (autograft), bone from another human (allograft), or a vertebral fiber-metal prosthesis.[64] The goal of surgery is to improve function, optimally without use of a brace, and to improve ambulation.

The ongoing concern of those providing care to patients with metastatic bone tumors is prevention of fracture. In a study of 54 individuals with skeletal metastasis while undergoing rehabilitation, all were found to have a low risk of fracture during rehabilitation. Fractures did occur while persons were in bed.[65] Therefore, rehabilitation was recommended for this group. Nurses should be aware of bony involvement in order to plan nursing care, especially transfers. Carefully executed care is not a guarantee against pathological fractures.[66] Equally important is thoughtful, ongoing pain management utilizing opioid and nonsteroidal anti-inflammatory medication.[67]

Symptom Management and Supportive Care

Pain

Pain is often the presenting symptom of a bone sarcoma and, at times, a soft tissue sarcoma. It may be severe enough to interfere with sleep. Pain management may begin with nonsteroidal anti-inflammatories, progress to mild opiates such as codeine, and eventually need opiates such as morphine or methadone. Administering these medications on an outpatient basis and with concurrent treatment such as chemotherapy and radiation is a complex endeavor. Multiple phone calls are needed to assess the effectiveness of pain medication as well as medication side effects. Attention must be given to the patient's other responsibilities—career, home responsibilities such as child care, driving a vehicle. The use of walking aids may also be ordered to take weight off the involved limb for pain relief and to prevent a fracture.

Limitations of Mobility

The tumor may limit motion of a joint and the ability to use the limb. Assistive devices such as a sling, crutches, or a cane may be necessary to support the involved area and prevent fracture. A wheelchair may facilitate out-of-home activities such as going to a shopping mall or to the park. These devices may, however, cause other disabilities such as the inability to work, attend school, clean house, use public transportation, or go to the grocery store. The nurse or other health care provider may then need to supply the individual with such interventions as handicapped license plates to park closer to stores, a letter to the patient's employer requesting light duty, arrangements for a home aide to assist with housekeeping, and possibly encouragement to the patient to arrange transportation with family members. Because treatment may lead to additional limitations of mobility, continued assessment of the patient's mobility must be made, with appropriate interventions made as needed.

Continuity of Care: Nursing Challenges

One of the ongoing issues in the care of orthopedic oncology patients is negotiating continuity of care from the insurance plan. Multiple contacts and at times contacts with this insurance carrier are needed. Oncology nurses, especially in the outpatient setting, are frequently the insurance contact. Many states have one or two orthopedic oncology centers with expert surgeons, oncologists, radiologists, pathologists, and nurses. The insurance carrier, however, may not allow radiographic studies to be done at the center but will allow surgery. Physical therapy, either at home or on an outpatient basis, may be approved only by the insurance provider. Although it is time consuming, it is nevertheless important that communication lines between the insurance provider and the patient and his or her family remain open.

Hospitalizations are becoming shorter. Discharge planning starts before admission and is a daily consideration. Modifying goals to being able to walk to the bathroom rather than walking long distances and flexing the knee to 90° allows lengths of stay to be shorter. Installing a hospital bed on the first floor of the home may also facilitate early discharge. Insurance carriers, however, are less familiar with the need of this population. Additional verbal and written communication may be required to justify even shortened lengths of stay. Utilizing home nurses and home transfusion services are other methods to return the patient home.

Certain patients, especially the elderly, are too weak, immobile, or in too much pain to be discharged to the home. Alternative plans such as having the patient go to a family member's home or transfer to a skilled nursing facility or rehabilitation facility may be necessary. Again, obtaining approval of the insurance carrier is crucial.

Many treatments are administered in ambulatory areas, including the vast majority of radiation treatment, biopsies, and much of chemotherapy. Coordinating appointments around friends' and family's schedules, work schedules, school schedules, and other doctor and treatment appointments is difficult but crucial if multidisciplinary treatments are to stay on track.

Home care, as previously mentioned, is available for nearly all treatments—for example, initiating and discontinuing chemotherapy infusion pumps, setting up continuous passive movement devices to facilitate range of motion after limb salvage surgery, and assisting the patient in doing complex dressing or even monitoring wounds. Making the decision to use these services entails obtaining insurance carrier and patient approval, and understanding the cost and quality of the services. For example, arranging for a home nurse to carry out a wound assessment twice a week is not necessary if the patient is in the chemotherapy clinic twice a week and could have a wound check there.

Frequent phone calls is another method to assess status of pain, wound drainage, and other problems relating to self-care if the patient and family are able to accurately describe these problems.

Conclusion

The treatment of bone and soft tissue sarcomas is complex. The overall survival rates have improved since the late 1970s. Progress can be attributed to factors such as improved staging, adjuvant chemotherapy, and pulmonary resections. With the advent of limb salvage surgery, fewer patients are having amputations, without altering their survival rates. It is hoped that ongoing studies of chemotherapy, surgery, radiation, and molecular genes will continue to show improved survival rates for bone and soft tissue sarcoma.

References

1. Greenlee RT, Murray T, Bolden S, et al: Cancer Statistics, 2000. *CA Cancer J Clin* 50:7–33, 2000
2. Hansen M: Molecular genetic consideration in osteosarcoma. *Clin Orthop* 270:237–246, 1991
3. Araki N, Uchida A, Kimura T, et al: Involvement of the retinoblastoma gene in primary osteosarcomas and other bone and soft tissue tumors. *Clin Orthop* 270:271–277, 1991
4. Mazanet R, Antman K: Sarcomas of soft tissue and bone. *Cancer* 68:463–473, 1991
5. Swan J, Weber D, Kolosec F, et al: Combined MRI and MRA for limb salvage planning. *J Comput Assist Tomogr* 17:339–342, 1993
6. Shives T: Biopsy of soft tissue tumors. *Clin Orthop* 289:32–35, 1993
7. Eary J, Bruckner J, Howlett A, et al: FDG PET scan assessment of histologic grade of sarcoma. *Proceedings of Combined*

Meeting of American European Musculoskeletal Tumor Societies 181, 1998 (abstract)

8. American Joint Committee on Cancer: *Manual for Staging of Cancer* (ed 5). Philadelphia, Lippincott-Raven, 1997, pp 143–156

9. Schajowicz F: *Tumors and Tumor-like Lesions of Bone: Pathology, Radiology and Treatment* (ed 2). New York, Springer-Verlag, 1994

10. Enneking WF, Spanier S, Goodman M: A system for surgical staging of musculoskeletal sarcomas. *Clin Orthop* 153: 105–119, 1980

11. Unni K: *Dahlin's Bone Tumors* (ed 5). New York, Lippincott-Raven, 1996, pp 143–217

12. Scully S, Temple H, O'Keefe R, et al: The surgical treatment of patients with osteosarcoma who sustain a pathological fracture. *Clin Orthop* 324:227–232, 1996

13. Eckardt J, Asazamongkolkul A, Yang R, et al: Expandable endoprosthetic reconstruction for limb salvage and as a limb equalization technique in the skeletally immature patient. *Proceedings of Combined Meeting of American European Musculoskeletal Tumor Societies* 54, 1998

14. Krajbich J: Modified Van Nes rotationplasty in the treatment of malignant neoplasms in the lower extremities of children. *Clin Orthop* 262:74–77, 1991

15. Cammisa F, Glasser D, Phil M, et al: The Van Nes tibial rotationplasty. *J Bone Joint Surg (Am)* 72A:1541–1547, 1990

16. Tsuchiya H, Tomita K, Munematusu K, et al: Limb salvage using distraction osteogenesis. *J Bone Joint Surg (Br)* 79: 403–411, 1997

17. Malawer M, Chou L: Prosthetic survival and clinical results with use of large segment replacements in treatment of high-grade sarcoma. *J Bone Joint Surg (Am)* 77A:1154–1165, 1995

18. Piasecki P: The nursing role in limb salvage surgery. *Nurs Clin North Am* 26:33–41, 1991

19. Markovich G, Dorr L, Klein N, et al: Muscle flaps in total knee arthroplasty. *Clin Orthop* 321:122–130, 1995

20. Evans G, Black J, Robb A, et al: Adjuvant therapy, the effects on microvascular lower extremity reconstruction. *Ann Plast Surg* 39(2):141–144, 1997

21. Zohman G, Boardman L, Eckardt J, et al: Stride analyses after proximal tibial replacement. *Clin Orthop* 339:180–184, 1997

22. Buck B, Malinin T, Brown M: Bone transplantation and human immunodeficiency virus. *Clin Orthop* 249:129–136, 1989

23. Enneking WF, Mindell ER: Observations on massive retrieved human allografts. *J Bone Joint Surg (Am)* 73A: 1123–1142, 1991

24. Gebhardt M, Flugstad D, Springfield D, et al: The use of bone allografts for limb salvage in high-grade extremity osteosarcoma. *Clin Orthop* 270:181–196, 1991

25. Piasecki P: Update in orthopaedic oncology. *Orthop Nurs* 11(6):36, 38–43, 1992

26. Power R, Wood D, Tomford W, et al: Revision osteoarticular allograft transplantation in weight-bearing joints. *J Bone Joint Surg (Am)* 73B:595–599, 1991

27. Tomford W, Thongphasuk J, Mankin H, et al: Frozen musculoskeletal allografts. *J Bone Joint Surg (Am)* 72A:1137–1150, 1990

28. Dealy M, Pazola K, Heistein D: Care of the adolescent undergoing an allograft procedure. *Cancer Nurs* 18:130–137, 1995

29. Simon M, Springfield D: *Surgery for Bone and Soft Tissue Tumors.* Philadelphia, Lippincott-Raven, 1998

30. Goorin A, Shuster J, Baker A, et al: Changing pattern of pulmonary metastases with adjuvant chemotherapy in patients with osteosarcoma: results from the multiinstitutional osteosarcoma study. *J Clin Oncol* 9:600–605, 1991

31. Snyder C, Saltzman D, Ferrell K, et al: A new approach to the resection of pulmonary osteosarcoma metastases. *Clin Orthop* 270:247–253, 1991

32. Michael J, Gailey R, Bowker J: New developments in recreational prostheses and adaptive devices for the amputee. *Clin Orthop* 256:64–75, 1990

33. Williamson V: Amputation of the lower extremity: An overview. *Orthop Nurs* 11(2):55–65, 1992

34. Lane J, Kroll M, Rossbach P: New advances and concepts in amputee management after treatment for bone and soft tissue sarcoma. *Clin Orthop* 256:22–28, 1990

35. Bartusch SL, Sanders B, D'Alessio J, et al: Clonazepam for the treatment of lancinating phantom limb pain. *Clin J Pain* 12(1):59–62, 1996

36. Cheng E, Dusenberg K, Winters M, et al: Soft tissue sarcomas: preoperative versus postoperative radiotherapy. *J Surg Oncol* 61:90–99, 1996

37. Issels R, Prenninger S, Nagele A, et al: Ifosfamide plus etoposide combined with regional hyperthermia in patients with locally advanced sarcomas. *J Clin Oncol* 8:1818–1829, 1990

38. Burk C, Belasco J, O'Neill J, et al: Pulmonary metastases and bone sarcomas. *Clin Orthop* 262:88–92, 1991

39. Garcia A: Ifosfamide induced Fanconi syndrome. *Ann Pharmacother* 29:590–591, 1995

40. Wornom I, Bochman S: *Bone and cartilaginous tissue,* in Cohen I, Piegelman R, Lindblad W (eds): *Wound Healing.* Philadelphia, Saunders, 1992, pp 356–383

41. Raymond K: Surface osteosarcoma. *Clin Orthop* 270:140–148, 1991

42. Glasser D, Lane J: Stage IIB osteogenic sarcoma. *Clin Orthop* 270:29–39, 1991

43. Bacci G, Picci P, Ferrari S, et al: Prognostic significance of serum alkaline phosphatase measurements in patients with osteosarcoma treated with adjuvant or neoadjuvant chemotherapy. *Cancer* 71:1224–1230, 1993

44. Bacci G, Picci P, Pignatti G, et al: Neoadjuvant chemotherapy for non-metastatic osteosarcoma of the extremities. *Clin Orthop* 270:87–98, 1991

45. Healy J, Meyer P, Gorlick R, et al: Intensive preoperative chemotherapy for osteogenic sarcoma. *Proceedings of Combined Meeting of American European Musculoskeletal Tumor Societies* 54, 1998

46. Wilkins R, Pritchard P, Burgert E, et al: Ewing's sarcoma of bone: experience with 140 patients. *Cancer* 58:2551–2555, 1991

47. Wexler L, DeLaney T, Tsokos M: Ifosfamide and etoposide plus vincristine, doxorubicin and cyclophosphamide for newly diagnosed Ewing's sarcoma family of tumour. *Cancer* 78:901–911, 1996

48. O'Connor M, Pritchard D: Ewing's sarcoma. *Clin Orthop* 262:78–87, 1991

49. Waterhouse D, Cohn S: *Diagnostic and Therapeutic Advances in Pediatric Oncology.* Boston, Kluwer Academic, 1997

50. Rosenthal H, Terek R, Lane J: Management of extremity soft tissue sarcoma. *Clin Orthop* 289:66–72, 1993

51. Rydholm A, Gustafon P, Rooser B, et al: Limb-sparing surgery without radiotherapy based on anatomic locale of soft tissue sarcoma. *J Clin Oncol* 9:1757–1765, 1991

52. O'Connor M, Pritchard D, Gunderson M: Integration of limb-sparing surgery, brachytherapy and external beam irra-

diation in treatment of soft tissue sarcoma. *Clin Orthop* 289: 73–80, 1993

53. Shiu M, Hilaris B, Harrison H, et al: Brachytherapy and functional saving resection of soft tissue sarcoma arising in limb. *Int J Radiat Oncol Biol Phys* 21:1485–1492, 1991

54. Pisters P, Patel S, Varma D, et al: Preoperative chemotherapy for stage IIIB extremity soft tissue sarcoma: long term results from a single institution. *J Clin Oncol* 15:3481–3487, 1997

55. Elias A: Chemotherapy for soft tissue sarcoma. *Clin Orthop* 289:94–105, 1993

56. Weinstein J: Differential diagnosis and surgical treatment of pathological spine fractures, in Eilert R (ed): *Instructional Course Lecture*, vol 41. Rosemont, IL, American Association of Orthopedic Surgeons, 1992, pp 301–315

57. Brown K: Cauda equina syndrome. *Orthop Nurs* 17(5):31–37, 1998

58. Frassica F, Gitelis S, Sim F: Metastatic bone disease: general principles, pathophysiology, evaluation and biopsy, in Eilert R (ed): *Instructional Course Lecture*, vol 41. Rosemont, IL, American Association of Orthopedic Surgeons, 1992, pp 293–300

59. Trail Z, Richards M, Moore N: Magnetic resonance imaging of metastatic bone disease. *Clin Orthop* 312:76–88, 1995

60. Lehing A, Ackery D, Bayly R, et al: Strontium-89 therapy for pain palliation in prostatic skeletal malignancy. *Br J Radiol* 64:816–822, 1991

61. Porter A, McEwan A, Powe J, et al: Results of a randomized phase III trial to evaluate the efficacy of strontium-89 adjuvant to local field external beam irradiation in management of endocrine resistant prostate cancer. *Int J Radiat Oncol Biol Phys* 25:805–813, 1993

62. Sim F: Metastatic bone disease of the pelvis and femur, in Eilert R (ed): *Instructional Course Lecture*, vol 41. Rosemont, IL, American Association of Orthopedic Surgeons, 1992, pp 317–327

63. Hipp J, Springfield D, Hayes W: Predicting pathological fracture risk in the management of metastatic bone defects. *Clin Orthop* 312:120–135, 1995

64. Hammerberg K: Surgical treatment of metastatic spine disease. *Spine* 17:1148–1153, 1992

65. Bunting R: Rehabilitation of cancer patients with skeletal metastases. *Clin Orthop* 312:76–88, 1995

66. Piasecki P: Nursing care of the patient with metastatic bone disease. *Orthop Nurs* 15(4):25–33, 1996

67. Twycross R: Management of pain in skeletal metastases. *Clin Orthop* 312:187–196, 1995

CHAPTER 47

Bladder and Kidney Cancer

Lynne M. Early, RN, MSN, CETN, OCN®
Rita M. Poquette RN, MSN, FNP, CS

Introduction

The two urinary tract cancers discussed in this chapter, bladder and kidney cancer, are relatively rare as they account for only about 6% of all cancers. Advances in the detection and therapeutic management of bladder and kidney cancer are described in this chapter. This chapter also provides the oncology nurse a basis for the care and management of the individual with bladder or kidney cancer.

BLADDER CANCER

Epidemiology

Bladder cancer is the second most common genitourinary cancer after prostate cancer, accounting for approximately 6% of cancers in the United States. It is the fourth leading cancer and seventh leading cause of cancer deaths in men, and eighth leading cancer and tenth leading cause of cancer deaths in women. Bladder cancer will be diagnosed in approximately 54,200 Americans in 1999 and will account for an estimated 12,100 deaths.[1] It occurs four times more often in men than in women, and is two times more common in whites than in blacks.[2] The average age at diagnosis is 65.

Etiology

There are hypothesized etiological risk factors associated with bladder cancer development. Currently, researchers believe that bladder tumors are a result of a combination of genetic events, including oncogene activation and anti-oncogene inactivation.[3] Cigarette smoking, which has been demonstrated to initiate and promote these events, is a risk factor that accounts for approximately 47% of bladder cancer deaths among men and 37% among women.[1] Sorahan and associates[4] concluded that the risk of bladder cancer associated with cigarette smoking was related to the lifetime consumption of cigarettes and the duration of smoking.

Occupational exposures to aniline dyes and aromatic amines, most commonly betanaphthylamine and benzidine, have also been related to an increased risk for bladder cancer. Occupations connected with this risk include textile workers, rubber industry workers, hairdressers, painters, printers, janitors, cleaners, and miners.[3] Ingestion of other physical agents, such as coffee, alcohol, saccharine, and phenacetin, have been weakly linked to bladder cancer.[2] There is a high incidence of squamous cell carcinoma of the bladder in many African countries, most notably Egypt. This is linked to exposure to the parasite *Schistosoma haematobium* that can be found in the water of these countries.

Pathophysiology

The urinary bladder is lined by transitional epithelium, often called the *urothelium*. About 90%–95% of bladder tumors in North America are transitional cell carcinoma that arise in the epithelial layer of the bladder. The epithelial layer rests on the basement membrane. Approximately 5% of bladder tumors originate below the basement membrane and include squamous cell carcinoma and adenocarcinoma.[5]

The growth rate of bladder tumors varies depending on the histological type, tumor grade, and depth of bladder wall invasion. Tumors have potential to spread to regional lymph nodes, the pelvis, and other adjacent structures, particularly the sigmoid colon, the rectum, the prostate, as well as the uterus and vagina. Hematogenous spread occasionally occurs resulting in metastatic spread to the bones, liver, and lungs.[6]

Clinical Manifestations

Hematuria is the most common presenting symptom of bladder cancer. It may be grossly visible or apparent only on microscopic urinalysis. The degree of hematuria does not relate to the stage or extent of the disease. Additional symptoms of bladder cancer may be voiding irritability, including dysuria, urinary frequency, and urgency. Symptoms of advanced disease or metastasis may manifest as flank, rectal, pelvic, or bone pain; bowel habit changes; decreased appetite or weight loss; lower extremity edema; and/or fever.[7]

Assessment

Physical Examination and Diagnostic Studies

There are no early signs of bladder cancer on physical examination. An invasive mass in the trigonal area occasionally may be revealed by rectal examination. Diagnostic tests establish the presence of a bladder mass. For bladder cancer the most useful diagnostic tests include urine cytology, flow cytometry, excretory urogram, cystoscopy, ultrasound, computerized tomography (CT), and magnetic resonance imaging (MRI). Exfoliative urinary cytology is a relatively simple diagnostic tool in the assessment of bladder cancer, particularly high-grade malignancies or carcinoma in situ. The collection of a total voided specimen is best obtained in the late morning or early afternoon. Bladder washings obtained through saline irrigation of the bladder produce even more reli-

Table 47-1 Jewett/Marshall Bladder Staging System

Stage 0	Carcinoma in situ (CIS) or superficial papillary tumor confined to the mucosa with invasion
Stage A	Papillary tumor invading the lamina propria
Stage B1	Tumor with superficial muscle invasion
Stage B2	Tumor with deep muscle invasion
Stage C	Invasion of the perivesical fat
Stage D1	Involvement of adjacent viscera and/or pelvic nodes
Stage D1	Involvement of nodes above the aortic bifurcation or distant spread

Adapted with permission from Carroll PR: Urothelial carcinoma—cancers of the bladder, ureter, and renal pelvis, in Tanagho EA, McAninch JW (eds): *Smith's General Urology* (ed 14). Norwalk, CT: Appleton and Lange, 1995, pp 354–355.[13]

able results.[8] Flow cytometry is a technique used to examine the DNA content of urine cells after being stained with DNA-specific fluorescein dye. Aneuploidy, or large numbers of DNA per cell, is typically an indication of bladder cancer. Flow cytometry has been useful in providing prognostic information beyond grading and staging.[9] The excretory urogram is done on initial diagnosis for the evaluation of hematuria. It is used to visualize the urinary tract and identify filling defects of the upper tracts or bladder, including the presence of hydronephrosis.[10] A cystoscopy is a diagnostic procedure used to visualize and evaluate a bladder tumor. Once the tumor is visualized, a biopsy is taken to assess the presence or absence of muscle invasion. Multiple biopsy specimens of the surrounding bladder wall, bladder neck, and trigone may be taken to diagnose carcinoma in situ or atypia. Bimanual palpation is performed under anesthesia when muscle invasion and/or extravesical extension is suspected.[9] Both abdominal and transurethral ultrasound have been used to define the local extension and degree of bladder wall involvement. Advocates for using CT scans in staging bladder cancer feel that they aid in defining extension beyond the bladder, lymph node involvement, or distant metastasis.[9] The MRI is also successful in detecting bladder cancer through visualization of multiple planes. There may be a greater reliability in identifying tumors at the base or dome of the bladder and extravesical extension with the use of the MRI.

Prognostic Indicators

Tumor markers may be useful in the prediction of the response to treatment, the recurrence, and the progression of bladder cancer. The identification of multiple markers may provide more accurate information because of the various mechanisms resulting in tumor recurrence or progression. One such marker is the *p53* gene, a cell cycle regulatory protein. Research is beginning to demonstrate evidence that the aberration of *p53* in bladder

tumors may decrease prognosis, but the addition of adjuvant chemotherapy may increase survival.[11] Another marker is the blood group antigen. The presence of blood group antigens A, B, and H on the surface of the bladder cancer cells has been shown to be advantageous in defining prognosis. Tumors expressing these blood group antigens are often associated with a better prognosis than tumors not displaying these antigens.[5] Epidermal growth factor (EGF), a potent mitogen and tumor promoter, has been found to be overexpressed in late-stage bladder cancer. The activation of epidermal growth factor receptor (EGF-R), possibly by EGF, initiates a cascade of molecular events that could prove to play a role in tumor persistence, recurrence, and adverse prognosis.[11] Beta-human chorionic gonadotropin (beta-hCG), normally regarded as a marker for testicular cancer, has been found to be increased in bladder cancer and associated with more advanced disease and decreased prognosis.[12]

Classification and Staging

There are two staging systems for bladder cancer: the Jewett-Marshall system (Table 47-1),[13] modified by Marshall, and the TNM system developed by the American Joint Committee for Cancer Staging (Table 47-2).[14] A compilation of these systems is depicted in Figure 47-1.[13] The classification and staging of tumors provides information to estimate prognosis and to assist in treatment decisions. The TNM system provides a more accurate classification and definition of tumor types than the Jewett-Marshall system. Although many physicians continue to use the Jewett-Marshall system because of their familiarity with it, the TNM classification system promotes collaboration in cancer research and facilitates comparison of data among national and international clinical investigators.

The grade or degree of cell differentiation of bladder tumors predicts the speed of recurrence, progression to invasion, and metastases. The grades for bladder cancer are usually referred to as grade I, II, III, or IV, with IV indicating poor differentiation. The grade of the tumor is also an important factor that affects the choice of treatment and the prognosis.

Therapeutic Approaches and Nursing Care

Carcinoma in Situ

Carcinoma in situ (CIS) is a noninvasive lesion(s) that has a high potential for invasion and recurrence. This type of bladder tumor requires aggressive follow-up after initial diagnosis and treatment in order to provide surveillance for tumor recurrence and invasive disease. Transurethral resection (TUR) and fulguration are the most

Table 47-2 TNM Bladder Classification

T = PRIMARY TUMOR

TX	Primary tumor cannot be assessed
T0	No evidence of primary tumor
Tis	Carcinoma in situ
Ta	Noninvasive papillary carcinoma
T1	Tumor invades submucosa/lamina propria
T2a	Tumor invades superficial muscle
T2b	Tumor invades deep muscle
T3	Tumor invades perivesical fat
T4	Tumor invades adjacent organs

N = REGIONAL LYMPH NODES (BELOW AORTIC BIFURCATION)

NX	Regional lymph nodes cannot be assessed
N0	No regional lymph node metastasis
N1	Metastasis in single node less than 2 cm
N2	Metastasis in single node more than 2 cm but less than 5 cm, or multiple nodes less than 5 cm
N3	Metastasis in nodes more than 5 cm

M = DISTANT METASTASES

MX	Presence of distant metastasis cannot be assessed
M0	No distant metastasis
M1	Distant metastasis

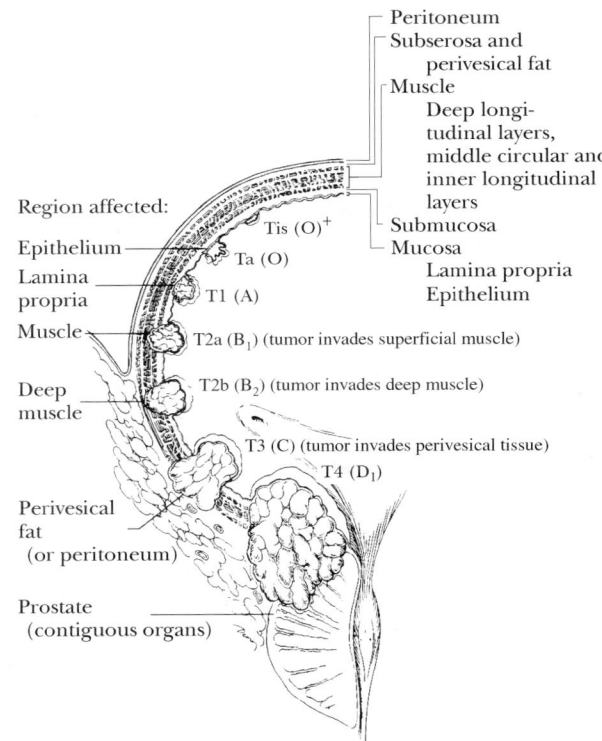

Figure 47-1 Staging of bladder cancer. (Reprinted with permission from Caroll PR: Urothelial carcinoma: Cancers of the bladder, ureter, and renal pelvis, in Tanagho EA, McAninch JW (eds): *Smith's General Urology* [ed 14]. Norwalk, CT, Appleton and Lange, 1995, p 355.)[13]

common and conservative forms of management of CIS. The TUR to obtain tissue for diagnosis often is sufficient in removing the tumor or tumors present. Radical cystectomy is indicated for high-grade, poorly differentiated CIS.[15] Radiotherapy has not proven to be of value in the treatment of CIS.[16] Intravesical treatment with chemotherapeutic agents such as thiotepa, mitomycin C, doxorubicin, or with immunotherapeutic agents such as bacillus Calmette-Guérin (BCG) have demonstrated effectiveness when administered to patients with multiple tumors or prophylatically following TUR and/or fulguration.[3]

BCG has shown superior protection from tumor recurrence and prevention of disease progression as compared to thiotepa, mitomycin C, and doxorubicin. BCG is a live, attenuated culture preparation of the bacillus Calmette-Guérin strain of mycobacterium bovis. Unlike conventional intravesical chemotherapeutic agents that attack tumor cells directly, BCG is a biological response modifier that is believed to exert its antitumor effect by stimulating various immune responses within the host.[17] The frequency and dosage of BCG varies slightly from institution to institution, but most commonly is administered weekly for six treatments at a dosage of 120 mg per instillation.

Nseyo and associates[18] describe an overall increase in disease-free survival from 65%–83% in patients with CIS who received three additional treatments at three months after initial therapy and maintenance treatments every six months for a total of three years. The side effects of BCG treatment include dysuria, urinary frequency, and cystitis with or without hematuria. Cystitis occurs in 90% of those treated with intravesical BCG and is accompanied by hematuria 25% of the time. Cystitis lasting more than 48 hours can be treated with 300 mg isoniazid daily until the symptoms resolve.

Nurses play an integral role in assessing the patient for side effects and holding treatment until side effects from the previous treatment have resolved. Sepsis can also be a side effect of treatment and can be diagnosed on clinical presentation with high fever, shaking chills, and hypotension. Antibiotics should be initiated promptly if BCG systemic infection is suspected.[17]

Superficial, Low-grade Tumors

More than 75% of individuals with bladder cancer present initially with superficial tumors (stages T0, Tis, Ta, and T1).[19] Superficial tumors of the bladder remain in the epithelium and lamina propria. Invasive tumors do not develop in approximately 80% of these cases.[20] However, high-grade tumors invading the lamina propria are at high risk for muscle invasion.[21] The standard treatments of superficial tumors are TUR and fulguration with or without intravesical chemotherapy, laser therapy, or cystectomy. The overall five-year survival rate of patients with superficial bladder cancer treated with TUR alone is approximately 80%.[5] Superficial bladder cancer recurs following TUR 40%–60% of the time.[5] Intravesical chemotherapy is often given as adjuvant therapy to prevent or treat local recurrence.[20]

Intravesical treatment. Intravesical therapy with chemotherapeutic and immunotherapeutic agents have shown effectiveness in the treatment of superficial bladder cancer. To date there is no uniform consensus on the choice of drug and the duration or schedule of treatment. Treatment with BCG has delayed progression of disease, reduced recurrences, and prolonged survival. It is considered the most successful adjuvant treatment for superficial bladder cancer. A typical regimen of BCG begins one to two weeks after biopsy or TUR of tumor and is repeated once a week for six treatments. A single six-week course of intravesical BCG may not be sufficient and additional treatments are required. Most patients tolerate BCG reasonably well, although side effects are expected as patients become sensitized to BCG.[18]

Other intravesical therapies. Interferons, bropirimine, and keyhole-limpet hemocyanin are immunotherapeutic agents currently being investigated for intravesical treatment of superficial bladder cancer. Photo-mediated photodynamic therapy (PDT) is another intravesical therapy currently being evaluated. These agents have shown effectiveness for prophylaxis and treatment of recurrent superficial bladder cancer. PDT is also being evaluated in individuals with refractory CIS who have failed intravesical chemotherapy or immunotherapy with BCG. The technique of PDT is systemic injection of the photosensitizing agent, Photofrin, followed by its activation intravesically by use of whole bladder laser-generated light source.[3] An immune response is initiated due to intense local inflammation and endothelial damage. The side effects of PDT are urinary frequency, urgency, nocturia, bladder spasms, and suprapubic pain in varying degrees. Permanent bladder contracture is experienced in 4%–24% of patients post-PDT.[17]

Partial (or segmental) cystectomy. Partial cystectomy is recommended for individuals with diffuse unresectable tumors that are located away from the bladder neck or base as well as for tumors that have not responded to intravesical therapy. The success of a partial cystectomy is much higher with stage T1 and grade I or II disease. Ten to fifteen percent of individuals are appropriate candidates for this procedure. The tumor recurrence rate after a partial cystectomy is as high as 78%. A radical cystectomy is indicated for recurrent superficial tumors.[22]

Invasive Tumors

Invasive bladder cancer represents muscle invasion (stages T2–T4) and requires aggressive therapy.[22] The treatment for muscle invasive bladder cancer focuses on bladder preservation or bladder reconstruction.[23] The various types of treatment are surgery, radiation, chemotherapy, or a combination of these options.[24] Thirty to fifty percent of patients with muscle invasive bladder cancer will develop recurrence and distant metastasis.

Radical cystectomy. Radical cystectomy with bilateral lymphadenectomy is the standard treatment for muscle

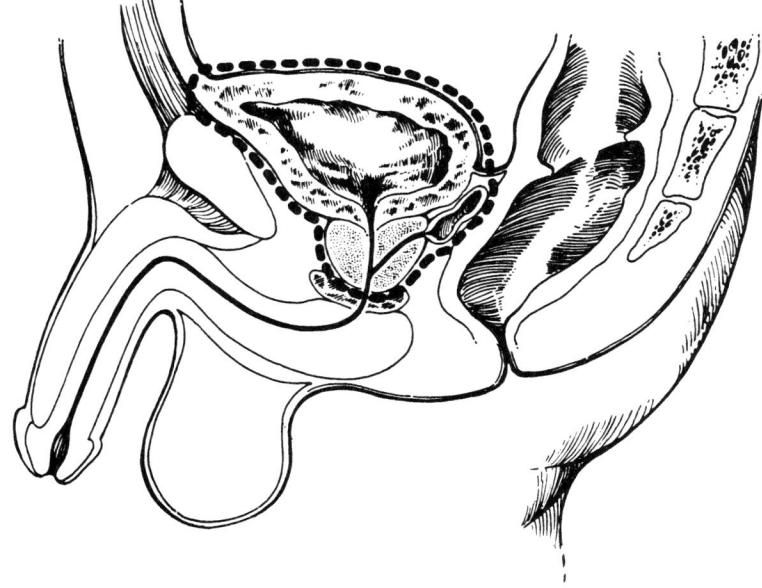

Figure 47-2 Surgical boundaries of radical cystectomy in a man. The specimen includes the bladder, the prostate, and the seminal vesicles. (Reprinted with permission from Swanson D: Cancer of the bladder and prostate: The impact of therapy on sexual function, in von Eschenbach AC, Rodriguez D (eds): *Sexual Rehabilitation of the Urologic Cancer Patient.* Boston, Hall, 1981, p 102.)[25]

invasive bladder cancer. This is the most effective treatment for the local control of tumor recurrence, precise pathological staging, and optimal survival for men and women.[21] In men, a radical cystoprostatectomy with a pelvic lymphadenectomy is the procedure of choice. This involves the excision of the bladder with perivesical fat, the attached peritoneum, the entire prostate, prostatic urethra, and seminal vesicles (Figure 47-2).[25] In women, a radical cystectomy or anterior exenteration includes the removal of the bladder with perivesical fat, proximal urethra, ovaries, fallopian tubes, uterus, cervix, vaginal cuff, anterior pelvic peritoneum, and pelvic and iliac lymph nodes (Figure 47-3A).[25] In both men and women, the entire urethra is removed if there is evidence of disease within the urethra (Figure 47-3B).[25]

Cystectomy with urinary diversion. A urinary diversion is performed to divert the urine stream away from the original lower urinary tract. There are several types of urinary diversions including the incontinent ileoconduit and the continent urinary reservoir cutaneous or orthotopic (urethrostomy).

Ileal conduit. Since the early 1950s the Bricker ileoconduit has been the cornerstone of diverting urinary flow in the absence of bladder function. This procedure involves isolation of a section of terminal ileum. The proximal end is closed and the distal end is brought out through an opening in the abdominal wall at a site selected prior to surgery. The ileal segment is sutured to the skin, creating a stoma. The ureters are implanted into the ileal segment, urine flows into the conduit, and peristalsis propels the urine out through the stoma (Figure 47-4).[26] Ureteral stents or a red Robinson catheter may be placed into the conduit to allow free flowing urine in the early postoperative period. The stents or catheter is usually left in place for five to seven days. Other portions of the bowel also have been used to create the conduit. Construction of any of these conduits requires the person to wear an external appliance to collect the urine.

Complications related to the ileoconduit construction include a flushed and recessed stoma and placement of the stoma in skin creases, scars, or over bony prominences. This results in difficulties with appliance adherence and management. Late complications include stomal stenosis, stone formation, and peristomal hernias. Chronic pyelonephritis and kidney deterioration may occur due to urinary reflux, ureteroileal obstruction, or urinary infection.

Continent urinary reservoir. In recent years, continent urinary reservoirs have become the procedure of choice when it is necessary to remove the bladder. They were developed in an attempt to better substitute the functions of the original urinary tract. Ideally, voiding of urine should be under voluntary control at convenient intervals. The upper renal tracts should be protected from both urine reflux and obstruction. With the creation of

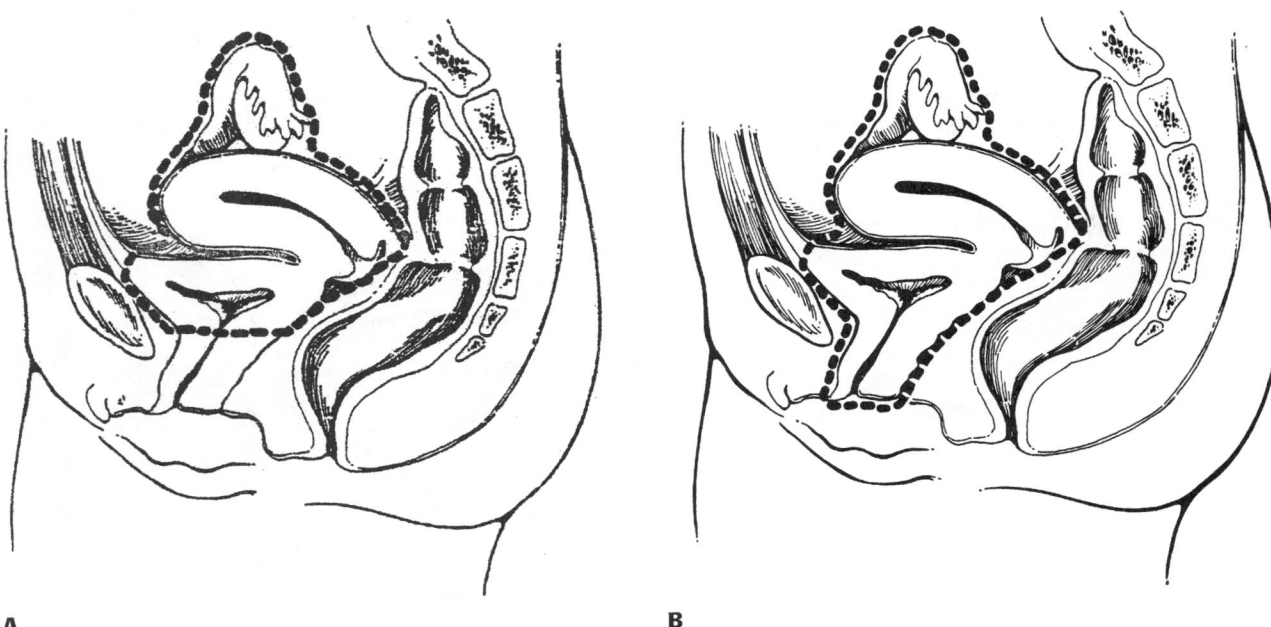

A

B

Figure 47-3 (A) Surgical boundaries of a radical cystectomy in a woman. The specimen includes the proximal urethra, bladder, uterus, ovaries, and fallopian tubes. (B) Surgical boundaries of radical cystectomy in a woman. The specimen includes the bladder and entire urethra, uterus, ovaries, fallopian tubes, and the anterior wall of the vagina. (Reprinted with permission from Swanson D: Cancer of the bladder and prostate: The impact of therapy on sexual function, in von Eschenbach AC, Rodriguez D (eds): *Sexual Rehabilitation of the Urologic Cancer Patient.* Boston, Hall, 1981, p 103.)[25]

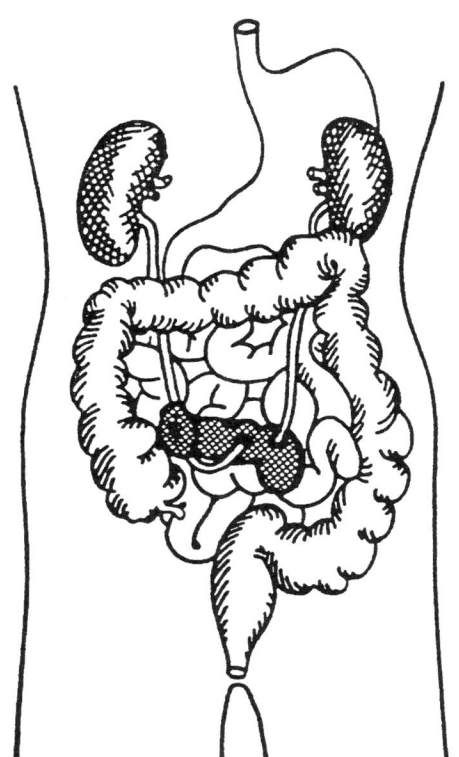

Figure 47-4   Urostomy (ileal conduit). Fifteen- to twenty-cm ileal segment, stoma exits through the rectus abdominis muscle, and the ureters reimplant at the base of the conduit. (Reprinted from American Cancer Society and United Ostomy Association: *Urostomy: A guide.* Atlanta, American Cancer Society, revised October 1990.)[26]

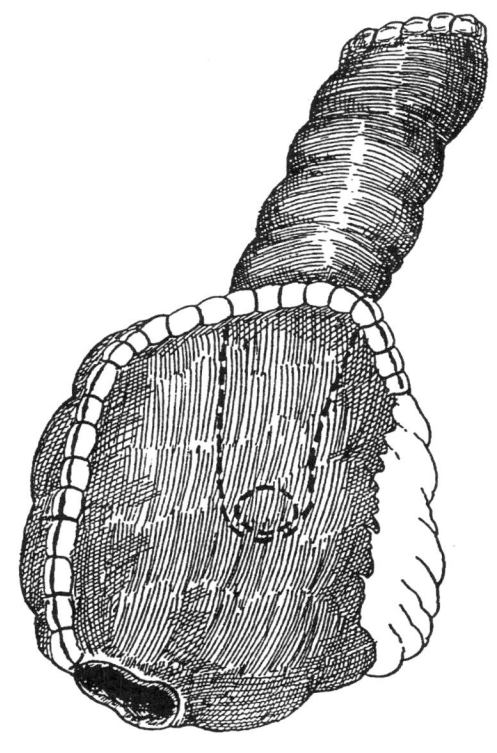

Figure 47-5   Completion of T-pouch. Most mobile and dependent portion of reservoir is anastomosed to urethra after ureteroileal anastomosis. (Reprinted with permission from Stein JP, Lieskovsky G, Ginsberg DA, et al: The T-pouch: an orthotopic ileal neobladder incorporating a serosal lined ileal antireflux technique. *J Urol* 159:1836–1842, 1998.)[27]

an antireflux mechanism, the continent urinary reservoir is designed to be a low-pressure pouch that is able to store at least 300–400 mL of urine.

There are several types of continent urinary reservoirs currently being constructed such as the T-pouch,[27] Kock pouch, Studer pouch,[28] Indiana pouch,[29] Mainz pouch, and the ileocecal pouch with appendostomy (ICPA).[30] Figure 47-5 illustrates a completed T-pouch. The surgical principles of the various pouches are discussed extensively in the literature. The differences between the reservoirs are the segment of intestine used to fashion the pouch, the surgical technique chosen to construct the antireflux and continence mechanisms, and the location of the urinary outlet (stoma or urethra).

At the time of surgery, catheters or tubes are placed to drain the urinary reservoir continuously. A flat latex drain called a *Penrose drain* is passed through a stab wound on the abdomen and covered with a drainage bag to collect fluid. The tube or catheters and Penrose drain remain in place for three weeks from the time of surgery.

The natural mucus production of the intestine will continue in the reservoir in varying degrees. To prevent mucus obstruction postoperatively, the tube or catheter is to be irrigated every four hours and as needed with 30–60 mL of normal saline. Three weeks following surgery, the reservoir is checked radiologically for extravasation. If no extravasation is present, the tube or catheters are removed. The individual is immediately taught self-catheterization or voiding technique.

Late complications may include difficulty catheterizing, incontinence including urinary leakage at the stoma or urethra, electrolyte abnormalities, afferent limb stenosis or prolapse, stone formation, pyelonephritis and/or hydronephrosis.[31]

Postsurgical sexuality.   A radical cystectomy with urinary diversion, performed in the traditional manner, particularly if accompanied by a lymphadenectomy, can affect many aspects of sexual functioning such as potency in men and narrowing and dryness of the vagina in women. The etiology of physiological sexual dysfunction in men is similar to that associated with treatment for prostatic cancer. Walsh[32] has described and developed the nerve sparing procedure that can preserve erectile potency in selected individuals without compromising cancer control. In a retrospective study conducted at

Johns Hopkins Hospital, Schoenberg and associates[33] discovered that recovery of sexual function in men following a nerve-sparing cystoprostatectomy was related to age: 20% of 70–79 year olds, 43% of 60–69 year olds, 47% of 50–59 year olds, and 62% of 40–49 year olds regained potency.

The insertion of a penile prosthesis may be selected for the treatment of erectile dysfunction in men who are impotent after radical cystectomy. There are several types, all of which continue to be refined. The semirigid prostheses are malleable plastic rods that are inserted into the corpus cavernosa. The result is a permanent semierection that is not painful and does not interfere with daily activities. The Jonas prosthesis is an example of the semirigid type. There are also several types of inflatable prostheses that make it possible to control erectile function. The single component inflatable prosthesis has inflating and deflating cylinders inserted into the corpus cavernosa and a pump bulb implanted in the scrotum. When the man wishes to have an erection, the pump bulb is repeatedly squeezed and released to pump fluid from a connected reservoir into the penile cylinders until an erection is achieved. To deflate the erection, finger pressure is exerted on the release valve located just below the pump bulb. This is not painful and does not interfere with daily activities. The AMS 700 inflatable penile prosthesis is an example of this type (Figure 47-6).[34]

In women, removal of the ovaries and uterus will result in sexuality changes similar to those following hysterectomy and oophorectomy for gynecological malignancies. These changes may include vaginal dryness, decreased libido related to hormonal changes and psychological influences such as loss from the removal of female reproductive organs. Physiological changes may occur due to shortening and narrowing of the vaginal wall. This may result in an alteration in sensation related to scar tissue and impairment of the ability to achieve orgasm and permit insertion of the penis into the vagina.[21] Informing the individual to use ample lubrication and to experiment with different positioning techniques during intercourse may decrease pain and discomfort and enhance activity. Hormone replacement in an adequately screened individual may be appropriate.

In both men and women, the psychological impact of a stoma and external appliance may contribute to sexual dysfunction. The change in body image can affect relationships with others and alter libido. As nurses, we can assist these individuals through these changes and provide suggestions to improve their quality of life.

Definitive radiotherapy.

External beam radiotherapy of approximately 60 Gy delivered in fractions to the pelvis in five to eight weeks is an alternative to radical cystectomy in select patients.[16] Although there has been controversy about the efficacy of definitive radiotherapy for invasive bladder cancer, studies have shown its ability in 20%–40% of selected cases to completely eradicate and permanently control tumors, while preserving bladder and sexual function.[19] For many individuals, however, the disease often

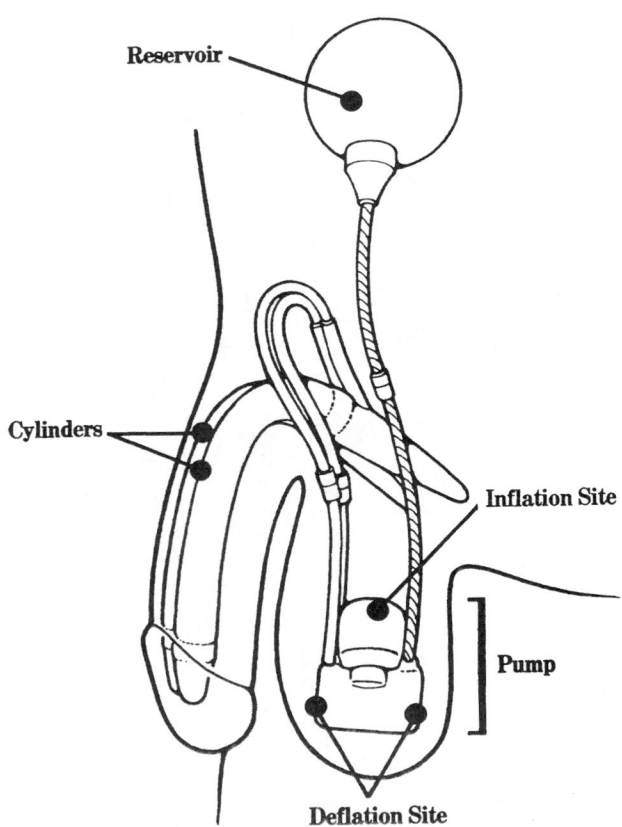

Figure 47-6 Inflatable penile prosthesis. (AMS 700 CX™ Penile Prosthesis, courtesy of American Medical Systems, Inc., Minnetonka, Minnesota.)[34]

recurs after years of local control. The differences between response rate and survival when comparing radiation and surgery are a result of the difference in clinical and pathological staging and patient selection.[24]

Treatment with concurrent chemotherapy and radiotherapy has been associated with improved rates of local control compared with radiotherapy alone.[35] The cytotoxic drug serves as a radiosensitizing agent.[24] In particular, cisplatin and radiotherapy have demonstrated a 40% five-year survival rate; however, there is significant morbidity. The toxicities include decreased bladder function, cystitis, hematuria, and adhesions.[19]

The most common approach includes radiation to the entire bladder, the perivesical soft tissues, and pelvic lymphatics, while minimizing the dose to the rectum and anus. The exact tumorcidal dose is unknown, but many successful protocols recommend giving 65 Gy at a daily single dose of 180–200 cGy to the tumor region and a lesser dose of 47–55 Gy to the whole bladder and perivesical area.

The acute (and self-limiting) side effects of fractionated treatment are dysuria, diarrhea, and urinary frequency in 50%–70% of patients. These can usually be treated symptomatically, and radiotherapy usually does not have to be interrupted. Long-term complications can occur as early as three years after radiation treatment and include chronic urinary frequency or hematuria and incontinence.[29] These chronic problems can significantly affect an individual's quality of life; therefore management is focused on the reduction of symptoms.

Chemotherapy.   The goals of chemotherapy are to control the disease, downstage inoperable tumors, preserve the bladder, and eradicate micrometastasis and therefore increase disease-free survival and cure patients with invasive bladder cancer.[36] Because of the frequency of distant metastasis, chemotherapy given preoperatively to decrease the presumed micrometastasis is under evaluation in clinical trials. Bladder cancer is a chemosensitive malignancy and has demonstrated objective responses in about 50% of treated patients.[37] In clinical trials, chemotherapy is used as a neoadjuvant (prior to surgery or radiotherapy) or an adjuvant (following surgery or radiotherapy) treatment of invasive bladder cancer. Results from clinical studies with combined-modality treatment of methotrexate, vincristine, doxorubicin (Adriamycin), and cisplatin (MVAC) have shown the best outcomes.[38] Cisplatin as a single agent and/or in combination regimens is the cornerstone of invasive bladder cancer therapy.[39]

New agents in clinical trials are revealing equivalent response rates to MVAC but with less toxicity. These agents include antifolates (trimetrexate and piritrexim), gemcitabine, taxanes (paclitaxel, docetaxel), ifosfamide, 5-FU, and gallium. However, MVAC continues to be the standard for the neoadjuvant and adjuvant therapy of muscle-invasive and metastatic bladder cancer. Improved response rates and increased length of survival will rely on the clinical trials of these agents alone and in combination regimens.[40]

Results and Prognosis

Survival rates for bladder cancer depend on the stage of the disease. The five-year survival rates (adjusted for normal life expectancy) as reported by the American Cancer Society can be seen in Table 47-3.[41]

Table 47-3 Approximate Five-Year Survival Rates for Bladder Cancer

Stage	Survival Percentage
Localized	94
Regional	49
Distant	6
All stages	82

Reprinted from American Cancer Society: *Cancer Facts and Figures—1999*. Atlanta, American Cancer Society, January 1999.[41]

Nursing Care of Individuals with Bladder Cancer

Preoperative Nursing Care

The decision for the type of urinary diversion is based on the stage of the disease, past medical and surgical history, performance status and motivation, lifestyle, and prognosis. Most urinary diversions have similar preoperative nursing considerations.

Support to the individual and family is essential to the overall treatment of patients with bladder cancer. Bowel preparation begins with a low-residue diet two days before surgery. On the day before surgery, the patient receives antibiotics, cathartics, and a clear-liquid diet. Teaching begins preoperatively with a description of the surgical procedure to be performed; the appearance of the abdomen after surgery, including location of tubes, drains, and midline incision; and pre- and postoperative care routines, including the progression of the return of bowel function after surgery, ambulation, diet, and pain control. Printed materials with explicit directions and illustrations are especially helpful preoperatively. It is important, if possible, to involve another family member or significant other. If indicated, the nurse can arrange for a preoperative visit by someone that has undergone and adjusted well to a similar surgery.[42,43]

The selection of a stoma site is an important preoperative consideration. The stoma site is selected and marked before surgery by the enterostomal therapy nurse. The type of urinary diversion to be performed will indicate to some extent the stoma site selected. Any diversion that requires wearing an external appliance for the collection of urine, such as an ileoconduit, must have an adequate abdominal surface for the adherence of the appliance and must be visible to the individual. A continent urinary reservoir does not require an external collecting device, but the stoma must be accessible by the patient. It is necessary to discuss with the patient the personal habits pertaining to work and recreational activities before selecting a site. The abdomen is examined while the patient is in a supine, sitting, and standing position. This is done to find an area of approximately 3-in. diameter over the abdominal rectus muscle that is free of wrinkles, bony prominences, scars or creases, and belt lines. A scratch mark or tattoo with subcutaneous methylene blue dye is performed at the selected site to prevent removal of the mark after the surgical scrub preparation.[43]

General Postoperative Care

Postoperative care will vary slightly depending on the method used to create the urinary diversion. As with all patients who have undergone major abdominal surgery, prophylactic anticoagulation measures and incentive spirometry may be used to prevent pulmonary emboli or respiratory complications. A nasogastric tube or gastrostomy tube is left in place until intestinal peristalsis resumes. Serum electrolytes and creatinine should be monitored postoperatively for the development of metabolic abnormalities. Intravenous access is necessary for the delivery of fluids, blood transfusions, antibiotics, pain medication, and any other essential medications in the initial postoperative period.[43]

The inner lining of the continent urinary reservoir and conduit produces mucus. An ileoconduit should have continuous flow of urine into the external appliance. The appliance is then connected to a bedside drainage bag for accurate measurement of output. The ureteral stents or red Robinson catheter may be irrigated if decreased urinary output is noted. During the first three weeks after surgery, the continent reservoir's urinary catheter must be irrigated every four hours and as needed to prevent mucus obstruction. Urinary drainage should be continuous. A sign of an obstructed catheter would be decreased output from the urinary catheter and increased output from the abdominal Penrose drain.[44]

Nursing Care Following Urinary Diversion with an Ileoconduit

Stoma characteristics. Viability of the stoma is assessed by its color. This should be checked regularly, especially in the early postoperative period. Normal color of the stoma is deep pink to deep red. The intestinal stomal tissue can be compared with the mucosal lining of the mouth. The stoma may bleed when rubbed because of the capillaries at the surface.[45]

A stoma with a dusky appearance ranging from purple to black, or necrotic, indicates impairment of circulation and should be reported to the surgeon. A necrotic stoma may develop from abdominal distention causing tension on the mesentery, from twisting of the conduit at the time of surgery, or from arterial or venous insufficiency. Necrotic tissue below the level of the fascia indicates conduit infarction and potential intra-abdominal urine leak. Prompt recognition and surgical re-exploration is necessary.

Stoma edema is normal in the early postoperative period as a result of surgical manipulation. This should not interfere with stoma functioning, but a larger opening will need to be cut in the appliance to prevent pressure or constriction of the stoma. Most stomas decrease in size four to six weeks following surgery with minor changes over one year. Teaching the individual to continue to measure the stoma with each change of appliance should alleviate the problem of the person wearing an appliance with an aperture too large for the stoma. The stoma needs only a space of ⅛-in diameter to allow for expansion during peristalsis.[45]

Ideally, a urinary stoma is located in the lower right quadrant, and protrudes ½–¾ in above the skin surface to allow the urine to drain efficiently. Table 47-4 describes various stoma types and their specific problems and appliances.[46]

Pouching a urinary stoma. The continuous outflow of urine from a conduit requires the individual to wear an appliance at all times. In the early postoperative period, any one of the many disposable pouches may be used. The selection of the particular type of pouch may be governed by the availability in the facility or by the surgeon's choice.

The skin around the stoma should be clean and thoroughly dry before positioning the appliance over the stoma. Although not always possible, an effective pouch should adhere at least three days. If no leakage occurs, the same pouch can remain adhered to the skin for up to ten days. It should then be changed for hygienic reasons and to observe the peristomal area. Table 47-5 describes common peristomal skin problems and their management.[47]

Today, the materials and design of appliances are continually updated to provide the consumer with the best protection and easiest care. The enterostomal therapy nurse, product representatives, and the ostomy/wound management buyers guide[48] are excellent resources for available products.

Teaching the patient continuing care of a conduit. The initial care rendered to the patient with a new conduit is extremely important both physiologically and psychologically. Before the individual is able to actively

Table 47-4 Stoma Types and Their Specific Problems and Appliances

Stoma Type	Appliance Needed	Problems Seen
Nipple or bud	Any pouch	Minimal
Flush	May need convex skin barrier with belt	Skin irritation and insecurity Inability to see stoma when applying the pouch Occlusion of the stoma by the pouch Decreased wearing time causing higher costs
Retracted	Rigid faceplate or convex skin barrier with belt	As above
Prolapsed	Flexible skin barrier so as to not constrict base of stoma	Ischemia or erosion of exposed bowel

Reprinted with permission from Carroll MD, Barbour S: Urinary diversion and bladder substitution, in Tanagho EA, McAninch JW (eds): *Smith's General Urology* (ed 13). Norwalk, CT, Appleton and Lange, 1992, p 436.[46]

Table 47-5   Common Peristomal Skin Problems and Their Management*

Problem	Cause	Management
Fungal infections—*Candida albicans* (Monilia)	• Urine accumulating under barrier (seen more frequently with diabetes mellitus and concurrent antibiotic use)	• Apply nystatin powder • Dry skin thoroughly (use hair dryer) • Prevent leakage under wafer
Allergic contact dermatitis	• Sensitivity to solvents, adhesives, detergents, wafers	• Identify irritant (skin patch test) and discontinue product • Apply hydrocortisone cream (avoid prolonged use) • Avoid solvents and soaps
Mechanical trauma	• Frequent or "excessive" pouch changing leading to skin stripping • Pressure from belts • Overuse of adhesive strips around the faceplate or barrier	• Minimize pouch changes • Encourage gentle skin care • Consider nonadhesive pouches (used with belt) • Minimize use of sealants and adhesives
Pseudoverrucous skin lesions	• Urine contact with skin over extended time	• Ensure that the barrier and pouch are the correct size

*The patient should see an enterostomal therapist nurse, if available.

Reprinted with permission from Carroll PR, Barbour S: Urinary diversion and bladder substitution, in Tanagho EA, McAninch JW (eds): *Smith's General Urology* (ed 14). Norwalk, CT: Appleton and Lange, 1995, p 458.[47]

participate in self-care, the nurse or enterostomal therapist can teach by example. Procedures are "talked through" as they are being performed. The individual should be given the opportunity to handle the equipment and do as much of the needed care as possible. All the procedures necessary for continuing care of the stoma should be written down, including addresses where future supplies may be purchased. As the individual's condition improves, he or she should be encouraged to verbalize concerns and fears. A visit from a person who has been rehabilitated with a similar diversion and names and telephone numbers of resource people to call if emergencies arise are additional methods of support and reassurance for the individual. The United Ostomy Association and the American Cancer Society are excellent resources.

Follow-up care.   A periodic reevaluation of the stoma, peristomal skin, and the function of the conduit can avoid many complications of a urinary diversion. An appliance opening too large for the stoma will result in peristomal skin exposure to urine. This leads to maceration and denudation of the skin, and the formation of hypertrophic lesions and poor adherence of the appliance. Reestablishing proper appliance fitting will eliminate these problems.

Mucus will always be present in varying amounts in the urine. The mucus will have a straw-like appearance. Excessive mucus may be produced by an inflamed mucosa such as from an infection. Increasing fluid intake to 2 liters/day will act as a natural irrigant.

Alkaline urine can cause encrustations around the stoma. This may cause stoma stenosis and bacterial infections. Individuals in some settings are advised to take 500–2000 mg of vitamin C per day, along with at least a quart of acidic fruit juice such as orange, grapefruit, or cranberry juice, to create an acidic urine and lower

bacterial counts. However, research has not been able to support efficacy of this intervention.

Stenosis, or narrowing, can occur in the stoma at the level of the skin, muscle, or fascia. Narrowing interferes with urinary drainage and can lead to urinary stasis, dilatation of the ileal segment, and/or infection. Surgical intervention is usually indicated for treatment.[49]

The kidneys and their collecting system, the renal pelvis and ureters, form the urinary component of a conduit. Ureteral angulation, stenosis, obstruction, or lithiasis leads to infection and hydronephrosis with possible irreparable renal damage. Periodic evaluation by means of excretory pyelography or loopography can detect this before damage occurs. A urine analysis and culture may be indicated. The specimen should be collected by removing the bag, cleaning the stoma with an antiseptic wipe, and inserting a 14-Fr female catheter through the stoma. A prepared ileoconduit specimen kit may be used. The end of the catheter is placed into a specimen cup, and time is allowed to collect adequate amount of urine.

Nursing Care of the Individual with a Continent Urinary Reservoir

The patient remains in the hospital for seven to ten days postoperatively. It is during this period that initial recovery and teaching begins. Discharge instructions for a continent urinary reservoir are presented in Table 47-6.[50] The nurse can use these instructions as a guide for teaching the individual.

Three weeks after surgery, the individual will be readmitted to the hospital for an overnight stay or may be seen in the outpatient clinic. Laboratory tests, a physical

Table 47-6   Continent Urinary Reservoir to the Skin or Urethra: Home Care of Tubes and Drains

PURPOSE:
The catheter drains the urinary reservoir of urine and mucus. Flushings are done to prevent the catheter from being plugged. Mucus and small blood clots can plug the catheter. There is a drain in the lower abdomen. Its purpose is to drain fluid from the belly.

SUPPLIES:
Kit for catheter flushing and drain care:
- One roll of 2″ paper adhesive tape
- Large package of 4 × 4 gauze dressings
- Urinary leg bag
- Urinary drainage bag
- Irrigation set
- 2 quarts normal saline
- Nonsterile specimen cup

RECIPE FOR NORMAL SALINE:
Mix 2 teaspoons of table salt in 1 quart of distilled water.

INSTRUCTIONS FOR IRRIGATION OF THE CATHETER:
1. Flush the catheter with 60 mL of normal saline every 4 hours during the day.
2. If the flow slows, if there is more fluid from the drain, or if you have pain, flush the catheter. It could be plugged.

NOTE: If the catheter or drain falls out or slips out, call your physician immediately.

INSTRUCTIONS FOR DRAIN CARE:
A clear plastic bag will be covering the drain to collect the draining fluid.
1. You may shower with the bag on.
2. Empty the bag when it becomes ⅓ to ½ full, or at least once daily.
3. Measure the output. Record the date, time, and amount.
4. If the draining fluid is a very small amount, or nothing at all, you may remove the bag. The bag is removed by peeling the adhesive, or waxy, surface off your skin.
5. You may then shower and allow the water to run over the drain. Clean your skin around the drain with soap and water. Rinse and pat dry. Apply a clean, dry gauze dressing pad over the drain. Tape in place.

Data from USC/Kenneth Norris Jr. Cancer.[50]

examination, and history of current condition are taken and reviewed. A radiographic study of the pouch will be taken to confirm that there is no extravasation of urine outside the pouch. The radiographic study is not necessary if the output from the Penrose drain has been less than 100 cc over the prior 24 hours. The catheter and ureteral stents are then removed.

The individual with a cutaneous continent urinary reservoir is taught to intubate/catheterize the pouch using a 20-Fr coudé red-rubber catheter every 2 hours during the day and every 3 hours at night for the first week after the catheter has been removed. The frequency of catheterization is increased gradually by 1 hour each week until the pouch is being intubated and drained approximately every 6 hours and not at all at night. The Penrose drain is removed prior to discharge home. The individual is instructed to wear a medical alert identification (ID) to inform health care personnel of care needed in case of an emergency. Table 47-7 describes instructions for home care of an individual with a continent urinary reservoir to the skin and a sample inscription for the medical alert ID.[51]

The individual with a continent urinary reservoir to the urethra is instructed on voiding technique, schedule of voiding, and Kegel exercises. The individual is taught to void by sitting on the commode, bearing down, double

Table 47-7   Training for Continent Urinary Reservoir to the Skin

HOME CARE INSTRUCTIONS: This is a clean procedure, not a sterile one.

SUPPLIES:
- A coudé-tip red rubber catheter, 20 Fr
- Povidone-iodine solution (Betadine)
- Water-soluble lubricant (e.g., K-Y Jelly). DO NOT USE Vaseline or petroleum jelly
- Clean paper towels
- Stoma covering (e.g., female panty liner cut in half or into thirds), or 2 × 2 gauze and paper tape, or Austin Medical (AM) patch
- Resealable plastic bags

CATHETERIZATION TECHNIQUE:
1. Wash hands prior to catheterizing.
2. Clean stoma with povidone-iodine solution or cleanser of choice on tissue or wipes to remove mucus and bacteria.
3. If needed, lubricate your catheter for easier insertion.
4. Insert the catheter into the stoma until urine begins to flow.
5. When urine stops flowing, push the catheter in a little more and/or pull it out slightly to ensure that all urine has drained.

   NOTE: If the urine flow is slow or absent, you may remove the catheter and rinse under warm water to remove mucus plugs, then reinsert the catheter as in step 4. You may also leave the catheter in place and irrigate with 60 mL of normal saline to remove mucus.

6. Pinch the catheter and remove.
7. Place covering over stoma. Your stoma will always be moist from mucus and the use of a waterproof covering will protect your clothing.

CATHETERIZATION SCHEDULE:

1st week	Catheterization should be done every 2 hours during the day and every 3 hours at night.
2nd week	Catheterize every 3 hours during the day and every 4 hours at night.
3rd week	Catheterize every 4 hours during the day and every 5 hours at night.
4th week	Catheterize every 5 hours during the day and every 6 hours at night.
5th week	Catheterize every 6 hours during the day and not at all during the night.

Table 47-7 Training for Continent Urinary Reservoir to the Skin (continued)

IRRIGATION SCHEDULE:

1. Flush the pouch once a day, following your catheterization procedure, for 2 months after your discharge from the hospital. Use a 60-mL syringe full of normal saline, or use a new turkey or meat baster to irrigate.
2. To make normal saline solution: Add 2 teaspoons of table salt to 1 quart of distilled water.
3. After two months, you can flush if you notice an increase in mucus or a change in the odor of your urine, or urine that does not come out easily.
4. Pressure or discomfort can be felt when the pouch is overdistended. If this happens, catheterize your pouch. Never go longer than 7–8 hours without catheterization.

CATHETER CARE:

1. Clean used catheters in warm, soapy water, then rinse with tap water. Be sure to rinse the inside and outside of the catheter.
2. Place the catheter on a clean paper towel to air dry.
3. Place the clean, air-dried catheter in a clean, covered plastic container or resealable plastic bag. A Tupperware celery container works well.
4. Make a kit to use away from home.

> *TRAVEL KIT:* Place two dry, clean catheters into double-bagged, resealable plastic bags. In the outer bag keep extra stoma dressings and Betadine wipes. Place this equipment into a cosmetic or tobacco pouch. Strips of paper tape may be adhered to the outer plastic bag to eliminate carrying a roll of tape.

5. When catheterizing in a public restroom:
   a. Remove old dressing from stoma.
   b. Swab stoma off with Betadine wipe.
   c. Insert catheter and drain pouch completely.
   d. Pinch-off catheter and remove.
   e. Dry catheter with toilet tissue and place dirty catheter into the outside resealable bag to be cleaned when you return home.

NOTE: Patients with a urinary pouch to the skin (stoma present) need to wear a Med-Alert band. Recommended inscription: Stoma, Continent Urinary Reservoir. Use 20-Fr coudé catheter every 4–6 hours. Do not use a Foley catheter.

Data from USC/Kenneth Norris Jr. Cancer Hospital.[50]

Table 47-8 Discharge Instructions for Self-Catheterization

PURPOSE: Three weeks after surgery the catheter is removed and you begin urinating on your own. The urethra (where the urine exits the body) could become plugged with mucus and stop urine from being passed. If this should occur, you would have to insert a catheter through the urethra into the pouch to drain it. Self-catheterization is taught before surgery so that you will know how to pass a catheter into your continent urinary reservoir.

EQUIPMENT:

- A moist towelette or soap and water
- A dry hand towel
- Water-soluble lubricant
- 18-Fr coudé catheter

INSTRUCTIONS:

1. Wash your hands thoroughly with soap and water and dry.
2. Position yourself either in front of the toilet or sitting on the toilet.
3. Clean the urethral opening.
   For women: with one hand, separate the labia (skin folds) and wash from front to back with soap and water or a moist towelette.
   For men: hold the penis up with one hand and wash the tip of the penis with soap and water or a moist towelette. You should wash in a circular motion starting at the urethra opening and moving away from the opening.
4. Lubricate the catheter end that will go into your urethra. Use a water-soluble lubricant such as K-Y Jelly. Do not use Vaseline or petroleum jelly.
5. Insert the catheter into the urethra until the urine begins to flow.
   For women: approximately 1–1.5 inches.
   For men: approximately 6–8 inches.
   Then insert the catheter about 1 inch farther and hold it there until urine stops running.
6. Take this opportunity to flush your reservoir. Leaving the catheter in place, flush the catheter with 60 mL of normal saline.
7. Slowly withdraw the catheter, stopping each time more urine drains out.
8. Pinch the catheter and remove.
9. Check the color, odor, and clarity of the urine to be aware of any changes that you may need to report to your doctor or nurse. For example, cloudy, foul-smelling, or bloody urine should be reported.

CATHETER CARE:

1. Wash the catheter with warm, soapy water.
2. Rinse with clear water, including through the center of the catheter.
3. Dry the catheter. Allow it to sit out on a clean surface so that the center of the catheter can air dry.
4. Store the catheter in a clean, dry container of your choice.

Data from USC/Kenneth Norris Jr. Cancer Hospital.[50]

voiding, and applying gentle pressure on the lower abdomen (Credé maneuver). The voiding schedule is the same as continent urinary reservoir to the skin; however, gradual increase may be by ½ hour instead of 1 hour. Kegel exercises are then taught to increase the strength of the pelvic floor muscle and therefore eliminate urinary incontinence. It takes a motivated person at least 3 months to obtain control during the day and night.[52] The individual is reinstructed on clean intermittent self-catheterization (Table 47-8) in the event that they experience urinary retention due to a mucus plug while at home. Table 47-9 presents discharge instructions for the training of the continent urinary reservoir to the urethra.

Follow-up care. Many complications of a urinary reservoir can be avoided by a periodic reevaluation. Radio-logical studies are used to confirm the integrity of the pouch, test the competence of the antireflux mechanism, and ensure complete emptying of the reservoir. Intravenous pyelogram is performed to view the upper tracts. Renal function is evaluated by laboratory tests including urea nitrogen, serum creatinine, urinary pH, and specific gravity or osmolality. If the urine is tested for culture and sensitivity, it is important to remember that the continent reservoirs are not closed sterile systems, as is the bladder.

Table 47-9   Training for Continent Urinary Reservoir to the Urethra

SUPPLIES:
Kit:
- Incontinent absorbent undergarment, chux
- 18-Fr coudé-tip red rubber catheter, K-Y Jelly, Betadine wipe prep
- Urinal (for men)

INSTRUCTIONS:
1. You will start to leak urine after removing the catheter. Try to empty the reservoir by sitting down on the commode, bearing down (like having a bowel movement), and/or using gentle pressure over the lower abdomen with your hands (Credé maneuver). Empty the reservoir as completely as possible.
2. Urinate on a schedule of every 2 hours during the day and every 3 hours at night. Try to increase the time between urination every week by ½–1 hour until you reach 4–6 hours during the day and 6–7 hours at night. If leaking starts before your scheduled time, you may empty the pouch early.
3. You will need to strengthen your muscle that will close the urethra and hold urine in the pouch. These exercises are called Kegel exercises.
   a. The Kegel exercise is a voluntary contraction and relaxation of the pelvic floor muscles to close the urethra and prevent urine leakage.
   b. Directions:
      (1) Relax belly (abdominal) muscles when doing the exercises.
      (2) Do the contractions while sitting, standing, and lying.
      (3) Slow-twitch muscle contractions: Contract and relax pelvic muscle 10 times in a row.
         - 1st week hold contractions for 3 seconds, relax for 6 seconds.
         - 2nd week hold contractions for 5 seconds, relax for 10 seconds.
         - 3rd week hold contractions for 7–10 seconds, relax for 14–20 seconds.
      (4) Fast-twitch muscle contractions:
      NOTE: Do the exercises every other hour during the day or at least 4–6 times per day until you do not leak urine.
         - Contract and relax the pelvic floor muscles quickly 5 times in a row after slow-twitch contractions.
4. Your continent urinary reservoir has to learn to expand and hold urine. IT TAKES TIME AND PATIENCE.
5. The drain has also been removed. Drainage from the site may be thick and look creamy to brown in color. Clean the site once a day with mild soap and water, rinse, and pat dry. Apply clean, dry 4 × 4 gauze dressing over site until there is no more drainage from the site. Change the dressing during the day when it is wet.
6. You may need to insert a catheter if you are unable to pass urine. [Refer to self-catheterizing instructions (Table 47-8)].

Data from USC/Kenneth Norris Jr. Cancer Hospital.[50]

The reservoirs are colonized with bacteria, and their presence does not necessarily indicate an infection. Cutaneous reservoir specimens are collected after cleaning hands (clean gloves for health care professionals), cleansing stoma with a betadine swab, and using a new sterile catheter to drain the urine into a specimen container. Specimens collected from reservoirs to the urethra are performed in the same way as for an original bladder.

KIDNEY CANCER

Epidemiology

The two major types of kidney cancer are renal cell cancer and cancer of the renal pelvis. Renal cell cancer is the more common of the two, accounting for approximately 3% of all cancers and 85% of all kidney cancers.[53] There were an estimated 30,000 new cases of kidney cancer and 11,900 deaths caused by this disease in the United States during 1999.

The four major variables related to kidney cancer incidence are race, gender, age, and geographic location. Renal cancer occurrence is equivalent between whites and blacks. The rate of kidney cancer is one-third greater in Hispanics than in white Americans.[54] There is a 2:1 male predominance in renal cell cancer. The average age at diagnosis is between 50 and 70 years of age.[55] Geographically, there is a high rate of kidney cancer in Scandinavian countries and a low incidence in Japan. The United States and most Western European countries appear to have an intermediate risk.[56]

Etiology

There are many risk factors associated with the cause of kidney cancer. The risk factor that has been linked persistently to kidney cancer by both cohort studies[56–58] and epidemiological case control studies[59–61] is cigarette smoking. For renal cell cancer, a consistent relationship between the number of cigarettes smoked and the risk of cancer has not been established. But for cancer of the renal pelvis there does appear to be a strong association between the number of cigarettes smoked and the risk of cancer.[62] It is not clear how cigarette smoking might induce kidney cancer, but studies have shown numerous mutagenic chemicals in the urine of cigarette smokers.[58] Occupational exposures linked to kidney cancer include shoemakers; leather tanners; and workers exposed to petroleum products, cadmium, and asbestos.[54] Heavy use of analgesics, specifically aspirin, phenacetin, or acetaminophen, have been shown to increase the risk of cancer of the renal pelvis.[56,62] A possible association between analgesics and renal cell cancer has been reported but not conclusively proven.[59,62] A strong connection between renal cell cancer and obesity in women was first identified in 1974.[60] Others have found similar associations, but there remains the question of whether the increased incidence in women is related to obesity or to hormonal (estrogen) influences.[62] An increased incidence of acquired cystic disease of the kidney and of renal cell carcinoma has been reported in patients undergoing dialysis. A 1990 study reported the risk of renal cell cancer in patients undergoing dialysis to be 57–134 times higher than in the general population.[63]

Epidermal and other growth factors have also been linked to renal cell carcinoma. Many patients have systemic effects—such as pyrexia, cachexia, abnormal liver function, hypercalcemia, and polycythemia—believed to be associated with abnormal growth factors.[6]

Genetic factors have been related to the development of renal cell cancer. Several rare familial types of renal cell cancer are characterized by kidney diseases such as horseshoe kidneys, acquired renal cystic disease, polycystic kidney disease; and autosomal dominant inheritance, and von Hippel-Lindau (VHL) disease. Individuals with familial renal cell cancer have been found to have a translocation of the short arm of chromosome three and the long arm of chromosome eight.[54]

Pathophysiology

Renal cell carcinoma arises from the tubular epithelial cells that are found in the parenchyma of the kidney and recognized as an adenocarcinoma. Histologically, renal cell tumors are clear cell, glandular cell, or mixed cell. Tumors usually arise as a solitary, unilateral mass.[55] The sizes of the renal tumors vary from a few centimeters to remarkably large tumors, filling the peritoneal space. The tumor is usually yellow or gray in color with noted areas of ischemia, hemorrhage, and necrosis. These tumors can be localized, spread by direct extension to the renal vein and into the vena cava or perinephric fat, or spread through the vasculature or lymphatics to distant sites.[54] The most common sites of metastatic spread are the lungs, bone, lymph nodes, and the brain.[64]

Tumors of the renal pelvis generally arise from the epithelial tissue anywhere in the renal pelvis.[55] These tumors often have independent, multifocal origins. The mucosal lining of the renal pelvis and ureter are composed of transitional epithelium, similar to that of the urinary bladder. Thus, the majority of renal pelvis cell types are transitional cell or squamous cell.[56] The renal pelvis tumors may extend into the ureter and through the muscular coats. Metastatic renal cell carcinoma is present in approximately 50% of cases at the time of diagnosis.[65] Papillary renal tumors account for approximately 5%–10% of the malignant renal cell cancers.[55]

Renal cell carcinoma has a considerable association with certain paraneoplastic syndromes (see Chapter 35). Approximately 10%–40% of patients with renal cell carcinoma will develop paraneoplastic syndromes during the course of their disease. Paraneoplastic syndromes associated with renal cell carcinoma are hypercalcemia (10%–20%), hypertension (25%), erythrocytosis (1%–8%), hyperglycemia (10%–20%), cachexia (33%), fever (20%–30%), anemia (20%–40%), amyloidosis (3%–5%), and nonmetastatic hepatic dysfunction or Stauffer syndrome (3%–20%). Typically, the paraneoplastic syndromes will resolve after a nephrectomy.[66] Hypercalcemia may resolve with medical management.[67] The reappearance of paraneoplastic manifestations after nephrectomy may signify disease recurrence.[66]

Clinical Manifestations

Renal cell carcinoma may exhibit a variety of signs and symptoms. The most common presentations are hematuria (in 50%–60% patients), pain (40%), and a palpable flank or abdominal mass (30%–40%).[53] These three manifestations comprise the classic triad and occur simultaneously in approximately 10%–20% of patients. This usually signifies advanced disease since the well-protected anatomical position of the kidney often delays the identification of a tumor. Other findings may include fever, night sweats, weight loss, anemia, or presence of a varicocele in a male patient. The renal cell tumors tend to invade the renal vein creating a thrombus at the area of invasion.[55]

Most tumors of the renal pelvis present with microscopic or macroscopic hematuria. Both hematuria and flank pain may occur due to the passage of blood clots or by the obstruction of the ureteropelvic junction. A palpable mass may be present from a tumor that has extended outside of the kidney or from massive hydronephrosis.[6]

Assessment

Renal Cell Carcinoma

Diagnostic tests establish the presence of renal masses and differentiate solid renal mass lesions from benign renal cysts.[6] For renal cell carcinoma the most useful diagnostic tests include computerized tomography (CT), magnetic resonance imaging (MRI), DNA flow cytometry, excretory urogram or intravenous pyelogram, renal ultrasound, and renal arteriography.

The CT scan is used to diagnose and stage renal cell carcinoma. It provides data about the size and character of the primary tumor, local extent of the cancer, renal vein and inferior vena caval thrombus, lymph node involvement, and adjacent organ metastasis.[9] The MRI detects local tumor invasion and renal vein or inferior vena cava involvement without the need for contrast. Flow cytometry adds information for predicting the prognosis of renal cell cancer. Aneuploid tumors were found to be more likely to progress to invasive lesions than diploid tumors.[68] An excretory urogram evaluates the entire urinary tract. The excretory urogram and the renal tomography are screening tests for suspicious renal mass lesions. Both tests are only 70%–75% accurate in differentiating benign cysts from malignant lesions.[69] Ultrasound evaluation can distinguish between cystic, solid, and complex masses.[32] This modality is noninvasive, easy to perform, and requires minimal physical expenditure from the patient.[70] Historically, renal arteriography has been a standard part of the diagnosis of a suspicious renal mass. Contrast-enhanced CT scans have, in some cases, replaced the need for a renal arteriography. This study is still used, however, to obtain information about the renal vasculature.[68]

Cancer of the Renal Pelvis

The most useful diagnostic studies for establishing a diagnosis of cancer of the renal pelvis are an excretory urogram, retrograde urogram, and urinary cytology. The urine cytology can detect from 20%–30% of low-grade renal pelvic cancers and 60% of higher-grade lesions. An ultrasound may identify a mass density in the central portion of the kidney. A CT scan can detect the presence of a soft tissue mass in the renal hilum. The MRI and CT scan can confirm the presence of regional lymph node involvement.[47]

Classification and Staging

Renal Cell Carcinoma

The system most widely used for classifying renal cell carcinoma is Robson's modification of the system described by Flocks and Kadesky (Figure 47-7).[71] The Robson classification system is limited since it does not clearly differentiate stages that might have significantly different prognoses.[72] The tumor, node, metastases (TNM) system

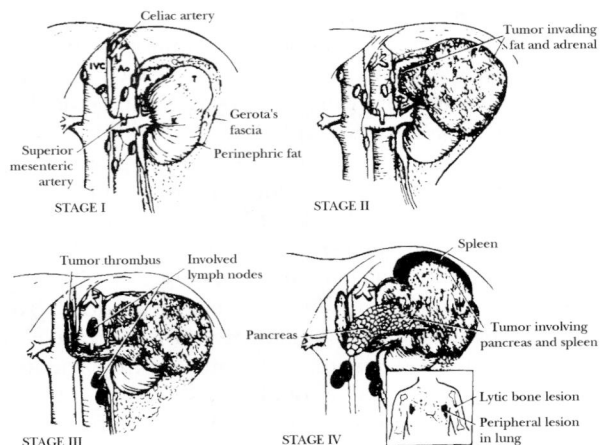

Figure 47-7 Robson staging system for renal cell carcinoma. In stage A, IVC is inferior vena cava; Ao, aorta; A, left suprarenal gland; T, tumor; K, left kidney. (Reprinted with permission from Dreicer R, Williams RO: Renal parenchymal neoplasms, in Tanagho, EA, McAninch JW (eds): *Smith's General Urology* [ed 14]. Norwalk, CT, Appleton and Lange, 1995, p 376.)[71]

(Table 47-10), proposed by the American Joint Committee on Cancer, more accurately defines tumor size, extent of local invasion, vein involvement, and presence of lymph node metastases.[54]

Cancer of the Renal Pelvis

Staging of renal pelvic cancers is based on an accurate assessment of the degree of tumor infiltration and parallels the staging system developed for bladder cancer.[47] Table 47-11 outlines the TNM system for staging cancer of the renal pelvis.

Treatment of Renal Cell Carcinoma

Surgery

A radical nephrectomy (Figure 47-8)[71] is the most effective, often curative, treatment for renal cell cancer. It generally involves the removal of the kidney, proximal ureter, Gerota fascia, adrenal gland, and lymph nodes. Approximately 5%–7% of individuals have renal vein or caval thrombus on presentation.[22] The treatment of

Table 47-10 TNM Staging System for Cancer of the Kidney

T = PRIMARY TUMOR	
TX	Primary tumor cannot be assessed
T0	No evidence of primary tumor
T1	Tumor 7 cm or less in greatest dimension limited to the kidney
T2	Tumor more than 7 cm in greatest dimension limited to the kidney
T3	Tumor extends into major veins or invades adrenal gland or perinephric tissues but not beyond Gerota fascia
T3a	Tumor invades adrenal gland or perinephric tissues but not beyond Gerota fascia
T3b	Tumor grossly extends into renal vein(s) or vena cava below the diaphragm
T3c	Tumor grossly extends into renal vein(s) or vena cava above the diaphragm
T4	Tumor invades beyond Gerota fascia
N = REGIONAL LYMPH NODES (BELOW AORTIC BIFURCATION)	
NX	Regional lymph nodes cannot be assessed
N0	No regional lymph node metastases
N1	Metastasis in single regional lymph node
N2	Metastasis in more than one regional lymph node
M = DISTANT METASTASES	
MX	Presence of distant metastasis cannot be assessed
M0	No distant metastasis
M1	Distant metastasis

Table 47-11   TNM Staging for Cancer of the Renal Pelvis and Ureter

T = PRIMARY TUMOR

TX	Primary tumor cannot be assessed
T0	No evidence of primary tumor
Tis	Carcinoma in situ
Ta	Noninvasive papillary carcinoma
T1	Tumor invades subepithelial connective tissue
T2	Tumor invades the muscularis
T2a	Tumor invades superficial muscle
T3	(For renal pelvis only) Tumor invades beyond muscularis into peripelvic fat or the renal parenchyma
T3	(For ureter only) Tumor invades beyond muscularis into periureteric fat
T4	Tumor invades adjacent organs, or through the kidney into the perinephretic fat

N = REGIONAL LYMPH NODES (BELOW AORTIC BIFURCATION)

NX	Regional lymph nodes cannot be assessed
N0	No regional lymph node metastasis
N1	Metastasis in single lymph node less than 2 cm in greatest dimension
N2	Metastasis in single lymph node more than 2 cm but less than 5 cm, or multiple nodes less than 5 cm in greatest dimension
N3	Metastasis in nodes more than 5 cm in greatest dimension

M = DISTANT METASTASES

MX	Presence of distant metastasis cannot be assessed
M0	No distant metastasis
M1	Distant metastasis

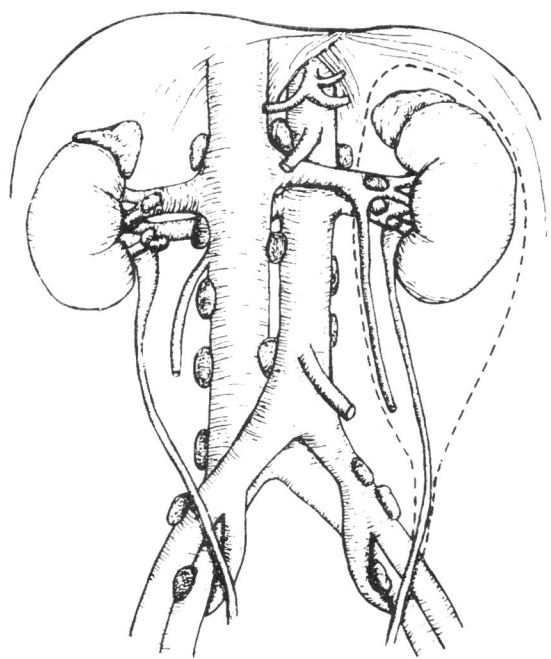

Figure 47-8 Boundaries of a left radical nephrectomy. Dotted line represents both the surgical margin and Gerota fascia. (Reprinted with permission from Drecier R, Williams RO: Renal parenchymal neoplasms, in Tanagho EA, McAninch JW (eds): *Smith's General Urology* [ed 14]. Norwalk, CT, Appleton and Lange, 1995, p 381.)[71]

choice is excision of the renal carcinoma and vena cava thrombus.[23] Cardiopulmonary bypass with circulatory arrest and hypothermia have been used with extensive vena cava or right atrium invasion.[73]

Regional lymphadenectomy remains controversial. Proponents believe that this offers a survival advantage when performed with a radical nephrectomy. Others argue that the staging value, in terms of predicting survival, is limited since the cancer can spread via the venous system bypassing the lymphatics.[23]

Radiotherapy and Chemotherapy

Radiotherapy after nephrectomy for control of microscopic disease has controversial results. Several studies have shown postoperative radiotherapy controlling local disease but not affecting overall survival.[74] Adjuvant chemotherapy has not demonstrated any improvement in survival rates or decreased possibility of relapse.[53]

Treatment of Advanced Renal Cell Carcinoma

About 30% of individuals with renal cell carcinoma present with metastasis at the time of diagnosis. Another 50% will develop metastasis after radical nephrectomy.[75] The goal of therapy in advanced renal cell cancer is palliation

of symptoms. Therapy may include nephrectomy and adjuvant therapy including radiotherapy, chemotherapy, and/or immunotherapy. Spontaneous regression occasionally occurs with this tumor.[53]

Radiation is an important modality in the palliation of patients with metastatic renal cell cancer. Despite the belief that this is a radioresistant tumor, effective palliation by the use of external beam radiation of metastatic disease to the bone, brain, and lungs is reported in up to two-thirds of individuals.[6] In a study performed by Dibiase and associates,[75] it was concluded that radiotherapy was found to be an effective palliation for metastatic disease.

Adjuvant or palliative nephrectomies are treatment options for individuals with metastatic renal cell carcinoma. An adjuvant nephrectomy is performed to improve survival, and a palliative nephrectomy can control symptoms of the primary renal tumor. These symptoms may be pain, bleeding, or endocrinopathies.[76]

Angioinfarction of the kidney is done with or without a nephrectomy to decrease the vascularity before surgery. It may lessen tumor bleeding, pain, or other systemic symptoms in patients with unresectable tumors.[6]

Chemotherapy has not demonstrated a response in renal cell carcinoma. Vinblastine and floxuridine have shown minimal antitumor effect. Further investigation with new chemotherapeutic agents and combination chemotherapy regimens is necessary.[53]

Various biological therapies have been evaluated in the treatment of metastatic renal cell carcinoma since it was first reported in 1983. Alfa-interferon has shown a response rate of up to 29% in individuals without bulky pulmonary and/or soft tissue metastasis, excellent performance status, and no weight loss.[54,73] This response rate was achieved with intermediate doses ranging from 3–20 million units administered subcutaneously or intramuscularly three times per week. These responses are rarely complete or durable.[55,78] The antitumor responses have also been achieved using high doses of interleukin 2 (IL2) with or without large numbers of lymphokine-activated killer (LAK) cells.[79] The response rates are similar to alfa-interferon, but durable complete remissions have been reported. Several clinical investigations are currently under way testing the synergistic effect of IL2 and alfa-interferon when administered as combination therapy.[55] Clinical trials have shown favorable response rates and much lower toxicity as the agents are administered at lower dosages.[80,81] Common side effects of IL2 and alfa-interferon include flu-like symptoms, fatigue, cognitive dysfunction, myelosuppression, abnormal liver function, and anorexia.[82–86] Interleukin 2 has the additional side effects of nausea and vomiting, diarrhea, stomatitis, fluid retention, hypotension, tachycardia, skin rash, erythema, and phlebitis at injection site[65,83]

Treatment of Cancer of the Renal Pelvis

Treatment for renal pelvic cancers is based on tumor grade and stage. The traditional treatment has been nephroureterectomy. This involves the removal of the kidney, all perinephric tissue, regional lymph nodes, the ureter, and a small cuff of the bladder. Radiation therapy and chemotherapy have not proven to be effective in controlling residual tumor, local recurrence, or unresectable disease.[47] New treatment strategies for cancer of the renal pelvis include percutaneous or ureteroscopic resection of the tumors followed by laser irradiation or supplemental intracavitary BCG or epidoxorubicin.[86]

Results and Prognosis

Survival rates for renal cell cancer depend on the stage of the disease. For patients with tumor confined to the kidney (T1–T2) the five-year survival is approximately 89%; for T3 tumors it is approximately 62%; for metastatic disease (T4, or any T with M1 or greater) the five-year survival is low, ranging from 10%. The overall five-year survival is 61%.[1] The five-year survival rates (adjusted for normal life expectancy) as reported by the American Cancer Society can be seen in Table 47-12.

Table 47-12 Approximate Five-Year Survival Rates for Kidney Cancer

Stage	Survival Percentage
Localized	89
Regional	62
Distant	10
All stages	61

Reprinted with permission from American Cancer Society: *Cancer Facts and Figures—1999.* Atlanta, American Cancer Society, January 1999.[41]

Nursing Care of Individuals with Cancer of the Kidney

Individuals who are undergoing diagnostic procedures or treatments for cancer of the kidney are extremely anxious. Some individuals equate the loss of a kidney with imminent death. Others worry that the remaining kidney will not be able to meet the body's total need for urine elimination. In the preoperative period, the nurse should assess the individual's knowledge and feelings about the disease and its treatment to help the patient set realistic goals for dealing with the malignancy and its treatment. In addition, the preparation of the individual prior to surgery and the postoperative nursing care is similar to that of individuals undergoing a laparotomy or other pelvic surgery. Nursing management includes pain control, prevention of atelectasis and pneumonia, monitoring for potential pneumothorax if a chest tube has been placed, monitoring renal function, preventing paralytic ileus, assessing for hemorrhage, and wound care. Discharge planning and individual instructions are essential and should include a family member or caregiver when possible. Prior to discharge the nurse should discuss with the individual the importance of liberal fluid intake of at least 2 liters per day and to avoid excess protein in the diet. Individuals who are prone to hypertension should have their blood pressure monitored for changes. An elevation of blood pressure may indicate compromised renal function or renal insufficiency due to an increased extracellular fluid volume because of decreased normal kidney excretion of NA+ and water or an increased production of aldosterone and NA+ retention resulting in hypertension. Patients should be taught to report any symptoms of respiratory distress, hemoptysis, pain, or fracture of extremity. These symptoms may signify metastasis. Finally, the individual should be reassured that life with one kidney can be normal.

Follow-up Care

The risk of metastasis is dependent on the pathological stage of the disease. Levy and associates[64] have designed surveillance protocols related to the stage of the tumor. The standard tests that are performed on follow-up surveillance include physical examination, serum alkaline phosphatase level and liver function, annual chest x-ray, and CT scan. There is not a standard guideline on when each of these tests should be performed, however, and this may vary for each institution. Bone and brain studies are indicated by site-specific symptoms such as change in mental status or fracture, presence of metastasis at another site, or elevated alkaline phosphatase levels.

Conclusion

The two urinary tract cancers discussed in this chapter are relatively rare, together accounting for only about 6% of all cancers. Smoking is an etiologic factor for both types of cancers, as are certain genetic factors. Surgery is the treatment of choice for cure in the United States for most bladder and kidney cancers. However, radiation therapy is the mainstay of treatment for bladder cancer in many countries.

Advances in treatment include the reemergence of intravesical BCG to prevent tumor progression for superficial bladder cancer, improved surgical procedures for invasive bladder cancer such as the continent urinary diversions following cystectomy, and neoadjuvant and adjuvant combined-modality treatment for invasive bladder cancer. Late-stage kidney cancer has recently shown improved response rates and lower toxicity to treatment with a combination of alfa-interferon and IL2. Clinical trials have also opened an avenue for patients with bladder and kidney cancer who have not responded to standard therapy.

Continued research efforts in the development of tumor markers sensitive and specific to the diagnosis and monitoring of bladder or kidney cancer is essential. Identifying patients earlier in their disease process and preventing disease advancement is another area of research investigation. Research is also currently focusing on the identification of systemic regimens that can effectively treat patients with more advanced disease while conserving bladder or kidney function and avoiding extensive surgery.

References

1. American Cancer Society: *Cancer Facts and Figures—1998.* Atlanta, American Cancer Society, 1999.
2. Droller M: Bladder Cancer: State-of-the-Art Care. *CA Cancer J Clin* 48:269–284, 1998
3. Kelly LP, Miaskowski C: An overview of bladder cancer: treatment and nursing implications. *Oncol Nurs Forum* 23: 459–468, 1996
4. Sorahan T, Lancashire RJ, Sole G: Urothelial cancer and cigarette smoking; findings from a regional case-controlled study. *Br J Urol* 74:753–756, 1994
5. Scher HI, Shipley WU, Herr HW: Cancer of the bladder, in DeVita VT, Hellman S, Rosenberg SA (eds): *Cancer: Principles of Oncology* (ed 5). Philadelphia, Lippincott-Raven, 1997, pp 1300–1322
6. Raghavan D, Shipley WU, Garnick MG, et al: Biology and management of bladder cancer. *N Engl J Med* 322: 1129–1138, 1990
7. Fradet Y, Cordon-Cardo C: Tumor markers in the management of bladder cancer, in Raghavan D, Scher HI, Leibel SA, et al (eds): *Principles and Practice of Genitourinary Oncology.* Philadelphia, Lippincott, 1997, pp 231–238
8. Hossan E, Striegel A: Carcinoma of the bladder. *Semin Oncol Nurs* 9:252–266, 1993
9. Flynn SD, Kacinski B, Peschel RE: Pathology and staging of urothelial cancer, in Ernstoff MS, Heaney JA, Peschel RF: *Urological Cancer.* Malden MA, Blackwell Science, 1997, pp 229–240
10. Droller MJ, Gospocbrowicz MK: Staging of bladder cancer, in Volgolzang NJ, Scardino PT, Shipley WU, et al (eds): *Comprehensive Textbook of Genitourinary Oncology.* Philadelphia, Williams and Wilkins, 1996, pp 359–370
11. Stein JP, Grossfeld GD, Ginsberg, et al: Prognostic markers in bladder cancer: a contemporary review of the literature. *J Urol* 160:645–659, 1998
12. Narayan P: Immunology of genitourinary tumors, in Tanagho EA, McAninch JW (eds): *Smith's General Urology* (ed 14). Norwalk, CT, Appleton and Lange, 1995, pp 334–352
13. Carroll PR: Urothelial carcinoma: Cancers of the bladder, ureter, and renal pelvis, in Tanagho EA, McAnirch JW (eds). *Smith's General Urology* (ed 14). Norwalk, CT, Appleton and Lange, 1995 pp 354–355
14. Fleming ID, Cooper JS, Henson DE, et al (eds): *American Joint Committee on Cancer: Manual for Staging of Cancer* (ed. 5). Philadelphia, Lippincott, 1998
15. Hall MC, Dinney CP: Radical cystectomy for stage T3b bladder cancer. *Semin Urol Oncol* 14:78–80, 1996
16. Zietman AL, Shipley WU, Heney, et al: The case for radiotherapy with or without chemotherapy in high-risk superficial and muscle-invading bladder cancer. *Semin Urol Oncol* 15:161–168, 1997
17. Nseyo UO, Lamm DL: Immunotherapy of bladder cancer. *Semin Surg Oncol* 13:342–349, 1997
18. Nseyo UO, Lamm DL: Therapy of superficial bladder cancer. *Semin Oncol* 23:598–604, 1996
19. Sternberg CN: Neoadjuvant chemotherapy in locally advanced bladder cancer. *Semin Oncol* 23:621–632, 1996
20. Smith JA: Surgical management of superficial bladder cancer (stages Ta/T1/CIS). *Semin Surg Oncol* 13:328–334, 1997
21. Stein JP, Skinner DG: Radical cystectomy in women. *Urol Clin North Am* 5:37-64, 1997
22. Lyne JC, Bahnson RR: Surgical management of invasive urothelial cancer, in Ernstoff MS, Heaney JA, Peschel RF (eds): *Urological Cancer.* Cambridge, MA, Blackwell Science, 1997, pp 272–292
23. Messing EM, Caralona C: Urothelial tumors of the urinary tract, in Walsh PC, Retile AB, Vaughan ED, et al (eds): *Campbell's Urology.* Philadelphia, Saunders, 1998, pp 2327–2382
24. Raghavan D, Huben R: Management of bladder cancer. *Curr Probl Cancer* 19:1–64, 1995
25. Swanson D: Cancer of the bladder and prostate: The impact of therapy on sexual function, in von Eschenbach AC, Rodriguez D (eds): *Sexual Rehabilitation of the Urologic Cancer Patient.* Boston, Hall, 1981, p 102-103

26. American Cancer Society and United Ostomy Association: *Urostomy: A guide.* Atlanta, American Cancer Society, revised October 1990

27. Stein JP, Lieskovsky G, Ginsberg, et al: The T pouch: an orthotopic ileal neobladder incorporating a serosal lined ileal antireflux technique. *J Urol* 159:1836–1842, 1998

28. Studer UE, Ackermann D, Casanova GA, et al: Three year experience with an ileal low pressure bladder substitution. *Br J Urol* 63:43–52, 1988

29. Rowland RG, Mitchell ME, Bihrle R, et al: Indiana continent urinary reservoir. *J Urol* 137:1136–1139, 1987

306. Stein RG: Continent urinary diversion and the ileal cecal pouch with appendostomy: a review with nursing care. *J WOCN* 22:51–57, 1995

31. Skinner DG, Lieskovsky G, Skinner EC, et al: Urinary diversion. *Curr Probl Surg* 24:407–471, 1987

32. Walsh PC: Anatomic radical retropubic prostatectomy, in Walsh PC, Retile AB, Vaughan ED, et al (eds): *Campbell's Urology.* Philadelphia, Saunders, 1998, pp 2565–2588

33. Schoenberg MP, Walsh PC, Breazeale DR, et al: Local recurrence and survival following nerve sparing radical cystoprostatectomy for bladder cancer: 10-year follow-up. *J Urol* 155:490–494, 1996

34. American Medical Systems, Inc. Minnetonka, Minnesota

35. Serretta V, Greco GL, Pavone C, et al: The fate of patients with locally advanced bladder cancer treated conservatively with neoadjuvant chemotherapy, extensive transurethral resection and radiotherapy: 10-year experience. *J Urol* 159:1187–1191, 1997

36. Pronzato P, Vigani A, Pensa F, et al: Second line chemotherapy with ifosfamide as outpatient treatment for advanced bladder cancer. *Am J Clin Oncol* 20:519–521, 1997

37. Milikan R, Dinney CP: The role of chemotherapy in the management of the patient with T3b bladder cancer. *Semin Urol Oncol* 14:81–85, 1996

38. Kish JA, Wolf MK, Schellhammer PF, et al: Continuous-infusion 5-fluorouracil and cisplatin for advanced/recurrent transitional cell cancer of the bladder: a southwest oncology group trial. *Am J Clin Oncol* 20:327–330, 1997

39. Roth BJ: Chemotherapy for advanced bladder cancer. *Semin Oncol* 23:633–644, 1996

40. Roth BJ, Bajorin DF: Advanced bladder cancer: the need to identify new agents in the post-m-vac (methotrexate, vinblastine, doxorubicin and cisplatin) world. *J Urol* 153:894–900, 1995

41. American Cancer Society: *Cancer Facts and Figures—1999.* Atlanta, American Cancer Society, January 1999

42. Stein JP, Cote RJ, Freeman JA, et al: Indications for lower urinary tract reconstruction in women after cystectomy for bladder cancer: a pathological review of female cystectomy specimens. *J Urol* 154:1329–1333, 1995

43. Reilly NJ: Cancer of the bladder, in Karlowicz (ed): *Urologic Nursing: Principles and Practice.* Philadelphia, Saunders, 1995, pp 243–270

44. Smith DB: Psychosocial adaptation, in Hampton BG, Bryant RA (eds): *Ostomies and Continent Diversions: Nursing Management.* Philadelphia, Mosby Year-Book, 1992, pp 1–28

45. Erwin-Toth P, Doughty DB: Principles and procedures of stomal management, in Hampton BG, Bryant RA (eds): *Ostomies and Continent Diversions: Nursing Management.* Philadelphia, Mosby Year-Book, 1992, pp 29–94

46. Carroll MD, Barbour S: Urinary diversion and bladder substition, in Tanagho EA, McAninch JW (eds): *Smith's General Urology* (ed 13). Norwalk, CT, Appleton and Lange, 1992, p 436

47. Carroll PR, Barbour S: Urinary diversion and bladder substitution, in Tanagho EA, McAninch JW (eds): *Smith's General Urology* (ed 14). Norwalk, CT: Appleton and Lange, 1995, p 458.

48. Anonymous: The 1998 ostomy/wound management buyers guide. *Ostomy/Wound Mgmt* 44:10–198, 1998

49. Hampton BG: Peristomal and stomal complications, in Hampton BG, Bryant RA (eds): *Ostomies and Continent Diversions: Nursing Management.* Philadelphia, Mosby Year-Book, 1992, pp 105–126

50. USC/Kenneth Norris Jr. Cancer Hospital, Division of Patient Care Services, 1997

51. Greig B: A new option for cystectomy patients. *RN* 53:34–40, 1990

52. Meaglia JC, Joseph AC, Cheng M, et al: Post-prostatectomy urinary incontinence: response to behavioral training. *J Urol* 144:674–676, 1990

53. Motzer RJ, Bander NH, Nanus DM: Renal-cell carcinoma. *N Engl J Med* 335:865–875, 1996

54. Franklin JR, Figlin R, Belldegrun A: Renal cell carcinoma: basic biology and clinical behavior. *Semin Urol Oncol* 14:208–215, 1996

55. Bukowski RM, Novick AC: Clinical practice guidelines: renal cell carcinoma. *Cleve Clin J Med* 64:Suppl 1 1–48, 1997

56. Ross RK, Paganini-Hill A, Landolph J, et al: Analgesics, cigarette smoking and other risk factors for cancer of the renal pelvis and ureter. *Cancer Res* 49:1045–1048, 1989

57. Weir JM, Dunn JE: Smoking and mortality: a prospective study. *Cancer* 25:105–112, 1970

58. Doll R, Petro R: Mortality in relation to smoking: 20 years' observations on male British doctors. *BMJ* 2:1525–1536, 1976

59. McLaughlin JK, Mandel JS, Blot WJ, et al: A population based case-control study of renal cell carcinoma. *J Natl Cancer Inst* 72:275–284, 1984

60. Wynder E, Mabuchi K, Whitmore W: Epidemiology of adenocarcinoma of the kidney. *J Natl Cancer Inst* 53:1619–1634, 1974

61. LaVecchia C, Negri E, D'Avanzo B, et al: Smoking and renal cell carcinoma. *Cancer Res* 50:5231–5233, 1990

62. Pagnini-Hill A, Ross RK, Henderson BE: Epidemiology of renal cancer, in Skinner DG, Lieskovsky G (eds): *Diagnosis and Management of Genitourinary Cancer.* Philadelphia, Saunders, 1988, pp 32–39

63. Ishikawa I, Saito Y, Shikura N, et al: Ten-year retrospective study on the development of renal cell carcinoma in dialysis patients. *Am J Kidney Dis* 16:452–458, 1990

64. Levy DA, Slaton JW, Swanson DA, et al: Stage specific guidelines for surveillance after radical nephrectomy for local renal cell carcinoma. *J Urol* 159:1163–1167, 1998

65. Letizia M, Conway AM: Interleukin-2 therapy for renal cell cancer: indications, effects, and nursing implications. *Crit Care Nurs* 16:20–35, 1996

66. Gold PJ, Fefer A, Thompson JA: Paraneoplastic manifestations of renal cell carcinoma. *Semin Urol Oncol* 14:216–222, 1996

67. Walther MM, Patel B, Choyke PL, et al: Hypercalcemia in patients with metastatic renal cell carcinoma: effect of nephrectomy and metabolic evaluation. *J Urol* 158:733–739, 1997

68. Ljungberg B, Larsson P, Stenling R, et al: Flow cytometric deoxyribonucleic acid analysis in stage I renal cell carcinoma. *J Urol* 146:697–699, 1991

69. Boswell WD: Diagnostic imaging in genitourinary cancer, in Skinner DG, Lieskovsky G (eds): *Diagnosis and Management*

of Genitourinary Cancer. Philadelphia, Saunders, 1988, pp 237–263

70. McClennan BL: Oncologic imaging-staging and follow-up of renal and adrenal carcinoma. *Cancer* 67:1199–1208, 1991

71. Drecier. R, Williams RO: Renal parenchymal neoplasms, in Tanagho EA, McAninch JW (eds): *Smith's General Urology* (ed 14). Norwalk, CT, Appleton and Lange, 1995, pp 376–381

72. Fleming ID, Cooper JS, Henson DE, et al (eds): *American Joint Committee on Cancer: Manual for Staging of Cancer* (ed 5). Philadelphia, Lippincott, 1998

73. Mattos RM, Libertino JA: Survival of patients with renal cell carcinoma invading the inferior vena cava. *Semin Urol Oncol* 14:223–226, 1996

74. Maulard-Durdux C, Dufour B, Hennequin Y, et al: Postoperative radiation therapy in 26 patients with invasive transitional cell carcinoma of the upper urinary tract: no impact on survival? *J Urol* 155:115–117, 1996

75. DiBiase SJ, Valicenti RK, Schultz D, et al: Palliative irradiation for focally symptomatic metastatic renal cell carcinoma: support for dose escalation based on a biological model. *J Urol* 158:746–749, 1997

76. Novick AC: Current surgical approaches, nephron-sparing surgery, and the role of surgery in the integrated immunological approach to renal-cell carcinoma. *Semin Oncol* 22:29–33, 1995

77. Muss HB: The role of biological response modifiers in metastatic renal cell carcinoma. *Semin Oncol* 15:Suppl 5 30–34, 1988

78. Fyfe G, Fisher RI, Rosenberg SA, et al: Results of treatment of 255 patients with metastatic renal cell carcinoma who received high-dose recombinant interleukin-2 therapy. *J Clin Oncol* 13:688–696, 1995

79. Rosenberg SA, Klotze MT, Muul LM, et al: Observations on the systemic administration of autologous lymphokine-activated killer cells and recombinant interleukin-2 with metastatic cancer. *N Engl J Med* 313:1485–1492, 1985

80. Atkins MB, Spatano KA, Fisher RI, et al: Randomized phase II trial of high-dose bolus interferon alfa-2b in advanced renal cell carcinoma. *J Clin Oncol* 11:661–670, 1993

81. Ravaud A, Negrier S, Cany L, et al: Subcutaneous low-dose recombinant interleukin 2 and alpha-interferon in patients with metastatic renal cell carcinoma. *Br J Cancer* 69:1111–1114, 1994

82. Sandstrom SK: Nursing management of patients receiving biological therapy. *Semin Oncol Nurs* 12:152–162, 1996

83. Bender CM: Cognitive dysfunction associated with biological response modifier therapy. *Oncol Nurs Forum* 21:515–523, 1994

84. Skalla K: The interferons. *Semin Oncol Nurs* 12:97–105, 1996

85. Wheeler VS: Interleukins: the search for an anticancer therapy. *Semin Oncol Nurs* 12:106–114, 1996

86. Ponchietti R, Neri B, Dilror F, et al: Endoluminal instillation of epidoxorubicin as adjuvant treatment for upper urinary tract urothelial tumors. *Anticancer Res* 16:537–539, 1996

CHAPTER 48

Breast Cancer

Dianne D. Chapman, RN, MS
Michelle Goodman, RN, MS

Introduction

Breast cancer is the most common cancer in women and the leading cause of death for women age 40–44. It is second to lung cancer as the leading cause of all cancer deaths in women. The incidence of breast cancer increases rapidly with age until menopause, after which time it increases more slowly with advancing years.[1,2] Over 70% of all breast cancer occurs in women who are age 50 or older. The National Institutes of Health consensus development conference statement emphasized that in the next decade, more than 1.8 million women (175,000 in 1999) in the United States will be newly diagnosed with invasive breast cancer and, of that number, 30% will die of their disease.[3] Screening methods, particularly mammography, have become more precise, permitting earlier diagnosis that in part accounts for the dramatic increase in the incidence of breast cancer between 1982 and 1987, and likely is also responsible for the current slight decrease in mortality figures.[1,2] However, more research in the area of chemoprevention, systemic therapies, and access to preventive health care and early detection for the socioeconomically disadvantaged are needed to change the current mortality rates from this disease.[4]

In 1963, the lifetime risk of breast cancer was about 5.5%, or 1 in every 18 women with an estimated life span of 72 years.[5] Current statistics indicate that the average woman in her early 60s has a projected lifetime risk of almost 14% of developing breast cancer. Breast cancer incidence varies across the country, but in general is about one in every eight women.[6] This increasing incidence is predominantly in women under age 55 and in black women. Possible reasons for this increased incidence are that there are more women who are living longer into the cancer-prone years, there is better statistical reporting, and there are better screening methods. In addi-

tion, changes in dietary and socioeconomic habits, and increasing exposure to carcinogens, may contribute to this increased incidence of breast cancer.[6,7]

While the incidence of breast cancer has increased over the past 30 years, the mortality rate has recently demonstrated a slight decrease (-1.7% from 1990–1995),[2] reflecting better cure rates for earlier-staged lesions. This apparent progress may in part be related to a better understanding of the natural history of breast cancer, as well as reflect the benefit of early detection methods. The utilization of screening tools and community awareness of the signs and symptoms of breast cancer has probably been influential in reducing the average size of a breast tumor at diagnosis (2.74 cm in 1983 to 2.17 cm in 1991).[6] This decrease is more evident among white women than black women (Figure 48-1). The most recent information confirms the continuation of this trend.[8–10] Speculations to explain the survival disparity among black women include diagnosis at a more ad-

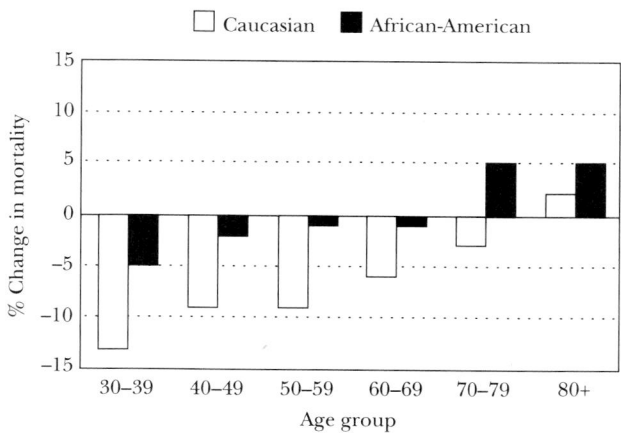

Figure 48-1 Breast cancer mortality 1989–1993.

vanced stage of disease and tumors with poor prognostic indicators.[8] It is imperative that nurses be acquainted with various cultural and economic barriers that may keep women from utilizing screening tools and benefiting from community education programs.

Historically, breast cancer has been considered a disease that remains localized until some time in which metastasis occurs via the lymph nodes and later spreads beyond regional nodes to distant sites. The possibility that hematogenous spread would occur early, prior to lymph node involvement, was proposed nearly two decades ago and supports the concept that breast cancer is a systemic disease at the time of clinical diagnosis.[11]

It is now widely accepted that breast cancer is not one disease but rather protean, differing in histological, biological, and immunologic characteristics. Phenotypic heterogeneity exists within individual breast neoplasms such that drug resistance, both intrinsic and acquired, occurs, rendering unresponsive cell lines unopposed and capable of establishing metastatic sites. Whether the individual with breast cancer survives the disease is determined by numerous factors, but the outcome primarily depends upon the intrinsic growth rate of the tumor, which varies dramatically; the age of the woman at diagnosis; and numerous biological parameters that ultimately define the natural history of the disease.

The interdisciplinary team utilizes various clinical, histological, and pathological findings to define, as precisely as possible, the particular characteristics of a breast cancer that will determine the most appropriate treatment plan for a given patient. This approach integrates the physical examination with the histopathological characteristics of the tumor, and incorporates the patient's personal bias based on her emotional needs and physical preferences. As a member of this team, the nurse must be aware of the factors affecting the selection of the treatment plan and appropriately educate the patient regarding the various treatment strategies in order to prevent and manage complications of the disease and its treatment.

Etiology

Risk Assessment

Experimental and clinical data indicate that the development of breast cancer is not a chance event. The genesis of breast cancer seems to be a multiphasic process involving many factors that are influential in the ongoing duel between tumor growth potential and host resistance.

Attempts are being made to reveal the etiology of breast cancer through an intense study of its epidemiology. As populations are identified in whom the incidence of the disease is increased, a genetic, hormonal, or biochemical factor may be identified that is considered significant in etiology. Epidemiological features, when statistically correlated with incidence of disease, designate a particular factor as a "risk factor." Each risk factor merely serves as one piece of the puzzle because there are so many different factors that either increase or decrease a woman's risk of developing breast cancer. Table 48-1 groups current risk factors for breast cancer according to their degree of importance in our understanding of the etiology of breast cancer.

Hormonal Factors

The hormone environment has long been recognized as a major factor in the development of breast cancer. This is well demonstrated in that gender is the most significant risk factor for the development of the disease. Women are 100 times more likely to develop breast cancer than men. Additionally, after a diagnosis of breast cancer has been made, the relationship of the tumor estrogen recep-

Table 48-1 Risk Factors

PRIMARY	
Female	
Age > 50	
Country of origin:	North America
	Northern Europe
Family history:	Personal history of breast cancer
	Two or more first-degree relatives with breast cancer
	Bilateral/premenopausal breast cancer in first-degree relative
	Known *BRCA1* or *BRCA2* mutation
Biopsy histology:	Atypical hyperplasia
	Carcinoma in situ (DCIS and LCIS)

SECONDARY
Postmenopausal obesity
Early menarche (< 12) coupled with late menopause (>55); onset of regular cycles within 1 year of menarche
First full-term pregnancy > 30 years of age
Use of oral contraceptive prior to age 20 and persisting for 6 or more years
Ionizing radiation to chest with exposure occurring prior to age 35
Benign breast disease

OTHER
Nulliparous
Estrogen replacement therapy
Alcohol
Diet

tor with the response to hormonal manipulation strongly suggests a hormonal connection. The significance of early menarche (before age 12), nulliparity or parity after age 30, and late menopause (after age 55) are well-known events that are considered risk factors for development of breast cancer. All of these events are linked to the type and duration of exposure to endogenous hormones that may have an impact on the development of breast cancer.

Pregnancy (full term) has been reported to exert a deterrent effect on the development of breast cancer. This is generally thought to be based on the change in the hormonal milieu. The exact mechanism is unknown, but speculation includes the effects of the alteration of prolactin and/or estriol. Prolactin has been recognized as having a direct effect on the growth of human breast epithelial tissue and is associated with the generation of mammary tumors in the rat. The decrease in prolactin levels during pregnancy may account for this protective effect.[12] Furthermore, there is a significant increase in estriol compared with estrone and estradiol during pregnancy. Estriol is considered to have a protective effect on cancer genesis, while estrone and estradiol may act as an initiator or a promoter on breast tissue.[13–16]

This preventive effect may be more pronounced with pregnancies at a young age (less than 20 years) and is enhanced by subsequent pregnancies.[17] Additionally, the benefit conferred on these women continues to be a positive factor throughout their lifetime. Lactation and breast-feeding have historically been considered protective mechanisms for breast cancer development. Although the theory remains controversial and the benefit may only be related to parity, there have been several studies that correlate a progressive risk reduction in premenopausal women with the number of breast-feeding years.[18–21]

A correlation between breast cancer and abortion, whether spontaneous or elective, has been suggested. An initial study in this country compared reproductive histories with women diagnosed with breast cancer and those of a matched control group. The study was small and indicated a positive correlation between abortion and risk of breast cancer.[22] Two other studies noted a positive correlation within certain groups.[23,24] A large Danish study used population registries to investigate this correlation and found no increased risk of breast cancer.[25] Since abortion is such a highly charged emotional issue, it is important for the nurse to properly assess reported modifiers of risk. All studies, especially those incorporating controversial issues, should meet the standards of validity and reliability.

The role that endogenous estrogens may play in the development of breast cancer suggests that exogenous therapy may be instrumental in the development of breast cancer. Animal studies have shown that exogenous estrogens, some progesterones, and some estrogen/progesterone combinations cause mammary tumors in rats and mice.[26] Exogenous hormones are given in various instances, but the primary reasons are pregnancy prevention in childbearing years and prophylaxis for heart disease, osteoporosis, and amelioration of hot flashes in menopausal women. Information on the use of hormone therapy[27] is limited in its consistency because of the disparity of dosages and duration as well as the current inability to assess cohort lifetime effects as well as multigenerational effects.

Oral contraceptives have been marketed since the 1960s. The question of a connection between oral contraceptives (OC) and breast cancer has resulted in inconsistent and controversial reports. Although studies investigating OC are often difficult to interpret, some basic risk information has been extrapolated. In general, nulliparous women who began using contraceptives before age 18 and continued uninterrupted use for more than eight years have a minimal increased risk of developing breast cancer. Long-term use may cause an initial increase in risk and result in a decreased risk in subsequent years.[28] It has been suggested that the risk may be more significant for black women, but further studies must be done to determine if a racial difference exists.[29–34] The literature also suggests the use of OC during the middle reproductive years seems to pose no additional risk. Another increase in risk has been associated with the use of OC during the perimenopausal years. The risk possibly may be due to delaying menopause by creating and maintaining a hormonal environment that mimics that of a menstruating woman.[12]

The question of risk in relation to hormone replacement therapy (HRT) is equally murky, with little replicated evidence of increased risk. A review of the literature has demonstrated that HRT users either exhibit no increase or a minimal increase in risk attributable to dosage and duration of use. In summarizing the results, it appears that the risk is negligible for most users and increases slightly for those using HRT before 1958, long-term users (eight years or more), and those who have also used OC.[35–42]

Current evidence suggests either no effect on breast cancer risk from HRT or an elevation in risk of less than two-fold with very long-term use or relatively high doses. Any potential effect of HRT on breast cancer risk must be considered with the therapy's established protective effect against osteoporotic fractures and increased risk of endometrial cancer, and probable decreased risk for coronary artery disease.[7]

The concern surrounding prescribing HRT for breast cancer survivors will undoubtedly become an increasingly problematic issue for clinicians. The number of survivors has steadily increased, including a growing population of women who are "forced" into a medical menopause through chemotherapeutic agents. The premenopausal women who experience an acute, early menopause seem to report more severe symptoms than premenopausal women who experience gradual, natural hormonal decreases over time. Although a majority of these women will enjoy disease-free survival, their quality of life may likely be compromised by somatic complaints (hot flashes, dyspareunia, labile mood swings)[43] and physical manifestations (heart disease and/or osteoporosis).[44,45] Hormone replacement therapy is known to remedy or reduce these problems, but physicians are reluctant to prescribe it. Giving breast cancer survivors estrogen therapy is a controversial issue, since the current standard of practice generally precludes prescribing these hormonal agents.[46–50]

Several articles have addressed the problem and the need for quantitative data; prospective randomized studies are required to begin to answer this complicated issue. One such study has begun but preliminary data is not yet available. Vassilopoulou-Sellin and Theriault[48] have initiated a study to determine if HRT constitutes a cancer recurrence risk versus the benefit of reducing bone demineralization, thereby preventing or arresting the disabling effects of osteoporosis. Eligible patients for this study are selected from those with stage I or II disease who are disease-free for at least two years if their tumors are estrogen receptor-negative, or ten years if their tumors are estrogen receptor-positive or unknown. The differences in the interval reflects the historical hypothesis that suggests that exposure to estrogen stimulates cancer growth. Although large, randomized trials would be the best source of information for this controversy, the feasibility and ethics of such studies may preclude implementation through cooperative groups.

Family History

Along with age and gender, family history of breast cancer is a contributing factor to the potential risk of developing the disease. Many people, including physicians, erroneously estimate risk factors. This is due to the wide range of risk associated with a family history of breast cancer dependent upon the age and known risk factors of the patient, the ages and number of first- and second-degree relatives with unilateral or bilateral breast cancer, and the presence of autosomal dominant gene mutations. Many studies have tried to extrapolate risk based on personal and family history.[46,51–54] Claus and associates,[55] using data from the Cancer and Steroid Hormone Study, developed a model that gives age-specific risk for a woman with a family history of one or more relatives. The Claus study provided confirmation that the risk of breast cancer not only is related to a positive family history but also is strongly correlated to the number and ages of affected relatives and can vary significantly. Examples of this variance are illustrated by a woman with a lifetime risk of 44% because she has two first-degree relatives diagnosed with cancer in their thirties versus a woman with a lifetime risk of 11% because two first-degree relatives were diagnosed in their seventies.[54]

The issue of lifetime risk is inferred in virtually all of these studies and is assumed to be true. The question of lifetime risk was addressed by examining data from 9000 women to determine if risk associated with family history remained stable or varied with age. Roseman and colleagues[56] found that family history may not be a determinant for women over age 60 and the Claus study[55] suggests that risk decreases with age for those with an autosomal dominant allele. Aside from those with genetic mutations, risk does seem to increase with age.[53]

Most women (approximately 70%) who develop breast cancer have no known risk factors. Familial and hereditary breast cancer account for a very small proportion of the diagnosed cases (23% and 7%, respectively). The majority of breast cancers are considered to be sporadic, which is defined as no history of breast cancer through two generations. Familial or polygenic breast cancer is described as a family history of one or more first-degree relatives with breast cancer. Hereditary or genetic breast cancer is defined as a positive family history, often with related cancers (e.g., ovarian), consistent with an autosomal dominant factor that includes early onset (less than age 40), an excess of bilaterality, male breast cancer, and other multiple cancers. Two autosomal dominant gene mutations have been isolated, one on the long arm of chromosome 17 and another on the long arm of chromosome 13. The ultimate goal of gene mapping is to be able to identify a crucial gene, characterize it, and thereby gain an understanding of the molecular predisposition of breast cancer in families. This information should conceivably lead to new methods of breast cancer therapy.

Many of the genes responsible for inherited familial cancers seem to be tumor suppressor genes that are actively involved in suppressing malignant growth during the cell cycle. When these genes undergo mutation(s), the effect is a loss of heterozygosity, which alters the normal function, causing abnormal proliferation, resulting in neoplastic and malignant cell growth.[57,58]

Epidemiologists and physician researchers began to look for patterns within families having an abnormal incidence of breast cancers among the members. Using linkage analysis, two breast/ovarian cancer susceptibility gene mutations (*BRCA1* and *2*) have been mapped and cloned. The first mutation identified, known as *BRCA1* (BReast CAncer #1) lies on the long arm of chromosome 17 (17q12-21) and *BRCA2* is located on the long arm of chromosome 13 (13q12-13).[58–62] Mutations to genes occur through physical, environmental, or genetic influences resulting in abnormal cell proliferation and culminating with neoplastic development.

Inheritance of the *BRCA1* and *BRCA2* susceptibility genes are associated with a strong penetrance (likelihood that the effect of the mutation will result in the disease) for families with multiple breast and ovarian cancers. These gene mutations follow an autosomal dominant pattern, meaning the mutation can be passed from either parent to a child and each child (male or female) has a 50% likelihood of inheritance. Because the science of genetics is constantly evolving, risk estimates can vary dependent upon locus of the mutation or ethnicity and should be interpreted with care. Women who have inherited a mutation on *BRCA1* or *BRCA2* generally have an 85% risk of developing breast cancer by age 70. The risk for developing ovarian cancer varies from 26%–85% for *BRCA1* to 10% or less for *BRCA2*.[63–66] The BRCA2 mutation seems to be associated with male breast cancer and early-onset female breast cancer.[67,68]

Some populations that have been isolated due to geographic, cultural, or religious considerations may exhibit a "founder effect"—that is, a deleterious mutation exists within one person and has been passed through the group and continues to be identified within the group. The Ashkenazi Jewish population exhibits this founder effect, which is estimated to affect 1 person in 40, considerably higher than the aforementioned heterogenous groups, estimated to affect 1 in 1000. Three mutations have been identified that are linked with Ashkenazi Jewish heredity, two on *BRCA1* and one on *BRCA2*. The risk of developing breast cancer for this group is estimated to be 56% by age 70. The risk for ovarian cancer is estimated to be 16%.[69] These figures are considerably lower than those listed above for more heterogenous populations. The disparities cannot be confirmed but may reflect the more general population of mutation carriers rather than the highly penetrant, linkage groups originally noted in the literature. Of note, men who carry the mutated *BRCA1* do not seem to be at an increased risk for developing breast cancer (less than 1%).[62] Although this inherited gene mutation identifies only a very small proportion of the breast cancer population (5%–8%), the hope is that the information gleaned from this and other inherited genes will provide additional information to understand the complex puzzle of sporadic breast cancer, affecting approximately 70% of those diagnosed.[63]

Another tumor suppressor gene, *p53*, also may become a promising marker for predicting breast cancers. This gene mutation has been identified in breast cancer and is often associated with a poor prognosis.[70,71] The *p53* gene has also been identified in various tissues ranging from normal to peritumoral.[72,73] These findings suggest that *p53* mutations may be present in varying degrees as the cells evolve from normal to malignant and, therefore, *p53* could conceivably become an important marker for assessing risk, evaluating prognosis, and testing respone to therapeutic modalities.[74]

For the woman who has breast cancer, there is a 2%–14% risk of developing a second primary breast cancer.[75] Some variabilities that may alter the risk of developing a contralateral breast cancer are early age of onset, having a first-degree relative with early onset or bilateral disease, or a genetic mutation. Treatment with chemotherapy and/or hormones for breast cancer may reduce the development of a second breast cancer.[51,58,59]

An increased risk of breast cancer also may be associated with primary ovarian or endometrial cancer, but this risk is low, estimated at less than two times the normal.

Diet

The wide range of variance in breast cancer rates worldwide and dramatic increases in migrant populations may reflect one or several factors that influence the risk of breast cancer. The risk of breast cancer is greatest in developed countries, especially those of North America and northern Europe. The risk is lowest in developing third-world countries. Apart from a genetic influence, diet has been investigated as the most plausible variant.

Japan is known to have a low incidence of breast cancer. However, when Japanese women migrate from Japan to Hawaii where the incidence of breast cancer is high, they experience a significant increase in breast cancer incidence. By the second generation, the incidence rate parallels that of daughters of Japanese women born in Hawaii, suggesting a dietary influence. Diet, however, may not be the only factor in cancer genesis of migrants. The new culture may provide accessibility to risk factors that may not have been an issue in the country of origin. Changes in exercise habits, alcohol and drug use, hormone therapy, and smoking may take place, which could confound the diet correlation.

Diets high in fats have been implicated in countries that have shown a sudden increase in incidence rates, as well as in high-risk countries. Reports of positive correlations with meat and dairy products have been issued, but additional case studies have largely failed to support the data.[76,77]

A potential answer to these questions may be provided by the Women's Health Initiative, sponsored by the National Institutes of Health. This study has begun to accrue approximately 100,000 women representing multicultural and multisocioeconomic backgrounds. The study will examine the effects of reducing dietary fat, adding calcium supplements, and hormone replacement to determine if any intervention reduces the expected incidence of breast and colorectal cancer, osteoporosis, and heart disease. This will be accomplished through clinical trials, observational studies, and community educational programs.[78,79]

There is still controversy regarding at which time of life dietary habits may be most influential in the development of breast cancer. Looking at current diet regimens in relation to breast cancer would not be helpful if perimenarchal diet were the determining factor. The possible significance of diet at this time of a woman's life corresponds to a cellular environment of accelerated growth and development of the breasts. These mammary tissues may potentially be altered by or sensitized to hormones produced by an excess of dietary fat.[80]

The relationship of dietary fats and breast cancer is largely based on consistent findings in animal studies. Rats ingesting a high-fat diet demonstrated an increase in breast malignancies compared with those on a low-fat diet, but other studies in animals suggest that the risk is associated with the amount of calories ingested rather than a specific food type.[81] It has been speculated that this connection may be linked to the amount and ratios of hormones produced by the endocrine system. The proliferation of breast tissue may be altered by changes in estrogen, pituitary, and thyroid function, which are sensitive to dietary changes.

Obesity

Obesity confers a slight increased risk overall but demonstrates more of a risk for those women who are postmenopausal than for any other age group.[82-84] A history of weight gain in early adult life may be associated with an increased risk. Although further studies are needed for confirmation, this weight gain may affect risk most if it occurs during the third decade.[85,86] Obese women, in general, may be more at risk for recurrence, but this may be explained by detection bias owing to the large amount of body fat that could obscure clinical findings.

A possible explanation of the discrepancy between pre- and postmenopausal risk may be linked to hormonal influences. Obesity during childbearing years has been associated with a decrease in the level of progesterone, which reduces cell proliferation in the breast. Obese postmenopausal women have no ovarian function and have both higher rates of conversion of androstenedione to estrogen in adipose tissue and lower levels of sex hormone-binding globulin than do thinner women.[83] Additionally, the enzyme responsible for converting estrone to estradiol is present in adipose breast tissue, and the rate of conversion has been positively correlated to body weight.

Alcohol

According to meta-analysis,[87,88] the literature favors a positive association between alcohol and breast cancer risk. The biological mechanisms of the association are not known. Whether the increased risk involves exposure to circulating cytotoxic by-products of alcohol, its effect on hepatic function, a possible alteration in the cell membrane permeability in breast tissue, or other mechanisms is yet to be determined. The most compelling evidence suggests that the relationship between alcohol and breast cancer risk is greatest for women who consume more than two drinks per day (hard liquor, beer, or wine).[88-90] However, this connection is not strong enough at this point to conclude a causality exists between the use of alcohol and breast cancer. Women who consume alcohol should be counseled regarding the potential cancer risks versus benefits based on known and family risk factors.

Radiation

The carcinogenic effect from both low- and high-dose ionizing radiation has been well documented. Survivors of the atomic bombs exhibited an increase in breast as well as other cancers. A risk of breast cancer has been associated with radiation therapy for a broad spectrum of health problems including chronic mastitis, tuberculosis, tinea capitis, thymus disorders, and adult and childhood cancers.[91] The risk increases with dosage, especially if a woman is exposed in the period of young adulthood. Mantle radiation for Hodgkin's disease is associated with an increased risk relative to age during treatment. Hancock and associates reviewed 885 women and calculated a relative risk of 4.1 overall and a relative risk of 136 for women treated before age 15. This risk remains increased for those radiated before the age of 30 and negligible for those treated after 30.[92,93]

The concern about the effects of radiation has generated some apprehension regarding the potential harm of repeated mammograms and chest radiographs. The doses for these procedures are extremely small, and the potential benefit far outweighs the risk. A mammogram emits a dose of 0.15 cGy, and a chest film generates approximately 0.002 cGy to each breast.[93] The radiation exposure from a mammogram is similar to the radiation exposure incurred from flying 400 miles in an airplane.

Nonproliferative Disease

Approximately 70% of biopsies reflect cellular changes that impart no risk or a very small risk to the patient and are often referred to as *fibrocystic change*. These include usual, moderate, or florid hyperplasia, sclerosing adenosis, and papillomatosis. In addition, some nonproliferative changes are recognized to bestow a very slight or no increased risk to the patient. These are adenosis, apocrine change, duct ectasia, and usual mild epithelial hyperplasia.[94]

Apocrine change is often accompanied with the diagnosis of a cyst. These cells may form tufted or papillary clusters instead of the characteristic single cell layer. Adenosis and duct ectasia refer to an increase in the number of cells in a gland and a dilation of a duct. Epitheliosis or mild epithelial hyperplasia is associated with common configurations seen with a slightly increased number of cells at the basement membrane.[95]

Proliferative Disease

The presence of proliferation on a pathology slide indicates a presence of increased cell growth. According to Page and DuPont, the term *proliferative breast disease* "indicates that proliferative alterations are noted by histology and that they indicate a disease by their demonstrated link to an increased risk of subsequent carcinoma"[96 p.119]. These risks have been categorized as slight, which is associated with one and one-half to two times the normal risk; moderate, which is associated with four to five times the normal risk; and high, which is associated with eight to ten times the normal risk.[95]

Proliferative disease without atypia falls into the slightly increased risk category. This classification includes examples of common types of epithelial hyperplasia, which may be subcategorized as mild, moderate, or florid. The degree refers to the number of cells present relative to the basement membrane of a lobular unit or duct. Since two cells are usually present above the basement membrane, the presence of three or more cells is described as mild hyperplasia. The presence of five or more cells constitutes moderate hyperplasia, and an increased progression of these changes characterizes florid hyperplasia. Twenty percent of breast biopsies contain moderate or florid hyperplasia. The presence of papilloma and sclerosing adenosis also falls in the slight risk category.[93–97]

The moderate risk category includes atypical ductal hyperplasia and atypical lobular hyperplasia. These risk statistics are not lifetime estimates, but are limited to approximately 18 years after biopsy, which is the limit of most benign breast disease follow-up. Atypical hyperplasia has some, but not all, of the characteristics of carcinoma in situ.[96] Carcinoma in situ is associated with high risk (eight to ten times normal risk).[95]

Carcinoma in Situ

Carcinoma in situ has been referred to as a *precancerous condition*. This definition reflects the potential capabilities of the cells rather than the histopathological characteristics. The nomenclature of carcinoma in situ refers to a localized process describing cells that are still within the site of origin. A malignant change has occurred without evidence of invasion in the basement membrane.[98] A carcinoma in situ that remains in the breast is capable of transforming to an invasive cancer but does not necessarily do so.

Ductal carcinoma in situ (DCIS) and lobular carcinoma in situ (LCIS) are characterized by an eight-fold to ten-fold increased risk of developing invasive cancer.[99,100] DCIS lesions are often singular, and conservative treatment with local excision is an accepted treatment. DCIS is the most common form of noninvasive breast cancer in women, but occurs in approximately 5% of male breast cancer.[101] Lobular carcinoma in situ may be associated with increased risk within both breasts. LCIS is found predominately in premenopausal women, with an average age of 44–47 years.[101] LCIS is usually not detected by palpation or mammography, and is most often an incidental microscopic finding when breast tissue is removed for another reason.[95] Current evidence suggests that LCIS functions as a marker of increased risk for developing an invasive ductal or lobular cancer. Mastectomy for LCIS should be considered a prophylactic procedure rather than therapeutic.[102] Mastectomy with close follow-up of the other breast has often been the treatment of choice, but clinicians increasingly feel LCIS may be treated with local excision and close follow-up that employs mammograms twice a year and clinical exam every three to four months. Improvements in mammography sensitivity have made this approach more feasible. Women who are unable or unwilling to comply with frequent monitoring may opt for a unilateral or bilateral mastectomy with or without reconstruction.

Prevention of Breast Cancer

While it is conceivable to determine the possibility of developing breast cancer based on risk factors, it is virtu-ally impossible to predict with certainty who will or will not develop breast cancer in a lifetime. The unknown etiology of breast cancer coupled with conflicting data regarding the identification of risk factors as well as how these risk factors influence the genesis of breast cancer makes preventive action difficult. To prevent an event from occurring, one must know the cause. Unfortunately, there is a paucity of information regarding the origin of breast cancer. As mentioned earlier in this chapter, some elements have been recognized to be primary risk factors in the development of breast cancer and others may be secondary or possible risk factors. Even this information is limited at best, because 70% of the women with breast cancer have no identifiable risk factors.

Research concerning prevention and early detection of breast cancer is critically important in the reduction of mortality from this disease. Of the more than 184,000 women diagnosed yearly, only 50% will be diagnosed with stage I disease, and approximately 30% of all women with breast cancer will subsequently die of their disease. Current evidence has indicated that the disease is often present in the breast six to eight years before it becomes mammographically or clinically evident. Newer, even more sophisticated methods of detecting breast cancer or preventing further proliferation of these undetectable pathological breast cancers are becoming the forefront of clinical research efforts. As nurses, our role in educating the public, promoting research, and recruiting women into these research studies cannot be overemphasized.

Chemoprevention

Chemoprevention is the use of a chemical agent to prevent or alter the development of cancer. The development of a chemoprevention agent should be based on a disease model that identifies progressive development over several years and involves multiple factors that can be reversed. These interventions must be based on a biological rationale and have minimal toxic effects.[103–105]

Chemoprevention for breast cancer has been proposed to possibly alter the course of disease for those with known risk factors. Several dietary micronutrients have been touted for their presumed protective capabilities in animal studies, but they remain controversial for human use. Vitamin A and its retinoid derivatives offer some promise for chemoprevention, but dosage is limited due to hepatic toxicity. Vitamin A can affect the growth and differentiation of epithelial tissue. Breast cancer is considered a disease of the breast epithelial cells, and the retinoids may have the capacity to alter the oncogenic course.[106] A study of the synthetic retinoid 4-HPR in preventing breast cancer in high-risk women and preventing a second primary cancer in the contralateral breast has recently closed after accruing almost 3000 women. This synthetic analog is less hepatotoxic than other retinoids.[107] Vitamins A, E, and C in foods act as antioxidants, which defend against free radicals and aid in stimulating the immune response. It is difficult, however, to attribute these qualities to specific micronutrients because of the multiple components of vegetables and fruits.[106,108]

The influence of hormones in breast cancer is uniformly recognized. Because of this known association, physicians and scientists have long entertained the possibility of an antiestrogen that may prevent breast cancer. A new category of agents that mimic the effects of estrogen in selected tissues and act as estrogen antagonists in other tissues are being referred to as *SERMs*—*selective estrogen receptor modulators*. Tamoxifen, introduced in the 1970s, was the first SERM and is the most widely used drug for breast cancer in the United States. It was first introduced as a treatment for advanced breast cancer in postmenopausal women.[109] Since then, tamoxifen has been found to be effective in the treatment of premenopausal women with advanced disease.[110] It has also been found to increase disease-free survival in node-negative, estrogen receptor (ER)-positive disease,[111] as well as node-positive disease.[112] Women taking tamoxifen for primary breast cancer have experienced a reduction in the expected incidence of contralateral breast cancer. This strengthens the possibility of a chemoprotective effect, and led to its use in a large U.S. prevention trial through the National Surgical Adjuvant Breast and Bowel Program (NSABP).

This breast cancer prevention study, NSABP P-1, was a randomized study using the standard daily dose of 20 mg of tamoxifen versus a placebo to determine if breast cancer can be prevented in women with known high risk.[113] This study was to have lasted for five years before data was to be available, but preliminary information indicated that the risk reduction was 45% for the tamoxifen group. This result was felt to be significant enough that the reports were published early to allow all high-risk women the opportunity to select this documented risk reduction.[114,115] The study did result in morbid events, which, though few, occurred more often in the tamoxifen group. Early-stage endometrial cancer was diagnosed twice as often in the tamoxifen group and this group also had an increased incidence of thromboembolus. These events were generally attributable to women over age 50. There were no instances of liver cancer, a rare occurrence in animal studies.[114,115] This study is being followed by NSABP P-2, a prevention trial examining the effects of breast cancer risk reduction and relative side effects using tamoxifen versus raloxifene, and has been named the *STAR* (*study of tamoxifen and raloxifene*) trial. The preliminary reports of raloxifene indicate similar properties as tamoxifen but do not seem to exert an estrogenic effect on the endometrium.[116]

The eligibility for the STAR trial is essentially the same as the P-1 trial, except women must be postmenopausal. If women are currently taking HRT, they must stop for three months prior to enrollment. The goal is to enroll 22,000 women with no prior history of breast cancer. As with the P-1 trial, the participants will be expected to comply with the schedule for daily medication, clinical examinations, and mammography.

Side effects are an important consideration when any drug is taken electively. The common tamoxifen toxicities reported are similar to menopausal symptoms: hot flashes, vaginal discharge, and irregular menses. Rare events include ocular changes, thromboembolic disease, and second primary cancers of the liver and endometrium, as mentioned previously. The side effects of raloxifene are similar, without the expected increase in endometrial cancer.

Although tamoxifen is considered an antiestrogen and, therefore, an antagonist, it may also act as an agonist. As an antagonist, tamoxifen competes with estradiol for the receptor sites in the nucleus. This mechanism causes an estrogen blockade and impedes growth of malignant cells. Although the exact action of the drug is unknown, several explanations have been postulated. Tamoxifen may alter the growth factors that regulate breast cell proliferation,[117] bind to cytoplasmic antiestrogenic binding sites thereby increasing intracellular drug levels,[118] inhibit the amount of free estrogen available to the cell,[119] stimulate natural killer cells, or affect the endocrine regulation of breast cancer cells.[120]

Tamoxifen also exhibits agonist activity, which was recognized in the early trials. This agonist mechanism suggests beneficial action regarding osteoporosis and cardiovascular disease, both of which are significant factors of morbidity and mortality in postmenopausal women.[121]

The recent dramatic outcome of the P-1 trial will potentiate the investigation of additional SERMs as more sources of tumor modulation are acknowledged. Other prevention studies will be introduced as more sources of tumor modulation are recognized. Toremifene is another SERM that seems to increase bone density and confers a better LDL/HDL cholesterol ratio, inferring a protective effect on coronary heart disease.[122]

Nurses across the country are instrumental in the identification of women who are eligible for prevention trials, the education of the public, recruitment of women to the study, and compliance with the treatment, as well as in the assessment of toxicity and data collection. Timely accrual of eligible participants will provide information on the action and efficacy of the various chemoprevention agents and provide innovative insights into the causal pathway of breast cancer.

Surrogate Endpoint Biomarkers

We know that cancer is a heterogenous disease, and it has recently been hypothesized that all diseases are the result of an evolving process of altered cells accumulating genetic mutation, either inherited or acquired. Identifying biomarkers that appear early in cell alterations theoretically would allow for repair of these alterations and prevention of disease. Endpoints may indicate later effects, e.g., dysplasia, or, more desirable, earlier alterations such as cell proliferation. The ability of these mutated cells to express malignancy may develop from the genetic disposition of *SEBs* (*surrogate endpoint biomarkers*). Interrupting the cascade of cellular changes early in the continuum is a necessary endpoint that replaces incidence reduction outcomes in prevention clinical trials. The incidence reduction data often takes several years (5+) to become definitive and adds considerable expense to the clinical trials. An effective SEB should be a factor in the causal pathway of breast cancer. The identified SEB should be altered in the presence of a chemoprotective agent and should ultimately reduce the incidence of breast cancer. The modulation of proliferative rate, extent of atypical ductal hyperplasia, and carcinoma in situ are examples of planned studies for breast cancer. Some cellular changes that occur along histopathological pathway to malignancy have been identified as probable indicators of neoplasia. Certain proteins and genes are abnormally expressed or regulated in breast cancer.[123] Other studies are directed at breast density on mammograms and chemopreventative interventions.[124] Changes in DNA, markers of cellular proliferation and apoptosis (programmed cell death) are under consideration. Studies that do identify modulation of a known biomarker will enable the practitioner to shift the care paradigm by offering interventions directed at preventing the onset of breast cancer rather than hoping for early detection using standard methods of clinical and mammographic examinations.

Exercise

The role of exercise in the prevention of breast cancer has not been widely studied. The endorsement of exercise is usually presented in the context of reducing or counteracting known risk factors. Women who exercise tend to have less body fat, which affects their hormone milieu. Strenuous exercising alters ovarian function, which may delay menarche or create irregular menses or an amenorrheic state. Exercising may reduce the risk of breast cancer for postmenopausal obese women by reducing the amount of free estrogen stored in body fat.

The few studies that have looked at exercise as a protective agent have been generally inconclusive. This is possibly related to the presence of confounding risk factors, inaccurate activity measures, or alteration of activity over time.[124–126] Recently, two papers have suggested that exercise confers a direct protective effect on the development of breast cancer. Bernstein and associates[127] found that young women (menarche to early middle age) who vigorously exercised three to eight hours or more per week experienced a 58% reduction in risk. Mittendorf and colleagues[128] conducted a large case-controlled study that showed a modest effect for young women who reported any strenuous activity and a 50% reduction for those who vigorously exercised daily. Conversely, a population based case-control study by Chen and associates did not find any correlation between exercise and a protective effect against breast cancer.[129] While more studies are necessary, these similar findings support the hypothesis that physical activity may reduce the risk of breast cancer.

Prophylactic Mastectomy

A prophylactic mastectomy, the removal of the majority of breast tissue—including total breast, tail of Spence, and nipple areola complex—may be warranted in certain high-risk women; however, controversy exists over how much risk is enough to justify performing this procedure. Women for whom a prophylactic mastectomy may be indicated have been identified as those with some or all of the following conditions.[121]

1. A family history of documented hereditary breast cancer consistent with an autosomal dominant factor. Women who are presumed to be gene carriers may have a breast cancer risk ranging from 50%–85% depending on family history.
2. A personal risk of at least 50% for developing breast cancer.
3. A proven history of breast cancer in one breast and extreme nodularity or cystic changes in the opposite breast. The incidence of a second breast cancer in the opposite breast is estimated to be 15%–20%.
4. Chronic cystic mastitis or a diagnosis of atypical hyperplasia with repeated surgical biopsies.
5. An overwhelming fear of breast cancer such that the possibility of developing breast cancer interferes with her daily life.

Since prophylactic mastectomies have been done for various reasons, not only for high risk, it is difficult to quantify the reduction in breast cancer risk.[130,131] The most complete study to date was conducted by Hartmann and colleagues.[132] The retrospective study investigated women who had prophylactic mastectomies performed at Mayo Clinic. The women were evaluated according to a risk profile and the results showed a 90% risk reduction for those who had a moderate or high risk for developing breast cancer. This is important information for women considering the surgery based on risk. Breast cancer has been known to occur in the chest wall, axillary region, and abdomen. It is therefore important for a woman to realize some risk of developing breast cancer exists after a prophylactic mastectomy. While the risk reduction for *BRCA1* or *BRCA2* carriers may be included in these statistics, the actual risk reduction for that subpopulation is unknown at this point

The patient must be presented with a clear, in-depth evaluation of her current and potential risk, stressing that a 50% risk also carries a 50% possibility of not developing the disease. It is important for the woman to take adequate time in weighing the risk versus benefit of this procedure. The complications are similar to those for a mastectomy. However, if reconstruction is added to this procedure, capsular contracture is another possibility.

Optimally, women at high risk for breast cancer should be followed by close surveillance utilizing mammograms and frequent clinical examinations, preferably through a comprehensive breast center. Provided such surveillance is feasible, this alternative is an important, even reassuring, alternative for the woman considering prophylactic mastectomy.

Multidisciplinary Breast Centers

The increasing public awareness of breast cancer treatment options and the recognized controversies in breast cancer detection and management, together with oncologists' and institutions' commitment to provide optimum care, have spearheaded the concept of the multidisciplinary breast center. The design of these centers is essentially a response to the fact that treatment of breast cancer has become a complicated process necessitating specialized, collaborative management that is often beyond the scope of an individual practitioner. The purpose and goals of a multidisciplinary breast center include, but are not limited to, the following:

1. To provide a comprehensive interdisciplinary evaluation and planning in the management of all aspects of breast disease.
2. To provide prompt and timely evaluation and diagnosis of potential breast disease implementing current methodology and state-of-the-art diagnostic tools.
3. To participate in and support national protocol studies that investigate new surgical and adjuvant treatment modalities as well as to maintain a patient database for retrospective and prospective in-house studies.
4. To provide risk assessment, genetic counseling referrals, and surveillance of women at high risk for breast cancer, thereby minimizing the anxiety associated with the knowledge that one has an increased risk for developing the disease as well as reducing the risk of patients being lost to follow-up.
5. To provide educational materials and the opportunity to learn about early detection measures (e.g., breast self exam (BSE)) and the possibility of participating in breast cancer prevention studies as well as research studies aimed at early detection and management of malignant breast cancer.
6. To provide educational opportunities for medical students, Fellows, general practitioners, nurses, and others involved in the care of the woman with breast disease as well as to provide a mechanism for peer review of the oncologist in practice.
7. To provide highly specialized assessment and diagnostic procedures that enable prompt decision making in the evaluation of a breast mass, which conceivably minimizes unnecessary surgical biopsies.
8. To provide the woman and family with the necessary information to allow her to make an informed decision regarding her choices for treatment in a prompt and timely manner.
9. To offer educational programs to the community that include instruction in BSE and information on risk factors and the importance of utilizing the current methods available to promote early detection.

Ideally, the comprehensive breast center should have a full complement of disciplines available to provide an expert opinion regarding assessment of diagnostic and histopathological data; prognostic indicators; genetic assessment and evaluation; and surgical diagnostic and treatment options including systemic chemoendocrine therapy, radiation treatment, and surgical reconstructive techniques when warranted. A psychooncologist and social worker provide counseling regarding body image issues, sexual concerns, and anticipated changes in lifestyle for those patients dealing with a potentially life-threatening disease.

The oncology clinical nurse specialist is often viewed as the coordinator of the comprehensive breast center. It is imperative that this professional possess specialized knowledge in all aspects of breast cancer and its treatment as well as a compassionate, yet controlled, approach to the evaluation of a suspected breast cancer. It is not uncommon for women to telephone the breast center, frantic with fear and apprehension, expressing a need to be seen as soon as possible. Regardless of the schedule, this is exactly what needs to occur if possible. Such understanding and prompt attention to the woman's needs and concerns will help establish a trusting and caring relationship, which is vital considering the possible diagnostic outcome. This approach to patient management is critical to the success of a comprehensive breast center.

The nurse coordinator ensures that all materials (slides, x-rays) necessary for a comprehensive evaluation are present at the time of the consultation. The nurse informs the patient and family of the sequence of events once the appointment is established. This includes which doctor(s) the patient will see and when, how materials will be reviewed, and the critical role the patient plays in the decision-making process. Emphasis is placed on the fact that often there is more than one approach to management of the problem and that once informed of her options, the patient is the ultimate decision maker. The nurse can be instrumental in ensuring that information is delivered in a manner that will enhance the patient's understanding and ability to make an informed decision.

In addition to facilitating the process of informed consent and decision making, the nurse is also instrumental in providing BSE instruction to all patients. The nurse also will be called on to answer questions regarding diagnostic tests, therapy regimens, clinical trials, postoperative events, and potential complications of treatment. The nurse may see patients postoperatively in the hospital to provide continuity of care as well as instruction concerning general postoperative care including infection precautions. Ideally, the nurse coordinator will be able to provide exercise instruction prior to surgery and evaluate the patient's understanding and potential for compliance during the period following hospitalization. Additionally, the nurse utilizes every opportunity to lecture to professionals and the public concerning breast cancer as a health issue and the methods available for early detection. In addition, time should be set aside specifically to accept or return phone calls concerning questions related to breast cancer risk specifically as well as other pertinent issues.

The design of a comprehensive breast center should reflect the goals of providing a complete, efficient, yet personal evaluation of the patient. The exam rooms should be large enough to accommodate the patient, family or significant other, as well as the team of physicians. The clinical area should have additional smaller consult rooms where the patient may be seen by individual consultants based on her individual concerns and needs.

A physician conference room should be available to provide an area for viewing films, pathology slides, and reports. Facilities for performing diagnostic tests and outpatient surgery suites that are located on site facilitate a quick and efficient diagnostic process.

These centers are successful because they meet a growing need for a multidisciplinary and comprehensive approach to the care of the woman with breast disease and because they are philosophically based on the premise that women are entitled to all the information available to make an informed decision regarding their choice of treatment.

Genetic Counseling Programs

As science and biotechnology continue to identify chromosomal abnormalities that confer a high probability for developing breast cancer, the need to provide more comprehensive risk assessment for families as well as genetic counseling and testing will direct practitioners and the public to seek genetic counseling programs. The information emanating from the Human Genome Project will possibly overwhelm and definitely challenge a primary care physician in assessing and referring patients for genetic assessment. The primary physician will often be responsible for referring a patient for further evaluation and, therefore, must possess a basic working knowledge of the personal and familial histories that may suggest a genetic link. According to Peters and Stopfer,[133] genetic counseling should assist the patient and family in understanding the medical information pertinent to the disease(s), comprehending how heredity causes or predisposes one to the disease, and the personal risk of developing it, as well as in creating a plan for follow-up that may include several treatment modalities.

Creating and implementing a breast genetic counseling program must include the following: a database and an assessment model based on known and accepted risk factors; genetic counselor(s) who carefully interview, screen, and educate the patient and family; a psychosocial support staff to address the emotional and physical consequences of the counseling and testing process; and clinicians, nurses, and researchers who share clinical responsibilities[134] and actively participate in treatment protocols and prevention trials for breast cancer. Additionally, once risk has been established, the patient and family members should receive specific recommendations tailored to the needs of the individual (see Table 48-2).

Technological advances historically precede the ethical and moral issues that may arise from this data. The staff should carefully address confidentiality, informed consent, potential discrimination, and insurance issues. The institution's risk management team may play an active or consultant role, providing advice and counsel for current problems and future dilemmas. The Ethical, Legal, and Social Implications branch of the Human Genome Project has a principal role in addressing the basic rights of the individual seeking counseling and the role of the government, as well as a role in exploring the moral and religious conflicts that will arise.

The American Society of Clinical Oncology (ASCO)[135] issued a position paper regarding genetic testing for cancer susceptibility. The ASCO paper recognizes that identifying those with the highest risk will certainly increase early detection and may ultimately lead to the prevention of many cancers. However, ASCO cites the importance of addressing the actual and potential risks of testing without extensive patient or family counseling and education and endorses testing within a research protocol format that includes a national registry, long-term outcomes, and psychological ramifications.

Very sensitive, often previously unknown, information may come to light that can challenge and alter relationships forever. DNA testing irrefutably identifies maternity and paternity. A man may discover that one or more of his children have another father. As the demand for testing increases, it is imperative that people become skilled in the assessment and interpretation of the results.

An oncology nurse who receives additional education in the field of genetics will provide a wealth of information for the patient and family. All those who seek genetic counseling for breast cancer may or may not necessarily be at high risk. It is important for the staff to educate the patient and family as well as the referring physician regarding family and personal history assessments.

Pathophysiology

Cellular Characteristics

The majority of primary breast cancers are adenocarcinomas located in the upper outer quadrant of the breast (Figure 48-2). The most common types of breast tumors are summarized in Table 48-3. Infiltrating ductal carcinoma may take various histological forms: well differentiated and slow growing; poorly differentiated and infiltrating; or highly malignant and undifferentiated with many mitoses. Adenocarcinoma can occur at any age, but highly malignant varieties with rapidly dividing cells affect more women in their early 50s. The overall ten-year survival rate is 50%–60%.

Invasive lobular carcinoma occurs in the same age

Table 48-2 Cancer Risk Evaluation Program: Breast and Ovarian Screening Guidelines

LOW RISK ≤ 15% LIFETIME CUMULATIVE RISK

Follow standard ACS recommendations

Mammography	Baseline at age 35 Every other year age 40–50 Every year age 50 and on
Clinical breast exam	Every year
Breast self-examination	Every month

MODERATE RISK 15%–30% LIFETIME CUMULATIVE RISK

Start following the standard ACS guidelines at any age when breast cancer risk is ≥ to the risk of an average 50-year-old woman (1 in 50 or 2%)

HIGH RISK ≥ 30% LIFETIME CUMULATIVE RISK

Mammography	Baseline at age 30 Next mammogram depending on informativeness
Clinical breast exam	Every 6 months
Breast self-examination	Every month

KNOWN *BRCA1/BRCA2* MUTATION CARRIERS

Mammography	Baseline at age 25 Every 6–12 months thereafter	Pelvic exam every 6 months Transvaginal ultrasound every year
Clinical breast exam	Every 6 months	CA-125 every 6 months
Breast self-examination	Every month	
Consider prophylactic mastectomy		**Consider prophylactic oophorectomy after childbearing**

Cancer Risk Evaluation Program, University of Pennsylvania Cancer Center. Reprinted with permission. These are guidelines that may change as new data become available, and must be individualized.

range as ductal carcinoma, accounts for 10%–15% of all breast cancers, and is frequently bilateral. The prognosis is similar to ductal carcinoma.

Tubular carcinoma is fairly uncommon and represents a well-differentiated adenocarcinoma of the breast. These cancers typically occur in women age 55 and older. The presence of microcalcification is characteristic and facilitates early mammographic discovery. Axillary metastasis is uncommon.

Medullary carcinomas account for 5%–7% of malignant breast tumors, occurring most commonly in younger women (less than age 50). These tumors may be quite large and circumscribed and may be bilateral.

Mucinous or colloid carcinoma is uncommon, occurring in women age 60–70. This tumor type is characterized by the presence of large pools of mucin interspersed with small islands of tumor cells. Metastasis to axillary lymph nodes occurs in about one-third of patients and distant metastasis occurs late.

Inflammatory breast cancer occurs infrequently and accounts for less than 4% of breast cancers. Inflammatory breast cancer often presents with skin edema, redness, warmth, and induration of the underlying tissue and is often mistaken for cellulitis. Even though it appears to be localized it is associated with a poor prognosis.

Other malignant tumors of the breast include sarcomas, papillary carcinoma, apocrine, invasive cribriform, and Paget's disease.

Patterns of Metastasis

Breast cancer is considered to be a heterogenous, highly variable disease. Even among women with the same histological type, clinical stage, and treatment, some will be cured while others have emergence of metastatic disease within six months of therapy. The development of aberrant cell clones, with diverse growth rates and metastatic potential, may in part account for the differences seen in clinical behavior. Research concerning the role of angiogenesis in tumor growth and its specific relevance in transformation, progression, and metastasis of breast cancer is ongoing. While the process of metastasis is a complex and poorly understood phenomenon, there is evidence to suggest that angiogenesis (neovascularization) of the tumor plays an important role in the biologi-

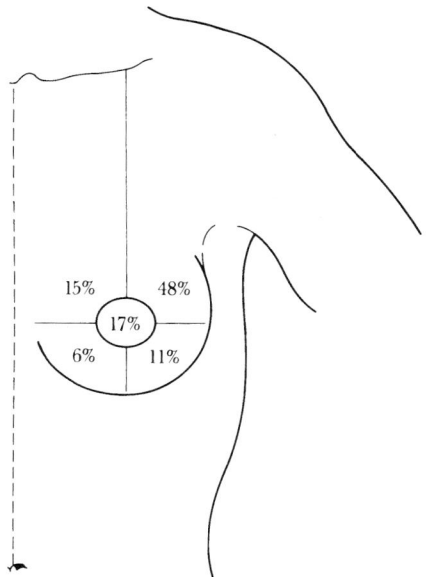

Figure 48-2 Incidence of breast cancer according to location.

with metastatic disease to bone often complain of bone pain or in the case of liver metastases, anorexia, weight loss, malaise, and occasionally right upper quadrant pain. Central nervous system (CNS) metastases may present with specific neurological symptoms such as headache that is more severe in the morning or relate to specific neurological damage such as cranial nerve palsies (double vision), motor dysfunction, or spinal cord symptoms.

Clinical Manifestations

Diagnostic Studies

Routine mammography may reveal a large spectrum of breast pathology ranging from equivocal benign conditions, to those that may mimic suspicious or malignant processes, to those that are considered malignant until proven otherwise. The appearance of these lesions is often a coincidental finding on a screening mammogram of an asymptomatic woman. However, if there is a palpable abnormality, additional diagnostic tools will be utilized to isolate the abnormality and provide more specific information for the clinician.

The diagnostic evaluation of breast lesions may be a simple one-step procedure or it may progress to a multi-level process. There are several noninvasive and low–invasive diagnostic tools that aid the clinician in identifying lesions within the breast. A series of steps may be taken before determining which lesions actually need open (excisional) biopsy. Figures 48-3 and 48-4 describe the steps involved in the diagnostic evaluation of a nonpalpable and a palpable breast mass.

Clinical manifestations that are more suspicious of malignant disease are nipple retraction or elevation,

cal aggressiveness of breast cancer.[136,137] Breast cancer metastasizes widely and to almost all organs of the body, but primarily to the bone, lungs, nodes, liver, and brain. The first sites of metastases are usually local or regional involving the chest wall or axillary supraclavicular lymph nodes or bone. Women with estrogen receptor-negative disease are more likely to have recurrences in visceral organs whereas women with estrogen receptor-positive disease more often have recurrences in skin and bone. Patients with metastatic disease generally present with symptoms specific to that organ. For instance, women

Table 48-3 Histological Types of Invasive Breast Cancers

Histological Type	Percentage of Occurrence	Clinical Features	Metastatic Pattern	Prognosis
Infiltrating ductal carcinoma	75	Stony hardness to palpation Prominent lump Malignant cells have invaded through the walls of the duct May have a spiculated appearance on mammogram	Axillary lymph nodes (common) Bone Lung Liver Brain	Poor
Infiltrating lobular carcinoma	5–10	Diffuse, ill-defined thickness Multicentric Bilaterality (30%)	Axillary lymph nodes (common) Occult lymph node micrometastasis may occur	Poor
Tubular	2	May be quite large	Axillary lymph nodes (uncommon) Distant metastases uncommon	Favorable
Medullary	5–7	Well circumscribed Rapid growth rate Bilaterality	Approximately 40% of cases demonstrate lymph node involvement at diagnosis	Favorable
Mucinous (Colloid)	3	Slow growing, bulky	Axillary lymph node involvement in less than 1/3 of cases at diagnosis	Favorable

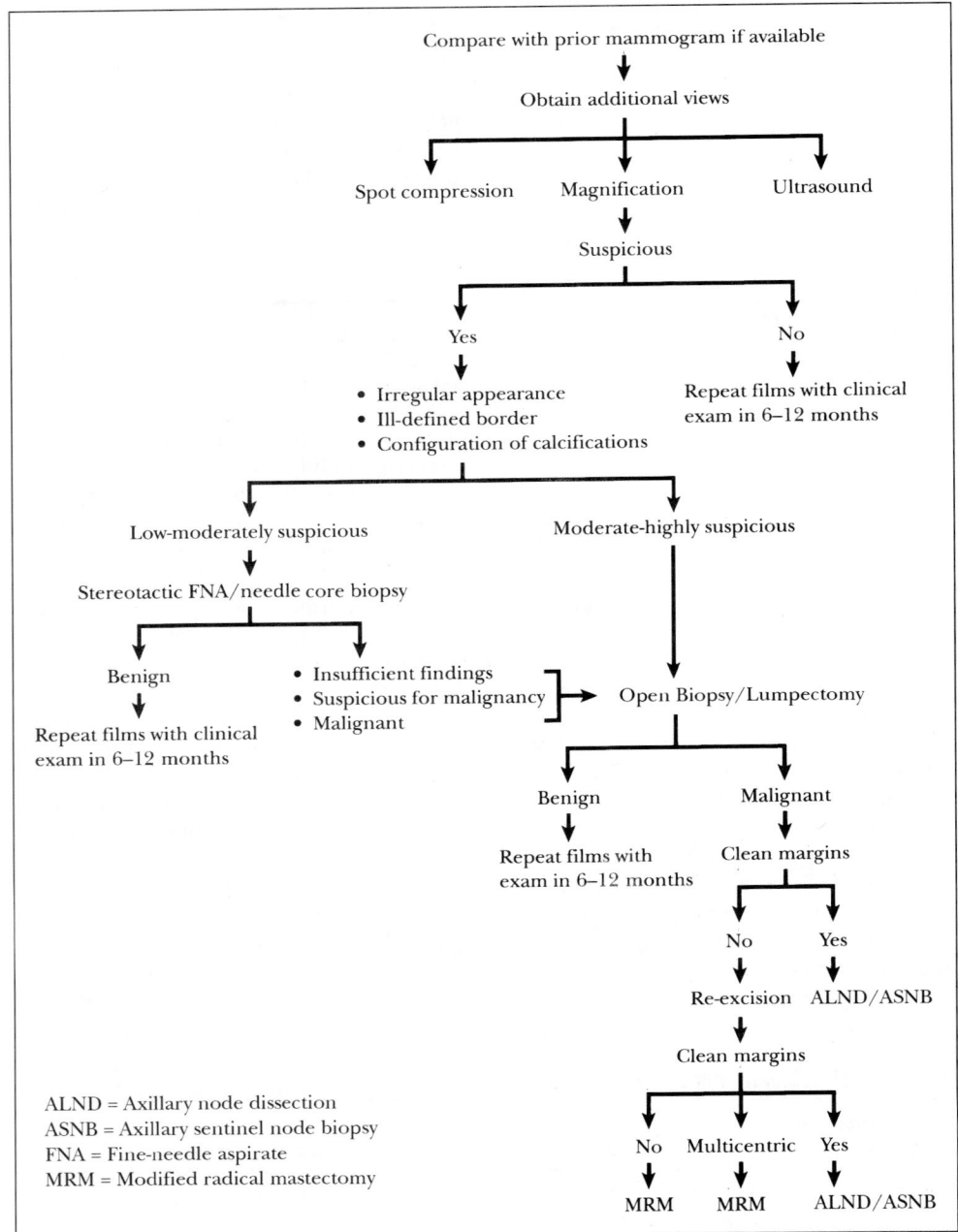

Figure 48-3 Evaluation of a nonpalpable mass found on mammogram.

which may be due to tumor fixation or infiltration into the underlying tissues. Skin dimpling or retraction also may be present and is possibly due to invasion of the suspensory ligaments and fixation to the chest wall. Heat and erythema of the breast skin may be related to inflammation, but they are also signs of inflammatory breast carcinoma. Skin edema, or *peau d'orange*, the French term for "skin of the orange" (Figure 48-5), is characteristic of malignant disease. The edema is thought to be due to the invasion and obstruction of dermal lymphatics by tumor. Ulceration of the skin with secondary infection

may be present. The presence of isolated skin nodules indicates invasion of blood vessels and lymphatics. This often results in implantation of tumor emboli in adjacent tissues and indicates that distant metastases are likely.[138] Clinical presentation may also include, or be limited to, signs of local or distant metastatic disease.

Mammograms

Screening mammograms. Screening mammograms are used for routine breast surveillance for the asymptom-

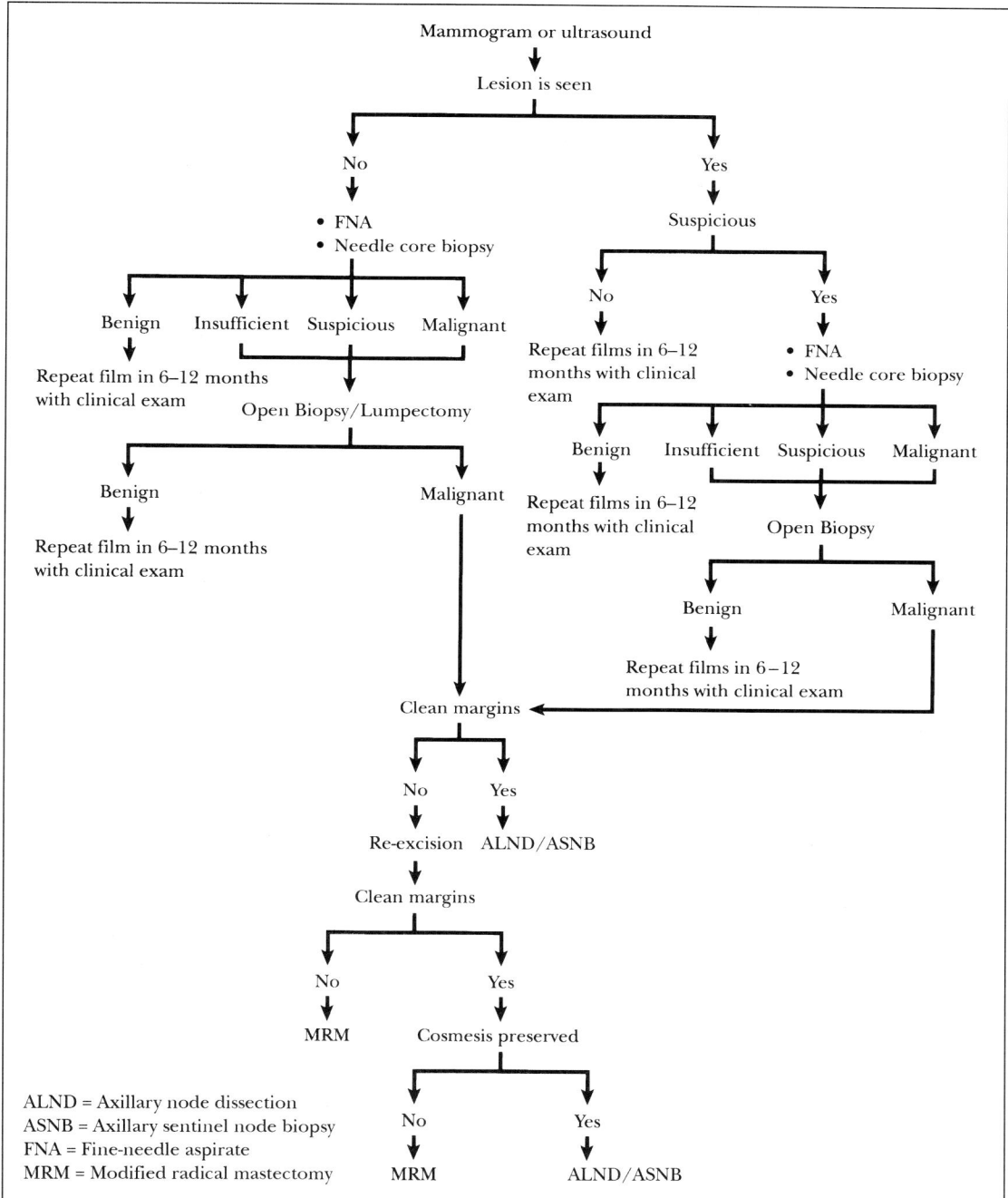

Figure 48-4 Evaluation of a palpable breast mass.

atic patient. The goal of screening mammography is to detect a malignancy before it becomes clinically apparent. It is important to have an appreciation for what mammography can accomplish. A 10-mm tumor containing 10^9 or 1 billion cells may be palpable by clinical examination. Mammography can improve this by about six or seven doublings, or approximately 20% of the life of the tumor. Detection at 10^7 by mammography or 10^9 by palpation (usually by a trained professional) occurs still earlier than

the discovery of a tumor of the size ordinarily encountered in clinical practice.[139]

Clinical detection through the use of BSE generally occurs when a tumor is approximately the size of a walnut, and is by no means early in the biological history of the cancer. Therefore, mammography is an important consideration in the triad of early detection of breast cancer.

The routine screening mammogram provides a high-sensitivity study at the lowest possible cost. A highly sensi-

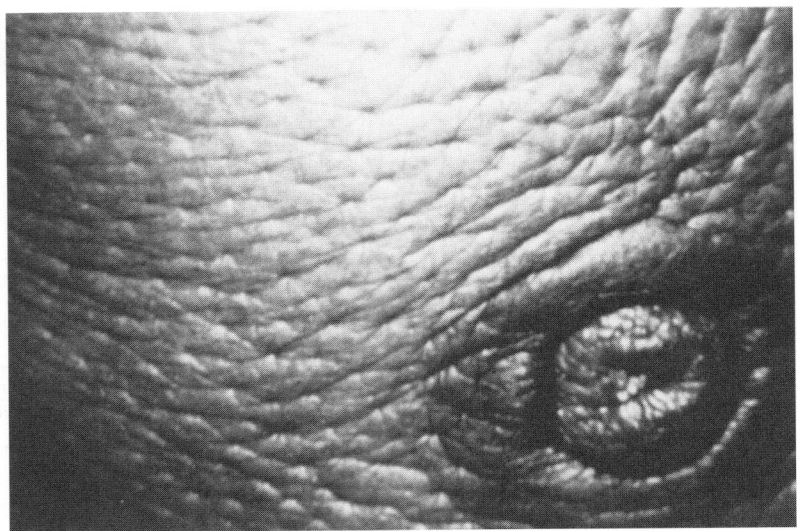

Figure 48-5 *Peau d'orange;* characteristic of lymphatic and dermal invasion by adenocarcinoma (inflammatory carcinoma).

tive study enables the radiologist to detect any discrete abnormality, thereby reducing the false-negative reports. Film-screen mammography allows a high-quality image with a minimum of radiation. Although xeromammography has been used in the past, it is no longer utilized.

A woman should consider the institution where the mammogram is performed. Since 1994, all facilities except Veterans Hospitals must comply with standards regarding equipment, personnel, record keeping, and must be certified by the Federal Drug Administration (FDA) through an FDA-accredited body, such as the American College of Radiology.[140] One can call 1-800-ACR-LINE for current information on accredited hospital and clinics.

The screening mammogram usually consists of four views, two per breast (Figures 48-6 and 48-7). A mediolateral oblique and a craniocaudal view of each breast enables the technologist to image as much breast as possible (i.e., the axillary tail and pectoralis muscle).

A screening mammogram allows the radiologist to detect characteristic benign and malignant masses. Benign masses include cysts, fibroadenomas, and inframammary lymph nodes, all of which have defined borders. Malignant lesions may present as spiculated or ill-defined masses, architectural distortion, asymmetric densities, and microcalcifications (Figures 48-8 and 48-9). Additionally, subtle abnormalities may be noted by the radiologist that require further studies to determine if pathology exists.[138]

Diagnostic mammograms. A diagnostic mammogram is performed when the patient reports specific symptoms, suspicious clinical findings exist, or an abnormality has been found on a screening mammogram. A diagnostic film uses additional views of the affected breast as well as the possibility of localized compression and magnification views to increase the specificity of identi-

Figure 48-6 Screening mammography of an asymptomatic breast from above (craniocaudal view).

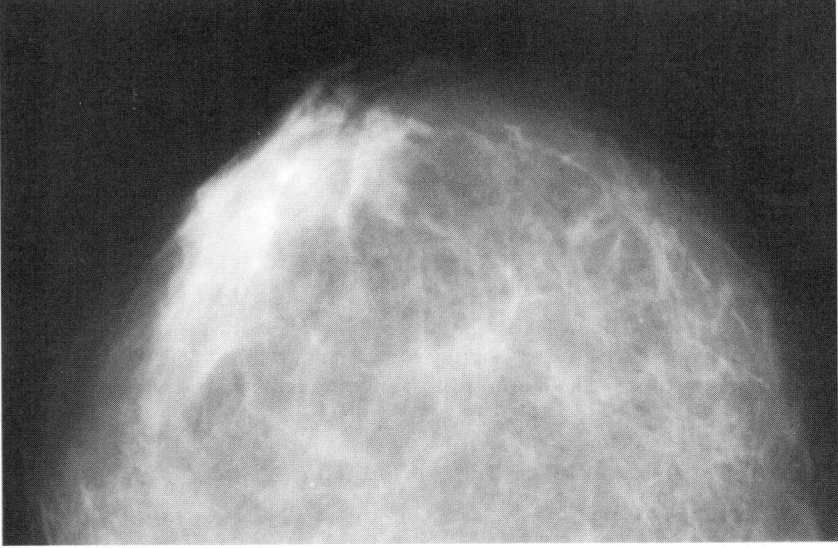

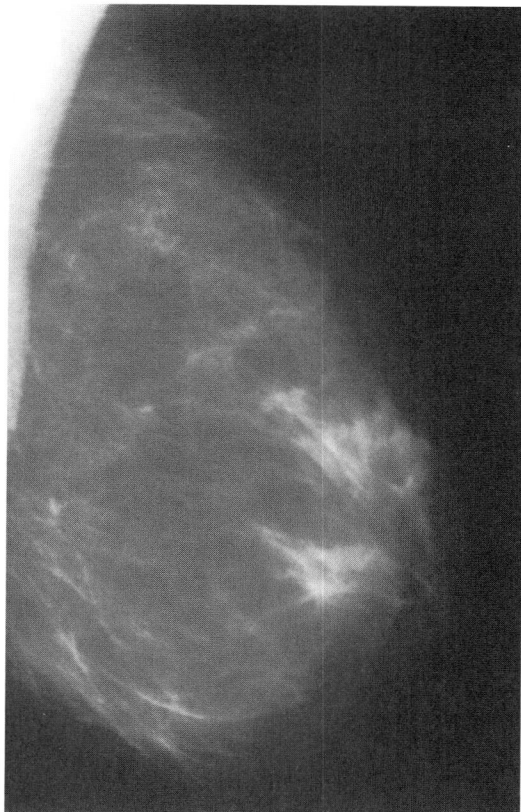

Figure 48-7   Screening mammography of an asymptomatic breast from the side (mediolateral view). Note the inclusion of the axilla and the pectoralis muscle, which ensures that the entire breast is imaged.

fying the abnormality.[141] The area in question is locally compressed and/or magnified, which enables the radiologist to comment more accurately on the lesion (Figures 48-10 and 48-11). The radiologist should be present during the diagnostic study. The ongoing evaluation of the

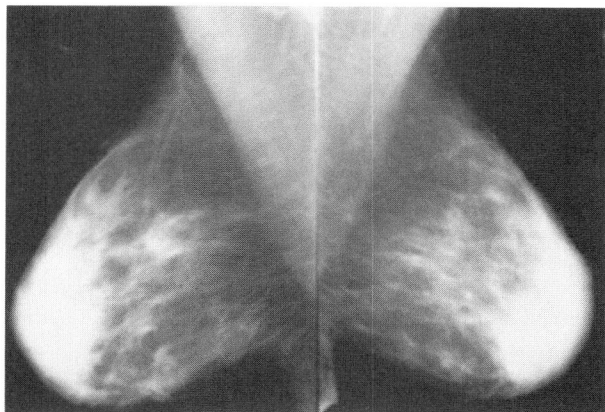

Figure 48-8   The mediolateral views show the appearance of an asymmetric density.

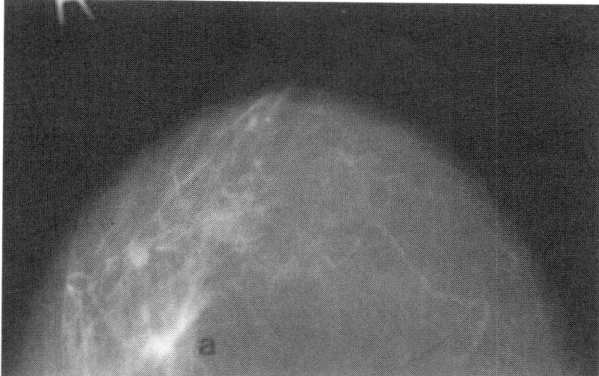

Figure 48-9   A craniocaudal view demonstrates the presence of spiculated nodules.

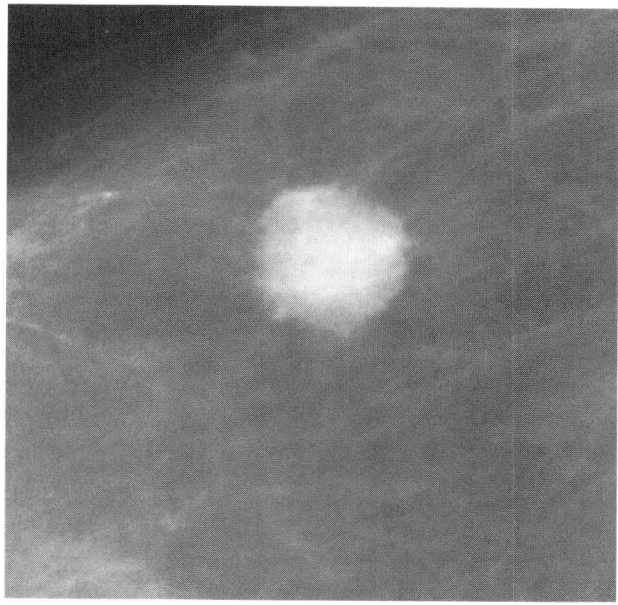

Figure 48-10   Magnification of the nodule provides a more accurate picture of the irregular border noted on screening mammogram. Note that the border is not clearly defined, but appears fuzzy or hazy, which is especially demonstrated on the left side. The irregular appearance makes this nodule suspicious for cancer.

additional films is crucial for rendering a diagnosis or recommending a plan of care.

Diagnostic mammography provides the radiologist with additional detail to render a more specific diagnosis, which may preclude the need for an open biopsy. However, if the diagnosis is nonspecific and the lesion has a low-suspicion threshold and is felt to be benign, the radiologist may recommend repeat films in six months to ensure the area in question has not changed. This approach must be discussed with the patient as some people are uncomfortable waiting to be reexamined

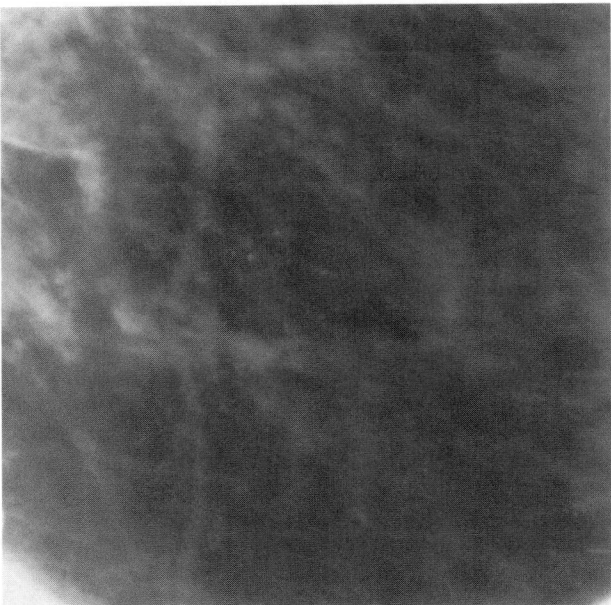

Figure 48-11   New microcalcifications were seen on a routine mammogram. The radiologist requested magnified views, which revealed a small area of clustered microcalcifications (top) as well as microcalcifications that tend to branch (below). Both are suspicious for cancer.

mammographically and may prefer to have the abnormality sampled or excised.

Digital mammography records the radiographic image in a digital format that can be stored in a computer. This image can be displayed on a monitor or transferred to film. The advantages of digital technology over film-screen mammography are that (1) digital technology allows for more variations in exposure, (2) the radiologist's performance is increased by virtue of a second look, (3) differences in tissue contrast are more easily seen, (4) images can be transmitted and easily stored.[142,143]

Computer assisted diagnosis (CAD) utilizes a software program to target potentially suspicious lesions for the radiologist to review and interpret. The computer identification involves an algorithm from a preset database generated from probability tables. There are several promising outcomes that may result from this method of imaging. The specificity of the image is enhanced by real-time evaluation on a screen, allowing for manipulation of contrast that enhances detection and permits more rapid interventional procedures. Additionally, this real-time evaluation will improve mobile systems in remote areas. Expert consultation may be immediately accessed via satellite.[144]

Digital imaging has its limitations and potential problems. Whole breast images equal to the quality of film-screen mammography is not yet possible, and interpretation and comparison using both types of imaging need more study. Cost is a major limiting factor for digital imaging and computer-assisted diagnosis. The basic digi-

tal mammographic unit is in the range of $250,000 compared to a standard film-screen unit price of $90,000. Additional expense will be incurred as accessory equipment is acquired to fully utilize the capabilities of digital imaging.

Sonogram

A sonogram or ultrasound is used to determine whether a lesion is solid or cystic. It can also be used to guide interventional procedures such as cyst aspiration, abscess drainage, fine-needle aspiration (FNA), needle core biopsies, or presurgical localization.[145,146] Ultrasounds are appropriate to investigate palpable lesions in young women whose breasts have the dense fibroglandular tissue that may obscure a lesion in the breast. Ultrasounds are also useful in pregnant women, who need to be spared radiation, when an abscess or galactocele is suspected, or in recently lactating women whose breasts are extremely dense.

While sonograms are useful in determining if a lesion is solid or cystic, their sensitivity and specificity are not of the same caliber as mammograms. They should generally not be used for screening purposes (Figure 48-12).

Magnetic resonance imaging

Magnetic resonance imaging (MRI—or magnetic resonance mammography (MRM)—of the breast is a relatively new procedure that may allow for earlier detection based on the ability of this test to determine smaller lesions and finer detail. MRI has become a highly accurate

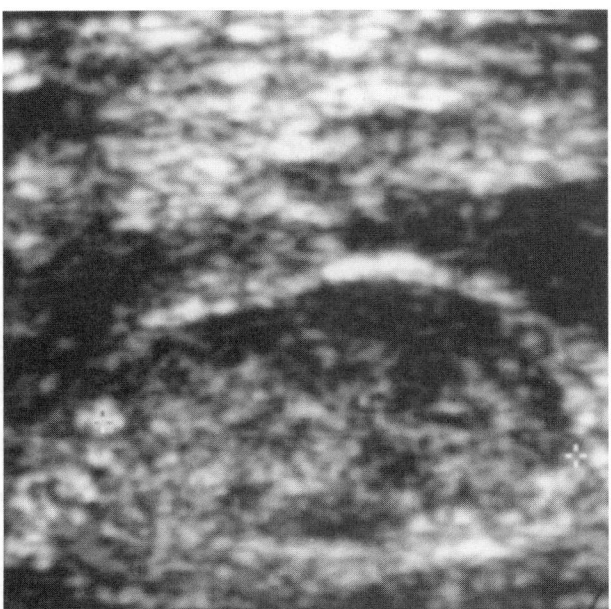

Figure 48-12   An ultrasound of a palpable mass reveals the characteristics of a fibroadenoma (between the crosses), which is a benign nodule.

though costly tool, now that specificity is enhanced by contrast infusion. It is superior to ultrasound in imaging the parenchyma, axilla, or chest wall and may aid in staging.[147] MRI evaluates the rate at which the contrast initially enters the breast tissue. Malignant lesions tend to exhibit an increased enhancement within the first two minutes. It is limited in the detection of calcifications, which excludes its use for many nonpalpable lesions. MRI may be best thought of as a complement to mammography and clinical exam to distinguish between a benign or malignant lesion in the high-risk population, with the hope of preventing benign biopsies. MRI may also be utilized to identify occult lesions, recurrences, as well as to evaluate implant integrity.[142,148,149]

Positron emission tomography

Positron emission tomography (PET) employs metabolic activity to image the breast tissue. The glucose radiopharmaceutical, 2-deoxy-2-[18F]-fluoro-D-glucose (FDG), has been reported most useful as a metabolic tracer that quantifies the overconsumption of glucose by a tumor cell.[142,150]

PET may be superior to MRI in identifying viable tumor versus scar tissue, benign and malignant axillary nodes, and tumors greater than 1 cm. It may also be utilized to locate primary, regional, and systemic metastases, and may play a future role in chemotherapy planning. The major limitations of PET are the high cost of the scanners and their limited availability, as well as the short half-life of the radiopharmaceuticals.[148] Currently, PET has been approved, by insurance carriers, for a few cancers and continues to be evaluated in the research setting. It will not be available as a screening tool until more definitive data becomes available.

Scintimammography

Scintimammography uses a variety of radioisotopes to image the breast. The most promising to date are thallium-201 (TI-201) and technetium-99M sestamibi (MIBI). This imaging tool is best known from the media reports that lauded it as the breakthrough needed to reduce unnecessary biopsies of the breast. While initial reports with small study numbers show sensitivity ranging from 89%–95% and specificity ranging from 72%–87%, larger prospective trials need to be conducted to determine its diagnostic and prognostic role before widespread clinical use is advocated.[151–155]

Fine-needle aspiration

Fine-needle aspiration (FNA) is employed when an abnormality is known to be solid or to determine if the palpable mass is a cyst. FNA may also be used to confirm a clinically apparent positive diagnosis. FNA is a simple office procedure that can be performed with or without local anesthetic using a small 20- or 22-gauge needle and 10-cc or larger syringe.

If the lump in question is a cyst, it should disappear after the aspiration is completed. The decision to discard the cyst contents or send to cytopathology involves several factors: the clinical evaluation of the mass, the appearance of fluid (straw-colored, green, cloudy are typical presentations), the number of previous aspirations, and the risk of breast cancer. Some practitioners routinely send any fluid aspirated from the breast while others may have a different threshold for discarding the aspirates. Cysts may return in the same area or in other areas of the breast and the patient may have repeated aspirations over time. If a previously aspirated cyst refills more than once in a short period of time (six to eight weeks), the decision to excise may be made, based on the patient's history of previous aspirations and personal risk of breast cancer. If a lump is solid, it is still possible to obtain a sample by making several passes into the lesion using the same entry point. This method will retrieve small cell samples from several sites within the lesion and reduce the false-negative result.

The usefulness of FNA cytology can vary and the practitioner must have confidence in the skill of the cytopathologist, must realize that the sample may not render a definitive diagnosis, and must know that a malignant cytology cannot distinguish between in situ or invasive cancers.

It should be mentioned that a lesion that does not demonstrate a malignant histology might still remain clinically suspicious to the physician. In cases such as these, a biopsy will often be recommended.

Core needle biopsy

The core needle biopsy is generally used for presumably solid, palpable masses that have some suspicion for cancer. Core needle biopsies are performed with a spring-action "gun" that automatically advances the needle to the lesion and obtains a specimen. The needle gauge is larger than FNA, 14g or 16g, thereby producing a small core of tissue.[156] The gun may be used several times to ensure an adequate sampling. The core needle biopsy is thought to be superior to FNA because the diagnosis is based on pathology interpretation, rather than cytopathology, a definitive diagnosis is usually rendered, and in situ cancers can be distinguished from invasive cancers.[157–159]

Stereotactic needle-guided biopsy

The increasing acceptance of mammography as a diagnostic tool has fostered advances in minimally invasive biopsy techniques. The stereotactic needle-guided biopsy (SNB) is mainly used to target and identify mammographically detected nonpalpable lesions in the breast.[160] SNB is appropriate for sampling most nonpalpable lesions; however, it is less suitable for very small lesions or areas of calcification, superficial lesions, or those on the extreme medial or lateral area of the breast.[161,162]

While mammography offers the best detection of

early breast cancer, it often cannot distinguish between benign or malignant tumors. Approximately 60%–80% of recommended biopsies are for benign abnormalities. The stereotactic biopsy permits diagnosis of benign disease without the trauma or scarring of an open biopsy. This procedure has been improved over time to yield sufficient tissue for diagnosis more than 97% of the time when performed by an experienced practitioner. It also results in a definite cost saving over excisional biopsy.[163–166]

The basic principle of stereotactic biopsy is to immobilize the breast from fixed horizontal and vertical coordinates to calculate the exact position of the lesion within a three-dimensional field.[161] The procedure takes place in a specially equipped operating room and generally takes about an hour. The room contains breast-imaging equipment and an examination table that has an opening at the front end through which the breast is suspended as the patient lies in a prone position (Figure 48-13). This positioning is necessary to examine and target the precise area to be sampled.

After proper placement is confirmed by stereoradiographs or digital mammograms, the breast is locally anesthetized and a small incision is made to penetrate the subcutaneous fibrous tissue. A needle (14g–20g) is placed in a spring-loaded biopsy gun that is mounted and stabilized. Because the gun emits a loud "pop," it is helpful to fire the gun before placing the needle to reduce the risk of startling the patient.[166]

The needle is inserted several times, which allows two or three core biopsy samples to be taken. Histology samples are then sent to the pathology department, and results are usually reported in one to two days. Cytology specimens may also be taken at this time.

Stereoradiographs are taken again to identify the exact area from which the samples are taken to ensure adequate sampling. If microcalcifications are the target, a specimen radiograph is used to confirm removal.[160]

After the procedure, pressure with or without an ice pack is applied for five minutes. The area is then cleaned and a sterile bandage is applied. The patient may shower the next day, but should avoid bathing for two days. The patient is then given instructions regarding notification of results.[166]

Wire localization biopsy

The preparation for the wire-localized biopsy is somewhat similar to the stereotactic method. The difference lies in the goal of the procedure. The aim of this biopsy procedure is to radiographically assist the surgeon in locating the nonpalpable lesion for the purpose of excisional biopsy and to minimize the volume of tissue removed to avoid unnecessary deformity. The character of the abnormality is identified after biopsy. See Figure 48-14.

The wire-localized biopsy targets the area via mammography usually using a 90-degree view to determine the depth of the abnormality along with possible craniocaudal and/or mediolateral oblique views. Once the area is anesthetized, a double-lumen needle is inserted into the area that has been calculated by the planes of the mammograms. Multiple lesions may be localized at one time using several wires.[167] A set of repeat mammograms is then taken to ensure proper placement.

Once proper placement has been determined, the outer needle is removed, leaving a thin hook wire marking the area of concern (Figure 48-15). This wire is then

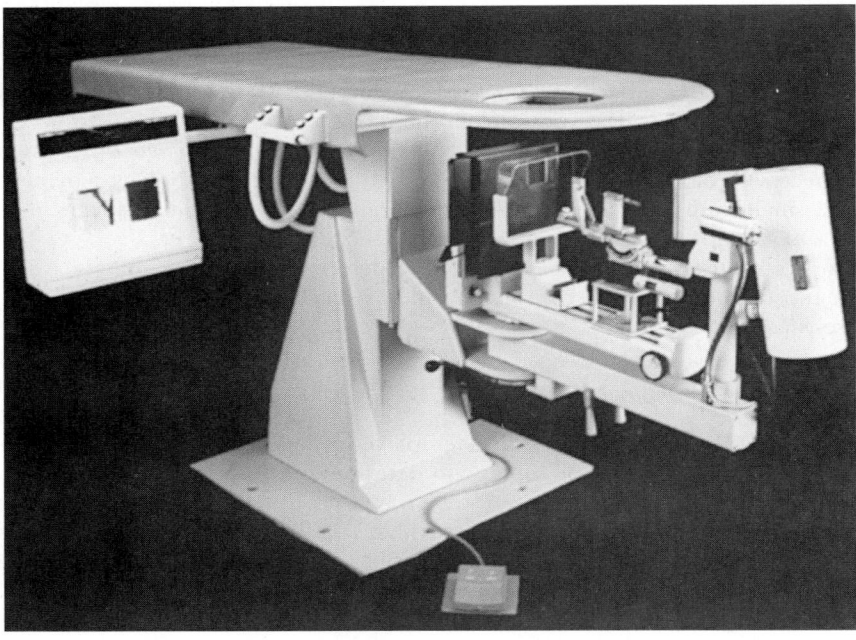

Figure 48-13 The stereotactic table allows for localization of the nonpalpable lesion between the Plexiglas plates below the opening from which the breast hangs down. Some machines allow for the procedure to be done in a sitting position, which is less favorable due to the possibility of syncope. (Photo courtesy of Fisher Imaging, Denver, CO.)

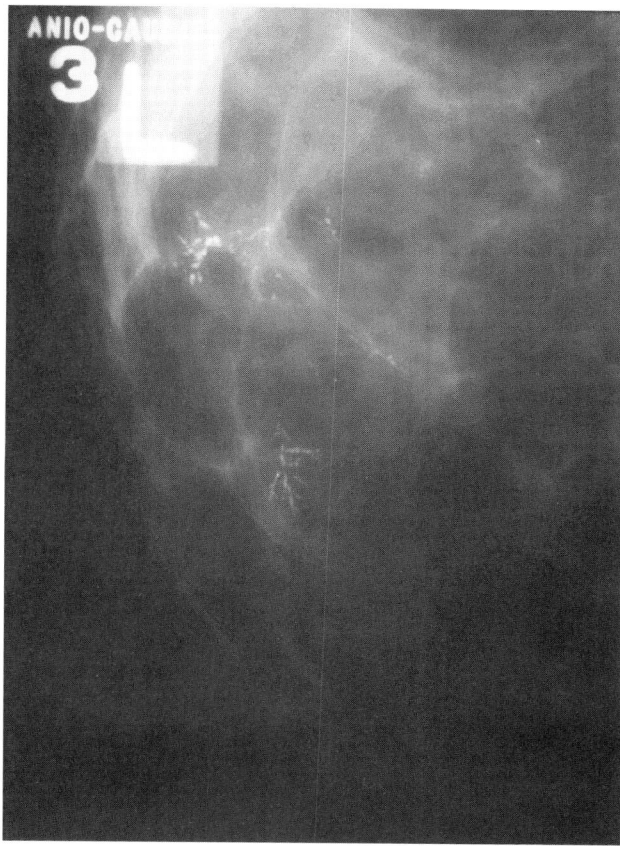

Figure 48-14   Magnification view of two areas of suspicious microcalcifications.

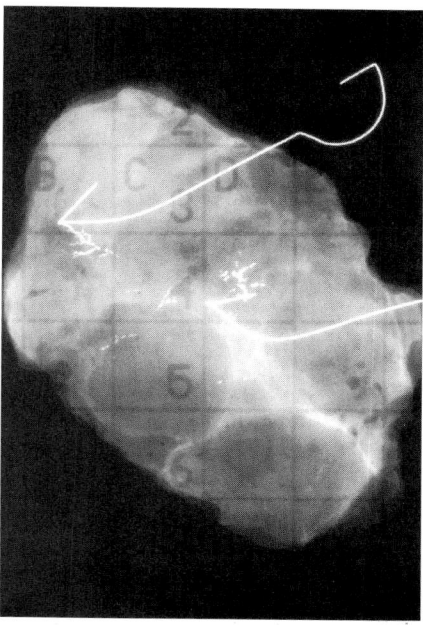

Figure 48-15   Specimen mammogram: Hook-wires were placed in each area of calcification. They were removed with good margins of surrounding tissue.

taped to the skin of the breast to prevent dislodgment. The patient is sent to the operating room with the mammograms that note the area to be excised.[167] After the biopsy, a specimen mammogram of the tissue is taken to ensure the abnormality has been removed.

Excisional biopsy/lumpectomy

The excisional biopsy is the most invasive diagnostic procedure. There are several reasons for recommending an excisional biopsy: (1) sonogram findings show the lesion to be solid and indeterminate, (2) the cytology and/or histology results are insufficient, (3) the clinical or mammographic findings are suspicious, or (4) the patient with a probable low-risk lesion requests a biopsy to allay her anxiety.

The objective of this biopsy is to remove the lump or area identified, along with a small amount of surrounding normal tissue. The potential for breast conservation should be considered during the planning for the biopsy. This is done by placing the incision above the lesion, using the most appropriate incision to follow the lines of tension and avoiding tunneling. After the tumor is removed, the skin is closed without approximating breast tissue or fat. This method results in less deformity at the

biopsy site. The excised tissue is identified and sent to pathology for histopathological diagnosis.

An incisional biopsy that removes only part of the lesion is rarely performed. If the tumor is very large and a diagnosis is needed, FNA or core-needle biopsy is usually sufficient and an incisional biopsy is not necessary.

Prognostic Indicators

When breast cancer is diagnosed and determined to be localized without evidence of metastatic spread, it is critical to identify patients who are at a substantial risk of recurrence either locally or systemically. Identification of variables that are associated with disease recurrence may make it possible to design the most appropriate treatment for the individual based on the biological aggressiveness of the cancer. Most women with node-negative disease, representing approximately 60% of women diagnosed with breast cancer today, will be cured by surgery alone. Thirty percent will develop recurrent disease within ten years of initial therapy. The identification of various prognostic indicators helps to define the natural history of breast cancer, establish prognosis with increasing accuracy, and most importantly, identify these subsets of women who may be cured by local therapy alone as opposed to those who would most benefit from adjuvant systemic therapies. For the majority of early breast cancers that are cured by local therapies alone, systemic treatment offers no benefit.

Valuable parameters for determining the prognosis for patients with breast cancer include the status of the axillary lymph nodes, size of the tumor, the invasive nature of the neoplasm, multicentricity, nuclear grade, hormone receptor levels, and histological type.

Cell proliferative indices, DNA ploidy, *HER2/neu* oncogene, and vascular endothelial growth factor protein are areas of investigation and are currently considered to be of high prognostic value in breast cancer, especially for women who have node-negative disease.

Axillary lymph node status

The involvement of axillary nodes by tumor has long been recognized as a key feature in determining prognosis in breast cancer (Figure 48-16). Clinical assessment of the axillary nodes carries a 30% false-positive and false-negative rate. Pathological staging of the lymph nodes is mandatory. However, in one study, 17% of stage I breast cancer patients initially diagnosed with no evidence of metastatic disease in lymph nodes had occult axillary metastatic disease when reexamined pathologically.[168] Once involvement is determined, important issues are whether the metastases are microscopic or macroscopic, the number of nodes involved, the levels of involvement, and whether the lymph node capsule has been invaded.[168] Extranodal extension is significant prognostically only

when the metastases are confined to one to three nodes.[169] Staging of axillary nodes requires pathological view of at least four axillary nodes.[170]

Seventy percent of patients with negative nodes survive ten years. Prognosis worsens as the number of positive lymph nodes increases. Recurrence of disease is seen in approximately 75% of women with many positive nodes. Metastases to the internal mammary nodes have the same significance as those to the axillary nodes. Internal mammary node metastasis occurs more readily in patients who have medial lesions. Internal mammary nodes are not commonly sampled but are invaded in 10% of patients when axillary nodes are negative. This may help to explain the recurrence patterns in some axillary node-negative women.[171] Table 48-4 demonstrates the correlation between survival and number of involved nodes in a large population of women.[172]

Tumor size

Prior to the more widespread use of mammography, less than 8% of women with node-negative breast cancer had tumors that were less than 1 cm in diameter with a relative overall five-year survival of nearly 99%. Patients with tumors measuring 1–3 cm have a relative five-year survival of approximately 91%, while those with tumors measuring more than 3 cm have a five-year survival of 85%.[173] Recurrence rates for patients with tumors greater than 3 cm is more than 50%, however.

Table 48-5 demonstrates a clear relationship between

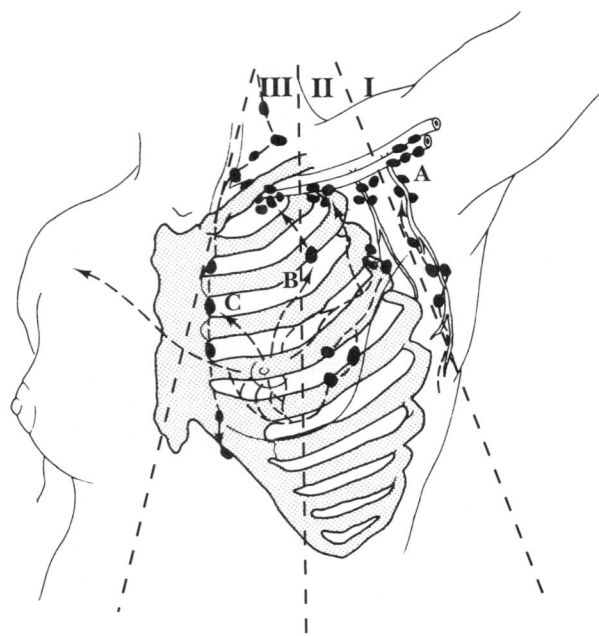

Figure 48-16 Lymphatics of the breast leading to (A) axillary nodes, which are distributed over a large area from the lateral aspects of the breast proper to the axillary vessels; (B) interpectoral chain leading to interpectoral node (circle detail) and to high nodes in the axilla; and (C) chain of the internal mammary leading frequently to nodes in second interspace and to supraclavicular and cervical nodes. The levels of lymph nodes (I, II, III) are defined by the pectoralis minor muscle.

Table 48-4 Recurrence Rates in 20,547 Women with Breast Cancer According to the Number of Histologically Involved Axillary Nodes

Number of Positive Nodes	Recurrence at 5 Years
0	25%
1–3	40%
4–6	49%
7–9	58%
10 +	78%

Data from Nemoto T, et al.[172]

Table 48-5 Tumor Size and Recurrence-free Survival in Node-negative Breast Cancer Without Chemotherapy

Tumor Size (cm)	Recurrence-free Survival (%)	
	10 years	20 years
≤ 1.0	91	88
1.1–2.0	77	72
2.1–3.0	75	71
3.1–5.0	62	59

Data from Rosen PP, et al.[174]

systemic risk of recurrence and tumor size.[174] In addition, the presence of peritumoral vascular invasion is a marker of both local recurrence and future distant metastases. Consideration of other prognostic indicators is often necessary to determine the appropriate approach to systemic therapies.

Hormone receptor status

Normal breast epithelium has hormone receptors and responds specifically to the stimulatory effects of estrogen and progesterone. A majority of breast cancers will retain estrogen receptors and for these tumors estrogen will retain proliferative control over the malignant cells. The major benefit to knowing a woman's hormone receptor status concerns its value in predicting which patients will respond to hormone manipulation. Tumors that are more well differentiated or are of a lower grade tend to be positive for estrogen and progesterone receptors (ER and PR) and have a better than 75% response rate for endocrine therapy, in comparison to tumors that are positive only for ER whose response rate is under 35%. Tumors that lack receptor activity will not respond to hormonal therapy and tend to be tumors with higher histologic grades. Postmenopausal women tend to be ER positive while premenopausal women tend to be ER negative.

Cell proliferative indices and DNA ploidy

Research indicates that assessment of cell proliferative potential may have important prognostic significance, especially in node-negative breast cancer. Using flow cytometry, it is possible to measure DNA content and proliferative activity (S-phase fraction) of a tumor. Patients whose tumors have an abnormal amount of DNA are aneuploid. Those with normal DNA are diploid. A high S-phase fraction consistently predicts a poorer outcome compared to those patients with a low S-phase calculation.

Tumors that are ER negative tend to have a high S-phase fraction reflecting a more aggressive metastatic potential.

Histopathological considerations

The more differentiated the tumor cells, the better the prognosis. Tumors are generally classified according to their histopathological grade, which takes into account the nuclear pattern and morphology and mitotic activity. Tumors that are well differentiated (grade I), have ductal/glandular features, uniform nuclear shape and staining characteristics, and low mitotic counts are low grade. Those tumors without these features and with markedly pleomorphic hyperchromic nuclei and abundant mitotic activity as evidenced by a high S-phase fraction are considered high-grade carcinomas. Such factors as nuclear size and shape, mitotic figures, and degree of tubule formation determine differentiation and likewise predict ag-

gressiveness and metastatic potential of tumor cells. Approximately 10% of patients have low-grade tumors and, of these patients, greater than 90% have ER positive tumors; the majority have diploid DNA, low mitotic activity and smaller tumors. Other important histopathologic considerations of tumor behavior are the amount of tumor necrosis, lymphatic/vascular invasion, and the extent of involvement of the surgical resection margin. Evidence of tumor involvement of either the microcapillary or lymphatic channels is considered nearly as predictive of recurrence as lymph node involvement.

Molecular and biological factors

Overexpression of vascular endothelial growth factor (VEGF) is thought to be involved in tumorigenesis and metastasis in primary breast cancer. Increased expression of VEGF is associated with decreased overall survival in women with node-negative breast cancer.[175,176] The degree of intratumoral vascularization in primary breast cancer is a significant independent prognostic indicator that correlates with metastasis and shortened survival.[177,178] Primary tumors and metastases will not grow beyond 2 mm in diameter without an enhanced vascular supply. Chemical signals (cytokines) from tumor cells are thought to stimulate resting vascular endothelial cells into a rapid growth phase thereby supporting the growth and spread of the tumor. VEGF is an angiogenic factor that stimulates proliferation of vascular endothelial cells. Tumor-induced neovascularization appears to be a critical step in the oncogenic and metastatic cascades and may have important implications for the evaluation and treatment of women with breast cancer, especially those with node-negative disease. Research in the development of monoclonal anti-VEGF antibody is an exciting development in breast cancer. Clinical trials are currently underway to test the safety and efficacy of rHuMAb VEGF as monotherapy and in combination with chemotherapy.

Under normal circumstances *p53* is a tumor suppressor gene that codes for a nuclear transcription factor that is involved with cell cycle regulation and programmed cell death. The loss of functioning of this tumor suppressor gene may be associated with increased aggressive tumor behavior. Mutation of the *p53* gene appears to be an independent prognostic marker of early relapse and could be an important factor to identify node-negative patients who have a poor prognosis and would therefore benefit from adjuvant systemic therapy.[179,180]

The *HER2/neu* proto-oncogene encodes for a transmembrane protein that appears to be a receptor for a peptide growth factor. Amplification of the *HER2/neu* gene occurs in approximately 30% of women with breast cancer resulting in overexpression of the gene product. It appears that amplification and/or overexpression of *HER2/neu* is associated with a worse disease-free and overall survival for women whose tumors overexpress this proto-oncogene, especially those with node positive disease. Further in women with metastatic breast cancer, high levels of *HER2/neu* correlated with poor response to endocrine therapy, and a favorable response to chemotherapy, especially cisplatin, doxorubicin and paclitaxel.[181,182]

Cathepsin D is a lysosomal enzyme that is synthesized in normal tissues but that may be overexpressed and secreted in certain breast cancers and appears to have a direct role in invasion and metastasis.[183] High cathepsin D levels increase the probability of recurrence (60% at five years) and poor survival in aneuploid node-negative breast cancer.[183,184]

Classification and Staging

Once a breast cancer has been diagnosed, a complete evaluation of the disease is initiated to establish stage of disease and the most appropriate approach to treatment. Such planning and evaluation are optimally orchestrated through the auspices of a comprehensive breast center where all disciplines consult with the patient and family concerning her decisions regarding therapy.

In the initial evaluation, the diagnostic mammogram is utilized to look for evidence of tumor multicentricity or for evidence of bilaterality. The history and physical exam; routine blood work including complete blood counts, liver function tests, and serum calcium; and a chest x-ray are completed prior to the initial planning session. A bone scan is generally considered part of the basic work-up if the tumor is larger than 1 cm or if the patient has elevated alkaline phosphatase. Bone films are only indicated if there is a suspicious area suggesting tumor involvement. Likewise, a liver scan would only be indicated if liver function tests were abnormal or if the primary tumor were inflammatory in nature or larger in size.

Following the pretreatment evaluation, the patient is clinically staged on the basis of the characteristics of the primary tumor, the physical examination of the axillary nodes, and the presence or absence of distant metastases. As previously mentioned, the clinical evaluation is inaccurate and, because of the prognostic significance of axillary node involvement, a pathological stage is necessary to determine stage of disease.[170,185]

The pathological staging recommended by the American Joint Committee on Cancer (AJCC)[186] is presented in Table 48-6. This system is relatively complicated and can be simplified in terms of the most critical components, that is, whether nodes are involved and whether distant metastases are known to be present.

Stage I	Tumor 0–2 cm in size; negative lymph nodes and no evidence of metastasis
Stage II	Small tumor with positive lymph nodes or a larger tumor with negative lymph nodes
Stage III	More advanced locoregional disease with suspected but undetectable metastases
Stage IV	Distant metastases are present

Therapeutic Approaches and Nursing Care

Women today are discriminating health consumers who actively seek information regarding their treatment options. It is not uncommon for the nurse to be called upon to advise where a woman might go for a consultation concerning how a suspicious mass should be investigated. If one is available in the area, the woman should be referred to a comprehensive breast center for an opinion. Women should not delay in seeking medical attention; indeed, most women view the need for a definitive diagnosis as a psychological emergency. Fortunately, nurses and physicians who specialize in breast cancer realize this and generally mobilize resources to provide a swift and accurate assessment of the breast problem. While a breast cancer diagnosis causes significant emotional, social, economic/vocational upheaval, such distress eases over time as therapy is planned and carried out. Most women actively participate in the decision-making process and are able to clearly articulate their need for information throughout treatment planning and months of therapy. To be a supportive advocate for the woman and her family, the nurse must be knowledgeable concerning the options for therapy, the goals of therapy, the measures to minimize complications of treatment, and the various resources that may need to be mobilized throughout the treatment period and beyond.

For rehabilitation to be optimal, the nurse should pay careful attention to the woman's expressed need for information at each juncture of treatment. Seeking information is a valuable coping device and yet rarely useful unless the woman recognizes the need for it. The right amount of accurate information will help the woman formulate questions and will facilitate decision making, decrease anxiety, and enhance overall adjustment to the illness and treatment.[187]

How well a woman adjusts psychologically and socially to the diagnosis and treatment will depend upon her previous coping strategies and emotional stability. In addition, social support has consistently been found to influence a woman's adjustment through treatment.[188] The threat to emotional, social, sexual, and physical well-being is multifaceted, and the relative impact of these factors on adjustment varies from patient to patient and assumes varying degrees of importance at different stages of treatment.

A strong source of social support will be extremely valuable throughout all phases of treatment. While the most important sources of social support are the woman's spouse, her family, and friends, other sources of support may also be needed to maintain a strong social network.[189] The roles of the psycho-oncologist, the social worker, and various support groups are important resources in the care of these women and their families.

The patient's need for information will vary considerably throughout each phase of treatment. It is not uncommon for the treatment plan to include surgery, radiation,

Table 48-6   AJCC Pathological Staging System

PRIMARY TUMOR (T)

Tx   Primary tumor cannot be assessed

T0   No evidence of primary tumor

Tis*   Carcinoma in situ: intraductal carcinoma, lobular carcinoma in situ, or Paget's disease of the nipple with no tumor

T1   Tumor 2 cm or less in greatest dimension
     T1a—0.5 cm or less in greatest dimension

T   T1b—more than 0.5 cm, but not more than 1 cm in greatest dimension

1   T1c—More than 1 cm, but not more than 2 cm in greatest dimension

T2   Tumor more than 2 cm, but not more than 5 cm in greatest dimension

T3   Tumor more than 5 cm in greatest dimension

T4†   Tumor of any size with direct extension to chest wall or skin
     T4a—Extension to chest wall

PRIMARY TUMOR (T)

T4†   T4b—Edema (including *peau d'orange*) or ulceration of the skin of the breast or satellite skin nodules confined to the same breast
     T4c—Both (T4a and T4b)
     T4d—Inflammatory carcinoma

REGIONAL LYMPH NODES (N)

NX   Regional lymph nodes cannot be assessed (e.g., previously removed)

N0   No regional lymph node metastasis

N1   Metastasis to movable ipsilateral axillary lymph node(s)

N2   Metastasis to ipsilateral axillary lymph node(s) fixed to one another or to other structures

N3   Metastasis to ipsilateral internal mammary lymph node(s)

DISTANT METASTASIS (M)

MX   Presence of distant metastasis cannot be assessed

M0   No distant metastasis

M1   Distant metastasis (includes metastasis to ipsilateral supraclavicular lymph node(s))

STAGE GROUPING

Stage 0	Tis	N0	M0
Stage I	T1	N0	M0
Stage IIA	T0	N1	M0
	T1	N1	M0
	T2	N0	M0
Stage IIB	T2	N1	M0
	T3	N0	M0
Stage IIIA	T0	N2	M0
	T1	N2	M0
	T2	N2	M0
	T3	N1,N2	M0
Stage IIIB	T4	Any N	M0
	Any T	N3	M0
Stage IV	Any T	Any N	M1

*Paget's disease associated with a tumor is classified according to the size of the tumor.

†Chest wall includes ribs, intercostal muscles, and serratus anterior muscle, but not the pectoral muscle.

and chemotherapy. For many women the time of active treatment lasts at least six months and most do not feel rehabilitated for up to a year following their diagnosis. If reconstruction is planned, this rehabilitation phase will be extended.

Primary Breast Cancer

Local-regional disease

Intraductal carcinoma or DCIS generally presents as clustered microcalcifications on mammography and rarely carries a risk of axillary node involvement. Options for treatment include total mastectomy, wide excision followed by radiation, or wide excision alone. Because ductal carcinoma in situ frequently extends beyond the area of microcalcification, a wide excision should include tumor-free margins around the area. Invasive carcinoma develops in about 20% of patients within ten years when excisional biopsy alone is selected as definitive treatment.[190,191]

While it is true that nearly 60% of women diagnosed with breast cancer today will have localized node-negative breast cancer and therefore be highly curable, most women with primary breast cancer, stages I–II, will have metastatic disease from which they will die, regardless of local or systemic treatment.[192,193] Further, numerous clinical trials have demonstrated that breast-conserving treatments consisting of removal of the primary tumor by lumpectomy with radiation therapy results in a survival rate that is comparable to that of more extensive local therapy such as mastectomy or modified radical mastectomy.[194] Currently more than one-third of women with breast cancer in the United States are managed by lumpectomy and radiation therapy. Breast conserving surgery would not be appropriate for women with larger tumors, tumors involving the nipple areola complex, tumors with extensive intraductal disease appearing to be multicentric, and for women who are unable or unwilling to undergo adjuvant radiation therapy. Breast conservation is reserved for women with small, localized disease.

An extensive intraductal component is a predictor of recurrence and generally considered a contraindication to conservative surgery. Selection of the most appropriate surgical procedure is critical to local control of the primary cancer. With local failure and recurrent disease comes deteriorating survival from systemic disease.[195] The cosmetic result of breast-preserving surgery is generally considered to be acceptable as body image is maintained. Scar tissue may form causing some contracture over time, but most women find the cosmetic result acceptable, especially when wearing a bra.

Complications following breast-preserving surgery include arm edema, seroma formation and wound infection, shoulder dysfunction, upper extremity weakness, fatigue, and limitations in mobility.

A modified radical mastectomy involves the removal of all breast tissue and nipple areola complex, and level I and II axillary node dissection (see Figure 48-16). The pectoralis muscle is preserved. A horizontal incision is made because it is cosmetically more acceptable. Modified radical mastectomy is indicated for larger, multicentric disease or where cosmesis is otherwise not achievable. Modified radical mastectomy may also be employed as definitive treatment following local recurrence in patients who fail conservative surgery and radiation. In general, patients with noninvasive or locally invasive tumors have excellent prognoses following salvage mastectomy. However, patients with predominantly invasive recurrent tumors are at significant risk for further relapse.

Postoperative complications following mastectomy include wound infection, flap necrosis, and seroma formation. A transverse incision is associated with less skin flap necrosis. Seromas occur in about 10% of patients and generally resolve following aspiration. Antibiotics may be indicated. Nursing care of the postmastectomy patient centers on wound care, with special attention to maintaining functioning wound drains. If drains become blocked, the wound is more likely to develop a seroma/hematoma leading to infection and possibly flap necrosis. To maintain suction and an adherent flap, drains may be "milked" to remove small clots. Drains are usually removed within two to four days following surgery. Patients may be discharged with drains intact.

Postmastectomy exercises to maintain shoulder and arm mobility may begin as early as 24 hours after surgery. The woman is instructed to maintain the affected arm in the adducted position but to perform limited exercises involving the wrist and elbow. Flexing fingers and touching the hand to the shoulder are encouraged. Squeezing a ball is discouraged, as it increases blood flow and, if done too vigorously, leads to swelling in the early postoperative period (Tables 48-7 and 48-8).

Prior to discharge, the patient should have clear instructions regarding wound care. Initial care of the wound involves maintaining a clean incision with dressing changes daily if indicated. A return appointment is usually made to assess the wound and if necessary remove stitches. At that time the patient should receive specific instructions regarding postmastectomy exercises. A mild analgesic may be indicated to promote arm mobility during exercises and to prevent shoulder dysfunction.

Complaints of a stiff shoulder are common and are due primarily to postoperative immobility. It is not uncommon for a tightness to develop under the axilla extending to the elbow. This cord-like substance is thought to be sclerosed lymphatics that gradually dissipate two to three months after surgery. Range of motion (ROM) exercises and massage therapy are beneficial. Care of the axilla involves avoiding the use of depilatory creams, strong deodorants, and shaving under the arm for approximately two weeks following surgery.

Instructions regarding breast self-exam and follow-up are usually given during the first outpatient visit after surgery. Introducing the patient to various prostheses and mastectomy bras can occur in the hospital, but women are generally more ready to receive this information once

Table 48-7   Postmastectomy Exercises

When to Begin	Purpose	Exercises: Perform Exercises 5–10 Times Each, Three Times a Day
Postoperatively days 1–5	Prevent and/or reduce swelling	• Position arm against your side in a relaxed position. Elbow should be level with your heart, and the wrist just above the elbow when resting. • Rotate wrist in a circular fashion. • Touch fingers to shoulder and extend arm fully.
After drains are removed	Promote muscle movement without stretching	• While standing, brace yourself with your other arm and bend over slightly, allowing your affected arm to hang freely. Swing the arm in small circles and gradually increase in size. Make 10 circles—rest—repeat in the opposite direction. • Swing arm forward and back as far as you can without pulling on the incision. • While standing, bend over slightly and swing arms across the chest in each direction. • While sitting in a chair, rest both arms at your side. Shrug both shoulders, then relax. • While sitting or standing, pull shoulders back, bring the shoulder blades together.
After sutures are removed	To stretch and regain full range of motion. To gain mobility of your shoulder, you must move it in *all* directions, several times a day	• While lying in bed with arm extended, raise arm over your head and extend backwards. • While lying in bed, grasp a cane or short pole with both hands across your lap. Extend arms straight up and over your head and return. • Repeat, rotating the cane clockwise and then counterclockwise while over your head. • While standing, extend arm straight over your head and down. • Extend your elbow out from your side at a 90° angle—hold it for 10 seconds—relax. • Extend your arm straight out from your side even with your shoulder—extend arm straight up toward the ceiling. • Stand at arms' length facing a wall. Extend arms so your fingertips touch the wall. Creep fingers up the side of the wall, stepping forward as necessary. Repeat the procedure going down the wall—keep arms extended. • Stand sideways to the wall. Extend arm out so fingers touch the wall. Creep up the wall a little more each day. • Use hand and arm normally (see Table 48-8).
After 6 weeks	To strengthen arm and shoulder and to regain total use of arm and shoulder	• Begin water aerobics. • Begin overall fitness program. • Begin aerobics, Jazzercise, or other resistive exercises. • Avoid using weights as these may increase arm edema and subsequent swelling.

the surgery is behind them. Most are not advised to wear a prosthesis until the wound has healed completely (six to ten weeks). During this period, the woman may want to meet with a Reach to Recovery or Y-ME volunteer who will assist her in learning about resources in her area for purchasing a prosthesis. There are many different kinds of prosthesis; some are foam filled, liquid silicone filled, or are the more permanent, self-adhering variety. It is important that the prosthesis fit properly and that the weight is similar to the remaining breast. Insurance pays

for most prostheses provided a prescription or letter demonstrating medical necessity is submitted.

The woman alone or together with her husband or spousal designate should have the opportunity to discuss any physical or emotional concerns regarding sexual relations. Evidence is mounting to support the contention that, while the diagnosis of breast cancer and the loss of a breast are certainly emotionally distressing for all concerned, they do not result in an increased prevalence of psychiatric disorders or sexual dysfunction.[196,197] The

Table 48-8 Patient Information—Hand and Arm Precautions

Do not permit injections (chemotherapy), blood samples, or vaccinations to be done on your affected arm unless approved by your physician.

When trimming cuticles, take extra care not to tear hangnails. Professional manicures *are* recommended.

Wear heavy gloves when gardening and digging or handling thorny plants.

Always use a thimble when sewing to avoid pinpricks, and wear rubber gloves while washing dishes.

Protect your arm from burns, especially from small appliances such as irons or frying pans, and from the sun.

Be sure your hand and arm are well protected with an elbow-length mitt when reaching into a hot oven.

Always have blood pressure measurements taken on the opposite arm.

Avoid arm constriction from tight elastic, sleeves, or jewelry.

Do not carry a heavy purse or other objects—especially grocery bags or luggage—with your affected arm.

Avoid strenuous upper body aerobics unless arm is supported by a properly fitted antilymphedema compression sleeve. Lifting weights of any kind is not recommended.

Apply a good lanolin cream several times daily if your skin appears dry.

Treat cuts and scratches by washing the area well and applying an antiseptic. Contact your physician if signs of infection, redness, warmth, or swelling occur.

woman's overall psychological health, relationship satisfaction, and prior sexual relations are far stronger predictors of sexual health than the extent of breast surgery. As a group, however, younger women have consistently been found to experience more episodes of depression, anger, resentment, sexual problems, and fears of recurrence compared to older women.[198,199]

Axillary and sentinel lymph node dissection

Axillary lymph node dissection (ALND) is not a therapeutic procedure as the overall survival, disease-free survival, and rate of distant metastasis is the same for those patients who have axillary dissection as for those who do not.[200] The principal reason to perform an axillary node dissection is to help determine prognosis, risk for recurrence, and whether adjuvant chemotherapy—specifically a doxorubicin-containing regimen—is indicated. Because lymph node dissection is responsible for significant morbidity associated with breast surgery, there is increasing interest in finding alternative methods to obtain prognostic information. Lymphatic mapping and sentinel node biopsy are two of the most promising techniques.[201]

The first node in the lymphatic basin that receives primary lymphatic flow is the sentinel lymph node. The histological characteristic of the sentinel lymph node is

thought to predict the histological characteristics of the remaining lymph nodes in the axilla. Sentinel lymph node mapping involves the injection of a radioactive substance or blue dye into the area around the tumor, which later drains into the ipsilateral axilla. The axilla is explored through a small incision and the lymph node that takes up the blue dye or technetium-labeled sulfur colloid—that is, the sentinel node—is excised. If the sentinel node is positive for tumor then the patient undergoes an axillary dissection, but only if doing so contributes to decisions regarding therapy. If the sentinel node is negative, the remaining axilla is negative 92%–95% of the time.[202] Many women, especially those with small primary tumors and clinically negative axillary lymph nodes could potentially be spared an axillary dissection if the sentinel node is found to be negative. Axillary node dissection would then be reserved for women for whom more information is needed to determine the need for chemotherapy and for those with larger primary tumors.

Axillary lymph node dissection is not without complications. Despite its advantages, ALND is associated with pain, numbness, swelling, weakness and stiffness, lymphedema, and a decreased quality of life.[203,204] As detection of breast cancer at very early stages becomes the norm, women will no longer be willing to accept pain, lymphedema, and decreased arm mobility as a result of axillary node dissection. Already, women with newly diagnosed breast cancer are seeking surgeons who perform sentinel node biopsy. Clearly more information about the safety and efficacy of sentinel node biopsy is needed so that more women can potentially be spared unnecessary axillary dissection and avoid the risk of lymphedema, without sacrificing disease-free and overall survival.

Radiation and chemotherapy

The role of radiation in the treatment of localized breast cancer has evolved over the years and is now standard treatment. In fact with an equivalent survival rate and preservation of the breast, conservative surgery plus radiation is now considered preferable to mastectomy for the majority of women. The major criteria for selecting patients for breast-conserving surgery and radiation therapy (RT) are (1) the size of the tumor and the feasibility of resecting the primary tumor without causing major cosmetic deformity, and (2) the likelihood of tumor recurrence in the breast. Local failure following breast-conserving surgery and radiation occurs in 13% of patients at ten years[205] and is considered not only as a marker of occult circulating distant metastases but also as a source of new distant metastases and subsequent mortality. Every effort should be made to decrease the local failure rate, mainly by obtaining clear surgical margins and possibly by adding chemotherapy and antiestrogen therapy.[206]

When radiation and chemotherapy are given following breast-conserving surgery the patients experience higher survival rates overall.[207] For women who are at high risk for local or regional recurrence (patients with large tumors invading the skin of the breast or the chest wall or those with many positive axillary nodes), radiation and chemotherapy are indicated postmastectomy. Research reveals that women experienced fewer local and regional recurrences and overall survival was improved when cyclophosphamide, methotrexate, and fluorouracil (5-FU)—or CMF—are given simultaneously with radiation therapy commencing after cycle 3 of CMF.[208,209] According to Overgaard and colleagues,[209] survival at ten years was 54% among those women given radiotherapy and CMF and 45% among those who received CMF alone. In patients whose tumors overexpress the *HER2* proto-oncogene and are eligible for herceptin therapy, herceptin therapy may be given weekly during the radiation because of enhanced radiation effect when herceptin is given with the radiation.

The role of RT postmastectomy is less certain owing to the risks associated with radiation to the chest wall particularly when given for left-sided breast cancer. There appears to be a higher risk for fatal myocardial infarction 10–15 years later compared with adjuvant radiation for right-sided cases.[210] Postmastectomy radiotherapy is routinely considered for premenopausal patients with involved axillary nodes, particularly those with four or more involved nodes and/or tumors larger than 5 cm. The value of specific nodal irradiation in patients who undergo adequate axillary dissection is much less clear, especially considering the potential long-term complications of lymphedema.[211]

Radiation generally begins within three to four weeks following chemotherapy especially if a doxorubicin-containing regimen is used. If CMF or methotrexate, 5-FU, and leucovorin are used, radiation commences usually following day 8 of cycle 3 to minimize the additive toxic effects of the radiation, methotrexate, and 5-FU. Radiation doses to the breast are delivered using supervoltage equipment and tangential fields to minimize lung and heart exposure. The whole-breast dose ranges from 45–50 Gy delivered in about six weeks. Whether a boost is given depends upon the type of local excision and risk for local recurrence. The morbidity of a boost of moderate size and dose delivered either by electron beam or interstitial implantation is small.[212] The cosmetic result following partial mastectomy and radiation therapy is generally considered to be good.

Women commonly experience fatigue, some nausea, but primarily skin changes and arm and breast swelling. Some immediate side effects of RT are transient breast edema, erythema, and dry or wet desquamation. Later effects include telangiectasia, which is seen less often, and arm edema that usually results from radiating the axilla for multiple positive nodes. Breast edema is unique to patients undergoing breast-preserving surgery and radiation and usually appears during the treatment or within the first six months of treatment. Breast edema is more common in women who have had an axillary dissection where more than 11 nodes are removed and in those also receiving adjuvant chemotherapy. Skin reactions occur in all patients and generally present as itching, dryness, scaling, redness, and tenderness. The breast may feel sore and warm to touch. Patients are instructed not to use soap to wash the area and to pat dry. Dry desquamation can progress to a moist desquamation with infection.

Arm edema occurs more commonly in patients who have axillary dissection followed by RT to the axilla. Symptomatic pneumonitis characterized by a dry cough and low-grade fever is infrequent, but can appear within two to three months of therapy and is more common in women receiving methotrexate and 5-FU concurrently. Brachial plexopathy manifesting as paresthesias, with or without arm and hand weakness, may be transient or permanent, but is an infrequent complication. Rib fractures and cardiac complications are also rare and relate to dose and whether concurrent chemotherapy is also given.

Breast Reconstruction

Initially, surgery was regarded as a primary curative modality with the emotional and psychological effects being virtually ignored or regarded as the "price a woman must pay." Consequently, many women experienced feelings of loss, depression, and alterations in body image. These responses may be lessened now that breast reconstruction has come to be regarded as a viable and acceptable component in the treatment of breast cancer. In the past decade, improved procedure techniques and advances in the manufacture of implants have enabled many women to retain their self-confidence and body image, thereby enhancing their quality of life. Prior to the advent of plastic surgery for the treatment of breast cancer, many women found the external prostheses cumbersome and consequently felt it necessary to alter their activity and/or selection of clothing due to fear of displacement or discomfort of the prosthesis.

Despite the recent findings equating the two surgical procedures (mastectomy versus lumpectomy plus radiation) in terms of survival, many women either choose or are advised to have a mastectomy. This decision may be based on a variety of circumstances including histological findings, emotional or body image issues, financial considerations, or accessibility of medical resources.

A woman who presents with diffuse microcalcifications or multicentric disease throughout the breast is not considered a suitable candidate for breast preservation. Some patients are troubled by the fact that, although the cancer appears to have been removed, an occult lesion may remain, and consequently they will choose to remove the breast. Additionally, cosmesis may be compromised because too great a proportion of breast tissue needs to be removed to ensure clear margins. Patients who are responsible for a substantial portion of their medical bills may forego the cost of radiation treatments and choose mastectomy. Other women find that suitable medical facilities for radiation treatments may require extensive travel time or are geographically unavailable.

Implants are considered to be safe and effective treatment despite recent media comments to the contrary.[213,214] Citing the potential harmful effects of silicone implants revealed in an ongoing investigation, the FDA imposed a moratorium on the use of silicone implants for augmentation and issued guidelines to limit their use for reconstruction. To qualify for placement of silicone implants, certain criteria must now be met. The surgeon informs the patient of the possible side effects as well as documents that the patient fulfills an "urgent need" that has been predetermined by the FDA. Additionally, the patient is enrolled in a registry to aid in the long-term tracking of these patients.

Initially, the criteria were very stringent, but the revised guidelines issued in August 1992 expanded the eligibility regulations. The patient must be 18 years of age or older. Women who have experienced cancer, other disease, or trauma may have immediate or delayed reconstruction. Implants may be placed in any woman who currently has silicone implants and needs replacement or revision for medical or health reasons resulting from augmentation or mastectomy surgery. Women with congenital defects or severe asymmetry are considered candidates for silicone implants. Additionally, women who require augmentation of the unaffected breast for any of the preceding reasons may have an implanted silicone prosthesis. In 1998, a statement was issued by the FDA announcing the permitted use of silicone implants for reconstruction, but not for augmentation. Additional information on current guidelines issued by the FDA is available from the American Society for Aesthetic and Plastic Surgery or the American Society of Plastic and Reconstructive Surgeons at 1-800-635-0635.

The patient exclusion criteria include pregnancy or lactation, tissue abnormalities, and increased risk due to other treatment or psychological issues. Women who demonstrate active infection, lupus, scleroderma, or uncontrolled diabetes are not candidates for the procedure. Patients experiencing radiation damage, problems with vascularization, or who have inadequate tissue available are not ideal candidates, and the extent of the problem may render the person ineligible. The surgeon may declare any patient unsuitable who possesses any other physical or psychological condition that will compromise compliance and/or success of the surgical procedure. Because of the adverse publicity of silicone gel implants, many women and physicians are choosing saline-filled implants, which reduces the risk of silicone contamination if rupture should occur. These implants, however, do not have the same suppleness and natural feel of silicone gel implants. Alternative implants that are filled with a radiolucent material compatible with surrounding tissue and absorbable by the body are still investigational.[214,215]

Although implants are considered a viable and acceptable choice, other avenues continue to be explored. Autologous transplants have provided a suitable alternative to the inert prosthesis in certain circumstances. These procedures, considered below, include latissimus dorsi flap, transverse rectus abdominis muscle (TRAM) flap, and free transfer of abdominal or gluteal tissue.[216]

The timing of the consultation is very important because of the myriad of considerations to be addressed prior to surgery. In the past the general rule of thumb was to delay reconstruction, sometimes waiting months to years. Currently, surgeons who recognize that the psychological trauma associated with the loss of a breast may be lessened by more timely reconstruction will, after careful assessment, offer the patient immediate reconstruction. Immediate reconstruction is often preferred to reduce the potential morbidity of the process as the woman avoids an additional general anesthesia. However, the woman's general health and/or treatment plan may indicate that a delay in reconstruction be considered.

The ideal candidate is one who has early-stage disease. However, the absolute limiting factor of this surgery is a medical condition that may compromise the patient's safety during or postsurgery.[162] Heavy smokers may be advised to quit smoking or significantly reduce daily use to ensure an adequate blood supply. The surgeon will also attempt to identify those who may be subject to additional problems such as hypotension or hypoxia, which may compromise circulation and affect the success of the surgical procedure.[215] Patients who present with extensive local or metastatic disease may need further evaluation regarding chemotherapy and/or radiation therapy, which may necessitate a minor or significant delay in reconstruction due to immunosuppression and skin changes.

During the initial consultation the surgeon additionally evaluates and addresses the patient's and family's expectations of surgery. This may be done through the use of "before and after" pictures as well as the surgeon's frank explanation of the expected outcome. A patient with realistic expectations is well informed and more likely to accept the expected imperfections when these aspects are known prior to surgery. The goals of reconstructive surgery are to achieve "acceptable" symmetry and softness, correct any deformity caused by prior treatment, and construct an adequate nipple areola complex.

Silicone Implants

Silicone implants are used for reconstruction when the surgeon has ascertained that adequate skin is or will be available postmastectomy. The surgery is usually done in stages: the implant is placed during one procedure, the nipple-areola complex is constructed during another procedure, and there is some additional subsequent surgery to attain the desired cosmetic result.

An ideal candidate for a silicone implant is a woman who is small-breasted with a minimum of ptosis on the contralateral breast. If the patient's opposite breast needs revision to achieve symmetry, an implant placement and/or mastopexy will be performed at the same time.

The procedure entails incising part of the mastectomy or using the mastectomy incision to form a pocket beneath the chest wall muscles and inserting the silicone prosthesis. Placing the implant beneath the chest wall muscle helps counteract the expected firmness due to capsular contraction and supports the implant.[162]

Complications that may arise include progressive contracture, hematoma, infection, and flap necrosis. Contracture is an expected sequela of silicone implants and is the result of scar tissue enveloping the prosthesis. However, some patients will experience increasing contracture that alters and deforms the breast. Anecdotal information suggests that deep tissue massage from a massage therapist that begins after placement and continues for approximately one year may help to prevent disfiguring contracture. New implants are being designed with an attempt to reduce the incidence of contracture, which has decreased from 35%–55% to 2%–11%. However, approximately 5% of implants need to be removed due to severe contracture.[217,218]

Saline Tissue Expanders

Saline expanders are used when an inadequate supply of skin is available at the mastectomy site or when a large and/or ptotic breast is required. Tissue expansion is the most frequently used reconstructive procedure.[162] The expanders are placed behind the chest wall muscles using the lines of the mastectomy incision. They have a filling port that is either located remotely or on the anterior of the implant. After allowing sufficient time for wound healing, a series of injections is performed as an office procedure. The saline expanders, which are partially filled at the time of insertion, usually require 60–200 cc injections on a weekly or biweekly basis. The expansion continues until the device is overinflated by approximately 50%, usually in six to eight weeks,[190] but may take as long as six months.[218] The overfilled expander is left in place for several months to allow for accommodation of the stretched tissue. This overfilling helps to promote a more natural, supple contour of the reconstructed breast (Figure 48-17). The expander is then removed and a permanent prosthesis of lesser fluid volume is placed.[218]

Contracture is a complication that may hinder or prevent further expansion. Deflation can occur spontaneously or as a result of needle puncture. Expanders with remote ports are less likely to be accidentally deflated.

Permanent Saline Prostheses

Class action litigation and the influence of wary consumers have led to the widespread use of saline implants over those containing silicone, although studies have failed to directly correlate collagen disease with silicone implants. The surgery for the permanent saline prosthesis is usually done in stages: the expander is placed during the mastectomy, the permanent implant is placed after desired expansion has been attained, the nipple areola complex is constructed during another procedure, and some additional surgery may be needed subsequently to attain the desired cosmetic result.

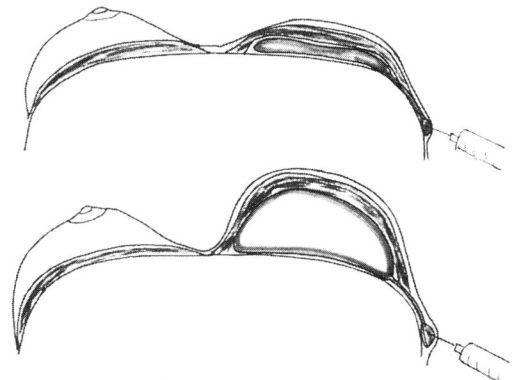

Figure 48-17   The horizontal view illustrates the overexpansion that is needed to allow for a more natural suppleness when the permanent prosthesis is implanted. (Courtesy of Dr. Craig Bradley, MD, Senior Attending, Plastic and Reconstructive Surgery, Rush Presbyterian St. Luke's Medical Center, Chicago.)

Exchanging the expander for the permanent prosthesis is an outpatient procedure. Just prior to surgery, the patient stands before a mirror as saline is removed to match the opposite breast. In the operating room, the surgeon incises along the mastectomy scar, and opens the wound with cautery to expose the expander. Cautery is used to protect the wall of the expander. The expander is removed and the volume of saline is measured to determine the size of the permanent implant. The permanent implant is placed behind the muscle in the pocket created by the expander. Placing the implant beneath the chest wall muscles helps counteract the expected firmness due to capsular contraction and supports the implant.[162]

The complications that may arise are the same as those mentioned above for silicone implants—progressive contracture, hematoma, infection, and flap necrosis. Hematomas occur infrequently and are most often surgically drained. Infections happen rarely and are most often successfully treated with antibiotics or removal of the implant in extreme cases. Flap necrosis can be serious and, if extensive, may necessitate the removal of the prosthesis. Usually, the necrosis involves a small amount of tissue that is excised.[215,218]

Latissimus Dorsi Flap

The latissimus dorsi is a large, fan-shaped muscle that is considered expendable because alternative muscle groups are able to adduct the humerus and posteriorly rotate the shoulder.[162] The latissimus dorsi flap is used when inadequate skin is available at the mastectomy site or if additional tissue is needed to fill the supraclavicular hollow and create an anterior axillary fold following a radical mastectomy (Figure 48-18). An ellipse of skin along with the latissimus dorsi muscle is rotated onto the mastectomy site. The viability of the tissue is maintained

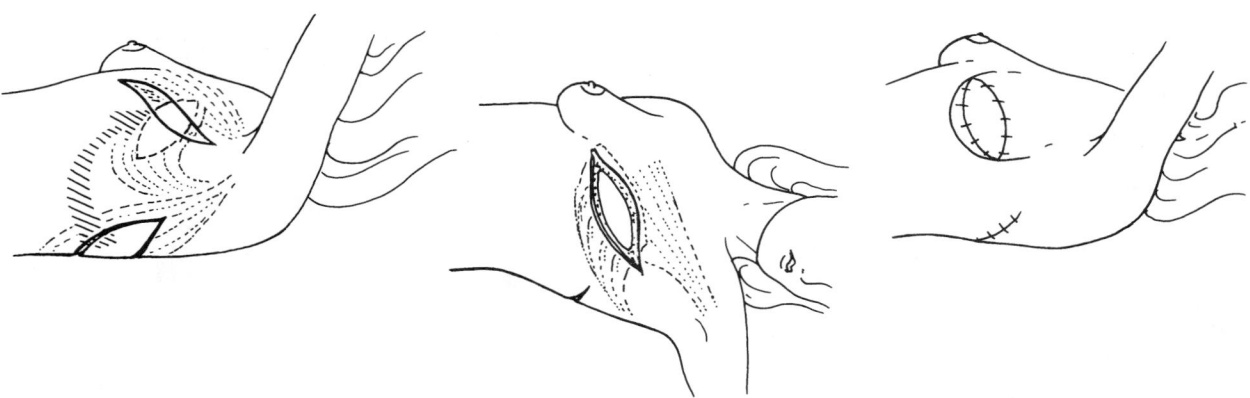

Figure 48-18 A diagram of the lastissimus dorsi procedure. (Courtesy of Dr. Craig Bradley, MD, Senior Attending, Plastic and Reconstructive Surgery, Rush Presbyterian St. Luke's Medical Center, Chicago.)

through the thoracodorsal vessels. The latissimus dorsi flap may also include a prosthesis for symmetrical cosmesis.[218]

Flap necrosis is rare due to the abundant vascularization of the area. The donor defect is often unnoticeable relative to the scar being beneath the bra-line.[162] This surgery takes three to four hours, approximately double the time needed for an implant procedure.

TRAM Flap

The transverse rectus abdominis muscle (TRAM) flap has been commonly referred to as the *tummy tuck*. During this procedure a low transverse ellipse incision is made and abdominal muscle and fat are tunneled under the abdominal skin to the mastectomy site. This procedure begins immediately after the mastectomy and lasts for approximately 4–6 hours. Tissue viability and perfusion are retained by the abdominal rectus muscle (Figures 48-19, 48-20, and 48-21).

Possible complications are hernia at the donor site, which can be remedied by the placement of synthetic mesh, and flap necrosis, which may be largely avoided by careful selection of the candidates. Obese patients (more than 20% overweight), those with circulatory problems, diabetes mellitus, prior history of liposuction or low back pain, smokers, and those over age 65 generally are not considered eligible for this procedure.[215]

Free Flap

The free flap represents the newest technique in reconstructive surgery. This procedure entails removing a portion of the skin and fat from the lower abdomen and grafting it to the mastectomy site with microvascular anastomoses. This is a complicated procedure that demands microsurgical technique from two teams of surgeons—one to remove the flap and one to prepare

the recipient vessels. The free TRAM flap has been reported to reduce complications, require shorter hospitalizations, and enhance the cosmetic outcome over pedicled tissue.[219] The time allotted for this procedure is usually four to six hours.[216] Its success depends on the reliability of the anastomoses of the vessels to ensure adequate nourishment of the tissues. The main complication is failure to maintain sufficient perfusion in the postoperative period. Tissue death will ensue within six hours if flow is interrupted and cannot be sustained.[216] The flow within the flap is monitored hourly by Doppler flow and clinical appearance for the first 24 hours, and every two hours for three to four days. Patients are discharged within four to five days. They are given detailed instruction for wound care and flap assessment. Anticoagulant therapy may also be used postoperatively to ensure integrity of flow.[218]

Gluteus Maximus Free Flap

If a TRAM flap is unavailable or inadequate in size, a portion of the buttock skin and muscle can be an alternative donor source, although this site is rarely used.[218] The skin and muscle are taken from the lower crease where the scar is less visible. Complications include posterior thigh numbness, slight gait alteration, possible flap necrosis, and a slight risk of infection. This surgery takes three to six hours to complete and requires a hospital stay of approximately four to five days with resumption of full activity in three to six months.[215,218]

Nipple-Areolar Construction

The nipple-areola complex is the final phase of the reconstruction process. The symmetry and cosmetic result of the breast mound should be satisfactory before this procedure is performed. The nipple should closely match the opposite side in size and pigment.

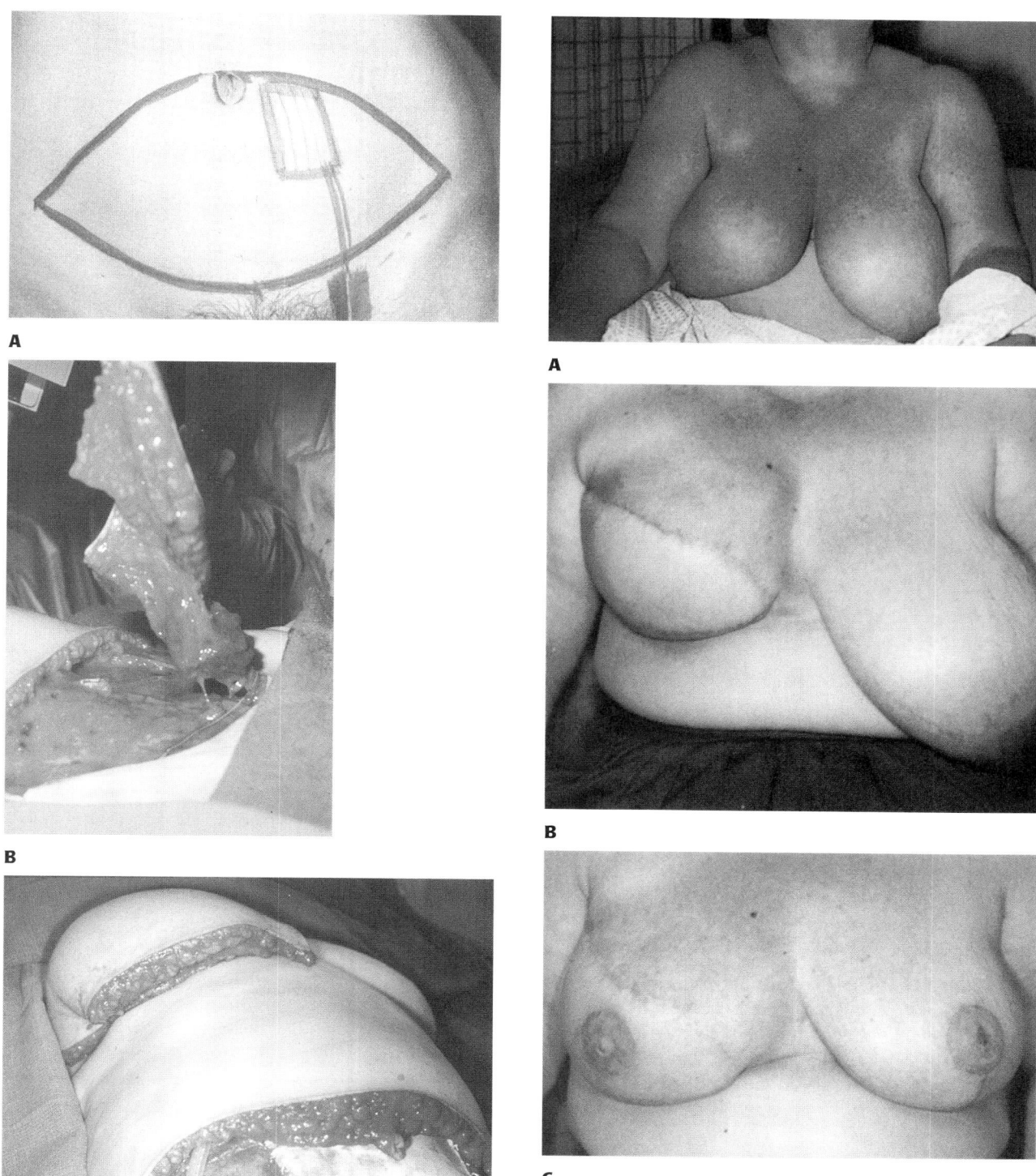

Figure 48-19 Three pictures illustrate (A) mapping the amount of tissue to be taken, (B) lifting the flap from the abdomen, and (C) the new mound prior to closing the incisions. Note that the abdomen needs placement of a reinforcement material (white area) to prevent hernia or other complications. (Courtesy of Dr. Craig Bradley.)

Figure 48-20 Three pictures illustrate a large woman (A) before the procedure, (B) after the mastectomy and latissimus dorsi flap, and (C) after mastopexy was performed to reduce the size of the other breast. Note the appearance of the tattooed nipple, which closely resembles the reduced breast. (Courtesy of Dr. Craig Bradley, MD, Senior Attending, Plastic and Reconstructive Surgery, Rush Presbyterian St. Luke's Medical Center, Chicago.)

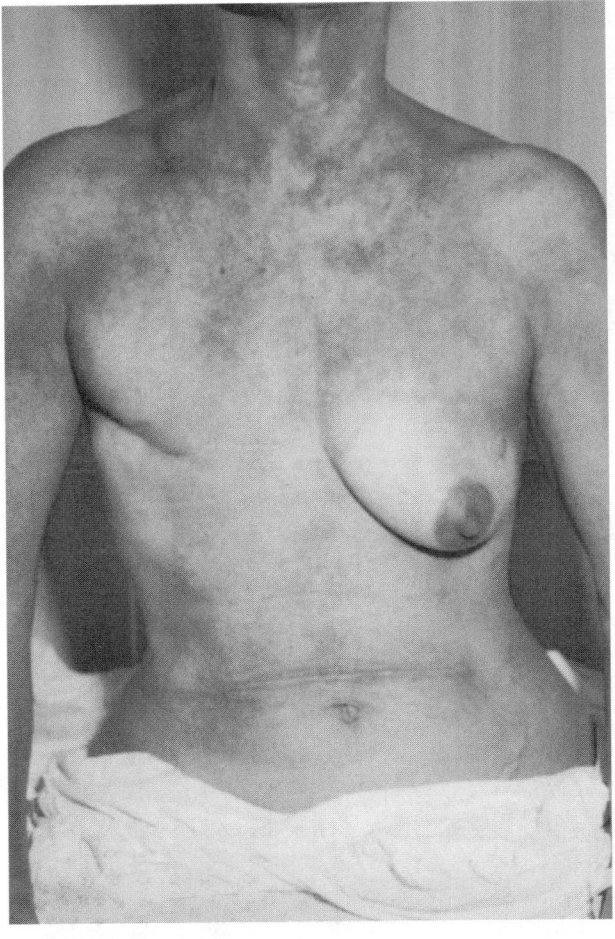
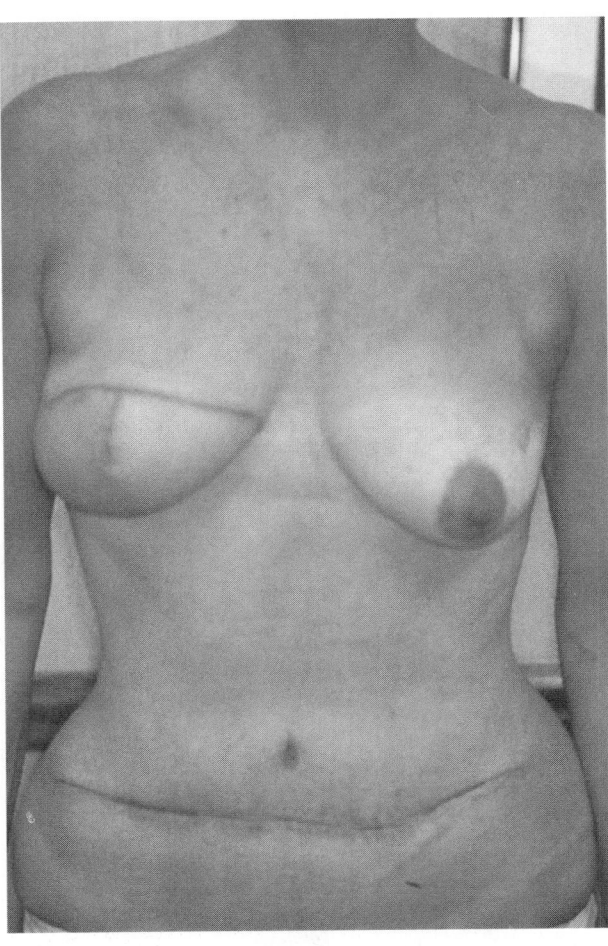

A

B

Figure 48-21 First picture shows a patient (A) after mastectomy and before the TRAM flap. The second and third pictures show the (B) anterior and (C) lateral view of the same patient shortly after the procedure. The scars will fade with time. (Courtesy of Dr. Craig Bradley, MD, Senior Attending, Plastic and Reconstructive Surgery, Rush Presbyterian St. Luke's Medical Center, Chicago.)

Tissue may be taken from the opposite breast if there is an adequate supply or if mastopexy has been performed. Previously, the nipple was often "banked" to the patient's thigh or groin to be used later. This method has fallen out of favor due to the risk of introducing potentially malignant tissue to the disease-free breast.

Tattooing is the primary method for creating the darker pigment of the areola.[216] Another option is a skin graft from the inner thigh. However, grafts are uncomfortable and can fade, requiring tattooing, so most women prefer to forgo this surgery and have the area tattooed.[215] See Figures 48-22 and 48-23.

Maintaining projection is a challenge that has been met by construction of pedicle flaps. These techniques employ folding the skin to achieve a slightly protuberant nipple. The most popular methods are the skate flap and c-v flap technique, in which the skin is raised and folded to achieve a natural nipple profile.[218]

Complications are rare with this reconstruction, but those that may occur are failure to maintain suitable projection of the nipple, graft failure, and fading of the pigmented areas.

Systemic Adjuvant Therapy

Early Stage I and II Breast Cancer

Much of the research in breast cancer has concentrated on finding optimal regimens of systemic therapy that can potentially destroy circulating tumor cells. The need for such research is paramount considering that nearly 90% of women newly diagnosed with breast cancer are potentially curable. Of that number, nearly 60% will have node-negative disease. The results of prospective clinical trials suggest that the rate of disease recurrence in patients with node-negative breast cancer can be reduced 20%–50% by adjuvant therapy.[190,219,220] This led to the conclusion at the

NIH Consensus Development Conference on Early Stage Breast Cancer that, although "the majority of patients with node-negative breast cancer are cured by breast-conserving treatment or total mastectomy and axillary node dissection, the rate of local and distant relapse following local therapy for node-negative breast cancer is decreased by both combination cytotoxic chemotherapy and by tamoxifen"[221 p.4]. See Table 48-9.

The Early Breast Cancer Trialists' Collaborative Group involved a worldwide meta-analysis of the results of randomized trials involving 75,000 women with early (stage I and II) breast cancer and results were updated in 1992.[222] This large statistical analysis demonstrated that overall optimal use of adjuvant therapy can significantly improve long-term survival in women with stage I and II breast cancer and has the potential to save more lives from this disease than any other malignancy. In women under age 50, adjuvant chemotherapy alone reduces the annual odds of recurrence by 27%. Adjuvant chemotherapy is less effective in postmenopausal women older than 50. Treatment for this group reduces the annual odds of recurrence 22% and the annual odds of death 14%.

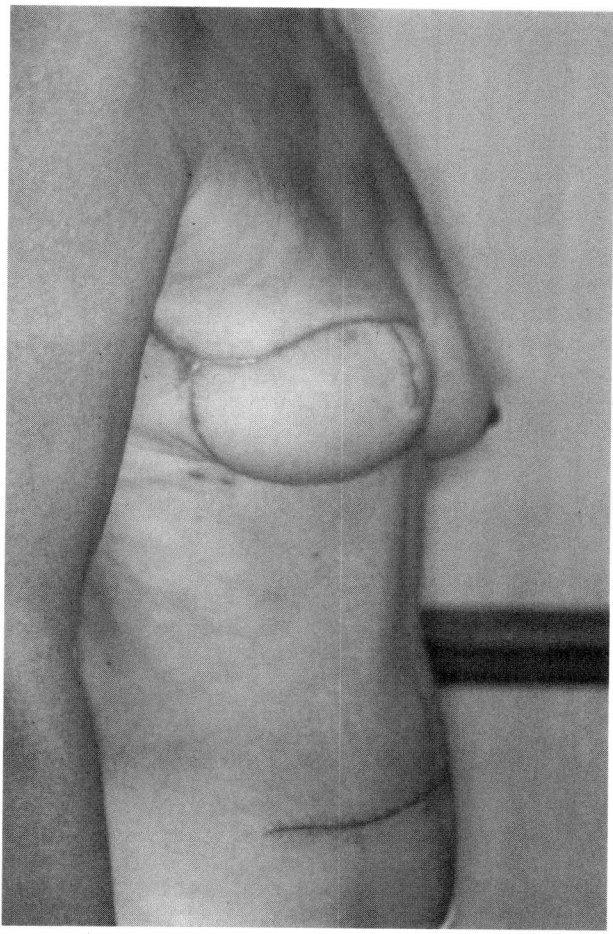

C

Figure 48-21 (Continued)

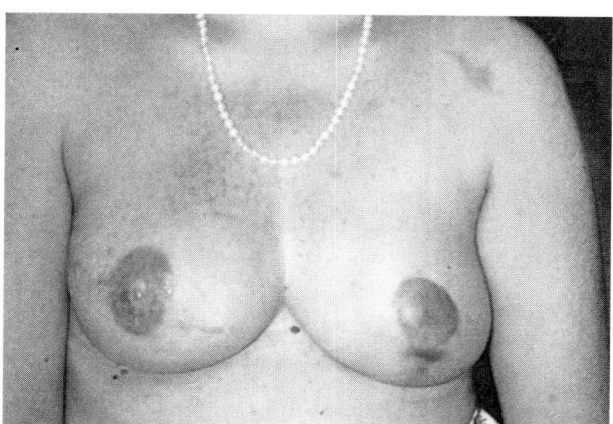

Figure 48-22 Right breast reconstruction following a modified radical mastectomy. Unilateral nipple tattoo on the right is compared to the patient's own unaffected nipple on the left following mastoplexy. (Courtesy of Dr. Craig Bradley, MD, Senior Attending, Plastic and Reconstructive Surgery, Rush Presbyterian St. Luke's Medical Center, Chicago.)

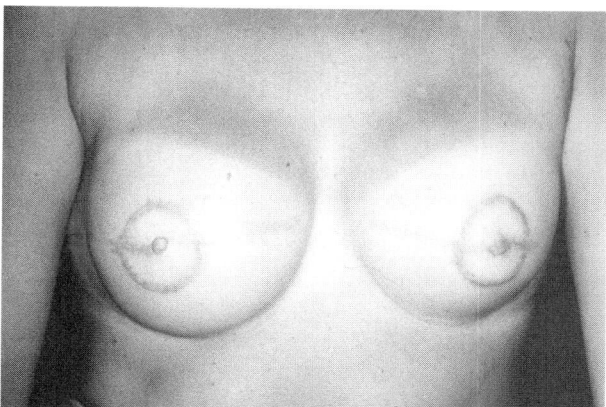

A

B

Figure 48-23 Two pictures illustrate bilateral nipple reconstruction (A) shortly after tattooing and (B) a few months later.

In addition, tamoxifen as well as ovarian ablation was shown to significantly reduce the incidence of contralateral breast cancer. Adjuvant tamoxifen is beneficial not only for women age 50–69 and those age 70 or more but also for those under 50.[223] The ability of adjuvant chemotherapy to increase disease-free intervals has been observed in clinical trials, but its effect on overall survival has not been demonstrated until recently. The meta-analysis demonstrates a clinically relevant reduction in tumor mortality due to adjuvant chemotherapy.

For patients with tumors less than 1 cm in diameter, the chance of recurrence is less than 10% at ten years. It may be reasonable not to offer these patients systemic adjuvant therapy. However, in certain subsets of women with node-negative breast cancer, the incidence of metastatic disease approaches 50%.[224] Combination chemotherapy can effectively reduce the annual odds of recurrence by at least 30% in this population. To accomplish this, 70% of patients will receive therapy unnecessarily because they have been cured by surgery alone.

Currently, there are important prognostic indicators that help to determine a woman's risk of recurrence, such as ploidy, proliferative indices, and tumor grade, but no one parameter is predictive of recurrence. Most clinicians agree that many women with node-negative breast cancer should receive adjuvant chemotherapy, especially those with larger tumors. Women with the lowest risk of recurrence are those with tumors less than 1 cm, a low-grade malignancy, positive estrogen/progesterone receptors, negative HER2/neu status, and a low proliferative rate. In contrast, those with tumors larger than 2 cm, a high-grade malignancy, negative estrogen/progesterone receptors, positive HER2/neu status, and a high rate of proliferation are most at risk for tumor recurrence.

For women with limited breast cancer there are a number of regimens known to be effective. One regimen involves methotrexate followed in one hour by 5-FU (M-F). Leucovorin calcium (L) is begun 24 hours after the methotrexate. This regimen has been compared to standard cyclophosphamide, methotrexate, and 5-FU (CMF) therapy, and it was found that both regimens offer at least a 30% risk reduction for recurrence. The M-F + L appears to be less toxic in terms of myelosuppression and hair loss and does not have the leukemogenic potential of an alkylating agent-containing regimen. In premenopausal women, M-F + L does not affect gonadal function.

Adjuvant tamoxifen significantly reduces the risks of recurrence and death in women in all age groups. Tamoxifen is a viable choice in women who present with advanced tumors when chemotherapy is contraindicated. See Figure 48-24. The benefit is greatest when tamoxifen is administered for about five years and when it is given to women with estrogen-receptor positive tumors.

Women with tumor involving the lymph nodes are recognized as having a greater likelihood for distant recurrence and death. Adjuvant chemotherapy, especially for premenopausal women age 50 and younger, is widely accepted. CMF for six months has been the standard approach to node-positive breast cancer.[188,189] When compared to the combination of doxorubicin and cyclophosphamide (AC) every three weeks for four cycles, patients receiving AC did as well as those who received CMF for six months. While patients receiving AC experienced more immediate and profound hair loss, they experienced less nausea over time, visited health professionals one-third as often, and completed their therapy in less time compared to those receiving CMF. Another option as adjuvant therapy for the woman with node positive breast cancer is the combination of cyclophosphamide orally for 14 days, epirubicin and 5-fluorouracil (CEF) day 1 and 8 every 28 days for 6 cycles.

For women with localized disease that also carries with it less favorable prognostic indicators, the addition of four cycles of paclitaxel to four cycles of AC has been found to improve both disease-free survival and overall survival rates.[225] In women whose tumors overexpress the HER2/neu proto-oncogene, the addition of weekly herceptin during the duration of the paclitaxel is thought to increase the sensitivity and efficacy of the paclitaxel, due to the synergism between the two agents.[226,227] Research further indicates that there is an increased dose-response effect of adjuvant therapy with an anthracycline-containing regimen in patients with HER2 overexpression but not in patients with no or minimal HER2 overexpression.[228,229]

Locally Advanced Breast Cancer

Efforts to improve outcome in more advanced, node-positive patients have focused on the development and application of new drugs in combination with systemic therapy. Dose intensification may effectively increase intracellular drug concentration. With the addition of colony stimulating factors, it may be possible to ameliorate the dose-limiting toxicity of myelosuppression, possibly preventing the need for dose reductions or treatment delays. Giving optimal doses at regular frequent intervals is also an important strategy in preventing resistance and ultimate recurrence of disease.

Preoperative chemotherapy has in the past been confined to the management of locally advanced disease. However, the goal of treating patients with operable breast cancer using neoadjuvant chemotherapy is two-

Table 48-9 Systemic Adjuvant Therapy: Node Negative Breast Cancer

	Number of Patients	Reduction in Recurrence (%)	Mortality (%)
Tamoxifen	12,900	26	17
Chemotherapy	2700	26	18

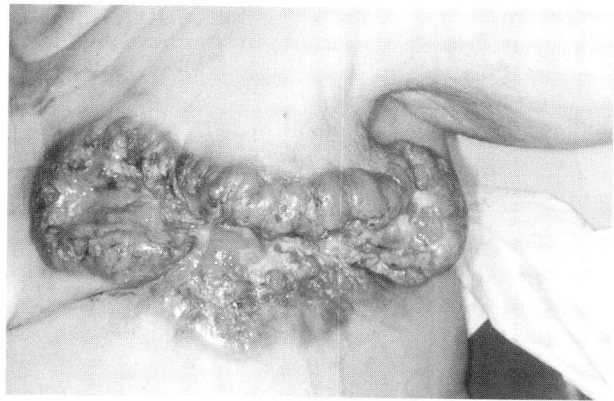

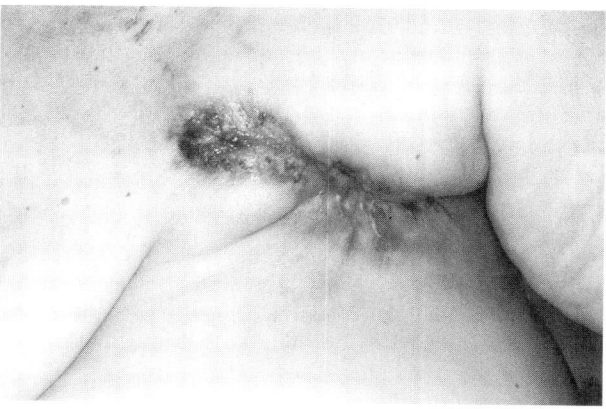

Figure 48-24 Two pictures depict a patient with a long-neglected breast cancer (A) who was placed on Tamoxifen 20 mg/qd and (B) illustrates the improvement after six months of therapy.

fold: the early treatment of "micrometastases" in the hope of improving survival and to achieve reduction of stage to allow for breast conservation in patients who would otherwise be treated with mastectomy.[230] In terms of survival, there is no apparent advantage to preoperative chemotherapy as compared with postoperative chemotherapy.[234]

Locally advanced breast cancer is associated with a high risk of developing distant metastases. The larger the size of the primary tumor and the greater the number of histologically positive lymph nodes, the greater the risk of metastasis and death.[232,233] These tumors, by virtue of their size (greater than 5 cm), are usually not amenable to treatment by breast-conserving surgery, and modified radical mastectomy is generally the treatment of choice if surgery is possible. Clinical characteristics of locally advanced disease include large or unresectable primary tumors, fixed axillary nodes, and the classic inflammatory carcinoma. While distant metastases are presumed to be present, they are not clinically apparent at staging.

If the tumor is fixed to the chest wall, inflammatory carcinoma is present, significant ulceration exists, or the axillary nodes are fixed to one another or other structures, the situation is generally considered to be inoperable due to the almost certain risk of recurrence.[236] The presence of supraclavicular lymph nodes is considered distant metastasis rather than locally advanced breast cancer; however, in the absence of more distinct distant metastasis, these patients are often grouped with locally advanced breast cancer.

The prognosis of patients with locally advanced disease is rarely improved by local therapy alone, and while many physicians approach these patients with a purely palliative intent, the role of systemic therapy is becoming more widely accepted. Results are superior when chemotherapy and radiation are included in the treatment plan.[234,235] The use of primary (neoadjuvant) chemotherapy has resulted in significant tumor regression in 60%–90% of women.[234] The advantage of this approach includes in vivo assessment of response. Significant tumor shrinkage may permit resection in previously unresectable disease, allowing for less extensive surgical procedures. Primary chemotherapy also provides immediate treatment to presumed metastasis that would otherwise be delayed by local therapy. Primary chemotherapy also avoids the postsurgery growth spurt of metastatic disease observed in the laboratory. Combined modality therapy employing chemotherapy, surgery, and radiation may result in complete disappearance of disease in many patients including those with inflammatory cancer.[236]

High-dose chemotherapy with peripheral blood stem cell autologous bone marrow transplant and hematopoietic growth factor support is currently an option for treatment for women with high-risk advanced disease. There is no evidence, however, that this results in any better palliation in women with refractory breast cancer than that obtained with standard-dose chemotherapy.[193] It is unclear whether the 15%–25% rate of long-term cancer-free survival is the result of high-dose therapy or simply a consequence of the selection of patients.[237,238]

Metastatic Breast Cancer

Despite improved screening techniques and increased awareness of breast cancer as a major health threat, approximately 10% of women diagnosed with breast cancer have metastatic disease at clinical presentation. Approximately 30% of women diagnosed with an early-stage node-negative disease and roughly 60% with node-positive disease will relapse despite adjuvant therapy.[239] The majority of patients who relapse (80%) do so within two years of the diagnosis. Excessive physical examination and testing (x-ray, CT, MRI) to identify disease recurrences and metastases in order to institute aggressive treatment has not altered the clinical course of women with metastatic breast cancer.

Most recurrences or metastases are diagnosed on the basis of symptoms and physical findings. Often a biopsy of a local recurrence will turn out to be cancer and the metastatic work-up ensues. Instead of an obvious physical finding a patient may complain of loss of appetite and a slightly swollen abdomen, which on CT scan reveals liver metastasis. An assessment of the extent of disease is made to first document the recurrence of disease and second to determine the most appropriate therapeutic approach. The goal of treatment is to control the symptoms and provide the best quality of life possible given the fact that currently metastatic breast cancer is not curable.

Often the manner in which the disease presents will determine the extent of the metastatic work-up. Typically a chest x-ray, bone scan, and serum chemistries are done initially to identify any abnormalities and the need for further investigation of extent of disease. For example, if the alkaline phosphatase is elevated along with other indicators of liver dysfunction a CT scan of the liver might be included in the metastatic work-up. Tumor markers (CEA, CA-15-3) may be done as a baseline as they generally parallel the clinical course. If the tumor has not been tested for overexpression of the *HER2/neu* proto-oncogene, the biopsy or archival tumor specimen is sent to pathology so that analysis of *HER2/neu* gene amplification and expression can be carried out.[240] Only women whose tumors are *HER2* positive would be candidates for herceptin therapy.

The median survival time for stage IV disease is two to three years; however, reports of five-year survival range from 12%–35% and ten-year survival from 5%–22%.[241] Race may influence survival in breast cancer. Black women tend to be diagnosed with more advanced disease than white women,[242] and they have a 29% higher death rate.[243] Differences in economic status, social factors, access to medical care, education levels, awareness of early detection measures, and willingness to comply with medical recommendations may contribute to this difference in survival.[244] There is no evidence that breast cancer in black women is in some way biologically different from that of white women. For example white women are as likely as blacks to have tumors that overexpress the *HER2/neu* proto-oncogene, which is clearly a reflection of the inherent biology of the cancer. Underserved minorities require intensive community screening programs aimed at education and assurance of access to care.

Routes of Metastasis

Breast cancer most commonly metastasizes to bone (more than 50% of patients), specifically the spine, ribs, and proximal long bones. Patients will commonly complain of localized, deep-seated, unrelenting pain. Pathological fracture of the proximal femur may occur spontaneously despite efforts to protect the weakened bone. Likewise, persistent back pain may herald a compression fracture and possible neurological impairment. Hypercalcemia may reflect bone resorption due to tumor growth and resultant osteoclastic stimulation. Bone marrow metastasis occurs frequently in patients with extensive multifocal bone disease, generally presenting as bone marrow failure or as fleeting nocturnal pain.[245]

Loss of appetite and abnormal liver function tests are early symptoms of liver involvement. Late symptoms include pain, abdominal distention, nausea, emesis, periodic fever, jaundice, and generalized weakness. Pulmonary involvement may begin as a subtle, nonproductive cough or shortness of breath. Lymphangitic pulmonary spread is an ominous sign of rapidly progressive disease. Pleural effusions can progress slowly over time and respond temporarily to drainage and sclerosing. Renal involvement generally presents as oliguria and/or uremia in a woman with deteriorating mental status. Brain metastasis usually occurs in the supratentorial region, multiple sites, or as carcinomatous meningitis presenting as cranial nerve palsies, altered mentation, seizures, and/or focal paresis. Local cancer spread to the chest wall usually presents as a painless subcutaneous nodule along the mastectomy scar and adjacent chest wall areas. These lesions may respond well to local therapy, but distant disease is presumed to be present.

If the disease recurs locally after breast-conserving surgery plus radiation, mastectomy may be indicated, provided the cancer recurs locally in the breast tissue and not in the skin. Disease that recurs in the skin of the breast is considered to be metastatic and a marker for metastatic (e.g., distant) disease. Likewise, evidence of disease in a supraclavicular node or recurrence in the scar or chest wall after mastectomy generally indicates metastatic spread beyond the breast and systemic therapy is warranted.

The management of patients with metastatic breast cancer is aimed at judicious use of local and systemic measures that control and/or palliate symptoms and improve quality of life. The initial choice of therapy is generally the one that is the least toxic and carries with it the highest response rate. See Figure 48-25. The basic strategy is to achieve optimal control of the disease and temporize for as long as possible. Local and systemic therapies are added periodically as needed until they have outworn their usefulness. For many women, especially those with hormone receptor positive disease, this can mean many years of quality of life. Table 48-10 describes combination and single-agent chemotherapy commonly used in metastatic breast cancer.

It may be difficult for a woman with metastatic disease to understand why her doctor is not recommending more aggressive treatment. The idea that a new or different treatment is introduced only with evidence of disease or troublesome symptoms causes some women to ask why the treatment was not given to prevent the problem before it occurred. The answer is based on the desire not to make the woman more ill than her disease is making her and the knowledge that these therapies, including chemotherapy, have only a small effect on the median survival of women with metastatic disease. The goal is to get as much mileage out of each therapy as possible

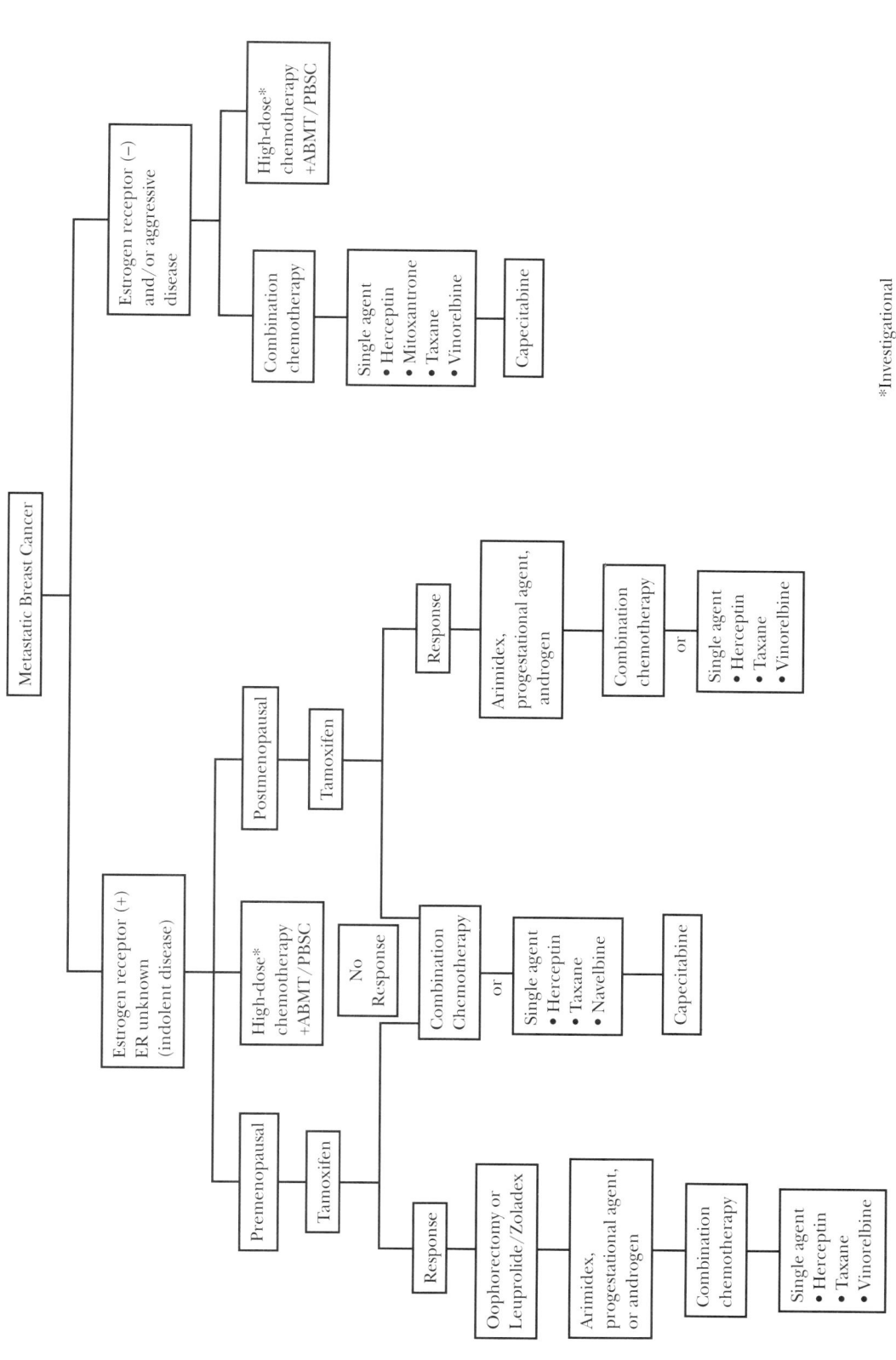

Figure 48-25 Metastatic breast cancer: systemic approaches to management.

*Investigational
ABMT = Autologous bone marrow transplant
PBSC = Peripheral blood stem cell transplant

Table 48-10 Cytotoxic Therapy for Advanced Breast Cancer

Acronym/Brand	Drugs	Dose (mg/m²)	Response Rate (%)	Median Duration of Response (months)
CMF ± P	Cyclophosphamide Methotrexate 5-fluorouracil Prednisone	100, PO days 1 to 14 40, IV days 1 and 8 600, IV days 1 and 8 40, PO days 1 to 14; repeat every 28 days	49–59	5–8
FAC	5-fluorouracil Doxorubicin Cyclophosphamide	500, IV days 1 and 8 50, IV day 1 500, IV day 1; repeat every 21 days	50–75	6–10
AC	Doxorubicin Cyclophosphamide	40, IV day 1 200, PO days 3 to 6; repeat every 21 days	40–80	6–12
CAF	Cyclophosphamide Doxorubicin 5-fluorouracil	100, PO days 1 to 14 30, IV days 1 and 8 500, IV days 1 and 8	60–80	10–12
Taxol	Paclitaxel	175, IV every 21 days	30	6
Taxotere	Docetaxel	100	41	6

Adapted from Ravdin PM, Osborne CK: Breast cancer, in Wittes RE (ed): *Manual of Oncologic Therapeutics,* Philadelphia, Lippincott, 1995.[185]

without compromising quality of life unless temporarily and absolutely necessary. However, an exception involves the patient who is asymptomatic or minimally symptomatic, is desirous of therapy, and is not likely to require significant palliation for three to six months. In this situation it is entirely appropriate and optimal that the woman be introduced to innovative and experimental treatment protocols including high-dose chemotherapy and bone marrow transplant. Such therapies are available in cancer centers and cooperative cancer study groups.

Chemotherapy

Women who have a disease-free interval of less than two years, have hormone receptor negative disease, are refractory to hormone therapy, or have aggressive disease in the liver or pulmonary system are candidates for chemotherapy.[185]

Combination chemotherapy results in higher response rates compared to single agents. Response rates vary from 50%–70% and can last for 9–12 months. The rate of complete response (percentage of individuals in whom all evidence of disease disappears) consistently has been only 10%–20% of cases.[245]

Currently, cyclophosphamide–methotrexate–5-FU plus leucovorin; cyclophosphamide–epirubicin–5-FU; or cyclophosphamide–doxorubicin–5-FU; or a taxane-containing regimen are among the more commonly used treatment approaches. Doxorubicin-containing regimens have shown a 10%–20% better response rate, but currently offer no significant survival advantage over combinations not containing doxorubicin. For women who are elderly and prefer a regimen that does not cause hair loss or significant nausea or vomiting, herceptin or methotrexate–5-FU plus leucovorin are available. For women who experience disease recurrence on therapies that include doxorubicin or a taxane, vinorelbine or liposomal-encapsulated doxorubicin HCl (Doxil®) are a second- and third-line choice with minimal toxicity.[246] Another choice includes capecitabine which offers a 20% response rate and is preferred because it is taken orally.[247]

Individuals with slow-growing disease and those with rapidly progressing disease will benefit from chemotherapy. The response of women to cytotoxic agents is not significantly related to the predominant site of disease. Women with visceral metastases as well as those with bony involvement will respond. Although radiological evidence of bone healing may take as long as six months, subjective improvement occurs within a shorter time. For women that have lytic bony disease, pamidronate given as an infusion over two hours once a month has been useful to promote bone healing; prevent new disease in bone; and decrease the fracture rate, the need for palliative radiation, and the use of narcotic analgesics in patients with metastatic disease in bone.[248,249]

Endocrine Therapy

Antiestrogen therapy

Women who have ER-positive breast cancer demonstrate a consistently superior survival after recurrence compared to women who are ER negative. It is generally accepted that the greater the ER content, the greater the response rate. Similarly, the presence of both the ER and the progesterone receptor (PR) on the tumor confers a higher response rate than the presence of only the ER. Choice of hormonal therapy is based on several factors. For the patient who has had no prior hormonal manipulation, or who is more than a year out from adjuvant tamoxifen, the use of the antiestrogen tamoxifen represents the standard of care.

Selective estrogen receptor modulators (SERMs) are a class of drugs that bind the ER and modulate the functions mediated by this receptor system. Tamoxifen is a nonsteroidal antiestrogen that binds competitively to the ER present in tumor cells. By blocking the binding of estrogen, it blocks cell cycle transit in G1 and inhibits tumor growth. Raloxifene is similar to tamoxifen in its antibreast cancer activity as well as in its proestrogenic effects on bone and serum lipids. One difference may be its neutral effects on the uterus, in contrast with tamoxifen, which is well established as a uterotrophic agent that increases the risk of uterine cancer. Raloxifene also appears to act as an antiosteoporosis agent. Little is known regarding the cardioprotective effects of raloxifene.

Evidence demonstrates that tamoxifen and toremifene are equally effective as front-line treatment of hormone receptor positive or unknown metastatic breast cancer.[250,251] A new antiestrogen, faslodex, downgrades the ER, but does not bind the DNA, therefore it has no estrogenic activity. Side effects are minimal. No vaginal dryness, hot flashes, changes in serum lipids, or change in endometrial thickness has been reported.

Undesirable consequences of the estrogen-like effects include stimulation of the endometrium. There is concern that tamoxifen may act as a promoter of endometrial cancer due to its estrogen agonist effects.[219] Fornander and associates,[252] in a study of 1846 women of whom 931 were randomized to therapy with 40 mg of tamoxifen daily, observed a relative risk of 2.7 in those receiving tamoxifen as compared with controls. Further analysis using 20 mg per day of tamoxifen has not revealed a strong association between tamoxifen, endometrial cancer, and duration of therapy.[252] Moreover, the benefits of tamoxifen in lives saved exceeds the incidence of endometrial cancer.[253] About 20% of women on tamoxifen report severe hot flashes, compared with 3% of the placebo group. Vaginal discharge and irregular menses are also associated with tamoxifen therapy. Ocular toxicity (retinopathy or keratophy) has been reported in women taking conventional doses of tamoxifen, but in general ocular toxicity is not a clinically significant danger of tamoxifen therapy.[254] After tamoxifen withdrawal, ocular abnormalities are usually found to be reversible. Currently the recommendation is to continue treatment unless visual symptoms are present. Patients might benefit from routine eye examination, especially those with other preexisting ophthalmologic conditions.

In premenopausal women tamoxifen is equivalent to ovarian ablation (via either surgery, radiation, or chemically through the use of LHRH agonists). Women who respond initially to tamoxifen and subsequently become resistant are likely to respond to Zoladex injections.

Aromatase inhibitors

The conversion of adrenal androgens to estrogens occurs primarily in adipose, muscle, ovarian, brain, and liver tissue, and is the primary source of estrogen in postmenopausal estrogen-dependent breast cancer. Aromatase inhibitors reversibly bind to the aromatase enzyme that is responsible for the conversion of androstenedione to estrone. The use of second-generation aromatase inhibitors (either anastrazole or letrozole) has become the treatment of choice for postmenopausal women whose disease no longer responds to tamoxifen. The steroidal aromatase inactivator exemestane is of particuler interest as it irreversibly binds to and inactivates aromatase. These drugs are more effective and less toxic compared to megestrol acetate and aminoglutethimide.[255,256] These agents are also being investigated as adjuvant treatment and first-line treatment for breast cancer. Aromatase inhibitors prevent the peripheral aromatization of other steroids to estrogen, primarily in body fat. The aromatase enzyme acts at the last step in the estrogen-synthesis pathway, catalyzing the conversion of androgens to estrogens. Another option is exemestane (Aromasin) a steroidal aromatase inactivator indicated for the treatment of advanced breast cancer in women who have recurred following tamoxifen therapy.

Androgens

Androgens are most effective in women who are five or more years postmenopause. The overall response rate is 20%. Androgens block pituitary gonadotropin secretion thereby opposing endogenous estrogens. Androgen therapy may be added to oophorectomy in women under age 35, but response rates are low. In the postmenopausal woman, androgens are indicated for the treatment of soft tissue or bone metastases and may result in "tumor flare" with initiation of treatment. Danazol is a synthetic steroid and is more commonly used because it has less virilizing effects (hirsutism, hair loss, acne, deepening of the voice, and increased libido) compared to testosterone or fluoxymesterone (Halotestin®). Generally, because of the toxicity profile, androgens are reserved for use after most other forms of hormonal manipulation are exhausted.

Progestins

The precise mechanism of action of progestins is unclear but they appear to inhibit the stimulator effect of estradiol on tumor growth. Megestrol acetate is a progestational agent with a response rate of 26%–30% and a median duration of up to 22 months.[242] The standard dose of megestrol acetate is 160 mg a day. This drug is generally tolerated as well as tamoxifen and is comparable in efficacy but it is usually used only after the patient has failed on tamoxifen. The mechanism of action of megestrol acetate is thought to include interference in binding of estrogen to the estrogen receptor, and interference of the aromatization of androgens to estrogens. Megestrol acetate effectively decreases follicle stimulating hormone (FSH) and luteinizing hormone (LH) as well as estradiol levels.

Antiprogestins including RU486 (mifepristone) and Onapristone are investigational agents. Each is thought to bind to both the progesterone receptor and the glucocorticoid receptor. RU486 is generally well tolerated and associated with some nausea, hot flashes, and dizziness. Studies using these agents in breast cancer are hindered by the societal implications of its use as an abortifacient in Europe. The most important side effect is weight gain, which occurs in up to 50% of patients. This weight gain is related primarily to increased food intake and increases with higher doses. Other side effects include hot flashes, vaginal bleeding, hypercalcemia, tumor flare, and thrombophlebitis.

Male Breast Cancer

It was estimated that 1300 new cases of breast cancer would be diagnosed in men in 1999 and 400 men would die of their disease.[257] Male breast cancer accounts for less than 1% of all breast cancers.[257] A higher incidence of male breast cancer is found in Jewish men compared with non-Jewish men. The anatomic structures of the male breast are the same as those of the female breast. It is the hormonal stimulation present in the female breast but absent in the male's that accounts for the developmental and physiological differences between the male and female breast. This lack of hormonal stimulation also may explain the comparatively low incidence of male breast cancer. However, the disease in both sexes is similar in terms of epidemiology, natural history, and response to therapy. Family history of breast cancer is present in about 30% of males with breast cancer.[258,259] Various factors contributing to the development of male breast cancer include undescended testes, orchiectomy, orchitis, late puberty, infertility, obesity, hypercholesterolemia, and estrogen use.[260] The *BRCA2* appears to be associated with male breast cancer, and is localized to chromosome 13q.

The incidence of breast cancer is increased in men who have undergone sex-change procedures. The administration of estrogens results in lobular development and enlargement of the male breast. Hormonal imbalance (androgen deficiency) and gynecomastia are characteristic of Klinefelter syndrome, and the incidence of breast cancer is increased 20-fold to 66-fold, with a risk of breast cancer of 3%.[261]

The administration of DES to men with carcinoma of the prostate has been associated with male breast cancer, but is a rare occurrence. While it is true that large numbers of men receiving DES for prostatic carcinoma do not exhibit an increased incidence of breast cancer, it is important to note that the life expectancy of these men is relatively short, and breast cancers may indeed be present but not yet manifested.

Breast cancer occurs most frequently in men age 50–70 with the peak incidence occurring at age 60. It appears that after 40 years of age, the Sertoli cells (elongated cells in the seminiferous tubules) secrete increasing amounts of estrogens. The majority of male breast cancers (75%) are known to be ER positive and approximately 30% will respond to hormonal manipulation. They typically arise from ductal elements and present as infiltrating ductal carcinoma, which is commonly fixed to underlying fascia and skin. Nipple retraction and a bloody discharge may be present.

A moderately tender, centrally located subareolar mass is usually the first symptom that brings the man to seek medical attention. Pectoral fixation, involvement of skin, nipple changes, and discharge are commonly present because of limited breast disease and delay in seeking medical attention. These factors may account for the increased frequency of widespread disease and early invasion of local and regional lymphatics. Ulceration may occur early in the course of the disease and carries a relatively poor prognosis. A bloody discharge from the nipple and nipple inversion may be present. Because of its relatively central location, male breast cancer can be expected to metastasize to the internal mammary nodes. The lungs and bony skeleton are the most common metastatic sites.

Because of the low incidence and relatively small number of patients, it is difficult to conduct controlled clinical trials to aid in establishing appropriate therapy. The treatment of male breast cancer is based on the treatment of female breast cancer. The modified radical mastectomy has been the mainstay of therapy. The skin and underlying fascia are frequently involved, requiring skin grafting. Adjuvant radiotherapy, hormonal manipulation, and chemotherapy are also part of the approach to treatment.

With evidence of extensive disease, hormonal manipulation (orchiectomy, arimidex, or tamoxifen) is indicated unless the disease is life-threatening or aggressive, in which case chemotherapy would be indicated. The response rate to chemotherapy is about 44%.[262]

Orchiectomy appears to remove the source of estrogen and androgen in recurrent male breast cancer and can result in a prompt remission. With recurrent disease, further hormonal manipulation using tamoxifen, arimidex, and progestin may be helpful. Arimidex, tamoxifen, and other forms of hormone manipulation are relatively ineffective without orchiectomy. However, Buserelin, or goserelin acetate, effectively reduces testosterone to castration levels and may be an important alternative to men who refuse orchiectomy.

Symptom Management and Supportive Care

Women with breast cancer often experience debilitating menopausal symptoms as a consequence of chemotherapy, hormone therapy, or as a function of aging. In fact many premenopausal women who receive chemotherapy will experience ovarian failure and early menopause, especially if a larger cumulative dose of an alkylating agent is included in the treatment regimen. The probability of premature menopause occurring and being permanent increases for women over age 35. For most, menses cease during therapy or become erratic over two to three years, and amenorrhea occurs. Levels of follicle stimulating hormone (FSH) increase gradually and remain elevated for two to five years. FSH levels greater than 30 ng/L are usually considered diagnostic for ovarian failure. Estradiol levels decrease and testosterone levels decrease by 60%, which may account for the reports of lessened sexual desire and arousability.[263,264]

Premenopausal women who receive chemotherapy should be clearly informed of their risk for temporary or permanent ovarian failure. Women experiencing ovarian failure generally experience less subjective desire and arousability, vaginal dryness, vulvar/vaginal soreness, a burning pain, and light spotting after intercourse. Women should be encouraged to use a water-soluble lubricant (Astroglide or K-Y Jelly) during vaginal intercourse to minimize discomfort.

Other menopausal symptoms that commonly occur in women receiving chemotherapy or hormonal therapy include hot flashes, night sweats, and irregular menses. Hot flashes and profuse perspiration may be most troublesome at night and may interfere with sleep. Some women may benefit from lowering the thermostat in the home, especially where they sleep. Avoiding highly seasoned foods, caffeine, and alcohol may minimize the frequency of hot flashes. Dressing in loose-fitting cotton clothing and in layers, so a sweater or jacket can be removed during a hot flash, is advised. Women can try vitamin E, 400–800 IU per day, or if this is ineffective, Bellargel-S®, one tablet twice daily[265] may be prescribed. A low-dose clonidine patch (Catapress Transderm®) may effectively control hot flashes. Side effects of clonidine include a dry mouth, headache, irritability, and dizziness.[266] Although no significant changes in blood pressure or pulse have been noted with low-dose clonidine, the patient's blood pressure should be checked once or twice a week during the first few weeks on clonidine therapy. Another option for the management of hot flashes is venlafaxine (Effexor) 12.5 mg twice daily.[267]

The possibility that hormone replacement therapy might be appropriate and safe for breast cancer survivors has yet to be adequately researched.[268] Awareness of the underlying pathophysiology of menopause, the patient's perceptions, and response to symptoms are important for the nurse to adequately manage the symptoms of menopause.[269,270] Research indicates that breast cancer survivors generally appear to exhibit levels of physical, emotional, and social well being that are similar to age-matched healthy women and are superior to those seen for patients with other chronic diseases. Likewise there appears to be little disturbance in sexual functioning for most women who are in a partnered relationship.[271]

Weight gain is a troublesome side effect of therapy and is commonly felt by patients to occur because of water retention. In fact, it is due to increased caloric intake.[272] It appears that menopausal status, nodal status, and adjuvant treatment are significant predictors of weight gain. Further, women who receive cyclophosphamide orally with methotrexate and 5-FU have been found to gain more weight than women who receive adjuvant doxorubicin and cyclophosphamide.[273] Women commonly relate their weight gain following breast cancer to their tamoxifen treatment, however research indicates that the moderate weight gain observed in this patient population is comparable to the general aging disease-free population and may not be related to the tamoxifen.[274] Significant correlations do exist between weight gain and subjective feelings of unhappiness, worry, and increased distress regarding appearance when these women are compared to women who lost or maintained their weight. Factors contributing to weight gain include prednisone, oral cyclophosphamide, taste changes, increased appetite, depression, mild nausea that is relieved by eating, and psychological distress.[272,275,276]

Women need to receive nutritional counseling regarding the avoidance of weight gain at the outset of therapy. Some women gain as much as 15 pounds, which they find very difficult to lose once therapy is over. This adds to their increased distress and is avoidable with counseling.

Fatigue is a common subjective complaint associated with adjuvant therapy, and symptoms such as total body tiredness, forgetfulness, and wanting to rest increase over time throughout therapy[276] and are more profound during chemotherapy compared to radiation therapy.[277] Women should be encouraged to interject rest periods into their normal schedule and, if possible, to begin a regular exercise program such as walking or water aerobics. In addition to combating fatigue, exercise helps to minimize nausea associated with treatment. Nausea and vomiting with chemotherapy is predictable based on the type of chemotherapy or hormone therapy treatment. Patients on methotrexate and 5-FU experience less nausea and vomiting than women receiving CMF. Oral cyclophosphamide is associated with more prolonged nausea compared to intravenous cyclophosphamide. Women on higher doses of doxorubicin and cyclophosphamide experience intense nausea and vomiting for 48–72 hours following therapy if appropriate antiemetics are not employed.

Most women will usually not experience nausea and vomiting on the first day of their therapy especially when given a serotonin antagonist such as ondansetron or granisetron plus 20 mg of dexamethasone over 45 minutes as a single dose. However, the nausea and vomiting are worse on the second and third day posttreatment. Therefore, patients need a clear plan for managing these unpleasant symptoms for at least 72 hours posttreatment. Ondansetron, 8 mg orally every six to eight hours, prochlorperazine, 15-mg spansules, and lorazepam, 1 mg every 12 hours for two days following therapy, are effective in minimizing these symptoms.

Doxorubicin and cyclophosphamide (AC) are commonly used in curable breast cancer, which means many women experience total alopecia within two to three weeks of beginning therapy. This is highly distressing and contributes greatly to feelings of loss and body image changes. Women need to be aware of when and how hair loss will occur and have a plan to manage hair loss. Some women prefer shaving their heads or cutting the hair very short to minimize the constant and annoying shedding of their hair. The American Cancer Society's "Look Good, Feel Better" program is an excellent support and resource for women experiencing not only hair loss but body image changes in general.

Women on methotrexate–5-FU therapy do not lose significant amounts of hair and rarely require a wig. Women receiving CMF experience gradual thinning over the six to eight months of therapy and may require a wig only toward the end of treatment. Hair begins to grow back within a month of ending therapy at a rate of about ¼ in. per month. Women, especially younger ones, often are able to go without a wig or head covering within four months of therapy. Large earrings, a little more makeup, and hair mousse enable a woman to feel attractive and stylish in the early recovery period.

Chronic Lymphedema

Lymphedema is the accumulation of a protein-rich lymph fluid resulting in an increased interstitial colloid oncotic pressure that attracts water molecules, creating a chronic buildup of fluid in the extremity. The increase in size of the arm contributes to pain, immobility, cellulitis, and even lymphosarcoma. Lymph is an excellent culture medium, and infections such as cellulitis and lymphangitis can flourish. Prevention of lymphedema is of primary concern because any fluid accumulation that is unchecked only leads to further edema. The longer the edema persists, the more difficult it is to manage. Once lymphedema is established it can be managed, but it cannot be entirely cured.

The overall incidence of lymphedema in breast cancer is 20%.[278] The extent of the surgery including axillary dissection is a primary factor in the occurrence of lymphedema. Lymphedema occurs in as much as 22% of women following radical mastectomy and only about 7% of women who have modified radical mastectomy. Breast-conserving surgery such as partial mastectomy or lumpectomy results in lymphedema in about 2%–8% of cases.[279] Because of research concerning the role of adjuvant chemotherapy in early-stage breast cancer, some would argue that an axillary lymph node dissection (ALND) be performed only when the primary tumor is larger than 5 mm. Others contend that there is no survival benefit associated with ALND and women with larger tumors should be spared any potentially damaging effects of ALND since adjuvant chemotherapy is going to be given regardless of whether there are positive nodes.

Axillary lymph node dissection, which is associated with pain, numbness, swelling and weakness/stiffness of the ipsilateral arm and/or shoulder, is a diagnostic and staging procedure, not a therapeutic procedure. If newer, more advanced sampling procedures (e.g., sentinel node biopsy) prove to be diagnostic as well as provide accurate staging with minimal morbidity compared to ALND, then these procedures should be done over the ALND. Sampling procedures contribute less to physical morbidity because they involve less nerve damage and a smaller surface area of tissue damage. Lymphedema leads to physical impairment and diminished quality of life due to an inability to throw objects, zip a dress, go jogging, or sleep without discomfort. Pain in the affected arm has at least a moderate impact on the daily life functioning of 25% of breast cancer patients.[280]

In a study of 222 women who had had an ALND in the past six months, just over half of the patients experienced pain-related discomfort and disability.[281] Younger women tended to report more intense pain than older women; those with a greater extent of axillary dissection, that is more than 13 nodes removed, reported more pain than women who had fewer nodes removed. Overall the researchers found that women who undergo ALND for breast cancer experience enduring surgery-related symptoms, the most predominant of which is numbness. Obviously more invasive surgery to the axilla causes greater damage to surrounding tissue and nerves, including the intercostobrachial nerve, therefore more pain and numbness would be anticipated. Surgeons should be encouraged to preserve the intercostobrachial nerve whenever possible.

Lymphedema can develop weeks, months, or years after axillary dissection. Lymph node dissection, radiation therapy, infection and delayed wound healing, obesity, and age all are considered risk factors for lymphedema. Lymphedema is most common in women who have had axillary dissection followed by radiation in excess of 46 Gy.[282] The most common causes of late or chronic edema are infection and tumor recurrence, or tumor enlargement in the axilla.

Prevention includes avoidance of medical procedures such as blood draws, IVs, injections, and blood pressure measurements on the affected arm. Avoid heavy lifting and vigorous, repetitive movements of the arm against resistance. Anything that increases blood flow to the affected arm contributes to the incidence and degree of lymphedema. Heat, strenuous exercise, or lifting objects weighing more than 5–10 pounds will contribute to lymphedema. Women who have had an axillary dissection are instructed not to lift weights, for instance, because that repetitive strenuous motion increases blood flow and can contribute to edema. Likewise they should not carry a suitcase or grocery bags because the arm as it hangs down has increased blood flow and muscle strain that ordinarily would promote lymph drainage, but does not because of the dependent nature of the arm as it carries the heavy object. Heavy handbags with shoulder straps should not be carried on the affected arm. Tight jewelry impedes venous blood flow and contributes to swelling. The patient is instructed to avoid cuts, bruises, sunburns or sports injuries, insect bites, and pet scratches or bites. An electric razor should be used to shave under the arm, especially since the area is usually numb. The woman is instructed to keep the wrist higher than the elbow and the elbow higher than or even with the heart whenever possible. A compression sleeve may be recommended for the arm while traveling on long airplane flights. It is important that the patient or significant other inspect the arm and hand daily for warmth, redness, swelling, or pain. Any rashes, blistering, or redness of the arm or increased temperature, pain, or discomort should be reported immediately to the medical care team.

The most effective treatment for lymphedema is a combination of manual lymph drainage, compression bandaging, and exercise. The first step is manual lymph drainage. This procedure stimulates the healthy lymphatics and increases lymph transport of the involved extremity.[283] The arm is then wrapped with compression bandages to decrease reabsorption of fluid back into the extremity. The arm is wrapped so that it is most snug distally to promote a graded fluid drainage. Initially the arm is wrapped 24 hours a day until the appropriate size is reached and then only at night. The exercise component involves strengthening exercises and aerobic exercises. Strengthening exercises create a muscle-pumping action that increases lymph flow. Aerobic activity elevates the heart rate and respiratory rate, further stimulating the lymph transport. Diet should include a well-balanced, low-sodium, high-fiber diet. The patient is encouraged to achieve or maintain ideal body weight.

The lymphedematous arm is cosmetically unattractive and can be functionally useless. The arm can cause tremendous strain on the neck and shoulder muscles, which can result in pain. The woman may have difficulty adjusting her wardrobe to provide for the increasing size of her arm. Furthermore, the edematous arm can rarely be concealed adequately and can renew feelings of disfigurement and depression associated with the mastectomy that the woman may have resolved before the lymphedema occurred. When function of the arm is affected the woman may not be able to work or perform activities of daily living. These limitations may not have been imposed on the woman following her mastectomy. Efforts should be make to discuss the goals and rationale of management with the woman, thereby enlisting her cooperation and participation in the planned treatment regimen. Many times it is appropriate to refer women with lymphedema to a lymphedema specialist who can design a program to minimize fluid accumulation early, at the first sign of fluid accumulation. To find the nearest lymphedema center, contact the National Lymphedema Network at http://www.lymphnet.org.

Continuity of Care

Support Systems

Women with breast cancer may find a need for different support systems as they maneuver through the different phases of their diagnosis, treatment, and survival. Initially, the prediagnosis worry is often shared with friends and family who then continue to provide ongoing support.

Many people find support through their faith and the people with whom they worship. Health professionals, often called upon to demonstrate support and encouragement during emotionally difficult times, may or may not be always up to the task. Many people have found comfort, validation, and information by joining a support group. Support groups are recognized as valuable sources of hope, encouragement, and education for the individual with breast cancer as well as other chronic diseases.[284]

Although the prognosis for breast cancer is constantly improving, the psychological impact of the disease may result in feelings of anxiety, depression, suicidal ideation, insomnia, and fear of recurrence and death. These directly affect the patient's ability to function.[285–287] Seeking out and participating in a support group often helps to reduce and alleviate some of these feelings of loss of control and vulnerability.

Most cancer support groups rely on mutual aid or interdependence to attain a common goal, and individual participation is usually grounded in the needs of the individual and what goals she hopes to accomplish. Cella and Yellen[289] identify basic needs most people are seeking: hope, honesty, emotional freedom, and the ability to discuss death and dying. Cella and Yellen also recognize that support groups help each person retain their social identity and provide educational, emotional, and environmental support.

Many successful groups such as Alcoholics Anonymous use the common bond shared by its members to provide a forum where essential needs can be addressed that include assistance, personal insights, support, and belonging. Groups may also stress needs and goals that are more specific to the concerns of its members, e.g., type of surgery or current disease status. Spouses find comfort and freedom to ask questions and hear the experiences of other men. Spanish-speaking women are able to be more expressive and forthcoming speaking in their native language. Women who have been treated with mastectomy have concerns and questions that differ from a woman who has had breast preservation. Women with metastatic disease have needs and issues beyond those who are disease-free.

Another recent advance in information and support exists through on-line web pages, which allow women who are isolated by geographic or physical constraints to communicate with others even on an international basis. Valuable information is provided by a wide spectrum of health care workers as well as patients and families, whose sharing of stories and experiences can create a helpful and inspiring chronicle.

Nursing Challenges

Possibly the greatest challenge in the care of the patient with breast cancer is to recognize rehabilitation goals throughout the trajectory or natural history of the disease as the individual woman experiences it. When the woman is first diagnosed with breast cancer, her initial fear of the disease is eased with the task of formulating a plan of care by consulting with a team of experts including a surgeon, plastic surgeon, medical oncologist, radiation oncologist, and clinical nurse specialist. When managed through the auspices of a comprehensive breast center, she and her family come to value the combined efforts of the team assembled to help manage her disease. With a thorough explanation of the disease and treatment plan, she may choose to proceed or to seek other opinions before making her decision. The task of seeking other opinions for treatment is worthwhile because it allows the individual to learn more about her disease and to feel confident in her decision once she has had time to evaluate all treatment options. But this time may also be particularly stressful because of the number of treatment options among which she is expected to choose. The nurse can be particularly helpful at this time to clarify the differences among the various approaches to management, to explain why such differences exist, and to give the woman and her family the opportunity to explore all options including appropriate research studies. Throughout this time the nurse concentrates on helping the woman find information and make contact with individuals who will help her make her own decision regarding treatment.

Once the plan of care is decided, the nurse formulates rehabilitation goals that are accomplished by further education regarding what the woman can expect and by teaching the woman self-care measures. Initially these goals will include postoperative care of the wound and appropriate exercises to regain optimal function of the arm and shoulder. Such instructions are written with personalized directions regarding how to perform the exercises and minimize pain through adequate use of analgesics. Some women will benefit from the assistance of a physical therapist trained specifically in the rehabilitation of the woman who has had a mastectomy. Often women have no difficulty performing their exercises. Some, however, are reluctant to exercise to the point of discomfort and need additional support and encouragement. Still others will exercise more than is recommended and experience pain and arm swelling in the postoperative period. Women need frequent follow-up in the postoperative period to be certain they are progressing to the best of their abilities.

In the initial six weeks following mastectomy, the patient will be instructed not to wear a prosthesis. Instead she usually wears a soft cotton form in her bra that will not irritate the incision. During this time she can be fitted for a prosthesis and explore the type she prefers. Because women need referrals to stores that specialize in these garments and breast forms, nurses must keep up-to-date records on such specialty stores since surgeons rarely will address this issue with their patients. The American Cancer Society's "Look Good, Feel Better" program is especially helpful to these women to help them look and feel their best. The Y-ME organization is another invaluable resource for women experiencing breast cancer and looking for advice concerning prostheses.

When chemotherapy is incorporated into the treatment plan, the nurse instructs the patient and family regarding the side effects of chemotherapy and management strategies. Depending on the plan, this can include prevention and management of nausea and vomiting, ways to minimize fatigue, managing hair loss, oral hygiene, and prevention of infection. Eventually other problems may arise including difficulty sleeping, complaints of fatigue and lack of energy, as well as menopausal symptoms. The nurse maintains close contact with the woman usually by telephone since most if not all patients are treated on an outpatient basis.

The primary goal for the woman with localized breast cancer is to finish therapy and resume her life goals and activities she enjoyed prior to her illness. For most women this process takes about a year, at which time the individual is likely to feel more energetic with fewer sleepless nights. Often the hair has grown back and she feels more like herself. She may begin to inquire about breast reconstruction if she has not already done so. Most women should realize this is major surgery and will again require an extended time period for recovery. It is often associated with a six-month period of fatigue and complaints of exhaustion. This is normal, however, and should not in any way discourage a woman from having the reconstructive procedures done.

While most women fear recurrence of their disease, seeing the physician (surgeon and/or medical oncologist) every three months for the first year, every six months for two years, yearly after that usually is frequent enough to be reassuring. Some patients may prefer to be seen more frequently. If the cancer does recur it is devastating. The disappointment and fears are often more intense than with the initial diagnosis. The patient feels betrayed by everyone, especially her own body. Most breast cancer patients work very hard to achieve wellness and to comply with all their doctors and nurses recommendations. When the disease comes back, the woman feels she has little control and begins initially to lose hope in her ability to once again be courageous. At this time many will need the counsel of a psycho-oncologist trained specifically in the care of the cancer patient. The recurrence is as devastating to the family as it is to the woman and they too will need to talk about their fears as therapy is once again discussed. Other supports include the woman's religious organization and an appropriate patient support group.

Goals for the person with recurring cancer center on helping her and her family understand the treatment goals and recognize how the treatment is helping. Remaining hopeful and supportive throughout with emphasis on the success of therapy and numerous options available is reassuring. Few women will need home care at this time since most recurrences are not debilitating unless the individual is elderly and the disease recurs in the brain or liver. When the disease begins to effect a woman's ability to perform activities of daily living, the need for home care should be introduced to determine the woman's options for insurance coverage. The family needs to be encouraged to identify their needs and whether they need assistance in her care on a daily basis or two or three times per week. Establishing a relationship with a nursing service that also has a hospice component is worthwhile because there is a smooth transition when hospice is deemed appropriate. Hospice should be introduced as an option for care once treatment is felt to be strictly palliative and the woman is thought to have less than six months to live.

Bereavement counseling is a component of hospice care and usually continues for at least a year. The nurse also can play a pivotal role in helping the family through the grieving process.

References

1. Mettlin C: Global breast cancer mortality statistics. *CA Cancer J Clin* 49:138–144, 1999
2. Landis SH, Murray T, Bolden S, Wingo PA: Cancer statistics. *CA Cancer J Clin* 49:8–11, 1999
3. Conference Statement: Treatment of Early Stage Breast Cancer. Bethesda, MD, National Institutes of Health, 1990
4. Kirkman-Liff B, Kronenfeld J: Access to cancer screening devices for women. *Am J Public Health* 82:733–735, 1992
5. Shimkin MB: Cancer of the breast. *JAMA* 183:358–361, 1963
6. American Cancer Society: *Cancer Facts and Figures—1996.* Atlanta, American Cancer Society, 1996
7. Kelsey JL, Gammon MD: The epidemiology of breast cancer. *CA Cancer J Clin* 41:146–165, 1991
8. Moormeier J: Breast cancer in black women. *Ann Intern Med* 124:897–905, 1996
9. Wojik BE, Spinks MA, Optenberg SA: Breast cancer survival analysis for African American women and white women in an equal-access health care system. *Cancer* 822:1310–1318, 1998
10. Wingo PA, Ries LA, Parker SL, et al: Long term cancer survival in the United States. *Cancer Epidemiol Biomarkers Prev* 7:271–282, 1998
11. Fisher B: Biology and clinical considerations regarding the use of surgery and chemotherapy in treatment of primary breast cancer. *Cancer* 40:574–587, 1977
12. Henderson BE, Bernstein L: Endogenous and exogenous hormonal factors, in Harris JR, Lippman ME, Morrow M, Hellman S (eds): *Diseases of the Breast.* Philadelphia, Lippincott-Raven, 1996, pp 185–200
13. Hulka BS, Liu ET, Lininger RA: Steroid hormones and the risk of breast cancer. *Cancer* 74:1111–1124, 1994 (suppl 3)
14. Zumoff B: Hormone profiles in women with breast cancer. *Obstet Gynecol Clin North Am* 21:751–772, 1994
15. Potten CS, Watson RJ, Williams GT: The effect of age and menstrual cycle upon proliferative activity of the normal human breast. *Br J Cancer* 58:163–170, 1988
16. Bernstein L, Ross RK: Endogenous hormones and breast cancer risk. *Epidemiol Rev* 15:48–65, 1993
17. Bruzzi P, Negri E, LaVecchia C, et al: Short term increase in risk of breast cancer after full term pregnancy. *Br J Med* 297:1096–1098, 1988
18. Yang CP, Weiss NS, Band PR, et al: History of lactation and breast cancer risk. *Am J Epidemiol* 138:1050–1056, 1993
19. Yoo KY, Tajima K, Karoishi T, et al: Independent effect of lactation against breast cancer: a case-control study in Japan. *Am J Epidemiol* 135:726–733, 1992
20. Land CE, Hayakawa N, Machado SG: A case-control interview study of breast cancer among Japanese A-bomb survivors. II. Interactions with radiation dose. *Cancer Causes Control* 5:167–176, 1994
21. Newcomb PA, Stover BE, Longnecker MP, et al: Lactation and a reduced risk of premenopausal breast cancer. *N Engl J Med* 330:81–87, 1994
22. Daling JR, Malone KE, White E, et al: Risk of breast cancer among young women: relationship to induced abortion. *J Natl Cancer Inst* 86:1584–1592, 1994
23. Daling JR, Brinton LA, Voight LF, et el. Risk of breast cancer in white women following an induced abortion. *Am J Epidemiol* 144:373–380, 1996
24. Newcomb PA, Storer BE, Longnecker MP, et al: Pregnancy termination in relation to risk of breast cancer. *JAMA* 275:283–287, 1996
25. Melbye M, Wohlfahrt J, Olsen JH, et al: Induced abortion and the risk of breast cancer. *N Engl J Med* 336:81–85, 1997
26. Petitti DB: Animal models of sex steroid hormones and mammary cancer: lessons for understanding studies in humans, in Institute of Medicine, Division of Health Promotion and Disease Prevention: *Oral Contraceptives and Breast Cancer.* Washington, DC, National Academy Press, 1991, pp 152–164
27. Vessey MP: Effect of endogenous and exogenous hormones on breast cancer. *Verh Dtsch Ges Pathol* 81:493–501, 1997
28. Malone KE, Daling JR, Weiss NS: Oral contraceptives in relation to breast cancer. *Epidemiol Rev* 15:80–97, 1993
29. Holmberg L, Lund E, Bergstrom R, et al: Oral contraceptives and prognosis in breast cancer: effects of duration, latency, frequency, age at first use and relation to parity and body mass index in young women with breast cancer. *Eur J Cancer* 30A:351–354, 1994
30. Rookus MA, vanLeeuwen FE: Oral contraceptives and risk of breast cancer in women aged 20–54 years. *Lancet* 344:844–851, 1994
31. Brinton LA, Daling JR, Liff JM, et al: Oral contraceptives and breast cancer risk among younger women. *J Natl Cancer Inst* 87:827–835, 1995
32. LaVecchia C, Negri E, Francaschi S, et al: Oral contraceptives and breast cancer, a cooperative Italian Study. *Int J Cancer* 60:163–167, 1995
33. Palmer JR, Rosenberg L, Rao RS, et al: Oral contraceptive use and breast cancer risk among African-American women. *Cancer Causes Control* 6:221–231, 1995
34. Mayberry RM: Age specific patterns of association between breast cancer and risk factors in black women, ages 20 to 39 and 40 to 54. *Ann Epidemiol* 4:205–213, 1994
35. Schlesselman JJ: Net effect of oral contraceptive use on the risk of cancer in women in the U.S. *Obstet Gynecol* 85:793–801, 1995
36. Bergkvist L, Adami HO, Persson I, et al: The risk of breast cancer after estrogen and estrogen-progestin replacement. *N Engl J Med* 321:293–297, 1989
37. Dupont WD, Page DL, Rogers LW: Influence of exogenous estrogens, proliferative breast disease and other variables on breast cancer risk. *Cancer* 63:948–957, 1989
38. Mills PK, Beeson L, Phillips RL, et al: Prospective study of exogenous hormone use and breast cancer in Seventh Day Adventists. *Cancer* 64:591–597, 1989
39. Colditz GA, Egan KM, Stampfer MJ: Hormone replace-

ment therapy and risk of breast cancer: results from epidemiologic studies. *Am J Obstet Gynecol* 168:1473–1480, 1993

40. Maguire PJ: Estrogen replacement therapy and breast cancer. *J Reprod Med* 38:183–185, 1993

41. Zumoff B: Biological and endocrinological insights into the possible breast cancer risk from menopausal estrogen replacement therapy. *Steroids* 58:196–204, 1993

42. Wilklund I, Holst J, Kurlberg J, et al: A new methodological approach to the evaluation of quality of life in postmenopausal women. *Maturitas* 14:211–224, 1992

43. Schover LR: Sexuality and body image in younger women with breast cancer. *Monogr Natl Cancer Inst* 16:177–182, 1994

44. Theriault RL, Sellin RV: A clinical dilemma: estrogen replacement therapy in postmenopausal women with a background of primary breast cancer. *Ann Oncol* 2:209–217, 1991

45. Davidson J: The need for a randomized trial of hormone replacement therapy in women with breast cancer. *Med J Aust* 157:429–433, 1991

46. Henderson IC: Risk factors for development of breast cancer. *Cancer* 71:2127–2140, 1993 (suppl)

47. Marchant DJ: Estrogen replacement therapy after breast cancer. *Cancer* 71:2169–2176, 1993

48. Vassilopoulou-Sellin R, Theriault RL: Randomized prospective trial of estrogen-replacement therapy in women with a history of breast cancer. *Monogr Natl Cancer Inst* 16: 153–159, 1994

49. Sattin RW, Rubin GL, Webster L, et al: Family history and the risk of breast cancer. *JAMA* 253:1908–1913, 1985

50. Cobleigh MA, Berris RF, Bush T, et al: Estrogen replacement therapy in breast cancer survivors. *JAMA* 272: 540–545, 1994

51. Bernstein JL, Thompson WD, Risch N, et al: The genetic epidemiology of secondary breast cancer. *Am J Epidemiol* 136:937–948, 1992

52. Gail MH, Brinton LA, Byar DP, et al: Projecting individualized probabilities of developing breast cancer for white females who are being examined annually. *J Natl Cancer Inst* 81:1879–1886, 1989

53. Kelsey JL, Horn-Ross PL: Breast cancer: magnitude of the problem and descriptive epidemiology. *Epidemiol Rev* 15: 7–16, 1993

54. Kelsey JL, Whittemore AS: Epidemiology and primary prevention of cancers of the breast, endometrium and ovary: a brief overview. *Ann Epidemiol* 4:89–95, 1994

55. Claus EB, Risch N, Thompson WD: Autosomal dominant inheritance of early-onset breast cancer: implications for risk prediction. *Cancer* 73:643–651, 1994

56. Roseman DL, Straus AK, Shorey W: A positive family history of breast cancer: does its effect diminish with age? *Arch Intern Med* 150:191–194, 1990

57. Frank TS: Introduction to molecular oncology, in Fechner RE, Rosen PP (eds): *Anatomic Pathology.* Chicago, American Society of Clinical Pathologists Press, 1997, vol 2, pp 227–237

58. Wolman SR, Heppner GH, Wolman E: New directions in breast cancer research. *FASEB J* 11:535–543, 1997

59. King MC, Rowell S, Love SM: Inherited breast and ovarian cancer. What are the risks? What are the choices? *JAMA* 269:1975–1980, 1993

60. Mikki V, Swensen J, Slattuck-Eidens D, et al: A strong candidate for the breast and ovarian cancer susceptibility gene BRCA1. *Science* 266:66–71, 1994

61. Futreal PA, Quingyron L, Shattuck-Eidens D, et al: BRCA1 mutations in primary breast and ovarian carcinomas. *Science* 266:120–122, 1994

62. Weber B: Genetic testing for breast cancer. *Sci Am* 3:12–21, 1996

63. Frank TS, Manley SA, Olopade OI, et al: Sequence analysis of *BRCA1* and *BRCA2*: correlation of mutations with family history and ovarian cancer risk. *J Clin Oncol* 16:2417–2425, 1998

64. Ford D, Easton DF: The genetics of breast and ovarian cancer. *Br J Cancer* 72:804–812, 1995

65. Ford D, Easton DF, Bishop DT, et al: Risks of cancer in BRCA1-mutation carriers. *Lancet* 343:692–695, 1994

66. Easton DF, Bishop DT, Ford D: Genetic linkage analysis in familial breast and ovarian cancer. *Am J Hum Genet* 52: 678–701, 1993

67. Wooster R, Neuhauser SL, Mangion J, et al: Localization of breast cancer susceptibility gene (BRCA2) to chromosome 13q 12–13. *Science* 265:2088–2090, 1994

68. Thorlacius S, Tryggvadottir L, Olafdottir G, et al: Linkage to BRCA2 in hereditary male breast cancer. *Lancet* 346: 544–545, 1995

69. Streuwing JP, Hartge P, Wacholder S, et al: The risk of cancer associated with specific mutations of BRCA1 and BRCA2 among Ashkenazi Jews. *N Engl J Med* 336: 1401–1408, 1997

70. Harris C, Holstein M: Clinical implications of the p53 tumor supression gene. *N Engl J Med* 329:1318–1327, 1993

71. Saitoh S, Gunningham J, Devries EMG, et al: p53 gene mutations in breast cancer in midwestern U.S. women: null as well as missense-type mutations are associated with poor prognosis. *Oncogene* 9:2869–2875, 1994

72. Aguilar F, Harris C, Sun T, et al: Geographic variation of p53 mutational profile in non-malignant human liver. *Science* 264:1317–1319, 1994

73. Nees M, Homann N, Sicher H, et al: Expression of mutated p53 occurs in tumor-distant epithelia of head and neck cancer patients. A possible molecular basis for development of multiple tumors. *Cancer Res* 53:4189–4196, 1993

74. Chang F, Syrjanen S, Syrjanen K. Implications of the p53 tumor-suppressor gene in clinical oncology. *J Clin Oncol* 13:1009–1022, 1995

75. Berstein JL, Thompson WD, Risch N, et al: Risk factors predicting the incidence of second primary breast cancer among women diagnosed with a first primary breast cancer. *Am J Epidemiol* 136:925–936, 1992

76. Berstein JL: Risk factors predicting the incidence of a second primary breast cancer. *Dis Abstract Int* 54:195, 1993

77. Wilett WC, Hunter DJ: Prospective studies of diet and breast cancer. *Cancer* 74:1085–1089, 1994 (suppl)

78. Hunter DJ, Speigelman D, Adami H-O, et al: Cohort studies of fat intake and the risk of breast cancer: a pooled analysis. *N Engl J Med* 334:356–361, 1996

79. Pinn VW: The role of the NIH's Office of Research on women's health. *Acad Med* 69:698–702, 1994

80. Goldbohm RA, van den Brandt PA, Brants HA, et al: Validation of a dietary questionnaire used in a large-scale prospective cohort study on diet and cancer. *Eur J Clin Nutr* 48:253–265, 1994

81. Howe GR: Dietary fat and breast cancer risk: an epidemiologic perspective. *Cancer* 74:1078–1084, 1994 (suppl 3)

82. Cummings NB: Women's health and nutritional research: U.S. governmental concerns. *J Am Coll Nutr* 12:329–336, 1993

83. Deslypere JP: Obesity and cancer. *Metabolism* 44:24–27, 1995 (suppl 3)

84. Huang Z, Hankinson SE, Colditz GA, et al: Dual effects of weight and weight gain on breast cancer risk. *JAMA* 278: 1407–1411, 1997

85. Stoll BA: Timing of weight gain in relation to breast cancer risk. *Ann Oncol* 6:245–248, 1995

86. Lyman GH, Cox CE, Timing of weight gain and breast cancer risk. *Cancer* 6:243–249, 1995

87. Longnecker MP: Alcoholic beverage consumption in relation to risk of breast cancer: meta-analysis and review. *Cancer Causes Control* 5:73–82, 1994

88. Smith-Warner SA, Spiegelman D, Yaun SS, et al: Alcohol and breast cancer: a pooled analysis of cohort studies. *JAMA* 279:535–540, 1998

89. Giovannucci E, Stampfer MJ, Colditz GA, et al: Recall and selection bias in reporting past alcohol consumption among breast cancer cases. *Cancer Causes Control* 4:441–448, 1993

90. Plant ML: Alcohol and breast cancer: a review. *Int J Addict* 27:107–128, 1992

91. John EM, Kelsey J: Radiation and other environmental exposures and breast cancer. *Epidemiol Rev* 15:157–162, 1993

92. Smita B, Robinson LL, Oberlin O, et al: Breast cancer and other second neoplasms after childhood Hodgkin's disease. *N Engl J Med* 334:745–751, 1996

93. Hancock SL, Tucker MA, Hoppe RT: Breast cancer after treatment of Hodgkin's disease. *J Natl Cancer Inst* 85:25–31, 1993

94. Page DL, Dupont WD: Anatomic markers of human malignancy and risk of breast cancer. *Cancer* 66:1326–1335, 1990

95. Page D, Simpson JF: Benign, high-risk and premalignant lesions of the breast, in Bland K, Copeland EM (eds): *The Breast: Comprehensive Management of Benign and Malignant Diseases* (ed 2). Philadelphia, Saunders, 1998, vol 1, pp 191–213

96. Page DL, Dupont WD: Anatomic indicators (histologic and cytologic) of increased breast cancer risk. *Breast Cancer Res Treat* 28:157–166, 1993

97. Dupont WD, Parl FF, Hartman WH, et al: Breast cancer risk associated with proliferative breast disease and atypical hyperplasia. *Cancer* 71:1258–1265, 1993

98. Frykberg RE, Bland KI: Current concepts on the biology and management of in situ (Tis, stage 0) breast carcinoma, in Bland K, Copeland EM (eds): *The Breast: Comprehensive Management of Benign and Malignant Diseases* (ed 2). Philadelphia, Saunders, 1998, vol 2, pp 1012–1043

99. Page DL, Dupont WD: Indicators of increased breast cancer risk in humans. *J Cell Biochem* 16G:175–182, 1992

100. Morrow M, Schmitt JS: Lobular carcinoma in situ, in Harris J, Lippman ME, Morrow M, Hellman S (eds): *Diseases of the Breast*. Philadelphia, Lippincott-Raven, 1996, pp 369–373

101. Camus MG, Joshi MG, Mackarem G, et al: Ductal carcinoma in situ of the male breast. *Cancer* 74:1289–1293, 1994

102. Bilimoria MM, Murrow M: The woman at increased risk for breast cancer: evaluation and management strategies. *CA Cancer J Clin* 45:263–278, 1995

103. Kelloff GJ, Johnson JR, Crowell JA, et al: Approaches to development and marketing approval of drugs that prevent cancer. *Cancer Epidemiol Biomarkers Prev* 4:1–10, 1995

104. Love RR: Prevention of breast cancer in premenopausal women. *Monog Natl Cancer Inst* 16:L61–65, 1994

105. Kelloff GJ, Boone CW, Steele VE, et al: Mechanistic considerations in chemopreventive drug development. *J Cell Biochem* 20:1–24, 1994 (suppl)

106. Lippman SM, Benner SE, Hong WK: Chemopreventive strategies for the control of cancer. *Cancer* 72:984–990, 1993 (suppl 3)

107. Noguchi M, Rose DP, Miyazaki I: Breast cancer chemoprevention: clinical trials and research. *Oncology* 53:175–181, 1996

108. Lippman SM, Benner SE, Hong WK: Cancer chemoprevention. *J Clin Oncol* 12:851–873, 1994

109. Cole MP, Jones CT, Todd ID: The new anti-estrogenic agent in late breast cancer: an early clinical approach of ICI 46474. *Br J Cancer* 25:270–275, 1971

110. Sawka CA, Pritchard KI, Paterson HG, et al: Role and mechanism of action of tamoxifen in premenopausal women with metastatic breast carcinoma. *Cancer Res* 46: 3152–3156, 1986

111. Fisher B, Constantino J, Redmond C, et al: A randomized clinical trial evaluating tamoxifen in the treatment of patients with node-negative breast cancer who have estrogen-receptor positive tumors. *N Engl J Med* 320:479–484, 1989

112. Cummings JF, Gray R, Tormey DC, et al: Adjuvant tamoxifen versus placebo in elderly women with node-positive breast cancer: Long term follow-up and causes of death. *J Clin Oncol* 11:29–35, 1993

113. NSABP Protocol P-1: A Clinical Trial to Determine the Worth of Tamoxifen for Preventing Breast Cancer. Pittsburgh, National Surgical Adjuvant Breast and Bowel Project, 1992

114. Wickerham DL, Constatino J, Fisher B, et al. Initial results from NSABP Protocol P-1; A Clinical Trial to Determine the Worth of Tamoxifen for Preventing Breast Cancer in Women at Increased Risk. Presented at the 34th annual meeting of the American Society of Clinical Oncology Plenary Session, Los Angeles, May 16–18, 1998

115. NSABP Protocol P-2: A Study of Tamoxifen and Raloxifene for the Prevention of Breast Cancer. Pittsburgh, National Surgical Adjuvant Breast and Bowel Project, 1999

116. Delmas P, Bjarnason N, Mitlak B, et al: Effects of raloxifene on bone mineral density, serum cholesterol concentrations and uterine endometrium inpost-menopausal women. *N Engl J Med* 337:1641–1647, 1997

117. Jaiyesimi IA, Buzdar AU, Decker DA, et al: Use of tamoxifen for breast cancer: twenty-eight years later. *J Clin Oncol* 13: 513–529, 1995

118. Knabbe C, Lippman ME, Wakefield LM: Evidence that transforming growth factor is a hormonally regulated negative growth factor in human breast cancer cells. *Cell* 48: 417–428, 1987

119. Jordan VC, Fritz NF, Tormey DC: Long-term adjuvant therapy with tamoxifen: effects on sex hormone binding globulin and antithrombin III. *Cancer Res* 47:4517–4519, 1987

120. Vogel VG: Prevention of breast cancer: clinical considerations in breast cancer prevention, in Harris JR, Lippman MC, Morrow M, Hellman S (eds): *Diseases of the Breast*. Philadelphia, Lippincott-Raven, 1996, pp 341–354

121. Vogel VG: High-risk populations as targets for breast cancer prevention trials. *Prev Med* 20:88–100, 1991

122. Powles TJ: Status of antiestrogen breast cancer prevention trials. *Oncology* 12:28–31, 1998

123. Pike MC, Spicer DV. The chemoprevention of breast cancer by reducing sex steroid exposure. *J Cell Biochem* 17G: 26–36, 1993 (suppl)

124. Paffenbarger RS Jr, Lee I-M, Wing AL: The influence of physical activity on the incidence of site specific cancers in college alumni, in Jacobs MM (ed): *Exercise, Calories, Fat and Cancer*. New York, Plenum, 1992

125. Dogan JF, Brown C, Barrett M, et al: Physical activity and

the risk of breast disease in the Framingham Heart Study. *Am J Epidemiol* 139:662–669, 1994

126. Ainsworth BE, Sternfeld B, Slattery ML, et al: Physical activity and breast cancer: evaluation of physical assessment methods. *Cancer* 83(3):611–620, 1998. (suppl)

127. Bernstein L, Henderson BE, Hanisch R, et al: Physical exercise and reduced risk of breast cancer in young women. *J Natl Cancer Inst* 86:1403–1408, 1994

128. Mittendorf R, Longnecker MP, Newcomb PA, et al: Strenuous exercises in young adulthood and risk of breast cancer. *Cancer Causes Control* 6:347–353, 1995

129. Chen CL, White E, Malone KE, et al. Leisure-time physical activity in relation to breast cancer among young women. *Cancer Causes Control* 8:77–84, 1997

130. Ziegler LD, Kroll SS: Primary breast cancer after prophylactic mastectomy. *Am J Clin Oncol* 14:451–454, 1991

131. Berger K, Bostnick JB: Preventive mastectomy for the woman at risk, in Berger K, Bostwick JL (eds): *A Woman's Decision: Breast Care Treatment and Reconstruction* (ed 4). St Louis, Quality Medical Publishing, 1994, pp 288–298

132. Hartmann L, Schaid DJ, Woods JE, et al: Efficacy of prophylactic mastectomy in women with a family history of breast cancer. *N Engl J Med* 340:77–84, 1999

133. Peters JA, Stopfer JE: Role of the genetic counselor in familial cancer. *Oncology* 10:159–166, 175, 1996

134. Lynch HT: Genetic counseling in cancer: a status report—part 2. *Oncology* 10:131–134, 1996

135. Statement of the American Society of Clinical Oncology: Genetic listing for cancer susceptibility. Philadelphia, American Society of Clinical Oncology, 1996

136. Durant JR: How to organize a multidisciplinary clinic for the management of breast cancer. *Surg Clin North Am* 70: 977–983, 1990

137. Gasparini G, Harris AL: Clinical importance of the determination of tumor angiogenesis in breast carcinoma much more than new prognostic tool. *J Clin Oncol* 12:765–782, 1995

138. Hayes DF: Angiogenesis and breast cancer. *Hematol Oncol Clin North Am* 8:51–69, 1994

139. Dodd GD: American Cancer Society Guidelines from past to present. *Cancer* 72:1429–1432, 1993

140. Garms R: Mammography quality standards act of 1992. *J Oncol Manage* 3:64–65, 1994

141. Bassett LW, Manjikian V, Gold RH: Mammography and breast cancer screening. *Surg Clin North Am* 70:775–800, 1990

142. Adler DD, Wahl RL: New methods for imaging the breast: techniques, findings, potential. *Am J Radiol* 164:19–30, 1995

143. Schmidt RA, Nishikawa RM: Clinical use of digital mammography: the present and the prospects. *J Digit Imaging* 81:74–79, 1995 (suppl)

144. Adler DD, Wahl RL: New methods for breast cancer imaging, in Harris JR, Lippman ME, Murrow M, Hellman S (eds): *Diseases of the Breast.* Philadelphia, Lippincott-Raven, 1996, pp 84–98

145. Venta LA, Dudiak CM, Salomon CG, et al: Sonographic evaluation of the breast. *Radiographics* 12:29–50, 1994

146. Mendelson EB: Interventional breast ultrasonography, in Dershaw DD (ed): *Interventional Breast Procedures.* New York, Churchill-Livingston, 1996, pp 129–153

147. Rosato EL. Examination techniques: roles of the physician and patient in evaluating breast diseases, in Bland K, Copeland EM (eds): *The Breast: Comprehensive Management of Benign and Malignant Diseases* (ed 2). Philadelphia, Saunders, 1998, vol 1, pp 615–623

148. Orel SG, Schnall MD, Powell CM, et al: Staging of suspected breast cancer: effect of MRI imaging and MR-guided biopsy. *Radiology* 196:16–28, 1995

149. Harms SE, Flamig DP, Evans WP, et al: MR imaging of the breast current status and future potential. *Am J Radiol* 163: 1039–1047, 1994

150. Crowe JP, Adler LP, Shenk RR, et al: Positron emission tomography and breast masses: comparison with clinical mammographic and pathologic findings. *Ann Surg Oncol* 1(2):132–140, 1994

151. Kotz D: Scintimammography: magic bullet or false promise? *J Nucl Med* 36:15–20, 1995

152. Stuntz ME, Khalkhali I, Moss JF, et al: Breast imaging techniques and their application in breast disease. *Breast J* 1: 285–294, 1996

153. Waxman A, Nagaraj N, Ashok G, et al: Sensitivity and specificity of TC-99m meltoxy isobutal isonitrile (MIBI) in the evaluation of primary carcinoma of the breast: comparison of palpable and non-palpable lesions with mammography. *J Nucl Med* 35:22, 1994 (abstr)

154. Khalkhali I, Cutrone J, Mena I, et al: Scintimammography (SSM) versus mammography: the complementary role of TC-99 sestamibi prone breast imaging for the diagnosis of breast carcinoma. *Radiology* 196:421–426, 1995

155. Picolo S, Lastoria S, Mainolfi C, et al: Role of TC-99M. MDP scintigraphy in the diagnosis of primary breast cancer. *J Nucl Med* 35:22, 1994 (abstr)

156. Evans WP. Core biopsy: guns and needles. In DD Dershaw (ed), *Interventional Breast Procedures.* New York: Churchill Livingstone, 1996, pp 55–87

157. Rubin E, Simpson JF: *Breast Specimen Radiography.* Philadelphia, Lippincott-Raven, 1998

158. Bassett LW. Breast imaging, in Bland K, Copeland EM (eds): *The Breast: Comprehensive Management of Benign and Malignant Diseases* (ed 2). Philadelphia, Saunders, 1998, vol 1, pp 648–697

159. Elvecrog EL, Lechner MC, Nelson MJ: Nonpalpable breast lesions; correlations of stereotaxic large-core needle biopsy and surgical biopsy results. *Radiology* 188:453–455, 1993

160. Robinson DS, Sundaram MD. Stereotactic imaging and breast biopsy, in Bland K, Copeland EM (eds): *The Breast: Comprehensive Management of Benign and Malignant Diseases* (ed 2). Philadelphia, Saunders, 1998, pp 689–703

161. Dowlatshahi K, Danaher M, Snider H, et al: Diagnosis of non-palpable lesions by stereotaxic needle biopsy and interval mammography. *Proc Am Soc Clin Oncol* 12:A118, 1993 (abstr)

162. Silen W, Matory E, Love S (eds): *Atlas of Techniques in Breast Surgery.* Philadelphia, Lippincott-Raven, 1996

163. Lieberman L: Stereotaxic biopsy techniques, in Dershaw DD (ed): *Interventional Breast Procedures.* New York, Churchill-Livingstone, 1996, pp 129–153

164. Gisvold JJ, Goellner JR, Grant CS, et al: Breast biopsy: a comparative study of stereotaxically-guided core and excisional technique. *Am J Radiol* 162:815–820, 1994

165. Mikhael RA, Nathan RC, Weiss M, et al: Stereotactic core needle biopsy of mammographic breast lesions as a viable alternative to surgical biopsy. *Ann Surg Oncol* 1:363–367, 1994

166. Lieberman L, Fahs MC, Dershaw DD, et al: Impact of stereotactic core breast biopsy on cost of diagnosis. *Radiology* 195:633–637, 1995

167. Dershaw DD: Needle localization for breast biopsy, in Dershaw DD (ed): *Interventional Breast Procedures.* New York, Churchill-Livingstone, 1996, pp 129–153

168. Leis HP: Prognostic parameters for breast carcinoma, in Bland KI, Copeland EM (eds): *The Breast: Comprehensive*

Management of Benign and Malignant Disease. Philadelphia, Saunders, 1991, pp 331–346

169. Mambo NC, Gallagher HS: Carcinoma of the breast: the prognostic significance of extranodal extension of axillary disease. *Cancer* 39:2280–2285, 1977

170. Kinne DW: Staging and follow-up of breast cancer patients. *Cancer* 67:1196–1197, 1991

171. Donegan WL: Prognostic factors: stage and receptor status in breast cancer. *Cancer* 70:1755–1764, 1992

172. Nemoto T, Vana J, Bedwani RN, et al: Management and survival of female breast cancer: results of a national survey by the American College of Surgeons. *Cancer* 45:2917–2924, 1980

173. Carter CL, Allen C, Henson DE: Relation of tumor size, lymph node status, and survival in 24,740 breast cancer cases. *Cancer* 63:181–187, 1989

174. Rosen PP, Groshen S, Kinne DW, et al: Factors influencing prognosis in node-negative breast carcinoma analysis of 767 T1N0M0/T2N0M0 patients with long-term follow-up. *J Clin Oncol* 11:2090–2100, 1993

175. Senger DR, Van De Walter L, Brown LF, et al: Vascular permeability factor in tumor biology. *Cancer Metastasis Rev* 12:303–324, 1993

176. Linderholm B, Tavelin B, Grankvist K, et al: Vascular endothelial growth factor is of high prognostic value in node-negative breast carcinoma. *J Clin Oncol* 16: 3121–3128, 1998

177. Weidner N, Folkman J, Pozza F, et al: Tumor angiogenesis: a new significant and independent prognostic indicator in early-stage breast carcinoma. *J Natl Cancer Inst* 84:1875–1887, 1992

178. Gasparini G, Toi M, Miceli R, et al: Clinical relevance of vascular endothelial growth factor and Thymidine phosphorglase in patients with node-positive breast cancer treated with either adjuvant chemotherapy or hormone therapy. *Cancer J Sci Am* 5:101–111, 1999

179. Falette N, Paperin M, Treilleux I, et al: Prognostic value of P53 gene mutations in a large series of node-negative breast cancer patients. *Cancer Res* 58:1451–1455, 1998

180. Iacopetta B, Grieu F, Powell B, et al: Analysis of p53 gene mutation by polymerase chain reaction single strand conformation polymorphism provides independent prognostic information in node-negative breast cancer. *Clin Cancer Res* 4:1597–1602, 1998

181. Mehta RR, McDermott JH, Hieken TJ, et al: Plasma c-erbB-2 levels in breast cancer patients: prognostic significance in predicting response to chemotherapy. *J Clin Oncol* 16:2409–2416, 1998

182. Baselga J, Norton L, Albanell J, et al: Recombinant humanized anti-HER2 antibody (Herceptin™) enhances the antitumor activity of paclitaxel and doxorubicin against HER2/neu overexpressing human breast cancer xenografts. *Cancer Res* 58:2825–2839, 1998

183. Rochefort H, Capony F, Garcia M: Cathespin D in breast cancer: from molecular and cellular biology to clinical application. *Cancer Cells* 2:383–388, 1990

184. Isola J, Weitz S, Visakorpi T, et al: Cathepsin D expression detected by immunohistochemistry has independent prognostic value in axillary node-negative breast cancer. *J Clin Oncol* 11:36–43, 1993

185. Ravdin PM, Osborne CK: Breast cancer, in MacDonald JS, Haller DG, Mayer RJ (eds): *Manual of Oncologic Therapeutics* (ed 3). Philadelphia, Lippincott-Raven, 1995, pp 153–161

186. American Joint Committee on Cancer: *AJCC Cancer Staging Manual.* (5 ed). Philadelphia, Lippincott-Raven, 1997

187. Fisher B, Constantino J, Redmond C, et al: A randomized clinical trial evaluating tamoxifen in the treatment of patients with node-negative breast cancer who have estrogen receptor positive tumors. *N Engl J Med* 320:479–484, 1989

188. Bonadonna G: Conceptual and practice advances in the management of breast cancer: the David A. Karnofsky memorial lecture. *J Clin Oncol* 7:1380–1397, 1989

189. Bonadonna G, Valagussa P, Rossi A, et al: Ten year results with CMF-based adjuvant chemotherapy in resectable breast cancer. *Cancer Res Treat* 5:95–115, 1985

190. Moore MP, Kinne DW: The surgical management of primary invasive breast cancer. *CA Cancer J Clin* 45:279–289, 1995

191. Marcial A: Primary therapy for limited breast cancer. *Cancer* 65:2159–2164, 1990

192. Fremgen AM, Bland KI, McGinnis LS, et al: Clinical highlights from the National Cancer data base, 1999. *CA Cancer J Clin* 49:145–158, 1999

193. Hortobagyi GN: Treatment of breast cancer. *N Engl J Med* 339:974–984, 1998

194. Morris AD, Morris RD, Wilson JF, et al: Breast conserving therapy vs mastectomy in early stage breast cancer: a meta-analysis of 10 year survival. *Cancer J Sci Am* 3:6–12, 1997

195. Dooley WC: Surgery for breast cancer. *Current Opin Oncol* 10:504–512, 1998

196. Schover LR: The impact of breast cancer on sexuality, body image and intimate relationships. *CA Cancer J Clin* 4:112–119, 1991

197. Psychological Aspects of Breast Cancer Study Group: Psychological response to mastectomy: a prospective comparison study. *Cancer* 69:189–196, 1987

198. Vinokur AD, Threatt BA, Vinokur-Kaplann D, et al: The process of recovery from breast cancer for younger and older patients: changing during the first year. *Cancer* 65:1242–1254, 1990

199. Schover LR: Sexuality and body image in younger women with breast cancer. *Monogr Natl Cancer Inst* 16:177–182, 1994

200. Haffty BG, Ward B, Pathare P, et al: Reappraisal of the role of axillary lymph node dissection in the conservative treatment of breast cancer. *J Clin Oncol* 15:691–700, 1997

201. Giuliano AE, Jones RC, Brennan M, et al: Sentinal lymphadenectomy in breast cancer. *J Clin Oncol* 15:2345–2350, 1997

202. Albertini JJ, Lyman GH, Cox C, et al: Lymphatic mapping and sentinel node biopsy in the patient with breast cancer. *JAMA* 276:1818–1822, 1996

203. Hack TF, Cohen L, Katz J, et al: Physical and psychological morbidity after axillary lymph node dissection for breast cancer. *J Clin Oncol* 17:143–149, 1999

204. Maunsell E, Brisson J, Deschenes L: Arm problems and psychological distress after surgery for breast cancer. *Can J Surg* 36:315–320, 1993

205. Harris JR, Lippman ME, Marrow M, et al: *Diseases of the Breast.* Philadelphia, Lippincott-Raven, 1996, p 159

206. Fortin A, Larochelle M, Laverdiere J, et al: Local failure is responsible for the decrease in survival for patients with breast cancer treated with conservative surgery and postoperative radiotherapy. *J Clin Oncol* 17:101–109, 1999

207. Recht A, Come SE, Henderson JC, et al: The sequencing of chemotherapy and radiation therapy after conservative surgery for early stage breast cancer. *N Engl J Med* 334:1356–1364, 1996

208. Ragaz J, Jackson SM, Le N, et al: Adjuvant radiotherapy and chemotherapy in node positive premenopausal women with breast cancer. *N Engl J Med* 337:956–962, 1997

209. Overgaard M, Hansen PS, Overgaard J, et al: Postoperative

radiotherapy in high risk pre-menopausal women with breast cancer who receive adjuvant chemotherapy. *N Engl J Med* 337:949–955, 1997

210. Paszat LF, Mackillop WJ, Groome PA, et al: Mortality from myocardial infarction after adjuvant radiotherapy for breast cancer in the surveillance, epidemiology, and end-results cancer registries. *J Clin Oncol* 16:2625–2631, 1998

211. Brennan MJ, DePompolo RW, Garden FH: Focused review: postmastectomy lymphedema. *Arch Phys Med Rehabil* 77: S74–S80, 1996

212. Romestaing P, Lehingue Y, Carrie C, et al: Role of a 10-Gy boost in the conservative treatment of early breast cancer: results of a randomized clinical trial in Lyon, France. *J Clin Oncol* 15:963–968, 1997

213. Duffy MJ, Woods JE: Health risks of failed implants: a 30-year clinical experience. *Plast Reconstr Surg* 95:1129–1131, 1995

214. Olof N, Li Y, Staffan J, et al: Risk of connective tissue disease and related disorders among women with breast implants: a nation-wide retrospective cohort study in Sweden. *BMJ* 316:417–422, 1998

215. Berger K, Bostwick III J: *A Woman's Decision—Breast Care Treatment and Reconstruction (ed 2).* St. Louis, Quality Medical Printing, 1995

216. Mackay GJ, Bostwick III J: Breast reconstruction: reconstructive breast surgery, in Harris JR, Lippman ME, Morrow M, et al: *Diseases of the Breast.* Philadelphia, Lippincott-Raven, 1996, pp 601–619

217. Baker RR, Niederhubert J: Breast reconstruction, in Baker RR, Niederhuber J (eds): *The Operative Management of Breast Disease.* Philadelphia, Saunders, 1992, pp 117–129

218. Hugo NE, Sultan MR: Breast reconstruction, in Kinne DW (ed): *Multidisciplinary Atlas of Breast Surgery.* Philadelphia, Lippincott-Raven, 1998, pp 147–171

219. Fisher B, Constantino J, Redmond C, et al: Randomized clinical trial evaluating tamoxifen in the treatment of patients with node-negative breast cancer who have estrogen-receptor-positive tumors. *N Engl J Med* 320:479–484, 1989

220. Mansour EG, Gray R, Shatila AH, et al: Efficacy of adjuvant chemotherapy in high-risk node-negative breast cancer. *N Engl J Med* 320:485–490, 1989

221. Door FA (ed): Proceedings of the NIH Consensus Development Conference on Early Stage Breast Cancer. *Monogr Natl Cancer Inst* 1–9, 1990

222. Early Breast Cancer Trialists Collaborative Group: Systemic treatment of early breast cancer by hormonal cytoxic or immune therapy: Parts I and II. *N Engl J Med* 339:1–15, 71–85, 1992

223. Early Breast Cancer Trialists Collaborative Group: Tamoxifen for early breast cancer: an overview of the randomised trials. *Lancet* 351:1451–1467, 1998

224. Winchester DP: Adjuvant therapy for node-negative breast cancer. *Cancer* 67:1741–1743, 1991

225. Henderson IC, Berry D, Demetri G, et al: Improved disease-free and overall survival from the addition of sequential paclitaxel but not from the escalation of doxorubicin dose level in the adjuvant chemotherapy of patients with node-positive primary breast cancer. *Proc Am Soc Clin Oncol* 17: 101:390, 1998 (abstr)

226. Baselga J, Seidman AD, Rosen PP, et al: HER2 overexpression and paclitaxel sensitivity in breast cancer: therapeutic implications. *Oncology* 11:43–48, 1997 (suppl 2)

227. Slamon D, Leyland-Jones B, Shak S, et al: Addition of Herceptin to first-line chemotherapy for HER2 overexpressing metastatic breast cancer markedly increases anti-cancer activity: a randomized multinational controlled phase III trial. *Proc Am Soc Clin Oncol* 17:98a, 1998 (abstr)

228. Thor AD, Berry DA, Dubman DR, et al: ErbB-2, p53, and efficacy of adjuvant therapy in lymph node-positive breast cancer. *J Natl Cancer Inst* 90:1346–1360, 1998

229. Paik S, Bryant J, Park C, et al: erB-2 and response to doxorubicin in patients with axillary lymph node-positive, hormone receptor negative breast cancer. *J Natl Cancer Inst* 90:1361–1370, 1998

230. Brenin DR, Morrow M: Breast-conserving surgery in the neoadjuvant setting. *Semin Oncol* 25:13–18, 1998

231. Fisher B, Bryant J, Wolmark N, et al: Effect of preoperative chemotherapy on the outcome of women with operable breast cancer. *J Clin Oncol* 16:2672–2685, 1998

232. Duggan D: Local therapy of locally advanced breast cancer. *Oncology* 5:67–72, 1991

233. Carter CL, Allen C, Henson DE: Relation of tumor size, lymph node status and survival in 24,470 breast cancer cases. *Cancer* 63:181–187, 1989

234. Swain S, Lippman M: Systemic therapy of locally advanced breast cancer: review and guidelines. *Oncology* 3:21–28, 1989

235. Osborne CK, Clark GM, Ravdin P: Adjuvant systemic therapy of breast cancer, in Harris J, Lippman M, Morrow M (eds): *Diseases of the Breast.* Philadelphia, Lippincott-Raven, 1996, pp 548–578

236. Hortobagyi GN, Buzdar AN: Locally advanced breast cancer: a review including the M.D. Anderson experience, in Ragaz T, Ariel T (eds): *High Risk Breast Cancer.* Berlin-Heidelberg, Springer Verlag, 1991, pp 382–413

237. Rahman ZU, Frye DK, Buzdar AU, et al: Impact of selection process on response rate and long term survival of potential high-dose chemotherapy candidates treated with standard-dose doxorubicin containing chemotherapy in patients with metastatic breast cancer. *J Clin Oncol* 15: 3171–3177, 1997

238. Tallman MS, Rademaker AW, Jahnke L, et al: High dose chemotherapy, autologus bone marrow or stem cell transplantation and posttransplant consolidation in patients with advanced breast cancer. *Bone Marrow Transplant* 20: 721–729, 1997

239. Honig SF: Hormonal therapy and chemotherapy, in Harris JR, Lippman ME, Morrow M, Hellman S (eds): *Diseases of the Breast.* Philadelphia, Lippincott-Raven, 1996, pp 669–718

240. Press MF, Bernstein L, Thomas PA, et al: HER-2/neu gene amplification characterized by fluorescence in situ hybridization: poor prognosis in node-negative breast carcinomas. *J Clin Oncol* 15:2894–2904, 1997

241. Boring CC, Squires TS, Heath CW: Cancer statistics for African-Americans. *CA Cancer J Clin* 42:7–14, 1992

242. Ries LA, Kosary CL, Hankey BF, et al: *SEER Cancer Statistics Review. 1973–1994 (NIH Pub. No. 97-2789).* Bethesda, MD, National Cancer Institute, 1997

243. Elledge RM, Clark GM, Chamnes GC, et al: Tumor biologic factors and breast cancer prognosis among white, Hispanic, and black women in the United States. *Int J Cancer* 86:705–709, 1994

244. Phillips JM, Cohen MZ, Moses G: Breast cancer screening and African American women: fear, fatalism, and silence. *Oncol Nurs Forum* 26:561–571, 1999

245. Canellos GB: Systemic therapy of breast cancer. *Med J Aust* 148:88–91, 1988

246. Vogel CL, Nabholtz JM: Monotherapy of metastatic breast cancer: a review of newer agents. *Oncologist* 4:17–33, 1999

247. Blum J, Buzdar A, LoRusso P, et al: A multicenter phase II trial of Zeloda (capecitabine) in paclitaxel-refractory metastatic breast cancer. *Proc Am Soc Clin Oncol* 17:125a, 1998 (abstr)

248. Hortobagyi GN, Theriault RL, Porter L, et al: Efficacy of pamidronate in reducing skeletal complications in patients with breast cancer and lytic bone metastases. *N Engl J Med* 335:1785–1791, 1996

249. Powles TJ, McCloskey E, Paterson AH, et al: Oral clodronate and reduction in loss of bone mineral density in women with operal primary breast cancer. *J Natl Cancer Inst* 90:704–708, 1998

250. Pyrhonen S, Valavaara R, Modig H, et al: Comparison of toremifene and tamoxifen in post-menopausal patients with advanced breast cancer: a randomized double-blind, the 'nordic' phase III study. *Br J Cancer* 76:270–277, 1997

251. Gershanovich M, Garin A, Baltina D, et al: A phase III comparison of two toremifene doses to tamoxifen in post-menopausal women with advanced breast cancer. *Breast Cancer Res Treat* 45:251–262, 1997

252. Fornander T, Rutquist LE, Wilking N: Effects of tamoxifen on the female genital tract. *Ann NY Acad Sci* 622:469–476, 1991

253. Jordan VC, Assikis VJ: Endometrial carcinoma and tamoxifen: clearing up a controversy. *Clin Cancer Res* 1:467–472, 1996

254. Longstaff S, Siguardsson H, O'Keeffe M, et al: A controlled study of the ocular effects of tamoxifen in conventional dosage in the treatment of breast carcinoma. *Eur J Cancer* 25:1805–1808, 1989

255. Plourde PV, Dyroff M, Dowsett M, et al: Arimidex: a new oral, once a day aromatase inhibitor: *Steroid Biochem Molec Biol* 53:175–179, 1995

256. Hortobagyi BN, Buzdar AU: Anastrozole (Arimidex), a new aromatase inhibitor for advanced breast cancer: mechanism of action and role in management. *Cancer Invest* 16:385–390, 1998

257. Cancer.org/statistics/99bcff/who.html Accessed 2/6/00

258. Rosenblatt K, Thomas D, McTiernan A, et al: Breast cancer in men: aspects of familial aggregation. *J Natl Cancer Inst* 83:849–853, 1991

259. Donegan WL: Cancer of the breast in men. *CA Cancer J Clin* 41:339–352, 1991

260. Thomas DB, Jiminez LM, McTiernan A, et al: Breast cancer in men: risk factors with hormonal implications. *Am J Epidemiol* 135:734–739, 1992

261. Evans DB, Crichlow RW: Carcinoma of the male breast and Klinefelter's syndrome: is there an association? *CA Cancer J Clin* 37:246–251, 1987

262. Patel HZ, Buzdar AU, Hortobagi GN: Role of adjuvant chemotherapy in male breast cancer. *Cancer* 64:1583–1585, 1989

263. U.S. Congress Office of Technology Assessment: *The Menopause, Hormone Therapy and Women's Health.* Washington, DC, U.S. Government Printing Office, May 1992

264. Goodman M: Menopausal symptoms, in Groenwald SL, Frogge MH, Goodman M, Yarbro CH (eds): *Cancer Symptom Management.* Sudbury, MA, Jones and Bartlett, 1996, pp 77–93

265. Bergmans M, Merkos J, Corbey R, et al: Effect of bellargel regard on climacteric complaints: a double blind placebo controlled study. *Maturitas* 9:227–234, 1987

266. Magamani M, Kelver M, Smith E: Treatment of menopausal hot flashes with transdermal administration of Clonidine. *Am J Obstet Gynecol* 156:561–565, 1987

267. Loprinzi CL, Pisansky TM, Fonseca R, et al: A pilot evaluation of venlafaxine HCl for the therapy of hot flashes in cancer survivors. *J Clin Oncol* 16:2377–2381, 1998

268. Cobleigh MA: Hormone replacement therapy in breast cancer survivors. *Diseases of the Breast: Updates* Lippincott-Raven, Philadelphia, 1:1–12, 1997

269. Knobf MT: Natural menopause and ovarian toxicity associated with breast cancer therapy. *Oncol Nurs Forum* 25:1519–1527, 1998

270. Goodman M: Menopausal symptoms in Yarbro CH, Frogge MH, Goodman M (eds): *Cancer Symptom Management* (ed 2). Sudbury, MA, Jones and Bartlett, 1999, pp 95–111

271. Ganz P, Rowland JH, Desmond K: Life after breast cancer: understandng women's health-related quality of life and sexual functioning. *J Clin Oncol* 16:501–514, 1998

272. Grindel CG, Cahill CA, Walker A: Food intake of women with breast cancer during the first 6 months of chemotherapy. *Oncol Nurs Forum* 16:401–407, 1989

273. Goodwin PJ, Ennis M, Pritchard KI: Adjuvant treatment and onset of menopause predict weight gain after breast cancer diagnosis. *J Clin Oncol* 17:120–129, 1999

274. Kumar NB, Allen K, Cantor A, et al: Weight gain associated with adjuvant tamoxifen therapy in stage I and II breast cancer: fact or artifact? *Breast Cancer Res Treat* 44:135–143, 1997

275. Knobf MT: Physical and psychological distress associated with adjuvant chemotherapy in women with breast cancer. *J Clin Oncol* 4:678–684, 1986

276. Knobf M, Mullen J, Xistris D, et al: Weight gain in women with breast cancer receiving adjuvant chemotherapy. *Oncol Nurs Forum* 10:28–33, 1983

277. Woo B, Dibble SL, Piper BF, et al: Differences in fatigue by treatment methods in women with breast cancer. *Oncol Nurs Forum* 25:915–920, 1998

278. Maunsell E, Brisson J, and Deschenes L: Arm problems and psychological distress after surgery for breast cancer. *Can J Surg* 36:315–320, 1992

279. Kalinowski B: Lymphedema, in Yarbro CH, Frogge MH, Goodman M (eds): *Cancer Symptom Management* (ed 2). Sudbury, MA, Jones and Bartlett, 1999, pp 457–486

280. Tasmuth T, Von Smitten K, Hietanen P, et al: Pain and other symptoms after different treatment modalities of breast cancer. *Ann Oncol* 6:453–459, 1995

281. Hack TF, Cohen L, Katz J, et al. Physical and psychological morbidity after axillary lymph node dissection for breast cancer. *J Clin Oncol* 17:143–149, 1999

282. Larsen D, Weinstein M, Goldberg I, et al: Edema of the arm as a function of the extent of axillary surgery in patients treated with stage I-II carcinoma of the breast treated with primary radiotherapy. *Int J Radiat Oncol Biol Phys* 16:1575–1582, 1986

283. Pillion M: Commentary: the physical therapist's role in treating lymphedema. *Oncol Nurs Forum* 26:508–509, 1999

284. Wolter J: Support programs, in Harris JR, Lippman M, Morrow M, Hellman S (eds): *Diseases of the Breast.* Philadelphia, Lippincott-Raven, 1996, pp 948–951

285. Katz AH, Maida CA: Health and disability self-help organizations, in Powell TJ (ed): *Working with Self-help.* Silver Springs, MD, National Association of Social Workers, 1990, pp 141–155

286. Cella DF, Yellen SB: Cancer support groups: the state of the art. *Cancer Prac* 1:56–61, 1993

287. Riessman F, Carroll D: Self-help and the new health agenda, in Reismann F, Caroll D (eds): *Redefining Self-help.* San Francisco, Josey Bass, 1995, pp 83–108

CHAPTER 49

Central Nervous System Cancers

Karen Belford, RN, MS, AOCN, CCRN

Introduction

Cancer of the central nervous system (CNS) includes primary and metastatic tumors of the brain and spinal cord. The incidence of these tumors is thought to be increasing, particularly metastatic tumors. CNS cancers are not uncommon and are associated with significant morbidity and mortality. Whether benign or malignant, primary or secondary, CNS tumors can drastically affect an individual's life and impede the ability to function. Knowledge of the various tumor types and their differences, associated neuroanatomy and neurophysiology, and the many issues related to treatment is essential to provide accurate assessment, ongoing intervention, and supportive management for these individuals.

BRAIN TUMORS

Epidemiology

Primary CNS cancers represent approximately 2% of all reported malignancies. An estimated 34,345 new cases of primary benign and malignant brain tumors were expected to be diagnosed in the United States in 1998.[1] Of these brain tumors, an estimated 17,400 will be malignant.[2] However, any intracranial tumor, regardless of its histological behavior, can potentially invade and displace critical areas of the brain causing devastating effects. Brain tumors are found in persons of all ages, with a peak incidence occurring in the first, fifth, sixth, and seventh decades. The incidence is slightly higher in men than in women with the exception of meningiomas, which occur more often in women. Brain cancer is the second most common cancer diagnosed in children, second only to leukemia.

Malignant CNS tumors are responsible for approximately 2.5% of all cancer-related deaths. An estimated 13,300 deaths in 1998 were attributed to primary malignant brain and other nervous system tumors.[2] The majority of these deaths result from malignant gliomas. In women age 15–34, CNS neoplasms are the fourth-leading cause of cancer mortality. In men age 15–34 they are the third, and in men age 35–54 years, CNS cancers are the fourth-leading cause of cancer-related mortality.[2] Most intracranial tumors, however, occur in individuals older than age 45.[3] Over the past three decades, the incidence of primary brain tumors appears to have increased in the elderly.[4] The average age of onset of glioblastoma and meningioma is approximately 62. The increasing incidence of most types of brain tumors with age could result from the length of exposure required for cells to become malignant or to an aging immune system's decreasing ability to protect against disease. It also may be attributed to possible environmental carcinogens found in industrialized nations, improved diagnostic capabilities, better access to specialized care, changing attitudes toward the care of the elderly, medical support programs,[5] and the increasing size of the elderly population.[4] The increased incidence is truly established only for primary central nervous system lymphoma (PCNSL).

Historically, it has been difficult to estimate the true epidemiology of CNS tumors. Fifteen cell types can potentially give rise to CNS tumors[3] and many of these tumors consist of more than one cell type. The most common primary brain tumor is the malignant glioma, accounting for more than half of all primary CNS cancers. The most prevalent CNS malignancy is the metastatic brain tumor, which is increasing in frequency and occurs ten times more often than primary brain tumors. Brain metastasis is the most common structural neurological complication of systemic cancer.[6]

Etiology

Genetic Factors

Specific causes and risk factors for CNS tumors have not been identified. Fewer than 5% of CNS tumors are associated with specific genetic disorders. The National Familial Brain Tumor Registry seeks to document that some brain tumors can occur as a familial disorder and thereby gain further insight into the etiology of these tumors by evaluating affected families.[7] Individuals with specific autosomal dominant disorders (i.e., neurofibromatosis, tuberous sclerosis, Li-Fraumeni syndrome, Turcot syndrome, and von Hippel-Lindau disease) have a higher incidence of brain tumors than the general population.

Neurofibromatosis type 1 (NF-1), also called von Recklinghausen's disease, occurs in 1 out of 3000 individuals.[8] The most common brain tumors associated with NF-1 are optic nerve gliomas, astrocytomas, ependymomas, meningiomas, and neurofibromas, reported in 4%–45% of individuals with NF-1.[9,10] Neurofibromatosis type 2 (NF-2) occurs less frequently and is characterized by an increased incidence of schwannomas, meningiomas, ependymomas, and astrocytomas.[9,11] Tuberous sclerosis, or Bourneville disease, has a reported incidence of one in 10,000 to one in 50,000. Approximately one-half of individuals with the disorder develop subependymal giant cell astrocytomas.[12] The Li-Fraumeni syndrome has been studied in more than 100 families and is associated with an increased incidence of many different types of cancer including astrocytomas and primitive neuroectodermal tumors (PNETs).[11] Gliomas, medulloblastomas, and pituitary adenomas have been observed in individuals with Turcot syndrome, a syndrome of CNS tumors in individuals with adenomatous polyposis coli (APC). Approximately 5% of families with APC have this syndrome.[8] Finally, those with von Hippel-Lindau disease are at risk for developing cerebellar hemangioblastomas.[13]

As with other cancers, CNS tumor pathogenesis is a multistep process in which tumor suppressor gene inactivation and oncogene activation and overexpression play a part, along with alterations in cell cycle progression, abnormalities in signal transduction pathways, glial cell invasion, and angiogenesis.[11] Genetic changes during the pathogenesis of CNS tumors can occur either at the chromosomal level or at the gene expression level. The changes at the genetic level can result from the loss of a major portion of a chromosome or from mutations within a single gene.[14] In astrocytic tumors, abnormalities have been identified, frequently involving various chromosomes.[11,15] Recent advances in molecular biology have identified both the expression of activated oncogenes and the inactivation of tumor-suppressor genes in a variety of brain tumors.[16] The *p53* tumor suppressor gene is frequently altered and is implicated in both the initiation and progression of astrocytic tumors.[14] Growth factors also appear to be involved in the pathogenesis of astrocytomas. Mutation of growth factors or their receptors may result in tumor cell proliferation and transformation. These include epidermal growth factor receptor (EGFR), which is amplified in glioblastoma patients, and platelet-derived growth factor receptor (PDGFR), which is overexpressed in astrocytomas. Vascular endothelial growth factor (VEGF) is overexpressed in malignant gliomas and can induce angiogenesis, which is an important factor in CNS tumor growth.

Chemical and Environmental Factors

Although many chemicals are carcinogenic in animals and produce brain tumors, the possible association of chemical exposure and brain tumors has not been established and is limited to a few occupations. Agricultural workers exposed to multiple chemicals in pesticides, herbicides, and fertilizers have had a higher than expected incidence of gliomas.[16,17] Several studies suggest a relationship between brain tumors and such industries as synthetic rubber, petrochemical, aeronautics, and nuclear energy.[18,19] Increased risk of gliomas and meningiomas has been associated with precision metal work.[16,20] Workers exposed to polyvinyl chloride may be at increased risk for gliomas. Other substances that may be implicated in the development of brain tumors are organic solvents, phenols, formalin, polycyclic aromatic hydrocarbons, and N-nitroso compounds.[16,18,21]

Viral Factors

Viruses have been directly implicated in the development of CNS tumors in animals. However, individuals with acquired immune deficiency syndrome (AIDS)-related PCNSL have been found to have a high rate of infection with the Epstein-Barr virus (EBV), and evidence of EBV has been isolated from the tumor tissue. It is not understood why PCNSL is often associated with acquired immunosuppression. Individuals with human immunodeficiency virus (HIV) have an increased risk for developing PCNSL[22] and possibly gliomas.[23]

Radiation

Therapeutic irradiation of the head has been linked to the subsequent appearance of brain tumors. This has been seen in individuals who have received radiation therapy (RT) during childhood for treatment of acute lymphoblastic leukemia[24] and tinea capitis[25] and in adults who have received cranial irradiation for treatment of pituitary adenomas.[26,27] An increased incidence of tumors, including PCNSL, has been found following immunosuppressive therapy.[28]

Electromagnetic Fields

Although disputed, epidemiological studies have suggested a possible association between exposure to extremely low-frequency electromagnetic fields (ELF-EMFs) and increased incidence of cancer.[29] While empirical evidence is inconsistent, several occupational studies have suggested a higher than expected incidence of brain tumors, specifically gliomas, among electricians, electronics and communications workers,[16,30] railway workers, and welders.[31] Occupational exposure may be just a fraction of the total ELF-EMF exposure. Exposure to ELF-EMFs is almost universal today in industrialized nations. Other ELF-EMF sources outside the workplace include residential heating, electrical appliances in the home, hand-held radios, cellular telephones, electric power lines, and transformers. Residential studies have focused primarily on ELF-EMFs and the two most common cancers in children—leukemia and brain tumors. While the evidence has been inconsistent, recent studies do not show that EMFs in residential settings increase the risk of brain tumors.[32,33]

Pathophysiology

Anatomy and physiology

The nervous system contains two types of cells: neurons and glial cells. The neurons are the basic anatomic and functional unit of the nervous system. The glial cells provide structural support, nourishment, and protection for the neurons. Approximately 40% of the brain and spinal cord is composed of glial cells. In the CNS, glial cells are subdivided into four main types: astrocytes, oligodendrocytes, ependymal cells, and microglia. In the peripheral nervous system (PNS), Schwann cells form myelin sheaths.[34] Unlike neurons, glial cells in the adult nervous system retain their capacity to divide. They can undergo anaplasia and are the major source of primary tumors of the CNS. The specific tumor type is derived from the glial cell of origin. For example, astrocytomas arise from astrocytes, and ependymomas arise from ependymal cells.

The brain is divided into three main areas: the cerebrum, the brain stem, and the cerebellum. The cerebrum contains the two cerebral hemispheres and the diencephalon. The cerebral hemispheres are connected by a large area of white matter, the corpus callosum, which allows each portion of one hemisphere to connect with its corresponding portion of the other hemisphere. It essentially allows communication between the two hemi-

spheres.[35] Each cerebral hemisphere is divided into four lobes: frontal, parietal, temporal, and occipital (Figure 49-1). The diencephalon is composed of the thalamus, hypothalamus, and basal ganglia. The pituitary gland is connected to the hypothalamus. The brain stem is made up of the midbrain, pons, and medulla. The cerebellum has two hemispheres and is connected to the brain stem by the cerebellar peduncles. The functions of these areas are listed in Table 49-1.[36,37]

Cranial nerves. The 12 pairs of cranial nerves (CNs) are part of the PNS. They have fiber pathways entering and exiting the brain. Cranial nerves I and II are located in the cerebral hemispheres, cranial nerves III and IV in the midbrain, cranial nerves V–VIII in the pons, and cranial nerves IX–XII in the medulla (Figure 49-2). They are responsible for motor and sensory function of the head and neck; their functions are listed in Table 49-2. Symptoms of cranial nerve dysfunction (cranial nerve palsy) can provide valuable information for localizing an intracranial tumor.

Meninges. The meninges are the membranes covering the brain and spinal cord. The cranial meninges are shown in Figure 49-3. There are three layers of meninges: the dura mater, arachnoid, and pia mater. The outermost layer, the dura mater, lines the interior of the skull. The outer layer of the dura is the periosteum of the cranial bone.[34] There is a potential space between the dura and the skull called the *epidural space*. The inner dural layer extends throughout the skull and folds in on itself to create anatomic compartments. The falx cerebri, the tentorium cerebelli, and the falx cerebelli are three such folds. The falx cerebri, a double fold of dura, descends vertically between the two cerebral hemispheres

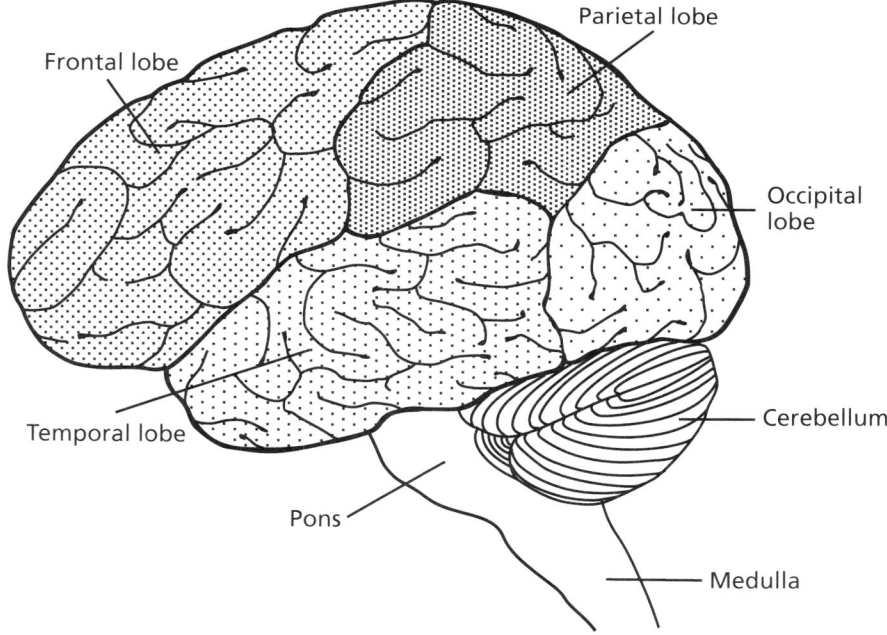

Figure 49-1 Lobes of the cerebral hemispheres.

Frontal lobe

Parietal lobe

Occipital lobe

Temporal lobe

Cerebellum

Pons

Medulla

Table 49-1 Clinical Manifestations of Intracranial Tumors

Location	Function	Abnormality

Frontal lobes	Intellect
	Personality
	Judgment
	Abstract thinking
	Mood and affect
	Long-term memory
	Voluntary motor activity (contralateral)
	Secondary urinary control
	Language expression (dominant side)
		Intellectual deterioration
		Personality changes
		Impaired judgment
		Emotional lability, flat affect
		Memory loss
		Muscle weakness or paralysis
		  Babinski's sign
		  Increased deep tendon reflexes
		Incontinence
		Expressive aphasia (Broca's aphasia)
		Seizures

Parietal lobes	Sensory integration (contralateral) Sensory interpretation (contralateral) Ability to carry out and understand special constructs	Decrease or loss of sensation (pain, temperature, pinprick, light touch, proprioception, vibration, two-point discrimination, stereognosis, graphesthesia) Inability to write, calculate Construction apraxia Seizures
Temporal lobes	Hearing Short-term memory Language comprehension (dominant side) Interpretation of memory Emotion	Hearing changes, hallucinations Memory loss Receptive aphasia (Wernicke's aphasia) Intellectual impairment Emotional lability Seizures
Occipital lobes	Vision Visual interpretation	Visual field defects (contralateral homonymous hemianopsia), blindness Hallucinations Inability to identify objects or symbols or meaning of written words Seizures
Thalamus	Sensory relay station Conscious awareness of pain Sleep–wake cycle Focusing of attention Emotion	Sensory abnormality Neuropathic pain Inattentiveness Emotional lability Hydrocephalus, increased ICP
Hypothalamus	Coordination of autonomic nervous system function Temperature regulation Regulation of water metabolism Regulation of hormone secretions Regulation of appetite Control of thirst center Regulation of part of sleep–wake cycle Mediation of affective and sexual behavior	Abnormalities in sweating, vasodilation, hypotonia, pulse Hypo or hyperthermia Abnormalities in absorption of free water Endocrine dysfunction Increase or decrease appetite Increase or decrease thirst Flat affect Emotional lability
Basal ganglia	Fine motor control	Weakness or paralysis Intention tremors, Parkinsonism

Brain stem
  midbrain
  pons
  medulla
	Point of origin for cranial nerves III through XII
	Vital reflex centers
	Maintenance of consciousness
		Cranial nerve dysfunction
		Abnormalities of reflex activities (heart rate, respirations, blood pressure, coughing, sneezing, swallowing, vomiting)
		Change in level of consciousness

Cerebellum	Coordination Fine motor control Balance (ipsilateral)	Ataxia, dysarthria Action tremor, nystagmus, Loss of balance, wide-based gait Hydrocephalus

Modified from Wegmann JA.[37]

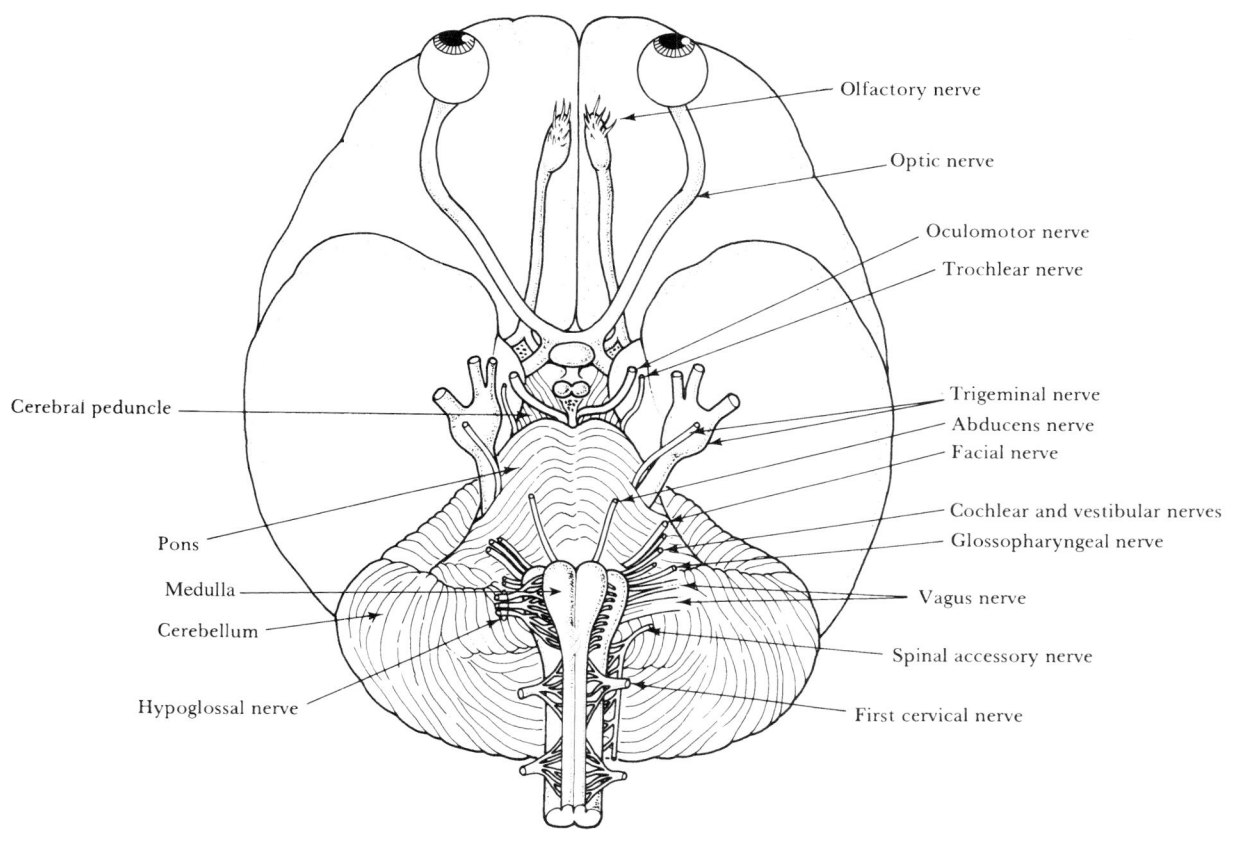

Figure 49-2 Cranial nerves from the base of the brain. (Modified from Wegmann JA).[37]

to partially separate the two hemispheres. The tentorium cerebelli, a tentlike double fold of dura running between the occipital lobes of the cerebrum and the cerebellum, divides the skull into the supratentorial space and the infratentorial space. Structures and tumors that lie above the tentorium (cerebral hemispheres, diencephalon, and basal ganglia) are located in the supratentorial compartment, and those lying below the tentorium (cerebellum and brain stem) are in the infratentorial compartment, also known as the posterior fossa (Figure 49-4).[37] An opening in the tentorium—the tentorial notch—allows the brain stem, blood vessels, and nerves to pass through the tentorium. A third fold of dura, the falx cerebelli, separates the two lobes of the cerebellum.

The middle meningeal layer, the arachnoid, is a thin, delicate, transparent membrane that loosely surrounds the brain. There is a potential space between the dura and the arachnoid—the subdural space—which is a common site of hematomas. The pia mater is the innermost meningeal layer. It is a meshlike, vascular membrane that adheres directly to the surface of the brain, dipping down between the convolutions of the brain surface. The pia mater and the arachnoid together are referred to as the *leptomeninges*. The space between the arachnoid and the pia mater, the subarachnoid space, is where cerebrospinal fluid (CSF) circulates.

Ventricular system. The ventricular system consists of a series of interconnected chambers and pathways responsible for the production and circulation of CSF around the brain and spinal cord (Figure 49-5).[38] The majority of CSF is formed in the choroid plexuses. Approximately 20–25 mL of CSF are produced hourly, and the volume of CSF found in the ventricular system at any one time is 125–150 mL. There are expanded areas of the subarachnoid space called *cisterns* where CSF may be aspirated. The major cisterns are the cisterna magnum, located between the medulla and the cerebellar region, and the lumbar cistern, between vertebrae L-2 and S-2.[34]

Cerebrovascular circulation. The cerebral arterial circulation is the body's most complex vascular network. The brain receives approximately 20% of the body's resting cardiac output. This large amount of blood flow reflects the brain's tremendous metabolic requirements, particularly for oxygen and glucose.[39] An adequate cerebral blood flow (CBF) is necessary to deliver oxygen, glucose, and other nutrients to the brain, and to remove carbon

Table 49-2 Examination of Cranial Nerves

Cranial Nerve	Major Function	Method of Testing	Desired Response
I. Olfactory	Smell	Inhalation of commonly recognized aromatic substance such as cloves; avoid use of ammonia or alcohol as these stimulate the trigeminal nerve and evoke a pain response	Correct identification of the substance with each nostril
II. Optic	Vision	Direct ophthalmoscopy; use finger movement and eye charts to test visual acuity and fields	Note the appearance of the optic disc, vessels, and retina; correct eye movement and chart identification with each eye separately
III. Oculomotor	Movement of eyes in four of the six cardinal directions of gaze (inward, upward, downward, and outward); pupillary constriction and accommodation; elevation of upper eyelid	Individual follows the examiner's finger with the eyes while not moving head to test eye movement; check pupil response to light; observe for ptosis of the eyelid	Movement of eyes should be equal in the cardinal directions of gaze; pupils react equally and briskly to light; consensual response and accommodation to light is present; eyes are symmetrical at rest and move conjugately
IV. Trochlear	Movements of eyes (downward and inward)	Individual follows the examiner's finger with the eyes to test eye movement	Movement of eyes should be equal
V. Trigeminal	Muscles of mastication and eardrum tension; general sensations from anterior half of head including face, nose, mouth	Individual clamps the jaw, opens the mouth against resistance and masticates to check motor division of the nerve; touch both sides of the person's face, checking for pain, touch, and temperature response; gently touch the person's cornea with a cotton wisp to check the corneal reflex	Jaw movement is strong and symmetrical; correct identification of sensations; rapid blinking
VI. Abducens	Lateral movement of eyes	Individual follows the examiner's finger to test eye movement (oculomotor, trochlear, and abducens are tested together)	Movement of eyes should be equal
VII. Facial	Muscles of facial expression and tension on ear bones; lacrimation and salivation; taste to anterior two-thirds of tongue	Observe for facial symmetry and the individual's ability to contract muscles to check motor division; individual tastes sweet, sour, salty, and acidic flavor	Individual smiles, frowns, wrinkles nose and brow, closes eyes tightly with symmetry; correct identification of tastes
VIII. Acoustic (cochlear and vestibular)	Hearing; balance and equilibrium	Test hearing ability with the use of whispered voice and tuning fork at various distances from the ear to check the cochlear nerve; check the vestibular nerve by having the individual stand on one foot with eyes closed	Recognition of sound; maintenance of balance
IX. Glossopharyngeal	Gag and swallowing, salivation, taste to posterior third of tongue	Have individual say "ah"; check the gag reflex by touching the pharynx with a tongue depressor; have individual taste different flavors	Soft palate and uvula elevate in the midline; gag response is present; correct identification of tastes
X. Vagus	Gag and swallowing, laryngeal control, parasympathetic to thoracic and abdominal viscera	Check the individual's swallowing ability; ask individual to cough and speak; glossopharygeal and vagus nerves are examined together because of overlapping innervation of the pharynx	No dysphagia present; speak without hoarseness or weakness
XI. Spinal accessory	Movement of head and shoulders	Ask the individual to elevate the shoulders, turn the head, and resist the examiner's attempts to pull the chin back to midline; check the symmetry of the trapezius and sternocleidomastoid muscles	Equal bilateral strength; atrophy may indicate nerve dysfunction
XII. Hypoglossal	Movement of tongue	Ask the individual to protrude the tongue and move from side to side and up and down	Absence of deviations atrophy, or tremors

Modified from Wegmann JA.[37]

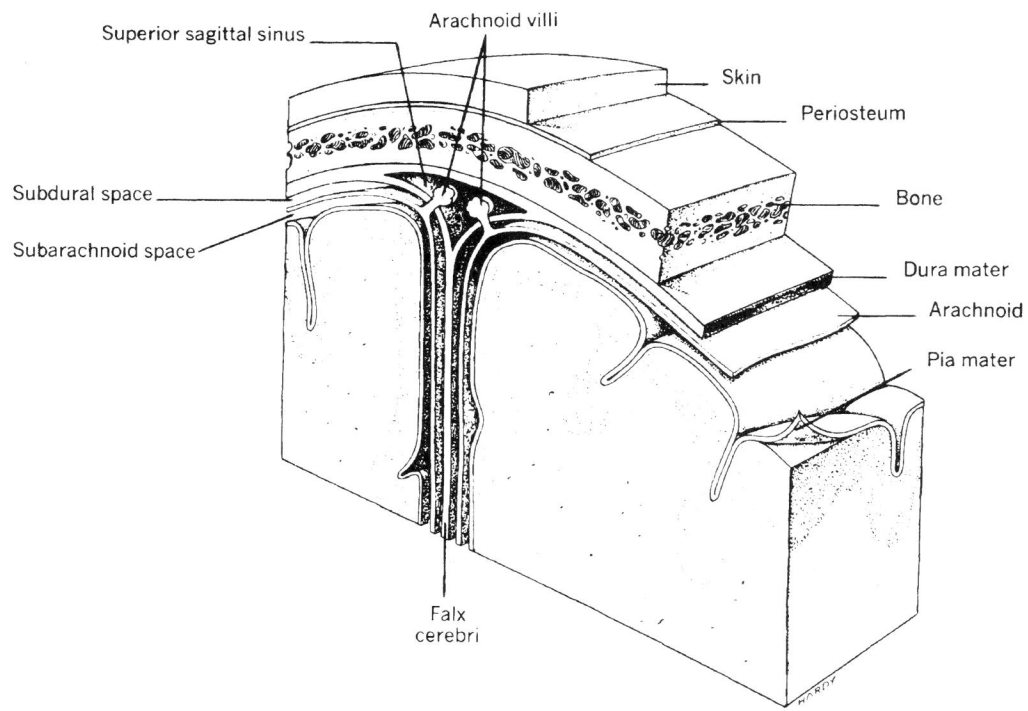

Figure 49-3 The cranial meninges. (Reprinted with permission from Hickey JV: Overview of neuroanatomy and neurophysiology, in Hickey JV (ed): *The Clinical Practice of Neurological and Neurosurgical Nursing* (ed 4). Philadelphia, Lippincott, 1997, pp 35–79.[34] Originally published in Chaffee EE, Lytle IM: *Basic Physiology and Anatomy*. Philadelphia, Lippincott, 1980).[36]

dioxide and other metabolic products from the brain. The CBF must remain relatively constant because the CNS has little ability to store oxygen and glucose in its tissue. A brief circulation failure may result in temporary or permanent loss of neurological function.

Blood flow to the brain is supplied by the two internal carotid arteries (anterior circulation) and the two vertebral arteries (posterior circulation). The internal carotids bifurcate to form the anterior and middle cerebral arteries, which supply blood to the frontal, temporal, and parietal lobes. They also have subdivisions, which supply the basal ganglia and part of the diencephalon. The vertebral arteries enter the base of the skull through the foramen magnum and unite to form the basilar artery, which subdivides into the posterior cerebral arteries. The vertebral arteries and their branches supply the cerebellum, the brain stem, the spinal cord, the occipital lobes, the inferior and medial aspects of the temporal lobes, and a portion of the diencephalon.[34] These major vessels become interconnected at the circle of Willis. An intact circle of Willis (Figure 49-6) may provide collateral circulation to the brain.

The cerebral venous circulation consists of veins located on the surface of the brain and vascular channels or sinuses located between the two dural layers. The superior sagital sinus is one of the dural venous sinuses and is a major site of CSF reabsorption. The cerebral veins drain into the cerebral sinuses, empty into the jugular veins,

and return blood to the heart. Obstruction of venous outflow can result in increased intracranial pressure (ICP).

Physiology of Intracranial Pressure

ICP is the pressure exerted within the skull and meninges by brain tissue, CSF, and cerebral blood volume (CBV). The skull and meninges form a rigid compartment holding these three major components: brain tissue (comprising 80% of the total volume), CSF (constituting 10%), and the blood volume (accounting for the remaining 10%). According to the Monro-Kellie hypothesis, the rigid vault formed by the skull and meninges is filled to capacity with essentially noncompressible contents, which remain relatively constant, and therefore is unyielding to any increases in volume. If any one component increases in volume, a concomitant decrease in the volume of one or both of the remaining components must occur to maintain normal ICP. If the reciprocal compensation does not occur, ICP rises. The normal ICP is 0–15 mm Hg or 80–180 cm H_2O.

The mechanism by which this secondary decrease in volume occurs is called *compensation*. Brain tumors increase the brain mass, and often the accompanying edema can further increase the volume. To maintain a normal ICP, the compensatory mechanisms reduce the

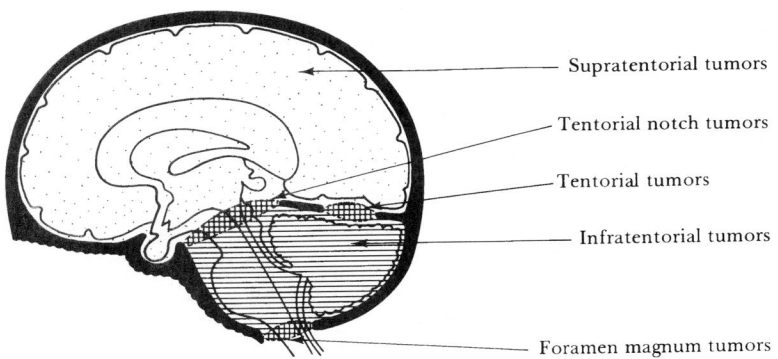

(a) Diagrammatic midsagittal section

Figure 49-4 Localization of intracranial tumors.

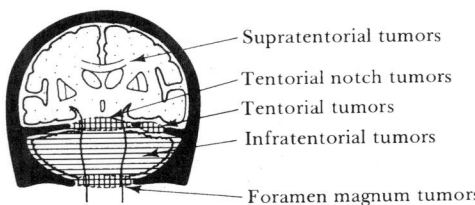

(b) Diagrammatic coronal section

amount of CSF, blood volume, or both. The volume of CSF is decreased by displacing CSF from the cranial subarachnoid space to the spinal subarachnoid space, and by increasing the amount of CSF absorbed into the venous circulation by the arachnoid villi. When ICP is elevated for prolonged periods, the choroid plexuses can decrease the amount of CSF they produce. The CBV decreases by shunting the venous blood away from the affected area into the venous sinuses. These compensatory mechanisms are finite and eventually become exhausted. Once all the compensatory mechanisms are depleted, relatively small increases in volume result in large increases in ICP.

Small volume increments can be compensated far more readily than large volume increments. Increases in volume made over long periods can be accommodated more easily than a comparable quantity introduced within a much shorter interval. An individual with an acute subdural hematoma, a rapidly enlarging lesion, will develop signs and symptoms of increased ICP much more rapidly than a person with a large, slow-growing, low-grade brain tumor. The individual with the slow-growing tumor may not exhibit clinical signs and symptoms until the compensatory mechanisms have been exhausted.

Another important concept relating to ICP is autoregulation, which provides a constant cerebral blood flow (CBF) despite fluctuations in systemic arterial pressure (SAP) by adjusting the diameter of blood vessels. However, when the SAP falls below 60 mm Hg or above 160 mm Hg, or when ICP is sustained above 30 mm Hg, the autoregulatory mechanisms fail and the CBF becomes passively dependent on changes in SAP.[40,41]

The autoregulatory mechanism also responds to cer-

tain metabolic factors. The cerebral blood vessels vasodilate in response to increased $PaCO_2$ and decreased pH, leading to an increased CBF and CBV. A decreased $PaCO_2$ and increased pH lead to constriction of cerebral blood vessels, resulting in a decreased CBF and CBV. The cerebral blood vessels are less sensitive to changes in the PaO_2. Vasodilation leading to an increased CBF and CBV generally does not occur until the PaO_2 falls to the hypoxic range.

Another consideration relating to ICP is the cerebral venous system. The cerebral veins do not have valves as do other venous vessels in the body. Any condition that obstructs or compromises the venous outflow may also increase CBV because more blood is backed up in the intracranial cavity.[40] Activities such as coughing, sneezing, or performing the Valsalva maneuver increase intrathoracic and intraabdominal pressures that increase ICP by decreasing cerebral venous outflow via the jugular veins.[41] Rotation and extreme flexion or extension of the neck may also obstruct venous outflow and arterial inflow. Positive end-expiratory pressure (PEEP) treatments, hip flexion, and lying on the abdomen also increase thoracic and abdominal cavity pressures.[37] Elevating the head of the bed facilitates venous drainage.

Gliomas

Gliomas are the most common primary brain tumor in adults and include the astrocytomas, oligodendrogliomas, ependymomas, and mixed gliomas.

Astrocytomas. The majority of gliomas are astrocytomas, accounting for approximately 60% of all primary

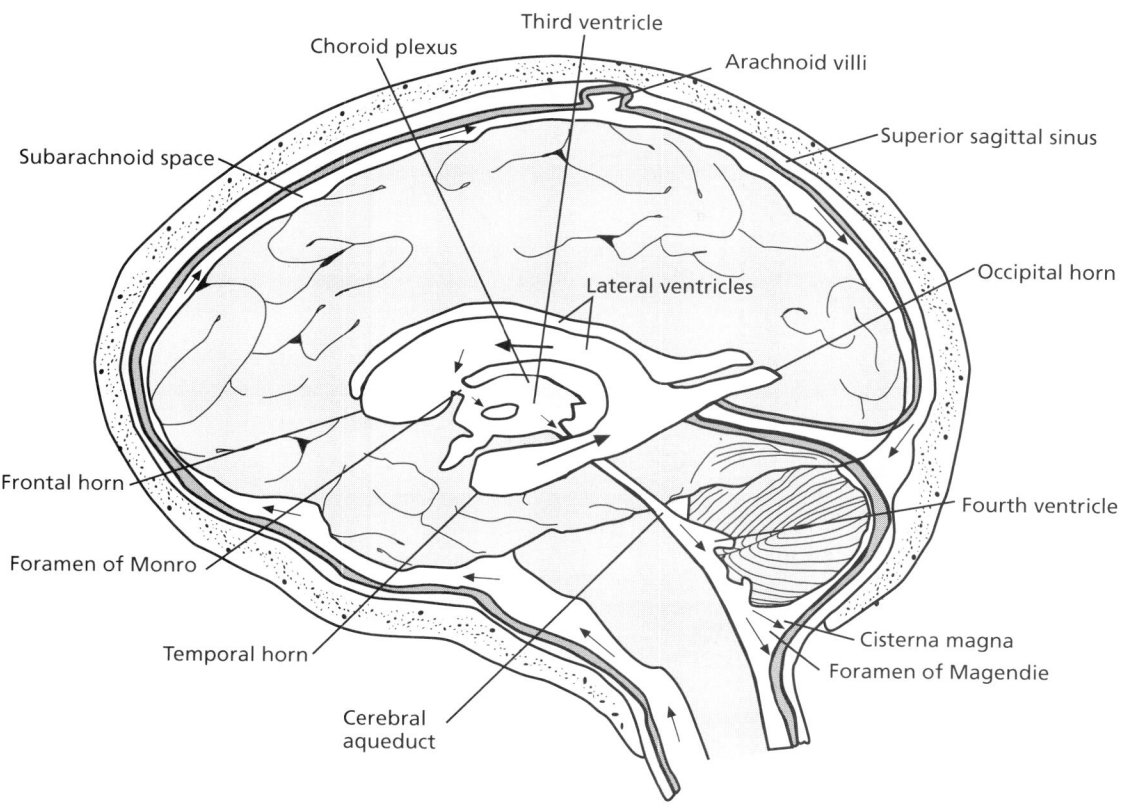

Figure 49-5 Circulation of cerebrospinal fluid.

brain tumors. Astrocytomas arise from the star-shaped supportive cells of the CNS, the astrocytes. These tumors are graded to describe their degree of malignancy. Grade is based on the tumor's microscopic appearance and indicates its similarity to normal cells, its tendency to spread, and its growth rate. A four-grade system describes these tumors as grade I through grade IV. In this system grade I tumors tend to be benign and grade IV tumors are the most malignant. A three-grade system divides this group of tumors into astrocytoma, anaplastic astrocytoma, and glioblastoma multiforme (GBM). The three-tiered grading system has been shown to be closely related to prognosis and today is widely used in grading astrocytomas.[42]

The prognosis for individuals with a specific tumor grade may be difficult to predict on the basis of grade alone. Clinically, astrocytomas with similar histological features may behave in a dissimilar fashion. There is a remarkable diversity of cells between different areas of the same tumor and between similar tumors of different individuals,[43] especially in those with the tumor GBM. Location of astrocytic tumors may also have important implications for treatment and prognosis. Tumors located in vital or inaccessible areas may be difficult to treat despite their histologically benign character.

Increasing grades of malignancy within the astrocytoma group are often associated with patient age. Low-grade astrocytomas are more common in individuals age

20–40, anaplastic astrocytomas in individuals age 30–50, and GBM, the most malignant glioma, in those age 50 or older.[42,44] Low-grade astrocytomas rarely occur in those over 50, whereas glioblastomas can occur in younger individuals and children. There is a slightly higher incidence of astrocytomas in males than in females.

Low-grade astrocytomas generally arise in the cerebral hemispheres. The lobar distribution of these tumors is similar to the amount of white matter present in each lobe, with the highest frequency occurring in the frontal lobes. Low-grade astrocytomas show an increased cellularity and have mild nuclear pleomorphism compared with normal brain tissue. Other features of anaplasia such as mitotic activity, vascular proliferative changes, and necrosis are absent. Some astrocytomas may be cystic, and microcalcifications can be present. These tumors are slightly discolored yellow or gray and have indistinct margins with the surrounding brain.[42] They are diffusely infiltrative tumors, although their invasion is largely limited to white matter. These tumors account for approximately 10% of primary brain tumors and up to 25% of all the gliomas.[14]

Controversy exists with regard to the optimal management of low-grade astrocytomas.[45] Large symptomatic and progressive tumors are usually surgically resected. Most individuals with low-grade astrocytomas are prescribed RT, although the timing of treatment is debated.[46] Some

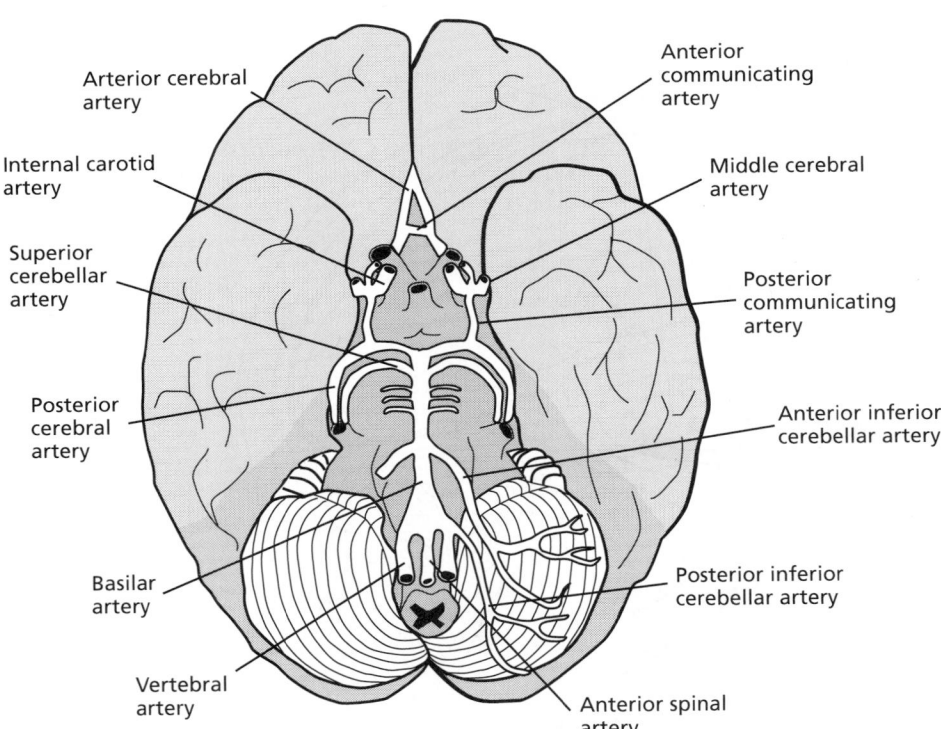

Figure 49-6 Circle of Willis.

low-grade astrocytomas present with well-controlled seizures and are relatively small, asymptomatic, and indolent lesions. Many individuals with these tumors can be safely observed and closely monitored without surgery or other treatment. Intervention would be indicated if the tumor progressed, the radiographic appearance changed (such as the development of new contrast enhancement), or the individual developed new or uncontrolled symptoms.[47] Delayed treatment postpones the risks of surgery and the side effects of RT. However, much of the available retrospective literature suggests a survival benefit of aggressive surgical resection. The general recommendation is to have as complete an excision of tumor as possible without compromising function.[48] These astrocytomas are rarely cured because they cannot be completely excised. In addition, a large percentage of these tumors undergo malignant transformation to a higher tumor grade over time. Some individuals with low-grade astrocytomas may survive for many years, whereas others experience a malignant course with short survival time. The latter group of individuals die as a result of their tumor's malignant transformation into a higher grade, rather than succumbing to a low-grade astrocytoma.[49] No specific therapy has been identified that can reliably prevent malignant transformation of a low-grade astrocytoma.[50] Median survival for individuals with low-grade astrocytoma is approximately 5–7.5 years.[46]

The high-grade gliomas are the anaplastic astrocytoma and GBM. They account for approximately half of all primary brain tumors. The histological features of

the anaplastic astrocytoma are similar to the low-grade astrocytomas but are more abundant and exaggerated. Cellularity is increased, as are nuclear and cellular pleomorphism. Mitotic activity and proliferative vascular changes are found within the tumor. Necrosis is not present. The GBM has these characteristics plus necrosis, which distinguishes it from anaplastic astrocytoma. Glioblastomas infiltrate the brain extensively but rarely spread to distant locations. Anaplastic astrocytomas account for less than one-third of the gliomas, whereas the GBM is the most common adult primary brain tumor and represents more than 50% of the gliomas. Individuals with anaplastic astrocytoma have a better prognosis than those with glioblastomas. With conventional therapy median survival for anaplastic astrocytoma is approximately three years, compared with 12 months for GBM.[51,52] Standard treatment for these high-grade gliomas includes surgery, RT, and chemotherapy.

Oligodendrogliomas. Oligodendrogliomas represent between 3%–7% of all primary brain tumors and less than 10% of the gliomas, although the actual incidence is largely underestimated.[53] Oligodendrogliomas arise from the oligodendrocyte cell, which is responsible for the development and maintenance of the myelin sheath. About 50% of these tumors contain oligodendrocytes, astrocytes, and ependymal cells and are referred to as *mixed gliomas*. Oligodendrogliomas frequently occur in middle-aged individuals, with a peak incidence between 25–49 years.[3]

These tumors typically present as well-defined, spongy,

vascular masses, usually located in the frontal or temporal lobes of the cerebral hemispheres. Approximately 50% of oligodendrogliomas have calcifications within the tumor and adjacent brain tissue,[54] and up to 20% are cystic.[3] Like astrocytomas, oligodendrogliomas vary in malignancy. Pure oligodendrogliomas are relatively low-grade, well-differentiated, and have cells that appear to be only slightly abnormal. They tend to be slow-growing and are often present for many years before diagnosis. Malignant forms, or anaplastic oligodendrogliomas, have highly abnormal-looking cells and usually grow more quickly. Anaplastic features include high cellularity, nuclear pleomorphism, frequent mitosis, areas of necrosis, and proliferation of blood vessels.[48]

Clinically, these tumors present in the same fashion as other similarly located tumors. However, two features separate the oligodendrogliomas: the antecedent (prodromal) history, averaging seven to eight years, tends to be longer, and seizures are more common, occurring in 70%–90% of patients by the time of diagnosis.[3,54] The standard treatment for oligodendrogliomas has been surgery, when a good neurological outcome is possible, and RT. Large symptomatic, unresectable, or incompletely resected tumors should be treated with RT.[55] Postoperative RT may be held for completely resected well-differentiated tumors.[48] Oligodendrogliomas have been found to be chemosensitive tumors. The PCV (procarbazine, lomustine [CCNU], and vincristine) regimen is particularly effective[54] and has become standard therapy for these tumors, although responses have also been seen with carmustine (BCNU). The PCV regimen has been tried as neoadjuvant therapy with good responses. Responses to PCV have also been reported in low-grade oligodendrogliomas.[56]

The unique response of this tumor to chemotherapy has led to additional clinical trials to determine the most effective treatment. Oligodendrogliomas have also shown responses to melphalan, diaziquone (AZQ), thiotepa, dacarbazine (DTIC), 7 dibromodulcitor, temazolamide, and regimens containing cisplatin.[15] Median survival for low-grade tumors is approximately ten years,[48] although survival has been reported as high as 13 years.[46] For anaplastic oligodendrogliomas, median survival is approximately three to five years.[48]

Ependymomas. Ependymomas represent less than 5% of all adult primary brain tumors and 9% of the gliomas.[57] They occur in all age groups but are most often seen in young adults and children. Ependymomas arise from the ependymal cells, which form the lining of the ventricles and the central canal of the spinal cord.

The majority of intracranial ependymomas are infratentorial and usually arise from the fourth ventricle. Supratentorial tumors develop from the ependymal lining of the third and lateral ventricles or may be located deep in the cerebral hemispheres without visible connection to the ventricles. Ependymomas may be differentiated and low-grade or anaplastic and high-grade. The characteristic histological pattern of low-grade ependymomas consists of epithelial-like arrangements of cells around an irregular open space or a radiating, tapering process of tumor cells surrounding a blood vessel.[57] In addition to the typical pattern of low-grade tumors, malignant or anaplastic ependymomas also have cellular pleomorphism, necrosis, mitoses, and multinucleation.[58]

High-grade and infratentorial tumors are more likely to spread through the CSF pathways. Signs and symptoms vary depending on the location of the tumor. Ependymomas are often associated with obstructive hydrocephalus, and a ventriculoperitoneal shunt may be required to relieve the increased ICP.

Standard treatment of ependymomas is surgery and RT. Maximal surgical resection should be performed when possible since outcome is closely associated with extent of surgical resection. Individuals with totally resected tumors have the best prognosis.[48] Individuals with infratentorial tumors have higher survival rates than those with supratentorial tumors.[59] Low-grade tumors are treated with local radiation unless there is evidence of disseminated disease. Craniospinal radiation is reserved for those individuals with either radiographic or pathologic evidence of craniospinal seeding. It does not appear that the routine use of prophylactic craniospinal or whole-brain radiation therapy (WBRT) leads to an improvement in survival.[48] There is an increasing tendency to also treat malignant ependymomas locally because the majority recur at the primary site. Chemotherapy is used primarily for recurrent tumors. A variety of agents used alone or in combination have been investigated, including CCNU, BCNU, carboplatin, cisplatin, procarbazine, vincristine, and cyclophosphamide. Five-year survival rates in individuals treated with surgery and radiation range from 33%–80%.[48]

Meningiomas

Meningiomas, the most common benign brain tumor, account for up to 20% of all adult intracranial tumors. They arise from the cap cells of the arachnoid layer of the meninges and are often located near major venous sinuses, large cerebral blood vessels, and the skull base.[60,61] They may occur as single lesions or in multiple sites. Meningiomas occur twice as often in women as in men and tend to occur late in life, with a peak incidence in the sixth decade for men and the seventh decade for women. The incidence of meningiomas is also higher in individuals with breast cancer.[62,63]

Most meningiomas are differentiated with low proliferative capacity, limited invasiveness, and have well-defined borders. The traditional classification divides meningiomas into various subtypes, but this distinction has little prognostic significance with the possible exception of the malignant meningioma, which contains abundant mitoses, nuclear pleomorphism, necrosis, high nuclear to cytoplasmic ratio, loss of normal architecture, and invasion of surrounding brain tissue.[64] Malignant meningiomas account for less than 10% of all meningiomas,[11] occur more often in men, are frequently multifocal, cause systemic metastases in up to 24% of patients,[62,65] and generally have a high recurrence rate.

Meningiomas produce symptoms by compression of surrounding brain tissue rather than by infiltration as the gliomas do. Individuals may present with seizures, headache, increased ICP, focal neurological deficits such as altered mental status and hemiparesis, and cranial neuropathies. The precise clinical features vary depending on the exact location of the tumor.

The primary treatment modality for meningiomas is surgery, with the extent of surgical resection the primary factor influencing the recurrence rate. Factors that impede the possibility of complete resection are tumor location, size, consistency, vascular and cranial nerve involvement, and, in the case of recurrence, prior surgery, radiotherapy, or both. A better understanding of neuroanatomy and improved neurosurgical techniques allow many previously unresectable meningiomas to be surgically excised today. The risk of recurrence for completely resected benign meningiomas is small and postoperative radiation is usually not recommended. Radiation is indicated for individuals with inoperable, partially resected, and recurrent meningiomas. Postoperative radiation prolongs the interval to recurrence, prevents tumor regrowth, and improves the survival of some individuals with incompletely resected tumors.[3] Incompletely resected individuals who received postoperative radiation have been reported to have a 20-year progression-free survival of more than 90%.[66] Those with malignant meningiomas should receive adjuvant radiation regardless of the extent of resection.[67,68] Chemotherapy for malignant meningiomas using varied regimens has been generally unsuccessful. There have been occasional responses to alfa-interferon.[60]

Hormones and growth factors may influence the growth of meningiomas. Approximately 30% of meningiomas have estrogen receptors, and 70%–80% have progesterone receptors.[62,69] Treatment with antiestrogens such as tamoxifen has been ineffective,[62,70] but antiprogesterone agents have shown promise.[62,71] The expression of platelet derived growth factor (PDGF) and its receptor is a common event in meningiomas.[11] Inhibitors to these growth factors need further investigation in these tumors. Current studies are under way to investigate the possibility of such medical therapy as treatment for meningioma.

Vestibular Schwannomas (Acoustic Neuromas)

Vestibular schwannomas, traditionally called *acoustic neuromas*, are benign tumors arising from the Schwann cells at the vestibular portion of the eighth cranial nerve (vestibulocochlear or acoustic nerve). They account for less than 10% of all intracranial tumors and commonly occur in individuals age 30–60. These are very slow-growing tumors whose symptoms are related to compression and stretching of cranial nerves, causing interference with their function.[72] As the tumor expands from its origin on

the vestibular nerve, it extends into the area between the cerebellum, pons, and medulla known as the *cerebellopontine angle*. The cochlear, trigeminal, and facial nerves are compressed. As the tumor continues to grow, it ultimately compresses the cerebellar peduncles, cerebellum, brain stem, and cranial nerves IX, X, and XI (glossopharyngeal, vagus, and spinal accessory nerves).[62] The most common presenting symptom is a unilateral sensorineural hearing loss. Other initial symptoms are tinnitus, vertigo, and disequilibrium. Late clinical features are facial palsy, facial numbness, headache, ataxia, diplopia, dysphagia, and hydrocephalus.[62,64] Schwannomas have occasionally been reported to occur in other locations in the brain, causing different symptoms related to their intraparenchymal location.[73]

Diagnostic tests include audiometry and brain stem auditory evoked potentials followed by magnetic resonance imaging (MRI) with gadolinium. Surgery and radiosurgery are the primary treatment modalities for most individuals with vestibular schwannomas. The goal of surgery is to completely remove the tumor while preserving facial nerve function and hearing. Factors that predict the success of postoperative hearing preservation are preoperative hearing level and tumor size.[74] Because most of these tumors lie around the vestibular portion of the eighth cranial nerve, the nerve may be severed during surgery in order to remove the entire tumor.[75] Vertigo occurs as a result. When Wiegand and Fickel[76] surveyed postoperative acoustic neuroma patients, 90% reported some degree of vertigo. While 8% rated vertigo as a severe handicap, many individuals eventually accommodate to this problem. For those tumors not completely resected or in individuals who do not undergo surgery, radiosurgery may be used.

Primary Central Nervous System Lymphomas

PCNSL is an aggressive non-Hodgkin's lymphoma that arises within and is confined to the CNS.[77] Until recently, PCNSL has been a rare tumor, accounting for only 2% of all intracranial cancers.[78,79] However, it is increasing in both immunocompetent and immunosuppressed individuals. The number of cases of PCNSL in otherwise healthy individuals has increased sevenfold in recent years.[80] This increase cannot be attributed only to new and improved diagnostic techniques, the adoption of a uniform classification system, or a similar rise in the number of systemic lymphomas diagnosed.[78,81] PCNSL is often associated with acquired or congenital immunosuppression. The highest incidence occurs in patients with AIDS, where PCNSL develops in up to 6% of cases.[77,82] This number may actually be higher because up to 50% of AIDS-related PCNSLs are diagnosed only at autopsy.[83] PCNSL is the second most common brain lesion and the fourth most common cause of death in AIDS patients.[79] Other populations at risk include organ transplant recipients, individuals with collagen vascular diseases, and those with congenital immunodeficiencies.

PCNSL is almost always disseminated within the CNS.

The sites involved may be the brain, leptomeninges, eyes, and (rarely) the spinal cord. Ninety-five percent of patients diagnosed with PCNSL have a brain lesion, and 50% of these lesions are multifocal. The lesions are often periventricular and involve the leptomeninges. As a result, seeding within the CSF often occurs. Positive cytology is found in approximately one-third of patients at diagnosis, and an additional one-third have a suspicious cytology.[84] The eyes are a direct extension of the nervous system and are involved in up to 20% of patients at diagnosis. PCNSL may develop in the eye only. Eventually more than one-half of these patients will go on to develop PCNSL lesions in the brain.[85]

These lymphomas are primarily of B-cell origin and are of the intermediate- to high-grade type. PCNSL is a stage I_E lymphoma, i.e., it is confined to a single extranodal site. These patients show no evidence of a systemic lymphoma. The EBV has been found in pathology specimens of AIDS patients with PCNSL, but it is not yet known what role this plays in the development of PCNSL.

Most PCNSLs involve the frontal lobes. Common symptoms include change in level of consciousness, personality changes, headache, nausea/vomiting, hemiparesis or hemiplegia, visual disturbances, and occasionally seizures. Diagnostic workup includes MRI, CSF analysis, ophthalmologic exam, and a workup to rule out systemic lymphoma. In immunocompetent individuals, PCNSL has a typical appearance on MRI that can help distinguish it from other processes. The lesions are usually multifocal, uniformly enhance with contrast, and are located near the ventricles, basal ganglia, and corpus callosum. If a diagnosis is made from positive CSF cytology or a positive biopsy of the vitreous of the eye, a brain biopsy is unnecessary. PCNSL does not respond well to standard chemotherapy regimens used in systemic lymphoma.[86] The most successful treatments to date in immunocompetent individuals have been with intra-Ommaya and high-dose intravenous (IV) methotrexate followed by focal RT and high-dose cytarabine,[87] blood-brain barrier (BBB) disruption with mannitol followed by intraarterial and systemic chemotherapy without RT,[88] and the combination of PCV chemotherapy,[89] yielding a mean survival of approximately 3.5 years. The combination of cranial RT with chemotherapy, particularly methotrexate, carries an increased risk of delayed neurological toxicity, especially in older individuals. In a follow-up report of individuals treated with intra-Ommaya and high-dose methotrexate, cranial irradiation, and high-dose cytarabine, nearly 80% of one-year survivors over age 60 developed progressive leukoencephalopathy.[87] The behavior of PCNSL in the immunosuppressed population differs from that in immunocompetent individuals, thereby creating specific diagnostic and therapeutic challenges.

Brain Metastases

Brain metastases occur in 20%–40% of individuals with cancer.[48] The incidence of brain metastases is increasing as patients are living longer, there is better control of systemic cancer, and the incidence of cancers that commonly metastasize to the brain—e.g., lung and breast—continues to rise. Other factors contributing to this phenomenon are advances in neuroimaging, use of routine staging tests that assess the CNS, and perhaps the sanctuary effect provided by the BBB, which may isolate the nervous system tissue from the antitumor effects of systemic chemotherapy.[90] Brain metastases generally occur in individuals with systemic disease, although as the primary cancers are better controlled, brain metastases may be the only symptomatic site of the cancer.[91]

Brain metastases occur at three sites: the brain parenchyma itself, the skull and dura, and the leptomeninges. Parenchymal brain metastases are found most frequently and occur ten times more often than primary brain tumors.[48] Approximately 150,000–170,000 new cases will be diagnosed annually.[92] The majority of brain metastases are a result of hematogenous spread from the primary tumor. Although most cancers can metastasize to the brain, melanoma and cancers of the lung, breast, kidney, colon, and thyroid have a particular propensity to do so.[93] The lung is the most common site of origin. If the primary tumor is not pulmonary, it may have metastasized to the lungs before reaching the brain. In addition, the majority of metastatic brain tumors of unknown primary cancer are of the lung. From the lungs, cancer cells may enter the pulmonary veins and reach the left atrium and ventricle. Tumor cells transported in this manner are widely dispersed and are ultimately deposited in the arterial circulation, where the tumor cells can readily travel to the brain.[36] Breast and lung cancers are prevalent in the population, whereas melanoma accounts for only 1% of all cancers diagnosed. Yet melanoma has the highest propensity of all systemic cancers to metastasize to the brain. Almost 40% of patients with melanoma develop brain metastases,[94,95] making it, despite the rarity of melanoma as a primary tumor, the third most frequent cause of brain metastases.

When neurological symptoms of brain metastases develop, the individual often has widespread systemic disease. Brain metastases are characterized by severe peritumoral edema, which contributes to the neurological symptoms. The presenting signs and symptoms of metastatic brain disease are dependent upon the lesion's location in the brain and can be identical to those of other space-occupying lesions. Most brain metastases occur in the cerebral hemispheres. Symptoms include signs of increased ICP (headache, nausea, and vomiting), change in level of consciousness, diminished cognitive function, personality changes, hemiparesis, language problems, and seizures. Seizures occur as the initial presenting symptom in 15%–20% of patients. Seizures are particularly common in metastatic melanoma, occurring 50% of the time, primarily because these lesions tend to be hemorrhagic.[94,96]

The majority of metastatic brain lesions occur in the cerebral hemispheres (80%), with 15% found in the cerebellum and 5% in the brain stem.[48] Between 50%–70% of individuals with brain metastases have multiple lesions.[48,97] Multiple metastatic lesions are often found in melanoma and lung cancer whereas single lesions often occur in colon, breast, and renal cell cancers.[97,98] With early diagnosis and management, brain metastases often respond to therapy. Most individuals benefit from palliative treatment; an increasing number of patients experience a prolonged remission or, rarely, are cured of their cerebral disease. Neurological function may be preserved and quality of life maintained. Thus, systemic cancer, rather than neurological disease, usually limits life expectancy.[90,99]

For many years WBRT had been the standard treatment for both single and multiple brain metastases. Patchell and associates[100] compared surgery plus WBRT with WBRT alone in a randomized prospective study in patients with single metastases. Those undergoing surgery plus WBRT lived longer, maintained a higher performance status and improved quality of life for a longer period of time, and had fewer recurrences compared to those receiving WBRT alone. Surgery is now considered the first therapeutic option for single brain metastases when feasible.[93,94] Postoperative RT is often recommended. Patients with multiple lesions (2–4) may also be considered for surgery. Bindel and colleagues[101] compared a group of individuals who had multiple lesions resected to a group that had some lesions left unresected. Survival in patients who had all metastases resected was longer than the group who had lesions left unresected, and there was no difference in surgical mortality or morbidity. Unfortunately, nearly 50% of patients are not candidates for surgery because of the inaccessibility of the tumor(s), extensive systemic disease, or other factors. These individuals are generally treated with radiosurgery. Retrospective comparisons suggest that survival is comparable for individuals treated with radiosurgery when compared to the combination of surgery and WBRT,[92,102] although no prospective randomized trials have been performed comparing the two.[93] Some physicians advocate radiosurgery instead of surgery. Multiple metastases have been treated effectively with radiosurgery. However, radiosurgery is contraindicated for large tumors. Radiosurgery can be followed by WBRT to decrease the likelihood of regional relapse,[103] but the value of this remains unclear. At times, radiosurgery may be used as a planned boost therapy after WBRT or may be used to treat recurrences or new metastases after prior WBRT. For individuals whose extent of systemic or intracranial cancer makes them poor candidates for either surgery or radiosurgery, WBRT may be indicated as a palliative measure.[92] Currently, a randomized trial is under way comparing WBRT with or without a radiosurgery boost.[104]

Chemotherapy is rarely used as primary therapy for brain metastases.[48] Many tumors that metastasize to the brain such as non–small cell lung cancer, melanoma, and unknown primary, are often resistant to chemotherapy.[48,105] Adjuvant chemotherapy may be considered for individuals with more chemosensitive tumors (e.g., germ cell, breast, and small cell lung cancers).

Tumors that metastasize to the bone, particularly metastatic tumors of the breast, prostate, and lung, may infil-trate the skull or dura by direct extension and may compress the venous sinuses or underlying brain tissue. Signs and symptoms include headache, a palpable mass, seizures, and other common symptoms of a parenchymal brain mass. Treatment may be radiation therapy or surgical resection.

Leptomeningeal metastasis, once thought to be a rare complication of cancer, is increasing in frequency. Leptomeningeal metastasis, or meningeal carcinomatosis, is a diffuse or multifocal seeding of cancer cells throughout the meninges and CSF. The seeding pattern of growth covers the surface of the brain and spinal cord.[106] Leptomeningeal metastasis is usually an indication of progressive systemic cancer.

Although the exact incidence of leptomeningeal metastasis is difficult to determine, studies have found an overall incidence of up to 8%.[97] While any systemic cancer can seed the meninges, the most common cancers leading to meningeal carcinomatosis are leukemia, lymphoma, melanoma, and breast, lung, and gastrointestinal (GI) cancers. The incidence of meningeal involvement from leukemia has decreased, while leptomeningeal metastases from breast and lung cancer are increasing. Clinical manifestations are headache, mental status changes, gait disturbances, hydrocephalus, cranial nerve palsies, back pain, radiculopathies, weakness, and paresthesias. Diagnosis is established by close examination of the CSF and MRI of the brain and spinal cord. Repeated lumbar punctures (LPs) are often required to identify malignant cells in the CSF. Other CSF findings are elevated CSF pressure, increased white blood cell (WBC) count, elevated protein, and decreased glucose. Treatment includes radiation to symptomatic areas only because radiation to the entire neuroaxis leads to bone marrow depression. This is followed by chemotherapy administered directly into the CSF. Chemotherapy can be injected directly into the lateral ventricle of the brain by using an Ommaya reservoir, thus ensuring optimal consistent CSF levels. Common chemotherapeutic agents include methotrexate, cytarabine, and thiotepa. Reports of median survival range from 7–24 weeks.[97]

Pattern of Spread

The pattern of spread of brain tumors differs from that of other cancers. While brain tumors may spread to other parts of the CNS, metastases outside the brain and spinal cord are rare. Metastases outside the CNS may occur when tumor cells are transferred to the scalp, cerebral blood vessels, or dural sinus during an operative procedure. Once they invade the cerebral blood vessels, tumor cells enter the circulation. The CNS does not contain lymphatic vessels,[97,107] but once the tumor cells have traveled outside the CNS, they can spread by way of the lymphatic system.[108] The spread of glial tumor cells through ventriculopleural and ventriculoperitoneal shunts has also been reported.

Brain tumors grow by expansion, infiltration, or both.

While gliomas rarely metastasize to distant sites outside the CNS, they do invade locally. Glioma cells are sometimes found at intracranial sites distant from the main tumor, making many of these lesions seem multifocal. Brain tumors may seed the CSF and spread through the subarachnoid space. Seeding occurs along the surface of the brain and spinal cord, and "drop metastases" can occur. Some tumors, including PCNSLs, ependymomas, and medulloblastomas, seed the CSF more often than others.

Most metastatic brain tumors develop from hematogenous spread of tumor cells, usually through the arterial circulation. In some cases tumor cells may reach the brain by way of Batson's plexus, which is a valveless system of veins that runs the length of the vertebral column from the pelvic veins to the large venous sinuses of the skull.[36]

Clinical Manifestations

The clinical manifestations of a brain tumor can vary tremendously from one individual to another and among different types of tumors. The particular signs and symptoms with which an individual presents are dependent on the location, size, type, method of expansion, and rate of tumor growth. Intracranial tumors produce signs and symptoms by creating a mass effect and increasing ICP, by infiltrating and damaging normal brain tissue, or both. The clinical manifestations can be divided into three major categories: generalized effects of increased ICP, focal effects, and effects caused by displacement of brain structures. Often a combination of these effects produces signs and symptoms simultaneously.

Generalized Effects of Increased Intracranial Pressure

Brain tumors increase ICP by their size, cerebral edema, or obstruction of CSF pathways. The presence of increased ICP and the speed at which it develops can be variable. In some locations of the brain, a very small tumor can lead to marked elevations of ICP. For example, a relatively small tumor near the third or fourth ventricle can obstruct the CSF flow. In other areas of the brain, however, large, extensive tumors may not initially cause ICP to rise, as in some tumors of the frontal or temporal lobes. A rapidly developing tumor with extensive edema will raise ICP sooner than a slower-growing lesion with little edema.

Signs and symptoms result from the effects of increasing pressure on nerve cells, blood vessels, and the dura. Sustained increases in ICP ultimately cause nerve cell damage and cell death. An expanding tumor (or other space-occupying lesion) can create a vicious cycle of intracranial hypertension (Figure 49-7). After the brain's normal compensatory mechanisms have been exhausted, the increased ICP results in a decreased CBF. The CBF drops because the autoregulatory system fails. Failure of the

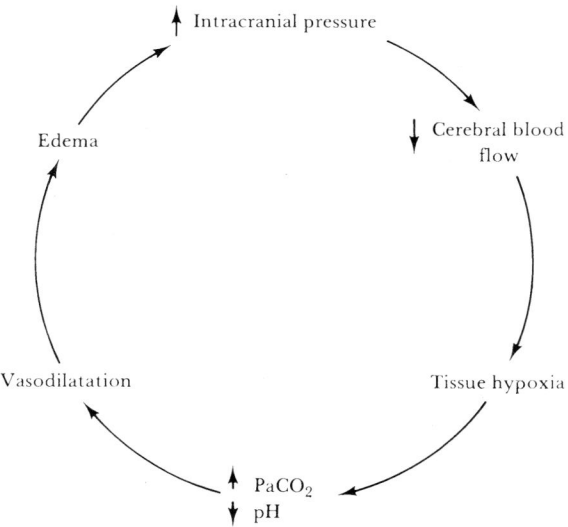

Figure 49-7   Cycle of intracranial hypertension.

autoregulatory system means that CBF will now fluctuate passively with the SAP, unlike the healthy brain where CBF is relatively constant. Increases in systemic blood pressure (SBP) will now directly affect ICP. A reduction in the brain's blood supply leads to tissue hypoxia because the brain does not receive sufficient oxygen. The diminished blood supply also interferes with the removal of CO_2 and lactic acid. These metabolic by-products act as potent vasodilators. Vasodilation of the cerebral blood vessels leads to further edema. As a result, the total volume within the cranium increases, ICP rises further, and the cycle repeats itself.[36]

The signs and symptoms of increased ICP include change in the level of consciousness or cognition, headache, pupillary changes and papilledema, motor and sensory deficits, vomiting, and changes in vital signs. Increased ICP may cause additional effects by displacing brain tissue.

Level of consciousness can be an extremely sensitive index of neurological status[35] and ranges from alert and oriented, restless, confused, unable to follow simple commands, lethargic, to comatose. An individual may have short-term memory loss, impaired judgment, difficulty concentrating, or may be forgetful. He or she may be drowsy or exhibit personality changes or diminished cognitive ability. Sleeping more is the most commonly reported early sign of the tumor. Many of the initial changes have a gradual onset and can be so subtle that they are evident only to the family or a skilled observer.[36] Families may report that the individual just isn't himself or herself. If the increased ICP is not treated, the level of consciousness deteriorates further.

Headache is a common presenting symptom in individuals with intracranial tumors. The location and characteristics of the headache must be evaluated to distinguish them from other common types of headache (migraine, tension, and muscle contraction). The brain parenchyma itself does not contain pain sensors. The headache pain is attributed to pressure or traction on pain-sensitive structures such as the dura, venous sinuses, blood vessels, and cranial nerves.

The headache is usually bilateral in the frontal, temporal, or retroorbital areas. Typically, the pain occurs in the early morning, subsides after arising, and recurs the following morning. The pain can be described as dull, sharp, or throbbing. Some individuals complain of an uncomfortable feeling in the head rather than a headache. Bending over, coughing, or performing a Valsalva maneuver often aggravates or initiates the pain. The headaches gradually increase in frequency, duration, and severity until, in their later stages, they are almost constant and may be associated with other signs and symptoms of increased ICP.[97]

Papilledema is considered a cardinal sign of increased ICP, but it may be a late finding. The edema of the optic disk results from compression around the optic nerve impeding the outflow of venous blood. A trained individual using an ophthalmoscope should assess the presence of papilledema. Other visual signs and symptoms can occur including blurry vision, visual field deficits, and changes in pupillary size and reaction to light.

Motor signs of increased ICP include hemiparesis or hemiplegia on the contralateral (opposite) side of the tumor, diminished reflexes, or the development of pathological reflexes. Decorticate and decerebrate posturing can occur in the late stages of increased ICP when the diencephalon and brain stem become compressed. Decorticate posturing is an abnormal flexion of the arms with extension of the legs. Decerebrate posturing is an abnormal extension of the arms and legs. Sensory symptoms consist of impaired sensation, inability to interpret sensory information, or both.

Vomiting as a sign of increased ICP occurs more commonly in children and in individuals with infratentorial tumors.[3] Vomiting may be preceded by nausea, or it may be sudden, unexpected, and projectile. It is not related to food ingestion. Increased pressure on the vomiting center of the medulla is believed to precipitate this symptom.[36]

Changes in vital signs occur late in the course of increased ICP. They result from increased pressure on the vasoactive centers of the medulla in the brain stem. SBP rises and diastolic blood pressure (DBP) drops, thus widening the pulse pressure. Bradycardia and an abnormal respiratory pattern (usually slowed and irregular respirations) develop. This combination of hypertension, bradycardia, and abnormal respirations, referred to as *Cushing's triad*, is a very late sign of increased ICP. By the time Cushing's triad is identified, the patient is usually already comatose.

Focal Effects

Intracranial tumors also cause localized or focal signs and symptoms of neurological dysfunction. Specific anatomic areas in the CNS have unique functions, and the neurological deficits produced are directly related to the particular area involved. Performing a careful neurological examination and possessing knowledge of neuroanatomy and neurophysiology can assist in identifying the location of a lesion based on the neurological findings (see Table 49-1).

Tumors of the frontal lobe can cause a variety of symptoms, including inability to concentrate, inattentiveness, difficulty with abstraction, impaired memory, personality changes, quiet flat affect, inappropriate behavior, lack of social control, indifference, emotional lability, and loss of initiative. To complicate the situation, the individual may be unaware that his or her behavior has changed or is inappropriate.[109] Tumors in the posterior portion of the frontal lobe where the motor strip is located can result in hemiparesis or hemiplegia on the contralateral side of the tumor. Deep tendon reflexes increase on the paretic side, and a positive Babinski sign is present. Broca's area is located in the frontal lobe. Damage to this area in the dominant hemisphere results in the inability to express oneself in words even though the individual may comprehend speech and language. Broca's aphasia has been referred to as *expressive aphasia* and can be extremely frustrating for individuals.

Most people have one cerebral hemisphere that is more developed or dominant than the other with respect to language. In right-handed and most left-handed individuals, the dominant hemisphere is the left. This is important to distinguish because the left side of the brain controls language and the right hemisphere (nondominant side in the majority of people) is the nonverbal or perceptual hemisphere, which processes temporospatial information.

Parietal lobe tumors affect sensory and perceptual functions more than motor function, although mild hemiparesis is sometimes seen with these tumors.[3] Tumors in either lobe can cause mild to severe disturbances. Common symptoms include impaired sensation, paresthesias, loss of two-point discrimination, inability to recognize an object by feeling its size and shape (astereognosis), inability to locate or recognize parts of the body (autotopagnosia), loss of awareness or denial of a motor or sensory defect in the affected body part (anosognosia), inability to write (agraphia) or to calculate numbers (acalculia), and inability to execute learned movements in the absence of weakness or paralysis (apraxia).

Tumors of the temporal lobe can cause impairment of recent memory, aggressive behavior, and psychomotor seizures. Psychomotor seizures are described as visual, auditory, or olfactory hallucinations and may begin with an aura. These seizures may be characterized by automatisms and behavioral changes. Involvement of the dominant side can lead to an inability to recall names (dysnomia), impaired perception of verbal commands, and Wernicke's or receptive aphasia. In this type of aphasia the patient speaks easily, appears to be making an effort to communicate, and is easily engaged in conversation. However, little meaning is conveyed. The individual does not understand what is being said. He or she may speak in phrases or complete sentences, but the listener is usually unable to make sense of the content. *Receptive aphasia* can make patient teaching extremely difficult. The meeting point of the temporal, occipital, and parietal lobes is called the *interpretive area*. Cognitive function will be significantly impacted by damage to this area in the dominant hemisphere.[109]

Occipital lobe tumors produce visual symptoms, including homonymous hemianopsia (visual loss in half of each visual field on the contralateral side of the lesion) and visual hallucinations. Tumors located in this area can also interfere with the ability to interpret what is seen. Tumors located in or near the thalamus can lead to hydrocephalus, mild sensory disturbances, paresthesias, neuropathic pain, emotional lability, and sleep pattern disturbances. Hypothalamic tumors typically lead to endocrine dysfunction. These tumors can also affect water metabolism, appetite, sexual behavior, and regulation of temperature, sleep–wake cycle, and the autonomic nervous system.

Brain stem tumors can produce dire consequences, since the centers that control respiration and heart rate are located here. The points of origin of cranial nerves III through XII are also located here, and dysfunction is common. Multiple nerve fiber tracts in the brain stem allow transmission of nerve impulses between the cerebral hemispheres and the spinal cord.

Tumors located in the cerebellum have a classic presentation. Individuals may have a wide-based ataxic gait, a dysarthric speech pattern, and nystagmus. They may exhibit clumsiness, balance difficulty, or tremors. Symptoms of increased ICP such as early morning headache and vomiting are often present.

Seizures, another common clinical manifestation in both primary and metastatic brain tumors, are seen primarily with supratentorial tumors. They may occur in 70%–90% of individuals with low-grade astrocytomas and oligodendrogliomas, and in 20%–30% of individuals with other tumor types. They may be the initial presenting symptom in a number of patients, sometimes occurring months to years before the clinical diagnosis is made. Seizures can also occur as a treatment-related complication.

The cerebral edema and alterations in the normal electrical potential of cells caused by the tumor result in hyperactive cells. This hyperactivity, in turn, produces abnormal, paroxysmal discharges or seizure activity that can be focal or generalized.[110] Focal or partial seizures involve a particular area of the brain, whereas generalized seizures involve both cerebral hemispheres. Focal seizures can aid in localizing the tumor, depending on the pattern of seizure activity.

Displacement of Brain Structure

The cranial cavity is divided into the supratentorial and infratentorial compartments by the infolding of the rigid dura mater. Normally pressure is distributed equally between the compartments. A growing tumor mass and the associated edema cause pressure to increase within the compartment. Initially the brain's compensatory mechanisms attempt to accommodate the pressure by decreasing the amount of CSF, blood volume, or both within the brain. Once these mechanisms are exhausted, the increased pressure can cause the brain tissue in the high-pressure compartment to protrude into the lower-pressure compartment. This process, called *herniation*, is a life-threatening neurological emergency.[36]

The shifting brain tissue compresses other neural tissue and structures, further increases the edema, causes ischemia from damage to blood vessels, and can obstruct CSF pathways, leading to hydrocephalus. These compressive, ischemic, vascular, and obstructive changes all add to and aggravate the original problem of increased ICP. The potentially reversible complications of an expanding tumor become irreversible.[36]

There are two major classifications of herniation: supratentorial and infratentorial. The clinical manifestations of the two types differ. Supratentorial herniation generally causes a change in the level of consciousness and ocular, motor, and respiratory signs, whereas infratentorial herniation leads to a loss of consciousness and respiratory and cardiac changes. The expanding tumor mass is capable of displacing tissue distant from the tumor site. The resulting neurological signs and symptoms may not have true localizing value.[36]

There is usually an orderly progression of abnormal clinical signs. Careful neurological assessment in patients at risk for herniation may facilitate early identification of this potentially life-threatening complication. However, herniation can occur with little warning. A sudden change in the ICP or contents (as in an acute hemorrhage or the performance of an LP) will rapidly lead to brain stem compression.

Supratentorial tumors, located above the tentorium cerebelli, can lead to cingulate, uncal, or central transtentorial herniation. Herniation of the cingulate gyrus under the falx cerebri compresses the contralateral frontal lobe and the anterior cerebral arteries. Such herniation can cause bilateral frontal lobe ischemia, urinary incontinence, leg weakness, and mental status changes. The diencephalon is shifted to the contralateral side, compresses itself and the third ventricle, and leads to diminished consciousness.[97]

Uncal herniation, usually occurring with expanding temporal lobe tumors, forces the medial portion of the temporal lobe (the uncus) into the tentorial notch. The midbrain is compressed laterally. The herniated uncus compresses the third cranial nerve, the posterior cerebral artery, and the diencephalon. Compression of the third cranial nerve, the oculomotor nerve, initially causes the ipsilateral pupil to sluggishly react to light. With further compression the pupil dilates and becomes unreactive. With midbrain compression, the motor pathways of the cerebral peduncle produce a contralateral hemiparesis. Sometimes uncal herniation compresses the opposite cerebral peduncle against the opposite tentorial notch (opposite the side of herniation). This is called *Kernohan's notch* and causes a hemiparesis that is ipsilateral (same) to the side of the lesion (and to the third cranial nerve palsy). This is a false localizing sign that may lead to confusion in determining the location of the lesion. The tumor is on the same side as the third nerve palsy.[36] A positive Babinski sign may be seen with the hemiparesis. The enlarging mass also shifts the diencephalon, leading to a progressive loss of consciousness beginning with drowsiness and proceeding to stupor and finally to coma.[97] Compression of the posterior cerebral artery can cause ischemia or infarction of the ipsilateral occipital lobe. Later findings in uncal herniation include decorticate followed by decerebrate posturing, and impaired oculocephalic and oculovestibular reflexes. Oculocephalic reflexes are tested by holding the patient's eyelids open and briskly rotating the head from side to side or by briskly flexing and extending the neck (doll's eyes phenomenon). Oculovestibular reflexes are tested by injecting ice water into the external ear canal. In the comatose patient, testing these reflexes assesses for the presence of brain stem function.

Central or transtentorial herniation results from the downward displacement of the cerebral hemispheres and basal ganglia onto the diencephalon and midbrain, which are then forced through the tentorial notch. Initially, there will be a change in the level of consciousness or behavior. The person becomes drowsy, inattentive, or agitated. Pupil size is reduced. There may be deep sighing or yawning with respirations.[35] As the tumor continues to displace tissue downward, the individual becomes stuporous and eventually progresses to coma. Pupils become nonreactive, eye movements disconjugate, and as the brain stem becomes compressed, decorticate posturing deteriorates to decerebrate in response to noxious stimuli. Oculocephalic and oculovestibular reflexes may be absent.

Both central and uncal herniations cause changes in the respiratory pattern. Irregular depth and rhythm often are more significant than changes in respiratory rate alone. Initially, respirations may be irregular with occasional pauses, sighs, or gasps. Later respiratory pattern changes include Cheyne-Stokes breathing, sustained hyperventilation, ataxic breathing, apnea, and finally, respiratory arrest.[36] The classic vital sign changes of Cushing's triad are seen during the terminal phase of herniation.

Tumors of the posterior fossa can lead to an infratentorial herniation causing displacement of the cerebellum either upward through the opening in the tentorium cerebelli or downward through the foramen magnum. In upward transtentorial herniation, the cerebellum compresses the midbrain. Obstruction and blockage of CSF pathways may occur. The individual may lose consciousness immediately. This may be accompanied by hyperventilation; pinpoint, fixed, and unequal pupils; upward-gaze paralysis; vomiting; and decerebration.[35]

Downward cerebellar tonsillar herniation is more common and results in the downward protrusion of the cerebellar tonsils through the foramen magnum. The lower brain stem is compressed; when the compression is acute, it can cause sudden loss of consciousness followed by respiratory arrest. This may be precipitated by events causing a sudden rise in ICP such as sneezing, coughing, or performing a Valsalva maneuver. The outflow of CSF from the fourth ventricle becomes blocked, leading to obstructive hydrocephalus. Other signs include lower cranial nerve dysfunction, suboccipital headache, vomiting, and neck pain. Altered consciousness with resulting coma may be an early sign. Later signs of medullary compression include abnormal respiratory patterns, fluctuating blood pressure and heart rate, and cardiac dysrhythmias. In both types of infratentorial herniation, respiratory arrest, cardiac arrest, or both will occur if untreated. Figure 49-8 illustrates the herniation syndromes.

Assessment

Assessment of the individual with a known or suspected brain tumor begins by obtaining the individual's medical history. The description and duration of symptoms, when they occur, the presence of exacerbating or relieving factors, and the order of their appearance are important pieces of information. This is followed by a complete neurological examination. An initial neurological assessment is essential because it provides a baseline knowledge of the individual's neurological function. Future assessments will be evaluated in comparison with the initial examination, allowing the detection of any changes or abnormalities.

The neurological exam begins with an assessment of the patient's level of consciousness and mental status. In most instances the first, earliest, and most sensitive indicator of dysfunction will be a change in the level of consciousness, which is the ability of the person to interact appropriately within the context of the immediate environment.[35] The individual whose level of consciousness is impaired must be sufficiently stimulated to be able to appropriately describe the degree of alteration. Various levels of alteration may occur, ranging from full consciousness to deep coma. Common descriptions include alert and oriented, confused, lethargic, stuporous, obtunded, semicomatose, and comatose. Many institutions have included components of the Glasgow coma scale, a tool that assesses neurological function in comatose patients, as part of their vital sign or neurological assessment forms.

Conversing with and observing the individual evaluates mental status and cognitive ability. One should note the person's behavior, appearance, mood, and affect. Observation of actions, posture, facial expressions, and responses to the conversation and environment provide information regarding general cerebral function. Orientation, general knowledge, recent and remote memory, attention span, immediate recall, abstract reasoning, and judgment are also part of the assessment of cognitive function. Language is evaluated for content, flow of speech, speech patterns, and comprehension. The presence of aphasia (the inability to understand or express one's own language), agnosia (the inability to recognize common objects through the senses of sight, touch, and sound), and apraxia (the inability to perform a skilled

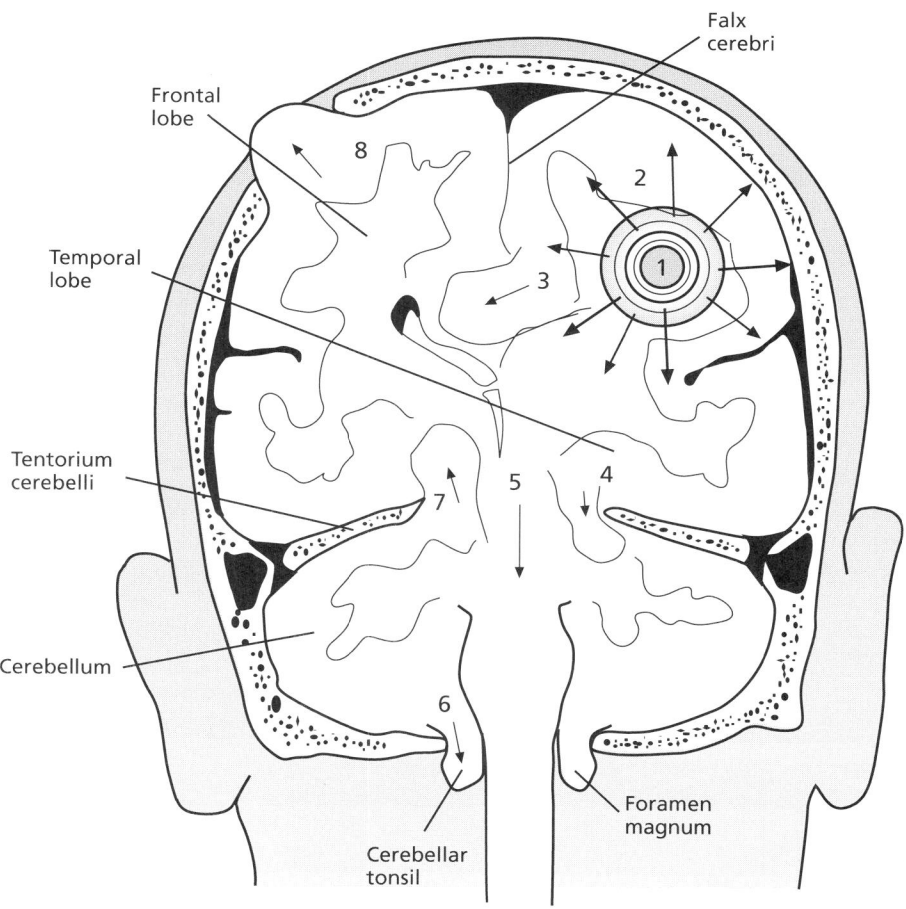

Figure 49-8 Herniation syndromes. (1) Tumor. (2) Edema. (3) Cingulate herniation. (4) Uncal herniation. (5) Central transtentorial herniation. (6) Downward cerebellar tonsillar herniation. (7) Upward herniation of the cerebellum. (8) Herniation through a cranial defect.

motor act in the absence of weakness or paralysis) is noted. Mental status changes often go unnoticed by patients. For this reason, family members, significant others, or work colleagues may initially identify a problem. They can often provide valuable information regarding the onset and progression of symptoms.

Motor and sensory function are also evaluated. A motor exam assesses whether the individual moves normally or abnormally, what the level of response is, and the strength of both the upper and lower extremities against gravity and resistance. A motor exam also tests gait, posture, and reflexes. Deep tendon reflexes (DTRs) and superficial reflexes are examined. Sensation is assessed by introducing various stimuli to different parts of the body with the eyes closed. Light touch, pain, temperature, and position sense are evaluated bilaterally.

Assessment of cerebellar function focuses on the ability to coordinate movement and to maintain normal muscle tone and equilibrium. The person is asked to perform the finger-to-finger, finger-to-nose, hand patting, Romberg, and tandem walking tests.

Testing of cranial nerve function can be the most intimidating portion of the neurological assessment. The 12 pairs of cranial nerves, their function, method of testing and desired response are listed in Table 49-2.

The performance of the initial assessment is as important for the individual newly diagnosed with a brain tumor as it is for the person with recurrent or progressive disease. Changes in the neurological assessment, the development of new symptoms, or both can indicate increased ICP, recurrent disease, or side effects of treatment. The presence and severity of generalized and focal signs and symptoms are documented. The history of the symptoms is important to ascertain from the patient and family. Any change in symptom characteristics should be identified, along with possible exacerbating or relieving factors. Seizures are another area that warrants investigation. The nurse determines whether the individual has had seizures, the frequency and pattern of occurrence, and whether the person experiences an aura before the seizure.

Diagnostic Studies

Developments in neuroimaging have dramatically improved the ability to diagnose, localize, and treat individuals with brain tumors. Computerized tomography (CT) and MRI are the standard imaging techniques. Although useful in some situations, CT has largely been replaced by

MRI.[111] Positron emission-tomography (PET) and single-photon emission computed tomography (SPECT) are being used to distinguish tumor from radiation necrosis and to increase the understanding of the metabolism of malignant tumors.[111]

Computerized tomography. CT scan allows differentiation between bone, brain tissue, and CSF.[35,112] CT is highly sensitive to blood within the brain and is the technique of choice for evaluating the presence of acute hemorrhage. A CT scan can be used to evaluate skull metastases and other bony pathology[113] since bony structures are extremely well visualized on CT. It can be conducted more rapidly than MRI, an important consideration in emergency situations or when sedation may be contraindicated.[37,114]

Magnetic resonance imaging. MRI is the more definitive and preferred imaging study for the individual with a brain tumor. It provides much better resolution than CT scans and more clearly differentiates between solid tumor, edema, and fluid collection. MRI provides superior definition of the borders of a brain tumor, and the extent of the tumor and its invasiveness can be better demonstrated by MRI than by CT (Figure 49-9).[114] The

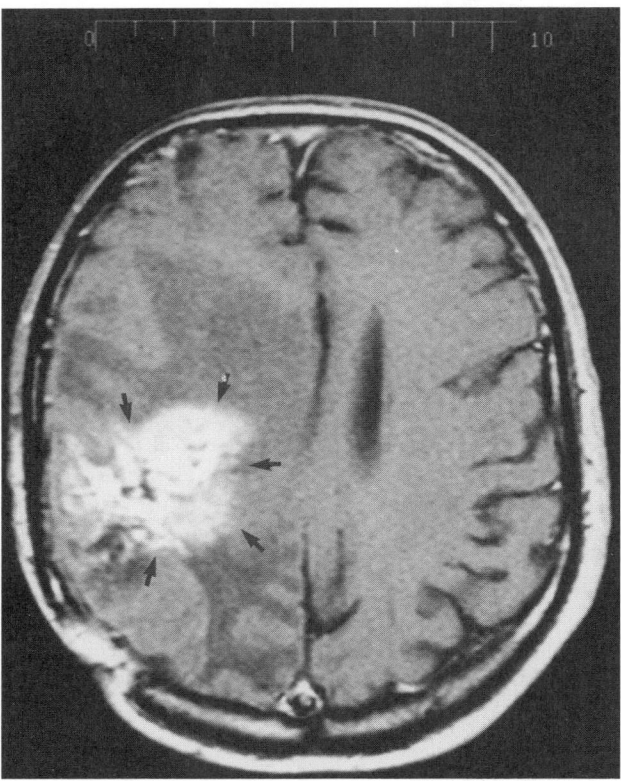

Figure 49-9 MRI of the brain. The image illustrates a large contrast-enhancing lesion with surrounding edema in the right parietal lobe, eventually diagnosed a glioblastoma multiforme. (Reprinted with permission from Memorial Sloan-Kettering Cancer Center, Department of Neurosurgery.)

use of paramagnetic agents such as gadolinium-DTPA allows contrast scanning with minimal risk of allergic complications or renal toxicity,[11] results in remarkable improvement in the image resolution, and illustrates BBB breakdown.[112,115]

MRI also demonstrates an increased sensitivity for small (< 1 cm) lesions[36] and can detect CT-occult tumors.[90] An MRI may be positive when the CT is negative; this may sometimes be seen with low-grade tumors and PCNSL lesions. A MRI may show multiple metastatic lesions that the CT demonstrated only as a single one. MRI is also superior to CT scan in imaging the posterior fossa because bone artifact is not present in MRI. It can also more readily identify leptomeningeal metastases (Figure 49-10).

Positron emission tomography. PET is a functional imaging technique that may also be used in individuals with brain tumors, specifically malignant gliomas. This technique provides dynamic information on CBF and metabolism rather than the precise anatomic localization seen in MRI. PET combines the properties of nuclear scanning with physical characteristics of positron-emitting isotopes of naturally occurring atoms.[37,113] Radioactive isotopes produced in a cyclotron are incorporated into a chosen brain metabolite and injected intravenously. These isotopes disintegrate and form a positively charged electron (a positron). The positron travels until it comes together with an electron and then converts into a pair of photons traveling in opposite directions. A ring of collimators surrounding the individual's head records these events, computers calculate measurements, and a reconstruction algorithm produces an axial view of brain uptake. Also, by monitoring the arterial concentration of radioactivity via an arterial line, the absolute metabolic rate of areas in the brain can be calculated.[113]

Most PET studies have used ^{18}F-fluorodeoxyglucose (FDG), a fluorinated glucose analog to measure glucose metabolism, which is increased in tumor cells.[111,116] The amount of FDG uptake correlates with the degree of malignancy, i.e., low-grade gliomas tend to have lower uptake (hypometabolic) and malignant gliomas have higher uptake (hypermetabolic). In addition to determining tumor grade, this technique has become the standard imaging modality to distinguish between tumor recurrence and radiation necrosis.

Single-emission photon computed tomography. SPECT is used for the imaging of functional neuroanatomy. This technique involves the IV administration of isotopes taken up by the brain and tumor cells. These isotopes emit photons that are detected by a rotating gamma camera. Regions of intense thallium uptake usually represent solid active tumor recurrence, whereas low thallium uptake generally represents radiation necrosis. This technique has also been shown to be effective in distinguishing the presence of infiltrating tumor from solid tumor.[113]

Angiography. Cerebral angiography may be used to confirm that the lesion in question is a vascular malforma-

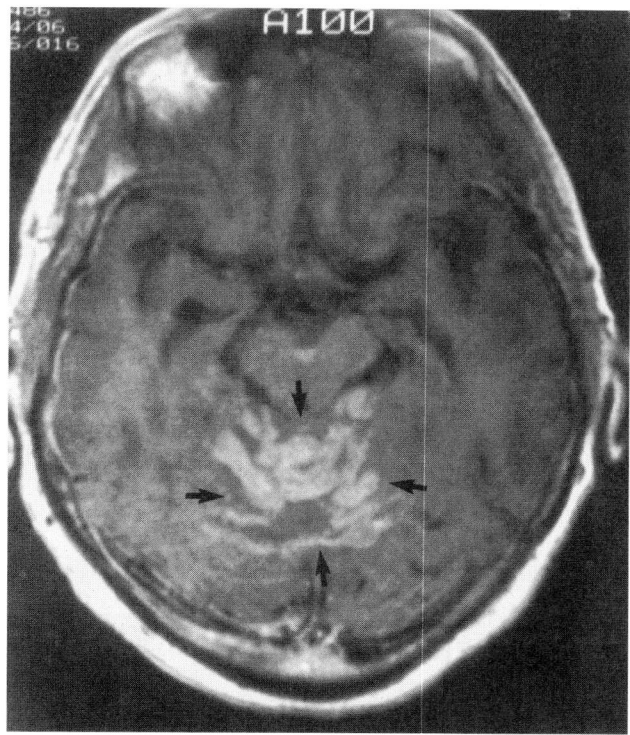 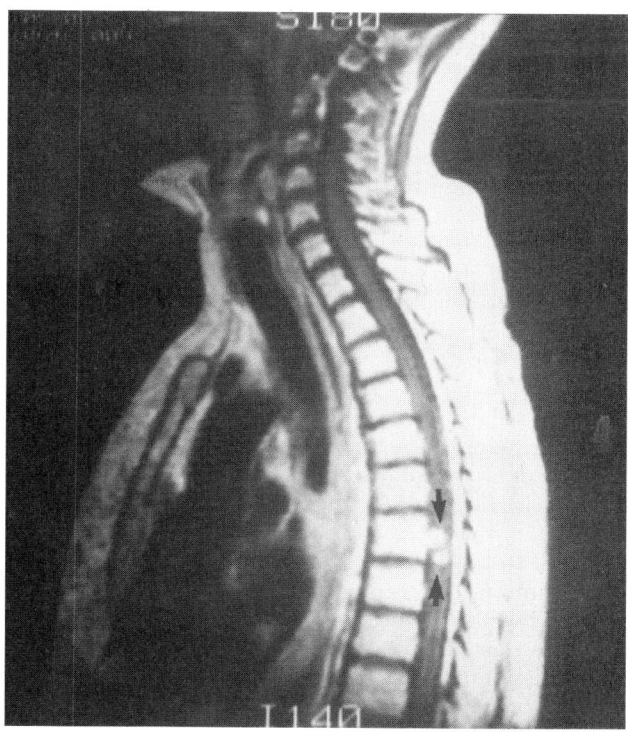

Figure 49-10   Leptomeningeal metastases. (Left) MRI of the brain with gadolinium. This image illustrates diffuse meningeal enhancement, depicting meningeal carcinomatosis. (Right) MRI of the cervicothoracic spine with gadolinium. This view illustrates nodular leptomeningeal tumors or "drop metastases." (Reprinted with permission from Memorial Sloan-Kettering Cancer Center, Department of Neurology.)

tion or an aneurysm rather than a neoplasm. In other situations, e.g., with large meningiomas, angiography may be useful before surgery to determine the blood supply so that it can be embolized during the angiography procedure, obliterated during the surgical procedure, or both.[3] Cerebral angiography involves percutaneous puncture of the femoral artery with injection of radiopaque medium to visualize the cerebral vasculature. It allows the circle of Willis and the large blood vessels that enter the cerebrum to be visualized by serial imaging of the transit of the contrast medium through the vasculature.[35,112] Neurological and neurovascular assessments are performed frequently after the procedure to identify signs and symptoms of weakness, stroke, seizures, or interrupted vascular integrity. Invasive cerebral angiography is being used much less frequently because of the increasing availability of less invasive MR angiography (MRA).

Lumbar puncture.   CSF is often examined for malignant cells in individuals with tumors such as medulloblastomas, ependymomas, and PCNSL that have the propensity to seed the subarachnoid space and spread throughout the CSF pathways. CSF studies are also evaluated in individuals with known or suspected leptomeningeal metastases. An LP should be performed after neuroimaging studies such as MRI and CT scan, especially in an individual with a suspected tumor, because of the risk of herniation.[3]

Prognostic Indicators

The prognosis for an individual with a brain tumor varies considerably depending on the specific type and location of the tumor. Generally, the prognosis for an intracranial malignant glioma, the most common adult primary brain tumor, is dismal. However, several important prognostic factors have been identified that may affect the eventual outcome. Young age, lower histological grade, and high performance status are favorable prognostic indicators for astrocytomas. In adults, younger patients do better and live longer than older patients even when adjusted for the other prognostic factors. Individuals younger than age 40 with a GBM have a 50% 18-month survival rate, compared with 20% for those age 40–60 and 10% for those older than 60.[116] Age appears to be a more important prognostic indicator than even histology.[51]

The more aggressive tumors, or those with a higher histological grade, have a poorer prognosis. As mentioned previously, individuals with anaplastic astrocytoma have a significantly better prognosis than those with GBM. The median survival for anaplastic astrocytoma is approximately 36 months with 30% having a five-year survival, compared with 12 months for glioblastoma. The nonanaplastic oligodendrogliomas have a median survival of approximately ten years, although survival for as many as 13 years has been reported.[46] The median survival for those with the higher-grade oligodendroglioma, the anaplastic oligodendroglioma, decreases to three to five years.[48]

The prognosis of individuals with high-grade gliomas, as with most of the CNS tumors, decreases as their functional status decreases. Those who have severe neurological deficits or are debilitated generally do not tolerate treatment as well as those with a higher performance status. They are generally more susceptible to complications as well. Individuals with high-grade astrocytomas whose Karnofsky Performance Status (KPS) is greater than 70 have been reported to have a 34% 18-month survival, compared with 13% for those with a KPS less than 60.[51]

The extent of surgical resection may be another important prognostic factor. Most of the retrospective studies have demonstrated a delay in tumor recurrence and an increased survival for those individuals undergoing a complete surgical resection compared with those having a partial resection or biopsy alone. Although this may not be universally accepted, the recent trend in the literature has been to support the strategy of removing as much tumor as possible in both malignant gliomas[117] and low-grade gliomas.[118] The extent of tumor resection is also an important prognostic indicator for other types of tumors. For example, completely excised meningiomas and acoustic neuromas have lower recurrence rates.

Other favorable prognostic factors have been suggested for many brain tumors but may not be universally accepted. They include a long duration of symptoms before diagnosis, the presence of seizures, a normal neurological examination, a cystic component to the tumor, location of the tumor (frontal lobe), and small preoperative tumor size.

Approximately 2% of patients with glioblastoma have been reported to survive at least five years.[119–121] In these patients, long-term survival was associated with young age, good preoperative and postoperative KPS, extensive tumor resection, multimodality therapy, and a prolonged relapse-free period. Currently, no clinical or pathological characteristics identify GBM patients destined for long-term survival;[120] however, the importance of patient age may suggest that the biological feature of GBM, such as a specific set of genetic abnormalities, could be the main determinant of survival.[121]

Brain metastases are generally associated with a poor prognosis. However, more favorable outcomes are associated with a high KPS, absent or controlled primary tumor, age under 60, metastatic spread limited to the brain, and a single surgically accessible lesion.

Classification and Staging

CNS neoplasms represent a diverse heterogeneous group of primary and metastatic tumors of the brain and spinal cord. The classification of CNS tumors is based on the premise that each type of tumor results from the abnormal growth of a specific cell type. The consistent naming and grouping of similar tumor types are extremely important when gathering information and statistics on the incidence, etiology, effectiveness of treatment, and prognosis of CNS tumors. Several classification systems are presently in use for CNS tumors, particularly the astrocytomas, which contributes to the complexity in grading and understanding these tumors.

The most critical feature in the classification of CNS tumors is histopathology.[37,122] Recently, the World Health Organization (WHO) revised its classification of CNS tumors. This system first characterizes a tumor histologically by its cell of origin and then designates a grade based on its similarity to normal cells. Grading assesses the degree of malignancy or aggressiveness of the tumor cells by comparing the cellular anaplasia, differentiation, and mitotic activity with normal counterparts.[123,124] Tumor classification has clinical implications, dictates the choice of therapy, and predicts prognosis.

Therapeutic Approaches and Nursing Care

Conventional treatment of the high-grade gliomas is usually a combination of surgery, RT, and chemotherapy. Low-grade gliomas and most benign tumors are generally treated with surgery and, in some cases, RT. The therapy for recurrent tumors is based on the previous types of therapy the individual has already received.

Surgery

Surgery remains the initial treatment for the majority of individuals with brain tumors. Recent technical advances in neuroanesthesia, neuroimaging, and instrumentation have made the surgical treatment of brain tumors safer and more effective. The goal of surgery is often multipurpose: to establish a diagnosis by providing tissue for histological examination; to provide relief of symptoms by quickly reducing the tumor bulk; and to alleviate ICP and the mass effect caused by compression or infiltration of brain tissue. Surgical reduction of tumor can prolong survival.[15] Tumor removal also provides room for edema that may develop with RT and tumor recurrence.[125] Decreasing the tumor burden may also increase the effectiveness of adjuvant therapies by decreasing the number of tumor cells that must be treated, altering cell kinetics, removing radioresistant hypoxic cells, and removing areas of the tumor inaccessible to chemotherapy.[126] Low-grade tumors can transform to higher-grade tumors. Reducing the tumor bulk decreases the number of tumor cells remaining that may be at risk for genetic transformation. Surgical intervention is also often indicated in cases of metastatic brain tumors.

When evaluating an individual for surgery, many factors must be considered: size and location of the tumor, relationship of the tumor to functional brain regions, presence of widespread or multiple sites of disease, and the individual's age and neurological status. For example, a tumor with well-defined margins or one that is encapsulated in the nondominant hemisphere lends itself to an extensive resection. A rapidly growing infiltrative tumor that extends across the midline and is located in a deep vital structure or within the motor or sensory cortex may not be completely excised. In these cases a biopsy or partial resection may be a safer option than a radical procedure. An individual with a single accessible brain metastasis may be a better surgical candidate than one with multiple metastatic lesions. PCNSL, a tumor often widely disseminated throughout the CNS, is not usually surgically resected. This tumor is often best managed by biopsy and adjuvant therapy.

Biopsy. The goal of biopsy is to provide the neuropathologist with a representative sampling of the lesion with which to establish a histological diagnosis. Different biopsy procedures may be performed. A needle biopsy is usually CT- or MRI-guided and is obtained through a burr hole drilled in the skull. An open biopsy, by way of a craniotomy, increases the accuracy of tissue samples, since the tumor can be visualized. Repeated tissue samples are obtained through a small cortical incision.[43] Stereotactic biopsy is the most precise means of obtaining a tissue sample and is the most widely used method today. Stereotaxis precisely locates areas in the brain using three-dimensional coordinates without direct visual access. Using a stereotactic frame (Figure 49-11),[127] the patient's head is secured to the head ring with four percutaneous skull pins to provide rigid skull fixation. A localizing cage composed of vertical and diagonal graphite rods is secured in the head ring and a CT or MRI is performed. The lesion is referenced to the nine x- and y-coordinates of the localizing cage, and these points are transformed to three-dimensional space. The localizing cage is removed, and in the operating room a sterile arc guidance system is fixed to the head ring. The center of the arc depicts the target lesion, which can be approached from any angle or point on the arc quadrant. The biopsy probe or needle is accurately directed to within 1–2 mm of the target.[115,117] In this way, the needle or probe can be guided to the target along the safest pathway, i.e., one that avoids major vascular and functional structures.[125]

Regardless of the biopsy procedure used, the possibility of sampling error exists. Stereotactic biopsy reportedly has a diagnostic accuracy of greater than 95%, an overall morbidity rate of 3.2%, and a mortality rate of 0.6%.[128] Potential complications after a brain biopsy include hemorrhage at the biopsy site, exacerbation of cerebral edema, development of a new neurological deficit, seizures, and infection.

Because they report discomfort with the head frame during placement, patients usually require premedication. In adults, stereotactic biopsy is generally performed under local anesthesia. This may decrease complications associated with general anesthesia but requires patient cooperation to perform the procedure. The need for patient cooperation with these systems discourages their use in pediatric patients and patients with dementia,[129] who typically require general anesthesia. Associated mortality and morbidity may be decreased with stereotactic procedures, and hospital stays may be shorter, leading to decreased hospitalization costs.

Stereotactic resection. The concepts of stereotaxis and radical surgery are combined to remove tumors in computer-assisted stereotactic resection. The surgeon is guided by three-dimensional reconstructions of the operative region generated from preoperative imaging studies. Specific coordinates on the preoperative images (CT, MRI, or both) are matched to landmarks on the patient's head (stereotactic registration), allowing the surgeon to identify specific points on the image as corresponding to identical points in the operative field.[93] Stereotactic craniotomies may be useful for small deep tumors or multiple brain metastases.

Craniotomy. The aim of brain tumor surgery is to remove the tumor completely and ultimately provide a cure. Surgical cure is often not possible, however, as in the case of most gliomas. Reduction of tumor bulk or partial resection during a craniotomy decompresses the brain and becomes the next goal. Partial tumor resection will generally improve the person's neurological condition by decreasing local compression and ICP. This should be the first therapeutic modality for most tumors. Determining where the tumor ends and normal brain begins is another factor adding to the complexity of tumor removal. Preoperative imaging studies are unable to precisely define the margins of a solid tumor, the surrounding areas of infiltrating tumor cells and peritumoral edema, and the normal adjacent brain.[126] Recent advances in neurosurgical and monitoring techniques allow most individuals with brain tumors today to safely undergo successful resections. Many tumors traditionally considered unapproachable are being biopsied, partially resected, and sometimes completely removed with success. These advances include intraoperative monitoring and interactive, image-guided stereotactic systems.

Intraoperative monitoring includes intraoperative ultrasound (IOUS) and brain mapping techniques. IOUS gives the surgeon immediate feedback during the craniotomy and depicts images that assist in the maximal resection of the tumor. A major advantage of ultrasound is its ability to portray an image of the tumor and operating field in real time, allowing visual tracking of changes in the tumor and shifts in the surrounding brain during the operation. IOUS helps to define the tumor's borders by delineating both the tumor and its transition toward normal tissue and differentiating edema from solid tumor and normal brain.[126,130] IOUS is also useful in planning the route or approach through normal tissue to reach the tumor.[126]

Brain mapping is useful in surgery in the dominant hemisphere, the motor and sensory regions, and the

A Head ring fixed to skull

B Localizing rods attached to head ring during scanning

C Scan and localizing landmarks for data processing

D Calculated coordinates verified on simulator

E Surgical biopsy performed

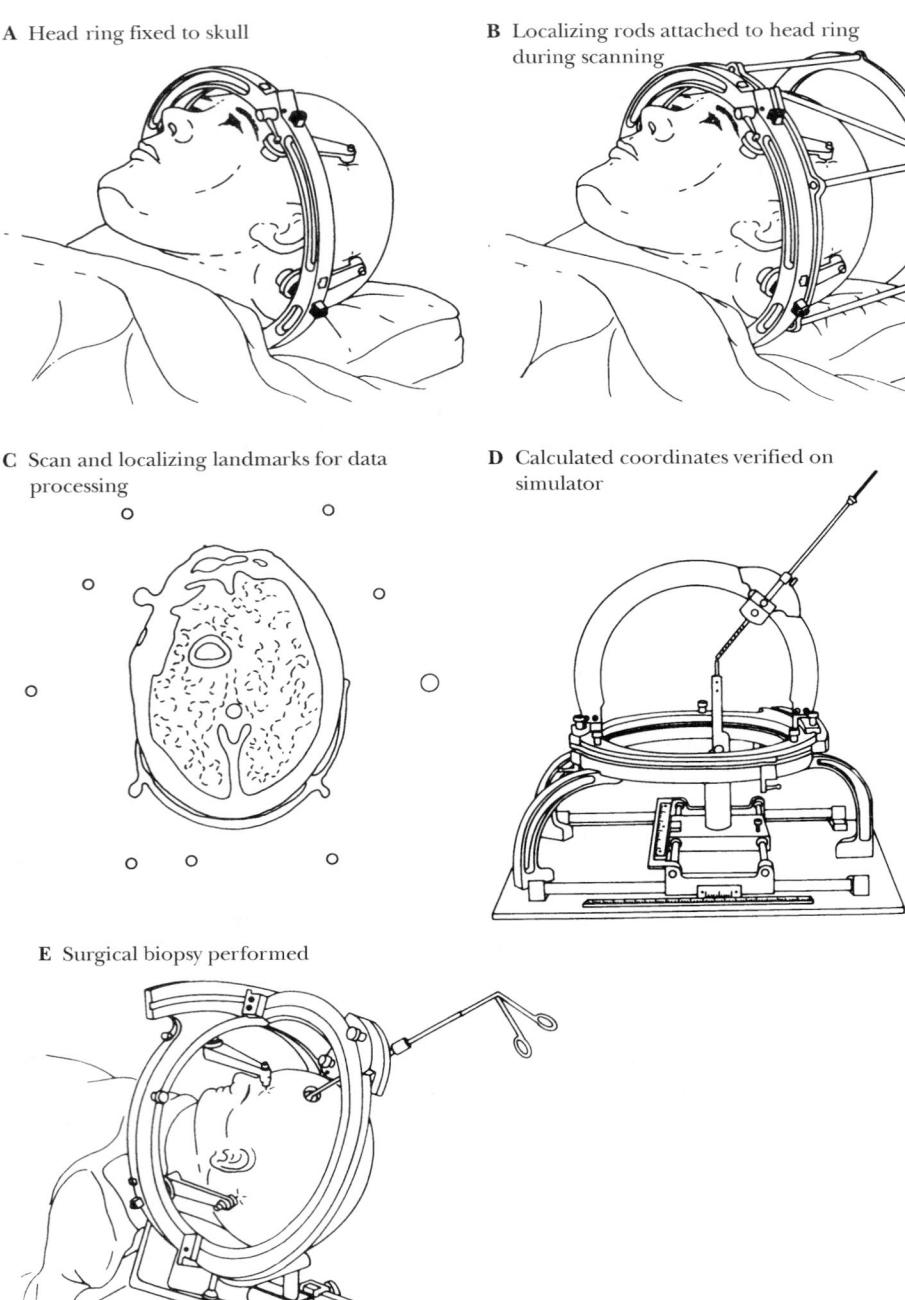

Figure 49-11 Stereotaxic surgery. Diagrams show the sequence of steps using the BRW stereotaxic guidance system. A: The head ring is fixed to the skull. B: The localizing rod system is attached to the head ring for scanning. C: A sample localizing scan from which x-y coordinates of nine localizing rod and intracranial target images are determined for computation by the calculator. D: Computed arc settings are verified for correct trajectory and depth to target on the simulator. E: Arc guidance system is attached to the head ring, and intracranial procedure is performed. (Reprinted with permission from Heilbrun MP, Roberts TS, Apuzzo MLJ, et al: Preliminary experience with Brown-Roberts-Wells (BWR) computerized tomography stereotaxic guidance system. *J Neurosurg* 59:217–222, 1983.[127])

speech centers. Brain mapping techniques use either direct stimulation of the cerebral cortex or sensory evoked potentials (SEPs). Both techniques can facilitate a more complete tumor resection, with decreased morbidity in some individuals. In direct cortical stimulation, the dura is opened and electrodes are placed on the surface of the brain. By stimulating the electrodes, the motor cortex and, in awake patients, the speech centers can be located. Once these functional areas are located, the resection continues and the tumor is removed, keeping the mapped

areas intact and reducing the neurological deficits. During SEP monitoring, sensory structures are stimulated and the electrical responses of the areas are analyzed on a monitor.[131] This technique permits mapping of the somatosensory, auditory, and visual cortex.

Interactive, image-guided, stereotactic systems provide neurosurgeons with precise preoperative and intraoperative patient information. They can improve the accuracy of localizing lesions and aid in defining tumor margins. This allows the surgeon to perform a safe, more effective, and less invasive tumor excision, which translates into improved patient outcomes. Before surgery, the patient undergoes a CT or MRI and markers or fiducials which will be visible on the images, are applied to the patient's head. A computer transforms the data into a three-dimensional image for use in the operating room. In the operating room, the patient's fiducials or coordinates are integrated to the image. A pointing device, such as the viewing wand, is used to quickly communicate surgical locations to a computer system.[129] At any time during the surgery, the surgeon can place the probe on a structure and, by viewing the screen, determine its location in relation to surrounding structures and the angle of the approach to the tumor (trajectory).[126]

Surgery also provides access for other adjuvant therapies. A stereotactic surgical procedure may be used to place radioactive sources within the tumor. Chemotherapy wafers may be implanted surgically within a tumor cavity to slowly and continuously release chemotherapy directly into the brain. Ommaya reservoirs may be placed to deliver chemotherapy directly into the CSF.

Nursing care.

Nursing interventions for patients undergoing neurosurgical procedures begin preoperatively in the outpatient setting. A baseline neurological examination is essential and includes assessment of general cerebral function, including level of consciousness and cognitive function, motor and sensory function, coordination, gait, and cranial nerves. Patient and family preoperative teaching consists of education in the planned surgical procedure, postoperative routines, measures to prevent complications, and medications that will be administered. Patients must be instructed to refrain from taking aspirin, aspirin-containing products, and nonsteroidal, anti-inflammatory agents preoperatively. Postoperative recovery practices vary among institutions. Neurological assessment is conducted on an ongoing basis to identify any variations that may signify potential complications such as increased ICP. If there are no complications, patients undergoing craniotomy are usually hospitalized for three to five days, while those having a stereotactic biopsy require a 24–48 hour hospital stay. Some patients will initially be cared for in a postoperative step-down or an intensive care unit. Others will not require intensive monitoring beyond the postanesthesia care unit. Many institutions use care maps or critical pathways to delineate the inpatient and outpatient care required during the perioperative period. This process may require multiple outpatient visits to complete the diagnostic workup and preoperative teaching.[131] Postoperatively, patients may have new or worsened neurological deficits. The plan of care must be individualized, reflecting the specific deficits. Safety measures assume the utmost importance for all personnel involved in the patient's care. Family members may not truly understand the severity of the potential risks related to deficits such as impaired judgment, memory loss, weakness or paralysis, and visual field disturbances, and will require frequent reinforcement.

Postoperative complications.

The postoperative management focuses on the early identification of neurological deterioration. Timely interventions may prevent or limit permanent neurological dysfunction. Complications after neurosurgery include intracranial bleeding, cerebral edema, further neurological impairment, electrolyte imbalance, infection, seizures, venous thromboembolism, and hydrocephalus. Hemorrhage at the operative site can occur within hours after surgery. Bleeding may also occur from traction on the bridging veins between the brain and the dura, leading to a subdural hematoma.[36] Additional areas where bleeding may occur are the epidural space, the subarachnoid space, or within the ventricles. Patients usually present with a new or worsening of a preoperative neurological deficit or seizures and often require surgery to evacuate the hematoma.

Postoperative cerebral edema is especially severe when there is residual tumor, but it occurs even after complete tumor removal. It results from the surgical manipulation of the surrounding brain tissue, changes in regional blood flow, or brain injury caused by excessive retraction.[126] The amount of edema varies in each individual but generally reaches its maximum peak at 48–72 hours postoperatively. Neurological deficit occurs in approximately 10% of patients.[132] Cerebral edema is treated with corticosteroids, usually dexamethasone, careful fluid management, and osmotherapy when necessary. Other techniques for controlling ICP are hyperventilation, CSF drainage, and the use of anesthetic agents. Activities that can exacerbate ICP should be avoided. The head of the bed is generally elevated 30°. Patients are assessed frequently to identify increased ICP. The signs and symptoms of cerebral edema may be similar to those of intracranial bleeding: decreased level of consciousness, progressive focal neurological deficit, increased ICP, seizures, and possible herniation.

Electrolyte imbalance—namely, hyponatremia—can occur and may be treated with fluid restriction. Some patients require fluid restriction to 1500 mL/day after craniotomy, although most patients are kept euvolemic. Hyponatremia can decrease the seizure threshold, exacerbate cerebral edema, and increase neurological deficits. Infection is often prevented by the prophylactic use of antibiotics for 24–48 hours postoperatively.

Seizures are managed with prophylactic anticonvulsants and maintenance of therapeutic serum levels. It is generally accepted that all patients undergoing supratentorial craniotomy receive seizure prophylaxis. Phenytoin (dilantin) is the most commonly used agent. A CT scan is indicated after a postoperative seizure to rule out hematoma, increased cerebral edema, or pneumocephalus. Other etiologies of seizures include low magnesium or calcium levels, hypoglycemia, hypoxemia, alcohol withdrawal, or meningitis.

Venous thromboembolism is a particular concern in neurosurgery patients because of the length of surgery, immobility of some postoperative patients, hemiparesis, and tumor-related hypercoagulable states.[126] Early ambulation is encouraged whenever possible. The incidence of this complication is reduced by the use of pneumatic compression devices. The use of postoperative prophylactic anticoagulation remains controversial. This complication may occur early or late in the postoperative period.

Postoperative hydrocephalus may be caused by tumor, periventricular swelling, or intraventricular blood. When severe, it is usually treated with ventriculostomy or ventriculoperitoneal shunting.

Radiation Therapy

Radiation therapy plays a central role in the treatment of adult brain tumors.[133] Early randomized studies by the Brain Tumor Cooperative Group (BTCG) firmly established the role of postoperative RT in patients with malignant gliomas, the most common adult primary brain tumor. Individuals who received postoperative RT had a significantly prolonged survival compared with those who received only postoperative supportive care.[134] These studies were so convincing that all subsequent clinical trials evaluating adjuvant therapy for malignant brain tumors have included RT in all treatment arms.[135] RT also has an important role in the treatment of patients with low-grade gliomas, inoperable, partially resected, or recurrent benign brain tumors, and metastatic brain tumors.

Conventional radiotherapy. Radiotherapy for malignant gliomas historically was delivered to the whole brain (WBRT). This was due in part to the belief in the diffuse nature of these tumors and that treatment failure was due to inadequate tumor coverage. Neuroimaging studies have shown that the majority of tumors recur within 1–2 cm of their original location. In addition, many individuals who survive for extended periods after WBRT develop significant treatment-related morbidity. Therefore, partial brain irradiation or local field radiotherapy (LFRT) is now accepted as the standard treatment approach.[136,137] The radiation is delivered to the tumor and a 3-cm margin of tissue surrounding the perimeter[133,136,138] in divided doses (fractions), generally once daily over five to six weeks to deliver 60 Gy to the involved field.[48] Alternative doses, fractions, and schedules have not improved the outcome[48] and in many cases have led to increased toxicity. WBRT is usually reserved for multifocal disease.

Other primary brain tumors may be treated with RT. Benign brain tumors such as meningiomas and pituitary adenomas are often surgically cured. In tumors that cannot be completely excised or that recur despite aggressive resection, RT is an important adjuvant therapy. Completely resected benign meningiomas and pituitary adenomas have a low risk of recurrence, and postoperative RT is not generally recommended. In contrast, the risk of recurrence in partially resected tumors is much higher, and studies have suggested that postoperative RT may delay recurrence, prevent tumor regrowth in some patients and provide a cure, and improve survival. A dose of 54 Gy is recommended for benign tumors. Individuals

with malignant meningiomas generally receive postoperative RT, regardless of the extent of resection, and the dose is increased to 60 Gy.[3]

RT is administered to most individuals with low-grade gliomas,[46] although no consensus exists regarding its appropriate timing.[48] Some advocate immediate postoperative RT, while others delay RT until tumor progression occurs. Shaw and associates[139] reported a prolonged survival in individuals with low-grade astrocytomas who received postoperative RT. The rationale for early intervention is based on the poor long-term survival in these individuals, the likelihood that low-grade tumors will transform into high-grade tumors, and the decreased morbidity of modern RT.[140,141] Others, though, have reported no increase in survival in individuals who received postoperative RT.[142,143] Those in favor of observation alone base their opinion on the lack of proven benefit, the potential long-term effects of RT in these patients,[115,117] and because some low-grade gliomas are remarkably indolent.[46] Immediate postoperative RT to prevent neurological deterioration may be appropriate for patients with poor prognostic factors (older age, bulky residual disease, astrocytoma pathology versus oligodendroglioma). Delayed RT to avoid or postpone the possibility of the neurotoxic effects of RT may be appropriate for patients with favorable prognostic factors (younger age, complete resection, oligodendroglioma pathology).[46,48] The standard radiation dose for these tumors is generally 54 Gy.[3,48]

Three-dimensional conformal radiation therapy. In many centers, the RT treatment plan for primary brain tumor patients uses three-dimensional treatment planning. Three-dimensional conformal radiation therapy (3D-CRT) is a new method of high-precision RT. It utilizes MRI, CT information, or both and powerful computer technology to plan and deliver external beam radiation treatments that shape the prescription dose distribution to conform to the anatomic boundaries of the tumor in its entire three-dimensional configuration.[136] This treatment plan requires reproducible and precise head immobilization.[144] Comparative two-dimensional and three-dimensional treatment planning studies in brain tumor patients have demonstrated a 30% reduction in the amount of normal brain irradiated when the 3D-CRT method is used.[136,145]

Alternative fractionation. Alternative forms of fractionation are hyperfractionation and accelerated fractionation. In hyperfractionation two or more treatments are administered daily using fraction sizes that are smaller than conventional dose fractions to increase the total dose given over the same period of time. It is known that damage to normal brain tissue is related not only to a higher total radiation dose but also to the size of the fraction administered and to the amount of brain irradiated. If the amount of each fraction is lowered or the volume of tissue radiated is decreased, an increase in the total dose may not cause excessive damage. This approach allows a higher dose to be given to the tumor while maintaining the normal brain tissue at or below tolerance levels.[133] In accelerated fractionation, conventional dose fractions are administered two to three times daily and reduce the overall treatment time. This fractionation scheme may be appropriate for individuals with a shorter life expectancy, such as the elderly.

Radiosensitizers. Malignant gliomas are radioresistant. It is believed that the radioresistance of gliomas may be due in part to the presence of hypoxic tumor cells. Hypoxia protects the tumor cells from the effects of RT. The radiation dose would have to be greatly increased to obtain the same effect in hypoxic cells that is achieved in fully oxygenated cells. This large amount of radiation, however, would cause unacceptable side effects and damage to normal brain tissue. Radiosensitizers are chemicals that increase the lethal effects of radiation. Hypoxic cell sensitizers sensitize the hypoxic tumor cells without increasing the radiation effect on the well-oxygenated normal tissue. One group of agents, the halogenated pyrimidines, has been studied in malignant gliomas.

The halogenated pyrimidines, iododeoxyuridine (IrdU) and bromodeoxyuridine (BrdU), are incorporated into DNA because of their similarity to thymidine.[146] Only actively dividing tumor cells incorporate these drugs. As a result of this substitution, the rapidly dividing tumor cells are more sensitive to the damaging effects of radiation. Therefore, there is increased tumor cell kill without increasing damage to the less rapidly dividing normal brain tissue.[147] In one study of individuals with anaplastic astrocytoma who received IudR with RT, 33% have survived for five years.[147] In another study by Sullivan and colleagues,[148] a 33% two-year survival was reported for individuals with glioblastoma who received hyperfractionated RT with BudR. Levin and associates[149] reported 50% of patients with anaplastic astrocytoma alive at four years after treatment with BrdU and RT followed by chemotherapy. The median survival of those who were treated with limited-field RT in that study was 5.2 years. The above results are encouraging and reports of randomized studies comparing BrdU-sensitized RT with nonsensitized RT in individuals with malignant gliomas are awaited.

Hydroxyurea as a radiosensitizer has also been used in individuals with malignant gliomas. Prados and colleagues reported 66% of individuals with anaplastic gliomas treated with combined modality treatment with RT, hydroxyurea, and adjuvant chemotherapy alive at 4 years.[150] There did not seem to be an advantage for those with GBM.

Conventional doses of radiation fail to locally control the majority of malignant gliomas. Techniques that allow focal dose escalation to the tumor while decreasing the radiation exposure to normal brain tissue include interstitial brachytherapy and stereotactic radiosurgery.

Interstitial brachytherapy. Brachytherapy involves the temporary high-activity or permanent low-activity implantation of radioactive sources directly into the brain tumor. Catheters are placed into the tumor using stereotactic surgical techniques, and the radiation seeds or pellets are then placed in the catheters. The implants are removed either after a few days, several months, or left in permanently, depending on the source used. Iodine 125 (^{125}I) is the most commonly used source for both temporary and permanent implants in North America.[151] The area of tumor receives the highest dose, since the sources are directly within the area to be irradiated. Surrounding normal brain tissue is spared because there is a rapid falloff in dose as the distance from the radiation source increases.[133] The advantage to interstitial brachytherapy is that the effect on normal tissue is greatly reduced, thus decreasing some of the resulting side effects.

Only about 30% of individuals with malignant gliomas are usually eligible for brachytherapy. Individuals with tumors that are large or multifocal, that cross the midline, that are inaccessible or located in functionally vital areas, or whose performance status is low are not candidates for this form of therapy. The initial studies using brachytherapy demonstrated an increased survival in individuals with recurrent GBM. These results led to trials with ^{125}I implants as a component of primary therapy along with conventional external beam RT. Gutin and associates[152] reported a median survival from diagnosis of 88 weeks in a group of newly diagnosed individuals with GBM who received conventional RT followed by brachytherapy boost as part of initial treatment. Survival in these patients was further prolonged if they underwent resection at the time of recurrence.[153] In a similar trial, Wen and colleagues[116] reported a median survival of 18 months. A significant finding was the increased two-year survival of 39% and 34%, respectively. Brachytherapy is generally not recommended in anaplastic astrocytomas since similar survivals have been reported with conventional RT and chemotherapy.

Permanent sources implanted at the time of initial surgery are becoming increasingly common. An advantage of this approach is that the tumor burden can be decreased at the same time, irradiation to high doses occurs over a long period of time, and the rate of subsequent radiation necrosis may be lower.[151,154]

Hyperthermia. Hyperthermia has been investigated in conjunction with interstitial brachytherapy. While heat is cytotoxic to both normal and malignant cells, several characteristics of brain tumor cells may make them more susceptible to heat damage. Hypoxic cells, acidic cells, and cells in the S phase are sensitive to heat; heat inhibits the repair of sublethal radiation damage and, therefore, has an additive effect when combined with RT; heat may also augment the effect of some chemotherapeutic agents.[155]

Various methods can be used to produce the heat, including radio frequency, microwave antennae, ultrasound, and electromagnetic techniques. However, the inability to homogeneously heat the tumor mass and the ineffective monitoring of intratumoral and normal brain temperatures have been limitations of this method.[155] Sneed and associates[156] reported a median survival of 47 weeks in a group of patients with recurrent GBM treated with brachytherapy and hyperthermia. In a prospective randomized trial comparing the benefit of hyperthermia to brachytherapy boost, mean survival was increased from 84 weeks to 118 weeks for newly diagnosed individuals with GBM.[52] The two-year survival improved from 15% to 31%.

Stereotactic radiosurgery. Stereotactic radiosurgery uses an imaging-compatible stereotactic device to precisely localize an intracranial target and delivers a high radiation dose in a single session without delivering significant radiation to the surrounding normal brain tissue.[136] This technique is performed using a modified linear accelerator, gamma knife unit, or cyclotron. Radiosurgery was initially used for small arteriovenous malformations (AVMs), benign brain tumors, and brain metastases. Malignant tumors were not considered appropriate for radiosurgery because of their invasiveness and large size. Recently, however, the use of radiosurgery in the treatment of primary and recurrent malignant brain tumors has increased. Shrieve and associates[138] reported on a group of individuals with recurrent GBM treated with radiosurgery. The median survival was 10.2 months, with a 19% two-year survival. In another study, 69 newly diagnosed individuals with GBM received radiosurgery as a boost following surgery and external beam RT. Median survival was 19.7 months, and two- and three-year survival rates were 31% and 20%.[133,157] Unfortunately, the majority of individuals with malignant gliomas would not be eligible for this type of therapy because of their tumor size or tumor shape. The Radiation Therapy Oncology Group (RTOG) is evaluating the role of radiosurgery in the initial management of those with malignant gliomas. Individuals are randomized to receive either radiosurgery followed by external RT and BCNU or external RT and BCNU alone.

There has not been a randomized trial comparing radiosurgery and brachytherapy in the treatment of either primary or recurrent GBM. Although the outcomes for brachytherapy and radiosurgery are similar, radiosurgery offers several advantages. Radiosurgery is a noninvasive single-day procedure usually performed in an outpatient setting. Thus the risk of hemorrhage and infection and a prolonged hospitalization can be avoided. The risk of radiation exposure to personnel does not exist. Radiosurgery can be used for lesions that may be unsuitable for brachytherapy because of their location. Radiosurgery may also be used to retreat patients with small, previously irradiated lesions.[136] In many centers that have the capability to perform either procedure, stereotactic radiosurgery has become the preferred treatment for recurrent GBM except in cases of large or irregularly shaped tumors.[158] For larger tumors that cannot be treated with radiosurgery, brachytherapy may be possible.

Stereotactic radiotherapy. Stereotactic radiotherapy uses the planning technology and precision of stereotac-

tic radiosurgery but delivers the treatment using standard fractionation doses. Stereotactic radiosurgery hardware and software and head frames that can be relocalized daily in a nontraumatic and reproducible fashion are used.[136] Standard fractionation avoids the toxicities associated with large single doses, and tumors located near critical structures may be more successfully treated with the precision of the stereotactic technique. This approach is being used for some benign tumors and gliomas.

Brain metastases. Radiation is standard treatment for metastatic brain tumors. Up to 50% of individuals with metastatic brain tumors will not be surgical candidates because the lesion may be surgically inaccessible or widespread systemic disease may be present. These individuals and those with multiple metastases typically undergo RT. Patients who undergo surgery generally receive postoperative WBRT. In a randomized study by Patchell and colleagues,[159] postoperative WBRT did not increase survival as compared to those undergoing surgery alone. It did reduce the recurrence rate at the original site, prevent the subsequent development of brain metastases at sites other than the original metastasis, and decrease the deaths resulting from neurological causes. WBRT has been preferred over partial field RT because multiple metastases may be present even if some are too small to be detected on imaging studies. Typical radiation treatment schedules for metastatic brain tumors consist of a total dose of 30–40 Gy delivered over 10–20 fractions.[48] Lower daily fractions and a more protracted course may be indicated in individuals with a better prognosis.[97] As with primary tumors, response rates vary with the histological characteristics of the primary tumor. For example, metastases from breast and small cell lung cancers respond better to RT than metastases from melanoma, renal, or colon cancers.[37,97]

Many metastatic brain lesions are now being treated with stereotactic radiosurgery.[92] Unlike surgery, few lesions are inaccessible to radiosurgical treatment because of their location in the brain. Because the tumors are generally small in size and tend not to invade adjacent brain tissue, the individual with brain metastases is an ideal candidate for radiosurgery.[104] Uncontrolled primary disease, uncontrolled or progressing nonbrain-metastases, tumors larger than 4 cm, tumors associated with significant mass effect and neurological symptoms, and, in some cases, low KPS scores are considered contraindications to radiosurgery.[92] Median survival for patients with brain metastases treated with radiosurgery has generally been reported at seven to ten months,[92] although Young and colleagues[160] found more than 30% of patients surviving beyond one year and 15%–20% beyond two years. Radiosurgery may be used alone, with WBRT, or may be used to treat recurrent or new metastases after prior WBRT. Multiple lesions may be treated as long as they are small. The disadvantages of radiosurgery are cost, increased risk of radiation necrosis, and failure to control micrometastases elsewhere in the brain.[160,161]

Side effects. Side effects of RT can be classified as acute, subacute, and delayed. The acute reactions occur during the course of treatment and are temporary. They are manifested as signs of increased ICP or worsening of neurological deficits. They result from an increase in cerebral edema; the administration of corticosteroids usually decreases or alleviates symptoms. Steroids are generally administered during the course of therapy to prevent this. Other acute adverse effects are nausea, vomiting, anorexia, fatigue, alopecia, and skin irritation. Alopecia lasting several months occurs after 54 Gy; it is often permanent after 60 Gy.[144] Acute reactions have been reported to occur in one-third of patients undergoing stereotactic radiosurgery and include headaches, nausea, vomiting, dizziness and vertigo (more commonly with acoustic neuromas), worsening neurological deficit, and seizures.[162]

The subacute reactions generally develop one to three months after completion of therapy. These, too, are of a temporary nature. Symptoms include anorexia, sleepiness, lethargy, and an increase in neurological deficits. These effects are thought to result from the temporary disruption of myelin formation, which helps speed the relay of nerve signals. It takes approximately six weeks for myelin to repair.

Delayed effects of RT usually occur 6–24 months after completion of treatment. These effects are irreversible and often progressive. They result from direct injury to brain tissue and blood vessels. Leukoencephalopathy, degeneration of the white matter, occurs at the tumor site and surrounding irradiated brain. The risk of developing leukoencephalopathy increases with a higher total dose, higher dose per fraction, and with the concomitant use of neurotoxic chemotherapeutic agents, particularly methotrexate. The clinical manifestations range from mild cognitive neurological impairment to dementia to death. The onset and progression can be quite variable. Radiation necrosis occurs more commonly after brachytherapy and radiosurgery but can occur after conventional RT as well. Those at increased risk for long-term radiation effects are children less than age 2 and adults over 50. Long-term effects can be initially managed to some degree with corticosteroids and surgery to remove necrotic tissue. Other long-term effects include loss of vision, development of secondary malignancies, and endocrine disturbances. The major complication of both brachytherapy and radiosurgery is the development of symptomatic radiation necrosis requiring prolonged administration of steroids and reoperation. The rate of reoperation is 30%–40%, usually within six months.

Nursing care. Nursing management of the individual receiving RT includes neurological assessment and evaluation of side effects, and patient and family education regarding treatment schedules, routines, the possible side effects, and the management of these effects. Additional interventions focus on the specific irradiation method used. The most common method, conventional external beam, is usually provided on an outpatient basis. Assistance may be necessary for transportation arrangements. Most patients will be on steroids to reduce the cerebral edema that occurs during brain irradiation. Education

is necessary regarding their many adverse effects. Brain irradiation causes the skin to become dry and peel, and moist desquamation may occur, most often behind the ears.[163] Individuals should be instructed on appropriate skin care and creams, and they must avoid sun exposure. Extreme fatigue occurs during and after treatment, and patients require support and encouragement to manage this distressing symptom.

Chemotherapy

Although it does not produce a cure, chemotherapy plays an important adjuvant role in the treatment of adult primary brain tumors. The most widely studied group of tumors has been the malignant glioma because it is the most common adult primary brain tumor and accounts for the majority of deaths in individuals with brain tumors. Many studies have evaluated a variety of single chemotherapeutic agents and multiple drug regimens. BCNU, CCNU, procarbazine, and vincristine remain the most commonly used agents both for newly diagnosed and recurrent malignant gliomas.[164] Historically it has been difficult to accrue large numbers of individuals with primary brain tumors into clinical trials. Early trials often contained heterogeneous patient populations and failed to separate participants according to prognostically significant variables such as age, tumor histology, and performance status. A younger person with a malignant glioma will generally respond better than an older individual with the same tumor. A person with an anaplastic astrocytoma has a better prognosis than a person with a GBM, and those with a higher performance status generally do better than those with a low performance status.

Of the malignant gliomas, GBM responds the least well to chemotherapy, anaplastic astrocytoma responds somewhat better, and oligodendrogliomas may be the most chemosensitive.[15] Unfortunately, no one prognostic factor or clinical feature reliably predicts which individuals will benefit most from adjuvant chemotherapy. In a meta-analysis by Fine and associates,[135] the results from 16 randomized clinical trials were evaluated to find out if adjuvant chemotherapy did indeed improve survival in individuals with malignant gliomas. They found a statistically significant survival advantage for those who received adjuvant chemotherapy. An increase in survival of 10% at one year and 8.6% at two years was described for those individuals who received chemotherapy in addition to RT.

The delivery of adequate concentrations of intravenous chemotherapy to tumors within the CNS is limited by the presence of the blood-brain barrier (BBB). The BBB is made of a continuous lining of endothelial cells that are connected by tight junctions.[36] The passage of substances across the lipid membranes of endothelial cells depends on molecular weight, lipid solubility, and ionization state.[165] Large, water-soluble, charged particles and compounds bound to plasma proteins are unable to penetrate the BBB. This vascular barrier normally protects the brain by limiting the entry of potentially toxic substances into brain tissue. Unfortunately, the BBB also effectively prevents the majority of chemotherapeutic agents from entering brain tissue. If the BBB did not exist, it is possible that CNS toxicity rather than myelosuppression or gastrointestinal toxicity would be the dose-limiting factor for most chemotherapeutic agents[3] because more drug would reach brain tissue.

Although the BBB can be a potential obstacle to the delivery of chemotherapy to these tumors, the most malignant brain tumors are often associated with marked disruption of this barrier. Water-soluble contrast agents administered with CT or MRI are able to cross the normally impermeable BBB and enter the brain in the region of the tumor. The surrounding normal brain, however, continues to exclude the contrast material because its BBB remains intact. Thus, the enhancing masses seen on CTs and MRIs represent regions of tumor with a substantially disrupted BBB. Malignant cells, however, often infiltrate adjacent tissue and spread to distant sites. Contrast enhancement usually does not occur in the surrounding normal brain that typically contains micrometastatic disease.[166] The BBB is therefore at least partially intact in many brain tumors, particularly in the periphery of the tumor and around infiltrating tumor cells.

Initial chemotherapeutic agents studied in individuals with malignant gliomas were lipid-soluble agents such as the nitrosoureas that readily cross the BBB, mainly BCNU.[167] After years of study and many trials, no other chemotherapeutic agent or combination of agents has been shown to be more effective than BCNU for those with GBM. Other agents that have shown some activity against gliomas include procarbazine, cisplatin, carboplatin, etoposide, cyclophosphamide, vincristine, iproplatin, nimustine, CCNU, paclitaxel, tamoxifen, and hydroxyurea.[165–170] In some studies the combination of PCV has been found to be more effective than BCNU alone for those with anaplastic astrocytoma. Levin and colleagues[54] demonstrated an increased median survival of 151 weeks in individuals with anaplastic astrocytoma treated with PCV as opposed to 82 weeks for those who received BCNU. This regimen (PCV), as opposed to BCNU, is being increasingly used as adjuvant chemotherapy for persons with anaplastic astrocytoma.

Anaplastic oligodendrogliomas have been found to be chemosensitive tumors. The PCV combination has been the most widely studied regimen for these tumors, and positive results have been obtained for both newly diagnosed and recurrent tumors. This regimen is now the treatment of choice.[171] A multi-institutional trial is underway evaluating intensive PCV chemotherapy followed by high-dose thiotepa and autologous stem cell transplantation. Mixed gliomas[172,173] and nonanaplastic oligodendrogliomas[174] also appear to respond to these agents. Other drugs these tumors seem to respond to include BCNU, diaziquone (AZQ), and melphalan.[175]

Unfortunately, the addition of adjuvant chemotherapy has added little improvement to the survival of individuals with malignant brain tumors, particularly those with GBM. New approaches have been explored in an attempt to increase the efficacy of the currently available chemotherapeutic agents by circumventing the BBB and delivering more drug to the tumor. These include IV continuous-infusion chemotherapy, intrathecal or intraventricular chemotherapy, intraarterial chemotherapy, high-dose chemotherapy with autologous bone marrow or stem cell rescue, and interstitial chemotherapy. These strategies can selectively deliver higher concentrations of chemotherapy to the tumors. Unfortunately, the neurotoxicity of these approaches may correlate with the drug levels in the normal brain surrounding the tumor.[166]

Continuous infusion. As mentioned previously, water-soluble contrast agents used to image tumors on CT or MRI scans are able to pass through the disrupted BBB near the area of tumor, producing contrast enhancement at the outer ring of the tumor. The inner portion of the tumor does not initially enhance. Bolus infusions of water-soluble agents with short plasma half-lives might treat the contrast-enhancing tumor ring but may never reach therapeutic concentrations within the center of the tumor. The observation that contrast enhancement, after hours of sustained blood levels, can reach the center of the tumor suggests that continuous infusions of water-soluble chemotherapeutic agents might result in a more uniform drug distribution within brain tumors.[166] A combination of BCNU and cisplatin (a lipid- and water-soluble agent) continuously administered over three days demonstrated an objective response greater than 60% with some complete radiographic responses noted.[176] A randomized study comparing this type of regimen to standard therapy of RT and BCNU is being evaluated.

Intrathecal/intraventricular. The instillation of chemotherapy directly into the CSF is an important method of administering chemotherapy for individuals with leptomeningeal metastases, leukemic or lymphomatous meningitis, PCNSL, and primary CNS tumors such as medulloblastomas where the subarachnoid space is involved. An LP for intrathecal chemotherapy administration has been performed safely in select persons. However, chemotherapy instilled directly into the ventricular CSF by way of the Ommaya reservoir has been found to produce better drug distribution throughout the CSF and more consistent drug levels. Thus, the Ommaya reservoir is the preferred method of delivering chemotherapy into the CSF. It allows for greater ease of administration and less discomfort for the patient. Complications occurring with the use of this device include infection, catheter blockage, catheter leakage, and, after the administration of chemotherapy, a chemical meningitis.

Intraarterial. Intraarterial chemotherapy involves the catheterization of the carotid or vertebral arteries, which provide the arterial supply to brain tumors for the administration of chemotherapeutic agents. Agents that have been evaluated in this approach include BCNU, cisplatin, carboplatin, CCNU, and methotrexate. This method can increase the amount of chemotherapy delivered to the tumor up to ten times[177] while decreasing the systemic toxicity. This method of drug delivery has significant toxicities. Shapiro and associates[178] reported on the large BTCG study evaluating intraarterial BCNU as one treatment arm that was discontinued early because of unacceptable toxicity. Fifteen percent of patients developed ipsilateral vision loss, and 10% had severe neurotoxicity. Moreover, survival rates were worse for those treated with intraarterial BCNU than for those who received conventional IV BCNU.

Blood-brain barrier disruption.

Another approach to intraarterial chemotherapy is to transiently disrupt the BBB with an osmotic agent such as mannitol just before the administration of the intraarterial chemotherapy. Hypertonic mannitol causes a loss of fluid from the capillary endothelial cells, causing the endothelial cells to shrink and the tight junctions to break, resulting in osmotic shrinkage.[36,37] Large molecular-sized materials or water-soluble agents may then diffuse through the opened junctions into the surrounding brain. Neuwelt and colleagues[179] treated GBM patients with IV cyclophosphamide followed by intraarterial mannitol, methotrexate, and oral procarbazine, and the median survival achieved was 17.5 months. Gumerlock and associates,[180] in a more recent study, treated GBM patients with the same regimen and described a 22-month median survival rate. BBB disruption can be associated with significant toxicity, however. This procedure is performed monthly for 12 cycles under general anesthesia. In addition to the risks of general anesthesia, intraarterial chemotherapy with BBB disruption produced worsening of neurological deficits in up to 56% and seizures in up to 44% of patients. One reason for this toxicity is that mannitol also increases the permeability of normal capillaries, which significantly increases the vulnerability of the normal brain tissue to the toxic effects of chemotherapy. Newer methods of selectively altering the BBB are being investigated.

Autologous transplantation.

High-dose chemotherapy followed by autologous bone marrow or stem cell rescue has also been evaluated in individuals with malignant gliomas. Most of the studies have used BCNU alone or in combination with other agents, including thiotepa and etoposide, as the preparative regimen. BCNU is the most effective agent to date for GBM, and its delayed and cumulative bone marrow depression is the dose-limiting toxicity. BCNU also has a steep dose-response curve, and these factors make it a good agent to consider for dose intensification followed by bone marrow or stem cell rescue.[165] Although some long-term survivors were noted, median survival for newly diagnosed patients undergoing this procedure was 12–17 months. This approach was associated with significant morbidity, including fatal pulmonary toxicity, hepatotoxicity, and progressive neurological deterioration.[171]

Interstitial.

Interstitial chemotherapy involves the use of biodegradable polymers impregnated with chemotherapeutic agents and is a promising approach in chemotherapy delivery for brain tumors. These polymers are placed intraoperatively in the walls of the tumor cavity after resection and continuously release high local concentrations of chemotherapeutic agents. Chemotherapy delivered directly to the tumor bypasses the variably disrupted BBB, results in high local drug concentrations, and minimizes systemic toxicity. Implantation of BCNU wafers was found to prolong median survival to 46 weeks in a group of patients with recurrent high-grade gliomas.[181] A follow-up randomized, double-blind, placebo-controlled clinical trial was conducted in patients with malignant glioma.[182] In this study the polymers containing BCNU modestly improved survival and did not cause significant adverse effects. This technology is being studied with higher doses of BCNU and alternative chemotherapeutic agents. This new route of administration may allow the use of new and established chemotherapeutic agents that previously could not be efficiently, safely, or effectively delivered to the brain.

Progress in the development of new chemotherapeutic agents for malignant brain tumors has been slow. Neoadjuvant chemotherapy is being increasingly used to evaluate new agents.[183] This approach allows the precise evaluation of tumor response without the confounding effects of RT.[177] Several promising new agents for malignant gliomas have entered clinical trials. Temozolomide, a new oral alkylating agent, has been tested in newly diagnosed and recurrent malignant gliomas and has demonstrated some objective responses. Other agents being studied include topotecan, a topoisomerase I inhibitor with excellent CNS penetration, and difluoromethylornithine (DFMO), a nonalkylating oral agent with activity against malignant gliomas.[11,164]

Nursing care.

Nursing management of the individual receiving chemotherapy depends on the method of chemotherapy administration and the specific agents used, and includes assessment and evaluation of side effects, patient and family education regarding treatment schedules, routines, possible side effects, and interventions to enhance tolerance and maintain functional ability. Potential side effects of BCNU, one of the most commonly administered agents, include pain and burning at the intravenous site, facial flushing, brown skin discoloration, nausea, vomiting, delayed myelosuppression, and pulmonary fibrosis. The PCV regimen is the most commonly administered combination. Side effects of procarbazine include nausea, vomiting, diarrhea, mental status changes, myelosuppression, hepatotoxicity, and hypertensive crisis with tyramine-containing foods; myelosuppression, nausea, vomiting, nephrotoxicity, and hepatotoxicity can occur with CCNU; and vincristine causes peripheral neuropathies, constipation, myelosuppression, alopecia, nausea, and vomiting.

Biotherapy

To date, biotherapy has had little success in the treatment of malignant brain tumors. Methods investigated include the use of cytokines (interferons, interleukins, and tumor necrosis factor), adoptive immunotherapy with lympho-kine-activated killer (LAK) cells and interleukin-2 (IL-2), and monoclonal antibodies. Research continues to grow in this area as improved methods of administration are developed and new agents are identified. These agents may be used in combination with other treatment modalities. Additional areas of investigation that appear promising include gene therapy, antiangiogenesis, inhibition of signal transduction, and growth factor inhibitors.

Gene therapy.   There are two main components to gene therapy, the delivery system and the therapeutic gene. The most commonly used delivery system (vector) are viruses, which will insert their genes only into dividing cells, making them particularly useful in brain tumors. Brain tumors also appear to be a good choice for gene therapy because they are relatively localized and rarely metastasize outside the CNS, and because well-established methods of drug delivery directly into the tumor (stereotactic injection, Ommaya reservoir, and intraarterial injection) already exist. The initial gene therapy trials for high-grade gliomas began in 1991 and used a mouse retrovirus to carry one of the herpes simplex virus genes, the thymidine kinase (TK) gene, into tumor cells. The tumor cell becomes genetically like the herpes virus, divides, and produces more such cells. When an antiviral agent, ganciclovir, is administered, the tumor cells are killed. While the initial gene therapy trials are encouraging, many questions remain, including how to improve the gene transfer and how to reach more tumor cells. Another trial is underway using an adenovirus as the vector-producing cell for the herpes simplex virus TK gene. Future studies are planned with the goal of transferring the *p53* gene (a tumor suppressor gene) into tumor cells, using an adenoviral vector.[11] The tumor suppressor gene, carried to the tumor by a virus, can restore normal function to existing but altered tumor suppressor genes or replace missing genes.[184]

Antiangiogenesis.   Angiogenesis is the growth of new blood vessels. Tumor growth is dependent on the development of a new vascular supply. Endothelial proliferation is a characteristic feature of astrocytomas. The inhibition of tumor-associated new vessel growth (antiangiogenesis) could retard tumor growth and become a potentially useful treatment modality. Agents in clinical trials include thalidomide and TNP-470. Other agents under investigation include angiostatin and endostatin, platelet factor 4, squalamine, and suramin.[184]

Signal transduction inhibition.   Inhibition of signal transduction is another area of research. The inhibition of protein kinase C (PKC) is one such strategy. Malignant gliomas express very high PKC activity when compared to nonmalignant glial cells.[170] Tamoxifen inhibits PKC activity and growth in some malignant glioma cell lines,[170] suggesting a role for agents such as tamoxifen in the adjuvant therapy of individuals with malignant gliomas.[169]

Other agents, bryostatin and UCN-01, are being studied for this purpose.

Growth factor inhibition.   Inhibitors of growth factors involved in the role of tumorigenesis are also being investigated. Leflunomide (SU101), an inhibitor of PDGF, is one such agent being evaluated in a randomized trial in malignant gliomas.

SPINAL CORD TUMORS

Epidemiology

Primary spinal cord tumors occur less frequently than primary brain tumors, accounting for only 15% of all primary CNS tumors. Approximately 2700 of these tumors are diagnosed each year. They occur most often in individuals age 20–60, and with the exception of meningiomas, which occur more often in women, spinal cord tumors are found with equal frequency in men and women. Metastatic tumors are much more common than primary spinal cord tumors and reportedly occur in 5%–10% of individuals with systemic cancer.

Etiology

The etiology of the majority of primary spinal cord tumors is unknown. Individuals with NF-1 may develop neurofibromas of the spinal cord,[185] spinal nerve root tumors (schwannomas) may be present in those with NF-2, and individuals with von Hippel-Lindau disease are at risk for developing spinal hemangioblastomas.[18]

Pathophysiology

Anatomy and Physiology

The spine is a flexible column formed by a series of vertebrae, each stacked one upon another to support the head and trunk. The vertebral column shown in Figure 49-12 consists of 33 vertebrae: 7 cervical, 12 thoracic, 5 lumbar, 5 sacral, and 4 coccygeal. The five sacral vertebrae fuse to form the sacrum, and the four coccygeal vertebrae fuse to form the coccyx.

The spinal cord, housed within the vertebral column, is an elongated mass of nerve tissue less than 1 inch in diameter and approximately 17–18 inches in length. It arises from the medulla oblongata, beginning at the top of the first cervical vertebra, and extends down to the lower border of the first lumbar vertebra, where it ends in a tapered, conelike structure called the *conus medullaris*. The spinal cord is about 10 inches shorter than the vertebral column, and the lower segments of the spinal cord, therefore, are not aligned opposite corresponding vertebrae. Thus, the lumbar and sacral spinal nerves have very long roots. These roots descend in a bundle from the conus, and because of its resemblance to the tail of a horse, this formation is called the *cauda equina*.[38]

There are 31 pairs of spinal nerves exiting from the spinal cord through the intervertebral foramina: 8 cervical, 12 thoracic, 5 lumbar, 5 sacral, and 1 coccygeal. The intervertebral foramina are narrow, and the nerves may easily be compressed at this site by a protruding disk or arthritic spurring.[39] Each spinal nerve has a dorsal root by which afferent (sensory) impulses enter the cord and a ventral root by which efferent (motor) impulses leave the spinal cord. The dorsal roots convey sensory input from skin segments that represent specific areas of the body known as *dermatomes*.[186] Interruption of one sensory nerve root may result in paresthesias or pain in that dermatomal area. The ventral roots convey motor impulses from the spinal cord to the body, innervating specific areas of muscle groups called *myotomes* (Table 49-3).

The cranial meninges are contiguous within the spinal canal to support and protect the spinal cord. The spinal dura is a continuation of the inner layer of the cerebral dura. The outer dural layer ends at the foramen magnum, being replaced by the periosteal lining of the vertebral canal. The spinal dura encloses the spinal nerves and

terminates at the level of the sacrum. The arachnoid layer of the spinal meninges is a continuation of the cerebral arachnoid. The pia mater in the spinal cord is thicker, firmer, and less vascular than that of the brain.[34] The spinal meninges are illustrated in Figure 49-13.

A cross section of the spinal cord shows that it is arranged as a butterfly-shaped area of gray matter surrounded by white matter. The gray matter consists of cell bodies, axon, and dendrites. The white matter consists of longitudinally running fiber tracts. The white matter in each half of the cord is divided into columns (funiculi). These columns are further divided into tracts, which are the sensory and motor pathways of the spinal cord. Impulses are conducted up the spinal cord via ascending tracts (sensory) to the brain, and the descending tracts conduct impulses from the brain down to the spinal cord (motor). The specific motor and sensory symptoms seen in spinal cord tumors depend on the tumor's involvement of these specific tracts.

Extradural Tumors

Spinal cord tumors are also classified by their cell of origin and anatomic location. The major anatomic consideration of spinal cord tumors relates to the tumor's location in relation to the spinal dura mater (Figure 49-14). Extradural tumors lie outside the dura. Most of these tumors are caused by metastatic cancer to the vertebral column, a common site of bone metastasis. Metastases can occur in multiple contiguous vertebrae and in multiple sites of the vertebral column. Metastatic spinal cord tumors most often originate from cancers of the breast, lung, prostate, and kidney and from multiple myeloma. Less common are cancers of the GI tract, thyroid, and melanoma. However, other tumor types can lead to vertebral body metastases as well. The neurological symptoms seen with extradural tumors result from compression rather than invasion of the spinal cord. The spinal cord is usually compressed anteriorly, which leads to edema and ischemia of the spinal cord and mechanically distorts and damages the nervous tissue. Spinal cord compression (SCC) occurs either by direct extension of the tumor into the epidural space, by vertebral collapse and displacement of bone into the epidural space, or by direct extension through the intervertebral foramina. The thoracic spine is the most frequent location of epidural SCC, followed by the lumbosacral and cervical spine. Lung and breast cancer most often cause thoracic compression, whereas prostate, renal, and GI tumors are more likely to affect the lower thoracic or lumbosacral vertebrae.

Lymphomas may be a cause of SCC because they can extend directly through the intervertebral foramina. Other tumors such as sarcoma and chordoma may arise as primary extradural tumors. The chordoma is a slow-growing but highly invasive tumor. It often occurs in the sacrum but can also be found in the cervical spine and

Table 49-3   Motor Nerve Roots (Myotomes) and Areas They Innervate

Spinal Cord Segment	Muscle Action
C-1 to C-4	Flexion, lateral flexion, extension, and rotation of neck
C-3 to C-5	Diaphragm (inspiration); elevation of upper thorax and scapula
C-5 to C-6	Shoulder movement; flexion of elbow
C-5 to C-7	Forward thrust of shoulder
C-5 to C-8	Adduction of arm from front to back
C-6 to C-8	Extension of forearm and wrist
C-6 to T-1	Thumb and index finger (C-6), middle finger (C-7), ring finger (C-8), and pinky finger (T-1)
C-7 to T-1	Flexion of wrist
T-1 to T-12	Control of thoracic, abdominal, and back muscles
L-1 to L-3	Flexion of hip
L-2 to L-4	Extension of leg; adduction of thigh
L-4 to S-2	Flexion, abduction, and rotation of thigh; flexion of lower leg; extension, flexing and spreading of toes
L-4 to L-5	Dorsal flexion of foot
L-5 to S-2	Plantar flexion of foot
S-2 to S-4	Perineum and sphincters

Figure 49-12   The spinal cord lying within the vertebral column. Spinal nerves are numbered on the left side, and the vertebrae are numbered on the right side. (Reprinted with permission from Hickey JV: Overview of neuroanatomy and neurophysiology, in Hickey JV (ed): *The Clinical Practice of Neurological and Neurosurgical Nursing* (ed 4). Philadelphia, Lippincott, 1997, pp 35–79.[34] Originally published in Chaffee EE, Lytle IM: *Basic Physiology and Anatomy*. Philadelphia, Lippincott, 1980).[36]

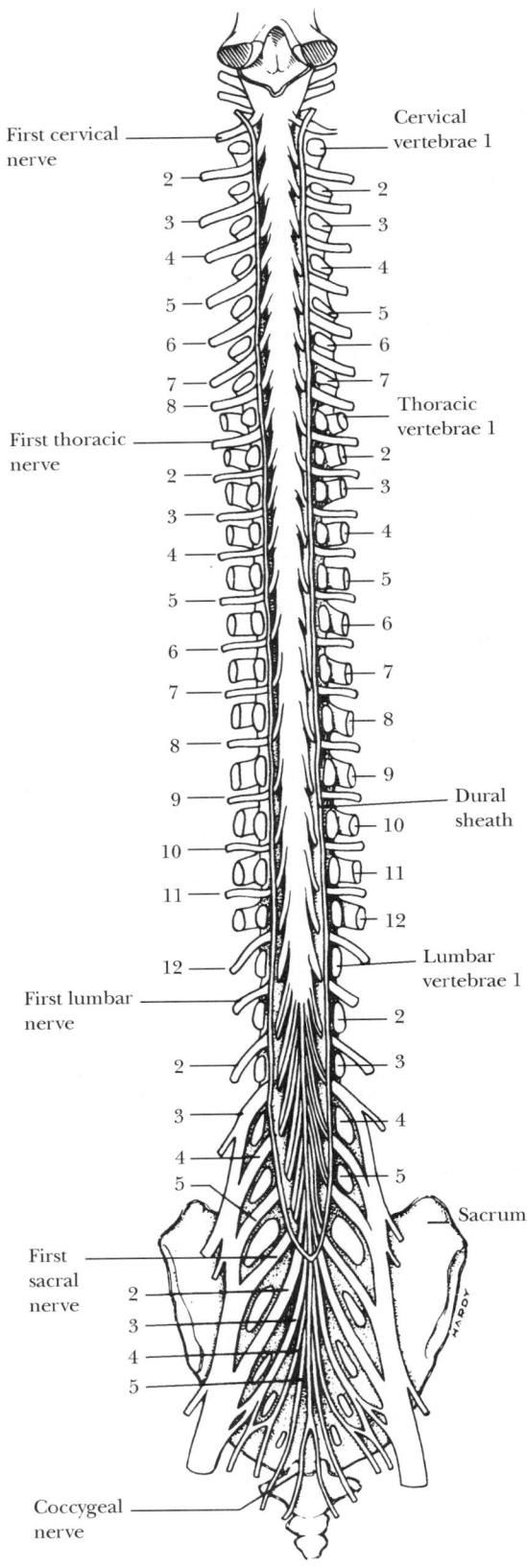

intracranially at the base of the skull. This tumor erodes bone and soft tissue extensively, and even though it is histologically benign, it is difficult to remove in its entirety.[187]

Epidural SCC is a relatively common neurological complication of cancer and is considered an oncological emergency. The incidence of SCC may actually be increasing because patients are living longer and the incidence of cancers that commonly spread to the bone is rising. Epidural SCC usually occurs late during the course of metastatic cancer, although it can be the first sign of cancer.[97]

Intradural Tumors

Intradural tumors arise from the nerve roots or coverings of the spinal cord (intradural, extramedullary) or develop in the spinal cord itself (intradural, intramedullary). The intradural, extramedullary tumors account for almost 90% of primary spinal cord tumors. Schwannomas are the most common extramedullary tumor and often are located in the lumbar spine on one of the many nerve roots of the cauda equina.[185] Meningiomas are the second most frequently occurring extramedullary tumor. They commonly occur in the thoracic spine. Both spinal schwannomas and meningiomas can often be completely removed by surgery and recurrence is rare with complete resection. Sarcomas can also arise as extramedullary tumors. Other less common intradural extramedullary tumors are vascular tumors, chordomas, and epidermoids.[3]

The intradural, intramedullary tumors arise from the same cell as their intracranial counterparts; however, the grade of malignancy is often lower, making the majority of primary spinal cord tumors benign. The majority of intramedullary tumors are ependymomas, followed next by astrocytomas. Less common histologies include hemangioblastomas and various hemangiomas, oligodendrogliomas, gangliogliomas, and medulloblastomas.[3] Most ependymomas are located in the lumbosacral area. Spinal cord ependymomas located in the cauda equina can often be removed without functional sacrifice.[59] Treatment usually includes maximal surgical resection and RT. Ependymomas that involve the CSF are treated with craniospinal RT. Chemotherapy is usually reserved for recurrent tumors.[188] Astrocytomas are distributed more evenly throughout the spinal cord. Surgical resec-

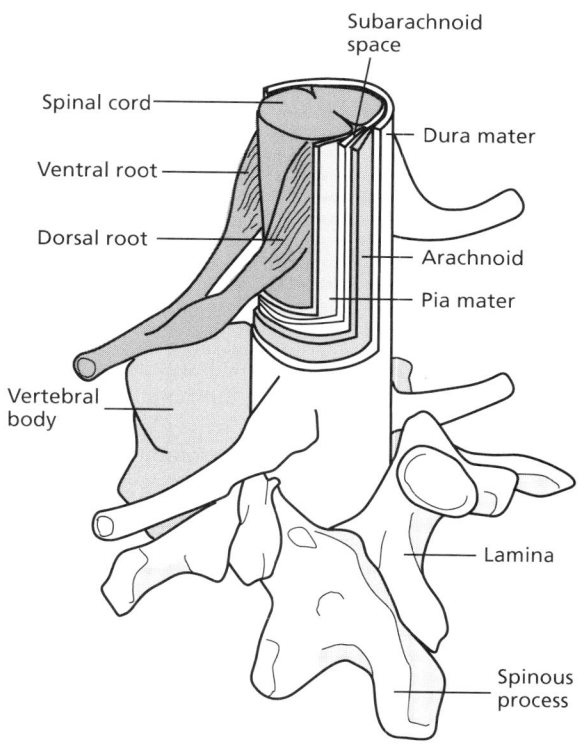

Figure 49-13   Spinal meninges.

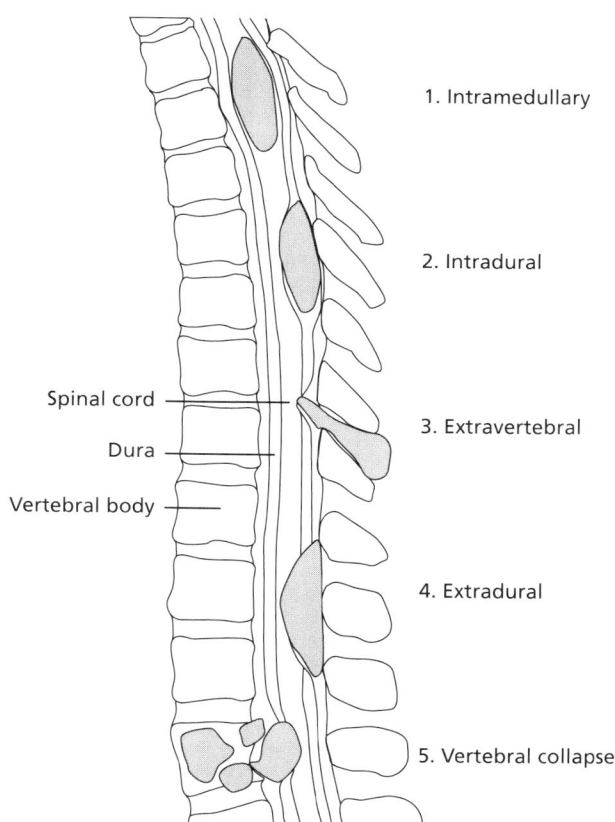

1. Intramedullary

2. Intradural

3. Extravertebral

4. Extradural

5. Vertebral collapse

Figure 49-14   Anatomic location of spinal cord tumors.

tion is often attempted followed by RT. Up to 20% of spinal cord astrocytomas are malignant. These high-grade tumors are generally treated only with RT. Hemangioblastomas are vascular tumors evenly distributed throughout the spinal cord except for those associated with von Hippel-Lindau syndrome, in which they are predominantly located in the cervical cord.[185]

Spinal cord tumors are also anatomically described based on their location in relation to the vertebral column. Approximately 50% of spinal tumors are located in the thoracic spine, 30% are located in the lumbosacral region, and 20% involve the cervical spine. Knowledge of the specific level of involvement is helpful in understanding the signs and symptoms in relation to the specific dermatomes and myotomes involved.

Pattern of Spread

The most common mechanism of spread for extradural spinal metastases is thought to be by way of hematogenous arterial spread. A second mechanism is by direct invasion through the intervertebral foramina by a paravertebral mass. Another possible mechanism of metastatic epidural spinal cord metastases is by retrograde venous spread from the primary site by way of Batson's plexus.[189]

Intradural, intramedullary metastases may occur through CSF pathways. Ependymomas can involve the CSF. A higher incidence of distant spread has been re-

ported in high-grade spinal astrocytomas. This increased propensity for dissemination of malignant spinal cord astrocytomas compared to intracranial astrocytomas is thought to result from the close proximity of tumor cells to the subarachnoid space and CSF pathways.[190] Primary spinal cord tumors rarely metastasize outside the CNS.

Clinical Manifestations

The clinical manifestations associated with spinal cord tumors result from compression and, much less frequently, invasion of the spinal cord. Extramedullary tumors affect the cord by compression, causing traction on or irritation of the spinal nerve roots, displacement of the spinal cord itself, interference with the spinal blood supply, or obstruction of CSF circulation. Intramedullary tumors invade and destroy the spinal cord itself. When spinal cord compression occurs, the normal physiology involved in providing an adequate blood supply, maintaining stable cellular membranes, and facilitating afferent and efferent impulses for specific sensory, motor, and reflex functions of the spinal cord and related spinal nerves is altered.[191] Edema results, causing additional deficits.

The clinical manifestations seen with spinal cord tumors are dependent on the tumor's rate of growth and the level of the spinal cord affected. A slow-growing benign tumor better allows the cord to accommodate the mass. Tumors can be present for years, compressing the cord into a thin, ribbonlike structure without causing significant neurological deficits. On the other hand, the spinal cord cannot accommodate a sudden mass or rapidly growing lesion such as a hematoma or a malignant or metastatic tumor. The spinal cord has little ability to compensate such lesions that increase pressure and create extensive edema causing sudden neurological dysfunction. The signs and symptoms of spinal cord tumors are pain, motor weakness, sensory impairment, and autonomic dysfunction involving bowel and bladder function.

Pain is the most common presenting symptom of a spinal cord tumor. In epidural metastases, back or neck pain may be present for weeks or months, and intradural tumors can cause pain for years before the correct diagnosis is established. Often the pain is initially dismissed as arthritis, back strain, or disc disease, and until other more obvious neurological manifestations appear, the diagnosis of a spinal cord tumor is usually not considered. Back or neck pain in cancer patients, especially those with tumor types that commonly metastasize to bone, should be evaluated for spinal metastases.

The pain may be localized or radicular. Localized pain and tenderness are common over the involved area, particularly with epidural metastases. Radicular pain may be described as bandlike and follows the distribution of the spinal nerve roots (dermatomes). The pain can vary from mild to severe and from dull to sharp or burning, and almost always becomes more severe with time. Pain may be worse at night; a recumbent position often aggravates it. Pain that is aggravated by movement and relieved with immobility may indicate spinal instability. Activities that produce a Valsalva maneuver such as sneezing, coughing, and straining increase the spinal pressure and cause intensification of pain.

Weakness is the most readily identified objective finding and may follow the appearance of sensory symptoms. The level of impairment determines the muscle groups involved (myotomes). The weakness is often associated with hyperreflexia, spasticity, and a positive Babinski sign. It will eventually progress to complete paraplegia unless treatment is initiated. Specific motor symptoms will vary depending on where the tumor is located on a cross section of the spinal cord. A lateral tumor will affect voluntary movement in the arms and legs, muscle tone, coordination, and posture. Tumors in the anterior cord will affect voluntary movement of the trunk muscles, equilibrium, and posture.

Specific sensory deficits will depend on where the tumor is located on a cross section of the spinal cord. A lateral tumor will affect pain and temperature, causing symptoms of coldness, numbness, and tingling. Awareness of vibration and proprioception of body parts are affected if the posterior aspect is involved. Touch and pressure on the opposite side of the body will be affected if the tumor is anterior. Compression affects function below the lesion; therefore, it is important to determine the highest functional level. A sensory assessment begins at the toes and moves upward to determine the level at which function remains, which is generally the level of the tumor. However, there may be a discrepancy between the level of remaining function and apparent tumor location. The lesion may actually be one or two vertebrae above the level of compression. A narrow band of hyperesthesia directly above often accompanies the tumor level.[191]

The effects may be symmetrical and bilateral, asymmetrical, and even unilateral. A combination of sensory and motor deficits may also be seen. A loss of touch, vibration, position sense, and motor ability on the same side as the lesion with contralateral loss of pain and temperature is called the Brown-Séquard syndrome. This occurs in approximately 20% of patients.[3]

Later symptoms are bowel dysfunction, bladder dysfunction, or both, and include constipation, fecal incontinence, urgency, difficulty in initiating urination, urinary retention, and urinary incontinence. These symptoms may be present earlier with an intramedullary tumor.

Assessment

Assessment of the individual with a known or suspected spinal cord tumor begins by obtaining a history. The description and duration of symptoms (when they occur), the presence of exacerbating or relieving factors, and the order of their appearance must be established. A neurological examination, especially of motor and sensory function, gait, and reflexes is performed. The possible presence of bowel or bladder dysfunction must be established, and a pain assessment is performed. This initial assessment provides the baseline from which all future assessments will be compared. The neurological assessment should attempt to initially determine where the tumor is likely to be located (cervical, thoracic, or lumbar). This is facilitated with an understanding of anatomy and physiology.

Diagnostic Studies

MRI is the diagnostic procedure of choice for the evaluation of both intramedullary and extramedullary spinal cord tumors (Figure 49-15). It provides superb anatomic detail of the spinal cord, is noninvasive, and has fewer risks than myelography. MRI is also helpful for planning radiation therapy and surgery.

CT myelography had been the standard method for identifying the location and level of spinal cord and nerve root compromise resulting from spinal tumors. Contrast medium is injected into the subarachnoid space, usually

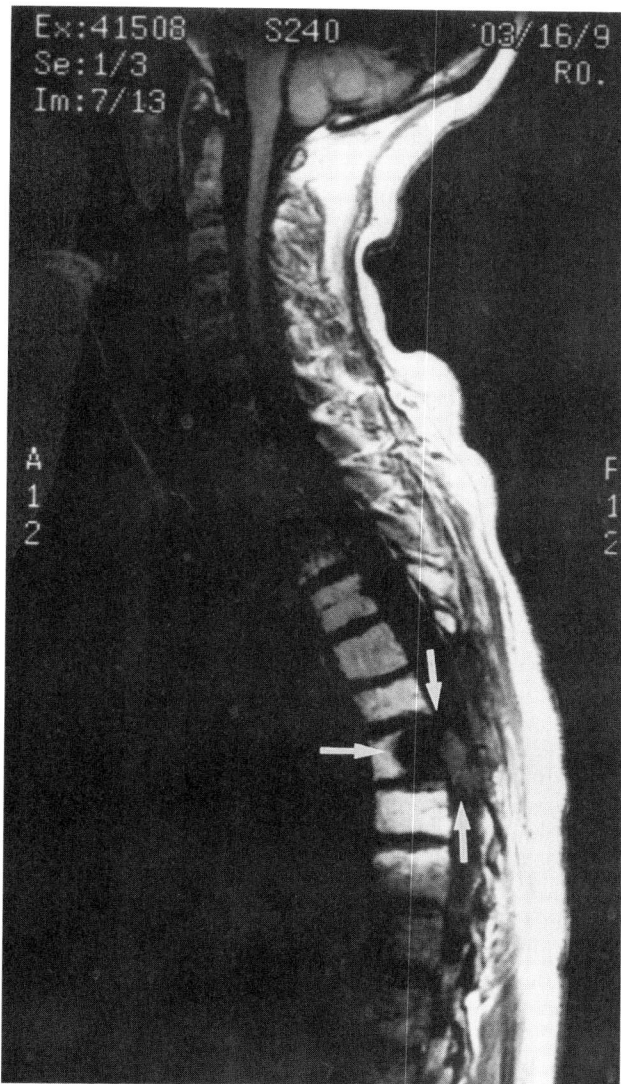

Figure 49-15 Tumor involving the spinal cord. This sagittal view of a cervico-thoracic MRI of the spine with gadolinium demonstrates an extradural metastatic lesion involving the T7 vertebral body causing spinal cord compression. (Reprinted with permission from Memorial Sloan-Kettering Cancer Center, Department of Neurosurgery.)

a good MRI image, or if MRI is contraindicated. This procedure also allows for examination of the CSF.

After a CT myelogram has been performed, the individual must be assessed for any neurological changes and positioned appropriately (usually supine, with the head of the bed elevated at a prescribed level). Possible complications include allergic reaction to the contrast agent, meningeal irritation, headache, nausea, vomiting, infection, and seizure.

Spine x-rays may be performed in individuals suspected of epidural metastases. It is estimated, however, that 30%–50% of the vertebral body must be destroyed before changes are seen on a plain radiograph.[97] Bone scans are sensitive in identifying vertebral disease, but they are not always specific and may identify pathology other than cancer.

Prognostic Indicators

The prognosis is far better for intradural spinal cord tumors than for extradural. The majority of extradural spinal tumors result from metastatic disease, which generally carries a poorer prognosis because of the more advanced stage of disease. Many survive less than a year, and death is often a result of the widespread systemic cancer rather than the epidural tumor. However, subgroups of patients—e.g., those with breast cancer, limited systemic disease, and radiosensitive tumors—survive for longer periods.

Rapid onset and quick progression are worse prognostic factors for recovery. Tumors causing neurological dysfunction that develop over hours to days carry a worse prognosis than those that evolve more slowly. When SCC develops rapidly, neurological recovery is less likely after treatment. The outcome of SCC relates to the neurological status at the time of treatment. The severity of weakness is the most significant prognostic factor for neurological recovery. Eighty percent of those who are ambulatory at the time of diagnosis remain so after treatment. As the neurological dysfunction increases, the likelihood of recovery diminishes. Only 30%–45% of patients who are initially paraparetic and nonambulatory become ambulatory, and those who are paraplegic at diagnosis are likely to remain so, with only 5% regaining the ability to walk.[189] In addition, those who do not regain or retain ambulation have a substantially shorter survival than those who do. The shorter survival results, in part, from complications of paraplegia.[97]

Favorable prognostic factors for the intradural tumors include extent of surgical resection, histological grade, and, as in extradural tumors, slow onset of neurological dysfunction. Schwannomas, meningiomas, and ependymomas have a low recurrence rate if completely resected. The same cannot be said for astrocytomas. The available literature has failed to demonstrate a significant correlation between prognosis and degree of surgical resection.[192,193] A higher-grade spinal astrocytoma carries a

by means of a lumbar puncture, and CT images of the spinal cord and vertebral column are taken to determine if a partial or complete obstruction is present. When the level of a complete block identified by lumbar myelography is uncertain, a cisternal myelogram should be performed to determine the extent of the lesion or to identify multiple levels of involvement. MRI has largely replaced CT myelography, although it may be useful where the complete extent of a block is unable to be determined by MRI or the individual has stabilization hardware already in the spine, which may interfere with obtaining

poorer prognosis as in brain tumors. Those with malignant astrocytomas of the spinal cord generally do not survive longer than eight months.[194]

Classification and Staging

Spinal tumors are classified by their cell of origin and their anatomic location. The types of spinal cord tumors are similar to those tumors found in the brain. Histologically, however, they tend to be less malignant. The major anatomic consideration of spinal cord tumors relates to the tumor's location in relation to the spinal dura mater.

Therapeutic Approaches and Nursing Care

Surgery

In the treatment of spinal cord tumors, the goals of surgery include provision of a diagnosis and partial or complete removal of the tumor. It is the primary treatment modality for most intradural, extramedullary tumors. Schwannomas and meningiomas can often be completely resected with modern microsurgical techniques and neurosurgical instruments. As in brain tumor surgery, intraoperative monitoring assists the surgeon in maximizing the resection while protecting the spinal cord. In most cases these tumors can be removed through a posterior (laminectomy) approach. The uncommon tumor directly anterior to the spinal cord must sometimes be approached anteriorly.[3] The risk of recurrence is estimated to be approximately 10% for complete resections, while recurrence rates increase to approximately 20% for incompletely resected tumors.[192] Recurrences are generally treated with repeat surgical resection unless the tumor extends beyond what is surgically accessible.

Surgery is the initial treatment for intramedullary tumors (ependymomas and astrocytomas) with the exception of the malignant astrocytomas. The determining factor in the successful surgical treatment of these tumors is the degree of tumor infiltration of the surrounding spinal cord. As with intracranial glial tumors, indistinct tumor margins and microscopic infiltration can prevent complete tumor removal. Attempts at complete removal often risk loss of neurological function. Astrocytomas are less clearly demarcated from the surrounding spinal cord tissue than ependymomas.[185] Some astrocytomas are treated with biopsy only, followed by RT. For well-delineated astrocytomas, surgical removal can provide long-term tumor control and, sometimes, cure. Ependymomas of the spinal cord have a longer natural history than astrocytomas. Recurrence of ependymomas may be delayed up to 12 years, whereas astrocytomas that recur generally do so within three years.[194,195]

In extradural tumors, surgery is generally indicated only in cases where the cause of SCC is unknown, there is spinal instability or bone collapse into the spinal canal, a recurrence cannot be retreated with additional RT, the tumor is known to be radioresistant, or the individual is rapidly deteriorating neurologically, perhaps during the course of RT. Two common surgical procedures are posterior decompressive laminectomy and anterior vertebral body resection.

A laminectomy generally only decompresses the spinal cord. The surgeon is often unable to remove the bulk of the tumor during this approach because the tumor is usually located anterior to the spinal cord. If the tumor has invaded posterior to the epidural space, a modified approach can sometimes allow considerable tumor removal. In a vertebral body resection, most or the entire tumor can be removed, and the resected vertebra is replaced with either bone or a synthetic substance such as methylmethacrylate. The spinal column is often further stabilized anteriorly, for example, with Steinmann pins or plates screwed into intact bone, or posteriorly with instruments such as Harrington rods or hooks.[97] Stabilization procedures require intact bone above and below the site of compression to accept, support, and maintain the fixation devices.[192] Patients with spinal instability typically must remain in bed until they can undergo a stabilization procedure or be fitted for a brace.

Complications related to surgical intervention include standard surgical risks (stroke, hematoma formation, deep vein thrombosis, pulmonary embolism, and infection) as well as the development of neurological deficits, CSF leak, and wound dehiscence. The individual with significant or long-standing preoperative neurological deficits is likely to have no improvement or even progression after surgery. The most significant complication to treat is a new neurological deficit in which the neurological function often may not return. The onset of a new deficit is typically related to vascular insult of or manipulation to the spinal cord during surgery.[95] A CSF leak may develop because the dura is not completely sealed or a tear was not repaired. A CSF leak is usually treated with lumbar drainage for several days. If the leakage continues, surgery may be required to repair the leak. A CSF leak increases the risk of infection and may lead to meningitis. Many individuals who develop SCC late in the course of their cancer may be debilitated and have often been on steroids. As a result, wound healing is poor and they are at risk for wound dehiscence.[97]

Radiation Therapy

RT is generally not recommended for completely resected intradural (intramedullary and extramedullary) spinal cord tumors. Both intramedullary and extramedullary tumors may be treated with RT if incompletely resected or on recurrence if repeat surgical resection is not feasible. Malignant tumors routinely receive RT. Doses of 50–55 Gy are generally used in these tumors.[3] Ependymomas are radiosensitive tumors. In patients with ependymomas who received adjuvant RT, five- and ten-year survival rates range from 60%–100% and 68%–95%, respectively.[195,196] The five- and ten-year survival rates for low-grade astrocytomas who received RT range from 60%–90% and 40%–90%.[194] For those individuals with a high-grade astrocytoma, RT is the only therapy available, and even so, the prognosis is poor.

RT and steroids are the most widely used therapy for extradural tumors. The treatment technique depends on the region of spinal involvement. The sensitivity of the spinal cord to radiation limits the prescribed dose. Spinal cord tolerance has been considered to be approximately 45–50 Gy delivered in 180-cGy fractions, 35–37.5 Gy in 250-cGy fractions, and 30–33 Gy in 300-cGy fractions.[189] The usual dose administered is 30 Gy in 300-cGy fractions.[97] Often, higher doses are administered for the initial treatments, especially if there is evidence of neurological dysfunction.

Spinal RT does not cause acute clinical symptoms. The major complication of spinal cord radiation—radiation myelopathy—results from demyelination and white matter necrosis or intramedullary microvascular injury. Radiation myelopathy may present as a subacute or more severe delayed reaction. A transient subacute myelopathy is clinically manifested by momentary electrical shock-like paresthesias or numbness radiating from the neck down to the extremities, and it is precipitated by flexing the neck (Lhermitte's sign). This syndrome develops after an average of three to four months following treatment and resolves within three to six months without the need for intervention.[3] Occasionally, it may persist for several years.[97]

The more severe delayed radiation myelopathy generally occurs 12–28 months following RT, but can take up to four years to appear. The clinical manifestations are irreversible; they begin with weakness and can progress to a complete functional loss from the level of the radiation portal down. It is estimated that for doses in the range of 57–61 Gy with conventionally fractionated RT, the incidence of myelopathy is 5%.[197] For doses above 65 Gy, the incidence increases to 50%. The number of individuals who develop this late myelopathy might be higher were it not for the fact that many succumb to their primary disease before the myelopathy becomes clinically evident. Risk factors for myelopathy include both the total dose and the dose per fraction.

Chemotherapy

Chemotherapy does not play a large role in the treatment of spinal cord tumors. It may be considered for metastatic extradural tumors in individuals with chemosensitive tumors. There have been no trials of chemotherapy for primary spinal cord tumors. It is possible that drugs active against intracranial gliomas may be effective against these same histologies in the spinal cord. Anecdotal patients have been treated with nitrosourea-based regimens.[3]

Symptom Management and Supportive Care

Individuals with CNS tumors frequently suffer from disabling symptoms that dramatically affect their ability to function. Many of these symptoms are directly related to the tumor. Neural structures are destroyed or compressed, leading to increased ICP or SCC. Other symptoms, however, are only indirectly related to the cancer. These include side effects of medications used for symptom relief, such as corticosteroids and anticonvulsants, and the psychological symptoms resulting from the devastating effects of the nervous system tumor itself (e.g., aphasia, paralysis, incontinence, cognitive dysfunction).[198] The care of these individuals continues to shift to the home and community, regardless of prognosis. Supportive nursing measures assume importance in all areas of patient care.[36] Table 49-4 describes common nursing diagnoses, suggests causes of the problems, and offers some of the associated nursing interventions for the care of these individuals.

Brain tumors increase ICP by their size, cerebral edema, or obstruction of CSF pathways. Cerebral edema can often be managed with corticosteroids such as dexamethasone. Dramatic improvements in neurological function are often seen along with reduction in ICP within hours to days following the initiation of steroids, particularly in those individuals with tumors producing substantial edema.[96] Malignant intracranial tumors typically cause disruption of the BBB. The leaky blood vessels allow extravasation of plasma proteins into the surrounding area, which then pulls water into the area as well. Although the mechanism is unclear, the steroids act to reestablish the BBB,[78] thus decreasing edema.

In situations where ICP is acutely elevated, corticosteroids alone are insufficient and osmotic diuretics, also referred to as *hyperosmolar agents*, are required. The high concentration of the drug causes water to be drawn from the normal tissue. The principle of water diffusion depends on the presence of a semipermeable membrane. The direction of flow is from the hypoconcentrated to the hyperconcentrated solution. When a hyperosmolar drug, usually mannitol, is given, the flow of fluid is from the brain to the blood. The extracellular fluid of the brain is hypotonic in relation to the hyperconcentration created by the drug in the blood. The fluid crosses the semipermeable cell membrane, moving into the blood and decreasing the edema in the brain.[40] Diuresis occurs within one to three hours and lasts up to approximately eight hours. An indwelling urinary catheter, strict recording of intake and output, and monitoring of electro-

Table 49-4 Nursing Management of an Individual with a CNS Tumor

Nursing Diagnosis	Possible Cause	Nursing Interventions
Altered cerebral tissue perfusion	Tumor size Cerebral edema Obstruction of CSF pathways Decreased cranial venous outflow Increased intraabdominal and intrathoracic pressure Increased systemic arterial blood pressure	Neurological assessment Corticosteroid administration ICP monitoring Avoid cumulative activities Ventriculostomy Elevate head of bed Avoid head rotation, neck flexion, and extension Avoid hip flexion and prone position Avoid Valsalva maneuvers, isometric muscle contractions, coughing, emotional arousal
High risk for seizures	Disturbance of intracranial contents Electrolyte abnormality	Prophylactic anticonvulsants Institute seizure precautions Maintain safe environment Be aware of concurrent medications that interfere with anticonvulsant action, absorption, or both Correct electrolyte abnormalities

Impaired cognition
  Memory
  Judgment
  Thought processes
	Frontal tumor
	Cerebral edema
	Hydrocephalus
	Radiation therapy
	Medication effects
		Maintain safe environment
		Reorient individual
		Utilize calendars, clocks, labels, photographs, etc. as visual cues or reminders
		Maintain as close to normal function as possible
		Encourage use of remaining functional ability
		Encourage social activities
		Instruct family members
		Provide written instructions

Impaired physical mobility
  Hemiparesis
  Hemiplegia
  Paraparesis
  Paraplegia
  Ataxic gait
  Level of consciousness
	Frontal tumor
	Parietal tumor
	Spinal tumor
	Spinal RT
	Steroids
		Maintain maximal activity level
		Provide assistance as necessary for ambulation, transfer, ADLs
		Encourage proper footwear (nonskid soles that enclose the foot)
		Maintain safe environment
		Keep needed objects close at hand
		Physical and occupational therapy
		Range of motion exercises
		Teach proper use of assistive devices (brace, cane, walker)
		Institute measures to prevent complications such as DVT, pressure ulcer, foot drop, pneumonia
		Develop specific interventions to compensate for deficits
		Instruct patient and family in safety measures and above techniques
		When preparing for discharge, obtain necessary equipment for home (wheelchair, bed, commode, walker, guardrail for bathroom, stool for shower)
		Assess home for physical setup and safety (stairs, rugs)

Alteration in sensory/ perceptual ability	Occipital tumor Parietal tumor Frontal tumor Spinal cord tumor Peripheral neuropathy	Monitor sensory function Identify highest level of intact sensory function Instruct patient and family on methods of compensation (checking position of involved areas visually, turning head completely to scan area) Occupational therapy for assistive devices Instruct patient and family in safety measures, proper clothing, and footwear

Knowledge deficit
  Disease
  Treatment
  Medications
  Discharge
	New diagnosis
	Anxiety
		Provide education to patient and family appropriately
		Encourage questions
		Clarify misconceptions
		Refer to resources as needed
		Provide written materials and written instructions

Alteration in comfort
  Headache
  Back pain
	Intracranial tumor
	Increased ICP
	Spinal cord compression
	Steroid withdrawal
		Assess for verbal and nonverbal indicators of pain
		Have patient rate pain using 0–10 scale, if possible
		Administer analgesics, steroids, or other nonnarcotic agents and evaluate effectiveness
		Encourage relaxation techniques or meditation
		Encourage diversional activities

High risk for impaired skin integrity	Immobility Sensory changes Poor nutrition	Assess skin condition frequently Position changes Frequent, thorough skin care Use of pressure relieving devices Maximize nutrition Instruct patient and family on measures to prevent skin breakdown (proper positioning techniques, lotion, massage, bathing, nutritious snacks, and meals)

Table 49-4 Nursing Management of an Individual with a CNS Tumor (continued)

Nursing Diagnosis	Possible Cause	Nursing Interventions
Alteration in urinary elimination Retention	Immobility Spinal cord tumor	Monitor intake and output Assist into effective position to void Assess for bladder distention Encourage increased fluids Intermittent catheterization If necessary, instruct patient or family member in catheterization technique
Incontinence	Overflow due to retention Frontal tumor Spinal cord tumor Diminished LOC	Assess for urinary retention Skin care Attempt toileting schedule Bladder training
Alteration in bowel elimination Constipation	Decreased mobility Spinal cord tumor Narcotics Steroids Inadequate diet	Assess bowel sounds and normal pattern of elimination Institute bowel regimen Encourage increased fluids and foods high in fiber Allow sufficient time and privacy Assist to proper position

Anxiety
  Individual
  Family
	New diagnosis
	Treatment protocols
	Functional loss
	Anticipatory grieving
	Poor prognosis
		Assess for verbal and nonverbal signs of anxiety
		Allow individual, family, or both, to verbalize feelings and source of anxiety
		Provide emotional support
		Keep individual and family updated on treatment plans, condition, etc.
		Refer to appropriate resources as necessary

Other possible nursing diagnoses
  Self-care deficit
  High risk for falls
  Alteration in nutrition
  Ineffective individual
    coping
  Ineffective family
    coping
  Alteration in comfort:
    nausea and vomiting
  Alteration in oral
    mucosa
  Fatigue
  Altered protective
    mechanisms:
    myelosuppression
  Anticipatory grieving		

lytes are necessary. Corticosteroids are administered concurrently. Other methods to help control increased ICP include fluid restriction, hyperventilation, sedation, and control of temperature. Valsalva maneuvers, isometric muscle contractions, coughing, sneezing, straining, and the use of positive-end expiratory pressure (PEEP) should be avoided as they can further aggravate increased ICP. A decrease in venous outflow will increase the total blood volume within the intracranial space, leading to elevated ICP. Head and neck positions that impair venous outflow include jugular compression, head rotation, neck flexion, and neck extension. The head of the bed should be elevated to promote venous drainage. Lying prone and flexing the hips should also be avoided because these positions increase intraabdominal and intrathoracic pressures, also leading to elevations in ICP. When turning or positioning in bed, the head and neck should be maintained in a neutral position. Alert individuals should be instructed not to turn themselves. Many patients unintentionally perform a Valsalva maneuver or grab the side rails tightly (isometric muscle contraction) when turning.[36]

Unfortunately, many nursing interventions, although necessary, can further aggravate increased ICP. These include turning and positioning, range-of-motion exercises, suctioning, and pulmonary hygiene. Although many of these activities cannot be avoided, they can be better spaced over time. It is a common practice to group these activities together. For example, when a patient is bathed, he or she is turned several times, receives range-of-motion exercises and pulmonary toileting, and is repositioned. The patient is probably suctioned, medicated, and may have a dressing or two changed before the nurse leaves the room to attend to other patients or responsibilities. While this is often considered necessary to manage time and remain efficient and organized, it is not always in the best interest of the patient with increased ICP. Spacing the activities and care can decrease sustained elevations of increased ICP.

Blocked CSF pathways lead to hydrocephalus and increases in ICP. A ventriculoperitoneal shunt or temporary ventriculostomy may be required. A tumor compressing the ventricle that may be completely removed will probably not require shunting. An unresectable tumor causing hydrocephalus will often require placement of a ventriculoperitoneal shunt. A ventriculostomy is indicated when the etiology of the hydrocephalus is believed to be of a temporary nature. Patients with a ventriculostomy require correct head positioning in relation to the level of the drainage system. The drainage system drip chamber level is ordered by the physician and is usually positioned level with the external auditory meatus. The level is changed based on the patient's clinical condition and the amount of CSF drainage. The procedure of leveling the drip chamber at, above, or below the external auditory meatus minimizes the risk of both excessive CSF drainage leading to collapse of the ventricles and insufficient CSF drainage leading to hydrocephalus. The level of the drip chamber is continuously monitored, the amount and consistency of CSF are assessed hourly, and the patient is evaluated for any neurological changes and signs of infection.

Individuals with spinal cord tumors also receive corticosteroids, especially when SCC has developed. Once the condition is determined or even clinically suspected, corticosteroids are initiated immediately, often in high doses. Steroids decrease the edema of the spinal cord and rapidly relieve back pain in many patients. Dexamethasone is the most commonly used steroid. For patients without neurological symptoms except for pain, low doses of steroids can be administered—usually 4 mg four times daily. The dose can be increased if pain persists, new symptoms develop, or a definitive diagnosis is made. For patients with severe pain or with neurological symptoms, high doses are given, usually 100 mg as an IV bolus followed by 24 mg every six hours for several days.[97] The dose should be tapered as the patient is treated with other treatment modalities, usually beginning within several days.

More than 95% of individuals with SCC report pain. While the addition of steroids provides pain relief for many individuals, others require additional analgesics. Effective analgesia needs to be established early on and dosages adjusted as the steroids and treatment further reduce the pain. The variety of available analgesics and the different methods of administration assist the nurse in providing adequate pain relief for spinal cord-compressed individuals.

Neurological symptoms of SCC other than pain usually evolve quickly. If prompt treatment is not initiated, weakness leading to paralysis will occur. If diagnosis and treatment are delayed until the patient becomes paraplegic, functional recovery is rare. However, patients who are ambulatory at the onset of treatment will most likely retain that ability. Individuals are taught to report signs and symptoms to ensure prompt treatment. The goal of treatment is to preserve and maintain existing neurological function. Patient assessment is therefore crucial throughout this period to evaluate neurological status.

This assessment includes monitoring motor, sensory, bowel, and bladder function. Changes in the neurological exam or the development of new deficits must be followed up immediately.

Glucocorticoid hormones are the most widely used drugs in neurooncology.[189] Unfortunately, they have many unwanted side effects. Some of the common side effects, while distressing to the individual, are considered mild. These include insomnia, fatigue, increased appetite, hiccups, blurry vision, behavioral changes, acne, edema, abdominal bloating, and the characteristic moon face (caused by the redistribution of fat). Other effects can be more serious: GI bleeding, bowel perforation, hyperglycemia, hallucinations, psychosis, myopathy manifested by proximal leg weakness, opportunistic infections, osteoporosis, and acute adrenal insufficiency resulting from steroid withdrawal. Individuals receiving steroids should be observed for these effects. Immunosuppression caused by prolonged steroid administration can lead to opportunistic infections, particularly *Pneumocystis carinii pneumonia* (PCP). For this reason many individuals on prolonged steroids also receive PCP prophylaxis with either trimethoprim and sulfamethoxazole (Bactrim) or pentamidine. PCP prophylaxis generally continues for one month after the steroids have been discontinued.

Ongoing assessment is necessary because neurooncology patients often receive steroids for prolonged and repeated periods of time. Patients and families need to be educated regarding the medications, including the absolute necessity of taking the prescribed dose, the side effects to observe for and interventions to take, and indications to call their physician. Sudden withdrawal of steroids can lead to adrenal insufficiency. Symptoms of this condition include fatigue, muscular weakness, joint pain, fever, anorexia, nausea, and orthostatic hypotension.[36] Steroid dosages are tapered slowly to prevent these symptoms of withdrawal. Patients should be given written instructions about the schedule of the steroid taper and should be monitored for increased neurological symptoms as the dose is decreased. Some individuals may become steroid-dependent and do not tolerate even a slow taper. It is also important to be familiar with the drug interactions of steroids and other medications the individual may be taking. Drugs such as dilantin, phenobarbital, and perhaps carbamazepine (Tegretol) increase the metabolic clearance of steroids and may decrease their therapeutic effect. Therefore, some individuals on stable doses of steroids may develop increased symptoms when they are coincidentally started on these medications[198] and may need to have their steroid dose increased.

Common anticonvulsants used to prevent seizures in individuals with primary and metastatic brain tumors include dilantin, phenobarbital, Tegretol, and valproate (Depakene). These agents all cause drowsiness and cognitive dysfunction. Worsening neurological symptoms occur at toxic therapeutic levels. These effects can add to already existing neurological dysfunction. Patients receiving these agents should have periodic blood levels assessed for therapeutic range. However, seizures may be controlled at levels below the therapeutic range; conversely, seizures may occur despite therapeutic levels. Also, some individuals may not exhibit signs of toxicity at high therapeutic levels. Individuals should be encouraged to obtain and wear a medic alert bracelet, especially if the patient has a seizure history.

Many individuals with CNS cancers experience anxiety and depression. The psychological impact of the diagnosis, with its relatively poor prognosis, can be devastating. Anxiety and depression, while considered a natural response to the illness with its disabling neurological deficits, is sometimes overlooked. The presence of excessive anxiety or depression should be evaluated. Antidepressants and antianxiolytics may help improve the psychological symptoms. Counseling can be of benefit to the individuals and families each grieving the loss of the "person they once knew." The debilitating effects of CNS cancers are not limited to obvious neurological deficits; perhaps more devastating are the effects on the "persona." The personality of the individual is often permanently changed due to the disease, treatment, or both.

Continuity of Care: Nursing Challenges

Discharge planning for the individual with a CNS tumor should begin on the day of hospital admission and evolve during the hospitalization. An accurate assessment of neurological deficits and functional limitations is made. A family member or caregiver should be involved in discharge teaching as brain tumors frequently cause cognitive disabilities including memory loss, poor concentration, and aphasia. Anxiety alone may impair an individual's ability to retain new information. The patient and family may be faced with many new issues in the home care setting, and they are assisted in setting realistic goals. For example, the paraplegic patient will not be able to walk up stairs. Rehabilitation potential is always viewed with hope and optimism; however, the attitude of realistic hope must be conveyed to the individual and family.[36] Rehabilitation for the CNS-impaired individual has undergone tremendous change. A modified program of home physical therapy is often available for those with CNS cancers even though they may be considered to have a shortened survival. Some individuals may benefit from speech therapy as well. Rehabilitation is especially important for the individuals with low-grade primary CNS tumors because many of these individuals have extended periods of time between recurrences. Vocational rehabilitation may be necessary.

The home should be assessed for its physical setup and safety. Maintaining a safe environment must be constantly reinforced. At some point during the course of the disease, the individual with a brain tumor often has cognitive impairment. Continuous supervision may become necessary to prevent harm. Stairs, rugs, and the shower are often a potential source of injury for individuals with both brain and spinal cord tumors. Obstacles should be cleared from common pathways to avoid falls. The individual may need to remain on the ground floor, making room changes necessary. Reality-orientation devices (clocks, calendars, written instructions, photographs) need to be readily visible. Daily roles and routines may need to be altered to accommodate the individual who now has neurological deficits. A thorough assessment of health care benefits, family, community, and agency support is essential.

Once the individual with a CNS tumor is discharged, coordination of care assumes an even greater role. Just as the primary nurse in the inpatient setting coordinated the patient's care among the many disciplines involved, the nurse in the outpatient setting must do the same. Follow-up appointments, diagnostic tests, travel arrangements, treatment schedules, special instructions, side effects of medications and treatments, home care issues, insurance company issues, and communication between the various disciplines involved are some of the many issues the outpatient nurse manages daily. It is important that the patient and family know the person who is familiar with the patient history and disease management. This provides a sense of continuity and can often allay anxiety. Many of these individuals develop progressive disease, and as their neurological deficits increase, they will require additional support. Many may travel a great distance for their cancer therapy. These individuals then must have a local physician who can provide emergency care and manage the day-to-day issues and problems that arise. For example, many individuals on steroids develop diabetes and require frequent insulin dosage adjustments as the steroids are being tapered.

Many persons with CNS tumors can rapidly deteriorate as their disease advances. Their neurological function, physical status, and support systems will need to be reevaluated frequently. Adjustments in the plan of care may be necessary. Coping mechanisms of caregivers are evaluated as they deal with the increasing disability as the disease progresses. There may be issues related to young children at home, employment, and finances. New goals and plans should be formulated. Family members may need to take on added responsibilities such as physical care of the individual, medication administration, and assessment of their condition. Additional resources may need to be accessed, such as other family members, friends, community agencies (e.g., Visiting Nurse Service, American Cancer Society, or Cancer Care), local community programs, and support groups. Life expectancy at home may not be of long duration. The person with progressive CNS involvement generally is at a terminal stage, and hospice care is an appropriate resource for families for both physical and emotional concerns.[199]

Conclusion

Malignancies of the CNS present tremendous challenges for individuals, families, and caregivers. Because the clinical manifestations, course of treatment, and complications vary with the type and site of tumors, individuals with CNS cancers require a highly individualized plan of care. Supportive care takes on a role of utmost importance and encompasses the entire course of illness from diagnosis through the terminal phase of disease. Even with advances in overall therapeutic modalities, successful treatment of CNS cancers remains elusive.[199] Outcomes can range from cure to permanent disability to life prolonged by a few days, weeks, or months. The ongoing physical and emotional support necessary for both the individual and the family create a challenging role for oncology nurses. The neurological symptoms and complications produced by CNS cancers are, unfortunately, profoundly disabling and severely affect quality of life. Assisting the individual to manage problems of daily living, maintain normal function to the best of his or her ability, and attain quality of life are our ultimate goals.

References

1. The Central Brain Tumor Registry of the United States (CBTRUS). *1997 Annual Report*, 1998
2. Landis SH, Murray T, Bolden S, et al: Cancer statistics, 1998. *CA Cancer J Clin* 48:6–29, 1998
3. Levin VA, Leibel SA, Gutin PH: Neoplasms of the central nervous system, in DeVita VT, Hellman S, Rosenberg SA (eds): *Cancer: Principles and Practice of Oncology* (ed 5). Philadelphia, Lippincott-Raven, 1997, pp 2022–2082
4. Riggs JE: Rising primary malignant brain tumor mortality in the elderly. *Arch Neurol* 52:571–575, 1995
5. Modan B, Wagener DK, Feldman JJ, et al: Increased mortality from brain tumors: a combined outcome of diagnostic technology and change of attitude toward the elderly. *Am J Epidemiol* 135:1349–1357, 1992
6. Sawaya R, Ligon BL, Bindal AK, et al: Surgical treatment of metastatic brain tumors. *J Neurooncol* 27:269–277, 1996
7. American Brain Tumor Association (ABTA): *A Primer of Brain Tumors*, 1996
8. Watkins D, Rouleau GA: Genetics, prognosis and therapy of central nervous system tumors. *Cancer Detect Prev* 18:139–144, 1994
9. Bondy M, Wiencke J, Wrensch M, et al: Genetics of brain tumors: a review. *J Neurooncol* 18:69–81, 1994
10. Bohnen NI, Radhakrishnan K, O'Neill BP, et al: Descriptive and analytic epidemiology of brain tumors, in Black PM, Loeffler JS (eds): *Cancer of the Nervous System*. Cambridge, Blackwell Science, 1997, pp 3–24
11. Prados MD, Berger MS, Wilson CB: Primary central nervous system tumors: advances in knowledge and treatment. *CA Cancer J Clin* 48:331–360, 1998
12. National Brain Tumor Foundation (NBTF): *Brain Tumors: A Guide*, 1994
13. Martz CH: von Hippel-Lindau disease: a genetically transmitted multisystem neoplastic disorder. *Semin Oncol Nurs* 8:281–287, 1992
14. Sehgal A: Molecular changes during the genesis of human gliomas. *Semin Surg Oncol* 14:3–12, 1998
15. Shapiro WR, Shapiro JR: Biology and treatment of malignant glioma. *Oncology* 12:233–246, 1998
16. Berleur MP, Cordier S: The role of chemical, physical, or

viral exposures and health factors in neurocarcinogenesis: implications for epidemiologic studies of brain tumors. *Cancer Causes Control* 6:240–256, 1995
17. Musicco M, Filippini G, Bordo BM, et al: Gliomas and occupational exposure to carcinogens: case-control study. *Am J Epidemiol* 116:782–787, 1982
18. Thomas LT, Waxweiler JR: Brain tumors and occupational risk factors: a review. *Scand J Work Environ Health* 12:1–15, 1986
19. Keyser A: Epidemiology of neuro-oncological disease, in Twijnstra A, Keyser A, Ongerboer de Visser BW (eds): *Neuro-Oncology*. Amsterdam, Elsevier, 1993, pp 1–12
20. Preston-Martin S, Mack W, Henderson BE: Risk factors for gliomas and meningiomas in males in Los Angeles County. *Cancer Res* 49:6137–6143, 1989
21. Bondy ML, Wrensch MR: Epidemiology of primary malignant brain tumors. *Bailliere's Clin Neurol* 5:251–270, 1996
22. Schiff D, Suman VJ, Yang P, et al: Risk factors for primary central nervous system lymphoma. *Cancer* 82:975–982, 1998
23. Chamberlain MC: Gliomas in patients with acquired immune deficiency syndrome. *Cancer* 74:1912–1914, 1994
24. Neglia JP, Meadows AT, Robinson LL, et al: Second neoplasms after acute lymphoblastic leukemia in childhood. *N Engl J Med* 325:1330–1336, 1991
25. Ron E, Modan B, Boice JD, et al: Tumors of the brain and nervous system after radiotherapy in childhood. *N Engl J Med* 319:1033–1039, 1988
26. Tsang RW, Laperriere NJ, Simpson WJ, et al: Glioma arising after radiation therapy for pituitary adenoma. *Cancer* 72:2227–2233, 1993
27. Alexander MJ, DeSalles AA, Tomiyasu U: Multiple radiation-induced intracranial lesions after treatment for pituitary adenoma. *J Neurosurg* 88:111–115, 1998
28. DeAngelis LM: Primary central nervous system lymphoma as a secondary malignancy. *Cancer* 67:1431–1435, 1991
29. Heath CW: Electromagnetic field exposure and cancer: a review of epidemiologic evidence. *CA Cancer J Clin* 46:29–44, 1996
30. Sahl JD, Kelsh MA, Greenland S: Cohort and nested case-control studies of hematopoietic cancers and brain cancers among electric utility workers. *Epidemiology* 4:104–114, 1993
31. Floderus B, Persson T, Stenkind C, et al: Occupational exposure to electromagnetic fields in relation to leukemia and brain tumors: a case-control study in Sweden. *Cancer Causes Control* 4:465–476, 1993
32. Gurney JG, Mueller BA, Davis S, et al: Childhood brain tumor occurrence in relation to residential power line configurations, electric heating sources, and electric appliance use. *Am J Epidemiol* 143:120–128, 1996
33. Preston-Martin S, Navid W, Thomas D, et al: Los Angeles study of residential magnetic fields and childhood brain tumors. *Am J Epidemiol* 143:105–119, 1996
34. Hickey JV: Overview of neuroanatomy and neurophysiology, in Hickey JV (ed): *The Clinical Practice of Neurological and Neurosurgical Nursing* (ed 4). Philadelphia, Lippincott, 1997, pp 35–79
35. Leahy NM: *Quick Reference to Neurological Critical Care Nursing*. Rockville, MD, Aspen, 1990
36. Chaffee EE, Lytle IM: *Basic Physiology and Anatomy*. Philadelphia, Lippincott, 1980
37. Wegmann JA: Central nervous system cancers, in Groenwald SL, Frogge MH, Goodman M, Yarbro CH (eds): *Cancer Nursing: Principles and Practice* (ed 3). Sudbury, MA, Jones and Bartlett, 1993, pp 959–983
38. Gilman S, Newman SW: *Manter and Gatz's Essentials of Clini-*

cal Neuroanatomy and Neurophysiology (ed 8). Philadelphia, Davis, 1992

39. Marshall SB, Marshall LF, Vos HR, et al: *Neuroscience Critical Care.* Philadelphia, Saunders, 1990

40. Hickey JV: Intracranial pressure theory and management of increased intracranial pressure, in Hickey JV (ed): *The Clinical Practice of Neurological and Neurosurgical Nursing* (ed 4). Philadelphia, Lippincott, 1997, pp 295–328

41. Andrus C: Intracranial pressure: dynamics and nursing management. *J Neurosci Nurs* 23:85–92, 1991

42. Bruner JM: Neuropathology of malignant gliomas. *Semin Oncol* 21:126–138, 1994

43. Adams BA, Clancey JK, Eddy M: Malignant glioma: current treatment perspectives. *J Neurosci Nurs* 23:15–19, 1991

44. Burger PC, Scheithauer BW, Vogel FS: *Surgical Pathology of the Nervous System and Its Coverings* (ed 3). New York, Churchill Livingstone, 1991

45. Lote K, Egeland T, Hager B, et al: Survival, prognostic factors, and therapeutic efficacy in low-grade glioma: a retrospective study in 379 patients. *J Clin Oncol* 15:3129–3140, 1997

46. Leighton C, Fisher B, Bauman G, et al: Supratentorial low-grade glioma in adults: an analysis of prognostic factors and timing of radiation. *J Clin Oncol* 4:1294–1301, 1997

47. Macdonald DR: Low-grade gliomas, mixed gliomas, and oligodendrogliomas. *Semin Oncol* 21:236–248, 1994

48. National Comprehensive Cancer Network: NCCN adult brain tumor practice guidelines. *Oncology* 11:237–277, 1997

49. Abdulrauf SI, Edvardsen K, Ho KL, et al: Vascular endothelial growth factor expression and vascular density as prognostic markers of survival in patients with low-grade astrocytoma. *J Neurosurg* 88:513–520, 1998

50. Piepmeier JM, Christopher S: Low-grade gliomas: introduction and overview. *J Neurooncol* 34:1–3, 1997

51. Wen PY, Fine HA, Black PM, et al: High-grade astrocytomas, in Wen PY, Black PM (eds): *Neurologic Clinics: Brain Tumors in Adults.* Philadelphia, Saunders, 1995, pp 875–900

52. Sneed PK, Stauffer PR, McDermott MW, et al: Survival benefit of hyperthermia in a prospective randomized trial of brachytherapy boost +/– hyperthermia for glioblastoma multiforme. *Int J Radiat Oncol Biol Phys* 2:287–295, 1998

53. Daumas-Duport C, Varlet P, Tucker ML, et al: Oligodendrogliomas. Part 1: patterns of growth, histological diagnosis, clinical and imaging correlations: A study of 153 cases. *J Neurooncol* 34:37–59, 1997

54. Levin VA, Silver P, Hannigan J, et al: Superiority of postradiotherapy adjuvant chemotherapy with CCNU, procarbazine, and vincristine (PCV) over BCNU for anaplastic gliomas: NCOG 6G61 final report. *Int J Radiat Oncol Biol Phys* 18:321–324, 1990

55. Macdonald DR: New therapies of primary CNS lymphomas and oligodendrogliomas. *J Neurooncol* 24:97–101, 1995

56. Mason WP, DeAngelis LM: Procarbazine, CCNU, vincristine (PCV) chemotherapy for benign oligodendrogliomas. *Neurology* 44:A262, 1994 (abstr) (suppl 2)

57. Schiff D, Wen PY: Uncommon brain tumors, in Wen PY, Black PM (eds): *Neurologic Clinics: Brain Tumors in Adults.* Philadelphia, Saunders, 1995, pp 953–974

58. Cohen ME, Duffer PK: Ependymomas, in Cohen ME, Duffer PK (eds): *Brain Tumors in Children* (ed 2). New York, Raven, 1994, pp 219–239

59. McLaughlin MP, Marcus RB, Buatti JM, et al: Ependymomas: results, prognostic factors and treatment recommendations. *Int J Radiat Oncol Biol Phys* 40:845–850, 1998

60. DeMonte F: Current management of meningiomas. *Oncology* 9:83–96, 1995

61. Schrell UMH, Fahlbusch R, Adams EF: Meningiomas and neurofibromatosis for the oncologist. *Curr Opin Oncol* 6:247–253, 1994

62. Black PM: Benign brain tumors, in Wen PY, Black PM (eds): *Neurologic Clinics: Brain Tumors in Adults.* Philadelphia, Saunders, 1995, pp 927–954

63. Rubenstein AB, Schein M, Reichenthal E: The association of carcinoma of the breast with meningioma. *Surg Gynecol Obstet* 169:334–336, 1989

64. Black PM: Brain tumors. *N Engl J Med* 324:1555–1564, 1991

65. Younis GA, Sawaya R, DeMonte F, et al: Aggressive meningeal tumors: review of a series. *J Neurosurg* 82:17–27, 1995

66. Goldsmith BJ, Wara WM, Wilson CB, et al: Postoperative irradiation for subtotally resected meningiomas: a retrospective analysis of 140 patients treated from 1967–1990. *J Neurosurg* 80:195–201, 1997

67. Wilson CB: Meningiomas: genetics, malignancy, and the role of radiation in induction and treatment. *J Neurosurg* 81:666–674, 1994

68. Dziuk TW, Woo S, Butler EB, et al: Malignant meningioma: an indication for initial aggressive surgery and adjuvant radiotherapy. *J Neurooncol* 37:177–188, 1998

69. Carroll R, Glowacka D, Dashner K, et al: Progesterone receptor in meningiomas. *Cancer Res* 53:1312–1316, 1993

70. Goodwin JW, Crowley J, Stafford B, et al: A phase II evaluation of tamoxifen in unresected or refractory meningiomas: a Southwest Oncology Group study. *J Neurooncol* 15:75–77, 1993

71. Lamberts SWJ, Tanghe HLJ, Avezaat CJJ, et al: Mifepristone (RU 486) treatment of meningiomas. *J Neurol Neurosurg Psychiatry* 55:486–490, 1992

72. Campbell C: Acoustic neuroma: nursing implications related to surgical management. *J Neurosci Nurs* 23:50–60, 1991

73. Beskonakh E, Cayh S, Turgut M, et al: Intraparenchymal schwannomas of the central nervous system: an additional case report and review. *Neurosurg Rev* 20:139–144, 1997

74. Koos WT, Day JD, Matula C, et al: Neurotopographic considerations in the microsurgical treatment of small acoustic neurinomas. *J Neurosurg* 88:506–512, 1998

75. Young JS: Acoustic neuroma: postoperative vertigo and the mechanisms of compensation. *J Neurosci Nurs* 24:194–198, 1992

76. Wiegand D, Fickel V: Acoustic neuroma: the patient's perspective: subjective assessment of symptoms, diagnosis, therapy, and outcomes in 541 patients. *Laryngoscope* 99:179–186, 1989

77. DeAngelis LM: Primary central nervous system lymphoma. *Recent Results Cancer Res* 135:155–169, 1994

78. Eby NL, Grufferman S, Flannelly CM, et al: Increasing incidence of primary brain lymphoma in the US. *Cancer* 62:2461–2465, 1988

79. O'Neill BP, Illig JJ: Primary central nervous system lymphoma. *Mayo Clin Proc* 64:1005–1020, 1989

80. Cote TR, Manns A, Hardy CR, et al: Epidemiology of brain lymphoma among people with or without acquired immunodeficiency syndrome. *J Natl Cancer Inst* 88:675–679, 1996

81. Selch MT, Shimizu KT, DeSalles AF, et al: Primary central nervous system lymphoma. *Am J Clin Oncol* 17:286–293, 1994

82. Rosenblum ML, Levy RM, Bredesen DE, et al: Primary central nervous system lymphoma in patients with AIDS. *Ann Neurol* 23:513–516, 1988

83. Forsyth PA, Yahalom J, DeAngelis LM: Combined-modality therapy in the treatment of primary central nervous system lymphoma in AIDS. *Neurology* 44:1473–1479, 1994

84. DeAngelis LM: Current management of primary central nervous system lymphoma. *Oncology* 9:63–71, 1995

85. DeAngelis LM, Yahalom J, Heinemann MH, et al: Primary CNS lymphoma: combined treatment with chemotherapy and radiotherapy. *Neurology* 40:80–86, 1990

86. Cheng AL, Yeh KH, Uen WC, et al: Systemic chemotherapy alone for patients with non-acquired immunodeficiency syndrome-related central nervous system lymphoma. *Cancer* 82:1946–1951, 1998

87. Abrey LE, DeAngelis LM, Yahalom J: Long-term survival in primary CNS lymphoma. *J Clin Oncol* 16:859–863, 1998

88. Neuwelt EA, Goldman DL, Dahlborg SA, et al: Primary CNS lymphoma treated with osmotic blood-brain barrier disruption: prolonged survival and preservation of cognitive function. *J Clin Oncol* 9:1580–1590, 1991

89. Chamberlain MC, Levin VA: Primary central nervous system lymphoma: a role for adjuvant chemotherapy. *J Neurooncol* 14:271–275, 1992

90. O'Neill BP, Buckner JC, Coffey RJ, et al: Brain metastatic lesions. *Mayo Clin Proc* 69:1062–1068, 1994

91. Posner JB: Brain metastases: 1995. A brief review. *J Neurooncol* 27:287–293, 1996

92. Young RF: Radiosurgery for the treatment of brain metastases. *Semin Surg Oncol* 14:70–78, 1998

93. Lang FF, Sawaya R: Surgical treatment of metastatic brain tumors. *Semin Surg Oncol* 14:53–63, 1998

94. DeAngelis LM: Management of brain metastases. *Cancer Invest* 12:156–165, 1994

95. Delattre JY, Krol G, Thaler HT, et al: Distribution of brain metastases. *Arch Neurol* 19:579–592, 1978

96. Byrne TN, Cascino TL, Posner JB: Brain metastasis from melanoma. *J Neurooncol* 1:313–317, 1983

97. Posner JB: *Neurologic Complications of Cancer.* Philadelphia, Davis, 1995

98. Sitton E: Central nervous system metastases. *Semin Oncol Nurs* 14:210–219, 1998

99. Posner JB: Surgery for metastases to the brain. *N Engl J Med* 322:544–545, 1990

100. Patchell RA, Tibbs PA, Walsh JW, et al: A randomized trial of surgery in the treatment of single metastases to the brain. *N Engl J Med* 322:544–545, 1990

101. Bindel RK, Sawaya R, Leavens ME, et al: Surgical treatment of multiple brain metastases. *J Neurosurg* 79:210–216, 1993

102. Oben A, Moriarty TM, Loeffler JS: Radiosurgery for metastases. *J Neurooncol* 27:279–285, 1996

103. Chang SD, Adler JR, Hancock SL: Clinical uses of radiosurgery. *Oncology* 12:1181–1192, 1998

104. Vermeulen SS: Whole brain radiotherapy in the treatment of metastatic brain tumors. *Semin Surg Oncol* 14:64–69, 1998

105. Bucholtz JD: Central nervous system metastases. *Semin Oncol Nurs* 14:61–72, 1998

106. Wujcik D: Meningeal carcinomatosis: diagnosis, treatment, and nursing care. *Oncol Nurs Forum* 10:35–40, 1983

107. Freilich RJ, DeAngelis LM: Primary central nervous system cancer, in Wen PY, Black PM (eds): *Neurologic Clinics: Brain Tumors in Adults.* Philadelphia, Saunders, 1995, pp 901–914

108. Willis D: Intracranial astrocytoma: pathology, diagnosis and clinical presentation. *J Neurosci Nurs* 23:7–14, 1991

109. Schnell S, DeLeon MEM: Anatomy of the central nervous system. *Semin Oncol Nurs* 14:2–7, 1998

110. Hickey JV, Armstrong T: Brain tumors, in Hickey JV (ed): *The Clinical Practice of Neurological and Neurosurgical Nursing* (ed 4). Philadelphia, Lippincott, 1997, pp 501–526

111. Byrne TN: Imaging of gliomas. *Semin Oncol* 21:162–171, 1994

112. Hickey JV: Diagnostic procedures and laboratory tests for neuroscience patients, in Hickey JV (ed): *The Clinical Practice of Neurological and Neurosurgical Nursing* (ed 4). Philadelphia, Lippincott, 1997, pp 81–101

113. Schwartz RB: Neuroradiology of brain tumors, in Wen PY, Black PM (eds): *Neurologic Clinics: Brain Tumors in Adults.* Philadelphia, Saunders, 1995, pp 723–756

114. Jaeckle KA: Neuroimaging for central nervous system tumors. *Semin Oncol* 18:150–157, 1991

115. Arbour RA: Stereotactic localization and resection of intracranial tumors. *J Neurosci Nurs* 25:14–21, 1993

116. Wen PY, Alexander E III, Black PM, et al: Long term results of stereotactic brachytherapy used in the initial treatment of patients with glioblastomas. *Cancer* 73:3029–3036, 1994

117. Berger MS: Malignant astrocytomas: surgical aspects. *Semin Oncol* 21:172–185, 1994

118. Berger MS, Rostomily RC: Low grade gliomas: functional mapping resection strategies, extent of resection, and outcome. *J Neurooncol* 34:85–101, 1997

119. Chandler KL, Prados MD, Malec M, et al: Long-term survival in patients with glioblastoma multiforme. *Neurosurgery* 32:716–720, 1993

120. Morita M, Rosenblum MK, Bilsky MH, et al: Long-term survivors of glioblastoma multiforme: clinical and molecular characteristics. *J Neurooncol* 27:259–266, 1996

121. Salvati M, Cervoni L, Artico M, et al: Long-term survival in patients with supratentorial glioblastoma. *J Neurooncol* 36:61–64, 1998

122. American Joint Committee on Cancer: *AJCC Cancer Staging Manuel* (ed 5). Philadelphia, Lippincott-Raven, 1997

123. O'Mary SS: Diagnostic evaluation, classification, and staging, in Groenwald SL, Frogge MH, Goodman M, Yarbro CH (eds): *Cancer Nursing: Principles and Practice* (ed 4). Sudbury, MA, Jones and Bartlett, 1997, pp 175–199

124. Kleihues P, Burger PC, Scheithauer BW: Histological typing of tumours of the central nervous system, in *World Health Organization, International Histological Classification of Tumours.* Berlin, Heidelberg, Springer-Verlag, 1993, pp 5–10

125. Harbaugh KS, Black PM: Strategies in the surgical management of malignant gliomas. *Semin Surg Oncol* 14:26–33, 1998

126. Sawaya R, Rambo WM, Hammond MA, et al: Advances in surgery for brain tumors, in Wen PY, Black PM (eds): *Neurologic Clinics: Brain Tumors in Adults.* Philadelphia, Saunders, 1995, pp 757–771

127. Heilbrun MP, Roberts TS, Apuzzo MLJ, et al: Preliminary experience with Brown-Roberts-Wells (BRW) computerized tomography stereotaxic guidance system. *J Neurosurg* 59:217–222, 1983

128. Krieger MD, Chandrasoma PT, Zee CS, et al: Role of stereotactic biopsy in the diagnosis and management of brain tumors. *Semin Surg Oncol* 14:13–25, 1998

129. League D: Interactive, image-guided, stereotactic neurosurgery systems. *AORN J* 61:360–370, 1995

130. Gooding GA, Edwards MS, Rabskin AE, et al: Intraoperative real-time ultrasound in the localization of intracranial neoplasms. *Radiology* 146:459–461, 1983

131. Bohan EM: Neurosurgical management of patients with central nervous system malignancies. *Semin Oncol Nurs* 14:8–17, 1998

132. Rambo WM, Sawaya RE: Neurosurgical treatment of brain tumors. *Cancer Bull* 45:320–325, 1993

133. Shrieve DC, Loeffler JS: Advances in radiation therapy for brain tumors, in Wen PY, Black PM (eds): *Neurologic Clinics: Brain Tumors in Adults.* Philadelphia, Saunders, 1995, pp 773–793

134. Walker MD, Alexander E, Hunt WE, et al: Evaluation of BCNU and/or radiotherapy in the treatment of anaplastic gliomas. *J Neurosurg* 49:333–343, 1978

135. Fine HA, Dear KB, Loeffler JS, et al: Meta-analysis of radiation therapy with and without adjuvant chemotherapy for malignant gliomas in adults. *Cancer* 71:2585–2597, 1993

136. Leibel SA, Scott CB, Loeffler JS: Contemporary approaches to the treatment of malignant gliomas with radiation therapy. *Semin Oncol* 21:198–219, 1994

137. Vick NA, Paleologos NA: External beam radiotherapy: hard facts and painful realities. *J Neurooncol* 24:93–95, 1995

138. Shrieve DC, Alexander E III, Wen PY, et al: Comparison of stereotactic radiosurgery and brachytherapy in the treatment of recurrent glioblastoma multiforme. *Neurosurgery* 36:275–284, 1995

139. Shaw EG, Daumas-Duport C, Scheithauer BW, et al: Radiation therapy in the management of low-grade supratentorial astrocytomas. *J Neurosurg* 70:853–861, 1989

140. Shaw EG, Scheithauer BW, O'Fallon JR: Management of supratentorial low-grade gliomas. *Oncology* 7:97–111, 1993

141. Shaw EG: Low grade gliomas—to treat or not to treat? The radiation oncologist's perspective. *Arch Neurol* 47:1138–1139, 1990

142. Recht LD, Lew R, Smith TW: Suspected low-grade glioma: Is deferring treatment safe? *Ann Neurol* 31:431–436, 1992

143. Philippon JH, Clemenceau SH, Fauchon FH, et al: Supratentorial low-grade astrocytomas in adults. *Neurosurgery* 32:554–559, 1993

144. Larson DA, Wara WW: Radiotherapy of primary malignant brain tumors. *Semin Surg Oncol* 14:34–42, 1998

145. Thorton AF, Hegarty TJ, Ten Haken RK, et al: Three-dimensional treatment planning of astrocytomas, a dosimetric study of cerebral irradiation. *Int J Radiat Oncol Biol Phys* 20:1309–1315, 1991

146. Prados MD, Scott CB, Rotman M, et al: Influence of bromodeoxyuridine radiosensitization on malignant glioma patient survival: a retrospective comparison of survival data from the Northern California Oncology Group (NCOG) and Radiation Therapy Oncology Group (RTOG) trials for glioblastoma multiforme and anaplastic astrocytoma. *Int J Radiat Oncol Biol Phys* 40:653–659, 1998

147. Urtasun RC, Kinsella TJ, Farnan N, et al: Survival improvement in anaplastic astrocytoma combining external radiation with halogenated pyrimidines: final report of RTOG 86-12, phase I–II study. *Int J Radiat Oncol Biol Phys* 36:1163–1167, 1996

148. Sullivan FJ, Herscher LL, Cook JA, et al: National Cancer Institute (phase II) study of high-grade glioma treated with accelerated hyperfractionated radiation and iododeoxyuridine: results in anaplastic astrocytomas. *Int J Radiat Oncol Biol Phys* 30:583–590, 1994

149. Levin VA, Prados MD, Wara WM, et al: Radiation therapy and bromodeoxyuridine chemotherapy followed by procarbazine, lomustine, and vincristine for the treatment of anaplastic gliomas. *Int J Radiat Oncol Biol Phys* 32:75–83, 1995

150. Prados MD, Larson DA, Lamborn K, et al: Radiation therapy and hydroxyurea followed by the combination of 6-thioguanine and BCNU for the treatment of primary malignant brain tumors. *Int J Radiat Oncol Biol Phys* 40:57–63, 1998

151. McDermott MW, Sneed PK, Gutin PH: Interstitial brachytherapy for malignant brain tumors. *Semin Surg Oncol* 14:79–87, 1998

152. Gutin PH, Prados MD, Phillips TL, et al: External irradiation followed by an interstitial high activity iodine-125 implant "boost" in the initial treatment of malignant gliomas:

NCOG study 6G-82-2. *Int J Radiat Oncol Biol Phys* 21:601–606, 1991

153. Prados MD, Gutin PH, Phillips TL, et al: Interstitial brachytherapy for newly diagnosed patients with malignant gliomas: the UCSF experience. *Int J Radiat Oncol Biol Phys* 24:593–597, 1992

154. Halligan JB, Stelzer KJ, Rostomily RC, et al: Operation and permanent low-activity ^{125}I brachytherapy for recurrent high-grade astrocytomas. *Int J Radiat Oncol Biol Phys* 35:541–547, 1996

155. Laperriere NJ, Bernstein M: Radiotherapy for brain tumors. *CA Cancer J Clin* 44:96–108, 1994

156. Sneed PK, Larson DA, Gutin PH: Brachytherapy and hyperthermia for malignant astrocytomas. *Semin Oncol* 21:186–197, 1994

157. Addesa AE, Shrieve DC, Alexander A III, et al: Stereotactic radiosurgery as primary adjuvant treatment for glioblastoma: the JCRT update. *Proc Am Soc Clin Oncol.* 14:144, 1995 (abstr 274A)

158. Alexander E, Loeffler JS: Radiosurgery for primary malignant brain tumors. *Semin Surg Onc* 14:43–52, 1998

159. Patchell RA, Tibbs PA, Regine WF, et al: Postoperative radiotherapy in the treatment of single metastases to the brain. *JAMA* 280:1485–1489

160. Young RF, Jacques DB, Duma C, et al: Gamma knife radiosurgery for treatment of multiple brain metastases: a comparison of patients with single versus multiple lesions. *Radiosurgery* 1:92–101, 1995

161. Sneed PK, Lamborn KR, Forstner JM, et al: Radiosurgery for brain metastases: is whole brain radiotherapy necessary? *Int J Radiat Oncol Biol Phys* 43:549–558, 1999

162. Werner-Wasik M, Rudoler S, Preston PE, et al: Immediate side effects of stereotactic radiotherapy and radiosurgery. *Int J Radiat Oncol Biol Phys* 43:299–304, 1999

163. Strohl RA: Radiation therapy in tumors of the central nervous system. *Semin Oncol Nurs* 14:26–33, 1998

164. Prados MD, Russo C: Chemotherapy of brain tumors. *Semin Surg Oncol* 14:88–95, 1998

165. Lesser GJ, Grossman SA: Tumor review: the chemotherapy of adult primary brain tumors. *Cancer Treat Rev* 19:261–281, 1993

166. Lesser GJ, Grossman SA: The chemotherapy of high-grade astrocytomas. *Semin Oncol* 21:220–235, 1994

167. Moynihan TJ, Grossman SA: The role of chemotherapy in the treatment of primary tumors of the central nervous system. *Cancer Invest* 12:88–97, 1994

168. Chamberlain MC, Kormanik P: Salvage chemotherapy with paclitaxel for recurrent primary brain tumors. *J Clin Oncol* 13:2066–2071, 1995

169. Mastronardi L, Puzzilli F, Couldwell WT, et al: Tamoxifen and carboplatin combinational treatment of high-grade gliomas. *J Neurooncol* 38:59–68, 1998

170. Couldwell WT, Hinton DR, Surnock AA, et al: Treatment of recurrent malignant gliomas with chronic oral high-dose tamoxifen. *Clin Cancer Res* 2:619–622, 1996

171. Conrad CA, Milosavljevic VP, Yung WK: Advances in chemotherapy for brain tumors, in Wen PY, Black PM (eds): *Neurologic Clinics: Brain Tumors in Adults.* Philadelphia, Saunders, 1995, pp 795–812

172. Glass J, Hochberg FH, Gruber ML, et al: The treatment of oligodendrogliomas and mixed oligodendrogliomas-astrocytomas with PCV chemotherapy. *J Neurosurg* 76:741–745, 1992

173. Kyritsis AP, Yung WKA, Bruner J, et al: The treatment of anaplastic oligodendrogliomas and mixed gliomas. *Neurosurgery* 32:365–371, 1993

174. Mason WP, DeAngelis LM: Procarbazine, CCNU, vincristine (PCV) chemotherapy (CT) for benign oligodendroglioma. *Neurology* 44:A262–A263, 1994

175. Peterson K, Cairncross JG: Oligodendroglioma. *Cancer Invest* 14:243–251, 1996

176. Grossman SA, Wharam M, Sheidler V, et al: Phase II study of continuous infusion carmustine and cisplatin followed by cranial irradiation in adults with newly diagnosed high-grade astrocytoma. *J Clin Oncol* 15:2596–2603, 1997

177. Armstrong TS, Gilbert MR: Chemotherapy of astrocytomas: an overview. *Semin Oncol Nurs* 14:18–25, 1998

178. Shapiro WR, Green SB, Burger PC, et al: A randomized comparison of intra-arterial versus intravenous BCNU, with or without intravenous 5-fluorouracil for newly diagnosed patients with malignant gliomas. *J Neurosurg* 76:772–781, 1992

179. Neuwelt EA, Howieson J, Frenkel EP, et al: Therapeutic efficacy of multiagent chemotherapy with drug delivery enhancement of blood-brain barrier modification in glioblastoma. *Neurosurgery* 19:573–582, 1986

180. Gumerlock MK, Belshe BD, Madsen R, et al: Osmotic blood-brain barrier disruption and chemotherapy in the treatment of high grade malignant glioma: Patient series and literature review. *J Neurooncol* 12:33–46, 1992

181. Olivi A, Brem H: Interstitial chemotherapy with sustained release polymer systems for the treatment of malignant gliomas. *Recent Results Cancer Res* 135:149–154, 1994

182. Brem H, Piantadosi S, Burger PC, et al: Intraoperative controlled delivery of chemotherapy by biodegradable polymers: safety and effectiveness for recurrent gliomas evaluated by a prospective multi-institutional placebo-controlled clinical trial. *Lancet* 345:1008–1012, 1995

183. Gruber ML, Glass J, Choudhri H, et al: Carboplatin chemotherapy before irradiation in newly diagnosed glioblastoma multiforme. *Am J Clin Oncol* 21:338–340, 1998

184. American Brain Tumor Association (ABTA): *A Primer of Brain Tumors*, Des Plaines, IL, ABTA, 1998

185. Maher de Leon ME, Schnell S, Rozental JM: Tumors of the spine and spinal cord. *Semin Oncol Nurs* 14:43–52, 1998

186. Barr ML, Kiernan JA: *The Human Nervous System* (ed 5). Philadelphia, Lippincott, 1988

187. Kornblith PJ, Walker MD, Cassady JR: *Neurologic Oncology.* Philadelphia, Lippincott, 1987

188. Schild SE, Nisi K, Scheithauer BW, et al: The results of radiotherapy for ependymomas: the Mayo Clinic experience. *Int J Radiat Oncol Biol Phys* 42:953–958, 1998

189. Grant R, Papadoppoulos SM, Sandler HM, et al: Metastatic epidural spinal cord compression: current concepts and treatment. *J Neurooncol* 19:79–92, 1994

190. Cohen AP, Wisoff JH, Allen JC, et al: Malignant astrocytomas of the spinal cord. *J Neurosurg* 70:50–54, 1989

191. Hickey JV, Armstrong TS: Spinal cord tumors, in Hickey JV (ed): *The Clinical Practice of Neurological and Neurosurgical Nursing* (ed 4). Philadelphia, Lippincott, 1997, pp 527–539

192. Abernathey CD: Spinal intradural extramedullary tumors, in Rengachary SS, Wilkins RH (eds): *Principles of Neurosurgery.* London, Wolfe, 1994, pp 38-1–38-8

193. Minehan KJ, Shaw EG, Scheithauer BW, et al: Spinal cord astrocytoma: pathological and treatment considerations. *J Neurosurg* 83:590–595, 1995

194. Linstadt DE, Wara WM, Leibel SA, et al: Postoperative radiotherapy of primary spinal cord tumors. *Int J Radiat Oncol Biol Phys* 16:1397–1403, 1989

195. Waldron JN, Laperriere NJ, Jaakkimainen L, et al: Spinal cord ependymomas: a retrospective analysis of 59 cases. *Int J Radiat Oncol Biol Phys* 27:223–229, 1993

196. Whitaker SJ, Bessell EM, Ashley SE, et al: Postoperative radiotherapy in the management of spinal cord ependymoma. *J Neurosurg* 74:720–728, 1991

197. Schultheiss TE: Spinal cord radiation "tolerance": doctrine versus data. *Int J Radiat Oncol Biol Phys* 19:219–221, 1990

198. Posner JB: Supportive care of the neuro-oncology patient, in Hildebrand J (ed): *Management in Neuro-Oncology.* Berlin, Springer-Verlag, 1992, pp 89–99

199. Wegmann JA: CNS tumors: supportive management of the patient and family. *Oncology* 5:109–113, 1991

CHAPTER 50

Cervical Cancer

Paula R. Klemm, RN, DNSc, OCN®

Introduction

Cervical cancer predominantly occurs during the reproductive years when women are more likely to receive regular gynecologic care, including Papanicolaou (Pap) smear testing. The majority of cervical lesions are diagnosed in the preinvasive stages of intraepithelial neoplasia when the disease is curable. Like many other malignancies, cervical cancer can be cured if diagnosed in early stages. Unfortunately, in developing nations and in ethnic minorities in the United States, cervical cancer remains a major problem because of the lack of regular screening and access to care.

Epidemiology

Cervical cancer is a significant cause of morbidity and mortality for women worldwide ranking second only to breast cancer.[1-4] Globally, almost 500,000 (and perhaps as many as 900,000) women are diagnosed and 300,000 die of cervical cancer each year. The five-year survival rate, worldwide, is about 40%.[4,5] Overall, the highest incidence of invasive cervical cancer is reported in the developing nations, particularly in Latin America, India, and Southeast Asia. Cervical neoplasia accounts for the highest rate of cancer mortality among Black South African women.[1,6-8] In the United States, invasive cervical cancer accounts for 17% of all gynecologic malignancies and 18% of all gynecologic deaths.

According to the American Cancer Society, 12,800 new cases of invasive cervical cancer were diagnosed in the United States in 1999, and approximately 4800 women died of the disease.[9] The incidence of invasive cervical cancer has steadily decreased as a result of the Pap smear, which can diagnose the disease in a preinvasive state. The number of deaths from cervical cancer has decreased in women over age 45, while mortality in women under 35 years has increased.[10,11] A bimodal distribution of cases has been noted, with peaks at age 35–39 and age 60–64.[12] However, cervical cancer remains a significant health problem in women age 65 and older who account for only 25% of cases but 40% of deaths.[13,14]

Though the incidence of invasive cancer has decreased by nearly 50%, the incidence of carcinoma in situ (CIS) has climbed dramatically since 1945. Women in their twenties are most often diagnosed with cervical dysplasia; those age 30–39 with in situ cancer; and those over age 40 with invasive cancer.[15]

Etiology

Many personal risk factors have been associated with precancerous lesions of the cervix.[16,17] A higher incidence of the disease occurs in poor women (especially in rural areas), the uninsured, ethnic minorities (especially Hispanics); smokers; elderly African Americans; and women who become sexually active prior to age 17, have many sexual partners, and are multiparous. An association has been noted between increased cervical cancer mortality and employment. Women who work in manufacturing, personal services, farm work, or are nurses aides have higher mortality rates.[18-24]

Cervical dysplasia, CIS, and cervical cancer have been designated as AIDS-defining illnesses by the Center for Disease Control. Women with human immunodeficiency virus (HIV) infection are at higher risk for developing squamous intraepithelial lesions (SIL) of the cervix.[25-27] In HIV-infected females, cervical cancer may manifest itself in unusual ways, be more aggressive, and run a more fulminant course.[28-32] Conversely, cervical carcinoma is infrequent in women who are nulliparous, and those who are lifetime celibates or lifetime monogamous.[17,33-36] Females exposed to diethylstilbestrol (DES) in utero have a higher incidence of clear-cell adenocarcinoma of the cervix and vagina.[37]

Human papillomaviruses (HPV) are highly infectious members of the family of DNA tumor viruses that can cause cellular hyperproliferation and a variety of warty infections. In women, the genital variety of HPV is called *papilloma acuminata* and is sexually transmitted. More than 70 distinct types of HPV have been identified but only some are associated with genital warts, precancerous lesions, or invasive cervical carcinoma.[38-41] Over 20 types of HPV have been associated with high-grade cervical intraepithelial lesions or invasive cancer. HPV 16, 18, 45, and 56 are associated with invasive cancer and account for more than 80% of all invasive cervical neoplasms.[39,42-44] HPV 18 is associated with 15%–50% of invasive cervical cancer lesions. It is the most common papillomavirus found in women with adenocarcinoma of the cervix, while HPV 16 is more commonly associated with squamous carcinomas.[15,45,46] High viral load appears to increase the risk of developing high-grade disease and, ultimately, progression to invasive cancer.[40] Recent research has indicated that the *E6* gene from HPV-mediated carcinogenesis binds to the tumor suppressor *p53* and interferes with normal cell proliferation.[47]

Crum and Newkirk[44] reported that women who had positive human papillomavirus DNA (HPV DNA) findings were 11 times more likely to develop cervical intraepithelial neoplasia (CIN) II/CIN III. More recently, researchers reported that the combination of Pap smear and HPV DNA analysis was more effective than Pap smear alone in diagnosing cervical neoplasia in HIV-1 infected women.[27]

Herpes simplex virus type 2 (HSV2) has been shown to be carcinogenic in animals. Women with cervical cancer usually have higher HSV2 specific antibody titers than controls, but several prospective studies have failed to show an association between development of HSV2 antibodies and development of cervical cancer.[46,48] Still, HSV2 may be a contributing factor in the development of cervical neoplasia.[49,50]

Males play a role in the etiology of cervical cancer. Women married to men whose previous spouses had cervical cancer seem to be at a higher risk of developing cervical cancer.[17] The male partner's age at first coitus, smoking habits, visitation of prostitutes, history of penile cancer, and number of sexual partners also may affect the female partner's relative risk.[17,51,52] Women married to men who are sailors, laborers, textile workers, chemical workers, gardeners, or sports workers have higher mortality rates from cervical cancer.[17] Women who work as maids, cleaners, and cooks may have a slightly elevated risk of developing invasive disease.[53] These findings are most likely related to women's being directly exposed to occupational carcinogens or indirectly exposed via sexual contact with men in the cited occupations.

Several factors may lower a woman's risk of developing preinvasive lesions as precursors to invasive cervical cancer. These include barrier-type contraception, vasectomy, recommended daily allowances of vitamin A, beta carotene, vitamin C, limiting the number of sexual partners, and initiating sexual activity at a later age.[17,54–57]

Santin and associates[58,59] found that a combination of retinoic acid and radiation had a powerful antiproliferative effect on tumor cells. Others reported that a combination of interferon-alfa, retinoic acid, and radiotherapy showed therapeutic benefit in the treatment of advanced cervical cancer.[60]

Pathophysiology

Cellular Characteristics

Histologically, 80%–90% of cervical tumors are squamous, 10%–20% are adenocarcinomas, and a very small number are of other types including adenosquamous, glassy cell, sarcomas, and melanomas.[46,61] Adenocarcinomas generally occur in younger women and impose a greater risk because the tumor arises within the endocervical mucous-producing gland cells. The tumor can become quite bulky before it becomes clinically evident. The bulkiness makes the tumor harder to treat, and thus has a high rate of local recurrence.[46,62] Adenocarcinomas appear to be increasing in prevalence and are more difficult to detect than squamous carcinoma.[62,63] There is no consistent definition of this histological type, no uniform reporting method, and no clear cut histological pattern for correlation of cytological features.[62] Oral contraceptives may be associated with higher rates of adenocarcinoma in younger women. This may be especially true if oral contraceptives are used during adolescence when the cervix has not fully matured. Prognosis seems to be related to tumor volume and nodal metastasis.[62]

Progression of Disease

The cervix—the lower part of the uterus—extends from the isthmus into the vagina and is divided into two major parts: the endocervix and the exocervix. The endocervix is contiguous to the exocervix, which includes the external os and extends to the vaginal fornix. Squamous epithelial cells line the outside surface of the cervix and the vagina, while columnar epithelial cells line the rest of the cervix and the uterus. The *squamocolumnar junction* (or transformation zone) refers to the area where the columnar epithelium of the endocervix joins the squamous epithelium of the exocervix at the os[10,64,65] (Figure 50-1). Cancer of the cervix is a culmination of a progressive disease that begins as a neoplastic alteration of the squamocolumnar junction. Over time, these abnormal cells can progress to involve the full thickness of the epithelium and invade the stromal tissue of the cervix. The initial preinvasive or premalignant changes are called *cervical intraepithelial neoplasia* (CIN).

The terminology used to describe cervical smears has changed since the original Papanicolaou numeric system was introduced. Originally, Pap smear findings were divided into five classes (I to V) that described atypical changes in cervical cells. In the mid-1960s the term *cervical intraepithelial neoplasia* was coined to better define epithelial cervical abnormalities. CIN classification demonstrates the progression of the disease process rather than delineating distinctly different abnormalities. As such, each step in the cervical disease spectrum merges imperceptibly into the next.[11] CIN is divided into three categories: CIN I, CIN II, and CIN III.

The term *CIN I* is used to describe dysplasia or atypical changes in the cervical epithelium involving less than one-third the thickness of the epithelium. *CIN II* describes neoplastic changes involving up to two-thirds the thickness. *CIN III* or *carcinoma in situ* (CIS) describes a lesion that has neoplastic changes involving up to full thickness of the epithelium with no areas of stromal invasion or

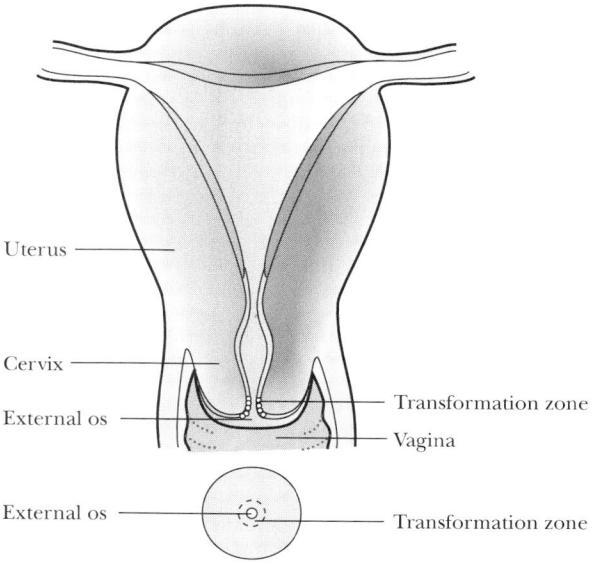

Figure 50-1   Cervical transformation zone

metastases[10,36,66] (Figure 50-2). Once the disease progresses beyond the basement membrane and invades the cervical stroma, the disease is considered invasive or malignant.

In 1988, a workshop sponsored by the National Cancer Institute (NCI) was held in Bethesda, Maryland to address problems inherent in the Papanicolaou system that has been described by some as diagnostic chaos.[67,68] The goal was to review existing terminology and to make recommendations for a more effective method of reporting. The outcome of this conference was the Bethesda system that is now used to report cervical/vaginal cytological diagnoses.[68,69]

The Bethesda system (TBS) (Table 50-1) was proposed in 1988, updated in 1991 and 1992, and addresses the following elements: (1) a statement of the adequacy of the cytological specimen (satisfactory, less than optimal, unsatisfactory); (2) a general categorization of the diagnosis (within normal limits, other); and (3) a descriptive diagnosis that includes several new terms: *atypical squamous cells of undetermined significance (ASCUS), low-grade squamous intraepithelial lesion (LSIL), high-grade squamous intraepithelial lesion (HSIL),* and *atypical glandular cells of undetermined significance (AGUS).* The descriptive diagnosis allows cytopathologists to list reactive and reparative changes (e.g., changes secondary to inflammatory processes, treatment (chemotherapy, radiotherapy), or contraceptive devices). By 1992, 85% of cytology laboratories were utilizing TBS terminology. As a result of the strict format used in reporting cytologic abnormalities, the number of women identified with abnormal Pap smears has increased.[67,70–72]

LSIL includes cellular changes associated with HPV or mild dysplasia (CIN I). HSIL includes lesions formerly designated as moderate dysplasia (CIN II) and severe dysplasia or CIS (CIN III). The use of the word *grade* as it is used with the SIL terminology does not imply invasive carcinoma. Both the ASCUS and AGUS classifications represent minor degrees of cellular abnormality. However, controversy exists with regard to the ASCUS classification. ASCUS classifications should be applied when a definitive diagnosis cannot be made. The rate of ASCUS should be less than 5% of abnormal Pap smears.[40,67,72] Exact interpretation of ASCUS often differs among clinicians and there is no consensus on management of

women in this category.[40,67,73] The NCI is currently conducting the ASCUS/LSIL Triage Study (ALTS) to help determine the best management options. AGUS includes both atypical lesions (which may or may not be preinvasive in nature) and preinvasive lesions (adenocarcinoma in situ).

While the use of TBS is becoming more widespread, there is still opposition to it. Some clinicians argue against using only one diagnostic category (SIL) with two subcategories (low-grade and high-grade SIL) for all intraepithelial lesions, even though qualifying terms may be added to the cytologic reports.[74,75] Several researchers have questioned the inclusion of CIN II and CIN III in the high-grade SIL category.[74] They felt that lumping CIN II and III together implied similar management, which may not be the case. Others have expressed the fear that women may be overdiagnosed and given unnecessary treat-

Table 50-1 Bethesda System for Reporting Cervical/Vaginal Cytological Diagnoses

Statement on specimen adequacy
- Satisfactory for interpretation
- Less than optimal
- Unsatisfactory

General categorization
- Within normal limits
- Other: See descriptive diagnoses

Descriptive diagnoses
- Infection
  - Fungal
  - Bacterial
  - Protozoan
  - Viral
- Other

Reactive and reparative changes
- Inflammation
- Effects of therapy
- Atrophic vaginitis
- Radiation
- Intrauterine contraceptive device
- Other

Cell abnormalities
- Squamous cell
  - Atypical squamous cells of undetermined significance (ASCUS)
  - Low-grade squamous intraepithelial lesion associated with HPV, mild dysplasia
  - High-grade squamous intraepithelial lesion, moderate to severe dysplasia
  - Squamous cell carcinoma
- Epithelial cell
  - Presence of endometrial cells, cytologically benign in postmenopausal woman
  - Atypical glandular cells of undetermined significance (AGUS)
  - Endocervical adenocarcinoma
  - Endometrial adenocarcinoma
  - Extrauterine adenocarcinoma
  - Adenocarcinoma not otherwise specified

Other malignant neoplasms

Hormonal evaluation (applies to vaginal smears only)

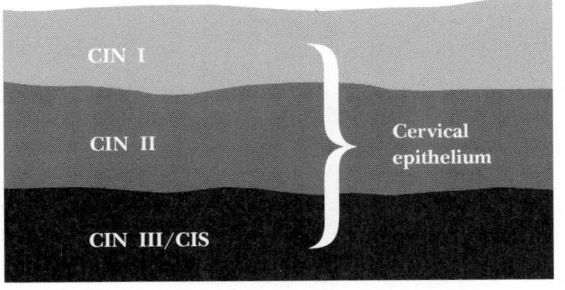

Figure 50-2 Atypical changes in the cervical epithelium

ment.[74,76] The terms *CIN* and *SIL* are both seen in the literature. A comparison of the three nomenclatures is presented in Table 50-2.

Patterns of Spread

Each type of SIL lesion can regress, persist, or become invasive. High-grade SIL (CIN III) is more likely to progress than the milder forms, which may regress spontaneously to normal. Because there is no way to predict which lesions will become invasive and which will not, all patients should be treated as soon as lesions are discovered. SIL is generally considered a venereal disease that has a prolonged incubation period.[77,78]

Several descriptive classification systems have been used to describe squamous cell carcinoma (SCC) lesions. One system uses three grades (grade 1, well differentiated; grade 2, moderately well differentiated; grade 3, poorly differentiated) to denote cell differentiation. Others have divided SCC into three groups known as *large-cell keratinizing, large-cell nonkeratinizing,* and *small cell.*[46,62] A third classification system divides the lesions into small-cell carcinoma (poorly differentiated) and large cell carcinoma (keratinizing or nonkeratinizing).[46,61,62]

Once invasive, cervical cancer spreads by four routes: (1) direct extension, (2) via lymphatics, (3) hematogenous spread, and (4) intraperitoneal implantation. Direct extension is the most common route and the lesion may spread in any direction. The lesion begins on the endocervix and spreads throughout the entire cervix, into the parametrium, and through the vesicovaginal and rectovaginal septae into the bladder and rectum. The upper vagina and corpus of the uterus may also become involved.[62]

Involvement of the lymph nodes in the spread of cervical cancer is fairly predictable and includes the obturator, external iliac, and hypogastric nodes. The secondary group of lymph nodes involved are the parametrial, inferior gluteal, and presacral nodes.[62] Lymph node involvement can be correlated with stage of disease.[10]

Hematogenous spread through the venous plexus and the paracervical veins occurs less frequently than lymphatic spread but is relatively common in the more advanced stages. The most common sites of metastasis are the lungs, mediastinal and supraclavicular nodes, liver, and bone.

Clinical Manifestations

Cervical cancer is usually asymptomatic in the preinvasive and early stages, although women may notice a watery vaginal discharge. In the majority of cases the disease is discovered by Pap smear during routine examination. The later symptoms that often prompt the woman to seek medical attention in cervical cancer are postcoital bleeding, intermenstrual bleeding, or heavy menstrual flow. If this bleeding is chronic, the woman may complain of symptoms related to anemia. A common complaint in advanced cervical malignancy is that of a foul smelling, serous vaginal discharge.[10,46,62]

Other late symptoms, which are indicative of advanced disease, include pain in the pelvis, hypogastrium, flank, or leg. This is secondary to involvement of the pelvic wall, ureters, lymph nodes, or sciatic nerve roots. Urinary and rectal symptoms may indicate invasion of these structures by tumor. End-stage disease may be characterized by edema of the lower extremities due to lymphatic and venous obstruction. Massive vaginal hemorrhage and development of renal failure may result from local invasion of blood vessels and bilateral ureteral obstruction by tumor.[10,46,62]

Table 50-2 Cytologic Report Correlations

Class	CIN Terminology	Description	Bethesda Terminology
I		Smear normal, no abnormal cells	Normal

II		Atypical cells present below the level of cervical neoplasia	Other
			  Infection
			  Reactive and reparative changes
			  Squamous cell abnormalities
			  Atypical squamous cells of undetermined
			    significance (ASCUS)

III	CIN I, CIN II	Smear contains abnormal cells consistent with dysplasia. Mild: CIN I; severe: CIN II	SIL
			  Low-grade
			  High-grade

	CIN III	Smear contains abnormal SIL cells consistent with high-grade severe dysplasia: CIN III	
IV	CIS	Carcinoma in situ	SIL High-grade
V	ISC	Invasive squamous carcinoma	Squamous cell carcinoma

CIN, cervical intraepithelial neoplasia; SIL, squamous intraepithelial neoplasia; CIS, carcinoma in situ; ISC, invasive squamous carcinoma.

SQUAMOUS INTRAEPITHELIAL LESIONS

Assessment

The Pap smear is an effective, accurate, and economical screening technique to detect cervical neoplasia. However, about 40% of American women are not tested regularly and one-half of women age 65 or older have not received a Pap smear in the past three years.[41,78] Accuracy of the examination depends on the sampling method, staining, and microscopic examination.[62,72,79] Automated interpreters can be useful in the detection of cervical abnormalities and can lower false-negative rates. High-resolution video scanners distinguish between normal and abnormal cytologic specimens and can decrease mistakes due to human error.[80–83] Recently, the ThinPrep Pap test was approved as an alternative to the traditional Pap smear. It offers greater accuracy, but costs significantly more than the standard Pap test. Even so, proponents of ThinPrep argue that in the long term, ThinPrep is more cost-effective because it reduces the need for repeat tests and colposcopies.[84–89]

The American Cancer Society recommends that all women who are or have been sexually active or who are at least age 18 have an annual Pap test and pelvic examination. After a woman has had three or more consecutive normal annual examinations, the Pap test may be performed less frequently at the discretion of her physician.[41,46,90] A single Pap smear has up to a 20% chance of being false negative. This percentage falls to about 2%, however, when three consecutive smears are negative.[91,92] The American College of Obstetricians and Gynecologists, the National Cancer Institute, the American Academy of Family Physicians, and the American Medical Association recommend annual examinations that begin with the onset of sexual activity or at 18 years of age.

Sexually active women should have annual Pap smears. Women who are postmenopausal or have had hysterectomies as well as women over age 55 should also have annual Pap smears.[41] Those who have any pelvic symptoms such as pain, vaginal discharge, or abnormal bleeding should be evaluated by their physician promptly.

When the Pap smear report shows SIL, referral for biopsy, colposcopy, and/or treatment is indicated. Colposcopy is done on an outpatient basis, using a stereoscopic, binocular microscope that illuminates and magnifies the view of the cervix.[93] During this procedure the cervix is swabbed with an acetic acid solution that accentuates the abnormalities and differentiates between normal or metaplastic areas.[94] The epithelium of the cervix is visualized and the abnormal areas biopsied.

Therapeutic Approaches

It is critical that the extent of the disease is determined as accurately as possible before treatment begins. The Pap smear, colposcopy, and biopsy determine the extent and severity of the cervical lesion, differentiating between SIL and invasive carcinoma of the cervix. Treatment for SIL may include a direct cervical biopsy, electrocautery/cryosurgery, laser surgery, electrosurgery, cone biopsy, or hysterectomy.[46,61,93]

Cryosurgery, a commonly used method for outpatient treatment of SIL in the United States, makes use of a portable probe to induce freezing of cervical tissue. It is a cost-effective and painless treatment with low morbidity that can be performed in the office. Patients most often complain of a watery discharge for two to four weeks after treatment.

Approximately 80%–90% of SIL can be eradicated by laser.[46,62] The laser is mounted on the colposcope, and the beam is directed under colposcopic control. The advantage of using the laser is that significantly less disease-free tissue is removed with the entire lesion. Patients may experience a little more discomfort than with cryosurgery, but there is usually less vaginal discharge, and complete healing occurs in about two weeks.[10,61,93] One disadvantage of the laser is that it may cause thermal damage to tissue, making it difficult to rule out invasive cancer.[62]

Treatment of SIL using the loop electrosurgical excision procedure (LEEP), or loop diathermy excision, is an increasingly popular alternative. In selected patients this approach may allow for diagnosis and treatment of SIL during one outpatient visit. LEEP uses a thin wire loop and a low level of electricity to excise affected tissue with minimal ablation.[62,95–97]

Darwish and Gadallah described a one-step procedure for diagnosing and treating cervical lesions using a large loop excision of the transformation zone.[98] Thus, the usual two sessions (diagnosis at initial visit and punch biopsy during the second) can be avoided. The advantage of loop excision technique is that there is less likelihood of tissue ablation than with the use of other procedures such as the laser. Complications of loop excision therapy are similar to those seen with laser treatment.[95,96,99]

Conization involves removal of a cone-shaped piece of tissue from the exocervix and endocervix.[10,93,100] The exact size of the cone depends on the colposcopic findings. Performed under general anesthesia on an outpatient basis, conization can be used (1) for diagnosis, if no lesion of the cervix is noted and an endocervical tumor is suspected; (2) to determine the extent of the lesion if microinvasion is diagnosed on biopsy or if the entire lesion cannot be seen with the colposcope, (3) if there are discrepancies between the cytologic report (Pap smear) and the histologic appearance of the lesions on biopsy, and (4) when the patient cannot be relied upon for long-term follow-up.[78] Major immediate complications of conization include hemorrhage, uterine perforation, and complications of anesthesia. Delayed complications include bleeding, cervical stenosis, infertility, cervical incompetence, and increased chances of preterm (low birth weight) delivery. In general, complications of conization are related to the amount of endocervix that is removed.[93,100]

Total vaginal hysterectomy (TVH) may be employed for treatment of individuals with HSIL (CIN III). It is appropriate for individuals with HSIL who have completed childbearing. These individuals must be followed as closely for recurrence as those treated with more conservative measures.[10,100]

Ultimately, the therapy selected is based on the extent of the disease, the patient's wishes to preserve ovarian and reproductive function, and the physician's recommendation. Women with LSIL who wish to maintain optimum fertility can be considered for electrocautery, laser therapy, or cryosurgery. High-grade SIL also can be treated in this manner as long as the woman is aware that there is a slightly higher incidence of recurrence with this treatment method.[10]

Continuity of Care: Nursing Challenges

The primary nursing responsibilities for women with SIL focus on education. This educational process includes defining the disease, explaining treatment, teaching the importance of close follow-up, and modifying high-risk behaviors.

If the biopsy indicates SIL, the woman may erroneously think that she has invasive cancer. The nurse assures the patient that she does not have cancer and that SIL is an easily treated premalignant condition. In women treated for SIL, self-esteem may drop and anxiety increase during the initial and postsurgical visits. In addition, women may fear losing sexual function.[100] The nurse helps the woman to understand the type of treatment recommended, explains the nature and purpose of treatment, and the side effects of the therapy.

Nonadherence following abnormal Pap tests have been shown to be as high as 40%. In one study, social support was strongly related to adherence to treatment regimens in a group of African American women, while tangible support was related to adherence in Latino women.[101] In another study, educational programs, transportation assistance and reminders helped improve follow-up after abnormal Pap tests.[102]

Following treatment, the nurse instructs the woman on how to care for herself at home. Douching, tampons, and sexual intercourse are prohibited for at least two to four weeks, depending on the treatment. A return visit must be scheduled for two to four weeks, then every three months for a year, and every six months thereafter. The importance of this follow-up must be stressed because there is a possibility of treatment failure or recurrence of the SIL. Minimal bleeding and vaginal discharge may be present for a week or longer after biopsy, cryosurgery, or laser and for several weeks following conization.

Information concerning sexual functioning and fertility should be discussed with women undergoing treatment for SIL, although electrocautery, cryosurgery, laser therapy, and conization rarely cause physiologic sexual dysfunction.[95,103] Most women report no change in libido, orgasm, coital frequency, or overall satisfaction with their

Table 50-3   Risk Factors and Preventive Measures for Preinvasive Lesions of the Cervix

Risk Factors	Preventive Measures
HSV2	Pap smear per ACS guidelines
HPV	Annual pelvic examination
Abnormal transformation zone	Barrier contraception
Sex prior to age 17	Limit number of sexual partners
Multiple sexual partners	Sex after age 17
History of smoking	Stop smoking
Chemicals in cigarette smoke	Hygienic environment for sexual activity
Spouse whose previous wife had cervical cancer	Assess occupational risk
Maternal use of DES	Educational programs targeted at high-risk groups (ethnic minorities, poor women, uninsured, smokers, elderly women)
Immunosuppression	
Multiparous	
Socioeconomic status	
Race/ethnic background	
Spouse with cancer of penis	

HSV2, herpes simplex virus type 2; HPV, human papilloma virus.

sex life. Fertility is usually maintained, but difficulty with conception may occur. Nurses should take time to educate women about reducing risk factors (e.g., HIV, multiple sexual partners) and preventive measures (e.g., smoking reduction, minimizing the number of sexual partners, and barrier protection) related to preinvasive disease. Table 50-3 summarizes issues specifically related to nursing management.

INVASIVE DISEASE

Assessment

A thorough clinical examination under anesthesia includes cervical biopsies, endocervical curettage, cystoscopy, and proctosigmoidoscopy. Additional diagnostic tests include chest and skeletal radiographs, intravenous pyelograph, barium enema, complete blood count (CBC), and blood chemistries. If liver enzymes are elevated, a liver scan (or computerized tomography (CT) scan) is indicated.[46,61,62,93,104] Ureteral obstruction has been found in 30% of patients with stage III disease and up to 50% of women with stage IV disease.[65]

Lymphangiogram may be indicated in selected individuals. Its use has been controversial, however, due to a false-positive rate between 20%–40% and a false-negative rate between 10%–15%.[12,62,66,71]

Additional studies that are helpful in defining the extent of disease but do not alter clinical staging include

Table 50-4 Clinical Staging for Carcinoma of the Cervix

Stage	Description
0	Carcinoma in situ, intraepithelial carcinoma
I	The carcinoma is strictly confined to the cervix
IA	Invasive cancer identified only microscopically. All gross lesions even with superficial invasion are stage IB cancers. Invasion is limited to measured stromal invasion with maximum depth of 5 mm and no wider than 7 mm.
IA1	Measured invasion of stroma no greater than 3 mm in depth and no wider than 7 mm.
IA2	Measure invasion of stroma greater than 3 mm and no greater than 5 mm in depth, and no wider than 7 mm.
IB	Clinical lesions confined to the cervix or preclinical lesions greater than stage IA.
IB1	Clinical lesions no greater than 4 cm in size.
IB2	Clinical lesions greater than 4 cm in size.
II	The carcinoma extends beyond the cervix but has not extended to the pelvic wall. The carcinoma involves the vagina but not as far as the lower third.
IIA	No obvious parametrial involvement.
IIB	Obvious parametrial involvement.
III	The carcinoma has extended to the pelvic wall. On rectal examination, there is no cancer-fee space between the tumor and the pelvic wall.
	The tumor involves the lower third of the vagina. All cases with hydronephrosis or nonfunctioning kidney are included unless they are known to be due to other causes.
IIIA	No extension to the pelvic wall.
IIIB	Extension to the pelvic wall and/or hydronephrosis of nonfunctioning kidney.
IV	The carcinoma has extended beyond the true pelvis or has clinically involved the mucosa of the bladder or rectum. A bullous edema as such does not permit a case to be allotted to state IV.
IVA	Spread of the growth to adjacent organs.
IVB	Spread to distant organs.

FIGO, International Federation of Gynecology and Obstetrics, 1995

CT and magnetic resonance imaging (MRI). Computerized axial tomograms may be used to determine the extent of pelvic disease, to define radiotherapy portals, and to evaluate lymph node status. However, CT and MRI are not effective in detecting small metastases.[46] The main use of CT is to help identify enlarged lymph nodes in the pelvis and paraaortic areas.[62] MRI offers no advantage over CT in evaluating lymph node metastasis or assessing the parametrium.[62] Researchers have found, however, that MRI offers improved evaluation of tumor size, stromal invasion, and extent of disease as compared to CT.[105] Both CT and MRI were able to evaluate lymph node metastasis (86% each). MRI has been used to assess the response of cervical cancer to neoadjuvant chemotherapy, but was not as precise as surgical staging in these cases.[106] Verification of tumor volume (the most important prognostic factor for survival of the patient with cervical cancer) by MRI may help the physician to determine the best treatment modality.[107] Positron emission tomography (PET) may be able to detect disease not seen on CT or MRI. In addition PET, if used in conjunction with CT and MRI, may be better able to determine extent of local disease and nodal involvement.[62]

Clinical staging is not changed on the basis of surgical findings, but treatment may be altered. In selected cases where lymphangiogram or CT are equivocal, a selected pelvic and periaortic lymphadenectomy may be performed. Surgical staging has been included in some investigational chemotherapy and radiation protocols to better define the extent of disease and select appropriate radiation therapy.[61,108]

Supraclavicular node biopsy is done if one of these nodes is palpable or if paraaortic nodes are positive. The left node is most often positive because this is where the thoracic duct enters into the subclavian vein. Positive supraclavicular nodes are often associated with a positive aortic node. In such cases a blind scalene node biopsy is recommended. If this is positive, systemic therapy is necessary. Following a thorough evaluation, the clinical stage is determined[62] (Table 50-4).

Tumor markers are not used extensively by oncologists, though several researchers have advocated their use. Borras and associates[109] found elevated carcinoembryonic antigen (CEA) levels in 33%, cancer antigen-19.9 (CA-19.9) in 32%, and CA-125 in 21.5% of women studied with invasive cervical carcinoma. Salman and colleagues[110] found elevated squamous call carcinoma (SCC) antigen levels in a study of women with gynecologic malignancies. Fifty-seven percent of the women with cervical cancer had elevated levels of SCC. By comparison, elevations in SCC were found in 100% of vulva/vaginal cancers and 90% of ovarian cancers. Takeshima and associates[111] found that SCC levels were elevated in 65% of women with cervical cancer who had extension of disease to pelvic lymph nodes. They suggested that SCC could be used as a predictor of nodal metastasis. Other researchers have indicated that SCC antigen and CA-125 are useful markers for the progression of disease because the markers increased about three months before clinical evidence of disease recurrence.[112,113] CA-125 is more likely to be elevated in women with adenocarcinoma.

Specimens from over 1000 women with cervical cancer from 22 countries were collected in order to determine if the association between genital HPV infection and cervical cancer is consistent worldwide. HPV DNA was detected in 93% of the malignancies.[45] DNA subtyping has been conducted to evaluate HPV-associated lesions.[62,114] Antibodies against HPV 16 have been found in the sera of women with cervical cancer. In one study, 44% of SIL lesions (CIN II/III) were found by HPV testing, although cytology was negative. However, 25% of SIL (CIN II/III) lesions were not detected by the HPV tests. In the future, HPV testing may play a role in the early detection and clinical management of disease, as a diagnostic tool for evaluating risk in the development of disease, or to help with immunologic monitoring in vaccination trials.[115–117]

Classification and Staging

Cervical cancer is staged clinically, with confirmation obtained from examinations completed with the patient under anesthesia. This allows for more accurate staging including visualization of the upper vagina and palpation of parametrial and lateral side wall tissues.[62] Evaluation under anesthesia usually occurs at the same time as the planned surgical intervention or when radiation implants are inserted. The clinical stage is not changed if disease recurs. The initial staging is one of the best prognostic indicators. Approximate overall five-year survival rates are about 70%. Status of lymph nodes is associated with overall survival. Five-year survival rates for women with negative nodes is 85%–90%. As the number of positive nodes increases, the survival rate decreases.[12]

Therapeutic Approaches

Once invasive cervical cancer is diagnosed and the stage is established, treatment is based on the woman's age, general medical condition, extent of the cancer, and the presence of any complicating abnormalities. Either surgery or radiation therapy can be used equally effectively for patients with early-stage disease. With either radio-

therapy or surgery, the five-year survival rate for stage I is 85%.[46,118] In the past 20 years, outcomes for locally advanced disease have improved with radiation therapy. This is related to more adequate placement of intracavitary brachytherapy, higher paracentral doses, and reduction of overall treatment time.[119] Radiotherapy can be used for all individuals, whereas surgery is indicated only for women who are considered good surgical candidates.[2,62] Key components include being treated in an institution with the appropriate personnel and equipment for either type of treatment and multidisciplinary planning.[71] In general, patients with stage IIb to IV are treated with radiotherapy.

Stage IA

Stage IA disease (microinvasive carcinoma) has been subdivided into IA1 and IA2. Stage IA1 (≤3-mm depth of invasion, horizontal dimension <7 mm, no lymphatic or vascular space involvement) should be treated by total abdominal hysterectomy (TAH) or total vaginal hysterectomy (TVH) if the patient is healthy and does not desire further childbearing. Conization can be done for those who are poor surgical risks or who wish to preserve fertility, as long as the biopsy margins are free of disease and the patient is followed closely.[2,46,61,66,93,120] Intracavitary radiation may also be utilized to treat cervical cancer in this stage.[62,120]

Stage IA2 disease is treated by TAH or TVH if invasion is less than 3 mm and there is no lymphovascular involvement. If the invasion is greater than 3 mm or there is lymphovascular invasion, the disease is managed the same as in stage IB. Five-year survival in patients with properly staged IA cervical cancer is close to 100%.[66,93,118] Conservative measures are recommended to treat stage IA1, but more aggressive measures (radical or modified radical hysterectomy with pelvic lymph node dissection) are indicated for stage IA2 because of the higher risk of lymphovascular involvement.[61,121,122]

Stages IB and IIA

In 1995 the Federation of Gynecology and Obstetrics (FIGO) divided stage IB into stage IB1 (lesions ≤4 cm in size) and IB2 (lesions >4 cm in size). The choice of therapy for patients with stage IB and IIA disease remains controversial, and the choice of surgery or radiation depends on the gynecologist and radiation oncologist involved as well as on the woman's condition and the characteristics of the lesion.

Stage IB and stage IIA disease can be treated with radical abdominal hysterectomy and pelvic lymphadenectomy or with definitive radiation, which may include external beam and/or intracavitary insertions.[123] Cure rates for stage IB using radiation or surgery are 80%–90%.[10,46,62]

Surgery is preferred to radiotherapy by some gynecologic oncologists since ovarian function can be preserved.

The vagina usually remains more pliable after surgery than with radiation, the overall treatment time is shorter, and long-term radiation complications to pelvic tissue can be avoided. Using radiation therapy has the advantages of avoiding major intraoperative and postoperative complications, and the patient can receive the therapy as an outpatient.[61,66]

Patients with bulky disease (barrel-shaped cervix) have a higher incidence of central recurrence, pelvic and paraaortic lymph node metastases, and distant dissemination. An increased dose of radiation to the central pelvis followed six weeks later by radical hysterectomy, or both, have been advocated in patients with bulky disease.[66] The use of combined radical surgery followed by radiation remains controversial because the patient faces complications associated with each treatment modality.[46]

Stages IIB, III, and IVA

Women with stages IIB, III, and IV cervical cancer are usually treated with high doses of external pelvic radiation followed by brachytherapy. The initial dose of external radiation may help reduce tumor load and facilitate placement of vaginal applicators to enhance the effects of brachytherapy.[62,118] Treatment is usually completed in about eight weeks.[46] The five-year survival rate of patients with stage IIB cancer is 60%–79%, while those with stage III have a survival rate of 25%–50%, and those with stage IV have a rate less than 10%.[62,66,124] The advantages of radiation over surgery for advanced disease are that radiation can be given on an outpatient basis, it avoids surgery, and is suitable for women who are poor surgical candidates.[62,66] However, Shingleton and Orr[62] assert that radical surgery for stage IIB disease may offer better cure rates than radiation.

The number of total pelvic exenterations has decreased dramatically in the past 20 years and today it is used only in a selected group of patients. Candidates for pelvic exenteration include women previously treated with radiation who have recurrent centralized disease not adherent to pelvic sidewalls and not involving lymph nodes. It is important to ensure they are psychologically able to adjust to the changes in body function and body image.[62,66,118] Unfortunately, inoperable disease is found about 60% of the time in candidates for pelvic exenteration.[125]

Surgical staging of advanced disease before initiating treatment is advocated in an attempt to gain a more precise evaluation of the extent of the disease.[108,125] Arguments for pretreatment laparotomy are that (1) the extent of the disease can be ascertained, (2) patients who have disease not curable by radiation may be offered palliative therapy, and (3) those patients most likely to benefit from extended field radiation are identified. Arguments against pretreatment laparotomy are that (1) surgical staging can cause morbidity and mortality, (2) many patients with paraaortic nodal metastases also have systemic disease not detected by surgery, (3) there is only minimal improvement in net survival, and (4) surviving patients have high morbidity. Some surgeons are using alternative extraperitoneal staging methods to determine the extent of disease. One approach involves making a small incision near the umbilicus and outside of the proposed radiation field. This allows sampling the aortic and/or common ileac nodes, collection of peritoneal fluids for cytology, and palpation of pelvic structures.[62]

At present, chemotherapy alone has not proved useful as initial therapy for women who are at high risk for recurrence, but it continues to be investigated. Chemotherapy is usually reserved for patients with recurrent disease or metastasis. Recently, interest in the use of neoadjuvant chemotherapy for advanced squamous cell carcinoma of the cervix has increased. Neoadjuvant chemotherapy is the use of chemotherapeutic agents to shrink tumors prior to surgery or radiotherapy.[126–129] Even though neoadjuvant chemotherapy may make more cervical tumors resectable, however, cure rates are not improved over definitive radiotherapy used alone.[130–139]

Recurrent or Persistent Disease

Approximately 35% of women with invasive cervical cancer will have recurrent or persistent disease.[10] Therefore, thorough, regular follow-ups after treatment are mandatory. Recurrent cervical cancer is difficult to diagnose. Clinical and cytological evaluation of an irradiated cervix is problematic because the cells and configuration of the cervix are distorted from the radiation. Therefore, histological confirmation of recurrence is essential.

Almost 80% of recurrences manifest within two years after therapy.[62,118] The signs and symptoms, however, may be subtle and varied. They may include unexplained weight loss, leg edema (excessive and often unilateral), pelvic or thigh and buttock pain, serosanguinous vaginal discharge, progressive ureteral obstruction, supraclavicular lymph node enlargement (usually of the left side), cough, hemoptysis, and chest pain. If the woman presents with the triad of weight loss, leg edema, and pelvic pain, the outlook is grim. Evaluation after histologic confirmation will usually include chest x-ray, intravenous pyelogram (IVP), CBC, and blood chemistries. Some physicians will include a CT scan, lymphangiography, or fluoroscopically directed needle biopsies to evaluate the status of the regional lymph nodes, liver, and kidneys. These procedures have replaced more elaborate operative procedures to provide histological confirmation of recurrence,[10] which may save the woman unnecessary surgery. In general, prognosis for women with central recurrence of disease is better than for those who experience recurrence in the pelvic wall.[46]

Following surgery or radiotherapy as primary treatment for patients with cervical cancer, about half of all recurrences are local (cervix, uterus, vagina, parametrium, and regional lymph nodes). The remaining cases involve distant metastases to the lung, liver, bone, mediastinal, or supraclavicular lymph nodes.[62]

The prognosis for patients with persistent or recurrent carcinoma of the cervix is dismal. One-year survival rates are 10%–15%.[10,12] Survival averages six to ten months once recurrent cervical cancer is diagnosed.[62] The aim of treatment in recurrent disease is palliation because control or cure is rare.

Surgery. When cervical cancer recurs centrally following radiotherapy, pelvic exenteration may be considered. Total pelvic exenteration includes radical hysterectomy, pelvic lymph node dissection, and removal of the bladder and rectosigmoid colon. Occasionally, a posterior exenteration (which preserves the bladder) or anterior exenteration (which preserves the rectum) can be performed.[10,62,140] Partial pelvic exenterations are usually not done because the bladder and rectum may have residual radiation effects and are prone to complications.

Because the goal of the surgery is curative, only a small percentage of women with recurrence are candidates for pelvic exenteration. Women with disease outside the pelvis or with the triad of unilateral leg edema, sciatic pain, and ureteral obstruction are not candidates for pelvic exenteration. Obesity, severe medical problems, and advanced age also may be reasons why this surgery is contraindicated.[10,12,62,118,125]

Extensive preoperative evaluation must be done to ensure that there is no disease outside the pelvis and that renal function is adequate. Studies usually performed include chest x-ray, IVP, blood chemistries, creatinine clearance, CT scan, bone scan, and liver-spleen scan. Some clinicians also order lymphangiography as well as an abdominal CT scan to evaluate the regional lymph nodes. If lymphadenopathy is present, a needle aspiration of the nodes may be done. If the aspirate is positive for malignancy, the woman may be spared an unnecessary laparotomy. A blind scalene node biopsy may be recommended to complete the evaluation. Preoperative evaluation of nutritional status is important in this population. Up to 60% of cancer patients may exhibit laboratory or clinical evidence of malnutrition.[62,141–143]

At laparotomy, the entire abdomen and pelvis is explored for metastases. A selective paraaortic lymphadenectomy, bilateral pelvic lymphadenectomy, and biopsies of the pelvic sidewalls are done and sent for frozen section. If any of these is positive, the exenteration is usually aborted because the disease is considered incurable.[10] However, some surgeons support the use of pelvic exenterations in patients with recurrent disease complicated by pelvic lymph node metastases.[144]

The use of the end-to-end anastomotic (EEA) stapling device has resulted in patients' not needing a permanent colostomy after pelvic exenteration.[140] The EEA also reduces the risk of anastomotic leaks, fistula formation, and late strictures, and decreases operative time. Permanent colostomy can also be avoided by using a segment of sigmoid colon as a rectal substitute.[62,145]

Immediate postoperative problems include pulmonary embolism, pulmonary edema, cerebrovascular accident, hemorrhage, myocardial infarction, sepsis, and small bowel obstruction. Long-term problems include fistula formation, urinary obstruction, infection, and sepsis. The use of pelvic exenteration has been limited to a highly select group of candidates, since reports indicate a five-year survival of 23%–50% and an operative mortality of approximately 9.8%.[12,46,62,66,92] Women under age 35 have a better prognosis when compared to those over age 35. Psychosexual and social rehabilitation of surviving patients is a major challenge.[62,146,147] Vaginal reconstruction at the time of exenteration and psychological support in the postoperative period can help patients adjust. Survival statistics are worse for women who have recurrent disease greater than 3 mm, bladder involvement, positive pelvic lymph nodes, and recurrence less than a year after previous treatment.[12]

Radiotherapy. In previously irradiated individuals, metastatic disease outside the initial radiation field may be treated cautiously with radiation to provide local control and relieve symptoms. In selected cases, radiation within previously treated areas may be used.[10,46,66] For women treated initially with surgery, full-dose radiotherapy using a combination of external and intracavitary implants may afford excellent palliation or even cure.[46,66]

Chemotherapy. In general, surgery or radiation will not be curative in women who have recurrent cervical cancer. Thus, chemotherapy may be the only hope for cure in these cases.[66,71] Chemotherapy for patients with cervical carcinoma is complicated because these patients frequently have decreased pelvic vascular perfusion, a limited bone marrow reserve, and poor renal function related to previous radiation or surgery, and ureteral obstruction from tumor or scarring.[10,12,61]

Response rates for patients with recurrent cervical cancer treated with single-agent and investigational chemotherapy[62] range from 0%–48%, with most less than 20%. In general, there is no long-term benefit, with responses lasting less than eight months with variable lengths of survival.[10,62] Response rates are higher in patients who have received no prior radiotherapy or chemotherapy. Documented activity has been shown for doxorubicin dibromoducitol, ifosfamide, CHIP (iproplatin), doxorubicin, vincristine, carboplatin, and topotecan.[62,148–150] Of the single agents, cisplatin remains the drug with the greatest antineoplastic activity, although carboplatin may be used as first-line treatment as well.[62,149–150] Even so, objective response rates with cisplatin only range between 17%–30% and provide no increase in survival time for patients.

Recently, gemcitabine has exhibited antitumor activity against cervical cancer in phase II clinical trials.[151] Topotecan has also shown efficacy against cervical cancer in phase II trials.[152] In a phase I clinical trial, Chen and colleagues[153] administered paclitaxel, cisplatin, and radiation therapy to women with advanced cervical cancer. A 93% response rate was reported, with 10 of 16 women having no evidence of disease at the time of the report. A combination of tirapazamine and cisplatin were recently given to 12 women with recurrent cervical cancer in a phase I trial. The regimen was well tolerated and 75% of participants showed clinical responses. Phase II studies are planned.[154]

Combination chemotherapy has not been proven more effective than single agents. Higher response rates may be achieved with combination therapy, but survival is not affected.[155,156] The drugs most commonly used are bleomycin, 5-FU, mitomycin C, methotrexate, cyclophosphamide, doxorubicin, and cisplatin. Complete response rates of up to 36% suggest some enhancement of effect using a combination of drugs. However, median survival rates range between 4–10.5 months.[62] Many clinical trials using combination chemotherapy have had relatively small sample sizes, making it difficult to determine their usefulness in treating advanced cervical cancer.[10,46,62,156–159]

Pelvic intraarterial chemotherapy using a variety of drugs (e.g., doxorubicin and cisplatin, cisplatin and bleomycin, cisplatin or carboplatin and doxorubicin in conjunction with radiation therapy or radical surgery has been studied in advanced cervical cancer. While some results have been promising, further investigation is warranted to define its role in treating cervical cancer.[136,160–163]

Chemotherapy has been used as a radiation sensitizer, particularly hydroxyurea.[62,164,165] This approach may be most useful in women who have large hypoxic tumors confined to the pelvis.[62] Results have also indicated that patients experienced an increased incidence of hematologic toxicity with hydroxyurea. Weekly low-dose cisplatin with radiation has been associated with a modest improvement in disease-free survival without any significant increases in toxicity.[66] A few studies have indicated that paclitaxel may act as a modest radiosensitizer.[153,166]

The use of chemotherapy and radiotherapy in the treatment of cervical cancer has been reported in the literature.[167–169] Recently, Koumantakis and associates[129] administered concurrent platinum chemotherapy and intracavitary brachytherapy to women with locally advanced cervical cancer prior to definitive treatment. Eighty-five percent of the sample was disease free at a mean of 2.8 years after therapy. Others have studied the effects of using 5-FU in conjunction with radiotherapy and found no therapeutic benefit.[131,170] Even though the benefits of combining radiation and chemotherapy remain marginal, their use is increasing.[171]

Initial treatment of cervical cancer with chemotherapy has been proposed for tumor debulking, spatial restoration, as a radiation sensitizer, and as adjuvant therapy.[172,173] Because radiotherapy works better on a smaller tumor volume, induction chemotherapy may debulk the tumor before other therapies are started. This might reduce the incidence of pelvic recurrence. Studies continue to support the use of chemotherapy in the initial treatment of cervical cancer.[157,158,174–176] Other studies have evaluated the efficacy of new protocols utilizing chemotherapy,[127,177] chemoradiation and surgery,[168] chemotherapy and radiation,[129,131,134,135,170,171,177,178] and surgery and radiation.[179–182]

Chemotherapy is not useful as adjuvant therapy after definitive treatment in high-risk women (e.g., women with positive nodes, bulky lesions, or adenocarcinomas). For women with bulky disease, treatment results with radiation have been disappointing. It had been hoped that the administration of chemotherapy prior to radiation might increase local control and survival as compared to the use of radiation alone. Results indicated a significant tumor response, but local control of disease and overall survival have not improved.[183,184]

Recent clinical trials to evaluate new treatments for cervical cancer include treatment with or without cisplatin and 5-FU; adjuvant simple hysterectomy versus radiation; adjuvant hysterectomy and weekly cisplatin; pelvic radiotherapy versus observation; radiotherapy with cisplatin, cisplatin, 5-FU, and hydroxyurea, or hydroxyurea alone; pelvic radiotherapy with concurrent chemotherapy versus pelvic and paraaortic radiotherapy; radiotherapy with intracavitary brachytherapy and chemotherapy using cisplatin and 5-FU; combination cisplatin and pentoxifylline, and paclitaxel; a carotenoid diet for treating cervical dysplasia; combination topotecan and paclitaxel; vinorelbine, paclitaxel, and radiotherapy; gemcitabine and 5-FU; isotretinoin and interferon; and tirapazamine and cisplatin.[185,186]

Adjuvant immunotherapy.   Interest in the use of immunotherapy for the treatment of cervical cancer has increased recently. Laboratory studies have indicated that interferon-alpha coupled with 13-cis-retinoic acid have inhibited growth in cervical cancer cells.[187–189] Clinical trials using this treatment option have shown some promise in the treatment of cervical cancer[190,191] and further clinical trials are underway.[192,193] Tumor necrosis factor,[194] monoclonal antibodies,[195] and interleukin 12[196] may play a role in the treatment of cervical cancer as well.

Complications of surgery.   Radical hysterectomy involves removal of the uterus, upper third of the vagina, entire uterosacral and uterovesical ligaments, all of the parametria, and pelvic node lymphadenectomy. This is a complex procedure because the organs removed are proximal to many vital body structures—the bladder, ureters, rectum, and great vessels of the pelvis.[62,118,123] The major complications of radical hysterectomy include ureteral fistulas, bladder dysfunction, pulmonary embolus, lymphocysts, pelvic infection, bowel obstruction, rectovaginal fistulas, and hemorrhage.[124]

Complications of radiotherapy.   Morbidity resulting from properly administered radiotherapy in cervical cancer is usually manageable. There are reported adverse reactions when poor technique is used, but these reactions occur infrequently in properly treated women. The higher the dose of radiation, the greater the rate of complications. Some morbidity attributed to radiation is secondary to uncontrolled tumor or compounded effects of multiple therapies and not a direct result of radiation alone. Major complication rates for stages I and IIA disease range from 3%–5%, and for stages IIB and III range from 10%–15%.[62,197]

The major complications related to radiotherapy include vaginal stenosis, fistula formation, sigmoid perforation or stricture, uterine perforation, rectal ulcer or proctitis, intestinal obstruction, fistulas, ureteral stricture, severe cystitis, pelvic hemorrhage, and pelvic abscess. Other problems related to radiation therapy include nausea, vomiting, diarrhea, and, rarely, radiation myelitis.

Sexual dysfunction secondary to vaginal atrophy, stenosis, and lack of lubrication is a known effect of the radiation therapy. Radiation causes thinning of the vaginal epithelium and the vagina may become shortened, less flexible, and partially obliterated. Vaginal intercourse may cause dyspareunia and bleeding.[62,198] Women who are not sexually active experience greater incidence of atrophy and stenosis than do sexually active women. The use of vaginal dilators and water-soluble lubricants can minimize the radiation effects.

Complications of chemotherapy. The complications of chemotherapy may manifest themselves in any organ system and depend on the agent, dose, and route utilized. In addition, chemotherapy may adversely affect psychological, emotional, and psychosocial aspects of the cancer patient's life. The reader is referred to the chapters on chemotherapy in this text for in-depth information related to these issues.

Continuity of Care: Nursing Challenges

Although mortality rates for cervical cancer have decreased over the past 40 years, the rates among ethnic minorities, poor women, and elderly women of all races are higher due to decreased utilization of screening methods in these populations.[1,6,199–204] Access to cervical cancer screening for African Americans, Hispanics, older women, and those who are economically disadvantaged should be a priority for health care professionals.

Barriers that discourage women from taking advantage of cervical screening include embarrassment, discomfort,[204,205] financial burden, fatalism, lack of access,[206] lack of transportation, population mobility, opposition

by partners,[6] lack of education,[206–208] lack of health insurance,[207] and age.[208]

Researchers have undertaken creative approaches to increase cervical cancer screening and follow-up for underserved groups including a screening program in a public hospital emergency room,[209] Pap smear screening offered in an inpatient setting,[210] the use of lay educators,[202] the use of nurse practitioners for cervical screening in medically underserved areas,[211] culturally based educational programs,[212–214] and interventions based on socioeconomic status.[215]

Nurses are in a unique position to educate women about the benefits of cervical cancer screening. It is through repeated, creative interventions with patients and their families that nurses can have an impact on the morbidity and mortality of cervical cancer. Given the complexity of treatment modalities provided in the hospital environment, outpatient setting, and in the home, continuity of care across health care settings should be a priority for all women with cervical malignancies. The availability of cancer related information and psychosocial support via the Internet should not be overlooked. Several sources for information on cervical cancer are listed in Chapter 85. In addition, prevention and/or control of side effects secondary to treatment are vital to maintaining patient quality of life during treatment. Table 50-5 summarizes issues related to the nursing management of women with premalignant and malignant cervical lesions.

Conclusion

Cervical cancer accounts for significant morbidity and mortality worldwide. Of the gynecologic malignancies, only cervical cancer has an effective screening method for early detection. The potential for cure is enhanced when the disease is diagnosed in early stages. Treatment modalities for women with invasive disease can be very aggressive and may result in a variety of illness-related demands on the woman and her family. Additionally,

Table 50-5   Treatment Modalities and Nursing Management of the Woman with Cervical Pre-invasive or Invasive Disease

Treatment Modalities	Nursing Management
Local therapies (e.g., laser cryosurgery, electrocautery, etc.) for preinvasive (SIL, CIN) disease	Explain the disease. Assure patient that SIL (CIN) is not cancer.
	Explain treatment and possible complications of treatment.
	Discuss possibility of treatment failure.
	Instruct in self-care after treatment (no douching, tampons, sexual intercourse for 2–4 weeks).
	Stress importance of follow-up care (next appointment, call physician if fever, bleeding develops).
	Assess concerns related to sexual function (changes in libido, orgasm, coital frequency, fertility).
	Assess for anxiety depression, changes in body or self image.
	Assess for psychological issues associated with sexually transmitted disease (guilt, blame, mistrust).

(continues)

Table 50-5 Treatment Modalities and Nursing Management of the Woman with Cervical Pre-invasive or Invasive Disease (continued)

Treatment Modalities	Nursing Management
Surgery	Instruct patient preoperatively in use of incentive spirometer, importance of turning, coughing, deep breathing, abdominal splinting, early ambulation, and use of antiemboletic stockings. Have patient do return demonstration as indicated.
	Review bowel preparation procedure.
	Review need for IV, urinary catheter, colostomy, ileal conduit as indicated.
	Begin ostomy teaching preoperatively as indicated.
	Stress availability of pain medication.
	Review use of patient-controlled analgesia as indicated.
	Explore nonpharmacologic pain relief measures with patient.
	Provide postoperative wound care.
	Encourage patient to participate in wound care as indicated.
	Assess concerns related to sexual function (changes in libido, orgasm, coital frequency, fertility).
	Assess cultural beliefs as they relate to treatment (blood transfusions, avoidance of drugs, dietary restrictions).
	Assess spiritual needs/concerns.
	Assess vital signs, body systems, lab values postoperatively.
	Assess for deep vein thrombosis.
	Assess nutritional status, lymphedema, skin integrity hazards of immobility, alternation in sleep/rest patterns.
	Assess psychosocial functioning.
Radiotherapy	Review treatment procedure (external beam, intracavitary, etc.).
	Review side effects of therapy (e.g., to skin, effect on blood values, vaginal stenosis as indicated).
	Explain mobility restrictions with intracavity, interstitial radiotherapy as indicated.
	Assess for deep vein thrombosis.
	Encourage diversional activities to relieve boredom.
	Emphasize availability of pain relief measures.
	Explore nonpharmacologic pain relief measures with patient.
	Assess concerns related to sexual function (changes in libido, orgasm, coital frequency, fertility).
	Assess cultural beliefs as they relate to treatment (blood transfusions, avoidance of drugs, dietary restrictions).
	Assess spiritual needs/concerns.
Chemotherapy	Explain treatment (rational for chemotherapy, name of chemotherapy agents, nadir, method of administration, side effects).
	Assess psychological status of patient.
	Assess for anxiety, depression, changes in body, self image.
	Assess effects of treatment on quality of life.
	Assess concerns related to sexual function.
	Assess cultural beliefs as they relate to treatment (blood transfusions, avoidance of drugs, dietary restrictions).
	Assess spiritual needs/concerns.
Clinical trials	Review information related to clinical trials if indicated.

when recurrences appear, expectations for cure may be unrealistic and effective palliation remains to be discovered. Risk factors in the development of preinvasive and invasive disease are well known and it may take many years for invasive disease to develop. Additional research should target improving the percentage of women who receive regular screening in order to diagnose the disease in its earliest stages.

References

1. Symonds RP: Screening for cervical cancer: different problems in the developing and the developed world. *Eur J Cancer Care* 6:275–279, 1997

2. National Institutes of Health Consensus Development Statement [online]. Available at http://text/nlm.nih.gov/nih/upload-v3/CDC. . .ements/Cervical/cervical.html# Conclusions Accessed on July 30, 1998

3. Klemm PR, Guarnieri C: Cervical cancer: a developmental perspective. *J Obstet Gynecol Neonatal Nurs* 25:629–634, 1996

4. Worldwide Cervical Cancer Issues. Available at http://nccc-online.org/worldcancer.htm Accessed on May 23, 1999

5. Alexy BB, Elnitsky C: Rural mobile health unit: outcomes. *Public Health Nurs* 15:3–11, 1998

6. Abrahams N, Wood K, Jewkes R: Barriers to cervical screening: women's and health workers perceptions. *Curationis* 20:50–52, 1998

7. Mashburn J, Scharo-DeHaan M: A clinician's guide to Pap smear interpretation. *Nurse Pract* 22:115–118, 124, 126–127, 1997

8. World Health Organization. Cervical cancer control in developing countries: memorandum from a WHO meeting. *Bull World Health Organ* 74:345–351, 1996

9. American Cancer Society. 1999 Facts and Figures. [online] Available <http://www.cancer.org/statistics/cff99/selectcancers.htm/#cervix> Accessed on January 18, 2000

10. DiSaia PJ, Creasman WT: *Clinical Gynecologic Oncology.* St. Louis, Mosby, 1993

11. Anderson M: The pathology of tumors of the cervix, in Blackledge GRP, Jordan JA, Shingleton HM (eds): *Textbook of Gynecologic Oncology.* Philadelphia, Saunders, 1991, pp 265–283

12. Hatch KD, Fu YS: Cervical and vaginal cancer, in Berek JS, Adashi EY, Hillard P (eds): *Novak's Gynecology* (ed 12). Baltimore, Williams & Wilkins, 1996, pp 1111–1153

13. Martin LM, Parker SL, Wingo PA, et al: Cervical cancer incidence and screening. *Cancer Pract* 4:130–134, 1996

14. Brooks SE: Cervical cancer screening and the older woman. *Cancer Pract,* 4:125–129, 1996

15. Parazzini F, Chatenoud L, La Vecchia C, et al: Determinants of risk of invasive cervical cancer in young women. *Br J Cancer* 77:838–841, 1998

16. Lovejoy NC, Anastasi JK: Squamous cell cervical lesions in women with and without AIDS: biochemical risk factors, prevention, and policy. *Cancer Nurs* 17:294–307, 1994

17. Lovejoy NC: Precancerous and cancerous cervical lesions: the multicultural "male" risk factor. *Oncol Nurs Forum* 21:497–504, 1994

18. Kenny JW: Risk factors associated with genital HPV infection. *Cancer Nurs* 19:353–359, 1996

19. Kenny JW: Ethnic differences in risk factors associated with

20. Sala M, Dosemeci M, Zahm SH: A death certificate-based study of occupation and mortality from reproductive cancers among women in 24 US states. *J Occup Environ Med* 40:632–639, 1998

21. Alterman R, Burnett C, Peipins L, et al: Occupation and cervical cancer: an opportunity for prevention. *J Womens Health* 6:649–657, 1997

22. Daly SF, Doyle M, English J, et al: Can the number of cigarettes smoked predict high-grade cervical intraepithelial neoplasia among women with mildly abnormal cervical smears? *Am J Obstet Gynecol* 179:399–402, 1998

23. Roteli-Martins CM, Panetta K, Alves VA, et al: Cigarette smoking and high-risk HPV DNA as predisposing factors for high-grade cervical intraepithelial neoplasia (CIN) in young Brazilian women. *Acta Obstet Gynecol Scand* 77:678–682, 1998

24. Olsen AO, Dillner J, Skrondal A, et al: Combined effect of smoking and human papillomavirus type 16 infection in cervical carcinogenesis. *Epidemiology* 9:346–349, 1998

25. Stratton P, Ciacco KH: Cervical neoplasia in the patient with HIV infection. *Curr Opin Obstet Gynecol* 6:86–91, 1994

26. Braun L: Role of human immunodeficiency virus infection in the pathogenesis of human papillomavirus-associated cervical neoplasia. *Am J Pathol* 144:209–214, 1994

27. HPV genotyping plus Pap test improves precancerous cervical lesion detection in HIV-positive women. Available at http://www.wcn.org/news/98/Sep/c109228e.asp Accessed on November 24, 1998

28. Suarez ZE, Siefert K: Latinas and sexually transmitted diseases: implications of recent research for prevention. *Soc Work Health Care* 28:1–19, 1998

29. Beral V, Newton R: Overview of the epidemiology of immunodeficiency-associated cancers. *J Natl Cancer Inst Monogr* 23:1–6, 1998

30. Biggar RJ, Rabkin CS: The epidemiology of AIDS-related neoplasms. *Hematol Oncol Clin North Am* 10:997–1010, 1996

31. Six C, Heard I, Bergeron C, et al: Comparative prevalence, incidence and short-term prognosis of cervical squamous intraepithelial lesions amongst HIV-positive and HIV-negative women. *AIDS* 12:1047–1056, 1998

32. Maiman M: Management of cervical neoplasia in human immunodeficiency virus-infected women. *J Natl Cancer Inst Monogr* 23:43–49, 1998

33. Munk C, Kjaer SK, Poll P, et al: Cervical cancer screening: knowledge of own screening status among women aged 20–29 years. *Acta Obstet Gynecol Scand* 77:917–922, 1998

34. Breslow RA, Sorkin JD, Frey CM, et al: Americans' knowledge of cancer risk and survival. *Prev Med* 26:170–177, 1997

35. Daling JR, Madeleine MM, McKnight B, et al: The relationship of human papillomavirus-related cervical tumors to cigarette smoking, oral contraceptive use, and prior herpes simplex virus type 2 infection. *Cancer Epidemiol Biomarkers Prev* 5:541–548, 1996

36. Roye CF: Condom use by Hispanic and African American teens and young adults who use hormonal contraception: implications for HIV prevention. *J Health Educ* 28:61–66, 1997 (suppl)

37. Lamb M, Moore M: Invasive cancer of the cervix, in Moore GJ (ed): *Women and Cancer: A Gynecologic Oncology Perspective.* Sudbury, MA, Jones and Bartlett, 1997, pp 95–127

38. Headly JA, Wardell DW: Neoplasms of the female pelvis, in Swearingen PL, Ross DG (eds). *Manual of Medical-Surgical*

Nursing Care: Nursing Interventions and Collaborative Management. St. Louis, Mosby, 1999, pp 634–645

39. Apgar BS: Human papillomavirus types and cervical cancer. *Hosp Pract* 31:39–40, 46, 1996

40. Lundberg GD: Abnormal Pap smears, ASCUS still Ob/Gyn puzzle. *JAMA* 276:1014–1016, 1996

41. Taking Aim at Cervical Cancer: Evaluating the Abnormal Pap. Available at http://www.med.upenn.edu/health/pf_files/penntoday/v8n1/wh_1.html Accessed on November 24, 1998

42. Kjaer SK, vanden Brule AJ, Bock JE, et al: Human papillomavirus—the most significant risk determinant of cervical intraepithelial neoplasia. *Int J Cancer* 65:601–606, 1996

43. Berumen J, Unger ER, Casas L, et al: Amplification of human papillomavirus types 16 and 18 in invasive cervical cancer. *Hum Pathol* 26:676–681, 1995

44. Crum CP, Newkirk GR: Abnormal Pap smears, cancer risk, and HPV. *Patient Care* 29:35–36, 38–40, 55–57, 61, 1995

45. Bosch FX, Manos MM, Munoz N, et al: Prevalence of human papillomavirus in cervical cancer: a worldwide perspective. International biological study on cervical cancer (IBSCC) study group. *J Natl Cancer Inst* 87:796–802, 1995

46. Eifel PJ, Berek JS, Thigpen JT: Cancer of the cervix, vagina, and vulva, in DeVita VT, Hellman S, Rosenberg SA (eds): *Cancer: Principles and Practice of Oncology* (ed 5). Philadelphia, Lippincott-Raven, 1997, pp 1433–1477

47. Rapp L, Chen LL: The papillomavirus E6 proteins. *Biochem Biophys Acta* 1378:1–19, 1998

48. Ferrera A, Baay MF, Herbrink P, et al: A sero-epidemiological study of the relationship between sexually transmitted agents and cervical cancer in Honduras. *Int J Cancer* 73:781–785, 1997

49. Olsen AO, Orstavik I, Dillner J, et al: Herpes simplex virus and human papillomavirus in a population-based case-control study of cervical intraepithelial neoplasia grade II-III. *APMIS* 106:417–424, 1998

50. DiPaolo JA, Woodworth CD, Coutlee F, et al: Relationship of stable integration of herpes simplex virus-2Bg/II N subfragment Xho2 to malignant transformation of human papillomavirus-immortalized cervical keratinocytes. *Int J Cancer* 76:865–871, 1998

51. Fox P, Arnsberger P, Zhang X: An examination of differential follow-up rates in cervical cancer screening. *J Community Health* 22:199–209, 1997

52. Eddy DM: Screening for cervical cancer. *Ann Intern Med* 113:214–226, 1990

53. Savitz DA, Andrews KW, Brinton LA: Occupation and cervical cancer. *J Occup Environ Med* 37:357–361, 1995

54. Creek KE, Geslani G, Batova A, et al: Progressive loss of sensitivity to growth control by retinoic acid and transforming growth factor-beta at late stages of human papillomavirus type 16-initiated transformation of human keratinocytes. *Adv Exp Med Biol* 375:117–135, 1995

55. Childers JM, Chu J, Voigt LF, et al: Chemoprevention of cervical cancer with folic acid: a phase III Southwest Oncology Group Intergroup study. *Cancer Epidemiol Biomarkers Prev* 4:155–159, 1995

56. Ahn WS, Lee JM, Namkoong SE, et al: Effect of retinoic acid on HPV titration and colposcopic changes in Korean patients with dysplasia of the uterine cervix. *J Cell Biochem Suppl* 28:133–139, 1997

57. Kwasniewska A, Charzewska J, Tukendorf A, et al: Dietary factors in women with dysplasia colli uteri associated with human papillomavirus infection. *Nutr Cancer* 30:39–45, 1998

58. Santin AD, Hermonat PL, Ravaggi A: Effects of retinoic acid combined with irradiation on the expression of major histocompatibility complex molecules and adhesion/co-stimulation molecules ICAM-1 in human cervical cancer. *Gynecol Oncol* 70:195–201, 1998

59. Santin AD, Hermonat PL, Ravaggi A, et al: Effects of retinoic acid on the expression of a tumor rejection antigen (heat shock protein gp96) in human cervical cancer. *Eur J Gynaecol Oncol* 19:229–233, 1998

60. Park TK, Lee JP, Kim SN, et al: Interferon-alpha 2a, 13-cis-retinoic acid and radiotherapy for locally advanced carcinoma of the cervix: a pilot study. *Eur J Gynaecol Oncol* 19:35–38, 1998

61. Savage EW Jr, Chapman G: Cervical dysplasia and cancer, in Hacker NF, Moore JG (eds): *Essentials of Obstetrics and Gynecology* (ed 3). Philadelphia, Saunders, 1998, pp 645–659

62. Shingleton HM, Orr JW: *Cancer of the Cervix.* Philadelphia, Lippincott, 1995

63. Rankow EJ, Tessaro I: Cervical cancer risk and Papanicolaou screening in a sample of lesbian and bisexual women. *J Fam Pract* 47:139–143, 1998

64. Thibodeau, GA: *The Human Body in Health and Disease.* St. Louis, Mosby, 1997

65. Cadman L: Lifelong protection from cervical cancer. *Community Nurse* 3:12–13, 1998

66. Bertelsen B, Hartveit F: Prognostic implications of cervical intraepithelial neoplasia in a single cervical smear: an age-matched case-control study of women with negative smear histories. *Gynecol Obstet Invest* 46:261–265, 1998

67. Henry M: The Bethesda system for cervical-vaginal nomenclature: inception and consequences. *Medical Laboratory Observer* 29:44–50, 1997

68. Koss LG: The New Bethesda System for reporting results of smears of the uterine cervix. *J Natl Cancer Inst* 82:988–991, 1990

69. Shepherd JC, Fried RA: Preventing cervical cancer: the role of the Bethesda system. *Am Fam Physician* 51:434–440, 1995

70. Jones HW: Impact of the Bethesda system. *Cancer* 76:1914–1918, 1995 (suppl)

71. Mahon SM: The Bethesda system for classification of Pap smears: the clinical experience of one cancer screening center. *Cancer Nurs* 18:458–466, 1995

72. Fontaine PL: Pap smears: controversies and challenges in interpreting abnormal results. *Consultant* 36:1976–1978, 1983–1984, 1986, 1989–1990, 1996

73. Robb JA: The "ASCUS" swamp. *Diagn Cytopathol* 11:319–320, 1994

74. Herbst AL: The Bethesda system for cervical/vaginal cytologic diagnoses: a note of caution. *Obstet Gynecol* 76:449–450, 1990 (editorial)

75. Bottles K, Reiter RC, Steiner AL, et al: Problems encountered with the Bethesda system: the University of Iowa experience. *Obstet Gynecol* 78:410–413, 1991

76. Vooijs GP: Does the Bethesda system promote or endanger the quality of cervical cytology? *Acta Cytol* 34:455–456, 1990

77. Cox JT: Epidemiology of cervical intraepithelial neoplasia: the role of human papillomavirus. *Clin Obstet Gynaecol* 9:1–37, 1995

78. Scott PM: Abnormal Pap smears: when is colposcopy needed? *J Am Acad Physician Assist* 9:71–72, 74,76, 1996

79. Shy K: Concepts in the application of cervical cytology, in Greer BE, Berek JS (eds): *Gynecologic Oncology: Treatment Rationale and Techniques.* New York, Elsevier, 1991, pp 13–32

80. Schiffman MH, Kiviat NB, Burk RD, et al: Accuracy and

interlaboratory reliability of human papillomavirus DNS testing by hybrid capture. *J Clin Microbiol* 33:545–550, 1995

81. Shea S, DuMouchel W, Bahamonde L: A meta-analysis of 16 randomized controlled trials to evaluate computer-based clinical reminder system for preventive care in the ambulatory setting. *J Am Med Inform Assoc* 3:399–409, 1996

82. Bartels PH, Bibbo M, Hutchinson ML, et al: Computerized screening devices and performance assessment: development of a policy towards automation. International Academy of Cytology Task Force summary. Diagnostic cytology towards the 21st century: an international expert conference and tutorial. *Acta Cytol* 42:59–68, 1998

83. Grohs DH: Impact of automated technology on the cervical cytologic smear. A comparison of cost. *Acta Cytol* 42:165–170, 1998

84. van Ballegooijen J, Beck S, Boon ME, et al: Rescreen effect in conventional and PAPNET screening. *Acta Cytol* 42:1133–1138, 1998

85. ThinPrep gains momentum as Pap test alternative. *Dis State Management* 4:5–6, 1998

86. Linder J, Zahniser D: ThinPrep Papanicolaou testing to reduce false-negative cervical cytology. *Arch Pathol Lab Med* 122:139–144, 1998

87. Linder J: Recent advances in thin-layer cytology. *Diag Cytopathol* 18:24–32, 1998

88. Bolick DR, Hellman DJ: Laboratory implementation and efficacy assessment of the ThinPrep cervical cancer screening system. *Acta Cytol* 42:209–213, 1998

89. Papillo JL, Zarka MA, St John TL: Evaluation of the Thin-Prep Pap test in clinical practice. A seven-month, 16,314 case experience in northern Vermont. *Acta Cytol* 42:203–208, 1998

90. Schwartz PE, Merino MJ, McCrea Curnen MG: Clinical management of patients with invasive cervical cancer following a negative Pap smear. *Yale J Biol Med* 61:327–338, 1988

91. Ross SH: Cervical cancer prevention. *Nurs Spectrum* 7:12–14, 1998

92. Novak-Smith P, Davidson SA: Gynecologic cancers, in Gates RA, Fink RM (eds): *Oncology Nursing Secrets.* Philadelphia, Hanley & Belfus, 1997, pp 169–179

93. Hatch K, Helm CW: Cancer of the cervix—surgical treatment, in Blackledge GRP, Jordan JA, Shingleton HM (eds): *Textbook of Gynecologic Oncology.* Philadelphia, Saunders, 1991, pp 313–327

94. Penna C, Fallani MG, Maggiorelli M, et al: High-grade cervical intraepithelial neoplasia (CIN) in pregnancy: clinicotherapeutic management. *Tumori* 84:567–570, 1998

95. Mitchell MF, Tortolero-Luna G, Cook E, et al: A randomized clinical trial of cryotherapy, laser vaporization, and loop electrosurgical excision for treatment of squamous intraepithelial lesions of the cervix. *Obstet Gynecol* 92:737–744, 1998

96. Rebane B: What you should know about LEEP. Available at http://oncolink.upenn.edu/specialty/gyn_onc/cervical/leep.html Accessed on July 30, 1998

97. Hulman G, Pickles CJ, Gie CA, et al: Frequency of cervical intraepithelial neoplasia following large loop excision of the transformation zone. *J Clin Pathol* 51:375–377, 1998

98. Darwish A, Gadallah H: One step management of cervical lesions. *Int J Gynaecol Obstet* 61:261–267, 1998

99. Tabbara S, Saleh ADM, Andersen WA, et al: The Bethesda classification for squamous intraepithelial lesions: histologic, cytologic, and viral correlates. *Obstet Gynecol* 79:338–346, 1992

100. Spinell A: Preinvasive diseases of the cervix, vulva, and vagina, in Moore GJ (ed): *Women and Cancer: A Gynecologic Oncology Perspective.* Sudbury, MA, Jones and Bartlett, 1997, pp 58–94

101. Crane LA: Social support and adherence behavior among women with abnormal pap smears. *J Cancer Educ* 11:164–173, 1996

102. Block B, Branham RA: Efforts to improve the follow-up of patients with abnormal Papanicolaou test results. *J Am Board Fam Pract* 11:1–11, 1998

103. Andersen BL: Stress and quality of life following cervical cancer. *J Natl Cancer Inst Monogr* 21:65–70, 1996

104. Flannery M: Nursing care of the client with genital cancer, in Itano JK, Taoka KN (eds): *Core Curriculum for Oncology Nursing* (ed 3). Philadelphia, Saunders, 1998, pp 524–551

105. Yamashita Y, Harada M, Torashima M, et al: Dynamic MR imaging of recurrent postoperative cervical cancer. *J Magn Reson Imaging* 6:167–171, 1996

106. Vives A, Castelo-Branco C, Iglesias X, et al: Is MRI helpful in evaluating the response of cervical cancer to neoadjuvant chemotherapy? *Acta Obstet Gynecol Scand* 74:467–471, 1995

107. Manfredi R, Maresca G, Smaniotto D, et al: Cervical cancer response to neoadjuvant therapy: MR imaging assessment. *Radiology* 209:819–824, 1998

108. Chu KK, Chang SD, Chen FP, et al: Laparoscopic surgical staging in cervical cancer: preliminary experience among Chinese. *Gynecol Oncol* 64:49–53, 1997

109. Borras G, Molina R, Xercavins J, et al: Tumor antigens CA 19-9, CA 125, and CEA in carcinoma of the uterine cervix. *Gynecol Oncol* 57:205–211, 1995

110. Salman T, el Ahmady O, Tony O, et al: Clinical value of squamous cell carcinoma antigen (SCC-A) in Egyptian gynecologic cancer patients. *Anticancer Res* 17:3083–3086, 1997

111. Takeshima N, Hirae Y, Katase K, et al: The value of squamous cell carcinoma antigen as a predictor of modal metastasis in cervical cancer. *Gynecol Oncol* 68:263–266, 1998

112. Gocze PM, Vahrson HW, Freeman DA: Serum levels of squamous cell carcinoma antigen and ovarian carcinoma antigen (CA 125) in patients with benign and malignant diseases of the uterine cervix. *Oncology* 51:430–434, 1994

113. Cecchini L, Iossa A, Bonardi R, et al: Comparing two modalities of management of women with cytologic evidence of squamous or glandular atypia: early repeat cytology or colposcopy. *Tumori* 83:732–734, 1997

114. Stoian M, Repanovici R: Identification of antibodies against human papillomavirus type 16 E4 and E7 proteins in sera of patients with cervical neoplasias. *Rev Roum Virol* 45:185–192, 1994

115. Park JS, Park DC, Kim CJ, et al: HPV-16-related proteins as the serologic markers in cervical neoplasia. *Gynecol Oncol* 69:47–55, 1998

116. Meschede W, Zumbach K, Braspenning J, et al: Antibodies against early proteins of human papillomaviruses as diagnostic markers for invasive cervical cancer. *J Clin Microbiol* 36:475–480, 1998

117. Sotlar K, Selinka HC, Menton M, et al: Detection of human papillomavirus type 16 E6/E7 oncogene transcripts in dysplastic and nondysplastic cervical scrapes by nested RT-PCR. *Gynecol Oncol* 69:114–121, 1998

118. Fowler J, Montz FJ: Malignancies of the uterine cervix, in Cameron RB (ed): *Practical Oncology.* Norwalk, CT, Appleton and Lange, 1994, pp 364–376

119. Lanciano R, Thomas G, Eifel P: Over 20 years of progress in radiation oncology: cervical cancer. *Semin Rad Oncol* 7:121–126, 1997

120. Horng SG, Tseng CJ, Lai CH, et al: Conservative treatment for cervical cancer IAI: four cases report. *Chang Keng I Hsueh* 20:318–322, 1997

121. Orlandi C, Costa S, Terzano P, et al: Presurgical assessment and therapy of microinvasive carcinoma of the cervix. *Gynecol Oncol* 59:255–260, 1995

122. Morris M: Conization for microinvasive carcinoma of the cervix. *Contemp OB/GYN* 40:79–99, 1995

123. Guo WD, Hsing AW, Li JY, et al: Correlation of cervical cancer mortality with reproductive and dietary factors, and serum markers in China. *Int J Epidemiol* 23:1127–1132, 1994

124. Clarke-Pearson DL, Soisson AP, Wall LL: Surgical treatment of early-stage cervical cancer, in Greer BE, Berek JS (eds): *Gynecologic Oncology: Treatment Rationale and Techniques.* New York, Elsevier, 1991, pp 187–206

125. Plante M, Roy M: Operative laparoscopy prior to a pelvic exenteration in patients with recurrent cervical cancer. *Gynecol Oncol* 69:94–99, 1998

126. Berek JS, Hacker NF: *Practical Gynecologic Oncology.* Baltimore, Williams and Wilkins, 1994

127. Eddy GL, Manetta A, Alvarez RD, et al: Neoadjuvant chemotherapy with vincristine and cisplatin followed by radical hysterectomy and pelvic lymphadenectomy for FIGO stage Ib bulky cervical cancer: a Gynecologic Oncology Group pilot study. *Gynecol Oncol* 57:412–416, 1995

128. Nevin J, Bloch B, Van-Wijk L, et al: Primary chemotherapy with bleomycin, ifosfamide and cisplatinum (BIP) followed by radiotherapy in the treatment of advanced cervical cancer. A pilot study. *Eur J Gynaecol Oncol* 16:30–35, 1995

129. Koumantakis E, Haralambakis Z, Koukourakis M, et al: A pilot study on concurrent platinum chemotherapy and intracavitary brachytherapy for locally advanced cancer of the uterine cervix. *Br J Radiol* 71:552–557, 1998

130. Corn BW, Lanciano RM: Combined modality treatment for carcinomas of the uterine cervix and vulva. *Curr Opin Oncol* 6:524–530, 1994

131. Colombo A, Landoni F, Maneo A: Neoadjuvant chemotherapy to radiation and concurrent chemoradiation for locally advanced squamous cell carcinoma of the cervix: a review of the recent literature. *Tumori* 84:229–237, 1998

132. Kumar L, Grover R, Pokharel YH, et al: Neoadjuvant chemotherapy in locally advanced cervical cancer: two randomized studies. *Aust N Z J Med* 28:387–390, 1998

133. Benedetti-Panici P, Greggi S, Scambia G, et al: Long-term survival following neoadjuvant chemotherapy and radical surgery in locally advanced cervical cancer. *Eur J Cancer* 34:341–346, 1998

134. Shueng PW, Hsu WL, Jen YM, et al: Neoadjuvant chemotherapy followed by radiotherapy should not be a standard approach for locally advanced cervical cancer. *Int J Radiat Oncol Biol Phys* 40:889–896, 1998

135. Corn BW, Micaily B, Dunton CJ, et al: Concomitant irradiation and dose-escalating carboplatin for locally advanced carcinoma of the uterine cervix: an updated report. *Am J Clin Oncol* 21:31–35, 1998

136. Sugiyama T, Nishida T, Hasuo Y, et al: Neoadjuvant intra-arterial chemotherapy followed by radical hysterectomy and/or radiotherapy for locally advanced cervical cancer. *Gynecol Oncol* 69:130–136, 1998

137. Giardina G, Richiardi G, Danese S, et al: Weekly cisplatin as neoadjuvant chemotherapy in locally advanced cervical cancer: a well-tolerated alternative. *Eur J Gynaecol Oncol* 18: 173–176, 1997

138. Lacava JA, Leone BA, Machiavelli M, et al: Vinorelbine as neoadjuvant chemotherapy in advanced cervical carcinoma. *J Clin Oncol* 15:604–609, 1997

139. Tewari K, Cappuccini F, Gambino A, et al: Neoadjuvant chemotherapy in the treatment of locally advanced cervical carcinoma in pregnancy: a report of two cases and review of issues specific to the management of cervical carcinoma in pregnancy including planned delay of treatment. *Cancer* 82:1529–1534, 1998

140. Osborne RJ, Murphy KJ, DePetrillo AD: Pelvic exenteration, in Greer BE, Berek JS (eds): *Gynecologic Oncology: Treatment Rationale and Techniques.* New York, Elsevier, 1991, pp 207–226

141. Schulmeister L: Nutrition, in Otto SE (ed): *Oncology Nursing.* Baltimore, Mosby, 1994, pp 641–657

142. Hardin TC, Page CP: Nutritional care, in Weiss GR (ed): *Clinical Oncology.* Norwalk, CT, Appleton and Lange, 1993, pp 50–58

143. Rivadeneira DE, Evoy D, Fahey TJ, et al: Nutritional support of the cancer patient. *CA Cancer J Clin* 48:69–80, 1998

144. Torres-Lobaton A, Bastida-Blanco A, Marquez-Acosta G, et al: Pelvic exenteration for cancer of the uterine cervix (prognostic factors). *Gynecol Obstet Mex* 62:189–193, 1994

145. Hatch KD, Shingleton HM, Potter ME, et al: Low rectal resection and anastomosis at the time of pelvic exenteration. *Gynecol Oncol* 31:262–267, 1988

146. Shell JA: Impact of cancer of sexuality, in Otto SE (ed): *Oncology Nursing.* Baltimore, Mosby, 1994, pp 737–760

147. Andersen BL, Lamb MA: Sexuality and cancer, in Murphy GP, Lawrence W, Lenhard RE (eds): *American Cancer Society Textbook of Clinical Oncology.* Atlanta, American Cancer Society, 1995, pp 699–713

148. Coleman RL, Miller DS: Topotecan in the treatment of gynecologic cancer. *Semin Oncol* 24 S20–55, 1997 (suppl)

149. Ito H, Shigematsu N, Kawada T, et al: Radiotherapy for centrally recurrent cervical cancer of the vaginal stump following hysterectomy. *Gynecol Oncol* 67:154–161, 1997

150. Hempling RE, Eltabbakh GH, Piver MS, et al: The addition of bleomycin and dose-escalated ifosfamide to the combination of cisplatin plus ifosfamide does not improve survival in advanced or recurrent cervical cancer. *Am J Clin Oncol* 20:315–318, 1997

151. Carmichael J: The role of gemcitabine in the treatment of other tumors. *Br J Cancer* 78:21–25, 1998 (suppl 3)

152. Coleman RL, Miller DS: Topotecan in the treatment of gynecologic cancer. *Semin Oncol* 24:S20–55, 1997

153. Chen MD, Paley PJ, Potish RA, et al: Phase I trial of taxol as a radiation sensitizer with cisplatin in advanced cervical cancer. *Gynecol Oncol* 67:131–136, 1997

154. Aghahanian C, Brown C, O'Flaherty C, et al: Phase I study of tirapazamine and cisplatin in patients with recurrent cervical cancer. *Gynecol Oncol* 67:127–130, 1997

155. Keys H, Gibbons SK: Optimal management of locally advance cervical carcinoma. *J Natl Cancer Inst Monogr* 1996: 89–92, 1996

156. Romisch M, Meier W, Kimmig R, et al: 13-cis-retinoic acid and interferon-alfa-2a as palliative therapy in pretreated, recurrent squamous epithelial carcinoma of the cervix uteri and vulva. *Geburtshilfe Frauenheilkd* 56:520–524, 1996

157. Cervellino JC, Araugo CE, Sanchez O, et al: Cisplatin and ifosfamide in patients with advanced squamous cell carcinoma of the uterine cervix. A phase II trial. *Acta Oncol* 34: 257–259, 1995

158. Fanning J, Ladd C, Hilgers RD: Cisplatin, 5-fluorouracil, and ifosfamide in the treatment of recurrent or advanced cervical cancer. *Gynecol Oncol* 56:235–238, 1995

159. Curtin JP, Hoskins WJ, Venkatraman ES, et al: Adjuvant chemotherapy versus chemotherapy plus pelvic irradiation

for high-risk cervical cancer patients after radical hysterectomy and pelvic lymphadenectomy. *Gynecol Oncol* 61:3–10, 1996

160. Toita T, Sakumoto K, Higashi M, et al: Therapeutic value of neoadjuvant intra-arterial chemotherapy (cisplatin) and irradiation for locally advance uterine cervical cancer. *Gynecol Oncol* 65:421–424, 1997

161. Noguchi M, Murata R, Sagoh T, et al: Intraarterial chemotherapy combined with radiation therapy for advanced cancer of the uterine cervix. *Gan To Kagaku Ryoho* 25:1314–1317, 1998

162. Sugiyamy T, Nishida T, Hasuo Y, et al: Neoadjuvant intra-arterial chemotherapy followed by radical hysterectomy and/or radiotherapy for locally advanced cervical cancer. *Gynecol Oncol* 69:130–136, 1998

163. Kokubo M, Tsutsui K, Nagata Y, et al: Radiotherapy combined with transcatheter arterial infusion chemotherapy for locally advanced cervical cancer. *Acta Oncol* 37:143–149, 1998

164. Kasai S, Nagasawa H, Kuwasaka H, et al: TX-1877: design, synthesis, and biological activities as a BRM-functional hypoxic cell radiosensitizer. *Int J Radiat Oncol Biol Phys* 42:799–802, 1998

165. Stehman FB, Bundy BN, Thomas G, et al: Hydroxyurea versus misoidazole with radiation in cervical carcinoma: long term follow-up of a gynecologic oncology group trial. *J Clin Oncol* 11:1523–1526, 1993

166. Rodriguez M, Sevin BU, Perras J, et al: Paclitaxel: a radiation sensitizer of human cervical cancer cells. *Gynecol Oncol* 57:165–169, 1995

167. Kobayashi H, Kodaira T, Yamada T, et al: 18 years of conformation radiotherapy at Nagoya University Hospital. *Nagoya J Med Sci* 59:17–24, 1996

168. Thomas G, Dembo A, Ackerman I, et al: A randomized trial of standard versus partially hyperfractionated radiation with or without concurrent 5-fluorouracil in locally advanced cervical cancer. *Gynecol Oncol* 69:137–145, 1998

169. Colombo A, Landoni F, Cormio G, et al: Concurrent carboplatin/5FU and radiotherapy compared to radiotherapy alone in locally advanced cervical carcinoma: a case-control study. *Tumori* 83:895–899, 1997

170. Thomas G, Dembo A, Ackerman I, et al: A randomized trial of standard versus partially hyperfractionated radiation with or without concurrent 5-fluorouracil in locally advanced cervical cancer. *Gynecol Oncol* 69:137–145, 1998

171. Russell AH, Shingleton HM, Jones WB, et al: Trends in the use of radiation and chemotherapy in the initial management of patients with carcinoma of the uterine cervix. *Int J Radiat Oncol Biol Phys* 40:605–613, 1998

172. Zanetta G, Lissoni A, Pellegrino A: Neoadjuvant chemotherapy with cisplatin, ifosfamide and paclitaxel for locally advanced squamous-cell cervical cancer. *Ann Oncol* 9:977–80, 1998

173. Li YX, Weber-Johnson K, Sun LQ, et al: Effect of pentoxifylline on radiation-induces G2–phase delay and radiosensitivity of human colon and cervical cancer cells. *Radiat Res* 149:338–342, 1998

174. Minagawa Y, Kigawa J, Irie T, et al: Radial surgery following neoadjuvant chemotherapy for patients with state IIIB cervical cancer. *Ann Surg Oncol* 5:539–543, 1998

175. Ijaz T, Iefel PJ, Burke T, et al: Radiation therapy of pelvic recurrence after radical hysterectomy for cervical carcinoma. *Gynecol Oncol* 70:241–246, 1998

176. Look KY, Blessing JA, Gallup DG, et al: A phase II trial of 5-fluorouracil and high-dose leucovorin in patients with recurrent squamous cell carcinoma of the cervix: a Gynecologic Oncology Group Study. *Am J Clin Oncol* 19:439–441, 1996

177. Edelmann DZ, Anteby SO: Neoadjuvant chemotherapy for locally advanced cervical cancer—where does it stand? A review. *Obstet Gynecol Surv* 51:305–313, 1996

178. Adjuvant Chemo/Radiation Treatment of Cervical Cancer Improves Survival. Available at http://www.ama-assn.org/special/womh/newsline/reuters/03235365.htm Accessed on April 1, 1999

179. Chatani M, Nose T, Masaki N, et al: Adjuvant radiotherapy after radical hysterectomy of the cervical cancer. Prognostic factors and complications. *Strahlenther Oncol* 174:504–509, 1998

180. Estape RE, Angioli R, Madrigal M, et al: Close vaginal margins as a prognostic factor after radical hysterectomy. *Gynecol Oncol* 68:229–232, 1998

181. Virostek LJ, Kim RY, Spencer SA, et al: Postsurgical recurrent carcinoma of the cervix: reassessment and results of radiation therapy options. *Radiology* 201:559–563, 1996

182. Esassolak M, Yalman D, Ozsaran Z, et al: Postoperative adjuvant radiotherapy in stage IB carcinomas of the uterine cervix. *Radiography* 4:41–47, 1998

183. Tattersall MH, Lorvidhaya V, Vootiprux V, et al: Randomized trial of epirubicin and cisplatin chemotherapy followed by pelvic radiation in locally advanced cervical cancer. *J Clin Oncol* 13:444–451, 1995

184. Park TK: Adjuvant therapy in cervical cancer patients with high risk factors. *Yonsei Med J* 38:255–260, 1997

185. Treatment options for cervical cancer. Available at http://oncolink.upenn.edu/upcc/clin_trials/fall94/RUBIN.html Accessed on November 24, 1998

186. Cervical cancer clinical trials. Available at http://cancernet.nci.nih.gov/cgi_bin/cancerform Accessed on April 1, 1999

187. Massad LS, Turyk ME, Bitterman P, et al: Interferon-alpha and all-trans-retinoic acid reversibly inhibit the in vitro proliferation of cell lines derived from cervical cancers. *Gynecol Oncol* 60:428–434, 1996

188. Street D, Kaufmann AM, Vaughan A, et al: Interferon-gamma enhances susceptibility of cervical cancer cells to lysis by tumor-specific cytotoxic T cells. *Gynecol Oncol* 65:265–272, 1997

189. Tomoda K, Ohishi N, Kikkawa F, et al: Cationic multilamellar liposome-mediated human interferon-beta gene transfer into cervical cancer call. *Anticancer Res,* 18:1367–1371, 1998

190. Fleming GF, O'Brien SM, Hoffman PC, et al: Phase I study of treatment with oral 13-cis-retinoic acid, subcutaneous interferon alfa-2a, cisplatin and 24 hour infusion 5-fluorouracil/leucovorin. *Cancer Chemother Pharmacol* 39:227–232, 1997

191. Veerasarn V, Sritongchai C, Tepmongkol P, et al: Randomized trial radiotherapy with and without concomitant 13-cis-retinoic acid plus interferon-alpha for locally advanced cervical cancer: a preliminary report. *J Med Assoc Thai* 79:439–447, 1996

192. Phase II trial of IFN-A/13-CRA in patients with recurrent squamous cell carcinomas including those of the cervix, skin, head and neck, esophagus, lung, and penis. Available at http://cancernet.nci.nib.gov/cgi-bin/cancerphy_show?file=pro09410.html Accessed on April 1, 1999

193. Phase II study of IFN-A/13-CRA for recurrent and/or metastatic squamous cell carcinoma of the cervix. Available at http://cancernet.nci.nih.gov/prot/menu/dx00103.html Accessed on April 1, 1999

194. Kato M, Shinohara H, Goto S, et al: Clinical experience of EET therapy for 75 advanced cancer patients. *Anticancer Res* 18:3941, 1998

195. Karius D, Marriott MA: Immunologic advances in monoclonal antibody therapy: implications for oncology nursing. *Oncol Nurs Forum* 24:483–496, 1997

196. Phase II study of interleukin-12 (IL-12) in patients with advanced, recurrent, or inoperable carcinoma of the cervix. Available at http://cancernet.nci.nih.gov/prot/menu/dx00103.html Accessed on April 1, 1999

197. Eifel PJ, Levenback C, Wharton JT, et al: Time course and incidence of late complications in patients treated with radiation therapy for FIGO stage IB carcinoma of the uterine cervix. *Int J Radiat Oncol Biol Phys* 32:1289–1300, 1995

198. Burke LM: Clinical sexual dysfunction following radiotherapy for cervical cancer. *Br J Nurs* 5:239–244, 1996

199. Lovejoy NC: Multinational approaches to cervical cancer screening: a review. *Cancer Nurs* 19:126–134, 1996

200. Lovejoy NC, Roche N, McLean D: Life stress and risk of precancerous cervical lesions: a pretest directed by the Life Stress Model. *Oncol Nurs Forum* 24:63–70, 1997

201. Peragallo NP, Alba ML, Tow B: Cervical cancer screening practices among Latino women in Chicago. *Public Health Nurs* 14:251–255, 1997

202. Dignan M, Sharp P, Blinson K, et al: Development of a cervical cancer education program for Native American women in North Carolina. *J Cancer Educ* 9:235–242, 1994

203. Harmon MP, Castro FG, Coe K: Acculturation and cervical cancer: knowledge, beliefs, and behaviors of Hispanic women. *Women Health* 24:37–57, 1996

204. Jennings KM: Getting a Pap smear: focus group responses of African American and Latina women. *Oncol Nurs Forum* 24:827–835, 1997

205. Jubelirer SJ, Blanton MF, Blanton PD, et al: Assessment of knowledge, attitudes, and behaviors relative to cervical cancer and the Pap smear among adolescent girls in West Virginia. *J Cancer Educ* 11:230–237, 1996

206. Carpenter V, Colwell B: Cancer knowledge, self-efficacy, and cancer screening behaviors among Mexican-American women. *J Cancer Educ* 10:217–222, 1995

207. Price JH, Easton AN, Telljohann SK, et al: Perceptions of cervical cancer and Pap smear screening behavior by women's sexual orientation. *J Community Health* 21:89–105, 1996

208. Brooks SE: Cervical screening and the older woman. *Cancer Pract* 4:125–129, 1996

209. Mandelblatt J, Freeman H, Winczewski D, et al: The costs and effects of cervical and breast cancer screening in a public hospital emergency room. *Am J Public Health,* 87:1182–1189, 1997

210. Ruge A, Lee C, Brown WJ: Inpatient cervical screening: a survey of patient acceptability. *Aust J Public Health,* 19:96–97, 1995

211. Morris DL, McLean CH, Bishop SL, et al: A comparison of the evaluation and treatment of cervical dysplasia by gynecologists and nurse practitioners. *Nurse Pract* 23:101–102, 108–110, 113, 1998

212. Baldwin D, Johnson P, Cotanch P, et al: An Afrocentric approach to breast and cervical cancer early detection and screening. Washington, DC, American Nurses Association, 1996

213. Kagawa-Singer M: Addressing issues for early detection and screening in ethnic populations. *Oncol Nurs Forum* 24:1705–1711, 1997

214. Strickland CJ, Chrisman NJ, Yallup M, et al: Walking the journey of womanhood: Yakama Indian women and Papanicolaou (Pap) test screening. *Public Health Nurs* 13:141–150, 1996

215. Marcus AC, Crane LA, Kaplan CP, et al: Improving adherence to screening follow-up among women with abnormal Pap smear knowledge, attitudes and behavior. *Behav Res Cancer* 7:143–150, 1990

CHAPTER 51

Colorectal Cancer

Coni Ellis, MS, RN-CS, C, OCN®, CWOCN
Delores Ann Hubbard Saddler, RN, MSN, CGRN

Introduction

More than 131,000 new cases of colorectal cancer are diagnosed each year. More than 55,000 deaths occur annually as a result of this disease.[1] Colorectal cancer is the second leading cause of cancer death in men and women. It is the third most common malignancy in both men and women, surpassing lung and breast cancer in women and lung and prostate cancer in men.[3] Colon cancer is 2.5 times more common than rectal cancer.[2] Anal cancers account for fewer than 4% of all lower gastrointestinal (GI) cancers.[2] Colon, rectal, and anal cancers are each diagnosed and treated differently.

Colorectal cancer is the most extensively studied of the GI malignancies, particularly from the perspective of genetics, molecular, biological, environmental, and dietary aspects. Because colorectal cancer is silent until the advanced stage, screening and early detection have become the primary methods for reducing morbidity and mortality. Advances in endoscopy, interventional radiology, and surgical resection for primary as well as metastatic disease, and improvements in chemotherapy and radiation therapy regimens over the last ten years show increasing promise in helping control the mortality and morbidity of colorectal and anal cancers. Nurses, physicians in primary care, and members of the health care team can help increase awareness that screening is available and that prevention methods are effective and valuable. Over 30,000 lives could be saved each year if the general public, primary care physicians, and managed care companies were more aware of and promoted methods of early detection and treatment.[1,4] State-of-the-art treatment and care can be provided by health care professionals as genetic mapping, clinical trials, advancements in the management of side effects, and alternative methods of treatment and support are developed.

Epidemiology

Colorectal cancer accounts for approximately two-thirds of all cancers arising in the GI tract. The peak incidence is in the sixth and seventh decades. Approximately 7% of colorectal cancer occurs in persons less than age 40.[5] There is no difference in the overall incidence of colorectal cancer between men and women. Rectal and anal cancer is seen more frequently in men than in women.[2] Some differences in incidence and mortality rates among racial and ethnic groups may be the result of differences in socioeconomic status.[3] Among Blacks, the incidence of colon cancer has increased by 30% since 1973 and is now higher than in Whites.[2]

Colorectal cancer is one of the leading causes of cancer-related deaths in the Western world. About 70% of individuals who have colorectal cancer present with apparently localized disease while the remaining 30%

have advanced disease at diagnosis.[2] Twenty-five percent of these have distant metastatic disease and 5% locally advanced disease. Metastasis to adjacent organs or lymph nodes reduces the survival rate to approximately 67%.[2] If the cancer has spread to distant sites, survival becomes much less.[2] The Digestive Health Initiative, a national study published in 1997, estimated the five-year survival rate from colorectal cancer to be 52%–55%. The Digestive Health Foundation was established through the cooperative effort of the American Gastroenterological Association, the American Society for Gastrointestinal Endoscopy, and the American Association for the Study of Liver Disease to promote digestive health for all Americans by supporting educational initiatives and research into the causes, prevention, diagnosis, treatment, and cure of digestive and liver diseases.[1] Cancer statistics revealed that mortality rates decreased by about 1.9% per year for men and 1.5% for women between 1990 and 1994.[3] In 1999, the five-year survival rate for colorectal cancer increased to greater than 90% in the early localized stage, and to greater than 60% after spread to adjacent organs or nodes.[2] These facts indicate that despite the high incidence of colorectal cancer, there has been a slow but progressive decline in the mortality rate with over half of patients now achieving five-year disease-free status.

One-fourth of the colorectal cancer cases are found in the rectum while the remainder are located in some other part of the colon.[5] Seventy percent of all cancers in the large bowel occur in the right side of the proximal colon.[6] Pathological staging is still presently the most important determinant of prognosis.[7]

The incidence of colorectal cancer is high in industrialized regions like North America, northwestern Europe, and Australia. Incidence is low in less-developed regions such as Asia, Africa, and South America. High-risk countries all consume diets that are high in total fat, animal fat, and protein, and that are relatively low in fruit, vegetables, and fiber. Individuals moving from a low-risk country to a high-risk one assume the higher risk of their new country. In addition to diet, many lifestyle habits are related to a higher risk of colorectal cancer.[1] Approximately 6% of the American population will at some point develop colorectal cancer.[6]

Etiology

The incidence of colon cancer increases with age, generally occurring in the sixth or seventh decade of life. While age is a major factor in the incidence of colorectal cancer, lifestyle, diet, alcohol intake, inflammatory bowel conditions, radiation exposure, and related medical conditions are associated with an increased risk. A decrease in physical activity leads to a decrease in intestinal tract transit time and allows potential carcinogens to have longer contact with gut mucosa. There is a noted association between obesity, or increased caloric intake in excess of energy expenditure, and an increased risk for colon cancer.[2] Diets high in fat increase the production of and change the composition of bile salts. These altered salts are converted into potential carcinogens by intestinal flora. While the exact mechanism by which bile salts act as a promoter for colorectal cancer is unknown, researchers suggest that the process is mediated by diacylglycerol.[8] Phospholipids are converted to diacylglycerol by intestinal bacteria. Diacylglycerol then enters the epithelial cell of the colon and activates protein kinase C, which has a role in cell growth and tumor promotion. On the other hand, increased intake of dietary fiber plays a major role in decreasing the risk for colon cancer. The protective mechanism of dietary fiber is exerted in a number of ways. One such way is by increasing fecal bulk, which changes the bacterial composition of the feces and accelerates the transit time in the intestinal tract. Not all dietary fiber is beneficial. Wheat bran and cellulose are the most protective while oat and corn bran seem to have little protective capabilities.[8]

Heavy alcohol consumption has been considered to be a factor in the development of colorectal cancer.[9,10] Alcohol is thought to stimulate gastrointestinal cell proliferation and promote carcinogenesis secondary to an excess of unabsorbed carcinogens such as nitrosamines found in beer and whiskey.[11] Radiation therapy to the pelvis for treatment of other primary malignancies correlates with an increased risk for developing carcinoma of the colon and rectum.[12] Uterosigmoidostomy is performed for a number of malignant conditions. Reports in the literature show a 5%–10% increased incidence of colon carcinoma occurring 15 years after the initial surgery.[12] In these cases, the most common site of the colon cancer is distal to the surgical site where there has been chronic exposure of the intestinal mucosa to both urine and feces. Persons with a history of colorectal carcinoma are at increased risk of developing a second primary colon cancer. Women with a history of endometrial, ovarian, or breast cancer have an increased chance of developing colorectal cancer.[2] Patients who have had a cholecystectomy have also been noted to have a higher incidence of colon cancers.[2]

Other risk factors for colorectal cancer can be broadly classified as environmental and genetic. Environmental factors include occupational exposure to asbestos, acrylonitrile, ethyl acrylate, synthetic fibers, halogens, printing materials, and fuel oils.

Several genetic polyposis syndromes are associated with a high risk of colorectal cancer. Familial adenomatous polyposis (FAP) coli is an inherited autosomal dominant trait that results in the development of polyps throughout the colon and rectum. This process generally starts in late adolescence. Persons with this syndrome have a 100% risk of developing colorectal cancer.[13] Hereditary nonpolyposis colorectal cancer (HNPCC) is an inherited autosomal dominant condition characterized by the occurrence of colorectal cancer at an average age of 45 years.[14] Affected persons have one or few adenomatous polyps, but no polyposis. Hereditary nonpolyposis colon

cancer occurs as type A (Lynch type I) and type B (Lynch type II). Type A is familial, site specific, nonpolyposis colon cancer. Type B is also nonpolyposis colon cancer but is found in association with other forms of cancer such as breast, endometrial, gastric, and ovarian. Once an individual at risk for HNPCC develops cancer, a subtotal colectomy should be performed. Prophylactic hysterectomy and/or bilateral salpingo-oophorectomy should be considered for women with HNPCC diagnosed with cancer or who are genetic carriers.

A variant of FAP consists of multiple, flat adenomas that have an increased risk of becoming cancerous.[15,16] Other genetic premalignant polyposis syndromes associated with a high risk of colorectal cancer include hamartomatous polyposis syndromes [Peutz-Jeghers, juvenile polyposis, Cowden's disease (multiple hamartoma syndrome), and neurofibromatosis] and types of adenomatous polyposis (Gardener's syndrome and Turcot's syndrome).[2]

Hereditary nonpolyposis colorectal cancer arises from mutations in one of the four genes that participate in mismatch repair, the repair of defective DNA strands. When mismatch repair does not function, mutations occur in one or more of the genes that are important to the control of cell growth.[17] The mutated genes in cancer syndromes have been identified and reproduced and are now available for testing in humans. Unfortunately, the genes involved in common familial risk have not been identified. Colon cancer is known to be developed as the result of an accumulation of genetic mutations; for example, initially an epithelial cell of the colon acquires the characteristics of an adenoma that eventually acquires the characteristics of invasive cancer. With or without familial risk, colon cancers seem to develop from a similar set of genes and a similar progression of accumulated mutations.[17] The most commonly mutated genes in colon cancer are the adenomatous polyposis coli genes (responsible for FAP, the K-*ras* oncogene, the *p53* gene, the deleted in colon cancer gene, and the DNA mismatched pair genes [HNPCC]).

Adenomatous polyps identified as villous and tubovillous adenomas are more likely to undergo malignancy transformation than are tubular adenomas. The probability that cancer will be present in an adenoma is approximately 5%. An adenomatus polyp smaller than 1 cm can convert to an invasive cancer over a ten-year period.[1,4] Patients with a history of colorectal cancer are at increased risk of developing a second primary colon cancer or other malignancy, especially at the site where an anastomotic connection was made by the previous surgery. Patients with ulcerative colitis are also at an increased risk of developing colorectal cancer, depending on the extent of colitis, the development of mucosal dysplasia, and the duration of symptoms. Colorectal cancer risk is also higher than normal in patients with Crohn's disease, which is an inflammatory disease usually involving all layers of the intestinal mucosa. Although the risk is less, persons with Crohn's disease can develop adenocarcinoma at a younger age.

Some 95% or more of colon cancers develop outside of the above-described syndromes and are referred to as *sporadic* or *common* cancers. About 10% of adults in Western countries have a first-degree relative affected with colonic cancer. These persons have a two- to threefold increased risk of acquiring the disease. Multiple relatives with colon cancer or relatives with a diagnosis at a younger age further increase the risk.[18] Colon cancers are generally known to evolve through a multistep process involving a benign adenomatous polyp that eventually becomes cancerous. This entire process can take anywhere from 5 to 15 years. Early colorectal carcinomas confined to the mucosa or submucosa usually produce a polypoid mass. Cancers less than 1.5 cm have a noticeable absence of lymph node metastasis.[5] There is generally no risk of invasive malignancy in polyps less than 5 mm. There is a 1% risk in polyps 5–19 mm, a 10% risk in polyps 1–2 mm, and a 30%–50% risk in polyps over 2 mm.[5]

The incidence of anal cancer for single men is said to be six times higher than that for married men.[2] Specific to anal cancer, a history of genital warts has been observed, suggesting that papillomavirus may be a causative factor. Recent epidemiologic studies suggest that receptive anal intercourse is strongly associated with anal cancer.[2]

Prevention, Screening, and Detection

Two types of prevention are recognized for colorectal cancer: primary and secondary. Primary prevention involves decreasing fat intake and increasing the amounts of fruits and vegetables in the diet. In addition, total fiber intake should be between 20–30 grams a day. It is suggested that wheat bran is protective.[1] Because increased caloric intake is considered to be a risk factor, total caloric intake should not exceed energy requirements; i.e., it is important to maintain normal body weight.

As part of secondary prevention, the use of antioxidants—betacarotene, vitamin C, vitamin E, calcium, and nonsteroidal anti-inflammatory drugs (NSAIDs)—are called *chemopreventive measures.* Controlled studies have shown a reduction in the incidence of colorectal cancer with regular, long-term use of aspirin which promotes a change in polyp formation and alters mucosal proliferation.[2] The mechanism of chemopreventive actions for NSAIDs is related to a reduction in endogenous prostaglandin. Sulindac has induced regression of large bowel polyps in patients with FAP and calcium taken orally has been shown to decrease the risk of developing colon cancer.[2]

The early detection of colorectal cancer improves survival. Based on reports by the Congressional Office of Technology Assessment and the National Cancer Institute, the cost per year of lives saved by colorectal cancer screening renders the screening cost-effective and could save up to 30,000 lives per year.[1] The fecal occult blood test and periodic flexible sigmoidoscopy are two easy methods of screening. The American Cancer Society has recently modified its recommendation regarding screening for average- and increased-risk individuals[19] (see Table 51-1). At age 40, all individuals should have a digital rectal examination. For those whose risk is low and average, annual examinations, fecal occult blood testing, and flexible sigmoidoscopy every three to five years is recommended beginning at age 50. Guaiac-based fecal occult blood tests have been associated with many false-positive and false-negative results. Newer fecal occult blood tests, including a guaiac-based product called Hemoccult SENSA and immunochemical tests for hemoglobin (HemeSelect), seem to have a better sensitivity than the older tests.[2]

Digital rectal examinations are simple and can detect tumors up to 7 cm from the anal verge. Sigmoidoscopy is easy to perform, requires no sedation, and detects up to 50% of colorectal tumors within 60 cm from the anal verge. A colonoscopy is a more sensitive tool for detecting tumors throughout the entire colon. Biopsy specimens can be obtained and polyps removed during the actual procedure. The accuracy of the colonoscopy examination depends on the ability of the endoscopist to reach the cecum and to negotiate blind corners and mucosal folds. To achieve a satisfactory examination, patient teaching for preparation and support during the procedure itself are crucial.

Persons at high risk for colon cancer should have first-degree family members screened by annual flexible sigmoidoscopy between the ages of 10 and 12.[2] Individuals with one or more first-degree relatives with colon cancer before the age of 55 should have an annual fecal occult blood test and a colonoscopy or double-contrast barium enema every five years staring at age 35–40.[1] Persons with lower levels of risk (one relative with colorectal cancer diagnosed at an advanced age) should have standard screening with fecal occult blood tests and flexible sigmoidoscopy starting at age 40.[1,2] The Society of Gastroenterology Nurses and Associates supports routine screening by flexible sigmoidoscopy by trained nurses as a way to increase access to screening as a means of early detection. A positive Hemoccult blood test is an indication for a colonoscopy. If the subsequent colonoscopy finding is negative, no further colonoscopy exam is needed for another ten years.[4]

Over the last two decades, mortality rates for colorectal cancer in many developed countries have declined in women but not in men. A possible explanation for the decrease in women is the use of oral contraceptives and hormone replacement therapy. A 20%–40% risk reduction is reported among users of hormone replacement therapy. The apparent protection tended to be stronger among recent users.[20]

Laboratory tests for gene mutations are now available, thus making it possible to screen individuals at increased risk for developing colorectal cancer. Genetic analysis for populations at risk could result in measures to reduce risk

Table 51-1   American Cancer Society Guidelines for Screening and Surveillance for Early Detection of Colorectal Polyps and Cancer

Risk Category	Recommendation[†]	Age to Begin	Interval
AVERAGE RISK			
All people 50 years or older who are not in the categories below	One of the following: FOBT plus flexible sigmoidoscopy[‡] or TCE[¶]	Age 50	FOBT every year and flexible sigmoidoscopy every 5 y Colonoscopy every 10 y or DCBE every 5–10 y
MODERATE RISK			
People with single, small (<1 cm) adenomatous polyps	Colonoscopy	At time of initial polyp diagnosis	TCE within 3 y after initial polyp removal; if normal, as per average risk recommendations (above)
People with large (≥1 cm) or multiple adenomatous polyps of any size	Colonoscopy	At time of initial polyp diagnosis	TCE within 3 y after initial polyp removal; if normal, TCE every 5 y
Personal history of curative-intent resection of colorectal cancer	TCE§	Within 1 y after resection	If normal, TCE in 3 y; if still normal, TCE every 5 y
Colorectal cancer or adenomatous polyps in first-degree relative younger than 60 y or in two or more first-degree relatives of any ages	TCE	Age 40 or 10 y before the youngest case in the family, whichever is earlier	Every 5 y
Colorectal cancer in other relatives (not included above)	As per average risk recommendations (above); may consider beginning screening before age 50		
HIGH RISK			
Family history of familial adenomatous polyposis	Early surveillance with endoscopy, counseling to consider genetic testing, and referral to a specialty center	Puberty	If genetic test positive or polyposis confirmed, consider colectomy; otherwise, endoscopy every 1–2 y
Family history of hereditary non-polyposis colon cancer	Colonoscopy and counseling to consider genetic testing	Age 21	If genetic test positive or if patient has not had genetic testing, colonoscopy every 2 y until age 40 y, then every year
Inflammatory bowel disease	Colonoscopies with biopsies for dysplasia	8 y after the start of pancolitis; 12–15 y after the start of left-sided colitis	Every 1–2 y

*Approximately 70%–80% of cases are from average-risk individuals, approximately 15%–20% are from moderate-risk individuals, and 5%–10% are from high-risk individuals.

†Digital rectal examination should be done at the time of each sigmoidoscopy, colonoscopy, or DCBE.

‡Annual FOBT has been shown to reduce mortality from colorectal cancer, so it is preferable to no screening, however, the ACS recommends that annual FOBT be accompanied by flexible sigmoidoscopy to further reduce the risk of colorectal cancer mortality.

§This assumes that a perioperative TCE was done.

¶TCE includes either colonoscopy or DCBE. The choice of procedure should depend on the medical status of the patient and the relative quality of the medical examinations available in a specific community. Flexible sigmoidoscopy should be performed in those instances in which the rectosigmoid colon is not well visualized by DCBE. DCBE would be performed when the entire colon has not been adequately evaluated by colonoscopy.

DCBE = double-contrast barium enema; FOBT = fecal occult blood testing; TCE = total colon examination; y = years.

Reprinted with permission from Byers I, Levin B, Rothenberger D, et al: ACS Guidelines for Screening and Surveillance for Early Detection of Colorectal Polyps and Cancer. *CA Cancer J Clin* 47:154–160, 1997.[19]

and earlier identification of the colorectal malignancy. Unfortunately, persons at high risk who should be genetically tested are potentially more likely to lose insurance benefits. The role of the nurse and/or the genetic counselor in this situation is to provide the necessary information needed for the patient to be able to make an informed decision. Many patients pay out of pocket for genetic testing in order to avoid insurance cancellation or loss of employment. Genetic testing and clinical screening usually should not be undertaken until 10–12 years of age.[1]

Pathophysiology

The colon is made up of four layers: the mucosa, the submucosa, the muscularis, and the serosa. The mucosa and submucosa are divided by the muscularis. Reproduction of cells in the colon takes place in the crypts of Lieberkuhn located in the mucosal layer. As new cells are produced, old cells mature, migrate out of the crypt, and shed. Damage to the crypts will affect reproducing cells and the crypts become prone to errors and to the formation of early adenomas.[21]

The large intestine consists of the cecum, ascending colon, transverse colon, descending colon, sigmoid colon, and rectum. The ascending colon, descending colon, and rectum are considered extraperitoneal organs because the ascending and descending colon lie in the anterior pararenal space and are covered by a single layer of the posterior peritoneum. The rectum is surrounded by extraperitoneal perirectal fat in the pelvis. The transverse and sigmoid colon are suspended in the peritoneal cavity by the mesocolon that is formed by two layers of peritoneal linings. The cecum is attached to the ileocolic mesentery in the right iliac fossa. The arterial supply to the cecum, ascending colon, and transverse colon derives from the superior mesenteric artery, whereas the blood supply to the sigmoid colon, descending colon, and upper rectum is from the inferior mesenteric artery. The lower rectum is supplied by the internal iliac arteries. The superior mesenteric vein drains the cecum, ascending colon, and transverse colon. The artery and vein supplying and draining each segment of the colon accompany each other in the mesocolon. The venous system of the colon and upper rectum drains into the portal circulation.[21] The distal 5–7 cm of the rectum has a dual drainage.

Nodal spread from each segment of the colon follows the blood vessels in the mesocolon.[22] Invasion of the venous system yields a poor prognosis. Once tumor cells invade the vascular system, widespread dissemination of the disease follows; it is not amenable to surgical resection and the effect of chemotherapy and radiation therapy is limited. Local invasion into the neighboring structures is more common in the cecum and rectosigmoid areas. The liver is the most frequent site of metastatic involvement. Solitary pulmonary metastasis is rare. Other areas

of metastasis include the brain (cerebellum), bones, kidneys, and adrenals.[21] By the time of the diagnosis, approximately 25% of the colon cancers will have extended through the bowel wall; whereas cancers of the rectum will have spread through the wall in 50%–77% of patients and will have metastasized to lymph nodes in 50%–60% of cases.[2] Distal rectal cancers are likely to produce isolated pulmonary metastasis.[1] Implantation of tumor cells at other sites can occur as a result of surgical manipulation of the tumor, intraluminal spread, or the shedding of tumor cells into the peritoneum. Intraperitoneal seeding and carcinomatosis may occur even without lymphatic or visceral spread.

The most common histological type of colorectal cancer is adenocarcinoma. Others, which are rare, include lymphoma, sarcoma, melanoma, and carcinoid. Adenocarcinoma accounts for over 90% of all large bowel cancers. Mucin adenocarcinoma is a variant characterized by increased amounts of extracellular mucus in the tumor. Signet ring cell carcinoma is characterized by large amounts of intracellular mucin material that cause the cytoplasm to displace the nucleus.[2] Squamous cell carcinomas, carcinoid tumors, and adenosquamous and undifferentiated carcinomas have been found in the colon and rectum as well.[2] Whereas previously the most common sites of colon cancers were the sigmoid and descending colon, now the proximal colon is the site of highest incidence.

The anus is the terminal 4–6 cm of the gastrointestinal tract. It is responsible for maintaining continence. The anal canal is that region extending from the anal verge to the junction between squamous and columnar epithelium. Another way of describing this area is the area between the anal verge and the anorectal ring. The anorectal ring is easily palpable and corresponds to the junction of a portion of the levator muscle with the external anal sphincter. The spread of anal and perianal cancers can be predicted based on the anatomy since the tumor usually spreads by direct extension, through the lymphatic system, and via the bloodstream. Tumors may spread upward for 5–6 cm before ulcerating into the rectum.[21] Most anal cancers are squamous cell carcinomas. Other less-common cell types are cloacogenic, basaloid, transitional, and mucoepidermoid carcinomas.[2] Unusual tumors arising in the anal canal include small-cell carcinomas, melanomas, and lymphomas. Small-cell carcinomas of the anal canal are aggressive and signal early distant metastases.[3]

Adenocarcinomas of the colon and rectum develop initially in the mucosa. The tumor then locally invades into the lumen of the bowel wall. When it has traversed the muscularis mucosa and infiltrated the submucosa, it is termed *invasive*. Further infiltration by way of the lymph and vascular system occurs next and direct extension may occur into the peritoneal surfaces as well.

Depending on their location in the bowel, colorectal lesions may exhibit different characteristics. Tumors in the ascending colon present as cauliflower-like fungating masses that progress to become ulcerative and necrotic.

These are usually well differentiated and have a better prognosis. Tumors in the descending and sigmoid colon present as ulcerative tumors that tend to infiltrate the bowel wall and have a poorer prognosis than those in the ascending colon. Rectosigmoid tumors present as villous, frond-like lesions.

Clinical Manifestations

Clinical manifestations of tumors in the colorectum vary depending on location. Tumors in the ascending colon are usually large and bulky. Symptoms generally include anemia, a palpable mass in the right lower quadrant, and a vague, dull pain. Cancer of the transverse colon is generally noted by a change in bowel habits and blood in the stool. Symptoms of cancer of the descending and sigmoid colon again depend on the type of growth typical of this area. Cancer of the rectum is usually manifested as bright-red bleeding, symptoms of incomplete evacuation, and tenesmus. The sensation of a mass in the rectum is often mistakingly attributed to hemorrhoids or anal fissures and may require a rectal examination and biopsy for accurate diagnosis. A proctosigmoidoscopy will provide an adequate examination to secure biopsy and provide a baseline for surgical assessment. Instructing the patient, assisting with the examination, and providing support and privacy for the patient during the procedure are crucial to a successful examination.

Clinical signs and symptoms that may be present in patients with colorectal cancer include the following[2,23,24]

- Early cancer: Asymptomatic; vague abdominal pain and flatulence, minor changes in bowel movements with or without rectal bleeding

- Late cancer: Severe pain, anorexia and weight loss, sacral or sciatic pain, jaundice, pruritus, ascites, hepatomegaly, renal impairment

- Descending/sigmoid: Constipation alternating with diarrhea, abdominal pain, obstructive symptoms (nausea/vomiting), melena, perforation

- Ascending: Vague abdominal aching, discomfort, anemia, weakness, weight loss, right-sided abdominal mass, fatigue, palpitations, change in stool

- Rectal: Changes in bowel movement, rectal fullness, urgency, bleeding, tenesmus, jaundice, malaise, occult blood, pelvic pain

- Anal: Bleeding, discharge, rectal mass, tenderness on palpation, pain on defecation

- Transverse: Constipation alternating with diarrhea, bowel obstruction, melena

Carcinoma of the colon-rectum during pregnancy is rare, but has been noted. Prognosis is poor since diagnosis is generally made at an advanced stage of the cancer. Early diagnosis is difficult because symptoms of colorectal cancer (vomiting, constipation, anemia, rectal bleeding, abdominal pain and distention) can be related to pregnancy. Occasionally, diagnosis is not made until a cesarean delivery is done.[25]

Assessment

The nurse should obtain a complete history and, in coordination with the multidisciplinary team, a thorough physical examination. This assessment includes individual and family risk factors that could contribute to colorectal cancer such as the presence of inflammatory bowel disease, familial polyposis syndromes, familial nonpolyposis syndromes, familial adenocarcinomas, occupational history, dietary history, exposure to radiation therapy, and any surgical history. In addition, an evaluation of symptoms includes recent weight loss or gain, changes in appetite, changes in the size, shape, or caliber of stools, presence of nausea and/or vomiting, blood in the stools, abdominal pain, bloating, fatigue, palpitations, skin color changes, and unusual itching.

Initial tests include a baseline carcinoembryonic antigen (CEA) level, chest x-ray, computerized tomography scans (CT), colonoscopy, and air contrast barium enema. Other tests include chemical survey including liver and renal function tests, a complete blood count with platelet count, urinalysis, and biopsy of any detected tumors. The use of endoscopic ultrasound (EUS) to stage tumors of the rectum has been a necessary part of the initial workup for rectal cancers; it clarifies surgical options and contributes to choosing a sphincter-saving procedure. While it is superior to CT scan in evaluating the depth of wall invasion and the involvement of adjacent soft tissues, a major disadvantage of EUS is that microinvasion of the submucosa may not be noted.

An endoscopic biopsy of colorectal tissue can be obtained and the chromosomal patterns and division phases of the cells evaluated by flow cytometry. Flow cytometry measures DNA ploidy and growth rate of cells in the S-phase and chromosomal patterns based upon diploidy (the normal number of chromosomes) and aneuploidy (an abnormal number of chromosomes). A recent study demonstrated that detection of micrometastases by reverse transcriptase polymerase chain reaction (RT-PCR) amplification of CEA and messenger RNA (mRNA) in lymph nodes from patients with stage II colorectal cancer was now possible.[26] Thymidylate synthase, the target enzyme for fluorodeoxyuridine monophosphate, may be another predictor of prognosis for colorectal cancer.[27]

Use of biomarkers such as CEA and a CA19-9 is still debatable and should be correlated with clinical presentation. Recent research demonstrated that the observation of specific human leukocyte antigen associated with particular subsets of colorectal cancer strongly suggests that genetic susceptibility for the development of colorectal cancer does exist. Although this was a small study, the identification of antigens DQ5 and A1 may have useful predictive and diagnostic value.[28] In another study done in Japan, researchers concluded that preoperative elevation of the marker CD44v6 in the serum could possibly be a prognostic indicator for patients with colorectal cancer.[29]

Advances in diagnostic radiology have contributed to innovations in diagnosing colorectal cancer and related metastases. Spiral CT scans allow identification of all layers of the circumference and assist in the prognosis, surgical management, and adjuvant therapy.[6] Virtual colonoscopy is a new technology that allows a noninvasive diagnosis through the use of spiral CT volume imaging with virtual-reality computer technology. Colography is a new technique to process and display two-dimensional spiral CT images at cross sections and orthogonal angles to the center of the colon, potentially providing quicker and more accurate detection of polyps, even those less than 1 cm. Potential limitations of colography include the possibility of a false-positive diagnosis secondary to residual stool.[6] CT portography enables clinicians to see small tumors than cannot be appreciated on a conventional CT scan with contrast. Preoperatively, CT portography is used to detect small focal hepatic metastasis 1–2 cm in diameter. It works on the principle that hepatic metastases derive their blood supply from the hepatic artery while normal hepatocytes are supplied predominantly by the portal circulation.[30] During CT portography, contrast medium is infused through an angiography catheter that has been introduced into the superior mesenteric or splenic artery. Seconds after injection of the contrast, dynamic sequence CT scanning of the liver begins. As the dye passes into the portal vein, the normal hepatic parenchyma infused by the portal blood circulation is enhanced with contrast, while the hepatic metastases, which receive no blood via the portal route, are visualized as dark spots that indicate solid lesions.[30]

In addition to the above diagnostic tests, patients with recurrent or metastatic disease may have other tests to evaluate the extent of disease. Immunoscintigraphy has been shown to exhibit a high positivity rate in cases of local recurrence and can detect metastases simultaneously at multiple sites. Two types of immunoscintigraphy are available: satumomab pendetide and the CEA scan. The former is used to determine the extent of extrahepatic malignant disease and to detect pelvic tumors as well as extrahepatic abdominal metastasis. In patients with occult cancer, combining the CEA scan with conventional imaging techniques significantly increases diagnostic accuracy.[2] Another test commonly used to diagnose advanced disease is magnetic resonance imaging (MRI), which is generally used to detect recurrent rectal cancer or tumors too small to be evaluated on CT scan. The MRI may also be done for patients who are unable to tolerate the CT scanner or who are allergic to the contrast material. Fine-needle aspiration, with or without the above diagnostic tests, is generally indicated to confirm the recurrence of disease.

Classification and Staging

The prognosis for persons with colorectal cancer is directly related to the stage of the disease at the time of diagnosis. This is determined by the depth of penetration of tumor invasion into and through the intestinal wall, the number of regional lymph nodes involved, and the presence or absence of distant metastases. The size of the primary tumor is the most important clinical predictor of survival for patients with anal carcinoma.[2] The Dukes classification, which dates to 1930, is still used by some clinicians in staging colorectal cancer because of its ease and simplicity of use. The TNM classification system has been modified to correlate with the Dukes system. The modified Astler-Coller Dukes system is now the most widely used clinical and pathologic staging system for colorectal tumors. It is based on the depth of tumor invasion into and through the intestinal wall, the number of regional lymph nodes involved, and the presence or absence of distant metastasis.

Following surgical resection of colorectal tumors, pathologic stage is the single most important prognostic factor. The prognosis for early stages I and II disease is more favorable, whereas stages III and IV disease have a poorer prognosis.[21] In the TNM classification, each of the three subsets of tumor, nodal, and metastatic involvement does not make any assumptions about the status in another part of the system. The classification of colorectal cancer has been revised to have a more precise definition of the tumor and nodal involvement.[6] See Table 51-2.[2]

Table 51-2   TNM Staging of Colorectal Cancer

TNM Stage	Primary Tumor*	Lymph Node Metastasis**	Distant Metastasis†	Modified Astler-Coller
Stage 0	Tis	N0	M0	
Stage I	T1	N0	M0	A
	T2	N0	M0	B1
Stage II	T3	N0	M0	B2
	T4	N0	M0	B3
Stage IIIA	Any T	N1	M0	C‡
Stage IIIB	Any T	N2, N3	M0	
Stage IV	Any T	Any N	M1	D

*Tis = carcinoma in situ; T1 = tumor invades submucosa; T2 tumor invades muscularis propria; T3 tumor invades through the muscularis propria into the subserosa or into nonperitoneal pericolic or perirectal tissues; T4 = tumor perforates the visceral peritoneum or directly invades other organs or structures.

**N0 = no regional lymph node metastasis; N1 = metastases in one to three pericolic or perirectal lymph nodes; N2 = metastases in four or more pericolic or perirectal lymph nodes; N3 = metastases in any lymph node along the course of a named vascular trunk.

†M0 = no distant metastasis; M1 = distant metastasis.

‡C1 = T2 N1, T2 N2, T2 N3; C2 = T3 N1, T3 N2, T3 N3; C3 = T4 N1, T4 N2, T4 N3.

Reprinted with permission of PRR, Inc. Melville, NY.[2]

Therapeutic Approaches and Nursing Care

Surgical Options for Colon Cancer

Surgery is the primary treatment for colon cancer. The goal of surgery is to eliminate the disease in the colon, nodal basins, and contiguous organs. The tumor location, blood supply, and lymph node pattern in the involved region will define the extent of surgical resection. The various surgical options as well as their indications and major morbidities are briefly discussed below and illustrated in Figure 51-1.[31]

Right hemicolectomy involves removal of the distal 5–8 cm of the ileum, right ascending colon, hepatic flexure, and transverse colon proximal to the middle colic artery. This procedure is indicated for cecal, ascending colon, and hepatic flexure lesions. Major morbidities include ureteral injury, duodenal injury, and bile acid deficiency. Bile acid deficiency is rarely seen and only with extensive resection of the terminal ileum.

Right radical hemicolectomy involves the removal of the transverse colon (including resection of the middle colic artery at its origin) in addition to structures removed in the right hemicolectomy. Indications for this procedure are lesions of the hepatic flexure or transverse colon. In addition to the complications associated with right hemicolectomy, morbidities include anastomotic dehiscence and diarrhea.

Transverse colectomy is the segmental resection of the transverse colon. This procedure is indicated for mid transverse colon lesions. The major morbidity is anastomotic dehiscence. This procedure is rarely performed because of the difficulty of achieving a tension-free anastomosis with adequate blood supply as the marginal artery of Drummond is sacrificed. Surgeons prefer to perform an extended right radical hemicolectomy with an ileosigmoid anastomosis.

Left hemicolectomy includes the removal of the transverse colon distal to the right branch of the middle colic artery and the descending colon up to but not including the rectum, plus division and ligation of the inferior mesenteric artery (IMA). Indications for this procedure are left colon lesions. Anastomotic dehiscence is the major morbidity.

Low anterior resection involves the removal of the descending colon distal to the splenic flexure, sigmoid colon, upper two-thirds of the rectum, and ligation of IMA and inferior mesenteric vein either at the origin or just distal to the origin of the left colic artery. This procedure is indicated for lesions of the sigmoid colon and proximal rectum. Morbidities include anastomotic dehiscence and bowel ischemia secondary to inadequate flow through the marginal artery of Drummond.

Subtotal colectomy is the removal of the right, transverse, descending, and sigmoid colon with ileorectal anastomosis. This procedure is indicated for multiple synchronous colon tumors and distal transverse colon

lesions particularly in a patient with a clotted IMA. Morbidities include diarrhea, perineal excoriation, and anastomotic dehiscence.[32]

Surgical Options for Rectal Cancer

The successful management of rectal cancer has five goals: cure, local control, restoration of intestinal continuity, preservation of anorectal sphincter function, and preservation of the patient's sexual and urinary function. Because of the anatomic constraints of the bony pelvis, it may be difficult in some cases to achieve adequate sphincter, sexual, and urinary function without compromising cure and local control.[33]

Local control is an extremely important aspect of treatment. Up to 25% of the patients who die of rectal cancer will have local recurrence only, while another 50% will have local recurrence in addition to distant disease.[32] Patients with local recurrence after initial treatment for rectal cancer are rarely advantaged by additional surgery. Many of these patients with advanced disease experience significant problems with bone and nerve pain, hemorrhage, pelvic sepsis, and bowel and urinary obstruction.[32,33]

The radical surgical approach and standard treatment of patients with rectal cancer has been abdominoperineal resection (APR), which involves transabdominal resection of the rectum and mesorectum from the level of the inferior mesenteric vessels to the levator muscles, in combination with transperineal excision of the anus and distal rectum.[32] APR is currently indicated for tumors of the distal third of the rectum within 3 cm of the anal verge, tumors involving the anal-sphincter musculature, tumors of the rectovaginal septum, patients with poor continence preoperatively, and patients with diarrheal disorders.[32]

In recent years the use of adjuvant therapy, the introduction of circular stapling devices, and the demonstrated adequacy of 2-cm distal margins have allowed safe use of sphincter-preserving surgery for resection of midrectal and some distal rectal cancers.[32] Low anterior resection (LAR), as described earlier, is an operation in which the dissection and anastomosis are performed below the peritoneal reflection.

A coloanal anastomosis preserves the sphincter mechanism in patients with low-lying rectal tumors whose negative distal margin of resection is up to but does not include the anal-sphincter musculature. The operative dissection is similar to that of LAR and APR, with transection of the distal margin at the level of the levator ani muscles within the abdomen. Through a perineal approach, the remaining anal mucosa is stripped and an anastomosis is made between the colon and the anus to restore intestinal continuity.[32,34] Some surgeons will hand suture the anastomosis at this level rather than using a stapling device. To provide adequate bowel length and a tension-free anastomosis, the splenic flexure of the colon is completely mobilized. The vascular supply of the left colon is then

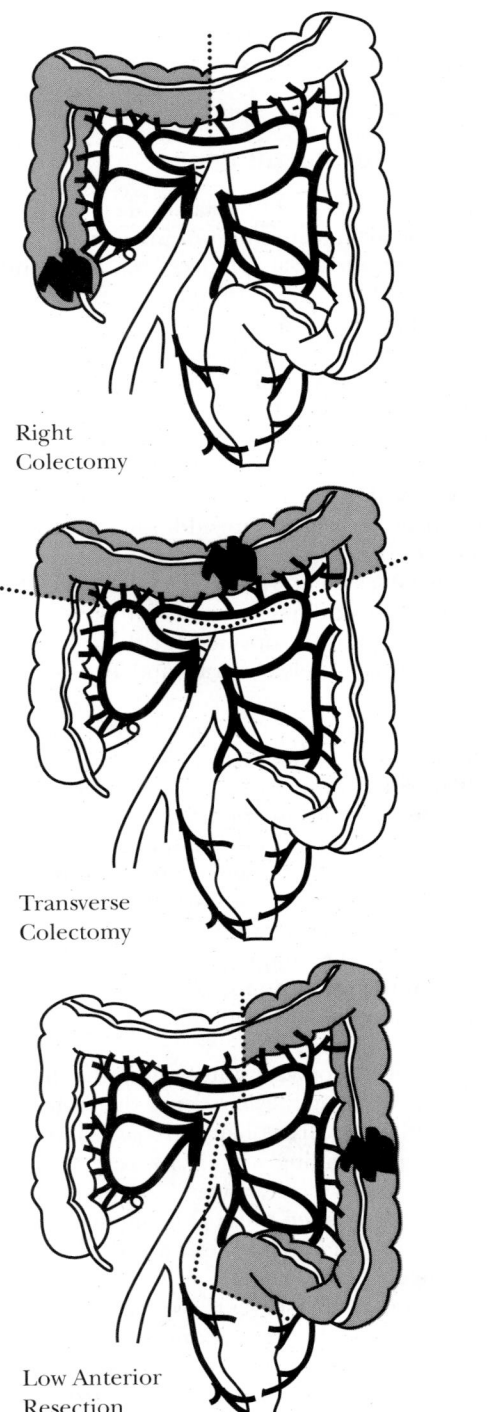

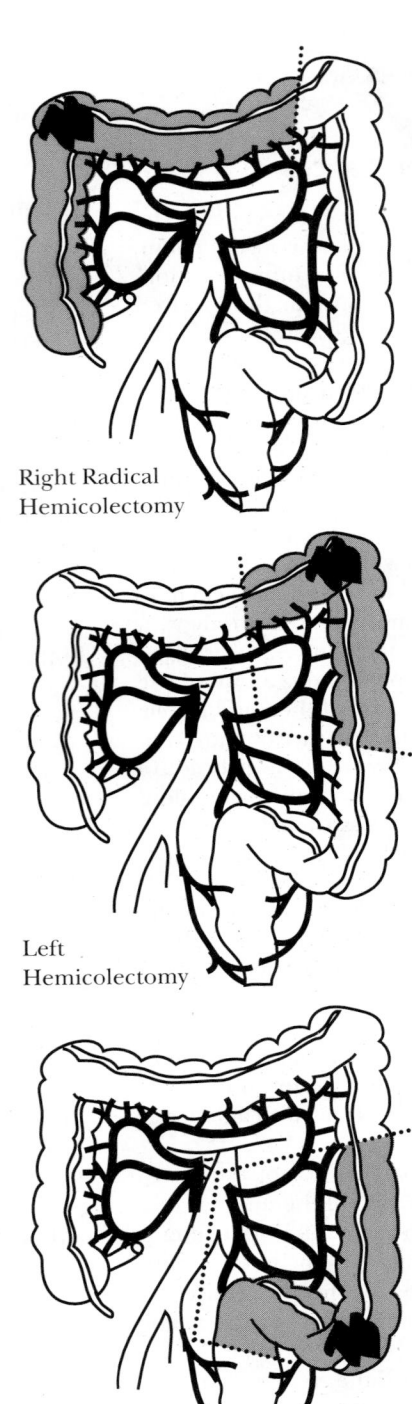

Figure 51-1 The procedure selected relates to the location and extent of the tumor.

Right Colectomy

Right Radical Hemicolectomy

Transverse Colectomy

Left Hemicolectomy

Low Anterior Resection

Subtotal Colectomy

based on the middle colic artery. The surgeon will then perform a protective diverting ileostomy in all patients who have coloanal anastomosis. Contraindications for an LAR or coloanal anastomosis include tumors involving the anal-sphincter musculature, tumors involving the rectovaginal septum, patients with poor continence preoperatively, patients with diarrhea disorders, and unfavorable anatomic constraints (e.g., obesity, narrow pelvis).

Complications of Colorectal Surgery

Table 51-3 identifies some of the complications of colorectal surgery.[35] The surgical procedures above may produce many different anatomic and functional alterations. Patients who have an APR will have a permanent sigmoid or descending colostomy, whereas, with a LAR or subtotal colectomy, the patient may have a temporary ileostomy.

Table 51-3   Complications of Colorectal Surgery

Complications	Signs and Symptoms
Anastomotic leak	Intraabdominal pain, pelvic abscess, peritonitis
Intraabdominal abscess	Recurring or persistent fever postoperatively, leukocytosis, no abdominal pain
Staphylococcal enteritis	Diarrhea, prostration, sepsis
Large-bowel obstruction	Constipation, abdominal pain, nausea/vomiting, abdominal distention
Injury to the genitourinary tract	Leakage of urine through the incision, oliguria, anuria
Sexual dysfunction	Impotence
Ostomy complications	Peristomal skin and stoma

Adapted with permission from Hoebler L, Irwinn MM: Gastrointestinal tract cancer: current knowledge, medical treatment, and nursing management. *Oncol Nurs Forum* 19:1403–1415, 1992.[35]

All of these patients will benefit from consultation with a Certified Wound, Ostomy, Continence Nurse (CWOCN, also known as an enterostomal therapist or ET nurse) from the first visit when they are told the diagnosis through the preoperative and postoperative phases. Nursing management is focused on early recognition of potential problems.

Radiation Therapy for Colorectal Cancer

When treated preoperatively by radiation, tumor cells are often well oxygenated because the blood supply to the tumor has not been surgically manipulated. Well-oxygenated cells are believed to have increased radiosensitivity, thus tumor cell killing by radiotherapy may be increased.[36] Despite these radiobiologic advantages, preoperative radiation has not affected overall rates of survival, distant recurrence, or cure rates.[37,38] However, locoregional tumor control rates have improved with preoperative radiation. Randomized studies have shown a significant decrease in local recurrence rates when preoperative doses of radiotherapy were higher than 34.5 Gy.[37–39] Additionally, one study reported a 91% sphincter preservation rate for patients with T3 and T4 lesions treated with 45 Gy of preoperative radiotherapy.[37] Local control and overall survival have been at acceptable levels with this approach, and 10% of patients in this series achieved a complete pathological response.[36]

The most common use of radiotherapy is following surgical resection. The advantages for the use of postoperative radiotherapy are that (1) adequate pathology data are available to evaluate the extent of disease, (2) patients who will not benefit from therapy are not treated, and (3) surgical treatment is not delayed. Despite the multiple research approaches, the rates of survival, local pelvic control, and extrapelvic recurrence have not been im-

proved consistently by postoperative radiation of 45–50 Gy.[37–39] In a large cohort study comparing preoperative to postoperative radiotherapy, a significant decrease in local recurrence was found in the group that received preoperative therapy compared to the postoperative group.[40] Table 51-4 describes the uses of radiation therapy for patients with colorectal cancer.[41]

Intraoperative radiation therapy (IORT) and stereotactic radiation therapy are innovative approaches to the treatment of colorectal cancer. IORT provides high-dose radiation therapy during an operative procedure directly to a localized area, such as an inoperable colorectal tumor, locally recurrent colorectal cancer, and residual disease after resection. High-energy radiation can be delivered while significantly reducing radiation exposure to adjacent tissues. To provide IORT, the facility must have a designated operating room or radiation suite, radiation equipment that is able to deliver electron or orthovoltage beams, computer planning equipment, and extensive coordination by the multidisciplinary health care team.

Patient selection for IORT is usually based upon the following criteria:

1. Surgery alone will not achieve local control.
2. External beam radiation therapy (EBRT) dose of 60–70 Gy or greater is needed for curative attempt.
3. IORT will be performed at the same time of a planned operative procedure.
4. IORT plus EBRT technique would theoretically result in a more suitable therapeutic ratio between cure and complications.

Table 51-4   Radiation Therapy for Colorectal Cancer

Preoperatively

- To reduce tumor size and increase potential for sphincter preservation
- To decrease risk of local failure and distant metastasis from cells shed at operation
- To decrease risk of late radiation enteritis since small bowel can be excluded from radiation field

Postoperatively

- For patients considered at high-risk of local recurrence
- When distant metastases are still a potential problem

Combined preoperative and postoperative radiation ("sandwich technique")

- To decrease potential of tumor dissemination
- To decrease potential of complications resulting from repopulation by residual cells if postoperative therapy is delayed by slow wound healing

Palliative radiation

- To treat symptoms of advanced cancer
- To control pain and bleeding

Reprinted with permission from Saddler D, Ellis C: Colorectal cancer *Semin Oncol Nurs* 15:63, 1999.[41]

5. There is no evidence of distant metastases or peritoneal seeding.[42]

As mentioned, IORT requires extensive preoperative planning and intraoperative collaboration between the radiation oncologist and surgeon. The procedure starts with the surgical exposure of the tumor. IORT may be delivered prior to excision of the tumor or after the mass is removed. Specialized electron cones are placed within the surgical cavity where a 15–20 Gy dose of radiation will be delivered. Potential complications and nursing implications will be reviewed in a later section of this chapter.

Stereotactic radiation (SRT) is a precise method for the delivery of focused radiation beams for small, well-defined lesions. It enables the radiation oncologist to treat a limited area within an organ and minimizes or prevents the radiation dose being delivered to adjacent normal tissue. Although SRT was initially developed to treat arteriovenous malformations and intracranial lesions, other applications are being studied.[43]

There are three primary treatment delivery methods for SRT:

1. Gamma knife: Cobalt 60 gamma radiation
2. Linear accelerator: high-energy photon
3. Heavy charged particle beams (e.g., proton, helium, neon)[44]

Investigational radiation therapy techniques

There are a number of other novel investigational approaches to treat GI cancers and enhance treatment results. These include the following:

1. *Altered fractionation schemes:* Hyperfractionation, increased number of fractions with smaller dose per fraction within the same overall time, and accelerated treatment in a shorter overall treatment time aim to improve the therapeutic ratio. This hyperfractionation approach has been studied with results less equivalent to conventional radiotherapy techniques in rectal cancers.[45] Recent data suggests that twice-daily radiation is better tolerated when delivered preoperatively rather than postoperatively.[46]

2. *Particle (neutron/proton) beam therapy:* Theoretical advantages with particle beam therapy include increased effect on hypoxic tumor cells and beneficial radiation repair and sensitivity profile of normal tissues. In small studies in highly specialized programs, however, these advantages have not been borne out and the use of particle beam therapy has even appeared detrimental.[47,48]

3. *Hyperthermia:* The benefits of the synergistic and additive interaction between heat (hyperthermia) and radiotherapy is being studied for treating colorectal cancers. Hyperthermia for colorectal cancer is still considered investigational.[49–51]

4. *Perioperative tumor bed brachytherapy with a mesh template:* This treatment involves the patient's wearing evenly spaced catheters placed into a mesh template in order to conform to the radiation target as defined by the surgeon. This approach reduces anesthesia time compared to conventional brachytherapy procedures because the brachytherapy catheters do not have to be individually secured with suture material.[52]

For rectal tumors, the rate of locoregional recurrence has been reduced by the use of radiation therapy. Preoperative radiation therapy has demonstrated a reduction in local tumor recurrence, but has not affected overall survival for patients with stage II or III rectal cancers. A combination of fluorouracil (5-FU) based chemotherapy and radiation given postoperatively is the most effective adjuvant therapy for patients with stage II or III rectal cancer. Radiation doses of 45–55 Gy are recommended in combination with 5-FU–based chemotherapy. Preoperative chemoradiation may be more effective than postoperative adjuvant treatment, especially in patients with T3 or T4 lesions. Such treatment may improve resectability and may have a lower frequency of complications compared to the postoperative treatment.[2] IORT can be used to treat advanced, recurrent, or inoperable rectal cancer. Unresectable rectal tumors may be treated with palliative radiation.

Injury to the bowel may occur as a result of radiation therapy. Some side effects of radiation may require surgical intervention (see Table 51-5), but most of the side effects generally subside when radiation therapy is stopped. Chronic radiation enteritis can lead to bowel mucosal thinning and inflammation, eventually resulting in ulceration. Radiation therapy is used as palliation for advanced rectal cancer symptoms. The pain from the local recurrence of rectal cancer is very difficult to control.

Advanced colorectal cancer is treated with 5-FU either by bolus injection or by continuous infusion. High doses of chemotherapy via implantable pumps as well as intrahepatic infusions are being studied.[2] 5-FU in combination with mitomycin and semustine have yielded response rates of only 25% and unfortunately have added side effects. The dose-limiting toxicities of continuous 5-FU infusion are mucositis and diarrhea. Palmar-plantar erythrodysesthesia (hand-foot syndrome) has also been noted with protracted infusions of 5-FU.[2]

Table 51-5 Side Effects of Colorectal Radiation Therapy

Side Effects	Signs and Symptoms
Proctosigmoiditis	Bleeding, tenesmus, and pain
Increased bowel motility	Cramping, loose watery stools
Chronic radiation enteritis	Ulcerations
Colon fibrosis and stricture	Large bowel obstruction
Nausea and vomiting	

Reprinted with permission from Saddler D, Ellis C: Colorectal cancer. *Semin Oncol Nurs* 15:63, 1999.[41]

Chemotherapy

Residual occult tumor cells can lead to treatment failure with surgery alone. These residual tumors are too small to detect with current diagnostic methods. Occult cells can be in the circulating system of the blood or lymph or may be present as microscopic cells at either local or distant sites.[7] Because of possible occult disease left after surgery, adjuvant therapy is delivered with the intent to target these microscopic, rapidly cycling foci of cancer cells and eradicate them before they become established. It is important to consider the risk-benefit ratio of adjuvant therapy and attempt to maintain a balance between maximum chance of cure/prolonged survival and tolerance of side effects.[7] It is more difficult for surgeons to obtain wide margins with resections of rectal cancer, which are associated with a higher incidence of regional recurrence. Thus, adjuvant therapy for patients with stages I and II rectal cancer must include an aggressive local approach to reduce the risk of local failure and increase overall survival. Patients with stage I colon cancer treated with surgery alone are not given adjuvant therapy because it is not necessary to increase survival. It is clear that patients with stage III disease colon cancer need adjuvant treatment. Adjuvant therapy for stage II colon cancer is still debatable.

For years, the standard adjuvant therapy for stage III colon cancer was 5-FU plus levamisole. In 1998, studies that added leucovorin to 5-FU demonstrated stabilization of the 5-FU-thymidylate-synthase complex, thereby increasing the period of tumor inhibition. While overall survival was not increased with leucovorin and 5-FU therapy, the response rate was increased significantly. The period of therapy with leucovorin and 5-FU was extended 6–12 months once results were noted to reduce the recurrence rate and improve survival. Studies to compare 5-FU and levamisole and the combination of 5-FU, leucovorin, and levamisole demonstrated that 12 months of adjuvant therapy had no significant improvement over six months, and that six months of triple drug therapy produced a significantly superior survival rate than 5-FU plus levamisole for the same time period. Thus, the current recommendation is that every patient with stage III colon cancer should be considered for adjuvant chemotherapy. This therapy should consist of one year of 5-FU plus levamisole or, more likely, 5-FU plus leucovorin for six months. For patients with stage II colon cancer, the answers are not as clear. The five-year survival rate without chemotherapy for this stage II colon cancer group is 75%–80%.[7]

Side effects from the combination of 5-FU and leucovorin include nausea, vomiting, diarrhea, mucositis, fever, leukopenia, thrombocytopenia, and hypotension. Oncology nurses are vital in managing the care of the patient receiving chemotherapy. The physical, psychosocial, and educational needs of the patient must be met. Educating the patient about adverse treatment effects helps them to manage symptoms and helps alleviate the serious or life-threatening treatment complications.

In 1996, irinotecan (Camptosar®) was made available as a second-line treatment option. In the United States, the current dose is 125 mg/m² for four consecutive weeks with a two-week rest period. Phase III studies demonstrated a favorable effect on survival, quality of life, and amelioration of disease-related symptoms. Based on these results, it has been suggested that irinotecan become the new standard of care for adjuvant therapy.[53] The major dose-limiting toxicities are diarrhea and neutropenia. Diarrhea can be severe, and a suggested approach to its management is a 4-mg loading dose of loperamide at the first sign of diarrhea, then 2 mg doses every 2 hours until diarrhea abates for at least 12 hours. Therapies using irinotecan in combination with other drugs are under study.[54]

Chemoradiation is the preferred treatment for anal cancers. Infusional 5-FU and mitomycin with radiation has been used as definitive therapy. Five-year survival rates above 70% have been noted.[2] A combination of 5-FU and radiation is the recommended postoperative adjuvant therapy for patients with stage II or stage III anal cancer.

Immunotherapy

In addition to levamisole, alpha and gamma interferon are being used as immunotherapy for advanced cancer of the colon and rectum. Interleukin-2 (IL-2) is being evaluated in clinical trials for efficacy against advanced colon cancer. Bacillus Calmette-Guérin (BCG) and autologous tumor cell vaccines are also being employed in the treatment of colorectal cancer. Another area of immunotherapy is the identification of antigens, such as CEA, CA19-9, and TAG 72 on the surface of colorectal cancer cells. The largest study is with murine monoclonal antibody 17-1A, which is marketed in Europe as Panorex. A U.S. intergroup trial is investigating the role of the antigen 17-1A in stage II colon cancer.[7]

New Drugs

Raltitrexed (Tomudex®) has shown some activity in advanced colon cancer. The drug is retained intracellularly for prolonged periods, which allows for intermittent dosing every 21 days. Raltitrexed is a strong selective inhibitor of thymidylate synthase. Phase III trials are comparing the effectiveness of this agent to 5-FU/leucovorin in patients with advanced colorectal cancers.[2]

Oral fluoropyrimidines are undergoing phase III trials in the United States and Europe. They include (1) UFT, a combination of uracil and tegafur, which is being given together with oral leucovorin (known as Orzel®), and (2) capecitabine (Xeloda®). Both UFT and capecitabine are metabolized to 5-FU.[2,7] These drugs offer the convenience of an orally administered therapy and potentially fewer toxic effects than conventional chemotherapeutic regimens.

The topoisomerase inhibitor irinotecan (CPT-11

Camptosar®) is effective in patients whose disease is refractory to 5-FU. Studies also demonstrated a survival benefit with the addition of irinotecan in patients who had already received 5-FU for palliative therapy. Consideration is underway to try 5-FU with irinotecan in place of leucovorin as an adjuvant approach.[7]

Eniluracil (776C85) plus oral 5-FU is a potent inactivator of dihydropyrimidine dehydrogenase (DPD), the initial catabolic enzyme of 5-FU. Eniluracil with 5-FU enables the absorption of 5-FU from the GI tract. Phase III studies are ongoing to compare this oral regimen to IV 5-FU and leucovorin.[2]

Oxaliplatin is a new diaminocyclohexane platinum compound that is under clinical investigation. It has demonstrated activity in patients who are resistant to 5-FU when used alone or in combination with 5-FU. Oxaliplatin's toxicity profile includes nausea, vomiting, and cumulative reversible neuropathy. When used with 5-FU or leucovorin, the efficacy of oxaliplatin increased to 30% and 50%, respectively.[7]

Angiogenesis inhibitors in clinical trials include thalidomide, a phase II drug used for patients with hepatomas; anti-VEGF antibody, which is a phase II/III drug that will be used for colorectal cancer as well as other tumor types; SU5416, a phase I/II drug for the treatment of colorectal cancer and other advanced malignancies; and endostatin, a phase I drug indicated for GI tumors. These drugs work by either inhibiting endothelial cells directly, blocking VEGF receptor signals, or blocking the activators of angiogenesis.

Symptom Management and Supportive Care

The care of the patient with colorectal or anal cancer can be complicated by several expected and unexpected developments. This section will discuss these symptoms and the care that should be provided for each.

Perineal Wound

The perineal wound or incisional site may be closed immediately following the removal of the rectum, anus, muscle, and fatty tissue, or it may be left open to heal by secondary intention. Primary closure of the perineal wound site at the time of surgery is the preferred technique, because it is more comfortable for the patient and requires much less care. Closed suction drains are inserted at the time of surgery and exit either through the incisional area or through a separate stab wound in the buttocks. The drains are removed on the third or fifth postoperative day. Primary closure is contraindicated when fecal spillage occurs, the bowel is perforated, an infected hematoma is present, or there is perineal disease such as abscess or fistula.[56]

Perineal wound healing by secondary intention prolongs the healing process, which may take as long as four months. The wound requires packing and meticulous care to promote granulation and to avoid infection or sepsis. Irrigations and sitz baths facilitate wound healing. The drainage and healing process must be carefully monitored by the nurses and any untoward signs and symptoms of infection must be reported to the primary surgeon. Nursing care can range from complex dressing changes to washing the area with soap and water, monitoring intake and output, and checking for patency of drainage tubes.

Bowel Obstruction

Bowel obstruction is a common complication in patients with abdominal or pelvic cancers, such as those arising from colon, ovary, and stomach. Although bowel obstruction may develop at anytime, it is more common and may evolve more rapidly in patients with advanced disease.

Bowel obstruction secondary to advanced colorectal carcinoma may be extrinsic or intrinsic. Extrinsic compression of the bowel may occur as a result of abdominal carcinomatosis or tumor studding along the bowel wall. Intrinsic compression of the bowel can result from growth and progression of the tumor within the lumen of the bowel itself.[57,58]

Signs and symptoms of bowel obstruction are nausea and vomiting, abdominal pain, progressive constipation, and the absence of bowel sounds over the affected area. Initially there is sporadic vomiting that increases progressively until its prevalence is in the range of 68%–100% of the time.[57] Vomiting can remain intermittent or become continuous. It develops early and in large amounts with obstruction of the gastric outlet or small intestine, but develops later in large bowel obstruction.[58] Biliary vomiting is almost odorless and indicates an obstruction in the upper part of the abdomen. The presence of foul-smelling, fecaloid vomiting can be the first sign of an ileal or colonic obstruction.

Diagnosis of a bowel obstruction is done with a radiologic assessment. An abdominal x-ray is taken in a supine or standing position to document dilated loops of bowel, air-fluid interfaces, or both. An x-ray following the ingestion of contrast dye can distinguish obstruction from metastases, radiation injury, or adhesions.[53] A more definitive examination can be done with colosigmoidoscopy.[59,60]

The usual treatment for symptom control is nasogastric suction and administration of parental fluids. This inpatient treatment decompresses the stomach and/or intestine and corrects fluid and electrolyte imbalance before surgery or while the decision for surgery is being made. To avoid the tube from becoming occluded, periodic flushing and or replacement are needed.

If the obstruction continues for more than a few days, gastrostomy tube is a much more acceptable and well-tolerated route for decompression than nasogastric intubation.[58] Intermittent venting of the gastrostomy tube allows the patient to continue oral intake and maintain an active lifestyle without the inconvenience of a nasogastric tube. The two options currently available are surgically placed gastrostomy and percutaneous endoscopic gastrostomy (PEG). Gastrostomy tube placed at the time of surgical exploration is the traditional method of long-term gastric decompression. It should be done whenever the surgeon's intraoperative impression is that complete bowel obstruction is imminent or may be prolonged or imminent. PEG is the insertion of a tube into the stomach through the abdominal wall under fluoroscopic or endoscopic guidance.[61] It can be performed safely as a venting procedure for patients with advanced cancer suffering from nausea and vomiting due to bowel obstruction.

Colicky pain occurs in 72%–76% of patients and continuous abdominal pain is present in more than 90% of cancer patients with bowel obstruction.[57] Pain may be due to abdominal distention, tumor mass, or hepatomegaly, as well as the obstruction itself.

Initially described 14 years ago, the pharmacological management of bowel obstruction due to advanced cancer focuses on the treatment of nausea, vomiting, pain, and other symptoms without the use of nasogastric tube or intravenous hydration. Palliative care units worldwide now use this approach. Somatostatin or octreotide acetate are newer drugs to minimize intestinal secretions. Antiemetic and pain regimens are well-established.[57] The average survival of patients who have inoperable bowel obstruction treated with drugs differs among studies: 3.7 months[57]; 13.4 days, with a range of 2–50 days.[62]

Fistula

Solid tumors may extend into the bowel from adjacent organs or may spread from the bowel to create fistulous openings to the skin, the vagina, or other organs.[63–65] Fistulas also may occur as a result of anastomotic breakdown following a surgical procedure on the bowel or as a complication of radiation therapy.[63,64]

Initial interventions for the patient with a fistula involving the intestinal tract include fluid and electrolyte stabilization and control of infection.[66–68] Specific fluid and electrolyte needs depend on the type and volume of fistula output; for example, small bowel fistulas usually produce high volumes of effluent containing significant amounts of sodium, potassium, and bicarbonate.[69] The patient with high-output fistula (over 500 cc in 24 hours) requires close monitoring of fluid-electrolyte balance with replacement titrated in response to type and volume of output and laboratory indices.[64] Initial management also involves careful evaluation for any intra-abdominal infectious process. Abscesses are drained via open surgical exploration and irrigation or via percutaneous catheter placement.[64,68,69]

Fistula closure is typically achieved either through medical management promoting spontaneous closure or through surgical resection or bypass of the fistulous tract.[63,66] Usually, conservative medical management is tried first, assuming there is no intraabdominal infection and that the distal bowel is patent. This conservative medical approach is based on studies indicating that in the absence of distal obstruction about 50% of fistulas will close spontaneously within four to six weeks and on the fact that surgical closure is frequently ineffective until the underlying factors contributing to fistula development have been corrected.[63,64,66] The two major principles on which conservative management is based are (1) provision of nutritional support and (2) bowel rest for the involved segment of the intestine.[63,65] The goal is to ensure the adequate intake and absorption of calories and protein to support the healing process while minimizing the volume of drainage through the segment of bowel containing the fistula.

Recently, a number of studies demonstrated a significant reduction in fistula output and in the time required for spontaneous fistula closure with the administration of somatostatin or its analog, octreotide acetate. Somatostatin is a naturally occurring intestinal hormone that reduces the volume of intestinal secretions.[66,68,69]

A major component of effective fistula management is the containment of the effluent and odor and the protection of the surrounding skin since these aspects of care have a profound impact on the patient's quality of life.[66] Many products and techniques are now available for achieving and maintaining these goals. For the standard pouching procedure see Table 51-6.[70] Hospitals and clinics who have Certified Wound, Ostomy, Continence Nurses (ET nurses) are able to provide expert patient consultation and to facilitate the education of the nursing staff in fistula management.

Stoma and Colostomy Management

Palliative care for patients with GI stomas must include attention to stoma site selection, stoma management, and maintenance of GI function. Careful selection of the stoma site by the Wound, Ostomy, Continence Nurse and surgeon is an important step toward ensuring the patient's quality of life after surgery. By assessing the patient's abdomen in a lying, sitting, and standing position the health care provider can ensure that the selected stoma site is within the rectus muscle and is in an area that can physically support ostomy equipment. It is important that the patient is able to visualize the proposed stoma site so self-care will be easier.[71] Scars, folds, bony prominences, belt and waistlines, and the umbilicus need to be avoided to ensure proper fit of the ostomy equipment. The anatomical location of the stoma influences the abdominal quadrant placement as well as the surgical technique.[56]

The stoma must be evaluated for viability, condition, size, and shape and whether all sutures are holding the everted stoma onto the abdomen. A red, shiny, moist, budded, or flush stoma with all sutures and peristomal skin intact is the desired outcome. Deviations from this should be reported to the surgeon as they may indicate early problems and require immediate surgical intervention.[72]

Table 51-6 Application of a Pouch

1. Select an appropriate pouch based on the type of drainage and abdominal contours.
2. If needed, have skin barrier powder, sealant, or paste available.
3. Empty the pouch and gently remove it by pushing down on the skin while lifting up on the pouch. Discard soiled pouch in a plastic bag/hazardous waste box. Save the clamp.
4. Using water, clean the stoma and peristomal skin area and pat dry. Shave or clip any hair in the pouching area.
5. Treat any peristomal skin damage with skin barrier powder and sealant.
6. Size the pouch opening using the stoma measuring guide or use the back of the barrier or pouch surface to make a pattern. The size of a new stoma may decrease in size for four to six weeks postop. For fistulas or flush stomas: size the opening to clear the fistula/stoma margins by ¼–½ inches; this helps prevent tunneling of the drainage under the barrier. For budded stomas: size the opening about ⅛ inch larger than the stoma.
7. Use skin barrier paste to fill any surface defects; apply a ring of paste around ileostomy stomas. A moist finger facilitates application and for later removal of a dry gauze.
8. Remove paper backing from pouch or barrier to expose adhesive surface; center pouch opening over stoma and gently press to ensure adherence.
9. If two-piece: snap pouch on the flange of barrier wafer.
10. Squirt some soapy water into pouch to facilitate emptying later.
11. Attach clamp.
12. For fistula: apply thin layer of skin barrier paste to any exposed skin edges and to caulk junction between wound edges and inner edge of pouch, and around flush stoma.
13. Change pouch every five to seven days and as needed for leakage.

Adapted with permission from Doughty D: Principles of fistulas and stoma management, in Berger A, Portenoy RK, Weissman DE (eds): *Principles and Practices of Supportive Oncology.* Philadelphia, Lippincott-Raven, 1998.[70]

Psychological support of the patient begins preoperatively with an explanation of the surgery to be performed and introduction to the pouching system and equipment. After surgery, support shifts to coping and adaptation, particularly when the patient first looks at his stoma, which can be very upsetting. The initial size of the stoma will depend upon the portion of the bowel segment involved and whether there was any bowel obstruction prior to surgery. The initial bowel edema gradually subsides following surgery, and the actual stoma size is established in six to eight weeks.[72] This is an important variable to remember when preparing the pouch opening to ensure proper sizing.

Initially the patient will have serosanguineous fluid in their pouch. The time the stoma will begin to function depends on the preoperative cleansing and prior obstruction. If this was an emergent surgery or poor cleansing was performed, stool would be present almost immediately. Once peristalsis returns and flatus is passed, then food is introduced. Stool will soon be expelled from the stoma. Usually, the more proximal a stoma is in the bowel, the sooner it functions and the more liquid the stool content.

The key principles in stoma management include the containment of the effluent and odor and the protection of the peristomal skin. The degree of skin protection

required is dictated by the characteristics of the effluent: effluent that is proteolytic, highly acidic, or highly alkaline (ileostomy, cecostomy, ascending colostomy) requires meticulous protection of peristomal skin, whereas nonenzymatic effluent with a pH that is essentially neutral primarily requires protection against pooling of drainage that can macerate the skin (descending/sigmoid colostomies).

Equipment costs vary but are reimbursable to some degree by Medicare and most private insurers. Certain agencies help with the costs for those who have particular needs; however, these groups differ across the country. A Wound, Ostomy, and Continence Nurse is usually aware of various groups who are of assistance in a specific region (see Table 51-7). Patient teaching proceeds in a stepwise fashion from the simple to the complex. Asking the patient what he/she wants to learn first may relieve some of his/her anxiety. With a family member or significant other present to serve as a backup caregiver when the patient is at home, the teaching usually proceeds from removing or applying the pouch closure clamp to looking at and cleansing the stoma to applying and emptying the pouch. The goal is for the patient to independently manage his pouch changing and stoma care prior to discharge.

The shorter length of stay in hospitals has made it difficult to include colostomy irrigation teaching prior to discharge. Individuals usually learn to perform colostomy irrigation and thus regulate evacuation from their clinic or home health nurse (see Table 51-8).[72]

Case managers coordinating the discharge plan for the patient should be encouraged to recommend home health agencies with Wound, Ostomy, and Continence Nurse consultants to ensure continuity of care and management of any peristomal complications. Many hospital-based Wound, Ostomy, and Continence Nurse consultants will also see outpatients for postdischarge care and instruction. Individualized patient education materials, mail order catalogs and a list of the supplies, names of community vendors, and support groups at the United Ostomy Association or the American Cancer Society are available to promote the patients' self-care.

Sexual Dysfunction

Early-stage colorectal cancer treated with removal of the rectum only may interfere with the individual's potential for orgasm, although erectile dysfunction is less common. However, the more extensive the surgery, the higher the reported incidence of sexual dysfunction, at least in males, on whom more research has been done than females. A study of 60 men who were sexually active prior to pretreatment and who received either high anterior resection, low anterior resection, or abdominoperineal resection found the latter group with APR had the highest percentage of sexual problems. Sixty-five percent became sexually inactive, 50% were unable to ejaculate, and 45% reported erectile dysfunction.[73]

Table 51-7 Pouching Products

Company	Pouching Systems	Accessory Products
Coloplast Marietta, GA 800-237-4555	One-piece and two-piece fecal and urinary pouches: flat and convex Pedi-pouches Wound pouch	Barrier paste Belts Stoma covers Irrigation sets
Convatec Bristol-Myers Squibb Princeton, NJ 800-422-8811	One-piece and two-piece fecal and urinary pouches: flat and convex Pedi-pouches Wound pouches	Skin sealant Stomahesive paste Stomahesive powder Stomahesive barriers Belts Irrigation sets
Hollister Libertyville, IL 800-323-4060	One-piece and two-piece fecal and urinary pouches: flat and convex Wound pouches	Skin sealant Premium paster Premium powder Premium and Flextend barriers Medical adhesive Pouch covers Irrigation sets
Marlen Bedford, OH 216-292-7060	One-piece and two-piece fecal and urinary pouches: flat and convex	Belts Double-faced discs
NuHope Pacoima, CA 800-899-5017	One-piece and two-piece fecal and urinary pouches: flat and convex	Hernia binders Nu-sorb Skin barrier Pouch covers

Patients with ostomies can become concerned with their body image as they worry about stoma appearance, stool collecting in the pouch, pouch leakage, sounds, and odors. These can all cause the person to feel unattractive and to have a diminished libido. Fear of rejection from their significant other can cause stress in the relationship and have a negative impact on the patient's self-concept. Support for the patient and significant other includes the following:

1. *Depression or anxiety:* Antidepressants may be useful but some drugs can interfere with erectile function; prescribing physicians should consult with a pharmacist.
2. *Fatigue:* Napping prior to sexual activity as well as avoiding heavy meals and alcohol can be helpful. Trying different positions during sexual activity that require minimal effort, such as the side-lying position, may be helpful.
3. *Pain:* Timing of medication is important to provide pain control without drowsiness. Relaxation techniques, warm baths or soaks, and massage may decrease pain and can be an opportunity for sexual foreplay when done as a couple.
4. *Nausea:* Meditating prior to sexual activity is often suggested. A light meal or crackers prior to activity may also be helpful. Usual accoutrements of sexual activity such as perfumes, colognes, and scented candles may have to be avoided if smells cause nausea.
5. *Odors:* Elimination ostomies should be emptied prior to sexual activity. Deodorizers or odor eliminators are

available if odors are a concern. Pouch covers are also available to shield the pouch contents.[74]

Other interventions for sexual dysfunction are discussed in Chapter 37.

Ureteral Obstruction

In 38% of cases, individuals with adenocarcinoma of the colon and rectum have ureteral obstruction.[69] Genitourinary signs and symptoms occur more frequently in individuals with metastatic colorectal carcinoma than when the primary tumor is genitourinary.[75] The five-year survival rate for individuals with genitourinary involvement from colorectal cancer approximates 30%.[76]

With advanced colorectal cancer, bilateral ureteral obstruction can occur as a result of direct tumor compression of the ureters. Individuals with ureteral obstruction present with oliguria and an elevated serum creatinine. A cystoscopy and bilateral retrograde pyelogram are the most reliable diagnostic tools for determining ureteral obstruction.[77] These exams also determine whether the obstruction is intrinsic to the ureter or extrinsic, as would be seen with an advancing colorectal lesion.

Treatment of ureteral obstruction may be accomplished at the time of the retrograde pyelogram. Urinary stents can be inserted into the ureters to establish patency and prevent further compression by the tumor. Stents can circumvent the need for a surgical procedure. If

Table 51-8 Instruction for Patient Teaching in Colostomy Irrigation

1. Gather supplies. Explain procedure to patient and provide for privacy and comfort.
2. Remove pouch or stomal covering.
3. Attach irrigation sleeve; place bottom of sleeve into toilet to direct returns, or close bottom of sleeve with rubber band, binder clip, or commercial tail closure. NOTE: Irrigation sleeves for two-piece systems are snapped onto the two-piece wafer with flange; other reusable sleeves are belted into place. Disposable adhesive sleeves also are available.
4. Prepare irrigating solution. Volume to be given is titrated for the patient and is based on the patient's tolerance and feelings of colonic distention ("fullness"). Initial irrigations usually are performed with 500 mL of solution or less to prevent overdistention and cramping. Routine irrigation for the average adult is performed using approximately 500–1000 mL of solution.
5. Close clamp on irrigating bag, and fill bag with desired amount of tepid water or prescribed irrigant. Open clamp and allow irrigating solution to flow to clear tubing of air. Suspend irrigating bag at approximately shoulder height or slightly higher.
6. Lubricate the cone tip; insert cone tip gently into stoma and hold tip securely in place to prevent backflow. Use water-soluble lubricant.
7. Open clamp and allow irrigation solution to flow in steadily; the desired time frame for instillation of fluid is 5 to 10 minutes.
8. When desired amount of irrigant has been delivered or when the patient senses colonic distention, close the clamp and remove the cone.
9. Wait approximately 30 to 45 minutes for returns. After initial returns are complete (usually 10 to 15 minutes), the individual has the option to close the bottom of the sleeve and move around.
10. When returns are complete, rinse and remove the irrigation sleeve.
11. Clean peristomal skin and apply pouch or desired stomal covering.
12. Prepare equipment for repeat use.

Adapted with permission from Hampton BG, Bryant RA (eds): *Ostomies and Continent Diversions.* St. Louis, Mosby Year-Book, 1992.[72]

the ureteral stents become occluded, they can be usually changed via cystoscopy. There are situations, however, when urinary stents cannot be utilized because of ureteral strictures or inability to visualize the ureters. In such cases, percutaneous nephrostomy tubes can be used to treat the obstruction. Nephrostomy tubes placed directly into the kidney via a percutaneous approach allow adequate urinary drainage from the renal pelvis.

Pulmonary Metastases

While endobronchial metastases are rare, colorectal carcinoma is one of the most common primary tumors with pulmonary metastases.[78] Colorectal tumors that metastasize to the lungs may present as solitary masses or multiple nodules. Individuals who experience pulmonary metastases from a colorectal primary may present with symptoms of dyspnea. It has been estimated that 85% of patients with pulmonary metastases are asymptomatic for pulmonary problems.[78]

Most colorectal metastases to the lungs are detected by routine chest x-ray. More definitive evaluation can be accomplished by a computerized tomography (CT) scan of the chest, which further defines the number and location of the lesions.

Pulmonary resection of the metastatic area provides the best long-term survival. Pulmonary wedge resection is undertaken if the lesion is isolated. Individuals with four or fewer metastatic pulmonary lesions have a better prognosis than individuals with four or more lesions.[79] Individuals with metastatic lung involvement from colon cancer have been found to have a 31% five-year survival rate after surgical resection of the metastatic lesion.[80]

Continuity of Care: Nursing Challenges

In today's health care environment, the delivery of care takes place in an accelerated fashion. The time span between presentation, physiological work-up, diagnosis, acute intervention, and follow-up treatment can be compressed into a month. Often there is a multitude of health care professionals involved in the individual's care, which makes communication and coordination of the treatment plan paramount. It has been estimated that 62% of whites and 53% of blacks diagnosed with colon cancer will attain the five-year survival rate.[76] Similarly, 60% of whites and 52% of blacks diagnosed with rectal cancer will be alive at the five-year mark.[76] Because the course of treatment for colorectal carcinoma, including follow-up, can span many years, there must be provision for continuity of care.

At the time of initial presentation, the individual's entry into the health care system is usually through the primary care physician either for a routine physical exam or because of troublesome symptoms. A physical exam and diagnostic testing ensues and once the appropriate results are evaluated, referral is made to a GI surgeon. Additional testing takes place, and should a colorectal biopsy be done, tissue pathology may already be available before the individual goes to the operating room. If a final tissue diagnosis is not available, the surgeon shares his or her suspicions with the individual prior to any surgical intervention. Close collaboration between the individual, family, primary care physician, and surgeon facilitates the flow of consistent information. Once the decision has been reached regarding operative intervention, the individual and family should be informed by the surgeon what to expect. The anticipated surgical preparation, day of surgery, length of surgery, potential complications, anticipated outcome, and length of hospital stay need to be reviewed. The patient and his family need to have a general understanding about the incision line, surgical drains, urinary catheter, nasogastric tube, potential for colostomy, and provisions for pain management. It is optimal to provide the patient and caregivers with the name and phone number of a specific health care professional for reassurance and reference should any questions or issues arise.

The average length of stay for someone who has had a surgical resection secondary to colorectal carcinoma is less than five days. At the time of admission, the appropriate referrals need to be made. Should the individual have a colostomy, the WOCN ET Nurse needs to be involved. A registered dietitian lends support for caloric calculations, hyperalimentation guidelines, and dietary specifics. Social service may be needed as dictated by the individual's home and support situation. Home care is also a consideration to meet specific health care needs once the individual is discharged.

Upon discharge the individual needs to be clear about when to call the physician for problems such as fever, chills, shortness of breath, or hemoptysis. Should any change occur with the incision such as erythema, drainage, or wound separation, the surgeon also needs to be notified. Information about discharge medications and resuming previous medications must be reviewed and clarified. Optimally, the specific name and number of the same health care professional should be given to the individual and family for questions or difficulties that may arise before the return appointment to the surgeon.

Upon return for the postoperative check, an overall physical assessment takes place and the final pathology is shared with the individual and family if the tissue diagnosis was not available at the time of discharge. The general plan for follow-up treatment can be discussed as well. While additional adjunctive therapy may not begin for another few weeks, the appropriate referrals to the radiation oncologist or medical oncologist need to be made in a timely fashion. Appointments with the appropriate physicians providing additional treatment could be made prior to departure from the surgeon's office.

Coordination of all these services and the provision for continuity of care is imperative. For the individual confronted with a diagnosis of cancer, recovery from surgery, and treatment follow-up, the nurse can provide invaluable assistance in organizing, scheduling, interpreting, and managing the treatment plan.

If the disease is advanced, palliation of symptoms is part of the spectrum of care. The individual and family should be educated regarding the gradual progression of the disease, what to expect from a physiological standpoint, and options available for the treatment of these symptoms. The individual and family can be offered the services and support of hospice. Options for interventions need to be explored so that an informed decision can be made. Most symptoms can be handled within the comfort of the individual's home if so desired. Should a hospital admission become necessary, however, decisions regarding life-support measures need to be explored with the individual and family.

Conclusion

Over the past 30 years there has been a downward trend in the incidence, morbidity, and mortality associated with colorectal carcinoma. Current screening mechanisms, diagnostic techniques, surgical interventions, and adjuvant therapy regimens have enabled individuals diagnosed with this malignancy to experience improved long-term survival and enhanced quality of life.

Factors that contribute to the pathogenesis of this disease are multifactorial. Age, genetics, diet, alcohol, environment, inflammatory bowel conditions, prior radiation therapy and surgery are risk factors for colorectal cancer. Genes are the focus of research at present. The presence or absence of certain genetic factors can increase the risk for the development of the malignancy.

Surgery continues to be the mainstay of therapy for colorectal adenocarcinoma. Some literature supports the premise that more extensive surgery leads to improved cure and long-term survival. Chemotherapy, radiation therapy, and immunotherapy continue to be utilized preoperatively, intraoperatively, and postoperatively to achieve better long-term survival.

Today's health care environment continues to change rapidly; more is accomplished on an outpatient basis and hospital lengths of stay dwindle. A multitude of specialties care for the individual with colorectal carcinoma. The coordination and quality of the care needs to be paramount as we move toward earlier diagnosis and better long-term survival for this disease.

The authors wish to acknowledge the contribution of Carolyn Ferrante in the development of this chapter.

References

1. Bond J, Levin B: *Prevention and Early Detection of Colorectal Cancer: A Clinical Update of the Digestive Health Initiative.* Washington, DC, Colorectal Cancer Education Company. American Digestive Health Foundation, 1997

2. Pazdur RL, Coia L, Wagman L, et al: Colorectal and anal cancer, in Pazdur RL, Coia W, Haskins L, Wagman L (eds): *Cancer Management: A Multidisciplinary Approach,* Melville, NY, PRR, 1999, pp 149–175

3. Landis SH, Murray T, Bolden S, et al: Cancer statistics in 1998. *CA Cancer J Clin* 48:6–30, 1998

4. American Gastroenterological Association: *Colorectal Cancer Screening: Clinical Guidelines and Rationale—Executive Summary.* Philadelphia, Saunders, 1997

5. Kelvin F: Diagnosis of colorectal cancer by conventional radiology, in Myers M (ed): *Neoplasms of the Digestive Tract: Imaging, Staging, and Management.* Philadelphia, Lippincott-Raven, 1998, pp 219–235

6. Meyers MA: Overview, colorectal carcinoma: Imaging, staging, and management, in Meyers MA (ed): *Neoplasms of the Digestive Tract: Imaging, Staging, and Management.* Philadelphia, Lippincott-Raven, 1998, pp 203–217

7. Peters M, Haller D. Therapy for early-stage colorectal cancer. *Oncology* 13:307–315, 1999

8. Waghorn A, Witold K: Colon and rectum, in McCulloch P, Kingsworth A (eds): *Management of Gastrointestinal Cancer.* London, BMJ Publishing Group, 1996, pp 321–365

9. Kune GA, Vitetta L: Alcohol consumption and the etiology

of colorectal cancer: a review of the scientific evidence from 1957 to 1991. *Nutr Cancer* 18:97–111, 1992

10. Newcomb PA, Storer BE, Marcus PM: Cancer of the large bowel in women in relation to alcohol consumption—a case control study in Wisconsin. *Cancer Causes Control* 4:405–411, 1993

11. Meyer F, White E: Alcohol and nutrients in relation to colon cancer in middle-aged adults. *Am J Epidem* 138:225–236, 1993

12. Mayer RJ: Tumors of the large and small intestine, in Isselbacher K, Braunwald E, Wilson J, Martin J, Fauci A, Kasper D: *Harrison's Principles of Internal Medicine* (ed 13). New York, McGraw-Hill, 1994, pp 1424–1429

13. Rosen N: Cancers of the gastrointestinal tract, in DeVita VT, Hellman S, Rosenberg SA (eds): *Cancer Principles and Practice of Oncology* (ed 5). Philadelphia, Lippincott-Raven, 1997, pp 971–980

14. Lynch H, Smyrk T, Watson P, et al: Genetics, natural history, tumor spectrum, and pathology of hereditary nonpolyposis colorectal cancer: an updated review. *Gastroenterology* 104: 1535–1549, 1993

15. Lynch H, Smyrk T, McGinn T, et al: Attenuated familial adenomatous polyposis (AFAP): a phenotypically and genotypically distinctive variant of FAP. *Cancer* 76:2427–2433, 1995

16. Stollman N, Raskin J: The flat adenoma. *Prac Gastroenterol* 21:9–15, 1997

17. Burt R: Update on genetic advances in colorectal cancer. *Prac Gastroenterol* 21:9–15, 1997

18. Burt R, Peterson G: Familial colorectal cancer: diagnosis and management, in Young G, Rozen P, Lein B (eds): *Prevention and Early Detection of Colorectal Cancer*. Philadelphia, Saunders, 1998, pp 171–192

19. Byers T, Levin B, Rothenberger D, et al: American Cancer Society guidelines for screening and surveillance for early detection of colorectal polyps and cancer: update 1997. American Cancer Society. *CA Cancer J Clin* 47:154–160, 1997

20. Franceschi S, LaVecchia C: Colorectal cancer and hormone replacement therapy: an unexpected finding. *Eur J Cancer Prev* 7:427–438, 1998

21. Savoca P, Wong W: Anal carcinoma: anatomy, staging, and prognostic variables, in Cohen A, Winawer S (eds): *Cancer of the Colon, Rectum, and Anus*. New York, McGraw-Hill, 1995, pp 1013–1020

22. Chuselp C: Pathways of nodal metastasis from cancer of the colon, in Meyers MA (ed): *Neoplasms of the Digestive Tract: Imaging, Staging, and Management*. Philadelphia: Lippincott-Raven, 1998, pp 257–267

23. Miaskowski C: *Oncology Nursing: An Essential Guide for Patient Care*. Philadelphia, Saunders, 1997

24. Strohl R: Nursing care of the client with cancer of the gastrointestinal tract, in Itano J, Taoka K (eds): *Core Curriculum for Oncology Nursing* (ed 3). Philadelphia, Saunders, 1998 pp 470–483

25. Colecchia G, Nardi M: Colorectal cancer in pregnancy. *Giornal di Chirurgia* 20:159–161, 1999

26. Liefers G, Cleton-Jansen A, Van De Velde C, et al: Micrometastases and survival in stage II colorectal cancer. *N Engl J Med* 339:223–228, 1998

27. Danenberg K, Metzer R, Groshen S, et al: Thymidylate synthase (TS) and thymidine phosphorylase are prognostic indicators of survival for colorectal cancer. *Proc Am Soc Clin Oncol* 16:257a, 1997 (abstr)

28. Chatzipetrou M, Tarassi K, Konstadoulakis M, et al: Human leukocyte antigens as genetic markers in colorectal carcinoma. *Dis Colon Rectum* 42:66–70, 1999

29. Yamane N, Tsujitani S, Makin M, et al: Soluble CD44 variant 6 as a prognostic indicator in patients with colorectal cancer. *Oncology* 56:232–238, 1999

30. Brandt B, DeAntonio P, Dezort M, et al: Hepatic cryosurgery for metastatic colorectal carcinoma. *Oncol Nurs Forum* 23: 29–37, 1996

31. Chang AE: Colorectal cancer, in Greenfield LJ, Mulholland MW, Oldham KT, Zelenock GB, Lillemoe KD (eds): *Surgery: Scientific Principles and Practice*. Philadelphia, Lippincott-Raven, 1997, pp 1139–1146

32. Hurd T, Gutman H: Cancer of the colon, rectum and anus, in Berger DH, Feig BW, Fuhrman GM (eds): *The M.D. Anderson Surgical Oncology Handbook*. Boston, Little, Brown, 1995, pp 160–177

33. Gold SC, Sakurai C: Colorectal cancer, in McCorkle R, Grant M, Frank-Stromborg M, Baird SB (eds): *Cancer Nursing: A Comprehensive Textbook* (ed 2). Philadelphia, Saunders, 1996, pp 652–673

34. Enker WE: Sphincter-preserving operations for rectal cancer. *Oncology* 10:1673–1684, 1996

35. Hoebler L, Irwinn MM: Gastrointestinal tract cancer: current knowledge, medical treatment, and nursing management. *Oncol Nurs Forum* 19:1403–1415, 1992

36. Perez CA, Brady LW, Roti JL: Overview, in Perez CA, Brady LW (eds): *Principles and Practice of Radiation Oncology* (ed 3). Philadelphia, Lippincott-Raven, 1998, pp 1–78

37 Marks G, Mohiuddunm M, Masoni L: The reality of radical sphincter preservation surgery for cancer of the distal 3 cm of rectum following high-dose radiation. *Int J Radiat Oncol Biol Phys* 27:779–783, 1993

38. Minsky BD: Sphincter preservation in rectal cancer. Preoperative radiation therapy followed by low anterior resection with coloanal anastomosis. *Semin Rad Oncol* 8:30–35, 1998

39. Rostock RA, Zajac AJ, Gallagher MJ: Radiation therapy in the treatment of colorectal cancer, in Ahlgren J, Macdonald J (eds): *Gastrointestinal Oncology* (ed 1). Philadelphia, Lippincott, 1992, pp 359–381

40. Mohiuddin M, Marks G: Long-term results of "selective sandwich" adjunctive radiotherapy for cancer of the rectum. *Am J Clin Oncol* 17:264–268, 1994

41. Saddler D, Ellis C: Colorectal cancer. *Semin Oncol Nurs* 15: 63, 1999

42. Grunderson LL, Willett CG, Harrison LB, et al: Intraoperative irradiation: current and future status. *Semin Oncol* 24: 715–731, 1997

43. Corn BW, Curran WJ Jr, Shrieve DC, et al: Stereotactic radiosurgery and radiotherapy: new developments and new directions. *Semin Oncol* 24:707–714, 1997

44. Iwamoto RJ: Emerging strategies in radiation therapy for colorectal cancer: intraoperative radiation therapy and stereotactic radiation therapy. *Colorectal Cancer: Balancing Therapeutic Interventions and Quality of Life Symposium*. Philadelphia, Meniscus Educational Institute, 1998, pp 14–23

45. Couke PA, Minimanoff RO: Adjuvant post-operative accelerated hyperfractionated radiotherapy in rectal cancer: a feasibility study. *Int J Radiat Oncol Biol Phys* 32:187–196, 1993

46. Couke PA, Cuttak JF: The rationale to switch from postoperative hyperfractionated accelerated radiotherapy to preoperative hyperfractionated accelerated radiotherapy in rectal cancer. *Int J Radiat Oncol Biol Phys* 32:181–188, 1995

47. Duncan W, Arnott SJ, Jack WJL, et al: Results of two random-

ized trials of neutron therapy in rectal adenocarcinoma. *Radiother Oncol* 8:191–197, 1987

48. Battermann JJ: Results of d + T fast neutron irradiation on advanced tumours of the bladder and rectum. *Int J Radiat Oncol Biol Phys* 8:2159–2164, 1982

49. Gonzales D, van Dijk JD, Blank LE: Radiotherapy and hyperthermia. *Eur J Cancer* 31A:1351–1355, 1995 (review)

50. Ichikawa D, Yamaguchi T, Yoshioka Y, et al: Prognostic evaluation of preoperative combined treatment for advanced cancer in the lower rectum with radiation, intraluminal hyperthermia, and 5-fluorouracil suppository. *Am J Surg* 171:346–350, 1996

51. Ohno S, Tomoda M, Tomisaki S, et al: Improved surgical results after combining preoperative hyperthermia with chemotherapy and radiotherapy for patients with carcinoma of the rectum. *Dis Colon Rectum* 40:401–406, 1997

52. Dibiase SJ, Rosenstock JG, Shabason L, et al: Tumor bed brachytherapy with a mesh template: an accessible alternative to intraoperative radiotherapy. *J Surg Oncol* 66:104–109, 1997

53. Pazdur R: Irinotecan: toward clinical end points in drug development. *Oncology* 12:13–21, 1998 (suppl 6)

54. Saltz L: Irinotecan in the first line treatment of colorectal cancer. *Oncology* 12:54–57, 1998 (suppl 6)

55. NCI Cancer Trials, Cancer trials: angiogenesis inhibitors in clinical trials (April 1999). Available at http://cancertrials.nci.nih.gov/NCI_CANCER_TRIALS/Zones/PressInfo/Angio/Table.html

56. Hampton BG: Gastrointestinal cancer: colon, rectum, and anus, in Groenwald SL, Frogge MH, Goodman M, Yarbro CH: *Cancer Nursing Principles and Practice* (ed 3). Sudbury, MA, Jones and Bartlett, 1993, pp 1044–1064

57. Baines M: The pathophysiology and management of malignant intestinal obstruction, in Doyle D, Hanks GWC, MacDonald N (eds): *Oxford Textbook of Palliative Medicine* (ed 2). Oxford, Oxford University Press, 1998, pp 526–534

58. Ripamonti C: Management of bowel obstruction in advanced cancer patients. *J Pain Sympt Manage* 1994, pp 193–200

59. Ziter FMH. Radiologic diagnosis: small bowel, in Welch JP (ed): *Bowel Obstruction*. Philadelphia, Saunders, 1990, pp 96–107

60. Markowitz SK: Radiologic diagnosis: colon, in Welch JP (ed): *Bowel Obstruction*. Philadelphia, Saunders, 1990, pp 108–118

61. George J, Crawford D, Lewis T, et al: Percutaneous endoscopic gastrostomy: a two year experience. *Med J Aust* 152:17–19, 1990

62. Ventafridda V, Ripamonti C, Caraceni A, et al: The management of inoperable gastrointestinal obstruction in terminal cancer patients. *Tumori* 76:389–393, 1990

63. Bryant R: Enterocutaneous fistulas: meeting the nursing challenge. *Progressions* 4:3–23, 1992

64. Benson D, Fischer J: Enterocutaneous fistula, in Fazio V (ed): *Current Therapy in Colon and Rectal Surgery*. Philadelphia, Decker, 1992, pp 372–376

65. Doughty D: *Gastrointestinal Disorders*. St. Louis, Mosby Year-Book, 1993, pp 245–253, 311–370, 324–337

66. Bryant R: Management of drain sites and fistulas, in Bryant R (ed): *Acute and Chronic Wounds: Nursing Management*. St. Louis, Mosby Year-Book, 1992, pp 248–287

67. Kimbrough T: Intraabdominal abscesses and fistulas, in Yamada T (ed): *Textbook of Gastroenterology*. Philadelphia, Lippincott, 1995, pp 2289–2298

68. Greenstein A: Enterocutaneous fistula, in Bayless T (ed): *Current Therapy in Gastroenterology and Liver Disease* (ed 4). St. Louis, Mosby Year-Book, 1994, pp 341–345

69. Pellegrini C, Gordon R: Abdominal abscesses and gastrointestinal fistulas, in Sleisenger M, Fordtran J (eds): *Gastrointestinal Disease: Pathophysiology, Diagnosis, Management* (ed 5). Philadelphia, Saunders, 1993, pp 1962–1976

70. Doughty D: Principles of fistulas and stoma management, in Berger A, Portenoy RK, Weissman DE (eds): *Principles and Practices of Supportive Oncology*. Philadelphia, Lippincott-Raven, 1998

71. Turnbull GW, Erin-Toth P: Ostomy care: foundation for teaching and practice. *Ostomy/Wound Management* 1A:235–305, 1999 (suppl)

72. Hampton BG: Peristomal and stomal complications, in Hampton BG, Bryant RA (eds): *Ostomies and Continent Diversions*. St. Louis, Mosby Year-Book, 1992, pp 105–128

73. Koukouras D, Spiliotis J, Scopa C, et al: Radical consequence in the sexuality of male patients operated for colorectal carcinoma. *Eur J Surg Oncol* 17:285–288, 1991

74. Bruner DW, Iwamoto RR: Altered sexual health, in Groenwald SL, Frogge MH, Goodman M, Yarbro CH (eds): *Cancer Symptom Management*. Sudbury, MA, Jones and Bartlett, 1998, pp 523–537

75. Lee LH, Khauli RB, Baker S, et al: Prognostic and therapeutic observations of manifestations in the genitourinary tract of adenocarcinoma of the colon and rectum. *Surg Gynecol Obstet* 169:511–518, 1989

76. Lim LH, Ko YT, Lee DH, et al: Determining the site and causes of colonic obstruction with sonography. *Am J Roentgenol* 163:1113–1117, 1994

77. Lieber MM: Urologic emergencies, in Wittes RE (ed): *Manual of Oncologic Therapeutics* (ed 1). Philadelphia, Lippincott, 1991, pp 336–338

78. McCormick PM, Martini N: A current view of surgical management of pulmonary metastases, in Economou SG, Witt TR, Deziel DJ, et al (eds): *Adjuncts to Cancer Surgery* (ed 1). Philadelphia, Lea and Febiger, 1991, pp 246–251

79. Avis F: Surgical treatment of isolated metastases to the liver, lungs, brain, in Wittes RE (ed): *Manual of Oncologic Therapeutics* (ed 1). Philadelphia, Lippincott, 1991, pp 308–309

80. Mountain CF, McMurtrey MJ, Hermes KF: Surgery for pulmonary metastases: a 20 year experience. *Ann Thorac Surg* 38:323–330, 1984

CHAPTER 52

Endocrine Malignancies

Rita Wickham, PhD, RN, AOCN
Kimberly Rohan, MS, RN

Introduction

During 1999, approximately 19,800 persons were diagnosed and 2000 people died from an endocrine malignancy in the United States.[1] Approximately 90% of these cancers occur in the thyroid. Endocrine malignancies arise from endocrine glands, which elaborate and secrete hormones (chemical signals) into the bloodstream to exert their effects at distant sites. Although most organs have some endocrine function, the classic endocrine glands include the pituitary, the thyroid, the parathyroids, and the adrenal glands, the gonads, and the islets of Langerhans.[2] This chapter will focus on malignancies arising in the thyroid, parathyroid, pituitary, and adrenal cortex and medulla, as well as multiple endocrine neoplasia (MEN) syndromes.

THYROID TUMORS

The thyroid, a small organ that normally weighs 15–20 grams, lies below the cricoid cartilage at the base of the neck and around either side of the trachea.[3] The functional units of the thyroid are follicles, composed of epithelial cells interspersed with parafollicular cells (also known as *C cells*). Groups of follicles are bound tightly together to form lobules. The follicular cells produce the thyroid hormones thyroxine (T_4) and triiodothyronine (T_3), and the C cells produce calcitonin. The thyroid synthesizes its hormones, all of which hold large amounts of iodine, in response to thyroid stimulating hormone (TSH) released by the anterior pituitary gland.

Virtually all body cells and tissues require thyroid hormones for optimal functioning.[3] Thyroid hormone is required for the production of growth hormone (GH), and acts as a growth factor to promote bone formation and skeletal maturation. Thyroid hormones also play a critical role in the maturation of the central nervous system (CNS) in infants and modulate the actions of the autonomic nervous system throughout life. Further, they play roles in oxidative metabolism, help maintain a steady body temperature by heat production or conservation, and positively affect carbohydrate and lipid metabolism, as well as the synthesis and degradation of body proteins.

Epidemiology

The incidence of thyroid cancer has been increasing over the last decade.[4] These malignancies usually occur between the ages of 25 and 65, but are most common in persons older than age 45 and in women, who are three times as likely as men to develop a thyroid tumor. Age is an important determinant of prognosis: five-year survival with thyroid cancer is 95% in patients younger than age 59, but only 64% in those older than age 70.[5]

Etiology

Ionizing radiation to the head and neck is the only clearly identified etiologic agent for papillary thyroid cancer.[4,6] Other factors, including benign thyroid disease, hormonal factors and reproductive factors in women, and a diet deficient in iodine, may play a role.[7-9] The carcinogenic risk of radiation is dose-dependent: minimal risk exists with exposure to very small doses (6.5–80 cGy), and risk increases linearly to a dose of 2000 cGy. At doses greater than 2000 cGy, the risk for thyroid cancer falls off as the thyroid cells die and the gland becomes sterile.[6,10] The carcinogenic effect of radiation has been demonstrated in adults who were treated as children with radiation for benign head and neck conditions such as enlarged thymus glands, tonsillitis, adenoid hypertrophy, pharyngitis, or acne.[4,7] Risk is inversely related to age, so infants and young children are more susceptible to the carcinogenic effect of radiation to the neck region than are older children.[8,9]

Carcinogenic effects of radiation may persist for as long as four decades after exposure, and this effect is also more pronounced in persons who received therapeutic or accidental radiation to the thyroid as younger children.[10,11] For instance, children who receive total body irradiation in preparation for allogeneic bone marrow transplant are at increased risk for papillary thyroid malignancy, and require regular follow-up for thyroid tumors.[12] Likewise, thyroid cancer has increased dramatically in children exposed to high levels of radioactive fallout from the Chernobyl nuclear plant disaster.[13] In addition, high rates of follicular and papillary tumors are noted in areas of endemic goiter, so iodine insufficiency may be a causative factor for thyroid malignancy, especially in women, adolescents, and young adults.[14,15]

Pathophysiology

Thyroid neoplasms include papillary, follicular, medullary, and anaplastic tumors. Papillary and follicular tumors arise from the follicle, medullary tumors from parafollicular cells, and anaplastic tumors arise from differentiated papillary or follicular tumors. Prognosis and therapy decisions are mainly related to whether the tumor is well or poorly differentiated.[4]

Papillary and Follicular Tumors

Papillary carcinomas include tumors consisting only of papillary cells and those consisting of mixed papillary and follicular cells, which behave similarly. Papillary tumors usually are multifocal and infiltrate local tissues, and 40% of patients have regional lymph node metastases at time of diagnosis.[14] Vascular invasion and metastasis to distant site, such as bone and lung, are more common in papillary tumors than in follicular tumors. Women are three times more likely than men to develop papillary carcinomas, which constitute 60%–70% of the thyroid malignancies in adults and children.[7] Papillary carcinomas are typically well differentiated, indolent, and have a good prognosis. However, males and older patients more often have aggressive tumors.[11,14] Patients may survive for decades even when they have metastatic disease.

Follicular thyroid cancer, which comprises approximately 20% of all cases, is more aggressive than papillary cancer. Age, tumor size, and blood vessel invasion are significant prognostic indicators.[16] Follicular cancer is most often diagnosed in persons in their fifties, but those younger than age 40 have the best prognosis.[6,11] Indicators of poor prognosis include large tumor size (> 6 cm) and blood vessel invasion. Hürthle cell carcinoma, which is a subtype of follicular carcinoma that occurs in older persons, may retain the ability to synthesize thyroid hormones and thus cause hyperthyroidism.[10,11]

Medullary Tumors

Medullary thyroid carcinomas (MTC) constitute 5%–10% of all thyroid neoplasm and occur equally in men and women older than age 50.[6] Eighty percent of cases of MTC are sporadic, while the remainder occur because of an inherited gene mutation that increases susceptibility for multiple endocrine neoplasia (MEN).[10,17] Fifty percent of patients have tumor spread to their cervical lymph nodes at time of diagnosis.[6,11] Regional lymph node spread is an ominous prognostic sign; ten-year survival is only 42% in patients with involved lymph nodes but is 90% in patients with negative regional lymph nodes. MTC tumors metastasize via the bloodstream and lymphatics to lung, liver, and bone.

Anaplastic Tumors

Five to ten percent of thyroid malignancies are anaplastic.[6,10,11,14] These tumors grow "explosively," and patients typically present with a rapidly growing firm or hard, ill-defined neck mass (because of invasion or extension into neck structures), dysphagia, and dysphonia. Males and females have approximately equal risk, and are usually in their sixties when an anaplastic tumor is diagnosed.[18] Completely resectable tumors have the best prognosis, but unfortunately this is not the usual case and most patients live for only 4–12 months following diagnosis. Metastatic sites may include lymph nodes, bone, and lung.[19] Radiation therapy and chemotherapy do not significantly alter survival rates, which are 1.0–7.1% at five years.[18]

Clinical Manifestations

Thyroid malignancies often do not cause symptoms until the disease is advanced. The patient may seek medical attention when they or someone else notices that their neck looks larger, or because a neck mass becomes painful and is noticeably enlarging. In other instances, local symptoms such as recent-onset dysphagia, dysphonia, or hoarseness may lead to seeking out medical attention.[20] A manifestation unique to MTC is diarrhea, which occurs in approximately 20%–30% of patients, secondary to hypersecretion of calcitonin by their tumor.[6]

Assessment

Diagnostic procedures for thyroid malignancies include history and physical examination, laboratory tests and imaging procedures (in some instances), and biopsy to confirm the diagnosis. The history may provide clues to the diagnosis, especially information about radiation exposure to the neck in early childhood. A thorough family history is important, especially if familial MTC or MEN2 is suspected.

At presentation, young patients with thyroid masses most often have painless anterior cervical adenopathy, whereas older individuals usually have regional lymph node metastasis, or rarely, distant metastasis.[21] Thyroid masses are commonly found by patients themselves or by an examiner during routine physical examination. Gentle palpation of the normal neck reveals thyroid lobes that are small, smooth, and free of nodules, and a thyroid that freely rises with swallowing. Any deviations from normal require further investigation.

Thyroid function tests are not included as part of the workup for thyroid cancer because most tumors do not alter the thyroid's functional capacity. One exception is elevated serum calcitonin levels, which are strongly suggestive of medullary hyperplasia or MTC.[22] Medullary tumor cells continue to secrete calcitonin, which may be a useful tumor marker to monitor the effectiveness of treatment and disease recurrence.[11] Postoperative calcitonin levels correlate with survival, and normalization is associated with long-term (as long as 15 years), complication-free survival. Patients whose calcitonin does not normalize survive for less than five years and often have extensive metastases.[17] Carcinoembryonic antigen (CEA) levels are occasionally elevated in MTC, but not other cell types. Current research is focusing on identifying other biochemical markers or gene mutations that might aid in the workup of thyroid tumors. For instance, *p53* status and MUC1 may in the future assist clinicians to determine the diagnosis and extent of disease.[23,24]

Ultrasonography or radionuclide scanning alone cannot distinguish benign and malignant nodules, but these or other imaging procedures—computerized tomography (CT), magnetic resonance imaging (MRI), positron emission tomography (PET)—may provide useful diagnostic information regarding primary or metastatic disease.[25] Ultrasonography, which distinguishes cystic, solid, and mixed lesions, is safe for children and pregnant women because it does not use ionizing radiation. Radionuclide scans following injection of radioiodine (usually ^{123}I) or technetium (^{99m}Tc) are used to visualize the thyroid. A suspicious nodule can trap and incorporate iodine, while ^{99m}Tc can only demonstrate a nodule's ability to trap iodine. However, ^{99m}Tc may be more sensitive than ^{131}I to identify metastatic lesions.[26] Most malignant nodules are nonfunctional and scan "cold," but a small percentage of functional (hot) nodules also prove to be malignant on biopsy.[27]

A patient who is discovered to have a thyroid nodule may receive a trial of TSH-suppressive drugs because these agents may cause benign nodules to shrink but will have no effect on malignant nodules.[10] The drugs, however, have adverse effects and suppression of growth does not guarantee the nodule is benign. Thus, biopsy and histopathologic examination of tumor tissue are ultimately necessary and fine-needle aspirate and biopsy (FNA) is the procedure of choice to confirm thyroid malignancy.[28,29] When done by an experienced and proficient surgeon, FNA biopsy is highly sensitive and accurately diagnoses thyroid malignancy 95% of the time. Under these circumstances, the false-negative rate is only 5%–10%. FNA thus helps eliminate unnecessary surgery for benign lesions and allows appropriate treatment when a malignant tumor is found. If the FNA is negative, it may be repeated with ultrasound guidance to confirm that the lesion is indeed benign.[30] Other advantages of FNA are that it is relatively inexpensive, can be performed in the outpatient setting, causes minimal complications, and sufficient tissue is obtained for DNA analysis, which may provide further information about the malignant potential of the tumor.

Classification and Staging

Histologic diagnosis and age are the two most important determinants of prognosis, which are incorporated into the American Joint Committee on Cancer (AJCC) staging system for thyroid cancer (Table 52-1).[31] Prognosis is most favorable for patients younger than age 40 whose tumors have not invaded local structures or blood vessels.[4]

Therapeutic Approaches and Nursing Care

Surgery

Treatment decisions regarding thyroid tumors are controversial, and complicated by the fact that most tumors are indolent. Because of this protracted clinical course, some

Table 52-1   AJCC TNM Staging for Thyroid Carcinomas

PRIMARY TUMOR (T)

All categories may be subdivided: (a) solitary; (b) multifocal tumor (the largest determines classification)

TX	Primary tumor cannot be assessed
T0	No evidence of primary tumor
T1	Tumor 1 cm or less in greatest dimension limited to the thyroid
T2	Tumor more than 1 cm but not more than 4 cm limited to the thyroid
T3	Tumor more than 4 cm in greatest dimension limited to the thyroid
T4	Tumor of any size extending beyond the thyroid capsule

REGIONAL LYMPH NODES (N)

Regional nodes are cervical and upper mediastinal lymph nodes

NX	Regional lymph nodes cannot be assessed
N0	No regional lymph node metastasis
N1	Regional lymph node metastasis
N1a	Metastasis in ipsilateral cervical lymph node(s)
N1b	Metastasis in bilateral, midline, or contralateral cervical or midiastinal lymph nodes

DISTANT METASTASIS (M)

MX	Presence of distant metastasis cannot be assessed
M0	No distant metastasis
M1	Distant metastasis

STAGING GROUPING

Papillary or Follicular

	Under 45 Years	45 Years and Over
Stage I	Any T, Any N, M0	T1, N0, M0
Stage II	Any T, Any N, M1	T2, N0, M0
		T3, N0, M0
Stage III		T4, N0, M0
Stage IV		Any T, Any N, M1

	Medullary	Undifferentiated
Stage I	T1, N0, M0	All cases are classified as Stage IV
Stage II	T2, N0, M0	**Stage IV** Any T, Any N, Any M
	T3, N0, M0	
	T4, N0, M0	
Stage III	Any T, N1, M0	
Stage IV	Any T, Any N, M1	

clinicians do not recommend treatment until the patient is symptomatic.[10] Surgery is the agreed upon treatment of choice for thyroid tumors, but there is no consensus regarding the extent of surgical resection for well-differentiated tumors. Studies comparing total, subtotal, and partial thyroidectomy have found that subtotal resection of tumors less than 1 cm in patients under age 45 results in similar recurrence and survival rates as more extensive surgery.[4,10,21] The risk of surgical complications is lower with lobectomy, but the risk for recurrence is 5%–10% higher than with total resection of the thyroid. When cure is possible, more aggressive surgery (near total thyroidectomy, tumor resection, and neck dissection) has been advocated for medullary and anaplastic tumors.[20]

Table 52-2 summarizes recommended therapeutic approaches in the management of thyroid tumors.

Postoperative complications of thyroidectomy include recurrent laryngeal nerve paralysis, vocal cord paralysis with subsequent respiratory embarrassment, thyroid storm, hemorrhage, and hypothyroidism.[32,33] Thyroid storm, or thyrotoxic crisis, is an acute episode of thyroid overactivity that is characterized by high fever, tachycardia, delirium, dehydration, and extreme excitability. Patients may experience temporary postoperative hoarseness, which is related to intubation and local swelling. Permanent hoarseness is rare but more serious, and is caused by damage to the laryngeal nerve during surgery that leads to vocal cord paralysis. Hemorrhage is another possible postoperative complication, so the nurse monitors for local hematoma (which may compromise the patient's airway) as well as for output from drains and symptoms of impending shock.

Postoperative nursing management also requires keen assessment for the signs and symptoms of tetany, for hypocalcemia, and for other complications (Table 52-3).[33–35] Calcium levels are monitored daily, because 1% of patients undergoing near-total thyroidectomies and as many as 6%–8% of those undergoing total thyroidectomies experience temporary or permanent hypoparathyroidism.[10,21] Hypothyroidism results in hypocalcemia, so patients must take exogenous thyroid hormone to prevent the clinical effects of hypothyroidism. Supraphysiologic doses of oral thyroxine are administered to suppress endogenous production of TSH, which is thought to be a growth factor for thyroid tumors.[32]

Radiation Therapy

Radioiodine therapy is used to treat some cases of papillary and follicular tumors but not medullary or anaplastic tumors, which do not concentrate and retain iodine. Four to six weeks after surgery, oral ^{131}I is administered to ablate any remaining functioning thyroid tissue, as well as residual local and metastatic tumor. A whole body scan is done two to three months after treatment to determine whether any tumor and functioning thyroid tissue remain, and is repeated at four- to six-month intervals as necessary.[6] If any tumor remains, ^{131}I is repeated until the whole body scan is negative.

Side effects of ^{131}I include nausea and vomiting, fatigue, headache, bone marrow suppression, salivary gland inflammation, and infrequently leukemia and radiation-induced pulmonary fibrosis.[36] Nursing care focuses on minimizing the patient's sense of isolation and providing radiation safety for staff and visitors. Patient and family education is extremely important to clarify misconceptions regarding ^{131}I treatment. (Figure 52-1)

External beam radiation occasionally results in local control of anaplastic tumors that do not take up ^{131}I, but tumors are usually radioresistant.[37] A clear indication for external beam radiation is to palliate painful bone metastases. In addition, there is only one report of successful

Table 52-2 Recommended Treatment Approaches for Thyroid Tumors

Tumor Type	Recommended Surgery	Comments	Postoperative
Papillary and follicular		Choice of surgery is based on age and size of nodule	Exogenous thyroid hormone (thyroxine) therapy is administered to suppress TSH
Stage I	Lobectomy	Lower incidence of complications Abnormal lymph nodes are biopsied and selectively resected	Papillary: [131]I may decrease recurrence
Stage II	Total thyroidectomy	5%–10% local recurrence Higher incidence of hypoparathyroidism Facilitates follow-up thyroid scanning	Follicular: Remaining disease may compromise effectiveness of ^{131}I ablative therapy
Stage III	Total thyroidectomy or lobectomy	See above	Local radiation therapy may be used to control symptoms
Stage IV	Total thyroidectomy and removal of lymph nodes/extrathyroid disease	See above	Patients are monitored for metastasis to lung and bone
			Treatment for metastases: [131]I, external beam radiation therapy, TSH suppression
Medullary	Total thyroidectomy with modified neck dissection if extrathyroidal disease present, unless patient has distant metastasis	Surgery is curative when disease is confined to the thyroid	Chemotherapy leads to occasional responses in metastatic disease
Anaplastic	Total thyroidectomy to reduce mass-induced symptoms	Tracheostomy is often necessary	Radiation therapy may be used for patients whose tumors are not surgically resectable or who cannot undergo surgery
			Chemotherapy may induce partial responses in some patients

Data from National Cancer Institute[4] and AACE.[32]

treatment with combined radiotherapy and chemotherapy.[38]

Chemotherapy

There are very few reports of chemotherapy for refractory, metastatic, and anaplastic thyroid cancers, and the results are generally discouraging. Doxorubicin has shown the greatest activity against thyroid malignancies.[39,40] Response rates vary, ranging from 14% to about 31% for anaplastic tumors and well-differentiated medullary tumors, respectively. Combination therapy with fluorouracil (5-FU) plus streptozotocin or dacarbazine for patients with metastatic medullary thyroid cancer resulted in partial responses or long-term stabilization of disease in 17 of 20 patients.[41] These agents may thus warrant further investigation.

PARATHYROID TUMORS

The parathyroid glands are located on the posterior thyroid, and lie at the surface or are imbedded in the thyroid. Most people have four glands, but the normal range is two to eight. Chief cells are the major functional cells of the parathyroid glands and produce parathyroid hormone (PTH), which is critical to maintain normal serum calcium balance. PTH is secreted to increase calcium resorption from bone when serum calcium is low; when the serum calcium level is high, it is not secreted.[42]

Epidemiology

More than 95% of parathyroid tumors are benign.[43] Carcinomas account for less than 0.1%–5% of primary hyperparathyroidism, and the literature regarding malignant parathyroid tumors is limited to case reports and small series.[44,45] Tumors occur equally in males and females, who are usually diagnosed in their forties and fifties.[8,43–45] Parathyroid tumors most commonly occur in individuals who have familial MEN1, and less frequently to MEN2A.[7]

Etiology

No definitive risk factors have been identified for the development of parathyroid carcinoma.[43] For instance, only rare individuals diagnosed with parathyroid adenoma or carcinoma have received radiation to or near the neck area.[46] One suggestion proposes a relationship between parathyroid carcinoma and chronic hypocalcemia caused by renal insufficiency, hypovitaminosis D, malabsorption of calcium in the gut, or PTH resistance.[7]

Table 52-3   Care Plan for Patient Undergoing Thyroid Surgery

Problem/Diagnosis	Nursing Observations/Actions	Comments
Potential for ineffective airway clearance related to: • Hematoma • Vocal cord paralysis	Assess respiratory status every hour for 12 hours, then every 4 hours for 48 hours Assess vital signs every 4 hours for 48 hours Observe for: • Hoarseness • Inability to speak • Retraction of neck muscles • Crowing respirations • Dyspnea • Cyanosis • Hematoma formation Keep head of bed elevated to > 45 degrees at all times Maintain neck support by placing hand behind neck with elbows raised when moving or sitting Turn, cough, and deep breathe every two hours	Notify MD immediately for: • Signs and symptoms of vocal cord paralysis • Respiratory distress • Patient reports of neck tightness, fullness, or pressure (indicates possible internal bleeding)
Potential for decreased serum calcium level related to impaired parathyroid function, secondary to removal or reimplantation	Observe for signs and symptoms of tetany every 4 hours for 7 days Monitor daily serum calcium Administer calcium gluconate, as ordered Teach patient to avoid foods that suppress calcium absorption (e.g., spinach, Swiss cheese, beets, bran, and whole grain cereals)	Symptoms of hypocalemia: • Numbness, tingling, cramps in extremities or around mouth • Stiffness, twitching, or spasms in hands or feet • Positive Chvostek sign • Positive Trousseau sign
Potential for thyrotoxic crisis (thyroid storm) related to partial thyroidectomy	Observe patient for signs and symptoms of thyroid storm every 4 hours In case of thyroid storm administer: • Prescribed IV fluid, vitamins, and glucocorticoid • Prescribed antithyroid medication (propylthiouracil) • Prescribed iodine medication Employ measures to reduce body temperature, such as cooling blanket, tepid sponge bath	Manifestations of thyroid storm: • Sudden increase in temperature • Extreme restlessness or irritability • Delirium • Tachycardia • Widening pulse pressure followed by hypotension • Nausea and vomiting, diarrhea, and warm, flushed skin Notify MD immediately if temperature rises to > 99°F orally or 100°F rectally (may be first sign of thyroid storm)

Data from Moore and Haughey,[33] Lehne,[34] and Giarelli.[35]

Pathophysiology

It is often difficult to establish that a tumor is benign or malignant, or even hyperplasia, because all appear histopathologically similar. However, adenomas usually involve only one parathyroid gland and are surrounded by a rim of normal parathyroid tissue. Hyperplasia occurs in multiple glands, while carcinomas may have more mitoses and may be surrounded by a thick and irregular capsule.[47] Ultimately, local infiltration, invasion into blood vessels, and metastases characterize malignant tumors. When discovered, carcinomas may be hard, lobulated, and larger than benign tumors, and 50% will have invaded adjacent structures.[48] Both benign and malignant parathyroid tumors are usually biochemically functional and hypersecrete PTH, which leads to hypercalcemia.[44]

Carcinomas tend to be indolent, so tumors may be discovered late. Recurrence of local disease can occur soon after surgical resection, but metastases can occur as long as 30 years after the initial diagnosis.[49] The recurrence of hypercalcemia or elevated serum PTH after sur-

What is ¹³¹I?

¹³¹I is radioactive iodine that goes to the thyroid gland and thyroid cancer cells. It is toxic to these cells, and the aim of treatment is to kill cancer cells. It will also kill normal thyroid cells.

Where will I go to get the ¹³¹I treatment?

You will have to go to the hospital to get this treatment. While in the hospital, you will wear only hospital gowns, robe, and slippers. Do not bring things from home.

How will I take the ¹³¹I?

You will be given a special container of ¹³¹I, and you will drink it through a straw.

Will I be able to have visitors while I am in the hospital?

You may have adult visitors while you are in the hospital, but because you will be radioactive there are some rules:

1. No pregnant women can visit.
2. Visitors will only be able to stay for 30 minutes or less for the first 48 hours.

Will I have any side effects from the ¹³¹I?

Possible side effects may include nausea and vomiting, tiredness, headache, a sore mouth, and a lowered white blood count after you get the treatment. Your nurse will give you medicine for the nausea or the headache if you have them, and your doctor may want you to get a blood test after you go home. You may also have a metallic taste in your mouth for several days after taking ¹³¹I.

Will I still be radioactive when I go home?

Yes, you will be radioactive for a few days. For three days after you go home, you should:

1. Sleep alone.
2. Not hold children close.

How can I help my body get rid of the ¹³¹I?

You need to drink as much fluid as you can (at least 2 quarts) for several days after getting the ¹³¹I. This can include water, juices, sodas, and so forth. The ¹³¹I will pass out of your body in your urine, so when you go to the bathroom you should:

1. Sit on the toilet to urinate so urine does not splash anywhere.
2. Flush the toilet three times after you pass urine.

How will my doctor know if the thyroid cancer is gone?

Your doctor will schedule you for a body scan in about three to six months. If the scan shows that there aren't any more thyroid cancer cells, you will not need any more ¹³¹I. If there are any thyroid cancer cells that show up on the scan, you will get another ¹³¹I treatment.

If you have any other questions, please write them down so you remember to ask your doctor or your nurse.

Figure 52-1 Teaching sheet for the patient receiving ¹³¹I treatment.

gery signals that a tumor, which may have been diagnosed as benign, is malignant. When parathyroid carcinoma is diagnosed, 20% of patients have cervical lymph node metastases and 16% have distant metastases—most commonly to the lungs, bone, or liver.[48]

Clinical Manifestations

Symptoms of hypercalcemic effects on the kidney, bone, and other organs and sometimes a palpable neck mass or hoarseness are manifestations of a parathyroid tumor. Typically, a patient's serum calcium is greater than 14 mg/dL (3.5 mmol/L).[8,43,44] Approximately 40% of patients have a palpable neck mass, while fewer than 10% have hoarseness when diagnosed.[43] Prolonged hypercalcemia may lead to rheumatologic symptoms, renal calculi, and calcification of the cornea and other soft tissues. In addition, patients may have neuromuscular, gastrointestinal (GI), and cardiovascular manifestations of moderate to severe hypercalcemia.

Assessment

The pathognomic signs and symptoms essentially confirm the diagnosis of parathyroid tumor. The patient may initially notice nonspecific symptoms such as fatigue, irritability, and difficulty concentrating. In some cases, these progress to symptoms of worsening hypercalcemia, which are characterized by nausea, anorexia, weight loss, and dehydration.[50]

When unexplained hypercalcemia is discovered, a search for parathyroid carcinoma begins with immunoassay for immunoassayable parathyroid hormone (iPTH). In the case of parathyroid tumor, levels are usually markedly increased.[51] The majority of patients do not have a palpable mass, so visualization procedures (ultrasonography, nuclear scan, CT, and MRI) are used to localize and evaluate tumor masses after surgery.[52] For instance, a 99m-technetium sestamibi (MIBI) radionuclide scan can aid in determining whether disease is confined to one or more glands, which may direct the extent of surgery.[53] Radiographs or bone scans are useful to confirm bone metastases, which occur in about 50% of patients.[51] Soft tissue radiography of the finger bones may be done, because subperiosteal bone resorption occurs in hyperparathyroid carcinoma. FNA to confirm the diagnosis before surgery is not recommended because of the risk of tumor spillage and local spread. Research continues to find more effective measures to confirm that a parathyroid tumor is malignant. For example, one recent study found that the expression of p27 is greatly reduced in carcinomas as compared to hyperplasia and benign adenomas.[47] It is likely that p27 is a tumor suppressor gene, which codes for a cyclin-dependent kinase that regulates the progression of a cell from G1 to the S phase of cell division. Assaying for reduced levels might therefore be useful in diagnosis.

Therapeutic Approaches and Nursing Care

Surgery

Surgery is the recommended treatment for parathyroid tumors, but even radical surgery may not change the course of the disease.[44] This is because the tumor's intrinsic biologic behavior is the most important prognostic determinant.[52] Radiotherapy and chemotherapy are ineffective to treat primary and metastatic disease.

The primary tumor is resected en bloc with the ipsilateral thyroid lobe and isthmus. The surgeon is careful to avoid rupture of the parathyroid capsule, which may result in local seeding of tumor.[43] Surgery for localized parathyroid adenomas and carcinomas may include unilateral neck dissection if local structures are involved.[52] Extensive surgery may be necessary to remove all tumor from the trachea, involved central lymph nodes, and any contiguous tissues to which the tumor adheres.[8,44] If the recurrent laryngeal nerve is involved, this too must be resected. Parathyroid tumors are usually indolent, and patients typically benefit from further resection of metastatic disease, such as lung metastases.[54] Recurrent disease is rarely curable.

The focus of postoperative nursing care is to monitor calcium levels, prevent hemorrhage, and teach the patient and family self-care management (see Table 52-3). After surgery, "hungry bone" syndrome—in which calcium and phosphorus are rapidly deposited into bone and symptomatic *hypocalcemia* occurs[44]—is evidence of successful tumor removal. The patient requires supplemental intravenous calcium and calcitrol until the remaining parathyroid glands recover. Serum calcium and PTH levels are monitored every three months for elevation, which signify recurrent local or metastatic disease. Hemorrhage is another potential and serious complication, particularly for patients undergoing parathyroid reexploration surgery.[55]

Chemotherapy

Parathyroid malignancy is so rare that there are no reported chemotherapy studies, but a few case reports document limited success and remissions of metastatic disease.[56,57] Combination regimens—including 5-FU, cyclophosphamide, and dacarbazine; or methotrexate, doxorubicin, cyclophosphamide, and lomustine—have been used. Overall, however, chemotherapy has been judged ineffective for parathyroid carcinomas. One potential pharmacologic method to decrease PTH production may be to immunize the patient with the bioactive portion of human and bovine PTH protein. A single case reported that a terminally ill patient who had exhausted standard therapy experienced rapid reversal of symptoms (confusion, anorexia, bone pain, immobility, and nausea and vomiting), as well as a decline in serum calcium from 14 mg/dL (3.5 mmol/L) to 10.1 mg/dL (2.52 mmol/L) after immunization.[58] The proposed mechanism of response was that the patient's immune system made antibodies to human and bovine PTH.

Palliative Care

Control of hypercalcemia in patients with parathyroid tumors is often difficult because it is caused by tumor recurrence. When surgery is not feasible, recurrent hypercalcemia is treated with the same drugs used to treat other instances of hypercalcemia. Calcitonin, bisphosphonates, or other antiresorptive therapies may be partially effective for a limited time, but calcium levels may remain persistently elevated despite attempts to inhibit the effects of tumor PTH.[8,43,44] Chronic, uncontrolled hypercalcemia, which leads to uncontrollable nausea, vomiting, and dehydration, remains the cause of death in most patients.

PITUITARY TUMORS

The pituitary, a 1-cm organ, lies at the base of the brain in the sella turcica, a bony cavity in sphenoid bone. It consists of the anterior and the posterior pituitary, which are anatomically and physiologically distinct. The anterior pituitary cells are hormone secreting or nonsecreting cells. Secreting cells differ, and each synthesizes a different hormone that controls the physiologic function of the thyroid, adrenal glands, gonads, or mammary glands. Secreting cells give rise to pituitary tumors.[59] The anterior pituitary also controls growth by secreting trophic hormones, including thyroid stimulating hormone (TSH), adrenocorticotropin, prolactin, and growth hormone (GH). TSH controls the rate of thyroxine secretion by the thyroid, adrenocorticotropin controls some adrenocortical hormones, prolactin promotes breast tissue development and milk production, and GH promotes growth and affects multiple metabolic processes. Secretion of trophic hormones is regulated by negative feedback loops that are influenced by the target organs and by the CNS, particularly the hypothalamus, which is connected to and communicates with the pituitary by the pituitary stalk. The hypothalamus plays a critical role in pituitary function by secreting releasing and inhibitory hormones that are carried through the hypothalamic-hypophysial portal vessels directly to the pituitary. Nonsecreting cells synthesize cytokines, which may play roles in regulating hypothalamo-pituitary-adrenal axis functions and in infection.[60]

Epidemiology

Approximately 10% of brain tumors are pituitary tumors.[61–63] These tumors usually remain small and hormonally silent incidentalomas, and as many as 11% of individuals are discovered to have an incidentaloma at autopsy or upon CT or MRI scans done for other reasons.[60] Female-to-male incidence varies by tumor type. Women are four times more likely than men to develop a prolactinoma, and are at three times greater risk to develop Cushing's disease, but acromegaly occurs equally in women and men.[61,62] Seventy percent of pituitary adenomas occur in persons age 30–50, but these tumors can also develop in children and teenagers.[64]

Etiology

The pathogenesis of pituitary tumors is unknown. Studies have shown that most pituitary tumors are monoclonal in origin, that is, they arise from repeated division of a single mutated cell, which probably arises from some key somatic mutation.[65] A pituitary tumor transforming gene (PTTG) has recently been cloned and is thought to play a role in tumorigenesis and progression.[66] PTTG is expressed in some nonfunctioning and functioning pituitary tumors, but not in normal pituitary tissues, and may thus be a useful marker for pituitary tumor aggressiveness. Many genetic mutations in tumor suppressor genes and oncogenes have been identified in pituitary tumors, which demonstrates that pituitary tumorigenesis is a multistep process. These alterations accumulate, causing tumors to become increasingly aggressive over time.[67] For example, mutations in the p53 gene are found only in invasive pituitary adenomas and carcinomas.[68] This is consistent with findings in other malignancies, in which p53 mutation is a late event that signifies a higher degree of malignancy.

Pathophysiology

Most pituitary tumors are localized, benign adenomas and are incapable of metastasizing. Adenomas consist of transformed cells and grow by expansion to cause mass effects. In addition, both benign and malignant tumors usually express altered gene products for neurotransmitters and hypothalamic hormones that cause physiological effects. True pituitary carcinomas, that is, malignant tumors that have the ability to metastasize, are rare.[69] Carcinomas may invade the subarachnoid space and metastasize to the brain and spinal cord through lymphatic or vascular channel, and to the liver and bone through the cervical lymphatics.[70]

Clinical Manifestations

In most cases, the signs and symptoms of pituitary adenomas result from secretion or depression of particular hormones, and to mass effects in fewer instances. A variety of tumors can arise, so a corresponding number of syndromes may occur. These relate to the hypersecretion of prolactin, growth hormone, adrenocorticotropic hormone (ACTH), or less commonly, to other hormones. Because prolactinomas arise most frequently, oligo- or amenorrhea, and galactorrhea are the most frequent hormone effects documented.[71] The most frequent symptoms of mass effects include headaches in 40%–60% of patients and visual changes (e.g., blurred vision, loss of peripheral vision or changes in particular visual fields, double vision, changes in visual acuity) in 60%.[64,71,72]

Hormone Effects

Prolactinomas. Prolactinomas constitute 60% of all functioning pituitary tumors.[63] Women are more likely to have small tumors (microadenomas), which cause galactorrhea, menstrual irregularities including amenorrhea, oligomenorrhea, or infertility, and in some instances osteoporosis. Men are more likely to have large tumors (macroadenomas), and high prolactin levels produced by the same tumor cause men to have decreased libido or impotence, and in some cases galactorrhea.[61,63] Women tend to notice their symptoms and seek medical attention earlier than men, who may attribute symptoms to advancing age.

Growth hormone-secreting tumors. Almost all cases of growth hormone GH-secreting tumors arise in the pituitary. These tumors induce acromegaly in adults and gigantism in prepubescent children. GH-secreting tumors progress slowly, and the average time from onset of symptoms to diagnosis is 6.5 years and may be as long as 10 years.[63,73] Early symptoms are nonspecific and include fatigue or lethargy, paresthesia, and headache. As tumors enlarge, excessive GH leads to enlargement of bone, organs, and soft tissues.[73] The result is arthropathies and neuropathies (from soft tissue swelling) that interfere with normal activities, and the characteristic disfigurement of the face (Figure 52-2). Other signs and symptoms include weight gain, excessive perspiration, insulin resistance, and decreased glucose tolerance leading to diabetes.[61,74] Cardiovascular disease, hypertension, upper airway obstruction, sleep apnea, and GI malignancy shorten life expectancy, and mortality is two to three times higher than in age-matched individuals.[63] Death often results from cardiac complications, cerebrovascular accidents, or infection.[73]

Cushing's syndrome. Sustained hypersecretion of ACTH by a pituitary adenoma is the major cause of Cushing's syndrome, resulting in 70%–80% of all cases.[75] The most frequent manifestations of Cushing's syndrome include the characteristic moon face, experienced by more than 90% of affected individuals, and 80%–90% have truncal obesity, hypertension, impaired glucose tolerance, and hypogonadism (menstrual irregularities, loss of libido) (Figure 52-3).[75,76] Other common symptoms in severe Cushing's syndrome include congestive heart failure (CHF), purple striae, muscular weakness, pedal edema, skeletal pain, and psychological changes.[61,77] In addition, women may also develop hirsutism. Less common symptoms are easy bruising, infection, poor wound healing, osteoporosis and fractures, polyuria, polydipsia, and renal calculi.

The onset of symptoms of Cushing's syndrome is often subtle, so there is usually a long period between symptom onset and diagnosis. Patients are often treated for individual symptoms such as obesity, menstrual irregularities, or depression before the pattern of symptoms is noted.[76] Cushing's is a severe disease, even if caused by a benign adenoma. As many as 50% of patients will die within five

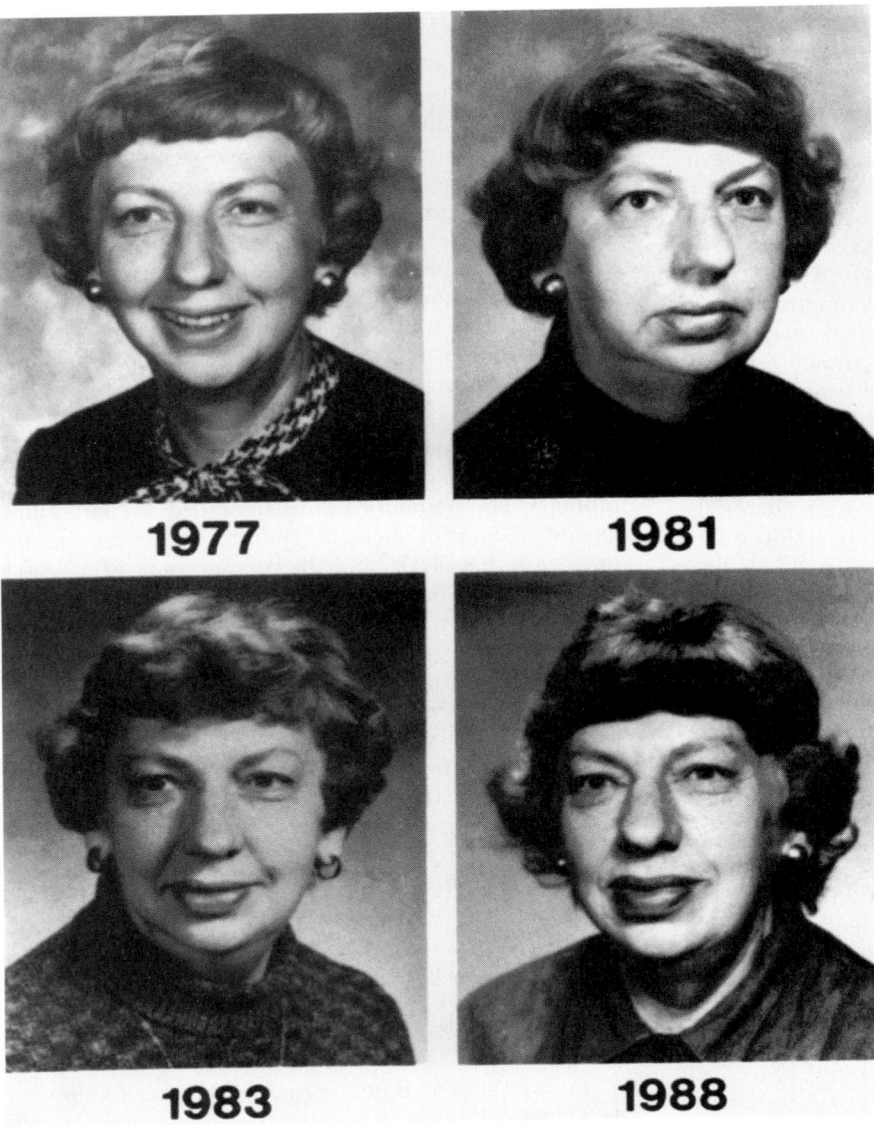

Figure 52-2 A 64-year-old woman with acromegaly. Photographs reveal gradual changes over 11 years. At the time she presented to a physician, she also had hypertension, arthropathy, and enlargement of her hands. (Reprinted with permission from Molitch ME: Clinical manifestations of acromegaly. *Endocrinol Metab Clin North Am* 21:597–614, 1992.)[73]

1977

1981

1983

1988

years from cardiovascular disease, infection, or suicide secondary to severe depression if treatment is not instituted.

Mass Effects

Many critical structures surround the sella turcica, and if the tumor enlarges beyond the sella or erodes bony structure to spread into the paracellar region, mass effects occur.[64,77] Tumors most commonly extend into the optic chiasm, which leads to compression of the optic nerve with resultant bilateral visual field loss that often begins with the superior temporal quadrants. If cranial nerves III, IV, and VI are compressed by lateral tumor extension, extraocular muscle function abnormalities, such as diplopia, may occur. Tumor extension superiorly through the diaphragm sellae may cause compression of the hypothalamus, pituitary stalk, or normal pituitary, leading to hypopituitarism.

Compression of the pituitary stalk leads to altered anterior pituitary control and sequential loss of hormone secretion, which begins with GH or the gonadotropins, luteinizing hormone and follicle stimulating hormone, followed by depressions of TSH and corticotropin.[61,77] The end result is hormone insufficiency. Altered secretion of posterior pituitary hormones causes increased appetite, diabetes insipidus (DI), or other effects.[64]

Enlargement beyond the sella can cause signs of increased intracranial pressure, headache, seizures, or cerebrospinal fluid (CSF) rhinorrhea. A rare cause of hypopituitarism is pituitary apoplexy, which occurs with hemorrhage into a large tumor. Infarction occurs, and may cause sudden headache, nausea, vomiting, loss of visual fields, blurred vision or even complete loss of vision, and altered level of consciousness.[78,79] Prompt surgical decompression may reverse neurologic problems and restore partial pituitary function.

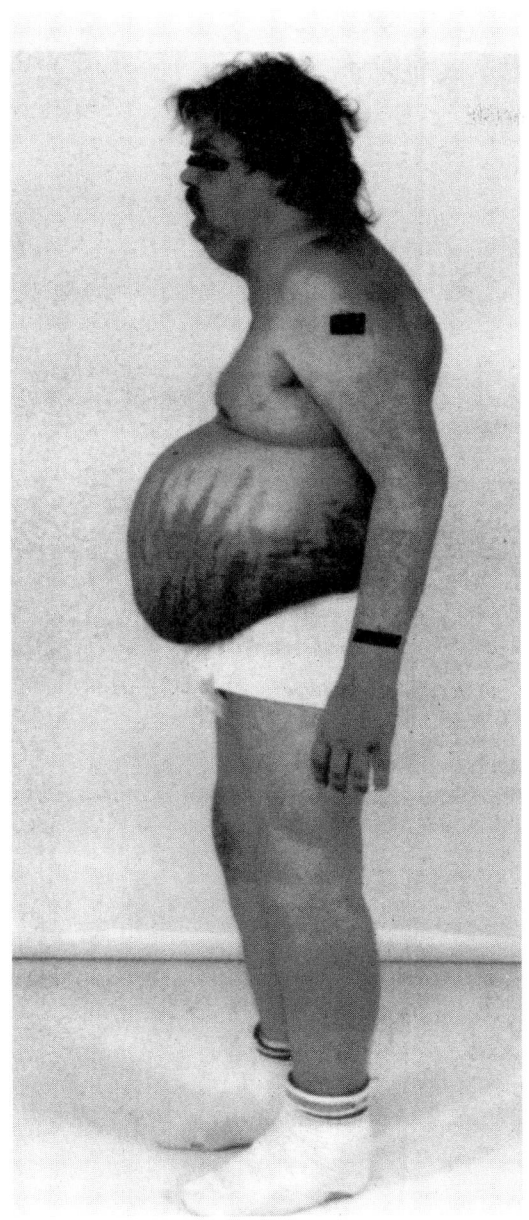

Figure 52-3 Side view of a patient with Cushing's syndrome. Note protuberant abdomen, marked abdominal striae, and buffalo hump. (Reprinted with permission from Gumowski J, Proch M, Kessler CA: Endocrinopathies of hyperfunction: Cushing's syndrome and aldosteronism. *AACN Clin Issues Crit Care Nurs* 3:331–347, 1992.)[75]

Assessment

Confirmation of a pituitary tumor includes the history and physical examination, endocrinologic testing, radiologic findings, and histopathologic examination. Because most pituitary tumors progress slowly, the history focuses on identifying subtle changes that have occurred over a long period.[69] The medication history is also important because many drugs, including dopamine antagonist antiemetics, tricyclic antidepressants, opioids, and antihypertensives, as well as physical conditions (e.g., chronic renal failure, cirrhosis, hypothyroidism, and exercise) can elevate serum prolactin, but to a lesser degree than elevations induced by tumors.[80,81] Physical examination includes testing of peripheral visual fields and cranial nerve function.

Diagnostic procedures for all patients with suspected pituitary tumor focuses on tests for the most frequent tumors, and may also include evaluation of gonadal, thyroid, and adrenal functioning. Thus prolactinomas are assessed at baseline and after therapy by serum prolactin levels.[63] In women, gonadal function evaluation includes luteinizing hormone, follicle stimulating hormone, and plasma estradiol, whereas plasma testosterone is assessed in men. When indicated, thyroid function tests, including T_3, T_4, and TSH are checked, and adrenal functioning is evaluated by sampling basal plasma or urinary steroids. More specific tests for stimulation and suppression of pituitary hormones are done in some cases to detect tumors and to evaluate response to therapy (Table 52-4).[61,73,77,82,83]

Radiologic tests may confirm abnormalities in and about the pituitary. Plain radiographs of the head can show only gross enlargement of the sella turcica. MRI and/or CT more clearly demonstrate in three dimensions the tumor size and extension preoperatively and after surgery.[63] Some tumors, such as those that cause Cushing's, may be so small as to elude detection. PET may also be useful to evaluate pituitary tumors.

Classification and Staging

Pituitary adenomas are classified by the hormone secreted, secretory ability, size, and invasiveness.[62] Most tumors are functioning, and secrete a given hormone and cause the corresponding clinical syndrome. Other tumors do not secrete an excessive amount of hormone, or secrete biologically inactive molecules or hormone precursors, and are thus considered to be nonfunctioning.[77] Prolactinomas are most common and account for 60% of all functioning tumors, GH-secreting tumors (acromegaly) occur in 20%, and ACTH-secreting tumors (Cushing's disease) in 10% of patients. Ten percent of tumors secrete more than one hormone, and 30% of pituitary tumors are nonfunctioning gonadotroph-cell adenomas.[63]

Microadenomas are tumors that are less than 10 mm in diameter, while macroadenomas are larger than 10 mm. Signs and symptoms often predict tumor size. For example, women of childbearing age are more likely to report symptoms of a prolactinoma whereas men may attribute decreased libido to normal aging. Thus women are more likely to have a microadenoma, while macroadenomas are diagnosed more often in men. ACTH-secreting

Table 52-4 Laboratory Tests for Pituitary Tumors

Diagnostic Test/Tumor	Normal Values	Test Procedure	Comments
Glucose tolerance test/ GH-secreting (acromegaly)	• Growth hormone = 2–6 ng/mL (in AM after 8 hr of sleep) • GH suppressed to < 2 ng/m after glucose tolerance test	• Fasting test (do in AM) • Administer 75–100 g of oral glucose (lemon juice may increase palatability) • Blood samples collected 1, 2, and 3 hr later	• In normal individuals GH causes increased blood glucose, which increases resistance to insulin; hypoglycemia leads to GH release and hyperglycemia to GH suppression • Acromegaly: GH not suppressed to < 0.5 mcg within 20–120 minutes • 60% of acromegalics have a paradoxical increase of GH
Urinary excretion of GH/GH-secreting (acromegaly)		• 24-hour urine collection • Store collection bottle in refrigerator to decrease bacterial growth	• Increased in some patients with acromegaly
Plasma insulin-like growth factor 1 (ILGF-1/ Somatomedin C)/GH-secreting (acromegaly)	• Normal values vary in males and females; children, adolescents, and adults	• Blood sample	• Normal values Males: preadolescent 60.8–724 ng/mL, adolescent 112.5–450 ng/mL, adult 141.8–389.3 ng/mL Females: preadolescent 65.5–841 ng/mL, adolescent 83.3–378.5 ng/mL, adult 54.0–328.5 ng/mL
Dexamethasone suppression test/ACTH-secreting (Cushing's syndrome)	• Serum cortisol suppressed to < 5 μ/dL • Fasting, 8 AM–noon, 5–25 μ/dL	• Administer 1 mg po dexamethasone at 11 PM • Draw plasma cortisol at 9 AM the following AM	• In normal individuals increased corticosteroid suppresses ACTH release and subsequently cortisol production • To confirm results, test may be repeated for 3 days while administering larger doses of dexamethasone • Sensitive test, but not specific for tumors only
Urinary free cortisol/ ACTH-secreting tumor	• 20–70 μ/24 hr • 25–95 ng/mg of creatinine	• Give dexamethasone 0.5 mg q 6 hr for 2 days • Then collect 24-hour urine sample (refrigerate)	• More specific than dexamethasone suppression test • Single best screening test for ACTH-secreting tumor • Spironolactone and quinacrine may affect accuracy
Plasma prolactin/ Prolactinoma	• Women (nonlactating): 0.48–0.9 IU/L or 0–15 ng/mL • Values increase during pregnancy • Values increase during lactation • Men: 0–15 ng/mL		• Values < 1 U/L are rarely clinically significant • Values < 2.5 U/L usually indicate nonfunctioning tumor • Values > 6 U/L usually indicate a macropro-lactinoma • Tests repeated because of normal variations in serum prolactin levels

Data from Lamberts,[74] Croughs,[77] and Corbett.[83]

tumors tend to be diagnosed while they are microadeno-mas, whereas 70% of GH-secreting tumors are macroade-nomas. Tumors are also characterized as intrasellar and extrasellar, depending on their ability to expand outside the sella turcica, and as noninvasive or invasive, depending on whether they can infiltrate into the dural and osseous walls.[60,62]

Therapeutic Approaches and Nursing Care

The goals of medical management are to normalize pituitary secretion, alleviate signs and symptoms of hormone hypersecretion, reduce tumor size to relieve compression on vital structures, preserve or restore residual anterior pituitary function, and prevent tumor recurrence.[62,63] The primary treatment approach depends on the tumor type, and may include surgery, radiation therapy, and drug therapy alone or in combination. Treatment decisions are based on the immediacy of need to relieve mass effect or endocrinologic abnormalities, the likelihood of long-term control from a particular therapy, and adverse effects of each therapy. If the tumor is small and not producing excess hormone, the physician may choose to monitor the patient with MRI or CT scans at yearly intervals.[69]

Surgery

Surgery is the treatment of choice for almost all tumors. An exception is prolactinomas, which are usually managed with medications. However, surgical resection is used if a patient is resistant to dopamine antagonists, has an invasive macroadenoma, or is experiencing compromised vision.[63] A potential benefit of surgery for patients with prolactinomas is that their serum prolactin levels will normalize and their symptoms will be alleviated without life-long medication.[84] The primary purposes of surgery are to resect or debulk large tumors compressing vital structures about the sella (optic chiasm or cranial nerves) and to confirm the histologic diagnosis.[69] In other instances surgery is done to evacuate a cyst about the tumor, to decompress a hemorrhagic tumor, or to reduce obstructive hydrocephalus.[77]

The surgical approach used most often is the transsphenoidal procedure, because the tumor can be removed and pituitary function preserved. The neurosurgeon makes an incision behind the upper lip, displaces the maxillary sinus and nasal septum, and then opens the sella and microsurgically resects the tumor (Figure 52-4).[64] The surgeon then packs the sella with adipose tissue harvested from the abdomen or other body site, muscle, and fibrin glue to decrease the risk of CSF leak. The septum and maxillary sinus are then reapproximated and the nares packed. An advantage of transsphenoidal surgery over the transcranial route is that the procedure is usually well-tolerated by elderly patients and those with cardiac or pulmonary disease or diabetes. In addition, body image is preserved because there is no visible scar; risks for infection and bleeding are lower; and the surgery is shorter and less traumatic, so patients are mobilized and discharged from the hospital earlier.[72,85,86]

Radiation Therapy

External beam radiation is used for patients who refuse or who cannot tolerate surgery, for tumor recurrence, in some cases of subtotal resection, or as part of the treatment plan with surgery.[77,87] Radiation plus surgery may increase rates of long-term control of pituitary adeno-

mas.[71] Stereotactic radiation therapy is used in some specialized treatment centers, in which a single fraction is administered directly to the tumor during surgery.[86] In most instances, standard radiation therapy is used and treatment fields are calculated to treat the tumor and minimize scatter to adjacent structures. Usual total doses are 4500–5400 cGy, given in 180- to 200-cGy daily fractions.[71] Lower doses may not control the tumor, and higher total doses or fractions greater than 200 cGy per day are more likely to cause complications. Potential disadvantages of radiation therapy are that a therapeutic effect is achieved too slowly in tumors that secrete excessive hormone, hypopituitarism or injury to the optic nerves/chiasm may occur, and in rare instances there is radiation-induced secondary CNS malignancy.[77] For instance, 38% of patients develop long-term complications, such as pituitary dysfunction or, less often, visual deterioration.[87] Radiation has limited effectiveness for prolactinomas.[63]

Drug Therapy

Antineoplastic chemotherapy is not used for pituitary tumors. Other drugs are indicated as first-line therapy for microadenomas or macroadenomas before surgery or radiation in some instances, and post-therapy in others. Dopamine agonists and octreotide are used to treat hormone oversecretion (Table 52-5). Bromocriptine, a long-acting dopamine agonist, is universally considered to be the primary therapy for prolactinomas. Sixty to seventy percent of treated patients experience decreased tumor size, normalization of serum prolactin level, and improved vision.[63] Dopamine agonists bind to D_2 dopamine receptors in the anterior pituitary, inhibit the synthesis and secretion of prolactin, and the proliferation of lactotroph cells in the pituitary.[63,77,88,89] Women who have small prolactinomas may be treated only with estrogen or oral contraceptives to restore ovulation and menses.[90] Estrogen is less expensive and prevents bone loss, which bromocriptine does not.

Octreotide is an effective agent to reduce GH secretion in patients with acromegaly.[73,88,89] Octreotide may be administered before surgery to reduce tumor size and increase resectability, and to strengthen diminished cardiac functioning.[91] One disadvantage of octreotide is that it is only available for parenteral administration, which is disagreeable to many individuals over time. Either dopamine agonists or octreotide may be helpful for gonadotropin secreting pituitary tumors.[77]

Nursing Care

Nursing care for patients with pituitary tumors begins during diagnosis and is an active part of surgical treatment and post-hospitalization follow-up. Patient teaching is particularly important during all phases. For example, during the diagnostic phase, the nurse explains the pur-

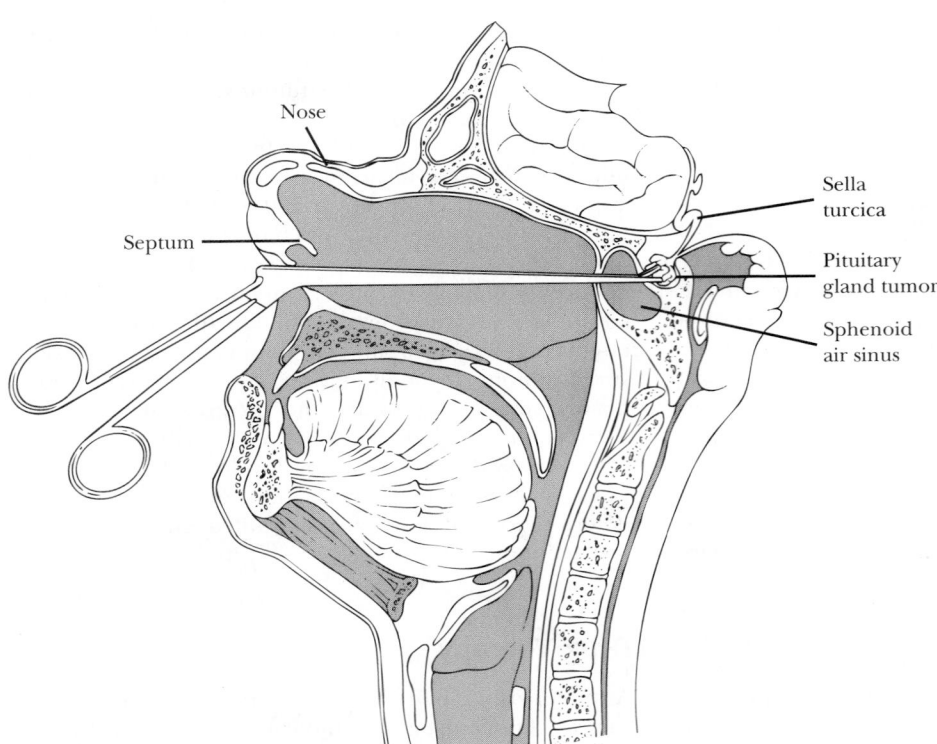

Figure 52-4 Transsphenoidal surgical resection of a pituitary tumor. The upper lip is retracted and an incision is made in the gingival mucosa. After displacing the septal cartilage, the surgeon removes the anterior wall of the sphenoid sinus and the floor of the sella turcica. The pituitary tumor is removed using the microsurgery technique in an attempt to preserve normal pituitary structure and function.

poses of tests and how they are done, and provides written teaching materials. Patients are cared for in a neurosurgical or surgical intensive care unit immediately after surgery. Nurses monitor patients for postoperative complications, which are usually transient but may be long lasting. The most common complication is surgical trauma-related transient swelling of the pituitary and pressure on the pituitary stalk or posterior pituitary.[85] This causes temporary diabetes insipidus (DI) with resultant excretion of large volumes of dilute urine and sodium retention. Manifestations of DI include urinary output of greater than 200 cc per hour for at least three hours, a decreased urine specific gravity (< 1.005), and increased serum sodium (> 145 mEq/L).[72] If this occurs, fluid losses are replaced, milliliter (mL) per mL each hour, until DI improves. Mild DI is usually managed with isotonic intravenous fluids, and vasopressin is administered in more severe cases.[70] The usual dose of vasopression is 5 units subcutaneously every four to six hours until urine volume becomes normal. If the patient develops *hyponatremia,* fluids are restricted until DI resolves, usually within ten days. Desmopressin (DDAVP), 0.1-ml intranasal, is administered once or twice a week in patients in whom DI persists.

Another major complication of transsphenoidal surgery is CSF fistula and leak, which can lead to meningitis or tension pneumocephalus.[85] The nurse monitors the patient for signs and symptoms of meningitis, and checks the patient's mustache-type dressing for glucose in any drainage, which indicates CSF fluid.[72] CSF leak presents as persistent postnasal drip, so the patient may also notice a salty taste in their mouth, may swallow frequently, and may notice increased drainage when they bend over. If CSF leak is confirmed, elevating the head of the bed and maintaining bed rest to decrease pressure is indicated.

Other major complications include prolonged epistaxis, vascular injury to the carotid artery, damage to cranial nerves III, IV, V, and VI, optic nerve or optic chiasm damage, anterior pituitary insufficiency, and death.[85,92,93] Damage to cranial nerves, optic nerves, or the optic chiasm may lead to complete or partial visual loss or visual field defects. In addition, sinusitis can occur from the intranasal trauma or if the nasal packing is left in too long. Thus the nasal packing is removed within 24–48 hours unless the patient has epistaxis. Other nursing assessments includes neurologic checks and visual field and acuity checks (e.g., blurred or double vision).[86]

Patients having transsphenoidal surgery may be discharged from the hospital in as few as three or four days and require clear, written discharge instructions regarding signs and symptoms of infection, medications to be taken, diet and activity restrictions. The patient is instructed to notify the surgeon for any fever greater than 101°F, any symptoms of meningitis (e.g., headache, stiff neck), persistent clear nasal drainage, persistent headache, visual changes, and excessive thirst.[86,93,94] The nurse also reinforces the importance of physician follow-up after the postsurgical period. Patients must be carefully monitored at regular intervals because complications of therapy, especially hypopituitarism and tumor recur-

Table 52-5 Drug Therapy of Pituitary Adenomas

Drug	Indication	Adverse Effects	Comments
Bromocriptine	Prolactinoma GH-secreting tumor (acromegaly) (may be helpful for gonadotrophin-secreting tumor)	• Dizziness • Headache • Nausea and vomiting • Orthostatic hypotension • Nasal congestion • Constipation • Peripheral vasoconstriction • Psychiatric reactions	• First-line treatment for prolactinoma • Normalizes plasma prolactin levels in 90% of patients • Headache, nausea, and orthostatic hypotension are most frequent and limit use in 10%–20% of patients • Menses resume within 2 months; use barrier birth control until then; birth control pills may be used after periods resume • Resistance occurs in about 10% • Side effects are less if doses are escalated gradually and taken with food • 5% continue to have side effects • May decrease GH secretion and acromegaly, improve glucose tolerance in acromegalic patients • Long-acting depot
Pergolide nesylate	Polactinoma GH-secreting tumor	• Suppression of GI motility and secretion • Flatulence and abdominal discomfort • Steatorrhea • Cholelithiasis	• Long-acting injection (administered once a month) available in Europe • Monitor patient for orthostasis and safety considerations with initial doses
Octreotide	GH-secreting tumor (acromegaly) (may be helpful for gonadotrophin-secreting tumor)		• Used similarly to bromocriptine • Parenteral drug administered 3 times per day • 100 mcg is usual dose, but optimal dose is variable and doses may be as high as 500 mcg • Injections may be painful • Used before surgery to shrink macroadenomas, then after surgery if elevated serum GH persists • 40%–50% of patients develop gallstones with long-term treatment, managed with drug-free interval or ureodeoxycholic acid (allow normal contraction of gall bladder)

Data from Lamberts[74] and Croughs.[77]

rence, can occur as late as 30 years after treatment. In addition, surgery and radiation therapy may result in moderate to severe memory loss that can affect patients' daily lives.[95]

There is little scientifically based knowledge of patients' response to the diagnosis and treatment of a pituitary tumor. One survey of patients with Cushing's disease found they experienced great distress from unexplained fatigue, depression, changes in appearance, and in decreased ability to work.[96] It is likely that patients with acromegaly or other pituitary tumors would experience similar feelings. Nurses can help patients cope by helping them find support, and by giving specific suggestions to conserve energy and to increase bone density, thereby decreasing the risk for fractures.[96]

ADRENAL TUMORS

The adrenal glands lie atop each kidney and comprise a cortex and a medulla, which are both critical to homeostasis. The adrenal cortex constitutes about 90% of the adrenal gland, and synthesizes several corticosteroids essential to life in response to signals from the pituitary gland or other systems.[97] The most important are the glucocorticoid cortisol (hydrocortisone) and the mineralocorticoid aldosterone, as well as small amounts of androgens (including testosterone) and estradiol. Corticosteroids play critical roles in many body processes, such as glucose, protein, and lipid metabolism, as well as in wound healing, myocardial contractility, and arteriolar tone. In addition, they oppose the inflammatory response by reducing the formation of inflammatory mediators (prostaglandins, leukotrienes, histamine, etc.), cause an overall general immunosuppression, specifically inhibit interleukins 1 and 2 (IL-1 and IL-2), and may inhibit the synthesis of antibodies and B lymphocytes.[97,98] Mineralocorticoids are critical to maintaining normal serum sodium balance and, to a lesser degree, potassium balance. The primary stimulus for the synthesis of aldosterone is fluid loss, but the pituitary plays a small role as well. Aldosterone induces the kidney to secrete renin and the further production of angiotensin. Adrenal cortical hormones are released slowly, but their actions are long-lived.

The adrenal medulla is actually part of the sympathetic nervous system (SNS), which is responsible for the "fight or flight" reaction. The functional cells of the medulla are chromaffin cells, which are modified postganglionic neurons. Chromaffin cells synthesize catecholamines, mainly epinephrine and norepinephrine, that have positive and inhibitory effects on almost all body tissues.[97] The medulla acts rapidly, and secretes catecholamines within seconds of encountering a stressful event (internal or external). When the stressor is abolished, catecholamine effects disappear rapidly as catecholamines return to sympathetic nerve endings via a reuptake mechanism. The medulla and the cortex thus act in concert, with medullary hormones rapidly responding to changes in the environment and the cortical hormones amplifying and sustaining the stress response.

Several types of adrenocortical tumors arise from the cortex, and pheochromocytomas arise from the medulla. Most of these tumors are benign, but both adenomas and carcinomas can alter quality of life and may be life-threatening. Because they occur in essentially different organs, adrenocortical tumors and pheochromocytomas will be discussed separately.

ADRENOCORTICAL TUMORS

Epidemiology

Adrenocortical carcinomas are extremely rare. The estimated risk of tumor development is approximately 0.6–2.0 new cases per million, and only 0.05%–0.2% of all malignant tumors in adults and less than 0.5% in children occur in the adrenal cortex.[99–101] Adrenocortical tumors have a bimodal peak occurrence, and are most frequent in children under age five and in adults in their forties and fifties. Females of all ages are more likely than males to develop adrenal tumors; children and women most often have hypersecreting tumors, whereas men more often have nonfunctioning tumors.[99,101] Adrenocortical tumors are most often sporadic, but some people have an increased risk to develop a tumor because of an inherited mutation in a predisposition gene(s) for Li-Fraumini syndrome, Wiedemann-Beckwith syndrome, Carney complex, or MEN1.[99]

Etiology

There are no known risk factors for adrenocortical tumors. Pathogenesis is a multistep process and is probably related to some chronic stimulation of the adrenal cortex by pituitary hormones that initiates a random mutation in a single cell. The support for this hypothesis is that adrenocortical tumor DNA is monoclonal.[99,102] It is not clear whether benign tumors progress to malignant ones or if each arises independently. It has been confirmed that the DNA of adrenocortical carcinomas becomes increasingly less stable as tumors become larger.[103] Genetic analysis of tumors confirm loss of heterozygosity (LOH) or allelic imbalance (AI) related to losses or gains of genetic material in multiple proto-oncogenes and tumor suppressor genes, most commonly 11q, 18p, 2q, 11p, and 4p. One mutation, LOH in 2p16 is frequent in carcinomas but never found in adenomas, which indicates this region is probably critical in malignant progression. Other genes that are highly expressed in carcinomas but rarely in adenomas are the multidrug resistance gene (MDR-1) and overexpression of an insulin-like growth factor.[104,105] Similarly, mutations of the p53 suppressor gene have been documented in adults and children with adrenal cortical carcinomas.[106,107]

Pathophysiology

Adrenocortical tumors may be functional or nonfunctional—that is, hormone secreting or nonsecreting. Functional tumors are further characterized by the hormone(s) they produce in excess. Thirty to fifty percent of adrenocortical carcinomas hypersecrete cortisol to cause Cushing's syndrome, 20%–30% secrete estradiol or testosterone to cause feminizing or masculinizing effects, respectively, and rare tumors secrete aldosterone to cause Conn syndrome.[99] Nonfunctional incidentalomas do not produce adrenocortical hormones, and are usually serendipitously discovered on radiologic scans done for unrelated reasons or at autopsy. For instance, as many as 5% of patients who undergo CT scans for other reasons are found to have an incidentaloma.[108]

It is often difficult to histopathologically differentiate adrenocortical adenomas and carcinomas. Tumors do not synthesize hormones as efficiently as normal adrenal glands, and tend to become large by the time they cause symptoms and are detected. As a rule, very large tumors are malignant. Adrenocortical carcinomas are highly aggressive, and 50%–70% of patients have locally advanced disease at presentation.[109] Up to one-third of all patients may have thrombus extension of tumor into the vena cava that may lead to ascites, nephrotic syndrome, hepatomegaly, or acute tricuspid valve failure, or that may be asymptomatic. Tumor thrombi are friable and gelatinous, and can result in massive hemorrhage, intravascular collapse, and death if preoperative planning does not take place.[110]

Clinical Manifestations

The signs and symptoms of adrenal cortical tumors vary depending upon the hormone or hormones secreted, or to symptoms from local mass effects. Of patients who have adrenocortical carcinomas, 50%–80% have an endocrine syndrome when they present (usually Cushing's syndrome) and 30%–40% have metastases.[99,111]

Benign or malignant adrenal cortical tumors are the cause of approximately 20%–25% of all cases of Cushing's syndrome and result in symptoms in multiple body systems (similarly to pituitary tumors). Patients with aldosterone hypersecreting tumors (Conn's syndrome) have hypertension, hypokalemia (serum potassium usually less than 3.5 mEq/L), hypernatremia, and suppressed renin activity.[75,112] Hypokalemia may cause the most serious effects, such as cardiac arrhythmias, abnormal changes on electrocardiogram (ECG), digitalis toxicity, weakness, polydipsia, and visual disturbances.

Women are likely to have virilizing tumors and have symptoms reflecting hypersecretion of androgen. Progressive hirsutism (increased hair on the face, trunk, and limbs) is the most frequent symptom. Acne, clitoral hypertrophy, menstrual abnormalities, deepening of the voice, frontal baldness, and increased libido may also occur.[113,114] Tumors that hypersecrete estradiol are the rarest adrenal tumors and generally occur in young to middle-aged men, who experience diminished libido, testicular atrophy, and gynecomastia.[115] Sex hormone-secreting tumors in children are manifested by pseudosexual precocious puberty in boys and virilization in girls, with the development of pubic hair, tall stature, accelerated growth and bone maturation, and clitoral or penile enlargement.[101] The most common symptoms of patients whose tumors do not hypersecrete hormones are fever, weight loss, symptoms related to the abdominal mass (pain or discomfort, abdominal fullness), and rarely symptoms from distant metastases.[111]

Assessment

Diagnosis of adrenocortical tumors is often protracted and delayed because symptoms are typically nonspecific and slowly progressive. In addition, these tumors are exceedingly rare and are thus not likely to be high on an initial list of differential diagnoses. Diagnosis is confirmed by correlating physical findings with laboratory values and localization procedures. Laboratory tests focus on abnormally high adrenal cortical hormones in the blood and high amounts of their metabolites in the urine. Even patients without symptoms of hormone overproduction should be evaluated by biochemical evaluation for hormone functioning tumors, because of the importance of early diagnosis of adrenocortical carcinoma.[108] Urinary excretion tests are frequently done because hormone metabolites are excreted in the urine, and these noninva-

sive tests are highly sensitive. No test is 100% sensitive or specific, so two or more tests may be done to confirm the diagnosis (Table 52-6).[83,114,116–119]

Localization or imaging procedures to examine the adrenal cortex may include CT or MRI.[99] CT scans are useful to visualize adipose tissue surrounding the adrenal glands; to define the size of large, unilateral, irregular masses; and to identify the homogeneity, calcification, areas of necrosis, and local invasion of masses. MRI, on the other hand, can confirm whether a tumor is invading into blood vessels (inferior vena cava, adrenal and renal veins) and can differentiate whether an adrenal mass is a primary adenoma or carcinoma, or a pheocromocytoma.

Classification and Staging

It is often difficult to determine whether an adrenocortical tumor is benign or malignant at initial diagnosis. If the patient does not have regional spread or distant metastases—to lung, liver, or peritoneum, and (rarely) brain or lung—no single finding confirms a diagnosis. While small tumors are more likely to be benign and large masses (greater than 100 g) malignant, there is considerable overlap and size alone is not a reliable indicator of pathology.[104] Several histologic features are characteristic of carcinomas and include a high mitotic rate (which correlates with poor prognosis), atypical mitoses, aneuploidy, high nuclear grade, hyperchromatic nuclei, low proportion of clear cells, grossly lobulated tumor, areas of necrosis, calcifications, capsular or vascular invasion, and steroid production.[99,111] Immunohistochemistry tests, such as MiB-1 activity and *p53* expression, may aid in diagnosis.[99] MiB-1 is an antibody that reacts with an antigen expressed only in proliferating cells (not in G_0). In one study, the majority (66%) of primary adrenocortical carcinomas were positive for *p53*, whereas all adenomas were *p53* negative.

Adrenocortical tumors are staged using the TNM system. Stage I tumors (up to 5 cm) and stage II tumors (greater than 5 cm) are considered localized. Advanced disease includes stage III (positive regional lymph nodes) and stage IV (metastases present). The overall prognosis of adrenocortical carcinomas is poor: median survival is 4–30 months, and fewer than 25% of patients survive for five years.[120] Of patients who have advanced disease at time of diagnosis, fewer than 50% survive for one year, and fewer than 10% are alive at ten years.[121]

Therapeutic Approaches and Nursing Care

Surgery

Surgery offers the only chance for cure of malignant adrenal tumors, so resection of local (and sometimes

Table 52-6 Laboratory Values of Adrenal Tumors

Tumor/Syndrome	Test	Implications/Comments
Cushing's disease	• Dexamethasone suppression test (see Table 52-4)	• Tumor-induced cortisol or metabolites will not be suppressed by feedback mechanisms • Plasma cortisol will be elevated the morning after administration
	• 24-hour urine for free cortisol	• Will be elevated to > 80–100 mcg
	• 2-day, high-dose dexamethasone suppression test	• Metabolites of adrenocortical steroids, 17 ketosteroids, are not suppressed; normal values vary with gender and age
	• Plasma ACTH immunoassay	• Suppressed to less than normal because of negative feedback loop (increased adrenal cortisol leads to decreased ACTH release by pituitary); normal: 6–76 ng/mL
Virilizing	Basal serum testosterone	• Elevated; nonsuppressible with dexamethasone administration (usually suppresses adrenocortical hormone production); normal: women = 20–90 ng/dL, men = 250–1000 ng/dL
Conn syndrome (aldosterone-secreting)	• Plasma aldosterone	• Elevated with tumor or hyperplasia, which increase production; normal: 7 AM supine < 16 ng/mL, 9 AM upright 4–316 ng/mL
	• Urinary aldosterone	• Elevated-> 20 mcg in 24 hours
	• Plasma renin activity	• Suppressed because increased plasma aldosterone has not been induced by low extracellular fluid volume-induction of renin/angiotensin system; normal: supine 0.5–1.6 ng/mL, upright 1.9–3.6 ng/mL
Pheochromocytoma	• Plasma catecholamines (dopamine, epinephrine, norepinephrine)	• Elevated by tumor production • Antihypertensives and antidepressants may invalidate test; confirm drug history
	• 24-hour urine for metanephrines or for normetanephrines	• Metabolites of catecholamines, elevated to 1.5 to 2 times greater than normal; normal: 0.0–0.9 μ/24 hr • Elevated to 1.5–2 times greater than normal • HCl is added to urine specimen bottle to maintain pH ≤ 3 • BP, height, and weight are recorded on laboratory requisition • Patient must be instructed to collect entire 24-hour collection, or results may be false negative

Data from Corbett[83] Müller 1990,[114] Derksen et al 1994,[116] Werbel and Ober,[117] Gerlo and Sevens,[118] Lenders et al.[119]

metastatic) disease is recommended whenever possible. Excisions of hormone-secreting tumors, hormone-non-secreting masses larger than 5 cm, and "suspicious" masses smaller than 5 cm is recommended, because surgery may increase the chance of cure or prolong survival for patients with localized disease.[99] En bloc resection offers the best chance of cure.[122] Large tumors and those suspected or confirmed to be malignant are resected during laparotomy, whereas adenomas smaller than 6 cm may be resected via laparoscopic adrenalectomy.[123] Even with surgery, almost 80% of patients develop recurrent regional disease or distant metastases.[111] Virtually all patients with stage III disease develop recurrent disease and metastases within five years of surgical resection.[99]

Chemotherapy

Chemotherapy is given in some instances for cortical tumors. Mitotane controls hormone hypersecretion in 75% of treated patients and is the usual first-line agent after resection of stage III and IV carcinomas.[39,111] Mitotane may act by reversing multidrug resistance mediated by MDR-1.[105] Phase II and other trials have demonstrated that response rates to mitotane are approximately 35%, but responses are rarely prolonged or complete, and survival does not increase.[124]

Mitotane often causes significant and unacceptable dose-related side effects.[99,111] Approximately 50% of patients experience neurologic effects including weakness, somnolence, confusion, lethargy, and headache.[105,124] In addition, most patients experience GI symptoms, which can include anorexia, nausea and vomiting, and diarrhea. Uncommon reactions include skin rash and toxic retinopathy with papilledema.[99] Side effects are greatest when 6–10 mg/day are administered, and smaller doses (1.5–3 mg/day) that have been used as adjuvant therapy after surgery are well tolerated and may decrease the risk for recurrence.[122] Fewer patients experience prolonged bleeding times, ataxia or dysarthria, or depression progressing to suicidal ideation.[120]

Antineoplastic therapy is indicated for patients whose tumors progress during mitotane therapy.[121] There are few prospective trials and anecdotal reports of chemotherapy alone or of chemotherapy plus mitotane. Cisplatin is the most widely tested antineoplastic agent and as single-agent therapy leads to response rates of about 30%. Cisplatin plus etoposide, with or without mitotane, is considered "standard" chemotherapy but does not generally result in greater response rates than cisplatin or mitotane alone (e.g., 33% versus 30%), and median survival is less than 12 months.[121]

In other reports, mitotane has been combined with other agents including cisplatin, doxorubicin, cyclophosphamide, etoposide, 5-FU, and streptozotocin.[120,125,126] In one small, prospective study of mitotane plus etoposide, doxorubicin, and cisplatin, more than 50% of patients who had locally advanced or metastatic disease experienced complete or partial responses that were sustained for approximately two years.[105] One negative aspect, however, was that the neurotoxicity of the chemotherapy regimen and mitotane were additive.

Symptom Management and Supportive Care

Because of delays in diagnosis, many patients with adrenal tumors have progressive disease that does not respond to treatment. Palliative treatment for these persons includes medications to reduce symptoms produced by hormone excess. Thus patients who have Cushing's syndrome may be treated with drugs that block steroid synthesis (aminoglutethimide, metyrapone, ketoconazole) or block steroid actions in target organs (mefipristone), which may control symptoms but not tumor growth.[111] Patients experiencing Conn syndrome may be treated with spironolactone, a potassium sparing diuretic, which is administered to correct tumor-induced hypokalemia.

PHEOCHROMOCYTOMA

Epidemiology

Pheochromocytomas arise from chromaffin cells (pheochromocytes). Eighty-five to ninety-five percent of tumors arise in the adrenal medulla, but they may also arise from the abdominal aortic paraganglia (and rarely within the thorax or urinary bladder) and are termed *paragangliomas*.[112,117] Both benign and malignant tumors synthesize, store, and release catecholamines, which are not regulated by the nervous system.[127] The unregulated release of massive amounts of catecholamines during stressful periods often causes life-threatening crises that may lead to death from myocardial infarction, cardiac arrhythmia or arrest, or shock.[128,129] While most patients are symptomatic, some individuals have pheochromocytomas that are discovered incidentally.[130]

Pheochromocytomas are rare tumors. The estimated incidence is less than five cases per million, and pheochromocytomas constitute only 0.3%–0.95% of all neuroendocrine tumors, and affect less than 1% of all hypertensive patients.[131,132] Approximately 90% of adults have a benign pheochromocytoma, but individuals younger than age 50 and children are at greater risk to have malignant tumors.[132] Males and females are at equal risk to develop a sporadic pheochromocytoma, most frequently in their thirties to fifties, and children frequently have a familial risk.[117,133,134] Pheochromocytoma is discovered during pregnancy in rare instances, and is dangerous to the mother and fetus, particularly during labor, induction of anesthesia, and within 72 hours of delivery.[135] Because labor increases abdominal pressure that may lead to catecholamine release, accurate diagnosis is critical before delivery so cesarean section delivery may be planned.[135]

Etiology

Almost nothing is known about the etiology of pheochromocytomas, but hyperplasia precedes tumor development. Approximately 90% of tumors occur sporadically, and the remainder occur as part of MEN2A, MEN2B, or another neuroectodermal syndrome. Loss of heterozygosity may occur at 1p, 22q, 17p, and 3p in tumor DNA, but it is not known which of these are tumor suppressor genes involved with the development of pheochromocytomas.[112] It has also been demonstrated that in comparison to normal adrenal tissue, tumor tissue has increased expression of three genes for catecholamine synthesizing enzymes, whereas one gene is expressed at a decreased level.[127]

Pathophysiology

Diagnosis of benign or malignant tumor depends on the absence or presence of metastases. Microscopic features have little predictive value for the biologic nature of the tumor, and both benign and malignant tumors may have aneuploid DNA, cellular hyperchromatism, and bizarre mitotic figures, as well as capsular and vascular invasion.[136] Although malignant tumors have been noted to be larger in some instances, differences have not been quantified and cannot be used to determine malignant status. Both benign and malignant pheocromocytomas hypersecrete the catecholamine norepinephrine, and less often epinephrine. Altered gene expression may explain why the predominant catecholamines in tumor (90% norepinephrine) and normal tissues (90% epinephrine) are reversed.[127,137]

In one small study, malignant pheochromocytomas were found to express telomerase while benign tumors did not.[138] This is not surprising because telomerase, an enzyme that prevents the progressive shortening of the telomeres on the chromosome tips that leads to cell aging and death, is expressed only in germ line and immortalized (malignant) cell lines. A problem in determining pathologic status is that after an initial diagnosis of benign or malignant tumor, a pheochromocytoma may recur in the tumor bed, regional lymph nodes, or as distant metastases as long as 10–15 years later.[129,132,136] Malignant tumors can metastasize to lymph nodes, bone, lung, liver, brain, and omentum.[128]

Clinical Manifestations

Intermittent catecholamine release usually causes the typical manifestations of pheochromocytoma, and tumors that produce large amounts of epinephrine cause many symptoms in all organ systems.[117,128,133,137,139] Hypertension (diastolic blood pressure (BP) greater than 110–120 mm Hg), persistent or paroxysmal (intermittent), is considered the hallmark or cardinal symptom, and is experienced by 82% of patients. Other frequently reported symptoms include sudden throbbing or pounding headache (58%), palpitations (48%), profuse and generalized perspiration (37%), and shortness of breath (28%). Some patients also experience, anxiety, nausea and vomiting, pallor, and chest or abdominal pain.

Symptoms usually occur during life-threatening crises, when excessive catecholamines are being released into the bloodstream, and are spontaneously triggered by changes in position, increased abdominal pressure, exercise, passing urine or stool, intercourse, pain, pressure on or palpation of the abdomen, trauma, labor, anesthesia, surgery, or chemotherapy.[128,134] In addition, anticholinergic drugs may cause perilous tachycardias, and other drugs such as dopamine antagonists (metoclopramide and phenothiazines), tricyclic antidepressants, and naloxone may precipitate extreme hypertension.[140] The most severe complication is pheochromocytoma crisis. This may lead to encephalopathy that can progress to coma, shock, and multiple organ system failure including renal and hepatic failure, disseminated intravascular clotting (DIC), seizures, and possibly death.[117] Crisis episodes vary and may last from a few minutes to an hour, and may occur daily or sporadically.[134] Afterward the patient may have tremor and feel short of breath, weak, or exhausted.

In rare instances patients (case reports) are normotensive, or present with other symptoms such as sudden presyncopal episodes accompanied by nausea, bradycardia (sinus node arrest or complete sinoatrial block), myocardial infarction, or cerebral vascular accident brought on by intermittent excess catecholamine secretion.[133,141] Patients may also experience increased glycolysis resulting in increased blood glucose and perhaps diabetes.[133] Patients are treated with oral agents when possible such as dihydralazine, phentalomine, labetalol, or nefedipine, captopril, sublingual nitroglycerin, or IV clonidine.[139]

Assessment

The diagnosis of pheochromocytoma is often delayed because hypertension is much more likely to be caused by other factors. Diagnosis is confirmed by correlating physical findings with laboratory values and localization procedures. Some clinicians advocate at least two 24-hour urine collections for total and fractionated catecholamines, metanephrines, and vanillylmandelic acid (VMA), and plasma epinephrine and norepinephrine.[131,136] However, urinary excretion tests for the catecholamine metabolite metanephrine, which is a direct tumor marker and indirect marker of catecholamine release, is most sensitive to detect pheochromocytomas (see Table 52-6).[118,119,128] Test accuracy may be affected by how the sample is collected and analysis technique. That is, if the collection period is less than or greater than 24 hours, the test result may be falsely negative or falsely positive, respectively. High-performance liquid chromatography and indexing urinary metanephrine levels by urinary creatinine levels increases test sensitivity and eliminates false positives related to food or drugs.[142] In addition, urinary catecholamine evaluation may also be inaccurate in patients who have advanced renal insufficiency.[134] Measurement of the serum catecholamines is not as useful because catecholamines have a short half-life and may not be measurable if obtained when the patient is not hypertensive.[142] Patients are followed after surgery with regularly scheduled measurements of plasma catecholamines and BP checks for the duration of their lives.[131]

Localization studies before surgery are imperative to prepare the patient for surgery and minimize the risk for cardiovascular morbidity during surgery.[143] Ultrasound, CT, MRI, and iodine[131]-meta-iodobenzylguanidine (MIBG) scans are all useful to localize pheochromocytomas, but there is no universal agreement regarding which should be included and the order of procedures. Ultrasonography can detect about 90% of tumors and is widely available and inexpensive, whereas a CT scan is highly sensitive and can more precisely image and localize tumors, and MRI can delineate tissue characteristics and extent of tumor localization.[128] MIBG injection is followed by a nuclear scan and is advantageous to determine the functional characteristics of a tumor and locate occult secondary or metastatic sites.[130]

Classification and Staging

As mentioned, most pheochromocytomas are benign in adults, and the presence of metastases is the only reliable indicator of malignancy. Patients with benign or malignant tumors may succumb from complications related to excessive catecholamine effects on normal systems, such as cardiovascular disease, hypertension, cerebral vascular accident, renal disease, or diabetes mellitus.[136]

Therapeutic Approaches and Nursing Care

Surgery

The treatment of choice for pheochromocytoma is surgery, which may cure resectable disease, and is also indicated to resect or debulk recurrent disease and metastases.[131] Surgery or other invasive procedures can precipitate severe and uncontrolled hypertension, so treatment to induce alpha-adrenergic blockade is commonly started at least one to two weeks before surgery or chemotherapy to control arterial hypertension and decrease the risk of crisis during surgery and of postoperative hypotension. Phenoxybenzamine or another selective postsynaptic alpha 1-adrenergic receptor antagonist (e.g., prazosin, terazosin) is administered.[136,143] Calcium channel blockers also prevent paroxysmal hypertension, do not cause overshoot or orthostatic hypotension, and may prevent cardiovascular complications.[143] If the patient has persistent tachycardia (pulse greater than 140 per minute), extrasystoles, or a history of arrhythmias, propranolol, atenolol, or metoprolol may be added only after the alpha blockade is complete to induce beta-adrenergic blockade (e.g., control tachycardia).

Preoperative nursing care focuses on ensuring adequate hydration, monitoring BP, and patient teaching.[137] The patient's weight is checked daily; they are prescribed a liberal salt diet and may be given one to two liters of IV fluids each day. In addition to concerns about hypertension, the nurse must be aware that the patient may also experience postural hypotension. Patient teaching includes avoidance of straining and rapid changes in position, and medication may be given to decrease stress.

Cardiovascular and hemodynamic status are monitored continuously during surgery, and hypertension and arrhythmias are treated promptly. During surgery IV nitroprusside, nitroglycerin, and pentalomine are administered to control hypertension, and esmolol, a short acting beta-blocker may be used to control tachyarrhythmias.[131] Immediate postoperative concerns include monitoring vital signs, hemodynamic status, fluid and electrolyte status, and urinary output.[137] The nurse also monitors for other postoperative complications such as bleeding and infection, which are rare, and pain. Patients may be hypotensive and receive IV fluid replacement for a few days after surgery, and may experience hypoglycemia. Blood pressure is usually normal by the time the patient is discharged from the hospital, but may remain elevated for four to eight weeks. A 24-hour urine collection for catecholamines is done about two weeks after surgery to monitor for residual disease (local or metastatic) and is checked annually for at least five years.[137]

Radiation Therapy

The indication for radiation therapy is to palliate metastatic disease.[128,134] Total doses of 3000–5000 cGy may reverse neurologic deficit from CNS metastases and provide symptomatic relief from metastases to lymph nodes or bone. In addition, some patients may experience long-term control of disease with radiation therapy.[144]

Chemotherapy

Chemotherapy is generally considered to be ineffective for pheochromocytomas,[112] but it has been suggested that patients may respond to effective drugs for other neuroendocrine neoplasms.[117] The reason for this is that few reports of chemotherapy for this tumor are found in the literature, perhaps because of the rarity of malignant pheochromocytomas.

Chemotherapy is a stressor and may precipitate severe hypertension as well as possible headache, vomiting, or chest pain within a few hours after administration. For example, hypertension was documented in two patients after treatment with cyclophosphamide, vincristine, and dacarbazine.[145] A possible explanation is that chemotherapy induces tumor lysis and rapid release of tumor-stored catecholamines into the circulation. Patients thus require adequate BP control before chemotherapy starts, and their hemodynamic status must be closely and continuously monitored, particularly during the first cycle of therapy.[145] Nifedipine 10-mg tablets are administered sublingually or orally to abort hypertensive crisis temporarily.

Symptom Management and Supportive Care

Some patients who have unresectable metastatic disease will experience recurrent hypertension, which is usually managed with phenoxybenzamine, propranolol, or labetolol.[137] Phenoxybenzamine, an irreversible, long-acting, alpha-adrenergic antagonist, has adverse effects including postural hypotension, tachycardia, miosis, nasal congestion, inhibited ejaculation, diarrhea, and fatigue. It is thus started at a low dose, which is gradually increased. Other patients may receive metyrosine, which prevents the conversion of catecholamine precursors to catecholamines. A benefit of metyrosine is that it allows the use of lower doses of alpha-adrenergic blockers, which minimizes the potential side effects of those agents.

MULTIPLE ENDOCRINE NEOPLASIA

Individuals affected with a multiple endocrine neoplasia (MEN) syndrome develop two or more characteristic benign or malignant endocrine tumors simultaneously or sequentially over their lifetimes (Table 52-7).[146–152] To

Table 52-7 Multiple Endocrine Neoplasia Syndromes

Syndrome	Major Organ Tumors	Presenting Symptoms/Comments
MEN1	Parathyroid (hyperplasia) 80%–100% Pancreas (insulinoma) 40%–85% Duodenum (gastrinoma, VIPoma) 25% Pituitary (prolactinoma, growth hormone-secreting adenoma) 30%–65% Neuroendocrine (carcinoids) other sites 5%–9%	• Presenting symptoms depend on organs involved and whether tumor secretes hormone. May include: Hypercalcemia, urolithiasis Hypoglycemia Peptic ulcer, diarrhea Galactorrhea, acromegaly • Other, less common tumors: thymus, stomach, carcinoid, lipoma, spinal cord ependymoma • Prediagnostic manifestations: 50% of patients have cutaneous manifestations, including angiofibromas, café-au-lait spots, pipomas, confetti-like hypopigmented macules, multiple gingival papules
MEN2 MEN2A	Thyroid (medullary thyroid carcinoma) 70% Adrenal medulla (pheochromocytoma) > 50% Parathyroid (adenoma) 15%–30%	• Presenting symptoms depend on organs involved and whether tumor secretes hormone. May include: Diarrhea Hypertension, palpitations Hypercalcemia, urolithiasis Diarrhea
MEN2B	Thyroid (medullary thyroid carcinoma) 100% Adrenal medulla (pheochromocytoma)	• Onset of MTC is 10 years earlier than MEN2A, most aggressive • Developmental abnormalities accompany syndrome: typical facies, marfanoid appearance, oral mucosa, conjunctiva, intestinal mucosa • Ganglioneuromas may cause difficult swallowing, vomiting, constipation, diarrhea • Parathyroid adenomas are noted to be rare to absent • Hypercalcemia, urolithiasis
Familial MTC	Thyroid (medullary thyroid carcinoma) 100%	• More benign than MEN2A or MEN2B, good prognosis

Data from Eng,[146] Komminoth et al,[147] Marx,[148] Darling et al,[149] Morrison and Nevin,[150] Ponder,[151] Eng et al.[152]

date, two broadly classified syndromes, MEN1 and MEN2, have been identified. Sporadic MEN syndromes are rarely diagnosed, and are almost always caused by an inherited gene mutation. MEN tumors produce the same symptoms as sporadic tumors but are characterized by cardinal features of all hereditary cancers: early age of onset of hyperplasia, benign or malignant neoplasia, multiple primary tumors that occur in particular combinations, portending physical signs in some individuals, distinctive pathologic features, more severe disease and poorer prognosis than sporadic tumors, and a mendelian pattern of tumor transmission.[153]

Patients with familial MEN1 or MEN2 develop tumors because of an inherited, autosomal-dominant mutated gene that codes for a particular tumor suppressor or proto-oncogene. This gene, present in the germ line of one parent, is passed on to affected offspring and is thus found in all of their cells. These individuals are predisposed to earlier and more frequent (but less than 100%) tumor development because these mutations have a high degree of expressivity but a variable rate of penetrance. For instance, it is estimated that 35% of the children who have the *MEN2* gene will develop clinically

significant disease.[154] Point mutations, which result in the substitution of a single nucleotide (codon) for another, cause missense mutations that change a single amino acid, and lead to activation and gain of function of a proto-oncogene or loss of function of a suppressor gene. A second mutation in the normal allele inherited from the unaffected parent occurs some time after birth and is necessary for tumor transformation. Mutations of several other genes that code for suppressor genes, oncogenes, and growth factors are undoubtedly involved in progression to malignancy.

Multiple Endocrine Neoplasia 1

The estimated incidence of MEN1 varies from 1:10,000 to 1:100,000.[155] The most frequent endocrine manifestations of MEN1 are diffuse or nodular parathyroid hyperplasia, anterior pituitary adenomas (most often prolactin or GH-secreting tumors), and enteropancreatic neuroendocrine tumors.[147,148,156] It is not possible to predict how these will present, but patients may have one, two, or all three tumors. Parathyroid neoplasms are diagnosed in 80%–100% of all patients at a mean age of 19, whereas 30%–65% of patients develop a single, pituitary adenoma that is usually clinically insignificant. These tumors, often diagnosed in patients in their forties, may or may not secrete hormones, and are frequently discovered only at autopsy.[156] Sixty-six percent of patients develop numerous microadenomas throughout the pancreas, and 30%–75% of these patients are symptomatic secondary to tumor secretion of one of the pancreatic peptides. Gastrin is the most frequently secreted peptide and causes hypersecretion of gastric acid (Zollinger-Ellison syndrome).[148] Fewer patients also develop carcinoids or neuroendocrine lung tumors, and other nonendocrine tumors (e.g., duodenum, stomach, thymus, adrenal hyperplasia, lipomas, spinal cord ependymomas).[147,155]

Manifestations of MEN1 vary depending on which organs are involved and whether tumors secrete hormones. Approximately 50% of affected individuals die at a younger age (mean 51 years) than non-MEN1 affected family members, and prognosis is affected by sites involved with tumor. For example, thymic tumors are aggressive, while pancreatic and duodenal tumors are usually low grade.[147] The majority of MEN1 patients who are not diagnosed early die from GI bleeding or metastatic pancreatic cancer in their sixties.[157]

Etiology

Linkage analysis located the gene for MEN1 on the long arm of chromosome 11, and it has now been confirmed to lie at 11q13. This gene was designated *Mu* among the original candidate genes, and has been cloned and codes for a protein that is called *menin*.[158] The function of the *MEN1* gene is not known, and at least 12 mutations (including frameshift, nonsense, in-frame deletions, and missense) have been identified. Genotype/phenotype implications of mutations in this large gene are not clear, and the implications for clinical management have not yet been defined.[159] Tumors occur because of a second mutation in the normal allele that results in the loss of that allele (loss of heterozygosity), suggesting that *MEN1* is a tumor suppressor gene. Inactivation of both alleles may not be sufficient to induce tumors, and other genes are likely to be involved.[148]

Multiple Endocrine Neoplasia 2

The estimated incidence of MEN2 is 1:500,000.[155] Individuals with MEN2 develop hyperplasia or tumors of the thyroid, parathyroid, and adrenal glands. MEN2A is most common and accounts for more than 90% of cases, while MEN2B accounts for about 5% of cases.[146] Some individuals develop only familial medullary thyroid cancer (FMTC).

MEN2A

The hallmark tumor of MEN2A is hyperplasia of thyroid C cells that progresses to MTC. The *RET* gene is not completely penetrant; 70% of carriers develop tumors by age 70, and more than 95% of patients develop only MTC.[146] Long-term prognosis depends upon the success of treatment for MTC. More than 50% of patients with MEN2A develop pheochromocytomas, most of which are benign and cause symptoms by overproducing hormones.[146,148] Hypertension is the most frequent symptom, as with sporadic pheochromocytoma, and is a major cause of death. Fifty to eighty percent of patients present with bilateral disease, and another 10% require adrenalectomy of the remaining gland within five years.[160] Parathyroid adenomas develop in 15%–30% of persons with MEN2A, but much later than in those with MEN1.[146] These tumors are not usually significant and patients appear physically normal.

MEN2B

The onset of MEN2B, which is more aggressive than MEN2A and FMTC, is approximately ten years earlier than MEN2A.[146,161] Virtually all patients with MEN2B develop MTC, and the average age of death is 21 in untreated patients.[150] Affected individuals may be identified by their typical physical appearance, including marfanoid appearance (85%), facial features, and proximal muscle wasting (Figure 52-5).[162] Patients often have musculoskeletal abnormalities including pes cavus, or an abnormally high arch of the foot (persons who have Marfan syndrome have pes planus, or flat feet), kyphosis, scoliosis, lordosis, and increased joint looseness.[150,154,162] Characteristic facial features include enlarged, blubbery lips from mucosal neuromas that are located throughout the entire GI tract, from anterior and dorsal tongue to colon. Neuromas can occur on other mucosal surfaces, such as the eyelids, which makes the patient look wide-eyed. In addition, the eyebrows are large, and an elongated face and prominent jaw are common.[150] Puberty is delayed in patients with MEN2B, and their reproductive rates are low secondary to mortality, impotence, and infertility. These findings support the idea that new mutations are common in MEN2B, and as many as 50% of cases of MEN2B arise from new mutations.[146,151]

Etiology

RET, a protooncogene located on the long arm of chromosome 10 (10q11.2), has been confirmed to be responsible for MEN2 and FMTC.[163] This proto-oncogene is expressed during fetal development of neural crest structures, and is expressed postnatally in neural crest-derived tissues including parathyroid glands, thyroid C cells, adrenal medulla, enteric ganglia, and the urogenital system.[146,154] *RET* is a dominant transforming gene for cancer/neoplasia, and a mutation results in a perma-

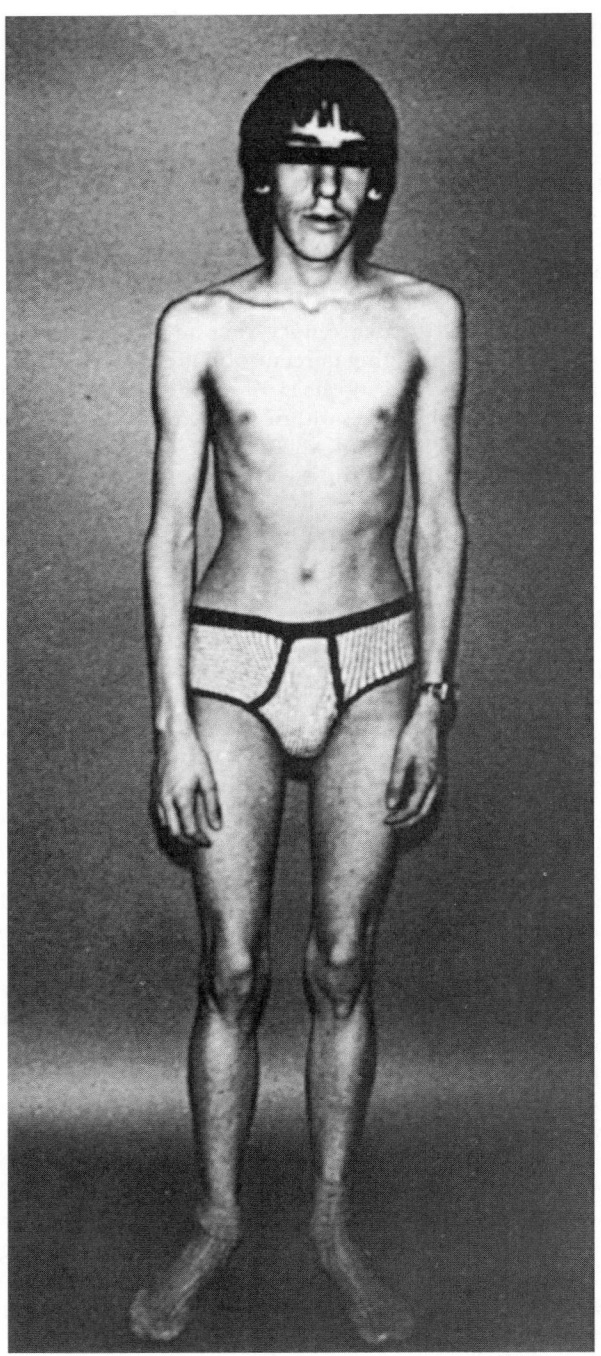

Figure 52-5 Typical appearance of a patient with MEN2B, demonstrating marfanoid habitus, thickening of the lips (ganglioneuromatomas), and elongated face. (Reprinted with permission from Frank K, Raue F, Gottswinter J, et al: The importance of early diagnosis and followup in sporadic MEN II. *Eur J Pediatr* 143:112, 1984.)[162]

in MEN2 families have mutations in *RET*.[152] Eight mutations account for all cases. For instance, 85% of all cases of MEN2A are associated with a mutation at codon 634 (TGC to CGC, which changes cysteine to arginine), and this mutation is strongly associated with the development of pheochromocytoma and hyperparathyroidism. In addition, a point mutation at codon 919 (ATG to ACG, which results in the substitution of threonine for methionine), is implicated in more than 95% of all cases of MEN2B.[146,152]

Assessment and Screening

Baseline and ongoing screening for affected individuals in families known to express MEN is the major focus of management. Current recommendations for MEN1 and MEN2 vary because of the differences in availability of genetic screening and therapy options. Annual screening may include serum tests for laboratory evidence of hypersecreting tumors, but negative tests do not guarantee that a person does not have the syndrome. Because tumors occur at varying ages, a negative test only indicates that they do not yet have detectable disease.[154]

MEN1 is most commonly diagnosed when patients are in their forties, but can be identified when patients are in their teens or twenties by periodic evaluations of serum hormones secreted by constituent tumors (calcium, parathyroid hormone, fasting gastrin, insulin, glucose, prolactin, and GH).[146,149] It is recommended that annual biochemical testing begin between ages 8–15. If a patient does not convert to positive by age 30, the risk of being a gene carrier decreases to 10%, but testing continues because the maximal age for conversion is not known.[148] In addition, patients may be clinically monitored for premonitory cutaneous manifestations of MEN1, such as multiple facial angiofibromas, collagenomas, café-au-lait macules, lipomas, and multiple gingival papules, which may aid in presymptomatic diagnosis. Clinical genetic testing is not standard because Mu is a large gene and identified mutations are spread across it, new mutations are being discovered, and there are no available testing "shortcuts" (e.g., protein truncation assay) because of the nature of gene mutations. In addition, MEN1 is a rare tumor, so there is limited demand for a genetic test, and confirmation would not lead to major therapeutic interventions.[156]

Genetic testing for *RET* mutations in family members with a known risk for MEN2A and MEN2B is the diagnostic method of choice.[164,165] DNA testing is simple and routine because the small number of *RET* mutations and the high likelihood that one of these will be detected in more than 90% of cases.[151,152] Confirmation of genetic status eliminates need for screening in noncarriers and identifies patients who should have an early thyroidectomy without waiting for abnormal biochemical tests. Advantages of genetic tests over previously used pentagastrin provocation are that the test is practical (only requires

nently activated mutant receptor that responds to its intrinsic tyrosine kinase enzyme activity.[159] Mutation of a single codon is sufficient to cause neoplastic transformation and gain of function, and more than 92% of patients

one blood sample), has no side effects, and is cost effective because repeated, expensive biochemical testing for all potential tumors is necessary only in carriers. Further, patients who require early surgery are identified when cure is most likely.[166] DNA analysis of *RET* gene for mutations is highly reliable, having no false-positive or false-negative results.[167] Persons in whom the mutation exists will require annual screening, as outlined above, starting in early childhood.[154]

Annual screening for MEN2A/FMTC gene mutation carriers—which includes plasma calcitonin after IV pentagastrin or calcium stimulation, BP, urinary or plasma catecholamines, serum calcium, and perhaps imaging of the adrenal glands—is recommended to start by age four to five and continue to age 20.[151] The recommended screening for older patients is controversial, and some clinicians opt to screen them at wider intervals until age 35.

Provocative tests for calcitonin involve the injection of pentagastrin or calcium and the measurement of serum calcitonin at baseline, two to three minutes, and five to ten minutes postinjection. Reproducible serum calcium elevations above a normal range indicate the need to proceed to total thyroidectomy, and patients whose calcitonin levels are borderline are retested within three to six months.[163] Calcitonin provocation tests are problematic in that both false negatives, which erroneously lull the patient into a sense of security, and false positives, which may result in an unnecessary total thyroidectomy, can occur.[165]

Therapeutic Approaches and Nursing Care

A multidisciplinary team—physicians, nurses, a genetic counselor, and a psychologist—that is knowledgeable and experienced in inherited cancer syndromes is required to care for patients with MEN syndromes.[155] Oncology nurses should be skilled in gathering a family history that includes the history of cancer at other sites and in constructing a pedigree.[153] These are useful in medical interpretation of risk and identification of the need for further diagnostic testing. In addition, knowledgeable nurses can play a key role in patient and family teaching, counseling, and support before and following genetic testing. Some of the issues surrounding genetic risk testing that the nurse should consider include family members' emotional responses and concerns, and potential areas of dissatisfaction, such as a lack of knowledge on the part of health care providers, who therefore cannot provide accurate information about genetic testing, support, and genetic counseling.[168] Waiting for the results of a genetic test is difficult, and finding out what the results are—whether normal or carrier—causes shock and anxiety that may decrease over time.

Treatment of constituent tumors may vary with MEN

syndromes as opposed to sporadic tumors. For instance, one major difference in the treatment of parathyroid hyperplasia or tumors is that most individuals with MEN1 have tumor in all four glands while those with sporadic tumors do not. Thus, the surgical exploration is always bilateral and includes extensive exploration of the tissues surrounding the thyroid so that all of the parathyroid tissue is located. Three and one-half parathyroid glands are removed, and the remaining half gland is autotransplanted to an accessible site (e.g., a neck muscle or the forearm) to maintain calcium homeostasis.[148] Tissue in these sites is easier to monitor and is important because even when the small amount of parathyroid appears normal, patients are most likely to experience remission and not cure. That is, hyperplasia and hyperparathyroidism recur in 67% of patients within eight years after surgery.[169] Thus, periodic screening of serum calcium will always be required in these patients.

MEN2-affected individuals undergo prophylactic thyroidectomy, usually no later than age four to five—especially MEN2A patients who have a mutation at codon 634 and MEN2B patients, whose disease is highly aggressive and often metastasizes by age six to ten.[150,161] Patients whose adrenal glands or thyroid are resected will require lifelong hormone replacement.

Conclusion

Several rare endocrine tumors occur and while most often they are benign, both benign and malignant tumors may cause significant morbidity, shorten life expectancy, and negatively affect quality of life. As with other malignancies, early detection of small tumors that are surgically resectable affords the best prognosis. The relative rarity of these tumors has hampered our ability to test the effectiveness of chemotherapy in most instances. Many endocrine tumors are detected late in their course, and cause the affected person's death because of mass effects or because of physiologic effects induced by hypersecretion of an endocrine hormone. Nursing care for patients with endocrine tumors requires knowledge of the hormones secreted, and of their effects on body systems, and in cases of inherited genes that increase tumor risk, knowledge of etiology. The focus of care is often on symptom assessment and management.

References

1. Landis SH, Murray T, Bolden, et al: Cancer Statistics, 1999. *CA Cancer J Clin* 49:8–30, 1999
2. Baxter JD, Frohman LA, Felig P: Introduction to the endocrine system, in Felig P, Baxter JD, Frohman LA (eds): *Endocrinology and Metabolism* (ed 3). New York, McGraw-Hill, 1995, pp 3–21

3. Goodman HM: Thyroid gland, *Basic Medical Endocrinology* (ed 2). New York, Raven Press, 1994, pp 46–70

4. National Cancer Institute: *PDQ Information for Health Care Professionals. Thyroid cancer.* Available at http://oncolink .upen.edu/pdq/101252.html (Accessed on December 18, 1998)

5. Steele G, Hessup LM, Winchester DP: Clinical highlights from the National Cancer Data Base. *CA Cancer J Clin* 45: 102–111, 1995

6. Grigsby PW, Luk KH: Thyroid, in Perez CA, Brady LW (eds): *Principles and Practice of Radiation Oncology* (ed 3). Philadelphia, Lippincott-Raven, 1997, pp 1157–1179

7. Stratakis CA, Chrousos GP: Endocrine tumors, in Pizzo PA, Poplack DG (eds): *Principles and Practice of Pediatric Oncology* (ed 3). Philadelphia, Lippincott-Raven, 1997, pp 947–976

8. Fraker DL: Radiation exposure and other factors that predispose to human thyroid neoplasia. *Surg Clin North Am* 75:365–375, 1995

9. Ron E, Lubin JH, Shore RE, et al: Thyroid cancer after exposure to external radiation: a pooled analysis of seven studies. *Radiat Res* 141:259–277, 1995

10. Fraker DL, Skarulis M, Livolsi V: Thyroid tumors. In DeVita VT, Hellman S, Rosenberg SA (eds): *Cancer Principles and Practice of Oncology* (ed 5). Philadelphia, Lippincott-Raven, 1997, pp 1629–1652

11. Wittes RE, Macdonald JS: Endocrine system, in Macdonald JS, Haller DG, Mayer RJ (eds): *Manual of Oncologic Therapeutics* (ed 3). Philadelphia, Lippincott, 1995, pp 237–245

12. Hallquist A, Hardell L, Degerman A, et al: Medical diagnostic and therapeutic radiation and the risk of thyroid cancer: a case-control study. *Eur J Cancer Prevent* 3:259–267, 1994

13. Bleuer JP, Averkin YI, Abelin T: Chernobyl-related thyroid cancer: what evidence for role of short-lived iodines? *Environ Health Perspect* 105:1483–1486, 1997 (suppl 6)

14. Mendelsohn G: Pathology of thyroid disease, in Mendelsohn G (ed): *Diagnosis and Pathology of Endocrine Diseases.* Philadelphia, Lippincott, 1988, pp 37–117

15. Galanti MR, Sparen P, Karlsson A, et al: Is residence in areas of endemic goiter a risk factor for thyroid cancer? *Int J Cancer* 61:615–621, 1995

16. Segal K, Arad A, Lubin E, et al: Follicular carcinoma of the thyroid. *Head Neck* 16:533–538, 1994

17. Hanna FWF, Cunningham RT, Ardill JES, et al: Prognostic factors in medullary carcinoma of the thyroid. *Endocrine-Related Cancer* 5:49–53, 1998

18. Tan RK, Finley RK, Driscoll D, et al: Anaplastic carcinoma of the thyroid: a 24-year experience. *Head Neck* 17:41–48, 1995

19. Farndon JR: Endocrine tumours, in McArdle CS (ed): *Surgical Oncology: Current Concepts and Practice.* London, Butterworths, 1990, pp 97–114

20. DeGroot LJ: Thyroid neoplasia, in DeGroot LJ, Besser GM, Burger HG, et al (eds): *Endocrinology* (ed 3). Philadelphia, Saunders, 1995, pp 834–854

21. Cady B: Neoplasms of the thyroid, in Holland JF, Frei E, Bast RC, et al (eds): *Cancer Medicine* (ed 3). Philadelphia, Lea & Febiger, 1993, pp 1138–1146

22. Lennquist S: The thyroid nodule: diagnosis and surgical treatment. *Surg Clin North Am* 67:213–232, 1987

23. Weiss M, Baruch A, Keydar I, et al: Preoperative diagnosis of thyroid papillary carcinoma by reverse transcriptase polymerase chain reaction of the MUCI gene. *Int J Cancer* 66:55–59, 1996

24. Ho YS, Tseng SC, Chin TY, et al: p53 gene mutations in thyroid carcinoma. *Cancer Lett* 103:57–63, 1996

25. Gallaway RJ, Smallridge RC: Imaging in thyroid cancer. *Endocrinol Metab Clin North Am* 25:93–113, 1996

26. Danese D, Centanni M, Farsetti A, et al: Diagnosis of thyroid carcinoma. *J Exp Clin Cancer Res* 16:337–347, 1997

27. Boigon M, Moyer D: Solitary thyroid nodules: separating benign from malignant conditions. *Postgrad Med* 98(2): 73–80, 1995

28. Hamburger JI: Diagnosis of thyroid nodules by fine needle biopsy: use and abuse. *J Clin Endocrinol Metab* 79:335–339, 1994

29. Chang HY, Lin JD, Chen JF, et al: The correlation of fine needle aspiration cytology and frozen section biopsies in the diagnosis of thyroid nodules. *J Clin Pathol* 50: 1005–1009, 1997

30. Dwarakanathan AA, Staren ED, D'Amore MJ, et al: Importance of repeat FN biopsy in the management of thyroid nodules. *Am J Surg* 166:350–352, 1993

31. American Joint Committee on Cancer: Thyroid gland, in *AJCC Cancer Staging Manual* (ed 5). Philadelphia, Lippincott-Raven, 1997, pp 59–61

32. American Association of Clinical Endocrinologists and American College of Endocrinology: *AACE Clinical Practice Guidelines for the Management of Thyroid Carcinoma.* Available at http://www.aace.com/clin/guides/thycancer.html (Accessed on June 6, 1999)

33. Moore S, Haughey BH: Surgical treatment for thyroid cancer. *AORN J* 65:710–725, 1997

34. Lehne RA: Drugs affecting calcium levels and bone mineralization. *Pharmacology for Nursing Care* (ed 3). Philadelphia, Saunders, 1998, pp 814–829

35. Giarelli E: Medullary thyroid carcinoma: one component of the inherited disorder multiple endocrine neoplasia type 2a. *Oncol Nurs Forum* 24:1007–1020, 1997

36. Baker KH, Feldman JE: Thyroid cancer: a review. *Oncol Nurs Forum* 20:95–104, 1993

37. Brierley JD, Tsang RW: External radiation therapy in the treatment of thyroid malignancy. *Endocrinol Metab Clin North Am* 25:141–157, 1996

38. Tennvall T, Lundell G, Hallquist A, et al: Combined doxorubicin, hyperfractionated radiotherapy, and surgery in anaplastic thyroid carcinoma. *Cancer* 74:1348–1354, 1994

39. McKittrick RJ, Stephens RL: Chemotherapy of endocrine tumors, in Perry MC (ed): *The Chemotherapy Source Book* (ed 2). Baltimore, Williams and Wilkins, 1996, pp 1201–1213

40. Droz JP, Schlumberger M, Rougier P, et al: Chemotherapy in nonmetastatic thyroid cancer: experience at the Institut Gustave-Roussy. *Tumori* 76:480–483, 1990

41. Schlumberger M, Abdelmoumene N, Delisle MJ, et al: Treatment of advanced medullary thyroid cancer with an alternating combination of 5FU-streptozocin and 5FU-dacarbazine. *Br J Cancer* 71:363–365, 1995

42. Goodman HM: Parathyroid cancer, *Basic Medical Endocrinology* (ed 2). New York, Raven, 1994, pp 175–202

43. Wu L-T, Chahinian AP, Baylin SB, et al: Neoplasms of the neuroendocrine system, in Holland JF, Frei E, Bast RC, et al (eds): *Cancer Medicine* (ed 4). Baltimore: Williams and Wilkins, 1997, pp 1571–1603

44. Shane E: Parathyroid carcinoma, in Bilezikian JP (ed): *The Parathyroids. Basic and Clinical Concepts.* New York: Raven, 1994, pp 575–581

45. Cordeiero AC, Montenegro FLM, Kulcsar MAV, et al: Parathyroid carcinoma. *Am J Surg* 175:52–55, 1998

46. Gillis D, Hirsch HJ, Landau H, et al: Parathyroid adenoma after radiation in an 8-year-old boy. *J Pediatr* 132:892–893, 1998

47. Erickson LA, Jin L, Wollan P, et al: Parathyroid hyperplasia, adenomas, and carcinomas: differential expression of p27[Kip1] protein. *Am J Surg Pathol* 23:288–295, 1999

48. Wang CA, Gaz RD: Natural history of parathyroid carcinoma: diagnosis, treatment and results. *Am J Surg* 149: 522–527, 1985

49. Sandelin K, Tullgren O, Farnebo LO: Clinical course of metastatic parathyroid cancer. *World J Surg* 18:594–599, 1994

50. Brown EM, Vickery AL: Weekly clinicopathological exercises: case 32-1996: a 44-year-old woman with a long history of intermittent hypercalcemia, a new mass, and hypercalcemic crisis. *N Engl J Med* 335:1213–1220, 1996

51. Fujimoto Y, Obara T: How to recognize and treat parathyroid carcinoma. *Surg Clin North Am* 67:343–357, 1987

52. Sloan DA, Schwartz RW, McGrath PC, et al: Diagnosis and management of thyroid and parathyroid hyperplasia and neoplasia. *Curr Opin Oncol* 7:47–55, 1995

53. Gupta VK, Yeh KA, Burke GJ, et al: 99m-technetium sestamibi localized solitary parathyroid adenoma as an indication for limited unilateral surgical exploration. *Am J Surg* 176:409–412, 1998

54. Obara T, Okamoto T, Ito Y, et al: Surgical and medical management of patients with pulmonary metastasis from parathyroid carcinoma. *Surgery* 114:1040–1049, 1993

55. Jaskowiak N, Norton JA, Alexander HR, et al: A prospective trial evaluating a standard approach to reoperation for missed parathyroid adenoma. *Ann Surg* 224:308–322, 1996

56. Bukowski RM, Sheeler L, Cunningham J, et al: Successful combination chemotherapy for metastatic parathyroid carcinoma. *Arch Intern Med* 144:399–400, 1984

57. Chahinian AP: Chemotherapy for metastatic parathyroid carcinoma. *Arch Intern Med* 144:1889, 1984 (letter)

58. Bradwell AR, Harvey TC: Control of hypercalcaemia of parathyroid carcinoma by immunisation. *Lancet* 353 (9150):370–373, 1999

59. Goodman HM: Pituitary gland, *Basic Medical Endocrinology* (ed 2). New York, Raven, 1994, pp 28–45

60. Nieuwenhuijzen Kruseman AC: Structure and function of the hypothalamus and pituitary, in Grossman A (ed): *Clinical Endocrinology* (ed 2). Boston, Blackwell Science, 1998, pp 83–89

61. Kamal T, Laws ER: Tumors of the pituitary gland, in Murphy GP, Lawrence W, Lenhard RE (eds): *American Cancer Society Textbook of Clinical Oncology* (ed 2). Atlanta, American Cancer Society, 1995, pp 411–427

62. Molitch ME: Hypothalamic and pituitary tumors: general principles, in Grossman A (ed): *Clinical Endocrinology* (ed 2). Boston, Blackwell Science, 1998, pp 129–137

63. Shimon I, Melmed S: Management of pituitary tumors. *Ann Intern Med* 129:472–483, 1998

64. Dolenc VV: Transcranial epidural approach to pituitary tumors extending beyond the sella. *Neurosurgury* 41: 542–552, 1997

65. Farrell WE, Clayton RN: Molecular biology of human pituitary adenomas. *Ann Med* 30:192–198, 1998

66. Zhang X, Horowitz GA, Heaney AP, et al: Pituitary tumor transforming gene (PTTG) expression in pituitary adenomas. *J Clin Endocrinol Metab* 84:761–767, 1999

67. Farrell WE, Clayton RN: Molecular biology of human pituitary adenomas. *Ann Med* 30:192–198, 1998

68. Thapar K, Scheitauer BW, Kovacs K, et al: p53 expression in pituitary adenomas and carcinomas: correlations with invasiveness and tumor growth fractions. *Neurosurgery* 38: 765–771, 1996

69. Molitch ME: Evaluation and treatment of the patient with a pituitary incidentaloma. *J Clin Endocrinol Metab* 80:8–11, 1995

70. McDermott MT: Nonfunctioning pituitary tumors, in McDermott MT (ed): *Endocrinology Secrets*. Philadelphia, Handley and Belfus, 1995, pp 99–101

71. Cornett MS, Paris KJ, Spanos WJ, et al: Radiation therapy for pituitary adenomas: a retrospective study of the University of Louisville experience. *Am J Clin Oncol* 19:292–295, 1996

72. Eisenberg AA, Redick EL: Transsphenoidal resection of pituitary adenoma: using a critical pathway. *Dimen Crit Care Nurs* 17:306–312, 1998

73. Molitch ME: Clinical manifestations of acromegaly. *Endocrinol Metab Clin North Am* 21:597–614, 1992

74. Lamberts SWJ: Acromegaly, in Grossman A (ed): *Clinical Endocrinology* (ed 2). Boston, Blackwell Science, 1998, pp 170–183

75. Gumowski J, Proch M, Kessler CA: Endocrinopathies of hyperfunction: Cushing's syndrome and aldosteronism. *AACN Clin Issues Crit Care Nurs* 3:331–347, 1992

76. von Werder K, Müller OA: Cushing's syndrome, in Grossman A (ed): *Clinical Endocrinology* (ed 2). Boston, Blackwell Science, 1998, pp 415–431

77. Croughs RJM: Pituitary tumors: diagnosis and treatment. *Anti-Cancer Drugs* 3:555–565, 1992

78. Nishizawa S, Ohta S, Yokoyama T, et al: Therapeutic strategy for incidentally found pituitary tumors ("pituitary incidentalomas"). *Neurosurgery* 43:1344–1348, 1998

79. Embil JM, Kramer M, Kinnear S, et al: A blinding headache. *Lancet* 350(9072):182, 1997

80. Delitala G: Hyperprolactinaemia: causes, biochemical diagnosis and tests of prolactin secretion, in Grossman A (ed): *Clinical Endocrinology* (ed 2). Boston: Blackwell Science, 1998, pp 138–147

81. Sarapura V: Prolactin-secreting pituitary tumors, in McDermott MT (ed): *Endocrinology Secrets*. Philadelphia, Hanley and Belfus, 1995, pp 102–105

82. Samuels MH: Cushing's syndrome, in McDermott MT (ed): *Endocrinology Secrets*. Philadelphia, Hanley and Belfus, 1995, pp 116–121

83. Corbett JV: *Laboratory Tests and Diagnostic Procedures with Nursing Diagnoses*. Stamford, CT, Appleton and Lange, 1996

84. Tyrell JB, Lamborn KR, Hannegan LT, et al: Transsphenoidal microsurgical therapy of prolactinomas: initial outcomes and long-term results. *Neurosurgery* 44:254–261, 1999

85. Ciric I, Ragin A, Baumgartner C, et al: Complications of transsphenoidal surgery: results of a national survey, review of the literature, and personal experience. *Neurosurgery* 40: 225–237, 1997

86. Counsell CM, Gilbert M, Snively C: Management of the patient with a pituitary tumor resection. *Dimen Crit Care Nurs* 15(2):75–81, 1996

87. Andrews DW: Pituitary adenomas. *Curr Opin Oncol* 6:53–59, 1994

88. McCutcheon IE: Management of individual tumor syndromes. Pituitary neoplasia. *Endocrinol Metab Clin North Am* 23:37–51, 1994

89. Levy A, Lightman SL: Diagnosis and management of pituitary tumours. *Br Med J* 308:1087–1091, 1994

90. Loriaux DL, Wild RA: Contraceptive choices for women with endocrine complications. *Am J Obstet Gynecol* 168: 2021–2026, 1993

91. Stevenaert A, Beckers A: Presurgical octreotide treatment in acromegaly. *Acta Endocrinol* 129(suppl 1):18–20, 1993

92. McEven DR: Transsphenoidal adenomectomy. *AORN* 61: 321–337, 1995

93. Smith-Rooker JL, Garrett A, Hodges LC: Case management of the patient with pituitary tumor. *Med Surg Nurs* 2: 265–274, 1993

94. Shiminski-Maher T: Patient/family preparation and education for complications and late sequelae of craniopharyngiomas. *Pediatr Neurosurg* 21:112–119, 1994 (suppl 1)

95. Guinan EM, Lowy C, Stanhope N, et al: Cognitive effects of pituitary tumours and their treatments: two case studies and an investigation of 90 patients. *J Neurol Neurosurg Psychiatry* 65:870–876, 1998

96. Gotch PM: Cushing's syndrome from the patient's perspective. *Endocrinol Metab Clin North Am* 23:607–617, 1994

97. Goodman HM: Adrenal glands, in *Basic Medical Endocrinology*. New York: Raven, 1994, pp 71–112

98. Vinson GP, Whitehouse BJ, Hinson JP: The adrenal cortex, in Grossman A (ed): *Clinical Endocrinology* (ed 2). Boston: Blackwell Science, 1998, pp 395–414

99. Latronico AC, Chrousos GP: Extensive personal experience. Adrenocortical tumors. *J Clin Endocrinol Metab* 82: 1317–1324, 1997

100. Vargas MP, Vargas HI, Kleiner DE, et al: Adrenocortical neoplasms: role of prognostic markers MIB-1, P53, and RB. *Am J Surg Pathol* 21:556–562, 1997

101. Wolthers OD, Cameron FJ, Scheimberg I, et al: Androgen secreting adrenocortical tumours. *Arch Dis Child* 80:46–50, 1999

102. Beuschlein F, Reincke M, Karl M, et al: Clonal compositions of human adrenal neoplasms. *Cancer Res* 54:4927–4932, 1994

103. Kjellman M, Roshani L, The BT, et al: Genotyping of adrenocortical tumors: very frequent deletions of the MEN1 locus in 11q13 and of a 1-centimorgan region in 2p16. *J Clin Endocrinol Metab* 84:730–735, 1999

104. Gicquel C, Bertagna X, Schneid H, et al: Rearrangements at the 11p15 locus and over expression of insulin-like growth factor-11 gene in sporadic adrenocortical tumors. *J Clin Endocrinol Metab* 78:1444–1453, 1994

105. Berruti A, Terzolo M, Pia A, et al: Mitotane associated with etoposide, doxorubicin, and cisplatin in the treatment of advanced adrenocortical carcinoma. *Cancer* 83:2194–2200, 1998

106. Reincke M, Karl M, Travis WH, et al: p53 mutations in human adrenocortical neoplasms: immunohistochemical and molecular studies. *J Clin Endocrinol Metab* 78:790–794, 1994

107. Wagner J, Postwine C, Tabin K, et al: High frequency of germline p53 mutations in childhood adrenocortical cancer. *J Natl Cancer Inst* 22:1707–1710, 1994

108. Ooi TC: Adrenal incidentalomas: incidental in detection, not significance. *Can Med J* 157:903–904, 1997 (editorial)

109. Hedican SP, Marshall FF: Adrenocortical carcinoma with intracaval extension. *J Urol* 158:2056–2061, 1997

110. Figueroa AJ, Stein JP, Lieskovsky G, et al: Adrenal cortical carcinoma associated with venous tumour thrombus extension. *Br J Urol* 80:397–400, 1997

111. Gicquel C, Baudin E, Lebouc Y, et al: Adrenocortical carcinoma. *Ann Oncol* 8:423–427, 1997

112. Norton JA: Adrenal tumors, in DeVita VT, Hellman S, Rosenberg SA (eds): *Cancer Principles and Practice of Oncology* (ed 5). Philadelphia, Lippincott-Raven, 1997, pp 1659–1677

113. Coonrod DV, Rizkallah TH: Virilizing adrenal carcinoma in a woman of reproductive age: a case presentation and literature review. *Am J Obstet Gynecol* 172:1912–1215, 1995

114. Müller J: Adrenocortical tumors: clinical and diagnostic findings. *Recent Results Cancer Res* 118:106–112, 1990

115. Paja M, Diez S, Lucas T, et al: Dexamethasone-suppressible feminizing adrenal adenoma. *Postgrad Med J* 70:584–588, 1994

116. Derksen J, Nagesser SK, Meinders AE, et al: Identification of virilizing adrenal tumors in hirsute women. *N Engl J Med* 331:968–973, 1994

117. Werbel S, Ober PO: Pheochromocytoma. Update on diagnosis, localization, and management. *Med Clin North Am* 79:131–153, 1995

118. Gerlo EAM, Sevens C: Urinary and plasma catecholamines and urinary catecholamine metabolites in pheochromocytoma: diagnostic value of 19 cases. *Clin Chem* 40:250–256, 1994

119. Lenders JWM, Keiser HR, Goldstein DS, et al: Plasma metanephrines in the diagnosis of pheochromocytoma. *Ann Intern Med* 123:101–109, 1995

120. Haake HR, Hermans J, van de Velde CJH, et al: Optimal treatment of adrenocortical carcinoma with mitotane: results in a consecutive series of 96 patients. *Br J Cancer* 69: 947–951, 1994

121. Bonacci R, Gigliotti A, Baudin E, et al: Cytotoxic therapy with etoposide and cisplatin in advanced adrenocortical carcinoma. *Br J Cancer* 78:546–549, 1998

122. Dickstein G, Shechner C, Arad E, et al: Is there a role for low doses of mitotane (o,p'-DDD) as adjuvant therapy in adrenocortical carcinoma. *J Clin Endocrinol Metab* 83: 3100–3103, 1998

123. Ushiyama T, Suzuki K, Kageyama S, et al: A case of Cushing's syndrome due to adrenocortical carcinoma with recurrence 19 months after laparoscopic adrenalectomy. *J Urol* 157:2239, 1997

124. Vassilopoulou-Sellin R, Guinee VF, Klein MJ, et al: Impact of adjuvant mitotane on the clinical course of patients with adrenocortical cancer. *Cancer* 71:3119–3123, 1993

125. Schlumberger M, Brugieres L, Gicquel C, et al: 5-fluorouracil, doxorubicin, and cisplatin as treatment for adrenal cortical carcinoma. *Cancer* 67:2997–3000, 1991

126. Bukowski RM, Wolfe M, Levine HS, et al: Phase II trial of mitotane and cisplatin in patients with adrenal carcinoma: a Southwestern Oncology Group study. *J Clin Oncol* 11: 161–165, 1993

127. Isobe K, Nakai T, Ykimasa N, et al: Expression of mRNA coding for four catecholamine-synthesizing enzymes in human adrenal pheochromocytomas. *Eur J Endocrinol* 138: 383–387, 1998

128. Lucon AM, Pereira MAA, Mendonca BB, et al: Pheochromocytoma: study of 50 cases. *J Urol* 157:1208–1212, 1997

129. Plouin P-F, Chatellier G, Fofol I, et al: Tumor recurrence and hypertension persistence after successful pheochromocytoma operation. *Hypertension* 29:1133–1139, 1997

130. Miyajima A, Nakashima J, Baba S, et al: Clinical experience with incidentally discovered pheochromocytoma. *J Urol* 157:1566–1568, 1997

131. Sandur S, Dasgupta A, Shapiro JL, et al: Thoracic involvement with pheochromocytoma: a review. *Chest* 115: 511–521, 1999

132. Vassilopoulou-Sellin R: Clinical outcome of 50 patients with malignant abdominal paragangliomas and malignant pheochromocytomas. *Endocr Rel Cancer* 5:59–68, 1998

133. Francis IR, Korobkin M: Pheochromocytoma. *Radiol Clin North Am* 34:1101–1112, 1996

134. Young WF: Pheochromocytoma: issues in diagnosis & treatment. *Compr Ther* 23:319–326, 1997

135. Smith CM, Wigent PJ: Pheochromocytoma in pregnancy: considerations for the advanced practice nurse. *J Perinat Neonat Nurs* 12(2):11–25, 1998

136. Goldstein RE, O'Neill JA, Holcomb GW, et al: Clinical experience over 48 years with pheochromocytoma. *Ann Surg* 53:S2–S5, 1998 (suppl 64)

137. Gavaghan M: Surgical treatment of pheochromocytomas. *AORN J* 65:1041–1071, 1997

138. Kubota Y, Naleada T, Sasagawa I, et al: Elevated levels of telomerase activity in malignant pheochromocytoma. *Cancer* 82:176–179, 1998

139. Tepel M, Zidek W: Hypertensive crisis: pathophysiology, treatment and handling of complications. *Kidney Int* 53:S2–S8, 1998 (suppl 64)

140. Agana-Defensor R, Proch M: Pheochromocytoma: a clinical review. *AACN Clin Issues Crit Care Nurs* 3:309–318, 1992

141. Zweiker R, Tiemann M, Eber B, et al: Bradydysrhythmia-related presyncope secondary to pheochromocytoma. *J Intern Med* 242:249–253, 1997 (case report)

142. Heron E, Chatellier G, Billaud E, et al: The urinary metanephrine-to-creatinine ratio for the diagnosis of pheochromocytoma. *Ann Intern Med* 125:300–303, 1996

143. Ulchaker JC, Goldfarb DA, Bravo EI, et al: Successful outcomes in pheochromocytoma surgery in the modern era. *J Urol* 161:764–767, 1999

144. Yu L, Fleckman AM, Chadha M, et al: Radiation therapy of metastatic pheochromocytoma: case report and review of the literature. *Am J Clin Oncol* 19:389–393, 1996

145. Wu L-T, Dicpinigaitis P, Bruckner H, et al: Hypertensive crises induced by treatment of malignant pheochromocytoma with a combination of cyclophosphamide, vincristine, and dacarbazine. *Med Pediatr Oncol* 22:389–392, 1994

146. Eng C: Seminars in medicine of the Beth Israel Hospital, Boston: The RET proto-oncogene in multiple endocrine neoplasia type 2 and Hirschsprung's disease. *N Engl J Med* 335:943–951, 1996

147. Komminoth P, Heitz PU, Klöppel G: Pathology of MEN-1: morphology, clinicopathologic correlations and tumour development. *J Intern Med* 243:455–464, 1998

148. Marx SJ: Multiple endocrine neoplasia type 1, in Vogelstein B, Kinzler KW (ed): *The Genetic Basis of Human Cancer.* New York, McGraw-Hill, 1998, pp 489–506

149. Darling TN, Skarulis MC, Steinberg SM, et al: Multiple facial angiofibromas and collagenomas in patients with multiple endocrine neoplasia type 1. *Arch Dermatol* 133:853–857, 1997

150. Morrison PJ, Nevin NC: Multiple endocrine neoplasia type 2b (mucosal neuroma syndrome, Wagenmann-Froboese syndrome). *J Med Genet* 33:779–782, 1996

151. Ponder BAJ: Multiple endocrine neoplasia type 2, in Vogelstein B, Kinzler KW (ed): *The Genetic Basis of Human Cancer.* New York, McGraw-Hill, 1998, pp 475–487

152. Eng C, Clayton D, Schuffenecker I, et al: The relationship between specific RET proto-oncogene mutations and disease phenotype in multiple endocrine neoplasia type 2: international RET mutation consortium analysis. *JAMA* 276:1575–1579, 1996

153. Anderson RJ, Lynch HT: Familial neuroendocrine tumors as a model for hereditary cancer. *Curr Opin Oncol* 9:45–54, 1997

154. Mulligan LM, Ponder BAJ: Genetic basis of endocrine disease: multiple endocrine neoplasia type 2. *J Clin Endocrinol Metab* 80:1989–1995, 1995

155. de la Chapelle A, Eng C: Molecular genetic diagnosis for hereditary cancer, in Perry MC (ed): *American Society of Clinical Oncology. 1999 Educational Book.* Alexandria, VA, American Society of Clinical Oncology, 1999, pp 445–453

156. Marx S, Spiegel AM, Skarulis MC, et al: Multiple endocrine neoplasia type 1: clinical and genetic topics. *Ann Intern Med* 129:484–494, 1998

157. Skogseid B, Rostad J, Oberg K: Multiple endocrine neoplasia type I. *Endocrinol Metab Clin North Am* 23:1–17, 1994

158. Chandrasekharappa SC, Guru SC, Manickam P, et al: Positional cloning of the gene for multiple endocrine neoplasia-type 1. *Science* 276:404–407, 1997

159. Falchetti A, Brandi ML: Genetic testing for multiple endocrine neoplasias. *Endocr Rel Cancer* 5:37–44, 1998

160. Casanova S, Rosenberg-Bourgin M, Farkas D, et al: Phaeochromocytoma in multiple endocrine neoplasia type 2 A: survey of 100 cases. *Clin Endocrinol* 32:532–537, 1993

161. Takami H: RET proto-oncogene mutation analysis for multiple endocrine neoplasia, type 2. *Arch Surg* 133:679, 1998 (letter and brief comm)

162. Frank K, Raue F, Gottswinter J, et al: The importance of early diagnosis and followup in sporadic MEN II. *Eur J Pediatr* 143:112–116, 1984

163. Vasen HFA, Vermey A: Hereditary medullary thyroid carcinoma. *Cancer Detect Prev* 19:143–150, 1995

164. Statement of the American Society of Clinical Oncology: genetic testing for cancer susceptibility. *J Clin Oncol* 14:1730–1736, 1996

165. Lynch HT: The Grosfeld et al article reviewed. *Oncology* 10:146–152, 1996

166. Heshmati HM, Graham H, Kohl S, et al: Genetic testing in medullary thyroid carcinoma syndromes: mutation types and clinical significance. *Mayo Clin Proc* 72:430–436, 1997

167. Lips CJM, Landsvater RM, Hoppener JWM, et al: Clinical screening as compared with DNA analysis in families with multiple endocrine neoplasia type 2a. *N Engl J Med* 331:828–835, 1994

168. Grosfeld FJM, Lips CJM, Beemer FA. Psychosocial consequences of DNA analysis for MEN type 2. *Oncology* 10:141–146, 1996

169. Burgess JR, Reuben D, Parameswaran V, et al: The outcome of subtotal parathyroidectomy for the treatment of hyperparathyroidism in multiple endocrine neoplasia type 1. *Arch Surg* 133:126–129, 1998

CHAPTER 53

Endometrial Cancer

Janet Ruth Walczak, RN, MSN, CRNP

Introduction

Endometrial cancer is the fourth leading cause of cancer in women and is the predominant cancer of the female genital tract (Table 53-1).[1] However it may be the most curable when the disease is diagnosed early. Endometrial carcinomas comprise 97% of all cancers of the corpus uteri and are the subject of this chapter. The remaining 3%, comprising uterine sarcomas, are not included in this chapter.[1,2]

Epidemiology

While in 2000 there were an estimated 36,100 new cases of endometrial cancer diagnosed in the United States, only approximately 6500 women died of the disease. Incidence and mortality rates have been relatively stable over the last decade with about 21 cases per 100,000 and mortality at 3 per 100,000.[3] Endometrial cancer is also among the five most frequent cancers in women despite race or ethnicity (except in Korean, Vietnamese, and Alaskan native women).[4] The low mortality rate in this disease reflects the fact that most women are diagnosed with localized disease (75% of white women and 51% of black women).[4,5] Survival rates for endometrial cancer by stage are 76% for stage I, 50% for stage II, 30% for stage III, and 9% for stage IV.[6]

Endometrial cancer is primarily a disease of postmenopausal women. The median age at diagnosis is 61 years, with the majority of women diagnosed between 50 and 59 years of age. Only about 5% of women will be diagnosed before age 40, and 20%–25% will be premenopausal.[5,6]

Etiology

Multiple risk factors have been associated with the development of endometrial cancer (Table 53-2). These include obesity (> 20 pounds overweight), nulliparity, late

Table 53-1 Leading Sites of Cancer in U.S. Women in 2000[1]

Site	Incidence
Breast	182,800
Lung and bronchus	74,600
Colon and rectum	66,600
Endometrium	36,100
Ovary	27,100

Table 53-2 Risk Factors for Endometrial Cancer

Obesity (> 20 pounds overweight)

Diabetes

Hypertension

Reproductive factors
  Nulliparity
  Menopause after age 52
  Failure to ovulate
  Irregular menses
  Excessive estrogen/inadequate progesterone

Estrogen replacement without adequate progesterone

Tamoxifen use

Family history of endometrial, colorectal, breast, or ovarian cancer

menopause (after age 52), diabetes, hypertension, infertility, irregular menses, failure of ovulation, a history of breast or ovarian cancer, adenomatous hyperplasia, prolonged use of exogenous estrogen therapy, and tamoxifen use. An obese, nulliparous woman who experiences menopause after age 59 appears to have a five-fold greater risk of developing endometrial cancer.[5,6] Additionally, Feldman and associates found that the nulliparous, diabetic woman over age 70 who presents with abnormal vaginal bleeding has an 87% risk of developing endometrial cancer or hyperplasia, while the woman who presents with abnormal bleeding and has none of the other factors has only a 3% risk.[7] Diabetes and hypertension are no longer considered independent risk factors but may be present as cofactors related to endocrine imbalances. Similarly, these factors tend to be more prevalent in older, obese women.[5,8]

Excessive endogenous estrogen metabolism or production or inadequate progesterone levels have been implicated in the development of endometrial cancer. Several hormonal aberrations can be linked to obesity. Increased body size plays a role in androgen conversion to estrogen.[2,9–11] Women who are more than 50 pounds overweight have a tenfold increase in risk.[2] Additionally, obese women with an upper body fat pattern have a 5.8-fold increase in risk over women who are nonobese or have a lower body fat pattern.[11,12] Fat cells are an excellent storage depot for estrogen, and the chronic slow release of estrogen from these cells may account for the increased risk. In obese postmenopausal women, secretion of serum sex hormone-binding globulin (SHBG) is depressed, leaving higher concentrations of free estradiol in the blood. Obese women have endocrine malfunctions such as inadequate progesterone levels that cause anovulatory cycles with irregular menses. Chronic anovulation, such as in polycystic ovarian disease, results in failure of progesterone to oppose chronic estrogen effects on the endometrium. Another source of endogenous estrogen can be feminizing ovarian tumors (e.g., granulosa cell tumors).[2,9,10]

Use of unopposed estrogen therapy has been linked to an increased incidence of endometrial cancer since the mid-1970s.[13] This problem can be virtually eliminated by cycling or combining estrogen and progesterone. Progesterone use should be a minimum of 12 days per month. However, despite the addition of progesterone, prolonged hormone replacement (greater than five years) has been associated with increased risk.[6,14,15] Tamoxifen, which acts as an antiestrogen on breast tissue, has a weak estrogenic effect on endometrial tissue and has been associated with thickening of the endometrium and changes from polyps to hyperplasia and cancer.[16–21] While there are conflicting data about the endometrial cancer risks associated with tamoxifen, recent data from the breast cancer prevention trial demonstrate a 2.53% increase in risk for endometrial cancer in women taking tamoxifen (95% confidence interval = 1.35–4.97). The greatest risk was in women over age 50. All endometrial cancers among the study group were diagnosed in stage I.[2,22,23]

Either exogenous or endogenous estrogen may lead to endometrial hyperplasia. While adenomatous hyperplasia is considered a risk factor of endometrial cancer, it is unclear if it is a precursor, unless atypia accompanies the hyperplasia.[7]

Women with a family history of endometrial cancer and colorectal cancer have an increased risk of developing endometrial cancer. Lynch II syndrome (nonpolyposis colorectal cancer) is associated with endometrial cancer as well as breast and ovarian cancer. In this group, endometrial cancer occurs in 4%–11% of women and at a time period about two decades earlier than would usually be expected. Overall, a family history of endometrial cancer is present in about 5% of all cases and a family history of colorectal cancer in about 2%.[2,14]

Prevention, Screening, and Early Detection

Two factors appear to have a protective effect against the development of endometrial cancer: oral contraceptives and cigarette smoking. Use of oral contraceptives, which since the 1970s have been comprised mostly of progesterone, decreases for at least 12 months the woman's risk of developing endometrial cancer, and this protection seems to persist for up to 15 years in nulliparous women. Similarly, smoking has been correlated with a reduction in risk, especially in women over age 50. However, the risks of developing lung cancer and other health problems well outweigh any protection gained against endometrial cancer.[6,24–28] A healthy lifestyle of a low-fat diet, regular physical activity, and maintaining normal weight may contribute to risk reduction and health promotion. Finally, treatment of endometrial hyperplasia, particularly the atypical type, can prevent progression to cancer. Usually a hysterectomy is performed. If future fertility is desired,

however, progestins can be given for about 12 days per month. Follow-up with repeat endometrial biopsies is indicated to evaluate response.[29]

Unfortunately, there is no sensitive and specific screening test for endometrial cancer. The Pap smear will only occasionally detect an endometrial cancer. Though endometrial biopsy is 90% effective in detecting a cancer and can be accomplished in the outpatient setting, it is not without morbidity and cost and should not at this time be used as a screen for the general population. The American Cancer Society and the American College of Obstetricians and Gynecologists currently recommend that women should have an annual pelvic examination and Pap smear, and that an endometrial biopsy should be obtained at menopause and periodically after that in women at high risk for endometrial cancer.[3,28] Special screening of the asymptomatic woman on tamoxifen or hormone replacement is not indicated; annual gynecologic examinations are recommended for these women as well as for the population at large.[5,23] Other screening techniques such as transvaginal ultrasonography, endometrial biopsy, and serum melatonin levels have been investigated but are not currently recommended as appropriate for screening in the asymptomatic woman.[2,14,30]

Pathophysiology

Cellular Characteristics

The uterine corpus is a muscular, hollow, pear-shaped organ with an endometrial lining composed of ciliated epithelial cells. Throughout the epithelium there are small, tubular glands that extend to the myometrium, or muscle wall of the corpus. Endometrial cancer develops in the tubular glands of the epithelial layer. Tumors that arise in the lower uterine segment involve the cervix sooner and have a higher incidence of pelvic and paraaortic lymph node involvement than do tumors that arise higher in the fundus. Similarly, tumors that have deep myometrial invasion tend to be more aggressive and have a poorer survival rate.[3,6]

Endometrial hyperplasia, primarily the atypical type, is a premalignant cytologic change that can progress to malignant. However, simple or complex hyperplasia without atypia rarely progresses to cancer.[22]

The majority of endometrial cancers are adenocarcinomas. Three types of adenocarcinomas account for more than 80% of histologic patterns: pure endometrioid adenocarcinoma, adenocarcinoma with a squamous metaplasia (formerly adenoacanthoma), and adenocarcinoma with squamous differentiation (formerly adenosquamous). The less frequent patterns include clear cell (mesonephroid) carcinoma, undifferentiated carcinoma, and papillary serous carcinomas. The clear cell and serous patterns are more aggressive than the other carcinomas.[3,6,24,26]

Progression of Disease and Patterns of Spread

Multiple factors affect the natural history and prognosis of endometrial cancer (Table 53-3). These include histological type and differentiation, stage of disease, myometrial invasion, peritoneal cytology, lymph node metastasis, and adnexal metastasis.[6,31]

Cancer usually starts in the fundus and may spread to involve the entire endometrium. Through direct extension and infiltration, the cancer spreads to the myometrium, endocervix, cervix, fallopian tubes, and ovaries. Adnexal spread is infrequent but is found at surgery in about 10% of women with clinical stage I disease. Recurrence appears in 38% of women with adnexal spread versus 11% of those without such involvement.[6]

Metastatic spread is usually to pelvic and paraaortic lymph nodes and has been positively correlated with tumor differentiation, stage of disease, and amount of myometrial invasion. Pelvic and paraaortic lymph node metastases can be present, even in women with stage I disease (Figure 53-1) when about 10% will have positive pelvic nodes, and stage II disease when 36% will have positive nodes.[6] Less common sites of metastases include the vagina, peritoneal cavity, omentum, and inguinal lymph nodes. Hematogenous spread often involves the lung, liver, bone, and brain. The size of the uterus, measured by uterine sound, has been used as an indicator of survival. However, because large uterine size can be secondary to concomitant disease, such as fibroids, uterine size is no longer included in the staging and prognosis of endometrial cancer.

Histological differentiation is one of the most sensitive indicators of metastases and prognosis. The less differentiated the tumor, the poorer the prognosis. Grade 1 tumors are highly differentiated, grade 2 tumors are moderately differentiated, and grade 3 tumors are mostly solid or undifferentiated carcinomas.[29,32] Overall five-year survival rates are 96% for patients with grade I tumors, 79% for those with grade II tumors, and 70% for those with grade III tumors.[5,6,29]

Another prognostic indicator, the degree of myometrial invasion, is generally classified as none (localized to the endometrium), superficial (invasion < 50%), or deep (> 50%).[5,6] The greater the invasion, the poorer the prognosis. Additionally, the less differentiated the tumor, the

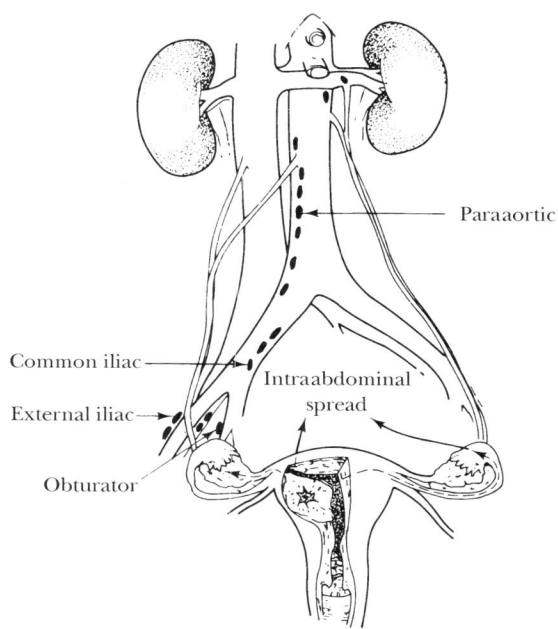

Figure 53-1 Spread pattern of endometrial cancer, with particular emphasis on potential lymph node spread. Pelvic and paraaortic nodes are at risk, even in stage I disease. (Reprinted with permission from DiSaia PJ, Creasman WT: *Clinical Gynecologic Oncology.* St Louis, Mosby, 1993.)[6]

greater the chance of myometrial invasion. Thus, the grade of the tumor is combined with the degree of myometrial invasion to estimate survival.

During laparotomy, samples of peritoneal fluid or washings of the peritoneal cavity are obtained for staging purposes, but the results also have prognostic significance. Women with positive peritoneal washings are at a higher risk for pelvic recurrence. Positive peritoneal washings have been reported in as many as 15% of women with stage I disease.[6] Recurrence developed in 34% of these individuals with stage I disease, compared with 10% among patients showing negative cytologic change.

Endometrial cancer tends to recur locally in the pelvis, regionally in the abdomen, or at distant sites outside the abdominal-peritoneal cavity. Patients with good prognostic indicators rarely have distant metastasis while women with poorer prognosis more frequently have distant metastasis.[22]

Clinical Manifestations

Fortunately, abnormal vaginal bleeding is an early symptom associated with endometrial cancer that usually causes women to seek medical attention promptly. Postmenopausal bleeding should always be evaluated, even though only 20% of women with this symptom will have cancer. Any serosanguinous vaginal discharge or new

Table 53-3 Prognostic Indicators

Indicator	Good Prognosis	Poor Prognosis
Stage of disease	I	II, III, IV
Histology	Adenocarcinomas: nonserous, non–clear cell	Serous or clear cell
Tumor differentiation	Grade 1	Grades 2, 3
Myometrial invasion	Superficial or none	Deep (> 50%)
Nodal metastasis	None	Present
Peritoneal cytology	Negative	Positive

heavy bleeding also needs evaluation. Premenopausal onset of irregular or heavy menstrual flow may be significant, especially if the patient is infertile with anovulatory cycles. Other more infrequent symptoms are pyometria and hematometria, particularly in the older woman, and lumbosacral, hypogastric, or pelvic pain in women with more advanced disease.[29,32]

Assessment

Patient and Family History

In women suspected of having endometrial cancer, a thorough history is taken. First, an in-depth description of the presenting symptom, such as postmenopausal bleeding, is obtained including onset of symptoms, duration, amount, intensity, color, consistency, and cramping. Other pertinent history information is focused on risk factors, such as reproductive history, estrogen use, weight change, tamoxifen use, and dietary habits. History questions should be focused on determining the extent of disease through a review of systems to identify symptoms such as abdominal pain, change in bowel or bladder function, and weight loss. Family and personal history of cancer, particularly breast, ovarian, endometrial, and colorectal cancer, should also be obtained.[22]

Physical Examination

Physical examination includes nodal surveillance (particularly supraclavicular and inguinal lymph nodes), lungs, abdomen for evidence of disease and organomegaly, and a complete pelvic examination (external genitalia, vagina, cervix, uterine size, adnexae and rectovaginal bimanual examination) to evaluate parametria and rectovaginal area.[22]

Diagnostic Studies

A Pap smear will only occasionally detect an endometrial cancer. A more reliable diagnostic technique is endometrial biopsy, which allows histologic rather than cytologic examination. Endometrial biopsy is 90% effective in detecting endometrial cancer and can be performed in the outpatient setting.[6] If the endometrial biopsy is negative and symptoms persist, a dilatation and curettage (D & C) and hysteroscopy are performed.

Other diagnostic tests include chest x-ray, stool guaiac, complete blood count (CBC), and blood chemistry profiles including liver function studies. Cystoscopy, barium enema, and proctoscopy are performed if bladder or rectal involvement is suspected. Though not routinely recommended, other studies that may be used to evaluate pelvic, abdominal, and nodal disease status include hysterography, hysteroscopy, lymphangiography, and com-

puterized axial tomogram scan.[2] Although magnetic resonance imaging (MRI) cannot distinguish benign from malignant neoplasms, it is effective in detecting the degree of myometrial invasion.[33-35] MRI may also be helpful to the gynecologist in determining who would benefit from pelvic and paraaortic node dissection and who should be referred to a gynecologic oncologist.[2]

Prognostic Indicators

Prognostic indicators in endometrial cancer are obtained through surgical staging and pathologic information. Good prognosis indicators include having risk factors that relate to endogenous or exogenous estrogen levels such as obesity, estrogen use without progesterone, nulliparity, and late menopause; estrogen-related risk factors; histologic grade 1 or 2, superficial myometrial invasion; no nodal metastasis; and stage I disease. In contrast, a poor prognosis involves histologic grade 3, deep myometrial invasion, nodal metastasis, high stage, and aggressive histologic behavior (usually clear cell or papillary serous).[2]

Classification and Staging

Endometrial cancer is staged surgically (Table 53-4), if medical condition and intraabdominal disease permit the woman to be a candidate for surgery. Staging helps to define primary tumor size and location as well as extent of spread beyond the uterus.[36] Approximately 73% of tumors are diagnosed in stage I, 12% in stage II, 12% in stage III, and 3% in stage IV.[6]

Surgical staging and treatment can involve an extensive evaluation of the abdominopelvic cavity and use of the following procedures: bimanual examination under anesthesia, peritoneal cytology, inspection and palpation of all peritoneal surfaces, biopsy of suspicious areas, selective pelvic and paraaortic lymphadenectomy, total abdominal hysterectomy (TAH), bilateral salpingo-oophorectomy (BSO), and possible omentectomy and resection of tumor implants.[37,38] Tissue from the primary tumor is obtained for analysis of estrogen and progesterone receptors, although the results are not used in the staging process.

Therapeutic Approaches and Nursing Care

Early-Stage Disease

The goals of treatment in stage I and II disease are for cure and long-term survival; thus nursing care must focus on management of side effects of treatment and promotion of health maintenance behaviors.

Table 53-4 Corpus Cancer Staging

CARCINOMA OF THE UTERINE CORPUS	HISTOPATHOLOGY: DEGREE OF DIFFERENTIATION

The Committee decided that corpus cancer should be surgically staged and as a result additional factors of prognostic importance are included in the staging. The Committee also decided to change the current definitions of tumor grading to coincide with the new recommendations of the International Society of Gynecological Pathologists. The recommended staging is as follows:

Cases of carcinoma of the corpus should be grouped with regard to the degree of differentiation of the adenocarcinoma as follows:

G1 5% or less of a nonsquamous or nonmorular solid growth pattern

G2 6%–50% of a nonsquamous or nonmorular solid growth pattern

G3 More than 50% of a nonsquamous or nonmorular solid growth pattern

STAGE

IA	G123	Tumor limited to endometrium
IB	G123	Invasion to < 1/2 myometrium
IC	G123	Invasion to > 1/2 myometrium
IIA	G123	Endocervical glandular involvement only
IIB	G123	Cervical stromal invasion
IIIA	G123	Tumor invades serosa and/or adnexa and/or positive peritoneal cytology
IIIB	G123	Metastases to pelvic and/or paraaortic lymph nodes
IVA	G123	Tumor invasion of bladder and/or bowel mucosa
IVB		Distant metastases including intraabdominal and/or inguinal lymph nodes

NOTES ON PATHOLOGICAL GRADING

(1) Notable nuclear aypia, inappropriate for the architectural grade, raises the grade of a grade I or grade II tumor by one.

(2) In serous adenocarcinomas, clear-cell adenocarcinomas, and squamous-cell carcinomas, nuclear grading takes precedence.

(3) Adenocarcinomas with squamous differentiation are graded according to the nuclear grade of the glandular component.

RULES RELATED TO STAGING

(1) Since corpus cancer is now surgically staged, procedures used previously for the differentiation of stages are no longer applicable (e.g., using dilatation and curettage findings to differentiate between stage I and stage II). (It is appreciated that there may be a small number of patients with corpus cancer who will be treated primarily with radiation therapy. If that is the case, the clinical staging adopted by FIGO* in 1971 would still apply but designation of that staging system would not be noted.)

(2) Ideally, the thickness of the myometrium should be measured along with the depth of tumor invasion.

*FIGO, International Federation of Gynecology and Obstetrics.
Data from FIGO News[36]

Surgery

Treatment of endometrial cancer includes surgical staging, TAH, BSO, selective pelvic and paraaortic lymphadenectomy, omentectomy, and peritoneal washings. Surgical staging is done initially on all women who are surgical candidates so that the radiation can be tailored to the individual's extent of disease. Many women with early-stage disease will not need additional therapy beyond the initial surgery. Thus time, effort, and morbidity associated with radiation therapy can be avoided. Also, the pathologist is better able to evaluate untreated tissue for the histologic indicators of prognosis (histologic type, grade, and myometrial invasion).

The woman undergoing surgery for endometrial cancer must be thoroughly informed preoperatively regarding the surgical procedure, recovery, and self-care issues (Table 53-5). Postoperative care includes fluid and electrolyte monitoring, progressive ambulation, and cardiopulmonary monitoring and intervention. Since many of these women may be overweight and over age 60, they may have concurrent medical problems such as hypertension, diabetes, or renal compromise that will require careful assessment and monitoring. Due to shortened hospital stays, discharge planning must begin early. Assessment includes identification of home care needs, ongoing monitoring needed, and follow-up care required. Because hysterectomy still is associated with loss of femininity, psychosocial support will be an important part of follow-up care. This may be particularly important when the woman is still of child-bearing age and premenopausal since the surgery itself will render her sterile and place her abruptly into menopause. Mobilization of support resources such as family, friends, social worker, spiritual counselor, and home care nurses may assist the woman in coping with these changes. For specific surgical oncology issues and nursing care, the reader is referred to Chapter 14.

Radiation

Selection of adjuvant radiation therapy for early endometrial cancer is determined by stage, histology, and cyto-

Table 53-5 Information Needs Related to Endometrial Cancer

Topic	Information
Health maintenance issues that affect risk	

Estrogen replacement therapy (ERT)	Indications:
	    Vaginal atrophy with infection or sexual dysfunction
	    Loss of pelvic support with incontinence
	    Postmenopausal osteoporosis
	    Perimenopausal emotional lability
	    Early surgical or radiation castration
	    Vasomotor instability
	    Lowered morbidity and mortality for cardiovascular disease
	Estrogen cycled with progesterone
	Annual pelvic exam
	Annual mammogram
	Seek medical attention if any abnormal vaginal bleeding occurs including postmenopausal bleeding (PMB)

Breast self-examination (BSE)	Importance of BSE in conjunction with ERT Determine schedule to aid in compliance Technique for performing BSE and demonstration of skill
Diet and weight control	Low-fat, calcium-rich diet Maintain weight within normal range Large amounts of caffeine and fiber may decrease calcium absorption Weight-bearing exercises to decrease bone loss (e.g., walking)
Abnormal vaginal bleeding	Seek medical attention for new onset of abnormal bleeding, including intramenstrual and PMB PMB and abnormal bleeding in the infertile patient with anovulatory cycles must be evaluated, even though only 20% of PMB is associated with malignancy Evaluation of abnormal bleeding includes pelvic exam and endometrial biopsy
Therapeutic interventions	
Surgery	Types of surgery planned, what will be removed, change in anatomy and function anticipated Clarify, reinforce informed consent Role in postoperative care to facilitate recovery, e.g., progressive ambulation, respiratory care Discharge planning related to self-care issues, need for assistance, and appointment for postoperative follow-up
Radiation	Type of therapy planned Associated morbidity, e.g., GI, GU Appointments for follow-up
Hormonal	Schedule for medications Expected side effects
Chemotherapy	Types of drugs and regimen planned Side effects and toxicities of drugs Inpatient versus outpatient versus home chemotherapy Duration of therapy Need for venous access device Regular appointments to monitor response
Psychosexual concerns	
Role functioning	Dispel myths related to perceived loss of femininity due to removal of uterus, tubes, and ovaries, e.g., weight gain, loss of sexual interest/enjoyment, aging, mental deterioration Help redefine self in terms other than reproduction

Sexual functioning	Review anatomy, physiology, and sexual functioning preoperatively
	Complete sexual assessment
	Alteration in sexual response secondary to hysterectomy:
	    Cervix contributes to but is not essential for orgasm
	    Uterus elevates during excitement phase and contracts rhythmically during orgasm
	Alteration in sexual functioning secondary to radiation:
	    Vaginal dryness and stenosis may result in patient who is not sexually active, unless vaginal dilators and lubricants are employed
	    Use of water-soluble lubricants during intercourse, such as Astroglide® or nonhormonal moisturizers used three times a week, such as Replens®

pathology. Patients with stage I, grade 1 or 2 disease, and no myometrial invasion require no further treatment after TAH or BSO. Indications for pelvic external beam radiation therapy (which allows treatment of all pelvic tissue including nodes and lymphatics) include disease localized to the pelvis, a high-grade tumor, or greater than 50% myometrial invasion. Women with stage Ic or IIa disease require whole pelvis radiation; stage IIb treatment adds intracavitary radiation to the regimen; stage III therapy includes whole pelvis, paraaortic (if paraaortic nodes are positive), and possibly whole abdominal radiation. Finally, stage IV treatment may include pelvic and abdominal radiation as well as chemotherapy.[2,6,14,22,31,38,39]

Women receiving radiation therapy should be taught prior to the initiation of therapy about the treatment plan, side effects, monitoring, and self-care issues (Table 53-5). During therapy, the patient is monitored closely for side effects of the treatment so that timely intervention can occur. Potential side effects of pelvic and abdominal radiation will be directly related to the organs or systems included in the radiation port. Potential side effects include nausea, diarrhea, urinary urgency or burning, myelosuppression, skin changes such as erythema, dryness, itching, burning, and desquamation. Sexual dysfunction can result due to atrophy and stenosis of the vagina from the radiation. The use of moisturizers will help minimize dryness. If the woman is sexually active, water-based lubricants can be used liberally during intercourse. If the woman is not sexually active, the use of vaginal dilators with the lubricants may help prevent vaginal stenosis. For specific radiation therapy issues and nursing care, the reader is referred to Chapters 16 and 17.

Advanced or Recurrent Disease

Treatment goals for stage III or IV, or for recurrent disease include controlling the disease and associated symptoms. Long-term survival is rare unless the disease is confined to the vagina. Palliation and supportive care are important nursing management goals so the patient's quality of life can be maximized.

Surgery and radiation

Endometrial cancer is difficult to treat if metastasis or recurrence has occurred.[40] Women with vaginal recurrences confined to the vagina can be treated successfully with surgery or radiotherapy. These individuals are usually considered cured and usually are long-term survivors. However, women with recurrences outside the upper vagina (pelvis or distant) require multimodal therapy and are rarely able to achieve long-term control. Radiotherapy has a limited role in the treatment of recurrent regional or distant disease, although palliative radiation can be used to control heavy vaginal bleeding in patients with advanced, incurable disease. Hormonal therapy or chemotherapy is essential to treat recurrent and advanced disease.[7]

Hormonal therapy

The most commonly used systemic therapy for recurrent endometrial cancer has been synthetic progestational agents. Response rates range from 30%–37%, and response seems to be related to histologic grade of the tumor, length of the disease-free interval, the woman's age, and presence of areas of squamous metaplasia within the primary tumor.[32] Receptor status can also predict which tumors will respond to progestins. Positive estrogen and progesterone receptor status correlates with a better response to progestin therapy regardless of the grade of the tumor. If both receptors are positive, there is a 77% response rate associated with progestin therapy, compared with only a 9% response rate if both receptors are negative.[2,41]

Oral preparations of megestrol acetate or intramuscular medroxyprogesterone acetate are effective agents against endometrial cancer.[32] The progestins are continued until the disease progresses. At that time, chemotherapy is considered.

Patient education about and close assessment and monitoring for side effects of the progestational agents are important components of care. The side effects include fluid retention, phlebitis, and thrombosis. Feelings of well-being as well as weight gain while taking progestins are also possible. Side effects are usually minimal unless high doses are employed.[32]

Chemotherapy

Cytotoxic agents have a limited role in the treatment of advanced endometrial cancer after women have failed to respond to hormonal therapy. Only a few agents have demonstrated activity equal to or greater than progestin therapy. Drugs that have shown activity in women who have not had prior chemotherapy include doxorubicin (37% response rate), cisplatin (up to 46%), ifosfamide (24.3%), and paclitaxel (35%).[42–45]

Combination chemotherapy using doxorubicin and cisplatin has become the standard of care following the results of a randomized trial that showed improved response rates for the combination over doxorubicin alone.[46] Studies of other combinations with additional drugs such as vinblastine and methotrexate have shown little additional improvement in response rates with increased side effects.[47,48] Currently, paclitaxel given in combination with cisplatin and doxorubicin is being compared with cisplatin and doxorubicin in a phase III randomized trial.[49] Newer approaches such as circadian-timed chemotherapy and the use of biologics need further study.[50,51]

Initially, the woman will need intensive education regarding the chemotherapy regimen, schedule, and side effects of the drugs (Table 53-5). Once treatment has been started, ongoing assessment and monitoring for treatment side effects will permit early recognition of problems and prompt intervention. Continuous psychosocial support is needed to assist the woman and her family in coping with the side effects of treatment, such as nausea, vomiting, hair loss, myelosuppression, and peripheral neuropathy. For specific issues and side effects of chemotherapy, the reader is referred to Chapters 19 and 20.

Symptom Management and Supportive Care

The woman with early stage endometrial cancer can expect long-term, disease-free survival. Since the majority of women with endometrial cancer fall into this favorable category, health maintenance will be a major focus of their ongoing care. It is important to note that this population of women will live their remaining lives without the health benefits of estrogen. Estrogen replacement therapy (ERT) is often raised as an important factor. For example, women with stage I disease, low-grade tumors, and no myometrial invasion, the benefits of ERT in decreasing the risk of cardiovascular disease and osteoporosis may outweigh the associated risk of breast cancer and recurrent endometrial cancer. A randomized study is currently under way to evaluate the effect of ERT on recurrence-free and overall survival in women with stage I or II endometrial cancer.[52] The American College of Obstetricians and Gynecologists issued a statement in 1993 that hormone replacement should be used in women with endometrial cancer using the same criteria as with general population but that special consideration should be given to the individual prognostic indicators and the risks that the woman is willing to accept.[53]

Additionally, as younger women develop endometrial cancer, conservative fertility sparing therapy for early-stage, low-grade disease needs to be prospectively evaluated for long-term outcomes. Another major area for assessment and intervention is knowledge related to health maintenance behaviors, therapeutic interventions, and psychosocial concerns. These issues are summarized in Table 53-5.

For those women who present with advanced disease or who have a recurrence, the challenges of care will vary according to the location and extent of disease present. Women with local, pelvic recurrence will have symptoms related to the structures that are involved, such as hematuria if the bladder is involved, fecal incontinence if a rectovaginal fistula is present, or pain if nerves are involved. Regional recurrence in the abdominal cavity can include ascites, a change in bowel habits due to compression or involvement of the bowel, or right upper quadrant pain from liver involvement. Finally, distant recurrence can involve respiratory compromise with lung metastases/effusions or central nervous system morbidity with brain metastases. The type of therapy used will depend on the specific recurrence. While surgery or radiation may be used in selected situations such as removing an isolated mass or treating an area that did not previously receive any radiation, chemotherapy is most often employed.

Information about the side effects of therapy and how to manage them; self-care issues such as care of a venous access device, nutritional intake, and pain control; and community resources for assistance including home care resources, support groups, and counseling are all important issues to consider. Quality of life is also an important issue to discuss with the woman and her family, particularly focusing on physical changes and functional status, psychosocial concerns such as changes in roles within the family, economic concerns, and spiritual and religious concerns. When the goal of treatment is supportive care, hospice care and bereavement counseling are the focus.

Continuity of Care: Nursing Challenges

For the vast majority of women with endometrial cancer, the major nursing challenges relate to compliance and regular follow-up. Since most patients will be cured with their primary surgery, regular follow-up will be the focus of their care. Follow-up usually involves regular pelvic examinations, at least quarterly in the initial years after diagnosis. Other tests and scans are performed as clinically indicated. Education about the importance of follow-up as well as a healthy lifestyle must be stressed. A healthy lifestyle includes weight reduction if appropriate, a diet low in fat, regular exercise, and regular screening for other cancers, including mammography.

For women who have advanced disease, mobilization of resources will be important in order to maximize care and quality of life. Coordination of care or case management is important to ensure that all physical and psychosocial needs are being addressed, either at time of discharge from the hospital or when care requirements change. Local ambulatory and home care resources, including nursing, social work, support groups, or spiritual counseling, can help the woman to remain at home during ongoing care for advanced disease whether the goal is cure, palliation, or comfort measures.

Conclusion

Though the majority of women are diagnosed with early-stage endometrial cancer, women still die from recurrent or advanced disease. Ongoing efforts strive to define appropriate screening techniques, adjuvant therapy, and new cytotoxic drugs and regimens to improve survival. Comprehensive, holistic nursing management will assist the woman and her family to achieve optimal health and quality of life.

References

1. Greenlee RT, Murray T, Bolden S, et al: Cancer statistics, 2000. *CA Cancer J Clin* 50:7–33, 2000
2. Rose P: Endometrial cancer. *N Engl J Med* 335:640–649, 1996

3. American Cancer Society: *Cancer Facts and Figures—1998.* American Cancer Society #5008.98, 1998

4. Parker SL, Davis JK, Wingo PA, et al: Cancer statistics by race and ethnicity. *CA Cancer J Clin* 48:31–48, 1998

5. Creasman WT: Endometrial cancer: incidence, prognostic factors, diagnosis, and treatment. *Semin Oncol* 24:140–150, 1997 (suppl 1)

6. DiSaia PJ, Creasman WT: *Clinical Gynecologic Oncology.* St. Louis, Mosby, 1993

7. Feldman S, Cook EF, Harlow BL, et al: Predicting endometrial cancer among older women who present with abnormal vaginal bleeding. *Gynecol Oncol* 56:367–381, 1995

8. Shoff SM, Newcomb PA: Diabetes, body size, and risk of endometrial cancer. *Am J Epidemiol* 148:234–240, 1998

9. Smith DB: Gynecological cancers: etiology and pathophysiology. *Semin Oncol Nurs* 2:270–274, 1986

10. Ewertz M, Schou G, Blice JD Jr: The joint effect of risk factors on endometrial cancer. *Eur J Cancer* 24:189–194, 1988

11. Goodman MT., Hankin JH, Wilkens LR, et al: Diet, body size, physical activity, and the risk of endometrial cancer. *Cancer Res* 57:5077–5085, 1997

12. Elliott EA, Matonoski GM, Rosenshein NB, et al: Body fat patterning in women with endometrial cancer. *Gynecol Oncol* 39:253–258, 1990

13. Persson I, Adami HO, Bergkvist L, et al: Risk of endometrial cancer after treatment with oestrogens alone or in conjunction with progestogens: Results of a prospective study. *Br Med J* 298:147–151, 1989

14. Yamada SD, McGonigle KF: Cancer of the endometrium and corpus uteri. *Curr Opin Obstet Gynecol* 10:57–60, 1998

15. Hulka BS: Replacement estrogens and risk of gynecologic cancers and breast cancer. *Cancer* 60:1960–1964, 1987

16. Fisher B, Costantino JP, Redmond CK, et al: Endometrial cancer in tamoxifen-treated breast cancer patients: findings from the National Surgical Adjuvant Breast and Bowel Project (NSABP) B-14. *J Natl Cancer Inst* 86:527–537, 1994

17. Fornander T, Rutquist LE, Cedarmark B, et al: Adjuvant tamoxifen in early breast cancer: occurrence of new primary cancers. *Lancet* 1:117–129, 1989

18. Cohen I, Beyth Y, Tepper R, et al: Adenomyosis in postmenopausal breast cancer patients treated with tamoxifen: a new entity? *Gynecol Oncol* 58:86–91, 1995

19. Cohen I, Rosen DJT, Shapira J, et al: Endometrial changes with tamoxifen: comparison between tamoxifen-treated and nontreated asymptomatic postmenopausal breast cancer patients. *Gynecol Oncol* 52:185–190, 1994

20. Barakat RR, Wong G, Curtin JP, et al: Tamoxifen use in breast cancer patients who subsequently develop corpus cancer is not associated with a higher incidence of adverse histologic features. *Gynecol Oncol* 55:164–168, 1994

21. Robinson DC, Bloss JD, Schiano MA: A retrospective study of tamoxifen and endometrial cancer in breast cancer patients. *Gynecol Oncol* 59:186–190, 1995

22. Greven KM, Corn BW: Endometrial cancer. *Curr Probl Cancer* 21:72–127, 1997

23. Fisher B, Costantino JP, Wickerham DL, et al: Tamoxifen for prevention of breast cancer: report of the National Surgical Adjuvant Breast and Bowel Project P-1 study. *J Natl Cancer Inst* 90:1371–1388, 1998

24. Franks AL, Kendrick JS, Tyler CW Jr: Postmenopausal smoking, estrogen therapy, and the risk of endometrial cancer. *Am J Obstet Gynecol* 156:20–23, 1987

25. The Cancer and Steroid Hormone Study of the Centers for Disease Control and the National Institute of Child Health and Human Development. *JAMA* 257:796–800, 1987

26. Hubbard JL, Holcombe JK: Cancer of endometrium. *Semin Oncol Nurs* 6:206–213, 1990

27. Parazzini F, LaVecchia C, Negri E, et al: Smoking and risk of endometrial cancer: results from an Italian case-control study. *Gynecol Oncol* 56:195–199, 1995

28. American College of Obstetricians and Gynecologists: *Routine Cancer Screening.* Technical Bulletin No. 128. Washington, D.C., 1993

29. Barakat RR, Park RC, Grigsby PW, et al: Corpus: epithelial tumors, in Hoskins RC, Perez CA, Young RC (eds): *Principles and Practice of Gynecologic Oncology* (ed 2). Philadelphia, Lippincott-Raven, 1997, pp 859–896

30. Grin W, Grunberger W: A significant correlation between melatonin deficiency and endometrial cancer. *Gynecol Obstet Invest* 45:62–65, 1998

31. Hacker NF: Uterine Cancer, in Berek JS, Hacker NJ (eds): *Practical Gynecologic Oncology.* Baltimore, Williams and Wilkins, 1989, pp 285–326

32. Burke TW, Eifel PJ, Muggia FM: Cancer of the uterine body, in DeVita VT Jr, Hellman S, Rosenberg SA (eds): *Cancer: Principles and Practice of Oncology* (ed 5). Philadelphia, Lippincott-Raven, 1997, pp 1478–1492

33. Yazigi R, Cohen J, Munoz AK, et al: Magnetic resonance imaging determination of myometrial invasion in endometrial carcinoma. *Gynecol Oncol* 34:94–97, 1989

34. Belloni C, Vigano R, delMaschio A, et al: Magnetic resonance imaging in endometrial carcinoma staging. *Gynecol Oncol* 37:172–177, 1990

35. Atsukawa H, Saski H, Tada S: A multivariate analysis of assessment of myometrial invasion of endometrial carcinoma by magnetic resonance imaging. *Gynecol Oncol* 54: 298–306, 1994

36. FIGO, International Federation of Gynecology and Obstetrics: Corpus Cancer Staging. FIGO News, *Int J Gynecol Obstet* 28:189–193, 1989

37. Shepherd JH: Revised FIGO staging for gynaecological cancer. *Br J Obstet Gynaecol* 96:889–892, 1989

38. Axelrod JH, Bundy B, Roy T, et al: Advanced endometrial carcinoma treated with whole abdominal irradiation: a Gynecologic Oncology Group (GOG) study. *Gynecol Oncol* 56: 135–136, 1995

39. Piver MS, Hempling RE: A retrospective trial of postoperative vaginal radium/cesium for grade 1–2 less than 50% myometrial invasion and pelvic radiation therapy for grade 3 or deep myometrial invasion in surgical stage I endometrial adenocarcinoma. *Cancer* 66:94–97, 1989

40. Edmonson JH, Krook JE, Hilton JF, et al: Randomized phase II studies of cisplatin and a combination of cyclophosphamide-doxorubicin-cisplatin (CAP) in patients with progestin-refractory advanced endometrial carcinoma. *Gynecol Oncol* 28:20–24, 1987

41. Thigpen T, Vance R, Lambuth B, et al: Chemotherapy for advanced or recurrent gynecologic cancer. *Cancer* 60: 2104–2116, 1987

42. Thigpen T, Buchsbaum HJ, Mangan C, et al: Phase II trial of adriamycin in treatment of advanced or recurrent endometrial carcinoma. *Cancer Treat Rep* 63:21–27, 1979

43. Seski JC, Edwards CL, Herson J, et al: Cisplatin chemotherapy for disseminated endometrial cancer. *Obstet Gynecol* 59: 225–228, 1982

44. Ball HG, Blessing JA, Lentz SS, et al: A phase II trial of taxol in advanced or recurrent adenocarcinoma of the endometrium: a Gynecologic Oncology Group study. *Gynecol Oncol* 62:278–281, 1996

45. Sutton GP, Blessing JA, DeMars LR, et al: A phase II Gynecologic Oncology Group trial of ifosfamide and mesna in

advanced or recurrent adenocarcinoma of the endometrium. *Gynecol Oncol* 63:25–27, 1996

46. Thigpen T, Blessing J, Homesley H, et al: Phase III trial of doxorubicin +/− cisplatin in advanced or recurrent endometrial carcinoma: a Gynecologic Oncology Group (GOG) study. *Proc Am Soc Clin Onc* 12:261, 1993, (abstr)

47. Long HJ, Langdon RM Jr, Cha SS, et al: Phase II trial of methotrexate, vinblastine, doxorubicin, and cisplatin in advanced/recurrent endometrial carcinoma. *Gynecol Oncol* 58: 240–243, 1995

48. Burke TW, Gershenson DM, Morris M: Postoperative adjuvant cisplatin, doxorubicin, cyclophosphamide (PAC) chemotherapy in women with high risk endometrial carcinoma. *Gynecol Oncol* 55:47–50, 1994

49. Fleming G, Ball H: A randomized study of doxorubicin plus cisplatin versus doxorubicin plus cisplatin plus 3 hour paclitaxel with G-CSF support in patients with primary stage III and IV or recurrent endometrial carcinoma: a Gynecologic Oncology Group (GOG) study no. 177, Philadelphia, 1993

50. Rossiello F, Nardone FDeC, Dell'Acqua: Interferon B increases the sensitivity of endometrial cancer cells to cell-mediated cytotoxicity. *Gynecol Oncol* 55:130–136, 1994

51. Gallion HH, Hrushesky WJ, Cibull M: A randomized study of doxorubicin plus cisplatin versus circadian timed doxorubicin plus cisplatin in patients with primary stage III and IV, recurrent endometrial carcinoma: a Gynecologic Oncology Group (GOG) study no. 139, Philadelphia, 1993

52. Barakat RR, Asbury R, Walder S: A randomized double-blinded trial of estrogen replacement therapy versus placebo in women with stage I or II endometrial adenocarcinoma: a Gynecologic Oncology Group (GOG) study no. 137, Philadelphia, 1997

53. American College of Obstetricians and Gynecologists: *Estrogen Replacement Therapy and Endometrial Cancer.* ACOG Committee Opinion no. 126, Washington DC, 1993

CHAPTER 54

Esophageal Cancer

Anita M. Reedy, RN, MSN, OCN®

Introduction

The esophagus is a tube that extends from the pharynx at the area of the cervical spine and ends at the junction connecting the esophagus to the stomach. It lies posterior to the trachea and is divided into the cervical (proximal) esophagus and the thoracic (mid and distal) esophagus (Figure 54-1).[1] Its function is to facilitate the swallowing process by peristaltic movements so that food and liquid can pass from the mouth to the stomach. The esophagus is made up of four layers; beginning with the innermost of the four, they include the (1) mucosal, (2) submucosal, (3) muscularis externa, and (4) adventitia layers.[2] The mucosal layer is convoluted, lined with epithelial tissue, and secretes mucus and other substances to keep the surface moist and flexible, features necessary to swallowing. Beneath the epithelium are the lamina propria, where the exocrine glands are located, and the muscularis mucosae, which is a thin layer of muscular tissue. Between the mucosa and submucosa are located major blood and lymphatic vessels. The submucosa, the second layer, consists of the submucus nerve plexus, an area rich in nerve fibers. The third layer, the muscularis propria, consists of both circular and longitudinal muscles as well as nerve tissue. The adventitia is the fourth and outer layer. There is no serosal layer in the esophagus.

Because of its location and function, the esophagus is subject to both internal and external factors that may affect its health. For example, the type and temperature of foods consumed, overflow of substances inhaled into the trachea, and acid refluxed from the stomach are all factors that are potentially harmful and damaging to the cells of the esophagus. One of the possible adverse outcomes of this cellular damage is the development of cancer of the esophagus.

Epidemiology

There are approximately 12,000 new cases of esophageal cancer diagnosed each year, which accounts for less than 1% of all cancers diagnosed.[3] There are almost the same number of deaths each year (11,200) as new cases. Esophageal cancer is more prevalent in men than in women and occurs more frequently in those over age 50. There are two major histologic types of esophageal cancer: squamous cell carcinoma (SCC) and adenocarcinoma (AC). SCCs are most often found in the proximal and midesophagus whereas ACs are most often found in the distal esophagus and esophagogastric junction. SCC is more prevalent among Asians and blacks while AC is more prevalent among whites.[4,5] SCC is the leading type of esophageal cancer in such countries as Japan, China, and Iran. In Western countries like the United States, there is an increasing incidence of AC such that adenocarcinoma of the esophagus is one of the most rapidly increasing types of cancer today. The reason for this change is not clear. In the United States, the incidence of esophageal cancer is higher in the eastern part of the country and in major urban centers.[4]

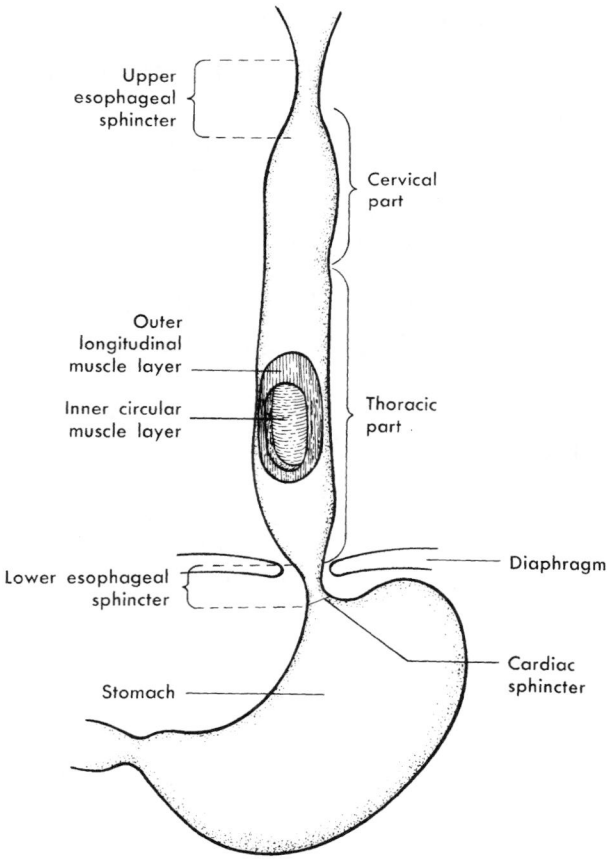

Upper esophageal sphincter

Cervical part

Outer longitudinal muscle layer

Inner circular muscle layer

Thoracic part

Lower esophageal sphincter

Diaphragm

Cardiac sphincter

Stomach

Figure 54-1 Normal anatomy of the esophagus with cutaway to show muscle layer. (Reprinted with permission from Given BA, Simmons SJ: Gastroenterology in Clinical Nursing St. Louis, MO, Mosby, 1999 p42.)[1]

Etiology

The cause of esophageal cancer is not completely known but is probably multifaceted. The major risk factors associated with the development of SCC are cigarette smoking and alcohol consumption. The most noted risk factor for AC is Barrett's esophagus,[3] which is a condition caused by injury from chronic reflux of gastric contents into the esophagus resulting in the squamous epithelium in the distal esophagus being replaced by columnar epithelium. Heitmiller and Sharma[6] noted that Barrett's esophagus was found in 64% of the patients with resected AC. Other risk factors for AC may be obesity and poor nutritional intake of substances such as vitamin A, vitamin C, magnesium, selenium, and zinc.[7]

Dietary links may play a role in developing both types

of esophageal cancer. Diets low in fruits and vegetables[4] and foods high in nitrosamine concentrations such as pickled and fermented foods may increase the risk. In contrast, foods high in vitamins C and E and selenium may inhibit esophageal cancer.

Another possible risk factor for developing esophageal cancer is viral infection. Human papilloma virus was found in up to 70% of patients with squamous cell carcinomas of the esophagus.[8] These viruses can disable tumor-suppressor genes such as the *p53* gene located on chromosome 17p13, which may lead to the overgrowth of tumor cells.[3] There may in fact be genetic components that contribute to the development of esophageal cancer. Both tumor suppressor genes such as *p53* and *APC and* proto-oncogenes including *EGFR* and *ERB-2* may be involved. The *p53* gene mutations are frequently found in high-grade dysplasia and adenocarcinoma[9] and may play a role in the tumor cell's resistance to chemotherapy.[10]

Prevention, Screening, and Early Detection Programs

There are no current recommendations in the United States for screening and early detection programs for esophageal cancer. The relatively small numbers of patients diagnosed with esophageal cancer each year may make it impractical to develop and utilize a mass screening program. Once cellular changes associated with Barrett's esophagus are detected, however, it is recommended that regular endoscopic surveillance be conducted in order to detect early, potentially curable neoplasms. Even in this high-risk group, it is not clear that endoscopic surveillance reduces mortality from esophageal cancer.[3]

Screening programs utilized in clinical practice usually concentrate on high-risk candidates with tobacco and alcohol use, poor dietary habits, and history of gastroesophageal reflux disease (GERD). Individuals must be educated to the role of tobacco, alcohol, and diet in the potential development of esophageal cancer. A person who reports frequent, chronic gastric reflux symptoms should be evaluated for the presence of Barrett's esophagus and medically managed with antireflux therapy.

Pathophysiology

Cellular Characteristics

The esophagus is lined with squamous epithelium, which is continuous until it reaches the grastroesophageal juncture where it is replaced with columnar tissue. Although there is a range of cell differentiation found in esophageal tumors, SCCs are generally better differentiated at diagnosis than ACs[11] and are most frequently found in the proximal or mid-esophagus. Cellular atypia usually precedes the development of SCC and is found more often in smokers than nonsmokers.[12] SCCs of the esophagus can be classified as polypoid, ulcerative, or infiltrative.[13] Tumor growth in the esophagus that is infiltrative in nature thickens the wall and leads to luminal narrowing. Frequently, the tumor is a polypoid mass that projects into the lumen of the esophagus. If not detected and removed, the tumor will grow until the esophagus is completely obstructed. Tumors that are ulcerative in nature are elevated with irregular, nodular edges. These ulcerative tumors expand into the submucosa and can be elevated to the point of obstruction. Some of these tumors will remain localized while others will extend throughout large areas of the esophagus.

ACs frequently arise from the columnar epithelium of the distal esophagus. The columnar epithelium cellular changes are most often attributed to Barrett's esophagus discussed in detail later in this chapter.

Progression of Disease

Because the esophagus does not have a serosal outer layer, it is easy for tumors to spread into adjacent tissues early in the disease. Frequently, the disease has spread to adjacent tissue and/or regional lymph nodes before it is detected. Tumors of the cervical esophagus can involve the left main stem bronchus, thoracic duct, aortic arch, or pleura. Tumors of the more distal areas of the esophagus can penetrate into the pericardium, pleura, descending aorta, and diaphragm. Invasion into these adjacent structures can make the tumor unresectable. The presence of a rich lymphatic system makes it easy for the tumor to metastasize to distant sites also making the tumor unresectable.

Patterns of Spread

The area surrounding the esophagus is rich in lymph nodes and vessels. These begin at the cervical esophagus and include the scalene, internal jugular, upper cervical, periesophageal, supraclavicular, and cervical nodes. Biopsy-proven, positive nodes in these areas are considered to be localized disease for cervical esophageal tumors but are considered distant disease for more distal tumors of the esophagus.

More distally located nodes surrounding the esophagus include the tracheobronchial, superior mediastinal, peritracheal, carinal, hilar, periesophageal, perigastric, pericardial, and mediastinal nodes. Positive nodes in these areas are considered localized disease for tumors of the thoracic esophagus but distant disease for tumors of the proximal esophagus.

The most distal nodes are the celiac axis nodes. When the celiac axis nodes are positive, it is considered localized disease for tumors of the distal and esophagogastric junction but distant disease for tumors of the proximal and mid esophagus.

Common distant metastatic sites beyond the esophageal area are the liver, lungs, pleura, and kidneys.[2] Other metastatic sites include bone, adrenal, peritoneum, and brain.[13]

Clinical Manifestations

Weight loss and dysphagia are the most common presenting symptoms of esophageal cancer.[12,14] The dysphagia is gradually progressive. Loss of appetite, malaise, and painful swallowing may also be present. An individual may be unable to swallow or clear salivary secretions if the esophagus is obstructed. There may also be pain if bone metastasis is present or the person may have elevated liver enzymes if liver metastasis is present.

Assessment

It is important to accurately determine the extent of the disease and the overall health status of the individual in order to provide the proper therapy. The first step in this assessment process is an extensive history and physical examination. Diagnostic studies and prognostic indicators all contribute to a comprehensive assessment for esophageal cancer.

History

The history should include information on any tobacco and alcohol use, diet, weight loss and over what period of time this loss has occurred, presence of dysphagia, pain especially with swallowing, heartburn, or gastric reflux, as well as the presence of comorbid conditions such as heart disease, pulmonary disease, and diabetes. Family history of cancer is also obtained. Performance status is a reliable indicator of general condition. For example, is the person able to carry on usual activities of daily living or is he staying in bed the majority of the day? Performance status usually correlates with length of time the individual has experienced dysphagia, weight loss, and other symptomatology. It is also important to determine the medications the individual is taking. Since alternative therapies are becoming more common, the use of any natural remedies the person may be taking to treat the disease or control symptoms should be included in the general history.

Physical Examination

Physical examination alone may not be particularly helpful in the detection of esophageal cancer. However, the overall assessment of the person's condition is useful to determine the ability to tolerate treatment. A thin, emaciated appearance could indicate the extent of the disease.

Other foci of the physical examination might include assessment for the presence of lymph nodes in the cervical and supraclavicular areas, focal tenderness, abdominal masses, or an enlarged or nodular liver.

Diagnostic Studies

Endoscopy with biopsy is the only definitive method for diagnosing the presence of esophageal cancer. Histologic examination of biopsied tissue will also determine cell differentiation. Cancer cells are classified as well differentiated, moderately differentiated, poorly differentiated, or undifferentiated. Most esophageal cancers are determined to be of the moderately differentiated grade.

Several tests and procedures can help determine the extent of the disease. The endoscopic ultrasound (EUS) and computerized tomography (CT) are used to identify tumor location, size, depth of invasion, and lymph node metastasis.[2] The location of the tumor at the time of endoscopy is noted by measuring the distance in centimeters from the front teeth (or incisors) to the tumor. The cervical esophagus is approximately 18 cm from the upper incisor teeth; the midthoracic esophagus extends approximately 24–32 cm from the upper incisor teeth; the distal thoracic esophagus and esophagogastric junction extend to approximately 40 cm from the incisors.

CT scans are particularly useful for detecting local lymph node involvement and distant metastatic disease.[15] They are effective in detecting metastasis to the liver and adrenals, and are also used to plan for radiation therapy and to monitor tumor response to treatment.[16] Areas of the chest, abdomen, and pelvis need to be radiographically examined for thorough assessment.

Positron emission tomography (PET) is a newer technology that utilizes the uptake of a glucose analog by tumor to detect the presence and extent of disease. Previously used in the assessment of lung cancer, research trials have shown PET to be more accurate than CT in detecting metastatic disease.[17,18]

Another method to determine the presence or absence of metastatic disease is the exploratory laparoscopy. Through small abdominal incisions, the area is visually explored for the presence of suspicious appearing nodes or tissue. If something suspicious is seen, a biopsy is taken so that a definitive diagnosis can be made.

Thorough staging involves the combination of all these diagnostic procedures to ensure the most accurate staging of the disease. This extensive assessment is extremely important in order to determine the best treatment approach.

Prognostic Indicators

Prognosis for patients with esophageal cancer is poor. This is partly due to the absence of a serosal layer in the esophagus that makes it easier for tumor to extend beyond the esophageal wall. Also, the rich lymphatic system in the esophageal area lends to early metastasis of the disease. Another factor contributing to the poor prognosis is the difficulty in eradicating the tumor at the primary site with surgery or radiation.[15]

Prognostic factors include stage, performance status, sex, age, anatomic location of the tumor, degree of weight loss, depth of tumor invasion, and involvement of lymph nodes.[4] Two key prognostic indicators for esophageal cancer are the depth of tumor invasion into or through the esophageal wall (T3 or T4) and the presence or absence of abdominal metastasis (M1).[19] Patients with T3N0 disease have a 50% chance of dying within five years of surgery.

Classification and Staging

Staging for esophageal cancer involves both clinical and pathologic staging of the disease. Clinical staging, conducted prior to treatment, involves disease that can be objectively examined. Included are history, physical examination, biopsy of the tumor, laboratory results, endoscopic examination, and radiologic imaging.[19]

Pathologic staging is based on surgical exploration, such as exploratory laparoscopy, and the examination of the surgically resected tissue and associated lymph nodes. Involvement of adjacent structures and detection of any distant metastatic sites must be documented in order to treat the disease appropriately.

Classification (Table 54-1) is based on the TNM system and includes size of the tumor and invasion into surrounding tissue, nodal involvement, and the presence or absence of metastasis.[19] *T* indicates presence and size of the primary tumor, *N* indicates presence and number of positive lymph nodes, and *M* indicates the presence of metastatic disease. The majority of people with esophageal cancer present with disease classified as either T3N1 (invasion of the adventitia and spread to regional nodes) or T4 (penetration into adjacent structures).[20]

Therapeutic Approaches and Nursing Care

Treatment for esophageal cancer is varied and depends on the stage of the disease and upon the general health status of the patient. For instance, tumor invasion into the aorta or tracheobronchial tree makes the tumor unresectable.[16] The presence of metastatic disease eliminates surgery (except for palliation) as an option. Presence of comorbid conditions may also preclude certain treatments. It is therefore important to have thorough staging and evaluation of the individual's condition as well as their understanding of the risks and benefits of various therapies before proceeding.

Nursing care is complex and sometimes difficult.[21] Aggressive measures for symptom control and support of

Table 54-1 AJCC TNM Staging System

Primary Tumor (T)	Staging Description
Tx	Cannot be assessed
T0	No evidence of primary tumor
Tis	Carcinoma *in situ*
T1	Tumor invades submucosa layer
T2	Tumor invades muscle layer
T3	Tumor invades adventitia
T4	Tumor invades adjacent structures

Regional Lymph Nodes (N)	Staging Description
Nx	Cannot be assessed
N0	No evidence of regional node metastasis
N1	Regional lymph node metastasis

Distant Metastasis (M)	Staging Description
Mx	Cannot be assessed
M0	No distant metastasis
M1	Distant metastasis

Stage Grouping

Stage 0	Tis	N0	M0
Stage I	T1	N0	M0
Stage IIA	T2	N0	M0
	T3	N0	M0
Stage IIB	T1	N1	M0
	T2	N1	M0
Stage III	T3	N1	M0
	T4	Any N	M0
Stage IV	Any T	Any N	M1
Stage IVA	Any T	Any N	M1a
Stage IVB	Any T	Any N	M1b

the patient and family throughout treatment need to be coordinated and implemented. The number and severity of side effects of treatment and the nursing care to manage these side effects depends on the extent of disease and the treatment given.

Barrett's Esophagus

There are vaying degrees of cellular dysplasia associated with Barrett's esophagus and, thus, varying approaches to its treatment. Barrett's esophagus with low-grade dysplasia may be treated with intensive medical antireflux therapy for 8–12 weeks and endoscopic examination repeated. If the condition persists, intensive antireflux therapy is continued with periodic surveillance; if the condition improves with therapy, periodic surveillance is conducted.[3]

The treatment for Barrett's esophagus with high-grade dysplasia is more controversial and involves two options. One option is a more conservative treatment similar to that for lower grades of dysplasia as described above; the second option is surgical resection. An important rationale supporting surgical resection is the prevalence of AC frequently found in tissue surgically removed from people with Barrett's esophagus who had high-grade dysplasia.[22] Photodynamic therapy has also been studied for the treatment of Barrett's esophagus, but it is not a commonly accepted approach to treatment at this time.[23]

Nursing care for people with Barrett's esophagus is focused on education about the disease process and the risk of the disease progressing to AC. The person must understand the importance of scheduled follow-up evaluations and appropriate treatment with antireflux medications. The care of the individual with a surgically resected esophagus is discussed in the following section.

Local and Locoregional Esophageal Cancer

Surgery alone

Surgical resection of the esophagus is the primary treatment for local and locoregional cancer for people with resectable disease and whose comorbid conditions do not prohibit surgical treatment. This has been the standard approach particularly in settings where clinical trials are not available. Several different resection approaches have been developed. The surgical approach selected depends on the location of the tumor and personal preference and expertise of the surgical team. The surgical approaches are radical esophagectomy, left thoracoabdominal approach, combined abdominal and right thoracotomy approach (Ivor-Lewis), and transhiatal approach.[4,24] The radical esophagectomy involves complete resection of the esophagus 10 cm above and below the tumor with resection of adjacent structures including arterial and venous supplies of the tumor as well as selected tissues. This radical procedure is associated with a high mortality rate. The combined abdominal and right thoracotomy is used for cancers of the upper and midesophagus because the approach allows better visualization of the involved area. The left thoracoabdominal and transhiatal approaches are used typically for cancers of the distal and gastroesophageal junction or for resection of Barrett's esophagus. The thoracoabdominal approach involves an incision across the left abdomen and thorax, then the distal esophagus and the proximal stomach are resected and anastomosed to the thoracic esophagus.

The transhiatal esophagectomy (Figure 54-2) has become more extensively used in recent years. Upper-midline abdominal and cervical incisions are made.[25] The intrathoracic esophagus is removed, the stomach is repo-

sitioned in the posterior mediastinum where the esophagus was located, and the gastric fundus is anastomosed to the cervical esophagus above the level of the clavicles. The advantages of this approach include the ability to avoid a thoracotomy with its attendant complications such as pain leading to ineffective breathing and atelectasis. Since the anastomosis site is in the neck as opposed to the chest, there is also a decreased risk of delayed detection should leakage at the anastomosis site occur. One disadvantage of transhiatal esophagectomy is the limited surgical view or exposure of the site, which makes it more difficult to mobilize the midesophagus and could increase the risk of bleeding. Nodal resection is completed at the time of surgery depending on the location of the tumor.[26]

Complications of surgery include esophageal leak at the anastomosis site, cardiac and pulmonary complications, and wound infection.[5] People who have undergone esophagectomy have an altered gastric passageway that changes the way they swallow and digest. A patient can experience gastric stasis, steatorrhea, diarrhea, early satiety, and regurgitation following esophagectomy.[27] Initially, people are fed by tube or vein following esophagectomy. After performing a swallowing test to determine whether there is leakage, the individual is advanced from a liquid to a soft to a regular diet as tolerated. Because the stomach is small as a result of the partial gastrectomy, the person must eat frequent small meals. This is quite often a struggle for people and they commonly lose weight after surgery until they are able to take in enough calories to maintain nutritional requirements. It is usually a trial-and-error process for the person to find the foods that can be eaten and tolerated best. Eventually the individual is able to eat in a more normal way and maintain or even regain some weight. However, there can be stenosis at the surgical site that may require mechanical dilatation at intervals following surgery. This stenosis and dilatation process can be very frustrating for the person who expected to be free of swallowing problems once recovered from surgery.

Initially there are drainage tubes at the incision site. The tubes are usually discontinued three to four days postsurgery.[28] The wound is then left open to air to heal. The patient also has a nasogastric tube in place until oral intake is initiated. The patient may also have a jejunostomy feeding tube in place until adequate nutrition can be taken orally.

Nursing care involves education of the person about what to expect following surgery. Expectations play a major role in how the patient and family view postsurgical status and progress. Aggressively evaluating weight and fluid balance postsurgery is important since these elements are being maintained via a feeding tube or intravenous route. Cardiac assessment is important following the surgical procedure since atrial fibrillation due to irritation of the vagus nerve during surgery may occur early in the postoperative period. It may be necessary to administer medications to control this dysrhythmia. Pulmonary assessment is also important to detect postsurgical fluid overload and the development of pneumonia. Once the

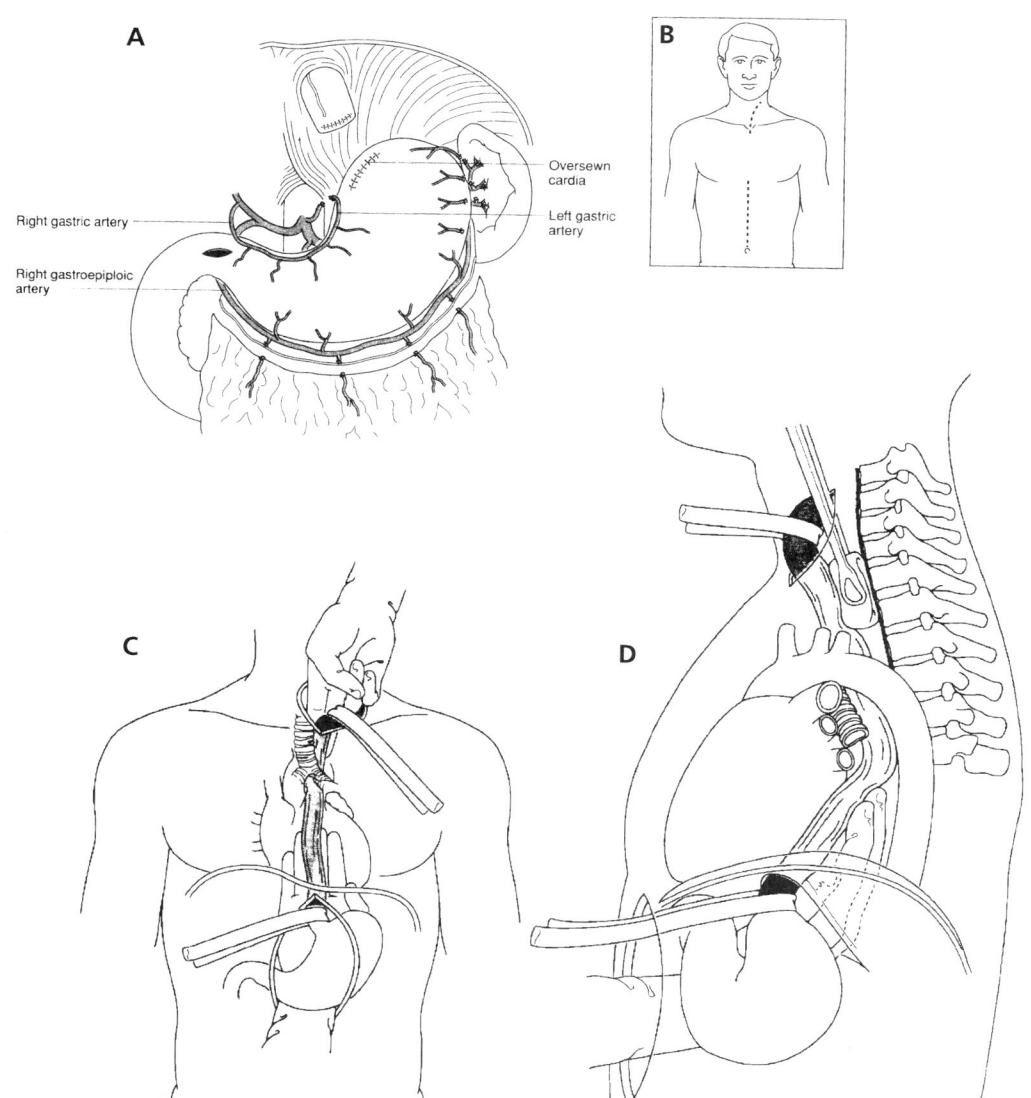

Figure 54-2 (A) Standard mobilization of the stomach for esophageal replacement either in the posterior mediastinal or substernal position. The left gastric artery and left gatroepiploic vessels have been divided. The mobilized stomach is based on the remaining right gastric and right gastroepiploic arteries that are preserved. A pyloromyotomy and generous Kocher maneuver are performed. (B) Left cervical incision and upper midline abdominal incision used for transhiatal esophagectomy and esophageal replacement with stomach in the posterior mediastinum. (C) Transhiatal mobilization of the thoracic esophagus from the posterior mediastinum using blunt dissection and traction on rubber drains placed around the esophagogastric junction and the cervical esophagus. The volar aspects of the fingers are kept against the esophagus to reduce the risk of injury to adjacent structures. (D) Lateral view showing transhiatal mobilization of the esophagus away from the prevertebral fascia using a half sponge on a stick inserted through the cervical incision and advanced until it makes contact with the hand inserted from below through the diaphragmatic hiatus. Arterial pressure is monitored as the heart is displaced forward by the hand in the posterior mediastinum. (Reprinted with permission from Orringer MB: Tumors, injuries, and miscellaneous conditions of the esophagus, in Greenfield LJ, Mulholland M, Oldham KT, Zelenock GB, Lillemoe KD (eds): *Surgery: Scientific Principles and Practice* (ed 2). Philadelphia, Lippincott-Raven, 1997, pp 694–735[25])

patient is extubated, usually 24 hours postsurgery, aggressive pulmonary management in needed.[28] Frequent turning, coughing, and deep breathing as well as spirometry is employed. After discharge from intensive care, physical therapy is initiated to gradually increase mobility. Pulmo-

nary complications are less likely with the transhiatal esophageal approach since a thoracotomy is not performed. Drainage tubes need to be maintained for patency and drainage assessed for signs of bleeding, infection, or anastomotic leak. Surgical wounds need to be monitored for signs and symptoms of infection. Once oral intake is initiated, assessment of the ability to swallow is important since the person may need encouragement to try different positions and approaches to swallowing. Initiating a nutritional consult to further educate the individual to dietary needs and possible supplements is helpful. The individual needs assurance that there will be gradual improvement in the ability to tolerate varied and larger quantities of food.

The patient may experience the dumping syndrome following surgery, which results from the unusually rapid passage of food from the mouth to the intestine due to removal of the esophagus. This syndrome improves with dietary correction including amount and frequency of meals. Dietary supplements such as Ensure®, which were helpful prior to surgery, often exacerbate the dumping syndrome postsurgery. Antidiarrheal drugs may also be useful. People should be encouraged to keep their follow-up appointments and to call the surgeon if there are problems after discharge.

Unfortunately the prognosis following the surgical treatment approach alone is poor. Most people die of distant metastasis within two years. Following surgical resection, the five-year survival is reported to be anywhere from 10%–20%.[11,29,30] Other approaches need to be explored to improve survival.

Combined therapy

Since the late 1970s clinical trials have been conducted to evaluate the use of multimodal or combined therapy in the treatment of esophageal cancer.[20] Strategies that have evolved to increase the survival rate in this population include chemotherapy and radiation alone without surgery, neoadjuvant chemotherapy given prior to surgery, and neoadjuvant chemotherapy and radiation therapy given concurrently prior to surgery.

Combined chemoradiation (without surgery) for the treatment of esophageal cancer has been shown to be more effective than radiation alone but still has a high rate of local recurrence and persistent disease. Consequently, combined chemoradiation alone should not be utilized with patients who have localized, potentially curable disease but rather should be reserved for patients who have comorbid conditions that make them nonsurgical candidates.

The neoadjuvant treatment approach is used to debulk or downstage the tumor thus facilitating surgical resection. Systemic therapy is also provided by this approach. The most active agents for treating esophageal cancer are cisplatin, fluorouracil (5-FU), vindesine, mitomycin, and paclitaxel. The most active single agent is cisplatin.[15,20] Vinblastine and methotrexate have also been used and docetaxel has been more recently incorporated into clinical trials for the treatment of esophageal cancer. These agents not only provide systemic treatment but also act as sensitizing agents for radiotherapy. Cisplatin and 5-FU, as combined therapy, have been shown to double or triple radiosensitivity.[29] Trials using various

cisplatin-based chemotherapy regimens without radiation prior to surgery in comparison to surgery alone showed that approximately 50% of tumors responded to chemotherapy; however, pathologic complete remissions were rare. No survival advantage was demonstrated by administering chemotherapy prior to surgery.[20]

The use of both chemotherapy and radiation followed by surgery may offer the most promising approach to treatment since the radiation allows for direct treatment of both the primary site and surrounding nodes along with the systemic treatment provided by chemotherapy. Accurate staging prior to treatment is used to identify areas of locoregional disease so the radiation port can be adjusted accordingly. Encouraging results from studies using this combined chemo-radiation-surgery approach have shown an increased response rate and an increased five-year survival over treatment with surgery alone.[12,21,31] In a clinical trial at Johns Hopkins, it was found that patients who had undergone combined chemoradiation and had no residual tumor (a complete remission) at surgical resection had the best prognosis.[29]

Various doses and schedules have been utilized to deliver cisplatin and 5-FU comcomitantly with radiation to patients with esophageal cancer. Some typical protocols follow. Cisplatin and 5-FU has been given for 15 days with 5-FU given over 16 hours on days 1–5 and cisplatin infused over 8 hours on day 7. This chemotherapy treatment was repeated in week 6 of the cycle. Radiotherapy was begun on the first day of the first course of therapy and given days 1–5, 8–12, and 15–19 for a total of 15 days. Radiation dose was 40 cGy per day using a three field technique (anterio-posterior, right-posterior, and left-posterior oblique fields).[11] Another regimen for delivering 5-FU and cisplatin has been to give cisplatin 100 mg/m² on days 1 and 21, and fluorouracil 600 mg/m² by continuous infusion on days 2–5 and days 22–25. With this regimen, a total radiation dose of 2000 cGy in 10–200 cGy fractions was given on days 8–19 followed by surgery.[26] Another treatment regimen used to administer cisplatin, 5-FU, and radiation is 5-FU 1000 mg/m²/day as a continuous infusion over 96 hours on days 1–4 and days 29–32 of irradiation. Cisplatin 100 mg/m² was administered on day 1 of irradiation only. Radiation was delivered in 25 (5 days/week) fractions over a 33-day period for a total dose of 45 Gy (39.6 Gy was given anteroposteriorly and 5.4 Gy through opposed lateral fields). One of the most effective treatment regimens is cisplatin 100 mg/m² given on day 1 and infusional 5-FU 1000 mg/m²/day for 4 or 5 days at three-week intervals.[20] Protracted infusion of low dose 5-FU given with cisplatin enhances the radiosensitizing effect because of the continual presence of the drug with each fraction of radiation given. Neoadjuvant 5-FU 300 mg/m²/day given as a continuous infusion for either 21 or 30 days along with cisplatin and vinblastine given concomitantly with a total of 44 to 45 cGy of radiotherapy is one treatment approach that has been researched.[26] One recently completed clinial trial at Johns Hopkins utilized protracted infusions of 5-FU 225 mg/m² over 28 days along with cisplatin 20 mg/m² on days

1–5 and 24–28 given concomitantly with radiation begun on day 1 of chemotherapy and given 5 days/week over the same 28-day period. This regimen has also been tested as neoadjuvant therapy.

The chemo-radiation-surgical approach offers the best hope for cure for esophageal cancer. Disease recurrence after this combined modality treatment approach is most often at a distant site such as the liver rather than at the site of the primary lesion.

While the combined approach results in a better tumor response and longer survival, it also has more associated toxicities and, thus, more complex nursing care is required. There are the postesophagectomy complications discussed above plus the toxicities associated with chemotherapy and radiation administered prior to surgery. One of the more serious complications of chemotherapy includes myelosuppression resulting in decreased white blood cells (WBCs), red blood cells (RBCs), and platelets. Routine monitoring of blood counts needs to be made so that the specific type of deficiency can be treated appropriately. Individuals may need transfusions of RBCs and platelets during the course of treatment. Colony stimulating factors, such as erythropoietin to stimulate RBC growth and oprelvekin to stimulate platelet growth, can also be administered. Sufficient iron stores must be available for stimulation of RBCs to be effective. Growth stimulating factors are usually given once or twice a week by subcutaneous injection either during a clinic visit or the patient can be taught to give the injections at home. The patient may need to be started on prophylactic antibiotics should neutropenia develop (usually absolute neutrophil count (ANC) < 1000/mm³). The patient will also need to monitor his temperature and should be advised to call should a fever of 100.5°F (38.3°C) or greater develop. Granulocyte colony stimulating factors, such as filgrastim, are also given to stimulate the growth of WBCs. This may be especially important for the patient who has experienced a neutropenic fever with previous chemotherapy treatments. Combining the use of growth factors and prophylactic antibiotics may enable the patient to tolerate chemotherapy treatments at higher and more effective doses. These medications are given daily via subcutaneous injections. The patient or family member will need to be taught how to give these injections. Growth stimulating factors are expensive and the patient's insurance benefits and financial status need to be taken into consideration before initiating treatments with these medications.

Gastrointestinal (GI) complications are another serious and common side effect of chemotherapy and radiation therapy. Prior to any treatment, people with esophageal cancer typically experience dysphagia and weight loss. In order to provide adequate nutritional support through treatment, it is often necessary to place a gastrostomy or jejunostomy feeding tube for aggressive supplementation. A nutritional consult will need to be made once the tube is placed and the person educated to the amount and type of feeding to be used. Caloric requirements are increased during treatment and often

an intake of 2000 calories or more is necessary to maintain weight.[28] Home nursing visits may need to be initiated once the tube is placed to educate the individual and family to the care of the tube as well as how to deliver the feedings. Chemotherapy, particularly cisplatin-based regimens, can cause nausea, vomiting, diarrhea, constipation, taste changes, mucositis, and loss of appetite. All of these side effects make it difficult to manage a patient's nutritional and fluid status. Antiemetics are utilized to prevent and control nausea and vomiting. The advent of the 5HT3 blockers such as granisetron and ondansetron have been particularly helpful for patients receiving highly emetogenic chemotherapies such as cisplatin. These antiemetics should be administered around-the-clock for 24–48 hours following administration of chemotherapy.[32] There are other antiemetics that can be utilized on an as-needed basis. Diarrhea and constipation management includes medications, adjusting activity level, as well as adjusting fluid intake particularly if the patient is nutritionally supported with tube feedings.

Quite often foods served at room temperature are better tolerated than heated foods and have less odors that people undergoing chemotherapy may find intolerable. Adding spices such as cinnamon or ginger may help improve the taste of foods. Tobacco and alcohol use should be avoided since they further irritate the GI lining.

Radiation side effects can include esophagitis, stenosis, and fistula formation that further contributes to difficulty swallowing, pain, and increased risk of aspiration.[33] Analgesics, which are usually required at some point in treatment, are more easily given topically or through a feeding tube since the patient may have difficulty swallowing. Topical and sustained-release analgesics through a feeding tube provide continuous blood levels of analgesia and improved pain control. Patients and their families must be educated about the use and side effects of analgesic medications and how to apply the topical medications or give them through the feeding tube. People are sometimes concerned about taking narcotics and need to be supported and educated about proper use and effectiveness.

Fatigue is present in nearly 100% of people with esophageal cancer who are receiving chemoradiation. It is often distressing to patients and their families because they may perceive that fatigue is an indicator of their disease status and because fatigue interferes with the routines of daily life. This type of treatment-induced fatigue may not be relieved by rest and people need to learn new ways to manage it. Exercise has been shown to be effective in decreasing fatigue in people with breast cancer.[34] It is important to maintain a balance between activity and rest. For example, daily walks and afternoon naps help establish a routine that can be managed by most people staying at home. Daily fatigue diaries can help identify times during the day when the person is most fatigued so that the day's activities can be adjusted accordingly. Priorities may need to be set and limits established since patients often do not feel up to their pretreatment activity level.

Anxiety, fear, worry, and depression are understandable and expected reactions to the diagnosis and treatment of esophageal cancer. Patients and their families may need counseling to help them cope with the challenges of therapy and outcomes of the disease. A social work or psychologic consult may be necessary. Financial burdens brought on by the cost of treatment or the inability to work may be a major source of stress. A social work consult may be helpful in assisting the individual and family to apply for disability benefits or other areas of financial assistance. Patients may find it beneficial to utilize self-care approaches such as massage therapy or other relaxation techniques to manage anxiety and stress. Patients and their families may also benefit by talking to others who have successfully undergone similar treatments for esophageal cancer.

Other side effects of chemotherapy include cardiac toxicity particularly associated with the taxanes and manifested by irregular cardiac rhythms. Hepatic toxicity is evidenced by an increase in liver enzyme levels. Pulmonary toxicity is particularly associated with mitomycin. Nephrotoxicity and ototoxicity can occur with cisplatin. Peripheral neuropathy is a side effect associated with cisplatin and the taxanes that is manifested by numbness and tingling of the fingers and toes. 5-FU can produce "hand/foot" syndrome, which is a redness and peeling of the skin that will resolve over time. The use of lotions and protection from the elements are usually adequate treatments. Alopecia, rashes, and dry skin are other common side effects associated with chemotherapy. While not a serious side effect, alopecia can be very difficult for people because of the visible change in appearance that results. Wigs, hats, or turbans may be utilized depending on cost and personal preference. Patients should be educated regarding which side effects to expect depending on their particular chemotherapy regimen and how to assess themselves for early signs of complications throughout treatment. Cardiac and pulmonary assessment need to be made during clinic visits and hospitalizations. If severe enough, side effects may limit the scope of the treatment plan.

In educating the individual and family about the disease process and side effects of treatments, verbal instruction, written information, and audio-visual material can be combined to help the patient and family assimilate the information. Frequent review of the educational information is necessary since high stress levels may make it difficult for the patient and family to remember much of the information initially provided. Often talking to someone else who has had the disease and experienced similar treatments may be helpful. Support groups where people can talk about their experiences and share with others can also be helpful.

Nonresectable or Metastatic Disease

Tumors may be considered to be nonresectable for various reasons. Patients may have comorbid conditions that preclude surgical resection. The location of the tumor may be such that resection is not feasible. This is the case with tumors located in the proximal cervical esophagus since anastomosis is not possible at this location. Presence of metastatic disease eliminates the option of surgery except as a palliative procedure. Treatment approaches utilized in patients with metastatic disease are palliative in intent. The type of treatment given depends on the type and location of the tumor, the overall condition of the person, accessibility, cost, and the individual's and physician's preference.[33]

Nonresectable tumors are often treated with radiation alone or radiation combined with chemotherapy. The combination of chemoradiation has shown to be more effective than radiation alone.[15] This is the treatment of choice in people with localized disease that is considered nonresectable either because of comorbid conditions or location of the tumor. The treatment of metastatic disease may involve chemotherapy and radiation. The chemotherapeutic agents have been discussed earlier in this chapter and are utilized in metastatic disease to decrease the size of the tumor in order to provide symptom relief. Radiation may be used to relieve dysphagia or, in this case, to relieve symptoms associated with conditions such as lytic bone lesions and brain metastases. The goal is palliative with the purpose of decreasing the size of the tumor in order to provide symptom relief.

Brachytherapy alone or in combination with external beam radiation is one treatment option for patients with nonresectable tumors or metastatic disease. Brachytherapy has been shown to improve dysphagia due to obstruction by the tumor. An advantage of brachytherapy is the ability to directly treat the nonresectable tumor while limiting exposure to surrounding tissue. Side effects of brachytherapy to the esophagus include ulceration, stricture, and fistula formation. Esophageal dilatation with surgical instruments can also help alleviate dysphagia but must be repeated frequently or performed in conjuction with other treatments such as radiation. It is also possible to place an esophageal stent that can be inserted during an outpatient visit and usually provides relief longer than dilatation. Stent placement is associated with less risk of perforation and bleeding than dilatation.

Laser therapy is another treatment option for people with tumors in locations amenable to laser therapy and for those who have a completely obstructed esophagus. The complication rate of laser procedure is low, with perforation and bleeding being the most common complications. Photodynamic therapy (PDT) is a more recent treatment option and can be used to treat total or partial obstructed esophageal lesions. A chemical sensitizer is given intravenously and selectively taken up by the tumor. The chemical sensitizer is activated in the presence of molecular oxygen by a light source of a specific wave length that then damages the tumor. The PDT process can be repeated as often as needed to open the obstructed esophagus. Complications of PDT include fistula and stricture formation. Sclerotherapy can also be used to treat total or partial obstructing tumors. Sclerotherapy is less expensive to use and has a relatively low complication rate.

Nursing care of the patient with advanced disease

involves the management of physiologic side effects of treatment as well as the psychosocial issues that are most often present. The patient and family must make difficult decisions about whether to take a particular treatment, when to stop treatment, financial matters associated with treatment, and how they wish the dying process to occur. Support through social work consult, open discussions with individuals and families, and referral to hospice care are all appropriate approaches that depend on personal preference, cultural differences, and social supports. Pain control and nutritional support are ongoing care needs.

Symptom Management and Supportive Care

Dysphagia and weight loss are the most common clinical symptoms associated with esophageal cancer.[2] Therefore, nutritional needs are often the most pressing initial problems to address. Assessment of swallowing capabilities of the individual and nutritional consults should be made. Patients who are able to swallow soft and liquid foods may be able to supplement their diet with high-calorie liquids such as Ensure® or Ensure Plus® or Scandi Shakes®. If the patient is unable to swallow adequately and maintain nutritional requirements, feeding tubes can be placed and the individual started on tube feedings as a means for complete nutrition. Nutrition can also be provided by parenteral infusions if alternative strategies fail. The patient may also be dehydrated, so fluid requirements must be taken into account.

Patients who have problems with nutritional intake and are fed through tubes often have other GI complications such as diarrhea or constipation. Often the type and amount of enteral solution and fluids will need to be adjusted. Patients may need to take medications to control diarrhea or constipation. Those persons with jejunostomy tubes may experience the dumping syndrome and the types, amounts, and frequency of feedings may need to be adjusted. Patients will need to be followed closely for weight changes and dehydration until tube feedings are adequately adjusted.

Individuals who have tumors that occlude the esophagus are not able to adequately clear their secretions. Consequently, they expectorate frequently. This is often frustrating and embarrassing for them. They may also be fearful of choking on the secretions, especially at night while sleeping. It may be helpful for the person to sleep with the head of the bed elevated so the risk of aspiration is decreased. Individuals with obstructing esophageal tumors need to have palliative treatment such as stent placement or dilatation as soon as possible to open up the area so secretions can be cleared adequately.

Tumors that are extensive can erode into surrounding tissue and vasculature causing hemorrhage. Emergency surgery may be required. Esophagothoracic fistulas may form especially after radiation to the site of the primary tumor. Esophageal tumors can also invade surrounding organs structures such as the lung and mediastinum causing pain and respiratory complications.

Distant metastatic disease can result in impairment of organ function such as hepatic failure. Elevated liver enzymes can lead to impaired mental function. The person with advanced esophageal cancer may also experience pain associated with bone metastasis. Supportive care includes home nursing, pain and nutritional management, respite care for the family, and hospice care.

Continuity of Care: Nursing Challenges

Nursing care depends upon the stage of the disease and treatment approach used. It should be individualized, often focusing on symptom management, and may need to cross many settings. These settings include inpatient, outpatient, home care, and hospice. In order to ensure that care is continuous, communication of the individual's condition and the plan of care is essential. One of the nurses' many challenges is to coordinate the patient's care and to meet the individual needs as the disease is treated or progresses.

Most patients receive the majority of their nonsurgical care for esophageal cancer as an outpatient. These patients need many supports in order to tolerate the often toxic treatments. Coordination and communication between providers (primary care provider, oncologist, home care provider, hospice, and primary clinic nurse) are essential and most often it is the responsibility of the primary clinic nurse to see that they take place. Again, nutritional status must be assessed during clinic visits. Tube feedings need to be initiated at any time the patient is unable to take adequate oral nutrition and hydration. This is particularly the case when radiation treatments are being utilized. Dietary consults and home nursing visits need to be initiated to determine proper fluid and nutritional intake and to ensure that the patient and family are able to manage the tube feedings. Trends in weight need to be followed with each clinic visit along with other GI complications such as nausea, vomiting, esophagitis, and loss of appetite. These need to be communicated to the appropriate provider so that proper treatments can be instituted.

Following surgical resection, some patients will be able to manage with minimal instruction and support. Others may require increasing levels of assistance and care. Many patients are capable of adequate oral intake by the time of discharge following esophagectomy and will only require a dietary consult prior to discharge and a follow-up appointment with the surgeon. However, other patients may not be able to swallow adequately and may need to go home with tube feedings. These patients need dietary consults, instruction on care of tubes and administration of tube feedings, and home nursing support as well as more frequent follow-up visits following discharge. Home nurses need to continue to assess the person's learning needs, home environment, support systems, and nutritional progress. Other supports may need to be initiated depending on the particular needs of the patient. These supports may include social work for emotional or financial issues or a consult with a swallowing therapist should the individual continue to experience difficulty with swallowing.

For those people who are appropriate for and opt for hospice care, frequent communications need to occur between the primary care provider and the hospice nurse pertaining to the person's overall condition, pain control, nutritional needs, and the individual's and family's wishes for ongoing care.

Conclusion

While the incidence of esophageal cancer is relatively low, it is one of the more rapidly increasing types of cancer today. The prognosis for esophageal cancer is generally poor; however, if the disease is diagnosed early there are options for treatment that may increase the likelihood for survival. While management of Barrett's esophagus is controversial, there is reason to consider prophylactic surgery for people with high-grade dysplasia in order to prevent the development of AC. For people with locoregional disease, the combined approach using neoadjuvant chemoradiation followed by esophagectomy appears to be the most effective treatment at the present time. For people with unresectable disease, there are various options to consider but the combination of radiation and chemotherapy seems to be superior. The person with metastatic disease also has several options for treatment and these depend on such factors as complications the person is experiencing and personal preferences.

Complications of esophageal cancer as well as of the treatments delivered are multifaceted and the nursing care required to manage them is complex. Thorough physical and psychosocial assessments must be made in order to develop a plan of care optimal for the patient and family. Symptom management is necessary in order to help the individual tolerate treatment. Coordination of various resources to provide care across the continuum and at the various stages of the disease is essential in addressing the needs of this population. Educating and supporting the individual and family so they can make informed decisions about treatments and life issues helps them to maintain some measure of control at one of the most difficult times in their lives.

References

1. Given BA, Simmons SJ: *Gastroenterology in Clinical Nursing* St Louis MO, Mosby, 1979, p 942
2. Vander AJ, Sherman JH, Luciano DS: *Human Physiology: The Mechanisms of Body Function* (ed 6). New York, McGraw-Hill, 1994
3. Spechler SJ: Barrett's esophagus and adenocarcinoma of the esophagogastric junction: epidemiology, surveillance, and management. *Proc Am Soci Clini Oncol* May 1997 (abstr)
4. Coia LR, Sauter ER: Esophageal cancer. *Curr Probl Cancer* 18:189–247, 1994
5. Blot WJ: Esophageal cancer trends and risk factors. *Semin Oncol* 21:104–109, 1994
6. Heitmiller RF, Sharma RR: Comparison of prevalence and resection rates in patients with esophageal squamous cell carcinoma and adenocarcinoma. *J Thorac Cardiovasc Surg* 12:130–136, 1996
7. Brown LM, Swanson CA, Gridley G, et al: Adenocarcinoma of the esophagus: role of obesity and diet. *J Natl Cancer Inst* 87:104–109, 1995
8. Suzuk L, Noffsinger AE, Hui YZ, et al: Detection of human papilloma virus in esophageal squamous cell carcinoma. *Cancer* 78:704–710, 1996
9. Moskaluk CA, Heitmiller R, Zahurak M, et al: p53 and p21 (WAF1/CIP1/SDI1) gene products in Barrett esophagus and adenocarcinoma of the esophagus and esophagogastric junction. *Hum Pathol* 27:1211–1220, 1996
10. Nabeya Y, Loganzo F, Maslak P, et al: The mutational status of p53 protein in gastric and esophageal adenocarcinoma cell lines predicts sensitivity to chemotherapeutic agents. *Int J Cancer* 64:37–46, 1995
11. Walsh TN, Noonan N, Hollywood D, et al: A comparison of multimodal therapy and surgery for esophageal adenocarcinoma. *N Engl J Med* 335:462–467, 1996
12. Klumpp TR, Macdonald JS: Esophageal cancer: epidemiology and pathology, in Ahlgren JD, Macdonald JS (eds): *Gastrointestinal Oncology.* Philadelphia, Lippincott, 1992, pp 71–80
13. Livinstone EM, Skinner DB: Tumors of the esophagus, in Berk JE (ed): *Gastroenterology.* Philadelphia, Saunders, 1985, pp 818–840
14. Held JL, Peahota A: Nursing care of patients with esophageal cancer. *Oncol Nurs Forum* 19:627–634, 1992
15. Kelsen DP, Ilson DH: Chemotherapy and combined-modality therapy for esophageal cancer (review). *Chest* 107: 224–232, 1995 (suppl 6)
16. Saunders HS, Wolfman NT, Ott DJ: Esophageal cancer. Radiologic staging: review. *Radiol Clin North Am* 35:281–294, 1997
17. Luketich JD, Schauer PR, Meltzer CC, et al: Role of positron emission tomography in staging esophageal cancer. *Ann Thorac Surg* 64:765–769, 1997
18. Block MI, Patterson GA, Sundaresan RS, et al: Improvement in staging of esophageal cancer with the addition of positron emission tomography. *Ann Thorac Surg* 64:770–777, 1997
19. Fleming ID, Cooper JS, Henson DE, et al: *AJCC Cancer Staging Manual* (ed 5). Philadelphia, Lippincott-Raven, 1997, pp 65–75
20. Forastiere AA, Heitmiller RF, Kleinberg L: Multimodality therapy for esophageal cancer. *Chest* 112:195–200, 1997 (suppl 4)
21. Medvec BR: Esophageal cancer: treatment and nursing interventions. *Semin Oncol Nurs* 4:246–256, 1988
22. Heitmiller RF, Redmond M, Hamilton SR: Barrett's esophagus with high-grade dysplasia: an indication for prophylactic esophagectomy. *Ann Surg* 224:66–71, 1996
23. Overholt BF, Panjehpour M: Photodynamic therapy in Barrett's esophagus: reduction of specialized mucosa, ablation of dysplasia, and treatment of superficial esophageal cancer. *Semin Surg Oncol* 11:372–376, 1995
24. Coleman, J: Esophageal, stomach, liver, gallbladder, and pancreatic cancers, in Groenwald SL, Frogge MH, Goodman M, Yarbro CH (eds): *Cancer Nursing: Principles and Practice* (ed 4). Sudbury, MA, Jones and Bartlett, 1997, pp 1082–1144

25. Orringer MB: Tumors, injuries, and miscellaneous conditions of the esophagus, in Greenfield LJ, Mulholland M, Oldham KT, Zelenock GB, Lillemoe KD (eds): *Surgery: Scientific Principles and Practice* (ed 2). Philadelphia, Lippincott-Raven, 1997, pp 694–735

26. Flood WA, Forastiere AA: Esophageal cancer. *Curr Opin Oncol* 7:381–386, 1995

27. Sigley T: Nutritional problems, in Ziegfeld CR, Lubejko BG, Shelton BK (eds): *Oncology Fact Finder: Manual of Cancer Nursing.* Philadelphia, Lippincott-Raven, 1998, pp 349–368

28. Quinn KL, Reedy AM: Esophageal cancer: therapeutic approaches and nursing care. *Semin Oncol Nurs* 15:17–25, 1999

29. Girvin GW, Matsumoto GH, Bates DM, et al: Treating esophageal cancer with a combination of chemotherapy, radiation, and excision. *Am J Surg* 5:557–559, 1995

30. Roth J, Putnam JB Jr, Rich TA, et al: Cancer of the esophagus, in DeVita VT Jr, Hellman S, Rosenberg SA (eds): *Cancer Principles and Practice of Oncology.* Philadelphia, Lippincott-Raven, 1996, pp 980–1054

31. Jones DR, Detterbeck FC, Egan TM, et al: Induction chemoradiotherapy followed by esophagectomy in patients with carcinoma of the esophagus. *Ann Thorac Surg* 64:185–192, 1997

32. Violette KM: Nausea and vomiting, in Ziegfeld CR, Lubejko BG, Shelton BK (eds): *Oncology Fact Finder: Manual of Cancer Nursing.* Philadelphia, Lippincott-Raven, 1998, pp 335–344

33. Reed CE: Comparison of different treatments for unresectable esophageal cancer (review). *World J Surg* 19:828–835, 1995

34. Mock V, Dow KH, Meares CJ, et al: Effects of exercise on fatigue, physical functioning, and emotional distress during radiation therapy for breast cancer. *Oncol Nurs Forum* 24:991–1000, 1997

CHAPTER 55

Gallbladder and Bile Duct Cancer

JoAnn Coleman, RN, MS, ACNP-CS, AOCN

GALLBLADDER CANCER

Introduction

The two most common malignancies of the biliary tree are adenocarcinoma of the gallbladder and bile duct (cholangiocarcinoma). Although there is some overlap in the diagnosis and treatment of these two cancers, they are distinct enough to require separate treatment. Carcinoma of the gallbladder, which we consider first, is a rare form of cancer and as such has a distinct etiology, pathophysiology, clinical presentation, and treatment. In most patients, the disease is not suspected clinically and is found at an advanced stage, often during surgery for cholelithiasis.

Epidemiology

Although gallbladder cancer is a rare form of cancer, it is the most common malignancy of the biliary tract and the fifth most common cancer of the gastrointestinal (GI) tract.[1] Approximately 6000 cases are diagnosed in the United States each year. The incidence of gallbladder cancer in the United States is 2.5 per 100,000 residents.[2] Wide variations in incidence exist throughout the world and in different regions of the United States. In the United States, gallbladder cancer incidence is highest in the southwestern regions, where the occurrence is most common among Native Americans and Hispanic Americans.[3] Other countries with high rates of gallbladder cancer include Israel, Mexico, Bolivia, Chile, and northern Japan. In contrast, gallbladder cancer rates are low in India, Nigeria, and Singapore.[4]

Women develop gallbladder cancer almost two times more often than men, which is similar to the incidence of gallstones.[3,5] Gallbladder cancer is rare in individuals under age 50, with most occurring among those in their late sixties and early seventies.[6]

Etiology

Several factors are associated with an increased risk for gallbladder cancer (Table 55-1). Gallstones are the most

Table 55-1   Risk Factors for Gallbladder Cancer

Gallstones (single gallstone usually larger than 3 cm)
Choledochal cyst
Anomalous pancreatobiliary duct junction
Carcinogens
Rubber plant workers
Azotoluene
Nitrosamines
Obesity
Estrogens
Typhoid carriers
Porcelain gallbladder (calcification of the gallbladder wall)
Gallbladder polyps

common etiologic factor, probably due to the high prevalence in the general population. More than 90% of individuals with gallbladder cancer have coexistent chronic cholecystitis (inflamed gallbladder) and cholelithiasis (gallstones). Gallbladder cancer is more likely to occur in individuals with a single large gallstone than with multiple smaller stones. It is presumed that the large gallstones have been present for a long period of time, causing chronic irritation of the gallbladder wall, and thus predisposing to the development of carcinoma.[4]

Individuals with a choledochal cyst may develop carcinoma throughout the biliary tree, but most tumors arise in the gallbladder. The chance of developing an associated gallbladder or bile duct cancer increases with age.[6] Recent studies have suggested that an anomalous pancreatobiliary duct junction (APBDJ) is associated with an increased incidence of gallbladder cancer in individuals with a choledochal cyst.[7,8] This common channel abnormality between the common bile duct and pancreatic duct allows reflux of pancreatic juice into the biliary tree. The question still remains whether it is the regurgitation of pancreatic juice or the relationship of the abnormal junction to bile stasis and the subsequent retention of carcinogens within the biliary tree that cause gallbladder cancer.[4]

Various chemical carcinogens have been suspected to cause biliary cancers because excretion via the bile is a common way of clearing toxic metabolites. An increased incidence of gallbladder cancer has been reported in rubber plant workers.[9] Further, animal studies have suggested that azotoluene and nitrosamines can cause gallbladder cancer, and an association between gallbladder cancer and obesity and estrogens has been suggested in epidemiological studies.[10]

Typhoid carriers have an increased risk of gallbladder and bile duct cancer. The higher incidence of gallbladder cancer in chronic typhoid carriers is also thought to result from chronic irritation.[11] Calcification of the gallbladder wall, the so-called porcelain gallbladder, is associated with sustained chronic cholecystitis and is associated with a 25%–60% incidence of gallbladder cancer.[12] Gallbladder polyps are also a risk factor for cancer. Polyps greater than 1 cm are most likely to become malignant and are an indication for cholecystectomy.[13] Adenomatous polyps of the gallbladder in individuals with Peutz-Jeghers syndrome are also associated with gallbladder cancer.[14]

Prevention, Screening, and Early Detection

At present there is no effective screening method for gallbladder cancer as it is such a rare tumor that is often confused with other biliary cancers. The presenting symptoms of gallbladder cancer usually occur with advanced disease, making early detection almost impossible. Effective ways to eliminate the formation of gallstones in the general population and especially in high-risk individuals would be beneficial for many reasons, one of which is decreased gallbladder cancer. Heightened awareness of the incidence of gallbladder cancer through education of high-risk individuals may lead to routine surveillance and early detection. Consideration may be given to more aggressive screening of high-risk individuals and early resection of the gallbladder in high-risk cases with any findings suggestive of gallbladder cancer.

Carcinoembryonic antigen (CEA) and alpha-fetoprotein (AFP) are serum markers that have been associated with gallbladder cancer.[15,16] These markers are not considered to be good screening tests since the incidence of elevated levels is low and their specificity is poor. When these tumor markers are elevated prior to resection for gallbladder cancer, changes may be important during follow-up for early identification of recurrent disease.[4]

The molecular and genetic events leading to the development of gallbladder cancer are considered to be different from those in extrahepatic biliary tract tumors. This information may lead to better screening tools.

Pathophysiology

Cellular Characteristics

The vast majority of gallbladder cancers are adenocarcinomas, which occur in 85% of patients, followed in frequency by papillary carcinoma and mucinous adenocarcinoma.[17] Cancers of the gallbladder can be one of several histological types including papillary, nodular, tubular, poorly differentiated, and combinations. Histological grades of gallbladder carcinoma include well differentiated, moderately differentiated, poorly differentiated, and undifferentiated.[4]

Progression of Disease

Since most individuals with cancer of the gallbladder present with disease at an advanced stage, it is difficult to know the exact progression of the disease. Gallbladder cancer is a locally invasive tumor that can extend directly into the gallbladder bed of the liver, extrahepatic bile ducts, duodenum or transverse colon, portal vein, hepatic artery, or pancreas. A tumor may originate anywhere in the gallbladder, although the site of origin may be difficult to determine because most gallbladder cancers have grown beyond the limits of resectability before they are discovered.[18]

Patterns of Spread

The patterns of spread predictably follow lymphatic and venous drainage of the gallbladder. Venous drainage of the gallbladder is directly into the adjacent liver, and the most common pattern of spread of gallbladder cancer is through direct extension into the liver. The lymphatic drainage of the gallbladder is to the cystic duct lymph nodes, periportal lymph nodes, and then to the celiac and superior mesenteric lymph nodes. These tumors can spread into and around the cystic duct and can extend into the common bile duct, causing biliary obstruction (Figure 55-1). Thus, jaundice may be the first clinical manifestation of a problem. Diffuse peritoneal seeding and distant metastasis are less common and occur late in the course of the disease.[19]

Clinical Manifestations

In its early stages, carcinoma of the gallbladder is usually asymptomatic. This fact contributes to the low curability rate of gallbladder carcinoma, since the lack of symptoms precludes the early diagnosis of the disease.

When signs and symptoms of gallbladder cancer manifest, they usually resemble those of benign gallbladder disease. Common symptoms are right upper abdominal quadrant pain, nausea, vomiting, fatty food intolerance, chills, and fever. A change in the pattern of pain and advanced age should raise the index of suspicion.[20] Individuals with gallbladder cancer commonly have advanced disease and present with nonspecific signs of malaise, anorexia, weight loss, abdominal distention, jaundice, and pruritus. Most individuals have multiple symptoms.

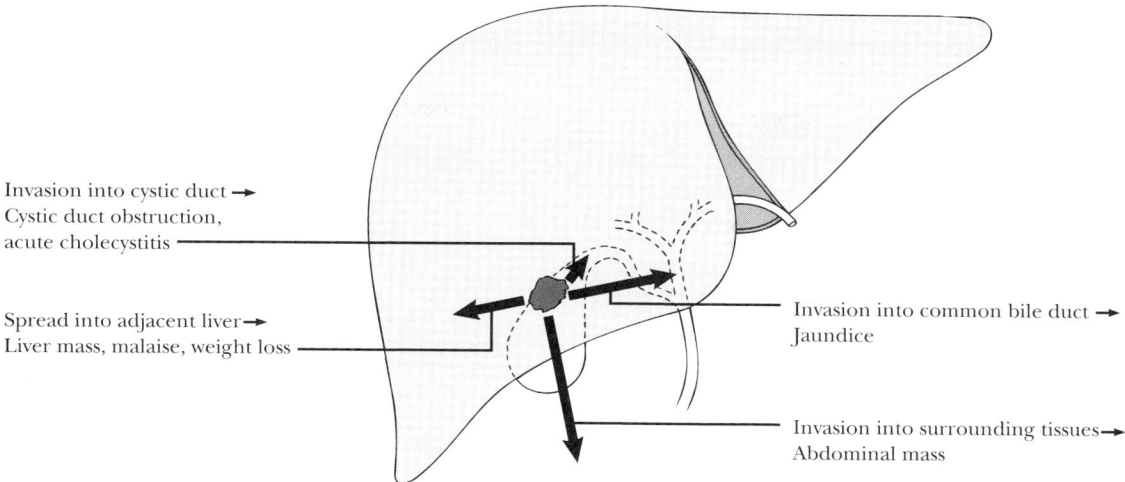

Figure 55-1 Tumor spread and presenting signs in gallbladder cancer. Gallbladder cancer commonly spreads by direct extension into surrounding tissues. This tumor extension results in the clinical presentations of jaundice, acute cholecystitis, abdominal mass, and weight loss. (Adapted with permission from Norwold DL, Dawes LG: Biliary neoplasms, in Greenfield LJ, et al (eds): *Surgery: Scientific Principles and Practice* (ed 2). Philadelphia, Lippincott-Raven, 1997, pp 1056–1067.)[19]

Almost half of individuals with gallbladder cancer will present with jaundice in addition to the clinical symptoms suggestive of biliary tract disease. Tumor invasion of the cystic duct can cause cystic duct obstruction, resulting in the development of acute cholecystitis. In advanced stages of the disease, individuals may present with a palpable mass in the right upper quadrant resulting from obstruction and distention of the gallbladder. Hepatomegaly, jaundice, cachexia, fever, and ascites may also be present as evidence of progressive disease and liver failure. Definitive diagnosis often is made at the time of surgery for jaundice or acute cholecystitis.[4,19]

Assessment

Patient and Family History

The individual may have had no previous symptoms or may have vague, chronic complaints of right upper quadrant pain. A change in the character of the symptoms may prompt that person to seek medical attention. Any individual who is at high risk for gallbladder cancer or who has a family history of the disease should receive a thorough evaluation.

Physical Examination

Jaundice with pruritus may be evident in individuals with an obstructing gallbladder cancer. In advanced carcinoma of the gallbladder, an individual with severe weight loss may have a visibly palpable gallbladder when supine.

Diagnostic Studies

With the exception of jaundice, no specific laboratory abnormalities may be present. Some individuals present with acute cholecystitis manifested by fever and leukocytosis on complete blood count (CBC). Other laboratory findings may include anemia, elevated sedimentation rate, and reduced serum albumin. In more advanced cases, elevated transaminase and coagulation abnormalities may reflect liver failure.

Ultrasonography (US), computerized tomography (CT) scan, magnetic resonance imaging (MRI), cholangiography, and angiography may all be helpful in evaluating individuals with suspected gallbladder cancer. US is used to identify a thickened gallbladder wall or a mass protruding into the gallbladder, either filling or replacing the gallbladder. It also may show tumor invasion of the liver or porta hepatis and may visualize adjacent adenopathy. A dilated biliary tree and hepatic metastasis may also be evaluated by ultrasound.[21] CT scan can demonstrate a gallbladder cancer as an intraluminal mass, a mass replacing the gallbladder, or a mass extending from the gallbladder. CT scan is also accurate in assessing the spread of the disease. Direct invasion of the liver or porta hepatis, involvement of adjacent lymph nodes, liver metastases, and invasion of adjacent structures can be evaluated by CT.[22] Limited experience exists with the use of MRI in the evaluation of gallbladder cancer. New magnetic resonance cholangiography and vascular enhancement techniques make it possible to visualize biliary obstruction, encasement of the portal vein, and hepatic involvement.[23]

Cholangiography can be useful for diagnosing gallbladder cancer in an individual with jaundice. Percutaneous transhepatic cholangiography (PTC) or endoscopic retrograde cholangiopancreatography (ERCP) may both be beneficial. The typical finding with either study is a long stricture of the common hepatic duct.[24] Angiography may be used to determine resectability through assessment of vascular encasement. However, new spiral CT scan and MRI techniques are useful radiological studies for staging gallbladder cancer by defining the presence of tumor in the gallbladder and encasement of the portal vein or hepatic artery.[25]

If radiological studies suggest that the gallbladder cancer may be resectable or if palliative surgery is considered, tissue diagnosis is not required before surgery. Whereas, if resection is not deemed possible due to extensive liver invasion, liver or peritoneal metastases, or encasement of the main portal vein, a biopsy of the tumor is necessary to help establish a diagnosis and confirm the stage of tumor. A percutaneous needle biopsy with US or CT scan guidance can assist in establishing the diagnosis. Brushings of obstructed bile ducts or bile cytology via PTC or ERCP has a low yield of sample for diagnosis.[26] Laparoscopy may also be used to obtain a biopsy of the liver, peritoneum, or tissue around the gallbladder.[27]

Prognostic Indicators

The histological grade has significant prognostic implications. The presence or absence of metaplasia is an important prognostic factor in gallbladder cancer. Individuals with metaplasia, which is more common in women, have a better prognosis.[28] Poorly differentiated infiltrating tumors have a strong association with gallstones, lymph node metastases, and direct extension into the liver.[17] Papillary cell tumors are less likely to directly invade the liver and have a lower incidence of lymph node metastasis. They are also less likely to have associated gallstones. Nodular forms of tumor are more likely to infiltrate early, to invade the liver, and to have lymph node metastases along with a higher incidence of gallstones. Tubular tumors are in the midrange with respect to their aggressive metastatic behavior.[4]

The degree of invasion by the tumor is predictive of survival. Tumors with the best prognosis are those found incidentally at the time of cholecystectomy for symptomatic gallstone disease.[29] This serendipitous finding emphasizes the importance of surgically opening the gallbladder at the time of cholecystectomy so any suspicious lesion can be examined immediately. Unfortunately, carcinoma is an incidental finding in approximately 1%–3% of all patients undergoing routine cholecystectomy for cholelithiasis and in 8%–10% of specimens from patients over age 70.[30]

Classification and Staging

The American Joint Committee for Cancer Staging has established the TNM classification presented in Table

55-2.[31] Alternative classification schemes are currently used in Europe and Japan. Histological grading on the basis of differentiation and the degree of invasion of the tumor are both important factors in staging gallbladder cancer and determining survival. Almost all known survivors of gallbladder cancer have had well-differentiated tumors. The higher the histological grade, the greater the association with advanced stage and rapid disease progression. No ideal staging system exists that ade-

Table 55-2 AJCC TNM Staging for Gallbladder Cancer

Primary Tumor (T)

TX   Primary tumor cannot be assessed

T0   No evidence of primary tumor

Tis Carcinoma in situ

T1   Tumor invades lamina propria or muscle layer
     T1a   Tumor invades lamina propria
     T1b   Tumor invades muscle layer

T2   Tumor invades perimuscular connective tissue; no extension beyond serosa or into liver

T3   Tumor perforates the serosa (visceral peritoneum) or directly invades one adjacent organ, or both (extension 2 cm or less into liver)

T4   Tumor extends more than 2 cm into liver, and/or into two or more adjacent organs (stomach, duodenum, colon, pancreas, omentum, extrahepatic bile ducts, any involvement of liver)

Regional Lymph Nodes (N)

NX   Regional lymph nodes cannot be assessed

N0   No regional lymph node metastasis

N1   Metastasis in cystic duct, pericholedochal, and/or hilar lymph nodes (i.e., in the hepatoduodenal ligament)

N2   Metastasis in peripancreatic (head only), periduodenal, periportal, celiac, and/or superior mesenteric lymph nodes

Distant Metastasis (M)

MX   Distant metastasis cannot be assessed

M0   No distant metastasis

M1   Distant metastasis

STAGE GROUPING

Stage 0	Tis	N0	M0
Stage I	T1	N0	M0
Stage II	T2	N0	M0
Stage III	T1	N1	M0
	T2	N1	M0
	T3	N0	M0
	T3	N1	M0
Stage IVA	T4	N0	M0
	T4	N1	M0
Stage IVB	Any T	N2	M0
	Any T	Any N	M1

quately correlates all aspects of gross and histological pathology of cancer of the gallbladder.

Therapeutic Approaches and Nursing Care

The individual and the stage of the tumor must be considered when deciding on the appropriate treatment for gallbladder cancer. An individual's general medical condition is more important than chronological age. When surgery is contemplated, several factors must be considered. Special attention must be given to any liver problems, as cirrhosis and portal hypertension will increase surgical risk. Obstructive jaundice may alter organ and immune function and should be treated preoperatively if liver resection is being considered.[32] Altered renal function, poor nutritional status, and sepsis are other parameters that increase the risk for a poor surgical outcome in individuals who are jaundiced.

Local invasion of the liver is a common finding that can sometimes be managed with a wedge resection of the liver. More extensive liver involvement may require a larger liver resection. Extension of the tumor into the colon may require a colon resection. Extension into the duodenum or pancreatic head can be resected with a pancreaticoduodenectomy. Multiple metastases in both lobes of the liver or peritoneum or distant metastases are considered contraindications to resection of the primary gallbladder tumor.

Surgery

Less than 25% of cancers of the gallbladder are resectable, but the most effective treatment for cancer of the gallbladder is resection of the primary tumor and areas where it has locally invaded.

Cholecystectomy is the primary treatment of stage I gallbladder carcinoma.[27] Many gallbladder cancers are found incidentally at the time of elective cholecystectomy. Reexploration to perform an extended resection may then be recommended within a few weeks of the original cholecystectomy.[33,34]

Treatment approach also depends on the depth of invasion of the gallbladder wall. If the tumor is limited to the mucosa, simple cholecystectomy is sufficient therapy and has a very good prognosis. Position of the tumor within the gallbladder wall may also dictate further therapy. If the tumor is next to the liver bed with minimal invasion, the recurrence rate may be high. Likewise, if the tumor is superficial and away from the liver, cholecystectomy may be an adequate operation.[35,36] If the tumor penetrates the serosa, a simple cholecystectomy is not adequate.

Laparoscopic removal of the gallbladder is not recommended. Tumor implantation at the trocar sites has been found when gallbladder cancer was removed laparoscopically. Laparoscopic manipulation of the tumor could also lead to tumor dissemination in the abdomen.[37]

When the cancer involves deeper layers of the gallbladder wall, the prognosis is grim. A radical or extended cholecystectomy has been recommended in the hopes of improving survival. The extended procedure consists of a cholecystectomy with a wide resection of the liver around the gallbladder bed and a major lymph node dissection[4] (Figure 55-2). If the tumor is near the cystic duct or if the bile duct is involved with tumor, a bile duct resection may be performed at the time of extended cholecystectomy. Studies have shown a five-year survival of 70%–85% with this extended cholecystectomy approach.[38,39] Even when the serosa is involved, extended cholecystectomy provides a better survival advantage over simple cholecystectomy. This extensive resection should be considered the therapy of choice for preoperatively recognized and potentially resectable gallbladder cancer.[40] More extensive resections that include both the liver and the duodenum or pancreas have been advocated by some researchers, but there is considerable morbidity and mortality with these radical operations.[41,42]

Survival after surgical resection depends on tumor stage and the operation performed. For stage I tumors, the five-year survival after routine cholecystectomy is greater than 85%. For stage II, III, and IV tumors, five-year survivals are approximately 25%, 10%, and 2%, respectively. Individuals with stage II tumors treated with an extended cholecystectomy may be expected to have a five-year survival of better than 65%.[4,43] The best survival for individuals with advanced tumors has been attained in Japan with more radical surgery, including removal of adjacent liver, lymph nodes, and/or involved adjacent viscera. Results from major hepatobiliary centers in the United States are revealing improved survival with reoperation after an incidental finding of gallbladder cancer after cholecystectomy and radial resection in patients with advanced disease.[44]

Postoperative care.   Routine postoperative care is necessary for an individual having a simple cholecystectomy. The surgery may be done on an outpatient basis or with a hospitalization of only a few days. For an extensive surgery involving the removal of any part of the liver or surrounding tissues, more intensive monitoring and assessment are needed. The nursing care for these individuals is the same as for anyone having a major liver resection. The main concerns in the care of an individual following hepatic surgery are control of hemorrhage, replacement of blood loss, prevention of infection and pneumonia, and appropriate supportive care. Postoperative complications include hemorrhage, biliary fistula, infection, transient metabolic consequences, subphrenic abscess, pneumonia, atelectasis, portal hypertension, and clotting defects. Knowledge of the potential complications, expected reactions, and anticipatory nursing care will aid greatly in the postoperative period.

Adjuvant treatment modalities are limited. It can be disconcerting to the individual to learn that there is little

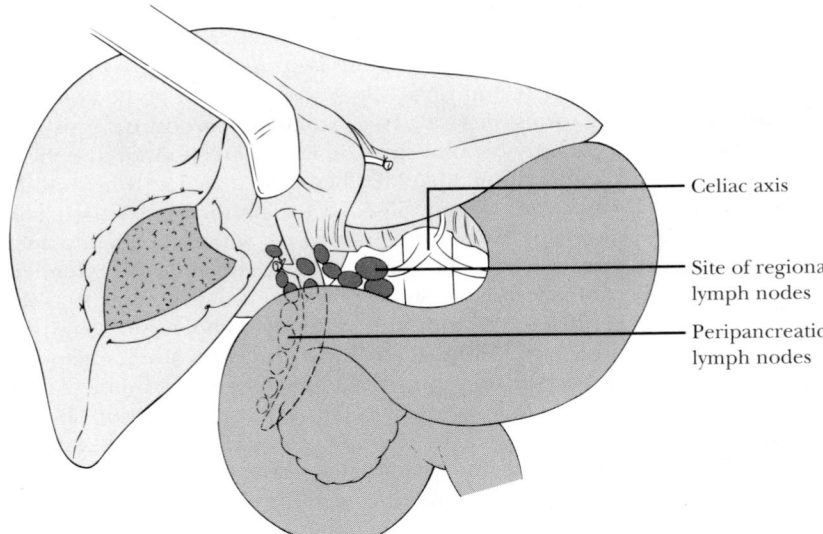

Figure 55-2 Treatment for invasive gallbladder cancer is cholecystectomy and a wedge resection of the liver along with a regional lymphadenectomy. The wedge resection of the liver is illustrated along with the lymph node regions that drain the gallbladder and that should be removed during the operation for gallbladder cancer. (Adapted with permission from Norwold DL, Dawes LG: Biliary neoplasms. In Greenfield LJ, et al (eds): *Surgery: Scientific Principles and Practice* (ed 2). Philadelphia, Lippincott-Raven, 1997, pp 1056–1067.)[19]

Celiac axis

Site of regional lymph nodes

Peripancreatic lymph nodes

treatment to offer with any proven benefit for advanced cancer of the gallbladder. The nurse should review and explain postoperative treatment options. Listening and supporting a patient during their perioperative care helps the individual and their family during a stressful time. Whereas hospitalization is often minimal after surgery, patients are faced with not only attempting to recover from a physical insult but also from the psychological impact of a cancer with a grim prognosis.

Palliative Therapy

Most therapies for gallbladder cancer are palliative.[27] The majority of gallbladder tumors are unable to be resected with negative margins. If a tissue diagnosis can be obtained through percutaneous liver biopsy or by laparoscopy, nonoperative palliation should be considered. Many individuals with gallbladder cancer will have obstructive jaundice, which can be relieved and managed with an endoscopic or percutaneous transhepatic biliary stent.[45] A complication with percutaneous transhepatic biliary stent is the development of acute cholecystitis, which subsequently may require percutaneous drainage of the gallbladder and intravenous antibiotics.[46] Recurrent jaundice and cholangitis are problems that may recur during the course of the disease due to tumor obstruction of the biliary tree or biliary stent. However, when a patient has a biliary stent placed that resolves jaundice and pruritus, an improvement in appetite, nausea, and quality of life also occur.[47]

Unfortunately, individuals who require nonoperative palliation usually do not survive more than three months. Pain should be treated aggressively to improve the individual's quality of life. Opiates are given as indicated. Radiation therapy may be helpful to palliate the pain.

Percutaneous celiac nerve block may also be helpful to reduce pain. Nerve blocks can be repeated.

Operative palliation may be used to obtain a tissue diagnosis, remove the gallbladder to prevent acute cholecystitis, relieve or prevent pain, and treat or prevent gastric outlet obstruction. A gastrojejunostomy bypass may be performed to relieve or prevent gastric outlet obstruction. The individual is then placed on acid antisecretory agents for the rest of his or her life.

The management of jaundice depends on the extent of the disease. If metastatic disease is found, the jaundice may be relieved by percutaneous transhepatic biliary catheter, which may be left in place or changed to an internal stent. If the tumor is locally unresectable without extension to adjacent organs (duodenum or pancreas), a Roux-en-Y choledochojejunostomy (anastomosis of a loop of jejunum to the common bile duct proximal to the obstruction) may be performed, which can be stented with transhepatic silastic biliary stents to relieve biliary obstruction. At the time of exploration, the tumor margins should be marked with radiopaque clips if external beam radiotherapy is being considered.[4] Nursing care is the same as for any abdominal surgery.

The addition of an internal-external percutaneous transhepatic biliary stent depends on the extent of the disease and the choice of the physician in treating jaundice. The individual and the family will need to be taught the care and flushing of the stent as it may be left in place for the rest of the person's life. The stent is usually flushed twice a day with sterile normal saline solution. Daily cleansing of the stent site is required. A patient may require right and left biliary stents to drain both lobes of the liver if tumor is obstructing the bifurcation of the biliary tree into the liver. Signs and symptoms of complications of the stent must be reviewed to enable the individual and family to notify the clinician promptly to avoid problems and unnecessary hospitalization. The use of an internal expandable stent to palliate obstructive jaundice is now favored for individuals with only a few months to live.[48] The stent can be easily placed by an interventional radiologist or endoscopist.

The majority of individuals with gallbladder cancer have unresectable disease at the time of diagnosis. Less than 15% of all individuals with gallbladder cancer are alive after five years. Individuals with unresectable stage III tumors have a median survival of six months. The median survival for an individual with stage IV gallbladder cancer with liver or peritoneal metastases at the time of presentation is only one to three months.[3]

Radiation Therapy

Radiation therapy has been used to treat individuals with resected gallbladder cancer as well as unresectable tumors. There has been no proven survival advantage with external beam radiation alone or after surgery. In unresectable cancer, external beam radiation has been used to help relieve pain or to relieve biliary obstruction. Intraoperative radiation has also been used, but the advantage of this technique combined with resection and/or external beam radiotherapy has not been proven and further trials regarding this modality are necessary.[49] Likewise, the role of radiation sensitizers, such as fluorouracil (5-FU), and the addition of leucovorin to intraoperative or external beam radiation therapy has yet to be conclusively studied in individuals with gallbladder cancer.[4] Overall, the data in support of using radiotherapy are meager but hopeful. The curative potential of an operation may be enhanced by postoperative radiotherapy.[50] Palliation, including relief from obstruction, may be achieved for a period in patients with advanced disease.

Chemotherapy

Chemotherapy agents for the treatment of gallbladder cancer have been limited due to poor tumor response. Mitomycin C and 5-FU have been most commonly used. In individuals suspected of having microscopic disease after resection, chemotherapy may be considered as adjuvant therapy, but its effectiveness has been difficult to document. Intraarterial and intraperitoneal delivery of chemotherapeutic agents has been tried with varying results.

Chemotherapy and radiation therapy have not been effective in the treatment of gallbladder cancer. Adjuvant therapy after cholecystectomy or extended resection has not been encouraging.[51] The rarity of gallbladder cancer limits the ability to perform prospective, randomized studies of therapy as the majority of cases present at an advanced stage. Surgical resection of gallbladder cancer has been the only form of therapy that has affected the natural history of the disease.[52]

Symptom Management

Individuals with advanced cancer of the gallbladder usually have disease involving the liver and biliary tree. Obstructive jaundice, liver abscess, and liver failure are potential complications. Management of any drain or percutaneous transhepatic biliary stent is taught to the individual and family. Teaching the signs and symptoms of potential problems resulting from the tumor or any tubes and drains may allow for earlier intervention and less hospitalization. Persistent pain, fever, chills, and recurrent jaundice may be symptoms of a liver abscess caused by obstructed bile ducts, or a malfunctioning endoscopic or percutaneous biliary stent.

With progressive liver failure, ascites and increased abdominal girth may cause pain, discomfort, and dyspnea. Supportive measures include aggressive pain management and proper body positioning. Ascites can be controlled by fluid and sodium restriction along with diuretic therapy. A peritoneal tap may be necessary to relieve abdominal distention and provide comfort and easier breathing. Intraabdominal spread of tumor can cause pain and palpable or visible tumor.

Nutritional intake is poor in the individual with gallbladder cancer and jaundice. Elevated bilirubin levels cause changes in taste, leading to a decrease in appetite and weight loss. Cold foods may be better tolerated. Food prepared with spices that enhance taste can be tried. Plastic silverware can be used if the individual complains of a metallic taste in the mouth. Small, frequent snacks and a change in the environment may be helpful. Nausea, vomiting, and anorexia can also hinder nutrition. Antiemetics prior to eating may assist in controlling nausea and vomiting. Megestrol acetate and cannabinoids may help to manage anorexia.

Liver failure usually develops as the disease progresses and follows a progression of lethargy and weakness to encephalopathy and hepatic coma. Renal failure is also common at this time. The nurse can assist the family by explaining what to expect as the symptoms develop. Individual and family support are the major goals of nursing care.

Continuity of Care: Nursing Challenges

Most individuals with gallbladder cancer present with advanced disease and rapid decline. Communication from the inpatient or outpatient nurse to home care and hospice nurses can be invaluable in providing quality care to an individual with a rapidly changing condition. The transition to hospice care with attention to individual and family needs is made easier when the nurses who know the most about the individual share information. The burden to the family and their experience with cancer can be greatly eased by anticipatory management and supportive care.

BILE DUCT CANCER

Introduction

Adenocarcinoma of the bile duct is also referred to as *cholangiocarcinoma*. It is a rare malignancy that can occur anywhere in the biliary tree. The spectrum of cholangiocarcinoma is best classified into three anatomic groups: (1) perihilar, (2) distal, and (3) intrahepatic. Perihilar lesions are the most common, accounting for approximately 70% of these tumors. Distal tumors are the second most common, and intrahepatic cholangiocarcinomas occur least frequently (Figure 55-3).[53] Cholangiocarcinoma occurs with conditions in which bile is stagnant, infected, or both, and with bile duct stone formation. The diagnosis of cholangiocarcinoma should be considered in every case of obstructive jaundice. Diagnosis and management of cholangiocarcinoma is often challenging and complex. Ideally, diagnosis of an early cholangiocarcinoma may reveal a small, localized tumor that may be amenable to an aggressive multidisciplinary approach.

Epidemiology

Approximately 15,000 new cases of liver and intrahepatic bile duct cancer are diagnosed annually in the United States.[2] Intrahepatic cholangiocarcinoma is much less common than liver cancer and also occurs less frequently than extrahepatic cholangiocarcinoma. Surveillance, Epidemiology, and End Results (SEER) data reports the total number of cancers of the extrahepatic bile duct to have been approximately 4000 in 1995.[3] The U.S. incidence approaches one per 100,000 people each year, with a higher incidence in specific groups at high risk for the disease.[54] The incidence of cholangiocarcinoma increases with age, with the mean age at presentation between 60 and 65 years. These tumors occur with a similar frequency in men and women.[55]

Increased frequency of cancers of the biliary tract have been reported in Southeast Asia, Japan, eastern Europe, Central and South America, and among American Indians and Hispanic Americans.[56-58]

Etiology

Several risk factors have been linked to cholangiocarcinoma (Table 55-3). Factors common to a number of these etiological parameters include biliary stasis, and infection with and without intrahepatic or common bile duct stones. Only a small proportion of individuals with cholangiocarcinoma typically have these risk factors.

Strong associations have been seen in individuals with cystic dilatation of the bile duct, including both choledochal cyst disease and Caroli's disease. Individuals with cholangiocarcinoma associated with choledochal cyst are usually diagnosed in the fourth decade of life.[59] The origin of choledochal cysts and subsequent formation of cholangiocarcinoma has been explained by an anomalous pancreatic biliary duct junction (APBDJ) where there is a high entry of the pancreatic duct into the extrahepatic biliary tree. This finding suggests that reflux of pancreatic exocrine secretions into the bile duct may lead to malignant transformation of the biliary epithelium.[60,61] Other factors that may lead to malignant transformation in choledochal cysts include bile stasis within the cyst, stone formation, chronic inflammation, and bacterial infection. These same factors may play a role in

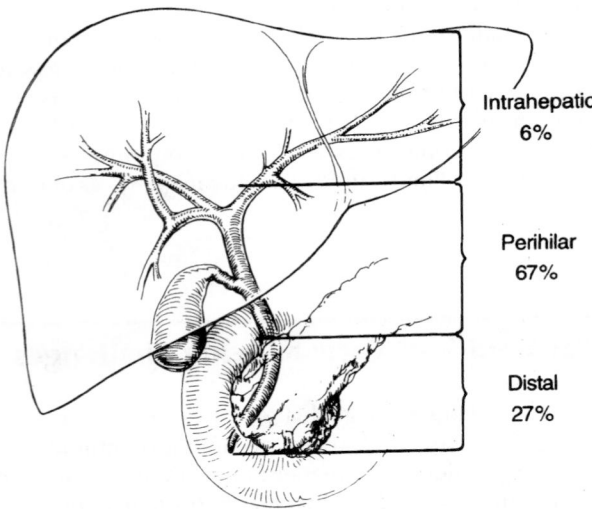

Intrahepatic 6%

Perihilar 67%

Distal 27%

Figure 55-3 Distribution of 294 cholangiocarcinomas into intrahepatic, perihilar, and distal subgroups. (Used with permission from Nakeeb A, Pitt HA, Sohn TA, et al. Cholangiocarcinomas: A spectrum of intraphepatic, perihilar, and distal tumors. *Annals of Surgery* 224:463–475, 1996.)[53]

Table 55-3	Risk Factors for Bile Duct Cancer
High Risk	**Possible Increased Risk**
Cystic dilation of bile duct	Asbestos
Choledochal cyst	Dioxin (Agent Orange)
Caroli's disease	Isoniazid
Clonorchiasis	Methyldopa
Hepatolithiasis	Nitrosamines
Sclerosing cholangitis	Opisthorchiasis
Thorium dioxide (Thorotrast)	Oral contraceptives
Ulcerative colitis	Polychlorinated biphenyls

the high incidence of cholangiocarcinoma in individuals with congenital dilatation of the intrahepatic bile ducts (Caroli's disease).[62]

In East Asia, a clear association has been recognized between cholangiocarcinoma and infection with the liver fluke *Clonorchis sinensis*.[63] Infection with the liver fluke is from consuming infected raw fish. The parasite usually occupies the intrahepatic bile ducts obstructing the flow of bile. Another liver fluke, *Opisthorchis viverrini*, is endemic to Thailand and is also associated with cholangiocarcinoma.[64] The combination of liver fluke infestation and a diet high in nitrosamines may explain the high incidence of cholangiocarcinoma in this region.[65] It has been suggested that the presence of *Opisthorchis viverrini* may induce DNA damage and mutation in the intrahepatic biliary epithelium.[66]

The cause-and-effect relationship between cholelithiasis and cholangiocarcinoma has not been established. Yet a recent study showed the risk of biliary tract cancer among women was significantly associated with a history of cholelithiasis and postmenopausal status.[67]

Individuals with hepatolithiasis, which is commonly found in Southeast Asia, have a 5%–10% risk of developing cholangiocarcinoma during their lifetime.[68,69] Bile stasis, infected bile, and cystic dilatation of the intrahepatic biliary tree may all be risk factors for development of bile duct cancer.[70]

Individuals with sclerosing cholangitis are also at increased risk for developing cholangiocarcinoma. Primary sclerosing cholangitis is an idiopathic disease characterized by multiple intrahepatic and extrahepatic inflammatory bile duct strictures that cannot be attributed to specific causes.[71,72] Cholangiocarcinoma that develops in individuals with sclerosing cholangitis is often manifested by rapid clinical deterioration and progressive jaundice.[73] The majority of individuals with sclerosing cholangitis have coexisting ulcerative colitis. The prevalence of cholangiocarcinoma in individuals with ulcerative colitis is significantly greater than the risk for the general population.[4] Ulcerative colitis is often quiescent in individuals who develop sclerosing cholangitis and can go unrecognized. The colitis precedes the cholangiocarcinoma by an average of five years.[74] Individuals with sclerosing cholangitis or ulcerative colitis who develop bile duct cancer are usually in their fifth decade, approximately 20 years younger than individuals without these risk factors.[75]

The radiocontrast agent thorium dioxide (Thorotrast) has also been shown to cause hepatic and bile duct malignancies. Thorotrast was used as a contrast agent for radiography from the late 1920s until the 1940s. Thorium dioxide emits energy as alpha particles and, when injected intravenously, is retained in the reticuloendothelial system for life. Cholangiocarcinomas have been diagnosed in individuals an average of 35 years after exposure.[76] A number of chemicals and several other drugs have been associated with cholangiocarcinoma, including asbestos, dioxin (Agent Orange), isoniazid, methyldopa, oral contraceptives, and polychlorinated biphenyls. Dietary nitrosamines, which are present in cured meats, have also

been suspected.[4] A clustering of persons with cholangiocarcinoma has been reported in certain geographical areas of the United States, underscoring the importance of environmental factors in the pathogenesis of cholangiocarcinoma.[77]

Prevention, Screening, and Early Detection

At present there is no effective screening for cancer of the biliary tree. Studies are needed to develop a serum or a bile marker for early detection of cholangiocarcinoma in high-risk individuals with hepatolithiasis, choledochal cysts, sclerosing cholangitis, and ulcerative colitis. Further genetic, dietary, occupational, and environmental analysis of clusters of people with cholangiocarcinoma may provide additional clues to the pathogenesis of these rare tumors.

The role of prevention is important as there is limited benefit from surgery in those patients and other therapies are even less effective. Early detection with timely resection is necessary to improve the survival rate of persons with biliary carcinoma. Screening and removal of stone-containing gallbladders may gain acceptance with the advent of innovative surgical techniques.

Pathophysiology

Cellular Characteristics

Cholangiocarcinomas arise from the epithelium of the intrahepatic and extrahepatic bile ducts. They appear as firm, gray-white tumors. Central necrosis may be observed. The majority of bile duct cancers are adenocarcinomas, with papillary adenocarcinoma and mucinous and mucin-producing adenocarcinomas the next largest groups of biliary cancer. Extrahepatic bile duct papillary adenocarcinomas have the best prognosis while mucinous adenocarcinomas have the poorest outcome.[3]

The tumors range from well differentiated to poorly differentiated varieties that exhibit glandular or acinar structures. Mucin is almost always found within the cytoplasm of the cells. Cells tend to be cuboidal or low columnar and resemble biliary epithelium, though bile production is not usually seen.[74]

Other histologic types of bile duct cancers include squamous, mucoepidermoid, leiomyosarcoma, rhabdomyosarcoma, cystadenocarcinoma, carcinoid, and granular cell carcinoma.[4] The pathologic determination of malignancy may be difficult, especially if there is cholangitis, hepatolithiasis, biliary obstruction, and stents. The pathologic diagnosis is supported by any additional finding of (1) a positive reaction to carcinoembryonic antigen (CEA), (2) nuclear size variation, (3) distended intracytoplasmic lumina, or (4) neural invasion. Most cholangiocarcinomas will stain positively for CEA as well as the carbohydrate antigens CA 50 and CA 19-9.[78,79] The relationship of oncogenes and tumor suppressor genes along with molecular genetic abnormalities are being investigated.[4,80]

Progression of Disease

Cholangiocarcinoma originating within the hepatic parenchyma usually is a solitary and large mass. Tumor invasion of the large portal or hepatic veins may occur. Intrahepatic tumors tend to present as solitary masses. Perihilar cholangiocarcinoma may present as an infiltrative mass that extends from the hilum into the parenchyma, as a sclerotic mass that encircles a large bile duct, or as a polypoid tumor that invades the lumen of a large bile duct.[74] Distal bile duct cancers tend to infiltrate locally.

In both the gallbladder and extrahepatic bile ducts, areas of dysplasia and carcinoma in situ may be found adjacent to invasive carcinoma, suggesting such a sequence in the development of these tumors.[29]

Patterns of Spread

Extrahepatic metastases occur more frequently through the lymphatic system than through the hematogenous route. Peripancreatic and hilar lymph nodes are involved in approximately half of the cases. Metastases to the liver or peritoneal cavity are common in cholangiocarcinoma. Perineural and periductal spaces and portal tracts tend to be invaded by tumor. Lung, bone, and other sites are much less likely to be involved. When the tumor causes chronic biliary obstruction, the liver may develop secondary biliary cirrhosis.[4]

Clinical Manifestations

The majority (more than 90%) of individuals with cholangiocarcinoma present with jaundice. Pruritus, mild abdominal pain, fatigue, anorexia, and weight loss occur less frequently. Cholangitis is rarely a presenting symptom, but commonly occurs following endoscopic or percutaneous biliary manipulation. Except for jaundice, the physical examination is usually normal. A mass may be palpable or the liver may be enlarged with intrahepatic biliary tumors. In an individual with a distal bile duct tumor, a distended, nontender gallbladder may be palpable. A person with perihilar cholangiocarcinoma typically presents with mild upper abdominal pain and unilobular hepatic enlargement as the tumor may be obstructing the intrahepatic biliary tree in either the right or left lobe of the liver.[4]

An individual who presents with upper abdominal symptoms or abnormal hepatic function without jaundice will require diagnostic studies to assist in the early diagnosis of bile duct carcinoma. Bile duct carcinoma without jaundice can be regarded as being in a relatively early stage, and likely to have a more favorable outcome than most bile duct carcinomas with jaundice.[81]

Assessment

Patient and Family History

The individual diagnosed with cholangiocarcinoma may have had subtle weight loss, malaise, indigestion, and vague abdominal pain; or there may have been no previous symptoms. Pruritus along with the appearance of tea-colored urine and clay-colored (acholic) stools may be noticed before jaundice is evident.

Cholangiocarcinoma is difficult to diagnose in the presence of primary sclerosing cholangitis. Rapid elevation of bilirubin associated with weight loss and abdominal discomfort in an otherwise stable person with primary sclerosing cholangitis should alert the clinician to the possibility of cholangiocarcinoma.[82–84]

Physical Examination

Apart from jaundice, the physical examination is usually normal in individuals with perihilar tumors. A mass may be palpable or the liver may be enlarged with an intrahepatic bile duct tumor. In an individual with a distal bile duct tumor, a distended, nontender gallbladder may be palpable.

Diagnostic Studies

Laboratory data. Laboratory evaluation reveals elevation of total serum bilirubin (greater than 10 mg/dL) in most individuals with cholangiocarcinoma at the time of presentation.[4] Marked elevations of alkaline phosphatase and gamma-glutamyl transferase levels reflect bile duct epithelial cell injury. Markers of hepatocyte injury such as alanine amino transferase and aspartate amino transferase may be only slightly elevated. Individuals with chronic biliary obstruction may have laboratory evidence of depressed hepatocyte function, such as low albumin or prolonged prothrombin time.

Serum tumor markers such as CEA and AFP are usually normal. Serum CA 19-9 and CA 50 may be elevated in individuals with cholangiocarcinoma, and they may be useful in screening those individuals at high risk of developing cholangiocarcinoma. The use of serum and bile tumor markers has been shown to improve the early detection of cholangiocarcinoma in persons with primary sclerosing cholangitis.[84–86] Other serum tumor markers are being investigated. High levels of interleukin 6 (IL-6) have been found in individuals with cholangiocarcinoma and correlate with tumor burden. In association with other tumor markers such as AFP, CEA, and CA 19-9, IL-6 may be useful in distinguishing among hepatic neoplasms.[87] Currently, no accurate screening test for bile duct cancer exists.

Radiologic evaluation. The goal of radiographic evaluation for individuals with cholangiocarcinoma is delineation of the extent of the tumor, including involvement of the bile ducts, liver, portal vessels, and distant metastases. An ordered sequence of studies will achieve this goal. Cholangiocarcinoma is suspected on the basis of an abnormal US or CT scan. An intrahepatic tumor is visualized as a liver mass, with or without peripherally dilated bile ducts. A perihilar cholangiocarcinoma produces a picture of dilated intrahepatic bile ducts, a normal or collapsed gallbladder, and a normal pancreas. A distal cholangiocarcinoma causes dilation of intrahepatic and extrahepatic bile ducts as well as the gallbladder, with or without a mass in the head of the pancreas. US and CT scan have comparable accuracy in depicting the level of biliary obstruction. CT is more useful than US for determining resectability because of its greater sensitivity in depicting the actual tumor mass, vascular invasion, spread to adjacent organs, and distant metastases.[88–91] However, a primary tumor mass often does not visualize on standard CT scan or US. The newer spiral CT techniques and even MRI are better at detecting the parenchymal extent of the tumor.[92] Magnetic resonance cholangiography is also being utilized as an effective, noninvasive method for the detection and extent of a bile duct tumor.[93–95]

After documentation of bile duct dilation, biliary anatomy is defined cholangiographically through either the percutaneous transhepatic or endoscopic retrograde route. The proximal extent of the tumor is the most important feature in determining resectability. In tumors of the perihilar region/hepatic hilum, percutaneous transhepatic cholangiography is favored because it best defines the proximal (uppermost) extent of tumor involvement. This approach also allows the preoperative placement of percutaneous transhepatic biliary catheters to drain the obstructed biliary tree for partial or complete relief of jaundice. For neoplasms involving the proximal common hepatic duct or the bifurcation of the bile duct, both the left and right hepatic ducts are intubated with transhepatic biliary catheters to drain both lobes of the liver.

For tumors of the distal common bile duct, the use of ERCP may allow visualization of both the proximal and distal extent of the tumor within the extrahepatic biliary tree. Decompression of the obstructed biliary tree can be performed by the placement of a biliary endoprosthesis. Angiography may be employed in some cases to assess tumor stage and resectability.

Biopsy/cytology. Percutaneous needle aspiration biopsy, brush or scrape biopsy, or cytological examination of bile may determine a tissue diagnosis.[96] The use of needle biopsy to establish a diagnosis may only be re-quired when the tumor is deemed unresectable. In this setting, punch biopsies from the lumen of the bile duct before placement of transhepatic biliary catheters may yield the best diagnostic information.[4] These techniques are not essential in persons with presumed bile duct cancer, as many individuals will ultimately be explored for resection or palliation.[53]

Classification and Staging

In the United States, cholangiocarcinoma is staged by the TMN classification of the American Joint Commission on Cancer (Table 55-4).[31] In this system, stage I tumors are confined to the bile duct mucosa or muscular layer, whereas stage II tumors invade periductal tissues. Stage III tumors have spread to regional lymph nodes and stage IV tumors either invade adjacent structures or have distant metastases. In Europe, the International Union Against Cancer classifies cholangiocarcinomas in a similar fashion. In Japan, a more complex system devised by the Japanese Cancer Society takes into account invasion of specific adjacent organs or blood vessels.

A combination of CT scan, cholangiography, and angiography are used to stage cholangiocarcinoma. CT scan findings of bilobar peripheral hepatic metastases or extrahepatic disease preclude curative resection. Atrophy of the lobe containing the tumor with hypertrophy of the other lobe is also a sign that resection may not be possible. Cholangiography findings of extensive bilobar intrahepatic duct involvement are another indicator of unresectability. Radiographic evidence of encased or occlusion of the common hepatic artery or main portal vein by tumor is also considered to be indicative of unresectability.

Therapeutic Approaches and Nursing Care

Surgery

Surgical resection remains the treatment of choice in bile duct carcinoma whenever feasible. Surgery is the appropriate option for prolonged survival and potential cure. Diagnostic imaging does not provide enough accuracy for a definitive decision about resectability. A histologically proven diagnosis of malignancy may not be possible to obtain and is not considered important to justify an operation. Therefore, laparotomy by specialized hepatobiliary surgeons should be considered in most cases.[97]

The type of surgical resection depends on the anatomic location of the tumor. A pancreaticoduodenectomy, or Whipple procedure, is usually the surgical operation for a distal bile duct carcinoma (see Chapter 63). The median survival rate has been reported to be 22 months. Intrahepatic cholangiocarcinoma is managed

Table 55-4   AJCC TNM Staging for Cholangiocarcinoma

Primary Tumor (T)

TX   Primary tumor cannot be assessed

T0   No evidence of primary tumor

Tis   Carcinoma in situ

T1   Tumor invades subepithelial connective tissue or fibromuscular layer
    T1a   Tumor invades subepithelial connective tissue
    T1b   Tumor invades fibromuscular layer

T2   Tumor invades perifibromuscular connective tissue

T3   Tumor invades adjacent structures: liver, pancreas, duodenum, gallbladder, colon, stomach

Regional Lymph Nodes (N)

NX   Regional lymph nodes cannot be assessed

N0   No regional lymph node metastasis

N1   Metastasis in cystic duct, pericholedochal and/or hilar lymph nodes (i.e., in the hepatoduodenal ligament)

N2   Metastasis in peripancreatic (head only), periduodenal, periportal, celiac, and/or superior mesenteric and/or posterior pancreaticoduodenal lymph nodes

Distant Metastasis (M)

MX   Distant metastasis cannot be assessed

M0   No distant metastasis

M1   Distant metastasis

STAGE GROUPING

Stage 0	Tis	N0	M0
Stage I	T1	N0	M0
Stage II	T2	N0	M0
Stage III	T1	N1	M0
	T1	N2	M0
	T2	N1	M0
	T2	N2	M0
Stage IVA	T3	Any N	M0
Stage IVB	Any T	Any N	M1

optimally with hepatic resection (see Chapter 58). The prognosis for resectable intrahepatic cholangiocarcinoma is more favorable than that for perihilar cholangiocarcinoma, with a median survival rate of 9–30 months.[98]

Incidental bile duct carcinomas may be found at the time of liver transplantation performed for primary sclerosing cholangitis.[99] Perihilar bile duct carcinomas may be removed with a hilar resection at the hepatic duct bifurcation combined with hepaticojejunostomy.

Percutaneous transhepatic biliary catheters may be inserted preoperatively in individuals undergoing surgical exploration for perihilar cholangiocarcinoma. The catheters assist in the technical aspects of hilar dissection by allowing palpation of the catheter within the biliary

tree to identify and dissect the hepatic duct bifurcation at the time of exploration. The catheters also aid in the reconstruction of the biliary tract during the removal of the tumor and facilitate placement of larger, softer Silastic transhepatic biliary stents at the time of surgery.[100]

Transhepatic biliary catheters may also be placed to facilitate the delivery of high doses of local radiation (brachytherapy). Radioactive seeds on long guidewires are placed directly adjacent to the site of the tumor through the transhepatic tubes (Figure 55-4).[72]

Perihilar cholangiocarcinoma may extend along either the right or left hepatic duct into the hepatic parenchyma. A hepatic lobectomy may be considered in addition to the hilar resection. The use of total hepatectomy and liver transplantation for intrahepatic and perihilar cholangiocarcinoma have been disappointing as a result of early and widespread recurrence and the critical shortage of available organs for transplant.[101]

Factors shown to be predictors of survival in patients with resection for bile duct carcinomas include negative margin status, preoperative albumin level, postoperative sepsis, serum bilirubin concentration, preoperative jaundice, and tumor grade. Nutritional status and underlying sepsis also may play an important role in the eventual outcome.[98,102]

Palliative Therapy

Although much progress has been made in the diagnosis and management of perihilar cholangiocarcinoma, complete surgical resection is usually impossible because of

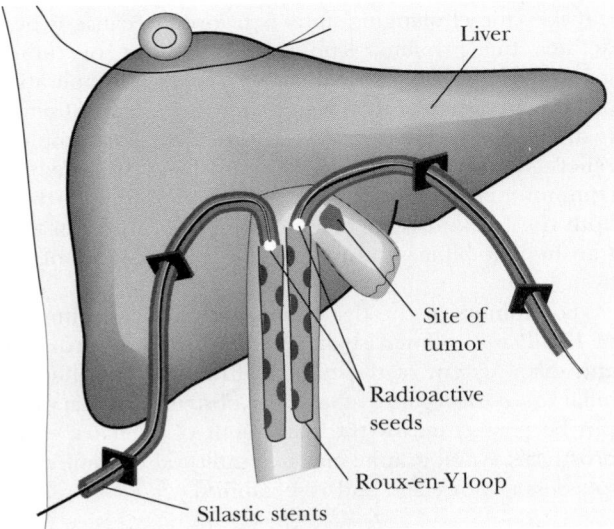

Figure 55-4   Transhepatic silastic stents can be used as conduits for delivering radioactive ^{192}Ir seeds to the site of tumor.

local tumor invasion. Most patients can only be managed by palliative drainage.[103]

Palliative therapy in patients with cholangiocarcinoma can include both nonoperative and operative procedures. Patients who need nonoperative palliation may have biliary decompression performed using stents placed by either percutaneous or endoscopic route.[4]

Patients who are found at laparotomy to have widespread intraperitoneal tumor will have their gallbladder removed to prevent the subsequent development of acute cholecystitis, which may result from the percutaneous transhepatic biliary stents obstructing the cystic duct.[46] Percutaneous transhepatic biliary stents are left in place and may be exchanged for larger-diameter, softer Silastic transhepatic stents by interventional radiology (Figure 55-5).[104]

Patients with locally advanced unresectable perihilar tumors may have a Roux-en-Y choledochojejunostomy with intraoperative placement of larger Silastic transhepatic stents. A segment III bypass to the left intrahepatic ducts may be performed for biliary decompression.[105] For distal bile duct tumors, a double bowel bypass, choledochojejunostomy, and gastrojejunostomy are usually the procedures of choice (see Chapter 63).

Adjuvant and Multimodality Treatment

Radiotherapy. Experience with adjuvant and multimodality treatment in randomized prospective trials is limited. There are reports in the literature combining external, internal, and intraoperative radiotherapy with systemic chemotherapy. In the reports, there are no clear data showing a real benefit of radiotherapy for survival of patients resected with intention of cure. The use of radiotherapy combined with chemotherapy may be possible in those patients with positive resection margins and unresectable tumors.[98,105–109] Neoadjuvant radiation and chemoradiation have also been investigated. The small number of patients in these studies makes it difficult to draw any conclusions.[110,111]

Most information on the use of radiation therapy is retrospective. At this time there are no prospective, randomized trials of the use of radiotherapy reported for bile duct carcinoma.

Chemotherapy. The use of chemotherapy alone, using 5-FU and multiple other chemotherapeutic drugs, has not been shown to improve survival in patients with either resected or unresected bile duct carcinoma. Other drugs—including hormones, antiestrogens, cholecystokinin, somatostatin, and antibiotics used as cytotoxic agents—have been tried as novel approaches.[4] Controlled human trials are necessary to determine if any of these have an impact on this tumor. Newer therapies such as photodynamic therapy, transarterial embolization, and intraluminal brachytherapy have also been employed in the treatment of patients with unresectable perihilar bile duct cancer.[113,114] Preoperative portal vein embolization has also been used to provide safer liver surgery and assist with resectability of these difficult perihilar tumors.[115]

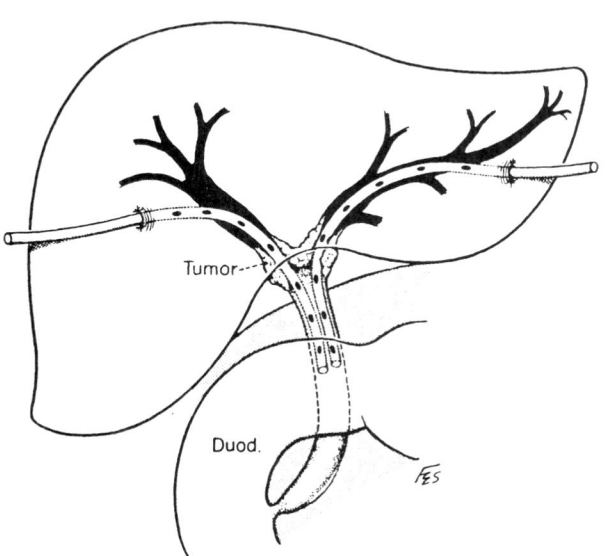

Figure 55-5 Transhepatic tubes are placed in both the right and left hepatic ductal system for palliation of an obstructing proximal tumor. The internal ends of the tubes are left in the distal common bile duct. (Used with permission from Rossi RL, Gordon M, Braasch JW: Intubation techniques in biliary tract surgery. *Surgical Clinics of North America* 60:297–312, 1980.)[104]

Symptom Management

The symptom management of individuals with advanced bile duct cancer parallels that of individuals with gallbladder cancer. Palliation of obstructive jaundice by endoscopic or percutaneous stents is a primary objective. Internal metallic, expandable stents placed in the biliary ducts to maintain lumen patency may be the optimal intervention for patients with only a couple of months to live. Liver abscess, due to obstruction of the biliary ducts, as well as liver failure are potential complications. The symptoms of persistent pain, fever, chills, and recurrent jaundice may indicate a liver abscess, which can be treated by percutaneous drainage and antibiotics. Malfunctioning endoscopic or percutaneous biliary stents can also present as fever, chills, and recurrent jaundice. Internal, metallic expandable stents may become occluded with debris or tumor. A percutaneous transhepatic biliary catheter may need to be placed to relieve the obstruction.

Erosion of tumor into a major blood vessel, such as the portal vein or hepatic artery, is another potential problem that can cause a massive bleed and death. Support for the family is important as the individual may meet a rapid demise unexpectedly. The nurse can assist the patient and family by explaining what to expect as symptoms develop.

Maintenance of nutrition is a challenge as individuals with obstructive jaundice have major interference of their taste buds and decreased appetite due to lack of bile in the GI system. Different food preparations or appetite stimulants can be tried to help bolster an individual's intake.

Individuals who succumb to progressive liver failure usually lapse into hepatic coma. Progressive liver failure must be recognized and supportive nursing care rendered. The major goals of nursing care in individuals with carcinoma of the biliary tree are recognition of overt as well as subtle symptoms and their impact as the disease progresses. Comfort measures are paramount in these patients. Family support is also important to help them cope with the inevitable loss of a loved one.

Continuity of Care: Nursing Challenges

Most individuals with bile duct cancer present at an advanced stage and rapidly decline. For those individuals who have surgical intervention, and whose length of survival may be extended, the outcome of the disease is the same. The nurse must be aware of how the individual and the family are coping. Not only the physical status of the patient but also the psychosocial welfare must be considered. Whatever treatment modality the patient embarks upon, there is always a reason to provide hope and encouragement. When the patient truly declines and enters the terminal stage of the disease, palliative care with emphasis on quality of life becomes paramount.

Conclusion

Significant advances in the pathogenesis, diagnosis, and treatment of malignancies of the biliary tract have been made in recent years. Most patients with carcinoma of the gallbladder and bile duct, however, continue to have a poor prognosis. Identification of the gene responsible for biliary anomalies and the development of serum or bile tumor markers may make early detection and prevention of these cancers for persons at risk possible. Dietary, occupational, environmental, and further genetic analysis of clusters of patients may provide more clues to the pathogenesis of these rare tumors.

Advances in technology will allow less invasive imaging diagnostic studies. Quality of life and length of survival will continue to be assessed in the palliated and aggressive surgically resected patients. New chemotherapeutic agents and novel therapies need to be tested. Safer surgeries and more effective adjuvant therapy are needed to improve the outlook for future patients with malignancies of the gallbladder and biliary tract. Further innovations

will require multidisciplinary collaboration to treat these patients based on the foundation of nursing care.

References

1. Donohue JH, Stewart AK, Menck HR: The National Cancer Data Base report on carcinoma of the gallbladder, 1989–1995. *Cancer* 83:2618–2628, 1998
2. *Cancer Facts and Figures–1999*. Atlanta, American Cancer Society, 1999
3. Carriaga MT, Henson DE: Liver, gallbladder, extrahepatic bile ducts, and pancreas. *Cancer* 75:171–190, 1995
4. Pitt HA, Dooley WC, Yeo CJ, et al: Malignancies of the biliary tree. *Curr Probl Surg* 32:11–36, 1995
5. Nagorney DM, McPherson GA: Carcinoma of the gallbladder and extrahepatic bile ducts. *Semin Oncol* 15:106–116, 1988
6. Jones RS: Carcinoma of the gallbladder. *Surg Clin North Am* 70:1419–1428, 1990
7. Chijiiwa K, Tanaka M, Nakayama F: Adenocarcinoma of the gallbladder associated with anomalous pancreaticobiliary ductal junction. *Am Surg* 59:430–434, 1993
8. Wang HP, Wu MS, Lin CC, et al: Pancreaticobiliary diseases associated with anomalous pancreaticobiliary ductal union. *Gastrointest Endosc* 48:184–189, 1998
9. Mancuso TF, Brennan MJ: Epidemiological consideration of cancer of the gallbladder, bile ducts and salivary glands in the rubber industry. *J Occup Med* 12:333–341, 1970
10. Hasegawa R, Ogawa K, Takaba K, et al: 3,2'-Dimethyl-4-aminobiphenyl-induced gallbladder carcinogenesis and effects of ethinyl estradiol in hamsters. *Jpn J Cancer Res* 83:1286–1292, 1992
11. Nath G, Singh H, Shukla VK: Chronic typhoid carriage and carcinoma of the gallbladder. *Eur J Cancer Prev* 6:557–559, 1997
12. Sons HU, Borchard F, Joel BS: Carcinoma of the gallbladder: autopsy findings in 287 cases and review of the literature. *J Surg Oncol* 28:199–206, 1985
13. Yamagiwa H: Mucosal dysplasia of gallbladder: isolated and adjacent lesions to carcinoma. *Jpn J Cancer Res* 80:238–243, 1989
14. Koichi W, Masao T, Koji T, et al: Carcinoma and polyps of the gallbladder associated with Peutz-Jeghers syndrome. *Dig Dis Sci* 32:943–946, 1987
15. Maxwell P, David RI, Sloan JM: Carcinoembryonic antigen (CEA) in benign and malignant epithelium of the gallbladder, extrahepatic bile ducts, and ampulla of Vater. *J Pathol* 170:73–76, 1993
16. Brown JA, Roberts CS: Elevated serum alpha-fetoprotein levels in primary gallbladder carcinoma without hepatic involvement. *Cancer* 70:1838–1840, 1992
17. Sumiyoshi K, Nagai E, Chijiiwa K, et al: Pathology of carcinoma of the gallbladder. *World J Surg* 15:315–321, 1991
18. Keller JW, Peacock JL, Smith JL: Cancer of the major digestive glands: pancreas, liver, bile ducts, gallbladder, in Rubin P (ed): *Clinical Oncology: A Multidisciplinary Approach for Physicians and Students* (ed 7). Philadelphia, Saunders, 1993, pp 597–615
19. Norwold DL, Dawes LG: Biliary neoplasms, in Greenfield LJ, Mulholland M, Oldham KT, Zelenock GB, Lillemoe KD (eds): *Surgery: Scientific Principles and Practice* (ed 2). Philadelphia, Lippincott-Raven, 1997, pp 1056–1067

20. Liu KJ, Richter HM, Cho MJ, et al: Carcinoma involving the gallbladder in elderly patients presenting with acute cholecystitis. *Surgery* 122:748–754, 1997

21. Bach AM, Loring LA, Hann LE, et al: Gallbladder cancer: can ultrasonography evaluate extent of disease? *J Ultrasound Med* 17:303–309, 1998

22. Soyer P, Gouhiri M, Boudiaf M, et al: Carcinoma of the gallbladder: imaging features with surgical correlation. *AJR Am J Roentgenol* 169:781–785, 1997

23. Kelekis NL, Semelka RC: MR imaging of the gallbladder. *Top Magn Reson Imaging* 8:312–320, 1996

24. Curley SA: Biliary tract cancer. *Cancer Treat Res* 90:273–307, 1997

25. Yoshimitsu K, Honda H, Kaneko K, et al: Dynamic MRI of the gallbladder lesions: differentiation of benign from malignant. *J Magn Reson Imaging* 7:696–701, 1997

26. Shukla VK, Pandey M, Kumar M, et al: Ultrasound-guided fine needle aspiration cytology of malignant gallbladder masses. *Acta Cytol* 41:1654–1658, 1997

27. Eckhauser FE, Raper SE, Mulholland MW, et al: Carcinoma of the gallbladder, in Neiderhuber JE (ed): *Current Therapy in Oncology.* St. Louis, Mosby-Year Book, 1993, pp 402–409

28. Yamamoto M, Nakajo S, Tahara E: Carcinoma of the gallbladder: the correlation between histogenesis and prognosis. *Virchows Arch A Pathol Anat Histopathol* 414:83–90, 1989

29. Henson DE, Albores-Saveedra J, Corle D: Carcinoma of the gallbladder: histologic types, stage of disease, grade, and survival rates. *Cancer* 70:1493–1497, 1992

30. Yamaguchi K, Tsuneyoshi M: Subclinical gallbladder carcinoma. *Am J Surg* 163:382–386, 1992

31. Fleming ID, Cooper JS, Henson DE, et al: AJCC Cancer Staging Manual (ed 5). Philadelphia, Lippincott-Raven, 1997, pp 104, 110

32. Pitt HA: The changing role of preoperative biliary decompression. *Perspect Gen Surg* 1:113–126, 1990

33. Shirai Y, Yoshida K, Tsukada K, et al: Inapparent carcinoma of the gallbladder: an appraisal of a radical second operation after simple cholecystectomy. *Ann Surg* 215:326–331, 1992

34. Fong Y, Heffernan N, Blumgart LH: Gallbladder carcinoma discovered during laparoscopic cholecystectomy: aggressive reresection is beneficial. *Cancer* 83:423–427, 1998

35. Donohue JM, Nagorney DM, Grant CS, et al: Carcinoma of the gallbladder. Does radical resection improve outcome? *Arch Surg* 125:237–241, 1990

36. Cubertafond P, Gainant A, Cucchiaro G: Surgical treatment of 724 carcinomas of the gallbladder: results of the French Surgical Association survey. *Ann Surg* 219:275–280, 1994

37. Lundberg O, Kristoffersson A: Port site metastases from gallbladder cancer after laparoscopic cholecystectomy. Results of a Swedish survey and review of published reports. *Eur J Surg* 165:215–222, 1999

38. Ogura Y, Mizumoto R, Isaji S, et al: Radical operations for carcinoma of the gallbladder: present status in Japan. *World J Surg* 6:337–342, 1991

39. Gagner M, Rossi RL: Radical operations for carcinoma of the gallbladder: present status in North America. *World J Surg* 15:344–347, 1991

40. Tsukada K, Hatakeyama K, Kurosaki I, et al: Outcome of radical surgery for carcinoma of the gallbladder according to the TNM stage. *Surgery* 120:816–821, 1996

41. Shirai Y, Ohtani T, Tsukada K, et al: Combined pancreaticoduodenectomy and hepatectomy for patients with locally advanced gallbladder carcinoma: long term results. *Cancer* 80:1904–1909, 1997

42. Paquet KJ: Appraisal of surgical resection of gallbladder carcinoma with special reference to hepatic resection. *J Hepatobiliary Pancreat Surg* 5:200–206, 1998

43. Pradeep R, Kaushik SP, Sikora SS, et al: Predictors of survival in patients with carcinoma of the gallbladder. *Cancer* 76:1145–1149, 1995

44. Bartlett DL, Fong Y, Fortner JG, et al: Long-term results after resection for gallbladder cancer. Implications for staging and management. *Ann Surg* 224:636–646, 1996

45. Vij JC, Govil A, Chaudhary A, et al: Endoscopic biliary endoprosthesis for palliation of gallbladder carcinoma. *Gastrointest Endosc* 43:121–123, 1996

46. Lillemoe KD, Pitt HA, Kaufman HS, et al: Acute cholecystitis occurring as a complication of percutaneous transhepatic drainage. *Surg Gynecol Obstet* 168:348–352, 1989

47. Luman W, Cull A, Palmer KR: Quality of life in patients stented for malignant biliary obstructions. *Eur J Gastroenterol Hepatol* 9:481–484, 1997

48. Lee BH, Choe DH, Lee JH, et al: Metallic stents in malignant biliary obstruction: prospective long-term clinical results. *AJR Am J Roentgenol* 168:741–745, 1997

49. Todoroki T, Iwasaki Y, Orii K, et al: Resection combined with intraoperative radiation therapy (IORT) for stage IV gallbladder carcinoma. *World J Surg* 15:357–366, 1991

50. Todoroki T: Radiation therapy for primary gallbladder cancer. *Hepatogastroenterology* 44:1229–1239, 1997

51. Collier NA, Blumgart LH: Tumours of the gallbladder, in Blumgart LH (ed): *Surgery of the Liver and Biliary Tract.* New York, Churchill Livingstone, 1994, pp 955–966

52. Wanebo HJ, Vezeridis MP: Treatment of gallbladder cancer. *Cancer Treat Res* 69:97–109, 1994

53. Nakeeb A, Pitt HA, Sohn TA, et al. Cholangiocarcinomas: A spectrum of intrahepatic, perihilar, and distal tumors. *Annals of Surgery* 224:463–475, 1996

54. Yeo CJ: Bile duct cancer, in Cameron JL (ed): *Current Surgical Therapy* (ed 5). Mosby-Year Book, 1995, pp 380–386

55. Chao TC, Greager JA: Carcinoma of the extrahepatic bile ducts. *J Surg Oncol* 46:145–150, 1991

56. Hsing AW, Gao YT, Devesa SS, et al: Rising incidence of biliary tract cancers in Shanghai, China. *Int J Cancer* 75:368–370, 1998

57. Tominaga S, Kuroishi T: Biliary tract cancer. *Cancer Surv* 19–20:125–137, 1994

58. Fraumeni JF, Devesa SS, McLaughlin JK, et al: Biliary tract cancer, in Schottenfeld D, Fraumeni JD (eds): *Cancer Epidemiology and Prevention.* New York, Oxford University Press, 1996, pp 683–691

59. Lipsett PA, Pitt HA, Colombani PM, et al: Choledochal cyst disease. A changing pattern of presentation. *Ann Surg* 220:644–652, 1994

60. Komi N, Takehara H, Kunitomo K: Choledochal cyst: anomalous arrangement of the pancreaticobiliary ductal system and biliary malignancy. *J Gastroenterol Hepatol* 4:63–74, 1989

61. Iwai N, Yanagihara J, Tokiwa K, et al: Congenital choledochal dilatation with emphasis on pathophysiology of the biliary tract. *Ann Surg* 215:27–30, 1992

62. Dagli U, Atalay F, Sasmaz N, et al: Caroli's disease; 1977–1995 experiences. *Eur J Gastroenterol Hepatol* 10:109–112, 1998

63. Watanapa P: Cholangiocarcinoma in patients with opisthorchiasis. *Br J Surg* 83:1062–1064, 1996

64. Shirai T, Pairojkul C, Ogawa K, et al: Histomorphological characteristics of cholangiocellular carcinomas in northeast Thailand, where a region infection with the liver fluke,

Opisthorchis viverrini is endemic. *Acta Pathol Jpn* 42:734–739, 1992

65. Haswell-Elkins MR, Satarug S, Elkins DB: *Opisthorchis viverrini* infection in northeast Thailand and its relationship to cholangiocarcinoma. *J Gastroenterol Hepatol* 7:528–548, 1992

66. Parkin DM, Ohshima H, Srivatanakul P, et al: Cholangiocarcinoma: epidemiology, mechanisms of carcinogenesis and prevention. *Cancer Epidemiol Biomarkers Prev* 2:537–544, 1993

67. Khan ZR, Neugut AI, Ahsan H, et al: Risk factors for biliary tract cancers. *Am J Gastroenterol* 94:149–152, 1999

68. Chen MF, Jan YY, Wang CS, et al: A reappraisal of cholangiocarcinoma in patients with hepatolithiasis. *Cancer* 71:2461–2465, 1993

69. Su CH, Shyr YM, Lui WY, et al: Hepatolithiasis associated with cholangiocarcinoma. *Br J Surg* 84:969–973, 1997

70. Chijiiwa K, Ichimiya H, Kuroki S, et al: Late development of cholangiocarcinoma after the treatment of hepatolithiasis. *Surg Gynecol Obstet* 177:279–282, 1993

71. Farrant JM, Hayllar KM, Wilkinson ML, et al: Natural history and prognostic variables in primary sclerosing cholangitis. *Gastroenterology* 100:1710–1717, 1991

72. Thuluvath PJ, Rai R, Venbrux AC, et al: Cholangiocarcinoma: a review. *Gastroenterologist* 5:306–315, 1997

73. Rosen CB, Nagorney DM: Cholangiocarcinoma complicating primary sclerosing cholangitis. *Semin Liver Dis* 11:26-30, 1991

74. Molmenti EP, Marsh JW, Dvorchik I, et al: Hepatobiliary malignancies: primary hepatic malignant neoplasms. *Surg Clin North Am* 79:43–57, 1999

75. Mir-Madjlessi SH, Farmer RG, Sivak MV: Bile duct carcinoma in patients with ulcerative colitis. Relationship to sclerosing cholangitis: report of six cases and review of the literature. *Dig Dis Sci* 32:145–154, 1987

76. Ito Y, Kojiro M, Nakashima T, et al: Pathomorphologic characteristics of 102 cases of thorotrast-related hepatocellular carcinoma, cholangiocarcinoma and hepatic angiosarcoma. *Cancer* 62:1153–1158, 1988

77. Nakeeb A, Matanowski GM, Coleman J, et al: Cholangiocarcinoma: an environmentally induced cancer. *Hepatology* 20:283A, 1994 (abstr)

78. Wolber RA, Greene CA, Dupuis BA: Polyclonal carcinoembryonic antigen staining in the cytologic differential diagnosis of primary and metastatic hepatic malignancies. *Acta Cytol* 35:215–220, 1991

79. Haglund C, Lindgren J, Roberts PJ, et al: Difference in tissue expression of tumour markers CA 19-9 and CA 50 in hepatocellular carcinoma and cholangiocarcinoma. *Br J Cancer* 63:386–389, 1991

80. Celli A, Que FG: Dysregulation of apoptosis in the cholangiopathies and cholangiocarcinoma. *Semin Liver Dis* 18:177–185, 1998

81. Sugiyama M, Atomi Y, Kuroda A, et al: Bile duct carcinoma without jaundice: clues to early diagnosis. *Hepatogastroenterology* 44:1477–1483, 1997

82. Rosen CB, Nagorney DM, Wiesner RH, et al: Cholangiocarcinoma complicating primary sclerosing cholangitis. *Ann Surg* 213:21–25, 1991

83. Van Laethem JL, Deviere J, Bourgeois N, et al: Cholangiographic findings in deteriorating primary sclerosing cholangitis. *Endoscopy* 27:223–228, 1995

84. Ramage JK, Donaghy A, Farrant JM, et al: Serum tumor markers for the diagnosis of cholangiocarcinoma in primary sclerosing cholangitis. *Gastroenterology* 108:865–869, 1995

85. Nichols JC, Gores GJ, Larusso NF, et al: Diagnostic role of serum CA 19-9 for cholangiocarcinoma in patients with primary sclerosing cholangitis. *Mayo Clin Proc* 68:874–879, 1993

86. Nakeeb A, Lipsett PA, Lillemoe KD, et al: Biliary carcinoembryonic antigen levels are a marker for cholangiocarcinoma. *Am J Surg* 171:147–153, 1996

87. Goydos JS, Brumfield AM, Frezza E, et al: Marked elevation of serum interleukin-6 in patients with cholangiocarcinoma: validation of utility as a clinical marker. *Ann Surg* 227:398–404, 1998

88. Soyer P, Bluemke DA, Reichle R, et al: Imaging of intrahepatic cholangiocarcinoma: I. Peripheral cholangiocarcinoma. *AJR Am J Roentgenol* 165:1427–1431, 1995

89. Soyer P, Bluemke DA, Reichle R, et al: Imaging of intrahepatic cholangiocarcinoma: II. Hilar cholangiocarcinoma. *AJR Am J Roentgenol* 165:1433–1436, 1995

90. Mittelstaedt CA: Ultrasound of the bile ducts. *Semin Roentgenol* 32:161–171, 1997

91. Baron RL: Computed tomography of the bile ducts. *Semin Roentgenol* 32:172–187, 1997

92. Soto JA, Barish MA, Ferrucci JT: Magnetic resonance imaging of the bile ducts. *Semin Roentgenol* 32:188–201, 1997

93. Worawattanakul S, Semelka RC, Noone TC: Cholangiocarcinoma: spectrum of appearances on MR images using current techniques. *Magn Reson Imaging* 16:993–1003, 1998

94. Mendler MH, Bouillet P, Sautereau D, et al: Value of MR cholangiography in the diagnosis of obstructive diseases of the biliary tree: a study of 58 cases. *Am J Gastroenterol* 93:2482–2490, 1998

95. Kuszyk BS, Soyer P, Bluemke DA, et al: Intrahepatic cholangiocarcinoma: the role of imaging in detection and staging. *Crit Rev Diagn Imaging* 38:59–88, 1997

96. Mansfield JC, Griffin SM, Wadehra V, et al: A prospective evaluation of cytology from biliary strictures. *Gut* 40:671–677, 1997

97. Pichlmayr R, Weimann A, Klempnauer J, et al: Surgical treatment in proximal bile duct cancer. A single-center experience. *Ann Surg* 224:628–638, 1996

98. Pitt HA, Nakeeb A, Abrams RA, et al: Perihilar cholangiocarcinoma. Postoperative radiotherapy does not improve survival. *Ann Surg* 221:788–798, 1995

99. Goss JA, Shackleton CR, Farmer DG, et al: Orthotopic liver transplantation for primary sclerosing cholangitis. A 12-year single center experience. *Ann Surg* 225:472–481, 1997

100. Ahrendt SA, Cameron JL, Pitt HA: Current management of patients with perihilar cholangiocarcinoma. *Adv Surg* 30:427–452, 1996

101. Jeyarajah DR, Klintmalm GB: Is liver transplantation indicated for cholangiocarcinoma? *J Hepatobiliary Pancreat Surg* 5:48–51, 1998

102. Washburn WK, Lewis WD, Jenkins RL: Aggressive surgical resection for cholangiocarcinoma. *Arch Surg* 130:270–276, 1995

103. Strasberg SM: Resection of hilar cholangiocarcinoma. *HPB Surg* 10:415–418, 1998

104. Rossi RL, Gordon M, Brasch JW. Intubation techniques in biliary tract surgery. *Surg Clin North Am* 60:297–312, 1980

105. Jarnagin WR, Burke E, Powers C, et al: Intrahepatic biliary enteric bypass provides effective palliation in selected patients with malignant obstruction at the hepatic duct confluence. *Am J Surg* 175:453–460, 1998

106. Minsky BD, Wesson MF, Armstrong JG, et al: Combined modality therapy of extrahepatic biliary system cancer. *Int J Radiat Oncol Biol Phys* 18:1157–1163, 1990

107. Foo ML, Gunderson LL, Bender CE, et al: External radiation therapy and transcatheter iridium in the treatment of extrahepatic bile duct carcinoma. *Int J Radiat Oncol Biol Phys* 39:929–935, 1997

108. Vallis KA, Benjamin IS, Munro AJ, et al: External beam and intraluminal radiotherapy for locally advanced bile duct cancer: role and tolerability. *Radiother Oncol* 41:61–66, 1996

109. Erickson BA, Nag S: Biliary tree malignancies. *J Surg Oncol* 67:203–210, 1998

110. Lee CK, Barrios BR, Bjarnason H: Biliary tree malignancies: the University of Minnesota experience. *J Surg Oncol* 65:298–305, 1997

111. McMasters KM, Tuttle TM, Leach SD, et al: Neoadjuvant chemoradiation for extrahepatic cholangiocarcinoma. *Am J Surg* 174:605–608, 1997

112. Hishinuma S, Ogata Y, Matsui J, et al: Preoperative radiotherapy for cancer of the extrahepatic bile duct. *Am J Clin Oncol* 21:203–208, 1998

113. Ortner MA, Liebetruth J, Schreiber S, et al: Photodynamic therapy of nonresectable cholangiocarcinoma. *Gastroenterology* 114:536–542, 1998

114. Vogl TJ, Balzer JO, Dette K, et al: Initially unresectable hilar cholangiocarcinoma: hepatic regeneration after transarterial embolization. *Radiology* 208:217–222, 1998

115. Shimamura T, Nakajima Y, Une Y, et al: Efficacy and safety of preoperative percutaneous transhepatic portal embolization with absolute ethanol: a clinical study. *Surgery* 121:135–141, 1997

CHAPTER 56

Head and Neck Malignancies

Lenore L. Harris, RN, MSN, AOCN

Symptom Management and Supportive Care

Airway Management

Tracheostomy tube products

Tracheostomy and laryngectomy care

Nutritional Management

Enteral therapy

Swallowing Rehabilitation

Pain Management

Speech Restoration

Psychosocial Support

Continuity of Care: Nursing Challenges

Quality-of-Life Issues

Conclusion

References

Introduction

Head and neck cancer accounts for a proportionately small percentage of all new cancer cases in the United States (males: 5%; females: 2%).[1] Due to the location of the tumor, the individual after treatment usually will have mild to severe impairment of aerodigestive function with associated changes in self-image. The changes in function for the individual often correspond in severity to the level of tumor invasion. The tumor may affect the respiratory and/or digestive pathways, with immediate and often long-lasting deficits following definitive treatment for the malignancy. There are other common changes in sensory function associated with this primary tumor site that affect the individual's sensory adaptation. The person may need to learn how to compensate for changes in taste, smell, hearing, balance, or vision. When the individual needs to cope with changes in appearance, it becomes important to assist in a healthy adaptation to alterations in how one is viewed by others and in what manner adjustments can be made to facilitate interactions in social settings.

The coordinated approach of the multidisciplinary team will be of paramount importance throughout the treatment and rehabilitation of the individual with head and neck cancer. Members of the team usually include the head and neck surgeon, radiation oncologist, medical oncologist, oral surgeon, pathologist, radiologist, dietitian, speech pathologist, plastic surgeon, advanced practice head and neck nurse, social worker, physical therapist, prosthetist, and home health nurse. A referral to pastoral care or psycho-oncology may be appropriate to promote adaptation. For the duration of the patient's follow-up, the work of the multidisciplinary team will be to assess for and manage complications, promote return of function, and strive to enhance quality of life. The goal for all is the healthful adaptation of the individual and his or her support system.

Epidemiology

Habitual use of any type of tobacco and excessive alcohol use have been found to promote the development of head and neck malignancies. Chronic irritation by these agents can affect any portion of the respiratory or digestive systems. According to the American Cancer Society (ACS),[2] incidence rates for men are twice as high as for women. Since the early 1980s, mortality rates for oral cavity and pharyngeal carcinomas have declined each year. In the same report, the ACS found that for patients with oral cavity or pharyngeal malignancies, one-year survival was 83%. The five-year survival for this group of patients was 53%, or the same as reported in 1997.[3] In 1999, the ten-year survival rate was 46%.

Studies have addressed incidence rates for head and neck cancer by race and ethnic group and are providing rationale for chemoprevention and survival studies. In an incidence study that included epidemiological conditions for the eleven largest cultural groups in the United States, black males were reported to have the highest overall incidence of oral cavity cancer (20.4 per 100,000 population). The same study reported that the fifth most frequent cause of cancer death in the Alaska Native population among males was nasopharyngeal cancer.[4] Studies that link head and neck malignancies more specifically to cultural conditions are needed in order to guide community outreach preventive endeavors.

Etiology

Tobacco abuse has been implicated for all head and neck tumor sites.[5] Every type of tobacco has been connected to dysplastic injuries and carcinogenic changes in all head and neck primary malignancy sites. These changes are associated with an increased incidence of patients developing second locoregional neoplasms and distant metastases resulting in the continuation of relatively low survival rates. Cigarettes, pipes, cigars, smokeless tobacco, and habitual use of marijuana are all considered to be physical carcinogens. The role of alcohol consumption has been often studied and is defined as having a synergistic effect with habitual tobacco use. It is important to note, however, that in a significant number of cases there is no sure evidence linking alcohol alone to an increased risk for the development of head and neck cancer. Risk factors for head and neck cancer will be discussed according to primary tumor site.

Carcinoma of the Nasal Cavity and Paranasal Sinuses

Exposure to tobacco, alcohol, chemicals such as nickel, and exposure to chemical inhalants such as those found in furniture making, shoe leather working, and textile work have been associated with an increased incidence of cancers of the nasal cavity and paranasal sinuses. In addition, chronic sinusitis has been linked with carcinoma of the maxillary sinus.[6]

Carcinoma of the Nasopharynx, Oropharynx

Nasopharyngeal carcinoma is a tumor category within the head and neck region that is unique epidemiologically in relationship to risk factors, cultural considerations, and course of disease. There are several key risk factors for malignancies of this site: (1) infection by the Epstein-Barr virus (EBV), which is applicable for all ethnic cultures; (2) routine inhalation of the nitrosamines in salt-cured, steamy foods such as meats, fish, eggs, and leafy vegetables, especially for Chinese and Asian cultural groups;[7] and (3) inhalation of toxic chemicals, for example, through woodworking. Genetic protein markers (antigens) on the surface of cells, which may be important in identifying risks for developing nasopharyngeal cancer are currently under study.

Carcinoma of the Major or Minor Salivary Glands

The statistical interpretation for risk factors for these sites has not yet been defined, but an inherited association has been inferred for malignancies of the parotid gland. Similar to nasopharyngeal malignancies, inhalation of toxic materials such as wood dust is associated with increased risk for salivary gland tumors.[8]

Carcinoma of the Oral Cavity

The synergistic effects of habitual use of both alcohol and tobacco have long been implicated in the etiology of oral cavity malignancies. Deficiencies in vitamin A and regular use of marijuana[9] have recently been connected to the development of oral cavity primary tumors. Insufficient oral hygiene has been linked to primary cancers of the oral cavity, as has the other extreme in oral care, frequent overuse of harsh mouthwash solutions. Both too much and too little oral hygiene will result in ongoing irritation to the mucosal sites involved. The dysplasia subsequent to oral mucosal irritation often precedes malignant changes.

A recent study of risk factors for oral epithelial dysplasia examined the effect of tobacco in nondrinkers who smoked and the role of alcohol in drinkers who were nonsmokers. The investigators found that oral dysplasia increased when greater than 20 cigarettes per day were smoked, regardless of alcohol use. The individuals in the nonsmoking group who did use alcohol showed no higher risk for the development of oral dysplasia than those who did not use either tobacco or alcohol. In this study, the role of alcohol strongly correlated only in relationship to the individual's use of tobacco.[10]

Carcinoma of the Lip

Tobacco use, especially with cigarettes, cigars, and pipes, directly exposes the lip to chronic irritation. Overexposure of the skin of the lip to the sun is another major risk factor for cancer of the lip. Squamous cell carcinoma (SCC) and basal cell carcinoma are the major nonmelanomatous skin cancers of the head and neck area. The lip is the most common site for oral cavity cancer. Lip malignancies occur most frequently on the lower lip. There is an increased incidence of SCC of the lip in persons who live in or work in rural areas and have daily ultraviolet exposure to the sun, including those employed in fishing or farming. The carcinogenic effect on the skin is compounded if the individual is fair-skinned. Women are reported to have a lower incidence of lip cancer than men. This has been explained by noting that women are more likely to regularly protect the lips from exposure to the sun with the use of sunscreen or lipstick.[11]

Carcinoma of the Larynx

The majority of individuals who develop laryngeal cancer have a long history of habitual tobacco use and alcohol abuse. Other etiologic factors may include constant irritation the vocal cords due to chronic laryngitis or an overprojection of the voice, which is termed *voice abuse*.

Carcinoma of the Hypopharynx

Plummer-Vinson syndrome, which is a type of chronic iron-deficiency anemia, is a risk factor for postcricoid tumors in nonsmoking women. It is felt that another metabolic deficiency, malabsorption of vitamin B12, may be a risk factor for this anatomic site. There may be a genetic effect for the development of hypopharyngeal cancer and the occurrence of multiple primary tumors, which is more common in this region.[12]

Prevention, Screening, and Early Detection Programs

Primary Prevention

Since habitual tobacco use in any form is strongly linked to the development of head and neck primary carcinomas of all primary tumor sites, educating the young in their formative years to never start using tobacco products is a key preventive action. Guest speakers at elementary school programs and extracurricular activities may be able to encourage resistance to the peer pressure to start smoking. It is important to employ nonthreatening, creative teaching techniques that highlight for children the risks of smoking. Since an individual can become dependent upon tobacco in a matter of months after a first cigarette, prevention from ever starting smoking is of major importance.

When early intervention methods are not successful and the individual has become a smoker, it should be the responsibility of the nurse, as well as the other members of the multidisciplinary team, to ask each patient about tobacco use at every office visit. In addition, it is important to take the time to document the tobacco use in the patient's record, also at every visit. The nurse is then able to sensitively convey to the patient, on an ongoing basis, the pathophysiological effects of tobacco products on, for example, posttreatment healing. Nursing care that is supportive and approachable encourages the patient who is ready to stop smoking to consult with the nurse, which then leads to an explanation of the variety of approaches available to assist with smoking cessation. Pharmacological assistance for smoking cessation is a focus for chemoprevention. The prescribed use of oral medications, such as bupropion HCl, with or without the nicotine patch, is under study with individualization of the interventions promoting success with tobacco cessation.

In light of the damaging synergistic effects to the respiratory and digestive tracts following habitual alcohol plus tobacco use, the individual's drinking history should be reviewed with the person in the same matter as is the use of tobacco products. Although tobacco is the main carcinogenic agent for persons with head and neck malignancies, alcohol use lowers inhibitions so that the individual uses more tobacco products. It is commonly accepted that the combined usage of tobacco and alcohol is synergistic for tissue damage and is strongly implicated in the development of laryngeal cancer.

Dietary patterns are under study and may have a role in head and neck cancer prevention. A variety of retinoids, such as beta-carotene, vitamin C, and vitamin E have been extensively studied with patients who have leukoplakia or erythroplakia of the oral cavity. Either of these types of premalignant lesions are problematic to treat locally, especially when the areas involved are widespread and diffuse and therefore unable to sustain a curative, localized therapy without causing loss in function. Since supplemental retinoids such as 13-cis retinoic acid (13 cRA) and beta-carotene have been shown in randomized trials to promote regression of oral premalignant lesions, maintenance retinoid therapy may be prescribed. Maintenance retinoid treatment over many months with daily oral doses results in 50% of the individuals less progression of mucosal changes to malignancy than for those individuals who did not receive maintenance therapy.[13] Research has revealed that a diet rich in fruits and vegetables, without processed red meats or eggs, is associated with a decreased risk for cancers of the oral cavity.[14]

Secondary Prevention and Screening Activities

For most adults, especially after age 40, the annual physical examination by the primary caregiver may be the most appropriate screening activity for premalignant changes and early diagnosis of a head and neck malignancy. Rarely does the individual recognize early symptoms of premalignant and malignant changes in the tissues of the nasal and paranasal sinuses, oral cavity, or pharynx. For early detection, the practitioner should carefully inspect the head and neck region, including (1) using the mirror to visualize the oral cavity, larynx, and pharynx, and (2) palpating the lymph node regions. The cardinal signs of laryngeal carcinogenic changes may be subtle, and for most persons do not prompt scheduling a physician visit. These symptoms could include hoarseness, difficulty swallowing, a sore throat that does not resolve, weight loss, and occasionally hemoptysis. For the smoker, such symptoms may be an everyday occurrence and therefore not alarming.

When an individual receives routine dental assessments every six months, the dentist or dental hygienist may be the first to note abnormalities in the oral cavity such as leukoplasia, erythroplasia, dysplagia, swelling, and pain upon palpation. A noninvasive screening method, which can be used for epithelial tissue, involves staining with toluidine blue those areas that are obviously abnormal. This method has been found to be relatively reliable as an early detection measure.[15]

On a broader scale, in 1994, the nonprofit National Oral Cancer Awareness Program (NOCAP) was established to raise both public and health care professional awareness of all components of oral cancer. The goals of this organization are to develop and provide resources that assist in increasing public awareness and screening for risk factors leading to earlier interventions, resulting in prevention or reduction of the incidence of oral cancer, and the subsequent mortality rate.[16] "Through with Chew" is a public education program of the American Academy of Otorhinolaryngology—Head and Neck Surgery that graphically teaches how regularly chewing tobacco can cause aggressive malignant changes that often result in the need for an extensive resection of the oral cavity. Health fairs, which are routinely held in many communities, provide another avenue for early detection of head and neck cancer.

Pathophysiology

Cellular Characteristics

Cancers of the head and neck originate in the epithelial tissue, and most are classified as squamous cell carcinomas (SCCs). The other main tumor type for this region is adenocarcinoma, which is known to originate from the major or minor salivary glands. SCCs are further assigned to macroscopic (observable pathological changes) or microscopic (changes visible with magnification) categories. Macroscopic tumors are diagnosed pathologically as either infiltrative (originating within the epithelium), exophytic (originating on the surface of the epithelium), or verrucous (wart-like) carcinomas. Head and neck tumors are graded sequentially and pathologically as either well differentiated, moderately well differentiated, or poorly differentiated. Prognosis for cure correlates directly with degree of loss of differentiation. Microscopic variants of SCCs are further classified as keratinizing (which includes well-differentiated and moderately well-differentiated changes) or nonkeratinizing (anaplastic), which incorporates the less common lymphoepithelioma, transitional cell, and spindle cell SCCs of the head and neck.[17]

Adenocarcinomas of the major and minor salivary glands include poorly differentiated, high- or low-grade mucoepidermoid, adenoid cystic, acenic cell, and malignant mixed (includes more than one of the adenocarcinoma tumor types). Although thyroid cancer may be considered to be a head and neck malignancy, it is discussed with endocrine conditions (see Chapter 52).

Prognostic Indicators

A number of molecular studies have attempted to link the overexpression or mutation of the most commonly altered protein, the *p53* cell-cycle regulation gene, with the development of SCC at specific head and neck sites.[18–21] Mutations of the *p53* gene site, which is located on chromosome 17, may actually be identified as a tumor suppressive gene that can protect cells from external damage.[22]

Progression of Disease

Head and neck tumors tend to recur locally.[23] Although the basement membrane, which underlies the squamous epithelium, provides an important natural barrier to local tumor cell invasion, primary head and neck lesions are locally invasive, and specific neoplastic receptors can advance tumor growth into the basement membrane. The incidence of spread to regional lymph nodes at diagnosis is high. Based upon location, there may be either early or late spread to one or more of the adjacent superficial or deep cervical lymph node chains (Figure 56-1). Lymph node involvement is predictable and based upon anatomic location of the tumor.[24] When there is involvement of distant lymph nodes, such as mediastinal nodes, the cancer is classified as metastatic.

A retrospective study by Leon and associates[23] found that, on average, 16% of all head and neck patients will develop a second head and neck neoplasm within nine years. In this study, the incidence of second primaries was 4% per year throughout the follow-up period. Locations of the second neoplasms were head and neck (40%), lungs (31%), esophagus (9%), and outside the aerodigestive tract (20%).

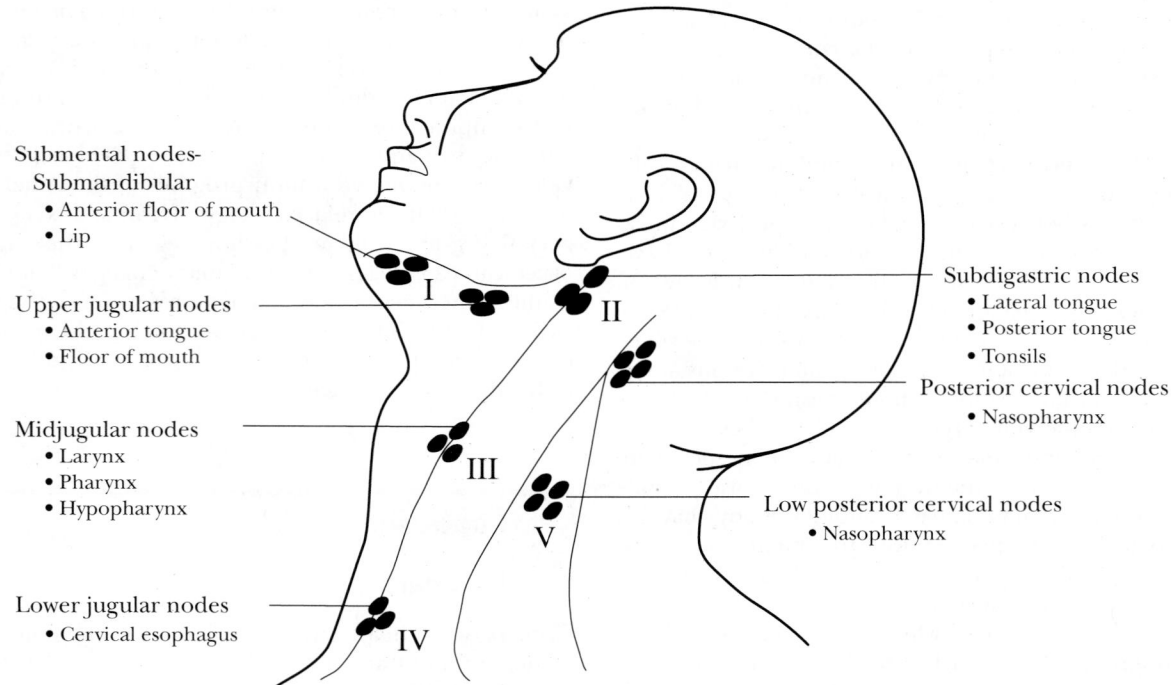

Submental nodes-
Submandibular
- Anterior floor of mouth
- Lip

Upper jugular nodes
- Anterior tongue
- Floor of mouth

Midjugular nodes
- Larynx
- Pharynx
- Hypopharynx

Lower jugular nodes
- Cervical esophagus

Subdigastric nodes
- Lateral tongue
- Posterior tongue
- Tonsils

Posterior cervical nodes
- Nasopharynx

Low posterior cervical nodes
- Nasopharynx

Figure 56-1 Lymphadenopathy of the head and neck area provides important clues to the location of the primary site.

Clinical Manifestations

The symptoms of the various head and neck cancers correspond to changes in function caused by tissue injury to the specific anatomic site. The usual symptoms for the major head and neck tumor sites are presented in Table 56-1. Common symptoms for all sites include weight loss and a persistent lump or mass. For most individuals with head and neck carcinomas, the symptoms are unilateral. Presence of a neck mass in association with any of the primary tumor sites indicates regional spread of the carcinoma.

Skull Base Malignancies

Although epidermoid, mucoepidermoid, and adenoid cystic adenocarcinoma skull base tumors are not common, presenting symptoms are important to mention since such tumors are often diagnosed in the head and neck setting. Symptoms of skull base tumors include otalgia, facial pain, epistaxis, headaches, changes in vision or hearing, and recurrent sinus infections. Abnormalities commonly correlate with cranial nerve (CN) involvement.

Table 56-1   Symptoms of Head and Neck Malignancies

Tumor Site	Symptoms
Oral cavity (including lip, floor of mouth, tongue, hard palate)	Loosening teeth/ill-fitting dentures, gingival swelling; hyperplasia; dysplasia; pain; nonhealing ulcerative or exophytic lesion; bleeding
Nose and paranasal sinuses	Unilateral obstruction of naris; nonhealing ulcer; intermittent epistaxis
Nasopharynx	Nasal obstruction; pain; otologic changes; may present without mucosal changes
Oropharynx (base of tongue, tonsil, soft palate)	Asymmetry; dull ache; pain; dysphagia; superficial, diffuse erythroplakia; referred otalgia; trismus
Trachea	Not a primary tumor site, but distant spread from larynx, lung, or esophagus
Larynx and hypopharynx Related to laryngeal area	Voice changes (early only when lesion is on vocal cord); leukoplakia or erythroplakia; stridor or dyspnea; skip lesions
Supraglottic	Dysphagia, odynophagia, aspiration, referred otalgia, tickling sensation in throat
Glottic	In addition to throat irritation and dysphagia, hoarseness is prevalent; dyspnea, and stridor with large tumors
Subglottic	Dyspnea, stridor, and hemoptysis are common
Salivary gland	Unilateral symptoms; impaired jaw mobility; neurological changes (numb lower lip)

Nasal Cavity, Paranasal Sinuses, and Nasopharyngeal Malignancies

In the United States, nasal cavity SCC occurs rarely, and the majority of nasal tumors are of a low grade. The most common paranasal sinus malignancies are those of the maxillary sinus. Symptoms of a malignancy of the nasal cavity or paranasal sinus may include nasal obstruction, epistaxis, localized pain, facial swelling, trismus, loosened teeth, localized mass, and facial nerve (CN VII) dysfunction. Malignant changes of the nasopharynx may present with symptoms similar to those of the nasal cavity such as epistaxis, nasal obstruction, and impaired CN VII function. Additional signs that herald malignant changes include enlarged but pain-free lymph nodes of the neck, tinnitus, recurrent otitis media, headache, and other symptoms associated with cranial nerve compression. See Table 56-2. Sinus cancers are associated with a poor prognosis due to early perineural and skull base invasion.

Oral Cavity and Oropharynx Malignancies

The structures of the oral cavity that may be affected by malignant changes include the lip, upper and lower buccal mucoses, upper and lower alveolar ridges, retromolar trigone (RMT), hard palate, anterior two-thirds of the tongue, and the floor of the mouth (FOM). The boundaries of the oral cavity are the upper and lower alveolar processes. The oral cavity extends from the anterior vermilion border of the lips superiorly to the posterior border of the hard palate and superior maxillary bone. Inferiorly, the oral cavity extends to the circumvallate papillae of the base of the tongue (BOT) and the FOM muscle. Lateral boundaries are the palatine arches or cheeks and include the muscle of the cheek.

Abnormalities of any of these structures may include a nonhealing ulcer versus a painless, firm mass, and may involve either leukoplakia or erythroplakia. The individual's first symptom may be that dentures no longer fit comfortably. Malignancies of the oropharynx are difficult to diagnose, as the same symptoms can readily be ascribed to nonmalignant conditions. Generalized symptoms may include mild but persistent dull ache and sore throat, referred otalgia, dysphagia with ongoing weight loss, and worsening airway obstruction. Because of the frequent delay of individuals in seeking diagnostic evaluations, it is common for the patient to have a large neck mass, perhaps with bilateral lymph node involvement, at the initial visit to the clinic.

Laryngeal Malignancies

Symptoms of laryngeal carcinomas are frequently defined in relationship to the region of the larynx where the tumor originated. The larynx is divided into three areas: supraglottic, glottic, and subglottic (see Table 56-1 for symptoms of malignant changes according to laryngeal region). Due to the persistent irritation the person has experienced over many years of habitual tobacco use or occupational exposure to irritants such as petroleum products or wood dust, presenting symptoms will usually be masked early on. The presence of a neck mass indicates regional lymph node spread. Presenting symptoms will be determined by the anatomic structures involved.

Hypopharyngeal Malignancies

Because of the anatomic location of the hypopharynx, tumors in this area are often detected late, after they have invaded muscle and adjacent structures. As with laryngeal carcinomas, early symptoms are often masked by years of chronic irritation to the area associated with tobacco and alcohol use. Pyriform sinus lesions may present with otalgia, which is usually described as dull ear pain. Voice changes and dysphagia tend to occur late, when there is advanced disease. Posterior pharyngeal wall lesions may present as a sore throat or with a feeling of mucous retention after swallowing.

Assessment

The nursing assessment includes obtaining a systematic, organized, and complete health history and documenting ongoing medical concerns, especially as they relate to the current head and neck problem. Because the individual may respond poorly to any evidence of criticism for tobacco or alcohol use by health care professionals, especially someone with a substance abuse history, this assessment involves sensitively obtaining the data needed. The nurse must utilize therapeutic psychosocial skills and elicit patient cooperation in order to obtain the necessary diagnostic data needed for treatment planning.

Patient and Family History

When the practitioner is obtaining the individual's history, it is important to stress the importance of recent or ongoing changes in sensation or function, and to establish what is now associated with this new occurrence of symptoms. In the elderly, certain alterations in the head and neck site are associated with aging and may be normal for those over age 65. These include decreased saliva formation, declining hearing acuity, decreasing olfactory and taste sensitivities, receding gingival tissue, changes in pharyngeal and laryngeal control resulting in weaker phonation, and an abnormal swallowing sequence with some aspiration.[26,27]

In addition to the elderly, individuals who are immunosuppressed should be provided special considerations in the evaluative process. Immunosuppressed persons such as those who have received organ, bone marrow, or stem cell transplants and are on immunosuppressants are obviously at risk for malignant changes to the head and neck. Persons with HIV or who have cancer at another site and are receiving chemotherapy are also immunosuppressed. There are few direct links of other disorders to head and neck cancer, with the exception of one condition called the *Plummer-Vinson syndrome* which is linked to tongue and postcricoid carcinomas. Plummer-Vinson is a hypochromic (iron-deficiency) anemia that develops mainly in premenopausal women. With this condition, before malignant changes occur, a thin web grows that coats the mucosal to submucosal esophagus. The patient experiences dysphagia related to the degeneration of esophageal muscle. Another rare type of cancer, nasopharyngeal, has been associated with EBV. Initially, this connection was found to occur specifically in Asian populations, but it is currently considered as a link regardless of race.[27]

As previously discussed, an individual's smoking and alcohol history contains significant risk factors. If these habits have been habitual for many years, the individual will need considerable assistance to become motivated to participate in a cessation program.

Physical Exam

Usually, squamous cell carcinomas are slow growing and well differentiated. As mentioned previously, it is common for the individual to adapt to the early changes, such as intermittent bleeding of a nonhealing ulcer, which is not painful and does not interfere with function. Because the initial symptoms may be silent, the person with a head and neck tumor may present with significant malignant changes, even though this person may have been compliant with regularly scheduled, routine, physical examinations. Since a large number of individuals with head and neck malignancies have poor nutritional status following years of habitual alcohol use, a complete nutritional assessment as well as a baseline chemistry profile and complete blood count (CBC) should be obtained. These tests provide important information for the treatment planning process, especially nutritional interventions.

In the limited amount of time practitioners have to provide comprehensive examinations, adequate attention needs to be provided for the survey of the head and neck region. Included in this examination should be a survey of the person's skin (color, contour), respiratory status, speech and swallowing, weight changes, facial symmetry, and hearing changes with or without otalgia. It is necessary to use the nasopharyngeal mirror as part of the assessment of nasal structure and mucosa. The examiner palpates the frontal and maxillary sinuses, then inspects the oral cavity, assessing for tongue symmetry (CN XII-hypoglossal). The symmetry of soft palate function is assessed (CN X-vagus), and the laryngeal mirror is used to visualize the larynx and hypopharynx. Then the neck is palpated bilaterally for lumps and lymphadenopathy along the five cervical node chains outlined in Figure 56-1.

As previously discussed, the most obvious sign of head and neck cancer is a mass or an ulcer that does not heal. Courses of antibiotics may have been prescribed for the person by the primary practitioner with minimal effect, which highlights the need to obtain a tissue diagnosis via excisional or needle biopsy at the time the initial abnormality is discovered.[28] Examination techniques are outlined in Table 56-2.

Diagnostic Studies

Various tests are necessary to provide key information prior to beginning treatment. The first test ordered after the initial physical examination will usually be the flexible fiberoptic nasopharyngoscopy with biopsies, performed by the head and neck specialist. This examination provides a thorough examination of the patient's nasal cavity, nasopharynx, oropharynx, and larynx. A topical anesthetic is given by nasal and oral spray prior to this exam, and the individual may be administered conscious sedation. It is important for the patient to remain responsive to verbal requests, as it is necessary to be able to make "a" and "e" sounds at the request of the examiner as part of the diagnostic process. Because of the topical anesthetic, the individual should have nothing by mouth until the gag reflex returns, which is usually within 30 minutes.

It may be necessary to perform a direct laryngoscopy (DL), also called a *panendoscopy*, with esophagoscopy in order to visualize the tumor. For this procedure, general anesthesia is required in order to evaluate the extent of the malignancy as well as to confirm the histological

Table 56-2   Examination Techniques by Cranial Nerve Distribution

Region	Evaluates	Assessment
Head	CN V–Trigeminal	
	Sensory: maxillary sinus, teeth	Place hands on temporal then masseter muscles to palpate muscle contractions for symmetry
	Motor: chewing action	
	CN VII–Facial	
	Motor: assess symmetry	Ask patient to lift both eyebrows, tightly close eyes, make exaggerated frown then wide smile, puff cheeks
	Sensory: taste	Taste test
Auditory	CN VIII–Acoustic	
	Sensory: hearing	Refer to audiologist to evaluate unilateral changes in hearing
	CN IX–Glossopharyngeal	
	Sensory: middle ear	
Nose and paranasal sinuses	CN I–Olfactory	
	Sensory: smell	Test smell with scratch card if possible, alcohol swab may be used
	Nasal structure	Inspect with headlight and nasal speculum
	Frontal sinuses	Palpate sinuses bilaterally for lumps, tenderness; transilluminate sinuses
	Maxillary sinuses	
	Ethmoid sinuses	
Mouth and pharynx	Parotid	Palpate for unilateral mass
	Mucosa	Inspect oral cavity for leukoplakia, erythroplakia, ulcer, mass
	CN IX–Glossopharyngeal	Test on both sides of back of tongue with tongue blade for gag reflex
	CN X–Vagus	Watch for rise of uvula/soft palate when patient says "ah"
	Mucosal changes	
Hypopharynx and larynx	CNX-Vagus	Apply local anesthetic spray to oropharynx, ask to breathe through mouth, stick out tongue, and repeat vowels "a" and "e" while examining, using laryngeal mirror and headlight or fiberoptic equipment
Neck		Palpate for masses, tenderness or pain, swelling along the cervical lymph node chains
	CNXI-Accesory	Gently hold neck and have patient turn head from side to side against resistance Direct patient to shrug shoulders against resistance

diagnosis. Since the pathologist's interpretation of histology type provides the tissue diagnosis, obtaining a biopsy of the abnormal mucosa is vital. An excisional or true-cut biopsy of a surface lesion may also be obtained. Biopsy by fine-needle aspiration (FNA) will be necessary to evaluate a salivary gland abnormality as well as to provide the tissue diagnosis for lymph node adenopathies. Following the DL, the patient will be prescribed voice rest, asked to take nothing by mouth for approximately one hour posttest, and will be provided symptom management interventions for the resulting sore throat.

Radiological studies are crucial in the evaluation of tumor size, invasion, and lymph node spread, as these conditions are not completely evaluable by physical examination alone. Plain x-ray films are important for assessing the soft tissues of the neck when there are differences in density, for studying the paranasal sinuses, and to define lateral and base of skull lesions. For malignancies of the pharynx (nasopharynx, oropharynx, and hypopharynx) as well as the sinuses, computerized tomography (CT) is superior to plain films for deciding whether the abnormality is the result of inflammation or tumor. The CT also can more clearly demonstrate cartilage invasion and extent of disease for most of the head and neck malignancies. However, the magnetic resonance imaging (MRI) technique is superior to CT for demarcating the depth of tumor invasion in soft tissues and separating malignant changes from those that represent inflammation. The MRI can take images in a variety of orientations without repositioning the patient.

Angiography is another radiological test which may be able to provide necessary information as part of pretreatment planning to define collateralization, especially when the tumor is adjacent to or invading the carotid artery.[29] Following the angiogram, frequent neurological checks and a pressure dressing will be ordered, along with activity restrictions that are critical to implement in order to prevent complications. When resection of the carotid artery is anticipated, a balloon test occlusion (BTO) with single photon emission computerized tomography (SPECT) scans, both before and after the BTO, may be necessary to assess cerebral contralateral blood flow.[30]

For T1 to T2 laryngeal tumors, videostroboscopy is used for early detection. Videolaryngoscopy will be necessary in order to assess larger lesions. If the individual has a hypopharyngeal or pyriform sinus malignancy, a barium sulfate cinefluoroscopy or upper GI is obtained in order to assess tracheao-esophageal function and also to detect the possible presence of a second primary tumor. Due to the risk of metastatic spread to the lungs of individuals with head and neck tumors, as well as the high incidence of a second malignancy in the lungs, plain chest x-rays and the more sensitive CT scan of the lungs are important pretreatment tests.[31] Head and neck cancers rarely metastasize early; a bone scan would therefore not be requested as part of the primary tumor workup unless there were symptoms suggestive of metastatic disease, such as bone pain.

Classification and Staging

Standardized classification of head and neck cancers is specific to each primary site, and provides a baseline for the evaluation of specific end points, including outcome and prognosis. As part of the staging process, the untreated individual will undergo certain diagnostic tests, depending on the site being evaluated. The American Joint Committee on Cancer (AJCC) staging criteria for cervical and regional lymph nodes is uniform for tumors of all head and neck primary sites (except for the nasopharynx) and is provided in Table 56-3.[32]

During the individual's pretreatment workup, the pathological classification of the tumor by histological grade takes place during the clinical tumor staging process. The histopathology subsets for SCCs, which are uniform for all primary sites, begin with GX (grade cannot be defined) and proceed according to differentiation, as G1 (well differentiated), G2 (moderately differentiated), or G3 (poorly differentiated). An example of the staging criteria for laryngeal cancer can be found in Table 56-4. A listing of primary head and neck tumor locations for all sites, with the exception of the thyroid, can be found in Table 56-5.

Therapeutic Approaches and Nursing Care

Primary treatment for the patient with a head and neck malignancy is intended to eliminate the tumor along with the potential for local recurrence or metastatic spread.

Table 56-3 AJCC Staging Criteria for Cervical Lymph Node Cancer

Stage	Description
NX	Regional lymph cannot be assessed
N0	No regional lymph node metastasis
N1	Metastasis in a single ipsilateral lymph node, 3 cm or less in greatest dimension
N2	Metastasis in a single ipsilateral lymph node, more than 3 cm but not more than 6 cm in greatest dimension; or in multiple ipsilateral lymph nodes, none more than 6 cm in greatest dimension; or in bilateral or contralateral lymph nodes, none more than 6 cm greatest dimension
N2a	Metastasis in a single ipsilateral lymph node more than 3 cm but not more than 6 cm in greatest dimension
N2b	Metastasis in multiple ipsilateral lymph nodes, none more than 6 cm in greatest dimension
N2c	Metastasis in bilateral or contralateral lymph nodes, none more than 6 cm in greatest dimension
N3	Metastasis in a lymph node more than 6 cm in greatest dimension

Table 56-4   AJCC Staging Criteria for Laryngeal Cancer

DEFINITIONS

Primary Tumor (T)

TX   Primary tumor cannot be assessed
T0   No evidence of primary tumor
Tis   Carcinoma in situ

Supraglottis

T1   Tumor limited to one subsite of supraglottis with normal vocal cord mobility
T2   Tumor invades mucosa of more than one subsite of supraglottis or glottis, or region outside the supraglottis without fixation of the larynx
T3   Tumor limited to larynx with vocal cord fixation and/or invades postcricoid area, medial wall of piriform sinus, or pre-epiglottic tissues
T4   Tumor extends through thyroid cartilage and/or extends into soft tissues of the neck, thyroid, and/or esophagus

Glottis

T1   Tumor limited to vocal cord(s) (may involve anterior or posterior commissures) with normal mobility
T1a   Tumor limited to one vocal cord
T1b   Tumor involves both vocal cords
T2   Tumor extends to supraglottis and/or subglottis, and/or with impaired vocal cord mobility
T3   Tumor limited to the larynx with vocal cord fixation
T4   Tumor invades through thyroid cartilage and/or extends to other tissues beyond the larynx (e.g., trachea, soft tissues of neck including thyroid, pharynx)

Subglottis

T1   Tumor limited to the subglottis
T2   Tumor extends to vocal cord(s) with normal or impaired mobility
T3   Tumor limited to the larynx with vocal cord fixation
T4   Tumor invades through cricoid or thyroid cartilage and/or extends to other tissues beyond the larynx (e.g., trachea, soft tissues of the neck including thyroid, esophagus)

Regional Lymph Nodes (N)

NX   Regional lymph nodes cannot be assessed
N0   No regional lymph node metastasis
N1   Metastasis in a single ipsilateral lymph node, 3 cm or less in greatest dimension
N2   Metastasis in a single ipsilateral lymph node, more than 3 cm but not more than 6 cm in greatest dimension, or multiple ipsilateral lymph nodes, none more than 6 cm in greatest dimension, or bilateral or contralateral lymph nodes, none more than 6 cm in greatest dimension
N2a   Metastasis in a single ipsilateral lymph node more than 3 cm but not more than 6 cm in greatest dimension
N2b   Metastasis in multiple ipsilateral lymph nodes, none more than 6 cm in greatest dimension

N2c   Metastasis in bilateral or contralateral lymph nodes, none more than 6 cm in greatest dimension
N3   Metastasis in a lymph node more than 6 cm in greatest dimension

Distant Metastasis (M)

MX   Distant metastasis cannot be assessed
M0   No distant metastasis
M1   Distant metastasis

Stage Groupings

0	Tis	N0	M0
I	T1	N0	M0
II	T2	N0	M0
III	T3	N0	M0
	T1	N1	M0
	T2	N1	M0
	T3	N1	M0
IVA	T4	N0	M0
	T4	N1	M0
	Any T	N2	M0
IVB	Any T	N3	M0
IVC	Any T	Any N	M1

Histopathologic Type

The predominant cancer is squamous cell carcinoma

Histopathologic Grade (G)

GX   Grade cannot be assessed
G1   Well differentiated
G2   Moderately differentiated
G3   Poorly differentiated

Location of Tumor

Supraglottis
    Suprahyoid epiglottis
    Infrahyoid epiglottis
    Aryepiglottic folds (laryngeal aspect)
    Arytenoids
    Ventricular bands (false cords)
Glottis
    Right true vocal cord
    Left true vocal cord
    Anterior commissure
    Posterior commissure
Subglottis
    Subglottis

Involvement of Neighboring Structures

    Oropharynx
    Hypopharynx
    Soft tissues of skin of neck

The treatment approach will include a consideration of the individual's important physiological functions, which may be impaired now due to the malignancy or are anticipated to become so as a result of ablative interventions. The goal is to preserve the highest level of function for the person, while still eradicating the cancer. In addition, an obvious concern for the person will be social acceptance, in light of the temporary or permanent changes to appearance. The patient should be informed of any expected cosmetic changes before treatment starts and

should meet with the prosthodontist, prosthetic specialist, and plastic surgeon early in the preoperative assessment phase. It comforts the patient to learn how carefully the team is working together for the best possible outcome.

Treatment approaches in head and neck oncology include surgery alone, radiation therapy alone, chemotherapy alone, or a combination of modalities. The application of combination therapy is discussed in the following section on surgery, according to the anatomical location of the tumor. Since chemotherapy, radiation

Table 56-5 Head and Neck Tumor Locations

Regions	Staging Site	Location of Primary Tumor
Lip and oral cavity	Nasopharynx	Posterior wall Lateral wall
	Oropharynx	Faucial arch Tonsillar fossa, tonsil Base of tongue Oropharyngeal wall
	Hypopharynx	Pyriform fossa Postcricoid area Posterior wall
Larynx	Supraglottis	Suprahyoid epiglottis Infrahyoid epiglottis Aryepiglottic folds Arytenoids Ventricular bands
	Glottis	(R) True vocal cord (TVC) (L) TVC Anterior commissure Posterior commissure
	Subglottis	Subglottis
Paranasal sinuses	Maxillary sinuses	(R) Maxillary sinus (L) Maxillary sinus
	Ethmoid sinuses	(R) Ethmoid sinus (L) Ethmoid sinus
Major salivary glands	Parotids	(R) Parotid gland (L) Parotid gland
	Submandibulars	(R) Submandibular gland (L) Submandibular gland
	Sublinguals	(R) Sublingual gland (L) Sublingual gland

therapy, hyperthermia, and concomitant chemoradiation are administered similarly across sites, adjuvant modalities will be discussed in more detail later in this chapter.

Surgery

Prior to surgery for any head and neck malignancy, the head and neck surgeon obtains a histopathic diagnosis through incisional, excisional, or needle biopsy while clinically staging the tumor. The importance of having the head and neck surgeon, who has expertise in this anatomical region, perform the biopsy includes minimizing any potential seeding of the tumor and preventing the compromise of an upcoming surgical approach. For stage I and stage II disease, when no cervical nodes are involved, surgical resection can often accomplish total removal of the tumor with clear margins. Surgery alone for early stage disease is often the standard of care. Radiation therapy alone is another consideration for stage I and II malignancies and is also a standard of care for early disease.

With stage III and IV malignancies, surgery often becomes an important part of combination therapy either before or after chemotherapy and/or radiation. When a wide resection is necessary, reconstructive procedures are of critical importance in order to achieve the best possible physiological and cosmetic results for the patient. Although pedicle flaps and grafts are often used to close defects, advances in newer reconstructive surgical techniques have been substantial in the last decade. When there is cervical lymph node spread from any of the head and neck regions to one side of the neck, either a radical neck dissection (RND) or a modified neck dissection (MND) may be performed. In the effort to achieve improved cosmetic and functional outcomes, clinical trials for patients who do not have palpable regional metastases may include selective neck dissection (SND) of nodes from levels I to IV.

Carcinoma of the nasal fossa and paranasal sinuses

Anatomy. The nasal cavity (Figure 56-2) is supported by the hard palate and soft palate (floor), divided by the septum, and topped by the ethmoid bone, which separates the superior aspect of the nasal fossa from the cranial cavity. Three curving, scroll-like bones form the lateral walls of the nasal cavity. These bones are the superior turbinate, middle turbinate, and inferior turbinate. Each of these bones has a tiny meatus (opening) for drainage to specific sinus regions. The masolacrimal duct drains into the inferior meatus. The middle turbinate meatus drains the maxillary, anterior ethmoid and frontal sinuses (Figure 56-3). The superior turbinate drains the posterior ethmoid and sphenoid sinuses. The four paired, paranasal sinuses are the maxillary, ethmoid, frontal, and sphenoid sinuses. Each pair of sinuses is named according to the skull bone housing it. The majority of sinus malignancies occur in the maxillary sinuses.

Treatment. Staging criteria for nasal cavity tumors have not yet been standardized by the AJCC. Small tumors may be treated by either surgery or radiation therapy. Tumor spread commonly occurs along the lateral walls of the nasal cavity. Local spread to the maxillary sinus or nasopharynx may be present upon initial diagnosis. In this situation, concomitant or sequential multimodal treatment can provide improved local and regional control.

For maxillary sinus lesions, when the tumor is confined to the sinus, a maxillectomy will usually be performed. Prior to surgery, a consultation with the maxillofacial prosthodontist will be scheduled. The prosthodontist will make impressions of the hard and soft palates and then create an obturator that will be used to fill the surgical defect. Following resection of the cancer, a skin graft may be required to cover the surgical defect. The graft also counters contraction of the tissue, which is a normal part of the healing process. The obturator will be wired into place in the operating room following resection, after the defect is packed with petroleum-based gauze or nonadhering intermediate reline resin.

The ability to speak and to complete the oral phases of swallowing are restored for the patient with placement

Figure 56-2   Structures of the nose and nasopharynx.

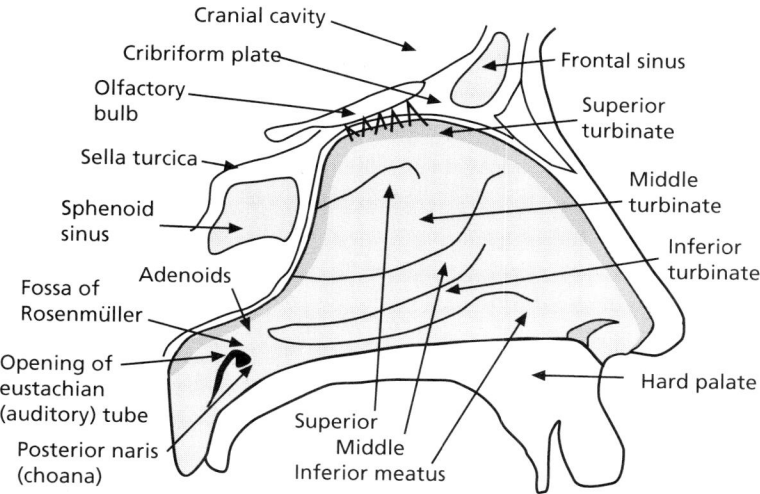

of the obturator, so there may be no need for a nasogastric tube postoperatively. After about five days, the surgeon removes the obturator and gauze and examines the surgical site. A removable obturator is designed by the prosthodontist. The patient is taught how to remove, clean, and replace the obturator. It can take up to six months of revisions before the fit of the obturator is satisfactory, depending upon the size of the defect, and the healing necessary following chemotherapy and radiation.[33] The patient is taught to remove the obturator after every meal and at bedtime. Once the obturator is removed, the patient irrigates the cavity with a solution of normal saline and baking soda, which cleanses the area without causing irritation.

One month post resection, the patient may be taught to use a 50% solution of 3% hydrogen peroxide and water to loosen crusting. A sponge-tipped applicator can be used to gently scrub the skin graft, followed by rinsing the oral cavity with salt and soda solution. Learning to protect the airway from aspiration by positioning is a part

of the process. Patients will be reminded that regular tooth brushing and flossing is a continuing part of oral hygiene. These individuals are at risk for infection, due to the decreased blood supply with postoperative tissue contraction. Nurses should use a mask and sterile gloves when irrigating the wound. The patient needs to be taught (1) to replace the irrigation solution daily, and (2) to regularly clean the irrigation system with soap and water.

If the sinus tumor has invaded the patient's orbit, a radical maxillectomy with orbital exeneration will need to be performed. Collaboration of the prosthodontist with the prosthetics specialist preoperatively addresses the management of appearance as well as speech and eating. Nursing care priorities following radical maxillectomy include inspecting the oral cavity for displacement of packing and securing emergency supplies such as forceps and tongue blades at the bedside. The head of the patient's bed should remain elevated to promote nasal drainage, minimize edema, and improve nasal breathing.

Figure 56-3   The paranasal sinuses.

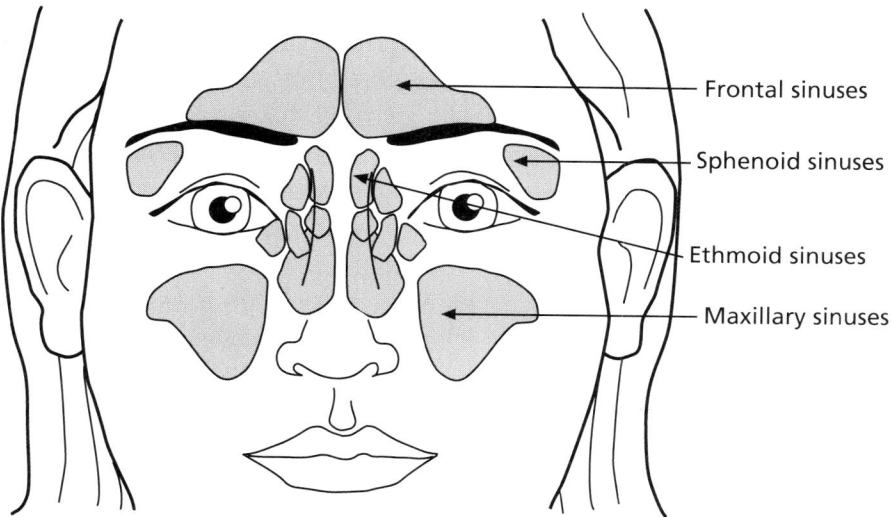

The patient will need time to accommodate proprioceptively to the loss of vision in one eye and is at increased risk for falls during the postoperative phase. Prior to discharge, the patient must be skilled in oral irrigation of the defect and be able to demonstrate an understanding of the symptoms of mucositis. The patient will be taught the importance of proper care of the prosthetic devise. The nurse stresses the need for meticulous oral care postoperatively, as well as during and after completion of any planned chemotherapy and radiation therapy. With large defects, the opening to the oral cavity may become markedly constricted. The patient will then be taught to perform stretching exercises at home. A device that can be used three to four times a day to progressively expand or maintain an adequate opening to the oral cavity may be necessary.

Carcinoma of the skull base

Anatomy.   Cranial base tumors are labeled according to the primary site of the tumor and the area of local spread. The skull base is divided into three regions— anterior, middle, and posterior. Structures located in the anterior region are the ethmoid sinuses, frontal sinuses, and the superior hemispheres of the orbits. In the middle region of the skull base are the greater and lesser wings of the sphenoid bone, the infratemporal bone, the infratemporal fossa, the optic apex, and the optic chiasm. The posterior skull base region contains the clivis, posterior fossa, jugular foramen, and interior auditory canal. Tumors may originate intracranially and extend into head and neck sites. Malignancies may also spread from the nasal fossa, paranasal sinuses, nasopharynx, or infratemporal fossa.

Treatment.   Surgical accessibility has dramatically improved in recent years, in part due to the improvements in preoperative radiological assessment. Often, large lesions are treated with a combined approach while small tumors can be treated with radiation therapy alone. Surgery is an integral part of treatment when the tumor invades the bone. Removal of the tumor and reconstruction of the surgical defect involves the skills of the head and neck surgeon, neurosurgeon, microvascular surgeon, and plastic surgeon. For nasal cavity, maxillary sinus, or ethmoid sinus lesions, the tumor is resected with an anterior fossa approach. Lesions originating in the nasopharynx may require a combined anterior/midfossa approach. Malignancy originating in the temporal bone and infratemporal fossa requires a midfossa approach. A posterior fossa approach is generally used for a temporal bone lesion. Important cranial nerves are located in this region: the glossopharyngeal (CN IX), vagus (CN X), and accessory (CN XI). Closure methods used will depend upon the type of reconstruction needed and may include a combination of skin grafts and composite flaps. Surgery usually lasts for over 12 hours. For patients with stage III or IV tumors, chemotherapy is often combined with radiation therapy. Radiation therapy may be given, in addition to the conventional methods, as part of radiosurgery or brachytherapy.

Potential complications following skull base surgery are many. In addition to the inability to remove the tumor, the patient is at risk for cerebral spinal fluid (CSF) leak, cerebral edema with increased intracranial pressure, artery thrombosis, dissection, or rupture, seizures, stroke, and infections such as meningitis. Systemic complications can include aspiration pneumonia, pulmonary edema, congestive heart failure, myocardial infarction, and sepsis. The individual may need rehabilitation for impaired vision and for defects in swallowing, hearing, mobility, and balance. Postoperatively, if there is nerve involvement, patients generally have considerable pain and will usually require scheduled narcotics to achieve an acceptable level of pain management. Pain medications may be supplemented with antidepressants and anticonvulsant therapy.

Nursing considerations include documenting the baseline neurological assessment preoperatively. Frequent postoperative neurological checks, beginning at 15-minute intervals, are performed in the critical care unit. As part of this evaluation, in addition to vital signs, cognition, pupillary response, hand grasps, reflexes, speech, and extremity mobility are assessed. Following sterile technique, the patient's incisional dressing is checked during each of these assessments for fresh CSF and blood. When either of these conditions occur, the surgeon is immediately notified. In addition to drainage on the dressing, other signs of CSF leakage, such as drainage from the nasal cavity or external ear, are confirmed by the *halo test*: A drop of drainage is placed on a dry dressing. If CSF is present, it will form a ring or halo around the center circle of serum.

Fluid balance is another critical ongoing assessment. Close monitoring of intracranial pressure (ICP) assists in detecting subtle changes requiring immediate interventions to correct bleeding or promote adequate ventilation. Headache is an early sign of increasing ICP. Wide fluctuations in blood pressure can occur postoperatively as a result of vasoconstriction and insufficient cerebral perfusion.

Carcinoma of the nasopharynx

Anatomy.   The nasopharynx is formed anteriorly by the posterior naris/choana and posteriorly by the adenoids, body of the sphenoid, and basilar process of the occipital bones (see Figure 56-2). Interiorly, the nasal passage merges with the oropharynx at the level of the soft palate. The eustachian tube orifice is just anterior to the fossa of Rosenmüller, which is also termed the *pharyngeal recess*. The fossa of Rosenmüller is the site of the majority of nasopharyngeal malignancies. Located just anterior to the fossa of Rosenmuller are the adenoids (pharyngeal tonsils). Lymphatic drainage is abundant and lymph node spread is common to both the ipsilateral and contralateral retropharyngeal nodes. Regional spread usually occurs early in the course of the disease.

Due to the abundant capillary lymphatic system, spread is first to the cervical triangle, upper/middle/lower jugular chains, or supraclavicular nodes. Blood supply is via the common carotid.

Treatment. Anti-EBV antibody titers are often obtained since EBV is a proven risk factor for nasopharyngeal cancer. Although the results of this test may not be conclusive, some studies suggest that high titers may correlate with advanced disease. The clinical exam during treatment for nasopharyngeal carcinoma must include a thorough assessment of all cranial nerves. Also, special attention is paid to the cervical lymph node chains and abnormal adenopathy is measured. Serous otitis media, with obstruction of the eustachian tube, is associated with treatment of nasopharyngeal malignancies. Prior to any radiation treatment, in anticipation of serous drainage during treatment, the surgeon may perform a myringotomy with ventilation tube insertion.[34]

Nasopharyngeal malignancies are usually treated with high-dose, external beam radiation therapy. Surgery is generally not recommended due to the difficult access to this location. Also, the inability to obtain clean margins along with difficulties in providing coverage for the defect enters into the decision not to operate. The delivery of radiation therapy to this site is complex, with critical attention paid to protection of the spinal cord from injury. Both sides of the patient's neck are usually treated with irradiation, even when there is no current evidence of lymph node spread. Radiation therapy will be necessary due to the high likelihood of undetectable neck disease. Radiation alone has been shown to control the patient's neck disease in certain situations. Neck dissection surgery is usually reserved for the patient with residual or recurrent disease. For recurrent, but localized disease, brachytherapy alone or in conjunction with a second course of conventional radiation therapy may be the best approach for treatment for a local recurrence.

Chemotherapy is often given in conjunction with radiation therapy for advanced T3 and T4 malignancies of the nasopharynx. (See section on chemotherapy below.) Combined treatment for this site is generally part of an investigational trial and may be given as a neoadjuvant, adjuvant, or concomitant administration. An intergroup study of stage III and IV disease has reported that chemoradiotherapy, when followed by adjuvant chemotherapy, provided a marked, statistically significant increase in both progression-free status and survival.[35] Nursing care during and following combination treatment includes symptomatic management of xerostomia, bone pain, otitis media, and wound care, and addresses interventions for rehabilitation that compensate for resultant cranial nerve dysfunctions.

Carcinoma of the oral cavity

Anatomy. The most common carcinomas of the oral cavity are those of the lip, tongue, and FOM (Figure 56-4). Descriptions of the primary tumor sites for this region are provided in Table 56-6. Oral cancers have been shown to be the least likely of the head and neck malignancies to spread to the cervical lymph nodes. As mentioned in the discussion of risk factors, the individual often ignores the first signs of malignant changes in the oral cavity. When the patient becomes aware of a painful, persistent ulcer, there may already be perineural or bone involvement. The tumor is generally either exophytic or infiltrative. Infiltrative tumors spread locally and aggressively. Anterior tongue lesions typically infiltrate to the FOM and become fixed. FOM lesions with close proximity to the periosteum of the mandible usually demonstrate bone invasion by the time of the diagnosis. Buccal lesions are known to spread superficially over a large area of the mucosa, but the tumor can also extend deeply into the pterygoid muscle (trismus) or buccinator muscle (skin

Figure 56-4   The oral cavity.

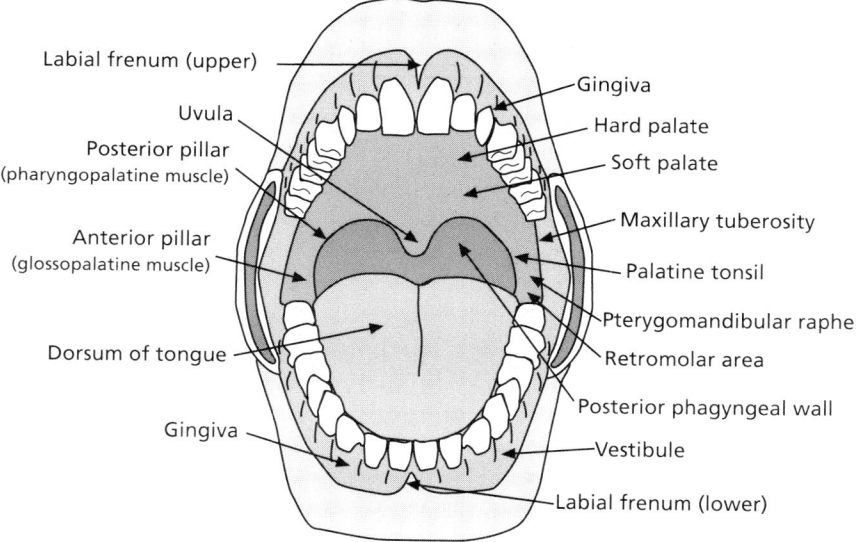

Labial frenum (upper)
Uvula
Posterior pillar (pharyngopalatine muscle)
Anterior pillar (glossopalatine muscle)
Dorsum of tongue
Gingiva

Gingiva
Hard palate
Soft palate
Maxillary tuberosity
Palatine tonsil
Pterygomandibular raphe
Retromolar area
Posterior phagyngeal wall
Vestibule
Labial frenum (lower)

Table 56-6 Structures of the Lip and Oral Cavity

Site	Description
Lip	From the vermilion border with the skin of the upper and lower lips; forms the opening to oral cavity; joined together by anterior commissures located laterally; ends with buccal mucosa
Buccal mucosa	Entire membrane that lines inner surface of cheeks; portion of lips interior from point of contact where upper and lower lips meet; includes mucosal attachment at upper and lower alveolar ridges; includes pterygomandibular raphe recess
Lower alveolar ridge	Mucosa covering mandibular alveolar process (houses teeth sockets); from buccal gutter to the free mucosa of FOM; extends posteriorly to ascending ramus (vertical portion) of mandible
Upper alveolar ridge	Mucosa covering maxillary alveolar process; from upper gingival buccal gutter; extends to hard palate; includes superior portion of pterygopalatine arch
Retromolar trigone (retromolar gingiva)	Mucosa attached and overlying ascending ramus of mandible; from posterior to last molar tooth to the apex; continues to the maxillary tuberosity
Floor of mouth	Semilunar area covering myelohyoid and hypoglossus muscles; from inner surface of lower alveolar ridge; reaching undersurface of tongue; extends to tonsillar pillar; frenulum of tongue separates (R) from (L) FOM; contains ostea of submandibular and sublingual salivary glands
Hard palate	Forms anterior portion of roof of mouth; covers palatine process of maxillary palatine bones; extends from inner surface of upper alveolar ridge to posterior edge of palatine bone
Oral tongue	Anterior two-thirds of tongue; mobile; from circumvallate papillae anteriorly; extends under tongue to junction of FOM; divided into four regions: tip, lateral borders, dorsum, undersurface

of cheek). RMT tumors may invade the pterygoid, resulting in trismus. Alveolar ridge tumors occur more frequently in the lower jaw than the upper. Local spread may be to the maxillary sinus or the maxilla. Lip malignancies are more common on the lower lip and are usually slow to spread.

Treatment. Stage I and II tumors of the oral cavity are treated with the endpoint of function as the determinant for whether surgery or radiation treatment should be the initial treatment of choice. The carbon dioxide laser may better preserve function for patients with early stage, transoral resections.[36] Management of early-stage

tumors with radiation therapy alone may provide improved functional and cosmetic results. Generally, for surgeries of the oral cavity and especially of the tongue, the larger the tumor, the greater the functional disability postoperatively for deglutition and speech.[37,38] The location of the lesion, relative to the preservation or restoration of oral competence, helps determine what the preferred treatment should be. For cancer of the lip, Mohs' micrographic surgical technique may be used for the resection of T1 or T2 tumors. Mohs' technique is employed when the tumor location has an increased incidence of deep invasion and/or local recurrence. The advantages of the Mohs' approach are the abilities to accomplish a total resection with clear margins and to provide improved cosmesis. Advanced tumors (stages III and IV) are usually managed with a combination of therapies, including surgery and radiation therapy (possibly with brachytherapy). With oral cavity tumors, depending upon the clinical stage, a continuous or discontinuous ipsilateral neck dissection is performed to prevent regional spread, followed by adjuvant radiation therapy.

Carcinoma of the oropharynx

Anatomy. The oropharyngeal region begins at the faucial arch (inferior surface of the soft palate, the uvula, and anterior border of the tonsillar pillar) and contains the lingual tonsils (pharyngeal tonsils), BOT (posterior one-third of the tongue), and the adjacent pharyngeal wall (Figure 56-5). All structures of the oropharynx have important roles in the aerodigestive functions of mastication, deglutition, phonation, and respiration. Malignancies of the oropharynx are relatively uncommon and difficult to diagnose clinically due to the hidden locations of most of the primary tumor sites. Carcinoma of the tonsil (tonsillar fossa or pillars) is the most common site for oropharyngeal malignancies.

Treatment. Stage I and II tumors of the oropharynx are managed similarly to early-stage oral cavity malignancies. The real or anticipated changes in function assist the multidisciplinary team in determining if surgery or radiation treatment will be the primary treatment modality. Tonsil malignancies are generally treated with radiation therapy due to the potential for fewer side effects. Cranial nerve paralysis and fistula formation as well as dysarthria and trismus may be complications of a surgical resection of the tonsil tumor. A surgical resection of the BOT carcinoma is the most difficult site of the oropharynx to manage postoperatively. Therefore, primary high-dose irradiation, often with brachytherapy, may be offered in order to avoid the severe functional impairments that follow BOT surgery. A higher level of tumor control may be able to be achieved with a local surgical resection plus a neck dissection. In addition to facial contour, speech and swallowing may be dramatically affected.

Nursing considerations for patients with oral cavity and oropharyngeal malignancies are similar. Preopera-

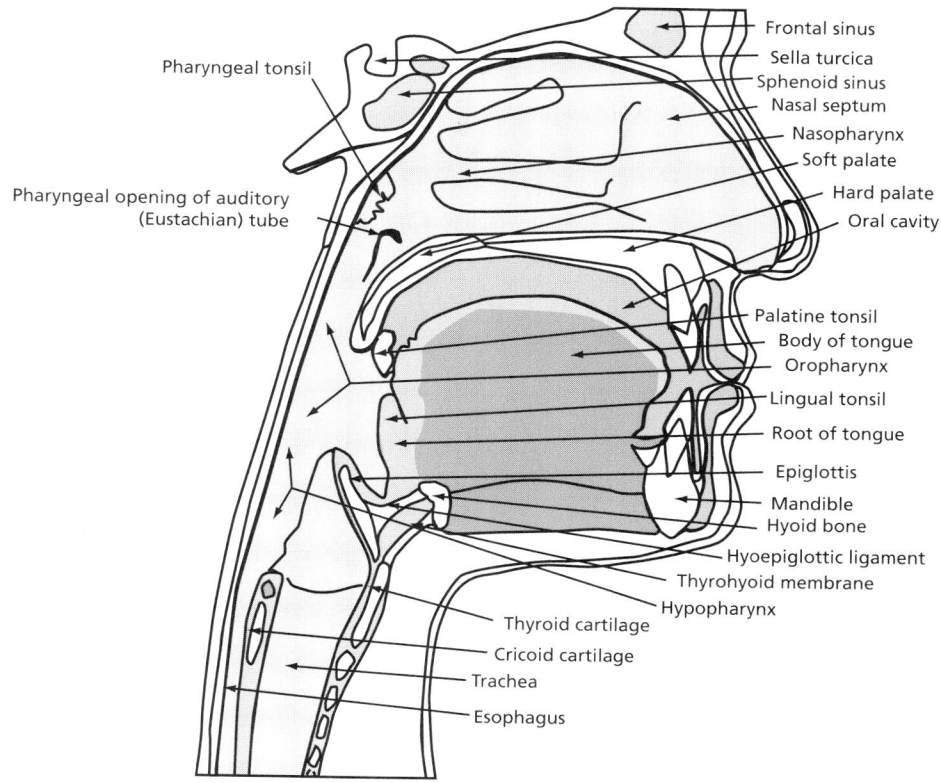

Figure 56-5 Structures of the oropharynx, hypopharynx, trachea, and larynx.

Labels (top to bottom, right side): Frontal sinus, Sella turcica, Sphenoid sinus, Nasal septum, Nasopharynx, Soft palate, Hard palate, Oral cavity, Palatine tonsil, Body of tongue, Oropharynx, Lingual tonsil, Root of tongue, Epiglottis, Mandible, Hyoid bone, Hyoepiglottic ligament, Thyrohyoid membrane, Hypopharynx

Labels (bottom, left side): Thyroid cartilage, Cricoid cartilage, Trachea, Esophagus

Labels (left side): Pharyngeal tonsil, Pharyngeal opening of auditory (Eustachian) tube

tive assessments and patient teaching are centrally important for persons scheduled for surgery. The individual needs to understand what functional changes are expected as a result of the resection. The patient should understand that it is anticipated that both a temporary tracheostomy tube and a temporary gastric tube will be placed at the time of surgery. It is important for the individual and family to know preoperatively what the options are for short-term and long-term management of the airway, nutritional support, wound care, pain management, and communication. Postoperatively, teaching will be reinforced and tailored depending upon the individual patient needs.[39]

For advanced (T4) BOT tumors, treatment is usually a total laryngectomy in conjunction with total resection of the tongue base. A laryngectomy is necessary when the adjacent preepiglottic space, which is separated only by a thin membrane from the tongue base, has tumor invasion. A total laryngectomy can provide total removal of the tumor. With advances in combination therapy, tumor control may be accomplished without the need for a laryngectomy. This organ-sparing procedure generally employs external beam irradiation given on a hyperfractionated (BID) schedule and may include brachytherapy as part of the treatment plan. However, when tumor involves the tongue base, en bloc removal of the jaw, tongue, and neck with a composite resection may become necessary. The mandible is not usually resected unless there is invasion to the bone.

Carcinoma of the salivary gland

Anatomy. The three paired salivary glands are the submandibulars, the sublinguals (submentals), and the parotids (Figure 56-6). The parotids are located in the preauricular areas, the sublinguals are within the FOM, and the submandibulars are positioned deep and inferior to the mandible.

Treatment. For patients with parotid tumors, a superficial parotidectomy with facial nerve dissection is performed. This procedure may be both diagnostic (with the biopsy confirming the histology) and therapeutic (removal of the tumor). Parotid tumors are known to spread directly to the mandible, upper neck, masseter muscles, skin, and infratemporal fossa. Frozen sections by surgical pathology determine when these structures are involved and need to be surgically sacrificed. The facial nerve (CN VII) travels horizontally, through the superficial lobe of the parotid. The segment of the gland below the facial nerve is called the *deep lobe* of the parotid. The head and neck surgeon will, when possible, carefully spare the facial nerve during the surgery. For a parotid resection, the head and neck surgeon will perform a nerve transposition to CN VII when possible. If the nerve is damaged or sacrificed, the surgeon may consider doing at a future time, a nerve crossover procedure, face lift, blepharoplasty, or microvascular free flap as is clinically warranted. For a parotid resection, the surgical approach is through a vertical incision anterior to the auricle, which extends

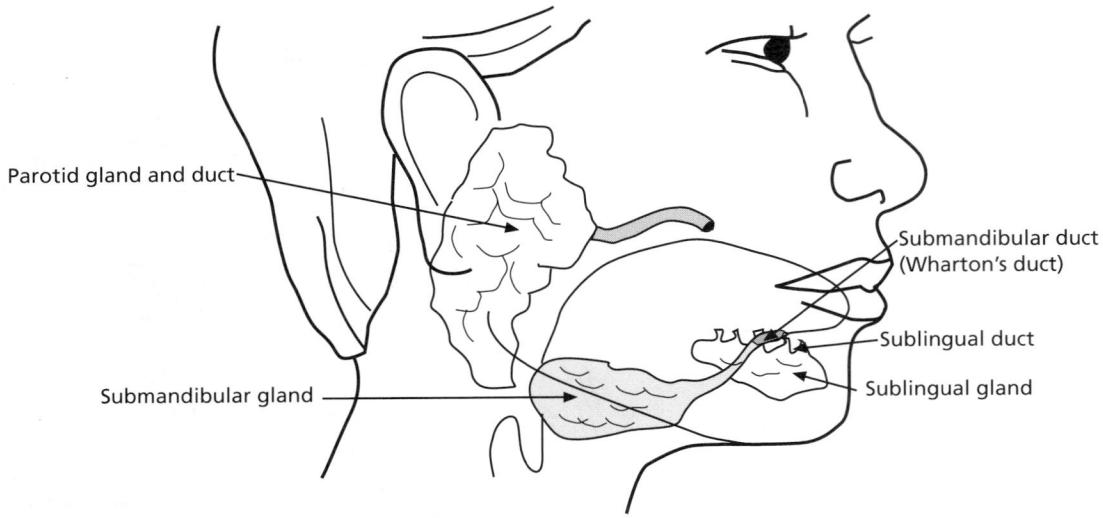

Figure 56-6   Major salivary glands and ducts.

into the creases of the lateral neck. Resulting scarring is usually minimal.

Advanced-stage salivary tumors have been shown to have a high incidence of recurrence when postoperative radiation treatment was not provided at the time of the patient's initial resection. Therefore, adjuvant radiation therapy is generally given to all postoperative patients. Radiation therapy is of prime importance when there are positive neck nodes, if the deep lobe of the parotid is involved, if there is facial nerve involvement, or when the tumor has high-grade tumor histology. Combination treatment with chemotherapy is also often part of the plan for patients with T3 or T4 tumors.[40]

Nursing care, when there has been facial nerve injury, includes interventions to protect the cornea of the affected eye from abrasion. Eye drops and ophthalmic ointments are generally prescribed to provide moisture to the cornea. As this individual will have facial numbness, protection for the skin from sun, wind, and cold damage should be stressed.[41,42]

Carcinoma of the larynx

Anatomy.   The larynx is vertically located between the epiglottis and cricoid cartilage (Figure 56-7). It lies between the carotid arteries and is posterior to the thyroid gland. The larynx is divided into three regions: the supraglottic, the glottis, and the subglottis. The supraglottic region begins inferior to the BOT and includes the epiglottis, aryepiglottic folds, arytenoid cartilages, and false vocal cords (FVC). The glottis includes the true vocal cord (TVC), rima glottis, and the glottic slit which separates the true vocal cords. The subglottis extends from the TVC to the cricoid cartilage. Innervation is by the recurrent and superior laryngeal nerves, which are branches of the vagus nerve (CN X). Glottic carcinoma is the most common site for laryngeal malignancies and the subglottic site is the least common.

Treatment for supraglottic carcinomas.   Early stage (T1 and T2) supraglottic lesions have been primarily treated by either supraglottic laryngectomy (horizontal partial laryngectomy) or by radiation therapy. Since the larynx is compartmentalized, the removal of the top portion (supraglottis) will allow the individual to be able to swallow and speak. In certain situations, endoscopic surgical management using a transoral excision, often with the carbon dioxide laser, may be employed to resect the tumor. A concern with laser treatment is not having the surgical specimen, during or after the procedure, for histological examination.[43–45] A tracheostoma is necessary in order to relieve airway obstruction due to postoperative edema and to provide easy access for assistance with bronchial hygiene. Preoperative teaching should address the patient's postoperative teaching requirements. Postoperative nursing care has an early focus on self-care and airway management. With a supraglottic laryngectomy, the true vocal cords and arytenoids are spared, allowing for speech. However, resection of the epiglottis results in aspiration due to the inability to protect the airway during deglutition.

Due to the likelihood of cervical spread, treatment of the patient's neck is the standard for supraglottic malignancies. Neck dissection surgery has undergone technical changes in recent years and today the operation is selected according to nodal involvement and removes the lymphatic pathways from one or both sides of the neck. The neck operation may be the radical neck dissection (RND), which removes the sternocleidomastoid muscle (SCM), jugular vein, and spinal accessory nerve. The modified neck dissection (MND) procedure is now commonly in use, which spares the SCM and spinal accessory nerve, and provides for improved shoulder function and cosmesis. If there is no evidence of nodal involvement, the sole treatment may be radiation therapy or selective neck dissection (SND) of level I to IV nodes. If there is regional spread to the neck, treatment will usually include

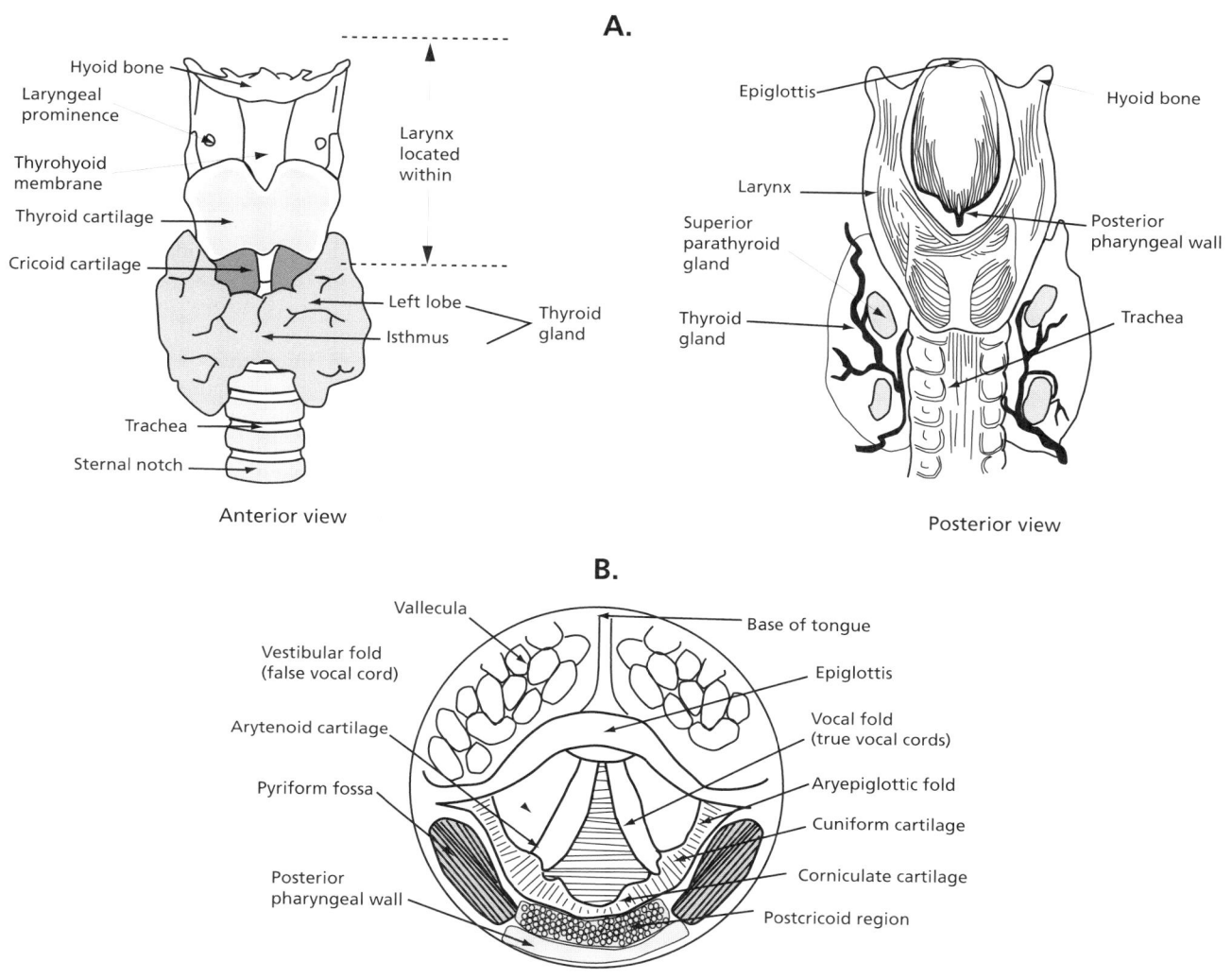

Figure 56-7   A. Larynx, trachea, thyroid, and parathyroid glands (anterior and posterior). **B.** Vocal cords and cartilages of the larynx and epiglottis (mirror view).

both a neck dissection operation and adjuvant radiation therapy. Following a neck dissection, patients are encouraged to participate in a home exercise program designed by the physical therapist to strengthen neck and shoulder muscles and expand the ranges of motion.[46]

For the postoperative supraglottic laryngectomy patient, the speech pathologist and nursing staff join forces to teach the patient the supraglottic swallowing technique. This is a series of steps that the individual takes to force the true vocal cords to occlude in order to protect the airway from aspiration. Normally, aspiration is prevented during the pharyngeal phase of swallowing by spontaneous, sequential actions: (1) the epiglottis closes to protect the laryngeal inlet, (2) the true vocal cords occlude (close), (3) the larynx rises and moves forward, (4) the cricopharyngeus opens in response to the laryngeal pull described in step 3, and (5) the bolus travels above the larynx to the open cricopharyngeus and on to the esophagus.

To promote relaxation of the cricopharyngeal sphincter, the surgeon may perform a cricopharyngeal myotomy. Laryngeal suspension, with the surgeon suturing the thyroid cartilage to the mentum of the mandible, may also provide protection from aspiration as the patient's larynx is then tilted posteriorly. Not every individual with a supraglottic tumor may be eligible for a supraglottic laryngectomy. Individuals with compromised pulmonary function due to chronic bronchitis or the effects of aging are generally not eligible for this surgery. Should the individual have continuing problems with aspiration, and especially if pneumonia develops, a total laryngectomy will be necessary and may be a life-saving procedure.[47,48]

The swallowing therapist works privately with the supraglottic patient for the first oral intake, and generally during each swallowing session, until a basic understanding of the supraglottic swallowing technique is achieved. Small bites of soft foods such as jello, applesauce, or mashed potatoes must be mastered first. Once the patient is able to swallow soft foods without significant aspiration, a cuffless tracheostomy tube is inserted. If aspiration is limited and a cuffed tube is in place, the cuff should be deflated whenever possible to permit the larynx to elevate with minimal resistance during swallowing a bolus of food. Patients tend to learn the supraglottic swallow more efficiently with a written outline of the steps to review.[49] Family members may need guidance in how to be supportive without encouraging unrealistic expectations for the patient. When soft foods are mastered, the patient progresses next to semisolid foods and then to liquids. Attention to tracheal suctioning should be ongoing. The edema in the laryngeal area from both the surgery and the attempts at swallowing will result in copious amounts of tracheal secretions.

Treatment for glottic carcinomas. Unlike supraglottic tumors, glottic carcinomas initially remain localized. Lymphatic supply is limited in this region, resulting in a lower percentage of early spread to the cervical neck nodes. Glottic tumors are also more likely to be detected early, since the individual promptly develops symptoms of hoarseness. In situ tumors may be treated with laser vaporization, microexcision, or radiation therapy. The advantage of laser excision and irradiation to the glottis over surgical treatment is the retention of a near normal voice. Of all of the resection procedures microexcision surgery, the voice changed the least. Also, microexcision allows for the surgical pathologist to examine tissue to histologically determine if there are areas of microinvasion. Patient's with T2 glottic carcinoma with a fixed, immobile, vocal cord may be treated with irradiation alone or by a vertical hemilaryngectomy. For the vertical hemilaryngectomy, the surgeon removes a part or all of the true vocal cord and false vocal cord, as well as the associated half of the thyroid cartilage. However, if the vocal cord is fixed and there is evidence of tumor extension or invasion, generally a total laryngectomy will be necessary.

In advanced cases of glottic carcinomas, patients with T3 or T4 tumors have usually been treated with either a total laryngectomy plus neck dissection and adjuvant radiation therapy or radiation therapy followed by surgical salvage as necessary for persistent disease. A total laryngectomy (TL) results in a complete separation of the pharynx from the trachea. The TL removes the cricoid and thyroid cartilage, both arytenoids, both true vocal cords, both false vocal cords, epiglottis, preepiglottic and paraglottic spaces, and the hyoid bone. Perioperative antibiotics are usually administered to prevent infection. Local control by surgery of advanced stage tumors of the glottis may be achieved in a variety of ways. When the tumor is associated with bulky neck disease or if there is tumor extension to the hypopharynx, treatment will usually be a total laryngectomy with surgical dissections of both sides of the neck, followed by adjuvant irradiation.

With a total laryngectomy plus neck dissection, there are increased risks for postoperative complications such as fistula formation, carotid rupture, wound infection, and pharyngeal stenosis. This is especially true when the tumor is recurrent and the individual has received prior radiation treatments to the tumor site. The healing of a fistula to the laryngeal region requires meticulous management of fistula drainage, with scheduled irrigations and packings of the wound. Salivary drainage from a fistula, when there is insufficient tissue coverage of the carotid, can result in the most dreaded critical complication, carotid artery rupture.[50] If the patient is at risk, the individual is placed on "carotid artery blowout precautions." Nursing interventions for carotid blowout include keeping the following at the bedside: gloves, a cuffed tracheostomy tube of the correct size, sterile saline, and towels for padding. Should a carotid rupture occur, the nurse, following standard precautions, assists the medical team in securing the airway with the inflation of the cuffed tracheostomy tube, engaging the suction, and applying pressure to the site (using saline-soaked gauze for intraoral bleeding and padding to neck for an external rupture). Later laryngeal complications, which can require a surgical repair, include tracheostomal stenosis and hypopharyngeal stricture.

Improvements in laryngeal tumor control by chemoradiation are steadily evolving with organ (larynx) preservation protocols becoming more widely utilized. Through larynx preservation, the individual experiences an improved quality of life by retaining the ability to speak. Initially, a temporary tracheostomy will be required. Although an individual's speech and swallowing abilities generally do not recover to the premalignancy baselines, functions are at least partially preserved.

Nursing care for laryngeal cancer patients includes ongoing attention to tracheostomy care and suctioning. Except for patients with early-stage disease, all individuals will have either a temporary or permanent tracheostomy in order to maintain an airway. Individuals with a total laryngectomy will require only a temporary laryngectomy tube, which is short and wide in comparison to the conventional tracheostomy tube. The laryngectomy tube helps to shape the stoma. Tracheostomy tube descriptions are provided in Table 56-7. Tracheostomy care interventions are summarized in Table 56-8.

Carcinoma of the hypopharynx and neck

Anatomy. The hypopharynx (see Figure 56-5), also referred to as the *laryngopharynx*, connects the oropharynx at the level of the hyoid bone to the esophageal introitus. The lower end is at the level of the sixth cervical vertebra. The regions of the hypopharynx are (1) the paired pyriform sinuses, (2) the posterior pharyngeal walls, and (3) the postcricoid area (lower pharyngeal wall). The majority of hypopharyngeal lesions originate in one of the pyriform sinuses. There are few obstacles to regional tumor advancement once cancer cells have penetrated the mucosa of the pharynx. The neck nodes are assigned to levels or groups (see Figure 56-1) and provide avenues for lymphatic drainage from the base of skull to the clavicle. The level of lymph node involvement is indicative of the location of the primary tumor.

Table 56-7 Tracheostomy Tubes: Components and Types

Component and Materials (Plastic (P), Silicone (S), or Metal (M))	Function
Obturator (P, S, M)	After removing inner cannula, use this to insert outer cannula; domed end smoothly guides the insertion Remove immediately after cannula is inserted to open the airway
Fenestrated inner cannula (P, M)	Removable rigid inner tube with holes on superior surface for air to travel to nose and mouth (for speech) Locks into place inside the outer cannula; removed for trach care cleaning
Unfenestrated inner cannula (P, M) Nondisposable	Locks inside outer cannula. Passageway for air exchange and tracheal secretions; removed for trach care cleaning
Disposable (DIC)	DIC is never reused, is changed during trach care, or every 8 hours
Cuffed outer cannula (P, S, M)	Provides seal when inflated, preventing airflow to mouth and nose so can only breathe through the tracheostomy tube May or may not have removable inner cannula; is inserted into the tracheostoma using the obturator
Cuffless outer cannula or laryngectomy tube (LT) (P, S, M)	May or may not have removable inner cannula; is inserted into the tracheostoma using the obturator; tube is shorter
Decannulation plug (P, S, M)	Used when trach is not in use for breathing and prior to permanent closure of a temporary tracheostomy Blocks air exchange through trach tube and forces breathing through the upper airway

Treatment. It would be unusual for T1 or T2 hypopharyngeal tumors to be detected early since the patient is not commonly aware of subtle abnormalities in function early in the disease process. Cervical lymph node metastasis is often present at the time of diagnosis due to the proximity of the tumor to the lymph node chains in the neck. Radiation therapy alone is frequently recommended for individuals with early-stage disease in order to preserve voice. In the event of recurrence, surgery, usually a laryngectomy, would be selected as the treatment of choice. A laryngectomy would be necessary in order to provide the necessary wide margins of resection as well as to prevent the ongoing aspiration of saliva and food. Ultimately, the treatment course depends upon lymph node spread and laryngeal involvement.

For individuals with T3 and T4 tumors, irradiation and chemotherapy may be offered preoperatively in order to preserve laryngeal function, or induction chemotherapy

may be used alone, preoperatively, in order to shrink the tumor to achieve operable status. Treatment for patients with advanced tumors would include a combination of total laryngectomy with partial or total pharyngectomy followed by radiation therapy. Because the majority of hypopharyngeal malignancies metastasize early to cervical lymph nodes, generally both sides of the patient's neck are treated. The patient will be offered radiation therapy even if there is no clinical evidence of neck disease. The individual will most likely undergo a neck dissection when there is measurable disease.[51]

Coverage of large hypopharyngeal postoperative defects will usually include a jejunal free flap with microvascular anastomoses and gastric pull-up. Nursing care after hypopharyngeal cancer surgery is complex, and patient recovery may be slow. Preoperative problems that the individual may need assistance with are many. The person may have, at the time of diagnosis, infections of the oral cavity with dental involvement. Oral care with rinses scheduled from three to four times per day will help to decrease bacteria counts within the oral cavity. The individual may also have problems with aspiration, resulting in pneumonia. Malnutrition is a common problem, which needs to be addressed in order to promote postoperative healing. Attentive tracheostomy suctioning and care will help to promote tissue oxygenation as well as improve pulmonary functioning. Postoperatively, the patient is at risk for wound infection (especially due to the contamination by salivary secretions), flap necrosis (with the potential for carotid rupture), swallowing dysfunction (due to injury to vagus or recurrent laryngeal nerve), and shoulder weakness (due to injury to the spinal accessory nerve).[52]

Surgical restoration: reconstruction and rehabilitation

Prior to removal of the individual's tumor, the head and neck surgeon anticipates the location and dimensions of the surgical defect. The surgeon's goal will be to promote the highest level of function and cosmesis following total resection of the tumor. The depth of the defect and need to protect underlying bone or cartilage will be considered along with the thickness, color, and texture needed for the overlying skin. In addition, the tissue to be used to cover the defect will need to be firm, have acceptable skin tone, especially for the face, and be applicable for a two- or three-dimensional repair.

As a part of preoperative teaching, the individual should be informed of the surgeon's plan to cover the surgical defect following tumor removal. Prior to surgery, it should be explained that certain conditions affect the successful neovascularization and delivery of sufficient blood flow through the flap or graft. The conditions associated with vasoconstriction include smoking, anticoagulation medications, small vessel disease related to diabetes, atherosclerosis, and delayed healing following prior radiation therapy. In addition, the individual should understand that the surgeon's final decisions will have

Table 56-8 Home Care Safety Precautions for Individuals with a Tracheostoma

Procedures	Rationale	Actions
Clean technique for suctioning and tracheostomy care	Prevent infection	Wash catheter and basins with hot water and mild liquid soap; store in clean covered container between use; catheter can be reused until discoloration occurs
		Weekly cleaning of suction machine and humidifiers or maintenance per manufacturer's guidelines
Change of outer cannula (need physician order)	Prevent infection and respiratory obstruction	Usually change weekly, beginning 2–3 weeks postoperatively: 1. Place trach ties on trach tube and obturator in clean outer cannula; apply water-soluble lubricant to the tip 2. Prepare 50% hydrogen peroxide + 50% saline solution in basin 3. Snip ties on indwelling trach tube 4. Remove trach tube in an arching outward, downward motion and place in peroxide solution 5. Patient coughs, clears stomal secretions with gauze, and inspects stoma 6. Insert lubricated clean outer cannula with obturator, guiding an arching, inward, and downward motion 7. Immediately remove obturator and secure trach ties or velcro 8. Insert inner cannula and luerlock 9. Patient relaxes, breathes deeply and slowly, and then suctions as necessary
Oral care	To prevent infection and promote healing	Oral rinses, as ordered, every 8 hours and as needed; set to lowest pressure when using oral power spray; report foul-smelling halitosis (may be infection)
Respiratory protection	To provide filtration of air, humidity, and airway protection	Use foam, crocheted, or moistened gauze trach covers; moisten center of cover to increase humidity of inspired air
		Use rubber or waterproof shield for showering, aiming water below stoma, and at lower chest

to be made during the surgery and will be based upon resection perimeters as well as the clinical tumor stage.

A small, superficial defect, when it is too large for primary closure, may be covered with a full thickness skin graft (epidermis and dermis). Full thickness grafts to cover facial defects are usually harvested from the preauricular or postauricular areas to cover defects of the nasal tip, eyelid, or auricle. Split thickness skin grafts (STSG) are nearly transparent, with a thickness between .006 and .02 inch. Frequently, the lateral thigh is the site for the STSG harvest. A STSG has limited use in facial reconstruction, as the thin graft is prone to shrink or shift as a result of contracting and wrinkling following radiation therapy.

Local flaps. Local skin flaps are created from partially or totally detached tissue and used to cover areas with partial to full thickness loss. Flaps may be organized according to the vascular supply for the site.

Random cutaneous flap. This flap contains musculocutaneous vessels at the base of the flap and, due to the proximity to the defect, matches the individual's skin in texture and color. The random flap can be advanced, tubed, rotated, or transposed to cover an adjacent area. Because the circulation, both arterial and venous, originates at the base of the flap, the flap cannot be bent or compromised in any way or neovascular perfusion at the attachment site will be compromised.

Arterial cutaneous flap. An arterial flap is also known as an *island flap.* The most common grafts of this type are the deltopectoral graft of the internal mammary artery and the midline forehead graft of the supratrochlear artery.

Distant flaps. With the advent of pedicled, *myocutaneous flaps* in the 1970s, it became possible to reconstruct large defects, especially of the oral cavity, and provide improved blood supply. The myocutaneous flap does not disrupt the local vasculature. In addition, muscle is incorporated into the flap to provide bulk following a large resection. Myocutaneous flaps are named for the muscle that is used in the repair. The tissue of the pectoralis myocutaneous flap incorporates a branch of the thoracoacromial artery. The pectoralis, latissimus dorsi, sternocledomastoid, and trapezius are the muscles used most often for one-stage reconstructive procedures. The main surgical limitation of the muscle flap procedure is the restriction in reach due to the constraint imposed by the pedicle. Problems with speech and swallowing are associated with this type of flap when used for oral cavity defects.[53] Function is usually impaired due to bulky muscle coverage and impaired sensation.

Free flap. During the 1980s, a reconstructive procedure based upon microvascular anastomoses of arteries and veins became more common as surgeons were trained in microsurgical techniques. Also, the necessary additional space for personnel and equipment could be accommodated in surgical suites. The free flap has become the chosen procedure for certain sites, including large defects of the oral cavity, nose, skin, and temporal bone. The free flap overcomes the limited reach and arc of rotation of the myocutaneous flap. The surgery has multiple, precise steps and involves two surgical teams (one to excise the tumor and another to harvest the graft). There are many advantages for this free tissue transfer operation. The free flap can be customized and harvested according to the needs and size of the defect. It can be composed of skin, muscle, bone, or nerve. Vascularity is generally improved for the repair to an irradiated site. Flexibility in flap placement can allow for improved anastomoses for motor and sensory innervation. When sufficient bone is used to reconstruct the maxillary or mandibular arches, it may be possible after the appropriate healing interval for the insertion of osteointegrated dental implants that support dentures.[54,55]

One of the most multifaceted free flaps is harvested from the lateral thigh. This site offers a large surface area with ample-sized vessels. It is usually hairless, and can be sculpted more freely into thin as well as thick portions. The flexibility of depth allows for the same flap to provide both the bulk needed for a base of tongue reconstruction and the pliable thin tissue to cover palate or pharyngeal wall defects.

Nursing care of flaps and grafts.

The nurse has the important responsibility to moniter the vascularization of the skin graft or flap through frequent observation, assessment, and documentation of the conditions of both the donor and recipient sites.

Skin grafts. Full thickness and split thickness skin grafts are secured by suturing the graft into the recipient defect. Full thickness grafts are usually harvested from areas of the body which have natural creases, such as the preauricular, supraclavicular, or lower lateral regions of the neck. STSG may also be taken from the lateral thigh. The recipient site, for example the floor of mouth, is generally bolstered in the operating room with gauze saturated with bismuth tribromophenate (XeroForm®). This bolus packing is not disturbed until it is removed in approximately five days. The nurse ensures that oral care is not provided until prescribed following removal of the bolus dressing. It is important that the patient's oral cavity be frequently inspected for drainage and odor, and assessed for signs and symptoms of infection during the time the bolus dressing is in place. Following removal of the packing, the patient is taught the importance of maintaining oral hygiene using a solution of 25% hydrogen peroxide and 75% water four times daily.

The donor site(s) for skin grafts are often covered in the operating room with a transparent adhesive film product that is occlusive to liquids and bacteria, but that provides a moist environment that promotes healing and allows for observation and assessment. The transparent dressing conforms to the patient's wound and may stay in place, undisturbed, for up to seven days. The donor site is likely to heal more quickly, with less scaring, in the moist environment that the transparent film provides. If

the surgeon uses a dry dressing, generally it is padded with a circular gauze dressing and stays in place for several days after surgery. The subsequent dressing changes are then accomplished using sterile technique. If the dressing becomes dry and adheres to the wound, saline-soaked gauze is placed over the area for several minutes in order to release it. Force should never be used to remove the dressing, as extreme pain and damage to viable tissue, bleeding, and disrupted healing will ensue.

In the past, donor sites were exposed to air and a heat lamp was used when drainage was present. Because heat promotes a dry environment, however, it may interfere with healing. With the use of a transparent film dressing instead of heat, the donor site heals autolytically and the dressing can more easily be removed with less discomfort for the patient. The patient is more likely to complain of pain at the donor site than at the recipient defect. Analgesics may be needed every three to four hours in order to keep the donor site discomfort at a tolerable level. It should be remembered that the weight of even pajamas on the donor graft might increase the individual's discomfort during the early postresection days.

Skin flaps. As previously explained, the blood flow to and from the flap provides avenues for nutritional support, oxygenation, thermoregulation, and transport of metabolic waste. If there is ischemia of the graft, there may be decreased perfusion pressure and lowered platelet activation following thrombus development at the level of the anastomoses. It is possible for obstructed lymphatic drainage to result in increased interstitial pressure from the resultant edema. Another factor to be closely monitored is the prevention of pressure on the flap from tracheostomy ties or dressings. Tracheostomy ties must not be tight to prevent constricture of blood flow and venous congestion in the flap. Venous congestion occurs when blood flow out of the flap is hindered. When myocutaneous flaps are used, the surgeon will carefully describe to the family as well as the staff how to maintain proper positioning to prevent tension or entanglement of the pedicle of the graft. The incision sites are to be kept clean, usually using a 50% hydrogen peroxide and 50% normal saline solution, at least every shift. Fibrin build-up on the suture line interferes with granulation and provides an avenue for infection.

Circulatory indicators, which are to be monitored postoperatively at least every two hours for two days and then every four hours through day 5 include:

1. *Temperature.* The nurse uses the front (nail side) of a finger to gently touch the flap (the finger pad is less sensitive) to assess the warmth of the skin. The flap should feel warm.

2. *Color.* In the immediate postoperative period, the flap may appear pale in response to epinephrine-containing anesthesia, but should become pale pink within no more than 24 hours.[56]

3. *Drainage.* The nurse assesses the amount and color of fluid accumulating in the wound and collecting from the surgical drains. Surgical drains can remain for up to six days postoperatively to evacuate serous fluids from the wound bed. If there is more than one drain, each is labeled for assessment purposes. For a closed-drain system such as the Jackson-Pratt, the nurse ensures that the tubing is patent and that a vacuum is maintained. A drain is removed when there is no greater than 50 mL of drainage over 24 hours. Ensuring that the drains are regularly monitored for an increased production of drainage is very important. Increase in drainage may herald the development of a hematoma, which must be reported immediately to the surgeon. For flap viability, a hematoma will be surgically drained immediately, either at the bedside or in the operating room.

4. *Capillary refill.* A quick estimate of perfusion is to apply gentle pressure to various areas of the flap and follow the blanching effect, observing for a return to normal color within two seconds. A deep reddish-blue hue usually means venous obstruction, which can lead to flap failure.

5. *Position.* Semi-Fowler to high-Fowler positions are maintained to promote drainage, reduce edema, and prevent hyperextension. A crease should not be allowed to form in the flap, nor should there be undue tension on the suture line.

6. *Medicinal leeches.* Medicinal leeches have been used to promote healing when arterial perfusion is intact but venous circulation is impaired and cannot be surgically corrected. Upon attachment, the leech supplies an anticoagulant and vasodilator to the wound in the process of withdrawing 5–10 mL of blood per 30-minute session. Leech therapy is generally not required for longer than seven days. If there is going to be a successful graft, the neovascularization usually corrects the venous congestion problem within three to seven days. Leech therapy is contraindicated if the patient has arterial occlusion or insufficiency or is immunosuppressed.[57]

7. *Additional interventions.* Other common methods to monitor circulation that may be necessary include Doppler scanning and pulse oximetry. If the flap shows signs of failure, vasodilating medications may be prescribed as well as hyperbaric oxygen treatments. Generally intravenous heparin has not been effective once thrombus has formed, but urokinase may be useful. Neutropenia has been shown to interfere with wound healing. In a recent study, granulocyte colony stimulating factor (GCSF) showed activity in healing a persistent wound at six months post laryngectomy.[58]

Chemotherapy

Combination therapy trials currently use cisplatin or methotrexate plus fluorouracil (5-FU), and generally include a total of three to four chemotherapy drugs. To date, combination treatment alone has not demonstrated better tumor control or survival. Small primary lesions are still best controlled with surgery and/or irradiation. It has been established that individuals with T3 or T4, N2 or N3

disease are subject to occult metastases. Goals for treatment with chemotherapy therefore include improving tumor kill for local, regional, and metastatic disease and in the process, increasing the patient's survival and quality of life.

Induction or neoadjuvant chemotherapy

Induction chemotherapy has significant activity in patients with recurrent and/or metastatic head and neck tumors. In a phase I study of 29 patients previously treated with chemotherapy, paclitaxel was administered for ten days sequentially at 21 mg/m²/day (total dose: 210 mg/m²).[59] Grade 3 to 4 neutropenia occurred in 50% of the patients. In another study, paclitaxel was combined with gemcitabine in 44 patients with recurrent or metastatic head and neck cancer[60] as six 21-day cycles of gemcitabine (1100 mg/m² over 30 minutes on days 1 and 8) with paclitaxel given over three hours immediately after the gemcitabine on day 1 (200 mg/m²). Grade 3 to 4 neutropenia occurred in 21% of the patients. Median time to progression was four months. Another approach to treating recurrent or metastatic tumors is with electroporation therapy, in which chemotherapy, usually bleomycin, is delivered directly into the tumor site via pulsed electric fields.[61]

It is often difficult to clinically assess response to chemotherapy for patients with advanced stage or recurrent tumors. Investigations of methods to measure metabolic activity may result in better predictions of tumor response to chemotherapy by identifying changes in tumor metabolism. Lowe and colleagues[62] have evaluated [F-18] fluorodeoxy-glucose (FDG) positron emission tomography (PET) before and after administration of taxol plus carboplatin in patients enrolled in a neoadjuvant organ preservation protocol. Pretreatment FDG-PET findings were confirmed by pathology review 90% of the time. Posttreatment pathology confirmation of residual tumor by FDG-PET achieved 90% sensitivity and 83% specificity. Future developments in FDG-PET may allow for consistent identification of tumor that is otherwise undetectable.

Neoadjuvant regimens have generally included up to four cycles of cisplatin and 5-FU plus up to three additional agents. Excellent tumor response has been able to be achieved; however, survival has not differed significantly from that achieved with conventional surgery plus radiation therapy. It has been demonstrated that when there is a complete response to chemotherapy, individuals generally will have improved survival over those who did not experience tumor shrinkage after chemotherapy. In addition, several trials have shown that those who received induction chemotherapy experienced a lower rate of distant metastases compared to those who did not receive chemotherapy.[63,64]

For those individuals with T3 or T4 glottic tumors who would otherwise receive a total laryngectomy, neoadjuvant chemotherapy trials are establishing that the larynx can be preserved with survival rates comparable to treatment with laryngectomy and radiation therapy.[65,66] In addition, some individuals with glottic carcinomas may feel that they cannot cope with a laryngectomy and request any treatment that will allow them to retain the ability for "normal" speech. They may feel this way even when understanding that the alternative treatment may have less effect on tumor containment.

Organ preservation investigational protocols vary in chemotherapy agents and dosages, irradiation fractionations, and courses of treatment, making it difficult to compare survival statistics. Treatment may consist of two courses of induction chemotherapy, generally utilizing a regimen based on cisplatin plus 5-FU. Other agents that are radiosensitizers and may be used include hydroxyurea, carboplatin, and paclitaxel. Tumor measurement often directly follows the second course. If the tumor has responded, another course of chemotherapy is usually given, followed by full course radiation therapy. If the tumor has not shrunk, the patient goes on to receive the standard surgery (usually including a laryngectomy) plus radiation therapy. The head and neck surgeon continues to work with the oncologist to jointly follow the induction chemotherapy and radiation therapy patients closely. When residual disease remains after completion of radiation therapy, the patient may be recommended for surgery. The surgeon may need to perform a neck dissection if there is nodal spread.

Chemoradiation

Clinical investigations involving concomitant chemoradiotherapy for individuals with stage II or III carcinomas of all head and neck primary sites have been based on the idea that certain antineoplastic agents are synergistic with radiation. For example, 5-FU[67,68] and the taxanes[69] are often given concomitantly to improve tumor response. Other agents include cisplatin,[70] carboplatin,[71] and methotrexate.[72,73] Combination chemotherapy with radiation therapy is associated with significant toxicities, especially mucositis and moist desquamation of the skin. In an attempt to minimize toxicity, chemotherapy and radiation may be given on an alternating basis. A focus for treatment protocols has been to design a schedule that can be accomplished without excessive myelosuppression or skin or mucosal toxicities. Trials for the management of individuals with locally advanced (T4), metastatic, or recurrent head and neck cancer have incorporated new agents such as paclitaxel with or without colony stimulating factors to manage myelosuppression.[74]

When aggressive chemoradiation protocols are planned, patients will have both a port-a-cath central venous catheter and an enteral feeding tube surgically placed. These interventions promote optimal support of the patient's nutritional needs and permit continuous infusion of chemotherapy on an outpatient basis. For those with stage II to III disease, the concomitant protocols have included six to seven cycles of five days of hydroxyurea and continuous infusion 5-FU along with twice daily (hyperfractionated) radiotherapy, followed by eight days of rest. When residual disease remains after treatment, definitive surgery is offered.[75]

Radiation Therapy

Squamous cell carcinoma cells are only moderately responsive to radiation therapy. Even so, radiation therapy alone is often curative for patients with early stage head and neck malignancies. A review by Nafoor and associates[76] of hyperfractionated radiotherapy for patients with supraglottic carcinoma (at median follow-up of 56 months) found local control for patients with N0 or N1 disease to be 86% and 74%, respectively, with relapse rates of 79% (N0) and 53% (N1). Voice preservation was 96% for patients with T1 lesions and 80% for those with T2 lesions. The best therapeutic approach for early glottic cancer remains controversial. Spector and colleagues[77] found no statistical differences in voice preservation, local control, or five-year survival rates among patients who received conservation surgery versus those who received high-dose radiation therapy.

The advantages for radiation alone, when compared to surgery alone, have generally included improved function and posttreatment cosmesis. As part of the decision process, the individual learns that, for radiation therapy, outpatient treatments will need to be given at a set time, once or twice a day, Monday through Friday, for a period of five to seven weeks, depending upon the protocol. Daily travel to and from the treatment center during this time period will be necessary. Other considerations include the health status of the patient, the anticipated success of local control based upon tumor histology, the expected voice quality after treatment, cost, and the patient's wishes. Tumor hypoxia (pO_2 below 2.5 mg Hg) may be assessed, and customized therapy could become necessary due to the poor response of hypoxic tumors to radiation therapy.[78]

In addition to early-stage tumors, unresectable malignancies may also be treated with radiation therapy alone. Large T3 and T4 tumors of the oral cavity, oropharynx, and glottis may be treated with radiation therapy only in order to preserve, as long as possible, normal pathways for speech and swallowing. At any time following receipt of 5000 or more cGy, if the tumor recurs and the patient needs surgery at that site, the patient will usually experience significant delays in postoperative healing.[79]

Treatment planning considerations will address the variety of radiation therapy options available and customize treatment according to the stage and histology of the individual's tumor. Treatment with the external beam approach will be planned using a three-dimensional grid and will administer higher doses to the tumor bed than to the adjacent areas that frame the tumor. Although the adjacent regions to be treated may not have clinically measurable disease, these areas will be subject to direct tumor spread. The total radiation dose delivered to head and neck malignancies increases in relationship to tumor size. Microscopic tumors are usually given 50 Gy. T1 lesions receive approximately 60 Gy, while T2 tumors may receive closer to 70 Gy. Near the end of the treatment course, external beam megavoltage irradiation will usually be administered. This action adds electron boost doses to specifically targeted superficial areas.

Brachytherapy and interstitial implantation

Brachytherapy for head and neck tumors generally places radioactive material in close proximity to or directly into the tumor, usually on a temporary basis, and is generally well tolerated. A commonly used radioisotope for this treatment is cesium-137, which may be used for both intercavitary and interstitial implants. Other radioisotopes that are used for head and neck tumors are iridium-192[80] and gold-198. The application of a specific radionuclide for brachytherapy is considered according to its half-life. For example, the half-life of cesium-137 is 30 years while iridium-192 has a half-life of 74 days.

Implants are most often placed in the operating room, under general anesthesia. When surgery is not an option, brachytherapy may be combined with external beam therapy in order to boost the total dose of radiation to the tumor.[81] Under certain conditions, implants may be placed in the patient at the radiation therapy center after the patient has been given a general anesthetic. There are several methods for inserting the implants. The holders for the radioisotopes may be inserted into the tumor in the operating room, with the actual placement of the isotopes occurring later in the patient's room. This is called *afterloading*. Outpatient brachytherapy can be accomplished in the radiation center by placement of the active or "hot" isotopes there. The "hot implant" is usually given one or two times, during the middle of the individual's external beam course.[82]

Primary tumor sites that are more often treated with implants are the tongue, lip, floor of mouth, skin, nasal vestibule, and buccal mucosa. Implants are generally uncomfortable. Base of tongue lesions, for example, may be treated with needles placed into the dorsum and through the tongue to the base of tongue region. Pain must be managed and the nutritional status monitored. Oral intake may be too uncomfortable for the patient. Also, the effect of brachytherapy on speech production should be anticipated and accommodations provided.

Hospital staff and family need to follow specific precautions to protect themselves from radioisotope exposure. All items the patient uses are to be saved and can be disposed of only when determined to be free of radioactive contamination. This includes the patient's disposable dishes, soiled tissues, and dressings. Direct care staff must wear precaution gowns and gloves as well as film badges. The Hospital Radiation Safety officer needs to be involved in both the admission and discharge processes in order to ensure that safe procedures are followed. The officer will usually provide a checklist to guide direct care interventions.

Hyperthermia with radiation

Using heat in combination with radiation therapy is expected to improve tumor kill over either treatment alone, as cell destruction is magnified. The goal is for the tumor to retain the applied heat and increase oxygen consumption, which in turn increases the tumor shrinkage response to irradiation. Hyperthermia is usually given while chemotherapy is infusing. The treatment is delivered one to two times per week using temperature sensors that have been inserted into the tumor. Blisters on the skin and localized pain or discomfort are the most common side effects reported.

Biologic Therapy

Biologic agents have been generally unsuccessful thus far in the treatment of patients with head and neck tumors. Clinical trials have studied the tumor response to BCG, alfa-interferon,[83] and interleukin 2 in combination with conventional chemotherapy agents such as cisplatin and 5-FU. The failure of biologic agents to produce a tumor response may be related to the depressed cellular and humoral immunity commonly found in head and neck cancer patients.

Nursing Management of Patients Receiving Radiation Therapy and Chemotherapy

Since the cumulative doses of radiation therapy are high, tissue damage to the mucous membranes and epithelium can be anticipated. Interventions need to be implemented during treatment to help prevent or minimize tissue damage.

Mucositis

Oral mucositis occurs due to radiation and/or chemotherapy-induced destruction of the rapidly regenerating surface squamous epithelial cells of the mucous membrane. It is a progressive, painful inflammation. Tissues of the buccal mucosa, soft palate, tonsillar pillars, lateral tongue, pharyngeal walls, and larynx are predisposed to this intense tissue response as early as the first week of treatment. When the oral cavity becomes inflamed, the complication is called *stomatitis*. The first clinical signs of inflammation are evident within 7–14 days when the patient is treated with radiation therapy alone.[84] Patients receiving chemoradiation generally experience an intensified mucosal reaction over those receiving either modality alone. Hydroxyurea and 5-FU are chemotherapy drugs that are commonly part of treatment, and both contribute to mucositis.[85]

Patients are taught to cleanse the oral cavity every three to four hours during the day and at night if possible. Cleansing the oral cavity with a soft bristle brush, using toothpaste with baking soda, as well as flossing regularly are important components of oral care. Despite rigorous oral hygiene, white or yellow patches may appear as a result of epithelial tissue destruction. A sore throat or mouth closely follows, and by the fourth to fifth week of treatment, the discomfort has been building and the tissue is vividly erythemic. Oral pain is often managed topically by a pharmaceutical mixture of anesthetic and anti-inflammatory medications along with an antacid, which provides a coating action to promote adherence to the tissues. Patients are taught to swish this mixture for two to three minutes then expectorate or swallow (if allowed) four times a day (e.g., after meals and at bedtime). Coating agents may also be topically applied in the event of breakthrough discomfort.

Patients are cautioned to only use the recommended mouth rinses and to avoid using rinsing solutions containing alcohol. Individuals also should be taught to avoid spicy and acid-containing fruits, vegetables, and juices (e.g., oranges, grapefruits, lemons, and tomatoes). The individual is taught that both hot and cold foods can induce pain. Systemic analgesics such as hydrocodone or acetaminophen alone or with codeine may be necessary on an around-the-clock schedule or as needed. Transdermal dosing may be required. There has been a decline in the use of topical viscous lidocaine or diphenhydramine since cardiovascular and neurological side effects have been reported.[86]

Infection

Individuals with mucositis/stomatitis are at risk for infections. Early detection may be compromised due to the immunosuppression associated with chemotherapy. Sterile technique, including the use of gloves and mask for all procedures, should be followed during hospitalization. When an infection is suspected, diagnostic cultures are obtained and the appropriate antifungal, antibacterial, or antiviral topical or systemic medication is initiated.

Xerostomia and taste changes

When the salivary glands are treated by radiation therapy, the patient's production of saliva may decrease by up to 50% during the first one to two weeks of treatment. As treatment progresses, the saliva becomes thick, tenacious, ropey, or even nonexistent. A dental evaluation should proceed the start of radiation therapy, with extractions as necessary. In the absence of meticulous oral care, a late effect following completion of radiation therapy is multiple radiation caries,[87] which may progress to osteoradionecrosis of the mandible or maxilla.[88]

The use of either tobacco or alcohol further dries and irritates the mucosa. Radiation injury may result in permanent, noncorrectable xerostomia. Absence of saliva and the management of tenacious secretions are uncomfortable conditions. The patient experiences burning sensations or ulcerations, difficulty swallowing, and oral friction that is associated with tongue adherence to the palate or buccal mucosa. Sodium bicarbonate toothpaste and swabs will help to thin the saliva and can partially correct the acidic effect of xerostomia. Diminished saliva flow results in changes to taste and smell, especially when taste or olfactory cells are in the radiation field. Taste changes are most often first reported by the second week of treatment. The alterations to the taste of salty and bitter foods are the most pronounced changes, while the taste of sweets is the least affected. Zinc sulfate may play a role in the radiation patient's perception of taste. In a randomized study of a small number of head and neck patients who received adjuvant radiation therapy, when a zinc supplement was initiated early, at the onset of taste changes, it was reported that those individuals experienced less change in taste than those who did not receive zinc supplementation.[89]

Nursing care includes multiple interventions to promote comfort and meet nutritional needs. Pilocarpine may be prescribed either at the start of or following radiation therapy. This drug increases the secretions from the remaining portions of the salivary gland. Antholetrithione may be prescribed to promote saliva secretion and may be administered with pilocarpine for its synergistic effect.[90] Patients are taught that they need to have adequate fluid intake to meet the increased needs during treatment, especially when experiencing diaphoresis as a side effect of pilocarpine. There are artificial saliva products available; however, the soothing effect is costly and only temporary. Xerostomia may be equally relieved with frequent small sips of water. Patients are advised to carry a water bottle with them. Hard candies and sugarless gum are other ways to moisten the oral mucosa. For those who wear dentures, it is usually recommended that they not be worn unless the dentist approves. There is a high risk of progressive tissue injury and necrosis in response to the wearing of ill-fitting dentures.[91]

Skin reactions

Basal cells normally rapidly divide in order to maintain uniform thickness of the epidermis. Radiation therapy interferes with this and, within the first two weeks of treatment, erythema of the skin develops. Erythema is seen even earlier if chemotherapy is also given. In addition, dermatitis and photosensitivity are side effects of 5-FU. Melanocytes, which provide the skin its color as well as protection from ultraviolet light, are also stimulated by irradiation, which can cause the skin in the treatment area to darken.

Dry desquamation—with itchy, flaky skin—generally begins in response to rapid turnover of basal cells at about the time that the radiation dose reaches 4000 cGy. Dry desquamation can also be in response to radiation damage to the sweat glands. Moist desquamation occurs when basal cell production cannot keep up with the demand for repair. This leads to the development of a serous exudate, which oozes or drips from the damaged surface of the skin. The skin becomes markedly erythematous and painfully sensitive. The skin is never able to fully recover from wet or dry desquamation. It will remain thinner than normal and the sebaceous and sweat glands as well as the hair cells may never recover. Individuals need to be taught that the damaged skin surfaces must be protected from sun, wind, heat, and cold.

Skin folds such as those found behind the ear, at the collar line and the creases of the neck, under the chin, and around the tracheostomy tube need to be closely monitored and protected. Loose clothing made of soft fabric should be worn. At the start of skin changes, the radiation therapy nurse may advise using an aloe vera gel or a lubricating cream that absorbs water. Use of any skin care product must have prior approval from the radiation oncologist. Then, application of the moisturizing cream to the involved skin should be provided at least four times a day. Diphenhydramine may be given to manage pruritus. For moist desquamation, the skin should be covered and protected at all times. Topical antibiotics such as 1% silver sulfadiazine (with monitoring for hypersensitivity), may be approved for use only during the weeks the patient is not receiving radiation therapy, since it leaves a residue on the skin.

The preferred coverage for moist desquamation is often a moisture- and vapor-permeable hydrogel or hydrocolloid dressing. These products have a high water content, can absorb some drainage, and are cool to the skin. It is advisable to refrigerate the dressings to enhance the cooling effect. With either of these dressings, a moist environment for healing is provided that also gently debrides the wound so the dressing can be removed for replacement with less pain. Hydrogel dressings are effective for up to 12 hours. As part of the dressing change, the skin is gently cleansed with gauze moistened with normal saline prior to application of the replacement hydrogel. The hydrogel dressing may be reinforced with a gauze dressing and supported by stockinet.[92]

The patient is taught to examine the skin twice daily, and interventions should begin as soon as skin reactions occur. The individual needs to know that skin reactions are to be expected and are not an indication of tumor progression. It should also be explained that the cumulative effects of radiation and chemotherapy on the skin continue on the weekends or weeks when treatment is not given, as well as for at least one month after treatment is concluded. The skin care regimen is to be followed until healing occurs, which is usually within 6–12 weeks.

Trismus

When the patient's treatment involves the oral cavity muscles for mastication or affects the posterior mandible, the opening of the oral cavity may become tightly restricted. Also, when grafts or neck surgery have diminished the circulation to the oral cavity, the patient is at risk for developing fibrosis of the muscles of the oral cavity as a late effect of treatment. This restriction may result in the inability of the individual to open the mouth. It is necessary to teach exercises that can stretch the interarch of the oral cavity over time. One method is to use increasing numbers of stacked tongue blades to stretch the opening, until there is a slight increase in discomfort, but not marked pain. This exercise should be done three or four times a day.

Fatigue

Most patients receiving radiation or chemotherapy describe a building fatigue, which gradually worsens during the treatment course. Individuals on chemoradiation protocols describe a more intense effect, especially when receiving hyperfractionated treatments. Although this condition is less discussed in the literature for the surgical patient, with multiple or expansive resections it should be expected that fatigue will be experienced. Fatigue can take months to resolve. Hematological and nutritional parameters should be monitored and corrected during this recovery time. Patients have stated that grouping activities and taking rest periods helps to cope with fatigue. Short walks when rested or hobbies such as music and art may also be helpful.

Symptom Management and Supportive Care

Airway Management

When the airway of the individual with head and neck cancer is compromised by tumor or postoperative edema, a tracheostomy may be required. The tracheostomy may be temporary or permanent. It may be placed in anticipation of airway obstruction or to manage the existing, compromised pulmonary function. Tracheostomy is usually performed in the operating room under general anesthesia, and may be done at the time of the panendoscopy.

The type of tracheostomy tube needed in the first postoperative days is a high-volume, low-pressure, cuffed tube. The brand of tracheostomy tube used depends upon what the physician prefers and what products the hospital carries. Customized tubes can be developed and available in advance of the operation for those who cannot be fitted with a standard-sized tube.

Tracheostomy tube products

Tracheostomy tubes are made of plastic, silicone, or metal. Plastic and metal tubes have an inner cannula, while silicone tracheostomy tubes have a single cannula. Components of the tracheostomy tube are described in Table 56-7.

Tracheostomy and laryngectomy care

Tracheostomy care includes providing ongoing attention to both the tracheostomy and the patency and cleanliness of the tracheostomy or laryngectomy tube. Sterile technique is followed in the hospital for patient protection from environmental organisms. Clean technique is taught and followed for self-care. *Tracheostomy care* is the generic term used regardless of the type of tube used. The laryngectomy tube is slightly shorter with less of an acute curve when compared to the tracheostomy tube.

Because there is no communication between the oral cavity esophagus and airway, there is no risk of aspiration or airway collapse with a laryngectomy. Once the stoma has matured, a laryngectomy tube is not necessary to maintain patency. The laryngectomy tube is otherwise of the same design with comparable management. During the postoperative period and during the ongoing treatment phase, the stoma site should be inspected and the tube cleaned at least every eight hours (see Table 56-8).

Individuals with altered airways have lost the ability for the nose to moisten, warm, or filter the air they breathe. This results in thick, tenacious, dry tracheal secretions that are a challenge to clear by coughing, and can result in mucous plugs that obstruct the tracheostomy tube and risk total blockage of breathing. Patients and their caregivers need to understand the importance of providing supplemental humidity. In the hospital, warm, humidified oxygen should be administered via tracheostomy collar when the patient is at rest. At home, the living area should have a large (ten-gallon) humidifier and, in the sleeping room, a small bedside humidifier for nighttime use. The laryngectomy patient should be taught that moistened gauze pads and foam or crocheted stoma covers, besides filtering the airway, collect the moisture of exhaled air and are sources of humidity. Instilling up to 5 mL of normal saline or spraying four to five puffs of normal saline into the stoma using a nasal atomizer are additional methods for increasing humidity.

Nutritional Management

Nutritional support is of paramount importance in providing the calories for healing following surgical resection and also during the extended time period required for intensive radiation or chemotherapy treatments. Ongoing consultation with the nutritionist is important upon the patient's admission and throughout treatment. Before the diagnosis of cancer, many head and neck patients already have nutritional deficits. When there is a prior condition of substance abuse or cirrhosis, the individual may have a long history of anorexia as well. Since head and neck malignancies do not usually cause pain, cancer-related weight loss is common, as the individual gradually accommodates to impairments in mastication and/or deglutition. Before treatment starts, there may already be significant, measurable, blood serum abnormalities. Magnesium is a marker to be tracked. Assessing protein levels at baseline and during treatment is standard. Since serum albumin has a half-life of 20 days, serum transferrin, with a half-life of ten days may be followed[93] along with the standard measurements of anemia.

Enteral therapy

Although an individual with a head and neck malignancy commonly has a functioning GI system, a portion of the person's upper tract can become temporarily or permanently obstructed. If this occurs, or the patient is unable to swallow for any reason, tube feedings will become necessary. Tube feedings are preferred over hyperalimentation unless intestinal function is impaired. Enteral feedings are administered through either a nasogastric feeding tube or a gastrostomy tube. The surgeon can place either the nasogastric or gastrostomy tube at the time of the panendoscopy or surgical resection. Another option is for the outpatient interventional radiologist to insert a gastrostomy tube with a smaller diameter by percutaneous puncture (PEG tube). The type of feeding tube chosen will depend upon the unique needs of the patient and duration of time the tube is needed.

Nasogastric tubes, made with or without stylets, small bore (8–12 French), flexible, and generally weighted. Small-bore tubes can be used for an extended time period with minimal irritation to the nasopharyngeal, esophageal, or gastric mucosa. It is recommended that only experienced staff insert stylet-containing tubes, due to the altered or sensitive mucosa and the risks for esophageal perforation or pulmonary insertion with lung puncture. The nasogastric tube can only be used after an x-ray of the abdomen has confirmed correct placement.

Standard gastrostomy tube placement may be preferred, as the feeding tube is not visible, does not pass through the irritated mucosa, and is larger in diameter, so it is less likely to become clogged. Tube feeding starts upon return of bowel sounds. For either the nasogastric or the gastrostomy tube, the patient assumes a sitting position or elevates the head of the bed. The usual check for residual feedings may not be possible with small-bore tubes. Feedings generally start at the slow rate of 25 to 30 mL/hour and may be advanced up to 25 additional mL/hr per day in order to provide the calories and volume needed.[94] Administration of tube feedings may be by gravity or pump and may be bolus (every four to six hours) or continuous flow. The dietitian monitors the nutritional status closely and recommends formula changes if the patient develops side effects, such as diarrhea. It is known that certain antibiotics cause diarrhea, but liquid medications containing sorbital, such as some formulations of acetaminophen plus codeine, can increase the incidence as well.[95]

Swallowing Rehabilitation

To perform deglutition is to transport liquid or a bolus of food through the patient's oral cavity, fauces, pharynx, esophagus, and into the stomach. Preservation and/or restoration of the swallowing function is a primary rehabilitation goal. The mobility of pharyngeal structures is assessed, noting hyoid elevation and displacement. Swallowing evaluations are structured collaboratively by the speech pathologist, radiologist, and advanced practice nurse. Function is studied by offering videofluoroscopy and a modified "cookie" barium swallow. The efficiency of the swallow will be examined during the management of paste and liquid consistencies. The presence or absence of aspiration, the amount of pharyngeal residue post-swallow, and the length of in-transit time are noted. Because inpatient stays are brief, the swallowing therapist assesses swallowing function when the patient returns for clinic visits.

In order for normal oral feedings to resume, the swallowing therapist and the surgeon will need to determine that the individual has acceptable function. When the physiology of the oral cavity has been compromised, for example by a resection of the tongue, the patient will need to learn methods for using the remainder of the tongue to propel a bolus of food back to and through the anterior faucial arches for the first phase of swallowing. When the sensory triggers for swallowing have been impaired due to damage to any of the cranial nerves—trigeminal (V), facial (VII), glossopharyngeal (IX), vagus (X), spinal accessory (XI), or hypoglossal (XII)—the swallowing triggers will be affected. Videofluoroscopy and the speech pathologist's evaluation will provide the diagnostic assessment data for the individual's four phases of swallowing,[96] as described in Table 56-9. Sievers[97] defines important nursing assessments of the dysphagic patient to be accomplished during a swallow: (1) auscultation of larynx, (2) evaluations for cough and voice impairment, (3) notations of gurgling with respiration, and (4) estimation of fatigue.

Kotz and colleagues[98] found that patients who have been treated with hydroxyurea in combination with hyperfractionated external beam radiation therapy on a larynx-sparing protocol have developed long-lasting deficits in pharyngeal function with impaired bolus transport. Kendall and associates[99] reported a general decrease in mobility of the pharyngeal structures following single-modality radiation therapy, with hyoid displacement occurring at the same level of elevation irregardless of bolus size. It has been reported that patients who have transport problems in movement of the bolus usually adapt and achieve improved function more successfully than those who have either impaired pharyngeal reflexes or inferior laryngeal sphincter function.[100]

Pain Management

The severing of superficial nerves during surgery may account for feelings of numbness over the operative area in the initial postoperative period. The subsequent edema results in feelings of pressure. When the jugular vein has been ligated or occluded, the increase in spinal fluid pressure may cause the patient to experience throbbing, pounding, and pressure sensations in the head. Postoperative pain control promotes comfort, permitting early ambulation, regular coughing, and deep breathing exercises. If there is a history of preoperative substance abuse, the nurse recognizes that opioid tolerance levels for this individual may vary from the norm, and that interventions for substance abuse are most helpful later, when the patient is more accustomed to the treatment protocol.

As mentioned previously, patients receiving radiation therapy alone, with or without chemotherapy, can experience high levels of discomfort due to mucosal and skin injury. Acetaminophen elixirs alone or with codeine may be helpful. It is preferable to use oral or enteral routes for pain management. In the case of intensely painful tissue reactions, however, fentanyl transdermal patches can be used to provide around-the-clock pain relief. When there is frequent use of pain medication, the nurse monitors bowel function. Should the patient report constipation for 48 hours, stool softener/laxative combinations should be taken daily and the amount of fluid intake, either by mouth or by feeding tube, increased.

Speech Restoration

When the patient has a total or partial laryngectomy or sustains laryngeal injury resulting in a weak or absent voice, the person may fear never speaking again. For the elderly patient, it is considered that in the normal course of time, at around age 65, voice quality, volume, and frequency change, resulting in a weaker voice. For all patients who have had partial laryngectomy surgeries, either the supraglottic or the hemilaryngectomy procedure, speech therapy will be required in order to strengthen the remaining portions of the larynx. Vocal cord adduction will have to be enhanced to improve voice quality, and the individual will be expected to learn to compensate for reduced laryngeal closure to avoid aspiration.

Total laryngectomy surgery eliminates the person's ability to speak. The laryngectomy patient will be able to participate in the selection of one or more restorative speech methods that will suit for day-to-day vocal for communication. Choices include:

Table 56-9	Phases of Swallowing
Phase	**Purpose**
Oral preparation	Movements of the lips, oral, and facial musculature, and the tongue in response to food (bolus) placement into oral cavity
Oral phase	Closure of the nasopharynx with soft palate retraction and elevation to propel bolus back to the posterior pharyngeal wall
Pharyngeal phase	Initiate the swallow to pass the bolus through the pharynx, involving laryngeal elevation and forward tilt
Esophageal phase	Laryngeal pull opens the cricopharyngeus and waves of peristalsis propel the bolus through the lower esophagus and into the stomach

Adapted with permission from Caplan S, et al: Speech therapy for verbal communication disorders and swallowing/dysphagia conditions and care, in Harris LL, Huntoon MB (eds): *Core Curriculum for Otorhinolaryngology and Head-Neck Nursing*. New Smyrna Beach, Society of Otorhinolaryngology and Head-Neck Nurses, 1998, pp 300–302.[49]

1. *Artificial larynx:* an electronic, vibrating device that resonates sound into the oral cavity, generating mechanical, robot-like speech; easy to learn.
2. *Esophageal speech:* swallowing air into the esophagus the person articulates instantly with the expulsion of air to form speech; "burping speech"; no equipment required; may take up to six months to learn.
3. *Tracheoesophageal puncture (TEP):* one-way plastic valve prosthesis that fits into a small tracheoesophageal slit; puncture is created while patient is under general anesthesia; provides for airflow from lung to esophagus to mouth when stoma is occluded; results in fluent, easy-to-learn speech; prevents aspiration; requires adequate stoma size, cricopharyngeal muscle, hand-eye coordination, and bimanual dexterity. The patient must learn to clean, maintain, and insert the prosthesis.[101]

With the choices available, the laryngectomy patient should be able to achieve satisfactory speech. The artificial larynx devices and esophageal speech are more commonly recommended. However, a recent retrospective study at the University of Illinois Hospital and Clinics and Westside Veterans Administration Hospital reviewed speech outcomes after tracheoesophageal puncture and followed individuals over a ten-year period. It was found that despite high alcohol abuse rates and low socioeconomic status, 66% of the individuals achieved long-term success with TEP speech.[102]

Psychosocial Support

When the person has a long history of smoking or drinking, the stress of what is felt to be a self-induced malignancy may hinder the recovery process. Depression, which is closely linked with anger, and also anxiety can contribute to noncompliance. It is important for those caring for these individuals to be supportive and to partner with the patient during the evolution of the treatment process. Knowledge reduces stress and promotes recovery.

Head and neck malignancies are devastating. Some of the key senses, including sight, taste, smell, hearing and sense of touch may be permanently impaired. When the social, emotional, and physical ways a person relates to others is changed by a deformity, the individual may feel isolated or rejected. During the first weeks of treatment the person is coping with self-image changes. Further, while coping with fatigue, the individual must learn complex self-care rituals such as dressing changes, tracheostomy care, and suctioning, as well as enteral feeding techniques. Although support from a significant other is important, the individual is taught and encouraged to perform all self-care activities if possible. A visit by a recovered patient with a similar diagnosis may be requested from the Lost Chord Club, American Cancer Society, or another community group. Such a visit may be well received about seven days after surgery.

In general, most patients will begin to incorporate their disfigurement into their concept of self early in the postoperative period. During this time, if the patient is not making progress with self-care, additional intensive teaching and coaching by the nurse should help achieve acceptance. When patients do not assume self-care early in the recovery period, the stage can be set for maladaptive, long-term anxiety and related continual difficulties with self-care management.[103]

Continuity of Care: Nursing Challenges

The management of care for the head and neck patient has been impeded by an increasing number of obstacles during the last decade. At many treatment centers, the specialized head and neck unit has disappeared in response to the increase in same-day surgeries and shorter hospital stays. In both the acute and ambulatory settings, a nurse is responsible for increasing numbers of patients and may be unable to spend an appropriate amount of time teaching the patient about surgery and self-care needs. In the early postoperative period, follow-up care needs to be coordinated with appropriate members of the rehabilitation team. Often appointments are not kept and recovery is less than optimal.

The costs of specialized therapies are also steadily increasing and insurance companies are often unwilling to pay for such services. Working with a case manager will help to secure services for the patient. It is important that patient discharge needs are identified early, prior to initiating surgical and therapeutic interventions. It can be anticipated if the patient will have an altered airway, need enteral feedings, require direct care needs and supervision, or will need special equipment at home. When the patient is to receive combined therapy, may be now possible for all chemotherapy and radiation treatments to be outpatient. Home infusion therapy continues to make rapid advances in methods and modes for chemotherapy administration. The home care nurse sees the patient nearly every day and is in a position to promote timely communication and coordination with all members of the team. In the process, self-care teaching and proper usage of equipment can be monitored and reinforced.[104]

Quality-of-Life Issues

By the late 1990s, quality of life outcomes, which measured the person's response to a variety of effects of treatment, became important parts of head and neck investigational protocols. Head and neck studies have addressed outcomes such as body image,[105] depression,[106] and sexuality.[107] In a recent study, Gritz and associates[108] followed 105 persons with newly diagnosed cancer of the head and neck region for 12 months following smoking cessation interventions. Those who had stop smoking had improvements in speech and swallowing, but experienced decreased marital/sexual functioning and increased alcohol use.

Quality-of-life assessments outcomes are part of most organ-preservation trials but are not yet standardized across studies. In a follow-up to the Department of Veterans Affairs Laryngeal Cancer Study Group publication reported earlier, survivors of the Veterans Affairs Laryngeal Cancer Study #268 of longer than nine years were surveyed with a 71% response (65 patients).[109] A better quality of life was achieved by the chemotherapy plus radiation therapy group versus the surgery plus radiation therapy group. Well-being was not related to preservation of speech but to less pain and lower levels of depression.

The combinations of treatment modalities studied have yet to clarify, for either early or advanced disease, what treatment course can best improve survival. In light of this, quality of life questions are becoming influential considerations within the treatment-planning process. For quality-of-life data to become truly meaningful, it will be necessary for universal comparisons to be made and for the same measurement scales to be utilized across treatment centers in similar ways. The measurement tools will need to be sensitive to the stage of disease and types of treatment. Methods for how and when to collect and record the data and analytic processes for interpretating the data need to be standardized in order to truly be able to use quality-of-life parameters in the head and neck clinical setting.

Conclusion

Head and neck patients today are experiencing the effects of better cosmetic results, improvements in physiological functioning and psychosocial understanding, and better management of symptoms. Improvements in equipment, materials, and medications are resulting in better, safer products. Public education efforts are geared toward informing the public about the risks associated with tobacco and alcohol use, especially concerning smokeless tobacco, second-hand smoke, and habitual drinking. Oncology nurses need to be involved at every level of prevention. Nursing research that provides outcomes for (1) adaptation strategies and (2) measurements to promote self-care and acceptance of disfigurement is necessary to help the individual with head and neck cancer achieve acceptable function and quality of life.

References

1. Landis SH, Murray T, Bolden S, et al: Cancer statistics, 1998. *CA Cancer J Clin* 48:6–25, 1998
2. American Cancer Society: Cancer facts and figures 1999: selected cancers, oral cavity and pharynx. American Cancer Society *www.cancer.org:pp* 7–8, 1999
3. American Cancer Society: Cancer facts and figures 1997. *American Cancer Society.* 13:1–32, 1997
4. Parker SL, Davis KJ, Wingo PA, et al: Cancer statistics by race and ethnicity. *CA Cancer J Clin* 48:31–48, 1998
5. Davidson BJ, Ellenhorn JDI, Shah JP: Head and neck cancer, in Harvey JC, Beattie EJ (eds): *Cancer Surgery.* Philadelphia, Saunders, 1996, pp 1–29
6. Jacobs CD: Etiologic considerations for head and neck squamous cancers, in Jacobs C (ed): *Carcinomas of the Head and Neck.* Boston, Kluwer Academic, 1990, pp 265–282
7. Armstrong RW, Imrey PB, Lye ML, et al: Nasopharyngeal carcinoma in Malaysian Chinese: salted fish and other dietary exposures. *Int J Cancer* 77:228–235, 1998
8. McEwen DR, Sanchez MM: A guide to salivary gland disorders. *AORN J* 65:559–567, 1997
9. Vokes EE, Weichselbaum RR, Lippman SM, et al: Head and neck cancer. *N Engl J Med* 328:184–194, 1993
10. Jaber MA, Porter SR, Scully C, et al: The role of alcohol in non-smokers and tobacco in non-drinkers in the aetiology of oral epithelial dysplasia. *Int J Cancer* 77:333–336, 1998
11. Visscher JG, Vanderwaal AM: Etiology of cancer of the lip: a review. *Int J Oral Maxillofac Surg* 27:199–203, 1998
12. Morita M, Kuwano H, Nashashima, et al: Family aggregation of carcinoma of the hypopharynx and cervical esophagus: special reference to multiplicity of cancer in the upper aerodigestive tract. *Int J Cancer* 76:468–471, 1998
13. Mayne ST, Lippman SM: Cancer prevention. Chemopreventive agents, in DeVita Jr VT, Hellman S, Rosenberg SA (eds): *Cancer: Principles and Practice of Oncology* (ed 5). Philadelphia, Lippincott-Raven, 1997, pp 585–617
14. Levi F, Pasche C, LaVecchia C, et al: Food groups and risk of oral and pharyngeal cancer. *Int J Cancer* 77:705–709, 1998
15. Sidransky D: Cancer of the head and neck, in DeVita Jr VT, Hellman S, Rosenberg SA (eds): *Cancer: Principles and Practice of Oncology* (ed 5). Philadelphia, Lippincott-Raven, 1997, pp 735–740
16. Bonner P: The national oral cancer awareness program. *Otolaryngol-Head Neck Nurs* 16(2):15–19, 1998
17. Barnes L: Pathology of the head and neck: general considerations, in Myers EN, Suen JY (eds): *Cancer of the Head and Neck* (ed 3). Philadelphia: Saunders, 1996, pp 17–29
18. Portugal LG, Goldenberg JD, Wenig BL, et al: Human papillomavirus expression and p53 gene mutations in squamous cell carcinoma. *Arch Otolaryngol Head Neck Surg* 123:1230–1234, 1997
19. Rowley NJR, Helliwell TR, Caslin A, et al: p53 protein expression in tumours from head and neck subsites, larynx and hypopharynx, and differences in relationship to survival. *Otolaryngology* 23:57–62, 1998
20. Pruneri G, Pignotaro L, Carboni N, et al: Clinical relevance of p53 and bcl-2 protein over-expression in laryngeal squamous cell carcinoma. *Int J Cancer* 79:263–268, 1998
21. Nogueira CP, Dolan RW, Gooey J, et al: Inactivation of p53 and amplification of cyclin D1 correlate with clinical outcome in head and neck cancer. *Laryngoscope* 108:345–350, 1998
22. Myers JN: Molecular pathogenesis of squamous cell carcinoma of the head and neck, in Myers EN, Suen JY (eds): *Cancer of the Head and Neck* (ed 3). Philadelphia, Saunders, 1996, pp 6–10
23. Leon X, Quer M, Diez S, et al: Second neoplasms in patients with head and neck cancer. *Head Neck* 21(3):204–210, 1999
24. Koch WM: Axillary nodal metastases in head and neck cancer. *Head Neck* 21(3):269–272, 1999

25. Yellowitz JA, Goodman HS, Farooq NS: Knowledge, opinions, and practices related to oral cancer: results of three elderly racial groups. *Spec Care Dentist* 17(3):100–104, 1997

26. Goodwin Jr WJ, Bakany T, Casiano RR: Managing geriatric patients, in Cummings CW, Fredrickson JM, Harker LA, et al (eds): *Otolaryngology Head and Neck Surgery* (ed 3). St Louis, Mosby, 1998, pp 314–326

27. Zagars GK, Norante JD, Smith JL, et al: Tumors of the head and neck, in Rubin P, McDonald S, Qazi R (eds): *A Multidisciplinary Approach for Physicians and Students* (ed 7). Philadelphia, Saunders, 1993, pp 319–362

28. Andresen HG, Cyr MH, Guadagnini JP, et al: General history, risk factors, and normal physical assessment, in Harris LL, Huntoon MB (eds): *Core Curriculum for Otorhinolaryngology and Head-Neck Nursing*. New Smyrna Beach, Society of Otorhinolaryngology and Head-Neck Nurses, 1998, pp 9–29

29. Curtin HD, Weissman JL: Radiologic evaluation of head and neck cancer, in Myers EN, Suen JY (eds): *Cancer of the Head and Neck* (ed 3). Philadelphia, Saunders, 1996, pp 50–59

30. Sievers AEF, Borcyckowski D: Nursing care of skull base surgery patients, in Donald PH (ed): *Surgery of the Skull Base*. Philadelphia, Lippincott-Raven, 1998, pp 119–136

31. Houghton DJ, McGarry G, Stewart I, et al: Chest computerized tomography scanning in patients presenting with head and neck cancer. *Clin Otolaryngol* 23:348–350, 1998

32. American Joint Committee on Cancer: *AJCC Cancer Staging Manual* (ed 5). Philadelphia, Lippincott-Raven. 1997

33. Martin JW, Austin JR, Chambers MS, et al: Postoperative care of the maxillectomy patient. *Otolaryngol Head Neck Nurs* 12(3):15–20, 1994

34. Wei WI, Sham JS: Cancer of the nasopharynx cancer, in Myers EN, Suen JY (eds): *Cancer of the Head and Neck* (ed 3). Philadelphia, Saunders, 1996, pp 284–285

35. Schantz SP, Harrison LB, Forastiere AA: Tumors of the nasal cavity and paranasal sinuses, nasopharynx, oral cavity, and oropharynx, in DeVita Jr VT, Hellman S, Rosenberg SA (eds): *Cancer: Principles and Practice of Oncology* (ed 5). Philadelphia, Lippincott-Raven, 1997, pp 741–802

36. Burkey BB, Garrett G: Use of the laser in the oral cavity. *Otolaryngol Clin North Am* 29:949–961, 1996

37. Truelson JM, Pearce AN: Tongue reconstruction procedures for treatment of cancer. *AORN J* 65(3):531–534, 1997

38. Altman K, Avery CM, Johnson PA: Reconstruction techniques in oral carcinoma. *Dental Update* 24(2):50–52, 1997

39. Cutright LH, Guadagnini JP: Oropharynx conditions and care, in Harris LL, Huntoon MB (eds): *Core Curriculum for Otorhinolaryngology and Head-Neck Nursing*. New Smyrna Beach, Society of Otorhinolaryngology and Head-Neck Nurses, 1998, pp 217–226

40. Sessions RB, Harrison LB, Forastiere AA: Tumors of the salivary glands and paragangliomas, in DeVita Jr VT, Hellman S, Rosenberg SA (eds): *Cancer: Principles and Practice of Oncology* (ed 5). Philadelphia, Lippincott-Raven, 1997, pp 830–847

41. Guadagnini JP, Means ME: Salivary, dental, TMJ and sleep apnea conditions and care, in Harris LL, Huntoon MB (eds): *Core Curriculum for Otorhinolaryngology and Head-Neck Nursing*. New Smyrna Beach, Society of Otorhinolaryngology and Head-Neck Nurses, 1998, pp 235–236

42. McEwen DR, Sanchez MM: A guide to salivary gland disorders. *AORN J* 65:571–572, 1997

43. Davis RK: Endoscopic surgical management of glottic laryngeal cancer. *Otolaryngol Clin North Am* 30:79–86, 1997

44. Osguthorpe JD, Putney FJ: Open surgical management of early glottic carcinoma cancer. *Otolaryngol Clin North Am* 30:87–99, 1997

45. Zeitels SM: Surgical management of early supraglottic cancer. *Otolaryngol Clin North Am* 30:59–78, 1997

46. Riley MA: Home exercises following neck dissection: the development of an instructional video. *The Journal* 9(1): 21–23, 1991

47. Myers EN: Management of cancer of the supraglottic larynx: evolution, current concepts, and future trends. *Laryngoscope* 106:559–567, 1996

48. Isaacs JH, Slattery WH, Mendenhall WM, et al: Supraglottic laryngectomy. *Clin ORL* 19:118–123, 1998

49. Caplan S, Hickey MM, Overmeyer CE, et al: Speech therapy for verbal communication disorders and swallowing/dysphagia conditions and care, in Harris LL, Huntoon MB (eds): *Core Curriculum for Otorhinolaryngology and Head-Neck Nursing*. New Smyrna Beach, Society of Otorhinolaryngology and Head-Neck Nurses, 1998, pp 300–302

50. Sinard RJ, Netterville JL, Garrett CG: Cancer of the larynx, in Myers EN, Suen JY (eds): *Cancer of the Head and Neck* (ed 3). Philadelphia, Saunders, 1996, pp 415

51. Sessions RB, Harrison LB, Forastiere AA: Tumors of the larynx and hypopharynx, in DeVita Jr VT, Hellman S, Rosenberg SA (eds): *Cancer: Principles and Practice of Oncology* (ed 5). Philadelphia, Lippincott-Raven, 1997, pp 802–829

52. Cyr MH, Higgins TS, McGuire MA: Laryngeal, hypopharyngeal conditions and care, in Harris LL, Huntoon MB (eds): *Core Curriculum for Otorhinolaryngology and Head-Neck Nursing*. New Smyrna Beach, Society of Otorhinolaryngology and Head-Neck Nurses, Inc, 1998, pp 275–290

53. Goding Jr GS: Skin flap physiology, in Cummings CW, Frederickson JM, Harker LA, et al (eds): *Otolaryngology Head and Neck Surgery* (ed 3). St Louis: Mosby, 1998, pp 145–170

54. Miller MJ, Robb GL, Schusterman MA: Microvascular reconstruction for cutaneous defects. *Clin Plast Surg* 24: 769–778, 1997

55. Marx RE, Morales MJ: The use of implants in the reconstruction of oral cancer patients. *Dental Clin North Am* 42: 177–202, 1998

56. Connor CD, Fosko SW: Anatomy and physiology of local skin flaps, Branham GH (ed) in *Facial Plast Surg Clin North Am*: 4:447–454, 1996

57. Adams JF, Lassen LF: Leech therapy for venous congestion following myocutaneous pectoralis flap reconstruction. *Otolaryngol Head Neck Nurs* 13(1):12–14, 1995

58. Cody DT, Funk GF, Wagner D, et al: The use of granulocyte colony stimulating factor to promote wound healing in a neutropenic patient after head and neck surgery. *Head Neck* 21:172–175, 1999

59. Shade RJ, Pisters KM, Huber MH, et al: Phase I study of paclitaxel administered by ten-day continuous infusion. *Invest New Drugs* 16:237–243, 1998–1999

60. Fountzilas G, Stathopoulos G, Nicolaides C, et al: Paclitaxel and gemcitabine in advanced non-nasopharyngeal head and neck cancer; a phase II study conducted by the Hellenic Cooperative Oncology Group. *Ann Oncol* 10:475–478, 1999

61. Hofmann GA, Dev SB, Dimmer S, et al: Electroporation therapy: a new approach for the treatment of head and neck cancer. *IEEE Trans Biomed Eng* 46:752–759, 1999

62. Lowe VJ, Dunphy FR, Varvares M, et al: Evaluation of chemotherapy response in patients with advanced head and neck cancer using [F-18]fluorodeoxyglucose positron emission tomography. *Head Neck* 19:666–674, 1997

63. The Department of Veterans Affairs Laryngeal Cancer Study Group: Induction chemotherapy plus radiation compared with surgery and radiation in patients with advanced laryngeal cancer. *N Engl J Med* 324:1685–1690, 1991

64. Jacobs C, Makuch R: Efficacy of adjuvant chemotherapy for patients with resectable head and neck cancer: a subset analysis of the head and neck contracts program. *J Clin Oncol* 8:838–847, 1990

65. de Serdio JL, Villar A, Martinez JC, et al: Chemotherapy as a part of each treatment fraction in a twice-a-day hyperfractionated schedule: a new chemoradiotherapy approach for advanced head and neck cancer. *Head Neck* 20:489–496, 1998

66. Carew JF, Shah JP: Advances in multimodality therapy for laryngeal cancer. *CA Cancer J Clin* 48:211–228, 1998

67. Vokes EE, Awan AM, Weichselbaum RR: Radiotherapy with concomitant chemotherapy for head and neck cancer. *Hematol Oncol Clin North Am* 5:753–767, 1991

68. Schlemmer HP, Becker M, Bachert P, et al: Alterations of intratumoral pharmocokinetics of 5-fluorouracil in head and neck carcinoma during simultaneous radiochemotherapy. *Cancer Res* 59:2363–2369, 1999

69. Herscher LL, Cook J: Taxanes as radiosensitizers for head and neck cancer. *Curr Opin Oncol* 11:183–186, 1999

70. Bachaud JM, David JM, Boussin G, et al: Combined postoperative radiotherapy and weekly cisplatin infusion for locally advanced squamous cell carcinoma of the head and neck: preliminary report of a randomized trial. *Int J Radiat Oncol Biol Phys* 20:243–246, 1991

71. Nishioka T, Shirato H, Fukuda S, et al: A phase II study of concomitant chemoradiotherpay for laryngeal carcinoma using carboplatin. *Oncology* 56:36–42, 1999

72. Gupta NK, Pointon RCS, Wilkinson PM. A randomized clinical trial to contrast radiation therapy with radiation and methotrexate given synchronously in head and neck cancer. *Clin Radiol* 38:575–581, 1987

73. Brizel DM, Albers ME, Fisher SR, et al: Hyperfractionated irradiation with or without concurrent chemotherapy for locally advanced head and neck cancer. *N Engl J Med* 338 : 1798–1803, 1998

74. Forastiere AA, Shank D, Neuberg D, et al: Final report of a phase II evaluation of paclitaxel in patients with advanced squamous cell carcinoma of the head and neck. An eastern cooperative oncology group trial. *Cancer* 82:2270–2274, 1998

75. Vokes EE: Interactions of chemotherapy and radiation. *Semin Oncol* 20:70–79, 1993

76. Nafoor BM, Spiro IJ, Wang CC, et al: Results of accelerated radiotherapy for supraglottic carcinoma: a Massachusetts General Hospital and Masachusetts Eye and Ear Infirmary experience. *Head Neck* 20:379–384, 1998

77. Spector JG, Sessions DG, Chao KS, et al: Management of stage II (T2N0M0) glottic carcinoma by radiotherapy and conservation surgery. *Head Neck* 21:116–123, 1999

78. Adam MF, Gabalski EC, Bloch DA, et al: Tissue oxygen distribution in head and neck cancer patients. *Head Neck* 21:146–153, 1999

79. Strohl RA: The etiology and management of acute and late sequelae of radiation therapy in persons with head and neck cancers. *Otolaryngol Head Neck Nurs* 13(4):23–27, 1995

80. Klein M, Menneking H, Langford K, et al: Treatment of squamous cell carcinomas of the floor of mouth and tongue by interstitial high-dose-rate irradiation using iridium-192. *Int J Oral Maxillofac Surg* 27:45–48, 1998

81. Harrison LB, Lee HJ, Pfister DG: Long term results of primary radiotherapy with/without neck dissection for squamous cell cancer of the base of tongue. *Head Neck* 20: 668–673, 1998

82. Dow KH: Principles of brachytherapy, in Dow KH, Hilderley LJ (eds): *Nursing Care in Radiation Oncology.* Philadelphia, Saunders, 1992, pp 16–29

83. Langer CJ, Schaebler D, Sauter E, et al: Phase II study of N-phosphonacetyl-L-aspartate, recombinant interferon-alpha, and fluorouracil infusion in advanced squamous cell carcinoma of the head and neck. *Head Neck* 20:385–391, 1998

84. Madeya ML: Oral complications from cancer therapy: part I-pathophysiology and secondary complications. *Onc Nurs Forum* 23:801–807, 1996

85. Beck SL: Mucositis, in Yarbro CH, Frogge MH, Goodman M, (eds): *Cancer Symptom Management* (ed 2). Sudbury, MA, Jones and Bartlett, 1999, pp 328–342

86. Madeya ML: Oral complications from cancer therapy: part I-pathophysiology and secondary complications. *Oncol Nurs Forum* 23:801–807, 1996

87. Barbour-Randall L: Radiation induced xerostomia: a review. *The Journal* 9:7–10, 1991

88. London SD, Park SS, Gampper TJ, et al: Hyperbaric oxygen for the management of radionecrosis of bone and cartilage. *Laryngoscope* 108:1291–1296, 1998

89. Ripamonti C, Zecca E, Brunelli C, et al: A randomized, controlled clinical trial to evaluate the effects of zinc sulfate on cancer patients with taste alterations caused by head and neck irradiation. *Cancer* 82:1938–1945, 1999

90. Maydeya MA: Oral complications from cancer therapy: part 2-nursing implications for assessment and treatment. *Oncol Nurs Forum* 23:308–323, 1996

91. Garg AK, Malo M: Manifestations and treatment of xerostomia and associated oral effects secondary to head and neck radiation therapy. *J Am Dent Assoc* 128:1128–1133, 1997

92. Myers JS, Warren T: Elastic net secures facial dressings comfortably. *Oncol Nurs Forum* 23:1484, 1996

93. Wenig BL, Goldenberg JD: Malnutrition from cancer, in Gates GA (ed): *Current Therapy in ORL and Head-Neck Surgery* (ed 6). St Louis, Mosby, 1998, pp 323–326

94. Dawson CJ, Hanrahan KA, Means ME, et al: Development of an enteral feeding protocol. *Otolaryngol Head Neck Nurs* 14(4):15–17, 1996

95. Reese JL, Means ME, Hanrahan K: The maze of variables associated with enteral feeding intolerance. *Otolaryngol Head Neck Nurs* 10(2):13–15, 1992

96. Barbour LA: Dysphagia, in Yarbro CH, Frogge MH, Goodman M, (eds): *Cancer Symptom Management* (ed 2). Sudbury, MA, Jones and Bartlett, 1999, pp 209–227

97. Sievers AEF: Nursing evaluation and care of the dysphagic patient, in Leonard R, Kendall K (eds): *Dysphagia Assessment and Treatment Planning, A Team Approach.* San Diego, Singular Publishing Group, 1997 pp 41–58

98. Kotz T, Abraham S, Beitler JJ, et al: Pharyngeal transport dysfunction consistent to an organ-sparing protocol. *Arch Otolaryngol Head Neck Surg* 125:410–413, 1999

99. Kendall K, McKenzie S, Leonard R: Structural mobility in deglutition after single modality treatment of head and neck carcinomas with radiotherapy. *Head Neck* 20:720–725, 1998

100. Dejonckere PH, Hordijk GJ: Prognostic factors for swallowing after treatment of head and neck cancer. *Clin Otolaryngol* 23:218–223, 1998

101. Harris LL, Kraege J: After t-e puncture: relearning to speak. *Am J Nurs* 86:55–58, 1986

102. Geraghty JA, Wenig BL, Smith BE, et al: Long-term follow-up of tracheoesophageal puncture results. *Ann Otol Rhinol Laryngol* 105:501–503, 1996

103. Dropkin MJ: Coping with disfigurement/dysfunction and length of stay after head and neck surgery. *Otolaryngol Head Neck Nurs* 15:22–26, 1997

104. Shellenbarger T, Narielwala S: Caring for the patient with laryngeal cancer at home. *Home Healthc Nurs* 14:80–90, 1996

105. Burgess L: Clinical outcome focus—facing the reality of head and neck cancer. *Nurs Standard* 8(32):30–34, 1994

106. D'Antonio LL, Long SA, Zimmerman GJ, et al: Relationship between quality of life and depression in patients with head and neck cancer. *Laryngoscope* 108:806–811, 1998

107. Siston AK, List MA, Schleser R, et al: Sexual functioning and head and neck cancer. *J Psychosoc Oncol* 15(3/4): 107–119, 1997

108. Gritz ER, Carmack CL, deMoor C, et al: First Year after Head and Neck Cancer: Quality of Life. *J Clin Oncol* 17: 352–360, 1999

109. Terrell JE, Fisher SG, Wolf GT: Long-term quality of life after treatment of laryngeal cancer. The veterans affairs laryngeal cancer study group. *Arch Otolaryngol Head Neck Surg* 124:964–971, 1998

CHAPTER 57

Leukemia

Debra Wujcik, RN, MSN, AOCN

Introduction

Leukemia is the name given to a group of hematologic malignancies affecting the bone marrow and lymph tissue. First described by the German pathologist Virchow in 1847 as simply "white blood," the term *leukemia* now includes abnormalities of proliferation and maturation in lymphocyte and myeloid (nonlymphocyte) cell lines. The acute leukemias are marked by an abnormal proliferation of immature blood cells with a short natural history (one to five months), while the chronic leukemias have an excessive accumulation of more mature-appearing but still ineffective cells and a slower, progressive course (two to five years). The excessive proliferation of the leukemia cells results in an overcrowding of the bone marrow, causing a decreased production and function of normal hemopoietic cells.

In the last decade, much has been learned about the biology of leukemia through cytogenetic and molecular analysis. This has led to an era of risk-adapted therapy where the identification of specific genetic abnormalities determines the aggressiveness of treatment and the expected prognosis.[1,2]

Epidemiology

Leukemia represents 3% of the cancer incidence in the United States, with an estimated 30,800 new cases and 21,700 deaths expected in 2000.[3,4] Approximately one-half of the cases are acute and the remaining cases are chronic, but the number of new cases per year is greater in adults (24,200) than in children (2600). The most common types of leukemia in adults are acute myelogenous leukemia (AML) and chronic lymphocytic leukemia (CLL), while acute lymphocytic leukemia (ALL) accounts for 80% of all childhood leukemias.[3,4] The incidence of leukemia rose steeply in the years between 1900 and the 1940s. Since then the incidence of AML has continued to increase steadily, both in the United States and developing countries, suggesting the influence of occupational and environmental exposure.[5]

Etiology

The cause of leukemia is not known. The etiologic factors most commonly considered are genetic predisposition, radiation, chemicals, drugs, and viruses.

Genetic Factors

The relationship of genetic factors to the incidence of leukemia has been suggested in certain high-risk families and specific hereditary syndromes. There is some evidence of familial clustering with a four-fold to sevenfold increased risk in individuals with a family member diagnosed with leukemia.[6,7] Additionally, 10%–20% of monozygous twins of individuals with leukemia develop the disease.[6–8]

Certain genetic disorders are associated with increased incidence of leukemia. Children with Down's syndrome (trisomy 21) have an 18-fold to 20-fold increased incidence of acute leukemia.[8,9] Other disorders with chromosome abnormalities or fragilities also associated with acute leukemia are Bloom's syndrome, Fanconi's anemia, Kleinfelter's syndrome, and Ellis-Van Creveld syndrome.[5]

Acquired clonal chromosomal abnormalities are found in 55%–78% of adult patients with acute leukemia and in 90% of secondary leukemias.[2] Evidence suggests some who appear to have normal cytogenetics (karyotyping) actually have submicroscopic aberrations of genetic material that can be detected only by molecular genetic techniques such as Southern Blot analysis. The cytogenetic and molecular analysis of leukemia gene abnormalities will be discussed further.

Radiation

Populations exposed to ionizing radiation have an increased incidence of leukemia, especially AML. Japanese survivors of the atomic bomb experienced a 20-fold increased incidence of AML and chronic myelogenous leukemia (CML). There appeared to be a direct relationship between increased incidence and distance from the center of the explosion. The peak incidence was at five to seven years following exposure, and increased risks continued for 20 years.[10,11] In addition, early radiologists exposed to excessive irradiation experienced a higher incidence of leukemia.[12] Also, patients treated for benign disorders such as ankylosing spondylitis, menorrhagia, and other gynecologic disorders have increased risk of AML.[13] Radiation remains the most conclusively identified leukemogenic factor in human beings.

Chemicals

Chronic exposure to certain chemicals has been associated with an increased incidence of pancytopenia and subsequent AML. Benzene, an aromatic hydrocarbon, is produced by natural processes and by industry (unleaded gasoline, rubber cement, cleaning solvents).[14,15] It was first implicated in the development of acute leukemia in Turkish cobblers in the early 1900s. Since then other populations have been identified as being at risk, including workers with explosives, distillers, dye users, painters, and shoemakers.

Drugs

Drugs that have demonstrated a relationship to the etiology of acute leukemia include certain alkylating agents, the antibiotic chloramphenicol, and phenylbutazone.[16,17] AML is the most frequently reported second cancer following aggressive chemotherapy and is associated with treatment for Hodgkin's disease, multiple myeloma, ovarian cancer, non-Hodgkin's lymphoma, and breast cancer. Recently the epipodophyllotoxin etoposide and topoisomerase II inhibitors have been implicated as a leukemogenic.[18-20]

Secondary leukemias induced by alkylators are characterized by chromosome translocations such as t(9;22) or t(4;11), while leukemias arising after epipodophyllotoxin therapy are identified by 11q abnormalities. Therapy-related leukemia now represents 20%–25% of all AML patients and overall median survival is four to eight months.[21] The time of greatest risk appears to be the first ten years after treatment.

Viruses

The role of viruses in the etiology of human leukemia remains unclear. The enzyme reverse transcriptase is present primarily in C-type viruses, a group of RNA viruses that can cause leukemia in animals. This enzyme reverses the usual transcription of genetic information from DNA to RNA, allowing the RNA tumor virus to produce oncogenic DNA within the host cells. There is evidence of horizontal transmission of this leukemogenic virus from cat to cat.[22] Reverse transcriptase has been detected in human leukemic blood cells, but not in normal blood cells.

Adult T-cell leukemia in Japan and the Caribbean is associated with the human T-cell leukemia virus (HTLV-I). There is evidence for a role of HTLV-I in the etiology of adult T-cell leukemia in the United States.[23] HTLV-II has been identified in a rare form of hairy cell leukemia and is also prevalent in intravenous drug addicts.[9,24]

Classification

Leukemias are classified as either chronic or acute and as either myeloid or lymphoid. In chronic leukemia the predominant cell is mature-appearing although it does not function normally. The disease has a gradual onset, prolonged clinical course, and a relatively longer survival time. The predominant cell in acute leukemia is undifferentiated or immature, usually a "blast" cell. The abrupt onset and rapid disease progression result in a short survival time. However, as progress is made in the treatment of children with acute lymphocytic leukemia and longer survival occurs, it may no longer be appropriate to describe acute leukemia as having a short survival.

Figure 57-1 presents the major classification of leukemia according to the type of cell that predominates and the location of arrested cellular maturation. All cell lines arise from the same totipotent stem cell. From this cell, which has the potential to differentiate into a variety of cells, the myeloid and lymphocyte series are derived. The myeloid stem cell is pluripotent and gives rise to erythrocyte, thrombocyte, granulocyte, and monocyte progenitors, or committed cells. These are immature forms that mature into fully functional red blood cells, platelets, and white blood cells. The lymphoid stem cell matures in the thymus to form T-cell progenitors, or in the bone marrow to form B-cell progenitors.

The type of leukemia is named according to the point at which cell maturation is arrested. Although the terms *lymphocytic* and *myelogenous* (nonlymphocytic) leukemia are most commonly used, further specification within each class (e.g., *promyelocytic, myelocytic*) describes the exact point at which arrest of maturation seems to occur.

In 1976 the French-American-British (FAB) Cooperative Group developed criteria for the classification of the acute leukemias[25] (Table 57-1). The purpose was to provide a systematic, objective system that would be feasible in most hematologic laboratories. The system, based on morphology and number of cells, was later revised and updated and is still used today to distinguish lymphoid and myeloid lineages and to assign initial treatment.[26-28] The additional information obtained through cytogenetics, identification of surface markers, and histochemical staining provides important therapeutic and prognostic information.

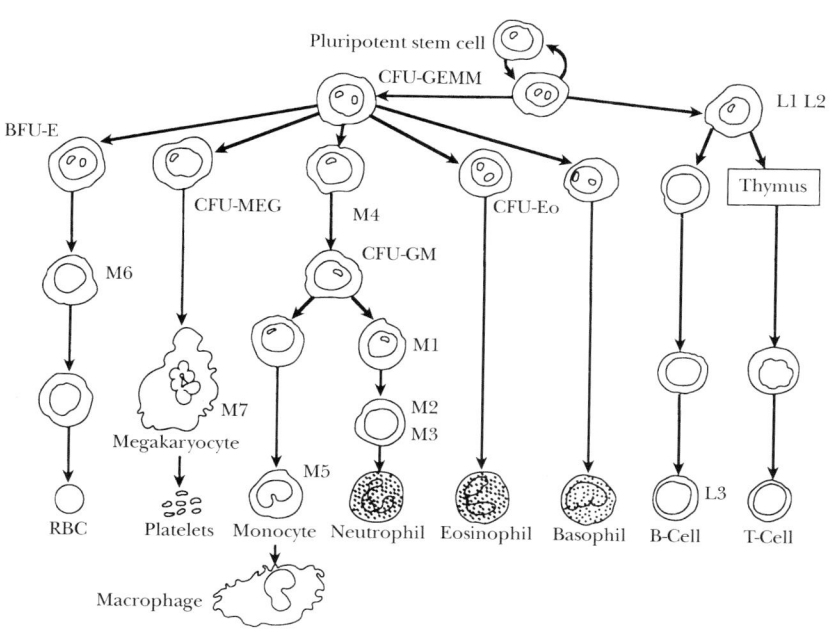

Figure 57-1 Hematopoietic cascade with FAB classifications of acute nonlymphocytic leukemia and acute lymphocytic leukemia at proposed levels of arrested cell maturation. BFU = burst-forming unit; CFU = colony-forming unit; GM = granulocyte, macrophage; GEMM = granulocyte, erythrocyte, macrophage, megakaryocyte; Epo = erythropoietin; MEG = megakaryocyte; Eo = eosinophil; E = erythrocyte; M1 = undifferentiated myelocytic; M2 = myelocytic; M3 = promyelocytic; M4 = myelomonocytic; M5 = monocytic; M6 = erythroleukemia; M7 = megakaryocytic; L1 = childhood; L2 = adult; L3 = Burkitt's type.

Pathophysiology

In the normal bone marrow, efficient regulatory mechanisms ensure that cell proliferation and maturation are

Table 57-1 French-American-British (FAB) Classification of Acute Leukemia

Myeloid	Lymphocytic
M0 Minimally differentiated	
M1 Undifferentiated myelocytic	L1, childhood (Pre B- and T-cell)
M2 Myelocytic	
M3 Promyelocytic	L2, adult (Pre B- and T-cell)
M4 Myelomonocytic	L3, Burkitt's type (B-cell)
M5 Monocytic	
M6 Erythroleukemia	
M7 Megakaryocytic	

Data from Bennett et al.[25]

adequate for the needs of the individual. In leukemia, control is missing or abnormal. The results are (1) arrest of the cell in an early phase of its maturation process, causing the accumulation of immature cells; (2) an abnormal proliferation of these immature cells; and (3) crowding of other marrow elements, resulting in inhibited growth and function of these elements and eventual replacement of the marrow by leukemic cells.

Manifestations of leukemia are related to three factors: (1) excessive proliferation of immature leukocytes within blood-forming organs such as the bone marrow, spleen, and lymph nodes, resulting in destruction of tissue; (2) infiltration of proliferating leukocytes into various organs of the body; and (3) decrease in the number of normal leukocytes, erythrocytes, and thrombocytes as a result of crowding of the bone marrow by proliferating leukemic cells. Table 57-2 summarizes possible leukemic manifestations, although these vary considerably with each type of leukemia.[29] The presenting manifestations, complications, course of disease, and treatment for each major type are discussed separately (Table 57-3).

Assessment of Acute Leukemia

Factors that influence the symptoms and physical findings are (1) the type of leukemic cell, (2) the degree

Table 57-2 Manifestations of Leukemia

Etiology	Manifestation
Granulocytopenia	Fever
	Abdominal pain
	Respiratory infection
	Perirectal abscess
	Adenopathy
	Mucositis
Thrombocytopenia	Purpura, petechiae, ecchymoses
	Bleeding gums
	Epistaxis
	Retinal hemorrhage
	Intracranial bleeding
Anemia	Fatigue or malaise
	Pallor
	Dyspnea
Leukemia infiltrates	Pain or swelling in bones and joints
	Hepatomegaly
	Splenomegaly

of leukemic cell burden (early-stage or advanced disease), (3) the involvement of organs or systems outside of the bone marrow or peripheral circulation, and (4) the depression of normal marrow elements by the leukemic process. Since the presenting symptoms of AML and ALL are similar, the assessment parameters of acute leukemia are discussed first. The classification and treatment of AML and ALL are discussed individually. Then the chronic leukemias, CML and CLL, are discussed separately.

Patient History

Acute leukemia presents with a large and rapidly growing population of leukemic cells. Usually, signs and symptoms have been present for less than three months, and perhaps for only a few days. Although the diagnosis cannot be made from the patient's history alone, many of the findings are typical and essential in guiding the diagnostic workup.[9]

The most common complaints of the patient are non-specific—e.g., fatigue, malaise, weight loss, and fever. The presenting symptoms are the manifestations of the effects of leukemic cells on the normal marrow elements. Infections are recurrent in the common sites such as the skin, gingiva, perianal tissue, lung, and urinary tract. The patient may complain of sore throat and describe fever with or without signs of localized infection. Unexplained bleeding may occur with nosebleeds, gingival bleeding, midcycle menstrual flow, or heavy bleeding with menses. Symptoms of progressive anemia include fatigue, palpitations, shortness of breath, and anorexia. Pain may arise from several sources: bones such as the sternum, enlarged lymph nodes, and hepatosplenomegaly.

Neurological complaints are frequent and may signal either leukemia infiltration (especially in ALL) or intracerebral hemorrhage. These include a history of headache, vomiting, visual disturbances, or seizures.

Review of the individual's past medical history may be noncontributory. However, it is of etiologic importance to note a history of recurrent infections or bleeding tendencies as well as the type and time of any drug exposure to try to document the approximate onset of leukemia. Similarly, the occupational (especially chemical and radiation) exposure and family history of genetic abnormalities or cancer contribute to the total epidemiologic picture.

An essential part of the initial history that serves as a baseline for understanding the individual and planning care is the psychosocial profile. Questions that elicit details concerning past and present coping strategies with illness or other crises should be asked. Determination of significant others can be made by asking such questions as: "Who can you talk to most easily about your illness?" Finally, the nurse must ascertain how the patient and family perceive the illness and what their previous experience with hospitalization has been.

Physical Examination

The physical findings of acute leukemia usually relate directly to the effects of pancytopenia. Vital signs may demonstrate fever, tachycardia, and tachypnea. The skin and mucous membranes generally appear pale, with readily apparent ecchymoses or petechiae. Generalized or localized adenopathy may be present due to leukemic infiltration or infection.

A comprehensive physical examination validates findings elicited in a complete history and review of symptoms. Ophthalmoscopic examination may reveal retinal capillary hemorrhage or papilledema due to leukostatic or thrombocytopenic-induced bleeding and/or increased intracranial pressure. An oral infection with *Candida albicans* may be present. Examination of the lungs and heart may reveal the effects of anemia (cardiac murmurs) or infection (abnormal lung sounds). Abdominal palpation may demonstrate hepatosplenomegaly or enlarged kidneys due to leukemic infiltration, especially in children with ALL. Perirectal tissue may be tender and swollen and the only evidence of an abscess or a fistula. Finally, gentle palpation of bones and joints may reveal swelling and elicit pain.

Diagnostic Studies

Laboratory and radiographic studies are essential for proper diagnosis. It is important to distinguish between AML and ALL, since the treatment and prognosis differ markedly. An ongoing explanation to the patient and family of the plan and purpose of the exhaustive diagnos-

Table 57-3 Comparative Features of the Leukemias at Presentation

Description	Median Age	Initial Remission Rate	Median Survival with Treatment	Splenomegaly	Infection	Adenopathy	Hemoglobin	White Blood Cell Count	Platelets
Acute myelogenous leukemia	50–60	60%–70%	10–15 mo	No	Yes	No	Low	Variable	Low
Acute lymphoblastic leukemia	4	Adult 65%–85%; children 90%	Adult 2 yr; children 5 yr	Yes	Yes	Yes	Low	Variable	Low
Chronic myelogenous leukemia	49	90%	3 yr	Yes	No	No	Low	100,000–300,000/mm³ granulocytes	Normal or low
Chronic lymphocytic leukemia	60	90%	4–6 yr	Yes	Yes	Yes	Low	20,000/mm³ lymphocytes	Low

tic workup will facilitate cooperation, decrease anxiety, and create an atmosphere of confidence and trust.

The diagnosis is suggested by the peripheral smear but requires a full examination of the bone marrow. The white blood cell count may be low, normal, or high, and 90% of patients have blast cells present in the peripheral blood. Neutropenia (absolute granulocyte count less than 1000 cells/mm³) is frequent, and thrombocytopenia is present in 40% of patients. Blood chemistry studies may reveal hyperuricemia and increased lactic dehydrogenase as well as altered serum and urine muramidase (greatly increased with monocyte and myelomonocytic leukemia, but normal to low in lymphoblastic leukemia). If acute promyelocytic leukemia (M_3) is suspected, laboratory evaluation should include plasma fibrinogen, fibrin split products, and prothrombin time.

Bone marrow contents are usually hypercellular, with 60%–90% blasts in the differential blood count. Auer rods are diagnostic of AML, as are special stains (Sudan black and peroxidase).

Improved techniques of cytogenetics (chromosome analysis) can provide information confirming the diagnosis and specific classification of the leukemia. More than two-thirds of patients with de novo acute leukemia exhibit nonrandom chromosome abnormalities.[30] These abnormalities in the leukemic cells serve as tumor markers that disappear during remission and reappear with recurrence of the leukemia.[31]

Cytogenetic analysis is performed at the time of diagnosis and is rapidly becoming the standard for establishing diagnosis and prognosis in acute leukemia.[9] These chromosome abnormalities are described as translocations, inversions, or loss or gain in chromosome number. Specific aberrations are related to a favorable or unfavorable outcome[2,30,32,33] (Tables 57-4 and 57-5). The results of chromosome analysis are usually available within four weeks. Since this is also the time the patient is recovering

from induction therapy, this information is useful in planning further treatment.

Structural chromosomal abnormalities produce protein products of genes that are inappropriately activated or altered. Gene activation occurs when the transcription regulatory elements of one gene become juxtaposed (placed side by side) to another gene. Under the control of the new promoter/enhancer region, the expression pattern is disrupted, leading to leukemogenesis.[30,32] Gene fusion occurs when segments from two genes become fused to create a new structure. Most chromosomal aberrations result in gene fusions. Genetic alterations in AML give rise to fusion genes. The majority of genetic alterations seen in ALL result in transfer of regulatory elements from one gene to another causing dysregulated expression from an otherwise normal gene. Further information is provided by differentiating primary alterations (one karyotype abnormality) from secondary (extra alterations thought to be later genetic events). Secondary alterations may be present at diagnosis or appear at the time of relapse.[30]

Additional information is obtained from immunologic studies. There are more that 100 antigen groups known as *clusters of differentiation (CDs)* on the surface of hematopoietic cells.[9] Monoclonal antibodies reactive to immature cells can identify the predominant cell type and stage of arrested development in the leukemic cell line. The use of surface marker antigens in patients with ALL has revealed the presence of markers for both lymphoid and myeloid cells.[34] Mixed lymphoid and myeloid surface markers are found in 21% of patients with de novo ALL.[35] These hybrid leukemias may be biphenotypic where one cell line expresses characteristics of two lineages, or bilineal where two distinct populations may express either myeloid or lymphoid characteristics separately.[9] In general, patients with mixed lineage leukemia have a poor response to

Table 57-4 Chromosomal and Molecular Abnormalities in Acute Myelogenous Leukemia

Abnormality	Karyotype	FAB	Molecular Change	Complete Response Rate
Transcription	t(6;11)(q27;q23)	M4, M5	AF6(6q27)	Low
	t(8;21)(q22;q22)	M2	ET0(8q22)	High
	t(10;11)(p12;p23)	M4, M5	AF10(p12)	Low
	t(11;17)(q23;q21)	M5	ALL I(11q23)	Low
	t(11;19)(q23;p13)	M4, M5	ELL(19p13.1)	Low
	t(15;17)(q22;q11)	M3	PML-RARα	High
	t(16;16)(p13;q22)	M4Eo	MYHI I(16p13)	High
	t(3;3)(q23;q26)	M1, M2, M4, M6	Gene activation	Low
	t(9;11)(p22;q23)	M5a	AF9(9p22)	Low
Inversion	inv(16)(p13;q22)	M4Eo	MYHI I (16p13)	High
	inv(3)(q21;q26)	M0, M1, M4, M5, M6, M7	Gene activation	Low
Loss or deletion	5			Low
	7			High
	del(16)(q22)	M4Eo		

treatment and should be considered for other investigational therapies.

ACUTE MYELOGENOUS LEUKEMIA

Classification

Acute myelogenous leukemia (AML), also referred to as acute nonlymphocytic leukemia (ANLL), is a disease of the pluripotent myeloid stem cell. The malignant clone arises in the myeloid, monocyte, erythroid, or megakaryocyte lines. The exact event that triggers the malignant transformation is not known.

The leukemic cells have more abundant cytoplasm and granulation in the cytoplasm is usually but not always present. Auer rods, which are abnormal lysosomal granules, are present and pathognomonic for AML. Multiple nucleoli are present and tend to vary in size.

As previously stated, the type of leukemia is named for the predominant cell. The most common myeloid leukemia is acute myelocytic leukemia (M_1). Acute promyelocytic leukemia (APL) (M_3) is associated with an increased risk of disseminated intravascular coagulation. This is due to the release of procoagulants from granules within the leukemic promyelocyte, especially during remission induction therapy.[36] Patients with acute monocytic (M_5) or myelomonocytic (M_4) leukemia often exhibit extramedullary leukemic infiltration with gingival hypertrophy, cutaneous leukemia, and liver, spleen, and lymph enlargement.[9]

Erythroleukemia (M_6), which was first described by DiGugliolmo, has both a chronic and acute form.[5] As the erythroleukemia progresses, the morphologic picture resembles that of myelocytic or myelomonocytic leuke-

Table 57-5 Chromosomal and Molecular Abnormalities in Acute Nonlymphocytic Leukemia

Abnormality	Karyotype	FAB	Molecular Change	Complete Response Rate
B-lineage translocations	t(8;14)(q24;Q32)	L 3	IGH, cMYC	Moderate
	t(1;19)(q23;p13)	L 1	EZA, PBX1	Low
	t(17;19)(q22;p13)	L 1	EZA, PBX1	Low
	t(9;22)(q34;q11)	L 1	cABL, BCR	High
	t(4;11)(q21;q23)	L 1	MLL, AF4	High
T-lineage translocations	t(8;14)(q24;q11)	L 3		Low

mia. Megakaryocytic leukemia (M_7) is quite rare and less responsive to chemotherapy.[37]

By the time an individual is diagnosed with AML, the bone marrow and peripheral blood contain up to 10^{12} leukemic cells.[38] The accumulation within the bone marrow space results in inhibition and crowding out of normal marrow stem cells and infiltration of other organs by myeloblasts. Anemia, thrombocytopenia, and neutropenia result. If the disease is left untreated, death occurs within a few months due to infection or uncontrolled bleeding.

Treatment

The goal of antileukemic treatment for AML is the eradication of the leukemic stem cell. Complete remission is defined as the restoration of normal peripheral counts and less than 5% blasts in the bone marrow.[34] Treatment regimens capable of inducing a complete remission are composed of several drugs, each of which is known to be effective against leukemic myeloblasts. The course of therapy is divided into two stages: (1) induction and (2) postremission therapy.

Induction Therapy

The goal of induction therapy is to cause severe bone marrow hypoplasia. At diagnosis the leukemic cells are proliferating more slowly than normal myeloid precursors. Therefore, the myeloid stem cells repopulate the depleted marrow faster than leukemic cells. The cornerstone for remission induction is the cell cycle-specific antimetabolite cytosine arabinoside plus an anthracycline (daunorubicin, doxorubicin, mitoxantrone, amsacrine, or idarubicin).[39-42] It is theorized that a drug that is not cycle specific will have a synergistic effect when given sequentially with a cell cycle-specific drug by causing proliferating cells to enter the cell cycle concurrently. Cytosine arabinoside is administered continuously for seven days and the anthracycline is given for three days. The continuous infusion of cytosine arabinoside ensures that slowly cycling leukemia cells are adequately exposed to the drug during the synthesis phase of the cell cycle.[43] This protocol is called *7 + 3*, but variations include five-day or ten-day infusions of cytosine arabinoside. Bishop[40] summarized the results of eight clinical studies, reporting a complete response rate of 64%, with the best results in the protocols with seven days of cytosine arabinoside. Idarubicin is the most common anthracycline used.[9,40]

The impact of the chemotherapy is assessed at one week after the completion of therapy with a bone marrow biopsy and aspiration on the 14th day. If residual leukemia is present, a second course is begun. Bone marrow recovery usually takes 14–21 days after the end of the chemotherapy with median time to complete recovery at 28–32 days. Complete response rates are now observed in

65%–80% of patients. Unfortunately, in spite of improving remission rates, only 20% of patients remain in complete remission. Relapse occurs in the remaining cases within one to two years.[40,44] Thus, postremission therapy is essential.

Postremission Therapy

By the addition of postremission therapy, the median duration of remission can be increased from 4-8 months to 10–60 months, and disease-free survival (DFS) of four years from 30%–40%.[45] Leukemia cells have certain biologic properties that can be distinguished from normal cells. Certain chromosomal aberrations are detected by polymerase chain reactions (PCR) or by fluorescence in situ hybridization (FISH). RNA transcript errors are detected by reverse transcription PCR (RT-PCR). Patterns of antigen coexpression are detected by flow cytometry.[46] All of these are used to detect minimal residual disease (MRD).

Postremission therapies include consolidation, intensification, maintenance, and allogeneic or autologous bone marrow transplant.[9,40,47] None has emerged as the clear-cut, optimal therapy (Figure 57-2).

Consolidation therapy consists of one or two courses of very high doses of the same drugs used for induction. Up to 30 times induction doses of cytosine arabinoside are used to consolidate the remission.[44] Although the patient is in a healthier state for this part of the treatment, the toxicities are substantial, with extended myelosuppression, cerebellar dysfunction, dermatitis, hepatic dysfunction, and conjunctivitis. The longest remissions appear to occur after two or more courses of consolidation therapy, with a median remission of one to two years.[40]

Intensification may be initiated immediately following remission induction (early intensification) or several

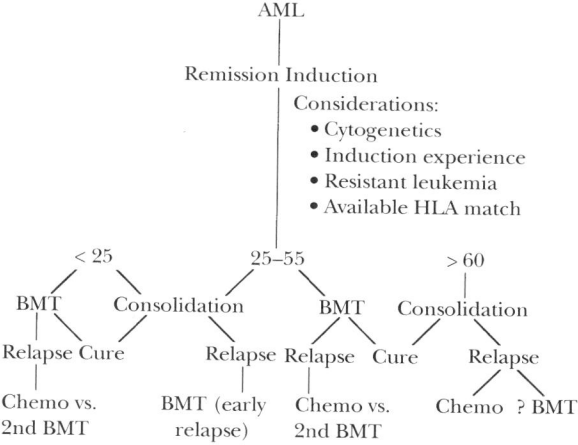

Figure 57-2 Treatment considerations and options for patients with acute myelogenous leukemia.

months later (late intensification). Different drugs are used with the hope that they will not be cross-resistant with the induction drugs. Mitoxantrone is less cardiotoxic and has less extramedullary toxicity than daunorubicin. With a steep dose-response curve, mitoxantrone is good for dose intensification.[31] Another combination being used for postinduction therapy is ICE (idarubicin, cytosine arabinoside, and etoposide).[48]

Maintenance therapy is treatment with lower doses of the same or other drugs given monthly for a prolonged period of time. Maintenance therapy is not currently recommended in the treatment of AML.[40,47]

Because microscopic disease is being treated in postremission therapy, it is difficult to know how much treatment is enough. Investigation continues to determine the optimal curative treatment.

Patients who relapse after induction and postinduction chemotherapy have a 30%–60% likelihood of achieving a second remission.[9] Leukemic cells acquire increasing resistance to chemotherapy. The cellular kinetics change due to an increased growth fraction and shortened generation time, resulting in a decreased doubling time.[31] The second and subsequent remissions are influenced by prior treatment, length of remission, and the initial response to therapy. Patients who relapse quickly or who have resistant leukemia should be considered for clinical trials or bone marrow transplant.

The role of bone marrow transplant (BMT) in the treatment of AML remains controversial.[49] The first issue is the availability of an HLA-matched donor. In the general population, a potential donor exists in less than 40% of cases. Other options may include a matched unrelated donor BMT obtained through the National Marrow Donor Program. There are increased risks of graft-versus-host disease (GVHD) and lack of engraftment from these histocompatible but unrelated cells. A purged autologous BMT may be performed in a young patient with no HLA match. In patients less than age 30, BMT may offer a higher cure rate than standard treatment. In patients in the fourth decade, the results of chemotherapy versus BMT vary. Transplant centers usually do not admit patients over age 55.

Because allogeneic BMT carries the risk of GVHD, interstitial pneumonia, and infection with cytomegalovirus, the decision for BMT is not easy. The question of the optimal timing for transplant remains unanswered. Patients who relapse after allogeneic BMT can be treated with a second BMT or an infusion of donor buffy coat to stimulate the graft-versus-leukemia effect.[50] (See Chapter 21 for an in-depth discussion of bone marrow transplantation.)

Another consideration in the treatment of AML is the significance of prognostic indicators, which may be useful in determining the best course of therapy. For example, patients with unfavorable factors such as older age or multiple chromosomal abnormalities may be treated with high-dose or investigational drugs. A patient who had a poor response to initial therapy and other medical problems is unlikely to benefit from reinduction therapy.

Such patients may benefit from a less aggressive approach, with transfusion support and oral hydroxyurea to control the white blood cell (WBC) count. In a younger patient with an unfavorable morphologic subtype, BMT may be preferred to consolidation therapy.

A newer strategy for treating patients with risk factors, early relapse, or resistant leukemia is drug therapy to overcome multidrug resistance (MDR). MDR is the phenomenon by which a cancer becomes resistant to multiple drugs that have little similarity in their chemical structure and mechanism of action.[51] MDR can be kinetic in origin, which means that the malignant cells are resistant at the onset of the disease. It can also be acquired when drugs that were initially effective are no longer effective. Acquired MDR is associated with P-glycoprotein, which acts as a pump to transport drugs in and out of malignant cells. P-glycoprotein is associated with the MDR phenotype. The MDR1 message or its P-glycoprotein product is expressed in approximately 25% of cases of newly diagnosed AML. In addition, more than 70% of cases with relapsed AML express P-glycoprotein.[52,53]

The anthracyclines, specifically daunomycin and doxorubicin, are associated with acquired MDR.[52] One strategy to overcome P-glycoprotein resistance is to use cyclosporine, a lipophilic endoecapeptide with immunosuppressive properties. Cyclosporine restores daunorubicin sensitivity in drug-resistant tumor cell lines.[53]

Strategies altering cellular kinetics to overcome de novo MDR are being explored. High-dose therapy with etoposide by continuous infusion for 29–69 hours along with cyclophosphamide for 3-4 days produced a complete remission (CR) in 42% of 40 patients with AML, including six patients with resistance to high-dose cytosine arabinoside.[54] Hematopoietic colony-stimulating factors (CSF) such as granulocyte (G-CSF), granulocyte-macrophage (GM-CSF), and interleukin-3 (IL-3) can enhance recruitment of cells into synthesis phase and optimize the cytotoxicity of cytosine arabinoside.[31,43]

APL is biologically distinct from other subtypes of AML. All-trans retinoic acid (RA), a derivative of vitamin A, is now used to induce remissions through differentiation.[55,56] The break point for the chromosome region abnormality characteristic in APL, t(15;17)(q22;q12), is clustered near the location of the retinoic acid receptor-alpha. The administration of RA seems to induce terminal differentiation and subsequent death of the previously arrested leukemic cells. Recently, RA was approved for remission induction in patients with APL who are refractory to chemotherapy or who have relapsed after prior chemotherapy. Once remission is obtained, treatment switches to chemotherapy because patients quickly develop resistance to RA.[36] Patients unable to tolerate conventional chemotherapy (older or with concomitant illness) also benefit from RA therapy. The most commonly used dosage is 45 mg/m²/day administered orally in two evenly divided doses for remission induction. About one-half of patients experience the complications of disseminated intravascular coagulopathy, but few hemorrhagic deaths occur. Common side effects include headache, dry skin, xerostomia, cheilitis (cracking at the corners of the lips), and bone pain.[57]

A small subset of APL patients carry a different fusion gene *PLZF-RARα* from the t(11;17)(q23;q12). Patients with these cells do not differentiate in the presence of RA and have a poor prognosis.[58]

ACUTE LYMPHOCYTIC LEUKEMIA

Acute lymphocytic leukemia (ALL) is a malignant disease of the lymphoid progenitors. The abnormal clone originates in the marrow, thymus, and lymph nodes, but the exact etiologic event is unknown. The leukemic lymphoblast is nongranular, with little cytoplasm. The round nucleus resembles a normal lymphoblast. Although the defect does not involve the myeloid cell lines, the secondary effect of the high leukemic cell burden on the bone marrow interferes with normal hematopoietic activity.

Classification

The FAB classification for ALL is based upon several cell properties: size ratio of nucleus to cytoplasm; number, size, and shape of nucleoli; and amount and basophilia of the cytoplasm[25,28] (see Table 57-1). In childhood ALL, 85% have L1 morphology, whereas the majority of adults with ALL have L2 morphology. Patients with L3 ALL, which resembles Burkitt's lymphoma, are rare.

Another classification system for ALL is based upon immune features.[9] Four subtypes are identified by the presence of certain markers on the cell surface. T-cell leukemias make up 20% of all ALL. Common ALL (cALL) is the most frequent and least differentiated ALL.[59] It is identified by the common ALL antigen (cALLa), recently renamed *CD 10*.[34] T-cell antigens such as CD5 and CD7 identify other T-ALL. Both cALLa and T-cell antigens contain another marker, terminal deoxynucleotidyl transferase (TdT). Other surface and cell immunoglobulins denote the rare B-cell ALL, which accounts for 80% of ALL. Finally, about one-fourth are pre pre-B (formally null) leukemias that do not have any identifiable surface markers.

Lymphoblasts have a propensity for organ infiltration and may remain sequestered in sanctuary sites even after remission has been achieved. Leukemic cells infiltrate into the central nervous system (CNS) early in the disease.[60] Because drugs used for treatment penetrate poorly into the cerebrospinal fluid, the leukemic cells are sheltered from the cytotoxic effects of the drugs. Over time, the leukemic cells proliferate and cause relapse. Cells can also be harbored in the testes. In addition, 80% of patients have lymphadenopathy and/or splenomegaly at the time of diagnosis due to the infiltration of these organs by leukemic cells.[9]

The prognosis for long-term survival is more favorable for individuals with ALL than AML since drugs are available that are uniquely effective against lymphocytes—e.g., prednisone. CNS prophylaxis is used in ALL and has proven successful.

As with AML, long-term survival and cure for individuals with ALL is possible only if a complete remission is achieved. This is documented by a bone marrow aspirate containing less than 5% lymphoblasts and the disappearance of all peripheral manifestations of the disease.

Treatment

In contrast to AML, current chemotherapeutic regimens proven effective against ALL contain drugs that are selectively toxic to lymphoblasts and relatively sparing of normal hematopoietic stem cells. Therefore, the patient experiences hypoplasia that is less severe and of shorter duration with greater leukemic cell kill. In addition, relapses may be more effectively treated because the marrow is better able to recover.

The focus of therapy for ALL is to eradicate all leukemic cells from the marrow and lymph tissue and eliminate any residual foci of disease within the CNS. Treatment is divided into three stages: (1) induction, (2) CNS prophylaxis, and (3) postremission therapy (Figure 57-3).

Induction Therapy

Although current therapy for ALL induces complete remission in 65%–85% of adults, only 20%–30% are cured of the disease.[9,61] Induction regimens usually comprise five drugs including vincristine, prednisone, an anthracycline, cyclophosphamide and/or asparaginase.[61,62] Be-

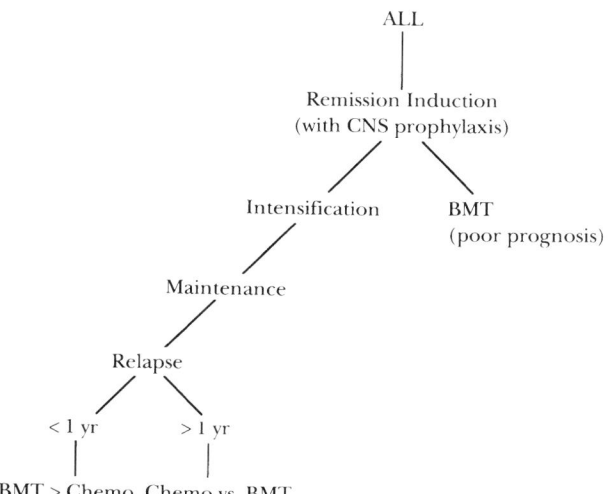

Figure 57-3 Treatment considerations and options for patients with acute lymphocytic leukemia.

tween 35%–40% achieve long-term, disease-free survival.[60] Therapy usually begins in the hospital, but hypoplasia is shorter than with AML treatment. Once remission is documented, the therapy is completed on an outpatient basis.

CNS Prophylaxis

Meningeal leukemia is present at diagnosis in about 5%–10% of patients and is known to occur in up to 35% of patients with ALL in the absence of CNS prophylaxis.[9,61] By comparison, in patients with AML the incidence is less than 5%. Leukemic lymphoblasts enter the leptomeninges either by direct extension from the blood of the meningeal vessels or by seeding from thrombocytopenic bleeding. The cells extend deeply into the cerebral sulci and nerve sheaths, causing a mechanical obstruction of the cerebral spinal fluid (CSF). If unchecked, hydrocephaly and death occur. Signs and symptoms of CNS leukemia include headache, blurred vision, nausea/vomiting, and cranial nerve palsies.[59]

CNS prophylaxis should start within a few weeks of the initiation of therapy. Treatment usually includes intracranial radiation and intrathecal methotrexate.[60,63] Cranial radiation delivered in fractionated doses of 200 cGy up to a total dose of 2400 cGy produces predictable penetration of leukemic cells regardless of CSF dynamics. This therapy can also kill or sterilize cells not undergoing cell division. There are recognized side effects, however, including somnolence, chemical meningitis, paraparesis, and leukoencephalopathy.[59]

Postremission Therapy

As in AML, even after complete remission, patients with ALL harbor remaining leukemic cells. Relapse occurs in two to three months if there is no continuing therapy. Prolonged chemotherapy may lead to a 40% overall cure rate, but the type and duration are not completely defined.[60] Currently many patients receive some type of intensification with high-dose chemotherapy or the use of multiple new drugs.[61,64] Methotrexate and 6-mercaptopurine may be added to the drugs used during induction. Maintenance therapy often continues for two to three years.

The outlook for patients in whom relapse occurs during therapy is quite poor, and younger patients with an HLA-matched donor should be immediately referred for BMT.[63] If relapse occurs after the completion of therapy, treatment is continued with high-dose methotrexate, tenoposide, and cytarabine, or high-dose cytosine arabinoside with an anthracycline or amsacrine. Second remission can be achieved in up to 72% of cases.[9] An analysis of eight studies using high-dose cytosine arabinoside in relapsed patients with ALL revealed a mean CR of 38%.[64] This same researcher reviewed 19 other studies that combined high-dose cytosine arabinoside (HDCA) with an-

thracyclines, vincristine, and/or prednisone and determined the CR rates to be 36%–63%.[65] Idarubicin and HDCA induced second remissions in 65% of adults with ALL.[47]

Chromosomal aberrations (summarized in Table 57-5) are also important in planning treatment for ALL.[60] Because patients treated with allogeneic BMT show a trend toward longer survival if the transplant is performed during the first remission,[49] it is important to identify patients with an unfavorable prognosis in the early stages of disease.

MYELODYSPLASTIC SYNDROMES

Myelodysplastic syndromes (MDS) are a group of hematologic disorders with an increased risk of transformation to AML. They are characterized by a change in the quantity and quality of bone marrow products. Hematologic disorders that preceded acute leukemia were first reported in the late 1940s and referred to as *preleukemia anemia*.[66] Other terms used are *preleukemia, hematopoietic dysplasia, refractory anemia with excessive myeloblasts, subacute myeloid leukemia, oligoblastic leukemia,* and *dysmyelopoietic syndromes*.[67]

Currently MDS are divided into five subtypes according to the FAB group classification: refractory anemia (RA), refractory anemia with ringed sideroblasts (RARS), refractory anemia with excessive blasts (RAEB), refractory anemia with excessive blasts in transformation (RAEB-t), and chronic myelomonocytic leukemia (CMML).[68] The FAB classification is limited in usefulness because it does not include such variables as a wide range of marrow blast cells within certain subgroups, marrow cytogenetics, and the degree of morbidity-associated cytopenias. Table 57-6 lists each type, along with diagnostic criteria, risk of evolution into acute leukemia, and average survival time.[67,68]

An International Prognostic Scoring System (IPSS) for MDS has been developed that categorizes risk as low, intermediate-1, intermediate-2, and high risk[69,70] (Table 57-7). Therapeutic decision making is guided by the patient's IPSS risk category, age, and performance status.

MDS are believed to occur as the result of an altered stem cell. The cause is unknown. Chromosome abnormalities are present at the level of the stem cell in 50% of patients with primary MDS and 75% of patients with therapy-related MDS. None are exclusively associated with MDS but common abnormalities involve chromosomes 5, 7, 8, 11, 12, and 20[67–69] (Table 57-8).

Approximately 30% of patients diagnosed with AML initially present with preleukemic syndrome.[9] MDS may be considered to be different stages of the same disease. Even if the evolution to acute leukemia never occurs, life-threatening anemia, thrombocytopenia, and/or neutropenia invariably occur. The defect is usually noted in the erythrocyte line first, then in the granulocytes and megakaryocytes.

Table 57-6 Classification of Myelodysplastic Syndrome with Percentage of Blast Cells, Leukemia Risk, and Average Survival

Category	BLASTS (%) Blood	BLASTS (%) Bone Marrow	Risk of Evolution to Acute Leukemia (%)	Survival (months)
RA	< 1	< 5	0–25	18–71
RARS	< 1	< 5	8	14–76 +
RAEB	< 5	≥ 5	20–44	7–16
RAEB-t	> 5	20–30	27–60	2.5–20
CMML	< 5 > 10^9 monocytes	1–20	14	9–60

RA = refractory anemia; RARS = refractory anemia with ringed sideroblasts; RAEB = refractory anemia excess blasts; RAEB-t = refractory anemia with excess blasts in transformation; CMML = chronic myelomonocytic leukemia.
Data from Kouides and Bennett[67]; Bennett et al.[68]

As with other hematologic disorders, chromosome aberrations are proving to be significant. Chromosome region 12–13 contains myeloid leukemia factor-2 gene (*MLF2*) that has the same structure as myeloid leukemia factor-1 gene (*MLF1*) on region 3q25.1. *MFL1* is associated with several subtypes of AML and MDS.[70] Another variable in MDS is the inability to repair DNA damage. The p53 protein is a tumor suppressor gene with a central link between DNA damage events, control of the cell cycle, and net cellular metabolism. When stimulated by certain types of DNA damage, p53 triggers pathways that culminate in apoptosis. Loss of p53 function may determine the net drug resistance of a malignant cell population. Loss of p53 function is associated with secondary MDS more than de novo MDS.[71] Several agents are being studied for their ability to overcome drug resistance by blocking P-glycoprotein activity. These include verapamil, quinine, cyclosporine, and its nonimmunosuppressive analog PSC 833. The mutation and abnormal expression of *ras* oncogenes are also detected in 10%–15% of MDS and are common in patients undergoing transformation to leukemia.[70]

The observation of increased programmed cell death (apoptosis) in the presence of rapid hyperproliferation of marrow cells has caused a major advance in understanding the pathogenesis of MDS.[72–74] Increased apoptosis may be related to apoptosis-related gene products such as *MYC*, which enhances apoptosis, and *BCL-2*, which diminishes apoptosis. Other cytokines that may be involved are TNF alpha, transforming growth factor beta, and interleukin 1-beta converting enzyme. This finding explains the opposing clinical findings of most MDS patients—marrow hypercellularity and peripheral blood pancytopenia.[75] Researchers are looking for new ways to interfere with this pathway.

Eighty to ninety percent of patients diagnosed with MDS are older than age 50. The incidence is slightly higher in males than females.[75] A bone marrow biopsy and aspirate usually reveal dyshematopoiesis in all cell lineages. Ringed sideroblasts, abnormal nuclear shapes, cytoplasmic abnormalities, and maturation defects of red blood cells (RBCs) indicate dyserythropoiesis. Evidence of dysmegakaryocytopoiesis includes atypical shapes; multiple, small nuclei; and increased or decreased numbers of platelets. Dysgranulocytopoiesis is seen with hypogranular cells, nuclear abnormalities, and maturation defects of granulocytes. A hypocellular bone marrow with one or more of these lineage defects provides a diagnosis of MDS.

About half of patients with MDS develop AML. Historically patients with MDS do not respond as well to antileukemic therapy as do those with de novo AML. However,

Table 57-7 International Prognostic Scoring System for Myelodysplastic Syndromes

Score	Subgroup	Median Survival (Years)	Bone Marrow Blasts (%)	Karyotype	Cytopenias
0	Low	5.7	< 5	Good	0–1
0.5–1.0	Intermediate-1	3.5	5–10	Intermediate	2–3
1.5–2.0	Intermediate-2	1.2	11–30	Poor	
≥ 2.5	High	0.4	> 30		

Karyotype: Good = normal, -Y, del(5q), del(20q); Intermediate = other abnormalities; Poor = complex (> 3 abnormalities) or chromosome 7 abnormalities; Cytopenias = anemia, thrombocytopenia, and/or neutropenia.

Table 57.8 Chromosomal Abnormalities in Myelodyspastic Syndromes

Abnormality	Description	Comment
Loss or deletions Monosomy 7	Loss of one of two chromosomes 7	Target for environmental or occupational toxins. DNA damaging agents associated with de novo AML
del 5q	Loss of small arm of chromosome 5	Associated with elderly women with macrocytic anemia; relatively benign
del 11q	Loss of small arm of chromosome 11	Associated with ringed anemia MDS
del 20q	Loss of small arm of chromosome 20	Associated with ringed anemia MDS
Chromosomal gain Trisomy 8	Gain of one extra chromosome 8	Poor prognosis and short survival
Rearrangements 3q	inv(3)(q21;q26) t(3;5)(q26;q34) t(3;3)(q21;q26)	40% therapy related; poor response to chemotherapy and poor survival
12p	t(5;12)(q33;p12)	Associated with topisomerase II activators; 50% RAEB, 50% RAEB-T, 10% CMML

a subset of patients with MDS (RAEB and RAEB-t) do respond to AML-type chemotherapy.[76] Survival for MDS ranges from several months to years, with median survival of 28 months. Poor prognostic indicators include excessive blast cells in the bone marrow, small clusters of immature myeloid precursors, pancytopenia, and complex chromosome abnormalities.[69,70] Death usually occurs within two years from complications related to bone marrow depression or transformation to acute leukemia.

Treatment for MDS is as aggressive as the course of the disease.[77] Serial bone marrow and peripheral blood examinations allow the physician to monitor the pace of the disease. Treatment for high-risk or intermediate-2 patients includes bone marrow ablation, suppression, or differentiation. Ablation of the abnormal clone of cells is accomplished with BMT, which is curative if from an HLA-matched donor and the patient is less than age 55. Success with BMT is limited by the morbidity and mortality of the procedure.[77] High-dose chemotherapy for ablation can induce remission in 40%–60% of patients, but it is of short duration.[75]

Agents to stimulate differentiation of cells so that they can mature and die include retinoic acids, vitamin D3, and interferon-alfa. A newly developed retinoid, CD437, inhibits AML cell growth independent of retinoic acid receptor based pathways, and activates multiple pathways that may reverse the premature apoptosis problem.[78]

Options for the low-risk or intermediate-1 group focus on the cytopenia. Supportive therapy includes replacement of RBCs if the hematocrit is less than 28%–30% or platelets if the level is less than 50,000/mm³. Antibiotics are used to treat infection and hematopoietic growth factors to avoid recurrent infections.

CHRONIC MYELOGENOUS LEUKEMIA

Chronic myelogenous leukemia (CML), also called *chronic granulocytic leukemia*, is a disorder of the myeloid stem cell characterized by marked splenomegaly and an increased production of granulocytes, especially neutrophils.[79] Approximately 90% of patients with CML have a diagnostic marker, the Philadelphia chromosome (Ph¹). The G group chromosome, number 22, is missing a portion of the long arm (q), which has been translocated to the long arm of number 9.[80,81] The significance of the marker is that a proto-oncogene is activated. When the proto-oncogene ABL is translocated from chromosome 9 to 22, a new oncogene, BCR-ABL, is formed. This gene produces a protein that is associated with triggering growth factor receptors.[82] It is speculated that this gene may induce uncontrolled growth of leukemic cells. Patients with Ph¹-negative CML have been found to have activation of this same gene even though no visible chromosome change is present.[83] In addition, as long as the marker is present, the patient is not cured of the disease.

There is no known specific cause for CML except exposure to ionizing radiation.[81] The peak incidence is in the third and fourth decades, and both sexes are affected equally.[79]

The natural course of CML is divided into a chronic and terminal phase. The initial chronic phase is characterized by excessive proliferation and accumulation of mature granulocytes and precursors. There is an absence of lymphadenopathy, but 90% of patients have palpable splenomegaly. Within 30–40 months, the disorder transforms into a terminal phase consisting of accelerated and blastic phases. The accelerated phase includes progressive leukocytosis with increasing myeloid precursors (including blasts), increasing basophils, splenomegaly, weight loss, and weakness. There is increasing resistance to therapy, and serial cytogenetic studies indicate progressive chromosomal abnormalities.[81]

The blastic phase resembles AML, with 30%–40% of the bone marrow cells being blasts or promyelocytes. A crisis occurs as blast cell counts rise rapidly, often exceeding 100,000/mm³. Leukostatic lesions caused by the high cell count result in occlusion in the microvasculature of the CNS or lungs. The majority of patients have myeloblastic transformation, but some have lymphoblastic transformation, evidenced by the presence of TdT or cALLa. Median survival after the onset of the terminal phase is three months.[80]

Assessment

CML in up to 20% of affected individuals is diagnosed in the absence of any symptomatology.[81] Most patients, however, present with a history that reflects the gradual accumulation of a white blood cell mass that is 10–150 times normal.

Patient History

The initial symptoms or illness typically are related to massive splenomegaly due to infiltration of the spleen by leukemic cells: left upper quadrant pain, early satiety, and vague abdominal fullness may be the presenting complaints. Leukemic infiltration of joints may also cause bone and joint pain. A history of malaise, fatigue, weight loss, and fever caused by a gradually worsening hypercatabolic state may precede more acute symptoms of anemia.[79]

To a lesser extent than with acute leukemia, epidemiologic clues may be provided by a complete past medical and family history, such as a history of exposure to ionizing radiation or a positive family history for leukemia.

Physical Examination

The vast majority of people are diagnosed during the chronic phase of their disease. The anemic individual appears pale and examination of the eyes, ears, nose, and throat may reveal leukemic infiltration. Splenomegaly and hepatomegaly are common.

The physical examination of the patient in blast crisis is similar to that for the patient with acute leukemia. In blast crisis, blastic transformation of the leukemic granulocytes has replaced the bone marrow, causing an acute illness with pancytopenia, infection, and hypercatabolism. Rapid diagnosis and treatment to reduce the number of proliferating blasts are essential.

Diagnostic Studies

A complete blood count in the chronic phase reveals anemia and severe leukocytosis (WBC > 100,000 mm³). The differential count of the leukocytes demonstrates WBCs in every stage of maturation, with a predominance of more mature cells. The presence of functional but leukemic granulocytes in these individuals accounts for the low incidence of infection during the chronic phase.

There is usually moderate anemia and thrombocytosis. The anemia is normocytic and normochromic with a median hemoglobin of 9–10 g/dL.[81]

Other laboratory studies reveal high serum B_{12} levels and a low leukocyte alkaline phosphatase level (LAP).[80] Both may return to normal with successful therapy. Bone marrow biopsy demonstrates hyperplasia, with a myeloid to erythroid ratio of 15:1 and normal to increased megakaryocytes (platelet precursors). If the abnormal Ph^1 chromosome is found in the granulocytic, erythrocytic, and megakaryocytic series of the marrow, the diagnosis of CML is confirmed.[80]

Another tool has become useful in confirming the diagnosis of CML. Polymerase chain reaction (PCR) probes are used to separate RNA from viable cells for analysis.[84] This process of reverse transcripterase-PCR (RT-PCR) is used to detect the fusion genes that result from chromosome translocations. In the case of patients with CML, RT-PCR detects the *BCR-ABL* fusion gene. In some cases, the PCR data showed the presence of the *BCR-ABL* fusion gene after successful response was indicated by the Ph chromosome negativity. Hypermetaphase fluorescent in situ hybridization (FISH) is a newer technique thought to be more sensitive in detecting the Ph chromosome.[85]

Treatment

The only chance for cure of CML is with ablation of the Ph^1 chromosome and absence of the *BCR-ABL* fusion gene. Currently this occurs after high-dose therapy followed by allogeneic BMT. CML is a chronic disease and usually is suppressed by chemotherapy with hydroxyurea or busulfan. Late in the disease or at blastic crisis, investigational drugs are used. Interferon is approved for patients in chronic phase CML.[86,87]

Chronic Phase

The standard therapy during the chronic phase is single-agent oral chemotherapy.[79] Busulfan, an alkylating agent, is active against primitive hematopoietic stem cells. The WBC count begins to drop 10–14 days after starting therapy. To prevent prolonged or severe myelosuppression, treatment is stopped if the WBC is less than 20,000/mm³. Long-term side effects include skin hyperpigmentation and pulmonary or retroperitoneal fibrosis. Hydroxyurea is cytostatic to cycling cells and inhibits ribonucleotide reductase. It acts on late progenitor stem cells causing rapid disease control, but it requires frequent monitoring of blood levels. Since hydroxyurea does not have the long-term toxicities on pulmonary and bone marrow tissue, it may be a better choice if a future BMT is a possibility.[79] Although both of these drugs decrease the leukemic cell mass and improve the quality of life, the progression to a terminal, refractory stage is not altered.

Interferon-alfa (IFN) is approved for previously untreated or pretreated patients with chronic-phase, Ph-positive CML. It is recommended that therapy begin within one year of diagnosis. The dose is 9 million international units (MIU) daily, administered subcutaneously or intramuscularly.[85,88] There is evidence that doses less than 5 MIU significantly reduce the response rate. Therefore doses of IFN are not decreased or held unless WBCs are less than 2000/mm³ or platelets are less than 50,000/mm³. Patients who achieve a hematologic response (defined as a normalization of blood counts) and a cytogenetic response (absence of the *ABL-BCR* gene) should continue with treatment until disease progression. Those who achieve only hematologic response should continue for up to two years to maximize the possibility of achieving a cytogenetic response.[87]

Side effects associated with IFN therapy in this population are similar to others previously reported. The most common are flu-like symptoms such as fever, chill, malaise, fatigue, headache, and myalgias.[89,90] Lowered blood counts occur with neutropenia (22%), thrombocytopenia (27%), and anemia (15%) that quickly reverses when therapy is held.[87] A large study compared IFN with standard chemotherapy.[91] The overall response rate for patients treated with IFN was 30% compared to 5% for standard chemotherapy. Median survival with IFN versus chemotherapy was 72 months and 52 months, respectively, and time to progression of disease was more than 72 months with IFN compared to 45 months with chemotherapy.

About 30% of patients with CML do not respond to IFN due to resistance and intolerable side effects. Recent studies demonstrate the addition of low-dose cytosine arabinoside overcomes resistance with no increased side effects.[92,93]

Terminal Phase

CML is a chronic neoplasm with a 100% incidence of blastic transformation.[80] Serial cytogenetic analyses can reveal signs of blastic transformation three to four months before clinical signs are evident. Bone marrow aspirations are required, however, which are costly and uncomfortable for the patient.[80] The current trend is to treat the accelerated phase by continuing chronic phase therapy until evidence of the blastic phase appears. Because the transformation from benign to malignant appears to be random in length, it is difficult to predict survival, although life expectancy is less than one year.

Blast crisis requires intensive chemotherapy, similar to that used in the treatment of AML. If the transformation is myeloblastic, therapy includes cytosine arabinoside, an anthracycline, and thioguanine. If lymphoblastic transformation has occurred, vincristine and prednisone are added. Patients who develop lymphoblastic transformation are more responsive to treatment and live longer.[83,94]

Although BMT remains the only chance for cure, only about 25% of patients with CML have an HLA-matched, related donor.[95] The best results have been obtained in patients receiving allogeneic BMT during the chronic phase, with 55%–70% being disease free at three to five years.[94] Transplants from unrelated, matched donor transplants and autologous transplants are being evaluated as other options.[96,97]

The proposed sequence of treatment for patients with CML is outlined in Figure 57-4.[94] Patients less than age 50 in chronic phase are immediately evaluated for an allogeneic BMT. Older patients with a high WBC receive hydroxyurea until the WBC is less than 20,000/mm³. Therapy is then changed to IFN which continues until complete cytogenetic response or, if no response, for six months. Then the patients without an allogeneic donor, those who do not respond to initial therapy, and those who relapse after therapy are considered for a matched, unrelated donor transplant, autologous BMT, or other investigational therapy. Interferon is not usually helpful in patients with advanced disease. However, effectiveness is noted in patients with advanced disease when interferon is given after cytotoxic therapy has decreased the tumor load.[88] Adoptive immunotherapy with donor lymphocyte infusions is being used to treat relapse after BMT.[98,99]

CHRONIC LYMPHOCYTIC LEUKEMIA

A progressive accumulation of morphologically normal but functionally inert lymphocytes is found in chronic lymphocytic leukemia (CLL). As the disease progresses, the abnormal lymphocytes accumulate in the bone marrow, spleen, liver, and lymph nodes. The median age at diagnosis is 70 years; the majority of cases are male.[100]

The pathologic cells are usually small lymphocytes with markers of B lymphocytes and surface IgM or IgD. The malignant cells express a characteristic phenotype with antigens such as CD5, CD19, CD20, and CD23.[100] Approximately one-half of individuals with CLL experience frequent viral and fungal infections due to hypogammaglobulinemia. For more than 95% of patients the diagnosis is an incidental finding during routine examination. Anemia, lymphadenopathy, or infection may be present. Coomb's positive autoimmune hemolytic anemia occurs in 25% of patients.[38]

The clinical course is variable, and, as with other hematologic malignancies, many attempts have been made to correlate a staging system with prognosis.[100] The two most commonly used systems are Rai and Binet. The Rai staging system, accepted in the United States, has five levels based on the extent of tissue involvement and compromise of bone marrow function. The Binet system distinguishes among three groups—A to C—on the basis of worsening prognosis; it is used in Europe. The International Workshop on CLL (IWCLL) attempt to combine the two systems is not widely accepted (Table 57-9). In general, treatment is withheld until the patient shows

Figure 57-4 Proposed treatment approach for patients with chronic myelogenous leukemia. BMT = bone marrow transplant; IFN-A = interferon-alfa; Ph = Philadelphia chromosome; MUD = matched unrelated donor. (Reprinted with permission from Kantarjian HM, Deisseroth A, Kurzrock R, et al: Chronic myelogenous leukemia: A concise update. *Blood* 82:691–703, 1993.)[94]

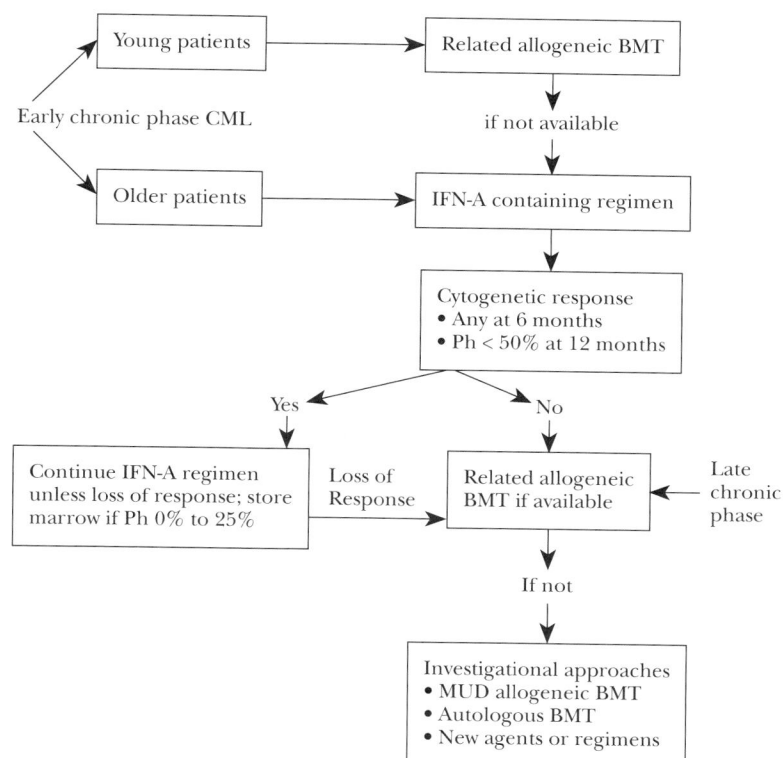

evidence of hemolytic anemia, cytopenia, disfiguring or painful lymphadenopathy, symptomatic organomegaly, or marked systemic symptoms.

Assessment

One-fourth of individuals with CLL are diagnosed during a routine physical examination. Clues that alert the clinician early on, however, may be provided by a complete health history.

Patient History

Early CLL may be asymptomatic. However, because CLL is a disease of immunoglobulin-secreting cells, a history of

Table 57-9 Three Systems for the Classification of Chronic Lymphocytic Leukemia

Rai	Binet	IWCLL*	Prognosis
0	A	A(0), A(I), A(II)	Good: > 10 yr
I	B	B(I), B(II)	Intermediate: < 7 yr
II	C	C(III), C(IV)	Poor: < 2 yr
III			
IV			

*International Workshop on Chronic Lymphocytic Leukemia.
Data from Cheson et al.[104]

recurrent infections, especially of the skin and respiratory tract, may be elicited. The onset, location, duration, and response to treatment for infection should be documented.

Progressive infiltration and accumulation in nodal structures and the bone marrow gradually produce the symptoms that are typical of more advanced disease. Vague complaints of malaise, anorexia, and fatigue are common, as is noticeable and bothersome lymphadenopathy. Splenomegaly may cause early satiety and abdominal discomfort. The past medical history should focus on the documentation of any underlying autoimmune or immune-deficiency diseases, bleeding tendencies, and infectious episodes.

Physical Examination

The individual with early CLL appears well. Splenomegaly may be the only clinical finding. In advanced disease there may be evidence of infection, fever, and rashes. Lymphadenopathy occurs in 60% of patients, especially in the cervical, axillary, inguinal, and femoral nodes. The nodes are described as mobile, discrete, and nontender.[101]

Diagnostic Studies

Peripheral blood examination reveals lymphocytosis with normal or immature lymphocytes. The lymphocyte count is greater than 20,000/mm³ in early disease and may be over 100,000/mm³ in advanced disease.[100] Protein electrophoresis documents the hypogammaglobulinemia that occurs in approximately 50% of patients. Bone marrow aspirate reflects the lymphocytosis seen peripherally, with varying degrees of infiltration. The severity of infiltration depends on the severity of the disease. Although early CLL causes patchy or focal infiltrates of the mature-appearing lymphocytes, progressive disease leads to a "packed marrow" with few normal hematopoietic cells.

As in the other hematologic disorders, cytogenetic analysis is important for diagnosis and prognosis. Chromosomal abnormalities are present in 50% of patients with CLL. Early stage disease is indicated by 20% abnormalities while 70% are present in later disease.[100,102,103]

Treatment

A consensus group sponsored by the National Cancer Institute has published guidelines for diagnosis and treatment of CLL.[104] In general, treatment consists only of observation until the patient is symptomatic with cytopenias or organomegaly.[102,105] The rate of progressive lymphocytosis directs the frequency of observation and start of therapy. The lymphocyte doubling time (LDT) is important to assess. For patients with a LDT of less than 12 months, the median survival is 12 months.[100]

Chlorambucil and cyclophosphamide are two alkylating agents used to treat CLL, providing a response rate of 60%, with complete remission in 10%–20% of patients.[102,105] Corticosteroids are used to control leukocytosis and immune-mediated cytopenias. When the patient no longer responds to steroid therapy, splenectomy may provide relief of symptoms. Radiation therapy may be used to treat lymphadenopathy or painful splenomegaly.

For untreated patients with advanced disease (stage III or IV) and anemia or thrombocytopenia, treatment with a purine analog is recommended.[106] This includes cyclophosphamide, vincristine, doxorubicin, and prednisone. Fludarabine, with an 80% response rate, is the newest agent approved for use in B-cell CLL. Fludarabine is given as a daily 30-minute infusion for five days and is generally well tolerated.[80,102] For patients refractory to fludarabine alone, cyclophosphamide is added.[105] Targeted molecular therapy is the newest strategy for treating CLL using agents such as UCN-01, topoisomerase I inhibitors, bryostatin, flavoperidol, and Campath 1-H.[106]

HAIRY CELL LEUKEMIA

Etiology

An unusual variant of the chronic leukemias is termed hairy cell leukemia (HCL), so named for the prominent cytoplasmic projections on circulating mononuclear cells.

HCL is also called *leukemic reticuloendotheliosis.* Clinically, HCL may be difficult to distinguish from CLL or malignant lymphoma. No genes have been found directly related to HCL.[103] The distinguishing characteristics are massive splenomegaly and little or no adenopathy. The characteristic hairy cells stain positively for tartrate-resistant acid phosphatase.[38] Two-thirds of individuals with HCL have pancytopenia, with symptomatic anemia, bleeding, and infection.

Treatment

The goal of therapy in HCL has progressed from palliation to cure with the use of nucleoside analogs and interferon. Historically, patients without cytopenias required no immediate treatment. Because infection is the primary cause of death, however, patients with HCL are monitored closely. Splenectomy has been the treatment of choice for patients with marked pancytopenia, recurrent infections, massive splenomegaly, or rapid disease progression and may allow prolonged survival of up to 15 years. However, complete remissions have been obtained in HCL with 2'-deoxycoformycin and 2-chlorodeoxyadenosine.[103,107,108] Normalization of peripheral blood counts occurs with absence of hairy cells in the bone marrow and long-term results are positive.[109] Recombinant interferon-alfa is considered the treatment of choice for those in whom the disease progresses.[80,106] Administered daily by intramuscular or subcutaneous injection, interferon-alfa decreases the need for transfusions, reduces risk of infection, and improves overall quality of life.

Supportive Therapy

The increase in the length and quality of survival experienced by most individuals with leukemia is due not only to advances in antileukemic therapy but also to improved blood product and antimicrobial support and specialized nursing care. The complex means of providing effective supportive care include medical management to maintain physiologic homeostasis as well as an interdisciplinary approach to the health care plan.

Effective nursing participation in the supportive care of any patient with leukemia depends on an understanding of the staging and natural history of each of the leukemias. From this base of knowledge the nurse contributes to the care of the patient with leukemia in each of the areas of education, physical care, symptom management, and psychosocial adaptation.

Education

Providing information related to the disease process and treatment is clearly a standard in oncology nursing.[110] The nurse caring for the patient with AML has the unique opportunity of providing information to the patient and family because the patient is usually hospitalized throughout the course of therapy. The teaching plan for all patients includes pertinent information about the diagnosis, strategies for self-care in the prevention and treatment of side effects both in the hospital setting and at home, and methods to facilitate coping and adaptation to the illness.

For all patients with leukemia it is helpful to include the basic physiology of the bone marrow in the teaching plan. A hematologic malignancy is not as easy to understand as the concept of a solid tumor. Describing the bone marrow as the center of the bone where all blood products are made is a simple start. Further explanation includes the type, function, and abnormalities of the blood cells (Figure 57-5). From this base, individualized instruction related to the specific leukemia is given. Educational materials can be obtained from the Leukemia Society, American Cancer Society, and the National Cancer Institute. Information for contacting these organizations is found in Chapter 85.

Physical Care

The physical care needs of patients with leukemia require nurses who are skilled in physical assessment. Patients with AML receive intensive therapy aimed at producing bone marrow aplasia for several weeks. Those with ALL have defective lymphocytes producing altered immuno-competence. The drugs received are cytotoxic. The hypogammaglobulinemia associated with CLL increases the patient's susceptibility to viral and fungal infections. In any type of leukemia the incidence of infection is high, but the usual signs and symptoms of infection are diminished or absent. Therefore, the nurse must regularly conduct a thorough physical examination in order to detect any evidence of infection. Subtle changes in vital signs and mentation may indicate early sepsis. Oozing of blood from gums and intravenous sites may be the first sign of disseminated intravascular coagulation. Cerebellar toxicity related to chemotherapy may be manifested as slightly altered responses in the neurological examination. Each of these situations may be life-threatening, and the astute skills of the experienced nurse may be the crucial factor in initiating appropriate treatment.

In addition to having good assessment skills, the nurse caring for the patient with acute leukemia must be experienced in the use of right atrial catheters (RACs) and vascular access devices (VADs).[11] Patients undergoing aggressive induction therapy in the hospital often have a double or triple lumen RAC placed prior to the start of therapy. The RAC is used for blood sampling as well as for the infusion of fluids, chemotherapy, antibiotics, total parenteral nutrition, and blood products.[111] Patients who require ongoing treatment but less frequent blood sampling and no simultaneous infusion of multiple fluids may have a VAD placed subcutaneously.[112,113] The advantages, disadvantages, and nursing procedures associated with RAC and VAD are beyond the scope of this chapter. How-

Figure 57-5 Patient teaching sheet for blood cell function.

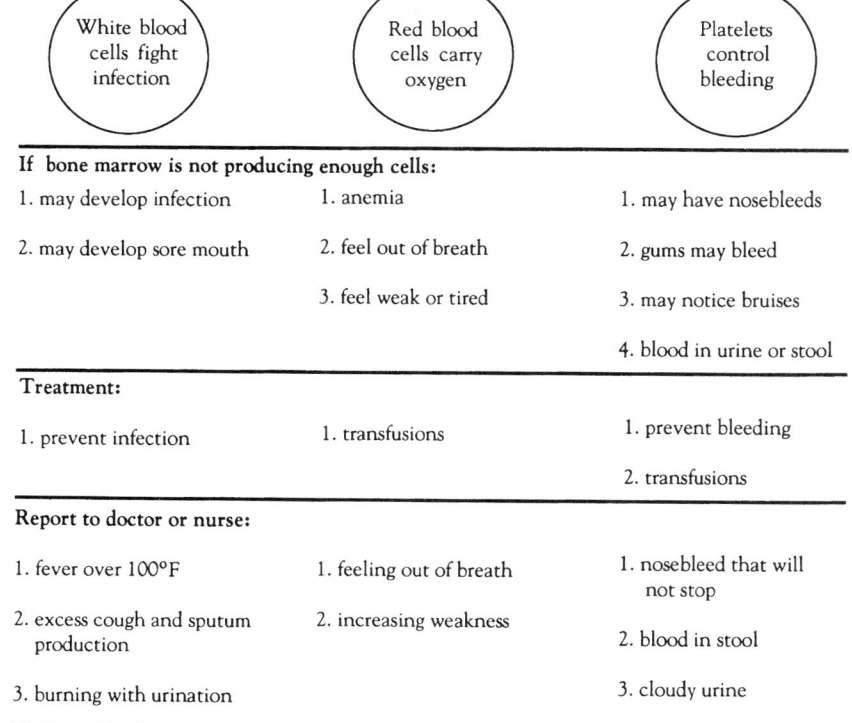

White blood cells fight infection	Red blood cells carry oxygen	Platelets control bleeding
If bone marrow is not producing enough cells:		
1. may develop infection	1. anemia	1. may have nosebleeds
2. may develop sore mouth	2. feel out of breath	2. gums may bleed
	3. feel weak or tired	3. may notice bruises
		4. blood in urine or stool
Treatment:		
1. prevent infection	1. transfusions	1. prevent bleeding
		2. transfusions
Report to doctor or nurse:		
1. fever over 100°F	1. feeling out of breath	1. nosebleed that will not stop
2. excess cough and sputum production	2. increasing weakness	2. blood in stool
3. burning with urination		3. cloudy urine

ever, since most patients with acute leukemia have one of these devices, it is important for the nurse to become familiar with them.

Symptom Management

Certain side effects associated with antileukemic therapy and disease-related complications can best be ameliorated if detected early and treated promptly. Knowing which side effects are expected and when they may occur allows the nurse to focus care appropriately.

Bone marrow depression

The desired effect of cytotoxic therapy is bone marrow hypoplasia. The duration of pancytopenia is variable, depending on the type of therapy and the person's ability to recover. However, individuals with acute leukemia in the induction phase or individuals with CML in blast crisis may remain severely hypoplastic for months.

Neutropenia. It takes nine to ten days for immature cells formed in the bone marrow to become mature granulocytes. Because granulocytes circulate for only six to ten hours, any interruption in their production quickly places the patient at risk for developing an infection. Infection is the major complication for leukemia patients, with up to 20%–30% mortality.[114,115] Neutropenia is commonly defined as an absolute neutrophil count less than 1000/mm³. Since the neutrophils are responsible for phagocytosis, neutropenia eliminates one of the body's first lines of defense against infection. The patient with leukemia is particularly at risk due to a rapid drop in WBC with the initiation of therapy, a continuing decrease until the nadir (lowest point) is reached, and a prolonged time for recovery.[116]

Approximately 60% of neutropenic individuals develop infection. One-third have documented bacteremia, another third have documented infection without bacteremia, and the rest have apparent infection with no microbiologically documented pathogen. The most frequent cause of bacteremia is coagulase-negative staphylococci and viridans streptococci.[114] The risk of infection rises as the neutrophil count decreases, with 100% incidence of infection if the neutrophil count remains less than 100/mm³ for three weeks. Other factors that add to the risk of infection are corticosteroids, hospital environment, antibiotic usage leading to increased colonization, and mucosal alteration.[117]

Adrenal corticosteroids are frequently used as part of the chemotherapeutic regimen or as supportive therapy. Steroids cause lysis of lymphocytes, suppression of antibody production, protein malnutrition, and suppression of inflammatory responses. As a result, the use of corticosteroids predisposes the patient to infection.

Most infections are due to organisms endogenous to the host or present in the environment.[116] The most common sites of infection are the alimentary tract (pharynx, esophagus, anorectum), sinuses, lungs, and skin.[117,118] The alimentary mucosa is directly damaged by the chemotherapy and the neutropenia allows colonization with yeasts and/or gram-negative bacilli. Perianal infection occurs in 25% of patients with AML. The only signs may be induration, erythema, and pain on defecation. Pneumonia can be caused by gram-negative organisms such as *Pseudomonas aeruginosa, Klebsiella pneumonia,* or *Escherichia coli.* The most common gram-positive organism causing infection is *Staphylococcus epidermidis.*[117,118]

More serious infections associated with prolonged neutropenia are fungal infections such as *Candida tropicalis, Aspergillus* spp, *Fusarium* spp, and *Trichosporon* spp or protozoa such as *Pneumocystis carinii.*[115,119] When these infections occur during severe aplasia and immune depression, recovery of the blood counts is the best hope for survival.

Empiric antibiotic therapy is used to treat high-risk (neutropenic and febrile) patients until an infecting organism is identified. Early empiric antibiotic therapy includes drugs to cover both gram-negative and gram-positive organisms. The usual combinations include an aminoglycoside plus an extended-spectrum cephalosporin or a broad-spectrum antipseudomonal penicillin.[120,121] A trend toward initial broad-spectrum monotherapy continues to be evaluated.[120]

Amphotericin B is used to treat life-threatening fungal infections in myelosuppressed, immunosuppressed individuals. It is indicated if fever continues for five to seven days after the start of antibiotic therapy, if there is no identified source of infection, and continued neutropenia is expected.[119,122] Common side effects of this toxic therapy include fever, chills, and rigors, nephrotoxicity, headache, anorexia, vomiting, and anemia. Because anaphylaxis is a risk, a test dose of 1 mg is administered over 30 minutes. If the patient does not experience cardiopulmonary or mental changes, the starting dose is given. Fever is not a contraindication when the patient has recurrent fevers prior to the therapy. The dose is escalated daily until the desired dose is reached, and therapy continues for weeks to months, depending on the organism being treated and the patient's response.

Symptom management includes the following interventions to prevent or treat fever, chills, or rigors: premedication with corticosteroids, acetaminophen, or diphenhydramine, and adding 10–15 mg hydrocortisone sodium succinate to the infusion. Intravenous meperidine 25–50 mg is given at the onset of chills or as a premedication. Increasing room temperature, adding extra covers, using relaxation and hypnosis, and isometric leg and arm movements are other suggested comfort measures.[123] Potential nephrotoxicity due to a decreased glomerular filtration rate requires close monitoring of blood urea nitrogen, creatinine, sodium, and magnesium as well as evaluation of fluid balance.[124] Peripheral phlebitis can be avoided by adding heparin to the solution. The anemia associated with amphotericin B is reversible and problematic only in that it compounds the existing myelosuppression.

There are currently a number of clinical trials evaluating the administration of amphotericin B in lipid vehicles.[115,124] The lipid vehicles do not enhance efficacy of the drug but seem to reduce the toxicities, thus allowing higher doses to be administered.[125] Randomized studies comparing the formations are not complete.

Some centers place patients on prophylactic fluconazole and itraconazole to prevent disseminated infections in patients expected to have prolonged neutropenia.[115] The Center for Disease Control, however, has issued a formal recommendation discouraging empirical vancomycin in the febrile neutropenic patient due to the increased risk of developing vancomycin resistant enterococci.[126]

Because the neutropenic patient does not produce an adequate inflammatory response to infection, the usual signs and symptoms are absent.[116] Fever is usually the first sign of infection that leads to closer inspection of high-risk areas (perirectal area, oral mucosa, IV sites). Patients are often unable to produce sputum; thus, the early indications of pneumonia are shortness of breath or cough. Vital signs are assessed every four hours. At the onset of fever over 100°F in the neutropenic patient, blood, urine, and sputum cultures are obtained and empiric antibiotic therapy is initiated. The importance of prompt reporting of fever and initiation of therapy cannot be overemphasized since delay of only a few hours can allow the patient to go into septic shock.

Prevention of infection focuses on restoring host defenses, decreasing invasive procedures, and decreasing colonization of organisms. Treatment and remission induction will restore normal defenses against infection. Decreasing invasive procedures includes avoiding the use of Foley catheters. If catheterization is necessary, the smallest lumen possible should be used, and the catheter should be anchored. Other measures are meticulous care of IV or RAC exit sites and aseptic technique for any invasive procedures.

To decrease the number of gram-negative organisms, uncooked fruits and vegetables are avoided, especially salads. *P. aeruginosa* can be decreased by removing aerators from faucets, using ice machines in which the ice falls directly into the cup, and by frequently changing stagnant water sources such as oxygen humidifiers. Proper hand-washing techniques by everyone in contact with the patient can eliminate the main source of gram-positive organisms. Fungi that are found in food or the air can also be decreased by cooking foods and eliminating live plants or flowers from the patient's room. A private room is necessary, and visitors are restricted. All of these measures are to be practiced by the health care team and taught to the patient and family.[116,127] Further information is provided in Chapter 30.

In certain circumstances such as BMT, total reverse isolation may be used. The patient is kept in a sterile laminar air-flow room. Nonabsorbable antibiotics are used to sterilize the alimentary canal. Normal skin flora is decreased by frequent cleansing with hexachlorophene or an iodine-base soap.

Granulocyte transfusions may be indicated for patients with profound neutropenia and documented infec-tions not responding to antibiotics.[119,128] However, the hazards of this therapy (increased alloimmunization and refractoriness to platelet transfusions) and its high cost make it a controversial therapy.

Hematapoietic growth factors (HGFs) have been used in the treatment of patients with leukemia in supportive care and for priming effects.[129,130] Both granulocyte (G-CSF) and granulocyte-macrophage (GM-CSF) have been administered to patients after completion of standard induction therapy to shorten the period of neutropenia. Because myeloid leukemia cells have receptors for CSFs and have demonstrated increased growth in response to CSFs in vitro, supportive use of HGFs are recommended for high-risk patients only, such as those older than age 60. There is concern about administering myeloid CSFs to patients with AML.

Erythrocytopenia. Individuals undergoing intensive chemotherapy develop a tolerance for chronic, low-grade anemia. However, in severe cases of hypoplasia, sudden blood loss due to bleeding, or symptomatic anemia, support with transfusions of RBCs is provided. Premedication with acetaminophen and diphenhydramine can decrease the febrile response to antibodies to white cells that occurs after multiple transfusions. Leukocyte-poor RBCs may be used to decrease the antibody production against antigens on the leukocytes.[131–133]

Thrombocytopenia. Thrombocytopenia is the abnormal decrease in the number of circulating platelets. The potential for bleeding occurs when levels are less than 50,000 platelets/mm³, and spontaneous bleeding occurs at levels of less than 20,000 platelets/mm³.[133] The first evidence of bleeding may be petechiae or ecchymoses on the skin of dependent limbs or on mucous membranes or oozing from gums, nose, or IV site.

Random donor platelets are given to keep the platelet count above 20,000/mm³. Once antibodies to the platelets develop, refractoriness to random donor platelets occurs. When blood counts one hour posttransfusion reveal poor increments, the patient may require HLA-matched, single-donor platelets.[133] Because chills and fever can destroy circulating platelets, the patient is premedicated with acetaminophen and diphenhydramine.[132] Additional measures used to prevent bleeding include maintaining skin integrity, preventing trauma, and avoiding medications that have the potential to induce or prolong bleeding. Stool softeners will prevent the Valsalva maneuver and rectal tears. Further detail is given in Chapter 31.

Complications

Certain complications of the specific leukemic process or therapy may be singled out as untoward but not unexpected side effects. Knowledge of these occurrences assists the nurse in anticipating problems in high-risk individuals. These complications include leukostasis, disseminated intravascular coagulation, retinoic acid-APL (RA-APL) syndrome, oral complications, and cerebellar toxicity.

Leukostasis. Individuals with extremely high numbers of circulating blasts are at risk of leukostatic-induced hemorrhage. This occurs most often in patients with ALL. Leukostasis occurs as leukemic blasts accumulate and invade vessel walls, causing rupture and bleeding. Because of the extensive capillary network and the limited vasculature space of the brain, intracerebral hemorrhage is the most common and most lethal manifestation of this complication. Therefore, early detection of patients at risk (WBC greater than 50,000 cells/mm³) and immediate efforts to reduce the number of circulating cells are imperative. Treatment consists of high doses of cytotoxic drugs to reduce the burden of circulating cells. Leukapheresis and cranial irradiation may be used to provide immediate treatment.[9]

Disseminated intravascular coagulation. Disseminated intravascular coagulation (DIC) is most frequently associated with acute promyelocytic leukemia, although it may occur with any acute leukemia.[134] During induction therapy there is excessive release of procoagulants from granules within the leukemic promyelocyte. (See Chapter 39 for a discussion of the pathophysiology of DIC.)

Correction of the coagulopathy in DIC depends on the successful treatment of the leukemia. Therapy usually includes heparin and replacement of plasma factors and platelets. Nursing care focuses on the prevention of injury, administration of prescribed therapy, and monitoring of the appropriate laboratory results.[131]

Retinoic acid-APL syndrome. Another toxicity associated with treatment of APL is RA-APL syndrome. This syndrome appears clinically similar to the capillary leak syndrome associated with interleukin-2 therapy and is characterized by fever, respiratory distress, pulmonary infiltrates on chest x-ray, and weight gain. The incidence of RA-APL is 40% and the etiology is unknown. Early identification and treatment with high-dose intravenous steroids has decreased the mortality associated with this syndrome.[135] Nursing care is focused on early detection of fluid retention (with measurement of weight, abdominal girth, orthostatic blood pressure, intake and output), fever (vital signs), and pulmonary distress.[134]

Oral complications. Oral complications of leukemia may be the result of the disease or the therapy. Gingival hypertrophy due to massive infiltration by leukemic cells is associated with acute myelomonocytic and monocytic leukemia.[9] The gingiva may be swollen, necrotic, and/or superinfected. The most effective treatment is therapy for the leukemia. Stomatitis due to the direct toxicity of chemotherapeutic agents such as the anthracyclines or methotrexate, combined with prolonged neutropenia and antibiotic therapy, renders the patient at high risk for oral infection.

Oral care consists of regular cleansing with a solution of one quart of water with one teaspoon each of salt and sodium bicarbonate or 1.5% hydrogen peroxide, treatment of infection with nystatin mouth rinses, and appropriate analgesia as needed.[136]

Cerebellar toxicity. Cerebellar toxicity is a CNS toxicity associated with the administration of high-dose cytosine arabinoside (HDCA). Conventional dosages are 100–200 mg/m², whereas HDCA is greater than 3 g/m². The incidence of neurotoxicity is 11%–28% at dosages of 3 g/m² and as high as 67% in dosages up to 4.5 g/m².[137] This toxicity is also age-related, with an increased risk in patients over age 50. The syndrome may begin with signs of ataxia and nystagmus and progress to dysarthria (difficulty in articulating words) and adiadochokinesis (inability to perform rapid alternating movements). This toxicity may be irreversible if not detected early. Therefore, it is essential that prior to each dose of HDCA the nurse completes a full neurological assessment.[138] Any changes are reported and the dosage is held until the physician evaluates the patient.

Psychosocial Support

Individuals and their significant others are at risk for ineffective coping during the diagnostic workup for malignancy and during subsequent treatments.[139] A primary objective of supportive care must be to facilitate the most effective coping mechanisms for the individual and family as well as to enable the patient to live as full and normal a life as possible. Several factors should be taken into consideration as the nurse coordinates the care plan for psychological and physical rehabilitation.

The age of the individual at the time of diagnosis may vary from infancy to old age. Issues may range from concern about fertility or the risk of a second malignancy in the young adult to fear of job stigma in the middle-aged individual. The elderly patient may be dealing with increasing physical decline in addition to the debilitating effects of cancer. Assessment of the individual's needs and degree of stress will facilitate the planning of suitable intervention.[140]

The stage and "curability" of the disease are other factors to be considered. It is imperative that the nurse understand the implications of the planned therapy and assist the patient in making appropriate decisions. For example, a young mother undergoing intensive chemotherapy for AML may need to make the necessary arrangement for child care and housekeeping for six to eight weeks. A patient undergoing BMT may need to discuss with his or her employer the need to be on extended sick leave. The emotional ups and downs related to multiple remission inductions and relapses are exhausting to the patient and family. As survival with leukemia increases, patients must deal with many issues such as fear of relapse, return to an independent state, and an uncertain future.[29,141] Ongoing support from the health care team is essential to overcome these fears.

Education and reassurance by consistent nursing staff can help the individual regain a sense of control and hopefulness.

Conclusion

The care of the individual with a diagnosis of leukemia requires a multidisciplinary approach that considers many factors. The classification of acute or chronic and myeloid or lymphoid determines diverse treatment plans and prognoses that are quite variable. The age of the patient and the stage of the disease determine the aggressiveness of therapy. Newer diagnostic studies allow the identification of both favorable and high-risk subsets of patients. As research continues, more durable cure rates may be achieved.

The role of the nurse providing direct care for patients with leukemia includes education, physical care, symptom management, and psychosocial support. In addition, contributions to research studies are essential. Although the nurse has an indirect impact on the prognosis through correct administration of therapy and management of side effects, the direct result of continuous support and education is an improved quality of life.

References

1. Bloomfield CD, Herzig GP, Caligiuri MA: Introduction: acute leukemia: recent advances. *Semin Oncol* 24:1–3, 1997
2. Mrozek K, Heinonen K, de la Chapelle, et al: Clinical significance of cytogenetics in acute myeloid leukemia. *Semin Oncol* 24:17–31, 1997
3. *Cancer Facts and Figures 2000.* Atlanta, American Cancer Society, 1999, p 4
4. Greenlee RT, Murray T, Bolden S, et al: Cancer statistics, 2000. *CA Cancer J Clin* 50:7–33, 2000
5. Hutton JJ: The leukemias and polycythemia, in Stein JH (ed): *Internal Medicine* (ed 5). St. Louis, Mosby, 1998, pp 682–691
6. Maguire-Eisen ME, Edmonds KS: Leukemias, in Clark JC, McGee RF (eds): *Core Curriculum for Oncology Nursing.* Philadelphia, Saunders, 1992, pp 480–487
7. Sandler DP: Epidemiology and etiology of acute leukemias: an update. *Leukemia* 6:3–5, 1992 (suppl)
8. Sandler DP: Epidemiology of acute leukemia in children and adults. *Semin Oncol* 24:3–16, 1997
9. Scheinberg DA, Maslak P, Weiss M: Acute leukemias, in Devita VT, Hellman S, Rosenberg SA (eds): *Cancer: Principles and Practice of Oncology* (ed 5). Philadelphia, Lippincott, 1997, pp 2293–2320
10. Preston DI, Kusumi S, Tomonaga M, et al: Cancer incidence in atomic bomb survivors: part III. Leukemia, lymphoma, and multiple myeloma, 1950–1987. *Radiat Res* 137:S68–S97, 1994 (suppl)
11. Kamada N, Tanaka K, Oguma N, et al: Cytogenetic and molecular changes in leukemia among atomic bomb survivors. *J Radiat Res* 32:257–265, 1991
12. Matanowski GM, Seltser R, Sartwell PE: The current mortality rates of radiologists and other physician specialists: specific causes of death. *Am J Epidemiol* 101:199–210, 1975
13. Inskip PD, Kleinerman RA, Stovall M, et al: Leukemia, lymphoma, and multiple myeloma after pelvic radiotherapy for benign disease. *Radiat Res* 135:108–124, 1993
14. Paustenbach DJ, Bass RD, Price P: Benzene toxicity and risk assessment, 1972–1992: implications for future regulation. *Environ Health Perspect* 101:177–200, 1993 (suppl 6)
15. Snyder P, Kalf GF: A perspective on benzene leukemogenesis. *Crit Rev Toxicol* 24:177–209, 1994
16. Dougan L, Woodleff AJ: Acute leukemia associated with phenylbutazone treatment. *Med J Aust* 1:217–219, 1965
17. Brauer MJ, Dameshek W: Hypoplastic anemia and myeloblastic leukemia following chloramphenicol therapy. *N Engl J Med* 277:1003–1005, 1967
18. Whitlock JA, Greer JP, Lukens JN: Epipodophyllotoxin-related leukemia. *Cancer* 68:600–604, 1991
19. Pedersen-Bjergaard J, Daugaard G, Hansen SW, et al: Increased risk of myelodysplasia and leukemia after etoposide, cisplatin, and bleomycin for germ-cell tumors. *Lancet* 338:359–363, 1991
20. Domer PH, Head DR, Renganathan N, et al: Molecular analysis of 13 cases of MLL/11q23 secondary acute leukemia and identification of topoisomerase II consensus-binding sequences near the chromosomal breakpoint of a secondary leukemia with the t(4;11). *Leukemia* 9:1305–1312, 1995
21. Karp JE, Smith ME: The molecular pathogenesis of treatment induced (secondary) leukemias: Foundations for treatment and prevention. *Semin Oncol* 24:103–113, 1997.
22. Ben David Y, Bernstein A: Friend views induced erythroleukemia and the multistage nature of cancer. *Cell* 66:831–834, 1991
23. Farias de Carvalho SM, Pombo de Oliveira MS, Thuler LC, et al: HTLV-I and HTLV-II infections in hematologic disorder patients, cancer patients and healthy patients from Rio de Janeiro, Brazil. *J Acquir Immune Defic Syndr Hum Retrovirol* 15:238–242, 1997
24. Rosenblatt JD, Plaeger-Marshall S, Giorgi JV, et al: A clinical, hematologic, and immunologic analysis of 21 HTLV-II-infected intravenous drug users. *Blood* 76:409–417, 1990
25. Bennett JM, Catovsky D, Daniel MT, et al: Proposals for the classification of the acute leukemias. *Br J Haemat* 33:451–458, 1976
26. Bennett JM, Catovsky D, Daniel MT, et al: Criteria for the diagnosis of acute leukemia of megakaryocyte lineage (M7). *Ann Intern Med* 103:460–462, 1985
27. Bennett JM, Catovsky D, Daniel MT, et al: Proposed revised criteria for the classification of acute myeloid leukemia. *Ann Intern Med* 103:626–629, 1985
28. Catovsky D, Matukis E, Buccheri V, et al: A classification of acute leukemia for the 1990s. *Ann Hematol* 62:16–21, 1991
29. Yeager KA, Miaskowski C: Advances in understanding the mechanisms and management of acute myelogenous leukemia. *Oncol Nurs Forum* 21:541–548, 1994
30. Caligiuri MA, Strout MP, Gilliland DG: Molecular biology of acute myeloid leukemia. *Semin Oncol* 24:32–44, 1997
31. Arlin ZA, Heddeman W, Feldman E, et al: Further thoughts on "cell kill" in acute leukemia. *Acta Haematol* 85:1–5, 1991
32. Strout MP, Caligiuri MA: Developments in cytogenetics

and oncogenes in acute leukemia. *Curr Opin Oncol* 9:8–17, 1997

33. Faderl S, Kantarjian HM, Talpaz M, et al: Clinical significance of cytogenetic abnormalities in adult acute lymphoblastic leukemia. *Blood* 91:3995–4019, 1998

34. Devine S, Larsen RA: Acute leukemia in adults: recent developments in diagnosis and treatment. *CA Cancer J Clin* 44:326–352, 1994

35. Matutes E, Morilla R, Farahat N, et al: Definition of acute biphenotypic leukemia. *Haematologia* 82:64–66, 1997

36. Fenaux P, Chomienne C, Degos L: Acute promyelocytic leukemia: biology and treatment. *Semin Oncol* 24:92–102, 1997

37. Peterson BA, Ellis EG: Uncommon subtypes of acute non-lymphocytic leukemia: clinical features and management of FAB M^5 M^6 M^7. *Semin Oncol* 14:425–434, 1987

38. Champlin R, Golde DW: The leukemias, in Braunwald E, Isselbacher KJ, Petersdorf RG, Wilson JD (eds): *Harrison's Principles of Internal Medicine* (ed 14). New York, McGraw-Hill, 1998, pp 1541–1550

39. Berman E, Heller G, Santorsa J, et al: Results of a randomized trial comparing idarubicin and cytosine arabinoside with daunorubicin and cytosine arabinoside in adult patients with newly diagnosed acute myelogenous leukemia. *Blood* 77:1666–1674, 1991

40. Bishop JF: The treatment of adult acute myeloid leukemia. *Semin Oncol* 24:57–69, 1997

41. Hansen OP, Pederson-Bjergaard J, Ellegaard J, et al: Adarubicin plus cytosine arabinoside versus daunorubicin plus cytosine arabinoside in previously untreated patients with acute myeloid leukemia: a Danish national phase III trial. *Leukemia* 5:510–516, 1991

42. Vogler WR, McCarley DH, Stagg M, et al: A phase III trial of high dose cytosine arabinoside with or without etoposide in relapsed or refractory acute myelogenous leukemia. *Leukemia* 9:1847–1853, 1994

43. Brach MA, Henschler R, Martelsman R, et al: To overcome pharmacologic and cytokinetic resistance to cytarabine in the treatment of acute myelogenous leukemia by using recombinant interleukin-3. *Semin Hematol* 28:39–43, 1991

44. Wolff SN, Marion J, Stern RS, et al: High dose cytosine arabinoside and daunorubicin as consolidation therapy for acute non lymphocytic leukemia in first remission: a pilot study. *Blood* 65:1407–1411, 1985

45. Schiller G, Gajewski J, Territo M, et al: Long-term outcome of high dose cytarabine based consolidation therapy for adults with acute myelogenous leukemia. *Blood* 80:2977–2982, 1992

46. Baer MR: Assessment of minimal residual disease in patients with acute leukemia. *Curr Opin Oncol* 10:17–22, 1998

47. Arlin ZA, Feldman ET, Finger LR, et al: Short course high dose mitoxantrone with high dose cytarabine is effective therapy for adult lymphoblastic leukemia. *Leukemia* 5:712–714, 1991

48. Bassan R, Barbui T: Remission induction therapy for adults with acute myelogenous leukemia: towards the ICE age. *Haematologica* 80:82–90, 1995

49. Zittoun RA, Mandelli F, Willemze R, et al: Autologous or allogeneic bone marrow transplantation compared with intensive chemotherapy in acute myelogenous leukemia. *N Engl J Med* 332:217–223, 1995

50. Barrett AJ, Locatelli F, Treleave JG, et al: Second transplants for leukemia relapse after bone marrow transplantation: high early mortality but favorable effect of chronic GVHD on continued remission, a report by the EBMT Leukaemia Working Party. *Br J Haematol* 79:567–574, 1991

51. Dalton WS, Miller TP: Multidrug resistance. *PPO Updates* 5:1–13, 1991

52. Maslak P, Hegewisch-Becker S, Godfrey L, et al: Flow cytometric determinations of the multi-drug resistant phenotype in acute leukemia. *Cytometry* 17:84–93, 1994

53. List AF, Spier C, Greer J, et al: Phase I/II trial of cyclosporine as a chemotherapy-resistance modifier in acute leukemia. *J Clin Oncol* 11:1652–1660, 1993

54. Brown RA, Herzig RH, Wolff SN, et al: High dose etoposide and cyclophosphamide without bone marrow transplantation for resistant hematologic malignancy. *Blood* 76:473–479, 1990

55. Degos L, Dombret H, Chomienne C, et al: All-trans retinoic acid as a differentiating agent in the treatment of acute promyelocytic leukemia. *Blood* 85:2643–2653, 1995

56. Warrell RP, Frankel S, Miller WH, et al: Differentiation therapy of acute promyelocytic leukemia treated with tretinoin (all-trans retinoid acid). *N Engl J Med* 324:1385–1393, 1991

57. Roche Laboratories: Vesanoid® (tretinoin) capsules (package insert). Nutley, NJ, 1995

58. Chen Z, Tong J-H, Dong S, et al: Retinoic acid regulatory pathways, chromosomal translocations, and acute promyelocytic leukemia. *Genes Chromosomes Cancer* 15:147–156, 1996

59. Henderson ES: Acute leukemia: general considerations, in Williams WJ, Beutler E, Erslev AJ, Lichtman MA (eds): *Hematology*. New York, McGraw-Hill, 1990, pp 236–251

60. Kantarjian HM: Adult acute lymphocytic leukemia: critical review of current knowledge. *Am J Med* 97:176–184, 1994

61. Laport GF, Larson RA: Treatment of adult acute lymphoblastic leukemia. *Semin Oncol* 24:70–82, 1997

62. Copelan EA, McGuire EA: The biology and treatment of acute lymphoblastic leukemia in adults. *Blood* 85:1151–1168, 1995

63. Preti A, Kantarjian HM: Management of adult acute lymphocytic leukemia: present issues and key challenges. *J Clin Oncol* 12:1312–1322, 1994

64. Hoelzer D: Acute lymphoblastic leukemia in adults, in Hoffman R, Benz EJ, Shattel SI, Furie B, Cohen HJ (eds): *Hematology: Basic Principles and Practice*. New York, Churchill Livingstone, 1991, pp 793–804

65. Hoelzer D: High-dose chemotherapy in adult acute lymphoblastic leukemia. *Semin Hematol* 28:84–89, 1991

66. Hamilton-Paterson JL: Preleukemia anemia. *Acta Haematol* 2:309–316, 1949

67. Kouides PA, Bennett JM: Morphology and classifcation of myelodysplastic syndromes. *Hematol Oncol Clin North Am* 6:485–499, 1992.

68. Bennett JM, Catovsky D, Daniel MT, et al: The French-American-British (FAB) Cooperative Group: proposals for the classification of the myelodysplastic syndromes. *Br J Haematol* 51:189–199, 1982

69. Sanz G, Sanz M, Greenberg P: Prognostic factors and scoring systems in myelodysplastic syndromes: recent advances in myelodysplastic syndromes. *Haematologica* 83:358–376, 1998

70. Karp J: Molecular pathogenesis and targets for therapy in myelodysplastic syndromes (MDS) and MDS-related leukemias. *Curr Opin Oncol* 10:3–9, 1998

71. Koeffler HP: Introduction: myelodyplastic syndromes. *Semin Hematol* 33:87–94, 1996

72. Raza A, Mundle S, Iftikhar A, et al: Simultaneous assessment of cell kinetics and programmed cell death in bone marrow biopsies of myelodysplastics reveals extensive apoptosis as the probable basis for ineffective hematopoiesis. *Am J Hematol* 489:143–154, 1995

73. Raza A, Mundle S, Shetty V, et al: A paradigm shift in myelodysplastic syndromes. *Leukemia* 10:1648–1652, 1996

74. Magill MK, Macfarlane E, McMullin MF: Intramedullary apoptosis may simply be a correlate of ineffective hematopoiesis. *Br J Haematol* 97:17–23, 1997 (suppl 1)

75. Koides PA, Bennett JM: Understanding the myelodysplastic syndromes. *Oncologist* 389–401, 1997

76. Estey E, Pierce H, Kantarjian H, et al: Treatment of myeloblastic syndromes with AML-type chemotherapy. *Leuk Lymphoma* 11:59–63, 1993

77. National Cancer Center Network: NCCN practice guidelines for the myelodysplastic syndromes. *Oncology* 12:53–80, 1998.

78. Hsu CA, Rishi AK, Su-Li X, et al: Retinoid induced apoptosis in leukemic cells through a retinoic acid nuclear receptor-independent pathway. *Blood* 89:4470–4479, 1997

79. Cortez JE, Talpaz M, Kantarjian HM: Chronic myelogenous leukemia: a review. *Am J Med* 100:555–570, 1996.

80. Morrison VA: Chronic leukemias. *CA Cancer J Clin* 44:353–377, 1994

81. Hughes TD, Goldman JM: Chronic myeloid leukemia, in Hoffman R, Benz EJ, Shattil SJ, Furie B, Cohen HJ (eds): *Hematology: Basic Principles and Practice.* New York, Churchill-Livingstone, 1991, pp 854–869

82. Fitzgerald PH, Morris CM: Ph-negative chronic myeloid leukemia: the nature of the breakpoint junction and mechanism of ABL transposition. *Leuk Lymphoma* 6:277–287, 1992

83. Deisseroth AB, Andreef M, Champlin R, et al: Chronic leukemias, in Devita VT, Hellman S, Rosenberg SA (eds): *Cancer: Principles and Practice of Oncology* (ed 5). Philadelphia, Lippincott-Raven, 1997, pp 2321–2343

84. Lee MS, Kantarjian H, Talpaz M, et al: Detection of minimal residual disease by polymerase chain reaction in Philadelphia chromosome-positive chronic myelogenous leukemia following interferon therapy. *Blood* 79:1920–1923, 1992

85. O'Brien S, Kantarjian H, Talpaz M: Practical guidelines for the management of chronic myelogenous leukemia with interferon alpha. *Leuk Lymphoma* 23:247–252, 1996

86. Morra E, Lazzarino M, Aliména G, et al: The role of interferon in the treatment of chronic myelogenous leukemia: results and prospects. *Leuk Lymphoma* 6:305–315, 1992

87. Roche Laboratories: Roferon®-A (interferon alfa-2a, recombinant) (package insert). Nutley, NJ, 1995

88. Kantarjian HM, Giles FJ, O'Brien SM, et al: Clinical course and therapy of chronic myelogenous leukemia with interferon-alpha and chemotherapy. *Hematol Oncol Clin North Am* 12:31–80, 1998

89. Moldawer NP, Figlin R: The interferons, in Rieger PT (ed): *Biotherapy: A Comprehensive Overview.* Sudbury, MA, Jones and Bartlett, 1995, pp 69–92

90. Rieger PT: Interferon-alpha: a clinical update. *Cancer Pract* 3:356–365, 1996

91. Italian Cooperative Study Group on Chronic Myeloid Leukemia: Interferon alfa-2a as compared with conventional chemotherapy for treatment of chronic myeloid leukemia. *N Engl J Med* 330:820–825, 1994

92. Thaler J, Ililbe W, Apfelbeck U, et al: Interferon-alpha-2C and LDARA-C for the treatment of patients with CML: results of the Austrian multi-center phase II study. *Leuk Res* 21:75–80, 1997

93. Guilhot F, Chastang C, Michallet M, et al: Interferon alfa-2b combined with cytarabine versus interferon alone in chronic myelogenous leukemia. *N Engl J Med* 337:223-229, 1997

94. Kantarjian HM, Deisseroth A, Kurzrock R, et al: Chronic myelogenous leukemia: a concise update. *Blood* 82:691–703, 1993

95. Pasweg JR, Rowlings PA, Horowitz MM: Related donor bone marrow transplantation for chronic myelogenous leukemia. *Hematol Oncol Clin North Am* 12:81–92, 1998

96. McGlave P: Unrelated donor transplant therapy for chronic myelogenous leukemia. *Hematol Oncol Clin North Am* 12:93–106, 1998

97. Bhatia R, Forman J: Autologous transplantation for the treatment of chronic myelogenous leukemia. *Hematol Oncol Clin North Am* 12:151–172, 1998

98. Jones RJ: Biology and treatment of chronic myeloid leukemia. *Curr Opin Oncol* 9:3–7, 1997

99. Porter DL, Antin JH: Infusion of donor peripheral blood mononuclear cells to treat relapse after transplantation for chronic myelogenous leukemia. *Hematol Oncol Clin North Am* 12:123–150, 1998

100. Zwiebel JA, Cheson BD: Chronic lymphocytic leukemias: staging and prognostic factors. *Semin Oncol* 25:42–59, 1998

101. Silbar R, Stahl R: Chronic lymphocytic leukemia and related diseases, in Williams WJ, Beutler E, Erslev AJ, Lichtman MA (eds): *Hematology.* New York, McGraw-Hill, 1990, pp 1005–1025

102. Cheson BD: Therapy for previous untreated chronic lymphocytic leukemia: a reevaluation. *Semin Hematol* 35:14–21, 1998

103. Montserrat E: Chronic proliferative disorders. *Curr Opin Oncol* 9:34–41, 1997

104. Cheson BD, Bennett JM, Grever M, et al: National Cancer Institute-sponsored working group for chronic lymphocytic leukemia. Revised guidelines for diagnosis and treatment. *Blood* 87:4990–4997, 1996

105. Keating MJ: Chronic lymphocytic leukemia in the next decade: where do we go from here? *Semin Hematol* 35:27–33, 1998

106. Byrd JC, Rai KR, Sausville EA, et al: Old and new therapies in chronic lymphocytic leukemia: now is the time for reassessment of therapeutic goals. *Semin Oncol* 25:65–74, 1998

107. Cheson BD, Sorenson JM, Vena DA, et al: Treatment of hairy cell leukemia with 2-chlorodeoxyadenosine via the Group C protocol mechanism of the National Cancer Institute: a report of 979 patients. *J Clin Oncol* 16:3007–3015, 1998

108. Casselith PA, Cheuvart B, Spiers AS, et al: Randomized comparison of pentostatin versus interferon alpha-2a in previously untreated patients with hairy cell leukemia: an intergroup study. *J Clin Oncol* 13:974–982, 1995

109. Flinn KJ, Kopecky MK, Foucar D, et al: Long term results in hairy cell leukemia (HCL) treated with pentostatin. *Am Soc Hematol* 90:2575, 1995 (abstr)

110. Somerville ET: Knowledge deficit related to chemotherapy, in McNally JC, Stair JC, Somerville ET (eds): *Guidelines for Cancer Nursing Practice.* Philadelphia, Saunders, 1985, pp 57–61

111. Hadaway LC: Comparison of vascular access devices. *Semin Oncol Nurs* 11:154–166, 1995

112. Winslow MN, Trammell L, Camp-Sorrell D: Selection of vascular access device and nursing care. *Semin Oncol Nurs* 11:167–173, 1995

113. Intravenous Nurses Society: The registered nurses' role in vascular access device selection. *J Intravenous Nurs* 20:71–72, 1997

114. Freifeld AG, Walsh TJ, Pizzo PA: Infections in the cancer patient, in DeVita VT, Hellman S, Rosenberg SA (eds): *Cancer Principles and Practice of Oncology* (ed 5). Philadelphia, Lippincott-Raven, 1997, pp 2659–2704

115. Bodey GP: What's new in fungal infections in leukemic patients. *Leuk Lymphoma* 11:127–135, 1993

116. Wujcik D: Infection, in Yarbro CH, Frogge MH, Goodman M (eds): *Cancer Symptom Management* (ed 2). Sudbury, MA, Jones and Bartlett, 1999, pp 307–327

117. Chanock SJ, Pizzo PA. Infectious complications of patients undergoing therapy for acute leukemia: current status and future prospects. *Semin Oncol* 24:132–140, 1997

118. Wade JC, Schimpff SA: Epidemiology and prevention of infection in the immunocompromised host, in Rubin RH, Young LS (eds): *Clinical Approach to Infection in the Immunocompromised Host* (ed 3). New York, Plenum, 1994, pp 5–40

119. Meunier F: Infections in patients with acute leukemia and lymphoma, in Mandell D, Bennett JE, Dolin B (eds): *Principles and Practice of Infectious Diseases* (ed 4). New York, Churchill-Livingstone, 1995, pp 2675–2686

120. deLalla F: Antibiotic treatment of febrile episodes in neutropenic patients: clinical and economic considerations. *Drugs* 53:789–804, 1997

121. Freifeld AG: The antimicrobial armamentarium. *Hematol Oncol Clin North Am* 7:813–839, 1993

122. Viscoli C, Castagtnola E, Machetti M: Antifungal treatment in patients with cancer. *J Intern Med* 740:89–94, 1997

123. Holtzclaw RJ, Rutledge DN: The use of amphotericin B in immunocompromised patients with cancer: pharmacodynamics and nursing implications. Part 2. *Oncol Nurs Forum* 17:737–742, 1990

124. Mayer J, Doubek M, Varlick J: Must we really fear toxicity of conventional amphotericin B in oncological patients? *Support Care Cancer* 7:51–55, 1999

125. Gulati M, Bajad S, Singh S, et al: Development of liposomal amphotericin B formulation. *J Microencapsul* 15:137–151, 1998

126. Hughes T, Armstrong D, Bodey GP, et al: 1997 Guidelines for the use of antimicrobial agents in neutropenic patients with unexplained fever. Infectious Disease Society of America. *Clin Infect Dis* 25:551–573, 1997

127. Bruce JL, Grove SK: Fever: pathology and treatment. *Crit Care Nurs* 12:40–49, 1992

128. Frelreich EJ: White cell transfusions born again. *Leuk Lymphoma* 11:161–165, 1993

129. Ohno R, Tomonoage M, Kobayaski T, et al: Effect of granulocyte colony stimulating factor after intensive induction therapy in relapsed or refractory acute leukemia. *N Engl J Med* 323:871–877, 1990

130. Buchner T, Wolfgang H, Wormann B, et al: Hematopoietic growth factors in acute myeloid leukemia: supportive and priming effects. *Semin Oncol* 24:124–131, 1997

131. Pruett J: Bleeding, in Yarbro CH, Frogge MH, Goodman M (eds): *Cancer Symptom Management* (ed 2). Sudbury, MA, Jones and Bartlett, 1999, pp 285–306

132. Gobel B: Bleeding disorders, in Groenwald SL, Frogge MH, Goodman M, Yarbro CH (eds): *Cancer Nursing Principles and Practice* (ed 4). Sudbury, MA, Jones and Bartlett, 1997, pp 604–639

133. Webb IJ, Anderson KC: Transfusion support in acute leukemia. *Semin Oncol* 24:141–146, 1997

134. Wujcik D: Update on the diagnosis of and therapy for acute promyelocytic leukemia and chronic myelogenous leukemia. *Oncol Nurs Forum* 23:478–487, 1996

135. Frankel SR, Eardley A, Lauwers G, et al: The "retinoic acid syndrome" in acute promyelocytic leukemia. *Ann Intern Med* 117:292–296, 1992

136. Beck SL: Mucositis, in Yarbro CH, Frogge MH, Goodman M (eds): *Cancer Symptom Management* (ed 2). Sudbury, MA, Jones and Bartlett, 1999, pp 328–323

137. Chabner BA: Cytadine analogues, in Chabner BA, Longo DL (eds): *Cancer Chemotherapy and Biotherapy* (ed 2). Philadelphia, Lippincott-Raven, 1996, pp 213–233

138. Wilkes GM: Neurological disturbances, in Yarbro CH, Frogge MH, Goodman M (eds): *Cancer Symptom Management* (ed 2). Sudbury, MA, Jones and Bartlett, 1999, pp 344–381

139. Doublisky J: Ineffective individual coping, in McNally JC, Stair JC, Somerville ET (eds): *Guidelines for Cancer Nursing Practice*. Philadelphia, Saunders, 1985, pp 66–72

140. Much JM, Barsevick AM: Depression, in Yarbro CH, Frogge MH, Goodman M (eds): *Cancer Symptom Management* (ed 2). Sudbury, MA, Jones and Bartlett, 1999, pp 594–617

141. Levinson JA, Lesko LM: Psychiatric aspects of adult leukemia. *Semin Oncol Nurs* 6:76–83, 1990

CHAPTER 58

Liver Cancer: Primary and Metastatic Disease

Jennifer Rychcik, MS, FNP, ACNP, CS, CETN, OCN®

Introduction

Primary and metastatic liver cancer present a significant challenge to the multidisciplinary health care team. The challenge is primarily due to the advanced stage of disease at initial diagnosis, since the hepatic parenchyma may be impaired. When hepatic reserve is reduced, surgery may not be an option. Therefore, early diagnosis is crucial to successful management. High-risk patient populations, such as those with hepatitis B or C infection, should be followed particularly closely to detect any signs of liver cancer early.

In the United States, metastatic liver cancer is more common than primary liver cancer. Colorectal carcinoma is the single most common primary malignancy that usually results in hepatic metastases. Neuroendocrine tumors are the next most common sources of metastatic deposits in the liver. Metastatic liver cancer is usually more amenable to surgical resection than primary liver cancer.

The discussion in this chapter is targeted at hepatocellular carcinoma, one of the most common primary liver malignancies worldwide and metastatic colorectal carcinoma, and neuroendocrine tumors that develop hepatic metastases. Other sources of metastases to the liver include breast, lung, and other gastrointestinal (GI) malignancies.

Epidemiology

Primary Liver Cancer

Approximately 90%–95% of primary liver cancer is hepatocellular carcinoma.[1] The incidence of hepatocellular carcinoma varies greatly in different areas of the world. This variance is a result of the epidemiological pattern of hepatitis B virus and hepatitis C virus causing chronic liver disease. There are approximately 300 million carriers of hepatitis B virus and greater than 170 million chronic hepatitis C virus carriers who are at risk for developing cirrhosis and/or hepatocellular carcinoma.[2]

The underlying history of hepatocellular carcinoma differs geographically. For example, in Africa hepatitis B virus and aflatoxin exposure are correlated with an increased incidence of hepatocellular carcinoma.[3] In contrast, hepatocellular carcinoma among people in Japan is more commonly the result of hepatitis C virus induced cirrhosis. Hepatocellular carcinoma is considered endemic in Southeast Asia and Subsaharan Africa. Another endemic area for hepatitis B virus is southern Italy, where it is assumed that transmission occurrs in the perinatal period.[4] Hepatocellular carcinoma occurs at an earlier age in Asia than in the West.[5] Increased incidence in Asia and Africa are associated with the high number of hepatitis B virus carriers and mycotoxin contamination of food, stored grains, drinking water, and soil.[6]

The rise in hepatocellular carcinoma incidence may continue for years because there is a long latency period for the development of cancer and many people are still infected with the hepatitis C virus, hepatitis B virus, or both.[7] In 5% of the population affected with the virus, the infection can become chronic and potentially result in cancer.[8,9] The development of hepatocellular carcinoma is significantly increased in people with the multiple risk factors of hepatitis C virus and hepatitis B virus who were also chronic alcohol users.[10] A five-fold increase in the incidence has been demonstrated.[11]

Hepatocellular carcinoma is less common in northern Europe and North America, where the hepatitis virus is also less common. Yet it represents the fourth most common gastrointestinal cancer in the United States. In North America and Europe, the population at risk are adults, including health care workers, heterosexuals, homosexuals, intravenous drug users, and immigrants from high prevalent countries. In 2000, there are an estimated 15,300 new liver and intrahepatic bile duct cancer cases and 13,800 people are approximated to die from the disease.[12]

Liver Metastases

Metastases to the liver can be defined as either synchronous or metachronous. *Synchronous metastases* are those present in the liver at the time of initial diagnosis. *Metachronous metastases* are those appearing following the surgical resection of the primary tumor.

Colorectal carcinoma is the third most common cancer diagnosed in the United States.[13] At the time of initial surgical resection of colorectal cancer, 15%–25% of patients are found to have synchronous metastases to the liver.[14] Approximately half of individuals with colorectal cancer who undergo surgical resection of the primary tumor will eventually develop metastatic disease.

Various tumor types of neuroendocrine tumors can also produce liver metastases, such as small bowel carcinoid tumors, bronchogenic carcinoid tumors, and islet cell tumors, which include gastrinoma and glucagonoma.[15] Neuroendocrine tumors less likely to develop liver metastases are appendiceal carcinoid tumors and insulinomas. A longer survival is noted with neuroendocrine hepatic metastases as compared to primary liver cancer. The incidence of liver metastases resulting from noncolorectal nonneuroendocrine tumors is not clearly demonstrated in the literature. Primary malignancies of the lung, pancreas, stomach, breast, and gallbladder commonly metastasize to the liver and other areas of the body. Other carcinomas including ocular melanoma, renal, and GI stromal tumors may develop liver metastases; however, there is no demonstrated impact of resection on survival.

Etiology and Risk Factors

Primary Liver Cancer

Hepatocellular carcinoma is associated with chronic hepatitis B and C virus infection, macronodular cirrhosis, schistosimias and other parasitic infections, environmental carcinogens (e.g., polychlorinated biphenyls, chlorinated hydrocarbon solvents, vinyl and polyvinyl chlorides, organochloride pesticides), and organic material (e.g., aflatoxins). Smoking has also been associated with the development of hepatocellular carcinoma.[16,17]

Aflatoxins are molds that grow on food and are produced as metabolites by strains of *Aspergillus flavus* and *Aspergillus parasiticas*. Individuals are exposed to aflatoxin by ingestion of contaminated foodstuffs or through products of animals fed with aflatoxin-contaminated grains.[18] *Aspergillus* fungus, also referred to as aflatoxin B1, is a known carcinogen that increases the risk of developing hepatocellular carcinoma.[19] Aflavus mold and aflatoxin products are found in grains stored in unrefrigerated conditions, mostly in hot, humid areas of the country.[20] *A. flavus* and *A. parasiticus* also contaminate other food supplies—e.g., corn, peanuts, milo, sorghum, and rice—in some areas of the country. In Taiwan, aflatoxins are found mostly in peanuts and corn.

Other carcinogens for hepatocellular carcinoma are natural products produced by plants, fungi, and bacteria. Individuals throughout the world ingest serecio plants, bush trees, and cycad plants containing the carcinogens pyrollizidine alkaloids, tannic acid, and safrole.

Interestingly, the hepatitis B virus is thought to be the second most potent carcinogen only following tobacco. A tumor suppressor gene, the *p53* oncogene on chromosome 17, has been associated with the hepatitis B virus and eventual development of hepatocellular carcinoma. An unfavorable outcome is associated with the presence of *p53* oncogene and hepatocellular carcinoma. The transforming growth factor alpha has also been proposed as a cofactor.[21–23]

Blood transfusion is a known risk factor. Posttransfusion hepatitis C infection can develop into hepatocellular carcinoma in approximately 30 years, whereas hepatitis B can develop into hepatocellular carcinoma in about 40–50 years following transfusion. However, this interval to development can vary greatly among populations.[24,25]

Other risk factors for the development of liver cancer are hepatitis-associated cirrhosis, alcoholic cirrhosis, autoimmune chronic active hepatitis, cryptogenic cirrhosis, and hepatitis C associated cirrhosis. Once cirrhosis develops, hepatocellular carcinoma will develop in 1.9%–6.7% of patients with the hepatitis C virus infection.[26] This is important as there are an estimated 3.9 million people in the United States affected with hepatitis C virus.[27] The hepatitis B virus is lower in the United States with approximately 1 to 1.25 million people affected.[8,9,28]

Hepatitis B and C virus is involved with the oncogenic process by exposing the individual to a persistent viral infection that produces inflammation, fibrosis, increased cell turnover, necrosis, and cirrhosis.[29–32] With prolonged infection, the hepatitis B virus genome may be incorporated into the chromosomes of the hepatocytes. This can produce instability of the genome resulting in mutations, deletions, translocations, and rearrangements at numerous locations where the viral genome is randomly inserted into the DNA of the hepatocyte.[31] Therefore, a strong link exists between hepatitis B virus, cirrhosis, and hepatocellular carcinoma.[31–33] A prospective study of hepatitis B virus carriers demonstrated a 200-fold increase in risk for development of hepatocellular carcinoma.[34] Individuals with hepatitis B virus combined with chronic alcohol consumption can develop hepatocellular carcinoma 8–10 years earlier than control groups.[35]

Within the male population, the onset of hepatocellular carcinoma usually occurs between age 40 and 60. The predominance of hepatocellular carcinoma in males versus females may be the result of there being more male smokers and drinkers.[36,37] Alcoholic cirrhosis plays a large role in hepatocellular carcinoma. Greater than 50% of the cases of hepatocellular carcinoma in western Europe and North America are associated with alcoholic cirrhosis.[38]

Certain metabolic conditions also place an individual at risk for hepatocellular carcinoma. These include Wilson disease, hemochromatosis, alpha1-antitrypsin deficiency, porphyria cutanea tardia, tyrosinemia, and glycogen storage diseases.[39,40] In children, congenital cholestatic syndrome (Alagille syndrome) is associated with a familial type of hepatocellular carcinoma.

The development of liver tumors may be associated with use of estrogens, androgens, and oral contraceptives. An association between the use of oral contraceptives and the development of benign hepatic adenomas is suspected, but the risk of an adenoma forming into a carcinoma in women taking oral contraceptives is unclear.[41,42]

Hepatocellular carcinoma in children is rare.[43] The prognosis for hepatocellular carcinoma in children is poor. Overall, the resectability rate is low. In Taiwan, hepatocellular carcinoma ranks as the fifth most common childhood malignancy where hepatitis B virus is endemic.[44,45] The hepatitis B vaccination is now being administered in Taiwan with the hope that incidence of hepatocellular carcinoma will decrease.

Liver Metastases

Individuals with a primary malignancy of the breast, lung, gastrointestinal tract, neuroendocrine tumors, gastrointestinal sarcoma, or ocular melanoma are most commonly at risk for the development of metastasis in the liver. The liver is the most frequent site of metastasis for all cancers.

Primary tumors that drain into the portal circulation, which is responsible for supplying approximately two-thirds of the liver's blood supply, have a greater chance of developing hepatic metastases than other malignancies. However, tumors that drain into the systemic circulation also may develop hepatic metastases, including primary tumors of the breast, lung, and ocular melanoma.

Following liver resection, a close follow-up program should be established. This would include a computerized tomography (CT) scan of the abdomen and pelvis every 3 months for two years, then every 6 months. A chest x-ray should also be performed. At five years following resection, if there are no signs of recurrence, then the individual is considered "cured."[46]

Prevention, Screening, and Early Detection

Prevention of the development of hepatocellular carcinoma is aimed toward the etiologic factors, which include, but are not limited to, chronic hepatitis B or C virus infection, alcoholic cirrhosis, and aflatoxin exposure. Vaccination for hepatitis B and C virus is targeted at specific populations depending on the geographic location. In the Far East, vaccination against the hepatitis B virus is focused on preventing perinatal transmission. In Africa, vaccination programs are focused on the childhood population, as this is the population with the greatest risk.[46] In Taiwan, vaccination programs decreased the incidence of hepatitis B in children from 10% to 1%, thus also reducing the incidence of hepatocellular carcinoma.[47] Currently, in the United States, the recommendation is that all newborns be vaccinated against the hepatitis B virus in the hope of preventing future cases of hepatocellular carcinoma.

There still remains difficulty in the development of a vaccine targeted at hepatitis C virus. The hepatitis A vaccine is also available. This is recommended for individuals traveling to high-risk foreign countries.

Due to the number of individuals who remain infected with hepatitis B and C infection in the latency period, it may be many years before there is a reduction in the incidence of hepatocellular carcinoma. Therefore, prevention of the hepatitis B and C virus is most important. If an individual is infected, the treatment measures include antiviral therapy to prevent chronic infection.

Chemoprevention is thought to be the novel prevention approach for the future. Alfa-interferon in combination with ribavirin has been noted to decrease the risk in the progression to hepatocellular carcinoma in patients with Childs' A and early Child's B hepatitis C virus related cirrhosis.[48–50] Interferon delays the onset of hepatocellular carcinoma by the following mechanisms: (1) activating the immune system by increasing the activity of cell destruction, (2) inhibiting the division of cells, and (3) slowing the hepatocyte degeneration and thus genetic abnormalities that may cause hepatocellular carcinoma.[46]

When hepatitis C infection is treated with interferon, approximately 50% of patients regain normal liver function; however, patients may relapse as a result of the virus not being completely cleared systemically.[51] Also, alcohol abuse has been noted to impair cellular immunity and inhibit the efficacy of interferon therapy. Interferon therapy has also been used in treatment of chronic hepatitis B infection to cause destruction of the replicating virus.[52]

Other preventive measures include health education targeted at high-risk populations, such as improvements in food and grain storage to decrease the exposure to aflatoxins. Use of condoms and avoiding needle sharing can also prevent hepatitis transmission. In addition, in some parts of the world, there is a practice of using the same needles for multiple injections in immunization programs, which should be abandoned. Continued screening of blood products is essential to decrease the incidence of posttransfusion hepatitis. Initiating educational programs targeted at children, teenagers, and adults regarding the risks of chronic alcohol consumption is imperative to decrease the development of hepatocellular carcinoma.

Ultrasonography of the liver is a beneficial screening tool in a high-risk population.[53] It is a simple, inexpensive, and noninvasive imaging modality. Ultrasound scanning forms images by the reflection of high-frequency sound waves from the surface of the tissue to identify a potential carcinoma. It allows for evaluation of smaller lesions, which will permit a limited surgical resection and best attempt at cure.[54] However, screening can create false negatives. Unfortunately, nodules identified by ultrasonography may represent an early hepatocellular carcinoma or regenerative macronodules. This is what ultimately creates difficulty in making an accurate diagnosis.[55]

In the high-risk person, tumor markers are also an important aspect in screening. Therefore, it is recommended individuals who are hepatitis B and C carriers and those individuals with cirrhosis have alpha-fetoprotein levels performed and ultrasound screening every six months.[56]

Normal Anatomy and Physiology

The liver is the largest organ within the body weighing 1200 to 1600 g.[57] It is located under the right diaphragm and is divided into right and left lobes. The right lobe, is larger than the left. (See Figure 58-1). The falciform ligament separates segment 4 from 2 and 3. The caudate lobe, segment 1, has its own portal and hepatic venous drainage and is neither part of the right or left lobe. The ligament teres is a fibrous cord that stems from the umbilicus to the inferior surface of the liver. The coronary ligament is the attachment of the inferior surface of the diaphragm.

The right and left hepatic lobe is further divided into segments. The right lobe is divided into four segments: anterior-inferior (segment V), posterior-inferior (seg-

Figure 58-1 Normal anatomy of the liver. Specific segments of the liver are referred to by their roman numeral. Top drawing is an anterior view. Center view is posterior and demonstrates the gallbladder system. The lower view is also an anterior view illustrating the rich vascular network. (Reprinted with permission from Choti MA. The liver, in Soidena JO, Schlossberg L (eds): *The John Hopkins Atlas of Human Functional Anatomy* (4th Ed). Baltimore. The John Hopkins University Press, 1997, pp 138.)[57]

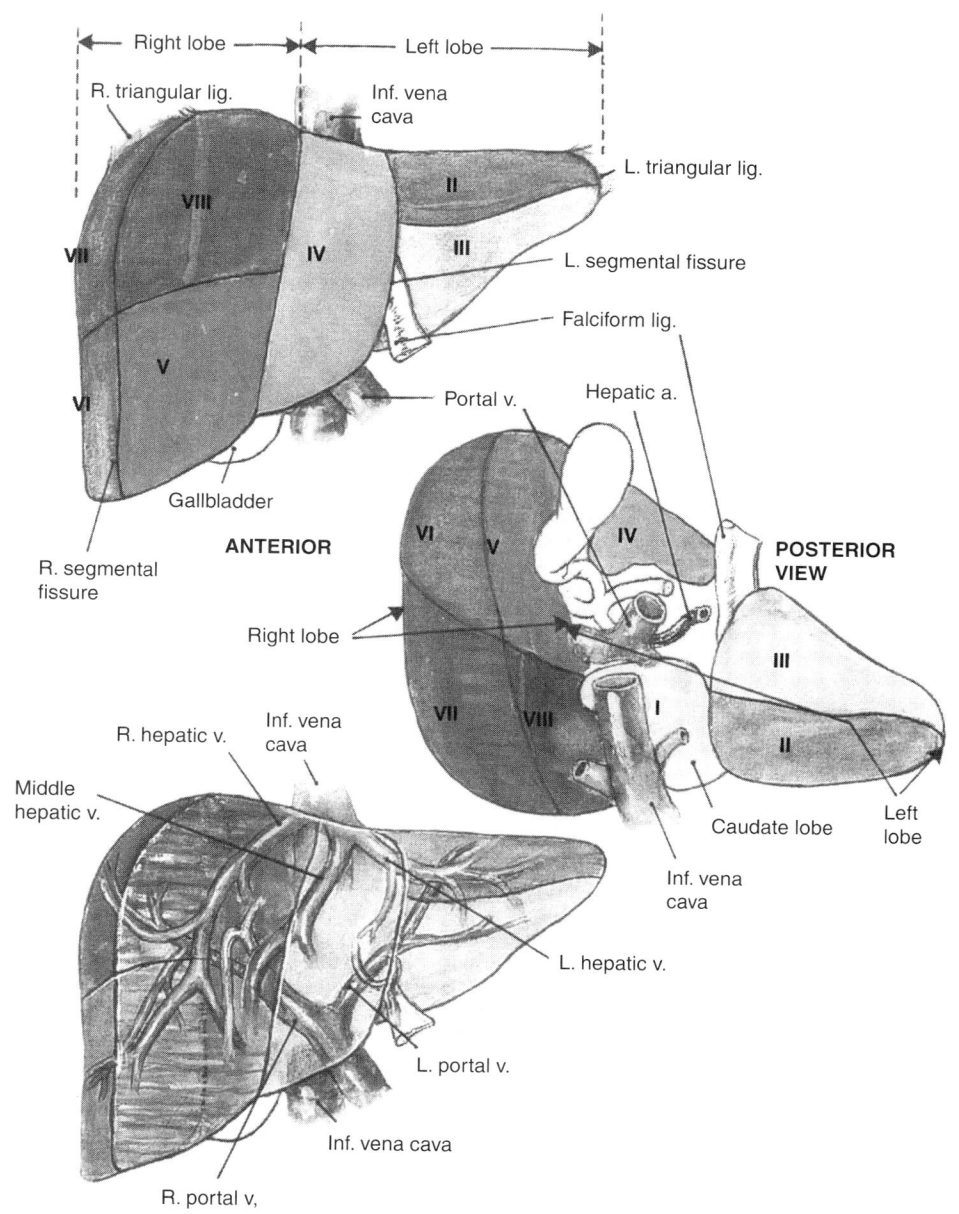

ment VI), superior-inferior (segment VII), and superior-anterior (segment VIII) with its branching portal structures. The left lobe is divided into the left medial segment and two segments lateral to the left of the falciform ligament, the superior component and inferior component. In addition, a capsule that encompasses blood vessels, lymphatics, and nerves covers the liver. This is referred to as "Glisson's capsule."

The liver receives its blood supply from both arterial and venous sources. Two-thirds of the normal hepatic blood flow comes from the portal vein and one-third from the hepatic artery. The hepatic artery branches from the abdominal aorta and supplies the liver with oxygenated blood from the systemic circulation. The portal vein supplies the liver with deoxygenated blood from

the superior mesenteric and splenic veins. The portal vein divides into two trunks on entrance to the liver to supply blood to both lobes. The hepatic veins then drain into the inferior vena cava.

Small ducts, referred to as "bile canaliculi," carry bile produced by the hepatocytes and drain into the common bile duct. The common bile duct empties into the sphincter of Oddi, which is an opening into the duodenum. Bile transported from the liver is concentrated and stored in the gallbladder.

The liver performs many functions:

• **Production of bile:** The liver assists with intestinal digestion and absorption of fats, cholesterol, and fat-soluble vitamins by secreting 700 to 1200 mL of bile per day. Bile is composed of bile salts, cholesterol, bilirubin, electrolytes, and water. Bile is formed by the hepatocytes and secreted into the canaliculi.[58] Bile salts are conjugated bile acids and necessary for emulsification and absorption of fats. These are absorbed in the terminal ileum and returned to the liver via the portal circulation for reabsorption. The recycling of bile salts is referred to as enterohepatic circulation.[58]

- **Metabolism of bilirubin:** Bilirubin is a byproduct of old red blood cells that undergo destruction by macrophages in the liver referred to as "Kupffer cells." Within these cells, the hemoglobin is separated into heme and globin. The globin is broken down into amino acids that are recycled and new proteins are produced. The heme portion is converted to biliverdin by cleaving iron. The iron attaches to transferrin in the plasma and is stored in the liver or utilized by the bone marrow to produce new red blood cells. Biliverdin is converted to bilirubin and released into the plasma. Within the plasma, the bilirubin binds to albumin (referred to as unconjugated or indirect bilirubin). Unconjugated bilirubin forms conjugated (direct) bilirubin by unconjugated bilirubin moving into the hepatocyte and uniting with glucuronic acid. Conjugated bilirubin is water-soluble and is secreted in the bile via the gastrointestinal tract.

- **Synthesis of coagulation factors:** The liver synthesizes prothrombin, fibrinogen, and factors I, II, VII, IX, and X. Vitamin K is essential for synthesis of clotting factors; the absorption of vitamin K is dependent on sufficient bile production in the liver. Therefore, if vitamin K is deficient, the production of clotting factors will be reduced.

- **Fat metabolism:** Triglycerides within the liver are hydrolyzed into glycerol and free fatty acids which produce metabolic energy or adenosine triphosphate (ATP). In addition, they can be released into the systemic circulation as lipoproteins and transported to adipose cells for storage.[59] The synthesis of phospholipids and cholesterol by the liver is necessary for the production of bile salts, steroid hormones, and components of plasma proteins.[58,59]

- **Protein metabolism:** Amino acids are metabolized in the liver by a process known as "deamination." Amino acids are converted to carbohydrates by removing ammonia, which is converted to urea and excreted by the kidneys. The liver also produces plasma proteins, albumin, and globulin. Albumin maintains the plasma oncotic pressure and fluid balance between the interstitial and vascular compartments. A decrease in oncotic pressure can contribute to edema and ascites. The globulins bind to the daily hormonal output from the thyroid and adrenal cortex. Binding of these substances maintains low blood levels of hormones. A decrease in hepatic protein levels can lead to an excess level of these hormones. The liver enzymes including aspartate aminotransferase (AST), alanine aminotransferase (ALT), lactate dehydrogenase (LDH), and alkaline phosphatase[58] synthesize several nonessential amino acids.

- **Carbohydrate metabolism:** Glycogenolysis and gluconeogenesis occur within the liver to maintain normal blood glucose levels. Following meals, glucose is metabolized into glycogen and stored. If hypoglycemia occurs, glycogen is broken down into glucose and is released into the systemic circulation. When glycogen stores are deficient, the liver will convert amino acids and glycerol to glucose. If hyperglycemia occurs, glucose is stored as glycogen or converted to fat.[58,59]

- **Storage of vitamins and minerals:** The liver stores vitamins A, D, E, K, and B12. Vitamin B12 and D are stored for several months and vitamin A for several years.[59] Iron in the form of ferritin is stored in the liver and is released for red blood cell production as necessary. Copper is also stored and released during excessive intake and depletion.

- **Detoxification:** Endogenous and exogenous substances are detoxified within the liver, such as ammonia, alcohol, barbiturates, amphetamines, steroids, and hormones, including estrogen, aldosterone, antidiuretic hormone, and testosterone, and excess accumulation is prevented. Ammonia is another substance processed by the liver. Despite detoxification, substances may be toxins. For example, the end products of alcohol metabolism are acetaldehyde and hydrogen. Excessive intake of alcohol and for an extended period of time will cause damage to the hepatocytes and inadequate liver function will result.[58]

- **Regeneration:** Liver function will continue to occur with up to 80% of the liver resected.[60] The process of regeneration (hypertrophy and hyperplasia) occurs over several months and continues until the total mass amount of the liver is replaced. The time period for regeneration is also dependent on the age of the individual, nutritional status, presence of liver damage, and extent of resection.[61]

Pathophysiology

Cancer of the liver may be a primary tumor or a secondary tumor originating from another site that metastasized to the liver. Prior to initiating treatment, differentiation of primary liver cancer from metastatic liver cancer is critical.

Cellular Characteristics

Primary liver cancer

Primary liver cancer is adenocarcinoma of two cell types: 90% are hepatocellular carcinomas arising from the liver and 7% are cholangiocarcinomas arising from the bile ducts. The remainder are hepatoblastoma, angiosarcoma, or sarcoma.[62,63] Fibrolamellar hepatocellular carcinoma, a variant of hepatocellular carcinoma, occurs and primarily affects adolescent females.[62,63]

The macroscopic appearance of hepatocellular carcinoma is nodular, massive, or diffuse. The nodular type consists of multiple, discrete nodules. The massive type consists of a single, large tumor mass with satellite nodules. The diffuse type is comprised of small nodules distributed throughout the majority of the liver. The tumor may be multifocal as typically noted in cirrhotic livers or may develop as a single lesion that produces satellite lesions. Hepatocellular carcinomas are soft and friable leading to the possibility of tumor rupture or hemorrhage.[64,65] A well-differentiated hepatocellular carcinoma, which produces bile, may have a yellow or green color, whereas areas of hemorrhage or necrosis may produce a red, purple, brown, or black coloration. Hepatocellular carcinomas can range from slow growing well-differentiated tumors to rapidly growing and moderately to poorly differentiated.[64]

Cholangiocarcinomas develop along the bile duct and extend directly into the liver. They may be nodular or diffuse type tumors; however, they typically appear as a solitary grayish-white mass. Cholangiocarcinomas are a firm, fibrous tumors that may secrete mucin, but do not produce bile.

Extrahepatic disease occurs in approximately 50% of the patient population with primary liver cancer, commonly invasion of the portal vein. The hepatic veins or diaphragm may also be invaded by tumor. Regional lymph node metastasis is uncommon.

Liver metastases

The development of hepatic metastases may occur because the liver is the first visceral organ that malignant cells of gastrointestinal origin encounter after release into the capillaries, postcapillary venules, and the portal circulation. For a tumor cell to form a metastasis, it must express a complex phenotype that begins invasion of the surrounding normal stroma either by a single tumor with increased motility or by a group of cells from the primary tumor. Once the invading cells penetrate the vascular or lymphatic channels, cancer cells may grow there or a single cell or clumps of cells may detach and be transported within the circulatory system. Tumor emboli must survive the host's natural defenses and turbulence of the circulatory system in order to finally rest in the capillary bed of a receptive organ, extravasate into the organ parenchyma, proliferate, and establish a micrometastasis. Growth of these new small tumors requires the development of a vascular supply (angiogenesis) and combatting continuous invasion of host defense cells. Failure to complete one or more steps of this intricate metastatic process (e.g., inability to grow progressively in a distant organ's parenchyma) will eliminate the migrating cancer cells. In order to produce clinically relevant metastases, the tumor must exhibit a complex phenotype that is regulated by transient or permanent changes in different genes at DNA and mRNA levels. Malignant tumors contain heterogeneous subpopulations of cells with a wide range of genetic, biochemical, immunologic, and biologic characteristics.[65]

Progression of Disease

With the progression of liver cancer, a multitude of complications arise. Hepatic failure will ultimately ensue. One theory states that if the portal vein is occluded early in the course of the disease, then collateral branches of the hepatic circulatory system will be unable to compensate and necrosis, rupture, and hemorrhage will result. Ascites and esophageal varices are a common sequelae of primary and metastatic liver cancer.

Clinical Manifestations

Hepatocellular carcinoma is usually asymptomatic in the early stage of the disease. Symptoms typically appear at an advanced stage, which first prompts a patient to seek medical advice. The most common symptom is upper abdominal pain resulting from compression of tumor on the extrahepatic structures. Fifty percent of patients develop dull, achy upper abdominal pain. The pain begins as dullness and progresses to become more severe in later stages of disease. Severe pain may also occur with tumor rupture or hemorrhage. Weight loss is common and may be the earliest presenting symptom. Intermittent nausea and/or vomiting occur secondary to delayed gastric emptying. Wasting and anorexia may also occur from decreased total protein and serum albumin along with a decreased metabolism of nutrients and an increase in tumor metabolism. Fever may occur from tumor volume and the development of cholangitis and/or sepsis. Fatigue and weakness result from accumulation of waste products and an increase in tumor metabolism.

Jaundice may be due to obstruction or as a result of massive liver involvement and dysfunction. Clay-colored stools are due to decreased bile. When jaundice is present, the prognosis is poor; however, jaundice could also be related to a malignant obstruction of the biliary system. It is important to recognize this obstruction since palliation may prolong survival. Nintey percent of patients will die within ten weeks of presentation.

In some cases, surgical resection is possible to relieve obstructive jaundice and biliary stents may also be used. The overall survival rate is similar to those patients with and without clinical jaundice. Hematemesis may occur due to esophageal varices from underlying liver disease with portal hypertension. Bone pain from bony metastases occurs in a small percentage of the patient population. Respiratory symptoms are rare, but may occur with elevation of the hemidiaphragm from hepatomegaly or pain from rib metastases. Paraneoplastic syndromes may also be accompanied by these other symptoms: erythrocytosis, hypoglycemia, hypercholesterolemia, hypercalcemia, leukocytosis, carcinoid-like syndrome, coagulation abnormalities, porphyria, and sexual changes.

Metastatic disease in the liver typically remains asymptomatic. However, the development of symptoms discussed earlier for hepatocellular carcinoma may develop with extensive liver involvement.

Manifestations of end-stage liver cancer include massive ascites, hepatic encephalopathy, hepatorenal syndrome, and infection. Massive ascites occurs due to a decrease in the synthesis of plasma proteins. Lower extremity edema may also be noted. Portal hypertension or portal vein thrombosis may be a causative factor for the ascites. Hepatic encephalopathy results from inadequate detoxification of ammonia, and mental confusion is a common finding. Hepatorenal syndrome is associated with portal hypertension and vasoconstriction of the arterioles. Infection results from the development of spontaneous bacterial peritonitis or cholangitis secondary to obstruction within the biliary system.

Assessment

Patient and Family History

To assess for primary liver cancer or metastases, the history should include identifying possible risk factors, such as hepatitis B or C virus infection, cirrhosis, or exposure to toxins. The history should also include identifying possible risk factors for the development of cancer that have the potential to produce hepatic metastases. These include identifying a history of genetic syndromes that increases an individual's risk for the development of primary liver cancer, colorectal cancer, or breast cancer. Other disease states should also be considered, for example, the presence of inflammatory bowel disease and risk for the development of colorectal carcinoma. Most importantly, investigating a family history of cancer and recognizing the development of various carcinomas within each generation will provide information regarding a possible genetic mutation. This may prompt genetic counseling that can assist in screening the individual at risk of developing other carcinomas.

Physical Exam

Typically, with the diagnosis of hepatocellular carcinoma hepatomegaly is most commonly assessed on physical examination. A hepatic bruit may be present secondary to compression of tumor on the hepatic artery. Ascites and/or peripheral edema may be evident resulting from portal hypertension either due to coexisting cirrhosis or tumor invasion of the portal vein. Jaundice may be present in addition to pruritus; however, this may be manifested late

in the course of the disease process. Splenomegaly also may be present from portal hypertension. Muscle wasting may be assessed. Patients are more at risk for bleeding due to a decrease in vitamin K absorption, increase in prothrombin time (PT) and partial thromboplastin time (PTT), and varices from portal hypertension. A persistent elevation in temperature can occur as a result of tumor necrosis. Sexual changes may also be identified including testicular atrophy and gynecomastia. Menstrual disorders may erupt. Patients with cirrhosis may present with any number of these symptoms; however, the development of a malignancy should be investigated if a patient experiences a sudden exacerbation in symptoms or deterioration in overall health. Patients with hepatic metastases rarely develop these symptoms discussed above until there is extensive liver involvement.

Diagnostic Studies

Laboratory studies

If the liver cancer is at an early stage, the hematological profile and liver function tests will most likely demonstrate normal findings. The tumor must involve a significant volume of the liver parenchyma before liver function is affected, unless cirrhosis is a concomitant condition that has already compromised function. However, aspartate amino-transferase may be slightly elevated in hepatocellular carcinoma whereas alkaline phosphotase may be slightly elevated in metastatic disease. In advanced hepatic disease, a decrease in the platelet and white blood cell counts may indicate hypersplenism. Prothrombin time, partial thromboplastin time, and albumin levels will reflect the hepatic synthetic function.

Alpha-fetoprotein (AFP) is a tumor marker specific to hepatocellular carcinoma and is elevated in the serum in approximately 60% of individuals.[66,67] Alpha-fetoprotein does not correlate to tumor size or growth rate. Testing for AFP is limited because it lacks specificity except when elevated to at least about 70%.[39] Individuals with hepatocellular cancer who have a normal AFP level will ultimately have a better prognosis.[68]

The tumor marker carcinoembryonic antigen (CEA) is produced in large quantities by colorectal cancer. CEA may be elevated in metastatic colorectal carcinoma; however, as with AFP, a small percentage of tumors do not secrete CEA.[69]

Imaging

Imaging modalities used to detect and characterize hepatic lesions have improved dramatically over the past decade. Once an initial diagnosis is made, the selection of various imaging modalities to evaluate the extent of primary and metastatic disease will depend on the plan of treatment. This plan may vary from no treatment, which may not warrant an extensive evaluation of disease, to a plan for systemic chemotherapy in which it is pertinent to evaluate all sites of disease for eventually determining a response to treatment. Individuals being considered for surgical resection will undergo a comprehensive evaluation to rule out extrahepatic disease. Initially, to evaluate a patient for the presence of extrahepatic disease, CT of the abdomen and pelvis is the most frequently utilized imaging modality. A CT scan of the abdomen and pelvis will identify additional disease within the abdomen, and a CT scan of the chest will identify pulmonary metastases. However, controversy exists between performance of chest x-ray versus chest CT to rule out thoracic metastases. A chest CT is more sensitive in detecting metastatic lesions. Lesions greater than 1 cm in diameter are noted approximately 95% of the time.[70,71]

Helical CT scanning is more advantageous in hepatic imaging in comparison to standard CT. Helical CT captures images during the optimal time frame of contrast enhancement to identify hepatic lesions.[72,73] Advances in helical CT include larger anatomic coverage and rapid scanning time during a single breath-hold.

With the development of the specialized hepatic helical CT scanner, the liver is sequentially imaged twice, first in the arterial and then during the portal phase with one single bolus injection of contrast.[74] This specialized CT enables extensive evaluation of hypovascular and hypervascular tumors.

In the past, hypervascular tumors have been difficult to detect on imaging because the tumors enhance rapidly and will thus appear as normal hepatic parenchyma. Hepatocellular carcinomas and other hepatic metastases including pancreatic islet cell tumors, carcinoid tumors, melanomas, renal carcinomas, breast carcinomas, and sarcomas are hypervascular lesions. Due to their greater arterial blood supply, contrast enhancement occurs during the hepatic arterial phase. (See Figure 58-2.) In contrast, colorectal metastases are typically hypovascular. These are best seen as nonenhancing lesions on portal-phase imaging.[75–78] With the presence of cirrhosis, identifying a primary hepatic lesion is more difficult due to scarring of the liver. Also, with hepatic arterial phase imaging, we are further able to quantify benign lesions, such as hemangiomas.

Lipiodol CT has been commonly used in Japan for the past decade. Lipiodol, an oily contrast material, is injected into the hepatic artery and the scan performed 7–14 days following injection. Lipiodol is rapidly cleared by the normal hepatic parenchyma but is retained within the malignant tumor. Lipiodol CT is most useful to detect hypervascular lesions.[79] The disadvantage of this approach is the need for an arteriogram to administer Lipiodol, the increased cost, and the number of false positives.

The arteriogram is most useful for hypervascular tumors, such as hepatocellular carcinoma. Hepatic arteriography is an imaging modality used to delineate hepatic anatomy and the presence of vascular invasion or enhancement of the tumor. Computed tomography arterial portography (CTAP) may be performed prior to surgical resection or other treatments including hepatic arterial chemotherapy or chemoembolization. CTAP involves performing a CT during injection of contrast via the

celiac or superior mesenteric arteries and enhancement of the hepatic parenchyma via the portal venous circulation.[80] CTAP has been shown to be sensitive in determining resectability of hepatic lesions; however, it has a high false-positive rate. The specificity of CTAP is also limited in the evaluation of a patient for surgical resection of hepatic metastases.[81] It is therefore not recommended for routine use as the high false-positive rate may affect a surgeon's decision not to perform resection in a patient who is potentially resectable.[82,83]

Magnetic resonance imaging (MRI) provides information regarding tumors and vascular anatomy. It details the patency of the hepatic and portal veins. Approved contrast agents for use with MRI are the gadolinium chelates.[84,85] Allergic reactions with gadolinium chelate contrast agents are rare, and patients who have an allergy to iodinated contrast may receive these agents. Newer contrast agents, which specifically target liver cells or the reticuloendothelial system are now becoming available. These new agents, utilize paramagnetic particles that are selectively absorbed by liver cells, thus increasing the sensitivity of MRI.

Detection of hepatocellular carcinoma with MRI varies depending on differentiation of the lesion. With gadolinium contrast imaging, the tumor is enhanced at the arterial phase. No matter what type of imaging, it is more difficult to detect a mass in a cirrhotic liver secondary to the disturbance in the architecture of the liver, which includes fibrosis, necrosis, or regenerating nodules. There is controversy as to whether CT or MRI is a better imaging modality for the detection of either primary liver cancer or metastatic disease.

Sonogram, or ultrasound, of the abdomen may be the initial imaging modality used to diagnose primary liver cancer. Ultrasound can detect the extent of vascular invasion from a primary tumor and, most importantly, invasion of the portal vein. Invasion of the portal vein or occlusion may be the only radiological finding in hepatocellular carcinoma. Sonography is more sensitive in identifying portal vein invasion than CT scan.

The appearance of a hepatocellular carcinoma on sonogram will depend on the tumor size, pattern of growth, cellular composition, degree of necrosis, and extent of cirrhosis. On ultrasonography, the lesions may vary in echogenity from hyperechoic, isoechoic, to hypoechoic.[86] Some may be more heterogeneous due to the presence of necrosis, fatty change, or hemorrhage.[87] Hepatocellular carcinomas less than 3 cm in diameter are often hypoechoic and homogenous without necrosis, whereas larger tumors are more heterogeneous with necrosis. Hepatic metastases may have a hypoechoic halo surrounding a focal lesion.[88]

Future developments in imaging for detection of hepatocellular carcinoma include three-dimensional ultrasound, second harmonic imaging, and ultrasound contrast agents. These newer imaging techniques may further increase the specificity and sensitivity of detecting early hepatocellular carcinomas and further differentiate nodules from hepatocellular carcinoma.

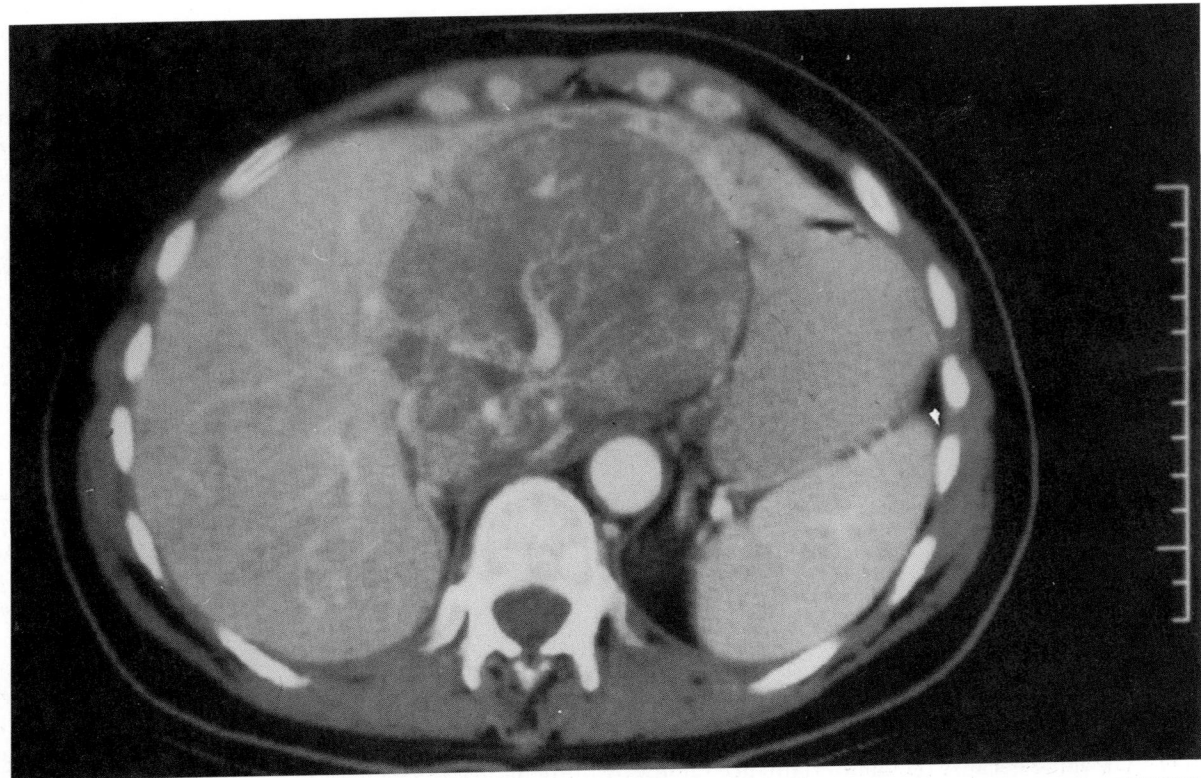

Figure 58-2   CT scan with contrast enhancement. Large hepatocellular carcinoma involving the left medial segment of the liver. (Photo courtesy of The Johns Hopkins Hospital.)

Nuclear medicine imaging is another modality used for preoperative evaluation. Radionuclide imaging uses various physiological and biochemical properties of tumors that identify areas of recurrence. Hepatic scintigraphy is an example; however, lesions less than 2.5 cm in diameter are difficult to detect. Single-photon emission computed tomography (SPECT) imaging, while not ideal, has increased the detection of smaller lesions.

Positron emission tomography (PET) is an advanced imaging technique that evaluates cell metabolism using a glucose analog, F-fluorodeoxyglucose (FDG), as a tracer. With some tumor cells, including colorectal carcinoma, there is an increase in glucose metabolism.[89] PET can be used to detect primary colorectal carcinoma and recurrent disease.[89–91] PET can be an accurate imaging modality for differentiating hepatic metastases, although it is not effective for lesions less than 1 cm. Because small lesions are difficult to detect, lesions containing active macrophages may produce false-positives.[92]

Immunoscintigraphy is a new advanced technique in cancer detection. CEA scanning is an imaging modality reported to have a sensitivity of 59% and a specificity of 84% in detecting recurrent disease.[93]

Needle biopsy

Fine needle aspiration biopsy (FNAB) is rarely used preoperatively in resectable tumors. It is thought that a needle biopsy can violate the tumor capsule and create tumor spillage and spread of the cancer; thus if curative surgical resection is an option, a needle biopsy should be avoided.[94] FNAB may be performed with ultrasound or CT guidance. The risk of a fine-needle biopsy is hemorrhage.[95] Prior to the performance of FNAB, a platelet count, PT, and PTT are necessary. If an individual's platelet count is low, platelets may need to be administered before the procedure. If a patient's PT/PTT are prolonged, fresh frozen plasma may need to be administered to decrease the risk of hemorrhage.

Classification and Staging

A staging system for primary liver cancer is used to quantify the tumor size, location, extent of disease, and presence of metastasis[96] (Table 58-1). Staging provides a universal language and systematic method for clinicians to communicate with one another about the disease and to measure the disease progression or response. If the liver is the site of metastatic deposits from another primary tumor, then the staging system for that particular primary tumor will be used to evaluate the liver involvement.

Table 58-1 AJCC Classification and Staging of Liver Cancer

PRIMARY TUMOR (T)

TX	Primary tumor cannot be assessed
T0	No evidence of primary tumor
T1	Solitary tumor 2 cm or less in greatest dimension without vascular invasion
T2	Solitary tumor 2 cm or less in greatest dimension with vascular invasion, or multiple tumors limited to one lobe, none more than 2 cm in greatest dimension without vascular invasion, or a solitary tumor more than 2 cm in greatest dimension without vascular invasion
T3	Solitary tumor more than 2 cm in greatest dimension with vascular invasion, or multiple tumors limited to one lobe, none more than 2 cm in greatest dimension with vascular invasion, or multiple tumors limited to one lobe, any more than 2 cm in greatest dimension, with or without vascular invasion
T4	Multiple tumors in more than one lobe or tumor(s) involve(s) a major branch of portal or hepatic vein(s) or invasion of adjacent organs other than the gallbladder or perforation of the visceral peritoneum

REGIONAL LYMPH NODES (N)

NX	Regional lymph node status cannot be assessed
N0	No regional lymph node metastasis
N1	Regional lymph node metastasis

DISTANT METASTASIS (M)

MX	Distant metastasis cannot be assessed
M0	No distant metastasis
M1	Distant metastasis

STAGE GROUPING

I	T1	N0	M0
II	T2	N0	M0
IIIA	T3	N0	M0
IIIB	T1	N1	M0
	T2	N1	M0
	T3	N1	M0
IVA	T4	Any N	M0
IVB	Any T	Any N	M1

Therapeutic Approaches and Nursing Care

Treatment Planning and Evaluation

Various treatments for primary liver cancer and liver metastases include surgical resection, transplantation, ablative and/or interstitial therapies, regional therapies, systemic chemotherapy, and radiation therapy. Surgical resection continues to remain the only potentially cura-

tive treatment option for patients with liver cancer. All of these treatment options may affect normal hepatic parenchyma and, ultimately, liver function. Surgically unresectable patients have other surgical treatment options available, including cryosurgery, radiofrequency ablation, or liver transplantation. Other therapies include chemotherapy, radiation therapy, chemoembolization, percutaneous ethanol injection, or percutaneous acetic acid injection. The treatment option selected depends on various factors: extent of tumor, comorbid disease, liver function and reserve, individual preference, performance status, nutritional status, and age.

Prior to initiating a treatment modality, laboratory studies include a complete blood count to identify anemia, liver function tests to determine hepatic function, coagulation tests to recognize abnormalities in clotting mechanisms, and tumor markers. Anemia may need to be corrected with transfusion of packed red blood cells (PRBC) and coagulopathies corrected with fresh frozen plasma (FFP). Fluid and electrolyte imbalances should be addressed prior to treatment.

Prior to hepatic resection, a thorough evaluation is of extreme importance. Various imaging modalities are performed to evaluate the extent of disease and the potential for resection, and any possibility of extrahepatic disease must be ruled out. An extensive workup prior to hepatic resection is done to prevent unnecessary laparotomy. Unresectable disease rates can range between 40%–70% of the cases.[97] Other factors affecting treatment choice must be considered, such as cardiac and pulmonary diseases that can increase the rate of morbidity and mortality following surgical therapy. Age is not an absolute contraindication to surgical resection or aggressive treatment.

Prior to initiation of definitive therapy, vitamins A, C, D, and B complex may be administered to decrease the distressing effect of jaundice. Pruritus may accompany jaundice, which results from the accumulation of bile salts causing irritation of the cutaneous sensory nerve fibers. Relief can be obtained by meticulous skin hygiene in addition to utilization of oil-based lotions, antihistamines, and/or cholestyramine. Deodorant soaps should be avoided as their use may intensify the pruritus. Pruritus will dissipate with resolution of the jaundice.

Nutritional imbalances may need correction prior to initiation of therapy. It is relatively common for patients with primary liver cancer to have had significant weight loss and a decrease in albumin and total proteins.

Surgery

Primary liver cancer

Surgical resection offers the best option for cure of hepatocellular carcinoma. Hepatocellular carcinoma is difficult to surgically resect due to large tumor volumes at the time of presentation and hepatic dysfunction. Hepatic dysfunction resulting from cirrhosis occurs in at least 75% of the patient population.[98] Hepatic resection in the cirrhotic patient also presents a challenge to the surgeon due to an inadequate hepatic reserve, bleeding tendencies, and a malnourished and immunocompromised state.[99] Only approximately 15%–30% of individuals with liver cancer are surgical candidates at time of initial presentation. The remaining individuals usually have unresectable disease, presence of metastatic disease, extensive cirrhosis, insufficient hepatic reserve, and poor performance status.[100]

Contraindications to surgical resection include ascites, renal insufficiency, prolonged PT and PTT, and jaundice without evidence of biliary obstruction secondary to tumor. Prior to hepatic resection, a metastatic workup should be completed to rule out known areas of spread, which include regional lymph nodes, lungs, adrenal glands, peritoneal surfaces, and bone.

The type of incision used to perform liver resection is usually a subcostal approach, as this approach can be extended further if the tumor is bulky or it invades the diaphragm. Types and extent of resection depends on tumor location. Resections will be as extensive as needed to eradicate the tumor. Surgeons attempt to avoid transfusion intraoperatively and postoperatively, as this has been thought to increase the tumor recurrence rate; however, this remains unproven.[101]

The type and extent of hepatic resection is dependent on the disease. Resections can be classified into major and minor hepatic resections. Major resection includes hepatic lobectomy or extended hepatic lobectomy, also referred to as trisegmentectomy. A minor resection includes nonanatomic wedge resections or anatomic resection of a specific segment(s). A more difficult resection is a lesion located within the posterior segment of the right lobe, due to location of the hepatic veins. Therefore, typical resections include a right or left hepatic lobectomy, trisegmentectomy, and segmentectomy or nonanatomic wedge resections. The Cavitron ultrasonic surgical dissector has been demonstrated to provide a controlled dissection of the hepatic parenchyma with clearly identified structures, thus decreasing operative blood loss.

Total hepatectomy with orthotopic liver transplantation may also be a treatment option for individuals with smaller lesions who are otherwise deemed unresectable as a result of advanced cirrhosis. The choice between surgical resection and transplantation remains controversial.[102,103] However, resection should be the first line of therapy due to organ shortage.[104]

Patients with both hepatitis B and hepatitis C virus infection, versus those with only one virus infection, are noted to possess higher mortality and morbidity rates following hepatic resection.[105,106] The mortality rate is also increased in patients undergoing surgical resection in the presence of cirrhosis, ranging from 3%–15%.[107,108] Five year survival rates for hepatocellular carcinoma range from 30%–40%.[106–108]

Liver metastases

Initial resection. Surgical resection for metastatic lesions in the liver is now considered an optimal treatment option in selected cases of isolated disease. Improvements in surgical technique and postoperative care have improved outcomes in recent years. Morbidity and mortality for metastatic liver cancer surgery have dramatically decreased with perioperative mortality rates now 1%–2%.

Surgical resection is a recommended treatment option for colorectal metastases to the liver. To plan the surgical resection, it is important to determine the number, size, and location of hepatic metastases. Survival rates following resection of metastases range from 22%–48%.[109–113]

The literature has reported that individuals with hepatic lesions not initially amenable to surgical excision may undergo neoadjuvant chemotherapy to reduce tumor bulk. This may convert the patient to a surgical candidate. In one study, however, no benefit in survival was demonstrated with the neoadjuvant administration of fluorouracil (5-FU), oxaliplatin, and folinic acid.[117] Presently, the role of neoadjuvant chemotherapy in treating liver metastases is unknown.

Interestingly, a resectable synchronous metastatic liver lesion may be discovered intraoperatively at the time of resection of the primary tumor. Usually, the surgeon will perform the resection of the primary tumor and biopsy the metastasis with a plan to perform resection of the metastasis at a later date. In this case, intraoperative ultrasonography should be performed at the time of colon resection to confirm resectability. However, there are times when the liver metastasis is a wedge-shaped, well-defined tumor amenable to resection at the time of initial surgery. Metastatic lesions as small as 5 mm can be palpated intraoperatively; however, this is more challenging in a cirrhotic liver.[115,116] Contraindications to hepatic resection are extrahepatic metastases, unresectable metastatic disease, presence of hepatic nodes, and four or more metastatic nodules within the liver.[117,118]

Repeat surgical resection. It is important to diagnose recurrence of liver metastases early to allow for the possibility of repeat resection.[119] For primary colorectal cancer, close follow-up to identify recurrent asymptomatic metastatic disease includes CEA every three months for two years, then every six months thereafter if the CEA level was elevated preoperatively.[120] Abdominal CT scan and chest x-ray should also be performed at regular intervals, typically 3 to 6 months. Among patients with colorectal cancer who have undergone a prior liver resection for metastases, approximately 50%–60% of recurrences will occur within the liver.[119,121–124] Repeat hepatectomy is possible because the liver regenerates almost to its original mass within four to six weeks.[125]

Repeat resection of metastases in the liver is technically more difficult secondary to adhesions and to the cut surface of the previous resection to neighboring organs. Regeneration of the liver also changes the shape of the organ and vascular structures creating a more difficult resection. In some instances, there may be increased bleeding.[126] Operative mortality is relative to initial hepatic resection, although the morbidity rates are higher.

The Repeat Hepatic Metastases Registry noted a 20% higher postoperative morbidity compared to the first resection.[127,128] Nonetheless, repeat resection for metastases should be considered a treatment option if the metastatic disease is resectable.

Intraoperative palpation and ultrasonography

Prior to performing definitive hepatic resection, intraoperative examination and evaluation of the extent of disease within the abdomen and liver is crucial. Inspection and palpation should include the site of primary tumor and the pelvis, especially if the primary diagnosis was rectal carcinoma. The peritoneal surfaces and periportal nodal region should be inspected and palpated. The presence of enlarged nodes within the periportal region directly affects probablity of survival, with a five-year survival rate of approximately 4%. Thus, the presence of periportal nodal metastases is a relative contraindication to hepatic resection.[129]

Intraoperative ultrasound (IOUS) provides the highest rate of sensitivity in the detection of hepatic lesions.[130] IOUS is an important aspect of hepatic surgery as it can provide a surgeon with additional information to detect small lesions not detected preoperatively.[131-133] IOUS and surgical palpation together are considered to be the best methods for staging liver disease.[134,135] In addition, IOUS is a vital aspect of the operation because approximately 50% of lesions are located deep within the liver and are nonpalpable, particularly hepatocellular carcinoma. IOUS can identify lesions initially thought to be metastatic tumors on the basis of preoperative imaging but are found to be benign on intraoperative ultrasound.[136] Even with advanced imaging modalities, approximately 20%–30% of hepatic tumors detected during IOUS and palpation were not noted by preoperative imaging modalities.[131,132]

Therefore, IOUS should be performed to assess hepatic metastases and determine if resection can be accomplished with clear margins.[137,138] It also helps define the relationship of the tumor with the portal or hepatic veins and the hepatic venous structures. This decreases the risk of injuring intrahepatic vessels, minimizes blood loss, and facilitates the decision about where venous structures should be resected. IOUS is pertinent for identifying liver anatomy and location of tumor specific to segments and lobes.[139,140] Tumor thrombi in the portal branches can be identified. Also, ultrasonography can be used to monitor cryogenic ablation of tumor.

To perform IOUS, it is important to first identify vasculature, then primary and secondary lesions.[141] IOUS should be performed following laparotomy and mobilization and bimanual palpation of the liver. It is important to perform IOUS procedure prior to dissection to prevent interrupting sound transmission.[142] Typically, it takes approximately 15–25 minutes to perform. Laparoscopic ultrasound is a form of IOUS that may be used to assist in identifying unresectable disease and decrease the need for patients to have exploratory laparotomy.

Postoperative care

Following major hepatic resection, the patient typically requires close monitoring in an intensive care setting for a period of 24 hours to manage intravascular volume and perfusion changes. Fluid resuscitation and/or transfusion may be necessary.

Individuals with cirrhosis are at increased risk for complications during the postoperative period compared to the noncirrhotic individual. Knowledge of the potential complications, signs of impending problems, and aggressive treatment are vital in caring for a patient postoperatively.

Monitoring liver function tests, phosphate, and glucose frequently until a downward trend in transaminases is noted is important. Hypophosphatemia is commonly seen as a normal pattern postoperatively and replacement of phosphate may be necessary. Liver function tests rise immediately postoperatively and usually return to normal within seven to ten days postoperatively. Elevations depend on the extent of liver resected and intraoperative ischemic time. If liver function tests are extraordinarily high early postoperatively, this may represent an injury to vascular inflow or outflow in the retained segment. In this case, a doppler ultrasound of the liver should be performed to rule out portal vein thrombosis. In addition, it is important to monitor an individual's glucose level, as this may also be indicative of hepatic failure. Decreased albumin levels are also noted following liver resection, which are related to protein loss in the abdomen. No benefit from administration of albumin has been noted.[143] The patient's diet is slowly advanced with resolution of a postoperative ileus. Drainage tubes, if placed, are discontinued when the output tapers off and no bile leak is evident.

In the event the patient develops ascites, this may interfere with nutritional intake and ventilation. Therefore, it is important to restrict sodium to 1000–1500 mg per day and water to 1500 mL per day. Addition of a loop diuretic and spironolactone will likely decrease the patient's weight by 0.5–1.0 kg. With this particular intervention, the patient's potassium, BUN, and creatinine should be monitored closely and potassium replaced as necessary.

Following hepatic resection, potential complications include; hemorrhage, biliary leak or biloma, subphrenic abscess, infection, pneumonia, pleural effusion, transient metabolic consequences, portal hypertension, clotting defects, and hepatic failure. See Table 58-2.

Hemorrhage. The liver is a vascular organ and with hepatic resection, a raw surface area of the liver could produce bleeding in the first 24 hours postoperatively. This may be indicated by hypotension, tachycardia, and increasing abdominal girth. A decrease in hematocrit and hemoglobin will be evident. Intraabdominal hemorrhage will require immediate exploratory laparotomy to repair the bleeder. During this time, nursing observations and assessment should include frequent vital signs and central venous pressure monitoring; assessing skin for adequate

Table 58-2 Postoperative Complications Following Liver Resection

Liver-Related Complications
Hemorrhage
Bile Fistula
Biloma
Subphrenic Abscess
Ascites
Liver Failure
Portal Hypertension
Coagulopathy

Infections
Wound
Urinary Tract Infection
Pneumonia

perfusion; measuring abdominal girth; assessing for bleeding from incision site; assessing urine, stool, and serial hemoglobin and hematocrit. In addition, cirrhotic individuals should be evaluated for overt and subclinical signs of bleeding disorders as a result of an increased risk in bleeding complications.

Biliary leak or biloma. Wound drains, typically Jackson-Pratt drains, are placed to prevent bile accumulation. A subhepatic drain is placed and a small amount of bile may be noted from necrosis on the edge of the liver. When no drains are present or when the bile leak is not by placed drains, a collection of bile may develop, called a biloma. Fever, pain, and a distended abdomen may also indicate a leak or biloma. The drain remains until a leak is no longer noted. If the leak persists, the patient may require further percutaneous drainage.

Subphrenic abscess. Perihepatic infection or necrotic remaining liver may precipitate a subphrenic abscess. Warning signs include a sharp, piercing right upper quadrant pain and low-grade fever. Typically, with short length of stays, patients will be at home and notify the physician of these symptoms as they appear late in the postoperative course. Auscultation of the base of the lungs may detect fluid and possible abscess.

Infection. Individuals with cirrhosis are at increased risk for infection following hepatic resection as a result of decreased protein stores. The mortality rate associated with infection is high. Continued assessment of vital signs, wound healing, and drain patency is crucial. Aggressive intervention is required early.

Pleural effusion and pneumonia. Pleural effusion is common following liver resection, most often seen after right hepatectomy. In most cases, patients are asymptomatic and should not be treated. Aggressive pulmonary toilet with incentive spirometry and deep breathing can prevent pneumonia. Individuals are reluctant to perform respiratory exercises due to the pain experienced with a subcostal incision. In addition, frequent ambulation and

administration of analgesics prior to conducting respiratory exercises are important nursing measures.

Transient metabolic consequences. A transient elevation in liver function tests is evident postoperatively. Concern arises when an upward versus downward trend is noted in the bilirubin and liver function tests. If accompanied by jaundice and signs of hepatic failure, mechanical obstruction and portal vein thrombosis must be ruled out.

Portal hypertension. Portal hypertension results from the surgical rerouting of the portal venous flow through a small remnant liver. This leads to sequestration in the splanchic circulation. Fortunately, the liver has a great potential for increasing blood flow if it has adequate time to compensate. Central venous pressure monitoring is a reliable indicator of blood volume. Bleeding from puncture site, wound, or cavity requires immediate attention.

Clotting defects. A slight rise in the prothrombin time may be noted postoperatively. Severe coagulatopathies may develop and may need to be treated with fresh frozen plasma. The nurse can detect complications from deficiencies in clotting mechanisms by observing puncture sites, monitoring abdominal girth, and testing urine and stool for blood.

Hepatic failure. Hepatic failure following hepatic resection can occur as a result of portal vein thrombosis or insufficient hepatic parenchyma. Insufficient parenchyma is more frequent in a cirrhotic individual. A continued rise in bilirubin and liver function tests will occur if hepatic failure is developing. In addition, the patient may display mental confusion with an increase in serum ammonia levels. Other systems may be compromised also. Frequent monitoring of mental status, vital signs, and laboratory studies are important nursing measures.

Adjuvant therapy

There is a significant role for adjuvant therapy following hepatic resection. Clinicians are more apt to administer adjuvant chemotherapy to those who have never received chemotherapy. In addition, individuals may be administered systemic chemotherapy to reduce the risk of recurrence if it has been a year or longer since the last chemotherapy was received. No randomized trials have demonstrated the impact of systemic chemotherapy following liver resection, however, retrospective studies have demonstrated an improved survival. Continued investigation including single and multi-institutional studies addressing administration of adjuvant systemic chemotherapy, regional chemotherapy, or both following hepatic resection are currently being conducted.[144]

Prognostic factors

Primary liver cancer. The prognosis for a person with hepatocellular carcinoma is determined by the cellular differentiation of the tumor in addition to the extent of the underlying disease.[145] Well-differentiated tumors have a favorable prognosis. The status of the accompanying hepatitis also has been noted to affect the recurrence of hepatocellular carcinoma and is identified as a prognostic factor.[146,147]

Pathological factors affecting prognosis for disease-free interval and overall survival include the differentiation of the tumor, growth pattern of hepatocellular carcinoma, and size of the tumor. Large tumors (greater than 5 cm) have a poor prognosis.[148,149] Multiplicity of tumors is also noted to affect overall prognosis.[150] Therefore, pathologically, a well-differentiated tumor, fibrolamellar tumor, absence of vascular invasion, and tumors less than 5 cm in diameter have a better outcome. Size of tumor-free margin, and presence of capsule fibrosis were noted to improve survival and decrease incidence of venous invasion.[151] Recurrence following resection of a hepatocellular carcinoma usually occurs at the previous margin of resection or as a new primary tumor within the residual liver. Intrahepatic metastases develops via the portal vein and/or multicentric nodules.[152–155] Approximately 67% of recurrences are intrahepatic without vascular invasion and are small in size and number. Intrahepatic recurrence of hepatocellular carcinoma at five years has been reported at 80%.[156] The resectability rate of recurrent hepatocellular carcinoma is less than 30%.[126] The five-year survival rate in one study was 30% following repeat hepatectomy, arterial chemoembolization, and percutaneous ethanol injection.[156,157]

Liver metastases. The most important prognostic factors are complete resection, negative margins, absence of periportal nodes, extrahepatic disease, number of metastases, stage of primary, and disease free interval.[158–166]

Those patients who do not undergo any treatment for hepatic metastases have a mean survival rate of 8.7 months and a three-year survival is rare.[167,168] A mean survival rate of approximately 15 months can be obtained with administration of systemic chemotherapy to treat hepatic metastases.[169]

Prognostic factors following second hepatic resection include the number of recurrent lesions and disease-free interval. The Repeat Hepatic Metastases Registry finds that the five-year survival rate is better in those patients with an interval of more than one year between two surgical resections versus an interval of less than one year (62% vs. 26%).[170]

Recurrent liver cancer. Treatment options for recurrence include repeat hepatic resection, percutaneous ethanol injection, and chemoembolization, which may improve long-term survival in hepatocellular carcinoma recurrence.[171–173]

Treatment options for recurrence of hepatic metastases are similar to initial therapy, and are dependent on the origin of the primary tumor. Systemic chemotherapy is also an option. Recurrence rates are similar to hepatocellular carcinoma.

Cryosurgery

Cryosurgery is an alternative surgical therapy that attempts a cure for unresectable hepatic tumors. It can be used for primary or metastatic disease of the liver. The technique is used to treat various skin malignancies, but its use has expanded to include deep tissues within a closed system. Cryosurgery is a method in which tissue is destroyed using liquid nitrogen at subzero temperatures. Cryosurgery to treat liver lesions has expanded with the development of new technology, most importantly, IOUS, which has minimized the destruction of normal hepatic tissue while allowing for maximal destruction of the entire tumor.[174] To ensure destruction of tumorous tissue, a rapid-freeze, slow-thaw, and then repeated freeze–thaw cycles should be performed. Cryosurgery affects the tissue by causing both direct and indirect cellular damage.[175,176] Direct cellular damage is a result of physiochemical effects and indirect cell damage results from the loss of structural integrity and vascular channels. As the temperature drops, crystals form both intracellularly and extracellularly. (See Figure 58-3.) Cryosurgery creates a hyperosmolar environment and draws water from inside the cells, which can result in cell shrinkage, destruction of cell membranes, and denatured proteins.[177] Cell damage continues during the thawing process.

Most hepatobiliary surgeons perform two cycles as part of cryotherapy. A rapid-freeze, slow-thaw, and then repeated freeze–thaw cycles will ensure destruction of tumorous tissue.[178] Cancerous cells and their survival are dependent on the cooling rate during freezing.[179] Cryoprobes vary in shape and size. Flat probes are used to treat small surface lesions or on the area surrounding the margin of resection or if there is concern regarding positive margins. Trocar probes are used for deeper lesions. A 3 mm probe will produce a cryolesion of approximately 3 cm in diameter; a 5 mm probe approximately a 4-5 cm cryolesion, and a 10 mm probe a 6 cm or larger cryolesion. Cryoprobes are placed with IOUS to confirm positioning. Liquid nitrogen at −196°C is circulated through the cryoprobes with freezing across the conductive tip of the probes.[180] It is important for the normal liver to be entered prior to the tumor. Cryosurgery usually is performed via an open laparotomy. Cryosurgery may also be performed laparoscopically, however, long-term studies are needed to determine for efficacy and impact on survival.[181,182] Exploration of the abdomen is performed in addition to palpation of the liver. A biopsy of all lesions should be performed to confirm malignancy.

Freezing time ranges from 5 to 20 minutes which is dependent on the size of the cryolesion as well as the interval thawing period between two freeze cycles of 10 to 20 minutes. Ultrasound is used to monitor progression of the iceball and tumor encased within the iceball. A 5–10 mm margin should be obtained. On ultrasound, the normal frozen liver appears hypoechoic as compared to the normal liver not frozen. The treated tumor remains hyperechoic after thawing and normal tissues are hypo-

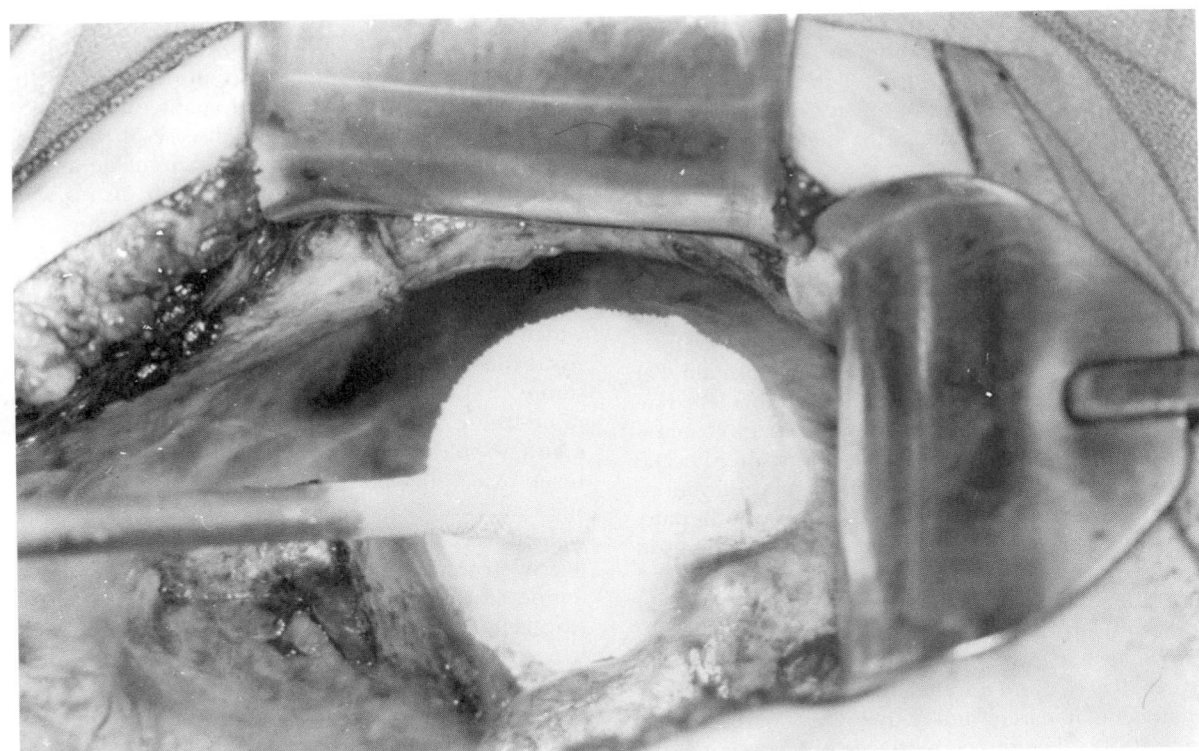

Figure 58-3 Cryosurgery utilizes extreme temperature of liquid nitrogen through a probe to freeze the tumor. A ball of ice is formed during cryo-assisted surgical resection of liver cancer. (Photo courtesy of The Johns Hopkins Hospital.)

echoic. Following the second cycle, the probe tip is heated with warmed gaseous nitrogen circulating though it and probes are removed when warmed and withdrawal is permitted.[183,184]

Limitations of cryosurgery include the inability to freeze lesions located in close proximity to major portal veins, vena cava, or hepatic veins. Complications postoperatively following hepatic cryosurgery are uncommon. Potential complications include cracking of frozen liver with subsequent hemorrhage, right-sided pleural effusion, subphrenic or hepatic abscess, bile collection, biliary fistula, thrombocytopenia, myoglobinuria, and acute renal failure (breakdown of products producing myoglobinuric state). Cryoshock phenomenon, which is associated with multisystem organ failure and disseminated intravascular coagulation, has been described but is exceedingly uncommon.[183,184] Bile duct injury is a possibility when tumors are centrally located near the bifurcation.

Following extensive cryosurgery, alkalination of urine is useful to prevent acute tubular necrosis from precipitation of myoglobin in the renal tubules. Maintaining adequate renal blood flow and hemodynamic stability are crucial. Pyrexia is common up to five days postoperatively, and in most cases, no infection is identified.[185–188] Because frozen tissue undergoes necrosis within a week, a CT scan in five to seven days following cryoablation should be performed to obtain a baseline appearance of the cryo-

lesion. It demonstrates necrosis with gas bubbles in the lesions. A gradual shrinkage of the cryoablated tumor will be evident over several months. The clinician can continue with percutaneous ethanol injection if imaging does not demonstrate complete tumor necrosis.[189] Follow-up CT scans should be performed every three months and gradual shrinkage of the cryolesion should be noted over time. An increase in size or change in shape may demonstrate recurrence. It is important to note that cryosurgery offers no clear advantage or disadvantage over standard surgical resection. Effect on overall survival requires long-term study.

Radiofrequency ablation

Another type of ablative therapy is radiofrequency ablation, which uses thermal energy to produce cell destruction when cells are heated greater than 45°C. With ablation, the proteins within the cell are denatured and cell membranes lose their integrity as a result of melting of the lipid component.[190–192] Specially designed probes deliver electrical energy to a spherical tissue volume, which results in tissue heating and destruction over 3.5–4.0 cm in diameter. Tumor size is an important factor. New multi-wire arrays with larger heat distribution are being designed to enable the treatment of larger tumors.[193,194] As with cryotherapy, ultrasonography is typically used to target accurate placement of the probe tip. Also it can be performed percutaneously or as a surgical procedure with open laparotomy or laparoscopically.

Dynamic CT is important in post-treatment evaluation to identify nonenhancing foci that demonstrate tumor necrosis. A post-treatment peripheral ring enhancement can be detected on imaging but it is unknown if the ring is indicative of postnecrotic edema or residual viable tumor.

Liver transplantation

Total hepatectomy with orthotopic liver transplantation may lower recurrence rates and improve survival for a select population.[195,196] Transplantation is an appropriate treatment option for a small hepatocellular carcinoma not amenable to resection. Orthotopic liver transplantation is not an option for patients with liver metastases. Liver transplantation is the only treatment option that can cure hepatocellular carcinoma and underlying liver disease, and is comparable if not better in outcome to hepatic resection. Unfortunately, transplantation is becoming a difficult treatment option as waiting lists are becoming longer and demand is exceeding donor organ availability.[197] This presents a dilemma in the management of the individual with a cancer diagnosis as there may be an extended time between diagnosis and transplantation. Further, the operative mortality rate for transplantation is higher than with surgical resection.[198] Contraindications to liver transplantation include patients with portal vein thrombosis secondary to invasion of tumor. It is currently premature to offer liver transplantation to patients with stage III or IV hepatocellular carcinoma.

Transplantation for stages I and II hepatocellular carcinoma in the presence of cirrhosis has demonstrated survival rates equal or superior to resection.[199,200] Following transplant, variables affecting recurrence are tumors larger than 5 cm, multiple tumors, bilobar involvement, and vascular invasion.[201–204] Cirrhotic patients have been noted to have a higher recurrence rate.[205,206] Due to high-dose immunosuppression, there is a concern regarding the impact and development of micrometastases.[207,208] The best indication for a successful transplantation is a small (< 3 cm) hepatocellular carcinoma.[208] A low AFP level is a positive prognostic factor.

Postoperative care following transplantation is similar initially to hepatic resection. However, the most important aspect of postoperative care in liver transplantation is the administration of immunosuppressive therapy to prevent organ rejection. Support provided to patients is critical because they are overwhelmed with the number of medications that must be taken on a daily basis. Studies of post-transplant improvement in emotional well-being has found that male spouses demonstrate more family cohesion with less conflict, whereas female spouses experience a higher level of stress. At one year, their overall quality of life improved.[209]

Chemotherapy

Systemic therapy

Primary liver cancer. Doxorubin remains the standard systemic treatment for hepatocellular carcinoma, with a response rate of less than 20%.[210] Etoposide, mitoxantrone, and cisplatin have been studied and have not been shown to provide a significant response. Results from recent phase II trials with advanced hepatocellular carcinoma have shown no response rate greater than 10% with single agents.[210]

Recently, combination immuno-chemotherapy using multiple agents including cisplatin, interferon, doxorubicin, and 5-FU were noted to have response rates of more than 25%; however, further investigation is necessary.[211] Antiestrogen therapy with tamoxifen has been studied in randomized trials and have shown no benefit. Current trials are pending utilizing an antiestrogen androlon and a lutenizing hormone goserelin (Zoladex®).[211]

Liver metastases. Systemic treatment of metastatic disease is based on utilizing chemotherapy regimens that are proven in the management of each specific primary cancer. Colorectal cancer commonly metastasizes to the liver and is discussed here. There have been a number of trials of chemotherapeutic agents for the treatment of hepatic metastases from colorectal cancer. Most widely used is 5-FU, which has been the first-line systemic chemotherapeutic agent in the treatment of colorectal carcinoma for the past 40 years.[212] This therapy can be administered by bolus or continuous infusion, producing a response rate of 15%–29%.[213] In comparing bolus 5-FU versus continuous infusion, a better response rate and slight increase in overall survival for advanced colorectal carcinoma was demonstrated.[214,215]

Clinical trials conducted over the past decade have demonstrated a therapeutic benefit using the combination of 5-FU and leucovorin for treating metastatic colorectal carcinoma.[216,217] Therefore, the standard therapy presently for metastatic disease is 5-FU and leucovorin. This treatment alone produces a median survival of 10–12 months.[218,219] When used following curative resection, clinical trials have demonstrated a delay in recurrence and improvement in overall survival.[220,221]

Levamisole may be used in combination with 5-FU for one year following curative resection, however, since leucovorin has been noted to enhance the rate of metabolism of 5-FU, it is less likely used. In addition, 5-FU and leucovorin are administered for 6 months versus one year of 5-FU and levamisole.

Until recently, there has been no good second-line treatment in the event the tumor fails to respond to 5-FU. Irinotecan, also referred to as CPT-11 or camptostar, is a semisynthetic derivative of campothecin that is considered the best treatment option as second-line therapy.[222] Clinical trials have demonstrated irinotecan to be active in metastatic colorectal cancer resistant to 5-FU with an 11%–23% response rate and an overall median survival of nine months.[223-225] Interestingly, a study performed with patients receiving irinotecan versus best supportive care demonstrated that except for diarrhea, toxicities were well managed and individuals experienced a quality of life benefit in addition to a survival advantage.[222] Therefore, systemic chemotherapy may affect overall survival in a small number of patients with metastic colon cancer; however, there are few long-term survivors.

Hepatic arterial infusion chemotherapy

Regional chemotherapy via hepatic artery infusion is a treatment option that is used mostly for unresectable hepatic colorectal metastases. The principle in the delivery of hepatic arterial infusion (HAI) chemotherapy is that normal hepatic parenchyma derives its blood supply from the portal system whereas metastatic lesions derive their afferent blood supply from the hepatic artery.[226,227] Therefore, high doses of chemotherapeutic agents are directed into the hepatic artery, increasing the concentration of the drug to which the tumor is exposed while limiting systemic exposure and toxicity. The systemic toxicities are limited because the chemotherapeutic agents delivered have a short half-life and are extracted by the liver on the first pass. Most commonly, floxuridine is used for HAI.

Regional chemotherapy delivers drugs via the hepatic artery with an implantable pump. Preoperative angiography with selective injection of the celiac and superior mesenteric arteries should be performed prior to hepatic pump placement to demonstrate arterial and venous phases. The standard anatomy is classified as the common hepatic artery arising from the celiac artery.[228] The common hepatic artery then gives rise to the gastroduodenal artery (GDA) and is separated into two branches 2 cm or more distally into the right and left hepatic arteries.[228] Variant anatomy that may be noted includes the common hepatic artery dividing into three branches, a replaced right or left hepatic artery, or the common hepatic arising from the superior mesenteric artery (SMA).[228,229]

The patient then undergoes exploratory laparotomy via right subcostal incision and exploration of the abdomen to rule out extrahepatic metastases. To perform the procedure, typically an implantable pump is placed in the subcutaneous pocket on the lower abdominal wall. Alternatively, the catheter can be attached to a subcutaneously implanted port. The GDA is ligated and used for cannulation. Fluroscein injection is performed intraoperatively with an ultraviolet lamp to determine adequate perfusion of both lobes of the liver. Routinely, cholecystectomy is performed at the time of pump implant. Postoperatively, a nuclear scan is used to assess the pump perfusion. Bilobular flow must be documented and extrahepatic perfusion ruled out.

Surgical expertise is a key factor to the implantation of hepatic arterial pumps, especially when variant anatomy of the liver is present. An inadequate surgical technique can result both in gastroduodenal ulceration and inadequate liver perfusion.[230,231] In addition, medical on-

cologists must be familiar with the management of HAI chemotherapy in terms of determining the need for decreased dosage versus discontinuation of therapy since HAI treatment may trigger the beginning of sclerosing cholangitis. Medical management includes close follow-up of biweekly laboratory tests, noting rising liver function tests. CEA levels are also performed monthly. Fluoropyrimidines, e.g., 5-FU and floxuridine (FUDR), are utilized to treat hepatic metastases. Regional chemotherapy is delivered for two-week periods. Therefore, the tumor cells are exposed to the drug throughout the vulnerable phase of their mitotic cycle. These particular drugs are metabolized by the liver with the liver extracting greater than 90% of FUDR on the first passage.[232]

Regional chemotherapy can produce varying side effects related to the toxicity of the specific drug. In the early stages of hepatic intraarterial floxuradine (FUDR), a high incidence (10%–56%) of gastroduodenal ulceration occurred.[233-235] With increased expertise in surgical technique, this complication is seen less frequently now.

Other complications from HAI chemotherapy can include partial or complete thrombosis of the hepatic artery, leakage of infusion arterial from the artery, occlusion or displacement of the catheter, hemorrhage, infection of the device or catheter, and acalculous cholecystitis.[236]

Another complication of regional chemotherapy with the delivery of FUDR is "chemical hepatitis," which is demonstrated by a rise in liver enzymes and bilirubin.[233] Bilirubinemia and strictures of the bile duct may indicate biliary sclerosis, which can be reversed with a biliary stent.[237] To determine if biliary obstruction is a result of nodal metastases in the porta hepatitis or stricturing of the bile ducts, a cholangiography should be conducted. If biliary obstruction is a result of nodal metastases in the porta hepatitis, cholangiography will reveal a focal area of compression of the ducts and dilatation of the ducts above the level of the lesion. In addition, with discontinuation of the chemotherapeutic agent, jaundice will not improve and only continue to progress.

To detect sclerosing cholangitis, it is important to frequently monitor serum bilirubin. A slight elevation of serum bilirubin should initiate temporary discontinuation of FUDR treatment. Also, dexamethasone has been given to normalize alkaline phosphotase and persistent bilirubin elevation in those patients undergoing hepatic arterial chemotherapy. Interestingly, increased tumor response rates were also noted with addition of dexamethasone. Also, patients may experience diarrhea as a result of extensive liver involvement secondary to impaired fluoropyrimidine hepatic metabolism.[238] Overall, complications of HAI therapy can vary and chemotherapy may need to be discontinued.[239]

HAI chemotherapy can also be given as adjuvant therapy following hepatic resection for metastases from colorectal cancer. Emerging data from randomized trials suggest a potential benefit of combined regional and systemic chemotherapy following liver rejection for metastatic colorectal cancer.[239-244] However, hepatectomy is rarely performed following intraarterial chemotherapy unless it has reduced the tumor volume enough to be surgically resectable.[245] It may be difficult to quantify the size and number of lesions due to the steatosis (fatty degeneration), which can result from intraarterial therapy. It must also be determined if there is enough functional hepatic parenchyma to prevent postoperative hepatic failure. Technically, it is more difficult to perform hepatectomy because the hepatic artery has been ligated previously and multiple collateral vessels may have developed.[246]

Hepatic arterial chemotherapy has also been utilized as a therapeutic modality following cryoablation, with a slight increase in overall survival as compared to those patients who only underwent cryotherapy.[247]

Radiation Therapy

Radiation therapy may be used to treat unresectable hepatocellular carcinoma in combination with systemic chemotherapy or chemoembolization. Radiolabeled antibodies given intravenously to target tumor cells have also been utilized. Radiation therapy is delivered in fractionated doses to allow for destruction of tumor cells and recovery of normal surrounding tissue.

Radiation therapy is not widely used for hepatocellular carcinoma, because the normal liver is extremely sensitive to radiation injury. Radiation is usually delivered in doses of 1900–3100 cGy to decrease tumor burden, improve hepatic function, and provide palliative relief for pain.[248] A response rate of 15%–30% has been demonstrated and a short survival benefit has been provided with radiation therapy.[249,250] Radiation doses greater than 2500 cGy may produce radiation hepatitis.[251] Other side effects may include nausea, vomiting, anorexia, fatigue, and skin irritation.

Alternative Therapies

Chemoembolization

Chemoembolization is a local regional approach that may be utilized as a treatment option, although patients with cirrhosis may experience severe toxicity and liver dysfunction. A majority of tumors receive blood flow from the hepatic artery and normal hepatic parenchyma receives its blood supply from the portal vein.[252] Through a catheter placed into the hepatic artery, chemoembolization is administered to treat hypervascular tumors, e.g., hepatocellular carcinoma and neuroendocrine tumors, rather than colorectal metastases, which are hypovascular tumors with no demonstrated benefit.

Prior to the procedure, a tissue diagnosis should be obtained in addition to CT or MRI to exclude extrahepatic disease. Laboratory studies include complete blood count, liver function tests, tumor markers, partial thromboplastin time, and prothrombin time. Education should include side effects related to postembolization syndrome.

The chemoembilization procedure involves insertion of a catheter via the femoral artery. An arteriogram is performed to determine the arterial blood supply to the liver as well as the patency of the portal vein. A catheter is then introduced into the right or left hepatic artery depending on which lobe contains the most tumor. The radiologist injects the chemoembolic material and iodized oil.[253] Chemotherapy is mixed with Lipiodol in its aqueous form. This forms an emulsion, which suspends droplets of chemotherapy in an oil matrix. When embolic particles are added, this increases the response rate. Embolization causes impedance to the arterial blood flow, increasing the exposure of chemotherapy to the lesion and decreasing the nutrition provided to the tumor causing tumor necrosis. A gelatin sponge and chemotherapy is then injected. The gelatin sponge blocks the hepatic artery flow that induces ischemic necrosis of bulky tumors and it prevents unfavorable portal or systemic embolization. The sponge also retains iodized oil for period of time and maintains the high concentration of chemotherapeutic agents. The drug concentration is 10–25 times higher than that achieved by infusion.[254,255] To prevent pulmonary oil embolism, use no more than 15 mL of iodized oil. Vigorous hydration should be administered in addition to antiemetics. Various institutions administer antibiotics to decrease the risk of infection and abscess formation pre- and postprocedure.[256–258]

The patient is usually admitted for a period of twenty-four hours. A noncontrast CT is performed 24 hours postprocedure. A mild to moderate increase in transaminases is noted five to seven days following embolization. Follow-up includes liver function tests, tumor markers, and repeat imaging in three to six weeks following the procedure. The patient may undergo repeat procedure to the other lobe in four to six weeks.

Small nodular lesions (adenomatous hyperplasia or early hepatocellular carcinoma) are at times more difficult to treat with chemoembolization as they do not typically demonstrate tumor necrosis as clearly as overt hepatocellular carcinoma. Therefore, its use may be limited in this particular patient population.[259]

It has been thought that combining chemoembolization with percutaneous ethanol injection will achieve complete tumor necrosis and be effective against capsular invasion and small daughter nodules. The cumulative survival rate was higher with the combination treatment than chemoembolization alone.[260,261] Percutaneous ethanol injection is performed usually two to four weeks following embolization and injected in both the edge and center of tumor.

Contraindications to treatment include severe thrombocytopenia, leukopenia, cardiac problems, or renal insufficiency. Patients at high risk for hepatic failure are those with tumor involving greater than 50% of the liver, an elevated AST, and bilirubin greater than 3 mg/dL.[262] Hepatic encephalopathy, ascites, coagulopathy, and jaundice are absolute contraindications. A relative contraindication for chemoembolization is portal vein thrombosis. Patients with class C cirrhosis should not undergo chemoembolization due to the high mortality rate.[256]

Side effects include right upper quadrant pain, epigastric pain, and nausea and vomiting. Fever is common within the first 24–48 hours and is thought to be related to tumor necrosis. If a fever is accompanied by chills, leukocytosis, and if pain persists, blood cultures are indicated.[263] Complications such as encephalopathy, biloma formation, hepatic abscess, septicemia, gallbladder infarction, splenic infarction, or pulmonary oil embolism can occur.[264]

Various chemotherapeutic agents are used in chemoembolization. Most common are cisplatin alone or in combination with doxorubicin and mitomycin.[265] An epirubicin emulsion has also been administered. The literature has not demonstrated a significant difference between doxorubicin emulsion versus epirubicin emulsion.[266] A drug that has also been used for hepatocellular carcinoma is mitoxantrone, as it has similar activity to doxorubicin.[267]

Zinostatin stimalamer is another chemotherapeutic agent that has been administered, although it required four injections to achieve an anticancer effect.[268] Spherex has also been utilized to cause hepatic artery occlusion without embolization. Spherex acts as a vascular occluding agent to cause vascular thrombosis. Combined with doxorubicin and cisplatin, an objective tumor response was noted in 63% of patients.[269]

The response rate of chemoembolization depends on the tumor size and extent of hepatic dysfunction. Tumor response can be as high as 88% with 60%–80% survival at one year, 40%–60% survival at two years, and 15%–30% survival at three years.[270] A higher therapeutic response was noted with chemoembolization and ethanol injection versus chemoembolization alone.[271]

Chemoembolization may be performed prior to or following hepatic resection. It is thought that the administration of chemoembolization preoperatively will prevent the recurrence of hepatocellular carcinoma[256] and also assist with hepatic resection.[272] The benefit is questionable and further investigation is necessary.[273–275]

Percutaneous ethanol injection

Percutaneous ethanol injection is an appropriate treatment for small hepatocellular carcinomas in patients with hepatic dysfunction for whom surgical therapy is not an option. It is effective in patients with lesions smaller than 3 cm and may be administered prior to hepatic resection.[276–281]

Ethanol is effective in generating tumor necrosis and usually spreads to the periphery of the tumor within a 1–3 cm radius surrounding the injection site. The ethanol diffuses easily as a result of neoplastic tissue being softer in consistency than the surrounding cirrhotic tissue. To reduce the incidence of pain experienced secondary to alcohol injection, the needle should remain in place for a period of 10–30 seconds and then withdrawn slowly. A single treatment with large volumes of alcohol could produce alcohol intoxication as a complication. In a limited number of patients, a chemical thrombosis may develop in the portal branch; however, this disappears in one to two months.

A CT scan is performed 24 hours postprocedure. A complete response is noted when there are no areas of enhancement within the lesion. In addition, AFP levels should decrease. Transient changes are noted with various levels including transaminases, bilirubin, d-dimer, blood cells, platelets, hemoglobin, and fibrinogen. These transient changes are due to hepatic necrosis, hemolysis, and localized thrombosis. Contraindications to performing percutaneous ethanol injection is PTT less than 40%, platelets less than 40,000, advanced cirrhosis, extrahepatic disease, thrombosis of main vein or portal branches, and biliary tree dilatation.[282]

The five-year survival rates for 628 patients with lesions less than 5 cm and cirrhosis were 48% with treatment versus 17% for no treatment.[280] Combination therapy can include Lipiodol arterial embolization and percutaneous ethanol injection therapy.[281,283,284]

Percutaneous acetic acid injection

Percutaneous acetic acid injection may also be administered to treat small hepatocellular carcinomas. It works by dissolving lipids and extracting collagen to cause death of the tumor cells. Some studies demonstrate that patients who receive percutaneous acetic acid have better survival rates compared with those who receive percutaneous ethanol injection.[285,286]

Therapeutic Modalities

Non-colorectal non-neuroendocrine liver metastases

Research is scarce in demonstrating advantages for the treatment of hepatic metastases resulting from non-colorectal or non-neuroendocrine metastases, which includes sarcomas, ovarian, breast, cervical, renal, and adrenal cancers. In one particular study, surgical resection of breast cancer, melanoma, and sarcoma was noted to have a five-year survival of 26%, resected genitourinary carcinomas had 6% five-year survival, and resection for gastrointestinal tumors demonstrated the poorest survival.[287] Renal cell carcinomas that are metastatic to the liver have been resected with a more favorable prognosis than other lesions.[288]

Metastatic neuroendocrine tumors

A number of tumor types will produce hepatic metastases. Most likely tumors are small bowel carcinoid tumors, bronchogenic carcinoid tumors, and islet cell tumors, which include gastrinoma and glucoganoma. Pancreatic neuroendocrine tumors possess varying degrees of malignancy.[289] Insulinomas are 90% benign and about 10% spread to the lymph nodes and liver. Other neuroendocrine tumors include glucagonoma, gastrinoma, and vasoactive intestinal polypeptide VIPoma. Neuroendocrine tumors can produce functional hormones, resulting in syndromes that can be quite disabling to patients.[290]

Treatment options for metastatic tumors include hepatic resection, cryosurgery, transplantation, chemoembolization, and systemic chemotherapy. Hepatic resection to debulk the tumor is usually performed in symptomatic and asymptomatic patients.[291,292] In approximately 90% of cases, however, it is difficult to perform resection due to multifocal disease.[289] Cryosurgery may therefore be the best option to provide palliation.[293–295] Liver transplantation is an option for metastatic neuroendocrine tumors that can provide palliation and long-term cure.[296–298]

Chemoembolization is another option. Chemoembolization is an effective treatment to control symptoms for hypervascular symptomatic hormone-secreting tumors.[299,300] Prior to chemoembolization, octreotide can be delivered to patients to prevent carcinoid crisis. Systemic chemotherapy is an option for both metastatic islet cell tumors and carcinoid tumors. The response rate with doxorubicin and streptozocin has been reported to be as high as 69% for treatment of metastatic islet cell tumors; the treatment for metastatic carcinoid tumor is slightly lower.[301]

Gene Therapy

Many clinical trials are being conducted to evaluate gene therapy for liver cancer. These include tumors caused by viral and nonviral vectors.[302] Cancer vaccines are under investigation presently and may be effective inducing and reinforcing a host immune response to the tumor. Gene therapy with tumor necrosis factor alpha has been investigated against hepatocellular carcinoma. There is a potential for prolonged survival periods.[303]

Symptom Management and Supportive Care

Manifestations of end-stage liver disease include massive ascites, hepatic encephalopathy, hepatorenal syndrome, and infection. In addition, the individual may experience pain, bleeding diathesis, weight loss, weakness, and pneumonia. Hepatic failure will ultimately result. Efforts should be directed toward relief of symptoms. The individual and family should be kept abreast of various treatment options directed at palliation and maintaining quality of life.

Pain is a difficult problem to manage in the late stages of the disease. Pain becomes severe, worsening at night, with radiation to the right scapular or subscapular areas resulting from hepatomegaly. Position, activity, coughing, and deep breathing will worsen the pain. Aggressive pain management is critical.

Ascites may become severe with advanced disease. Palliation measures include fluid and sodium restriction, diuretic therapy, and paracentesis. Albumin administration offers little benefit.

Anorexia and vomiting may present in the late stages of the disease. Antiemetics, vitamin supplementation, antidepressants and tranquilizers may provide relief. Presentation of food may stimulate the individual's appetite. Significant weakness, muscle atrophy, and immobility can lead to pulmonary congestion, atelectasis, pneumonia, and death.

Jaundice with pruritus may be present and difficult to control. Hepatic encephalopathy can develop when hepatic dysfunction progresses and toxins accumulate within the body. Pain medications may also contribute to encephalopathy due to the inability of the liver to metabolize drugs. Bleeding disorders may result from liver dysfunction. Dehydration and infection can accelerate hepatic failure.

Anticipatory management of rapidly developing symptoms and individual and family support are major goals of nursing care in advanced disease. Education and psychological support are vital components of holistic care for the individual facing uncertainty with their cancer diagnosis. Education targeted at the disease process, progression, and prognosis will empower patients and families to make decisions regarding their care.

Continuity of Care

A number of treatment modalities continue to evolve in the treatment of primary liver cancer and metastatic disease. With improved treatment options, tumor response and prolonged survival has resulted. To best educate patients, the oncology nurse should be knowledgeable about evolving treatments. In addition, communication with other clinicians is important. The nurse may also be involved with research and evaluation of new treatments to determine their impact on survival.

Awareness of symptoms and management is necessary to provide support. Anticipatory management is necessary when an individual fails or no longer desires aggressive therapy. The nurse can assist in the transition to the terminal phase of the disease through caring and support and initiating hospice services at the appropriate time.

Conclusion

Ultimately, the oncology nurse plays a vital role in assessment and management of the individual with primary liver cancer and metastatic disease. The goal of the oncology nurse is to enhance cancer care services the patient receives across the continuum, and assure the quality of care, and outcome. In order for this goal to be met, the nurse must utilize various assessment and patient/family education tools applicable to the practice of oncology nursing.

References

1. LaBreque DR: Neoplasia of the liver, in Kaplowitz N (ed): *Liver and Biliary Diseases* (ed 2). Baltimore, Williams and Wilkins, 1996, pp 391–436

2. Hepatitis C: *Wkly Epidemiol Rec* 72:65–72, 1997

3. Falkson G, Cnaan A, Schutt AJ, et al: Prognostic factors for survival in hepatocellular carcinoma. *Cancer Res* 48:7314–7318, 1993

4. Giacchino R, Navone C, Facco F, et al: HBV-DNA-related hepatocellular carcinoma occurring in childhood: report of three cases. *Dig Dis Sci* 36:1143–1146, 1991

5. Nagorney DM, Gigot JF: Primary epithelial hepatic malignancies: etiology, epidemiology, and outcome after subtotal and total hepatic resection. *Surg Oncol Clin North Am* 5:283–300, 1996

6. Khakoo SI, Grellier LFL, Soni PN, et al: Etiology, screening, and treatment of hepatocellular carcinoma. *Med Clin North Am* 80:1121–1145, 1996

7. El-Serag HB, Mason AC: Rising incidence of hepatocellular carcinoma in the United States. *N Engl J Med* 340:745–750, 1999

8. McQuillan GM, Alter MJ, Everhart JE: Viral hepatitis, in Everhart JE (ed): *Digestive diseases in the United States: Epidemiology and Impact.* Washington, DC, Government Printing Office, 1994, pp 127–156 (NIH pub. no. 94-1447)

9. McQuillan GM, Townsend TR, Fields HA, et al: Seroepidemiology of hepatitis B virus infection in the United States: 1976–1980. *Am J Med* 87:5–10, 1989 (suppl 3A)

10. Fattorich G: Progression of hepatitis B and C to hepatocellular carcinoma in western countries. *Hepatogastroenterology* 45:1206–1213, 1998

11. Benegnu L, Fattorich G, Noventa F, et al: Concurrent hepatitis B and C virus infection and risk of hepatocellular carcinoma in cirrhosis. *Cancer* 74:2442–2448, 1994

12. American Cancer Society: Cancer Facts and Figures 1999. Atlanta, American Cancer Society, 1999

13. Landis SH, Murray T, Bolden S, et al: Cancer statistics, 2000. *CA Cancer J Clin* 50:7–33, 2000

14. Zavadsky KE, Lee YT: Liver metastases from colorectal carcinoma: incidence, resectability, and survival results. *Am J Surg* 60:929–933, 1994

15. Declore R, Friesen SR: Gastrointestinal neuroendocrine tumors. *J Am Coll Surg* 178:188–211, 1994

16. Tsukuma H, Higama T, Tanaka S, et al: Risk factors for hepatocellular carcinoma among patients with chronic liver disease. *N Engl J Med* 328:1797–1801, 1993

17. Blum HE: Does hepatitis C virus cause hepatocellular carcinoma? *Hepatology* 19:251–255, 1994

18. DeCampos M, Olszyma-Marzys AE: Aflatoxin contamination in grains and grain products during the dry season in Guatemala. *Bull Environ Contam Toxicol* 22:350–356, 1979

19. Bosch FX, Monoz N: Prospects for epidemiological studies on hepatocellular as a mode for assessing viral and chemical interactions, in Bartsch H, Hemminiki K, O'Neill IK (eds): *Methods for Detecting DNA Damaging Agents in Humans: Applications in Cancer Epidemiology and Prevention.* Lyon, IARC: Scientific publications 89 IARC, 1988, pp 427–438

20. Bhoola KKD: Cellular interactions and metabolism of aflatoxin: an update. *Pharmacol Ther* 65:163–192, 1995

21. Hsia CC, Axiotis CA, DiBisceglie AM, et al: Transforming growth factor-alpha in human hepatocellular carcinoma and coexpression with hepatitis B surface antigen in liver. *Cancer* 70:1049–1056, 1992

22. Saegusa M, Takano Y, Kishimoto H, et al: Comparative analysis of p53 and c-myc expression and cell proliferation in human hepatocellular carcinomas: an enhanced immunohistochemical approach. *J Cancer Res Clin Oncol* 119:737–744, 1993

23. Jaskiewicz K, Bonarch L, Izycka E: Hepatocellular carcinoma in young patients: histology, cellular differentiation, hepatitis B virus infection, and oncoprotein 53. *Anticancer Res* 15:2723–2726, 1995

24. Kiyosawa K, Sodeyama T, Taneka E, et al: Interrelationship of blood transfusion, non-A, non-B hepatitis and hepatocellular carcinoma: analysis by detection of antibody to hepatitis C virus. *Hepatology* 12:671–675, 1990

25. DiBisceglie AM, Goodman ZD, Ishak KG, et al: Long-term clinical and histopathological follow-up of chronic post transfusion hepatitis. *Hepatology* 14:969–974, 1991

26. DiBisceglie AM: Hepatitis C and hepatocellular carcinoma. *Hepatology* 26:34–38, 1997 (suppl 1)

27. Alter MJ: Epidemiology of hepatitis C. *Hepatology* 26:62–65, 1997 (suppl 1)

28. DiBisceglie AM, Rustgi VK, Hoofnagle JH, et al: NIH conference: hepatocellular carcinoma. *Ann Intern Med* 108:390–401, 1998

29. Beasley RP: Hepatitis B virus: the major etiology of hepatocellular carcinoma, in Fortner JC, Rhoads JE (eds): *Accomplishment in Cancer Research.* Philadelphia, Lippincott, 1988, pp 80–106

30. Ince N, Wands JR: The increasing incidence of hepatocellular carcinoma. *N Engl J Med* 340:798–799, 1999

31. Alberti A, Pontissi P: Hepatitis viruses as aetiological agents of hepatocellular carcinoma. *Ital J Gastroenterol* 23:452–456 1991

32. Chen CJ, Llang KY, Chang YC, et al: Effects of hepatitis B virus, alcohol drinking, cigarette smoking, and familial tendency on hepatocellular carcinoma. *Hepatology* 13:398–406, 1991

33. Villa E, Melegari M, Scaglioni PP, et al: Hepatocellular carcinoma: risk factors other than hepatitis B virus. *Ital J Gastroenterol* 23:457–460, 1991

34. Beasley RP: Hepatitis B virus: the major etiology of hepatocellular carcinoma. *Cancer* 61:1942–1956, 1988

35. Ohnishi K, Ilda S, Iwama S, et al: The effect of chronic habitual alcohol intake on the development of liver cirrhosis and hepatocellular carcinoma: relation to hepatitis B surface antigen carrier. *Cancer* 49:672–677, 1982

36. Naccarato R, Farinati F: Hepatocellular carinoma, alcohol, and cirrhosis: facts and hypotheses. *Dig Dis Sci* 36:1137–1142, 1991

37. Kubo S, Tamori A, Nishiguchi S, et al: Effect of alcohol abuse on polyamine metabolism in hepatocellular carcinoma and noncancerous tissue. *Surgery* 123:205–211, 1998

38. Imberti D, Fornari F, Sbolli G, et al: Hepatocellular carcinoma in liver cirrhosis: a prospective study. *Scand J Gastroenterol* 28:540–544, 1993

39. Colombo M: Hepatocellular carcinoma. *J Hepatol* 15: 225–236, 1992

40. Okuda K: Hepatocellular carcinoma: recent progress. *Hepatology* 15:948–963, 1992

41. Neuberger J, Forman D, Doll R, et al: Oral contraceptives and hepatocellular carcinoma. *Brit Med J* 292:1355–1357, 1986

42. Prentice RL, Thomas DB: On the epidemiology of oral contraceptives and disease. *Adv Cancer Res* 49:285–401, 1987

43. Ni CH, Chang MH, Hsu HG, et al: Hepatocellular carcinoma in childhood. *Cancer* 68:1737–1741, 1991

44. Beasley RP: Hepatitis B virus as the etiologic agent in hepatocellular carcinoma: epidemiologic considerations. *Hepatology* 2:215–216, 1982

45. Chen WJ, Lee JC, Hung WT: Primary malignant tumor of liver in infants and children in Taiwan. *J Pediatr Surg* 23: 457–461, 1988

46. Addleston A: Modern vaccines: hepatitis. *Lancet* 335: 1142–1145, 1990

47. Chang MH, Chen CJ, Lai MS, et al: Universal hepatitis B vaccination in Taiwan and the incidence of hepatocellular carcinoma in children. *N Engl J Med* 336:1855–1859, 1997

48. Nishiguchi S, Kuroki T, Nakatani S, et al: Randomized trial of effects of interferon-alpha on incidence of hepatocellular carcinoma in chronic active hepatitis C with cirrhosis. *Lancet* 346:51–55, 1995

49. Harper SE, Grenstag JL: Can interferon alpha treatment prevent hepatocellular carcinoma in patients with chronic hepatitis C infection and compensated cirrhosis? *Hepatology* 23:930–933, 1996

50. Mazzella G, Accogli E, Sottili S, et al: Alpha interferon treatment may prevent hepatocellular carcinoma in hepatitis C virus related cirrhosis. *J Hepatol* 24:141–147, 1996

51. Schloger LK, Bodenheimer H Jr: Tackling liver cancer with interferon. *Lancet* 346:1049–1050, 1995

52. Perrillo RP, Schiff ER, Davis GL, et al: A randomized controlled trial of interferon alpha-2b alone and after prednisone withdrawal for the treatment of chronic hepatitis B. *N Engl J Med* 323:295–301, 1990

53. Sherman M, Peltekian KM, Lee C: Screening for hepatocellular carcinoma in chronic carriers of hepatitis B virus: incidence and prevalence of hepatocellular carcinoma in a North American urban population. *Hepatology* 22:432–438, 1995

54. Larcos G, Sorokopud H, Berry G, et al: Sonographic screening for hepatocellular carcinoma in patients with chronic hepatitis or cirrhosis: an evaluation. *Am J Roentgenol* 171:433–435, 1998

55. Ganne-Larrie N, Beargrand M: Prevention of the occurrence of hepatocellular carcinoma in patients with cirrhosis. *Hepatogastroenterology* 45:1291–1295, 1998

56. Kubos S, Kinoshita H, Hirohashi K: High malignancy of hepatocellular carcinoma in alcoholic patients with hepatitis C virus. *Surgery* 121:425–429, 1997

57. Choti MA: The liver, in Zuideno SD, Schlossberg L (eds): The Johns Hopkins Atlas of Human Functional Anatomy (4th ed) Baltimore. The Johns Hopkins University Press, 1997, p. 138

58. Huether SE: Structure and function of the digestive system, in Huether SE (ed): *Pathophysiology: The Biologic Basis for Disease in Adults and Children* (ed 3). St. Louis: Mosby Year Book, 1998, pp 1323–1377

59. Hudak CM: Anatomy and physiology of the gastrointestinal system, in Hudak CM, Gallo BM (eds) : *Critical Care Nursing:*

A Holistic Approach (ed 6). Philadelphia, Lippincott, 1994, pp 803–817

60. Schwartz SI: Primary hepatic neoplasm, in Bayless TM (ed): *Current Therapy in Gastroenterology and Liver Disease* (ed 4). St Louis: Mosby, 1994, pp 585–588

61. Bisgard HC, Thorgeirsson SS: Hepatic regeneration: the role of regeneration in pathogenesis of chronic liver disease. *Clin Lab Med* 16:325–329, 1996

62. Aahlgren JD, Wanebo HJ, Hill MC: Hepatocellular carcinoma, in Ahlgren JD, Macdonald JS (eds) : *Gastrointestinal Oncology.* Philadelphia, Lippincott, 1992 pp 417–436

63. Wanebo HJ, Falkson G, Order SE: Cancer of the hepatobiliary system, in DeVita VT, Hellman S, Rosenberg SA (eds): *Cancer: Principles and Practice of Oncology* (ed 5). Philadelphia, Lippincott-Raven, 1997, pp 1087–1127

64. Curley SA, Levin B, Rich TA: Liver and bile ducts, in Abeloff MD, Armitrage JO, Lichter AS, Niederhuber JE (eds): *Clinical Oncology.* New York, Churchill Livingstone, 1995, pp 1305–1372

65. Radinsky R, Lee E: Molecular determinants in the biology of liver metastasis. *Surg Oncol Clin North Am* 5:215–222

66. Sitzmann JV: Hope for cure through earlier detection of hepatocellular carcinoma. *Ann Surg Oncol* 6:133–134, 1998

67. Izzo F, Cremona F, Ruffalo F, et al: Detection of hepatocellular carcinoma during screening of 1125 patients with chronic hepatitis virus infection. *J Chemother* 9:151–152, 1997

68. Sheu JC, Sung JC, Chen DS, et al: Growth rate of symptomatic hepatocellular carcinoma and its clinical implications. *Gastroenterology* 89:259–266, 1985

69. Moertel CG, Fleming TR, MacDonald JS, et al: An evaluation of the carcinoembryonic antigen (CEA) test for monitoring patients with resected colon cancer. *JAMA* 270: 943–947, 1993

70. Zerhoun EA, Stitik FP, Siegelman SS, et al: CT of the pulmonary nodule: a cooperative study. *Radiology* 160: 319–327, 1986

71. Povoski SP, Fong Y, Sgouros SC, et al: Role of chest CT in patients with negative chest x-rays referred for hepatic colorectal metastases. *Ann Surg Oncol* 5:9–15, 1998

72. Urban BA, Fishman EK, Kuhlman JE, et al: Detection of focal hepatic lesions with spiral CT: comparison of 4 and 8 mm interscan spacing. *AJR Am J Roentgenol* 160: 783–785, 1993

73. Bluemke DA, Fishman EK: Spiral CT of the liver. *AJR Am J Roentgenol* 160:787–792, 1993

74. Baron RL, Oliver JH, Dodd GD, et al: Hepatocellular carcinoma: evaluation with biphasic, contrast-enhanced, helical CT. *Radiology* 199:505–511, 1996

75. Van Leeuwen MS, Noordzji J, Feldberg MA, et al: Focal liver lesions: characterization with triphasic spiral CT. *Radiology* 201:327–336, 1996

76. Miller FH, Butler RS, Hoff FL, et al: Using triphasic helical CT to detect focal hepatic lesions in patients with neoplasms. *AJR Am J Roentgenol* 171:643–649, 1998

77. Togo S, Shimada H, Kanemura E, et al: Usefulness of three-dimensional computed tomography for anatomic liver resection: sub-segmentectomy. *Surgery* 123:73–78, 1998

78. Jacobs JE, Birnbaum BA: Computed tomography imaging of focal hepatic lesions. *Semin Roentgenol* 30:308–323, 1995

79. Kodo M: Morphological diagnosis of hepatocellular carcinoma: special emphasis on intranodular hemodynamic imaging. *Hepatogastroenterology* 45:1226–1231, 1998

80. Matsui O, Kadoye M, Suzuki M, et al: Dynamic sequential

computed tomography during arterial portography in the detection of hepatic neoplasms. *Radiology* 146:721–727, 1986

81. Karl RC, Choi J, Yeatman TJ, et al: Role of computed tomographic arterial portography and intraoperative ultrasound in the evaluation of patients for resectability of hepatic lesions. *J Gastrointest Surg* 1:152–157, 1997

82. Fortunsto L, Clair M, Hoffman J, et al: Is CT portography (CTAP) really useful in patients with liver tumors who undergo intraoperative ultrasonography (IOUS)? *Am Surg* 61:560–565, 1995

83. Soyer P, Bluemke DA, Fishman EK: CT during arterial portography for preoperative evaluation of hepatic tumors: how, when and why? *AJR Am J Roentgenol* 163:1325–1331, 1994

84. Luaffer RB: Magnetic resonance contrast media: principles and progress. *Magn Reson Q* 6:65–84, 1990

85. Schnall M: Magnetic resonance imaging of focal liver lesions. *Semin Roentgenol* 30:347–361, 1995

86. Kruskal JB, Kane RA: Imaging of primary and metastatic liver tumors. *Surg Oncol Clin North Am* 5:231–257, 1996

87. Menu Y: Hepatocellular carcinoma: radiological findings. *Hepatogastroenterology* 45:1232–1235, 1998

88. Nisenbaum HL, Roweling SE: Ultrasound of focal hepatic lesions. *Semin Roentgenol* 30:324–346, 1995

89. Kim EE, Chung SK, Haynie TP, et al: Differentiation of residual or recurrent tumors from post-treatment changes with F-18 FDG PET. *Radiographics* 185:149–155, 1992

90. Falk PM, Gupta NC, Thorson AG, et al: Positron emission tomography for preoperative staging of colorectal carcinoma. *Dis Colon Rectum* 37:153–156, 1994

91. Schiepers C, Penninckx F, Deradder N, et al: Contribution of PET in the diagnosis of recurrent colorectal cancer: comparison with conventional imaging. *Eur J Surg Oncol* 21:517–522, 1995

92. Vitola JV, Delbeke D, Sandler MP, et al: Positron emission tomography to stage suspected colorectal carcinoma to the liver. *Am J Surg* 171:21–26, 1996

93. Takenoshita SI, Hashizume T, Asao T, et al: Immunoscintography using 99mTc-labeled anti-CEA monoclonal antibody for patients with colorectal cancer. *Cancer Res* 5:471–476, 1995

94. Scheele J, Altendorf HA: Tumor implantation from needle biopsy of hepatic metastases. *Hepatogastroenterology* 37:335–337, 1990

95. Rajender Reddy K, Jeffers LJ: Evaluation of the liver: Biopsy and laparosocopy, in Schiff ER, Sorrell MF, Maddrey WC (eds): *Schiff's Diseases of the Liver*. Philadelphia, Lippincott-Raven, 1999, pp 245–266

96. Fleming ID, Cooper JS, Henson DE, Hutter KVP, et al: AJCC Cancer Staging Manual (ed 5), Philadelphia, Lippincott-Raven, 1997, p 98

97. Gibbs JF, Weber TK, Rodriguez-Bigas MA, et al: Intraoperative determinants of unresectability for patients with colorectal hepatic metastases. *Cancer* 82:1244–1249, 1998

98. Johnson PJ, Williams RI: Cirrhosis and the etiology of hepatocellular carcinoma. *Hepatology* 4:140–147, 1987

99. Shanbhogue RLK, Bistrian BR, Jenkins RL, et al: Resting energy expenditure in patients with end-stage liver disease and in normal population. *J Parenter Enteral Nutr* 11:305–308, 1987

100. Fan ST: Problems of hepatectomy in cirrhosis. *Hepatogastroenterology* 45:1288–1290, 1998

101. Matsumata T, Ikeda Y, Hayashi H, Kamakura T, et al: The association between transfusion and cancer-free survival after curative resection for hepatocellular carcinoma. *Cancer* 72:1866–1871, 1993

102. Bismuth H, Chiche L, Adam R, et al: Liver transplantation versus resection for hepatocellular carcinoma in cirrhosis. *Ann Surg* 218:145–151, 1993

103. Marcos-Alvarez A, Jenkins RL, Washburn WK, et al: Multimodality treatment of hepatocellular carcinoma in a hepatobiliary specialty center. *Arch Surg* 131:292–298, 1996

104. Philosophe B, Greig PD, Hemming AW, et al: Surgical management of hepatocellular carcinoma: resection or transplantation? *J Gastrointest Surg* 2:21–27, 1998

105. Chen MF, Jeng LB, Lee WC, et al: Surgical results in patients with dual hepatitis B and C-related hepatocellular carcinoma compared with hepatitis B or C-related hepatocellular carcinoma. *Surgery* 123:554–559, 1998

106. Takenaka K, Kawahara N, Yamamoto K, et al: Results of 280 liver resections for hepatocellular carcinoma. *Arch Surg* 131:71–84, 1996

107. Colombo M: Hepatocellular carcinoma in cirrhotics. *Semin Liver Dis* 13:374–383, 1993

108. Al-Hadeedi S, Choi TK, Wong J: Extended hepatectomy for hepatocellular carcinoma. *Br J Surg* 77:1247–1250, 1990

109. Sugihara K, Hojo K, Moriya Y, et al: Pattern of recurrence after hepatic resection for colorectal metastases. *Br J Surg* 80:1032–1035, 1993

110. Gayowski TJ, Iwatsuki S, Madariaga JR, et al: Experience in hepatic resection for metastatic colorectal cancer: analysis of clinical and pathologic risk factors. *Surgery* 116:703–711, 1994

111. Rees M, Plant G, Wells J, et al: One hundred and fifty hepatic resections: the evolution of techniques towards bloodless surgery. *Br J Surg* 83:1526–1529, 1996

112. Nordlinger B, Jaeck D, Guiguet M, et al: Surgical resection of hepatic metastases: multicentric retrospective study by the French association of surgery, in Nordlinger B, Jaeck D (eds): *Treatment of Hepatic Metastases of Colorectal Cancer*. Paris, Springer France, 1992, pp 129–146

113. Van Ooijen B, Wiggers T, Meijer S, et al: Hepatic resections for colorectal metastases in the Netherlands: a multi-institutional 10-year study. *Cancer* 70:28–34, 1992

114. Bismuth H, Adam R, Levi F, et al: Resection of nonresectable liver metastases from colorectal cancer after neoadjuvant chemotherapy. *Ann Surg* 224:509–522, 1996

115. Busch E, Kemeny MM: Colorectal cancer: hepatic-directed therapy: the role of surgery, regional chemotherapy, and novel modalities. *Semin Oncol* 22:494–508, 1995

116. Kobayashi A, Imamura H, Miyagawa S, et al: Extended right posterior segmentectomy for metastatic liver tumors. *Surgery* 121:698–703, 1997

117. D'Angelica M, Brennan MF, Fortner J, et al: Ninety-six five year survivors after liver resection for metastatic colorectal cancer. *J Am Coll Surg* 185:554–559, 1997

118. Kalakos EA, Kim JA, Young DC, et al: Determinants of survival following hepatic resection for metastatic colorectal cancer. *World J Surg* 22:399–405, 1998

119. Bismuth H, Adam R, Navarro F, et al: Re-resection for colorectal liver metastases. *Surg Oncol Clin North Am* 5:353–363, 1996

120. Nordlinger B, Vaillant JC, Guiget M, et al: Survival benefit of repeat liver resections for recurrent colorectal metastases: 143 cases. *J Clin Oncol* 12:1491–1496, 1994

121. Stone MD, Cady B, Jenkins RL, et al: Surgical therapy for recurrent metastases from colorectal cancer. *Arch Surg* 125:718–721, 1990

122. Cady B, Jenkins RL, Steele GDJ, et al: Surgical margin in hepatic resection for colorectal metastasis: a critical and improvable determinant of outcome. *Ann Surg* 227: 566–571, 1998

123. Fong Y, Blumgart LH, Cohen A: Repeat hepatic resections for metastatic colorectal cancer. *Ann Surg* 220:657–662, 1994

124. Vaillant JC, Balladur P, Nordlinger et al: Repeat liver resection for recurrent colorectal metastases. *Br J Surg* 80: 340–344, 1993

125. Chu QD, Vezeridis MP, Avradopoulos KA, et al: Repeat hepatic resection for recurrent colorectal cancer. *World J Surg* 21:292–296, 1997

126. Elais D, Lasser PH, Hoang JM, et al: Repeat hepatectomy for cancer. *Br J Surg* 80:1557–1562, 1993

127. Fernandez-Trigo V, Shamsa F, Sugarbaker PH, et al: Repeat liver resections from colorectal metastases. *Surgery* 117: 296–304, 1995

128. Adam R, Bismuth H, Castaing D, et al: Repeat hepatectomy for colorectal liver metastases. *Ann Surg* 225:51–62, 1997

129. Choti MA, Bulkley GB: Management of hepatic metastases. *Prog Liver Transpl* 5:65–80, 1999

130. Rafaelsen SR, Kronburg O, Larsen C, et al: Intraoperative ultrasonography in detection of hepatic metastases from colorectal cancer. *Dis Colon Rectum* 38:355–360, 1995

131. Clarke MP, Kane RA, Steele G Jr, et al: Prospective comparison of preoperative imaging and intraoperative ultrasonography in the detection of liver tumors. *Surgery* 106:849–855, 1989

132. Machi J, Isomoto H, Kurohisi T, et al: Accuracy of intraoperative ultrasonography in diagnoising liver metastasis from colorectal cancer: evaluation with postoperative follow-up results. *World J Surg* 15:551–557, 1991

133. Knol JA, Marn CS, Francis IR, et al: Comaprison of dynamic infusion and delayed computed tomography, intraoperative ultrasound, and palpation in the diagnosis of liver metastases. *Am J Surg* 165:81–87, 1993

134. Paul MA, Sibinga Mulder MA, Cuesta AC, et al: Impact of intraoperative ultrasonography on treatment strategy for colorectal cancer. *Brit J Surg* 81:1660–1663, 1994

135. Plant GR: Intra-operative ultrasonography, in Gosgrove D, Meire H, Dewbury K (eds): *Abdominal and General Ultrasound*. Edinburgh, Churchill Livingstone, 1993, pp 243–250

136. Takayama T, Makuuchi M, Kosuge T: Liver diseases: clinical application of intraoperative ultrasound, in Lygidakes NJ, Makuuchi M (eds): *Pitfalls and Complications in the Diagnosis and Management of Hepatobiliary and Pancreatic Diseases*. Stuttgart, Georgia, Thieme, 1993, p 17

137. Fuhrman GM, Curley SA, Hohn DC, et al: Improved survival after resection of colorectal liver metastases. *Ann Surg Oncol* 2:537–541, 1995

138. Boutkan H, Luth W, Meyer S, et al: The impact of intraoperative ultrasonography of the liver on the surgical strategy of patients with gastrointestinal malignancies and hepatic metastases. *Eur J Surg Oncol* 18:342–346, 1992

139. Kruskal JB, Kane RA: Intraoperative ultrasonography of the liver. *Crit Rev Diagn Imaging* 36:175–226, 1995

140. Kokudo N, Bandai Y, Imanishi H, et al: Management of new hepatic nodules detected by intraoperative ultrasonography during hepatic resection for hepatocellular carcinoma. *Surgery* 119:634–640, 1996

141. Takayama T, Makuuchi M: Intraoperative ultrasonography and other techniques for segmental resections. *Surg Oncol Clin North Am* 5:261–269, 1996

142. Soyer PH, Mosnier H, Choti MA, et al: Intraoperative and laparoscopic sonography of the liver. *Eur Radiol* 7: 1296–1302, 1997

143. Grundmann R, Heistermann S: Postoperative albumin infusion therapy based on colloid osmotic pressure: a prospectively randomized trial. *Arch Surg* 120:911–915, 1985

144. Nuzzo G, Giulante F, Giovanni I, et al: Resection of hepatic metastases from colorectal cancer. *Hepatogastroenterology* 44: 751–759, 1997

145. Calvet X, Bruix J, Gines P, et al: Prognostic factors of hepatocellular carcinoma in the west: a multivariate analysis in 206 patients. *Hepatology* 12:753–760, 1990

146. Ko S, Nakajima Y, Kanehiso H, et al: Significant influence of accompanying chronic hepatitis status on recurrence of hepatocellular carcinoma after hepatectomy: result of multivariate analysis. *Ann Surg* 224:591–585, 1996

147. Sasaki Y, Imaoka S, Matsutani S, et al: Influence of co-existing cirrhosis on long-term prognosis after surgery in patients with hepatocellular carcinoma. *Surgery* 112: 515–521, 1992

148. Yuki K, Hirohashi S, Sakamoto M, et al: Growth and spread of hepatocellular carcinoma: a review of 240 consecutive autopsy cases. *Cancer* 66:2174–2179, 1990

149. Izumi R, Shimizu K, Li T, et al: Prognostic factors of hepatocellular carcinoma in patients undergoing hepatic resection. *Gastroenterology* 106:720–727, 1994

150. Toyosaka A, Okamoto E, Mitsunobu M, et al: Pathologic and radiographic studies of intrahepatic metastases in hepatocellular carcinoma: the role of efferent vessels. *HPB Surg* 10:97–104, 1996

151. Nzeako UC, Goodman ZD, Ishak KG: Hepatocellular carcinoma in cirrhotic and noncirrhotic livers: a cliniohistopathologic study of 804 North American patients. *Am J Clin Pathol* 105:65–75, 1996

152. Matsumata T, Kanematsu T, Takenaka K, et al: Patterns of intrahepatic recurrence after curative resection of hepatocellular carcinoma. *Hepatology* 9:457–460, 1989

153. Ouchi K, Matsubara S, Fukuhara et al: Recurrence of hepatocellular carcinoma in the liver remnant after hepatic resection. *Am J Surg* 166:270–273, 1993

154. Nayao T, Inoue S, Yoshimi F, et al: Postoperative recurrence of hepatocellular carcinoma. *Ann Surg* 211:28–33, 1990

155. Belghiti J, Panis Y, Farges O, et al: Intrahepatic recurrence after resection of hepatocellular carcinoma complicating cirrhosis. *Ann Surg* 214:114–117, 1991

156. Farges O, Regimbeau JM, Belghiti J: Aggressive management of recurrence following surgical resection of hepatocellular carcinoma. *Hepatogastroenterology* 45:1275–1280, 1998

157. Nagasue N, Yukaya H, Chang YC, et al: Assessment of pattern and treatment of intrahepatic recurrence after resection of hepatocellular carcinoma. *Surg Gynecol Obstet* 171:217–222, 1990

158. Doci R, Gennari L, Bignami P, et al: One hundred patients with hepatic metastases from colorectal cancer treated by resection: analysis of prognostic determinants. *Br J Surg* 78:797–801, 1991

159. Taylor I, Mullee MA, Campbell MJ: Prognostic index for the development of liver metastases in patients with colorectal cancer. *Br J Surg* 77:499–501, 1990

160. Scheele J, Stangl R, Altendorf-Hofmann A, et al: Resection of colorectal liver metastases. *World J Surg* 19:59–71, 1995

161. Ohlsson B, Stenram U, Tranberg KG: Resection of colorectal liver metastases: 25-year experience. *World J Surgery* 22:268–277, 1998

162. Taylor M, Forster J, Langer B, et al: A study of prognostic factors for hepatic resection for colorectal metastases. *Am J Surg* 173:467–471, 1997

163. Gayowsky TJ, Iwatsuuki S, Madariaga JR, et al: Experience in hepatic resection for metastatic colorectal cancer: analysis of clinical and pathologic risk factors. *Surgery* 116: 703–711, 1994

164. Scheele J, Stangle R, Altendorf-Hofmann A, et al: Resection of colorectal liver metastases. *World J Surg* 19:59–71, 1995

165. Hananel N, Garzon J, Gordon PH: Hepatic resection for colorectal liver metastases. *Am Surg* 61:444–447, 1995

166. Scheele J, Rudroff C, Altendorf-Hofmann A: Resection of colorectal liver metastases revisted. *J Gastrointest Surg* 1: 408–422, 1997

167. Nagorney DM: Opinion: resection of hepatic metastasis for colorectal cancer. *J Surg Oncol* 2:74, 1991 (suppl)

168. Sheiner PA, Brower ST: Treatment of metastatic cancer to the liver. *Semin Liver Dis* 14:169–177, 1994

169. Lise M, DaPian PP, Nitti D, et al: Colorectal metastases to the liver: present results and future strategies. *J Surg Oncol* 2:69–73, 1991 (suppl)

170. Fernandez-Trigo V, Shamsa F, Sugarbaker PH, et al: Repeat liver resections from colorectal metastasis. *Surgery* 117: 296–304, 1995

171. Neeleman N, Anderson R: Repeated liver resection for recurrent liver cancer. *Br J Surg* 83:893–901, 1996

172. Lee PH, Lin WJ, Tsang YM, et al: Clinical management of recurrent hepatocellular carcinoma. *Ann Surg* 222: 670–676, 1995

173. Sato M, Watanabe Y, Iseki N, et al: Chemoembolization and percutaneous ethanol injection for intrahepatic recurrence of hepatocellular carcinoma after hepatic resection. *Hepatogastroenterology* 443:1421–1426, 1996

174. Ravikumar TS, Buenaventura S, Salem R, et al: Intraoperative ultrasonography of liver: detection of occult liver tumors and treatment by cryosurgery. *Cancer Detect Prev* 18: 131–138, 1994

175. Bischof J, Christov K, Rubinsky B: A morphological study of cooling rate response in normal and neoplastic human liver tissue: cryosurgical implications. *Cryobiology* 30: 482–492, 1993

176. Gage AA: Cryosurgery in the treatment of cancer. *Surg Gynecol Obstet* 174:73–92, 1992

177. Ravikumar TS, Sotomayor R, Goel SD: Cryosurgery in the treatment of liver metastases from colorectal cancer. *J Gastrointest Surg* 1:426–432, 1997

178. Gage AA, Baust J: Mechanisms of tissue injury in cryosurgery. *Cryobiology* 37:171–186, 1998

179. Rubinsky B, Lee CY, Onik G: The process of freezing and the mechanism of damage during hepatic cryosurgery. *Cryobiology* 27:85–97, 1990

180. Kane RA: Ultrasound-guided hepatic cryosurgery for tumour ablation. *Semin Interven Radiol* 10:132–142, 1993

181. Lezoche E, Paganini AM, Feliciotti F, et al: Ultrasound-guided laparoscopic cryoablation of hepatic tumors: preliminary report. *World J Surg* 22:829–836, 1998

182. Heniford BT, Arca MJ, Iannitti DA, et al: Laparoscopic cryoablation of hepatic metastases. *Semin Surg Oncol* 15: 194–201, 1998

183. Ravikumar TS, Kane R, Cady B, et al: A 5-year study of cryosurgery in the treatment of liver tumors. *Arch Surg* 126:1520–1523, 1991

184. Steele G, Ravikumar TS, Benotti PN: New surgical treatments for recurrent colorectal cancer. *Cancer* 65:723–730, 1990

185. Zoro LM, Staren ED: Cryosurgical ablation of unresectable hepatic tumors. *AORN* 64:231–244, 1996

186. Adam R, Akpinar E, Johann M, et al: Place of cryosurgery in the treatment of malignant liver tumors. *Ann Surg* 225: 39–50, 1997

187. Brandt BT, DeAntonio P, Dezort MA, et al: Hepatic cyrosurgery for metastatic colorectal carcinoma. *Oncol Nurs Forum* 23:29–38, 1996

188. Yeh KA, Fortunato L, Hoffman JP, et al: Cryosurgical ablation of hepatic metastases from colorectal carcinomas. *Am Surg* 63:63–68, 1997

189. Ohto M, Yoshikawa M, Saisho H, et al: Nonsurgical treatment of hepatocellular carcinoma in cirrhotic patients. *World J Surg* 19:42–46, 1995

190. Lounsberry W, Goldschmidt V, Linke C: The early histologic changes following electrocoagulation. *Gastrointest Endosc* 41:68–70, 1995

191. McGahan J, Brock J, Tesluk H: Hepatic ablation with use of radiofrequency electrocautery in the animal model. *J Vasc Interv Radiol* 3:291–297, 1992

192. McGahan J, Schneider P, Brock J: Treatment of liver tumors by percutaneous radio frequency electrocautery. *Semin Interv Radiol* 10:143–149, 1993

193. Rossi S, DiStasi M, Buscarini T, et al: Percutaneous RF intersititial thermal ablation in the treatment of hepatic cancer. *Am J Radiol* 167:759–768, 1996

194. Nagata Y, Hiraoka M, Nishimura Y, et al: Clinical results of radiofrequency hyperthermia for malignant liver tumors. *Int J Radiat Oncol Biol Phys* 38:359–363, 1997

195. Busitil RW, Farmer RG: The surgical treatment of primary hepatobiliary malignancy. *Liver Transplant Surg* 2:114–130, 1996

196. Penn I: Hepatic transplantation for primary and metastatic cancers of the liver. *Surgery* 110:726–735, 1991

197. Williams R, Rizzi P: Treating small hepatocellular carcinomas. *N Engl J Med* 334:728–729, 1996

198. Figueras J, Jaurrieta E, Valls C: Survival after liver transplantation in cirrhotic patients with and without hepatocellular carcinoma: a comparative study. *Hepatology* 25: 1485–1489, 1997

199. Trinchet JC, Beaugrand M: Treatment of hepatocellular carcinoma in patients with cirrhosis. *J Hepatol* 27:756–765, 1997

200. Ranjan D, Johnston TD: Liver transplantation for hepatocellular carcinoma. *Hepatogastroenterology* 45:1369–1374, 1998

201. Carr BI, Flickinger JC, Lotze MT: Hepatobiliary cancers, in DeVita VT Jr, Hellman S, Rosenberg SA (eds): *Cancer: Principles and Practice of Oncology* (ed 5). Philadelphia, Lippincott-Raven, 1997, pp 1087–1113

202. Lohmann R, Bechstein Wo, Langrehr JM, et al: Analysis of risk factors for recurrence of hepatocellular carcinoma after orthopopic liver transplantation. *Transplant Proc* 27: 1245–12466, 1995

203. Mazzaferro V, Regalia E, Doci R, et al: Liver transplantation for the treatments of small hepatocellular carcinoma in patients with cirrhosis. *N Engl J Med* 332:693–697, 1996

204. Mazziotti A, Grazi GL, Cavallari A: Surgical treatment of hepatocellular carcinoma on cirrhosis: a western experience. *Hepatogastroenterology* 45:1281–1287, 1998

205. Busuttil RW, Farmer DG: The surgical treatment of primary

hepatobiliary malignancy. *Liver Transplant Surg:* 114–130, 1996 (suppl)

206. Otto G, Heuschen U, Hofmann WT, et al: Is transplantation really superior to resection in the treatment of small hepatocellular carcinoma? *Transplant Proc* 29:489–491, 1997

207. Johnson PJ: Why can't we cure primary liver cancer? *Eur J Cancer* 31A:1562–1564, 1995

208. Bismuth H, Chiche L, Adam R, et al: Liver resection versus transplantation for hepatocellular carcinoma in cirrhotic patients. *Ann Surg* 218:145–151, 1993

209. Tarter RE: Quality of life following liver transplantation. *Hepatogastroenterology* 45:1398–1403, 1998

210. Okada S: Chemotherapy in hepatocellular carcinoma. *Hepatogastroenterology* 45:1259–1263, 1998

211. Okada S: Chemotherapy for hepatocellular carcinoma, in Okuda K, Tabor E (eds): *Liver Cancer.* London, Churchill Livingstone, 1997, pp 441–447

212. Rougier P, Bugat R, Douillard JY, et al: Phase II study of irinotecan in treatment of advanced colorectal cancer in chemotherapy naïve patients and patients treated with fluorouracil-based chemotherapy. *J Clin Oncol* 15:251–260, 1997

213. Leichman CC, Fleming TR, Muggia FM, et al: Phase II study of fluorouracil and its modulation in advanced colorectal cancer: a southwest oncology group study. *J Clin Oncol* 13:1303–1311, 1995

214. Meta-Analysis Group in Cancer: Efficacy of intravenous continuous infusion of fluorouracil compared with bolus administration in advanced colorectal cancer. *J Clin Oncol* 16:301–308, 1998

215. Wilke HJ: Comparing irinotecan with best supportive care and infusional 5-fluorouracil: a critical evaluation of the results of two randomized phase III trials. *Semin Oncol* 26:21–23, 1999

216. Stevenson HC, Green I, Hamilton JM, et al: Levamisole: known effects on the immune system, clinical results, and future applications in the treatment of cancer. *J Clin Oncol* 9:2052–2066, 1991

217. Advanced Colorectal Cancer Meta-Analysis Project: Modulation of fluorouracil by leucovorin in patients with advanced colorectal cancer: evidence in terms of response rate. *J Clin Oncol* 10:896–903, 1992

218. Nordic Gastrointestinal Tumor Adjuvant Project: Expectancy or primary chemotherapy in patients with advanced asymptomatic colorectal cancer: A randomized trial. *J Clin Oncol* 10:904–911, 1992

219. Fuchs CS, Mager RJ: Adjuvant chemotherapy for colon and rectal cancer. *Semin Oncol* 22:472–487, 1995

220. Krook JE, Moertel CG, Gunderson LL, et al: Effective surgical adjuvant therapy for high-risk rectal carcinoma. *N Engl J Med* 324:709–715, 1991

221. Zaniboni A: Adjuvant chemotherapy in colorectal cancer with high-dose leucovorin and fluorouracil: impact on disease-free survival and overall survival. *J Clin Oncol* 15:2432–2441, 1997

222. Cunningham P, Glimelius BA: Phase III study of irinotecan (CPT-11) versus best supportive care in patients with metastatic colorectal cancer who have failed 5-fluorouracil therapy. *Semin Oncol* 26:6–12, 1999 (suppl 5)

223. Van Custem E, Rougier P, Droz JP, et al: Clinical benefit of irinotecan (CPT-11) in metastatic colorectal cancer resistant to 5-FU. *Proc Am Soc Clin Oncol* 16:268a, 1997 (abstr 950)

224. Rothenberg ML, Eckhardt JR, Kuhn JG, et al: Phase II trial of irinotecan in patients with progressive or rapidly recurrent colorectal cancer. *J Clin Oncol* 14:1228–1235, 1996

225. Conti JA, Kemeny NA, Saltz LB, et al: Irinotecan is an active agent in untreated patients with metastatic colorectal cancer. *J Clin Oncol* 14:709–715, 1996

226. Watkins E, Khazei AM, Nahra KS: Surgical basis for arterial infusion chemotherapy of disseminated carcinoma of the liver. *Surg Gynec Obstet* 130:581–605, 1970

227. Lin G, Lunderquist A, Hagerstrand I, Boijsen E, et al: Postmortem examination of the blood supply and vascular pattern of small liver metastases in man. *Surgery* 96:517–526, 1984

228. Campbell KA, Burns RC, Sitzmann JV, et al: Regional chemotherapy devices: effect of experience and anatomy on complications. *J Clin Oncol* 11:822–826, 1993

229. Daly J, Kemeny N, Sigurdson E, et al: Regional infusion for colorectal hepatic metastases: a randomized trial comparing the hepatic artery versus the portal vein. *Arch Surg* 122:1273–1277, 1987

230. Mavlight GM, Patt YZ, Haynie TP, et al: Differential tumor progression in patients with bilobar hepatic metastases and dual arterial supply: evidence supporting the advantage of intra-arterial over intravenous route of drug delivery. *Sel Cancer Ther* 5:37–45, 1989

231. Hohn DC, Stagg RJ, Price, DC, et al: Avoidance of gastroduodenal toxicity in patients receiving hepatic arterial 5-fluoro-2′-deoxyuridine. *J Clin Oncol* 3:1257–1260, 1985

232. Ensminger WD, Rosowsky A, Raso V, et al: A clinical-pharmacological evaluation of hepatic arterial infusions of 5-fluoro-2′deoxyuridine and 5-fluorouracil. *Cancer Res* 38:3784–3792, 1978

233. Kemeny N, Daly J, Oderman P, et al: Hepatic artery pump infusion: Toxicity and results in patients with metastatic colorectal carcinoma. *J Clin Oncol* 2:595–600, 1984

234. Martin JK Jr, O'Connell MJ, Wieand HS, et al: Intra-arterial floxuridine vs. systemic fluorouracil for hepatic metastases from colorectal cancer. *Arch Surg* 125:1022–1027, 1990

235. Kemeny MM, Goldberg DA, Browning S, et al: Experience with continuous regional chemotherapy and hepatic resection as treatment of hepatic metastases. *Cancer* 55:1265–1270, 1985

236. Kemeny MM, Hogan JM, Goldberg DA, et al: Continuous hepatic artery infusion with an implantable pump: problems with hepatic artery anomalies. *Surgery* 99:501–504, 1986

237. Kemeny MM, Baltifora H, Douglas W, et al: Sclerosing cholangitis after continuous hepatic artery infusion of FUDR. *Ann Surg* 202:176–181, 1985

238. Kemeny N, Seiter K, Conti JA, et al: Hepatic arterial floxuridine and leucovorin for unresectable liver metastases from colorectal carcinoma. *Cancer* 73:1132–1142, 1994

239. Hohn D, Melnick J, Stagg R, et al: Biliary sclerosis in patients receiving hepatic arterial infusions of floxuridine. *J Clin Oncol* 3:98–102, 1985

240. Curley SA, Roh MS, Chase JL, et al: Adjuvant hepatic arterial infusion chemotherapy after curative resection of colorectal liver metastases. *Am J Surg* 166:743–748, 1993

241. Patt YZ: Regional hepatic arterial chemotherapy for colorectal cancer metastatic to the liver: the controversy continues. *J Clin Oncol* 11:815–819, 1993

242. Kemeny N, Huang Y, Cophen AM, et al. Hepatic arterial infusion of chemotherapy after resection of hepatic metastases from colorectal cancer. *N Eng J Med* 341:2039–2948, 1999

243. O'Connell MJ, Nagorney DM, Bernata AM, et al: Sequen-

tial intrahepatic fluorodeoxyuridine and systemic fluoro-uracil plus leucovorin for the treatment of metastatic colorectal cancer confined to the liver. *J Clin Oncol* 16: 2528–2533, 1998

244. Kemeny N, Conti JA, Sigurdson E, et al: A pilot study of hepatic artery floxuridine and combined with systemic 5-fluorouracil and leucovorin: a potential adjuvant program after resection of colorectal metastases. *Cancer* 71: 1964–1971, 1993

245. Ogita S, Tokiwa K, Shimotake T, et al: Intraarterial chemotherapy with lipiodol got initially unresectable hepatoblastomas in children. *Reg Cancer Treat* 3:106–109, 1992

246. Elias D, Lasser P, Rougier P, et al: Frequency, technical aspects, results, and indications of major hepatectomy after prolonged intra-arterial hepatic chemotherapy for initially unresectable tumors. *J Am Coll Surg* 180:213–219, 1995

247. Preketes AP, Caplehorn JRM, King J, et al: Effect of hepatic artery chemotherapy on survival of patients with hepatic metastases from colorectal carcinoma treated with cryotherapy. *World J Surg* 19:768–771, 1995

248. Ciezki J, Macknis RM: The palliative role of radiotherapy in the management of the cancer patient. *Semin Oncol* 22: 82–90, 1995

249. Sitzmann JV: Conversion of unresectable to resectable liver cancer: an approach and follow-up study. *World J Surg* 19: 790–794, 1995

250. Dhir V, Swaroop VS, Mohandas KW, et al: Combination chemotherapy and radiation for palliation of hepatocellular carcinoma. *Am J Clin Oncol* 15:304–307, 1992

251. Sitzmann JV, Abrams R: Improved survival for hepatocellular cancer with combination surgery and multimodality treatment. *Ann Surg* 217:149–154, 1993

252. Cho K, Andrews J, Williams D, et al: Hepatic arterial chemotherapy: role of angiography. *Radiology* 173:783–791, 1989

253. Lynes AC: Percutaneous hepatic arterial chemotherapy and chemoembolization. *Cancer Nurs* 16:283–287, 1993

254. Konno T: Targeting cancer chemotherapeutic agents by use of lipiodol contrast medium. *Cancer* 66:1897–1903, 1990

255. Egawa H, Maki A, Mori K: Effects of intraarterial chemotherapy with a new lipophilic anticancer agent, estradiol-chlorambulic (KM 2210), dissolved in lipiodol on experimental liver tumor in rats. *J Surg Oncol* 44:109–114, 1990

256. Bismuth H, Morino M, Sherlock D, et al: Primary treatment of hepatocellular carcinoma by arterial chemoembolization. *Am J Surg* 163:387–394, 1992

257. Castells A, Ayusu C, Bru C, et al: Transarterial embolization for hepatocellular carcinoma: antibiotic prophylaxis and clinical meaning of postembolization fever. *J Hepatol* 22: 410–415, 1995

258. Rimola A: Infections in liver disease, in McIntyre N, Benhamou JP, Bircher, et al (eds): *Oxford Textbook of Clinical Hepatology* (vol 2). Oxford, Oxford Medical Publications, 1991, pp 1272–1284

259. Takayasu K, Wakao F, Moryama N, et al: Response of early-stage hepatocellular and borderline lesions to therapeutic arterial embolization. *AJR Am J Roentgenol* 160:301–306, 1993

260. Yamamoto K, Masuzawa M, Kato M, et al: Evaluation of combined therapy with chemoembolization and ethanol injection for advanced hepatocellular carcinoma. *Semin Oncol* 24:50–55, 1997 (suppl 6)

261. Bronowicki JP, Boudjema K, Chone L, et al: Comparison of resection, liver transplantation, and transcatheter oily chemoembolization in the treatment of hepatocellular carcinoma. *J Hepatol* 24:293–300, 1996

262. Charnsangavej C: Chemoembolization of liver tumors. *Semin Invest Radiol* 10:150–160, 1993

263. Rospond RM, Mills W: Hepatic artery chemoembolization therapy for hepatic tumors. *AORN J* 61:573–576, 1995

264. Gane-Carru N, Beaugrand M: Intra-arterial chemoembolization in patients with hepatocellular carcinoma. *Hepatogastroenterology* 45:1242–1247, 1998

265. Soulen MC: Chemoembolization of hepatic malignancies. *Oncology* 8:77–93, 1994

266. Oi H, Kishimoto H, Matsushita M, et al: Antitumor affect of transcatheter oily chemoembolization for hepatocellular carcinoma assessed by computed tomography: role of iodized oil. *Semin Oncol* 24:56–60, 1997 (suppl 6)

267. Civalleri D, Pellicci R, Decaro G, et al: Palliative chemoembolization of hepatocellular carcinoma with mitoxantrone, lipiodol, and gelfoam: a phase II study. *Anticancer Res* 16: 937–942, 1996

268. Hirashima N, Sakakibara K, Itazu I, et al: Zinostatin stimalamer—transcatheter arterial embolization for hepatocellular carcinoma: a comparison with lipiodol-transcatheter arterial embolization. *Semin Oncol* 24:91–96, 1997 (suppl 6)

269. Carr BI, Zlejko A, Bron K, et al: Phase II study of spherex (degradable starch microspheres) injected into the hepatic artery in conjunction with doxorubicin and cisplatin in the treatment of advanced-stage hepatocellular carcinoma: interim Analysis. *Semin Oncol* 24:97–99, 1997 (suppl 6)

270. Yoshioka H, Sato M, Sonomura T: Factors associated with survival exceeding 5 years after transcatheter arterial embolization for hepatocellular carcinoma. *Semin Oncol* 24: 29–37, 1997

271. Bartolozzi C, Lencioni R, Caramella D, et al: Treatment of large HCC: transcatheter arterial chemoembolization combined with percutaneous ethanol injection versus repeated transcatheter arterial chemoembolization. *Radiology* 197:812–818, 1995

272. Wu C, Ho Y, Ho W, et al: Preoperative transcatheter arterial embolization for resectable large hepatocellular carcinoma: a reappraisal. *Br J Surg* 82:122–126, 1995

273. Paye F, Jagot P, Vilgrain V, et al: Preoperative chemoembolization of hepatocellular carcinoma: a comparative study. *Arch Surg* 133:767–772, 1998

274. Lenhart T, Herfarth C: Chemoembolization for hepatocellular carcinoma: what, when and for whom? *Ann Surg* 224: 1–3, 1996

275. Elli M, Cristaldi M, Mezzabotta M: Transcatheter arterial chemoembolization in cytoreduction of inoperable hepatocarcinomas. *Hepatogastroenterology* 44:522–524, 1997

276. Vilanma R, Bruix J, Bru J, et al: Tumor size determines the efficacy of percutaneous ethanol injection for the treatment of small hepatocellular carcinoma. *Hepatology* 16: 353–357, 1992

277. Livraghi Y, Bolondi L, Lazzaroni S, et al: Percutaneous ethanol injection in the treatment of hepatocellular carcinoma in cirrhoisis. *Cancer* 69:925–929, 1992

278. Ravikumar TS: Interstitial therapy for liver tumors. *Surg Oncol Clin North Am* 5:365–371, 1996

279. Castells A, Bruix J, Bru C, et al: Treatment of small hepatocellular carcinoma in cirrhotic patients: a cohort study comparing surgical resection and percutaneous ethanol injection. *Hepatology* 18:1121–1126, 1993

280. Livraghi T, Giorgio A, Marin G, et al: Hepatocellular carcinoma and cirrhosis in 746 patients: long-term results of percutaneous ethanol injection. *Radiology* 197:101–108, 1995

281. Tateishi H, Oi H, Masuda N, et al: Appraisal of combination treatment of hepatocellular carcinoma: long-term follow-up and lipiodol-percutaneous ethanol injection therapy. *Semin Oncol* 24:81–90, 1997 (suppl 6)

282. Taavitsainen M, Vehmas T, Kauppila R: Fatal liver necrosis following percutaneous ethanol injection for hepatocellular carcinoma. *Abdom Imaging* 18:357–359, 1993

283. Livraghi T: Percutaneous ethanol injection in the treatment of hepatocellular carcinoma in cirrhosis. *Hepatogastroenterology* 45:1248–1253, 1998

284. Livraghi T, Bolondi L, Boscarini L, et al: No treatment, resection, and ethanol injection in hepatocellular carcinoma: a retrospective analysis of survival in 391 patients with cirrhosis. *J Hepatol* 22:522–526, 1995

285. Ohnishi K, Yoshioka H, Ito S, et al: Prospective randomized controlled trial comparing percutaneous acetic acid injection and percutaneous ethanol injection for small hepatocellular carcinoma. *Hepatology* 27:67–72, 1998

286. Ohnishi K, Ohyama N, Ito S, et al: Small hepatocellular carcinoma: treatment with US-guided intratumoral injection of acetic acid. *Radiology* 193:747–752, 1994

287. Harrison LE, Brennan MF, Newman E, et al: Hepatic resection for noncolorectal nonneurodendocrine metastases: a fifteen-year experience with 96 patients. *Surgery* 121:625–632, 1997

288. Schwartz S: Hepatic resection for noncoloretcal nonneuroendocrine metastases. *World J Surg* 19:72–75, 1995

289. Ihse I, Persson B, Tibblin SD: Neuroendocrine metastases of the liver. *World J Surg* 19:76–82, 1995

290. Johnson LB, Krebs T, Wong-You-Cheong J, et al: Cryosurgical debulking of unresectable liver metastases for palliation of carcinoid syndrome. *Surgery* 121:468–470, 1997

291. Que FG, Nagorney DM, Batts KP, et al: Hepatic resection for metastatic neuroendocrine carcinomas. *Am J Surg* 169:35–43, 1995

292. Chen H, Hardacre JM, Uzar A, et al : Isolated liver metastases from neuroendocrine tumors: does resection prolong survival? *J Am Coll Surg* 187:88–93, 1998

293. McCall JL, Booth MW, Morris DL: Hepatic cryotherapy for metastatic liver tumours. *Br J Hosp Med* 54:378–381, 1995

294. McEntee GP, Nagorney DM, Kvol LK, et al: Cytoreductive hepatic surgery for neuroendocrine tumors. *Surgery* 108:1091–1096, 1990

295. Bilchik AJ, Sarantou T, Foshag LJ, et al: Cryosurgical palliation of metastatic neuroendorine tumors resistant to conventional therapy. *Surgery* 122:1040–1048, 1997

296. Cozzi PJ, Englund R, Morris DL: Cryotherapy treatment of patients with hepatic metastases from neuroendorine tumors. *Cancer* 76:501–509, 1995

297. Lang H, Oldhafer KL, Weinmann A, et al: Liver transplantation for metastatic neuroendocrine tumors. *Ann Surg* 225:347–354, 1997

298. Le Treut P, Delpero JR, Dousset B, et al: Results of liver transplantation in the treatment of metastatic neuroendocrine tumors: a 81-case French multicentric report. *Ann Surg* 225:355–364, 1997

299. Rusniewski P, Rougier P, Roche A, et al: Hepatic arterial chemoembolization in patients with liver metastases of endocrine tumors. *Cancer* 71:2624–2630, 1993

300. Perry LJ, Stuart K, Stokes KR, et al: Hepatic arterial chemoembolization for metastatic neuroendocrine tumors. *Surgery* 166:1111–1117, 1994

301. Moertel CG, Lefkopoulo M, Lipsitz S, et al: Streptozocin, doxorubicin, streptozocin-fluorouracil, or chlorozotocin in the treatment of advanced islet-cell carcinoma. *N Engl J Med* 326:519–523, 1992

302. Nabel G, Chang A, Nabel E: Clinical protocol: immunotherapy of malignancy by in vitro gene transfer into tumors. *Hum Gene Ther* 3:399–401, 1992

303. Cau G, Kuriyama S, Du P, et al: Complete regression of established murine hepatocellular carcinoma by in vivo tumor necrosis factor alpha gene transfer. *Gastroenterology* 112:501–510, 1997

Lung Cancers

Rebecca J. Ingle, RN, MSN, CS, FNP

Biotherapy

Photodynamic Therapy

Symptom Management and Supportive Care

Cough

Hemoptysis

Dyspnea

Pain

Fatigue

Gastrointestinal Disturbances: Nausea and
Vomiting, Anorexia and Cachexia, and Elimination

Psychosocial Issues

Continuity of Care: Nursing Challenges

Conclusion

References

Introduction

Lung cancer is the most frequent cause of cancer death in men and women in North America. At the beginning of the twentieth century, lung cancer was a rare disease; over the next 40 years it reached epidemic proportions for men, and is now considered to be an epidemic among women.[1-4] Although many factors have been associated with this major national and worldwide health problem, cigarette smoking has been estimated to cause 80%–90% of all lung cancer deaths.[1,3,5]

Despite the use of multimodality treatments for lung cancer, overall cure rates remain a discouraging 14%.[6] There is reason for cautious optimism, however, with the clinical investigation of several new promising chemotherapeutic agents, new diagnostic techniques, and improving feasibility of primary and secondary prevention measures that must receive preferential emphasis if progress is to be made in the control of this deadly disease.

Epidemiology

In 1999, 171,600 new cases of lung cancer and 158,900 deaths from lung cancer were estimated to have occurred.[6] These alarming numbers are in stark contrast to the 956 cases reported in 1920.[7] Today, lung cancer kills more women than any other cancer in the United States (Figure 59-1), and U.S. women lead the world in age-adjusted death rates for lung cancer per 100,000 population.[6] Although the mortality rate for men with lung cancer began to decline in the mid-1980s, lung cancer continues to cause over 2.5 times more deaths in men than prostate cancer, the second leading cancer killer among men in the United States (Figure 59-2).[6] Peak exposure to tobacco among women occurred in the 1960s, more than a decade later than for men. Because lung cancer incidence and mortality rates are highest about 35 years after peak exposure, the mortality rates in women will not decline until after the year 2010, when incidence rates plateau.[1,8]

Although lung cancer death rates for American Indians are currently lower than for blacks or whites, tobacco use in American Indian men is more than 50% higher than for other racial or ethnic populations.[9] Mortality rates among black men are slightly higher than for white men, but are comparable among black and white women.[2] The highest incidence of lung cancer is in the elderly, peaking at 75 years of age, probably due to longer lifetime carcinogen exposure.[1]

Etiology

Cigarette Smoke

The causal relationship between lung cancer and cigarette smoking has been well established.[1,4,7,10] The risk of lung cancer development in heavy smokers is estimated to be 10–25 times the risk of nonsmokers.[1,7] Risk from smoking is determined by multiple factors: number of cigarettes smoked per day, duration of smoking, age at which smoking began, inhalation patterns, and tar content of cigarettes.[1,2,7,11-13] Several studies have shown that reducing tar exposure can reduce the risk of lung cancer.[12] However, others have documented that when smokers choose a lower-tar content cigarette they often compensate by inhaling more deeply, thereby negating the benefit of less tar.[14] Age at beginning to smoke appears to be related more to duration of smoking than to an increased susceptibility at a younger age.[2]

Chyou and colleagues[10] were able to compute attributable risk due to cigarette smoking in a large cohort of men. Attributable risk estimates how much risk might be reduced if cigarette smoking was discontinued or never initiated. Their findings showed an attributable risk of 85% among current smokers, and they estimated that if current smokers had quit smoking, 60% of their risk for lung cancer could have been eliminated.[10] Others concur that benefit from smoking cessation begins five years after quitting and increases steadily over time, although the risk for lung cancer among former smokers will remain higher than the risk for lifetime nonsmokers.[2,8,11,13]

Cigarette smoke is known to contain over 4000 chemical compounds that insult the bronchial epithelium when smoke is inhaled. Tar, the most carcinogenic compound, causes basal cell hyperplasia, then dysplasia with displacement of the normal, healthy ciliated and mucus-secreting cells. With repeated exposure to smoke a lung cell may undergo neoplastic transformation.[8]

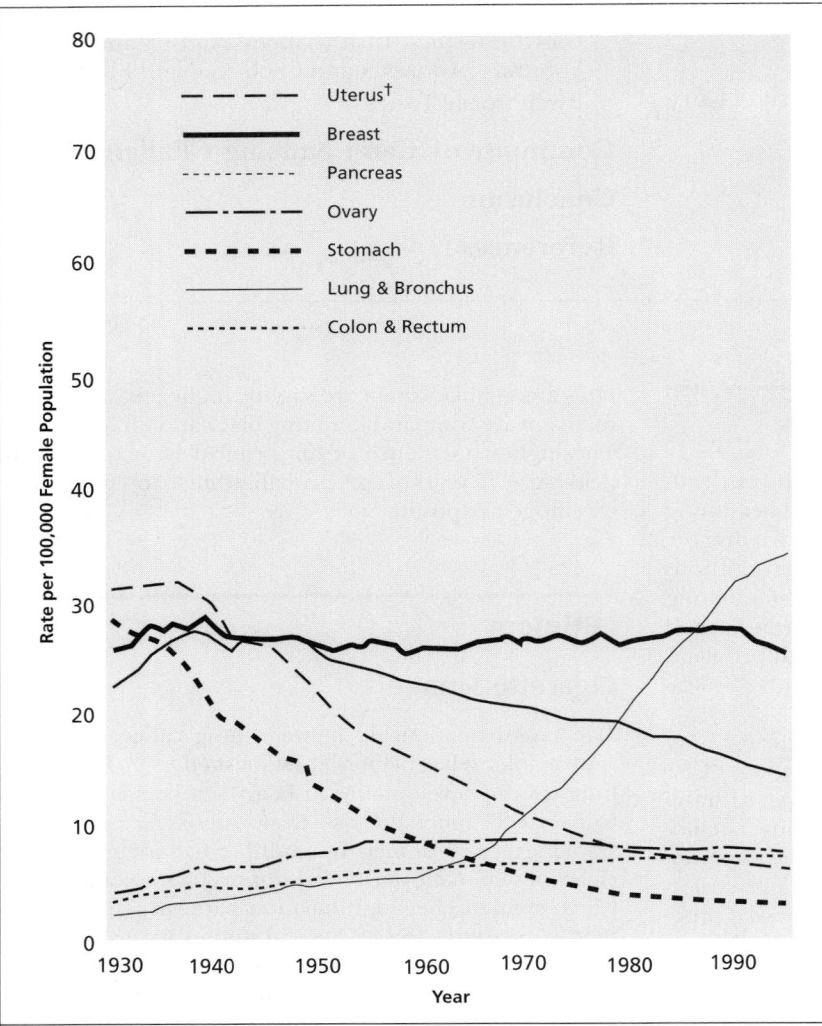

Figure 59-1 Age-adjusted cancer death rates* for females by site, United States, 1930–1995. (Reprinted from Landis SH, Murray T, Bolden S, et al: Cancer statistics, 1999. *CA Cancer J Clin* 49:8–31, 1999.)[6]

Note: Due to changes in the ICD coding, numerator information has changed over time. Rates for cancer of the uterus, ovary, lung & bronchus, and colon & rectum are affected by these coding changes.
*Rates are per 100,000 population and are age-adjusted to the 1970 US standard population.
†Uterine cancer death rates are for uterine cervix and uterine corpus combined.
Data source: Vital Statistics of the United States, 1998.

Tobacco smoke is a complete carcinogen, containing both initiator and promoter substances. Initiators can cause irreversible gene mutations. Repeated exposure to promoters may cause a cell to exhibit malignant behaviors, although cellular repair may occur if promoters are withdrawn. Eventually tumor progression ensues and the cellular damage is irreversible.

Passive Smoke

Considerable attention has been given in the past two decades to the effects of environmental tobacco smoke (ETS), also called *sidestream smoke, involuntary smoke,* or *passive cigarette smoke.*[12] Sidestream smoke contains nearly all of the carcinogens contained in mainstream smoke inhaled by smokers, but because it is not filtered, greater numbers of carcinogens are inhaled passively.[15] Even though ETS increases the risk for lung cancer less than active smoking, a causal relationship has been firmly established and the Environmental Protection Agency (EPA) considers ETS to be a human carcinogen.[16,17] In a study of exposure to passive smoke in the household, Janerich and colleagues found that the risk of lung cancer doubled for persons exposed to 25 or more years of passive smoke during childhood and adolescence. Exposure to ETS accounts for 17% of lung cancers among nonsmokers.[18] In contrast, the risk for lung cancer did not increase in adult nonsmokers exposed to ETS at home or in the workplace. Other epidemiological studies have shown statistically significant increased risks for persons living with smoking spouses.[15] These data

Figure 59-2   Age-adjusted cancer death rates* for males by site, United States, 1930–1995. (Reprinted from Landis SH, Murray T, Bolden S, et al: Cancer statistics, 1999. *CA Cancer J Clin* 49:8–31, 1999.)[6]

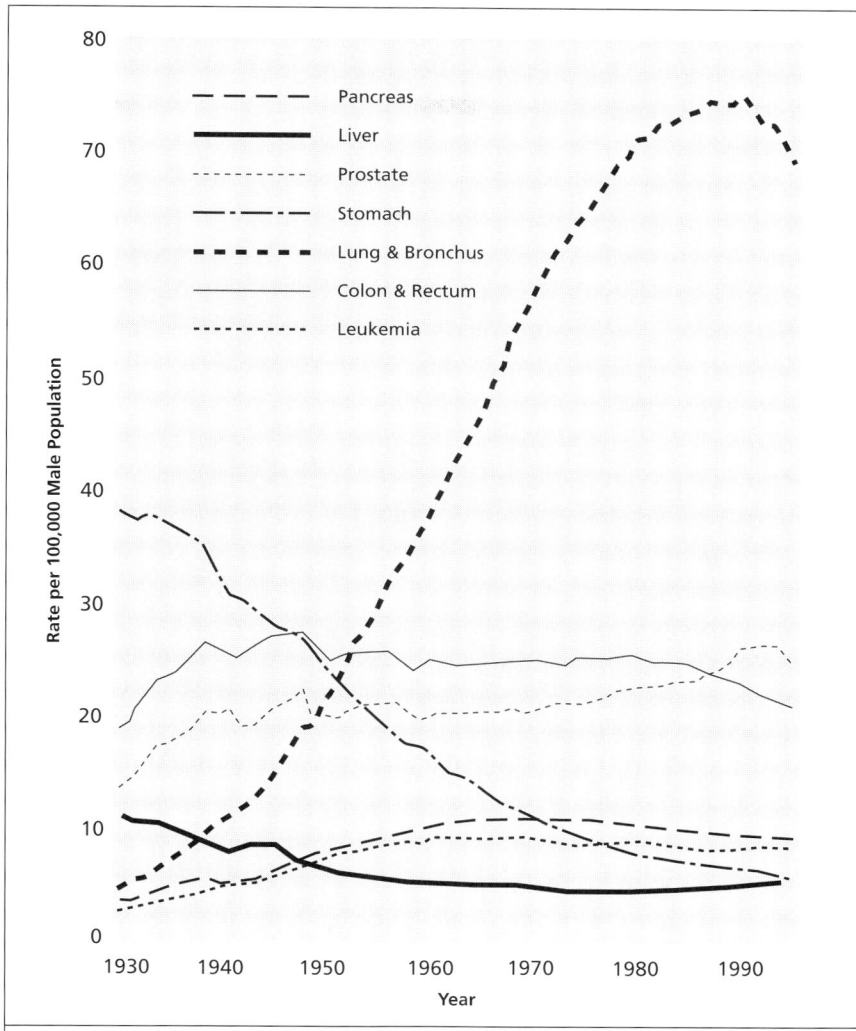

Note: Due to changes in the ICD coding, numerator information has changed over time. Rates for cancer of the liver, lung & bronchus, and colon & rectum are affected by these coding changes.
*Rates are per 100,000 population and are age-adjusted to the 1970 US standard population.
Data source: Vital Statistics of the United States, 1998.

suggest that 30% of all lung cancers are caused by exposure to ETS.[12]

Asbestos

Asbestos exposure is the most common occupational etiology of lung cancer,[1] causing 3%-4% of all cases.[19] *Asbestos*, a general term describing fibrous silicates with different properties, is divided into two types of fibers: chrysotile and amphibole. Although the sharp, needle-like amphibole asbestos bodies are more likely to cause disease due to deeper penetration into the lung,[12] both types have been implicated in lung cancer development.

In a study of 158 Japanese subjects exposed to asbestos, squamous cell carcinoma was seen most frequently and small-cell lung cancer was rare.[20]

Asbestos and smoking have a synergistic effect on lung cancer promotion. Compared with nonexposed nonsmokers, the incidence of lung cancer is increased five-fold in nonsmokers exposed to asbestos and a startling 80-fold to 90-fold in exposed smokers.[1]

Radon

Radon gas is an inert, natural product of uranium decay. Its effects were studied initially in underground uranium mine workers. During the radioactive decay process, radon products emit heavily ionizing alpha particles that, when inhaled, deliver intense radiation to the bronchial epithelium.[13,19] Radon particles act as both initiators and promoters, causing nonlethal events in cell nuclei. Synergy with cigarette smoke has been reported.[12]

Because radon is present in rock and soil and is known to seep into homes and office buildings through basements and crawl spaces, it has become an environmental concern. The amount of radon in a home is dependent upon ventilation and distance from the source. Although the residents of over 1 million U.S. homes have radon exposure similar to that of uranium miners, insufficient data exist at this time to predict their risk of developing lung cancer.[1,19] Nevertheless, the EPA estimates that over 14,000 lung cancer deaths per year are caused by radon, mostly in smokers.[2]

Occupational Agents

An increased incidence of lung cancer has been documented in individuals working with arsenic, copper, silica, lead, zinc, gold, chloromethyl ether, diesel exhaust, chromium, coal, hydrocarbons, nickel, ionizing radiation, cadmium, and beryllium.[2,11,13] Fur handlers and vineyard workers are also known to have increased risk.[13] Evidence linking these occupational agents to cigarette smoking is limited, and no conclusions can be drawn.

Indoor Air Pollution

In developing countries, exposure to carcinogenic cooking oil aerosols has been associated with lung cancer.[3,4] Indoor environments may be contaminated with other harmful pollutants including radon, cigarette smoke, building materials, household aerosol products, combustion devices, and the entry of outdoor air contaminants.[2] Data regarding risk are inconclusive.

Dietary Factors

Although the relationship of diet to lung cancer requires further investigation, early evidence suggested an inverse relationship between lung cancer risk and consumption of vitamin A or beta-carotene, vitamin C, vitamin E, and selenium.[2,3,19] It was proposed that these nutrients may prevent carcinogenesis by acting as scavengers of free oxygen radicals produced by tobacco smoke, solvents, and pollutants.[2,19] However, clinical trials of oral beta-carotene administered in populations at high risk for lung cancer were ceased in early 1996 due to the finding of increased lung cancer in the population receiving beta-carotene.[21] Hennekens and colleagues found neither harm nor benefit relative to incidence of malignancies

in a 12-year study of beta-carotene supplementation in healthy men.[22] Other nutrients such as watercress are also being investigated as inhibitors of a tobacco-specific carcinogen.[1]

Prevention, Screening, and Early Detection Programs

Primary Prevention

Primary prevention of lung cancer depends on identifying successful strategies for smoking prevention and cessation. If smoking were totally eliminated, 85% of lung cancers would disappear. Multiple economic, political, and social factors continue to impede progress toward this goal. Smoking dates back to the ancient Mayan civilization. Its medicinal qualities, addictive properties, and use through the years in ritual and ceremony have made acceptance of its harmful properties more difficult.

After automobiles, cigarettes are the second most heavily advertised product in the United States.[23] Women, children, and persons in developing countries have become primary targets of cigarette company marketing.[12] Cigarette smoking was considered to be socially unacceptable for women prior to the 1920s. As marketing strategies associated smoking with beauty, thinness, and independence, large numbers of women began to smoke. Today's death rate from lung cancer in women is 500% higher than that of 1935. Over 22 million women in the U.S. smoke, including 25% of those who are pregnant.[24]

Perhaps the most vulnerable groups targeted by cigarette advertisers are children and adolescents. Cartoon characters such as Old Joe Camel appeal to children, and have been found to be as familiar to small children as Mickey Mouse.[25] In 1998 the tobacco industry agreed to a ban on the use of cartoon characters in marketing and advertising, although familiar human characters such as the Marlboro Man may still be used. Of the 1 million Americans who become smokers each year, most are children or adolescents. Ninety percent of smokers begin smoking before age 20,[12,24] and most are girls.[3] Tobacco companies take advantage of adolescent vulnerability, spending over $4 billion a year in advertisement and promotional fees related to cigarettes and smoking.[12]

As antismoking efforts have gained acceptance in developed countries, tobacco companies have sought to develop new markets in underdeveloped countries. Tobacco is a prized export of the United States, and American cigarettes are a status symbol in some countries.[8] In these countries, little emphasis is placed on the harmful effects of smoking, and warning labels on cigarette packages may not be required.

In the United States, higher smoking rates are seen in individuals of a lower socioeconomic status, particularly women, although male blue-collar workers continue to be the heaviest smokers. Smoking is more common among blacks than whites. Though fewer cigarettes are smoked by black Americans, smoking cessation rates are also lower.[26] Education appears to be inversely related to smoking rates.[8,24]

Efforts to prevent smoking must focus on antismoking education, legislation, and taxation of cigarettes. Given the propensity for young people to smoke, education must begin early. Many nonprofit organizations, including the American Cancer Society, the American Lung Association, and the American Heart Association, promote smoking prevention programs through the distribution of a variety of educational materials about smoking. Nurses should incorporate education about smoking across the continuum of care, working within communities to promote healthy lifestyle behaviors. School-based programs to promote a tobacco-free environment should be encouraged. Educational efforts that target high-risk populations should emphasize the association between smoking and lung cancer. Repetition of the message may help individuals to internalize its meaning.

Antismoking legislation appeared in the 1960s following the 1964 surgeon general's report on the dangers of smoking. Laws were passed requiring health warnings on cigarettes, and cigarette advertisements in the broadcast media were banned. During the 1970s, 1980s, and 1990s, significant progress was made to limit and/or ban smoking in the workplace, on airplanes, in U.S. government buildings, and in other public places. In 1995 President Clinton approved a Food and Drug Administration regulatory plan to restrict seductive advertising directed at minors and to reduce easy access to cigarettes by banning vending machines except in areas of adult entertainment, banning free sample distribution, eliminating the sale of "singles" and "kiddie packs," and requiring proof of age to purchase cigarettes. The tobacco industry opposed the regulations and immediately filed lawsuits attempting to block the actions, accusing the president of government meddling in private choice decisions.[27]

Over the next few years legislation for a national comprehensive tobacco control plan was initiated but because of a strong tobacco lobby discussions were officially halted in June 1998. Later that year the tobacco industry agreed to a $206 billion deal to settle all pending state lawsuits. In addition to monies provided to each state over 25 years, the tobacco companies agreed to eliminate billboard and cartoon character advertising and to limit sponsorship of sporting events. They also agreed to fund antismoking campaigns and a research foundation for reduction of teen smoking. While each state lost the right to sue the tobacco industry, individual and class action lawsuits are still permitted. The agreement was predicted to raise the price of a pack of cigarettes by about 40 cents.

Almost all states have passed legislation prohibiting the sale of tobacco to minors, and campaigns are under way to impose a high excise tax on each pack of cigarettes sold.[12] Increasing the cost of cigarettes and enforcing age restrictions are thought to be the most effective strategies in reducing the number of minors who smoke.[28]

Secondary Prevention

Smoking cessation

While primary prevention is the most effective means of controlling lung cancer, the elimination of all tobacco products is not a realistic goal. Smoking cessation, as secondary prevention, can reduce the risk for lung cancer in a smoker, depending on how much and how long the person smoked. Up to 90% of smokers say they would like to quit, and as many as 60% have made serious attempts to stop smoking.[29–31] Those who are successful usually have a strong desire to quit, use behavioral techniques, and are supported in their efforts by family, friends, and/or health care providers.[30–32]

In 1996 the Agency for Health Care Policy and Research (AHCPR), an agency of the U.S. Department of Health and Human Services, published clinical practice guidelines for smoking cessation.[33] A multidisciplinary panel of tobacco addiction and smoking cessation experts compiled and reviewed data from over 3000 research articles and abstracts. Specific step-by-step strategies for primary care clinicians, including those discussed in the following sections, are provided in the guidelines.

Cromwell and colleagues[34] performed an analysis of the 15 recommended smoking cessation strategies in the AHCPR guidelines to determine their relative cost effectiveness. They found that smoking cessation strategies were extremely cost effective, particularly when more aggressive, costly interventions such as intensive counseling and the nicotine patch were used.[34]

Because it has been shown that smokers respond to direct, unequivocal messages from nurses and physicians to quit smoking, such messages should be given at every opportunity.[31,35,36] Failure to ask about smoking may give the false impression that smoking cessation is not a priority. Fiore has proposed that smoking status be the "new vital sign," measured each time vital signs are taken in the outpatient follow-up setting.[37] Two simple questions asked by the care provider—"Do you smoke now?" and "Have you ever smoked in the past?"—offer many opportunities to promote smoking cessation and to reinforce attention to the issue. Such brief intervention has been associated with 5% quit rates lasting more than one year.[29,30,35]

Smokers must believe that they are personally vulnerable before they are ready to quit. The nurse can point out that symptoms such as cough, bronchitis, or decreased energy are associated with smoking.[30] If cancer has already been diagnosed, benefits of cessation should be discussed. These include decreased rate of cancer recurrence, less risk of second primary tumors, improved tolerance of therapy, and lower risk of pulmonary infections.[29]

Smoking cessation behaviors have been described as occurring in stages,[38] each with opportunities for nursing intervention. The first stage is precontemplation, during which there is no plan to quit smoking. The smoker does not recognize the risks of smoking to self or others. During this stage, the nurse can assess the smoker's knowledge, beliefs, and attitudes about smoking and can raise risk awareness through education.

During the following stage of contemplation, the smoker expresses a desire to quit within the next six months and may ask for educational materials. Fears associated with quitting such as nicotine withdrawal, weight gain, and fear of failure may be verbalized. The nurse can express support and respect for the addiction while personalizing the benefits of quitting. It may be helpful to identify specific barriers to quitting and to suggest strategies for overcoming those barriers. Help the smoker set a quit date and reinforce the idea that smoking, as a learned behavior, can be unlearned.

Preparation is the third stage, during which the smoker plans to stop smoking within the next month. Behavioral therapy during this stage may help the smoker to identify reasons for smoking and for wanting to quit, to substitute alternative behaviors as a distraction from smoking behaviors, to learn to cope with urges and withdrawal symptoms, and to develop and implement a plan of action. Referral to a structured, behavioral smoking cessation program is appropriate in this stage, although as many as 95% of smokers prefer to quit without a structured program.[29,30] The smoker should consider nicotine or pharmacological replacement therapy, and pertinent educational materials should be provided. The nurse should arrange for follow-up by mail, telephone, or visits.

Action, the fourth phase, involves efforts to quit and prevent relapse. Relapse is common, and usually occurs during the first week after cessation when nicotine withdrawal symptoms are most pronounced. Smokers often quit several times before they achieve long-term success. The nurse provides nonjudgmental support, framing the relapse as a "rehearsal" for the next cessation attempt.

The last phase, maintenance, begins when the smoker has been smoke-free for six months or longer. The risk for relapse lessens, although stressful life events may trigger a relapse.[29] Follow-up with physician and nurse counseling in frequent face-to-face contacts contributes to maintenance of smoking cessation.[35] Lerman and colleagues propose the use of biological markers as a motivation for success.[38] Other investigators have demonstrated that measuring carbon monoxide (CO) levels and correlating them with physical symptoms such as nausea, headaches, and reduced exercise tolerance has tripled quit rates as compared with a standard nursing educational intervention.[39] Measurement of cotinine, a more sensitive indicator of tobacco exposure, is another potential motivational intervention for smoking cessation.[40] In addition, markers of abnormal cytological changes such as the CVP2D6 enzyme have been related to lung cancer susceptibility and show promise as a component of smoking cessation programs.[38]

Smoking cessation rates after behavioral interventions alone have been discouraging, as low as 13% at six months and lower than 5% at one year.[36,38] Success rates of 20% or more for a particular program are considered a good outcome.[30] Nicotine withdrawal symptoms often contribute to relapse. Symptoms, including irritability, restlessness, craving to smoke, impatience, hunger, wakefulness,

anxiety, lowered heart rate, headache, and altered bowel habits, peak several days after cessation and last up to four weeks.[8,12,30] Nicotine replacement using chewing gum or the transdermal patch has been shown to relieve withdrawal symptoms and has improved success rates to as high as 27.5% at one year when combined with smoking cessation counseling.[31,41]

The best candidates for nicotine replacement are smokers who are physically addicted to nicotine. The Fagerstrom Test for Nicotine Dependence, a brief, eight-item scale, can be used to measure degree of addiction.[42] When nicotine gum or patch replacement therapy is used, careful instructions are given regarding usage to avoid adverse effects. Nicotine replacement can be very expensive; cost information should be provided to the individual smoker.

New research findings reported by Fowler and colleagues give clues about the addictive properties of smoking.[43] They found that the brains of living smokers had significantly lower levels of the enzyme monoamine oxidase B (MAO B) than the brains of nonsmokers and former smokers. MAO B helps break down dopamine, a neurotransmitter involved in feelings of pleasure associated with many substances of abuse, including nicotine. Because nicotine stimulates the release of dopamine, it is thought that this action is synergistic with that of low levels of MAO B in boosting dopamine levels, thereby enhancing the addictive effects of the nicotine. The causative substance of lower levels of MAO B in smokers has not been identified, although it is known that it is not nicotine.[43] These findings have exciting implications for potential smoking cessation strategies.

Bupropion (Zyban), an antidepressant with dopaminergic properties, has been approved as the first nonnicotine replacement drug for the relief of withdrawal symptoms[44] and has demonstrated efficacy superior to placebo in increasing and sustaining smoking cessation rates.[45] Side effects are generally mild and include dry mouth, insomnia, and headache. It is contraindicated in persons with a seizure disorder or persons on any other medications that contain bupropion because the risk for seizures is dose dependent.

The dose of bupropion should begin at 150 mg per day for the first three days, then 150 mg twice daily. A smoking quit date should be set by the client within the first two weeks of treatment, and treatment should continue for 7–12 weeks.

Chemoprevention

Chemoprevention as a secondary prevention measure appears to show promise for current or former smokers. Chemoprevention, also called *chemoprophylaxis*, is treatment with agents that may prevent or reverse the promotion phase of carcinogenesis.[46–48] It is based on the concept of field cancerization, which holds that the entire area of epithelium exposed to carcinogens such as cigarette smoke is susceptible to cancer development, and that individuals who develop one malignancy are at high risk for developing a second primary tumor (SPT) later in the same epithelial field.[46] Survivors of small cell lung cancer may have a cumulative risk of 50% at ten years for SPT development.[46-49] The risk for SPTs in non-small cell lung cancer patients may exceed 10%, and in one study 26% of persons with laryngeal cancer developed a secondary lung cancer.[48,50] The leading cause of death in early-stage lung cancer is SPTs.[47]

Chemoprevention agents are being investigated as a means of preventing primary or secondary cancer development after carcinogen exposure. The most commonly studied groups of chemoprevention agents are the retinoids and carotenoids, which, as synthetic analogues of vitamin A, regulate normal and malignant cell growth and differentiation. In a landmark 1990 chemoprevention trial at MD Anderson, Hong and colleagues studied the effects of 13-cis retinoic acid (13-cRA) versus placebo in patients with head and neck cancers.[51] Although the agent had no effect on recurrence, patients receiving 13-cRA had significantly fewer SPTs. Low-dose 13-cRA has been well tolerated with significantly less toxicity compared with high-dose 13-cRA.[47]

Dietary intake of beta-carotene and vitamin A has been associated with a decreased risk of lung cancer. Studies have shown a stronger correlation of decreased risk of lung cancer with vegetable consumption as compared with equivalent carotenoid intake, suggesting that other dietary factors play a role in risk reduction.[46] However, a large-scale randomized trial of beta-carotene plus retinol versus placebo in smokers and asbestos-exposed smokers was stopped when it was discovered that the individuals receiving beta-carotene were experiencing a higher rate of lung cancer development.[21] This confirmed similar findings in an earlier Finnish study showing an increase in lung cancer in smokers who had been given beta-carotene prophylactically.[52] Another carotenoid, lycopene, has been found to inhibit proliferation of lung cancer cells in culture.[53]

The most common end point for chemoprevention trials has been the appearance of a malignancy, which often takes many years to develop. In order to more quickly evaluate promising new chemopreventive agents, investigators are searching for cell markers that might verify the effects of these agents before a malignancy actually develops. These markers could also be used to identify high-risk individuals, who might benefit from chemoprevention by the detection of early changes associated with carcinogenesis.[46,48,49,54] Markers under investigation include suppressor oncogenes such as *p53* and the retinoblastoma gene *RB*, dominant oncogenes such as *RAS* and *MYC*, and several growth factors.[49] Ideally a marker should have a causal relationship with the cancer rather than just an associated change.[55]

Screening and Early Detection

In the early 1970s the National Cancer Institute (NCI) Early Lung Cancer Group screened 30,000 male smokers with chest radiograph and sputum cytology. The results of these large trials showed that even though lung cancers identified by the screening methods were more frequently at an early stage, long-term survival rates did not improve.[28,32,54,56] European trials have confirmed that screening can detect lung cancer at an earlier stage but does not improve survival. Therefore, mass screening for lung cancer using currently available techniques is not recommended. However, scientific trials are under way to identify mutated genes in lung cancer cells that may represent early events in carcinogenesis and offer opportunities for interventions to cure or reverse the disease.[54,57] Tockman and colleagues developed a monoclonal antibody that successfully identified sputum abnormalities in 20 of 25 subjects who later developed lung cancer.[58] Ongoing trials are further evaluating these findings.

Two groups of oncogenes are involved in lung cancer development and are included in the early detection research. Dominant oncogenes, whose expression promotes neoplastic growth, include the *RAS* and *MYC* families. The *RAS* oncogenes appear to function early in the process of carcinogenesis and may be a good target for early detection. However, their screening usefulness will be limited since only about 15% of lung cancers exhibit a *RAS* mutation. Expression of the *MYC* oncogene is a late event and thus might not be effective as a target for early detection.[54]

The recessive oncogenes, or tumor-suppressor genes, inhibit cellular growth. When they are absent or reduced, neoplastic growth can occur. Mutations of the *RB* suppressor gene are present in over 90% of small-cell lung cancers. Difficulties in defining this gene have limited its usefulness as an early detection marker.[54]

Pathophysiology

Cellular Characteristics

During normal embryogenesis, a branched tracheobronchial tree forms by the tenth week. It is lined with a single layer of cells from which the respiratory mucosa develops. All lung cancers are thought to arise from a pluripotent stem cell originating from this primitive endodermal structure, eventually differentiating into multiple different histological subtypes.[19,56]

Normally the bronchial epithelium is composed of pseudostratified columnar cells, some of which are ciliated. Others are mucus-secreting goblet cells. Basal cells and neuroendocrine cells containing secretory granules complete the epithelial stratification, which has a protective function. Repeated carcinogenic irritation to the bronchial epithelium may cause increased rates of cellular replication. Healthy ciliated cells are replaced with a proliferation of basal cells, eventually resulting in hyperplasia, dysplasia, or carcinoma in situ.[59]

Bronchogenic cancers have been grouped into two

broad categories: small cell lung cancer (SCLC) and the non-small cell lung cancers (NSCLC), which include squamous cell carcinoma, adenocarcinoma, and large cell carcinoma. Each of these subtypes has distinct cellular characteristics upon which diagnosis and management are based. Because all types of lung cancer arise from a pluripotent stem cell, many tumors are heterogeneous, containing cells from more than one histological type, which makes accurate classification more difficult.[19,59] A discussion of cellular characteristics of each subtype follows.

Small cell lung cancer

SCLC was recognized as an epithelial tumor in 1926. Prior to that time it was believed to be a sarcoma.[60] SCLC invades the submucosa and is thought to arise from Kulchitsky cells, which are neuroendocrine cells that secrete peptide hormones. Most SCLC tumors are centrally located, developing around a main bronchus as a whitish-gray growth that invades surrounding structures, eventually compressing the bronchi externally.[1,11,13,60,61] Necrosis and areas of hemorrhage are frequently seen, although SCLC usually does not cavitate. Responsible for 25% of all lung cancers, SCLC is an aggressive tumor and often is metastatic at the time of diagnosis. Its doubling time, shorter than that of any other lung cancer type, is slightly less than two months.[1,13]

The World Health Organization has classified SCLC into three subtypes: (1) oat cell, which accounts for 90% of cases; (2) intermediate; and (3) combined (oat cell with adenocarcinoma or squamous cell carcinoma component).[60,61] This classification was intended to show a link between small cell and large cell carcinomas, although the clinical significance of the subtypes is controversial. In many instances, no difference in subtypes is seen relative to response to treatment or survival.[60] Other classifications have been proposed, each striving for diagnostic and clinical significance.[61]

Although morphologically the cells of each subtype differ from each other, all SCLC cells are several times larger than a mature lymphocyte, have scant cytoplasm, and show multiple atypical mitoses.[60,61] Many genetic abnormalities have been identified, including absence of two suppressor genes, the retinoblastoma *(RB)* gene and the *p53* gene. There is evidence that suppression of the *RB* gene may play a role in the initiation or progression of SCLC. Mutations of the *p53* gene appear to occur in response to cigarette smoke and radon exposure.[62]

Amplification of the *MYC* family of proto (dominant) oncogenes, including *MYC*, *N-MYC*, and *L-MYC*, has also been observed in SCLC.[11,13,60,62] Amplification is the process in which the DNA is duplicated many times, thereby activating the proto-oncogene and releasing it from normal growth-controlling mechanisms.[62] While *MYC* amplification is not thought to be a primary contributor to the pathogenesis of lung cancer, *C-MYC* amplification has been correlated with a shorter duration of survival in SCLC patients. Amplification of *MYC*, which occurs in up to 24% of SCLC tumors, occurs less frequently in NSCLC cells.[60,62]

It has long been recognized that about 70% of SCLCs produce neuroendocrine markers, including neuron-specific enolase, L-dopa decarboxylase, chromogranin A, synaptophysin, and bombesin.[11,13,62] While these markers are not specific to SCLC, they help explain many of the paraneoplastic syndromes that occur in SCLC patients. Early identification of neuroendocrine markers may aid in the diagnosis and management of SCLC, and may have prognostic significance.[11]

Lung cancer cells can produce autocrine growth factors, which are peptide hormones that stimulate their own growth by binding to their own receptors. The most common autocrine growth factor is gastrin-releasing peptide (GRP). Studies have shown that the growth factor receptor sites can be blocked by a monoclonal antibody developed in the laboratory against bombesin, a GRP analog from frog skin.[60,63] Figure 59-3 illustrates autocrine growth in lung cancer cells and the mechanism of mono-

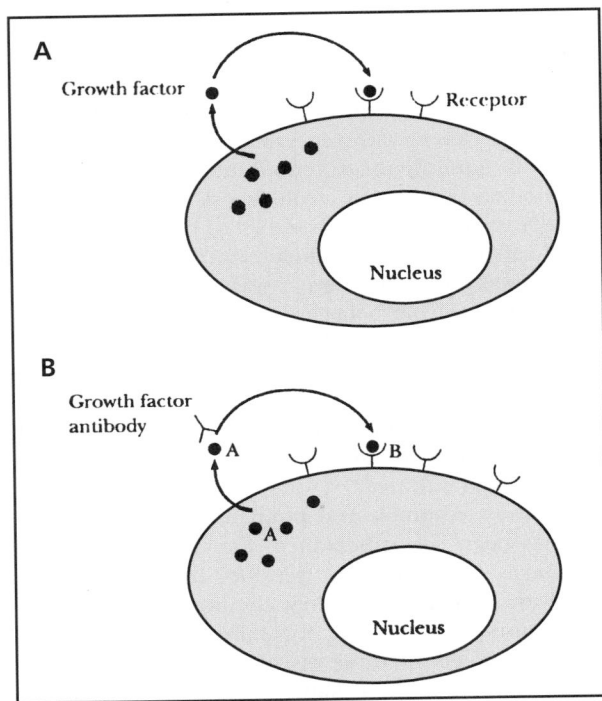

Figure 59-3 (A) Autocrine growth in lung cancer. The cell produces peptide hormones or growth factors (represented as dark circles) that are secreted from the cell, bind to receptors on its surface, and stimulate their own growth. (B) Blocking autocrine growth with antibodies in lung cancer. The figure diagrammatically shows the mechanism that has been successfully used to interrupt the autocrine growth loop. The monoclonal antibody directed against growth factors (A) prevents the growth factor from binding to its receptor (B) and thereby blocks the autocrine growth of the cell. (Reprinted from *Lung Cancer,* Vol. 12, Johnson BE, Kelley MJ, Biology of small cell lung cancer, S5–S16, 1995 (suppl), with kind permission from Elsevier Science Ltd., P.O. Box 800, Oxford OX51DX , UK.)[63]

clonal antibody blockage, which inhibits growth of the SCLC cells.[63]

Non-small cell lung cancer

Squamous cell carcinoma. Squamous cell carcinomas constitute 30% of all lung cancers and are more common in males than in females.[64] These tumors arise from the basal cells of the bronchial epithelium and usually present as masses in large bronchi. Growth into adjacent structures, cavitation, and extension centrally are common, causing atelectasis and pneumonitis.[13] When detected early, squamous cell cancers are often resectable.

Squamous tumors may be well differentiated or poorly differentiated. Well-differentiated tumors may show pearly formation, while poorly differentiated tumors are characterized by keratinization. Other cellular characteristics of squamous cell carcinomas include intercellular bridges and inflammation.[1] Because cells of these tumors are easily shed, sputum cytologies may be positive at an early stage, long before a lesion can be detected on a chest radiograph.[19]

Squamous cell carcinoma has a doubling time of 90–100 days.[1] Because it is a relatively slow-growing tumor, several years may elapse between the development of a carcinoma in situ and clinical detection. In about 8% of cases, mutations in the *RAS* family of oncogenes are seen.[62] Squamous cell cancers have been associated with ectopic production of a parathyroid hormone-type substance, causing hypercalcemia.

Adenocarcinoma. Adenocarcinoma is the most common lung cancer in males, in females, and in nonsmokers, accounting for 40% of all tumors.[1,19] Its increasing incidence in recent years has been attributed to more accurate histological distinction between adenocarcinoma and undifferentiated large cell carcinoma. Adenocarcinoma arises from the bronchial epithelium and may form in lung scars or fibrous tissue. Adenocarcinoma usually presents as a single peripheral nodule, although rapidly progressive multifocal disease may be present at diagnosis. This malignancy may be quite silent initially, producing few symptoms,[13] and is often detected radiographically before sputum cytologies are positive.[1]

Most adenocarcinomas form glands and produce mucin. They tend to metastasize early through hematogenous spread, and nearly half of the tumors are considered to be unresectable at the time of diagnosis.[1] Areas of metastasis commonly include the brain, liver, bone, and adrenal glands. Adenocarcinomas have the longest doubling time of all lung cancers, approximately six months.[1]

Mutations of the *K-RAS* oncogene are seen in approximately one-third of adenocarcinoma cases and represent about 90% of all mutations seen in these tumors.[56,62] In several studies, identification of the *K-RAS* oncogene in all non-small-cell lung cancers has been associated with shortened survival and therefore may prove to be an important prognostic marker for adenocarcinoma.[56,62]

The World Health Organization (WHO) has classified adenocarcinomas of the lung by four histological subtypes: (1) acinar, (2) papillary, (3) solid carcinoma with mucus formation, and (4) bronchoalveolar, although there is controversy regarding whether the latter should be considered a separate entity. Bronchoalveolar tumors show little glandular change, usually present as solitary or multiple peripheral lesions, and are slow-growing tumors.[1,19]

Large cell carcinoma. Large cell carcinoma is the least common type of lung cancer, representing approximately 10%–15% of cases.[19] Although large-cell carcinoma is larger than adenocarcinoma, other features common to the two types have sometimes precluded accurate diagnosis. Often diagnosis is made by eliminating other cell types.

Large cell tumors usually arise as peripheral nodules and metastasize early, often to the gastrointestinal (GI) tract. The average doubling time is about three months. The tumor cells have abundant cytoplasm and enlarged nuclei.[1] Ras mutations are found in about 23% of large cell cancer cases.[62]

Large cell carcinomas are classified by the WHO into two types: (1) clear cell and (2) giant cell. The rare giant cell tumors have the poorest prognosis. In general, large cell tumors have the same prognosis as adenocarcinomas of the lung.[19]

Progression of Disease

Repeated carcinogenic exposure results in epithelial cell transformations that progress from a benign to a malignant phenotype. Manifested initially as atypical metaplasia, then carcinoma in situ, and finally invasive carcinoma of the lung, invasion of deeper tissues follows until the malignancy is clinically detectable. A lung tumor has undergone about 30 doublings, or three-quarters of its natural history, by the time it is large enough to be detected on chest radiograph or sputum cytologies.[1] Many tumors metastasize in the preclinical phase, as evidenced by the dismal 14% overall cure rates for lung cancer.[6]

Patterns of Spread

Lung cancers spread by direct extension, lymphatic invasion, and hematogenous routes. In SCLC, metastasis to distant sites has already occurred in up to 63% of cases at the time of diagnosis.[60] The most common metastatic sites for SCLC are the bone, liver, central nervous system, lymph nodes, pleurae, and subcutaneous tissue, although metastases to nearly every organ system have been found.[11]

Non-small cell lung cancers are more likely to spread initially by direct extension or lymphatic invasion. Tumors may grow into and around the bronchial lumen, extending in plaque-like fashion or completely occluding the lumen. Other pulmonary structures may be compressed, including vasculature, lymphatic channels, nerves, and alveolar tissue. Extension to the pleurae, chest wall, and diaphragm may occur. Rich mediastinal lymphatic drainage offers routes for tumor invasion into the bronchopulmonary, mediastinal, and supraclavicular lymph nodes. Once vascular invasion occurs, metastasis is seen most frequently to bone, liver, adrenal glands, pericardium, and the brain.[19]

Clinical Manifestations

Clinical manifestations of lung cancer are dependent upon the location of the tumor and the extent of spread. Only 6% of patients are asymptomatic at the time of diagnosis.[13] Symptoms may be divided into three categories: local-regional symptoms, symptoms due to extrathoracic involvement, and systemic symptoms with or without paraneoplastic syndromes (see Chapter 35). A summary of symptoms associated with lung cancer is presented in Table 59-1.

Local-Regional Symptoms

Lung tumors may be present for as long as five years before symptoms are experienced. The most common symptoms of local-regional disease include cough, dyspnea, hemoptysis, wheezing, chest pain, and postobstructive pneumonia. Cough occurs in 75% of patients and often is attributed to a cold, especially if fever is present. It is not uncommon for a patient to be treated empirically with several courses of antibiotics before further diagnostic investigation is done. Hemoptysis is seen in 50%–70% of patients and should always raise the suspicion of a malignancy.[13,56]

Although peripheral tumors cause chest pain in as many as 50% of patients, central tumors are more likely to cause symptoms associated with airway obstruction, such as wheezing, stridor, dyspnea, atelectasis, and pneumonia.[65] As the tumor grows, intrathoracic involvement of adjacent structures produces other symptoms, particularly those related to nerve involvement. Involvement of the left recurrent laryngeal nerve may produce hoarseness, a poor prognostic sign, and phrenic nerve involvement may cause hiccups.[66] Apical tumors may involve the cervical and first thoracic nerves, producing shoulder and arm pain; first and second rib destruction; and Horner's syndrome, characterized by ptosis, pupil contraction, miosis, enophthalmos, and ipsilateral decreased sweating.[65] Pleural effusions are seen commonly with pleural involvement.[19] Bloody pleural fluid is likely due to metastasis and is a poor prognostic sign.[65] Pericardial effusions due to pericardial invasion may also be seen. As a lung tumor with mediastinal involvement grows, it may eventually compress the superior vena cava, causing superior vena cava syndrome (see Chapter 42).

Symptoms Due to Extrathoracic Involvement

Signs and symptoms of extrathoracic metastases depend upon the site of involvement. Bone pain due to metastases occurs in approximately 37% of patients. Pathological fractures are rare.[60] Central nervous system metastases produce symptoms 90% of the time, including headache, seizures, confusion, gait disturbances, and personality changes.[60,66] Liver involvement may manifest in jaundice, hepatomegaly, abdominal pain, and GI disturbances. Although adrenal metastases are fairly common, signs of adrenal insufficiency are rarely seen.

Systemic Symptoms with or without Paraneoplastic Syndromes

Systemic symptoms of lung cancer include generalized weakness and fatigue, anorexia, cachexia, weight loss, and anemia. The mechanisms for these symptoms are poorly understood. They occur with equal frequency among the various types of lung cancer.

Lung cancer has been associated with many paraneoplastic syndromes (Table 59-2), with manifestations unrelated to the spread of cancer. Some syndromes are related to ectopic hormone production; others involve

Table 59-1 Clinical Manifestations Associated with Lung Cancer

Local-regional manifestations	Cough
	Dyspnea
	Hemoptysis
	Wheezing
	Chest pain
	Stridor
	Hoarseness
	Hiccups
	Atelectasis
	Pneumonia
	Pancoast syndrome
	Horner's syndrome
	Pleural effusion
	Pericardial effusions
	Superior vena cava syndrome
Manifestations of extrathoracic involvement	Bone pain
	Headache
	Central nervous system disturbances
	Gastrointestinal disturbances
	Jaundice
	Hepatomegaly
	Abdominal pain
Systemic symptoms	Weakness
	Fatigue
	Anorexia
	Cachexia
	Weight loss
	Anemia
	Symptoms associated with paraneoplastic syndromes

Table 59-2 Paraneoplastic Syndromes Associated with Lung Cancer

Type of Cancer	Associated Paraneoplastic Syndrome
Small cell lung cancer	Ectopic ACTH (Cushing syndrome)
	Syndrome of inappropriate antidiuretic hormone (SIADH) secretion
	Lambert-Eaton myasthenic syndrome (LEMS)
Non-small cell lung cancer	Humoral hypercalcemia of malignancy
	Hypertrophic pulmonary osteoarthropathy
	Nephrotic syndrome
All lung cancers	Hypercoagulable state
	Erythrocytosis, granulocytosis
	Neurological syndromes
	Dermatologic syndromes (acanthosis nigricans)

autoimmune mechanisms. Some syndromes are specific to a particular type of lung cancer, while other syndromes may be associated with all lung cancers.

Small cell lung cancer is associated with paraneoplastic syndromes more frequently than the non-small cell tumors. Cushing's syndrome, resulting from ectopic secretion of adrenocorticotropic hormone (ACTH), is seen in 5% of SCLC patients and manifests in edema, proximal myopathy, elevated cortisol levels, hypokalemia, and hyperglycemia.[11] The syndrome of secretion of inappropriate antidiuretic hormone (SIADH) results from ADH secretion by the tumor. The incidence of SIADH in SCLC is 5%–10%. Symptoms include hyponatremia and low serum osmolality, characterized by mental status changes, lethargy, seizures, and confusion.

Although the Lambert-Eaton myasthenic syndrome (LEMS) was documented by Lambert in 6% of patients with SCLC,[67] others report a lower incidence.[68,69] LEMS is thought to be an autoimmune disorder in which the release of acetylcholine by the motor nerve terminals is impaired. Symptoms include proximal muscle weakness, especially in the pelvis, thighs, arms, and shoulders; dry mouth; and double vision.[70,71] LEMS may be the presenting symptom of SCLC.

Humoral hypercalcemia of malignancy, the most frequent paraneoplastic syndrome in NSCLC, commonly is associated with squamous cell carcinomas. It is caused by ectopic production of a parathyroid hormone-like substance.[66] Hypertrophic pulmonary osteoarthropathy, a paraneoplastic condition associated with periostitis of the long bones and clubbing of the fingers and toes, can cause pain, tenderness, and swelling in the joints.[65]

Assessment

Patient and Family History

An accurate health history is an important means of gathering information needed to establish a diagnosis. This part of the health assessment will help guide decisions regarding diagnostic testing and can give early clues to the diagnosis.

The patient is asked first to describe the problem(s) prompting the health care visit. Questions eliciting a full description of each complaint or symptom should be asked, helping the person to describe the onset, duration, location, character, severity, frequency, and measures that aggravate or alleviate each symptom. The nurse should ascertain how the symptoms have had an impact on the quality of the patient's life.

An assessment of past history and family history should also be included, related particularly to smoking, prior respiratory problems, lung cancer history, and exposure to other carcinogens known to increase the risk of lung cancer. Smoking history for all family members should include age of starting to smoke, number of years as a smoker, average amount smoked per day, and type of tobacco smoked. Although a genetic link to lung cancer is not firmly established, a family history of lung cancer may increase a person's risk for developing the disease.

After a determination of coping abilities, strengths, and available supportive resources is gleaned from a thorough psychosocial history, a review of systems completes this part of the health assessment.

Physical Exam

The physical exam, the second component of the assessment process, focuses on a thorough examination of the pulmonary and lymphatic systems. The systematic assessment should include inspection, palpation, percussion, and auscultation. A detailed discussion of the physical examination is provided in Chapter 9.

Inspection can provide information about the pattern of respirations, symmetry and integrity of the thorax, and thoracic configuration. Dyspnea, although a subjective observation, is a general indication of inadequate respiration. Pleuritic chest pain may be manifested by rapid, shallow breathing. Intercostal retractions on inspiration indicate obstruction to air inflow, while bulging interspaces on expiration are associated with outflow obstruction; either may be an indication of tumor.[72] Stridor is a manifestation of extrathoracic airway obstruction. The use of accessory muscles for breathing, labored, prolonged expiration, and wheezing may indicate obstruction of intrathoracic airways.

Clubbing of the fingers; skin changes consistent with weight loss; visible signs of Horner, Pancoast, and SVC syndromes; and joint swelling consistent with hypertrophic pulmonary osteoarthropathy are also noted.

Palpation is used to assess areas of tenderness, thoracic expansion, tactile fremitus, position of the trachea, and abnormal areas identified by inspection. Asymmetrical thoracic excursion may be indicative of pulmonary pathology. Decreased tactile fremitus may be associated with pleural effusion and tumors of the pleural cavity, while increased tactile fremitus may indicate a lung mass.[73] Tracheal deviation from midline may be a result of tumor growth, lymphadenopathy, or pleural effusion.[65,72]

Percussion is used in the thoracic exam to determine the presence or distribution of air, fluid, or areas of consolidation in the lungs, and to delineate the boundaries of other organs. In a normal lung, percussion produces resonant sounds that are loud, low in pitch, and long in duration. Short dull sounds heard on percussion indicate the presence of consolidation, masses, and pleural effusions.[73]

Auscultation of the lungs with a stethoscope gives the examiner information about the flow of air throughout the tracheobronchial tree. The lungs are systematically assessed by auscultating the apices and the posterior, lateral, and anterior chest. Absent or decreased breath sounds can be heard when normal lung tissue is replaced by tumor, or when the patient has a pleural effusion. Wheezing and rhonchi may be heard in the presence of bronchial obstruction. A pleural friction rub may be indicative of an inflammatory response to invading tumor. Any abnormal or adventitious breath sounds are described relative to pitch, intensity, quality, and duration of inspiratory and expiratory phases.

Diagnostic Studies

When a lung malignancy is suspected, diagnostic studies are crucial in making an accurate determination of tumor type, location, and extent of disease. Selection of appropriate tests will provide the necessary information for making treatment decisions. The nurse should become familiar with each test so that education and guidance can be provided to the patient and family.

Imaging studies

Chest radiograph. The chest radiograph is probably the most helpful diagnostic study for lung cancer. Peripheral nodules usually can be detected when 1 cm or larger in size.[1,65] Central lesions may manifest as a variety of radiographic changes, such as atelectasis or hilar changes.[1] Mediastinal changes on radiograph may suggest lymphadenopathy or pleural effusions, and an elevated diaphragm may be seen with phrenic nerve involvement.[56,65]

Digital radiography is increasingly being used for thoracic imaging. A reusable phosphor plate can be read digitally by computer, and the data can be transmitted electronically to viewing stations.[74]

Computed tomography, positron emission tomography, and magnetic resonance imaging. Computerized tomography (CT), introduced in the late 1970s, has greatly improved the precision of lung cancer staging.[56] Lesions not seen on chest radiograph can be detected on CT and previously identified lesions can be more clearly defined. The chest CT can be particularly helpful in evaluating mediastinal lymph nodes that, if enlarged, should be evaluated further in the staging process before treatment decisions are made.[19,56] Upper abdominal scanning is done along with the chest CT scan to evaluate the liver and adrenals for signs of metastasis.

Scanning with positron emission tomography (PET), a more costly newer imaging technique using radionuclides, has not been widely accepted but is promising. Initial studies in lung cancer showed greater sensitivity and specificity for hilar and mediastinal nodes than CT scanning.[74]

Magnetic resonance imaging (MRI) of the chest does not offer an advantage over CT scanning and is not used routinely as part of the diagnostic workup. However, MRI may be superior in evaluating the perihilar and paravertebral regions and may be employed when CT scan results are not definitive.[1,19,56]

Tissue diagnostic studies

Sputum cytology. When lung cancer is suspected, the sputum cytology test can be a simple, cost-effective means of obtaining a pathological diagnosis. Early-morning sputum samples are collected for three to five days; deep coughing is recommended since coughing dislodges cancer cells into the sputum. The diagnostic yield for sputum cytologies is up to 80% for central tumors but drops to below 20% for small peripheral tumors.[56] Squamous cell carcinomas are the most frequent type diagnosed by sputum cytology; adenocarcinomas are least often diagnosed by this test. Although the false-positive rate is extremely low at less than 1%, the false-negative rate can be as high as 43%. Therefore, a negative sputum cytology does not rule out malignancy.[1]

Bronchoscopy. Fiberoptic bronchoscopy is a procedure in which a flexible bronchoscope is passed through the trachea into the bronchi to collect samples for cytological or histological examination. When central lesions can be visualized, the diagnosis can be made more than 90% of the time from biopsies, brushings, and washings.[19] Even peripheral lesions and suspicious areas where no lesion is seen can be evaluated through the use of needles, cytology brushes, or biopsy forceps introduced via a bronchoscope. Sputum cytology yields are often higher after bronchoscopy.

Recent advances have included the measurement of tumor markers in the bronchoalveolar fluid obtained by bronchoscopy[1] and use of the bronchoscope to sample mediastinal lymph nodes.[28] Complications from bronchoscopy, including hypoxemia, arrhythmias, and mild hemorrhage, are rare.[75]

Fine-needle aspiration. Percutaneous fine-needle aspiration is used when lung lesions cannot be visualized by bronchoscopy but are accessible percutaneously. A needle guided by CT or fluoroscopy is inserted into the lesion for aspiration of cells. A positive diagnosis can be made up to 95% of the time.[76] Pneumothorax is the most common complication, with an increased risk in persons with chronic obstructive pulmonary disease.[1]

Mediastinoscopy. Mediastinoscopy is an invasive procedure used primarily for staging, although it can also be used diagnostically. Mediastinoscopy allows for direct visualization and palpation of mediastinal lymph nodes. A small incision is made in the suprasternal fossa through which the surgeon inserts a finger to evaluate the size and consistency of the lymph nodes; a mediastinoscope is then passed to view and biopsy the nodes.[72]

Mediastinoscopy is indicated in patients who have enlarged mediastinal lymph nodes on CT scan because up to 45% of the time those nodes will be benign.[77] Accurate nodal assessment is vital in determining which patients are candidates for surgery or multimodality protocols. Even when the CT scan is negative for enlarged lymph nodes, mediastinoscopy may be performed if risk factors for occult mediastinal involvement are present.

Video-assisted thoracoscopic surgery. Video-assisted thoracoscopic surgery (VATS) has been used in recent years for the staging and diagnosis of lung cancer. Small thoracotomy incisions are made through which thoracoscopic instruments are inserted (Figure 59-4).[76] Visualiza-

tion of the chest and mediastinum and assessment of pleural effusions are superior to that achieved using older scopes, which may help improve diagnostic accuracy. Although VATS will probably not replace mediastinoscopy, it may prove to be highly effective in evaluating suspicious peripheral nodules. In some centers VATS is being used successfully to perform resections such as lobectomies[76] and has been associated with significantly less pain than thoracotomy.[78]

Thoracotomy. On rare occasions thoracotomy is necessary to make a diagnosis of lung cancer. Adequate tissue samples are almost always obtained by thoracotomy, although morbidity and mortality are higher than with mediastinoscopy.[65]

Prognostic Indicators

Small cell lung cancer

The most favorable prognostic factor in SCLC is limited-stage disease. In addition, there appears to be some benefit in extensive-stage disease when metastases are limited to a single organ and when there is no liver or brain involvement.[60] Ambulatory performance status, female gender, and a normal serum lactic dehydrogenase (LDH) are also favorable prognostic factors for SCLC.[1] In some studies, weight loss and impaired immunocompetence as measured by delayed hypersensitivity skin testing have been unfavorable prognostic factors.[60] Cushing's syndrome has been associated with a poorer clinical outcome. Data regarding the effects of SIADH and other paraneoplastic syndromes are inconclusive.[79]

Studies have shown that the tumor marker neuron-specific enolase (NSE) is a promising prognostic indicator. Other markers under investigation include thymidine kinase and tissue polypeptide antigen (TPA).[79] Although amplification of the *MYC* oncogene has been associated with more aggressive tumor growth, the clinical significance of this finding is yet to be defined.[56]

SCLC has the poorest survival rates of all lung cancer types. Untreated, survival averages 6–12 weeks.[80] With treatment for limited- and extensive-stage disease, two-year survivals of 12%–21% and 1%–4%, respectively, can be expected.[1]

Non-small cell lung cancer

Stage of disease is the most significant prognostic factor for NSCLC, with early-stage cancers responding better to treatment and demonstrating longer survival.[81] The presence of mediastinal lymph node metastases usually indicates a very poor prognosis, although patients with ipsilateral node involvement may be curable with multimodality treatment.[82] Factors associated with shortened survival include weight loss, poor performance status, male gender, elevated serum LDH, and bone or liver metastases. Although diploid tumors have been associ-

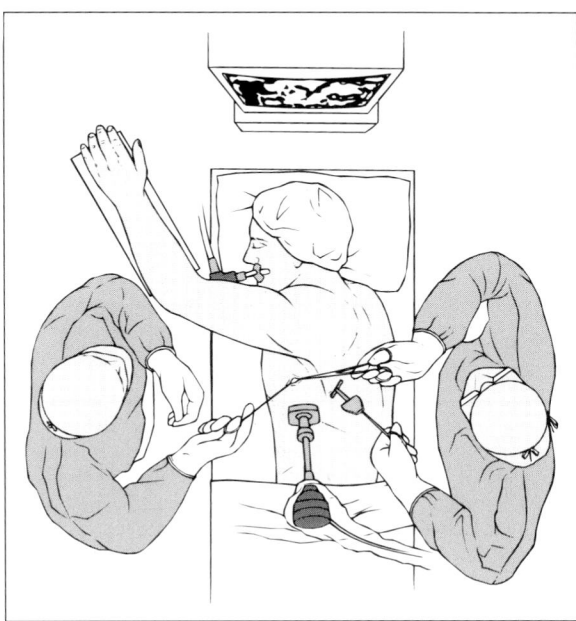

Figure 59-4 A video-assisted, left-sided thoracoscopic procedure. Two surgeons working with thoracoscopic instruments through a small thoracotomy incision using a video monitor (VATS). (Reprinted with permission from Sugarbaker DJ, Strauss GM: Advances in surgical staging and therapy of non-small cell lung cancer. *Semin Oncol* 20:163–172, 1993.)[76]

ated with longer survival, aneuploidy may have a negative survival impact on squamous cell carcinomas.[19]

Several neuroendocrine markers have been studied relative to their prognostic value for NSCLC, including NSE, chromogranin, and Leu-7. A positive NSE is associated with improved response to treatment in patients with adenocarcinoma but has had no effect on survival.[19] Point mutations of the *K-RAS* oncogene also appear to be an important prognostic factor for NSCLC, especially adenocarcinoma. Their presence has been associated with resistance to radiation and chemotherapy treatment, high risk for relapse, and shortened survival.[19,56] Although up to 50% of NSCLC cases are associated with *p53* genetic mutations, their prognostic significance is unclear.[83-86]

Survival rates for NSCLC depend upon the extent of disease at diagnosis and the treatment modalities used. Five-year survival for resectable tumors may exceed 70%, whereas rates for locally advanced and metastatic NSCLC are, at best, 0%-30% at five years.[60]

Classification and Staging

Non-small Cell Lung Cancer

In 1996 revisions in the International System for Staging Lung Cancer were adopted by the American Joint Commission on Cancer (AJCC) and the Union International Contre le Cancer (UICC).[87] The changes provide greater specificity in identifying patient groups relative to prognosis and treatment options. The system continues to use the *TNM* letters. *T* designates primary tumor and is divided into categories relative to size, location, and invasion. *N*, with three categories, represents regional lymph node status. *M* designates the absence or presence of distant metastases (Table 59-3).[88] Lung cancer is now divided into eight instead of six stages (Table 59-4),[87] each of which is distinct relative to treatment and five-year survival statistics. Intrapulmonary ipsilateral disease in a lobe different from the site of the primary tumor is now classified as M1 disease. Accurate staging is crucial in determining appropriate curative or palliative treatment for the patient with lung cancer.

Small Cell Lung Cancer

Although the AJCC has always recommended that SCLC be staged using the TNM classification system, most clinicians use the simple two-stage system. Since most SCLC patients have metastatic disease at the time of diagnosis, this system describes the extent of disease as either "limited" or "extensive." Limited-stage disease is defined as tumor confined to one hemithorax and regional lymph nodes with or without pleural effusion. It is meant to include all tumor that can be encompassed within a single radiotherapy portal. Extensive-stage disease refers to tumor that has spread beyond the boundaries of limited

Table 59-3 AJCC TNM Definitions for Lung Cancers

Primary Tumor (T)

TX	Primary tumor cannot be assessed, or tumor proved by the presence of malignant cells in sputum or bronchial washings but not visualized by imaging or bronchoscopy
T0	No evidence of primary tumor
Tis	Carcinoma in situ
T1	Tumor 3 cm or less in greatest dimension, surrounded by lung or visceral pleura, without bronchoscopic evidence of invasion more proximal than the lobar bronchus (i.e., not in the main bronchus)*
T2	Tumor with any of the following features of size or extent: More than 3 cm in greatest dimension Involving main bronchus, 2 cm or more distal to the carina Invading the visceral pleura Associated with atelectasis or obstructive pneumonitis that extends to the hilar region but does not involve the entire lung
T3	Tumor of any size that directly invades any of the following: chest wall (including superior sulcus tumors), diaphragm, mediastinal pleura, or parietal pericardium; or tumor in the main bronchus less than 2 cm distal to the carina but without involvement of the carina; or associated atelectasis or obstructive pneumonitis of the entire lung
T4	Tumor of any size that invades any of the following: mediastinum, heart, great vessels, trachea, esophagus, vertebral body, carina; or tumor with a malignant pleural effusion**

Regional Lymph Nodes (N)

NX	Regional lymph nodes cannot be assessed
N0	No regional lymph node metastasis
N1	Metastasis in ipsilateral peribronchial and/or ipsilateral hilar lymph nodes, including direct extension
N2	Metastasis in ipsilateral mediastinal and/or subcarinal lymph node(s)
N3	Metastasis in contralateral mediastinal, contralateral hilar, ipsilateral or contralateral scalene or supraclavicular lymph node(s)

Distant Metastasis (M)

MX	Presence of distant metastasis cannot be assessed
M0	No distant metastasis
M1	Distant metastasis

*Note: The uncommon superficial tumor of any size with its invasive component limited to the bronchial wall, which may extend proximal to the main bronchus, is also classified as T1.

**Note: Most pleural effusions associated with lung cancer are due to tumor. However, there are a few patients in whom multiple cytopathological examinations of pleural fluid are negative for tumor. In these cases, fluid is nonbloody and is not an exudate. When these elements and clinical judgment dictate that the effusion is not related to the tumor, the effusion should be excluded as a staging element and the patient should be staged as T1, T2, or T3.

disease. This system has been meaningful in identifying groups of SCLC patients that differ from each other relative to survival length. The TNM system is sometimes helpful in identifying the rare SCLC surgical candidate.

Table 59-4 Stage Grouping*

Stage	TNM Subset		
0	Carcinoma *in situ*		
1A	T1	N0	M0
1B	T2	N0	M0
IIA	T1	N1	M0
IIB	T2	N1	M0
	T3	N0	M0
IIIA	T3	N1	M0
	T1	N2	M0
	T2	N2	M0
	T3	N2	M0
IIIB	T4	N0	M0
	T4	N1	M0
	T4	N2	M0
	T1	N3	M0
	T2	N3	M0
	T3	N3	M0
	T4	N3	M0
IV	Any T any N M1		

*Staging is not relevant for occult carcinoma, designated TXN0M0

Reprinted with permission from Mountain CF: Revisions in the International System for Staging Lung Cancer. *Chest* 111:1710-1717, 1997.[87]

Therapeutic Approaches and Nursing Care

Surgery

Surgical resection is considered standard treatment for stage I and stage II NSCLC and is performed with the intent to cure the patient. Over 50,000 operations for lung cancer are performed each year in the United States.[89] Despite advances in early diagnosis, 50% of all lung cancer cases are inoperable at diagnosis, and another 25% of patients have tumors that cannot be completely resected.[90] The five-year survival rates following surgical resection exceed 50% for stage I and 35% for stage II tumors.[19] Decreased survival has been shown for stage I patients who had any symptom at the time of diagnosis.[91]

Controversy exists regarding the appropriate treatment for stage IIIA patients, particularly those who have ipsilateral mediastinal lymph node involvement (N2 disease). Mediastinal lymph node involvement is a poor prognostic sign, especially when diagnosed preoperatively.[19] However, carefully selected patients with N2 disease have achieved cure rates of up to 29% after complete surgical resection.[92] Most surgeons consider individuals with stage IIIB and stage IV lung cancer to be inoperable, which includes tumors that invade the mediastinum, heart, great vessels, trachea, esophagus, or carina, and any tumors that present with distant metastases.[90] In selected cases, solitary metastatic lesions can be resected, particularly lung and brain lesions.[92] Resection of solitary brain lesions is associated with prolonged survival and improved quality of life, and five-year survival is 5%–10%.[56]

Surgical resection may be an option for the limited number of SCLC patients who present with a small, solitary mass, no lymph node involvement, and no distant metastases. Since many SCLC cancers recur in the chest, surgery is thought to offer increased cure benefit when combined with radiation and chemotherapy in those patients with T1 N0 M0 disease.[90,92]

Because of the high risk of complications following thoracic surgery, candidates should be carefully selected. Cardiopulmonary status is evaluated to determine whether the patient can tolerate pulmonary resection. Pulmonary function tests are done. Increasing emphasis is being given to cardiac studies to more accurately identify patients at risk for postoperative cardiopulmonary complications. In general, if the ratio of the forced expiratory volume in 1 second (FEV_1) to forced vital capacity (FVC) is below 75% of the predicted value, postoperative complications increase dramatically. Unacceptable morbidity and mortality are associated with FEV_1/FVC ratios of less than 50% of the predicted value.[19] The patient's ability to perform pulmonary toilet measures and upper extremity range-of-motion exercises postoperatively should be evaluated in a preoperative education session.

Surgical procedures

Pneumonectomy.   Although it was the standard surgical lung cancer procedure for many years, pneumonectomy is now performed only if a tumor cannot be completely excised by lobectomy.[19] Pneumonectomy is chosen when the tumor involves the proximal bronchus, is widespread throughout the lung, or is fixed to the hilum.[56,90]

Pneumonectomy can be a simple or radical procedure. A simple pneumonectomy involves removal of the affected lung with suturing or stapling of the bronchus. The radical procedure includes removal of the mediastinal lymph nodes. After either procedure, mediastinal shift is prevented by allowing the empty thoracic space to consolidate gradually with fluid (Figure 59-5A). The average mortality rate for pneumonectomy is 6%.[19]

Lobectomy.   Lobectomy is the most common surgical procedure performed for primary lung cancer confined to a single lobe of the lung. It includes dissection and excision of the affected lobe from the remaining lung tissue, with closure of the bronchial stump (Figure 59-5B). Two chest tubes are placed in the pleural cavity on the operative side to drain fluid, blood, and air. The remaining lung tissue expands to fill the space left by the resected lobe. Because noncancerous lung tissue is conserved, morbidity with lobectomy is lessened and the mortality rate, at 3%, is half that of pneumonectomy.[19,56]

Sleeve resection with bronchoplastic reconstruction.   When the tumor is confined to the bronchus or pulmonary artery and there is no evidence of metastasis, the affected area can be removed and the bronchus re-

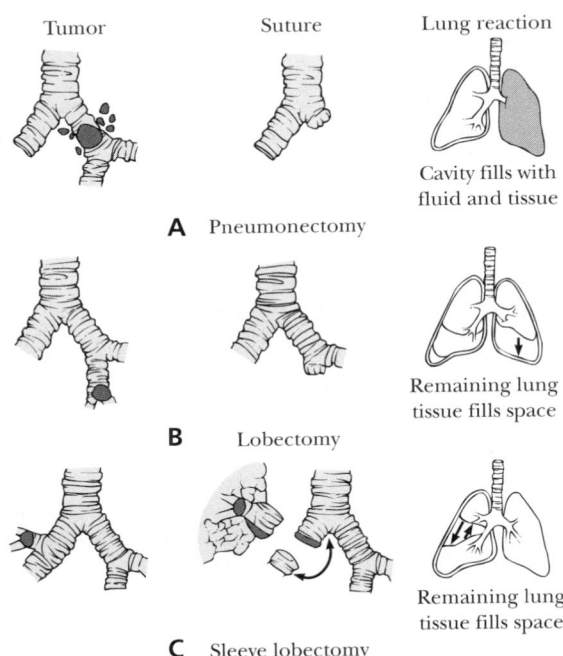

Tumor — Suture — Lung reaction

A Pneumonectomy

Cavity fills with fluid and tissue

B Lobectomy

Remaining lung tissue fills space

C Sleeve lobectomy

Remaining lung tissue fills space

Figure 59-5 Approaches to lung resection (a) Pneumonectomy: The lung alone is removed (simple pneumonectomy) or the lung and involved adjacent nodes are removed (radical pneumonectomy). (b) Lobectomy: A single pulmonary lobe is resected. (c) Sleeve lobectomy: The tumor-bearing lobe is resected together with a segment of the main bronchus, followed by an end-to-end anastomosis. Classic indication is a cardinoma of the right upper lobe bronchus.(From Elpern EH: Lung cancer, in Groenwald SL, Frogge MH, Goodman M, Yarbro CH (eds): *Cancer Nursing: Principles and Practice* (ed 3). Sudbury, MA, Jones and Bartlett, 1993, pp 1174–1199.)[64]

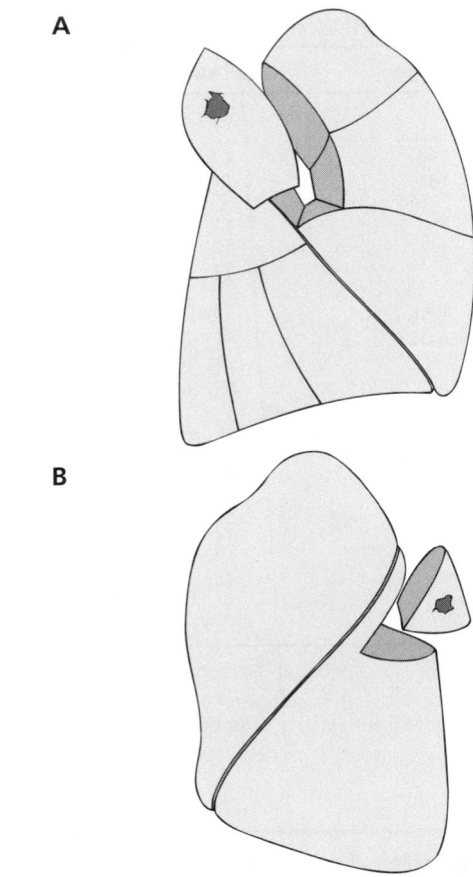

A

B

Figure 59-6 (A) Segmentectomy. Partial removal of a lobe of the lung. (B) Wedge resection. Removal of a small area of disease.

attached with cure rates comparable to those for pneumonectomy for similar patients.[19] Sleeve resection can also be successfully combined with lobectomy (Figure 59-5C). This lung-conserving operation improves the quality of life and reduces morbidity and mortality.

Segmental resection (segmentectomy). Segmental resection is the partial removal of a lobe of the lung, including the bronchovascular segment supplying the resected area (Figure 59-6A). The role of this procedure has yet to be clearly defined. A well-designed trial by the Lung Cancer Study Group of limited resection versus lobectomy in stage I NSCLC showed a threefold increase in local recurrence in the limited resection group, although mortality and morbidity were equal in both groups.[93] At the present time, limited resections are reserved for those patients with cardiopulmonary compromise who are not suitable candidates for more extensive surgery.[91,92] The mortality rate for segmental resection averages 1%.[56]

Wedge resection. Wedge resection, the most conservative surgical approach, is done to remove small periph-

eral nodules or as the procedure of choice in individuals whose physical condition will not permit more extensive surgery. The procedure involves removing the small area of disease without removing the bronchovascular segment of the lobe (Figure 59-6B). As with the other limited resection procedures, mortality is low at 1% but local recurrence rates average 15%, three times higher than with lobectomy.[19,92]

Types of incisions. Pulmonary resection can be accomplished through a variety of operative approaches, depending on the size and location of the tumor and the type of procedure to be performed. The most common approach is the posterolateral thoracotomy, in which a curved incision is made from the submammary fold to slightly below the scapula along the underlying rib. This incision gives the surgeon access to both the lung and the mediastinum.[90]

The anterolateral thoracotomy incision extends from the sternal border between the fourth and fifth intercostal spaces to the midaxillary line. Limited exposure of the lung lessens its usefulness.

The median sternotomy, which is used to gain access

to both lungs and/or to tumor in the mediastinum, has been associated with less postoperative pain than with other procedures.[90,94] An incision is made from the sternal notch to the xiphoid or umbilicus. The sternum is then split with an oscillating saw and spread with retractors to provide maximum exposure. After the resection, the sternum is closed with heavy steel wires.

The axillary incision, from the anterior to the posterior axillary line, is used in patients with lateral peripheral lesions easily accessible by this approach.

Complications

Complications associated with surgical resection of the lung are largely dependent upon the physical status of the patient, the extent of disease, and the surgical procedure performed. Perioperative complications may include air leak, bleeding, atelectasis, and the myriad other well-known intraoperative complications.

The most common postoperative complications are pain and atelectasis. Postthoracotomy incisional pain can be severe and is aggravated by the presence of chest tubes. Inadequate pain control prevents effective coughing and mobilization, and atelectasis may result. Complications that cause impaired gas exchange include pneumothorax, bronchospasm, pulmonary embolus, bronchopleural fistula, and adult respiratory distress syndrome.

Infection and sepsis may also complicate the postoperative course. Wound infections may develop at the incision or chest tube insertion sites; empyema and pneumonia are not uncommon, especially with prolonged intubation. Invasive monitoring devices, urinary catheters, and a generally compromised physical state also increase the risk of infection. Some surgeons recommend preoperative bronchoscopy cultures to assess the bacterial flora of the patient so that appropriate treatment can be initiated before infection manifests.[94]

Cardiac arrhythmias and myocardial infarction may occur postoperatively, and preoperative digitalization is sometimes employed as a preventive measure.[91,94] Sequential compression devices on the lower extremities both during and after surgery help to prevent pulmonary emboli.

Nursing care

Surgery for lung cancer is a major procedure with the potential for significant morbidity and discomfort for the patient. Meticulous nursing care is essential in preventing postoperative complications and in promoting comfort. A plan of care or critical pathway should be developed based on nursing diagnoses and appropriate nursing interventions.

Knowledge deficit. The patient must be fully engaged in the treatment process to increase the chance for successful recovery. Preoperative education about the surgical procedure and what the patient will experience before, during, and after surgery are provided, with particular emphasis on the patient's participation in pulmonary toilet activities. Demonstration and return demonstration of cough, deep breathing, and splinting techniques are included. Anticipatory guidance about the intensive care unit, monitoring devices, and ventilatory support is provided to minimize fear and anxiety related to the initial postsurgical period. Ongoing education about self-care measures to be used after discharge is provided throughout the hospitalization.

Alteration in comfort. Pain is assessed frequently to evaluate the effectiveness of analgesics. Intravenous or epidural infusion of narcotic analgesics is necessary for control of incisional pain, which is severe initially and has been shown to last as long as four years in up to 50% of cases.[89] Teaching the patient position changes and exercises to do in bed can also promote comfort and help to prevent "frozen shoulder," which occurs when pain impairs mobility in the arm and shoulder on the operative side. Range-of-motion exercises should be encouraged.

Nausea due to anesthesia or analgesic medications can occur. Antiemetics should be offered and their effectiveness evaluated.

Potential for impaired gas exchange. Postsurgical complications can be life-threatening, and their early recognition by the nurse can ensure appropriate intervention. Vital signs and arterial blood gases are monitored. Sputum production is assessed for amount, color, and consistency. Patency of chest tubes is assessed, and drainage amount measured and recorded. The patient is encouraged to cough and deep breathe frequently, using incentive spirometry or respiratory treatments to help mobilize secretions.

Potential for infection. The incision and chest tube insertion sites are inspected regularly for signs of infection, including erythema, induration, and drainage. Preventive nursing measures regarding wound management are instituted. Attention to signs and symptoms of other types of infections are a regular part of the nursing assessment.

Alterations in bowel elimination. Both diarrhea and constipation can occur in the postoperative period. Diarrhea is most often related to enteral feedings or stress and may be treated with antidiarrheal agents and by addressing the causative factors. Consulting a dietitian can be helpful in developing a nutritional plan that is less likely to cause diarrhea. Constipation may result from narcotic analgesics, immobility, and decreased dietary intake. Dietary fiber should be increased, and a bowel protocol established early in the postoperative course.

Potential for ineffective coping/anxiety. Fear and anxiety are normal manifestations of the stress associated with lung cancer and surgery. The patient and family members are encouraged to express their feelings and concerns. Realistic information and reassurance are given, and referrals to other members of the health care team, including the social worker, clinical nurse specialist, case manager, or chaplain, are made as appropriate. Discharge planning should begin on admission, utilizing available resources in the institution and the community to facilitate a smooth transition to the use of self-care measures in the home.

Radiation Therapy

Non-small cell lung cancer

Radiation therapy (RT) is an important treatment in the management of individuals with NSCLC. The usual dosage of external beam chest irradiation is 50–60 Gy delivered in fractions of 1.8–2.0 Gy five days a week over five to six weeks.[95] Although surgery offers the best chance for cure for stage I and stage II disease, RT offers a potentially curative alternative in patients who refuse surgery or are not surgical candidates.[96] Postoperative RT is not commonly used for early-stage NSCLC because even though it decreases the incidence of local recurrence, it has not improved overall survival.[19,56]

Postoperative RT is the standard of care for selected stage IIIa patients undergoing surgical resection, and it is thought to prolong disease-free survival, although not long-term survival.[19] RT is also the standard treatment for patients with unresectable stage III disease. When used alone, however, the effectiveness of RT is limited, with median survival of eight to ten months and five-year survival of 5%–7%.[97,98] In an effort to improve survival rates in patients with regionally advanced NSCLC, new methods of fractionation of RT dosages are being tested. With continuous hyperfractionated accelerated RT (CHART), three fractions per day of less than 1.8 Gy each are given over 12 consecutive days with an interval of at least six hours between fractions. The total CHART dosage is greater than standard dosages, and the short interval between fractions prevents cancer cell repopulation. The lower dosage per fraction enhances normal repair of sublethal tissue damage.[95,98] Several studies have shown impressive one- and two-year survival rates with CHART compared with conventional RT.[97,98] Esophagitis is the most common toxicity, occurring at around day 18 when treatment is completed. CHART and conventional RT have been found to have comparable long-term physical and psychological morbidity.[99]

Multimodality treatment of stage III patients combining chemotherapy and radiation therapy is a current area of considerable interest. A landmark study by Sause and colleagues showed a statistically significant survival advantage for unresectable stage III patients treated with chemotherapy followed by RT versus standard RT alone or hyperfractionated radiation therapy.[100] Chemotherapy treatment for NSCLC is discussed in greater detail later in this chapter.

Small cell lung cancer

SCLC is quite sensitive to both radiation and chemotherapy. Most oncologists consider thoracic RT in combination with chemotherapy for limited-stage disease to be the standard of care.[60,98] Combined-modality treatment results in lower recurrence rates and appears to confer a modest survival advantage over chemotherapy alone.[98] The usual dosage of chest RT for SCLC is 45–50 Gy over three to four weeks. Conventional and hyperfractionation schedules have been used. Concurrent or alternating treatment appears to improve response rates over sequential chemotherapy and RT, although toxicity is more intense with concurrent therapy.[101,102]

Prophylactic cranial irradiation (PCI) in limited-stage SCLC is an area of considerable debate. Because of the potentially serious long-term side effects of PCI, including dementia, gait disturbances, and intellectual impairment, benefit must be weighed against risk.[103] Some argue that because there is a 50% chance of central nervous system recurrence with SCLC, PCI is worth the risk of toxicity, particularly if (1) it is given only to individuals who have a complete response to initial therapy; (2) it is not given concurrently with any drugs; and (3) standard or lower dosages are used.[98]

Others argue that because PCI reduces brain recurrence but does not improve overall survival, the associated morbidity does not justify brain irradiation unless a metastatic brain lesion develops.[104] Figure 59-7 illustrates this point. Group A patients who received PCI were compared

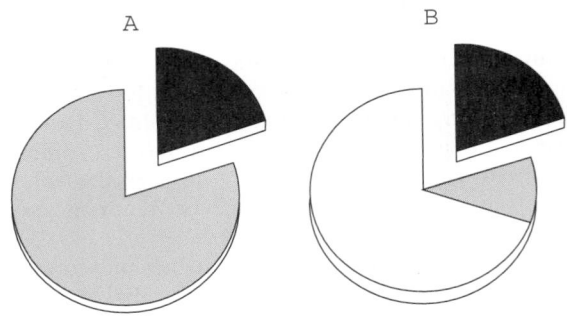

☐ Asymptomatic patients who have had cranial irradiation (RT or PCI)

■ Symptomatic brain metastases in spite of cranial irradiation (RT or PCI)

Figure 59-7 Schematic presentation of two different scenarios in the management of SCLC. Each cycle represents the groups of complete responders (CR) with small cell lung cancer. (A) All CR patients receive prophylactic cranial irradiation (PCI) and approximately 20% relapse in the brain, with very limited chances of further palliation (black area). (B) Cranial irradiation is withheld until a manifest brain relapse occurs. This happens in 30% of CR patients, of whom 40% achieve a complete symptomatic alleviation of some duration. Approximately 20% are left with symptomatic brain metastases (black area). (Reprinted from *Lung Cancer*, Vol. 12, Kristjansen PEG, Hansen HH, Prophylactic cranial irradiation in small cell lung cancer: an update, S23–S40, 1995 (suppl), with kind permission from Elsevier Science Ltd., P.O. Box 800, Oxford OX51DX, UK.)[104]

with group B patients who received cranial RT only when a brain metastasis developed. The ultimate outcomes were the same. Twenty percent of patients were left with unresolved symptomatic brain metastases, although most patients in group B were spared the toxicity of PCI. PCI is not recommended for patients who do not have a complete response to therapy because it does not reduce the risk of brain recurrence in those patients. Chest irradiation in extensive-stage SCLC offers no survival advantage and is not recommended.[60]

Palliative radiation therapy

RT can be used as an effective palliative treatment for many of the distressing symptoms caused by metastatic lung cancer. Duration and toxicity of the treatment relative to expected survival of the patient should always be considered and treatment decisions individualized.

Bone metastases can be irradiated to alleviate pain, prevent pathological fractures, and prevent spinal cord compression. Individuals with superior vena cava syndrome (SVCS) often experience relief within one to two days after RT is initiated. Radiation to metastatic brain lesions can also promote improved function and symptomatic relief. Stereotactic radiosurgery for metastatic brain lesions in NSCLC has shown promise in improving survival and quality of life.[105]

One of the most common indications for palliative RT is major airway obstruction by endobronchial lesions. External beam irradiation and brachytherapy have been used. Most recently, high-dose-rate (HDR) brachytherapy has been used to palliate symptoms of obstruction such as cough, hemoptysis, and dyspnea.[106] During the HDR brachytherapy procedure a catheter is placed bronchoscopically beyond the distal margin of the tumor (Figure 59-8). A radioactive source is delivered into the tumor via the catheter providing a high dose of therapy in a short period of time, usually minutes.[107] The one-time treatment can be given safely in the outpatient setting. Although side effects of HDR brachytherapy are usually minimal, pneumothorax and bronchoesophageal fistulae have been reported, and in one study, massive fatal hemoptysis was reported in 6 of 12 patients.[108]

Side effects of radiation therapy

Side effects of RT are generally related to the area being irradiated and are experienced by most patients. The most common side effects of chest RT include skin irritation; esophagitis, manifested by dysphagia; radiation pneumonitis, manifested by dry cough, dyspnea on exertion, and fever; pericarditis, with chest pain, electrocardiogram abnormalities, and a pericardial friction rub; and fatigue. Acute side effects usually begin during the second to third week of therapy;[60] long-term effects such as pericarditis may not develop for more than a year after therapy completion.[95] Larson and colleagues reported that outcomes related to weight, body mass index, and multidimensional functional status were no different for

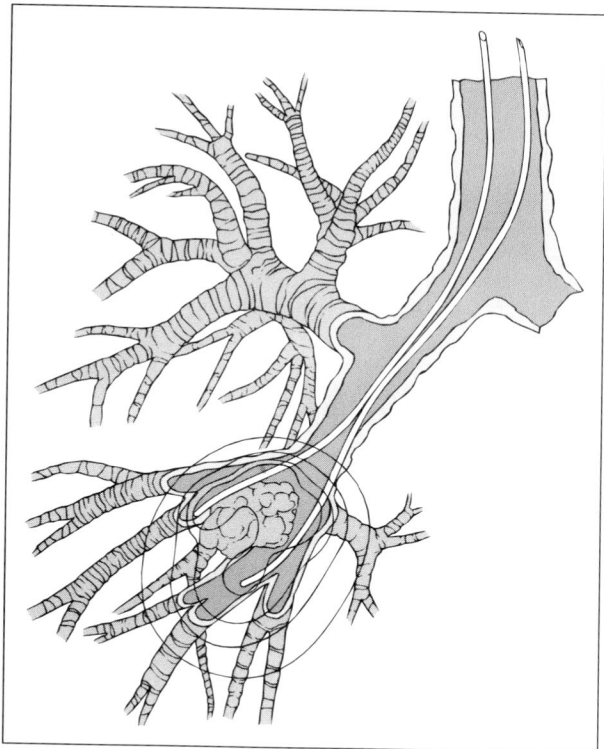

Figure 59-8 Lung implant for delivery of radiation. Two brachytherapy catheters surround the tumor and deliver a high dose of radiation directly to the tumor. (Used with permission from the Nucletron Oldelft Corporation, Columbia, MD.)

persons over age 65 than for younger patients after RT for lung cancer.[109] This study suggests that age should not be the only determinant of ability to manage demanding treatment. Weight loss after RT for lung cancer is common, and was found to be greater in men, current smokers, and the elderly.[110] These findings can be used to identify individuals at high risk for weight loss and to guide early nutritional intervention. Nursing care of the person receiving RT is discussed in detail in Chapter 17.

Chemotherapy

Non-small cell lung cancer

Fifty to seventy-five percent of all patients with NSCLC will present with regionally advanced or metastatic disease and are not candidates for surgery.[111,112] Eighty percent of those who present with resectable disease relapse with distant metastases.[49] If progress is to be made in survival rates of individuals with NSCLC, improvements in systemic treatment must be realized. Although adjuvant chemotherapy for stage I and stage II disease has not shown a survival benefit and is not the standard, continued clinical trials with new drugs are currently under way.[49,113]

Chemotherapy is used to treat stage III and stage IV

patients. Response rates of 50%–70% are seen in stage III patients when chemotherapy is added to surgery or RT, and some chemotherapeutic agents act as radiation sensitizers.[112,113] A survival advantage has been demonstrated in stage III individuals treated with chemotherapy followed by RT versus RT alone.[100] Cisplatin-based chemotherapy protocols are the standard of treatment.[112]

Neoadjuvant therapy—chemotherapy with or without RT prior to surgery—has been an area of interest in recent years for patients with stage III disease. Neoadjuvant therapy is based on the premise that eradicating micrometastatic disease and debulking the tumor prior to surgery may improve the chance of a complete resection and cure. Survival rates after neoadjuvant therapy have been higher than with other treatments.[100,114–116] However, sample sizes in neoadjuvant trials have been small and further clinical trials are needed before neoadjuvant therapy for stage III disease can be considered the standard of care.[117,118] Although neoadjuvant treatment shows promise, it can be quite difficult for the patient, with increased operative complications and higher morbidity and mortality.

Although multimodality treatment is the emerging standard of care for stage III NSCLC, patients with distant metastases (stage IV) have traditionally been treated with either chemotherapy alone or supportive care.[119] Agents used in the past ten years have included ifosfamide, vinblastine, vindesine, cisplatin, etoposide, and mitomycin. Given the intrinsic resistance to chemotherapy manifested by NSCLC cells, use of these drugs has been repeatedly questioned. Response rates with chemotherapy average 15%, and median survival time is only 25–30 weeks.[120,121]

Palliation of symptoms, quality of life, and length of survival, in addition to response rates, must be evaluated when chemotherapy is given for metastatic NSCLS. Chemotherapy has been compared with best supportive care (BSC) in many clinical trials. In these trials BSC has included measures for pain control, symptom management, palliative RT, and antibiotics, but no chemotherapy.[49] Chemotherapy extended survival and also improved symptoms such as cough, hemoptysis, bone pain, malaise, and weight loss.[110,122] A cost analysis performed by the National Cancer Institute of Canada revealed that chemotherapy saved health care dollars when compared with BSC because symptoms improved and patients spent less time in the hospital.[110] With the widespread use of improved antiemetic drugs, chemotherapy has become a more acceptable option for patients with advanced NSCLC.

Despite skepticism over the past few decades about the relative efficacy of chemotherapy in NSCLC, a number of promising new chemotherapeutic agents are available (Table 59-5). Many of these agents have mechanisms of action different from those of standard drugs. Some have shown more activity as a single agent than standard combination chemotherapy. A discussion of each new agent follows.

Table 59-5 Promising New Chemotherapeutic Agents Used in the Treatment of NSCLS

Camptothecin analog	Irinotecan (CPT-11)
Taxanes	Paclitaxel
	Docetaxel
Vinca alkaloid	Vinorelbine
Antimetabolites	Gemcitabine

Camptothecin analogs. The camptothecins, including topotecan and irinotecan (CPT-11), are plant alkaloids extracted from a large-leafed tree common in southeastern China. They exert their cytotoxic action by inhibiting topoisomerase I, an enzyme necessary for DNA replication.[113]

Results of topotecan clinical trials in patients with NSCLC have not been encouraging.[123] CPT-11, studied extensively in Japan, has shown promising activity in NSCLC. Response rates of up to 41% as a single agent and 54% when combined with cisplatin have been reported.[112] Dose-limiting toxicities include diarrhea and myelosuppression. Nausea, vomiting, alopecia, anorexia, stomatitis, and anemia have also been reported.[123] Because the diarrhea can be life-threatening, the importance of patient education about the recommendations for diarrhea management cannot be overemphasized.

Taxanes. Paclitaxel and docetaxel exert their effects by stabilizing microtubules so that the cell cannot progress beyond the G_2 or M phase of the cell cycle into cell division.[112,113] Using paclitaxel as a single agent, response rates of over 20% have been seen.[49] In a landmark study by Langer and colleagues, paclitaxel and carboplatin together in advanced NSCLC yielded an astonishing 62% response rate, with 9% complete responses.[124] The one-year survival rate was 54%. The regimen was fairly well tolerated: severe myelosuppression was less than 22% with the use of filgrastim. Response rates of over 50% have been reported in other phase II trials of paclitaxel and carboplatin[125], although Belani and colleagues reported a response rate of only 21.6% in a phase III trial.[126] In addition to myelosuppression, other reported side effects have included anemia, thrombocytopenia, neuropathy, myalgias, and arthralgias. Paclitaxel alone may also cause nausea and vomiting, stomatitis, diarrhea, and a rare hypersensitivity reaction.[112]

Docetaxel has also shown promise, with single agent response rates of up to 33% in early trials.[119,123] Docetaxel has been studied in combination with cisplatin, with response rates of 25%–53%.[125] Side effects are similar to those of paclitaxel, including neutropenia, skin reactions, hypersensitivity, neuropathy, edema, stomatitis, alopecia, and weakness. Symptomatic third-space fluid collections have been minimized with the routine use of corticosteroids.[118,127]

Vinorelbine. Vinorelbine, the newest drug in the vinca alkaloid class, inhibits cellular replication by interfering with the assembly of microtubules. In patients with advanced NSCLC, vinorelbine in combination with cisplatin has shown a survival advantage over vindesine and cisplatin and vinorelbine alone.[122,128] Neutropenia is the dose-limiting toxicity. Other side effects include nausea, vomiting, and diarrhea, although neurotoxicity has been less severe than with the other vinca alkaloids.[112]

Antimetabolites. Gemcitabine is a new antimetabolite that, in combination with cisplatin, has been approved for first-line treatment of persons with inoperable, locally advanced, or metastatic NSCLC. There is evidence of synergy with cisplatin, and and reported response rates for the combination have been 29%–54%.[125,127] As a single agent, gemcitabine has consistently shown response rates of about 20%.[125] A relatively mild side effect panel including minimal myelosuppression, a flu-like syndrome, alopecia, and rash—make it an attractive drug to combine with other more myelosuppressive regimens.[49,113,118,119]

Small cell lung cancer

SCLC is initially much more sensitive to chemotherapy than NSCLC. Chemotherapy, with or without RT, has been the mainstay of treatment for many years. Despite complete response rates of up to 90% in limited-stage disease, long-term survival at five years is 10% at best, and almost 0% for patients with extensive-stage SCLC.[121] Eventual resistance to chemotherapy is acquired over time and is currently an area of vigorous investigation.

Several chemotherapy regimens have emerged as effective options for treatment (Table 59-6), although a single best regimen is yet to be defined. In the 1970s and 1980s the CAV regimen (cyclophosphamide, doxorubi-

cin, and vincristine) was most commonly used, with high response rates and occasional cures.[129] Later, etoposide emerged as an extremely active agent in SCLC and became the cornerstone of new regimens. Currently, etoposide and cisplatin (EP regimen) are standard induction therapy for SCLC. They appear to be synergistic, have comparable efficacy to CAV, and combined side effects are less severe than with CAV.[129,130]

More recently, carboplatin and etoposide have been reported to exhibit activity equal to that of EP, with significantly less nausea, vomiting, nephrotoxicity, mucositis, neurotoxicity, neutropenia, and sepsis events.[131] The CODE regimen (cisplatin, vincristine, doxorubicin, etoposide), currently under investigation, has shown promise when combined with RT in patients with extensive SCLC, with response rates of 94% and two-year survival of 30%.[129] Because myelosuppression is the dose-limiting toxicity for many of the drugs active in SCLC, the use of hematopoietic growth factors has shortened the duration of neutropenia and enabled safer administration of higher-dose regimens, although to date no study has shown a clear survival advantage when growth factors were used.[132]

Newer drugs, including gemcitabine,[133] paclitaxel,[134] docetaxel,[135] topotecan,[136] and irinotecan[137] are active in SCLC with relatively high response rates. The optimal use of these agents is yet to be defined.

Many of the drugs used in the treatment of SCLC are poorly tolerated by elderly individuals. Potential nephrotoxicity with the EP regimen is a concern, and tolerance for myelosuppression may be decreased. The elderly often are excluded from clinical trials because of the fear that they will experience undue toxicity. In this group of patients, oral etoposide has been shown to be an excellent alternative to more aggressive therapy, with overall response rates of up to 85%.[138] Neutropenia is still a concern, although less so than with other therapies.

Chemotherapy for SCLC is usually given for four to six months. Maintenance chemotherapy beyond this time is not recommended because it does not improve survival.[60] Although autologous bone marrow transplantation in patients with SCLC has been studied for over a decade, results are inconclusive.[130]

Complications of chemotherapy

Complications associated with chemotherapy for lung cancer are many and are dependent upon the drugs given. Side effects may be acute or chronic. Acute side effects include myelosuppression, nausea, vomiting, diarrhea, mucositis, constipation, anorexia, alopecia, skin changes, hemorrhagic cystitis, hypersensitivity reactions, myalgias, and arthralgias. Potential long-term effects include organ toxicities such as cardiomyopathy, hepatotoxicity, nephropathy, peripheral neuropathy, pulmonary toxicity, ototoxicity, and infertility.[139] Specific aspects of nursing care related to side effects are described in Chapter 20.

Table 59-6   Chemotherapy Regimens Commonly Used for Small Cell Lung Cancer

Regimen	Drug Names
CAV	Cyclophosphamide, doxorubicin, vincristine
EP CAV alternating with EP	Etoposide, cisplatin
Oral EP	Oral etoposide, cisplatin
EC	Etoposide, carboplatin
CAE	Cyclophosphamide, doxorubicin, etoposide
CAVE	Cyclophosphamide, doxorubicin, vincristine, etoposide
CODE	Cisplatin, vincristine, doxorubicin, etoposide
ICE (VIP)	Ifosfamide, cisplatin, etoposide

Many patients with lung cancer are symptomatic at diagnosis and present in a debilitated state. Chemotherapy usually adds to debilitation, at least temporarily, and some of the side effects can be life-threatening.

Education for the patient and family about chemotherapy begins early. Emphasis is placed on teaching self-management of side effects since most side effects will be experienced in the home setting. Early referrals to supportive resources are made, encouraging the patient to attend to the emotional as well as the physical aspects of the illness. Because accessibility of the health care providers is extremely important and reassuring to the patient during treatment, phone numbers for the nurse and physician should be provided.

Biotherapy

In general, results of clinical trials with biological therapies have not been encouraging. Response rates with alfa-interferon alone in both SCLC and NSCLC have been less than 15%.[49] Beta-interferon is thought to be synergistic with RT, and in one study produced an overall response rate of 81% in 25 patients with stage III NSCLC.[112] Continued clinical trials to evaluate efficacy and toxicity of this combination are under way. Alfa-interferon with cisplatin or carboplatin does not appear to be superior to chemotherapy alone,[113] although data from current trials are pending. Interleukin 2, studied as a treatment for NSCLC, has resulted in poor response rates with significant toxicity.[113,140]

Because lung cancer is known to impair both cellular and humoral immunity, restoration of immune function has been targeted in recent studies. Intrapleural bacillus Calmette-Guerin (BCG) was studied with no observed improvement in treated patients. Likewise, treatment with levamisole, an immunomodulator, did not produce results more favorable than in the control arm of the study.[140]

The hematopoietic growth factors have been the most useful biological response modifiers in the treatment of lung cancer. Both granulocyte (G) and granulocyte-macrophage (GM) colony-stimulating factors (CSFs) decrease myelosuppression, febrile episodes, and number of hospital days when given in conjunction with chemotherapy. Although the CSFs do not affect survival, their impact on cost and quality of life has been profound.[56]

Photodynamic Therapy

Photodynamic therapy (PDT) has been used in an investigational setting to treat cancer of the esophagus and lung cancer.[141] The patient receives an injection of Photofrin (porfimer sodium), a photoactive drug. A few days later light generated from a laser is aimed through a bronchoscope to the tumor on the bronchial surface. The cancer cells absorb the Photofrin which is activated by the light from the laser. This process kills the cancer cells with minimal damage to normal cells. A bronchoscopy is done a few days later to remove any cellular debris and mucus that is too thick for the patient to expectorate. If residual tumor is seen at that time, the PDT procedure may be repeated.

PDT is most useful in early-stage lung cancer. Several studies in Japan showed that 90% of small, superficial tumors can be completely eradicated with PDT.[141] Complete response rates have been as high as 89%. PDT is not used to treat regional lymph nodes and is not effective for bronchial stump recurrences.

Photodynamic therapy requires careful instructions regarding exposure to bright light or direct sunlight. Risk for intense sunburn and photosensitivity exists for 30 days after the injection. It is important to take precautions to shield the skin and eyes from exposure. Patients are instructed to bring a hat, sunglasses, and gloves to the hospital for the first treatment. Protective clothing and dark sunglasses are worn even on cloudy days. Under no circumstances should skin be exposed to the sunlight within the 30 day period. After the 30 day period a small amount of skin on the hand may be exposed to the sun for 10 minutes. If swelling, redness, or blistering of the area occur, in the next 24 hours the patient should continue to take precautions for an additional 2 weeks. If no reaction occurs after 24 hours the patient may gradually increase exposure to the sunlight.

PDT has been compared with yttrium aluminum garnet (YAG) laser therapy in treating bronchial obstruction from intraluminal tumors. While both treatments are equally effective, relief of obstruction is quicker with YAG laser therapy. YAG should be used in acute cases of bronchial obstruction. The porfimer sodium used with PDT can cause skin photosensitivity for up to several months. However, time to treatment failure has been slightly longer after PDT than after YAG laser therapy.[141]

Brachytherapy continues to be the treatment of choice for patients with advanced obstructive bronchial tumors invading the submucosa. Studies combining PDT with external beam radiation have shown promise in achieving better local control than RT alone.

Complications for PDT and YAG laser therapy are similar. Fatal hemorrhage, respiratory failure, or cardiac arrest occurs in 1.5% of patients. Less severe complications occur in less than 0.5% of cases.[142]

Symptom Management and Supportive Care

Suffering has been defined as a negative state that results from events or situations perceived to be physically or psychologically painful, uncomfortable, or distressing.[116,143–145] Lung cancer is synonymous with suffering for many people. Up to 90% of patients report some degree of suffering relative to physical, emotional, or psychosocial dysfunction. While the nursing care challenges are significant, so too are the opportunities for meaningful intervention. Sarna found that systematic use by nurses of a structured symptom assessment tool was associated with decreased symptom distress over time in persons with advanced lung cancer.[146] Symptom management and supportive care for this population of patients, discussed in the following, require finely honed nursing skills.

Cough

A chronic cough may result from stimulation of irritant receptors in the bronchial mucosa through tumor infiltration. Hypersecretion of mucus also may cause coughing. Persistent coughing may increase pain, prevent adequate rest, and promote fatigue, and it can cause rib fractures when bone metastases are present.[64] The dry, irritating cough must be distinguished from the productive cough. Although it may be appropriate to suppress a dry, persistent, and debilitating cough, this should not be attempted at the expense of removal of secretions.

The goal of nursing interventions is to promote comfort. Narcotic medications, specifically codeine preparations, are generally used for cough suppression. Inspired air is warmed and humidified and cigarette smoking discouraged. Deep breathing and effective coughing techniques are taught and reinforced as necessary. Tracheal suctioning is to be used only if the individual's cough is ineffective in removing secretions. A chronic, nonproductive cough in a patient with underlying chronic obstructive lung disease may respond to inhaled bronchodilators.[64]

Hemoptysis

Mild hemoptysis is common and is caused by erosion of the pulmonary vasculature by tumor. If the volume of bleeding is less than 50 mL in 24 hours, the patient usually is treated conservatively on an outpatient basis.[64] If hemoptysis is exacerbated by coughing, cough suppressants may be prescribed. Although death from exsanguination is rare, the fear of bleeding to death is often expressed by patients. Accurate information and reassurance should be provided.

Hospitalization and careful monitoring are required for patients with profound hemoptysis. Bleeding of over 200 mL in 24 hours requires immediate attention. The patient should be positioned with the suspected bleeding lung in a dependent position to prevent blood spillage into the unaffected lung.[64] Emergency surgery may be required.

Dyspnea

Dyspnea and the sensation of smothering can be a terrifying experience for the patient, and is much more common in advanced lung cancer than was previously recognized.[147] Dyspnea may be associated with destruction of lung tissue by tumor, pleural effusions, airway obstruction by endobronchial lesions, and increased mucus production. Palliation of dyspnea can be achieved in many cases with appropriate treatment.

Helping the patient cope with and manage dyspnea is a primary goal of nursing care. Teach the patient to assess patterns of occurrence including precipitating factors, duration, and relief measures. Help plan coping strategies including interventions such as relaxation techniques, controlled coughing techniques, oxygen administration, or position changes. Help the patient identify ways to conserve energy and minimize fatigue.[148,149]

Dyspnea in the individual with lung cancer is often associated with pleural effusion. Not all pleural effusions are malignant, and etiology should be established before palliative treatment is initiated. Large volumes of fluid can be removed by thoracentesis or by an implanted pleural port attached to a Tenckhoff catheter, which results in lung reexpansion unless the lung has become trapped by tumor.[150]

When pleural effusions reaccumulate, as is often the case, pleurodesis is the recommended therapy.[151,152] A chest tube is inserted to completely drain the pleural space; then a sclerosing agent is instilled into the pleural space to obliterate the space and prevent reaccumulation of fluid. Agents used for pleurodesis include bleomycin, talc, doxycycline, and minocycline.[151] Tetracycline, formerly the most frequently used sclerosing agent, is no longer available in the injectable form. Because pleurodesis is a painful procedure, appropriate analgesics should be administered by the nurse. In cases of recurrent effusion, a pleuroperitoneal shunt can be inserted to divert fluid from the chest cavity to the abdomen[151] (see Chapter 36).

Pain

Pain is experienced by most individuals with lung cancer, and the prevalence increases as the disease advances.[153] Chest pain occurs in half of all patients with lung cancer and may be caused by mediastinal extension of tumor, pleural effusions, bronchial obstruction, or infection.[148] Bone pain is common, as is pain related to metastases to other distant sites. Many patients with lung cancer experience pain for more than a year prior to death. While not all patients experience pain as suffering, adequate pain control is clearly a key goal in promoting quality of life. Guidelines for cancer pain management have been published by the Agency for Health Care Policy and Research[154] and promote a well-researched approach to pain management with pharmacological and nonpharmacological interventions. Narcotic analgesics commonly used include morphine, hydromorphone, and fentanyl. Nonsteroidal anti-inflammatory drugs have been effective for metastatic bone pain.[155]

The key to pain management is its accurate assessment. Visual analog scales, multidimensional instruments such as the McGill Pain Questionnaire, and pain flow sheets are helpful in assessing pain and evaluating the effectiveness of interventions. Wilkie and colleagues investigated if coaching patients to communicate pain in ways that clinicians recognize would reduce the discrepancy between patients' self-report of sensory pain and nurses' assessment of pain.[153] A trend toward improvement in percent agreement between patients and nurses was reported. A continued larger study now under way may have implications for patient education relative to communication of pain (see Chapter 28).

Fatigue

Fatigue and weakness have been the most commonly reported aspects of physical suffering in both general and lung cancer populations,[146,156] and disability related to fatigue and weakness has been reported to be the source of greatest suffering among persons with lung cancer.[143] Serious disruptions in physical functioning occur as the disease progresses. Difficulty with household chores, interference with work, reduced energy, and problems with ambulation and recreation are reported commonly.[157,158] These disruptions are often stressful and are a burden borne by the whole family. Anticipating difficulties can help the nurse prepare the patient and family for the course ahead of them.

The individual's feeling of fatigue is influenced by many factors—physiological, pathological, psychological, and behavioral. Significant correlations have been reported between pain and fatigue in individuals with lung cancer, as well as between fatigue and mood states as measured by the Profile of Mood States.[159] Regular assessments for fatigue should be performed regardless of age, stage of disease, or treatment. Interventions to control factors contributing to fatigue, such as pain, should be planned and implemented so that energy is restored rather than depleted. Patients' satisfaction with their level of functioning is the ultimate goal for quality of life (see Chapter 32).

Gastrointestinal Disturbances: Nausea and Vomiting, Anorexia and Cachexia, and Elimination

Nausea and vomiting related to the disease process in the person with lung cancer have several etiologies, including GI obstruction, liver metastases, increased intracranial pressure from brain metastases, and narcotic analgesics. Metabolic disturbances related to paraneoplastic syndromes also may cause nausea. Often, treatment of the underlying causes can alleviate the symptoms. The array of effective antiemetic drugs in use today may also relieve nausea and promote comfort.

Anorexia and cancer cachexia are common manifestations of lung cancer.[160] The disease process itself, treatment complications, and psychological factors may all

contribute to anorexia. Pain, fatigue, and dyspnea also interfere with the desire to eat. The cancer cachexia syndrome—manifested by weight loss, anorexia, taste changes, emaciation, and muscle wasting—is poorly understood. The patient may experience an increase in the basal metabolic rate and alterations in protein, fat, and carbohydrate metabolism.

As many as 50% of all individuals with lung cancer lose weight prior to their diagnosis, which is generally considered to be a poor prognostic factor.[161] Weight loss from cachexia is thought to first occur in the skeletal muscle and then adipose tissue, which helps explain the rapid impairment of functional status. In a study by Sarna and colleagues, weight loss in persons with lung cancer was greater in adults under age 65, in patients with SCLC, and in those receiving chemotherapy.[160] Those who had experienced greater weight loss at the initiation of the study reported greater functional impairment and symptom distress. These findings can help the nurse identify individuals at high risk for weight loss and initiate early support strategies.

Because eating and enjoyment of food are equated with health and wellness in our society, anorexia and weight loss can be particularly distressing to the patient and family. A thorough nutritional assessment and appropriate nutritional counseling and education can help to promote an improved quality of life. In addition to nursing strategies known to promote appetite, the drug megestrol acetate has been found to improve appetite and contribute to weight gain when administered orally to individuals with cancer.[155]

Constipation may occur as a result of any combination of factors such as medication side effects, inactivity, poor fluid intake, and lack of dietary fiber.[148] The patient taking opioid analgesics is at high risk for constipation. Information obtained in the nursing assessment includes normal bowel patterns and any deviation from that pattern, medications, dietary factors that might affect elimination, and measures that relieved constipation in the past. The abdomen is examined for the presence of bowel sounds and any sign of distention.

Natural laxatives and dietary measures such as increased fiber and fluids can be recommended for mild constipation. For moderate to severe constipation, stronger laxatives, enemas, or digital disimpaction may be needed. The key to managing constipation is prevention. Many health care settings have implemented prophylactic bowel protocols developed by the multidisciplinary team.

Psychosocial Issues

Given the current lack of success with curative treatment for lung cancer, many patients and their families will be confronted with the myriad stressors and traumas that accompany a rapidly progressive fatal disease. Therefore, attention to psychosocial issues and care takes on great importance.[147]

The goal of nursing care relative to psychosocial issues

is to foster appropriate coping responses of the patient and family members.[162] Identifying factors that have an impact on psychosocial adjustment can help guide nursing interventions. Klemm reported that patients who experienced greater demands of illness, including physical symptoms, issues of family functioning, and treatment issues, had lower psychosocial adjustment scores.[163] Findings from a study of causal attribution, perceived control, and adjustment in patients with lung cancer suggest that when coping with a difficult disease like lung cancer it is the discovery of meaning in the disease that gives one a sense of mastery, regardless of whether the meaning or attributed cause of the cancer is external or internal. Helping the patient to talk and make sense of his or her experience may be the primary nursing intervention in promoting that sense of mastery.[164]

Fear and anxiety are common among individuals with lung cancer and have been associated with high degrees of suffering.[143] They may occur at various times throughout the illness, and one may precipitate the other. Specific fears may include fear of pain, fear of abandonment, fear of recurrence, fear of dependency, and fear of death.[162] Reassurance about the effectiveness of pain control measures can be of help to the patient and family. Fear of abandonment and separation from family, friends, and health care workers is pervasive. The patient should be encouraged to verbalize feelings of loss and grief related to unfulfilled desires and dreams, and leaving loved ones.

The recurrence of lung cancer can be a greater crisis than the initial diagnosis. Hope, often synonymous with life and living, is not as strong, and the patient and family may be at high risk for depression during this time.[162,165] Social withdrawal is common due to the disability associated with lung cancer,[166] and fears of inability to care for oneself and becoming dependent on loved ones may be particularly anxiety-provoking. Anxiety may be alleviated somewhat by emphasizing benefits of palliative treatment and by recognizing and affirming healthy, intact parts of the patient.[162]

Often the fear of dying is not as profound as the fear of suffering in the process of dying. An assessment of resources available to the patient and family and referral to supportive resources such as hospice or home health care may be appropriate. The patient should be allowed to explore fears, concerns, and wishes regarding death. Attentive listening and guidance can provide comfort and emotional healing. Sometimes just the quiet, accepting presence of the nurse can help ease the pain associated with fear and anxiety.

Major depression has been reported with greater frequency in persons with lung cancer than in healthy people.[166] Correlates of depression have included psychiatric history and the presence of metastatic disease. It is sometimes difficult for the clinician to distinguish between biological and psychological etiologies for depression in individuals with lung cancer. Side effects from the disease or treatment such as extreme fatigue, anorexia, and sleep disorders may be confused with symptoms of depression, and vice versa. Brain metastases cause symptoms that are

mistaken for psychological distress. In SCLC, ectopic corticotropin production can produce manic episodes.[166] All possibilities should be considered when the patient presents with altered mood or behavior.

Although the database relating to psychological distress in persons with lung cancer is small, experience with this population indicates that the needs are great. Unfortunately, current lung cancer educational materials do not adequately address psychosocial issues and require tenth-grade or higher-level reading skills.[167] Early intervention using a multidisciplinary team approach can ensure that the patient and family receive thorough education on all aspects of the disease and treatment, referrals for counseling and support groups, and information about other resources that promote psychological, social, and spiritual well-being.

Continuity of Care: Nursing Challenges

With the current chaos in health care delivery systems, challenges to continuity of care have never been greater. Central to the challenge is seamless access to high-quality care for the patient and family and a systematic flow of information to all care providers from diagnosis until resolution of the illness. Access to care can be impeded by competition for patients and territoriality among agencies. In addition, individuals without insurance or with restricted coverage may have to go without much-needed services or pay out of pocket.[168] The nurse caring for the patient with lung cancer is often at the organizational hub of the care continuum and can play a major role in ensuring that appropriate communication and coordination of care take place and that, through collaboration, effective negotiation around barriers to care can occur.

Today, most treatment for lung cancer is administered in the outpatient setting. The complexity of treatment requires that the nurse not only be skilled technically but also be able to perform a comprehensive patient and family assessment to develop a plan of care for the patient to follow at home.[169] Education about self-care must be provided and other care resources coordinated. Many larger cancer centers utilize a comprehensive approach to the treatment of lung cancer by having practitioners from multiple disciplines collaborate on a treatment and follow-up plan.[170] State-of-the-art services, including rehabilitation and support services, can be tailored to the individual needs of the patient.

It is the nurse in the ambulatory care setting who is positioned to facilitate continuity of care over a period of months or years. Since transitions into new care settings can be particularly stressful for the patient as the illness progresses, the outpatient or office nurse can be a familiar and comforting touchstone, providing reassurance and preventing feelings of abandonment and despair. Often a referral to home health care or hospice is appropriate for the person with lung cancer. Arranging opportunities for contact with the new agency before the transition actually takes place creates a linkage between the care settings and promotes a feeling of control and orientation for the patient and family. Most home care nurses are trained to administer chemotherapy in the home setting, and all are required to manage the complex symptoms and side effects that are associated with lung cancer and its treatment. Communication back to the referring physician is vital in maximizing opportunities for successful management of care in the home.

When medical care for the person with lung cancer shifts from curative to palliative, the patient and family must choose a care setting. Home or hospice care can provide familiar surroundings, feelings of normalcy, involvement of family, and less cost,[148] although not all individuals have family members or friends who are willing or able to provide care. Although hospice has proved to be an extremely effective model for terminal care, referrals to a hospice often are not made until the final days or hours of life. The difficulty lies in predicting when death will occur, since Medicare reimbursement requires that a hospice patient have a life expectancy of six months or less. A case manager or other nurse responsible for coordination of care can help to make more timely referrals to hospice because of familiarity with the patient and improved communication among all care providers.

Regardless of the setting, self-care should be promoted along the continuum of care. Most effects of lung cancer and its treatment will be experienced in the home, and the patient and family must be taught how to manage them. A learning needs assessment should be conducted, with particular attention to willingness, desire, and ability to learn. Barriers to learning, such as illiteracy and environmental and social factors, should be assessed. Supportive resources for self-care should be provided as required by the individual situation. Patients will be able to manage less self-care as the disease progresses, and family members will require education with demonstration of care techniques, return demonstration, and opportunities for questions and verbalization of feelings about caring for the one who is ill.

Conclusion

Despite discouraging survival statistics for lung cancer, there is reason for optimism as one considers the disease trajectory. Emphasis on primary and secondary prevention will decrease the incidence and prevalence. Discoveries in chemoprevention and early identification of premalignant lung cells increase our hope for effective early intervention. Promising new chemotherapeutic agents and multimodality treatments are improving cure and control rates. Increasingly effective strategies for palliative care, including pain control, symptom management, and emotional support, are serving to promote comfort and well-being during the final days of life. The nurse has opportunities at every juncture of the patient's care for clinical practice, education, and research. Each

role will have increasing importance as the fight against this epidemic disease escalates.

References

1. Lee-Chiong TL, Matthay RA: Lung cancer in the elderly patient. *Clin Chest Med* 14:453–472, 1993
2. Samet JM: The epidemiology of lung cancer. *Chest* 103: 20S–29S, 1993 (suppl)
3. Dumas L: Lung cancer in women. *Nurs Clin North Am* 27: 859–869, 1992
4. Gilliland FD, Samet JM: Lung cancer. *Cancer Surv* 19: 175–195, 1994
5. American Cancer Society: *Cancer Facts and Figures—1996*. Atlanta, American Cancer Society, 1996
6. Landis SH, Murray T, Bolden S, et al: Cancer statistics, 1999. *CA Cancer J Clin* 49:8–31, 1999
7. Nathan FE: Introduction. *Semin Oncol* 20:103–104, 1993
8. Franklin RA: Smoking. *Nurs Clin North Am* 27:631–642, 1992
9. Parker SL, Davis KJ, Wingo PA, et al: Cancer statistics by race and ethnicity. *CA Cancer J Clin* 48:31–48, 1998
10. Chyou P, Nomura AM, Stemmermann GN: A prospective study of the attributable risk of cancer due to cigarette smoking. *Am J Public Health* 82:37–40, 1992
11. Glover J, Miaskowski C: Small cell lung cancer: pathophysiologic mechanisms and nursing implications. *Oncol Nurs Forum* 21:87–95, 1994
12. Potanovich LM: Lung cancer: prevention and detection update. *Semin Oncol* 9:174–179, 1993
13. Seale DD, Beaver BM: Pathophysiology of lung cancer. *Nurs Clin North Am* 27:603–613, 1992
14. Wynder E, Kabat GC: The effect of low yield cigarette smoking on lung cancer risk. *Cancer* 62:1223–1230, 1988
15. Tredaniel J, Boffetta P, Saracci R, et al: Exposure to environmental tobacco smoke and risk of lung cancer: the epidemiological evidence. *Eur Respir J* 7:1877–1888, 1994
16. U.S. Environmental Protection Agency: Respiratory Health Effects of Passive Smoking: Lung Cancer and Other Disorders. EPA/600/6-90/006 F. Washington, DC, Office of Research and Development, 1992
17. Burns DM: Environmental tobacco smoke: the price of scientific certainty. *J Natl Cancer Inst* 84:1387–1388, 1992
18. Janerich DT, Thompson WD, Varela LR, et al: Lung cancer and exposure to tobacco smoke in the household. *N Engl J Med* 323:632–636, 1990
19. Ginsberg RJ, Kris MG, Armstrong JG: Non-small cell lung cancer, in DeVita VT, Hellman S, Rosenberg SA (eds): *Cancer: Principles and Practice of Oncology* (ed 4). Philadelphia, Lippincott, 1993, pp 673–722
20. Kishimoto T, Okada K: The relationship between lung cancer and asbestos exposure. *Chest* 94:486–490, 1988
21. Omenn GS, Goodman GE, Thornquist MD, et al: Effects of a combination of beta carotene and vitamin A on lung cancer and cardiovascular disease. *N Engl J Med* 334: 1150–1155, 1996
22. Hennekens CH, Buring JE, Manson JE, et al: Lack of effect of long-term supplementation with beta carotene on the incidence of malignant neoplasms and cardiovascular disease. *N Engl J Med* 334:1145–1149, 1996
23. MacKenzie TD, Bartecchi CE, Schrier RW: The human costs of tobacco use: part II. *N Engl J Med* 330:975–980, 1994

24. Ernster VL: Women and smoking. *Am J Public Health* 83: 1202–1203, 1993 (editorial)
25. Fischer PM, Schwartz MP, Richards JW, et al: Brand logo recognition by children, aged 3 to 6 years: Mickey Mouse and Old Joe the camel. *JAMA* 266:3145–3153, 1991
26. Stotts RC, Glynn TJ, Baquet CR: Smoking cessation among blacks. *J Health Care Poor Underserved* 2:307–319, 1991
27. Carroll-Johnson RM: Smoke screen. *Oncol Nurs Forum* 22: 1331, 1995 (editorial)
28. Aisner J, Belani CP: Lung cancer: recent changes and expectations of improvements. *Semin Oncol* 20:383–393, 1993
29. Rose MA: Intervention strategies for smoking cessation: the role of oncology nursing. *Cancer Nurs* 14:225–231, 1991
30. Risser NL: Prevention of lung cancer: the key is to stop smoking. *Semin Oncol Nurs* 12:260–269, 1996
31. Miller NH: Tips for smoking cessation. *Heart Dis Stroke* 2: 5–7, 1993
32. Stanislaw A, Wewers ME: A smoking cessation intervention with hospitalized surgical cancer patients: a pilot study. *Cancer Nurs* 17:81–86, 1994
33. The Agency for Health Care Policy and Research Smoking Cessation Clinical Practice Guideline. *JAMA* 275:1270–1280, 1996
34. Cromwell J, Bartosch WJ, Fiore MC, et al: Cost-effectiveness of the clinical practice recommendations in the AHCPR Guideline for Smoking Cessation. *JAMA* 278:1759–1766, 1997
35. Manley M, Epps RP, Husten C, et al: Clinical interventions in tobacco control: a National Cancer Institute training program for physicians. *JAMA* 266:3172–3173, 1991
36. Hollis JF, Lichtenstein E, Vogt TM, et al: Nurse-assisted counseling for smokers in primary care. *Ann Intern Med* 118:521–525, 1993
37. Fiore MC: The new vital sign: assessing and documenting smoking status. *JAMA* 266:3183–3184, 1991
38. Lerman C, Orleans CT, Engstrom PF: Biological markers in smoking cessation treatment. *Semin Oncol* 20:359–367, 1993
39. Risser NL, Belcher DW: Adding spirometry, carbon monoxide, and pulmonary symptom results to smoking cessation counseling: a randomized trial. *J Gen Intern Med* 5: 16–22, 1990
40. Velicer WF, Prochaska JO, Rossi JS, et al: Assessing outcome in smoking cessation studies. *Psychol Bull* 111:35–41, 1992
41. Hurt RD, Lowell CD, Fredrickson PA, et al: Nicotine patch therapy for smoking cessation combined with physician advice and nurse follow-up. *JAMA* 271:595–600, 1994
42. Heatherton TF, Kozlowski LT, Frecker RC, et al: The Fagerstrom test for nicotine dependence: a revision of the Fagerstrom tolerance questionnaire. *Br J Addict* 86:1119–1127, 1991
43. Fowler JS, Volkow ND, Wang GJ, et al: Inhibition of monoamine oxidase B in the brains of smokers. *Nature* 379: 733–736, 1996
44. Ascher JA, Cole JO, Colin JN, et al: Bupropion: a review of its mechanism of antidepressant activity. *J Clin Psych* 56: 395–401,1995
45. Hurt RD, Sachs DPL, Glover ED, et al: A comparison of sustained-release bupropion and placebo for smoking cessation. *N Engl J Med* 337:1195–1202, 1997
46. Huber MH, Lee JS, Hong WK: Chemoprevention of lung cancer. *Semin Oncol* 20:128–141, 1993
47. Lippman SM, Benner SE, Hong WK: Chemoprevention strategies in lung carcinogenesis. *Chest* 103:15S–19S, 1993 (suppl)
48. Goodman GE: Chemoprophylaxis strategies in high-risk groups with an emphasis on lung cancer. *Chest* 103: 60S–62S, 1993 (suppl)
49. Bunn PA: Future directions in clinical research for lung cancer. *Chest* 106:399S–407S, 1994 (suppl)
50. Christenson P, Joergensen K, Munk J, et al: Hyperfrequency of pulmonary cancer in a population of 415 patients treated for laryngeal cancer. *Laryngoscope* 97: 612–614, 1987
51. Hong WK, Lippman SM, Itri LM, et al: Prevention of second primary tumors with isotretinoin in squamous-cell carcinoma of the head and neck. *N Engl J Med* 323:795–801, 1990
52. The effect of vitamin E and beta carotene on the incidence of lung cancer and other cancers in male smokers. The Alpha-Tocopherol, Beta Carotene Cancer Prevention Study Group. *N Engl J Med* 330:1029–1035,1994
53. Levy J, Bosin E, Feldman B, et al: Lycopene is a more potent inhibitor of human cancer cell proliferation than either alpha-carotene or beta-carotene. *Nutr Cancer* 24: 257–266, 1995
54. Szabo E, Birrer MJ, Mulshine JL: Early detection of lung cancer. *Semin Oncol* 20:374–382, 1993
55. Singh DK, Lippman SM: Cancer chemoprevention—part 1: retinoids and carotenoids and other classic antioxidants. *Oncology* 12:1643–1658, 1998
56. Feld R, Ginsberg RJ, Payne DG, et al: Lung, in Abeloff MD, Armitage JO, Lichter AS, Niederhuber JE (eds): *Clinical Oncology.* New York, Churchill-Livingstone, 1995, pp 1083–1152
57. Mulshine JL, Treston AM, Brown PH, et al: Initiators and promoters of lung cancer. *Chest* 103:4S–9S, 1993 (suppl)
58. Tockman MS, Gupta PK, Myers JD, et al: Sensitive and specific monoclonal antibody recognition of human lung cancer antigen on preserved sputum cells: a new approach to early lung cancer detection. *J Clin Oncol* 6:1685–1693, 1988
59. Chia MM, Gazdar AF, Carbone DP, et al: Biology of lung cancer, in Murray JF, Nadel JA (eds): *Textbook of Respiratory Medicine* (ed 2). Philadelphia, Saunders, 1994, pp 1485–1503
60. Ihde DC, Pass HI, Glatstein EJ: Small cell lung cancer, in DeVita VT, Hellman S, Rosenberg SA (eds): *Cancer: Principles and Practice of Oncology* (ed 4). Philadelphia, Lippincott, 1993, pp 723–758
61. McCue PA, Finkel GC: Small-cell lung carcinoma: an evolving histopathological spectrum. *Semin Oncol* 20:153–162, 1993
62. Richardson GE, Johnson BE: The biology of lung cancer. *Semin Oncol* 20:105–127, 1993
63. Johnson BE, Kelley MJ: Biology of small cell lung cancer. *Lung Cancer* 12:S5–S16, 1995 (suppl)
64. Elpern EH: Lung cancer, in Groenwald SL, Frogge MH, Goodman M, Yarbro CH (eds): *Cancer Nursing: Principles and Practice* (ed 3). Sudbury, MA, Jones and Bartlett, 1993, pp 1174–1199
65. Epps ME: Diagnostic testing for patients with lung cancer. *Nurs Clin North Am* 27:615–629, 1992
66. Holmes CE, Livingston R, Turrisi A: Neoplasms of the thorax, in Holland JF, Frei E, Bast RC, Kufe DW, Morton DL, Weichselbaum RR (eds): *Cancer Medicine* (ed 3). Malvern, PA, Lea and Febiger, 1993, pp 1285–1336
67. Pancrazio JJ, Viglione MP, Tabbara IA, et al: Voltage-dependent ion channels in small-cell lung cancer cells. *Cancer Res* 49:5901–5906, 1989
68. Nesbitt JC, Lee JS, Komaki R, et al: Cancer of the lung,

in Holland JF, Bast RC, Morton DL, Frei E, Kufe DW, Weichselbaum RR (eds): *Cancer Medicine* (ed 4). Baltimore, Williams and Wilkins, 1997, pp 1723–1803

69. Marchioli CC, Graziano SL: Paraneoplastic syndromes associated with small cell lung cancer. *Chest Surg Clin North Am* 7:65–80, 1997

70. Sanders DB: Lambert-Eaton myasthenic syndrome: pathogenesis and treatment. *Semin Neurol* 14:111–117, 1994

71. Struthers CS: Lambert-Eaton myasthenic syndrome in small cell lung cancer: nursing implications. *Oncol Nurs Forum* 21:677–683, 1994

72. Assessment of the respiratory system, in Malasanos L, Barkauskas V, Stoltenberg-Allen K (eds): *Health Assessment* (ed 4). St. Louis, Mosby, 1990, 297–324

73. Patient assessment, in DesJardins T, Burton GG (eds): *Clinical Manifestations and Assessment of Respiratory Disease* (ed 3). St. Louis, Mosby-Year Book, 1995, pp 3–118

74. Shaffer K: Imaging and medical staging of lung cancer. *Hematol Oncol Clin North Am* 11:197–213, 1997

75. Thompson AB, Rennard SI: Diagnostic procedures not involving the pleura, in Baum GL, Crapo JD, Celli BR, Karlinsky JB (eds): *Textbook of Pulmonary Diseases* (ed 6). Philadelphia, Lippincott-Raven, 1998, pp 239–253

76. Sugarbaker DJ, Strauss GM: Advances in surgical staging and therapy of non-small-cell lung cancer. *Semin Oncol* 20: 163–172, 1993

77. Rea HH, Sherland JE, House AJS: Accuracy of computed tomographic scanning in assessment of the mediastinum in bronchial carcinoma. *J Thorac Cardiovasc Surg* 81:825–829, 1981

78. Mentzer SJ, DeCamp MM, Harpole DH, Sugarbaker DJ: Thoracoscopy and video-assisted thoracic surgery in the treatment of lung cancer. *Chest* 107:298S–301S, 1995

79. Buccheri G, Ferrigno GB: Prognostic factors in lung cancer: tables and comments. *Eur Respir J* 7:1350–1364, 1994

80. Souhami RL, Law K: A report to the lung cancer subcommittee of the United Kingdom coordinating committee for cancer research. *Br J Cancer* 61:584–589, 1990

81. Shepherd FA: Treatment of advanced non-small cell lung cancer. *Semin Oncol* 21:7–18, 1994 (suppl 7)

82. Stitik FP: The new staging of lung cancer. *Radiol Clin North Am* 32:635–647, 1994

83. Sidransky D, Hollstein M: Clinical implications of the p53 gene. *Annu Rev Med* 47:285–301, 1996

84. Mitsudomi T, Lam S, Shirakusa T, et al: Detection and sequencing of p53 gene mutations in bronchial biopsy samples in patients with lung cancer. *Chest* 104:362–365, 1993

85. Lee J, Yoon A, Kalapurakal S, et al: Expression of p53 oncoprotein in non-small-cell lung cancer: a favorable prognostic factor. *J Clin Oncol* 13:1893–1903, 1995

86. Salgia R, Skarin AT: Molecular abnormalities in lung cancer. *J Clin Oncol* 16:1207–1217, 1998

87. Mountain CF: Revisions in the International System for Staging Lung Cancer. *Chest* 111:1710–1717, 1997

88. American Joint Committee on Cancer: *AJCC Cancer Staging Manual* (ed 5). Philadelphia, Lippincott-Raven, 1997

89. Lederle FA, Niewoehner DE: Lung cancer surgery: a critical review of the evidence. *Arch Intern Med* 154:2397–2400, 1994

90. Langston WG: Surgical resection of lung cancer. *Nurs Clin North Am* 27:665–679, 1992

91. Harpole DH, Herndon JE, Young WG, et al: Stage I non-small cell lung cancer: a multivariate analysis of treatment methods and patterns of recurrence. *Cancer* 76:787–796, 1995

92. Pearson FG: Current status of surgical resection for lung cancer. *Chest* 106:337S–339S, 1994 (suppl)

93. Ginsberg RJ, Rubinstein L: The comparison of limited resection to lobectomy for T1N0 non-small cell lung cancer: LCSG 821. *Chest* 106:318S–319S, 1994 (suppl)

94. Beattie EJ, Harvey JC, Pisch J: Lung, in Beattie EJ, Bloom N, Harvey J (eds): *Thoracic Surgical Oncology*. New York, Churchill-Livingstone, 1992, pp 27–185

95. Stewart GS: Trends in radiation therapy for the treatment of lung cancer. *Nurs Clin North Am* 27:643–651, 1992

96. Sibley GS: Radiotherapy for patients with medically inoperable stage I nonsmall cell lung carcinoma. *Cancer* 82: 433–438, 1998

97. Belani CP: Multimodality management of regionally advanced non-small-cell lung cancer. *Semin Oncol* 20:302–314, 1993

98. Hazuka MB, Turrisi AT: The evolving role of radiation therapy in the treatment of locally advanced lung cancer. *Semin Oncol* 20:173–184, 1993

99. Bailey AJ, Parmor MKB, Stephens RJ: Patient-reported short-term and long-term physical and psychologic symptoms: results of the Continuous Hyperfractionated Accelerated Radiotherapy (CHART) Randomized Trial in non-small-cell lung cancer. *J Clin Oncol* 16: 3082–3093, 1998

100. Sause WT, Scott C, Taylor S, et al: Radiation Therapy Oncology Group (RTOG) 88-08 and Eastern Cooperative Oncology Group (ECOG) 4588: preliminary results of a phase III trial in regionally advanced, unresectable non-small cell lung cancer. *J Natl Cancer Inst* 87:198–205, 1995

101. Turrisi AT: Innovations in multimodality therapy for lung cancer: combined modality management of limited small-cell lung cancer. *Chest* 103:56S–59S, 1993 (suppl)

102. Williams TE, Turrisi AT: Role of radiotherapy in the treatment of small cell lung cancer. *Chest Surg Clin North Am* 7: 135–149, 1997

103. Harris DT: Prophylactic cranial irradiation in small-cell lung cancer. *Semin Oncol* 20:338–350, 1993

104. Kristjansen PEG, Hansen HH: Prophylactic cranial irradiation in small cell lung cancer: an update. *Lung Cancer* 12: S23–S40, 1995 (suppl)

105. Kim Y, Kondziolka D, Flickinger J, et al: Stereotactic radiosurgery for patients with nonsmall cell lung carcinoma metastatic to the brain. *Cancer* 80:2075–2083, 1997

106. Gustafson G, Vicini F, Freedman L, et al: High dose rate endobronchial brachytherapy in the management of primary and recurrent bronchogenic malignancies. *Cancer* 75:2345–2350, 1995

107. Jordan LN, Mantravadi R: Nursing care of the patient receiving high dose rate brachytherapy. *Oncol Nurs Forum* 18:1167–1171, 1991

108. Khanavkar B, Stern P, Alberti W, et al: Complications associated with brachytherapy alone or with laser in lung cancer. *Chest* 99:1062–1065, 1991

109. Larson PJ, Lindsey AM, Dodd MJ, et al: Influence of age on problems experienced by patients with lung cancer undergoing radiation therapy. *Oncol Nurs Forum* 20: 473–480, 1993

110. Brown JK: Gender, age, usual weight, and tobacco use as predictors of weight loss in patients with lung cancer. *Oncol Nurs Forum* 20:466–472, 1993

111. Evans WK: Management of metastatic non-small-cell lung cancer and a consideration of cost. *Chest* 103:68S–71S, 1993

112. Feigal EG, Christian M, Cheson B, et al: New chemotherapeutic agents in non-small-cell lung cancer. *Semin Oncol* 20:185–201, 1993

113. Shepherd FA: Future directions in the treatment of non-small cell lung cancer. *Semin Oncol* 21:48–62, 1994 (suppl 4)

114. Faber LP: Current status of neoadjuvant therapy for non-small cell lung cancer. *Chest* 106:355S–358S, 1994 (suppl)

115. Rosell R, Gomez-Codina J, Camps C, et al: A randomized trial comparing preoperative chemotherapy plus surgery with surgery alone in patients with non-small cell lung cancer. *N Engl J Med* 330:153–158, 1994

116. Roth JA, Fossella F, Komaki R, et al: A randomized trial comparing perioperative chemotherapy and surgery with surgery alone in resectable stage IIIa NSCLC. *J Natl Cancer Inst* 86:673–680, 1994.

117. Einhorn LH: Neoadjuvant and adjuvant trials in non-small cell lung cancer. *Ann Thorac Surg* 65:208–211, 1998

118. Sweeney CJ, Sandler AB: Treatment of advanced (stages III and IV) non-small-cell lung cancer. *Curr Probl Cancer* 22:81–132, 1998

119. Livingston RB: Current management of unresectable non-small cell lung cancer. *Semin Oncol* 21:4–13, 1994

120. Johnson DH, Einhorn LH: Paclitaxel plus carboplatin: an effective combination chemotherapy for advanced non-small-cell lung cancer or just another Elvis sighting? *J Clin Oncol* 13:1840–1842, 1995 (editorial)

121. Doyle LA: Mechanisms of drug resistance in human lung cancer cells. *Semin Oncol* 20:326–337, 1993

122. Vokes EE: Integration of vinorelbine into chemotherapy strategies for non-small-cell lung cancer. *Oncology* 9:565–582, 1995

123. Eckardt J, Eckhardt G, Villalona-Calero M, et al: New anti-cancer agents in clinical development. *Oncology* 9:1191–1199, 1995

124. Langer CJ, Leighton JC, Comis RL, et al: Paclitaxel and carboplatin in combination in the treatment of advanced non-small-cell lung cancer: a phase II toxicity, response, and survival analysis. *J Clin Oncol* 13:1860–1870, 1995

125. Bunn PA: Triplet chemotherapy combinations with new agents: is there a rationale? *Semin Oncol* 25:55–61, 1998 (suppl 9)

126. Belani CP, Natale RB, Lee JS, et al: Randomized phase III trial comparing cisplatin/etoposide versus carboplatin/paclitaxel in advanced and metastatic non-small cell lung cancer (NSCLC). *Proc Am Soc Clin Oncol* 17:455a, 1998

127. Carney DN: New agents in the management of advanced non-small cell lung cancer. *Semin Oncol* 25:83–88, 1998 (suppl 9)

128. Viallet J, Ayoub J, Rousseau P, et al: Vinorelbine (Navelbine) in the adjuvant and neoadjuvant treatment of non-small cell lung cancer. *Semin Oncol* 21:64–72, 1994 (suppl 10)

129. Johnson DH: Recent developments in chemotherapy treatment of small-cell lung cancer. *Semin Oncol* 20:315–325, 1993

130. Blackstein ME: Advances in chemotherapy for small cell lung cancer. *Semin Oncol* 21:38–42, 1994

131. Kosmidis PA, Samantas E, Fountzilas G, et al: Cisplatin/etoposide versus carboplatin/etoposide chemotherapy and irradiation in small cell lung cancer: a randomized phase III study. *Semin Oncol* 21:23–30, 1994

132. Clark R, Ihde DC: Small-cell lung cancer: treatment progress and prospects. *Oncology* 12:647–658, 1998

133. Postmus PE, Schramel FMNH, Smit EF: Evaluation of new drugs in small cell lung cancer: the activity of gemcitabine. *Semin Oncol* 25:79–82, 1998 (suppl 9)

134. Ettinger DS, Finkelstein DM, Sarma R, et al: Phase II study of paclitaxel in patients with extensive disease small cell

135. Smyth JF, Smith IE, Sessa C, et al: Activity of docetaxel in small cell lung cancer. The early clinical trials groups of the EORTC. *Eur J Cancer* 30A:1058–1060, 1994

136. Schiller JH, Kim K, Hutson P, et al: Phase II study of topotecan in patients with extensive-stage small cell carcinoma of the lungs: an Eastern Cooperative Group trial. *J Clin Oncol* 14:2345–2352, 1996

137. Fujita A, Takabatake H, Tagaki S, et al: Pilot study of irinotecan in refractory small cell lung cancer. *Gan To Kagaku Ryoho* 22:889–893, 1995

138. Johnson DH: Treatment of the elderly patient with small-cell lung cancer. *Chest* 103:72S–74S, 1993 (suppl)

139. Pate RW: The role of chemotherapy in the treatment of lung cancer. *Nurs Clin North Am* 27:653–663, 1992

140. Fishbein GE: Immunotherapy of lung cancer. *Semin Oncol* 20:351–358, 1993

141. Lam S: Photodynamic therapy of lung cancer. *Semin Oncol* 21:15–19, 1994

142. Gelb AF, Epstein JD: Laser in treatment of lung cancer. *Chest* 86:662–666, 1984

143. Benedict S: The suffering associated with lung cancer. *Cancer Nurs* 12:34–40, 1989

144. Cassell E: The Nature of Suffering and the Goals of Medicine. New York, Oxford University Press, 1991

145. Cassell E: The nature of suffering: physical, psychological, social and spiritual aspects, in Starck P, McGovern J (eds): *The Hidden Dimension of Illness: Human Suffering.* New York, National League for Nursing Press, 1992, pp 1–10

146. Sarna L: Effectiveness of structured nursing assessment of symptom distress in advanced lung cancer. *Oncol Nurs Forum* 25:1041–1048, 1998

147. Bernhard J, Ganz PA: Psychosocial issues in lung cancer patients (part 1). *Chest* 99:216–223, 1991

148. Turner JT: Nursing care of the terminal lung cancer patient. *Nurs Clin North Am* 27:691–702, 1992

149. Wickham RS: Managing dyspnea in cancer patients. *Dev Support Cancer Care* 2(2):33–40, 1998

150. Blendowski C, Haapoja IS: Pleural access port: a creative alternative to repeated thoracentesis. *Dev Support Cancer Care* 2(2):41–44, 1998

151. Keller SM: Current and future therapy for malignant pleural effusion. *Chest* 103:63S–67S, 1993 (suppl)

152. Sahn SA: Malignant effusions. *Emerg Med* 23(5):119–126, 1991

153. Wilkie DJ, Williams AR, Grevstad P, et al: Coaching persons with lung cancer to report sensory pain. *Cancer Nurs* 18:7–15, 1995

154. Management of Cancer Pain Panel: *Management of Cancer Pain.* U.S. Department of Health and Human Services, Agency for Health Care Policy and Research publication No. 94–0593. Rockville, MD, 1994

155. Schmitt R: Quality of life issues in lung cancer: new symptom management strategies. *Chest* 103:51S–55S, 1993 (suppl)

156. Kuuppelomaki M, Lauri S: Cancer patients' reported experiences of suffering. *Cancer Nurs* 21:364–369, 1998

157. Sarna L: Functional status in women with lung cancer. *Cancer Nurs* 17:87–93, 1994

158. Sarna L: Fluctuations in physical function: adults with non-small cell lung cancer. *J Adv Nurs* 18:714–724, 1993

159. Blesch KS, Paice JA, Wickham R, et al: Correlates of fatigue in people with breast or lung cancer. *Oncol Nurs Forum* 18:81–87, 1991

160. Sarna L, Lindsey AM, Dean H, et al: Nutritional intake, weight change, symptom distress, and functional status over time in adults with lung cancer. *Oncol Nurs Forum* 20: 481–489, 1993

161. Dewys WD, Begg C, Lavin PT, et al: Prognostic effect of weight loss prior to chemotherapy in cancer patients. *Am J Med* 69:491–497, 1980

162. Houston SJ, Kendall JA: Psychosocial implications of lung cancer. *Nurs Clin North Am* 27:681–690, 1992

163. Klemm PR: Variables influencing psychosocial adjustment in lung cancer: a preliminary study. *Oncol Nurs Forum* 21: 1059–1062, 1994

164. Berckman KL, Austin JK: Causal attribution, perceived control and adjustment in patients with lung cancer. *Oncol Nurs Forum* 20:23–30, 1993

165. Cooley ME: Quality of life in persons with non-small cell lung cancer: a concept analysis. *Cancer Nurs* 21:151–159, 1998

166. Bernhard J, Ganz PA: Psychosocial issues in lung cancer patients (part 2). *Chest* 99:480–485, 1991

167. Sarna L, Ganley BJ: A survey of lung cancer patient-education materials. *Oncol Nurs Forum* 22:1545–1550, 1995

168. Beddar SM, Aikin JL: Continuity of care: a challenge for ambulatory oncology nursing. *Semin Oncol Nurs* 10: 254–263, 1994

169. Rostad M: Advances in nursing management of patients with lung cancer. *Nurs Clin North Am* 25:393–403, 1990

170. An update on the new USC/Norris Lung Cancer Management Center. *Cope*, July/August 1995, pp 16–17

CHAPTER 60

Malignant Lymphomas

Connie Henke Yarbro, MS, RN, FAAN

Introduction

The malignant lymphomas constitute a diverse group of neoplasms that arise from the uncontrolled proliferation of the cellular components of the lymphoreticular system. This complex network of specialized cells and organs defends the body against infection. Malignancies of the immune system may present locally; however, the majority are widespread at the time of diagnosis, presumably because of the natural ability of the immune cells to circulate. Based on histological characteristics, the lymphomas are divided into two major subgroups—Hodgkin's disease (HD) and non-Hodgkin's lymphoma (NHL). Some suggest that the term *lymphocytic lymphoma* be ascribed to the latter because it emphasizes the essential role that lymphocyte transformation has in its ontogeny. However, both terms are equally acceptable, and since NHL is used most frequently in practice and in the literature, it is selected for this chapter.

Lymphomas are among the most studied human tumors, and determination of their immunophenotypes, gene rearrangements, cytogenetic abnormalities, and oncogene activation are providing valuable clues about the inherent mechanisms of the neoplastic process itself. Also, some are considered to be among the most curable of all malignancies. Impetus for this clinical success is provided by therapeutic advances using combination chemotherapy, chemotherapy plus radiation therapy, and ablative chemotherapy followed by bone marrow transplantation in patients with refractory disease.

Despite a number of shared superficial similarities, the distinctions between HD and NHL are important because their clinical courses, prognoses, and treatments are substantially different. Indeed, controversy truly begins at the cellular level with an unresolved debate about their respective cells of origin. Although several distinct T-cell lymphomas have been identified, B-cell neoplasms account for the majority of non-Hodgkin's lymphomas. A variety of candidates have been proposed for the originating cell in HD, including lymphocytes (T and B), monocytes-macrophages, and interdigitating reticulum cells.[1] At least some Reed-Sternberg cells of HD have a B lymphocyte as the cell of origin based on immunoglobulin gene rearrangements, and several sites of loss of heterozygosity have been identified.[2] The Epstein-Barr virus (EBV) seems to be related to transformation in some but not all cases of HD.[3]

The clinical behavior of the malignant lymphomas is highly variable. Some patients follow a rapid downhill course, with progressive generalized adenopathy, fever, night sweats, splenomegaly, and infiltration of the bone marrow, lungs, liver, and other organs with proliferative neoplastic cells. Death occurs within one to two years of diagnosis and usually results from infection, hemorrhage due to tumor-induced destruction of the bone marrow, or systemic failure of vital organ function. Other individuals follow a more indolent course in which the disease is apparently limited to the lymph nodes for many years.

Eventually the malignant process becomes more aggressive, and invasion of extranodal organs requires a revision in management strategies.

Recent statistical analysis indicates that the incidence of lymphomas, particularly NHL, is escalating, and it has now become the fifth most common cancer in the United States. Incidence in 1999 is estimated at 64,000 newly diagnosed cases and the annual mortality rate is expected to reach 27,000.[4] A major factor contributing to this increase is the established association between NHL and the acquired immunodeficiency syndrome (AIDS) caused by the retrovirus known as human immunodeficiency virus (HIV). Advances in antiviral therapy and treatment or prophylaxis against opportunistic infections have resulted in the prolonged survival of AIDS patients, and a substantial increase in secondary NHL has been noted in the AIDS population. Gail and associates[5] estimated that 8%–27% of all 1992 cases of NHL would be attributable to this syndrome. There is, in addition to the NHL in the AIDS population, an independent and dramatic increase in NHL that began before the AIDS epidemic, the cause of which is unknown.[6] Thus, this malignancy truly has the potential to become an increasing burden and challenge to health care systems well into the twenty-first century.

In an effort to help oncology nurses effect optimal patient care and education, this chapter provides comprehensive information about the etiology, classifications, clinical manifestations, staging, diagnosis, and therapeutic management of HD and NHL. Treatment and disease-related complications as well as important issues related to survivorship are also addressed.

The Immune System and Neoplasia

The immune system is a highly integrated, complex mechanism that has evolved to help the body protect itself against foreign tissues and invading microbes such as viruses, bacteria, fungi, and parasites. It distinguishes such threats from normal tissue by recognizing invasive antigens or foreign molecules as "nonself" and seeks to eliminate or destroy them by mounting an appropriate response via the formation of antigen-specific protein antibodies.[7] The organs of the immune system are scattered throughout the body and are generally referred to as *lymphatic* or *lymphoid* organs because they are concerned with the growth, development, and deployment of T and B lymphocytes. These white blood cells are the key operatives of immune function and the primary cellular component of malignant lymphomas. The lymphoid organs, as illustrated in Figure 60-1, include the spleen, bone marrow, thymus, lymph nodes, tonsils, adenoids, appendix, and clumps of lymphoid tissue in the small intestine known as Peyer's patches. The blood and lymphatic vessels that transport lymphocytes also can be considered part of this system.

Lymph is derived from interstitial fluid and flows through lymphatic vessels transporting immune cells and

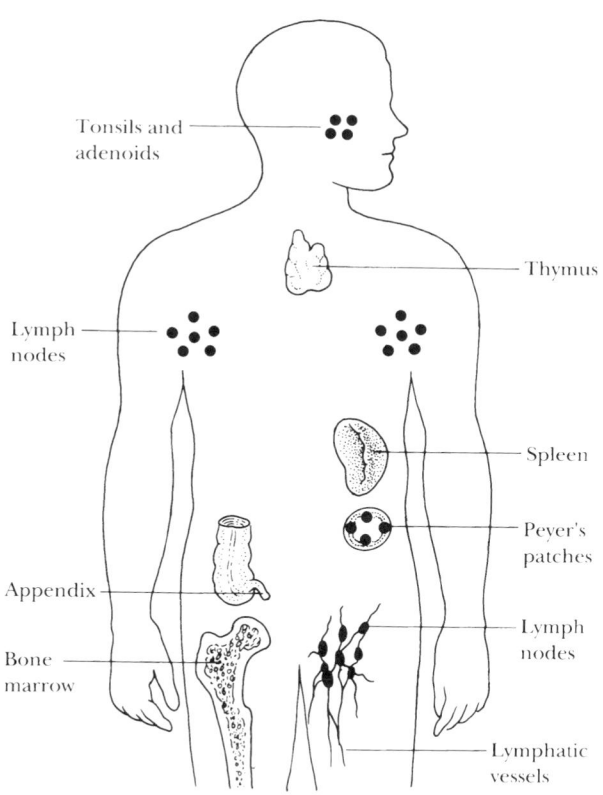

Figure 60-1 Organs of the immune system (Illustrated by J. Thommen.)

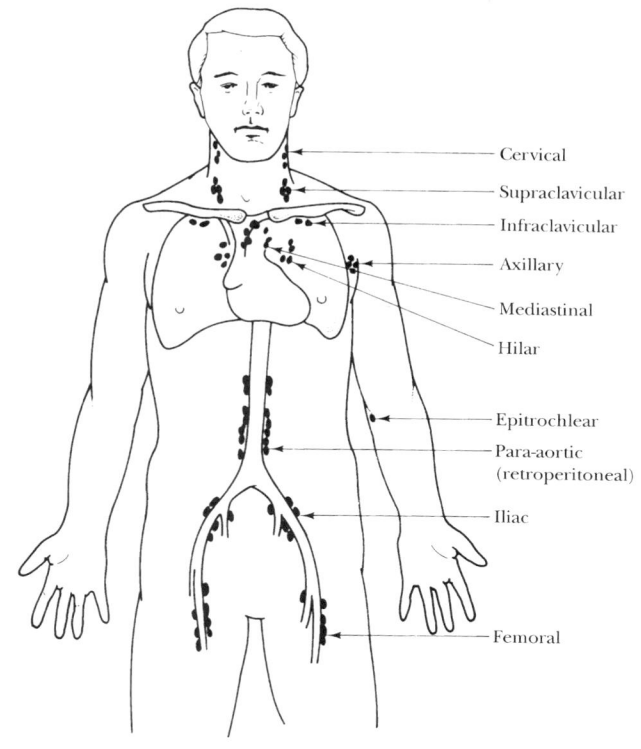

Figure 60-2 Major lymph node groups

foreign antigens to the circulatory system via the thoracic duct. Along its course, detritus is filtered out of lymph by the lymph nodes. These small, encapsulated clusters in the neck, axilla, abdomen, and groin (Figure 60-2) have a very specific structure and contain specialized compartments that facilitate lymphocyte maturation and differentiation. T lymphocytes are selectively concentrated in the paracortical regions of the lymph node and within the periarterial lymphoid sheaths of the spleen. Small numbers of T cells are also found within the follicles, where they facilitate B-cell differentiation. On the other hand, B lymphocytes are concentrated in the follicles and medullary cords of the lymph nodes and in the follicles of the spleen. The lymphoid follicles represent the proliferative site of the B-cell system, and the medullary cord region represents its secretory component. Monocytes circulate in the peripheral blood, while histiocytes are preferentially found in the subcapsular and medullary sinuses of the lymph nodes and the red pulp of the spleen. Figure 60-3 depicts normal lymph node architecture and the areas associated with lymphoid localization and malignant transformation.

Lymphomas are preeminently a malignancy of the lymphocyte, and the process by which a lymphoid neoplasm is generated may be thought of as a series of cellular changes in which a normal lymphoid cell (or cell clone) becomes refractory to the regulation of its differentiation

and proliferation. These changes are, of necessity, genetic, whether induced by mutation, chromosomal translocation/deletion, or insertion of foreign genes (e.g., viral genes) into the cell. Translocations generally result in altered expression of an adjacent gene. Deletions may cause loss of genes necessary for appropriate cellular regulation and differentiation. Mutations could stimulate either of these effects, while viruses are likely to enhance modification of adjacent genes by viral promotion/enhancement or of distant genes via viral transactivation.

Once transformed, the new clone of malignant cells follows the behavior pattern of the stage at which lymphocyte alteration took place. For example, if the function of the maturing lymphocyte is secretion of an antibody protein, the tumor cells will continue to secrete the normal protein, albeit in abnormal quantities. In this case a faulty regulatory mechanism and not abnormal cell proliferation is responsible for the neoplastic change. However, if the function at the time of transformation is for the lymphocytes to form maturing nodules in the lymph nodes, their excessive production will result in nodular lymphoma.

The association of certain malignancies with congenital or acquired immunodeficiency diseases and the bimodal distribution of cancer in the very young and the very old suggests that an immature or debilitated immune system predisposes to neoplasia.[8] Malignant lymphomas are linked strongly with congenital immunodeficiency disorders such as Wiskott-Aldrich syndrome, Klinefelter

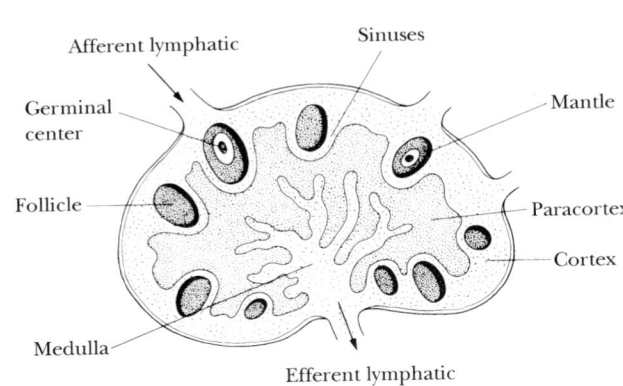

B-CELL LYMPHOMAS
Follicle
- Nodular lymphoma
- Large-cell lymphoma (sonic)
- Burkitt's lymphoma

Germinal Center/Mantle Zone
- Lymphocytic lymphoma
- Mantle zone lymphoma (intermediate differentiation)

Medulla
- Chronic lymphocytic leukemia
- Well-differentiated lymphocytic lymphoma
- Waldenström's macroglobulinemia

T-CELL LYMPHOMAS
Paracortex
- Peripheral T-cell lymphoma
- Mycosis fungoides
- Sézary syndrome
- Acute lymphoblastic leukemia
- T-cell lymphoblastic lymphoma

Miscellaneous Malignancies
Sinus Region
- Malignant histiocytosis
- Kt-1 large-cell lymphoma

Figure 60-3   Sites of lymphocyte transformation in the lymph node (Illustrated by J. Thommen.)

syndrome, and ataxia telangiectasia. The chronic inflammatory process activated by many autoimmune diseases (e.g., rheumatoid arthritis, systemic lupus erythematosus, and Sjögren syndrome) predisposes an individual to lymphomas of extranodal origin. Renal, cardiac, and other organ transplants also have been found to increase risk.[9] Such tumors usually occur in the first year following transplant; they are rapidly progressive and frequently involve the central nervous system. Definitive cause of these lymphomas is unknown, but viral infection, drug-induced immunosuppression, and chronic antigenic stimulation from the graft may be contributing factors.

Maturation of the Lymphocyte

The origin of the lymphocyte can be traced to a pluripotent stem cell in the bone marrow that has the potential to develop into any of the cells that normally circulate in the blood. At each step along the path of differentiation, a cell loses its capacity to proceed along an alternate route. In the first step, the stem cell matures so that it is either the precursor of the lymphocyte series or of all the other cellular series of the blood (erythrocyte, megakaryocyte, polymorphonuclear neutrophil, or monocyte). The lymphocyte precursor then develops into one of a number of types of mature lymphocytes. Figure 60-4 demonstrates the maturation sequence of the immunocompetent lymphocyte.

Lymphocytes are responsible for the two arms of the immunologic defense system: the humoral arm, which consists of plasma cells that produce circulating antibodies against foreign antigens, and the cellular arm, which consists of circulating lymphocytes that have developed specificity against foreign antigens. These two arms of the immune process are distinct, but they function jointly in defending the host against foreign proteins. An early step in the differentiation of the maturing lymphocyte occurs when the cell is programmed either by the bone marrow (bursa equivalent) or by the thymus to become a B lymphocyte or a T lymphocyte, respectively. Humoral immunity is provided by the B lymphocytes, which, when exposed to an appropriate foreign antigen, mature into plasma cells and produce antibodies against that antigen. T lymphocytes, when similarly exposed to a foreign antigen, develop into killer lymphocytes that will attack and destroy the foreign antigen without benefit of an antibody intermediary, thus providing cellular immunity. In addition, some T lymphocytes develop specific regulator roles in which they either suppress or stimulate immune functions (suppressor cells and helper cells).

Eighty percent of lymphomas manifest B-cell origin, and most patients initially present with disease involving bone marrow or lymph nodes. Nonlymphoid tissue extension is also common, particularly in the thyroid, gastrointestinal tract, salivary glands, and conjunctiva. Diagnosis is usually straightforward because of characteristic monoclonal immunoglobulin elevations and/or distinct morphological features. In general, B-cell neoplasms tend to

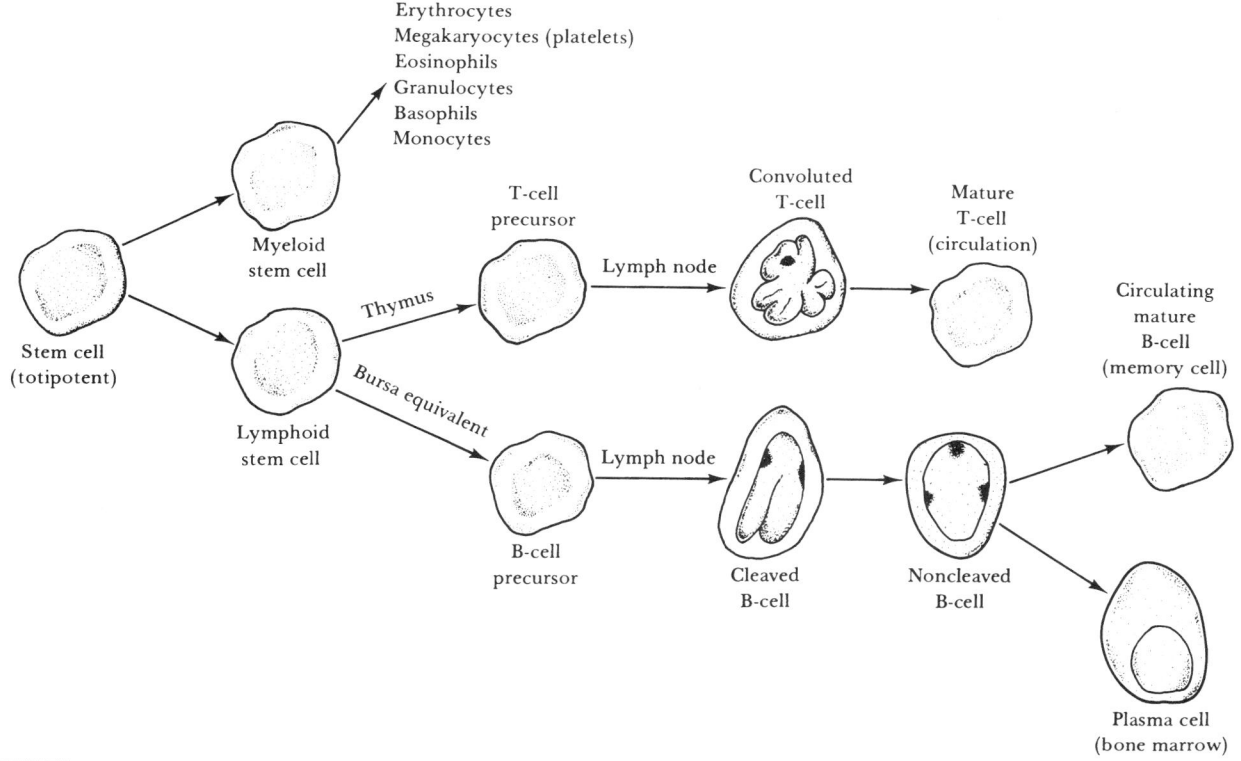

Figure 60-4 Maturation sequence of the lymphocyte (Illustrated by J. Thommen.)

follow a more indolent course than those induced by T-cell transformation.[10]

Lymphomas derived from T lymphocytes are a complex group of diseases with marked biological and clinical heterogeneity. These neoplasms usually arise in bone marrow, thymus, lymph nodes, and skin. They may produce abnormal amounts of lymphokines or may markedly activate histiocytes (macrophages) throughout the body. These activated cells often destroy normal blood cells causing anemia, thrombocytopenia, and/or leukopenia.[11] T-cell lymphomas are generally more aggressive and grow more rapidly than their B-cell counterparts.

HODGKIN'S DISEASE

Historical Perspective

In 1832, Dr. Thomas Hodgkin, an English physician, described clinical data and postmortem findings of seven patients with a relentlessly progressive, ultimately fatal tumorous enlargement of the lymph nodes, liver, and spleen.[12] His recognition that these pathological changes represented a primary proliferation inherent in the nodal tissues themselves rather than a reactive, inflammatory process was extremely important and insightful. Prior to that time, lymphomas often had been mistaken for a common infectious disease, tuberculosis of the lymph nodes.

More than three decades after Hodgkin's paper was presented, Samuel Wilks rediscovered the original manuscript and, after further clinical clarification and elaboration, he attached the eponym *Hodgkin's disease* in 1865.[13] A review of the original tissues nearly 100 years later demonstrated that Hodgkin's cases actually represented examples of what we now call Hodgkin's disease as well as non-Hodgkin's lymphoma. All lymphomas were called HD until around the turn of the century when the giant, multinucleated cells in the nodal material of HD patients were characterized by Reed[14] and Sternberg,[15] and their names have been associated with the pathognomonic cell of HD ever since. Subsequently, those lymphomas demonstrating the Reed-Sternberg cell were classified as *HD* and those in which the cell was absent were called *lymphosarcoma* or *reticulum* cell sarcoma and later *NHL*. Although the nature and origin of the Reed-Sternberg cell remain uncertain, it is clear that this cell is useful in prognosis since lymphocytic malignancies that are similar in pathological appearance behave differently according to the presence or absence of this cell. Today, diagnosis of HD requires two components. First, the presence of Reed-Sternberg cells must be verified. Second, the diagnostic cells must be identified within an appropriate cellular background that is composed of a polymorphous mixture of apparently normal inflammatory cells in various proportions.

Epidemiology

Hodgkin's disease currently accounts for approximately 11% of the malignant lymphomas and less than 1% of all cancers. However, because a disproportionate number of HD victims are young adults, it is viewed as a particularly serious problem. The American Cancer Society estimates that in 1999, 7200 new cases (3800 male and 3400 female) and 1300 deaths will occur.[4] The disease has a world-wide distribution, and its most prominent epidemiological feature pertains to the distinct age-related incidence patterns that have been observed. In developed countries the incidence of HD is clearly bimodal. In these areas the disease is infrequent in children under 10 years old. Incidence rises rapidly in adolescence and has its first peak among young adults age 20–30. Subsequently, it falls until after age 45; then the incidence of new cases begins to climb steadily. This second upslope continues throughout the seventh and eighth decades. Similar bimodality appears to exist in less developed countries except that the young adult age peak is shifted closer to childhood. Of interest is the fact that as underdeveloped geographical areas become increasingly progressive, their incidence patterns of HD change as well. Histological category and anatomic distribution also vary with age. The nodular sclerosis form of the disease predominates in young adults, while mixed cellularity is more common in middle age and lymphocyte-depleted HD is the predominant histology in the elderly.[16]

It has been suggested that HD is really two separate entities and that the first incidence peak may represent a disease of viral etiology, more common in middle-class than in lower-class families and more common in developed than in undeveloped countries.[16] These characteristics are consistent with a virus that is widely disseminated under conditions of poor hygiene and that, if contracted, rarely leads to severe illness. Such a pattern favors the evolution of a subclinical or asymptomatic process in low socioeconomic groups and undeveloped countries because children in such circumstances are antigenically exposed at a very early age, when they are resistant and able to develop immunity. In middle-class families and developed nations, however, improved hygiene delays such exposure until adolescence or young adulthood. Indeed, the general level of home hygiene has been found to correlate inversely with incidence—the better the general sanitation, the higher the risk of HD among children in the household. The second incidence peak of HD in those over age 45 appears to be relatively similar across all societal groups.[17]

Etiology

Although many theories have been proposed, the etiology of HD remains unclear. Because of clinical manifestations such as fever, chills, and leukocytosis, and because of histological similarity to a granulomatous process, an infectious source has long been a topic of speculation. The Epstein-Barr virus (EBV) is now recognized as being associated with several forms of lymphoma. It was initially described in Burkitt's lymphoma in Africa. Subsequently it was described in association with AIDS-related NHL and more recently EBV antigens have been found in the Reed-Sternberg cells of HD.

The exact manner in which EBV interacts to transform lymphocytes to malignant growth has not yet been elucidated. EBV is the etiological agent of infectious mononucleosis, in which it infects B lymphocytes and causes them to proliferate. This polyclonal proliferation is subsequently brought under control by T lymphocytes in subjects with a normal immune system. Presumably, with immune suppression, EBV-induced proliferation is not controlled and subsequently the polyclonal proliferation is transformed by unknown mechanisms into a malignant monoclonal proliferation.

EBV is identified in Reed-Sternberg cells more commonly in children than in adults, more commonly in underdeveloped countries than in the United States, and more commonly in some histological types of HD than in others.[18–20] This is consistent with the hypothesis that there may be different etiologies of HD in adults and children and with different histological types. EBV is detected more frequently in HIV associated than in non-HIV associated HD.[21]

Genetic and occupational predispositions for HD may also exist. Familial patterns have been documented, and HD clearly occurs with increased frequency in first-degree relatives of HD patients.[22,23] Although such findings might also be expected to lend support to the notion of an infectious vector, increased incidence has not been documented in marital partners or health care professionals caring for HD patients.[17] In contrast to other forms of cancer, evidence is sparse that chemical exposures are a significant factor in the development of HD. The possible role of viruses, especially EBV, remains an important consideration.[24]

Pathophysiology

Cellular Abnormalities

Although humoral immunity appears to remain relatively intact, patients in all stages of HD exhibit a molecular defect characterized by markedly reduced cellular immunity. This deficit is manifested by impaired delayed hypersensitivity skin reactions and reduced T-cell proliferation following antigenic stimulation. They also display increased susceptibility to infectious complications from opportunistic pathogens such as herpes zoster, cytomegalovirus, and *Pneumocystis carinii.*[25]

Elucidation of the biochemical mechanisms of HD has been difficult and data are sometimes conflicting. The *BCL-2* oncogene is able to prevent apoptosis and this promotes malignant growth because cells with genetic damage continue to proliferate rather than die as is normally the case. In nodular NHL there is a translocation t(14;18) which activates *BCL-2*. Activation of *BCL-2* is seen in some cases of HD but the t(14;18) translocation is seen only rarely. However, EBV infection may activate *BCL-2* and it has been suggested that in at least some cases of HD the pathogenesis involves EBV infection, subsequent activation of *BCL-2*, followed by suppression of apoptosis.[26,27] This mechanism seems common in most forms of HD, but is probably not the case in the nodular lymphocyte predominant form.[28,29] Thus there are probably at least two mechanisms involved in the development of HD and this is consistent with the data showing that EBV may be involved in virtually all pediatric cases and most adult cases in underdeveloped countries but is far less frequent in developed countries.[30]

Clinical Manifestations

A typical HD patient presents with a slow, insidious, superficial lymphadenopathy. Characteristic nodes of variable size (from 1 cm to several centimeters) are firm, rubbery, and freely movable. Occasionally their size varies spontaneously over a period of several days. The enlarged nodes may be unilateral or bilateral, and most are located in the cervical and supraclavicular areas. Axillary and inguinal involvement is reported in less than 10% of the patients. A second common presentation, mediastinal adenopathy, is often recognized during routine chest x-ray. Overall, the adenopathy is usually painless unless lymph node growth is rapid. However, pain does occur in about 20% of the cases following ingestion of alcohol.

Constitutional symptoms of fever, malaise, night sweats, weight loss (greater than 10% of normal body weight), and pruritus appear in about 40% of affected individuals. These manifestations, called *B symptoms*, are more common in patients with advanced disease.

The spread of HD is via contiguous nodal groups, and the pattern is quite predictable. In general, symptomatology and prognosis are related to the location and number of disease sites. Local pressure symptoms may arise from enlarged mediastinal nodes causing cough, dyspnea, dysphagia, pleural effusions, and, in extreme situations, superior vena cava syndrome. An enlarged spleen may result in left upper quadrant pain. Jaundice may evolve due to hepatic extension or extrahepatic bile duct obstruction. Retroperitoneal adenopathy often induces gastrointestinal and genitourinary dysfunction, abdominal pain, and ascites. Bone pain and fractures may be caused by secondary skeletal involvement of the vertebrae, ribs, and sternum. Herpes zoster infections are a relatively frequent finding and usually indicate impending epidural involvement. Exfoliative dermatitis and intense pruritus develop when the lymphatics of the skin are involved; indeed, they are often the first subjective symptoms to be reported.[31]

Assessment

The diagnosis of HD can be established only by biopsy of involved tissue, usually a lymph node. Cervical nodes are preferable to axillary and inguinal nodes because the latter often reveal evidence of chronic inflammatory changes. Occasionally, multiple biopsies are necessary for proper evaluation since reactive hyperplasia of nodes adjacent to those involved with tumor may provide equivocal results. It is important to remember that there are many causes of lymphadenopathy, especially in younger individuals. These include upper respiratory infections (bacterial or viral), infectious mononucleosis, allergic reactions, and other nonspecific causes. Older persons with cancers of the head and neck also may present initially with enlarged cervical nodes.

When an abnormal node is palpated during routine physical examination or when the patient reports such a complaint, a careful history and physical examination should be performed. If there is evidence of a recent infection or other nonmalignant process, the physician may choose to delay biopsy and observe the clinical course. In most cases, lymphadenopathy of infectious origin will usually resolve in a few days or weeks. When the adenopathy persists or the etiology is not apparent, a biopsy is generally indicated. Because a family history of HD increases the risk to other siblings, this, too, may be a factor in the decision process. In the absence of fever or overt systemic complaints, the detection of an enlarged lymph node in the neck of an older person is an indication that a careful search of the mouth, pharynx, and larynx for the presence of a malignant process should be made. Once a diagnosis is confirmed, it is necessary to obtain accurate histological typing and staging of the disease in order to determine the precise prognosis and selection of therapy.

Histopathology

Hodgkin's disease is distinguished from other lymphomas by the presence of the Reed-Sternberg cell. This is a large, bizarre cell with two or more mirror-image nuclei, each containing a single, prominent nucleolus. Unlike most cancers, this characteristic cell represents only a small fraction of the cells in a malignant lymph node. Normal lymphocytes, plasma cells, and fibrous stroma comprise the bulk of palpable tissue. Although Reed-Sternberg cells are essential for the diagnosis of HD, they also have been reported in other conditions such as lymphoid hyperplasia, infectious mononucleosis, nonlymphoid malignancies (carcinomas and sarcomas), and phenytoin therapy.[32]

The classic histopathologic classification of HD, established in 1966 by an international conference in Rye, New York,[33] is being replaced by an updated classification that incorporates recent immunologic and molecular data, and is part of the Revised European-American Lymphoma (REAL) classification.[17,34] The major difference is that the old classification of lymphocyte predominant HD has been divided into two groups based on immunologic and morphologic differences. One group is nodular with or without diffuse areas and the other is almost always diffuse throughout. Five distinct subtypes of HD are enumerated: nodular sclerosis, nodular lymphocyte-predominant, diffuse lymphocyte-predominant, mixed cellularity, and lymphocyte-depleted. Each category has well-defined characteristics and manifests certain features of natural history (Table 60-1). Prior to the availability of highly curative chemotherapy and radiation therapy, these subtypes also implied notable differences in expected survival. However, recent therapeutic advances have rendered each of them potentially curable, though not to the same degree.

Nodular sclerosis HD (NSHD), with its unique age incidence (15–34) and its different sex incidence (females more commonly than males), has a singular histological makeup that does not fit into the spectrum presented by the other types. In NSHD, the lymph node is divided into nodules by sclerosing bands of collagen. Lymphocytes within these collagen-bound nodules may be of various types, from predominantly small lymphocytes to large histiocytic forms. A variation of the Reed-Sternberg cell, the lacunar cell, is an identifiable feature of this subtype. Most patients are asymptomatic at presentation and exhibit stage I or II disease. They also tend to be clustered in the urban areas of developed countries. Anterior mediastinal involvement is exceedingly common and ultimately may involve cervical, supraclavicular, and upper abdominal lymph nodes as well as the spleen. Bulky mediastinal disease often contributes to metastatic infiltration of the lung parenchyma.

Nodular lymphocyte-predominant HD (NLPHD) has recently emerged as a distinct entity that has a high risk of transformation into NHL. Some investigators feel it might even be better classified as a variant of NHL. There is usually expression of B-cell antigens and the Reed-Stern-

berg cells are variants from their usual histology. The median age is the mid-thirties, the disease is often localized, and the prognosis is excellent with 90% entering remission and 90% alive at 10 years. Late relapses are more common than in other forms of HD and often represent transformation to NHL.

Lymphocyte-rich classic HD (LRHD) shows classic Reed-Sternberg cells against a background of lymphocytes usually in a diffuse pattern, although rarely nodular. Immunologic studies fail to show the B-cell antigens of NLPHD. It has clinical features and an intermediate prognosis more like mixed cellularity disease.

Mixed cellularity HD (MCHD) is intermediate between nodular lymphocyte-predominant and lymphocyte-depleted in terms of histology and prognosis. Disorderly fibrosis may be seen, but the broad fibrous bands indicative of the NSHD subtype are absent. There is a wide age range that peaks in the group aged 30–40, and male cases predominate. More than 50% of the patients have stage III or IV disease and the majority manifest B symptoms. Extranodal abdominal extension is common.

Lymphocyte-depleted HD (LDHD) is the most aggressive of the five REAL classifications. It is marked by a paucity of small lymphocytes and an increased number of Reed-Sternberg cells. Two slightly different variants have been identified—reticular and diffuse fibrosis. Reticular LDHD patients often present with bone marrow infiltration and peripheral lymphadenopathy. Those with diffuse fibrosis are more likely to exhibit lymph node and visceral involvement. Patients in this group are usually elderly males with advanced-stage disease and B symptoms. Prior to the advent of combination therapy, LDHD carried a very poor prognosis. It is interesting to note that in some retrospective histological studies, up to one-third of LDHD tumors have been reclassified as NHL.

Staging

After the diagnosis of HD has been established on the basis of lymph node biopsy and the histological type has been determined in accordance with the outlined criteria, the next step in patient management is the careful determination of the extent of the disease. This process is referred to as *staging* and it indicates the degree of systemic progression and the intensity of treatment that will be required; it also allows the clinician to draw an inference with regard to disease progression and prognosis.

Beginning in 1970, most HD patients were staged according to the Ann Arbor Classification System.[35] Over time, however, adherence to its guidelines became less strict due to (1) new features of recognized prognostic importance, (2) questions concerning the need for staging laparotomy, and (3) advances in diagnostic imaging techniques that facilitated recognition of occult disease sites. In an effort to address these issues, a meeting was convened in Cotswolds, England, in 1989. Specialists in attendance approved criteria for a new system that re-

Table 60-1 REAL Classification of Hodgkin's Disease

Histology	Frequency (%)	Features
Nodular sclerosis	60–80	Adolescents and young adults usually stage I or II; females predominate
Nodular lymphocyte-predominant	6–9	Adults in thirties usually stage I or II; males predominate
Diffuse lymphocyte-predominant	3–6	Presentation and survival-like mixed cellularity
Mixed cellularity	15–30	Males predominate; B symptoms common; intermediate prognosis
Lymphocyte-depleted	< 1	Older males predominate; widespread dissemination; poor prognosis

tained the original Ann Arbor framework but included modifications incorporating designations for number of sites and bulk of disease.[36]

Lymph node involvement in just one area is designated as stage I disease. Involvement of two or more areas confined to one side of the diaphragm constitutes stage II. In stage III, lymph node groups above and below the diaphragm are affected. The spleen may be involved (stage III$_S$), which often precedes widespread hematogenous dissemination. In HD, stage III is subdivided further into stage III$_1$ for disease limited to the upper abdomen (spleen and splenic, hilar, celiac, and/or porta hepatic nodes), and stage III$_2$ for disease involving the lower abdomen (periaortic, pelvic, or inguinal nodes). Stage IV is marked by diffuse extralymphatic progression that may affect, for example, the liver, bone marrow, lung, and skin. A subscript $_E$ in stages I, II, and III indicates localized extranodal extension from a nodal mass, and designation of a stage as either *A* or *B* indicates the absence (A) or presence (B) of unexplained weight loss greater than 10% of body weight in the preceding six months and/or fever of greater than 38°C and/or night sweats. Subscript $_X$ is indicative of bulky disease. This Ann Arbor Cotswolds staging system applies to both Hodgkin's and non-Hodgkin's lymphoma and can be summarized as follows:

Stage I   Involvement of a single lymph node group or single extralymphatic site (I$_E$).

Stage II   Involvement of two or more node groups on the same side of the diaphragm. If a single extralymphatic site is involved designate as II$_E$.

Stage III   Involvement of node groups on both sides of the diaphragm. May be divided into disease of the upper (III$_1$) or lower (III$_2$) abdomen. If spleen is involved designate III$_S$; if extralymphatic site is involved designate III$_E$.

Stage IV   Involvement of the liver, bone marrow, lung, or diffuse extralymphatic disease.

The adoption of this classification schema implies a dual system of stage designation according to both clinical and pathological criteria. Clinical staging (CS) rests on history, physical examination, initial diagnostic biopsy, laboratory tests, and radiographic evidence. Pathological staging (PS) adds definitive, histopathological information obtained through biopsy of strategic sites. It is customary to specify whether a stage is determined on the basis of clinical signs alone (e.g., an abdominal lymphangiogram) or on the basis of pathological examination of a biopsy section. Thus, a patient may be referred to as having "clinical" stage III (CS III) or "pathological" stage III (PS III), depending on the strength of the evidence. The nurse should be familiar with the essential procedures and terms used in diagnostic staging in order to help a patient follow the sequence and understand the significance of the evaluative workup.

The staging evaluation for HD usually includes, in addition to a careful history and physical examination and routine laboratory work, the following diagnostic procedures:

- surgical lymph node biopsy evaluated by classic histologic technique and immunophenotyping
- chest and abdominal computerized tomography (CT) and magnetic resonance imaging (MRI) as necessary to evaluate lymph nodes, spleen, and liver
- bipedal lymphangiogram if HD presents with inguinal or femoral nodal involvement
- bilateral needle biopsy of iliac crests in clinical stages IB, IIB, III, IV, or elevated alkaline phosphatase
- evaluation of suspected extranodal disease by biopsy or by imaging by two techniques

A controversial component of the staging process is the exploratory laparotomy, an extensive surgical procedure that includes splenectomy, wedge and needle liver biopsies, anterior iliac crest bone marrow biopsy, and extensive biopsy and dissection of abdominal lymph nodes. Although surgical mortality is quite uncommon, morbidity may include wound infection, subphrenic abscess, pulmonary embolus, stress ulcer, gastrointestinal bleeding, and wound dehiscence. In addition, splenectomy patients face the lifelong risk of a septic event from encapsulated organisms. Since these risks are not insignificant, a case has been made for chemotherapy in early-stage disease but reserving radiation therapy for specific indications such as a mediastinal mass greater than one-third the chest diameter.[37] With more recent movement toward a combined modality approach, especially in patients with bulky stage II disease or confirmed stage III$_2$ A disease, the need for laparotomy to define possible sites of occult intraabdominal disease has become limited.

Therapeutic Approaches

The initial treatment plan for HD is crucial in determining eventual outcome because the overwhelming majority of patients, even those in the most advanced disease stages, are potentially curable if optimal therapy is employed. A comprehensive approach is essential and requires input from a variety of disciplines (radiology, surgery, pathology, medical oncology) working together collaboratively as an interdisciplinary team.

Association with multiple physicians and the complexity of the staging procedures often cause a patient to feel confused and overwhelmed. In many cases the nurse may be the only constant contact this individual has with the diagnostic and treatment teams. Therefore, it is essential that psychological support be provided as the individual adjusts to the full ramifications of a malignant diagnosis. The diverse procedures to which the patient will be subjected may require clarification and repeated explanations. These should be given with understanding, empathy, compassion, and tact.

The management of HD since the discovery of curative chemotherapy over 30 years ago has traditionally been radiation for early-stage disease (stages I and II) and chemotherapy for more advanced stage disease (stages III and IV), with multimodal therapy in certain unique situations. However, the demonstration that chemotherapy is at least as effective as radiotherapy in early-stage HD has led to a reevaluation of this traditional approach.[38] As the long-term complications of radiotherapy have been better delineated and as nonalkylating agent chemotherapy (ABVD) has been shown to be as effective and less toxic than alkylating agent therapy (MOPP), there has been a move toward chemotherapy of early-stage disease.[37] The major long-term complication of concern is acute leukemia secondary to radiation or alkylating agent therapy; together radiating and alkylating agents are synergistic in causing leukemia.

Radiation therapy is curative in most patients with limited disease. Several important factors affect its effectiveness: skilled use of linear accelerators, careful field simulation, administration of tumoricidal doses, and comprehensive follow-up. The radiation fields commonly employed in HD may be divided into three volumes: the mantle, the paraaortic, and the pelvis (Figure 60-5). In order to achieve high cure rates, each of these fields generally must be extended to include adjacent, clinically negative nodal sites. Carefully constructed field shapes and blocks are used to protect the lungs, heart, spinal cord, larynx, kidneys, iliac crests, and gonads. All standard radiation treatments employ an opposed field, usually anterior-posterior, technique to provide homogenous dose distribution and to minimize potential radiation damage.

For stage I A and II A disease above the diaphragm, without bulky mediastinal extension, mantle irradiation to a total dose of 3500–4400 cGy over a period of four to six weeks is advocated. Paraaortic lymph nodes are usually included except in those with mediastinal involvement or those with lymphocyte predominant histology. Stage III$_1$ A patients having only splenic involvement may be treated with total or subtotal nodal irradiation. Generally, total nodal irradiation is considered inappropriate for stage III$_2$ A individuals. When bulky mediastinal disease is known to be present, both radiation and chemotherapy are unequivocally required. In addition, the combined approach is usually indicated for patients with adverse prognostic factors such as B symptoms, bulky masses, or disease involving nodes in the lower abdomen.

Whereas radiotherapy is curative in local and regional HD, chemotherapy may be curative in both early and advanced disease. The use of both modalities together is sometimes required for cure, but because multimodality therapy is associated with a much higher complication rate, especially second malignancies, there is controversy as to when to combine these modalities.[39,40]

Because of their high response and durable remission rates, the MOPP regimen (Table 60-2) and the ABVD regimen (Table 60-3) have become the benchmarks for combination chemotherapy in HD. Both regimens are routinely administered in 28-day cycles for a minimum of six cycles. As a rule, chemotherapy is continued for two cycles after complete remission is documented. Each combination can be expected to produce remissions in more than 80% of previously untreated patients, and 60%–70% of those who achieve complete remission will be alive with no evidence of disease after ten years, presumably cured.

Overall, either MOPP or ABVD can be expected to produce a complete remission in more than half of the patients who have recurrent disease after treatment with the other combination. At present, there is no evidence

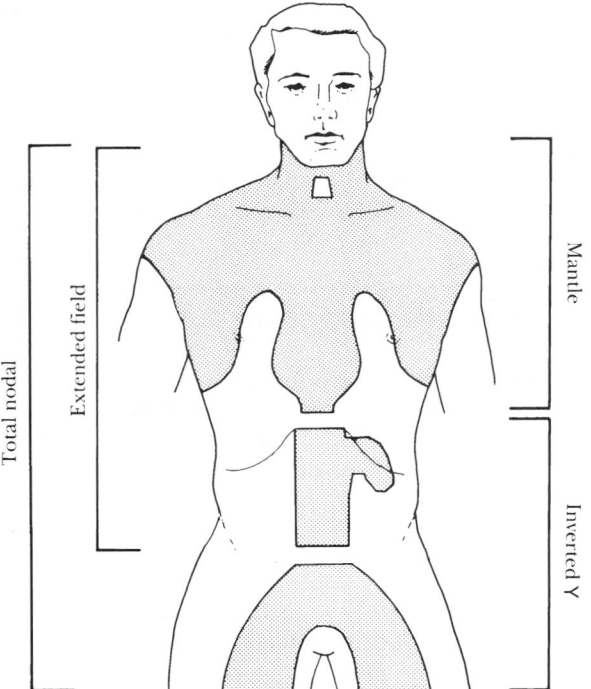

Figure 60-5 Standard radiation fields for Hodgkin's disease. Mantle—from mandible to diaphragm. Lungs, heart, spinal cord, and humeral heads are shielded. Inverted Y—from diaphragm to ischial tuberosities, including the spleen if not removed; spinal cord, kidneys, bladder, rectum, and gonads are shielded. Extended Field—involves mantle zone and uppermost inverted Y zone; does not include the pelvic, inguinal, or femoral nodes. Total Nodal—mantle zone and complete inverted Y zone.

Table 60-2 The MOPP Regimen for Hodgkin's Disease

Drug	Dosage	Schedule
Nitrogen mustard	6 mg/m² IV	Days 1 and 8
Vincristine (Oncovin)	1.4 mg/m² IV	Days 1 and 8
Procarbazine	100 mg/m² PO	Days 1 through 14
Prednisone (cycles 1 and 4 only)	40 mg/m² PO	Days 1 through 14

Repeat cycle every 28 days for a minimum of six cycles. Complete remission must be documented before discontinuing therapy.

Table 60-3   The ABVD Regimen for Hodgkin's Disease

Drug	Dosage	Schedule
Doxorubicin	25 mg/m² IV	Days 1 and 15
Bleomycin	10 units/m² IV	Days 1 and 15
Vinblastine	6 mg/m² IV	Days 1 and 15
Dacarbazine (DTIC)	375 mg/m² IV	Days 1 and 15

Repeat cycle every 28 days for a minimum of six cycles. Complete remission must be documented before discontinuing therapy.

that maintenance therapy adds to cure for patients in remission. It is important to note that recent studies indicate ABVD may actually be superior to MOPP because it minimizes the leukemogenesis and permanent male sterility associated with regimens containing alkylating agents.[41]

The drugs used in MOPP and ABVD have been combined in various ways. The underlying principle of increasing the number of drugs in a combination is the Goldie-Coldman hypothesis, which postulates that multiple drugs reduce the chance of failure due to development of drug resistance by tumor cells.[42] Combining MOPP and ABVD has been shown to improve failure-free survival in randomized trials, but there is no improvement of overall survival compared to ABVD alone.[43,44] A seven-drug regimen (BEACOPP) that substitutes cyclophosphamide for nitrogen mustard and omits vinblastine has been used in Europe, but to date no regimen has clearly shown to have an advantage in regard to long-term survival.

The success of aggressive chemotherapeutic regimens is quite dependent on the dosage and timing of drug administration because even minor alterations can have a substantial impact on efficacy. The reduction of doses and omission of drugs to avoid nausea and vomiting, with its attendant loss of curative potential, is truly a poor bargain for any patient. Nursing can play a pivotal role in promoting patient compliance by providing emotional support, effective symptom management, and reassurance about the finite nature of the treatment program.

Refinements in treatment protocols have led to the identification of specific subsets of patients who appear to benefit from combined chemotherapy and radiation therapy.[45] Some patients present with what has been called *bulky disease*, usually defined as adenopathy greater than one-third the width of the chest on x-ray examination. This pattern of disease has a high recurrence rate after radiotherapy alone and poses some risk in exploratory laparotomy because the mediastinal mass may complicate anesthesia.[46–48] These patients are best managed with multimodal therapy.

Residual or recurrent disease poses a unique challenge. Those who relapse following radiation can sometimes be treated with chemotherapy, and, under certain circumstances, additional radiation may be possible. In the past it was not unusual to treat the patient again

with a standard regimen,[49] but more recently high-dose regimens have been used.[50] When relapse occurs after chemotherapy, the extent of the disease-free interval is an important prognostic factor. When relapse occurs less than 12 months after initial remission or patients are refractory to initial therapy, the prognosis is grave and conventional salvage regimens are rarely effective.

High-dose chemotherapy (HDC) with stem cell rescue, utilizing either autologous bone marrow or peripheral stem cells, has been investigated as an alternative to conventional salvage therapy.[51] Results tend to be better in relapsed patients than in initially refractory patients,[52] probably because of the degree of tumor chemosensitivity. There is evidence that HDC with stem cell rescue is effective, with disease-free survival of 75% at two years, although treatment-related complications account for a 13% mortality.[53] There are three independent prognostic variables: the number of prior chemotherapy regimens, prior radiotherapy, and extranodal disease at the time of high-dose therapy. Of these the number of prior chemotherapy regimens is the most important. HDC has led to three- and four-year disease-free survival rates exceeding 50% in several studies.[50] The preparative regimen used and the role of total body radiation remain under study. Cytoreductive therapy prior to HDC has been recommended by some, but its use is unproven. The apparent benefit of cytoreductive pretreatment may be due to the selection of better prognosis patients.[50] It is likely that high-dose therapy will be used increasingly in the future and will be applied earlier in the disease in order to treat patients before tumors acquire resistance to chemotherapeutic agents.

NON-HODGKIN'S LYMPHOMAS

Historical Perspective

The non-Hodgkin's lymphomas are a diverse group of neoplasms derived from the different developmental and functional subdivisions of the lymphoreticular system. Although these malignancies have many features in common, they also reflect the diversity of their normal counterpart cells and exhibit a wide range of immunological and biological characteristics. There is no precise definition of NHL that is universally accepted, and although many meet the criteria that have been proposed for neoplasia, others lurk in a nebulous area between benign lymphoproliferation and true malignancy. Furthermore, the classification of lymphomas has long been a controversial issue.[54]

In the past, pathologists used a variety of terms (e.g., *giant follicle lymphoma, lymphosarcoma,* and *reticulum cell sarcoma*) to categorize these tumors, and "pseudoleukemia" became a catchall for a host of conditions that exhibited lymphadenopathy and splenomegaly. Recent technological refinements have enabled pathologists and clinicians to classify NHL according to a number of individual determinants including cytoarchitecture (follicular versus diffuse), cell size (small or large), nuclear characteristics (cleaved or noncleaved, convoluted or cerebriform), and immunological ontogeny (T-cell or B-cell lymphocytes). Today the most accurate definition of lymphoma type is one that includes each of these elements and genetic markers as well.[55]

Epidemiology

In the United States, NHL is diagnosed nearly six times as often as HD, and its death rate is 13 times greater. American Cancer Society statistics for 1999 indicate that 56,800 new cases and 25,700 deaths will occur.[4] Age-adjusted incidence is somewhat higher in males than in females (32,600 to 24,200), and whites are affected more than blacks. Age-specific analyses reveal a preadolescent peak, a late teenage drop, and then a logarithmic rise with increasing age that persists into the eighth decade.

Because of the many available classification schemes for NHL, it is difficult to compare the incidence or frequency of the histological subtypes of lymphoma in different parts of the world. However, a rising incidence appears to be noted internationally; there has been a onefold to twofold increase in most Western countries since 1960. Part of this rising incidence may be due to the increased frequency of NHL in patients with AIDS and patients whose immune function is suppressed for purposes of organ transplantation.[56]

Etiology

The heterogeneity of NHL suggests that a variety of factors including viral infections, genetic abnormalities, and immune disturbances interact in the pathogenesis. The most convincing evidence of a viral etiology of malignant lymphoma has come from the studies of adult T-cell leukemia/lymphoma (ATL). A unique RNA retrovirus, human T-cell leukemia/lymphoma virus type I (HTLV-I), has been isolated from lymphocytes of patients with ATL in endemic areas of southwestern Japan, the Caribbean, and southeastern United States. ATL is primarily a disease of adults over age 40. Its manifestations include a high frequency of cutaneous infiltration, hepatosplenomegaly, lymphadenopathy, and hypercalcemia.[57]

Epstein-Barr virus (EBV), a DNA herpes virus, is the most likely etiologic agent for another form of NHL, Burkitt's lymphoma (BL). This neoplasm is confined almost exclusively to endemic areas of Africa and New Guinea, and, indeed, evidence of EBV infection is found in 96% of African cases of BL. In Africa, BL is a malignancy of childhood. The mean age at presentation is 7 years, and males are affected twice as often as females. The children usually present with large extranodal tumors involving the bones of the jaw (72%) and abdominal organs (56%), particularly the ovaries, kidneys, and retroperitoneum. Although the etiology of BL is unknown, a current hypothesis focuses on an acute malarial infection as the environmental factor that interacts with a susceptible host immune system to predispose an individual to EBV-induced lymphoma.[58,59] Recently, EBV has been linked to neoplastic proliferation in a variety of congenital, iatrogenic, and acquired immunodeficient conditions.[56,60,61]

Environmental factors and exposure to chemicals in the workplace also are implicated in the pathogenesis of NHL. Pesticides and fertilizers have been suspected because of increased lymphoma incidence among midwestern farmers born after 1900 and dying before age 65. Vinyl chloride workers in the U.S. tire manufacturing industry exhibit increases, as do anesthetists, chemists, and workers in petroleum refining, asbestos, and herbicide industries. Japanese survivors of the atomic bomb and patients receiving ionizing radiation for congenital disorders and HD also face increased neoplastic potential.[62]

One form of lymphoma, gastric lymphoma of mucosa-associated lymphoid tissue (MALT), has recently been reported to be due to the same bacteria that induces gastric ulcers, *Helicobacter pylori*. In its early stages it may be cured by eradication of the bacteria with antibiotics.[63] The full implications of this exciting observation are not yet understood.

Pathophysiology

Cellular Abnormalities

A consideration of the molecular pathogenesis of both B- and T-cell origin in NHL reveals several consistent features. In most cases, chromosomal translocations facilitate the identification of the genetic lesion responsible for oncogenesis. Nearly all individuals with BL have one of three translocations involving the *MYC* proto-oncogene. These include chromosomes 8 and 14 (t 8;14), chromosomes 2 and 8 (t 2;8), and chromosomes 8 and 22 (t 8;22). Eighty-five percent of follicular lymphomas and 20% of diffuse lymphomas have the characteristic t(14;18) translocation that activates the *BCL-2* gene that suppresses apoptosis.[64] Mantle cell lymphomas, also called *centrocytic* or *intermediate lymphomas*, have a characteristic t(11;14) translocation that activates the *BCL-1* gene causing cyclin D1 protein overexpression, leading to very rapid proliferation and resistance to cure by conventional chemotherapy.[65]

Cytogenetic analysis of lymphoma cells has identified other abnormalities as well. Deletions on chromosome 6 are found in a significant portion of patients with large-cell lymphoma. Such a loss of chromosomal material may lead to deleterious effects via the elimination of functional suppressor or growth inhibitory genes. Gains of one or more whole chromosomes are common, and trisomy of chromosomes 2,3,7,18, and 21 have been described.[66] At present the sequence of events that explains the transformation of a normal lymphocyte into a lymphomatous cell is unknown. Optimally, a better understanding of the genetic mechanisms of malignancy will translate eventually into new strategies of treatment based on the biology of the disease.[67]

Clinical Manifestations

NHLs encompass a spectrum of neoplasms ranging from indolent tumors, which can occasionally undergo spontaneous regression, to rapidly progressive tumors, which may be fatal within weeks if untreated. They are often generalized diseases and can involve almost any organ or tissue, thus resulting in a wide array of systemic manifestations. Although usually NHL presents with enlarged lymph nodes, between one-fourth and one-half of the cases are extranodal.[68] These extranodal lymphomas may present as gastrointestinal problems resembling peptic ulcer, bone lesions, testicular tumors, pulmonary tumors, brain tumors, and even tumors in the thyroid and breast. Cutaneous presentations are also frequent. Although extranodal lymphoma may not be seen during initial evaluation, it generally is confirmed in more than 50% of cases at autopsy. Malignancies originating in Waldeyer's ring of the nasopharynx have a particular propensity for gastric extension. Common clinical signs are pain, abdominal mass, and anorexia and, less commonly, nausea, vomiting, bleeding, diarrhea, or obstruction. Some of the clinical features may be caused by chemical mediators produced by the lymphoma cells, by metabolic changes resulting from a high rate of cell death in the tumor, or by secondary events such as opportunistic infections, immunosuppression, and paraneoplastic electrolyte abnormalities.

On occasion lymphomas may present as oncologic emergencies such as cardiac tamponade, superior vena cava syndrome, or increased intercranial pressure or they may develop sepsis or tumor lysis syndrome during therapy.[69] In contrast to HD, 80% of patients with NHL present to their physicians with advanced disease (stage III or IV). Systemic B symptoms (fever, night sweats, and/or weight loss) are the initial complaint in as many as 20% of the cases. Although their presence signifies advanced disease, it is not as predictive of prognosis as in HD.

Pulmonary parenchymal disease is related most often to lymphatic tumor spread from hilar and mediastinal nodes, and cough, dyspnea, and chest pain are quite indicative of lung infiltration. Central lymphatic obstruction or pleural seeding with tumor may result in superior vena cava syndrome or pleural effusion. Lytic bone lesions are seen in the femurs, pelvis, vertebrae, ribs, and skull. Lymphomas occasionally infiltrate the skin as red or purplish nodules, primarily in the head and neck region, while tumorous replacement of the bone marrow can result in a leukemia-like picture in the peripheral blood.

Liver involvement often occurs without signs or symptoms, and, unlike the situation in HD, splenic extension need not occur concomitantly.

Solitary brain lymphomas are being reported with increasing frequency. They are often associated with AIDS or iatrogenic immunosuppression. These mass lesions may induce headaches, seizures, and changes in mental status. Another common central nervous system manifestation is leptomeningeal spread, which results in cranial nerve palsies, meningeal irritation, and increased intracranial pressure.[70]

Assessment

Because every enlarged lymph node does not necessarily represent NHL, careful histological evaluation is the most important first step toward initiating proper care of the patient. When a lymphoma is suspected, the pathologist should be notified so that special processing procedures including cytogenetics, surface markers, immunohistochemistry stains, and molecular biological studies can be used in addition to routine histology of biopsied specimens. Since NHL occurs more commonly in extranodal sites than HD, needle biopsies may be more diagnostically helpful; widespread visceral extension or occult retroperitoneal disease may require open biopsy or laparotomy for confirmation.

A careful history and physical examination should be precise in evaluating abnormal clinical manifestations and the length of time they have been present. This is particularly important in patients who present with vague constitutional complaints or with derangements referable to more than one organ system. In general, the principles governing assessment of NHL are the same as those previously identified for HD.

Histopathology

Few areas of pathology have evoked as much controversy and confusion as the classification of NHL, and the lack of consistent standardization makes international analysis and comparison extremely difficult. The first widely accepted classification was proposed by Rappaport and associates[71] in 1956. This scheme distinguishes lymphomas on the basis of two morphological features: (1) pattern of growth (nodular or diffuse depending on the macrostructure of the lymph node); and (2) the degree of cytological differentiation of the predominant malignant cell. Tumors composed of cells similar in size and morphology to normal lymphocytes are considered *well-differentiated*, whereas those composed of irregularly shaped lymphocytes are referred to as *poorly differentiated*. If tumor cells are two to three times larger than small lymphocytes and have abundant cytoplasm, they were called *histiocytes* because of their resemblance to macrophages. *Undifferen-*

tiated lymphomas are composed of intermediate-sized cells that fail to demonstrate evidence of either lymphoid or histiocytic origin. *Mixed lymphomas* are tumors formed by poorly differentiated lymphocytes and histiocytes.[71] Over the years, the Rappaport classification has been popular with clinicians because it is reproduced easily and correlated well with clinical observations and was simple to understand and use. It gave little insight into the underlying pathophysiology, however, which led to many attempts to replace it. One of the first was by Lukes and Collins,[72] who proposed an immunologic classification system that provided important correlations with the pathophysiology of the lymphoreticular system. Their approach relates lymphoma cell morphology to the sequential stages in the histogenesis of normal B and T lymphocytes (see Figure 60-3), and their observations were reinforced by the identification of specific T- or B-cell markers on the cell surfaces.

By the late 1970s, in addition to the schemes of Rappaport and Lukes and Collins, four other classifications were in use throughout the world. The alternatives included classifications by the British National Lymphoma Group, Dorfman, the World Health Organization, and Kiel. A study funded by the National Cancer Institute developed what was hoped would become an international standard of classification for NHL. The Working Formulation[73] was proposed as a means of translation among the various systems to facilitate clinical comparisons and therapeutic trials. This scheme classified the lymphomas into low, intermediate, and high grade and assigned letter designations from A to J that corresponded roughly with decreasing survival. The low grade lymphomas were predominantly B-cell tumors; intermediate-grade lymphomas included B-cell and some T-cell neoplasms; immunoblastic malignancies were predominantly B cell in origin, while the lymphoblastic group usually was composed of T-cell tumors. Although the diagnosis of NHL in the Working Formulation was based solely on morphological features, it had predictive value for survival. However, because of their biological behavior and clinical course, most treatment protocols continued to recognize only two major groups: low grade and high grade.

Recently, yet another classification of NHL has been proposed, the Revised European-American Lymphoma (REAL) classification.[34] This system offers some advantages in that it includes several types of lymphoma (e.g., Mantle cell lymphoma and MALT lymphoma) not included by the Working Formulation and because it has incorporated more biological markers that correlate with pathophysiology. The major classifications in the Working Formulation and their pathological counterparts in the Rappaport and the REAL classification systems are compared in Table 60-4. In spite of the complexity of the various classifications, the concept of low-, intermediate-, and high-grade lymphomas remains useful for clinical purposes, although it is still necessary to consider the

Table 60-4 Non-Hodgkin's Lymphoma Nomenclature: Comparative Classifications

Working Formulation	Rappaport System	Real Classification*
LOW-GRADE		
A Small lymphocytic	Diffuse, well-differentiated lymphocytic	Chronic lymphocytic leukemia
B Follicular, small cleaved	Nodular, poorly differentiated lymphocytic	MALT** Follicle center cell, follicular grade I
C Follicular, mixed small cleaved, and large cell	Nodular, mixed lymphocytic and histiocytic	Follicle center cell, follicular grade II
INTERMEDIATE-GRADE		
D Follicular, large cell	Nodular histiocytic	Follicle center cell, follicular grade III
E Diffuse, small cleaved	Diffuse, poorly differentiated lymphocytic	Mantle cell***
F Diffuse, mixed small and large	Diffuse, mixed lymphocytic and histiocytic	Follicle center cell, diffuse small cell Large B cell rich in T cells
G Diffuse, large cell	Diffuse histiocytic	Diffuse large B cell
HIGH-GRADE		
H Immunoblastic, large cell	Diffuse histiocytic	Diffuse large B cell
I Lymphoblastic	Lymphoblastic	Precursor B lymphocytic
J Small, noncleaved Burkitt's	Undifferentiated, Burkitt's and non-Burkitt's	Burkitt's High-grade B cell Burkitt's-like

*The REAL classification separated B-cell and T-cell lymphomas. Most of the T-cell lymphomas are not shown here except for chronic lymphocytic leukemia.

**Malt tumors are extranodal indolent, usually follicular but some were previously classified in groups A, B, C, E, and rarely F.

***Mantle cell tumors are defined by *BCL-1* overexpression and sometimes have a morphology similar to groups AB and F.

implications of MALT and mantle cell lymphomas and the importance of the site of the tumor—e.g., central nervous system or skin.

Low-grade Lymphomas

The low-grade lymphomas in the Working Formulation occur predominantly in older individuals (median age is 55 years), and they affect males and females equally. The majority of patients are asymptomatic. The usual presenting problems are connected with a painless, progressive, often symmetrical generalized lymphadenopathy. Except for liver and bone marrow involvement, extranodal extension is uncommon.

Like normal lymphocytes, low-grade, B-cell lymphomas often circulate; thus, patients generally present with widespread stage III or IV disease. Some patients describe a history of lymph nodes that wax and wane in size for many years prior to diagnosis. Host immunity has been invoked to explain this phenomenon, and, in some cases, clinical regression has been preceded by a viral or bacterial infection.

Most low-grade lymphomas have a long natural history (median survival is seven to nine years) that appears to be largely unaffected by treatment. As the disease progresses, patients may complain of increasing fatigue, malaise, low-grade fever, night sweats, and weight loss. Eventually the general pace of the disease accelerates and the majority of indolent lymphomas transform from low-grade to intermediate- or high-grade malignancies. Treatment strategies must then be modified to be appropriate for aggressive lymphomas. Death usually results from progressive growth and eventual lymphoma replacement of hematopoietic and lymphoid tissues, thereby producing multiple systemic dysfunctions. Although the overall picture for these lymphomas seems optimistic, the disease is usually fatal; median survival generally is less than one year after such transformation.

Up to one-third of gastric lymphomas are of the MALT type, are thought to be secondary to chronic gastritis due to *H. pylori,* and in their early polyclonal stages are curable by eradication of this bacterium using conventional therapy. As the disease progresses to a monoclonal lymphoma, it it low grade initially and highly responsive to the chemotherapy or radiotherapy. Occasionally, this lymphoma may become more aggressive.[74] MALT lymphomas also occur in the orbit, the lung, and the thyroid.

Intermediate-grade Lymphomas

The intermediate-grade lymphomas in the Working Formulation include an uncommon tumor with a follicular architecture and predominantly large lymphocytes that has a more aggressive clinical course than that of the other more indolent of follicular lymphomas. Most patients have advanced disease at the time of diagnosis. Peripheral blood involvement is unusual. The REAL classification specifies three grades of follicular tumors, a nomenclature that replaces the Working Formulation terminology of follicular, small cleaved; follicular, mixed small cleaved, and large cell; and follicular, large cell. Immunologically, these are neoplasms of B lymphocytes, and almost all cases exhibit translocations of chromosomes 14 and 18, which leads to expression of the *BCL-2* antiapoptosis gene.

Most cases of the diffuse small cleaved cell lymphomas are now classified as mantle cell lymphomas on the basis of a translocation (11;14) that leads to a deregulation of *BCL-1* also known as PRAD1 or cyclin D1. This is a disease of older adults with a male predominance and patients usually have widespread disease at presentation.[55] Mantle cell lymphoma is intermediate in its aggressiveness with a median survival of three to five years.

The diffuse large-cell and mixed-cell lymphomas in the Working Formulation occur mainly in adults, and, although nodal presentation is common, these subtypes frequently involve extranodal progression to the gastrointestinal tract, skin, and bone. Privileged sites such as the testes and central nervous system also may be involved. If left untreated, mixed- and large-cell diffuse NHLs are rapidly fatal. However, these malignancies are responsive to chemotherapy and a significant chance for cure exists. Diffuse large-cell NHL comprise over one-third of all adult lymphomas.

High-grade Lymphomas

There are a number of diffuse large-cell lymphomas that are highly aggressive. These include the following: T-cell immunoblastic or anaplastic large-cell lymphoma sometimes called *malignant histiocytosis;* precursor T lymphoblastic lymphoma (convoluted) and precursor B lymphoblastic lymphoma; primary thymic lymphoma; and angioimmunoblastic T-cell lymphoma. Adult T-cell lymphoma/leukemia induced by HTLV-1 may show a histology of diffuse small cleaved cells, mixed small and large cells, diffuse large cells, or immunoblastic cells. Burkitt's and Burkitt's-like lymphomas show a population of small noncleaved cells.

Burkitt's lymphoma occurs endemically in tropical Africa and New Guinea, where it is associated with EBV. This lymphoma is more common in males than females, and the average age at onset is 7 years. Massive involvement of the jaw, ovaries, kidneys, liver, mesentery, and central nervous system is a prominent feature. Cases of BL in the United States are not associated with EBV and arise in slightly older children (age 11). Involvement of the ileocecal region of the bowel is common and often results in obstruction and intussusception. Children older than age 13 at onset have a poorer prognosis. In general, Burkitt's tumors are highly sensitive to chemotherapeutic agents, and their response is often dramatic and enduring. Burkitt's-like lymphoma is a relatively uncommon entity.

Typically, aggressive lymphomas exhibit rapid tumor

growth and a high mitotic index. Without treatment, survival is usually less than 18 months. However, because these neoplasms respond better to chemotherapy than the indolent, low-grade lymphomas, they have a greater potential for cure, especially if complete remissions are sustained for at least two years.

A variety of factors other than the histology of the lymphoma influence the prognosis of aggressive lymphoma. The most important ones are poor performance status, B symptoms, anemia, high serum lactic dehydrogenase (LDH), bone marrow involvement, liver involvement, large (greater than 10 cm) abdominal mass, and older than 65. These prognostic factors have been developed into an international prognostic index utilizing five pretreatment characteristics that remained independently significant: age (over 60 versus under 60), extent of disease (stage I or II versus stage III or IV), performance status (0–1 versus 2 or more), number of extranodal sites (none versus one or more), and LDH (normal versus elevated).[75]

Mycosis Fungoides (Cutaneous T-cell Lymphoma)

Among the miscellaneous group of lymphomas, the best characterized is a rare disorder referred to in older literature as *mycosis fungoides* and in current reviews as *cutaneous T-cell lymphoma (CTCL)*. Involvement of the skin is a hallmark of this malignancy that results from the clonal proliferation of T lymphocytes. CTCL tends to be initially indolent, but it may evolve into a widely disseminated malignancy. The disease occurs in middle age, and males are affected more often than females. Histologically, there is infiltration of the epidermis and upper dermis with neoplastic T cells that have an extremely unusual cerebriform nucleus. Clinically, the lesions exhibit three distinct cutaneous stages. The initial premycotic stage is characterized by superficial inflammatory skin eruptions and generalized pruritus. In this stage, CTCL may be confused with other dermatological disorders such as psoriasis and eczema. Eventually the disease progresses through an aggravated plaque stage to one with nodular tumors. In most patients with extensive disease, extracutaneous manifestations and visceral dissemination develop and ultimately lead to a fatal outcome. A variety of CTCL, the Sézary syndrome, presents with generalized exfoliative erythroderma and circulating leukemia-like cerebriform lymphocytes. The full implication of detecting circulating neoplastic cells has not been fully determined. In general, however, CTCL patients with a high percentage of circulating Sézary cells have a shorter survival compared to those with a lower percentage.[76]

Staging

Once a histological diagnosis of NHL has been confirmed by biopsy, a careful, comprehensive staging work-up is essential to determine the extent of the disease, the bulk of the tumor mass, and the imminence of potential complications. The work-up enables the physician to provide an accurate prognosis and to plan effective treatment. Both the condition of the patient and the histopathological classification of the tumor direct the type and speed of staging procedures to be performed. For example, an individual with a rapidly progressive, high-grade lymphoma whose natural history can be measured in weeks requires immediate initiation of therapy with only essential procedures performed beforehand. On the other hand, an indolent, low-grade lymphoma can be staged at the convenience of the patient and physician.

Baseline studies for all patients should include complete history and physical examination with particular emphasis on all lymphoid tissue including liver, spleen, Waldeyer's ring, and lymph nodes. Special attention should be given in the history to B symptoms. Also required are complete blood count, blood chemistries including liver and kidney function tests, erythrocyte sedimentation rate, uric acid, serum immunoglobulins, LDH, and beta-2 microglobulin. Bone marrow biopsy should be a part of the evaluation. This is an important evaluative component because there is a high incidence of marrow involvement in stage III and IV disease in the low-grade lymphomas and an equal distribution of stage I and II versus stage III and IV with less marrow involvement in the intermediate- and high-grade groups.[55]

Unlike HD, where the disease sites are more predictable and orderly, the multiplicity of potential NHL locations and the variety of their clinical presentations forestall the adoption of a single radiological scheme. All patients require a chest x-ray to facilitate detection of hilar adenopathy, mediastinal mass, parenchymal lung infiltration, or pleural/pericardial effusions. A CT scan of the chest is advised when the x-ray is suspicious. Abdominal and pelvic CT should be performed on all individuals because nodal and extranodal masses in these regions occur frequently in some subgroups. The CT scan is replacing lymphangiography (LAG) in many patients because of its usefulness in detecting upper retroperitoneal and mesenteric nodes, as well as hepatic and splenic extension.

Additional studies that may be appropriate in certain circumstances include biopsy of the liver and removal of the spleen for pathological study. However, surgical evaluation of the abdomen should be undertaken only if it clearly makes a major difference in the treatment selection. In patients with extensive gastrointestinal disease, a staging laparotomy can be helpful in reducing the risk of perforation and/or bleeding complications. Refinements in endoscopic technology may eliminate the need for gastrectomy and its associated sequelae during the initial treatment phase of gastric lymphomas.[77]

After clinical evaluation is complete, patients are classified according to the criteria previously outlined for HD in the Ann Arbor–Cottswolds staging system. It is important to note that this system is not as useful in directing the management of NHLs because these malignancies are characterized by early hematogenous dissemination and their natural history is poorly described by staging criteria based primarily on anatomic distribution. However, the clinical stage within each histological subtype does appear to carry reliable prognostic significance. In the aggressive lymphomas, when the international index derived from prognostic factors is utilized in conjunction with stage, there is a threefold variation in five-year survival in the four risk groups identified by the system.[75]

Therapeutic Approaches

The treatment of NHL usually requires a multidisciplinary approach to effect an optimal cure rate. This approach is determined by several key factors: histology of the tumor, stage of the disease, and physiological performance status of the patient. The histological grades of the Working Formulation represent a spectrum of survival in untreated patients that ranges from just weeks in the highly aggressive lymphomas to years in the indolent grades. Thus, the primary determinant in any treatment program is the natural history of the histological subtype.

The second major consideration is the extent of disease. Unlike HD, with its organized progression via contiguous nodal groups, most NHLs are widely disseminated at diagnosis. Therefore, in order to be of any practical use, their staging must always be modified according to histology.

Evaluation of individual performance status is the final component in treatment planning. Because the primary goal for many lymphomas is cure, the majority of therapeutic regimens are quite toxic. However, the observed toxicities are nearly always dose-related and predictable. Although the patient's physical status, age, and underlying medical problems should be taken into consideration when planning aggressive therapy, it is important to remember that advanced age per se is not a contraindication to using an effective program.

Indolent Lymphomas

There is no area of lymphoma treatment that is more controversial than what, if any, approach can alter the natural history of indolent or low-grade NHL and induce long-term, disease-free survival. This concern is quite understandable because the natural history of these malignancies has been such that, despite any therapeutic intervention, most patients live with their disease and eventually die from it. Some physicians advocate a policy of "watchful waiting" until systemic symptoms require intervention. When symptoms develop, patients are managed with sufficient chemotherapy or radiotherapy to control the disease, at which point the program of watchful waiting is resumed. It has been shown that this approach in asymptomatic patients does not reduce their survival.[78]

An alternate approach is the use of intensive combination chemotherapy regimens to induce a complete remission. The patient is then observed until the time of recurrence. These regimens almost never produce a cure as in the treatment of aggressive lyhmphoma. Total-body irradiation will produce a complete remission, but the average duration is only two to three years and it is doubtful if this is superior to combination chemotherapy. This approach does not increase the survival rate in comparison to watchful waiting.[79]

The development of new agents such as fludarabine and monoclonal antibodies may improve the treatment of indolent NHL, and maintenance therapy with interferon may keep patients in remission longer.[80,81] At the present time, however, other than the control of symptoms, there seems little that can be done to alter the natural history of this disease, unless high-dose therapy with stem cell rescue proves effective. Given the long, benign course of this disease, even though it is ultimately fatal, a conservative approach may be best.

High-dose chemotherapy (HDC) with stem cell rescue is as yet unproven in indolent NHL. Several phase II trials have been encouraging but the acute toxicity is high, the follow-up is short, there are late toxicities of concern, and randomized trial data are not available. Many questions remain. The role of irradiation with high-dose therapy has not been clearly delineated. Indolent NHL often transforms into an aggressice diffuse large-cell tumor and it remains uncertain whether HDC should be given early in the course of the disease or after there has been a transformation. Data are conflicting on this question. Since indolent NHL often involves the bone marror and shows circulating stem cells, the question of in vitro purging has been raised, but not resolved. At the present time, HDC with stem cell rescue in indolent NHL remains a question to be resolved in randomized trials.[50,80,82,83]

Aggressive Lymphomas

Patients with unfavorable histology (intermediate- and high-grade lymphomas) have a much more aggressive disease process, which usually results in a rapid, downhill progression. Thus, there is no place for administration of single agents in the primary treatment plan. Historically, radiation therapy (RT) has been used with moderate success in those with stage I and II disease.

The recognized treatment of choice for advanced-stage, aggressive NHL is combination chemotherapy. Over the past 20 years, therapeutic regimens of increasing intensity have evolved (Table 60-5). The initial combination of an alkylating agent, a vinca alkaloid, and a corticosteroid (CVP or COP) has been enhanced by the addition of doxorubicin and other agents, resulting in such protocols as CHOP, BACOP, and C-MOPP. These are usually given as monthly cycles for six to nine months and produce long-term remissions in 35%–45% of cases. The

Table 60-5 Selected Chemotherapeutic Regimens for Lymphomas

Regimen	Dose and Route	Day	Frequency
CHOP			Repeat every 21 days
C—cyclophosphamide	750 mg/m² IV	1	
H—doxorubicin (Adriamycin)	50 mg/m² IV	1	
O—vincristine (Oncovin)	1.4 mg/m² IV (max 2.0 mg)	1	
P—prednisone	100 mg PO	1–5	
CVP			Repeat every 21 days
C—cyclophosphamide	400 mg/m² PO	1–5	
V—vincristine (Oncovin)	1.4 mg/m² IV	1	
P—prednisone	100 mg/m² PO	1–5	
BACOP			Repeat every 28 days
B—bleomycin	5 u/m² IV	15, 22	
A—doxorubicin (Adriamycin)	25 mg/m² IV	1, 8	
C—cyclophosphamide	650 mg/m² IV	1, 8	
O—vincristine (Oncovin)	1.4 mg/m² IV	1, 8	
P—prednisone	60 mg/m² PO	15–28	
ProMACE-MOPP			Repeat every 28 days
Pro—prednisone	60 mg/m² PO	1–14	
M—methotrexate*	1500 mg/m² IV (over 12 hours)	15	
A—doxorubicin (Adriamycin)	25 mg/m² IV	1, 8	
C—cyclophosphamide	650 mg/m² IV	1, 8	
E—etoposide	120 mg/m² IV	1, 8	
Followed by MOPP after maximal response			
ProMACE-CytaBOM			Repeat every 21 days
Pro—prednisone	60 mg/m² PO	1–14	
A—doxorubicin (Adriamycin)	25 mg/m² IV	1	
C—cyclophosphamide	650 mg/m² IV	1	
E—etoposide	120 mg/m² IV	1	
Cyta—cytarabine	300 mg/m² IV	8	
B—bleomycin	5 u/m² IV	8	
O—vincristine (Oncovin)	1.4 mg/m² IV	8	
M—methotrexate*	120 mg/m² IV bolus	8	
COMLA			Repeat every 91 days
C—cyclophosphamide	1500 mg/m² IV	1	
O—vincristine (Oncovin)	1.4 mg/m² IV (max 2.0 mg)	1, 8, 15	
M—methotrexate	120 mg/m² IV (bolus)	22, 29, 36, 43, 50, 57, 64, 71	
L—leucovorin	25 mg/m² PO × 4	24 hours after methotrexate	
A—cytarabine	300 mg/m² IV	Same as methotrexate	
M-BACOD			Repeat every 21 days
M—methotrexate*	3000 mg/m² IV (over 40–60 minutes)	14	
B—bleomycin	4 u/m² IV	1	
A—doxorubicin (Adriamycin)	45 mg/m² IV	1	
C—cyclophosphamide	600 mg/m² IV	1	
O—vincristine (Oncovin)	1 mg/m² IV	1	
D—dexamethasone (Decadron)	6 mg/m² PO	1–5	
m-BACOD			Repeat every 21 days
m—methotrexate*	200 mg/m² IV (over 15 minutes)	8, 15	
B—bleomycin	4 u/m² IV	1	
A—doxorubicin (Adriamycin)	45 mg/m² IV	1	
C—cyclophosphamide	600 mg/m² IV	1	
O—vincristine (Oncovin)	1.4 mg/m² IV	1	
D—dexamethasone (Decadron)	6 mg/m² PO	1–5	

*Leucovorin rescue is given for 24 hours after each methotrexate dose.

IV = intravenously; PO = by mouth.

major problems associated with these combinations involve tumor regrowth between cycles and central nervous system relapse.

Methotrexate and cytosine arabinoside have the ability to cross the blood-brain barrier and have been incorporated into second-generation regimens such as M-BACOD, m-BACOD, ProMACE/MOPP, and COP-BLAM. These combinations use methotrexate with leucovorin rescue or cytosine arabinoside to prevent lymphomatous extension to the central nervous system. In an attempt to defeat the intrinsic drug resistance of tumor cell populations, they also utilize multiple drugs and a staggered dose schedule for myelotoxic and nonmyelotoxic agents.

Attempts to refine programs with even more intense protocols have led to third-generation combinations such as MACOP-B, ProMACE/CYTABOM, and COP-BLAM III. The two major principles that have influenced their design are the Goldie-Coldman[42] hypothesis and the Hryniuk[84] dose-intensity hypothesis. The former theory proposes that a larger fraction of patients will be cured if they are exposed to the largest number of agents at full doses as early as possible in the treatment course. The latter theory proposes that the best results will occur when a maximum rate per week of drug delivery is maintained.

The second- and third-generation regimens for aggressive NHL were developed and tested in nonrandomized trials. Before they could be accepted as standard therapy it was necessary to compare them to CHOP, which was the accepted standard. This was done in a series of randomized studies with rather surprising results. CHOP was either superior to or equivalent to the more intensive regimens.[85–87] It was concluded that CHOP was the best treatment for intermediate-grade and high-grade NHL.

High-dose chemotherapy with stem cell rescue was suggested as appropriate for patients who had slow responses to initial therapy and thus were at high risk of early relapse. When this approach was compared in a randomized fashion to conventional CHOP in patients who achieved only a partial remission after three cycles of CHOP, no difference in disease-free survival was noted.[88] It was concluded that high-dose marrow ablative chemoradiotherapy with autologous bone marrow transplantation did not improve the outcome in patients with aggressive NHL that responds slowly to first-line CHOP chemotherapy.

Salvage Therapy

In contrast to indolent lymphomas that remain responsive to conventional therapy for substantial periods of time, the outlook for relapsed aggressive lymphomas is dismal. Despite the fact that most of the tumors are sensitive to chemotherapeutic combinations at the time of relapse, refractoriness to treatment develops rapidly after treatment is initiated and cure is rarely possible with recurrent aggressive NHL using conventional chemotherapy.

With the advent of HDC followed by autologous bone marrow transplantation (ABMT), a substantial number of relapsed patients with aggressive lymphoma are achieving durable, second complete remissions.[50,89,90] The confirmation of phase II studies in a randomized trial has made HDC standard therapy for relapsed NHL.[90] The induction regimen usually consists of high-dose cyclophosphamide followed by total body irradiation, and it appears that other agents such as cytosine arabinoside and etoposide can be added without significant increase in toxicity.[91] Usually patients are given several courses of conventional chemotherapy and those with a good response are then placed on the HDC stem cell rescue protocol. Several questions remain. The management of patients who fail to achieve complete remission during their first course of CHOP is not well established. The management of patients whose disease is resistant to chemotherapy at the time of relapse is unclear. It has not been determined whether the HDC should be given at the time of relapse or earlier in the course of the disease.

There is a role for HDC in high-grade NHL including lymphoblastic lymphoma and small, noncleaved cell lymphoma. Clinical trials indicate that allogeneic bone marrow transplantation may provide an alternative to conventional chemotherapy for those with poor-prognosis BL.[92] Because of the low incidence of these tumors, very few studies are available, but a few reports indicate excellent response and survival rates after HDC.[50]

Complications of Treatment

Radiotherapy often causes complications during treatment (acute) or following the completion of treatment (subacute or late). The most common reactions associated with mantle irradiation are loss of taste, dry mouth, redness of skin, dysphagia, loss of hair at the nape of the neck, nausea, and vomiting. Because the amount of saliva is decreased, these individuals are at increased risk of dental caries. Therefore, instructions in proper dental hygiene, which includes routine examination and cleaning every four to six months, should always be given.

Inverted-Y port irradiation usually results in nausea, vomiting, anorexia, diarrhea, and malaise. Bone marrow depression may occur and must be monitored by frequent complete blood counts. Total nodal irradiation leads to all the side effects noted previously and particularly to severe bone marrow depression.

The various combinations of chemotherapy used in the treatment of HD and NHL will invariably result in acute and chronic side effects. The nature of these responses depends on the drugs used, but many are common to most anticancer agents. The most frequent side effect is nausea and vomiting. Although the severity of this reaction varies from one individual to another, it is generally transient and can often be effectively controlled by antiemetics. Depending on the particular drug regimen administered, other reactions can include alopecia, myalgia, chills, fever, euphoria, fluid retention, stomatitis, gastrointestinal disturbances, hemorrhagic cystitis, and mental depression. The most serious side effect produced by all combination regimens is bone marrow suppression, which renders the individual susceptible to infection and hemorrhage.

Symptom Management and Supportive Care

Consequences of Survival

Oncological advances in diagnostic technology, therapeutic regimens, and supportive interventions have shown great progress in the past two decades, and many lymphoma patients face a future in which long-term survival is a reasonable expectation. However, the cost of such progress is yet to be determined. While acute toxicities of established treatment modalities are well documented, clinical evaluation studies are just beginning to investigate the delayed effects and iatrogenic risks associated with surgery (splenectomy/laparotomy), radiation therapy, and chemotherapy. The delayed toxicities tend to produce lifelong problems and may vary in severity from relatively minor to potentially fatal.[93]

It is important to stress that no organ system is immune to alteration. An extension of injury to the lungs is common in mantle irradiation, and it may develop as early as one to three months after RT is completed. Resulting complications can include pneumothorax, radiation pneumonitis, pulmonary fibrosis, and superimposed pulmonary and parenchymal infections. In addition, nitrosoureas, high-dose busulfan, and bleomycin are known to induce fibrotic lung damage.[94]

Tumors on the right side of the superior mediastinum have the potential to obstruct the return of blood to the heart from the superior vena cava. This produces a characteristic syndrome of edema in the upper half of the body that is associated with prominent collateral circulation. Lung cancer, especially the oat cell variety, is the most common cause of this complication, but the lymphomas represent the second most common precipitating factor. This is an oncologic emergency that necessitates prompt therapy aimed at relieving pressure on the superior vena cava. External beam radiation therapy has been the traditional approach, especially in the management of an acute-onset syndrome.[95]

Both RT and chemotherapy promote toxic effects on the heart and peripheral blood vessels. Acute and chronic pericarditis are not uncommon, and a patient often presents with a spectrum of symptoms ranging from cough and chest pain to edema, paradoxical pulse, cardiac tamponade, and hemodynamic compromise. Coronary artery disease and cardiomyopathy are also seen following extensive mediastinal radiation. Similar risks have been noted with doxorubicin, whose cumulative dose effect often is potentiated when drug administration follows RT.[96]

The multiagent regimens used most in HD appear to induce little nephrotoxicity. However, glomerulonephritis is considered a paraneoplastic syndrome of this malignancy. Despite improvements in shielding techniques, radiation damage to the kidneys is possible in retroperitoneal NHL. Limiting the radiation dose to 2000 cGy or less may minimize the risk of a functional deficit. Cyclophosphamide induces topical damage to the bladder, and hemorrhagic cystitis is a potentially serious complication of all chemotherapeutic regimens using this drug.[97]

Because both chemotherapy and radiotherapy are immunosuppressive, bacterial as well as other unusual infections may occur. The most common gram-negative organisms in individuals with lymphoma are *Escherichia coli, Pseudomonas aeruginosa,* and *Klebsiella.* Various species of *Staphylococcus* are also becoming increasingly prevalent in these patients. Although fever as a presenting complaint may be attributable to the lymphoma itself, fever in a patient who has been treated (especially one who is neutropenic) must always be considered a sign of potentially life-threatening sepsis until proven otherwise. Thus, appropriate cultures should be obtained and empiric antibiotic therapy must be started immediately. In addition, patients who have undergone splenectomy face a lifelong risk of activation by encapsulated organisms.

The two fungal infections diagnosed most often are candidiasis and aspergillosis. *Pneumocystis carinii* is a rare protozoal infection in immunologically normal individuals, but it is frequently pathogenic in lymphoma patients. Currently it is recognized as one of the leading causes of death in the AIDS population.

Herpes zoster is a troublesome complication that is often seen in individuals with HD and NHL. It results from the reactivation of latent foci of chickenpox virus, presumably secondary to the immunosuppression caused by the lymphoma and/or its treatment. The virus is usually localized, but on occasion a life-threatening fulminant process may occur. This infection may be seen at any time during the course of illness, from initial treatment to relapse.

Chronic progressive radiation myelopathy is a disabling neurological problem rarely associated with mantle radiation. Symptoms include paresthesias, weakness, and bowel/bladder dysfunction. Peripheral neuropathies are associated with vincristine and vinblastine.

Rare as a presenting symptom but commonly seen in progressive lymphoma, compression of the spinal cord represents a complication that is dreaded because of its potential to cripple with paraplegia a person who might otherwise have many productive years remaining. This oncologic emergency develops swiftly, with weakness of the lower extremities, increased tendon reflexes, positive Babinski signs, and the development of a sensory "level" below which sensation is lost. Precise localization of the compression by myelogram is essential. Recently, MRI has offered the promise of a noninvasive diagnostic technique, but myelography remains the current diagnostic standard. Early diagnosis is critical to prevention of neurological impairment. Patients who have already developed compromised neurological status usually do not have a return of function after treatment.[98] Consequently the nurse must be sensitive to complaints of leg weakness or bowel and bladder dysfunction, especially in patients with back pain.

Two of the most devastating complications associated with lymphoma treatment are sterility and carcinogenesis. Because many of the patients are younger than age 40 when initially diagnosed, these tragic consequences not only confer physical alterations but also create severe psychological distress, as the individual is forced to face a lack of procreative potential and another malignant threat to life.

During RT, men will experience transient aspermia, but recovery of spermatogenesis has been documented when careful testicular shielding is employed. Women who have not had an oophoropexy or shielding of the ovaries may undergo artificial menopause. At the time of exploratory laparotomy, surgical fixation of the ovaries to the uterus is often performed in young female patients to preserve their ovarian function.

Transient and sometimes permanent male sterility is a recognized complication of induction chemotherapy for lymphoma. As a group, the alkylating agents are the most toxic to the testicular germ cells. In general, reversible changes occur up to a given threshold level; irreversible germinal aplasia develops once that threshold has been exceeded. Individuals with HD who are treated with MOPP have a greater than 80% likelihood of developing germinal aplasia, azoospermia, and testicular atrophy with elevated serum follicle-stimulating hormone levels.[99] Chapman and colleagues[100] reported 100% infertility during the first 12 months after therapy in 74 men who received this regimen. Return of active spermatogenesis was seen in only 4 of 64 men 15–51 months after therapy stopped. ABVD, an alternative chemotherapy program for HD, may be as effective as MOPP, but it is less toxic to germinal epithelial cells. The use of combination chemotherapy in women also produces ovarian dysfunction, with those older than age 35–40 being the most susceptible. In the case of MOPP therapy, only 40%–50% of the women experienced ovarian failure.[99] Clearly, the complications of gonadal dysfunction may result in considerable psychosocial problems in both men and women being treated for cure.[6] Thus, reproductive counseling and procreative alternatives are essential components of nursing care to consider for this patient population.[101]

Second malignancies may develop after curative treatment for lymphoma.[102] Acute nonlymphocytic leukemia is the most common and well-recognized long-range complication of exposure to radiation or alkylating anticancer drugs. Cumulative risk varies according to the intensity and nature of the treatment and the period of observation. It may range from less than 1% to well over 10%.[103] If both radiation and chemotherapy are used, the risk of subsequent leukemia is greatest. It is generally believed that the alkylating agents are more leukemogenic than other anticancer drugs; thus, a regimen such as ABVD might be associated with a lower rate of leukemia than MOPP.

Supportive Care

Supportive care of the lymphoma patient begins at diagnosis with an explanation of the disease, a description of the steps that will be taken for staging and treatment, and the effort to evoke in the patient a feeling of confidence in the multidisciplinary team responsible for care. Regardless of whether the primary treatment is radiotherapy or chemotherapy, it is certain that the clinical course will be lengthy and highly toxic. The individual must be prepared to cope with this reality. The person who presents with constitutional symptoms and receives several cycles of chemotherapy often becomes completely asymptomatic. Because symptoms are relieved, the patient might question why he or she should proceed with a treatment program that causes adverse side effects. This follow-up period is crucial if a positive outcome is to be achieved. The nurse can play a major role by providing the understanding and emotional support the patient needs and by making sure the patient understands that although small foci of disease cause no symptoms, they will, if untreated, lead to recurrence.

After the primary treatment there will be a prolonged period (months to years) during which the patient must be observed for a recurrence of disease. This is a particularly trying period because the individual has already, in his or her own mind, been very close to death by virtue of having dealt with the diagnosis of cancer. The treatment has (as a rule) produced complete remission, but each visit to the clinic now carries with it the threat that the disease may have relapsed and the nightmare must begin all over again. The nurse must be aware that whereas the treatment team views this as a "routine" visit for a patient who has responded very well to therapy, the individual perceives every word or facial expression as a potential clue that the cancer has recurred. Although the outlook for survivors of lymphomas is positive, long-term sequelae and survivorship issues must be addressed by both survivors and health care providers. These issues include psychosocial adjustment, employment and economic issues, rehabilitation, education, and periodic follow-up and screening for second malignancies.[104,105] See Chapters 69–71 for a review of cancer survivorship issues.

Conclusion

The lymphomas comprise more than a dozen separate neoplasms that exhibit a wide gamut of clinical presentations ranging from slow, indolent growth to rapidly fatal progression. Some lymphomas are highly curable with appropriate therapy, while others show no increase in survival following treatment. These malignancies are separated from each other on the basis of subtle differences and require expert interpretation and evaluation. Megavoltage radiotherapy and combination chemotherapy have provided improved management techniques, leading to the expectation of cure in well over 50% of all individuals with lymphoma. However, the skillful application of the complex and toxic treatments requires a precise delineation of histological type and extent of disease in accordance with rigorously established principles of staging.

Although the etiology of the lymphomas remains elusive, tantalizing hints are provided by the suggestion of EBV-induced Burkitt's lymphoma and other lymphomas, the virus-like epidemiological pattern of nodular sclerosing Hodgkin's disease, the clear association between malfunction of the immune defense system and the development of non-Hodgkin's lymphoma, and the identification of altered genes involved in the cell cycle and apoptosis.

Effective diagnosis, staging, and multimodal management of the lymphomas require the collaborative efforts of multiple health care disciplines. The contributions of the nurse are vital to the achievement of a positive outcome. It is the nurse who, to a greater extent than others on the team, must respond to the patient's deepest need for support and understanding; it is the nurse who must meet the patient's need for careful explanation of the complex diagnostic and therapeutic methods designed to deal with a life-threatening malignancy; and it is the nurse who constantly must be alert to the possible complications of both the disease and its treatment.

The ultimate goal of any therapeutic regimen should be to return the individual to as healthy a lifestyle as possible. Because the cohort of cancer survivors continues to increase, the scope of nursing practice must expand as well. Now that cure is no longer beyond our grasp, emphasis must shift to rehabilitation, where attention that complements the goals of acute care can be directed toward each individual's functional, psychological, vocational, and economic limitations. Although many iatrogenic effects cannot always be anticipated or reversed, early identification of rehabilitation issues and timely intervention by an expert caregiver can help minimize potential disability and enhance overall quality of life. Patients who have struggled to overcome their cancer experience and those who supported them make such efforts meaningful and worthwhile.

References

1. Urba WJ, Longo DL: Hodgkin's disease. *N Engl J Med* 326: 678–687, 1992
2. Hasse U, Tinguely M, Oppliger E, et al: Clonal loss of heterozygosity in microdissected Hodgkin and Reed-Sternberg cells. *J Natl Cancer Inst* 91:1581–1583, 1999
3. Kadin ME: Pathology of Hodgkin's disease. *Curr Opin Oncol* 6:456–463, 1994
4. Landis SH, Murray T, Bolden S, et al: Cancer Statistics, 1999. *CA Cancer J Clin* 49:8–31, 1999
5. Gail MH, Pluda JM, Rabkin CS, et al: Projections of the incidence of non-Hodgkin's lymphoma related to acquired immunodeficiency syndrome. *J Natl Cancer Inst* 83:695–701, 1991
6. Carli PM, Boutron MC, Maynadie M, et al: Increase in the incidence of non-Hodgkin's lymphomas: evidence for a recent sharp increase in France independent of AIDS. *Br J Cancer* 70:713–715, 1994
7. Workman ML: The lymphoid system and its role in maintaining immunocompetence. *Semin Oncol Nurs* 14:248–255, 1998
8. Appelbaum JW: The role of the immune system in the pathogenesis of cancer. *Semin Oncol Nurs* 8:51–62, 1992
9. Opelz G, Henderson R: Incidence of non-Hodgkin's lymphoma in kidney and heart transplant recipients. *Lancet* 342:1514–1516, 1993
10. Parker JW, Lukes RJ: Neoplasms of the immune system, in Stites DP, Terr AI (eds): *Basic and Clinical Immunology.* Norwalk, CT, Appleton and Lange, 1991, pp 599–631
11. Rahr VA, Tucker R: Non-Hodgkin's lymphoma: understanding the disease. *Cancer Nurs* 13:56–91, 1990
12. Hodgkin T: On some morbid appearances of the absorbent glands and spleen. *Med Chir Tran* 17:68–114, 1832
13. Wilks S: Cases of enlargement of the lymphatic glands and spleen, or Hodgkin's disease. *Guy's Hosp Rep* 11:56–67, 1865
14. Reed DM: On the pathological changes in Hodgkin's disease, with especial reference to tuberculosis. *Johns Hopkins Rep* 10:133–196, 1902
15. Sternberg C: Über eine eigenartige unter dem Bilde der Pseukoleukamie verlaufende: tuberculose des lymphatischen apparates. *Z Heilkd* 19:21–90, 1898
16. Cole P, MacMahon B, Aisenberg A: Mortality from Hodgkin's disease in the United States: evidence for the multiple etiology hypothesis. *Lancet* 2:1371–1376, 1968
17. DeVita VT, Mauch PM, Harris NL: Hodgkin's disease, in DeVita VT, Hellman S, Rosenberg SA (eds): *Cancer: Principles and Practice of Oncology* (ed 5). Philadelphia, Lippincott-Raven, 1997, pp 2242–2283
18. Ambinder RF, Browning PJ, Lorenzana I, et al: Epstein-Barr virus and childhood Hodgkin's disease in Honduras and in the United States. *Blood* 81:462–467, 1993
19. Preciado MW, De Matteo E, Diez B, et al: Presence of Epstein-Barr virus and strain type assignment in Argentine childhood Hodgkin's disease. *Blood* 86:3922–3929, 1995
20. Armstrong AA, Alexander FE, Paes RP, et al: Association of Epstein-Barr virus with pediatric Hodgkin's disease. *Am J Pathol* 142:1683–1688, 1993
21. Siebert JD, Ambinder RF, Napoli VM, et al: Human immunodeficiency virus-associated Hodgkin's disease contains latent, not replicative, Epstein-Barr virus. *Hum Pathol* 26:1191–1195, 1995
22. Grufferman S, Delzell E: Epidemiology of Hodgkin's disease. *Epidemiol Rev* 6:76–106, 1984
23. Robertson SJ, Lowman JT, Grufferman S, et al: Familial Hodgkin's disease. *Cancer* 59:1314–1319, 1987
24. Haluska FG, Brufsky AM, Cannellos GP: The cellular biology of the Reed-Sternberg cell. *Blood* 84:1005–1021, 1994

25. Slivnick DJ, Nawrocki JF, Fisher RI: Immunology and cellular biology of Hodgkin's disease. *Hematol Oncol Clin North Am* 3:205–220, 1989

26. Hell K, Lorenzen J, Fischer R, et al: Hodgkin cells accumulate mRNA for *bcl-2*. *Lab Invest* 73:492–496, 1995

27. Bhagat SK, Medeiros LJ, Weiss LM, et al: *bcl-2* expression in Hodgkin's disease: correlation with the t(14;18) translocation and Epstein-Barr virus. *Am J Clin Pathol* 99:604–608, 1993

28. Alkan S, Ross CW, Hanson CA, et al: Epstein-Barr virus and *bcl-2* protein overexpression and not detected in the neoplastic cells of nodular lymphocyte predominance Hodgkin's disease. *Mod Pathol* 8:544–547, 1995

29. Schlaifer D, March M, Krajewski S, et al: High expression of the *bcl-x* gene in Reed-Sternberg cells of Hodgkin's disease. *Blood* 85:2671–2674, 1995

30. Weinreb M, Day PJR, Niggli F, et al: The consistent association between Epstein-Barr virus and Hodgkin's disease in children in Kenya. *Blood* 87:3828–3836, 1996

31. Seiz AM, Yarbro CH: Pruritus, in Yarbro CH, Frogge MH, Goodman M (eds): *Cancer Symptom Management* (ed 2). Sudbury, MA, Jones and Bartlett, 1999, pp 148–160

32. Strum SB, Dark JK, Rappaport H: Observations of cells resembling Sternberg-Reed cells in conditions other than Hodgkin's disease. *Cancer* 26:176–190, 1970

33. Craver LF, Hall TC, Rappaport H, et al: Report of the nomenclature committee. *Cancer Res* 26:1311, 1966

34. Harris NL, Jaffe ES, Stein H, et al: A revised European-American classification of lymphoid neoplasms: a proposal from the International Lymphoma Study Group. *Blood* 84:1361–1392, 1994

35. Carbone PP, Kaplan HS, Musshoff K, et al: Report of the committee on Hodgkin's disease staging. *Cancer Res* 31:1860–1861, 1971

36. Lister TA, Crowther D, Sutcliffe SB, et al: Report of a committee convened to discuss the evaluation and staging of patients with Hodgkin's disease: Cotswolds meeting. *J Clin Oncol* 7:1630–1636, 1989

37. Golomb HM: Management of early stage Hodgkin's disease: a continuing evolution. *Semin Oncol* 25:476–482, 1998

38. Longo DL, Glatstein E, Duffey PL, et al: Radiation therapy versus combination chemotherapy in the treatment of early stage Hodgkin's disease: seven year results of a prospective randomized trial. *J Clin Oncol* 9:906–917, 1991

39. Longo DL: The case against the routine use of radiation therapy in advanced-stage Hodgkin's disease. *Cancer Invest* 14:353–360, 1996

40. Prosnitz LR, Wu JJ, Yahalom J: The case for adjuvant radiation therapy in advanced Hodgkin's disease. *Cancer Invest* 14:361–370, 1996

41. Santoro A, Bonadonna G, Valagussa P, et al: Long-term results of combined chemotherapy-radiotherapy approach in Hodgkin's disease: superiority of ABVD plus radiotherapy versus MOPP plus radiotherapy. *J Clin Oncol* 5:27–37, 1987

42. Goldie JH, Coldman AJ, Guaduskus GA: Rationale for the use of alternating non-cross-resistant chemotherapy. *Cancer Treat Rep* 66:439–449, 1982

43. Somers R, Carde P, Henry-Amar M, et al: A randomized study in stage IIIB and IV Hodgkin's disease comparing eight courses of MOPP versus an alternation of MOPP with ABVD. *J Clin Oncol* 12:279–287, 1994

44. Cannellos GP, Anderson JR, Propert KJ, et al: Chemotherapy of advanced Hodgkin's disease with MOPP, ABVD, or MOPP alternating with ABVD. *N Engl J Med* 327:1478–1484, 1992

45. Henkelmann GC, Hagemester FB, Fuller LM: Two cycles of MOPP and radiotherapy for Stage III, A and III, B Hodgkin's disease. *J Clin Oncol* 6:1293–1302, 1988

46. Schomberg PJ, Evans RG, O'Connell MJ, et al: Prognostic significance of mediastinal mass in adult Hodgkin's disease. *Cancer* 53:324–328, 1984

47. Prakash U, Abel MD: Mediastinal mass and tracheal obstruction during general anesthesia. *Mayo Clin Proc* 63:1004–1011, 1988

48. Leopold KA, Canellos GP, Rosenthal D, et al: Stage IA–IIB Hodgkin's disease. Staging and treatment of patients with large mediastinal adenopathy. *J Clin Oncol* 7:1059–1065, 1989

49. Fisher RI, DeVita VT, Hubbard SP, et al: Prolonged disease-free survival in Hodgkin's disease with MOPP reinduction after first relapse. *Ann Intern Med* 90:761–763, 1979

50. Laport GF, Williams SF: The role of high dose chemotherapy in patients with Hodgkin's disease and non-Hodgkin's lymphoma. *Semin Oncol* 25:503–517, 1998

51. Jones RJ, Piantadosi S, Mann RB, et al: High-dose cytotoxic therapy and bone marrow transplantation for relapsed Hodgkin's disease. *J Clin Oncol* 8:527–537, 1990

52. Ager S, Wimperis JZ, Tolliday B, et al: Autologous bone marrow transplantation for Hodgkin's disease—a five-year single centre experience. *Leuk Lymphoma* 13:263–272, 1994

53. Nademanee A, O'Donnell MR, Snyder DS, et al: High-dose chemotherapy with or without total body irradiation followed by autologous bone marrow and/or peripheral blood stem cell transplantation for patients with relapsed and refractory Hodgkin's disease: results in 85 patients with analysis of prognostic factors. *Blood* 85:1381–1390, 1995

54. Koeppen H, Vardiman JW: New entities, issues, and controversy in the classification of malignant lymphoma. *Semin Oncol* 25:421–434, 1998

55. Shipp MA, Mauch PM, Harris NL: Non-Hodgkin's lymphomas, in DeVita VT, Hellman S, Rosenberg SA (eds): *Cancer: Principles and Practice of Oncology* (ed 5). Philadelphia, Lippincott-Raven, 1997, pp 2242–2283

56. DeMario MD, Liebowitz DN: Lymphomas in the immunocompromised patient. *Semin Oncol* 25:492–502, 1998

57. Purtilo DT, Stevenson M: Lymphotropic viruses as etiologic agents of lymphoma. *Hematol Oncol Clin North Am* 5:901–923, 1991

58. Urba WJ, Longo DL: Burkitt's lymphoma, in Moosa AR, Schimpff SC, Robson MC (eds): *Comprehensive Textbook of Oncology*, vol 2 (ed 2). Baltimore, Williams and Wilkins, 1991, pp 1296–1301

59. Wright DH: Pathogenesis of non-Hodgkin's lymphoma: clues from geography, in Magrath IT (ed): *The Non-Hodgkin's Lymphomas*. Baltimore, Williams and Wilkins, 1990, pp 122–134

60. Shapiro RS: Epstein-Barr virus-associated B-cell lymphoproliferative disorders in immunodeficiency: meeting the challenge. *J Clin Oncol* 8:371–373, 1990 (editorial)

61. Joncas JH, Russo P, Brochu P, et al: Epstein-Barr virus polymorphic B-cell lymphoma associated with leukemia and with congenital immunodeficiencies. *J Clin Oncol* 8:378–384, 1990

62. Urba WJ, Longo DL: Lymphocytic lymphomas: epidemiology, etiology, pathology, and staging, in Moosa AR, Schimpff SC, Robson MC (eds): *Comprehensive Textbook of*

Oncology, vol 2 (ed 2). Baltimore, Williams and Wilkins, 1991, pp 1268–1276

63. Roggero E, Zucca E, Pinotti G, et al: Eradication of *Helicobacter pylori* infection in low-grade gastric lymphoma of mucosa-associated lymphoid tissue. *Ann Intern Med* 122: 767–769, 1995

64. Yang E, Korsmeyer SJ: Molecular thanatopsis: a discourse on the *BCL2* family and cell death. *Blood* 88:386–401, 1996

65. Segal GH, Masih AS, Fox AC, et al: CD5 expressing B-cell non-Hodgkin's lymphomas with *bcl-1* gene rearrangement have a relatively homogeneous immunophenotype and are associated with an overall poor prognosis. *Blood* 85: 1570–1579, 1995

66. Levine EG, Bloomfield CD: Cytogenetics of malignant lymphomas, in Wiernik PH, Canellos GP, Kyle RA, Schiffer CA (eds): *Neoplastic Diseases of the Blood* (ed 2). New York, Churchill-Livingstone, 1991, pp 689–700

67. Peng JW, Lee EC: Cytogenetics, in Magrath IT (ed): *The Non-Hodgkin's Lymphomas*. Baltimore, Williams and Wilkins, 1990, pp 77–95

68. Doll DC: Introduction: Extranodal lymphomas. *Semin Oncol* 26:249–250, 1999

69. Hogan DK, Rosenthal LD: Oncologic emergencies in the patient with lymphoma. *Semin Oncol Nurs* 14:312–320, 1998

70. Maher EA, Fine HA: Primary CNS Lymphoma. *Semin Oncol* 26:346–356, 1999

71. Rappaport H, Winter WJ, Hicks EB: Follicular lymphoma: a reevaluation of its position in the scheme of malignant lymphomas, based on a survey of 253 cases. *Cancer* 9:792, 1956

72. Lukes RJ, Collins RD: Immunologic characterization of human malignant lymphomas. *Cancer* 34:1488–1503, 1974

73. The Non-Hodgkin's Lymphoma Pathologic Classification Project: National Cancer Institute Sponsored Study of Classifications of Non-Hodgkin's Lymphomas. Summary and description of a Working Formulation for clinical usage. *Cancer* 49:2112–2135, 1982

74. Crump M, Gospodarowicz M, Shepherd FA: Lymphoma of the gastrointestinal tract. *Semin Oncol* 26:324–337, 1999

75. Shipp M, Harrington D, Anderson J, et al: The international non-Hodgkin's lymphoma prognostic factors project: a predictive model for progressive non-Hodgkin's lymphoma. *N Engl J Med* 329:987–994, 1993

76. McFadden ME: Cutaneous T-cell lymphoma. *Semin Oncol Nurs* 7:36–44, 1991

77. Maor MH, Velasquez WS, Fuller LM, et al: Stomach conservation in Stages IE and IIE gastric non-Hodgkin's lymphoma. *J Clin Oncol* 8:266–271, 1990

78. Horning SJ, Rosenberg SA: The natural history of initially untreated low-grade non-Hodgkin's lymphomas. *N Engl J Med* 311:1471–1475, 1984

79. Young RC, Longo DL, Glatstein E, et al: The treatment of indolent lymphomas: watchful waiting versus aggressive combined modality treatment. *Semin Hematol* 25:11–16, 1988 (suppl)

80. Vose JM: Current approaches the management of non-Hodgkin's lymphoma. *Semin Oncol* 25:483–491, 1998

81. Zinzani PL, Bendandi M, Tura S: FMP regimen (fludarabine, mitxantrone, prednisone) as therapy in recurrent low-grade non-Hodgkin's lymphoma. *Eur J Haematol* 55: 262–266, 1995

82. Morrison VA, Peterson BA: High-dose therapy and transplantation in non-Hodgkin's lymphoma. *Semin Oncol* 26: 84–98, 1999

83. Weiss RB: Introduction: dose intensive therapy for adult malignancies. *Semin Oncol* 26:1–5, 1999

84. Hryniuk W, Bush H: The importance of dose intensity in chemotherapy of metastatic breast cancer. *J Clin Oncol* 2: 1281–1287, 1984

85. Fisher RI, Gaynor ER, Dahlberg S, et al: Comparison of a standard regimen (CHOP) with three intensive chemotherapy regimens for advanced non-Hodgkin's lymphoma. *N Engl J Med* 328:1002–1006, 1993

86. Gordon LI, Harrington D, Andersen J, et al: Comparison of a second-generation combination chemotherapeutic regimen (m-BACOD) with a standard regimen (CHOP) for advanced diffuse non-Hodgkin's lymphoma. *N Engl J Med* 327:1342–1349, 1992

87. Cooper IA, Wolf MM, Robertson TI, et al: Randomized comparison of MACOP-B with CHOP in patients with intermediate grade non-Hodgkin's lymphoma. The Australian and New Zealand Lymphoma Group. *J Clin Oncol* 12: 769–778, 1994

88. Verdonck LF, van Putten WL, Hagenbeek A, et al: Comparison of CHOP chemotherapy with autologous bone marrow transplantation for slowly responding patients with aggressive non-Hodgkin's lymphoma. *N Engl J Med* 332: 1045–1051, 1995

89. Phillip T, Armitage JO, Spitzer G, et al: High dose therapy and ABMT after failure of conventional chemotherapy in one hundred adults with intermediate or high grade non-Hodgkin's lymphoma. *N Engl J Med* 316:1493–1498, 1987

90. Philip T, Guglielmi C, Hagenbeek A, et al: Autologous bone marrow transplantation as compared with salvage chemotherapy in relapses of chemotherapy sensitive non-Hodgkin's lymphoma. *N Engl J Med* 333:1540–1555, 1995

91. Gribben JG, Goldstone AH, Linch DC, et al: Effectiveness of high-dose combination chemotherapy and autologous bone marrow transplantation for patients with non-Hodgkin's lymphomas who are still responsive to conventional-dose therapy. *J Clin Oncol* 7:1621–1629, 1989

92. Troussard X, Leblond V, Kuentz M, et al: Allogeneic bone marrow transplantation in adults with Burkitt's lymphoma or acute lymphoblastic leukemia in first complete remission. *J Clin Oncol* 8:809–812, 1990

93. Ruccione K, Weinberg K: Late effects in multiple body systems. *Semin Oncol Nurs* 5:4–13, 1989

94. Wickham R: Pulmonary toxicity secondary to cancer treatment. *Oncol Nurs Forum* 13:69–76, 1986

95. Baker GL, Barnes HJ: Superior vena cava syndrome: etiology, diagnosis, and treatment. *Am J Crit Care* 1:54–64, 1992

96. Kaszyk LK: Cardiac toxicity associated with cancer therapy. *Oncol Nurs Forum* 13:81–88, 1986

97. Lydon J: Nephrotoxicity of cancer treatment. *Oncol Nurs Forum* 13:68–77, 1986

98. Wilson JK, Masaryk TJ: Neurologic emergencies in the cancer patient. *Semin Oncol* 16:490–503, 1989

99. Yarbro CH, Perry MC: The effect of cancer therapy on gonadal function. *Semin Oncol Nurs* 1:3–8, 1985

100. Chapman R, Rees L, Sutcliffe SB, et al: Cyclical combination chemotherapy and gonadal function: retrospective study in males. *Lancet* 1:285–289, 1979

101. Kaempfer SH, Wiley FM, Hoffman DJ: Fertility considerations and procreative alternatives in cancer care. *Semin Oncol Nurs* 1:25–34, 1985

102. Jacquillat C, Khayat D, Desprez-Curely JP, et al: Occurrence of non-Hodgkin's lymphoma after therapy for Hodgkin's disease. *Cancer* 53:459–462, 1984

103. Fraser MG, Tucker MA: Second malignancies following cancer therapy. *Semin Oncol Nurs* 5:43–55, 1989

104. Callaghan M: Hodgkin's disease. *Semin Oncol Nurs* 14:262–272, 1998

105. Fernsler J, Fanuele JS: Lymphomas: long-term sequelae and survivorship issues. *Semin Oncol Nurs* 14:321–328, 1998

CHAPTER 61

Multiple Myeloma

Carol A. Sheridan, RN, MSN, AOCN
Maria Serrano, RN, MSN, CS, NPC, AOCN

Introduction

Waldenstrom macroglobulinemia, monoclonal gammopathy of undetermined significance (MGUS), and multiple myeloma constitute the group of diseases classified as *plasma cell disorders*. These disorders are characterized by the overproduction of immunoglobulins.[1] In these diseases the malignant cell is the plasma cell, the functional mature cell that differentiates and develops from the B lymphocyte.[2,3] Multiple myeloma is considered a chemosensitive disease at the time of initial presentation. Despite response rates in the 40% range, patients eventually relapse, requiring other therapeutic interventions.[2] In the past decade there have been advances in the biologic characterization of the growth and survival of multiple myeloma cells within the marrow microenvironment. There has also been the identification of common chromosomal abnormalities. These advances and the advent of high-dose therapy with stem cell support have led to an improvement in the event free survival (EFS) and overall survival (OS). Results of randomized clinical trials have produced enthusiasm and cautious optimism in this universally chronic and fatal disease.[4,5] Multiple myeloma, the most common malignant plasma cell disorder, can affect the hematologic, skeletal, renal, and nervous systems.[4]

Epidemiology

Within the United States, multiple myeloma represents 1% of all hematologic malignancies.[1] Although the incidence of multiple myeloma appears to be increasing in the United States, there is some evidence that the increased incidence may be due to earlier and improved diagnosis in older, high-risk populations. The onset of multiple myeloma is late, with peak occurrence between the fifth and seventh decades of life.[6,7] The median age at diagnosis is 65, but 2% of all cases occur before age 40.[1,6] Differences in disease incidence can be noted based on sex and race. Within the United States, multiple myeloma is more common among blacks than among whites by a 2-to-1 margin.[1] For all racial groups there is a male predominance, with a male to female ratio of 3:2, although black females have a higher incidence than white males.[6] This racial difference persists in the five-year relative cancer survival rates. For all white Americans diagnosed during the years 1974–1976 and 1989–1994, there was a statistically significant increase in the five-year relative survival rates (24%–28%, $p < 0.05$). There was a slight improvement in the five-year relative survival rates for blacks diagnosed with multiple myeloma during this period, but it did not reach statistical significance (27%–30%).[8]

Two explanations have been put forward for these racial differences. First, blacks have a higher circulating level of immunoglobulin G (IgG), representing a greater opportunity for B-cell malignant transformation.[1] The second explanation has to do with a general increased exposure to pollutants (air, water, food) over time, promoting chronic antigenic stimulation of the immune system.[9] The black community within the United States is clearly at higher risk for morbidity and mortality associated with multiple myeloma. Worldwide, some Asian populations have the lowest incidence rates.[2]

Etiology

The exact etiology of multiple myeloma is unknown, although a variety of factors have been associated with the development of the disease. In an attempt to better understand the etiologic factors, Potter[10] used an animal model and demonstrated that only specific strains of mice developed plasmacytomas following mineral oil injections. An analogous case for genetic linkage was made by Maldonado and Kyle,[11] who documented an increased frequency of plasma cell disorders among close relatives of individuals with multiple myeloma. First-degree relatives of patients with multiple myeloma appear to have a higher incidence of the disease.[3] Chromosomal abnormalities have also been documented in mice that underwent experimentally induced plasma cell disease.

Recent studies suggest a viral etiology. Human herpes virus-8 (HHV-8) has been identified in bone marrow stromal cells of patients with multiple myeloma.[12] The significance of this finding as an etiologic agent has yet to be confirmed. In humans with multiple myeloma, chromosomal translocations have been identified. These translocations frequently involve the Ig gene locus and have led to the identification of potential oncogenes. In particular, *RAS* mutations are associated with aggressive disease and a poor prognosis.[13] Other chromosomal abnormalities involve the loss of chromosome 13 and the jumping translocation of chromosone 1q. Both of these chromosomal abnormalities are commonly associated with poor outcome.[14] Through continued investigation, scientists may soon be able to identify individual or common mechanisms by which these different genes contribute to the malignant transformation of the plasma cell.

Risk Factors

Chronic low level exposure to radiation has been associated with a two-fold to six-fold increase in the incidence of multiple myeloma, which may develop as late as 20 years after the radiation exposure.[7] Chronic antigenic stimulation, such as recurrent infections and drug allergies, may be part of the medical history in individuals who develop multiple myeloma. Occupational exposure to low-dose ionizing radiation, wood, textile, rubber, metal, petroleum products, and chemicals used as herbicides has been associated with the development of multiple myeloma.[7,15,16] No clear evidence demonstrating a common environmental or chemical etiologic factor has been established. In all such instances, further study is warranted to demonstrate a definitive risk relationship.

Prevention/Early Detection

In the absence of known causative agents, identified tumor markers, or definitive diagnostic tests, the ability to apply prevention and early detection strategies remains illusive. Clinicians providing primary care who know the risk factors associated with multiple myeloma can utilize this knowledge to maintain a "high index of suspicion" when evaluating individuals who present with signs and symptoms that may be indicative of multiple myeloma.[1,6,13]

Pathophysiology

The pluripotent stem cell resides within the bone marrow and has the ability to self-replicate or to differentiate into either the myeloid or lymphoid stem cell. The lymphoid stem cell is the earliest lymphoid cell. It resides within the bone marrow and retains the ability to self-replicate or to differentiate into either T lymphocytes or B lymphocytes. T lymphocytes regulate the immune response and participate in cell-mediated immunity. B lymphocytes mature into plasma cells that manufacture and secrete large quantities of immunoglobulins. B lymphocytes are responsible for humoral immunity.

Five classes of immunoglobulins are secreted: IgG, IgA, IgM, IgD, and IgE. IgM is the first immunoglobulin produced during a primary immune response and the first immunoglobulin produced in infants.[1] IgA is the primary immunoglobulin in saliva, tears, and the secretions of the gastrointestinal and respiratory tract. IgA plays a primary role in protecting these mucous membranes and vital organ systems by maintaining the first line of defense.[16] IgD and IgE are trace immunoglobulins found in the plasma. IgD acts as a cell-surface receptor that binds with antigen and triggers further B-lymphocyte differentiation and production. IgE can be elevated in response to parasitic infections and allergic response such as hay fever and asthma. It is thought that IgE binds to receptors on basophils and mast cells and may stimulate these cells to release vasoactive substances, as part of the allergic response.[1,16] IgG is the primary immunoglobulin in the serum. It has four subclasses (IgG1–4) with slightly different physiologic properties. IgG1 and IgG3 bind complement and mononuclear cells better than IgG2 and IgG4. When IgG1 and IgG3 are overproduced in multiple myeloma, the hyperviscosity syndrome may result. IgG is the only immunoglobulin that can cross the placenta and therefore confers passive immunity to newborns. In adults, IgG constitutes the largest proportion of immunoglobulin, followed by IgA and IgM.

The immunoglobulins are composed of four polypeptide chains, two heavy and two light. The heavy chains take their names from the class of immunoglobulin: IgG (gamma), IgA (alpha), and IgM (mu). The light chains are either lambda (λ) or kappa (κ).[7,17] Each immunoglobulin has a dual function: one function is the specific antibody that binds to complement or antigen; the other function is the constant region or Fc fragment that binds to membrane receptors.[16]

The plasma cell is derived from the B lymphocyte and is the functionally mature cell producing immunoglobulins; it has been thought to be the identifiable malignant cell in multiple myeloma.[17] Pilarski and colleagues demonstrated the expression of myeloid and megakaryocytic antigens on the plasma cell clone, leading the investigators to hypothesize that myeloma development may be programmed into cells prior to B-cell differentiation.[18]

A final proposed model for myeloma development involves genetic and molecular defects in the early development of myeloma. A large number of chromosomal changes have been identified, and as many as one-third of all myeloma patients had chromosomal changes in one report.[7] With flow cytometry and fluorescence in situ hybridization (FISH) analysis, investigators could detect the presence of cytogenetic abnormalities in as many as 80%–90% of patient samples regardless of disease status.[19] These hypotheses require further investigation and may prove useful in developing future successful therapies.

Regardless of the exact location of the malignant change in multiple myeloma, there is abnormal overproduction of one immunoglobulin called the M protein; the M refers to monoclonal antibody, myeloma protein, or malignant protein. Although an excessive amount of immunoglobulin is being produced, the M protein is unable to effectively produce antibody necessary for maintaining humoral immunity. Approximately 80%–90% of all multiple myeloma patients will show evidence of the aberrant M protein in the serum.[3]

Role of Cytokines

The exact site of the malignant transformation that causes multiple myeloma remains unknown. There have been advances in our understanding of the role many cytokines play in the development and growth of multiple myeloma (Table 61-1).[7,16,18]

Interleukin-6 (IL-6) has been identified by both in vitro and in vivo studies as one of the major growth factors involved in the development of multiple myeloma.[20] The paracrine growth function of IL-6 has been demonstrated. It is produced by the bone marrow stromal cells as well as by monocytes.[7,21] Reibnegger and associates demonstrated that serum IL-6 levels controlled C-reactive protein production and were prognostic in multiple myeloma patients.[22,23] An elevated IL-6 level was associated with increased C-reactive protein levels and associated with increased severity of multiple myeloma (i.e., hypercalcemia and poor survival). Interleukin-6 has also been shown to be a survival factor by inhibiting apoptosis of

Table 61-1 Cytokines Currently under Investigation in the Pathogenesis of Multiple Myeloma

Interleukin-1B (IL-1B)

Interleukin-3 (IL-3)

Interleukin-5 (IL-5)

Interleukin-6 (IL-6)

Interleukin-10 (IL-10)

Tumor necrosis factor (TNF)

Granulocyte-macrophage colony-stimulating factor (GM-CSF)

Alfa-interferon

myeloma cells.[24,25] Other cytokines such as tumor necrosis factor (TNF) and interleukin-1B (IL-1B) have been shown to increase the bone marrow stromal cell production of IL-6.[7] Both IL-1B and TNF have been identified as the so-called osteoclast-activating factors (OAFs) responsible for the bone resorption and destruction associated with multiple myeloma.[1,7]

Investigational in vitro studies have demonstrated that IL-3, IL-5, and granulocyte-macrophage colony-stimulating factor (GM-CSF) has a synergistic effect with IL-6, promoting myeloma cell production. Future research directed at these early progenitor growth factors might increase our knowledge regarding the exact pathogenesis of multiple myeloma.

Interleukin-10 has been identified as a differentiating factor promoting B cells into cells responsible for immunoglobulin production.[20] In vitro results demonstrate an increase in myeloma cell proliferation in short-term cultures of bone marrow cells from individuals with multiple myeloma. The exact role of IL-10 in vivo requires further investigation.

Alfa-interferon in vitro has been demonstrated to promote the growth of IL-6 dependent myeloma cells in culture.[20] The exact role and use of alfa-interferon in the treatment of multiple myeloma remains controversial. Future laboratory and clinical studies will clarify the exact role that cytokines play in the pathogenesis and progression of multiple myeloma.

Clinical Manifestations

The most frequent symptom at presentation is bone pain. Once symptoms are present, untreated individuals with multiple myeloma have a median survival of seven months.[3] This can be extended with standard therapy to a median survival of two to three years.[3,26] Individuals with multiple myeloma may have a long prodromal, indolent, or asymptomatic period. Once symptoms occur, however, systemic therapy becomes necessary. Patients may eventually enter a period in which their disease becomes refractory or unresponsive to conventional therapy, at which time investigational therapies are warranted.[6] The clinical course of the disease is complicated by pathological fractures, pain, hypercalcemia, spinal cord compression, anemia, fatigue, thrombocytopenia, recurrent bacterial infections, and renal failure.

Skeletal Involvement

From 68% to 80% of individuals with multiple myeloma present with destructive, painful osteolytic lesions at the time of diagnosis.[9,27,28] Symptoms associated with these lesions include hypercalcemia (20%–40% of patients), pathological fractures with acute and chronic pain, decreased mobility, and an inability to fully participate in activities of daily living.[28–30] The bone lesions can be of three distinct types: (1) a solitary osteolytic lesion, (2) diffuse osteoporosis, and (3) multiple discrete osteolytic "punched-out" or "cannonball" lesions. The pathophysiology of the bone destruction is thought to be myeloma cell production of osteoclast activating factor (OAF). Once thought to be a single substance, OAFs have now been identified as a class of bone-resorbing factors (cytokines) produced by lymphocytes and monocytes.[31] Several OAFs have been purified and molecularly cloned, including lymphotoxin, TNF, the interferons, and IL-1.[1] Although the precise relationships and interactions between these cytokines have not been described, IL-IA, IL-IB, TNF, and IL-6 have been associated with an increase in both myeloma proliferation and osteoclast activity.[20,32,33]

Myeloma-associated bone lesions occur as a result of increased osteoclast activity and are most readily diagnosed by roentgenograms or bone surveys.[34] Magnetic resonance imaging (MRI) is the test of choice for evaluating and diagnosing spinal cord compression.[4] If untreated, myeloma-induced osteolytic lesions can lead to compression fractures of the spine with irreversible neurological sequelae, refractory hypercalcemia compromising renal function, and possibly death.

Infection

As with most malignancies, 50%–70% of all multiple myeloma patients will die as a result of bacterial infection.[3,35] The two most common sites of infection are the respiratory and urinary tracts.[9,36] Common infectious organisms include *Staphylococcus aureus*, *Streptococcus pneumoniae*, *Escherichia coli*, *Pseudomonas*, and *Klebsiella*. In the 1980s, Savage and associates[37] demonstrated a biphasic pattern of infection in the person with multiple myeloma. *Streptococcus pneumoniae* and *Haemophilus influenzae* occurred early in the disease (within eight months of diagnosis) or in patients who responded early to chemotherapy, whereas infections caused by nonencapsulated gram-negative bacilli and *S. aureus* typically occurred in neutropenic patients or those individuals with unresponsive or refractory disease.[3,38] Gram-negative organisms account for approximately 50% of all infections in patients with multiple myeloma.[39]

A number of mechanisms have been identified as responsible for the immunosuppression and infection associated with multiple myeloma. These include a deficiency in the normal amount and function of immunoglobulins, neutropenia associated with plasma cell replacement in the bone marrow, qualitative defects in neutrophil and complement system functioning, and decreased physical activity as a result of symptoms and syndromes caused by the disease.

Bone Marrow Involvement

A normocytic, normochromic anemia clinically manifested by fatigue and weakness occurs in over 60% of patients at initial diagnosis.[7,40] The anemia is initially caused by the excessive replacement of erythrocyte precursors with plasma cells in the bone marrow. Anemia can also be caused by increased red blood cell destruction. The M protein can coat normal erythrocytes, causing the red cells to line up similar to a roll of coins (rouleaux formation). This formation results in capillary sludging with associated hemolysis.[1,40] A multifactorial model for multiple myeloma–associated anemia has been postulated (Table 61-2).[3,6] It includes the replacement of erythrocyte precursors in the bone marrow with plasma cells; an increase in erythrocyte destruction; elevated levels of circulating immunoglobulins (IgG, IgA) with an increase in plasma volume, resulting in a falsely lowered hematocrit by approximately 5%–6%; chronic renal failure; low erythropoietin levels (< 100 mU/mL); low iron stores (< 50 μg/dL); and the in vivo activity in animals of IL-6 as a growth factor for multiple myeloma inducing anemia and thrombocytosis.[20,41]

As the myeloma cell burden increases or if the patient is treated with systemic chemotherapy, qualitative as well as quantitative defects in neutrophil and platelet function can occur. Impaired serum opsonic activity can be observed in the neutrophils of multiple myeloma patients, this can result in a quantitative defect in the function of circulating neutrophils.[39] Qualitative platelet defects occur in approximately 33% of patients with IgA myeloma

Table 61-2 Multifactorial Basis for Multiple Myeloma–Associated Anemia

Replacement of erythrocyte precursors with plasma cells

Increased erythrocyte destruction (rouleaux formation)

Elevated levels of immunoglobulins increase plasma volume, and result in falsely lowered hematocrit

Chronic renal failure

Low erythropoietin levels (< 100 mU/mL)

Low iron stores (< 50 μg/dL)

Interleukin-6 (IL-6)

and 15% of patients with IgG multiple myeloma.[42] Bleeding can be caused by a decrease in the number of circulating platelets, by the M protein's effect on clotting factors, or by nonspecific coating of platelets with immunoglobulins.[1] The final result is platelet dysfunction and bleeding.

Renal Insufficiency

At initial diagnosis, renal insufficiency is present in 20%–25% of patients with multiple myeloma. During the course of the disease and its treatment, 50% of these individuals will experience renal failure, 2%–3% will present with renal failure severe enough to require dialysis, and 15% will die as a result of renal insufficiency.[6] The presence of renal insufficiency as a negative prognostic indicator in multiple myeloma has been well established.[43,44] Multiple myeloma can cause intrinsic renal lesions as well as renal failure precipitated by the sequelae of the disease (infection, hypercalcemia, and dehydration).[30]

"Myeloma kidney" is the principal type of lesion associated with renal failure. In myeloma kidney, the renal tubules are filled with damaging, dense casts surrounded by multinucleated giant cells. These large, dense, tubular casts lead to the formation of precipitates in the tubules that can obstruct and rupture the tubular epithelium. Interstitial inflammation, dilatation, atrophy, fibrosis, and tubular degeneration can finally result in a damaged nephron that does not function.[1,7,43] The tubular casts have been shown to contain characteristic light-chain immunoglobulins (Bence Jones proteins), which may be directly toxic to the renal tubular epithelium regardless of the presence of tubular casts.[9,44] The excretion of large amounts of Bence Jones proteins in the face of clinical dehydration with a low urine pH contributes to the risk of precipitation of light-chain proteins in the renal tubule and possibly coprecipitation with calcium, further exacerbating acute renal failure.

Another renal lesion that occurs in approximately 10%–30% of myeloma patients is caused by amyloid deposits[1,4] that can be found in the tubular basement membranes, renal blood vessels, interstitium, or glomerulus. Evidence of albuminuria and nephrotic syndrome strongly suggests amyloidosis, an adverse prognostic factor that can occur in up to 10% of myeloma patients.[1,43,44]

Infection is the leading cause of death in multiple myeloma patients. Any episode of sepsis associated with hypotension or the use of nephrotoxic antibiotics (aminoglycosides with or without concurrent cephalosporins) should alert the clinician to closely monitor the individual for signs and symptoms of renal insufficiency.[45]

The treatment of renal insufficiency associated with multiple myeloma should be directed toward preventing or correcting the predisposing factors (dehydration, hypercalcemia, infection, hyperuricemia) and reducing the concentration and/or risk for precipitation of light-chain proteins in the renal tubules.

One study demonstrated that aggressive approaches

to treatment resulted in 51% of the patients achieving normal renal function.[46] More recent studies demonstrate that recovery of renal function occurs in approximately 50% of multiple myeloma patients treated with hydration, treatment of the underlying factors, plus or minus dialysis.[44] The recovery of renal function usually occurs within four months but can occur as late as 17 months after dialysis support.[44] The prognosis for multiple myeloma patients with renal insufficiency has clearly improved, with one year survival rates between 40%–70%.

Metabolic Syndromes

Hypercalcemia as a clinical sequela of multiple myeloma has been described earlier. Untreated hypercalcemia in multiple myeloma patients can precipitate renal insufficiency by reducing the glomerular filtration rate, altering renal blood flow, changing the kidney's ability to concentrate urine, and precipitating calcium in the tubules or renal interstitium.

Hyperuricemia occurs in multiple myeloma patients as a result of a large tumor burden with an increased rate of cell death. Uric acid–induced nephropathy is caused by the precipitation and crystallization of uric acid in the distal tubules, where the urine pH is low and the concentration of uric acid is high.[45] This syndrome can be exacerbated in patients who are dehydrated. If untreated, elevated uric acid levels will lead to further kidney damage.

Hyperviscosity Syndrome

Although rare (< 5% of multiple myeloma patients), hyperviscosity syndrome can occur in individuals with IgM myeloma and occasionally in those with IgA, IgG1, and IgG3 myeloma.[1,47] It is caused by a high concentration of proteins that increase serum viscosity and result in vascular sludging. Initial clinical signs (blurred vision, irritability, headache, drowsiness, confusion) may indicate neurological impairment. Vascular sludging may also occur within the kidney, further compromising renal perfusion and increasing the risk of renal insufficiency. Plasmapheresis can be life-saving and is the treatment of choice for hyperviscosity syndrome.[36]

Peripheral Neuropathy

Peripheral neuropathies have been recognized as part of the clinical sequelae associated with multiple myeloma.[48] In some cases the hyperviscosity syndrome has been identified as the causative factor.[48] Bosch and Smith recently postulated an autoimmune mechanism, with the IgM monoclonal antibody directed at peripheral nerve antigens.[49] Although evidence of this mechanism is devel-

oping, a definitive causal relationship between monoclonal proteins and peripheral neuropathies has not been established.

Assessment

Physical examination findings may include bone pain, with or without a decrease in range of motion, an inability to bear weight, or signs and symptoms of spinal cord compression. This may be indicative of skeletal involvement, which can be diagnosed by conventional radiographs, MRI, or bone surveys.[1,7,9] Individuals with multiple myeloma may present with changes in mental status that could be related to hypercalcemia, hyperviscosity syndrome, or renal insufficiency. Routine chemistry laboratory values may be significant for elevations in blood urea nitrogen (BUN), creatinine, uric acid, and calcium. Serum protein immunoelectrophoresis (SPEP) can confirm the monoclonal spikes, and immunoelectrophoresis (IPEP) can also confirm the presence of M protein in the urine.[1,4] Individuals with multiple myeloma may appear pale and fatigued, and may show evidence of anemia on peripheral blood counts and evidence of plasmacytosis on bone marrow biopsy.[1,3]

The diagnosis of multiple myeloma can be confirmed by bone marrow biopsy with histological confirmation of increased (greater than 10%) numbers of plasma cells and the presence of the M protein in either the serum or the urine. Osteolytic "punched-out" lesions may or may not be present at initial diagnosis. The diagnostic workup for multiple myeloma is designed to determine the extent of involvement of other organs (Table 61-3). Serum B_2 microglobulin, platelet count, and the presence of either renal failure and/or infection have been identified as having a role in predicting prognosis when diagnosing, staging, and treating myeloma patients.[27,50]

A number of negative prognostic factors have been identified in the literature (Table 61-4).[1,4,16,27] Clinicians should consider these prognostic factors along with performance status and comorbid conditions when presenting treatment options to patients and their families.

Table 61-3   Diagnostic Work-up for Multiple Myeloma

Diagnostic Exams	Purpose
Bone marrow aspirate/biopsy	Check % of plasma cells
Serum protein electrophoresis Immunoelectrophoresis	Check for the presence of M protein
Serum chemistry	Check for evidence of hypercalcemia, renal dysfunction
Complete blood count	Check for evidence of anemia, thrombocytopenia
Skeletal survey	Check for evidence of osteolytic bone lesions

Table 61-4 Negative Prognostic Findings in Multiple Myeloma

Infection

High labeling index

Elevated B_2 microglobulin

Renal insufficiency (hypercalcemia, hyperuricemia)

Plasmacytosis (> 30%) in the bone marrow

Classification and Staging

Staging for multiple myeloma incorporates both the Durie/Salmon system that was proposed in 1975 and the labeling index proposed by Durie and associates in the 1980s[51,52] (Table 61-5). This staging system integrates clinical and laboratory findings associated with multiple myeloma. In 1980 Durie and associates identified a process to quantitate the total-body myeloma cell mass.[52] This number is calculated by dividing the total-body M component synthetic rate per myeloma cell. In examining a large series of individuals with multiple myeloma, the authors identified three stages of the disease.

Table 61-5 Myeloma Staging System

Criteria	Estimated Myeloma Mass (Cells × 10^{12}/m²)
Stage I	
All of the following:	
Hemoglobin value > 10 g/dL	
Normal serum calcium	
Normal bone structure	
Low M-protein production	< 0.6 (low burden)
IgG value < 5 g/dL	
IgA value < 3 g/dL	
Urine kappa or lambda < 4 g/24 hr	
Stage II	
Overall data fits in neither stage I nor stage III	0.6–1.20 (intermediate burden)
Stage III	
One or more of the following:	
Hemoglobin value < 8.5 g/dL	
Serum calcium value > 12 mg/dL	
More than 3 lytic bone lesions	
High M-protein production	> 1.20 (high burden)
IgG value > 7 g/dL	
IgA value > 5 g/dL	
Urine kappa or lambda > 12 g/24 hr	
Subclassification	
A = creatinine value < 2.0 mg/dL	
B = creatinine value ≥ 2.0 mg/dL	

IgA, Immunoglobulin A; IgG, immunoglobulin G.
Data from National Cancer Institute. PDQ@cancernet.aci.nih.gov. 1999

First, stage I, or low cell mass, consists of less than 0.6×10^{12} cells/m². Stage II, or intermediate cell mass, reflects more than $0.6–1.2 \times 10^{12}$ cells/m². Finally, stage III, or high cell mass, consists of greater than 1.2×10^{12} cells/m².[1,4] Further staging is done based on renal status at the time of diagnosis. Group A consists of individuals with a normal renal function (creatinine level less than 2.0 mg/mL), and group B consists of individuals with evidence of renal dysfunction (creatinine level greater than 2.0 mg/mL).

In addition to renal function, infection, C-reactive protein, B_2 microglobulin, and abnormal karyotype have been identified as prognostic in predicting response and overall survival.[53,54] The identification of the kinetic features of the predominant clone in the individual with myeloma is useful for both prognosis and treatment. The labeling index (LI) is the percentage of myeloma cells incorporating thymidine during a one-hour flash label.[3] To calculate the total number of myeloma cells in the compartment, one multiplies the LI by the total myeloma cell mass.

Individuals with a high cell mass and an LI greater than 3% have a poor prognosis, with a median survival of less than six months.[3,5,21] In the future, these prognostic factors may be considered by clinicians when offering standard, intensive, or investigational therapy given the toxicity, morbidity, and overall survival.

Therapeutic Approaches and Nursing Care

Chemotherapy

Patients with indolent, asymptomatic multiple myeloma are typically not treated with systemic therapy until clinical symptoms occur. There is no clinical evidence that initiating antineoplastic therapy in asymptomatic patients increases response rates or improves overall survival. There is widespread agreement that with the onset of symptoms (anemia, bone pain, and hypercalcemia), systemic antineoplastic therapy consisting of melphalan and prednisone is the first line of therapy.[16,50,55,56] The response rate is 50%–60%, with a median survival of 24–36 months.[3,6,16,46,50] Melphalan is usually administered on an intermittent schedule (8 mg/m²/day for four days) along with prednisone (75 mg/day for seven days).[7,50] The treatment cycle is repeated every four weeks. This intermittent schedule allows patients to recover from the immunosuppressive effects of the drugs, is associated with less acute toxicity, and requires fewer blood draws to monitor blood counts. This chemotherapy protocol can be safely administered on an outpatient basis and allows the myeloma patient to remain part of the family system and continue participating in the community.

Both agents are administered orally. Due to the uncertain absorption of melphalan from the gastrointestinal tract, patients should be encouraged to take this antineoplastic agent on an empty stomach, unlike prednisone, which the patient should be instructed to take with meals.[6,57,58] Alternately, patients may take a H_2-histamine receptor antagonist designed to control gastric secretions and prevent the gastric distress associated with steroids.[4] Patients are monitored closely for signs of renal impairment (increased BUN and creatinine, proteinuria), and the dose of melphalan may need to be reduced based on the severity of renal toxicity. It is also important to closely monitor serial blood counts because the bone marrow–suppressive effects of melphalan may be cumulative in older patients. Although the addition of prednisone increases the response rate, it does not confer any benefit toward long-term survival; it is useful, however, in preventing bone resorption that could contribute to hypercalcemia and pathological fractures.[1] If the individual's myeloma is unresponsive, the melphalan dose may be escalated by 20% every five weeks provided there is no evidence of hematopoietic toxicity.[6]

It has been demonstrated that VAD—vincristine (0.4 mg/24–hour continuous infusion × four days), doxorubicin (Adriamycin 9 mg/m² /continuous infusion × four days), and dexamethasone (odd-number cycles 40 mg PO days 1–4, 9–12, 17–20; even-number cycles 40 mg PO days 1–4 only)—could be safely administered as first-line therapy, with an improved response rate (84%) and improved median survival (44 months).[59] VAD is administered every 28 days. This regimen has the added benefit of efficacy as both initial therapy and therapy for resistant disease.[4,58] Using it as initial therapy, a higher response rate (55%) has been reported in newly diagnosed patients.[5] Unfortunately, this did not result in improved overall survival when compared with melphalan/prednisone.

Clinically, VAD is beneficial to patients as first-line therapy because it can be used in patients with myeloma-associated renal dysfunction and has been shown to rapidly induce remission, which may translate into a decrease in symptoms associated with hypercalcemia, renal failure, or bone disease. Although initial response rates are slightly improved, clinicians must administer the VAD regimen with caution in patients older than 60 because there is some evidence that the elderly experience more toxicity associated with high-dose steroid administration.[7,16,50] The VAD regimen has gained widespread acceptance as treatment for resistant or refractory myeloma, with reported response rates between 65% and 75%.[3,7,16,50,58] Clinicians must monitor the total dose of doxorubicin and treat patients to a maximum tolerated dose of 450 mg/m². Patients will most likely require an implantable intravascular device or peripherally inserted central catheter (PICC) line to enable safe administration of these vesicants and close monitoring of blood counts. Depending on the patient's performance status and the available community services, this regime may require a four-day hospital stay or a referral to a skilled home care agency for safe administration of VAD in the home. Patients are closely monitored for signs and symptoms of steroid toxicity: severe dyspepsia, fluid and sodium reten-

tion, corticosteroid myopathy, acute pancreatitis, insulin-dependent hyperglycemia, and steroid psychosis. Patient and family education will include signs and symptoms of steroid-induced gastritis; if these persist or worsen (including nausea and vomiting with or without hematemesis), the treatment team should be contacted. Steroid gastritis that is not prevented, identified early, and appropriately treated can proceed to gastric ulceration and bleeding.

Steroid-associated sodium and fluid retention is of particular concern, especially in elderly individuals with multiple myeloma who may have concurrent diseases like congestive heart failure. Monitoring the patient for weight gain and peripheral edema is imperative because these may precede rales and pulmonary compromise. Individuals with underlying insulin-dependent and non-insulin-dependent diabetes should be closely evaluated for signs and symptoms of steroid-induced hypoglycemia. Any one of these toxicities mandates at least a 50% reduction, if not complete discontinuation, of dexamethasone.

Severe neurologic toxicities (paresthesias or constipation) require at least a 50% reduction in the vincristine dose. In the face of progressive toxicity (paralytic ileus), vincristine must be discontinued. Prolonged thrombocytopenia and granulocytopenia require a 50%–100% reduction in the dose of doxorubicin. If the doxorubicin cannot be administered due to prolonged bone marrow suppression, the entire cycle may be delayed for one week and therapy resumed once the platelet count is above 50,000/mm³ and the absolute neutrophil count (ANC) is over 750. Hepatic toxicity characterized by a bilirubin greater than 2.0 requires reduction or discontinuation of both doxorubicin and vincristine, depending on the severity. If the bilirubin is greater than 5.0, both doxorubicin and vincristine are discontinued.

If drug resistance emerges, cyclophosphamide is another, structurally different, alkylating agent that is cross resistant with melphalan. Cyclophosphamide is also administered orally on an intermittent schedule. Patients are encouraged to increase their oral intake to avoid possible exacerbation of underlying renal dysfunction. Patients who may be concurrently receiving allopurinol should be carefully monitored, as this agent may enhance bone marrow suppression in patients receiving cyclophosphamide.

Thirty to forty percent of myeloma patients will not respond to first-line therapy, while those who initially respond will eventually relapse.[1,9] Consequently, second-line combination chemotherapy regimens have been developed. The most consistently effective second-line therapy, resulting in a 70% response rate with projected survival greater than one year, is the combination of vincristine, doxorubicin, and dexamethasone (VAD) previously described.[6,60] In an effort to minimize toxicity, increase response rates, and improve overall survival, investigators continue to combine agents such as doxorubicin and carmustine (BCNU); vincristine, carmustine, doxorubicin, and prednisone (VBAP); and vincristine, cyclophosphamide, doxorubicin, and prednisone (VCAP). To date, clinical trials of these combinations have been equivocal; further studies are warranted to identify new agents or combinations of agents that increase response rates without increases in toxicity.[55,56,60,61]

Interferon

In view of the equivocal results with combination chemotherapy for refractory multiple myeloma, it is not unreasonable for investigators to examine alternatives such as alfa-interferon.[62] The specific mechanism of action of interferon in multiple myeloma is unknown but is thought to be multifactorial. Interferon exerts its biological effects by stimulating the host cells to indirectly affect tumor cells, specifically by inhibiting plasma cell growth and the ability of myeloma stem cells to self-replicate.[6,63] Despite this indirect effect on tumor cells, clinical investigators have demonstrated minimal to no effect in previously treated myeloma patients.[58] However, alfa-interferon has been proposed as a strategy to prolong remission duration and survival in multiple myeloma patients who initially respond to cytotoxic therapy.[64,65] Investigators have used interferon for maintenance therapy in patients who have responded to 12 courses of induction chemotherapy. The investigators concluded that they were able to prolong response and survival with minimal toxicity.[66]

In contrast, the Southwest Oncology Group reported a randomized prospective trial involving 522 previously untreated individuals with multiple myeloma who were randomized to three chemotherapy regimes with differing glucocorticoid doses.[60] A total of 193 patients achieved remission and were randomized to receive 3 million units of alfa-interferon three times per week of observation. The investigators drew two conclusions: (1) that higher-dose glucocorticoids increase the frequency of response to chemotherapy and prolong survival in myeloma; and (2) that there was no significant difference in overall survival between the interferon group and observation.

Browman and associates reported on a smaller-perspective randomized trial that involved 402 newly diagnosed individuals with multiple myeloma who received melphalan and prednisone (M-P) as induction therapy.[63] In this trial, 176 responders were randomized to either 2 million units of alfa-interferon subcutaneously three times per week (n = 85) or no maintenance (n = 91). The conclusions include a statistically significant improvement in response duration and overall survival for interferon compared with no maintenance therapy. A second observation was that interferon toxicity caused 58% of the patients to reduce their dose, and 14% of the patients had to discontinue interferon treatment.

The toxicity associated with alfa-interferon requires thorough assessment and consistent interventions to manage side effects (flu-like syndrome, anorexia, fatigue, hepatotoxicity, thrombocytopenia, and neurological tox-

icity).[62,63] The patient is closely monitored by the treatment team for evidence of interferon toxicity. The dose-reduction schedule (50%–100%) and plan to discontinue interferon are dependent on the individual's response to the severity of the toxicity. Nurses play a key role in assessing and grading treatment-related toxicities and in assisting patients and their families in managing side effects.

Oken and associates report findings similar to those above from an Eastern Cooperative Oncology Group (ECOG) study in which 608 previously untreated individuals with multiple myeloma were randomized to three treatment arms.[67] First vincristine, BCNU, melphalan, cyclophosphamide, and prednisone (VBMCP); second, VBMPC and interferon (interferon 5 MU/m²; 3×/week); third, in patients under age 70, cyclophosphamide 600 mg/m² was substituted for prednisone 100 mg/m² PO day 1–4 for cycles 3 and 5 of VBMCP (VBMCP and high-dose cyclophosphamide (HiCy)). The VBMCP/interferon arm had a higher complete response rate with a trend toward failure-free survival, but without an increase in survival. Clinically these improved response rates associated with maintenance therapy in individuals with multiple myeloma can translate into clinical improvement in symptoms associated with the disease (bone lesions, pain, renal dysfunction) and an overall improvement in the individual's functional ability and quality of life.

Some investigators have raised concerns regarding the controversial role of alfa-interferon in multiple myeloma. Laboratory data suggest that alfa-interferon is a potent myeloma cell growth factor. It induces the autocrine production of IL-6, thus promoting further myeloma cell growths.[3,21] With equivocal results from a number of large randomized trials, the burden of proof rests with scientists and clinicians to define the specific safe role for alfa-interferon in treating multiple myeloma.[68,69]

Radiation

Radiation therapy has long been recognized as an important therapeutic option to palliate symptoms associated with multiple myeloma. Approximately 70% of patients will eventually benefit from this therapy.[58] Multiple myeloma is considered a disseminated disease with evidence of distant organ involvement at the time of diagnosis. However, in rare instances (fewer than 5%) the disease may be localized and present as a solitary bone plasmacytoma.[9] On biopsy the individual's bony lesion will show evidence of plasma cells. Bone marrow aspiration and biopsy, peripheral counts including complete blood counts (CBCs), and serum chemistry will be unremarkable and show no evidence of other organ involvement (i.e., renal). Although this clinical presentation is rare, Dimopoulos and colleagues reported 45 cases followed over ten years where megavoltage irradiation (at least 3000 cGy) to the solitary lesion was curative.[70] Persistent myeloma protein was an adverse prognostic factor, and the reemergence of the myeloma protein heralded recurrence requiring systemic therapy.

Multiple myeloma remains an extremely radiosensitive malignancy, and historically the goal of radiation therapy has been palliative. Radiation therapy has been effective in arresting local bone disease prior to the point of fracture, but it does not lead to bone repair and healing. This nonoperative approach to managing painful bony lesions is aimed at symptom relief for the individual, maintaining functional ability and promoting the individual's overall satisfaction with quality of life.[71]

Hemibody irradiation has been used in individuals with refractory or advanced multiple myeloma.[9] It involves a technique in which a single dose of radiation (500–800 cGy) is administered to a large body area at one time. The benefit of this approach is that it allows for the potential treatment of both halves of the body sequentially in doses that are higher than could be delivered with total-body irradiation.[63] This approach provides pain relief within 24–48 hours, and this time frame should be considered by clinicians when ordering and administering narcotic analgesics to manage pain. Treatment toxicity may be significant and dependent on the treatment field (upper hemibody field: head to the fourth lumbar vertebrae; midbody field: the abdomen and pelvis from the top of the diaphragm to the obturator foramina; and the lower hemibody: the torso below the iliac crest and extending to the ankles).[72] Providing patient education and managing symptoms such as nausea, vomiting, diarrhea, and bone marrow toxicity may include coordinating or administering premedications (corticosteroids, antiemetics, and narcotic analgesics) so that the individual will be able to comfortably complete his or her therapy in the radiotherapy department.[73]

Bone Marrow Transplantation

Bone marrow transplantation (syngeneic, allogeneic, autologous) and peripheral stem cell support have been attempted in the treatment of multiple myeloma.[74–83] Age restrictions for both donor and recipient previously limited the use of this technology in individuals over age 60. More recently high-dose therapy with transplant (bone marrow and peripheral blood progenitor cells) support has been safely and effectively employed in patients over age 65.[84]

Jagannath and colleagues treated 55 previously treated myeloma patients with myeloablative chemoradiation and unpurged autologous bone marrow transplant.[74] They identified two pretransplant variables that were associated with negative patient outcomes: a pretransplant elevated B_2 microglobulin level (greater than 3 mg/liter) and the presence of non-IgG isotype myeloma. Response rates improved when investigators purged autologous marrow.[74,80]

Gahrton and colleagues reported a series of 90 myeloma patients who received allogeneic bone marrow transplant in 26 European centers.[76] The complete remission after bone marrow transplant was 43%, with a median

duration of relapse-free survival of 48 months for complete responders. One clinically significant finding was that bone lesions were largely unaffected by the cytotoxic therapy used in the bone marrow transplant setting. Two posttransplant factors were useful in predicting individuals with better long-term survival: complete remission after transplant and grade 1 graft-versus-host disease. Gahrton and colleagues were the first to hypothesize a possible graft-versus-myeloma effect similar to the graft-versus-leukemia effect.[76] Five years later, Trict and associates reported a case demonstrating direct evidence of graft-versus-myeloma effect in a 40-year-old individual with multiple myeloma who received a matched unrelated T-cell-depleted transplant after conditioning with total-body irradiation, thiotepa, and cyclophosphamide. The patient also received allogeneic peripheral blood mononuclear cells (stem cells) without further chemotherapy. The patient experienced severe acute and chronic graft-versus-host disease with complete response duration greater than 14 months.[81]

Throughout the early 1990s investigators continued to design clinical trials aimed at improving response rates and duration of responses. Tura and Cavo reviewed allogeneic bone marrow transplant data and reported remission rates of 50%–60%.[77] Despite high mortality rates (40%–50%), Tura and Cavo suggested that allogeneic transplant be used earlier in the disease treatment as consolidation therapy, postulating that this might improve the number of long-term, disease-free survivors.

Some investigators and treatment centers incorporate hematopoietic growth factors (granulocyte colony-stimulating factor [G-CSF], granulocyte macrophage colony-stimulating factor [GM-CSF]) into clinical trials with transplant and stem cell support regimes to shorten the duration and depth of neutropenia after cytotoxic therapy. Investigators are reporting dramatic decreases in mortality rates (less than 5%) in autologous bone marrow transplant.[80]

Two studies have shown that high-dose therapy with transplant support offers patients superior outcomes over conventional therapy.[5,82] Attal and colleagues reported the results of a European prospective randomized trial of autologous bone marrow transplant or conventional chemotherapy in multiple myeloma.[82] Two hundred previously untreated myeloma patients younger than age 65 were randomly assigned to two treatment groups. The conventional dose treatment consisted of alternating cycles of VMCP/BVAP or high-dose therapy with autologous bone marrow transplant (Table 61-6). The investigators reported an 81% response rate in the high-dose group and a 57% response rate in the conventional chemotherapy group ($p < 0.001$). Complete response rates were disappointing in both groups: high-dose (22%) and conventional (5%). Treatment-related mortality (less than 10%) was similar in the two groups. This study did not include the use of hematopoietic growth factors after transplant to shorten the duration of neutropenia, and the investigators are considering the use of these agents in future treatment regimes.

Table 61-6 Treatment Schema of European Bone Marrow Transplant Trial in Multiple Myeloma

CONVENTIONAL TREATMENT—VMCP/BVAP*

VMCP:
Vincristine	1 mg IV; day 1
Melphalan	5 mg/m² PO; days 1–4
Cyclophosphamide	110 mg/m² PO; days 1–4
Prednisone	60 mg/m² PO; days 1–4

BVAP:
Vincristine	1 mg IV; day 1
Carmustine	30 mg/m² IV; day 1
Doxorubicin	30 mg/m² IV; day 1
Prednisone	60 mg/m² PO; days 1–4

Recombinant alfa-interferon (3 million U/m² SQ 3 times/week from cycle 9 until relapse).

HIGH-DOSE AS ABOVE

Autologous bone marrow was collected after cycle 4 (200 million nucleated cells/kg body weight).

All patients received between 4 and 6 cycles of VMCP/BVAP; if their WHO (World Health Organization) performance status was < 3 and a transplant facility was available, the individual was transplanted.

Preparative regimen: Melphalan 140 mg/m²
Total-body irradiation (8 Gy 4 fractions over 4 days with no lung shields)

Unpurged autologous bone marrow was readministered.

Alfa-interferon was administered from cycle 9 until relapse; after bone marrow transplantation hematologic recovery occurred (granulocyte count > 1500/mm³; platelet count > 75,000/mm³).

*Alternating cycles (every 3 weeks for 12 months; total 18 cycles).
Data from Attal M, Harousseau JL, Stopp AM, et al[82]

The second trial, reported by Barlogie and associates, involved 116 previously untreated patients. This was a pair-matched comparison of patient's enrolled in their "total therapy program" (including tandem transplants) compared to patients who were "conventionally" treated on Southwest Oncology Group trials (SWOG).[80] Both overall and event-free survival were improved in the "total therapy treated" patients. Overall survival was 62 months versus 48 months in the conventionally treated patients ($p = 0.01$). Event-free survival was improved, 49 months in the total therapy group versus 22 months in the conventional therapy group ($p = 0.0001$). One factor that has become evident is that treatment with conventional agents has a negative impact on the ability to mobilize and harvest an adequate amount of stem cells.[85] With this knowledge many clinicians are now looking to earlier identify patients who may be candidates for autotransplantation. This would allow for earlier mobilization and collection of adequate stem cells prior to exposure to alkylating agents.[86–88]

A number of questions remain unanswered regarding the appropriate use of transplantation in the treatment of multiple myeloma. Future clinical trials will attempt to determine the best time to do transplant (first remission versus at the time of disease progression). What type of transplant should be done (autologous bone marrow or peripheral stem cells versus allogeneic bone marrow or peripheral stem cells)? Have we identified all the prognostic factors that will identify the "best" patients or the patients most likely to benefit? As we learn more about the body's natural immune response and the specific pathogenesis of myeloma, we may be able to take advantage of new classes of cytotoxic agents: topoisomerase inhibitors, suramin, paclitaxel, retinoids, B-cell–directed immunotoxins, graft-versus-myeloma effect, and vaccinations with idiotypes.[80,82,89,90]

Antiangiogenesis Factors

Strategies to maintain complete response (CR) rates and extend event-free survival (EFS) and overall survival (OS) have recently taken advantage of not only induction/consolidation/high-dose therapy platforms, but newer modalities in an attempt to control minimal residual disease (MRD). Recently clinical trials have begun in an attempt to take advantage of our limited knowledge of angiogenesis and the role it plays in malignant disease. Thalidomide has reentered clinical trials and has shown activity in the treatment of multiple myeloma.[91,92]

Bisphosphonates

This class of agents acts by binding to the surface of damaged bone and inhibits further bone destruction. This can allow for bone repair and interfere with painful boney metastasis, pathologic fractures, and the ability to maintain osseous structure and function.[6] Bisphosphonates (etidronate, clodromate, pamidronate) are effective treatment for hypercalcemia, but more recently have shown benefit in preventing sequelae associated with metastatic bone lesions.[93]

Long-Term Sequelae

The risk of developing a secondary malignancy or treatment-related malignancy after primary treatment for cancer has been recognized by the oncology community since the 1970s.[1] Reported risks for treatment-related malignancies range between 1.3-fold and 20-fold in comparison to the general public.[94] Recognizing this risk, oncology clinicians must monitor multiple myeloma patients for evidence of acute leukemia.[9] The precise pathogenesis of this leukemia remains obscure, but two hypotheses have been proposed. First, the chronic long-term administration of alkylating agents (melphalan and cyclophosphamide) causes significant damage within the pluripotent stem cell compartment. The second hypothesis is that there is an inherent defect in the early bone marrow progenitor cells that causes the development of both malignancies (multiple myeloma and acute leukemia). Ongoing studies continue to show a low but significant risk for post–bone marrow transplant malignancies.[95] As myeloma patients continue intensive regimes requiring transplant support, clinicians will need to incorporate the risk for the development of acute leukemia into the informed consent process, the management, and the long-term follow-up of these patients. Secondary acute leukemia can be refractory to treatment. Treated patients have a dismal median survival of four to eight months.[96]

Symptom Management and Supportive Care

Multiple myeloma remains a disease that primarily strikes older adults. Despite advances in the therapeutic options, and improvements in CR, EFS, OS, few patients are cured and most must adjust to the chronic nature of the disease. In planning the nursing care it is imperative that the entire treatment team be knowledgeable of the patient's realistic prognosis. Initially and throughout the treatment trajectory, it is critical to include the patient and his or her family when discussing therapeutic goals and treatment options. Goals can range from intensive treatment, preventing or delaying life-threatening complications, prolonging disease-free survival, palliation, or terminal care. Regardless of the goal, a symptom management approach to nursing care with a review of systems is useful in organizing assessments and interventions (Table 61-7).[97]

Neurological

The most frequent symptom that myeloma patients present with is pain. Bone destruction from the myeloma results in osteoporosis and pathological fractures of long bones or vertebrae that may result in spinal cord compression that requires aggressive assessment and management of both acute and chronic pain.[71,98,99] Acute pain is characterized by a specific trauma (fracture) and is of short duration (less than six months), whereas chronic pain has no specific obvious initiation point and may occur over a protracted period. Interventions for pain include assessment and documentation of the individual's severity of pain (0–10 scale), proper positioning of affected limbs, use of supports and braces (cervical collar, back brace, sling) to prevent additional stress on bones, and consultation with physical and occupational therapists. Interventions to treat and manage pain should incorporate the effective and appropriate utilization of narcotics, nonnarcotic analgesics, and nonpharmacological therapies (massage, heat, cold, relaxation, and immobilization).[100,101]

Mental status changes can be an initial sign of hypercalcemia, hyperviscosity syndrome, or drug toxicity. Any change in mental status requires closer assessment to determine etiologic factors so that appropriate treatment can be promptly initiated. The nurse also plans for prevention of injury and maintaining the patient in a safe environment.[102] Depression, anxiety, and insomnia are but a few of the psychological responses that patients may exhibit in response to their disease and treatment.[103] Cognitive strategies (cognitive restructuring, assisting with problem solving, giving information in small amounts, listening, and expressing care and concern) are recommended to assist in the adaptation to a cancer diagnosis.[104]

Table 61-7   Nursing Care of the Patient with Multiple Myeloma

System	Signs and Symptoms	Patient Education
Neuromuscular	Pain (acute/chronic) Hypercalcemia Hyperviscosity syndrome Spinal cord compression Pathological fractures Depression	Pain control measures Signs and symptoms of hypercalcemia Prevention of pathological fractures Cognitive strategies Counseling
Protective mechanisms	Anemia Neutropenia Thrombocytopenia	Exercise Energy conservation activities Prevention of infection Prevention of bleeding Self-administration of prescribed hematopoietic growth factors
Respiratory	Pneumonia	Prevention of pooling of pulmonary secretions Increase gas exchange Use of incentive spirometer
Gastrointestinal	Constipation	Preventive measures Change in fluid and dietary intake
Genitourinary	Renal insufficiency	Increase fluid intake Allopurinol administration Recognition of signs of urinary tract infection

Protective Mechanisms

Infection is the leading cause of death in patients with multiple myeloma. The supportive care of cancer patients with anemia, thrombocytopenia, and neutropenia is well documented in the nursing literature, and guidelines for the care of patients with anemia, infection, and bleeding are provided in Chapters 21 and 22.[105–107] Guidelines for the care of neutropenic patients are principally aimed at the early recognition and/or prevention of infection. The care of the thrombocytopenic patient is directed toward preventing bleeding; and care of the anemic patient is directed toward early recognition and treatment to prevent contributing to the fatigue–weakness state that may be a component of the disease and/or its treatment.[108] A recent review of the literature identified four areas of intervention that nurses can utilize in managing and or studying fatigue in multiple myeloma: exercise, attention-restoring activities, preparatory education, and psychosocial techniques.[109]

Blood product support will consist mainly of packed red blood cell and platelet transfusions. The clinical use of hematopoietic growth factors in the prevention of febrile neutropenia after myelosuppressive chemotherapy, in the treatment of anemia in cancer patients receiving chemotherapy, in patients undergoing peripheral blood progenitor cell (PBPC) collection, and in patients receiving bone marrow transplant is now established as supportive therapy in managing individuals with multiple myeloma.[110–112]

The 1996 guidelines by the American Society of Clinical Oncology for the use of hematopoietic colony–stimulating factors adds two important risk factors (poor performance status and more advanced cancer) for consideration in the older population (over age 60) of individuals with multiple myeloma.[113] Clinicians may use these and other risk factors when assessing patients prior to ordering hematopoietic growth factors for primary prophylaxis of febrile neutropenia after myelosuppressive chemotherapy.

Respiratory

The respiratory system is the most frequent site of infection in myeloma patients. As a result, nursing care is directed toward teaching patients and their families activities to decrease pooling of pulmonary secretions and increase gas exchange (e.g., coughing and deep breathing exercises, use of incentive spirometers, avoiding family members with signs and symptoms of upper respiratory infection). Patients and families are instructed about the symptoms that are important to report to the clinician immediately, such as fever, cough, sore throat, and sputum production. Due to the underlying defect in humoral immunity induced by multiple myeloma, patients should be instructed not to receive vaccines with live organisms or be in close contact with others who may have received live organism vaccines that may be shedding organisms

(i.e., children immunized with oral polio and MMR).[114] Protection against pneumococcal infection is appropriate to discuss with patients. All patients with multiple myeloma, and in particular those over age 65, should be protected with a single dose of the 23-valent pneumococcal vaccine.[115]

Gastrointestinal

Multiple myeloma patients are at risk for constipation as a result of decreased physical activity due to bone pain/pathologic fractures, treatment of pain with narcotic analgesics, dehydration, and the use of vincristine. Although not considered a life-threatening clinical problem, this condition can influence nutritional intake, comfort, and quality of life.[116] Nursing management includes the assessment of past and present bowel habits, changes in fluid and dietary intake, medication administration, activity changes, and patient and family education.

Genitourinary

Renal insufficiency or failure can be exacerbated as a result of the primary disease, fluid and electrolyte abnormalities (hyperuricemia, hypercalcemia), dehydration, and/or infection.[117,118] Nonsteroidal anti-inflammatory drugs (NSAIDs) frequently used in the treatment of bone pain have been associated with the development of acute renal failure in multiple myeloma.[119] A thorough drug history, including use of over-the-counter products, is imperative. Patient education regarding the strategies to avoid renal compromise is critical. NSAIDs should be cautiously used in multiple myeloma patients given the significant risk for acute renal failure.[16,44] Nursing care is directed at preventing or quickly reversing renal insufficiency. Maintaining adequate hydration, along with the administration of allopurinol, will protect the kidneys from uric acid nephropathy.[120] The nurse closely monitors the patient for early signs and symptoms of urinary tract infection (fever, dysuria, frequency, urgency) and educates patients and families to recognize these symptoms and report them promptly to the physician.

Continuity of Care

The majority of the care that a person with multiple myeloma receives will occur as an outpatient. One of the greatest challenges that face both the family and the health care team is providing continuity of care. There will be many providers involved in one person's care. Case management approaches will provide some structure for the health care team. The amount of self-care and family administered care can become a daunting task. The family and patient need time, support, and reinforcement to begin to master the many signs and symptoms they

Table 61-8   Patient Education Support Services

Counseling and Support	Public, Patient Resources
Bone Marrow Transplant Family Support Network P.O. BOX 845 Avon, CT 06001 800-826-9376	American Cancer Society (ACS) 1599 Clifton Road, NE Atlanta, GA 30329-4251 404-329-7623 (patient services) 800-ACS-2345 www.cancer.org (Web site)
Cancer Care, Inc. 275 Seventh Avenue New York, NY 10001 212-712-8354 www.cancercare.org (Web site)	International Myeloma Foundation 2129 Stanley Hills Drive Los Angeles, CA 90046 800-452-CURE www.myeloma.org (Web site)
National Coalition for Cancer Survivorship (NCCS) 1010 Wayne Avenue, Suite 505 Silver Spring, MD 20910 301-650-8868	Leukemia Society of America 600 Third Avenue New York, NY 10016 212-573-8484 800-955-4LSA www.leukemia.org (Web site)

must report. In addition, they will need assistance learning the physical skills and tasks of care.

A number of patient and family support organizations are available to assist patients with multiple myeloma to learn about and to cope with their disease[121] (Table 61-8). These organizations provide individual and group support, and provide written materials regarding the disease and its treatment. Many of these organizations can be accessed via the Internet.

Conclusion

The last decade has witnessed dramatic improvements in the overall response rates for patients with multiple myeloma. The utilization of combination chemotherapy, high-dose therapy with transplant support, earlier recognition of complications, and appropriate utilization of support therapies have all contributed to increasing patient survival. Evidence-based guidelines that address the initial diagnostic workup, ongoing surveillance, and supportive care have been established by the National Comprehensive Cancer Network (NCCN) and should guide clinical practice, clinical trials, and areas for future nursing research.[16]

We are witnessing increasing utilization of new technologies to better determine etiologic factors contributing to the development of multiple myeloma. The nursing care of multiple myeloma patients and their families offers the nurse an opportunity to care for patients experiencing both acute and chronic sequelae of disease. Nursing care can have a direct effect in early recognition of complications and managing toxicity. Patient and family education can lead to the early recognition and identification of complications, contributing to overall improvement in quality of life. Future areas for nursing

research include clinical demonstration projects that produce evidence that specific nursing interventions contribute to the patients' quality of life and event-free and overall survival.[122]

References

1. Bubley GJ, Schnipper LE: Multiple myeloma, in Murphy GP, Lawrence W, Lenhard RE (eds): *American Cancer Society Textbook of Clinical Oncology.* Atlanta, American Cancer Society, 1995, pp 470–485

2. Stevenson F, Anderson KC: Introduction: immunotherapy for multiple myeloma—insights and advances. *Semin Hematol* 3(1):1–2, 1999

3. Hussein M: Multiple myeloma: an overview of diagnosis and management. *Cleve Clin J Med* 61:285–298, 1994

4. Sheridan CA: Multiple myeloma. *Semin Oncol Nurs* 12:1–12, 1996

5. Barlogie B, Jagannath S, Vesole DH, et al: Superiority of tandem transplantation over standard therapy for previously untreated multiple myeloma. *Blood* 89:789–793, 1997

6. Bataille R, Harousseau JL: Multiple myeloma. *N Engl J Med* 336:1657–1664, 1997

7. Gautier M, Cohen MJ: Multiple myeloma in the elderly. *J Am Geriatr Soc* 42:653–664, 1994

8. American Cancer Society: Cancer Facts and Figures—1999. Atlanta, American Cancer Society, 1999, p 23

9. Shulman LN: Plasma cell diseases and related disorders, in Hadin RI, Lux SE, Stossel TP (eds): *Blood Principles and Practice of Hematology.* Philadelphia, Lippincott, 1995, pp. 885–913

10. Potter M: Plasmacytomas in mice. *Semin Oncol* 13:275–281, 1986

11. Maldonado JE, Kyle RA: Familial myeloma: report of eight families and a study of serum proteins in their relatives. *Am J Med* 57:875–884, 1974

12. Liu P, Leong T, Quam L, et al: Activating mutations of N- and K-ras in multiple myeloma show different clinical associations: analysis of the Eastern Cooperative Oncology Group phase III trial. *Blood* 88:2699–2706, 1996

13. Sawyer JR, Tricot G, Mattox S, et al: Jumping translocations of chromosomal 1q I multiple myeloma: evidence for a mechanism involving decondensation of pericentromeric, heterochromatin. *Blood* 91:1732–1741, 1998

14. Michaeli J, Choy CG, Zhang X: The biologic features of multiple myeloma. *Cancer Invest* 15:76–84, 1997

15. Anderson KC, Hamblin TJ, Traynor A: Management of multiple myeloma today. *Semin Hematol* 36:3–8, 1999

16. Gallucci BB, McCarthy D: The immune system, in Reiger PT (ed): *Biotherapy: A Comprehensive Overview.* Sudbury, MA, Jones and Bartlett, 1995, pp 15–42

17. Varterasian ML: Biologic and clinical advances in multiple myeloma. *Oncology* 9:417–424, 1995

18. Pilarski LM, Mant MJ, Ruether BA: Pre-B cells in peripheral blood of multiple myeloma patients. *Blood* 66:416–422, 1985

19. Tricot G, Sawyer JR, Jagannath S, et al: Unique role of cytogenetics in the prognosis of patients with myeloma receiving high-dose therapy and auto-transplants. *J Clin Oncol* 15:2659–2666, 1997

20. Klein B: Cytokine receptors, transduction signals, and oncogenes in human multiple myeloma. *Semin Hematol* 32:4–19, 1995

21. Klein B, Zhang XG, Luz Y, et al: Interleukin-6 in human multiple myeloma. *Blood* 85:863–872, 1995

22. Reibnegger G, Krainer M, Herold M, et al: Predictive value of interleukin-6 and neopterin in patients with multiple myeloma. *Cancer Res* 51:6250–6253, 1991

23. Pelliniemi TT, Irjala K, Mattila K, et al: Immunoreactive interleukin-6 and acute phase proteins as prognostic factors in multiple myeloma. *Blood* 85:765–771, 1995

24. Chauhan D, Kharbanda S, Ogata A, et al: Interleukin-6 inhibits Fas-induced apoptosis and SAP kinase activation in multiple myeloma cells. *Blood* 89:227–234, 1997

25. Rettig M, Ma HJ, Vescio RA, et al: Kaposi's sarcoma associated herpesvirus infection of bone marrow dendritic cells from myeloma patients. *Science* 276:1851–1854, 1997

26. MacLennan IC, Drayson M, Dunn J: Multiple myeloma. *BMJ* 308:1033–1036, 1994

27. Kyle RA: High dose therapy in multiple myeloma and primary amyloidosis: an overview. *Semin Oncol* 26:74–83, 1999

28. Brage ME, Simon MA: Evaluation, prognosis, and medical treatment considerations. *Orthopedics* 15:589–596, 1992

29. Bataille R, Boccadoro M, Klein B, et al: C-reactive protein and B₂ microglobulin produce a simple and powerful myeloma staging system. *Blood* 80:733–737, 1992

30. Kaplan M: Hypercalcemia of malignancy: a review of advances in pathophysiology. *Oncol Nurs Forum* 21:1039–1048, 1994

31. Moscinski LC, Ballester DF: Recent progress in multiple myeloma. *Hematol Oncol* 12:111–123, 1994

32. Carter A, Merchau S, Silvian-Draxler I, et al: The role of interleukin-1 and tumor necrosis factor in human multiple myeloma. *Br J Haematol* 74:424–431, 1990

33. Bataille R, Chappard D, Klein B: Mechanisms of bone lesions in multiple myeloma. *Hematol Oncol Clin North Am* 6:285–295, 1992

34. Niesvizky R, Warrell RP: Pathophysiology and management of bone disease in multiple myeloma. *Cancer Invest* 15:85–90, 1997

35. Jacobson DR, Zolla-Pazner S: Immunosuppression and infection in multiple myeloma, in Wiernik PH (ed): *Neoplastic Diseases of the Blood.* New York, Churchill Livingstone, 1991, pp 415–426

36. Lawrence J: Critical care issues in the patient with hematologic malignancy. *Semin Oncol Nurs* 10:198–207, 1994

37. Savage DG, Lindenbaum J, Garrett TJ: Biphasic pattern of bacterial infection in multiple myeloma. *Ann Intern Med* 96:47–50, 1982

38. Berthaud V, Milder J, el-Sadr W: Multiple myeloma presenting with *Hemophilus influenzae* septic arthritis: case report and review of the literature. *J Natl Med Assoc* 85:626–628, 1993

39. Shaikh BS, Lombard RM, Appelbaum PC, et al: Changing patterns of infections in patients with multiple myeloma. *Oncology* 39:78–81, 1992

40. Duff TP: The many pitfalls on the diagnosis of myeloma. *N Engl J Med* 326:394–396, 1992

41. Barlogie B, Beck T: Recombinant human erythropoietin and the anemia of multiple myeloma. *Stem Cells* 11:88–94, 1993

42. Rao AK, Carvalho ACA: Acquired qualitative platelet defects, in Colman RW, Hirsh J, Marder VJ, et al (eds): *Hemostasis and Thrombosis Basic Principles and Clinical Practice.* Philadelphia, Lippincott, 1994, pp 685–704

43. Kyle RA: Multiple myeloma and other plasma cell disorders, in Hoffman R, Benz EJ, Shattile SJ, et al (eds): *Hematology Basic Principles and Practice.* New York, Churchill Livingstone, 1995, pp 1354–1374

44. Clark AD, Shetty A, Soutar R: Renal failure and multiple myeloma: pathogenesis and treatment of renal failure and management of the underlying myeloma. *Blood Rev* 13:79–90, 1999

45. Brasfield K: Renal disorders, in Thelan LA, Davie JK, Urden LD, Lough ME (eds): *Critical Care Nursing.* St. Louis, Mosby, 1994, pp 603–620

46. Alexanian RJ, Barlogie B, Dixon D: Renal failure in multiple myeloma pathogenesis and prognostic implications. *Arch Intern Med* 150:1693–1695, 1990

47. Paterson WP, Caldwell CW, Doll DC: Hyperviscosity syndromes and coagulopathies. *Semin Oncol* 17:210–216, 1990

48. Sidoti SP, Cherpack FJ: Neurologic involvement of multiple myeloma: Literature review and case report. *J Am Podiatr Med Assoc* 81:220–223, 1991

49. Bosch EP, Smith BE: Peripheral neuropathies associated with monoclonal proteins. *Med Clin North Am* 77:125–139, 1993

50. Oken MM: Multiple myeloma: prognosis and standard treatment. *Cancer Invest* 15:57–64, 1997

51. Durie BGM, Salmon SE: A clinical staging system for multiple myeloma. *Cancer* 36:842–854, 1975

52. Durie BG, Salmon SE, Moon TE: Pretreatment tumor mass cell kinetics and prognosis in multiple myeloma. *Blood* 55:364–372, 1980

53. Weh HJ, Gutensohn K, Selbach J, et al: Karyotype in multiple myeloma and plasma cell leukemia. *Eur J Cancer* 29:1269–1273, 1993

54. Barlogie B, Jagannath S, Epstein J, et al: Biology and therapy of multiple myeloma in 1996. *Semin Hematol* 34:67–72, 1997

55. Boccadoro M, Marmont F, Tibalto M, et al: Multiple myeloma: VMCP/VBAP alternating combination chemotherapy is not superior to melphalan and prednisone even in high-risk patients. *J Clin Oncol* 9:444–448, 1991

56. Gregory WM, Richards MA, Malas JS: Combination chemo-

therapy versus melphalan and prednisone in the treatment of multiple myeloma: an overview of published trials. *J Clin Oncol* 10:334–342, 1992

57. Skidmore-Roth L: *1996 Nursing Reference.* St. Louis, Mosby, 1996, pp 880–881

58. Salmon SE, Cassady JR: Plasma cell neoplasms, in Devita VT, Hellman S, Rosenberg SA (eds): *Cancer Principles and Practice of Oncology.* Philadelphia, Lippincott-Raven, 1997, pp 2344–2387

59. Samson D, Gaminara E, Newland A, et al: Infusion of vincristine and doxorubicin with oral dexamethasone as first-line therapy for multiple myeloma. *Lancet* 2:882–885, 1989

60. Salmon SE, Crowley JJ, Grogan TM, et al: Combination chemotherapy, glucocorticoids and interferon alfa in the treatment of multiple myeloma: a Southwest Oncology Group study. *J Clin Oncol* 12:2405–2414, 1994

61. Oken MM: Standard treatment for multiple myeloma. *Mayo Clin Proc* 69:781–786, 1994

62. Rödjer S, Vikrot O, Wahlin A, et al: Effect of interferon alpha-2b in advanced multiple myeloma. *J Intern Med* 227: 45–48, 1990

63. Browman GP, Bergsagel D, Sicheri D, et al: Randomized trial of interferon maintenance in multiple myeloma: a study of the National Cancer Institute of Canada Clinical Trials Group. *J Clin Oncol* 13:2354–2360, 1995

64. Camba L, Durie BG: Multiple myeloma: new treatment options. *Drugs* 44:170–181, 1992

65. Borden EC: Innovative treatment strategies for non-Hodgkin's lymphoma and multiple myeloma. *Semin Oncol* 21:14–22, 1994

66. Mandellia F, Avvisati G, Amador S, et al: Maintenance treatment with recombinant interferon alpha-2b in patients with multiple myeloma responding to conventional chemotherapy. *N Engl J Med* 322:1430–1434, 1990

67. Oken MM, Leong T, Kay NE, et al: The effect of adding interferon or high-dose cyclophosphamide to VBMCP to treat multiple myeloma: results from an ECOG phase III trial. *Blood* 86:441a, 1995

68. Ludwig H, Cohen AM, Polliack A, et al: Interferon-alpha for induction and maintenance in multiple myeloma: results of two multicenter randomized trials and summaries of other studies. *Ann Oncol* 6:467–472, 1995

69. Westin J: For the nordic myeloma study group interferon alpha 2 in addition to melphalan prednisone for initial and maintenance treatment in multiple myeloma: a randomized Nordic trial. *Blood* 86:441a, 1995

70. Dimopoulos MA, Goldstein J, Fuller L, et al: Curability of solitary bone plasmacytoma. *J Clin Oncol* 10:587–590, 1992

71. Anderson MG: The lymphomas and multiple myeloma, in Baird SB, McCorkle R, Grant M (eds): *A Cancer Source Book for Nurses.* Atlanta, American Cancer Society, 1991, pp 286–295

72. Dudjak LA: Alternatives in dose fractionation and treatment volume, in Dow KG, Hilderley LJ (eds): *Nursing Care in Radiation Oncology.* Philadelphia, Saunders, 1992, pp 285–294

73. Hilderley LJ: Radiotherapy, in Groenwald SL, Frogge MH, Goodman M, Yarbro CH (eds): *Cancer Nursing: Principles and Practice* (ed 3). Sudbury, MA, Jones and Barlett, 1993, pp 235–269

74. Jagannath S, Barlogie B, Dicke K, et al: Autologous bone marrow transplantation in multiple myeloma: identification of prognostic factors. *Blood* 76:1860–1866, 1990

75. Anderson KC, Barut BA, Ritz J, et al: Monoclonal antibody-

76. Gahrton G, Tura S, Ljungman P, et al: Allogeneic bone marrow transplantation in multiple myeloma. *N Engl J Med* 325:1267–1273, 1991

77. Tura S, Cavo M: Allogeneic bone marrow transplantation in multiple myeloma. *Hematol Oncol Clin North Am* 6: 425–435, 1992

78. Copelan EA, Biggs JC, Szer J, et al: Allogeneic bone marrow transplantation for acute myelogenous leukemia, acute lymphocytic leukemia, and cyclophosphamide (BuCy2). *Semin Oncol* 20:33–38, 1993 (suppl 4)

79. Ballester OF: Allogeneic bone marrow transplantation for multiple myeloma. *Semin Oncol* 20:67–71, 1993 (suppl 6)

80. Barlogie B, Jagannath S, Vesole D, et al: Autologous and allogeneic transplants for multiple myeloma. *Semin Hematol* 32:31–44, 1995

81. Trict G, Vesole DH, Jagannath S, et al: Graft-versus-myeloma effect: proof of principle. *Blood* 87:1196–1198, 1996

82. Attal M, Harousseau JL, Stoppa AM, et al: A prospective, randomized trial of autologous bone marrow transplantation and chemotherapy in multiple myeloma. *N Engl J Med* 335:91–97, 1996

83. Cunningham D, Paz-Ares L, Milan S, et al: High-dose melphalan and autologous bone marrow transplantation as consolidation in previously untreated myeloma. *J Clin Oncol* 12:759–763, 1989

84. Siegel DS, Desikan KR, Mehta J, et al: Age is not a prognostic variable with autotransplants in multiple myeloma. *Blood* 93:51–54, 1999

85. Powles R, Raj N, Milan S, et al: Outcome assessment of a population based group of 195 unselected myeloma patients under 70 years of age offered intensive treatment. *Bone Marrow Transplant* 20:435–443, 1997

86. Kwak LW, Thielemans K, Massaia M: Idiotypic vaccination as therapy for multiple myeloma. *Semin Hematol* 36:34–37, 1999

87. Gertz MA, Lacy MQ, Inwards DJ, et al: Factors influencing platelet recovery after blood cell transplantation in multiple myeloma. *Bone Marrow Transplant* 20:375–380, 1997

88. Mehta J, Singhal, S Desikan K, et al: High dose therapy and stem cell support in myeloma, in Devita VT, Hellman S, Rosenberg SA (eds): Update *Cancer Principles and Practice of Oncology* 13(8):1–12, 1999

89. Schlossman RL, Anderson KC: Bone marrow transplantation in multiple myeloma. *Cancer Invest* 15:65–75, 1997

90. Mehta J, Singhal S: Graft versus myeloma. *Bone Marrow Transplant* 22:835–843, 1998

91. Singhal S, Mehta J, Eddlema P, et al: Marked anti-tumor effect from anti-angiogenesis (AA) therapy with thalidomide in high risk refractory multiple myeloma. *Blood* 92: 318a, 1998 (suppl 1)

92. Barlogie B, Desikan R, Munshi N, et al: Single course DT PACE anti-angiochemotherapy effects CR in plasma cell leukemia and fulminant multiple myeloma. *Blood* 92:273b, 1998 (suppl 1)

93. Berenson JB, Lichtenstein A, Porter L, et al: Efficacy of pamidronate in reducing skeletal events in patients with advanced multiple myeloma. *N Engl J Med* 334:488–493, 1996

94. Bhatia S, Ramsay NKC, Steinbuch M, et al: Malignant neoplasms following bone marrow transplantation. *Blood* 87: 3633–3639, 1996

95. Deeg HJ, Witherspoon RP: Risk factors for the develop-

ment of secondary malignancies after marrow transplantation. *Hematol Oncol Clin North Am* 7:417–423, 1993

96. Wujcik D: Leukemia, in Groenwald SL, Frogge MH, Goodman M, Yarbro CH (eds): *Cancer Nursing: Principles and Practice* (ed 3). Sudbury, MA, Jones and Bartlett, 1993, pp 1149–1173

97. McDaniel RW, Rhodes VA: Symptom experience. *Semin Oncol Nurs* 11:232–234, 1995

98. Held JL, Peahota A: Nursing care of the patient with spinal cord compression. *Oncol Nurs Forum* 20:1507–1514, 1993

99. Struthers C, Mayer, Fisher G: Nursing management of the patient with bone metastasis. *Semin Oncol Nurs* 14:199–209, 1998

100. Coyle N, Cherny N, Portenoy RK: Pharmacologic management of cancer pain, in McGuire DB, Yarbro CH, Ferrell BR (eds): *Cancer Pain Management* (ed 2). Sudbury, MA, Jones and Bartlett, 1995, pp 89–130

101. Spross JA, Burke MW: Non-pharmacologic management of cancer pain, in McGuire DB, Yarbro CH, Ferrell BR (eds): *Cancer Pain Management* (ed 2). Sudbury, MA, Jones and Bartlett, 1995, pp 159–205

102. Kanak MF: Interventions related to patient safety. *Nurs Clin North Am* 27:371–395, 1992

103. Valente SM, Saunders JM, Cohen MZ: Evaluating depression among patients with cancer. *Cancer Pract* 2:65–71, 1993

104. Hagopian GA: Cognitive strategies used in adapting to a cancer diagnosis. *Oncol Nurs Forum* 20:759–763, 1993

105. McNally JC, Stair J: Potential for infection, in McNally JC, Somerville ET, Miaskowski C, Rostad M (eds): *Guidelines for Oncology Nursing Practice*. Philadelphia, Saunders, 1991, pp 191–202

106. Alexander EJ: Potential for injury related to thrombocytopenia, in McNally JC, Somerville ET, Miaskowski C, Rostad M (eds): *Guidelines for Oncology Nursing Practice*. Philadelphia, Saunders, 1991, pp 203–207

107. Rostad M: Potential for injury related to anemia, in McNally JC, Somerville ET, Miaskowski C, Rostad M (eds): *Guidelines for Oncology Nursing Practice*. Philadelphia, Saunders, 1991, pp 208–215

108. Nail LM, Winningham ML: Fatigue and weakness in cancer patients: the symptom experience. *Semin Oncol Nurs* 11:272–278, 1995

109. Ream E, Richardson A: From theory to practice: designing interventions to reduce fatigue in patients with cancer. *Oncol Nurs Forum* 26:1295–1303, 1999

110. Desikan KR, Barlogie B, Jagannath S, et al: Comparable engraftment kinetics following peripheral blood stem cell infusion mobilized with granulocyte colony stimulating factor with or without cyclophosphamide in multiple myeloma. *J Clin Oncol* 16:1547–1553, 1998

111. Alegre A, Diaz-Mediavilla J, San-Miguel J, et al: Autologous peripheral blood stem cell transplantation for multiple myeloma: a report of 259 cases from the Spanish registry. *Bone Marrow Transplant* 21:133–140, 1998

112. Weaver CH, Zhen B, Schwartzberg LS, et al: Phase I–II evaluation of rapid sequence tandem high-dose melphalan with peripheral blood stem cell support in patients with multiple myeloma. *Bone Marrow Transplant* 22:245–251, 1998

113. The American Society of Clinical Oncology Health Services Committee: Update of recommendations for the use of hematopoietic colony-stimulating factors: evidence-based clinical practice guidelines. *J Clin Oncol* 14:1957–1960, 1996

114. Wong DL: Health promotion of the infant and family, in Wong DL, Wilson D (eds): *Nursing Care of Infants and Children*. St. Louis, Mosby, 1995, pp 514–573

115. Prevention of Pneumococcal disease: recommendations of the advisory committee immunization practices (ACIP). *MMWR Morb Mortal Wkly Rpt* 46:1–24, 1997

116. Canty SL: Constipation as a side effect of opioids. *Oncol Nurs Forum* 21:739–745, 1994

117. Moore JM: Tumor lysis syndrome, in Gross J, Johnson BL (eds): *Handbook of Oncology Nursing*. Sudbury, MA, Jones and Bartlett, 1994, pp 691–700

118. Kreamer K, Lynch MP: Hypercalemia, in Preston FA, Cunningham RS (eds): *Clinical Guidelines for Symptom Management in Oncology*. New York: Clinical Insights Press, 1998, pp 12–25

119. Shilberg O, Douer D, Ehrenfield S, et al: Naproxen associated fatal acute renal failure in multiple myeloma. *Nephron* 55:448–449, 1990

120. Hubbard SM, Galassi A: Chemotherapy, in Gross J, Johnson BL (eds): *Handbook of Oncology Nursing*. Sudbury, MA, Jones and Bartlett, 1994, pp 55–94

121. Cancer Resources in the United States. *Oncol Nurs Forum* 25:1785–1799, 1998

122. Skeel RT: Measurement of outcomes in supportive oncology, in Berger AM, Portenoy RK, Weissman DE (eds): *Principles and Practices of Supportive Oncology*. Philadelphia, Lippincott-Raven, 1998, pp 875–888

CHAPTER 62

Ovarian Cancer

Virginia R. Martin, MSN, RN, AOCN

Introduction

There has been remarkable progress in the understanding and management of ovarian cancer. It is known that there is a genetic basis for hereditary ovarian cancer and screening efforts can target those at high risk; the role of cytoreductive surgery and accurate staging of the disease is now well defined; and there is effective adjuvant chemotherapy treatment for advanced disease. Yet considerable work remains before the origin and biology of the disease are completely understood and, more importantly, before specific and sensitive tests to detect the disease in its early curable stages can be developed. For years ovarian cancer has been characterized as the silent killer. Patients with ovarian cancer have recently formed a powerful voice through coalition and advocacy groups, which speak for research funding and other issues. For example, the Ovarian Cancer Coalition more accurately describes the early stages of ovarian cancer by its motto: "It whispers . . . so listen." The advocacy conference held in 1998 by the Ovarian Cancer National Alliance titled their program "SILENT NO MORE." Clearly, both groups are working diligently to actively change public and professional views about the disease.

The ovaries are located in the pelvis lateral to the uterus, and slightly posterior and caudal to the fallopian tubes (Figure 62-1).[1] Due to endocrine stimulation, the ovaries change size, shape, position, and histology during the monthly menstrual cycle and during their lifetime.[1-3]

Epidemiology

Ovarian cancer is the most lethal of the gynecologic cancers. The incidence is about one-half that of endometrial cancer; however, its mortality rate in the Western world exceeds that of cervical and endometrial cancers combined. In 1999, 25,500 new cases are predicted in the United States and 14,500 deaths.[4] It represents only 4% of all cancer in women, but, more notably, is the fourth leading cause of cancer death in women. Over a lifetime, 1 in 70 women will develop ovarian cancer, considerably less than the 1 in 8 incidence for breast cancer. The lifetime risk of this disease for the general population is 1.5%; however, three-fourths of those individuals will have advanced disease at diagnosis.[5] Ovarian cancer occurs primarily in women age 40–70, it is uncommon in women less than age 40, and the median age of occurrence is 55.[6] The incidence rate increases sharply in women as they age until the eighth decade of life when incidence plateaus, as depicted in Figure 62-2.

Ovarian cancer has a wide variation in international incidence rates, with the highest rates in North America, Scandinavian countries, and Israel. The lowest incidence is in Japan and in developing countries. In the United States incidence is slightly higher among white and Hawaiian races, intermediate in blacks, Hispanics, and Asian Americans, and lowest in Native Americans.[7] There has been little change in incidence in the United States over the last three decades.

Etiology

Hormonal, environmental, and genetic factors all play a role in the development of ovarian cancer. The major risk and preventive factors for ovarian cancer are summarized in Table 62-1. The factors that attract the most attention are those that relate to hormonal and reproductive factors.

Hormonal

The monthly ovulatory cycle in women and how it affects the ovarian epithelium is the focus of the hormonal etiology and the risk of ovarian cancer. It is postulated to be the direct function of the number of ovulatory cycles in a woman's life span.[8,9] It is hypothesized that the uninterrupted cell division and regeneration of the ovarian epithelium, which provide opportunity for mutation and malignant transformation without pregnancy-induced rest periods, contribute to neoplasia of the ovary.[8,9] In 1983 this theory was expanded by investigators who theorized that the ovarian epithelium repeatedly invaginates throughout life to form clefts and inclusion cysts within the ovary and suggested that, under excessive gonadotropin stimulation of the ovarian stroma and resulting stimulation by estrogen or estrogen precursors, the epithelium may undergo proliferation and malignant transformation.[10] In addition to incessant ovulation and gonadotropin stimulation, androgens and progesterone may be implicated in the etiology of ovarian cancer.[11]

Parity, infertility, and lactation

Pregnancy has been associated with a protective effect in ovarian cancer risk. Women who are multiparas have a 10%–30% reduction in ovarian cancer compared to nulliparas.[7] A large prospective study showed a 45% decrease in ovarian cancer risk in parous women, it also demonstrated a 16% decrease with each subsequent birth.[12] Most studies now show there is no significant effect of the age at menarche, age at first birth, or age at menopause with regard to risk of ovarian cancer.[13] Infertility may be associated with risk since childless women who have been pregnant have the same risk as nulliparas.[14] There is an increased risk among women who have used fertility drugs. Drugs such as clomiphene increase the risk of ovarian cancer twofold to threefold when used more than 12 cycles.[15] There is also evidence that pelvic inflammatory disease, which may result in infertility, may stimulate proliferation of the surface epithelium of the ovary and increase the risk for those women.[7] Lactation is known to suppress ovulation in some

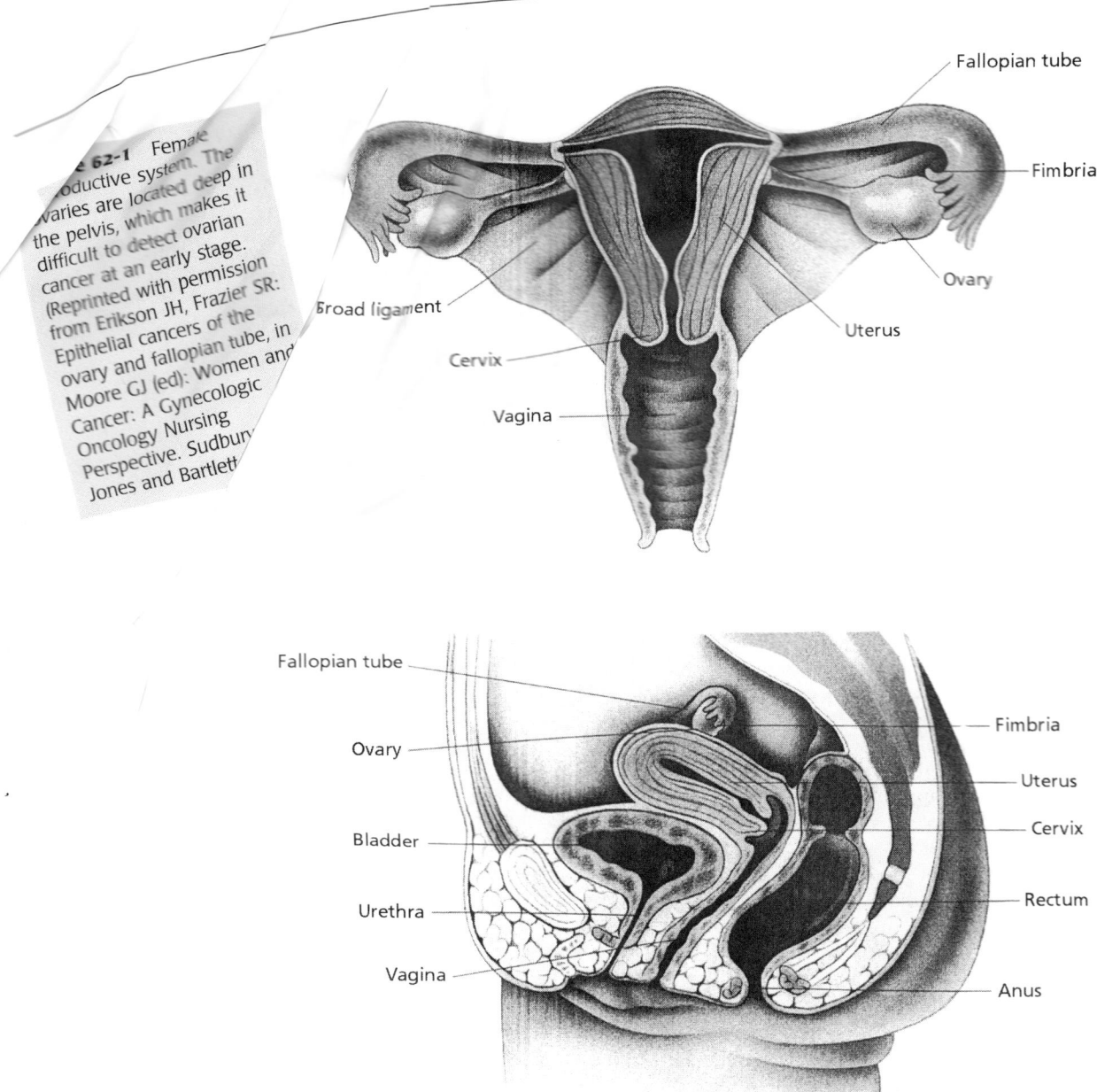

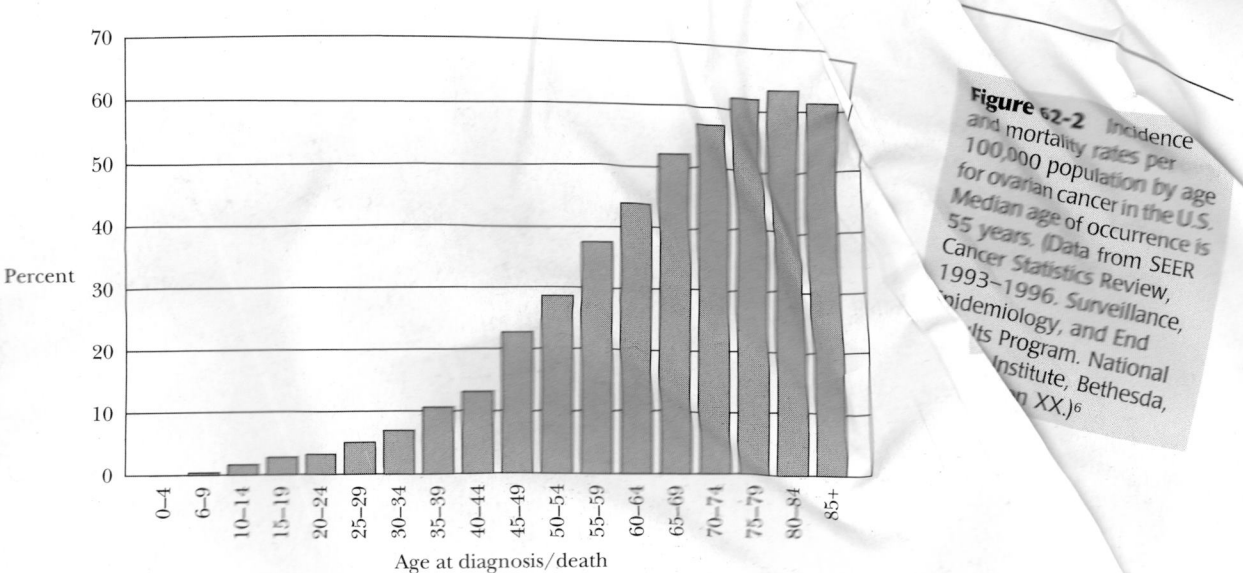

Risk Factors and Preventive Factors	Preventive Factors
	Parity
	Lactation
	Oral contraceptives
	Tubal ligation
	Oophorectomy

Figure 62-1 Female reproductive system. The ovaries are located deep in the pelvis, which makes it difficult to detect ovarian cancer at an early stage. (Reprinted with permission from Erikson JH, Frazier SR: Epithelial cancers of the ovary and fallopian tube, in Moore GJ (ed): Women and Cancer: A Gynecologic Oncology Nursing Perspective. Sudbury, MA. Jones and Bartlett, 1997.)[1]

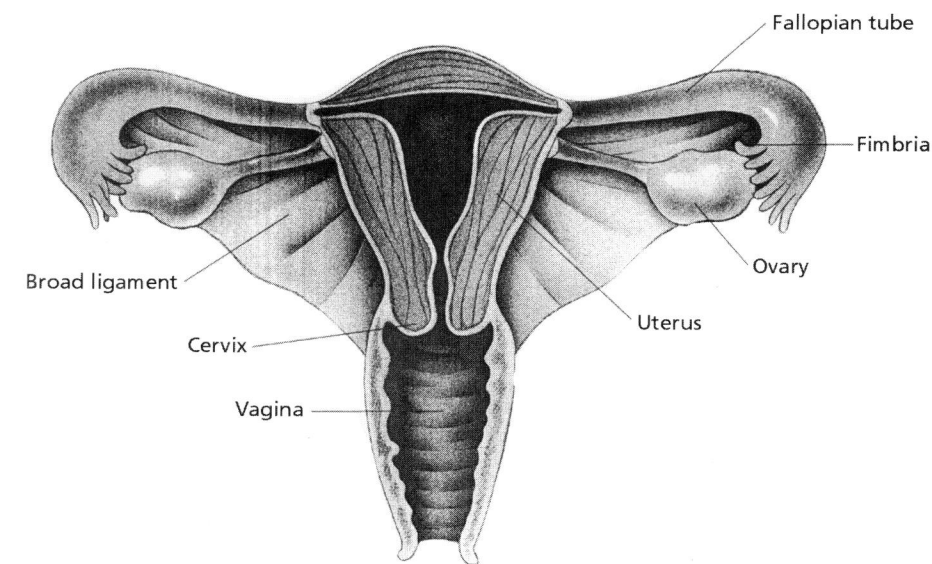

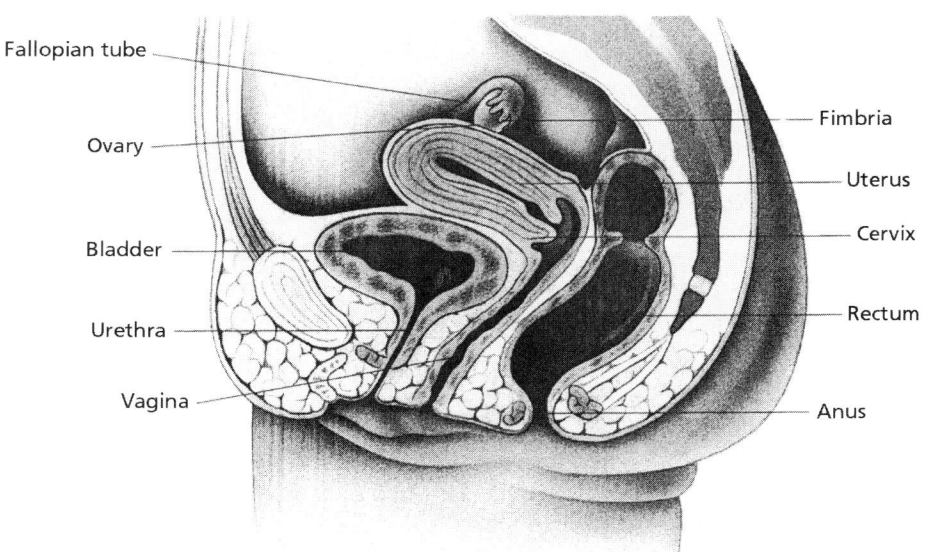

women and pregnancy with lactation appears protective. Whittemore reported that the risk of ovarian cancer decreased 1% for each month of lactation, with the most significant protective effect in the first six months after delivery.[14]

Exogenous hormones

Combined oral contraceptives decrease a woman's risk of ovarian cancer by 30%–60% depending on the duration of use.[7] In a meta-analysis report, five years of contraceptive use by nulliparous women reduces their risk to that of parous women and ten years of oral contraceptive use in women with a positive family history can reduce their risk to a level below that of women with a negative family history.[16] It is theorized that the progestin

in the oral contraceptives induces damaged ovarian cells to die before they turn malignant.[17] Hormone replacement therapy (HRT), even long-term use, does not appear to influence a woman's ovarian cancer risk.[18]

Endogenous hormones

It appears that women with low serum gonadotropin levels (FSH and LH) are at an increased risk of ovarian cancer, as are women with high androstenedione and dehydroepiandrosterone (DHEA) levels.[19] Further, women with a history of polycystic ovary syndrome and elevated androstenedione levels may be at an increased risk of ovarian cancer.[20] These findings do not support the hypothesis that gonadotropin stimulation is an etiologic factor in ovarian cancer; instead, it is theorized that oral

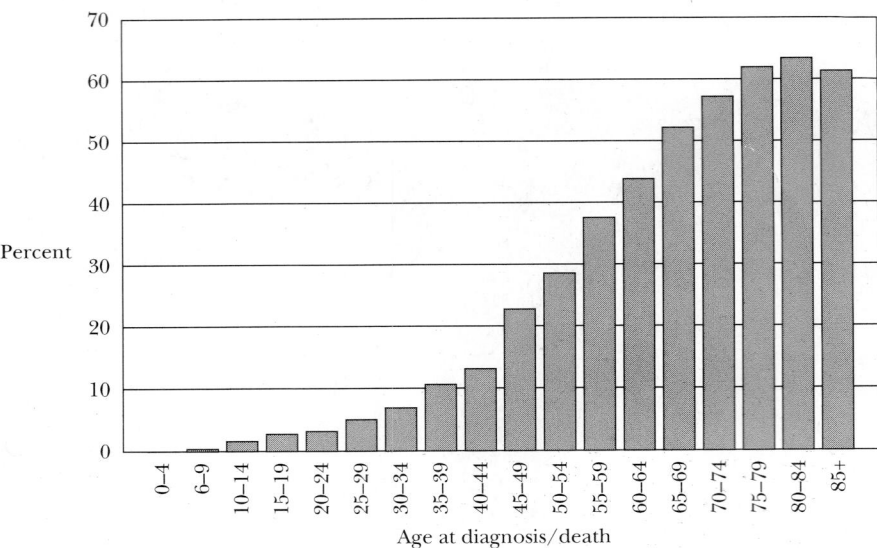

Figure 62-2 Incidence and mortality rates per 100,000 population by age for ovarian cancer in the U.S. Median age of occurrence is 55 years. (Data from SEER Cancer Statistics Review, 1993–1996. Surveillance, Epidemiology, and End Results Program. National Cancer Institute, Bethesda, MD, Section XX.)[6]

contraceptives and gonadotropins may act through changing androgen levels.[11] Women with endometriosis experience a variety of hormone and immunologic abnormalities and are thus at increased risk, as are women with more total ovulatory cycles in their lifetime.[21] Women who have more ovulatory cycles are at higher risk for having *p53* positive tumors if they develop ovarian cancer, which lends support to the theory that a higher number of ovulatory cycles may lead to increased DNA damage.[22]

A tubal ligation or hysterectomy physically interrupts the utero-ovarian circulation thereby decreasing the risk of ovarian cancer.[23] It appears that because the route from the vagina to the ovaries is disrupted, exposure to exogenous toxins is likely to be diminished. The role of hormones in the etiology of ovarian cancer likely reflects a composite of factors. For example, among younger women with fewer menstrual cycles, aside from a family history, exposure to androgens may be the dominant

factor, whereas among older women, continuous uninterrupted ovulation and the greater number of menstrual cycles may be the most critical factor.[7]

Environmental

Industrialized countries, with the exception of Japan, have a higher incidence of ovarian cancer, which could lead to the yet unproven conclusion that environmental factors are somehow related to the etiology of ovarian cancer. Multiple dietary influences have been studied. Galactose metabolism has been proposed as a risk factor for ovarian cancer based on data that galactose is toxic to oocytes. Galactosemic women have premature menopause and increased gonadotropin levels. One study[24] has supported this theory but others have not.[25,26] Selenium may have a protective effect against ovarian cancer.[27] Increased activity and vigorous physical exercise may increase the number of anovulatory cycles, which may provide a protective effect against ovarian cancer. However, in direct contrast to this finding, women reporting regular leisure physical activity have a 1.5-fold greater risk, and women who vigorously exercise (more than four times a week) have been found to have a 2.5-fold greater risk of developing ovarian cancer.[28] Daly and associates theorize that the rigorous activity has a negative effect on circulating estrogen feedback and produces increased serum gonadotropins.[7] Cosmetic talc use in dusting the perineum, in feminine hygiene sprays, or on sanitary napkins, condoms or diaphragms, has also been suggested as a possible risk. Studies have reported a significant risk of ovarian cancer with the use of talc.[29–31] In another study, however, a significant association between the use of talcum powder and the risk of developing ovarian cancer was not demonstrated even with prolonged exposure.[32] More research in the area of exercise, diet, and other potential environmental factors related

Table 62-1 Risk Factors and Preventive Factors in Ovarian Cancer

Risk Factors	Preventive Factors
Nulliparity	Parity
Use of infertility drugs	Lactation
Pelvic inflammatory disease	Oral contraceptives
Low serum gonadotropin	Tubal ligation
Use of talc	Oophorectomy
Family history of breast or ovarian cancer	
Living in industrialized western countries	
Being of Jewish descent	

to ovarian cancer needs to be done before conclusions can be drawn.

Genetics

Among the factors associated with increased risk of ovarian cancer, nothing alters the magnitude of the risk more than a family history of ovarian cancer.[7] The closer the degree of the familial relationship and the younger the age of the relative at diagnosis, the higher the risk of developing ovarian cancer.[33] Three separate syndromes of genetic predisposition for ovarian cancer exist: (1) familial ovarian cancer, (2) hereditary breast-ovarian cancer (HBOC), and (3) hereditary nonpolyposis colorectal cancer (HNPCC). Familial ovarian cancer accounts for 5%–10% of the overall incidence; however these other hereditary categories have a lifetime risk of developing the disease that approaches 50%.[34] The most understood hereditary cancer syndromes are HBOC syndrome and HNPCC or the Lynch II syndrome. Genetic predisposition to cancer is known to be the result of germ-line mutations. In HBOC syndrome, germ-line mutations of *BRCA1* and *BRCA2* have been identified.[35] In HNPCC, another set of genes involved in DNA mismatch repair have been identified: *hMSH2, hMLH1, hPMS2, hMSH3,* and *hMSH6*.[35]

Hereditary ovarian cancer is recognized to occur via an autosomal dominant mode of inheritance.[36–38] A link has been identified between a locus on chromosome 17q and breast cancer.[39] This same locus on chromosome 17q is responsible for HBOC syndrome.[40] The gene is known as *BRCA1*.[41] *BRCA1* is a tumor suppressor gene whose normal function is to inhibit the development of cancer. Mutations in this *BRCA1* gene destroy its protective function and increase the chance of developing breast or ovarian cancer. A second breast cancer susceptibility locus on the long arm of chromosome 13q has been identified as *BRCA2* gene.[42,43] *BRCA2* is associated with ovarian cancer, breast cancer, prostate cancer, head and neck cancer, malignant melanoma, and pancreatic cancer. The lifetime risk of ovarian cancer for persons with *BRCA1* mutations is in the range of 40%–66%.[44,45] The risk for ovarian cancer in families with *BRCA2* mutations is lower and ranges from 10%–20%.[44,45]

The other type of hereditary syndrome identified with ovarian cancer is HNPCC. Ovarian cancer occurs in about 5%–10% of HNPCC patients with a germ-line mutation.[46]

Women of Ashkenazi Jewish descent have been found to have high rates of *BRCA1* and *BRCA2* mutations.[47] One percent of Ashkenazi Jews tested positive for *BRCA1* and *BRCA2* mutations, much higher than the general population.[48]

The number of family members with ovarian cancer defines the degree of risk in the familial category. If one family member has ovarian cancer, there is a two-fold to three-fold increased risk of ovarian cancer, leading to a lifetime risk of 5%.[49] If two or more family members have ovarian cancer, the lifetime risk increases to 7%.[49] Familial

risk does not approach the significant elevation of risk that occurs with hereditary ovarian cancer.

Prevention, Screening, and Early Detection

The ovaries are located anatomically deep in the pelvis, (see Figure 62-1) which is why it is difficult to detect ovarian cancer at an early stage. An ovarian tumor can grow undiscovered until it becomes large. There are three different techniques available for early detection: the pelvic exam, serum tumor marker (CA-125), and a transvaginal ultrasound. None of these are sufficiently sensitive or specific to be recommended for screening of the general population.

Studies have been done using various screening measures such as surgery, CA-125, pelvic exam, and ultrasound. No conclusive recommendations for screening were reached.[50–55] There are several studies currently under way that may be able to answer some of the questions that still remain about screening healthy women for ovarian cancer. The National Institutes of Health is conducting a 16-year study on 74,000 women over 60 years of age, randomizing them to a control group for observation or a screening group with a clinical exam, ultrasound and CA-125.[56] A large study in Europe at St. Bartholomew's Hospital is following 120,000 postmenopausal women older than age 50 in a three-year study using a control group and study group in women with abnormal transvaginal ultrasounds.[53] When completed, these studies will provide more concrete information on the value of our current screening methods.

Pelvic Examination

An annual physical exam, including a pelvic examination with bimanual rectovaginal exam, is part of routine health care for women. The palpation of the ovaries during this exam is not established as a useful screening procedure for ovarian cancer. Pap smear should be performed although this test does not provide valuable screening information in this disease. The size of the ovaries in premenopausal women can change. Palpation of a pelvic mass on pelvic exam is abnormal in postmenopausal women and is an indication for a diagnostic ultrasound.

CA-125

CA-125 is a tumor antigen commonly elevated in ovarian cancer. Eighty percent or more of epithelial ovarian cancers have been found to have serum CA-125 titers greater than 35 U/mL, whereas just 1% of healthy women have serum CA-125 titers at this level.[57] However, population screening studies found that only about 50% of primary ovarian carcinomas confined to the ovary (stage I) are associated with elevated CA-125 levels.[58–60] Thus, early studies concluded that serum CA-125 determinations, while encouraging, are not sufficiently sensitive or specific enough to recommend CA-125 as a single test for population screening, particularly for premenopausal women.[58–63] Therefore, the marker CA-125 is not helpful in the screening of the general population, although 75%–90% of women diagnosed with ovarian cancer will have an elevated CA-125 level.[57,64] An elevated CA-125 level in asymptomatic women may indicate the presence of cancer; but if the CA-125 level is normal in women with an ovarian mass it does not rule out ovarian cancer. CA-125 can be elevated in multiple benign or other malignant diseases (Table 62-2).[65] If elevated prior to diagnosis, it is an important indicator of early treatment failure during front-line therapy. Further, CA-125 is of proven value in confirmation of disease relapse, and is used during treatment as a tool to evaluate response to therapy.[55,66,67]

Ultrasound

Although transabdominal ultrasound provides information on the characteristics of an ovarian mass and the presence or absence of ascites, it does not provide a

Table 62-2 Conditions Associated with an Increased CA-125 Level

Ovarian cancer

Endometriosis

Fibroids

Hemorrhagic ovarian cysts

Menstruation

Pelvic inflammatory disease (acute)

Pregnancy (first trimester)

Acute pancreatitis

Colitis

Chronic active hepatitis

Cirrhosis

Diverticulitis

Pericarditis

Renal disease (serum creatinine > 2.0)

Polyarteritis nodosa

Sjögren syndrome

Systemic lupus erythematosus

Other malignancies: bladder, breast, endometrium, lung, liver, non-Hodgkin's, lymphoma, pancreas

Used with permission from Rosenthal A, Jacobs I: Ovarian Cancer Screening. *Semin Oncol* 25:315–323, 1998.[65]

definitive diagnosis. Ultrasound is unable to differentiate between a benign, functional, or malignant mass.

The transabdominal method has been replaced by the transvaginal method, which allows a closer evaluation of the ovaries via the probe placed in the vagina. Transvaginal ultrasound permits superior visualization with increased efficiency, comfort, and greater patient acceptance.[68] Additionally, color Doppler imaging is used with ultrasound to measure the blood flow patterns in ovarian vessels. An increase in the blood flow resistance is found with a malignancy. Although more sensitive, any type of ultrasound screening is expensive, lacks specificity, and requires multiple studies to evaluate abnormal findings. Ultrasound also has a low positive predictive value and may lead to excessive numbers of surgical procedures.[65]

Routine screening with pelvic examination, CA-125, and ultrasound is not recommended for the general population. However, intensive screening using a combination of the methods available should be used for women with familial or hereditary risk factors. Pedigree analysis, linkage studies, and/or DNA testing are done to determine genetic risk.[46] The process of determining genetic risk begins with information about the availability of DNA testing. Genetic counseling is mandatory prior to DNA testing and at the time of disclosure of the findings. It is the clinician's role to provide detailed information regarding the inheritance and natural history of ovarian cancer as well as advantages and limitations of genetic testing, surveillance, and management strategies.

If a patient does not have an increased genetic risk based on the DNA testing, then that individual should return to general population screening recommendations. If the patient has positive findings confirming genetic predisposition, an intensive screening program is initiated. Screening and surveillance with baseline and interval multiple serum tumor markers and pelvic transvaginal ultrasound screening are recommended. For women with HBOC syndrome the recommendations include a semiannual breast and pelvic exam, annual mammogram, monthly breast self-examination, baseline multiple tumor markers, and tumor markers at six-month intervals.[35] For HNPCC syndrome, all of the above is recommended plus pelvic ultrasound, endometrial screening for cytology and histology, and annual colonoscopic exam.[35] Women should be counseled to eat a balanced diet, restrict fat and carbohydrate intake, and maintain a reasonable weight. High-risk women may also elect to take medicine to suppress ovulation, or consider prophylactic oophorectomy. In spite of prophylactic oophorectomy, the risk for a primary peritoneal carcinomatosis remains 2%–5%.[69–71]

Video laparoscopy is an excellent method to examine the undersurfaces of the diaphragm, the peritoneum, serosal surfaces, and the pelvic contents. Members of autosomal dominant hereditary cancer syndrome families are encouraged to participate in studies to detect early precancerous and cancerous changes in their ovaries through programs that test and evaluate the screening methods now available.[46]

It was previously recommended that women in HBOC and HNPCC syndrome families take combined estrogen-progestin oral contraceptives before plans for conception and between pregnancies.[35] Oral contraceptives have been linked to an increased risk for breast cancer among younger women so it is no longer recommended for the HBOC syndrome families. Oral contraceptives are recommended for HNPCC families not genetically at risk for breast cancer.[35]

Women with hereditary ovarian cancer are usually diagnosed at an earlier age (early forties and younger) than women with sporadic ovarian cancer. The mean age for developing ovarian cancer in HBOC families was 51 years, compared to 43 years for HNPCC syndrome.[46] The youngest age observed was 26 years for HBOC, and 24 years for HNPCC syndrome.[46] Therefore, genetic counseling of high-risk females should begin in their teenage years.

At present the recommendations for the general population is for any woman over age 18 to see a physician yearly for a thorough physical examination that should include a bimanual rectovaginal examination. With the tests currently available, routine screening for ovarian cancer is not recommended.[49] Asymptomatic women may consider discussing with their practitioner the use of oral contraceptives and tubal ligation for increased protection. Although a very personal decision, another method of risk reduction is parity.

Pathophysiology

Biology

The most common type of ovarian cancer develops predominantly from the malignant transformation of a single cell type, the surface epithelium.[46] The exact mechanism of transformation is not clear; however, ovarian cancer appears to arise from the accumulation of mutations in multiple combinations of genes.[72] These changes involve inherited or acquired activation of cellular proto-oncogenes and somatic or germ-line inactivation of tumor suppressor genes.[72] The tumor suppressor gene most extensively studied in solid tumors is *p53*. The *p53* gene product plays a role in normal cellular proliferation by regulating gene transcription and apoptosis.[73] Mutations of *p53* have been identified in 30%–79% of epithelial ovarian cancers.[74,75] Cytogenic characterization of surgical ovarian tumors have revealed extensive and complex structural chromosome abnormalities involving numerous chromosomes including 1, 3, 6, 11, 14, 17.[76–80] Multiple sites of loss of heterozygosity have been observed in ovarian tumors and cell lines. Both allelic loss and mutations of *p53* are seen and do not correlate with prognosis in this disease.[79,81]

Although progress continues in the biology of ovarian

cancer, little is known about all the molecular events that lead to the development of ovarian cancer and many more genes involved remain to be discovered as well as the clinical significance of the genes. It is known that penetration of the tumor cells through the basement membrane is a prerequisite for metastatic disease. This phenomenon is also under genetic control; the specific genes have yet to be determined. The combination of genetic changes that determine the malignant phenotype with its ability to invade and metastasize account for the lethality of the disease.

The most common type of ovarian cancer is the epithelial type, which accounts for 85%–90% of the disease. Germ cell or sex-cord stromal cell tumors constitute the majority of nonepithelial tumors. Ovarian tumors range from benign, to tumors of low malignant potential, to invasive cancer. Epithelial cancer is further classified according to its behavior, either as borderline or invasive, and the cell type. Serous or mucinous types are the most common classifications of epithelial tumors. The epithelial type originates from the cells on the surface of the germinal epithelium or the mesothelium of the ovary. The remaining tumors arise from the germ or stromal cells. Germ cells are precursors of the ova; the most common type of malignancy is dysgerminoma. Sex-cord stromal cells secrete hormones and connect the different components of the ovary together; the most common tumor is the granulosa cell tumor.

Metastasis in epithelial ovarian cancer can often occur by direct extension. It penetrates the capsule of the ovary and invades the structures next to it. It can also spread by lymphatic dissemination, most frequently the pelvic or aortic lymph nodes. Rarely it spreads by blood-borne metastases. The continuous circulation of the peritoneal fluid in the peritoneal cavity facilitates the widespread dissemination of the malignant cells. This may be referred to as *peritoneal seeding*. Disease spreads to the liver, diaphragm, bladder, or intestines by this route (Figure 62-3).[82]

Prognostic Factors

In terms of patient characteristics, age and performance status correlate with outcome. A patient with a good performance status (ECOG 0–2) is more likely to respond to treatment and experience less toxicity and better outcome.[83–85] The Gynecology Oncology Group (GOG) has reported age as a prognostic variable in 2000 patients on six trials.[86] Patients older than 69 had a poorer survival compared to those under age 50. Better prognostic indicators are needed in this disease. The standard prognostic indicators are subjective and far from sufficient to predict prognosis. Abnormalities of oncogenes, such as *p53*, *MYC*, *RAS*, *ERB-2*, and tumor suppressor genes have been reported to have prognostic importance and the expression of certain growth factors may also be associated with poor prognosis.[87] It is still too early to completely understand the significance of these findings related to the

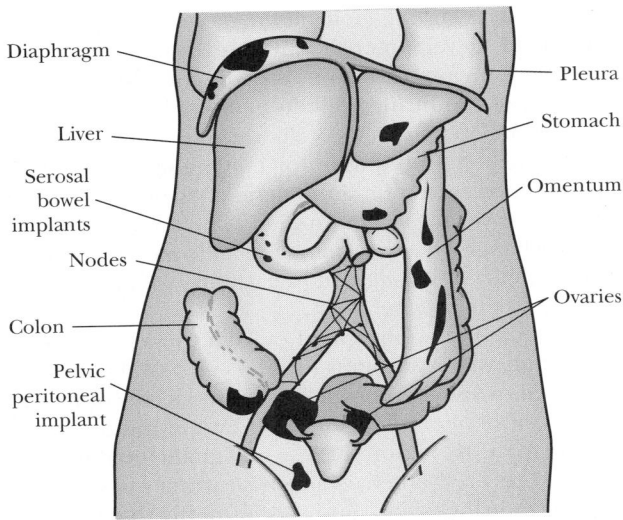

Figure 62-3 Typical sites of metastases. (Adapted with permission from DiSaia PJ: Diagnosis and Management of Ovarian Cancer. *Hosp Pract* 22: 235–250, 1987.)[82]

development of ovarian cancer or the progression of the disease and apply the findings to clinical practice. Other prognostic factors under investigation include DNA ploidy, and proliferation activity (S-phase fraction), tumor markers, flow cytometry, and factors regulating transformation and growth.

Clinical Manifestations

Ovarian cancer occurs most frequently in women over age 50. Most patients with the disease are 50–59 years old and approximately 70% of patients present with advanced stage III or IV disease. The initial signs and symptoms are often dismissed or ignored. Abdominal bloating or discomfort is the most common sign and symptom, followed by vaginal bleeding, gastrointestinal symptoms, or

Table 62-3 Common Signs and Symptoms of Ovarian Cancer

Early Signs	Late Signs
Lower abdominal pressure: discomfort or pain	Ascites
	Pleural effusion
Abdominal distention	Anorexia
Change in bowel or bladder habits	Nausea or vomiting
	Abdominal, pelvic, ovarian, omental mass
Early satiety	
Indigestion, dyspepsia	
Back pain	

urinary tract symptoms. A recent study of 50 female ovarian cancer patients reported the following symptoms by more than one-half of the participants: fatigue, abdominal swelling, indigestion, lower abdominal pressure or heaviness, abdominal pain, back pain, early satiety, and constipation.[88] See Table 62-3. In Gilda Radner's book, *It's Always Something*, she described the frustrations she encountered getting to the diagnosis of ovarian cancer.[89] The popularity of this book has helped other women become aware of the importance of recognizing their symptoms early and insisting that medical professionals interpret these symptoms appropriately. Another woman with ovarian cancer has developed and published a business card with the symptoms listed and would like it to be made available in physicians' offices to increase awareness of the disease (Figure 62-4).[90]

Assessment

During a physical assessment, the most important finding is the presence of an ovarian mass. A mass is considered suspicious if it is immobile and painless, if it is irregular, if there is bilateral ovarian involvement, or if any other mass is found on exam.[1] In premenopausal women enlarged ovaries are common due to functioning ovarian cysts or benign ovarian cysts. It is common practice for the physician to observe an ovarian mass through several menstrual cycles since it could typically regress in one to

Ovarian Cancer Symptoms

- Bloating, a feeling of fullness, gas
- Frequent or urgent urination
- Nausea, indigestion, constipation, diarrhea
- Menstrual disorders, pain during intercourse
- Fatigue, backaches

TAKE ACTION if any symptoms last more than 2-3 weeks.
Ask for a combination pelvic/rectal exam, CA-125 blood test, and a transvaginal sonogram.

Ovarian Cancer Facts

- Occurs in 1 out of 55 women, at any age.
- Most women are diagnosed when the chance of survival for 5 years is about 20%. Early detection improves survival rates.
- Symptoms are subtle, persistent, and usually increase over time.
- A Pap smear is not an effective detection method.

Ovarian Cancer National Alliance (OCNA)
202–452–5910   http://www.ovarian.org

Figure 62-4 Ovarian Cancer Facts and Symptoms. Source: Ovarian Cancer National Alliance.

three cycles. If the mass measures 8 cm or less on exam, observation is indicated. If the mass is greater than 10 cm or enlarges beyond 5 cm while under observation, further evaluation is indicated.[1] A physician may also prescribe oral contraceptives for these patients expecting the mass to disappear. Masses that persist need investigation including a CA-125 and a transvaginal ultrasound. Ultrasound should reveal if the mass has irregular borders, presence of solid components with papillary projections, or bilateral involvement or multiple dense irregular septae. If any of these characteristics are present a malignancy is suspected.[1]

During the process of malignant transformation, vascular endothelial cell growth is stimulated. This results in irregular blood vessels without a progressive decrease in the caliber of the vessels. Transvaginal Doppler measures blood flow and a high impedance is normal (greater than 1.0).[91,92] The resistance measured in malignancy is higher.

After these studies document an abnormality, a computerized tomography (CT) scan of the abdomen and pelvis with oral and intravenous contrast is ordered to assess the entire area. Particular attention is paid to the lymph nodes in the retroperitoneal and paraaortic areas. A barium enema or colonoscopy may be ordered if cancer is present or suspected or if the patient has symptoms. A chest x-ray, mammogram, and a baseline CA-125 completes the metastatic work-up prior to surgery. The patient should be referred to a gynecologic oncologist. Research has demonstrated that patients experience increased disease-free and overall survival when a gynecologic oncologist is part of the management team.[93–95]

Classification and Staging

There are over 30 types of ovarian cancer classified by their cells of origin. The World Health Organization (WHO) and the International Federation of Gynecology and Obstetrics (FIGO) histologic classification is presented in Table 62-4.[96] The classification system reflects the cell type, the location of the tumor, and the degree of malignancy.

Ovarian cancer is a surgically staged disease and the International Federation of Obstetrics and Gynecology (FIGO) staging system is the system used universally (Table 62-5).[97] FIGO stage is the most important prognostic variable, hence the need for rigorous surgical staging. Table 62-6[98] outlines survival based on FIGO stage.[99] The volume of residual tumor after surgery is another very important prognostic variable, with an inverse relationship between the size of residual tumor and patient outcome.[99] Griffths and colleagues defined optimally debulked primary cytoreductive surgery as no tumor larger than 1.5 cm present.[100] An even better outcome has been demonstrated by several studies for patients with tumors less than 0.5 cm left behind.[101–102] The Gynecologic Oncol-

Table 62-4 World Health Organization Classification of Malignant Ovarian Tumors

Common Epithelial Tumors

Malignant Serous Tumors
Adenocarcinoma, papillary, papillary cystadenocarcinoma
Surface papillary carcinoma
Malignant adenofibroma, cystadenofibroma

Malignant Mucinous Tumors
Adenocarcinoma, cystadenocarcinoma
Malignant adenofibroma, cystadenofibroma

Malignant Endometrioid Tumors
Carcinoma
    Adenocarcinoma
    Adenoacanthoma
    Malignant adenofibroma, cystadenofibroma
Endometrioid stromal sarcomas
Mesodermal (müllerian) mixed tumors; homologous and heterologous
Clear cell (mesonephroid) tumors, malignant
    carcinoma and adenocarcinoma
Brenner tumors, malignant
Mixed epithelial tumors, malignant
Undifferentiated carcinoma
Unclassified

Sex-Cord Stromal Tumors

Granulosa-Stromal Cell Tumors
Granulosa cell tumor
Tumors in the thecoma-fibroma group
Fibroma
Unclassified

Androblastomas: Sertoli-Leydig Cell Tumors
Well differentiated
Tubular androblastoma, Sertoli cell tumor (tubular adenoma of Pick)
Tubular androblastoma with lipid storage, Sertoli cell tumor with lipid storage (folliculoma lipidique of Lecene)
Sertoli-Leydig tumor, hilus cell tumor of intermediate differentiation
Poorly differentiated (sarcomatoid) with heterologous elements
Gynandroblastoma
Unclassified

Lipid (Lipoid) Cell Tumors

Germ Cell Tumors
Dysgerminoma
Endodermal sinus tumor
Embryonal carcinoma
Polyembryoma
Choriocarcinoma
Teratomas
    Immature
    Mature dermoid cyst with malignant transformation
    Monodermal and highly specialized
        Struma ovarii
        Carcinoid
        Struma ovarii and carcinoid
        Others
Mixed forms

Gonadoblastoma
Pure
Mixed with dysgerminoma or other form of germ cell tumor

Table 62-5 Staging for Ovarian Cancer: International Federation of Obstetrics and Gynecology.

Stage	Description
Stage I	Growth limited to the ovaries
Stage IA	Growth limited to one ovary, no ascites; no tumor on the external surface, capsule intact
Stage IB	Growth limited to both ovaries, no ascites; no tumor on the external surface, capsules intact
Stage IC*	Tumor stage IA or IB but with tumor on the surface of one or both ovaries, with capsule ruptured, with ascites present containing malignant cells, or with postitive peritoneal washings
Stage II	Growth involving one or both ovaries with pelvic extension
Stage IIA	Extension or metastases to the uterus or tubes
Stage IIB	Growth involving one or both ovaries with pelvic extension
Stage IIC*	Tumor either stage IIA or IIB with tumor on the surface of one or both ovaries, with capsules ruptured, with ascites present containing malignant cells, or with positive peritoneal washings
Stage III	Tumor involving one or both ovaries with peritoneal implants outside the pelvis or positive retroperitoneal or inguinal nodes; superficial liver metastases equal stage III; Tumor limited to the true pelvis but with histologically verified malignant extension to small bowel or omentum
Stage IIIA	Tumor grossly limited to the true pelvis with negative nodes but with histologically confirmed microscopic seeding of abdominal peritoneal surfaces
Stage IIIB	Tumor of one or both ovaries with histologically confirmed implants of abdominal peritoneal surfaces, none exceeding 2 cm diameter; nodes negative
Stage IIIC	Abdominal implants greater than 2 cm in diameter, or positive retroperitoneal or inguinal nodes
Stage IV	Growth involving one or both ovaries with distant metastases; if pleural effusion is present, there must be positive cytologic test results to allot a case to stage IV; parenchymal lower metastases equals stage IV

*To evaluate the impact on prognosis of the difference criteria for allotting cases to stage IC or IIC, it would be of value to know whether rupture of the capsule was spontaneous or caused by the surgeon, and what the source of malignant cells detected was peritoneal washings or ascites.
Reprinted with permission from Changes in the definition of clinical staging for carcinoma of the cervix and ovary. *Am J Obstet Gynecol,* 156–236, 1987.[97]

Table 62-6 Five-year Survival of Ovarian Cancer Patients

Stage	Five-Year Survival (%)
I	85
II	60
III	30
IV	18

Data from Partridge EE[98]

entiated tumors are grade II, and poorly differentiated are grade III. As the tumor grade increases, the survival rate decreases within each cell type. Grade is especially important in determining treatment, for example grades I and II tumors need no further therapy.[103] Numerous studies have shown a high degree of intraobserver and interobserver variability associated with grading. Pathologists are interested in developing a more quantitative and reproducible grading system, such as molecular markers or DNA cytometry.[104–106] A newer grading system that is reproducible, simple, and useful for all histologic subtypes and clinical stages of ovarian cancer has been developed.[107] With the new system, tumors are graded on architectural patterns, nuclear pleomorphism, and mitotic activity. The new tumor grade system correlates with survival in early and advanced disease for all histologic cell types except clear cell.[107]

However staging is commonly documented using the FIGO staging system that was revised in 1987 (see Table 62-5).[97] Surgical staging during cytoreductive surgery provides the basis of treatment decisions for ovarian cancer.

Therapeutic Approaches and Nursing Care

Surgery

Surgery is the mainstay of treatment in ovarian cancer. The aim of surgery is to provide a definitive diagnosis, determine the exact stage, and remove as much tumor as possible to improve survival and relieve symptoms. The National Institute of Health (NIH) consensus conference concluded that aggressive efforts at maximal cytoreduction are important since minimal residual tumor is associated with improved survival.[49] The surgical procedure includes total abdominal hysterectomy, bilateral salpingoophorectomy, peritoneal cytology, omentectomy, scraping of the undersurface of the right diaphragm, multiple peritoneal biopsies, pelvic and paraaortic lymph node sampling, and multiple random biopsies. A vertical midline incision from the symphysis pubis to above the umbilicus is essential. The goal is to leave no tumor greater than 1 cm, i.e., optimally debulked disease.

A gynecologic surgical oncologist is specially trained to perform ovarian cancer surgery. The gynecologic on-

ogy Group (GOG) defines optimally debulked disease as no tumor larger than 1 cm left behind.

Although histologic subtype is important to determine, only clear cell and mucinous types of tumors are of independent prognostic significance. Grade is more important prognostically than histologic subtype although there is no universally accepted grading system. Well-differentiated tumors are grade I, moderately differ-

cologists are concerned about adequate surgical staging in ovarian cancer. In a study of 785 women diagnosed with stage I and II ovarian cancer, only 10% of the women received optimal debulking surgery according to the NIH treatment guidelines.[108,109] The study revealed that women over age 65 received incomplete surgical staging compared with those under age 65.[109]

The gynecologic surgeon should discuss with the patient and family the goals of surgery, potential outcomes, and complications. Surgery is the initial approach to treatment in stages I–III of ovarian cancer. Surgical debulking is more controversial in stage IV disease. In a study by Curtin and associates, optimal debulking resulted in a 40-month median survival in stage IV patients versus an 18-month median survival in those suboptimally debulked.[110] There is an apparent survival benefit for women with stage IV disease who are aggressively debulked. This approach is supported by the NIH consensus conclusions, which stress the importance of aggressive surgical debulking.[49]

Surgery also has a role at other times in the ovarian disease process. Procedures can include interval debulking, secondary surgical cytoreductive surgery, second-look surgery, laparoscopic surgery, and palliative surgery. Interval cytoreduction is the surgical attempt to debulk the tumor after a limited course of chemotherapy, usually two to four courses. Interval cytoreduction is used in women who did not have a primary debulking operation and are responding or stable during induction chemotherapy. Studies have demonstrated that interval cytoreductive surgery improved progression-free interval and median survival.[111]

Secondary cytoreductive surgery used at time of relapse is an approach whose value is unknown at this time. Second-look surgery, or exploratory surgery at the end of primary treatment, remains controversial. Second-look surgery is not appropriate for stage I and II disease but it remains an option for stages III and IV disease. The patient with stage III or IV disease who had cytoreductive surgery followed by standard chemotherapy and is in a complete remission with a normal CA-125 and a negative CT scan is a potential candidate for second-look surgery. The goal would be to explore the entire abdomen and pelvis and do a series of biopsies to provide the most accurate assessment of the response to induction chemotherapy. Unfortunately, a negative second-look surgery does not mean the patient is cured. In fact, negative second-look surgery may be followed by a relapse in up to 50% of patients.[112] Additionally, if a patient is found to have disease at second-look, the treatment available at this time is not effective in obtaining a cure.[112,113]

Second-look surgery does not improve survival with currently existing salvage modalities and should be confined to those patients willing to participate in research protocols evaluating second-line therapy.[114] Current recommendations support the use of second-look surgery as part of treatment protocols; however, it is not considered a standard approach outside of clinical trials.

Laparoscopy surgery is not standard but is an acceptable alternative in a research setting. At this time there is no prospective data to support its use.[108] Controversy exists because this type of surgery may facilitate rupture of the ovary mass and several studies have documented the adverse effect of rupture in early stage ovarian patients.[115,116] Neoadjuvant chemotherapy treatment prior to surgery continues to be investigated especially in stage IV disease. The goal of neoadjuvant therapy is to shrink the tumor so the debulking surgery can be more effective.

Palliative surgery in ovarian cancer is often involved when a bowel obstruction occurs. It is an important component in improving a patient's quality of life and providing relief of adverse symptoms in this setting.

Treatment of Epithelial Ovarian Cancer

Early stage disease

Once surgery has been performed, the early stage I and II disease patients are further classified into the low-risk (favorable) category or high-risk (unfavorable) category by grade, cytology, presence or absence of ascites, differentiation of the tumor, rupture of the capsule, or growth outside the ovaries (Table 62-7).[117] Early-stage, low-risk (IA, IB, well or moderately well differentiated) patients require no further treatment after a comprehensive staging surgery.[103,118,119] Their five-year survival is greater than 90%.[103]

The perspective on treatment for the high-risk group began to evolve with a GOG trial of 81 patients randomized to melphalan versus observation that resulted in a five-year survival of 91% and 98% and defined the good prognosis patients who required no further therapy.[102] High-risk (IC, high grade IA2 or IB2, II), early-stage disease has a 25%–40% recurrence rate and the role of immediate treatment and type of therapy remains controversial. Those in the high-risk group have a 30%–40% risk of relapse and a 25%–30% chance of dying within the first five years after surgery.[120] The high-risk group

Table 62-7 Classification of Risk of Early-Stage Ovarian Cancer

Favorable or Low Risk	Unfavorable or High Risk
Stage IA or IB disease with well or moderately well-differentiated tumor	Stage IA or IB with poorly differentiated tumor All stage II
No ascites	Ascites
No tumor on external surface of the ovary	Tumor on external surface of ovary
Negative peritoneal cytology	Positive peritoneal cytology
Growth confined to ovaries	Growth outside the ovaries Ruptured capsule

Adapted with permission from Ozols RF, Rubin SC, Thomas G, et al: Epithelial ovarian cancer, in Hoskins et al (eds): *Principles and Practice of Gynecologic Oncology (ed 2).* Baltimore, Lippincott-Raven, 1997, pp 919–986.[117]

was treated with therapy in a trial randomizing them to either melphalan or p32, an intraperitoneal (IP) radioisotope; the result was an equivalent five-year survival of 80% in both arms.[103] Melphalan's risk of a second malignancy and severe myelosuppression eliminated this drug from further trials and p32 was the preferred treatment. The high-risk patients were then randomized in the next set of trials to IP p32 versus cisplatin and cyclophosphamide (CP). This trial has reported an 84% five-year survival rate for CP versus 76% for p32 and concluded that although there are no statistically significant differences between the two treatments, the better progression-free interval for CP supports platinum-based regimens.[121] Because p32 was difficult to administer and bowel complications occurred, the standard became a platinum-based regimen for the high-risk group.[121]

Cisplatin and CP were replaced with carboplatin and paclitaxel after the results of the GOG-111 trial. A recently completed GOG trial is looking at whether three cycles versus six cycles of the regimen is significant, however, it is too early to interpret data. The current GOG trial is studying three weeks of carboplatin and paclitaxel followed by observation versus 24 weeks of a weekly injection of paclitaxel.[122] The GOG, Italian, Norwegian, and Scandinavian clinical trials groups all came to the same conclusion that treating this group of patients with combination chemotherapy with a platinum-based regimen is optimal.[123–125] Several studies have compared chemotherapy versus whole abdominal radiation in early-stage patients, but the results were conflicting.[126–128] The role of radiotherapy in high-risk early stage disease is still not clear. In conclusion, awaiting the results of the current clinical trials, the treatment of the high-risk group of early-stage disease patients remains under investigation but includes combination chemotherapy with a platinum-based regimen.

Advanced disease

Advanced stage disease is routinely managed with a combination of surgery and postoperative chemotherapy. Complete cytoreductive surgery is feasible about 50% of the time and maximizes survival in patients with advanced ovarian cancer. Survival appears to be directly affected by the initial cytoreductive surgery in advanced disease.[100] Numerous studies have demonstrated a clear clinical benefit for patients in the optimal category having a higher complete response rate, a prolonged progression-free survival, and an improved median survival.[108] Therefore, the goal of cytoreductive surgery in this stage also is to minimize the residual tumor to less than 1 cm in maximum diameter.

Chemotherapy, especially the anthracyclines, platinum-based compounds, and the taxanes, are critically important in ovarian cancer treatment.[129–132] Five meta-analyses incorporating data from 45 randomized trials, including 10,000 patients, helped clarify the role of platinum-based chemotherapy. The conclusions were that immediate platinum-based therapy was better than non-

platinum-based therapy, platinum in combination was better than single agent when used at the same doses, and there was no difference between carboplatin and cisplatin either as single agents or when substituted for one another in combination regimens.[133] Substitution of carboplatin, a less toxic analog, for cisplatin has been compared in multiple combination regimen clinical trials.[134–136] Results obtained by the Southwestern Oncology Group and the National Cancer Institute of Canada showed no survival differences.[134,135] However, the European trial had a higher complete remission rate for the cisplatin arm.[136]

Anthracyclines were included in the early combination regimens in this disease. Controversy still exists as to whether the inclusion of anthracyclines is superior to nonanthracycline containing regimens. Two meta-analyses in the 1990s focused on including doxorubicin. One showed the three-drug regimen with cyclophosphamide/doxorubicin/cisplatin was superior to two-drug regimen cyclophosphamide and cisplatin. There was improvement for two- and five-year survival; it was 6% better.[137] Two subsequent trials confirmed these results.[138,139] A trial reported in 1996 randomized 1500 patients to either carboplatin versus the standard doxorubicin combination and no difference in survival was noted.[140] These mixed results have led to a current European study that is comparing paclitaxel/carboplatin versus paclitaxel/epirubicin/carboplatin, which may lead to a better understanding of the value of anthracyclines in ovarian cancer therapy.

In the early 1990s came the development of a new class of drugs, the taxanes. The first drug from this group to be used in clinical trials, paclitaxel was very active in women with advanced recurrent ovarian cancer.[141] Due to the drug's activity in recurrent disease, it was quickly included in clinical trials using it as initial therapy in comparison to the standard combination at that time, cisplatin and cyclophosphamide.

Two pivotal clinical trials in the mid 1990s occurred. First, in the GOG-111 trial, one arm with the standard cyclophosphamide and cisplatin was compared to paclitaxel and cisplatin. All patients on this clinical trial had suboptimal surgical debulking or stage IV disease. With the paclitaxel arm, there was improvement in response rate of 73% versus 60%, and in median survival of 38 months versus 24 months.[122] This trial has a minimum follow-up of 60 months and there is a 28% reduction of progression and a 34% reduction in risk of death for the paclitaxel arm. A large clinical trial that confirmed these findings was titled "OV-10," an Ovarian Group from Canada and Europe. Of the 600 patients enrolled in this trial, 35% had low-volume disease at entry or were optimally debulked. The treatment arms consisted of cyclophosphamide and cisplatin versus paclitaxel and cisplatin, paclitaxel this time being given at 175 mg/m² over three hours, also a change from GOG-111.[142] Similar to GOG-111, the response rate was significantly improved in the paclitaxel arm, 77% versus 66% for the cyclophosphamide arm, and the median time to progression was 16.6 months versus 12 months.[141] In both studies, the cisplatin and paclitaxel regimen was superior; there were also similar results achieved with 24-hour versus three-hour paclitaxel. There was, however, significant neurotoxicity noted in the three-hour paclitaxel regimen, with 18% grade III. The GOG also compared cisplatin/paclitaxel versus paclitaxel alone versus cisplatin alone. The combination regimen was superior in terms of response rate.[143]

As a result of these pivotal clinical trials, the standard for ovarian cancer treatment with chemotherapy was changed to a platinum compound and paclitaxel.[143] Clinical guidelines have been published to support the use of this regimen.[144] An updated analysis of multiple research trials shows a significantly improved overall survival for cisplatin-paclitaxel as first-line treatment of advanced ovarian cancer. The regimen was also found to be superior in response rates, time-to-progression, and a clinically important improvement in median survival.[145]

Three trials have now been completed using carboplatin/paclitaxel compared to cisplatin/paclitaxel.[146-148] The most recent GOG-158 trial debulked stage III patients compared cisplatin and paclitaxel (R1) versus carboplatin and paclitaxel (R2). Patients were randomized to second-look surgery or no second-look surgery at the time of enrollment. The results showed no difference in median survival (21.7 months for R1 versus 22 months for R2) and no difference in recurrence-free survival in the second-look surgery patients versus the no second-look surgery patients (45.2% versus 51%). The study concludes that carboplatin/paclitaxel is not less effective than cisplatin/paclitaxel, carboplatin/paclitaxel is less toxic and easier to administer, and second-look surgery does not influence recurrence free survival.[148] The dose of carboplatin still needs to be defined since area-under-the-curve (AUC) dosing in these pending studies varies from 5.0–7.5. Jakobsen and associates and Gore and colleagues conclude that dosing AUC greater than 5.0 does not demonstrate a clinically significant advantage.[149,150] The next phase of clinical trials for the optimally debulked patient includes cisplatin and a 24-hour infusion of paclitaxel versus 24-hour infusion of paclitaxel day 1, plus intraperitoneal cisplatin day 2, followed by intraperitoneal paclitaxel on day 8.

Paclitaxel administration has posed several nursing challenges, the most significant being hypersensitivity reactions. Prevention of the hypersensitivity reaction involves a premedication regime, including dexamethasone, the evening before and morning of treatment. Most patients who have hypersensitivity reactions experience itching, shortness of breath, a tightness in the chest, and perhaps back pain. The infusion is stopped immediately and routine anaphylactic measures are employed. The infusion may be restarted at half the rate. Olson and associates found that in the case of paclitaxel hypersensitivity, rapid retreatment was safe and cost effective.[151] Their retreatment schema is presented in Figure 62-5.

Optimal duration of therapy with paclitaxel has yet to be determined. There is no evidence that additional treatments beyond the standard six cycles adds to survival

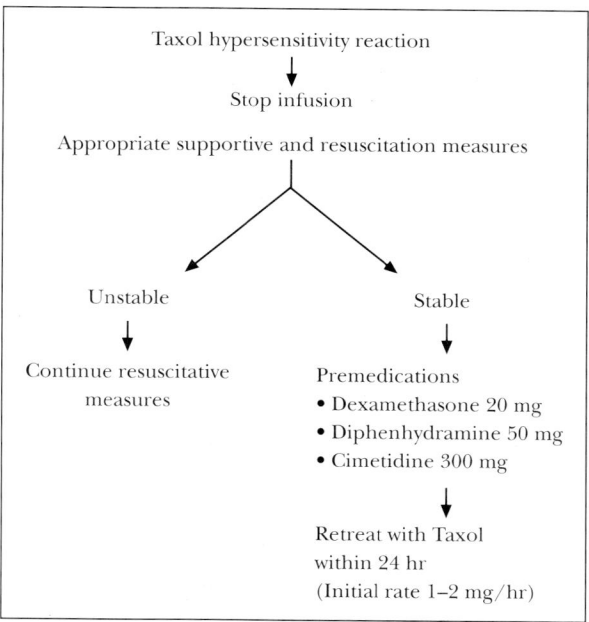

Figure 62-5 Retreatment schema with paclitaxel (Taxol) for patients with hypersensitivity reactions. (Reprinted with permission from Olson JK, Sood AK, Sorosky JI, et al: Taxol hypersensitivity: rapid retreatment is safe and cost effective. *Gynecol Oncol* 68:25–28, 1998.)[151]

benefit. New agents demonstrating cytotoxic activity in this disease include gemcitabine, topotecan, doxil, oral etoposide, and docetaxel. The next phase of clinical trials will begin to add these agents to the platinum and paclitaxel standard, either using a three-drug regimen (i.e., paclitaxel/carboplatin/gemcitabine) or sequential doublets (i.e., paclitaxel/topotecan followed by platinum analog/gemcitabine) to extend the survival in ovarian cancer.

To summarize, the majority of women with clinically curable ovarian cancer will receive primary debulking surgery, chemotherapy, and possibly a second-look surgery. Depending upon the response to therapy, the woman may not require maintenance therapy.

Maintenance therapy

Once a patient has completed primary therapy and achieves a complete remission there is controversy regarding the role of maintenance therapy. Between 50%–75% of advanced disease patients who achieve a clinical complete remission following primary therapy will ultimately relapse.[53] Maintenance or consolidation therapy is commonly used to decrease the relapse rate and increase survival. Maintenance therapy considerations include high dose, intraperitoneal, radioactive isotope of phosphorous (32P), hormone, whole-abdominal radiotherapy, or prolonged chemotherapy. Interest in maintenance therapy has intensified due to the results of a recent study evaluating a group of patients with recurrent platinum-sensitive disease that then achieved a complete response with additional platinum therapy. This group received monthly platinum therapy for one year, followed by maintenance (every eight weeks) chemotherapy.[152] The study group had a significant longer disease-free interval compared to those who refused or discontinued therapy (35 months versus 6 months). The findings indicate that maintenance therapy is safe and may extend disease-free interval. The overall ten-year survival for ovarian cancer approximates 20%; therefore, continued effort must be directed at improved results with primary therapy.[153]

Intraperitoneal therapy

Intraperitoneal (IP) therapy can provide a large pharmacologic advantage, that is the high ratio of the peak peritoneal drug levels compared to plasma levels. The drugs administered via the IP route will also enter the systemic circulation and achieve a 50%–75% uptake of IV administration exposure via the lymphatic channels or by passive diffusion. Therefore, because ovarian cancer predominantly is confined to the abdomen, there has been a great deal of interest in pursuing the IP method of drug administration. Numerous phase I and II trials have studied single agents including methotrexate, fluouracil, doxorubicin, carboplatin, cisplatin, and paclitaxel. The most experience is with cisplatin IP and has led to two conclusions concerning intraperitoneal therapy. First, IP therapy is unlikely to benefit patients other than those with small-volume disease because drug penetration into the larger tumor nodules is limited.[154] In a clinical trial at Memorial Sloan Kettering Cancer Center, patients with microscopic disease had a 41% complete response rate compared to a 5% complete response rate in patients with tumor nodules greater than 1 cm.[155] The second conclusion is that patients with tumors that were previously resistant to intravenous cisplatin were not able to be successfully treated by IP platinum.[154] Markman and associates documented a 33% complete response rate in patients who had a prior response to intravenous platinum versus a 3% response rates in those who had previously experienced recurrence.[155] The trials that followed included a GOG/SWOG trial for optimal stage III patients with no tumor greater than 2 cm. These patients received IP or IV cisplatin (100 mg/m²) and IV cyclophosphamide (600 mg/m²).[156] More than 600 women were enrolled and the IP complete response rate was 47% compared to an IV rate of 36%; median survival was 49 months versus 41 months. The subsequent GOG trial randomized patients to six months of IV cisplatin (75 mg/m²) and paclitaxel 135 mg/m² over 24 hours versus two doses of carboplatin (AUC = 9) followed by six cycles of IP cisplatin (100 mg/m²) and IV paclitaxel 135 mg/m² over 24 hours.[157] There was a statistically significant difference in overall survival of 27.6 months versus 22.5 months, but no significant improvement in overall survival. The results of these two trials justify more prospective randomized trials. The current GOG trial

for optimally debulked patients includes IP therapy as discussed previously in advanced disease.

Another area of interest is the use of IP therapy during a consolidation phase of treatment. Barakat and associates completed a phase II trial of IP cisplatin and etoposide as consolidation therapy in advanced disease.[158] At 36-month follow-up, 39% of patients who had consolidation therapy with three courses had recurrence compared to 54% of those in the observation arm.[158] Other current trials of intraperitoneal therapy include a SWOG/GOG study where patients with a surgically defined complete response after systemic chemotherapy are randomized to IP alfa-interferon or no further therapy. Similarly, in Europe those patients achieving a surgically confirmed complete response are then getting IP cisplatin.

In conclusion, the role of IP therapy is not yet established. IP therapy is not considered standard therapy at this time, but possibly plays a role as part of consolidation or maintenance therapy or as part of initial therapy in patients with small-volume yet advanced disease.[154] IP therapy is also a reasonable strategy for early-stage, high-risk patients.[154]

Radiotherapy

Early trials suggested that control of pelvic disease was superior with radiotherapy. When compared to chemotherapy, the survival rates were similar but the complications were higher in patients who had whole-abdominal radiation (WAR) therapy. Clinical trials have demonstrated that abdominopelvic or WAR radiotherapy is superior to limited pelvic radiotherapy. WAR is toxic treatment since the entire abdomen is included in the field; however, the current technique and new fractionation schedules appear to reduce toxicity.[159] It appears that WAR therapy has no role in curative management of the optimally debulked early-stage, low-risk ovarian cancer patient. Possible roles for radiotherapy include following chemotherapy for early-stage, high-risk patients as part of consolidation therapy; for advanced disease patients with minimal or no residual disease; in the salvage setting with minimal residual disease; and in palliative therapy.[159] Patients with platinum-resistant tumors were studied to determine palliative benefit of radiation therapy. Forty-seven patients received palliative therapy and 39% obtained relief of their symptoms for longer than 12 months; 30% obtained relief of their symptoms for 6–12 months. The authors concluded that radiation could provide effective and durable palliation of symptoms in platinum-refractory ovarian cancer patients.[160]

High-dose therapy

The interest in pursuing high-dose therapy for ovarian cancer is based on the knowledge of dose response relationship (in vitro) as well as the established correlation between cisplatin dose and dose response.[161] Overall, ovarian cancer is highly sensitive to chemotherapy, yet most patients suffer from disease recurrence. Up to this time, almost all trials have failed to show any significant impact of higher-dose cisplatin on survival in patients with ovarian cancer. In addition, randomized trials of different AUC doses of carboplatin have failed to demonstrate any significant advantage for higher AUC doses.[149,150] Thus far, high-dose therapy in refractory or recurrent disease is not worth the toxicity because it does not offer any advantage over standard therapy. Patients with platinum-resistant, bulky disease are not appropriate for bone marrow transplant. In the future, there may be a role for transplant in consolidation therapy or as part of initial therapy with previously untreated advanced ovarian cancer patients with minimal disease.[161] The clinical trials of high-dose therapy being conducted today must prove a significant improvement in long-term survival in patients with small-volume disease and those who are chemosensitive. High-dose therapy for ovarian cancer is recommended in the context of a clinical trial only.

Drug resistance

Drug resistance in ovarian cancer is a major problem. Fifty to seventy-five percent of ovarian cancer patients achieve a complete response but then go on to relapse and develop resistance to further chemotherapy. About 20% of patients are even intrinsically resistant to chemotherapy. Understanding the molecular basis for multidrug resistance (MDR) is important for the design of new treatment strategies.[162-164] Some of the identified mechanisms of MDR resistance include host factors (altered pharmacokinetics), host-tumor factors, cellular factors, DNA repair, tolerance to DNA repair, and altered cellular target.[162] Decreased drug accumulation, metabolic drug inactivation, and repair or tolerance to drug-induced cellular injury contributes to resistance at the cellular level.[162] Resistance is a multifactorial problem in this disease especially as it relates to alkylating agents and platinum compounds.[53]

Ovarian cancer drug resistance has been associated with decreased susceptibility to apoptosis. A recent study has identified the *BCl-xl* gene in ovarian cancer and it may be responsible for the resistance to chemotherapy-induced apoptosis.[165] Gene therapy, both related to tumor biology and overcoming drug resistance, is a promising new strategy for improving survival in this disease. Progress has been made in MDR, from in vitro studies to the thorough study of cell lines from relapsed patients; an understanding of why ovarian cancer cells become resistant to treatment is progressing.[162]

Disease recurrence

An elevated level of the tumor marker CA-125 is predictive of a recurrence of ovarian cancer. The median time for CA-125 to be elevated is two to four months prior to obvious symptoms or definitive clinical disease progression.[166,167] Thus, a rising CA-125 level has clouded

the definition of time of recurrence since the patient is often without clinically detectable disease. There is no evidence that immediate chemotherapy is beneficial in recurrence. Patients follow this tumor marker closely and usually want treatment as soon as it is elevated. A rising CA-125 level is definitely associated with increased stress in the patient. An alternative approach may be to use the drug tamoxifen, a nontoxic but active drug until clinical evidence of disease recurrence exists.[144,168,169] Many clinicians feel that there is no reason to start chemotherapy in patients with a serologic marker of recurrence as long as the patient is asymptomatic, has a normal pelvic exam, and is without evidence of definitive disease recurrence.

Patients with documented recurrent disease frequently respond to salvage therapy; however, the duration of response is brief. Roland and colleagues found that the tumor response to initial paclitaxel/platinum therapy was predictive of tumor response to second-line treatment.[170] These authors found that the current salvage therapy appears of little benefit to resistant tumors and also noted a 24% increase of significant complications with salvage therapy. Most clinicians feel that patients must be categorized into one of three of the following categories prior to salvage therapy: (1) drug-sensitive—time to recurrence is longer than six months; (2) drug-resistant—time to recurrence is less than six months; or (3) drug-refractory—no response to initial therapy. See Table 62-8. In treatment of recurrence, the drug-sensitive patients have a high response rate to drugs used in the initial regimen and the longer the treatment-free interval, the higher the chance of response when recurrence is treated.[171] There is no evidence at this time that rechallenging patients with their original primary treatment is any better than using new agents. Recurrent disease treatment might start with single-agent paclitaxel or single-agent carboplatin. There is no evidence that combination chemotherapy is better unless the disease-free interval is greater than 12–18 months.[172] The drug-sensitive patient will probably have a higher response rate to new drugs as well. They are usually treated with a new agent. The patients who progress while on treatment, called the *drug refractory group*, should be offered investigational therapy. All patients should be considered candidates for clinical trials.

The challenge is that second-line treatment is benefi-

Table 62-8 Category of Response and Time to Recurrence for Ovarian Cancer

Category of Response	Time to Recurrence
Drug sensitive	> 6 months
Drug resistant	< 6 months
Drug refractory	No response to therapy

cial but cannot produce cure. Several chemotherapy agents demonstrate cytotoxic activity in recurrent disease patients, but the response is not durable. The likelihood of benefit must be weighed against the toxicity of the treatment. The patients most likely to benefit from second-line treatment include those with small-volume disease, a good performance status, a long treatment-free interval, serous histology, and a low number of sites of disease. New drugs being explored include gemcitabine, topotecan, oral etoposide, vinorelbine, docetaxel, and doxil. See Table 62-9 for a list of the agents and their respective response rates.[170] Tamoxifen in recurrent ovarian cancer produced an overall response rate of 11%.[173]

Some critical parameters for choosing treatment for recurrent disease are prior responses, quality of life, toxicity profile, age, comorbid illness, or patient preference. Overall the standard approach is to treat for two cycles and reevaluate to determine if there has been a clinical benefit before continuing further. If there is no response, palliative support is used through to the end stages of the disease.[171]

Future direction of therapy

Future directions for treatment of ovarian cancer include research aimed at screening and prevention, finding a molecular basis for ovarian cancer, and identifying high-risk individuals. Advanced disease treatment research will explore new treatment protocols utilizing new agents, three-drug combinations, or sequential doublets with the newer agents, and will come to a final conclusion

Table 62-9 New Active Agents in Recurrent Ovarian Cancer

Agent	Response (%)	Comment
Prior treatment did not include paclitaxel		
Paclitaxel	19–40	Multiple studies
Topotecan	14–23	Lower response rates in platinum-resistant patients
Vinorelbine	22	Duration of response > 19 weeks
Gemcitabine	29	Activity in platinum-resistant patients
Docetaxel	40	Neutropenia and fluid retention common
Prior treatment with paclitaxel and platinum		
Liposomal doxorubicin	26	Median survival 11 months
Oral etoposide	27–35	Higher response rate in platinum-sensitive patients

Reprinted with permission from McGuire WP, Ozols RF: Chemotherapy of advanced ovarian cancer. *Semin Oncol* 25:345, 1998.[171]

regarding the benefit of high-dose therapy and its place in the treatment schema. Newer treatment strategies may be directed at immunotherapy, vaccine therapy, or gene therapy. The health care team will continue to be challenged to keep pace as new treatments for ovarian cancer are brought into the clinical arena and new patient care strategies unfold.

Primary Treatment of Other Ovarian Tumors

Ovarian germ cell tumors

These tumors are uncommon and occur in women in their teens and twenties.[172] The critical distinction to make in diagnosis is between dysgerminoma tumors and all others called nondysgerminoma. Dysgerminoma is analogous to seminoma and is a radiosensitive tumor; it may be associated with pregnancy. The signs and symptoms of germ cell tumors include abdominal pain and a palpable pelvic or abdominal mass. Some 10% of patients present with acute abdominal pain usually caused by rupture, hemorrhage, or torsion of the ovarian mass.[172] Abdominal distention, fever, and vaginal bleeding are less common signs and symptoms. An abnormal HCG or alpha-fetoprotein level or both may be found and the level of the marker CA-125 may be elevated. The staging system used for germ cell tumors is identical to epithelial ovarian cancer.

Initial treatment is surgery for both definitive diagnosis and treatment. A vertical midline incision is done and the type of surgical procedure depends on the findings when the abdomen is explored. All attempts will be made to save the uterus and the other ovary if one goal is to preserve childbearing. At a minimum, it is important to remove the tumor and inspect the entire peritoneal cavity. Any suspicious lesions should be biopsied and if metastatic disease is present, cytoreductive principles apply as in epithelial ovarian cancer.

Treatment after surgery for nondysgerminoma includes three cycles of bleomycin, etoposide, and platinum (BEP) chemotherapy. Dysgerminoma patients will have the same chemotherapy but only if disease is greater than stage IA. Stage IA patients are followed with observation only. Most cases of dysgerminoma are curable and have a good prognosis.

Sex-cord stromal tumors

Sex-cord stromal tumors are a classification of ovarian tumor that constitutes 5%–8% of ovarian malignancies. These tumors consist of granulosa and theca cells as well as Sertoli and Leydig cells; the most common type is granulosa cell. Granulosa-theca cell tumors are low grade and secrete estrogen or testosterone. The symptoms include irregular periods in premenopausal women and vaginal bleeding in postmenopausal women. Sertoli-Leydig tumors are low-grade malignancies that occur usually in the third or fourth decade of life. These tumors present with signs of virilization due to androgen production. The staging process is the same as with epithelial tumors and if diagnosed early, treatment consists of surgery alone. The surgical procedure depends on the extent of the tumor, and the age of the patient, and whether fertility preservation is important. If chemotherapy is indicated, it is usually a combination such as BEP or cisplatin, bleomycin, and vinblastine. Prognosis is good, with five-year disease-free rates of 85%–90%.[53]

Ovarian cancer of low malignant potential

Epithelial tumors comprise 90% of all ovarian cancers. Of the epithelial tumors, 10%–15% will have low malignant potential (LMP) or be borderline tumors or atypical proliferating epithelial tumors. Borderline or low malignant potential designation means that although the cells of the tumor appear malignant, the cells have not invaded the underlying tissue. These tend to occur in younger patients, in earlier stages, and have an excellent overall survival rate of 80%–90%.[173,174] These are intermediate tumors, between cystadenomas and frankly invasive. Lu and colleagues found bilateral and advanced borderline tumors were multifocal in origin, whereas epithelial ovarian cancer is unifocal.[175] In 1971 FIGO called this group *low malignant potential*, and in 1973, WHO labeled this group *borderline tumors*.[176,177] The surgical procedure and staging is similar to epithelial ovarian cancer. Overall, the most important characteristic to note is that they are not invasive. Surgery alone cures the majority, and adjuvant therapy is not indicated.

Extraovarian peritoneal carcinoma

Primary peritoneal carcinomas are characterized by their diffuse involvement of the peritoneal surfaces with a neoplasm appearing identical to papillary serous carcinoma but without a primary ovarian tumor. This disease can occur in women with intact ovaries or after an oophorectomy. These tumors are frequently advanced at presentation. Surgical cytoreductive surgery is less successful due to the diffuseness of the metastasis. The tumors are sensitive to platinum-based therapy after surgery.

Symptom Management and Supportive Care

Nursing care and support of patients with ovarian cancer involves three major phases: (1) during surgical therapy, (2) during chemotherapy, and (3) during advanced disease. The nurse is critical for delivery and management of care, patient education, as an advocate for the patient, and for emotional support.

In the first phase of care, nursing care focuses on preparing the patient for surgery, on the acute postoperative period and the prevention of complications, and on the psychosocial support for a cancer diagnosis. Initially the nurse will explain the plan with the patient and em-

phasize the prevention of possible postoperative complications (Table 62-10). Preadmission testing is done and the patient is given a bowel prep to cleanse the bowel entirely prior to surgery. The family must be educated about the operative procedure itself and the length of time it takes. Nursing clinical pathways, a step-by-step outline of the components of care, can be developed to ensure all aspects of care are considered.[178] These tools help increase efficiency and decrease costs by providing specific outcomes to follow. The phase of diagnosis and surgical intervention usually covers five to seven days in the hospital and a short recuperative break before the next phase of treatment, chemotherapy. However, many clinicians administer the first course of treatment during the postoperative period.

The second phase of nursing care is the chemotherapy treatment plan. The nursing care focus is mainly one of education and information regarding the treatment regimen, and support and assessment for potential problems from chemotherapy toxicities. The specifics of nursing care in this phase depend on the treatment administered to the patient. The current standard for chemotherapy involves paclitaxel and a platinum compound. Possible side effects include alopecia, an allergic reaction, myelosuppression, nausea, vomiting, arthralgias, and myalgias. If a woman receives information about side effects of treatment and how to manage them, she is more likely to successfully reduce physical and emotional distress from treatment effects.[179] Nurses provide vital links to patients through telephone triage roles in the ambulatory or office setting for questions, problems, or support during this phase of care.

Unfortunately, the majority of patients with advanced ovarian cancer recur. Nurses are critical caregivers during this final phase of care. Ovarian cancer, which is usually spread throughout the abdomen, can cause dysfunction in many different organ systems. Women often present with a multitude of gastrointestinal complaints at diagnosis and these symptoms continue or reoccur during treatment or recurrence. Metastases can appear in any organ and site; the most frequently occurring metastatic sites

---

Table 62-10   Common Problems Following Laparotomy for Tumor Debulking

Bleeding/hemorrhage

Thromboembolic event

Infection/sepsis

Fluid and electrolyte imbalance

Atelectasis/pneumonia

Bowel dysfunction

Bladder dysfunction

Reprinted with permission from Eriksson JH, Frazier SR: Epithelial cancers of the ovary and fallopian tube, in Moore GJ (ed): *Women and Cancer: A Gynecologic Oncology Nursing Perspective.* Sudbury, MA, Jones and Bartlett, 1997, pp 205–256.[1]

include the intestines, liver, diaphragm, or lungs. The major problems nurses confront in caring for women with advanced recurrent disease include ascites, intestinal obstruction, malnutrition, lymphedema, or a pleural effusion. Each of these potential problems will be discussed along with the nursing management strategies.

Ascites

One-third of women with ovarian cancer will present with ascites at diagnosis; two-thirds of women will have ascites present at death.[180] The parietal peritoneum lines the abdominopelvic wall, the diaphragm, and the visceral peritoneum that covers the abdominal organs and encloses the peritoneal cavity.[181] Fluid is normally present in a small volume to constantly lubricate the cavity and prevent abdominal organs from adhering to abdominal walls.[181] Ascites occurs when the fluid produced is greater than the amount of fluid cleared, usually caused by tumor obstructing lymphatic channels or the tumor itself producing excessive fluid.[182] A fluid increase of greater than 500 cc produces symptoms that include weight gain, abdominal bloating, feeling full after small meals, indigestion, and/or lack of appetite.[181] Early symptoms of ascites progress if there is no intervention to eliminate its source. Profound ascites will have a devastating effect on the individual's ability to function. Gastrointestinal function, nutrition, ambulation, breathing, sleeping, and psychosocial sequelae are all affected by ascites. Nursing assessment could reveal any or all of the following physical findings: abdominal skin, shiny or tense; everted umbilicus; diminished bowel sounds; dullness over flank area; or midabdomen tympany.[183,184] The presence of ascites in the abdomen may create a compression phenomenon that could contribute to bowel obstruction.

A diagnosis of ascites is confirmed with an abdominal flat plate x-ray or abdominal ultrasound. Paracentesis is used most often to remove the fluid without altering the hemodynamic equilibrium of the peritoneum. Blood chemistries should be drawn, specifically serum protein, potassium, and sodium, and the ascitic fluid may be sent for gross inspection, cytology, cell count, chemistries, and microbiology. Paracentesis is a temporary measure, and unless the underlying reason for fluid accumulation is addressed, the ascites fluid recurs.

Several other approaches for ascites fluid removal include intraperitoneal infusion therapy or peritoneovenous shunting, which is used less frequently. Intracavitary or intraperitoneal infusion therapy involves direct instillation of a drug into the abdominal cavity through a temporary or implanted catheter. Radioactive colloids, chemotherapy, or biologic response modifiers can be administered through the intraperitoneal route. Once a catheter is placed it is a means for draining the fluid. A Tenckhoff catheter or an abdominal port is commonly utilized.

Another method for removing excess ascites fluid is peritoneovenous shunting. This is a continuous shunt to rechannel ascites fluid from the peritoneal cavity to the superior vena cava and eventually into the venous circulation. The shunt consists of a length of tubing, one end of which is placed in the peritoneal cavity; the other is tunneled subcutaneously and inserted into the superior vena cava.[185] The ascites fluid flows upward into the superior vena cava via a one-way valve that opens with each inhalation as the intraperitoneal pressure increases and the intrathoracic pressure decreases.[185,186] Shunt malfunctions such as kinking or occlusion, pulmonary edema from rapid intravascular infusion of large quantities of fluid, disseminated intravascular coagulation, infection, and pulmonary embolus are all potential complications of this procedure.[181,185,186] Shunting is reserved for untreatable disease and is appropriate to use if the time to reaccumulation of ascites is less than one month. Shunting is usually reserved for those with a reasonable life expectancy where symptom relief is anticipated.[188] Mild diuretics are often prescribed but are usually not effective in diminishing ascites fluid.

Nursing care includes educating the patient to notify the physician or nurse when fluid starts to reaccumulate by measuring their weight daily or abdominal girth daily or weekly. A bowel regimen may be needed to relieve constipation. Nursing care is aimed at relieving symptoms associated with ascites and minimizing further accumulation of the fluid. Instruct patients to alternate activity with rest periods to conserve energy. Encourage the patient to lay on her left side with her feet elevated to alleviate pressure on the internal organs, improve vascular return from the lower extremities, facilitate lymphatic flow, and improve diuresis.[187] Ascites can make it physically uncomfortable to eat; so small frequent snacks or meals are suggested. An adequate protein intake and calories are needed to help increase low serum albumin levels. Families should offer calorie-rich beverages and encourage adequate fluids especially after the paracentesis procedure to restore fluid and electrolyte balance. Fluid restrictions may be imposed in some circumstances to minimize ascites reaccumulation. Ascites affects self-esteem, body image, and the ability to function. Assisting patients to take an active part in the management of ascites will lessen anxiety and help restore control.

Intestinal Obstruction

Approximately one-quarter to one-half of patients with ovarian cancer experience some degree of intestinal obstruction during their disease.[189] With more advanced stages, there is a higher probability of occurrence of obstruction. Tumor or adhesions cause extrinsic compression of the bowel. Obstruction can involve either the small or large intestine, can be acute or chronic, partial or complete. Signs and symptoms are dependent on the location of the obstruction and are summarized in Table 62-11.[183] A bowel obstruction with ovarian cancer most frequently tends to be an insidious process that progresses

Table 62-11 Signs and Symptoms of Intestinal Obstruction

Location	Signs and Symptoms
Small intestine	Colicky pain Vomiting Severe dehydration Minimal or absent distention
Lower small intestine	Less acute presentation Moderate vomiting Dehydration Some distention Lack of feces or flatus Severe electrolyte imbalances
Large intestine	Insidious Pronounced distention Lack of feces or flatus Overflow diarrhea Vomiting

Data from Martin.[183]

over weeks to months. An acute presentation of obstruction, such as perforation, is a rare complication.[183] The accumulation of fluid in the bowel near the obstruction, the increased gas from swallowed air, and the overgrowth of bowel flora can all contribute to the compression problem.[185]

The most common presenting symptom is colicky abdominal pain. Abdominal distention usually occurs once the obstruction is established. Stools gradually become more infrequent and vomiting can occur with small bowel obstruction. If intestinal strangulation with ischemia is found, fever, rebound tenderness, and leukocytosis may be present.[185] A diagnosis is made based on presenting signs, physical findings, and a flat and upright x-ray film of the abdomen. The film will reveal dilated loops of bowel, increased gas and fluid accumulation, and multiple air-fluid levels.[185] Further testing might include an upper GI with small bowel follow-through or a barium enema, an endoscopy, or a CT scan. A thorough assessment of the patient by the nurse includes evaluation for pain, fever, distention, nausea, vomiting and quality of emesis, bowel pattern, and fluid status.[183]

Medical treatment consists of relieving the distention, correcting the fluid imbalances, and removing the source of obstruction.[183] Initial treatment may involve decompression of the bowel with a nasogastric tube or long intestinal tube or simple bowel rest for 24–48 hours without oral intake.[183,184] Intravenous fluids are administered simultaneously, if needed. Analgesics, antiemetics, and anticholinergics are prescribed to manage pain, nausea, and vomiting. If there is no significant improvement, surgery is considered.[185]

Decisions about surgery for advanced cancer are always difficult. Quality-of-life considerations and potential complications after surgery are significant factors that must be weighed against possible gains since as many

as one-third of patients with a bowel obstruction will develop another bowel obstruction from their advanced disease.[185,190] Alternatively, the mortality rate from an ischemic bowel is 30% and patients who develop perforation, peritonitis, or bowel strangulation will likely require emergency surgery.[191] As part of an assessment for surgery, certain prognostic factors should be considered: the patient's age, tumor burden, nutritional status, and whether they could tolerate additional chemotherapy after surgery to prevent further recurrence.[1] Surgery may involve lysis of the adhesions or a bypass procedure with a proximal diverting colostomy or ileostomy if the obstruction is in the colon. The goals of surgical intervention are to alleviate the obstruction, remove ischemic and necrotic tissue, prevent gangrene, and prevent sepsis. Long-term medical management for patients who are not surgical candidates is achieved with placement of a gastrostomy tube. A gastrostomy tube is comfortable and patients can maintain adequate hydration with small, low-residue fluid meals. Additionally, total parental nutrition may be initiated for temporary or permanent nutritional supplement. In advanced ovarian cancer, conservative management of a bowel obstruction through restricted oral intake is indicated and can be achieved while the patient is at home. Patients are instructed to begin small amounts of clear liquids after several hours of bowel rest and slowly advance their diet as tolerated. A low-fiber diet may be indicated because of profound narrowing of the small or large intestine.

Malnutrition

Anorexia and cachexia both lead to malnutrition.[192,193] The anorexia-cachexia syndrome can be caused by a bowel obstruction or dysfunction; excessive protein or fluid loss from the bowel; gastrointestinal symptoms such as nausea, vomiting, diarrhea, or early satiety; complications of chemotherapy; or psychologic factors.[1] Unfortunately, the anorexia-cachexia symptom progresses as the ovarian cancer progresses.

Weight loss in cancer patients can influence both response to therapy and duration of survival.[194] In an Eastern Cooperative Oncology Group (ECOG) analysis of 3047 cancer patients on nine treatment protocols, median survival was significantly shorter for patients with weight loss compared with patients with no weight loss.[195] In a study of 105 patients evaluating the effects of dietary counseling and food intake on body weight, response rate, survival, and quality of life, Oversen and associates indicated that even modest weight losses were correlated with lower quality-of-life scores.[196] The patient should be evaluated first for reversible causes of decreased appetite such as xerostomia and depression.

Anorexia-cachexia is a major concern for nurses because the impact on patients is tremendous, coupled with disease and treatment side effects, physical weakness, fatigue, altered physical appearance, and loss of control over everyday life. Additionally, anorexia is most distressing to patients and their family members because those who have prepared the food may feel that they, not the food, are what is being rejected and tremendous struggles can develop over eating.[188] An assessment of anorexia-cachexia involves subjective and objective measures including a food diary, daily weights, tools to assess nutritional status and appetite, and blood tests. Early intervention is essential. The oral route of intervention is preferred because it is known that significant atrophy of intestinal villi occurs within days of decreased enteral stimulation.[194] Provide information on maintaining a well-balanced, high-calorie diet, enlist the help of a dietitian, and use nutritional supplements. Instruction includes tips on enhancing the flavor of foods, attention to the likes and dislikes of the patient, and avoiding foods with disturbing odors or tastes. Management of symptoms interfering with appetite may also be necessary.

Pharmacologic intervention for anorexia-cachexia include corticosteroids, appetite stimulants, metoclopramide, or cannabinoids. Corticosteroids produce short-term improvements in appetite but are associated with adverse effects. Megestrol acetate has been successfully used to stimulate the appetite and increase weight gain in breast cancer patients; the dose is 20 mL (800 mg)/day.[197–200] Dronabinol has proved efficacious in reversing anorexia in AIDS patients but has been less studied in patients with advanced cancer.[188] Nurses should assess food intake every four weeks and allow 8–12 weeks for weight gain. Successful intervention for anorexia-cachexia must focus on both the physiologic and psychologic factors influencing the development of the problem.

Total parental nutrition (TPN) should be reserved for those patients who are undergoing aggressive surgery, chemotherapy, or radiotherapy with severe gastrointestinal toxicity, or those severely malnourished patients receiving active therapy. It is a difficult decision to initiate TPN that must be made with consensus of the entire medical team regarding ethical appropriateness for a given patient.

Lymphedema

In ovarian cancer, lymphedema is usually secondary due to obstruction or blockage of the lymph system caused by tumor or trauma to the lymphatic channels.[201] The dominant site for lymphedema in ovarian cancer is in the lower extremities because of blockage of the pelvic or inguinal lymph nodes. In the early stages of obstruction, compensatory mechanisms such as collateral lymphatic flow occurs, but often it is insufficient and the consequence is excessive accumulation of a protein-rich fluid in the tissue spaces. Patients experience discomfort or pain, a fullness or heaviness of the extremity, numbness, weakness, and limited mobility. Clothing becomes increasingly tight and ambulation more difficult. Assessment is usually by patient self-report and the measurement of the swollen limb. CT scan or magnetic resonance imaging (MRI) can confirm a diagnosis of lymphedema and characterize it by degree: mild (stage

I), moderate (stage II), or severe (stage III).[202] Management of lymphedema is related to the primary treatment of the cancer. With systemic chemotherapy, the lymph node involvement will shrink and the fluid will subsequently drain.

The stages of lymphedema, a description of the swollen limb's appearance and physical findings, and treatment are found in Table 62-12. Complex decongestive physiotherapy is a five-part regimen critical to successful management of lymphedema. The regimen consists of skin care, manual lymphatic drainage (MLD), bandaging the affected limbs, exercises, and wearing a compression garment.[203] The mainstay of symptomatic lymphedema treatment is MLD performed by a physical therapist trained in lymphedema management. MLD is light stimulation of the dermal lymphatomes and the lymphatic vessels and it is not to be confused with deep massage, which concentrates on the muscles.[202,204] By stimulating the lymphatic vessels, a therapist is able to redirect the protein-rich fluid around the affected area and increase the reabsorption of lymphatic fluid. Compression therapy is also applied at the end of the one-hour session, wrapping the extremity with a low-pressure stretch bandage while carefully distributing pressure from distal to proximal.[204] Patients are also instructed to perform exercises to increase flexion of the muscle, which creates resistance against the bandage to stimulate additional lymphatic flow. Patients are treated daily for four to five weeks during the initial phase. Then maintenace therapy frequency is determined by patient's response and therapist's judgment. Compression garments should be worn continuously between treatments. Meticulous instructions regarding skin care are a component of the therapy plan, since skin of the edematous limb is at risk for breakdown and infection. If MLD no longer helps, gradient pressure pneumatic pumps may be prescribed. The pumps require a two-hour per day commitment and should be provided by a company that requires therapists and home counseling.

Nurses should teach the caregiver and patient to report early swelling or problems with edema. When edema develops, the nurse should provide the patient with strategies to manage this discomforting and disabling problem. Limitations of mobility are difficult for patients to deal with since many people try to maintain their normal activities despite progressive disease. In the absence of a response to systemic chemotherapy, there is little other drug therapy to offer except for antibiotics as required for infectious processes. Diuretics are of limited benefit in the treatment of edema due to advanced disease.

Pleural Effusion

Pleural effusions are an accumulation of fluid in excess of the normal 25 cc of fluid within the intrapleural space.[205] About 25%–30% of patients with metastatic ovarian cancer develop pleural effusions.[1,206,207] Pleural effusions develop when the flow of pleural fluid from the parietal pleura to the visceral pleura is interrupted by tumor. The effusion may be exudate or transudate in nature.[204] The

Table 62-12   Management of Lymphedema

Stages of Lymphedema	Findings	Treatment
Stage I (reversible)	Skin smooth textured	Elevate extremity
	Pitting edema	Compression garment
	2–3 cm difference between limb circumference	Massage
	Limb feels heavy, throbbing	Physical therapy
Stage II (chronic, does not reverse spontaneously)	Limb is swollen	Same as stage I; if ineffective begin complex decongestive physiotherapy
	Edema NOT pitting	
	Skin stretched, shiny	
	Tissue soft	
	3–5 cm difference in limb circumference	
⌐)	Extreme increase in swelling until the limb is column shaped, NOT pitting	Aggressive treatment
	Hand or foot massively swollen	May use gradient
	Skin dark or purple colored	Pneumatic pressure
	⌐retched, tissue firm	Pump therapy
	⌐d	Pain management
	⌐through the skin	
	⌐rcumference	

⌐ion for several days. As the drainage diminishes, ⌐ space is obliterated using a sclerosing agent ⌐ fluid reaccumulation. In women whose ⌐adequately drained or in whom the ⌐ but who have a reasonable life ⌐s or a pleuroperitoneal shunt

⌐pleural effusion can ⌐dvanced disease ⌐g informa- ⌐his dis- ⌐nxiety ⌐ator of ⌐elpful in ⌐agery, pro- ⌐ng, listening ⌐ge of motion ⌐lessness include ⌐ning over a table, ⌐ote lung expansion ⌐er.[210] Patients have to ⌐ing and plan frequent ⌐ort.

⌐escribing the concerns of women ⌐ound increased distress because of ⌐e frame to confront life-threatening ⌐ap expressed overwhelming feelings of ⌐d uncertainty while facing mortality and

⌐o effective screening methods, it is ⌐ages of disease that ovarian cancer is ⌐of treating ovarian cancer during the long and ⌐by the nurse. The trajectory of primary ⌐d disease is an area for ⌐d then management of the complications ⌐setting. The acute care phase of care in an ⌐treatment is usually during the early phase of the ⌐setting or briefly during a crisis of treatment ⌐vanced disease. Nurses are in the key position to ⌐cate patients on the prevention and control of the ⌐the effects from treatment or disease progression so that ⌐the patients' quality of life can be maintained. The plan ⌐for continuity of care must include seamless access to ⌐necessary care as needs arise and information must flow ⌐between caregivers irrespective of their practice settings.

⌐er ⌐g on ⌐Can- ⌐Wellness ⌐Internet ⌐prompted. She ⌐an like herself, ⌐rth of a newslet- ⌐nting ovarian can- ⌐culation of ten, but ⌐five years. The news- ⌐g with treatment side ⌐als available for patients ⌐ss for subscribing to this ⌐marillo, Texas, 79114-7948.

redefining goals and expectations. Steginga and Dunn studied 150 women with gynecologic cancers.[212] Eighty-one percent reported psychosocial difficulties as their main worries or problems at diagnosis and during treatment. Over time, this percentage fell to 39%, but such problems continued to be listed as a persistent problem. Forty-eight percent of the study group reported distressing physical effects as their main worries or concerns. Support from family was ranked the most important social support.[213] Women with gynecologic cancer reported family was important in contributing to their positivity on quality of life (QOL). Nursing assessment of social structure is important to identify those without support and begin efforts to enhance their network. Nurses were cited by the study participants as being most helpful when providing emotional and practical support.

Another group of authors found significant psychological distress that impaired physical function.[214] For these women, relief came from psychologic counseling and support and improvement in their physical symptoms. Ersek and colleagues studied ovarian cancer survivors who described the negative aspects of treatment and impact on work, relationships, and their ability to enjoy life.[215] Guidozzi used a questionnaire to evaluate the impact of ovarian cancer and its management on the woman's quality of life and found a profound impact on the individual's activities of daily living, support, and outlook.[216] The psychosocial sequelae of ovarian cancer may include psychosocial discomfort (anxiety, anger, guilt, and depression), changes in life patterns (alterations in physical abilities and functioning and changing social relationships), and fears, concerns, and anxiety about specific treatment and survival. Gynecologic cancers also potentially affect sexual functioning by body image changes and physiologic disturbances. Nurses are key to helping women with ovarian cancer by providing both physical and emotional care during the disease trajectory and improving quality of life.

Ovarian Cancer Patient Resources

Following the path established by the successful breast cancer and AIDS advocacy groups, ovarian cancer now has a public voice. The Ovarian Cancer National Alliance (OCNA), formed in 1997, is an organization with the mission to unite organizations and individuals in the fight to overcome ovarian cancer. The National Ovarian Cancer Coalition (NOCC) was founded by a group of ovarian cancer survivors in April 1995. It now has over 2000 members and 23 state chapters nationwide. The mission of NOCC is to raise awareness about ovarian cancer and to promote education about the disease. The alliance and coalition were successful in 1998 in having September of that year designated the first National Ovarian Cancer Awareness Month. President Clinton designated September 13–19, 1998 as the first Ovarian Cancer Awareness Week. OCNA held the initial national advocacy confer-

ence on ovarian cancer titled "Silent No More" in September 1998, with other founding partner and member organizations.

Earlier, in 1994, the National Cancer Institute (NCI) had held the first consensus development conference devoted to screening, prevention, diagnosis, and treatment of ovarian cancer. Funding increased steadily for women's health from 1987–1996.[217] Now ovarian cancer research and education initiatives seem to be close to getting an appropriate share of NCI monies budgeted for women's health. Bills remain before Congress asking for $90 million dollars for ovarian cancer research and one Special Program of Research Excellence (SPORE grant) application has been approved.[217]

The Web sites *www.ovarian.org* and *www.ovariancancer.org* offer a multitude of information that includes a chat forum and an "Ask the Experts" page. Other general information resources include American Cancer Society, National Cancer Institute Cancer Information Service; Society of Gynecologic Oncologists; Gilda Radner Familial Ovarian Cancer Registry; and Gynecologic Cancer Foundation Information Hotline. Resources focusing on support include CancerCare; National Coalition for Cancer Survivorship; Gilda's Club; SHARE; and the Wellness Community. Addresses, phone numbers, and Web addresses are provided in Table 62-13.

A new diagnosis of an unfamiliar disease led one woman to launch her own network of women who was desperate to talk with another woman, specifically a survivor, which led to the newsletter titled *Conversations* for women fighting cancer.[218] *Conversations* started with a circulation that has grown considerably over the last year. The newsletter is filled with tips for dealing with side effects, and the latest clinical trials for women seeking treatments. The address for this newsletter is P.O. Box 7948, A

Continuity of Care

Because there are no reliable methods, often in the late stages of disease when discovered. Consequently chronic course concentration treatment in advance or home inpatient disease or a ed si

Table 62-13 Resources for Ovarian Cancer Information and Support

National Ovarian Cancer Coalition
2335 East Atlantic Boulevard, Suite 401
Pompano Beach, Florida 33062
1-888-ovarian
www.ovarian.org

Ovarian Cancer National Alliance
PO Box 33107
Washington, DC 20033-0107
202-452-5910
www.ovariancancer.org

Gynecologic Cancer Foundation Information Hotline
1-800-444-4441
www.sgo.org

Women's Cancer Network
312-644-6610
www.wcn.org

CancerCare, Inc.
1-800-813-HOPE

National Coalition for Cancer Survivorship
www.cansearch.org

Gilda's Club: Gilda Radner Ovarian Cancer Familial Registry
212-647-9700
1-800-OVARIAN
www.ovariancancer.org

The Wellness Community
1-888-793-WELL

National Cancer Institute
Cancer Information Service
1-800-4-CANCER
www.cancernet.nci.nih.gov

NEWSLETTERS

Conversations
P.O. Box 7948
Amarillo, Texas 79114-7948
806-355-8565

Ovarian Plus
P.O. Box 498
Paauilo, Hawaii 96776-0498
1-800-776-1696

SHARE
212-719-1204
www.sharecancersupport.org

Society of Gynecologic Oncologists
www.sgo.org

Sandra G. Davis Ovarian Cancer Research Program
713-792-2765

The ambulatory or office nurses are critical links to support and guide these ovarian cancer patients. For example, the patient typically uses self-care measures to monitor the reaccumulation of ascites fluid and the nurse is informed when weight gain or discomfort reaches an unacceptable level. The nurse consults with the physician and a plan is developed to relieve the existing problem. In other instances, surgical intervention for a partial intestinal obstruction may not be possible in an advanced disease case and then it is the nurse who helps the patient and family cope with the problem until the end of life.

Addressing the emotional needs is as important a component of nursing care as managing the symptoms. Helping the patient and family cope with the end of life is central to the role and skills of the oncology nurse. Dealing with anxiety and depression and preventing feelings of abandonment or despair are a few of the psychosocial needs of both the patient and family during the final stages of the disease. Involvement of the hospice team when appropriate will add support at a critical phase of need for the patient and family. At each phase and step along the trajectory of ovarian cancer care, collaboration between health care team members and the patient and family is critical.

Conclusion

Ovarian cancer is achieving broader public attention through education by coalition and advocacy groups which have also been active in lobbying the federal government to dedicate more research dollars to ovarian cancer studies. The increase in overall survival for breast cancer was directly related to the improvements in screening, early detection, changes in treatment, and dramatic increases in funding. The same needs to be done for ovarian cancer. The problems related to the care of women with advanced disease will continually challenge nurses in any setting. Nurses need to remain aware of the symptoms of ovarian cancer and educate others. The most important challenge is to erase the historical association of ovarian cancer as the silent killer and remember the words of the National Ovarian Cancer Coalition: "It whispers . . . so listen."

References

1. Eriksson JH, Frazier SR: Epithelial cancers of the ovary and fallopian tube, in Moore GJ (ed): *Women and Cancer: A Gynecologic Oncology Nursing Perspective.* Sudbury, MA, Jones and Bartlett, 1997, pp 205–256
2. Barber HRK: *Ovarian Carcinoma: Etiology, Diagnosis, and Treatment* (ed 3). New York: Springer-Verlag, 1993, p 25
3. Sadler TW: *Langman's Medical Embryology* (ed 6). Baltimore: Williams and Wilkins, 1990, p 260
4. Landis SH, Murray T, Bolden S, et al: Cancer Statistics 1999. *CA Cancer J Clin* 49:8–31, 1999
5. Petterson F: Annual report of the results of treatment of gynecologic cancer. Stockholm: International Federation of Gynecology and Oncology, 1988
6. SEER Cancer Statistics Review, 1993–1996. Surveillance, Epidemiology, and End Results Program. National Cancer Institute, Bethesda, MD, Section XX

7. Daly M, Obrams GI: Epidemiology and risk assessment for ovarian cancer. *Semin Oncol* 25:255–264, 1998

8. Fathalla MF: Incessant ovulation—a factor in ovarian neoplasia? *Lancet* 2:163, 1971

9. Casagrande JT, Louie EW, Pike MC, et al: "Incessant ovulation" and ovarian cancer. *Lancet* 2:170–173, 1979

10. Cramer DW, Welch WR: Determinants in ovarian cancer risk. II. Inferences regarding pathogenesis. *J Natl Cancer Inst* 49:717–721, 1983

11. Risch HA: Hormonal etiology of epithelial ovarian cancer, with a hypothesis concerning the role of androgens and progesterone. *J Natl Cancer Inst* 90:1774–1786, 1998

12. Hankinson SE, Colditz GA, Hunter DJ, et al: A prospective study of reproductive factors and risk of epithelial ovarian cancer. *Cancer* 76:284–290, 1995

13. Adami HO, Hsieh CC, Lambe M, et al: Parity, age at first childbirth, and risk of ovarian cancer. *Lancet* 344:1250–1254, 1994

14. Whittemore AS: Characteristics relating to ovarian cancer risk: implications for prevention and detection. *Gynecol Oncol* 55:515–519, 1994

15. Rossing MA, Daling JR, Weiss NS, et al: Ovarian tumors in a cohort of infertile women. *N Engl J Med* 52:161–183, 1994

16. Gross TP, Schlesselman JJ: The estimated effect of oral contraceptive use on the cumulative risk of epithelial ovarian cancer. *Obstet Gynecol* 83:419–424, 1994

17. Research Reports. Progestin may prevent ovarian cancers by triggering death of damaged ovarian cells. *Oncology* 12:1666–1667, 1998

18. Hempling RE, Wong C, Piver MS, et al: Hormone replacement therapy as a risk factor for epithelial ovarian cancer: results of a case-contol study. *Obstet Gynecol* 89:1012–1016, 1997

19. Helzlsouer KJ, Alberg AJ, Gordon GB, et al: Serum gonadotropin and steroid hormones and the development of ovarian cancer. *JAMA* 274:1926–1930, 1995

20. Schildkraut J, Schwingl PJ, Bastos E, et al: Epithelial ovarian cancer risk among women with polycystic ovarian syndrome. *Obstet Gynecol* 88:554–559, 1996

21. Brinton LA, Gridley G, Persson I, et al: Cancer risk after a hospital discharge of endometriosis. *Am J Obstet Gynecol* 176:572–579, 1997

22. Schildkraut JM, Bastos E, Berchuck A: Relationship between lifetime ovulatory cycles and overexpression of mutant p53 in epithelial ovarian cancer. *J Natl Cancer Inst* 89:932–938, 1997

23. Hankinson SE, Hunter DJ, Colditz GA, et al: Tubal ligation, hysterectomy, and risk of ovarian cancer: a prospective study. *JAMA* 270:2813–2818, 1993

24. Cramer DW, Muto MG, Reichardt JK, et al: Characteristics of women with a family history of ovarian cancer. I. Galactose consumption and metabolism. *Cancer* 74:1309–1317, 1994

25. Risch HA, Jain M, Marrett LD, et al: Dietary lactose intake, lactose intolerance, and the risk of ovarian cancer in southern Ontario (Canada). *Cancer Causes Control* 5:540–548, 1994

26. Herrinton LJ, Weiss NS, Beresford SA, et al: Lactose and galactose intake and metabolism in relation to the risk of epithelial ovarian cancer. *Am J Epidemiol* 141:407–416, 1995

27. Helzsouer KJ, Alberg AJ, Norkus EP, et al: Prospective study of serum micronutrients and ovarian cancer. *J Natl Cancer Inst* 88:32–37, 1996

28. Mink PJ, Folsom AR, Sellers TA, et al: Physical activity, waist-to-hip ratio, and other risk factors for ovarian cancer: a follow-up study of older women. *Epidemiology* 7:38–45, 1996

29. Harlow BL, Cramer D, Bell DA, et al: Perineal exposure to talc and ovarian cancer risk. *Obstet Gynecol* 80:19–26, 1992

30. Cramer D, Welch WR, Scully RE, et al: Ovarian cancer and talc—a case control study. *Cancer* 50:372–376, 1982

31. Wong C, Hempling RE, Piver MS, et al: Perineal talc exposure and subsequent epithelial ovarian cancer: a case control study. *Obstet Gynecol* 93:372–376, 1999

32. Cramer DW, Liberman RF, Titus-Ernstoff L, et al: Genital talc exposure and risk of ovarian cancer. *Int J Cancer* 81:351–356, 1999

33. Eltabbakh GH, Piver MS: Ovarian cancer: the myths and facts. *Quality of Life—A Nursing Challenge* 6:83–87, 1998

34. Schildkraut JM, Thompson WD: Familial ovarian cancer: a population-based case-control study. *Am J Epidemiol* 128:456–466, 1988

35. Lynch HT, Casey MJ, Shaw TG, et al: Hereditary factors in gynecologic cancer. *Oncologist* 3:319–338, 1998

36. Lynch HT, Krush AJ: Carcinoma of the breast and ovary in three families. *Surg Gynecol Obstet* 133:644–648, 1971

37. Lynch HT, Krush AJ, Lemon HM, et al: Tumor variation in families with breast cancer. *JAMA* 222:1631–1635, 1972

38. Lynch HT, Guirgis HA, Albert S, et al: Familial association of carcinoma of the breast and ovary. *Surg Gynecol Obstet* 138:717–724, 1974

39. Hall JM, Lee MK, Neuman B, et al: Linkage of early-onset breast cancer to chromosome 17q21. *Science* 250:1684–1689, 1991

40. Narod SA, Feunteun J, Lynch HT, et al: Familial breast-ovarian cancer locus on chromosome 17q12-q23. *Lancet* 388:82–83, 1991

41. Miki Y, Swensen J, Shattuck-Eidens D, et al: A strong candidate for the breast and ovarian cancer susceptibility gene BRCA1. *Science* 266:66–71, 1994

42. Wooster R, Neuhausen SL, Mangion J, et al: Localization of a breast cancer susceptibility gene, BRCA2, to chromosome 13q12–13. *Science* 265:1088–2090, 1994

43. Wooster R, Bignell G, Lancaster J, et al: Identification of the breast cancer susceptibility gene BRCA2. *Nature* 378:789–792, 1995

44. Easton DF, Bishop DT, Ford D, et al: Genetic linkage analysis in familial breast and ovarian cancer: results from 214 families. *Am J Hum Genet* 52:678–701, 1993

45. Easton DF, Ford D, Bishop DT, et al: Breast and ovarian cancer incidence in BRCA1 mutation carriers. *Am J Hum Genet* 56:265–271, 1995

46. Lynch HT, Casey MJ, Lynch J, et al: Genetics and ovarian carcinoma. *Semin Oncol* 25:265–280, 1998

47. Beller U, Halle D, Catane R, et al: High frequency of BRCA1 and BRCA2 germline mutations in Ashkenazi Jewish ovarian cancer patients, regardless of family history. *Gynecol Oncol* 60:505–514, 1997

48. Streuwing JP, Hartge P, Wacholder S, et al: The risk of cancer associated with specific mutations of BRCA1 and BRCA2 among Ashkenazi Jews. *N Engl J Med* 336:1401–1408, 1997

49. National Institutes of Health Consensus Development Conference Statement. Ovarian cancer: screening, treatment, and follow-up. April 5–7, 1994. *Gynecol Oncol* 55:S4–S14, 1994

50. VanNagell JR, Higgins RV, Donaldson ES, et al: Transvaginal sonography as a screening method for ovarian cancer: a report of the first 1000 cases screened. *Cancer* 65:573–577, 1990

Table 62-12   Management of Lymphedema

Stages of Lymphedema	Findings	Treatment
Stage I (reversible)	Skin smooth textured	Elevate extremity
	Pitting edema	Compression garment
	2–3 cm difference between limb circumference	Massage
	Limb feels heavy, throbbing	Physical therapy
Stage II (chronic, does not reverse spontaneously)	Limb is swollen	Same as stage I; if ineffective begin complex decongestive physiotherapy
	Edema NOT pitting	
	Skin stretched, shiny	
	Tissue soft	
	3–5 cm difference in limb circumference	
Stage III (severe)	Extreme increase in swelling until the limb is column shaped, NOT pitting	Aggressive treatment
	Hand or foot massively swollen	May use gradient
	Skin dark or purple colored	Pneumatic pressure
	Skin stretched, tissue firm	Pump therapy
	Rough textured	Pain management
	Lymph leaks directly through the skin	
	> 5 cm difference in limb circumference	

Data from Martin.[183]

two major pathophysiologic processes associated with exudative effusion involve an inflammatory process or neoplastic disease. Dyspnea caused by the accumulating effusion is the most commonly reported symptom.[205,208,209] Sharp pleuritic chest pain, if present, may or may not be accompanied by a pleural rub.[205,208] Other symptoms associated with a pleural effusion include fever (if inflammatory), dry irritating cough, and hypoxia.[205] Effusions are diagnosed by a posterior, anterior, and lateral chest x-ray. On physical exam, findings include decreased breath sounds and dullness to percussion, most often in the lung base.

Once the diagnosis of pleural effusion is made, a thoracentesis may be needed to remove the excess fluid if it is causing significant impairment. An ultrasound is often used to locate the fluid for removal during a thoracentesis. The patient must be prepared for the procedure and the possible complications which include pain, infection, pneumothorax, or pulmonary edema. The nurse must observe for any pain or discomfort, increased respiratory rate or dyspnea, increased pulse rate, vertigo, or uncontrollable cough during the procedure.[1] The fluid is removed and sent for diagnostic studies. A chest x-ray is performed after the procedure to rule out a pneumothorax. The fluid will usually rapidly reaccumulate in four to five days, unless the underlying cause of the problem, the ovarian cancer, is effectively treated with systemic chemotherapy. Insertion of a chest tube or thoracostomy and the addition of a sclerosing agent or pleurodesis may be performed if pleural fluid reaccumulates. The sclerosing procedure requires hospitalization; the chest tube is inserted at the bedside and the tube is connected to suction for several days. As the drainage diminishes, the pleural space is obliterated using a sclerosing agent to prevent the fluid reaccumulation. In women whose effusion cannot be adequately drained or in whom the lung does not reexpand, but who have a reasonable life expectancy, open pleurodesis or a pleuroperitoneal shunt may be considered.[188]

The severe dyspnea caused by a pleural effusion can be controlled in sedentary patients with advanced disease with oxygen and/or morphine.[188] By providing information concerning palliative measures to manage this distressing side effect, the nurse can help lessen anxiety because pleural effusion is an undeniable indicator of disease progression. Relaxation exercises are helpful in decreasing anxiety and may include guided imagery, progressive relaxation with controlled breathing, listening to relaxing music, mild massage, and range of motion exercises.[210] Exercises to help with breathlessness include sitting upright and leaning forward, leaning over a table, or resting elbows on knees to promote lung expansion and help the patient breathe easier.[210] Patients have to modify their activities of daily living and plan frequent rest periods for increased support.

Stress and Support

One qualitative study describing the concerns of women with ovarian cancer found increased distress because of the compressed time frame to confront life-threatening issues.[211] The group expressed overwhelming feelings of helplessness and uncertainty while facing mortality and redefining goals and expectations. Steginga and Dunn studied 150 women with gynecologic cancers.[212] Eighty-one percent reported psychosocial difficulties as their main worries or problems at diagnosis and during treatment. Over time, this percentage fell to 39%, but such problems continued to be listed as a persistent problem. Forty-eight percent of the study group reported distressing physical effects as their main worries or concerns. Support from family was ranked the most important social support.[213] Women with gynecologic cancer reported family was important in contributing to their positivity on quality of life (QOL). Nursing assessment of social structure is important to identify those without support and begin efforts to enhance their network. Nurses were cited by the study participants as being most helpful when providing emotional and practical support.

Another group of authors found significant psychological distress that impaired physical function.[214] For these women, relief came from psychologic counseling and support and improvement in their physical symptoms. Ersek and colleagues studied ovarian cancer survivors who described the negative aspects of treatment and impact on work, relationships, and their ability to enjoy life.[215] Guidozzi used a questionnaire to evaluate the impact of ovarian cancer and its management on the woman's quality of life and found a profound impact on the individual's activities of daily living, support, and outlook.[216] The psychosocial sequelae of ovarian cancer may include psychosocial discomfort (anxiety, anger, guilt, and depression), changes in life patterns (alterations in physical abilities and functioning and changing social relationships), and fears, concerns, and anxiety about specific treatment and survival. Gynecologic cancers also potentially affect sexual functioning by body image changes and physiologic disturbances. Nurses are key to helping women with ovarian cancer by providing both physical and emotional care during the disease trajectory and improving quality of life.

Ovarian Cancer Patient Resources

Following the path established by the successful breast cancer and AIDS advocacy groups, ovarian cancer now has a public voice. The Ovarian Cancer National Alliance (OCNA), formed in 1997, is an organization with the mission to unite organizations and individuals in the fight to overcome ovarian cancer. The National Ovarian Cancer Coalition (NOCC) was founded by a group of ovarian cancer survivors in April 1995. It now has over 2000 members and 23 state chapters nationwide. The mission of NOCC is to raise awareness about ovarian cancer and to promote education about the disease. The alliance and coalition were successful in 1998 in having September of that year designated the first National Ovarian Cancer Awareness Month. President Clinton designated September 13–19, 1998 as the first Ovarian Cancer Awareness Week. OCNA held the initial national advocacy conference on ovarian cancer titled "Silent No More" in September 1998, with other founding partner and member organizations.

Earlier, in 1994, the National Cancer Institute (NCI) had held the first consensus development conference devoted to screening, prevention, diagnosis, and treatment of ovarian cancer. Funding increased steadily for women's health from 1987–1996.[217] Now ovarian cancer research and education initiatives seem to be close to getting an appropriate share of NCI monies budgeted for women's health. Bills remain before Congress asking for $90 million dollars for ovarian cancer research and one Special Program of Research Excellence (SPORE grant) application has been approved.[217]

The Web sites *www.ovarian.org* and *www.ovariancancer.org* offer a multitude of information that includes a chat forum and an "Ask the Experts" page. Other general information resources include American Cancer Society, National Cancer Institute Cancer Information Service; Society of Gynecologic Oncologists; Gilda Radner Familial Ovarian Cancer Registry; and Gynecologic Cancer Foundation Information Hotline. Resources focusing on support include CancerCare; National Coalition for Cancer Survivorship; Gilda's Club; SHARE; and the Wellness Community. Addresses, phone numbers, and Internet addresses are provided in Table 62-13.

A new diagnosis of an unfamiliar disease prompted one woman to launch her own network of support. She was desperate to talk with another woman like herself, specifically a survivor, which led to the birth of a newsletter titled *Conversations* for women fighting ovarian cancer.[218] *Conversations* started with a circulation of ten, but has grown considerably over the last five years. The newsletter is filled with tips for dealing with treatment side effects, and the latest clinical trials available for patients seeking treatments. The address for subscribing to this newsletter is P.O. Box 7948, Amarillo, Texas, 79114-7948.

Continuity of Care

Because there are no effective screening methods, it is often in the late stages of disease that ovarian cancer is discovered. Continuity of care during the long and chronic course of treating ovarian cancer is an area for concentration by the nurse. The trajectory of primary treatment and then management of the complications in advanced disease is often centered in the outpatient or home setting. The acute care phase of care in an inpatient setting is usually during the early phase of the disease treatment or briefly during a crisis of treatment or advanced disease. Nurses are in the key position to educate patients on the prevention and control of the side effects from treatment or disease progression so that the patients' quality of life can be maintained. The plan for continuity of care must include seamless access to necessary care as needs arise and information must flow between caregivers irrespective of their practice settings.

Table 62-13 Resources for Ovarian Cancer Information and Support

National Ovarian Cancer Coalition
2335 East Atlantic Boulevard, Suite 401
Pompano Beach, Florida 33062
1-888-ovarian
www.ovarian.org

Ovarian Cancer National Alliance
PO Box 33107
Washington, DC 20033-0107
202-452-5910
www.ovariancancer.org

Gynecologic Cancer Foundation Information Hotline
1-800-444-4441
www.sgo.org

Women's Cancer Network
312-644-6610
www.wcn.org

CancerCare, Inc.
1-800-813-HOPE

National Coalition for Cancer Survivorship
www.cansearch.org

Gilda's Club: Gilda Radner Ovarian Cancer Familial Registry
212-647-9700
1-800-OVARIAN
www.ovariancancer.org

The Wellness Community
1-888-793-WELL

National Cancer Institute
Cancer Information Service
1-800-4-CANCER
www.cancernet.nci.nih.gov

NEWSLETTERS

Conversations
P.O. Box 7948
Amarillo, Texas 79114-7948
806-355-8565

Ovarian Plus
P.O. Box 498
Paauilo, Hawaii 96776-0498
1-800-776-1696

SHARE
212-719-1204
www.sharecancersupport.org

Society of Gynecologic Oncologists
www.sgo.org

Sandra G. Davis Ovarian Cancer Research Program
713-792-2765

The ambulatory or office nurses are critical links to support and guide these ovarian cancer patients. For example, the patient typically uses self-care measures to monitor the reaccumulation of ascites fluid and the nurse is informed when weight gain or discomfort reaches an unacceptable level. The nurse consults with the physician

and a plan is developed to relieve the existing problem. In other instances, surgical intervention for a partial intestinal obstruction may not be possible in an advanced disease case and then it is the nurse who helps the patient and family cope with the problem until the end of life.

Addressing the emotional needs is as important a component of nursing care as managing the symptoms. Helping the patient and family cope with the end of life is central to the role and skills of the oncology nurse. Dealing with anxiety and depression and preventing feelings of abandonment or despair are a few of the psychosocial needs of both the patient and family during the final stages of the disease. Involvement of the hospice team when appropriate will add support at a critical phase of need for the patient and family. At each phase and step along the trajectory of ovarian cancer care, collaboration between health care team members and the patient and family is critical.

Conclusion

Ovarian cancer is achieving broader public attention through education by coalition and advocacy groups which have also been active in lobbying the federal government to dedicate more research dollars to ovarian cancer studies. The increase in overall survival for breast cancer was directly related to the improvements in screening, early detection, changes in treatment, and dramatic increases in funding. The same needs to be done for ovarian cancer. The problems related to the care of women with advanced disease will continually challenge nurses in any setting. Nurses need to remain aware of the symptoms of ovarian cancer and educate others. The most important challenge is to erase the historical association of ovarian cancer as the silent killer and remember the words of the National Ovarian Cancer Coalition: "It whispers . . . so listen."

References

1. Eriksson JH, Frazier SR: Epithelial cancers of the ovary and fallopian tube, in Moore GJ (ed): *Women and Cancer: A Gynecologic Oncology Nursing Perspective*. Sudbury, MA, Jones and Bartlett, 1997, pp 205–256
2. Barber HRK: *Ovarian Carcinoma: Etiology, Diagnosis, and Treatment* (ed 3). New York: Springer-Verlag, 1993, p 25
3. Sadler TW: *Langman's Medical Embryology* (ed 6). Baltimore: Williams and Wilkins, 1990, p 260
4. Landis SH, Murray T, Bolden S, et al: Cancer Statistics 1999. *CA Cancer J Clin* 49:8–31, 1999
5. Petterson F: Annual report of the results of treatment of gynecologic cancer. Stockholm: International Federation of Gynecology and Oncology, 1988
6. SEER Cancer Statistics Review, 1993–1996. Surveillance, Epidemiology, and End Results Program. National Cancer Institute, Bethesda, MD, Section XX

7. Daly M, Obrams GI: Epidemiology and risk assessment for ovarian cancer. *Semin Oncol* 25:255–264, 1998

8. Fathalla MF: Incessant ovulation—a factor in ovarian neoplasia? *Lancet* 2:163, 1971

9. Casagrande JT, Louie EW, Pike MC, et al: "Incessant ovulation" and ovarian cancer. *Lancet* 2:170–173, 1979

10. Cramer DW, Welch WR: Determinants in ovarian cancer risk. II. Inferences regarding pathogenesis. *J Natl Cancer Inst* 49:717–721, 1983

11. Risch HA: Hormonal etiology of epithelial ovarian cancer, with a hypothesis concerning the role of androgens and progesterone. *J Natl Cancer Inst* 90:1774–1786, 1998

12. Hankinson SE, Colditz GA, Hunter DJ, et al: A prospective study of reproductive factors and risk of epithelial ovarian cancer. *Cancer* 76:284–290, 1995

13. Adami HO, Hsieh CC, Lambe M, et al: Parity, age at first childbirth, and risk of ovarian cancer. *Lancet* 344:1250–1254, 1994

14. Whittemore AS: Characteristics relating to ovarian cancer risk: implications for prevention and detection. *Gynecol Oncol* 55:515–519, 1994

15. Rossing MA, Daling JR, Weiss NS, et al: Ovarian tumors in a cohort of infertile women. *N Engl J Med* 52:161–183, 1994

16. Gross TP, Schlesselman JJ: The estimated effect of oral contraceptive use on the cumulative risk of epithelial ovarian cancer. *Obstet Gynecol* 83:419–424, 1994

17. Research Reports. Progestin may prevent ovarian cancers by triggering death of damaged ovarian cells. *Oncology* 12:1666–1667, 1998

18. Hempling RE, Wong C, Piver MS, et al: Hormone replacement therapy as a risk factor for epithelial ovarian cancer: results of a case-contol study. *Obstet Gynecol* 89:1012–1016, 1997

19. Helzlsouer KJ, Alberg AJ, Gordon GB, et al: Serum gonadotropin and steroid hormones and the development of ovarian cancer. *JAMA* 274:1926–1930, 1995

20. Schildkraut J, Schwingl PJ, Bastos E, et al: Epithelial ovarian cancer risk among women with polycystic ovarian syndrome. *Obstet Gynecol* 88:554–559, 1996

21. Brinton LA, Gridley G, Persson I, et al: Cancer risk after a hospital discharge of endometriosis. *Am J Obstet Gynecol* 176:572–579, 1997

22. Schildkraut JM, Bastos E, Berchuck A: Relationship between lifetime ovulatory cycles and overexpression of mutant p53 in epithelial ovarian cancer. *J Natl Cancer Inst* 89:932–938, 1997

23. Hankinson SE, Hunter DJ, Colditz GA, et al: Tubal ligation, hysterectomy, and risk of ovarian cancer: a prospective study. *JAMA* 270:2813–2818, 1993

24. Cramer DW, Muto MG, Reichardt JK, et al: Characteristics of women with a family history of ovarian cancer. I. Galactose consumption and metabolism. *Cancer* 74:1309–1317, 1994

25. Risch HA, Jain M, Marrett LD, et al: Dietary lactose intake, lactose intolerance, and the risk of ovarian cancer in southern Ontario (Canada). *Cancer Causes Control* 5:540–548, 1994

26. Herrinton LJ, Weiss NS, Beresford SA, et al: Lactose and galactose intake and metabolism in relation to the risk of epithelial ovarian cancer. *Am J Epidemiol* 141:407–416, 1995

27. Helzsouer KJ, Alberg AJ, Norkus EP, et al: Prospective study of serum micronutrients and ovarian cancer. *J Natl Cancer Inst* 88:32–37, 1996

28. Mink PJ, Folsom AR, Sellers TA, et al: Physical activity, waist-to-hip ratio, and other risk factors for ovarian cancer: a follow-up study of older women. *Epidemiology* 7:38–45, 1996

29. Harlow BL, Cramer D, Bell DA, et al: Perineal exposure to talc and ovarian cancer risk. *Obstet Gynecol* 80:19–26, 1992

30. Cramer D, Welch WR, Scully RE, et al: Ovarian cancer and talc—a case control study. *Cancer* 50:372–376, 1982

31. Wong C, Hempling RE, Piver MS, et al: Perineal talc exposure and subsequent epithelial ovarian cancer: a case control study. *Obstet Gynecol* 93:372–376, 1999

32. Cramer DW, Liberman RF, Titus-Ernstoff L, et al: Genital talc exposure and risk of ovarian cancer. *Int J Cancer* 81:351–356, 1999

33. Eltabbakh GH, Piver MS: Ovarian cancer: the myths and facts. *Quality of Life—A Nursing Challenge* 6:83–87, 1998

34. Schildkraut JM, Thompson WD: Familial ovarian cancer: a population-based case-control study. *Am J Epidemiol* 128:456–466, 1988

35. Lynch HT, Casey MJ, Shaw TG, et al: Hereditary factors in gynecologic cancer. *Oncologist* 3:319–338, 1998

36. Lynch HT, Krush AJ: Carcinoma of the breast and ovary in three families. *Surg Gynecol Obstet* 133:644–648, 1971

37. Lynch HT, Krush AJ, Lemon HM, et al: Tumor variation in families with breast cancer. *JAMA* 222:1631–1635, 1972

38. Lynch HT, Guirgis HA, Albert S, et al: Familial association of carcinoma of the breast and ovary. *Surg Gynecol Obstet* 138:717–724, 1974

39. Hall JM, Lee MK, Neuman B, et al: Linkage of early-onset breast cancer to chromosome 17q21. *Science* 250:1684–1689, 1991

40. Narod SA, Feunteun J, Lynch HT, et al: Familial breast-ovarian cancer locus on chromosome 17q12-q23. *Lancet* 388:82–83, 1991

41. Miki Y, Swensen J, Shattuck-Eidens D, et al: A strong candidate for the breast and ovarian cancer susceptibility gene BRCA1. *Science* 266:66–71, 1994

42. Wooster R, Neuhausen SL, Mangion J, et al: Localization of a breast cancer susceptibility gene, BRCA2, to chromosome 13q12-13. *Science* 265:1088–2090, 1994

43. Wooster R, Bignell G, Lancaster J, et al: Identification of the breast cancer susceptibility gene BRCA2. *Nature* 378:789–792, 1995

44. Easton DF, Bishop DT, Ford D, et al: Genetic linkage analysis in familial breast and ovarian cancer: results from 214 families. *Am J Hum Genet* 52:678–701, 1993

45. Easton DF, Ford D, Bishop DT, et al: Breast and ovarian cancer incidence in BRCA1 mutation carriers. *Am J Hum Genet* 56:265–271, 1995

46. Lynch HT, Casey MJ, Lynch J, et al: Genetics and ovarian carcinoma. *Semin Oncol* 25:265–280, 1998

47. Beller U, Halle D, Catane R, et al: High frequency of BRCA1 and BRCA2 germline mutations in Ashkenazi Jewish ovarian cancer patients, regardless of family history. *Gynecol Oncol* 60:505–514, 1997

48. Streuwing JP, Hartge P, Wacholder S, et al: The risk of cancer associated with specific mutations of BRCA1 and BRCA2 among Ashkenazi Jews. *N Engl J Med* 336:1401–1408, 1997

49. National Institutes of Health Consensus Development Conference Statement. Ovarian cancer: screening, treatment, and follow-up. April 5–7, 1994. *Gynecol Oncol* 55:S4–S14, 1994

50. VanNagell JR, Higgins RV, Donaldson ES, et al: Transvaginal sonography as a screening method for ovarian cancer: a report of the first 1000 cases screened. *Cancer* 65:573–577, 1990

51. VanNagell JR, DePriest PD, Gallion HH, et al: Ovarian cancer screening in asymptomatic postmenopausal women by transvaginal ultrasound. *Cancer* 68:458–462, 1991

52. DePriest PD, VanNagell JR, Gallion HH, et al: Ovarian cancer screening in asymptomatic postmenopausal women. *Gynecol Oncol* 51:205–209, 1993

53. Ozols RF, Schwartz PE, Eifel PJ: Ovarian cancer, fallopian tube carcinoma, and peritoneal carcinoma, in DeVita VT, Hellman S, Rosenberg SA (eds): *Cancer Principles and Practice of Oncology.* (ed 5). Philadelphia, Lippincott-Raven, 1997, pp 1502–1539

54. Einhorn N, Sjovall K, Knapp RC, et al: Prospective evaluation of serum CA 125 levels for early detection of ovarian cancer. *Obstet Gynecol* 80:14–18, 1992

55. Jacobs I, Davies AP, Bridges J, et al: Prevalence of screening for ovarian cancer in postmenopausal women by CA-125 measurement and ultrasonography. *BMJ* 306:1030–1034, 1993

56. Kramer BS, Gohagan J, Prorok PC, et al: A National Cancer Institute sponsored screening trial for prostatic, lung, colorectal, and ovarian cancers. *Cancer* 71:589–593, 1993 (suppl 2)

57. Bast R, Klug T, St John E, et al: A radioimmunoassay using a monoclonal antibody to monitor the course of epithelial ovarian cancer. *N Engl J Med* 309:883–887, 1993

58. Bast RC, Xu FJ, Yu YH, et al: CA 125: The past and the future. *Int J Biol Markers* 13:179–187, 1998

59. Jacobs I: Combinations of markers in screening for ovarian cancer. *Int J Gynecol Obstet* 46:83–86, 1994

60. Woolas RP, Xu FJ, Jacobs IJ, et al: Evaluation of multiple serum markers in patients with stage I ovarian cancer. *J Natl Cancer Inst* 85:1748–1751, 1993

61. Berek JS, Bast Jr RC: Ovarian cancer screening: the use of serial complementary tumor markers to improve sensitivity and specificity for early detection. *Cancer* 76:2092–2096, 1995

62. Cane P, Azen C, Lopez E, et al: Tumor marker trends in asymptomatic women at risk for ovarian cancer: relevance for ovarian cancer screening. *Gynecol Oncol* 57:240–245, 1995

63. Skates SJ, Xu FJ, Yu YH, et al: Toward an optimal algorithm for ovarian cancer screening with longitudinal tumor markers. *Cancer* 76:2004–2010, 1995

64. Nagele F, Petru E, Medl M, et al: Preoperative CA 125; an independent prognostic factor in patients with stage I epithelial ovarian cancer. *Obstet Gynecol* 86:259–264 (1995)

65. Rosenthal A, Jacobs I: Ovarian cancer screening. *Semin Oncol* 25:315–323, 1998

66. Van Der Burg MEL, Lammes FB, Van Putten WLJ, et al: Ovarian cancer: the prognostic value of the serum half life of CA 125 during induction chemotherapy. *Gynecol Oncol* 30:307–312, 1988

67. Rustin GJS, Nelstrop AE, McClean P, et al: Defining response of ovarian carcinoma to initial chemotherapy according to serum CA 125. *J Clin Oncol* 14:1545–1551, 1996

68. Wardle FJ, Collins W, Pernet AL, et al: Psychological impact of screening for familial ovarian cancer. *J Natl Cancer Inst* 85:653–657, 1993

69. Tobacman JK, Tucker MA, Kase R, et al: Intra-abdominal carcinomatosis after prophylactic oophorectomy in ovarian cancer-prone families. *Lancet* 11:795–797, 1982

70. Piver MS, Jishi MF, Tsukada Y, et al: Primary peritoneal carcinoma after prophylactic oophorectomy in women with a family history of ovarian cancer: a report of the Gilda Radner Familial Ovarian Cancer Registry. *Cancer* 71:2751–2755, 1993

71. Struewing JP, Watson P, Easton DF, et al: Prophylactic oophorectomy in inherited breast/ovarian cancer families. *J Natl Cancer Inst Monogr* 17:33–35, 1995

72. Bast Jr RC, Boyer CM, Jacobs I: Cell growth regulation in epithelial ovarian cancer. *Cancer* 71:1597–1601, 1993

73. Harris CC, Hollstein M: Clinical implications of the p53 tumor-suppressor gene. *N Engl J Med* 329:1318–1327, 1993

74. Kohler MF, Marks JR, Wiseman RW, et al: Spectrum of mutation and frequency of allelic deletion of the p53 gene in ovarian cancer. *J Natl Cancer Inst* 85:1513–1519, 1998

75. Kupryjnczyk J, Thor AD, Bauchamp R, et al: P53 gene mutations and protein accumulation in human ovarian cancer. *Proc Natl Acad Sci U S A* 90:4961–4965, 1993

76. Ferrell R, Anderson D, Chidambaram A, et al: A genetic linkage study of familial breast-ovarian cancer. *Cancer Genet Cytogenet* 38:241–248, 1989

77. Whang-Pen J, Knutsen T, Douglass E, et al: Cytogenetic studies in ovarian cancer. *Cancer Genet Cytogenet* 11:91–106, 1984

78. Wake N, Hreshchysen M, Piver S, et al: Specific cytogenetic changes in ovarian cancer involving chromosomes 6 and 14. *Cancer Res* 40:4512–4518, 1980

79. Okmota A, Sameshima Y, Yokoyama S, et al: Frequent allelic losses and mutations of the p53 gene in human ovarian cancer. *Cancer Res* 51:5171–5176, 1991

80. Panani A, Ferti-Passantonopoulou A: Common marker chromosomes in ovarian cancer. *Cancer Genet Cytogenet* 16:65–71, 1985

81. Marks JR, Davidoff AM, Kerns BJ, et al: Overexpression and mutation of p53 in epithelial ovarian cancer. *Cancer Res* 51:2979–2984, 1991

82. DiSaia PJ: Diagnosis and Management of Ovarian Cancer. *Hosp Pract* 22: 235–250, 1987

83. Omura GA, Brady MF, Homesley HD, et al: Long term follow up and prognostic factor analysis in advanced ovarian carcinoma: the Gynaecological Oncology Group Experience. *J Clin Oncol* 9:1138–1150, 1991

84. van Houwelingen JC, ten Bokkel Huinink W, van der Burg ATM, et al: Predictability of the survival of patients with ovarian cancer. *J Clin Oncol* 7:769–773, 1989

85. Voest EE, van Houwelingen JC, Nejit JP: A meta-analysis of prognostic factors in advanced ovarian cancer with median survival and overall survival measured with the log (relative risk) as main objectives. *Eur J Cancer Clin Oncol* 28A:1328–1330, 1989

86. Thigpen T, Brady MF, Omura GA, et al: Age as a prognostic factor in ovarian carcinoma. The Gynaecological Oncology Group Experience. *Cancer* 71:606–614, 1993 (suppl)

87. van der Zee AGT, Hollema H, Suurmeijer AJH, et al: Value of p-glycoprotein, glutathione s-transferase pi, c-erbB-2, and p53 as prognostic factors in ovarian carcinomas. *J Clin Oncol* 13:70–78, 1995

88. Igoe BA: Symptoms attributed to ovarian cancer by women with the disease. *Nurse Pract* 22:122–144, 1997

89. Radner G: *It's Always Something.* New York: Avon Books, 1989

90. Ovarian Cancer National Alliance. 1627 K St, NW, 12th floor, Washington, D.C.

91. Brooks SE: Preoperative evaluation of patients with suspected ovarian cancer. *Gynecol Oncol* 55:S80–S90, 1994

92. Karlan BY, Platt LD: The current status of ultrasound and color Doppler imaging in screening for ovarian cancer. *Gynecol Oncol* 55:S28–S33, 1994

93. Mayer AR, Chambers SK, Graves E, et al: Ovarian cancer staging: does it require a gyencologic oncologist? *Gynecol Oncol* 47:223–227, 1992

94. Nguyen HN, Averette HE, Hoskins W, et al: National survey of ovarian carcinoma. Part V. The impact of physicians specialty on patients survival. *Cancer* 72:3663–3670, 1993

95. Eisenkop SM, Spirtos NM, Montag TW, et al: The impact of subspecialty training on the management of advanced ovarian cancer. *Gynecol Oncol* 47:203–209, 1992

96. Scully RE. Tumors of the ovary and maldeveloped gonads, in Rosai J, Sobun LH (eds): *Atlas of Tumor Pathology.* Armed Forces Institute. Washington, D.C.

97. Changes in definition of clinical staging for carcinoma of the cervix and ovary. *Am J Obstet Gynecol* 156:263–264, 1987

98. Partridge EE, Phillips JL, Menck HR: The national cancer database report on ovarian cancer treatment in the United States hospitals. *Cancer* 78:2239–2246, 1996

99. Friedlander ML: Prognostic factors in ovarian cancer. *Semin Oncol* 25:305–314, 1998

100. Griffths CT, Park LM, Fuller AF: Role of cytoreductive surgery in the management of advanced ovarian cancer. *Cancer Treat Rep* 63:235–240, 1979

101. Hogberg T, Carstensen J, Simonsen E: Treatment results and prognostic factors in a population-based study of epithelial ovarian cancer. *Gynecol Oncol* 48:38–49, 1993

102. Eisenkop S, Nalick R, Teng N: Peritoneal implant excision or ablation during cytoreductive surgery. The impact on survival. *Gynecol Oncol* 45:97, 1993 (abstract)

103. Young RC, Walton L, Ellenberg SS, et al: Adjuvant therapy in stage I and II epithelial ovarian cancer. Results of two prospective randomized trials. *N Engl J Med* 322:1021–1027, 1990

104. Bertelson K, Holund B, Anderson E: Reproducibility and prognostic value of histologic type and grade in early epithelial ovarian cancer. *Intl J Gynecol Cancer* 3:72–79, 1993

105. Baak JP, Langley FA, Talerman A, et al: Interpathologist and intrapathologist disagreement in ovarian tumor grading and typing. *Anal Quant Cytol Histol* 8:354–357, 1986

106. Hernandez E, Bhagavan BS, Parmley TH, et al: Interobserver variability in the interpretation of eptihelial ovarian cancer. *Gynecol Oncol* 17:117–123, 1984

107. Shimizu Y, Kamai S, Amada S, et al: Toward the development of a universal grading system for ovarian epithelial carcinoma. *Cancer* 82:893–901, 1998

108. Boente MP, Chi DS, Hoskins WJ: The role of surgery in the management of ovarian cancer: primary and interval cytoreductive surgery. *Semin Oncol* 25:326–334, 1998

109. Munoz KA, Harlan CC, Trimble EL: Patterns of care for women with ovarian cancer in the United States. *J Clin Oncol* 15:3408–3415, 1997

110. Curtin JP, Malik R, Venkatraman ES, et al: Stage IV ovarian cancer: impact of surgical debulking. *Gynecol Oncol* 64:9–12, 1997

111. Van Der Burg MEL, Van Lent WJ, Buyse M, et al: The effect of debulking surgery after induction chemotherapy on the prognosis in advanced epithelial ovarian cancer. *N Engl J Med* 332:629–634, 1995

112. Rubin SC, Hoskins WJ, Hakes TB, et al: Recurrence after negative second look laparotomy for ovarian cancer: analysis of risk factors. *Am J Obstet Gynecol* 159:1094–1098, 1988

113. Nicoletto MO, Tumolo S, Talamini R, et al: Surgical second look in ovarian cancer: a randomized study in patients with laparoscopic complete remission—a Northeastern Oncology Cooperative Group—Ovarian Cancer Cooperative Group Study. *J Clin Oncol* 15:994–997, 1997

114. Potter ME, Hatch KD, Soong SJ, et al: Second look laparotomy and salvage therapy: a research modality only question. *Gynecol Oncol* 44:3–9, 1992

115. Webb MJ, Decker DG, Mussey E, et al: Factors influencing the survival in stage I ovarian cancer. *Am J Obstet Gynecol* 116:222–228, 1973

116. Purola E, Nieminim U: Does rupture of cystic cancer during operation influence the prognosis? *Ann Chir Gynaecol* 57:615–617, 1968

117. Ozols RF, Rubin SC, Thomas G, Robboy S: Epithelial ovarian cancer, in Hoskins WJ, Perez CA, Young RC (eds): *Principles and Practices of Gynecologic Oncology* (ed 2). Philadelphia, Lippincott-Raven, 1997, pp 919–986

118. Schwartz PE: Surgical management of ovarian cancer. *Arch Surg* 116:99–106, 1981

119. Young RC, Decker DG, Wharton JT, et al: Staging laparotomy in early ovarian cancer. *JAMA* 250:3072–3076, 1983

120. Young RC, Pecorelli S: Management of early ovarian cancer. *Semin Oncol* 25:335–339, 1998

121. Young RC, Brady MF, Nieberg RM, et al: Randomized clinical trial of adjuvant treatment of women with early (FIGO I-IIA High Risk) ovarian cancer—GOG #95. Abstract #1376. *Proc Am Soc Clin Oncol* April 1999

122. McGuire WP, Hoskins WJ, Brady MR, et al: Cyclophosphamide and cisplatin compared with paclitaxel and cisplatin in patients with stage III and IV ovarian cancer. *N Engl J Med* 334:1–6, 1996

123. Bolis G, Colombo N, Pecorelli S, et al: Adjuvant treatment for early epithelial ovarian cancer. Results of two randomized clinical trials comparing cisplatin to no further treatment or chromic phosphate (p32). *Ann Oncol* 6:887–893, 1995

124. Vergote IB, Vergote-De Vos LN, Abeler VM, et al: Randomized trial comparing cisplatin with radioactive phosphorous or whole abdomen irradiation as adjuvant treatment of ovarian cancer. *Cancer* 69:741–749, 1992

125. Trope C, Kaern J, Vergote I, et al: Randomized trial of adjuvant carboplatin versus no treatment in stage I high risk ovarian cancer by the Nordic Ovarian Cancer Study Group (NOCOVA). *Proc Am Soc Clin Oncol* 16:352a, 1997

126. Dembo A, Bush R, Beale F, et al: Ovarian carcinoma: improved survival following abdominopelvic irradiation in patients with a completed pelvic operation. *Am J Obstet Gynecol* 134:793–800, 1979

127. Dembo AJ, Bush R, Belae FA, et al: The Princess Margaret Hospital study of ovarian cancer: stages I, II, and asymptomatic presentations. *Cancer Treat Rep* 63:249–254, 1979

128. Smith JP, Rutledge FN, Delclos L: Postoperative treatment of early ovarian cancer of the ovary: a random trial between postoperative irradiation and chemotherapy. *Natl Cancer Instit Monogr* 42:149–153, 1975

129. Young R, Chabner B, Hubbard S, et al: Advanced ovarian adenocarcinoma: a prospective clinical trial of melphalan (L-PAM) versus combination chemotherapy. *N Engl J Med* 299:1261–1266, 1978

130. Omura G, Blessing JA, Ehrlich CE, et al: A randomized trial of cyclophosphamide and doxorubicin, with or without cisplatin, in advanced ovarian carcinoma. *Cancer* 56:1725, 1987

131. Decker DG, Fleming TR, Malkasian GD, et al: Cyclophosphamide plus cis-platinum in combination: treatment program for stage II or IV ovarian carcinoma. *Obstet Gynecol* 60:481–487, 1982

132. Neijt JP, ten Bokkel Huinink WW, van der Burg ME, et al: Randomized trial comparing combination chemotherapy regimens CHAP-5 versus CP in advanced ovarian carcinoma. *J Clin Oncol* 5:1157–1168, 1987

133. Stewart LA for the Advanced Ovarian Cancer Trials Group

(AOCTG). Chemotherapy in advanced ovarian cancer: an overview of randomized clinical trials. *BMJ* 303:884–893, 1991

134. Alberts DS, Green S, Hannigan EV, et al: Improved therapeutic index of carboplatin plus cyclophosphamide versus cisplatin plus cyclophosphamide: final report by the Southwest Oncology Group of a phase III randomized trial in stages III and IV ovarian cancer. *J Clin Oncol* 10:706–717, 1992

135. Swenerton K, Jeffrey J, Sturat G, et al. Cisplatin-cyclophosphamide versus carboplatin-cyclophosphamide in advanced ovarian cancer: a randomized phase III study of the National Cancer Institute of Canada Clinical Trials Group. *J Clin Oncol* 10:718–726, 1992

136. ten Bokkel Huinink WW, van der Burg MEL, van Oosterom AT, et al: Carboplatin in combination therapy for ovarian cancer. *Cancer Treat Rev* 15:9–15, 1988

137. The Ovarian Cancer Meta-Analysis Project: Cyclophosphamide plus cisplatin versus cisplatin plus cyclophosphamide, doxorubicin, and cisplatin chemotherapy of ovarian carcinoma. *J Clin Oncol* 9:1668–1674, 1991

138. Ahern RP, Gore ME: Impact of doxorubicin on survival in ovarian cancer. *J Clin Oncol* 13:726–732, 1995

139. Fanning J, Bennett TZ, Hilgers RD: Meta-analysis of cisplatin, doxorubicin, and cyclophosphamide chemotherapy of ovarian carcinoma. *Obstet Gynecol* 80:954–960, 1993

140. Torri V: Randomized study of cyclophosphamide doxorubicin and cisplatin (CAP) vs. single agent carboplatin in ovarian cancer patients requiring chemotherapy: interim results of ICON2. *Proc Am Soc Clin Oncol* 15:280, 1996 (abstr)

141. Trimble EL, Adams JD, Vena D, et al: Paclitaxel for platinum-refractory ovarian cancer: results from the first 1,000 patients registered to National Cancer Institute Treatment Referral Center 9103. *J Clin Oncol* 11:2405–2410, 1993

142. Piccart MJ, Bertelsen K, Stuart G, et al: Is cisplatin-paclitaxel the standard in first-line treatment of advanced ovarian cancer: The EORTC-GCCG, NOCOVA, NCI-C and Scottish intergroup experience. *Proc Am Soc Clin Oncol* 16: A1258, 1997 (abstr)

143. Muggia FM, Braly PS, Brady MR, et al: Phase III trial of cisplatin or paclitaxel, versus their combination in suboptimal stage III and IV epithelial ovarian cancer: Gynecologic Oncology Group study #132. *Proc Am Soc Clin Oncol* 16: A1257, 1997 (abstr)

144. Ozols RF: Ovarian cancer practice guidelines. *Oncology* 11: 95–105, 1997

145. Stuart G, Bertelsen K, Mangioni C, et al: Updated analysis shows a highly significant improved overall survival (os) for cisplatin-paclitaxel as first-line treatment of advanced ovarian cancer. Mature results of the EORTC-GCCG, NOCOVA, NCI-C, CTG and Scottish intergroup trial. *Proc Am Soc Clin Oncol* 17:361, 1998 (abstr)

146. Neijt JP, Hansen M, Hansen SW, et al: Randomized phase III study in previously untreated epithelial ovarian cancer FIGO Stage IIB, IIC, III, IV, comparing paclitaxel-cisplatin and paclitaxel-carboplatin. *Proc Am Soc Clin Oncol* 16:352a, 1997 (abstr)

147. DuBois A, Richter B, Warm M, et al: Cisplatin/paclitaxel vs. carboplatin/paclitaxel as first-line treatment in ovarian cancer. *Proc Am Soc Clin Oncol* 17:361a, 1998

148. Ozols RF, Bundy BN, Fowler J, et al: Randomized phase III study of cisplatin (CIS)/paclitaxel (PAC) versus carboplatin (CARBO)/PAC in optimal stage III epithelial ovarian cancer (OC): a Gynecological Oncology Group Trial (GOG158). *Proc Am Soc Clin Oncol* 18:356a, 1999 (abstr)

149. Jakobsen A, Bertelsen K, Anderson JE, et al: Dose-effect study of carboplatin in ovarian cancer. A Danish Ovarian Cancer Group Study. *J Clin Oncol* 15:193–198, 1997

150. Gore M, Mainwaring P, A'Hern R, et al: Randomized trial of dose-intensity with single-agent carboplatin in patients with epithelial ovarian cancer. *J Clin Oncol* 16:2426–2434, 1998

151. Olson JK, Sood AK, Sorosky JI, et al: Taxol hypersensitivity: rapid retreatment is safe and cost effective. *Gynecol Oncol* 68:25–28, 1998

152. Eltabbakh GH, Piver MS, Hempling RE, et al: Prolonged disease-free survival by maintenance chemotherapy among patients with recurrent platinum-sensitive ovarian cancer. *Gynecol Oncol* 71:190–195, 1998

153. Thigpen JT, Vance RB, Khansur T: Second-line chemotherapy for recurrent carcinoma of the ovary. *Cancer* 71: 1559–1564, 1993

154. Markman M: Intraperitoneal therapy of ovarian cancer. *Semin Oncol* 25:356–360, 1998

155. Markman M, Reichman B, Hakes T, et al: Responses to second-line cisplatin-based intraperitoneal therapy in ovarian cancer: Influence of a prior response to intravenous cisplatin. *J Clin Oncol* 9:1801–1805, 1991

156. Alberts DS, Liu PY, Hannigan EV, et al: Intraperitoneal cisplatin plus intravenous cyclophosphamide versus intravenous cisplatin plus intravenous cyclophosphamide for stage III ovarian cancer. *N Engl J Med* 335:1950–1955, 1996

157. Markman M, Bundy B, Benda J, et al: Randomized phase III study of intravenous cisplatin/paclitaxel versus moderately high dose IV carboplatin followed by paclitaxel and intraperitoneal cisplatin in optimal residual ovarian cancer: an intergroup trial (GOG, SWOG, ECOG). *Proc Am Soc Clin Oncol* 17:361a, 1998 (abstr)

158. Barakat R, Almadrones L, Venkatraman E, et al: A phase II trial of intraperitoneal cisplatin and etoposide as consolidation therapy in patients with stage II–IV epithelial ovarian cancer following negative surgical assessment. *Gynecol Oncol* 64:294, 1997

159. Lanciano R, Reddy S, Corn B, et al: Update on the role of radiotherapy in ovarian cancer. *Semin Oncol* 25:361–371, 1998

160. Gilblum D, Mychalczak B, Alomadrones L: Palliative benefit of external-beam radiation in the management of platinum refractory epithelial ovarian cancer. *Gynecol Oncol* 69: 36–41, 1998

161. Stiff PJ, Bayer R, Kerger C, et al: High-dose chemotherapy with autologous transplantation for persistent/relapsed ovarian cancer: a multivariate analysis of survival for 100 consecutively treated patients. *J Clin Oncol* 15:1309–1317, 1997

162. Auersperg N, Edelson MI, Mok SC, et al: The biology of ovarian cancer. *Semin Oncol* 25:281–304, 1998

163. Ozols RF: Treatment of recurrent ovarian cancer: increasing options-"recurrent" results. *J Clin Oncol* 15:2177–2180, 1997

164. Lehnert M: Clinical multidrug resistance in cancer: a multifactorial problem. *Eur J Cancer* 32A:927–944, 1996

165. Liu JR, Fletcher B, Page C, et al: BCl-xl is expressed in ovarian carcinoma and modulates chemotherapy induced apoptosis. *Gynecol Oncol* 70:398–403, 1998

166. Niloff JM, Knapp RC, Lavin PT, et al: The CA-125 assay

as a predictor of clinical recurrence in epithelial ovarian cancer. *Am J Obstet Gynecol* 155:56–60, 1986

167. Zanaboni F, Presti M, Scarfone G, et al: CA-125 reliability in predicting ovarian cancer recurrence. *Tumori* 75:69–71, 1989

168. Markman M, Iseminger K, Hatch KD, et al: Tamoxifen in platinum-refractory ovarian cancer. A gynecologic oncology group ancillary report. *Gynecol Oncol* 62:4–6, 1996

169. van der Velden J, Gitsch G, Wain GV, et al: Tamoxifen in patients with advanced epithelial ovarian cancer. *Int J Gynecol Cancer* 5:301–305, 1995

170. Roland PY, Barnes MN, Niwas S, et al: Response to salvage treatment in recurrent ovarian cancer treated initially with paclitaxel and platinum based combination regimens. *Gynecol Oncol* 68:178–182, 1998

171. McGuire WP, Ozols RF: Chemotherapy of advanced ovarian cancer. *Semin Oncol* 25:340–348, 1998

172. Williams SD: Ovarian germ cell tumors: an update. *Semin Oncol* 25:407–413, 1998

173. Aure JC, Hoeg K, Kolstad P: Clinical and histologic studies of ovarian carcinoma. Long term follow up of 990 cases. *Obstet Gynecol* 37:1–9, 1971

174. Trimble CL, Trimble EL: Management of epithelial ovarian tumors of low malignant potential. *Gynecol Oncol* 55: 552–561, 1994

175. Lu KH, Bell DA, Welch WR, et al: Evidence for multifocal origin of unilateral and advanced human serous borderline ovarian tumors. *Cancer Res* 58:2328–2330, 1998

176. Ingelman-Sandberg A: Classification and staging of malignant tumours of the female pelvis. *Acta Obstet Gynecol Scand* 50:1–7, 1971

177. Serov SF, Scully RE, Solun LH: Histologic typing of ovarian tumours, in *International Histologic Classifiscation of Tumours no. 9*. Geneva, World Health Organization, 1973

178. Tucci RA, Bartels KL: Ovarian cancer surgery: a clinical pathway. *Clin J Oncol Nurs* 2:65–66, 1998

179. Ferrell BR, Dow KH, Leigh S, et al: Quality of life in long-term cancer survivors. *Oncol Nurs Forum* 22:915–922, 1995

180. Olopade OI, Ultmann JE: Malignant effusions. *CA Cancer J Clin* 41:166–179, 1991

181. Walczak JR, Heckman CS: Ascites, in Yarbro CH, Frogge MH, Goodman M (eds): *Cancer Symptom Management* (ed 2). Sudbury, MA, Jones and Bartlett, 1999, pp 405–415

182. Puls LE, Duniho T, Hunter JE, et al: The prognostic implication of ascites in advanced-stage ovarian cancer. *Gynecol Oncol* 61:109–112, 1996

183. Martin VH: Managing symptoms associated with ovarian cancer, in *Negotiating Optimal Ovarian Cancer Care: A Clinicians Guide*. (Monograph) Balacywood, PA. Meniscus Ltd. Educational Institute, 1999, pp 18–26

184. Kraemer K., Lynch MP: Ascites, in Preston FA, Cunningham RS (eds): *Clinical Guidelines for Symptom Management in Oncology*. New York, Clinical Insights Press, 1998, pp 115–119

185. Kelvin JF, Scagliola J: Metastases involving the gastrointestinal system. *Semin Oncol Nurs* 14:187–198, 1999

186. Bain VG, Minuk GY: Jaundice, ascites, and hepatic encephalopathy, in Doyle D, Hanks GWC, MacDonald N (eds): *Oxford Textbook of Palliative Medicine*. Oxford, Oxford University, 1993, pp 337–348

187. Kehoe C: Malignant ascites: etiology, diagnosis, and treatment. *Oncol Nurs Forum* 18:523–530, 1991

188. Abrahm JL: Promoting symptom control in palliative care. *Semin Oncol Nurs* 14:95–109, 1998

189. Drakes TP: Resolution of bowel obstruction due to newly diagnosed inoperable advanced ovarian cancer with medical therapy. *West J Med* 155:76–77, 1991

190. Chang AE, August DA: Acute abdomen, bowel obstruction, and fistula, in Abeloff MD, Armitage JO, Lichter AS, Niederhuber JE (eds): *Clinical Oncology*. New York, Churchill Livingstone, 1995, pp 583–597

191. Summers RW, Lu CC: Approach to the patient with ileus and obstruction, in Yamada T (ed): *Textbook of Gastroenterology* (ed 2). Philadelphia, Lippincott, 1995, pp 796–812

192. Rust DM: Anorexia and cachexia, in Yasko JM (ed): *Management of Symptoms Associated with Chemotherapy*. Bala Cynwyd, PA, Meniscus Health Care Communications, 1998, pp 35–54

193. Grant MM, Rivera LM: Anorexia, cachexia, and dysphagia: the symptom experience. *Semin Oncol Nurs* 11:266–271, 1995

194. Cunningham R: Nutrition in Cancer: An overview *Semin Oncol Nurs*, May 2000 (in press)

195. Dewys WD, Begg C, Lavin PT, et al: Prognostic effect of weight loss prior to chemotherapy in cancer patients. *Am J Med* 69:491–497, 1980

196. Oversen L, Allingstrup L, Hannibal J, et al: Effect of dietary counseling on food intake, body weight, response rate, survival, and quality of life in cancer patients undergoing chemotherapy: a prospective, randomized study. *J Clin Oncol* 11:2043–2049, 1993

197. Tchekmedyian NS, Hickman M, Heber D: Treatment of anorexia and weight loss with megestrol acetate in patients with cancer or acquired immunodeficiency syndrome. *Semin Oncol* 18:35–42, 1991 (suppl 2)

198. Loprinzi CL, Ellison NM, Schard DJ, et al: Controlled trial of megesterol acetate for the treatment of anorexia and cachexia. *J Natl Cancer Inst* 82:1127–1132, 1990

199. Schmoll E, Wilke H, Thole R, et al: Megestrol acetate in cancer cachexia. *Semin Oncol* 18:32–34, 1991 (suppl 2)

200. Bruera E, MacMillan K, Kuehn N, et al: A controlled trial of megestrol acetate on appetite, caloric intake, nutritional status, and other symptoms in patients with advanced ovarian cancer. *Cancer* 66:1279–1282, 1990

201. Joyce M, Cunningham RS: Metastases that interfere with circulation. *Semin Oncol Nurs* 14:230–239, 1998

202. Ascherl P: Lymphedema. *Soc Gynecol Oncol Nurs J* 8:9–11, 1998

203. Kalinowski BH: Lymphedema, in Yarbro CH, Frogge MH, Goodman M (eds): *Cancer Symptom Management* (ed 2). Sudbury, MA, Jones and Bartlett, 1999, pp 457–486

204. Cutter K, Atkins B: Freedom from lymphedema. *Soc Gynecol Oncol Nurs J* 6:11–13, 1996

205. Shuey KM: Heart, lung, and endocrine complications of solid tumors. *Semin Oncol* 10:177–188, 1994

206. Rubin SC, Sutton GP: *Ovarian Cancer*. New York, McGraw-Hill, 1993, pp 361–373

207. Kerr VE, Cadman E: Pulmonary metastasis in ovarian cancer: analysis of 357 patients. *Cancer* 56:1209–1213, 1985

208. McCoy AM, Mierzewski A: Acute oncologic disorders, in Kinney MR, Packa DR, Dunbar SB (eds): *AACN's Clinical Reference for Critical Care Nursing* (ed 3). St. Louis, Mosby, 1993, pp 1077–1097

209. Harwood KV: Dyspnea, in Yarbro CH, Frogge MH, Goodman M (eds): Cancer Symptom Management (ed 2). Sudbury, MA, Jones and Bartlett, 1999, pp 45–57

210. Smith EL: Pulmonary metastasis. *Semin Oncol Nurs* 14: 178–186, 1998

211. Powell L, Midler A, Steiner A: Concerns of women with

ovarian cancer: a qualitative investigation. *Quality of Life—A Nursing Challenge* 6:92–101, 1998

212. Steiginga SK, Dunn J: Women's experiences following treatment for gynecologic cancer. *Oncol Nurs Forum* 24: 1403–1410, 1997

213. Zacharis D, Gilg C, Foxall M: Quality of life and coping in patients with gynecologic cancer and their spouses. *Oncol Nurs Forum* 21:1699–1706, 1994

214. Kornblith AB, Thaler HT, Wong G, et al: Quality of life of women with ovarian cancer. *Gynecol Oncol* 59:231–242, 1995

215. Ersek M, Ferrell BR, Dow KH, et al: Quality of life in women with ovarian cancer. *West J Nurs Res* 19:334–350, 1997

216. Guidozzi F: Living with ovarian cancer. *Gynecol Oncol* 50: 202–207, 1993

217. Burnett CB: Ovarian cancer: advocacy, quality of life, and politics. *Quality of Life—A Nursing Challenge* 4:73–77, 1996

218. Melancon C: From victim to victor: a personal perspective of ovarian cancer. *Quality of Life—A Nursing Challenge* 4: 78–81, 1996

CHAPTER 63

Pancreatic Cancer

JoAnn Coleman, RN, MS, ACNP-CS, AOCN

Introduction

Pancreatic cancer accounts for 2% of new cancer cases in the United States as well as worldwide.[1] During the past two decades, the incidence has peaked and plateaued,[2,3] with a current estimate of 29,000 new cases of pancreatic cancer each year and an equal number of deaths from pancreatic cancer in the United States.[1] The disease has a poor prognosis and is considered by many to be one of the deadliest malignancies. Less than 20% of affected individuals survive one year after diagnosis, and the overall five-year survival is only 3%.[4]

Pancreatic cancer is one of the most difficult tumors to detect or diagnose because of the anatomic location of the pancreas. It is also difficult to treat due to the biologic nature of the tumor. Its onset is insidious, with signs and symptoms that occur late, are vague and misleading, and mimic other diseases. The individual with pancreatic cancer typically will ignore the initial signs and symptoms or rely on self-treatment for months until jaundice or other prominent and intolerable signs appear.

Recent advances in basic science and improved technology have provided a better understanding of the pathogenesis and clinical management of cancer of the pancreas.[5] It is hoped that a growing understanding of the biology and molecular genetics and the influence of growth factors on the progression of pancreatic cancer will provide opportunities for advances in prevention, earlier tumor detection, and more effective and novel therapies.

Table 63-1 Risk Factors for Pancreatic Cancer

Demographic Factors	Advancing age
	Black race
	Male gender
	Jewish religion
	Geography
Environmental Factors	Tobacco
	Radiation
Dietary Factors	Carbohydrate
	Cholesterol
	Meat
	Salt
	Dehydrated food
	Fried food
	Refined sugar
	Soybeans
	Nitrosamines
Occupational Factors	Chemists
	Coal gas workers
	Metal industries
	Aluminum milling
	Leather tanning
	Textile industry
	Building trades
	Transportation
	Butchers
	Flour industry
	Ethylene chlorhydrin
	Halogenated hydrocarbons
	Chlorinated water
	DDT
Host Factors	Diabetes
	Chronic pancreatitis
	Genetic syndromes

Epidemiology

The demographics of pancreatic cancer have been widely investigated (Table 63-1). Age is the strongest risk factor for pancreatic cancer, with the peak incidence between ages 60 and 80.[6] Although cancer of the pancreas can occur in individuals younger than age 40, it is uncommon.[7] Pancreatic carcinoma is almost equal among males and females.[1] The incidence of pancreatic cancer is slightly higher in blacks and among members of the Jewish religion. Geography has been considered a possible risk factor. The incidence rates of pancreatic cancer are highest in Western and industrialized countries, and lowest in underdeveloped nations. Studies have been inconclusive regarding the risk of pancreatic cancer and socioeconomic status and migrant status.[6]

Etiology

Numerous environmental factors may be associated with increased risk of pancreatic cancer. Cigarette smoking is the risk factor with the strongest association with pancreatic cancer.[8-10] The risk increases with the number of cigarettes smoked, but risk decreases after cessation of smoking.[11] Alcohol and coffee consumption have been implicated, but there is insufficient evidence to confirm these observations.[12-17] Exposure to radiation has also been investigated as a risk for pancreatic carcinogenesis. Persons irradiated in infancy for skin hemangioma have been reported to have an increased risk of pancreatic cancer.[18]

Many epidemiologic studies have examined the role of diet and pancreatic cancer, but the relationship remains unclear.[19,20] A number of studies have reported an association between pancreatic cancer and increasing ingestion of carbohydrate, cholesterol, meat, salt, dehydrated food, fried food, refined sugar, soybeans, and nitrosamines. The studies do not support an association with pancreatic cancer and excess intake of dietary fat or beta carotene.[19] A decreased risk or perhaps a protective effect has been reported for fiber, vitamin C, fruits, vegetables, preservative-free foods, raw foods, and the use of pressure cooking and microwave cooking.[6]

Obesity as a risk factor for pancreatic cancer suggests that energy balance may play an important role in pancreatic carcinogenesis.[21]

Numerous studies have examined certain occupational exposures. Cancer of the pancreas has been reported to occur among chemists and coal gas workers and among individuals working in metal industries, aluminum milling, and the leather tanning industry. There have been reports of increased risk associated with exposure to welding materials, paint thinners, refuse and detergents, and floor cleaning agents as well as petroleum products. Butchers, transportation workers, and workers in flour mills where pesticides were used more frequently than other segments of the industry are occupations considered to be a possible risk. Workers exposed to DDT during the manufacturing process were at risk. Those workers exposed during production of ethylene chlorhydin, halogenated hydrocarbons, and consumption of chlorinated water have also been implicated between exposure and disease.[6]

The relationship between diabetes and pancreatic cancer is inconclusive.[9,10,22] Studies demonstrate no consistent association of diabetes with cancer of the pancreas, except in cases where diabetes was diagnosed immediately before the cancer diagnosis.[23] Diabetes is more commonly an early symptom of pancreatic cancer rather than a causative influence. In addition, data indicate that pancreatic cancer occurs with increasing frequency among persons with long-standing diabetes.[24]

A relationship between chronic pancreatitis and pancreatic cancer has been suggested for pancreatitis that occurs within the ten years before the diagnosis of pancreatic cancer.[25] Some form of chronic pancreatitis may represent an indolent manifestation of cancer of the pancreas.[26-29] Other conditions possibly associated with pancreatic cancer are thyroid and other endocrine tumors, cystic fibrosis, and pernicious anemia.[6]

Peptic ulcer surgery and cholecystectomy have also been linked to pancreatic cancer. The initial symptoms of pancreatic cancer can mimic biliary tract disease, which in turn may lead to cholecystectomy and pancreatic cancer.

Genetics

With advances in the understanding of human genetics, it is now known that cancer of the pancreas is a disease of acquired and inherited mutations in cancer-causing genes. The development of cancer of the pancreas has been associated with the activation of the oncogene, *K-RAS*, the inactivation of multiple tumor suppressor genes, and DNA mismatch repair.[30] Specifically, the *p16* tumor suppressor gene is inactivated in approximately 95% of pancreatic cancers.[31,32] The second most important tumor suppressor gene is *p53*, which is inactivated in 50%–70% of pancreatic cancers.[33] The *DPC4* (deleted in pancreatic cancer on locus 4) gene is specific for pancreatic cancer and is inactivated in approximately 50% of pancreatic cancers.[34] The *BRCA2* gene is inactivated in only 7% of pancreatic cancers, but is noteworthy because the mutations in *BRCA2* associated with pancreatic cancer are inherited mutations.[35]

K-RAS is the most frequently activated oncogene in pancreatic cancer. More than 90% of pancreatic cancers harbor activating mutations in *K-RAS*, and most of these mutations are in codon 12 of the gene. The localization of these mutations to a single codon makes them relatively easy to detect.[36]

The DNA mismatch repair genes are the last group of cancer-causing genes that have been found to play a role in the development of pancreatic cancer. When these DNA repair genes do not function appropriately, errors in DNA replication are not repaired. Approximately 4% of pancreatic cancers have been found to contain genetic alterations in DNA mismatch repair genes. This subgroup of cancers may arise through a pathway separate from that of the usual ductal carcinomas and therefore may have a more favorable prognosis.[37]

Cancer of the pancreas clusters within families. There are two broad groups of familial aggregation of pancreatic cancer: those associated with known syndromes and those without such an association.[38] Six genetic syndromes are associated with an increased risk of developing pancreatic cancer. (See Table 63-2.)

Hereditary pancreatitis is a rare disease characterized by recurrent episodes of severe epigastric pain and hyperamylasemia, with an onset usually before age 10. Individuals affected with this disease are at increased risk for the development of pancreatic pseudocysts, pancreatic exocrine insufficiency, chronic pancreatitis, diabetes mellitus, and pancreatic cancer.[39]

Hereditary nonpolyposis colorectal cancer (HNPCC) can predispose some families to the development of pancreatic cancer, but the contribution of this syndrome to the numbers of individuals with pancreatic cancer appears to be small.[40] *BRCA2* has been found to be associated not only with an increased risk of breast cancer but also cancer of the ovaries, prostate, colon, and pancreas.[35,41]

Familial atypical multiple mole melanoma syndrome (FAMMM) is characterized by multiple nevi, atypical nevi, and multiple melanomas. The gene responsible for the FAMMM syndrome is the *p16* tumor suppressor gene.[42]

The ataxia-telangiectasia syndrome is associated with disabling cerebellar ataxia, oculocutaneous telangiectasia, and humoral and cellular immune deficiencies. The *ATM* gene is responsible for this syndrome and individuals that carry this genetic mutation are also at increased

Table 63-2 Genetic Syndromes Predisposing to Pancreatic Cancer

Hereditary pancreatitis

Hereditary nonpolyposis colorectal cancer (HNPCC)

Familial breast cancer (linked to *BRCA2* tumor suppressor gene)

Familial atypical multiple mole melanoma syndrome (FAMMM)

Ataxia-telangiectasia syndrome

Peutz-Jeghers syndrome

risk for the development of cancers of the breast, ovaries, biliary tract, stomach, and pancreas.[43]

The Peutz-Jeghers syndrome is characterized by hamartomatous polyps of the gastrointestinal tract and by mucocutaneous melanin deposition. These individuals are at an increased risk of developing multiple cancers and have a 100-fold greater incidence of pancreatic cancers than expected.[44] The gene responsible for this syndrome has been found on a region of chromosone 19p.[45]

Studies of families without a genetic syndrome in which an aggregation of pancreatic carcinoma exists help researchers understand the genetic alterations associated with the development of cancer of the pancreas. A recent analysis of familial pancreatic tumor data looked at similarities and differences between familial and sporadic cases. There was no difference in the age at which pancreatic cancer was diagnosed between the two groups of cases, with both groups having a mean age of 65 years.[30]

Growth Factors

Various growth factors and their receptors are important in the regulation of pancreatic cancer cell growth. Overexpression of specific growth factors and their receptors may contribute to the biologic aggressiveness of pancreatic cancer.[46]

The epidermal growth factor receptor (EGFR) binds a family of peptides that includes epidermal growth factor (EGF), transforming growth factor *a* (TGF-*a*), heparin-binding EGF-like growth factor, amphiregulin, betacellulin, and epiregulin. These growth factors may all contribute to pancreatic cell growth. Overexpression of EGFR has been linked to enhanced metastatic potential and increased tumor invasiveness.[47]

The transforming growth factor *B*(TGF-*B*) polypeptide family has been implicated in the development of pancreatic cancer. Overexpression of TGF-*B* enhances tumor development by promoting tumor angiogenesis, altering extracellular array/matrix, and enhancing adhesiveness that facilitates tumor metastasis.[46] Overexpression of TGF-*B* has been associated with a shorter postoperative survival or worse prognosis in individuals with pancreatic adenocarcinoma.[48]

The fibroblast growth factor (FGF) family consists of many polypeptide growth factors that have an affinity for heparin, which results in changes in cell differentiation and tissue repair.[49] A current hypothesis is that FGFs enhance pancreatic cell growth and may contribute to abnormal epithelial–mesenchymal interactions inside the growing tumor.[50]

The insulin-like growth factor I (IGF-I) is also overexpressed in pancreatic cancer cells and enhances the growth of those cells.[51]

Other analyses that evidence genetic alterations in pancreatic cancer-causing genes are karyotyping, comparative genomic hybridization (CGH), and allelotyping. Karyotyping can help to identify specific chromosomes lost or gained in pancreatic cancer. Comparative genomic

hybridization has been used to screen for gains or losses of chromosomes material within the tumor DNA. Finally, allelotyping has allowed for improved exactness in determining genetic material. Examination of pancreatic adenocarcinomas has revealed high frequencies of losses at specific chromosome arms.[38]

Prevention, Screening, and Early Detection

Prevention of pancreatic cancer will require definitive identification of factors demonstrated to cause or place individuals at a high risk of developing pancreatic cancer. Then reduction or elimination of these risk factors may prevent cancer of the pancreas. This is an insidious disease with little that is known about the best treatment, much less the cause.

The general hypothesis currently being tested is that adenocarcinoma of the pancreas represents a multistep disease involving progressive, acquired genetic rearrangements in cancer-causing genes. These mutations are detectable in stool, duodenal fluid, pancreatic juice samples, bile, and blood, and they may become an accurate screening marker for pancreatic cancer to easily detect persons at risk.[52,53]

Pathophysiology

Pancreatic cancer is most commonly an adenocarcinoma that originates from the cells lining the pancreatic duct.[52] Tumors of the pancreas develop in both the endocrine and the exocrine parenchyma (See Table 63-3). Approximately 90% of tumors arise from the exocrine pancreas, which contains two major types of epithelium: acinar and ductal. The acinar cells of the pancreas produce digestive enzymes, whereas the cells lining the pancreatic duct are responsible for the secretion of fluid and electrolytes and the conveyance of pancreatic juice to the duodenum.

Cellular Characteristics

Adenocarcinomas of the pancreas usually are whitish-yellow, hard, nodular, poorly defined, firm masses surrounded by dense reactive fibrous tissue. Tumors may vary from well differentiated to undifferentiated and exhibit variable gland formation, irregular cell size, and variable nuclear changes. Because of the tumor's infiltrative nature, visualizing the complete extent of the disease is difficult. Many ductal adenocarcinomas of the pancreas infiltrate into vascular spaces, lymphatic spaces, and perineural spaces, which can be appreciated only on microscopic examination.[53]

Lesions in the pancreatic ducts and ductules frequently are first found on histologic examination in resected pancreatic specimens. Precursor lesions may progress from flat duct lesions, to papillary duct lesions without atypia, to papillary duct lesions with atypia, and finally to infiltrating adenocarcinoma of the pancreas.[54–56] (See Figure 63-1)

Adenosquamous carcinoma of the pancreas is a rare variant of ductal adenocarcinoma that shows both glandular (adeno) and squamous differentiation. This variation is more common in individuals who have received previous chemotherapy or radiation therapy. The biologic behavior of adenosquamous carcinoma is the same as the typical ductal adenocarcinomas. Adenosquamous carcinoma has an especially poor prognosis.[53]

A small percentage of pancreatic cancers are classified as acinar cell carcinomas that have a distinct histologic appearance and an unusual clinical presentation. Most individuals with acinar cell carcinoma have biliary or gastrointestinal obstruction because of the tumor. Individuals with acinar cell carcinoma fare better than those with ductal adenocarcinoma.[57] Giant cell carcinoma accounts for approximately 5% of primary nonendocrine pancreatic malignancies. Giant cell carcinomas arise with equal frequency in the head, body, and tail regions of the pancreas. These pancreatic carcinomas are associated with a poorer prognosis than ductal adenocarcinomas.[53]

Cystic neoplasms of the pancreas, arising from the exocrine pancreas, are classified as either benign serous cystadenomas, potentially malignant mucinous cystadenomas, or malignant cystadenocarcinomas.[58] Most serous cystic neoplasms are benign and the prognosis for individuals with resected mucinous cystadenomas is excellent.[59]

Intraductal papillary-mucinous neoplasms (IPMN) are relatively newly reported neoplasms that occur with equal frequency in both sexes. Most individuals with this tumor are found to have mucin oozing from the ampulla of Vater during endoscopic assessment.[60,61] Patients with

Table 63-3	Pathology of Exocrine Pancreatic Cancer

Solid tumors
  Ductal adenocarcinomas
  Adenosquamous carcinoma
  Acinar cell carcinoma
  Giant cell carcinoma

Cystic tumors
  Serous cystic neoplasms
  Mucinous cystic neoplasms
  Intraductal papillary mucinous neoplasms (IPMN)
  Solid and cystic papillary neoplasms (Hamoudi tumor)

IPMN usually have favorable outcomes after resection, but metastases can occur.

Solid and cystic papillary neoplasms of the pancreas, also called *Hamoudi tumors*, occur primarily in women in their third and fourth decades of life. These tumors have solid, cystic, and papillary components when viewed microscopically. Most individuals are cured after surgical resection, although metastases have been reported.[62]

The most common tumor sites that may metastasize to the pancreas are breast, lung, colorectum, melanoma, and renal cell carcinoma. Systemic neoplasms such as leukemia and lymphoma can involve the pancreas. The pancreas may be the presenting site for these cancers.[53] Most pancreatic lymphomas are non-Hodgkin's lymphomas. Pancreatic lymphomas are rare, but early recognition is important because of their dramatic response to chemotherapy.[63]

Endocrine or islet cell tumors constitute the remainder of pancreatic malignant tumors. These uncommon tumors account for approximately 5% of all pancreatic neoplasms. Many islet cell tumors secrete excessive hormones, resulting in significant clinical manifestations. Nonfunctional islet cell tumors do not produce obvious clinical manifestations and are usually detected because of their space-occupying characteristics or as an incidental finding.[64]

Islet cell tumors arise from the endocrine parenchyma. The tumors usually occur as small, well-circumscribed, reddish-orange tissue that rarely extends beyond the pancreas. On microscopy, islet cell tumors are well vascularized and encapsulated, usually compressing adjacent parenchyma. Fibrosis and calcification may be seen. Malignant islet cell tumors are difficult to distinguish because they closely resemble normal islet cells and retain secretory or synthetic functions. The presence of metastases is the most reliable criterion for establishing malignancy.[64] Chapter 52 presents a more detailed discussion of endocrine tumors.

Progression of Disease

Tumors of the head of the pancreas are those arising to the right of the left border of the superior mesentric vein. The uncinate process is part of the head of the

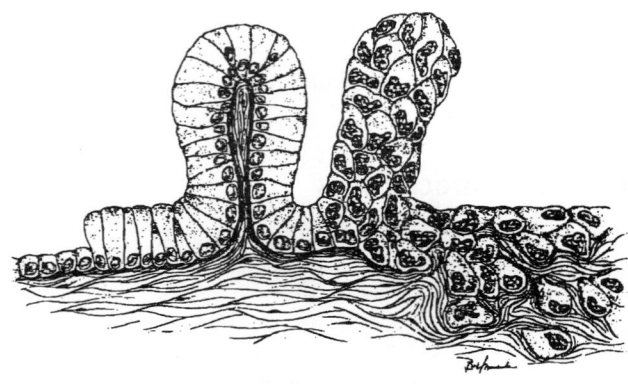

Figure 63-1 Progression from normal duct epithelium (left) to low-grade pancreatic intraepithelial neoplasia (PanIN) to high-grade PanIN to infiltrating cancer (right). (Used with permission from Wilentz RE, Hruban RH. Pathology of cancer of the pancreas. *Surgical Oncology Clinics of North America.* 7(1) 43–65, 1998. p 47.)[55]

pancreas. Tumors of the body of the pancreas are those arising between the left border of the superior mesenteric vein and the left border of the aorta. Tumors of the tail of the pancreas are those arising between the left border of the aorta and the hilum of the spleen.

Pancreatic cancer arises in the head, neck, or uncinate process of the pancreas in 60%–70% of cases. About 15% of tumors develop in the body and tail of the gland, and the remaining 20% diffusely involve the entire gland.[38]

Tumors in the head of the gland are often detected at a small size (2–3 cm). The bile duct is invaded early in the course of the disease, causing obstruction of the distal common bile duct. This obstruction accounts for easily recognized symptoms, such as jaundice, which enable detection of smaller tumors. Extension beyond the pancreas is the rule rather than the exception. Ductal adenocarcinomas usually infiltrate into vascular perineural and lymphatic spaces. These tumors tend to invade local structures, such as the duodenum and retroperitoneum, either directly or along the course of autonomic nerves of the celiac plexus. Some degree of perineural invasion is present in 90% of cases. The portal or superior vein may also be invaded. Venous invasion or encasement by tumor growth may result in obstruction, thrombosis, ascites, and portal hypertension. Vascular encasement and neural infiltration can contribute to severe back pain. Involvement of the mesenteric vessels may preclude resection of these tumors.

In the body and tail of the pancreas, tumors are often larger than 5 cm before they produce symptoms. Tumors of the body and tail of the pancreas can invade the splenic vein resulting in thrombosis and gastric varices.[38]

Patterns of Spread

At the time of detection, the tumor may be fixed to tissues behind the pancreas or to the vertebral column. The tumor may directly invade surrounding organs, such as kidney, spleen, or diaphragm. Invasion of the celiac nerve plexus may account for unrelenting pain. Other sites of local invasion, which tends to occur later, include the superior mesenteric and splenic arteries, transverse colon, stomach, kidneys, and left adrenal gland.[65] Obstruction of the portal vein and tributaries can lead to portal hypertension and esophageal varices.

Characteristically, tumors of the pancreas grow slowly, with late signs and symptoms of pathology. At the time of diagnosis, 90% of cases have perineural invasion, 70%–80% have lymphatic spread, 50% have venous involvement, and 20%–25% have duodenal invasion. The liver, peritoneum, and regional lymph nodes are the most commonly involved structures.[66] Supraclavicular nodes (Virchow nodes) may be involved more frequently with carcinoma of the body and tail of the pancreas. Metastatic deposits reach the liver through the portal bloodstream or lymphatics. Peritoneal seeding by metastatic deposits also occurs. The frequency of lymph node metastasis correlates with the size of the primary tumor.[67]

Clinical Manifestations

The early signs and symptoms of pancreatic cancer are vague, nonspecific, and gradual, which often contributes to a delay in diagnosis by both the individual and the physician. Specific symptoms usually develop late and only after invasion or obstruction of a nearby structure. Careful assessment and extensive inquiry into the character, onset, duration, and modulators of presenting signs and symptoms is important. Manifestations of disease differ according to the location of the tumor (see Table 63-4). A clinical suspicion of pancreatic cancer must be high to identify the presence of a tumor. Individuals that have resectable pancreatic cancer tend to present with few symptoms.

Weight loss and clinical wasting are classic symptoms of cancer of the pancreas, particularly when the tumor is located in the head of the gland. Initially the weight loss may not cause concern and may be attributed to gastric maladies. As the cancer advances, significant weight loss is common and often accelerated by pain, anorexia, flatulence, nausea, and vomiting. Duodenal obstruction, with nausea and vomiting, is a late manifestation of pancreatic cancer. Tumor involvement of the pancreas prevents secretions of the digestive pancreatic enzymes and may diminish insulin production. Malabsorption can lead to diarrhea, constipation, steatorrhea, and muscle weakness.[68] New onset diabetes may be the first clinical feature in approximately 10%–20% of individuals.[69] The onset of glucose intolerance in an elderly person with vague gastrointestinal symptoms should alert the clinician to the possibility of pancreatic cancer.[68] Meta-

Table 63-4 Clinical Manifestations of Cancer of the Pancreas

Location of Tumor	Stage	Clinical Manifestation
Head	Early	Weight loss
		Jaundice
		Pain
		Anorexia
		Diarrhea
		Weakness
		Indigestion
		Depression
Body	Late	Palpable mass
		Severe pain
		Early satiety
		Indigestion
		Vomiting
		Weight loss
Tail	Late	Severe pain
		Indigestion
		Anorexia
		Weight loss
		GI bleeding
		Splenomegaly

bolic disturbances such as hyperglycemia, glycosuria, and hypoalbuminemia may occur.

A combination of factors probably causes the weight loss associated with pancreatic cancer. An increase in resting energy expenditure,[70] a decrease in consumption of calories, and fat malabsorption exist in individuals with pancreatic cancer.[71]

Pain is often vague and nonspecific. A dull, intermittent, diffuse, upper abdominal or back discomfort is initially experienced by most individuals. The discomfort may be attributed to other causes such as indigestion or gaseous distention. The discomfort or pain may become more distinctive. It may progress to continuous mid-epigastric pain and frequently radiates to the back or right upper quadrant of the abdomen, often most pronounced during the evening or night. It may be colicky, dull, or vague. The intensity of the pain is affected by activity, eating, and posture. The pain is often ameliorated when the individual sits or leans forward, called *proning*, or lies in the fetal position.[72] The pain can be caused by invasion of the tumor into the splanchnic plexus and retroperitoneum, as well as by obstruction of the pancreatic duct.

Pain is a more prevalent symptom in individuals with tumors in the body and tail of the pancreas. These tumors are larger at presentation and are located in the retroperitoneum, which contributes to nerve involvement, resulting in pain. Although intractable pain is associated with pancreatic cancer, it seldom is an early manifestation. Recent studies suggest that fewer than one-third of individuals with cancer of the pancreas report moderate to severe pain. Severe pain usually indicates invasion of splanchnic nerves, suggestive of advanced disease.[73]

Acute pancreatitis may be the presenting sign of a pancreatic neoplasm. This is caused by the partial obstruction of the pancreatic duct. Consideration must be given to the diagnosis of a pancreatic tumor in patients who are initially seen with pancreatitis, especially when there is no obvious cause for acute pancreatitis, such as gallstones or alcohol abuse.[38]

Head of Pancreas

When carcinoma involves the head of the pancreas, the signs and symptoms often appear earlier than a tumor in the body or tail of the pancreas (Figure 63-2). A classic triad of symptoms is seen in individuals with cancer of the head of the pancreas: jaundice, pain, and weight loss.

Jaundice, caused by obstruction of the distal common bile duct as it passes through the head of the pancreas, is the presenting symptom in most cases of cancer of the head of the pancreas. Regardless of whether jaundice is the initial symptom or follows the onset of pain, it is the symptom that invariably causes individuals to seek medical attention. Jaundice accompanied by abdominal pain is far more common than painless jaundice.[74] Obstructive jaundice leads to severe pruritus, dark urine, and clay-colored stools. Jaundice does not necessarily indicate extensive disease and unresectability.

Other symptoms are less common and nonspecific. These include weakness, food intolerance, and anorexia. Two unusual symptoms include depression and superficial thrombophlebitis. Depression and anxiety may be part of the initial presentation of pancreatic cancer, independent of pain and other somatic symptoms. These symptoms predate the diagnosis of a pancreatic tumor in approximately 50% of individuals. A triad of depression, anxiety, and feelings of impending doom has been described.[75] This increased incidence of depression is significantly higher than that seen in individuals with other intraabdominal malignancies.[76] The triad of depression, anxiety, and feelings of doom may indicate the presence of neuroendocrine agents in pancreatic cancer that circulate and target the central nervous system. Thromboembolism (Trousseau syndrome) occurs in fewer than 5% of individuals with pancreatic cancer.[77]

Body of Pancreas

Tumors in the body of the pancreas produce signs and symptoms late in the disease process, making early detection virtually impossible. By the time it is brought to the attention of a clinician, the tumor may be large enough to palpate. Severe epigastric pain usually is the predominant symptom. The individual may experience intense epigastric pain three to four hours after a meal. This is caused by the space-occupying tumor displacing the stomach or by encroachment at the ligament of Treitz. The pain often is excruciating and accompanied by vomiting. Relief is brought about by sitting up, leaning forward, or lying on the right side with both knees drawn up to the chest. These episodes of pain are short in duration and are most severe at night.[72] Cancer located in the body and tail produce more pain and weight loss than lesions in the head of the pancreas.[78] There is no jaundice with tumors of the body and tail of the pancreas. An enlarged spleen may be found on palpation, caused by tumor pressing on the splenic vein and resulting in splenic vein thrombosis and splenomegaly.

Tail of Pancreas

Cancer in the tail of the pancreas has the most silent and insidious progression of disease. Individuals with carcinoma of the tail of the pancreas may complain of left upper quadrant abdominal pain, generalized weakness, vague indigestion, anorexia, and unexplained weight loss. Metastatic disease is usually present when cancer in the tail of the pancreas is diagnosed. Upper gastrointestinal bleeding, splenomegaly, and signs of portal hypertension and ascites may result from thrombosis of the portal system or extensive liver damage. In rare cases a bruit may be ascultated in the left upper quadrant of the abdomen from splenic artery compression or involvement by tumor.[79]

In advanced carcinoma of the pancreas, hepatomeg-

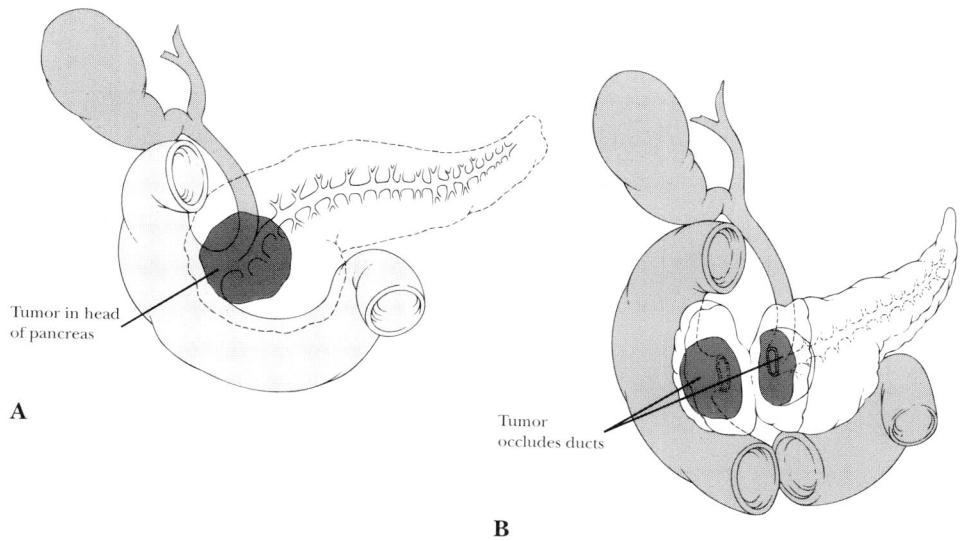

Figure 63-2   Pancreatic cancers originate in the duct and when they are located in the head of the pancreas (A) they will occlude the distal common bile duct (B). Note the proximity of the pancreatic duct and common bile duct, explaining the characteristic cutoff on cholangiography at the "knee" of the distal bile duct. (Used with permission from Bastidas VA, Neiderhuber JE. Pancreas in Abeloff MD, Armitage JD, Lichter AS, Neiderhuber JE (eds): *Clinical Oncology*. New York, Churchill Livingstone, 1995, pp 1373–1403.)[65]

aly and a palpable gallbladder (Courvoisier sign) may also be found. There may be evidence of cachexia, muscle wasting, and a nodular texture of the liver consistent with metastatic disease. Other physical findings that serve as markers in disseminated tumor include left supraclavicular adenopathy (Virchow node), periumbilical lymphadenopathy (Sister Mary Joseph nodes), and drop metastases in the pelvis encircling the perirectal region (Blumer shelf).[38]

Assessment

Patient and Family History

Careful attention to an individual's presenting symptoms and risk factors, and a heightened awareness of the possibility of pancreatic cancer by the clinician are important. Eliciting a family history of pancreatic cancer or related genetic syndromes could help to detect genetic abnormalities and perhaps aid in better treatments for family members in the future.

Physical Examination

Physical examination of the pancreas is virtually impossible because it is an inaccessible organ, lying behind the stomach and in front of the vertebral column. It has been called the *hermit organ* because of its hidden location in the abdomen. There are few signs on presentation except in those individuals presenting with obstructive jaundice.

A palpable liver is the most common finding on physical exam in 30%–50% of individuals. A hard, well-defined, mass palpable in the left upper quadrant of the abdomen is found in individuals presenting with lesions in the body and tail of the pancreas but is uncommon in lesions in the head of the pancreas. Any finding of lymphadenopathy on physical examination may warrant a lymph node biopsy.

Diagnostic Studies

A number of diagnostic studies are available to assist in the identification of pancreatic cancer, to accurately define the extent of disease, to direct appropriate therapy, and to avoid unnecessary interventions in a cost-efficient fashion. (Table 63-5) If definitive diagnosis cannot be made with these studies, exploratory laparotomy may be necessary.

As more knowledge of the molecular genetic abnormalities in pancreatic cancer accumulates, the importance of specific oncogenes and tumor suppressor genes will be elucidated and may play a role in the staging of the disease.

Diagnostic procedures

Ultrasonography (US) of the abdomen can be used as an initial diagnostic test when pancreatic cancer is suspected, especially for lesions in the head of the pancreas. It is a marginal study for visualization of the body, tail, and uncinate process of the pancreas. US can detect intrahepatic and extrahepatic bile duct obstruction, a pancreatic mass, liver metastases greater than 1 cm in

Table 63-5 Techniques for Assessment of Cancer of the Pancreas

Imaging	Laboratory	Tumor Markers	Surgery
Ultrasound	Total bilirubin	CA 19-9	Laparoscopy
Computerized tomography	Alkaline phosphatase	CA 494	Percutaneous fine-needle aspiration biopsy
Magnetic resonance imaging	Gamma glutamyl transpeptidase	CA 50	
Cholangiography	Alanine aminotransferase (ALT)	DU-PAN-2	
Endoscopic	Aspartate aminotransferase (AST)	CA 125	
Percutaneous	Hemoglobin	CA 72-4	
Angiography	Hematocrit	SPAN-1	
Endoscopic ultrasound	Albumin		
Positive emission tomography (PET)	Total protein		
Magnetic resonance cholangiopancreatography	PT, aPTT		
	Glucose		

diameter, and ascites. It is not sensitive in defining local nodal spread or involvement of the major blood vessels in the area.[74,80] US has largely been replaced by computerized tomography (CT).

A high-quality spiral or helical CT with thin-cut examination is the noninvasive diagnostic and staging procedure of choice for the jaundiced individual with a suspected pancreatic malignancy, especially in older individuals. The CT is limited to detecting lesions greater than 5 mm, even with resolution. CT is as sensitive as US in defining biliary structures and is superior in defining the level of obstruction. It can also demonstrate the presence of a pancreatic mass and enlarged lymph nodes adjacent to the pancreas, as well as detect liver metastases, local vascular invasion, or thrombosis. Likewise, CT is more accurate in the diagnosis of unresectability. CT findings that indicate the tumor is unlikely to be resected for cure include liver metastases, ascites, vascular invasion, and tumor spread to adjacent retroperitoneal structures.

Pancreatic cancer usually appears as a hypoechoic mass that differs in consistency from the normal surrounding tissue. The use of intravenous iodine contrast enhances the imaging of the pancreas and liver. The preferred method of pancreatic CT scanning is a dual-phase CT in which the arterial phase is performed after administration of intravenous contrast.[81] Both venous and arterial phase imaging is necessary for the most complete evaluation of the pancreas and its adjacent structures. Improved CT imaging has diminished the role of visceral angiography and endoscopic retrograde cholangiopancreatography (ERCP) in the diagnosis and staging of cancers of the pancreas.

Magnetic resonance imaging (MRI) has not been shown to be superior to CT in detection and staging of pancreatic cancer. CT is usually more cost-effective and less time consuming.[81] MRI may be used if CT is inconclusive.[82] It may also be used if there is a contraindication to CT, as with an allergy to iodine contrast. Fast spin echo, or turbo spin echo, and the use of gadolinium—a high-resolution intravenous contrast agent—allow faster and enhanced MRI results.[83,84]

Cholangiography is indicated in the evaluation of the jaundiced individual to define the site of biliary obstruction, by either the endoscopic or the percutaneous approach. Using ERCP, both biliary and pancreatic ductal systems can be visualized. In addition to delineating the site of obstruction, biopsy specimens for cytologic analysis can be obtained. A diagnostic ERCP may be important if the differential diagnosis includes chronic pancreatitis and clinical deterioration. In most cases of pancreatic carcinoma, the pancreatic ductal system will be obstructed with the finding of a long, irregular stricture in an otherwise normal pancreatic duct, a finding not usually seen in pancreatitis. ERCP may be most useful to evaluate the nonjaundiced individual with vague gastrointestinal symptoms in whom an early nonobstructing cancer is suspected or in the person with obstructive jaundice presumed to have pancreatic cancer but in whom no mass is evident on CT.[38,74]

The percutaneous transhepatic approach to the biliary tree is technically easier if there is a dilated biliary tree and is most helpful in defining the proximal biliary system in cases of bile duct cancer (cholangiocarcinoma).[85] PTC with percutaneous transhepatic biliary drainage (PTBD) is usually reserved for those individuals who fail endoscopic biliary drainage.[86]

Preoperative angiography is performed selectively to determine vascular invasion and to delineate the important vascular anomalies that might alter the operative approach.[87] The study may also be done when the CT scan suggests vascular abnormalities or in persons who have undergone previous operative palliation or chemoradiation. Assessment of the vascular anatomy may be difficult because of previous operation or radiation-induced scar formation.[38] Modern CT scanning has replaced angiography in the identification of pancreatic tumors.[88]

Endoscopic ultrasonography (EUS) is useful in staging pancreatic tumors as it can establish the size of the tumor, its extension into adjacent structures, local and regional nodal involvement, and any vascular involvement such as the celiac axis, superior mesenteric artery, and the mesenteric venous structures.[89,90] EUS is most useful in the detection of small pancreatic lesions, less than 3 cm in size, which are not visualized on CT or ERCP.[91] EUS was also found to be superior to dynamic, nonspiral CT, and to MRI for staging pancreatic tumors.[92] EUS is useful in the assessment of the pancreas in the case of failed ERCP, or in the evaluation of ductal structures seen at ERCP with a brush cytology sample negative for malignancy.[93] The development of EUS-guided fine-needle aspiration is a safe and effective approach of confirming the diagnosis of a pancreatic malignancy.[94] Although EUS is a promising modality in the staging of pancreatic malignancy it is highly operator dependent and is not widely available.[95]

Positron emission tomography (PET) scanning is a newer technique that uses the increased metabolism of glucose by pancreatic cells as the basis of imaging.[96] PET scanning is limited at this time because of the expensive and sophisticated nature of this technology.

The use of ultrafast magnetic resonance cholangiopancreatigraphy (MRCP) has been reported to provide higher quality images of the pancreas with a potential for greater accuracy in the diagnosis and staging of pancreatic cancer. This imaging modality may provide the information previously obtained with CT, angiography, and ERCP in a single examination.[97]

Laparoscopy and direct visualization are best used for staging cancer of the pancreas. Laparoscopic examination allows direct visualization of intraabdominal contents and can identify hepatic and peritoneal metastases not visualized by other modalities. Biopsy of metastatic peritoneal or omental lesions or liver implants can be performed at the same time. Enlarged lymph nodes can also be sampled with needle biopsy. The use of laparoscopic ultrasound has also been used for the detection of metastases not seen on the surface of the liver, vascular invasion, or deep lymph node involvement. This minimally invasive procedure can help prevent an unnecessary laparotomy for diagnosis and staging of pancreatic cancer, particularly in individuals with advanced disease and limited survival. Laparoscopy can be performed as an outpatient procedure, or it may be done as an initial procedure at the time of proposed resection to evaluate for resectability.[98–100] Peritoneal washings at the time of laparoscopy have detected micrometastases in individuals who had no other evidence of metastatic spread. This finding predicted advanced disease in which the individual would not benefit from aggressive surgical therapy.[101]

Percutaneous fine-needle aspiration biopsy (FNAB) of pancreatic tumors is useful in selected individuals, especially when guided by CT or US. This technique is safe and reliable, but it is not indicated in individuals who are candidates for resection or surgical palliation.[102,103] FNAB may not be useful in potentially resectable tumors because a negative result cannot exclude malignancy, and

it is the smaller and more curable tumors that are most likely to be missed by the needle. There have also been reports of neoplastic cells seeding along the tract of the needle, raising concerns regarding tumor dissemination within the abdominal cavity.[104,105] The pancreas is a vascular organ with a rich lymphatic network. Unnecessary manipulation can disseminate a cancer that already has a high propensity for local invasion and vascular permeation.[74] FNAB is primarily used in an individual with an unresectable cancer based on preoperative staging in whom nonoperative palliation is appropriate. The results of the biopsy may then help to direct palliative chemoradiation therapy. This technique is also useful in individuals with cancer in the head of the pancreas who are not surgical candidates and for whom neoadjuvant protocols are being considered. FNAB may be most useful in individuals whose clinical presentation and imaging studies do not suggest pancreatic adenocarcinoma. Uncommon pancreatic malignancies may be treated differently after diagnosis by FNAB, such as pancreatic lymphoma, which is best managed with chemotherapy, and pancreatic islet cell carcinoma may need further testing and consideration for aggressive surgery for tumor debulking.[106]

Laboratory tests

Routine laboratory tests are generally within the normal range, except for those individuals presenting with obstructive jaundice. Increased serum total bilirubin, alkaline phosphatase, gamma glutamyl transpeptidase, and often elevated levels of hepatic aminotransaminases are found. Normochromic anemia and hypoalbuminemia may reflect chronic neoplastic disease and its nutritional sequelae. When liver function tests abnormalities occur in individuals with cancer of the body and tail of the pancreas, it indicates metastatic disease with liver involvement. Coagulation parameters should be checked in persons with deep jaundice because prolonged absence of bile from the gastrointestinal tract leads to malabsorption of fat soluble vitamins and decreased production of vitamin K-dependent clotting factors.[38]

New-onset diabetes mellitus may be found in an individual with elevated glucose levels, which may or may not be controlled with oral hyperglycemic agents. A pancreatic problem should be investigated in an individual with previously controlled diabetes who exhibits any unexplained changes in glucose control.

Tumor markers

No serum tumor marker is sufficiently sensitive or specific to be considered cost-effective and 100% reliable for screening of pancreatic cancer. A wide variety of serum tumor markers have been proposed for use in the diagnosis and follow-up of pancreatic carcinoma. The carbohydrate antigen 19-9 (CA 19-9) is tumor-associated, not tumor-specific, and has been a useful tool in the diagnosis and management of individuals with pancreatic cancer.[107] Several factors can influence interpretation of CA 19-9:

reference value, positive Lewis blood phenotype, jaundice, and prior use of interferon.[107–109] There is a lack of consensus concerning a useful reference value for the diagnosis of carcinoma of the pancreas. A reference value of CA 19-9 greater than 90 U/mL reaches an accuracy of 85% for diagnosis; the accuracy improves to 95% with a level greater than 200 U/mL.[110] CA 19-9 is not produced by individuals without the Lewis antigen (5%–10% of the Western population). Jaundice in an individual can cause a false increase in serum levels of Ca 19-9.[111] It has also been found that interferon significantly elevates CA 19-9.

CA 19-9 has not proved useful as a screening test as it is normal in early stage, potentially curable tumors.[112] Use of CA 19-9 combined with either US, CT, or ERCP improves diagnostic accuracy.[113] Elevated CA 19-9 levels may be useful in differentiating benign diseases from pancreatic cancer.[114] After resection of pancreatic cancer, CA 19-9 levels fall and the antigen may be useful for prognosis and follow-up surveillance for tumor recurrence. A high preoperative CA 19-9 level usually indicates a large pancreatic neoplasm and greater probability of unresectability.[115,116] CA 19-9 level is used to monitor response to treatment since increasing levels of CA 19-9 reflect progression of disease. Stable or declining levels of CA 19-9 are associated with a stable tumor burden and an improved prognosis.[117,118]

Several other tumor markers have been evaluated, either alone or in combination, to screen for pancreatic cancer. CA 494 is specific for differentiation between chronic pancreatitis and pancreatic cancer.[119] Other tumor markers (CA 50, DU-PAN-2, CA 125, CA 72-4, and SPAN-1) have been evaluated but thus far have not been as reliable as CA 19-9 in the diagnosis and monitoring of pancreatic cancer. The use of molecular genetic markers as a mechanism for screening for genetic abnormalities in individuals with pancreatic cancer is rapidly evolving.

Classification and Staging

The goal of staging cancer of the pancreas is to determine the optimal treatment for each individual, with minimal risks and in a cost-effective manner. The aim is to determine whether the individual has potentially resectable disease, locally advanced disease, or metastatic disease, because therapeutic options and ultimate prognosis differ.[114] The definition of "resectability" can vary and reflects both the expertise and philosophy of the individual surgeon and institution.[95]

At this time, there is no consensus to the appropriate approach to staging of pancreatic cancer. Academic centers experienced in treating pancreatic cancer have reported various approaches using combinations of diagnostic tests.[99,120–123] The choices for staging techniques will depend on availability and local expertise in a particular modality to accurately classify patients and determine appropriate therapy.[95]

The staging of pancreatic carcinoma is based on the tumor-node-metastases (TNM) system. Four stages have been described for use in the diagnosis of exocrine cancer of the pancreas by the American Joint Committee on Cancer (Table 63-6).[124] These parameters represent the most important factors influencing resectability and prognosis of exocrine tumors of the pancreas.

Therapeutic Approaches and Nursing Care

Every individual diagnosed with cancer of the pancreas should be carefully evaluated prior to initiation of any therapy. An individual must also be adequately prepared physiologically and psychologically before undergoing

Table 63-6 AJCC TMN Classification System for Staging of Cancer of the Pancreas

Primary Tumor (T)

TX	Primary tumor cannot be assessed
T0	No evidence of primary tumor
Tis	In situ carcinoma
T1	Tumor limited to the pancreas, 2 cm or less in greatest dimension
T2	Tumor limited to pancreas, more than 2 cm in greatest dimension
T3	Tumor extends directly to any of the following: duodenum, bile duct, or peripancreatic tissues
T4	Tumor extends directly to any of the following: stomach, spleen, colon, or adjacent large vessels

Regional Lymph Nodes (N)

NX	Regional lymph nodes cannot be assessed
N0	No regional lymph node metastasis
N1	Regional lymph node metastasis -pN/a Metastases in a single regional lymph node -pN/b Metastases in multiple regional lymph nodes

Distant Metastasis (M)

MX	Distant metastasis cannot be assessed
M0	No distant metastasis
M1	Distant metastasis

Stage Groupings

Stage 0	Tis	N0	M0
Stage I	T1	N0	M0
	T2	N0	M0
Stage II	T3	N0	M0
Stage III	T1–3	N1	M0
Stage IVA	T4	Any N	M0
Stage IVB	Any T	Any N	M1

any therapy. Historically, the poor prognosis of individuals with pancreatic cancer has caused many clinicians to have a dismal outlook and thus be reluctant to treat the disease aggressively. However, recent reports on surgical outcomes are encouraging,[120,125–127] and the overall current perspective on the disease is changing.

Surgery, radiotherapy, and chemotherapy are the principal treatment modalities used for pancreatic cancer. Surgical resection still remains the best therapeutic option even though few individuals are cured. Most surgical procedures are palliative as nonresectable pancreatic cancer predominates. Only about 10% of malignancies of the head of the pancreas are resectable and potentially curable at surgery.[128] The three-year and five-year survival after resection of the head of the pancreas are only 35% and 21%, respectively.[120] The resection and survival rates for tumors in the body and tail of the pancreas are much lower.

Available therapeutic interventions include surgery, usually in combination with radiation therapy, and chemotherapy with single agents or in combination for either cure or palliation. Various regimens of chemotherapeutic agents alone or in combination with radiation therapy are also used for nonoperative cancer of the pancreas. Experimental vaccines and drugs that target the genes involved with pancreatic cancer are also being investigated and will soon be a routine part of multimodal therapies. Palliation for longer periods is usually achieved with combined modalities.

Once a diagnosis has been made, the extent of the tumor involvement established, and complete assessment of the individual's physical status made, a treatment plan will be presented to the individual. If surgery is an option, the individual's physical ability to undergo general anesthesia and a major abdominal operation must be considered; advanced age is not necessarily a negative factor.[125,129] Nutritional status, hematologic status, liver function, concomitant disease, and skill of the principal clinicians all contribute to the choice of therapy.

Prior to surgery a biliary stent to alleviate jaundice can be placed through the obstructing lesion by either the endoscopic or the percutaneous approach. In previous studies the use of biliary stents preoperatively has not been shown to improve overall operative risk.[130,131] Current studies suggest that the use of routine preoperative biliary stenting leads to an increase in postoperative surgical complications.[132,133] In selected individuals with severe malnutrition, sepsis, and/or correctable medical conditions, or in whom there is a time delay before surgery, preoperative biliary drainage may be useful. Theoretically, the internal drainage of biliary secretions may provide an immunologic advantage, leading to decreased perioperative complications of sepsis. An endoscopic stent or a percutaneously placed biliary catheter can be used in the operative management of individuals with pancreatic cancer either for resection or for palliation. An ERCP with stent placement, is performed under conscious sedation and the person can be discharged the same day. Antibiotics are usually administered intrave-

nously as prophylaxis against cholangitis due to manipulation within the biliary tract. The benefit of an internal stent for drainage that there is no external tube to manage. The individual needs to be taught the signs and symptoms of possible complications of the stent, such as recurrent jaundice and cholangitis (shaking chills and fever). Any manifestation of these signs or symptoms needs to be reported to the clinician immediately, since the individual is prone to bacteremia and sepsis.

The individual having a PTC with placement of a PTBD catheter needs to be taught about the procedure as well as the care and management of the external biliary catheter. This interventional radiological procedure is performed under conscious sedation. An internal-external catheter is placed. Prophylactic antibiotics are given to prevent biliary sepsis. Individuals are usually monitored for 24 hours to assess patency of the catheter and ensure bile drainage. Initially, the biliary catheter is attached to a bile bag, for external drainage, to allow the obstructed biliary tree to decompress. The bile bag is removed and the biliary catheter is capped off to allow internal drainage and the free flow of bile into the bowel.

Care of a percutaneously placed biliary catheter in order to maintain a properly functioning catheter is an important aspect of patient teaching. Signs and symptoms of any complications, such as fever, chills, recurrent jaundice, bleeding at the exit site or through the biliary catheter, dislodgment of the catheter from its original site, or inability to flush the catheter, must be reported immediately to the clinician to prevent problems. Teaching protocols are important for consistent and correct information. Written instructions given to the individual as a handout or video to take home are also very helpful.[130–133]

Cure is the objective if the tumor is small, localized, not fixed to other structures, and if there is no evidence of regional or distant metastases. Complete resection of the tumor will be performed and supplemented with adjuvant therapy.

Control or palliation is the goal of therapy if the tumor is unresectable or has metastasized to regional or distant nodes or to other organs. Unfortunately, 90% of all cases of pancreatic carcinoma are diagnosed as unresectable. In a significant number of individuals, operative palliation for obstructive jaundice and/or gastric outlet obstruction may be indicated for optimal long-term management. Other treatments aimed at palliating devastating symptoms may include radiotherapy, chemotherapy, percutaneous pain block, percutaneous or endoscopic biliary decompression to relieve obstruction and pressure, and gastric decompression for gastric outlet obstruction. Nutritional supplementation to achieve adequate total protein levels helps to decrease surgical risk, puts the individual in a better metabolic state for having any treatment modality, and increases the overall general state of well-being.

It is important to understand the individual's goal and plan of therapy, method of family coping, and pattern of communication. When all members of the health care team, along with the individual, agree upon a course of treatment, communication is enhanced and issues or problems can be identified and addressed. Illness has a special meaning to each person. Living with cancer of the pancreas and dealing with the knowledge that the disease has a poor prognosis, regardless of what treatment is undertaken, can create many unforeseen problems.

Surgery

Surgical resection of pancreatic cancer still remains the best therapeutic option and the only opportunity for cure. Most surgical procedures for cancer of the pancreas are palliative. Only about 10% of carcinomas of the head of the pancreas are resectable and potentially curable at surgery. The survival rate for tumors in the body and tail is much lower. There is limited prospective research evaluating surgical procedures for cancer of the pancreas.

Recent reports from institutions with large series of patients have reported increasing survival periods following resection and operative mortality rates that have decreased to less than 5%.[114,120,125] Decreased complications are attributed to refinements in surgical technique, anesthesia, critical care, and preoperative and postoperative care. Other reasons for improved surgical outcome include the operation's being performed by surgeons who are experienced in the surgical management of pancreatic carcinoma, concentration of patients in centers of excellence, and improved methods to diagnose and treat complications.[134,135] Most surgical results report collective overall outcomes; however, individuals with small (less than 2 cm) tumors have five-year survival rates of 30%, and survival rates increase for those with no residual disease or without lymphatic involvement.[114] The crux of the problem is late detection of pancreatic tumors. Until advances in early detection and diagnosis are made, curative surgery will be limited to very few candidates and palliative measures will continue as the mainstay of therapy.

When cure is the objective, the surgical approach most used for neoplasms of the head of the pancreas is a pancreaticoduodenectomy (Whipple procedure). Total pancreatectomy may be performed for tumor involving the entire gland, tumor that extends across the neck and body of the gland, or when the pancreatic remnant is too soft and friable to allow a safe pancreatic-enteric anastomosis. An extended or radical pancreaticoduodenectomy has also been performed as an alternative or modification of the original regional pancreatectomy. The regional pancreatectomy has been found to have higher morbidity and mortality rates, with no improvement in survival over the standard pancreaticoduodenectomy.[136] Controversy exists over the advantages, disadvantages, and long-term results of each operation.[137] (See Table 63-7.)[138] To determine the best operation for resectable pancreatic cancer, data from prospective randomized studies comparing standard versus radical pancreaticoduodenectomy in individuals are being evaluated.

Despite sophisticated preoperative staging methods, many individuals with adenocarcinoma of the head of the pancreas that preoperatively appears to be resectable are found to have metastatic or locally invasive disease. During surgical exploration, it is possible to encounter local spread of tumor into adjacent major vascular structures (portal vein, superior mesenteric vein, superior mesenteric artery, or abdominal aorta). The tumor can encase and grow into these vessels precluding surgical resection. The tumor may also have metastasized to the liver or peritoneal surfaces. If unresectable or metastatic disease is discovered, surgical palliation may provide a single procedure that can treat or prevent the major symptoms of obstructive jaundice, duodenal obstruction, and pain.

Pancreaticoduodenectomy (Whipple procedure). The Whipple procedure is the most commonly performed operation for carcinoma of the head of the pancreas. (Figure 63-3A).[140] The classic Whipple procedure includes resection of the distal stomach, gallbladder, distal common bile duct, head of the pancreas, and duodenum. Gastrointestinal continuity is restored by anastomosing the common bile duct and the remaining pancreas to the jejunum proximal to the gastrojejunostomy. Some surgeons anastomose the remaining pancreas to the back of the stomach because they believe it is safer and decreases the potential for pancreatic fistula formation.[139] The gastrojejunostomy is performed to allow alkaline bile and pancreatic juices to enter the jejunum before acidic gastric secretions.[140] This decreases the potential of ulceration at the gastrojejunostomy. The distal gastrojejunostomy also reduces reflux of intestinal contents into the bile duct and pancreas. The risk of ulceration has been greatly reduced by the use of postoperative prophylactic acid antisecretory agents such as H2-receptor antagonists or proton pump inhibitors.[141]

A modification of the original or classic Whipple procedure, called a *pylorus preserving pancreaticoduodenectomy,* is preferred by some surgeons. (Figure 63-3B) This procedure preserves the entire stomach, including the pylorus, and a small cuff of proximal duodenum. It has the advantage of maintaining a normal gastric reservoir and environment, avoiding potential nutritional problems associated with the classic Whipple procedure such as weight loss, dumping syndrome, diarrhea, and anastomotic ulcer at the gastrojejunostomy site. This procedure requires less time and is technically easier to perform.[142] Delayed gastric emptying that may occur following this operation generally resolves over time with conservative treatment (gastric decompression, parenteral or enteral nutrition, and prokinetic agents). Erythromycin, a motilin agonist, also has been used to improve gastric emptying after surgery.[143] Concern continues that the pylorus preserving pancreaticoduodenectomy is not an adequate cancer operation because of limited surgical margins and inadequate removal of lymph nodes in the area draining the cancer, which may compromise cure. Studies are being conducted to compare the two procedures with respect to morbidity and survival.

Pancreatic fistula and delayed gastric emptying are

Table 63-7 Comparison of Types of Pancreatic Resections for Malignancy

	Indications	Tissues Removed	Potential Advantages	Potential Disadvantages
Classic pancreaticoduodenectomy (Whipple)	Periampullary or localized carcinoma of head, neck, or uncinate process of pancreas	Head, neck, and uncinate process Duodenum Gastric antrum and pylorus Common bile duct Gallbladder Lymph nodes in pancreaticoduodenal groove	Pancreatic remnant may prevent diabetes and malabsorption Better cancer operation compared with pylorus preserving	Partial pancreatic resection may leave residual tumor in body or tail of gland Issue of multicentricity Dumping syndrome secondary to loss of pylorus Nutritional problems Leak at pancreatic anastomosis
Pylorus-preserving pancreaticoduodenectomy (Whipple)	Periampullary or localized carcinoma of head, neck, or uncinate process of pancreas	Head, neck, and uncinate process Duodenum (except most proximal portion) Common bile duct Gallbladder Lymph nodes in pancreaticoduodenal groove	Pancreatic remnant may prevent diabetes and malabsorption Normal gastric reservoir Less disruption of digestion compared with classic Whipple Reduced marginal ulceration at duodenojejunostomy	Partial pancreatic resection may leave residual tumor in body or tail of gland Leak at pancreatic anastomosis Delayed gastric emptying
Extended or radical pancreaticoduodenectomy	Periampullary or localized carcinoma of head, neck, or uncinate process of pancreas	Head, neck, and uncinate process Duodenum Gastric antrum and pylorus Common bile duct Gallbladder Extensive lymph node and retroperitoneal tissue dissection Vascular resection may be included	Extensive regional nodal dissection Pancreatic remnant may prevent diabetes and malabsorption Better cancer operation?	Partial pancreatic resection may leave residual tumor in body or tail of gland Leak at pancreatic anastomosis Dumping syndrome secondary to loss of pylorus Nutritional problems Chylous leak Longer operation with potential for increased blood loss and complications
Total pancreaticoduodenectomy (may be classic or pylorus-preserving)	Diffuse carcinoma of entire gland or a multicentric tumor	Entire pancreas Duodenum (gastric antrum and pylorus) Common bile duct Gallbladder Spleen Peripancreatic nodes Lymph nodes in pancreaticoduodenal groove	Excision of entire pancreas may remove multifocal tumor More complete peripancreatic nodal dissection No pancreatic enteric anastomosis	Insulin-dependent diabetes and complete exocrine absence Need for insulin and enzyme replacement Postsplenectomy state
Distal pancreatectomy	Carcinoma localized to body or tail of gland	Distal pancreas Spleen Peripancreatic lymph nodes	Pancreatic remnant may prevent diabetes and malabsorption No pancreatic or billiary enteric anastomosis	Limited resection may leave residual tumor Postsplenectomy state

Reprinted with permission from Sauter PK, Coleman J: Pancreatic cancer: a continuum of care. *Seminars in Oncology Nursing* 15:36–47, 1999[138]

the most common serious complications after a pancreaticoduodenectomy. The pancreas, attached to the jejunum, is technically the most difficult of the anastomoses. If the pancreas does not heal properly, a pancreatic fistula may develop. Although fistulae and leaks were previously associated with significant mortality because pancreatic juices eroded into major blood vessels, the incidence and severity of pancreatic anastomotic leaks appear to have

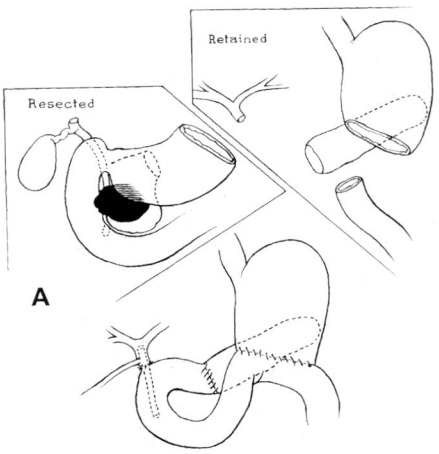

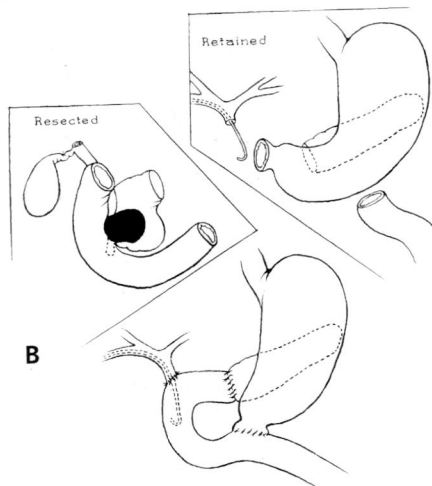

Figure 63-3 Classic pancreaticoduodenectomy (**A**) and pylorus-preserving pancreaticoduodenectomy (**B**), showing the resected specimens, the structures retained, and one method of reconstruction by way of pancreaticojejunostomy. (Used with permission from Yeo CJ, Cameron JL: The pancreas, in Hardy JD (ed): *Hardy's Textbook of Surgery* (ed 2) Philadelphia, PA Lippincott-Raven, 1988, p 695–725.)[140]

Table 63-8 Complications after Pancreaticoduodenectomy
Pancreatic fistula
Delayed gastric emptying
Wound infection
Intraabdominal abscess
Hemorrhage
Diabetes
Pancreatic exocrine insufficiency

decreased with improved surgical technique, intravenous nutritional support, modern antibiotics, and appropriate wound drainage systems.[129,144] The use of the somatostatin analog octreotide, which decreases pancreatic secretions, may also be useful in the management of postoperative pancreatic fistulae.[145–147] Intraabdominal infection, gastrointestinal bleeding, wound infection, diabetes, and pancreatic exocrine insufficiency occur less frequently.[144] (See Table 63-8.)

It is important for the nurse to know exactly what surgical procedure was performed in order to know what to assess from various drains and tubes placed at the time of surgery. Bile duct-to-jejunum anastomosis may be stented with either a preoperatively placed percutaneous transhepatic biliary catheter or with an operatively placed T-tube for decompression of the jejunum and to allow the free flow of bile. This stent also provides direct access into the biliary tree to assess for an anastomotic leak, obstruction, or stricture. Likewise, wound drains are placed adjacent to the pancreatic and biliary anastomoses to enable rapid assessment of bile or pancreatic juice leakage or bleeding. The use of various feeding tubes placed at the time of surgery depends on the preference of the surgeon.

Nutritional assessment is important to establish that the person has adequate protein and calories for wound healing. Most individuals will receive postoperative adjuvant therapy; therefore, good nutritional status along with physical and psychological readiness are essential. Immediate postoperative pain management can be successfully provided by intravenous or epidural patient-controlled analgesia (PCA).

Extended (radical) pancreaticoduodenectomy. This operation consists of a pancreaticoduodenectomy or sometimes a total pancreatectomy, along with an extensive retroperitoneal lymph node and soft-tissue resection. Resection of the superior mesenteric vein, portal vein, or superior mesenteric artery may also be included. The extended pancreaticoduodenectomy has been supported by some Japanese and European researchers since lymph node involvement is an important prognostic factor in individuals with carcinoma of the head of the pancreas. There are no published prospective randomized studies that demonstrate a consistent survival advantage for individuals undergoing extended pancreaticoduodenectomy.[38]

Total pancreatectomy. A total pancreatectomy includes an en bloc resection of the distal stomach, duodenum, gallbladder, and distal common bile duct, along with the entire pancreas, spleen, and a wide margin of peripancreatic tissue including lymph nodes. Total pancreatectomy eliminates the problem of residual tumor at the margins of the pancreas, tumor spillage when the pancreas is divided, and pancreatic fistula. This operation has shown no reduction in mortality or morbidity nor evidence of any increase in survival when it is performed routinely.[124,148–150] Individuals who have total pancreatectomy develop pancreatic endocrine and exocrine insufficiency and become brittle diabetics with glucose levels that are difficult to control. Pancreatic enzyme supplementation is necessary for a lifetime. This operation is usually reserved for selected cases, particularly when there is evidence of tumor throughout the entire pancreas or when the pancreas is considered to be unsafe for anastomsis. Reasons for an unsafe anastomosis are that the pancreas is too soft and friable, or acute edematous pancreatitis develops during surgery after manipulation of the gland.[136]

Distal pancreatectomy.

In rare cases, tumors of the body and tail of the pancreas are detected early enough to be considered curable. In these cases a distal pancreatectomy with a splenectomy is performed. The prognosis is poor, with few persons surviving for more than two years. Lesions of the body and tail rarely cause gastrointestinal obstructive symptoms and as a result are not recognized until the tumor has become unresectable.[151,152] Most individuals with adenocarcinomas of the body or tail of the pancreas are unresectable and survive for only a short period. The only change in the management of these individuals has been a diminished need for exploratory laparotomy to establish tissue diagnosis.[79] The use of laparoscopy and FNAB to determine metastatic or unresectable disease spares these individuals an unnecessary laparotomy.

Palliative procedures.

Only about 10% of individuals with pancreatic cancer are resectable for cure at the time of presentation. Therefore, palliation of symptoms to maximize quality of life is the primary goal for most individuals who are not curable.[153] These individuals present challenging management problems because optimal palliation of symptoms is difficult. Obstructive jaundice, duodenal obstruction, and pain are the most frequent symptoms requiring aggressive intervention using operative and nonoperative techniques.[68] Management can be tailored to the individual's clinical presentation, prognosis, and overall medical condition.[153] A choice must be made between operative and nonoperative palliation. Operative palliation is used for those who are deemed appropriate surgical candidates, have a good performance status, and are expected to survive for longer than six months. Individuals in poor health or those not expected to live for a prolonged time should be considered for nonoperative palliation.[68]

Conventional surgical palliation for an individual with a tumor in the head of the pancreas is done to relieve obstructive jaundice, avoid or treat duodenal obstruction, palliate tumor-associated pain, and improve quality of life. Operative procedures designed for palliation include biliary-enteric drainage, gastrojejunostomy, and chemical splanchnicectomy. Individuals with body and tail lesions of the pancreas are less likely to have jaundice or duodenal obstruction, and pain is the major symptom.

Obstructive jaundice is the most common presenting symptom in the majority of cancers of the head of the pancreas.[154,155] If untreated, obstructive jaundice results in progressive liver dysfunction, culminating in liver failure and early death. In addition, the pruritus associated with obstructive jaundice can be unbearable and is seldom responsive to medications. The jaundiced individual usually experiences anorexia, nausea, and progressive malnutrition.[153] Relief of jaundice can provide improvement in an individual's overall well-being.

The surgical options for palliation of obstructive jaundice include an internal biliary bypass by means of a choledochojejunostomy (common bile duct to jejunum) or a cholecystojejunostomy (gallbladder to jejunum). Bypass of the obstructed biliary tree to the jejunum is preferred and is necessary if the gallbladder is surgically absent.

Minimally invasive surgery is now being used for palliation of biliary and duodenal obstruction with laparoscopic cholecystojejunostomy and gastrojejunostomy.[156-158] The preliminary results have shown technical success, low morbidity, and satisfactory outcomes. Palliative pancreaticoduodenectomy may also offer some advantages to those individuals with seemingly unresectable disease. This major operation would be performed on selected individuals considered to have low perioperative morbidity and mortality.[159]

Nonoperative palliation of obstructed jaundice by either percutaneous or endoscopic drainage methods is also effective. Placement of a stent through the area of biliary obstruction allows the free flow of bile. Compared with operative decompression, a biliary stent reduces the length of initial hospitalization, is associated with lower complication rates and lower procedure-related mortality, and is significantly less expensive.[160]

Endoscopically placed biliary stents offer an advantage over the percutaneous technique, with fewer procedure-related complications and better patient acceptance. The major complication is stent occlusion associated with recurrent jaundice and sepsis. This can require stent replacement every three to four months.[161,162] Prolonged stent patency is now being achieved with the use of large-diameter expandable metallic stents. These metallic stents appear to stay patent for a time that closely approximates the length of survival of the individual.[163] Endoscopic stents are also preferred for individuals with ascites.

Percutaneous biliary drainage is indicated when endoscopic biliary drainage is unsuccessful and with recurrent jaundice following surgical bypass.[163] An internal–external drainage catheter is placed by an interventional radiologist. The biliary catheter requires daily maintenance by the individual or caregiver. Daily catheter flushing and dressing of the catheter entry site are needed. The presence of the external catheter is a constant reminder to the individual of the disease. Bile leakage around the catheter, skin irritation, catheter dislodgment, and catheter occlusion may also occur. In individuals with ascites, leakage of ascitic fluid around the catheter almost always occurs and is difficult to control. Because all catheters placed within the biliary tree eventually will occlude, percutaneous biliary catheters are exchanged approximately every three months to prevent development of catheter obstruction, recurrent jaundice, or cholangitis. This exchange can be easily performed as an outpatient procedure. Complications related to percutaneous biliary drainage are transient bacteremia or sepsis, hemobilia, and bile peritonitis.

Duodenal obstruction occurs in a significant number of individuals when unresectable disease progresses. Obstruction from cancer in the head of the pancreas typically occurs at the duodenal C loop causing nausea and vomiting. A large tumor in the body or tail of the pancreas will usually obstruct the junction of the duodenum and jejunum at the ligament of Treitz.[153] A retrocolic gastrojejunostomy can be performed to treat or prevent gastric outlet obstruction. Controversy exists as to the value of the procedure as a prophylactic measure because the individual's morbidity or mortality is not increased when gastrojejunostomy is performed as either a therapeutic or a prophylactic measure.[164] If an individual is not a surgical candidate because of recurrent tumor or is in the terminal stage of disease, duodenal obstruction can be alleviated by placement of a percutaneous endoscopic gastrostomy (PEG) decompression tube. This tube is not used for feeding, but it is effective in relieving gastric distention and may improve the comfort of the individual in the terminal stages of the disease.

Endoscopically placed metallic stents within the native duodenum at the site of tumor infiltration or at the site of an obstructed gastrojejunostomy has provided an alternative nonoperative option for individuals with malignant duodenal obstruction. This novel approach continues to be assessed as an appropriate palliative management device to allow a person to resume enteral nutrition until death.[162,165,166]

Pain is the most significant symptom for individuals with pancreatic cancer. For many individuals, pain is poorly managed and remains so until death. The severity and persistence of pain correlate with the stage of the disease. For most individuals with pancreatic cancer who are not surgical candidates, the appropriate use of oral agents can successfully manage pain.[167,168] Chemical splanchnicectomy (alcohol nerve block) is an alternative therapy available to those individuals who do not benefit from oral analgesia or cannot tolerate oral intake due to gastric outlet obstruction. It is performed using a spinal needle to inject alcohol on each side of the aorta at the level of the celiac axis (Figure 63-4).[169] Percutaneous celiac nerve block, with either fluoroscopic or CT guidance, can be performed to reduce pain and to reduce the need for oral narcotics. Nerve blocks can be done as an outpatient procedure or at the time of surgery for those individuals undergoing a palliative operation. Percutaneous nerve blocks can be repeated in individuals with previous blocks that have subsequently worn off.[169,170] Orthostatic hypotension is the most common complication after the block. Intraoperative injection of alcohol into the celiac nerves has been shown to both relieve pain and prevent the development of pain. Improvement

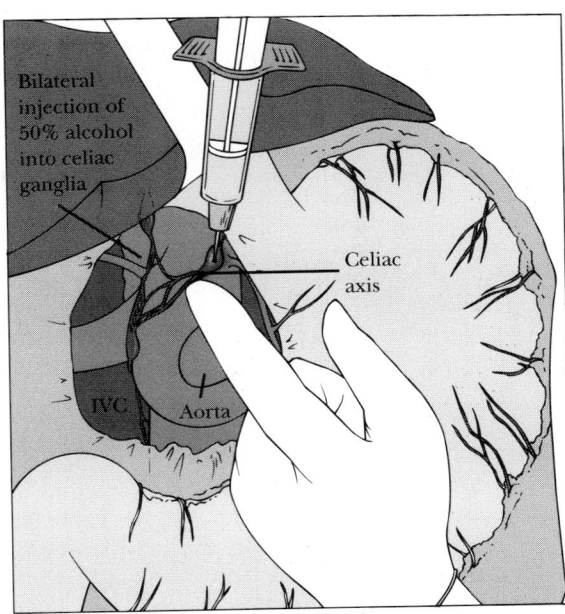

Figure 63-4 Chemical splanchnicectomy was performed using a syringe and a 20- or 22-gauge spinal needle. Solution (20 cc) was injected on each side of the aorta at the level of the celiac axis. (Used with permission from Lillemoe KD, Cameron JL, Kaufman HS, et al: Chemical splanchnicectomy in patients with unresectable pancreatic cancer: A prospective randomized trial. *Ann Surg* 217:447–457, 1993.)[169]

in pain control is associated with prolonged survival and enhanced quality of life.[169,170]

Another modality used for control of pain due to unresectable pancreatic cancer is external beam radiation therapy. Finally, transthoracic splanchnicectomy[171] and endoscopic chemical splanchnicectomy with the aid of US guidance[164] have been performed to relieve pain due to unresectable pancreatic cancer in selected individuals.

Postoperative care

Postoperative medical and nursing management of individuals who undergo pancreatic resection is critical for reducing surgical morbidity and mortality. Careful assessment, anticipatory management, and complete patient and family teaching will greatly enhance recovery and rehabilitation.[172] Hemorrhage, hypovolemia, and hypotension pose the greatest threats in the immediate postoperative period.

Following a pancreatic resection, individuals may be admitted to an intensive care unit, where hemodynamic monitoring is performed. Stabilizing and maintaining fluid requirements are essential. Careful attention is given to signs of bleeding, security and patency of wound drains, and pain management. Pain management can be achieved with opiates delivered by intravenous or epidural patient controlled analgesia (PCA). Following endotracheal extubation, aggressive pulmonary toilet is needed to reduce the risk of respiratory problems. Ideally, patients should be out of bed and sitting in a chair within a few hours following extubation.

Hemorrhage in the early postoperative period can be life-threatening. Hemorrhage can occur from failure of surgical hemostasis, from leakage at the anastomosis, or from generalized coagulopathy. Abdominal distention, shock, hematemesis, bloody drainage from gastrointestinal decompression tubes, wound drains, or bloody stool warrant immediate attention. Successful management requires correction of coagulation abnormalities and prompt reoperation if a surgical cause is suspected.

Hypovolemia can develop from fluids lost during extensive surgery, through decompression tubes and wound drains, or from the shift of fluid from the vascular space to the interstitial space (third spacing). Low levels of circulating plasma proteins secondary to malnutrition and hypoalbuminemia usually account for the third spacing syndrome. The first phase of fluid compartment shifting begins immediately after surgery and can last 48–72 hours. Signs of fluid shift are

- Decreased blood pressure
- Increased pulse rate
- Low central venous pressure
- Decreased urine output
- Increased specific gravity
- Low levels of serum albumin
- Hemoconcentration

When the plasma protein is replaced and levels return to normal, fluid reabsorption follows. Urine output will dramatically increase and will greatly exceed intake. The individual is closely monitored for signs of circulatory overload. The reabsorption phase will reach equilibrium within 24–48 hours.

Hypotension is a potential postoperative complication that is believed to result from severance of the sympathetic nerve fibers of the mesenteric complex. Vital signs and urine output should be monitored frequently to detect alterations. Vasopressor drugs and liberal intravenous fluids may be administered.

Pulmonary complications following surgery usually result from immobility and inadequate lung expansion secondary to pain and splinting. In addition, those individuals who are malnourished and protein-deficient are susceptible to pneumonia. The importance of vigorous pulmonary hygiene and early ambulation cannot be over-emphasized. Parenteral nutrition may also be needed to correct nutritional deficiencies.

Careful attention is given to wound drains for any sudden change in amount, color, or consistency of drainage. Abdominal wound drains are observed for evidence of bile or clear pancreatic juice that would suggest anastomotic leakage. Pancreatic juice that changes color to milky or brown with a foul odor suggests a pancreatic fistula. The somatostatin analog octreotide may be given to reduce pancreatic secretion to allow the pancreatic anastomosis to heal.[145–147]

Prolonged ileus and delayed gastric emptying are also potential complications. These generally resolve by taking a conservative approach with nasogastric suction, maintenance of parenteral or enteral nutrition, and the use of prokinetic agents, such as metoclopramide, or a motilin agonist, such as erythromycin.[143] The surgical incision must be examined routinely for any signs of infection as this complication can be synergistic with a pancreatic fistula or delayed gastric emptying.[144]

Following resection of the pancreas, exocrine and endocrine functions will be temporarily or permanently altered, depending on the amount of viable pancreatic tissue remaining. In the immediate postoperative period, laboratory tests are useful for monitoring protein, fat, and glucose levels. Prior to discharge, the patient and family must become familiar with and be able to recognize the signs and symptoms of exocrine and endocrine abnormalities such as hyperglycemia, hypoglycemia, steatorrhea, stupor, and lethargy.

Endocrine function, the secretion of insulin, and the production of glucagon may be altered after a pancreatic resection. Usually, a nondiabetic individual will not develop diabetes after a pancreaticoduodenectomy (occurring in less than 10% of cases).[173] Individuals who have a total pancreatectomy will develop significant hyperglycemia and are usually managed in the immediate postoperative period with an insulin drip infusion. Endocrinology consultants should be contacted soon after surgery to assist with glucose management and insulin adjustment, particularly when the individual is taking oral foods and fluids. Serum glucose levels are monitored at least every six hours, and a sliding-scale insulin dose is administered as needed if the individual can take nothing by mouth. These individuals generally require only moderate amounts of insulin and are not prone to ketoacidosis. However, they are particularly brittle and easily develop life-threatening hypoglycemia.[174] Discharge teaching and home therapy programs including self-administration of insulin, knowledge of signs and symptoms of hyper- or hypoglycemia, diabetic diet, meticulous hygiene, and the importance of routine follow-up with an endocrinologist or a medical physician for diabetes management are the same as for individuals with diabetes. Inability to control glucose levels could indicate recurrence of disease.

Alteration of exocrine function by removal of pancreatic tissue can result in a malabsorption syndrome characterized by an inability to use ingested forms of fat and protein. The caloric requirements of the individual following surgery exceed 3000 calories per day; therefore, adequate nutritional intake is essential to recovery. Oral ingestion of food is the best means of maintaining essential nutrients, but ileus or delayed gastric emptying may prohibit this mode. Parenteral or enteral alimentation may be necessary to replace calories lost as a result of the surgically induced malabsorption of fats and proteins until the individual can be advanced to an oral diet.

Pancreatic enzymes are replaced with oral enzyme supplements, which contain lipase, amylase, and trypsin. The most frequently used forms are pancreatin and pancrelipase. Pancreatin and pancrelipase supplements are made from extracts of hog or beef pancreas enriched with bile salts and plant and fungal enzymes. The usual therapeutic dose is three to six tablets with each meal and one to two tablets with a fatty snack. The enzymes are taken with or during the meal.[175] It may require several adjustments before the most appropriate dosage for each person is determined, because eating patterns and individual responses vary.[176]

When the individual is able to tolerate food, several small feedings consisting of foods that are low in fat and high in carbohydrates and protein are tolerated better than large meals. Restrictions include overindulgence (which places a great demand on the pancreas), caffeine, and alcohol. It is advantageous for the clinical dietitian to consult with the individual to select the most agreeable diet plan based on individual needs and lifestyle. The individual and family should be instructed on how to monitor the individual's tolerance to the diet and pancreatic enzyme replacement therapy. The stool should be examined daily for the characteristic signs of steatorrhea: frothy, floating, foul-smelling stool with greasy, fat particles floating in the water, crampy abdominal pain, or bloating. If these are observed, it should be reported to the physician or nurse for dietary and/or pancreatic enzyme dosage adjustment.[175] The individual should be informed that steatorrhea will decrease but may not be eliminated.

Chemotherapy

Because most individuals present with unresectable cancer of the pancreas and are already in a debilitated state, benefit from antineoplastic therapy is unlikely. Individuals with pancreatic cancer exhibit precarious physiologic conditions, which makes it difficult to differentiate the side effects of therapy from the natural progression of the disease. Response to therapy is also difficult to evaluate. The use of chemotherapy and radiation therapy both alone and in combination has shown a marginal improvement in survival, often with relatively high toxicity rates and some negative impact on quality of life.

Several chemotherapeutic agents have been used as single agents in the treatment of pancreatic cancer: fluorouracil (5-FU), mitomycin C, streptozocin, ifosfamide, and doxorubicin. The results have been minimally effective with single agents. It was hoped that combinations of chemotherapeutic agents with regimens such as SMF (streptozocin, mitomycin C, 5-FU) and FAM (5-Fluorouracil doxorubicin mitomycin C) would produce higher response rates. Unfortunately, combination chemotherapy has shown no survival advantage over treatment with single agents. Chemotherapy as adjuvant treatment for pancreatic cancer is still being investigated. The high rate of mortality associated with metastatic disease indicates that systemic therapy is needed as part of multimodality

treatment. Current applications of chemotherapy have failed to produce significant results.

A more realistic objective of treatment with chemotherapy may be improvement in quality of life, with prolonged survival being a secondary benefit. Drug efficacy in pancreatic cancer may be better judged by the alleviation of tumor-related symptoms than by measuring tumor shrinkage. A new cytotoxic agent, gemcitabine, has been evaluated in the treatment of individuals with unresectable pancreatic cancer. Clinical benefit response is a novel approach to assess the clinical effectiveness of gemcitabine based on marked improvement in pain control, analgesic consumption, and performance status. Prolonged survival is a secondary benefit. The drug has been found to be well tolerated, with a relatively mild toxicity profile. This new therapeutic paradigm for measuring response may serve as a model for the development of other effective therapies for individuals with advanced pancreatic cancer.[177,178]

Other chemotherapeutic agents are currently being studied for a role in the palliation of persons with pancreatic adenocarcinoma. Inhibitors of angiogenesis (TNP-470) is one group of compounds offering promise in cancer research. These drugs block angiogenesis, the development of new blood vessels. Solid tumors cannot grow beyond the size of a pinhead (1–2 cubic mm) without causing the formation of new blood vessels to supply the nutritional needs of the tumor. By blocking the development of new blood vessels, the hope is to cut off the supply of oxygen and nutrients to the tumor thus preventing the continued growth and spread of the tumor.[179,180]

Matrix metalloproteinases (MMP) are a family of enzymes capable of degrading the components of the extracellular matrix. A high concentration of MMP enzymes has been detected in tumors and are considered to be important in invasion and metastasis. Tissue inhibitors of matrix metalloproteinases (TIMPs) bind to and inactivate MMP. Studies that use TIMPs have shown a reduction in tumor growth and metastases by the use of matrix metalloproteinase inhibitors (MMPI).[181] Marimastat, the first of the new class of MMPI, inhibits MMP by chelating the zinc molecule in the catalytic site of the enzyme. It is an oral agent that appears to be well tolerated with only minor dose-limiting side effects.[182]

Perillyl alcohol is a nontoxic, naturally occurring substance that may enhance tumor apoptosis by increasing the ability of the tumor cell to activate and respond to transforming growth factor B.[183]

The demonstration of estrogen binding by normal and neoplastic pancreatic cells, as well as evidence that pancreatic tumors may be hormonally sensitive, led to the clinical use of tamoxifen in individuals with pancreatic cancer.[184] A question to be answered is what concentration of tamoxifen is needed to be effective.[185]

Clinical trials of these newer agents are currently underway in individuals with carcinoma of the pancreas. It is hoped that new chemotherapeutic agents, new sequencing of therapies, or new drug combinations will improve outcomes.

Radiation Therapy

Radiation therapy has been used for both palliation and curative therapy of pancreatic cancer. Directed radiation to the pancreas is difficult because of the limited radiation tolerance of adjacent organs in the upper abdomen, including the kidney, liver, stomach, small bowel, and spinal cord.[186] The technique usually used to treat pancreatic cancer is external beam radiotherapy. More specialized methods of radiotherapy have been used, such as intraoperative radiotherapy[187,188] and brachytherapy,[189] but no benefit over external beam irradiation has been found.

Radiation therapy in combination with surgery has been used to improve local disease control and survival. Radiation therapy is given postoperatively as tumor may still remain in adjacent tissue and lymph nodes. It may also be given preoperatively to reduce tumor size to permit subsequent resection. For those individuals with unresectable pancreatic cancer, radiation therapy can palliate signs and symptoms of local disease, especially pain.[190]

The benefit of using adjuvant combined chemotherapy and radiation therapy after surgical resection for pancreatic cancer was demonstrated by the Gastrointestinal Tumor Study Group (GITSG).[191] Radiation therapy is directed at the region from which the tumor was resected or where the greatest tumor burden lies, and chemotherapy is used to address the smaller or microscopic tumor burden that may remain. The use of external beam radiation combined with 5-FU significantly increased survival when compared with controls who had curative resection without adjuvant therapy. Likewise, for individuals with locally unresectable disease, the use of chemoradiation provides modest benefit.[192] Adjuvant therapy is now recommended for all individuals with pancreatic cancer.

The use of radiation sensitizing agents is now being studied. Paclitaxel is thought to enhance the effect of radiation therapy through reoxygenation of hypoxic tumor cells; as oxygenated cells are more sensitive to the toxic effects of radiation than are hypoxic cells.[193] Preliminary data also demonstrate that gemcitabine may be a potent radiation sensitizer of human pancreatic cancer cells. It appears that DNA synthesis is prolonged in tumor compared with normal tissues when gemcitabine is combined with irradiation.[194]

Newer combinations and means of administering radiation therapy and chemotherapy may provide better local control and survival for individuals with resectable and locally unresectable disease. The development of more promising neoadjuvant and adjuvant therapies, such as combining chemoradiation with immunotherapy, may further enhance survival of individuals with pancreatic cancer.

Hormone Therapy

Estrogens and androgens may affect pancreatic cancer growth.[195] The role of these hormones in human pancreatic cancer remains unclear.

Two gastrointestinal hormones, cholecystokinin (CCK) and gastrin, may have an influence on the growth of pancreatic adenocarcinoma.[195] Further studies of both CCK and gastrin alone or in combination with other agents are needed to determine their possible roles in the therapy of pancreatic cancer.

Gene Therapy

Novel treatment strategies that use gene transfer technology is a new field that has become possible through recent developments in molecular biology. Modern gene therapeutics, incorporating the use of recombinant DNA technology and more efficient gene delivery systems, have led to the development of anticancer protocols.

Immunotherapeutic strategies that use recombinant DNA technology constitute the largest group of anticancer gene therapies. Immunotherapy has the potential to provide an alternative systemic treatment for adenocarcinoma of the pancreas. This is an important consideration in the treatment of pancreatic cancer as most individuals with pancreatic cancer present with locally unresectable or metastatic disease. Even in those individuals who have surgery that removes all evidence of gross disease, most die of locally recurrent or metastatic disease within five years, and almost all eventually die as a direct result of their disease. Any effective treatment regimen against pancreatic cancer must address both its aggressive local growth and its propensity to metastasize.[196]

Immunotherapy has an advantage over chemotherapy and radiation because it can act specifically against the tumor without causing normal tissue damage. Vaccines are a form of immunotherapy. Pancreatic cancer vaccines have been developed using the whole tumor cell as the antigen source because it is not known which proteins expressed by pancreatic cancers are recognized by the immune system. Research is currently underway to study the genetic modification of pancreatic tumor cells to better present their tumor antigens to the immune system, which it is hoped will result in potent activation of a systemic antitumor immune response. Beyond this, tumor-associated antigens mixed with defined adjuvant therapy administered systemically are being developed that will result in new and more potent vaccines. Antigen-based vaccines may eliminate the need for the genetic manipulation of tumor cells.[95]

Currently, a phase I trial evaluating a cytokine-secreting pancreatic adenocarcinoma vaccine is being evaluated. Preliminary results from this trial using a granulocyte/macrophage colony stimulating factor-secreting allogenic whole cell vaccine in individuals with resected pancreatic adenocarcinoma have indicated no treatment related toxicity and measurable improvements in cell-mediated immunity.[197]

The impact of gene therapy and vaccine strategies on survival in individuals with pancreatic cancer is presently unknown. An effective treatment for pancreatic cancer may incorporate cytoreductive modalities to enable curative resection and systemic protection with immunotherapeutic approaches.

Symptom Management

The individual who has had surgery for pancreatic cancer usually dies of locally recurrent disease and/or metastatic disease. The most common harbingers of imminent death are recurrence of pain, jaundice from obstruction or intrahepatic metastases, and the development of ascites. These symptoms require symptomatic or palliative treatment. Likewise, the individual who is diagnosed with advanced cancer of the pancreas, either locally or due to metastases, may present with the following:

- Pain

- Obstructive jaundice, which can lead to intrahepatic abscess

- Infection

- Ascites

- Liver failure

- Hemorrhage

- Malnutrition from bowel obstruction

- Anorexia

- Early satiety

- Cachexia

- Nausea and vomiting

- Change in bowel habits (constipation or diarrhea)

- Dyspnea

The goal of palliative therapy is to reduce the debilitating symptoms of the disease and to improve the quality of remaining life. This is best accomplished by treating the individual with respect to his or her wishes and not just treating the tumor.[198]

Relief of pain is a primary objective, particularly in advanced disease. The pain syndrome associated with cancer of the pancreas is usually related to the anatomic location of the tumor in the organ and subsequent impingement on other structures: tissues, blood vessels, bile or pancreatic ducts, or body organs. The complex nerve fibers and ganglions that affect the pancreas and related organs and structures contribute to the pain associated with pancreatic cancer.[199] Pain associated with tumors in the head of the pancreas may be due to pancreatitis. Tumors located in the body and tail of the pancreas often present later, are larger, and tend to cause pain by invading the stomach, retroperitoneum, and nerves.

The nature of pain will evolve and change throughout the progression of the disease. Treatment approaches must address the current, specific complaints of pain using all available modalities.[200] Eliminating the source of the pain is the first objective, as in bile duct decompression or relief of duodenal obstruction. The most effective approach to pain therapy in individuals with advanced disease is to prevent the pain from peaking by routinely administering the selected relief measures. Oral, parenteral, or transdermal opiates, sedatives, nerve blocks, relaxation therapy, and proper positioning may provide pain relief. Radiotherapy in combination with chemotherapy has also been used to reduce pain. Concomitant use of analgesics, celiac nerve blocks, and radiotherapy should be considered as palliative treatments. An aggressive pain treatment plan should be devised and started immediately. The goal of pain management should be to permit an acceptable level of functioning and to allow the individual to die as free of pain as possible. Continuous pain assessment facilitated by good communication and trust between the individual and the clinician is necessary for effective pain management.

Nutritional status affects an individual's quality of life in regard to self-image, ability to perform activities of daily living, and overall life satisfaction. An individual's ability to socialize and interact with friends and family is affected by his or her ability or desire to eat.[201] Malnutrition, cachexia, muscle weakness, and fatigue all contribute to depression, causing a cycle of difficulties. Reduced activity and bedrest lead to constipation and more muscle wasting.

Nutritional support may pose a difficult problem as a result of the obstructive nature of advanced pancreatic cancer. Supportive nutritional efforts for individuals undergoing active treatment can decrease complications, shorten hospital stays, reduce costs, and improve the individual's sense of well-being. Oral feedings should be maintained as long as the individual can meet caloric requirements. Frequent, small feedings and supplemental mixtures may be tolerated better than larger meals. Antiemetics prior to eating may assist in controlling nausea and vomiting. Metoclopramide, megestrol acetate, and cannabinoids are some of the pharmacologic agents used to manage anorexia by stimulating the appetite.[202–204] Individuals with pancreatic cancer complain of sensory changes that interfere with food intake. The sense of smell may be profoundly affected. Sensitivity to food odors as well as aversions to perfumes and soaps can also occur. Serving food cold instead of hot may be helpful in decreasing the aroma. Cooking odors can be minimized by using covered pots, boiling bags, or a kitchen fan. Taste changes are common, particularly complaints that food has a metallic taste. The use of plastic eating utensils and nonmetal cooking containers can help alleviate this problem. The use of parenteral nutrition in end-stage disease is controversial due to the high cost, high risk of complications, and lack of proven benefit.[203,204]

If the individual is diagnosed with a bowel obstruction, the cause must be elicited. Bowel obstruction can be from a mechanical or a functional problem. Immediate management consists of nasogastric suction for control of nausea and large-volume emesis along with hydration by intravenous fluids. Bowel obstruction caused by tumor may necessitate the placement of a gastric tube for decompression. The tube can be placed surgically or endoscopically. The use of metallic expandable stents as a palliative measure to maintain duodenal opening and allow unobstructed flow through this part of the small bowel is being tried. Removal of a nasogastric tube and allowing small amounts of liquids by mouth are the most humane course. Somatostatin has also been used in treating individuals with bowel obstruction, as it reduces intestinal secretions and the dose can be titrated to control the volume of secretions. Prokinetic agents should not be used in individuals with known bowel obstruction.

Opiate-induced bowel obstruction must also be considered. This can be avoided by the aggressive use of laxatives and an established bowel regimen along with appropriate education of the individual and family for symptoms suggestive of bowel obstruction: pain, nausea, vomiting, abdominal distention, and change in bowel elimination.

The administration of continuous subcutaneous opiate infusions by means of a PCA pump has the advantage of delivering analgesics to individuals with impaired gastrointestinal function and for whom oral analgesics are not appropriate. The pump can also provide optimal analgesia in those individuals who develop a bowel obstruction and are not able to take food or liquids by mouth.[198]

The cause of constipation can usually be delineated by a careful bowel history and abdominal examination. Prevention of opioid-induced constipation can best be accomplished by the use of an established bowel program.[205] Diarrhea is associated with tumors in the head of the pancreas; its management depends on identifying the cause. Malabsorption may result from steatorrhea and pancreatic exocrine insufficiency. Lactose intolerance may also be seen. Treatment consists of a diet high in protein and carbohydrate and replacement of pancreatic enzymes.

Individuals with cancer of the pancreas frequently have liver involvement, resulting in abdominal distention from malignant ascites. The treatment is difficult, but symptom control can be accomplished with the careful use of diuretics. Spironolactone and furosemide can reduce ascites, improve the person's comfort, and decrease the need for paracentesis.[198] Dyspnea may result not directly from the tumor itself but from disease complications, as seen in an individual with ascites and a diminished lung capacity. Individuals with dyspnea from pancreatic cancer will have a shortened survival.[206]

Jaundice due to ductal obstruction or liver damage is a debilitating symptom that occurs in the majority of individuals with pancreatic cancer. It causes severe pruritus and dry skin. The individual should be instructed to use soap sparingly, preferably using mild soaps and oil-based lotions, calamine lotion, or cocoa butter, or to bathe in sodium bicarbonate to relieve pruritus.

Palliation of obstructive jaundice can be provided with endoscopic or percutaneous procedures. Insertion of internal biliary stents by endoscopy can relieve jaundice and its concomitant symptoms. Percutaneously placed internal–external biliary drainage catheters also can provide relief of jaundice. The catheter and insertion site must receive daily care and routine flushing. Unrelieved biliary obstruction can cause recurrent infection in the biliary tree as well as lead to liver abscess that can cause pain and sepsis. Liver abscesses are treated by percutaneous insertion of a drain and intravenous antibiotics.

Jaundice not relieved by biliary decompression is usually a sign of liver failure. Liver failure results in progressive weakness, lethargy, encephalopathy, and eventual coma with imminent death of the individual. Renal failure usually occurs as the liver fails (hepatorenal failure). The individual is more prone to coagulation problems and bleeding as the liver continues to fail. Hemorrhage may also occur from metastatic tumor eroding into blood vessels in the liver or local tumor eroding into nearby vessels. These individuals die of massive internal hemorrhage.

Almost 90% of individuals with pancreatic cancer die within a year of diagnosis. The course of the disease can be rapid. It is important that the individual and family understand that some form of treatment or another medication will always be available to make the person as comfortable as possible.

Continuity of Care: Nursing Challenges

Whatever the course of treatment chosen by the individual, both physiological and psychological preparation are necessary. By discerning patterns of family support, coping, and communication, the nurse can adopt a teaching style that suits the individual. Listening is vital to good communication in order to understand and be sensitive to the individual's needs. Education by the nurse can increase compliance as well as prepare the individual and family for side effects of both the disease and its treatment. The nurse is the constant figure of hope, understanding, and support through all the diagnostic tests, from the time an individual is told of the diagnosis of cancer of the pancreas, continuing through whatever treatment modalities are performed as the disease progresses, assisting with symptom management, and helping the individual and his or her family in the terminal stages of the disease.

The individual with terminal pancreatic cancer can be cared for at home by family or a caregiver with hospice support. The hospice nurse assists the individual and the caregiver in the terminal stages of the disease by educating them as to what to expect and helps to manage symptoms. Individuals in the terminal stage of pancreatic cancer may not wish to eat, may become extremely cachectic, and may have decreased or no urine output as hepatorenal failure ensues. Helping the family and especially the caregiver to deal with the eventuality of the disease is a primary nursing concern.

Conclusion

Much research is now being done on all aspects of pancreatic cancer. Discoveries in the field of molecular genetics hold promise for earlier detection. The ability to predict tumor biology in order to customize the treatment of individuals with pancreatic cancer brings hope for improved survival. New vaccines aimed at activating an individual's immune system to fight his or her cancer are currently being developed and tested.

There has been a reduction in morbidity and mortality associated with surgical resection for pancreatic cancer. This has led to more aggressive surgical therapy. These changes, along with improved responses to multimodality therapy and the potential for earlier diagnosis, lead to cautious optimism in the treatment of pancreatic cancer.

References

1. *Cancer Facts and Figures—1999.* Atlanta, American Cancer Society, 1999
2. Devesa SS, Blot WJ, Stone BJ, et al: Recent cancer trends in the United States. *J Natl Cancer Inst* 87:175–182, 1995
3. Neiderhuber JE, Brennan MF, Menck HR: The National Cancer Data Base report on pancreatic cancer. *Cancer* 76: 1671–1677, 1995
4. Landis SH, Murray T, Bolden S, et al: Cancer statistics, 1998. *CA Cancer J Clin* 48:6–29, 1998
5. Sauter PK, Coleman J: Pancreatic cancer: a continuum of care. *Semin Oncol Nurs* 15:36–47, 1999
6. Gold EB, Goldin SB: Epidemiology of and risk factors for pancreatic cancer. *Surg Oncol Clin N Am* 7:67–91, 1998
7. Ivy EJ, Sarr MG, Reinman HM: Nonendocrine cancer of the pancreas in patients under forty years. *Surgery* 108: 481–487, 1990
8. Zheng W, McLaughlin JK, Gridley G, et al: A cohort study of smoking, alcohol consumption, and dietary factors for pancreatic cancer. *Cancer Causes Control* 4:447–482, 1993
9. Kalapothaki V, Tzonou A, Hseih CC, et al: Tobacco, ethanol, coffee, pancreatitis, diabetes mellitus, and cholelithiasis as risk factors for pancreatic carcinoma. *Cancer Causes Control* 4:375–382, 1993
10. Friedman GD, van den Eeden SK: Risk factors for pancreatic cancer: an exploratory study. *Int J Epidemiol* 22:30–37, 1993
11. Chyou PH, Nomura AM, Stemmermann GN: A prospective study of the attributable risk of cancer due to cigarette smoking. *Am J Public Health* 82:37–40, 1992
12. Bouchardy C, Clavel F, La Vecchia C, et al: Alcohol, beer and cancer of the pancreas. *Int J Cancer* 45:842–846, 1990
13. Lyon JL, Mahoney JK, French TK, et al: Coffee consumption and the risk of cancer of the exocrine pancreas: a case control study in a low-risk population. *Epidemiology* 3:164–170, 1992
14. Adami HO, McLaughlin JK, Hsing AW, et al: Alcoholism and cancer risk: a population-based cohort study. *Cancer Causes Control* 3:419–425, 1992
15. Bueno de Mesquita HB, Maisonneuve P, Moerman CJ, et al: Lifetime consumption of alcoholic beverages, tea and coffee and exocrine carcinoma of the pancreas: a population-based case control study in the Netherlands. *Int J Cancer* 50:514–522, 1992
16. Ji BT, Chow WH, Dai Q, et al: Cigarette smoking and alcohol consumption and the risk of pancreatic cancer: a case-control study in Shanghai, China. *Cancer Causes Control* 6: 369–376, 1995
17. Silverman DT, Brown LM, Hoover RN, et al: Alcohol and pancreatic cancer in blacks and whites in the United States. *Cancer Res* 55:4899–4905, 1995
18. Lundell M, Holm LE: Risk of solid tumors after irradiation in infancy. *Acta Oncol* 34:727–734, 1995
19. Gold EB: Epidemiology of and risk factors for pancreatic cancer. *Surg Clin North Am* 75:819–843, 1995
20. Howe GR, Burch JD: Nutrition and pancreatic cancer. *Cancer Causes Control* 7:69–82, 1996
21. Silverman DT, Swanson CA, Gridley G, et al: Dietary and nutritional factors and pancreatic cancer: a case-control study based on direct interviews. *J Natl Cancer Inst* 90: 1710–1719, 1998
22. Gullo L, Pezzilli R, Morselli-Labate AM: Diabetes and the risk of pancreatic cancer. *New Engl J Med* 331:81–84, 1994
23. O'Mara BA, Byers T, Schoenfeld E: Diabetes mellitus and cancer risk: a multisite case-control study. *J Chronic Dis* 38: 435–441, 1985
24. Everhart J, Wright D: Diabetes mellitus as a risk factor for pancreatic cancer: a meta-analysis. *JAMA* 273:1605–1609, 1995
25. Lowenfels AB, Maisonneuve P, Cavallini G, et al: Pancreatitis and the risk of pancreatic cancer. *New Engl J Med* 328: 1433–1437, 1993
26. Bueno de Mesquita HB, Maisonneuve P, Moerman CJ, et al: Aspects of medical history and exocrine carcinoma of the pancreas: a population-based case-control study in the Netherlands. *Int J Cancer* 52:17–23, 1992
27. Ekbom A, McLaughlin JK, Karlsson BM, et al: Pancreatitis and pancreatic cancer: a population-based study. *J Natl Cancer Inst* 86:625–627, 1994
28. Karlsson BM, Ekbom A, Josefsson S, et al: The risk of pancreatic cancer following pancreatitis: an association due to confounding? *Gastroenterology* 113:587–592, 1997
29. Ji BT, Hatch MC, Chow WH, et al: Anthropometric and reproductive factors and the risk of pancreatic cancer: a case-control study in Shanghai, China. *Int J Cancer* 66:432–437, 1996
30. Hruban RH, Petersen GM, Ha PK, et al: Genetics of pancreatic cancer. From genes to families. *Surg Oncol Clin North Am* 7:1–23, 1998
31. Caldas C, Hahn SA, daCosta LT, et al: Frequent somatic mutations and homozygous deletions of the p16 (MTS1) gene in pancreatic adenocarcinoma. *Nat Gen* 8:27–32, 1994
32. Schutte M, Hruban RH, Geradts J, et al: Abrogation of the Rb/p16 tumor-suppressive pathway in virtually all pancreatic carcinomas. *Cancer Res* 57:3126–3130, 1997
33. Rozenblum E, Schutte M, Goggins M, et al: Tumor-suppressive pathways in pancreatic carcinoma. *Cancer Res* 57:1731–1734, 1997
34. Schutte M, Hruban RH, Hedrick L, et al: DPC4 gene in various tumor types. *Cancer Res* 56:2527–2530, 1996
35. Goggins M, Schutte M, Lu J, et al: Germline BRCA2 gene mutations in patients with apparently sporadic pancreatic carcinomas. *Cancer Res* 56:5360–5364, 1996
36. Hruban RH, van Mansfeld AD, Offerhaus GJ, et al: K-ras oncogene activation in adenocarcinoma of the human pancreas. A study of 82 carcinomas using a combination of mutant-enriched polymerase chain reaction analysis and

allele-specific oligonucleotide hybridization. *Am J Pathol* 143:545–554, 1993

37. Goggins M, Offerhaus GJA, Hilgers W, et al: Pancreatic adenocarcinomas with DNA replication errors (RER+) are associated with wild-type K-ras and characteristic histopathology. Poor differentiation, a syncytial growth pattern, and pushing borders suggest RER+. *Am J Pathol* 152:1501–1507, 1998

38. Yeo J, Cameron JL: Pancreatic cancer. *Curr Prob Surg* 36:59–152, 1999

39. Whitcomb DC, Gorry MC, Preston RA, et al: Hereditary pancreatitis is caused by a mutation in the cationic trypsinogen gene. *Nat Gen* 14:141–145, 1996

40. Kinzler KW, Vogelstein B: Lessons from hereditary colorectal cancer. *Cell* 87:159–170, 1996

41. Phelan CM, Lancaster JM, Tonin P, et al: Mutation analysis of the BRCA2 gene in 49 site-specific breast cancer families. *Nat Genet* 13:120–122, 1996

42. Goldstein AM, Fraser MC, Struewing JP, et al: Increased risk of pancreatic cancer in melanoma-prone kindreds with p16 INK4 mutations. *New Engl J Med* 333:970–974, 1995

43. Lynch HT, Smyrk T, Kern SE, et al: Familial pancreas cancer: a review. *Semin Oncol* 23:251–275, 1996

44. Giardiello FM, Welsh SB, Hamilton SR, et al: Increased risk of cancer in Peutz-Jeghers syndrome. *New Engl J Med* 316:1511–1514, 1987

45. Hemminki A, Tomlinson I, Markie D, et al: Localization of a susceptibility locus for Peutz-Jeghers syndrome to 19p using comparative genomic hybridization and targeted linkage analysis. *Nat Gen* 15:87–90, 1997

46. Kroc M: Role of growth factors in pancreatic cancer. *Surg Oncol Clin North Am* 7(1):25–41, 1998

47. Lemoine NR, Hughes CM, Barton CM, et al: The epidermal growth factor receptor in human pancreatic cancer. *J Pathol* 166:7–12, 1992

48. Friess H, Yamanaka Y, Buchler M, et al: Enhanced expression of transforming growth factor beta isoforms in human pancreatic cancer correlates with decreased survival. *Gastroenterology* 105:1846–1856, 1993

49. Mason IJ: The ins and outs of fibroblast growth factors. *Cell* 78:547–552, 1994

50. Leung HY, Gullick WJ, Lemoine NR: Expression and functional activity of fibroblast growth factors and their receptors in human pancreatic cancer. *Intl J Cancer* 59:667–675, 1994

51. Bergmann U, Funatomi H, Yokoyama M, et al: Insulin-like growth factor I overexpression in human pancreatic cancer: evidence for autocrine and paracrine roles. *Cancer Res* 55:2007–2011, 1995

52. Poston GJ, Gillespie J, Guillou PJ: Biology of pancreatic cancer. *Gut* 32:800–812, 1991

53. Kataria R, Bhatnagar V, Agarwala S, et al: Clinical course and management of pancreatoblastoma in children. *Trop Gastroenterol* 19:67–69, 1998

54. DeGuiseppe JA, Yeo CJ, Hruban RH: Molecular biology and the diagnosis and treatment of adenocarcinoma of the pancreas. *Adv Anat Pathol* 3:139–155, 1996

55. Wilentz RE, Hruban RH: Pathology of cancer of the pancreas. *Surg Oncol Clin North Am* 7(1):43–65, 1998

56. Brat DJ, Lillemoe KD, Yeo CJ, et al: Progression of pancreatic intraductal neoplasias to infiltrating adenocarcinoma of the pancreas. *Am J Surg Pathol* 22:163–169, 1998

57. Klimstra DS, Heffess CS, Oertel JE, et al: Acinar cell carcinoma of the pancreas. A clinicopathologic study of 28 cases. *Am J Surg Pathol* 16:815–837, 1992

58. Fernandez-del Castillo C, Warshaw AL: Cystic tumors of the pancreas. *Surg Clin North Am* 75:1001–1016, 1995

59. Talamini MA, Pitt HA, Hruban RH, et al: Spectrum of cystic tumors of the pancreas. *Am J Surg* 163:117–124, 1992

60. Kawarada Y, Yano T, Yamamoto T, et al: Intraductal mucin-producing tumors of the pancreas. *Am J Gastroenterol* 87:634–638, 1992

61. Z'graggen K, Rivera JA, Compton CC, et al: Prevalence of activating K-ras mutations in the evolutionary stages of neoplasia in intraductal papillary mucinous tumors of the pancreas. *Ann Surg* 226:491–500, 1997

62. Nishihara K, Nagoshi M, Tsuneyoshi M, et al: Papillary cystic tumor of the pancreas. Assessment of their malignant potential. *Cancer* 71:82–92, 1993

63. Webb TH, Lillemoe KD, Pitt HA, et al: Pancreatic lymphoma. Is surgery mandatory for diagnosis or treatment? *Ann Surg* 209:25–30, 1989

64. Bieligk S, Jaffe BM: Islet cell tumors of the pancreas. *Surg Clin North Am* 75:1025–1040, 1995

65. Bastidas JA, Neiderhuber JE: Pancreas, in Abeloff MD, Armitage JO, Lichter AS, Neiderhuber JE (eds): *Clinical Oncology.* New York, Churchill Livingstone, 1995, pp 1373–1400

66. Cubilla AL, Fitzgerald PJ: Cancer of the exocrine pancreas: the pathological aspects. *CA Cancer J Clin* 35:2–18, 1985

67. Nagakawa T, Kobayashi H, Ueno K, et al: The pattern of lymph node involvement in carcinoma of the head of the pancreas. A histologic study of the surgical findings in patients undergoing extensive nodal dissections. *Intl J Pancreatol* 13:15–22, 1993

68. Lillemoe KD: Current management of pancreatic carcinoma. *Ann Surg* 221:133–148, 1995

69. Rosa JA, Van Linda BM, Abourizk NN: New-onset diabetes mellitus as a harbinger of pancreatic carcinoma. A case report and literature review. *J Clin Gastroenterol* 11:211–215, 1989

70. Falconer JS, Fearon KC, Plester CE, et al: Cytokines, the acute-phase response, and resting energy expenditure in cachectic patients with pancreatic cancer. *Ann Surg* 219:325–331, 1994

71. Perez MM, Newcomer AD, Moertel CG, et al: Assessment of weight loss, food intake, fat metabolism, malabsorption, and treatment of pancreatic insufficiency in pancreatic cancer. *Cancer* 52:346–352, 1983

72. Ventafridda GV, Caraceni AT, Sbanotto AM, et al: Pain treatment in cancer of the pancreas. *Eur J Surg Oncol* 16:1–6, 1990

73. Hudis C, Kelsen D, Niedzwieck D, et al: Pain is not prominent in most patients with early pancreatic cancer. *Proc Am Soc Clin Oncol* 10:326, 1991

74. Moossa AR, Gamagami RA: Diagnosis and staging of pancreatic neoplasms. *Surg Clin North Am* 75:871–890, 1995

75. Green AI, Austin CP: Psychopathology of pancreatic cancer. A psychobiologic probe. *Psychosomatics* 34:208–221, 1993

76. Fras I, Litin EM, Pearson JS: Comparison of psychiatric symptoms of carcinoma of the pancreas with those in some other intra-abdominal neoplasms. *Am J Psychiatry* 123:1553–1562, 1967

77. Dhami MS, Bona RD: Thrombosis in patients with cancer. *Postgrad Med* 93:131–140, 1993

78. Raijman I, Levin B: Exocrine tumors of the pancreas, in Go VLM, Dimagno EP, Gardner JD, Lebenthal E, Reber HA, Scheele GA (eds): *The Pancreas: Biology, Pathobiology, and Disease* (ed 2). New York, Raven, 1993, pp 889–913

79. Nordback IH, Hruban RH, Boitnott JK, et al: Carcinoma of the body and tail of the pancreas. *Am J Surg* 164:26–31, 1992

80. Brand RE, Matamoros A: Imaging techniques in the evalua-

tion of adenocarcinoma of the pancreas. *Dig Dis* 16:242–252, 1998

81. Bluemke DA, Fishman EK: CT and MR evaluation of pancreatic cancer. *Surg Oncol Clin North Am* 7:103–124, 1998

82. Semelka RC, Kelekis NL, Molina PL, et al: Pancreatic masses with inconclusive findings on spiral CT: is there a role for MRI? *J Magn Reson Imaging* 6:585–588, 1996

83. Ichikawa T, Haradome H, Hachiya J, et al: Pancreatic ductal adenocarcinoma: preoperative assessment with helical CT versus dynamic MR imaging. *Radiology* 202:655–662, 1997

84. Trede M, Rumstadt B, Wendl K, et al: Ultrafast magnetic resonance imaging improves the staging of pancreatic tumors. *Ann Surg* 226:393–407, 1997

85. Tan HP, Smith JS, Garberoglio CA: Pancreatic adenocarcinoma: an update. *J Am Coll Surg* 183:164–184, 1996

86. Kaufman SL: Percutaneous palliation of unresectable pancreatic cancer. *Surg Clin North Am* 75:989–999, 1995

87. Biehl TR, Traverso LW, Hauptmann E, et al: Preoprative visceral angiography alters intraoperative strategy during the Whipple procedure. *Am J Surg* 165:607–612, 1993

88. Savader BL, Fishman EK, Savader S, et al: CT arterial portography vs pancreatic arteriography in the assessment of vascular involvement in pancreatic and periampullary tumors. *J Comput Assist Tomogr* 18:916–920, 1994

89. Rosch T, Lorenz R, Braig C, et al: Endoscopic ultrasound in pancreatic tumor diagnosis. *Gastrointest Endosc* 37:347–352, 1991

90. Rosch T, Braig C, Gain T, et al: Staging of pancreatic and ampullary carcinoma by endoscopic ultrasonography. Comparison with conventional sonography, computed tomography, and angiography. *Gastroenterology* 102:188–199, 1992

91. Snady H, Cooperman A, Siegel J: Endoscopic ultrasound compared with computer tomography with ERCP in patients with obstructive jaundice or small peri-pancreatic mass. *Gastrointest Endosc* 38:27–34, 1992

92. Muller MF, Meyenberger C, Bertschinger P, et al: Pancreatic tumors: evaluation with endoscopic US, CT, and MR imaging. *Radiology* 190:745–757, 1994

93. Scheiman JM, Jednak M: Innovations in pancreatic evaluation: endoscopic ultrasound and MRI. *Pract Gastroenterol* 22:17–28, 1998

94. Wiersema MJ, Vilmann P, Giovannini M, et al: Endosonography-guided fine-needle aspiration biopsy: diagnostic accuracy and complication assessment. *Gastroenterology* 112:1087–1095, 1997

95. Yeo CJ: Pancreatic cancer: 1998 update. *J Coll Surg* 187:429–442, 1998

96. Keogan MT, Tyler D, Clark L, et al: Diagnosis of pancreatic carcinoma: role of FDG PET. *AJR Am J Roentgenol* 171:1565–1570, 1998

97. Barish MA, Soto JA: MR cholangiopancreatography: techniques and clinical applications. *AJR AM J Roentgenol* 169:1295–1303, 1997

98. John TG, Greig JD, Carter DC, et al: Carcinoma of the pancreatic head and periampullary region. Tumor staging with laparoscopy and laparoscopic ultrasonography. *Ann Surg* 221:156–164, 1995

99. Conlon KC, Minnard EA: The value of laparoscopic staging in upper gastrointestinal malignancy. *Oncologist* 2:10–17, 1997

100. Andren-Sandberg A, Lindberg CG, Lundstedt C, et al: Computed tomography and laparoscopy in the assessment of the patient with pancreatic cancer. *J Am Coll Surg* 186:35–40, 1998

101. Fernandez-del Castillo C, Warshaw AL: Pancreatic cancer. Laparoscopic staging and peritoneal cytology. *Surg Oncol Clin North Am* 7:135–142, 1998

102. Murr MM, Sarr MG, Oishi AJ, et al: Pancreatic cancer. *CA Cancer J Clin* 44:304–318, 1994

103. DiMagno EP: Preoperative staging of pancreatic ductal cancer in the USA. *Int J Pancreatol* 16:112–114, 1994

104. Rashleigh-Belcher HJ, Russell RC, Lees WR: Cutaneous seeding of pancreatic carcinoma by fine-needle aspiration biopsy. *Br J Radiol* 59:182–183, 1986

105. Weiss SM, Skibber JM, Mohiuddinn M, Rosato FE: Rapid intra-abdominal spread of pancreatic cancer. Influence of multiple operative biopsy procedures. *Arch Surg* 120:415–416, 1985

106. Centeno BA: Fine needle aspiration biopsy of the pancreas. *Clin Lab Med* 18:401–427, 1998

107. Ritts RE, Pitt HA: CA 19-9 in pancreatic cancer. *Surg Oncol Clin North Am* 7:93–101, 1998

108. Steinberg W: The clinical utility of the CA 19-9 tumor-associated antigen. *Am J Gastroenterol* 85:350–355, 1990

109. Plebani M, Basso D, Panozzo M, et al: Tumor markers in the diagnosis, monitoring and therapy of pancreatic cancer: state of the art. *Int J Biol Markers* 10:189–199, 1995

110. Forsmark CE, Lambiase L, Vogel SB: Diagnosis of pancreatic cancer and prediction of unresectability using tumor-associated antigen CA 19-9. *Pancreas* 9:7311–734, 1994

111. Fabris C, Basso D, Piccoli A, et al: Role of local and systemic factors in increasing serum glycoprotein markers of pancreatic cancer. *J Med* 22:145–156, 1991

112. Satake K, Takeuchi T: Comparison of CA 19-9 with other tumor markers in the diagnosis of cancer of the pancreas. *Pancreas* 9:720–724, 1994

113. Ritts RE, Nagorney DM, Jacobsen DJ, et al: Comparison of preoperative CA 19-9 levels with results of other diagnostic imaging modalities in patients undergoing laparotomy for suspected pancreatic cancer or gallbladder disease. *Pancreas* 9:707–716, 1994

114. Warshaw AL, Fernandez-del Castillo C: Pancreatic carcinoma. *New Engl J Med* 326:455–465, 1992

115. Tian F, Alpert HE, Myles J, et al: Prognostic value of serum CA 19-9 levels in pancreatic adenocarcinoma. *Ann Surg* 215:350–355, 1992

116. Lundin J, Roberts PJ, Kuusela P, et al: The prognostic value of preoperative serum levels of CA 19-9 and CEA in patients with pancreatic cancer. *Br J Cancer* 69:515–519, 1994

117. Willett CE, Daly WJ, Warshaw AL: CA 19-9 is an index of response to neoadjuvant chemoradiation in pancreatic cancer. *Am J Surg* 172:350–352, 1996

118. Bluemke DA, Abrams RA, Yeo CJ, et al: Recurrent pancreatic adenocarcinoma: spiral CT evaluation following the Whipple procedure. *Radiographics* 17:303–313, 1997

119. Friess H, Buchler M, Auerbach B, et al: CA 494: a new tumor marker for the diagnosis of pancreatic cancer. *Int J Cancer* 53:759–763, 1993

120. Yeo CJ, Cameron JL, Lillemoe KD, et al: Pancreaticoduodenectomy for cancer of the head of the pancreas: 201 Patients. *ANN Surg* 221:721–733, 1995

121. Brugge WR, Lee MJ, Kelsey PB, et al: The use of EUS to diagnose malignant portal venous system invasion by pancreatic cancer. *Gastrointest Endosc* 43:561–567, 1996

122. Gloor B, Todd KE, Reber HA. Diagnostic workup of patients with suspected pancreatic carcinoma: the University of California-Los Angeles approach. *Cancer* 79:1780–1786, 1997

123. Holzman MD, Reintgen KL, Tyler DS, et al: The role of laparoscopy in the management of suspected pancreatic and periampullary malignancies. *J Gastrointest Surg* 1:236–244, 1997

124. Spitz FR, Abbruzzese JL, Lee JE, et al: Preoperative and postoperative chemoradiation strategies in patients treated with pancreaticoduodenectomy for adenocarcinoma of the pancreas. *J Clin Oncol* 15:928–937, 1997

125. Cameron JL, Pitt HA, Yeo CJ, et al: One hundred and forty-five consecutive pancreaticoduodenectomies without mortality. *Ann Surg* 217:430–438, 1993

126. Yeo CJ, Cameron JL, Sohn TA, et al: Six hundred fifty consecutive pancreaticoduodenectomies in the 1990's: pathology, complications, and outcomes. *Ann Surg* 226:248–260, 1997

127. Yeo CJ, Sohn TA, Cameron JL, et al: Periampullary adenocarcinoma: analysis of 5-year survivors. *Ann Surg* 227:821–831, 1998

128. Raijman I, Levin B: Exocrine tumors of the pancreas, in Go VLW, Dimagno EP, Gardner JD, Lebenthal E, Reber HA, Scheele GA (eds): *The Pancreas: Biology, Pathobiology, and Disease* (ed 2). New York, Raven, 1993, pp 889–913

129. Sohn TA, Yeo CJ, Cameron JL, et al: Should pancreaticoduodenectomy be performed in octogenarians? *J Gastrointest Surg* 2:207–216, 1998

130. Pitt HA, Gomes AS, Lois JF, et al: Does preoperative percutaneous biliary drainage reduce operative risk or increase hospital cost? *Ann Surg* 201:545–553, 1985

131. Lygidakis NJ, van der Heyde MN, Lubbers MJ: Evaluation of preoperative biliary drainage in the surgical management of pancreatic head carcinoma. *Acta Chir Scand* 153:665–668, 1987

132. Heslin MJ, Brooks AD, Hochwald SN, et al: A preoperative biliary stent is associated with increased complications after pancreaticoduodenectomy. *Arch Surg* 133:149–154, 1998

133. Povoski SP, Karpch MS, Conlon KL, et al: Positive intraoperative bile cultures at the time of pancreaticoduodenectomy are associated with preoperative biliary drainage and subsequent development of postoperative infectious complications and mortality. *Gastroenterology* 114:A537, 1998

134. Gordon TA, Burleyson GP, Tielsch JM, et al: The effects of regionalization on cost and outcome for one general high-risk surgical procedure. *Ann Surg* 221:43–49, 1995

135. Sosa JA, Bowman HM, Gordon TA, et al: Importance of hospital volume in the overall management of pancreatic cancer. *Ann Surg* 228:429–438, 1998

136. Yeo CJ, Cameron JL: Alternative techniques for performing the Whipple operation. *Adv Surg* 30:293–310, 1996

137. Yeo CJ, Cameron JL: Pancreatic cancer: current controversies, in Schein M, Wise L (eds): *Clinical Controversies in Surgery*. Basel, Karger Landes, 1998, pp 70–77

138. Morris DM, Ford RS: Pancreaticogastrostomy: Preferred reconstruction for Whipple resection. *J Surg Res* 54:122–125, 1993

139. Takao S, Shimazu H, Maenohara S, et al: Modified Pancreaticogastrostomy following Pancreaticoduodenectomy: Current Management. *Am J Surg* 165:317–321, 1993

140. Yeo CJ, Cameron JL. The pancreas, in Hardy VD (ed): Hardy's *Textbook of Surgery* (ed 2). Philadelphia, Lippincott-Raven, 1988, pp 695–725

141. Grace PA, Pitt HA, Tompkins RK: Decreased morbidity and mortality after pancreaticoduodenectomy. *Am J Surg* 151:141–149, 1986

142. Yeo CJ: Pylorus-preserving pancreaticoduodenectomy. *Surg Oncol Clin North Am* 7:143–156, 1998

143. Yeo CJ, Barry MK, Sauter PK, et al: Erythromycin accelerates gastric emptying after pancreaticoduodenectomy. A prospective, randomized, placebo-controlled trial. *Ann Surg* 218:229–238, 1993

144. Yeo CJ: Management of complications following pancreaticoduodenectomy. *Surg Clin North Am* 75:913–924, 1995

145. Buchler M, Friess H, Klempa I, et al: Role of octreotide in the prevention of postoperative complications following pancreatic resection. *Am J Surg* 163:125–131, 1992

146. Pederzoli P, Bassi C, Falconi M, et al: Efficacy of octreotide in the prevention of complications of elective pancreatic surgery. Italian Study Group. *Br J Surg* 81:265–269, 1994

147. Montorsi M, Zago M, Mosca F, et al: Efficacy of octreotide in the prevention of pancreatic fistula after elective pancreatic resections: a prospective, controlled, randomized clinical trial. *Surgery* 117:26–31, 1995

148. Warshaw AL, Swanson RS: Pancreatic cancer in 1988. Possibilities and probabilities. *Ann Surg* 208:541–553, 1988

149. Cameron JL, Crist DW, Sitzmann JV, et al: Factors influencing survival after pancreaticoduodenectomy for pancreatic cancer. *Am J Surg* 161:120–125, 1991

150. Bakkevold KE, Kambestad B: Morbidity and mortality after radical and palliative pancreatic cancer surgery. Risk factors influencing the short-term results. *Ann Surg* 217:356–368, 1993

151. Dalton RR, Sarr MG, van Heerden JA, et al: Carcinoma of the body and tail of the pancreas: is curative resection justified? *Surgery* 111:489–494, 1992

152. Brennan MF, Moccia RD, Klimstra D: Management of adenocarcinoma of the body and tail of the pancreas. *Ann Surg* 223:506–512, 1996

153. Lillemoe KD, Barnes SA: Surgical palliation of unresectable pancreatic carcinoma. *Surg Clin North Am* 75:953–968, 1995

154. Singh SM, Longmire WP, Reber HA: Surgical palliation for pancreatic cancer. The UCLA experience. *Ann Surg* 212:132–139, 1990

155. Lillemoe KD, Sauter PK, Pitt HA, et al: Current status of surgical palliation of periampullary carcinoma. *Surg Gynecol Obstet* 176:1–10, 1993

156. Fletcher DR, Jones RM: Laparoscopic cholecystojejunostomy as palliation for obstructive jaundice in inoperable carcinoma of the pancreas. *Surg Endosc* 6:147–149, 1992

157. Nathanson LK: Laparoscopy and pancreatic cancer: biopsy, staging and bypass. *Baillieres Clin Gastroenterol* 7:941–960, 1993

158. Rhodes M, Nathanson L, Fielding G: Laparoscopic biliary and gastric bypass: a useful adjunct in the treatment of carcinoma of the pancreas. *Gut* 36:778–780, 1995

159. Lillemoe KD, Cameron JL, Yeo CJ, et al: Pancreaticoduodenectomy. Does it have a role in the palliation of pancreatic cancer? *Ann Surg* 223:718–728, 1996

160. Watanapa P, Williamson RC: Surgical palliation for pancreatic cancer: developments during the past two decades. *Br J Surg* 79:8–20, 1992

161. Cotton PB: Nonsurgical palliation of jaundice in pancreatic cancer. *Surg Clin North Am* 69:613–627, 1989

162. Lichtenstein DR, Carr-Locke DL: Endoscopic palliation for unresectable pancreatic carcinoma. *Surg Clin North Am* 75:969–988, 1995

163. Kaufman SL: Percutaneous palliation of unresectable pancreatic carcinoma. *Surg Clin North Am* 75:989–999, 1995

164. Lillemoe KD: Palliative therapy for pancreatic cancer. *Surg Oncol Clin North Am* 7:199–216, 1998

165. Keymling M, Wagner HJ, Vakil N, et al: Relief of malignant

duodenal obstruction by percutaneous insertion of a metal stent. *Gastrointest Endosc* 39:439–441, 1993

166. Maetani I, Ogawa S, Hoshi H, et al: Self-expanding metal stents for palliative treatment of malignant biliary and duodenal stenoses. *Endoscopy* 26:701–704, 1994

167. Saltzburg D, Foley KM: Management of pain in pancreatic cancer. *Surg Clin North Am* 69:629–649, 1989

168. Levy MH: Pharmacologic treatment of cancer pain. *N Engl J Med* 335:1124–1132, 1996

169. Lillemoe KD, Cameron JL, Kaufman HS, et al: Chemical splanchnicectomy in patients with unresectable pancreatic cancer. A prospective randomized trial. *Ann Surg* 217:447–457, 1993

170. Lee MJ, Mueller PR, van Sonnenberg E, et al: CT-guided celiac ganglion block with alcohol. *AJR Am J Roentgenol* 161:633–636, 1993

171. Worsey J, Ferson PF, Keenan RJ, et al: Thorascopic pancreatic denervation for pain control in irresectable pancreatic cancer. *Br J Surg* 80:1051–1052, 1993

172. Coleman J: Supportive management of the patient with pancreatic cancer: role of the oncology nurse. *Oncology* 10:23–25, 1996 (suppl)

173. Doty JE, Fink AS, Meyer JH: Alterations in digestive function caused by pancreatic disease. *Surg Clin North Am* 69:447–465, 1989

174. Ashley SW, Reber HA: Surgical management of exocrine pancreatic cancer, in Go VLW, Dimagno EP, Gardner JD, Lebenthal E, Reber HA, Scheele GA (eds): *The Pancreas: Biology, Pathobiology, and Disease* (ed 2). New York, Raven, 1993, pp 913–930

175. Ottery F: Supportive nutritional management of the patient with pancreatic cancer. *Oncology* 10:26–32, 1996 (suppl)

176. Held-Warmkessel J, Volpe H, Waldman AR: Treatment for pancreatic cancer. *Clin J Oncol Nurs* 2:127–134, 1998

177. Rothenberg M, Burris H III, Andersen J, et al: Gemcitabine: effective palliative therapy for pancreas cancer patients failing 5-FU *Proc Am Soc Clin Oncol* 14:198, 1995 (abstr)

178. Rothenberg ML: New developments in chemotherapy for patients with advanced pancreatic cancer. *Oncology* 10:18–22, 1996 (suppl)

179. Ingber D, Fujita T, Kishimoto S, et al: Synthetic analogues of fumagillin that inhibit angiogenesis and suppress tumor growth. *Nature* 348:555–557, 1990

180. Konno H, Tanaka T, Kanai T, et al: Efficacy of an angiogenesis inhibitor, TNP-470, in xenotranplanted human colorectal cancer with high metastatic potential. *Cancer* 77:1736–1740, 1996 (suppl)

181. Khokha R: Supression of the tumorigenic and metastatic abilities of murine B16-F10 melanoma cells in vivo by the overexpression of the tissue inhibitor of the metalloproteinases-1. *J Natl Cancer Inst* 86:299–304, 1994

182. Parsons SL, Watson SA, Brown PD, et al: Matrix metalloproteinases. *Br J Surg* 84:160–166, 1997

183. Mills JJ, Chari RS, Boyer IJ, et al: Induction of apoptosis in liver tumors by the monoterpene perillyl alcohol. *Cancer Res* 55:979–983, 1995

184. Wong A, Chan A: Survival benefit of tamoxifen therapy in adenocarcinoma of the pancreas. A case-control study. *Cancer* 71:2200–2203, 1993

185. Miller AR, Robinson EK, Lee JE, et al: Neoadjuvant chemoradiation for adenocarcinoma of the pancreas. *Surg Oncol Clin North Am* 7:183–197, 1998

186. Abrams RA, Grochow LB: Adjuvant therapy with chemo-
therapy and radiation therapy in the management of carcinoma of the pancreatic head. *Surg Clin North Am* 75:925–938, 1995

187. Dobelbower RR, Konski AA, Merrick HW, et al: Intraoperative electron beam radiation therapy (IOEBRT) for carcinoma of the exocrine pancreas. *Int J Radiat Oncol Biol Phys* 20:113–119, 1991

188. Zerbi A, Fossati V, Parolini D, et al: Intraoperative radiation therapy adjuvant of resection in the treatment of pancreatic cancer. *Cancer* 73:2930–2935, 1994

189. Mohiuddin M, Rosato F, Barbot D, et al: Long-term results of combined modality treatment with I-125 implantation for carcinoma of the pancreas. *Int J Radiat Oncol Biol Phys* 23:305–311, 1992

190. Dobelbower RR, Battle JA: Radiotherapy, in Howard JM, Idezuki Y, Ihse I, Prinz RA (eds): *Surgical Diseases of the Pancreas* (ed 3). Baltimore, Williams & Wilkins, 1998, pp 587–595

191. Gastrointestinal Tumor Study Group: Further evidence of effective adjuvant combined radiation and chemotherapy following curative resection of pancreatic cancer. *Cancer* 59:2006–2010, 1987

192. Gastrointestinal Tumor Study Group: Therapy of locally unresectable pancreatic carcinoma: a randomized comparison of high dose (6000 rads) radiation alone, moderate dose radiation (4000 rads + 5-fluorouracil) and high dose radiation + 5-fluorouracil. *Cancer* 48:1705–1710, 1981

193. Milas L, Hunter NR, Mason KA, et al: Role of reoxygenation in induction of enhancement of tumor radioresponse by paclitaxel. *Cancer Res* 55:3564–3568, 1995

194. Lawrence TS, Chang EY, Hahn TM, et al: Radiosensitization of pancreatic cancer cells by 2′,2′-difluoro-2′-deoxycytidine. *Int J Radiol Oncol Biol Phys* 34:867–872, 1996

195. Andren-Sandberg A, Backman PL: Hormonal therapy and immunotherapy, in Howard JM, Idezuki Y, Ihse I, Prinz RA (eds): *Surgical Diseases of the Pancreas* (ed 3). Baltimore, Williams & Wilkins, 1998, pp. 613–622

196. Clary BM, Lyerly HK: Gene therapy and pancreatic cancer. *Surg Oncol Clin North Am* 7:217–237, 1998

197. Jaffee EM, Schutte M, Gossett J, et al: Development and characterization of cytokine-secreting pancreatic adenocarcinoma vaccine from primary tumors for use in clinical trials. *Cancer J Sci Am* 4:194–203, 1998

198. Walsh D: Palliative management of the patient with advanced pancreatic cancer. *Oncology* 10:40–44, 1996 (suppl)

199. Alter CL: Palliative and supportive care of patients with pancreatic cancer. *Semin Oncol* 23:229–240, 1996

200. Foley KM: Supportive care and the quality of life of the cancer patient, in DeVita VT, Hellman S, Rosenberg SA (eds): *Cancer: Principles and Practice of Oncology* (ed 4). Philadelphia, Lippincott, 1993, pp 2417–2448

201. Padilla GV: Psychological aspects of nutrition and cancer. *Surg Clin North Am* 66:1121–1135, 1986

202. Walsh D: Palliative care: management of the patient with advanced cancer. *Semin Oncol* 21:100–106, 1994 (suppl)

203. Watanabe S, Bruera E: Anorexia and cachexia, asthenia, and lethargy. *Hematol Oncol Clin North Am* 10:189–206, 1996

204. Albrecht JT, Canada TW: Cachexia and anorexia in malignancy. *Hematol Oncol Clin North Am* 10:791–800, 1996

205. Portenoy RK: Constipation in the cancer patient: causes and management. *Med Clin North Am* 71:303–311, 1987

206. Krech RL, Walsh D: Symptoms of pancreatic cancer. *J Pain Symptom Manage* 6:360–367, 1991

CHAPTER 64

Prostate Cancer

Jeanne Held-Warmkessel, RN, MSN, CS, AOCN

Introduction

Each year, thousands of men are diagnosed with prostate cancer. Nurses in all practice settings will care for men with a potential or actual prostate cancer diagnosis. Up-to-date information is required by nurses to educate and care for these patients. This chapter will present current information regarding screening, early detection, diagnosis, and management of prostate cancer.

Epidemiology

Prostate cancer is the most commonly diagnosed solid tumor in American males and the second-leading cause of cancer-related deaths. In 1999, an estimated 179,300 new cases of prostate cancer were diagnosed and 37,000 men died from the disease.[1] The incidence of prostate cancer increased in the years between 1976 and 1994.[2] It now appears that the number of cases diagnosed each year since then has stabilized. Prostate-specific antigen (PSA) screening is largely responsible for the initial increase and eventual decline in the number of newly diagnosed patients. With the onset of PSA testing availability, large numbers of men were diagnosed. As time passed, the pool of potential patients dwindled and fewer men were potentially diagnosable and the incidence of disease fell.[3,4] Prior to 1990, the death rate from prostate cancer was on the rise.[5] The death rate from prostate cancer fell from 26.5 to 17.3 deaths per 100,000 men in the years 1990–1995.[6] Possible causes of the reduced death rate include screening over the prior 20 years, improved documentation of cause of death, changes in treatment modalities, and diagnosis of disease at an earlier, more treatable stage.[5]

Black males have the highest incidence of prostate cancer, with a mortality rate twice that for white males. Among black Africans living in Africa, there is wide variability in the incidence of prostate cancer.[2] Racial and ethnic groups living in the United States with a lower prostate cancer incidence include men of Korean descent with prostate cancer ranked as the fifth most common cause of cancer. Japanese men who emigrate to the United States soon have a similar incidence of prostate cancer as compared to white men living in the United States even though Japanese men living in Japan have the world's lowest incidence of prostate cancer.[2,7,8]

Prostate cancer is a major health problem throughout the world. Countries with rates higher than the United States include Trinidad, Tobago, and Switzerland. Countries with rates lower than the United States in addition to Japan include Singapore and the Russian Federation.[2]

Etiology

The cause of prostate cancer is unknown. Risk factors have been identified and relate primarily to lifestyle, age, and heredity.

Lifestyle factors include nutrition and exposure to carcinogens. Fat consumption appears to be related to the risk of the development of prostate cancer[9,10] or the diagnosis of cancer at an advanced stage.[11] Diets higher in animal fat may alter the hormonal environment and predispose a man to an increased cancer risk.[12] Reducing the consumption of animal fats may offer some protection from developing prostate cancer.[13] Increasing fiber consumption may also be beneficial.[14] Fat consumption may account for the higher incidence of prostate cancer among black men.[10] The issue of the role of vitamins and the risk of prostate cancer remains inconclusive.[9] Beta-carotene may have a protective role as may vitamins A and D.[15–17] Vitamin A as a chemoprevention agent is currently being investigated in clinical trials. Vitamin A is an essential fat-soluble vitamin that promotes normal cellular growth.

Exposure to carcinogens such as cigarette smoke, cadmium, or zinc may play a role in prostate cancer development.[18] Further research is needed into the roles diet, animal fat, fiber, vitamins, and trace elements play in prostate carcinogenesis.

The use of bilateral vasectomy for birth control may increase the risk of prostate cancer.[18] The risk appears to be greater for men who had a bilateral vasectomy more than 20 years ago.[19,20] The age-related relative risk of prostate cancer after vasectomy is 1.66.[19] If the vasectomy was done 22 years ago or more, the relative risk is 1.85.[19] The etiology by which vasectomy may promote prostate cancer development is poorly understood but may relate to prostatic gland fluid stasis, which occurs postvasectomy as it does with aging. Many other studies have failed to demonstrate an increased risk of prostate cancer in men who have had a vasectomy.[21–23] Nurses should inform their patients who wish to undergo vasectomy control that the procedure may increase the risk of prostate cancer; however, more research is needed to determine the etiologic relationship between vasectomy and carcinogenesis.[24] Men who do select this procedure should consider participating in annual prostate cancer screenings provided by their family doctor.

Prostate cancer is a disease of the older male. Before age 50, clinically evident prostate cancer is rare. The incidence after age 50 increases on a yearly basis to reach approximately 1000 cases per 100,000 males age 65–69.[25] By age 80–84, the incidence per 100,000 males is greater than 3000.

Hereditary-linked prostate cancer is characterized by an early onset of disease and the presence of an autosomal dominant pattern of inheritance.[26] The risk of cancer for a particular individual is greater if the family member with cancer is a first-degree relative (father, brother) and greatest if both first-degree and second-degree relatives (grandfather, uncle) had prostate cancer.[27] Also, family history is a greater risk factor for patients younger than age 55 than it is for older patients (70–85 years)[28] and for black and white men than for Asian American men.[29]

Black males have the highest incidence of prostate cancer in the world[9]—averaging 30%–50% higher incidence with poorer survival rates than whites.[1] Multiple factors may cause this higher incidence including higher prevalence of high-grade prostatic intraepithelial neoplasia (PIN), a possible cancer precursor, and the reluctance of black males to participate in screening programs.[30,31] Generally poor attitudes toward the system of health care by black males is an additional barrier to health care. Additionally, black males have more advanced tumors at the time of diagnosis and the tumors may have a more aggressive nature.[32,33] It was thought that when patients have equal access to the same health care system, the survival rates for both groups would be similar.[33] However, in a study of health maintenance organization patients black men had poorer survival because of more aggressive disease.[34]

Testosterone levels are regulated by the hypothalamus and the anterior pituitary gland. The hormones from these glands cause the testicles to produce testosterone. The enzyme 5-alpha-reductase in the prostate converts testosterone into dihydrotestosterone (DHT), which has a potent direct effect on prostate development.[2,9] Research into the influence of hormones on prostate cancer development has been inconclusive.[9] Men without androgens do not develop prostate cancer.[2] A study of four different ethnic groups revealed that in all groups, older men have lower testosterone levels than younger men but the DHT: testosterone ratio was different among ethnic groups.[35] The ratios were highest in blacks and next highest in white men. These ratios are comparable to the incidence of disease in these groups and may be related to 5-alpha-reductase activity and the differences in enzyme activities among racial groups.[35] Testosterone levels were higher in black men but the results were not statistically significant.[35]

Multiple genetic changes may play a role in the development of prostate cancer, the development of PIN, the incidence of localized disease, and a tumor's metastatic potential. The change from androgen dependence to androgen independence is associated with additional genetic alterations. Changes occur in oncogene expression, deletion of chromosome arms, suppression of apoptosis and inactivation of tumor suppressor genes.[36,37] Variants of the human *SRD5A2* gene are found in high-risk black males.[38] This gene is responsible for 5-alpha-reductase activity and this alteration may help explain the higher incidence of prostate cancer in this group.

Prevention, Screening, and Early Detection

As the etiology of prostate cancer is unknown, specific recommendations regarding prevention cannot be made. Rather, based upon the known risk factors, several suggestions can be proposed. Consuming a low-fat, high-fiber diet may reduce the risk of developing prostate cancer. Maintaining normal weight for height would also seem reasonable. Obtaining vitamins and trace minerals from vegetable sources and avoiding known carcinogens such as cigarette smoke may also reduce one's risk of prostate cancer. Participating in screening would also be an important intervention.

The Prostate Cancer Prevention Trial (PCPT) opened to accrual in 1993 and closed in 1996 after 18,059 men without prostate cancer were randomized. The men received either placebo or 5 mg finasteride daily for seven years. Finasteride is a 5-alpha-reductase inhibitor that interferes with the formation of dihydrotestosterone.[39] Each year, the participants undergo digital rectal exam (DRE) and analysis of PSA. In seven years, at the end of the drug intervention, the men will have prostate biopsies performed.[40] This study will help answer questions about the ability of finasteride to prevent prostate cancer.[39] Other agents that have been investigated for the chemoprevention of prostate cancer include fenretinide and aromatase inhibitors.[41,42]

Screening for prostate cancer involves the use of DRE, PSA level, and, if appropriate, evaluation of the gland using transrectal ultrasound (TRUS). DRE involves palpation of the prostate gland. The posterior and lateral glandular tissue is evaluated by the examiners' finger.[43] It is the most commonly performed screening exam for prostate diseases[44] and assists in evaluating for lesions, texture, and symmetry of the gland. Limitations to DRE include failure to locate tumors in the anterior and midline of the prostate, where approximately 40% of cancers may be found.[45,46] DRE is recommended as part of an annual physical exam for men beginning at age 50 who are expected to live ten years or more.[47] Those with higher risk factors, such as black men, should begin screening at a younger age. It is also important that the man being screened is educated as to the risks versus the benefits of screening.[47]

PSA is a glycoprotein found in normal prostate tissue. The protein is found in higher concentrations within the gland than in the blood. A barrier of three tissue layers lies between the blood and the PSA found in prostate ducts.[48] Anything that destroys this natural tissue barrier allows PSA to enter the bloodstream, where it can be collected and evaluated in a laboratory. Procedures that can falsely elevate PSA levels, such as biopsy, urethral instrumentation, catheterization, and possibly rectal examination, should be avoided prior to obtaining PSA blood specimens.[49]

The normal reference range for PSA is 0–4 ng/mL.[3] The human prostate gland continues to grow in the adult male after the completion of puberty. As the prostate increases in size, the PSA also increases. Benign prostatic hyperplasia (BPH) tissue can therefore be expected to produce a higher serum concentration of PSA both in the absence and presence of prostate cancer. Also, conditions other than prostate cancer can give rise to elevated PSA levels. Men with prostate cancer have been found to have higher PSA levels even when variables such as tumor volume, stage, age, and tumor grade are controlled.[50] In order to identify race-related and age-related PSA values, 3475 men (1802 white, 1673 black) were randomly selected from a pool of 14,826 military men to form a study group. The goal was to identify the PSA ranges in white

Table 64-1 Summary of Recommendations Regarding Prostate Cancer Screening

Test	Frequency	Beginning at Age	How Test Is Performed
Digital rectal exam	Annual	50*	The examiner's gloved and lubricated finger is inserted into the rectum while the patient bends over the examining table
Prostate exam	Annual	50	

*High-risk patients may begin screening at an earlier age.

Normal Results		Significance
DRE	No palpable abnormality	Able to detect abnormal gland symmetry and texture and abnormal lesions
PE	prostate gland symmetry, texture, and no masses felt	

Age	PSA Range—Whites (PSA Results (normal 0–4.0 ng/mL))	PSA Range—Blacks
40–49	0–2.5 ng/mL	0–2.0 ng/mL
50–59	0–3.5 ng/mL	0–4.0 ng/mL
60–69	0–3.5 ng/mL	0–4.5 ng/mL
70–79	0–3.5 ng/mL	0–5.5 ng/mL

Results are age and race related. All abnormal results require additional diagnostic studies.
Data from vonEscenbach et al[47]; Morgan, et al[51]

and black men. As a result of their study, the authors recommended a new range for PSA values based on patient age and race.[51] The new ranges will improve the usefulness of PSA in identifying important cancers in younger and older patients in both races (see Table 64-1). PSA tests are not foolproof. About 25% of cancers do not secrete PSA and an elevated PSA does not mean that a man has cancer. As mentioned above, benign prostatic conditions can also increase PSA levels.

Total PSA includes free PSA and conjugated PSA. Free PSA has been evaluated for its ability to enhance differentiation of benign and malignant disease. It has been found to be both useless and useful in different trials.[52–54] In one study, free PSA levels were lower in patients with prostate cancer than in patients without prostate cancer, but free PSA was not more useful than total PSA.[52] Other studies have determined that free PSA is useful in reducing the number of biopsies of benign disease.[53,54] For cancer detection, the amount of free PSA from total PSA should be 25% when the total PSA ranges between 4–10 ng/mL and DRE evaluation indicates benign disease.[54] The use of free PSA may also be helpful when evaluating men with PSA values of 2.6–4.0 ng/mL and a benign prostate exam.[55] Free PSA can be used with individual patients to help determine the need for biopsy or follow-up biopsy.[54,56] Patients with more than 25% free PSA are more likely to have benign disease and those with 25% or less free PSA need to undergo biopsy to assess for cancer.

PSA density describes the ratio of serum PSA to prostate volume as determined by TRUS.[57] Research has demonstrated TRUS is of most use with PSA levels of 4–10 ng/mL[54] and in conjunction with additional tests when making a decision about biopsy.[56]

PSA velocity is how much PSA values increase over time. An increase of 0.75–0.80 ng/mL/year is significant[58–61] and may be useful in identifying cancers. Specimens should be obtained over a two-year period to detect a trend in PSA changes.[62,63]

Finasteride is a 5-alpha-reductase inhibitor used to treat BPH. It reduces PSA levels by 50%.[64] A PSA level of 2 ng/mL should be used when screening for prostate cancer in men taking finasteride.[37]

TRUS is used to follow up abnormal DRE or elevated PSA levels. The test can evaluate prostate volume and identify suspicious areas of 5 mm or larger for biopsy.[65] Its role in screening programs is not yet defined.[66] An ultrasound probe is inserted into the rectum and can reveal hypoechoic areas and other abnormalities in the prostate. Needle biopsies of suspicious areas are then obtained under ultrasonic guidance. Three additional directed biopsies from each lobe of the prostate are routinely obtained.

No area of cancer research continues to be as hotly debated as the issue of whether there should be mass public screenings to detect prostate cancer. A 1994 study reviewed the pathologic features of 583 localized prostate cancers for the number that were clinically unimportant, clinically important, curable, or clinically important advanced.[67] The patients had either clinically-detected or cystoprostatectomy-detected cancers. Tumors detected by cystoprostatectomy were smaller, more likely to be confined to the prostate, and less likely to contain poorly differentiated cells. Most of these lesions were felt to be clinically unimportant. Tumors that had been clinically detected and then removed by radical prostatectomy were more likely to be clinically important. Fifty-five of the 583 patients had nonpalpable tumors but elevated PSA. The cancers in the latter group were of higher grade, and 40% of them extended outside the prostatic capsule. Patients with tumors palpable by DRE were more likely to be advanced than nonpalpable tumors (34% versus 11%). Another study determined that 84% of cancers detected by PSA were clinically significant.[68,69]

Additional support for the ability of PSA to detect clinically important cancer comes from the Physician's Health Study.[70] During ten-year follow-up, only 8.7% of the men with an elevated PSA did not develop clinical prostate cancer. In fact, it was determined that one PSA assessment would have found 80% of the important prostate cancers that became apparent in five years and would also have found approximately 50% of those that were identified in ten years. The authors therefore concluded that PSA is a valid tool for screening cancer.

Contradicting this evidence are data from the American Cancer Society National Prostate Cancer Early Prostate Detection Program.[71] The study involved 2999 healthy men age 55–70, who were followed annually for five years or until a cancer was diagnosed in the prostate. The annual exam included DRE, TRUS, and PSA. Biopsies were obtained via TRUS when a suspicious area was detected during the test. Biopsies from 265 men were evaluated and were diagnostic for prostate cancer in 177 men. Seven men were diagnosed as having PIN and the remainder as having atypical glands, atypical hyperplasia, or benign hyperplasia. The men with cancers were found to have early, low-grade tumors.[71]

The number of important cancers diagnosed by PSA screening has increased.[72–76] Until recently, however, there have been no controlled trials to demonstrate that screening saves lives. The first and only study to demonstrate that screening has an impact on prostate cancer was reported as an abstract.[77] A prospective randomized trial of 46,289 men was conducted in Canada. Men assigned to the screening arm underwent PSA (0–3 ng/mL was defined as normal) and DRE on the first evaluation. If either test was abnormal, TRUS was performed. On follow-up, TRUS was completed if PSA increased above 3 ng/mL or increased by 10 percent from the last visit. In the unscreened arm of 38,160 men, there were 138 prostate cancer-related deaths and six prostate-cancer related deaths in the screening arm of 8129 men. This was a statistically significant difference.[77] Additional trials are needed to validate this finding. Until then, the American Cancer Society (ACS) guidelines should be utilized. Black males, because of their higher risk of prostate cancer, should be encouraged by nurses to participate in annual prostate cancer screening provided by their family physicians. Men who have first-degree relatives with prostate cancer should also be educated regarding the need to participate in earlier screening.

The cost of screening to both the individual and society cannot be ignored. From a financial perspective, do the dollars spent on screenings prolong life or prevent unnecessary deaths? Presently, there are no research trials that can answer the question of whether prostate cancer screening is cost effective.[78] Screening identifies not only clinically important cancers that require treatment but clinically insignificant prostate cancers that may not shorten survival or threaten the patient's life. The individual needs to understand that treatment may not influence survival and may cause important side effects including impotence and incontinence.

Pathophysiology

The prostate gland, which is approximately the size of an inverted, triangularly shaped walnut, sits beneath the bladder and anterior to the rectum. The section of the urethra that passes through the prostate is known as the *prostatic urethra*. Draining into the prostatic urethra are the prostatic ducts. Prostatic fluid drains into the prostatic ducts from the glandular elements of the prostate. This fluid aids in the fertilization process[79] (Figure 64-1).

The prostate gland is composed of three major sections: the central zone, the peripheral zone, and the transitional zone. The larger peripheral zone that surrounds the central zone is the most common site for cancer.[37]

The prostate is well vascularized. Its major blood supply originates from the inferior vesical artery.[37] Venous drainage is through the inferior hypogastric venous system and the presacral prevertebral venous plexus; lymphatic drainage is via the external and internal iliac groups and obturator lymph nodes. These nodes and lymphatics then drain into the common iliac and preaortic lymph nodes.

Cellular Characteristics

The vast majority (95%) of prostate cancers are adenocarcinomas. Of the 5% of prostate cancers that are not adenocarcinomas, greater than 90% are transitional cell carcinomas. A rare squamous cell carcinoma may also occur and is the third most common type. All prostate cancers arise from glandular epithelial cells.[80]

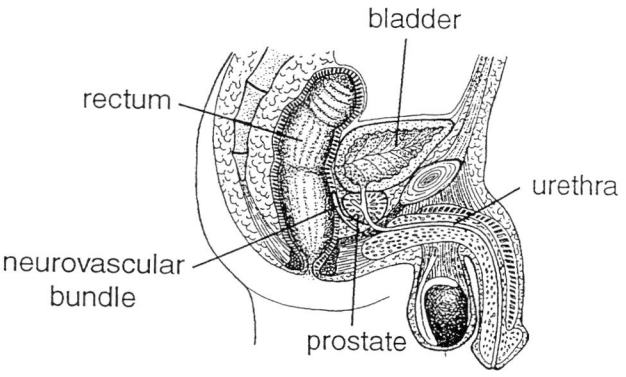

Figure 64-1   Prostate anatomy.

Epithelial cells proceed through a variety of stages on their way to becoming malignant. As already mentioned, premalignant changes in prostate tissue is termed *prostatic intraepithelial neoplasia (PIN)*.[81] PIN is further categorized as low grade or high grade[82,83] and may be present for ten or more years before cancer is diagnosed.[84] Presently, it is not possible to determine if PIN will evolve into cancer in a particular patient because the exact biology of PIN has yet to be determined. High-grade PIN should be further evaluated for the presence of invasive cancer.[82]

Prostate tissue specimens are subjected to a type of pathologic scoring based on cellular architecture known as the *Gleason score*. The majority of the tumor is occupied by cells with one type of histologic feature that is given a number (grade) of 1 to 5 based upon the severity of the cellular changes. The lower numbers are assigned to cellular patterns that are similar to prostatic tissue (well differentiated). The higher numbers are cellular patterns with more bizarre architectural features that look less like normal prostatic tissue (poorly differentiated).[85] This primary number is added to a secondary number, which reflects the second most common type of cellular structure using the same grading format. The sum of the two numbers gives the total Gleason score. Not all studies utilize the summed format. Tumors graded 1–3 are considered well differentiated and those graded 4 or 5 are considered poorly differentiated carcinomas. When the entire prostate gland is available for pathologic review, the volume of tissue and the Gleason grade may be able to predict the presence of extracapsular spread and lymph node metastases.[86] When the Gleason grade is 4–5 (poorly differentiated), the risk of nodal metastases increases when the volume of cancer is more than 3.2 cc.[87] The risk of nodal metastases is less than 1% when the cancer volume is less than 3.2 cc. Nodal metastases are correlated with Gleason grade, PSA and clinical stage.[88]

Prostate cancers can also be divided into those that are clinically important (significant) and those that are clinically unimportant.[89] Clinically important cancers include features such as large tumor volume, Gleason grade 3–5 (moderate to poor differentiation), an invasive, proliferative pattern of growth, elevated PSA, and origination in the peripheral zone.[89] These cancers threaten the patient's life because they progress to fatal metastatic cancers. Cancers that do not threaten the patient's life are termed *indolent* and considered clinically unimportant. These indolent cancers, which comprise the vast majority of prostate cancers, are small with a Gleason's grade of 1–2 (well differentiated), are noninvasive in their pattern of growth, do not elevate the PSA, originate in the transitional zone, and tend to fail to progress into invasive metastatic cancers.[89]

Progression of Disease

Prostate cancer is generally characterized by a slow pattern of growth. The tumor grows locally along tissue planes such as the prostatic capsule and may penetrate through junctional areas of the capsule.[65] These junctional areas include the bladder neck, ejaculatory ducts and prostatourethral area.[65] Cancers of the prostate apex and base are more likely to have spread beyond the capsule due to inherent structural weaknesses in these areas.[65] Perineural invasion may accompany capsular invasion.[90] Surrounding structures such as the bladder may be involved with tumor growth. When lymphatic metastases occur, they may involve the obturator, presacral, presciatic, internal, and external iliac nodes.[37] After lymph node metastases, the next most commonly involved metastatic site is bone, especially the lumbar spine, pelvis, femur, and skull. The cells spread to these distant sites via the bloodstream after gaining access to the Batson plexus of presacral veins.[63] Other distant sites of metastases include the lungs, bladder, and liver.

Clinical Manifestations

Prostate cancer is usually asymptomatic in its early stages. As the disease progresses, patients may present with urinary tract obstructive symptoms similar to BPH, such as frequency, incomplete bladder emptying, hesitancy, nocturia, and urgency.[91] Symptoms may be abrupt in their onset but otherwise are similar to BPH. Other symptoms may include a change in erectile capability. Advanced prostate cancer may be evidenced by the appearance of ureteral obstruction caused by ureterovesical junction compression by tumor or nodal metastases.[92] Hydronephrosis can then ensue, threatening function of the associated kidney. Back pain may reveal the presence of vertebral body metastases with the potential for spinal cord compression.[93] There may also be local pain due to the presence of the cancer in the prostate gland and invasion into surrounding structures, and referred pain to the legs and abdomen. Bone pain can be problematic and is related to the presence of additional skeletal metastases. The hip, legs, neck, shoulders, and ribs are the next most common areas to be affected.[92] Additional symptoms related to advanced prostate cancer growth include weight loss, rectal obstruction from local growth, coagulation deficits related to the release of procoagulant into the bloodstream from the prostate cancer cells, hypercalcemia, leg edema from nodal metastases, and pancytopenia from marrow metastases.[92,93]

Assessment

Patient and Family History

Nursing assessment of patients at risk for or with a diagnosis of prostate cancer should begin with questioning the patient about past medical problems or prior diagnoses of prostate disorders. The presence of a prostate cancer diagnosis in first- and second-degree relatives should be ascertained, and exposure to potential prostate carcinogens or risk factors needs to be determined.

The nurse should evaluate the patient's voiding pattern and ask if the patient has problems with dysuria, frequency, nocturia, hematuria, and other signs of bladder outlet obstruction (Table 64-2).

Physical Exam

The patient is examined for evidence of local and distant metastases. The pelvic and suprapubic areas should be percussed and palpated for bladder distention. A postvoid residual measurement may be ordered by the physician or nurse practitioner to evaluate the volume of residual urine in the bladder. Inguinal nodes are assessed, and the patient is queried regarding bone pain, specifically back pain. If back pain is present, the patient is questioned about signs of spinal cord compression, such as numbness, tingling, and other indications of sensory loss, motor weakness, or bowel or bladder incontinence.[95] Other potential areas of pain include the rectum and local pelvic area. The patient is asked for information about any pain medications he has been using, their effectiveness, and side effects. The patient's legs should be examined for edema and its severity and for indications of deep vein thromboses, such as unilateral leg edema, pain, local heat, and redness. The skin should be checked for petechiae and ecchymoses. The patient is weighed and asked how much weight he has lost since the illness began.

Diagnostic Studies

Once a presumptive diagnosis of prostate cancer is made, the patient will have a PSA level drawn and a DRE performed if these tests have not previously been ordered. As PSA levels reflect the severity of the patient's disease,[91] it may be drawn before and after therapeutic interventions and then periodically to monitor the status of the cancer. Additional blood tests include serum chemistries, including calcium, liver function tests, blood urea nitrogen (BUN), creatinine, and complete blood count (CBC). A urine analysis is performed and a chest x-ray is completed. Magnetic resonance imaging (MRI) scans of the abdomen and pelvis may be done to evaluate local and nodal metastasis and to determine the proper treatment for the patient. A bone scan is frequently performed to evaluate bone pain and may be performed as part of the staging workup. Bone scans are usually negative in patients with a PSA of less than 8 ng/mL.[96] TRUS may be used to assist in evaluating the extent of localized prostate cancer.[96] In patients being considered for curative surgery and who have a Gleason score of greater than 7 ng/mL, a laparoscopic pelvic lymph node dissection may be performed to evaluate the presence of nodal metastasis.

Prognostic Indicators

PSA levels may reflect the extent of disease and the amount of cancer found in the prostate gland.[91] For example, PSA levels in stage A disease average 3.1 ng/mL; A_2—12.1 ng/mL; B_1—12.3 ng/mL; B_2—25 ng/mL; B_3—40 ng/mL; C—102 ng/mL; and D_2—563 ng/mL.[97] PSA levels are used to monitor the effectiveness of treatment and to monitor the patient for disease recurrence. Unfortunately, not all prostate cancers produce PSA, and other diagnostic studies, such as MRI or computerized tomography (CT) scan or ProstaScint scan, may be needed to monitor disease status. Baseline blood levels are obtained before and after treatment and usually are monitored every three months after treatment for one year and then every 6–12 months. Levels greater than

Table 64-2 Questions Useful in Assessing Urinary Symptoms Associated with Prostate Cancer and Other Urologic Disorders

Symptom	Assessment
Dysuria	Does the patient have difficulty initiating urination? If so, how often?
	Does the patient have difficulty maintaining or ending the urine stream?
	Does the patient need to apply pressure to the bladder to initiate urination?
	Does dribbling occur at the end of urination?
	Is there pain on urination? If so, how does the pain feel? Does it persist or is it intermittent?
	Are there bladder spasms?
Frequency	How often does the patient need to urinate?
	What is the volume of each voiding?
	Does the patient void and then need to void again a few minutes later?
	Is there a reduction in the urine volume produced?
Nocturia	How many times does the patient get out of bed each night to urinate?
	Is there incontinence at night?
Hematuria	Is there blood in the urine? Clots?
	What is the color of the urine?
Other	Does the urine have an odor?
	Is particulate matter present in the urine?
	When did the patient void most recently?
	Can the patient feel his bladder through the abdominal wall?
	Is there flank pain?
	How many urinary tract infections has the patient had in the last 12 months?
	Has there been a change in the strength of penile erections?

Data from Black and Matassarin-Jacobs.[94]

Table 64-3 American Joint Committee on Cancer Staging for Prostate Cancer

Primary Tumor, Clinical (T)

TX Primary tumor cannot be assessed

T0 No evidence of primary tumor

T1 Clinically inapparent tumor not palpable nor visible by imaging
  T1a Tumor incidental histologic finding in 5% or less of tissue resected
  T1b Tumor incidental histologic finding in more than 5% of tissue resected
  T1c Tumor identified by needle biopsy (e.g., because of elevated PSA)

T2 Tumor confined within prostate*
  T2a Tumor involves one lobe
  T2b Tumor involves both lobes

T3 Tumor extends through the prostate capsule**
  T3a Extracapsular extension (unilateral or bilateral)
  T3b Tumor invades seminal vesicle(s)

T4 Tumor is fixed or invades adjacent structures other than seminal vesicles: bladder neck, external sphincter, rectum, levator muscles, and/or pelvic wall

  *Note: Tumor found in one or both lobes by needle biopsy, but not palpable or reliably visible by imaging, is classified as T1c.

  **Note: Invasion into the prostatic apex or into (but not beyond) the prostatic capsule is not classified as T3, but as T2.

Primary Tumor, Pathologic (pT)

pT2*** Organ confined
  pT2a Unilateral
  pT2b Bilateral

pT3 Extraprostatic extension
  pT3a Extraprostatic extension
  pT3b Seminal vesicle invasion

pT4 Invasion of bladder, rectum

  ***Note: There is no pathologic T1 classification.

Regional Lymph Nodes (N)

NX Regional lymph nodes cannot be assessed

N0 No regional lymph node metastasis

N1 Metastasis in regional lymph node or nodes

Distant Metastasis ** (M)**

MX Distant metastasis cannot be assessed

M0 No distant metastasis

M1 Distant metastasis
  M1a Nonregional lymph node(s)
  M1b Bone(s)
  M1c Other site(s)

  ****Note: When more than one site of metastasis is present, the most advanced category is used. pM1c is most advanced.

STAGE GROUPING

Stage	T	N	M	G
Stage I	T1a	N0	M0	G1
Stage II	T1a	N0	M0	G2, 3–4
	T1b	N0	M0	Any G
	T1c	N0	M0	Any G
	T1	N0	M0	Any G
	T2	N0	M0	Any G
Stage III	T3	N0	M0	Any G
Stage IV	T4	N0	M0	Any G
	Any T	N1	M0	Any G
	Any T	Any N	M1	Any G

80 ng/mL reflect a large disease burden and, often, metastatic cancer.

After undergoing primary therapy for any stage of prostate cancer, an increasing PSA level reflects disease progression.[98] After undergoing curative resection for prostate gland-confined cancer, PSA levels should be undetectable.[63,99] Doses of 5040–5400 cGy external beam radiation therapy are used to treat prostate cancer. PSA levels should be normal 3–18 months after completion of therapy. Failure of PSA to normalize often reflects localized disease recurrence.[100] Therefore, PSA is a highly useful tool for the monitoring of disease response to therapy and monitoring the patient for cancer relapse.

Classification and Staging

A commonly used staging system for prostate cancer is the American Urologic Association (AUA) system,[37] which was originally developed by Whitmore and then updated by Jewett. The tumor-node-metastasis (TNM) (Table 64-3) system was developed by the American Joint Committee on Cancer (AJCC) Chicago, Illinois and is also frequently used. Table 64-4 presents a comparison of these two staging systems.

Small cancers found on transurethral resection of the prostate for BPH are often asymptomatic and are staged as A. When the cancer involves less than both lobes of the gland, it is considered B_1 disease. B_2 cancer involves both lobes of the prostate. After the cancer has invaded into or beyond the prostate capsule, stage C disease is present. With metastases to distant sites, the patient has stage D cancer.[37] Survival is stage dependent. Patients with stage A disease have survival at ten years of 95%; stage B at ten years—80%; stage C at ten years—60%; stage D (nodal metastases)—40%; and stage D (distant metastases)—10%.[87]

Therapeutic Approaches and Nursing Care

Treatment options available for a particular patient are based upon patient preference, PSA, age, life expectancy,

Table 64-4 Comparison of the TNM and Whitmore-Jewett Staging Systems for Clinically Localized Prostate Cancer

TNM	Whitmore-Jewett	Description
	STAGE	
TX	*	Tumor cannot be assessed
T0	*	No evidence of tumor
T1a	A1	Tumor found incidentally at TURP (<5% of resected tissue)
T1b	*	Tumor found incidentally at TURP (<5% of resected tissue)
T1c	B0	Nonpalpable tumor identified by means of an elevated serum PSA value†
T2a	B1	Tumor involves half of a lobe or less
T2b	B1	Tumor involves more than half a lobe but not both lobes
T2c	B2	Tumor involves both lobes
T3a	C1	Unilateral extracapsular extension
T3b	C1	Bilateral extracapsular extension
		Tumor invades one or both seminal vesicles
T4a	*	Tumor invades the bladder neck, external sphincter, or rectum
T4b	*	Tumor invades the levator muscles or is fixed to the pelvic side wall

*No corresponding stage.

†In the TNM staging system, the tumor should not be visible on transrectal ultrasonography.

Reprinted with permission from Oesterling J, Fuks Z, Lee CT, et al: Cancer of the prostate, in DeVita VT, Hellman S, Rosenberg SA (eds): *Cancer: Principles and Practice of Oncology* (ed 5). Philadelphia, Lippincott-Raven, 1997, p 1334.[37]

general medical condition, tumor grade (Gleason score), and tumor volume (stage).[96] A patient may be offered watchful waiting (periodic observation), surgery, radiation therapy, combination therapy, hormonal manipulation, chemotherapy, or investigational drugs administered in a clinical trial setting.

Watchful Waiting or Periodic Observation for Early-Stage Prostate Cancer

Prostate cancer is a heterogenous disease. The current challenge lies in differentiating the clinically significant diagnosable cancer from the clinically insignificant tumor.[101] As indicated previously, prostate cancer is often slow growing. Men with small-volume, well-differentiated cancers may die with, rather than from, prostate cancer. In the male population of the United States as a whole, there exists a group of 8 million men over age 50 with a potentially diagnosable prostate cancer. Of these 8 million men, 7.9 million will have an autopsy-discoverable

cancer.[89] The remaining 100,000 men have a clinically diagnosable cancer.[89] Clinically diagnosable prostate cancer, untreated, will continue to grow and threaten the life of the patient. Latent or clinically unimportant cancers do not threaten the patient's life. Of men age 50 or older, approximately one-third will have malignant cells in their prostate.[102] As men age beyond 50, the incidence of cancer cells in the prostate increases. However, only 2%–3% of men who develop malignant cells in their prostate will die of the disease.[102] For men with early stage A and B₁ prostate cancer, this observation has led some physicians to offer periodic observation as a method of cancer management. Periodic observation involves monitoring PSA level and physical examination every three to six months to determine if there has been clinical disease progression.

For patients over age 70, watchful waiting may be an appropriate treatment option.[103] Research has yet to demonstrate that for the approximately 60% of men who present with stage A or B cancer, treatment is more beneficial than watchful waiting.[104] For men under age 70, a physician may often be reluctant to offer watchful waiting. There is also evidence that for younger men with moderately or poorly differentiated localized prostate cancer, treatment may offer a survival advantage.[103] For patients older than 70, treatment that produces side effects such as incontinence may be less beneficial.[103]

Treatment for localized prostate cancer may be presented as a means of preventing metastatic disease from developing.[102] However, there is no evidence that this is true. Currently for men in their forties and fifties, even with well-differentiated cancers, definitive treatment is almost always offered. Prostate cancer may behave in a more aggressive manner because of higher-grade tumors in younger men, and for this reason alone, definitive treatment is offered. Also, younger men have the potential to live longer and thus develop metastases that may be life-threatening.

The option of watchful waiting may not gain widespread support without evidence from prospective randomized trials. Until such results are known, scientifically proven therapy with surgery or radiation therapy will be offered to patients with localized prostate cancer. Several studies have been conducted that address the concept of watchful waiting, both in Sweden and in the United States. However, some of the studies contain methodological flaws. Even though flawed, these studies are often cited as evidence that watchful waiting is an appropriate option in selected patients. A Swedish study followed 223 patients with stage A or B prostate cancer.[105] Urinary symptoms were managed with transurethral prostatic resection (TURP), and if disease progression occurred, hormonal manipulation was initiated. At the ten-year mark, 124 of the original 223 patients were dead, but for only 8.5% of the patients was the cause of death related to the prostate cancer.[105]

Aus and associates studied mortality of patients with prostate cancer registered at the Swedish Cancer Registry from 1961–1990.[106] A group of 536 patients were identified and 514 were included in the report. The other patients were lost to follow-up (2), treated (16), or identified at autopsy (14). Patients were monitored every 6–12 months. Endocrine therapy was administered to 63% (324 patients). The other 185 patients were managed with deferred treatment. There were 301 men with M0 disease, 50% of whom died due to prostate cancer. Sixty-five patients lived longer than ten years and had a prostate cancer-related mortality rate of 63%. Compared to the whole group of M0 patients with a 50% mortality rate, this was a statistically significant finding (p < 0.05).[106] These results indicate that at diagnosis, younger patients have a greater risk of dying of prostate cancer after ten years. Additionally, patients who live longer than ten years may have a local disease at diagnosis and would be the group most likely to benefit from curative treatment.

Albertsen and colleagues performed a retrospective cohort study of men age 65–75 diagnosed in Connecticut with localized prostate cancer from 1971–1976.[107] The cohort consisted of 451 men with an average age of 70.9 years. At time of diagnosis, the patients were TA1, TA2, TAx, or TBx based on chart content and pathologic information. Treatment when offered consisted of hormonal manipulation. Follow-up continued for 15.5 years, at which time 40 men (9%) were still alive. In only 34% of the cases of these who had died could the cause of death be attributed to prostate cancer. In 8%, the cause could not be determined and 49% had causes of death other than prostate cancer listed on the death certificate. The Gleason score was the most powerful predictor of death in this study. With a Gleason score of 8–10, 46% of men were dead in ten years and 51% were dead in 15 years. The death rates at 10 and 15 years respectively for Gleason score 5–7 were 24% and 28%, and for Gleason score 2–4, the mortality rate was 9% at both intervals. Men with high Gleason scores lost six to eight years of life and those with a Gleason score of 5–7 lost about four to five years of life. Men with low-grade tumors did not experience loss of life years.

Fleming and colleagues examined the literature to identify risks and benefits of currently available therapy for men over age 60.[103] Men with well-differentiated tumors and men over age 75 were identified as benefiting from watchful waiting. The research also concluded that patients with moderately to poorly differentiated tumors should undergo treatment, as longer survival (3.5 years) may be achieved.

Another study evaluated data from 828 patients who participated in six nonrandomized trials. The men received observation and delayed hormone therapy for localized stage A and B cancer.[108] The cancers were graded 1 (well differentiated, Gleason score 2–4), 2 (moderately differentiated, Gleason score 5–7), or 3 (poorly differentiated, Gleason score 8–10). Grade 3 patients had a poorer survival ratio and at ten years, 34% of these men were alive and 26% were free of metastatic disease. The authors concluded that for grade 1–2 clinically localized cancer in men with a life expectancy of less than ten years, observation and delayed hormonal manipulation is an option for selected patients.

In a more recent study, 113 patients in a program of watchful waiting were evaluated for outcome. Patients were placed on the program for four reasons: patient preference, physician preference, medical problems that reduced expected life survival, and contraindications to radiation therapy.[109] Disease progression was defined as increased T classification or palpable disease.[109] Patients had rapid disease progression by two years on the study. In patients with T1 disease, 40% progressed and in T2 disease, 51% progressed. At three years of follow-up, almost 60% in both groups progressed. The Gleason score did not predict clinical progression.

Based on these studies, it is easy to understand the conflict and confusion around the issue of watchful waiting. One study that may potentially shed light on this issue is the Prostate Cancer Intervention versus Observation Trial (PIVOT). This trial compares radical prostatectomy to observation in men with clinically localized prostate cancer.[110]

Surgery

Transurethral resection of the prostate (TURP)

Prostate cancer is not cured by TURP. Rather, the procedure is used to treat symptoms of bladder outlet obstruction and in some patients, provides pathologic evidence that a cancer, previously unsuspected, is present. Using a transurethral resectoscope and electrocautery, the hypertrophic prostate is removed in pieces called *chips*. The procedure is done under spinal anesthesia or general anesthesia with the patient in the dorsal lithotomy position. Potential immediate postoperative complications include clot retention, bleeding, and infection. The bladder is kept as free of blood and clots as possible using continuous saline irrigation through a three-way indwelling catheter. Bladder spasms can be problematic and patients may require analgesics and antispasmodics. After the bleeding decreases, bladder irrigation is discontinued. As the urine becomes more normal in appearance, the catheter is removed. Rarely, patients may have difficulty initiating urination after catheter removal and may require recatheterization.

Nursing aspects of managing patients include preoperative education as to routine aspects of anesthesia, such as coughing, deep breathing, and early ambulation. The patient needs to know he will have a catheter after surgery and bladder irrigation for approximately 24 hours or less. Pain management approaches using oral and rectal medications are discussed. The patient must drink large volumes of fluid, such as water, to promote urine formation. Accurate recording of intake and output is required until discharge. Large amounts of fluid may be absorbed through the cut prostatic capillaries during surgery resulting in volumetric overload. This is referred to as the *TUR syndrome* and may occur in the first 24 hours postoperatively. TUR syndrome is common, occurring in 10%–15% of men who undergo TURP.[111] As a result of fluid shifts, electrolyte disturbances and hypoosmolality may precipitate neurologic and hypovolemic symptoms.[112] Supportive therapy is used to manage the patient. The nurse must monitor the patient for changes in mental status and cardiac and renal function. The patient needs to be aware that late complications, such as incontinence, impotence, and bladder neck contraction requiring urethral dilation may occur.[65] Patients may have problems with recurrent bladder outlet obstruction; approximately 5% of men need to undergo repeat TURP. (Table 64-5 presents an overview of the management of the TURP patient.)[94,112,113]

Radical prostatectomy

The use of radical prostatectomy has increased since 1985.[114,115] In 1984, 8.9% of patients with a newly diagnosed prostate cancer underwent radical prostatectomy. By 1990, the incidence of radical prostatectomy had increased to 21.4%.[116] The majority of procedures are done in younger men (age 59 or younger) with localized disease as opposed to regional disease. More procedures are done in the Pacific region and the fewest in the mid-Atlantic and New England regions.[117] The increasing use of radical prostatectomy is related to the use of PSA to screen asymptomatic men.[118]

The procedure involves removal of the prostate gland, ejaculatory ducts, seminal vesicles, and possibly the lymph nodes. Radical prostatectomy is usually done on patients staged with T1 or T2 disease.[65] With T3 disease, it may be more difficult to obtain tumor-free margins. The patient should be informed preoperatively by the physician about the potential for postoperative incontinence and impotence. Incontinence may occur after indwelling catheter removal and continues to be a problem for about 10% of men postoperatively.[119] Risk factors identified for the development of postoperative incontinence include age over 65, development of anastomotic stricture, and stage T1a or T1b disease.[119] Fifty incontinent men were evaluated for the impact of incontinence after radical prostatectomy on their quality of life.[120] Twenty-six percent reported that moderate to severe incontinence had a serious impact on their quality of life. Not only were physical activities reduced, so were activities of daily living. In spite of the inconvenience of incontinence, 68% of the men would still select the surgical intervention. Persistent incontinence requires urologic evaluation for bladder neck contracture, stricture, bladder dysfunction, or sphincter dysfunction.[119]

The autonomic nerves that control erectile function lie next to the prostate. Surgery may damage or sever these nerves. Currently, however, the right, left, or both neurovascular bundles may be preserved[121] (see Figure 64-1). Walsh developed and continues to refine the method of sparing the neurovascular bundles responsible for an erection.[122] With this nerve-sparing procedure, it is possible to spare potency; however, there will not be prostatic fluid and therefore no emission and ejaculation. It is recommended for patients with stage T1 or T2 disease

who are eligible to undergo radical prostatectomy. The nerve-sparing procedure was performed in 503 men who were able to maintain an erection before surgery.[123] Sixty-eight percent of the patients were potent after surgery. Factors identified that promote sexual function after surgery are age less than 50, stage of disease, and the preservation of neurovascular bundles. In younger men (age 50 and younger), lower stage and surgical procedure were the factors associated with potency. When one bundle is intact in patients younger than 50, potency is preserved. In patients over 70, only 22% will regain potency postoperatively, even if both neurovascular bundles are spared. If disease is more advanced and there is involvement of the prostatic capsule or seminal vesicles at the time of surgery, resection may involve removal of or damage to the nerves. In the patients with B_2 or C disease, 51% had one bundle left intact. Age again becomes important with men under 50 regaining potency and older patients having a reduced likelihood of potency.

A meta-analysis of the literature available on erectile dysfunction after surgery and radiation therapy indicates that the patients who were potent preoperatively were more likely to remain potent postoperatively. Also, patients were more likely to be potent after radiation therapy than surgery (probability 0.69 versus 0.42, $p < 0.0001$).[124]

Incontinence and impotence can place a heavy burden on male patients and their families. Increasingly research is addressing concerns related to quality of life (QOL). Compared with normal age-matched men living in the same location, men who have undergone treatment for localized prostate cancer are more likely to have problems related to sexual, urinary, or bowel function.[125] QOL issues may be amenable to nursing interventions, such as patient education, and nurses need to accept responsibility for the assessment, management, and evaluation of these patient concerns.

Preoperative nursing care is similar to that provided to patients undergoing other surgical procedures of the abdomen and pelvis.[126] Many patients undergoing radical prostatectomy will be over age 50, and special attention should be paid to the patient's comorbid factors such as cardiopulmonary status. Additional routine preoperative care includes administering a bowel preparation to evacuate the colon, starting prescribed intravenous therapy, and ensuring that the patient eats or drinks nothing after midnight. Elderly patients should understand that they may have longer postoperative recovery times.

Intraoperatively, the prostate and its surrounding structures are removed via a perineal or retropubic incision.[65] One or more drains may be placed during surgery, and frequent dressing changes may be required to control drainage, reduce bacterial growth, and reduce the risk of skin maceration and resultant infection. The nurse must monitor incision and drainage sites for infection.

Depending upon the surgical approach and degree of intraoperative findings, such as disease greater than expected, the patient may be immobilized on the operating room table for several hours. He is thus at risk

Table 64-5 Nursing Management of the Patient Undergoing a TURP

Nursing Diagnosis	Etiology	Outcome	Nursing Management
Knowledge deficit Surgery	Lack of prior experience with surgery	Patient will verbalize an understanding of preoperative and postoperative course	1. Assess patient's understanding of cancer diagnosis, planned surgery to remove obstructing section of prostate gland around prostatic urethra compressing urethra and impeding release of urine from the bladder, expected outcome that patient will be able to void with reduced difficulty, potential complications of surgery including incontinence. 2. Educate patient regarding: <ul><li>care of indwelling catheter</li><li>continuous bladder irrigation (CBI)</li><li>drinking fluids</li><li>ambulating first day postop</li><li>coughing and deep breathing</li><li>pain management with belladonna and opium suppositories for bladder spasms, oral narcotics for pain</li><li>signs/symptoms of urinary tract infection (UTI) to report to physician after surgery—pain, burning, frequency, hematuria</li><li>need to notify physician after discharge of inability to void, continued incontinence, bright red urine, numerous clots, chills, fever, decreased stream size and force</li></ul>
Incontinence	The urinary sphincter may be injured during surgery—may persist up to three months in elderly	The patient will be able to manage incontinence	<ul><li>methods for managing incontinence (see Table 64-6)</li></ul>
Indwelling catheter care	The patient is unable to void after indwelling catheter is removed postop and requires recatheterization and discharge home with indwelling catheter	The patient will demonstrate the skills necessary to maintain an indwelling catheter at home	3. Educate patient to: <ul><li>wash around urinary meatus with soap and water, rinse and dry the area twice daily</li><li>utilize leg bag during day, how to attach, disconnect, empty and cleanse bag to maintain a clean environment inside the equipment</li><li>utilize straight drainage at night, how to cleanse bag to maintain a clean environment inside the equipment</li><li>maintain a clean bag environment by rinsing the equipment, washing it with soapy water, rinsing well, and allowing it to air dry</li></ul>
Altered urinary elimination related to TURP and indwelling catheter	The patient has undergone TURP and requires catheter to maintain prostate urethra patency and elimination of urine and blood Clots have formed in the bladder, occluding the catheter/tubing lumen. As the bladder fills, clots slide down the outside of the catheter and out the meatus	The catheter will remain patent. Urine output will be ≥ 30 mL/h	1. Maintain accurate I&O 2. Empty urinary drainage bag when ⅔ full 3. Maintain CBI at rate to keep urine clear using NSS 3-liter irrigation bags. Do not allow bags to empty. Keep NSS running at all times to maintain pink-colored drainage. CBI is usually discontinued 24 hr postop, but may by required for a longer period if some bleeding or clot formation persists beyond the first 24 h 4. Monitor for clots in the tubing, monitor for clot retention with subsequent bleeding around the catheter. Assess for bladder distention. Notify physician of clot retention. Irrigate Foley manually with saline until free of clots. Do not forcefully irrigate catheter—notify surgeon 5. Maintain IV fluids at prescribed rate of infusion 6. Encourage fluid intake, usually 2000 ml/24 h 7. Maintain catheter tubing patency by unkinking tubing 8. One to two days postop, the catheter is removed. Accurately measure the first and each subsequent voiding until discharge. Notify physician if patient does not void in 8 h

Table 64-5   Nursing Management of the Patient Undergoing a TURP (continued)

Nursing Diagnosis	Etiology	Outcome	Nursing Management
Bleeding related to TURP	The prostate is highly vascularized. Cauterization during the surgery does not seal all the bleeding capillaries, therefore bleeding occurs in the postoperative period	The patient will have prompt recognition of and immediate intervention for increased bleeding. Bleeding will decrease daily	1. Monitor hemoglobin and hematocrit values. Notify physician of ≥ 1 g reduction in hemoglobin 2. Maintain traction with tape on catheter applied during surgery to assist in control of venous bleeding in prostatic bed 3. Monitor color of urine. There should be a noted reduction in the amount of blood in the urine daily. If increased blood is present, notify physican 4. Do not remove water from overfilled indwelling catheter balloon, as this helps to control bleeding 5. Do not remove indwelling catheter until physician orders its removal. Premature removal may result in bleeding 6. Monitor for bladder distention, which increases bleeding by pulling on capillaries
Potential for infection related to surgery and indwelling catheter	The presence of an indwelling catheter may promote bladder infection. The patient has undergone surgery under general anes-thesia and may develop postop atelectasis, which may develop into pneumonia	The patient will not develop a fever or other sign of infection	1. Encourage q1h coughing and deep breathing 2. Use aseptic technique when emptying drainage bag and attaching new bladder irrigation bags 3. Perform meatal care twice daily with soap and water 4. Maintain catheter patency. Observe for clots, chips of tissue, mucus that can obstruct catheter lumen. Keep catheter and tubing straight and free of kinks. Keep drainage bag off floor. Hang with hook from bed 5. Notify physician of temp ≥ 38.5°C, tachycardia, tachypnea, decreased BP, other signs of infection 6. Obtain urine, blood, or other cultures as prescribed
Altered comfort related to pain, bladder spasms, or both	Pain or bladder spasms may be due to surgery, bladder distention, infection, clots, or the catheter balloon	The patient will verbalize an acceptable level of analgesia	1. Assess quantity, quality, and duration of pain 2. Check for bladder distention, kinked tubing, freely flowing drainage. Palpate bladder after turning off CBI. Restart CBI if patient not distended. Otherwise, notify physician 3. Administer prescribed narcotic for pain 4. Administer belladonna and opium suppository, oxybutynin, or propantheline for bladder spasms 5. Gently irrigate indwelling catheter if prescribed. Never force irrigation fluid—notify physician 6. Remind patient not to tug or pull at the catheter. If the patient should pull out the catheter, notify physician immediately
Potential for urethral stricture formation related to surgery	The urethra may heal with stricture formation if catheter is removed prematurely	The patient will have a patent urethra	1. The catheter is never to be removed without a physician's order 2. Monitor for signs of stricture, such as small urine stream, straining to void, and difficulty voiding
Potential for urinary retention after catheter removal	The patient is not able to void after catheter is removed	The patient will not develop urinary retention	1. The patient should void when he feels the urge and not wait, as this may produce urinary distention, which may cause retention
Constipation related to antispasmodics used to manage bladder spasms	Anticholinergic drugs cause constipation. Straining can cause bleeding	The patient will have an easy bowel movement	1. Administer stool softeners/laxatives to reduce constipation and promote easy colon evacuation 2. Educate patient not to strain on bowel movement
Potential for altered fluid and electrolyte balance	Fluid balance and electrolyte alterations occur during surgery	The patient will have prompt recognition of signs and symptoms of altered fluid and electrolyte balance	1. Monitor electrolytes, BUN, creatinine. Notify physician of abnormal results 2. Assess patient for changes in mental status, vital signs, for tremor, vomiting, headache 3. Monitor patient for change in renal or cardiac function

Data from Black et al[94], Gravenstein et al[112], Held et al.[113]

for the usual postoperative complications. The nurse needs to encourage coughing, deep breathing, use of analgesics, and moving around in bed to promote lower extremity venous return to the heart. Compression stockings are usually used in the postoperative period to reduce the risk of thrombophlebitis and potentially fatal pulmonary embolus. In the presence of thrombophlebitis or suspected/proven pulmonary emboli, anticoagulant therapy is initiated with a heparin bolus and a heparin drip is started.

An indwelling urinary catheter is placed in the operating room and will remain in place postoperatively. Attention is needed to reduce the risk of infection with thorough hand washing, use of aseptic technique when emptying the drainage bag, and monitoring the catheter for patency. In addition to maintaining the indwelling catheter, the nurse must monitor the amount of hematuria.

In the initial postoperative period, a nasogastric tube may be placed to control gastric distention and remove gastric secretions. Management includes monitoring the type and amount of drainage, providing mouth care to promote oral comfort, and maintaining tube patency. Drains will collect serosanguineous drainage for four to five days postoperatively.[127] A sudden increase in the amount of drainage, the presence of increased bleeding, or the appearance of urine in the drains requires prompt physician notification.

Postoperatively, it is crucial that the patient maintain a urine output of greater than 30 mL/hr.[113] In addition to monitoring for hematuria and clots, maintaining a patent catheter, and ensuring an accurate intake and output, the nurse should assess the bladder for urinary retention and administer parenteral fluids. Also, the catheter taped to the patient's upper leg must be maintained securely to avoid catheter movement and tugging on the newly anastomosed urethra. The catheter provides support to the healing urethra and must not be removed without a physician's order.

Bladder spasms can be annoying and painful. They may be caused by kinking of the catheter, bladder distention, or from the catheter itself.[94] Bladder spasms are commonly managed by administering antispasmodics such as oxybutynin, and, if not contraindicated, belladonna and opium (B&O) suppositories.

Hematuria is common for the first 24 hours after surgery.[127] Frank bleeding and clots are abnormal and require physician notification. Frequent monitoring of vital signs is needed to assess the patient for signs of excess blood loss and temperature elevation, which may indicate a wound or urinary tract infection.

The patient is discharged with an indwelling catheter and needs to be educated in meatal care, attachment of a leg drainage bag, change to straight drainage bag at bedtime, cleaning technique, and signs of urinary tract infection that would require physician notification. After the catheter is removed two to three weeks postoperatively, incontinence may be a problem for days, weeks, or months. A variety of management options are available.

Simple devices, such as penile clamps or incontinence pads, may be suggested. Reducing the volume of fluid consumed after dinner may control problems with nighttime incontinence. Frequent emptying of the bladder (e.g., every hour) may provide a patient with enough control over his incontinence that he finds occasional incontinence tolerable. Instructing the patient to use Kegel exercises to strengthen the muscles also may be beneficial.

Incontinence is a problem not only for patients undergoing prostate surgery but also for many other adults. The problem is so severe that the Agency for Health Care Policy and Research released urinary incontinence guidelines in 1992.[128] The guidelines provide an in-depth discussion of incontinence and its management (Table 64-6).

An additional burden placed on postprostatectomy men is the development of altered sexuality. See Chapter 37 for an in-depth discussion of sexual dysfunction and suggestions for nursing management. Table 64-7 presents "Helpful Hints for Starting Sexual Activity After Prostate Surgery."

Cryosurgery

Cryosurgery to treat prostate cancer was revived in the 1990s due to the development of TRUS and improved surgical techniques that permit access to the prostate through a percutaneous approach.[142] Probes deliver a substance, such as liquid nitrogen, to freeze the tissues and are inserted percutaneously into the prostate. The urethra is kept warm with an indwelling urinary catheter that circulates warm water (44°C).[143] Iceballs form at the end of the probes freezing the prostate tissue and killing the cancer cells. Freezing must be rapid for good cell kill.[144] The procedure is monitored using TRUS. Candidates for cryoablation include patients who are not candidates for radical prostatectomy or radiation therapy. Advantages include less pain, bleeding, and incontinence.[143] Possible complications include bleeding, infection, incontinence, fistula formation, urethral obstruction, urethral strictures, numbness of the penis, and possibly impotence.[143] Also, not all the cancer cells may be killed.

Cryosurgery of the prostate remains an investigational procedure. In one research study, 83 patients had cryosurgical ablation of the prostate performed.[145] The first 12 patients were treated using TRUS guidance only and 83% of the patients had positive biopsies postprocedure. The other 71 patients had TRUS and temperature monitoring during the procedure and had a 90% negative biopsy rate. Complications included urethral sloughing, incontinence, impotence, and bladder neck contractures.[145] Long-term follow-up of these and other cryosurgery patients and additional research trials are needed to determine the role of this procedure in the treatment of prostate cancer.

Nursing care includes preoperative teaching regarding the bowel preparation with polyethylene glycol and home

Table 64-6 Assisting Patients to Manage Urinary Incontinence After Prostate Surgery

After prostate surgery, continence is maintained by the external urinary sphincter. It is this striated urethral sphincter that prevents urinary leakage after prostate surgery.[129] Damage to the muscle controlling the sphincter or damage to its nerve supply can result in postoperative incontinence. The retropubic approach to prostatectomy may result in a lower rate of incontinence by avoiding injury to the cavernous nerves of the pelvic plexus.[130,131] After radical prostatectomy, 92% of patients achieve urinary control, 8% experience stress incontinence, and 6% wear one or fewer incontinence pads per day. Approximately 1% of men are incontinent after a TURP.[132]

Evaluation

Diagnostic studies are performed to evaluate incontinence after a history and physical exam are performed. Cystourethroscopy is used to evaluate the integrity of the external urinary sphincter under direct visualization. A voiding cystourethrogram looks for anatomic abnormalities while urodynamic studies evaluate physiology.[133]

Management

Diapers, liners—These devices absorb urine. There are a variety available on the market. Liners are useful for light to moderate incontinence. Adult diapers are needed for heavy urine loss. All devices should be changed frequently to avoid odor and skin maceration. Fungal infections can occur, and in summer, diapers can be hot and uncomfortable.[134] Cost can become a factor when absorbent products need to be changed frequently; for people with a limited income, this can be a financial burden. Bulky items may be noticed under clothing.

Drip collectors—The penis is placed inside the collector which is worn underneath clothing in a garment holder designed to hold the disposable collecting device.[134]

Condom catheters—Latex self-adhesive condom-shaped external urine collecting device. Problems include adhesive loss, skin breakdown, and urinary tract infections. The skin needs to be cleansed daily and monitored daily for irritation and infection.[128]

Indwelling catheters—Closed sterile system that includes a catheter with a retaining water-filled balloon inserted into the urethra attached to a collection bag. Often left in place after surgery, these devices require daily cleansing and skin care to reduce the risk of infection and skin necrosis. These are not useful for long-term management of incontinence unless no other approach is successful.

Penile clamps—External urethral compressive device that occludes the urethra to reduce incontinence. The position of the clamp must be changed every 3 hr to prevent skin necrosis. Other complications include pain, edema, penile and urethral erosion, and urethral obstruction.[128]

Ostomy pouch—Useful for a small or retracted penis. Clip the hair around where the adhesive is applied and attach pouch to a collection bag.

Fluid restriction—The patient who experiences incontinence mostly at night should restrict fluids after dinner to reduce the bladder urine volume and thus the risk of incontinence. Otherwise, 2 quarts of fluids per day are encouraged.

Timed voiding—At predetermined intervals, the patient empties the bladder. To develop a schedule, the patient needs to keep a diary for three or four days to identify times of incontinence. A schedule is then developed for the patient to void prior to the times identified as being at risk for incontinence.[128]

Kegel exercises—The pelvic floor muscles are crucial to maintaining continence. These muscles can be strengthened with exercise. The exercise consists of contracting the pelvic floor muscles by squeezing the pubococcygeus muscle.[128] Squeezing this muscle closes the urethra. The abdominal, pelvic, and thigh muscles must not be contracted during the exercises. Contracting the muscles involved in a bowel movement by pulling them in and holding for 10 seconds, followed by a 10-second rest, and repeated 30 to 80 times a day for a minimum of 6 weeks, can result in better bladder control.

Biofeedback—Used in conjunction with Kegel exercises and timed voiding, biofeedback helps the patient become attuned to his physiology. Instruments help the person learn about bladder control.

Bladder dysfunction (detrusor instability)—Symptoms include frequency, urgency, urge incontinence.[135] Treatment includes fluid restriction and medications:

Anticholinergics

Propantheline—blocks bladder contractions, dose 7.5 mg to 30 mg 3 to 5 times a day;[128] cost—inexpensive; effect—may reduce incontinence in up to 53% of patients; side effects—urinary retention, dry mouth, blurred vision, nausea, constipation, confusion, drowsiness. Hyoscyamine is a newer drug.

Oxybutynin—also relaxes smooth muscle, dose 2.5 to 5 mg 3 to 4 times a day; effect—may reduce incontinence in up to 56% of patients; side effects—dry skin, blurred vision, nausea, constipation.[128]

Muscarinic receptor antagonist—tolterodine

Tolterodine—dose 2 mg 2 times a day PO—muscarinic receptor antagonist, new drug—expensive, lower incidence of dry mouth, better tolerated and as effective as oxybutynin.[136,137]

Antidepressants

Imipramine—anticholinergic properties, dose 10 to 25 mg 1 to 3 times a day; side effects—rare; effect—up to 77% of patients may have reduced incontinence.[128]

Sphincter incompetence—Symptoms include dribbling and stress incontinence.[135] Treatment includes alpha-adrenergic agonist drugs and surgery. The drugs increase sphincter resistance:

Phenylpropanolamine—dose 50 mg twice a day; effect—up to 45% of patients are drier; side effects—nausea, dry mouth, rash, itching, restlessness, insomnia.[128]

Surgery—goal is urethral compression.[133] Artificial urinary sphincter—useful in patients with normal detrusor function and an incompetent sphincter[132] and after failure of previously discussed methods.[128] Approximately 80% of patients treated will be dry or almost dry requiring no incontinence pads.[132] Complications include infection, device malfunction, bleeding, erosion of cuff site, and urethral injury.[128] Injections of collagen or polytetrafluoroethylene may be useful in patients who are not surgical candidates.

Data from Black et al[94], Urinary Incontinence Guideline Panel[128], Walsh[129], Steiner et al[130], Walsh et al[131], Marks et al[132], Foote, Leach[133], Thayer[134], Freedman, Love[135], Appell[136] Abrams et al.[137]

Table 64-7　Helpful Hints for Men Starting Sexual Activity After Prostate Surgery

With removal of the prostate, men may notice changes in their sexual functioning. Some men and their partners benefit from understanding these changes and learn how to adapt to them. Beginning with some definitions of the changes, methods of ways to adapt to these changes will be described.

Erection—stiff penis due to increased blood flow

Potency—ability to cause vaginal penetration

Orgasm—sexual climax or pleasure with ejaculation of semen

Semen—mixture of sperm, prostate secretions, and seminal vesicle fluid

Sperm—reproductive cells produced by testes

Radical prostatectomy—removal of prostate, seminal vesicles, and surrounding tissues to remove cancer. With removal of the prostate and seminal vesicles, the ejaculate will be reduced and may be retrograde into the bladder resulting in a dry ejaculation. The urine will become cloudy from the sperm. Orgasms may still occur without ejaculation but with the contractions that occur as part of ejaculation. Impotency can result from surgery or radiation therapy. This can be partial or complete inability to obtain an erection. Some men will regain potency postoperatively, especially those under age 50.

Nerve-sparing radical prostatectomy—Depending on the size and location of the tumor, the surgeon spares one or both nerve bundles responsible for an erection. In the majority of men under 50 potency returns after wound healing occurs and all edema from the surgery subsides. This can take up to two years. Older men, over age 70, will probably not regain an erection.

Orgasms after prostate surgery may be weaker but are rarely completely absent. Alternative methods of obtaining pleasure need to be pursued if there is impotency.

In order to begin sexual activity after prostate surgery, wound healing must be complete; therefore, the urologist's permission is needed. This may occur six weeks to three months after surgery. Open, honest discussion of sexual issues with one's physician, nurse, and partner will help explore avenues of sexuality not previously considered. Open communication with the partner is the cornerstone of sexual recovery. Explore alternative methods of pleasure such as kissing, stroking, cuddling, massage, gentle rubbing, and fondling. Consider sexual counseling with a therapist if open discussion with the partner and other methods of pleasure are not successful. Couples need to understand that there is more to sexuality and pleasure than penis-vagina intercourse. The intimacy that develops between two partners who love each other will permit exploration. Beginning exploration produces trust and more intimacy that promotes the desire to find ways to pleasure the partner that may not have been previously considered. Failure to communicate desires and needs to one's partner is the greatest barrier to regaining sexual relations. It must also be understood that cancer of the prostate cannot be transmitted during sex or in the sperm. Cancer of the prostate is not a sexually transmitted disease.

Alternate methods of obtaining an erection include external and internal devices. Men in stable relationships with a previously good sex life are the best candidates. However, many of these couples have been able to substitute other sexual activity if erections are not able to penetrate the vagina.[138]

External Devices

Suction apparatus—vacuum erection device fits over the penis and air is removed by pumping it out with the device. Blood flows into the penis, making it rigid. A band is placed at the base of the penis to prevent blood from leaving the penis after the device is removed. After intercourse, the band is removed.[139]

Injections of drugs into the spongy penile tissue increase blood flow to the area and produce an erection. Side effects include penile fibrosis and priapism. Drugs include prostaglandin E (alprostadil) and papaverine.[112]

Drug impregnated pellets that are placed into the urethra also produce an erection.[140] Side effects include hypotension, urethral pain and burning, penile pain, and dizziness.

Internal Devices (implanted penile prostheses)

Semirigid—a variety of devices are available. The rod is placed in the spongy tissue of the penis but away from the urinary sphincter so that voiding is not affected. Heavy athletic undergarments will conceal the crotch bulge. Many of the devices available have a metal core that allows the device to be bent upward for sexual activity and downward for everyday activities.[139]

Self-containing prosthesis, semirigid—a self-contained device with a pump behind the head of the penis that is pumped to fill the rod with fluid from a reservoir. As the rod fills, an erection is produced. After sexual activity, a release valve drains the fluid back into the reservoir. Many of these devices can be placed under local anesthesia. Semirigid rods are the most commonly implanted penile prostheses. Success rates run about 95% for semirigid devices.[112]

Inflatable penile prosthesis—consists of inflatable rods, reservoir, tubing, and pump. The reservoir for the fluid which fills the inflatable rods is placed in the abdomen with the pump in the scrotum. When the pump is activated manually, the fluid exits the reservoir and enters the rods, producing an erection. To release the fluid and deflate the rods at the end of intercourse, the release valve is activated. Mechanical problems occur in 10% to 20% of devices placed.[112,138]

Medication—Sildenafil 100 mg PO 1 hr prior to sexual activity. Effective in men with both neurovascular bundles intact.[141] Side effects include headache, color vision abnormalities. Contraindications—nitrates. Deaths have been reported in men taking both medications.

Data from Black et al[94], Schrover[138], Schrover[139], Costabile et al[140], Zippe.[141]

care of the suprapubic urinary catheter.[143] Postoperative care includes monitoring vital signs, intake & output (I&O), administering IV fluids, assessing the suprapubic catheter site, and pain management. Sequential compression stockings may be used to promote venous return. Ambulation is promoted on the first postoperative day. The patient must drink large amounts of fluid each day (2.5 liters) and report signs of infection to the physician after discharge. Home care may be needed to assist with bladder retraining and care of the catheter.

Radiation Therapy

External beam radiation therapy may be administered in curative doses to treat men with early prostate cancer

(T1, T2) confined to the gland itself. Radiation therapy is an available option if a patient wishes to avoid surgery or is not a surgical candidate due to preexisting medical problems. There is no evidence that either radiation therapy or surgery is superior in early stage disease (T1a–T2b).[146] No randomized trials have been completed to compare surgery and radiation therapy in patients with the same stage of disease.[146] Radiation therapy may also be used for stage T3 or T4 disease.[147] The dose of radiation administered is 62–74 Gy over seven to eight weeks.[148] Factors predicting postradiation treatment failure are the pre- and postradiation PSA levels and tumor classification.[149]

The radiation portal includes the prostate, periprostatic tissue, and pelvic lymph nodes. Treatment is usually given to a wide pelvic field to 45 Gy and then the treatment area is reduced to the prostate and surrounding area to complete the prescribed dosage.[147] Radiation therapy also can be administered in the postoperative setting after radical prostatectomy. Common indications include positive surgical margins, "close" surgical margins, and seminal vesicle involvement.[150] Patients who relapse after prostatectomy may also benefit from radiation therapy.[151] In one study of 23 patients who relapsed after prostatectomy, radiation doses administered ranged from 60–65 Gy. This allowed 74% of patients to achieve tumor control with 45% having five-year, relapse-free survival. Patients with locally advanced disease benefit from goserelin administered concurrently with radiation therapy.[152] Both local control and survival are improved. Radiation is also useful in managing complications of advanced prostate cancer including hematuria, urinary obstruction, ureteral obstruction, and pelvic pain. Some patients with recurrence after radiation therapy may be eligible to receive additional treatment with brachytherapy.[151]

Side effects of radiation therapy include fatigue, urinary frequency and burning, impotence, urinary incontinence, diarrhea, and rectal bleeding.[153,154] Diarrhea can be problematic, as a part of the colon and rectum lie within the radiation field. The patient needs dietary counseling at the initiation of therapy. Teaching includes a low-residue diet and management of diarrhea through regulation of the quantity of fiber consumed. Antidiarrheals, such as loperamide HCl, may be used to control diarrhea. Severe diarrhea may require opioid therapy.

The skin in the perineal area is thin and easily damaged by radiation therapy. Skin integrity is maintained through frequent perineal care, including gentle washing of the rectal area with soap and water after each bowel movement and applying a radiation-approved gel such as Natural Care Gel (Bard Patient Care Division) or a cream after treatment. All gels and creams should be washed off before treatment each day. The patient needs to avoid ointments and products that are difficult to remove until radiation therapy is completed. Silver sulfadiazine cream may be useful in promoting wound healing after radiation is completed.

Symptoms of radiation cystitis can be managed through the use of urinary antispasmodics such as oxy-butynin, urinary analgesics such as phenazopyridine, frequent voiding, and management of urinary tract infections with antibiotic therapy. Fluids should be consumed in large volumes and caffeine should be avoided.

Altered sexual functioning probably is related to damage to the blood supplying the corpora cavernosa.[155] Potency is maintained in approximately 30%–50% of patients receiving radiation[156,157] and may be related to age, with older men being at greater risk of impotency. Impotence begins months to years after completion of therapy. Cigarette smoking may have a negative affect on potency.[155] Diabetes, hypertension, and myocardial infarction are also known to decrease potency.[157,158]

Proctitis and rectal bleeding require medical management, including sigmoidoscopy, fulguration of bleeding vessels, and hydrocortisone enemas. Blood transfusions may be required if bleeding causes the hemoglobin to drop to 8 gm/dL.

Urethral strictures from inflammation are managed with periodic dilation or transurethral incision of the stenosis.[159] Repeated dilation may be needed. The incidence of urinary complications from radiation therapy is low and is related to the dose of radiation delivered and the volume of the radiation portal; the higher the dose and the larger the volume of tissue treated, the greater the risk of complication development.[153] In a study of 1000 patients undergoing radiation therapy for prostate cancer, 7.7% developed urinary complications and only 0.5% needed surgery.[159]

Leg edema may occur following radiation therapy. Management includes leg elevation when sitting out of bed, leg exercises to promote venous and lymph return, compression stockings, and elevating the scrotum with a folded towel.[113]

Brachytherapy

Recent improvements in the methods of using brachytherapy to treat prostate cancer are related to new technology and better knowledge of brachytherapy radiobiology.[160] Prostatic brachytherapy involves the placement of radioactive seeds directly into the prostate. Iodine-125 and palladium-103 seeds are frequently used sources of radiation.[148,161] A high dose of radiation is delivered to a smaller volume of tissue with reduced doses delivered to surrounding normal structures such as the bladder and rectum. Implants may be permanent or temporary. With the patient under general anesthesia, in the lithotomy position, a template is placed on the perineal area and needles are placed into the target tissue. Radioactive seeds are left in place. Early-stage patients may be offered brachytherapy as a single-modality therapy, or it can be used in locally advanced disease as a boost to the primary therapy.[160]

After insertion of the source, the principles of time, distance, and shielding should be utilized as iodine-125 emits gamma radiation. Side effects include discomfort from the needle and seed insertion, dysuria, hematuria for 24 hours, and in rare cases, infection.[113,162] Urine should be strained to locate any dislodged radioactive seeds.[162] Routine predischarge instructions for patients with permanent implants include teaching the patient to avoid close contact with children and pregnant women. A condom should be worn during sexual intercourse for the two months following implantation in case a radioactive seed is lost during intercourse.[162] In this way the seed can be safely retrieved. The patient poses no danger as a radioactive source and the patient and his family must understand this concept before discharge to avoid issues related to self-imposed isolation for fear of exposing others to radiation. Palladium-103 has a shorter half-life than iodine-125 and therefore produces fewer urinary and rectal side effects.[161]

Hormonal Therapy

Advanced prostate cancer is frequently managed by altering the patient's hormonal status. Tumors comprise a heterogenous population of cells. Three different cell populations constitute both normal and malignant prostate tissues: androgen dependent, androgen sensitive, and androgen independent.[163] When the androgen source is eliminated from androgen-dependent cells, they die, and the androgen-sensitive ones no longer divide.[164] Androgen-independent cells do not respond to the loss of hormones and continue to grow. The adrenal gland also produces hormones, which will continuously support hormone-independent cells.[36]

The vast majority of androgen is produced by the testes. Androgen secretion is dependent on luteinizing hormone-releasing hormone (LHRH) released from the hypothalamus. LHRH stimulates the pituitary gland to produce luteinizing hormone (LH), which in turn stimulates the testes to produce testosterone (androgen).[165] The goal of hormone therapy for prostate cancer is to reduce the level of circulating androgens, causing the death of androgen-dependent cells and inhibiting the growth of androgen-sensitive cells, thereby reducing tumor size. Hormonal manipulation is not curative therapy but can provide many patients with symptom control and palliation.

There are surgical and medical approaches to reducing serum testosterone levels. The oldest method is bilateral orchiectomy. Testosterone levels are reduced quickly as 90%–95% of testosterone production is eliminated with removal of the testicles.[166]

Estrogen administration blocks LHRH and LH, resulting in reduced testosterone secretion. Diethylstilbestrol is a commonly used estrogen. The potential for cardiovascular side effects makes estrogen therapy less favorable in light of newer therapies available, which include LHRH agonists and antiandrogens. There is an estrogen compound in the oral antineoplastic, estramustine.

LHRH agonists initially increase testosterone levels, but after several days of therapy, testosterone levels fall to castration level. The surge of testosterone production after initiation of an LHRH agonist is called a *flare*. During a flare, patients need to be aware that symptoms can worsen and require prompt medical intervention. Pain may increase as well as symptoms of bladder outlet obstruction. Serious complications include spinal cord compression. Flutamide, an antiandrogen, may be administered prior to the initiation of an LHRH agonist to reduce the flare. Antiandrogens prevent the binding of testosterone to receptors on prostate cells.[167] Combining antiandrogenic therapy with an LHRH agonist, such as leuprolide or goserelin, is called *total androgen ablation (TAA)* or *maximal androgen blockade (MAB)*. TAA may improve survival and increase the amount of time before tumor progression.[165] When a patient is suitable for hormonal manipulation, combination therapy is an often-used treatment option.[168] However, a recent meta-analysis of 22 MAB studies failed to demonstrate that MAB was superior to castration alone in terms of prolonging survival.[169] Hormonal manipulation may also be used with radiation therapy in patients with T2–T3 disease.[170] Compared to radiation alone, patients receiving hormonal manipulation and radiation therapy have better local, distant, and PSA outcomes.

All hormonal manipulations have the potential to produce side effects. The most common ones are hot flashes, impotence, and decreased libido.[171] Patients on hormonal therapy may have problems with altered self-esteem, such as feelings of emasculation.[157] The loss of sexual potency may be a crisis for the patient and his sexual partner. Sensitive discussions allowing verbalization of feelings are encouraged before and during treatment.

Leuprolide and goserelin injections are administered on a monthly basis. The depot formulations are administered every three to four months. Leuprolide is given as an intramuscular injection. The drug is available in a prefilled syringe. Special instructions are provided by the manufacturer for mixing the drug and diluent. On the other hand, goserelin is given as a subcutaneous injection into abdominal fat as follows:[171] (1) Ice, a topical anesthetic cream (Emla Disc®) or a small bleb of local anesthetic may be applied to the injection site to reduce the discomfort produced by the large-gauge needle. (2) Ascertain that the drug pellet is visible in its see-through chamber. (3) Cleanse the skin with alcohol and stretch the skin tautly. (4) Firmly grasp the syringe and insert the needle into the fat. (5) After the bevel enters the skin, move the syringe so the needle is parallel to the skin and insert the needle up to the hub and then back up 1 cm. (6) Press the plunger. (7) Withdraw the needle, apply pressure to the needle site, and examine the see-through chamber to confirm that the pellet has been administered. (8) Discard the syringe according to hospital policy. (9) Again, apply ice to the injection site to reduce some of the discomfort associated with the large-gauge needle. (Bleeding is minimal.)

Patients will respond well to hormonal therapy 70%–89% of the time and responses can be several years in duration.[157] Progression of disease may be managed with palliative radiation therapy or second-line hormonal manipulation. LHRH agonists need to be continued in nonorchiectomy patients to maintain testosterone castration levels.[172]

Hormone-refractory prostate cancer may respond to the withdrawal of flutamide.[173] Discontinuing flutamide in 36 patients receiving flutamide plus an LHRH agonist resulted in ten patients having reduced PSA levels and improved clinical symptoms. Aminoglutethimide and hydrocortisone or ketoconazole and hydrocortisone combination therapy may be tried, or hydrocortisone may be used as a single agent.[172] Adrenal suppression occurs with aminoglutethimide; therefore, hormonal replacement with hydrocortisone is required (20 mg, twice a day). Hydrocortisone alone, however, lowers testosterone levels, and as a single agent may be appropriate treatment for hormone-refractory men.

Chemotherapy

For a patient with hormone-refractory prostate cancer, antineoplastic therapy may be an option. Over the past several years, research has produced several drug regimens that enhance the quality of life of patients with hormone refractory prostate cancer (HRPC). However, none of these drug combinations improve survival. A review of 26 drug trials conducted from 1987 to 1991 failed to demonstrate the effectiveness of chemotherapy.[174] Remissions in the trials averaged 8.7%, indicating that, for the most part, hormone-refractory prostate cancer is also chemotherapy resistant. Multidrug resistance is a possible explanation for the failure of patients to respond to chemotherapy.

When evaluating the response rates and research protocols used in HRPC, several factors must be taken into consideration. The trials need to disclose the hormone therapy the patient has received and control for ongoing hormonal therapy, as the withdrawal of antiandrogens during the research study may affect PSA levels rather than the agent being investigated.[173,175] PSA is often used as a method to measure research outcome. PSA values need to be clearly described in the methodology section of the research report with respect to partial and complete response and the length of time the response needs to be maintained in addition to how frequently blood levels are evaluated.[176] PSA results can be reduced by drug effect without evidence of a corresponding reduction in tumor size and therefore is used with caution as means of evaluation of tumor response in drug trials.[177,178] Likewise, soft tissue disease and bone metastases may not reflect response to treatment as patients may not have adequate disease to measure on a CT scan and bone disease is slow to demonstrate response on a bone scan.[176–179]

Recently, palliative endpoints (specifically pain) have

been used to assess treatment outcome.[180,181] For example, different tools were used in the trials to evaluate the effect of mitoxantrone and prednisone on HRPC. In one trial, 27 men with HRPC received IV mitoxantrone 12 mg/m² every three weeks with prednisone 5 mg BID.[180] Hormonal therapy was continued throughout the trial. The patients completed a present pain intensity (PPI), a visual analog scale (VAS), and the European Organization for Research and Treatment of Cancer (EORTC) 32-item quality of life tool. A palliative complete response (CR) was defined as symptom absence for six weeks. A palliative partial response (PR) was at least a 50% reduction in analgesic score without a PPI increase or a PPI decrease without an analgesic score increase.[180] The CR rate was 36% with one additional PR. Side effects included neutropenia, nausea, anorexia, constipation, and alopecia. This trial demonstrated that mitoxantrone and low-dose prednisone can reduce pain and that pain assessments and quality of life indicators can be used to evaluate drug outcome.

Another potentially useful drug combination is oral etoposide and oral estramustine. This combination has been administered with doses of estramustine ranging from 10–15 mg/kg/day in divided doses to a fixed dose of 140 mg TID.[182–185] Oral etoposide is administered in divided doses at a total dose of 50 mg/m²/day for 21 days of a 28-day cycle. Overall response rates range from 36%–53%.[182–184] Good pretreatment performance status may predict improved survival; however, this finding needs to be evaluated in phase III trials. Side effects from combination of oral etoposide and oral estramustine include nausea, alopecia, neutropenia, neutropenic fever, fatigue, deep vein thrombosis, and pedal edema.

Suramin, a polysulfonated naphthylurea, has undergone extensive study to determine the best dosing and drug administration schedule.[186–189] The goal of these research studies has been to find a method of dosing and scheduling to maintain suramin plasma levels between 100–300 mcg/mL, the lower number being the nontherapeutic level and the upper number the toxic level. A phase III trial is currently underway to determine the safest and most effective dose of suramin.[190] Suramin side effects include adrenal insufficiency requiring hydrocortisone replacement of 30–40 mg/day, polyradiculopathy, malaise, fatigue, anorexia, renal insufficiency, rash, edema, and hematologic and liver toxicity.[191] As the drug has been studied, more toxicities have been identified and include mineralocorticoid insufficiency, suramin keratosis, acute renal toxicity/failure, and coagulopathy managed with vitamin K supplements.[192–196]

Hydrocortisone has been administered with suramin to manage adrenal insufficiency and has been a potentially confounding variable in suramin response rates.[197] Another variable that required prospective control was flutamide withdrawal. After control of these two variables, the response rate to suramin in this trial of patients with HRPC was 19%.

Other drugs potentially useful in HRPC include oral

cyclophosphamide, estramustine in combination with docetaxel or ketoconazole plus doxorubicin.[198-201] Phase III trials are needed to compare the current standard of mitoxantrone plus steroid to these other drug combinations to identify the best combination to improve quality of life and perhaps affect survival.

Symptom Management and Supportive Care

Patients with advanced prostate cancer may experience a number of symptoms requiring nursing management. Problems include bone pain, spinal cord compression (SCC), leg or scrotal edema, coagulation disorders, and bladder or urethral obstruction.

Bone pain management includes a thorough assessment of location, onset, duration, and precipitating and alleviating factors. Analgesics useful in the management of bone pain include nonsteroidal anti-inflammatory drugs (NSAIDS) and narcotics, including opioids.[202,203] Routine long-acting narcotics supplemented by immediate-release, short-acting narcotics is a useful regimen. Doses are titrated to achieve maximal analgesia with minimal side effects. Expected narcotic side effects include constipation that requires management with routine laxatives and stool softeners. Additional side effects may include dry mouth, nausea, vomiting, and sedation. NSAID side effects include gastric distress, dizziness, and drowsiness. Higher doses produce more side effects but without enhancing analgesia. Other agents useful in the management of bone pain include the radionuclides strontium-89 and samarium-153.[204] Myelosuppression is the dose-limiting toxicity. Bisphosphonates may also be useful in the management of bone pain, but their use outside clinical trials is currently not recommended due to lack of data supporting their efficacy.[205] Radiation therapy is also effective in the management of bone pain.

All patients with bone metastasis are at risk for SCC. Prompt diagnosis and intervention are required to reduce the risk of permanent disability. Patients with SCC frequently have back pain. There may be a radicular component with the pain encircling the chest or abdomen. Leg weakness, sensory changes, and alterations in bowel or bladder function may be present. Diagnosis of SCC is made by MRI or myelogram. Treatment includes the use of dexamethasone, radiation therapy, and, in selected cases, surgery.[206,207] Pretreatment performance status is a useful predictor of patient outcome. Of patients who are ambulatory at diagnosis, 75% will remain so but only 28% of paraplegic patients become ambulatory.[207] Nursing management focuses on preserving function, promoting restoration of lost function, and assisting the patient to adapt to changes in his ability to perform activities of daily living while monitoring for changes in neurologic functioning.

Leg and scrotal edema are distressing symptoms produced by advanced prostate cancer. A deep vein thrombosis (DVT) must always be considered as a potential cause of unilateral or bilateral leg edema. Additional causes include lymphedema and medical conditions such as hypoalbuminemia or fluid overload. Elevation of the affected area may be useful but is often difficult to maintain. Diuretics reduce intravascular fluid volume without reducing edema.[208] Compression stockings may be needed to reduce the edema.

In addition to DVT, a coagulation disorder found in patients with advanced prostate cancer is disseminated intravascular coagulation (DIC), which is characterized by the consumption of clotting factors and platelets resulting in concurrent hemorrhage and clotting. Patients experience bleeding from multiple body areas, abnormal laboratory results, and clotting throughout the body.[209] Nursing management includes frequent assessment of all body systems, administration of blood products, IV fluids, and medications, and monitoring of laboratory results.

Bladder outlet obstruction evidenced by the inability to void may be managed by intermittent or indwelling urinary bladder catheterization, TURP, or urethral stent. Ureteral stents or percutaneous nephrostomy tubes are used in the treatment of ureteral obstructions. Nursing management includes monitoring for infection and bleeding and educating the patient about catheter care.

Gradually, as the disease progresses and symptoms worsen, patients will find that they are less able to perform their usual activities of daily living. A palliative care team approach is useful in managing the progressive symptoms associated with advancing prostate cancer. A hospice referral provides optimum end-of-life care.

Conclusion

As the incidence and prevalence of prostate cancer continues to rise, it is imperative that nurses, particularly those in advanced nursing practice roles, become active in early detection programs that target high-risk individuals, especially black males. Participation in public education programs in the workplace will further demonstrate the nurse's role as educator and patient advocate. Helping families to understand the controversies involved in the management of prostate cancer continues to be a nursing priority.

References

1. Landis SH, Murray T, Bolden S, et al: Cancer Statistics, 1999. *CA Cancer J Clin* 49:8–31, 1999
2. Haas GP, Sakr WA: Epidemiology of prostate cancer. *CA Cancer J Clin* 47:273–287, 1997
3. Potosky AL, Miller BA, Albertsen PC, et al: The role of increasing detection in the rising incidence of prostate cancer. *JAMA* 273:548–552, 1995

4. Wingo PA, Landis S, Ries LAG: An adjustment to the 1997 estimate for new prostate cancer cases. *CA Cancer J Clin* 47:239–242, 1997

5. Mettlin CJ, Murphy GP: Why is the prostate cancer death rate declining in the United States? *Cancer* 82:249–251, 1998

6. Surveillance, Epidemiology and End Results (SEER) Program: Age-adjusted U.S. cancer death rates. *J Natl Cancer Inst* 89:12, 1997

7. Parker SL, Davis KJ, Wingo PA, et al: Cancer statistics by race and ethnicity. *CA Cancer J Clin* 48:31–48, 1998

8. Shimizu H, Ross RK, Bernstein L, et al: Cancers of the prostate and breast among Japanese and white immigrants in Los Angeles County. *Br J Cancer* 63:963–966, 1991

9. Keeley FX, Gomella LG: Epidemiology of prostate cancer, in Ernstoff MS, Heaney JA, Peschel RE (eds): *Prostate Cancer*. Malden, MA: Blackwell Science, 1998, pp 2–14

10. Whittemore AS, Kolonel LN, Wu AH, et al: Prostate cancer in relation to diet, physical activity and body size in blacks, whites, and Asians in the United States and Canada. *J Natl Cancer Inst* 87:652–661, 1995

11. Rose DP: Dietary fatty acids and cancer. *Am J Clin Nutr* 66:998S–1003S, 1997 (suppl)

12. Ross RK, Henderson BE: Do diet and androgens alter prostate cancer risk via a common etiologic pathway? *J Natl Cancer Inst* 86:252–254, 1994

13. Giovannucci E, Rimm EB, Colditz GA, et al: A prospective study of dietary fat and risk of prostate cancer. *J Natl Cancer Inst* 85:1571–1579, 1993

14. Ross JK, Pusateri DJ, Shultz TP: Dietary and hormonal evaluation of men at different risks for prostate cancer: fiber intake, excretion, and composition, with in vitro evidence for an association between steroid hormones and specific fiber components. *Am J Clin Nutr* 51:365–370, 1990

15. VanPoppel G, Goldbohm RA: Epidemiologic evidence for beta-carotene and cancer prevention. *Am J Clin Nutr* 62:1393S–1402S, 1995 (suppl 6)

16. Hanchette CL, Schwartz GG: Geographic patterns of prostate cancer mortality: evidence for a protective effect of ultraviolet radiation. *Cancer* 70:2861–2869, 1992

17. Kadmon D, Thompson TC: Chemoprevention in prostate cancer, in Vogelzang NJ, Scardino PT, Shipley WU, et al (eds): *Comprehensive Textbook of Genitourinary Oncology*. Baltimore, Williams and Wilkins, 1996, pp 657–667

18. Pienta KJ, Esper PS: Risk factors for prostate cancer. *Ann Intern Med* 118:793–803, 1993

19. Giovannucci E, Ascherio A, Rimm EB, et al: A prospective cohort study of vasectomy and prostate cancer in U.S. men. *JAMA* 269:873–877, 1993

20. Giovannucci E, Tostesone TD, Speizer FE, et al: A retrospective cohort study of vasectomy and prostate cancer in U.S. men. *JAMA* 269:878–887, 1993

21. Nienhuis H, Goldaere M, Seagroatt V, et al: Incidence of disease after vasectomy: a record linkage retrospective cohort study. *Br Med J* 304:743–746, 1992

22. Moller H, Knudsen LB, Lynge E: Risk of testicular cancer after vasectomy: cohort study of over 73,000 men. *Br Med J* 309:295–299, 1994

23. John EM, Whittemore AS, Wu AH, et al: Vasectomy and prostate cancer: results from a multiethnic case-control study. *J Natl Cancer Inst* 87:662–669, 1997

24. Mahon SM, Casperson DS: Focus on oncology: vasectomy and the risk of prostate cancer. *J Urol Nurs* 12:599–602, 1993

25. Carter HB, Piantadosi S, Isaacs JT: Clinical evidence for and implications of the multistep development of prostate cancer. *J Urol* 143:742–746, 1990

26. Carter BS, Beaty T, Steinberg G, et al: Mendelian inheritance of familial prostate cancer. *Proc Natl Acad Sci USA* 89:3367–3371, 1992

27. Carter BS, Bova GS, Beaty TH, et al: Hereditary prostate cancer: epidemiologic and clinical features. *J Urol* 150:797–802, 1993

28. Walsh PC, Partin AW: Family history facilitates the early diagnosis of prostate carcinoma. *Cancer* 80:1871–1874, 1997

29. Whittemore AS, Wu AH, Kolonel LN, et al: Family history and prostate cancer risk in black, white and Asian men in the United States and Canada. *Am J Epidemiol* 141:732–740, 1995

30. Skar WA, Grignon DJ, Haas GP, et al: Epidemiology of high grade intraepithelial neoplasia. *Pathol Res Pract* 191:838–841, 1995

31. Catalona WJ, Richie JP, Ahmann FR, et al: Comparison of digital rectal examination and serum prostate-specific antigen in the early detection of prostate cancer: results of a multicenter clinical trial of 663 men. *J Urol* 151:1283–1290, 1994

32. Powell IJ: Prostate cancer and African-American men. *Oncology* 11:599–605, 1997

33. Optenberg SA, Thompson IM, Friedrichs P, et al: Race, treatment, and long-term survival from prostate cancer in an equal-access medical care delivery system. *JAMA* 274:1599–1605, 1995

34. Robbins AS, Whittemore AS, VanDenEeden SK: Race, prostate cancer survival, and membership in a large health maintenance organization. *J Natl Cancer Inst* 90:986–990, 1998

35. Wu AH, Whittemore AS, Kolonel LN, et al: Serum androgen and sex hormone-binding globulins in relation to lifestyle factors in older African-American, white and Asian men in the United States and Canada. *Cancer Epidemiol Biomarkers Prev* 4:735–741, 1995

36. Scher HI, Issacs JT, Fuks Z, et al: Prostate, in Abeloff MD, Armitage JO, Lichter AS, Niederhuber JE (eds): *Clinical Oncology*. New York, Churchill Livingstone, 1995, pp 1439–1472

37. Oesterling J, Fuks Z, Lee CT, et al: Cancer of the prostate, in DeVita VT, Hellman S, Rosenberg SA (eds): *Cancer: Principles and Practice of Oncology* (ed 5). Philadelphia, Lippincott-Raven, 1997, pp 1322–1386

38. Reichardt JKV, Makridakis N, Henderson BE, et al: Genetic variability of the human SRD5A2 gene: implications for prostate cancer risk. *Cancer Res* 55:3973–3975, 1995

39. Guess HA, Gormley GJ, Stover E, et al: The effect of finasteride on prostate specific antigen: review of available literature. *J Urol* 155:3–9, 1996

40. Swan DK, Ford B: Chemoprevention of cancer: review of the literature. *Oncol Nurs Forum* 24:719–727, 1997

41. Pienta KJ, Esper PS, Zwas F, et al: Phase II chemoprevention trial of fenretinide in patients at risk for adenocarcinoma of the prostate. *Am J Clin Oncol* 20:36–39, 1997

42. Kelloff GJ, Lubet RA, Lieberman R, et al: Aromatase inhibitors as potential cancer chemopreventives. *Cancer Epidemiol Biomark Prev* 7:65–78, 1998

43. Thomas RD, Clejan S: Digital rectal examination-associated alteration in serum prostate-specific antigen. *Am J Clin Pathol* 97:528–534, 1992

44. Waldman AR, Osborne DM: Screening for prostate cancer. *Oncol Nurs Forum* 21:1512–1517, 1994

45. Littrup PJ, Lee F, Mettlin C: Prostate cancer screening: current trends and future implications. *CA Cancer J Clin* 42:198–211, 1992

46. McNeal JE, Price HM, Redwine EA, et al: Stage A versus stage B adenocarcinoma of the prostate: morphological comparison and biological significance. *J Urol* 139:61–65, 1988

47. vonEschenbach A, Ho R, Murphy GP, et al: American Cancer Society guideline for the early detection of prostate cancer: update 1997. *CA Cancer J Clin* 47:261–264, 1997

48. Ploch NR, Brawer MK: How to use prostate-specific antigen. *Urology* 43:27–35, 1994 (suppl)

49. Brawer M, Catalone W, McConnell J: Prostate cancer: is screening the answer? *Patient Care* 26:55–68, 1992

50. Moul JW, Sesterhenn IA, Connelly RR, et al: Prostate specific antigen values at the time of prostate cancer diagnosis in African American men. *JAMA* 274:1277–1281, 1995

51. Morgan TO, Jacobsen SJ, McCarthy WF, et al: Age-specific reference ranges for serum prostate-specific antigen in black men. *N Engl J Med* 335:304–310, 1996

52. Murphy GP, Barren RJ, Erickson SJ, et al: Evaluation and comparison of two new prostate carcinoma markers. *Cancer* 78:809–818, 1996

53. Catalona WJ, Smith DS, Wolfert RL, et al: Evaluation of percentage of free serum prostate-specific antigen to improve specificity of prostate cancer screening. *JAMA* 274:1214–1220, 1995

54. Catalona WJ, Partin AW, Slawin KM, et al: Use of the percentage of free prostate specific antigen to enhance differentiation of prostate cancer from benign prostatic disease. *JAMA* 279:1542–1547, 1998

55. Catalona WJ, Smith DS, Ornstein DK: Prostate cancer detection in men with serum PSA concentrations of 2.6 to 4.0 ng/mL and benign prostate exam. *JAMA* 277:1452–1455, 1997

56. Pannek J, Partin AW: Prostate-specific antigen: what's new in 1997. *Oncology* 11:1273–1278, 1997

57. Benson MC, Whang IS, Pantuck A, et al: Prostate specific antigen density: a means of distinguishing benign prostatic hypertrophy and prostate cancer. *J Urol* 147:815–816, 1992

58. Brawer MK: How to use prostate-specific antigen in the early detection or screening for prostatic carcinoma. *CA Cancer J Clin* 45:148–164, 1995

59. Carter HB, Pearson JD, Metter EJ, et al: Longitudinal evaluation of prostate specific antigen levels in men with and without prostate disease. *JAMA* 267:2215–2220, 1992

60. Oesterling JE, Chute CG, Jacobsen SJ, et al: Longitudinal changes in serum PSA (PSA velocity) in a community-based cohort of men. *J Urol* 149:412A, 1993 (abstract)

61. Smith DS, Catalona WJ: Rate of change in serum prostate specific antigen levels as a method for prostate cancer detection. *J Urol* 152:1163–1167, 1994

62. Carter HB, Pearson JD, Waclawiw Z, et al: Prostate-specific antigen variability in men without prostate cancer: effect of sampling interval on prostate-specific antigen velocity. *Urology* 45:591–596, 1995

63. Kadmon D, Weinberg AD, Williams RH, et al: Pitfalls in interpreting prostate specific antigen velocity. *J Urol* 155:1655–1657, 1996

64. Stenman UH, Alfthan H: Scandinavian BPH study group: effect of long term treatment with finasteride on free and total PSA in serum. *J Urol* 155:698A, 1996 (abstract)

65. Narayan P: Neoplasms of the prostate gland, in Tanagho E, McAninch J (eds): *Smith's General Urology* (ed 14). Norwalk, CT, Appleton and Lange, 1995, pp 392–433

66. Coley CM, Barry MJ, Mulley AG: Screening for prostate cancer. *Ann Intern Med* 126:480–484, 1997

67. Ohori M, Wheeler TM, Dunn JK, et al: The pathologic features and prognosis of prostate cancer detectable with current diagnostic tests. *J Urol* 152:1714–1720, 1994

68. Epstein JI, Walsh PC, Carmichael M, et al: Pathologic and clinical findings to predict tumor extent of nonpalpable (stage T1c) prostate cancer. *JAMA* 271:368–374, 1994

69. Epstein JI, Walsh PC, Brendler CB: Radical prostatectomy for impalpable prostate cancer. The Johns Hopkins experience with tumors found on transurethral resection (stages T1A and T1B) and on needle biopsy (stage T1C). *J Urol* 152:1721–1729, 1994

70. Gann PH, Hennekens CH, Stampfer MJ: A prospective evaluation of plasma prostate-specific antigen for detection of prostate cancer. *JAMA* 273:289–294, 1995

71. Mostofi FK, Murphy GP, Mettlin C, et al: Pathology review in an early prostate cancer detection program: results from the American Cancer Society—National Prostate Cancer Detection Project. *Prostate* 27:7–12, 1995

72. Lodding P, Aus G, Bergdahl R, et al: Characteristics of screening detected prostate cancer in men 50 to 66 years old with 3 to 4 ng/mL prostate specific antigen. *J Urol* 159:899–903, 1998

73. Mettlin CJ, Murphy GP, Babaian RJ, et al: Observations on the early detection of prostate cancer from the American Cancer Society National Prostate Cancer Detection Project. *Cancer* 80:1814–1817, 1997

74. Newcomer LM, Stanford JL, Blumenstein BA, et al: Temporal trends in rates of prostate cancer: declining incidence of advanced stage disease, 1974 to 1994. *J Urol* 158:1427–1430, 1997

75. Reissigl A, Horninger W, Fink K, et al: Prostate carcinoma screening in the county of Tyrol, Austria: experience and results. *Cancer* 80:1818–1829, 1997

76. Smith DS, Humphrey PA, Catalona WJ: The early detection of prostate carcinoma with prostate specific antigen. *Cancer* 80:1852–1856, 1997

77. Labrie F, DuPont A, Candas B, et al: Decrease of prostate cancer death by screening: first data from the Quebec prospective and randomized study. *Proc Am Soc Clin Oncol* 17:2A, 1998 (abstract)

78. Benoit RM, Naslund MJ: The economics of prostate cancer screening. *Oncology* 11:1533–1543, 1997

79. Guyton AC: *Textbook of Medical Physiology* (ed 8). Philadelphia, Saunders, 1991, pp 885–898

80. Verhagen APM, Ramaekers FCS, Aadlers TW, et al: Colocalization of basal and luminal cell-type cytokeratins in human prostate cancer. *Cancer Res* 52:6182–6187, 1992

81. Bostwick DG: Prostatic intraepithelial neoplasia (PIN). *Urology* 34:16–22, 1989

82. Bostwick DG, Amin MB, Dundore P, et al: Architectural patterns of high-grade prostatic intraepithelial neoplasia. *Hum Pathol* 24:298–310, 1993

83. Sakr WA, Grignon DJ, Crissman JD, et al: High grade prostatic intraepithelial neoplasia (HGPIN) and prostatic adenocarcinoma between the ages of 20–69: an autopsy study of 249 cases. *In Vivo* 8:439–443, 1994

84. Skar WA, Haas GP, Cassin BF, et al: The frequency of carcinoma and intraepithelial neoplasia of the prostate in young male patients. *J Urol* 150:379–385, 1993

85. Gleason DF: Classification of prostatic carcinomas. *Cancer Chemother Rep* 50:125–128, 1966

86. Gleason DF: Histologic grading of prostate cancer: a perspective. *Hum Pathol* 23:273–279, 1992

87. McNeal JE, Villers AA, Redwine EA, et al: Histologic differentiation, cancer volume, and pelvic lymph node metastasis in adenocarcinoma of the prostate. *Cancer* 66: 1225–1233, 1990

88. Bluestein DL, Bostwick DG, Bergstralh EJ, et al: Eliminating the need for bilateral pelvic lymphadenectomy in selected patients with prostate cancer. *J Urol* 151:1315–1320, 1994

89. Scardino PT, Weaver R, Hudson MA: Early detection of prostate cancer. *Hum Pathol* 23:211–223, 1992

90. Bastacky SI, Walsh PC, Epstein JI: Relationship between perineural tumor invasion on needle biopsy and radical prostatectomy capsular penetration in clinical stage B adenocarcinoma of the prostate. *Am J Surg Pathol* 17:336–341, 1993

91. Garnick MB: Prostate cancer: screening, diagnosis and management. *Ann Intern Med* 118:804–818, 1993

92. Surya BV, Provent JA: Manifestations of advanced prostate cancer: prognosis and treatment. *J Urol* 142:921–928, 1989

93. Payne R: Pain management in the patient with prostate cancer. *Cancer* 71:1131–1137, 1993 (suppl)

94. Black J, Matassarin-Jacobs E (eds): *Medical-Surgical Nursing: Clinical Management for Continuity of Care* (ed 5). Philadelphia, Saunders, 1997, pp 1571–1624, 2293–2385

95. Held JL, Peahota A: Nursing care of the patient with spinal cord compression. *Oncol Nurs Forum* 20:1507–1516, 1993

96. Baker LH, Hanks G, Gershenson D, et al: NCCN prostate cancer practice guidelines. *Oncology* 10(11):265–288, 1996

97. Stamey TA, Kabalin JN: Prostate-specific antigen in the diagnosis and treatment of adenocarcinoma of the prostate. I. Untreated patients. *J Urol* 141:1070–1075, 1989

98. Andriole GL: Serum prostate-specific antigen: expanding its role as a measure of treatment response in patients with prostate cancer. *J Clin Oncol* 11:596–597, 1993

99. Morton RA, Steiner MS, Walsh PC: Cancer control following anatomical radical prostatectomy: an interim report. *J Urol* 145:1197–1200, 1991

100. Ritter MA, Messing EM, Shanahan TG, et al: Prostate-specific antigen as a predictor of radiotherapy response and patterns of failure in localized prostate cancer. *J Clin Oncol* 10:1208–1217, 1992

101. Corless CL: Evaluating early-stage prostate cancer. *Hematol Oncol Clin North Am* 10:565–579, 1996

102. Garnick MB: The dilemmas of prostate cancer. *Sci Am* 270: 72–81, 1994

103. Fleming C, Wasson JH, Albertsen PC, et al: A decision analysis of alternative treatment strategies for clinically localized prostate cancer. *JAMA* 269:2650–2658, 1993

104. Wasson J, Cushman C, Bruskewitz R, et al: A structured literature review of treatment for localized prostate cancer. *Arch Fam Med* 2:487–493, 1993

105. Johansson JE, Adami HO, Andersson SO, et al: High 10-year survival rate in patients with early, untreated prostate cancer. *JAMA* 267:2191–2196, 1992

106. Aus G, Hugosson J, Norlen, L: Long-term survival and mortality in prostate cancer treated with noncurative intent. *J Urol* 154:460–465, 1995

107. Albertsen PC, Fryback DG, Storer BE, et al: Long-term survival among men with conservatively treated localized cancer. *JAMA* 274:626–631, 1995

108. Chodak GW, Thisted RA, Gerber GS, et al: Results of conservative management of clinically localized prostate cancer. *N Engl J Med* 330:242–248, 1994

109. McLaren DB, McKenzie M, Duncan G, et al: Watchful waiting or watchful progression? *Cancer* 82:342–348, 1998

110. Wilt TJ, Brawer MK: The Prostate Cancer Intervention Versus Observation Trial (PIVOT). *Oncology* 11:1133–1139, 1997

111. Ghanem AN, Ward JP: Osmotic and metabolic sequelae of volumetric overload in relation to the TURP syndrome. *Br J Urol* 66:71–78, 1990

112. Gravenstein D: Transurethral resection of the prostate (TUPR) syndrome: a review of the pathophysiology and management. *Anesth Analg* 84:438–446, 1997

113. Held JL, Osborne DM, Volpe H, et al: Cancer of the prostate: treatment and nursing implications. *Oncol Nurs Forum* 21:1517–1529, 1994

114. Mettlin C, Murphy G, Menck H: Trends in treatment of localized prostate cancer by radical prostatectomy: observations from the Commission on Cancer National Cancer Database 1985–1990. *Urology* 43:488–492, 1994

115. Lu-Yao GL, Greenberg ER: Changes in prostate cancer incidence and treatment in USA. *Lancet* 343:251–254, 1994

116. Mettlin C, Jones G, Murphy G: Trends in prostate cancer care in the United States, 1974–1990: observations from the patient care evaluation studies of the American College of Surgeons Commission on Cancer. *CA Cancer J Clin* 43: 83–91, 1993

117. Lu-Yao GL, McLerran D, Wasson J, et al: An assessment of radical prostatectomy: time trends, geographic variation, and outcomes. *JAMA* 269:2633–2636, 1993

118. Kantoff PW, Talcott JA: The radical prostatectomy series: apples are not oranges. *J Clin Oncol* 11:2243–2245, 1994

119. Eastham JA, Scardino PT: Radical prostatectomy, in Walsh PC, Retik AB, Vaughn ED, Wein AJ (eds): *Campbell's Urology* (ed 7). Philadelphia, Saunders, 1998, pp 2547–2564

120. Herr H: Quality of life of incontinent men after radical prostatectomy. *J Urol* 151:652–654, 1994

121. Waxman ES: Sexual dysfunction following treatment for prostate cancer: nursing assessment and intervention. *Oncol Nurs Forum* 20:1567–1571, 1993

122. Walsh PC: Anatomic radical prostatectomy: evolution of the surgical technique. *J Urol* 160:2418–2424, 1998

123. Quinlan DM, Epstein JI, Carter BS, et al: Sexual function following radical prostatectomy: influence of preservation of neurovascular bundles. *J Urol* 145:998–1002, 1991

124. Robinson JW, Dufour MS, Fung TS: Erectile functioning of men treated for prostate carcinoma. *Cancer* 79:538–544, 1997

125. Litwin MS, Hays RD, Fink A, et al: Quality of life in men treated for localized prostate cancer. *JAMA* 273:129–135, 1995

126. Maxwell M: Cancer of the prostate. *Semin Oncol Nurs* 9: 237–251, 1993

127. Klimaszewski AD, Karlowicz KA: Cancer of the male genitalia, in Karlowicz KA (ed): *Urologic Nursing: Principles and Practice*. Philadelphia, Saunders, 1995, pp 271–308

128. Urinary Incontinence Guideline Panel: *Urinary Incontinence in Adults: Clinical Practice Guidelines*. AHCPR Publication No. 92-0038. Rockville, MD, Agency for Health Care Policy and Research, 1992

129. Walsh PC: Radical retropubic prostatectomy, in Walsh PC, Retik AB, Vaughan ED, Wein AJ (eds): *Campbell's Urology* (ed 7). Philadelphia, Saunders, 1998, pp 2565–2588

130. Steiner MS, Morton RA, Walsh PC: Impact of anatomic radical prostatectomy on urinary continence. *J Urol* 145: 512–515, 1991

131. Walsh PC, Quinlan DM, Morton RA, et al: Radical retropubic prostatectomy: improved anastomosis and urinary continence. *Urol Clin North Am* 17:679–684, 1990

132. Marks JL, Light JK: Management of urinary incontinence after prostatectomy with the artificial urinary sphincter. *J Urol* 142:302–304, 1989

133. Foote J, Yun S, Leach GE: Postprostatectomy incontinence: pathophysiology, evaluation and management. *Urol Clin North Am* 18:229–241, 1991

134. Thayer D: How to assess and control urinary incontinence. *Am J Nurs* 94:42–47, 1994

135. Freedman A, Hahn G, Love N: Follow-up after therapy for prostate cancer. *Postgrad Med* 100(3):125–136, 1996

136. Appell RA: Clinical efficacy and safety of tolterodine in the treatment of overactive bladder: a pooled analysis. *Urology* 50:90–96, 1997 (suppl)

137. Abrams P, Freeman R, Anderstrom C, et al: Tolterodine, a new antimuscarinic agent: as effective but better tolerated than oxybutynin in patients with an overactive bladder. *Br J Urol* 81:801–810, 1998

138. Schrover LR: *Sexuality and Cancer: For the Man Who Has Cancer, and His Partner.* Atlanta, American Cancer Society, 1997

139. Schrover LR: Sexual rehabilitation after treatment for prostate cancer. *Cancer* 71:1024–1030, 1993

140. Costabile RA, Spevak M, Fishman IJ, et al: Efficacy and safety of transurethral alprostadil in patients with erectile dysfunction following radical prostatectomy. *J Urol* 160:1325–1328, 1998

141. Zippe CD, Kedia AW, Kedia K, et al: Treatment of erectile dysfunction after radical prostatectomy with sildenafil (Viagra). *Urology* 52:963–966, 1998

142. Schmidt JD, Doyle J, Larison S: Prostate cryoablation: update 1998. *CA Cancer J Clin* 48:239–253, 1998

143. Brenner ZR, Krenzer ME: Update on cryosurgical ablation for prostate cancer. *Am J Nurs* 95(4):44–48, 1995

144. Leininger SM: Managing patients with cryosurgical ablation of the prostate and liver. *Medsurg Nurs* 6:359–386, 1997

145. Wong WS, Chinn DO, Chinn M, et al: Cryosurgery as a treatment for prostate carcinoma. *Cancer* 79:963–974, 1997

146. American Urologic Association Prostate Cancer Clinical Guidelines Panel: *Report on the Management of Clinically Localized Prostate Cancer.* Baltimore, American Urologic Association, 1995

147. Porter AT, Littrup P, Grignon D, et al: Radiotherapy and cryotherapy for prostate cancer, in Walsh PC, Retik AB, Vaughan ED, Wein AJ (eds): *Campbell's Urology* (ed 7). Philadelphia, Saunders, 1998, pp 2605–2626

148. Maher KE: Male genitourinary cancers, in Dow KH, Bucholtz JD, Iwamoto RR, Fieler VK, Hilderley LJ (eds): *Nursing Care in Radiation Oncology* (ed 2). Philadelphia, Saunders, 1997, pp 184–219

149. Crook JM, Bahadur YA, Bociek RG, et al: Radiotherapy for localized prostate cancer: the correlation of pretreatment prostate specific antigen and nadir prostate specific antigen as assessed by systematic biopsy and serum prostate specific antigen. *Cancer* 79:328–336, 1997

150. Lillis P, Thompson IM: Should asymptomatic progression following definitive local treatment for prostate cancer be treated? *Hematol Oncol Clin North Am* 10:703–712, 1996

151. Perez C, Cosmatos D, Garcia DM, et al: Irradiation in relapsing carcinoma of the prostate. *Cancer* 71:1110–1122, 1993

152. Bolla M, Gonzalez D, Warde P, et al: Improved survival in patients with locally advanced prostate cancer treated with radiotherapy and goserelin. *N Engl J Med* 337:295–300, 1997

153. Llawton CA, Won M, Pilepich M, et al: Long-term treat-ment sequelae following external beam irradiation for adenocarcinoma of the prostate: analysis of RTOG studies 7506 and 7706. *Int J Radiat Oncol Biol Phys* 21:935–940, 1991

154. Shipley WU, Zietman AL, Hanks GE, et al: Treatment-related sequelae following external beam radiation therapy for prostate cancer: a review with update in patients with T1-2 tumors. *J Urol* 152:1799–1805, 1994

155. Goldstein I, Feldman MI, Deckers PJ, et al: Radation-associated impotence: a clinical study of its mechanism. *JAMA* 251:903–910, 1984

156. Gittes RF: Carcinoma of the prostate. *N Engl J Med* 324:236–245, 1991

157. Keller JW, Sahasrabudhe DM, McCune CS: Urologic and male genital cancers, in Rubin P, McDonald S, Qazi R (eds): *Clinical Oncology: A Multidisciplinary Approach for Physicians and Students* (ed 7). Philadelphia, Saunders, 1993, pp 419–452

158. Helgason AR, Adolfsson J, Dickman P, et al: Factors associated with waning sexual function among elderly men and prostate cancer patients. *J Urol* 158:155–159, 1997

159. Pilepich MV, Krall J, George FW, et al: Treatment-related morbidity in phase III RTOG studies of extended-field radiation for carcinoma of the prostate. *Int J Radiat Oncol Biol Phys* 10:1861–1867, 1984

160. Porter A, Blasko J, Grimm P: Brachytherapy for prostate cancer. *CA Cancer J Clin* 45:165–178, 1995

161. Cash JC, Dattoli MJ: Management of patients receiving transperineal palladium-103 prostate implants. *Oncol Nurs Forum* 24:1361–1367, 1997

162. Greenberg S, Peterson J, Hansen-Peters I, et al: Interstitially implanted I-125 for prostate cancer using transrectal ultrasound. *Oncol Nurs Forum* 17:849–854, 1990

163. Isaacs JT, Lundmo PI, Berges R, et al: Androgen regulation of programmed cell death of normal and malignant prostatic cells. *J Androl* 13:457, 1992

164. Martikainen P, Kyprianou N, Tucker RW, et al: Programmed death of nonproliferating androgen-independent prostatic cancer cells. *Cancer Res* 51:4693–4700, 1991

165. Crawford ED, Nabors WL: Total androgen ablation: American experience. *Urol Clin North Am* 18:55–63, 1991

166. Schroder FH: Endocrine treatment of prostate cancer, in Walsh PC, Retik AB, Vaughan ED, Wein AJ (eds): *Campbell's Urology* (ed 7). Philadelphia, Saunders, 1998, pp 2627–2644

167. McLeod DG: Antiandrogenic drugs. *Cancer* 71:1046–1049, 1993

168. LaBrie F, Belanger A, Simard J, et al: Combination therapy for prostate cancer. *Cancer* 71:1059–1067, 1993 (suppl)

169. Prostate Cancer Trialists' Collaborative Group: Maximal androgen blockade in advanced prostate cancer: an overview of 22 randomized trials with 3283 deaths in 5710 patients. *Lancet* 346:265–269, 1995

170. D'Amico AV: What is the optimal patient selection for combined androgen ablative and radiation therapy? The role of combined modality staging. *Hematol Oncol Clin North Am* 10:643–651, 1996

171. Taylor TK: Endocrine therapy for advanced stage D prostate cancer. *Urol Nurs* 11:22–26, 1991

172. Smith DC: Secondary hormonal therapy. *Semin Urol Oncol* 15:3–12, 1997

173. Scher HI, Kelly WW: Flutamide withdrawal syndrome: its impact on clinical trials in hormone-refractory prostate cancer. *J Clin Oncol* 11:1566–1572, 1993

174. Yagoda A, Petrylak O: Cytotoxic chemotherapy for ad-

vanced hormone-resistant prostate cancer. *Cancer* 71: 1098–1109, 1993

175. Kelly WK, Scher HI: Prostate specific antigen decline after antiandrogen withdrawal: the flutamide withdrawal syndrome. *J Urol* 149:607–609, 1993

176. Kelly WK, Slovin S, Scher HI: Clinical use of posttherapy prostate-specific antigen changes in advanced prostate cancer. *Semin Oncol* 23:8–14, 1996 (suppl)

177. Thalmann GN, Sikes RA, Chang S-M, et al: Suramin-induced decrease in prostate specific antigen expression with no effect on tumor growth in the LNCaP model of human prostate cancer. *J Natl Cancer Inst* 88:794–801, 1996

178. Dreicer R: Metastatic prostate cancer: assessment of response to systemic therapy. *Semin Urol Oncol* 15:28–32, 1997

179. Newling D, Fossa SD, Andersson L, et al: Assessment of hormone refractory prostate cancer. *Urology* 49:46–53, 1997 (suppl)

180. Moore MJ, Osoba D, Murphy K, et al: Use of palliative end points to evaluate the effects of mitoxantrone and low-dose prednisone in patients with hormonally resistant prostate cancer. *J Clin Oncol* 12:689–694, 1994

181. Tannock IF, Osoba D, Stockler MR, et al: Chemotherapy with mitoxantrone plus prednisone or prednisone alone for symptomatic hormone-resistant prostate cancer: a Canadian randomized trial with palliative endpoints. *J Clin Oncol* 14:1756–1764, 1996

182. Pienta KJ, Redman BG, Hussain M, et al: Phase II evaluation of oral estramustine and oral etoposide in hormone-refractory adenocarcinoma of the prostate. *J Clin Oncol* 12: 2005–2012, 1994

183. Dimopoulos MA, Panopoulos C, Bamia C, et al: Oral estramustine and oral etoposide for hormone-refractory prostate cancer. *Urology* 50:754–758, 1997

184. Pienta KJ, Redman BG, Bandekar R, et al: A phase II trial of oral estramustine and oral etoposide in hormone refractory prostate cancer. *Urology* 50:401–407, 1997

185. Smith DC, Dunn RL, Strawderman MS, et al: Change in serum prostate-specific antigen as a marker of response to cytotoxic therapy for hormone-refractory prostate cancer. *J Clin Oncol* 16:1835–1843, 1998

186. Jodrell DI, Reyno LM, Sridhara R, et al: Suramin: development of a population pharmacokinetic model and its use with intermittent short infusions to control plasma drug concentration in patient with prostate cancer. *J Clin Oncol* 12:166–175, 1994

187. Eisenberger MA, Sinibaldi VJ, Reyno LM, et al: Phase I and clinical evaluation of a pharmacologically guided regimen of suramin in patients with hormone-refractory prostate cancer. *J Clin Oncol* 13:2174–2186, 1995

188. Reyno LM, Egorin MJ, Eisenberger MA, et al: Development and validation of a pharmacokinetically based fixed dosing scheme for suramin. *J Clin Oncol* 13:2187–2195, 1995

189. Kobayashi K, Vokes EE, Vogelzang NJ, et al: Phase I study of suramin given by intermittent infusion without adaptive control in patients with advanced cancer. *J Clin Oncol* 13: 2196–2207, 1995

190. Vogelzang NJ, Small EJ, Halabi S, et al: A phase III trial of

3 different doses of suramin (SUR) in metastatic hormone refractory prostate cancer (HRPC): safety profile of CALGB 9480. *Proc Am Soc Clin Oncol* 17:347A, 1998 (abstr)

191. Eisenberger MA, Sinibaldi V, Reyno L: Suramin. *Cancer Pract* 3:187–189, 1995

192. Kobayashi K, Weiss RE, Vogelzang NJ, et al: Mineralocorticoid insufficiency due to suramin therapy. *Cancer* 78: 2411–2420, 1996

193. Kenner JR, Sperling LC, Waselenko J, et al: Suramin keratosis: a unique skin eruption in a patient receiving suramin for metastatic prostate cancer. *J Urol* 158:2245–2246, 1997

194. Figg WD, Cooper MR, Thibault A, et al: Acute renal toxicity associated with suramin in the treatment of prostate cancer. *Cancer* 74:1612–1614, 1994

195. Smith A, Harbour D, Liebmann J: Acute renal failure in a patient receiving treatment with suramin. *Am J Clin Oncol* 20:433–434, 1997

196. Konety BR, Getzenberg RH: Novel therapies for advanced prostate cancer. *Semin Urol Oncol* 15:33–42, 1997

197. Dawson NA, Cooper MR, Figg WD, et al: Antitumor activity of suramin in hormone-refractory prostate cancer controlling for hydrocortisone treatment and flutamide withdrawal as potentially confounding variables. *Cancer* 76: 453–462, 1995

198. Raghaven D, Cox K, Pearson BS, et al: Oral cyclophosphamide for the management of hormone-refractory prostate cancer. *Br J Urol* 72:625–628, 1993

199. Natale RB, Zaretsky S: Phase I/II trial of estramustine (E) with taxotere (T) or vinorelbine (V) in patients (pts) with metastatic hormone-refractory prostate cancer (HRPC). *Proc Am Soc Clin Oncol* 17:338A, 1998 (abstr)

200. Sella A, Kilbourn R, Amato R, et al: Phase II study of ketoconazole combined with weekly doxorubicin in patients with androgen-independent prostate cancer. *J Clin Oncol* 12:683–688, 1994

201. Vogelzang NJ: Editorial comment. *Urology* 50:406–407, 1997 (editorial)

202. Eisenberg E, Berkey CS, Carr DB, et al: Efficacy and safety of nonsteroidal antiinflammaroty drugs for cancer pain. *J Clin Oncol* 12:2756–2765, 1994

203. Payne R: Mechanisms and management of bone pain. *Cancer* 80:1608–1613, 1997

204. Merterns WC, Filipczak LA, Ben-Josef E, et al: Systemic bone-seeking radionuclides for palliation of painful osseous metastases: current concepts. *CA Cancer J Clin* 48: 361–374, 1998

205. Body JJ, Bartl R, Burckhardt P, et al: Current use of bisphosphonates in oncology. *J Clin Oncol* 16:3890–3899, 1998

206. Loblaw DA, Laperriere NJ: Emergency treatment of malignant extradural spinal cord compression: an evidence-based guideline. *J Clin Oncol* 16:1613–1624, 1998

207. Huddart RA, Rajan B, Law M, et al: Spinal cord compression in prostate cancer: treatment outcome and prognostic factors. *Radiother Oncol* 44:229–236, 1997

208. Hardy JR: Lymphoedema-prevention rather than cure. *Ann Oncol* 2:532–533, 1991 (editorial)

209. Shuey K: Platelet-associated bleeding disorders. *Semin Oncol Nurs* 12:15–27, 1996

CHAPTER 65

Skin Cancer

Suzanne M. Mahon, RN, DNSc, AOCN
Susan G. Yackzan, RN, MSN, AOCN

Introduction

The skin is a large and very visible organ that serves both protective and aesthetic functions. Historically, these visible characteristics have served as indicators of social status and class. Until the second decade of the twentieth century, smooth, pale skin was valued as an indication of belonging to the more wealthy, leisure class. Those who worked as laborers and field hands had darker skin, tanned from exposure to the sun. During this century, outdoor leisure activities have become associated with a higher social status. This change in perception has led more people to seek tanned, bronze-colored skin. This change may also be one of the biggest factors contributing to the rise in the incidence of skin cancer.

The term *skin cancer* is often used to describe several types of malignancies that occur in the skin. Basal cell carcinoma (BCC) and squamous cell carcinoma (SCC) are often combined and described as nonmalignant melanoma skin cancer (NMSC). Malignant melanoma (MM) is usually referred to separately because of the differences in this malignancy when compared to NMSC in terms of treatment and prognosis. Most MMs are cutaneous; however, unusual presentations in the eye and viscera may occur. This chapter will focus on the cutaneous skin cancers.

Oncology nurses can have a significant impact on the morbidity and mortality associated with NMSC and MM. As educators, nurses can influence the public to practice primary and secondary prevention strategies. As clinicians, nurses can perform risk assessments and screening examinations to promote early detection of malignancies, ensure appropriate management of biopsies, administer therapies safely, manage symptoms, and provide appropriate psychosocial care. As researchers, nurses can improve strategies for education, management of symptoms, and knowledge acquisition through clinical trials.

Epidemiology

The incidence of skin cancer continues to grow in both the United States and throughout the world. Skin cancers account for approximately one-third of all diagnosed cancers. In the United States alone, the American Cancer Society (ACS) estimates there are approximately 1 million cases of the highly curable BCCs and SCCs detected annually.[1] Of the NMSCs, cases of BCC predominate over SCC by about five to one in males and ten to one in females.[2] Accurate figures on the incidence of these NMSCs are difficult to obtain as many countries do not register these malignancies. In addition, these lesions are often removed in primary care practices and are treated without laboratory verification of the clinical diagnosis.[3] It is clear, however, that the incidence of these cancers has increased over the last few decades and that the increased incidence of NMSC is related to cumulative sun-exposure behaviors.

The annual incidence of the more serious form of skin cancer, MM, is estimated to be 44,200 new cases in 1999 according to the ACS.[1] The annual incidence of MM has risen steadily from a risk of one out of 1500 persons in 1930 to one out of 75 persons in the year 2000, as shown in Figure 65-1.[4,5] From a public health perspective it is vital that public awareness of MM be improved. Better means are needed to identify high-risk persons and to detect MM early; more specific therapies are also needed. The incidence of MM continues to rise with age, thus lifetime prevention and early detection strategies are critical to decrease the morbidity and mortality associated with MM (Figure 65-2).[5]

Clearly, the dramatic rise in MM is real and not due to artifact. MM incidence is increasing worldwide at a faster rate than any other cancer.[6] This increase is not due to better surveillance techniques. It is hypothesized that the increase in MM incidence is related to the fact that people are going outdoors more often than in the past and are exposing themselves not only to sunlight but also increasingly to artificial ultraviolet radiation (UVR).[7] Incidence rates are approximately 20 times higher among whites as compared to blacks.

The mortality rate from the highly curable BCCs and SCCs is approximately 1900 persons per year according to ACS estimates.[1] These deaths are largely preventable as most NMSC are visible for long periods of time prior to metastasis. An estimated 7300 persons die annually from MM.[1] The decreasing mean thickness of MMs at the time of diagnosis has resulted in an overall increased survival with localized MM from about 50% in the 1950s to almost 90% in 2000. It is important to note however, that the absolute number of thicker MMs has also increased. The mortality rate from MM continues to increase, although not at the same rate as the incidence of new cases[5,6] (see Figures 65-1 and 65-2).

Etiology

The etiology of skin cancer is multifactorial in nature. The likelihood that an individual might develop skin cancer during his or her lifetime depends both on constitutional factors and environmental exposures. Constitutional factors include the genotypic and phenotypic characteristics of an individual.[3] Different skin cancers are associated with different risk factors (Table 65-1).[2,6,8–10]

Genotypic Factors

Skin color is one of the most important genotypic features that places a person at risk for developing skin cancer. MM is very rare in blacks.[8,11] Persons who are light or fair complected, have a tendency to freckle, or burn easily are at higher risk. The development of melanocytic nevi in childhood is strongly related to characteristics of pigmentation associated with poor sun tolerance.[12]

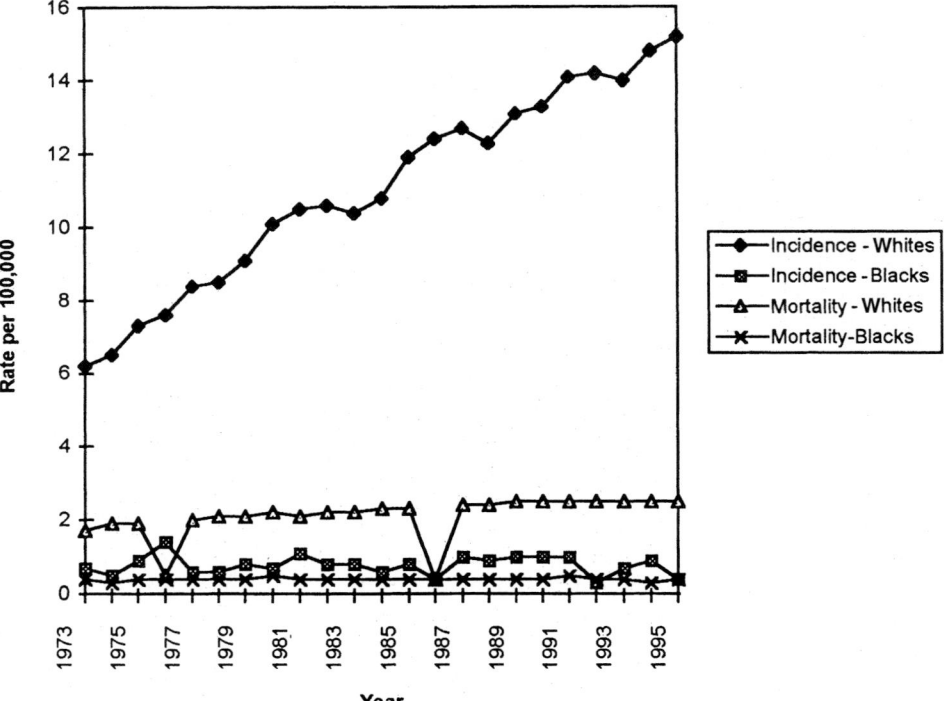

Figure 65-1 Incidence and mortality rates for malignant melanoma, United States, 1973–1995. (Ries LAG, Kosary CL, Hankey BF, et al: *SEER Cancer Statistics Review, 1973–1995.* Bethesda, MD, National Cancer Institute, 1998.)[5]

The epidermis of blacks has been shown to have a natural sun protection factor (SPF) of 13.4 with the melanin in the epidermis filtering twice as much ultraviolet B (UVB) as the epidermis of a white person.[11] This protection, however, is not complete, and both NMSC and MM can develop in black persons. SCC is the most frequently seen skin cancer in blacks. BCCs in blacks are almost always pigmented. Further, up to 67% of MMs in the black population arise in non-sun-exposed skin such as on the palmer and plantar surfaces and even the mucous membranes. Blacks have proportionately greater percentages of the acral lentiginous type of MM and also tend to have poorer prognoses than do whites with MM.

Large congenital melanocytic nevi are also considered a significant risk factor associated with the development of MM and are estimated to occur in 1% of newborns.[13] This increase in risk has been reported to range from 0%–42%. In most studies, the larger the nevus, the higher the lifetime risk.[14,15] Surgical removal of these large nevi is thought to decrease but not eliminate these individuals'

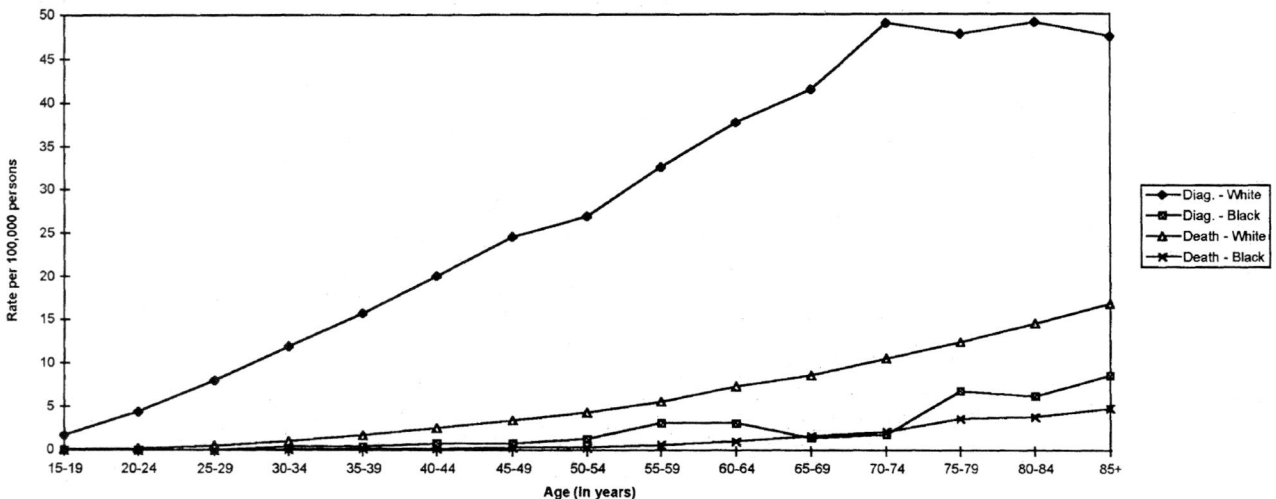

Figure 65-2 Age specific rates—incidence and mortality for malignant melanoma, United States, 1973–1995. (Ries LAG, Kosary CL, Hankey BF, et al: *SEER Cancer Statistics Review, 1973–1995.* Bethesda, MD, National Cancer Institute, 1998.)[5]

Table 65-1 Risk Factors for Skin Cancer

Risk Factor	Risk Factor for NMSC	Risk Factor for MM
Actinic keratoses*	+	+
Arsenic ingestion (well water, insecticides, medical)	+	
Chronic exposure to tar, soot, shale, or petroleum	+	
Cigarette or pipe smoking	+	
Congenital nevus		+
Family history of melanoma*		+
Geographic area where childhood was spent	+	+
History of NMSC in a first-degree relative	+	
History of three or more blistering sunburns before the age of 20 years*	+	+
Immunosuppression	+	+
Increasing age	+	+
Ionizing radiation (therapeutic or occupational)	+	
Large number of dysplastic nevi		+
Large number of melanocytic nevi		+
Male gender	+	+
Personal history of BCC	+	+
Personal history of MM	+	+
Personal history of SCC	+	+
Red or blond hair*	+	+
Scar related to heat burn, chemical burn	+	
Skin color	+	+
Tendency to freckle especially on the upper back area*	+	+
Three or more years of outdoor summer jobs during teenage years*	+	+
Xeroderma pigmentosum		+

*The presence of any one or two of these factors increases a person's risk for the development of MM threefold to fourfold and three or more of these factors increases the risk almost 20-fold according to data from Rigel DS: Malignant melanoma: incidence issues and their effect on diagnosis and treatment in the 1990s. *Mayo Clin Proc* 72:367–371, 1997.[6]

Data from Rhodes AR[2]; Rigel DS[6]; Marks R[8]; Hill L[9]; Goldsmith LA[10].

and especially dysplastic nevi, clinicians can identify individuals at high risk for developing MM and implement aggressive screening and intervention programs. Higher nevus counts are associated with an increased risk of MM with at least a tenfold greater risk for individuals who have 100 or more moles.

Dysplastic nevi may develop throughout life and show clinical features similar to normal moles and MMs (see Color Plates 9 and 10 [Figures 65-3 and 65-4]). These features include a size greater than 6–8 mm, irregular borders, variable pigmentation, and irregular surface characteristics. The identification of truly dysplastic nevi is more difficult to perform clinically than many epidemiologists realize, however, and requires in most cases a pathologic diagnosis.[16] Dysplastic nevi occur in approximately 10% of the general population and the risk of progression to MM is not clear in this group.[13]

Another important genotypic feature includes family history. Approximately 10% of patients with MM describe a history of an affected family member.[17] People with a family history of MM and/or dysplastic nevi, or who have a large number of nevi themselves, are at a very high risk of developing an MM over a lifetime. A hereditary predisposition to MM is sometimes associated with an earlier age of onset.[18] Sex distribution between males and females is usually about equal to those with a hereditary predisposition to MM.[19] In general, those with a hereditary predisposition to MM have malignancies that are clinically and histopathologically similar to those without such a family history.[20] Patients from these families are, however, often diagnosed with thinner lesions and generally have a better prognosis. This may be related to heightened awareness and increased surveillance. A second primary MM does develop in 17%–20% of patients from these families who survive their first MM.[21]

As the Human Genome Project continues, it is likely that a number of susceptibility loci will be identified, for which genetic testing will ultimately be available. Presently a susceptibility gene has been clearly linked to chromosome 9p (a tumor suppressor gene), chromosome 1p, and CDKN2A.[17,22–25] An understanding of the genetics of MM is just beginning. It is speculated that a genetic predisposition to MM may be present on a number of genes. Penetrance may be variable, thus, the gene may not be expressed consistently. It is also thought that the gene is transmitted in an autosomal dominant fashion, but the impact of environmental factors on the subsequent development of MM is not fully understood.[18] Therefore, at this time, even if the location of one or more susceptibility genes is known, the usefulness of genetic testing is not clear. As genetic testing becomes available and the ramifications of testing are better understood, a number of education and counseling issues will emerge.

A personal history of BCC or SCC is associated with a much higher risk of MM. The increase in relative risk has been reported to be anywhere from 2.8–17.0.[26] A personal history of a NMSC is associated with a much higher risk of developing a second NMSC, especially in persons with a history of significant sun exposure.

risk for developing MM because approximately 50% of the MMs arise in extracutaneous sites. Therefore lifetime screening is important.

The number of melanocytic nevi (moles) is correlated with risk. This includes common acquired nevi, atypical nevi, and dysplastic nevi.[3] On the basis of nevus numbers

The importance of the immune system in controlling skin cancers, particularly MM, is not completely understood.[7] Persons with chronic immunosuppression are at higher risk for developing MM. Renal transplant recipients may have a fourfold increased risk for developing MM.[27] The risk may be as much as eight times higher in persons who have been successfully treated for cancers such as lymphoma.

Age itself is also a risk factor for both NMSCs and MMs (see Figure 65-2).[2] It is difficult to separate the interaction of age from cumulative exposure to sunlight.

Environmental Factors

Frequent and prolonged exposure to UVR over years will induce cellular changes in human skin. Ultraviolet radiation can act as an initiator, a promoter, a cocarcinogen, and an immunosuppressive agent.[28] Episodic high exposure resulting in sunburn, especially when it occurs in childhood, may be critical.[3,6,16,28]

There are two adverse consequences associated with UVR. First, UVR exposure leads to direct tissue and cellular damage. Second, exposure to UVR also results in local and systemic immunosuppression.[7] The effects of UVR are both acute and chronic.[29] Acute changes include sunburn and discomfort. Chronic effects include photoaging, premalignant and malignant growths, and immunosuppression.[16,30]

Solar keratoses, which are a direct result of chronic sun exposure, are major risk factors for NMSC as well as a risk factor for MM. Data suggest that NMSCs are associated with cumulative sun exposure, whereas MM is associated with short, intense episodes of sun exposure, especially those involving sunburns.[9] Exposure to sunlight is the only environmental factor consistently linked to MM in most studies.[3] The exact relationship between sunlight exposure and risk of MM is not completely clear, but is probably a causal relationship that includes a complex relationship between dose response, latent period, body site, genetics, and other unknown factors.[13,28]

Some occupations may be associated with a higher risk of developing MM. Persons who earn a higher salary and are employed in typical white collar occupations may be at higher risk for developing MM than those who have more chronic occupational outdoor exposure to UVR.[31] These risks may be related to the fact that persons from this socioeconomic group have the financial means to travel to sunny climates on vacation, where they intermittently expose themselves to intense UVR resulting in sunburn, especially those associated with pain and blistering. This is probably related to the combination of reflected UVR from disturbed water and the cooling effect of water, which leads to a false sense of security. The same is true of cloudy days. Clouds give a false sense of security that is similar to the cooling effect of the water because clouds reduce the warming sensation of the sun. Another reason for the higher rate of MMs and NMSCs in this socioeconomic group is that people in these occupations may

have better health insurance, a higher awareness of health issues, and ultimately better detection of lesions.[31] An association between high paying jobs and MM may be due to confounding factors in recreational patterns rather the occupational choice.[28]

Certain times of life with high sun exposure confers higher risks for developing different types of skin cancer. Early sun exposure, particularly in childhood and adolescence, is associated with a much higher risk for developing BCC and is estimated to confer a tenfold elevated risk for developing SCC.[30,32,33] Sun exposure in the ten years prior to diagnosis may be important in accounting for many cases of SCC and is associated with a 2.5-fold increased risk when compared to those without this exposure.[32] Sun exposure during childhood and adolescence seems to have a substantial influence on the risk of developing MM.[34,35] Continued exposure in adulthood increases the risk for NMSC. For MM, the risk seems to increase with intermittent sun exposure on areas of skin only occasionally exposed.

The ocular structures can also be affected by UVR.[16] Repeated and prolonged exposure of the conjunctiva will lead to thickening and hypervascularity. There also appears to be a positive correlation between increased cataract formation, decreased latitude, increased UVB, and total sunlight exposure.

UVR includes radiation wavelengths ranging from 200 nm to more than 18,000 nm.[36] Damage to the skin comes from UVR in the 200–400 nm range. There are several types of UVR in this range. The two that have been studied the most in relation to the development of NMSC and MM are ultraviolet A (UVA) and ultraviolet B (UVB). UVA are longer waves (320–400 nm), resulting in deeper skin penetration. It is estimated that 50%–55% of UVA penetrates the dermis.[36] Although UVA has significant risks, the risks are probably greatest in association with UVB.[37] UVB waves are the shortest (220–290 nm), make up about 5% of the sunlight striking the earth, and are probably the most biologically important component of UVR from the sun. Of UVB that reaches the skin, 85% is absorbed primarily in the epidermis, with only 10%–15% transmitted to the deeper dermal layers.[36] Ultraviolet C (UVC) is largely blocked by the ozone layer. The physiologic effects of UVA and UVB on the skin are different and are summarized in Table 65-2.[29,36–38]

Erythema associated with a sunburn is due to excessive UVB. The minimal erythema dose (MED) is the amount of UVR necessary to cause the skin to change to shades of red or pink. MED is highly variable and depends on an individual's skin type, skin thickness, amount of melanin in the skin, and whether the UVR is short or long wave.[16] The erythema is due to an increase in blood flow to the affected skin that begins about four hours after exposure with peak erythema occurring 8–24 hours after exposure. The appearance of the erythema suggests that a threshold of UV damage has been reached sufficient to activate prostaglandin and other inflammatory pathways.

Wavelengths of UVR that produce the largest amount of erythema are also the most efficient at producing py-

Table 65-2 Effects of Ultraviolet Light on the Skin

Effect	UVA (320–400 nm)	UVB (290–320 nm)
Immediate pigment darkening (usually fades within a few hours) due to photo-oxidation of melanin already in epidermis	Yes	Not as evident
Number of functioning melanocytes	No change	Increased number
Photosensitivity reactions	May occur quickly	May occur
Delayed tanning (occurs 36–72 hours after exposure)	Yes	Yes
Production of vitamin D from cholesterol precursors in the skin	None	Yes
Site of absorption	55% in dermis	Primarily the epidermis; 10%–15% in dermis
Radiant heat	Little to none	Moderate to large amount
Sunburn	Seldom evident except after large doses	May occur very quickly
Thickening of the stratum corneum	No	Yes
Carcinogen	Potentiates the effects of UVB	Yes
Distribution of melanosomes	Within dendrites of melanocytes only in basal cell layer	Within keratinocytes throughout the epidermis
Photoaging	Yes	Yes
Etiologic cause of NMSC	Role not completely clear	Yes
Immunosuppression	Yes	Yes
Etiologic cause of MM	Role not completely clear	Yes
Pathologic changes in the dermis	Yes	Yes

Data from National Institutes of Health[29]; Stewart DS[36]; Farmer KC, Naylor MF[37]; Pathak MA.[38]

rimidine dimers. The inference is that the wavelengths that produce maximum erythema are most likely to be the wavelengths that produce the maximum number of carcinogenic mutations.

Two different types of tanning occur in response to UVR exposure. Immediate tanning is a transient grayish, brown discoloration of the skin induced by UVA. It begins during exposure and is maximal at the end of exposure. Immediate tanning lasts a few hours to about 36 hours after exposure. Delayed tanning occurs 48–72 hours following UVR exposure, peaks in seven to ten days, and can persist several days to months.

Photodamage (dermatoheliosis) is a spectrum of skin changes affecting the epidermis and the dermis. This includes the formation and growth of flat, brown spots on the skin (solar lentiges), fine and deep wrinkling, blackheads, telangiectasias, a yellow, sallow color to the skin, and loss of elasticity.[30] These changes can be prevented by the consistent and adequate application of sunscreen.

There appears to be an inverse relationship between increasing latitude and MM mortality. The closer a person lives to the equator, the higher the risk. For every decrease in latitude of two degrees there is an associated 10% increase in the death rate from MM.[8]

Wavelengths of UVR that produce the largest amount of erythema are also the most efficient at producing py-

rimidine dimers. It has been noted that there is a rough correlation between pyrimidine dimer yield and susceptibility to sun-induced erythema. Of the UVR that reaches the earth's surface, wavelengths that are 290–310 nm are the most efficient for the production of pyrimidine dimers. The maximum wavelength for erythema to be seen in humans is estimated to be 298.5 nm.[7,28] The inference is that the wavelengths that produce maximum erythema are most likely to be those that produce the maximum number of carcinogenic mutations.

Stratospheric ozone depletion may also be a causative factor associated with both NMSC and MM. Ozone depletion may lead to increased terrestrial UVB levels for many populations. It has been estimated that for every 1% decrease in ozone there is a 2% increase in UVB penetration to the earth. This increased UVB penetration is predicted to result in an additional 1%–3% increase per year in NMSC.[29] It has also been estimated that for each percentage decrease in the amount of ozone, MM incidence increases about 1%.[27]

Photosensitizing agents have also been associated with the development of skin cancer, as well as premature skin aging, reduced immunity, blood vessel damage, and allergic reactions.[39] Photosensitivity is defined as a chemically induced change in the skin that makes an individual unusually sensitive to light. Rashes, sunburn, or other adverse effects may occur from exposure to UVR of an intensity or duration that would not normally affect that individual. Many medications have photosensitizing agents such as antihistamines, oral contraceptives and estrogen, nonsteroidal and anti-inflammatory drugs, phenothiazines, psoralens, sulfonamides, sulfonylureas, thiazide diuretics, tetracylines, tricyclic antidepressants, many chemotherapeutic agents, antiparasitic drugs, and oral hypoglycemics.[37,39,40] Persons who are taking a photosensitizing medication need to reduce UVR exposure whenever possible.

Prevention

Primary and secondary prevention are both important in regard to skin cancer. Primary prevention strategies are the steps taken to keep the malignancy from developing. In the case of skin cancer, primary prevention efforts include properly applying sunscreen, wearing protective clothing, and decreasing UVR exposure. Public

education programs are an excellent means of addressing these primary prevention strategies. Secondary prevention efforts include the attempts to detect skin cancer(s) early in asymptomatic persons. Table 65-3 provides an overview of primary and secondary prevention strategies for both NMSCs and MMs and appropriate patient education points.

Primary Prevention

Public education programs

Public education programs need to include not only information about skin cancer and reducing UVR exposure, but also a behavioral component that ensures long-term adaptation of healthy behaviors.[41,42] All public education programs and health messages are most successful if they reflect regional and individual differences as well as the social context of culture and/or ethnicity.[10]

To reap the most benefits, public education programs need to be started early in a child's life with the goal

Table 65-3 Primary and Secondary Prevention for Skin Cancer

Strategy	Patient Education	Strengths	Limitations
Risk assessment (secondary prevention)	Define and interpret individual risks for developing skin cancer	Patients who understand their personal risk for developing skin cancer may be more motivated to practice prevention strategies	Time-consuming Patient must be motivated to assist with and try to understand assessment Requires skilled health care providers
Reduce ultraviolet radiation exposure (primary prevention)	Decrease sun exposure between 10 A.M. and 3 P.M. Instruction that UVR is present on cloudy days Infants 6 mo of age and under should not have direct UVR exposure	Decrease carcinogen exposure	Personal practices may be difficult to change
Avoid use of indoor tanning devices (primary prevention)	Large amounts of UVA are potentially carcinogenic Tanned skin is not healthy, rather it is a sign of injured skin Use of indoor tanning devices may lead to premature aging of skin and cataract formation	Large source of carcinogen exposure which can be avoided	Personal practices may be difficult to change—many persons believe they look healthier with a tan
Use chemical sunscreens correctly and consistently (primary prevention)	Use an SPF of at least 15–20 that is waterproof Apply a test dose to check for allergies Apply liberally (about an ounce for an adult in a swim suit) to all exposed skin surfaces 15–30 min prior to sun exposure Reapply sunscreen every 90 min and more frequently after toweling off	When used correctly, sunscreen will block most of the UVB exposure and a variable amount of UVA	Some consider sunscreens expensive and inconvenient to use Many persons do not apply products prior to exposure, apply in inadequate amounts and do not reapply when indicated, thereby limiting the effectiveness of the agents Personal practices may be difficult to change—many persons believe they look healthier with a tan May not apply on children less than 6 mo of age

Table 65-3 Primary and Secondary Prevention for Skin Cancer (continued)

Strategy	Patient Education	Strengths	Limitations
Apply zinc oxide (a physical block) to sun-exposed areas (primary prevention)	Apply a visible, liberal coat to sun-exposed areas Block is effective as long as a visible coat is seen on skin	Excellent for areas with a tendency to burn such as the nose, backs of ears Is more waterproof than chemical sunscreens	Unsuitable to be applied to all sun-exposed areas because of the amount of product necessary
Wear protective clothing (primary prevention)	Protective clothing with a tighter weave can provide an effective physical block against UVR Shirts with sleeves and hats with wide brims provide more protection	Provides a means to directly reduce direct UVR to skin surfaces Relatively inexpensive Easy to apply	Patients may forget to wear hats or not see the benefits of protective clothing as worth the effort
Take extra precaution to reduce UVR exposure when taking photosensitizing medications (primary prevention)	Teach patients about classes of photosensitizing medications and the need for extra protection	Reduces severe sunburns and UVR exposure	Patients may forget to take precautions or underestimate the dangers of photosensitizing medications
Practice monthly skin self-examination (secondary prevention)	Demonstrate technique on the patient Point out any potential problems that require extra monitoring Teach patients to perform in a well-lit area and to pay attention to hard-to-see areas as well as sun-exposed areas	Inexpensive Can be done in privacy of own home Patient may be able to note an early interval change	Patients often forget to do examination or do not see the value of self-examination Some areas of body may be difficult for patient to adequately examine Patients may lack confidence in ability to detect a change
Annual professional examination (secondary prevention)	Opportunity to review many primary prevention strategies Teach skin self-examination Detect lesions that may not be immediately obvious to the patient	May detect subtle, early changes in lesions	May result in removal of borderline lesions Dependent on the skill of the examiner Most cost-effective in higher risk patients—cost effectiveness in the general population is not known

of the individual's adopting attitudes and practices that minimize UVR exposure. A number of such programs have demonstrated that even preschoolers can learn and practice behaviors that reduce UVR exposure.[42–45] Further evidence suggests that in order to get children to change practices and attitudes, their parents must first adapt more healthy behaviors.[46]

Short-term goals and outcomes for primary prevention programs should include an increase in knowledge about the importance of sun protection and a decreased desire for a suntan.[8] Until these are achieved primary prevention strategies will not be implemented effectively.

Medium-term goals of primary prevention programs should include an increased use of hats, clothing, shade, and sunscreens that results in a decreased number of sunburns.[8] Truly effecting these changes in behavior so that they are practiced from childhood through adulthood can be very complicated and difficult to accomplish.

Ultimately, the long-term goals of primary prevention programs (which may not be evident for decades) include a decrease in the number of NMSCs and MMs and a decrease in mortality, especially from MM. Since most cases of BCC and SCC are induced by natural or artificial sources of UVR, primary prevention may truly be theoretically possible.[2] The exact role of UVR in the development of MM is not as clear, although it is speculated that primary prevention strategies are still important.

Sunscreens

There are two types of sunscreens: chemical sunscreens that provide protection by absorbing UVR and physical sunscreens that block UVR from reaching the skin.

Chemical sunscreens. The primary goal of protecting the skin from UVR is not just to avoid a sunburn. Studies demonstrate that incremental damage occurs with each exposure to UVR regardless of whether there is clinical evidence of erythema.[28,29,37,47] It is impractical and impossible to think that humans can avoid sun exposure completely; therefore prevention with sunscreens and other protective clothing is necessary.

Epidemiologic studies suggest that recent UVR exposure may be more important than cumulative UVR exposure. Thus, even older individuals and those with high cumulative sun exposure histories can benefit from sunscreen use by preventing the promoting influence of recent sun exposure and by avoiding new initiating mutations. Sunscreen clearly reduces further actinic damage in patients with such damage when used consistently and adequately. These results can be evident in as little as two years.[47] Children and younger individuals benefit by avoiding the initiating mutations caused by UVR. It has been estimated that regular use of sunscreens (at least SPF 15) to the face, ears, neck, and upper extremities during the first 18 years of life could lead to a 78% reduction in the lifetime incidence of BCC and SCC.[2]

The level of protection offered by a chemical sunscreen is indicated by SPF. Chemical sunscreens contain one or more chemicals in a carrier base, which may be a gel, lotion, cream, or ointment. Some formulations are clear; others are available in milky or colored formulations. Chemical sunscreens are designed to be applied in a thin film to all exposed skin. Depending on the chemicals used, a laboratory SPF of 2–50 can be obtained.

Sunscreens are rated for their UVR absorption under strict and ideal laboratory conditions. In a laboratory, a sunscreen with an SPF of 15 will absorb 92% of UVB, an SPF of 30 will absorb 96.7% of UVB, and an SPF of 40 will absorb 97.5% of UVB.[37] The effectiveness of a particular sunscreen agent on an individual depends on body site, degree of normal skin color, thickness of the epidermis, time of day, time of year, cloud cover, ozone levels, reflection, and scatter. In practice, most health care professionals will recommend an SPF of at least 15 and consider the patient's formulation preference (gel, lotion, etc.). It is also usually recommended that the sunscreen be broad-spectrum, to block some UVA as well. Waterproof sunscreens are usually preferred.

Sunscreens of sufficient SPF can substantially limit or prevent DNA damage and pyrimidine dimer formation. Chemical sunscreens usually contain a variety of products that protect primarily against UVB and to a lesser extent against UVA. Current products used in sunscreens include PABA esters, benzophenones, and cinnamates. Each family has a different absorption spectrum and these agents are used in combination to provide broader protection. In 1990, Parsol 1789 was released which absorbs the longer UVA rays.[30]

Many recommend that the maximum SPF not exceed 30 because of costs and reactions associated with additional active ingredients. Other studies suggest that an SPF of no less than 30 is necessary to prevent immunosuppression.[48] There is no published evidence of harm from using higher SPF sunscreens.[37] In many cases, these irritations that occur with sunscreen use may be related to the quantity and quality of fragrances, preservatives, emulsifiers, film formulations, thickening agents, solvents, and other ingredients added to sunscreens. A test dose should be applied to check for sensitivity reactions to the active agents in chemical sunscreens.

Sunscreens need to be applied 15–30 minutes before exposure, liberally and uniformly, and then should be allowed to dry. Products that are applied too thinly or rubbed vigorously into the skin will not provide the indicated protection.[49] Even if an appropriate sunscreen is selected, the technique of application greatly affects the effectiveness of the product.[50] It should be reapplied every 90 minutes. Eyelids are commonly not covered due to concerns of skin irritation or stinging. Another facial area commonly missed are the ears. Sunscreen is now available in lipstick form to protect the lips.[38] These products should also be applied liberally and reapplied frequently like chemical sunscreens.

Physical sunscreens. Physical sunscreens contain molecules such as zinc oxide, talc, or titanium dioxide in an ointment base. They are available in white and neon colors and flesh tones. These preparations physically block UVR from reaching the dermis and epidermis. Physical sunscreens are effective and useful in protecting selected areas of the body such as the nose, cheeks, ears, and shoulders if applied thickly, but they are considered cosmetically unappealing by many.[16]

Protective clothing

The effectiveness of hats and shirts should not be underestimated. A brim size of 10 cm can lead to a reduction of 70% of UVR exposure to the head and neck.[8] The weave of the material used in hats and clothing is very important. In general, synthetic materials provide better protection against UVA than cotton materials. Densely woven material provides a reflective barrier to UVR. On average, most clothes such as hats and summer wear offer an SPF of 2–6.5, although sun-protective clothing is available that offers an SPF of up to 30.[9]

Protection of the ocular structures is also important. Some sunglasses can offer protection against both UVA and UVB.[51]

Reducing UVR exposure

Outdoor exposure. It is estimated that approximately 60% of the total UVB is received from 10 A.M. to 2 P.M. When possible, avoiding prolonged exposure during this time is recommended. Shade from trees and canopies can further reduce this exposure.[3]

In the United States, the National Weather Service (NWS) has developed an ultraviolet index (UVI) as an initial step in a national program of public education about the dangers of UVR.[48] The program was initiated in 1991. The public is informed by television and radio news and by newspapers of the day's solar ultraviolet intensity rating (a scale of 0 [minimal] to 10+ [very high]) and is given instructions on how to decrease UVR.[52] The long-term effectiveness of this program is not yet known.

Artificial UVR exposure. Indoor tanning represents a relatively new area that public education programs need to target. Preliminary evidence suggests that there is an increase in MM risk for persons who regularly use artificial sources of UVA.[51]

Every day, more than 1 million Americans use tanning parlors that are largely unregulated. This is a $2.5 billion business with an estimated 24,000 salons in the United States. The most frequent users are adolescents and young adults, especially women. The UVA from these tanning parlors is often five times more UVA per time unit than solar UVA.[29] Indoor tanning beds typically emit approximately 95% UVA and 5% UVB, which the parlors market as a "safe tan" because sunburning seldom occurs.[36] In reality there is no known benefit from exposure to artificial UVA and tanning actually represents the body's response to injury.

Secondary Prevention

Early detection of BCC and SCC is important to prevent the disfiguring effects of these tumors and their treatment. Early detection of MM is an approach to control that, if used effectively and consistently, can have a relatively rapid impact on decreasing the mortality rate from MM.[8] This is the approach taken by most nations when implementing a public health control and awareness program for MM, even though the evolution of MM is not completely understood and it may not be completely preventable.[2] Table 65-4 provides an overview of approaches to screening. There are inherent strengths and weakness associated with each approach and providers who design screening programs need to select one that is consistent with the goals of the program and the resources of the providers and their institution.

Screening programs

A panel sponsored by the American Academy of Dermatologists and the Centers for Disease Control and Prevention identified skin cancer control issues as a priority.[10] MM meets the criteria for a disease amenable to screening because it is a serious disease that is increasingly common, has an asymptomatic period, an available screening tool exists, and the disease can be detected and treated early. The panel concluded that primary care providers need to assume a major responsibility for skin cancer detection. These health care providers have an excellent opportunity either as part of a total physical examination or during focused examinations to assess for suspicious lesions and to refer for further evaluation when appropriate.

Data suggests, however, that total skin examinations are infrequently performed and documented in the primary care setting.[53] First, primary care physicians do not consistently examine the entire skin surface. Patients who are most likely to receive a skin examination from a primary care provider are those who request such an examination. Although managed care promotes health promotion and wellness services, in reality fewer patients may actually receive a total skin examination on a regular

basis unless there is a clearly defined program directed toward screening, education, and prevention.[53–56]

The effectiveness of screening programs is also closely related to the skill of the provider performing the screening examination. In general, dermatologists and health professionals with special training in detecting skin lesions are better able to diagnose MM than primary care providers.[55] Over the last four decades there has been a gradual improvement in the diagnostic accuracy of dermatologists in detecting MM. In programs with trained skin cancer screening specialists, reports suggest an overall sensitivity of 81%, a specificity of 99%, and a positive predictive value of 73% for the detection of MM.[8] Those who are not trained specifically in skin cancer detection and diagnosis have rates substantially lower than these figures.

A common criticism of skin self-examination is that people will be burdening the medical system with benign lesions, although research has not substantiated this criticism.[2] It is also important to note that a total skin examination and skin self-examination detect NMSCs. The high prevalence of these types of skin cancers suggests that a total skin examination will result in a higher yield of positive finds than screening of any other organ system. A properly conducted skin examination may be considered time consuming by some, although it can be performed effectively in approximately five minutes. A risk assessment and total skin examination will identify persons at increased risk for developing NMSC and MM who may benefit from increased and more intensive surveillance. Often these persons who are at higher risk for developing NMSC and MM can be referred to special clinics for pigmented lesion where intensive surveillance and education services are available.

When skin cancer screening programs are designed, provisions for diagnostic and treatment services for those with positive screens need to be made available. Of great concern is the disposition of persons who have a positive screen.[57] Ultimately the goal of such programs is that patients follow through with the recommended care. The usefulness and justifiability of any screening program depends on the extent to which those with a positive screen can be followed and treated. If the financial resources necessary for such follow-up care and treatment are not calculated into the total budget for such screening programs, they will not achieve the intended goal.

Screening checklists

In clinical practice, decisions must be made regarding when to refer patients for further evaluation of suspicious skin lesions. Ideally, a screening checklist should detect abnormalities, without overreferring for benign lesions. A variety of checklist systems have been devised to make decisions for referral when screening for skin cancer. Two of the more common checklists are the American ABCDE system and the seven-point checklist (Table 65-5).

The seven-point checklist is reported to be a sensitive screening tool for MM.[58] The scale emphasizes changes

Table 65-4 Approaches to Screening for Skin Cancer

Approach	Characteristics	Strengths	Limitations
Skin self-examination	Regular (usually monthly) examination of all skin surfaces	Note interval changes Convenient Inexpensive	Patients often forget to do examination Some areas of body may be difficult for patient to adequately examine Patients may lack confidence in ability to detect a change
Opportunistic screening (case-finding)	Sporadic examination of patients who present for other health reasons	Earlier detection of lesions that patient may be unaware of	Dependent on the skill of the health provider All skin surface areas may not be examined
Professional skin examination	Annual examination of all skin surfaces by a trained health professional with the goal of detecting skin cancers early	Trained professional may be able to detect a subtle sign or change Examination is focused on finding early changes or skin cancers Safe; noninvasive Usually includes an extensive educational component on ways to prevent skin cancer	Dependent on the skill of the health provider May result in increased removal of borderline lesions
Mass screening	Regular population-based screening of asymptomatic patients at a defined clinical site on a specific date	Large numbers of persons may be examined in a relatively short period of time Trained professionals may be able to detect a subtle sign or change Examination is focused on finding early changes or skin cancer	Dependent on the skill of the health provider May result in increased removal of borderline lesions May be difficult to ensure patients with suspicious lesions receive adequate follow-up
Surveillance	Regular examination (usually every 3–6 mo) of patients with a high risk of developing skin cancer May include medical photography of suspicious lesions	Earlier detection of tumors Usually includes an extensive educational component on ways to prevent skin cancer	May result in increased removal of borderline lesions More expensive
Genetic testing	DNA studies to determine if a patient who has a hereditary predisposition to malignant melanoma carries susceptibility genes	More accurately select patients who will benefit from intense surveillance Usually includes extensive education on ways to reduce the risk of developing malignant melanoma	Expensive Patient may be psychologically disturbed by the results Results may be inconclusive A negative test does not mean the patient may not go on to develop malignant melanoma Results do not tell if, when, or where the patient will go on to develop malignant melanoma

in a lesion, particularly a change in size, shape, or color. The usefulness of this tool in detecting BCC and SCC is not reported. In this checklist, the recommendation is that the presence of one or more major features is an indication for referral. Suspicion for MM should be very high in the presence of two or more major features, but low when only minor features are identified. No studies have been located that compare the efficacy of these two scales.

Pathophysiology

Normal Skin Structures

The skin is the largest organ of the body and is responsible for vital functions such as protection from injury, maintenance of homeostasis, and regulation of temperature. It is a structure made up of two layers, the epidermis and

Table 65-5 Components of Two Screening Checklists for the Early Detection of Skin Cancer

American System	Seven-Point Checklist
A Asymmetry	Major Features
B Border irregularity	• Change in size
C Color irregularity	• Change in color
D Diameter > 6 mm	• Change in shape
E Elevation	Minor Features
	• Diameter > 7 mm
	• Sensory change
	• Oozing/crusting/bleeding
	• Inflammation

dermis (Figure 65-5). The epidermis is composed of stratified, or layered, epithelial cells, the majority of which are keratinocytes that are replaced every 15–30 days. There are four layers of keratinocytic cells named for either their morphology or position: the stratum corneum (outermost layer), the stratum lucidum, the stratum granulosum, and the stratum spinosum.[59] Beneath these four layers is the stratum germinativum, or germinative layer, which has basal cells that, in response to growth-stimulating signals, undergo mitosis. Following mitosis, the newly produced cells are outwardly displaced from the germanitive layer and move toward the superficial layers. As they do so, they lose their nuclei and thus their proliferative ability and they begin to manufacture keratin. Upon reaching the stratum corneum, the epithelial cells are flat, dead cells filled with keratin.

Basal cells grow in a single column on top of a basement membrane. Also in this germanitive layer, atop the basement membrane, are cells known as *melanocytes* that are derived from the neural crest in embryology. Most migrate to the skin but they also populate the mucous membranes, uveal tract, meninges, and the stria vascularis of the inner ear. Melanocytes of the retinal pigmented epithelium arise from the outer layer of the optic cup.[60]

Melanocytes synthesize melanin, the primary skin pigment. Melanin absorbs radiation and accumulates as granules or melanosomes. In melanocytes unexposed to UVR, the melanosomes form a protective supranuclear cap around the nucleus of the cell. Subsequent exposure to UVR initiates the transfer of melanosomes through dendrites of the melanoctye to dendrites in the more superficial layers of the epidermis. Although blacks have the same number of melanocytes as those with lighter skin, their melanocytes have more numerous and larger melanosomes that contain more melanin and are transferred singly. In light-skinned persons, the melanosomes are small, are less numerous, contain less melanin, and are transferred in clusters. MMs arise from melanocytes.[36]

Immediately beneath the basement membrane lies the second layer of the skin, the dermis. It is a supportive, connective tissue network containing the vascular and lymphatic vessels, nerves, glands, hair follicles, and collagen-producing fibroblasts that give the skin much of its strength.[61] The dermis is also divided into two layers distinguished largely by the organization of the cells, nerves and vascular vessels, and the connective tissue.[59] The upper layer is known as the *papillary dermis* because it forms projections (papilla) into the epidermis. It is usually no more than two times the thickness of the epidermis.[59] The lower layer, the *reticular dermis*, is beneath the papillary dermis and is composed primarily of bundles of collagen. The reticular dermis lies above the subcutaneous fat and fascia that attaches the dermis to underlying structures.

Figure 65-5 Anatomy of the skin demonstrating Clark's and Breslow's staging criteria.

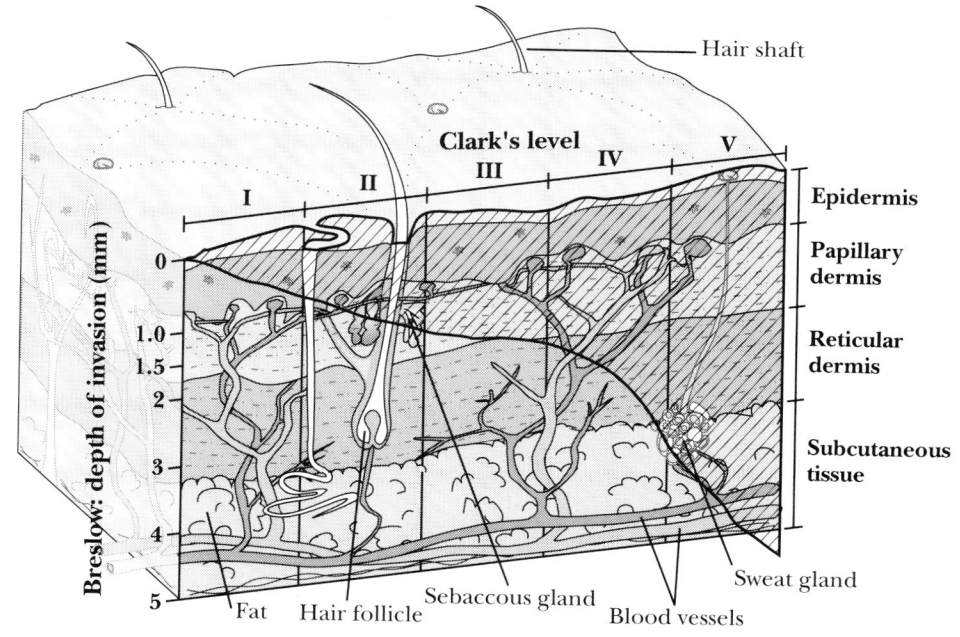

Malignant Change

Nonmelanoma skin cancers

Basal cell carcinoma.   BCC results when a malignant transformation of the basal cells occurs. Regardless of their location within a tumor, these malignant basal cells retain their ability to divide beyond the basal layer. They show no sign of keratinization and can accumulate into a bulky tumor.[62] A universal property of BCCs is the presence of both epidermal and dermal components within the tumors. BCCs transplanted beyond the skin without dermal tissue do not survive.[62] This may explain the usual slow-growing, nonmetastatic nature of BCCs.

Squamous cell carcinoma.   SCC is a tumor of the epidermis that arises from the malignant transformation of the keratinocytes. It can occur anywhere on the skin or mucous membranes where there is squamous epithelium.[61] Unlike BCC, SCC can rapidly progress to local tissue destruction by filling the epidermis, invading the dermis, and then infiltrating other tissues. SCC has the potential to metastasize depending largely on location, depth, and size of the tumor.[63,64] Metastases from SCC are more likely with larger and deeper cutaneous lesions.[63] Tumors originating in the dorsa of the hands or in the head and neck are also more likely to metastasize.

Malignant melanoma

Most MM occurs in cutaneous sites after malignant transformation of melanocytes. The initial site of MM is known as the *primary tumor.* MM may also occur in any melanocyte-containing tissue including the meninges, the mucosa of the gastrointestinal (GI) and respiratory tract, the uveal tract, and the vagina. MM may arise from preexisting lesions or may occur in apparently healthy skin.[65]

Most MMs exhibit two growth phases: radial and vertical. In the radial phase, cells grow in a radial fashion from the primary site and do not metastasize.[66] This phase may continue for an extended period of time in superficial spreading, lentigo maligna, and acral lentiginous MMs or may be of very short duration as in nodular MM. Eventually, the MM enters a vertical growth phase in which the cells invade down into and through the dermis and have the potential to metastasize. Although there are exceptions, MM tends to recur or metastasize in the stepwise manner of local recurrence, regional metastases, and distant metastases.[67]

Local recurrence is the reappearance of MM within 5 cm of the excised primary site. It may be considered extension of the primary tumor or the first sign of metastases.[66] Usually occurring within five years, the risk of local recurrence is 3.2% and is related to tumor thickness.[67] Lesions thicker than 4 mm, that are ulcerated, that are located on the foot, hand, ear, or scalp, or that presented with nodal metastases are at increased risk for local recurrence.

Intransit or satellite metastases occur anywhere between the primary site (beyond 5 cm) and the regional lymph nodes. They are usually multiple, small, bluish, or amelanotic nodules,[67] and represent tumor emboli that were in the lymph channels draining the primary lesion. Regional lymph node metastases most commonly involve the ilioinguinal, axillary, intraparotid, and cervical nodes. Positive regional lymph nodes are highly predictive of visceral metastases.

Distant metastases usually involve nonvisceral sites including the skin, subcutaneous tissue, and distant lymph nodes. The next most common sites (in descending order) are the lungs, liver, brain, bone, and small intestine. Brain metastases are the initial site of metastases in 20% of patients and 50% of patients with other metastatic sites eventually get brain metastases.[68] With polymerase chain reaction (PCR) technique, it has been demonstrated that up to 95% of patients with distant organ sites of metastases have circulating tumor cells and are theoretically likely to develop other metastases.

MM may rarely present as metastatic disease with an unknown primary site. It is thought that these patients may have had a primary cutaneous tumor at one time that regressed, a visceral primary MM, or a clear cell sarcoma (malignancy of the soft tissue).[67]

Clinical Manifestations

Skin cancers have a wide variety of clinical presentations and signs and symptoms (Table 65-6). Tables 65-7 and

Table 65-6   Signs and Symptoms of Skin Cancer

Nonmelanoma Skin Cancer	Malignant Melanoma
Nonhealing sore or ulcer	New pigmented nevus
Scaling red or pink patch that does not heal	New unpigmented nevus
	A nevus that is asymmetrical
Enlarging pink papule or nodule	A preexisting lesion that has developed notched or faded borders
New nodule with or without scaling, erosion, ulceration, or crusting	
	A preexisting lesion that has developed irregular borders
Pearly papule with telangiectasia	
	An unusual or prominent nevus that stands out from the rest of the nevi on the body
	A nevus that is persistently itching, tender, or bleeding
	A nevus that has grown in size or is greater than 6 mm
	A nevus that has changed in color or has multiple colors
	A preexisting nevus that has a change in surface (elevation, erosion, crusting, ulceration)

Table 65-7 Characteristics of Premalignant and Nonmalignant Melanoma Skin Cancers

Type	Characteristics	Location	Other Features
Solar keratosis	Raised red papule or patch with roughened surface	Light exposed surfaces such as face, dorsum of hand, bald scalp	Premalignant lesions with variable degrees of dysplasia
		May occur on trunk	Increased risk for NMSC
Actinic chelilitis	Well-defined white patches (leukoplakia)	Lips, especially the lower lips	Range from epidermal dysplasia to invasive squamous cell carcinoma
		Usually seen in men age 40–70	
Bowen disease	Solitary lesion usually a well-defined, slightly raised red plaque with an adherent scale	Predominantly on the legs, backs of hands, finger, and face	Carcinoma in situ with full-thickness dysplasia
		May occur on non-sun-exposed areas	When Bowen's disease occurs on non-sun-exposed areas it is associated with an increased frequency of internal malignancy
Paget disease	Solitary red, slightly raised well-defined plaque	Nipple and areola	Epidermis is infiltrated by variable numbers of large cells
Squamous cell carcinoma	Nodule or ulcer	Sun-exposed areas including ears, lower lips, backs of hands, forearms	Grows more rapidly than BCC
	May have a crusted surface		Well to poorly differentiated variants
Basal cell—rodent ulcer	Small papule that subsequently ulcerates	Face	Locally invasive
	Ulcer margin is well-defined slightly raised with rolled, pearl-colored margin		Rarely metastasizes
	Most common skin cancer		Accounts for 70%–75% of BCC
Basal cell—cystic type	Central part of tumor does not break down until late in evolution	Face especially the inner canthus of the eye	Often not detected early because it is mistaken for a benign cyst
			Accounts for about 5% of BCC
Basal cell—pigmented	Features similar to rodent ulcer except margins are heavily pigmented	Usually the face	Often misdiagnosed as malignant melanoma
			Accounts for about 1%–3% of BCC
Basal cell—morphoeic type	Begins as a slightly elevated plaque	Usually the face	Often misdiagnosed because it spreads insidiously
			Accounts for 2%–4% of BCC
Basal cell—superficial	Red plaque with adherent scale	Usually the trunk	After a number of years it may become invasive
	Slightly raised minute well-defined margin that is rolled, pearly, and has telangiectasia		Accounts for 13%–15% of BCC
Basal cell—nevus syndrome (Gorlin syndrome)	Multiple lesions	Presence of palmar and planter pits	Dominantly inherited
	Multisystem disorder		Begins in childhood

Data from Du Vivier A[69]; Sober AJ, Burstein JM[70]; Tong AKF, Fitzpatrick TB[71]; McCormack CJ, Kelly JW, Dorevitch AP.[72]

65-8 outline many of the common clinical characteristics of both NMSCs and MMs.[13,69–72] Many of these characteristics are shared among the malignancies and are difficult to distinguish with the naked eye. The signs and symptoms of the various skin cancers can be variable. SCC seems to be difficult to diagnose clinically.[57] BCCs have more distinctive features making the clinical diagnosis easier. Distinguishing between dysplastic nevi and true MM can be very challenging. MM often presents on the lower extremities in women and on the trunk in men. The classic signs in a preexisting nevus include darkening or irregular color, increasing size, nodularity, ulceration, pruritus, and bleeding. A biopsy is necessary to determine the histopathologic characteristics of these different malignancies and to provide guidance for further treatment and follow-up recommendations.

Table 65-8   Characteristics of Malignant Melanoma Skin Cancers

Type	Characteristics	Location	Other Features
Dysplastic nevus syndrome	Large number of atypical nevi with irregular margins and variable pigmentation	Sun-exposed and non-sun-exposed areas	Increased risk of developing MM May be sporadic or have a hereditary predisposition
Congenital nevus	May be giant or small Present at birth or shortly after birth	May occur anywhere on the body	Giant congenital nevus is rare occurring in about 1 of 20,000 births with a lifetime risk of malignant transformation of 2%–40% Small congenital nevus occurs in 1 of 100 births and lifetime risk of malignant transformation is not known
Lentigo maligna (Hutchinson freckle)	Flat pigmented lesion that gradually enlarges Light tan to brown or black with irregular notched borders	Usually on the face, neck, or arms of the elderly	Begins as MM in situ and may take 5–50 yr to become invasive Usually occurs in the seventh decade Accounts for 5% of MM Three times more common in females
Superficial spreading malignant melanoma	Slightly raised lesion with an irregular border and variable, unevenly distributed pigmentation with shades of red, blue, brown, purple, and black	May be found anywhere on the body but usually on the upper back of men and women and the lower extremities of females	Most common of the MMs (about 70%–75%) With early diagnosis the five-year survival rate approaches 95% Long phase of horizontal growth prior to vertical growth and metastasis Usually occurs in fifth decade Equally common in men and women
Acral lentinginous malignant melanoma	Initially the lesion is flat with irregular margins and pigmentation. The lesion rapidly becomes raised and nodular	Soles, palms of hands, nailbeds, and oral mucosa	Early vertical growth and rapid metastasis May occur in Asians and blacks Accounts for 5%–10% of MM
Nodular malignant melanoma	Lesion is raised, nodular, and sometimes ulcerated Borders are irregular and color variegated Occasionally the tumor has no apparent visible pigmentation (amelanotic MM)	May occur on any part of the body, but most commonly on the legs and trunk	Does not seem to have a horizontal growth phase. It grows vertically quickly with metastasis Twice as common in men Usually occurs in the fifth decade

Data from Swetter SM[13]; Du Vivier A[69]; Sober AJ, Burstein JM.[70]

Assessment

Patient and Family History

A risk assessment is the first step in any secondary prevention or cancer screening program. Assessment should include all of the factors identified in Table 65-1.[2,6,8–10] In particular, it is important to try to obtain an accurate history of sun exposure. This includes quantifying information about severe sunburns (especially in childhood), occupational history, use of indoor tanning devices, and overall cumulative exposure. In reality, however, it is very difficult to quantify lifetime exposure to UVR.[27] The history should also include a family history with particular

emphasis on the number of cases of NMSCs, MMs (including specific pathology when available), dysplastic nevus syndrome, and other genetic diseases such as Gorlin syndrome or xeroderma pigmentosum. Finally, the assessment should include detailed information about any lesions that have been removed in the past. Particular attention should be given to determining if the patient has had any of the following lesions: dysplastic nevi, congenital melanocytic nevi, actinic keratosis, Bowen's disease, solar keratoses, BCC, SCC, or MM. In some cases, pathology reports must be ordered to provide a more accurate assessment and to ultimately provide better screening recommendations.

Once the assessment is complete, screening recommendations can be discussed in light of the individual's risks. Those with higher risk profiles will need screening more often than annually and may possibly need medical photography. Prophylactic removal of suspicious lesions may be indicated. It is important to communicate to the patient that an accurate risk assessment provides more appropriate screening recommendations. It is also important for the patient to understand that the presence or absence of risk factors is not an absolute guarantee that the patient will or will not go on to develop malignancy. The risk assessment offers an opportunity to teach the patient about appropriate primary prevention strategies.[71] Risk assessment counseling also offers an opportunity to correct misconceptions about risk and offer reassurance about the benefits of early detection and primary prevention.

Before beginning the physical examination it is also important to determine if the patient has noted any change in a lesion or if the patient has any concerns about a lesion(s). If such a history is elicited, further information should be obtained about any changes in size, shape, color, or other physical characteristics and when these changes were noted (see Table 65-6).

Physical Examination

Technical aspects

The mainstay for the early detection of both NMSC and MM is the physical examination. Clearly the number of both NMSCs and MMs detected is greatly increased when the examiner is focused on that particular task and has a working knowledge of the different types of skin lesions (see Tables 65-7 and 65-8) as well as the signs and symptoms of skin cancer (see Table 65-6). It is estimated that diagnostic methods that involve inspection alone are about 60%–80% effective in identifying MM.[6] Primary care providers need to be aware of high-risk persons and high-risk anatomic sites since only 20% of MM occur on sun-exposed body surfaces in contrast to 85% of NMSC.[29] Those who practice in the pediatric setting need to emphasize primary prevention strategies.

To be effective, the examination should be carried out in a well-lit room and include all skin surfaces. Dermatologic visual diagnosis is a skill that must be practiced to increase proficiency and appears to be based more on visual pattern recognition than on mastery of complex rules of logic.[35]

The physical examination of the skin should be performed systematically.[73] The areas to be assessed are the same as that of skin self-examination (see Chapter 9, Figure 9-11). The patient should be taught the importance of and rationale for a total skin examination. All concealing cosmetics should be removed. In order to make the patient as comfortable as possible, only one area of the skin should be exposed at a time.

The lighting in the room should be carefully selected. Ideally, a total skin examination would be conducted in daylight, but this is impractical. A combination of incandescent and fluorescent light is probably best. Fluorescent light accentuates blue to yellow colors and incandescent brings out red colors. The combination can help bring out the wide range of colors sometimes seen in skin cancers. Tangential lighting will aid in the recognition of subtle elevations.[73]

During the examination, all findings should be carefully documented on an anatomic chart. Characteristics to be documented include location, color(s), size (measured in millimeters), border characteristics, and the presence or absence of elevation, telangiectasias, crusting, or ulceration. If the patient is being seen for follow-up screening, the anatomic chart from the most recent examination should be used for comparison to determine if any characteristics of the lesions have changed.

Photography of lesions allows the clinician to accurately document the location and clinical characteristics for future reference. Total body photography is very important to assist in the identification of early MM in patients with dysplastic nevus syndrome. It usually requires about 24 different views.[73] In some cases, measuring tapes may be placed on the skin prior to photography to assess for changes in size.

Dermoscopy (epiluminescence microscopy, incident light microscopy, or surface microscopy) is now being used as an adjunct to the physical examination in some clinical practices. The technique is not new but until recently was of limited use in the United States because of the timely and costly technical aspects and lack of available formal training in its use.[74,75] Recently, improvements in the technique and equipment, consensus about terminology, and research validation have made the procedure more attractive. The diagnostic accuracy of the instrument directly depends on the training and expertise of the clinician using the instrument.

Dermoscopy involves the application of oil to the surface of the lesion in question followed by examination. The oil eliminates some of the light reflection of skin and makes the surface of the skin more transparent.[74] After application of the oil, the lesion is gently compressed with a transparent material such as a glass slide. Various tools for visual examination are then used. These tools can be as simple as a hand-held microscope (called a *dermatoscope*), a surgical stereomicroscope, or computerized equipment that may include digital video cameras. This procedure may aid in the early detection of MM by assisting in distinguishing malignancy from benign pigmented skin lesions.[74]

Physical characteristics of lesions

Most BCCs begin as a small, firm, well-demarcated, dome-shaped papule (see Color Plate 11 [Figure 65-6] and Table 65-7). A wide range of colors may be present from pearly white to pink to red. Telangiectasias may or may not be present on the surface. Some lesions will have scaling plaques. As lesions progress, the center usually ulcerates and the borders develop a raised or rolled appearance.

The physical characteristics of SCC may not be as distinct (see Table 65-7). SCC often begins as a red, raised, firm papule. Crusting and ulceration is often seen (see Color Plate 12 [Figure 65-7]). It is not uncommon for the patient to report that the lesion is tender or painful.

A wide range of clinical characteristics may be noted in MM (see Table 65-8). It is often difficult to distinguish a dysplastic nevus from an MM. Within the different classifications of MM, a range of clinical characteristics may be seen (see Color Plates 13–16 [Figures 65-8–65-11]). Physical characteristics include asymmetrical, faded, or jagged borders; two or more colors in a lesion or a lesion that is a different color than the rest of the pigmented lesions on a patient; diameter greater than 5 mm; nodular surface characteristics; and bleeding or ulceration.

Diagnostic Studies

Biopsy of the suspicious lesion is necessary for histologic examination. On occasion, the lesion may be so small that boundaries of excision are much the same as they would be for a biopsy and the entire diagnostic and treatment phases may be carried out in one step. This is only prudent for small lesions when the lesion and disease-free margin can be obtained.

Table 65-9   Biopsies for Suspicious Skin Lesions

Type	Indication	Purpose	Method	Healing	Advantage	Disadvantage
Punch	BCC Pigmented lesions	Incisional or excisional depending on size of lesion and instrument	Lesion is cut with a circular cutting instrument (punch). The cylinder of tissue is lifted and the base is transected with small scissors Specimen should not be removed with toothed forceps that may crush the tissue and may interfere with pathologic examination of tissue Punch sizes range from 1.5–6 mm	By second intention or suture	Simple, easy to perform	Small specimen size may lead to difficult histopathologic examination Large (5–6 mm) punch biopsies may leave round, cosmetic defects
Shave	BCC	Removal of tissue that extends above the plane of surrounding skin	Injection of local anesthetic under the skin is used to elevate the lesion above the plan of surrounding tissue Scalpel or hand-held razor blade is used to shave off lesion Shave is made at depth between papillary and reticular dermis	By second intention	Simple Good cosmetic effect	Not enough tissue for histopathologic examination of suspected SCC or melanoma Nevi may return with central pigmentation
Saucerization	BCC Pigmented lesions SCC	Removal of tissue extending through dermis and down into subcutaneous fat	Scalpel or hand-held razor blade used to undercut the lesion at a 45° angle to the skin Incision carried down to fat	By second intention	Simple Provides complete dermal specimen	May result in hypopigmented, hyperpigmented, or hypertrophic scar Limited to areas of the skin that can close by second intention without cosmetic defect
Elliptical incision or excision	BCC Pigmented lesions SCC	Removal of large or deep lesions Removal of specimens with changes extending into the fascia	Scalpel is used to cut a fusiform or football-shaped incision with the lesion in the center Specimen is undercut with either scissors or scalpel and removed Blunt dissecting scissors are used to undermine the edges of the wound to maximize tissue healing and cosmesis	Sutures Some sites with concave surfaces such as facial areas heal better by second intention	Provides complete specimen for histopathologic examination Good cosmetic effect	More time-consuming and difficult Requires postsurgical wound care More discomfort and risk to the patient

Data from Robinson et al[76].

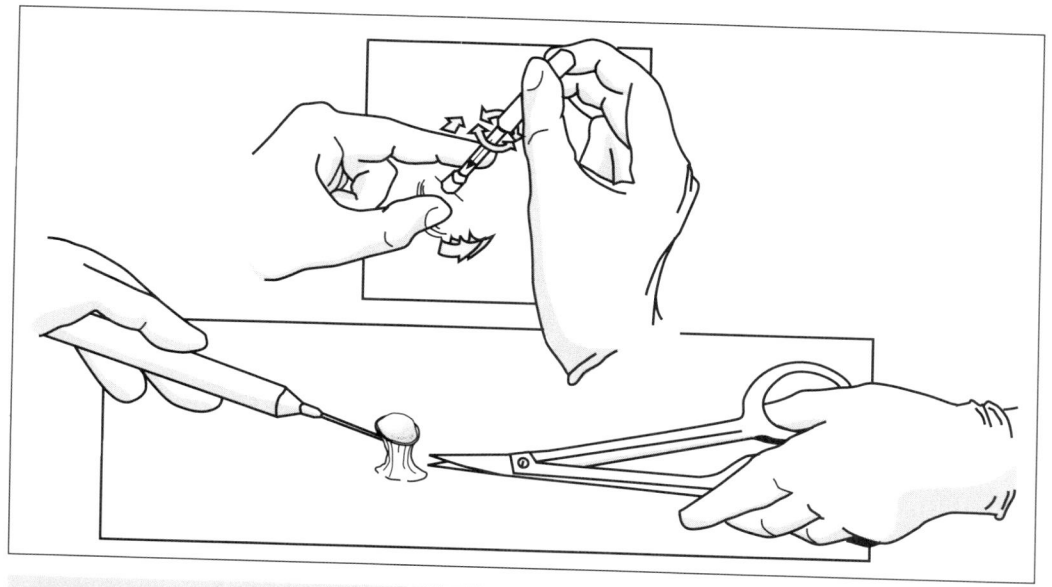

Figure 65-12 Punch biopsy of a lesion.

Biopsies can be accomplished using several techniques: punch, shave, saucerization, and incisional or excision elliptical biopsies[76] (see Table 65-9 and Figures 65-12, 65-13, 65-14, and 65-15). It should be noted that although BCCs may be biopsied using any of those techniques, SCCs and lesions suspected of being MM should only be biopsied using methods that remove the necessary tissue for complete dermatopathologic examination without disturbing margins so lesions may be correctly staged. Ocular MMs usually are not biopsied to avoid sight damage. Potential complications from biopsies include infec-

tion, bleeding, hyperpigmentation, hypopigmentation, adhesions, scarring, and problems with wound closure.

Patients diagnosed with MM should undergo diagnostic testing to rule out metastatic sites. Before therapy is prescribed, the extent of disease must be determined. A chest x-ray, complete blood count (CBC), and liver function tests including lactic dehydrogenase (LDH) should be obtained. Liver scans or ultrasounds may be indicated for persistent elevations in LDH to rule out liver metastases.[77] Further studies may include computerized tomography (CT) scans, bone scans, magnetic resonance

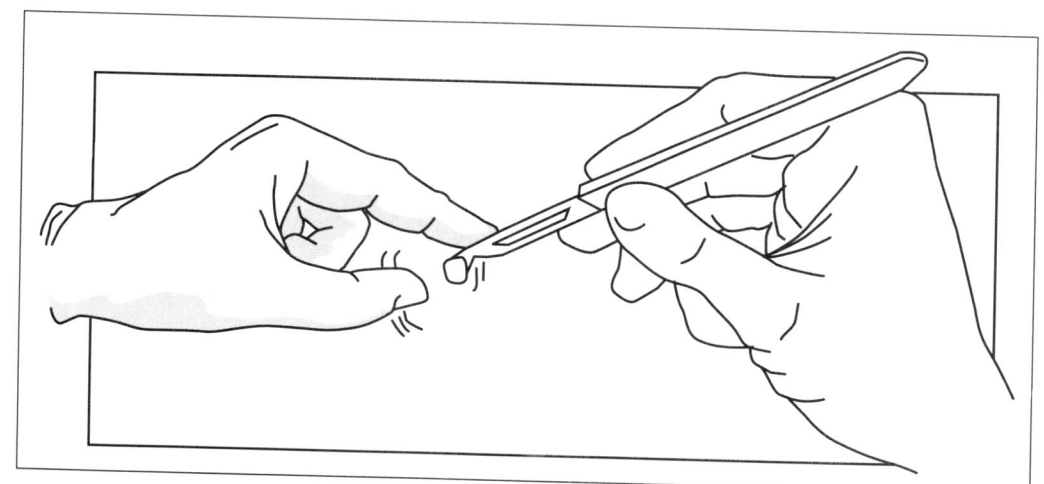

Figure 65-13 Shave biopsy of a lesion.

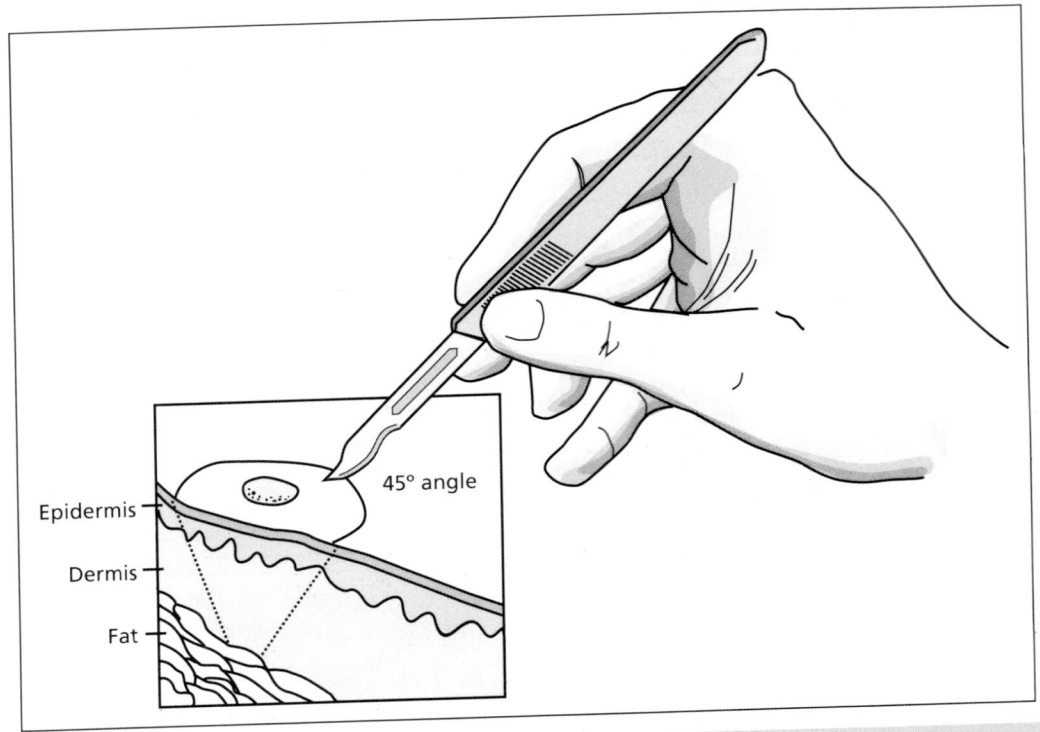

Epidermis

Dermis

Fat

45° angle

Figure 65-14 Saucerization biopsy of a lesion.

imaging (MRI), and positron emission tomography-(PET). More extensive workup is necessary if the patient complains of symptoms related to other body systems. For example, because MM may metastasize to the GI tract, patients with MM and GI symptoms should have further studies to rule out metastases.

Prognostic Indicators

Nonmalignant melanoma skin cancers

BCC is usually slow-growing. Complete excision of a primary BCC suggests a 95% cure rate and complete excision using Mohs' surgery may further increase the

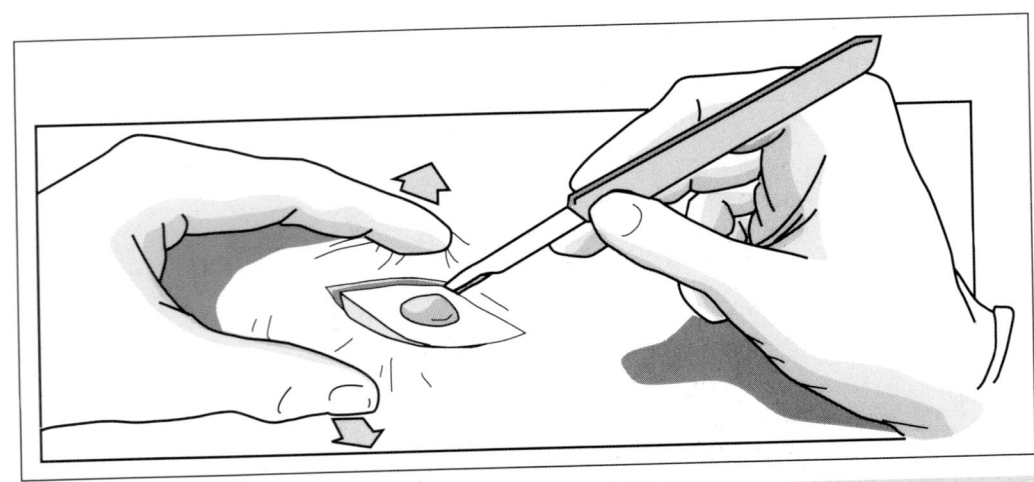

Figure 65-15 Incisional or excisional biopsy technique.

cure.[71] The risk of developing a second BCC in patients with a complete resection of their primary lesion may be as high as 45%.[78] Primary lesions that are large and involve underlying structures are more likely to have metastasized, in which case the prognosis is poor. For metastatic lesions, the one-year survival rate is less than 20% and the five-year survival rate is 10%.[71]

The course of SCC ranges along a continuum from slow-growing, locally invasive tumors to rapidly growing, widely invasive ones.[63] Discussion of prognosis is, therefore, difficult. Overall, the five-year survival rate for SCC is 90% and its metastatic rate is 3%–6%.[71] Its metastatic potential, in some cases, appears to be related to the cause, location, and morphologic characteristics of the tumor. SCC arising in areas of sun-damaged skin rarely metastasize. SCC of the lower lip has a metastatic rate of approximately 15%.[71] SCC originating in the oral mucosa, on the penis, and on the vulva tend to be more invasive at diagnosis and have a higher rate of metastases.

Malignant melanoma

Prognosis of MM may be based on several factors including Clark's and Breslow's microstaging, histologic evaluation, anatomic location, and extent of spread at time of diagnosis. Presence or absence of nodal involvement is the most powerful predictor of survival. The most important prognostic factors by stage of MM are: stages I and II—tumor thickness, presence of ulceration, and anatomic site of primary tumor; stage III—similar to stages I and II with the addition of extent of nodal disease; and stage IV—the number and location of metastatic sites.[79]

Tumor thickness has a direct correlation with the risk of metastatic spread of MM: the thicker the lesion, the greater the risk of metastases and the poorer the prognosis. A lesion less than 0.75-mm thick is likely to be lethal in less than 5% of patients.[8] Tumors that are 4 mm or more in thickness at the initial (primary) excision have probably metastasized and are likely to be lethal in more than 50% of patients.[8] There are, however, some relatively thin MMs that grow aggressively.[79] The extent of tumor depth (Clark's level) also has a direct correlation with prognosis, with deeper lesions being worse. Ulcerated lesions are associated with a worse prognosis and tend to predict metastatic involvement.[79] MM occurring on the upper or lower extremities has a better prognosis than those occurring on the trunk, head, and neck. Lesions on the anterior chest particularly predict a better prognosis and those on the scalp particularly predict a poorer one. Lesions on the heels and palms are more aggressive.[66] Females appear to have a better prognosis than males, although this may be because most MMs in females occur on the lower extremities whereas in males most occur on the trunk. Age may also be an important factor with younger men (less than 50) having an advantage over older men with stage III disease.[79]

Nodal involvement for stage III MM is an additional prognostic indicator. The number and percent of positive nodes is important, and as they increase the prognosis becomes worse.[79] In the case of metastatic MM (stage IV), a greater number of metastatic sites and the presence of visceral metastases negatively affects prognosis. Median survival is seven months for patients with one metastatic site, four months for two sites, and two months for greater than two sites.[66] There are also other prognostic factors, which are listed in Table 65-10.[79]

Patients who present with lymph node metastases and an unknown primary site are a unique category. Their five-year survival rate after total lymph node dissection approximates that of patients with thin, primary lesions.[66]

Classification and Staging

Nonmalignant Melanoma Skin Cancers

Clinical staging is accomplished by inspection and palpation of lesions and involved lymph nodes plus imaging studies of any underlying bony structures.[80] Pathologic staging is accomplished by the examination of completely resected tumors and lymph nodes. The TNM categories for both clinical and pathologic classifications of NMSC are the same and are grouped as stages I–IV (Table 65-11). The histologic grade of specimens is described as grades (G) I–IV. G1 is a well-differentiated tumor, G2 is a moderately differentiated tumor, G3 a poorly differentiated tumor, and G4 an undifferentiated one. GX denotes a grade that cannot be assessed.[81]

Table 65-10   Additional Tumor Factors Affecting Prognosis of Patients with Melanoma

Factor	Indication of Poor Prognosis
Tumor regression	Tumors < 1.0 mm with notable regression
Mitotic rate	Increasing mitotic rates
Host cellular response	Diminished lymphoid infiltrates
Microscopic satellites	Presence of satellites
Tumor cell type	Tumors without spindle cells
Tumor volume	Increasing volume
Cross-sectional profile	Polypoid or verrucous configuration
Volume-weighted mean nuclear volume	Increasing nuclear volume
Nucleolus organizer regions	Increasing AgNOR counts*
DNA content	Increasing DNA aneuploidy
Proliferation cell index	Increasing indices (in some cases)

*AgNOR = silver-staining nucleolus organizer region.
Reprinted with permission from Ahmed I: Malignant melanoma: Prognostic indicators. *Mayo Clin Proc* 72:356–361, 1997 (Table 3, p 359.)[79]

Table 65-11 American Joint Committee on Cancer Staging for Nonmelanoma Skin Cancers

Stage 0 (Tis-N0-M0)	• Carcinoma in situ
	• No regional lymph node or distant metastasis
Stage I (T1-N0-M0)	• Tumor 2 cm or less in greatest dimension
	• No regional lymph node or distant metastasis
Stage II (T2-N0-M0 or T3-N0-M0)	• Tumor more than 2 cm but no more than 5 cm in greatest dimension (T2) or tumor more than 5 cm in greatest dimension (T3)
	• No regional lymph node or distant metastasis
Stage III (T4-N0-M0 or any T-N1-M0)	• Tumor invades deep extradermal structure (i.e., cartilage, skeletal muscle, or bone) or any tumor size with regional lymph node metastasis
Stage IV (any T-any N-M1)	• Any tumor size, any regional lymph node metastasis, and distant metastasis

Malignant Melanoma

Tumors are described using two systems, Clark's level and Breslow's measurement (see Figure 65-5). The Clark's level describes the lesion based on the depth of invasion into the dermis and subcutaneous fat. Level I (in situ) lesions do not penetrate the basement membrane. Level II lesions extend through the basement membrane and into the papillary dermis. Level III lesions reach into the reticular/papillary junction, and Level IV lesions invade the reticular dermis. Thickness of the dermis may vary depending on anatomic site and individual differences and may affect the accuracy of Clark's level. The success of this method of microstaging depends on the ability of the examiner to correctly recognize the microscopic anatomy of the skin.[65] The level of invasion is directly correlated to the metastatic potential of the lesion.[66]

Tumor thickness is described by the Breslow method. The lesion is measured with an ocular micrometer and is defined as the distance from the epidermis to the deepest identifiable layer of contiguous MM cells.[65] Measurements are reported in millimeters. The thicker the lesion, the higher the metastatic potential.

The American Joint Committee on Cancer (AJCC) has adopted a TNM system that incorporates both Breslow and Clark methods to clinically stage MM[80] (Table 65-12). If the data is not in agreement, the least favorable of the two should be used to assign staging.[66,82] Lesions that have been distorted by previous procedures and cannot be measured are assigned "TX." If no primary can be found, the tumor is assigned "T0." The extent of tumor should be assigned after excision only.

Therapeutic Approaches and Nursing Care

Initially, treatment of both NMSC and MM relies on biopsy and histopathologic evaluation of the suspicious le-

Table 65-12 American Joint Committee on Cancer Staging for Malignant Melanoma Skin Cancers

Primary Tumor (pT)

pTX	Primary tumor cannot be assessed
pT0	No evidence of primary tumor
PTis	Melanoma in situ (atypical melanocytic hyperplasia, severe melanocytic dysplasia), not an invasive malignant lesion (Clark level I)
pT1	Tumor 0.75 mm or less in thickness and invades the papillary dermis (Clark level II)
pT2	Tumor more than 0.75 mm but not more than 1.5 mm in thickness and/or invades to papillary-reticular dermal interface (Clark level III)
pT3	Tumor more than 1.5 mm but not more than 4 mm in thickness and/or invades the reticular dermis (Clark level IV)
pT3a	Tumor more than 1.5 mm but not more than 3 mm in thickness
pT3b	Tumor more than 3 mm but not more than 4 mm in thickness
pT4	Tumor more than 4 mm in thickness and/or invades the subcutaneous tissue (Clark level V) and/or satellite(s) within 2 cm of the primary tumor
pT4a	Tumor more than 4 mm in thickness and/or invades the subcutaneous tissue
pT4b	Satellite(s) within 2 cm of the primary tumor

Regional Lymph Nodes (N)

NX	Regional lymph nodes cannot be assessed
N0	No regional lymph node metastasis
N1	Metastasis 3 cm or less in greatest dimension in any regional lymph node(s)
N2	Metastasis more than 3 cm in greatest dimension in any regional lymph node(s) and/or in-transit metastasis
N2a	Metastasis more than 3 cm in greatest dimension in any regional lymph node(s)
N2b	Intransit metastasis
N2c	Both (N2a and N2b)

Note: Intransit metastasis involves skin or subcutaneous tissue more than 2 cm from the primary tumor but not beyond the regional lymph nodes.

Distant Metastasis (M)

MX	Distant metastasis cannot be assessed
M0	No distant metastasis
M1	Distant metastasis
M1a	Metastasis in skin or subcutaneous tissue or lymph node(s) beyond the regional lymph nodes
M1b	Visceral metastasis

Stage Grouping

Stage 0	pTis	N0	M0
Stage I	pT1	N0	M0
	pT2	N0	M0
Stage II	pT3	N0	M0
Stage III	pT4	N0	M0
	Any pT	N1	M0
	Any pT	N2	M0
Stage IV	Any pT	Any N	M1

sion. In the case of MM in particular, removal of the entire lesion for histopathologic evaluation is the method of choice. This enables the pathologist to most accurately assess the Breslow and Clark's measurement levels to give prognostic indicators and guide the definitive surgical excision.

Nonmalignant Melanoma Skin Cancers

Complete removal of the lesion, including tumor-free margins, is the goal of treatment. Skin cancers usually begin as small, locally invasive lesions that can be easily removed with a variety of methods with minimal morbidity.[83,84] Extensive or recurrent skin cancer, however, requires complex surgical or radiation therapy, is expensive and difficult to treat, and treatment outcome is less certain. Treatments for NMSC include surgical excision, electrosurgery, Mohs' micrographic surgery, cryosurgery, radiation therapy, and chemotherapy. Surgical excision, Mohs', and radiation therapy are the most frequently used methods of treatment. Laser removal, curettement, cryotherapy, electrodessication, and topical chemotherapy are less frequently used treatments. Surgical excision and Mohs' micrographic surgery result in a complete specimen that can be examined by a pathologist. Laser removal, cryosurgery, and electrosurgery should only be used when the diagnosis is certain and the lesion is small because there will not be a specimen for histopathologic diagnosis and evaluation for free margins.

Surgery

Surgical excision with tumor-free margins is the absolute goal. Primary closure or repair with skin graft or flaps usually produces good cosmetic results.[71] BCCs with tumor present in the lateral margins at the time of surgical excision may result in recurrence. The recurrences usually present early and can be surgically excised again. Positive deep BCC margins result in deep recurrences at the tumor site, invasion of other structures, and may be delayed. SCCs should be removed with margins of 3–5 mm.[71,83] Tumors larger than 2 cm, invasive tumors, and those on high-risk areas (scalp, ears, nose, eyelids, or lips) should be removed with margins of 6 mm.[71,83] SCCs previously treated with radiation therapy should be excised with the entire radiation scar to try to remove multiple foci in the radiation field.[71,83]

Electrosurgery. Electrosurgery uses heat to cut tissue. It is fast, efficient, and relatively inexpensive.[76] When combined with curettage, electrosurgery may be useful in the removal of distinct, superficial, or nodular BCCs. After the tumor is anesthetized, a sharp curette is used to scoop out the gelatinous carcinoma. Bleeding is stopped and the perimeter of tissue is destroyed by using electrocautery or electrodessication. The wound is explored again with a curette to ensure complete removal of the lesion. Two or three cycles of curettage followed by electrodessication may be used.

Mohs' micrographic surgery. Originally called *chemosurgery*, this procedure is used for tumors that are recurrent, those with indistinct margins, and those that are in a location where wide margins of healthy skin removal would be surgically or cosmetically unacceptable.[85] In this procedure, the tumor is excised under local anesthesia using horizontal frozen sections that are microscopically examined during the surgery (Figure 65-16). Any margins of areas with residual tumor can continue to be selectively excised while normal tissues are preserved, until clear margins are obtained. For removal of primary skin cancer, Mohs' offers a 95%–99% chance for complete removal without recurrence.[76,84]

Cryosurgery. Cryosurgery uses freezing temperatures to destroy tissue and may follow shave excisions. A cryogen such as carbon dioxide, nitrous oxide, or liquid nitrogen must be used. The cryogen can be swabbed or sprayed on the lesion. Another method involves the use of a cryoprobe. It is cooled and then applied to the lesion for seconds or minutes. The deepest part of the tumor must reach at least $-50°C$ during freezing. Thick lesions may be debulked with excision or curettage before cryosurgery or repeated cycles may be employed to improve results. Cryosurgery for SCC is only used for superficial tumors and carcinoma in situ.[71] Cryosurgery is not used on tumors in hair-bearing areas, periorbital areas, and vermilion borders of the lips (related to risk of scar retraction). Nor is it indicated for recurrent tumors, deeply invasive and ulcerated lesions, tumors with indistinct borders, and those that are morphea-like.

Radiation therapy

Radiation therapy is the treatment of choice for some small lesions in areas that would be difficult to excise including the eyelids, ear pinna, nasolabial fold, alar nasi, and lips. SCCs have a tendency to follow embryonal planes of closure, therefore tumors may invade deeply and not be amenable for cure with other treatments. Radiation therapy can penetrate through tissue and help destroy deeper tumors.[63] Total dose is divided into several fractions over several weeks to promote cure while causing minimal damage to normal tissue.

Chemotherapy

Topical and intralesional fluorouracil (5-FU) have been used to treat BCCs. Topical applications are usually prescribed twice a day for several weeks for small, superficial tumors in persons who are unable to tolerate other treatments. Recurrence in patients treated with 5-FU versus other therapies is higher.[71] This high recurrence rate may be due to the use of 5-FU with large tumors in which the 5-FU fails to penetrate the depth of the lesion.[86] Intralesional 5-FU has been used in nodular lesions. Intralesional interferon has been used as an investigational treatment for both BCCs and SCCs.

Severe irritation may occur with topical 5-FU. Patients should apply the chemotherapy with a cotton-tipped applicator or latex glove to avoid contact with other skin

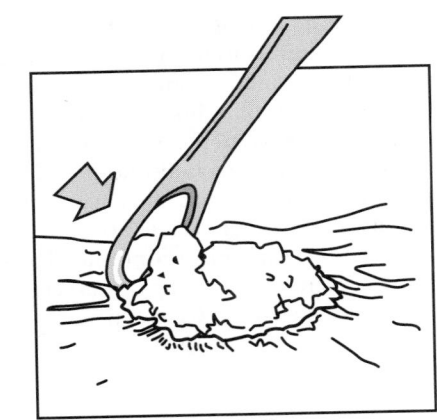

1. Tumor is debulked by curettage

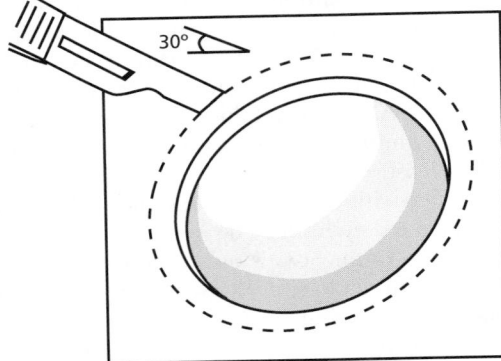

2. Wound base is excised

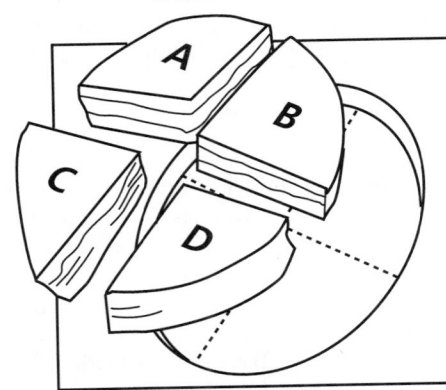

3. Excised wound base is divided and sectioned

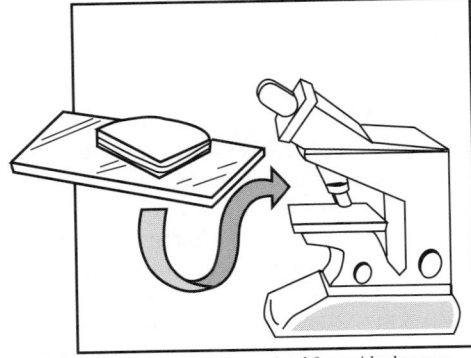

4. Each section is examined for residual tumor

Figure 65-16 Mohs' micrographic surgical technique.

surfaces. In general a dressing is not applied, but if the physician requests a dressing, it should be gauze with tape instead of adherent-type dressings. Topical 5-FU can lead to a significant photosensitizing reaction and patients must be instructed to avoid UVR exposure.

Retinoids

The synthetic retinoids, isotretinoin and etretinate, have been used in the prevention and treatment of skin cancers. Although the mechanism of action is unclear and they do not usually cure cancer, they have caused regressions when given at high dosages (1.5 mg/kg/day or more).[87] Retinoids are an active area of study as chemoprevention agents against skin cancer. In some studies, however, they have caused toxicities resulting in patient withdrawal.[87]

Malignant Melanoma

The treatment of MM is based on the appearance and stage of progression of the disease. An algorithm of treatment for primary MM is described in Figure 65-17.[65] Primary lesions should be completely excised with disease-free margins. Surgery techniques that do not remove the lesion in the entirety of its depth with disease-free margins should not be used. Surgical excision or Mohs' micrographic surgery are acceptable techniques and have been discussed in previous sections.

There is no standard treatment for patients with local or intransit metastases, although surgical excision should be considered. Immunotherapy, chemotherapy, and radiation therapy may also be of use.

Recommendations for treatment of metastatic MM are made based on the number and location of metastases. Solitary lesions or those of a limited number may be amenable to surgical excision that can result in significant palliation and even long-term survival. For patients with multiple metastatic sites in multiple organs, chemotherapy and immunotherapy may be utilized.

Surgery

Surgical excision. Complete surgical excision should be wide and should include disease-free margins, although the size of the margins is a subject of controversy. Three- to five-cm margins were advocated in the past for all size lesions. However, local recurrences of thin MM (less than 1-mm deep) are rare regardless of the surgical margin. It is now recommended that 1-cm margins are adequate for thin (less than 1-mm) primary lesions.[88] Lesions deeper than 1–4 mm should have 2–3 cm margins with exceptions based on cosmetic effect.[65] Controversy exists about required margins for lesions thicker than 4 mm. Three- to five-cm margins around the primary site and including the underlying fascia have been recommended.[65,88] Others argue that for tumors greater than 4 mm in thickness, wider excisions may decrease the rate

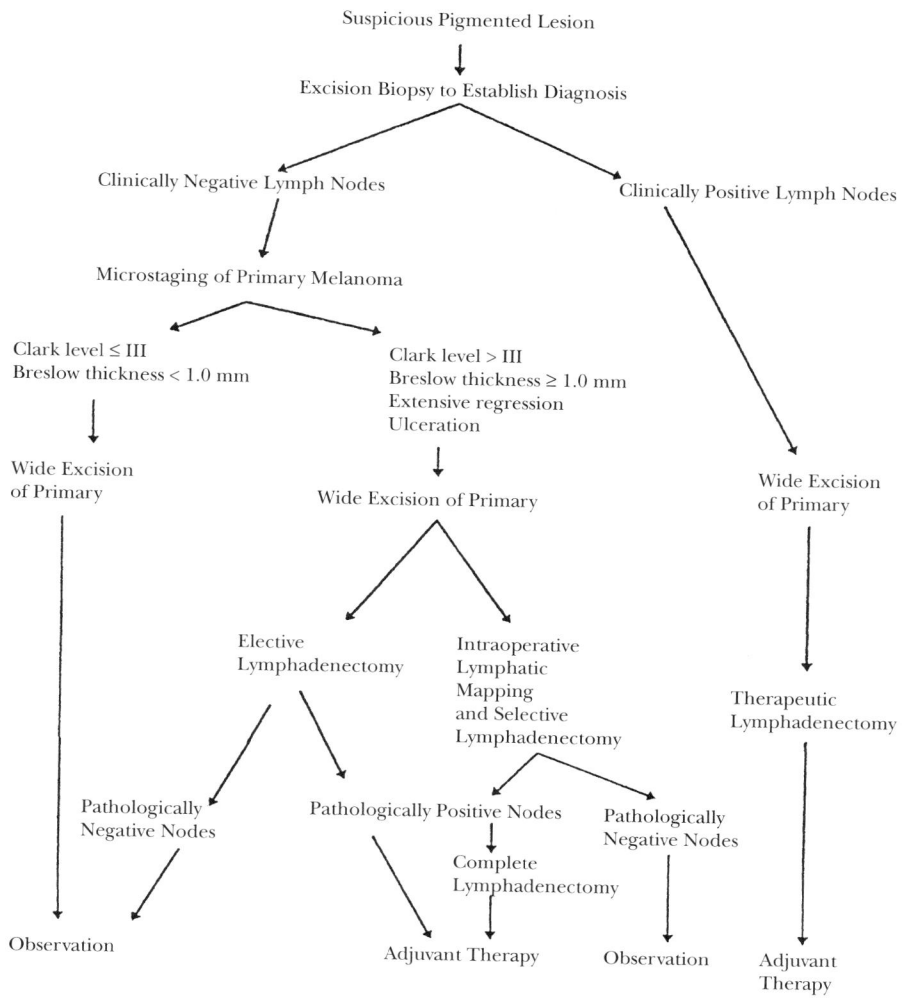

Figure 65-17 Algorithm for the management of primary melanoma. (Adapted with permission from Morton DL, Essner R, Kirkwood JM, et al: Malignant melanoma, in Holland JF, Bast Jr RC, Morton DL, Frei III E, Kufe DW, Weichselbaum RR (eds): *Cancer Medicine*, vol 2 (ed 4). Baltimore, Williams and Wilkins, 1997, pp 2467–2499.)[65]

of local recurrence but are unlikely to influence survival.[89] Amputation of the digit at the interphalangeal joint is necessary for subungual MM and larger lesions may require more proximal amputation.[65] Ear MMs may be successfully excised using a wedge excision of the helix with margins of 2 cm, without ear amputation.[65] Defects can usually be repaired by primary closure although skin flaps may be necessary.

Lymph node dissection. Elective lymph node dissection (ELND) remains a very controversial issue. Its use has been based on the theory that MM metastasizes in a predictable pattern from the primary lesion through the lymphatics to the regional lymph nodes.[66] Theoretically, the removal of regional lymph nodes should eliminate the most likely source of metastasis. However, the majority of patients (80%) with stage I or II MM have lymph nodes that are uninvolved at the time of excision and might be subjected to an unnecessary procedure with potential complications and no benefit.[65,66] Studies are ongoing, but it appears that ELND may have some benefit in patients with stage IA–IIA lesions of intermediate thickness

(0.76–4.0 mm) but little or no benefit for those with stage IA thin MM lesions (less than 0.76 mm, Clark's level II).[65,89] ELND usually does not improve the survival of patients with tumors greater than 4 mm since they have a high incidence of distant as well as local metastases.[89]

Decisions about the therapeutic advantage of ELND may also take other prognostic indicators into consideration. MM of the heels and palms, for example, although often intermediate in size, may be an indication for ELND owing to the aggressive nature of lesions in these anatomic sites.[66] Similarly, ulcerated lesions, superficial spreading MM, and nodular MM in men (and especially older men) may be indicators for the use of ELND.

Therapeutic lymph node dissection (TLND) should be performed when lymph nodes are positive by physical examination or by biopsy.[89] TLND is often more extensive than ELND, involving both superficial and deep nodes. Modified dissections are usually recommended in the neck to preserve cosmesis and function.[89] Infection, flap necrosis, seroma, and nerve dysfunction are all potential side effects of lymphadenectomy. Lymphadema may also occur. With axillary node dissection, lymphadema is limited to the affected arm. Cervical lymphadenectomy has low morbidity. With inguinal node dissection, there is a reported incidence of extremity edema in up to 39% of patients.[88] The majority of these patients exhibit mild lymphadema and up to 10% exhibit debilitating edema.[66]

Lymphatic mapping and selective lymph node dissection.
A technique that identifies patients who would benefit from lymphadenectomy is lymphatic mapping. It is based on the premise that the first or "sentinel" lymph nodes draining a primary MM lesion can be identified and sampled. Decisions about further intervention (removal of all of the nodes) can be made based upon that data.

Lymphoscintography may first be used to identify the draining basin and therefore improve the identification of the sentinel lymph nodes.[88] Extremity lesions usually drain into regional lymph basins in either the axilla or groin.[66] Trunk, head, and neck lesions may flow to more than one lymph node basin. Lymphoscintography involves the injection of radiolabeled substances into the site of the primary MM. Hand-held gamma detectors are used to pick up the tracer and identify the draining nodes.[65,88] This procedure alone cannot indicate the presence or absence of tumor cells in the identified lymph nodes.

Intraoperative identification of the sentinel lymph node can be accomplished by the injection of patent blue-V or isosulfan blue dye, 0.5–1.0 mL, into the primary MM site on either side of the biopsy scar before closure.[88] Injections may be repeated every 20 minutes due to the rapid venous drainage of the dye.[66] An incision is made over the identified lymph node basin draining that area. As the injected blue dye stains the lymphatic channel and then stains the draining lymph nodes, sentinel nodes can be identified. The sentinel node(s) can then be excised and examined by frozen section.[65] If positive, complete lymphadenectomy follows.

Twenty percent of patients with stage I MM are positive for regional lymph node metastasis using this method. They can be treated with lymphadenectomy while the other 80% can be spared the complications of the procedure.[66] The incidence of wound infection, seroma, and necrosis following selective lymph node dissection is less than 5%.

Chemotherapy

Since the 1970s, dacarbazine (DTIC) has been the standard of comparison for all other antineoplastic agents used to treat MM. In patients with soft tissue metastases, overall response rates of 20% have been documented with single agent DTIC.[68,90] Subcutaneous, lymph node, and pulmonary metastases are the most likely to respond to DTIC; however, it has been ineffective against brain metastases. Complete remissions are rare and the duration of response can approach one year. Side effects of DTIC vary with the dose and may include mild hematologic toxicity, nausea and vomiting, photosensitivity, and

liver toxicity. Nitrosoureas, vinca alkaloids, cisplatin, paclitaxel, and docetaxel have also been used in the treatment of MM.

Combination regimens of several different chemotherapies have been the subject of clinical trials, some showing modest improvement over single-agent DTIC. Of particular note is a regimen including DTIC, BCNU, cisplatin, and tamoxifen. Initial response rates with this regimen were as high as 50%.[91] Other investigators have replicated this combination with resulting response rates of 27%–62%.[90,91]

Dose intensification with and without stem cell support is an area of investigation in the treatment of MM. There is some indication of a dose responsive nature of MM with a few chemotherapeutic agents, particularly cisplatin.

When a relatively confined area is the target of treatment, regional rather than systemic administration of chemotherapy may be an avenue of approach. In this manner, systemic side effects can be diminished or avoided and higher concentrations of drugs can be delivered to the tumor site. Liver metastases from MM, for example, may be treated by intrahepatic infusion of chemotherapy with or without chemoembolization. A treatment for intransit metastases of MM in the extremities is regional perfusion, which is usually combined with hyperthermia. Arterial inflow and venous outflow vessels in the targeted area are isolated and cannulated and collateral circulation of the area is interrupted. Venous blood is collected from the cannulated veins and is pumped through an oxygenator, warmed, and pumped back through the cannulated artery. The chemotherapy can be injected into the blood at several points in the system increasing the exposure of the tumor to the chemotherapy. Melphalan is the most commonly used chemotherapy with regional perfusion although other chemotherapies such as nitrogen mustard and cisplatin have also been used. The overall response rate of this therapy is 65% and the overall complete remission rate is 44%.[91] Despite the attempts to contain the chemotherapy to the targeted area, there may be some systemic effect of the drugs as evidenced by the occurrence of severe hypotension in 10% of patients and the experience of a reaction similar to adult respiratory distress syndrome (ARDS) in 16% of patients receiving melphalan.[91]

Hormonal therapy

There appears to be a relationship between estrogen and MM. Incidence, progression, and regression have all been associated with times of peak estrogen activity such as pregnancy.[65] It has been hypothesized that MM may be estrogen-dependent and estrogen receptors have been discovered on some MM tumors. In a tamoxifen-containing, multidrug chemotherapy regimen, initial investigators noted an unusual increase in deep vein thromboses and deleted tamoxifen from the regimen.[91] With the deletion of tamoxifen, however, the response rate decreased from near 50% to 10%. When tamoxifen was added back to the regimen, the response rate increased. The mechanism of action of tamoxifen in multidrug regimens is not completely understood but a hypothesis has been made that tamoxifen may act against chemoresistance of the tumor.

Radiation therapy

Radiation therapy may be of use in the treatment of MM. Although it is rarely chosen as the primary mode of therapy, it may be the treatment of choice for patients who cannot undergo surgery because of physical limitations or for patients whose lesions are not amenable to surgery. Radiation therapy may serve as an adjuvant treatment when combined with surgical resection for patients with lesions at particularly high risk of recurrence, such as those with head and neck lesions.[90] In those cases, radiation therapy would follow surgical excision. Radiation therapy may also be used for palliation of symptoms of metastases such as pain or obstruction.

Immunotherapy

The potential immunoresponsive nature of MM has been suggested by both clinical and histopathologic observations. Clinically, MM is a disease with a highly variable nature. The course of the disease may wax and wane over time.[68] Spontaneous regressions of disseminated disease, although rare, have been documented and regressions in up to 30% of primary MMs have been noted.[68,92] Rarely, and usually in association with bacterial infections, spontaneous regressions have occurred in distant metastatic sites.[68] In addition, there is evidence of increased incidence of MM in immuncompromised individuals. These observations all point to a host immune response on MM. Lymphoid infiltrates are regularly found on histopathologic examination of MM specimens, suggesting an activated host response directly at the tumor site.[68]

Immunotherapy is an active area of research in the treatment of MM. Several agents, alone or in combination, have been examined. In many cases, these agents are used in combined modality regimens with chemotherapy. The two areas of most promise are the use of immunotherapy as adjuvant treatment for high-risk patients with surgical resection and for treatment of patients with metastatic disease. In either case, it is most effective as a treatment for patients with small tumor burden.[92]

Immunotherapy of MM may be broadly classified as either specific or nonspecific.[92] Specific immunotherapy agents target the tumor selectively. Monoclonal antibody therapy is an example. Nonspecific immunotherapy agents, e.g., interferon, are used to stimulate the immune system as a whole.

Interferon. Trials of alfa-inteferon (IFN) as a treatment for MM began in the late 1970s. It is thought to have both direct effects on malignant cells and to indirectly affect them by augmenting and stimulating the host immune response.[93] IFN has been found to have synergistic activity with several chemotherapy agents and with other immunotherapy agents. It may be administered by subcutaneous, intravenous, and intralesional routes. The presence of visceral disease is a predictor of poor outcome because of larger tumor burden. Central nervous system (CNS) disease is not well treated with IFN because of poor penetration of IFN into the CNS.[93]

One of the most exciting treatment advances for MM occurred with trials of IFN for patients with resected stage IIB or III disease. A study by the Eastern Cooperative Oncology Group (ECOG) was the pivotal trial introducing this strategy. In this study, intensive intravenous IFN (20 MU/m[2]/day) was administered to patients for one month followed by subcutaneous IFN (10 MU/m[2] three times per week) for 11 months. There was considerable toxicity experienced with this regimen. Fifty percent of subjects required dose adjustments in the first month and more than 50% during the final 11 months.[94] However, a significant increase in relapse-free survival was demonstrated and there was a trend toward increased overall survival.[94]

Interleukin-2. Interleukin-2 (IL-2) causes the stimulation of several aspects of the immune system. It is another example of a nonspecific immunotherapy treatment for MM. In clinical trials, IL-2 has been given alone and in combination with lymphokine-activated killer cells (LAK) and with tumor infiltrating lymphocytes (TIL). It is thought to have some synergistic activity when given in combination with IFN and it is part of many chemotherapy and hormonal therapy combination regimens for MM.

Clinical trials of IL-2 have employed different dosage ranges and administration routes. High-dose therapy (up to 720,000 IU/kg) given by intravenous bolus has resulted in a range of response rates from 5%–22%.[95] In a pivotal study of high-dose IL-2, significant, life-threatening toxicities were observed, including sepsis, respiratory distress, and hypotension, and necessitated intensive monitoring during administration.[95,96] IL-2 by continuous infusion is more toxic and therefore regimens employing this administration method must use lower doses. In this manner, life-threatening toxicities from the therapy have been decreased but response rates have also been lower in some trials.[95]

Bacille Calmette-Guérin. Bacille Calmette-Guérin (BCG) is a nonspecific immunotherapy agent used to treat MM. It may be administered intralesionally or as an epilesional scarification. When administered intralesionally, a 26-gauge needle is used and the BCG is directly injected into the site of disease. Complete saturation of the tumor is attempted.[94] Epilesional scarification is done by scratching the skin over the tumor nodules into a 5-cm square grid. BCG droplets are placed onto the grid, dried, and covered for 24 hours.[97]

The action of BCG in the lesion is hypothesized to be twofold. Its presence in the tissue causes a local inflammatory response at the site. The process of this local inflammation is thought to be the primary mechanism of destruction of tumor cells.[97] Its presence in the tissue also causes an immune response including cytokine production and lymphocyte activation that causes further destruction of the tumor.[97]

Injection of lesions is easily accomplished on the skin surfaces and can actually be done to any epithelial surface accessible by instrumentaton (e.g., bronchus, bladder, etc.). Injection into MM lesions has resulted in regression of other sites of disease, both regional and distant.[97] This may be the result of activation of the systemic immune response or, if the regression is in areas of lymphatic drainage of the BCG from the injected lesion, it may be a direct response to the BCG.

Prior to therapy, patients are skin tested with other microbial antigens such as mumps, Candida, and streptokinase.[97] Patients who show a delayed hypersensitivity reaction to those antigens are more likely to respond to BCG. This skin testing serves as a measure of immune competence. Also prior to treatment, purified protein derivative (PPD) skin tests are administered to assess the patient's prior sensitization to mycobacterial antigens. Patients who are PPD positive are at risk for acute and life-threatening hypersensitivity reactions following BCG administration. Doses of BCG are varied based on the patient's PPD status, the patient's immunocompetence, and the strain of BCG used.

Side effects of BCG administration include local reactions, systemic reactions, and long-term effects on organs. Local reactions include necrosis and ulceration, which may occur within seven to fourteen days. Healing may take eight to ten weeks. Acute systemic reactions include fevers and flu-like symptoms. Hypersensitivity reactions are possible and the risk increases with subsequent injections. BCG are living bacillus organisms and may, therefore, cause bacteremia. Long-term toxicities include the development of granulomas in the visceral organs, especially the lung.[97]

Monoclonal antibodies.   Several antigens on the surface of MM cells have been identified. These include melanotransferrin, GD3, GD2, and MM chondroitin sulfate (mCSP).[98] Monoclonal antibodies can be developed for those antigens and, when used to treat MM, cause a direct antigen/antibody cytotoxicity or complement-mediated cytotoxicity.

Monoclonal antibodies can be given systemically, intralesionally, and intravascularly during isolated limb perfusion, and intrathecally.[98] They are commonly conjugated with chemotherapy, toxins, or radionucleides to increase their cytotoxicity.

Vaccines.   MM vaccines are a form of specific active immunotherapy. Vaccines are manufactured using a variety of techniques and may contain autologous antigens (from the patient's own tumor). More commonly, allogeneic preparations of antigens derived from multiple MM cell lines are used. In either case, the vaccine is administered to the patient to stimulate the immune system to actively seek out and destroy the MM cells.

MM vaccines may inhibit metastasis and are most effective for patients who have had complete resections of all sites of disease.[68] In patients with unresected MM sites, best results are seen if metastases are less than 2 cm in diameter.[68] In those patients, slowed tumor growth is a more common result.[68]

Time to response with vaccines is very different than experience with chemotherapy. Vaccines are weak antigens and have no direct cytotoxicity, and patients must be repeatedly immunized for prolonged periods. Since they work by stimulating an immune response, they may require six to eight months to induce a remission.[68] After initial immunization, the disease may actually progress for four to eight weeks before tumor effects occur.[97] Patients who exhibit stimulation of humoral and cell-mediated responses are more likely to have a response to vaccine therapy.[97] Positive responses to vaccines are usually durable over months to years.[97]

Because vaccines are weak antigens, they may be given in combination with immune adjuvants to boost the immune response. There are several types of immune adjuvants, including microorganisms (*Corynebacterium parvum*, BCG); subcellular microbial products and fractions (detoxified endotoxin or DETOX); haptens; immunogenic proteins; immunomodulators (Levamisole, interleukins); IFN; thymic hormones; and colony stimulating factors (GM-CSF, G-CSF).[99]

Vaccines have a very low toxicity profile. When combined with immune adjuvants, the toxicity profile may be more intense depending on the specific adjuvant employed.

Continuity of Care: Nursing Challenges

Skin cancer is a unique area of oncology practice in that a great number of subspecialty disciplines are often involved. These may include prevention and detection specialists as well as surgical, medical, and radiation oncologists. In addition, treatment of these cancers may also involve the services of other specialists such as geneticists, dermatopathologists, vascular surgeons, and immunologists. Oncology nurses often assume the responsibility of communicating to the patient what the role of each of these specialists is in the patient's care and providing clarification about treatment. Communication and documentation between these disciplines is vital to ensure a positive outcome for the patient.

Follow-up After Screening Examinations

Follow-up after screening examinations is important, regardless of whether the screen was positive. Follow-up includes written communication to the patient and primary care provider(s) about the outcome of the screening and primary prevention recommendations. This includes information about the interval when screening should be repeated.

Those patients who have a hereditary predisposition to developing MM may benefit from in-depth education about the physiology of the skin, genetic transmission, and the benefits of employing more sophisticated screening techniques such as medical photography. Information about the benefits and limitations of genetic testing should be presented. Such information should also be communicated with primary care providers. Information about primary prevention strategies and chemoprevention should also be provided when available. Written reminders for follow-up screening examinations at more frequent intervals may be helpful in motivating the patient to follow up with screening. Patients from these families often need reassurance. They need to understand that primary prevention efforts may prevent or delay the onset of the malignancy and regular, thoughtful screening may result in the detection of lesions at an earlier stage, when treatment is most effective.

Follow-up Care After Treatment

The risk of developing a second BCC after resection is estimated to be 45%.[78] Clearly patients with NMSC need to have life-long screening for development of second primary malignancies. These patients need to be reassured that with early detection a second primary malignancy is also curable, and that primary prevention efforts may be effective in preventing or delaying the development of a second NMSC.

The risk of recurrence of MM is a function of tumor thickness and other prognostic factors. A second primary MM is estimated to occur in about 5% of persons who have already been diagnosed with MM.[6] These patients need to understand the importance of and rationale for life-long follow-up for both recurrence and a second primary malignancy. If this follow-up is to be provided by a primary care physician, specific instructions need to be given to both the patient and physician that outline the interval and specific tests to completed.

Psychosocial Care

Although NMSC are relatively common, little has been written about the psychological impact of its diagnosis and treatment.[100] Some patients delay treatments because they have a misconception that all cancer is uniformly fatal, despite the excellent prognosis for nonmetastatic NMSC. The NMSC often requires wide surgical excisions that are potentially disfiguring to obtain a good long-term prognosis. Careful psychological preparation may be necessary to help a patient accept such a treatment and postoperative follow-up should consider assessment of adjustment, self-esteem, and socialization. If this assessment indicates difficulties with adjustment, referral to a mental health professional may be indicated.

Patients diagnosed with MM may face similar problems with disfiguring surgery. Often these patients also face issues related to undergoing extensive cytotoxic therapy, anxiety related to long-term follow-up and fears of recurrence, and ultimately concerns related to having a potentially fatal disease. Continuous assessment of these concerns is indicated and, again, in some cases referral to a mental health professional may be helpful to improve quality of life for these patients.

Another area of psychological care for patients diagnosed with MM relates to fear of genetic susceptibility in relatives and particularly children. Education about primary and secondary prevention strategies and correction of misconceptions can be an effective intervention. Referral to a mental health professional with expertise in genetics and related counseling may help patients to better cope with these fears.

Conclusion

There is much to be learned about skin cancer. As its incidence increases at an alarming rate, there is much work to be done in the areas of public education and awareness of prevention. Because the skin is an organ which is visible, these malignancies lend themselves to early detection. Programs staffed by qualified practitioners could be an important means of reducing the morbidity and mortality associated with both NMSC and MM. Treatment of early lesions is relatively straightforward and usually effective, but further research is needed to improve the outcomes of recurrence and second primaries. Especially in the case of MM, treatment is often unsuccessful and new therapies are needed. Genetics represent a promising area of research and there is much to be learned about both the genetic predisposition for these cancers and the use of gene therapy as a targeted treatment for them.

References

1. American Cancer Society: *Cancer Facts and Figures—1999.* Atlanta, American Cancer Society, 1999
2. Rhodes AR: Public education and cancer of the skin. What do people need to know about melanoma and nonmelanoma skin cancer? *Cancer* 75:613–636, 1995
3. Marks R: An overview of skin cancers, incidence and causation. *Cancer* 75:607–612, 1995
4. Rigel DS: Malignant melanoma: perspectives on incidence and its effects on awareness, diagnosis, and treatment. *CA Cancer J Clin* 46:195–198, 1996
5. Ries LAG, Kosary CL, Hankey BF, et al: *SEER Cancer Statistics Review, 1973–1995.* Bethesda, MD, National Cancer Institute, 1998

6. Rigel DS: Malignant melanoma: incidence issues and their effect on diagnosis and treatment in the 1990s. *Mayo Clin Proc* 72:367–371, 1997

7. Naylor MR, Farmer KC: The case for sunscreens: a review of their use in preventing actinic damage and neoplasia. *Arch Dermatol* 133:1146–1154, 1997

8. Marks R: Prevention and control of melanoma: the public health approach. *CA Cancer J Clin* 46:199–216, 1996

9. Hill L, Ferrini RL: Skin cancer prevention and screening: summary of the American College of Preventive Medicine's Practice Policy Statements. *CA Cancer J Clin* 48:232–235, 1998

10. Goldsmith LA, Koh HK, Bewerse BA, et al: Full proceedings from the National Conference to Develop a National Skin Cancer Agenda. American Academy of Dermatology and Centers for Disease Control and Prevention, Washington DC, April 8–10, 1995. *J Am Acad Dermatol* 35:748–756, 1996

11. Halder RM, Bridgeman-Shah S: Skin cancer in African Americans. *Cancer* 75:667–673, 1995

12. Luther H, Altmeyer P, Garbe C, Ellwanger U, et al: Increase of melanocytic nevus counts in children during 5 years of follow-up and analysis of associated factors. *Arch Dermatol* 132:1473–1478, 1996

13. Swetter SM: Malignant melanoma from the dermatologic perspective. *Surg Clin North Am* 76:1287–1298, 1996

14. Williams ML, Sagebiel RW: Melanoma risk factors and atypical moles. *West J Med* 160:343–350, 1994

15. Marghoob AA, Schoenbach SP, Kopf AW, et al: Large congenital melanocytic nevi and the risk for the development of malignant melanoma. *Arch Dermatol* 132:170–175, 1996

16. Council on Scientific Affairs: Harmful effects of ultraviolet radiation. *JAMA* 262:380–384, 1989

17. Haluska FG, Hodi S: Molecular genetics of familial cutaneous melanoma. *J Clin Oncol* 16:670–682, 1998

18. Grange F, Chompret A, Guilloud-Bataille M, et al: Comparison between familial and nonfamilial melanoma in France. *Arch Dermatol* 131:1154–1159, 1995

19. Bishop JA, Bataille V, Pinney E, et al: Family studies in melanoma: identification of the atypical mole syndrome (AMS) phenotype. *Melanoma Res* 4:199–206, 1994

20. Goldstein AM, Tucker MA: Genetic epidemiology of familial melanoma. *Dermatol Clin* 13:605–612, 1995

21. Lucchina LC, Barnhill RL, Duke DM, et al: Familial cutaneous melanoma. *Melanoma Res* 5:413–418, 1995

22. Cannon-Albright LA, Kamb A, Skolnick M: A review of inherited predisposition to melanoma. *Semin Oncol* 23:667–672, 1996

23. Easton D: The role of atypical mole syndrome and cutaneous naevi in the development of melanoma. *Cancer Surveys* 26:237–249, 1996

24. Greene MH: Genetics of cutaneous melanoma and nevi. *Mayo Clin Proc* 72:467–474, 1997

25. Meyer LJ, Zone JH: Genetics of cutaneous melanoma. *J Invest Dermatol* 103:112S–116S, 1994 (suppl)

26. Marghoob A, Slade J, Salopek TG, et al: Basal cell and squamous cell carcinomas are important risk factors for cutaneous malignant melanoma screening implications. *Cancer* 75:704–714, 1995

27. Liu T, Soong S: Epidemiology of malignant melanoma. *Surg Clin North Am* 76:1205–1222, 1996

28. Elwood JM: Malignant melanoma and sun exposure. *Semin Oncol* 23:650–666, 1996

29. National Institutes of Health: Sunlight, ultraviolet radiation, and the skin. *NIH Consensus Statement* 7(8):1–29, 1989.

30. Kaminester LH: Photoprotection. *Arch Fam Med* 5:289–295, 1996

31. Pion IA, Rigel DS, Garfinkel L, et al: Occupation and the risk of malignant melanoma. *Cancer* 75:637–644, 1995

32. Gallagher RP, Hill GB, Bajdik CD, et al: Sunlight exposure, pigmentation factors, and risk of nonmelanocytic skin cancer. I. Squamous cell carcinoma. *Arch Dermatol* 131:164–169, 1995

33. Gallagher RP, Hill GB, Bajdik CD, et al: Sunlight exposure, pigmentary factors, and risk of nonmelanocytic skin cancer. I. Basal cell carcinoma. *Arch Dermatol* 131:157–163, 1995

34. Katsambas A, Nicolaidou E: Cutaneous malignant melanoma and sun exposure. *Arch Dermatol* 132:444–450, 1996

35. Shenefelt PD: Skin cancer prevention and screening. *Primary Care* 19:557–574, 1992

36. Stewart DS: Indoor tanning: the nurse's role in preventing skin damage. *Cancer Nurs* 10:100–106, 1987

37. Farmer KC, Naylor MF: Sun exposure, sunscreens, and skin cancer prevention: a year-round concern. *Ann Pharmacother* 30:662–673, 1996

38. Pathak MA: Sunscreens: progress and perspectives on photoprotection of human skin against UVB and UVA radiation. *J Dermatol* 23:783–800, 1996

39. Department of Health and Human Services: *Medications that Increase Sensitivity to Light.* Bethesda, MD, DHHS, Pub. No. 292-810 (40270), 1990

40. DeLeo VA: *Photosensitivity Diseases.* Tokyo, Igaku-Shoin, 1992

41. Rossi JS, Blais LM, Redding CA, et al: Preventing skin cancer through behavior change. Implications for interventions. *Dermatol Clin* 13:613–622, 1995

42. Boutwell WB: The Under Cover Skin Cancer Prevention Project. *Cancer* 75:657–660, 1995

43. Loescher LJ, Buller MK, Buller DB, et al: Public education projects in skin cancer. *Cancer* 75:651–656, 1995

44. Loescher LJ, Emerson J, Taylor A, et al: Educating preschoolers about sun safety. *Am J Public Health* 85:939–943, 1995

45. Buller DB, Buller MK, Beach B, et al: Sunny days, healthy ways: evaluation of a skin cancer prevention curriculum for elementary school-aged children. *J Am Acad Dermatol* 35:911–922, 1996

46. Rodrigue JR: Promoting healthier behaviors, attitudes, and beliefs toward sun exposure in parents of young children. *J Consult Clin Psychol* 64:1431–1436, 1996

47. Naylor MF, Boyd A, Smith DW, et al: High sun protection factor sunscreens in the suppression of actinic neoplasia. *Arch Dermatol* 131:170–175, 1995

48. Fitzpatrick TB: The skin cancer cascade: from ozone depletion to melanoma—some definitions and some new interpretation, 1996. *J Dermatol* 23:816–820, 1996

49. Stern RS: Sunscreens for cancer prevention. *Arch Dermatol* 131:220–221, 1995

50. Loesch H: Pitfalls in sunscreen application. *Arch Dermatol* 130:665–666, 1994

51. Koh HK, Geller AC, Miller DR, et al: Prevention and early detection strategies for melanoma and skin cancer. Current status. *Arch Dermatol* 312:436–443, 1996

52. Centers for Disease Control: Media dissemination of and public response to the Ultraviolet Index—United States, 1994–1995. *MMWR Morb Mortal Wkly Rep* 46:370–373, 1997

53. Fenderman DG, Concato J, Caralis PV, et al: Screening for skin cancer in primary care settings. *Arch Dermatol* 133:1423–1425, 1997

54. Weinstock MA, Goldstein MG, Dube CE, et al: Basic skin

cancer triage for teaching melanoma detection. *J Am Acad Dermatol* 34:1063–1066, 1996

55. Grin CM, Kopf AW, Welkovich B, et al: Accuracy in the clinical diagnosis of malignant melanoma. *Arch Dermatol* 126:763–766, 1990

56. Wender RC: Barriers to effective skin cancer detection. *Cancer* 75:691–698, 1995

57. De Rooij MJM, Rampen FHJ, Schouten LJ, et al: Volunteer melanoma screenings. Follow-up, compliance, and outcome. *Dermatol Surg* 23:197–201, 1997

58. Healsmith MF, Bourke JF, Osborne JE, et al: An evaluation of the revised seven-point checklist for the early diagnosis of cutaneous malignant melanoma. *Br J Dermatol* 130: 48–50, 1994

59. Holbrook KA, Wolff K: The structure and development of skin, in Fitzpatrick TB, Eisen AZ, Wolff K, Freedberg IM, Austen KF (eds): *Dermatology in General Medicine*, vol 1 (ed 4). New York, McGraw-Hill, 1993, pp 97–145

60. Mosher DB, Fitzpatrick TB, Hori Y, et al: Disorders of pigmentation, in Fitzpatrick TB, Eisen AZ, Wolff K, Freedberg IM, Austen KF (eds): *Dermatology in General Medicine*, vol 1 (ed 4). New York, McGraw-Hill, 1993, pp 903–995

61. Vargo NL: Basal and squamous cell carcinomas: an overview. *Semin Oncol Nurs* 7:13–25, 1991

62. Carter DM, Lin AN: Basal cell carcinoma, in Fitzpatrick TB, Eisen AZ, Wolff K, Freedberg IM, Austen KF (eds): *Dermatology in General Medicine*, vol 1 (ed 4). New York, McGraw-Hill, 1993, pp 840–847

63. Schwartz RA, Stoll Jr HL: Squamous cell carcinoma, in Fitzpatrick TB, Eisen AZ, Wolff K, Freedberg IM, Austen KF (eds): *Dermatology in General Medicine*, vol 1 (ed 4). New York, McGraw-Hill, 1993, pp 821–839

64. Walsh DS: Molecular genetics of skin cancer. *Adv Dermatol* 13:167–204, 1997

65. Morton DL, Essner R, Kirkwood JM, et al: Malignant melanoma, in Holland JF, Bast Jr RC, Morton DL, Frei III E, Kufe DW, Weichselbaum RR (eds): *Cancer Medicine*, vol 2 (ed 4). Baltimore, Williams and Wilkins, 1997, pp 2467–2499

66. Morton DL, Essner R: Skin cancers: melanoma, in Harvey JC, Beattie EJ (eds): *Cancer Surgery*. Philadelphia, Saunders, 1996, pp 505–521

67. Barnhill RL, Mihm MC, Fitzpatrick TB, et al: Neoplasms: malignant melanoma, in Fitzpatrick TB, Eisen AZ, Wolff K, Freedberg IM, Austen KF (eds): *Dermatology in General Medicine*, vol 1 (ed 4). New York, McGraw-Hill, 1993, pp 1078–1115

68. Morton DL, Barth A: Vaccine therapy for malignant melanoma. *CA Cancer J Clin* 46:225–244, 1996

69. Du Vivier A: *Atlas of Skin Cancer*. New York, Gower, 1991

70. Sober AJ, Burstein JM: Precursors to skin cancer. *Cancer* 75:645–650, 1995

71. Tong AKF, Fitzpatrick TB: Neoplasms of the skin, in Holland JF, Bast Jr RC, Morton DL, Frei III E, Kufe DW, Weichselbaum RR (eds): *Cancer Medicine*, vol 2 (ed 4). Baltimore, Williams and Wilkins, 1997, pp 2433–2464

72. McCormack CJ, Kelly JW, Dorevitch AP: Differences in age and body site distribution of the histological subtypes of basal cell carcinoma. A possible indicator of differing causes. *Arch Dermatol* 133:593–596, 1997

73. Kopf AW, Salopek TG, Slade J, et al: Techniques of cutaneous examination for the detection of skin cancer. *Cancer* 75:684–690, 1995

74. Argenyi ZB: Dermoscopy (epiluminescence microscopy) of pigmented skin lesion. Current status and evolving trends. *Dermatol Clin* 15:79–95, 1997

75. Sober AJ: Digital epiluminescence microscopy in the evaluation of pigmented lesions: evaluation of pigmented lesions: a brief review. *Semin Surg Oncol* 9:198–201, 1993

76. Robinson JK, Arndt KA, LeBoit PE, Wintroub BU: *Atlas of Cutaneous Surgery*. Philadelphia, Saunders, 1996

77. Lawler PE: Cutaneous malignant melanoma. *Semin Oncol Nurs* 7:26–35, 1991

78. Marghoob A, Kopf AW, Bart RS, et al: Risk of another basal cell carcinoma developing after treatment of a basal cell carcinoma. *J Am Acad Dermatol* 28:22–28, 1993

79. Ahmed I: Malignant melanoma: prognostic indicators. *Mayo Clin Proc* 72:356–361, 1997

80. Fleming ID, Cooper JS, Henson DE, et al (eds): *AJCC Cancer Staging Manual* (ed 5). Philadelphia, Lippincott-Raven, 1997

81. Otto SE: *Oncology Nursing* (ed 3). St. Louis, Mosby, 1997

82. Harris MN, Shapiro RL, Rosea DF: Malignant melanoma. Primary surgical management (excision and node dissection) based on pathology and staging. *Cancer* 75:715–725, 1995

83. Fleming ID, Amonette R, Monaghan T, et al: Principles of management of basal and squamous cell carcinoma of the skin. *Cancer* 75:699–704, 1995

84. Ratner D, Grande DJ: Mohs' micrographic surgery: an overview. *Dermatol Nurs* 6:269–273, 1994

85. Motley RJ: The technique of micrographic surgery for excising skin tumours. *J Wound Care* 4:380–382, 1995

86. Shupack JL, Stiller MJ, Webster GF: Cytotoxic agents and dermatologic therapy, in Fitzpatrick TB, Eisen AZ, Wolff K, Freedberg IM, Austen KF (eds): *Dermatology in General Medicine*, vol 2 (ed 4). New York, McGraw-Hill, 1993, pp 2872–2883

87. Peck GL, DiGiovanna JJ: Retinoids, in Fitzpatrick TB, Eisen AZ, Wolff K, Freedberg IM, Austen KF (eds): *Dermatology in General Medicine*, vol 1 (ed 4). New York, McGraw-Hill, 1993, pp 2883–2908

88. Karakousis CP: Surgical treatment of malignant melanoma. *Surg Clin North Am* 76:1299–1312, 1996

89. Urist MM. Surgical management of primary cutaneous melanoma. *CA Cancer J Clin* 46:217–224, 1996

90. Ho RCS: Medical management of stage IV malignant melanoma. *Cancer* 75:735–741, 1995

91. Nathan FE, Berd D, Mastrangelo MJ: Chemotherapy of melanoma, in Perry M (ed): *The Chemotherapy Source Book* (ed 2). Baltimore, Williams and Wilkins, 1996, pp 1043–1069

92. Oratz R, Bystryn JC: Immunotherapy of malignant melanoma. *Dermatol Clin* 9:669–682, 1991

93. Kirkwood JM: Melanoma, in DeVita VT, Hellman S, Rosenberg SA (eds): *Biologic Therapy of Cancer* (ed 2). Philadelphia, Lippincott, 1995, pp 388–406

94. Kirkwood JM, Strawdrman MH, Ernstoff MS, et al: Interferon alfa-2b adjuvant therapy of high-risk resected cutaneous melanoma: the Eastern Cooperative Oncology Group Trial EST 1684. *J Clin Oncol* 14:7–17, 1996

95. Marincola FM, Rosenberg SA: Melanoma, in DeVita VT, Hellman S, Rosenberg SA (eds): *Biologic Therapy of Cancer* (ed 2). Philadelphia, Lippincott, 1995, pp 250–260

96. Rosenberg SA, Yang JC, Topalian SL, et al: Treatment of 283 consecutive patients with metastatic melanoma or renal cell cancer using high-dose bolus interleukin 2. *JAMA* 271:907–913, 1994

97. Morton DL, Barth A: Intralesional therapy, in DeVita VT,

Hellman S, Rosenberg SA (eds): *Biologic Therapy of Cancer* (ed 2). Philadelphia, Lippincott, 1995, pp 691–704

98. Houghton AN, Chapman PB: Melanoma, in DeVita VT, Hellman S, Rosenberg SA (eds): *Biologic Therapy of Cancer* (ed 2). Philadelphia, Lippincott, 1995, pp 576–586

99. Akporiaye ET, Hersh EM: Immune adjuvants, in DeVita

VT, Hellman S, Rosenberg SA (eds): *Biologic Therapy of Cancer* (ed 2). Philadelphia, Lippincott, 1995, pp 635–646

100. Holland JC: Skin cancer and melanoma, in Holland JC, Rowland JH (eds): *Handbook of Psychooncology, Psychological Care of the Patient With Cancer.* New York, Oxford University Press, 1989, pp 246–249

CHAPTER 66

Stomach Cancer

Katherine G. O'Connor RN, MS, ANP

Scope of the Problem

Gastric cancer is a significant health problem worldwide. The high mortality associated with this malignancy is due to the late stage of disease on presentation and the lack of effective adjuvant therapies.[1] Although diagnostic techniques and surgical treatments have improved the detection of gastric cancer, the mortality remains high. Early gastric cancer without lymph node metastasis is highly curable, whereas advanced-stage gastric cancer is associated with a poor prognosis.[2]

Epidemiology

There has been a continuing decline in the incidence and death rate from gastric cancer in the United States over the past 50 years.[3] Presently, an estimated 13,500 people die annually from gastric cancer in the United States, which translates to approximately six deaths per 100,000 cases.[4] In the United States, gastric cancer is the thirteenth most prevalent malignancy and ranks eighth as the most common cause of cancer-related deaths.[4] Worldwide, gastric cancer is the second most common cause of cancer-related deaths, surpassed only by the great increase in lung cancer during the 1970s.[5] While there has been a decrease in the incidence of distal gastric cancer, proximal gastric cancer incidence has increased and carries a poor prognosis despite surgical resection.[6,7] Gastric cancer ranks in the top five causes of cancer-related deaths for U.S. minority populations.[8]

The incidence of gastric cancer is highest in Japan, Chile, and Costa Rica.[5,9] Nordic countries, such as Scandinavia, have shown an increased prevalence in recent decades, with an incidence rate two to three times that found in the United States. With the highest incidence rates of gastric cancer in Japan, officials have implemented aggressive screening programs that have led to earlier diagnosis, improved surgical outcomes, and increased survival. Males have a greater incidence of gastric cancer than females; no country shows a greater incidence of women over men developing this disease.[5] Black Americans, Native Americans, and Hispanics are twice as likely to develop gastric cancer than whites in the United States.[9] The average age of onset is during the fifth to seventh decade of life.

Etiology

Several conditions are strongly linked with the development of gastric cancer, including dietary intake, infection with *Helicobacter pylori*, socioeconomic class, and prior gastric resection for benign peptic ulcer disease. Other factors associated with an increased risk of gastric cancer include patients with blood group A, those with a history of pernicious anemia which is associated with achlorhydria, and those with atrophic gastritis. Cigarette smoking in combination with alcohol intake also has been proven to place one at a higher risk for adenocarcinoma of the cardia.[5,10]

Dietary intake has been one of the most widely studied risk factors for the development of gastric cancer. N-nitroso-compounds found in smoked, pickled, preserved, and cured foods all have been implicated as contributing links to the development of this disease.[5,8–11] Salts contain caustic properties that may cause chronic atrophic gastritis, and hypertonic salts may cause delayed gastric emptying. Dietary salts facilitate the conversion of nitrates to carcinogenic nitrosamines in the stomach. With delayed emptying of gastric contents, there is a greater exposure time of the stomach to the nitrosamine compounds, possibly contributing to the development of cancer.[12] Conversely, diets high in vitamins A and C, fresh fruits, and vegetables are associated with a lower incidence of gastric cancer. Ascorbic acid and beta carotene function as antioxidants and nitrate neutralizers, decreasing the stomach's susceptibility to *H. pylori* gastritis.[5,13]

Low socioeconomic class has been reported to be a risk factor in the development of gastric cancer, but no specific link has been identified. Researchers suggest that this is related to dietary factors and environmental issues associated with poor housing conditions, including overcrowding and unsanitary settings, which may facilitate the transmission of *H. pylori* infection.[14] Advances in refrigeration and freezing techniques have replaced salting and smoking as primary methods of food preservation and this has contributed to the decline in the incidence of gastric cancer.[10]

In recent years there has been a strong correlation between the development of distal stomach cancers and individuals who are infected with *H. pylori*, especially in China.[5] It is estimated that up to one-third of the U.S. population is infected with this *H. pylori* organism, which is more commonly transmitted in childhood years.[14] *H. pylori* is a spiral-shaped, gram-negative bacillus that has been found to inhabit the gastric tissue between the mucous layer and the underlying epithelium. It is known to cause atrophic gastritis and intestinal metaplasia followed by chronic gastritis, which is an early inflammatory process precursor to gastric cancer.[5,12–15]

Initially, when the *H. pylori* organism enters the stomach, acute inflammatory changes and mild to moderate dyspepsia occur over a time period of days to weeks. This inflammatory reaction gradually converts to a chronic reaction with the presence of neutrophils, eosinophils, monocytes, and lymphocytes, with the ultimate development of lymphoid follicles. After 10 to 15 years, atrophic gastritis occurs involving the mucosa of the antrum, initially but then gradually developing throughout the entire gastric mucosa.[14]

The eradication of *H. pylori* with an intensive antibiotic regimen is necessary in patients with gastric or duodenal ulcers since elimination of the bacteria prevents recurrent ulcer disease. In addition to having a strong association with the development of adenocarcinoma, infection with *H. pylori* has been implicated in the development of regional low-grade gastric mucosa-associated lymphoid tissue (MALT) lymphoma. The *H. pylori* infection has been observed in a large number of the MALT lymphomas, and more than half of the local nonbulky tumors will demonstrate complete histologic regression after eradication of the organism.[13]

Chronic peptic ulcers not related to infection with the *H. pylori* bacteria have a small incidence of developing into a gastric tumor. However, patients who have undergone past gastric resection for benign peptic ulcers have an increased incidence of gastric remnant carcinoma, which is defined as a cancer that arises in the remaining gastric tissues five or more years after resection for benign peptic ulcer disease.[16] The development of this malignancy may be due to the absence of normal gastric acid secretions, which permits the proliferation of bacteria, inflammatory reaction, and chronic atrophic gastritis reaction known to be a precursor for the development of adenocarcinoma. Other theories propose that gastric remnant carcinoma may be the result of duodenogastric reflux[16] or Epstein-Barr virus.[5,12,17,18] Careful screening of patients with known past gastric resection with endoscopy and biopsy may detect early carcinogenic changes, thus allowing for curative surgical resection.[16,17]

Prevention, Screening, and Early Detection

In high incidence areas such as Japan, mass screening programs for gastric cancer have successfully increased survival rates. Screening tests usually include the upper gastrointestinal series and endoscopy, which has a 90% sensitivity and specificity. Regular screening with endoscopy has been recommended to patients who have undergone gastric resection for benign peptic ulcer disease to detect early carcinogenic changes.[16,17]

Since the early symptoms of gastric cancer are vague, it is not unusual for misdiagnosis or a delay in treatment to occur. Although the incidence of gastric cancer is decreasing, aggressive preventive health care in high-risk populations is essential to maintain the decreasing incidence and mortality.

Pathophysiology

Cellular Characteristics

Approximately 95% of all gastric cancers are adenocarcinomas.[11] The remaining 5% are comprised of leiomyosarcomas, lymphomas, carcinoid tumors, squamous cell carcinomas, or other rare cancers.[8,9,19] It is essential to distinguish between gastric lymphomas and gastric adenocarcinomas because the staging, treatment plan, and prognosis will differ depending on the specific tumor pathology. Those diagnosed as adenocarcinomas are divided further into four subcategories: papillary, tubular, mucinous, and signet-ring cell carcinomas.

Historically, the majority of gastric cancers were located in the antrum. However, over the past three decades there has been an increase in the incidence of tumors found in the cardia or upper third of the stomach.[8] Approximately 10% of tumors involve the entire stomach, aggressively spreading through the submucosal layers, producing a nondistendible rigid organ. This is referred to as "linnitis plastica" and is usually a metastatic disease that carries a very poor prognosis.[8]

The most widely used histologic classification system for gastric tumors is the Lauren system, which recognizes two distinct histologic types: intestinal and diffuse. The intestinal histologic type is more commonly found in underdeveloped countries, occurs in men more frequently than women, presents in the older population, and is usually detected in the distal stomach (antrum and lesser curvature). *H. pylori* infection is associated with the intestinal histologic type.[13] The diffuse histologic type is characterized by poorly differentiated cells, lack of organized gland formation, and is composed of signet-ring cells. Diffuse histologic type tumors usually have extensive submucosal spread and early metastasis with a more aggressive clinical course. The incidence is equal among men and women, and diffuse histologic type usually occurs at a younger age than the intestinal type.[12]

Medical reports from Japan, where mass screening programs are in place for diagnosing early gastric cancers, describe the pathology of the stomach tumors that are confined to the mucosa. These tumors are small, discrete, single or multiple lesions; they infrequently metastasize to local lymph nodes and are associated with a much improved five-year survival rate.[12]

Macroscopically, early gastric carcinomas, all being T1 lesions, are classified using types:

Type I: polypoid—protrudes above the mucosal surface as a nodular or papillary growth

Type IIa: elevated—flat elevation, slightly thickens the mucosa by two or more times

Type IIb: flat—mass is at the same level as non-neoplastic gastric tissue

Type IIc: depressed—mass is slightly below level of non-neoplastic tissue

Type III: excavated—ulcer-like, are often mistaken for benign ulcers

These early gastric cancer lesions more commonly develop in the distal stomach, along the lesser curvature. (Figure 66-1)[20] Early cancers may be up to 10 cm in diameter, have any degree of differentiation, and may be associated with regional lymph node involvement. In Japan, probably as a result of early detection, aggressive treatment, and extensive experience with the disease, nearly all patients with early gastric cancer who undergo gastrectomy are cured.

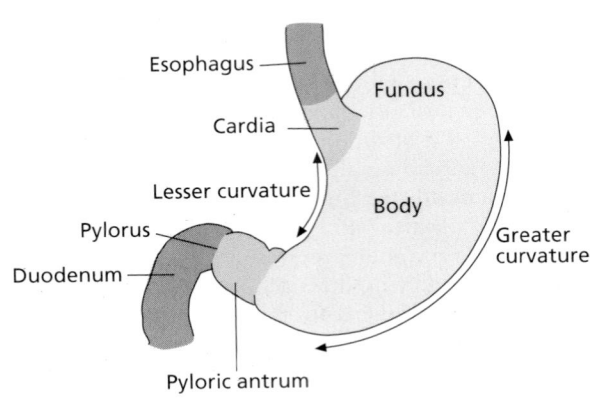

Figure 66-1 Divisions of the stomach.

Progression of Disease

Gastric cancer often progresses to an advanced stage before the patient develops obvious symptoms and seeks medical attention. Patients usually present with stage III tumors and complain of early satiety, postprandial fullness, rapid weight loss, anorexia, and fatigue, which is often secondary to anemia and obstruction. Vague abdominal pain is a common complaint with most gastric tumors and dysphagia is a common complaint with proximal tumors. Presentation with massive gastrointestinal bleeding is uncommon.[21] As the disease advances, weight loss is profound and problems with nutrition become significant.

The pattern of metastatic spread of gastric cancer is by direct extension and lymph node metastases. Pattern of spread is closely correlated with the size and location of the primary tumor. Gastric cancer has the ability to metastasize through direct extension to adjacent organs such as the esophagus, pancreas, liver, transverse colon, and mesocolon.[12] Lesions of the distal stomach most commonly metastasize to subpyloric, inferior gastric, and celiac axis lymph nodes. Tumors of the proximal stomach will often metastasize to splenic, pancreatic, pericardial, and superficial diaphragmatic lymph nodes. Lymphatic spread of gastric cancer along the intrathoracic lymph channels may be manifested clinically by a metastatic lymph node in the left supraclavicular fossa (Virchow node) or in the left axilla (Irish node). Tumor spread to the lymphatics in the hepatoduodenal ligament can extend along the falciform ligament and result in subcutaneous periumbilical deposits in the lymph nodes known as "Sister Mary Joseph's node." Krukenberg tumor, which is metastatic disease to the ovary, and Blumer shelf, a large peritoneal implant in the cul de sac palpable on digital rectal examination, are clinical findings representing evidence of diffuse peritoneal spread of disease.

Clinical Manifestations

Patients with early gastric cancers are essentially asymptomatic. Those with symptoms report nonspecific complaints similar to peptic ulcer disease or other gastrointestinal ailments including reflux, indigestion, early satiety, nausea and vomiting, abdominal pain, weight loss, dysphagia, and anorexia. The majority of patients with advanced stage disease report experiencing symptoms for less than 12 months. Ascites, hepatomegaly, and a palpable epigastric mass are significant findings for advanced disease, along with pulmonary, osseous, adrenal, and cutaneous metastasis.[9,11]

Assessment

On presentation to the health care provider, a complete history and physical examination, complete blood count, and blood chemistries with liver function tests are performed. The history can provide valuable findings to direct the sequence of diagnostic studies. It may be necessary to perform radiographic, endoscopic, and surgical intervention to establish the diagnosis of gastric carcinoma.

There is no specific serum tumor marker for gastric cancer. The carcinoembryonic antigen level (CEA) is elevated in only approximately 25%–30% of patients with gastric cancer; therefore, monitoring of patients with an elevated CEA level may only be beneficial for assessing response to treatment or as an indicator of recurrent disease. Assessing CEA level is not helpful for screening purposes.[9]

Patient and Family History

To establish a clinical picture, a complete assessment of the individual's nutritional status, physical examination, social, and family history should be obtained. Particular attention should be directed to the following:

1. Oral intake (food and fluids) including amounts, frequency, calories, and supplements
2. Symptoms associated with eating including pain, dysphagia, distention, nausea, vomiting, fullness
3. Changes in appetite or dietary habits including food intolerances, aversions, volumes, consistency of foods ingested
4. Weight including current weight, usual weight, weight six months and one year ago; intentional and unintentional weight loss
5. Bowel patterns and habits including frequency, consistency, color, flatulence
6. Medications including over the counter, prescribed, vitamins, and homeopathic remedies
7. Past medical and surgical history including childhood and adult illnesses

Physical Examination

The initial work-up of a presumed gastric cancer includes a complete physical examination from which physical manifestations of metastatic disease can be detected. Particular attention should be given to palpation of the abdomen for masses and or hepatomegaly, and lymph node beds, particularly the supraclavicular and axillary lymph nodes. Palpate around the umbilicus for nodules indicative of metastatic disease. A large ovarian mass palpable on pelvic exam or a large anterior shelf palpable on rectal examination are indicative of metastatic peritoneal deposits. The presence of ascites and/or jaundice are also indicative of advanced or metastatic disease.

Diagnostic Studies

A computerized tomography (CT) scan is the most common diagnostic study used to evaluate abdominal malignancies. Scanning of the chest, abdomen, and pelvis is performed for staging the extent of disease, including extragastric extension, lymph node involvement, and peritoneal or hepatic metastasis. This scan, however, has little specificity in determining the depth of tumor penetration (T stage) of the gastric wall and approximately 25% of patients will be found to be understaged by this method at the time of surgery.[22,23]

The barium swallow/upper gastrointestinal series is a noninvasive radiology procedure used to visualize the anatomic structures of the alimentary tract. Using double-contrast, hypotonic radio-opaque material, this test helps to identify polypoid masses, ulcerative lesions, and nondistendible lesions suggestive of gastric cancer. It has limited capability for determining the depth of lesions and lymphadenopathy associated with malignancy.

The flexible upper gastrointestinal endoscopy is the procedure of choice for diagnostic purposes. This invasive procedure allows for the direct visualization of the gastric mucosa, biopsy of visible lesions, exfoliative cytology, and brush biopsies. With multiple biopsies and brushings, the endoscopy accurately detects more than 95% of gastric cancers.[22]

While executing the endoscopy, a simultaneous endoscopic ultrasound (EUS) of the gastric mucosa is performed by the gastroenterologist. The EUS is one of the newest technologic advances in imaging and allows the physician to evaluate tumor depth (T stage) through the layers of the stomach wall and the presence of lymph node involvement, allowing for more accurate disease staging[23,24] (Figure 66-2). The major disadvantage to this study is that the EUS cannot distinguish between benign and malignant tumors; this determination can only be determined by pathologic study of the biopsy specimens.[23] The depth of tumor invasion has a great impact on prognosis, the prognosis being directly proportional to the stage of disease.

The presence of *H. pylori* can be diagnosed by either invasive or noninvasive diagnostic tests. Endoscopic evaluation and biopsy of the gastric mucosa is an invasive procedure that allows for direct visualization and pathologic evaluation of tissue samples for the physical presence of the organism. Another study is the rapid urease test that detects *H. pylori* by the presence of urease, which is not a normal gastric finding. The bacteria produces

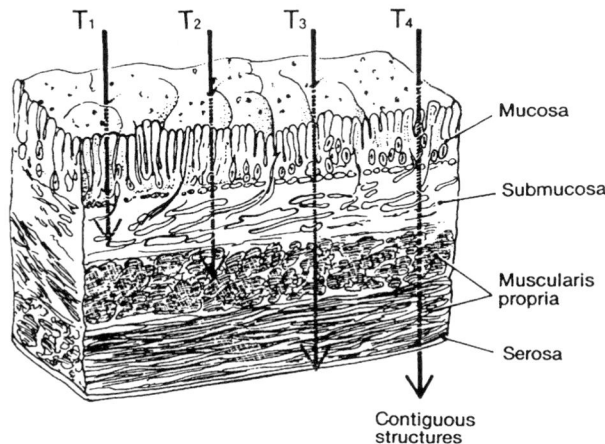

Figure 66-2 Depth of tumor through the gastric wall (T-stage). (Reprinted with permission from Alexander RH, Kelsen DG, Tepper JC: Cancer of the stomach, in DeVita VT, Hellman S, Rosenberg SA (eds): *Principles and Practice of Oncology* (ed 5). Philadelphia, Lippincott-Raven, 1997, p 1031.)[24]

large amounts of urease, which neutralizes the normal acidity of the gastric environment, allowing the organism to proliferate and survive. When the biopsy tissue is applied to a combination urea substrate and pH-sensitive marker in the tester kit, the urease is detected by its ability to convert urea to ammonia, which causes a change in color. Noninvasive methods of detecting *H. pylori* include carbon-labeled breath testing, which indirectly detects urease production, and elevated immunoglobulin G and immunoglobulin A antibodies from immunologic response in blood testing.[14,15]

Gastric acid studies should be part of the evaluation of any gastric ulcer since benign ulcers do not occur in achlorhydria. Benign ulcers treated aggressively with proton pump inhibitors or H2 blocking agents, when taken as prescribed, usually heal within six to eight weeks. If an ulcer persists despite aggressive therapy, a repeat biopsy should be performed to rule out gastric carcinoma because many almost 15% of ulcers are malignant.[8]

Prognostic Indicators

The Japanese lead the world in the early diagnosis and radical surgical treatment for gastric cancer. With localized gastric cancer, approximately 50% of patients can be cured. Japanese survival statistics are consistently better for individuals with nodal metastasis when compared with similar individuals in the United States. Strong predictors of outcome in gastric cancer have been shown to be lymph node metastasis or the number of positive nodes at the time of surgery. The risk of recurrence after surgical resection is related to the stage of disease based on the TNM classification system for gastric cancer; patients with later-stage disease (T3 or T4 lesions) and those with lymph node metastasis are at a higher risk.[25]

Table 66-1 TNM Classification System for Gastric Cancer

T1	Tumor invades lamina propria or submucosa
T2	Tumor invades muscularis propria or subserosa
T3	Tumor penetrates serosa
T4	Tumor invades adjacent organ structures
N0	No metastases in lymph nodes
N1	Metastasis in perigastric lymph node(s) within 3 cm of primary tumor
N2	Metastasis in perigastric lymph node(s) >3 cm from primary tumor, or in lymph nodes along left gastric, common hepatic, splenic, or celiac arteries
M0	No evidence of distant metastasis
M1	Evidence of distant metastasis

Staging				
IA	T1	N0	M0	
IB	T1	N1	M0	
	T2	N0	M0	
II	T1	N2	M0	
	T2	N1	M0	
	T3	N0	M0	
IIIA	T2	N2	M0	
	T3	N1	M0	
	T4	N0	M0	
IIIB	T3	N2	M0	
	T4	N1	M0	
IV	T4	N2	M0	
	Any T, N	M1		

Classification and Staging

The current method of staging gastric cancer is based on the guidelines of the American Joint Committee on Cancer (AJCC).[26] (Table 66-1). This system categorizes the stage of disease using a TNM designation whereby T refers to the depth of tumor invasion through the gastric wall regardless of tumor size (see Figure 66-2), N represents the extent of lymph node involvement, and M indicates the presence or absence of metastatic disease.

Therapeutic Approaches and Nursing Care

Once the diagnosis of gastric cancer is established, a thorough explanation of the disease, treatment options, and expected outcomes should be provided to the individual and family. The plan of therapy is dependent on the patient's health status, the stage of disease, and current advances in surgery, radiation, and chemotherapy. The particular treatment must be individualized to the patient's nutritional status and concurrent cardiovascular, respiratory, renal, and hematologic status. The pa-

tient's potential for rehabilitation is another important consideration. The treatment plan selected is dependent on the location and extent of the lesion and the presence of lymphatic spread.

In the absence of metastatic disease, localized gastric tumors are treated with aggressive surgical resection. However, since the majority of patients present with advanced disease, only approximately 30% are eligible for curative resection.[19] Advanced tumors that are unresectable are treated with combined modality treatment such as chemotherapy and surgical palliation. Combination chemotherapy has demonstrated transient improvement in control of the disease. Palliative surgical procedures include resection, gastric bypass, laser fulguration, and placement of a gastric drainage tube or insertion of a jejunal feeding tube.

Surgery

Surgical resection is the only effective therapy for curing gastric cancer, and is also an effective approach for palliation.[27,28] Consideration for surgical intervention is given to all patients with a good performance status and no major medical contraindications to surgery. Necessary considerations by both the health care team and the individual include morbidity, nutritional issues, and postoperative rehabilitation.

Prior to surgical intervention, it is necessary to correct abnormal hematologic conditions (such as anemia) and establish an adequate hydration and nutritional status. Patients should receive blood transfusions for significant anemia or oral iron supplementation for borderline anemia. Improving nutritional status requires extensive planning since weight loss, emaciation, and malnutrition can adversely affect postoperative healing and recovery. Improvement of the nutritional status through enteral feeding is the preferred route, but more aggressive measures using hyperalimenatation may be necessary in some cases.

The choice of the surgical resection procedure is based on location and extent of disease.[29] Gastric neoplasms should not be considered unresectable or incurable based on the size of the tumor, but may be determined unresectable based on the involvement of other organs, vital blood vessels, and distant metastasis. Lymphatic spread is recognized as a major prognostic indicator of this disease,[12,30,31] although great controversy exists over the extent of lymph node dissection that should take place. In Japan, where the incidence of gastric cancer is very high, extensive lymph node dissection is utilized during surgery and cure rates are higher than in the United States.[27] Nonetheless, it should be noted that due to mass screening programs throughout Japan for the past 25 years, gastric cancer is often detected at an early stage, allowing for improved survival rates. Researchers in the United States have studied this difference and concluded that a more extensive lymphadenectomy does not necessarily improve survival; it in fact may increase the morbidity associated with surgery.[27] The benefits from an extended lymph node dissection, total gastrectomy for tumors of the antrum or body of the stomach, and prophylactic splenectomy are being investigated.[28]

The initial surgical approach often will be a diagnostic/staging laparoscopic procedure to evaluate the primary tumor, obtain tissue for pathologic diagnosis, and detect metastatic tumor deposits. Laparoscopy also spares patients with unresectable or metastatic disease an unnecessary larger operation with extended recovery time, expediting their entry into adjuvant therapy.[32]

At the time of laparoscopy, those patients with stage I or stage II disease then advance to an exploratory laparotomy and open surgical procedure to examine the stomach and regional lymph nodes, and to evaluate for evidence of extragastric extension of tumor or metastasis. With confined disease, the surgeon proceeds with en bloc resection of the tumor and appropriate locoregional lymphadenectomy. Those with stage III or stage IV disease are referred for neoadjuvant chemotherapy before resection unless there is bleeding or a visible lesion that could potentially cause a gastric outlet obstruction that may be surgically relieved prior to chemotherapy.

Total gastrectomy

A total gastrectomy may be performed for a resectable lesion in the midportion or body of the stomach. Linitis plastica is usually treated with a total gastrectomy because of the extensive tumor involvement of the stomach wall. The entire stomach is excised en bloc, along with resected duodenum, a section of abdominal esophagus, supporting mesentery and lymph nodes.[33] Reconstruction of the alimentary tract is achieved with the use of a jejunal segment anastamosed to the remaining esophagus. A jejunal loop is brought up and an end-to-side Roux-en-Y jejunojejunostomy is placed distally to provide flow for bile and pancreatic secretions. It is important for the surgical team to try to obtain adequate tissue margins around the tumor site that are free of malignant cells; this is a standard of surgical oncology. However, this margin free of cancer may not be possible in some cases due to the size of the tumor, surrounding vasculature, and location of the tumor.

Radical subtotal gastrectomy

Lesions located in the middle and distal portions of the stomach are treated with a radical subtotal gastrectomy. A Billroth I or Billroth II operation will be performed. (See Figure 66-3).[34] The Billroth I, or gastroduodenostomy, involves resection of the distal stomach, pylorus, first portion of the duodenum, and supporting lymph and vasculature. The remaining stomach is then anastamosed to the duodenum. The Billroth I involves a limited amount of resection, and as a result generally produces a lower cure rate than the Billroth II. The Billroth I procedure is utilized primarily when the patient is debilitated and needs restricted intraoperative time.[24]

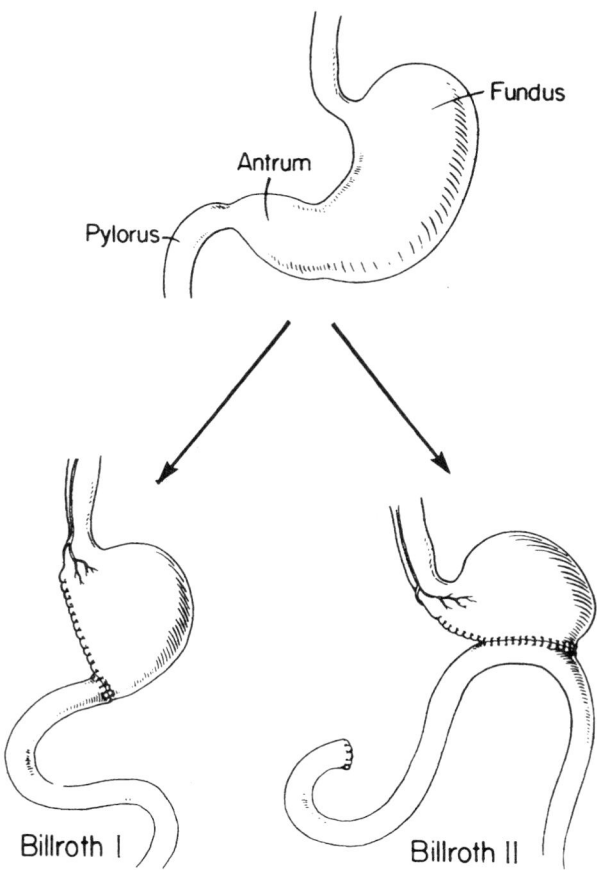

Figure 66-3 Reconstruction after gastrectomy. The Bilroth I involves limited resection. The Bilroth II is a wider resection of about 75% of the stomach. (Reprinted with permission from Seymour NE: Operations for peptic ulcer and their complications, in Feldman M, Scharschmidt BF, Sleisenger MH (eds): *Sleisenger and Fordtran's Gastrointestinal and Liver Disease: Pathophysiology, Diagnosis, and Management* (vol 1, ed 6). Philadelphia, Saunders, 1998, p 700.)[34]

A Billroth II procedure is a wider resection that includes removing approximately 75% of the stomach, thereby decreasing the possibility of nodal or metastatic recurrence. The Billroth II involves removal of the antrum, pylorus, first part of the duodenum, supporting vasculature, and all visible and palpable lymph nodes. The remaining stomach is anastamosed end-to-side to the jejunum. The duodenal stump is then oversewn with sutures. Gastric emptying is altered by both the Billroth I and II, as well as with a total gastrectomy. There is also potential for a duodenal stump leak following the Billroth II procedure.[24]

Proximal subtotal gastrectomy

A proximal subtotal gastrectomy may be performed for a resectable tumor located in the proximal portion of the stomach or cardia. In many cases, a total gastrectomy or an esophagogastrectomy will be performed in place of this surgery to achieve a more extensive resection. Following resection of the stomach and distal esophagus, the esophagus is anastamosed to the duodenum of jejunum. Potential complications include pneumonia, anastamotic leak, infection, reflux aspiration, and esophagitis.[24]

Palliative surgical procedures

Unfortunately, many patients with gastric cancer are not candidates for extensive curative resection. Often the symptoms of advanced gastric cancer are so severe that they significantly affect a person's quality of life and will require palliative surgical intervention. Gastric outlet obstruction, bleeding, and severe pain are common problems of advanced gastric cancer that are not well controlled without surgery. Gastric perforation is an emergency situation requiring surgery.

If the patient is an acceptable surgical risk, resection can be the most effective palliative treatment for advanced gastric cancer. The difficulty with performing a major operation such as a total gastrectomy in the setting of metastatic disease is that this extensive procedure is associated with a high rate of mortality and complications, while ultimately providing no true survival benefit. Surgery also delays the patient from beginning systemic therapy. Although the survival time with palliative surgery is disappointing, it appears to be slightly longer than when no procedure is performed. The main benefit to a palliative resection is evident in the patient's quality of life. Relief of gastrointestinal symptoms, such as vomiting, can be achieved through palliative surgery. Placement of an esophageal stent can restore the patient's ability to swallow, particularly liquids, and aids in preventing aspiration of saliva. Palliative procedures such as gastric or esophageal bypass, gastrostomy, or jejunostomy temporarily alleviate symptoms but do not affect long-term survival. Laser surgery has been shown to benefit patients with obstructing tumors of the esophagus and the gastroesophageal junction with satisfactory results.[28]

Postoperative care

Nursing measures for the individual with gastric cancer who undergoes surgical resection do not differ from those individuals who undergo gastric surgery for benign disorders. The nurse must be acutely aware of the postoperative status of the patient and must employ nursing measures necessary to maintain or improve the person's preoperative condition. Pneumonia, wound infection, deep venous thrombosis, anastamotic leak, hemorrhage, sepsis, and reflux aspiration are the common postoperative complications following gastric surgery. Occasionally a patient will develop a bezoar formation, which is ingested fibrous food clumping, causing a gastric outlet obstruction. A bezoar can be dissolved with enzymes, such as papain, or broken up through endoscopic intervention.

Weight loss is one of the greatest problems for patients with gastric cancer and for those who have had a gastric resection.[34] Preoperatively, inadequate food intake occurs from tumor bulk or compression; postoperatively, patients are unable to ingest high carbohydrate or normal size meals leading to inadequate food intake. With decreased stomach size, foods may be inadequately absorbed due to the organ's inability to properly break down, churn, and mix foods. In response to this, an enteral feeding tube may be placed during surgery for nutritional support. This is particularly advantageous for those individuals who have already had significant weight loss and are at greater risk for further weight loss with adjuvant therapy. The involvement of a registered dietitian is beneficial for determining enteral feeding solutions, for calculating and monitoring caloric requirements, as well as for patient and family teaching.

Surgical resection can lead to additional nutritional problems. Anemia following gastrectomy can result from iron, vitamin B12, or folate deficiency. Iron malabsorption may occur because of decreased gastric acid secretion as the gastric acids convert the iron molecule into a substance that is more easily absorbed by the body. Iron absorption is further compromised in those patients who have undergone the Billroth II (gastrojejunostomy) reconstruction because the duodenum, where iron is normally absorbed, has been surgically resected.[35] Vitamin B12 deficiency is a complication that typically occurs several weeks after a gastrectomy due to the loss of parietal cells, which secrete intrinsic factor needed to facilitate the absorption of vitamin B12. Folate deficiency is directly related to poor nutritional intake and/or malnutrition. Management of these surgically induced problems include oral iron and folate replacements and monthly vitamin B12 injections.

Many patients experience problems with their oral food intake after gastric resection. The most commonly reported occurrence is known as "postparandial dumping syndrome." This syndrome begins with the rapid emptying of hypertonic/hyperosmolar chyme into the intestine approximately 10–20 minutes after eating. This influx causes a rapid shift of fluid from the vasculature into the small intestine causing severe gastrointestinal and vasomotor symptoms. The symptoms include abdominal fullness and pain accompanied by vomiting, cramping, flushing, diarrhea, dizziness, and palpitations, all of which disappear once the bowels have emptied.

Most cases of dumping syndrome are remedied with dietary management, which consists of the patient's eating small, frequent meals of high-protein and low-carbohydrate foods. Patients should ingest minimal fluids with meals to reduce the volume ingested, reduce the possibility of triggering the syndrome, and thus allow for greater caloric intake from solid foods. Those who have undergone a proximal gastric resection or total gastrectomy should remain in the upright sitting position for at least one hour after meals because they no longer have a cardiac sphincter that prevents reflux of gastric contents into the upper esophagus and possibly into the lungs causing an aspiration pneumonia. Patients with persistent dumping syndrome that does not respond to dietary modifications may require surgical modification to reconstruct the pylorus, or revise the gastrojejunostomy to maintain their weight and adequate hydration.[35,36]

Radiation Therapy

Research into the benefits of radiation therapy for patients with gastric cancer is ongoing, but radiation has not been shown to have a significant role in the treatment of gastric cancer. Radiation is often used as an adjuvant treatment with chemotherapy (fluorouracil [5-FU]) in patients with locally advanced, unresectable gastric cancer because gastric adenocarcinomas are generally radiosensitive. Radiation therapy given for palliation purposes can provide quality of life benefits to patients with bulky proximal obstruction, chronic gastrointestinal bleeding secondary to tumor infiltration, and symptomatic pain relief.[9]

For adjuvant therapy purposes, the area of irradiation extends from the diaphragm to the umbilicus, including the gastric area in the left upper quadrant and the nodal beds in the right upper quadrant of the abdomen. The treatments are given by anterior and posterior fields over a five-week period for a maximum total of 4500 cGy. A boost of 500–1000 cGy may be given to the gastric area if there is bulky disease present. Advances in the field of radiation therapy have made it possible to deliver decreased doses to the extremely radiosensitive small intestine, while providing the necessary dose to the involved gastric area.

Specific attention must be given to the nutritional status of the patient with gastric cancer who is receiving radiation therapy. Excessive weight loss is the main dose-limiting toxicity that can lead to a delay or cessation of radiation treatment. Most patients receiving this treatment develop acute gastrointestinal symptoms including diarrhea, abdominal cramping, nausea, and gastritis. All of these reactions usually resolve within two weeks after completion of radiation treatments.[37] See Chapter 17 for additional information on the management of radiation toxicities.

Chemotherapy

A strong emphasis has been placed on the development of more effective systemic chemotherapy regimens because metastatic disease is a common problem with gastric cancer, either at presentation or later in the clinical course.[38] The risk of recurrence is directly related to the stage of the disease after pathologic review, with patients at advanced stage disease (T3 or T4) and those with lymph node metastasis being at higher risk for recurrence.[25] Palliative chemotherapy is offered to those with surgically unresectable disease for control of symptoms and improved quality of life.

Adjuvant treatment with chemotherapy is not the standard approach for all patients undergoing surgical resection; it is reserved for patients diagnosed with advanced-stage disease. There is no single-agent chemotherapeutic regimen that alone has been able to demonstrate a major impact on survival from gastric cancer. Single agents, such as 5-FU, doxorubicin, cisplatin, etoposide, and mitomycin-c, have been shown to have moderate activity in gastric cancer.[38] However, it is more common to administer combination therapy for improved response rates. Commonly used regimens during the late 1980s and early to mid 1990s include FAM (5-FU, doxorubicin, mitomycin), FAMTX (5-FU, doxorubicin, high-dose methotrexate), and EAP (etoposide, doxorubicin, cisplatin). The toxicities associated with FAM and EAP are such that they outweigh the benefit of their use.[9,37,38] For elderly patients and those with cardiac risks, ELF (etoposide, leucovorin, and 5-FU) is a well-tolerated regimen demonstrating promising results in those individuals with locally advanced disease.[39,40] However, response rates were lower in patients with peritoneal carcinomatosis. Current treatment consists primarily of fluorouracil-based therapy with cisplatin, either on day 1 and 2, or in daily divided low doses. This regimen is well tolerated with few side effects.

For those patients receiving chemotherapy, nursing assessment is an essential part of patient care. Stomatitis is an indication of toxicity for those individuals receiving 5-FU. If stomatitis develops early in the course of treatment, it may be necessary to withhold treatment with this drug until the sores resolve or, depending on the degree of toxicity (grade 3 and grade 4 being most significant), doses may need to be reduced for future chemotherapy cycles. Nursing staff should encourage meticulous oral hygiene including rinsing with sodium bicarbonate-saline solution four to six times daily. Patients should be instructed to notify their physician if mouth sores develop. These sores are quite painful for patients and are capable of preventing patients from eating and drinking, which compromises their nutritional status further. Symptoms may be improved with local analgesic preparations.

Patients with known cardiac dysfunction need further monitoring while undergoing chemotherapy with doxorubicin or 5-FU. Doxorubicin is known to have dose-related cardiotoxicity at cumulative doses of 550 mg/m², and therefore a baseline echocardiogram is essential, as well as routine echocardiograms at specified intervals to monitor the left ventricular ejection fraction (LVEF). Should a significant change in LVEF occur over time, the chemotherapy regimen may need to be changed to alternate agents. Those individuals receiving 5-FU as part of their chemotherapy regimen may require telemetry monitoring, as this drug may cause vasoconstriction and electrocardiogram (ECG) changes. Patients should be instructed to notify the nursing staff of chest pain or angina-like pain.

New therapies that may increase the potentially curative resection rates and decrease the risk of recurrence after surgery are currently being closely studied. These new approaches include preoperative (neoadjuvant) systemic chemotherapy and treatment with intraperitoneal adjuvant chemotherapy. Neoadjuvant regimens focus on reducing tumor burden preoperatively to allow a more complete resection of microscopic and macroscopic disease leading to lower rates of recurrence. Conversely, there is potential for drug resistance to develop from exposing tumors to the chemotherapy agents before surgery, thus blocking potential effects of the subsequent chemotherapy given postoperativley. Some oncologists argue that neoadjuvant therapy delays local control of the primary tumor by surgery and therefore should not be considered.

Another approach for chemotherapy administration being studied is regional therapy delivered through an intraperitoneal (IP) catheter.[41] The intraperitoneal catheter is surgically placed with the tip of the catheter lying in the peritoneum. The port of the catheter is accessed with a needle and then the chemotherapy is delivered directly into the peritoneal cavity. The drug is dispersed throughout the peritoneum and then absorbed by the body over the course of a few days. Intraperitoneal therapy is directed at treating both peritoneal and hepatic metastasis, common sites of recurrence for gastric cancer. Patients should be instructed that it is common to feel bloated after this therapy as 2–3 liters of fluid are instilled into the abdominal cavity. Intraperitoneal therapy is not associated with severe nausea and vomiting.

Symptom Management and Supportive Care

Advanced gastric cancer can result in rapid deterioration of an individual's health. Medical and nursing management is aimed at controlling symptoms and maintaining optimal functioning. As gastric cancer progresses or recurs, nutritional problems usually become a serious problem. Without aggressive nutritional support, patients may be unable to receive further chemotherapy, cannot maintain strength, and cannot fully perform activities of daily living. Many of the advanced-stage problems are due to the dysfunction of the stomach, either from the lack of gastric secretions or the presence of tumor within or surrounding the stomach causing gastric outlet or intestinal obstruction. Nursing personnel and dietitians should make every effort to monitor the patient's nutritional intake and provide measures to supplement intake whenever possible.

Patients with progressive gastric cancer require supportive physical care depending on their symptoms. Common complications of advanced gastric cancer include pneumonia, deep vein thrombosis from immobility, pulmonary emboli, sepsis, and anastamotic rupture. Any of these complications could potentially lead to death.

Many individuals and families feel a strong and long-lasting sense of regret, anger, and guilt as they often ignored early symptoms or self-treated prior to seeking medical evaluation. Providing the individual and family an opportunity to verbalize these feeling is an important nursing measure, as well as dispelling misconceptions and promoting a realistic sense of hope.

Continuity of Care

The nurse provides comprehensive care to the individual with gastric cancer. Providing information and clarifying and explaining the multiple treatment modalities can help the individual and the family understand their options and make informed decisions. The nurse can help the individual and the family deal with physical problems and obtain assistance for emotional and economic issues. Strong nurse-to-nurse communication across the various disciplines can ensure a smooth transition, as many of the patients with this disease receive combined modality therapy. Nursing staff must be aware of the entire disease management treatment plan for individuals with gastric cancer. The nurse remains an advocate for the patient no matter what treatment options are chosen. To help prevent or treat complications that may hinder treatment, nurses must constantly evaluate and reevaluate patients with this disease for signs and symptoms of problems. Finally, compassionate care for the individual with gastric cancer can help to alleviate the physical and emotional pain of such a devastating illness.

Conclusion

Gastric cancer has been steadily decreasing in incidence in the United States, but the disease continues to be a significant challenge in many parts of the world, particularly Japan. Improvements in food preparation and mass screenings may contribute to the decline in incidence and mortality. The outcomes of treatment for early gastric cancer are positive when aggressive surgery and close follow-up surveillance is in place, yet the prognosis for stage III and IV disease remains poor because the unresectable disease is difficult to treat with chemotherapy or radiation. Less aggressive surgical procedures can be used to control or palliate advanced disease. Nutritional management is often one of the greatest challenges in the course of gastric cancer.

References

1. Whooly BP, Conlon KC: Palliative surgery, in Berger AM, Portenoy RK, Weissman DE (eds): *Principles and Practice of Supportive Oncology.* Philadelphia, Lippincott-Raven, 1998, pp 627–637
2. Smith JW, Brennan MF: Surgical treatment of gastric cancer. *Surg Clin North Am* 72:333–345, 1992

3. Hanks JB, Jones RS, Minasi JS: Tumors of the stomach and duodenum, in Ritchie Jr WP (ed): *Shackelford's Surgery of the Alimentary Tract* (vol 2, ed 4). Philadelphia, Saunders, 1996, pp 88–95

4. *Cancer Statistics—1999*. Atlanta, American Cancer Society, 1999

5. Neugut AI, Hayek M, Howe G: Epidemiology of gastric cancer. *Semin Oncol* 23:281–291, 1996

6. Volpe CM, Driscoll DM, Moloro SM, et al: Survival benefit of extended D2 resection for proximal gastric cancer. *J Surg Oncol* 64:231–236, 1997

7. Kitamura K, Yamagachi T, Sawai K, et al: Chronologic changes in the clinicopathologic findings and survival of gastric cancer patients. *J Clin Oncol* 15:3471–3480, 1997

8. Luk GD: Tumors of the stomach, in Feldman M, Scharschmidt BF, Sleisenger MH (eds): *Sleisenger and Fordtran's Gastrointestinal and Liver Disease: Pathophysiology, Diagnosis and Management* (vol 1, ed 6). Philadelphia, Saunders, 1998, pp 733–757

9. Haskell CM, Lavey RS, Ramming KP: Stomach, in Haskell CM (ed): *Cancer Treatment* (ed 4). Boston, Little, Brown, 1995, pp 452–463

10. Bruckner HW, Kondo T: Neoplasms of the stomach, in Holland JF, Frei E, Bast RC, Kufe DW, Morton DL, Weichselbaum RR (eds): *Cancer Medicine* (vol 2, ed 3). Philadelphia, Lea & Febiger, 1993, pp 1395–1425

11. Tabbarah HJ: Gastrointestinal tract cancers, in Casciato DA, Lowitz BB (eds): *Manual of Clinical Oncology* (ed 3). Boston, Little, Brown, 1995, pp 145–182

12. Fenoglio-Preiser CM, Nofsinger AE, Belli J, et al: Pathologic and phenotypic features of gastric cancer. *Semin Oncol* 23: 292–306, 1996.

13. Wisniewski RM, Peura DA: *Helicobacter pylori*: beyond peptic ulcer disease. *Gastroenterologist* 5:295–305, 1997

14. Schwesinger WH: Is *Helicobacter pylori* a myth or the missing link? *Am J Surg* 172:411–417, 1996

15. Cutler AF: Diagnostic tests for *Helicobacter pylori* infection. *Gastroenterologist* 5:202–212, 1997

16. Newman E, Brennan MF, Hochwald SN, et al: Gastric remnant carcinoma: just another gastric cancer or a unique entity? *Am J Surg* 223:292–297, 1997

17. Greene FL: Management of gastric remnant carcinoma based on the results of a 15-year endoscopic screening program. *Ann Surg* 223:701–708, 1996

18. Yanamoto N, Tokunaga M, Uemura Y, et al: Epstein-Barr virus and gastric remnant carcinoma. *Cancer* 74:805–809, 1994

19. Staley CA: Gastric carcinoma, in Bears DH, Feig BW, Fuhrman GM (eds): *The M.D. Anderson Surgical Oncology Handbook*. Boston, Little, Brown, 1995, pp 120–141

20. Dempsey DT, Ritchie Jr WP: Anatomy and physiology of the stomach, in Ritchie Jr WP (ed): *Shackelford's Surgery of the Alimentary Tract* (vol 2, ed 4). Philadelphia, Saunders, 1996, p 4

21. Lawrence M, Shiu MH: Early gastric cancer: twenty-eight-year experience. *Ann Surg* 213:327–334, 1991

22. Conlon KC, Karpeh MS: Laparoscopy and laparoscopic ultrasound in the staging of gastric cancer. *Semin Oncol* 23: 347–351, 1996

23. Catalano MF: Endoscopic ultrasonography for esophageal and gastric lesions. *Gastroenterologist* 5:3–9, 1997

24. Alexander R, Kelsen DG, Tepper JC: Cancer of the stomach, in DeVita VT, Hellman S, Rosenberg SA (eds): *Principles and Practice of Oncology* (ed 5). Philadelphia, Lippincott-Raven, 1997, pp 1021–1050

25. Kelsen D: Introduction: gastric cancer. *Semin Oncol* 23: 279–280, 1996

26. American Joint Committee on Cancer: *The AJCC Cancer Staging Manual* (ed 5). Philadelphia, Lippincott-Raven, 1997

27. Brennan MF, Karpeh MS: Surgery for gastric cancer: the American view. *Semin Oncol* 23:352–359, 1996

28. Lawrence Jr W, Zfass A: Gastric neoplasms, in Murphy GP, Lawrence Jr W, Lenhard Jr RE (eds): *American Cancer Society Textbook of Clinical Oncology* (ed 2). Atlanta, American Cancer Society, 1995, pp 281–292

29. Boland CR: Gastrointestinal and pancreatic neoplasms, in Kelley WN (ed): *Textbook of Internal Medicine* (ed 3). Philadelphia, Lippincott-Raven, 1997, pp 768–782

30. Roukos D, Kappas AM, Encke A: Extensive lymph node dissection in gastric cancer: is it of therapeutic value? *Cancer Treat Rev* 22:247–252, 1996

31. Kelsen DG: Adjuvant and neoadjuvant therapy for gastric cancer. *Semin Oncol* 23:379–389, 1996

32. Burke EC, Karpeh MS, Conlon KC, et al: Laparoscopy in the management of gastric adenocarcinoma. *Ann Surg* 225: 262–267, 1997

33. Harrison LE, Karpeh MS, Brennan MF: Proximal gastric cancers resected via transabdominal-only approach: results and comparison to distal adenocarcinoma of the stomach. *Ann Surg* 225:678–685, 1997

34. Seymour NE: Operations for peptic ulcers and their complications, in Feldman M, Scharschmidt BF, Sleisenger MH (eds): *Sleisenger and Fordtran's Gastrointestinal and Liver Disease: Pathophysiology, Diagnosis, and Management*. Philadelphia, Saunders, vol I, pp. 696–710, 1998

35. Huether SE, McCance KL, Tarmina MS: Alterations in digestive function, in McCance KL, Huether SE (eds): *Pathophysiology: The Biologic Response for Disease in Adults and Children* (ed 2). St. Louis, Mosby, 1994, pp 1320–1375

36. Eagon JC, Miedema BW, Kelly KE: Post gastrectomy syndromes. *Surg Clin North Am* 72:445–462, 1992

37. Minsky BD: The role of radiation therapy in gastric cancer. *Semin Oncol* 23:390–396, 1996

38. Kelsen D, Atiq OT, Saltz L, et al: FAMTX versus etoposide, doxorubicin, and cisplatin: a random assignment trial in gastric cancer. *J Clin Oncol* 10:541–548, 1992

39. Wils J: The treatment of advanced gastric cancer. *Semin Oncol* 23:397–406, 1996

40. Cascinu S, Labianca R, Alessandri P, et al: Intensive weekly chemotherapy for advanced gastric cancer using fluorouracil, cisplatin, epi-doxorubicin, 6S-leucovorin, glutathione, and filgrastim: a report from the Italian group for the study of digestive tract cancer. *J Clin Oncol* 15:3313–3319, 1997

41. Kelsen D, Karpeh MS, Schwartz, G, et al: Neoadjuvant therapy of high-risk gastric cancer: a phase II trial of preoperative FAMTX and postoperative intraperitoneal fluorouracil-cisplatin plus intravenous fluorouracil. *J Clin Oncol* 15: 1818–1828, 1996

CHAPTER 67

Testicular Germ Cell Cancer

Shelley M. Poirier, MS, RN, OCN®
Susan M. Rawl, PhD, RN

Introduction

Germ cell tumors (GCT) are the most common solid malignancy in men age 15–35. Approximately 95% of tumors arising in the testis are GCT. The American Cancer Society estimates that there will be approximately 7600 new cases of testicular germ cell cancers diagnosed in the United States in 1998.[1] More than 90% of patients with newly diagnosed GCT are cured of their disease.[2,3] A direct correlation exists between early diagnosis, intervention, and lower cancer staging at time of presentation. The optimal management of patients with GCT usually requires an interdisciplinary approach by medical, surgical, and (in the case of seminoma) radiation oncologists.

Epidemiology

Testicular cancer accounts for approximately 1% of all male cancers. For unknown reasons, the worldwide incidence has more than doubled over the past four decades[4] with the greatest numbers being reported in Scandinavia, Germany, and New Zealand.[5] The incidence of testicular cancer in blacks and Asians is rare, and although it can occur at any age, it most frequently affects men age 20–30. Testicular cancer occurs less frequently in adolescents with an increased incidence noted over age 40 and again after the age of 60.

Germ cell tumors are composed of seminoma and nonseminomatous cell types. Seminoma is the most common singular cell type, although mixed germ cell tumors are most common. True seminomas do not differentiate; they retain germ cell characteristics. Nonseminomatous tumors include teratoma, endodermal sinus tumor (yolk sac carcinoma), choriocarcinoma, and mixed cell types. Any seminoma associated with an increased alpha-fetoprotein (AFP) is considered to be a nonseminomatous tumor.

Less than 10% of all GCT arise outside the gonads. These rare tumors occur, in descending order, most frequently in the retroperitoneum, mediastinum, and pineal gland and have a poorer prognosis than a primary testicular cancer.[6]

Etiology

The cause of germ cell tumors is unknown, but several risk factors have been suggested for the development of this malignancy. These include prior history of testicular cancer, cryptorchidism, genetics, familial, environmental factors, and hormones.

Men who developed a GCT in one testis are 500 times more likely than the normal male population to develop testicular cancer in the contralateral testis.[7,8] This occurs in approximately 1%–2% of males diagnosed with testicu-

lar cancer. Synchronous presentation of bilateral testicular cancers is uncommon and should suggest an infiltration process (e.g., leukemia, lymphoma).

Cryptorchidism (undescended testes) is associated with a 20-fold to 40-fold increased risk of developing testicular germ cell cancer compared to the normal male population. Once thought to eliminate the risk for testicular cancer in patients with cryptorchidism, orchiopexy remains controversial as 25% of testicular cancers in patients with cryptorchidism occurs in the normal, undescended testis. It has been suggested that in order to receive the best outcome from the orchiopexy, it should be done by age 6, but this still does not eliminate the risk for subsequent GCT. Klinefelter's syndrome is associated with an increased incidence of mediastinal GCT.[9] Males with Down's syndrome or patients with testicular feminization are also thought to be at an increased risk. Germ cell tumors are nearly always hyperdiploid, implying early chromosomal changes preceding the process of carcinogenesis.[10]

A familial tendency for the development of testicular germ cell cancer has been reported. One such report suggests a ten-fold increase in risk for development of GCT in male siblings of testicular cancer patients with a four-fold increase in risk for father–son transmission.[11] Environmental concerns include drug exposures such as diethylstilbesterol (DES) in utero. Male offspring of mothers treated with DES exhibited several developmental abnormalities, including testicular hypoplasia and cryptochidism, but direct evidence of DES induced germ cell cancer is lacking.[12–14] Increased levels of gonadotropins also seem to play a role in the formation of GCT. To date, there remains no substantial data to prove a viral etiology.

Prevention, Screening, and Early Detection

Testicular self-examination (TSE), not unlike breast self-examination (BSE), should be done routinely. Given the nature of testicular GCT, early diagnosis can lead to a more favorable outcome. Cure rates are highest for early stage disease and decrease significantly for more advanced disease. Given the reproductive potential of these males, those experiencing infertility problems should be evaluated since approximately 80% of patients analyzed for reproductive capacity prior to initiation of therapy are oligospermic. This is mainly thought to be a side effect of the malignancy itself although the exact cause remains unknown.[15]

Educational programs beginning during the individual's teens should incorporate specific instructions on how to perform TSE. These exams should be performed after a warm shower/bath when the scrotum is relaxed and abnormalities can be more easily identified. While standing, each testicle should be examined for lumps, swelling, and any changes by rolling the testicle between the thumb and fingers. Any abnormalities should be reported to a health care provider immediately. The American Cancer Society and the National Cancer Institute (NCI) provide pamphlets explaining testicular cancer and TSE.

Massive screening campaigns for testicular cancer have not been felt to be economically feasible because of the rarity of this disease. Nonetheless, public awareness through education is important.

Pathophysiology

As mentioned earlier, germ cell tumors are divided into two main histological categories: seminomas and nonseminomas. Seminomas include classic and spermatocytic whereas nonseminomas include embryonal, yolk sac, choriocarcinoma, and teratoma. The tumor markers followed in testicular cancer are AFP and beta–human chorionic gonadotropin (BHCG). An elevated BHCG (but not AFP) in a patient diagnosed with seminoma can be managed clinically as a seminomatous GCT, but an elevated AFP in a "pure seminoma" connotes nonseminomatous germ cell tumor (NSGCT). Yolk sac carcinomas generally secrete only AFP; choriocarcinoma secretes only BHCG, and embryonal cancer may secrete both AFP and BHCG. Teratomas are benign tumors that do not secrete markers.

GCT, like other cancers, start from the transformation of a single cell and evolve from its subsequent abnormal growth pattern. They are believed to be more responsive to chemotherapy because of their high tumor cell doubling time. The spread of these cancers is generally predictable with initial spread to the retroperitoneal lymph nodes. Once spread has occurred to the lymphatics, vascular spread follows. The lungs are the most common distant organ affected by this pattern of invasion. Approximately 95% of GCT will arise in the testicle.

Clinical Manifestions

The most common presenting symptom of testis cancer is a painless swelling or enlargement of the testis. This symptom is often ignored because many patients may attribute this finding to recent trauma. Painful enlargement occurs in 30%–50% of patients. Often these latter individuals with painful scrotal enlargement may be initially treated for epididymitis or testicular torsion, thus delaying the diagnosis of testicular cancer. Other presenting symptoms include back pain, secondary to retroperitoneal adenopathy, and gynecomastia that can be unilateral or bilateral and is associated with increased BHCG. Those with advanced disease may exhibit cough, dyspnea, chest pain, and shortness of breath. Symptoms related to metastatic disease are rare at time of presentation.

Assessment

Patient and Family History

A thorough patient and family history are important components for establishing a plan of care. As mentioned previously, a prior history of testicular cancer represents a 500-fold chance of developing testicular cancer over the normal male population. Patient histories of trauma, cryptorchidism, epididymitis, gynecomastia, back pain, and infertility should all be noted.

Individuals thought to be at greater risk for the development of germ cell cancer include those with Klinefelter syndrome and Down's syndrome. Others at increased risk include patients with testicular feminization syndrome and hermaphrodites.

According to Horwich,[16] there is a significant familial risk for the development of testicular cancer. In this case-controlled study, the cumulative risk for development of testicular cancer was 2.2% before age 50, and 9.8% when compared to the general population.

Physical Examination

A physical examination should incorporate a careful inspection of the scrotum. A mass that cannot be separated from the testis is indication for further evaluation, as are irregularities of tissue or nodularities. Transillumination of the mass will diagnose a hydrocele; approximately 20% of patients with GCT will have an associate hydrocele. Ultrasound is the diagnostic test of choice to diagnose testicular masses. Lymph nodes should be examined, especially the abdominal and supraclavicular lymph nodes. In general, adenopathy is not observed in the absence of prior surgical violation of the scrotum. Breasts should be examined for gynecomastia.

Diagnostic Studies

Ultrasound is used predominantly and reliably to diagnose a testicular mass. It can provide information about testicular masses and surrounding tissues but cannot tell if a mass is malignant. Nonetheless, 95% of masses within the testicles are malignant. Seminomatous masses will appear hypoechoic when compared to adjacent tissue, whereas nonseminomatous masses may have an echo pattern that is hypoechoic, hyperechoic, or isoechoic.

Chest x-rays are valuable in determining if a patient has gross metastases. If the chest x-ray is normal, a chest computerized tomographic (CT) scan is warranted to rule out metastases within the lung or mediastinum. Abdominal CT scans will provide information regarding retroperitoneal/pelvic disease.

Serum markers BHCG and AFP are elevated in 85% percent of patients with disseminate nonseminomatous germ cell tumors. These are the only markers with diagnostic value in this disease; although lactate dehydrogenase (LDH) is frequently elevated in patients with advanced disease. A fine-needle biopsy or transcrotal approach orchiectomy of the testicular mass is contraindicated because of an increased risk of local recurrence or metastatic spread of disease to inguinal lymph nodes.

Prognostic Indicators

Extent of disease and histology at the time of diagnosis determines stage and prognosis. Virtually all patients with stages I (testis alone) and II (testis and retroperitoneal lymph nodes) seminomatous and nonseminomatous tumors should survive their disease. Approximately 70% of testicular GCT present with either stage I or II disease. The remaining patients present with stage III, disseminated disease (Table 67-1). Patients with low serum markers or no evidence of pulmonary or mediastinal disease have a good prognosis. Patients with low tumor markers and/or limited disease will have an excellent chance of cure if treated appropriately. Most patients with disseminated testicular cancer fall into the minimal or moderate disease category at time of diagnosis, which is associated with over a 90% cure rate with cisplatin-based combination chemotherapy. The prognosis is closely correlated with increased stage and tumor burden (Table 67-2 and 67-4).

Classification and Staging

Several systems exist for the classification and staging of testicular cancer. A frequently used staging system in Europe is the Royal Marsden Hospital Staging Classification,[17] which includes seminomas and nonseminomatous tumors (Table 67-3). In the United States, staging systems used are somewhat institutionally dependent. In 1997, the International Germ Cell Collaborative Group developed a new staging system that has become the standard (Table 67-4).

Therapeutic Approaches and Nursing Care

Nonseminomatous Germ Cell Tumors

Nonseminomatous germ cell tumors comprise about 60% of all GCT and serve as an extraordinary example of a

Table 67-2 Indiana University Staging System for Disseminated Disease

Minimal Disease
1. Elevated markers after retroperitoneal lymph node resection
2. Cervical nodes ± retroperitoneal disease < 10 cm
3. Unresectable, but retroperitoneal disease < 10 cm
4. Minimal pulmonary disease (< 5 pulmonary metastases per lung and largest < 2 cm in size with ± retroperitoneal disease < 10 cm)

Moderate Disease
5. Retroperitoneal disease > 10 cm as only anatomic site of disease
6. Moderate pulmonary metastasis (5–10 pulmonary metastases per lung and largest < 3 cm, or mediastinal mass < 50% intrathoracic diameter, or solitary pulmonary metastasis and size > 2 cm with ± retroperitoneal disease < 10 cm)

Advanced Disease
7. Advanced pulmonary metastasis (mediastinal mass > 50% intrathoracic diameter or > 10 pulmonary metastasis per lung field or pulmonary metastasis > 3 cm with ± retroperitoneal disease < 10 cm; also any NSGCT or seminoma mediastinal primary of > 50% intrathoracic diameter)
8. Retroperitoneal disease > 10 cm, plus pulmonary metastasis ± supraclavicular disease
9. Hepatic, bone, or CNS metastasis

multidisciplinary approach to successful cancer management. Early-stage disease primarily is approached surgically. Subsequent stages are treated with cisplatin-based chemotherapy with possible postsurgical resection of remaining tumor. Cisplatin-based combination chemotherapy has had a dramatic impact upon the treatment of advanced disease. This success has had a subsequent impact upon the treatment of patients with earlier disease. Stage I and early stage II disease can be managed well with primary surgery, but other options for selected patients are emerging. A discussion of the management of GCT patients follows.

Stage I

Stage I germ cell testis cancer is defined as disease that is confined to the testis (see Table 67-1). The choice of management for stage I NSGCT is one of the most controversial topics in urologic oncology. A retroperitoneal lymph node dissection (RPLND) following orchiectomy has been the time-honored approach to the treatment of testicular cancer confined to the testis. Recently, however, this approach for patients with early-stage NSGCT has been challenged.[19] Current treatment options following orchiectomy include surgery with a RPLND or surveillance.

The rationale for surgery is well grounded. RPLND in low-volume testis cancer is useful for staging because approximately 30% of patients with clinical stage I testis cancer are, in fact, pathological stage II. Surgery alone provides cure in approximately 90% of patients with pathological stage I and 70% of pathological stage II testis

Table 67-1 Testicular Cancer Staging

Stage I	Tumor limited to testes
Stage II	Tumor has spread beyond testes and involves the retroperitoneal lymph nodes
Stage III	Disseminated disease—hematological spread to lung, liver, bone, and supradiaphragmatic region

Table 67-3   Royal Marsden Hospital Staging Classification

		Seminoma	Nonseminomatous Tumors
Stage I	No evidence of metastases	Tumor confined to testes	Tumor confined to testes
Stage II	Abdominal node disease Tumor spread beyond testes	IIA disease < 2 cm diameter IIB disease 2–5 cm diameter IIC disease > 5 cm diameter	IIA < 6 LN < 2 cm diameter IIB > 6 LN > 2 cm diameter IIC massive retroperitoneal disease
Stage III	Supradiaphragmatic node metastastes	Supradiaphragmatic nodal disease	Tumors are disseminated
Stage IV	Extralymphatic metastastes	Involvement of lung, bone, and liver	

Adapted from Prow.[17]

cancer with less than 1% chance of local recurrence. Individuals who undergo a staging RPLND and are found to have pathologically negative lymph nodes are classified as pathological stage I. Ten percent of pathological stage I males will develop recurrent disease.[20] Most relapses will occur in the lungs since the lymph nodes within the retroperitoneum have been surgically removed. With close monthly follow-up during the first year and every two months of the second year, virtually all individuals who develop recurrent disease will have minimal disease, for which the cure rate with cisplatin-based chemotherapy is 99% or greater.[21] Therefore, RPLND is advantageous for two reasons: for staging and as a therapeutic modality.

The RPLND involves selection of a surgical approach to best visualize the nodal involvement. Normal abdominal surgical preparations are made preoperatively. A nasogastric tube and indwelling catheter are anchored. Central and arterial lines may be utilized to maximize feedback during and after surgery. Routine postoperative care is essential to a full recovery. Discharge is usually on the fifth postoperative day.[22] Postoperative evaluation occurs in approximately four to six weeks. Recommendations for follow-up include serum markers and chest x-rays monthly the first year, every other month the second year, every six months in years 3–5, and yearly thereafter.

The major objections to RPLND have been related to sexual dysfunction and fertility. Males who undergo full bilateral lymphadenectomy universally lose emission and the ability to ejaculate with resultant loss of fertility.[23] In an attempt to minimize ejaculatory dysfunction, "nerve-sparing" RPLND has been successfully refined. Donohue and colleagues demonstrated that the unilateral dissection is an acceptable alternative in individuals with grossly negative nodes.[24] Unilateral RPLND generally involves surgical dissection of lymph nodes on the same side as the primary lesion with limited intervention on the contralateral side. This innovation preserves the contralateral sympathetic efferent nerves and normal ejaculatory function in 75%–100% of males with testicular cancer.[25]

Because improvements in combination chemotherapy during the past 20 years have resulted in cure for most men who experience recurrent disease, the need for RPLND has been questioned.[26] The strategy of surveil-lance followed by chemotherapy for the 30% who relapse has gained acceptance. With meticulous follow-up in centers with extensive experience with testicular tumors, cure rates have approached those seen in pathological stage I disease.[26]

Selection for surveillance must be considered carefully for individuals with clinical stage I testicular cancer. Individuals must have normal serum BHCG and AFP following orchiectomy, plus normal x-rays and scans. Since it is known that approximately 30% of these individuals will relapse, primarily within the retroperitoneum, individuals selected for this approach must be highly motivated and able (logistically and psychologically) to comply with consistent lifelong follow-up.[27]

Pathological stage IIA/B

Metastasis to the retroperitoneal lymph nodes renders a patient with pathological stage II disease with either microscopic (IIA) or gross (IIB) involvement. If no additional therapy is provided to pathological stage II patients postsurgery, approximately 30% of stage IIA and 40%–50% of stage IIB will relapse.[27] Virtually all of these patients will be cured with three or four cycles of chemotherapy depending upon stage at time of recurrence. Significant improvement in relapse rates have been seen with adjuvant cisplatin-based chemotherapy. Two immediate postoperative courses of adjuvant cisplatin-based chemotherapy—usually bleomycin, etoposide, and cisplatin (BEP)—after complete resection of stage II disease prevent relapse in nearly 100% of men diagnosed with testicular cancer (Table 67-5).

Surveillance after RPLND, rather than immediate postoperative chemotherapy, is also an option for patients with pathological stage II disease. Men who ultimately recur have the same chance for survival as patients given immediate adjuvant chemotherapy.[28] The only difference is that immediate postoperative chemotherapy consists of fewer courses of therapy compared to the standard three or four courses of chemotherapy doses given to the 30% of patients who later relapse.[26] The obvious benefits of not having chemotherapy are that the 70% of patients who are cured by surgery are spared the experience as well as the long-term toxicities associated with chemotherapy.

Table 67-4 International Germ Cell Consensus Classification

Nonseminoma Tumors	Seminoma
Good Prognosis	
Testis/retroperitoneal primary	Any primary site
and	*and*
No nonpulmonary visceral metastases	No nonpulmonary visceral metastases
and	*and*
Good markers—all of AFP < 1000 ng/mL BHCG < 5000 IU/L (1000 ng/mL) LDH < 1.5 × upper limit of normal	Normal AFP, any BHCG, any LDH
Intermediate Prognosis	
Testis/retroperitoneal primary	Any primary site
and	*and*
No nonpulmonary visceral metastases	Nonpulmonary visceral metastases
and	*and*
Intermediate markers—any of AFP ≥ 100 ng/mL and ≤ 1000 ng/mL or BHCG ≥ 5000 IU/L and ≤ 50,000 IU/L or LDH ≥ 1.5 × N and ≤ 10 × N	Normal AFP, any BHCG, any LDH
Poor Prognosis	
Mediastinal primary	No patients classified as poor prognosis
or	
Nonpulmonary visceral metastases	
or	
Poor markers—any of: AFP > 10,000 ng/mL or BHCG > 50,000 IU/L (10,000 ng/mL) or LDH > 10 x upper limit of normal	

Adapted from International Germ Cell Collaborative Group.[18]

Clinical stage IIB

Those individuals who have a nonpalpable (smaller than 3 cm transverse diameter) abdominal mass visualized on CT scan traditionally will have RPLND with complete resection followed by either observation or adjuvant chemotherapy. For patients with bulkier disease, primary chemotherapy is indicated. In patients who achieve a clinical complete remission, no further therapy is indicated. If a residual mass is present following three or four

Table 67-5 Testicular Germ Cell Cancer Chemotherapy Regimens

Adjuvant Chemotherapy
  Bleomycin 30 units, weekly for 8 weeks
  Cisplatin 20 mg/m², daily for 5 days
  Etoposide 100 mg/m², daily for 5 days—every 28 days for 2 cycles

Disseminated Disease Chemotherapy (BEP)
  Bleomycin 30 units, weekly for 9–12 weeks
  Cisplatin 20 mg/m², daily for 5 days
  Etoposide 100 mg/m², daily for 5 days—every 21 days for 3–4 cycles

Salvage Chemotherapy (VeIP)
  Vinblastine 0.11 mg/kg on days 1 and 2
  Ifosfamide 1.2 gm/m², daily for 5 days plus Mesna
  Cisplatin 20 mg/m², daily for 5 days—every 21 days for 4 cycles

Relapsed: Marker positivity, with or without radiographic evidence of disease
  The preferred regimen for relapsed disease would include ABMT. High-dose chemotherapy (carboplatin and etoposide) with autologous bone marrow transplant or peripheral stem cell rescue. Some patients would receive 1–2 cycles of either BEP or VeIP prior to ABMT.

BEP: bleomycin, etoposide, cisplatin

VeIP: vinblastine, ifosfamide, cisplatin

Modified from Brock D, Fox S: Testicular germ cell cancer, in Groenwald S, Frogge M, Goodman M, Yarbro C *Cancer Nursing: Principles and Practice*, 4e; Sudbury, Jones and Bartlett, 1997.[6]

cycles of BEP, surgical resection via RPLND should be performed. The surgical finding in such cases yield necrosis (40%–45%), teratoma (40%–45%), and cancer (10%). In patients who are found to have cancer in the resected residual specimen, two additional cycles of cisplatin and etoposide (PE) should be administered.

Disseminated disease

A palpable abdominal mass with lymph nodes larger than 5 cm or involvement of more than five lymph nodes is designated as stage IIC disease. Abdominal disease of this magnitude will prohibit initial surgical resection. Metastasis above the diaphragm, involvement of visceral organs, brain, or bone is classified as stage III. Approximately 70% of men with stage III disease will achieve a complete remission. For an additional 10%–20% of patients, serum markers will normalize but radiographic abnormalities will persist and surgery is required to achieve disease-free status.[29]

In men who present with advanced or bulky disease, chemotherapy is the mainstay of treatment. Following orchiectomy, initial cisplatin-based chemotherapy is recommended for cytoreduction and potential cure. The most widely used front-line regimen is BEP (see Table 67-5), consisting of bleomycin, etoposide, and cisplatin for three to four cycles, depending on whether an individual is deemed high or low risk for recurrence.[30] Chemotherapy should always be given on schedule (every three weeks), regardless of myelosuppression, in view of the typically rapid tumor cell doubling time. Likewise, cytokines are used when indicated to avoid dose reductions. Since cisplatin is not myelosuppressive, it is rarely necessary to reduce the dose or delay treatment.

Evaluation of men with disseminated GCT treated with BEP has led to various staging systems that estimate prognosis. The Indiana University Staging System (see Table 67-2) separated those patients with minimal and moderate disease who were considered a "good risk" with a greater than 90%–99% cure rate from those individuals with advanced disease considered at "poor risk" with a 50%–60% cure rate.[31] Treatment strategies in advanced disease have focused on minimizing toxicity for men who are a good risk and investigating innovative and intensive therapy for men who are a poor risk (see Figure 67-1).[6]

Research has shown that in men presenting with minimal to moderate disease, three cycles of BEP is the chemotherapy regimen of choice (see Table 67-5). Several nonparallel studies have suggested or proven that (1) three cycles of BEP are roughly equivalent to four cycles of EP; (2) three cycles of BEP are better than three cycles of EP alone; and (3) carboplatin plus etoposide is less effective than EP.[20,28–33] If bleomycin cannot be given for medical reasons in a patient with good-risk disease, the individual should receive four cycles of EP.

The present emphasis in the initial treatment of advanced disseminated poor-risk disease is the exploration of cisplatin-intense regimens and the incorporation of new innovative agents. Intensification of therapy has included both high-dose cisplatin as well as administering all five active agents within the same regimen (i.e., VIP/VeB—etoposide, ifosfamide, cisplatin, vinblastine, bleomycin).[34] Other intensification regimens have included high-dose carboplatin and etoposide with either bone marrow transplantation or peripheral stem cell rescue.[35–37]

Although cisplatin-based chemotherapy is not without morbidity, selective 5HT-3 antagonists and other supportive care aspects have made the cisplatin-based chemotherapy utilized in testicular cancer relatively well-tolerated. While alopecia is universal, with good assessment, cisplatin-induced renal damage and bleomycin-induced lung damage are rare. Aggressive pre- and posthydration ameliorates nephrotoxicity, and careful pulmonary evaluation will pinpoint toxicity early. Due to empirical antibiotic therapy, febrile neutropenic episodes rarely occur. Thrombocytopenia is not common. Other manageable side effects may include diarrhea, mucositis, constipation/paralytic ileus, peripheral neuropathy, and hypomagnesemia.

Thirty percent of men who present with disseminated disease will require surgery postchemotherapy.[22] A postchemotherapy RPLND (PC RPLND) is indicated if a residual mass remains. Most commonly a full bilateral nodal dissection is performed with the subsequent loss of emission and antegrade ejaculation. A small percentage of men will qualify for a nerve-sparing procedure that may spare ejaculatory function. Postchemotherapy surgery patients have a higher incidence of side effects than primary RPLND patients and are usually admitted postoperatively

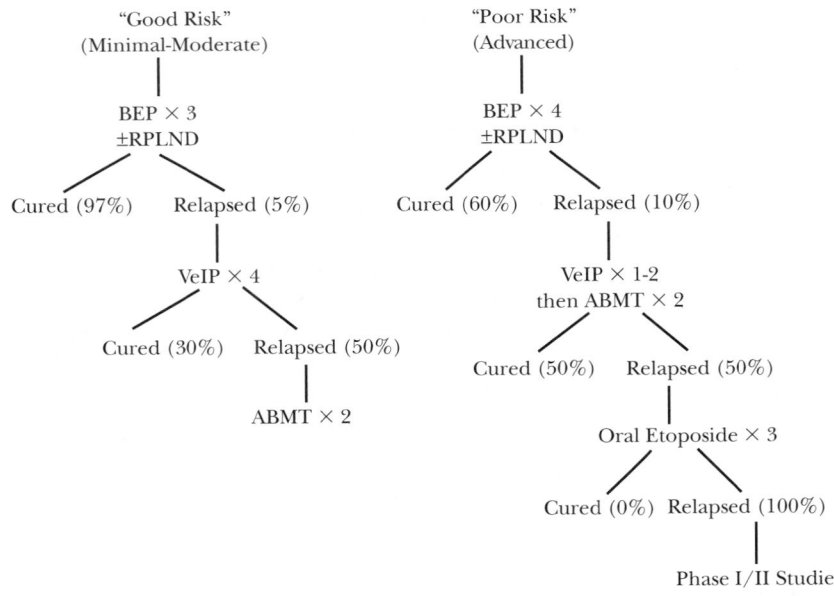

Figure 67-1 Treatment for disseminated testicular cancer. (Reprinted with permission from Brock D, Fox S: Testicular germ cell cancer. In Groenwald S, Frogge M, Goodman M, Yarbro C *Cancer Nursing: Principles and Practice,* 4e. Jones and Bartlett Publishers, Sudbury, MA 1997.)[6]

Relapsed: Marker positivity, with or without radiographic evidence of disease

ABMT: High-dose chemotherapy (carboplatin and etoposide) with autologous bone marrow transplant or peripheral stem cell rescue

BEP: bleomycin, etoposide, cisplatin

VeIP: vinblastine, ifosfamide, cisplatin

to an intensive care unit.[22] Side effects of PC RPLND include pulmonary toxicity from the combination of bleomycin and anesthesia; temporary rise in serum creatinine and tachycardia from necessary fluid restrictions; noncardiogenic pulmonary edema; and ileus.[22,38] Hospitalization usually lasts about six days. For individuals with residual disease above the diaphragm, thoracic surgery may be necessary. The scope of the thoracic surgery and potential for cure will depend on the amount and location of residual disease that is present postchemotherapy.

Late relapse testis cancer

Until recently, it has been generally accepted that if an individual were to relapse following surgical resection or chemotherapy-induced complete remission, it would occur within two years following completion of therapy. Late relapse in testicular cancer is defined as recurrence after greater than a 24-month, disease-free interval. As an increased number of case reports of late relapse appeared, retrospective analysis of several large series were undertaken in an attempt to determine the true rate of relapse.[39–43] These series consistently describe a relapse rate following a complete remission of 2%–4% with recurrences as late as 18 years. In general after surgery, individuals recurring with mature teratoma have done well. Men with marker positive neoplasms have tended to recur with bulky disease and have had a less favorable response even when surgery has been combined with chemotherapy.

Investigators at Indiana University retrospectively analyzed records of 81 men who had recurrence after two or more years.[44,45] Forty-seven percent of these men relapsed beyond five years with a median relapse of 6.2 years and the latest relapse being 32 years. Marker elevations were seen with 44 (54%) individuals having an elevated AFP and 27% an elevated BHCG. Fifteen men (19%) had a recurrence of teratoma and eight remain free of disease. Four additional men are currently disease free. Overall, 65 individuals received cisplatin-based chemotherapy and 17 (26%) achieved disease-free status with chemotherapy with or without the addition of aggressive surgery. Eleven (65%) of these 17 men have relapsed. Only two individuals treated with chemotherapy alone are presently disease free; both were chemotherapy naive. Another series demonstrated similar results, strongly suggesting that chemotherapy alone may be ineffective in patients with late relapse of GCT.[46]

The appearance of rapidly progressive, marker-positive cancer after more than two years has been puzzling. One possibility may be that residual, mature teratoma may have the ability to de-differentiate into malignant germ cell tumors after a length of time. The presence of teratoma in the original pathology may be a statistically significant predictor of late relapse. The tendency toward large-volume disease at the time of relapse may be a result of inadequate follow-up. Nurses need to educate patients that at least yearly medical evaluations should continue indefinitely for all men with a history of testicular cancer.

Seminomas

Pure seminomas account for approximately 40%–50% of all GCT of the testicles.[47] With the use of effective chemotherapy and radiotherapy, the overall cure rate for all stages is above 90%.[48] Unlike nonseminomatous testicular tumors, 80% of seminomas present as clinical stage I disease.[27] Seminomas are known to be exquisitely sensitive to radiotherapy. Both stage I and stage IIA/B are treated with external beam irradiation. Chemotherapy is the primary treatment of bulky stage IIC and disseminated disease. The management following chemotherapy remains controversial.

Stage I and IIA/B

A total dose of 25 Gy of radiotherapy is administered in 1.25–1.5 Gy daily fractions for individuals with stage I disease.[48] For stage IIA/B, a boost dose of an additional 5–10 Gy to the involved nodes with a 5-cm margin is recommended. Both anterior and posterior fields are treated. The area of treatment includes the paracaval and paraaortic nodes extending superiorly to the level of T-10/11 and extending inferiorly to include the bilateral common iliac and the ipsilateral external iliac nodes. Elective radiation to the mediastinum is no longer indicated.[49] If the scrotum has been incised at the time of orchiectomy, if tumor spill has occurred, or if positive margins are present, the radiation field may be extended to include the ipsilateral hemiscrotum. If an inguinal approach to orchiectomy is utilized, the scrotum and contralateral testis are shielded to limit scatter irradiation to the remaining testicle. The bladder is also shielded. Although surveillance may be an option following orchiectomy for stage I seminoma, excellent results with minimal side effects and morbidity make radiation the treatment of choice.

Oligospermia or azoospermia may occur as a result of radiation even when appropriate radiation shields are employed. Spermatogenesis recovery is dose dependent. Recovery of pretreatment sperm counts may occur between nine months to five years; most men recover within one year.[50] Other treatment-related side effects include mild nausea, myelosuppression, diarrhea, mild anorexia, and fatigue.

Long-term survival of more than 95% of men diagnosed with stage I disease is expected.[51–53] Eighty to ninety percent of men with evidence of retroperitoneal metastasis smaller than 5 cm (stage IIA/B) will be cured.[54]

Stage IIC

Treatment of bulky, localized retroperitoneal disease is controversial. Both chemotherapy and radiotherapy are effective. It is known that radiotherapy alone provides cure for 30%–60% of patients with stage IIC disease.[27] However, a direct correlation exists between the volume of disease and the anticipated cure rate with radiotherapy. Individuals who present with large abdominal masses (larger than 10 cm) have a high relapse rate with radiation alone. Initial combination cisplatin-based chemotherapy for men with bulky retroperitoneal disease allows for a greater than 90% cure rate.[47,48] In individuals with abdominal masses between 5–10 cm, equivalent results can be obtained with either radiotherapy or chemotherapy. A viable option may be to use chemotherapy for individuals with retroperitoneal disease greater than 5 cm and infradiaphragmatic radiation as a front-line, single-modality treatment for those individuals with less than 5-cm retroperitoneal disease, retaining chemotherapy for the 30%–40% that will eventually relapse.[27]

Stages III and IV

Initial radiotherapy for metastasis to distant sites and bulky abdominal masses produces survival rates of 20%–30% while cisplatin-based regimens will yield response rates of 60%–100%.[47,55–57] Stage IV, extranodal disease of the bone, lung, liver, or central nervous system has a cure rate of 60%–80% with chemotherapy. Bleomycin, etoposide, and cisplatin for three to four cycles in identical doses to those used in NSGCT are standard treatment (see Table 67-5).

Management of residual disease following chemotherapy remains debatable. Motzer and colleagues support biopsy following chemotherapy if the residual mass is greater than 3 cm with possible resection.[58] Other centers endorse close monthly observation versus surgery for two reasons. First, a retrospective review of patients at Indiana University revealed only a 10% incidence of significant pathological finding on biopsy with residual radiographic evidence of disease.[59] This incidence rate is identical to all patients (NSGCT and seminoma) who achieve a complete remission with chemotherapy alone. Second, following therapy a dense desmoplastic reaction may occur at the tumor site making surgery difficult, therefore increasing morbidity.[27]

Salvage Therapy in Recurrent Disease

Twenty to thirty percent of individuals will not achieve a complete remission with initial therapy, and 10% will relapse following a complete remission.[28,60,61] Men in this group are candidates for second-line or "salvage" therapy (Figure 67-1). Testicular cancer is one of the few cancers where second-line chemotherapy offers a chance of cure. Men who fail to achieve a complete response with salvage therapy have a dismal probability for long-term survival. Greater than 50% of individuals will relapse following a complete remission from salvage therapy.[62] Present therapeutic strategies for salvage treatment include chemotherapy, surgical salvage, phase II agents, and high-dose chemotherapy with bone marrow rescue.

Salvage chemotherapy

Evaluation for disease recurrence is a thought-provoking process. Occasionally individuals will be misdirected for salvage chemotherapy based on misleading radiographic evidence or rising serum markers (AFP, BHCG) that appear to demonstrate progressive disease. False elevations of serum markers due to marijuana use (BHCG), cross-reactivity with luteinizing hormone (BHCG), hepatitis (AFP), benign, growing teratoma, and pulmonary pseudonodules from bleomycin may all mimic presentation of metastatic disease. Likewise, persistent marker elevation may represent a cancer within the brain or remaining testis that can serve as sanctuary sites.

The combination of cisplatin, vinblastine (or etoposide, if not included in initial chemotherapy), and ifosfamide (VeIP) is the recommended front-line salvage regimen for recurrent disease when initial induction therapy was composed of cisplatin, etoposide (or vinblastine), and bleomycin (see Table 67-5).[63–65] This exposes the patient to two additional drugs that they have not yet seen. Loehrer and associates reported that 45% of patients achieved disease-free status and 23% remained free of disease with four cycles of VeIP.[66]

Phases I and II trials are in progress investigating agents for use in third-line chemotherapy. Oral etoposide is a schedule-dependent agent known to have activity in germ cell tumors.[67] Research has demonstrated a response in individuals who have failed to achieve a complete remission following salvage chemotherapy. Oral etoposide has also been shown to significantly prolong remission duration in men who have achieved a complete remission with salvage chemotherapy.[62,68] Recent evaluation of paclitaxel demonstrated a 26% response as second-line therapy in men who did not obtain disease-free status with six or less prior cycles of primary chemotherapy. VIP/VeB (etoposide, ifosfamide, cisplatin, vinblastine, and bleomycin) in combination is being investigated. Both paclitaxel and gemcitabine have minimal activity in recurrent GCT.

Surgical salvage

Individuals with persistently elevated serum markers, indicative of persistent viable disease following salvage chemotherapy, have not usually been considered surgical candidates because of the presumed systemic nature of the disease. However, some of these men do have locoregional tumors amenable to resection.[69] Approximately 20% of carefully selected individuals achieve long-term survival with salvage surgery.[63] Salvage surgeries should be performed at centers with significant experience with GCT management.

High-Dose Chemotherapy with Rescue

Individuals who recur following salvage chemotherapy or who do not respond to first-line cisplatin therapy are considered cisplatin-refractory. These individuals are incurable by standard chemotherapy. Autologous bone marrow and/or peripheral blood stem cell rescue in conjunction with high-dose chemotherapy have been and continue to be investigated in this population. High-dose chemotherapy has been found to offer a better response than conventional chemotherapy.

Initially researchers explored the use of etoposide in high doses without cisplatin.[70,71] Etoposide was investigated in high dosages for the treatment of testicular cancer primarily because of efficacy, but also for its manageable side effects. Although complete responses occurred with etoposide alone, remissions were brief and no overall improvement in survival was seen.

Subsequent research underscored the importance of combining etoposide with cisplatin due to synergy between the two drugs. Pico and colleagues demonstrated a continuous complete response in 31% of men with recurrent GCT using high-dose etoposide, cisplatin, and cyclophosphamide.[72] Unfortunately cisplatin, the most active agent in testicular cancer, is poorly suited to dose intensity due to the known side effects of nephrotoxicity and ototoxicity. Therefore, carboplatin, a second-generation platinum analog, is better suited for dose intensification because its toxicity is largely confined to myelosuppression. A number of preclinical and clinical studies suggested similar antitumor activity of carboplatin and cisplatin.[73] In 1989 Nichols and associates reported responses to high-dose etoposide and carboplatin in 14 of 33 men, including eight complete remissions and three men obtaining continuous disease-free survival for greater than one year.[65] All eligible individuals had extensive prior therapy and two-thirds were cisplatin-refractory. Other investigators at Indiana University have subsequently provided long-term follow-up for 40 individuals.[74,75] Overall, 60% of those men achieved an objective response with 30% in complete remission. Fifteen percent of the complete responders achieved and remained in remission beyond two years. A large national study confirmed these responses.[76]

A logical next step has been to incorporate high-dose chemotherapy with rescue earlier in the treatment of poor-risk individuals. Seigert and colleagues treated 55 men with conventional cisplatin, etoposide, and ifosfamide before initiating high-dose carboplatin.[77] Thirty-eight percent of individuals responded with disease-free survivals of 3–26 months. Motzer and associates reported the use of two to three cycles of VAB-6 (bleomycin, cyclophosphamide, actinomycin D, vinblastine, cisplatin) followed by high-dose carboplatin and etoposide with bone marrow support, with 56% obtaining a complete response.[78]

It is established that a small but definite cure rate exists for heavily pretreated, refractory individuals. However, it remains unclear whether high-dose chemotherapy will become a part of standard initial therapy in poor-risk individuals with testicular cancer.[79]

Sanctuary Sites

In advanced testis cancer, the central nervous system (CNS) and contralateral testicle are the most common sanctuary sites.[27] CNS metastasis, whether it is present at diagnosis or as a manifestation of relapse, is approached with curative intent. Chemotherapy poorly penetrates the blood-brain barrier. Whole-brain radiation therapy of 50 Gy over five weeks in combination with chemotherapy for systemic disease is recommended for individuals with CNS metastasis and disseminated disease. Those individuals relapsing with a single CNS focus without evidence of systemic relapse undergo resection followed by radiotherapy and two postoperative cisplatin-based chemotherapy regimens. Occult CNS metastases should be suspected if, in the presence of chest/abdominal radiological remission following therapy, new elevations or persistent tumor markers are present. In this situation, CT scan or magnetic resonance imaging (MRI) of the brain should be obtained even in the absence of clinical symptoms.

It is questionable if chemotherapy penetrates the testicle, which is why the testicle has long been considered a sanctuary site for tumor cells. Normally the testis primary tumor is surgically resected prior to treatment. In the presence of advanced disseminated disease and positive tumor markers, however, chemotherapy may be initiated prior to a tissue diagnosis. At the completion of chemotherapy the involved testis is removed. Whenever markers remain elevated following removal of the involved testicle (in the absence of radiographic evidence of disease) a second testis primary should be investigated.

Symptom Management and Supportive Care

The time of diagnosis and initiation of treatment are stressful. Education must begin early. Careful explanations of the nature of the disease, its treatment, goal of therapy, and side effects are essential.[79] Information must be provided and reinforced at various intervals along the treatment continuum. The patient's and family's anxiety levels may be elevated from perceived and real threats of mortality, alterations in life roles, and sexual identity, all of which require specialized attention. Consistent evaluations of the patient and family knowledge deficits are necessary to effectively provide educational interventions.

Surgery

An inguinal orchiectomy is performed as an outpatient procedure for both diagnostic and therapeutic purposes—to establish a histological diagnosis and to remove the tumor. Nursing interventions should focus on postoperative teaching regarding pain management, activity level, and incisional wound care. Individuals and family need to learn how to change the dry, sterile dressing and to recognize and report signs of infection and unusual bleeding. Men need to understand that neither sexual function nor fertility will be impaired or changed as a result of the orchiectomy. However, alterations in body image may result. Supportive interventions may be indicated to improve coping.

Care of the individual undergoing an RPLND, outside of the issues of fertility, is similar to other abdominal surgeries. However, for the person who has had chemotherapy, RPLND is associated with specific side effects, namely, adult respiratory syndrome with pulmonary fluid overload, ileus, and fertility issues. Each of these potential complications is specifically addressed in the following sections.

Pulmonary complications

Men who have received bleomycin at a cumulative dose of greater than 200 mg/m² are at greater risk of pulmonary fibrosis with subsequent respiratory failure or death during the postoperative recovery period.[80] Individuals with even mild bleomycin toxicity demonstrate to some degree arterial oxygen desaturation with high concentrations of inspired oxygen and an abnormal carbon monoxide diffusion capacity.[81] Special precautions are taken prior to surgery to safeguard patients, including baseline pulmonary function test, careful physical exam, radiographic imaging of the lungs, and alerting the anesthesiologist.

The day before surgery, individuals begin a clear liquid diet with nothing by mouth permitted after midnight. Intravenous fluid consisting of 50 cc/hour of synthetic volume expander and 25 cc/hour of D_5 1/2 NS begin before surgery. To minimize bleomycin lung toxicity, rigid fluid restrictions imposed during surgery and a reduction in inspired oxygen during surgery to an FiO_2 of 0.24 has been shown to prevent mortality.[80] Fluid restrictions continue postoperatively. However, following surgery 150–200 cc/hour of ice chips are usually allowed. A clear liquid diet is introduced when bowel sounds have been auscultated. Intravenous fluids are gradually decreased.

As a result of fluid restrictions, transient elevations of the serum creatinine and sinus tachycardia may occur. Kidney function is assessed through close monitoring of laboratory values, intake and output, and daily weight. Auscultation is routinely performed to assess cardiac function. Pulmonary function tests have been shown to return to baseline normal a median of four years after treatment.[82]

Gastrointestinal complications

Paralytic ileus, a common side effect of abdominal surgery, may be prolonged for two to four days after an RPLND depending on the extent of the abdominal resection performed and length of time under anesthesia. Men are started on a clear liquid diet the day before surgery and undergo bowel preparation usually consisting of ingesting magnesium citrate or a full mechanical bowel preparation. A nasogastric tube is placed during surgery and will remain in place until normal bowel sounds are present. After auscultation of normal bowel sounds, a clear liquid diet will be initiated, advancing to a regular diet as tolerated.

Fertility

The traditional bilateral RPLND results in the loss of antegrade ejaculation with resultant infertility from retrograde ejaculation. The ability to experience a normal orgasm is not impaired. Nerve-sparing modifications to the classic RPLND has steadily increased postoperative ejaculatory rates with virtually all patients maintaining ejaculatory function. Ninety-eight percent of men undergoing nerve-sparing RPLND will have fertility comparable to the preoperative state. Awareness and sensitivity to the individual's and family's educational needs and initiating appropriate interventions to provide for psychosocial adjustment to the real or possible fertility changes will promote coping and acceptance. Sperm banking prior to initiation of treatment may be an option depending on the stage of disease and sperm count at diagnosis. Sperm banking can take weeks to obtain sufficient viable sperm. Men need to be understand the risks of treatment delay, the cost of sperm collection, storage, and potential costs of reproductive assistance (e.g., in vitro fertilization (IVF)) if needed. Because of the aggressive nature of the disease, sperm banking may not be a viable option for some men due to their urgent need for therapy.

Radiation

The resultant toxicities of abdominal radiotherapy for testicular cancer are less severe than in the past due to lower effective doses, improved equipment, and computerized axial tomographic planning.[83] Sequelae that may be problematic include diarrhea, fatigue, nausea, fertility issues, myelosuppression, and occasionally, bladder irritation and peptic ulcers.

Gastrointestinal complications

Radiation to the abdominal and pelvic regions can cause diarrhea. Individuals should be instructed to manage radiation-associated diarrhea with a low-residue diet and over-the-counter antidiarrheals but to seek medical attention if diarrhea continues despite these interventions. Prescriptive antidiarrheal medication is often required to manage radiation-related diarrhea. A low-residue diet may be helpful and is designed to reduce the amount of fiber in the intestinal tract by restricting indigestible carbohydrates such as milk products, high fat-content foods, fruit and vegetables with seeds or skins, and high-fiber breads.

Unlike radiation to other parts of the body, nausea and vomiting are not unusual with the first radiotherapy treatment. Oral antiemetics administered one hour prior to the radiotherapy treatment and as needed usually control the associated mild nausea and vomiting.[84] Serotonin 5HT-3 antagonists used in combination with a steroid may be useful. Light meals prior to treatment should be encouraged.

Fertility

Radiotherapy does not effect libido or potency but can lead to impairment of spermatogenesis.[85] During radiotherapy gonad shields are in place; however, scatter radiation can occur to the remaining testis, decreasing sperm production or resulting in azoospermia.[86] Individuals and families need to know that recovery to pretreatment sperm levels may take 9–18 months or as long as five years.[87] The opportunity for sperm banking may be appropriate prior to radiation therapy.

Myelosuppression

Radiation to the paraaortic lymph nodes and the pelvis often produces myelosuppression. Weekly complete blood counts with differential and platelets are monitored. Acute complications are uncommon. Information should be provided on the importance of seeking medical assistance for fever when neutropenia is present. Instruction should be provided to avoid medication that could potentially mask a fever. Individuals should be made aware that fatigue may interfere with normal activities. Pacing activities and frequent rest periods will help the patient cope with fatigue. Also, instructions should be given to call the physician's office if bruising or unusual bleeding occurs since these could be a sign of thrombocytopenia, although transfusion is rarely performed.

Between 4%–10% of individuals will experience dyspepsia with radiotherapy.[88] Frequent small, low-fat meals, avoiding meals and snacks within one hour of bedtime, and the use of antacids may provide relief from dyspepsia. However, the use of over-the-counter antacids needs to be monitored since medical intervention for an active gastric ulcer may be indicated.[89]

Chemotherapy

The side effects of chemotherapy are specific to the drug combinations and the dosages administered, the volume of disease present, and history of prior therapy. Nursing management can best be approached with awareness and anticipation of potential side effects (Table 67-6).[90-98]

Psychosexual Issues and Counseling

Assessment and management of the reproductive and sexual concerns of cancer patients should be a routine part of nursing care, yet many nurses are reluctant to address these issues.[99] During diagnosis and treatment, concerns about future fertility are likely to be of secondary importance to survival.[100] Research indicates that the biological inability to father a child presents a serious challenge to a man's perception of his masculinity, his self-

esteem, and his intimate relationships.[101,102] Counseling men with GCT about therapeutic options to maintain their reproductive potential prior to treatment is a professional, ethical, and legal responsibility of health care professionals.[99] Recent technological advances in reproductive medicine, such as IVF, have made pregnancies possible even when sperm counts and motility are very low.

In addition to concerns about fertility, men are likely to be affected by the impact of the GCT diagnosis and treatment, and by the altered body image that results from treatment.[103] Long-term effects on sexual functioning also have been documented. Results of a study of 223 survivors at one year postdiagnosis indicated that 30% of patients reported distress about their sexual performance, 10% had erectile dysfunction, and 6% were anorgasmic.[102] In another study of 121 men, 11% were not sexually active at all, 9% were sexually active less than once per month, 10% reported erectile dysfunction, and 38% reported decreased pleasure at orgasm. Assessing sexual functioning and addressing these issues by providing appropriate counseling and referral is an important aspect of comprehensive care for these patients.

Partners and families of men with GCT also are likely to experience significant distress. At diagnosis and during treatment, partners and family members will have immediate fears about potential loss of the patient through death and concerns about the future. At any point during or after treatment, partners may have concerns about sexual activity. Misconceptions about "catching" the cancer through sexual contact or fear of hurting their partner during sex may exist, and partners may be hesitant to ask questions. Assessing and meeting the informational needs of families and partners of GCT patients is a nursing responsibility.

Continuity of Care: Nursing Challenges

Germ cell cancer is unique, compared to other cancers, in that recurrence is highly treatable and the efficacy of treatment is related to the volume of disease at the time of recurrence.[104] Surveillance and follow-up after GST treatment is necessary for the remainder of the patient's life.[105] As the cure rate for GST approaches 100%, patient adherence to surveillance recommendations will significantly affect overall mortality from this disease. Health care providers have experience with patients who refuse therapies or fail to comply with follow-up visits and eventually die from their disease.[106] Nurses can contribute to improving patient adherence by effectively educating them regarding their diagnosis, treatment options, and outcomes. Additional research is needed in this area to enhance our understanding of factors contributing to patient nonadherence to surveillance recommendations.

The nurse's role in early detection of GCT by providing community health education regarding testicular self-examination was mentioned earlier in this chapter. The

Table 67-6   Nursing Care and Educational Needs of Patients Receiving Chemotherapy for Testicular Cancer

Problem	Drug(s)	Nursing Interventions
Nausea/vomiting	Cisplatin Ifosfamide	• Administer prophylactic antiemetics with 5 HT-3 antagonist and high-dose dexamethasone[90] • Write down schedule for antiemetics regimen • Encourage and maintain adequate fluid intake • Consider supplemental IV hydration • Consider the use of music and relaxation therapy[91,92]
Constipation	Vinblastine Etoposide	• Assess bowel function prior to giving drug • Encourage fluids and teach high-fiber diet • Monitor bowel sounds • Instruct patient to report significant bowel changes • Administer stool softeners and laxatives
Myelosuppression	Ifosfamide Vinblastine Etoposide	• Monitor complete blood count • Instruct patient to report signs of infection, fever, bleeding, shortness of breath, severe weakness, tachycardia • Instruct patient on avoiding crowds and individuals with active infections, bleeding precautions, and good hand-washing technique • Inform patients with advanced disease that blood/platelet transfusions may be necessary • Monitor incisions, wounds, catheter, sites for infection • Obtain blood and urine cultures, chest x-ray prior to administering antibiotics • Administer antibiotics as prescribed or instruct patient to take the full course of the antibiotics
Nephrotoxicity	Cisplatin Ifosfamide	• Monitor serum electrolytes, creatinine and BUN daily intake and output[93] • Provide aggressive pre- and posthydration and increase oral intake • Avoidance of aminoglycosides for the treatment of granulocytopenic fever when receiving cisplatin[94]
Hemorrhagic Cystitis	Ifosfamide	• Obtain urinalysis daily; if >10 RBCs per high-powered field, alert physician and hold drug • Provide aggressive pre- and posthydration and instruct patient to increase oral intake • Administer Mesna, a uroprotectant, as directed
Integumentary changes	Ifosfamide Bleomycin Etoposide	• Prepare patient for hair loss, reinforcing its temporary nature[95] • Alert patient regarding skin hyperpigmentation and nail changes
Reproduction	Cisplatin Etoposide Bleomycin Ifosfamide Vinblastine	• Arrange for sperm banking if possible prior to chemotherapy • Reinforce that ejaculation/impotence will not change • Inform patients of azoospermia for at least 12 months with normal spermatogenesis returning in 50% of men within 2 years. Those treated with 3–4 cycles of BEP are at higher risk for persistent semen abnormalities.[16,21,96–98]
Neurological changes	Cisplatin Vinblastine Bleomycin	• Instruct reporting of numbness and tingling of hands and feet (i.e., Raynaud phenomenon) • Inform patients to wear gloves and dress warmly in cold weather • Instruct patients to report hearing changes[94] • Obtain baseline and serial audiometry for high-risk patients (i.e., > 50 years, total dose of > 400 mg cisplatin, abnormal renal function)[79,94]
Pulmonary complications	Bleomycin	• Assess for bibasilar rates, inspirational lag, and cough[16,22] • Evaluate men at high risk for fibrosis (i.e., smokers, decreased renal function, previous chest irradiation, and > 450 units of bleomycin)[16,96,98]
Body image changes		• Encourage patient to verbalize feelings about hair loss and changes in appearance • Teach patient self-care activities related to body image disturbance • Reinforce any attempts to attend to the body part • Reinforce any verbalizations of feelings about actual or perceived loss • Provide consultation with hair stylist or barber

Adapted from Brock et al.[6,22]

importance of educating GCT patients about their need to regularly perform TSE also is essential. Men who have testicular cancer in one testis are 500 times more likely to develop cancer in the contralateral testis. Contralateral testicular tumors have been found up to 25 years after the initial diagnosis, and the majority of these are found by TSE.[107]

The recent changes in health care delivery have modified certain aspects in the approach of care for testicular cancer. The shift from inpatient to primarily outpatient chemotherapy, the role of managed health care, the continued shortening of inpatient hospitalization following surgery, and the increasingly important role of home care has affected how care is provided to the individual with testicular cancer. A plan of care that can be individualized to identify specific patient issues, organize care, shorten planning time, and better utilize nursing time is essential. Management protocols developed for testicular cancer are a potentially useful method to manage individual needs within a multidisciplinary framework, to identify outcomes and necessary resources, and to direct interventions within the expected time frame. Pathways can be utilized by nursing, medicine, and support staff for specific aspects of treatment or across the health care continuum to provide individualized care that strikes a balance between quality care and cost-saving efficiency.[89]

Within these pathways health professionals need to integrate community resources that provide support to patients and families, not only to assist with coping but also for transportation, child care, and financial assistance for individuals in need of such assistance.

Home care can be of assistance with management of hydration including assessment of fluid intake and output, with phlebotomy to monitor lab results, with monitoring nausea and vomiting, with wound care, and with discharge postsurgery that may include administration of antibiotics. With the continued need for cost containment and the advent of managed care, home care nurses may experience a more primary role in treatment and education. Hospice in the home environment is a preferable option for those with terminal disease.

Conclusion

Although testicular cancer is a rare and devastating disease to the young population it affects, it also is one of the most highly curable malignancies. Testicular self-exam remains the best available tool for early diagnosis and treatment. Most males today can be successfully treated with adverse side effects vastly improved over therapy available 20 years ago. The high cure rate of testicular cancer can be attributed to dedicated clinical researchers who utilize combination modalities such as surgery, chemotherapy, radiation therapy, and bone marrow transplantation in the treatment of testicular cancer. Researchers continue to look for ways to improve current treatment modalities.

References

1. Landis SH, Murray T, Bolden S, et al: Cancer Statistics, 1998. *Ca Cancer J Clin* 48:10, 1998
2. Scher H, Bosl G, Geller N, et al: Impact of symptomatic interval on prognosis of patients with stage III testicular cancer. *Urology* 21:559–561, 1983
3. Bosl GJ, Vogelzang NJ, Goldman A, et al: Impact of delay in diagnosis on clinical stage of testicular cancer. *Lancet* 2:970–973, 1981
4. Bosl GJ, Bajorin D, Sheinfeld J, et al: Cancer of the testis, in DeVita VT, Hellman S, Rosenberg S (eds): *Cancer: Principles and Practice of Oncology* (ed 5). Philadelphia, Lippincott, 1997, pp 1397–1425
5. Bosl GJ, Motzer RJ: Testicular germ-cell cancer. *N Engl J Med* 337:242–253, 1997
6. Brock DL, Fox SM: Testicular germ cell cancer, in Groenwald S, Frogge M, Goodman M, Yarbro C (eds): *Cancer Nursing: Principles and Practice* (ed 4), Sudbury, MA, Jones and Bartlett, 1997, pp 1374–1389
7. Montie JE: Carcinoma in situ of the testis and bilateral carcinoma. *Urol Clin North Am* 20:127–132, 1993
8. Dieckmann KP, Boeckmann W, Brosig W, et al: Bilateral testicular germ cell tumors. *Cancer* 51:1254–1258, 1986
9. Nichols CR, Heerema NA, Palmer C, et al: Klinefelter's syndrome associated with mediastinal germ cell neoplasms. *J Clin Oncol* 5:1290–1294,1987
10. Chaganti RSK, Rodriquez E, Bosl GJ: Cytogenetics of male germ-cell tumors. *Urol Clin North Am* 20:55–66, 1993
11. Murty VVS, Chaganti RSK: A genetic perspective of male germ cell tumors. *Semin Oncol* 25:133–144, 1998
12. Cosgrove M, Benton B, Henderson B: Male genitourinary abnormalities and maternal diethylstilbesterol. *Urology* 117:220–222, 1977
13. Depue R, Pike M, Henderson B: Estrogen exposure during gestation and the risk of testicular cancer. *J Natl Cancer Inst* 71:1151–1155, 1983
14. Gill W, Schumaker G, Bibbo M: Structural and functional abnormalities in the sex organs of male offspring of mothers treated with DES. *Reprod Med* 16:147–153, 1976
15. Stephenson WT, Poirier SM, Rubin L, et al: Evaluation of reproductive capacity in germ cell tumor patients following treatment with cisplatin, etoposide, and bleomycin. *J Clin Oncol* 13:2278–2280, 1995
16. Horwich A: Testicular germ cell tumors: an introductory overview, in Horwich A (ed): *Testicular Cancer—Investigation and Management* (ed 2). New York: Chapman and Hall, 1996, pp 1–17
17. Prow DM: Germ cell tumors: staging, prognosis and outcome. *Semin Urol Oncol* 16:82–93, 1998
18. International Germ Cell Cancer Collaborative Group: International Germ Cell Consensus Classification: a prognostic factor-based staging system for metastatic germ cell cancers. *J Clin Oncol* 15:594–603, 1997
19. Donahue J, Thornhill R, Foster R, et al: Retroperitoneal lymphadenectomy for clinical stage A testis cancer (1965 to 1989): modifications of technique and impact on ejaculation. *J Urol* 149:237–243, 1993
20. Loehrer P: Testicular cancer, in Carbone P, Brain M (eds): *Current Therapy in Hematology-Oncology* (ed 4). Philadelphia: Dekker, 1992, pp 300–305
21. Roth B, Griest A, Kubilis P, et al: Cisplatin-based chemo-

therapy for disseminated germ cell tumors: long term follow-up. *J Clin Oncol* 6:1239–1247, 1988

22. Brock D, Fox S, Gosling G, et al: Testicular cancer. *Semin Oncol Nurs* 9:224–236, 1993

23. Donohue J, Rowland R: Complications of retroperitoneal lymphadenectomy. *J Urol* 125:338–340, 1981

24. Donohue J, Zachary J, Maynard B: Distribution of nodal metastasis in nonseminomatous testis cancer. *J Urol* 128:315–320, 1982

25. Donohue J, Foster R, Rowland R, et al: Nerve sparing retroperitoneal lymphadenectomy with preservation of ejaculation. *J Urol* 144:287–292, 1990

26. Foster R, Roth B: Clinical stage I nonseminoma: surgery versus surveillance. *Semin Oncol* 25:145–153, 1998

27. Roth B, Nichols C, Einhorn L: Neoplasms of the testis, in Holland J, Frei E, Bast R, Kufe D, Morton D, Weichselbaum R (eds): *Cancer Medicine,* vol 2 (ed 3). Philadelphia, Lea and Febiger, 1993, pp 1592–1619

28. Einhorn L, Williams S, Loehrer P, et al: Evaluation of optimal duration of chemotherapy in favorable prognosis disseminated germ cell tumors: a Southeastern Cancer Study Group protocol. *J Clin Oncol* 7:387–391, 1989

29. Keller J, Sahasrabudhe D, McCune C: Urologic and male genital cancers, in Rubin P (ed): *Clinical Oncology* (ed 7). Philadelphia, Saunders, 1993, pp 442–453

30. Sturgeon J, Herman J, Jewlett M, et al: A policy for surveillance alone after orchiectomy for stage I nonseminomatous testis tumors. *Proc Am Soc Clin Oncol* 4:1199, 1986 (abstr)

31. Loehrer P, Ahlering T, Pollack A: Testicular Cancer, in Pazdur R, Coia L, Hoskins W, Wagman L (eds): *Cancer Management: A Multidisciplinary Approach* (ed 1). Huntington, NY, PRR, 1996, pp 401–416

32. Levi J, Raghavan D, Harvey V, et al: Deletion of bleomycin from therapy for good prognosis advanced testicular cancer. *Proc Am Soc Clin Oncol* 5:97, 1986 (abstr)

33. Schmoll H, Schubert I, Arnold H, et al: Disseminated bulky disease: results of a phase II study with cisplatin/ultra high dose/VP-16/Bleomycin. *Int J Androl* 10:311–317, 1987

34. Loehrer P, Johnson D, Elson P, et al: Importance of bleomycin in favorable prognosis disseminated germ cell tumors: an Eastern Oncology Group study. *J Clin Oncol* 13:470–476, 1995

35. Droz J, Pico J, Ghosen M, et al: High complete remission and survival rates in poor prognosis nonseminomatous germ cell tumors with high-dose chemotherapy and autologous bone marrow transplant. *Proc Am Soc Clin Oncol* 8:130, 1989 (abstr)

36. Horwich A, Brada M, Nicholls J, et al: Intensive induction chemotherapy for poor risk nonseminomatous germ cell tumors. *Eur J Clin Oncol* 25:177, 1989

37. Wettlaufer J, Feiner A, Robinson W: Vincristine, cisplatin, and bleomycin with surgery in the management of advanced metastatic nonseminomatous testis tumors. *Cancer* 53:203–209, 1984

38. Bihrle R, Donahue J, Foster, R: Complications of retroperitoneal lymph node dissection. *Urol Clin North Am* 15:237–242, 1988

39. Terebelo H, Taylor G, Brown A, et al: Late relapse of testicular cancer. *J Clin Oncol* 1:566–571, 1983

40. Lianes P, Paz-Ares L, Rivera F, et al: Late recurrence in malignant germ cell tumors. *Ann Oncol* 3:165, 1992 (suppl 5)

41. Deleo M, Greco F, Hainsworth J, et al: Late recurrence in long-term survivors of germ cell neoplasms. *Cancer* 62:985–988, 1988

42. Chabner B, Cannellos G, Olweny C, et al: Late recurrence of testicular tumors. *N Engl J Med* 287:413, 1972

43. Blom J: Late recurrence of testicular tumor. *J Urol* 112:211, 1974

44. Nichols C, Baniel J, Foster R: Late relapse of germ cell tumors. *Proc Am Soc Clin Oncol* 13:1994 (abstr 497)

45. Baniel J, Foster R, Gonin R, et al: Late relapse of testicular cancer. *J Clin Oncol* 13:1170–1176, 1995

46. Gerl A, Clemm C, Hartenstein R, et al: Late relapse of nonseminomatous germ cell tumors (NSGCT) after cisplatin-based chemotherapy. *Proc Am Soc Clin Oncol* 13:229, 1994 (abstr)

47. Richie J: Detection and treatment of testicular cancer. *CA Cancer J Clin* 43:151–175, 1993

48. Hanks G, Peters T, Owen P: Seminoma of the testis: long-term beneficial and deleterious effects. *Int J Radiat Oncol Bio Phys* 24:913–919, 1992

49. Thomas G, Rider W, Dembo A, et al: Seminomas of the testis: results of treatment patterns and failures after radiation therapy. *Int J Radiat Oncol Bio Phys* 8:165–174, 1982

50. Bracken R: Cancer of the testis, penis and urethra: the impact of therapy on sexual function, in von Eschenbach A, Rodriguez D (eds): *Sexual Rehabilitation of the Urological Cancer Patient.* Boston, Hall, 1981, pp 108–127

51. Calman F, Peckman M, Hendy W: The pattern of spread and the treatment of metastases in testicular seminomas. *Br J Urol* 51:154–160, 1979

52. Cavelli F, Klepp O, Renard J, et al: A phase II study on oral VP-16-213 in nonseminomatous testis cancer. *Eur J Cancer* 17:245–249, 1981

53. Cavelli F, Sonntag R, Brunner K: Epipodophyllotoxin derivative (VP-16-213) in the treatment of solid tumors. *Lancet* 2:362, 1977

54. Gregory C, Peckman M: Results of radiotherapy for stage II testicular seminoma. *Radiother Oncol* 6:285–292, 1986

55. Einhorn L, Williams S: Chemotherapy of disseminated seminoma. *Cancer Clin Trials* 3:307–313, 1980

56. Vugrin D, Whitmore W, Batata M: Chemotherapy of disseminated seminoma with combination platinum and cyclophosphamide. *Cancer Clin Trials* 4:423–427, 1981

57. Wajsman Z, Beckley S, Pontes J: Changing concepts in the treatment of advanced seminomatous tumors. *J Urol* 129:303–306, 1983

58. Motzer R, Bosl G, Heelan R, et al: Residual Mass: an indication for further therapy in patients with advanced seminoma following chemotherapy. *J Clin Oncol* 5:1064–1070, 1987

59. Schulz S, Einhorn L, Conces D, et al: Management of postchemotherapy residual mass in patients with advanced seminoma. *J Clin Oncol* 7:1497–1503, 1989

60. Einhorn LH: Treatment of testicular cancer: a new and improved model. *J Clin Oncol* 8:1777–1781, 1990

61. Nichols C, Williams S, Loehrer P, et al: Randomized study of cisplatin dose intensity in poor risk germ cell tumors: a Southeastern Cancer Study Group and Southwest Oncology Group protocol. *J Clin Oncol* 9:1163–1172, 1991

62. Cooper M, Einhorn L: Maintenance chemotherapy with daily oral etoposide following salvage therapy in patients with germ cell tumors. *J Clin Oncol* 13:1167–1169, 1995

63. Einhorn LH: Salvage therapy for germ cell tumors. *Semin Oncol* 21:47–51, 1994

64. Motzer R, Cooper K, Geller N, et al: The role of ifosfamide plus cisplatin-based chemotherapy as salvage therapy for

patients with refractory germ cell tumors. *Cancer* 66: 2476–2481, 1990

65. Nichols C, Tricot G, Williams S, et al: Dose intensive chemotherapy in refractory germ cell cancer—a phase I–II trial of high dose carboplatin and etoposide with autologous bone marrow transplantation. *J Clin Oncol* 7:932–939, 1989

66. Loehrer PJ, Gonin R, Nichols CR, et al: Vinblastine plus ifosfamide plus cisplatin as initial salvage therapy in recurrent germ cell tumor. *J Clin Oncol* 16:2500–2504, 1998

67. Williams S, Einhorn L, Greco F, et al: Salvage chemotherapy for refractory germinal neoplasms. *Cancer* 46: 2154–2158, 1980

68. Miller J, Einhorn L: Phase II study of daily oral etoposide in refractory germ cell tumors. *Semin Oncol* 17:36–39, 1990

69. Murphy B, Breeden E, Donohue J, et al: Surgical salvage of chemo-refractory germ cell tumors. *J Clin Oncol* 11: 324–329, 1993

70. Mulder P, DeVries E, Koops H, et al: Chemotherapy with maximal tolerated doses of VP-16-213 and cyclophosphamide followed by autologous bone marrow transplantation for the treatment of relapsed or refractory germ cell tumors. *Eur J Cancer Clin Oncol* 24:675–679, 1988

71. Wolff S, Hohnson D, Hainsworth J, et al: High dose VP-16-213 monotherapy for refractory germinal malignancies: a phase II study. *J Clin Oncol* 2:271–274, 1984

72. Pico J, Droz J, Gouyette A, et al: 25 high dose chemotherapy regimens (HDCR) followed by autologous bone marrow transplantation (ABMT) in refractory or relapsed nonseminomatous germ cell tumors. *Proc Am Soc Clin Oncol* 5:111, 1986 (abstr)

73. Saxman S: Salvage chemotherapy in recurrent testicular cancer. *Semin Oncol* 19:143–147, 1992

74. Broun E, Tricot G, Fox E, et al: Long-term follow-up of salvage chemotherapy in relapse and refractory germ cell tumors using high dose carboplatin and etoposide with autologous bone marrow transplant. *Proc Am Soc Clin Oncol* 10:167, 1991 (abstr)

75. Broun R, Nichols C, Kneebone P, et al: Long term outcome of patients with relapsed and refractory germ cell tumors treated with high dose chemotherapy and bone marrow rescue. *Ann Intern Med* 117:124–128, 1992

76. Nichols C, Anderson J, Lazarus H, et al: High dose carboplatin and etoposide with autologous bone marrow transplantation in refractory germ cell cancer: an Eastern Cooperative Oncology Group protocol. *J Clin Oncol* 10: 558–563, 1992

77. Siegert W, Beyer J, Wersback V, et al: High dose carboplatin, etoposide, ifosfamide with autologous stem cell rescue for relapsed and refractory nonseminomatous germ cell tumors. *Proc Am Soc Clin Oncol* 10:163, 1991 (abstr)

78. Motzer R, Gulati S, Crown J, et al: High dose chemotherapy and autologous bone marrow rescue for patients with refractory germ cell tumors: early intervention is better tolerated. *Cancer* 69:550–559, 1992

79. Higgs DJ: The patient with testicular cancer: nursing management of chemotherapy. *Oncol Nurs Forum* 17:243–246, 1990

80. Goldiner P, Carlon G, Critkovic E, et al: Factors influencing postoperative morbidity and mortality in patients treated with bleomycin. *Br Med J* 1:1664, 1978

81. Lazo J, Chabner B: Bleomycin, in Chabner B, Longo D (eds): *Cancer Chemotherapy and Biotherapy: Principles and Practice* (ed 2). Philadelphia, Lippincott-Raven, 1996, pp 379–393

82. Osanto S, Bukman A, Van Hoek F, et al: Long-term effect of chemotherapy in patients with testicular cancer. *J Clin Oncol* 10:574–579, 1992

83. Boyer M, Raghavan D: Toxicity of germ cell tumors. *Semin Oncol* 19:128–142, 1992

84. Strohl R: Symptom management of acute and chronic reactions. *Oncol Nurs Forum* 15:429–434, 1988

85. Lind J, Irwin R: Genitourinary cancer, in Baird S, McCorkle R, Grant M (eds): *Cancer Nursing: A Comprehensive Textbook.* Philadelphia, Saunders, 1991, pp 477–480

86. Einhorn L, Richie J, Shipley W: Cancer of the testis, in DeVita VT, Hellman S, Rosenberg SA (eds): *Cancer: Principles and Practices of Oncology* (ed 4). Philadelphia, Lippincott, 1993, pp 1126–1151

87. Fossa S, Ous S, Abyholm T, et al: Post treatment fertility in patients with testicular cancer. *Br J Urol* 57:210–214, 1985

88. Marks L, Ansher M, Shipley W: Radiation therapy for testicular seminoma: controversies in the management of early stage disease. *Oncology* 6:43–52, 1991

89. Lyons J: Models of nursing care delivery and case management: clarification of terms. *Nurs Econ* 11:163–169, 1993

90. Fox S, Einhorn L, Cox E, et al: Ondansetron versus ondansetron, dexamethasone, and chlorpromazine in the prevention of nausea and vomiting associated with multiple-day cisplatin chemotherapy. *J Clin Oncol* 11: 2391–2395, 1993

91. Cotanch P, Strum S: Progressive muscle relaxation as antiemetic therapy for cancer patients. *Oncol Nurs Forum* 14: 33–37, 1987

92. Frank J: The effects of music therapy and guided imagery on chemotherapy-induced nausea and vomiting. *Oncol Nurs Forum* 12:47–52, 1985

93. Nichols C, Roth B, Einhorn L: Managing testicular cancer. *Contemp Oncol* 1:13–30, 1991

94. Schweitzer V, Hawkins J, Lilly D, et al: Ototoxic and nephrotoxic effects of combined treatment with cisdiaminedichloroplatinum and karamycin in guinea pig. *Otolaryngol Head Neck Surg* 92:38–49, 1984

95. Wagner L, Bye M: Body image and patient experiencing alopecia as a result of chemotherapy. *Cancer Nurs* 2: 365–369, 1979

96. Senturia Y, Peckham C, Peckham M: Children fathered by men treated for testicular cancer. *Lancet* 2:766–769, 1985

97. Roth B, Einhorn L, Griest A: Long-term complications of cisplatin based chemotherapy for testicular cancer. *Semin Oncol* 15:345–350, 1988

98. Stephenson W, Poirier S, Rubin L, et al: Evaluation of reproductive capacity in germ cell tumor patients following treatment with cisplatin, etoposide, and bleomycin. *J Clin Oncol* 13:2278–2280, 1995

99. Sweet V, Servy EJ, Karow AM: Reproductive issues for men with cancer: technology and nursing management. *Oncol Nurs Forum* 5:51–58, 1996

100. Brodsky MS: Testicular cancer survivors impressions of the impact of the disease on their lives. *Qualitative Health Res* 5:78–96, 1995

101. Reiker P: How should a man with testicular cancer be counseled and what information is available to him? *Semin Urol Oncol* 14:17–22, 1996

102. Reiker P, Fitzgerald E, Kalish L, et al: Psychosocial factors, curative therapies, and behavioral outcomes. A comparison of testis cancer survivors and a control group of healthy men. *Cancer* 64:2399–2407, 1989

103. Ofman US: Psychosocial and sexual implications of genitourinary cancers. *Semin Oncol Nursing* 9:286–292, 1993

104. Koch MO: Cost-effective strategies for the follow-up of

patients with germ cell tumors. *Urol Clin North Am* 25: 495–502, 1998

105. Coogan CL, Foster RS, Simmons GR, et al: Bilateral testicular tumors. *Cancer* 83:547–552, 1998

106. Gospodarowicz MK, Sturgeon FG, Jewett MAS: Early stage and advanced seminoma: role of radiation therapy, surgery, and chemotherapy. *Semin Oncol* 25:160–173, 1998

107. Celebi I, Tekgul S, Ozen H, et al: Sequential bilateral germ cell tumours of the testis. *Int Urol Nephrol* 27:183–187, 1995

CHAPTER 68

Vulvar and Vaginal Cancer

Carol Guarnieri, RN, MSN, AOCN
Paula R. Klemm, RN, DNSc, OCN®

Introduction

Approximately 5600 females in the United States were diagnosed with vaginal or vulvar cancer in 1999 and an estimated 1500 deaths occurred from these cancers that same year.[1] Even though vulvar and vaginal cancer occur infrequently, nursing care for these women is very challenging. Vulvar and vaginal cancer usually occur in older, postmenopausal women. Treatment with surgery and radiation therapy will typically affect sexuality and many women will face some degree of change in their body image. It is important for nurses to understand normal female genital anatomy because it is often affected or altered by treatment.

Both vulvar and vaginal cancer are frequently preceded by a preinvasive intraepithelial neoplasia and both can be curable if diagnosed in the early stages. Close follow-up care and education for women with preinvasive disease is crucial for early detection and to prevent progression to invasive disease.

VULVAR CANCER

Epidemiology

Vulvar carcinoma accounts for 3%–5% of all gynecologic cancers. It is a disease of elderly women, with peak incidence occurring in the seventh decade of life. Vulvar cancer rarely occurs in women under age 40.[2,3] Similar to cervical cancer, vulvar cancer can be preceded by a preinvasive intraepithelial neoplasia of the vulvar tissue. *Vulvar intraepithelial neoplasia (VIN)* is the term used to denote epithelial abnormalities of the vulva, which are divided into three categories (VIN I, II, or III) that differentiate the degree of epithelial involvement by neoplastic cells.[4] Although the incidence of VIN has dramatically increased during the past two decades, the incidence of invasive vulvar carcinoma has remained stable. While VIN can develop at any age, it is usually seen in women in their forties and fifties. Frequency of occurrence appears

to be increasing among younger women.[5,6] The stable incidence of invasive carcinoma of the vulva, even as the overall number of cases of preinvasive disease increases, could suggest that the treatment for VIN is effective in preventing an increase in the incidence of invasive disease.[7]

Etiology

The etiology of VIN and invasive vulvar cancer is largely unknown. Even the relationship of VIN to invasive vulvar disease remains unclear. The human papillomavirus (HPV), most commonly HPV type 16, is associated with VIN and invasive vulvar cancer. HPV has been found in 80%–90% of women with VIN, but HPV decreases to 30% in women with invasive disease. HPV positive tumors are higher in incidence among cigarette smokers than nonsmokers, more commonly found in younger women, and are multifocal in nature.[8,9] Recent research has shown that the *p53* tumor suppressor gene also may play a role in the etiology of squamous cell carcinoma. The *p53* gene plays an important role in the regulation of the cell cycle. In the absence of normal *p53* activity, proliferating cells must replicate their DNA. This puts the cell at a greater risk for DNA damage, which could contribute to the development of a cancer.[10,11]

Other risk factors for vulvar cancer include venereal warts, multiple sexual partners, and the presence of herpes simplex virus type 2. A history of chronic vulvar disease and previous malignancies of the lower genital tract are also seen in women with vulvar cancer. Preliminary reports suggest that immunosuppression may play an important role in vulvar cancer. Individuals who have had organ transplants or individuals who are human immunodeficiency virus (HIV) positive may be at an increased risk for vulvar cancer[12,13] (Table 68-1).

Prevention and Screening

Screening for vulvar cancer should be performed when a woman has a Papanicolaou (Pap) smear done. Careful

Table 68-1 Vulvar Cancer: Risk Factors and Preventive Measures

Risk Factors	Preventive Measures
Human papillomavirus	Pap smear per ACS guidelines
Herpes simplex virus type 2	Routine vulvar self-examination
History of smoking	Stop smoking
Venereal warts	Limit number of sexual partners
Multiple sexual partners	Use of barrier contraception
Immunosuppression	
Chronic vulvar disease	
Previous malignancies of lower genital tract	
Age > 60 yr	

examination of the vulva is critical. Screening should focus on women who smoke, women with HPV infection, and women who have other preinvasive disease of the cervix, vagina, or perianal area. Nurses are often excellent resources to help educate women (especially older women) that a regular pelvic examination following American Cancer Society (ACS) guidelines is crucial. Nurses can also teach women about performing vulvar self-examination, avoiding exposure to HPV, and the negative effects of smoking.

Women who are diagnosed with VIN or vulvar cancer at an early stage can benefit from early detection. If a woman has a lesion present, she should insist on a biopsy if the lesion persists despite treatment.[3] With early detection, treatment morbidity is often decreased because physicians may be able to perform less radical surgery to eradicate the disease. Stage I and II tumors have a low rate of recurrence.

Pathophysiology

Cellular Characteristics

VIN commonly presents in a multifocal pattern. Discoloration of the vulva with white, gray, red, or brown lesions is usual. The lesions may be macular or papular and often present with a roughened warty-like surface.[7] On examination, the tumor often appears as an ulcerated mass and usually remains confined to the vulva for a long period of time. Histologically, squamous cell carcinoma accounts for over 90% of the primary vulvar neoplasms. The remaining 10% of vulvar neoplasms include malignant melanoma, basal cell, adenocarcinoma and sarcoma.[4]

Progression of Disease

VIN is divided into three categories: VIN I, VIN II, and VIN III. The term *VIN I* is used to describe mild dysplasia.

VIN II describes moderate dysplasia. *VIN III* or carcinoma in situ (CIS) describes severe dysplasia and suggests full thickness changes of the epithelium. VIN III/CIS of the vulva does not appear to have the same malignant potential as preinvasive disease of the cervix. VIN III/CIS is most likely to progress to invasive disease if the woman is elderly (above 60), immunosuppressed, or has multifocal disease.

Patterns of Spread

The vulva includes the mons pubis, the labia majora and minora, the clitoris, the vestibule of the vagina, and the Bartholin glands. The mons pubis is the pad of fat anterior to the pubis symphysis and is covered by hair-bearing skin. The labia majora extends posteriorly from the mons into the vaginal opening. The labia minora are small folds of skin that lie between the labia majora and divide anteriorly to envelop the clitoris. The vestibule is the area into which the vagina opens. The bulbs of the vestibule are erectile tissue on each side of the vaginal opening. The vulva is surrounded by a network of lymphatics.[14]

Although primary disease can develop anywhere on the vulva, approximately 70% of tumors arise on the labia majora. The labia minora, clitoris, and perineum are also common sites. Vulvar cancer usually remains a localized disease with well-defined margins.[4]

The most common routes of metastatic spread are through direct extension or dissemination to regional lymph nodes. The pattern of lymphatic spread of vulvar cancer is usually predictable. From the superficial inguinal lymph nodes, the tumor usually spreads to the deep inguinal/femoral nodes and then to the pelvic lymph nodes[7,15] (Figure 68-1). Tumors involving the midline can metastasize to the groin nodes on both sides. Early stage tumors rarely metastasize to the contralateral lymph nodes. At diagnosis, the overall incidence of positive lymph nodes is approximately 45%. Inguinal node metastases can occur in 35%–40% of women, and the incidence of pelvic node metastases is 5%–10%.[7,16,17] In advanced stages, vulvar cancer may spread to the urethra, vagina, anus, rectum, and pubic bone. The most common site of distant metastasis is the lung.

Clinical Manifestations

The symptoms of VIN and invasive vulvar carcinoma are variable and insidious. Fifty percent of women with VIN are asymptomatic, whereas other women may complain of vulvar pruritus or burning or the presence of a lesion. Less common presenting symptoms include vulvar bleeding, discharge, or dysuria. Up to 20% of women with vulvar cancer are asymptomatic, with lesions detected only during routine pelvic examination.[18,19]

Delay in diagnosing a woman with vulvar cancer may occur because she is too embarrassed to seek medical

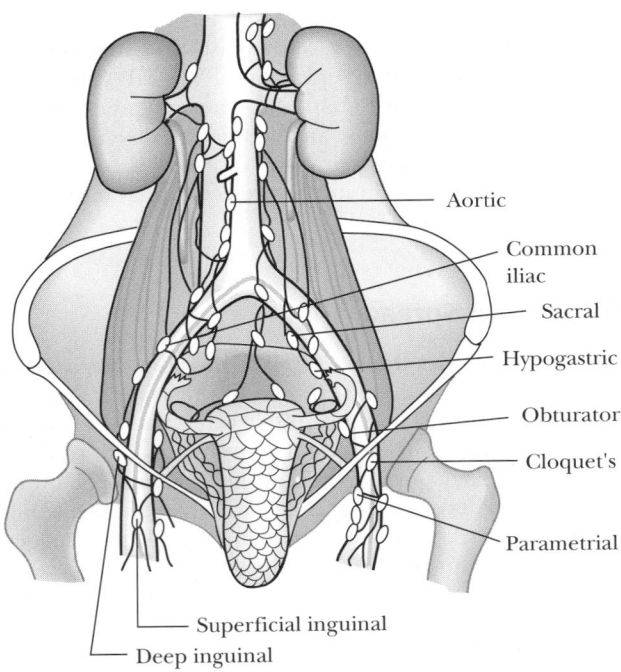

Aortic

Common iliac

Sacral

Hypogastric

Obturator

Cloquet's

Parametrial

Superficial inguinal

Deep inguinal

Figure 68-1 Lymphatics of the pelvis. (Reprinted with permission from Hammond CB: Gynecology: the female reproductive organs, in Sabiston Jr DC, Lyerly HK (eds): *Textbook of Surgery: The Biological Basis of Modern Surgical Practice* (ed 15). Philadelphia, Saunders, 1996.)[15]

assistance due to the intimate area of the body that is involved. As a result, the woman may have symptoms for 2–16 months before seeking medical attention.[20] A delay in definitive treatment may occur because symptomatic topical treatment for vulvar lesions can continue for up to 12 months or longer before the lesion is biopsied for definitive diagnosis, or because the health care provider fails to adequately assess a woman reporting symptoms of vulvar irritation.[17,21] Lesions are usually diagnosed and treated when they are small, which may suggest that women with vulvar cancer are being biopsied earlier.

Assessment

Patient and Family History

Women with VIN and invasive cancer should have a complete history that includes the duration and severity of signs and symptoms. Women with VIN or vulvar cancer may have a history of a previous malignancy in the lower genital tract. Detailed questioning about gynecological history is warranted. Since cigarette smoking and multiple sexual partners are risk factors, a smoking and sexual history should be taken. A family history related to cancer

is important; however, having a history of vulvar cancer in the family is not a potential risk factor.

Physical Examination

Careful inspection of the vulva during routine gynecologic examination is imperative since this remains the most productive diagnostic measure. The entire vulva, perineum, and perianal area should be evaluated. Lymph nodes in the groin should be palpated. A Pap smear should be done in order to rule out cervical cancer. Colposcopic examination may help to define the extent of the disease and thorough examination under anesthesia with multiple biopsies is important to determine the extent of disease. Needle aspiration biopsy of any suspicious lymph node can also be done at this time.[19]

Diagnostic Studies

All patients require a chest x-ray, complete blood count, and biochemical profile. Computerized tomography (CT) and magnetic resonance imaging (MRI) are used to evaluate nodal metastasis and possible distant metastasis. In selected cases, cystoscopy and proctosigmoidoscopy may also be necessary. If the disease is thought to be advanced and the patient states that she has pelvic pain, skeletal radiographs should be done to rule out bone metastasis.[16]

Prognostic Indicators

The five-year survival rate for vulvar cancer can be correlated with stage and nodal involvement. Groin lymph node status is the best indicator of survival. In women with negative nodes, the five-year survival rate is as high as 90%. Survival rate decreases as the number of positive nodes increases. Five-year survival rate is approximately 40% when three to four nodes are positive and decreases to 20% with six or more positive nodes.[18,22] In addition to nodal status, tumors that have evidence of HPV infection have a better prognosis. HPV negative tumors are correlated with a higher risk of recurrence and death rate from vulvar cancer than HPV positive tumors.[23]

Classification and Staging

The International Federation of Gynecology and Obstetrics (FIGO) staging is shown in Table 68-2. Surgical findings are incorporated into the staging evaluation. To make a diagnosis of invasive vulvar carcinoma, a wedge biopsy of the lesion is needed. The biopsy should be full thickness and include a margin of normal connective tissue. This biopsy will help in differentiating between stage I and stage II disease.[7] Biopsy of the nodes should also be done. In stage I and stage II, all lymph nodes are

Table 68-2 FIGO Staging of Vulvar Cancer

Stage	TNM	Clinical Findings
Stage 0		Carcinoma *in situ*, e.g., VIN 3, noninvasive Paget's disease.
Stage I	$T_1N_0M_0$ $T_1N_1M_0$	Tumor confined to the vulva, 2 cm or less in largest diameter, and no suspicious groin nodes.
Stage II	$T_2N_0M_0$ $T_2N_1M_0$	Tumor confined to the vulva more than 2 cm in diameter, and no suspicious groin nodes.
Stage III	$T_3N_0M_0$ $T_3N_1M_0$ $T_3N_2M_0$ $T_1N_2M_0$ $T_2N_2M_0$	Tumor of any size with: (1) adjacent spread to the urethra and/or the vagina, the perineum, and the anus, and/or (2) clinically suspicious lymph nodes in either groin.
Stage IV	$T_xN_3M_0$ $T_4N_0M_0$ $T_4N_1M_0$ $T_4N_2M_0$ $T_xN_xM_{1a}$ $T_xN_xM_{1b}$	Tumor of any size: (1) infiltrating the bladder mucosa, or the rectal mucosa, or both, including the upper part of the urethral mucosa, and/or (2) fixed to the bone and/or (3) other distant metastases.

TNM Classification

T: Primary Tumor

T_1 Tumor confined to the vulva, 2 cm in largest diameter.

T_2 Tumor confined to the vulva, > 2 cm in diameter.

T_3 Tumor of any size with adjacent spread to the urethra and/or vagina and/or perineum and/or anus.

T_4 Tumor of any size infiltrating the bladder mucosa and/or the rectal mucosa or including the upper part of the urethral mucosa and/or fixed to the bone.

N: Regional Lymph Nodes

N_0 No nodes palpable.

N_1 Nodes palpable in either groin, not enlarged, mobile (not clinically suspicious for neoplasm).

N_2 Nodes palpable in either or both groins, enlarged, firm and mobile (clinically suspicious for neoplasm).

N_3 Fixed or ulcerated nodes.

M: Distant Metastases

M_0 No clinical metastases.

M_{1a} Palpable deep pelvic lymph nodes.

M_{1b} Other distant metastases.

x = any T or N category; VIN = vulvar intraepithelial neoplasia.

negative. In stage III disease, the tumor has spread to adjacent areas of the urethra and/or the vagina, perineum, and the anus. Lymph nodes in the groin are clinically suspicious for tumor. Stage IV disease has tumor that has infiltrated to the bladder and/or rectal mucosa, and may be fixed to bone.[7]

Therapeutic Approaches and Nursing Care—VIN

Some controversy exists about the treatment of choice for patients with VIN. In the past, a total vulvectomy was done for the management of VIN. Presently, a more conservative surgical approach is usually undertaken. A wide local excision of the lesion or lesions may be all that is necessary. This helps maintain the sexual and reproductive function of the vulva and may help women avoid the adverse physical and psychological effects of more extensive surgery. The effectiveness of wide local excision in eradicating VIN varies from 83%–91%.[24] For multicentric disease, a skinning vulvectomy[21] (Figure

68-2) is performed in which the vulvar skin is excised while conserving the fat, muscle, and glands below the skin.[19] A split thickness skin graft reconstruction from the thigh or buttock is performed. The skinning vulvectomy has a success rate similar to other surgical treatment modalities.[25] The wide local excision and skinning vulvectomy provide excellent cosmetic and functional results.[24,25] A skinning vulvectomy may not be an option for elderly or debilitated women, since the healing of the skin graft after a skinning vulvectomy requires prolonged bed rest.

An alternative to excision of the vulvar lesion is to treat it locally with cautery, laser surgery, or cryosurgery. The advantages of these surgical techniques are outpatient management, sparing effect on surrounding tissue, and minimal scarring. However, the procedures can result in painful ulcers and require several sequenced treatments. Healing time can be prolonged. Comparative studies of excisional surgery and laser ablation demonstrate that both are equally effective in eradicating the disease, although some evidence exists to suggest that relapse occurs more quickly after laser ablation.[25] Topical 5% fluorouracil (5-FU) cream may be used to treat VIN. This topical treatment requires daily applications and can

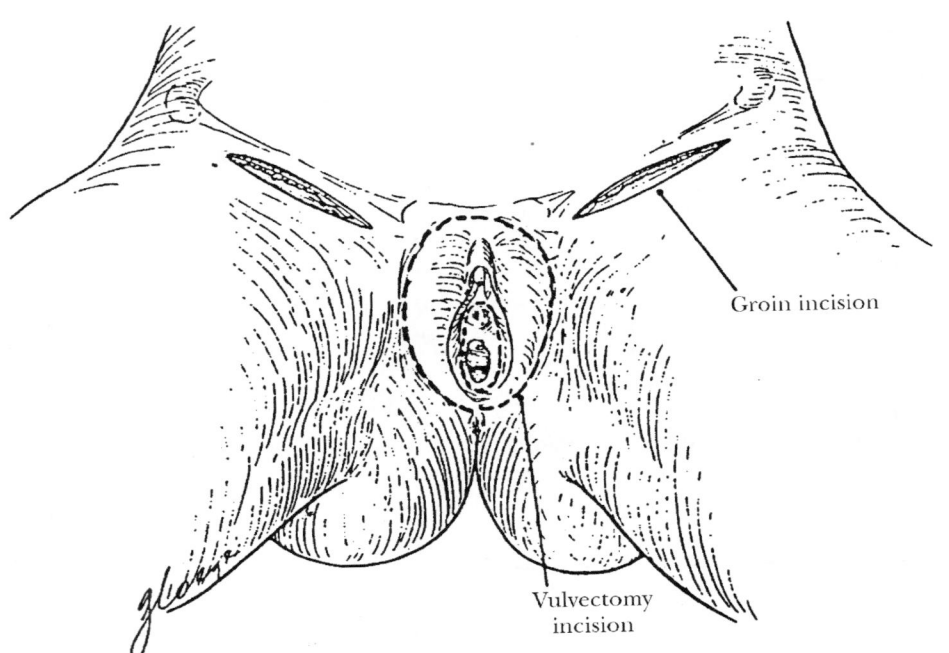

Groin incision

Vulvectomy incision

Figure 68-2 Skin incision for vulvectomy and separate groin incisions. (Reprinted with permission from Hacker NF: Vulvar Cancer, in Berek JS, Hacker NF (eds): *Practical Gynecologic Oncology*. Baltimore, Williams and Wilkins, 1989, p 404. © 1989 the Williams and Wilkins Co., Baltimore, MD.)

produce painful, slow-healing ulcers. Response rates to topical 5-FU therapy are variable, ranging from 75% response to complete failure.[25]

Continuity of Care: VIN

For women with VIN, education is an essential responsibility of nursing. Explaining the difference between VIN and invasive vulvar cancer is key. The nurse can help the woman understand the type of treatment recommended. Follow-up care by the nurse includes teaching the woman how to care for herself at home. When sexual intercourse is resumed in approximately four to six weeks following surgery, a water soluble lubricant can be used for comfort. Sexual satisfaction is possible and nurses can discuss with the woman methods to maintain sexual activity. Because of the uncertain malignant potential of VIN and its possibility to recur, close and long-term follow-up care should be stressed.

Therapeutic Approaches and Nursing Care–Invasive Disease

Surgery

The traditional treatment for women with cancer of the vulva has been surgical: en bloc dissection of the tumor along with contiguous skin, subcutaneous fat, regional inguinal and femoral nodes, and vulva (labia minora, labia majora, clitoris, and perineal body). Historically, physicians recommended routine pelvic node dissection be done on every individual. With a pelvic node dissection, wound closure was difficult to achieve. Many surgeons have abandoned the en bloc approach and are now performing the nodal dissections through separate groin incisions (see Figure 68-2). Many studies have since attested to the reduced morbidity of separate groin incisions without increasing recurrence rates.[14,26] In the absence of clinical suspicion of groin node involvement, unilateral lymphadenectomy may be sufficient.[14] The trend is away from the radical surgery that has been associated with disturbances in sexual function and body image. Now, there is more emphasis on individualized treatment for each women, taking into account age, location of disease, extent of disease, and psychosocial consequences.[3,26]

Stage I carcinoma of the vulva is treated with wide local excision and ipsilateral inguinofemoral lymphadenectomy. For patients with midline lesions, bilateral node dissections using separate groin incisions is recommended. Stage II vulvar cancer may require more extensive surgery. This usually involves a radical vulvectomy to obtain adequate tumor-free margins. A radical vulvectomy removes the labia minora and majora and the clitoris. Bilateral node dissections are usually performed.[7,27] With stage III disease, the tumor has spread to the urethra, vagina, anus, or to the lymph nodes in the inguinal area. For stage III disease, radical vulvectomy often involves removal of a portion of the distal urethra or vagina and may require excision of a portion of the anus. To prevent local recurrence, a course of radiation therapy alone or a combination of radiation therapy and chemotherapy is recommended.[18,28] Patients with stage IV disease may require pelvic exenteration in addition to a radical vulvectomy if the bladder or rectum is involved. A total pelvic exenteration removes the vagina, uterus, ovaries, fallopian tubes, bladder, and rectum. Patients will have a urinary conduit and colostomy. A neovagina is usually constructed. While the five-year survival rate for this surgery may be as high as 70%, there can be many complications, including a high psychological morbidity.[29] Women should be carefully selected for this surgery. Usually, elderly women are not candidates. If the tumor is fixed to the bone or distant metastases has occurred, treatment is usually palliative and mainly consists of radiotherapy.[14]

The major immediate complication after radical surgery is groin wound infection and breakdown. With the use of the separate incision approach for nodal resection, the incidence of wound breakdown decreased to about 44%, whereas with an en bloc operation, it was reported to be as high as 85%. Major wound breakdown occurs in about 14% of patients. With proper debridement and wound care, the groin area can granulate and reepithelialize within a few weeks. Wet-to-dry dressings are usually recommended. Whirlpool therapy is also effective for areas of extensive breakdown.[19] Other early postoperative complications include urinary tract infection, deep venous thrombosis, seromas in the femoral triangle, and pulmonary embolism.

The major late complication of radical surgery is chronic leg edema, which has been reported to occur in up to 30%–50% of women. The use of elastic stockings is recommended for 12 months after surgery to allow development of collateral pathways for lymph drainage. Recurrent cellulitis of the leg occurs in about 10% of women and usually responds to antibiotics. Urinary stress incontinence and genital prolapse occurs in about 10% of patients and may require corrective surgery. Numbness and paresthesia over the anterior thigh is common due to femoral nerve injury. This nerve injury usually resolves slowly.[7,14,19]

Radiation

The role of radiation therapy in the management of carcinoma of the vulva is still evolving. To reduce the need for extensive radical surgery, radiation therapy is being used more often in combination with surgery. Women who have undergone a resection of the primary lesion and are considered at high risk for recurrence due to inadequate resection margins or positive nodes may be good candidates for postoperative irradiation. Women with two or more positive groin lymph nodes or positive pelvic lymph nodes are considered to be at high risk for recurrence.[19] While the use of radiation therapy has decreased recurrence rates, it cannot be used as a replacement for groin node dissection. The Gynecologic Oncology Group (GOG) had to terminate a study early due to high recurrence rates among women who had radiation therapy alone to the groin.[30] Preoperative radiation in combination with chemotherapy for locally advanced cancer has been shown to be an effective approach that enables reducing the extent of radical surgery.[31,32]

Patients who receive external radiation to the vulva can develop severe erythema and swelling. Maintaining skin integrity and management of pain and discomfort is the aim of nursing care. Radiation cystitis may also occur with radiation treatment of the pelvis. If cystitis occurs, appropriate antibiotic therapy and antispasmodics are indicated to provide relief of symptoms. The woman should also be encouraged to increase fluid intake.[33] Severe late radiation effects, such as vulvar fibrosis, atrophy, or even necrosis may occur. To prevent severe radiation effects, the total dose for postoperative radiation therapy is 4500–5000 cGy if there is no macroscopic residual disease. Higher doses of irradiation (6000–7000 cGy) can be given to known areas of gross residual tumor. When chemotherapy is used in combination with radiation therapy, the maximum dose is usually 6500 cGy.[14]

Chemotherapy

The use of concurrent radiation and chemotherapy for initial therapy shows the promise of allowing a more conservative approach to surgery. The most common chemotherapy agents used are 5-FU, cisplatin, or mitomycin C.[7] The studies using concurrent radiation and chemotherapy have had small sample sizes and further research needs to be completed in order to fully define and develop the use of chemotherapy in the treatment of vulvar cancer. Chemotherapy with radiation therapy is usually well tolerated by most women. However, vulvar cancer patients, who typically are elderly and often have concurrent medical problems, should be closely monitored for evidence of side effects.[28,32]

Symptom Management and Supportive Care

Advanced/Recurrent Disease

About 80% of recurrences of vulvar cancer will develop within the first two years after initial treatment, which demands initial close follow-up. Patients with less than three positive nodes generally have a low incidence of recurrence, whereas high recurrence rates are correlated with more than three positive nodes.[22] Over half of the recurrences are local and in close proximity to the original lesion. In many instances, local recurrences can be successfully treated using wide local excision with adequate tumor-free margins. For treatment of advanced recurrent disease, pelvic exenteration may be an option for some women. For recurrent vulvar cancer, the five-year survival rate is 38%–50%.[17,29] Distant recurrence is difficult to treat, with an 8% survival rate at five years. A combination of radiation and chemotherapy may be used as a palliative treatment measure in metastatic disease.[7]

For the woman with advanced recurrent vulvar cancer, the physical symptoms can be distressing. The tumor can become very large, disfiguring, and painful. With a comprehensive assessment of the pain, an appropriate and effective pain management regimen can be developed. If the tumor becomes ulcerated, care should be taken to prevent infection. Meticulous skin care is important. Leg edema may become a problem for the woman with positive, enlarged lymph nodes. Elastic stockings are usually recommended. Massage and exercise of the legs may also help relieve discomfort. Skin care of the legs is essential to prevent infection and cellulitis. Moisturizing the skin can help.

Along with the physical symptoms, the patient and family may be at risk for ineffective coping. The nurse and health care team can help the patient and family cope with the many debilitating changes of advanced disease. Nurses in the hospital can make appropriate referrals to home care or hospice care. Continual education and reassurance can facilitate effective coping mechanisms to allow the patient to live as fully as possible.

Continuity of Care: Invasive Disease

Because cancer of the vulva primarily affects elderly women and radical surgery may be involved, a multidisciplinary approach to care for the patient is essential. The patient may face many short- and long-term complications. Preoperatively, nurses should educate the woman and her family about the extent of the surgery, changes that will occur, and the patient's participation in postoperative care. Sexual and reproductive counseling will be needed for every woman. Sexual satisfaction is low among postvulvectomy patients. Nurses can help with open discussions about sexual concerns with the woman and her partner. With shorter hospital stays, coordination of care from the hospital to home is imperative. Nurses in all settings can assist patients in dealing with the physical, psychological, and social implications of a radical vulvectomy.

VAGINAL CANCER

Epidemiology

Primary carcinoma of the vagina represents less than 2% of all gynecologic malignancies. Vaginal carcinomas should be classified as such only when the primary site of tumor growth is in the vagina. Any tumor that has extended to the cervical area and has reached the exter-

nal os should be classified as a cervical carcinoma.[7] Secondary spread to the vagina from sites such as cervix, vulva, endometrium, ovary, and rectum occurs more frequently than primary carcinoma of the vagina.[34]

The peak incidence of squamous carcinoma of the vagina, the most common cell type, usually occurs in women age 50–70. It is rare that women under age 40 are diagnosed with vaginal cancer. In contrast, the peak incidence for clear cell adenocarcinoma of the vagina, which is associated with maternal use of diethylstilbestrol (DES), most frequently occurs in women age 18–19.

Invasive squamous cell carcinoma of the vagina is often preceded by vaginal intraepithelial neoplasia (VAIN) just as cancer of the cervix and vulva are preceded by cervical and vulvar intraepithelial neoplasia, respectively. VAIN is much less common than cervical intraepithelial neoplasia (CIN), squamous intraepithelial lesions of the cervix (SIL), or VIN.[35] However, the incidence of VAIN is climbing and the mean age at diagnosis is decreasing.[16,36] VAIN is divided into three categories (I, II, III) with each higher number indicative of increasing epithelial involvement. Although the natural history of VAIN is not well defined, VAIN III lesions are premalignant. The majority of women with VAIN III will have a history of CIN (SIL) or invasive disease of the cervix.[37] Up to 30% of women with primary vaginal carcinoma will have a history of in situ or invasive cervical cancer treated at least five years earlier.[38]

Etiology

Incidence of squamous cell cancer of the vagina increases with age. Rates were thought to be higher in the black population, but a case-controlled study has failed to show this to be a variable independent of socioeconomic status. This study also showed limited education, low family income, a history of genital warts, and abnormal cervical Pap smears as risk factors.[35] Smoking cigarettes, the age of first intercourse, and the number of sexual partners are key risk factors in the development of cervical and vulvar cancer, but are not risk factors for vaginal cancer.[39]

There is an association between HPV and herpes simplex type 2 virus and vaginal cancer.[40,41] Another risk factor is a history of vaginal trauma linked to the use of vaginal pessaries. Long-term use of vaginal pessaries is thought to produce a chemical and physical irritation to the vaginal mucosa. Previous abdominal hysterectomy for benign disease has also been associated with an increased incidence of VAIN and vaginal cancer. Prior radiation therapy may also be a predisposing factor in primary vaginal carcinoma. This may be particularly important in young women who live long enough to develop a second neoplasm in the irradiated vagina (Table 68-3).

Since 1971, the study of adenocarcinoma of the vagina has focused on young women who were exposed to DES in utero and who seemed to have an unusually high incidence of vaginal cancer. DES was used in the manage-

Table 68-3 Vaginal Cancer: Risk Factors and Preventive Measures

Risk Factors	Preventive Measures
Human papillomavirus	Pap smear per ACS guidelines
Herpes simplex virus type 2	Decrease use of vaginal pessaries
Long-term use of vaginal pessaries	Use of barrier contraception
Abdominal hysterectomy for benign disease	
Prior radiation therapy to lower genital tract	
Lower educational level	
Lower socioeconomic status	
Genital warts	
Age > 60 yr	
Maternal use of Diethylstilbestrol	

ment of diabetic pregnancies, threatened abortion, habitual abortion, and other high-risk obstetric problems. From the late 1940s to 1970, an estimated 2 million pregnant women received DES. The risk of developing vaginal cancer in women exposed to DES in utero is about 1 in 1000 up to age 35 and is the highest if the hormone was taken before 12 weeks' gestation.[42,43] Of greater risk is the development of cervicovaginal dysplasia, which has been estimated to be as high as 18% in this population.[44] There have been several cases of women with a history of in utero DES exposure who developed non-clear cell adenocarcinoma of the vagina. These vaginal cancers were found in older women and were more advanced than the clear cell adenocarcinoma associated with DES.[45] With women developing cancer later in life, long-term surveillance of DES-exposed women is warranted.

Prevention and Screening

The incidence of vaginal cancer is 0.6 per 100,000 women.[31] Routine screening is probably not warranted given the low incidence. However, women should be encouraged to have a Pap smear following the ACS guidelines. At the time the Pap smear is done, inspection of the vagina should be performed. Because women who had cervical cancer, vulvar cancer, or a hysterectomy for benign disease have a higher incidence of vaginal cancer, it is recommended that a Pap smear surveillance for vaginal cancer be performed yearly.[31,46] For women who have a history of VAIN, follow-up examination should also include colposcopy as a part of every examination.[47] Presently, there are no molecular markers for early detection of vaginal cancer that are promis-

ing. In the future, chemoprevention with retinoids may prove advantageous.[47]

Pathophysiology

Cellular Characteristics

Squamous cell carcinoma makes up 80%–90% of all vaginal cancers.[34] Other histological types include verrucous, adenocarcinoma, melanoma, and sarcoma.[1,7] A lesion may appear to be red, white, or gray in color and have an ulcerated look.

Progression of Disease

The vagina is lined throughout by stratified squamous epithelium. Embryologically, the upper two-thirds of the vagina develops separately from the lower one-third. The upper two-thirds grows downward and shares its blood supply and lymphatic drainage with the cervix. The lymphatics drain to the internal and external iliac and obturator nodes and to the common iliac and lower paraaortic nodes. The lower one-third of the vagina grows upward and shares its blood supply and lymphatic system with that of the vulva. The lymphatics drain to the inguinal and femoral nodes. All the lymph nodes of the pelvis may at one time or another serve as potential sites of drainage from the vagina[15,16] (see Figure 68-1). Superiorly, the cervix protrudes into the vaginal vault and inferiorly the vagina meets the vulva. The bladder is positioned anterior to the vagina. The rectum and anus are posterior to the vagina[48] (Figure 68-3).

Similar to vulvar and cervical cancer, the preinvasive disease VAIN is divided into three categories. VAIN I describes mild dysplasia. VAIN II describes moderate dysplasia. VAIN III describes severe dysplasia and may be associated with microinvasive or invasive disease.[36]

Patterns of Spread

Vaginal cancers occur most commonly in the upper third of the vagina. Early reports indicated that most tumors developed on the posterior wall of the vagina. However, more recent reviews noted that lesions were more equally distributed on the posterior, anterior, and lateral walls.[49,50] The tumor may spread along the vaginal wall to involve the cervix or vulva. However, if the cervix is involved, the tumor is considered a primary cervical lesion. Anterior vaginal lesions can penetrate into the vesicovaginal septum during early stages. Posterior lesions can invade the rectum, but this is usually in the late stages. Even though the urethra, bladder, and rectum are in close proximity to the vagina, fewer than 10% of vaginal tumors invade these structures, even in the later stages of disease.[19,49,50]

The lymphatic drainage of the vagina consists of a vast,

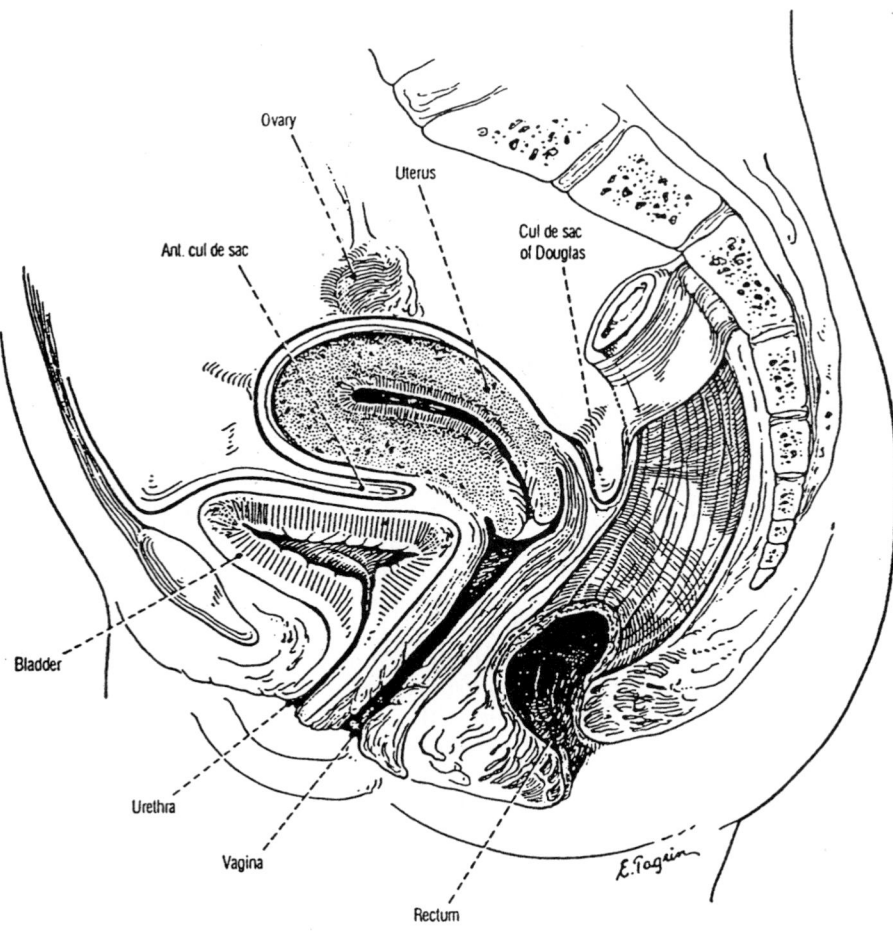

Figure 68-3 Sagittal section of the female pelvis. (Reprinted with permission from Bengton JM: The Vagina in, Ryan KJ, Berkowitz RS, Barbieri RL (eds): *Kistner's Gynecology Principles and Practice*. St. Louis, Mosby, 1996, p 82.)[48]

interconnecting network that facilitates drainage into any of the local nodal groups regardless of the location of the vaginal lesion. The incidence of lymph node metastasis is directly proportional to the stage of the vaginal cancer. The overall incidence of positive lymph nodes is about 30%.[38] With squamous cell carcinoma, metastasis to the lungs or supraclavicular nodes tends to occur in the more advanced stages. In clear cell carcinoma, metastasis to the lungs and supraclavicular nodes occurs more frequently.[51]

Extension or metastasis of other malignancies to the vagina occurs more frequently than primary cancer of the vagina. Spread of cervical cancer to the vagina is the most common, but cancers of the endometrium, ovary, urethra, bladder, rectum, and malignant trophoblastic disease may also spread or metastasize to the vaginal area.[21]

Clinical Manifestations

The most frequent initial symptom of invasive vaginal cancer is abnormal bleeding that may occur after coitus. Other symptoms may include foul-smelling discharge and pain in the lower pelvis.[33,49] With more advanced tumors,

if the tumor presses on the bladder, urinary retention, bladder spasms, and hematuria may occur. Tumors developing on the posterior vaginal wall may produce rectal symptoms such as tenesmus, constipation, or blood in the stool.[52] Because many lesions are asymptomatic, an abnormal Pap smear may be the diagnostic event that initiates the search for a definitive diagnosis.

Assessment

Patient and Family History

All women should have a complete history regarding the duration and severity of their signs and symptoms. Since exposure to DES in utero is a high risk factor for developing vaginal cancer, all women should be questioned about their mothers' possible use of DES. For some women, a primary vaginal cancer can actually be a second pelvic cancer. A detailed history of the previous cancer and its treatment are necessary. Information about a woman's exposure to HPV and herpes simplex type 2 should be obtained. Vaginal cancer does not have a genetic predisposition.

Physical Examination

Clinical diagnosis of a vaginal neoplasm is made by careful visual examination and palpation of the vagina. This examination helps to determine the location, number, and size of the lesions, which is essential information for planning appropriate therapeutic management. Pap smear is helpful for squamous carcinoma, but not for adenocarcinoma because it is often subepithelial. Colposcopy is particularly helpful for directed biopsies of abnormal vaginal areas.[7] The disease may then be evaluated and staged under anesthesia by the gynecologic oncologist and radiation therapist, and additional vaginal and cervical biopsies taken. Negative biopsies of the cervix are necessary to rule out cervical cancer and confirm the diagnosis of primary vaginal carcinoma.[35]

Diagnostic Studies

All patients require a chest x-ray, complete blood count, and biochemical profile. An intravenous pyelogram (IVP), barium enema, cystoscopy, and proctosigmoidoscopy may be helpful in determining extent of disease. An MRI or CT of the abdomen and pelvis is usually performed to assess local invasion and spread to the lymph nodes.[53]

Prognostic Indicators

Clinical stage is the most important prognostic indicator in vaginal cancer. A better prognosis is associated with early diagnosis, small tumor burden, and negative nodal involvement. Other prognostic factors include age of the patient and location of the lesion.[49] One research group divided their patients with vaginal cancer into two groups matched by stage of disease, age, and nodal status. Group I included patients with tumor in the proximal half of the vagina. The five-year survival for this group was 81%. Group II included patients with tumor in the mid to distal half of the vagina. Their five-year survival rate decreased to 41%.[54] There have been conflicting reports about the influence of histological grade and type on outcome. Several studies indicate a poor prognosis with an increasing grade of squamous cell carcinoma, while other studies have found no correlation between grade and prognosis.[7,49] Eighty percent of women whose disease recurs have pelvic recurrences within two years of primary treatment.[7]

Classification and Staging

The International Federation of Gynecology and Obstetrics (FIGO) staging is used (Table 68-4). Staging for vaginal cancer is achieved by clinical examination. Information from MRI or CT is not used to change the FIGO stage, but can be helpful in planning treatment. The

Table 68-4   FIGO Staging of Vaginal Cancer

Stage	Description
Stage 0	Carcinoma in situ, intraepithelial carcinoma.
Stage I	The carcinoma is limited to the vaginal wall.
Stage II	The carcinoma has involved the subvaginal tissues but has not extended onto the pelvic wall.
Stage III	The carcinoma has extended onto the pelvic wall.
Stage IV	The carcinoma has extended beyond the true pelvis or has clinically involved the mucosa of the bladder or rectum. Bullous edema as such does not permit a case to be allotted to stage IV.
Stage IVA	Spread of the growth to adjacent organs, direct extension beyond the true pelvis, or both.
Stage IVB	Spread to distant organs.

overall five-year survival rate for all stages of squamous cell vaginal carcinoma is 50%–65%. The survival rate is 80% for patients with stage I, 65% for those with stage II, 40% for those with stage III, and 15% for those with stage IV.[7,49,55,56] The ten-year survival rate in patients with adenocarcinoma is 79%. This may be related to the fact that females exposed to DES in utero have been followed closely due to their risk for developing adenocarcinoma, and are often diagnosed early in the disease. However, clear cell carcinoma has a greater tendency to recur late and develop metastases in distant sites more frequently than squamous cell carcinoma.[21,34]

Therapeutic Approaches and Nursing Care–VAIN

Location of the lesion, the size of the lesion, and whether it has a single focus or multiple foci are factors considered in determining the treatment option. Women with VAIN I usually do not require any treatment. These lesions often disappear without treatment. Women with VAIN II are usually treated with ablative treatment such as laser or 5-FU cream. With 5-FU cream, care must be taken to ensure direct contact with the entire lesion and to avoid contact with the vulva.[37,57] Laser therapy can cure between 69% and 80% of patients with vaginal intraepithelial lesions.[36,58] Both laser therapy and application of 5-FU cream are well tolerated by the patient. Commonly, patients will complain of a watery discharge for two to three weeks after treatment with laser.

Because VAIN III lesions are considered to be premalignant, local excision is appropriate for single lesions or for several lesions clustered in a single portion of the vagina.[7] For multifocal lesions or recurrent disease, or in poor surgical candidates, the treatment of choice is irradiation of the vagina with high-dose bradytherapy. Treatment is usually well tolerated and recurrence rates are low.[37,55]

Therapeutic Approaches and Nursing Care–Invasive Disease

Radiation

The anatomic position of the vagina, located between the urethra and bladder anteriorly and the rectum posteriorly, is the predominant factor in treatment planning. Radiation therapy is the most widely used treatment modality for all stages of vaginal cancer. Patients who have stage I small, superficial tumors may be treated with brachytherapy alone. A fractionated dose of 6000–7000 cGy to the whole vaginal mucosa is usually administered.[34] For women with larger stage I or stage II tumors, a combination of external beam therapy and brachytherapy is recommended.

In stages III and IV disease, tumors are large and may involve other organs. Again, a combination of external beam and brachytherapy is recommended. Careful treatment planning is critical for shielding the bladder and rectum during high-dose radiation therapy. A total dose of 7000 cGy of external beam and brachytherapy to the pelvis is usually given. The groin area is irradiated with a 5000-cGy dose in women with positive nodes. In general, radiation treatment provides good control of tumor with limited morbidity.[49,55,56] Women with stage III and IV vaginal tumors have a high recurrence rate; therefore in order to enhance the radiation therapy, radiosensitizers such as cisplatin, 5-FU, and hydroxyurea may be used.[59]

For women receiving radiation therapy to the vagina, vaginal fibrosis and scarring with a loss of blood supply and elasticity is a major adverse effect. Frequent intercourse can minimize these effects. For patients who are not sexually active, the use of a vaginal dilator with water-soluble lubricants or prescribed estrogen cream starting two weeks after treatment is an effective prophylactic measure to minimize functional loss.[33]

In the vulvar and groin area, desquamation of the skin from radiation therapy can be distressing to the patient. Educating the woman about meticulous skin care is imperative (Table 68-5). Application of corticosteroid and antibiotic cream can help prevent a skin infection. Once the radiation therapy is completed, the skin usually recovers quickly.

Table 68-5   Skin Care of the Woman Receiving Radiation Therapy to the Lower Pelvis

- Wash the treated area with a mild soap. Use warm water, not hot.
- Do not rub skin dry, pat skin dry with a towel. Try to keep the skin free from moisture.
- Do not apply creams, lotions, or powder to the treated area.
- Do not shave skin.
- If skin becomes reddened, tell your nurse or physician. Application of a corticosteroid and/or antibiotic cream may be indicated. Apply medicated cream after daily dose of radiation.

More serious complications include rectovaginal fistula, rectal ulceration, urethral stricture and small bowel obstruction. The patient should be closely monitored for these complications. Fortunately only a small percentage of women will develop these problems.[55]

Surgery

For a selected group of women, surgery may be an option. Because of the pelvic anatomy, curative surgery often means radical surgery. For superficial lesions in the upper part of the vagina, a radical vaginectomy or radical hysterectomy can be done.[60] With radical vaginectomy, vaginal reconstruction will be necessary for patients who wish to continue vaginal intercourse. For women who have had a reconstructed vagina, sexual intercourse or the use of vaginal dilators is also encouraged because the neovagina can be narrow. Open communication between the nurse and the patient about sexual concerns is essential. Sexual satisfaction can be achieved for women posttreatment for cancer of the vagina.

For treatment of larger tumors without involvement of the pelvic side walls, a more extensive surgery may be warranted, such as pelvic exenteration.[50] However, many women with vaginal cancer are elderly and have other medical problems that may preclude this surgery. For women with recurrent disease or those who have received prior radiation therapy for cervical cancer, a pelvic exenteration may be the only option to achieve a cure.[7] For any patient who receives surgery, extensive preoperative counseling, postoperative care, and rehabilitation is necessary.

Chemotherapy

For patients who have metastatic or recurrent vaginal cancer, or if surgery or radiation therapy cannot be done, chemotherapy may be an option. Very few studies using chemotherapy to treat vaginal cancer have been reported. One promising report using methotrexate, vinblastine, doxorubicin, and cisplatin for advanced or recurrent vaginal cancer showed objective tumor regression in all patients.[61] Presently the major role of chemotherapy in vaginal cancer treatment is as a radiosensitizer.[59,62] More research is needed to better define the role of chemotherapy in vaginal cancer. 5-FU and cisplatin are the most common chemotherapeutic agents used concurrently with radiation therapy. Mitomycin C has also been used with radiation therapy with some success.[34]

Symptom Management and Supportive Care

Advanced/Recurrent Disease

Unfortunately, women with stage III and IV vaginal cancer have a high recurrence rate. The symptoms of advanced vaginal cancer depend upon the location of the tumor.

In tumors located anteriorly, the woman may experience urinary problems such as hematuria and urinary tract infections. Palliative radiotherapy can reduce hematuria from an ulcerating lesion. In addition to radiation therapy to treat the ulcerating lesion, the patient may need continuous bladder irrigation to decrease the bleeding. Repeated urinary tract infections may be indicative of fistula formation and the patient may experience urinary incontinence, dysuria, and painful bladder spasms. For some women, surgery might be the best treatment choice to close the fistula.[63] For women who are too ill or when the tumor is too extensive, symptomatic treatment with appropriate antibiotics and antispasmodics is used. For larger draining fistulas, a urinary-vaginal prosthesis can be used to divert the drainage and to maintain the woman's skin integrity.

If the tumor grows posteriorly, constipation and blood in the stool may occur. For mild constipation, the use of stool softeners and laxatives may be all that is necessary. If complete obstruction occurs, surgery or radiation therapy is usually warranted. A rectovaginal fistula may occur and can cause distressing fecal incontinence. If the fistula is small, measures to keep the stool well-formed may help the healing process. The use of vaginal tampons can help to control fistula discharge. For larger fistulas, a simple loop colostomy should be considered to provide relief of symptoms.[63]

Continuity of Care: Invasive Disease

Women with cancer of the vagina face both physical and emotional challenges. Nurses should educate women diagnosed with VAIN about the importance of regular follow-up visits. A pelvic examination with colposcopy should be done yearly.

The majority of the women with vaginal cancer will be treated with radiation therapy. Since radiation therapy to the lower pelvis can cause vaginal fibrosis, the radiation oncology nurse addresses changes in body image, alteration in sexuality, and coping mechanisms with the woman. Because most patients with vaginal cancer are elderly, the probability of hospitalization or the need for home health care is high. The radiation therapy nurse can be key in helping facilitate communication between settings. Surgery for vaginal cancer can be extensive and radical. Nurses should understand the surgical implications and help the woman and her family develop a plan for care and rehabilitation.

Conclusion

While the emphasis is on individualized treatment for the woman who is diagnosed with vulvar or vaginal cancer, the treatment may be considered aggressive and can be disfiguring. Multimodal treatment has led to decreased recurrence rates. Excellent communication across health care disciplines is necessary in order to achieve a successful and comprehensive approach for the patient. Nurses must consider the social, sexual, and spiritual needs of all the patients. With the demand for shorter hospital stays, home care with family involvement is usually necessary. To further improve the quality of care for women with vulvar or vaginal cancer, more nursing research on the management of treatment-related symptoms and care of the patient with advanced disease is essential.

References

1. American Cancer Society [online]: Available at <*http://www.cancer.org*> (accessed on June 14, 1999)
2. Edwards CL, Balat O: Characteristics of patients with vulvar cancer: an analysis of 94 patients. *Eur J Gynaecol Oncol* 17: 7–12, 1996
3. Edwards CL, Tortolero-Luna G, Linares AC, et al: Vulvar intraepithelial neoplasia and vulvar cancer. *Obstet Gynecol Clin North Am* 23:295–324, 1996
4. Rollason TP: Vulva and vagina: pathology of malignant tumors, in Blackledge CRP, Jordan JA, Shingleton HM (eds): *Textbook of Gynecologic Oncology.* Philadelphia, Saunders, 1991, pp 390–411
5. Hording U, Junge J, Poulsen H, et al: Vulvar intraepithelial neoplasia III: a viral disease of undetermined progressive potential. *Gynecol Oncol* 56:276–279, 1995
6. vanBeurden M, ten Kate FJ, Smits HL, et al: Multifocal vulvar intraepithelial neoplasia grade III and multicentric lower genital tract neoplasia is associated with transcriptionally active human papillomavirus. *Cancer* 75:2879–2884, 1995
7. Eifel PJ, Berek JS, Thigpen JT: Cancer of the cervix, vagina, and vulvar, in Devita VT, Hellman S, Rosenberg SA (eds): *Cancer: Principles and Practice of Oncology* (ed 5). Philadelphia, Lippincott-Raven, 1997, pp 1433–1477
8. Hildesheim A, Han CL, Brinton LA, et al: Human papillomavirus type 16 and risk of preinvasive and invasive vulvar cancer: results from a seroepidemiological case-control study. *Obstet Gynecol* 90:748–754, 1997
9. Madeleine MM, Daling JR, Carter JJ, et al: Cofactors with human papillomavirus in a population-based study of vulvar cancer. *J Natl Cancer Inst* 89:1516–1523, 1997
10. Sliutz G, Schmidt W, Tempfer C, et al: Detection of p53 point mutation in primary human vulvar cancer by PCR and temperature gradient gel electrophoresis. *Gynecol Oncol* 64:93–98, 1997
11. Chambers SK: Molecular biology of gynecologic cancers, in Devita VT, Hellman S, Rosenberg SA (eds): *Cancer: Principles and Practice of Oncology* (ed 5). Philadelphia, Lippincott-Raven, 1997, pp 1427–1432
12. Hording U, Junge J, Daugaard S, et al: Vulvar squamous cell carcinoma and papillomaviruses: indications for two different etiologies. *Gynecol Oncol* 52:241–246, 1994
13. Baker VV: Vulvar: pathogenesis and epidemiology of vulvar cancer, in Shingleton HM, Fowler WC Jr, Jordan JA, Lawrence WD (eds): *Gynecologic Oncology—Current Diagnosis and Treatment.* Philadelphia, Saunders, 1996, pp 239–245
14. Soutter WP, Lambert H, McIndoe GAJ: Carcinoma of the vulvar and its putative precursors, in Peckham M, Pinedo HM, Veronesi U (eds): *Oxford Textbook of Oncology.* New York, Oxford University Press, 1995, pp 1383–1394

15. Hammond CB: Gynecology: the female reproductive organs, in Sabiston DC, Lyerly HK (eds): *Textbook of Surgery: The Biological Basis of Modern Surgical Practice* (ed 15). Philadelphia, Saunders, 1996, pp 1490–1505

16. Berek JS, Hacker NF: *Practical Gynecologic Oncology.* Baltimore, Williams and Wilkins, 1994

17. Chan KK, Helm CW: Invasive vulvar cancer, in Shingleton HM, Fowler WC, Jordan JA, Lawrence WD (eds): *Gynecologic Oncology—Current Diagnosis and Treatment.* Philadelphia, Saunders, 1996, pp 264–271

18. Rosen C, Malmstrom H: Invasive cancer of the vulva. *Gynecol Oncol* 65:213–217, 1997

19. Hacker NF: Vulvar cancer, in Berek JS, Adashi EY, Hillard PA (eds): *Gynecology* (ed 12). Philadelphia, Williams and Wilkins, 1996, pp 1231–1260

20. Rubin D: Gynecologic cancer: cervical, vulvar, and vaginal malignancies. *RN* 5:56–63, 1987

21. DiSaia PJ, Creasman WT: *Clinical Gynecologic Oncology.* St. Louis, Mosby, 1993

22. Homesley HD, Bundy BN, Sedles A, et al: Assessment of current International Federation of Gynecology and Obstetrics staging of vulvar carcinoma relative to prognostic factors for survival (a Gynecologic Oncology Group Study). *Am J Obstet Gynecol* 164:997–1010, 1991

23. Monk BJ, Burger RA, Lin F, et al: Prognostic significance of human papillomavirus DNA in vulvar carcinoma. *Obstet Gynecol* 85:709–715, 1995

24. Wolcott HD, Gallup DG: Wide local excision in the treatment of vulvar carcinoma in situ: a reappraisal. *Am J Obstet Gynecol* 150:695–698, 1984

25. Warwick A, Luesley DM: Vulvar intraepithelial lesions, in Shingleton HM, Fowler WC, Jordan JA, Lawrence WD (eds): *Gynecological Oncology—Current Diagnosis and Treatment.* Philadelphia, Saunders, 1996, pp 259–263

26. Nash JD, Curry S: Vulvar cancer. *Surg Oncol Clin North Am* 7:335–346, 1998

27. Siller BS, Alvarez RD, Conner WD, et al: T2-3 vulvar cancer: a case control study of triple incision versus en bloc radical vulvectomy and inguinal lymphadenectomy. *Gynecol Oncol* 57:335–339, 1995

28. Leiserowitz GS, Russell AH, Kinney WK: Prophylactic chemoradiation of inguino-femoral lymph nodes in patients with locally extensive vulvar cancer. *Gynecol Oncol* 66:509–514, 1997

29. Miller B, Morris M, Levenback C, et al: Pelvic exenteration for primary and recurrent vulvar cancer. *Gynecol Oncol* 58:202–205, 1995

30. Keys H: Gynecologic Oncology Group randomized trials of combined technique therapy for vulvar cancer. *Cancer* 71:1691–1696, 1993

31. Lupi G, Raspagliese F, Zucali R, et al: Combined preoperative chemoradiotherapy followed by radical surgery in locally advanced vulva carcinoma, a pilot study. *Cancer* 77:1472–1478, 1996

32. Landoni F, Maneo A, Zanetta G, et al: Concurrent preoperative chemotherapy with 5-fluorouracil and mitomycin C and radiotherapy (FUMIR) followed by limited surgery in locally advanced and recurrent vulvar carcinoma. *Gynecol Oncol* 61:321–327, 1996

33. Chamorro T: Cancer of the vulva and vagina. *Semin Oncol Nurs* 6:198–205, 1990

34. Helm CW, Chan KK: Vaginal cancer, in Shingleton HM, Fowler WC, Jordan JA, Lawrence WD (eds): *Gynecologic Oncology—Current Diagnosis and Treatment.* Philadelphia, Saunders, 1996, pp 109–116

35. Blake P: Carcinoma of the vagina, in Peckham M, Pinedo HM, Veronesi U (eds): *Oxford Textbook of Oncology.* New York, Oxford University Press, 1995, pp 1378–1382

36. Audet-Lapointe P, Body G, Vauclair R, et al: Vaginal intraepithelial neoplasia. *Gynecol Oncol* 36:232–239, 1990

37. MacLeod C, Fowler A, Dalrymple C, et al: High-dose-rate brachytherapy in the management of high-grade intraepithelial neoplasia of the vagina. *Gynecol Oncol* 65:74–77, 1997

38. Davis KP, Stanhope CR, Garton GR, et al: Invasive vaginal carcinoma: analysis of early stage disease. *Gynecol Oncol* 42:131–136, 1991

39. Brinton LA, Nasca PC, Mallin K, et al: Case-control study of in situ and invasive carcinoma of the vagina. *Gynecol Oncol* 38:49–54, 1990

40. Sugase M, Matsukurat T: Distant manifestations of human papillomaviruses in the vagina. *Int J Cancer* 72:412–415, 1997

41. Merino MJ: Vaginal cancer: the role of infectious and environmental factors. *Am J Obstet Gynecol* 165:1255–1259, 1991

42. Auclair CA: Consequences of prenatal exposure to diethylstilbestrol. *J Gynecol Nurs* 8:35–39, 1979

43. Herbst AL, Anderson S, Hubby MM, et al: Risk factors for the development of diethylstilbestrol-associated clear cell adenocarcinoma: a case-control study. *Am J Obstet Gynecol* 154:814–822, 1986

44. Robboy SJ, Noller KL, O'Brien P, et al: Increased incidence of cervical and vaginal dysplasia in 3980 diethylstilbestrol-exposed young women. Experience of the National Collaborative Diethylstilbestrol Adenosis Project. *JAMA* 252:2979–2983, 1984

45. DeMars LR, Van Le L, Huang I, et al: Primary non-clear-cell adenocarcinoma of the vagina in older DES-exposed women. *Gynecol Oncol* 3:389–392, 1995

46. Wharton JT, Tortolero-Luna G, Linares AC, et al: Vaginal intraepithelial neoplasia and vagina cancer. *Obstet Gynecol Clin North Am* 23:325–345, 1996

47. Kalogiroud D, Antoniou G, Karakitsos P, et al: Vaginal intraepithelial neoplasia (VAIN) following hysterectomy in patients treated for carcinoma in situ of the cervix. *Eur Gynaecol Oncol* 18:188–191, 1997

48. Bengton JM: The vagina, in Ryan KJ, Berkowitz RS, Barbieri RL (eds): *Kistner's Gynecology Principles and Practice.* St. Louis, Mosby, 1996, pp 80–93

49. Kirkbride P, Fyles A, Rawlings GA, et al: Carcinoma of the vagina: experience at the Princess Margaret Hospital (1974–1989). *Gynecol Oncol* 56:435–443, 1995

50. Stock RG, Chen ASJ, Seski J: A 30-year experience in the management of primary carcinoma of the vagina: analysis of prognostic factors and treatment modalities. *Gynecol Oncol* 56:45–51, 1995

51. Aho M, Vesterinen E, Meyer B, et al: Natural history of vaginal intraepithelial neoplasia. *Cancer* 68:195–197, 1991

52. Hatch KD, Fu YS: Cervical and vaginal cancer, in Berek JS, Adashi EY, Hillard PA (eds): *Gynecology* (ed 12). Philadelphia, Williams and Wilkins, 1996, pp 1111–1154

53. Kucera H, Vavra N: Radiation management of primary carcinoma of the vagina: clinical and histopathological variable associated with survival. *Gynecol Oncol* 40:12–16, 1991

54. Ali MM, Huang DT, Goplerud DR, et al: Radiation alone for carcinoma of the vagina: variation in response related to the location of the primary tumor. *Cancer* 77:1934–1939, 1996

55. Chyle V, Zagars GK, Wheeler JA, et al: Definitive radiotherapy for carcinoma of the vagina: outcome and prognostic factors. *Int J Radiat Oncol Biol Phys* 35:891–905, 1996

56. Fine BA, Piver MS, McAuley M, et al: The curative potential

of radiation therapy in the treatment of primary vaginal carcinoma. *Am J Clin Oncol* 19:39–44, 1996

57. Nolke S, Hanjani P: Intraepithelial neoplasia of the lower genital tract. *Semin Oncol Nurs* 6:181–189, 1990
58. Diakomanolis E, Rodolakis A, Sakellaropoulos G, et al: Conservative management of vaginal intraepithelial neoplasia (VAIN) by laser CO_2. *Eur J Gynaecol Oncol* 17:389–392, 1996
59. Yordan E, Deppe G, Malviya V, et al: Chemotherapy of the vulvar and vaginal malignancies, in Deppe G (ed): *Chemotherapy of Gynecologic Cancer*. New York, Wiley-Liss, 1990, pp 107–118
60. Morley GW, Peter WA: Microinvasive carcinoma of the vagina, in Coppleson M (ed): *Gynecology Oncology*. New York, Churchill-Livingstone, 1992, pp 501–504

61. Long HJ, Cross WG, Wiegand HS, et al: Phase II trial of methotrexate, vinblastine, doxorubicin, and cisplatin in advanced/recurrent carcinoma of the uterine cervix and vagina. *Gynecol Oncol* 57:235–239, 1995
62. Perez CA: Vagina, in Perez CA, Brady LW (eds): *Principles and Practice of Radiation Oncology*. Philadelphia, Lippincott, 1992, pp 1258–1272
63. Regnard CFB, Comiskey MC: Advanced cancer: the hospice approach, in Shingleton HM, Fowler WC, Jordan JA, Lawrence WD (eds): *Gynecologic Oncology—Current Diagnosis and Treatment*. Philadelphia, Saunders, 1996, pp 397–415

Cancer Survivor

CHAPTER 69

Psychosocial Responses to Cancer

Andrea M. Barsevick, DNSc, RN, AOCN
Judie Much, MSN, CRNP, AOCN
Carole Sweeney, MSN, RN, AOCN

Introduction

The Need for Psychosocial Care

The prevailing Western view is that cancer is a chronic treatable disease. Societal expectations for the individual with cancer include his or her accepting the diagnosis, seeking care, complying with treatment, and having a "fighting" spirit. To the individual living through the experience, however, cancer is greatly feared. It usually occurs without warning, may have an uncontrollable spread, may be incurable beyond a certain point, is assumed to be accompanied by pain and discomfort, and is a threat to quality of life.

Persons with cancer are not confronted with a single stressor but, rather, with a series of stressors. The stress is not limited to diagnosis and treatment; it continues throughout survival, with long-term physiological alterations, fears of relapse and death, dependence on caregivers, survivor guilt, and negative effects on families. It is paramount for the individual with cancer and for those with whom he or she shares a life to develop skills for managing the stresses associated with the cancer experience.

Cancer affects the functioning of the entire family unit. Its impact has been likened to dropping a stone into a pond.[1] The ripple effect changes family members and forces them to adjust their routines and basic functions, including eating, sleeping, working, and communicating with each other. No family emerges unchanged.[2] Because of the transition of health care from the hospital to the home, individuals with cancer rely on their families to assist them with complex medical regimens. Both family members and patients may have difficulty adjusting to role changes and lifestyle adaptations. If the cancer progresses, the family's role becomes more central. Families who are able to share their feelings and the work of caregiving may have less difficulty coping with the changes than families whose members function in isolation from one another.

In this chapter, we address the stressful challenges faced by individuals and families dealing with cancer by using a model of family-based care and a model of the stress-coping process. We use a research base to describe factors influencing family members as they cope with the stress of cancer, interventions to enhance coping efforts, and common problems encountered by individuals and families affected by cancer. We also address professional responses to cancer.

A Model of Family-Based Care

As the environment of health care has changed in recent years, the family's involvement in the care of a loved one with cancer has expanded dramatically. When nurses cared for patients primarily at the hospital bedside, the focus of care was the nurse-patient dyad. With the shifting of care to outpatient settings and to people's homes, family members now play an increasingly important role in cancer care. Families drive loved ones to appointments, communicate with health care providers, administer drugs and monitor their effects, assess health care problems and seek medical advice, assist with activities of daily living, and discuss issues of diagnosis and prognosis.

Defining a "family"

A *family* is a self-defined group of two or more individuals who may or may not be related by blood lines but who claim a special relationship and function in support of one another.[3,4] The structure of the family unit is extremely heterogeneous in American culture. Its members may include spouse, children, parents, grandparents, siblings, step-family, in-laws, cousins, homosexual partners, and unmarried partners. Variations in family structure include single-parent families, unmarried couples, step-parent families, and homosexual couples with adopted children or children from past relationships. The oncology nurse who is getting to know a family unit must begin by inquiring about the makeup of that particular family and the nature of the relationships involved.

Family assessment

Availability of support. As the nurse becomes acquainted with the family, initial dealings with the family include an assessment of the family's structure, including key family members, whether they live together, and the nature of their kinship. It is necessary to determine whether the family has meaningful ties that can provide support and assistance when needed. These ties might include relatives, neighbors, social or religious groups, or community organizations. If social ties are not in place, it is important for the nurse to understand why.

Patterns of family-based care. To assess the family support system, the nurse attempts to understand established patterns of family-based care. Schumacher has described three patterns of care: self-care, caregiver, and collaborative.[5]

Self-care occurs when the individual with cancer manages his or her care independently. The individual may curtail some usual activities, but it is not necessary for someone else to take on those activities. In the self-care pattern, potential caregivers often assume a standby role, ready to become involved if necessary. Otherwise, caregiver involvement is limited to established role responsibilities and activities.

A pattern of illness care in which there is a *primary caregiver* may be necessary when the person with cancer is very ill and has limited ability to function independently.[5] In the caregiver pattern, the caregiver "does everything" for the individual. This pattern of care can be difficult and distressing for both the individual with cancer and the caregiver, and is generally quickly given up as the patient's condition improves.

The most frequent pattern of care is described as

collaborative.[5] In the collaborative pattern, there is joint involvement in care. *Collaborative care* may involve task specialization or task sharing. Specialization occurs when some illness care tasks are carried out primarily by one member of the dyad, while other tasks are carried out by the other person. This approach is beneficial in that a caregiver becomes involved without violating the autonomy of the person with cancer. In task sharing, activities are carried out together, producing a synergistic effect. Together the partners accomplish more than either could alone.

Patterns of caregiving are dynamic, changing in response to changes in the illness. Therefore, the oncology nurse must assess caregiver patterns at frequent intervals in order to maintain current understanding. Schumacher argues that a dyadic focus should be the norm during cancer treatment because illness care

> is an area of endeavor in which *both* ill person and family caregiver participate. An individualistic focus, whether it is on self-care by the ill individual or caregiving by a family member, tends to render invisible the important involvement of the role partner in illness management.[5, p.268]

Starting with a broader view of family-based care, then focusing on the relative involvement of the ill person and family member is more realistic and in keeping with the reality of family involvement today.

Stage-specific needs. Like individuals, families go through several stages of development. An oncology nurse encountering families in different developmental stages must be aware of and assess the special issues that occur at each juncture.[3,6,7] Table 69-1 provides a description of family developmental stages and the factors that need to be addressed at each stage.

Cancer trajectory. It is generally agreed that the trajectory or course of the individual's cancer can have a profound effect on family interaction and adjustment.[8-11] Families dealing with an initial diagnosis often cope with the illness by using a process called *normalization.*[12] The family members acknowledge the existence of their loved one's cancer. At the same time, they try to maintain, or minimize disruption of, their usual routines and "reframe" their experience in more positive terms.

Families coping with cancer recurrence may also try to keep the cancer in the background, but they have a much more difficult time doing so.[8,13] Couples dealing with a breast cancer recurrence may limit what they discuss about the cancer and when they discuss it.[13] They may focus on symptoms or treatment and not discuss the meaning of the recurrence. Couples often justify their avoidance of sensitive issues by explaining their need not to dwell on the negatives and to get on with their lives.

Still, the use of avoidant coping can come at high cost to the couple. Two studies report couples' dissatisfaction with their marriages, depressive mood, and high distress levels, despite their attempts to normalize the situation and get on with their usual activities.[8,13] Lewis and Deal's interviews with couples record numerous examples of one partner wanting to discuss the possibility of death from the disease and the other partner wanting to main-

Table 69-1   Family Assessment Needs Based on Stage of Development

Stage of Family Development	Nursing Assessment of Developmental Tasks
Transitional stage: Unattached young adult living alone	• Prediagnosis relationship with parents
Beginning family: Married couple without children	• Prediagnosis relationship with both sets of parents • Ability of couple to communicate and make joint decisions
Young family: Couple or single parent with infant and preschool children	• Prediagnosis status of partner relationship • Capacity to maintain sense of normalcy in family routines
Middle family: Couple or single parent with school-age and teenage children	• Prediagnosis status of partner relationship • Prediagnosis level of dependency of each child • Family's ability to prioritize expectations and activities collaboratively • Flexibility in reallocating roles and responsibilities • Support system to manage schedule conflicts, household tasks, and routine errands
Mature family: Couple or single adult with adult children	• Prediagnosis status of partner relationship • Prediagnosis relationship with adult children
Family in old age: Elderly couple or single adult	• Whether partner is still living • Physical and mental health of couple • Prediagnosis relationship with children, grandchildren, other family members • Willingness of family to respect patient choices • Appropriateness of home residence to accommodate disability

tain a positive, upbeat image of the disease trajectory. By taking into account the disease trajectory, the nurse can anticipate the kinds of cognitive and emotional reactions that families may display.

Family functioning. *Family functioning* refers to a set of attributes that characterize and explain how a family system typically appraises, and behaves during, a stressful situation.[14] *Cohesion* refers to the degree of emotional bonding each individual experiences within the family system. Family cohesion ranges from highly entangled (enmeshment) to little connection (disengagement). *Adaptability* refers to the family's flexibility in responding to new demands. *Hardiness* is defined as the family's ability to work together to solve problems, view change as beneficial, and become active in managing difficult situations. Families with higher levels of functioning tend to adapt better to the challenges of cancer. An evaluation of family functioning will enable the oncology nurse to gauge the family's ability to work together and to determine whether additional resources are needed to support the family.

Family-based interventions

Levels of family-based care. Family nursing care is provided on at least four different levels:[6]

1. *The oncology nurse views the family as a resource and support system but secondary in importance to the individual with cancer.* This situation might occur when the patient is able to manage all care independently, such as when the disease is in remission or treatment is not intense or demanding.
2. *Family members are viewed as separate rather than interacting or interrelated persons and are assessed as individuals.* This level of care might occur in a hospice situation when the nurse recognizes that family members have their own needs and problems resulting from terminal cancer in a family member. In this scenario, the nurse works with both the patient with cancer and family member(s), treating them as separate individuals with separate needs.
3. *The family is viewed as an interacting system in which the nurse works with the interacting unit.* Schumacher suggests that the nurse adopt an interactional focus in any situation in which a family caregiver is identified.[5] During active therapy, both the ill person and the family caregiver collaborate and participate in care. So it is most appropriate to work with the collaborating unit.
4. *The entire family is the focus of care.* Family dynamics, structure, function, and relationships are the focus of assessment and intervention. A psychiatric clinical specialist might engage in this level of care by conducting family therapy with a family experiencing difficulty adjusting to the cancer diagnosis in a family member.

Family-focused interventions. Interventions for families, including teaching and counseling, are not unlike those nurses typically use with individuals. However, the emphasis changes somewhat within a family context.[6] For example, nurses are more likely to engage in informal teaching in nurse-family interactions. Role modeling, demonstration, and experiential strategies are most effective in helping families to learn new competencies or to reframe their experience in more positive terms. Family intervention may involve coaching family members in the performance of a treatment procedure or in negotiations with a health care agency or insurer.

Informal teaching may take the form of *anticipatory guidance.* Information is provided about what to expect with regard to a future event, potential problem, or developmental phase. Anticipatory guidance or preparatory information effectively reduces anxiety and emotional distress and maintains adaptive functioning in unfamiliar health care situations.[15]

Counseling is an interactive process that helps families address and cope with needs, problems, and feelings that could interfere with adaptive behavior.[6] It also enables family members to use their competencies and resources more effectively. Acceptance, empathy, and congruency characterize the relationship between nurse and family members. Encouraging families to express and share their concerns with other family members is an essential part of this process. Assisting family members to restructure their thoughts and feelings in a more positive way is also a major component of counseling. Family counseling strategies also may encourage family members to interact differently with one another, by assuming caregiver roles or learning more effective ways to communicate.

A Model of the Stress and Coping Process

The stress and coping model of Lazarus and Folkman is the basis for this discussion of psychosocial issues related to cancer[16] (Figure 69-1). This model provides the clinician with a useful framework for understanding the complex psychosocial problems of individuals and families coping with cancer. It also provides a basis for gathering information to conduct a psychosocial assessment and

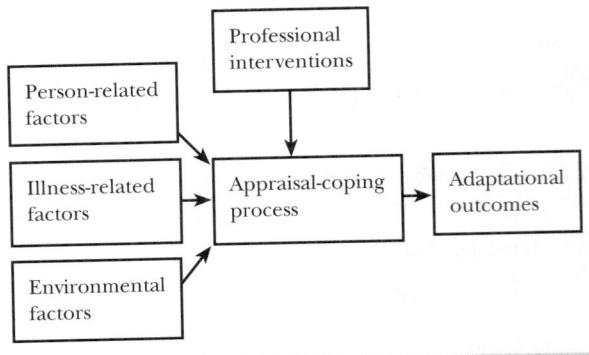

Figure 69-1 The stress-coping process.

for selecting and designing interventions to assist and support the individual's coping efforts.

The appraisal-coping process

Central to the model is the appraisal-coping process. Appraisal and coping are cognitive and behavioral processes people use to deal with a problem. *Appraisal* is a person's evaluation of the problem, including the definition of the problem; one's perception of it as a threat, loss, or challenge; and the resources available for dealing with it. *Coping* refers to the cognitive and behavioral strategies used to manage the stressful situation, including strategies directed toward management of the problem itself as well as those used to deal with the negative emotions that are aroused by the situation.

To describe appraisal and coping as a process means that we are describing what a person actually thinks and does within a specific context or situation. *Process* also suggests that thoughts and actions change as the situation unfolds, as information is obtained, and as the demands on the individual change. The dynamics and changes that occur are not random. A process can be likened to a sailboat on the sea. The captain watches the horizon, the weather, and the water conditions. On the basis of these, he decides on a course and constantly readjusts the rudder and fine-tunes the sails to stay on course. So it is with the coping process. The individual appraises a specific situation and puts in motion a set of coping strategies, constantly readjusting and fine-tuning the appraisal and coping strategies used as new information becomes available and as aspects of the situation change. Shifts in the information available to the individual lead to a reappraisal of what is happening, its significance, and what can be done. The reappraisal, in turn, determines subsequent coping efforts.

Coping serves two basic functions. *Problem-focused coping* efforts are directed at managing or altering the problem causing the stress, while *emotion-focused coping* strategies are directed at regulating emotional responses to the stressful situation. Problem-focused coping involves problem-solving efforts such as defining the problem, generating alternative solutions, weighing the alternatives with regard to their costs and benefits, choosing among them, and acting. Problem-focused coping also includes strategies for reducing environmental pressures or barriers, information-seeking, and learning new skills or behaviors. Emotion-focused coping includes strategies with the direct intent of reducing the emotional distress caused by the stressful problem. These include typical defense mechanisms such as denial, avoidance, distancing, or selective attention. Emotion-focused coping also may include expressions of emotion, including humor, hope, grieving, and anxiety, as expressing feelings is often necessary to reduce distress.

Problem- or emotion-focused coping strategies can be used successfully or unsuccessfully (Table 69-2). The success of a coping strategy is determined by its outcome

Table 69-2 Successful and Unsuccessful Coping

Strategy	Successful	Unsuccessful
Anger	Able to identify source Able to resolve Maintain sense of self	Depression, passivity, or aggression
Humor	Tension reducer Decreases social distance	Masks feelings Avoidance
Depression	Normal response	Persistent, pervasive feelings of loss Suicide
Anxiety	Gradual understanding Initially protective	Ignoring, refusing reality
Hopefulness	Comforting, sustaining Belief that future good exists	Limited choices Inability to mobilize energy

or intended outcome. The behavior of denial is *value neutral*, meaning that it is not inherently adaptive or maladaptive. Its adaptiveness is determined by what it can or does achieve. An example of successful use of denial as a coping strategy involves a woman who, after hearing the diagnosis of breast cancer, refuses to discuss her diagnosis in the first weeks of treatment. This protective behavior allows her to assimilate information at her own pace, preventing despair. Later, this same woman becomes active in advocating breast health and visits other women having surgery for breast cancer. If this woman's denial resulted in refusal or discontinuation of treatment, the potential negative outcome would have defined the coping behavior as *maladaptive*.

Adaptational outcomes

The principal importance of the appraisal-coping process is that it affects adaptational outcomes. An *outcome* is commonly defined as a relevant end result.[17,18] The main psychosocial outcomes of the appraisal and coping process in the health care context are the maximization of (1) physical health, (2) functioning in work and social living, and (3) psychological well-being. To the extent that the appraisal-coping process fosters one or more of these outcomes, it is adaptive; when it does not, it is maladaptive.

Factors influencing the process

The appraisal-coping process does not occur in a vacuum. It is influenced by a variety of person-related, illness-related, and environmental factors. Knowing which factors influence the stress and coping process can help the clinician identify persons who may be at risk for developing psychological or behavioral problems. Identifying these individuals is critical so that resources can be directed to persons with the greatest need for them. Being aware of these factors can also provide cues to the clinician about how to approach the individual or family.

Professional interventions

Professional interventions to support or enhance the appraisal-coping process are necessary if the individual's appraisal of the problem is inaccurate or distorted, if the individual has inadequate resources for dealing with it, or if the individual's coping efforts are inadequate or unlikely to achieve the desired outcome. Professional interventions may include preparatory information, teaching cognitive or behavioral skills, or providing supportive care.

Assessment of the Appraisal-Coping Process

Individuals and families faced with a potential or actual cancer diagnosis generally use the appraisal-coping process effectively to deal with the problems they encounter. They gather information from health care providers, make decisions about diagnostic and treatment options, manage their emotional distress, and effectively make use of support systems. Professional nursing assessment is indicated at two junctures: (1) the initial contact between nurse and patient/family when a baseline assessment is performed, and (2) when the nurse observes difficulties indicating a breakdown in the effectiveness of the appraisal-coping process. In keeping with the tenets of the stress and coping model, an assessment of the appraisal-coping process must be viewed as a snapshot of one point in time because the process is constantly changing.

At the initial contact between nurse and patient, the nurse can use the concepts of the appraisal-coping process as a basis for an initial assessment (Figure 69-2). The individual's perception of a problem is a major component of his or her appraisal of it.[19] A probable diagnosis of cancer will be appraised differently, depending on the specific circumstances of the individual facing the

---

What are the major problems you face related to your cancer?

↓

For each problem identified, ask yourself:

↓

- How difficult the problem is for you to handle;
- How you feel about this problem;
- What resources you have to help you deal with it;
- How you are coping with it;
- How you are coping with your feelings about it;
- What the desired outcome of your efforts to deal with this problem is.

Figure 69-2 Self-assessment of the appraisal-coping process.

---

diagnosis. To a young woman with small children, a diagnosis of breast cancer can be a devastating crisis not only because of the disease itself but also because of the threat it poses to her family. From her vantage point, the most stressful problem she faces may not be the diagnostic and treatment procedures but the uncertainty about her ability to care for her family in the immediate and long-term future. For an elderly woman who is the sole caregiver to her elderly mate, the stressful problem may be the diagnostic and treatment procedures that take her away from her responsibilities as caregiver. It is important for the nurse to understand the individual's unique perception of the problems he or she faces in order to provide targeted and individualized interventions.

An important aspect of the individual's perception of the problem is his or her feelings about it. A problem may be appraised as a threat, a loss, or a challenge, each suggesting different patterns of response based on perception.[16] Individuals who perceive a problem as a threat are likely to experience anxiety or fear; those perceiving loss may experience grief or depression; and individuals who view a problem as a challenge could experience positive feelings such as eager anticipation or hopefulness.

Another important aspect of appraisal is the individual's perception of the resources he or she has for dealing with the problem. To say a person is *resourceful* means that she or he has tangible items or competencies to draw on and is able to use them to manage difficult or complex situations. Tangible resources include people, information, equipment, and money. Internal resources include energy, positive beliefs, problem-solving skills, or social skills.

Factors Influencing the Appraisal-Coping Process

Person-Related Factors

Cultural background

A person's culture is the lens through which he or she perceives the world. Values, beliefs, and norms are culture-bound ideals that guide thinking, decision making, and actions[20] and explain many differences in behavior. When faced with the problem of cancer, persons from different cultures are likely to appraise and cope with it in diverse ways related to their specific cultural backgrounds.

The use of a stress and coping model requires that care be based on the individual's perception of the problem(s) he or she faces. Within a cultural context, the nurse must recognize that the individual's perceptions are culture-bound and culturally determined, as are the nurse's own. In a pluralistic society, nurses need to be prepared to work with individuals of varied cultural backgrounds and to ensure that nursing care is culturally appropriate. Where there is a cultural difference between the nurse and the individual under his or her care, differences in key areas may need to be acknowledged and addressed.[20] Communication may be a problem if there are discrepancies between the nurse and patient with regard to language or their conceptions of health and illness. Personal space may also be a problem or source of discomfort, as different cultures have different spatial needs. Time may be an issue because different cultures vary in their sense of urgency about time and in the degree to which they focus on the present or future.

Social organizations must also be considered. Every culture determines acceptable ways for families to interact with and assist one another. The use of family resources called for by the stress and coping model must be evaluated within the cultural context. Religious affiliation must be considered because cultural and religious values are often linked. Lastly, culturally determined health-seeking and sick-role behaviors must be considered as cultures often differ in their behavioral expectations of individuals who are seeking health care. The reader is referred to Chapter 7 for a detailed discussion on culture diversity and nursing implications.

Socioeconomic status

Differences in culture may be compounded by differences in socioeconomic status because minorities in the United States often have fewer financial and educational resources.[21-23] It has long been recognized that socioeconomic status has an important influence on morbidity and mortality due to cancer. Individuals with low annual incomes are three to seven times more likely to die of cancer than those with high annual incomes.[21] Not graduating from high school has been associated with death rates from cancer that are two to three times greater than college graduates. These factors are likely to have a profound effect on the appraisal and coping strategies used by persons of lower socioeconomic means. When examining psychological responses of persons with lower socioeconomic status, the clinician must recognize the influence of lack of education, unemployment, poor nutrition, lifestyle factors that increase risk, and difficulties with access to health care.

Illustrations of the influence of culture and socioeconomic status on people's appraisal of the problem of cancer are found in a study of a white working-class neighborhood in Philadelphia targeted for a cancer prevention program,[24] and in a study of a group of black women from eastern North Carolina who had advanced breast cancer.[25] In both settings, cancer was viewed as a powerful and unstoppable disease that was fatal and incurable. The people being studied could identify no particular cause for cancer, so they had no explanation for why one person fell victim to it and another did not. Another important concept in both settings was the desire not to tempt fate by engaging in cancer screening. For working-class Philadelphians, "to think about cancer, to try to prevent it, is to tempt fate."[24,p.16] One of the North Carolinians expressed it this way, "If you have a lump and it's not

bothering you, leave it alone. You don't want to get it started."[25,p.795] For the North Carolina women, fatalism, lack of knowledge of risk factors for breast cancer, lower educational levels, and a strong belief in the effectiveness of folk medicine contributed to late-stage presentation of disease.[25]

When culture and socioeconomic status constitute a barrier to care, the nurse should consult with the patient and family members to gain a better understanding of the health values and behaviors of their culture and incorporate these values whenever possible into the plan of care. Several textbooks are now available that describe the health beliefs, values, and behaviors of a number of cultural groups in the United States.[20,26] It also may be helpful to involve a person who is culturally, linguistically, and socially similar to the person in need of care. This individual could serve as an interpreter if there is a language barrier.

Age

Age is a sociodemographic factor that is predictive of psychological adjustment to cancer. Still, health care professionals have misunderstood its influence, believing that older people have greater adjustment difficulties.[27] In fact, research has demonstrated that younger people report greater adjustment difficulties in comparison to their older counterparts.[27] At 12-month and 4-year follow-ups, women under 65 who were treated for breast cancer experienced greater emotional distress, poorer mental health, and greater deterioration of psychological well-being than older women.[28,29] Younger individuals with a variety of cancers also reported more problems with physical health, finances, communication with providers, and home care than older people.[27] This research underscores the need for clinicians to pay careful attention to the problems identified by each individual under his or her care, particularly younger people, who often undergo more aggressive therapy with greater threats to their quality of life.

Psychological coping styles

Another important factor is the enduring beliefs or traits that constitute an individual's personality. *Beliefs* are personally formed or culturally shared cognitive ideas about reality that determine what is fact and shape the individual's understanding of reality.[16] *Traits* are relatively stable and enduring ways in which one individual differs from others and that exert generalized effects on behavior.[30] For example, the idea has been introduced that people differ in their preference for control in health situations.[31] Such beliefs can buffer or exaggerate the individual's appraisal and subsequent coping efforts in a stressful situation. When a situation is highly ambiguous, the individual with an internal locus of control is more likely to appraise it as controllable than the person whose locus of control is external.

Evidence suggests that individual differences in stable

coping styles serve as buffers in stressful situations. Traits such as personal control or optimism may give rise to an appraisal of challenge rather than threat or loss when a diagnosis of cancer is made. This could lower the individual's perceived stress during the diagnostic and treatment period in comparison to the stress experienced by those whose world view is pessimistic. Thus, traits can moderate an individual's appraisal of a problem. Another way that personality traits can influence the stress-coping process is by influencing the individual's choice of coping strategies. Although they may be distressed by the diagnosis of cancer, optimists have been found to make greater use of positive, adaptive coping strategies such as acceptance, positive reframing, and gaining comfort from religious beliefs and less use of denial or behavioral disengagement.[32] Likewise, information preference coping styles determine the extent to which individuals engage in and benefit from information-seeking behavior.[33] Individual differences or traits often are not immediately evident to the observer. However, measurement instruments are available that can aid the clinician.[34]

Illness-Related Factors

A history of comorbidity (whether psychiatric or medical) and the presence of more advanced disease increases the individual's risk for poor psychosocial outcomes after a cancer diagnosis. Still, these factors do not constitute a guarantee of problems. They *do* alert the professional to observe and question the individual so that coping difficulties do not result in poorer outcomes.

A history of previous psychiatric diagnosis, particularly depressive disorders, increases the risk of developing depression after a cancer diagnosis.[35] Among women with breast cancer, two-thirds of those with a history of depression reported significant distress 18 months after diagnosis, while only 14% of those without a psychiatric history reported distress.[36] Likewise, the presence of other comorbid conditions when cancer is diagnosed also seems to heighten the individual's risk for psychological problems. Research indicates that individuals with higher morbidity risk have poorer social and role functioning, poorer mental health, and perceptions of poorer health than individuals with low morbidity risk.[37] Severity of disease has also been associated with poorer psychological adjustment. Women with more extensive surgery for breast cancer and those with regional as opposed to local disease reported higher levels of psychological distress and poorer long-term adjustment than women with less severe disease.[36]

Environmental Factors

Social networks have been found to have a protective effect with regard to psychosocial outcomes. Married people live longer and have lower mortality rates for all major causes of death than persons who have never been married or who are separated, widowed, or divorced.[38] Individuals with cancer who have support from a spouse or a social network are diagnosed at an earlier stage and receive more complete treatment than individuals without a social network.[39,40]

Psychosocial Interventions

A critical question with regard to the psychosocial management of the individual with cancer is, "What specific intervention is most effective for the individual with a specific problem, and under which set of circumstances is it effective?" Answering this question is difficult because cancer encompasses different diseases with disparate etiologies and outcomes. Examining psychological interventions in the context of the magnitude of the disease and treatment process, Andersen concluded that those with advanced disease made more significant gains in quality of life with the help of psychosocial interventions.[41] Furthermore, they were more likely than individuals with localized disease to worsen without intervention.

Descriptive and intervention studies point to the effectiveness of crisis intervention and brief therapy models of intervention.[41] Both use similar approaches with regard to early assessment, present-day focus, limited goals, counseling direction, and prompt interventions. The components of this type of therapy include information about the disease and its treatment; an emotionally supportive context in which to address emotional concerns, including fears and anxieties; instruction in cognitive and behavioral coping strategies, including relaxation techniques; and focused interventions for specific problems such as sexual functioning in individuals with diseases affecting the sexual organs. Procedural variations such as whether the intervention is administered individually or in groups do not have an impact on the effectiveness of the intervention.

Andersen also addresses the probable mechanism for intervention effectiveness.[41] Interventions assist individuals to learn more about the stressor and to confront it in a positive coping state with active behavioral strategies. Using skills learned through the intervention process, the individual is able to reduce emotional distress, make a realistic appraisal of current and impending stresses, and enhance his or her self-efficacy and feelings of control early in the adjustment process. Gains have been found to continue and often increase during the first posttreatment year even when the therapy has been brief.

A variety of interventions are available to the oncology nurse, including education, counseling, storytelling, and relaxation. Each of these will be addressed.

Education

In addition to the obvious benefits of increased knowledge, education assists the individual with cancer to reduce his or her sense of helplessness and inadequacy related to uncertainty.[42] A meta-analysis of 116 psychoeducational intervention studies for cancer patients examined the effect of educational interventions on anxiety, depression, mood, nausea, vomiting, pain, and knowledge.[43] Educational topics included specific information on type and stage of disease, treatment types, and how to live with cancer. Beneficial effects were found across all seven outcomes. The most effective intervention for knowledge acquisition was printed material, although other educational methods were also effective. Education can be effective when targeted to an individual or to a group. It may consist of written or oral content, including videotape, audiotape, or didactic methods.

Counseling

The individual who is depressed or has difficulty coping with the disease is best managed with consistent emotional support and counseling within the context of a trusting relationship. The oncology nurse can help with problem solving, acknowledge the person's fears, and allow for control and decision-making based on the person's unique needs. The goals of this intervention are to improve the individual's self-worth, correct misconceptions about the past and present, and integrate the present illness into the individual's self-concept. Active listening is used by the nurse to build trust and acceptance.[44] Good communication sets a stable tone and is supportive of hope.[45] Counseling involves the provision of support by the nurse and the identification of other social supports for the individual, such as family, friends, other patients, support groups, and community resources. It optimizes past strengths, supports past coping efforts, and mobilizes resources. Experienced oncology nurses weave this approach into their everyday activities, including self-care activities, examinations, phone calls, and treatment visits. There is evidence that providing the opportunity for patients to air their feelings helps individuals cope with the cancer experience.[46–48]

Storytelling

Intervening in the individual's experience of cancer may cause the nurse to reach deep into the self for creativity. Storytelling can be an effective method of communicating with individuals for whom more direct methods of communication are ineffective.[49] Stories can be used to transmit knowledge, improve learning, and assist with problem solving.[50–52] Procedures and situations can be explained by way of stories containing metaphor and symbolism. Stories are perceived by individuals hearing or reading them as being "outside" themselves; therefore, the content or metaphor is easily taken in and is less likely to trigger a defensive response. Techniques that can be used include prescribing a story to be read, telling a story, or using a metaphor. In order for storytelling to be successful, the story must fit the situation and the information must be given in a natural manner and only after rapport has developed. When the intervention is successful, it can provide the patient and family with a new perspective with which to view their situation. Patients and families can also derive satisfaction from telling or writing their stories. Using this technique, an individual may be able to verbalize endings that are either desired or greatly feared. Stories also may be written in a journal or in letters that are kept.

Relaxation

Behavioral relaxation is helpful in dealing with conditioned nausea associated with chemotherapy administration.[53] Behavioral relaxation reduces anxiety and physiological arousal related to cancer stressors; it serves as a distraction, redirecting the individual's attention away from the stressful stimulus; and it promotes feelings of control and reduces feelings of helplessness.

Psychosocial Outcomes

The Importance of Outcomes

The stress and coping model used to guide the discussion of psychosocial problems defines outcomes as the final variable in the process. Coping strategies used by individuals and their families are value neutral; that is, they are not adaptive or maladaptive by virtue of any inherent properties. Their effectiveness is determined by the intended or actual outcome. Therefore, the type of nursing care required in a given set of circumstances is determined by the intended outcome(s) of that care, and the effectiveness of the nursing care provided is evaluated by the actual outcomes achieved. Without being aware of nursing outcomes, the nurse cannot be sure of the direction or the effectiveness of the care provided.[17]

More importantly, from a clinical standpoint articulation of intended outcomes provides a means for the oncology nurse to communicate with the patient and family and make mutual decisions about the type and direction of care. It helps them to set the direction and course for their work together. For example, if the patient's goal is to minimize symptom burden (desired outcome) so he or she can continue working during treatment, then the nurse identifies the information and skills training that will be necessary to achieve this outcome. If the patient is elderly and is likely to need additional physical care during treatment to maintain comfort and satisfaction, the nurse begins the process of identifying the resources available to supply the physical and emotional support needed.

Outcomes are a critical focus of oncology nursing practice because they define our practice. Medicine defines survival and tumor response as critical outcomes. As such, the effectiveness of any medical intervention is evaluated with regard to its effect on these two outcomes, and cure and survival rates remain the domain of medical practice. Likewise, nursing uses outcomes to define its domain of practice. This requires that oncology nurses measure, track, and report outcomes.

An even more critical reason for the emphasis on outcomes has to do with the atmosphere of cost containment and cost effectiveness in which oncology nurses practice today. As a group, nurses must be able to identify and quantify nursing's effect on patient outcomes in order to establish their worth and position in patient care. If nurses cannot document their positive role in patient outcomes, then the number of nurses involved in patient care may be reduced and their responsibilities turned over to lesser-skilled providers.

What Outcomes Are Important

The psychosocial care that oncology nurses provide to individuals with cancer is likely to influence a broad range of outcomes, including physical health, functional well-being, psychological well-being, and social well-being. Within each of these domains of outcomes are perhaps hundreds of individual factors that are measurable. But which of these individual outcomes or domains are of greatest importance to oncology nursing? How can we communicate about these outcomes in a language that is understandable to the lay public and that includes, in a meaningful way, a variety of outcomes?

Quality-of-life (QOL) is a health care construct that incorporates these diverse outcomes.[17,18] Cella defines QOL as the appraisal of and level of satisfaction with one's current state of well-being.[54] Quality-of-life is complex in that it cannot be evaluated adequately by means of a single indicator or dimension, instead requiring indicators from several domains to adequately represent it. It is also subjective; that is, it can only be understood from the perspective of the individual experiencing it. This is because the individual's own cognitive processes determine his or her evaluation of QOL, including illness and treatment perceptions, expectations of self and outcomes, and appraisal of risk or harm.

The dimensions or domains of QOL have not been firmly established.[54] However, four dimensions that are typically represented include physical, functional, psychological, and social well-being. Each of these domains is relevant to nursing and, in some cases, nursing interventions have been associated with improvements in quality of life.

Physical well-being

The *physical dimension* of QOL refers to perceived bodily dysfunction or disruption. Common examples in oncology are physical symptoms including pain, nausea, and fatigue. Our discussion of symptom management related to treatment in this chapter suggests that preparatory information reduces the number and severity of symptoms experienced.[55–57] The provision of psychological interventions for persons with advanced cancer has demonstrated positive outcomes.[37,58]

Functional well-being

Distinct from the physical dimension is the functional dimension of QOL. *Functional status* refers to the ability to perform activities related to one's personal care and role responsibilities.[54] It can refer to activities of daily living or the ability to carry out responsibilities related to family, home, or work. The use of preparatory information for individuals undergoing radiation treatment for prostate cancer has resulted in better functioning, particularly in recreational and leisure activities.[56,57]

Psychological well-being

Psychological well-being refers to emotional state, including both positive and negative moods. For many individuals with cancer, emotional distress is not a major problem.[59,60] However, blunting of positive emotions may occur.[54] The literature on psychosocial interventions indicates that a brief counseling or crisis intervention approach is beneficial to psychological well-being, especially in individuals with more advanced disease.[41] Whereas studies have shown that individuals with less advanced disease improved emotionally without intervention, those with more advanced disease who received no counseling worsened.[47,58]

Social well-being

Another dimension of QOL is *social well-being*, which includes social support, family functioning, and intimacy. Abundant research has demonstrated that the diagnosis of cancer (particularly advanced cancer) has a negative impact on the family.[13] Social support groups benefit people by reducing isolation and loneliness.[61,62] Counseling interventions have demonstrated beneficial effects on sexual functioning.[63]

Overall, psychosocial care of patients with cancer—including education, counseling, crisis intervention, social support, and behavioral skills training—has had favorable effects on many aspects of their QOL. Research has also shown that certain populations of individuals are more vulnerable to poor outcomes. These include individuals of low socioeconomic status, younger age, and more advanced disease. Nurses can begin to target their intervention efforts to individuals with these characteristics in order to make their services effective and efficient.

Common Problems of the Individual/ Family with Cancer

Making Decisions About Treatment

When counseling the patient in the pretreatment phase, there are two issues the oncology nurse must consider:

(1) role preference in treatment decision making, and (2) desire for information. With regard to treatment decisions, individuals with cancer typically have played a passive role.[64,65] Yet increasingly, patients are expressing a desire for greater participation in decision making about treatment, most notably women with breast cancer and persons with AIDS.

Three different role preferences have been identified among individuals with cancer.[66] Between 12% and 20% of cancer patients expressed a desire to take an active role in making the final selection of treatment. A second group of 32%–59% preferred passivity, allowing the physician to make the final decision about treatment. A third group of 28%–40% preferred to collaborate with the physician in making decisions.

It would seem to follow logically that individuals who wish to participate in decision making need sufficient illness- and treatment-related information to make informed decisions. But what of those who prefer a passive role in decision making? Do they need little or no information? When the desire for information of each of the role preference groups was examined, virtually all of the individuals who wanted to play an active or collaborative role also wanted detailed information about treatment alternatives, treatment procedures, and side effects.[64] There was also a group of persons desiring a passive role who wanted minimal information. However, a second group of passive patients wanted detailed medical information. Even though they were content to play a passive role in decision making, they still wanted to know what would be happening to them. These findings provide clear guidance to the oncology nurse in determining patient preference for involvement in decision making.

Preferences have been determined by asking individuals to sort five cards, consisting of written statements and an illustrative drawing, according to their preferred role in treatment decision making[64,67] (Figure 69-3). This approach is adapted easily for clinical use by simply asking individuals how involved they wish to be in making decisions about their treatment. For individuals who wish to participate, providing written information about specific aspects of their illness and treatment enhances retention

Figure 69-3 Preferred roles in treatment decision making. (Reprinted with permission from Newfeld KR, Degner LF, Dick JAM: A nursing intervention strategy to foster patient involvement in treatment decisions. *Oncol Nurs Forum* 20:631–635, 1993.[67])

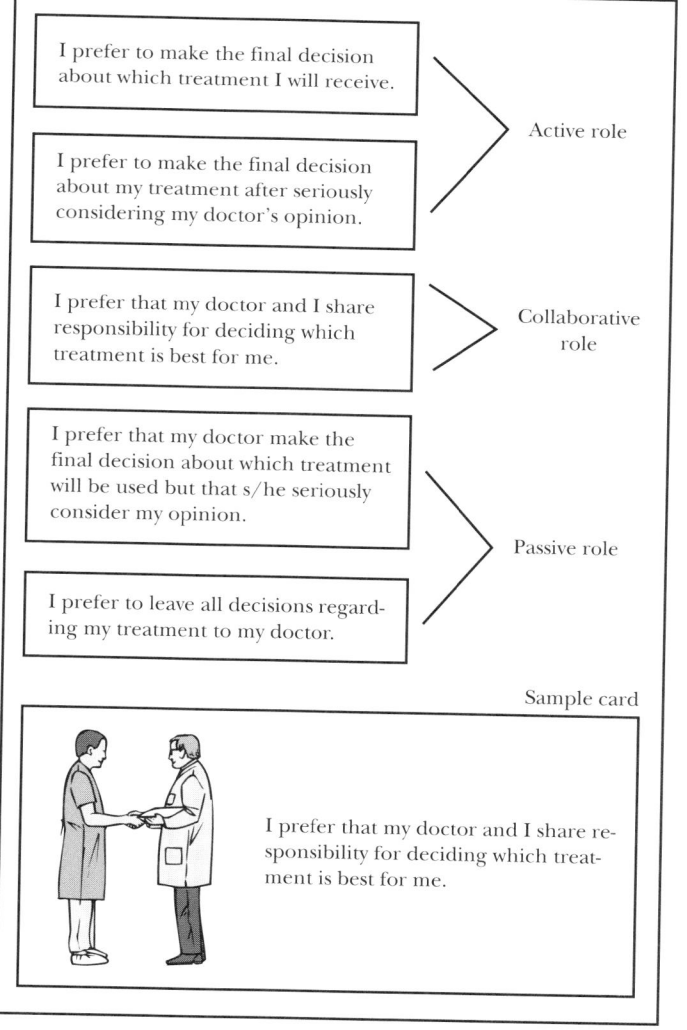

and recall of information and reduces anxiety.[67–69] Individuals have also benefited from "coaching" on how to ask questions and negotiate decisions.[70] To summarize, individuals desiring an active role should be encouraged to assert themselves and be furnished with detailed information about their care.

Research is less clear about how to deal with individuals who prefer a more passive role in decision making and who prefer minimal information. One might be tempted to say that passive individuals should have their information preferences respected. However, ample research demonstrates clear benefits to patients and families when information about what they should expect is provided.[55,56] For individuals who desire minimal information, there is some evidence that this preference is rooted in the individual's concern about the negative emotions that are likely to be aroused by an influx of information on a threatening topic such as cancer. It has been proposed that the professional must tease out the fears, anxieties, and concerns of these individuals and first teach them ways of coping with their negative emotions through relaxation techniques and cognitive restructuring procedures.[71] Once patients have mastered the skills for dealing with the negative emotions that are likely to be aroused, the nurse can begin the educational process.

Dealing with Uncertainty

Uncertainty is a common problem experienced by individuals and families dealing with cancer. The probabilistic nature of cancer diagnosis and treatment, the complexity of treatment and systems of care, the lack of information about diagnosis and treatment, and unpredictability of the disease course contribute to the uncertainty associated with cancer.[72] Uncertainty interferes with the formation of a realistic appraisal of a stressful problem because the individual is hampered in his or her efforts to recognize and classify information.

In a situation of uncertainty, *appraisal* involves the processes of inference and illusion. When using inference, the individual bases his or her appraisal on general knowledge and past experience by identifying examples from similar situations. The greater the similarity between the recalled event and the current situation, the greater the effect of recall on the formation of an appraisal.[72] *Illusions*, beliefs constructed in the absence of knowledge, may also be used to form an appraisal. The use of illusion can be valuable in protecting the individual when information is unavailable or when information is available but difficult to accept. The danger in using inference and illusion as a basis for making an appraisal of a threatening problem is that it may be flawed, distorted, or inaccurate. As shown in the example of the poor black women in North Carolina, the idea that a painless lump in the breast is best left alone has had enormous consequences, contributing to unnecessary disability and premature death.[25]

Under conditions of uncertainty, appraising a situation as threatening is likely to result in pessimism, elevated anxiety, or depression.[72] Coping efforts are directed at reducing the uncertainty and managing the emotion generated by an appraisal of threat. *Direct action* may be used to reduce uncertainty, although there is evidence that in catastrophic illnesses such as cancer, direct action is the least-used coping strategy. *Vigilance* in monitoring symptoms or health problems also may be used. However, the primary means for reducing uncertainty is *information seeking*, which is used to formulate probabilities and to create a framework for ordering illness-related experiences. Health care providers serve as information sources, and they also help to structure information. Significant others can also provide or reinforce expert information or they can interpret events. If these strategies are not effective in reducing uncertainty, then emotion-focused coping strategies are used to achieve this goal.

The goal of nursing is to reduce uncertainty whenever possible while recognizing that some aspects of uncertainty related to cancer may never be removed. Mishel, who has studied this phenomena extensively, suggests that one way that health care professionals reduce uncertainty is by providing credible authority.[72] *Credible authority* refers to the strength of the relationship and level of trust between an individual and a health care provider. Patients with cancer may rely on professionals to provide a logical structure for interpreting their experiences and to provide judgments and recommendations regarding the physical aspects of care, the efficacy of treatment, expectations about outcomes, and the performance of the health care system. The greater the nurse's credible authority, the greater his or her ability to reduce uncertainty related to cancer and its treatment.

The most common means of reducing uncertainty is by providing preparatory information about the specific aspects of the cancer experience. (See sections on Treatment and Care of Individuals with Cancer, for specifics about the process of preparing patients in a manner that enables them to cope more effectively with the experience.) Research has demonstrated that the most effective information is that which helps people to form a realistic mental image of the experience they are about to undergo.[56,73] Both the subjective and objective characteristics of the experience should be described. Subjective features include physical sensations and experiences that can be verified only by the person experiencing them. This information must be obtained from people who have experienced a particular type of treatment and its effects.[74,75] Objective features include the temporal and spatial characteristics of an experience, such as how long a procedure lasts and what the environment looks like.

Several guidelines may be followed in the provision of this type of information. Physical sensations should be described without evaluation. For example, patients may be told that after surgery, the incision will feel tender and sore and that they may feel pressure, aching, and pulling. They should be informed of the reasons for the sensations so they will be less likely to misinterpret them as evidence that something has gone wrong. This is especially true for individuals with cancer, because treatment-related symptoms can be confused with symptoms of the disease. Research has also shown that the use of emotionally charged words such as *pain* and descriptions of the magnitude of sensations such as the severity of pain are not helpful.[75]

Individuals who are properly informed are freed from the task of sorting through a large number of details about an experience to figure out the best way to handle it. Individuals are also less likely to misinterpret their experiences and choose inappropriate or inefficient methods of coping with them. This information has been found to have positive long-term effects on an individual's functional recovery from treatment procedures.[56,57]

Managing the Side Effects of Treatment

Cancer treatment, whether curative, palliative, or prophylactic, does not come without a cost.[76] Treatment results in a variety of adverse side effects that can be debilitating and long lasting, causing considerable distress for patients and their families. Not surprisingly, many of the interventions that have been found to be effective in managing these side effects are psychosocial in nature, given that many of the side effects are stress related.

In order to provide efficient and effective nursing assessment and interventions for side effects of treatment, nurses need to be aware of the frequency, onset, duration, and severity of the symptoms presented by their patients. For example, individuals receiving specific treatments can be asked about their experiences of treatment-related symptoms.[77] For example, symptoms associated with radiation therapy often occurred during the second and third weeks of treatment, with many affecting nutritional status (e.g., anorexia, nausea, fatigue, sore throat, changes in saliva, and diarrhea). The nurse must determine whether the experience of these symptoms compromises the patient's ability to maintain adequate intake of food or fluids. As such, a critical time for nursing assessment of this population is the second and third week of treatment. This information enables the nurse to allocate scarce nursing resources during the most critical time period without compromising patient care. At-risk individuals, such as insulin-dependent diabetics or individuals taking potassium-depleting diuretics, also can be scheduled for a symptom assessment at this time.

Various psychosocial interventions that prevent or alleviate treatment-related symptoms have been identified. Primary among these is preparatory information. Nursing interventions can be used to prepare individuals for treatment by informing them about what symptoms to expect, whether symptoms will increase or decrease in severity, and how long symptoms will last.[57] This information provides individuals with a standard for comparison with their own experience. The ability to anticipate side effects assists the individual in planning daily activities.

The effectiveness of preparatory information for individuals with treatment-related symptoms is underscored by an investigation by Burish et al.[55] They compared a general coping preparation procedure for individuals undergoing chemotherapy with a progressive muscle-relaxation training to determine the most effective means for reducing the conditioned side effects of chemotherapy and other types of treatment-related distress. The preparatory intervention consisted of one 90-minute class for patients and their families prior to the first chemotherapy treatment. A videotape presented the chemotherapy procedure provided information dealing with typical questions, and showed a patient successfully dealing with the experience. A question-and-answer period followed, and a written summary of the session was provided.

The progressive muscle-relaxation training consisted of one 30-minute session in which the individual was trained to tense and relax ten major muscle groups, followed by several minutes of relaxing imagery involving the use of a sequence of thoughts and mental pictures that facilitate or deepen relaxation. This training session was audiotaped so the individual could practice the relaxation techniques at home.

The preparatory information intervention was most effective, reducing conditioned side effects, increasing individuals' knowledge of the disease and its treatment, reducing negative emotions, and improving general coping ability. The relaxation intervention decreased negative moods and vomiting but did not have the other beneficial effects of the preparatory information. A combination intervention did not have any advantage over the preparatory intervention. Burish et al concluded that the preparatory information oncology nurses provide is more effective at relieving treatment-related side effects than a behavioral relaxation procedure, which requires special training to administer.[53]

Other interventions have also been identified that prevent or alleviate symptoms related to cancer treatment.[78] Stress reduction and distraction including relaxation, music, self-hypnosis, and massage have been effective for nausea and vomiting or pain.[79–85] Physical remedies have also been used: exercise to manage fatigue[86,87]; extremity wraps for shivering[88]; and hypnosis for mucositis.[89]

Responses of Families and Caregivers

Individuals with cancer are living longer with increasingly complex medical regimens. During periods of active treatment, patients frequently depend on their families for assistance with care, transportation, medical procedures, medication, and symptom management.[55] While the individual with cancer is under the family's care, a principal caregiver usually emerges. Most caregivers are older women caring for spouses or their parents. Caregivers often feel ultimately responsible for coordinating the care of the family member with cancer; they often feel that they must be available 24 hours a day. When the caregiver requires assistance, most often it is obtained from another family member, rarely from a health care professional. A variety of caregiver needs and issues have been identified. These needs are most acute following the patient's hospitalization.[90,91] A major concern of caregivers is their own health and how they will manage their many obligations. The caregiver who is employed often expresses concern about being able to maintain or return to his or her usual work pattern. Caregivers also report that providing emotional support to the individual with cancer is one of their most difficult tasks.[92] They report a lack of time to develop supportive social relationships for themselves. Caregivers are unwilling to discuss their concerns with the patient with cancer because of fears that it might be distressing and because of a need to protect him or her from becoming upset. The overwhelming demands and complexity of care for the individual with cancer can result in caregiver burden.[91–95]

In order to provide support to a husband or wife with cancer, a spouse must be able to see the situation from the other's perspective and to understand what he or she is experiencing. In an examination of the attitudes and experiences of Israeli spouses and patients about head and neck cancer, Chaitchik et al found that, overall, spouses had little knowledge about the way in which their husband or wife experienced the stress of cancer.[96] When relationships were examined between spouse and patient perceptions of health problems, social relationships, family functioning, work adjustment, or negative moods after diagnosis, few correlations were found between spouse and patient responses. However, when patients with low and high levels of information about their disease were compared, there was a significant correspondence between the perceptions of well-informed patients and spouses; whereas, for patients and spouses with limited information, there was no correspondence. The investigators concluded that the likely cause of low correspondence between patient and spouse responses was lack of information. When the individual with cancer knows little about his or her disease, the couple functions under highly restrictive conditions of denial, fear, isolation, and conjecture.

Other research points to differences in the types of issues that concern patients with cancer and their spouses. Patients receiving palliative care for advanced cancer reported that closeness with their partner was most important to their QOL,[97] whereas spouses indicated that coping successfully with marital situations was the major contributor to their QOL. The difference probably reflects a distinction between the roles of the ill or healthy partner: The ill person is coming to terms with eventual death, and the healthy partner is coping with the concrete necessities of providing for the patient.

Research suggests that nurses can play an important role in opening up channels of communication between the spouse and patient. The oncology nurse informs the patient and spouse of the diagnosis and can deepen the spouse's understanding of the situation by sharing the patient's perspective. This can be accomplished by conversing with the patient and spouse individually, then together. The nurse who knows the patient and spouse well describes for each partner individually how the other views the situation, thereby disclosing to the spouse the experience of the patient and suggesting to the patient the spouse's possible ignorance. In doing this, the nurse evokes in each party some degree of curiosity about the experience of the other, thus compelling them to overcome the fear and despair that typically block effective communication. When meeting with patient and spouse together, the nurse can help them adopt a terminology for describing disease phenomena. This process of informal teaching of patient and spouse may help both initiate a dialogue and then expand on it.

In addition to imparting information and supporting the communication efforts of patient and family, the oncology nurse plays other important supportive roles. In a study by Hull, 24-hour accessibility and availability of the hospice nurse was identified by family caregivers as critical in reducing their anxieties about caregiving.[98] Accessibility means that there is always a respected, knowledgeable professional who can make helpful suggestions for changes in care or who will come in person if needed. As more complex regimens are being implemented at home, the need for such resources will likely expand to include more individuals and families.

Changes in Sexual Functioning

Because of the seriousness of a cancer diagnosis, it is understandable that professionals often do not address sexual dysfunction resulting from treatment. In addition, the reluctance of Americans to discuss sexuality echoes the silence often maintained by both professionals and patients. The oncology nurse can play a pivotal role in preparing individuals for the effects of treatment on sexual functioning by (1) educating individuals about what to expect and how to cope with changes in sexual functioning, (2) identifying individuals who may have difficulty coping with these changes, and (3) making appropriate referrals. The need for timely professional nursing assessment is reinforced by research suggesting that approximately 50% of women receiving treatment for gynecological malignancies report sexual dysfunction during recovery and survival, despite satisfactory QOL in other domains.[99] Another study found that 50% of women with pelvic exenteration did not resume sexual activity, even though 70% had a potentially functional neovaginas.[100] The most common problems were self-consciousness about ostomies and being seen nude by one's sexual partner, vaginal dryness, and vaginal discharge. These findings suggest that realistic counseling and aggressive support could minimize sexual morbidity.

Sexual dysfunction in patients with cancer may be related to a variety of biological, psychological, and social factors. Diseases that affect the sexual organs, pelvis, or breasts are more likely to have consequences for sexual functioning than other cancers.[101] More invasive or disfiguring surgery and greater anatomical changes are more likely to result in sexual dysfunction. Hormonal changes including ovarian failure can result in loss of desire as well as problems with arousal. Not to be underestimated are the effects of chemotherapy on sexuality. Nausea and vomiting as well as hair loss affect body image and feelings of attractiveness. Low sexual desire, dyspareunia, and difficulty reaching orgasm are reported more frequently by women undergoing chemotherapy for breast cancer than by women who do not receive this treatment.[102] Also, concurrent medical conditions and treatments such as diabetes or the use of antihypertensive drugs can affect sexual functioning.

Psychological factors can also place an individual at risk for sexual difficulties. Negative moods, loss of personal control, cancer worries, relationship difficulties (such as poor communication or fear of rejection), and past psychiatric problems (including alcohol abuse) can contribute to sexual dysfunction.[103] Younger people, those without partners, and persons in relationships of shorter duration are at higher risk than older, longer married patients.[104] Sexual adjustment for older individuals with cancer may be jeopardized by diseases and treatment as well as the normal effects of aging.[104] People with traditional views of sexuality and gender role and those who are pessimistic about their future are more prone to sexual dysfunction after cancer treatment.[105]

Andersen suggests that the extent of disease and treatment plays a major role in determining who is at risk for sexual morbidity after a diagnosis of cancer.[63] More extensive disease is characterized by higher stage, more invasive or mutilating treatment, lack of reconstructive procedures, and continuing stressors from disease or treatment. A review of several studies of women treated for cancer of the cervix, endometrium, or ovary revealed that persons with extensive disease had a 90%–100% risk of sexual morbidity, whereas those with limited disease had a risk of 20%–30%.[63] However, individuals with limited disease who reported little disruption of overall QOL reported a substantial degree of disruption in sexual functioning. Furthermore, 30% of low-risk women reported that their partners had difficulty reaching orgasm, suggesting that partners of cancer patients need to be included in the plan of care for sexuality changes.

Assessment of sexual functioning must begin with information gathering and sexual history. Because health care professionals often feel uneasy about dealing with the topic of sexuality, a few general guidelines may be helpful. Privacy is important for discussions of sexuality. It is useful for the nurse to assume a nonjudgmental attitude and not react emotionally to the discussion of sensitive issues. Moving from less-sensitive to more-sensitive issues can also help both the nurse and patient manage anxiety. The nurse must be aware of timing to ensure that such a discussion is appropriate to the functional level and needs of the patient and partner.

Nurses are often wary about initiating discussions of sexuality with their patients because they feel they lack the necessary expertise to give advice. However, most discussions do not require a sexuality expert.[106,107] What the individual needs is a knowledgeable person who is willing to discuss sexuality issues, offer advice about how to manage immediate problems (such as vaginal dryness), and identify resources (such as a sex therapist or a physician who treats erectile dysfunction) for managing more difficult problems.

Three questions that can be incorporated into the general patient assessment at the beginning of treatment are recommended:[106]

1. *Has your cancer treatment interfered with being a spouse or parent?* This invites the individual to discuss his or her functional role in the family and how it has been altered by illness or treatment.
2. *Has your cancer treatment changed the way you view yourself as a man or a woman?* This addresses the individual's sexual self-image.
3. *Do you expect your sexual functioning/sex life to be changed by your cancer treatment?* This directly addresses sexual functioning.

The nurse who conducts a nonthreatening and nonjudgmental sexual history at the beginning of cancer treatment can do much to prevent and reduce the anxiety and guilt that can surround sexual concerns and problems. By initiating an early discussion of sexual issues, the nurse establishes both the legitimacy of these concerns and the willingness to discuss them. For example, a man anticipating an abdominoperitoneal resection who is encouraged to talk about sexual concerns in the preoperative period will probably be more comfortable initiating questions after treatment.

One approach to sexual rehabilitation is the PLISSIT model that describes four levels of intervention for sexuality issues.[108] At the first level, the nurse gives permission (P) to express sexual concerns. In some cases, the simple acknowledgment and discussion of a perceived change in sexual health may be sufficient to help the patient or partner resolve the problem. Providing limited information (LI) is the second level of the model. This may include information about sexual anatomy, the sexual response cycle, or specific sexual changes to be expected after treatment. The third level of intervention involves specific suggestions (SS) for communication of sexual concerns, alternative positions and techniques, the use of devices, and medical interventions to restore function or appearance. The fourth level, intensive therapy (IT), is the only one that is more appropriately referred to a trained professional.

Health professionals often concentrate only on issues relevant to the individual with cancer, overlooking those of the partner. Cancer and its treatment may have consequences for the sexual partner of the individual with cancer, though the needs of the partner have not been well researched.[102–107] Experts agree that more attention should be paid to the partner's responses and that both partners should be involved in treatment planning for sexual dysfunction to enhance recovery.[106]

Interventions for changes in sexual health generally combine education and counseling. A few empirical studies have addressed the effectiveness of such interventions.[109,110] The studies demonstrate that a brief therapy model is most effective in improving sexual outcomes, particularly for individuals with less extensive disease.[63] These interventions are characterized by early assessment of problems, present-day focus, limited goals, direction by the counselor, and prompt intervention. The interventions provide a supportive context for the discussion of varied concerns and information about specific problems related to disease and treatment, also focusing on the development of cognitive and behavioral coping skills. The therapeutic components of the interventions have a greater impact on outcome than their specific format. For example, Andersen found that both group and individual approaches were equally effective.[109] Likewise, involvement of sexual partners was not critical to the effectiveness of interventions for the individual with cancer. The research also indicates the need for interventions specifically focused on sexual functioning for individuals treated for cancer of the genitals.[63] This includes information about sexuality, an explanation of the anticipated changes in sexual functioning resulting from treatment, a discussion of medical interventions that could restore functioning or appearance, and specific suggestions and strategies to improve sexual functioning.

Problems of Cancer Survivors

Cancer survival rates have steadily improved over the past four decades and, between 1989 and 1994 have reached 62% for whites and 47% for blacks.[111] Increased survival means that more individuals complete treatment with the anticipation of being disease-free for an extended period of time. Still, survivors report a host of QOL problems, including difficulties with physical functioning, role adaptation, work productivity, social adaptation, and psychological distress.[112,113]

The experience of surviving cancer has been characterized as producing long-standing mental scars, despite a lack of major or severe psychopathology.[114–116] Cancer survivors easily recall emotions related to illness and recovery, continuing concerns about mortality, and an enduring sense of vulnerability.[116] Even after definitive cure, cancer survivors are less certain about living a long life and have greater anxiety and mood changes.[113] The anniversary of a cancer diagnosis can trigger reactions that include reexperiencing the diagnosis and nightmares or flashbacks about the experience.[112] One year after diagnosis, breast cancer survivors express concern about whether the cancer will recur or progress, not being able to care for themselves in the future, and how their families will manage without them if they die. They also report difficulty communicating with their health care providers and families about these fears and worries.[116,117]

Survivors often experience stress during reentry into the "well role."[113] The intense outpouring of emotional support experienced during treatment may not be sustained when the individual no longer looks and acts sick.

Friends and relatives engage in a sorting-out process, ultimately determining who remains close and who distances themselves from the survivor.[114] Likewise, marital stress that accumulates during treatment can produce marital disruption after the completion of therapy.[116] The issue of infertility caused by treatment can be a source of distress for childless couples.

Employment-related problems, including denial of insurance or other benefits, not getting job offers, conflict with supervisors or coworkers, and termination of employment, have been identified by almost 40% of cancer survivors.[116] Despite difficulties, approximately 80% return to work after diagnosis. Some survivors indicate that the experience of having had cancer has "locked" them into their jobs because of fears of lost medical coverage, pension rights, or other benefits. The Americans with Disabilities Act of 1990 has greatly increased the rights of workers with disabilities due to cancer.

Although it has not been well researched, survivors themselves have pointed to the need for education to restore and maintain their well-being. Survivors want to be informed of potential disruptions before they experience them. A number of specific learning needs have been identified for survivors.[118–120] They must be informed that fatigue or energy loss may be a problem for a year or more after therapy is completed, especially if the individual is elderly. Survivors also need information about the likelihood of marital stress after treatment is over. Likewise, employers may need information and input to understand the survivor's work-related limitations due to the cancer or its treatment. Fear of cancer recurrence is common, and education about the problem as well as strategies for overcoming it are necessary. In addition, survivors need information about how to cope with physical disabilities.

Professional Responses to Cancer

Like individuals and families dealing with cancer, oncology nurses use coping skills to adapt to the charged emotional environment in which they work. Professionals need to see the challenge of the cancer experience in a way that resonates with their beliefs about life, death, and illness, so that caring for this group of people does not become emotionally overwhelming. Generally, this adaptation occurs on both conscious and unconscious levels.[121]

Consciously, nurses engage their intellects to grasp the situation in which they find themselves, rejecting superstitions and myths about cancer. Examples of superstitions include beliefs about contagion and horrible deaths. Oncology nurses work with patients and families to solve problems, offer constructive feedback, and function under pressure with patients. Their emotional controls generally work effectively.

The unconscious, however, is less rational. Nurses may find themselves avoiding certain situations or responding to them irrationally. They may believe that verbalizing their anxiety and acknowledging their fear of cancer renders them both vulnerable and nonprofessional. In turn, feelings of embarrassment, shame, guilt, and anger focused at themselves for their weaknesses are kept hidden.

These feelings are normal adaptations to the professional life of an oncology nurse, just as it is normal for patients and families to experience a wide range of emotions. Until they have dealt with cancer extensively or experienced many losses, most nurses are not optimally equipped to deal with the stresses they experience.

In a process that parallels that experienced by patients and families, there is a time component involved in the resolution of feelings in the oncology nurse. Anxiety related to working with cancer patients is greatest at the beginning of work life and is usually stabilized after about 6 months. During this time, nurses may experience transient cancer-phobia; for example, they may experience feelings of panic about swollen lymph nodes, fearing it is lymphoma.[121] Stress levels of oncology nurses have been likened to those of recently widowed women. Stress levels returned to normal by the end of the first year.

As they accept their lack of control over this disease and acknowledge their emotional reactions to cancer, nurses may doubt their own sense of purpose. Questions such as "Why am I putting myself through this?" and "Why am I bothering if I can't cure this person?" are normal. With time, nurses should mourn the losses and discover an inner strength. Both personal and professional experiences combine, shaping the character of and influencing the choices nurses make. A minority of professional caregivers become stuck in reactive anxiety and depression that, with proper support, can resolve spontaneously in weeks or months. Conversely, some nurses may decide it is better to transfer to another type of nursing.

As patients and families choose coping behaviors that are successful or unsuccessful, so does the oncology nurse choose from various strategies. Two concepts, distancing and caring, can be examined from the standpoint of being "value neutral" forms of coping. Either strategy employed to excess can have negative consequences for both the caregiver and the patient.

Distancing is a response used by professionals, either consciously or unconsciously, to those in their care, often when a patient is dying. It may manifest as less time spent with a particular individual, ignoring a call light, failure to communicate, and an unwavering "professionalism" in emotionally charged situations such as when a patient or family is viewed as difficult. Distancing can be helpful in allowing the patient and family to test their own problem-solving skills in a controlled situation before having to handle the problems alone, or by setting appropriate limits about the amount of nursing time or resources that realistically can be provided. Distancing becomes unsuccessful when it occurs over a long period of time and results in increased loneliness and isolation of those for whom one is caring.

Professionals also use caring as a response to cancer. Benner and Wrubel define *caring* as an enabling condi-

tion of connection and concern.[122] Caring is communicated through acceptance and respect for thoughts, feelings, and needs. It implies access. Caring describes the quality of the nurse-patient interaction. Like distancing, caring can be given in excess, withheld, or used successfully as a technique to help the nurse and patient achieve goals.

Another way of thinking about caring and distancing is to describe boundaries. Caring is the essence of the therapeutic use of self, such as empowering the patient and family—through care, education, and guidance—to gain control over the situation in which they find themselves.[123] In order for caring to be successful, professional boundaries need to be maintained; otherwise, potentially negative outcomes (such as overinvolvement and burnout) can develop for both the patient and professional. A *boundary* is a psychological term referring to one's sphere of influence. Interactions start at the point where nurses' boundaries touch those of others. Boundaries can be rigid, diffuse, or clear. If the boundaries are *rigid*, there will be a psychological gap between the patient and caregiver. Most nurses have encountered a caregiver who never gets involved with the patient or family and seems untouched by the emotions around them.

If boundaries are *diffuse*, they overlap with the boundaries of others. Nurses may become enmeshed with their patients and overinvolved in their care. The nurse in this scenario often stays late, believes he or she is the only one who can care adequately for this individual, and provides personal opinions about medical care and treatment decisions. As an example, the nurse may promote chemotherapy for a similarly aged woman with children because that is what the nurse would want if she had cancer. The nurse has become overinvested emotionally.

When psychological boundaries are *clear*, nurses relate and are empathetic but they do not impose their choices on others. Rather, they help others decide what is in their best interest. Clear boundaries are those toward which all health professionals strive. In this context, caring is therapeutic.

Oncology nursing is full of situations that may compel nurses to violate the boundaries of others. Examples include patients of the same age, those who remind nurses of family members or loved ones, patients with circumstances similar to their own, those patients similar to favorite patients for whom they have cared, and colleagues who are patients.

It is normal for the oncology nurse to "cross" boundaries periodically, either by being too close or too aloof in a particular situation. When most interactions fall one way or the other, the nurse must consider the ramifications. Underinvestment leaves the nurse unfulfilled and the patient feeling alone and lost; it may result from repeated overinvestment in the past. Conversely, overinvestment can cause the patient to be overly reliant on the nurse for decision making and leave the nurse feeling overextended and burned out. It is important to remember that when nurses become like family to a patient, they lose their value as a professional resource.

In such situations, the nurse needs to ask the following questions:

- Is my job satisfaction related to how much a patient or family needs me?

- Do I feel no one can care for the patient as well as I can?

- Is it difficult for me to leave my patients at the end of the day?

If the answer to any of these questions is "yes," boundary difficulties may be present. Other questions need to be asked individually or of the institution as a whole:

- Are there "favorite" patients?

- What happens to those patients who are no one's favorite?

- Are nurses simultaneously maintaining professional and social relationships with patients and families?

- Are nurses assuming responsibility for some facets of care that might be better handled by families, social services, or community resources (e.g., buying gifts for patients or families, taking care of children while parents are hospitalized, or providing meals for patients and families after hospital discharge)?

Issues related to boundaries are best handled through open, honest communication and discussions. This can be done by informal discussion, staff development programs, standards for professional nursing practice, and departmental guidelines. The approach taken should consider the institutional norms, the individual setting, the desire to change, the resources available, and the degree of administrative support.

Barnsteiner and Gillis-Donovan reported on the method used by one urban pediatric center to develop standards for therapeutic relationships and culture modifications.[123] Staff representation and nursing leadership collected sufficient data to define and conceptualize the problem, and then went on to write policy, train staff regarding concepts, and educate other departments. Mental health clinical nurse specialists were employed to help resolve issues as they were identified (e.g., issues of loss and grief for staff, close identification with patients/families, etc.). Systems were put into place to help provide for the unique needs of patients and families so that an individual nurse would not need to provide for the patients.

Individually, nurses need to understand themselves and the dynamics of their family of origin; seek balance between their personal and professional lives; seek the counsel of their managers, peers, families, friends, or a mental health professional; take time to recognize their limitations and vulnerabilities; and let go of the illusion of controlling the whole situation.

Conclusion

Cancer threatens both quantity and quality of life for the person who is faced with complex treatment plans, uncertainty of recurrence, and the prospect of alterations in self-concept, roles, and relationships with others. The oncology nurse can play a significant role in helping individuals and their families cope with the many stresses they face by assessing their needs and concerns and by being flexible in providing both educational and emotional support. The ultimate goal is to help individuals adjust to and achieve control over the stresses of the cancer experience.

References

1. Sabo D: Men, death anxiety, and denial: Critical feminist interpretations of adjustment to mastectomy, in Clark C, Fritz J, Reid P (eds): *Clinical Sociological Perspectives on Illness and Loss.* Philadelphia, Charles Press, 1990, pp 71–84
2. Gorman L: The psychosocial impact of cancer on the individual, family, and society, in Carroll-Johnson RM, Gorman LM, Bush NJ (eds): *Psychosocial Nursing Care Along the Cancer Continuum.* Pittsburgh, Oncology Nursing Press, 1998, pp 3–25
3. Barhamand BA: Coping with cancer: Family issues, in Burke CC (ed), *Psychosocial Dimensions of Oncology Nursing Care.* Pittsburgh, Oncology Nursing Press, 1998, pp 28–52
4. Whall AL: Family system theory: Relationship to nursing conceptual models, in Whall AL, Fawcett J (eds): *Family Theory Development in Nursing: State of the Science and Art.* Philadelphia, F.A. Davis, 1991, 317–341
5. Schumacher KL: Reconceptualizing family caregiving: Family-based illness care during chemotherapy. *Res Nurs Health* 19:261–271, 1996
6. Friedman MM. *Family Nursing Research, Theory, and Practice* (ed 4). Stamford, CT, Appleton & Lange, 1998
7. Jassak PF: Families: An essential element in the care of the patient with cancer. *Oncol Nurs Forum* 19:871–876, 1992
8. Morse SR, Fife B: Coping with a partner's cancer: Adjustment at four stages of the illness trajectory. *Oncol Nurs Forum* 25:751–760, 1998
9. Kurtz ME, Kurtz JC, Given CW, Given B: Relationship of caregiver reactions and depression to cancer patients' symptoms, functional states, and depression: A longitudinal view. *Soc Sci Med* 40:837–846, 1995
10. Munkres A, Oberst MT, Hughes SH: Appraisal of illness, symptom distress, self-care burden, and mood states in patients receiving chemotherapy for initial and recurrent cancer. *Oncol Nurs Forum* 19:1201–1209, 1992
11. Northouse LL, Dorris G, Charron-Moore C: Factors affecting couples' adjustment to recurrent breast cancer. *Soc Sci Med* 40:69–76, 1995
12. Hilton BA: Getting back to normal: The family experience during early stage breast cancer. *Oncol Nurs Forum* 23:605–614, 1996
13. Lewis FM, Deal LW: Balancing our lives: A study of the married couple's experience with breast cancer recurrence. *Oncol Nurs Forum* 22:943–953, 1995

14. Cooley ME, Moriarty HJ: An analysis of empirical studies examining the impact of the cancer diagnosis and treatment of an adult on family functioning. *J Fam Nurs* 3: 318–347, 1997

15. Leventhal H, Johnson JE: Laboratory and field experimentation: Development of a theory of self-regulation, in Wooldbridge PJ, Schmitt MH, Skipper Jr JK, Leonard RC (eds): *Behavioral Science and Nursing Theory.* St. Louis, Mosby, 1983, pp 189–262

16. Lazarus RS, Folkman S: *Stress, Appraisal, and Coping.* New York, Springer, 1984

17. Brooten D, Naylor MD: Nurses' effect on changing patient outcomes. *Image J Nurs Schol* 27:95–99, 1995

18. Lang NM, Marek KD: Outcomes that reflect clinical practice. Proceedings of the State of the Science Conference sponsored by the National Center for Nursing Research, in *Patient Outcome Research: Examining the Effectiveness of Nursing Practice.* NIH publication No. 93-3411. Bethesda, MD, Public Health Service, National Institutes of Health, 1992

19. Aguilera DC: *Crisis Intervention Theory and Methodology* (ed 6). Philadelphia, Mosby, 1990

20. Giger JN, Davidhizar RE: *Transcultural Nursing: Assessment and Intervention.* Philadelphia, Mosby Year Book, 1991

21. Chen MS: Behavioral and psychosocial cancer research in the underserved. *Cancer* 74:1503–1508, 1994

22. Evans LA: Black and white differences: Narrowing the gap in cancer medicine. *In Vivo* 6:429–434, 1992

23. Kerner JF, Dusenbury L, Mandelblatt JS: Poverty and cultural diversity: Challenges for health promotion among the medically underserved. *Annu Rev Public Health* 14:355–377, 1993

24. Balshem M: Cancer, control, and causality: A working-class community. *Am Ethnol* 18:152–172, 1991

25. Mathews HF, Lannin DR, Mitchell JP: Coming to terms with advanced breast cancer: Black women's narratives from Eastern North Carolina. *Soc Sci Med* 38:789–800, 1994

26. Frank-Stromborg M, Olsen S (eds): *Cancer Prevention in Minority Populations: Cultural Implications for Health Care Professionals.* St. Louis, Mosby, 1993

27. Kahn SB, Houts PS, Harding SP: Quality of life and patients with cancer: A comparative study of patient versus physician perceptions and its implications for cancer education. *J Cancer Educ* 7:241–249, 1992

28. Mor V, Allen S, Malin M: The psychosocial impact of cancer on older versus younger patients and their families. *Cancer* 74:2118–2127, 1994

29. Vinokur AD, Threatt BA, Vinokur-Kaplan D, et al: The process of recovery from breast cancer for younger and older patients: Changes during the first year. *Cancer* 65: 1242–1254, 1990

30. Mischel W: *Personality and Assessment.* New York, Wiley, 1968

31. Marshall GN: A multidimensional analysis of internal health locus of control beliefs: Separating the wheat from the chaff? *J Pers Soc Psychol* 61:483–491, 1991

32. Carver CS, Pozo C, Harris SD, et al: How coping mediates the effect of optimism on distress: A study of women with early stage breast cancer. *J Pers Soc Psychol* 65:375–390, 1993

33. Hack TF, Degner LF, Dyck DG: Relationship between preferences for decisional control and illness information among women with breast cancer: A quantitative and qualitative analysis. *Soc Sci Med* 39:279–289, 1994

34. Strickland OL: Measures and instruments. Proceedings of the State of the Science Conference sponsored by the National Center for Nursing Research, in *Patient Outcome Research: Examining the Effectiveness of Nursing Practice.* NIH publication No. 93-3411. Bethesda, MD, Public Health Service, National Institutes of Health, 1992

35. Massie MJ: Depression, in Holland JC, Rowland JH (eds): *Handbook of Psychooncology: Psychological Care of the Patient with Cancer.* New York: Oxford University Press, 1990, pp 283–290

36. Maunsell E, Brisson J, Deschenes L: Psychological distress after initial treatment of breast cancer. *Cancer* 70:120–125, 1992

37. Andersen BL: Psychological interventions for cancer patients to enhance the quality of life. *J Consult Clin Psychol* 60:552–568, 1992

38. Berkman LF: The role of social relations in health promotion. *Psychosom Med* 57:245–254, 1995

39. Seeman TE, Berkman LF, Charpentier PA, et al: Behavioral and psychological predictors of physical performance: MacArthur studies of successful aging. *J Gerontol* 50: M177–183, 1995

40. Goodwin JS, Hunt WC, Samet JM: A population-based study of functional status and social support networks of elderly patients newly diagnosed with cancer. *Arch Intern Med* 151:366–370, 1991

41. Andersen BL: Psychological interventions for cancer patients to enhance the quality of life. *J Consult Clin Psychol* 60:552–568, 1992

42. Fawzy FI, Fawzy NW, Arndt LA, et al: Critical review of psychosocial interventions in cancer care. *Arch Gen Psychiatry* 52:100–113, 1995

43. Devine EC, Westlake SK: The effects of psychoeducational care provided to adults with cancer: Meta-analysis of 116 studies. *Oncol Nurs Forum* 22:1369–1381, 1995

44. McCabe MS: Psychological support for the patient on chemotherapy. *Oncology* 5:91–99, 1991

45. Penrod J, Morse JM: Strategies for assessing and fostering hope: The hope assessment guide. *Oncol Nurs Forum* 24: 1055–1063, 1997

46. Greer S: Psychological response to cancer and survivors. *Psychol Med* 21:43–49, 1991

47. Spiegel D: *Living Beyond Limits: New Help and Hope for Facing Life-threatening Illness.* New York, Times Books/Random House, 1993

48. Meyer TJ, Mark MM: Effects of psychosocial interventions with adult cancer patients: A meta-analysis of randomized experiments. *Health Psychol* 14:101–108, 1995

49. Heiney SP: The healing power of story. *Oncol Nurs Forum* 22:899–904, 1995

50. Cunningham M: The moral of the story, in Weaver M (ed): *Tales as Tools: The Power of Story in the Classroom.* Jonesborough, TN, National Storytelling Association Press, 1994, pp 11–14

51. MacDonald M: Making time for stories, in Weaver M (ed): *Tales as Tools: The Power of Story in the Classroom.* Jonesborough, TN, National Storytelling Association Press, 1994, pp 9–10

52. Schram P: Collections for the people of the story, in Weaver M (ed): *Tales as Tools: The Power of Story in the Classroom.* Jonesborough, TN, National Storytelling Association Press, 1994, pp 176–178

53. Burish TG, Tope DM: Psychological techniques for controlling the adverse side effects of cancer chemotherapy: Findings from a decade of research. *J Pain Symptom Manage* 7: 287–301, 1992

54. Cella DF: Quality of life: Concepts and definition. *J Pain Symptom Manage* 9:186–192, 1994

55. Burish TG, Snyder SL, Jenkins RA: Preparing patients for cancer chemotherapy: Effect of coping preparation and relaxation interventions. *J Consult Clin Psychol* 59:518–525, 1991

56. Johnson JE, Fieler VK, Jones LS, et al: *Self-Regulation Theory: Applying Theory to Your Practice.* Pittsburgh: Oncology Nursing Press, 1997, pp 1–91

57. Johnson JE: Coping with radiation therapy: Optimism and the effects of preparatory interventions. *Res Nurs Health* 19:3–12, 1996

58. Sarna L, McCorkle R: Burden of care and lung cancer. *Cancer Pract* 4:245–251, 1996

59. Barsevick AM, Pasacreta J, Orsi A: Psychological distress and functional dependency in colorectal cancer patients. *Cancer Pract* 3:105–110, 1995

60. Carver CS, Pozo D, Harria SD, et al: How coping mediates the effect of optimism on distress: A study of women with early stage breast cancer. *J Pers Soc Psychol* 65:375–390, 1993

61. Cella DF, Yellen SB: Cancer support groups: The state of the art. *Cancer Pract* 1:56–61, 1993

62. Spiegel D, Moore R: Imagery and hypnosis in the treatment of cancer patients. *Oncology* 11:1179–1195, 1997

63. Andersen BL: Predicting sexual and psychologic morbidity and improving the quality of life for women with gynecologic cancer. *Cancer* 71:1678–1690, 1993 (suppl 4)

64. Hack TF, Degner LF, Dyck DG: Relationship between preferences for decisional control and illness information among women with breast cancer: A quantitative and qualitative analysis. *Soc Sci Med* 39:279–289, 1994

65. Bilodeau BA, Degner LF: Information needs, sources of information, and decisional roles in women with breast cancer. *Oncol Nurs Forum* 23:691–696, 1996

66. Degner LF, Sloan JA: Decision-making during serious illness: What role do patients really want to play? *J Clin Epidemiol* 45:941, 1992

67. Neufeld KR, Degner LF, Dick JAM: A nursing intervention strategy to foster patient involvement in treatment decisions. *Oncol Nurs Forum* 20:631–635, 1993

68. Johnson JD, Roberts CS, Cox CE, et al: Breast cancer patients' personality style, age, and treatment decision making. *J Surg Oncol* 63:183–186, 1996

69. North N, Cornbleet MA, Knowles G, et al: Information giving in oncology: A preliminary study of tape-recorder use. *Br J Clin Psychol* 31:357, 1992

70. Kaplan SH, Greenfield S, Ware Jr JE: Assessing the effects of physician-patient interactions on the outcomes of chronic disease. *Med Care* 27:S110–S127, 1989

71. Miller SM, O'Leary A: Cognition, stress, and health, in Kendall PC, Dobson K (eds): *Psychopathology and Cognition,* New York, Academic Press, 1993, pp 159–189

72. Mishel MH: Reconceptualization of the uncertainty in illness theory. *Image J Nurs Schol* 22:256–262, 1990

73. McHugh NG, Christman NJ, Johnson JE: Preparatory information: What helps and why. *Am J Nurs* 82:780–782, 1982

74. Ward SE: The common sense model: An organizing framework for knowledge development in nursing. *Schol Inquiry Nurs Pract* 7:79–90, 1993

75. Leventhal H, Nerenz DR, Steele DJ: Illness representations and coping with health threats, in Johnston M, Wallace L (eds): *Stress and Medical Procedures.* New York, Oxford University Press, 1990, pp 219–252

76. Burish TG, Redd WH: Symptom control in psychosocial oncology. *Cancer* 74:1438–1444, 1994

77. King KB, Nail LM, Kreamer K, et al: Patients' descriptions of the experience of receiving radiation treatment. *Oncol Nurs Forum* 12:55–61, 1985

78. Smith MC, Holcombe JK, Stullenbarger E: A meta-analysis of intervention effectiveness for symptom management in oncology nursing research. *Oncol Nurs Forum* 21:1201–1210, 1994

79. Lerner M: Psychological approaches to cancer, in Lerner M (ed): *Choices in Healing: Integrating the Best of Conventional and Complementary Approaches to Cancer.* Cambridge, MA, MIT Press, 1994, pp 137–194

80. Lerman C, Rimer B, Blumberg B, et al: Effects of coping style and relaxation on cancer chemotherapy side effects and emotional responses. *Cancer Nurs* 13:308–315, 1990

81. Steggies S, Maxwell J, Lightfoot NE, et al: Hypnosis and cancer: An annotated biography: *Am J Clin Hypn* 39:187–200, 1997

82. Weinrich SP, Weinrich MC: The effect of massage on pain in cancer patients. *Appl Nurs Res* 3:140–145, 1990

83. Ezzone S, Baker C, Rosselet R, Terepka E: Music as an adjunct to antiemetic therapy. *Oncol Nurs Forum* 25:1551–1556, 1998

84. Beck SL: The therapeutic use of music for cancer-related pain. *Oncol Nurs Forum* 18:1327–1337, 1991

85. Lazlo J, Cotanch P: Managing chemotherapy-induced nausea and vomiting. *Cancer* 70:1007–1011, 1992

86. Mock V, Dow KH, Meares CJK, et al: Effects of exercise on fatigue, physical functioning, and emotional distress during radiation therapy for breast cancer. *Oncol Nurs Forum* 24:991–1000, 1997

87. Friedenreich CM, Courneya KS: Exercise as rehabilitation for cancer patients. *Clin J Sport Med* 6:237–244, 1996

88. Holtzclaw BJ: Control of febrile shivering during amphotericin B therapy. *Oncol Nurs Forum* 17:521–524, 1990

89. Syrjala KL, Cummings C, Donaldson GW: Hypnosis or cognitive behavioral training for the reduction of pain and nausea during cancer treatment: A controlled clinical trial. *Pain* 48:137–146, 1992

90. Hoskins CN, Baker S, Sherman D, et al: Social support and patterns of adjustment to breast cancer. *Schol Inquiry Nurs Pract* 10:99–133, 1996

91. McCorkle R, Wilkerson K: Home care needs of cancer patients and their families. *Final Report (NR01914).* Philadelphia, National Center for Nursing Research, 1991

92. Carey PJ, Oberst MT, McCubbin MA, et al: Appraisal and caregiving burden in family members caring for patients receiving chemotherapy. *Oncol Nurs Forum* 18:1341–1348, 1991

93. Siegel K, Raveis VH, Houts P, et al: Caregiver burden and unmet patient needs. *Cancer* 68:1131–1140, 1991

94. Jensen S, Given BA: Fatigue affecting family caregivers of cancer patients. *Cancer Nurs* 14:181–187, 1991

95. Given CW, Stommel M, Given B, et al: The influence of cancer patients' symptoms and functional states on patients' depression and family caregivers' reaction and depression. *Health Psychol* 12:277–285, 1993

96. Chaitchik S, Kreitler S, Rappoport Y, et al: What do cancer patients' spouses know about the patients? *Cancer Nurs* 15:353–362, 1992

97. Fuller S, Swensen CH: Marital quality and quality of life among cancer patients and their spouses. *J Psychosoc Oncol* 10:41–56, 1992

98. Hull MM: Hospice nurses: Caring support for caregiving families. *Cancer Nurs* 14:63–70, 1991

99. Andersen BL, Woods XA, Copeland LJ: Sexual self-schema

and sexual morbidity among gynecologic cancer survivors. *J Consult Clin Psychol* 65:221–229, 1997

100. Ratliff CR, Gershenson DM, Morris M, et al: Sexual adjustment of patients undergoing gracilis myocutaneous flap vaginal reconstruction in conjunction with pelvic exenteration. *Cancer* 78:2229–2235, 1996

101. Schover LR: The impact of breast cancer on sexuality, body image, and intimate relationships. *Cancer* 41:112–120, 1991

102. Schover LR, Yetman RJ, Tuason LJ, et al: Partial mastectomy and breast reconstruction. *Cancer* 75:54–64, 1995

103. Dobkin PL, Bradley I: Assessment of sexual dysfunction in oncology patients: Review, critique, and suggestions. *J Psychosoc Oncol* 9:43–75, 1991

104. Lamb MA: Effects of cancer on the sexuality and fertility of women. *Semin Oncol Nurs* 11:120–127, 1995

105. Andersen BL, Cyranowski JM: Women's sexuality: Behaviors, responses, and individual differences. *J Consult Clin Psychol* 63:891–906, 1995

106. Shell JA, Smith CK: Sexuality and the older person with cancer. *Oncol Nurs Forum* 21:553–558, 1994

107. Smith DB, Babaian R: The effects of treatment for cancer on male fertility and sexuality. *Cancer Nurs* 15:271–275, 1992

108. Hughes MK: Sexuality issues: Keeping your cool. *Oncol Nurs Forum* 23:1597–1600, 1996

109. Andersen BL: Predicting sexual and psychologic morbidity and improving the quality of life for women with gynecologic cancer. *Cancer* 71:1678–1690, 1993

110. Anderson BL: Stress and quality of life following cervical cancer. *Monogr Natl Cancer Inst* 21:65–70, 1996

111. Landis SH, Murray T, Bolden S, et al: Cancer statistics, 1999. *Cancer J Clin* 49:8–31, 1999

112. Schag CAC, Ganz PA, Polinsky ML, et al: Characteristics of women at risk for psychosocial distress in the year after breast cancer. *J Clin Oncol* 11:783–793, 1993

113. Ferrans CE: Quality of life through the eyes of survivors of breast cancer. *Oncol Nurs Forum* 21:1645–1651, 1994

114. Dow KH: The enduring seasons in survival. *Oncol Nurs Forum* 17:511–516, 1990

115. Northouse LL, Cracchiolo-Caraway A, Appel CP: Psychologic consequences of breast cancer on partner and family. *Semin Oncol Nurs* 7:216–223, 1991

116. Berry DL: Return to work experience of people with cancer. *Oncol Nurs Forum* 20:905–911, 1993

117. Schag CAC, Heinrich RL, Aadland RL, et al: Assessing problems of cancer patients: Psychometric properties of the Cancer Inventory of Problem Situations. *Health Psychol* 9:83–102, 1990

118. LaFortune Fredette S: Breast cancer survivors: concerns and coping. *Cancer Nurs* 18:35–46, 1995

119. Loescher LJ, Clark L, Atwood JR, et al: The impact of the cancer experience on long-term survivors. *Oncol Nurs Forum* 17:223–229, 1990

120. Tuls Halstead M, Fernsler JI: Coping strategies of long-term cancer survivors. *Cancer Nurs* 17:94–100, 1994

121. Lederberg MS: Psychological problems of staff and their management, in Holland JC, Rowland JH (eds): *Handbook of Psycho-oncology: Psychological Care of the Patient with Cancer.* New York, Oxford University Press, 1990, pp 631–646

122. Benner P, Wrubel J: *The Primacy of Caring: Stress and Coping in Health and Illness.* Menlo Park, CA, Addison-Wesley, 1989

123. Barnsteiner JH, Gillis-Donovan J: Being related and separate: A standard for therapeutic relationships. *Am J Matern Child Nurs* 15:223–228, 1990

CHAPTER 70

Physical, Economic, and Social Issues Confronting Patients and Families

Catherine J. Bradley, PhD
Barbara A. Given, PhD, RN, FAAN
Charles W. Given, PhD
Sharon Kozachik, RN, MSN

Introduction

Increased awareness of certain types of cancer (e.g., prostate, breast) and improved detection methods and treatment regimens have led to more—and younger—people being diagnosed, treated, and surviving cancer. Increasing numbers of patients with cancer are either cured or have longer disease-free survival. The five-year survival rate for all cancers is 58%,[1] meaning that approximately 8 million people have survived their initial diagnosis and episode of cancer treatment. In the 1930s, only about one in four patients diagnosed with cancer (25%) were alive five years later.

Survival rates are commonly used to monitor progress in the treatment of cancer. These rates include all persons who are in remission, disease free, or under treatment. While these rates are an indication of some improvement in the treatment of cancer, they are an inadequate measure of overall progress. The rates tell us nothing about the quality of survival or how cancer has affected the lives of patients and their families. For patients and their families, treatment decisions are only the beginning of long-term dilemmas that may lead to changes in employment, reorganization of family relationships, and diminished economic viability.

Who is considered a cancer survivor? The traditional medical definition of a *cancer survivor* is one who has remained free from disease five years or more after diagnosis. However, many reject this definition and argue that survival begins at diagnosis and continues for the rest of the person's life.[2] The National Coalition for Cancer Survivorship (NCCS) defines survivorship this way: "From the time of [the cancer's] discovery and for the balance of life, an individual diagnosed with cancer is a survivor." In the spirit of the NCCS definition, this chapter refers to survivorship as the period beginning once initial treatment of the primary cancer ends and continuing throughout the remainder of the person's life.

Given the attention placed on detection and treatment, it is clear that equal emphasis has not been placed on how the postdiagnosis and treatment period impacts patients and their families. No long-term treatment guidelines exist, and survivors are not followed into perpetuity by the health care system. In fact, once the initial treatment period ends, health care delivery is shifted from inpatient and specialty care to ambulatory treatment centers and the home setting. Thus, little is known about how patients and families adapt to the longer term survival periods.

Beyond the acute treatment period, patients' contacts with cancer specialists are limited. Therefore, nurses play a critical role in coordinating care in the survivorship phase. Nurses are left to recognize patients' and family members' needs, make appropriate referrals for care, and prepare patients and their families for situations they are likely to face as cancer survivorship begins. While these responsibilities may have always been part of routine practice, the scope and importance of discharge planning has increased with shorter hospital stays and expanded emphasis on outpatient treatments. Nurses may provide the only education patients and families receive on day-to-day care, symptom management and monitoring, coordination of services, and how to function at home and in their jobs after having been treated for cancer.

The extent of the study of cancer survival to date has been primarily on patients' functional status, which unfortunately tells us little about the psychosocial well-being[3] of patients. The goal of this chapter is to increase the reader's awareness of several important issues faced by patients with cancer and their families, as patients increasingly live beyond initial diagnosis and treatment. Nurses and other health care professionals should consider these issues as they assist patients in their transition from the active treatment and follow-up phase to a transition phase where direct contact with oncology specialists is sporadic at best. Emphasis is placed on the time period 3–5 years after diagnosis. The longer term issues, such as eventual health problems due to radiation scarring, that are likely to occur 10–20 years after treatment are not addressed in this chapter.

Consistent with Leigh, the family is referred to as the "unit of care" in this discussion.[4] Focus is placed on how cancer care professionals can guide patients and families into an immediate phase of problem solving and decision making about how they will integrate the effects of cancer into their lives. Several daunting situations face patients and families, including adjustment to physical disability, employment changes, insurance challenges, and ongoing medical care needs and associated costs. Special attention is given to these issues and suggestions and strategies are provided for nurses assisting patients and their families during the transition from acute cancer care to longer term survivorship.

Physical Disability: Implications for the Family

Physical disability is the root of many of cancer's long-term adverse consequences. Although improvements in cancer treatment have extended life expectancy, the treatment itself often leaves patients with functional deficits that can have long-term medical, psychosocial, vocational, and economic implications. Symptoms of fatigue, pain, low blood counts, and changes in weight or appetite may continue indefinitely.[4] And, as levels of impairment increase during the survivorship phase, psychological distress will likewise increase.[3,5] Thus, the extent of physical disability is an important predictor of how well patients and their families will transition into the survivorship phase.

Most patients will experience some disability as a result of cancer and its treatment. Patients' prior disposition will influence how they respond to treatment and the time until they recover following treatment. Those with compromised health or comorbid conditions (e.g., older adults) prior to diagnosis may have few reserves or little resilience to the effects of cancer and its treatment. The severity of their disability will ultimately influence a sequence of psychosocial events for patients and their families.

Patients' disabilities vary by individual characteristics, cancer site and stage, and treatment modality. Common disabilities and their causes are listed in Table 70-1. Fatigue, nausea, and severe deconditioning are perhaps the most common functional problems for all patients recovering from treatment.[6] These symptoms persist long after chemotherapy and radiation are administered. Some patients may require medications for many months or even years after the initial acute treatment phase. These medications may hinder patients' abilities to fully recover.

Once patients have moved from the acute treatment phase to home, nurses caring for these individuals must be aware of functional problems and make appropriate referrals for rehabilitation, palliative care, and long-term follow-up. Patient and family education can also play an important role in maintaining or restoring physical function. For example, maintenance of strength and range of motion in the upper extremity of the affected side following breast cancer surgery or aerobic exercise following bone marrow transplantation is vital to preventing further disability.[6] Compliance with these rehabilitative exercises will largely be the responsibility of patients and their families because the health care system is not designed to oversee patients long-term. Nurses must emphasize the importance of maintaining a routine of care and develop a means of communicating expectations for physical functioning that patients and families can understand, assess within the home, and communicate about to nurses and other health care providers.

Table 70-1 Functional Impairments Common in Patients with Cancer

Deficit	With Common Cause(s)
Impaired cognition and memory loss	Radiation, chemotherapy
Loss of motor control	Surgery, radiation
Cranial nerve deficits	Surgery, radiation for head and neck cancer
Speech difficulties	Surgery for head and neck cancer
Problems with swallowing and feeding	Surgery, pulmonary radiation for head and neck and esophageal cancers
Fatigue	All treatments
Severe deconditioning	Chemotherapy, surgery
Scarring and fibrosis	Surgery for breast cancer
Sensory loss, reduction in fine motor skills	All treatments
Loss of bowel and bladder control	Surgery for bladder cancer, prostate cancer

One method to communicate objectively and assess functional status is through the use of validated questionnaires. Measures of functioning include the Karnofsky Performance Scale, Functional Independence Measures, the Cancer Inventory and Problem Situations,[6] Functional Assessment of Cancer Treatment,[7] the Brief Pain Inventory,[8] and the Short Form-36.[9] Responses to these scales provide an indication of physical and to a lesser extent emotional functioning, but they may not adequately translate how disability has diminished patients' abilities to work, reduced their earnings, and perhaps altered their insurance benefits. These measures are calibrated using indicators that patients can understand. Based on functional status, a plan may be devised to promote recovery of physical functioning and to prevent further deterioration.

Nurses need to assess family members as well as patients to fully ascertain the impact of disability. The assessment measures noted above are not universally applicable to caregivers and family members. The health care system focuses health and wellness efforts on the cancer survivor, however the family caregivers who provide both direct care assistance and standby monitoring of cancer treatment effectiveness and side effects frequently have unmet health needs. Caregivers are not immune to chronic health conditions (e.g., diabetes, hypertension), may need to provide physically demanding tasks, such as lifting and turning, and have interrupted nocturnal sleep.

The family caregiver's attention is focused on providing comfort, symptom management, and emotional support to the patient with cancer, and in the process, the family caregiver's own physical and mental well-being may suffer. Braithwaite showed a correlation between caregiver burden and minor psychiatric symptoms.[10] Krach and Brooks found that caregiving responsibilities interfered with rest, and that caregivers reported experiencing headaches, nervousness, insomnia, weight changes, and unusual drowsiness.[11] In addition, Hoyert and Seltzer found that caregiving women reported poorer health and were more depressed than other women, and that female spousal caregivers report the poorest health and greatest levels of depression over those caring for a parent, child, or a non-caregiver.[12]

Successful rehabilitation and future survival often depend on patients' abilities to get the care they need. In this era of constrained costs and limited use of services, the spouse and family play essential roles in encouraging patients to return to their usual daily functioning, to engage in limited exercise, and to implement prescribed regimens of care. The health care environment places considerable responsibility on the family to become active participants in the care of the person with cancer. The effectiveness of this approach depends partially on patients' and families' understanding and awareness of the disease, their financial resources to obtain the care they need, and the structure of the health care system. Nurses can greatly enhance the ability of patients and family members to get the most possible support from the health care system.

Cancer Survival, Employment, and Vulnerable Populations

Cancer survivors often want and need to work and to perform in their customary roles, regardless of their physical and emotional limitations. Studies have shown that patients employed at the time of diagnosis are strongly motivated to return to work.[13–15] Going back to work may be one of the main objectives of rehabilitation and recovery and can be an important indication of how well patients are coping. However, the ability to return to work can vary by cancer site, treatment modality, and characteristics inherent to patients and their jobs.

Because job requirements are often related to workers' gender, education, and local economic conditions, certain groups of patients may be disproportionately and adversely affected by cancer- and treatment-related disability. To illustrate this point, one study found that functional limitations and health impairments have significant negative effects on employment for men.[16] Among employed men who reported having a neoplasm, 62% reported a functional disability, and 50% reported a work disability. Among employed women with a neoplasm, 67% had a functional disability, but only 38% had a work disability. Even though both genders reported approximately the same percentage of functional disability, disability prevented more men from working than women. Perhaps this is because more men are employed in physically demanding jobs than women.

In general, persons employed in physically demanding jobs are more likely to become unemployed due to the functional limitations resulting from cancer and its treatment than are people employed in sedentary jobs. These individuals may not be able to perform at their former pace or may have to exert greater effort in carrying out activities. Because of physical disability, fewer blue-collar workers return to their previous jobs than do white-collar workers.[15]

For those who perform physical work or whose work requires use of machinery, safety may be a serious concern. Some chemotherapeutic agents and radiation therapy cause paresthesia and neurological and cognitive deficits that may endanger the worker. For other patients, nerve damage to an extremity such as an arm or leg may result from surgical procedures or from radiation and interferes with job responsibilities. Unfortunately, these laborers are more likely to have low wages and are less likely to have adequate insurance coverage; thus, their inability to work can have dramatic consequences for their families if all members become uninsured due to job loss by the primary wage earner. Men, particularly men of minority races or ethnic groups, are more likely to be employed in physically demanding jobs and are more likely to report themselves as limited in their ability to work after a cancer diagnosis than are white men.[17]

Cancer survivors who are from an ethnic minority are also at a greater risk of being unemployed. This may be due to a number of factors including severity of illness and socioeconomic status. Being from an ethnic minority is associated with a poorer outcome and shorter cancer survival. Blacks are diagnosed at more advanced cancer stages than whites and have uniformly lower survival from cancer for every major site.[18] For example, in 1993 the mortality rate from cervical cancer, an easily detectable cancer in the preinvasive stage, in black women was more than two times greater than the rate among white women. In a study of women 3 months after their breast cancer diagnosis, black women were twice as likely as white women to be on medical leave.[19] Being on leave was associated with the need for assistance with transportation, limitations in upper body strength, and employment in jobs requiring physical activity.

Unemployment due to cancer has also been shown to vary by both disease site and treatment. Kornblith reports the following unemployment percentages by site among cancer survivors: 19% Hodgkin's disease, 25% leukemia, 19% breast cancer, 11% prostate, 22% colon, and 40% lung cancer.[15] Razavi et al found that patients treated for lymphoma often have difficulty returning to their jobs.[20] Of lymphoma patients in remission and able to work, only 54% actually returned to work. Anxiety, depression, and issues related to treatment were cited as reasons patients refused to reenter the workforce.[20] Because the incidence of Hodgkin's lymphoma peaks between ages 15 and 34 and after age 50, professional rehabilitation and return to function is extremely important for these individuals. Only 41% of patients with head and neck cancer return to work, which is most likely due to the nature of the surgery required and resulting disfigurement.[21]

One study conducted in The Netherlands examined changes in employment and earnings among adult five-year cancer survivors (n = 649).[21] This study provides several insights. Approximately one-third of the five-year cancer survivors had a change in their employment status from employed to either homemakers, retired, or unemployed. The percentage of patients that were employed part-time at the end of 5 years doubled from the time of diagnosis. Nurses need to consider the long-term implications of unemployment as they assist patients and families in planning for these likely events. To avoid unnecessary patient disability and unemployment, nurses can help develop a plan to ensure that patients get the maximum recovery and rehabilitation services available.

As noted by Mellete, little data exist on the employment experience of people with cancer who are able to work.[22] Some patients may be only temporarily disabled during and immediately after treatment, followed by eventual recovery to full functioning. In this scenario, patients and most likely members of their families will require minimal time away from work or alteration in their work.

Some patients become partially disabled and may need to take a leave of absence, switch to jobs that are less physically or emotionally demanding, or work fewer hours during the day or work fewer days during the week. These patients can be characterized as having reduced functional capacity due to the effects (e.g., arm limitations, lymphedema, altered memory, cognition, and concentration) of surgery, chemotherapy, or radiation. Patients may no longer be able to do their former jobs, which can lead to reduced earnings and a change in health care benefits. This transition is also likely to lead to adverse emotional consequences for patients and their families.

Other patients may become totally disabled and it is likely that one or more members of their families will be unable to work because patients require help in their day-to-day functioning. If previously employed, patients may leave the workforce altogether through early retirement or disability. Patients with colorectal or lung cancer and patients requiring bone marrow transplants often experience prolonged periods of disability. These patients and their families may have to adjust to their never being able to work again. As a result, their family roles and their income may be drastically altered.

Factors that influence postdiagnosis employment include:

- *Physical disability:* Common examples include diminished cognition, neurological damage, poor endurance, deformity, reduced range of motion, and incontinence.

- *Gender:* Men may be less likely than women to return to work because they are more often employed in physically demanding jobs.

- *Race:* Ethnic minorities are more likely to be employed in physically demanding jobs, earn lower wages, and are less likely to be diagnosed at an early stage and to get the care they need.

- *Job type:* Any person employed in a physically demanding job is less likely to be able to fully return to work, depending on the type of cancer, aggressiveness of treatment, and long-term morbidity. These individuals may also be less skilled and educated and have lower wages, making a job change extremely difficult.

Patients and families require guidance and counseling to address how disability will affect their lives, finances, and roles. Identifying problems with employment and intervening appropriately is a significant challenge for nurses.

In the following sections, specific problems (i.e., barriers to job reentry, inability to change jobs, early retirement, and problems specific to self-employment) that can occur at the work site, regardless of patient characteristics, job type, or disability are discussed.

Other Employment Considerations

Work Site Barriers to Job Reentry

Of survivors who report problems returning to work, many report instances of gross discrimination in which they were fired or laid off because of their cancer diagnosis. Others report that they were encouraged to leave, transferred to less desirable jobs, demoted, had difficulty finding a new job, and that their work responsibilities were unwillingly curtailed.[3,15] Nurses and other health care professionals must work with patients and their families to prepare them for possible discrimination and to help them develop strategies to thwart its effects. These strategies must be consistent with survivors' goals, expectations, and capabilities.

Breast cancer survivors identified four situations that hindered successful job reentry: (1) breach of confidentiality of medical information, (2) absence of support from coworkers and managers to assist in reentry and management of the stigma associated with cancer, (3) difficulty talking to colleagues about health, and (4) difficulty asking for and receiving assistance.[23] It is important to note that one cannot assume that employers or employees are aware of or adhere to federal regulations such as the Americans with Disabilities Act (1990). Common violations include disclosure of health history information and failure to provide reasonable accommodation for patients returning to work. However, the return to work does not have to be a negative experience. Some survivors report positive experiences of being relieved of difficult physical tasks, job sharing, modification of equipment, and flexible work schedules to accommodate medical appointments.[15]

Inability to Change Jobs

Examining whether a patient can return to work is insufficient. The inability to change jobs, or *job lock*, is another important outcome that may result from having been treated for cancer. Job lock is a reluctance to change jobs for fear of not finding comparable insurance coverage or an employer willing to hire someone with cancer. Lack of career mobility is part of many cancer survivors' experience.[3]

Job lock can lead to reduced worker productivity, less job satisfaction, and limited income. Also, some patients may stay in jobs they are no longer able to perform in order to preserve their insurance coverage. One study reported that 44% of breast cancer survivors felt "locked in" to their current job in order to retain their insurance coverage.[24] Particularly troubling is a situation in which patients survive cancer but they (or another wage earner in the household) cannot seek better employment for fear of job discrimination or losing insurance coverage.

Insurance-related reasons for not changing jobs include waiting periods, preexisting conditions, incomparable coverage, and higher premiums. Employers, particularly small firms, may not find persons (or their family members) with medical risks desirable because the employer's risk rating and premiums will dramatically increase. The risk of losing insurance coverage is greatest for workers with less experience and limited skills.[25]

Job lock can be a frustrating experience for cancer

survivors. These individuals may not be able to attain the career goals they have set for themselves. Until public policies such as health insurance portability are adopted, little can be done to remedy job lock. Coping strategies that refocus priorities away from career achievement to another meaningful goal are perhaps the only means to alleviate frustration. Job counseling and training for new skills may also be appropriate, in some cases.

Early Retirement

For many patients nearing retirement and with the financial means to do so, early retirement may be an option for coping with the cognitive and functional disabilities resulting from cancer and its treatment. However, this decision is not without consequences. Palmore et al found that when someone retires for health reasons, their income and standards of living dramatically decrease compared to other retirees, even after controlling for preretirement characteristics.[26] They also suffer more dissatisfaction with their living situations and experience decreased happiness.

Alternatively, cancer may provide patients with the opportunity to reflect on their lives in a positive way and help them to order their priorities so that the most can be made of the retirement experience. For a survivor choosing full or partial retirement, a realistic plan of care needs to be set that accommodates both goals and priorities. Nurses may need to advise patients not to make decisions too hastily. Patients may be tempted to make decisions when they are in the midst of aggressive treatment and before they know whether they can return to previous functioning levels. All patients should be encouraged to seek employment and financial counseling before making retirement decisions.

Self-Employment

Individuals who are self-employed, especially those in sole proprietorships, are not likely to have many options for job sharing, retirement, or working fewer hours. These individuals require special attention and counseling. Some may need to sell their business, hire someone to resume their previous responsibilities, or rely on other members of their families to take over the business either permanently or temporarily. This transition can cause worry, a sense of loss, and financial and emotional hardships. Because of the personal nature of owning and growing a business, letting go of some or all responsibilities and control may be extremely difficult. In addition, a number of legal concerns regarding ownership and decision making may need to be resolved.

Recommendations

Nurses need to urge patients and their family members to consider the possible effects cancer and its treatment

may have on their ability to work *prior* to receiving treatment. Many patients require treatments that can affect concentration and mental alertness. Some long-term treatments such as steroids can cause mood swings and depression. Patients may require pain, sleeping, and anti-emetic medication that may interfere with cognitive functioning. These treatments may last for months or years, and the treatment effects may remain for up to 6 months after treatment stops. This may decrease survivors' accuracy and efficiency or general ability to do cognitive work. In other situations, fatigue and lack of endurance prevent patients from being productive at their former work levels. Nurses can play a pivotal role in helping patients and families prepare for treatment and to anticipate what work-related adaptations might be needed. Such preparation minimizes lost work time and helps families plan to be available to provide care and to assist with recovery.

While employment issues can be quite formidable, nurses can aid patients first by making them aware of potential difficulties, and then by helping them think about solutions. For example, some coworkers may be willing to job share with the patient during the acute treatment phase. Some employers may be willing to assist the patient with internal placement in less physical and emotionally demanding jobs. If these changes are initiated by the survivor, chances are greater that he or she will feel more in control of the situation than if the change were imposed on him or her. Long-term strategies can be developed such as early retirement, finding a new job, or reducing the number of hours worked. Family members who were not previously working may need to work, or if they were working they may need to plan for time away from work to care for the patient. These strategies help patients and their families to become proactive and more prepared for inevitable changes.

The following section discusses the Americans with Disabilities Act and the Family Medical Leave Act, both of which may prove useful to cancer survivors and their family members. Other legislation may also be pertinent, but these two acts apply to the immediate concerns of taking time away from a job to seek care and possible job discrimination.

Legislative Protection

Fortunately, legislative protection exists for some of the challenges that may confront the cancer survivor in the workplace. It is essential that nurses and other health care professionals be aware of these protections and provide patients and families with information about their rights. Survivors and their family members are protected at the workplace by the Americans with Disabilities Act (ADA) and the Family Medical Leave Act (FMLA). Cancer is considered a disability under the ADA. The ADA requires employers to make "reasonable accommodation" for employees with a disability. Scheduling changes would be considered reasonable, for example, but turning a full-time job into a part-time job is not required.[27] The ADA specifies that employers may ask only job-related medical questions, prohibits employers from firing an employee with a disability without first making a reasonable accommodation on the job, and requires that employers treat all employees the same. Thus, an employer who provides insurance benefits to all employees, with the exception of a employee with a disability, violates the ADA requirement for equitable treatment of all employees. In addition, the ADA prohibits exclusion of an applicant for a job or from a training program because of disability.

The ADA has some noteworthy restrictions. It applies to employers with 15 or more employees, so persons with disabilities who are employed by small businesses are not protected. This may impose a greater hardship on those living in rural communities where small businesses are the principal employers. In addition, a 180-day statute of limitations on filing complaints from the date of discrimination exists. Patients with cancer must be proactive in making their needs known to their employer, becoming their own advocate to ensure their needs are met. If a court finds in favor of an employee, the remedy may include back pay, an injunction, and attorney's fees.

The FMLA gives employees the right to take time off due to their own illness or if they are caring for an ill dependent, without the threat of losing their jobs. Currently, this law provides for 12 weeks of unpaid leave per year for serious illness. A *serious health condition* is defined as one that incapacitates the patient for more than 3 consecutive days, requires a doctor's or other health care professional's care, or requires a regimen of continuous treatment. Cancer is a condition generally considered serious enough for FMLA to apply to both patients and family members needing to care for them.

The 12-week leave does not have to be taken all at once but can be taken in blocks of time. For example, taking several hours of leave per day over a period of weeks for treatments or follow-up tests receives the same protection as a more extensive leave of 12 consecutive weeks. During this time, the employer is required to continue providing health benefits. Taking blocks of time off may be particularly beneficial for patients requiring treatment over long periods of time. Nurses can help patients plan the time they will need to be away from their jobs to maximize FMLA's benefits.

An important limitation of FMLA is that it only applies to employers with 50 or more employees. Therefore, cancer patients and family members employed by most small businesses will not be covered. These individuals are likely to suffer greater hardships due to discrimination and may even lose their jobs because of their need for medical care and time away from work.

The literature indicates that up to three-fourths of cancer survivors have been able to resume employment at their previous levels.[15] Some studies show no differences in employment status between the cancer and noncancer populations.[13,14] Survivors of breast cancer, for example, were more likely to be working than women in a noncancer comparison group.[13] Nurses need to assist patients and their families to understand their rights and legal protections. This assistance may simply involve providing information to the patient or may require documenting a patient's illness and treatment for his or her employer. Table 70-2 summarizes the benefits and restrictions of the ADA and FMLA.

Cancer and its treatment lead to numerous workplace challenges for the survivor. These challenges can apply to family members as well and may lead to considerable hardship. In most situations, cancer survivors and their family members are faced with difficult decisions that can have serious emotional and financial implications. Fortunately, some patients report positive experiences at the work site, but many others report difficulty. The realities of disability and physical, emotional, and cognitive limitations need to be discussed with patients. Oncology nurses can play an important role in helping families plan for inevitable work challenges and the possibility of financial hardships before patients receive treatment. In addition, primary care nurses need to be aware of and plan for the long-term employment implications of the patient's cancer and its treatment.

Health Insurance Challenges

In the United States, insurance status continues to be closely tied to employment for individuals under age 65. Therefore, all of the problems associated with having been treated for cancer and employment—specifically, presence of physical disability, physically demanding job, minority race, low-income or low-skilled job—affect one's ability to obtain and keep insurance coverage. For example, in a study by Guidry et al, 26% of white patients and 46% of black patients lost insurance after they were diagnosed with cancer.[28] The difference in percentage was because African Americans were employed in lower paying and physically demanding jobs. Twenty-one percent of white patients were denied insurance coverage after changing jobs, whereas 55% of black patients were denied insurance coverage after changing jobs. Inability to work often translates to lack of insurance coverage for medical care and lost wages.

Survivors and their families have constant concerns about future health and the possibility of cancer recurrence and progression. Because medical costs are increasing, the need for adequate health insurance is critical. A lack of insurance is associated with physical, emotional, and financial burdens,[29,30] therefore health insurance coverage is extremely important to these individuals.

Any change in employment status is likely to lead to a change in health insurance coverage. For example, becoming unemployed, changing jobs, and working fewer hours can mean reduced coverage or loss of benefits. Studies among people with HIV infection show that advancing disease is associated with an increased likelihood of having public insurance. Fleishman found that over an 18-month period, 23% of the respondents to the

Table 70-2 Provisions of Americans with Disabilities Act and Family Medical Leave Act

For	Benefits	Restrictions
AMERICANS WITH DISABILITIES ACT, 1990		
Patients	• Requires reasonable accommodation for disability • Restricts employer inquiries to job-related medical questions • Provides for equitable insurance benefits • Prohibits exclusions from hiring decisions or training programs due to disability	• Applies to employers with 15 or more employees • 180-day statute of limitations
FAMILY MEDICAL LEAVE ACT, 1993		
Patients Family members	• 12 weeks of unpaid leave without losing job or benefits • Leave can be taken all at once or in blocks of time	• Applies to employers with 50 or more employees

AIDS Costs and Service Utilization Survey reported a change in insurance status, and 27% reported a change in employment status.[31] During the course of the study, 15% of the patients who initially reported having private insurance lost their coverage. Transitions from no insurance to public insurance occurred most frequently.

Transitions from private to public insurance may also occur in people with cancer. A change in patient insurance status (e.g., loses insurance, becomes insured, becomes disenrolled in Medicaid, changes policies) will likely lead to a change in health care provider and subsequently to a loss in continuity of care. A change in insurance status may also affect access to pharmaceuticals, particularly if the new insurer does not include certain drugs on its formulary.

Specific challenges to insurability include refusal, policy cancellation, higher premiums, and extended waiting periods.[32] For some patients, the price to obtain insurance is prohibitive once their health history is known. Persons with no insurance may have to exhaust their savings in order to become medically indigent and qualify for Medicaid. This process in itself can have serious psychosocial and long-term consequences for patients and their family members. In addition, some health care providers may not accept patients covered under Medicaid or who have no insurance. This may subsequently lead to fragmented care and perhaps worsening of disease.

Insurance coverage for cancer care often is not comprehensive. Coverage for anticancer drugs, investigational medications, and mental health and rehabilitation services and therapies are frequently lacking.[33] For patients over age 65, Medicare pays for a substantial portion of the care. However, only drugs administered in the physician's office and drugs administered by infusion pump are covered; oral drugs and injectable drugs that are self-administered by the patient are not covered. Medicare does not pay for prescription medications and other out-of-pocket expenditures. In addition, Medicare pays 80% of average wholesale price and the remaining 20% is the patient's responsibility.[34] Therefore, by the

time patients enter into the survivorship phase, they have already incurred many expenses. Insufficient funds may hinder the patients' ability to get the rehabilitation care they require in order to recover to the fullest extent possible.

Even though Medicare pays 80% of the average wholesale price of drugs administered in a physician's office or by infusion pump, this benefit is restrictive. For example, the use of a well-known chemotherapeutic agent for an indication not specified by the Food and Drug Administration (FDA) is prohibited by Medicare. This is particularly problematic because a General Accounting Office study found that one-third of the chemotherapy used was for an indication other than the one approved by the FDA. At least 56% of patients in this study received one "off-label" drug (a drug used for an indication not specifically approved by the FDA) as part of their treatment.[35,36] For patients who cannot receive state-of-the-art care due to health insurance and financial restrictions, survivorship may become difficult. These patients may lack access to medications. For example, drugs that can ease the effects of cancer treatments or that can slow disease progression may be financially prohibitive. Therefore, patients with insufficient insurance are more likely to experience adverse events, cancer recurrences, and disease progression due to the use of less effective therapies.

Under many managed care arrangements, specialists such as oncologists are paid on a discounted fee-for-service basis.[37] The primary care physician's income may be capitated and he or she may receive financial incentives to curtail referrals to specialists such as oncologists. Therefore, generally the managed care system reduces access to oncology specialists once the initial treatment phase is complete. In this arrangement, patients are likely to have discontinuity in their care and must take much of the responsibility for managing their symptoms and seeking treatment.

Medicaid is one option for financially indigent people meeting fairly stringent criteria that are set on a state-by-state and sometimes case-by-case basis. However, less than 45% of the population below the federal poverty level is eligible for Medicaid.[37] Medicaid is designed for acute care needs and is not meant to provide for patients' long-term chronic needs. For example, once patients are able to work (according to standards set by the state in which they reside) or are disease free for a specified period of time, Medicaid may cancel their coverage. Social Security Disability Insurance, a program offered under Medicare, is available to patients who are disabled depending on the site, stage, and type of cancer. This insurance is canceled if the patient is disease free for 3 years. Thus, survivors with this type of insurance soon find that their ongoing medical care needs are not covered by Medicare and that they are responsible for paying for their care out-of-pocket.

Understanding patients' insurance coverage can offer clues about access to care, utilization of services, and quality of care. Nurses are posed with considerable challenges in trying to understand the different plans and their limitations. Coordinating care while navigating through insurance provisions can be quite difficult, but it is critical to ensuring that patients have access to the most appropriate care available. Primary care nurses have a unique opportunity to devise a plan of care for survivors and to follow them over time. These nurses need to incorporate survivorship and rehabilitation issues into their conceptual framework of primary care that traditionally focuses on wellness. For example, nurses could educate patients to monitor their symptoms for possible cancer recurrences. Nurses could also help patients prevent long-term disability by developing regimens for rehabilitation and health maintenance. By doing so, nurses help patients and their families avoid long-term health care costs.

Cost-of-Care Considerations: Influences on Treatment Decisions and Long-Term Impact

Conservative estimates of medical care costs for cancer treatment show that the cost of care increased from $18.1 billion in 1985 to $41.1 billion in 1994.[38] Many of the recently adopted cancer treatment regimens are particularly expensive. Examples of these therapies include stem cell transplantation for hematological disorders, transplant procedures, paclitaxel for palliative chemotherapy, serotonin-antagonist antiemetics, and growth factors for supportive care during treatment.[38] With gaps in insurance plan coverage, and managed care organizations that have capitated payment systems, both patients and health care providers must understand the relative value of different treatment options. This is no easy task. Many new treatments may offer outcomes comparable to standard therapies or may provide only marginal gains in life expectancy and symptom relief. If the economic impact of cancer treatment on patients is not considered, many

may receive expensive therapies that offer little benefit or that leave them with limited resources to pay for future health care services.

Economic evaluation of cancer treatments has become more relevant in recent years. In 1996, the FDA announced an initiative to accelerate the approval process of cancer treatments.[39] This initiative allows the FDA to approve new products based on evidence of increased survival or improved quality of life. Thus, a survivor may undergo treatment and its side effects for the sake of quality-of-life improvements, realizing there is no chance for improved survival. As may be expected, many new and often expensive therapies are becoming available, and the challenge to health care providers and patients is to determine the *value* of the new therapies compared to standard treatment regimens.

Economic concerns are likely to have an important role in the treatment decisions of health care providers and patients. Cost-effectiveness analysis is an increasingly popular technique that compares the costs and effects among treatment strategies. *Effects* are health outcomes such as cases of disease prevented, years of life gained, or quality-adjusted life-years.[40] The quality-adjusted life-year incorporates patients' symptoms and disability over time, but does not consider family burden. Furthermore, the costs to keep the survivor alive in a compromised health state are typically estimated from the perspective of the payer (i.e., insurance provider), not the patient. The results of a cost-effectiveness analysis provide the incremental or additional cost of obtaining a unit of effect, such as a life-year, from one medical intervention compared to another. For example, autologous bone marrow transplantation costs $116,000 per life-year gained compared with standard chemotherapy[38] for patients with metastatic breast cancer.

Cost-effectiveness analysis is likely to effect survivors in two ways: (1) by making treatments more (or less) available, and (2) by offering an economic dimension to treatment choices. Managed-care organizations use economic evaluations to develop treatment practice guidelines and to make formulary decisions for the inclusion of medications. These practice guidelines and formulary decisions may dictate the type of treatment patients receive and the availability of certain medications. Patients need to know their options for obtaining "off-formulary" medications and alternative medical procedures. This information is relevant when making initial and long-term cancer treatment decisions. When patients consider the long-term consequences of the treatments available, they too need to consider its economic implications.

Cost-effectiveness analysis available in the literature can be evaluated using the criteria shown in Table 70-3. Perhaps the most important among these criteria are clarity of the research question, the inclusion of all pertinent costs and consequences (including those incurred by family members), and relevance to clinical practice. Regardless of the methodological rigor, if the study is not relevant to clinical practice and the alternatives are not reasonable comparisons (i.e., placebo may not be a reason-

Table 70-3 Twelve Criteria for Evaluating Cost-Effectiveness Analysis to Assist Patients with Treatment Decisions

Checklist	Comments
1. Well-defined research question	Is it clear what the researchers were trying to accomplish?
2. Alternative therapies well defined and explained	Is each alternative therapy and its sequelae fully explained?
3. Alternative therapies are reasonable comparisons	Is this something that would normally be used in routine practice? Or is the comparison to a therapy that is used rarely?
4. Target population well defined	Is the target population a high risk group? Is the target population the "typical" patient treated for the illness under consideration? Who was *excluded* from the analysis?
5. Statement of the perspective of the analysis	Was the analysis conducted from the perspective of the payer? Society? Patient?
6. All important costs and consequences identified for each strategy	Were all direct medical care costs and productivity costs (i.e., time away from work) fully estimated? Were all consequences including side effects, disabilities, and benefits included?
7. Sources for obtaining costs and outcomes stated	Are the sources credible? Are they applicable to other treatment settings?
8. Sensitivity analysis performed	Were other reasonable costs and survivorship outcomes considered in the analysis?
9. Results expressed as incremental costs and outcomes	Were the results expressed in terms of cost per life year gained for each alternative studied?
10. Study limitations are stated	Were any of the limitations stated a "fatal flaw" of the analysis?
11. Study conclusions have relevance to clinical practice	Were the results relevant to clinical practice? For example, if the study was conducted in a clinical trial setting, are the results applicable to routine practice and to survivorship?
12. Published in a peer-reviewed journal	Is the publication source credible?

patients understand their treatment alternatives and the costs and consequences of each alternative. For example, a cost-effectiveness analysis may be the only source of information that incorporates time away from work and lost wages, long-term medical care required and their costs, and quality-adjusted survival into a single study.

Ongoing Medical Care Needs of Survivors and Their Impact on Family Members

An understanding of the economic implications of medical treatment is important because the medical care needs of patients and families extend far beyond the initial treatment episodes and, as previously discussed, insurance benefits are often limited. Long-term treatment of individuals with cancer involves periodic medical visits to monitor patients' conditions and may require prolonged use of medications, medical supplies, durable medical equipment, and life style alteration to manage the symptoms and side effects (e.g., pain) of cancer and treatment. In addition, inpatient care to combat other concomitant conditions (e.g., bowel obstructions, fistulas) or cancer recurrences may be necessary.

Finding a balance between the long-term negative effects and costs of aggressive treatment and the anticipated benefits must be uppermost in the minds of those making treatment decisions. For example, increased use of palliative care may lower total costs by preventing or delaying hospitalization.[34] Patients with cancer, in particular, can benefit from the assistance of a nurse case manager, who provides assessment, education, and support, as well as referral to medical treatment, supportive services, and community resources. However, the health care system is changing and the burden of locating and paying for supportive services is often shifted to patients and their families. Therefore, the role of the nurse may be to identify where gaps exist in patients' care and to help them evaluate their alternatives.

Examples of ongoing care include medications, treatment for second malignant neoplasms, and rehabilitation. Rehabilitation can occur in many settings including inpatient, acute care, subacute rehabilitation, outpatient, and home. In addition, psychological counseling and participation in support groups for patients and family members is often an important part of the recovery process. Many communities have resources and advocacy groups that can be helpful to survivors and their families in locating the care they need.

Because patients and their family members are responsible for their care, they need to have an awareness of potential side effects and long-term problems associated with treatment so that difficulties can be quickly recognized and acted on before they become difficult to manage. For example, pain, compromised immunity, significant fatigue and endurance problems, and psychosocial problems are best addressed proactively. Nurses can take a leadership

able comparison), the study has limited application. In a practical sense, studies of cost-effectiveness can help patients understand why certain therapies are available and others are not and may be useful for helping patients make treatment decisions. Nurses can use these studies to help

role in assessing patients' needs and offering guidance for meeting long-term medical requirements.

For cancer survivors who require ongoing care and monitoring in the home setting, family members are frequently asked to provide both direct care, such as bathing, feeding, dressing changes, and medication administration, and indirect care, such as emotional support, transportation, and monitoring and standby care. Chronic illnesses such as cancer are not diagnosed during time periods that are predetermined by the individual. Because of this, the caregiving role is one that may be disruptive to family members' developmental needs.

Employed young and middle-aged adult caregivers must balance work roles with care-giving tasks. Stommel, Given, and Given documented that the work provided by family members during and immediately after the treatment phase can be equivalent to a part-time job.[41] They found that family caregivers were devoting up to 6 hours per day in the provision of care to their family member with cancer. Seventy-two percent of unpaid caregivers are women and most continue to be employed on a part or full-time basis outside of the home.[42]

Krach and Brooks found that the average amount of time spent in caregiving activities was 5 hours per week (range 1–30 hours per week).[11] Forty percent of their sample of employed caregivers reported that they received no assistance in the caregiving tasks from either formal or informal supports, and 48% of these employed caregivers reported missing an average of 4 days of work over a 6-month time period due to care-giving activities.

Caregivers who are employed in minimum wage positions may not have paid time off as part of their benefits and may not be employed in settings where the FMLA applies. Therefore, these caregivers may need to (1) arrange for secondary caregivers to stay with the patient when the primary caregiver is working, (2) take days off from work without pay, or (3) negotiate with their supervisors to rearrange work schedules so that they are able to be at home during times when the patient with cancer requires the greatest amount of care. Employed caregivers may not have enough time available for care-giving, and their job performance may be negatively impacted through decreased productivity and quality of work. Nurses need to be cognizant of the needs of these family members and must help them prepare for the immediate and ongoing requirements of caregiving. They can also assist family members by ensuring that patient appointments are not delayed and by being available for questions or care after normal working hours.

Improved life expectancy without full restoration to former health status leads to increased lifetime aggregate costs. For many patients and their families, cancer survivorship may bring financial problems. In addition to direct medical treatment costs, patients spend a significant amount of their earnings and savings for "ancillary" expenditures. These include travel, child care, parking, overnight expenses, insurance copayments, medications, and lost wages. These costs can be expected to continue, though at a lesser rate, during the survivorship phase.

Some patients may even be required to modify their homes to accommodate special beds, wheelchairs, or other durable equipment. Lost earnings due to the inability to work is also included in patients' expenses. Other family members may also be required to miss work.[43] Therefore, even those who are insured can be financially crippled by substantial gaps in coverage.

Persons with few financial resources are more likely to be diagnosed with cancer when the disease is advanced and treatment options are limited.[37] Because they have limited access to treatment, they may also have limited access to community services and ongoing care because referrals for these services are often made from within the medical care system. Financial problems may inhibit treatment, making cancer more costly in the long run. These patients are likely to experience greater morbidity and shorter survival.

Regardless of socioeconomic status, all families are likely to experience financial burdens due to gaps in insurance coverage, lost wages, and out-of-pocket expenditures. In a study of breast cancer survivors, Polinsky reported that 19% reported their income was inadequate to cover their medical care, 63% reported that they had inadequate insurance, and 44% worried about future health expenditures because they were concerned that they would not be able to afford the escalating cost.[24] Nurses, patients, and family members together must consider future care needs. Nurses can help patients and families devise a plan to prepare for future expenditures.

The Cultural Dimension of Survivorship

Many issues that patients with cancer and family caregivers face are dictated by their cultural affiliation, the predominant cultural affiliation of the community in which they reside, and their socioeconomic status. Cultural affiliation involves beliefs, opinions, attitudes, customs and rituals, and values, with multiple cultural identities existing within singular ethnic/racial groups. Self-identification as a cancer survivor depends on how the individual defines illness, health, life, and quality of life, as well as how the cause of cancer is viewed.

Beyond the cultural implications of cancer survival, caregivers are faced with their own unique social issues. Females have traditionally been socialized as the homemakers and nurturers and males have been traditionally socialized as the breadwinners. Becoming enculturated into the care-giving role may be difficult based on cultural expectations by gender.

Recommendations for Care

Throughout the care trajectory, family members will have to assume new roles and reorganize established and familiar roles due to the nature of the needs of the patient with cancer. When the patient is unable to participate in self-care activities, such as during chemotherapy, family caregivers will need to reassign or relinquish long-held roles in order to assist the patient and to ensure that care needs are being met. As the patient regains the ability to perform self-care tasks, the caregiver may be able, to some extent, reclaim previously reassigned and relinquished roles. The unpredictability and fluid nature of the caregiving role makes it difficult for family caregivers to plan for their own needs for social and leisure time. Nurses need to be aware of the toll that cancer takes on the family members, and provide information on support groups, resources, and respite services that are available in their community. Nurses also need to understand that culture and values can either complicate or enhance patient and family's survivorship experience.

Because of improved treatment regimens and longevity following a cancer diagnosis, an understanding of survivorship issues will become increasingly more important to patients, families, and health care professionals. To date, the oncology nursing literature has provided one of the few forums available to discuss survivorship issues. Nurses in cancer care need to continue examining survivorship issues as they develop plans of care because this

Table 70-4 Preparing for Survivorship—Relevant Patient Information

Patient Information

Name:	
Address:	
Age:	Gender: M/F
Diagnosis:	

Functional Status

Physical Limitations: 1. 2. 3. 4.	Overall Health Status: Excellent Very Good Good Fair Poor

Treatment Information

Recommended Treatment:	Duration:
Common Side Effects: 1. 2. 3. 4.	Duration:
Concomitant Medications:	

Employment Information

	Job Title:
Employer:	
Job Description (typical duties):	
Hours Worked Per Week:	
Caregiver Employer:	
Job Description (typical duties):	
Hours Worked Per Week:	

Insurance Information

Type of Insurance:	Description of Coverage:
Copayments (visits, medications, hospitalizations):	Is insurance coverage through patient's or caregiver's employer?
Restrictions in coverage (cancer specific):	

phase, whether short or long, is vitally important to those who have endured the diagnosis and treatment.

Oncology nurses must be sensitive to survivorship issues in their discharge plans and as they refer patients back to their primary care provider. Psychosocial assessment is as important as biomedical examinations. Programs geared toward the survivor must address not only the patients' physical activities, but also the daily demands (e.g., employment, insurance) they are likely to face once they leave the acute treatment phase. Table 70-4 provides a worksheet that can serve as a basis for devising such a plan. The worksheet in Table 70-5 can serve as a template for the actual plan.

Most cancer survivors will seek long-term care from primary care providers (physicians and nurse practioners).[44] Correct identification of patients with a cancer history is the first step toward making an accurate assessment of their needs. Information about the treatment regimen and potential long-term sequelae, including second malignancies, helps to prepare survivors to recognize the importance of monitoring symptoms[45] and being vigilant in their follow-up care. Cancer centers should make specific referrals and discharge plans that are pertinent to survivorship. Nurses can take a leadership role in the continuity of care for survivors.

Recommendations for nurses caring for cancer survivors can be summarized as follows:

- Educate patients and their families on the disease and its anticipated trajectory.

- Educate patients and their families on treatment modalities and long-term consequences.

- Educate patients and their families on common symptoms and adverse effects of treatment and provide strategies for their management.

- Foster a spirit of teamwork among patients, families, and health care providers.

- Help patients and their families anticipate and plan for time away from work and advise them to be prepared for long-term accommodations.

- Make patients and family members aware of their rights at work.

Table 70-5 Survivorship Worksheet

Employment
1. How much time should the patient plan to be away from work during the acute treatment phase?
2. Will the side effects of treatment affect the patient's ability to perform his or her job over the short-term? Long-term?
3. Will the side effects of medications interfere with the patient's ability to perform his or her job? How long will medications be administered?
4. What can be done to reduce the impact on the patient's job? Is job sharing an option?
5. Should the patient consider a job change? Different job? Fewer hours?
6. How much time should the caregiver plan to be away from work while the patient is undergoing treatment?

Insurance
1. Will patient's health insurance coverage be affected by a change in his or her employment?
2. If yes, is the patient a candidate for Medicaid or Social Security Disability Insurance?
3. If yes, will the patient have to change health care providers?

Estimate of Out-of-Pocket Expenses
Copayments (visits per month @ $xx.xx/per visit)
Deductible
Prescription Medication
Over-the-Counter Medication
Equipment
Transportation Costs
Childcare Costs
Lost Wages
Monthly Total

Alternative Therapies
1.
2.
3.

Rehabilitation Needs/Referrals
1.
2.
3.

Psychosocial Assessment (Patient)
Date:
Findings

Supportive Services/Referrals
1. Self-Advocacy Training
2.
3.

Psychosocial Assessment (Family Members)
Date:
Findings

Community Services/Referrals
1.
2.
3.

Other Resources (books, tapes, Web sites)
1.
2.
3.

Table 70-6   Web Sites and Telephone Numbers for Cancer Information

Organization	Web Site/Phone
National Cancer Institute (NCI)	http://www.nci.nih.gov/; 1-800-4-CANCER
National Coalition for Cancer Survivorship	http://www.cansearch.org/ 1-888-937-6227 (1-888-YES-NCCS)
NCI Publications List	http://cnetdb.nci.nih.gov/ cancerlit.shtml 1-800-4-CANCER
NCI Clinical Trials Information	http://cancertrials.nci.nhi.gov/ 1-800-4-CANCER
OncoLink	http://oncolink.upenn.edu
American Cancer Society	http://www.cancer.org/ 1-800-ACS-2345
Wellness Web	http://www.wellweb.com/ cancer/cancer.htm (212) 686-0901
Oncology Nursing Society	http://www.ons.org/ (412) 921-7373
Healthfinder	http://www.healthfinder.org/
Cancer Care, Inc.	1-800-813-HOPE
Leukemia Society of America	http://www.leukemia.org/ 1-800-955-4LSA
National Alliance of Breast Cancer Organizations	http://www.nabco.org/ (888) 80-NABCO 1-800-719-9154
National Brain Tumor Foundation	no Web site 1-800-934-CURE
Y-ME National Breast Cancer Organization	http://www.y-me.org/ 1-800-221-2141

- Become knowledgeable in studies of cost-effectiveness of alternative therapies so that treatment decisions incorporate economic concerns.

- Understand patients' insurance limitations and advocate for patients with their insurance providers, where possible.

- Assist patients and families in taking responsibility for their health care through self-advocacy, and make patients and their families aware of resources available to them.

- Develop a discharge plan for follow-up care.

- Become familiar with survivor groups (both general and disease-specific) that further assist patients and their families and help them to become advocates for their own health care.

Part of the nurse's challenge is to educate survivors to access information and resources appropriate to their needs, values, and beliefs.[32] Because such a diversity of resources exist, patients must be prompted to become active participants in their health care. Nurses should prepare patients and their family members to advocate for themselves in matters concerning their health. They need to feel empowered so that they can communicate effectively and access the care they need. It is critical that survivors have a sense of control in their lives and continue to face the challenges inherent in cancer and the health care system.

The NCCS stresses the need for rehabilitative services, psychosocial services, and a choice of interventions and training in cancer-related self-advocacy, information seeking, negotiation, communication, and problem-solving skills. For many patients, self-advocacy and problem solving are skills that must be acquired. Fortunately, many survivorship groups offer classes in communication, negotiation, information seeking, and problem solving. Referral to these groups may be appropriate for many patients. Table 70-6 lists Internet sites and toll-free telephone numbers that may be useful in locating resources that may be of benefit long-term.

Conclusion

Despite the many challenges, cancer survivorship is cause for celebration for patients and their families. Nurses can play an important role in guiding patients and their families through the survivorship phase. The most visionary institutions are those that will successfully combine state-of-the-art treatment programs with strong, active survivor programs.[32] The physical, economic, and social issues confronting patients and their families during the survival period are an integral part of cancer care.

References

1. American Cancer Society. *Cancer Facts and Figures*. Atlanta, American Cancer Society, 1998
2. Tamlyn-Leaman K: Adult cancer survivorship issues and challenges. *Can Oncol Nurs J* 5:45–47, 1995
3. Quigley KM: The adult cancer survivor: Psychosocial consequences of cure. *Semin Oncol Nurs* 5:63–39, 1989
4. Leigh S: Survivorship, in Sigler B, George LM (eds): *Psychosocial Dimensions of Oncology Nursing Care*. Pittsburgh, PA, Oncology Nursing Press, 1998, pp 130–148
5. Stafford RS, Cyr P: The impact of cancer on the physical function of the elderly and their utilization of health care. *Cancer* 801:1973–1980, 1998
6. Fow NR: Cancer rehabilitation: An investment in survivorship. As more people survive the disease, focus shifts on improving quality of life. *Rehabil Manage* 9:48–53, 1996
7. Cella D, Tulsky D, Gray G, et al: The functional assessment of cancer therapy scale: Development and validation of the general measure. *J Clin Oncol* 11:570–579, 1993
8. Twycross R, Harcourt J, Bergl S: A survey of pain in patients

with advanced cancer. *J Pain Symptom Manage* 12:273–282, 1996

9. Ware J, Sherbourne C: The SF-36 short-form health status survey. I. Conceptual framework and item selection. *Med Care* 30:473–483, 1992

10. Braithwaite V: Between stressors and outcomes: Can we simplify the caregiving process variables? *Gerontologist* 36:42–53, 1996

11. Krach P, Brooks JA: Identifying the responsibilities and needs of working adults who are primary caregivers. *J Gerontol Nurs* 21:41–50, 1995

12. Hoyert DL, Seltzer MM: Factors relating to the well-being and life activities of family caregivers. *Fam Relations* 41:74–81, 1992

13. Craig TJ, Comstock GW, Geiser PB: The quality of survival in breast cancer: A case-control comparison. *Cancer* 33:1451–1457, 1974

14. Van Tulder MW, Aaronson NK, Bruning PF: The quality of life of long-term cancer survivors of Hodgkin's disease. *Ann Oncol* 5:153–158, 1994

15. Kornblith AB: Psychosocial adaptation of cancer survivors, in Holland JC, Rowland J (eds): *Psycho-oncology*. New York, Oxford University Press, 1998, pp 223–241

16. Loprest P, Rupp K, Sandell SH: Gender, disabilities, and employment in the health and retirement study. *J Hum Resources* 30:S293–S318, 1995 (suppl)

17. Bound J, Schoenbaum M, Waidmann R: Race and education differences in disability status and labor force attachment in the health and retirement study. *J Hum Resources* 30:S227–S267, 1995 (suppl)

18. Hampton JW: The disproportionately lower cancer survival rate with increased incidence and mortality in minorities and underserved Americans. *Cancer* 83:1687–1690, 1998 (suppl)

19. Satariano WA, DeLorenze GN: The likelihood of returning to work after breast cancer. *Public Health Rep* 111:236–241, 1996

20. Razavi D, Delvaux N, Bredart A, et al: Professional rehabilitation of lymphoma patients: A study of psychosocial factors associated with return to work. *Support Care Cancer* 1:276–278, 1993

21. van der Wouden MC, Greaves-Otte JGW, Greaves J, et al: Occupational reintegration of long-term cancer survivors. *J Occup Med* 34:1084–1089, 1992

22. Mellete SJ: Cancer rehabilitation. *J Natl Cancer Inst* 85:781–784, 1993

23. Carter B: Surviving cancer: A problematic work re-entry. *Cancer Pract* 2:135–140, 1994

24. Polinsky ML: Functional status of long-term breast cancer survivors: Demonstrating chronicity. *Health Soc Work* 19:165–173, 1944

25. Cooper PF, Monheit AC: Does employment-related health insurance inhibit job mobility? *Inquiry* 30:400–416, 1993

26. Palmore E, Burchett B, Fillenbaum G, et al (eds): *Retirement: Causes and Consequences*. New York, Springer, 1985

27. Abeloff MD (ed): Lawyer tells cancer patients how to fight job discrimination. *Oncol News Int* 7:34–35, 1998

28. Guidry JJ, Aday L, Zhang D, Winn RJ: Cost considerations as potential barriers to cancer treatment. *Cancer Pract* 6:182–187, 1998

29. Glajchen M: Psychosocial consequences of inadequate health insurance for patients with cancer. *Cancer Pract* 2:115–120, 1994

30. Franks P, Nutting PA, Clancy CM: Health care reform, primary care, and the need for research. *JAMA* 270:1449–1453, 1993

31. Fleishman JA: Transitions in insurance and employment among people with HIV infection. *Inquiry* 35:36–48, 1998

32. Leigh S: Cancer survivorship: A consumer movement. *Semin Oncol* 21:783–786, 1994

33. Card IC: National coalition for cancer survivorship perspective. *Proceedings from the American Cancer Society Workshop on Children*. Atlanta, American Cancer Society, 1991

34. Bailes JS: Health care economics of cancer in the elderly. *Cancer* 80:1348–1350, 1997 (special section)

35. Boring CG, Squires TS, Tong T: Cancer statistics, 1992. *CA Cancer J Clin* 42:19–38, 1992

36. Leake AR: The economic impact of cancer. *Nurse Pract Forum* 6:207–214, 1995

37. Berkman BJ, Sampson SE: Psychosocial effects of cancer economics on patients and their families. *Cancer* 72:2846–2849, 1993 (suppl)

38. Brown M, Glick HA, Harrell F, et al: Integrating economic analysis into cancer clinical trials: The national cancer institute—American society of clinical oncology economics workbook. *J Natl Cancer Inst Monogr* 24:1–28, 1998

39. Beltz SE, Yee GC: Pharmacoeconomics of cancer therapy. *Cancer Control* 5:415–424, 1998

40. Gold MR, Siegel JE, Rusell LB, Weinstein MC (eds): *Cost-effectiveness, in Health and Medicine*. New York, Oxford University Press, 1996

41. Stommel M, Given CW, Given BA: The cost of cancer home care to families. *Cancer* 71:1867–1874, 1993

42. Robinson KM: Family caregiving: Who provides the care, and at what cost? *Nurs Econ* 15:243–247, 1997

43. Moore K: Out-of-pocket expenditures of outpatients receiving chemotherapy. *Oncol Nurs Forum* 25:1615–1621, 1998

44. Herold AH, Roetzheim RG: Cancer survivors. *Primary Care* 19:779–791, 1992

45. Fernsler J, Fanuele JS: Lymphomas: Long-term sequelae and survivorship issues. *Semin Oncol Nurs* 14:321–328, 1998

CHAPTER 71

Spiritual and Ethical End-of-Life Concerns

Elizabeth Johnston Taylor, PhD, RN

Introduction

I had to do a crash course in spirituality. I mean, you may be facing the end of your life. . . . I started going back to church and trying to investigate my feelings about God, and about what would happen after I die. . . . At one point you're facing death, and then the next point you're like facing, "What am I going to eat for breakfast tomorrow morning?" . . . That's what I think I came to terms with after crying for 6 months, that, you know, either this is it and you might as well die right now, or you can have a life. It's your choice. So I said, "OK, I'm going to have a life."

This statement about living with breast cancer by a 40-year-old woman poignantly describes a pervasive experience among cancer survivors: When diagnosed with cancer, individuals inevitably become more aware of their personal mortality. And when confronted with death, individuals typically confront spiritual and ethical questions. Such spiritual and ethical concerns can be summed up in the following two questions: "How shall I die?" and "How shall I live before I die?" These two fundamental end-of-life decisions confronting cancer survivors (albeit with varying degrees of awareness) are addressed in this chapter.

To prepare the reader for a discussion of these questions, a review of literature discussing the relationship between imminent death and spirituality in persons with cancer is presented. This discussion identifies factors within the cancer experience that help explain why imminent death can bring spiritual concerns into greater awareness. The chapter concludes by addressing ethical issues faced by patients with cancer at the end of their lives and identifies strategies for promoting spiritual well-being.

Definitions

Before a discussion using easily misunderstood terms such as *spirituality, religiosity,* and *ethics* proceeds, the terms must be defined. *Spirituality* refers to that dimension of being human that motivates meaning-making and self-transcendence—or intra-, inter-, and transpersonal connectedness.[1,2] In nursing literature that defines related terms such as spiritual distress, need, or well-being; one will find spirituality described as an integrating energy, a life principle, an innate human quality.[3-6] Spirituality prompts individuals to make sense of their universe and to relate harmoniously with self, nature, and others—including any god(s), as conceptualized by each person.

In contrast to spirituality, religiosity often is viewed as a narrower concept.[4,5,7,8] *Religion* is the representation and expression of spirituality. A religion offers an individual a specific world view and an explanation that seeks to provide answers to the questions of ultimate meaning; it also may recommend how one is to live harmoniously with self, others, nature, and god(s). Such explanations and recommendations are presented in a religion's belief system (e.g., myths/stories, doctrines, dogmas) and are remembered and appreciated with rituals and other religious practices or observances.[9] One's religion may or may not be of an institutional nature.

Ethics involves reflecting systematically about "oughts," theorizing about right conduct and how to live as a good person.[10] Thus, an ethical dilemma or conflict arises when a choice must be made between the lesser of evils or the best of goods. In addressing such ethical conflicts, certain frameworks (e.g., utilitarianism, deontology) and principles (e.g., respect for autonomy, beneficence, nonmaleficence, justice, veracity) are considered during the decision-making process.[10,11]

Spirituality and ethics are closely related. This relationship is brought to awareness by such questions as: What is it that determines our oughts? Where do the values and meanings behind our ethical principles originate? What is this instinctual motivation to do right, not wrong? Where does it come from? As one considers the supreme values and ultimate meanings accompanying ethical issues, one is essentially exploring spiritual elements. Thus, ethical questions inevitably lead to spiritual questions.

Spirituality and the Cancer Experience

Research and clinical observations suggest that there is heightened spiritual awareness among individuals surviving cancer.[12-17] This heightened awareness of personal spirituality may manifest itself as spiritual or existential distress[18-20] or increased spiritual well-being.[2,21-25] Several articles have been written by health care professionals regarding the spiritual and religious needs of individuals with cancer[26-28] and imply that individuals surviving cancer have unique spiritual needs.

However, few empirical studies exist that directly support these clinical observations about the pervasiveness of spiritual distress. One study found that 32 of 50 consecutive patients with cancer referred for a psychiatric consult were concerned with religious issues; these included recent loss of religious support, pressure to adopt a different religious position, conflict between religious views and view of illness, and preoccupation with the meaning of life and illness.[19] Other studies document that aspects of spirituality, such as meaningfulness and hopefulness, are threatened by the cancer experience, thereby creating the possibility of spiritual distress.[29-32]

In contrast, other research lends evidence to the possibility that the cancer experience may contribute to spiritual well-being. For example, Reed observed that terminally ill patients with cancer had greater spiritual perspective than did nonterminally ill hospitalized patients and healthy adults (N = 300).[23] Furthermore, various indicators of spiritual well-being have been found to be positively related to various indicators of psychosocial well-being among cancer survivors.[23,33-36]

The research reporting that individuals with cancer frequently use spiritual and religious strategies to cope with their cancer-related experiences also indicates the heightened spiritual awareness among individuals with cancer. Studies of individuals surviving cancer document religious faith or prayer as a top-ranked coping strategy.[12,17,37–41] Sodestrom and Martinson found that of 25 cancer patients, 88% used a variety of spiritual coping strategies; they also reported that these patients indicated an increase in the awareness and practice of their spiritual beliefs since diagnosis.[12]

In summary, the literature indicates that individuals surviving cancer characteristically become more aware of their spirituality. This increased awareness may be experienced as painful and negative, positive and pleasant, or some combination of the two. Indeed, within one individual, spiritual responses to cancer can be mixed and ambivalent.

The Relationship Between Spirituality and Imminence of Death

Why do some individuals surviving cancer have a heightened sense of spiritual awareness? The fundamental answer appears to lie in the realization of personal mortality and vulnerability that a cancer diagnosis creates. Even if a survivor believes that "Cancer is a word, not a sentence," the reality of eventual death becomes vivid for those diagnosed with cancer. Moberg expanded on this relationship between imminence of death and spirituality when he argued that both were integrally linked in three primary ways: "The avoidance of death is a spiritual phenomenon; the social meanings of death relate to spiritual issues; and the preparation for death is a spiritual task."[42,p.140]

Whereas the literature reviewed earlier indicated that the experience of surviving cancer can bring an increased awareness of personal spirituality, there is also evidence of a direct relationship between spirituality and imminence of death; that is, the closer to death an individual with cancer gets, the more she or he will become aware of and concerned with personal spirituality. This relationship between spirituality and imminence of death is empirically supported in a variety of ways. For example, Gotay found that praying, having faith, and hoping were used as coping strategies more by women with advanced cancer than by their counterparts with early-stage cancer.[40] Reed observed significantly greater religiousness among 57 terminally-ill patients with cancer than among the 57 healthy matched counterparts.[22] Filipp observed from a post-hoc analysis of data collected from individuals with cancer that those who were soon to die used the "search for meaning in religion" as a coping strategy more often than did survivors.[43] Also, health care professionals in oncology settings have written anecdotally of an increased spiritual awareness or sensitivity accompanying the end of life.[27,44,45]

What is it about the imminence of death that contributes to this increased spiritual awareness for persons with cancer? What are the "end-of-life" experiences that heighten one's sense of spirituality? Table 71-1 offers an

Table 71-1 Possible Contributors to Increased Spiritual Awareness in Persons with Cancer Facing Imminent Death

Experiences Inherent in Facing Imminent Death	Manifestations of Spirituality
Losses and changes	Search for meaning
Realization of mortality	Search for immortality (e.g., afterlife beliefs, leaving legacies)
Existential questions	Search for answers, meaning, and purpose
Powerlessness and vulnerability	Search for security, comfort; transcend self to seek a greater Power
Isolation or loneliness	Search for relatedness and love
Social disengagement	Engagement with greater Other, self-transcendence
Guilt or shame	Search for forgiveness and acceptance
Life review	Joy and meaning, or anger and questions

incomplete list of possible answers. Such experiences of cancer can contribute to greater spiritual awareness—spiritual pain, pleasure, or both.

Cancer survivors, especially those at the end of life, experience numerous and various losses and changes. These might include loss of mobility and independence, changes in social roles, loss of the future, and so forth. Social psychologists theorize that significant losses and changes cause individuals to search for meaning as a way to try to make sense of such a negative experience.[46–49] This process of searching for meaning often makes individuals reexamine their beliefs about their world, including religious beliefs.

A human response to the reality of death is to seek immortality.[46,48,50] Rather than accepting that their lives are finite or insignificant, humans are comforted by beliefs in an after-death life and by leaving legacies that benefit others. Leaving a legacy, whether it is a monetary endowment, an oral history, a work of art, or a baby blanket for a future grandchild, brings a sense of value and significance to a dying individual's life and work.

Anxiety and existential questions often arise for individuals confronting imminent death.[42,51,52] Indeed, it has been argued that death is the fundamental source of all anxiety.[53] The questions can be framed in a variety of ways and reflect varying degrees of intellectual honesty. For some survivors, such questions may be too painful to acknowledge. Blatant existential questions a nurse may hear from an intellectually bold cancer survivor might include: "What is the purpose of my death? What was the purpose for my life? Why was I born if I was meant to die?" These questions often directly challenge an individual's spiritual or religious assumptions.

At the end of life, a person with cancer may be especially overwhelmed by pain, fatigue, anger, depression, and other difficult aspects of suffering and dying. Such aspects of suffering and dying characteristically leave an individual feeling powerless and vulnerable. Indeed, many individuals with cancer are heard to say that their illness experience teaches them that they are "not in control" of their bodies, their world, or their future. While some respond to this lack of control with a sense of helplessness and perhaps hopelessness, others regain "control" by cognitively reframing the experience as positive (e.g., "Having cancer has taught me how to receive help from others" or "I've learned to take responsibility for the things I can change, and not to worry about the rest").[54–56] Powerlessness and vulnerability, and the subsequent emotional and cognitive responses to these states, reflect and draw from one's core, one's spirituality.

The experiences of suffering and dying also frequently contribute to isolation and loneliness. Whether one is institutionalized for death or surrounded at home by loved ones, dying can be a lonely experience. After all, no one can share the personal experience of irreversible death with a dying individual. Furthermore, the fear and denial of death prevalent in the United States causes people to distance or remove themselves from those who are dying,[46,49] contributing to the feelings of isolation and loneliness. The self-transcendent nature of spirituality that prompts individuals to love and relate to others is thus stressed. Another related aspect of dying is disengagement; a social death often precedes biological death.[51] Because the human spirit provokes or requires love and relationship, a dying person may seek such love and relationship with a spiritual being or God, instead of, or in addition to, human relationships. Derrickson calls this spiritual work of the dying reconciliation and reunion.[8]

Some individuals with cancer may become increasingly aware of their spirituality at the end of life because of a sense of guilt or shame.[27] Whereas some may believe that their cancer is punishment for past "sins,"[57] others may feel guilty or shamed because of illness-related factors. For example, a person may feel guilty for being angry and doubtful about God, or for being a burden to family caregivers. Regardless of whether the guilt is appropriate or logical, one's desire to resolve this spiritual distress with acceptance and forgiveness demands attention.

Fundamental "End-of-Life" Questions

How Shall I Die?

While this question is too disturbing for some to ask and answer openly, others consider it with directness and honesty. Whether an active or passive answer is given, a decision inevitably is made. For those who confront seriously the conditions of their death, several questions may be explicitly asked:

- *Where do I want to die?* At home? In a hospice? Somewhere else?

- *When do I want to die?* When "nature takes its course," or before certain other conditions like pain or dementia reach an unbearable threshold?

- *When should death be delayed, if at all?* If delayed, to what extent should "heroic" and resuscitation measures be used?

- *How do I want to die?* Alone or with loved ones present? Naturally or with assistance? What would constitute a good or dignified death for me?

Because life is valued as sacred by most humans, questions related to how one will die consequentially introduce ethical and spiritual issues. Is it right to hasten a death when suffering is unbearable, or even when it is bearable? Is it right to cause a death, or assist with a death, when life is present? These questions of suicide and euthanasia create debate not only for cancer nurses and other health care professionals, but for societies at large.

Suicide is the intentional taking of one's own life. *Euthanasia,* translated from Greek as an easy or good death, refers to the act of assisting or enabling a sufferer's death, preferably without pain. Because suffering is thereby relieved by death, euthanasia is often called "mercy killing"; euthanasia is sometimes referred to as assisted suicide or assisted death. However, some may differentiate between assisted suicide or death and euthanasia, reserving the term euthanasia to describe a self-inflicted death. (For example, the physician who gives the lethal dose in contrast to the physician who provides the patient with a lethal dose to self-administer.) *Active euthanasia* refers to direct intervention causing death, whereas passive euthanasia refers to letting a sufferer die by withholding or withdrawing life-sustaining care. Passive or active euthanasia is voluntary if the sufferer requests it.

End-of-life issues, debated for centuries, have received increased attention in contemporary American society, exemplified by organizations such as the Hemlock Society and Choice in Dying; self-help books such as *Final Exit,* which offer laypersons techniques for nonviolent death; news media coverage of physician-assisted suicides facilitated by pathologist Jack "Dr. Death" Kervorkian; and state initiatives proposing legalization of physician-assisted death. Oregonians' approval of the Death With Dignity Act in 1994 (and opposition of the repeal of the Act in 1997) may be just the beginning of a U.S. trend of states legalizing euthanasia.[58,59] Indeed, a recent poll of 1200 adults revealed that nearly two-thirds supported the legalization of physician-assisted suicide.[60] Half of these respondents also acknowledged that they could imagine wanting to be euthanized themselves. It is helpful to note that being religiously conservative, a member of a minority, and older than 55 years were factors related to negative attitudes regarding euthanasia.

Nurses' perspectives on end-of-life issues

The American Nurses' Association's (ANA) code for nurses begins by stipulating that "the nurse provides services with respect for human dignity and the uniqueness of the client."[61] It continues by asserting that "nurses individually and collectively have an obligation to provide comprehensive and compassionate end-of-life care, which includes the promotion of comfort and the relief of pain, and at times, foregoing life-sustaining treatments." The Oncology Nursing Society (ONS) is one of several nursing specialty organizations that have endorsed the ANA Code. Both nursing organizations support the role of the nurse as a patient advocate who is obligated to protect the moral and legal rights of care recipients.

In 1991, the ONS passed a resolution in recognition of the need for cancer nurses to examine, understand, and respond to current ethical issues related to oncology practice, and to promote decision making based on patient-centered values.[62] In 1996, a resolution recognizing factors that interfere with provision of humane end-of-life care and affirming oncology nurses' commitment to quality end-of-life care was presented to the ONS membership.[63] Again in 1997, ONS endorsed the ANA's position, which opposes active euthanasia and assisted suicide.[64] Assisted suicide and end-of-life decisions were identified as the two most important ethical issues by the Oncology Nursing Society Ethics Advisory Council and by 900 nurses surveyed by the ANA.[65]

Clearly, cancer nurses recognize the importance of addressing end-of-life issues; they are dedicated to understanding how nursing values and ethics can be implemented in clinical practice. Considering Oregon's Death With Dignity legislation and other states' attempts to introduce such legislation, oncology nurses must be informed and philosophically grounded, as soon they likely will encounter a decision regarding how involved they will be in assisting with euthanasia or assisted suicide if they have not already been challenged with such a decision.[58,59] In a research report that nurses have contested, Asch stated that 16% of 1139 critical care nurses surveyed indicated that they had participated in active euthanasia or assisted suicide at least one time during their careers.[66] Nurses' beliefs about euthanasia and assisted suicide presumably determine their clinical practice.

Although often intimately involved in caring for cancer survivors making end-of-life decisions, oncology nurses hold diverse perspectives about such controversial decisions. Several researchers have explored cancer nurses' attitudes about end-of-life issues.[67-70] Young et al found that ONS members who responded to a questionnaire about physician-assisted dying (N = 1210) held widely varying attitudes; that is, while some respondents stated that they believed it wrong and would refuse involvement, others indicated that it was a legitimate choice that they would support.[68] Furthermore, the researchers found that many nurses were willing to lay aside their personal beliefs about the wrongness of physician-assisted death to support a patient who requested it. Richardson also noted ambivalence among oncology nurses when she questioned them about voluntary active euthanasia; although some of the 200 nurses wrote about situa-

tions where they wished for a terminally ill person's rapid death, 40% indicated that they disagreed with voluntary active euthanasia for themselves or their loved ones.[70] When Davis' research team interviewed 80 nurses (many of whom were cancer nurses) about active euthanasia, only 17% justified it.[67] While the rationale for nurses who opposed active euthanasia included personal and professional integrity, sanctity of life, and religious beliefs, the nurses who supported active euthanasia typically cited patient autonomy, families' wishes, severe suffering, and terminal illness as reasons for supporting active euthanasia. Interestingly, the same arguments and ethical principles were cited by nurses both for and against active euthanasia.

It is important to note that private religiosity does significantly influence oncology nurses' attitudes about end-of-life options.[68,70] Richardson observed that nurses with "strong religious belief" disagreed with legalization of voluntary active euthanasia.[70] Young et al reported that Roman Catholic nurses accepted physician-assisted death significantly less than did Protestant, Jewish, atheist, or agnostic nurses.[68] Valente et al noted that "suicide was against their religion" for some cancer nurses.[69] These findings underscore the subtle yet strong influence nurses' religious views can have on clinical practice. In contrast, a large survey of British individuals grieving the recent loss of a loved one to terminal illness observed that religiosity did not contribute to beliefs about euthanasia and whether their loved one should have died earlier.[71] Perhaps religious mores are overridden when one is forced to confront end-of-life issues in personal reality. (In such cases, religiosity may be overruled by instinctual or more fundamental ethical-spiritual principles.)

Factors influencing end-of-life decisions

Compared with the general population, cancer survivors have been found to have a higher suicide rate.[72] Numerous factors appear to contribute to a cancer survivor's desire to end life with suicide or euthanasia;[69,73-75] these factors include medical, social, psychological, and spiritual concerns:

- Advanced illness, poor prognosis
- Inadequately managed severe physical symptoms (pain, fatigue, exhaustion)
- Delirium, disinhibition
- Hospitalization
- Preexisting psychopathology
- Family history of suicide or personal suicide history
- Hopelessness, helplessness
- Depression
- Loss of self-esteem, loss of control
- Fear of abandonment

- Anxiety
- Existential distress
- Caregiver (family or health care professional) fatigue

Pain and other symptom distress are the most frequently addressed factors contributing to cancer-related suicide or euthanasia. Indeed, cancer pain is a prevalent and typically controllable problem. Pain plays a large role in determining quality of life because of its impact on sleep, mood, fatigue, hopelessness, and so forth. Several cancer clinicians suggest that if pain and other distressing cancer symptoms are adequately managed, requests for ending life will be unnecessary and will abate.[73–76]

Few researchers have explored the relationship between symptom distress and the desire to die among individuals with cancer.[77] A study of 185 cancer survivors with pain found that 17% had suicidal ideation.[78] From surveying more than 4000 British individuals, Seale and Addington-Hall determined that dying individuals' requests for euthanasia increased as symptom distress and dependency increased.[71] For people dying of cancer, they found that the more pain was experienced, the more their relatives were likely to say that it would have been better if the patient had died earlier. A study of 48 persons with painful metastatic cancer also supports the contention that somatic symptom burden is associated with interest in a hastened death. Sullivan et al observed that 80% of these persons condoned active modes of hastening death and nearly half of them stated that if their pain became unbearable they would want information about suicide or a lethal prescription.[79]

Researchers are also beginning to discover sociocultural factors that influence a person's end-of-life decision making. In a study of 212 hospitalized persons with a terminal diagnosis, Mutran et al observed that having "unfinished business" and a fear of death contributed to a desire to have life prolonged.[80] However, contact with family moderated the effect of these two factors, especially for blacks. Several studies have also demonstrated that attitudes about life-prolonging treatments, advanced directives, and how open to be with dying persons vary considerably among American cultural groups.[81] Seale et al concluded after analyzing survey data from 3696 persons dying in the United Kingdom that Anglophones are particularly eager to maintain control and a sense of individualism during the dying process.[82]

Ethical considerations

The spiritual urge to be and do right is reflected in the debate about what is the ethical response to end-of-life decisions.[83–85] On one side, there are those who posit euthanasia and suicide as immoral killing. They argue that euthanasia devalues life and may lead to devaluation of other aspects of human life. Clinicians who oppose euthanasia argue that palliative care is a preferred alternative to euthanasia. They suggest that terminally ill individuals do not equate wanting to die with wanting to be

killed, or that the right to die translates to the duty to die.[75,86] Instead, the desire for euthanasia may actually be a response to fear—fear of loss of control, fear of pain, and so forth. Opponents further argue that euthanasia robs patients and their loved ones of the opportunity to allow the end of a life to be celebrated.

Those in favor of euthanasia contend that it can allow closure for a life. By having control over one's death, euthanasia allows one to have control over one's life. It allows death to occur with dignity, without the devaluing context of misery. The ethical principles of respecting the autonomy of the person, of self-determination and beneficence, and of promoting individual well-being are used by supporters of euthanasia.

Ogden synthesizes this debate by suggesting that palliation and euthanasia may both be ethical end-of-life options: "Are palliative care and euthanasia really opposites, or are they on a continuum of health care? Is there only one morally right way to die?"[77,p.82]

Regardless of how one decides to die, perhaps the proverb "One dies as one has lived" best summarizes how the person with cancer will respond to this debate.

How Shall I Live Before I Die?

Living at the end of life, of course, poses many challenges. Two primary end-of-life challenges that patients with cancer often deal with are spiritual and ethical in nature: (1) how to ascribe meaning to their life, illness, and death; and (2) how to relate to themselves and others (which might include a deity or other spiritual beings).

Meaning making

Unless a person expects cancer and perceives it to be a nonthreatening, positive experience, he or she will search for meaning.[24,87,88] It is exceptional if a person with cancer does not search for meaning to some degree. That is, all individuals will attempt to make sense of their cancer experience by trying to find answers to questions about what caused the cancer, what is responsible for bad things happening to people, why the cancer happened to them in particular, and what the significance or meaningfulness of the cancer is.

Perhaps the most frequent approach to meaning making is by attempting to attribute a cause to the cancer. Causes for cancer that individuals frequently consider include personal lifestyle factors (e.g., smoking or diet), environmental causes (e.g., polluted water or air), heredity, randomness, and stressors (e.g., work or poor family relations).[54,89] While some individuals immediately accept an explanation of cause with complete confidence, others are never certain as to what really caused their cancer.

Related to attributing a cause to cancer are the sensitive notions of responsibility and blame.[87,90,91] Individuals with cancer may find comfort in blaming themselves for their condition; this allows them to view their illness as controllable, thereby decreasing their sense of vulnerability.[92] Yet, blaming the self may create a sense of shame, guilt, and spiritual distress. Indeed, some people with cancer question, and sometimes accept, the cancer as punishment for previous wrongdoing or sin.[57] Studies have also found that cancer patients occasionally identify "God" or "God's will" as a cause of cancer.[93-95]

The need to make sense of cancer is often expressed in the question "Why me?" This question of selective incidence[90] asks not only why something bad has happened, but why it has happened to "me" in particular. Some people appear to find comfort in answering this question with "I was chosen [by a deity]," whereas others deny this could be possible and seek other answers for comfort. Some respond to the question with another question: "Why not me?" Regardless of the answer conjectured, the person has a spiritual need to maintain a sense of self-respect. A sense of self-respect is illustrated in the following contrasting statements made to the author by women with breast cancer: "I was chosen because I was strong; God knew He could use me as a witness through this cancer." "I don't know why it happened to me; things just happen—but I do know it's not because I deserved it."

Another aspect of meaning making is construing benefit or ascribing a positive significance to the negative experience of cancer.[96,97] This cognitive reframing explains why some survivors comment that they are better for having had cancer. Several types of construed benefits may be described by a survivor: For example, because of cancer, (1) personal values and purpose were reconsidered, (2) profound appreciation and joy for life and nature resulted, (3) spiritual sensitivity increased, and (4) self-knowledge and self-respect increased.[54]

For survivors with a belief in an omnipotent God who maintains whatever is in humankind's best interest, the suffering associated with cancer and death raises theodical questions (i.e., questions about the justification of God's ways when considering the problem of suffering). Foley identified twelve attitudes toward personal suffering by which individuals explain such theodical issues (Table 71-2). Regardless of a survivor's conjectures, answers to such theodical questions are ultimately unverifiable. This unknowing and mystery contributes to end-of-life spiritual and ethical struggles.

Relating

When patients with cancer face the end of life and reevaluate the meaning and values in their lives, they characteristically realize anew their intense appreciation for family and friends. This appreciation frequently is potentiated by the experience of receiving physical or emotional care from loved ones. As a result, people with cancer often attempt to restructure their lives so that more time can be spent with loved ones.

While receiving care and love from others has its joy, it also can create spiritual pain and ethical dilemmas. It is difficult to receive care and love when one cannot reciprocate. Hence, dependent cancer patients often per-

Table 71-2   Interpretations of Suffering

Theodical Theory	Example
Punishment	"My pain is the result of my sins."
Testing	"God is testing my loyalty to Him."
Bad luck	"The odds are against me."
Submission to the laws of nature	"It's nature taking her course, and I've got to grin and bear it."
Resignation to the will of God	"God willed it—even though I don't know why, so there is no way that I can avoid it."
Acceptance of the human condition	"Pain is a part of life."
Personal growth	"This suffering is making me a better person."
Defensiveness and denial	"I just don't think about it."
Minimization	"It could be worse."
Divine perspective	"If I could see things from God's perspective, I know I'd see a reason for this pain."
Redemption	"There is joy in my suffering because it has increased my appreciation for Christ's suffering."

Data from Foley.[98]

ceive that they are "being a burden" to their loved ones if not to society. Being a burden challenges one's sense of worth and purpose. It is this sense of being a burden that may bring an individual to conclude that suicide or euthanasia is appropriate.

Activities that can allow a person to return the gifts of love to others include praying for others; listening to others; sharing personal wisdom gained from the cancer experience with others; and creating legacy gifts such as poems, prose, taped oral histories, or crafts as functional ability permits. If such activities are valued and encouraged by those near to the care recipient, he or she will likely value the activity and find meaning and self-worth in doing it.

Because the cancer experience increases one's sense of the preciousness of each moment, it often teaches individuals to be more selective about the people with whom they spend time. Many individuals with cancer learn from their illness "who their friends really are." As a result, the friends and family members patients with cancer continue to value are those who are not only compassionate but emotionally and spiritually honest.

While individuals' relationships with others may change as a result of the cancer experience, so also may their relationship with their deity or spiritual beings. Indeed, many cancer survivors report intensified and satisfying relationships with God resulting from illness.[12,99] However, it is likely that cancer survivors' experiences with their deity or spiritual being are diverse. Relational experience with a deity may range from intensity and closeness to apathy and distance. For example, anger at a deity or spiritual being can facilitate closeness or distance. Some survivors' anger at God may help them to engage and struggle with God. These survivors may be heard to ask "Why?" and wonder if God is to blame. Others may not exhibit anger at God; they may believe God is not to blame, may be afraid to question God, or refrain from questions that challenge personal beliefs. Presumably, a survivor's experience with a deity or spiritual being is influenced by multiple factors such as culture, place in the cancer trajectory, previous spiritual responses to critical life experiences, and degree of spiritual development.[10,100–102]

Approaches to Making Spiritual and Ethical End-of-Life Decisions

When caring for a person confronted with any of these end-of-life decisions, the goal of nursing care is to facilitate and promote informed decision making. The nurse ultimately cannot make decisions for care recipients. A nurse can (1) encourage activities that increase the individual's sense of meaningfulness, self-awareness, and spiritual sensitivity; (2) offer a caring relationship and openness to dialogue; and (3) provide information about decision making and the issues confronted. In these ways the nurse facilitates the building of an environment for making informed decisions.

The following approaches can assist individuals in addressing spiritual and ethical end-of-life decisions. Each approach must include respect for the unique personal spiritual perspective and religious background of the patient with cancer. Various religious beliefs regarding death are summarized in Table 71-3.[103] Although an individual may state acceptance of a specific institutional religion, beliefs can vary widely within a religion. Even though an individual may acknowledge affiliation with one religion, he or she may be strongly influenced by another (e.g., the religion of parents or spouse). The following approaches that can assist one in resolving spiritual and ethical issues are presented because they are appropriate regardless of the individual's beliefs about religion.

Dedication to a Mission or Cause

The question of "How shall I make sense of my death, life, or illness?" can be answered by creating the answer, rather than by finding the answer.[104] One way to create a sense of meaningfulness and purpose is to dedicate oneself to a cause or mission.[105] This mission may be sociopolitical, artistic, or scientific in nature. For example, cancer survivors may become involved in advocating for cancer research funding, may become active in cancer support activities, may apply themselves to writing about the cancer experience, may begin to write the poetry they always had dreamed of writing but never did, may

Table 71-3 Religious Perspectives on Death and Afterlife

Baha'i Faith: Persons who recognize the Divine Manifestations (including Baha'u'llah) and obey their law and guidance will achieve salvation, which is a process of recognizing the reality of God and following God's guidance. Spiritual development continues after death; resurrection is spiritual not physical. Heaven and hell are not literal places, but spiritual conditions reflecting closeness to God. Cremation is not allowed because the body has been a temple for the spirit and must be respected. Suicide is forbidden, but those who do it are not beyond redemption.

Buddhism: At death a person's consciousness leaves the body and takes rebirth soon thereafter, unless and until Enlightenment is achieved. Place of rebirth depends on degree of virtuousness (especially just preceding death); there are numerous heavens and hells. Thus, someone who dies in an anguished or depressed state is apt to be propelled to a similarly unhappy situation subsequently.

Church of Jesus Christ of Latter-Day Saints (Mormons): When one's life ends, his/her spirit leaves the body and goes to a spirit world where one continues to grow spiritually and awaits resurrection and judgment. After resurrection (when the spirit is reunited with a perfected physical body), a person progresses to one of the three degrees of glory (heavens). Persons may obtain a lower degree of glory, or if they deny the Holy Ghost, be deprived of glory. Cremation is allowed. Christ is the judge of those who commit suicide.

Hinduism: Human beings are souls on an evolving spiritual journey; no soul is lost. At death, the soul enters one of seven heavens or seven nether worlds (relative planes of existence), to reap the results of their virtuous actions or to expiate through suffering the results of unrighteous actions. The soul then becomes reborn or reincarnated as a human. Cremation is common. Suicide is a heinous sin.

Islam: Those who live ethically and believe in the oneness of Allah will be worthy of heaven. There are five clear requirements of believers, which if not met mean hell after death: verbal testimony of belief in Allah (God) and Mohammed, His prophet; prayer five times per day; fasting during month of Ramadan; paying alms-tax; and at least one pilgrimage to the holy cities. After death there is a place where souls await fearfully the judgment. Cremation is not practiced, and suicide is considered a grave sin.

Judaism: A life where God's commandments, the mitzvot, are obeyed is more important than seeking heaven. There is variation among Jews regarding beliefs about heaven, but generally the concept of hell is not addressed. Traditionally, suicide has been considered a major offense. Cremation is not permitted (except by Reform Jews).

Roman Catholicism: Heaven is a condition of eternal fullness of life and intimacy with God, and is a gift that comes with salvation through Jesus Christ. Hell is a self-chosen alienation from God. At death, God accepts or rejects; a full resurrection and final judgment follow at the end of time. Purgatory is a condition of transition and adaptation for those entering heaven. Cremation and organ donation are permitted. Suicide is generally attributed to unbearable stress; thus victims are accordingly not refused Christian burial.

Protestants: After judgment, those who believed in Jesus Christ, repented, and were baptized will be saved and dwell with God in heaven. In contrast, the unrighteous will be cast in the (sometimes eternal) fires of hell. Heaven and hell are seen by some Protestants as literal, whereas others view them as metaphorical. A resurrection of spiritual and/or physical bodies will occur at the return of Jesus Christ to earth, which many believe occurs after a millennium. Cremation is generally permitted. Suicide is often considered to be a violation of God's desires, but God may show mercy to those who commit suicide.

Data from Johnson and McGee.[103]

become more involved in campaigning against smoking, and so forth. Dedication to a cause not only provides survivors with a sense of purpose and "something to live for," but exposes them to "the larger picture"—it offers them perspective. A side benefit may be that it also offers distraction from personal suffering.

Leaving a Legacy

Those who question how to confront mortality may find comfort and meaning in activities that leave a legacy. A poignant example of how one can leave a legacy was told to this author by a mother with breast cancer: "I'm cutting up my wedding dress. I'm going to make a christening dress with it. I figure, my son will marry someday, and someday have a child. When that grandchild that I'll never get to see is christened, he or she will be wearing my gown. In that way I can still be there for my offspring." Other ways people can leave legacies include writing or taping personal histories or messages for their descendants. A legacy can also be left for the world by the individual's dedication to a cause. Many people state that they "just want to leave the world a better place."

Storytelling

Individuals' questions about the meaning of their lives can be answered in part by telling life stories and reminiscing. Churchill and Churchill defined *storytelling* as "the forward movement of description of actions and events, which makes possible the backward action of self-understanding."[106,p.73] Stories of the past influence human thought and serve as a vehicle for transmitting beliefs and values, world views and frameworks for making meaning. Stories of the present enable a person to integrate the past with the present in order to find meaning for the future. Thus, stories assist people to make the past, present, and future meaningful.[107]

Storytelling promotes well-being in several ways. Encouraging people to tell their stories allows them to organize their thoughts and experiences, to reflect on their past, and to make sense of their life. Storytelling also allows them to share and connect with the listener, promoting intimacy. Finally, storytelling allows the individual to transmit values and leave a legacy.[108]

Although storytelling has typically been used as an intervention for the aged, it is therapeutic for others as well.[109,110] Pickrel outlined several activities for storytelling used in counseling the terminally ill, including diagramming one's life timeline with or without its peaks and valleys; family activities (e.g., members gather to discuss family memorabilia); creating a "This is your life" production; discussing life anecdotes; mind traveling (e.g., completing statements such as "I always wanted to . . ."); or creating a collage or artwork to depict one's life.[110]

Prayer, Meditation, and Journal Writing

Prayer can develop inward awareness and spiritual sensitivity. "To pray is to listen to and hear the self who is speaking." This speech is primary because it is basic and fundamental; it grounds us. In prayer we say who in fact we are—"not who we should be, nor who we wish we were, but who we are."[111,p.1] The inner awareness that prayer facilitates provides a basis for (self-) informed decision making about end-of-life issues.

Regardless of one's beliefs about religion, prayer (liberally defined) can be a resource to all. Of course, the philosophy and expression of prayer vary among religious traditions. Furthermore, the function and content of prayer will vary for an individual depending on the circumstances. One study of predominantly Christian North Americans identified four types of prayer expression; conversational and meditative types were more directly correlated with spiritual well-being than petitionary and ritualistic approaches.[112]

Although there is no evidence that sociocultural factors contribute to type of prayer experience, analyses of national opinion survey data demonstrate that culture, age, and gender are predictors of frequency of prayer. That is, women and blacks report praying more frequently than men and persons of other ethnicities, and prayer frequency directly increased with age.[100]

Considering that roughly 90% of North Americans pray,[112] it is no surprise that a number of studies have documented that patients with cancer use prayer as a coping strategy for managing illness, distressing symptoms, and anxiety-provoking medical procedures.[12,37,39,41] Prayer is also used among the critically and chronically ill for maintaining hope.[113,114] Indeed, some patients with cancer desire that nurses allow them time for prayer when they are hospitalized.[37]

During the terminal phase of life, individuals' prayers may reflect unique end-of-life issues.[115] Terminally ill patients often pray about salvation, that their deity will deem them worthy (e.g., for Heaven or for a better life when reincarnated). Some terminally ill individuals will pray about the circumstances of their death (e.g., that it will come soon, that it will be without pain). Likewise, the terminally ill often pray for the loved ones who will grieve their death.

In addition to the content of prayers reflecting end-of-life issues, individuals' prayers may change form. When the end of life brings severe emotional or physical distress, individuals may find comfort in very short repetitive prayers (e.g., "God, have mercy").[116] For survivors who are able, prayer may also be expressed while meditating, keeping a journal, or creating art. By keeping a journal or writing, the individual becomes reflective and aware.[117] Strength and insight can be gained by reading past entries. Similarly, when people express themselves in art (be it music, painting, poetry, quilting, or another art form), they can reflect on this creativity as an expression of the spiritual. They may seriously analyze it to learn from it, or simply bathe themselves in its beauty.[118]

Spiritual Mentoring

Cancer survivors who have become increasingly aware of their inner spirituality may benefit from interactions with a spiritual director, mentor, or soul friend.[119] Similar to a psychological counselor who addresses psychological issues with a patient, a spiritual mentor can assist with spiritual issues. A spiritual mentor provides comfort, encouragement, and companionship, as well as guidance and prodding.

A spiritual mentor preferably has training in spiritual direction or pastoral counseling, and has personally received spiritual direction.[119] Regardless of training, a spiritual mentor must have a high level of self-awareness and spiritual maturity, as well as listening skills, honesty, and openness. Although religious centers and retreat houses often offer the services of spiritual directors, a person may have to (or want to) find such a resource elsewhere.

The individual with cancer and his or her spiritual director need to mutually agree on the nature, purpose, and frequency of their meetings together. Those experienced in spiritual direction recommend meetings at least once every 6 weeks and suggest that visits be limited to topics that are most related to spiritual issues. Although directly uninvolved in this process of spiritual mentoring, the nurse can initiate the process by providing the person with information.

Cognitive Strategies

Janoff-Bulman asserts that individuals each have a set of assumptions about themselves and their world.[88] Specifically, individuals assume that the world is benevolent, meaningful, and that they have worth. Traumatic events such as a cancer diagnosis or recognition of an imminent death can shatter such assumptions. When individuals' assumptions about the world are shattered, they will work to reconstruct their world view so that it includes assumptions that are maturer and wiser, encompassing the trauma.

This work of reconstructing a world view involves a process of balancing thoughts about the painful subject with avoiding painful thoughts (approach versus avoidance).[88] Cognitive strategies that individuals use for reconstructing the assumptions include making comparisons (e.g., "It could be worse"), self-blame (e.g., "Because I caused it, I can prevent it from happening again"), and construing benefit and positive meaning from the suffering (e.g., "This cancer has made me a better person").

The individual must construe his or her own meanings for life's traumas and death. The nurse cannot do this cognitive work. However, a nurse can encourage a person to verbalize thoughts and feelings about the meaning of cancer.[120] Using therapeutic techniques such as clarification and summarization, the nurse can assist a person in identifying and appreciating cognitive strategies that provide comfort and meaning (e.g., "I hear how emotion-ally distressing cancer has been for you; however, I also hear how you have learned to find good things that have come from your cancer experience").

The nurse can also instruct the patient regarding the process of searching for meaning. By understanding that searching for meaning is normal and a process, the distress of not finding satisfactory meaning immediately may be allayed.[47] Some people with cancer suggest that it is beneficial to put boundaries on the rumination that can viciously circle about the "Why?" questions. Some survivors also recognized the helpfulness of releasing unanswerable "Why?" questions, and focusing on "How do I choose to respond?" These practical suggestions from cancer survivors complement Janoff-Bulman's suggestion that individuals need to use both a cognitive approach and avoidance when adapting to trauma.[88]

Confronting the Reality of Death

The influence of a death-denying society continues to have an impact on how individuals with cancer and their families and professional caregivers confront the realities of death. While some individuals may initiate discussions about their death, others cannot. Some may wish to talk about their death but are prevented from doing so by those around them (e.g., family or health care professionals). The oncology nurse must remain gentle, honest, and sensitive when discussing death-related topics with care recipients.

Recognizing the function and multifaceted nature of denial will also assist the nurse in addressing death at an appropriate level. Breznitz contends that denial, as a defense mechanism against a threat, protects an individual from additional threatening information.[121] Although denial serves a useful function, extreme denial prevents hopefulness and the ability to recognize positive outcomes of stress. Table 71-4 offers Breznitz's typology of denial, with examples from the context of cancer-related death.

Advance Directives

A recent intervention that presumably has increased patient-practitioner dialogues about death is the Patient Self-Determination Act (PSDA) passed by the United States Congress in 1990.[122-124] This legislation requires that all health care institutions receiving Medicare or Medicaid reimbursement ask the patients they admit if they have an advance directive. If patients do not, the institution is obligated to provide written information about such directives.

All fifty states and the District of Columbia now have laws regarding advanced directives (ADs). Most state statutes support two types of advance directives. An AD "is a statement made by a competent person that directs their medical care in the event that they become incompetent."[122.p.891] A Directive to Physician, or Living Will (a

Table 71-4 Seven Kinds of Denial

Kind of Denial	Example
Denial of information	"I don't really have cancer."
Denial of threatening information	"I have cancer, but it isn't a life-threatening kind."
Denial of personal relevance	"I have a life-threatening type of cancer, but I'm hardy; it isn't going to get me."
Denial of urgency	"I have a life-threatening type of cancer, but it's not going to affect me really until I get old anyway."
Denial of vulnerability or responsibility	"I have a life-threatening cancer, but I can cope with it and conquer it."
Denial of affect	"I have a life-threatening cancer, but it doesn't really scare me."
Denial of affect relevance	"I have a life-threatening cancer and I do get scared, but it's not because I think I'm going to die."

Data from Breznitz.[121]

less accurate term), allows individuals to state their wishes regarding medical treatment in the event they become unable to do so. A Durable Power of Attorney for Health Care allows an individual to designate an agent who will make health care decisions on his or her behalf in the event that he or she becomes incompetent. Dimond outlines the advantages of ADs for oncology nurses.[122] Advance directives provide clarification of individual's wishes and values, guidance for family members concerning patients' choices, direction for the health care team, and protection of patients' assets from depletion caused by futile, high-cost care.

In addition to informing patients about ADs, oncology nurses can also facilitate discussions about ADs and end-of-life issues between patients and their families. If a challenging end-of-life decision arises for a patient or family, the nurse may walk them through a decision-making or problem-solving process such as the "nursing process." For instance, the nurse can assist those involved with making the decision to identify the contributing factors (e.g., values, beliefs), specifically define the problem and the desired outcome, list the possible approaches to solving the problem, choose and implement the appropriate approach, and evaluate.

Hoffman discusses several problems related to ADs that clinicians can encounter in practice:[125]

- Patients can misconstrue what a Living Will means; they do not specify disbursement of assets.

- Advance directives do not address all possible medical situations; they generally address only terminal conditions due to illness or injury.

- The words *artificial* and *extraordinary* are often used in an AD; however, these words can be interpreted differently.

- A directive may not always be honored and implemented; technicalities can arise such as questions about the patient's competency when the AD was signed or the inability of the physician to determine the terminality of the patient's condition.

- An AD is a one-person statement, not a legally binding contract.

Conclusion

As death becomes imminent for a person with cancer, ethical and spiritual issues and questions arise. The oncology nurse can assist the person and his or her family to face and respond knowingly to such decisions. Addressing such concerns may not decrease morbidity or mortality, save health care dollars, or be evidenced by other outcome indicators; however, providing such care can certainly make a marked difference in the quality and worth of the lives of individuals with cancer, their family caregivers, and their nurses. Indeed, it is the awareness of our death that contributes to the life that is present; as Koestenbaum stated, "It is a better understanding of death that makes us into individuals."[126,p.31]

References

1. Golberg B: Connection: An exploration of spirituality in nursing care. *J Adv Nurs* 27:836–842, 1998
2. Reed PG: An emerging paradigm for the investigation of spirituality in nursing. *Res Nurs Health* 15:349–357, 1992
3. Haase J, Britt T, Coward D, et al: Simultaneous concept analysis of spiritual perspective, hope, acceptance and self-transcendence. *Image J Nurs Sch* 24:141–147, 1992
4. Emblen JD: Religion and spirituality defined according to current use in nursing literature. *J Prof Nurs* 8:41–47, 1992
5. Mansen TJ: The spiritual dimension of individuals: Conceptual development. *Nurs Diagn* 4:140–147, 1993
6. Wright KB: Professional, ethical, and legal implications for spiritual care in nursing. *Image J Nurs Sch* 30:81–83, 1998
7. Halstead MT, Mickley JR: Attempting to fathom the unfathomable: Descriptive views of spirituality. *Semin Oncol Nurs* 13:225–230, 1997
8. Derrickson BS: The spiritual work of the dying: A framework and case studies. *Hospice J* 11:11–30, 1998
9. Indinopulus TA, Wilson BC (eds): *What is Religion? Origins, Definitions, and Explanations.* Boston, Brill, 1998
10. Fowler JW: *Stages of Faith: The Psychology of Human Development and the Quest for Meaning.* San Francisco, Harper & Row, 1981
11. Beauchamp TL, Childress JF: *Principles of Biomedical Ethics* (ed 4). New York, Oxford University Press, 1994
12. Sodestrom KE, Martinson IM: Patients' spiritual coping strategies: A study of nurse and patient perspectives. *Oncol Nurs Forum* 14:41–46, 1987
13. Mermann AC: Spiritual aspects of death and dying. *Yale J Biol Med* 65:137–142, 1992

14. Taylor EJ, Mickley JR: Introduction. *Semin Oncol Nurs* 13: 1–2, 1997

15. Burns S: The spirituality of dying. *Health Prog* 72:48–54, 1991

16. Highfield MF: Spiritual health of oncology patients. *Cancer Nurs* 15:1–8, 1992

17. Halstead MT, Fernsler JI: Coping strategies of long-term cancer survivors. *Cancer Nurs* 17:94–100, 1994

18. Weisman AD, Worden JW: The existential plight in cancer: Significance of the first 100 days. *Int J Psychiatr Med* 7:1–15, 1976

19. Peteet JR: Religious issues presented by cancer patients seen in psychiatric consultation. *J Psychosoc Oncol* 3:53–66, 1985

20. Dobratz MC, Burns KM, Oden RV: Pain in home hospice patients: An exploratory descriptive study. *Hospice J* 5: 117–132, 1989

21. Highfield MF: Spiritual health of oncology patients: Nurse and patient perspectives. *Cancer Nurs* 15:1–8, 1992

22. Reed PG: Religiousness among terminally ill and healthy adults. *Res Nurs Health* 9:35–41, 1986

23. Reed PG: Spirituality and well-being in terminally ill hospitalized adults. *Res Nurs Health* 10:335–344, 1987

24. Coward DD: Self-transcendence: Making meaning from the cancer experience. *Qual of Life* 4:53–58, 1995

25. Fryback PB: Health for people with a terminal diagnosis. *Nurs Sci Q* 6:147–159, 1993

26. Highfield MF, Cason C: Spiritual needs of patients: Are they recognized? *Cancer Nurs* 6:187–192, 1983

27. Vastyan EA: Spiritual aspects of the care of cancer patients. *CA Cancer J Clin* 36:110–114, 1986

28. Taylor EJ: Spiritual self-care after a cancer diagnosis. *Coping* 9:30–31, 1995

29. O'Conner AP, Wicker CA, Germino BB: Understanding the cancer patient's search for meaning. *Cancer Nurs* 13: 167–175, 1990

30. Steeves RH: Patients who have undergone bone marrow transplantation: Their quest for meaning. *Oncol Nurs Forum* 19:899–905, 1992

31. Ersek M: The process of maintaining hope in adults undergoing bone marrow transplantation for leukemia. *Oncol Nurs Forum* 19:883–889, 1992

32. Post-White J, Ceronsky C, Kreitzer MJ, et al: Hope, spirituality, sense of coherence, and quality of life in patients with cancer. *Oncol Nurs Forum* 23:1571–1579, 1996

33. Smith ED, Stefanek ME, Joseph MV, et al: Spiritual awareness, personal perspective on death, and psychosocial distress among cancer patients: An initial investigation. *J Psychosoc Oncol* 11:89–103, 1993

34. Kaczorowski JM: Spiritual well-being and anxiety in adults diagnosed with cancer. *Hospice J* 5:105–116, 1989

35. Pace JC, Stables JL: Correlates of spiritual well-being in terminally ill patients with AIDS and terminally ill persons with cancer. *J Assoc Nurses AIDS Care* 8(6):31–42, 1998

36. Fehring RJ, Miller JF, Shaw C: Spiritual well-being, religiosity, hope, depression, and other mood states in elderly people coping with cancer. *Oncol Nurs Forum* 24:663–671, 1997

37. Reed PG: Preferences for spiritually related nursing interventions among terminally ill and nonterminally ill hospitalized adults and well adults. *Appl Nurs Res* 4:122–128, 1991

38. Johnson SC, Spilka B: Coping with breast cancer: The roles of clergy and faith. *J Relig Health* 30:21–33, 1991

39. Peteet JR, Stomper PC, Ross DM, et al: Emotional support for patients with cancer who are undergoing CT: Semistructured interviews of patients at a cancer institute. *Radiology* 182:99–102, 1992

40. Gotay CC: The experience of cancer during early and advanced stages: The views of patients and their mates. *Soc Sci Med* 18:605–613, 1984

41. Ferrell B, Taylor EJ, Grant M, et al: Pain management at home: Struggle, comfort, and mission. *Cancer Nurs* 16: 169–178, 1993

42. Moberg D: Spiritual well-being of the dying, in Lesnoff-Caravaglia G (ed): *Aging and the Human Condition.* New York, Human Sciences Press, 1982, pp 139–155

43. Filipp SH: Could it be worse? The diagnosis of cancer as a prototype of traumatic life events, in Montada S, Filipp SH, Lerner MJ (eds): *Life Crises and Experiences of Loss in Adulthood.* Hillsdale, NJ, Lawrence Erlbaum Associates, 1992, pp 23–56

44. Brown-Saltzman KA: Tending the spirit. *Oncol Nurs Forum* 21:1001–1006, 1994

45. Granstrom S: Spiritual care for oncology patients. *Top Clin Nurs* 7:39–45, 1985

46. Aries P: *The Hour of Our Death.* New York, Knopf, 1981

47. Marris P: *Loss and Change.* London, Routledge, 1986

48. VandeCreek L, Nye C: Trying to live forever: Correlates to the belief in life after death. *J Pastoral Care* 48:273–280, 1994

49. O'Gorman SM: Death and dying in contemporary society: An evaluation of current attitudes and the rituals associated with death and dying and their relevance to recent understandings of health and healing. *J Adv Nurs* 27:1127–1135, 1998

50. Parry JK, Ryan JK: *A Cross-Cultural Look at Death, Dying, and Religion.* Chicago, Nelson-Hall, 1995

51. Parkes CM, Loungani P, Young B: *Death and Bereavement Across Cultures.* London, Routledge, 1997

52. Bryant C: Said another way: Death from a spiritual perspective. *Nurs Forum* 26:31–34, 1991

53. Becker E: *The Denial of Death.* New York, Free Press, 1973

54. Taylor SE: Adjustment to threatening events: A theory of cognitive adaptation. *Am Psychol* 38:1161–1173, 1983

55. Taylor SE, Wood JV, Lichtman RR: It could be worse: Selective evaluation as a response to victimization. *J Soc Issues* 39:19–40, 1983

56. Rothbaum F, Weisz JR, Snyder SS: Changing the world and changing the self: A two-process model of perceived control. *J Pers Soc Psychol* 42:5–37, 1982

57. Mahon SM, Cella DF, Donovan MI: Psychosocial adjustment to recurrent cancer. *Oncol Nurs Forum* 17:47–52, 1990 (suppl)

58. Kirk K: How Oregon's Death With Dignity Act affects practice. *Am J Nurs* 98:54–55, 1998

59. Musgrave CF: Active euthanasia and assisted suicide: A perspective from an American Abortion and Dutch euthanasia scenario. *Oncol Nurs Forum* 25:1587–1591, 1998

60. Nathan Cummings Foundation: Spiritual beliefs and the dying process: Key findings. Available at: *http://www ncf org/ncf/publication rts/fetzer/fetzer_keyfindings html.* Accessed July 15, 1998

61. American Nurses' Association: *Code for Nurses with Interpretive Statements.* Washington, DC, American Nurses' Association, 1985

62. Oncology Nursing Society: Oncology Nursing Society's Support of the oncology nurse's role in dealing with ethical decision-making relative to client-centered care, and related legal issues. *Oncol Nurs Forum* 20:47, 1993 (suppl)

63. Oncology Nursing Society: Resolution for end-of-life care proposed. *Oncol Nurs Soc News* 10:8, 1995

64. Oncology Nursing Society: ONS Position Statement: Endorsement of the American Nurse's Association position statements on active euthanasia and assisted suicide. Available at: *http://www ons org/ons/cross/position/endorsement htm.* Accessed July 15, 1998

65. Ersek M, Scanlon C, Glass E, et al: Priority ethical issues in oncology nursing: Current approaches and future directions. *Oncol Nurs Forum* 22:803–807, 1995

66. Asch DA: The role of critical care nurses in euthanasia and assisted suicide. *N Engl J Med* 334:1374–1379, 1998

67. Davis AJ, Phillips L, Drought TS, et al: Nurses' attitudes toward active euthanasia. *Nurs Outlook* 43:174–179, 1995

68. Young A, Volker D, Rieger PT, et al: Oncology nurses' attitudes regarding voluntary, physician-assisted dying for competent, terminally-ill patients. *Oncol Nurs Forum* 20:445–451, 1993

69. Valente SM, Saunders JM, Grant M: Oncology nurses' knowledge and misconceptions about suicide. *Cancer Pract* 2:209–216, 1994

70. Richardson DS: Oncology nurses' attitudes toward the legalization of voluntary active euthanasia. *Cancer Nurs* 17:348–354, 1994

71. Seale C, Addington-Hall J: Euthanasia: Why people want to die earlier. *Soc Sci Med* 39:647–654, 1994

72. Fox BH, Stanek EJ, Boyd SC, et al: Suicide rates among cancer patients in Connecticut. *J Chronic Dis* 35:89–100, 1982

73. Foley KM: The relationship of pain and symptom management to patient requests for physician-assisted suicide. *J Pain Symptom Manage* 6:289–297, 1991

74. Cherny NI, Coyle N, Foley KM: The treatment of suffering when patients request elective death. *J Palliat Care* 10:71–79, 1994

75. Coyle N: The euthanasia and physician-assisted suicide debate: Issues for nursing. *Oncol Nurs Forum* 19:41–46, 1992 (suppl)

76. Baile WF, DiMaggio JR, Schapira DV, et al: The request for assistance in dying: The need for psychiatric consultation. *Cancer* 72:2786–2791, 1993

77. Ogden R: Palliative care and euthanasia: A continuum of care. *J Palliat Care* 10:82–85, 1994

78. Breitbart WS: Assessing suicide risk in cancer patients, in Holland JC, Lesko LM, Massie MJ (eds): *Current Concepts in Psycho-Oncology.* New York, Memorial Sloan-Kettering Cancer Institute, 1991, pp 115–119

79. Sullivan M, Rapp S, Fitzgibbon D, et al: Pain and the choice to hasten death in patients with painful metastatic cancer. *J Palliat Care* 13:18–28, 1997

80. Mutran EJ, Danis M, Bratton KA, et al: Attitudes of the critically ill toward prolonging life: The role of social support. *Gerontologist* 37:192–199, 1997

81. Ersek M, Kagawa-Singer M, Barnes D, et al: Multicultural considerations in the use of advance directives. *Oncol Nurs Forum* 25:1683–1690, 1998

82. Seale C, Addington-Hall J, McCarthy M: Awareness of dying: prevalence, causes, and consequences. *Soc Sci Med* 45:477–484, 1997

83. Dowd S, Davidhizar R: Euthanasia: A pragmatic view. *Elder Care* 10:16–19, 1998

84. Brock DW: Euthanasia. *Yale J Biol Med* 65:121–129, 1992

85. Fischer DS: Observations on ethical problems and terminal care. *Yale J Biol Med* 65:105–120, 1992

86. Sicola V, Hall J: "I wouldn't want to live": The myth about attitudes of terminal patients. *J Nurs Law* 4:31–43, 1997

87. Taylor EJ: Whys and wherefores: Adult patient perspectives of the meaning of cancer. *Semin Oncol Nurs* 11:32–40, 1995

88. Janoff-Bulman R: *Shattered Assumptions: Towards a New Psychology of Trauma.* New York, The Free Press, 1992

89. Berckman KL, Austin JK: Causal attribution, perceived control, and adjustment in patients with lung cancer. *Oncol Nurs Forum* 20:23–30, 1993

90. Janoff-Bulman R, Lang-Gunn L: Coping with disease, crime, and accidents: The role of self-blame attributions, in Abramson LY (ed): *Social Cognition and Clinical Psychology.* New York: Guilford Press, 1988, pp 116–147

91. Weiner B: *Judging Sin and Sickness: Foundations for a Theory of Social Behavior.* New York, Guilford, 1994

92. Meyerowitz B: Correlates of breast cancer. *Psychol Bull* 87:108–131, 1980

93. Gotay CC: Why me? Attributions and adjustment by cancer patients and their mates at two stages in the disease process. *Soc Sci Med* 20:825–831, 1985

94. Linn MW, Linn BS, Stein SR: Beliefs about causes of cancer in cancer patients. *Soc Sci Med* 16:835–839, 1982

95. Baider L, Sarell M: Perceptions and causal attributions of Israeli women with breast cancer concerning their illness: The effects of ethnicity and religiosity. *Psychother Psychosom* 39:136–143, 1983

96. Taylor SE, Lichtman RR, Wood JV: Attributions, beliefs about control, and adjustment to breast cancer. *J Pers Soc Psychol* 46:489–502, 1984

97. Thompson SC, Pitts J: Factors relating to a person's ability to find meaning after a diagnosis of cancer. *J Psychosoc Oncol* 11:1–21, 1993

98. Foley DP: Eleven interpretations of personal suffering. *J Relig Health* 27:321–328, 1988

99. Coward DD: The lived experience of self-transcendence in women with advanced breast cancer. *Nurs Sci Q* 3:162–169, 1990

100. Levin JS, Taylor RJ: Age differences in patterns and correlates of the frequency of prayer. *Gerontologist* 37:75–88, 1997

101. Highfield MF: Spiritual assessment across the cancer trajectory: Methods and reflections. *Semin Oncol Nurs* 13:263–270, 1997

102. Stepnick A, Perry T: Preventing spiritual distress in the dying client. *J Psychosoc Nurs* 30:17–24, 1992

103. Johnson CJ, McGhee MG (eds): *Encounters with Eternity: Religious Views of Death and Life After Death.* New York, Philosophical Library, 1986

104. Baird RM: Meaning in life: Discovered or created? *J Relig Health* 24:117–124, 1985

105. Yalom ID: *Existential Psychotherapy.* New York, Basic Books, 1980

106. Churchill LR, Churchill SW: Storytelling in medical arenas: The art of self-determination. *Lit Med* 1:73–79, 1982

107. Brody H: *Stories of Sickness.* New Haven, CT, Yale University Press, 1987

108. Taylor EJ: The story behind the story: The use of storytelling in spiritual caregiving. *Semin Oncol Nurs* 13:252–254, 1997

109. Tarman VI: Autobiography: The negotiation of a lifetime. *Int J Aging Human Dev* 27:171–191, 1988

110. Pickrel J: "Tell me your story": Using life review in counseling the terminally ill. *Death Studies* 13:127–135, 1989

111. Ulanov A, Ulanov B: *Primary Speech: A Psychology of Prayer.* Atlanta, John Knox Press, 1982

112. Poloma MM, Gallup GH Jr: *Varieties of Prayer: A Survey Report.* Philadelphia, Trinity Press International, 1991

113. Raleigh EDH: Sources of hope in chronic illness. *Oncol Nurs Forum* 19:443–448, 1992

114. Miller JF: Hope-inspiring strategies of the critically ill. *Appl Nurs Res* 2:23–29, 1989

115. Lucas MA: Praying with the terminally ill. *Hosp Progress* 59:66–70, 1978

116. Taylor EJ, Ersek M: Ethical and spiritual dimensions of cancer pain management, in McGuire D, Yarbro CH, Ferrell B (eds): *Cancer Pain Management* (ed 2). Sudbury, MA, Jones and Bartlett, 1994, pp 41–60

117. Cunningham AJ: Does cancer have "meaning"? *Advances in Mind-Body Medicine* 9:63–69, 1993

118. Bailey SS: The arts in spiritual care. *Semin Oncol Nurs* 13:242–247, 1997

119. Guenther M: *Holy Listening: The Art of Spiritual Direction.* Cambridge MA, Cowley, 1992

120. Wortman CB, Silver RC: Reconsidering assumptions about coping with loss: An overview of current research, in Montada L, Filipp S, Lerner MJ (eds): *Life Crises and Experiences of Loss in Adulthood.* Hillsdale, NJ, Lawrence Erlbaum Associates, 1992, pp 341–365

121. Breznitz S: The seven kinds of denial, Goldberger L, Breznitz S (eds): *Handbook of Stress: Theoretical and Clinical Aspects.* New York, Free Press, 1982, pp 257–286

122. Dimond EP: The oncology nurse's role in patient advance directives. *Oncol Nurs Forum* 19:891–896, 1992

123. Volker DL: Assisted suicide and the domain of nursing practice. *J Nurs Law* 5:39–50, 1998

124. Schulmeister L, Haisfield-Wolfe ME: Living wills, advance directives, and surrogate decision making. *Clin J Oncol Nurs* 2:148–150, 1998

125. Hoffman MK: Use of advance directives: A social work perspective on the myth versus the reality. *Death Studies* 18:229–241, 1994

126. Koestenbaum P: *Is There an Answer to Death?* Englewood Cliffs, NJ, Prentice-Hall, 1976

Issues in the Delivery of Care

CHAPTER 72

Quality of Care

Diane Scott Dorsett, PhD, RN, FAAN

Conceptual Foundations of Quality Care

Historical Context and Origins

Well over a century ago, Nightingale[1] said that the prime objective in nursing was "to put the patient(s) in the best condition for nature to act." Since then, both conceptually and operationally, care has become the essence of nursing. Over the past 20 years, a science of caring has emerged as a discrete theme in the nursing literature,[2–6] but only recently has care been accorded the importance recognized by Nightingale so long ago.

The relevance of care to society's health is becoming increasingly evident as demographic trends, such as an expanding elderly population, accelerate the incidence of chronic disease and as an increasingly advanced treatment technology extends life. Cure, once an important concept in the history of illness, when disease was primarily acute and infectious, has been replaced by the notion of prolonged remission with maximal quality of life.

As modern science ushers in a wave of biological modalities influencing prevention, detection, and treatment, and as oncology treatment becomes increasingly grounded in molecular biology and genetic modification, clinical health care providers will continue to face the reality of rigorous treatments and more critically acute, morbid episodes superimposed on the chronic illness itself. To wit, the Oncology Nursing Society (ONS) has published a position paper on the role of the oncology nurse in genetic counseling with cancer patients and families.[7]

Quality of care is challenged by a health care system that seeks to reduce hospital stay time and health care cost coverage and by a health care environment in which large segments of the most vulnerable members of society (nonwhite, poor, less educated), who have greater than average health care needs, also have less than equal access to health care. Furthermore, those disadvantaged who do gain access often receive health care of lower quality—especially when measured in terms of appropriateness, timeliness, comprehensiveness, and continuity.[8] As documented in a publication of the President's Commission for the Study of Ethical Problems in Medicine and Biomedical and Behavioral Research,[9] cancers of white Americans are detected earlier than those of nonwhites, and those of paying patients are found earlier than those of nonpaying ones.

Although the reasons for these trends are interwoven throughout the social, political, and economic fabric of American society, the outcome places a heavy burden not only on the underserved population but on all other segments of the society as well. Given today's challenges of specialization, complex technology, patterns of chronic illness, and restrictive health care environment, the quality care of cancer patients and their families demands an interdisciplinary team approach and the extension of the role of nursing in its total management.

In July 1997, the Oncology Nursing Society, a major voice in the effort to secure quality cancer care, issued a position paper as part of its first public venture into health policy formation.[10,11] This position asserted clearly that cost concerns in health care and its delivery have undercut quality in terms of access, available treatment options, support of specialty training, reduction in specialty care units, and treatment administration by nonqualified and untrained personnel. Further, ONS asserted that since the patient and family have a right to cancer care, access to services, reimbursement, and culturally competent, family-oriented care from well-trained and educated specialty practitioners, oncology nurses should be involved in all areas of cancer care and should be included with equal parity in the planning and implementation of cancer care services.[12]

In short, oncology nurses, by virtue of their knowledge, skills, and holistic (biopsychosocial) perspective of persons with cancer, are well-qualified practitioners to assume the case manager role. In today's health care system, the role of case manager is designed to contain cost, guide in the appropriate use of health resources, and secure quality outcomes for patients.[13] Based on its position paper on quality, the ONS board of directors in October 1998 approved the Patient Bill of Rights for Quality Cancer Care.[14]

Care and caring

To care is to respond to another in need because of pain, illness, or distress. Caring involves a sense of commitment and responsibility and, when taken to higher levels, can be considered a body of knowledge and skill known tacitly, empirically, or scientifically to accomplish change for the good. Although caring behavior is central to most public and private human activity, when defined for nursing, caring becomes a set of meaning-laden actions.[2,15] Early in the education of most nursing students, Virginia Henderson's classic definition of nursing is introduced:

> Nursing is primarily assisting individuals (sick or well) with those activities contributing to health, or its recovery (or to a peaceful death) that they perform unaided when they have the necessary strength, will or knowledge; nursing also helps individuals carry out prescribed therapy and be independent of assistance as soon as possible.[16]

Each state has its own legislation enacted to outline and define nursing as a profession, a discipline, and a practice. This legislation, usually called the Nurse Practice Act, is remarkably similar in wording throughout the country. Most legislate nursing as the diagnosis and treatment of human responses in health and illness—a broad definition, further operationalized in the interest of public safety by a regulated and standardized system of education, registration, certification, standards of practice, and quality assurance.

Following the broad, formative brushstrokes of Nightingale,[1] who recognized "the fundamental needs of the sick and principles of good care," the concise, comprehensive definition of nursing by Harmer and Henderson,[16] and the more recent legislative revisions that modernized nurse practice statutes in this country, nursing began to establish a taxonomy of nursing diagnoses.[17-19] Nursing diagnoses operationalize the statutory language identifying nursing practices as "human responses to an actual or potential health problem."[20]

Diagnostic taxonomies generally allow for a clear definition of professional purpose and for faster communication among the practitioners of a discipline, and they become the basis for a profession's research and development activity. As Herberth and Gosnell[18] advise, the next step is the integration of standards of practice and nursing diagnoses (Table 72-1) to foster relevant research, promote therapeutic interventions, and, ultimately, advance the quality of care.

Caring actions cannot be separated from intent, however, if the outcome is to be effective. It is not enough to practice according to a guiding set of rules and regulations. To achieve even an acceptable level of quality of care, one must have commitment, creativity, and a willingness to innovate. Knowing one's craft well is not enough. Caring requires understanding our patients and their beliefs, values, and cultural norms and tailoring care accordingly. Thus understanding and defining quality of care in terms of practices that enable health promotion and recovery from illness requires that caring be intrinsic to the process. Leininger[5] defined caring as behavioral attributes characterized by empathy, support, compassion, protection, succor, and education, firmly grounded in a comprehension of the needs, problems, values, and goals of the person or group being assisted.

Quality

The nature of *quality* is multifaceted and difficult to define, especially in relation to nursing care. Yet quality emerged as the most important issue in patient care services in the final two decades of the twentieth century.

Quality has become the focus of all cancer service provider groups, including the Commission on Cancer of the American College of Surgeons, the National Cancer Institute, the American Cancer Society, the College of American Pathology, the American College of Radiology, and, in joint affiliation, the American Nurses' Association and the Oncology Nursing Society.[21] Quality will continue to be a major tenet of practice in the new century.

Quality of care has been defined by the American

Table 72-1   Functional Health Pattern Categories and Nursing Diagnoses

Health perception—health management pattern
Health maintenance alteration
Health management deficit (total)
Health management deficit (specify)
Health seeking behavior
Noncompliance (specify)
Potential noncompliance (specify)
Potential for infection
Potential for physical injury
Potential for poisoning
Potential for suffocation

Nutritional-metabolic pattern
Alteration in nutrition: potential for more than body requirements or potential obesity
Alteration in nutrition: more than body requirements or exogenous obesity
Alteration in nutrition: less than body requirements or nutritional deficit (specify)
Ineffective breast feeding
Impaired swallowing
Potential for aspiration
Alterations in oral mucous membranes
Potential fluid volume deficit
Fluid volume deficit (actual) (1)
Fluid volume deficit (actual) (2)
Fluid volume excess
Potential or actual impairment of skin integrity or skin breakdown
Decubitus ulcer (specify stage)
Impaired skin or tissue integrity
Altered body temperature
Ineffective thermoregulation
Hyperthermia
Hypothermia

Elimination pattern
Alteration in bowel elimination: constipation or intermittent constipation pattern
Alteration in bowel elimination: diarrhea
Alteration in bowel elimination: incontinence or bowel incontinence
Altered urinary elimination pattern
Urinary incontinence: functional, stress, urge or total
Stress incontinence
Urinary retention

Self-perception—self-concept pattern
Fear (specify focus)
Anticipatory anxiety (mild, moderate, severe)
Anxiety
Mild anxiety
Moderate anxiety
Severe anxiety (panic)
Reactive depression (situational)
Hopelessness
Powerlessness (severe, low, moderate)
Self-esteem disturbance
Body image disturbance
Personal identity confusion

Role-relationship pattern
Anticipatory grieving
Dysfunctional grieving
Disturbance in role performance
Unresolved independence-dependence conflict
Social isolation
Social isolation (rejection)
Impaired social interaction
Altered growth and development: social skills (specify)

(continued)

Table 72-1 Functional Health Pattern Categories and Nursing Diagnoses (continued)

Role-relationship pattern (cont.) Translocation syndrome Altered family process Weak mother-infant attachment or parent-infant attachment Potential altered parenting	Pain self-management deficit Uncompensated sensory deficit (specify) Sensory-perceptual alterations: input deficit or sensory deprivation Sensory-perceptual alterations: input excess or sensory overload Unilateral neglect Knowledge deficit (specify) Uncompensated short-term memory deficit Potential cognitive impairment Impairment of thought processes Decisional conflict (specify) Altered parenting Parental role conflict Impaired verbal communication Altered growth and development: communication skills Potential for violence
Activity-exercise pattern Potential activity intolerance Activity intolerance (specify level) Fatigue Impaired physical mobility (specify level) Potential for disuse syndrome Total self-care deficit (specify level) Self-bathing—hygiene deficit (specify level) Self-dressing—grooming deficit (specify level) Self-feeding deficit (specify level) Self-toileting deficit (specify level) Self-care skills deficit Diversional activity deficit Impaired home maintenance management (mild, moderate, severe, potential, chronic) Potential joint contractures Ineffective airway clearance Ineffective breathing pattern Impaired gas exchange Decreased cardiac output Altered tissue perfusion Dysreflexia Altered growth and development	**Sexuality-reproductive pattern** Sexual dysfunction Altered sexuality patterns Rape trauma syndrome Rape trauma syndrome: compound reaction Rape trauma syndrome: silent reaction
	Coping—stress tolerance pattern Coping, ineffective (individual) Avoidance coping Defensive coping Ineffective denial Impaired adjustment Posttrauma response Family coping: potential for growth Ineffective family coping: compromised Ineffective family coping: disabling
Sleep-rest pattern Sleep-pattern disturbance	
Cognitive-perceptual pattern Pain Chronic pain	**Value-belief pattern** Spiritual distress (distress of human spirit)

Reproduced with permission from Gordon M: *Manual of Nursing Diagnosis 1988–1989*. St. Louis, Mosby.[19]

Federation of Clinical Oncologic Societies as the assurance that patients with cancer have access to a multidisciplinary team of cancer specialists, a full range of services (prevention, early detection, staging, treatment, palliation, supportive therapies, long-term follow-up, rehabilitation, psychosocial services, hospice), the coordination of those services, continuity of care, and cost-effective, high-quality care. Included as well are referral for specialty care, patient access to information and participation in decision making, high-quality diagnostic assessment, full insurance coverage for total care, access to clinical trials, effective symptom management, comprehensive rehabilitation services and devices, and the elimination of obstacles to access and third party coverage based on preexisting conditions, genetics, and other risk factors.

Quality in nursing, by definition, is a set of properties, attributes, and capacities essential to evaluation. In a generic sense, quality connotes a degree of excellence as measured by recognized standards that are characterized by utility, durability, stability, and flexibility; in the health care environment, quality incorporates certain correlates related to both clinical and organizational qualities. Beyers[22] defines these correlates of quality as cost, productivity, and risk.

The concept of quality of care is grounded in the integration of a sound body of knowledge and skill, standards of practice, and performance that promote excellence, a coordinated team approach, and a built-in capacity for innovation (research), all of which emerge from a deep sense of caring.

Quality of Care Model

A model of quality of care (Figure 72-1) has been designed to represent the major goals in cancer care and treatment and those structural factors that ensure the quality of care in terms of structure, process, and outcome.

Structure

The structures that have been developed to support quality care include Standards for Oncology Nursing Practice, the Classification of Nursing Diagnoses, and a

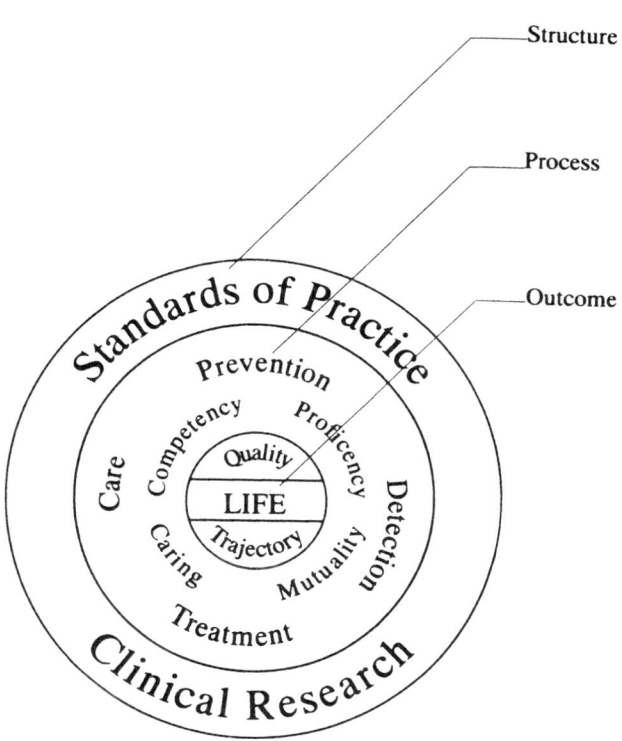

Structure

Process

Outcome

Figure 72-1 This model represents the major goals in cancer care and those structural factors that ensure quality of care in terms of process and outcome.

method for categorizing the NANDA Taxonomy into clinically useful groups. There are several paradigms in current use: Gordon's 11 functional health pattern categories, NANDA's human response patterns, and Maslow's hierarchy of human needs.[23] Since the 11 functional health pattern categories by Gordon are cited most often and are part of the ONS published standards of care, they will be used in this chapter to assess and synthesize the research component of care.

Another major structure that promotes quality of care is clinical research and the development of nursing technology to test and improve interventions and maximize positive results. Nursing research in cancer care can be built into every patient care environment on some level. For some, this might mean keeping up with the nursing research literature or participating in a journal club, or it might involve undertaking a small study of one's own or participating in a larger multisite research project. Research allows for the development of nursing technology as well: audiovisual patient teaching programs; drug dispensers that allow for safer self-administration of the many medications that cancer patients take at home; or measures that aid mobility, protect the skin and mucous membrane, or improve ventilation are examples of new developments that improve or refine care. As such innovations are developed, they need to be tested and the results shared with others.

Process

The second dimension of the quality of care model is represented by the process variables of cancer prevention, detection, treatment, and nursing care. This dimension brings together the nursing care–medical treatment complex because the components of this complex are mutually dependent in achieving the desired outcome. More often than not, nursing care revolves around medical treatment but, in the best sense, extends itself beyond the immediate goals of interest to the physician. Cell kill and reduced tumor size are important, but without attention to management of side effects and promotion of functional recovery, the effect is diminished at best and ineffective at worst. In this sense, medical response and care do not conflict. Care augments and enhances response and in the process humanizes the total outcome.

Outcome

With a structural base of standards and research, the processes of prevention, detection, treatment, and care lead to a broad concern with patient outcomes. The objectives of oncology care providers do not stop with the elimination of disease. Given the current status of cancer treatment, there is a documented 50% cure rate in all patients with a diagnosis of cancer.[24,25] Thus there are other outcomes of cancer care, such as quality of life, that are critical variables to measure and understand.

After 35 years of massive biomedical scientific effort, the lives of many patients with a diagnosis of cancer are now extended far beyond what was thought possible a generation ago. Paralleling the work on this frontier, the biopsychosocial scientific effort in nursing has promoted advances in the quality of the lives that medical science has extended. The amalgamation of life extension and quality of life makes clear the ultimate and optimal outcome of cancer care: maximal quality of life for cancer patients and their families.

Standards of Nursing Practice

The theoretical foundation for the science of caring is based on nursing principles of practice that must be continuously tested, refined, and verified by research. Central to the concept of quality care is a set of standards to define and guide its practice.

The publication of *Outcome Standards for Cancer Nursing Practice*[26] in 1979 and of its integration into the *Standards of Oncology Nursing Practice*[27] in 1987 were joint ventures of the Oncology Nursing Society (ONS) and the American Nurses' Association (ANA). Although the revision, *Statement on the Scope and Standards of Oncology Nursing Practice*,[28] is rooted in the ANA published standards of nursing practice,[29] the former is a separate statement developed in recognition of cancer as a major health problem and of the importance of oncology nursing as a specialty practice devoted to the care of cancer patients and their families.

There are 14 standards of oncology nursing practice

in the 1996 revision,[28] six of which address professional practice and eight that concern professional performance (Table 72-2). To complement the practice standards, the ONS published *Outcome Standards of Oncology Nursing Education*,[30] *Standards of Oncology Education*,[31] and a *Statement on the Scope and Standards of Advanced Practice in Oncology Nursing*.[32]

Standards of care are based on the nursing process.[28] When standards of care and standards of performance are integrated with the classification of nursing diagnoses further broken down into the 11 high-incidence problems in oncology nursing, the oncology nurse has a potent guide for providing quality care. See Table 72-3.

Table 72-2 Standards of Oncology Nursing Practice

Standards of Care

I. *Assessment:* The oncology nurse systematically and continually collects data regarding the health status of the client.

II. *Diagnosis:* The oncology nurse analyzes assessment data in determining nursing diagnoses.

III. *Outcome identification:* The oncology nurse identifies expected outcomes individualized to the client.

IV. *Planning:* The oncology nurse develops an individualized and holistic plan of care that prescribes interventions to attain expected outcomes.

V. *Implementation:* The oncology nurse implements the plan of care to achieve the identified expected outcomes for the client.

VI. *Evaluation:* The oncology nurse systematically and regularly evaluates the client's responses to interventions in order to determine progress toward achievement of expected outcomes.

Standards of Professional Performance

I. *Quality of care:* The oncology nurse systematically evaluates the quality of care and effectiveness of oncology nursing practice.

II. *Performance appraisal:* The oncology nurse evaluates his/her own nursing practice in relation to professional practice standards and relevant statutes and regulations.

III. *Education:* The oncology nurse acquires and maintains current knowledge in oncology nursing practice.

IV. *Collegiality:* The oncology nurse contributes to the professional development of peers, colleagues, and others.

V. *Ethics:* The oncology nurse's decisions and actions on behalf of clients are determined in an ethical manner.

VI. *Collaboration:* The oncology nurse collaborates with the client, significant others, and multidisciplinary cancer care team in providing client care.

VII. *Research:* The oncology nurse contributes to the scientific base of nursing practice and the field of oncology through the review and application of research.

VIII. *Resource utilization:* The oncology nurse considers factors related to safety, effectiveness, and cost in planning and delivering client care.

Reprinted with permission from *Statement on the Scope and Standards of Oncology Nursing Practice.* Pittsburgh, American Nurses' Association and the Oncology Nursing Society, 1996.[28]

Table 72-3 High-Incidence Problems in Cancer Nursing Practice

I. *Prevention and early detection:* Client and family possess adequate information about cancer prevention and detection.

II. *Information:* Client and family possess knowledge about disease and therapy in order to attain self-management, participate in therapy, optimal living, and peaceful death.

III. *Coping:* Client and family manage stress optimally according to their individual capacity and in accord with their value system.

IV. *Comfort:* Client and family manage factors that influence comfort.

V. *Nutrition:* Client and family manage nutrition and hydration optimally.

VI. *Protective mechanisms:* Client and family possess knowledge to prevent or manage alterations in protective mechanisms.

VII. *Mobility:* Client and family maintain optimal mobility.

VIII. *Elimination:* Client and family manage problems with elimination.

IX. *Sexuality:* Client and partner can manage threats to sexual function and satisfaction and maintain their sexual identity.

X. *Ventilation:* Client and family can anticipate factors that impair ventilatory function and maintain optimal ventilatory capacity.

XI. *Circulation:* Client and family can identify signs and symptoms of change in circulation, such as shortness of breath and fluid retention, and take measures to manage those changes.

Data from Oncology Nursing Society.[28]

Research and Evaluation in Quality of Care

Background and Context

Research-based clinical practice and quality care are the hallmarks of professional nursing. These important processes are founded on a theory-based body of knowledge, standards for practice, and valid and reliable measurements that allow for the evaluation of care and the expansion of the scientific foundation of practice.

Oncology nursing literature and the espousal of a scientific data-based practice came of age with the beginning publication of two journals, *Cancer Nursing* and *Oncology Nursing Forum*. In a review of research-based articles published in these journals through 1984, a total of 15 were found to evaluate nursing care programs.[33] All interventions tested were educative or of a supportive, counseling nature, perhaps reflecting Herberth and Gosnell's finding that over 40% of diagnoses involve knowledge deficit.[18] Most of the studies did not allow for control-group comparisons. Nine articles described tools designed to evaluate patient outcomes. Rarely was care measured directly, and most measures were constructed by the investigator because of the lack of sound instrumentation at that time. Few were tested for accuracy or consistency.

A distinct shift in the cancer nursing literature, noted from 1985 onward, seemed to coincide with the establishment of oncology nursing standards and their clinically useful format (patient outcome standards and high-incidence oncology nursing problems). Clearly, more authors attempted schema that integrated patients' clinical problems and deficits, nursing diagnoses, assessment parameters, causes, and interventions into plans for care that provided a useful guide for the practicing nurse and a methodical approach for quality assurance programs.

The following review of methods for measuring quality of cancer nursing care recognizes the seminal work of early researchers[34–38] but concentrates on studies published in the cancer nursing literature since 1995 that reflect more recent trends in the field.

Approaches to Measuring Quality of Care

There are three major approaches to measuring quality of care: (1) quality improvement programs, (2) clinical research that includes both program evaluation and experimental studies of interventions, and (3) measurement tools or instrument development—including the construction of quantitative scales, questionnaires, and inventories and qualitative measures—for establishing clinical indicators, predictors, and guidelines for assessment.

Quality improvement

The Joint Commission on the Accreditation of Health Care Organizations (JCAHO) publishes standards used in the United States for the accreditation of hospitals and other types of health care organizations (long-term care, psychiatric care, ambulatory health care, hospice care, and home care organizations).[39] These standards pertain to the structures, processes, and outcomes of patient care activities in all services provided by the organization, including nursing services. There are standards that address the provision, management, and monitoring of nursing services regardless of location or institutional type. The standards are concerned directly with the quality of nursing care: maintenance of established standards of nursing practice; the use of the nursing process; written documentation that care reflects optimal standards of practice; and monitoring and evaluation of care and the identification and resolution of problems.

Therefore, to operationalize a quality improvement program, the health care institution must maintain a sound system for documentation of nursing care activities and patient outcomes and must establish a system to review and assess regularly both quality and appropriateness. In addition to evaluation, there is the need for a system to rectify or resolve problems or breeches of quality

in all aspects of care: diagnostic, preventive, therapeutic, rehabilitative, supportive, and palliative.

Depending on the nature and specialization of the nursing care unit, there may be a need for a more precise definition of both patient outcomes and nursing practices to achieve those outcomes, or what is known as *clinical functions*. Oncology nursing is a prime example of the need for care and practice standards to be tailored to the unique needs and problems of the patient and for more precise operationalization of clinical functions such as assessment, evaluation of learning needs, provision of physical care, teaching, goal setting, nursing interventions based on nursing diagnosis, implementation of the medical plan of care and required medications and treatments, and the coordination of nursing goals and plans for care with those of other professional team members.[40]

In these specific cases, both health care institutions and accrediting organizations look to the professional specialty group to establish and promulgate those standards of nursing practice. Quality improvement structures look to organizations such as the ONS for current, state-of-the-art, research-based standards. On the basis of these published specialty guides, the hospital or agency customizes the standards further to be in line with the nature and character of its own caregiving environment. For example, nursing practice standards at one of the nation's five major cancer centers might differ from those in a small community hospital, where there may or may not be a discrete oncology unit or where there may or may not be a department of nursing research that focuses on oncology care. However, no matter how specialized or how large or small the institution might be, mandated quality improvement accords to every oncology patient the *right* to quality of care as defined by the ONS standards of nursing practice.

A clinical database can be established to provide a structured framework for the collection of data critical to formulating nursing diagnoses. Miaskowski and Nielsen[41] developed a cancer nursing assessment tool to evaluate the integrity of 15 functional systems at high risk because of cancer and its treatment. The assessment included teaching needs and discharge planning. Gray and associates[42] published a clinical database that provides description and analysis of age, metastatic sites, diagnoses, and associated symptoms of hospitalized patients with advanced cancer. Their study of 1103 patients generated more than 400 variables and provided important information on problem areas related to cancer metastasis. Since symptom management is the "cornerstone of care" in this patient group, the database facilitated the identification of relevant nursing diagnoses and related nursing practices that improved the measurement of quality of care.

On another level, two separate studies by Moore and colleagues[43] and McGee and colleagues[44] sought to establish nurse competencies and to measure proficiency in cancer nursing practice. The Moore team constructed an appraisal of practice behaviors instrument based on the five dimensions of the theoretical framework used by ONS to develop its standards of oncology nursing practice. Three classes enrolled in a master's-level oncology nursing graduate program were tested before and after each of the two years of their educational program for both frequency and self-assessed proficiency in achieving the ONS outcome standards of oncology practice. The instrument consists of 92 items divided among six subscales. Findings revealed that frequency of practice and proficiency were positively related and that students significantly increased in self-assessed proficiency as their educational program progressed. The investigators further suggest evaluation of the instrument in both academic and clinical settings to expand the database.

In contrast, McGee and associates[44] conducted a two-round Delphi survey to identify oncology clinical nurse specialist (OCNS) competencies. The initial pilot study amassed 363 competencies, which the investigators further divided into knowledge, skill, attitude, and human trait categories. Ranking by means for each category revealed that attitude and human traits were ranked highest in importance by the 47 respondents. Attitudes of greatest importance had to do with ethical practice, respect for humanity, responsibility for behavior, and commitment to continued learning. Identifying nursing diagnoses and commitment to cost-effective practices were ranked lowest in the category. The human traits most valued included accountability, common sense, caring, flexibility, and resourcefulness. Of lower importance were sympathy and abstract thinking. The highest number of competencies, 173, were amassed in the "skills" category, and knowledge ranked second in number of competencies, totaling 137.

In interpreting their results, McGee's group concluded that attitudes and human traits concerned with caring, commitment, and professionalism were most important to OCNS functioning. They considered their results to be consistent with Yasko's survey[45] of 185 OCNSs, who reported a decided "care orientation" described as "keeping the client comfortable, maintaining a therapeutic environment, providing emotional support, personalized care, friendliness, emotional acceptance and ensuring that clients understand their medical problems."

The information generated from these key studies helps to expand and facilitate attempts to improve quality of care. By integrating findings from these and future studies on acuity, audit assessment tools, safety guidelines, clinical databases, and nursing competencies and practice proficiency, quality assurance has moved into a new era.

Clinical research

Research offers a means of improving and refining practice to ensure optimal outcomes. The desired result of practice usually is defined as a valuable change in the patient for the better. In most institutional settings, this means cost-effective patient outcomes and consumer satisfaction, i.e., quality of life.

However, a recent survey by Rutledge and Engelking[46]

reported that more than half of both oncology staff nurses and clinical nurse specialists had found significant barriers to research utilization in their work settings. Most reported organizational barriers, primarily lack of time to read and lack of authority to implement research and change patient care. Poorly communicated research with convoluted statistical analyses was also cited. The most important barrier was the lack of clear implications of clinical research for practice.

Clinical research, in the context of evaluating quality of care, includes two major categories: (1) experimental studies of nursing interventions and (2) evaluations of programs of care. The program of research in most disciplines is shaped by the intellectual and practical problems and challenges encountered in carrying out its objectives and by the diagnostic and functional categories that constitute its focus.

In a review of research-based articles appearing in the cancer nursing literature between 1976 and 1984, Scott[33] found 122 articles representing 25% of all articles published. More than 60% of the studies were published after 1981, most concerned with side effects of treatment (26%) or with oncology nurses themselves (24%). Approximately 15% examined the impact of cancer on the family, and another 16% described phenomena about cancer patients. Only 12% were intervention-management studies, and fewer (7%) offered assessment-measurement approaches to evaluate care.

In a developmental sense, the era before 1985 may be viewed as a descriptive phase when the rich database that exists today was established. Clinical research, comprising both program evaluation and experimental studies of interventions, began slowly between 1980 and 1985, marked by the seminal work of Satterwhite, Pryor, and Harris;[47] Dodd and Mood;[48,49] Johnson;[50] Miller and Nygren,[51] Marty, McDermott, and Gold;[52] Watson;[53] and Heinrich and Schag.[54]

Since 1985, the advent year of data-based literature in oncology nursing publications, there has been a significant expansion of the cancer research literature. Over 40 experimental studies have been published addressing 5 of the 11 high-incidence problems: prevention/detection, information, coping, comfort, and protective mechanisms. Recent examples are presented in Table 72-4. Most of the studies address side effects of treatment and venous access device protocols, but a rapidly growing number of studies are focused on coping. The roles of support groups, exercise programs, nurse assessment, counseling and therapeutic touch, and educational interventions were examined utilizing randomized experimental methods. The results in general were significant and a tribute to the importance of the expanded role of the oncology nurse.

From 1984 to 1996, a total of 18 program evaluation reports (Table 72-5)[82-98] covering a wide range of outcome standards were published. The largest number (eight, 44%) evaluated programs designed to assist patients and families to cope with cancer. The next largest category (four, 22%), comfort, described multidisciplinary pain

Table 72-4   Experimental Studies of Oncology Nursing Interventions and Patient Outcomes by Functional Pattern Category

Problem/Author	Method	Findings	Implications
PREVENTION AND EARLY DETECTION			
BSE proficiency in older women (> 50 years) –Coleman et al[55]	N = 79 women; random assignment 2-group design to compare women who were taught BSE using self-modeling as well as breast model methods with women taught by use of breast model only. Subjects evaluated using pre- and posttesting method. First posttest immediately after the teaching; second posttest 3 months later	• Women taught by both methods performed BSE significantly more proficiently than those taught by model only	• Performance is not always related to a woman's reported self-confidence • Patients need to be evaluated directly to determine proficiency in BSE
Effect of knowledge on participation in prostate cancer screening –Weinrich et al[56]	N = 319 men, 82% black American, tested for whether prior knowledge, demographics, and type of educational program determined later follow-through with prostate cancer screening	• Predictors of who would obtain screening included age, marital status, education, prior knowledge, income, urinary symptoms, type of pre-educational program, and, to some degree, ethnicity	• Educational programs increase participation in prostate screening programs; at risk black population needs educational intervention
INFORMATION			
Effect of weekly radiation therapy newsletter on knowledge, self-care, and severity of side effects –Hagopian[57]	N = 103 radiation patients assigned to experimental (51) and control (52) groups. Experimentals had opportunity to read newsletter during treatment; controls did not. *Instruments:* Radiation Side Effects Profile, a knowledge test, and a demographics form; posttest-only design.	• Subjects who read newsletter scored significantly higher on knowledge test • All other correlations nonsignificant	• Majority of patients found newsletter to be helpful source of information • It cannot replace a caring professional
Effect of informational audiotapes on knowledge and self-care behaviors in RT patients –Hagopian[58]	N = 75 RT adults randomized into audiotape vs. standard care control groups using posttest measurement	• Experimental subjects were more knowledgeable and used more self-care measures and practiced more self-care behaviors than controls	• Audiotapes are a useful tool in radiation oncology patient teaching
Information amount and presentation in treatment selection and recall –Hughes[59]	N = 71 stage I & II breast cancer patients. Amount, location, and presentation determined by checklist observation with follow-up telephone survey	• Choice of treatment unrelated to amount and presentation during clinic visits • Treatment selection related to amount of information received *before* clinic visit • Patient recall of information about treatment and associated risks was poor	• Further research on both clinical implications and legal ramifications needed
Effect of demonstration-type preparation program on anxiety and cooperation during pediatric lumbar puncture –Mansson et al[60]	N = 30 children with leukemia/lymphoma, aged 4–17 years, divided into 3 groups of 10. Controls: no specific preparation; preparation using demo, doll, and book of photos of procedure. Preparation began 1 hour prior to LP. Child videotaped. Scales to measure anxiety and noncooperation	• Anxiety and noncooperation were strongly associated • Children under 8 years exhibited higher anxiety, noncooperation, and self-rated pain • Repeated preparations for subsequent LPs seemed effective	• Overall, children seemed to benefit from the attention. More research on clinical contacts with children needed

(continued)

Table 72-4 Experimental Studies of Oncology Nursing Interventions and Patient Outcomes by Functional Pattern Category (continued)

Problem/Author	Method	Findings	Implications
		INFORMATION (cont.)	
		• No significant differences found among groups	
		• Children's self-reported pain ratings generally higher than anxiety and noncooperation	
Efficacy of prostate cancer education intervention on black men –Collins[61]	N = 75 black men who participated in an education intervention; pretest, posttest method	• Correct responses increased from 23%–64%	• Intervention had a positive effect on short-term knowledge acquisition
Effect of smoking cessation intervention on patients tested for suspected lung cancer –Wewers et al[62]	N = 15 men and women provided smoking cessation intervention while hospitalized with verification of smoking status via saliva continine levels at 6 weeks postintervention	• 87% reported intent to quit; at postintervention time, 93% reported at least one cessation attempt with a 40% confirmation by saliva analysis of abstinence during prior week	• Idea and timing for intervention program have promise and indicate beginning effectiveness; need to fine-tune program and test again
		COMFORT	
Effect of music in decreasing cancer pain –Beck[63]	N = 15 outpatients with cancer receiving scheduled analgesics for pain; experimental repeated measures crossover design using McGill Pain Questionnaire and analog scales to measure mood and pain; from a menu of 7 types of music, subjects chose type of music preferred; controls listened to tape with low-frequency hum; tapes were 45 min in length; study conducted in 4 phases: baseline data for 3 days, randomized to E or C group for 3 days, crossover to alternate group for 3 days, baseline repetition for all subjects for 3 days; pain ratings taken before and after listening to tape	• When listening to music, 75% had < 20% response, 50% had < 40% or > 40% responses • When listening to hum, 20% had < 40% and > 40% responses and 53% had no change in pain • 60% listening to music reported some improvement in mood with music, with ⅓ responding with moderate to great improvement • Mood and pain were found to be unrelated • Although not statistically significant, overall music decreased pain 22%; hum decreased pain 11%	• Music therapy has promise as a pain reducing modality, but further refinements in methods and research required
Effect of distraction and imagery on reducing pain during painful procedures in children and on reducing anxiety in child's mother –Broome et al[64]	N = 14 children receiving lumbar punctures and their mothers; multiple case study design; children videotaped for first 3 visits to obtain baseline; distraction and imagery program not described; *instruments (child):* Child Medical Fear Scale, Observation of Behavioral Stress Scale, Baker-Wong FACES Scale; *instruments (mother):* Spielberger's State-Trait Anxiety Inventory (STAI), Parent Behavior Tool	• No change in children's fears or behavioral distress; children's pain ratings decreased significantly over time • Mothers' state of anxiety did not change • Mothers' behaviors were nondistressed and stable over time	• Research control of ability of child to relax and use distraction and frequency of parent-child practice need to be improved • Decrease in children's pain reports an important finding and corresponds with previous reports

Table 72-4   Experimental Studies of Oncology Nursing Interventions and Patient Outcomes by Functional Pattern Category (continued)

Problem/Author	Method	Findings	Implications
COMFORT (cont.)			
Music as diversional intervention to affect perception of nausea and vomiting in high-dose chemotherapy –Ezzone et al[65]	N = 33 subjects undergoing BMT; control and music intervention groups randomization; music intervention during 48 hours of chemotherapy	• Significant reduction in nausea distress and number of vomiting times in experimental group	• Music is effective adjunct to chemotherapy
Effect of walking on physical functioning and symptom intensity during radiation therapy –Mock et al[66]	N = 46 women with breast cancer undergoing RT randomly assigned to exercise and control groups; pre- and post-RT assessments of fatigue and symptoms distress plus symptoms were assessed at 3 weeks	• Exercise group scored significantly higher on physical functioning and lower on symptom intensity, especially fatigue, anxiety, and insomnia	• Nurse-prescribed exercise programs may help to facilitate recovery in women with breast cancer
Efficacy of ondansetron versus perphenazine with diphenhydramine in emesis-control with children undergoing BMT –Mehta et al[67]	N = 28 children age 4–17 randomized to one of two antiemetic regimens with crossover if 5 emeses over 12 hours; if still no control, subjects eliminated from study	• 67% on ondansetron (10 subjects) had < 2 emetic episodes with 0% control with the other regimen; 38% (5 subjects) of perphenazine with diphenhydramine were able to achieve control after crossover to ondansetron	• Clearly ondansetron offered superior antiemetic control
Efficacy of structured symptom assessment on symptom distress over time –Sarna[68]	N = 48 subjects with advanced lung cancer randomly assigned to structured assessment or usual care; Symptom Distress Scale completed monthly; scores regressed for level and rate of change in symptom distress	• Fatigue most common severe symptom; chemotherapy and structured assessment associated with less symptom distress over time; depression and functional limitation associated with higher distress	• Proactive approach using assessment, chemotherapy, treatment of depression, and approaches to enhance function form a collective approach to reduce symptom distress in advanced lung cancer
COPING			
Compare rehab treatment program results with usual-care group results of breast cancer patients: functional, physical, psychosocial adjustments –Mock et al[69]	N = 14 women with breast cancer randomized to either treatment or usual-care control groups. Performance, functioning, psychosocial adjustment, self-concept, body image, and dysphoria were measured pre-, mid-, and postprogram. Experimental program included walking and support group attendance	• Selective measures of performance, psychosocial adjustment, and symptom intensity revealed improved adaptation in experimental group	• Patients benefit from an exercise and support group rehab program
How support groups facilitate self-transcendence and emotional and physical well-being –Coward[70]	N = 16; Pilot intervention of women recently diagnosed with breast cancer participating in 90-minute group session for 8 weeks; quantitative measurement of physical and emotional well-being	• Association between self-transcendence and emotional well-being; only functional performance, mood and life satisfaction improved statistically	• Promising theory for clinical use
Improvement in depression, anxiety, and self-esteem with aerobic exercise –Segar et al[71]	N = 24 breast cancer survivors randomized to exercise, exercise + behavior mod or control group; pre-, post-, and crossover scores evaluated for depression, anxiety, and self-esteem	• Significantly less depression and anxiety in exercise groups; self-esteem did not change; 12 weeks later (crossover) controls achieved comparable improvements; women with physician recommendations exercised more	• Exercise seems to be of therapeutic value to breast cancer survivors • Physician recommendation is important to motivation

(continued)

Table 72-4 Experimental Studies of Oncology Nursing Interventions and Patient Outcomes by Functional Pattern Category (continued)

Problem/Author	Method	Findings	Implications
COPING (cont.)			
Patterns of functioning and psychosocial adjustment in midlife and older women with breast cancer who have or do not have adjuvant therapy after surgery –Wyatt and Friedman[72]	2 × 3 mixed design with treatment between-group factor and time within-group factor; baseline data at 1 week postsurgery; follow-up data at 6 weeks, 3 mo and 6 mo times; telephone and mail interviews	• No difference among groups and scores did not change significantly over time; functional and psychosocial needs were present and require intervention	
Efficacy of dialogue and therapeutic touch on pre- and postoperative anxiety and mood and P.O. pain from breast surgery –Samarel et al[73]	N = 29 women diagnosed with breast cancer divided between experimental and control groups; State-Trait Anxiety Scale, Affects Balance Scale, and Visual Analog Scale Pain administered 7 days before surgery and within 24 hours after hospital discharge	• Experimental group had lower preop anxiety than controls; no other measures significantly different	• Future research needs to fraction out placebo effects on control group
Efficacy of informational intervention based on Self-Regulatory Theory on life activity disruption and mood state during radiation therapy –Johnson et al[74]	N = 226 patients receiving RT for breast and prostate cancer divided between usual care group and experimental group receiving interventions at 4 different times; patients also categorized according to optimistic or pessimistic outcome expectation, amount of life disruption and mood state	• Experimental group had less disruption in life activities and in patients with pessimistic outlook, greater elevation in mood	• Self-regulation theory-based interventions may help patients cope with RT
PROTECTIVE MECHANISMS			
Comparison of two CVC dressing protocols on catheter infections in ABMT patients –Brandt et al[75]	N = 101 patients, with long-term tunneled CVCs inserted in OR, randomized into two groups: (1) dry, sterile gauze changed every 24 hours; (2) Opsite 3000 ™ transparent moisture vapor permeable dressing changed weekly	• No statistical difference in infection rate between groups • CVC sepsis occurred in 1 dry dressing and 5 Opsite subjects	• Both methods can be used safely
Comparison of chlorhexidine with water in preventing mucositis –Dodd et al[76]	N = 222 patients beginning mucositis-induced chemotherapy for 3 cycles. Randomized clinical trial of agents with results measured by Oral Assessment Guide with each chemotherapy cycle to determine any change in oral status	• No significant differences in incidence, days to onset, or severity	• Chlorhexidine is much less cost-efficient than water for preventing oral mucositis
Comparison of transparent adherent dressing (TAD) and dry sterile gauze dressing (DSGD) in preventing infection in long-term central catheters –Shivnan et al[77]	N = 98; TAD (51); DSGD (47); randomized, stratified design with assignment to DSGD changed daily or TAD changed every 4 days; data collected with investigator-designed demographic and assessment forms for skin irritation and intactness, dryness of dressing,	• DSGD group had significantly more skin irritation and wet dressings after showering, and had more exudate • Exit site infection occurred in 2 TAD and 1 DSGD subjects • No systemic infection occurred • One catheter-related sepsis occurred in TAD group	• TADs provide a safe, comfortable, and cost-effective alternative to DSGDs

Table 72-4 Experimental Studies of Oncology Nursing Interventions and Patient Outcomes by Functional Pattern Category (continued)

Problem/Author	Method	Findings	Implications
		PROTECTIVE MECHANISMS (cont.)	
	erythema, swelling, pain, and exudate; dressing comfort, ease of application, safety, change frequency, and satisfaction recorded	• TADs required significantly fewer dressings and less nursing time and were significantly less costly • Subjects reported greater satisfaction and comfort with TADs	
Effect of chlorhexidene gluconate (CHG) in reducing perirectal infections in patients with acute leukemia –Yeoman et al[78]	N = 40 acute or chronic leukemia patients; 16 randomized to CHG group, 24 to nonmedicated skin cleanser group; chi-square and t-tests used to analyze (1) incidence of skin breakdown and rectal infections, and their correlation, (2) positive history of rectal infections, fissures, hemorrhoids, (3) presence of hemorrhoids, (4) severity of diarrhea, and (5) duration and severity of granulocytopenia; *instruments:* Perirectal Skin Assessment Tool (PSAT), perirectal clinical examinations conducted by blinded evaluators for duration and severity of granulocytopenia, presence of hemorrhoids, severity of GI mucositis, signs of perirectal infection	• Treatment did not influence development of perirectal infections or degree or incidence of skin breakdown • Severity and duration of granulocytopenia significantly related to development of rectal infections • No other variable statistically significant influence	• Due to small sample size, replication is advisable • PSAT has some demonstrated validity and reliability • Need for strategies to prevent rectal infection in immunocompromised patients is clear
48-versus 24-hour change of IV administration sets in incidence of septicemia in neutropenic cancer patients –DeMoissac and Jensen[79]	N = 50 adult cancer patients receiving stem cell transplant; prospective randomized, 5 repeated measures trial; rates of infusate colonization, microorganisms identified and incidence of infusion-related septicemia measured	• Trend toward increased colonization in 48 hour group; overall, no differences detected between two time groups	• 48-hour standard is recommended except with blood products and parenteral nutrition
Effect of infusion rate on quality of transfused platelets and patient physical and subjective responses –Norville et al[80]	N = 26 children, age 3–20, with cancer and thrombocytopenia requiring platelet transfusion and 12 randomly selected platelet units in vitro with 4 infusion rates in vitro and 2 infusion rates in vivo; platelet count, morphology score, corrected count increment and patient responses measured	• No significant differences found in either in vitro or in vivo studies	• More rapid infusion rate preferred because it cuts infusion time by half
Efficacy of heparinized versus nonheparinized flush in preventing clot formation and persistent withdrawal occlusion (PWO) in Groshong catheters –Mayo et al[81]	N = 28 double-lumen Groshong catheters flushed with saline and N = 23 catheters maintained with a heparin flush; saline control group results obtained by retrospective chart audit	• PWO occurred significantly less frequently with the heparin flush; all 28 saline-flushed catheters developed an adherent clot in both lumens	• Flushing Groshong catheters with heparinized saline decreases intraluminal clot formation and catheter malfunction

TSE, testicular self-examination; *STAI,* State-Trait Anxiety Inventory; *PMR,* progressive muscle relaxation; *DMSO,* dimethyl sulfoxide.

Table 72-5 Care Program Evaluation Studies

Program/Author	Method	Results
PREVENTION AND DETECTION		
Family High Risk Program —Beck et al[82]	Health Family Tree Questionnaire; Family health survey to assess satisfaction with program, health practices, health history, and behavior; includes retrospective data	• No results
INFORMATION		
Patient Education Program —Nieweg et al[83]	Comparison of patient self-care of chemotherapy port infection rates with literature-based norms; weekly clinical assessments; no standardized evaluation methods used	• Empirically judged effective • Takes considerable time • Required teaching materials • Greater social support involvement • Less need for hospitalization • Greater patient freedom
COPING		
I Can Cope —McMillan et al[84]	First national evaluation of ICC in 8 areas: demographics, format, objectives, content, audiovisual materials, training, implementation, evaluation	• Wide variations in comparison to official facilitator's guide • Facilitators agreed with objectives and content • Wide participant levels • Topics most often requested include medical care, resources, emotional support, and stress management
Living with Cancer —Pillon and Joannides[85]	Based on anecdotal statements and empirical observation of a program conducted since 1979	• Program needs to be comprehensive, addressing problems of the entire family from diagnosis to disease-free state or death • Facilitators should include an oncology nurse and mental health clinician
We Can Weekend —Lane and Davis[86]	Postprogram participant evaluation; staff feedback; director evaluation of training sessions, staff, facilities, schedule, public relations, and supplies	• Recommended use of preprogram questionnaires to enable advance custom planning • Also use a postprogram questionnaire
Living With Cancer —Fredette and Beattie[87]	Precourse and postcourse knowledge test; precourse and postcourse personal needs assessment; postcourse interviews; written comments of specialist-observer; end-of-class and end-of-program evaluations	• Coping skills can be taught • Profiles "good coper" as one who pursues information and seeks opportunities to learn • Adaptive, resilient, optimistic, and assertive • Need further exploration into program design for those who desire less or differently structured programs • Teaching skills of coping was primary value of program
Cancer Caregivers Program —Cawley and Gerdts[88]	Committee-constructed evaluation tool: evaluates 8 dimensions of care in terms of time, instructor, handouts	• Provides steps in establishment of program • Evaluation tool developed and provided • No results
I Can Cope —Diekmann[89]	Postprogram mail questionnaire	• Demographic characteristics • Overall evaluation: valuable to help people learn about cancer • More research to improve impact on coping

(continued)

Table 72-5 Care Program Evaluation Studies (continued)

Program/Author	Method	Results
COPING (cont.)		
Bereavement Outreach Program Mosely et al[90]	No formal means of evaluation	• Excellent client response • Need to tailor program to institution
COMFORT		
Home Pain Management Program –Coyle et al[91]	Evaluated 123 patients with advanced disease for pain management at home	• Nurse becomes primary liaison • Successful pain management at home with use of analgesic and behavioral modes • Team as expert information resource in community
Continuous SC Infusion Pain Management Program –Coyle et al[92]	Evaluated 15 patients for quality of pain management	• Avoids repeated injection, need for intravenous access, analgesia delay, pain breakthrough
Pain Management Team –Ferrell et al[93]	No evaluation of effect of interventions on pain	• Patients visits: 7500 (750 patients) over course of 5 years • Community presentations: 300
Patient-controlled Analgesia (PCA) Service –Kane et al[94]	Patient questionnaire on discharge; nurse evaluation of 2 pumps regarding safety, ease of use, saving of time; bedside flow sheets to rate pain and sedation; daily patient evaluation by PCA team	• Use of pump gives excellent control of pain in postsurgical patients, has few problems, and frees nurse to care for patient • Further studies in chronic pain populations needed • Choice of one pump over another
NUTRITION		
Home Parenteral Nutrition Program –Konstantinides[95]	Patient teaching flow sheet; no formal evaluation methods presented	• Cost estimated between $55,000 and $70,000 for nutritional solutions, supplies, home visits, clinic follow-up, and laboratory costs • Guides for patient teaching, discharge planning, laboratory monitoring, and follow-up given
Protocol for Venous Access Port –Long and Ovaska[96]	$N = 26$ outpatients with venous access devices randomly assigned to sterile (12) or clean (14) group; sterile group used commercially prepared kit; compared occurrence of infection assessed by increase in WBC, febrile episode (> 100.4), drainage, pain, redness, swelling, warmth at port site	• After 6 months, no documented infection in either group • Institution changed to nursing protocol based on its cost-effectiveness
GENERAL FOCUS		
Day Hospital for Cancer Patients –Clark[97]	Economic feasibility measures	• One-year pilot project
Home Care Transfusion Program –Pluth[98]	Cost comparisons with patients receiving transfusions in different settings; client satisfaction; difficulties in implementation	• Cost-effective and beneficial to patients' quality of life

management programs. The rest were divided among prevention/detection (one, 6%), information (one, 6%), protection (one, 6%), and two economic feasibility studies (11%) of an adult day care hospital and a home transfusion program.

The therapeutic programs generally were well defined, as was the patient population. Most were service innovations based on the institution's database of patient needs and problems. In a majority of these studies, evaluation methods proved to be the weakest component. Although all programs were judged as valuable by the investigators, only half employed evaluation criteria developed before program initiation. Some measured quality by the number of clients seen or by unsolicited patient feedback. Others, however, made use of standardized surveys, questionnaires, interviews, and preprogram and postprogram comparisons of knowledge tests or needs assessments with baseline findings. Almost all investigative teams communicated willingness to share their programs with others but advised tailoring them to the unique needs of the institutions and their patient populations. Most suggested the need for further study and program modifications or refinements.

Although the program evaluations reflected significant effort in planning and execution by hardworking teams, it must be remembered that program evaluation generally requires an expert team of outside investigators to conduct the study. Two noteworthy examples include the Brown University evaluation of the Adult Day Care Hospital, Memorial Sloan-Kettering Cancer Center[99] and the University of Washington study of the effect of the Planetree Unit, a primary-nursing, family-centered care facility at California Pacific Medical Center (Pacific campus), San Francisco.

The overall picture of these studies suggests the beginning establishment of a clinical scientific base for practice. Clearly, much more research is needed in all areas of standards of practice. Research that replicates or builds on the work of others and that refines established interventions may be the most economic ventures. To address meaningfully the issue of quality of care, however, longitudinal studies expanding the clinical database and testing the effects of nursing intervention over time are critically needed. The oncology nursing research program, to have an impact on quality of care, will need not only to continue building the growing knowledge base in symptom management and patient education but also to turn attention to the issues of quality of life, recovery, transition, and the effects of the many new modalities on patients' lives and health.

Measurement tool development: quantitative

As psychometric theory advances and the results of nursing research build over time, better methods for measuring quality of care will emerge. Hartshorn,[100] Duffy,[101] and Lynn[102] emphasize the importance of using reliable and valid instruments in clinical research. Research-based practice should be precise enough to be replicable and to produce predictable patient outcomes. Results from studies employing poor instruments cannot be accepted or implemented. Indeed, many nursing studies that have taken considerable time and effort conclude with a long list of limitations to the generalizability of their findings and with an underdeveloped interpretation of important data because of faulty design, inadequate sampling technique, and use of untested measurement tools. Frank-Stromborg has written an excellent nursing research reference.[103]

The basic ingredients of sound quantitative measurement techniques include adequate reliability and validity of the instrument. Reliability tests both the stability (test–retest correlations) and the internal consistency (intercorrelations among items or alpha coefficient) of an instrument. Correlations of at least 0.8 in internal consistency and test–retest correlations ensure that the instrument is reliably measuring the construct it purports to measure and is stable in its ability to reproduce results in repeated testing of the sample. A third type of reliability, interrater reliability, is also important to ensure that all persons using a set of evaluation criteria have closely correlated results.[104]

Validity testing offers a way to assess the ability of the instrument to measure the construct of interest accurately and objectively. The three most important types of validity include construct, content, and criterion related (predictive or concurrent).[100,104] One of the most definitive signs of increasingly improved and sophisticated cancer nursing research is growing evidence that reliable and valid instruments are used.

Table 72-6 provides a partial list of cancer nursing measurement tools grouped by functional category, including the construct measured and whether evidence of reliability and validity testing are given.[105–121] Note that most of these instruments quantify patient attributes. The aim is to further establish a normative database or to

---

Table 72-6 Tools to Measure Patient Outcomes

Tool/Author	Construct	Findings	Implications
BMT Outpatient Nursing Treatment Record –Burns and Tierney[105]	Documentation method to enhance efficient and accurate communication in complex patient care environment	Reduction in written documentation time and verbal reports with easier assessment tracking	Staff satisfaction increased
Patient Assessment Record (PAR) –Allaster et al[106]	Nursing/toxicity assessment form for clinical trials	Form minimizes recording repetition while maintaining quality of toxicity data	Effective in enhancing toxicity documentation
McGill Pain Questionnaire –Camp[107]	Location, quality, pattern, increase, intensity, verbal–nonverbal symptoms; reliability established; validity established	Compared patient perceptions and nurse documentation; less than 50% of patients' pain perceptions were documented	Replication and assessment of pain management protocols
Hypercalcemia Knowledge Questionnaire (HKQ) –Coward[108]	Hypercalcemia risk factors and knowledge		Need for educational program to evaluate

(continued)

Table 72-6 Tools to Measure Patient Outcomes (continued)

Tool/Author	Construct	Findings	Implications
Derdiarian Behavioral System Model –Derdiarian[109]	Achievement, affiliation, aggressive–protective, dependence, elimination, ingestion, restoration, sexuality; based on Johnson Behavioral Symptom Model; reliability established; validity established	Defines imbalance in behavioral subsystems caused by illness; predicts direction and quality of change; sensitive to age, site of cancer, and stage of cancer	Further studies in larger samples
Oral Assessment Guide –Eilers et al[110]	Stomatitis or oral mucositis and mucosal changes in radiotherapy and chemotherapy patients: voice, swallow, lips, tongue, saliva, mucous membranes, gingivae, teeth, and dentures	Clinical guide to evaluate oral care protocols and toxic effects of treatment protocols and persons at risk	Further clinical use
Breast Self-Examination (BSE) Belief and Attitude Questionnaire –Lauver[111]	Remembering, competence, comfort, interference, efficacy; reliability established	Positive relationship between frequency of BSE and competence, remembering, and comfort	Replication in larger, heterogeneous population with test-retest reliability; further testing for methods to promote competence and remembering
Pain Assessment Tool (PAT) and Pain Flow Sheet (PFS) –McMillan et al[112]	Ongoing assessment of pain and its management	Pain intensity and level of sedation documented in 2-group study	Further research with both tools
Self-care and Symptom Report Interview –Rhodes et al[113]	Symptom distress, self-care activities, coping strategies regarding fatigue and weakness; based on Orem's self-care deficit theory	Lays foundation for tool to measure symptom occurrence and distress and to assess self-care efficacy	Ongoing development and testing
Linear Analogue Modification (LAM) of Profile of Mood States (POMS) –Sutherland et al[114]	Emotional distress; fatigue, anxiety, confusion, depression, energy, anger	Significant correlation between LAM and POMS in 29 subjects	To evaluate patients' ongoing emotional status as base for psychosocial interventions over time
Champion's Instrument and Williams's Breast Inventory –Williams[115]	Likert scale of 5 constructs of Health Belief Model, health history, and personal knowledge	Health motivation represents 18% of variance; barriers, 8%; age differences	Further testing of variables
Multidimensional Quality of Life Scale Cancer Version (MQOLS-CA) –Dibble et al[116]	Secondary analysis of gender differences in perception of QOL	For women, phychosocial well-being and physical competence, and for men, vitality and personal resources emerged as important in assessing QOL	Gender-specific questions need to be built into QOL scales to improve validity
Piper Fatigue Scale (PFS) –Piper et al[117]	To confirm multidimensionality of scale and to reduce number of items without compromising validity and reliability	Result: 22 items and 4 subscales: behavior, affect, sensory, and cognitive; some redundancy still remains	Additional revisions to increase ability to clinically measure an ubiquitous side effect of treatment
Schwartz Cancer Fatigue Scale (SCFS) –Schwartz[118]	Four factors accounting for 70% variance: physical, emotional, cognitive, temporal; 28 items	Cronbach alpha for total scale 0.96 with between 0.82–0.93 for subscales	Clinically relevent measure in assessing effect of fatigue treatment measures and for overall management
Family Inventory of Needs-Husbands (FIN-H) –Kilpatrick et al[119]	Information needs of husbands of women with breast cancer; to determine internal consistency, tet–retest reliability and internal validity	Established internal consistency and test–retest reliability; found 5 factors: pre- and postop care needs, communication with health professionals, family relationship issues, disease/treatment specifics, husband's practical involvement	Provides a valid, consistent tool for determining educational needs of husbands
Hope Assessment Guide –Penrod and Morse[120]	Hope	Conceptual model of hope provides good fit for assessment and intervention planning	Provides a background in processes of developing hope for the nurse
Pain Management Documentation Tool –Jadlos et al[121]	To assess acute and chronic pain after specific implemented pain management activities	Tool demonstrated consistency in documenting pain management activities	Use of pain assessment and pain management flow sheet with a pain protocol maximizes effect of the care process

measure the qualitative outcomes of nursing practice, or both.

Measurement tool development: qualitative

During the past ten years, an increasing interest in qualitative methods of research has become evident in the nursing literature. Measuring quality of care quantitatively does not readily capture the contextual nature and natural richness of the situational and interpersonal data that compose the nursing care environment.

Nursing literature generally reflects attempts at establishing patient databases composed of qualitative sets of indicators, predictors, and assessment parameters that form the foundations of patient concerns and nursing practices. For example, if we review the available quantitative tools, most are based on the identification of indicators grouped to facilitate diagnostic reasoning. However, less precision is found in scoring instrument results. Few scoring systems are based on large amounts of normative data, particularly those established in healthy populations that allow clear comparisons and interpretation of new data.

The most recognized qualitative approaches include case study, grounded theory, phenomenology, and ethnography, among others.[122] Qualitative research begins with carefully conceptualized and clearly articulated research questions to guide data collection and later interpretation. The motive is to understand an aspect of human experience and to shape a representation of it from the data. The results of the qualitative method may include (1) operationalizing a single concept, (2) developing a conceptual framework, (3) establishing guidelines for practice, (4) creating portraits, paradigm cases, or typologies, and (5) forming theory.

Although reliability testing and validity testing in the conventional sense do not have a place in the qualitative process, there are sound principles and methods to guide study design, data gathering, data analysis and management, data interpretation, and paradigm construction. These processes are no less rigorous than those of the quantitative approach. In many areas of quality of care research, the qualitative paradigm or a combination of the qualitative and quantitative paradigms may be the best approach.

The qualitative cancer nursing research literature represents a mixed bag of clinically relevant information that, for the purposes of understanding quality of care, may be categorized according to format and content considerations. The research articles have been grouped as either indicators, predictors, or guidelines for care.

Indicators are sets of variables that empirically describe an important clinical manifestation. They are derived generally from a review of published work on the subject or a descriptive exploratory or qualitative study, or both. For example, Saunders and Valente's article[123] on suicide in cancer patients brings together their wealth of empirical knowledge as well as general information about depression and suicide. One outcome is a useful "Brief

Suicide Assessment Guide" for practitioners. In contrast, Thorne[124] reported the results of her phenomenological study of the family cancer experience, providing important insights into family perceptions and coping strategies when a member has cancer. Therefore, information in a wide variety of content areas produced sets of clues to facilitate better understanding of many common clinical issues. Research on quality of life, family dynamics, and caregiver adjustment reflect an increased sophistication and utility of research-based guides to practice.

Predictors are variables that have been tested to determine their ability to predict a future event with some degree of accuracy. Predictors are critical to nursing's role in health promotion and prevention. For example, Hays's article[125] on predictors of hospice utilization identified specific patient and family parameters that, when taken into consideration early enough in the nursing plan of care, have a good chance of strengthening the family unit so that the patient can be maintained at home under quality care conditions for longer periods. Another illustration of the establishment of predictors is the research that has identified clusters of variables predicting the occurrence of anticipatory nausea and vomiting.[126,127]

Guidelines for care are organized, integrated schemata for practice. These presentations are readily identifiable by title descriptors such as nursing care, nursing interventions, nursing implications, the nursing role, nursing assessments, nursing management, and nursing plans for a variety of patient problems, specialized treatments, or situations. In most cases, guidelines are in tabular format, resembling the traditional nursing care plan (problem, care, scientific rationale) with updated language such as nursing diagnoses, nursing etiology, nursing interventions, and nursing evaluations by outcome criteria.

Table 72-7 provides a list of indicators, predictors, and assessment guidelines used in recent studies addressing quality of care.[127–280] These articles report studies of cancer-related disease and treatment problems, psychosocial adjustment, risk factors, and family response and coping.

Quality in Performance: Applications in Practice

No discussion of care is complete without a look at process—the performance of nursing care and its meaning for both patient and nurse. Although patient outcome has become the basis for care evaluation, the multiple forces impinging on a patient's condition often make this method of assessment partially precise at best. Outcomes are relative, and frequently are only partly related to the quality of nurse performance. More often, quality is deeply embedded in the rich, mutual interpretations of care and caring that constitute the nurse–patient bond. Measuring quality of care by documented patient outcome is only one aspect of the multipronged approach

Table 72-7 Indicators, Predictors, and Guidelines for Quality of Care

Indicators

Adaptive strategies with cancer diagnosis[127]
Adjustment of children to mother's breast cancer[128]
Beliefs about breast cancer and mammography[129]
Brain tumor support group content and support[130]
Cancer fatigue[131]
Coagulation values in central venous catheters[132]
Cognitive dysfunction in BRMT[133]
Cognitive/emotional disruption in patients after RT[134]
Information and decisions in breast cancer[135]
Nurses' ethical/moral experiences[136]
Pain with mammography[137]
Quality of life and hospice care[138]
Research-based practices by oncology staff nurses[139]
Self-esteem in women receiving chemotherapy[140]
Sexuality of elders with cancer[141]
Voluntary physician-assisted dying[142]
Wire localizations for nonpalpable breast lesions[143]
Quality of life and care during biological therapy[144]
Maintaining hope during BMT[145]
Quest for meaning after BMT[146-148]
Treatment effect on male fertility and sexuality[149]
Nursing diagnosis in an oncology population[150]
Spiritual health of oncology patients[151]
Patient/significant other's response to detection program[152]
Nurse knowledge/teaching/performance of breast exams[153]
Patterns of fatigue, activity, and rest[116,126,154-156]
Prostate cancer decisions[157]
Health promotion, screening, and detection[158,159]
Genetic discrimination in the workplace[160]
Nutritional assessment and weight loss in lung cancer[161]
Uncertainty, reappraisal, and distress in breast cancer[162-167]
Quality of life in cancer[127,168]
Pain[169,170]
Post-mastectomy reconstruction[171]
Partner and parental adjustment in cancer[172-180]
Body image in breast cancer[181]
Diarrhea[46,182,183]
Euthanasia[184,185]
Cancer economics[186]
Oral cavity toxicity in chemotherapy[187]
GYN cancer experience[188]
Hope[189,190]
Cancer patient concerns and information preferences[191,192]
Expectations regarding breast cancer care[193]
Risk taking and decisions of adolescent cancer survivors[194]

Predictors

Radiation skin reactions[195]
Attribution, control, and adjustment[196]
Constipation and opioids[197]
Delayed complications of BMT[198]
Discard volumes from heparinized Hickman catheters[199]
Family experience in breast cancer[200]
Family caregiver needs in home hospice[201]
Laminar air flow vs. reverse isolation in BMT[202]
Lung cancer experience[203]
Nurses' cancer pain management[204]
Obstacles to cancer care in disadvantaged[205]
Oral gram-negative bacilli in BMT[206]
Patient/nurse perceptions of BMT symptomology[207]
Precancerous and cancerous cervical lesions[208]
Side effects and self-care in patient chemotherapy[209]
Stress and development of breast cancer[210]
Strontium-89 treatment for prostate cancer[211]
Needs of home caregivers[212]

Fatigue mechanisms: tumor necrosis factor and exercise[213]
Sources of hope in chronic illness[214]
ARDS during interleukin-2 immunotherapy[215]
Precursors of cervical cancer[216]
Flushing protocols for central venous catheters[217]
Information seeking in HIV-positive homosexual/bisexual men[218]
Factors influencing successful return to workplace for cancer patients[219]
Effect of alkylating agent in acute nonlymphocytic leukemia[220]
Blood infusion[221]
DNA testing for cancer predisposition[222]
Menopause and ovarian toxicity in breast cancer[223]
Nausea and vomiting treatment algorithm[224]
Dihydropyrimidine dehydrogenase deficiency[225]
Pregnancy and cancer[226]
Symptom management[227]
Screening and detection[228]
Exercise[229]

Guidelines for Care

Acute myelogenous leukemia[230]
Acute tumor lysis syndrome[231]
Bacterial translocation with neutropenia[232]
Behavioral interventions in leukemia[233]
Bladder cancer[234]
Chronic myelogenous leukemia and acute promyelocytic leukemia[235]
Glial neoplasms[236]
Inpatient education and support programs[237]
Intravenous immunoglobulin[238]
Lambert-Eaton myasthenic syndrome[239]
Leukemia[240]
Patient involvement in treatment[241]
Producing videotapes for cancer education[242]
Social support and BSE[243]
Strategies to improve cancer education[244]
Testicular cancer[245]
Thyroid cancer[246]
Vena cava filters[247]
VIPoma[248]
Nursing implications for photodynamic therapy[249]
Care of patients with esophageal cancer[250]
Nursing of patients with multisystem organ failure[251]
Care of families[252]
Nursing care of irradiated skin[253]
Diversion activity to enhance coping[254]
Home care resources for rural families[255]
Nursing of patient receiving antimitotics in chemotherapy[256]
Bereavement care[257]
Pancreatic cancer[258]
Chemotherapy and IV therapy flowsheet[259]
Amifostine as pancytoprotectant[260]
Irinotecan hydrochloride-topoisomerase I inhibitor[261]
Stem cell transplant[262-264]
Hormone replacement therapy in breast cancer[265]
Hereditary colon cancer[266]
Osteoporosis in cancer survivors[267]
Interferon alfa-2b in melanoma[268]
Palliative care[269,270]
Leptomeningeal metastasis[271]
Pain[272-274]
Cancer risk assessment[275]
Prostate cancer screening[276]
Tamoxifen in breast cancer[277]
Thyroid cancer[278]
Transperineal palladium-103 prostate implants[279]
Nausea and vomiting[280]

required, an important indication that evaluation must go beyond the standard.

Determining the quality of a process is tricky but necessary for the search for excellence. There are four important patterns to the process of giving and receiving care. The first is *mutuality*. Care behavior and the caring attitude forge a mutual response between two people that is characterized by reciprocity and complementarity. The experience is shared and cooperative, and the roles of caregiver and care receiver are complementary in that there is a degree of dissimilarity in the nature of the role relationship that works in a nondissonant way, allowing for harmony. However, the degree of dissimilarity is important in that the effect of care can be compromised if patient–nurse perceptions are either too much alike or radically different.

Larson[281,282] laid a foundation for unraveling the intricacies involved in giving and receiving care. She interviewed two separate samples of patients and nurses to determine what nurse behaviors were most and least important in making cancer patients feel "cared for." Her assumption was that the optimal expectation of nursing care is for patients to feel cared for as a result of nursing actions. Feeling cared for was defined as a sensation of well-being and safety linked to the behavior of the nurse. Nurses and patients were asked to rank, in order of importance, 50 nurse caring behaviors categorized by six action themes: anticipation, accessibility, explanation–facilitation, provision of comfort, establishment of trust, and monitoring with follow-up. Findings revealed that patients and nurses held highly divergent opinions of what was most important. The highest-ranked behaviors reported by patients were those demonstrating competency, actions mostly concerned with monitoring and follow-up and with accessibility. Actions rated highest by nurses were more focused on meeting comfort and psychosocial needs, such as listening and touch. In an examination of the top ten responses of both groups, however, several mutual choices appeared: being quickly accessible, giving good physical care, putting the patient first, and listening. These choices indicated several important shared values.

Mayer[283] replicated Larson's study and found similar results. There was 100% agreement between samples of nurses in both studies regarding the most and least important caring behaviors. Comparisons of the two patient groups revealed 40% agreement for the most important behaviors and 80% for the least important. Across both studies and all samples, conventions of professional etiquette—such as appearance, cheerfulness, and polite social behavior—were viewed as least important. In Mayer's study, listening was again rated highest by nurses, and knowing how to give injections, intravenous infusions, and manage technical equipment remained most important to patients. Mayer concluded that patients seem to value the instrumental, technical caring skills whereas nurses are more attuned to expressive caring behaviors.

These results might reflect understandable differences in perception between the two groups. Patients seem to value those competencies and skills most concretely apparent and directly linked to their welfare. Nurses, on the other hand, may perceive expressive and instrumental dimensions of care as inextricably connected, similar to the mutuality of care and cure. Who can deny the effect when patient preparation, technical skill, and gentleness are integrated during administration of an uncomfortable, intrusive procedure? To emphasize one aspect without the others decontextualizes care and strips it of its healing quality.

As the site of cancer care increasingly moves into the home, the concept of caregiver will expand to include family members and others in charge of the patient's welfare. In light of this trend, congruence between caregiver and care recipient perceptions of quality of life was examined in 23 care dyads in a home hospice program.[284] The overall trend, although not statistically significant, was for patients to report a higher quality of life for themselves in comparison with their caregivers' assessments. Patients reported better sleeping and pain control than did caregivers, but much less fun and sexual satisfaction. Thus nurse caregivers are not alone in their struggle to interpret the patient's situation accurately.

The needs of family members as they care for their loved ones with cancer are emerging as an important dimension in quality of care. Dyck and Wright[285] found that almost half of their sample of next of kin said that nurses did not do anything for them as family members, nor did they expect anything. Their expectation, however, seemed to be a function of limitations in their knowledge of the role of the nurse and what was thought to be the appropriate focus—the patient. If the patient was competently cared for and the nurse kept the family accurately informed, families said they could not expect more. Yet a parallel analysis of their needs documented acceptance, support, and comfort as being very important to them. Furthermore, the traits they looked most for in nurses differed depending on the stage of the patient's illness. Competence was number one in the early diagnostic stage, friendliness when the disease recurred, and compassion during the terminal stage. The authors concluded that appropriate emphasis of a trait is contextually determined and a significant way that nurses may express "caring for" patients.

The second major pattern in the caregiving and care-receiving process is *context*. The contextual aspects of care have been highlighted repeatedly in these studies, with location of care and phase of illness emerging as two important determinants of the most appropriate clinical approach. Often, phenomenological studies provide the best look at contextuality.

For example, Thorne,[124] in studying helpful and unhelpful communications in care, refers to cancer as "a modern metaphor for human confrontation with existential uncertainty." She found that communication is important in shaping the illness experience. Patients in Thorne's study were able to recall communication with health care providers during their illness and distinguish between styles that were more and less helpful. She found that the more uncertain a patient's situation, the greater was the vulnerability to communication characterized by lack of concern. On the other hand, the providers' feelings of failure, vulnerability, and hopelessness were part of the total picture as well. Nurses did not figure prominently into this compilation of opinions about helpful and unhelpful communicators, although study subjects reported that physicians communicated more about the disease and nurses provided advice about treatment and the illness. More often, a communication was perceived to be helpful if it was thought to be intentionally supportive. The most frequent unhelpful type was described as advice that was intentionally unhelpful, when the person withheld information or abused his power. Moreover, most important to the caring process was content, style, and a manner perceived by the patient as intentionally designed to be useful, encouraging, and supportive.

Nine recent descriptive studies have cast a new and expanded light on the plight of caretakers, spouses, and parents during the cancer experience.[175–183] These studies highlight the importance of mutuality and context in determining the quality of nursing care performance. Yet two other patterns have emerged as major influences on quality of performance; these patterns are so mutually dependent that they are best considered as one: *competence* and *proficiency*.

Clinical practice involves constant interpretation and prediction based on complex, contextual information. The nurse's competence and proficiency grow with the ability to read the clinical situation based on past.

The fourth major pattern of the care process is *intention in caring*, which effectively coordinates the other patterns of mutuality, context, and competence/proficiency. Intention in caring requires awareness and a determined effort to provide quality care in any setting or to facilitate others as they provide care for cancer patients. It serves to enhance quality in practice by

- Recognizing that care is mutual—a cooperative venture between two human beings, based on a balanced complement of perceptions

- Considering the context of the care environment on the basis of an understanding of the shared meaning of the circumstances

- Encouraging pride in one's acquired competencies (knowledge, skills, attitudes, and traits) and having a desire to increase proficiency and become expert

Overall, intention in caring links the science and the art of nursing knowledge and skill. Its most overt manifestation in practice is known as *clinical judgment*. Intention in caring has increasingly emerged from a new level of self-confidence found in nursing and the public's view of the nurse as the true broker of quality oncology practice today.

Quality of Care for the Nurse

Increased attention has been given to the idea that being able to fully care for another means caring for yourself first. The National Family Caregivers Association (NCFA) has provided guidelines for family caregivers that have relevance for professional caregivers as well.[288] The Oncology Nursing Society also recognizes that oncology nurses need care as do their patients and families. The headline of a recent ONS publication[289] said, "Nurses need time for recreation, rest, and reflection." This advice is more crucial now than at any other time in oncology nursing history.

Conclusion

Every health care provider group today is struggling with the definition, provision, and evaluation of quality care. Nursing faces these challenges relying on its long tradition of empirically established caring skills and on the more recently compiled data from clinical research.

For two decades, experts in the quality assurance field have advocated a three-dimensional approach comprising structure, process, and outcome variables and their relatedness. Structural elements are those grounding fundamentals that provide a sense of shared purpose and criteria against which effectiveness can be measured. The structural elements include nursing's direction, definition, education, legislation, diagnostic taxonomy, standards of practice, research and technology, and programs of peer review and quality assurance.

Process is a much more elusive phenomenon in that it involves the performance of competencies characterized by knowledge, skills, human traits, and attitudes[49] under diverse and unique environmental conditions (contextuality) where the mutuality of caregiver and care receiver is central. Process is most manifest in the intention in caring of the care provider and in the proficiency with which competencies are revealed. Therefore, process is much more difficult to evaluate in comparison with the components of structure and outcome.

Oncology nursing has come closest to evaluating the process dimension by defining standards of performance that recognize several critical determinants of quality: continuously working to perfect the art, science, and skill of practice; participating as a contributing, valued member of the health care team; utilizing the problem-solving process in the planning, organization, and execution of care and in its evaluation through the conduct or utilization of research; and providing a health care service to patients on the basis of a host of both independent and interdependent interventions conducted in an autonomous way. The measurement of process is based generally on written documentation and periodic peer evaluation. Some attempts have been made to categorize[286] and to measure[43] proficiency, and the literature on caring as a science is expanding rapidly.

Outcome criteria have been defined in terms of patient outcomes, quality of life, and, for nursing to some degree, maximum life extension. These criteria are best represented by patient outcome standards and by a burgeoning literature focused on the quality of life of the individual with cancer and his or her family. As we gain knowledge about the quality of life, the purpose of nursing as a science of caring will more clearly be understood and will further enable us to foster, nurture, and strengthen its quality.

References

1. Nightingale F: *Notes on Nursing*. New York, Appleton-Century-Crofts, 1859
2. Benner P: Nursing as a caring profession. Working paper for the Academy of Nursing Annual Meeting, Kansas City, MO, October 16–18, 1988
3. Larson P: Cancer nurses' perceptions of caring. *Cancer Nurs* 9:86–92, 1986
4. Gaut DA: A philosophic orientation to caring, in Leininger MM (ed): *Care: The Essence of Nursing and Health*. Thorofare, NJ, Slack, 1984, pp 17–26
5. Leininger MM (ed): *Care: The Essence of Nursing*. Thorofare, NJ, Slack, 1984
6. Watson J: *Nursing: The Philosophy and Science of Caring*. Boston, Little, Brown, 1979
7. Oncology Nursing Society: The Role of the Oncology Nurse in Cancer Genetic Counseling. *Oncol Nurs Forum* 25:264, 1998
8. Dougherty CJ: *American Health Care: Realities, Rights, and Reforms*. New York, Oxford University Press, 1988
9. President's Commission for the Study of Ethical Problems in Medicine and Biomedical and Behavioral Research: *Securing Access to Health Care*, vol. 1. Washington, DC, U.S. Government Printing Office, 1983
10. Haylock PJ: Improving the quality of cancer care. *Oncol Nurs Forum* 24:949, 1997
11. Oncology Nursing Society: Position paper on quality cancer care. *Oncol Nurs Forum* 24:951–953, 1997
12. Oncology Nursing Society: Board approves revised scope of practice statement. *ONS News* 3:1–2, 1988
13. Bonvissuto C, Kostens J, Atwell S: Preparing health care organizations for successful case management programs. *J Case Management* 6(2):51–55, 1997
14. Oncology Nursing Society: Patients' bill of rights for quality cancer care. *Oncol Nurs Forum* 25:1301, 1998
15. Taylor C: *Philosophic Papers*, vols. 1 and 2. Cambridge, Cambridge University Press, 1985
16. Harmer C, Henderson V: *Principles and Practices of Nursing*. New York, Macmillan, 1956
17. Mundinger L: Nursing diagnoses for cancer patients. *Cancer Nurs* 1:221–226, 1978
18. Herberth L, Gosnell DJ: Nursing diagnosis for oncology nursing practice. *Cancer Nurs* 10:41–51, 1987
19. Gordon M: *Manual of Nursing Diagnoses: 1998–1999*. St. Louis, Mosby, 1999
20. American Nurses' Association: *Nursing: A Social Policy Statement*. Kansas City, MO, American Nurses' Association, 1980
21. Winchester DP: The assurance of quality for the cancer patient. Paper presented at the American Cancer Society Symposium on Advances in Cancer Management, Los Angeles, December 1988
22. Beyers M: Quality: The banner of the 1980s. *Nurs Clin North Am* 23:617–623, 1988
23. Ackley BJ, and Ladwig GB: *Nursing Diagnos Handbook: A Guide to Planning Care*. St. Louis, Mosby, 1997
24. National Cancer Institute: Five-year survival rates. *SEER Program*. Washington, DC, U.S. Government Printing Office, 1983
25. Henderson M: Introduction, in Roberts L (ed): *Cancer Today: Origins, Prevention, and Treatment*. Washington, DC, National Academy of Sciences Press, 1984
26. Oncology Nursing Society: *Outcome Standards for Cancer Nursing Practice*. Pittsburgh, Oncology Nursing Society, 1979
27. Oncology Nursing Society and American Nurses' Association: *Standards of Oncology Nursing Practice*. Kansas City, MO, American Nurses' Association, 1987
28. Oncology Nursing Society: *Statement on the Scope and Standards of Oncology Nursing Practice*. Pittsburgh: Oncology Nursing Society, 1996
29. American Nurses' Association: *A Plan for Implementation of Standards of Nursing Practice*. Kansas City, MO, American Nurses' Association, 1979
30. Oncology Nursing Society: *Standards of Oncology Nursing Education*. Pittsburgh, Oncology Nursing Society, 1995
31. Oncology Nursing Society: *Standards of Oncology Education*. Pittsburgh, Oncology Nursing Society, 1995
32. Oncology Nursing Society, *Statement on the Scope and Standards of Advanced Oncology Nursing Practice*. Pittsburgh: Oncology Nursing Society, 1997
33. Scott DW: *The Research Connection: Practice, Research, Theory*. Keynote address to American Cancer Society Nursing Research Conference, Honolulu, Hawaii, June 1985. Denver, American Cancer Society, 1986
34. Brown MH, Kiss ME: Cancer audit. *Cancer Nurs* 2:1–6, 1979
35. Legge JS, Reilly BJ: Assessing the outcomes of cancer patients in a home nursing program. *Cancer Nurs* 3:357, 1980
36. Valencius JC, Packard R, Widiss T: The ONS-ANA Outcome Standards for Cancer Nursing Practice: two models for implementation—implementation of the nutrition standard at City of Hope National Medical Center. *Oncol Nurs Forum* 7:137–140, 1980
37. Edlund BJ: Patient education: determining the effectiveness of an ostomy care guide in facilitating comprehensive patient care. *Oncol Nurs Forum* 8:43–46, 1981
38. Wood HA, Ellerhorst JM: Using site-specific nursing algorithms as an adjunct to oncology nursing guidelines. *Oncol Nurs Forum* 10:22–27, 1983
39. Joint Commission on the Accreditation of Hospitals: *Accreditation Manual for Hospitals* (AMH/88). Chicago, Joint Commission on the Accreditation of Hospitals, 1987
40. Patterson CH: Standards of patient care: the Joint Commission focus on nursing quality assurance. *Nurs Clin North Am* 23:625–638, 1988
41. Miaskowski CA, Nielsen B: A cancer nursing assessment tool. *Oncol Nurs Forum* 12:37–42, 1985
42. Gray G, Adler D, Fleming C, et al: A clinical data base for advanced cancer patients: implications for nursing. *Cancer Nurs* 11:77–83, 1988
43. Moore IM, Piper B, Dodd MJ, et al: Measuring oncology nursing practice: results from one graduate program. *Oncol Nurs Forum* 14:45–49, 1987

44. McGee RF, Powell ML, Broadwell DC, et al: A Delphi survey of oncology nurse specialist competencies. *Oncol Nurs Forum* 14:29–34, 1987

45. Yasko JM: A survey of oncology clinical nursing specialists. *Oncol Nurs Forum* 10:25–30, 1983

46. Rutledge DN, Engelking C: Cancer-related diarrhea: selected findings of a national survey of oncology nurse experiences. *Oncol Nurs Forum* 25:861–873, 1998

47. Satterwhite BA, Pryor AS, Harris MB: Development and evaluation of chemotherapy fact sheets. *Cancer Nurs* 3:277–284, 1980

48. Dodd MJ, Mood DW: Chemotherapy: helping patients to know the drugs they are receiving and their possible side effects. *Cancer Nurs* 4:311–318, 1981

49. Dodd MJ: Self-care for side effects in cancer chemotherapy: an assessment of nursing interventions. Part II. *Cancer Nurs* 6:63–67, 1983

50. Johnson J: The effects of a patient education course on persons with a chronic illness. *Cancer Nurs* 5:117–123, 1982

51. Miller MW, Nygren C: Living with cancer: coping behaviors. *Cancer Nurs* 1:297–302, 1978

52. Marty PJ, McDermott RJ, Gold RS: An assessment of three alternative formats for promoting breast self-examination. *Cancer Nurs* 6:207–211, 1983

53. Watson PJ: The effects of short-term postoperative counseling on cancer/ostomy patients. *Cancer Nurs* 6:21–29, 1985

54. Heinrich RL, Schag CC: A behavioral medicine approach to coping with cancer: a case report. *Cancer Nurs* 7:243–247, 1984

55. Coleman EA, Riley MB, Fields F, et al: Efficacy of breast self-examination teaching methods among older women. *Oncol Nurs Forum* 18:561–566, 1991

56. Weinrich SP, Weinrich MC, Boyd MD, and Atkinson C: The impact of prostate cancer knowledge on cancer screening. *Oncol Nurs Forum* 25:527–534, 1998

57. Hagopian GA: The effects of a weekly radiation therapy newsletter on patients. *Oncol Nurs Forum* 18:1199–1203, 1991

58. Hagopian GA: The effects of informational audiotapes on knowledge and self-care behaviors of patients undergoing radiation therapy. *Oncol Nurs Forum* 23:697–700, 1996

59. Hughes KK: Decision making by patients with breast cancer: the role of information in treatment selection. *Oncol Nurs Forum* 20:623–628, 1993

60. Mansson ME, Bjorkhem G, Wiebe T: The effect of preparation for lumbar puncture on children undergoing chemotherapy. *Oncol Nurs Forum* 20:39–45, 1993

61. Collins M: Increasing prostate cancer awareness in African American men. *Oncol Nurs Forum* 24:91–95, 1997

62. Wewers ME, Jenkins L, Mignery T: A nurse-managed smoking cessation intervention during diagnostic testing for lung cancer. *Oncol Nurs Forum* 24:1419–1422, 1997

63. Beck SL: The therapeutic use of music for cancer-related pain. *Oncol Nurs Forum* 18:1327–1337, 1991

64. Broome ME, Lillis PP, McGahee TW, et al: The use of distraction and imagery with children during painful procedures. *Oncol Nurs Forum* 19:499–502, 1992

65. Ezzone S, Baker S, Rosselet R, et al: Music as an adjunct to antiemetic therapy. *Oncol Nurs Forum* 25:1551–1556, 1998

66. Mock V, Dow KH, Meares CJ, et al: Effects of exercise on fatigue, physical functioning and emotional distress during radiation therapy for breast cancer. *Oncol Nurs Forum* 24:991–1000, 1997

67. Mehta NH, Reed CM, Kuhlman C, et al: Controlling condition-related emesis in children undergoing bone marrow transplantation. *Oncol Nurs Forum* 24:1539–1544, 1997

68. Sarna L: Effectiveness of structured nursing assessment of symptom distress in advanced lung cancer. *Oncol Nurs Forum* 25:1041–1048, 1998

69. Mock V, Burke MB, Sheehan P, et al: A nursing rehabilitation program for women with breast cancer receiving adjuvant chemotherapy. *Oncol Nurs Forum* 21:597–605, 1994

70. Coward DD: Facilitation of self-transcendence in a breast cancer support group. *Oncol Nurs Forum* 25:75–83, 1998

71. Segar ML, Katch VL, Roth RS, et al: The effect of aerobic exercise on self-esteem and depression and anxiety symptoms among breast cancer survivors. *Oncol Nurs Forum* 25:107–113, 1998

72. Wyatt GK, Friedman LL: Physical and psychosocial outcomes of midlife and older women following surgery and adjuvant therapy for breast cancer. *Oncol Nurs Forum* 25:761–768, 1998

73. Samarel N, Fawcett J, Davis MM, et al: Effects of dialogue and therapeutic touch on preoperative and postoperative experiences of breast cancer surgery: an exploratory study. *Oncol Nurs Forum* 25:1369–1376, 1998

74. Johnson JE, Fieler VK, Wlasowicz GS, et al: The effects of nursing care guided by self-regulation theory on coping with radiation therapy. *Oncol Nurs Forum* 24:1041–1050, 1997

75. Brandt B, DePalma J, Irwin M, et al: Comparison of central venous catheter dressings in bone marrow transplant recipients. *Oncol Nurs Forum* 23:829–836, 1996

76. Dodd MJ, Larson PJ, Dibble SL: Randomized clinical trial of chlorhexidine versus placebo for prevention of oral mucositis in patients receiving chemotherapy. *Oncol Nurs Forum* 23:921–927, 1996

77. Shivnan JC, McGuire D, Freedman S, et al: A comparison of transparent adherent and dry sterile gauze dressings for long-term central catheters in patients undergoing bone marrow transplant. *Oncol Nurs Forum* 18:1349–1356, 1991

78. Yeoman A, Davitt M, Peters CA, et al: Efficacy of chlorhexidene gluconate use in the prevention of perirectal infections in patients with acute leukemia. *Oncol Nurs Forum* 18:1207–1213, 1991

79. DeMoissac D, Jensen L: Changing IV administration sets: is 48 versus 24 hours safe for neutropenic patients with cancer? *Oncol Nurs Forum* 25:907–913, 1998

80. Norville R, Hinds P, Wilimas J, et al: The effects of infusion rate on platelet outcomes and patient responses in children with cancer: an in vitro and in vivo study. *Oncol Nurs Forum* 24:1789–1793, 1997

81. Mayo DJ, Horne MK, Summers BL, et al: The effects of heparin flush on patency of the Groshong catheter: a pilot study. *Oncol Nurs Forum* 23:1401–1405, 1996

82. Beck S, Breckenridge-Patter S, Wallace S, et al: The Family High-Risk Program: targeted cancer prevention. *Oncol Nurs Forum* 15:301–306, 1988

83. Nieweg R, Greidanus J, de Vries EGE: A patient education program for a continuous infusion regimen on an outpatient basis. *Cancer Nurs* 10:177–182, 1987

84. McMillan SC, Title MB, Hill D: A systematic evaluation of the "I Can Cope" program using a national sample. *Oncol Nurs Forum* 20:455–461, 1993

85. Pillon LR, Joannides G: An 11-year evaluation of a Living with Cancer program. *Oncol Nurs Forum* 18:707–711, 1991

86. Lane CA, Davis AW: Implementation: We Can Week-end in the rural setting. *Cancer Nurs* 8:323–328, 1985

87. Fredette S, La F, Beattie HM: Living with cancer: a patient education program. *Cancer Nurs* 9:308–316, 1986

88. Cawley MM, Gerdts EK: Establishing a cancer caregiver's program: an interdisciplinary approach. *Cancer Nurs* 11:266–273, 1988

89. Diekmann JM: An evaluation of selected "I Can Cope" programs by registered participants. *Cancer Nurs* 11:274–282, 1988

90. Mosely JR, Logan SJ, Tolle SW, et al: Developing a bereavement program in a university hospital setting. *Oncol Nurs Forum* 15:151–155, 1988

91. Coyle N, Monzillo E, Loscalzo M, et al: A model for continuity of care for cancer patients with pain and neuro-oncologic complications. *Cancer Nurs* 8:111–119, 1985

92. Coyle N, Mauskop A, Maggard J, et al: Continuous SC infusions of opiates for cancer patients with pain. *Oncol Nurs Forum* 13:53–57, 1986

93. Ferrell BR, Wenzl C, Wisdom C: Evolution and evaluation of a pain management team. *Oncol Nurs Forum* 15:285–289, 1988

94. Kane NE, Lehman ME, Drugger R, et al: Use of patient-controlled anesthesia in surgical oncology patients. *Oncol Nurs Forum* 15:29–32, 1988

95. Konstantinides NI: Home parenteral nutrition: a viable alternative for patients with cancer. *Oncol Nurs Forum* 12:23–29, 1985

96. Long MC, Ovaska M: Comparative study of nursing protocols for venous access ports. *Cancer Nurs* 15:18–21, 1992

97. Clark M: A day hospital for cancer patients: clinical and economic feasibility. *Oncol Nurs Forum* 13:41–45, 1986

98. Pluth NM: A home transfusion program. *Oncol Nurs Forum* 14:43–46, 1987

99. Lewis PM: Implementing practice and organizational models. *Cancer Nurs* 8:75–78, 1985 (suppl 1)

100. Hartshorn JC: Research-based practice: the need for, use and reporting of instrument reliability and validity. *Heart Lung* 16:100–101, 1987

101. Duffy ME: Research in practice: the time has come. *Nurs Health Care* 6:127, 1985

102. Lynn MR: Reliability estimates: use and disuse. *Nurs Res* 34:254–256, 1985

103. Frank-Stromborg M (ed): *Instruments for Clinical Nursing Research* (ed 2). Boston, Jones and Bartlett, 1997

104. Nunally JC: *Psychometric Theory.* New York, McGraw-Hill, 1978

105. Burns JM, Tierney DK: A daily flowsheet for an outpatient bone marrow transplant treatment center. *Oncol Nurs Forum* 23:1313–1316, 1996

106. Allaster RM, Frayne BK, Malpage AS, et al: Development of a comprehensive nursing/toxicity assessment form. *Oncol Nurs Forum* 23:1317–1324, 1996

107. Camp LD: A comparison of nurses' recorded assessments of pain with perceptions of pain as described by cancer patients. *Cancers Nurs* 11:237–243, 1988

108. Coward DD: Hypercalcemia knowledge assessment in patients at risk of developing cancer-induced hypercalcemia. *Oncol Nurs Forum* 15:471–476, 1988

109. Derdiarian AK: Sensitivity of the Derdiarian Behavioral System Model instrument to age, site, and stage of cancer: a preliminary validation study. *Sch Inq Nurs Pract* 2:103–127, 1988

110. Eilers J, Berger AM, Petersen MC: Development, testing and application of the oral assessment guide. *Oncol Nurs Forum* 15:325–330, 1988

111. Lauver D: Development of a questionnaire to measure beliefs and attitudes about breast self-examination. *Cancer Nurs* 11:51–57, 1988

112. McMillan SC, Williams FA, Chatfield R, et al: Validity and reliability study of two tools for assessing and managing cancer pain. *Oncol Nurs Forum* 15:735–741, 1988

113. Rhodes VA, Watson PM, Hanson BM: Patients' descriptions of the influence of tiredness and weakness on self-care abilities. *Cancer Nurs* 11:186–194, 1988

114. Sutherland HJ, Walker P, Till JE: The development of a method for determining oncology patients' emotional distress using linear analogue scales. *Cancer Nurs* 11:303–308, 1988

115. Williams RD: Factors affecting practice of BSE in older women. *Oncol Nurs Forum* 15:611–616, 1988

116. Dibble SL, Padilla GV, Dodd MJ, et al: Gender differences in the dimensions of quality of life. *Oncol Nurs Forum* 25:577–583, 1998

117. Piper BF, Dibble SL, Dodd MJ, et al: The revised Piper Fatigue Scale: psychometric evaluation in women with breast cancer. *Oncol Nurs Forum* 25:677–684, 1998

118. Schwartz AL: Patterns of exercise and fatigue in physically active cancer survivors. *Oncol Nurs Forum* 25:485–491, 1988

119. Kilpatrick MG, Kristjanson LJ, Tataryn DJ: Measuring the information needs of husbands and women with breast cancer: validity and reliability of the Family Inventory of Needs–Husbands. *Oncol Nurs From* 25:1347–1351, 1998

120. Penrod J: The lived experience of surviving breast cancer. *Oncol Nurs Forum* 24:1343–1351, 1997

121. Jadlos MA, Kelman GB, Marra K, et al: A pain management documentation tool. *Oncol Nurs Forum* 23:1451–1454, 1996

122. Ammon-Gaberson KB, Piantanida M: Generating results from qualitative data. *Image* 20:159–161, 1988

123. Saunders JM, Valente SM: Cancer and suicide. *Oncol Nurs Forum* 15:575–581, 1988

124. Thorne SE: Helpful and unhelpful communications in cancer care: the patient perspective. *Oncol Nurs Forum* 15:167–172, 1988

125. Hays JC: Patient symptoms and family coping. *Cancer Nurs* 9:317–325, 1986

126. Duigon A: Anticipatory nausea and vomiting associated with cancer chemotherapy. *Oncol Nurs Forum* 13:35–40, 1986

127. Hagopian GA: Cognitive strategies used in adapting to a cancer diagnosis. *Oncol Nurs Forum* 20:759–763, 1993

128. Armsden GC, Lewis FM: Behavioral adjustment of school-age children of women with breast cancer. *Oncol Nurs Forum* 21:39–45, 1994

129. Champion VL: Beliefs about breast cancer and mammography by behavioral stage. *Oncol Nurs Forum* 21:1009–1014, 1994

130. Leavitt MB, Lamb SA, Voss BS: Brain tumor support group: content themes and mechanisms of support. *Oncol Nurs Forum* 23:1247–1256, 1996

131. Winningham ML, Nail LM, Burke MB, et al: Fatigue and the cancer experience: the state of the knowledge. *Oncol Nurs Forum* 21:23–36, 1994

132. Pinto KM: Accuracy of coagulation values obtained from a heparinized central venous catheter. *Oncol Nurs Forum* 21:573–575, 1994

133. Bender CM: Cognitive dysfunction associated with biological response modifier therapy. *Oncol Nurs Forum* 21:515–523, 1994

134. Walker BL, Nail LM, Larsen L, et al: Concerns, affect and cognition disruption following completion of radiation treatment for localized breast or prostate cancer. *Oncol Nurs Forum* 23:1181–1187, 1996

135. Bilodeau BA, Degner LF: Information needs, sources of information and decisional roles in women with breast cancer. *Oncol Nurs Forum* 23:691–696, 1996

136. O'Connor KF: Ethical/moral experiences of oncology nurses. *Oncol Nurs Forum* 23:787–794, 1996

137. Nielsen B, Miaskowski C, Dibble SL: Pain and mammography: fact or fiction? *Oncol Nurs Forum* 20:639–642, 1993

138. McMillan SC: The quality of life of patients with cancer receiving hospice care. *Oncol Nurs Forum* 23:1221–1228, 1996

139. Rutledge DN, Greene P, Mooney K, et al: Use of research-based practices by oncology staff nurses. *Oncol Nurs Forum* 23:1235–1241, 1996

140. Carpenter JS, Brockapp DY: Evaluation of self-esteem of women with cancer receiving chemotherapy. *Oncol Nurs Forum* 21:751–757, 1994

141. Shell JA, Smith CK: Sexuality and the older person with cancer. *Oncol Nurs Forum* 21:553–558, 1994

142. Young A, Volker D, Rieger PT, et al: Oncology nurses' attitudes regarding voluntary, physician-assisted dying for competent, terminally ill patients. *Oncol Nurs Forum* 20:445–451, 1993

143. Kelly P, Winslow EH: Needle wire localization for nonpalpable breast lesions: sensations, anxiety levels, and informational needs. *Oncol Nurs Forum* 23:639–645, 1996

144. Rieker PP, Clark EJ, Fogelberg PR: Perceptions of quality of life and quality of care for patients with cancer receiving biological therapy. *Oncol Nurs Forum* 19:433–440, 1992

145. Ersek M: The process of maintaining hope in adults undergoing bone marrow transplantation for leukemia. *Oncol Nurs Forum* 19:883–889, 1992

146. Steeves RH: Patients who have undergone bone marrow transplantation: their quest for meaning. *Oncol Nurs Forum* 19:899–905, 1992

147. Ferrell B, Grant M, Schmidt GM, et al: The meaning of quality of life for bone marrow transplant survivors. Part I: the impact of bone marrow transplant on quality of life. *Cancer Nurs* 15:153–160, 1992

148. Ferrell B, Grant M, Schmidt GM, et al: The meaning of quality of life for bone marrow transplant survivors. Part 2: improving quality of life for bone marrow transplant survivors. *Cancer Nurs* 15:247–253, 1992

149. Smith DB, Babaian RJ: The effects of treatment for cancer on male fertility and sexuality. *Cancer Nurs* 15:271–275, 1992

150. MacAvoy S, Moritz D: Nursing diagnoses in an oncology population. *Cancer Nurs* 15:264–270, 1992

151. Highfield MF: Spiritual health of oncology patients: nurse and patient perspectives. *Cancer Nurs* 15:1–8, 1992

152. Vranicar-Lapka D, Barbour-Randall L, Trippon M, et al: Oncology patients' and their significant others' responses to a proposed cancer prevention/detection program. *Cancer Nurs* 15:47–53, 1992

153. Ludwick R: Registered nurses' knowledge and practices of teaching and performing breast exams among elderly women. *Cancer Nurs* 15:61–67, 1992

154. Berger AM: Patterns of fatigue and activity and rest during adjuvant breast cancer chemotherapy. *Oncol Nurs Forum* 25:51–62, 1998

155. Woo B, Dibble SL, Piper BF, et al: Differences in fatigue by treatment methods in women with breast cancer. *Oncol Nurs Forum* 25:915–920, 1998

156. Messias KKH, Yeagear KA, Dibble SL, et al: Patients' perspectives of fatigue while undergoing chemotherapy. *Oncol Nurs Forum* 24:43–48, 1997

157. O'Rourke ME, Germino BB: Prostate cancer treatment decisions: a focus group exploration. *Oncol Nurs Forum* 25:97–104, 1998

158. Bakkor DA, Lightfoot NE, Steggles S, et al: The experience and satisfaction of women attending breast cancer screening. *Oncol Nurs Forum* 25:115–121, 1998

159. Fitch MI, Greenberg M, Levstein L, et al: Health promotion and early detection of cancer in older adults: assessing knowledge about cancer. *Oncol Nurs Forum* 24:10, 1743–1748, 1997

160. Jacobs LA: At-risk for cancer: genetic discrimination in the workplace. *Oncol Nurs Forum* 25:475–480, 1998

161. Brown JK, Raake KJ: Nutritional assessment, intervention, and evaluation of weight loss in patients with non-small cell lung cancer. *Oncol Nurs Forum* 25:547–553, 1998

162. Mast ME: Survivors of breast cancer: illness uncertainty, positive reappraisal, and emotional distress. *Oncol Nurs Forum* 25:555–562, 1998

163. Steginga S, Occhipinti S, Wilson K, et al: Domains of distress: the experience of breast cancer in Australia. *Oncol Nurs Forum* 25:1063–1070, 1998

164. DeKeyser FG, Wainstock JM, Rose L, et al: Distress, symptom distress and immune function in women with suspected breast cancer. *Oncol Nurs Forum* 25:1415–1422, 1998

165. Pelusi J: The lived experience of surviving breast cancer. *Oncol Nurs Forum* 24:1343–1353, 1997

166. Longman AJ, Braden CJ, Mishel MH: Pattern of association over time of side-effects burden, self-help and self-care in women with breast cancer. *Oncol Nurs Forum* 24:1555–1560, 1997

167. Hoskins CN: Breast cancer treatment-related patterns in side effects, psychological distress, and perceived health status. *Oncol Nurs Forum* 24:1575–1583, 1997

168. Yarbro CH, Ferrans CE: Quality of life of patients with prostate cancer treated with surgery or radiation therapy. *Oncol Nurs Forum* 25:685–693, 1998

169. Burrows M, Dibble SL, Miaskowski D: Differences in outcome among patients experiencing different types of cancer-related pain. *Oncol Nurs Forum* 25:735–741, 1998

170. Riddell A, Fitch MI: Patients' knowledge and attitudes toward the management of cancer pain. *Oncol Nurs Forum* 24:1775–1784, 1997

171. Neill KM, Armstrong N, Burnett CB: Choosing reconstruction after mastectomy: a qualitative analysis. *Oncol Nurs Forum* 25:743–750, 1998

172. Morse SR, Fife B: Coping with a partner's cancer: adjustment at four stages of the illness trajectory. *Oncol Nurs Forum* 25:751–760, 1998

173. Kilpatrick MG, Kristjanson LJ, Tataryn DJ, et al: Information needs of husbands of women with breast cancer. *Oncol Nurs Forum* 25:1595–1601, 1998

174. Silveira JM, Winstead-Fry P: The needs of patients with cancer and their caregivers in rural areas. *Oncol Nurs Forum* 24:71–76, 1997

175. Hinds PS, Oakes L, Furman W, et al: Decision making by parents and healthcare professionals when considering continued care for pediatric patients with cancer. *Oncol Nurs Forum* 24:1523–1528, 1997

176. Douglass LG: Reciprocal support in the context of cancer:

perspectives of the patient and spouse. *Oncol Nurs Forum* 24:1529–1536, 1997

177. Meares CJ: Primary caregiver perceptions of intake cessation in patients who are terminally ill. *Oncol Nurs Forum* 24:1751–1765, 1997

178. Stetz KM, McDonald JC, Compton K: Needs and experiences of family caregivers during marrow transplantation. *Oncol Nurs Forum* 23:1422–1427, 1996

179. Compton K, McDonald JC, Stetz KM: Understanding the caring relationship during marrow transplantation: family caregivers and healthcare professionals. *Oncol Nurs Forum* 23:1428–1432, 1996

180. McDonald JC, Stetz KM, Compton K: Educational interventions for family caregivers during marrow transplantation. *Oncol Nurs Forum* 23:1432–1439, 1996

181. Cohen MZ, Kahn DL, Steeves RH: Beyond body image: the experience of breast cancer. *Oncol Nurs Forum* 25:835–841, 1998

182. Ippolitti C, Neumann J: Octreotide in the management of diarrhea induced by graft versus host disease. *Oncol Nurs Forum* 25:873–878, 1998

183. Hogan CM: The nurse's role in diarrhea management. *Oncol Nurs Forum* 25:879–886, 1998

184. Musgrave CF: Active euthanasia and assisted suicide: a perspective from an American abortion and Dutch euthanasia scenario. *Oncol Nurs Forum* 25:1587–1591, 1998

185. Matzo ML, Emanual EJ: Oncology nurses' practices of assisted suicide and patient-requested euthanasia. *Oncol Nurs Forum* 24:1725–1732, 1997

186. Moore K: Out-of-pocket expenditures of outpatients receiving chemotherapy. *Oncol Nurs Forum* 25:1615–1622, 1998

187. Berger AM, Eilers J: Factors influencing oral cavity status during high-dose antineoplastic therapy: a secondary data analysis. *Oncol Nurs Forum* 25:1623–1626, 1998

188. Steginga SK, Dunn J: Women's experiences following treatment for gynecologic cancer. *Oncol Nurs Forum* 24:1403–1408, 1997

189. Koopmeiners L, Post-White J, Gutknecht S, et al: How healthcare professionals contribute to hope in patients with cancer. *Oncol Nurs Forum* 24:1507–1513, 1997

190. Post-White J, Ceronsky C, Kreitzer MJ, et al: Hope, spirituality, quality of life in patients with cancer. *Oncol Nurs Forum* 23:1571–1579, 1996

191. Burman ME, Weinert C: Concerns of rural men and women experiencing cancer. *Oncol Nurs Forum* 24:1593–1600, 1997

192. Fieler VK, Wlasowicz GS, Mitchell ML, et al: Information preferences of patients undergoing radiation therapy. *Oncol Nurs Forum* 23:1603–1608, 1996

193. Lauver D, Angerame M: Women's expectations about seeking care for breast cancer symptoms. *Oncol Nurs Forum* 20:520–523, 1993

194. Hollen PJ, Hobbie WL: Risk taking and decision making of adolescent long-term survivors of cancer. *Oncol Nurs Forum* 20:769–776, 1993

195. Porock D, Kristjanson L, Nikoletti S, et al: Predicting the severity of radiation skin reactions in women with breast cancer. *Oncol Nurs Forum* 25:1019–1029, 1998

196. Berckman KL, Austin JK: Causal attribution, perceived control and adjustment. *Oncol Nurs Forum* 20:23–30, 1993

197. Canty SL: Constipation as a side effect of opioids. *Oncol Nurs Forum* 21:739–745, 1994

198. Buchsel PC, Leum EW, Randolph SR: Delayed complications of bone marrow transplantation: an update. *Oncol Nurs Forum* 23:1305–1312, 1996

199. Mayo DJ, Dimond EP, Kramer W, et al: Discard volumes necessary for clinically useful coagulation studies from heparinized Hickman catheters. *Oncol Nurs Forum* 23:671–675, 1996

200. Hilton BA: Getting back to normal: the family experience during early stage breast cancer. *Oncol Nurs Forum* 23:605–614, 1996

201. Steele RG, Fitch MI: Needs of family caregivers of patients receiving home hospice care for cancer. *Oncol Nurs Forum* 23:823–828, 1996

202. Zerbe MB, Parkerson SG, Spitzer T: Laminar air flow vs. reverse isolation: nurses' assessments of moods, behaviors and activity levels in patients receiving bone marrow transplants. *Oncol Nurs Forum* 21:565–568, 1994

203. Lindsey AM, Larson PJ, Sarna L, et al: The lung cancer experience: nutritional intake, weight, functional status, and other factors—comparison of variables and findings across three studies. *Oncol Nurs Forum* 20:465–493, 1993

204. O'Brien S, Dalton JA, Konsler G, et al: The knowledge and attitudes of experienced oncology nurses regarding the management of cancer-related pain. *Oncol Nurs Forum* 23:515–521, 1996

205. Underwood SM, Hoskins D, Cummins T, et al: Obstacles to cancer care: focus on the economically disadvantaged. *Oncol Nurs Forum* 21:47–52, 1994

206. Raybould TP, Carpenter AD, Ferretti GA, et al: Emergence of gram-negative bacilli in the mouths of bone marrow transplant recipients using chlorhexidine mouthrinse. *Oncol Nurs Forum* 21:691–696, 1994

207. Larson PJ, Viele CS, Coleman S, et al: Comparison of perceived symptoms of patients undergoing bone marrow transplant and the nurses caring for them. *Oncol Nurs Forum* 20:81–88, 1993

208. Lovejoy NC: Precancerous and cancerous cervical lesions: the multicultural "male" risk factor. *Oncol Nurs Forum* 21:497–504, 1994

209. Foltz AT, Gaines G, Gullotte M: Recalled side effects and self-care actions of patients receiving in-patient chemotherapy. *Oncol Nurs Forum* 23:679–683, 1996

210. Bryla CM: The relationship between stress and the development of breast cancer: a literature review. *Oncol Nurs Forum* 23:441–448, 1996

211. Altman GB, Lee CA: Strontium-89 for treatment of painful bone metastasis from prostate cancer. *Oncol Nurs Forum* 23:523–527, 1996

212. Hileman JW, Lackey NR, Hassanein RS: Identifying the needs of home caregivers of patients with cancer. *Oncol Nurs Forum* 19:771–777, 1992

213. St. Pierre BA, Kasper CE, Lindsey AM: Fatigue mechanisms in patients with cancer: effects of tumor necrosis factor and exercise on skeletal muscle. *Oncol Nurs Forum* 19:419–425, 1992

214. Raleigh EDH: Sources of hope in chronic illness. *Oncol Nurs Forum* 19:443–448, 1992

215. Farrell MM: The challenge of adult respiratory distress syndrome during interleukin-2 immunotherapy. *Oncol Nurs Forum* 19:475–480, 1992

216. Yoder L, Rubin M: The epidemiology of cervical cancer and its precursors. *Oncol Nurs Forum* 19:485–493, 1992

217. Kelly C, Dumenko L, McGregor SE, et al: A change in flushing protocols of central venous catheters. *Oncol Nurs Forum* 19:599–605, 1992

218. Lovejoy NC, Morgenrath BN, Paul S, et al: Potential predictors of information-seeking behavior by homosexual/bisexual (gay) men with a human immunodeficiency virus

seropositive health status. *Cancer Nurs* 15:116–124, 1992

219. Berry DL, Catanzaro M: Persons with cancer and their return to the workplace. *Cancer Nurs* 15:40–46, 1992

220. Uhlenhopp MB: An overview of the relationship between alkylating agents and therapy-related acute nonlymphocytic leukemia. *Cancer Nurs* 15:9–17, 1992

221. Cosca PA, Smith S, Chatfield S, et al: Reinfusion of discard blood from venous access devices. *Oncol Nurs Forum* 25:1073–1079, 1998

222. Loescher LJ: DNA testing for cancer predisposition. *Oncol Nurs Forum* 25:1317–1327, 1998

223. Knobf MT: Natural menopause and ovarian toxicity associated with breast cancer therapy. *Oncol Nurs Forum* 25:1519–1530, 1998

224. Johnson MH, Moroney CE, Gay CF: Relieving nausea and vomiting in patients with cancer: a treatment algorithm. *Oncol Nurs Forum* 24:51–57, 1997

225. Morrison GB, Bastian A, DelaRosa T, et al: Dihydropyrimidine dehydrogenase deficiency: a pharmacogenetic defect causing severe adverse reactions to 5-fluorouracil-based chemotherapy. *Oncol Nurs Forum* 24:83–88, 1997

226. Canty L: Breast cancer risk: protective effect of an early first full-term pregnancy versus increased risk of induced abortion. *Oncol Nurs Forum* 24:1025–1031, 1997

227. Kwekkeboom KL: The placebo effect in symptom management. *Oncol Nurs Forum* 24:1393–1399, 1997

228. Kagaura-Singer M. Addressing issues for early detection and screening in ethnic populations. *Oncol Nurs Forum* 24:1705–1711, 1997

229. Courneya KS, Friedenreich CM: Determinants of exercise during colorectal cancer treatment: an application of the theory of planned behavior. *Oncol Nurs Forum* 25:1715–1723, 1997

230. Yeager KA, Miaskowski C: Advances in understanding the mechanism and management of acute myelogenous leukemia. *Oncol Nurs Forum* 21:541–548, 1994

231. Stucky LA: Acute tumor lysis syndrome: assessment and nursing implications. *Oncol Nurs Forum* 20:49–59, 1993

232. Carter LW: Bacterial translocation: nursing implications. *Oncol Nurs Forum* 21:857–865, 1994

233. Caudell KA: Psychoneuroimmunology and innovative behavioral interventions in patients with leukemia. *Oncol Nurs Forum* 23:493–502, 1996

234. Kelly LP, Miaskowski C: An overview of bladder cancer: treatment and nursing implications. *Oncol Nurs Forum* 23:459–468, 1996

235. Viele CS: Chronic myelogenous leukemia and acute promyelocytic leukemia: new bone marrow transplant options. *Oncol Nurs Forum* 23:488–493, 1996

236. Armstrong TS, Gilbert MR: Glial neoplasms: classification, treatment and pathways for the future. *Oncol Nurs Forum* 23:615–625, 1996

237. Grassman D: Development of inpatient oncology education and support programs. *Oncol Nurs Forum* 20:669–676, 1993

238. Timmerman PR: Intravenous immunoglobulin in oncology nursing practice. *Oncol Nurs Forum* 20:69–75, 1993

239. Struthers CS: Lambert-Eaton myasthenic syndrome in small cell lung cancer: nursing implications. *Oncol Nurs Forum* 21:677–683, 1994

240. Wujcik D, Viele CS, Caudell KA: Leukemia management strategies: the next generation. *Oncol Nurs Forum* 23:477–487, 1996

241. Neufeld KR, Degner LF, Dick JAM: A nursing intervention strategy to foster patient involvement in treatment decisions. *Oncol Nurs Forum* 20:631–635, 1993

242. Meade CD: Producing videotapes for cancer education: methods and examples. *Oncol Nurs Forum* 23:837–846, 1996

243. Lierman LM, Powell-Cope G, Benoliel JQ: Using social support to promote breast self-examination performance. *Oncol Nurs Forum* 21:1051–1056, 1994

244. Doak LG, Doak CC, Meade CD: Strategies to improve cancer educational materials. *Oncol Nurs Forum* 23:1305–1312, 1996

245. Hawkins C, Miaskowski C: Testicular cancer: a review. *Oncol Nurs Forum* 23:1203–1211, 1996

246. Baker KH, Feldman JE: Thyroid cancer: a review. *Oncol Nurs Forum* 20:95–104, 1993

247. Sticklin LA, Walkenstein M: Vena cava filters: a nursing perspective. *Oncol Nurs Forum* 20:507–515, 1993

248. Meriney DK: Pathophysiology and management of VIPoma: a case study. *Oncol Nurs Forum* 23:941–948, 1996

249. Dachowski LJ, DeLaney TF: Photodynamic therapy. The NCI experience and its nursing implication. *Oncol Nurs Forum* 19:63–67, 1992

250. Held JL, Peahota A: Nursing care of patients with esophageal cancer. *Oncol Nurs Forum* 19:627–634, 1992

251. McFadden ME, Sartorius SE: Multiple system organ failure in patients with cancer. Part II: nursing implications. *Oncol Nurs Forum* 19:727–737, 1992

252. Jassack PF: Families: an essential element in the care of the patient with cancer. *Oncol Nurs Forum* 19:871–876, 1992

253. Sitton E: Early and late radiation-induced skin alterations: part II. Nursing care of irradiated skin. *Oncol Nurs Forum* 19:907–912, 1992

254. Radziewicz RM, Schneider SM: Using diversional activity to enhance coping. *Cancer Nurs* 15:293–298, 1992

255. Buehler JA, Lee HJ: Exploration of home care resources for rural families with cancer. *Cancer Nurs* 15:299–308, 1992

256. Lobert S: Antimitotics in cancer chemotherapy. *Cancer Nurs* 15:22–33, 1992

257. Cooley ME: Bereavement care: a role for nurses. *Cancer Nurs* 15:125–129, 1992

258. Stephens CD: Gemcitabine: a new approach to treating pancreatic cancer. *Oncol Nurs Forum* 25:87–93, 1998

259. Spath ML, Rimkus CF, Saenz DA: A chemotherapy and infusion therapy flow sheet for outpatient oncology settings. *Oncol Nurs Forum* 25:129–135, 1998

260. Viele CS, Holmes BC: Amifostine: drug profile and nursing implications of the first pancytoprotectant. *Oncol Nurs Forum* 25:515–523, 1998

261. Berg D: Irinotecan hydrochloride: drug profile and nursing implications of a toposomerase I inhibitor in patients with advanced colorectal cancer. *Oncol Nurs Forum* 25:535–543, 1998

262. Foelher R: Autologous stem cell transplant plus interleukin-2 for breast cancer: review and nursing management. *Oncol Nurs Forum* 25:563–568, 1998

263. Wagner ND, Quinones VW: Allogeneic peripheral blood stem cell transplantation: clinical overview and nursing implications. *Oncol Nurs Forum* 25:1049–1055, 1998

264. Herrmann RP, Leather M, Leather HL, et al: Clinical care for patients receiving autologous hematopoietic stem cell transplantation in the home setting. *Oncol Nurs Forum* 25:1427–1432, 1998

265. Snyder GM, Sielsch EC, Reville B: The controversy of hormone-replacement therapy in breast cancer survivors. *Oncol Nurs Forum* 25:699–706, 1998

266. Jacobs LA: Hereditary nonpolyposis colon cancer: genetic

basis, testing and patient-care issues. *Oncol Nurs Forum* 25: 719–725, 1998

267. Mahon SM: Osteoporosis: a concern for cancer survivors. *Oncol Nurs Forum* 25:843–851, 1998

268. Donnelly S: Patient management strategies for interferon alfa-2b as adjuvant therapy of high-risk melanoma. *Oncol Nurs Forum* 25:921–927, 1998

269. Brant JM: The art of palliative care: living with hope, dying with dignity. *Oncol Nurs Forum* 25:995–1004, 1998

270. Boyle DM, Abernathy G, Baker L, et al: End-of-life confusion in patients with cancer. *Oncol Nurs Forum* 25(8): 1335–1343, 1998

271. Kormanik PA, Chamberlain MC: Leptomeningeal metastasis: pathophysiology, treatment, and nursing management. *Oncol Nurs Forum* 25:1355–1362, 1998

272. Wakefield B, Johnson J, Kron-Chalupa J, et al: A research-based guideline for appropriate use of transdermal fentanyl to treat chronic pain. *Oncol Nurs Forum* 25:1505–1513, 1998

273. Wholihan D: A patient-education tool for patient-controlled analgesia. *Oncol Nurs Forum* 24:1801–1803, 1997

274. Skobel SW: Epidural administration: what nurses should know. *Oncol Nurs Forum* 23:1555–1560, 1996

275. Mahon SM: Cancer risk assessment: conceptual considerations for clinical practice. *Oncol Nurs Forum* 25:1535–1547, 1998

276. Gerard MJ, Frank-Stromborg M: Screening for prostate cancer in asymptomatic men: clinical, legal and ethical implications. *Oncol Nurs Forum* 25:1561–1569, 1998

277. Pasacreta JV, McCorkle R: Providing accurate information to women about tamoxifen therapy for breast cancer: current indications, effects and controversies. *Oncol Nurs Forum* 25:1577–1583, 1998

278. Giarelli E: Medullary thyroid carcinoma: one component of the inherited disorder multiple endocrine neoplasia type 2A. *Oncol Nurs Forum* 24:1007–1020, 1997

279. Cash JC, Dattoli MJ: Management of patients receiving transperineal palladium-103 prostate implants. *Oncol Nurs Forum* 24:1361–1367, 1997

280. Fessele KS: Managing the multiple causes of nausea and vomiting in the patient with cancer. *Oncol Nurs Forum* 23: 1409–1415, 1996

281. Larson P: Important nurse caring behaviors perceived by patients with cancer. *Oncol Nurs Forum* 11:46–50, 1984

282. Larson P: Comparison of cancer patients' and professional nurses' perceptions of important nurse caring behaviors. *Heart Lung* 16:187–192, 1987

283. Mayer DK: Oncology nurses' versus cancer patients' perceptions of nursing care behaviors: a replication study. *Oncol Nurs Forum* 14:48–52, 1987

284. Curtis AE, Fernsler JI: Quality of life of oncology hospice patients: a comparison of patient and primary caregiver reports. *Oncol Nurs Forum* 16:49–53, 1989

285. Dyck S, Wright K: Family perceptions: the role of the nurse throughout an adult's cancer experience. *Oncol Nurs Forum* 12:53–56, 1985

286. Benner P: *From Novice to Expert: Excellence and Power in Clinical Nursing Practice.* Menlo Park, CA, Addison-Wesley, 1984

287. Benner P, Wrubel J: *The Primacy of Caring: Stress and Coping in Health and Illness.* Menlo Park, CA, Addison-Wesley, 1989

288. Sobel D, Ornstein R: Sense of control and health. *Mind/Body Health Newsletter* 8(3):1–8, 1998

289. Oncology Nursing Society, *ONS News* 14:1, January 1999

CHAPTER 73

Patient Education and Support

Lawrence F. Padberg, PhD
Rose Mary Padberg, RN, MA

Introduction

Nearly all health care professionals place a high value on patient education. The importance of patient education has been stated and reinforced many times, but nearly always with an emphasis on the content to be taught. For example, the *Guidelines for Oncology Nursing Practice*[1] include patient teaching directives in each section. These directives outline in detail the *content* to be taught. Such treatment of patient education is appropriate within each of the segments. The overall guidelines for practice, however, do not include directives for the oncology nurse to understand the *processes* of teaching and learning that underlie the patient teaching directive. With this in mind, it is not unreasonable for the oncology nurse to place an emphasis on *what* to teach rather than on understanding *how* to teach. And yet cancer nurses, often with little or no formal preparation in teaching theory or processes, regularly perform patient teaching and most often perform it well, guided by common sense, colleagues' examples, trial and error, and their own good judgment.

Even so, it is important to consider that the area of patient teaching is dependent not only on special expertise in terms of the information to be given but also on understanding the different ways in which individuals learn, the variety of strategies for patient teaching that are available, how to match appropriate strategies to specific content and specific learners, and much more.

The primary focus of this chapter is on patient education and the related area of patient support programming. The issues that are addressed include understanding what patient education is and is not; understanding the many forms of patient support; a rationale for patient education and support drawn from an understanding of the multiple purposes assigned to them; theoretical perspectives and practical guidelines for patient teaching; difficulties in ensuring continuity of teaching and support across settings; key factors to be considered in developing materials or in conducting patient education; resources available for patient teaching and support and how they can be accessed.

A Definition of Patient Education

Patient education is "a planned learning experience using a combination of methods such as teaching, counseling, and behavior modification techniques which influence patients' knowledge and health behavior."[2] Though simply stated, this definition identifies three important elements. Patient education involves planned learning experiences. It is not haphazard or accidental. Patient education uses a combination of methods. There is no single way to conduct patient education. Rather, the health care provider involved in patient education has a variety of resources and techniques from which to draw for effective teaching. The methods can be shaped and tailored to best meet the needs, style, and capabilities of the learner and the educator, or particular conditions in the teaching–learning setting. Finally, patient education seeks to influence or modify a patient's knowledge and/or health behavior. The goal of patient education is to effect some change in the learner. While the health care provider serving as educator cannot always ensure that learning has occurred, that is the goal. To complete a teaching activity and confidently check off that the patient education responsibility has been fulfilled without assessing whether any change has occurred in the patient at best overlooks valuable information; at worst, it may falsely assume efficacy.

Patient Support

The literature on cancer patient support includes a varied set of activities, programs, and groups. Some writers define support in terms of small-group mutual aid structures,[3] while others discuss support within the context of other forms of psychosocial interventions, including psychotherapy.[4,5] There is a distinction between psychotherapy groups, which seek to effect individual change through personal exploration and reflection done within the context of a group, and social support groups, which seek to help the group members find meaning and a sense of belonging through participation in the group.[6] Group psychotherapy may have social support outcomes, though these are not the primary purpose. Similarly, social support groups may assist some members to achieve personal changes through personal exploration and reflection flowing from the participation in the social group, but again such outcomes are not the purpose of the social support group.

The phenomenon of social support groups used in health care originated early in this century,[3] and recent estimates indicate that up to 15 million Americans participate in various types of support groups to deal with physical and emotional distress.[7] Support group objectives include sharing information that assists members in coping with cancer, finding inspiration or hope from the experiences of others, and the catharsis of being able to express strong emotions within a supportive setting.[3,6] The ability to express emotions helps in managing intense, negative feelings; it may also help by assisting the individual to move from coping with the emotions to beginning to resolve some of the causes.[5]

Educational and psychosocial programming are closely linked. Some patient education programs designed for groups have social support purposes. And even programs designed only for educational purposes may have social support outcomes and may be seen by many health care professionals and many participants as support programs.[3] For example, the "I Can Cope" program of the American Cancer Society (ACS) is designed as a patient education program. In the evaluation of the program when it was first developed, however, two of the three patient outcomes assessed were in the psychosocial area (state of anxiety, and purpose and meaningfulness in life),[8] and "I Can Cope" is often discussed among cancer care providers as a support program. Often programs are developed to combine both clear educational and social support/psychosocial purposes.[9–11]

Support programs may be tailored for people with a specific type of cancer, or for those in a particular stage of the illness, or for family members alone. There are concerns that some groups of people are less likely to join support groups or programs, and that special effort is needed to reach such audiences. In general, women and individuals of higher socioeconomic standing are most likely to participate in support programs. It has been suggested that men join programs that are identified as informational, and that programs designed to provide education and skill training, along with having support purposes, may be more effective in attracting men.[6] Once recruited to support programs, however, men may benefit more than women since men in our society have fewer opportunities for expressing emotions and receiving supportive response.[5] Efforts to better serve people from lower socioeconomic backgrounds require special considerations; issues in the area of serving culturally diverse audiences are discussed later in this chapter.

Understanding the Purposes of Patient Education

At first the purposes of patient education seem clear: that patients understand their diagnoses, their treatment options, their responsibilities as part of treatment; that they understand symptoms that need to be reported; that they comply with treatment procedures; and ultimately that they do all they can to promote a return to health, to adapt to ongoing limitations, or to cope with the reality of a terminal condition.

The possible intended outcomes of patient education are numerous. The purposes just stated reflect a care provider's perspective of those actions for which the patient should be responsible in order to maximize the positive benefits of treatment. Another perspective is that of a patient and family who want to understand the diagnosis and treatment options in order to make autonomous decisions regarding treatment—including the option to accept no further treatment. Still another perspective might be to ensure the care provider's compliance with a professional standard, or to fulfill an obligation or responsibility to the patient. From an organizational perspective, the purpose of patient education might be stated in terms of meeting an accreditation standard, fulfilling a legal responsibility, or even avoiding any legal liability for leaving a patient uninformed.

A difficulty in thinking about patient education and in planning programs and activities is the complexity of the purposes attributable to it. Rather than trying to assign a narrow purpose to patient education, the health care provider should understand the complexity and think critically when attempting to define goals for any patient education activity.

Five rationales or perspectives supporting the need for patient education have been identified: patients' rights, professional standards, legal and agency mandates, benefits to patients, and benefits to society and/or health care agencies.[12] Of these, two are traditional views supporting patient education: first, benefit to patients, that is, providing the patient with certain knowledge and understanding necessary for beneficial treatment; second, satisfying professional standards, the duty of the health care provider to share information with the patient. Of course the view of what information is appropriate to share with the patient has changed over time. Notions of patients' rights to information and to autonomy in decision making, legal standards and questions of legal liability, and the broader view of societal gain through the cumulative impact of effective and efficient health care decisions resulting from patient education have developed only more recently as perspectives in health care. Whether traditional or recent, all five of these rationales support the importance of patient education.

Patients' Rights

The idea of patients' rights as a basis for patient education flows from philosophical principles recognizing individual autonomy and the right to self-determination. It might be assumed that in a democratic society such as the United States, with our political orientation toward maximizing individual freedoms, the perspective of individual autonomy as a basis for patients' rights should be a long-standing tradition. This perspective, however, has developed only in the latter half of the twentieth century.

It was only in 1972 that the American Hospital Association developed its formal statement on the rights of patients.[13] These include rights to information about diagnosis, treatment, prognosis, procedures and their medical consequences, and other areas. Over the past 25 years the rights of patients have become a cornerstone for contemporary health care, replacing the former paternalistic perspective that the health care professional knew what was best for the patient based on specialized knowledge and expertise. The recognition of patients' rights is reflected today in professional standards, in organizational standards and policies, and in laws related to health care practice.

In recent years issues related to cancer patients' rights have been broadened beyond the arena of treatment and direct health care. Cancer survivors, for example, often experience discrimination. In 1989 the National Coalition for Cancer Survivorship developed a statement of the rights of cancer survivors, *The Cancer Survivor's Bill of Rights*.[14] This statement includes areas that have direct implications for patient education. The first section discusses responsibilities of health care professionals, but the statement also deals with issues of employment opportunity, insurability, and the personal expectations and pressures often placed upon cancer survivors.

Professional Standards

The development of professional standards has reflected the changing perspectives regarding patients' rights. While professional standards in health care have long expressed the underlying philosophy of the Hippocratic oath—to do good and do no harm—recognition of and respect for a patient's right to full knowledge and self-determination have developed only more recently in conjunction with changing perspectives in the larger society. If the individual has the right to full knowledge regarding health status and a right to make self-determining health care decisions, then the health care professional has a responsibility to ensure that the patient has the knowledge base and appropriate support for such autonomy.

Clear guidelines regarding patient education responsibilities as part of professional standards, therefore, are relatively new. Fernsler and Cannon note that various American Nurses' Association documents that provide guidelines for the scope of professional practice give direction for nurses' responsibilities in patient education more through implication than through explicit statement.[12] The Oncology Nursing Society's *Outcome Standards for Cancer Patient Education* were first published in 1982.[15] The current guidelines[16] provide descriptive criterion statements organized around five areas: the responsibilities and qualifications of the oncology nurse; patient and family educational resources; the content of patient and family education; the teaching–learning process and application of theory; and the anticipated learning outcomes for patients and family.

Legal and Accreditation Requirements

States are responsible for establishing guidelines for professional practice through state law. State nursing practice acts, which delineate the responsibilities of and limitations on nursing practice, may include specific requirements for patient and family education or, more typically, may imply an obligation for patient teaching as a necessary part of fulfilling the duties and responsibilities of nursing practice.[12,17]

A specialized issue in legal responsibility for patient education is the area of informed consent. This concept has its roots in post–World War II reactions to the human experimentation conducted by the Nazis, leading to the development of the Nuremberg Code to provide standards for use by the Nuremberg military tribunal.[18] Central to this code is the use of voluntary consent to protect human subjects in experimentation. Such consent assumes not only the ability to consent and freedom from coercion but also that there is an understanding of the risks and benefits, that the subject is giving an informed consent.

The codification of informed consent can be traced through several well-known landmark documents, including the Declaration of Helsinki, adopted by the World Medical Association in Helsinki, Finland, in 1964, and the Belmont Report, developed by the National Commission for the Protection of Human Subjects of Biomedical and Behavioral Research in 1978.[18] General acceptance of informed consent principles has extended over time beyond human subjects in research settings to broader expectations for informed consent by patients for participation even in standard treatment.

In addition to legal obligations for patient education, a variety of accreditation or other certifying standards have developed specific requirements for patient education, with responsibilities assigned to nurses and other health professionals. In 1993 the Joint Commission on Accreditation of Healthcare Organizations (JCAHO) reorganized its standards for accreditation to bring stronger focus to the area of patient and family education. Combining standards previously found in many department-specific chapters, the 1993 accreditation manual included for the first time a chapter on patient and family education.[19] This chapter has been retained through several subsequent updates of the *Comprehensive Accreditation Manual for Hospitals*.[20]

Other agencies and organizations have joined this call for patient education as an integral part of health care. The Health Care Financing Administration (HCFA), which regulates Medicare and Medicaid reimbursement, mandates discharge planning and the patient and family education this implies.[21] In recognition of the JCAHO patient and family education standards, the HCFA accepts JCAHO-accredited institutions as also having met HCFA requirements.

The Association of Community Cancer Centers' *Standards for Cancer Programs* includes standards on patient and family education, as well as specific statements regarding the oncology nurse's responsibilities for patient and family education.[22]

Patient Benefits

Patient education goals obviously include increasing patients' knowledge and understanding of the disease and their own diagnoses. Patient education and support seek to ensure compliance with treatment, appropriate self-care, attention to symptoms or change of status, and timely and accurate reporting of symptoms or health changes. A major focus of much patient education and of most support programs is improving psychological status by reducing anxiety, relieving depression, and maintaining self-concept or self-esteem. The ultimate goal is that education and support can contribute to improved physical and emotional status.

While improved patient outcomes are the most readily acknowledged goals of patient education, empirical evidence for physical improvement outcomes is difficult to establish. Clinical research often faces difficulties in establishing control groups, avoiding confounding factors, and attaining sufficient sample size. Much of the literature on patient outcomes for education and support interventions deals primarily with aspects of psychosocial status. For example, in recently reported studies, education and orientation programs designed to prepare individuals for beginning treatment have been shown to reduce anxiety and overall stress and to improve satisfaction during the course of treatment.[23,24] A group program providing both psychosocial support and training in coping skills resulted in improved mood status and enhanced quality of life.[9] A group psychotherapy program for cancer patients experiencing depression helped to reduce anxiety and maladaptive somatic preoccupation as well as reducing depression.[4] An inpatient education and support program that included informational, emotional, and spiritual components increased knowledge of symptom management, decreased anxiety, reduced patients' sense of isolation, and increased their sense of control and comfort.[10] A computer-based educational and support system helped produce feelings of acceptance, motivation, understanding, and relief.[25,26]

There is less empirical information regarding education and support outcomes related to enhanced physical health status. Educational programs clearly serve to increase patient knowledge regarding self-care, symptom management, and monitoring and reporting changes in health status. As patient information needs are met, increased compliance with treatment regimens and reduced medical complications are achieved, thus contributing to reductions in preventable hospital readmissions and similar health benefits.[27] Emotional gains from education and support programs may influence the experience of physical symptoms. For example, a group psychotherapy program reduced physical symptoms of anorexia, nausea and vomiting, and fatigue. The investigators noted that such symptoms may be attributed to emotional sources and speculated about possible explanations for the effects of psychotherapy: that the symptoms are of emotional origin; that one's emotional state can influence perceptions of symptoms and thus the reporting of them; or that these two factors combine in some way.[28] A meta-analysis of 116 studies reported between 1976 and 1993 found that education and psychological interventions provided benefits in the areas of knowledge, psychosocial status (anxiety, depression, mood), and physical symptoms (nausea, vomiting, pain).[29]

It is difficult, however, to demonstrate that the benefits of patient education and support programs seen in the psychosocial area translate into medical gains. An association between participation in education and support programs and survival has been shown.[3,30] It is not clear, however, what factors contribute to the links between support and survival. In addition to the potential direct effect of emotional state on physical state, other explanations might be that individuals who have an improved

emotional outlook as a result of therapy or other support programs will monitor symptom changes more carefully, seek additional medical attention in a more timely manner, comply with treatment regimens more fully, or more easily manage difficult treatment regimens and thereby receive more rigorous treatment. Others have reported not being able to find a link between psychological factors and survival, suggested methodological concerns in studies reporting such findings, and noted that psychological effects are, at best, very small compared to medical factors related to survival.[31,32]

Benefits to Society and to Health Care Organizations

The benefits to society and to health care organizations represent a fifth broad purpose for patient education,[12] an area of benefit not often considered. While patient and family education contributes to the improved physical and psychosocial health status of individuals experiencing illness, benefits accruing to organizations or individuals beyond the patient and family include reduced hospital stays, reduced utilization of health care materials and resources, and reduced absenteeism from school or work. Health care agencies may see significant benefits from avoiding extending hospital stays beyond reimbursable limits, reducing need for expensive forms of care, satisfied patients providing referrals, and increasing patient volume.

The Teaching–Learning Process: Theory and Practice

A theoretical base for patient education is important because it provides the clinician with a guide for approaching individual patients and their needs, for selecting materials or methods when planning patient education activities, and for assessing the effectiveness or outcomes of those activities.[33,34]

The Health Belief Model

The health belief model is a value expectancy model based on the principle that action will be taken if an individual perceives a threat, believes that it is significant, and believes that something can be done regarding the threat.[35] The model is often applied within the context of health education, but the general principles also are useful in thinking about patient education.

An individual who is a patient already has experienced illness and therefore readily acknowledges individual susceptibility. The patient may not understand the severity of the illness, although in cancer patient education it is typical that individuals anticipate that any cancer experience is serious and life-threatening. Thus, patients usually are already aware of the "threat" represented by their illness. However, to assist patients in making decisions about how to respond to the acknowledged threat, the expectation principles of the health belief model still must be addressed. The patient must come to believe that possible actions are of value. The patient needs to be able to weigh the benefits of the actions compared with the barriers—are the potential benefits of treatment likely to be of greater value than the disadvantages such as the likely levels of pain, the disruptions of personal or family life, side effects of treatment, and costs to self or family? Finally, patient education must address the issue of efficacy, that the patient believes he or she can accomplish the actions required in order to undertake treatment. The health belief model can guide patient education: By understanding the issues, the patient makes a treatment decision and complies with the treatment regimen; and the health care provider identifies the education interventions needed to address these issues.

The PRECEDE Model

The PRECEDE model (Predisposing, Reinforcing, and Enabling Causes in Educational Diagnosis and Evaluation) attempts to provide a comprehensive consideration of factors predisposing, reinforcing, and enabling targeted health behaviors.[36] Predisposing factors include knowledge, attitudes, beliefs, and values about health behaviors. If an individual has had a relative die quickly from cancer in spite of extensive treatment and then is diagnosed with the same type of cancer, the individual may simply believe that his or her fate is to repeat the course of events in the same way. Interventions to assist the person in learning specific information about diagnosis, options for treatment, and potential outcomes may be wasted unless some action is taken to address and change the predisposing belief.

Predisposing factors may be positive or negative. The PRECEDE model assists the clinician in understanding potential predisposing factors that may support or inhibit patient readiness and motivation to learn.

Reinforcing factors support the continuation of the intended health behavior or reinforce resistance to the targeted behavior. Patient education interventions that help the patient to see progress, that strengthen understanding and respond to questions or concerns, that provide reminders for continuing intended behaviors, and that continue providing support are reinforcing factors.

Enabling factors are resources or other structures within an individual's environment that may affect the target health behavior, enabling or facilitating or, conversely, inhibiting or serving as barriers to the intended behavior. For example, adverse side effects of treatment may become significant inhibitors of patient compliance. Eliciting information from the patient regarding any possible side effects being experienced and appropriately intervening to manage those effects are important steps to ensure continued compliance with the treatment regi-

men. The PRECEDE model helps in directing attention to enabling factors, acting to best utilize positive factors and to minimize or eliminate negative factors.

Control Theory

A number of theories advanced in patient education are variations of personal control theory. The primary underlying perspective of control theory is an individual's perception or belief that specific outcomes are contingent upon the individual's own action or, alternately, other sources. Social learning theory,[37] or self-efficacy theory, is one widely utilized control theory. Perception of self-efficacy will affect the individual's decisions regarding behavior, level of effort, and persistence.

A sense of self-efficacy derives from four sources of information: personal mastery, vicarious experiences, verbal persuasion, and physiological feedback. Mastery learning, contract learning, and modeling are teaching techniques that are suggested to be useful in working from this theoretical perspective.[34,35] For example, development of personal mastery in teaching skills can be accomplished by teaching in small increments with repetitions at each level until mastery is achieved. An attempt to present a complex task in its entirety, thus allowing the patient to experience unsuccessful attempts to demonstrate the behavior, would diminish a sense of self-efficacy and make learning more difficult.

Another theoretical perspective in the general area of control theory is locus of control, that is, a view that behavior is a function of expectancy and reinforcement, with expectancy defined along an internal control–external control continuum. Variations of this perspective define locus of control in three domains: personally controlled, controlled by chance, or controlled by powerful others.[33] Patient education interventions based on a locus of control theory perspective need to assess patient beliefs regarding control.

Coping Theory

Another general category of theories applied to patient education is coping theory. Coping involves behavioral and/or cognitive responses to perceived stressors or threats intended to mediate or manage those stressors or threats. Lorig, drawing from the work of Lazarus and Folkman,[38] notes a variety of coping strategies used by individuals: confronting, distancing, self-control, seeking social support, accepting responsibility, escape-avoidance, problem solving, positive reappraisal, activity, distraction, self-talk, and prayer.[35] Lorig discusses approaches for patient education, or ways of understanding and interpreting patient actions, within each of these types of coping strategies. For example, confronting is a coping strategy that may be useful to patients experiencing difficulties caused by a nonsupportive spouse. A suggested approach consistent with a confronting coping strategy would be to provide the patients with teaching focused on reporting their own feelings, that is, confronting the stress or negative feelings they have, and moving them away from focusing on the question of spousal support.

Understanding coping strategies may help the health care professional provide appropriate teaching to give the patient tools to deal with the issues being faced, or provide teaching strategies that respond well to the coping style of the patient. Miller identified two coping styles for dealing with cancer or other major health threats—monitoring and blunting—that have implications for patient teaching.[39] *Monitors* are individuals who give high levels of attention to threatening health information. They tend to seek a great deal of information, to be more active in understanding their health condition, and to seek greater participation in decisions regarding their health status and treatment. In contrast, *blunters* are individuals who avoid information that presents threatening health information. They tend not to seek additional information and take less responsibility for health decisions. Distinguishing between patients as information seekers and nonseekers, and linking information seekers to more active involvement in care decisions, has been noted by other researchers.[40,41]

Health care professionals may react in less than optimal ways when presenting information to monitors and blunters or information seekers and nonseekers.[39,42] Because monitors display greater agitation and concern in response to threatening information, providers may avoid giving more information in an attempt to avoid further distress for the patient. On the other hand, because blunters tend to exhibit disinterest and take little initiative to seek more information, the health care professional may extend or increase the presentation of information regarding a negative health condition, trying to ensure that the person has heard the relevant and important information. In both cases the health professional's actions may not be well suited to the coping styles of the patients. Monitors may benefit from more complete and extensive information; more information may increase understanding and certainty and help the individual to process the information and thus cope with the diagnosis. Blunters appear to cope with the threat by avoidance and distraction; forcing them to hear and confront threatening information may increase their anxiety and emotional distress. Thus the monitor–blunter coping style framework may be helpful to the health professional in guiding how to react to individual patients and to provide information that is most helpful.

Adult Learning Theory

Another source of information and theoretical perspective that can inform patient education is the field of adult education and adult learning theory.[43] While there are a variety of learning theories that may be useful to draw from, much of adult education in recent years has been influenced by the work of Malcolm Knowles and the principles of *andragogy*, or adult education, that he proposed.[44] Knowles's principles of adult education can be helpful in considering the role of the nurse as an educator and the patient as a learner.[34] Adult learning theory also emphasizes task- or problem-oriented learning relevant to the needs and interests of the learner, a viewpoint that fits well with patient education.[27]

Knowles's perspective can be especially effective to assist in moving away from a paternalism that assumes the health care professional has total responsibility for determining goals and process for patient teaching, and in moving toward a position that respects patient autonomy and rights of self-determination, shares responsibility in setting educational goals by responding to needs as identified by the patient/learner, and utilizes the resources represented by the knowledge and experience that the patient/learner brings to the learning setting. Table 73-1 provides a summary of Knowles's four assumptions regarding adult learners and their implications for patient education.

Guidelines for Patient Teaching Practice

The nurse in clinical practice confronted with immediate patient education needs and seeking to respond as effectively as possible often looks first to practical guidelines rather than to a study of underlying theory. In response, much of the professional literature emphasizes practice tips and techniques either through case presentations or easy-to-use guides for practice. Morra provided a set of techniques for patient teaching that, combined with consideration of underlying principles drawn from theory, can assist the nurse in thinking about effective ways of meeting patients' needs (Table 73-2).[45]

Basic steps for conducting patient education include assessing educational needs, planning the teaching process, implementation, and evaluation. Assessing educational needs too often is done from the health care professional's perspective alone.[43] That is, the professional care provider can readily identify information about diagnosis, or treatment regimen, or potential side effects, or complications—all important information that should be conveyed to the patient and family. In addition, the experienced care provider is knowledgeable about typical psychosocial difficulties and can suggest resources for social and personal support. Effective needs assessment, however, must seek to identify needs as seen from the patient's perspective too.

Involvement of the patient in needs assessment can be complex. As Morra notes, patients often are not sufficiently knowledgeable even to formulate meaningful questions.[45] The care provider must be attentive to indications of knowledge gaps expressed by patients, be ready to ask questions, and give patients ample time to think through their concerns and questions. The period immediately following diagnosis can be an especially difficult time emotionally, complicating the process of giving im-

Table 73-1 Principles of Adult Learning and Their Implications for Practice

Principles	Assumptions and Implications
Adults are independent learners.	The process of moving from childhood to adulthood is a process of moving from dependence to increasing independence. There is a deep psychological need for adults to see themselves, as well as to have others see them, as generally independent or self-reliant. The educator working with adult learners must respect this independence and ability of the adult learner to control his/her own learning. Adults are responsible for what is to be learned and take an active role in their learning. The learning takes place between the learner and the material; the teacher is there only to facilitate the exchange.
Adults' past experiences are resources for learning.	Unlike children, adults have a reservoir of past experience that can be a resource for learning. Whenever possible, adults' past experiences should be drawn upon to enhance the learning process. Further, adults' self-images are often defined, at least in part, by their past experiences, and they have a deep investment in their value. Ignoring these past experiences in current learning can be interpreted as essentially rejecting a large part of the adult learner.
Adults' readiness to learn emerges from life's developmental stages.	The adult learner's readiness to learn develops from life's tasks and problems. As the adult years progress, there is a shift in career, social roles, personal responsibilities, etc. The transitions that evolve during life create opportunities for learning as the individual strives to better understand and cope. Such phases have been labeled as "teachable moments." The individual is both more highly motivated to learn, and the information is more readily understood when presented within this context.
Adults' learning is task- or problem-oriented	Adults will seek out various resources for specific learning (information or skills) to help them in answering a question or dealing with a problem. They are motivated in their learning to find answers or solve problems. Learning experiences will be most effective when they respond to adult learners' perceived needs.

Reprinted with permission from Padberg RM and Padberg LF: Strengthening the effectiveness of patient education: applying principles of adult education. *Oncol Nurs Forum* 17:65–69, 1990.[43] Adapted with permission from Knowles MS: *The Modern Practice of Adult Education: From Pedagogy to Andragogy* (ed 2). Upper Saddle River, NJ, Globe Fearon/Cambridge, 1980.[44]

portant information. McGinn, an oncology nurse who experienced cancer, noted the initial shock of hearing a cancer diagnosis—and hearing hardly anything else.[46] Complicating matters further, the patient later may feel too embarrassed to admit that he or she cannot remember the information given earlier and may be even less willing to ask questions in spite of feeling a loss of control and a need for information.

Assessing patient needs is an ongoing process; information often needs to be repeated and new needs and questions will arise as the individual progresses through treatment. Similarly, psychosocial needs vary from one person to another and change over time. Reassessing support needs at various points, therefore, should be done in the same way as reassessing educational needs.

Information and support needs change substantially as different stages of living with cancer are experienced.[47] The new challenges and issues that arise at each stage create new needs for knowledge, understanding, and coping. Once needs are identified, plans for patient teaching activities can be developed. Several of the guidelines shown in Table 73-2 relate to how educational activities should be planned. The plan should include several relatively short teaching sessions that focus on a single area or small amount of related information. Family members or others who are providing assistance and support to the individual are included in all teaching sessions. Multimedia approaches are used whenever possible.

Planning allows for selecting resources and identifying specific activities to address all of the needs identified; for approaching these teaching activities in an ordered

and prepared manner; for identifying who will be responsible for various teaching tasks; for establishing strategies to monitor or track the completion of teaching activities; and for planning how the achievement of learning outcomes will be assessed. Patient teaching responsibilities and activities should be included as components of any patient management planning tool or process. It is important to build into the plan easy access to care providers so that patients and families may readily ask questions, clarify information, and seek assistance when questions, concerns, and needs arise.

Patient teaching is not complete unless patient learning has been verified. Ongoing assessment incorporated in each teaching activity guides the teaching process: what information will need to be repeated, what concepts still need clarification, what new needs or questions have arisen. Evaluation is ongoing, a part of the teaching–learning process.

Much of patient/family teaching at the time of treatment focuses on aspects of self-care and, therefore, includes skill development as well as sharing knowledge. Competency in performing skills often is easier to assess than other learning since direct observation of skill performance can be used. Assessment of skill performance may require specialized resources such as skills labs or special demonstration models. For example, to provide a hands-on opportunity for mastectomy patients to practice caring for incisions and emptying drains, staff at a military medical center modified a CPR mannequin to simulate mastectomy surgery.[48]

Whether knowledge- or skill-oriented, the primary

Table 73-2 Guidelines for Patient Teaching

1. Present the most important material first.	The first material presented is best remembered. Stress the importance because people remember best the information they believe is most important.
2. Offer information.	Do not wait for patients to ask before giving information. Make it easy for the person to start a conversation. Open the door by asking a question such as "Is there anything going on right now you'd like to talk about?"
3. Combine sight and sound when presenting materials.	Most of the information a listener has stored in the brain has been received *visually*. Use printed explanations to accompany what you say. Remember that people respond to different methods of presenting printed materials, so combine different forms—questions and answers, pictures, charts, questions to ask, quizzes—all reinforcing one another.
4. Ask patients and family members what they want to know about their illness.	People remember best the information they are most interested in knowing.
5. Categorize.	Tell people the categories of information that you are going to discuss with them, then follow those categories. People remember better when the information is organized into parts that make sense and can be remembered as a set.
6. Don't be afraid to repeat information.	Patients forget about a third of what is said to them. Recall of instructions and advice is less than 50%. Remember that a person's intelligence seems to show no relation to ability to recall and remember.
7. Give information in small amounts whenever possible.	The proportion of information forgotten increases with the amount of information presented.
8. Involve family members and supportive friends as completely as possible.	Encourage family/friends to share and discuss information, to participate in care, and to support the patient. Share with them appropriate sources of information.
9. Try to give information when people are relatively calm.	Recall of information is related to level of anxiety, being poorest when anxiety is particularly high or low, and best when there is moderate anxiety. It is important to let people get over the initial shock of a cancer diagnosis before giving detailed information.
10. Speak plainly and use short sentences.	Many people find long sentences, fast speech, and unfamiliar terms hard to understand. Don't speak "medicalese." Words such as *palpate* or *palliate* are not everyday household words, no matter the age or education of your audience.
11. Ask for questions.	Encourage patients and family members to write down questions as they think of them for you to answer when you see them. Help them understand that you expect questions, no matter how simple or complex they might be. Stress that there is no such thing as a "stupid" question if it is bothering the patient.
12. Help the patient and family understand there are choices from the beginning.	Some are simple such as choosing the time for treatment. Others are more complex such as different therapies. However, there are choices, and if the patient and family are not involved, someone else is making the choices.
13. Be responsive to even the most searching and difficult question, such as second opinions or alternative treatments.	Answer them freely and fully. Make it known that seeking a second opinion is an accepted practice and that the majority of physicians respect an individual's right to further consultation.
14. Encourage patients and family members to ask the doctor questions that only the doctor can answer.	Many people, particularly many older people, have problems asking doctors questions; and often people have problems recalling what the doctor has said. Encourage them to ask questions, and ensure them that the doctor wants them to ask anything about which they are confused or worried. Encourage them to write down the answers and keep them in a notebook or tape-record them to review when they get home and for future reference. Suggest that patients bring someone with them when they meet with the physician; different people hear different things.
15. Ask questions yourself.	Ask patients to explain back to you what you have presented. Such feedback helps check whether they have heard the information as you intended.
16. Use silence.	Don't try to keep the conversation moving. Wait to allow the questions or comments that will advise you where to go next.
17. Take time to sit down.	Patients perceive a visit in which a health professional sits down as much longer than when the person is standing. Sitting close and at the person's level adds warmth to the visit.
18. Maintain eye contact.	It signals that you are willing to talk. Not looking at a person gives the sense that you don't want a conversation.
19. Body language affects communication.	Inappropriate facial expressions, nuances of body positions, and nervous habits can all convey impressions of disinterest or create barriers for open conversation. Often physical contact, such as holding a hand, can be appropriate and can help dissipate feelings of isolation or fear that cancer patients say they experience.
20. Don't worry about not saying the right thing.	The simple, sincere gesture of one person reaching out to another communicates comfort, hope, and support. You—the nurse—are in a unique position to offer it.

Adapted with permission from Morra ME: Making choices: The consumer's perspective. *Cancer Nurs* 8:54–59, 1985 (suppl 1).[45]

issue is that the level of learning needs to be assessed if there is to be any confidence that patient education has met its goals. When deficiencies are identified or new learning needs are identified as a result of assessment, this information serves as the new needs assessment findings for planning ongoing patient teaching activities.

Continuity Across Care Settings

An important issue in patient education is providing effective patient teaching across multiple care settings. While this is not a new issue, changing patterns of health care delivery have introduced a greater need for addressing how patient education is coordinated and communicated across settings. Efforts to decrease length of stay in acute care settings, the increased use of outpatient services for initial treatment as well as follow-up care, expanded use of home health agencies, and the growth in new health care systems such as health maintenance organizations (HMOs) are all major contributors to these changes. Patient education needs also have increased as larger numbers of people are living with cancer as a chronic illness and as greater attention is given to their psychosocial needs. With earlier discharge and increased use of outpatient treatment and follow-up care, families and patients often are expected to perform technical and monitoring procedures previously done only by professionals and to take greater responsibility for coordinating care.[49] Attention must be given to preparing patients and families for these responsibilities and to the coordination of ongoing support during the period of self-care.

Continuity in care and patient education typically is considered from the view of linkage between the initial treatment setting and ongoing contact through the physician's office, the outpatient clinic, or the home health agency. The accreditation standards for hospitals address this interrelationship of patient and family education, discharge planning, and continuity of care, calling for the sharing of discharge plans and instructions with all health care providers working with the patient.[20]

The concept of continuity of care includes not only coordination and consistency across multiple settings but also the ongoing access to care services. Typically, comprehensive care is provided during the period of hospitalization or initial outpatient treatment, but the availability of care often drops quickly after discharge. Yet care needs, including medical, psychosocial, and daily living, extend throughout the illness and recovery experience.[27] Informational needs often change, thus making reassessment of patient teaching needs important at various points during the continuum of care.[50] Benefits of effective patient teaching, referrals, and follow-up processes include shortened hospitalizations, a decrease in preventable hospital readmissions, increased compliance with medical regimens, decreased medical complications, and improved psychosocial status (decreased anxiety, improved coping, increased sense of competency in self-care, and increased knowledge of therapy).[27]

There are a variety of models available for strengthening continuity of care. A recent review of continuity of care strategies looked both at studies focusing on effective approaches for inpatient teaching and discharge planning and at studies looking at teaching and planning interventions across the continuum of care.[27] For example, a visiting nurse service has successfully implemented a nursing practice model in which a nurse specialist from the home health agency serves as the primary contact and case manager for the patient. This individual is available to the patient and family on a 24-hour basis. In addition to providing direct care, the nurse assists in making treatment decisions and facilitates contacts for the patient and family across various care settings.[51,52]

Effective continuity of care and patient education are most dependent on strong communication among health care providers across all care settings.[53,54] Ultimately, standardization of discharge planning, patient education, and outpatient and community follow-up processes is needed in order to ensure continuity of care.[27]

Developing Patient Education and Support Materials and Programs

Though patient education and support resources from government agencies, nonprofit organizations, health care institutions, and commercial sources are extensive, there are times when it is appropriate to develop materials or programs to meet special needs within a specific health care setting. Material and program development has been described as a six-step process that should continually repeat itself; that is, evaluation of the implemented program should provide feedback that can then be used to refine the program, progressing again through the development steps. The process described here is adapted from the developmental process presented in the National Cancer Institute Office of Cancer Communication's publication, *Making Health Communication Programs Work: A Planner's Guide.*[55] This process is shown graphically in Figure 73-1.

Step 1: Planning and Strategy Selection

This is the basic planning stage for educational materials development. Several key issues are included in this stage:

1. Clearly identify the issues, problems, or patient education goals to be addressed. It should be clear why a decision is made to develop materials or a program for a particular setting or purpose and that existing materials are not sufficient to address the need.

2. Identify the target audience. This might be done in many ways: by type of cancer or particular stage of the illness; whether the target group will be diverse or more

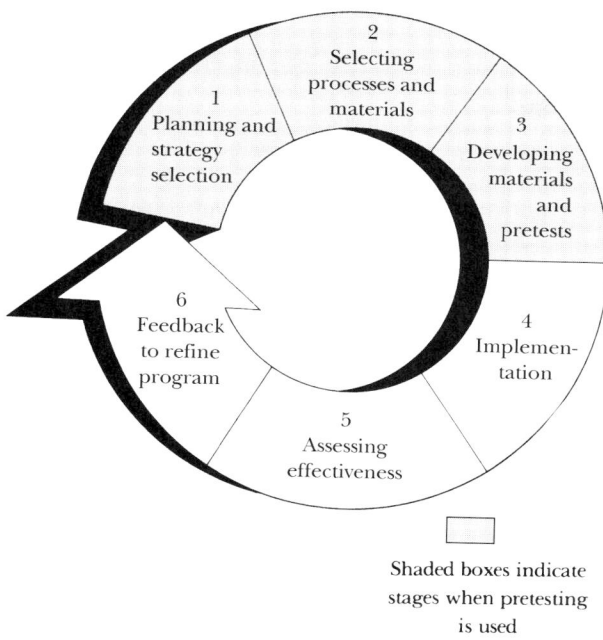

Shaded boxes indicate
stages when pretesting
is used

Figure 73-1 Steps in the development of patient education materials and resources. (Office of Cancer Communications, National Cancer Institute: *Making Health Communication Programs Work: A Planner's Guide.* NIH publication No. 92-1493. Washington, DC, U.S. Department of Health and Human Services, National Institutes of Health, 1992.)[55]

narrowly defined in terms of factors such as age, gender, or ethnic or socioeconomic factors; or the setting in which the audience will be found for the program or materials. Understanding the audience is important to guide later decisions regarding strategies to be used and to identify individuals for pretesting the materials.

3. Identify the intended outcomes, the goals of the materials or program. Measurable objectives should be established. Identify how they will be evaluated to determine the success of the materials or program.

4. Identify constraints—financial, time, personnel, setting—placed upon the development process and on the use of the materials once developed. These constraints will limit or guide later decisions.

Step 2: Selecting Processes and Materials

This is the stage in which the purposes, characteristics of the audience, and constraints identified in step 1 will guide decisions about the types of materials or program structure that will be used. Decisions must be made about the processes or channels for delivering the materials or program, about the specific structure or format of the program or materials, whether some existing materials will be used or modified, or all new materials will be developed. Consider what program structures or material

formats work best for the target audience or within the setting or location in which the program will occur.

Step 3: Developing Materials and Pretesting

At this stage the process moves from planning to development. The work of drafting and producing the actual materials must be done, with ongoing testing throughout the process. Involvement of expert reviewers to provide suggestions as development begins or to critique early materials can be especially useful both for shaping the content and for the style of presentation to be most effective. Also, those health care professionals who will use the materials or implement the program, and those who control decisions about adopting new materials or programs, should be involved. For example, if developing a new brochure for assisting patients in understanding a particular self-care technique, nurses involved in teaching these patients can provide guidance not only on the information that is needed but also on the types of questions that patients have, the time that is available for presenting the materials, the likely settings for this presentation, the opportunities for demonstration, and other particular conditions that will help guide the content and format.

Serving special populations

Other considerations during development include making materials or programs responsive to diverse populations or, if the materials are targeted for a particular audience, making them appropriate for that target group. For instance, examples and illustrations in culturally sensitive materials should reflect diversity in racial and ethnic character, age, socioeconomic and occupational identification, and religious identification. If the materials are being developed for use with a specific target audience, care must be taken to ensure that elements of the audience's standards and practices are properly presented and respected.

A special target audience may be defined in many ways, and tailoring materials for a special audience similarly may take many forms. Print materials developed for use with an elderly target group, for example, can be designed to use large font sizes and be double-spaced. Programs for older persons need to consider other issues such as the setting in which the program will be conducted and potential difficulties with acoustics and accessibility. Elders seeking to participate in education and support programs may be hampered by transportation problems; daytime programs held in settings linked to other programs and services for older persons enhance participation.

In general, materials and programs designed for older people need to be developed with an awareness of the physiological changes associated with aging that may reduce or limit hearing, vision, motor function, and cognitive processes. Possible economic and psychosocial changes that may affect older persons' ability to participate and benefit also should be considered.[56,57] At the same time, health care professionals must avoid thinking of older people, or any special population, in stereotypical terms. Again considering older people as a target group, while there are general patterns that the care provider should be aware of, variability among the elderly reflects the diversity of the overall population. The health professional should acknowledge the potential for individuals to experience cancer and their responses to cancer in divergent ways.[57,58]

Nurses whose practice settings serve people of diverse cultural backgrounds, and most practice settings do, need to be sensitive to cultural differences and to respond appropriately. Too often cultural diversity is described and discussed in the literature only in terms of racial or ethnic minority status. Culture, however, is a complex concept that includes a mix of beliefs, values, modes of dress, social relationships, behavioral norms, and other factors.[59] Cultural differences may affect many aspects of the interaction between health care professionals and their clients. The lack of common cultural background between health care professionals and clients has been suggested as a major contributor to problems in compliance.[60]

Strategies for effective culturally sensitive approaches to patient education and support are varied. Health care professionals serving populations from cultural backgrounds different from their own need to make linkages with key members of the target community, involving members of the community in the development of educational materials, programs, and community outreach strategies.[61,62] It is important that programs be placed in the community in locations that reach the target audience.[6,63] The Oncology Nursing Society's *Cancer Prevention in Minority Populations*[64] is a helpful resource for understanding cultural perspectives within many ethnic minority populations and the implications of these cultural views for effective health care.

In spite of the large volume of patient education materials available today from government agencies, nonprofit organizations, and commercial vendors, materials designed to reach special populations are often difficult to find. This is an area in which nurses and other health care professionals may find the greatest need for developing local materials. For example, health care organizations serving large numbers of persons for whom English is not their first language or who have little or no ability to speak or read English may find bilingual or non-English materials difficult to obtain. Only a small portion of publications from the National Cancer Institute or the American Cancer Society are available in non-English versions. Developing such materials requires special attention to cultural differences as well as a sophisticated understanding of the language of the target audience. Translating materials from English should be done by individuals who are sufficiently fluent to fully understand connotations of words, common expressions, and colloquial terms, and the application of formal and familiar forms of address.

Readability

One aspect of printed patient education materials that has received considerable attention in the nursing literature is reading level. It is estimated that 20% of Americans read below the fifth-grade level,[65] which has been identified as the minimum reading level for making good use of basic written materials.[66] Individuals with reading skills below this level are functionally illiterate, lacking the reading and writing skills needed for daily activities in contemporary society. Many adults, while not illiterate, still have low literacy skills. The 1992 National Adult Literacy Survey found that 90 million adult Americans, or 47%, demonstrated low literacy.[67] Although the reading level of print materials can be easily evaluated, and though the literacy issue has been discussed in the literature, the use of reading levels that are barriers for many within the general public still occurs.

A review of 137 consent forms for clinical oncology protocols in use at a major university medical center found that reading levels of the forms varied from grade 6 to grade 16.[68] The mean grade level was 11.1, and only 6% of the forms had a reading level at grade 6 or lower. A 1992 study of 51 publications provided by the ACS found that only one publication was written below the sixth-grade level.[69] Over half of the publications were written at the twelfth-grade level or higher, up to a level equivalent to graduate study. A more recent study assessed the reading levels of 30 commonly used patient education pamphlets provided by the ACS and the National Cancer Institute (NCI) and the educational attainment and actual reading levels of a group of cancer patients.[70] The 30 pamphlets ranged from grades 6 to 16 in reading level, with a mean grade level of 9.8. Only 27% of the patient group tested could be expected to understand all of the printed materials.

It should be noted that both the ACS and the NCI, as well as many other organizations that provide cancer patient education materials, are actively addressing problems with the level of literacy required for comprehending their materials. Currently, the ACS and the NCI review reading levels and modify materials to reach as broad an audience as possible as new materials are developed or as older publications are revised and updated. Both organizations also offer some publications specifically designed for use with low-literacy audiences.[65]

A variety of readability assessment scales are available. The readability formula used by the NCI's Office of Cancer Communication is the SMOG, selected because it provides ease of use with a high level of accuracy. Guidelines for using the SMOG readability test and a table for conversion of SMOG scores to approximate grade levels of reading ability are provided in Table 73-3. Readability scales generally assess the difficulty of vocabulary and sentence length and complexity. Readability tests designed for use on computers also may assess grammar, style, word usage, and punctuation as indicators of reading difficulty.[67]

Much of the literature addressing readability of mate-

Table 73-3   The SMOG Readability Formula

To calculate the SMOG reading grade level, begin with the entire written work that is being assessed, and follow these four steps:

1. Count off 10 consecutive sentences near the beginning, in the middle, and near the end of the text.
2. From this sample of 30 sentences, circle all of the words containing three or more syllables (polysyllabic), including repetitions of the same word, and total the number of words circled.
3. Estimate the square root of the total number of polysyllabic words counted. This is done by finding the nearest perfect square, and taking its square root.
4. Finally, add a constant of 3 to the square root. This number gives the SMOG grade, or the reading grade level that a person must have reached if he or she is to fully understand the text being assessed.

A few additional guidelines will help to clarify these directions:

- A sentence is defined as a string of words punctuated with a period (.), an exclamation point (!) or a question mark (?).
- Hyphenated words are considered one word.
- Numbers which are written out should also be considered, and if in numeric form in the text, they should be pronounced to determine if they are polysyllabic.
- Proper nouns, if polysyllabic, should be counted, too.
- Abbreviations should be read as unabbreviated to determine if they are polysyllabic.

Not all pamphlets, fact sheets, or other printed materials contain 30 sentences. To test a text that has fewer than 30 sentences:

1. Count all of the polysyllabic words in the text.
2. Count the number of sentences.

3. Find the average number of polysyllabic words per sentence as follows:

$$\text{Average} = \frac{\text{Total \# of polysyllabic words}}{\text{Total \# of sentences}}$$

4. Multiply that average by the number of sentences *short of 30.*
5. Add that figure to the total number of polysyllabic words.
6. Find the square root and add the constant of 3.

Perhaps the quickest way to administer the SMOG grading test is by using the SMOG conversion table. Simply count the number of polysyllabic words in your chain of 30 sentences and look up the approximate grade level on the chart.

SMOG Conversion Table*	
Total Polysyllabic Word Counts	Approximate Grade Level (+ 1.5 Grades)
0–2	4
3–6	5
7–12	6
13–20	7
21–30	8
31–42	9
43–56	10
57–72	11
73–90	12
91–110	13
111–132	14
133–156	15
157–182	16
183–210	17
211–240	18

*Developed by Harold C. McGraw, Office of Educational Research, Baltimore County Schools, Towson, Maryland.

Office of Cancer Communications, National Cancer Institute: *Making Health Communication Programs Work: A Planner's Guide.* NIH Publication No. 92-1493. Washington, DC, U.S. Department of Health and Human Services, National Institutes of Health, 1992.[55]

rials is focused on reading level. Other factors, however, also contribute to the readability or the reader's likelihood of comprehending information being presented. Beyond the level of the text itself, comprehension is enhanced by how blocks of text are placed on the page, the use of open space and wide margins, the use of headings and other organizers, choice of typeface, the use of graphics and illustrations, and other design factors. For example, low-literate women exhibited better comprehension of information on cervical cancer and condyloma when given a pamphlet with illustrations and a narrative text rather than a pamphlet with no illustrations and a bulleted text, even though the pamphlet with illustrations had a slightly more difficult reading level.[71] Tables 73-4 and 73-5 provide guidelines for both reducing the reading difficulty and enhancing comprehension through design, illustrations, and other visual effects. An excellent resource for developing materials that work well with persons with low literacy is *Teaching Patients with Low Literacy Skills* by Doak, Doak, and Root.[66] Reducing the

complexity of the text and using an effective format, graphics, and illustrations improve the readability for all readers, not just for those with low literacy.

Much of the discussion in the nursing literature regarding development of patient education materials focuses on printed materials. In general, locally produced materials make less use of more complex technologies such as audio- and videotapes, computer programs, or computer technologies that provide interactive video capabilities. Just as in the development of print materials, there are many factors that distinguish effective audiovisual programs from ineffective ones. Some are much the same as those that affect print materials—culturally sensitive content, use of vocabulary and sentence structures that are appropriate for the literacy level of the audience. Many of the guidelines for use of format, illustrations, and visual effects in print materials have comparable guidelines applicable to video or computer programs. But other factors also come into play. For example, the pace of presentation is very important since,

Table 73-4   Reducing Reading Difficulty of Written Patient Education Materials

1. Pick short words—2 syllables or less.
2. Use common words. For instance, replace the word *physician* with the word *doctor*.
3. Write in the active voice. Instead of writing, "The patient should," say, "You should."
4. Create short sentences—5 to 7 words.
5. Write in conversational style, as if you were talking to the person.
6. Give information in small amounts—one idea at a time.
7. Do not use initials and abbreviations. Even simple ones, such as days of the week and months of the year, can be a problem for this audience.
8. Do not change a word just for variety. If you start using the word *cancer,* do not change to *tumor.*
9. Avoid lists. They present a problem in comprehension for adults with low literacy skills. If you use them, break them up with easily understandable visual effects.

Reprinted with permission from Morra ME, Varricchio C: Teaching patients with limited reading skills. *Cancer Pract* 1:154–156, 1993.[65]

unlike the pace of print materials, which is set by the reader, the pace of an audio or video program is not directly controlled by the listener or viewer. Production of materials using such technology benefit greatly by having knowledgeable professionals who work with these media participate in the development.

Pretesting

The development stage for patient education and support materials and programs can also be enhanced by pretesting draft materials with selected groups that are representative of the intended target audience. A variety of techniques can be used for pretesting, and a variety of characteristics or qualities of the materials can be evaluated. Are the materials attractive so that people will try to read them? Is the format easily followed? Is the information organized in a logical pattern or sequence? Most important, is the material understood? Are the learning goals achieved? Individual interviews, focus groups, surveys, and pilot testing of materials are all mechanisms that can be used for pretesting.

It is important again at this stage to use feedback from health care professionals who will use the materials. Both health care professionals and representatives from the target audience can provide important, though different, types of feedback. The health care professionals' comments are likely to focus on factors that will affect practical usefulness. Are materials too lengthy to be presented in the time available? Will the materials complement other resources being used? Are they organized into categories of information or topical groupings that clinicians typi-

Table 73-5   Improving Readability with Pictures and Visual Effects

1. Make illustrations simple, direct, and lifelike. Use sketches and line drawings with heavy, clean lines. Make people look as human as possible.
2. When showing parts of the body, include sections that people will recognize, such as legs and arms. Do not show drawings only of the inside parts of the body.
3. Use visuals to show desired behavior. Show only the correct way to accomplish a task. Using visuals to demonstrate both right and wrong can be confusing.
4. Comic books that tell stories of real people, using human figures, can be useful teaching tools. Make sure the messages are short, with no more than 15 words in each balloon area.
5. Stylized visuals and abstract forms are not appropriate for this audience.
6. Do not use charts with many columns. Cut down the amount of statistical data.
7. Cartoons usually are not useful ways of communicating with low-literacy people. Cartoons often confuse, introducing figures that are irrelevant to the message.
8. Present one idea on a single page—or two pages if they are face-to-face. Simple ideas should not need more than two facing pages.
9. Two columns on a page are preferable. This ensures that the line will not be too long for a person to comprehend.
10. When using a series of steps, make them few. Place the steps in left-to-right order, down the page in the normal reading order. Number each step and place related text next to the visual, so that the reader does not need to move back and forth to other parts of the page.
11. Use an action title or caption to direct the reader on what to do. Make it brief—no more than 10 words. Tie captions directly into the visuals.
12. If you wish to emphasize something, underline it. Or use circles, arrows, larger print, or color to help the eye focus on critical points.
13. Do not use all capital letters, italics, or script. Avoid fancy typefaces. Avoid stylized symbols whenever possible. All of these are difficult for this audience to read. If possible, select 14-point type.
14. Have a clear idea in your mind why you are using a visual, and make sure the visual fits that objective. Make sure each visual has a distinct focus point.

Reprinted with permission from Morra ME, Varricchio C: Teaching patients with limited reading skills. *Cancer Pract* 1:154–156, 1993.[65]

cally use as they speak with patients and families? Do clinicians have available any special equipment required (if the program or materials use audiotapes, videotapes, or computers)? Will they consider using the materials or program in their practice setting?

An excellent resource for guiding development of patient education materials is the NCI's publication *Clear and Simple: Developing Effective Print Materials for Low-Literate Readers*.[67] Although intended to assist in developing materials for low-literacy audiences, the processes outlined and most of the issues discussed are applicable to any program or materials development activities.

Step 4: Implementation

At this point the educational and support material or program is ready for use with the target group in the settings for which it was designed. Close monitoring of the implementation, especially in the early stages, might involve several issues. Are the materials being provided to those for whom they were intended? Are enough copies available? Are the materials being used in the settings and for the purposes for which they were designed? Is there any initial feedback indicating major problems that need to be addressed? And, of special importance for future assessment and improvement of the materials or program, are evaluation procedures being followed as designed?

Step 5: Assessing Effectiveness

At this stage, evaluation information collected during program implementation is reviewed to gauge the level of effectiveness of the program or materials. Possible actions for addressing weaknesses and improving the program or materials are considered. The evaluation should be based upon information gathered as designed in step 1. The primary question to be addressed is whether the program or materials met the objectives. If materials were used in a manner different from that for which they were intended, or if the program was implemented differently than designed, what caused the changes? How did the changes affect effectiveness? What can be changed to improve the materials or program?

Step 6: Program Refinement

The final step is to use the results of the evaluation to revise and refine the materials or program. The development cycle in effect becomes a spiral, with the evaluation findings of one cycle being used as the starting point to again look at objectives and strategies, and strengthen evaluation procedures; to update, revise, or replace materials; to use feedback from users and target audience representatives to test the revised materials or program; to once again implement or use the materials or program,

including reevaluating outcomes; and to collect the evaluation information to plan for further refinement and a new cycle. This ongoing cycle also allows the materials or program to be continually updated with new information, to meet new needs within the target audience, or to adjust to changes in the professional settings in which the materials or programs are used.

Developing materials or programs locally can be challenging. Using a careful sequence of developmental steps ensures that the special effort and resources committed to the challenge are used well for the maximum gains possible.

Resources for Patient Education and Support

The number of resources for patient education and patient support in oncology has grown tremendously in recent years. Some resources are not new—the Cancer Information Service of the NCI has been in existence since 1975, and the ACS began its work of providing a wide range of public and patient education materials many years earlier. In recent years, however, there has been rapid growth in new materials, information services, and support programs. In part, new resources reflect changes in technology, particularly the opportunities for rapid data retrieval and response as well as widespread access to electronic databases using computer technology. In part, the growth in resources and programs reflects the success in treatment of cancer and the resulting change in perspective, from viewing cancer as a fatal illness to a chronic illness. The increased numbers of people living with cancer have created a need for a wide range of both information and support resources. Public demand for information and support programs also reflects a growth in a consumer-oriented perspective throughout our society. And in part, the growth of resources reflects increased awareness of the need for information and the ongoing efforts by many organizations to provide better information and easier access for larger audiences.

In spite of the growth in resources and specialized systems for obtaining information, in a recent study sponsored by the Oncology Nursing Society (ONS) of nurses in clinical practice,[72] nurses reported inadequate resources in many areas and difficulty in locating or accessing information when it is available. Nearly half of the nurses responding indicated that they often meet the gap between available resources and resource needs by using self- or institution-developed materials. Both nurses and their patients indicated a need for a central clearinghouse on available information. The researchers noted that it is unclear whether information is unavailable or nurses are unable to access available information.

Effective patient teaching is dependent not only upon process but also content. Accurate, effective instructional materials are essential. The following sections review a limited number of the major sources of information and support programs available for patients and their caregivers, both professional and nonprofessional.

American Cancer Society

The ACS is a nationwide, community-based organization that offers a wide range of programs and services focused on public understanding about cancer; research on prevention, early detection, and treatment of cancer; and education and support for both health professionals and cancer patients and their families. The ACS provides many public education efforts seeking to enhance public understanding of cancer, cancer prevention and treatment options, and cancer survivorship issues. In addition, the ACS provides direct information to individuals through two primary inquiry routes: the Resources, Information and Guidance system operated by local offices of the ACS, and the Cancer Resource Service provided by the national ACS office. The ACS also maintains an Internet site that serves as an easy link to its many information resources.

At the national level ACS staff can provide information regarding ACS publications, video programs, and other such material resources, and can arrange for materials to be provided to the inquirer. In addition, the national office can provide contact information for resources available at the local level.

Complementing the national ACS office, the local-level, volunteer-staffed network can provide access to print and audiovisual materials provided by the ACS and information regarding locally offered programs sponsored or supported by ACS. ACS also works in cooperation with other organizations and provides referrals to programs offered by other groups.

The national and local ACS offices provide complementary services, with the national service focused primarily on access to a wide variety of specialized informational materials and the local offices intended to make links to the many direct services and programs available at the local level. The ACS strives to provide a seamless system for delivering information and services so that an individual can access ACS services beginning at either level of entry.[73,74]

The ACS also provides extensive resources for health care professionals as well as for the public. These include a wide range of publications written for professionals, research grant programs, scholarship and fellowship programs, and many types of support provided through the national, division, and local offices to professional groups. The national ACS office can be contacted through a toll-free number: 1-800-ACS-2345 (1-800-227-2345). The numbers for contacting local and state offices of ACS can be found through local telephone directories.

The ACS Web site <http://www.cancer.org>, provides basic descriptive information and standard treatment options for all types of cancer, access to several thousand informational documents, information on ACS services and programs for patients and their families as well as for health care professionals, information and links to local ACS offices, and links to many other Internet cancer information resources. Several of the ACS programs designed for education and support of cancer patients and their families are widely used, four of which are described briefly here.

"I Can Cope"

This is a structured patient education program originally developed by oncology nurses with support from a local ACS office.[8] The success of the local program led to its adoption by the ACS on the national level in 1979. The ACS currently provides program materials as well as local training sessions for health care professionals to serve as program leaders.

"I Can Cope" is designed primarily as an educational program, but, as do many other educational programs, it also provides support for patients and families through group discussions and socialization.[3] As one of the oldest programs of its type available, it has been extensively evaluated.[75]

"Man to Man"

This initiative includes several programs designed for men experiencing prostate cancer. Information programs, group programs for the partners of men with prostate cancer, and a one-on-one visitation program are all options available through this initiative.

"Reach to Recovery"

This visitation program for women with breast cancer began in 1973. Cancer patients are put in contact with trained volunteers with similar backgrounds who also have experienced breast cancer. "Reach to Recovery," "Look Good . . . Feel Better," and several other programs and resources are components of ACS's Breast Cancer Network.

"Look Good . . . Feel Better"

This national program is designed to help women undergoing cancer treatment to maintain grooming and appearance. Changes in personal appearance can be important factors affecting self esteem, psychosocial well-being, and quality of life. "Look Good . . . Feel Better" was developed by the ACS in 1989 in cooperation with the Cosmetics, Toiletry and Fragrance Association Foundation and the National Cosmetology Association.

National Cancer Institute

As the primary federal agency with responsibility for research on cancer causes, treatment, and prevention, the NCI is heavily involved in providing the most recent, up-to-date information to both health care professionals and the general public. Within the NCI the Office of Cancer

Information, Communication and Education, established in 1998, has primary responsibility for these responsibilities. In recent years, the NCI has emphasized developing systems to improve access to comprehensive, state-of-the-art information, increasing the emphasis on quality-of-life issues, and strengthening information resources and access for underserved and hard-to-reach audiences.

The NCI has been described as having built the "deepest and broadest communication infrastructure" for making cancer research findings and state-of-the-art practices available for both health care professionals and the general public.[76] With the rapid growth of the Internet and of the number of people with computer access, NCI has developed an impressive array of electronic information resources along with a national information service that can be contacted by telephone. The major components of the NCI information system include the following.

PDQ

Developed in 1984 as "Physician Data Query," PDQ is the NCI's most up-to-date source of cancer information. PDQ provides three types of information: cancer information summaries, clinical trial and standard protocols, and directories.[77]

Cancer information summaries are concise statements on the prognosis, staging, and treatment of the major types of cancer, with statements on assessment and management of commonly encountered problems, screening summaries of evidence for selected types of cancer, summaries on selected investigational or newly approved drugs for treatment, and references and abstracts to key papers in the medical literature. The cancer information summaries are updated by five editorial boards; new and updated information is added to the database monthly.

The second major component of PDQ is the clinical trial and standard protocol reports. This component provides information on over 1600 active treatment, supportive care, screening, and prevention studies with objectives, entry criteria, regimen information, and participating investigators. NCI-funded studies, non-NCI studies that have been reviewed by a PDQ editorial board, and European studies approved by the European Organization for Research and Treatment of Cancer or the United Kingdom Cancer Research Campaign are included in this database. A number of standard therapy protocols also are listed as well as an archival file of protocols no longer accruing patients.

Finally, PDQ provides directories of physicians in clinical oncology practice, members of selected professional societies for physicians in oncology practice, clinical investigators for those protocols in the PDQ database, NCI grantees, and members of the NCI clinical trials cooperative groups. Over 22,000 physicians, 200 genetic counselors, and 8000 organizations active in cancer care are included.[78,79]

The NCI strives to make access to cancer information widely available. Both health care professionals and the general public can access PDQ directly through the NCI's

CancerNet Web site <http://cancernet.nci.nih.gov/pdqfull.html>. PDQ also serves as the basic information resource to support other NCI information sources such as the Cancer Information Service.

Following an extensive assessment of NCI information resources and a series of demonstration projects in the mid-1990s, the NCI initiated a major review and redesign of the structure of PDQ and how it is accessed.[80,81] The goals of this effort were to make the NCI information resources easier to use and more widely accessible. One result has been to minimize the distinctions between information available for "health care professionals" and "the general public." Recognizing that many within the general public seek and use the more detailed information previously identified as intended for health care professionals, the system will simply identify levels of information—one general and the other with more detail. The changes flowing from this redesign effort will be incorporated into the PDQ by the end of the year 2000.

CancerNet

CancerNet is the site established and maintained by NCI as the primary entry into the variety of information resources provided by NCI through electronic networks. Sikorski and Peters called it "as close as one can get to the epicenter of reliable cancer information."[76] CancerNet provides information from three major sources: PDQ, CancerLit Topic Searches, and CancerTrials.

CancerLit Topic Searches provides citations and abstracts from a bibliographic database of over 1.4 million citations from more than 4000 sources published since 1963. NCI indicates that the database is updated with over 8000 items monthly. NCI prepares monthly topic searches on about 90 topics and makes these searches (as well as the past six months of such searches) available to facilitate review of new information for users.

CancerTrials, initiated in early 1998, is a searchable database of over 1600 current trials open and approved for patient accrual. It includes trials in the areas of supportive care, screening, and prevention as well as those focused on diagnosis and treatment. Information on more than 9500 trials that have been closed also is maintained.

The CancerNet site also refers users to two other avenues for obtaining most of the information available through CancerNet: CancerMail and CancerFax. CancerMail provides for submitting requests for information by e-mail <cancermail@icicc.nci.nih.gov>. Submitting a request with the word *HELP* in the body of the message will result in a response providing a list of available information. By including the word *SPANISH* in the body of the message, the response will be provided in Spanish. CancerFax can be contacted at 301-402-5874 by use of a fax machine with a touch-tone telephone. Once connected, various voice prompts allow the caller to indicate the information being requested with numbered touch-tone responses. Most CancerFax information is available in both English and Spanish.

At times descriptive information about NCI's CancerNet, PDQ, CancerLit, CancerTrials or other resources and services may create a confusing picture of the internal structure of the databases and services offered. Fortunately, understanding the internal organization is not necessary. There are multiple entries to the information with explanations and directions for navigating and a variety of cross links. The CancerNet Web site address is <http://cancernet.nci.nih.gov>. CancerNet also is available through a gopher site, <gopher://gopher.nih.gov:70/11/clin/cancernet>.

Cancer Information Service

The Cancer Information Service (CIS) is a national network of 19 regional offices funded and coordinated by the NCI. Established in 1975, the CIS is contacted through the toll-free number 1-800-4-CANCER (1-800-422-6237); calls are routed to the appropriate regional center. The CIS centers are staffed by certified information specialists prepared to provide a wide variety of services and information.

The CIS is responsible for three types of services; the first is to provide up-to-date information in response to inquiries. Each CIS office accesses the NCI's PDQ database to provide information on treatment, detection, supportive care, and the full range of information available through PDQ. Second, each center in the network is responsible for maintaining a directory of cancer-related services and programs in the region it serves—such as local and regional cancer education programs, speakers, regional cancer centers, and voluntary health organizations. Thus they help link individuals to specific services. Third, each center's staff includes an outreach coordinator who is responsible for an outreach program designed to serve as a catalyst for cancer education initiatives in the region and for providing technical assistance for activities related to those initiatives. Such assistance might include providing state or regional statistical information, review of materials, program planning and evaluation assistance, or referral to appropriate individuals or organizations that can provide the particular expertise that is needed.[82]

As part of its information responsibilities, the CIS handles requests for printed materials produced or developed by the NCI. These materials are sent primarily to health care professionals and organizations, which in turn distribute such information to the general public. The CIS is a major user of the PDQ, drawing information from PDQ to fulfill its role of providing cancer diagnosis, treatment, clinical trial options, and other information to the public.[76,83]

At a time when so much emphasis is placed upon use of the Internet and computer-accessed information systems, it is important to keep in mind that there remain many people who do not have ready access to such resources and many others who are not knowledgeable about using computer-based systems or who prefer not to use them. The CIS, the local offices of the ACS, and other such services provide a human-to-human approach for patient and public information that remains very important to ensure that accurate and timely information is available to all.

Combined Health Information Database

The Combined Health Information Database (CHID) is a searchable bibliographic database developed and maintained cooperatively by several health-related federal government agencies. Initiated in 1982, the CHID became available to health care professionals outside the federal government and to the public in 1985. At the present there are 18 subfiles within the CHID, including one devoted to cancer patient education and another for cancer prevention and control. The cancer patient education subfile is maintained by the NCI; the cancer prevention and control subfile is found in a database maintained by the Centers for Disease Control and Prevention. In addition to journal articles and books, the database includes bibliographic citations and abstracts for a variety of special reports, pamphlets, audiovisuals, product descriptions, "hard-to-find information sources," and health promotion and education programs at state and local levels. The CHID provides source and availability information for many of these materials to help users obtain materials directly. New information is added to the CHID on a quarterly basis, and previously entered information is regularly reviewed for current availability.[84,85] The CHID Web site, CHID Online, is accessed at <http://chid.nih.gov>.

National Coalition for Cancer Survivorship

The National Coalition for Cancer Survivorship (NCCS) was founded in 1986 based on the perspective that all persons who experience cancer are cancer survivors from diagnosis onward, experiencing different stages or "seasons" along the continuum of survivorship. The NCCS seeks to be both an organization of individuals and a coalition of organizations working in the field of cancer services, research, and advocacy. It focuses on a wide range of issues related to quality of life for cancer survivors: providing referral to appropriate local support services; addressing barriers to employment and access to health insurance; and advocating for changes in health care delivery and policy to maximize cancer survivors' access to optimal treatment and support. The NCCS responds to individual inquiries, provides free consultation services to survivors on employment and insurance issues, provides support programs—often in cooperation with other organizations—for cancer survivors, and publishes a variety of information materials, especially in the areas of employment rights and health insurance. The coalition is particularly active as an advocacy group, testifying and advocating at local, state, and national levels on public policy issues affecting cancer survivors.

The NCCS has been a powerful voice, among both the general public and health care professionals, in changing views about cancer. The perspective of survivorship that underlies the philosophy of the NCCS was first outlined and promoted by Fitzhugh Mullan, a physician and cancer survivor.[47] The concept of survivorship is conveyed in a simple statement often cited in materials provided by NCCS: "From the time of discovery and for the balance of life, an individual diagnosed with cancer is a survivor." Mullan described "seasons" along the continuum of survivorship. At the medical or acute stage, which begins with diagnosis, the focus is on efforts to contain the illness. From the view of patient education and support, emphasis is on understanding the illness, treatment and treatment options, self-care, and quality-of-life issues, and particularly on fostering an understanding that people can and do survive a cancer diagnosis.

When the course of treatment has been completed, or a period of remission occurs, the season of watchful waiting emerges. The person with cancer must reintegrate into a life pattern more like that which preceded diagnosis. It is not unusual for there to be a letdown or sense of loss as a result of being less actively involved with the medical personnel who were regularly available during active treatment. Educational and support needs address a return to routine activities, coping with the fears of recurrence, the need for appropriate medical surveillance, and promoting wellness and healthy behaviors.

In the longer term, the individual moves to the season of permanent survival or cure. At this stage concerns about long-term effects of treatment, as well as social stigma and policy barriers that affect employment and insurability, become very important. Educational and support issues relate to these problems, seeking to empower cancer survivors to speak out for their rights. This activism for the rights of cancer survivors also builds support and understanding for other individuals at all stages of survivorship.

The view of cancer patients as survivors can be an effective strategy for thinking about the needs of patients at various stages of their experience with cancer. It is an important perspective for changing society's views of cancer, replacing unreasonable fears with understanding, and working to remove biases that place limits on the rights and opportunities of people with cancer.

The NCCS maintains a Web site available at <http://cansearch.org> that provides ready access to a wide range of information resources, both those provided by NCCS and those available from many other organizations. The Web site includes a guide to cancer resources at <http://cansearch.org/cansearch/cansearch.htm> that provides links to about 150 other Web sites with brief descriptions of these sites.[86]

Oncology Nursing Society

The ONS is a natural source of information for oncology nurses. In addition to its professional journals, the ONS maintains a Web site at <http://www.ons.org> that provides information for both nurses and patients and the general public. A component of the site designed especially for patient use is the Patient Information and Educa-

tion Resource (PIER). PIER provides access to over 400 reviewed patient education materials with a search feature.[87]

New Technologies and the Growth of Patient Education and Support

A large number of specialized organizations have developed that focus on providing education and support programs for cancer patients and their families, particularly in the area of cancers affecting women.[88] Some organizations—such as the ACS, the American Lung Association, and the Leukemia Society of America—have long and well-known records of work in the field of advocacy and support for cancer research, public education, and patient education and support. There are, however, many such groups, some of which have national prominence while others a more regional impact. In the past, there tended to be few groups that had the resources to achieve national recognition or to reach a national audience—or even to a large regional audience. In recent years, however, the tremendous growth in information technologies has facilitated widespread dissemination of information and has contributed to making even local or regional organizations potential sources of information on a national scale.

As an example of the wide range of information resources, a recent article on using Internet resources for strengthening oncology nursing provided a list of 32 clinical resources on the Internet.[89] The list included professional organizations, major cancer centers, organizations from the pharmaceutical industry, publishers, public advocacy organizations, universities, and other sources. The NCI's CancerNet Web site provides links to 40 additional Web sites offering cancer information, a listing of 58 NCI-designated cancer centers, a listing of FDA-certified mammography facilities, and two other Web sites that in turn provide links to all other government sites. The Web site of the National Coalition for Cancer Survivorship provides links to nearly 150 other sites, some of them identified as lists of links to additional sites on particular topics. In short, the development of information technology has made it possible for large and small organizations—and even individuals, if willing to give sufficient time to the project—to become visible resources within the electronic information network. A report on former surgeon general C. Everett Koop's effort to evaluate health-related sites on the Internet noted that there were, in mid-1998, over 12,000 health sites.[90]

In many ways this is a wonderful development for enhancing patient education and support. The convergence of consumer telecommunications, electronic mass media, and computer systems is creating information service opportunities unimagined by most people even a few years ago.[91] The new technologies have made possible systems and services such as PDQ and the opportunity for users, including both health care professionals and patients and families, to access such systems. Developing technologies such as the CD-ROM have created the possibility of interactive video programming that far exceeds the capabilities of older computer-based instructional programs.[92]

The increasing availability and use of information drawn from electronic resources and the reliance on talk and support groups as a source of nonprofessional information does raise, however, questions regarding the potential for misinformation being given.[93–95] Recognizing concerns about the uneven quality of information available on the Internet, guidelines for assessing the quality of such information have been discussed in the professional literature.[89,96] In general, such guidelines are similar to what might be applied to any written materials: Consider the credentials and credibility of the source of the information, and be cautious about information that does not clearly identify a source. Evaluate whether the person or organization providing information may have a particular perspective or bias. Assess the timeliness of the information; Web site information should clearly identify when it was developed and how often it is reviewed.

It is important that health care professionals and organizations assist patients and families in making use of the wide variety of information and support resources, but it is also important to provide assistance in assessing the quality and understanding the potential problems. A good example of a sensitive approach can be seen on the National Coalition for Cancer Survivorship Web site. Within its Online Guide to Cancer Resources available at <http://cansearch.org/canserch/canserch.htm>, information is provided about newsgroups, mailing lists, and chat rooms. There is a clear discussion about the openness of these features for anyone to participate and to provide information or ideas. In discussing the use of chat rooms, the NCCS information notes that many who participate are in the midst of coping emotionally with the illness, and that others will seek to find people in a weak moment in order to take advantage of them. The text is sensitive but straightforward in providing this warning, and represents an important attempt to help the user understand the potential problems related to electronic information and support sources.

The growth in information technology and electronic networks provides new, expanding opportunities for patient and family education and support. These resources may serve to empower cancer patients to be more active and in control of their search for information and support.[91] Health care professionals need to be aware of the growth of these resources and to continue to seek information and understanding regarding the best use of such resources for themselves and their patients.

Future Considerations for Patient Education and Support

Identifying future trends or long-term projections is difficult in any field. Yet some futurist speculation is important and necessary if we seek to prepare for the changes and new developments that will shape the realities of future practice. Others have noted trends in demographics, the influences of technology, and changing social patterns as factors affecting future patient education and cancer practice patterns.[97,98] Based on the review of literature and discussions with professionals working in patient education and support programs, the following emerge as four key areas of future change and challenge for education and support in oncology nursing practice.

Demographic Patterns and Their Implications

Some future aspects not only of patient education but also of many other areas of our society will be determined by demographics. It is clear that the population of the United States is shifting to a larger percentage of older people based on the aging of the "baby boomers." It is also clear that the future U.S. population will be more diverse than the current population due both to differences in birth rates across various ethnic and racial groups and to patterns of immigration. These two known demographic trends point to the likelihood of increases in cancer incidence since many types of cancer are closely linked to aging, and to an increasing need for culturally sensitive and appropriate public education programs, medical care delivery systems, and patient education and support programming and materials.

These demographic patterns, in conjunction with changing socioeconomic patterns—themselves caused in part by demography—have implications for patient support structures and economic factors affecting education and support opportunities. For example, smaller family sizes and the mobility of our society contribute to a loss of extended family structures supporting people experiencing cancer. The reduced ratio of younger workers to older nonworking people will put greater economic burdens on those working adults and reduce resources for older persons experiencing cancer or other illnesses. A higher growth rate seen in low-income populations, persons less likely to receive preventive health care or early diagnosis, raises the likelihood of increased health problems, greater need for health care services, and economic pressure on health systems serving such populations.

These changes will present challenges for creating effective support structures, for meeting these needs with limited economic resources, and for creating effective outreach activities to reach disadvantaged and underserved populations.

Changes in Technology

The potential benefits of new technologies, especially the advances in computer and telecommunications technology, have already been discussed. The primary benefits are the tremendously expanded access to large amounts of information and the potential for bringing education and support programs to individuals without regard to physical barriers or distance. In addition, technological developments may make possible much wider use of more effective media, especially as developments in video technology bring down the cost of video communications and increase flexibility for continually updating such materials.

Caution may be raised about creating systems that provide information but lose a human dimension. The effective use of technology, however, may provide opportunities for even greater personal communications among individuals experiencing cancer and between health care providers and those needing assistance. The opportunities for communication among people from many different settings without regard to geographic barriers through computer bulletin board technology has tremendous potential for providing certain types of social support.

Special challenges in the area of using technology will be keeping pace with new developments, assisting those who find the use of computers or other electronic equipment to be stressful or perplexing, and simply finding ways to assess, select, and manage the vast amount of resources that become available.

The Changing Patterns of Health Care Delivery Systems

Much has been written in recent years regarding the changes in health care systems. Efforts to reduce both frequency and duration of hospitalizations; restrictions imposed by third-party payers; emphasis on cost reduction; an increasing role played by for-profit organizations in an area formerly dominated by nonprofit organizations; growth in outpatient and home health services; the diversity of roles played by nurses and many other health professionals; and the creation of new delivery systems such as health management organizations are all among the many changes that have been experienced.

The changing health care delivery system presents two major challenges from a patient education and support perspective. First, nurses need to be alert to the need to be advocates for strong education and support programming to ensure that these services are retained and appropriately incorporated within newly evolving forms of health care delivery. Second, particular attention is needed to ensure continuity in patient education and support services across the diverse components of the delivery system.

Demonstrating Effectiveness of Patient Education and Support

This last area for consideration is related to each of the three already discussed. As changes in our population and social patterns call for new approaches in patient education and support, as technology provides new op-

portunities and new challenges, and as the health care system itself changes, there will be an ongoing need for research, development of new approaches, and careful evaluation to understand, document, and promote effective patient education and support.

Research and development in patient education and support obviously flow directly from the changes that have been described. There will be a need to find effective strategies to respond to new social conditions and to reach new and diverse audiences of people with cancer. There will be a need to find the best ways to use new technologies. And there will be a need to create patient education and support approaches that fit within the new delivery systems. Most important, the ongoing financial pressures that all of health care will continue to experience will create a demand for solid evidence that patient education and support are important components of the health care system that result in measurable positive outcomes. Patient education and support must be shown to be essential elements of the health care system, and the system must be built in a way that will ensure the time, the resources, and the financial support for these critical elements.

References

1. McNally JC, Somerville ET, Miaskowski C, Rostad M (eds): *Guidelines for Oncology Nursing Practice* (ed 2). Philadelphia, Saunders, 1991
2. Barlett EE: At last, a definition. *Patient Educ Counsel* 7: 323–324, 1985 (editorial)
3. Johnson J, Lane C: Role of support groups in cancer care. *Support Care Cancer* 1:52–56, 1993
4. Evans RL, Connis RT: Comparison of brief group therapies for depressed cancer patients receiving radiation treatment. *Public Health Rep* 110:306–311, 1995
5. Spiegel D: How do you feel about cancer now? Survival and psychosocial support. *Public Health Rep* 110:298–300, 1995 (commentary)
6. Cella DF, Yellen SB: Cancer support groups: the state of the art. *Cancer Pract* 1:56–61, 1993
7. Hermann JF, Cella DF, Robinovitch A: Guidelines for support group programs. *Cancer Pract* 3:111–113, 1995
8. Johnson J: The effects of a patient education course on persons with a chronic illness. *Cancer Nurs* 5:117–123, 1982
9. Cunningham AJ, Lockwood GA, Edmonds CV: Which cancer patients benefit most from a brief, group, coping skills program? *Int J Psychiatry Med* 23:383–398, 1993
10. Grassman D: Development of inpatient oncology educational and support programs. *Oncol Nurs Forum* 10:669–676, 1993
11. Gustafson DH, Taylor JO, Thompson S, et al: Assessing the needs of breast cancer patients and their families. *Qual Manage Health Care* 2:6–17, 1993
12. Fernsler JI, Cannon CA: The whys of patient education. *Semin Oncol Nurs* 7:79–86, 1991
13. American Hospital Association: *Statement on a Patient's Bill of Rights.* Chicago, American Hospital Association, 1973
14. Spingarn ND, Chasen NH: Working with your doctor and hospital system: becoming a wise consumer, in Hoffman

F (ed): *A Cancer Survivor's Almanac: Charting Your Journey.* Minneapolis, Chronimed, 1996, pp 55–65

15. Oncology Nursing Society Education Committee: *Outcome Standards for Cancer Patient Education.* Pittsburgh, Oncology Nursing Society, 1982

16. Oncology Nursing Society: *Standard of Oncology Education: Patient/Family and Public.* Pittsburgh, Oncology Nursing Society, 1995

17. Whitman NI, Graham BA, Gleit CJ, et al: *Teaching in Nursing Practice: A Professional Model* (ed 2). Norwalk, CT, Appleton and Lange, 1992

18. Nelson-Marten P, Rich BA: A historical perspective of informed consent in clinical practice and research. *Semin Oncol Nurs* 15:81–88, 1999

19. Joint Commission on Accreditation of Healthcare Organizations: AMH completes transition to important functions. *Perspectives: The Joint Commission Newsletter* 14(3):1, 7–8, 1994

20. Joint Commission on Accreditation of Healthcare Organizations: *Comprehensive Accreditation Manual for Hospitals.* Oakbrook Terrace, IL, Joint Commission on Accreditation of Healthcare Organizations, 1998

21. *Conditions of Participation for Hospitals,* codified at 42 C.F.R. §482

22. Association of Community Cancer Centers: *Standards for Cancer Programs.* Rockville, MD, Association of Community Cancer Centers, 1997

23. Poroch D: The effect of preparatory patient education on the anxiety and satisfaction of cancer patients receiving radiation therapy. *Cancer Nurs* 18:206–214, 1995

24. Wells ME, McQuellon RP, Hinkle JS, et al: Reducing anxiety in newly diagnosed cancer patients: a pilot program. *Cancer Pract* 3:100–104, 1995

25. Gustafson D, Wise M, McTavish F, et al: Development and pilot evaluation of a computer–based support system for women with breast cancer. *J Psychosoc Oncol* 11:69–93, 1993

26. McTavish F, Gustafson DH, Owens BH, et al: CHESS: an interactive computer system for women with breast cancer piloted with an under-served population. *Proc Annu Symp Comput Appl Med Care* 599–603, 1994

27. O'Hare PA, Yost LS, McCorkle R: Strategies to improve continuity of care and decrease rehospitalization of cancer patients: a review. *Cancer Invest* 11:140–158, 1993

28. Forester B, Kornfeld DS, Fleiss JL, et al: Group psychotherapy during radiotherapy: effects on emotional and physical distress. *Am J Psychiatry* 150:1700–1706, 1993

29. Devine EC, Westlake SK: The effects of psychoeducational care provided to adults with cancer: meta-analysis of 116 studies. *Oncol Nurs Forum* 22:1369–1381, 1995

30. Spiegel D: Cancer and depression. *Brit J Psychiatry* 168:109–116, 1996 (suppl 30)

31. Buddeberg C, Sieber M, Wolf C, et al: Are coping strategies related to disease outcome in early breast cancer? *J Psychosom Res* 40:255–264, 1996

32. Tross S, Herndon J, Korzun A, et al: Psychological symptoms and disease-free and overall survival in women with stage II breast cancer. *J Natl Cancer Inst* 88:661–667, 1996

33. Padilla GV, Bulcavage LM: Theories used in patient/health education. *Semin Oncol Nurs* 7:87–96, 1991

34. Rankin SH, Stallings KD: *Patient Education: Issues, Principles, Practices* (ed 3). Philadelphia, Lippincott, 1996

35. Lorig K: *Patient Education: A Practical Approach* (ed 2). Thousand Oaks, CA, Sage, 1996

36. Green LW, Kreuter MW: *Health Promotion Planning: An Educational and Environmental Approach* (ed 2). Mountain View, CA, Mayfield, 1991

37. Bandura A: *Social Foundation of Thoughts and Actions: A Social Cognitive Theory.* Englewood Cliffs, NJ, Prentice-Hall, 1986

38. Lazarus RS, Folkman S: *Stress Appraisal and Coping.* New York, Springer, 1984

39. Miller SM: Monitoring versus blunting styles of coping with cancer influence the information patients want and need about their disease. *Cancer* 76:167–177, 1995

40. Manfredi C, Czaja R, Price P, et al: Cancer patients' search for information. *Monogr Natl Cancer Inst* 14:93–104, 1993

41. Hack TF, Degner LF, Dyck DG: Relationship between preferences for decisional control and illness information among women with breast cancer: a quantitative and qualitative analysis. *Soc Sci Med* 39:279–289, 1994

42. Howe KG: Approaches (and possible contraindications) to enhancing patients' autonomy. *J Clin Ethics* 5:179–188, 1994

43. Padberg RM, Padberg LF: Strengthening the effectiveness of patient education: applying principles of adult education. *Oncol Nurs Forum* 17:65–69, 1990

44. Knowles MS: *The Modern Practice of Adult Education: From Pedagogy to Andragogy* (ed 2). Upper Saddle River, NJ, Globe Fearon/Cambridge, 1980

45. Morra ME: Making choices: The consumer's perspective. *Cancer Nurs* 8:54–59, 1985 (suppl 1)

46. McGinn KA: It's all in the timing. *ONS Patient Education SIG Newsletter* 6(1):1, 3, 1995

47. Mullan F: Seasons of survival: reflections of a physician with cancer. *N Engl J Med* 313:270–273, 1985

48. Young-McCaughan S: Care path and CPR mannequin have new roles in early discharge teaching. *Oncol Nurs Forum* 22:149–150, 1995 (letter)

49. Stevenson E, Crosson K: Patient education: history, development, and current directions of the American Cancer Society and the National Cancer Institute. *Semin Oncol Nurs* 7:135–142, 1991

50. Harrison-Woermke DE, Graydon JE: Perceived informational needs of breast cancer patients receiving radiation therapy after excisional biopsy and axillary node dissection. *Cancer Nurs* 16:449–455, 1993

51. Saunders JM, McCorkle R: Models of care for persons with progressive cancer. *Nurs Clin North Am* 26:365–377, 1985

52. Tornberg M, McGrath BB, Benoliel JQ: Oncology transition services: partnership of nurses and families. *Cancer Nurs* 7:131–137, 1984

53. Meili L: The community hospital perspective of clinical trials and the role of the nurse educator. *Semin Oncol Nurs* 7:280–287, 1991

54. Ferrell BR, Grant M, Chan J, et al: The impact of cancer pain education on family caregivers of elderly patients. *Oncol Nurs Forum* 22:1211–1217, 1995

55. Office of Cancer Communication, National Cancer Institute: *Making Health Communication Programs Work: A Planner's Guide.* NIH Publication No. 92-1493. Washington, DC, U.S. Department of Health and Human Services, National Institutes of Health, 1992

56. McDermott MK: Patient education and compliance issues associated with access devices. *Semin Oncol Nurs* 11:221–226, 1995

57. Boyle DM: Realities to guide novel and necessary nursing care in geriatric oncology. *Cancer Nurs* 17:125–136, 1994

58. Boyle DM, Engelking C, Blesch KS, et al: Oncology Nursing Society position paper on cancer and aging: the mandate for oncology nursing. *Oncol Nurs Forum* 19:913–933, 1992

59. Habayeb GL: Cultural diversity: a nursing concept not yet reliably defined. *Nurs Outlook* 43:224–227, 1995

60. Charonko K: Cultural influences in "non-compliant" behavior and decision making. *Holistic Nurs Pract* 6:73–78, 1992

61. Dignan M, Sharp P, Blinson K, et al: Development of a cervical cancer education program for Native American women in North Carolina. *J Cancer Educ* 9:235–242, 1994

62. Freeman WL: Making research consent forms informative and understandable: the experience of the Indian Health Service. *Camb Q Health Ethics* 3:510–521, 1994

63. Yancey AK, Tanjasiri SP, Klein M, et al: Increased cancer screening behavior in women of color by culturally sensitive video exposure. *Prev Med* 24:142–148, 1995

64. Frank-Stromborg M, Olsen SJ (eds): *Cancer Prevention in Minority Populations: Cultural Implications for Health Care Professionals.* St. Louis, Mosby-Year Book, 1993

65. Morra ME, Varricchio C: Teaching patients with limited reading skills. *Cancer Pract* 1:154–156, 1993

66. Doak CC, Doak LG, Root JH: *Teaching Patients with Low Literacy Skills* (ed 2). Philadelphia, Lippincott, 1996

67. National Cancer Institute, National Institutes of Health: *Clear and Simple: Developing Effective Print Materials for Low-Literate Readers.* NIH Publication No. 95-3594. Washington, DC, U.S. Department of Health and Human Services, National Institutes of Health, 1994

68. Grossman SA, Piantadosi S, Covahey C: Are informed consent forms that describe clinical oncology research protocols readable by most patients and their families? *J Clin Oncol* 12:2211–2215, 1994

69. Meade C, Diekmann J, Thornhill DG: Readability of American Cancer Society patient education literature. *Oncol Nurs Forum* 19:51–55, 1992

70. Cooley ME, Moriarty H, Berger MS, et al: Patient literacy and the readability of written cancer educational materials. *Oncol Nurs Forum* 22:1345–1351, 1995

71. Michielutte R, Bahnson J, Dignan MB, et al: The use of illustrations and narrative text style to improve readability of a health education brochure. *J Cancer Educ* 7:251–260, 1992

72. Griffiths M, Leek C: Patient education needs: opinions of oncology nurses and their patients. *Oncol Nurs Forum* 22:139–144, 1995

73. Black BL: Comprehensive, seamless, integrated program for cancer resources, information and guidance. Unpublished material, American Cancer Society, September 1995

74. American Cancer Society: Cancer Facts & Figures 1998. American Cancer Society Web site, available at <http://cancer.org/statistics/index.html>. Accessed December 21, 1999

75. McMillan SC, Tittle MB, Hill D: A systematic evaluation of the "I Can Cope" program using a national sample. *Oncol Nurs Forum* 20:455–461, 1993

76. Sikorski R, Peters R: Oncology ASAP. Where to find reliable cancer information on the Internet. *JAMA* 277:1431–1432, 1997

77. Hubbard SM, Martin NB, Thurn AL: NCI's Cancer Information Systems: bringing medical knowledge to clinicians. *Oncology* 9:302–307, 1995

78. National Cancer Institute, NCI Information Associates Program: About PDQ. *ProtoCall: The Newsletter of the NCI Information Associates Program* 1:8, 1995

79. National Cancer Institute: PDQ—NCI's Comprehensive Cancer Database, National Cancer Institute Web site, available at <http://cancernet.nci.nih.gov/pdqfull.html>. Accessed December 21, 1999

80. National Cancer Institute, International Cancer Information Center and Patient Education Section of Office of Cancer Communications: *PDQ Patient Information Interview Project: Final Report.* Bethesda, MD, National Cancer Institute, 1994

81. National Cancer Institute, International Cancer Information Center/Office of Cancer Communications: PDQ/PIF Demonstration Project. Unpublished material, May 1995

82. Thomsen C: Updates from the National Cancer Institute: Cancer Information Service update. Cancer Patient Education Network Conference, Washington, DC, September 1995

83. Morra ME, Van Nevel JP, Nealon EO, et al: History of the Cancer Information Service. *Monogr Natl Cancer Inst* 14:7–33, 1993

84. National Cancer Institute, Office of Cancer Communications: Combined Health Information Database. General Information about CHID. Unpublished material, National Cancer Institute. March 1995

85. National Institutes of Health, Centers for Disease Control and Prevention: CHID Online. The Combined Health Information Database. The Combined Health Information Database Web site, available at <http://chid.nih.gov>. Accessed December 21, 1999

86. National Coalition for Cancer Survivorship: NCCS Web site, available at <http://www.cansearch.org>. Accessed December 21, 1999

87. Gomez E: Web sites help oncology nurses to strengthen leadership positions, easily access resources. *ONS News* 13(12):11, 1998

88. McCabe MS, Varricchio CG, Padberg RM, et al: Women's health advocacy: its growth and development in oncology. *Semin Oncol Nurs* 11:137–142, 1995

89. Gomez EG, DuBois K, King CR: Improving oncology nursing practice through understanding and exploring the Internet. *Oncol Nurs Forum* 25:4–10, 1998 (suppl 10)

90. Schultz S: No miracle cure. *U.S. News & World Report* 125:65, 1998

91. Bartlett EE: The digital revolution and patient self-empowerment. *Patient Educ Counsel* 20:1–3, 1993 (editorial)

92. Agre P: Interactive computer technology. *Cancer Pract* 2:74–76, 1994

93. Harris KA: The informational needs of patients with cancer and their families. *Cancer Pract* 6:39–46, 1998

94. Keoun B: Cancer patients find quackery on the Web. *J Natl Cancer Inst* 88:1263–1265, 1996

95. Silberg WM, Lundberg GD, Musacchio RA: Assessing, controlling, and assuring the quality of medical information on the Internet: *caveant lector et viewer*—let the reader and viewer beware. *JAMA* 277:1244–1245, 1997

96. Davis LE, Arndt TS: On-line sources of drug information in oncology. *Highlights Oncol Pract* 15(2):26–41, 1998

97. Morra ME: Future trends in patient education. *Semin Oncol Nurs* 7:143–145, 1991

98. Boyle DM: New identities: the changing profile of patients with cancer, their families, and their professional caregivers. *Oncol Nurs Forum* 21:55–61, 1994

CHAPTER 74

Hospital Care

Sharon L. Krumm, PhD, RN

Introduction

Hospital-based oncology nurses constitute the largest segment of oncology nurses in practice today. However, in recent years hospitals have undergone significant changes, the magnitude of which has not previously been experienced. The practice of oncology nursing in hospitals is influenced by a number of issues arising from these changes. This chapter identifies some of the major issues and briefly discusses their influence on hospital-based oncology nursing practice. Oncology nurses, whether new graduates or experienced practitioners, need to understand these issues and how they influence their practices. With this understanding comes the ability to mold and shape one's practice and to make better practice-related decisions. The issues are divided into three broad topics: the practice environment, general professional issues, and oncology nursing practice issues. The discussion of these issues is informally presented with references, but it reflects the experience and observations of nearly thirty years of personal, hospital-based oncology nursing.

Practice Environment Issues

Managed Care

It should not surprise the reader that a discussion of the influences on hospital-based oncology nursing practice begins with the issues of health care reform and managed care. The federal government's failure to establish a national health care system has led to an increasingly market-driven environment. Large businesses' and the federal government's demands for reducing the cost of health care have resulted in shorter hospital stays, increased inpatient acuity, and the shifting of care to ambulatory settings. As a result of these demands, a significant number of patients, including Medicare and Medicaid recipients, are in some form of managed care organization (MCO); however, the percent of the population in an MCO varies by state and region. Managed care organizations influence hospital care by setting limits on reimbursement, defining treatment options and lengths of stay, and externally managing the care of patients. Between 1987 and 1997, the average patient acuity increased by 12% as measured by case mix index (CMI) and the length of stay decreased by 23% across the country.[1] Within our National Cancer Institute (NCI) Comprehensive Cancer Center, the length of stay decreased by two days within two years and the CMI is the highest of any department in our approximately 1000-bed academic medical center. Within this vortex of changes in health care, some hospitals have closed or merged; health care organizations, including hospitals, have reorganized first vertically and then horizontally; and operational reorganization or redesign within hospitals is the norm. Solu-

tions that worked in the past are ineffective as hospitals face unprecedented pressures and challenges.

Financial Pressures

Hospitals are under tremendous pressure to reduce the cost of providing care and to simultaneously maintain or increase revenues. These pressures can provoke hospital administrators to shift the allocation of resources from clinical care to other administrative services to ensure that referrals are enhanced; insurance information is obtained and verified for every aspect of care prior to and throughout hospitalization and at time of discharge; documentation and coding are quickly and accurately completed; confidentiality of patient information is protected; bills are submitted and collected in a timely manner; beds are utilized efficiently; care is efficiently managed across the continuum; and the demands of external regulators are met. Nurse staffing has always been a primary target for expense reductions, as nursing salaries constitute a significant percentage of a hospital's operating budget. In some hospitals the total number of nursing hours per patient per day (NHPPD) has been reduced. In others, the total hours may have remained at a constant level but the skill mix has changed, resulting in a reduction in the number of hours of professional, direct care, that is to say, of registered nurse hours of care. This reduction in professional NHPPD is a major concern for many health care providers and increasingly so to the consumers of care.

External Regulations

Among external regulators influencing hospital care are the Joint Commission on Accreditation of Health Care Organizations (JCAHO), the Occupational Safety and Health Administration (OSHA), the Health Care Finance Administration (HCFA), the American College of Surgeons (ACOS), the Foundation for the Accreditation of Hematopoietic Cell Therapy (FAHCT), the National Bone Marrow Registry (NBMR), and the Office of Inspector General (OIG). In addition, managed care organizations require that specific criteria be met before including hospitals in their networks or as part of their centers of excellence. The JCAHO and other external agencies are publishing "report cards" of survey results and analysis of specific outcomes data. While proffered as protection for patients and consumers of health care, these reports can be misinterpreted or misleading to patients and the public; and they may prompt hospitals to further divert sparse resources away from clinical care to prepare for or defend against these reports and surveys.[2] The Web site available at <www.healthgrades.com> provides access to a number of report cards and is an example of one way that this information is made available to the public.

The federal and state governments control many aspects of hospital care through executive orders, the budget process, legislation, and administrative regulations. However, the legislation recently enacted in California and being considered by other state legislatures, that, among other provisions, establishes the nurse-to-patient staffing ratios, is noteworthy in the potential scope of its direct influence and control of nurse staffing levels.[3] The Balanced Budget Act (BBA) of 1997 and legislation and regulations related to Medicare and state medical assistance programs continue to have significant control over hospitals' revenues. Hospitals' responses to these controls directly and indirectly affect nurses and patient care as hospitals manage resources to revenues.

Consumerism

This is an age of active consumer involvement in many areas of public and private life, and this consumerism extends to health care services and the providers of health care. Patients are more knowledgable, more demanding, and better consumers of health care than in the past. It is not unusual for patients to present themselves to their physicians and nurses filled with information gathered from the Internet and other sources. While hospitalized, many patients continue to use the Internet as a source of health and treatment-related information. The consumer movement has been especially effective in positively influencing cancer care. The National Coalition of Cancer Survivors, the highly successful Komen Foundation for Breast Cancer Education, and other advocacy groups have effectively lobbied policymakers and politicians and are partially responsible for the significant increase in the National Institutes of Health's (NIH) budget and positive attention to the issues of cancer in our country. These same consumers and patients arrive at hospital doorsteps with specific expectations and demands of our institutions and caregivers; and, unfortunately they often are not always satisfied that their expectations are met. Public and consumer expectations are shaped by how well we as health professionals educate them. Additionally, the media and popular culture shape these expectations and may fuel consumer dissatisfaction. The television programs *Chicago Hope*, *ER*, and "exposés" on network news programs are examples of how popular culture influences consumers' expectations.

Social Issues

As our population ages the incidence of cancer increases, as do other chronic illnesses that often must be concurrently managed. Because of the increasingly complex care needs of patients and the movement toward ambulatory and home care, there is greater demand on hospital nurses and other personnel to ensure that care is effectively managed across the continuum. Some hospitals and cancer centers are incorporating aspects of traditional and intensive ambulatory care within their inpatient units.

Many social issues directly or indirectly affect the work of our institutions, including hospitals. These issues include increasing violence; a more diverse population; decreasing numbers of potential employees with appropriate skill for unlicensed, nonprofessional hospital positions; and the risks of resistant organisms and infections, such as AIDS and hepatitis. Many hospitals have joined with their neighborhoods and community organizations to form coalitions or partnerships and are actively working to reduce the negative impact of these conditions. Further, hospital-based nursing practice provides certain safeguards against some of these conditions, including universal precautions, isolation facilities, appropriate air handling mechanisms, and a diverse workforce.

Academic Medicine

Academic medical centers face additional pressures in this environment. It is often these institutions that care for a greater percentage of patients who do not have adequate health insurance or who have a multitude of physical and social problems resulting from the effects of poverty. It has long been believed that academic medical centers are more expensive than other hospitals. Recent analysis of data demonstrated that a Whipple surgical procedure in our academic medical center costs less and has the same or better clinical outcomes than the same surgery performed in other settings, including community hospitals. More studies of this nature are needed to convince third-party payers not to exclude academic medical centers from their referral base or covered options. Academic physicians are feeling thinly stretched as they are coaxed to see additional patients and generate revenue for the hospital at the same time that they are striving for academic promotions that are based on research, grant acquisition, and publications. These are important issues for cancer care and for oncology nursing.

Many cancer centers, including those designated as "comprehensive" by the NCI, are located within or affiliated with academic medical centers. It has traditionally been within academic medical centers that new knowledge about cancer is discovered and translated or applied to medical and nursing care of patients. The loss of these institutions or a reduction in their ability to provide care or conduct research would threaten our profession and significantly reduce the quality of health care in this country.

Research and Technology

Ironically, cancer research has never been as well funded as it is today. The NCI's budget was significantly increased as part of the NIH's budget allocation from Congress. Industry, especially the pharmaceutical industry, and organizations such as the Oncology Nursing Foundation and the American Cancer Society are financially supporting research in unprecedented amounts. Proceeds from the settlement with the tobacco industry will be used by some organizations, including cancer centers, in many states to support cancer research. In Maryland, millions of dollars have been pledged from the state tobacco settlement to support cancer prevention and basic, translational, and applied cancer research. The genome project and advances in molecular biology and genetics are causes for optimism about the discovery of the causes of cancer, its prevention, and cure. Advances in technology are responsible for minimally invasive surgical procedures and enhanced radiation treatments. Further refinements and advances in imaging technologies continue to reduce the negative effects of cancer diagnosis and treatment. Finally, advances in information technology enable oncology nurses to remain at patients' bedsides while documenting their assessments and reviewing medications, radiology and pathology results; comparing the patients' progress with the plans of care or critical pathways, and communicating with other members of the health care team within and across care settings.

Professional Issues

Demographics

Hospital-based nurses, including oncology nurses, today average 43 years of age, which is older than in the past. This fact, coupled with decreasing enrollments in schools of nursing, portend an acute shortage of nurses, and oncology and critical care nurses are projected to be in especially short supply.[4-6] Further deepening the shortage of professional nurses is the trend among young women, traditionally the majority of the nursing workforce, to seek careers in law, medicine, and other professions that are viewed as more prestigious, powerful, and financially rewarding than nursing. Hospital nursing is especially vulnerable to this shortage as the number of job opportunities outside of the hospital continues to increase. As occurs when the supply of nurses does not meet the demand, hospital nurses' salaries have increased in recent years, with an average of $27.50 an hour for entry-level positions, and many hospitals are offering sign-on and retention bonuses.

The majority of hospital nurses are educated at the associate-degree level. However, the need for baccalaureate and master's-prepared nurses will continue to increase as the care requirements of patients become increasingly complex and must be managed throughout an episode and across the continuum of care. Within this academic medical center at Johns Hopkins, 74% of nurses are prepared at the baccalaureate- or master's-degree levels. This compares to a national average of 40%.[7]

Clearly most hospitals actively seek to retain their experienced nurses. The voluntary turnover rate among hospital nurses has increased to a national average of 16%. This is believed to reflect nurses' dissatisfaction with

their compensation and with organizational restructuring and redesign initiatives that have negatively affected the number of professional nurses staffing inpatient and intensive care units. Meanwhile, many hospitals are becoming increasingly dependent upon agency, traveling, and part-time nurses to staff their oncology units, intensive care units, and operating rooms. The use of unlicensed personnel to assist the professional nurse is common practice in most hospitals.

Unlicensed Assistive Personnel

Perhaps no issue is as onerous to professional nurses as is the use of unlicensed assistive personnel (UAP). With pressures to reduce expenses and redesign the delivery of care, most hospitals have added UAP and other multiskilled workers to their nursing staff while reducing the number of professional nurses. Although this trend appears to be decreasing and is being reversed in many hospitals, the issue of UAPs is clearly a pivotal one. Often the unlicensed and multiskilled workers represent a different generation, sex, ethnicity, race, and economic background from the professional nurses. This diversity is challenging to effectively integrate and manage on a patient care unit. Nurses raised and nurtured on primary nursing do not want to delegate care to another provider who does not have the same education and professional credentials. Nor do many nurses have sufficient experience to effectively delegate care. The satisfaction that oncology nurses derive from physically ministering to patients, assessing and planning care, attending to psychosocial needs, and educating patients and families is deeply rooted and must be respected, especially as new patient care roles are introduced. Fortunately, compelling research findings that demonstrate the relationships among appropriate numbers of professional nurses and positive patient outcomes and patient satisfaction are beginning to guide decisions about the role of UAP and the number of professional nurses staffing hospital units.[1,7,8]

Professional Development

As younger nurses enter the profession they reflect the values and mores of society and their generation. Hospitals have learned that recruitment and retention strategies must be aligned with these values. However, staffing and compensation programs need to reflect the reality of younger nurses who do not anticipate lifelong employment in a single institution and who value their professional development as well as their time away from work. The orientation and socialization of new graduates into the profession—the speciality of oncology, and often a subspeciality of bone marrow transplantation or surgical oncology—require thoughtful planning and, often, creativity. Hospitals must ensure that quality and standards of care are met and that educational resources are effectively used. Internships, extended orientation programs, and a variety of educational opportunities are often used to accomplish these objectives. In today's environment, however, where turnover is high, staffing often minimal, and clinical instructors or experts scarce or nonexistent, it is challenging to provide the orientation and mentoring that is needed.

Collective Bargaining

While union membership in other professions and occupations has remained the same or declined, there is increased interest in unionization among nurses and physicians. This interest is primarily ascribed to nurses' dissatisfaction with the cost-cutting strategies employed by hospitals and health plans across the country. Nurses have identified working conditions and patient welfare as the major focus of collective bargaining activities. The full impact of contract language that sets the nurse-to-patient ratios has not yet been fully realized, nor all of the consequences fully appreciated. Hospital administrators have taken notice of nurses' interest in unionization, however, and many are taking steps to ensure that the issues that encourage union activity are clearly and appropriately addressed.

Hospital Culture

There is a body of literature that describes the hospital culture that supports excellent patient care through excellent nursing practice. Much has been learned from the initial and subsequent studies of the "magnet" hospitals. We know that the following have positive effects on nursing care and patient outcomes:

- Interdisciplinary teams
- Effective communications among all levels of staff
- Highly visible nurse managers and administrators
- Participative management structures
- Professional practice/primary nursing focus
- Leadership development and empowerment
- Valuing nurses and nursing's contribution
- Enhancing nurse physician relationships and collaboration[8]

It is striking to note that much of oncology nursing's history and many of its values are deeply imbedded in these tenets.

Role Changes

Similar to staff nurses, the roles of nurse managers, directors of nursing, and nurse executives are changing in response to external demands and internal restructuring. In the recent past, nurse managers were often asked to manage more than one unit; today we see this trend being reversed. Directors of nursing and nurse executives commonly have broad spans of control, usually encompassing multiple services and nursing and nonnursing clinical departments. The range of knowledge and skills required in these positions have significantly expanded to include those of finance and business. Balancing the budget, meeting financial targets, and managing revenue streams are as much a part of the daily life of an oncology nurse manager or director of nursing as are staffing issues, patient outcomes, and staff development.

Simultaneously the roles of oncology advance practice nurses have been affected by many of the same factors influencing other nursing roles. Many hospitals have reduced the number of advanced practice nurses (especially clinical nurse specialists), converted them to case manager positions, or eliminated them altogether. Conversely, the number of acute care nurse practitioners (NPs) on clinical units has increased, especially in academic medical centers. This is partially due to the increased demands on faculty time and the restrictions on the use of house staff, resulting in the integration of nurse practitioners into traditionally medical practices and roles. When nurse practitioner role expectations are clearly defined for the nursing staff, effective communication and interactions, positive patient outcomes, and collaborative relationships have emerged. The reimbursement status of NPs varies from state to state, while regulations established by the OIG and Medicare also influence their scope of practice and ability to charge for their services.

As with other positions, clinical nurse specialists are being reemployed by hospitals to assist with the orientation and mentoring of new graduates and less experienced nurses, and to facilitate the delivery of quality patient care to increasingly complex and acutely ill patients and their families. Ideally, these clinical nurse specialists will continue to advance our profession as they have traditionally done—e.g., through research activities and publications that advance the practice of oncology nursing and patient care. The role of the oncology case manager, while continuing to evolve, appears to have demonstrated value in ensuring that care is efficiently and effectively delivered across care settings and that third-party payers are well informed, thereby ensuring appropriate reimbursement for services provided. Models of case management include the coordination of care by the case manager with physicians, utilization management nurses, staff nurses, social workers, external case managers, and patients and families.

With increased financial support for clinical trials and translational research, the number of research nurses has increased in many comprehensive cancer centers and other academic medical centers. This important role offers additional professional and personal opportunities for nurses. However, because research nurses are often recruited from the ranks of the most experienced clinical nurses, this often leaves a void in staffing inpatient units with experienced and expert nurses and in providing qualified mentors for less experienced nurses.

In general, when research nurses are part of or have close affiliation with the nursing department, they are more successful than when they are separate from the department of nursing. While there are exceptions, a strong relationship between research nurses and the department of nursing improves the recruitment, orientation, and credentialing of research nurses, enhances their professional development, and facilitates their interactions with other nurses. The relationship between the research nurse and the principal investigator is to be respected and recognized as central to the successful conduct of the research protocol or program. The nursing department, often in collaboration with staff in other offices who are responsible for and have oversight of clinical research, must ensure that training and continuing education meet internal standards and the requirements of external funding sources and regulators.

Professional Relationships

Other roles within the hospital setting, some of them nursing roles, are also changing. Oncology nurses and social workers have traditionally been close professional colleagues. With the advent of the case manager role, the responsibilities of social workers and their relationships with nurses are often redefined and renegotiated. Similarly, the roles of the utilization review and performance improvement nurses and transplant coordinators are often affected or changed by the case manager role. With thoughtful planning and effective communication, any potential negative effects of these role changes are minimally realized by oncology staff nurses, while the positive effects enhance their practice and improve patient care and clinical outcomes.

Practice Guidelines

Critical pathways, care maps, and clinical guidelines are frequently used to structure the process of patient care. When used effectively and combined with clinical outcomes data, they provide important information about how best to care for populations of patients with specific cancer and noncancer diagnoses. Increasingly, as with the American Society of Clinical Oncology (ASCO) and the National Cancer Centers Network (NCCN), guidelines are externally developed and sanctioned by professional associations or cancer organizations. The Oncology Nursing Society publishes guidelines for clinical practice issues such as chemotherapy administration and professional issues such as the use of UAP.[9,10] Ideally, these guidelines reduce variations in practice within programs or hospitals and provide standards for "best practices." They are not substitutes, however, for individualized care for patients, as nurses are always responsible for assessing patients and altering care as indicated by the patients conditions.

Oncology Nursing Practice Issues

Oncology nursing has been at the forefront of nursing practice from the beginning of the speciality and continues to be a leader in advancing the profession today. Hospital-based oncology nursing is the "proving ground" for much of our clinical practice, research, and education. It is within hospitals that students and novice oncology nurses learn how to assess and care for patients with cancer and their families; learn the meaning of professional nursing; ask and answer important questions about clinical practice and outcomes; learn to collaborate with physicians and members of other disciplines and their peers; learn how to be mentored and how to mentor others; and learn how to share the joys as well as the sorrows of caring for patients with cancer. It is within hospitals that oncology nurses learn the art of nursing care. And, it is there that experienced oncology nurses continue to learn and to expand their professional skills and knowledge and to share that knowledge with the larger nursing community.

The practice of oncology nursing within hospitals is affected by all of the issues previously discussed. Within the maelstrom of changes occurring within hospitals and health care in general, there is evidence that oncology nursing practice remains solidly grounded in its principles and commitment to holistic, quality care for patients and their families. While many hospitals have fewer resources to support professional activities, oncology nurses' contributions to professional organizations and professional publications are witnesses to this commitment. It is also within the context of these changes that oncology nurses are developing new and effective ways to provide care to their patients.

Care Delivery Models

An example of a new approach to care delivery is the Inpatient/Outpatient Continuum of Care (IPOP) for patients undergoing bone marrow transplantation (BMT) in the comprehensive cancer center at Johns Hopkins. This project originated with two nurse managers and the physician clinical director of the BMT program who were seeking to improve the continuity of care for individual patients. The rapid penetration of managed care into our market added motivation to reduce the length of stay and the expense of hospitalization as much as possible, without shifting the cost of care to the patients. An intensive ambulatory clinical program was established that requires that a caregiver be identified for each patient and the caregiver and patient receive extensive education about their treatment, self care, and how to recognize significant changes in the patients condition. A structured education program for the nursing staff, all of whom are inpatient BMT staff nurses, provides information about the multiple facets of this new approach to care and the ambulatory nursing care required by this group of patients. Patient and family living accommodations are provided in a local facility that meets stringent infection control standards.

IPOP is a highly successful program that exceeded its goals for length of stay and cost reductions, demonstrated quality clinical outcomes, increased patient satisfaction, ensured continuity of care between the inpatient and outpatient settings, and did not increase the patients' financial burden. The nurses find IPOP to be a challenging and rewarding practice. It is important to them to see patients and their families in IPOP who they cared for during an acute or critical care inpatient stay. Seeing the IPOP patient outside of the traditional sick role reinforces the nurses' sense of accomplishment. Because the initial IPOP program was so successful, similar programs have been developed for pediatric oncology patients (POPIN) and for adult patients with hematologic malignancies (HIPOP).

Oncology Nursing Research

Throughout the course of an inpatient stay, oncology nurses provide care and comfort to acutely and critically ill patients and their families within a multidisciplinary framework. A great deal of nursing care is based on the results of nursing research related to symptom management. For example, pain scores are often included with daily vital signs and standardized scales are used to record the patients' level of fatigue, their mental status and psychological discomfort, mucositis, and wound appearance. Nursing interventions for these symptoms are based on the results of research associated with these instruments that was conducted by oncology nurse researchers. In a recent nursing journal club meeting, a clinical nurse specialist reviewed an article on the treatment of fever. There were students, staff nurses, other advanced practice nurses, and nurse managers participating in this discussion of a significant problem for patients with cancer who are receiving chemotherapy. All of the nurses left the meeting more knowledgeable about the basis of appropriate pharmacological and nonpharmacological interventions for this symptom. The application or utilization of research in clinical care is strongly embraced by oncology nursing.

Complementary Approaches

Complementary or alternative approaches to care, such as massage and aroma therapy, are today more frequently included with traditional oncology nursing interventions than in the past. Nursing assessments and patient and family education include the patients' use of nutritional supplements and alternative practices, and how their use might affect the patient's prescribed medical care and treatment. It is not unusual to find cancer centers affiliated with or offering programs of complementary care.

Often oncology nurses are the primary referrers to and providers of this care. While today's nurses are more knowledgeable about these other approaches, often we do not have the answers to patients questions about their uses or the resources to obtain the answers. Further, some physicians and nurses are reluctant to endorse any treatment or intervention that is not supported by the results of clinical trials research. Studies, such as the use of accupressure during bone marrow infusion being conducted by nurses on our BMT unit, are beginning to provide this support.

Individualizing patients' care requires thoughtful planning that can begin before the patient is admitted to the hospital. Oncology case managers are often responsible for ensuring that the proposed care is financially covered and that the patient and family understand their insurance benefits. Upon discharge, nurses, social workers, and case managers collaborate to ensure that care following discharge is appropriately provided and will be reimbursed. Patient financial matters, including financial eligibility for certain procedures such as BMT, are more complex for patients with cancer and extend over a longer period of time than for most patient populations. The financial aspects of hospital and health care is challenging for oncology nurses who have not historically been prepared to address these issues with patients, families, and internal and external financial staff.

End-of-Life Issues

Discussions about advance directives often arise between patients and oncology nurses, as patients are asked if they have or would like to receive information about advance directives at the time of admission to the hospital. Unless the nurse is prepared through education and has reference materials and referral resources available, such discussions may be difficult. Often it is the oncology nurse who, having been a patient's primary nurse throughout multiple admissions or a critical event, understands the patient's wishes regarding life support measures. Nurses recognize the importance of reaching a consensus among the health care team, patient, and family about the use of such measures before an event occurs. In the highly technical hospital environment where discharges occur sooner and nurses, physicians, and support staff have more patients to care for, addressing this and other end of life issues can be difficult.

Although there has been a shift from hospital to hospice care for patients during the end stages of their diseases, oncology nurses continue to care for a significant number of dying patients. It is essential that oncology nurses are able to attend to patients' and families' needs during this stage of their illness in the manner that reflects each patient's individual dignity and worth. This is as essential for oncology nurses' sense of professional accomplishment and gratification as it is for patients and families. Some nursing units have established structured bereavement programs for patients' families. Support for nurses following the death of their patients varies among oncology units, but is critically important for the mental health and professional development of the nurse.

Professional Burnout

Oncology nurses are at risk for professional burnout because of the nature of their work with acutely ill patients with complex physical and psychological needs and their inherent characteristics and commitment to their patients. The added stresses of today's work environment further increase the risk of burnout. Nurse leaders as well as oncology nurses themselves should be alert to this possibility and develop interventions to prevent its occurrence or ameliorate its effect. This may be accomplished by promoting an appropriate balance between work, family, and leisure activities through scheduling patterns, and by recognizing and acknowledging the importance of the nurses' contributions to patients, families, and their peers. In some hospitals, oncology/psychiatric liaison nurses help identify early signs of burnout and offer specific suggestions for individual nurses or nursing units at risk.

Nursing Practice Models

Primary nursing has been the principle model of care delivery for oncology units. The introduction of UAP and multiskilled workers to the nursing team often forces modifications to the model. Many nurses and patients prefer this model, however, because it affords continuity of care and greater nursing satisfaction in seeing a patient through an episode of care. With organizational redesign, other models of care delivery have emerged, such as modular, team, and primary team. While some continue to struggle, other oncology nurses have successfully adapted to these models and find them as satisfying as the primary nursing model and with equivalent patient outcomes. Although it will take time for many of the dissatisfying issues regarding newer practice models to be resolved, changes will continue to occur.

Models of professional practice vary but usually include such common tenets as self-scheduling, some or all salaried staff, and self-governance through committee structures. Because nurses value autonomy in their practices, these models can enhance their sense of professional self worth. However, without sufficient numbers of nurses to consistently staff units at the appropriate and desired levels, it is more difficult to sustain these models.

An analysis of the adequacy of nurse staffing on an oncology unit must take into account a number of variables. These include the size of the unit, patient population (BMT, solid tumor, etc.), patient acuity, average length of stay, model of care delivery, integrated critical care or separate intensive care unit, level of experience of the nurses, skill mix, and the presence of other care providers such a social workers, spiritual counselors, physician extenders, residents, and fellows. Other considerations include the extent to which research is conducted on the unit, the appropriateness of research activity support, and the use of technology, especially information systems.

In a 1999 survey of NCI comprehensive cancer centers, Grant[11] found that an average of 9.16 NHPPD was provided by registered nurses among eight of these centers, and the average total direct care hours was 11.87. In an informal survey of community and other academic medical centers in our area at the same time, the average NHPPD on inpatient units ranged from 5 to 8.5. Again, caution must be used when interpreting these data without knowledge of the variables previously listed.

Conclusion

Hospital oncology nursing today is both favored and vexed. It is favored because it offers the richest possible environment for nurses to learn and become highly competent, self-actualized oncology nurses. It is vexed by the external health care environment that is assailing its historic foundations and causing significant, unsettling changes. The issues discussed in this chapter require our collective attention and expertise to ensure that hospital-based oncology nursing will continue to provide the quality of patient care and professional fulfillment and advancement that we value so highly.

References

1. Bartley J: Understanding the impact of changes in nurse staffing: A review of recent outcomes studies. *Nursing Watch,* Issue 4. Newsletter, The Advisory Board Company, Washington DC, July 29, 1999, p 2
2. Kumar J (ed): *"Hospital Report Card"* Web site to grade physicians, HMOs. Medical Staff Briefing, July 1999, p 5
3. Frustrated nurses turning to unions. Baltimore Sun. October 31, 1999, p 19A
4. HSM Group: *Research on Nursing Staff Shortages.* Washington DC, American Organization of Nurse Executives, February 1999
5. The Registered Nurse Population, 1996. Findings from the *National Sample Survey of Registered Nurses.* US Department of Health and Human Services; Health Resources and Services Administration, Bureau of Health Professions, Division of Nursing, Washington DC, 1996
6. Silber M. *The Johns Hopkins Hospital Study of Retention of Registered Nurses.* Clarksville MD, Silber & Associates, 1999
7. Aiken LH: *Accounting for variations in hospital outcomes: Implications for strategic planning.* A summary. The Johns Hopkins Hospital. Baltimore MD. June 10, 1999, pp 1-2
8. Sovie MD: Hospital restructuring's impact on outcomes (HRIO), A glimpse at the work in progress. The Johns

Hopkins Hospital. Baltimore MD. (personal communication), June 10, 1999, p 1

9. Oncology Nursing Society: Position statement on advanced practice in oncology nursing. Oncology Nursing Society, Pittsburgh PA, 1997

10. Oncology Nursing Society: Position statement on the role of unlicensed assistive personnel in cancer care. Oncology Nursing Society, Pittsburgh PA, 1997

11. Grant SM: *NCI Comprehensive Cancer Center Survey Fiscal Year 1999.* Dana Farber Institute, Boston MA, 1999

CHAPTER 75

Ambulatory Care

Virginia R. Martin, RN, MSN, AOCN
Deanna Xistris, APRN, MSN, AOCN

Introduction

Ambulatory care services are organized in the United States based on a complex mix of historical, philosophical, political, economic, and environmental factors. Historically, the system is based on a medical model and the emphasis has been on acute care and high-tech treatments with little attention to the broad public health picture, to environmental measures, or to the individual's personal response to health.[1-3] Most of the health care system has been organized around the physician's delivery of reimbursable clinical care to the individual who seeks care when ill.[1] Physicians, historically, have been in control of this model of care delivery.[1] However, current health care delivery has been profoundly affected by how Americans conceptualize health and disease.[1]

Today's changing health care delivery system has created a new highly competitive marketplace with economics now influencing health care decisions. Economic impact on the delivery system includes four primary changes or shifts: (1) from hospital care to ambulatory care settings; (2) from primary care to preventive care; (3) from indemnity insurance to a managed care insurance system; and (4) to the development of advances for the treatment of chronic health problems.[4,5] The economic drive to decrease length of stay in the hospital and the development of new technology that makes surgical procedures less invasive has resulted in procedures that once were performed in the hospital now being done in the outpatient arena. These forces have created demands on the ambulatory practice area to develop new programs, accommodate increased volume and acuity, and provide more efficiently for the patient's needs.

Cancer care has shifted with these changes and in many instances has been the pioneer in ambulatory care. The complex technology and cancer treatments and the management of crisis events or adverse effects once dealt with in the inpatient setting now are provided in outpatient settings. The current overall trends in oncology result in longer survival of cancer patients. It is estimated that 85%–95% of cancer care takes place in the ambulatory area.[6,7]

For the patient, the major advantages of ambulatory care are that it is much less disruptive, people are able to maintain their jobs and family life, and individuals potentially have more control of their own care in this setting. Unfortunately, rapid changes and economic constraints have stressed this area of ambulatory care delivery and created challenges to maintain those major advantages. This chapter will highlight the major issues in the oncology ambulatory setting for the nurse in practice as well as the patient.

Ambulatory Care Delivery Systems

Factors Influencing Delivery

Ambulatory care delivery is affected by multiple factors, which include environmental, support service, patient-related, and personnel-related factors. Important environmental factors that affect the delivery of ambulatory care include the layout of the clinic or office, the types of clinic services, hours of operation, the management structure, the scheduling system, and computerization. Support services critical to the delivery of care include having an on-site laboratory or using an off-site laboratory, how the medical records are kept, transportation support, supplies, housekeeping, and environmental maintenance and repair. The types of patients—medical, surgical, or radiation; adult or pediatric—the volume, the acuity, and the telephone call systems or other systems utilized for care constitute the patient-related factors. Personnel factors include the types of staff employed, the skill mix of the staff, and the support services such as social work, rehabilitation, pharmacy, and nutritional care.

Ambulatory Practice Settings and Services

There are six broad categories of ambulatory practice settings: university hospital–based, community hospital–based, health maintenance organization, physician group or private practice, federal health system, and the freestanding center.[1,4] Historically, the university hospital outpatient departments were set up to fulfill the obligation of academic centers to provide care for the indigent and uninsured. Today that focus has changed significantly to meet current care delivery models and demands. Community hospital outpatient departments were also traditionally a charitable function for the community. Today they include surgery centers, cardiac rehabilitation, drug and alcohol programs, work-site health promotion programs, hospice and community health programs, urgent care centers, and infusion centers. Physician groups or private practices remain the principal mode by which physicians provide ambulatory services. Today, the physicians group includes alignments into larger groups or affiliations with hospitals rather than the solo private practice groups of the past. Health maintenance organizations (HMOs) sometimes have a full complement of physicians as employed providers who deliver a stated range of services to a defined population through a prepaid fee. The HMO's focus is on prevention and maintenance, but some provide cancer care services.

Oncology outpatient care can be delivered in any of these settings. The available services include prevention, screening, and detection; medical/hematology oncology; chemotherapy; surgical oncology including outpatient surgery; radiation therapy; blood component therapy; patient and family education; discharge planning referral; nutrition support; group/individual counseling; physical therapy/rehabilitation; supply and prescription procurement; survivor services; treatment planning; and symptom management.[8,9] How the services are combined will define a practice setting. Typically medical oncology or hematology oncology programs are separate from radiation or surgical oncology programs. Some centers—for example, those designated by the National Cancer Institute (NCI) as comprehensive cancer centers and many community cancer centers—integrate all or as many components of care as possible into one setting. Other ambulatory cancer centers might provide a combination of two of the oncology services. Some types of ambulatory oncology sites may include chemotherapy and transfusion therapy centers, day hospitals, freestanding clinics, outreach or network programs, clinics for screening and prevention of cancer, and genetic screening programs. Clinical research can be conducted in the office, community, or the academic setting.

Medical oncology/hematology

The medical oncology or hematology practice usually includes or is physically connected to an infusion center or treatment room, as most of the practice involves the administration of chemotherapy with a specialized nursing staff. Some practices have satellite facilities for treatment as well. The practice may also include or have ready access to laboratory services. Medical oncology visits include new patient consultations, symptom management, chemotherapy treatment, immunotherapy, blood component therapy patients, long-term follow-up care, and unscheduled or urgent visits. The volume is high and the pace is quick.

Radiation oncology

There are two kinds of practice settings for radiation oncology, hospital-based or freestanding. The hospital-based radiation programs have the advantage of a wide range of support services available.[10] The hospital-based radiation oncology program also benefits from nursing resources and multidisciplinary care planning teams on site. The radiation therapy process consists of an initial consult visit, a treatment planning visit, the treatment itself (which is generally three to six weeks of daily visits), and follow-up after treatment. The staff includes the radiation oncologist, technicians, dosimetrist, and the most recent role to be implemented is the registered nurse.

Surgical oncology

Ambulatory surgery for cancer has grown tremendously in the last decade, with new technology and cost containment being the driving forces. The ambulatory surgery program can be hospital-based, linked directly to either the main operating room or a distinct section; freestanding; or a satellite facility associated with a hospital facility but some distance away.[11] Surgical oncology visits are usually high volume, intense, and brief.

Continuity of Care

As health care reform continues to unfold, the ambulatory care system will expand and evolve. Coordinating care is often one of the most important and difficult challenges in delivering care to the cancer patient. This is especially true with those patients who receive complex and intensive care as outpatients. Patients often have to travel to multiple delivery sites to receive complicated treatment or supportive care services. New programs are being designed with as much integration and combined services as possible to contain health care costs while providing more efficiently for patients' needs.

The role of the ambulatory care nurse in oncology is evolving and will continue to encounter many challenges as health care reform proceeds. Limited research has been done on the role of oncology nurses in the ambulatory setting and with the expansion in the amount and complexity of outpatient care delivered, nurses and administrators are critically in need of additional information.

The Ambulatory Care Nursing Role

The American Academy of Ambulatory Care Nursing (AAACN) was founded in 1978 to advance and influence the art and science of ambulatory care nursing practice and health care delivery systems to improve the health of individuals and communities. AAACN defines ambulatory care nursing to include "those clinical, management, educational, and research activities provided by registered nurses for and with individuals who seek care for health-related problems or concerns or seek assistance with health maintenance and/or health promotion. These individuals engage predominantly in self-care and self-managed health activities or receive care from family and significant others outside an institutional setting."[4]

Dimensions of the Staff Nursing Role

The historic role of the nurse in ambulatory care was to manage the patient flow, answer the phone, complete paperwork, and assist the physician.[5] The office-based nurse of the past was viewed as the handmaiden to the physician.[12] In the early 1980s, dramatic changes in ambulatory care also led to dramatic changes in the ambulatory nurse role.

In 1981, Verran developed a taxonomy of the domain of ambulatory nursing practice that was the first in a series of efforts to define and describe ambulatory nursing practice.[13] In 1985, Tighe and associates completed a study using Verran's framework to describe and compare the current role of oncology and nononcology nurses.[5] The findings supported the use of a taxonomy to describe, categorize, and quantify ambulatory nursing practice in oncology.[5]

In the same year, Brown asserted that the future of cancer care would be based in ambulatory care and that one of the major issues nurses would face in this setting would be the importance of improving quality of life for cancer patients.[14] The need for a change in the nursing role in ambulatory care from the traditional role was critical. Oncology patients would need a full assessment by nurses, a plan of care, and an evaluation of the effectiveness of the nursing interventions. Yet frequent limitations to carrying out the plan exist, such as the limited time, the large number of patients, and the functional tasks nurses must carry out that take away from nursing time.[14]

In 1991, Barhamand studied the role, benefits, and realities of the office-based oncology nurse as a multifaceted, independent practitioner.[15] Office-based nurses were found to have opportunities for enhanced nurse–patient relationships and professional independence with their role.[15] Tasks for the office-based nurse were profiled in four categories: nursing-related activities, administrative duties, clerical-related activities, and ancillary activities. Providing problem-solving via the telephone and psychological support for the patient were the most frequently reported (96% response) nursing-related tasks.[15] Within this category, Barhamand classified the tasks as routine (vital signs, weights), mid-skill (venipuncture, mixing chemotherapy), as requiring special skills (electrocardiograms, accessing venous access devices), or as requiring a higher level of independence (facilitation of a support group).

The Oncology Nursing Society (ONS) conducted a national survey that documented the salary, staffing, and professional practice patterns in ambulatory oncology

settings. Nursing activities included patient and family teaching; care of catheters, ports, and pumps; patient assessments; treatment delivery; toxicity management; and facilitation of support groups.[12,16]

Ambulatory care nursing services are episodic, less than 24 hours in duration, and occur as a single encounter or a series of encounters over days, weeks, months, or years. The context for ambulatory care nursing depicted in Figure 75-1 shows the relationship between the various components of the delivery system and the role of the nurse.[17] The characteristics or themes of ambulatory nursing practice were identified by focus groups of nurses.[4] The themes are similar to the role of nurses in many settings but certain key themes that reflect the ambulatory role can serve as a foundation to a specialty such as oncology nursing. See Table 75-1.

A recent survey described the scope and dimensions of the staff nurse role in the ambulatory setting and projected the development of activities that will be important for the future.[1,18,19] The authors also identified those core dimensions of the role that should be retained by the professional nurse and those that could be delegated to others. These core dimensions of the nurse's role are outlined in Table 75-2,[18] and enhance the understanding of current ambulatory practice. A significant

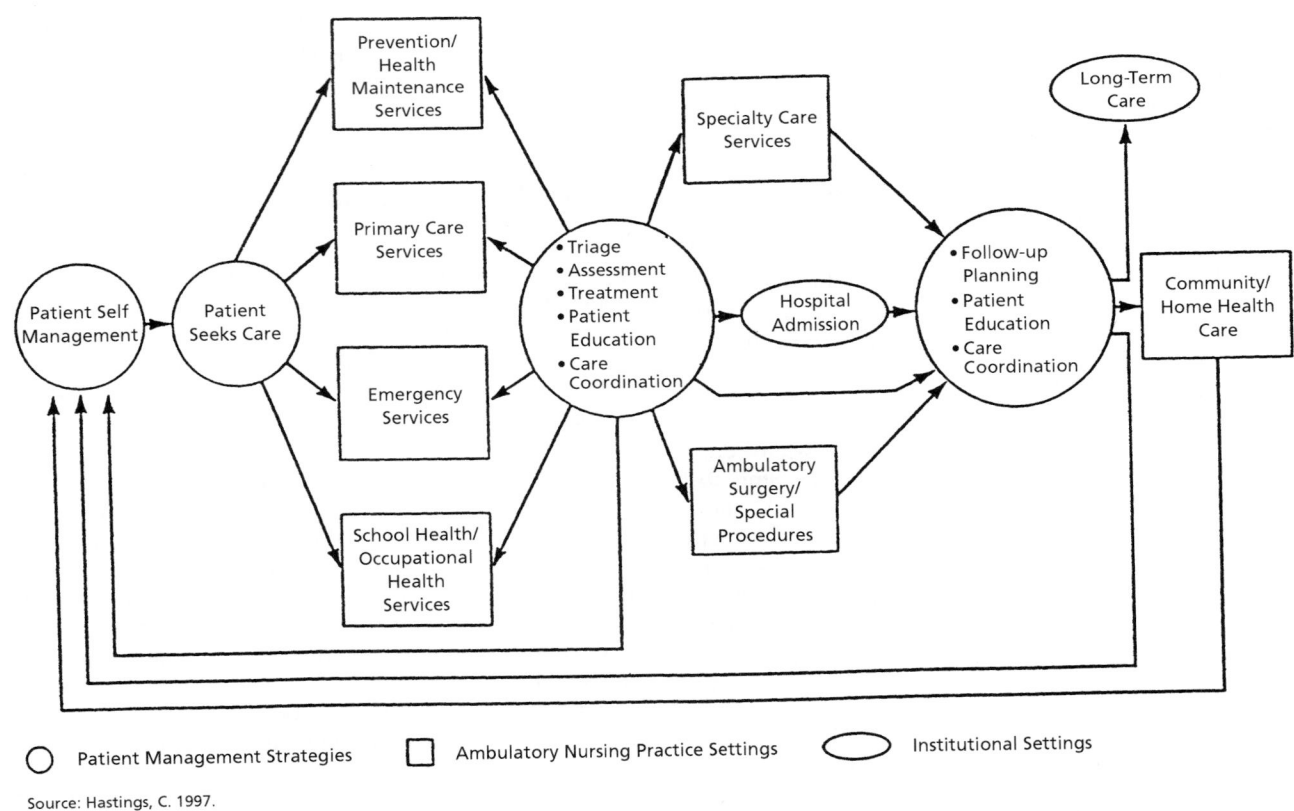

Source: Hastings, C. 1997.

Figure 75-1 The context for ambulatory care nursing. (Reprinted with permission from Hastings C: *The Context for Ambulatory Care Nursing.* Washington, DC, The Washington Hospital Center, 1997.)[17]

Table 75-1   Characteristics of Ambulatory Care Practice

Nursing autonomy

Patient advocacy

Skillful rapid assessment

Holistic nursing care

Client teaching

Wellness and health promotion

Coordination and continuity of care

Long-term relationships with clients and families

Telephone triage, advice, instruction

Patient and family control as major caregivers, users of the health care system and decision makers regarding compliance with care regimen

Collaboration with other health care providers

Case management

Reprinted with permission from AAACN: *Nursing in Ambulatory Care: The Future is Here.* Washington, DC, American Nurses Publishing, 1997, p 12.[4]

Table 75-2   Eight Core Dimensions of the Current Clinical Practice Role in Ambulatory Care

Factor I
Enabling Operations: maintain safe work environment, maintain traffic flow, search for space/equipment, set up room, locate records, order supplies, transport clients, provide emotional support, and take vital signs

Factor II
Technical Procedures: assist with procedures, prepare client for procedures, chaperone during procedures, inform client about treatment, witness signing consent forms, administer oral/IM medications, and collect specimens

Factor III
Nursing Process: develop nursing care plan, use nursing diagnosis, complete client history, assess client learning needs, conduct exit interview, evaluate client outcomes, and chart client encounters

Factor IV
Telephone Communications: telephone triage, call pharmacy with prescription, and call client with test results

Factor V
Advocacy: make clients aware of rights, promote positive public relations, act as a client advocate, and triage client to appropriate provider

Factor VI
Teaching: instruct client on medical/nursing regime and instruct client on home and self-care

Factor VII
Care Coordination: long-term supportive relationship, act as a resource person, coordinate client care, assess needs and initiate referrals, find resources in the community, and instruct on health promotion

Factor VIII
Expert Practice within Setting: expertise in advanced nursing practice, function as advanced nursing resource, serve as a preceptor for students, design and present in-depth education

Reprinted with permission from Hackbarth DP, Haas SA, Kavanagh JA, et al: Dimensions of the staff nurse role in ambulatory care: part I—methodology and analysis of data on current staff nurse practice. *Nurs Econ* 13:92, 1995.[18]

component of contemporary ambulatory care involves enabling operations and technical procedures, which encompass lower-level functions such as setting up rooms, searching for space and equipment, transporting clients, and collecting specimens. Nursing process, teaching, advocacy, and telephone communication are important role components that include higher-level professional nursing activities but were performed less frequently. Very complex and sophisticated activities such as care coordination and expert practice within setting dimensions were the least frequently performed dimensions of the current staff nurse role.

The barriers to higher-level clinical practice were identified to be lack of time, lack of support staff, excessive paperwork, administrative blocks to clinical practice, excessive number of patients, lack of monetary resources, and physician resistance.[18] Physical space was another barrier. Without adequate exam rooms, a place to keep files, secretarial support, or access to phone or computer, the nurses could not coordinate or provide care well. Thus, the role of the oncology nurse in ambulatory care has evolved from a simple role to a very diverse one. Staff nurses, advanced practice nurses, the nurse manager or administrator, and assistive personnel usually make up the ambulatory nursing team. The core role in the ambulatory clinic or office-based practice is that of the staff nurse.

Competencies

Competencies for the ambulatory staff nurse practice include proficient clinical nursing knowledge and skill, telephone triage skills, case management skills, computer skills, health education skills, basic leadership/supervi-

sion skills, quality improvement skills, and research skills.[4] Advanced practice roles, at the master's level, include the nurse practitioner, certified nurse midwife, certified registered nurse anesthetist, and clinical nurse specialist. Assistive personnel are a significant part of the health care delivery team in ambulatory care. In some settings, assistive personnel have been the major providers of ambulatory services. It is vital to distinguish a task that can be performed by clerical or assistive personnel from that of a nurse. The staff mix is dramatically influenced by the technology and complexity of therapies rendered in the ambulatory setting.

The physician's education and experience, the availability and role potential of the nurses in the work setting, the organizational structure of the agency, and the complexity of the work may also affect the role of the oncology nurse.[20] The many needs of the oncology patient coupled with the limited time in the ambulatory setting for patient–nurse interaction present a formidable challenge. Because of the myriad needs of oncology patients, the transitions from hospital to home and inpatient to outpatient must be carefully coordinated among health care providers.

Standards of Care

The AAACN established the first national guidelines or standards of ambulatory care nursing (Table 75-3).[21] These standards can be integrated with other specialty standards such as the ONS standards. Guidelines for practice in an ambulatory oncology facility were published in 1992.[22] Nursing practice standards specify how nurses should perform and provide the foundation for staff development programs and performance appraisal systems.

Table 75-3 AAACN Ambulatory Care Nursing Administration and Practice Standards

Standard I Structure and Organization of Ambulatory Care Nursing—Ambulatory care nursing is based on a philosophy committed to the delivery of efficient, cost-effective, and quality nursing care.

Standard II Staffing—Sufficient numbers of qualified nursing staff are available to meet patients' nursing care needs.

Standard III Competency—Nursing staff demonstrates knowledge and skills necessary to complete their assigned responsibilities.

Standard IV Ambulatory Nursing Practice—Registered nurses use the nursing process as a framework to determine the allocation and delivery of nursing care in the ambulatory setting.

Standard V Continuity of Care—Ambulatory care nurses facilitate continuity of care through the nursing process, interdisciplinary collaboration, and coordination of all appropriate health care services, including available community resources.

Standard VI Ethics and Patient Rights—Ambulatory care nurses recognize the dignity and worth of individuals, respect cultural, spiritual, and psychological differences, apply philosophical and ethical concepts that promote equality and continuity of care.

Standard VII Environment—Ambulatory care nurses facilitate the creation and maintenance of a hazard-free, safe, comfortable, and therapeutic environment for patients, visitors, and staff.

Standard VIII Research—Ambulatory care nurses conduct and participate in clinical and health care systems research. Research findings are disseminated and used to improve patient care and organizational effectiveness.

Standard IX Quality Management—The quality management process is coordinated and integrated with that of the organization and includes the continuous assessment, evaluation, and improvement of the quality and appropriateness of ambulatory care nursing. Ambulatory care nursing leaders set expectations, provide resources and training, foster communication and coordination and participate in improvement activities.

Reprinted with permission from AAACN: *1996 Ambulatory Care Nursing Administration and Practice Standards*. Pitman, NJ, Anthony J. Janetti, 1996.[21]

Models of Ambulatory Care Nursing

"Model of care delivery" is the phrase used to denote a method of organizing resources to provide patient care. Administrators are responsible for providing an appropriate level of care to meet the needs of the patient population.[20,23] The mission, philosophy, structure, and functioning of an organization should be considered in advance of designing a nursing model.[24] This analysis must be followed by looking at the internal environment, that is, how the organization's resources are configured. The resources consist of the physicians, nurses, other providers, as well as support staff, equipment, and space. Delineating the role of the nurse is the next step in the process of designing models of care delivery. The final step is the examination of the external environment and the literature or research. The medical model, functional model, primary nursing model, case management model, team nursing, collaborative practice, and community nursing models of care delivery have all been identified in ambulatory care.[15,19,24] The study by Haas and Hackbarth showed that the functional model is more likely to be used in the university setting whereas HMOs are more likely to use the medical model.[19]

A primary prevention model, a primary health care model, a case management model, and a paired partners model are all models for future care in the ambulatory setting.[19] The primary prevention model is focused on prevention and detection and in the current environment the opportunities for staff nurses in ambulatory care seem limitless. In the primary health care model, there is a role for the advanced practice nurse who can diagnose and treat minor illnesses, manage chronic illnesses in collaboration with physicians, as well as focus on prevention and wellness. The case management model begins with an assessment of who and what is to be managed and then articulates the components of the nurses' roles. Not every client needs a case manager, but those who do most likely have complex problems who are seen over long periods of time and have potential for complications (high risk, high volume). The paired partners model consists of professional nurses and other health care providers who work as a team and divide up the work in a setting. The division of labor is based on the staff's skills and knowledge, and the particular state's nurse practice act. The most appropriate level of provider is consistently assigned to provide the needed care.

A recent study questioned whether the role of the ambulatory oncology nurse in a regional cancer center is different from the nurse's role in the community outpatient clinic.[20] The study concluded that two models of ambulatory oncology nursing practice were found: (1) the nurse complement model and (2) the nurse substitute model.[20] In the complement model, the nurse serves as a complement to the medical oncologist. Nursing tasks include admission and discharge of the patient, starting the IV line, monitoring the drugs, and reporting problems. In the substitute model, the nurse works collaboratively with the physician. The nurse teaches the patient about the disease, treatment, and self-care, administers the drug, assesses the development of side effects, and manages the side effects.[23] Greater efficiencies in care for cancer patients were found at the site where the substitute model is used.[23]

There are a number of models of care delivery that can be adapted to the oncology ambulatory setting. It is the acuity of patients, not the delivery systems, which should determine staffing levels because practice expectations can add or subtract to the nurse workload.[24,25] Practice expectations such as patient assessment tools, standards, and practice guidelines clarify the scope and quality of nursing care received in the setting.[24]

Measurement of Patient Intensity and Classification Systems

In today's costly and competitive health care environment, managers must link patient needs with provider activities, resource use, and patient outcomes to effectively manage resources.[26] The ambulatory patient's needs differ from the patient in the hospital. Among these differences are that the usual patient visit is brief; a single visit may involve multiple distinct encounters; care can be discontinuous with patients returning for visits at irregular intervals; patients have widely different care needs from one visit to the next; telephone management and screening are important dimensions of some ambulatory services; and many visits involve no specific medical treatments or procedures.[26]

A patient classification system (PCS) measures patients' needs for care and care activities.[26] Managers need to forecast workload to prepare budgets and plan future programs. It is a method of sorting patients into levels for the purpose of predicting the demand for nursing time.[27] Patient classification systems that collect clinically meaningful patient data can be used for a framework for practice and patient outcomes, staffing and budgeting, restructuring and skill mix outcomes, data for use with clinical paths and protocols, and research.[27,28] Such sys-

tems remain institution specific because the rationale for ambulatory nursing services is still not universally understood and accepted.[26]

Most approaches to patient classification in ambulatory care have been focused on capturing physician resource use or largely for payment, including the ambulatory visit groups or the more recent ambulatory patient groups.[26] These classification approaches have not included nursing services as an important professional resource to be accounted for within these systems. There also have been various nursing approaches to patient classification in ambulatory care. Verran developed and tested the Ambulatory Care Client Classification Instrument (ACCCI), which acknowledged the importance of classifying task and time but more importantly the complexity associated with nursing care.[29] Hastings stated that the visit type rather than the patient classification was more important in ambulatory care.[30]

Parrinello and colleagues and Hastings and Muir-Nash both published their mixed results utilizing the ACCCI.[31,32] Tighe and associates and Joseph published adaptations of the Verran work.[5,33] A Patient Intensity System for Nursing in Ambulatory Care (PINAC) tool was tested in a variety of clinics in the early 1990s. This classification method combined classifications of the severity of illness, psychosocial needs, and complexity of care with the type of visit. The authors found it to be reliable and valid as well as practical and clinically meaningful.[26,34]

One classification method sorts clients into levels for the purpose of predicting the demand of nursing care time.[27] The process includes identifying the model of care delivery, then documenting how the work is organized and what professional nurses should be doing for the client population served, the number and level of acuity of the ambulatory care client population, and approximate time expenditure for each level of care. A four-level prototypical nursing intensity instrument is presented in Figure 75-2.[27]

Another approach to gathering productivity information is workload analysis of the time it takes to complete tasks and how frequently those tasks are performed. Four patient classification categories were developed and a patient was classified on entrance and exit to the system.

Level 1	**Level 2**	**Level 3**	**Level 4**
Short return visit for acute illness	Return visit for chronic illness	Initial visit or visit for procedure, teaching	Visit for prolonged therapy

Figure 75-2   Four Level Prototypical Nursing Intensity Instrument useful for sorting clients into levels to predict demand of nursing care time. (Reprinted with permission from Haas SA, Hackbarth DP. Dimensions of the staff nurse role in ambulatory care: part IV—developing nursing intensity measures, standards, clinical ladders, and QI programs. *Nursing Economics* 13:285–294, 1995.)[27]

Data was collated by clerical staff and utilized by the manager to ensure adequate levels of staffing.[35]

Many authors have documented the need for a patient intensity or classification system but no one system that can be applied across all settings has been developed. To individualize a patient classification system, it is important to fit the existing instruments to the practice perhaps by modification, to completely define the specific classification process to be undertaken, and to identify early what PCS will or will not do for the organization.[28]

The major difference in workload intensity in ambulatory care, including oncology, compared to the inpatient setting is that there is no predictable boundary or limit to those who need ambulatory care. Theoretically, there is a limit in appointments. In reality, however, drop-ins or extra patients commonly occur. The large numbers of patients seen in one day of ambulatory care and the variability and unpredictability in the care requirements of even a few patients can dramatically alter workloads and create bottlenecks and delays. The future of classification systems and measurement of nursing intensity depends on the development of an accurate model of data collection.[28] Research in this area is ongoing and is critical to monitoring productivity, for short- and long-range planning, evaluating trends, and monitoring quality improvement.

Telephone Triage

One of the ways formal communication is accomplished between the nurse and patient in ambulatory care is through the telephone. As a subspecialty in ambulatory care nursing, telephone nursing practice is defined as using the nursing process to provide care for individual patients or defined patient populations over the telephone (Table 75-4). An AAACN special interest group on telephone triage developed the Telephone Nursing Practice Administration and Practice Standards.[37] The

---

Table 75-4 Definition of Telephone Nursing

1. Telephone nursing service encompasses the following:
   Triaging
   Providing health information
   Prescription refill
   Referral/resource identification
   Nursing consultation
   Communicating test results

2. Delivery of telephone nursing services in ambulatory programs varies across service areas based on client populations, staff mix/skill levels, amount and type of specialty education of nurses.

3. Telephone nursing services follow physician/nurse-approved protocols and organized policies.

Reprinted with permission from Gulanick M, Green M, Crutchfield C, et al: Telephone nursing in a general medicine ambulatory clinic. *MEDSURG Nurs* 5:93–124, 1996.[36]

---

standards address the structure and organization of telephone nursing, staffing, competency, use of the nursing process in telephone nursing practice, continuity of care, ethics and patients rights, environment, research, and quality management.[37]

Interventions over the phone can be just as effective as outpatient visits for increasing compliance with health care and follow-up visits.[38] Watts and associates examined problems presented by patients in telephone contacts with clinical nurse specialists and concluded that a clinical nurse specialist resolved 80% of the patient problems over the phone.[39]

Nail and colleagues published a hallmark study on ambulatory cancer nursing in 1989.[40] In an ambulatory oncology practice over a six-month period, nurses gathered information on 1844 patient calls. The nurses collected data on the duration, initiator, purpose, nurses' assessment of urgency level, impact on nursing care plan, and changes made in health care services. Nurses functioned independently, handling 91% of the calls they received and using consultation with the MD for 52% of the calls.[40] This study followed patients in medical, gynecologic, and radiation oncology. Nurses in radiation oncology reported the fewest calls, which is reasonable given the fact that these patients make daily trips to the department for treatment. Patients in other services used the phone for more frequent contact. Mean length of time for a call was 6.65 minutes.[40] The study suggested the value of establishing specific hours to call in or return calls so the nurse is not interrupted while attending to other patient care responsibilities, and using triage calls for appointments, prescriptions, and insurance questions.

Telephone practice has been shown to positively affect patient satisfaction.[36] It nevertheless poses unique challenges since the nurse must make a judgement based on information provided by patient or family and any other auditory cues given. The telephone offers the means to identify, triage, and manage patient problems as well as educate and counsel patients and their significant others. Nurses must be able to quickly identify the nature of the call and must have an intuitive ability to accurately assess situations, narrow the range of possibilities, and identify the problem.[41] Nurses must also have skills for probing and creating an environment of trust over the phone.[4]

Telephone practice is not for novices. It requires critical thinking, professional judgment, evaluation, and cannot be delegated to nonprofessional staff. The potential risk to patients is significant and practices must have guidelines for decision making and methods to document all interactions.[4] Outcomes of telephone practice include improving patient access for information, support, and coordination of care; improving responsiveness to patient and family needs; enhancing communication among professionals providing patient and family care; expanding the responsibilities of the professional nurse within the clinic; and more appropriately using physician time.[36]

Telephone practice today ranges from triage and advice lines to health management call centers that provide decision support (symptom calls, self-care questions, referral services, and proactive contacts with patient populations), health education (screenings, maintenance, prevention, resource lines, and counseling), and care management of populations at risk.[36,42-44] These call centers have become an integral component in the continuity of care and facilitate a partnership with clients (caller/patients, payor, and providers). Customer service is the primary focus of these centers, but they also support three initiatives in care delivery: access, cost management, and quality of care.[42]

The major side effects from treatment and the emotional impact of the diagnosis of cancer lend itself to nurses counseling and educating over the phone. One of the most common uses of telephone triage is managing the patient's chemotherapy side effects. Many cancer nurses call outpatients receiving chemotherapy 24 or 48 hours after administration to ensure that the education provided on management of symptoms has been understood and that no problems have developed. Triaging patient problems via the telephone is a unique nursing skill. Telephone triage decision trees for neutropenia/fever, anemia/fatigue, thrombocytopenia, nausea/vomiting, diarrhea, constipation, stomatitis, anorexia, pulmonary, renal, hepatic, neuro, and cardiac toxicity are helpful in developing telephone protocols.[45] See Figure 75-3 for an example.

Any nursing workload measurement needs to include the number of telephone calls in addition to number of patient visits, the number and type of procedures done, and the number of treatments administered.[42] The call or encounter should reflect the assessment of actual or potential health problems that require further evaluation and intervention. Evaluation of the telephone role requires an audit tool for monitoring. Productivity measures in the telephone triage practice area must consider the customer service focus, access, cost management, and quality of care.[42] It is helpful to have preprinted brochures that explain telephone services, which calls are appropriate, which calls should go to 911, and which calls can wait for the next business day. Some practice settings require nurses to be available 24 hours/day to patients via pagers or cellular phones.

Educational programs should be designed to help nurses develop telephone skills. If telephone calls are a cost-effective alternative to other forms of care, nurses may, in the future, be able to negotiate reimbursement for telephone nursing care. Further research is needed to assess the scope and extent of nursing involvement in activities related to calls and to assess the outcomes of telephone-based ambulatory patient care.

There are important legal issues in telephone practice as well as in all other practice settings. Nurses should use standard protocols and procedures, and do accurate and concise documentation, with quality assessment reviews. The best defense against a malpractice claim is accurate documentation. (See Figure 75-4.) Narrative notes, flow charts, checklists, telephone ledgers, dictation, computer charting, and an imprinted stamp are all possible methods of documentation. Whatever documentation is used, however, it must be time efficient because outpatient nurses usually squeeze calls in between patient visits. Before the call is finished the nurse should determine if a follow-up plan is needed; and all telephone interactions

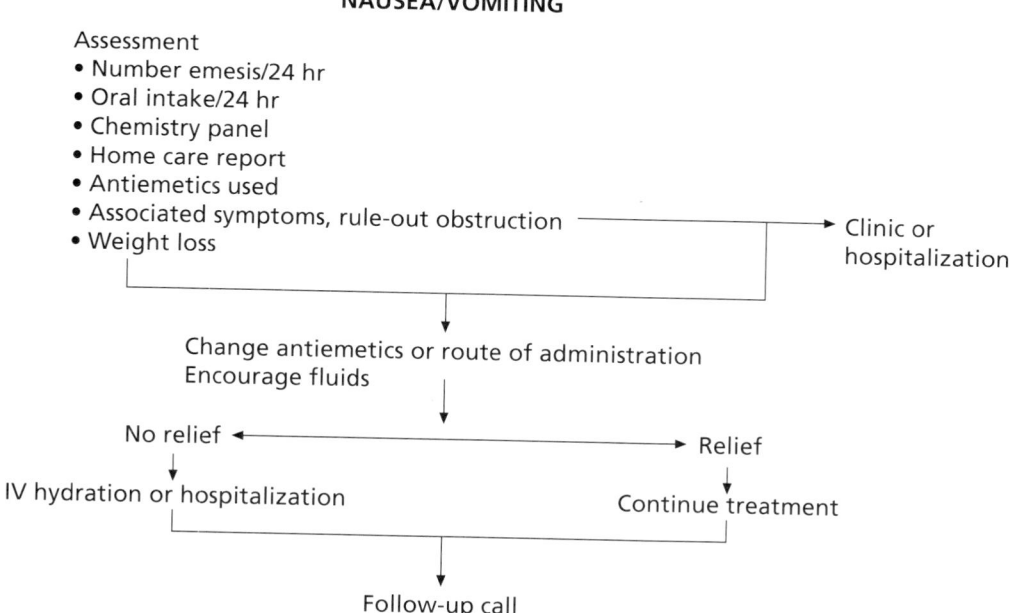

NAUSEA/VOMITING

Assessment
- Number emesis/24 hr
- Oral intake/24 hr
- Chemistry panel
- Home care report
- Antiemetics used
- Associated symptoms, rule-out obstruction ———→ Clinic or hospitalization
- Weight loss

Change antiemetics or route of administration
Encourage fluids

No relief ←———————→ Relief

IV hydration or hospitalization   Continue treatment

Follow-up call

Figure 75-3   An example of a telephone triage decision tree. (Reprinted with permission from Anastasia PJ, Blevins MC: Outpatient chemotherapy: telephone triage for symptom management. *Oncol Nurs Forum* 24:13–24, 1997.) [suppl 1][45]

FOX CHASE
CANCER CENTER
TELEPHONE DOCUMENTATION

Call received by:_____ Date_____ Time_____

Call initiated by: ☐ Patient ☐ Family ☐ Pharmacy ☐ Home Health RN ☐ Family MD ☐ Other

Patient name _____ Medical Record #:_____ Phone Number _____

Attending MD/Fellow: _____ Primary RN: _____

Allergies: _____ Treatment: ☐ Chemo ☐ XRT ☐ Surgery ☐ F/U

PURPOSE OF CALL: Patient Problem/Question:_____

_____

Prescription: _____

Tests/Appointments: _____

ACTION TAKEN: ☐ Handled by RN ☐ Secretary ☐ Physician/Fellow ☐ Other _____

_____
_____
_____

Prescription called ☐   Lab Results Given ☐   Physician Notified ☐ YES ☐ NO TIME_____

See Progress Notes _____   Dr. _____

Signature _____

Figure 75-4 Telephone documentation forms can facilitate accurate and concise communication.

must be communicated to the attending physician. For patient satisfaction, it is also important to provide a time when a patient can expect a call back. Some practices use call-in hours while others designate a time frame for the expected response.

Documentation

Documentation in the ambulatory setting must be accurate, concise, clear, objective, and quickly done.[46,47] A variety of tools have been developed to accommodate these documentation needs and often these tools include a component of self-report, which lends itself to the ambulatory setting.[46,47] History and initial visit forms if mailed to the new patient before the first visit can provide comprehensive summaries of care from the patient's perspective that will give the provider insight into their understanding of the disease. (See Figure 75-5 for an example). Follow-up forms can be in the checklist format since the volume of patients scheduled does not lend itself to the lengthy narrative format. Patients can also participate in follow-up self-report by listing problems or changes since the last visit on a questionnaire. Chemotherapy administration documentation is the most com-

monly used form of documentation in outpatient settings. It includes drug names and dosages, method of administration, date, site, observations during administration, documentation of nursing actions, patient response, laboratory values, patient teaching, and discharge status.[47] Documentation of key discussions on the telephone must be performed and the use of a quick checklist format is the preferred method. The administrative aspects of documentation of care include accreditation, legal ramifications, financial/reimbursement issues, quality improvement, and ethical issues.[47] The current health care environment makes documentation that the care was competently delivered a critical issue.

Treatment Centers

Chemotherapy/Infusion Centers

Health care trends continue to shift more oncology care to outpatient treatment. The challenge is to optimally use the resources available. Chemotherapy administration takes place in a treatment room, also called an *infusion room*, that is part of or attached to the physician practice or hospital, or is in a freestanding chemotherapy

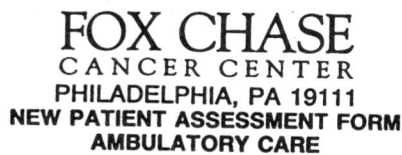

FOX CHASE
CANCER CENTER
PHILADELPHIA, PA 19111
NEW PATIENT ASSESSMENT FORM
AMBULATORY CARE

PART ONE TO BE COMPLETED BY PATIENT OR FAMILY MEMBER

To help plan your care, please complete this form while you are waiting for your appointment. The information will be kept confidential and used only by your doctors and nurses.

GENERAL INFORMATION

Instructions: Please circle all that apply.

1. Why did you come to Fox Chase Cancer Center today?

    Treatment   Follow-up care
    Second Opinion   Other _____

2. Have you received any treatment for your diagnosis?   YES   NO
    If YES was it:
    surgery   chemotherapy   radiation
    Can you tell us when the treatment was given? _____

3. Do you have any of the following health problems?   YES   NO
    if the answer is YES please circle all that apply:

    Diabetes   Gastrointestinal   Hepatitis   Stroke
    Seizures   High Blood Pressure   Urinary Infections   Arthritis
    Heart Disease   Headaches   Lung Problems
    Pneumonia   Angina
    OTHER _____

4. Have you had any previous surgeries?   YES   NO
    if the answer is YES please list:_____
    _____
    _____

5. Do you have problems with any of the following: *(please circle)*
    climbing stairs   nausea   tiredness   vomiting
    hearing   bladder control   breathing   sleeping
    walking   vision   diarrhea   stress
    constipation   speaking english transportation   child care
    household chores

6. Do you currently smoke cigarettes/cigars/pipes?   YES   NO
    Did you smoke in the past?   YES   NO
    For how long? _____

7. Do you drink alcohol presently/in the past?   YES   NO
    If YES, how much do you drink weekly? _____
                          daily? _____

8. Are you taking any medicine?   YES   NO
    if the answer is YES, please list all medicines you take:
    _____
    _____
    _____

Figure 75-5 New patient assessment forms can be mailed to patient prior to first visit.

PART TWO TO BE COMPLETED BY THE NURSE

PRESENTING PROBLEM:

Information • Comfort • Protective Mechanisms • Elimination • Coping • Nutrition
Mobility Mechanisms • Sexuality • Ventilation • Circulation

1._____ 2._____ 3._____

PATIENT TEACHING INTERVENTIONS:

Initial teaching   _____

Written material given   _____

NURSING NOTES:

_____

_____

_____

_____

_____

_____

_____

_____

_____

_____

_____

_____

_____

_____

SEE PROGRESS NOTES

REFERRAL INITIATED: YES   NO

Social Service   Physical Therapy   Palliative Care
Home Care   Pain Management   Other

Nurses' signature_____ DATE_____

Figure 75-5 New patient assessment form (continued).

center. Typical layouts include a combination of infusion chairs and beds, common space, and private space. Nurse staffing is based on the number of scheduled treatments and predicted patient procedures or interventions.

Measuring patient acuity is essential to predicting and implementing staffing requirements. There is no simple method to calculate this need. Managers gather data on treatment types and length, schedules are developed to provide order and control, and nurses are usually assigned in a patient/nurse ratio. In oncology care, these patterns are uncertain at best. On any given day, a person scheduled to receive routine treatment could have an unexpected adverse reaction that warrants individual nursing care. Intensive chemotherapy treatment protocols require additional nurses and resources that are difficult to plan. There must be some flexibility in the daily assignments to accommodate these unpredictable circumstances.

Radiotherapy Treatment Centers

Radiation treatment is administered as a set number of treatments over a few weeks, usually 5–6 weeks. This finite time for treatment is the main difference between the schedule at a chemotherapy treatment center compared with a radiation center. The average length of treatment is five days a week for five weeks for external radiotherapy. The needs of the patient during the entire treatment plan must be considered. Often transportation to and from the radiation facility is the first challenge. Before treatment begins a planning session is an important component so the patient knows what to expect. It is important to dispel misconceptions about treatment and carefully explain the process since patients may become frightened when left alone in the radiation treatment room. The initial appointment for simulation and treatment planning can take three to four hours and involves the physician, physicist, dosimetrist, and nurse. Daily treatments take about 30 minutes to set up and deliver the dose. While undergoing radiotherapy treatment patients need information about the treatment, general emotional support, and side effect management strategies.[48]

The registered nurse's role in radiotherapy includes assessment, education, and support. Often, the radiation nurse will maintain an appointment schedule specifically to educate, counsel, and manage patients. The goal for the patient is to continue treatment until it is finished, which can become difficult to achieve owing to side effects and fatigue. Nutritional support during radiotherapy is also integral to the care plan.

Radiotherapy can often be given as a part of a multimodal approach in cancer treatment. Implants, high-dose brachytherapy, and unsealed source therapy require extensive preplanning, insertion time, and close follow-up. Coordination of care becomes essential, as these patients need individualized planning of their treatment program. Some protocols involve timed radiotherapy treatment occurring between a chemotherapy infusion or after an infusion. Departments must communicate closely so that this can be achieved. Less common but more demanding is the oncologic emergency that must be immediately assessed and treated. The entire team must be mobilized within a few hours for the intensive treatment of a severe situation.

Scheduling Systems

One successful scheduling system for an oncology treatment center is divided into 15-minute blocks of time with nurse time and infusion chair time factored together. Several chairs or beds are held open each day for the unplanned patient visit and emergency problems. In addition, a block of time to allow for test results to be made available is included in the schedule. Chemotherapy regimens in this system are assigned an internal code ranging from 001 to 998 and each code is assigned to a particular therapy combination, which has its own guidelines for administration. For example, CAF (cyclophosphamide, doxorubicin, fluorouracil) is listed as a chair only procedure, nursing set up time for administering is listed as 30 minutes, total length of time is 120 minutes, and the guideline includes that schedulers are not to schedule CAF for later than 3:00 P.M. in the day. A month after the program's initiation, the center experienced improved patient flow and decreased wait times.[49]

Multiple waits can occur in all oncology treatment areas. Patients have to get laboratory results and drugs must be mixed based on these lab results. The next wait is for the nurse to treat the patient. Some scheduling factors remain outside the center's control, such as the patient's arriving on time for their scheduled visit. Also, the infusion centers are often connected to clinics or offices where patients see their physicians prior to treatment. These treatment appointments are made to follow office visits and are often delayed due to physicians' schedules not running according to plan. The timeliness of the pharmacy and lab are also factors.

A scheduling system like the one described above is effective in that it factors in both the treatment time and the nursing staff time. An optimal scheduling system would also be able to factor in the limitations on distinct resources within the department or from the patient's perspective. For example, if the physician's clinic time is only in the afternoon and the chemotherapy is a six-hour treatment, then the system must alert the scheduler of those limitations.

Oncology patient care scheduling is more complicated than routine outpatient scheduling. A blood count result that is abnormal on a scheduled treatment day will cause an entire regimen of scheduled events to be changed. Scheduling systems may often have to be customized to fit the unique needs of the center. The development of such custom-made systems is time consuming and complicated.

Another important practical aspect of scheduling is

limiting the number of patients with appointments who may not show up for their appointments. This decreases the efficient use of facilities and resources. Patient reminders, either by phone or by mail, result in a significantly smaller no-show rate.[50]

Scheduling and communication systems are major challenges facing health care. Technology is evolving faster than operational developments. The voice mail and e-mail systems enhance our communication but make it more difficult to monitor documentation. Order entry and scheduling systems are advanced but may not be coordinated with existing information systems, thus creating opportunity for errors. Keeping up with such technological changes are personnel intensive and costly, and are often prohibitive in our current environment of cost containment.

Patient Self-Care

Oncology treatments of chemotherapy, radiation, or surgery are accompanied by multiple side effects. The shift from inpatient to outpatient care has placed a tremendous burden on the patient and patient's caregiver to manage the treatment side effects. Management of these side effects and the symptoms associated with the disease process itself is also a key role for both the staff nurse and the advanced practice nurse in the ambulatory setting. Increasingly, advanced practice nurses are in the ambulatory setting delivering holistic services targeted to achieve both a positive response to therapy and optimal quality of life.[51]

Throughout oncology treatment, the most common side effects include fatigue, sleeping difficulty, nausea, decreased appetite, and changes in taste and smell.[51,52] The unique aspect of treating these symptoms in the ambulatory oncology setting is the necessity of preparing the patient and family for self-care at home through patient education. Easy access to the care team is critical should self-care activities become inadequate to afford comfort, if symptoms worsen, or if new symptoms occur. Without such a plan for easy access, distressed patients will assuredly go to the emergency room of the local hospital or show up in the office as unscheduled office visits. A patient's understanding of the situation he or she faces has been found to be a strong predictor of successful self-care.

Self-care activities to manage the side effects of chemotherapy were the focus of a recent research study.[52] Using a self-care diary to record their side effects, patients rated the severity of the side effects and reported the use and efficacy of self-care activities after treatment. The most common side effect was fatigue, which occurred in 81% of the patients.[52] More than one-third of the patients reported sleeping difficulty, nausea, decreased appetite, and changes in taste and smell. The self-care activities were rated as providing some to moderate relief of the

individual's side effects. Three other studies investigated self-care activity during radiotherapy.[53–55] Dodd[53] and Hanucharurnkul[54] found a significant relationship between an understanding of radiation therapy and self-care. Because patients in the ambulatory setting are responsible for their own care, a nursing system must be supportive and provide the essential education and emotional support that will enhance self-care.[48]

Unscheduled Patient Visits

Many patients are on aggressive therapy or research protocols and require expert medical intervention periodically. Some patients with cancer that experience the adverse effects of treatment go to the emergency room with problems. Others can have their problems handled over the phone. But many patient problems are handled by an unscheduled patient visit to the outpatient center.

One institution that lacked an emergency facility described their plan to set up a symptom evaluation area for the unscheduled patient visit.[56] An inpatient unit was the logical location and the plan assigned one RN to each symptom evaluation area room in combination with inpatient responsibilities. The scope of services, utilization guidelines, and disposition guidelines were developed. The authors reported seeing 1373 patients since opening, with an average number of encounters per month of 46.[56] Most were seen during the week and the average length of stay was two to three hours. The predominant reasons for admission were nausea, vomiting, fever, and pain. Sixty-nine percent of the patients admitted were discharged to home. The primary benefits of the plan were continuity of care for patients and the prevention of costly visits to the emergency room.[56] This is but one example of an innovative program initiated to meet patients' needs.

Some centers or offices block time in the daily schedule to accommodate unscheduled visits. Others have triage rooms available and are staffed to quickly assess the patient and intervene. A nurse practitioner is an excellent provider for evaluation and treatment of the unexpected patient with problems. Also, using the holistic approach, the nurse cannot only assess and intervene with the crisis but can add valuable insight into the patient and family's management of the illness or treatment. This model is affordable in most practice settings because advance practice nurses can be reimbursed for their services.[57]

Research

Clinical research contributes to the advancement of the treatment of cancer, management of side effects, and quality-of-life issues. Traditionally, clinical research trials were sponsored through the NCI and cooperative research study groups funded by the NCI and implemented in major clinical centers. In recent years, collaborative groups of researchers, including basic scientists, physicians, nurses, and the pharmaceutical and biotechnology industry have brought research into the community-based practice. In addition, many research institutions and agencies are looking to develop community networks to provide research opportunities in private practice settings that provide ambulatory cancer care. Pharmaceutical companies now contract directly with outpatient centers to participate in phase I and II trials. The driving force behind this trend is increased access to greater numbers of patients, a presumed decrease in the cost of research, and the availability of expert oncologists and oncology nurses in the ambulatory community-based settings. An example of a recent national study that relies heavily on the community-based ambulatory care setting for optimal patient accrual is the Women's Intervention Study (WINS), sponsored by the National Institutes of Health (NIH), and the National Surgical Breast and Bowel Project (NSABP) sponsored *STAR* chemoprevention of breast cancer study begun in July 1, 1999. The accrual goal is 22,000 women.

To successfully implement quality research in the ambulatory setting, there must be a commitment and capital investment in the development of a research team. The team includes the physician(s) and a principal investigator who is thoroughly educated in the trial and its related administrative matters; a research coordinator with the time and opportunity to obtain data as needed; clinical nurses who monitor the patient and deliver care; general health care personnel for the pharmacy and laboratory support; and administrative staff for medical record keeping, budgeting, data management, and meeting regulatory requirements.[58] The role of the clinical research nurse is increasingly recognized to be integral to the success of clinical trials in the ambulatory settings. The components of the research nurse role include data collection, clinical assessment, patient teaching, and acting as a liaison between the patient, the research team, and the physician.[12] Also critical to the success of clinical trials in the ambulatory setting is the quality of the data and the development and investment in skilled data managers and clinical research nurses.

Cost of Clinical Trials

The presumed or implied cost savings of community-based clinical research may be misleading. While the overall cost may be less, the expense to a given institution or practice setting may be considerable. Many clinical research trials have cost challenges beyond the obvious administrative and data management costs. Most troublesome is the overall cost of patient care, which is often increased with the clinical trial. The providers and the care setting must absorb that cost. A careful review of the total cost of a research trial must be done prior to

contracting to participate in the clinical study. Table 75-5 summarizes guidelines for office-based ambulatory programs considering expansion into research clinical trials.[58]

There are usually three kinds of costs attributed to clinical trials: (1) the administrative and data gathering costs; (2) the specific and unique costs of the treatment and the tests or procedures unique to the study project; and (3) the cost of clinical care of the patients. Traditionally, the institution or group sponsoring the trial has supported the first two categories. Less clear and more troublesome are the patient care and "associated costs" of clinical research because many insurance companies view clinical trials as "experimental and unproven" and deny payment for the usual medical costs associated with treatment.[59] Knowledge of probable and potential reimbursement problems is useful in obtaining payment. A pretreatment discussion with payers as to the rationale for enrolling the patients in a particular research protocol is essential. The education of both legislators and insurers to the expanded use of the ambulatory setting for investigational treatment is critical to increasing reimbursement.

Pursuing quality research is clearly necessary to advancing knowledge and clinical outcomes in cancer care. The challenge in today's health care environment is to blend this goal with practical issues often limited by reimbursement restraints.

Reimbursement

For the oncology nurse in the ambulatory setting, reimbursement challenges are encountered on a daily basis, often affecting many aspects of a patient's therapy. Payer approval or denial of a therapy for a given diagnosis and how the therapy is administered are often points of debate between the providers of care and both the private insurers (Blue Cross/Blue Shield, commercial carriers, HMOs, preferred provider organizations [PPOs]) and government insurers (Medicare and Medicaid).

Off-label drug use, administration method, and dosage of drug that differs from original Federal Drug Administration (FDA) approval for a given drug are challenges to reimbursement throughout the cancer care spectrum. Advanced technology (such as portable infusion pumps) and specialized clinicians have made it possible to provide complex and multimodality plans of treatment in the outpatient setting. However, regulatory guidelines at times can undermine the cost effectiveness that outpatient services are intended to provide. For example, patients who are prescribed growth factor support and are insured by Medicare are covered only if they go to an office or infusion center for the injection but are not covered if the injection is self-administered at home.

The Omnibus Budget Reconciliation Act (OBRA) of 1993 added a new section to the Social Security Act that

Table 75-5 Office-Based Clinical Research Guidelines

Basic Requirements

- An oncologist who has the potential to enroll more than 100 patients per year in clinical trials and can deliver a predictable accrual

- Enthusiastic physician support of the clinical initiative

- Clinicians with access to promising drugs not yet approved by the FDA

- Innovative trials that answer important clinical questions

- A sufficient number of trials available through contacts with the pharmaceutical industry

- An effective research staff

- Trials that fill clinical needs and have scientific merit

Criteria for Establishing Scientific Merit

- What is being studied?

- Are the objectives clearly defined?

- Are the objectives as measurable as possible?

- Are there enough patients in the study to give it statistical power?

- Do the planned assessments permit valid conclusions?

- Is the study designed appropriately for the proposed subjects?

- Does the study incorporate reasonable precautions to eliminate bias?

- Are the control groups appropriate?

- What is the degree of physician and nursing interest in the trial?

- Will the study sponsor be willing to modify the trial if portions require changes?

- What academic reputation can be gained by participation?

- What provisions are made in the contract regarding publication rights?

Questions To Ask To Ensure that a Proposed Trial Meets Ethical Guidelines

- What are the risks to the patients?

- Is the product safe and effective?

- Are there any issues, such as the use of placebos, that might affect institutional review board approval?

- Are qualified staff members available to conduct the trial?

- Can patient enrollment be achieved in the projected time period?

- Are federal protocols included or excluded in the study?

- Is the principal investigator fully committed in terms of time?

- Is the research laboratory personnel fully involved?

- Is there enough space (furniture, personnel) and equipment (copier, refrigerator to hold specimens) to handle new procedures?

- Are safety issues covered?

- Are measures in place to handle emergencies, such as adverse drug reactions?

Reprinted with permission from ONS guidelines on office based clinical trials. *Oncology* 13:162–165, 1999.[58]

extended coverage under Medicare B (physician reimbursement) to include certain self-administered oral cancer chemotherapeutic drugs. The issues of dispensing packets and patient instructions are state and federally regulated and remain a challenge in any ambulatory care settings, as does the lack of reimbursement for the monitoring and management of associated side effects and toxicity.

Rapid developments in the knowledge and technology available for the treatment of patients with cancer may create gaps between what the clinician deems "best treatment" and what the payer views as "allowable" for reimbursement. It is imperative that ambulatory care providers be fully aware of reimbursement strategies and approaches to avoid unnecessary denials of payment and unexpected costs to the patients. Denials may occur for a variety of reasons and insurance claims often require additional documentation. (See Table 75-6.)

Off-Label Drug Use and Unproven Methods

Off-label or unproven therapy has traditionally been defined as the use of a drug or treatment for a specific disease that is not listed in the package insert as an indication for therapeutic usage or, alternatively, not listed in the three compendia (Drug Evaluations by the America Medical Association, American Hospital Formulary Service Drug Information, or the United States Pharmacopeia Drug Information) as an acceptable indication. The Medicare Cancer Coverage Improvement Act (OBRA 1993) mandated coverage of off-label drug use if it appears in one of the three major compendia, if it

Table 75-6 Common Reasons for Reimbursement Denials

- Incorrect billing code (CPT code)

- Use of drug therapy that is not yet approved for the diagnosis under which the bill is submitted

- Insufficient documentation

- Complicated coverage and payment issues related to the use of an investigational drug

- Services related to the administration of complex chemotherapy regimens

Documentation to Support Reimbursement Claims

- Written documentation and/or medical records that provide the rationale for the prescribed therapy—justify the medical necessity

- Written documentation (chart review) that describes the elements of the billed service level

- Articles, preferably from "peer review journals," that support the use of drugs or biological agents for off-label use. Refer to major drug compendia, published articles, position papers from medical societies

- Letters from colleagues, expert "second opinions" that establish that the treatment requested is "the standard of practice" for the particular patient is supported by published clinical evidence, or if it is medically accepted in the community. HCFA's (Health Care Financing Administration) changeable interpretations of "medically inappropriate" is currently the most difficult issue in seeking payment resolutions.

Ambulatory Patient Classifications

HCFA has proposed a regulation that will dramatically change reimbursement for services and drugs in the outpatient setting, specifically oncology care.[60–62] The proposed change groups chemotherapy into four ambulatory patient classifications for reimbursement. Unfortunately, many of the older chemotherapy agents received the highest reimbursement classification and the newer, more expensive agents received the least amount of reimbursement. Also supportive care drugs, such as growth factors, were bundled in with the chemotherapy agent reimbursement and not reimbursed separately. Such classification limits reimbursement for state-of-the-art therapies. In addition, support drugs have been successful in minimizing side effects and reducing hospitalizations but under the proposal may not be reimbursed, which will have an obvious negative affect to patient care.[63] An important impact of this reduction in reimbursement may be the decrease in money available for nurses to staff the ambulatory setting. Radiation care reimbursement reductions have been proposed, which would mean radiation centers would need increased patient loads to remain solvent.

Reimbursement for Nursing Services

The ambulatory nurse is uniquely challenged with securing reimbursement for nursing services through a system defined primarily for physician rendered care (Medicare B). Currently, ambulatory nursing services are covered under the Medicare provision of services furnished "incident to" a physician's service. This includes the services of a physician's employee delivered in an ambulatory setting if the service is within the scope of the nurse's practice, if the physician is on site, and if the service is related to the physician's plan of care and the primary condition for which the patient is under medical care. This category of reimbursement limits nursing practice to physician supervision and does not allow for independent treatment or interventions for conditions that are within the defined scope of nursing practice, particularly at the advanced practice level.

Reimbursement Strategies

The economic issues related to patient care and treatment are integral to the oncology nursing role. For the ambulatory-based oncology nurse, this may mean assisting and educating patients to negotiate with representa-

tives of their insurance plans. Patients have a need and a responsibility to be informed of the financial issues related to their cancer treatment, particularly if involved in investigational therapy. Patients generally assume that their insurance covers any therapy they need, and are frequently frightened and angry to discover that this is not the case. Grassroots efforts have increased with such national groups as CAN ACT being formed by patients to put pressure on both private payers and legislators to develop and maintain a system of payment that ensures access to state-of-the-art care for the treatment of cancer as well as funding for ongoing cancer research.[64,65]

For office-based oncology nurses, the involvement with reimbursement issues is often more direct. The nurse can pursue various strategies to help patients and the practice obtain reimbursement and to overcome specific obstacles regarding the ambulatory care setting and investigational therapies (Table 75-7).[64] This can best be accomplished through collaboration among the physicians, the office manager, and the nurses.

The cost and billing issues of drug therapy pertain to all oncology care settings; however, they are felt most intensely in the ambulatory care setting. Without the billing staffs and finance departments that are present in a hospital structure, it falls to the physician and nurse to articulate to the patient how and why payment and financial issues can affect the plan of therapy. Bridging the gap between patients and payers is challenging and requires the clinicians to temper their natural patient advocacy role with financial sophistication and to have the tenacity to continue to challenge payers to provide the best available treatment.

Key to the process is communication that is effective between the health care providers and the payers.[66] A written, objective treatment plan with a clearly stated rationale is an essential component to ensuring the delivery of quality care. The benefits of such an approach

Table 75-7 Strategies for Obtaining Reimbursement

1. Accurately and thoroughly identify costs and allocate them to the most appropriate CPT code.

   Determine costs of drugs and medical supplies.

   Determine costs of administering therapy (time, special skills, services, and equipment, patient care, and other requirements of each therapy).

2. Advise, inform, and educate third-party payers on the appropriateness and necessity of newest modalities. In general, contact case managers, state Medicare directors, medical directors.

   Individual cases help document the scientific data, clinical outcomes, and cost benefits supporting a treatment decision.

3. Participate with professional societies to set standards of care that differentiate between state-of-the-art and experimental therapy.

Reprinted with permission from Xistris D, Houlihan N: Impact of reimbursement and health care reform on the ambulatory oncology setting. *Semin Oncol Nurs* 10:281–287, 1994.[64]

include increased cost efficiency, improved patient outcomes, and a higher level of patient satisfaction.[67]

Patient Perspective

Ambulatory cancer care from the patient perspective has never been more challenging. Ensuring continuity of care is the most challenging daily task of the ambulatory care nurse. Driven by insurance restrictions, patients may need to obtain tests at different diagnostic sites and may need referrals from primary care physicians before coming for care to the cancer specialist. These patients are usually not feeling well and are in the midst of difficult cancer treatments. Length of a hospital stay has never been shorter and the preparation for discharge and self-care is limited. Patients and their caregivers are assuming tremendous burdens that require nursing support and guidance. The relationship between the nurse and the patient in the ambulatory setting is unique. It is there that the patient is often diagnosed and treatment is planned. It is in this same ambulatory setting where treatment failure information is given and new plans are discussed. The visits are limited in duration but not in intensity, and the bonds formed between the patient and nurse are strong.

The challenges for the patient include navigation of the health care system and in meeting this challenge ambulatory nurses become the patient's closest ally. Advocacy for the patient is a major aspect of today's ambulatory nursing role. For example, coordinating weekly blood counts for treatment takes time and energy on the part of both the patient and nurse. Often the blood sample is obtained in a separate outpatient center and then the specimen is sent to a main laboratory center for processing. Getting the correct result to the oncologist and nurse is a process that often does not go smoothly for the patient. Technologists in settings not specific to oncology may have little experience with patients with limited venous access and often are not able to obtain blood results from access devices or difficult veins. Nurses must be proactive and obtain information about the expertise of the local laboratory and staff to prevent problems for the patient.

Open and ongoing communication back and forth among members of the health care team and the patient and family is essential. It fosters the trust relationship necessary for a well-coordinated plan of care.

Future

There will be roles for generalists, specialists, and critical care nurses in oncology ambulatory care in the future, as even more intensive technical procedures will be managed in the outpatient department. Nurses will assess and teach intensively over the phone, and there will be more electronic communication of activities. The future includes e-mail transmission of patient data between providers and more complex telephone communication activities. The expansion of research activities to test new drugs and protocols will continue. Advocacy activities—assisting patients to access health care, making them aware of their rights and negotiating on their behalf, and helping identify ethical dilemmas—will remain a major part of the ambulatory nursing role. Critical to the success of that role is communication between caregivers.

The recruitment and preparation of nurses for this specialty is also critical. Education programs must include this practice clinical setting in rotations for undergraduate and graduate nurses.

Many challenges lie ahead for the ambulatory oncology nurse and the patient as reimbursement decisions are made. The goal will be to obtain the best clinical care for the patient with cancer and maintain the professional nurse role in this specialty.

References

1. Haas SA, Hackbarth DP, Kavanagh JA, et al: Dimensions of the staff nurse role in ambulatory care: part II—comparison of role dimensions in four ambulatory settings. *Nurs Econ* 13:152–164, 1995
2. Ginsberg, E. Future of health care reform. The effects on physicians. *West J Med* 161:71–73, 1994
3. McKeown T. Man's health: the past and the future. *West J Med* 132:49–57, 1980
4. AAACN: *Nursing in Ambulatory Care: The Future is Here.* Washington, DC, American Nurses Publishing, 1997, pp. 1–53
5. Tighe MG, Fisher SG, Hastings C, et al: A study of the oncology nurse role in ambulatory care. *Oncol Nurs Forum* 12:23–27, 1985
6. Martin C: Incidence of emergency visits among oncology patients receiving outpatient chemotherapy: implications for care in a capitated market. *Cancer Control* 3:435–441, 1996
7. Shirkman N, Cloutier A, Tittle M, et al: Meeting the challenge of unscheduled outpatient visits. *Nurs Manage* 30:51–53, 1999
8. Lamkin L: Outpatient oncology settings: a variety of services. *Semin Oncol Nurs* 10:229–236, 1994
9. Houston DA, Houston GR: Administration issues and concepts in ambulatory care, in Buschel PC, Yarbro CH (eds): *Oncology Nursing in the Ambulatory Setting.* Sudbury, MA, Jones and Bartlett, 1993, pp 3–19
10. Iwamoto R, Gough S: Radiotherapy: ambulatory care models, in Buschel PC, Yarbro CH (eds): *Oncology Nursing in the Ambulatory Setting.* Sudbury, MA, Jones and Bartlett, 1993, pp 133–163
11. Moskowitz R: Day surgery for oncology patients, in Buschel PC, Yarbro CH (eds): *Oncology Nursing in the Ambulatory Setting.* Sudbury, MA, Jones and Bartlett, 1993, pp 165–183
12. Cooley ME, Lin EM, Hunter SW: The ambulatory oncology nurse's role. *Semin Oncol Nurs* 10:245–253, 1994
13. Verran J: Delineation of ambulatory care nursing practice. *J Ambulatory Care Manage* 4:1–13, 1981
14. Brown JK: Ambulatory services: the mainstay of cancer nursing care. *Oncol Nurs Forum* 12:57–59, 1985
15. Barhamand B: A survey of the role, benefits, and realities of the office-based oncology nurse. *Oncol Nurs Forum* 18:31–37, 1991

16. Oncology Nursing Society: *National Survey of Salary, Staffing, and Professional Practice Patterns in Ambulatory Oncology Clinics.* Pittsburgh, PA, ONS Nursing Press, 1992

17. Hastings C: *The Context for Ambulatory Care Nursing.* Washington, DC, The Washington Hospital Center, 1997

18. Hackbarth DP, Haas SA, Kavanagh JA, et al: Dimensions of the staff nurse role in ambulatory care: part I—methodology and analysis of data on current staff nurse practice. *Nurs Econ* 13:89–98, 1995

19. Haas SA, Hackbarth DP: Dimensions of the staff nurse role in ambulatory care: part III—using research data to design new models of nursing care delivery. *Nurs Econ* 13:230–241, 1995

20. Porter HB: The effect of ambulatory oncology nursing practice models on health resource utilization: part I, collaboration or compliance. *J Nurs Adm* 25:21–29, 1995

21. AAACN: *1996 Ambulatory Care Nursing Administration and Practice Standards.* Pitman, NJ, Anthony J. Jannetti, 1996

22. Kennedy GM, Fitch MI (eds): *Ambulatory Oncology Nursing Practice Guidelines: A Focus on Patient Outcome Standards.* Toronto, CA, Toronto-Sunnybrook Regional Cancer Center, 1994

23. Porter HB: The effect of ambulatory oncology nursing practice models on health resource utilization: part 2, different practice models—difference use of health resources? *J Nurs Adm* 25:237–244, 1994

24. Walter JM, Robinson SH: Nursing care delivery models in ambulatory oncology. *Semin Oncol Nurs* 10:237–244, 1994

25. Manthey M: Delivery systems and practice models: a dynamic balance. *J Nurs Manage* 22:28–30, 1991

26. Prescott PA, Soeken KL: Measuring nursing intensity in ambulatory care—part I: approaches to and uses of patient classification systems. *Nurs Econ* 14:14–21, 1996

27. Haas SA, Hackbarth DP: Dimensions of the staff nurse role in ambulatory care: part IV—developing nursing intensity measures, standards, clinical ladders, and QI programs. *Nurs Econ* 13:285–294, 1995

28. Medvec BR: Productivity and workload measurement in ambulatory oncology. *Semin Oncol Nurs* 10:288–295, 1994

29. Verran J: Testing a patient classification instrument for the ambulatory care setting. *Res Nurs Health* 9:279–287, 1986

30. Hastings CE: Classification issues in ambulatory care nursing. *J Ambulatory Care Manage* 10:50–64, 1987

31. Parrinello K, Brenner PS, Vallone B: Refining and testing a nursing patient classification instrument in ambulatory care. *Nurs Adm Q* 13:54–65, 1988

32. Hastings C, Muir-Nash J: Validation of a taxonomy of ambulatory nursing practice. *Nurs Econ* 7:142–149, 1989

33. Joseph AC: Ambulatory care: an objective assessment. *J Nurs Adm* 20:27–33, 1990

34. Prescott PA, Soeken KL: Measuring nursing intensity in ambulatory care—part II: developing and testing PINAC. *Nurs Econ* 14:86–91, 1996

35. Karr J, Fisher R: A patient classification system for ambulatory care. *Nurs Manage* 28:27–28, 1997

36. Gulanick M, Green M, Crutchfield C, et al: Telephone nursing in a general medicine ambulatory clinic. *MEDSURG Nurs* 5:93–124, 1996

37. AAACN: *Telephone Nursing Practice Administration and Practice Standards.* Pitman, NJ, Anthony J. Jannetti, 1997

38. Jones PK, Jones SL, Katz J: Improving follow-up among hypertensive patients using a belief model intervention. *Arch Intern Med* 147:1557–1560, 1987

39. Watts RJ, Dafoe DC, Martorelli RD, et al: Nurse-physician collaboration and decision outcomes in transplant ambulatory care settings. *ANNA J* 22:25–32, 1995

40. Nail LM, Greene D, Jones LS, et al: Nursing care by telephone: describing practice in an ambulatory oncology center. *Oncol Nurs Forum* 16:387–395, 1989

41. Brennan M: Nursing process in telephone advice. *Nurs Manage* 23:62–64, 1992

42. Becker CA: Rethinking performance measures for health manage call centers. *AAACN Viewpoint* 21:5–6, 1999

43. Morrisey J: On call Foundation Health Systems' sophisticated telephone triage center gains popularity with patients and physicians. *Mod Healthc,* 27(24):72–78, 1997

44. Kastens JM: Integrated care management: aligning medical call centers and nurse triage services. *Nurs Econ* 16:320–322, 1998

45. Anastasia PJ, Blevins MC: Outpatient chemotherapy: telephone triage for symptom management. *Oncol Nurs Forum* 24:13–24, 1997 (suppl 1)

46. Behrend SW, Sklaroff RB: The evolving profile of the office oncology nurse, in Buschel PC, Yarbro CH (eds): *Oncology Nursing in the Ambulatory Setting.* Sudbury, MA, Jones and Bartlett, 1993, pp 73–105

47. Behrend SW: Documentation in the ambulatory setting. *Semin Oncol Nurs* 10:264–280, 1994

48. Wengstrom Y, Forsberg C: Justifying radiation oncology nursing practice—a common literature review. *Oncol Nurs Forum* 26:741–750, 1999

49. Majidi F, Enterline JP, Ashley B, et al: Chemotherapy and treatment scheduling: the Johns Hopkins Oncology Center outpatient department. *Proc Annual Symp Comput Appl Med Care* 154–158, 1993

50. Koren ME, Bartel JC, Corliss J: Interventions to improve patient appointments in an ambulatory care facility. *J Ambulatory Care Manage* 17:76–80, 1994

51. Preston F, Cunningham R: *Clinical Guidelines for Symptom Management in Oncology—A Handbook for Advanced Practice Nurses.* New York, Clinical Insights, 1998

52. Nail LM, Jones LS, Greene D, et al: Use and perceived efficacy of self-care activities in patients receiving chemotherapy. *Oncol Nurs Forum* 18:883–887, 1991

53. Dodd MJ: Patterns of self-care in cancer patients receiving radiation therapy. *Oncol Nurs Forum* 11:23–27, 1984

54. Hanucharurnkul S: Predictors of self-care in cancer patients receiving radiotherapy. *Cancer Nurs* 1:21–27, 1989

55. Kubricht DW: Therapeutic self-care demands expressed by outpatients receiving external radiation therapy. *Cancer Nurs* 7:43–52, 1984.

56. Shirkman N, Cloutier A, Tittle M, et al: Meeting the challenge of unscheduled outpatient visits. *Nursing Manage* 30: 51–53, 1994

57. Camp-Sorrell D, Spencer-Csek P. Reimbursement for advance practice. *Oncol Nurs Forum* 22:31–34, 1995

58. ONS guidelines on office based clinical trials. *Oncology* 13: 162–165, 1999

59. Freedman M, McCabe M: Commentary—Assignment costs associated with therapeutic oncology research: a modest proposal. *J Natl Cancer Inst* 84:760–763, 1992

60. Mortenson LE, Edwards JJ, Bowers ML: Implementation of ambulatory payment classifications threatens viability of hospital outpatient cancer programs, use of new agents, and supportive care drugs. *Oncol Issues* 13:1–5, 1998

61. Niemeyer S: It pays to know your APCs and APGs. *Inside Ambulatory Care* 5:5–7, 1998

62. Meier E: Congress weighs health policy issues. Nurses, patients may see strong ripple effects. *AAACN Viewpoint* 21:1, 1999

63. Special symposium. *The changing healthcare environment: the effects of trends, reimbursement, and regulations on oncology care*

delivery. Syllabus of the 24th Annual ONS Congress. ONS, Pittsburgh, PA. 1999, p 84

64. Xistris D, Houlihan N: Impact of reimbursement and health care reform on the ambulatory oncology setting. *Semin Oncol Nurs* 10:281–287, 1994

65. Xistris D: Reimbursement of biotherapy: present status, future directions-perspectives of the office based oncology nurse. *Semin Oncol Nurs* 8:8–12, 1992

66. Mellody P, Owen MS: Improving managed care communications. *Negotiating optimal ovarian cancer care.* Bala Cynwyd, PA: Meniscus Limited Educational Institute, 1999, pp 27–31

67. Mastal P: New signposts and directions: indicators of quality in ambulatory care. *Nurs Econ* 17:103, 1999

CHAPTER 76

Home Care

Connie M. Yuska, RN, MS, CORLN
Patricia G. Nedved, RN, MSN, ACRN

Introduction

The home care industry has experienced great changes throughout the 1990s to the present. Changes occurring at the macro level of the health care delivery system present new challenges and opportunities to home care providers in every community. Merely a cottage industry 15 years ago, home care now is the fastest-growing sector of health care.[1] The cause of this dramatic increase was the implementation of prospective payment for hospital services in 1983. This change in payment methodology rapidly resulted in decreased lengths of hospital stays and subsequent increase in referrals for home health care.[2]

Current Home Care Challenges

Despite the rapid change occurring within the industry, two key goals of home health care have remained constant: (1) to provide health care services to patients in the home setting and (2) to provide education to the patient and family with the goal of attaining health and independence from formal care systems. Today's home health care strongly reflects the government-funded medical programs of Medicare and Medicaid that began in the 1960s. In addition, public health initiatives and changes in private insurance benefit regulation have provided constant challenges to the provider. The provision of home care services not only depends on the complex interaction between the patient, family, and available community resources, but on the availability of payment sources to fund the care as well.[3]

The average number of days a Medicare beneficiary spent in the hospital in 1994 was 7.4. This is approximately half the number (13 days) spent in the hospital in 1970.[4] These changes within the broader health care system have increased demand for home care services and have created competition within the home care industry. The rapid growth of home care has also resulted in increased demands from regulatory agencies and public and private insurers whose demands are changing the way care is provided.[5]

The Changing Patient Population

One of the most dramatic changes in home health care over the past few years has been the change in the type of patients who now receive care in the home. The level of patient acuity has increased dramatically and new categories of patients who can safely receive care at home have emerged. Many treatment modalities delivered in the hospital setting to oncology patients just a few short years ago are now safely and routinely administered in the home setting.

Increased patient acuity has resulted in patients who require more skilled nursing and complex assessments than in the past. In many cases, patients spend less time in the hospital, and they return home with only an introduction to the education they need to adequately care for themselves at home. Thus, the role of the home care nurse as teacher becomes even more critical. Teaching activities in the home consumes more of the nurse's time as patients and families assume a greater responsibility for patient care.[5] This increased focus on promotion of patient independence often results in a longer, more involved nursing visit.

The increase in the elderly population and changing societal conditions also have created new challenges for the home care nurse. Many elderly patients are socially isolated, living alone or with family members who are out of the home during the day, leaving no caregiver in the home. A population that is becoming more ethnically diverse also challenges the home care nurse to meet the needs of various ethnic groups.

The Response of Nursing

One exploratory, descriptive study designed to identify how the recent changes in the home care industry have affected nursing practice and the quality of health care services collected information from home care nurses regarding their perceptions of recent changes in their practice.[5] Researchers discovered that home care nurses are responding to health care system changes by altering the way they work with patients. The nurses in this study reported their patient care is more focused and the goals of returning the patient to self-care and early discharge from home care are prominent. In addition, nurses are aware of increased constraints by managed care companies on the number of visits allowed, which motivates nurses to structure their plan of care in a manner that expedites self-care.

Although nurses reported experiencing frustration when the standard dictated by the insurance company differs from that of the nurse, overall the nurses responded with positive feelings about the recent changes in the health care system and the impact those changes have had on home care nurses. There is a feeling that home health care has emerged stronger than ever. Home care has earned the respect of hospital colleagues, physicians, and insurance companies and the home care nurse has been at the center of that increased respect.

Changes in Covered Services

Another challenge to home care is the elimination of some previously covered services such as venipuncture. Coverage for venipuncture without another skilled need was eliminated as a covered service from the Medicare program in February 1998. Agencies responded to this change by referring their patients who only required venipuncture to the physician's office or other outpatient facility.

Coordination of Care

Effective coordination of the patient's care and communication with other health care team members remains a challenge inherent to home care. It is not uncommon for agencies to have a service territory that spans several hundred miles, numerous counties, and in some areas of the country, more than one state. With nurses, therapists, and home health aides all potentially visiting the patient, mechanisms must be established to effectively communicate changes in patient condition and treatment modalities. Recent advances in technology have made this task much easier. The nurse's home office often includes a computer and a fax machine and some home care agencies provide computers for each nurse. In addition, home care personnel regularly use pagers, cellular phones, and voice mail to stay in touch with patients, physicians, and agency managers.

Economic Issues

Financing Home Care

There are three primary payers for home care services: Medicare, Medicaid, and a variety of commercial payers. Different regulations govern care under each of these models. It is essential that the home care nurse have knowledge of the different payer requirements and consider these differences when planning care for the patient.

Medicare

Home care funding is provided by the federal government under a variety of programs created by the Social Security Act, including Medicare (Social Security Act Title XVIII), Medicaid (Social Security Act Title XIX), and the Older Americans Act (Pub. L. No. 89-73, 1965; Pub. L. No. 98-459, 1984). Medicare was enacted July 30, 1965, and became effective on July 1, 1966. It is a two-part program, commonly referred to as Part A and Part B. In Part A, beneficiaries receive certain insurance coverage for hospitalization and specifically defined home health care. In addition to Part A coverage, beneficiaries may purchase additional coverage under the Part B portion of the benefit. Part B coverage extends to physician services provided on an outpatient basis, pathology services, outpatient hospital services, and others. On July 1, 1981, Part A began to pay for home health services to beneficiaries who are covered by both Part A and Part B.[7]

To participate in the Medicare program for home care and to receive reimbursement for services delivered, the home care provider is guided by the Medicare Conditions of Participation. A basic understanding of the Conditions of Participation is essential for the nurse providing home care services. Many of the Conditions of Participation are also used by private payers as well. A review of the Conditions of Participation and all applicable state regulations should be provided in the orientation of every home care nurse. The Medicare-certified home health agency must demonstrate compliance with the Conditions of Participation on an ongoing basis through state surveys held at predetermined intervals based on the outcome of the previous survey.[8]

Under the Medicare model, several conditions must be present to establish eligibility for home care services. It is important for the nurse to understand these conditions since most payers generally follow Medicare guidelines. First, the patient must be *homebound*. This means the patient has a physical or medical condition that limits his or her ability to leave the house other than to receive medical care such as at the physician's office or the hospital. Second, the patient requires *skilled intermittent care* to treat the qualifying condition. Skilled intermittent services include nursing, physical therapy, or speech therapy. The patient may be eligible to receive other services such as occupational therapy, home health aide services, and medical social services if there is a "skilled need." Finally, a third condition is that the referring *physician must approve the plan of treatment in writing*. Additionally, the physician must certify that the patient is homebound and has a skilled need. The plan of treatment will include the services needed, the frequency of those services, and the duration of care to be provided.[9]

Home health agencies bill for Medicare services on a monthly basis. The initial plan of care is created and submitted to the physician for signature on the Health Care Financing Administration (HCFA) form and physician certification form, commonly referred to as the "485," a reference to the form number. After the first month of providing services, the home health agency transmits the bill to the fiscal intermediary. The agency *must* have the physician-signed 485 in their possession *before* billing Medicare for services. States have different regulations regarding the number of days the agency has to process the paperwork internally and produce a bill to Medicare. Likewise, any verbal orders received from physicians must be signed and returned to the agency before the bill is sent.[9] It is imperative that the nurse caring for the Medicare patient know and understand both federal and state requirements so that necessary documentation is turned into the agency to meet billing deadlines.

The Balanced Budget Act of 1997

In August 1997, the Balanced Budget Act (BBA) was signed into law. This law affects 39 million recipients of Medicare as well as insurers, providers, suppliers, and physicians. The act mandates the reduction of federal government spending on the Medicare program by $116.4 billion between fiscal years 1998 and 2002. To meet this mandate, numerous changes will have to be made in the way the program operates.

The BBA has a significant impact on the home health care industry. The savings from home health care is expected to total $16.2 billion and will be obtained through the introduction of an interim payment system (IPS), reduced cost limits, and a per beneficiary cap.[6] For the home care industry, these changes will be as significant as the implementation of Diagnostic Related Groups was for the hospital industry in the 1980s.

Coverage of home health services under Part A of Medicare was reduced to a maximum of 100 visits during an episode of illness after a three-day hospital stay or after receiving any covered services in a skilled nursing facility. Coverage for all other home health services will be reimbursed under Medicare Part B.

The BBA provides for dramatic changes in the reimbursement methodology for Medicare home health services. The IPS is in effect for those agencies with cost-reporting periods beginning on or after October 1, 1997. The interim payment system will remain in effect until a new prospective payment system (PPS) is implemented in October 2000. The overall impact to home care agencies is decreased cost limits and an aggregate per beneficiary limit.[6] The magnitude of this change is great and it forces agencies and individual nurses to operate very differently from only a few years ago. Agencies must change their thinking from "costs represent reimbursement" to "provision of service represents cost."

Managed Care

The home care market and, in particular, home infusion grew rapidly during the 1980s. Profit margins were at an all-time high. In the early 1990s, managed care introduced competition and price compression that negatively affected many home care providers. Successful home care agencies responded with detailed analysis of their operations and development of strategic plans to ensure future operational viability. Agencies that survive the tumultuous environment of the 1990s will be those that adjusted their marketing and operational strategies to compete in the new health care marketplace.

Pricing home care products and services effectively within the marketplace is one of the first steps the home care provider can take to ensure continued success. The home care nurse must be familiar with the most common pricing strategies in the marketplace so that resources and services can continue to be provided and reimbursed. This requires that the nurse have a basic knowledge of the definitions of common pricing models currently used for home care services. The eight models for reimbursement are listed in Table 76-1. It is important to remember that the use of any particular strategy will be dependent upon the degree of managed care penetration in a given market.

Managed care organizations (MCOs) have begun to articulate what they want from home care providers. The overarching goal of the managed care organization is to find effective ways to control overall cost while simultaneously providing high quality care. The MCO is interested in securing relationships with providers who share these

Table 76-1 Home Care Reimbursement Models

Methodology	Description
Fee for service	A specific fee for each product or service provided
Discounted fee for service	A fixed amount or percentage is subtracted from the list price fee
Per diem	A negotiated daily rate which is set for all of the products or services over the course of a day
Per case	A fixed dollar amount per episode or occurrence
Capitation	The provider receives a per-member, per-month flat fee
Risk sharing	Arrangement made with the managed care organization to share the cost for care on a select risk population
Outcomes-based pricing	Fixed dollar amount per case is received based on expected outcomes

values. In addition, the MCO may want to share the risk with the provider for the cost of providing high quality care. This arrangement mandates that the provider find ways to establish effective communication channels about the day-to-day condition and needs of the patient. The MCO also wants to partner with providers who can supply comprehensive home care services—skilled intermittent care, infusion, maternal child care, psychiatric care, durable medical equipment, private duty services, etc. If the provider cannot directly offer all of these services, it is in the best interest of the MCO to develop strong referral relationships with providers who can.

MCOs also want to partner with providers who can measure and effectively report outcomes of care. Providers should establish quality programs within their agencies and ensure that commitment to quality care is present throughout all levels of staff. The MCOs want to partner with providers who have both clinically effective programs and specialty niche programs such as infusion services for oncology care.

Patient satisfaction is another parameter measured by the MCO when considering a contract with a home care agency. Those agencies who not only measure and report patient satisfaction, but also participate in programs to provide benchmarking data are highly attractive to managed care organizations.

Finally, the attainment of accreditation through the Joint Commission on Accreditation of Healthcare Organizations (JCAHO) and certification for participation in the Medicare program are essential criteria for partnering with managed care organizations. Attaining these credentials provides a structure for the organization to follow that will signify quality not only to agency staff, but to the community and patients as well.

Providing high quality services at a lower cost challenges the home care provider to critically examine internal operations. Managers will need to examine their assumptions and beliefs, and ask several difficult questions: What skill level of staff is truly needed to perform certain activities? What level of support is needed to prevent field staff from performing clerical duties? What will the cost-benefit ratio be of introducing increased technology to the field staff? What is a reasonable productivity standard given the geographic region, the case mix and the skills of the staff? How can the number of visits be reduced while still ensuring acceptable outcomes?[10]

Managed care in the future

The next ten years are predicted to be the era of the megaprovider. Mergers and acquisitions of managed care companies will continue. For providers to survive, an understanding of some basic principles is necessary. Providers must realize that they cannot continue their old ways and they must change with the times. Change will continue to occur very quickly and they will need to learn to share the liability for the cost of care with others. Their internal operations and fiscal planning will need to accommodate this new risk sharing. They must also remember that effective care costs less than ineffective care. In the midst of such changes, however, decisions about clinical care will remain in the arena of the properly trained and educated clinicians.[11]

State-Funded Programs

Medicaid

Medicaid is a state-funded program designed to help needy citizens pay for health care. Coverage for home care services by the Medicaid program initially began with the passage of the 1965 Social Security Amendments. Medicaid is jointly funded by the federal government and individual states. The program also serves impoverished individuals who are blind, aged, or disabled. Additionally, it serves impoverished adult members of families with dependent children. Each state is responsible for setting standards for reimbursement and claims processing. This is administered through the development of policies and regulations at the state level which conform to the federal guidelines.[12]

Continuity of Care: Discharge Planning

Today's managed care environment and shorter hospital stays make discharge planning critically important in the development of a plan for a patient after a hospitalization. Discharge planning programs were developed in response to changes in the provision of and the payment for health care services. They were also developed as a result of changing illness patterns and changing patient support systems.[13] Thorough discharge planning can reduce costs and lower hospital readmissions. Discharge

planning is defined as activities that involve the patient and a team of individuals from various disciplines collaborating to facilitate the transition of a patient from one setting to another.[14] Such planning greatly affects the delivery of care and services by home health care agencies. In order to provide high-quality, efficient care, home care agencies must have thorough information regarding the patient's social situation, caregiver availability, payer information, diagnosis, and plan of care. Delivery of equipment and pharmaceutical supplies must also be coordinated. If any of this crucial information is missing, the continuity of care suffers. Discharge planning allows patients and family members to be involved in the process and also provides some choice for the patient.

Discharge planners work for the referral source on behalf of the patient and their family. Over the years JCAHO has increased its emphasis on comprehensive discharge planning. JCAHO requires that hospitals develop policies and procedures on discharge planning requiring early intervention for those patients with discharge needs. The development of an early discharge plan also contributes to a shortened hospital stay, resulting in a decreased cost per case. This also results in a home care referral of a patient who is often more acutely ill than in the past. Discharge planning is recognized as a key element in cost containment by third-party payers such as health maintenance organizations (HMOs) and preferred provider organizations (PPOs).[13]

Regulations do not allow employees of home health care agencies to act as a discharge planner for the referral source. However, the discharge planner and designated employees of home health care agencies do need to work together closely to provide the best services for a patient. Collaboration of disciplines across the care continuum, inclusion of the patient/family in care planning, and provision of adequate education for the patient/family to meet ongoing health care needs are areas designated by the JCAHO as essential for both hospitals and home care agencies to address.

Home Care Nurse Liaison

Because the discharge process is occurring more rapidly than in the past, home health care agencies may want to consider developing a home care *nurse liaison* role to facilitate the process of referral to the home care agency. The nurse liaison role provides a link between major referral sources and the home care agency. The nurse liaison works closely with the hospital or clinic discharge planner in organizing the care the patient will receive at home. Because acute care hospitals are just one point in the continuum of care, collaboration between the discharge planner and the home care nurse liaison is essential in planning the oncology patient's care across the continuum and throughout the patient's course of treatment. The nurse liaison can also communicate pertinent information about the patient's progress to staff in the physician's office.

In addition, the nurse liaison serves as a resource to the discharge planner for arranging home care services. The liaison also acts as an educator to discharge planners, hospital staff, and clinic employees regarding Medicare regulations for home care, products and services offered, and infusion therapy.

Using information provided by the discharge planner, the nurse liaison is better able to assess the patient's needs and to determine appropriateness for home care. The nurse liaison is able to offer suggestions to streamline care, while maintaining the care as high quality and cost effective.

One advantage of the nurse liaison role is the opportunity to meet with patients and their families prior to discharge from the acute care setting to discuss the home care plan and caregiver availability. Patients and family members will have an increased comfort level after meeting the nurse liaison and receiving information about the home care services. The process of including the patient and family in discharge planning demonstrates concern for them and affirms the patient's rights and responsibilities for his or her own health.[13] In addition, this discussion will help to allay patient and caregiver anxiety. Care coordination with the nurse liaison also helps to identify any area of confusion or conflict related to the home care plan. Family members will have a more realistic picture of the role they will play in the care of the patient. The nurse liaison will also discuss the plan of treatment with professionals from other disciplines whose services will also be included in the plan. Understanding and coordinating the various needs of the patient, including input from disciplines such as physical therapy, occupational therapy, speech therapy, nutrition support, and other departments, are necessary to establishing a comprehensive discharge plan.[13]

Nurse liaisons are also able to provide continuity of care for infusion services. Their role can include connecting patients to the ambulatory infusion pump in the hospital prior to discharge so there is no interruption in therapy. For instance, for a patient discharged on intravenous analgesics, the nurse liaison connects the patient to a home care pump and multidose bag of pain medication, thus ensuring continuation of therapy when the patient leaves. The start of home care in such a case coincides with the discharge from an acute care setting. At times, the nurse liaison may initiate home care in a specialty clinic setting. Continuous chemotherapy is mixed by the infusion pharmacist and sent to the clinic with an ambulatory infusion pump. The first administration of chemotherapy is initiated by the nurse liaison at the clinic. This approach provides greater continuity of care between settings.

The nurse liaison can also communicate clinical updates to the discharge planner. Initiating this communication allows the agency to maintain close contact with the referral source to alert discharge planners to a change in the medical condition and to the social situation of the patient. This communication will help to ensure greater continuity of care if the patient is readmitted to an acute care facility.

Three key elements in the creation of a discharge plan for home care are (1) interdisciplinary collaboration, (2) communication among caregivers, and (3) patient/family involvement in the creation of a treatment plan. Collaboration between the nurse liaison and the discharge planner will contribute to a seamless patient transition along the care continuum.

The Nurse Case Manager

The role of the nurse case manager (field nurse) is critical in the care delivery process. The nurse case manager (NCM) in home care is responsible for the coordination of the patient's home health care services. One of the greatest challenges in home care is to ensure that the plan of care is followed by all caregivers. This typically involves coordinating communication between each of the disciplines involved in the patient's care. The NCM is responsible for the retrieval of laboratory results and the communication of those results to both the physician and the infusion pharmacist. In addition, the NCM plays a critical role in communicating clinical changes.

The initial patient visit requires the NCM to evaluate many different areas. A comprehensive assessment should include an environmental, psychosocial, and physical assessment of the patient and his/her surroundings.

Environmental Assessment

A home environmental assessment is an essential part of a patient's plan of care. Ensuring that the patient's living environment is safe and that there is an appropriate area for the storage of medical supplies are basic to the initial assessment. The nurse should also view the living area for cleanliness including evidence of rodents or insects. In addition, the assessment of the physical environment must address such things as fire safety, electrical safety, bed and mobility safety, and bathroom safety. The outcome of the home assessment should be included in the development of the plan of care. The intent of the assessment is not to determine home care candidacy but to identify conditions or problems in the home that can be resolved.

Psychosocial Assessment

The NCM must evaluate the patient's psychosocial situation. This assessment includes meeting with the primary caregiver to describe the treatment plan and determine the caregiver's willingness and availability to assist in the plan of care. The nurse should assess the ability of both the patient and caregiver to learn tasks related to the patient's plan of care.

During the psychosocial assessment, the NCM should also evaluate the degree of potential caregiver burden that may be experienced by the patient's caregivers. This includes a discussion of the patient's safety needs as well as the patient's ability to participate in care. Caregiver burden should be continually evaluated and discussed with the patient and caregivers as the patient's condition changes.

Physical Assessment

The physical assessment occurs during the initial comprehensive visit and at each subsequent visit thereafter. The NCM should review the patient's medical history and family illness history with the patient and caregiver. A comprehensive review of all body systems should be completed. During the physical exam, the nurse should also review with the patient all of the medications ordered, their purpose, and potential side effects. In addition, the nurse should report any newly identified physical changes to the patient's physician and obtain any additional orders that are necessary based on the outcome of the assessment.

Ensuring the provision of adequate nutrition in the home can be a challenge to the nurse caring for the oncology patient. A baseline nutritional risk assessment is performed during the initial visit to identify the patient as being at no risk, at moderate risk, or at severe risk. Nutritional interventions are recommended for those who are at moderate and severe risk. The nurse should monitor the progress of the patient's nutritional status and implement changes to the plan as ordered.

In addition to assessment components, the initial visit also contains several other key elements. The nurse should review the patient's rights and responsibilities. A copy of the document is left in the home for reference. The patient should be notified of the agency's process for filing a complaint with regard to home care services. The patient will also sign a consent for treatment that allows the nurse to proceed with the plan of care. The nurse should also explain the patient's financial responsibility for services provided during the episode of care. Advanced directive options are reviewed with the patient and it needs to be determined whether the patient currently has an advanced directive in place. In addition, it is crucial that the nurse discuss measures to be taken in an emergency and develop an exigency plan with the patient. This will involve giving the patient and caregivers information regarding access to the home care agency 24 hours a day. The patient should also know how to access paramedics in the event of an acute situation. Each of these areas is integral to a complete assessment of the patient.

Documentation

Documentation is one of the most challenging aspects of home care for the professional caregiver. The increase in the acuity of patients admitted to home care has neces-

sitated clear, concise, accurate documentation. The documentation must demonstrate coordination and development of a care plan with the multiple services required for the patient. The clinical notes, orders, and all other documentation related to the patient's plan of care must be submitted to the home care agency within the time frame mandated by state guidelines.[14]

Home care agencies should develop a medical record policy that outlines guidelines for maintenance of the clinical record. It would behoove an agency to create a record policy that does not put unnecessary restraints on the agency. For example, time limits for forms requiring physician signature should not be more stringent than state law requires. Because orders may frequently be delayed in a physician's office or in the mail when sent out for signature, the agency should develop an internal tracking mechanism to control this process. Where state law allows, faxed physician signatures are useful for meeting state guidelines regarding timeliness. Other mechanisms to facilitate submission of documentation include electronic submission via a laptop computer or a handheld device.

Accurate documentation is essential to ensure reimbursement. Through documentation, the patient's need for home care is presented. Some payers require that the nurse's documentation be submitted before payment is issued. It is most important that the documentation reflect the clinical status of the patient as well as a description of the services being provided. Quality documentation should include observations written in measurable terms. Through documentation, the professional caregiver is directly accountable for reimbursement.[15]

Another reason for documentation is to substantiate coordination of services and document continuity of care. The medical record is a vehicle for different members of the interdisciplinary health care team to communicate with one another. One mechanism to facilitate this communication is through the use of discipline-specific care plans. Short- and long-term goals are established and expected outcomes are identified. The goals should be realistic and measurable. The plan of care and clinical notes inform other professionals of what has taken place in the care of the patient.

Additionally, the coordination of services should be documented in the clinical note. Coordination should be documented between caregivers, between the clinical staff and supervisory staff, with pharmacy staff, and with the physician's staff. Professional caregivers are required to report any clinical changes to the physician. A caregiver may be held liable if evidence of such communication with the physician cannot be produced. It is therefore imperative that clinical notes reflect evidence of anticipated plans, expected outcomes, and interdisciplinary communication.

In home care, the clinical record is the primary tool for assessing quality care. One way an agency can evaluate quality of care is to establish a quarterly record review. Standards for clinical record review should be defined and stated in measurable terms. The record will be evaluated to verify compliance with the defined terms. A quarterly record review may show deficiencies in care provided to a patient. If care is not documented, it can be presumed that it did not occur.

Documentation of patient/caregiver teaching must also be reflected in the clinical note. Written teaching tools are useful for patients and will serve as a reference for the patient and other caregivers. Teaching should continue until the patient/caregiver can verbalize understanding of the material. If the instruction involves teaching of a task, the education should continue until the patient/caregiver is able to successfully provide a return demonstration of the skill. Once the patient's understanding of the instruction has been documented, teaching in this area no longer constitutes a need for continued skilled care.

HCFA and some commercial payers require documentation of homebound status for reimbursement. The reason the patient is homebound must be documented at the initial comprehensive visit and at least weekly thereafter. All disciplines involved in the patient's home care should document the patient's homebound status. Coordination of care between the disciplines will ensure that various services do not document contradictory clinical information.

A key to successful documentation lies in the professional caregiver's ability to accurately describe why the patient requires home health care services and how the home health care will improve the patient's clinical status. When evaluating documentation an agency should explore the following questions: Was the care provided reasonable and necessary? Was the care provided ordered by the physician? Was homebound status documented? Was the patient's overall health status improved? Each of these questions are key to ensuring reimbursement and limiting liability for the home care agency.[15]

Challenges to Delivery of Care in the Home

Infection Control

The rising number of resistant organisms and the increasing number of intravenous access devices being used in the home are two of the key reasons for home care agencies to implement an infection control program. A comprehensive infection control program in home health care consists of activities related to direct patient care as well as activities that support the provision of such care. All of these activities are designed to reduce the transmission of infections among a facility's patients and staff members.[16] Infection surveillance needs to be defined by the agency to monitor the occurrence of nosohusial (home-acquired) infections, to recognize outbreaks of infection, and to reduce risk.

The word *surveillance* in this context means the ongoing systematic collection, analysis, and interpretation of health data essential to the planning, implementation, and evaluation of public health practice. Surveillance is also integrated with timely dissemination of these data to those who need to know.[17] Surveillance is pertinent to many areas of health care, including nosohusial infections.

Criterion

To date, there is no standard definition for a home-acquired or nosohusial infection. Therefore, agencies may need to collaborate with infectious disease physicians to develop their own definition.

An infection may be considered nosohusial in nature if it presents at least 48 hours after a patient is discharged from an inpatient setting. Incisional infections that develop within 30 days of surgery are considered nosocomial. Nosohusial infections are reported in the following categories: pneumonia, symptomatic urinary tract infection, eye infection, gastrointestinal infection, incisional site infection, decubitus ulcer infection, primary bloodstream infection, and vascular access site infection. A urinary tract infection related to a Foley catheter that has been in place longer than 30 days is generally not considered a nosohusial infection due to the increased prevalence of infections with chronic indwelling catheters.

Infection identification log

An infection identification log can facilitate the collection of data required for complete analysis and follow-up of actual or potential exposure to infection.[16] The collection tool usually includes specific diagnosis information that may influence an infection outcome. See Figure 76-1. For example, an oncology diagnosis with chemotherapy and resultant neutropenia is pertinent as it relates to a bloodstream infection.

Policies and procedures

A home health care agency must establish policies and procedures related to the specifics of infection prevention and transmission in the following areas:

- Handwashing
- Bag technique
- Disposal of sharps
- Disposal of biohazardous waste
- Personal protective equipment
- Transportation of biohazardous materials
- Needlestick and body fluid exposure
- Disinfection of equipment

It is also the obligation of a home health agency to develop guidelines related to patient-to-caregiver, caregiver-to-patient, and patient-to-patient transmission of

INFECTION SCREENING REPORT

Date of Report: _____   Completed by: _____

Patient Name: _____   Gender: ☐ Male ☐ Female Age: _____

Primary Diagnosis: _____   SOC Date: _____

☐ Lives alone   ☐ Lives with spouse/family/other

---

*Instructions: **The staff member observing the signs and symptoms should complete sections one and two and submit the report to the infection control practitioner.***

Section One: Patient Signs and Symptoms (Check all that apply)

Signs and Symptoms and Date Observed: _____

☐ Fever ≥ 100.5°F (oral)   ☐ Neutropenic

☐ Chills and rigors

☐ Elevated serum WBC   Date: _____   Results: _____ or ☐ Copy of lab results attached

☐ New culture order—Date obtained: _____   Site of culture: _____

☐ Culture results or ☐ Copy of lab results attached

  Results: ☐ positive ☐ negative

  Organism(s) isolated: ☐ Staph ☐ Strep ☐ E.Coli ☐ gm+ ☐ gm− ☐ Pseudomonas ☐ Klebsiella ☐ Other

  Drug resistant organisms: ☐ MRSA ☐ VRE ☐ MRSE ☐ N/A ☐ Other _____

☐ New antibiotic order Date: _____   Order: _____

Section Two: Potential Infection Site(s)

Catheter-associated UTI

☐ Insertion date: _____

☐ Change in character of urine (Check all that apply: ☐ increased sediment, ☐ cloudiness, ☐ foul odor, ☐ hematuria)

☐ New flank pain or suprapubic pain   ☐ WBC's in urine test

Bloodstream infection

☐ IV catheter-related bloodstream infection   ☐ IV infusate-related bloodstream infection

☐ Secondary to other infection site

  Primary site (e.g., pneumonia, peritonitis): _____

IV catheter-related infection (Check one: ☐ exit site ☐ pocket)

☐ Site (Check all that apply: ☐ redness, ☐ pain, ☐ swelling, ☐ tenderness, ☐ induration)

☐ Pain, tenderness, swelling of associated limb

☐ Purulent drainage—Describe: _____

☐ Date of catheter insertion: _____

☐ MD ordered catheter to be removed

Wound infection (Check One: ☐ wound ☐ drain site ☐ decubitus)

☐ Redness, tenderness   ☐ Swelling

☐ Purulent drainage—Describe: _____

☐ Post-operative wound   Date and type of surgery _____

Pneumonia

☐ Change in sputum (Check all that apply: ☐ color, ☐ purulence, ☐ thickness)

☐ Increase in rales and rhonchi   ☐ Decrease in breath sounds

☐ Pain in chest/thorax   ☐ Change or worsening mental status   ☐ Shortness of breath

Eye infection

☐ Pain   ☐ Redness   ☐ Purulent exudate

Gastrointestinal

☐ Sudden onset of nausea and vomiting

☐ Diarrhea

☐ Abdominal pain

☐ Rebound tenderness

Figure 76-1 Infection Screening Report.

(continued)

PNEUMONIA

Patient has crackles or dullness to percussion on physical exam of the chest not previously present, *and* at least 2 of the following:

1. New onset of purulent sputum (sputum that is green, yellow, or gray in color)
2. Fever, chills
3. Increasing dyspnea

SYMPTOMATIC URINARY TRACK INFECTION IN A PATIENT WITH A FOLEY IN PLACE >30 DAYS

Patient has at least 1 of these symptoms: fever (38°C or 101°F), urgency, frequency, dysuria, suprapubic tenderness *and* at least 1 of the following:

1. Positive dipstick of WBC or leukocytes
2. CVA tenderness on exam
3. Physician diagnosis of UTI
4. MD starts appropriate therapy for UTI

EYE INFECTION: CONJUNCTIVITIS

Patient has pain and redness of conjunctiva or eyelids or the presence of purulent exudate.

GASTROINTESTINAL INFECTION

Patient has at least 2 of these symptoms: nausea, vomiting, abdominal pain, diarrhea for >12 hours, fever > 38°C or 101°F *and,*

1. An enteric pathogen cultured from stool or rectal swab
2. C.difficile toxin detected in the lab
3. Household exposure or diagnosis of viral gastroenteritis

INCISIONAL SITE INFECTION

<30 days post-op report to hospital infection control staff the following signs and symptoms:

1. Pain, erythema, induration, poor healing, dehiscence, and purulent drainage (green or yellow in color)
2. Fever of >38°C or 101°F, chills

DECUBITUS ULCER INFECTION

Patient has at least 2 of these symptoms: redness, tenderness swelling of decub, wound edges, or enlargement in the size or depth of the ulcer, *and* 1 of the following:

1. Organisms cultured from fluid
2. Organisms cultured from blood
3. Presence of purulent exudate not previously present
4. New onset distinct, foul odor

PRIMARY BLOODSTREAM INFECTION

1. Patient has a recognized pathogen cultured from one or more blood cultures, and
2. Organism cultures from blood is NOT related to infection at another site.

OR

1. Patient has at least 1 of these symptoms: fever >38°C or 101°F, chills, hypertension and,
2. Common skin contaminant (Diptheroids, Staphylococci) is cultured from >2 blood cultures drawn on separate occasions or
3. Common skin contaminant is cultured from at least 1 blood culture from a patient with venous access; there is evidence of local site infection, and the MD institutes antimicrobial therapy.

VASCULAR ACCESS SITE INFECTION

1. Redness, warmth, tenderness, induration at the site
2. Purulent drainage at the site (green or yellow)
3. Fever of >38°C or 101°F

Figure 76-1 Infection Screening Report (continued).

CONFIRMED HOME CARE-ACQUIRED INFECTION REPORT

Confirmed Site of Infection:	*Culture Results (if available):*
☐ Catheter-associated UTI ☐ Bloodstream infection: 　☐ IV catheter-related bloodstream infection 　☐ IV infusate-related bloodstream infection 　☐ Secondary to other infection ☐ IV catheter-related infection 　☐ Exit site infection　☐ IV pocket infection ☐ Skin or soft tissue infection 　☐ Decubitus　　☐ Other ☐ Surgical site infection ☐ Wound drain or G-tube site infection ☐ Pneumonia ☐ Peritonitis ☐ Gastrointestinal infection	☐ Attach a copy of culture results 　OR complete as follows: Date obtained: _____ Site of culture: ☐ Urine ☐ Blood ☐ Wound drainage ☐ Sputum ☐ Other Organism(s) isolated: _____ _____ Multidrug-resistant ☐ Yes　☐ No If yes, describe: _____

UTI
☐ Indwelling foley　　　　　Date of original insertion: _____　Date of last insertion: _____
☐ Indwelling suprapubic catheter　Date of original insertion: _____　Date of last insertion: _____

IV-Related infection
☐ Central Venous Access Device　　Date of insertion: _____
　☐ Nontunneled CVC—Number of lumens: _____　☐ Hickman/Broviac—Number of lumens: _____
　☐ Implanted port—Number of lumens: _____
　　☐ Single lumen　☐ Double lumen　☐ Triple lumen
　☐ PICC—Number of lumens: _____
　☐ Other
☐ Peripheral Venous Access Device: Type: _____　Date of insertion: _____
　☐ Shortline　☐ Midline

Pneumonia
☐ Post-operative
☐ Immobility (non-post-op) including stroke. Cause of immobility: _____
☐ Ventilator dependent　☐ Tracheostomy tube　☐ Enteral feeding
☐ Respiratory Therapy (e.g., oxygen, nebulizer)　Type: _____

Surgical site infection
☐ Type of surgical procedure _____　☐ Date of surgical procedure _____

G-Tube site infection
☐ Date of g-tube insertion

Gastrointestinal infection
☐ Enteral feeding　Feedings prepared by: _____　Feedings provided by: _____

Peritonitis
☐ CAPD　　☐ Other _____

Eye infection
☐ Lacrimal inflammation　☐ Bacterial conjunctivitis　☐ Viral conjunctivitis

Previous hospital or long-term care admission (date of discharge) _____
Other risk factors: _____

To be completed by infection control practitioner
Screening Results: (Check one): ☐ Home care-acquired infection ☐ Nosocomial infection ☐ Community-acquired infection
Infection reported to, as applicable:
☐ Physician (Name and address): _____
☐ Hospital (Name and address:) _____
☐ Pharmacist (Name and date): _____
☐ Department of Health (Name and date): _____
Reviewed by: (Name and date) _____
Recorded for surveillance period of FY _____ Quarter _____

Figure 76-1　Infection Screening Report (continued). Reprinted with permission of Northwestern Memorial Home Health Care.

infections and, often times, resistant organisms. A policy to be considered is one for patients with a diagnosis of vancomycin-resistant enterococcus (VRE). Home care agencies may want to implement a policy of using disposable stethoscopes and patient-specific sphygmomanometers to prevent patient-to-patient transmission. The development of policies and procedures that describe proper clinical practice for certain devices, patient diagnoses, and surgical procedures is an essential component to any facility's infection control program.[16] Agencies will also need to consider their cost constraints and specific needs of their patient population and staff when developing policies and procedures related to infection control.

Policies need to be established regarding baseline and ongoing health assessments of direct caregivers. One option home care agencies may want to consider is the establishment of a protocol that directs employees to have a baseline physical exam upon hire. The exam should include a two-step Mantoux tuberculosis testing and an offer to receive the hepatitis B vaccine. In addition, flu vaccinations should be offered to all employees yearly. Professional caregivers must also comply with annual tuberculosis testing.

The fundamentals of the policies and procedures related to infection control should be reviewed during orientation of the home care nurse. The orientation should include a review of clinical practices and a demonstration of specific skills related to infection control. In addition, direct caregivers need to complete an annual skills competency lab. Competency assessments should be tailored to an agency's scope of care and services.[18] Several areas of the skills competency lab should address policies related to infection control practices. Staff should be required to demonstrate proper sterile technique within the laboratory setting. Mandatory inservice sessions on infection control and Occupational Safety and Health Administration (OSHA) testing should be conducted yearly to ensure continued staff competency.

Data collection and analysis

A measurement system used for infection reporting should be one that is common to the home health care industry. Commonly used measurement systems allow for benchmarking between agencies. One frequently utilized calculation for rates of infection is the number of infections per 1000 patient days. This final number can then be plotted on a graph in order to visualize and track the rate of infection in an agency over a period of time.

Infection control surveillance programs are critical to identifying areas in need of improvement. An infection control surveillance program is also a recommendation of the JCAHO. Infection monitoring and its results are crucial to determining clinical practice in the home setting. For example, the results of a central line infection study can lead to implementation of new policies regarding the frequency of sterile dressing changes in the home setting.

High-Technology Care and Infusion Therapy

Over the past several years, payers have looked for more cost-effective means to provide high technology care to their customers. Care delivery in the home setting has been found to be an acceptable alternative to hospitalization in many cases. As part of a development plan, home care agencies may need to consider the delivery of high-technology home care services to meet the increasingly complex needs of home care patients. High-technology care is now becoming routine, as new and more sophisticated therapies are able to be provided in the home.[19] To meet the needs of the community and the needs of the payers, while trying to remain viable in a rapidly changing home care environment, home care agencies need to provide more highly skilled care.

Agencies should first determine what types of patients qualify for their high-technology programs. This may include patients receiving any infusion therapy, i.e., antibiotics, total parenteral nutrition, chemotherapy, or intravenous pain management; patients receiving any type of respiratory therapy; patients with complex disease management, i.e., outpatient bone marrow transplant or solid organ transplant care; or patients receiving transfusion of any blood products. Demand for these services by patients, the medical community, and payors, will force agencies to investigate providing these services in the home and/or clinic setting.

To deliver quality home care, agencies first need to develop a set of competencies to test the nursing staff. One way to test the competency of staff is through self-evaluation upon hire and then through annual demonstration in a laboratory setting. Staff should also have a preceptor in the field during orientation so that return demonstration for each identified skill can be monitored and documented. Managers should also make visits at least annually with their staff to assess competency and to check skill performance of certain procedures.

Establishing patient acceptance criteria

Not all patients are appropriate for the administration of high-technology home care services. An assessment should be made by home care personnel for eligibility based on direct assessment and on input from referral sources and from patients and family members. Eligibility will then be determined based on clinical, financial, and social criteria.

The first step in admitting a patient for high-technology care will be to gather basic demographic, payer, and clinical data. A home health care agency can determine immediately if a patient resides in its geographical service territory. The specific type of care will need to be identified to ensure that it is offered by the agency and that policies and procedures specific to the therapy are in place.

Payment method will need to be determined and insurance benefits will need to be verified for both government and commercial payers. Once insurance benefits are verified, regulations need to be checked to ensure that the ordered therapy is a covered, billable item. Commercial and managed care payers may require precertification of the plan of care prior to initiating therapy. Negotiations for pricing on specific medications and supplies may need to occur with commercial payers and managed care organizations.

Some minimal discussion should take place with regard to the patient's social situation prior to the start of care. A more in-depth assessment will occur during the admission visit to home care but some basic questions should be posed prior to a start of care. Home health care employees will need to ensure the patient has access to a working telephone, has electricity and running water and a working refrigerator on the premises. Electricity may be required for the use of some infusion pumps and a refrigerator may be used to keep medications stored at the proper temperature.

Methods of delivery

When considering any type of infusion in the home, an assessment of the appropriate delivery mode and infusion device needs to occur. The length and type of therapy are the most critical elements to be evaluated when recommending the type of intravenous line to be used. Types of venous access devices used in the home setting range from peripherally to centrally inserted lines. In addition, the duration of device placement ranges from short-term to permanent usage. Total parenteral nutrition (TPN) and vesicant chemotherapies always require a centrally placed venous access line for administration. Short-term therapy or those treatments under two weeks in length may only require the use of a peripheral intravenous line (PIV). Both central lines and PIVs need to be changed according to the policy of the agency. Guidelines for venous access device care have been established by the Intravenous Nursing Society and can be adapted for agency use. See Table 76-2.

The care of oncology patients in the home may require several different high-technology services. At any point in a patient's episode of home care, they may receive any one or a combination of the following: chemotherapy administration, total parenteral nutrition, blood product transfusions, anti-infective therapy, and/or pain management. There are different considerations that need to be evaluated in the implementation of any of the above therapies.

Chemotherapy administration

Agencies commonly administer some chemotherapy agents in the home. It is important that the agency be fully aware of any related safety issues and develop policies and procedures to specifically address them. Staff must also be competent in chemotherapy administration.

Vesicant administration.   In order to aid in the prevention of an extravasation, agencies should develop agency specific standards of practice related to chemo-

therapy, and in particular vesicant administration. Standards of practice reflect competency or the expected nursing performance.[20] For example, an accepted practice for administering a vesicant may be the required use of a central venous catheter.[21]

In developing a standard of practice for managing extravasations, agencies must consider the many risk factors associated with a potential for extravasation. The skill of the nurse administering the vesicant is one potential risk factor. The nurse should be educated and then observed for clinical skill competency at least annually. Knowledge of central venous access devices (VADs) and chemotherapy administration must be demonstrated before the nurse gives a vesicant agent in the home setting. Specific components of the chemotherapy administration procedure, such as securing the needle into a port, taping connections into other central lines, and taping all tubing connections, should be clearly outlined in a written procedure.

Another way to reduce the risk of extravasation is to frequently check the site for a blood return. Although the frequency of performing blood return checks in the home setting is not outlined in the Oncology Nursing Society or Intravenous Nursing Society standards, agencies may want to establish a protocol wherein a blood return is verified twice daily for a continuous infusion of a vesicant drug.[22] Administration via a centrally placed intravenous line is the established practice for bolus injection of a vesicant. In the absence of a blood return in a central line, vesicant agents should not be administered until the potency of the line can be evaluated by radiography or until positive blood return is restored. Health care today challenges nursing agencies to develop innovative and safe procedures for the administration of complex chemotherapy regimens in the home.

Nonvesicant administration.   Nonvesicant chemotherapeutic agents may be administered via a well-established peripheral intravenous line. However, for any continuous infusion of chemotherapy, the preferred administration route is through a centrally placed VAD, which helps ensure a greater reliability of patency and a positive blood return.[22] If a nurse is present during a complete chemotherapy infusion, there is no need for an infusion pump. If the patient's chemotherapy protocol requires any type of continuous infusion, an infusion device should be used to control both the rate and amount of the infusion. There are many types of ambulatory, pole-mounted, and elastomeric pumps for agencies to consider for use. The length of therapy, the patient's payer source, the patient's mobility, and the volume of medication are all issues to be considered when choosing an appropriate infusion pump.

Safety considerations.   In addition to the safety issues specific to the administration of vesicants, there are general safety issues related to handling and disposing of chemotherapeutic agents in the home. As part of a policy addressing biohazardous materials, agencies should out-

Table 76-2 Practice Guidelines for Intravenous Access Devices

Peripheral Lines	Sterile Dressing Change	Saline Flush	Heparin Flush	Flush Frequency
Peripheral IV (PIV) • change site every 72 hours	72 hours	1–3 cc	1–3 cc (100 U/mL)	With use and every day
Midline • change every 6–8 weeks or as needed	Every week	3 cc	3 cc (100 U/mL)	With use and every day
Central Lines*				
Port-a-cath (PAC)	Every week and huber needle when accessed	5 cc	5 cc (100 U/mL)	With use and every month
Passport	Every week and huber needle when accessed	5 cc	5 cc (100 U/mL)	With use and every month
PICC	Every week	3 cc	3 cc (100 U/mL)	With use and every day
IJ	Every week	3 cc	3 cc (100 U/mL)	With use and every day
Groshong	Every week	5 cc	N/A	With use and every day
Hickman	Every week	3 cc	3 cc (100 U/mL)	With use and every day
Hohn	Every week	3 cc	3 cc (100 U/mL)	With use and every day
Vascath	Every week	10 cc	1.5 cc (5000 U/mL)	With use and every 72 hours

*All of the centrally placed devices can remain in place until the end of therapy or until complications arise.

line specific guidelines for handling chemotherapy. For instance, personnel should always wear chemotherapy gloves or double-glove with latex gloves when handling or administering chemotherapy. Nurses should also teach patients and family members to utilize the same safety practices if there is a leak or spill of chemotherapy, in which case the agency should be contacted immediately.

A chemotherapy spill kit should be on hand for immediate use if a chemotherapy spill occurs in the patient's home. The kit contains protective equipment to be used by the individual cleaning up the chemotherapy spill. Patients and family members should be instructed that any materials that come in contact with the chemotherapeutic agent should be disposed of in the chemotherapy biohazard container.

Agencies also need to develop policies and procedures related to the disposal of infusion equipment used to administer the chemotherapy. Any syringe, tubing, or bag utilized for the chemotherapy administration in the home should be disposed of in a puncture-resistant chemotherapy container. The container should then be sealed and disposed of by a licensed biohazardous waste disposal agent. If the container is returned to the infusion provider prior to disposal, the container should be returned to the delivery area of the building and held in the designated "dirty" area of the warehouse until pick-up of the container is arranged. Although local laws governing biohazardous waste disposal may differ, it is recommended that a licensed biohazardous waste hauler be utilized. The practice of using a waste hauler reduces potential risk to the community and the agency.

Patient and caregiver responsibility

Today's home infusion market forces agencies to re-evaluate infusion policies in all specialty areas to remain on the cutting edge of clinical practice. Agencies should consider developing a policy governing first-time dose administration of chemotherapy in the home. Traditionally, patients have received their first infusion of a chemotherapy regimen in a clinic, office, or the hospital.

There are additional responsibilities for a patient's caregiver when administering a first-time chemotherapy regimen in the home. If it is determined that a patient meets the agency's criterion for first-dose eligibility, the caregiver's responsibility must be determined and confirmed. If the chemotherapy is being given to a drug-naive patient, a caregiver *must* be available in the home during the infusion and for eight hours after the completion of the infusion. The caregiver needs to be able to access paramedics in the event of an emergency during the infusion. Upon completion of the chemotherapy infusion, the caregiver should observe for any potentially emergent side effects and be prepared to contact the appropriate medical personnel.

Total parenteral nutrition

Total parenteral nutrition has been administered safely in the home setting for many years. If TPN is indicated for a patient in the home, several considerations need to be considered. First, TPN must be administered via a central VAD due to the hyperosmolarity of the solution. Second, TPN should be administered with an infusion pump that features a dose-programming or ramping mode. Frequently, TPN is ordered to be given at an initial rate and then the rate is increased one or two hours after initiating the infusion. Some protocols include decreasing the TPN infusion rate during the last few hours of a treatment cycle.

In developing a teaching plan for the patient and family, the goal of the home care nurse should be to foster the independence of the patient or caregiver in TPN administration. The nurse should also establish a clearly defined emergency plan for the patient and family in the event of a pump failure or adverse clinical reaction. Patients should always be assured of having access to home care agency personnel 24 hours a day. But patients and families should also be taught to perform some basic troubleshooting techniques for the infusion pump that may be used prior to contacting health care personnel for assistance. This knowledge will help the family be more secure and independent during the TPN therapy.

Blood product transfusion

Many oncology patients require blood transfusions as a result of their disease process and/or as a result of bone marrow suppression secondary to chemotherapy. Some third-party payers provide coverage for patients to receive transfusion of blood products in the home, which avoids additional hospitalizations for a patient population that may be immunocompromised and at risk for developing a nosocomial infection.

The home care agency should establish criteria such as the following for accepting a patient for a blood transfusion in the home:

- An allergy history should be evaluated and a number or type of allergies should be established that would exclude a patient from home blood transfusions.

- There should be a second adult capable of contacting the emergency medical system via a working telephone in the home.

- Informed consent should be obtained prior to initiating the transfusion.

- There should be an anaphylactic kit containing appropriate supplies necessary in case of an adverse reaction (IV tubing, a bag of normal saline, IV diphenhydramine, IV hydrocortisone, and epinephrine).

The nurse should determine the physician's availability prior to a transfusion to obtain orders in the event of a reaction.[23]

Safety considerations. There are several safety considerations unique to transfusing blood products in the home. Coordination between the blood supplier, the transporter, and the nurse is crucial to delivering and administering a safe blood product transfusion in the home. Factors the agency must consider when ordering blood products include timely delivery to ensure transfu-

sion prior to product expiration, temperature control of the blood product, and compliance by delivery personnel with regulatory guidelines.

It is important for the individual who is coordinating the transfusion to ensure the appropriate type and cross match. It is also imperative that the coordinator and the nurse administering the transfusion check the blood product for the expiration date and time.

In addition, proper temperature of the blood product must be maintained prior to administration. This includes ensuring that the temperature is maintained both during transport as well as prior to the nurse's arrival in the home. Special temperature-controlled containers should be supplied. Generally, packed red blood cells are kept cool and platelets are maintained at room temperature. The agency's policy related to temperature control of blood products should be consistent with the recommendations of the agency's blood supplier.

The home care agency must ensure that delivery personnel are trained according to regulatory guidelines for transport and handling of blood products. The guidelines specify there must be a designated area in the transport vehicle where extreme temperature changes are avoided. Blood products should also be properly labeled and transported in a rigid container. All transfusion supplies should be disposed of in a puncture-resistant sharps container. The container should then be disposed of by a licensed biohazardous waste hauler.

Intravenous anti-infective therapy

Oncology patients frequently require intravenous anti-infective therapy. These medications may be administered to treat an existing infection or as prophylaxis to protect an immunocompromised patient. An alert, oriented patient or caregiver is essential to successful completion of a course of home anti-infective therapy.[24] Because of insurance or managed care benefit restrictions, patients and caregivers may have to learn the administration of these IV medications in as little as two or three home visits. Patients and caregivers should be instructed to check the medication labels for accuracy, use aseptic technique, and be aware of side effects specific to the medications. The patient or caregiver should also alert the health care provider when side effects occur.

As with other home therapies, a puncture-proof receptacle should be used for disposal of used needles. When the sharps container is full, the lid should be sealed and the container removed from the home by the home care agency to be disposed of by a biohazardous waste hauler.

The duration of anti-infective therapy is a significant factor to consider in the selection of an appropriate IV device. For therapies of less than seven days, a peripheral IV is sufficient unless poor venous access dictates otherwise. Anti-infective therapy lasting more than seven days may require the placement of a midline or a central VAD. All types of VADs are appropriate for anti-infective therapy. However, the insertion of implanted or tunneled devices may not be necessary for short-term therapy.

Gravity infusion of anti-infective agents is appropriate for dosing regimens of up to three times a day. Using programmable ambulatory infusion pumps for intermittent administration of four to six doses a day provides accurate and easy medication administration. These infusion pumps require a daily change of a cassette or bag. Programmable pumps eliminate noncompliance by missed doses. Some antibiotics can be administered by the IV push route. IV push administration greatly reduces infusion time and can lead to greater patient satisfaction.[25]

Pain control

The methodologies used to combat cancer pain are similar across the various health care settings. However, the home care nurse needs to use superior assessment skills to determine how well pain is controlled. Unlike the hospital, which can call upon professional caregivers around the clock, the home care nurse must rely on the patient or caregiver's report of pain control often over an extended period of time.

Patients with cancer can experience pain because of disease progression or due to side effects of cancer treatment. Intravenous pain control measures should be considered as an option when the dose required to relieve the patient's pain cannot be conveniently administered by another route. The IV route should be considered for long-term pain management in the home.

Short-term IV pain therapy in the home is usually administered through a peripheral intravenous line. If the IV pain control therapy will be longer term, it is best to place a central venous catheter for ease of administration. Most pain control agents can be given safely and effectively in the home. See Table 76-3.

Infusion pumps can be programmed to deliver a continuous base rate of a narcotic. A bolus infusion option is also available with these pumps. Patients are then able to self-administer an additional dose of medication during a period of heightened pain. If the pain management regimen prescribed allows for periodic supplemental bolus doses of agent, then the volume of cassettes or IV bags should be enough to cover the potential bolus use.

Pain medications can also be administered via devices implanted directly into the epidural space. Patients may experience decreased systemic side effects with intraspinal drug administration.[26] The epidural route for pain

medication is a viable, safe option for fast-acting relief for patients who have minimal response to medication delivered by other routes, who have uncontrollable side effects, or who have continuing intolerable pain despite increased doses.

Outpatient bone marrow transplant programs

Over the past decade, there has been an increased focus on the transmission of nosocomial infections to patients with compromised immune systems. As an unavoidable part of a bone marrow transplant protocol, the patient's immune system is severely compromised. To prevent secondary infections, portions of the care of the bone marrow transplant patient has moved to the outpatient setting. Immediately following transplantation, the patient can be cared for in hospital-affiliated apartments or hotels. This change in practice has created an expanded role for the home care nurse.

The home care nurse typically provides the posttransplant care in the affiliated hotels or apartments. Protocols may include twice-daily nursing visits for patient and caregiver teaching, obtaining laboratory specimens, IV electrolyte replacement, caring for central lines and pheresis catheters, transfusing blood products or IV anti-infectives for neutropenia, and administering growth factors and nutritional supplementation.

Infusion therapy in the home has become a frequently used alternative for oncology and bone marrow transplantation patients. Agencies need to continue to evaluate clinical programs and devise plans to provide cutting edge, cost-effective, high-technology services in the home.

Quality Improvement in Home Care

Quality improvement in home care plays an increasingly important role as home care visit numbers and expenditures for home care services continue to grow. Payers are more interested in the quality of care and in specific outcomes of care relative to the cost of that care. As patients participate more in their own care, they too are more interested in care outcomes, as are accrediting bodies such as the JCAHO and the Community Health Accreditation Program (CHAP) of the National League for Nursing. Finally, regulatory bodies such as state and federal government certification agencies have also become more focused on outcomes of care. This increased emphasis on quality outcomes of care is due to the increasingly competitive environment in the home care industry. An agency's quality results are a means to separate itself from others in the marketplace.[27]

Quality Outcome Indicators

The Center for Health Services and Policy Research at the University of Colorado Health Services Center conducted

Table 76-3 Intravenous Pain Control Agents Commonly Used in the Home

Agent	Mechanism of Action
Morphine	Well tolerated, fast-acting, short half-life
Hydromorphone	Fast-acting, longer half-life
Meperidine	Fast-acting, short half-life, should only be used in short-term pain management
Fentanyl	Fast-acting, may be given via epidural route

research that led to the development of a measurement tool for assessing home care. This study was conducted over a ten-year period and was funded by the Health Care Financing Administration (HCFA) and the Robert Wood Johnson Foundation. The result of the study was a system to measure outcome-based quality improvement (OBQI) in home care. Developed primarily for Medicare beneficiaries, this measurement system resulted in indicators that pertain to all adult patients.[27] The purpose of this research was to develop valid and reliable measures of patient outcomes that could be quantified and used to compare between home health agencies and specific types of patients.[27]

OASIS

The set of data items used in the OBQI system is now called the Outcome and Assessment Information Set (OASIS). The OASIS provides a foundation for several types of performance-based measures that can be used in reports that summarize outcomes, case mix, and resource consumption in home care. This data will greatly benefit individual home care agencies in their business-planning processes.[27]

Effective February 24, 1999, the use of OASIS became a requirement of the conditions of participation for home care agencies. Every Medicare certified home care agency must now collect the entire OASIS data set on each patient. This requirement does not, however, apply to patients under age 18 or obstetric patients. The requirement stipulates that the nurse must perform an initial assessment visit based on the physician's orders to determine the immediate care and support needs of the patient either within 48 hours of referral, within 48 hours after the patient's return home, or on a physician-specified start of care date. The regulation further specifies that the comprehensive assessment must include information on the patient's progress toward clinical outcomes and must be updated and revised as frequently as the patient requires, but no less frequently than every 62 days from the start of care date, when the patient's plan of care is revised for physician review, within 48 hours of the patient's return home from the hospital, and when the patient is discharged.[28] OASIS data are computerized, edited, coded, and transmitted to the state agency that will forward it on to HCFA.

The OASIS data will provide agencies with at least annual outcome results for a number of clinical outcomes: physiologic, cognitive, functional, and mental health. In addition, utilization outcomes such as hospitalization, emergent care, and discharge to the community will be reported. The case mix report provided in the OASIS data will help in the allocation or redeployment of agency staff. The case mix data will also describe patient characteristics, diseases, and disabilities of patients admitted to the agency over the past 12 months. This makes it possible for the agency to compare itself with national data and to assess its own performance during the previous year[27] (Table 76-4).

Finally, the agency will receive a report that documents negative outcomes or events for its patients. For example, the agency will be able to determine how many patients were admitted to the hospital for emergent care due to a fall in the home. This data gives the agency's quality improvement committee an opportunity to examine these patients' clinical records to determine if the untoward event may have been prevented with appropriate interventions. Over time, progressive agencies will learn to use the OASIS data for outcomes management, process improvement, and certain types of resource management.

ORYX

The JCAHO has also introduced its own outcome measurement system referred to as ORYX. All agencies accredited by JCAHO will collect outcome-related data and through an approved measurement system vendor, will report outcome findings to JCAHO on a quarterly basis. The agency is allowed to choose the outcomes they wish to measure, but regulations specify the percentage of patients to which the outcomes should pertain. These percentages and the number of measures chosen will increase each year.[27] It is clear that the outcome measurement movement is strong and growing in the home care industry. As care provided in the home continues to expand, these programs will go far in setting and maintaining standards of care across the industry. Moreover, the patient who is receiving care in the home can be assured that the care provided from an agency meets both local and national standards.

Quality Improvement Framework

The agency will benefit by developing a structured method to facilitate the process of quality improvement. This is generally accomplished through the establishment of a quality improvement committee to identify issues in care or service that can be improved. Since home care is only one segment of the overall patient experience, it is best that quality improvement initiatives be developed in collaboration with the hospital and the physician's office.

Once quality improvement initiatives are identified, leaders in the organization should establish a process improvement team to study the problem and recommend a process for improvement. Since most issues in home care involve more than one discipline or profession, most process improvement teams are cross-functional. As just mentioned, depending on the nature of the question to be addressed, it may be appropriate for a representative from the hospital or the physician's office to be a member of the team.

An issue that is commonly considered by an agency's process improvement team is management of cancer pain. If the home care agency identifies that patients are frequently admitted to the hospital for pain management

Table 76-4 Sample Performance Measurement Requirements for OASIS

Measure	Method of Collection	Outcome
Percent of patients admitted to an acute care hospital	OASIS data collection tool	Reason for rehospitalization researched and potential modification in plan of treatment made, resulting in decreased rehospitalizations
Percent of patients frequency of pain stabilized	OASIS data collection tool	Pain controlled due to comprehensive, consistent assessment and timely initiation of medication changes

in their quality improvement study, further investigation into the reasons may be warranted. The following professionals would be represented on the process improvement team: the field nurse, the clinical manager, the home care liaison, a representative from the hospital inpatient unit, and a nurse from the physician's office. The sponsor of the team may be the clinical director of home care and the leader may be the clinical manager or the field nurse. The director of quality improvement would facilitate the team. The team could then begin by identifying the reasons for readmission to the hospital for pain management rather than by merely instituting more aggressive interventions in the home setting.

If the leaders of the home care agency define the system within which quality improvement will occur, and support and facilitate the sharing of learning in the organization, improvement will be accelerated. Tools and methods for improvement should be easily accessible and used in the course of daily work. If a structured framework for quality improvement is developed and supported, continual improvement in home care can be accomplished.[29]

Ethical Concerns

Although the types of ethical issues encountered in the home setting are generally not much different from those encountered in other health care settings, there are several issues that are unique to home care. The emergence of managed care, the increase in technological advances, and an increased emphasis on providers to contain health care costs have created new ethical challenges for the home care provider.

Ethical Decision Making

Rawls proposed five criteria for judging proposed ethical principles. These criteria can serve as a guide when identifying and analyzing any ethical issue or dilemma:

1. *Universality:* the same principle must hold for everyone.
2. *Generality:* reference must not be made to specific people or situations.
3. *Publicity:* the situation or issue must be known and recognized by all involved.

4. *Ordering:* conflicting claims must be ordered without resorting to force.
5. *Finality:* the issue may override the demands of law and custom.[30]

The home care agency should develop a structure within the organization that can help to resolve ethical dilemmas. For most agencies, this structure is an ethics committee that is charged with examining the nature of the ethical issue and developing an action plan to reach resolution. The home care nurse can bring the issue to his or her manager and if the issue cannot be resolved at that level, the matter is taken to the ethics committee. These issues are often very detailed and complex and are not easily resolved.

New drugs and technological advancements in patient care have presented new quality of life issues for many oncology patients. Each individual patient must consider the following issues: ability to function independently, living conditions, changes in lifestyle, relationships with family or significant other, and emotional support. For some, these quality of life issues must be reconsidered daily as the clinical condition changes.[31]

Compliance

Issues surrounding compliance often present an ethical dilemma for the home care provider. The premise of providing home care is to return the patient to independence if possible. When an ethical issue arises, the nurse must include not only the patient but the family or other caregivers in tactical problem solving. The nurse will need to identify the moral values held by each person involved in the plan of treatment. The situation should be assessed and a potential course of action determined based on a decision-making process that considers what is best for the patient based on the values of the persons involved and their ethical principles.

The patient or caregiver who either refuses to learn a particular treatment or does not comply with the prescribed treatment plan presents a unique challenge to the home care nurse. In the hospital environment patients may be continuously monitored, and for the most part nurses are able to ensure proper administration of a treatment plan. Conversely, in home care, the nurse can only control the situation for the short period of time during the visit. The remainder of the care provided during the day is dependent upon the patient and/or their caregiver.

One particularly difficult case involved the family caregiver of an elderly woman with basal cell carcinoma of the face. The woman was extremely debilitated and dependent upon her caregiver for a majority of her care. The patient had a gastrostomy tube placed and there was an order to administer feedings of a nutritional supplement three times a day. Instead of the nutritional supplement, the nurse discovered the caregiver was administering soup through the gastrostomy tube. Needless to say, the patient's nutritional status was compromised. Upon the nurse's reporting the clinical status of the patient, the patient was readmitted to the hospital for nutritional support. The home care nurse had stressed the importance of providing the proper supplement to the patient, so it was indeed extremely frustrating when the patient's caregiver did not comply with the treatment regimen and the patient needed to be rehospitalized.

It is often helpful to develop a "contract" with a patient who the nurse suspects may be noncompliant with the treatment plan. The contract will specifically identify the treatment plan and the consequences if the patient does not comply with the plan. Of course, the physician should be apprised of and support this approach. In most cases, the result of noncompliance will be termination of home care services. Although this is a very difficult course of action to take and one of last resort, patients and families must accept responsibility for administering the treatment plan appropriately. In addition, they need to understand the consequence for overt failure to do so.

The Role of the Nurse

As technological advances and new drug therapies prolong life and present challenges to patients about their quality of life and the course of treatment, nurses need to recognize the implications of their interventions and their care. They must be actively involved in health care decisions that affect their patient's care, ensuring that the patient understands the result of the choice he or she is making. The home care nurse also needs to be actively involved with the agency ethics committee to share ethical situations with other health care professionals in order to provide a learning experience. The ethics committee can also develop agency policies and guidelines that address ethical issues (e.g., do-not-resuscitate decisions, informed consent, determination of competency, withholding life-sustaining treatment).[32]

Conclusion

Cost-containment initiatives in the health care industry have forced many health systems to look at alternate sites for the delivery of oncology care. One of those alternate sites is the patient's home. As technology advances, more cancer therapies and follow-up care are appropriately delivered in the home setting. Improved communication tools and monitoring systems make the organization and delivery of home care services more feasible than in the past. Moreover, delivering care to the oncology patient in the home provides the professional caregiver with a unique opportunity to witness the patient in his or her surroundings. The professional caregiver also can observe interactions with others that may assist in the development of the plan of care. Through working with the oncology patient in his or her own home, the professional caregiver is able to establish a relationship with the patient unlike that in any other setting.

References

1. Linne EB: Home care and managed care: the future approaches, in Linne EB (ed): *Home Care and Managed Care: Strategies for the Future*, Chicago, American Hospital Publishing, 1995, pp 1–12
2. Linne E: Growth trends in hospital home care 1980–90. *Ambulatory Care Trendlines*. 1(3) Chicago, American Hospital Association, 1992
3. Dieckmann J: Home health administration: an overview, in Harris M (ed): *Handbook of Home Healthcare Administration* (ed 2). Gaithersburg, MD, Aspen, 1997, pp 3–13
4. Gorvich M: Thirty years of Medicare: impact on the covered population. *Healthcare Financing Rev* 18:201–210, 1996
5. Ellenbecker CH, Warren K: Nursing practice and patient care in a changing home healthcare environment. *Home Healthc Nurse* 16:531–539, 1998
6. Harris M: The impact of the balanced budget act of 1997 on home healthcare agencies and nurses. *Home Healthc Nurse*, 16:435–437, 1998
7. Kohler C: Reimbursement, in Harris M (ed): *Handbook of Home Healthcare Administration* (ed 2). Gaithersburg, MD, Aspen, 1997, pp 585–606
8. Webb P: Medicare conditions of participation, in Harris M (ed): *Handbook of Home Healthcare Administration* (ed 2). Gaithersburg, MD, Aspen, 1997, pp 25–57
9. Randall D: The role of the medicare fiscal intermediary and the regional home health intermediary, in Harris M (ed): *Handbook of Home Healthcare Administration* (ed 2). Gaithersburg, MD, Aspen, 1997, pp 836–850
10. Smith NM: Managed care, in Harris M (ed): *Handbook of Home Healthcare Administration* (ed 2). Gaithersburg, MD, Aspen, 1997, pp 531–542
11. Christiansen K: A paradigm shift for the home care provider, in Linne EB (ed): *Home Care and Managed Care: Strategies for the Future*. Chicago, American Hospital Publishing, 1995, pp 13–19
12. Sherwin A: Legal issues of concern to home care providers, in Harris M (ed): *Handbook of Home Healthcare Administration* (ed 2). Gaithersburg, MD, Aspen, 1997, pp 653–670
13. Erb J: Discharge planning, in Harris M (ed): *Handbook of Home Healthcare Administration* (ed 2). Gaithersburg, MD, Aspen, 1997, pp 427–444
14. McKeenan K: *Continuing Care: A Multidisciplinary Approach to Discharge Planning* (ed 3). St. Louis, Mosby, 1981

15. DellaMonica E: Home health care documentation and recordkeeping, in Harris M (ed): *Handbook of Home Healthcare Administration* (ed 2). Gaithersburg, MD, Aspen, 1997, pp 119–129

16. Bellen V: A model for a comprehensive infection control program in home healthcare. *J Healthc Qual* 18(3):7–10, 1996

17. Centers for Disease Control and Prevention: *Definitions, APIC Infection Control and Applied Epidemiology: Principles and Practice, Appendix A*, Atlanta, CDC, 1996

18. Clarke C, Banacki C, Golden M: Implementing a competency system in home care, in Harris M (ed): *Handbook of Home Healthcare Administration* (ed 2). Gaithersburg, MD, Aspen, 1997, pp 160–181

19. DiTrapano VC, Williams JJ: High technology home care services, in Harris M (ed): *Handbook of Home Healthcare Administration* (ed 2). Gaithersburg, MD, Aspen, 1997, pp 250–270

20. Miaskowski C, Rostad M: Implementing the ANA/ONS standards of oncology nursing practice. *J Nurs Qual Assur* 4(3): 15–23, 1990

21. American Nurses Association, Task Force on Nursing Practice Standards and Guidelines: Working Paper. *J Nurs Quality Assurance* 5(3):1–17, 1991

22. Camp-Sorrell D: Developing extravasation protocols and monitoring outcomes. *J Intraven Nurs* 21:232–239, 1998

23. Benson K, Popovsky MA, Hines D, et al: Nationwide survey of home transfusion practices. *Transfusion* 38(1):90–106, 1998

24. Hammond D: Home intravenous antibiotics. *J Intraven Nurs* 21:81–95, 1998

25. Weinstein SM: *Plumer's Principles and Practice of Intravenous Therapy* (ed 6). Philadelphia, Lippincott-Raven, 1997

26. Grossman SA, Staats PS: Current management of pain in patients with cancer. *Oncology* 8(3):93–115, 1994

27. Shaughnessy P, Crisler K: Outcome-based quality improvement in Harris M (ed): *Handbook of Home Healthcare Administration* (ed 2). Gaithersburg, MD, Aspen, 1997, pp 377–386

28. Federal Register, vol. 61, no. 15, Monday, January 25, 1999/ Rules and Regulations, pp 3765–3784

29. Batalden P, Stoltz P: A framework for the continual improvement of health care: building and applying professional and improvement knowledge to test changes in daily work. *J Joint Commission* 19:424–452, 1993

30. Rawls J: *A Theory of Justice.* Cambridge, MA, Harvard University Press, 1971

31. Fitzig C: Ethical issues, in Harris M (ed): *Handbook of Home Healthcare Administration* (ed 2). Gaithersburg, MD, Aspen, 1997, pp 671–682

32. Haddad AM: Ethical considerations in home care of the oncology patient. *Semin Oncol Nurs* 12:226–230, 1996

CHAPTER 77

Hospice and Palliative Care

Jeanne Marie Martinez, RN, MPH, CHPN
Steven Wagner, RN, BSN, CRNH

Introduction

The late 1990s have seen a virtual revolution in what has become known as "end-of-life" care. This term currently encompasses what was previously referred to as death and dying, terminal care, palliative care, and hospice care. The current trend is to apply the principles of palliative care, which became the foundation for hospice programs, to inpatient and other health care settings where terminally and chronically ill patients receive care. This chapter will give a brief history and definition of hospice and palliative care, describe the scope of services provided by hospice programs, and discuss other strategies needed for optimal care at the end of life.

Hospice care was conceived in the 1960s and further developed in the 1970s to meet a simple objective: to facilitate a comfortable and natural death. However, the concept of a natural death runs counter to American society's values of youth, health, and technology, including medical technology. Death is a taboo topic.[1] This is reflected in today's complex medical system, which emphasizes technological intervention and aggressive treatment to prevent death. Hospice care was developed around the principles of palliative care: care focused on symptom management goals rather than care that attempts to correct or cure disease.

Palliative care, which has been defined as "the active total care of patients whose disease is not responsive to curative treatment,"[2] is symptom management, usually at the end-of-life, that encompasses physical, emotional, and spiritual symptoms and their interrelated suffering.

Development of the Hospice Concept

Developers of the hospice concept recognized that allowing a "natural death" requires preparation of the patient and family, changes in the focus of medical care, and redesign or circumvention of some aspects of the existing health care system.[2] An analogy for the scope of the change can be made to birthing and medical care in American society. In the 1960s birthing was treated primarily as a medical problem. Change in the practice of obstetrics was instituted largely by consumer demand from the women's movement, which sought to view birth as a life process over which each woman should have control, and by the growing realization of the importance of family participation. In response to this demand, obstetric medical practice changed in the 1980s to focus more on prenatal preventive care and education.[3] Attempts to deinstitutionalize the process in the United States included creating birthing centers that are more homelike and that can facilitate family participation.

Consumer groups also influenced hospice care in America. Initially, hospice was identified as a "movement" or as an "alternative" to mainstream medical care. When hospices first began to appear as organized programs, they were commonly volunteer programs composed of lay volunteers, nurses, and clergy, organized perhaps from a church basement or around someone's dining room table. Today this model is all but extinct, except that hospices retain the use of lay volunteers as part of the core team of interdisciplinary hospice services. The ideas for the American hospice were adapted directly from the original model at St. Christopher's Hospice in England, developed by Dame Cicely Saunders in 1968.

The National Hospice Organization developed the following definition of hospice:

> Hospice care is specialized care for terminally ill people. Hospice care is a medically directed, interdisciplinary team-managed program of services that focuses on the patient/family as the unit of service. Hospice care is palliative rather than curative, with an emphasis on pain and symptom control, so that a person may live the last days of life fully, with dignity and comfort, at home or in a home-like setting.[4]

The 1983 federal guidelines under the Health Care Finance Administration (HCFA) defining the Hospice Medicare Benefit have become the standard of hospice care in the United States. These guidelines were developed by hospice program planners to ensure that care was comprehensive and holistic, and included financial incentives to encourage home hospice care as a viable alternative to costly hospitalization.

The Role of Nurses in the Development of Hospice

The word *hospice*, or *hospitia*, was used during the Crusades in the Middle Ages to designate a place of temporary shelter for travelers or sick pilgrims.[4] In the late nineteenth century, "hospice" was applied to the care of the dying by Sister Mary Aikenhead, a colleague of Florence Nightingale, who opened Our Lady's Hospice in Dublin,[3,4] the first facility dedicated to care of the terminally ill.

Although Dame Cicely Saunders is best known as the founder and medical director of St. Christopher's Hospice, she began her career as a nurse and went on to become a medical social worker prior to attending medical school. Dame Saunders developed many of the current concepts in palliative care, including oral opioid administration on a scheduled rather than on an as-needed basis.[3]

It was Dame Saunders's visit to Yale University in 1963 that precipitated the interest of Florence Wald, dean of the Yale School of Nursing, in the concept of hospice care. Wald subsequently resigned as dean to participate in the development of the first American hospice, Connecticut Hospice Inc. Connecticut Hospice began serving home care patients in 1974, and in 1979 opened an independent 44-bed inpatient facility, the first U.S. facility to be designed as a hospice.[4]

In 1984 the Joint Commission on Accreditation of Hospitals (JCAH) published its first standards manual for hospice programs.[5] In 1992 some of the original hospice standards were incorporated into the Joint Commission on Accreditation of Healthcare Organizations (JCAHO) standards that apply to all dying patients in hospitals.[6]

A major factor influencing the development of palliative care was the groundbreaking work in the 1960s of Elisabeth Kübler-Ross, a psychiatrist at the University of Chicago. Dr. Kübler-Ross demonstrated how health care professionals, due largely to their own ineffectual coping with the subject of death, isolated dying patients. She helped to demystify the dying process by devising the radical teaching technique of interviewing dying patients in front of a group of health care professionals.[1] This not only provided an opportunity to learn firsthand from patients themselves but also provided role modeling for professionals on how to talk to patients. More than anyone else, Elisabeth Kübler-Ross opened the debate on care of the dying not only for the public but for health care professionals as well.

Principles of Palliative Care

The overall goal of palliative care is to manage symptoms and optimize quality of life on the patient's terms. Palliative care begins with an identification of the life goals of the patient within the context of his or her beliefs, values, relationships, and environment. Then the treatment plan can be developed to facilitate the most appropriate patient care. The following are some guiding palliative care principles:

- Death is regarded as a natural process, to be neither hastened nor prolonged.

- The patient and family is the unit of care.

- Invasive medical procedures and diagnostic tests are minimized, unless they are likely to result in the alleviation of symptoms.

- Use of "heroic," life-prolonging treatment measures are not recommended, unless to improve or maintain quality of life.

- When managing pain with opioid analgesics, the correct dose is the dose that provides pain relief without unacceptable side effects.

- The patient is the "expert" on whether pain and symptoms have been adequately relieved.

- Fluids and feeding are not forced or artificially induced. Patients eat if they are hungry or for the social benefit of sharing food.

Palliative care involves a shift in the treatment goals to providing relief of suffering.[3] Relief of suffering goes beyond merely identifying and treating physical symptoms. The emotional and spiritual (existential) components of suffering and pain are also addressed. Our current health system still consists largely of fragmented, specialized care episodes for specific problems rather than a holistic approach to illness.[3]

The "Revolution" in End-of-Life Care

The interest in end-of-life care has grown exponentially in a number of areas. The Project on Death in America developed in 1994 by philanthropist George Soros has provided millions of dollars in grants to support a variety of projects on the subject of death.[7] Some of these have been community-oriented projects, but many have been palliative care initiatives. The SUPPORT Study of 1995 was a large multihospital study which concluded that care of the dying in hospitals still suffers from ineffective communication and overtreatment of patients, in spite of advance directives.[8] Although the goals of end-of-life care are similar, most of the current palliative care initiatives and studies are physician and inpatient focused, whereas hospice promotes care in the home.

Hospice Care

Hospice care is an organized approach to caring for those who are at the end of illness through death, including bereavement support to the family. Hospice care provides an expertise in nursing care, medical care, spiritual support, and counseling that is focused on emotional support, symptom management, and improving quality (rather than quantity) of life. Most hospice care is provided in the patient's home, including the care and support needed to facilitate a home death when possible.

Unique in its design under Medicare hospice regulations, hospice care crosses over the continuum between home and inpatient settings (see Table 77-1). While enrolled in a hospice program, inpatient admission is principally for management of acute pain or other symptoms that cannot be controlled easily in the home. Inpatient admission is also used for short-term respite care. Often a hospice patient returns home after symptoms have been alleviated and the patient is medically stable. According to Medicare guidelines, at least 80% of an individual hospice's *aggregate* patient days of care under the hospice

Table 77-1 Comparison of Home Care and Home Hospice Care Under Medicare

Home Care	Home Hospice Care
Patient must have skilled care needs to qualify	Physician certification of terminal illness needed to qualify
Care primarily provided by RN	Care provided by the interdisciplinary team
Care focused on rehabilitation or resolution of a specific disease process	Holistic approach to care encompassing physical, emotional, and spiritual needs
Patient must be homebound	Patient is not required to be homebound
Medicare coverage at 80% level with a 20% copayment	Medicare coverage at 100% level with no copayment

Table 77-2 NHO Guidelines for Determining Appropriateness of Hospice Certification for All Diagnoses

Terminal prognosis as determined by attending physician

Patient and family aware of prognosis

Treatment goals are primarily directed toward relief of symptoms, not cure

Patient has progression of disease, which can be documented by physician assessment, including laboratory data or other studies

Patient has had multiple ER visits or hospitalizations over last six months

Recent decline in functional status due to terminal illness

Symptoms of impaired nutrition indicated by unintended weight loss greater than 10% over prior six months, serum albumin less than 2.5 g/dL or combination of cholesterol below 156 mg/dL and HCT less than 41 mg/dL

Recent decline in functional status demonstrated by Karnofsky Performance status less than or equal to 50%, ECOG of 3 or 4, or dependence in 3 or more ADLs

Patient refuses further curative medical treatment

benefit must be provided at home. Likewise, a maximum of 20% of aggregate days of care can be provided in the inpatient setting. If the maximum aggregate inpatient ratio of 20% is exceeded, the hospice will be denied reimbursement for the excess inpatient days.

Hospital inpatient care for hospice patients may be "scattered," so that patients are admitted to any general medical or oncology unit. Some hospices have designed specific units for inpatient care of hospice patients. These units attempt to simulate a comfortable, homelike environment. Care is focused on symptom management and limitation of invasive or painful procedures. Visiting policies are less restrictive; for example, pets may be allowed to visit.

Patient Criteria

For a patient to qualify for the Medicare hospice benefit, he or she must be eligible for Medicare Part A. Two physicians must certify that the patient is terminally ill and has less than six months to live.[9] This latter criterion is controversial for a number of reasons. Professionals who work with the dying know that there currently is no formula to accurately predict time of death. It could therefore be detrimental for physicians or nurses to attempt to give predictions about time of death to patients and family members.[1]

It has proven to be even more difficult to predict prognosis in noncancer end-stage patients. This difficulty in prediction has prompted the development of more specific medical criteria to be required to admit noncancer patients into hospice care under the Medicare hospice benefit. At the urging of the HCFA, guidelines were devel-

oped in 1995 by a National Hospice Organization (NHO) physician task force and were revised in 1996.[9] There are general guidelines for admission (Table 77-2) and comprehensive criteria for eight categories of noncancer, end-stage illness including cardiac, pulmonary, and liver disease; dementia (Table 77-3); and HIV. These criteria are currently being studied to assess their accuracy.[10]

Another criterion under Medicare and most state hospice regulations is that the patient sign a consent form or election statement declaring that hospice care is their choice of treatment and that they have the right to elect out of hospice at any time. Similar to advance directives, this regulation is meant to ensure that the patient has been told the nature of the disease state and chooses a palliative approach over experimental (or no) treatment. Finally, for home hospice in particular, the patient should identify a primary caregiver, that is a friend or family member willing to assume day-to-day patient care and be available for treatment decisions should the patient be unable to do so.

A Unique Reimbursement Structure

Hospice care was a prototype for what is now commonly referred to as *managed care*. Consistent with the managed care and case management approach, the Medicare hospice benefit is a capitated per diem reimbursement structure. Per diem is a system of reimbursement that pays a flat daily rate for all services provided to a patient, rather than paying for individual services or items on the traditional fee-for-service basis. The advantages of the per diem system are that it allows the hospice program to provide an individualized comprehensive approach to assess needs and prevent problems. Additional team ser-

Table 77-3 NHO Guidelines for Dementia

Patient requires assistance as demonstrated by all the following characteristics:

- Inability to ambulate independently
- Unable to dress without assistance
- Unable to bathe properly
- Incontinent of urine and stool
- Unable to speak or communicate meaningfully, i.e., ability to speak is limited to six words or fewer per day

Patient had one or more of the following medical complications related to dementia during the past year:

- Aspiration pneumonia
- Upper urinary tract infection
- Septicemia
- Decubitus ulcers: stage 3–4
- Recurrent fever after treatment with antibiotics
- Inability or unwillingness to take food or fluids sufficient to sustain life

vices are also provided as the patient's condition changes. A case management approach is the most efficient and effective way to enable a patient to stay at home. Similarly, there is an annual per-patient reimbursement cap that is applied on an aggregate basis to all patients served by a particular hospice. For example, an individual hospice program can be reimbursed $16,000 within a year for one patient if this amount can be balanced out by another patient whose hospice reimbursement did not exceed $10,738 in the same year. The exact amount of reimbursement varies based upon geographic area of the country.

The per diem payment for the Medicare hospice benefit is reimbursed on four levels, as defined by the HCFA: (1) a routine rate, (2) a continuous rate for home care, (3) an inpatient rate for acute care, and (4) an inpatient rate for respite care.[4] For a patient to qualify for the Medicare hospice benefit, certification by two physicians of a prognosis of six months or less is required. Recertification of the patient's appropriateness for hospice care is determined by the medical director of the hospice. The first and second recertification periods are 90 days each, followed by an unlimited number of 60-day periods of care (see Table 77-4). Only hospital care, pharmacy, or home services contracted with the hospice program will receive reimbursement under the benefit. The patient has the option at any time to rescind the hospice benefit and return to regular Medicare Part A coverage.[9]

The Nurse's Role in Management of Care

Direct patient care and physical assessment skills are important in the hospice nurse's role. The nurse often provides basic nursing care, such as skin care, care of central venous lines, monitoring compliance with medication regimens, and indwelling catheter management. The nurse assesses the patient's response to care approaches to determine what changes need to be made, and always assesses the effectiveness of symptom management in the context of the patient's emotional and spiritual issues. The nurse provides education and support to patients and family members, and identifies other resources and services needed for care (see Table 77-5).[11-13]

The interdisciplinary team—roles of the non-nurse team members

The care needs of the patient and family are multifaceted and require the attention of an interdisciplinary team to address the physical, emotional, and spiritual suffering that often result from a terminal illness. Core members of the hospice team are a physician, nurse, social worker, and chaplain or counselor. In addition, hospice care includes trained volunteers available for a variety of services and companionship at home. The complexity of care often requires the participation of other disciplines such as nursing assistant, physical therapy, occupational therapy, speech therapy, bereavement counselor, and dietician.

Table 77-4 Selected Guidelines: Medicare Hospice Benefit

Patient Eligibility

Terminal prognosis determined by two physicians

Patient and family aware of prognosis

Treatment goals are primarily directed toward relief of symptoms, not cure

Patient has progression of disease as evidenced by impaired nutrition and/or recent functional decline

Patient refuses curative or experimental treatment

Levels of Care

Routine Home Care—intermittent home visits based on patient need

Continuous Care—8- to 24-hour nursing care in the home for periods of medical crisis

Respite Care—inpatient care for maximum of 5 days to relieve family from caregiving

General Inpatient Care—inpatient care for acute medical problems related to the terminal illness

Home Services Provided at 100%

Intermittent home visits by interdisciplinary team members

Durable Medical Equipment (DME) and supplies

Medications for symptom management

Physician and nurse on-call 24 hours per day

Bereavement care for family

Benefit Periods (dependent upon physician recertification)

1st period = 90 days

2nd period = 90 days

Thereafter, subsequent periods of 60 days each.

There is no maximum benefit

The physician assuming primary responsibility for the patient's medical care may be the patient's attending physician or a hospice physician. Hospice programs encourage the attending physician to remain involved in the patient's care whenever possible, as this relationship is often particularly important to the patient. The role of the physician is to maximize symptom management and promote quality of life.[14] For home hospice care, physicians write orders, approve the care plan, and certify terminal status of the illness. In addition, physicians may provide home visits and must participate in required interdisciplinary team meetings. The hospice physician or medical director is required to provide any of the above functions the attending physician is unable to do, such as attend regular patient team meetings. Ideally, the hospice physician has an expertise in end-of-life care, pain and symptom management, and excellent communication skills. The hospice physician often is called upon to assist patients and families to understand the benefits of palliative care versus the burden of treatment and to under-

Table 77-5 Selected Principles and Approaches for Symptom Management of Patients at the End of Life

Problem	Principles	Management Approaches
Pain	The correct dose is the dose that relieves the patient's pain without unacceptable side effects.	Explore patients and family perceptions of pain and usage of pain medication.
	Respiratory depression can be avoided by careful dose titration.	Instruct patient and family on positive effects of pain management, i.e., control of pain, improved mood, and activity.
	Pain is a natural antagonist to opioids. (Even patients with severe lung disease can tolerate large doses of narcotics if the dose is escalated gradually).	Reinforce that addiction is rare and unimportant in the care of the terminally ill.
	Clinicians have shown slow movement from step 2 to step 3 on the WHO analgesic ladder.	Assess/document patient's goal for pain management.
	According to WHO, morphine is the drug of choice for severe cancer pain. There is no ceiling to effective opioid dosage.	Placebos are never appropriate.
	If PO medications are not possible, opioids can be given by buccal, sublingual, rectal, or SQ routes without resorting to IV or IM administration.	IM/SQ injections—morphine 30 mg PO is as potent as 10 mg IM/SQ.
	Continuous SQ infusions can be initiated at home with the help of home health or hospice nurses.	Can avoid pain and expense of injections with PO or SQ morphine.
	If central line access is already established, IV infusion may be the route of choice and usually can be initiated at home.	Titrate dose as needed.
		Utilize noninvasive comfort measures as appropriate, e.g., applications of ice, heat, gentle massage, relaxation techniques.
		Evaluate effectiveness of analgesia at regular intervals. Teach the patient and family about the medications and alternative measures.
		Avoid:
		meperidine—very low oral potency, toxic metabolite accumulation
		pentazocine—no more potent than codeine, high incidences of hallucinations and agitation (30% in cancer patients)
		methadone—extremely long half-life (48–72 hr) and short duration of analgesia (6–8 hr), makes dose titration difficult in severely ill patients. May be the least costly long-acting agent.
Dyspnea	Defined as unpleasant awareness of increased need to ventilate.	Oral morphine in low doses 5–10 mg every 4 hr helps to decrease air hunger.
	Anxiety is often a component of dyspnea.	Help patient decrease anxiety through use of an anxiolytic, e.g., a benzodiazepine.
	Avoid high-dose bronchodilators.	Position patient for maximum comfort by elevating head of bed.
	Theophylline toxicity is common as patients approach death.	Advise patient in methods to modify environment or activity to decrease physical exertion.
	Adrenergic agonists (metaproterenol, etc.) may exacerbate anxiety more than they alleviate dyspnea.	Oxygen may be effective in addition to oral opioids.
Seizures	Patients with recent history of seizures should receive therapeutic doses of phenytoin phenobarbital, carbamazepine, or valproic acid.	Options: If patient cannot swallow phenytoin: midazolam—5 to 10 mg/day by SQ infusion phenobarbital—20–60 mg oral, sublingual BID carbmazepine—600 mg per rectum or SQ BID-TID valproic acid—250 mg QID per rectum fosphenytoin—IM or IV 75 mg is equivalent to 50 mg phenytoin sodium.
		Instruct caregiver on seizure precautions.
		Protect patient from injury in event of seizure.
		Remove or pad objects near head of body.
		Instruct patient and family regarding needs for regular dosing and side effects of seizure medication.

Table 77-5 Selected Principles and Approaches for Symptom Management of Patients at the End of Life (continued)

Problem	Principles	Management Approaches

Diarrhea	Rule out fecal impaction, bowel obstruction, laxative overuse, and other drug side effects.	Maintain hydration according to patient's comfort level and tolerance of fluids. Bland low-residue diet. Protect skin with barrier cream.
		   ioperamide HCL—2–4 mg QID PRN
		   diphenoxylate HCL, atropine sulfate—2.5-2 mg QID PRN
		   natural psyllium fiber—1–3 tsp BID

Constipation	Nearly all patients on opioids require a maintenance laxative regimen to prevent constipation. As the dose of opioid is increased, the dose of laxative must be increased. Patients who are not eating still may require laxatives as waste continues to be produced in the bowel in form of secretion, bacteria, and desquamation. Avoid: • bulk laxatives—difficult for anorexic patients to take, and cause impaction if fluid intake is inadequate, not effective unless a patient is active and eating. • frequent enemas—useful for severe cases of constipation, however, oral medications are better tolerated for prophylaxis.	"Ladder" of increasing potency of laxatives: a. standard senna concentrate and docusate sodium or casanthranol and docusate sodium—1–2 tabs at hs. b. standardized senna concentrate and docusate sodium or casanthranol and docusate sodium—2 tabs BID c. standardized senna concentrate and docusate sodium or casanthranol and docusate sodium—3–4 tabs BID d. Lactulose—15cc BID e. Lactulose—30cc BID f. Lactulose—30cc TID-QID or along with b or c above. If a patient has not had a bowel movement in 24 hr, increase the laxative dose to the next higher level. If a patient has not had a bowel movement in 3 days, check for impaction and consider one of the following treatments once or twice daily until results are obtained: a. Milk of magnesia 30 cc at bedtime b. 2 bisacodyl suppositories c. Lactulose or sorbitol 30 cc q 1 hr until results
Upper Airway Congestion	Assess patient for potential causes such as aspiration. Position for comfort—usually with patient on side with head of bed elevated at least 30 degrees. Assess patient for fluid overload. Patients at end stage of disease find dehydration to be an advantage as they have less pulmonary secretions and decreased likelihood of vomiting.[11]	Scopolamine patch—change every 72 hours. In severe congestion 2 or more patches may need to be applied.[11] Anticholinergic such as ipratopium bromide can be helpful especially with lung cancer to reduce respiratory secretions.

Terminal Delerium	Rule out reversible causes for delerium.
	
	Review medications for contributing side effects, toxicity and drug interactions. Assess for physiological cause such as metabolic imbalance, hypoxemia, dehydration, hypercalcemia, renal or hepatic dysfunction.
	
	Protect patient from self harm. Pad side rails. Remove dangerous objects from reach. Use chemical and physical restraints with caution.
	
	Promote soothing environment by minimizing noxious physical, auditory, and visual stimuli.
		Use touch to help patient feel less anxious.
		
		Hold their hand, give a gentle massage, try either a cool or warm cloth to the forehead or back of neck.
		
		Play soothing music, preferably the type of music that the family identified as a patient favorite.
		
		Medication to ease delerium or agitation:
		  Haloperidol—can be given at doses of 1–5 mg for mild agitation, 5–10 mg moderate to severe agitation[12] every 30 minutes to 1 hour until calm and then every 6 hours as needed.
		  Cogentin—2 mg every four hours as needed for extra pyramidal symptoms. May also alternate Haloperidol with Lorazepam 2 mg oral or sublingual.
		  Chlorpromazine—25 mg–50 mg oral or by suppository every 6 hours as needed. Avoid doses above 50 mg because of side effect of severe hypotension.[13]

stand the expected disease progression. The hospice physician also serves as a resource to the interdisciplinary team and the medical community at large.

The social worker assists the patient and family in dealing with emotional and social difficulties created by the impending illness. The social worker assesses patient and family previous coping strategies, previous losses or trauma, cultural and age-specific factors that may affect their ability to cope with the terminal illness. The social worker also assists in providing emotional support, negotiates family conflict, and assesses financial and community resources.[15] He or she can also assist the family in exploring funeral plans, facilitate family communication, and help patient and family understand the grieving processes.

Volunteers give freely of their time and talents to assist other members of the hospice team in providing the necessary services of the program and promoting quality of life for the hospice patient and family. The participation of volunteers is mandated under the Medicare hospice benefit guidelines. Volunteers come from all sectors of the community and often serve as a representative sample of the social and cultural diversity of the community the hospice serves. The services provided by volunteers can also be varied. A large part of their role can be to provide a supportive presence or companionship for patients and families or to assist with activities of daily living such as shopping, homemaking, or respite care. Volunteers with special expertise may serve as consultants in areas such as legal matters, massage therapy, counseling, and bereavement support.

The volunteers may be invaluable in providing administrative support by answering and triaging phone calls, assisting with filing, fund raising, or organizing the hospice library. The role of volunteers is enhanced by the special training they are provided by the hospices. This training helps to ensure that the volunteer is sensitive to the special needs of hospice patients and their families.

Occupational therapists (OTs) assess functions with which patients need assistance and identify the most important needs to maintain independence and quality of life. The OT assists the patient to achieve or maximize the highest level of function in order to perform necessary activities of daily living or activities that will enhance patient goals. Meeting self-care needs are basic to a person's sense of well being. A therapist can provide invaluable assistance in supporting a patient's level of functioning to allow for completion of essential tasks that are important for the patient to complete prior to death. This may include energy conservation techniques or adaptive devices to complete these tasks. Such activities may include creating a lasting remembrance for loved ones or returning one last time to the family summer home. The OT is specially trained in making adaptive equipment or functional splints to improve independence and/or prevent injury.

Physical therapists (PTs) assess the patient's level of function and establish the goal of maximizing strength and mobility. The PT can promote safety in ambulation and the use of assistive walking devices such as cane, walker, and crutches. The PT has a special role in educating the patient and family in therapeutic exercises, transfer techniques, and gait training.

The chaplain is a counselor who helps assess the patient and family for spiritual needs and facilitates their being met. The hospice chaplain can be a valuable support whether the patient and family have established religious affiliations. Many priests, rabbis, and other clergy do not have expertise in caring for the terminally ill. The hospice chaplain specializes in this population. Questions arising from guilt or doubt and patient and family searching for meaning and purpose can be the special focus of the chaplain. Crises in faith and striving to bring meaning to suffering and death can be identified, brought to the surface, and resolved.

The role of the chaplain is often that of a gentle listener helping the patient initiate a life review, ask for pardon, and give thanks for what has brought meaning and joy in one's life. Referral or liaison with community clergy to facilitate religious rituals and sacraments meaningful to the individual and family can also help the patient prepare for death. In addition to spiritual counseling, the chaplain is often involved with discussion of ethical questions or may be a source of counsel and support to the team during periods of stress or conflict.[15,16]

Spiritual Care

The spiritual dimension of care can be defined as the beliefs, values, and existential concerns of each individual. For many, religious beliefs provide the basis for life values. Religion encompasses dogmas, creeds, rituals, and celebrations on the part of those who choose to participate in the life and worship of a particular sect.[17] It is helpful for health care providers to have a working knowledge of the important beliefs of the major religions common to their patient population. However, religion may be only one aspect of a person's spirituality. The full scope of the individual's beliefs and values cannot be assumed to fit neatly within the teachings of a particular religious group.

Individual assessment of spiritual beliefs, concerns, and issues is vital in assisting a patient with care during a serious illness and at the end of life. Although it may be deeply repressed in some individuals, spirituality is an essential characteristic of all human beings, even those who have no formal religious affiliation.[17] The reader is referred to Chapter 71 for additional information.

There is no standard approach for a comprehensive spiritual assessment. Assessment tools commonly include questions about religious affiliation and membership in a local parish, temple, or synagogue. However, a thorough assessment must inquire further into individual beliefs, sources of strength and spiritual sustenance, spiritual or religious fears, important prayers and/or rituals surrounding the dying process, and sources of spiritual conflict among family members.

Spiritual interventions will vary depending upon the concerns identified and the patient's time and energy. The skilled nurse, counselor, or chaplain helps the patient examine beliefs about an afterlife, resolve issues in relationships, and examine issues of a crisis of faith. Spiritual care should always include bridging contact with any involved community clergy or congregation identified by the patient or family as important. Often spiritual care involves resolving conflicts about religion and other beliefs among family members. All team members need to respect and understand the patient and family value system. Staff and volunteers are *never* to impose personal beliefs on any patient or family member. Spiritual support requires continuous assessment and intervention as needs change throughout the patient's illness and as death approaches.[18]

Dying at Home

Hospice care is uniquely characterized by its commitment to facilitating a person's death at home. It is common for patients and families in American society to respond initially to the idea of death at home with fear and anxiety. Many adults in this country have never seen anyone die.[19] In a society where death has been regarded as a medical problem requiring technological support, hospitalization, and professional care, we have lost the concept of death as a natural life event.[3] Patients' overriding concerns about death at home often revolve around being a burden to their family.[1] Family caregivers are concerned about their emotional ability to cope with a home death, sufficient caretaking ability, and the potential effects on other family members, particularly when children are in the home.

For most families, the ability to provide care for a home death will require professionals to teach families about the death event itself, immediate signs of death, management of symptoms and suffering, and how to access professional help when needed. When given enough time to work with a patient and family, hospice care is ideally structured to provide this support, education, and preparation. One of the most satisfying experiences for hospice nurses is to provide a full spectrum of hospice care that begins with a family who expresses anxiety about caring for a patient at home and continues through the death event, where family members in bereavement cannot say enough about what a wonderful experience it was for them. In her book *Dying at Home*, Andrea Sankar relates her experience with the home death of her mother:

> Home death is a powerfully significant experience despite the strain, exhaustion, and conflict that sometimes accompanies it. Its power lies in the fact that in the face of certain death, the caregiver can give the person life, that is, the continuation of life as a social being.[19]

Advantages of home death

The approach of death evokes feelings of loss in a dying person.[20] Loss of control may be the most overwhelming and distressing feeling, which is often further intensified by hospitalization. Terminal care and death at home can afford the patient and family control over their environment, as well as the comfort of being in the midst of familiar surroundings. The patient at home maintains the opportunity to interact with neighbors, children, and pets. If children are living in the same home as the dying person, there is often concern that this experience will be detrimental to them. However, the opposite effect is often true. Rather than being protected

from the illness and death, children can benefit from being involved in very concrete ways to better understand the dying process and work through their own grief.[19]

Another major loss for the patient is diminishment of their role as a contributing social being. Individuals have several roles that make up their identity. Loss of one's role in the workplace, for example, is a major adaptation for a chronically or terminally ill person. However, being cared for at home can afford the opportunity for an alert patient to maintain his or her family role. When possible, this person will continue to be included in family events and decision making.[19]

A final and obvious advantage of home death is that unwanted medical intervention is much less likely to occur than in a hospital or nursing home setting. The greatest potential risk for a home patient to receive unwanted medical intervention arises if the emergency medical system (EMS) is called, since this call can result in unplanned and unwanted resuscitation and, ultimately, ventilator care.

Disadvantages of home death

Caregivers, particularly those lacking social outlets or family support, may find the physical and emotional task of home care and home death too difficult. Home death must be prepared for within the context of a realistic plan of care.

Although most anticipated deaths occur quietly without physical distress, the occasional patient may have symptoms too difficult to manage at home, such as uncontrolled hemorrhage. For such a patient, hospitalization may be the better option, as long as the care provided is consonant with the patient's goals, and the patient and family receive appropriate emotional and spiritual support. Lack of resources to provide adequate home care is another reason home death can prove too burdensome.

When hospice care is initiated, a psychosocial assessment is completed by interviewing the patient and family in the home environment. This assessment addresses the emotional and physical health of the caregiver as well as the social and financial resources. Social resources include other family, friends, or neighbors willing to assume some of the patient care or other tasks. Financial resources include eligibility for Medicare hospice benefit or hospice benefits available from commercial insurance plans. Sometimes, life insurance policies can be accessed before death for a terminally ill patient to assist with the cost of home care or other needs.

This information, together with the nursing assessment of the patient, provides the basis for planning care and determining patient and family needs. However, even an in-depth assessment by experienced staff may not provide a reliable predictor for whether a patient will remain home to die. Hospices have provided care for a wide spectrum of families, from those with every resource who at the last minute access the EMS, to those with limited finances and inadequate coping histories who are able to provide good care at home through the death event. At each home visit, hospice staff must reevaluate the patient/family situation and revise plans as necessary.

Preparation of the patient and family

Once home death has been established as a desired goal, an individualized home care plan is developed with the patient and family. The patient and family need to know specifically what the hospice team can and will provide. Friends and other resources are also identified. The patient's primary caregiver may need encouragement to ask for help from these other resources, and it should be emphasized that when a person is terminally ill, friends and neighbors may also have difficulty coping with their own feelings. This may be due to their discomfort with not knowing how to help. Friends and neighbors are often grateful when a patient or family caregiver assigns them specific tasks, so they can be of help in a concrete way.

The primary caregiver is continually and carefully assessed to determine what direct care he or she wants to do and is capable of doing. Support to the primary caregiver and other family members includes acknowledging how physically and emotionally exhausting caring for someone ill at home can be. Caregivers need to feel okay about taking a break from their caregiver role and delegating that care.

Preparation for the death event

Families need to be prepared for the time immediately preceding and the actual time of the patient's death. The most difficult aspect of preparation is that each patient's death may not be completely predictable. However, there are some universal signs that families can anticipate and on which they can receive instruction. Table 77-6 is an example of a patient and family instruction sheet that lists many of the common signs seen in patients whose death is imminent. For family members who have cared for an ill person for a long time, or who are health care professionals themselves, it is important to emphasize that laboratory results and vital signs are unreliable indicators of the time of death.

The family is instructed to listen to the patient carefully, even if it appears that the patient is confused. Many times dying patients will speak in symbolic language.[21] A common example is a patient who talks about "going home." It may seem that the patient is confused if he or she already is home. Further conversation may indicate that "going home" refers to dying. It is not unusual for patients to report actually seeing or having conversations with a loved one who has died. Family members may be the most capable of interpreting some symbolic language for the patient. Patients may indicate when they feel they are ready to die. If this occurs, family members can be encouraged to allow the patient to "let go," that is, give the patient permission to die.[21] Although no one can be sure how much an individual has control over the time of his or her own death, having a family member tell the patient that it is all right to "let go" can add to the patient's peace of mind.[3] Emotional care of the patient and family around the time of death occurs based upon need and the hospice team's assessment of family dynamics.

Funeral arrangements

In most situations a home death will go more smoothly if the patient or family chooses a funeral home before the death occurs. Although it can be most helpful for complete funeral arrangements to be made prior to the death of the patient, family members may find this action

---

Table 77-6 Hospice Home Care Instruction Sheet: Signs and Symptoms of Approaching Death

The hospice team's goal is to help prepare you for some things that might occur close to the time of death. Although we can never predict exactly when a terminally ill person will die, we know when the time is getting close by a combination of signs and symptoms. Not all of these signs will appear at the same time, and some may never appear at all. All of the signs described are ways the body prepares itself for the final stages of life.

1. Your loved one may sleep more and might be more difficult to awaken. Hearing and vision may decrease.
   What to do: Plan your time and activities for times when he/she is more alert. Always talk as if the person can hear you, even if he/she appears to be in a coma. When providing care, explain what you are doing as you do it.
2. There may be a gradual decrease in need for food and drink. Your loved one will say he/she doesn't have an appetite or isn't hungry. This is the body's natural response to the dying process. It is telling the person that eating and drinking are no longer helpful—that the body can't use food and fluid properly anymore.
   What to do: Allow your loved one to choose when and what to eat or drink, even if this means little or nothing will be taken in. Liquids often are more easily tolerated than solid food.
3. Your loved one may become more confused or restless or experience visions of people and places.
   What to do: Remind him/her of the time and the day and who is there with them. Be calm and reassuring when talking to him/her.
4. Hands, arms, feet, and legs may become cooler, and the skin may turn a bluish color with purplish splotches.
   What to do: Use blankets for warmth. Do *not* use an electric blanket or heating pad.
5. Irregular breathing patterns may occur. There might be a space of time (10–30 seconds) when there will be no breathing at all. This is called *apnea*. There may be phlegm in the throat that is difficult to cough.
   What to do: Position the person on his/her side with head elevated.

Contact hospice team at any time for questions, or to discuss changes.

premature. Beyond choosing a funeral home, no other arrangements need be made prior to death.

The hospice team can be a resource to families about the different types of funeral homes available in their area. Important factors that differentiate funeral homes are religious affiliation, financial considerations, and policies about home removal of the body. The hospice team provides information on organ and body donation and on autopsy. These procedures usually are compatible with home death as long as the wishes of the patient and family are known in advance so arrangements can be made with the funeral home. Finally, the hospice team needs to be a resource to ensure that the family is aware of local ordinances or laws surrounding an expected home death.

Availability of the hospice team

Of utmost importance in supporting families through a patient's home death is instructing them on how to contact the hospice team at any time as needed. Families should be encouraged to call about any changes in the patient's status or for what may seem to them like minor questions. For the hospice team, emotional support of exhausted and anxious family members is just as important an intervention as a change in pain medication for the patient. Family members also need to be instructed to call the hospice immediately when the home death occurs. It is also important to remind families not to call the EMS, and to inform them of the possible consequences of such an action, such as attempted resuscitation. This instruction often needs to be repeated because many people call 911 or the emergency medical system (EMS) as a natural reaction to an "emergency."

Grief and Bereavement

Facilitating grief

As family members prepare for the death of a loved one at home, they are also preparing themselves for the loss. This is often referred to as *anticipatory grief*.[22] Family members who can give a dying person permission to "let go" are at the very same time letting go of the person themselves. Part of the hospice team's care is assisting the family during this anticipatory grief phase. A thorough assessment includes exploring with family members previous losses and coping mechanisms. The family is encouraged to identify and discuss unresolved issues with the dying person. This can be an opportunity to resolve certain issues, so that after death there are minimal or no regrets for the family. Even when conflict does not exist, family members can say things to the dying person that they may not have said or feel that they have not said enough previously.[3] The dying person and family members can honor the meaning of their relationship and their life together.[1] Asking a couple how they met or going through a family photo album with them is a good way to facilitate grieving and provide a therapeutic life review.

Bereavement support

Bereavement support is a required component of hospice care under Medicare and most state licensing regulations.[9] However, the specific structure of a hospice's bereavement program is not well defined. Each hospice program develops its own policies and mechanisms for bereavement care and follow-up.

Grieving is a normal reaction to loss and is manifested in a variety of ways, both physical and emotional. Some of these are loss of appetite, sleeplessness, heart palpitations, lack of energy, sadness, and anger. The following four tasks have been identified as necessary for the normal grieving process:

1. Accepting the reality of the loss
2. Experiencing the pain of grief
3. Adjusting to the environment in which the deceased is missing
4. Withdrawing emotional energy and placing it in another relationship[20]

The goal of bereavement care or counseling is to assist and support survivors as they move through the process of adjusting to the loss and move toward resolution.[20,22] Hospice programs generally follow survivors for one year, although there is no mandated standard time for follow-up. This period should be understood as a time frame in which the most acute grief occurs, not the period in which mourning is completed. Grief resolution is an individualized process that takes place gradually over varying periods of time.

Methods of bereavement care commonly include a bereavement assessment, contact of survivors at regularly scheduled intervals, and, as necessary, referrals for professional counseling for those with complicated or abnormal grief reactions. Bereavement support can also take the form of support groups, socials or teas, educational classes on specific topics, and/or memorial services conducted by the hospice program.[3]

Abnormal grief

Survivors unable to progress through the tasks of mourning have typically developed some form of abnormal or complicated grief.[20] Generally, abnormal or complicated grief will manifest itself in one of three ways. First, the grief reaction may be prolonged. Second, the grief reaction may be masked in behavioral or physical symptoms, even such seemingly unrelated symptoms as pain, sexual impotence, and behavioral "acting out." Finally, abnormal grief may be evident in exaggerated expressions of normal grief reactions, such as excessive anger, sadness, or depression.[20] Therapy for abnormal grief extends beyond the scope of the bereavement care services provided by most hospice programs. However, hospice staff should be able to identify abnormal grief and recommend referrals to specialists who treat such syndromes.

Unresolved grief has been associated with several physical and emotional illnesses, including increased risk of suicide.[20,22] Therefore, facilitation of anticipatory grieving and bereavement can be viewed as preventive health care for survivors. After a review of the literature on the effectiveness of grief counseling, Collin Murray Parkes, psychiatrist and consultant to St. Christopher's Hospice, concluded that "professional services and professionally supported voluntary and self-help services are capable of reducing the risk of psychiatric and psychoanalytic disorders resulting from bereavement."[22]

Current Issues and Challenges of Hospice Programs

Patients who live alone

The rising number of elderly who live alone combined with decreasing proximity of family has created a population of individuals at risk for nursing home placement. Hospice programs encourage patients to remain at home as long as safety and comfort can be maintained. However, the coverage provided by the hospice Medicare benefit and private insurance policies are based on the notion of family or friends providing the majority of care in the home. These government or private insurance benefits are not designed to provide extended custodial care to persons who live alone. The challenge is how to provide the hospice services to a population that does not have readily accessible family and friends who can provide care.

For patients who live alone the main concerns of hospice are legal liability, safety concerns, intensive staff resources, ethical issues of patient autonomy versus injury risk, potential for increased patient discomfort due to a sudden change in health status, and maintenance of the home environment.

Strategies to meet the challenges of caring for those who live alone involve a coordinated effort from all members of the interdisciplinary team and compliance by the patient with the mutually agreed upon plan of care. Specific strategies to meet this challenge include the following:

- Utilization of a written contract that specifies the resources and limitations of the plan of care

- Detailed home safety assessment and documentation of initial plan to address risks

- Coordination of resources such as friends, family, community, volunteers, and hospice staff

- Installation of a system for emergency phone contact

- Mobilization of community resources such as Meals on Wheels, homemaker services, delivery services, and support from church or volunteer agencies.[23]

Meeting the needs of culturally diverse populations

The earliest hospices in Connecticut, California, New Jersey, and Arizona were founded by and served a predominantly middle-class, white population. Black and Hispanic populations historically have been underserved by health care agencies, including hospice. The black population is better served than Hispanics, but not in proportion to their cancer-related death rates. Both of these minority populations are underrepresented among hospice staff and volunteers, even in urban hospice programs.[24] The reasons for this are complex but include the fact that black and Hispanic populations have less access to health care in general and are less likely to have medical insurance. Some religious beliefs and cultural values may also be a factor.[25]

Children represent another underserved population in the United States. Dedicated pediatric hospice services are rare. A 1992 survey by the National Hospice Organization indicated that although most hospices will provide pediatric services, actual representation of children cared for by hospice was only about 2% of total patients served.[26] For example, in the Chicago metropolitan area, which is served by more than 20 hospice programs and four large children's hospitals, there are no dedicated pediatric hospice services.

Patients with AIDS have presented a tremendous challenge to hospice care. However, the introduction of treatment with protease inhibitors has over the past several years greatly diminished the need for hospice care in this population.[27]

There are other groups of patients ("outliers") whose diagnoses and related social issues also challenge hospice care. Alzheimer's, amyotrophic lateral sclerosis (ALS), and other dementias are common examples. The Medicare hospice benefit was originally designed for the elderly cancer patient with an intact family available to provide most of the home care, supplemented by the support and resources of the hospice team.[3] However, we are rapidly facing an aging population with either no primary caregivers or immediate support persons who are too frail to provide care. The challenge for hospice is to broaden its scope to create effective care models for such divergent populations.[28] Residential and day care hospice components are two models currently being explored around the country.

Palliative Care Approaches

Communication

Honest, compassionate communication is the hallmark of good palliative and hospice care.[29] Poor communication about the dying process remains a major barrier to providing adequate care at the end of life, as well as a barrier to supporting patients and their families through treatment for chronic and progressive illnesses.

Good listening skills include body posture that conveys interest, sitting at a person's eye level, conveying adequate time to listen, and conveying an attitude of compassion. The sense of abandonment and isolation so feared by patients, and experienced by both patients and their family members, can be overcome with good listening skills.[30]

Communication also must be nonjudgmental and consistent with the health care plan. Nurses and other health care givers must be mindful not to impose personal opinions and values in a way that causes the patient and family to have doubt and conflict.

The ability of the nurse to foster a relaxed, friendly relationship with the patient, family, and other team members helps to promote confidence in achieving the goals of care. Interpersonal skills are invaluable in enabling the nurse to discuss such difficult issues as preparation for home death and funeral arrangements. The stressful nature of terminal illness tends to bring out the best and the worst in patients and families. An unhurried approach to care gives the patient and family time and encouragement to address their concerns.[30]

Quality-of-Life

The concept of quality-of-life (QOL) can be described as a comparison of the individual's expectations of life with the reality of his or her life situation. QOL is a complex concept; it is subjective and is usually determined in part by community and cultural values.[15] Beyond managing symptoms and providing emotional and spiritual support, optimal palliative care assists the patient in defining and promoting his or her own QOL. This may include the patient's desire to plan a trip, complete a project, or pursue activities for enjoyment or means of self-expression. Complementary therapies have begun to be explored as additional avenues to enhance QOL. These include meditation, therapeutic touch, massage therapy, and aromatherapy.[31] How helpful these various therapies are, how they work, and who they help are not yet well defined. Meditation may help patients achieve a sense of control and inner peace. The touch therapies provide an avenue for patients to feel physical pleasure and human presence.

End-of-life patients often are able to describe and appreciate a QOL not previously achieved. This can have a positive effect on the family, friends, and sometimes even the community. An example is the current best-selling book, *Tuesdays with Morrie*, the true story of a teacher, Morrie Schwarz, dying of ALS. Morrie takes us through his dying process and teaches us how he finds joy and purpose until the very end of his life.[32]

Care at the Time of Death—
The Inpatient Setting

The JCAHO has devised specific standards applicable to hospitals for the care of dying patients that are consistent with a holistic, palliative approach. The nurse can be instrumental in facilitating a palliative care approach on the patient unit. For the person expected to die, the primary care goal of palliative care is to create a private and comfortable environment for the patient with the physical symptoms of advanced disease under control. Emotional and spiritual care should be readily available. In addition, the family will receive education about the physiology of the dying process and what to expect regarding their own grieving. For the patient expected to die, the plan of care should be focused on the following areas:

- Patient and family goals for care are identified, with patient choices honored as much as possible

- Assessment of patient and family members' understanding of the patient's prognosis, status, and current coping strategies

- Advanced directives completed or reviewed, with documentation in place, where appropriate

- Identification of the decision maker for any patient unable to make his or her own decisions

- Identification and facilitation of religious, cultural, and personal practices that are important to observe before, at, or immediately after the time of death

- Assessment and treatment of a patient's symptoms by the least invasive method possible.

Special Considerations in Symptom Management

The nursing plan of care should be tailored to focus on symptom management and eliminating tests or treatments that are burdensome to the patient and offer no QOL benefit. Basic nursing care is important to facilitate a comfortable death. Excellent body hygiene, mouth care, and skin care are important basic components of care. Even for a patient who is comatose or noncommunicative, cleanliness and appearance are important issues of dignity for both patients and their family members. The nurse is in the position to model behavior for family and friends, such as speaking to and orienting a nonresponsive patient with the assumption that he or she may still be able to hear. Families need continual education about the status of the patient and adequacy of care being provided. Nurses need to explain how discomfort is assessed, why analgesics and other medications may be continued or discontinued, reasons for repositioning the patient, and for other care tasks being provided.

Prior to death, family members may benefit from participating in physical care of the patient such as offering ice chips or providing mouth care. Families can be encouraged to read to patients, play music, and say their good-byes to their loved one prior to death. Some family members will need permission *not* to participate in the care or the death vigil if they cannot tolerate doing so. It is important for nurses to understand that grieving is an individual process and not to judge family behavior. Nurses can assist family members in identifying what may be meaningful to them and in providing choices for family involvement.

At the time of death, even the most prepared family members may be in shock and in need of support. Family members should be allowed to spend time with the body of the deceased person after death. In some cultures, family participation in postmortem care may be an important ritual; this should be accommodated as important for the grieving process. An American ritual in hospitals is pronouncement of death, usually by a licensed physician or nurse. When the person is pronounced and the death verified, the nurse should ensure that the family has been told in concrete terms that their loved one has indeed died. Condolences are offered to family members by the staff in a sensitive manner. A chaplain visit or contact with clergy should be offered, if this need was not already anticipated.

Some family members may prefer to be given privacy with the deceased person, and others may prefer to have a staff member present in the room for support. If possible, all family members who want to should be allowed to come in to say good-bye before the deceased person's body is removed from the room. If this is not possible, some institutions allow for deceased persons' bodies to be taken to another room or area for viewing or visitation. The family needs assurance that the person's body will be handled in a dignified and respectful manner. It is ideal for family members to be given written information about grieving, grief support groups, or other counseling resources in the area before they leave the inpatient setting.

Stress of the Nurse in the Care of the Dying

Providing compassionate care to dying patients and their loved ones can create unique stressors for professional caregivers. Studies have shown that nurses and other hospice staff members tend to identify with younger patients (those under age 40) and to feel a greater sense of injustice when these patients die. Staff attitudes toward death can be greatly influenced by unresolved grief issues in their own personal and/or professional life.[33] Stress can be increased due to unrealistic expectations of ourselves, our coworkers, or the therapy we use to manage symptoms. The inability to relieve symptoms such as intractable pain and nausea can evoke feelings of impotence or helplessness. Supportive interactions with patients and their families can be emotionally draining, especially when long-standing problems in their interpersonal relationships are involved.[34]

Caregivers with high-stress jobs who cope successfully are able to recognize when signs of stress are developing within themselves, to acknowledge their own limits, and to initiate self-help techniques or seek the help of others.

Several methods for coping with stress have been used successfully by nurses and other professional caregivers (Table 77-7). Recently, some complementary therapies recommended to enhance patient QOL, such as massage therapy, have begun to be explored by nurses and others as effective means to reduce their own stress.

Legal and Ethical Issues Surrounding Palliative Care

Due to the population characteristics and specialized nature of terminal care, hospice programs have been innovators in encouraging patients to identify their own goals, particularly goals related to cardiopulmonary resuscitation (CPR), invasive procedures, and identification of family or friends to assist in decision making if the patient becomes incapacitated. However, the hospice nurse and other members of the team are directly affected by recent legislative and court decisions that can either hinder or enhance the ability to assist the family in meeting those goals.

Advance Directives

The federal Patient Self-Determination Act, enacted in December 1991, requires hospices, hospitals, and other health care agencies to provide patients, on admission, with written information about two key areas: (1) their right to accept or refuse treatment under state law, and (2) ways to execute advance directives such as a living will and a durable power of attorney for health care.[35] The purpose of this legislation is to ensure that patients' wishes are carried out in the event they become mentally incapacitated or are incapable of making or communicating their decisions. As with all other health care organizations receiving federal funds, hospice programs are mandated to provide information to facilitate completion of a living will or a durable power of attorney for health care. Hospice team members provide whatever information is needed to assist the patient in making an informed decision, especially when it affects the patient's decision not to have CPR, intravenous fluids, or tube feedings.

Patients with cancer, sepsis, pneumonia, renal failure, diabetes, or advanced age have a low chance of survival after CPR. An average of 4% of patients receiving CPR in a general acute-care setting survive. For those who do survive, subsequent QOL is compromised.[36] Hospice patients and families may need reassurance that their focus on comfort and QOL is being reinforced by their decision not to have CPR.

This same approach holds true when the decision not to have intravenous fluids or tube feedings is challenged. As death approaches, the patient may lose the ability to drink, which can result in dehydration if death does not

Table 77-7 Useful Methods for Coping with Stress

- Take responsibility for caring for yourself. Allow at least 15–20 minutes each day for quiet introspection. Assess your body for signs of stress, for example, muscle tension, headaches, insomnia, GI distress, and frequent illness. The body systems showing stress should be the focus for rejuvenation. For example, muscle tension may indicate a need for relaxation therapy.

- Reduce stress by prioritizing work. Make a conscious choice between those events worth your energy and those you need to delegate or otherwise not take on at all.

- Promote training and education not only for new staff but also for experienced team members. The continual development of our knowledge base promotes confidence. Special attention should be placed on identified stresses. If you are feeling overwhelmed, then dealing with family dynamics, reading, or attending a seminar on that subject could give you additional tools to improve future interactions.

- Take time off! Whenever possible get out of town, away from reminders of work.

- Take time for your hobby. Creative self-expression through arts, crafts, or hobbies can provide an additional outlet for release of stress.

- Focus on maintaining a healthy body through regular exercise and eating a balanced diet. Leave the clinical setting during lunch and go for a long walk or do something not work-related.

- Seek supportive interactions with individuals or in a group. Regular involvement with a support group can be helpful in providing an environment to share with others on the team who are under similar pressures. Such interactions serve to promote team building and problem identification. For a group to be successful, trust and an open, nurturing environment must be established. An experienced facilitator can be invaluable in attaining this goal. Group members make a contract with each other to be supportive and nonjudgmental and to keep all conversation in strict confidence.

- Give yourself permission to find the humor in certain situations that otherwise may be tragic or depressing. Share this humor with other members of the hospice team, being careful to keep it respectful of patients and families involved.

- Focus on the positive satisfying aspects of the role of hospice caregiver. Assisting a patient in the last few days of life can be very rewarding. Promoting comfort and quality-of-life issues involves nursing skills and principles of the highest order.

---

soon follow. However, fluid depletion has the following benign QOL effects:[37]

- Urine output is decreased, so there is less incontinence

- Gastric secretions lessen; therefore, episodes of vomiting decrease

- Pulmonary secretions lessen, resulting in less congestion

- Peripheral edema secondary to tumor subsides, resulting in decreased pain from nerve compression

- Although the sensation of dry mouth and thirst may increase, this can be relieved by good mouth care and small amounts of oral fluids.

In 1990, the U.S. Supreme Court delivered a decision that made it clear that life-and-death decisions depend on the availability of written evidence of the patient's wishes. Under the current Patient Self-Determination Act, individuals are not required to enact an advanced directive. However, failure to do so may later compromise the individual's ability to limit aggressive medical treatment. In general, the power of attorney for health care is more useful than the living will. A living will is applicable only when it pertains to a terminal illness and only for those issues identified in the living will document. This is limiting, as not every issue can be anticipated. The living will does not identify another person who can act as the agent for a disabled patient.[35]

Through the power of attorney for health care, the patient chooses an agent to act on the patient's behalf if the patient is no longer competent to make decisions.

This is especially important for individuals who have diagnoses such as AIDS, cancer metastases to the brain, or other medical problems in which eventual confusion or other mental status changes are an expected complication of the disease. By electing to assign an agent as the power of attorney, the patient is able to make clear his or her wishes regarding the removal of life support in the event of irreversible coma, the use of artificial feeding if unable to swallow, and any limitation on the decision-making powers of the agent. A patient may also identify restrictions to care, such as those prohibiting blood transfusions for religious reasons.

The health care team caring for the patient in accordance with these documents usually is protected from liability if it follows the patient's wishes. A copy of the living will or health care power of attorney must be placed in the patient's medical record.

Euthanasia and Assisted Suicide

The moral, ethical, and legal questions surrounding terminal illness and methods used to hasten death have their origins in ancient times. The word *euthanasia* is taken from the Greek *euthanasias*, meaning "good or easy death." For the ancient Greeks and others, euthanasia did not necessarily denote an act or method of hastening death. It was important to them that a person meet death voluntarily, with peace of mind and minimal suffering. This "good death" meant that the ill individual was meeting death in a condition of self-control. Toward this end, it was permissible for a person to shorten life intentionally.[38]

In modern times, euthanasia has come to mean the

intentional ending of the life of a terminally ill person for purposes of compassion. The modern concept is more accurately described as *active* euthanasia, for it is achieved by "doing something," such as giving the patient a lethal injection.[38] Euthanasia is not the same as refusing medical treatment that will not contribute reasonably to improved QOL or will likely be burdensome. Additionally, pain medication or other symptom management measures that are used to improve comfort but could lead to an early death should not be considered euthanasia.[38] The distinguishing factor is intent. If the intent is to relieve pain or manage symptoms and not to cause death, then the unintentional death by such care is not euthanasia. This is the principle of "double-effect."[38] On the other hand, physician-assisted suicide is providing the patient the means (usually medication) and knowledge with the intent of assisting him or her in hastening death.

In the past few years, the issues of euthanasia and legalized physician-assisted suicide for the terminally ill have emerged to be debated around the world, particularly in the United States. The issue of the "right" of a terminally ill individual to determine the timing and method of his or her own death came before the U.S. Supreme Court for the first time on January 8, 1997. The Court ruled that individuals did not have the "right" to euthanasia or physician-assisted suicide, but did have the right to "optimal palliative care."[39]

The Supreme Court decision is in accord with the National Hospice Organization's position against euthanasia and physician-assisted suicide, arguing that optimal pain and symptom management, along with emotional support, are still not widely enough available to dying patients outside of hospice programs.[39] It has been the general experience of those who provide optimal palliative care that their patients do not need or desire euthanasia. However, even experts in palliative care acknowledge that there may always be some patients whose symptoms cannot be completely controlled or who may request euthanasia in spite of the availability of optimal terminal care. A concern is that the legalization of assisted suicide for this very small group might encourage society to consider euthanasia an option for some non-terminal people, such as the disabled, those with AIDS, those without caregivers, or the poor.

Oregon's legalization of physician-assisted suicide

The many difficulties in enacting legalized physician-assisted suicide are now being played out in Oregon. On November 4, 1997, Oregon voters affirmed their support for assisted suicide by defeating a measure that sought to repeal it. To date, more than ten patients have apparently requested, and probably received, physician assistance with their deaths. This has raised controversy in a number of ways, including how to report these deaths on death certificates, guidelines for what to prescribe to assist a patient's death, and conflicts with state physician and pharmacist practice and ethics laws.[40] If physician-assisted suicide becomes more common, hospice programs will

have to decide their role, if any, in this care, and may need to create policies on how to handle such requests and the limits of their services.

Owing to this debate in our society, those in oncology, hospice care, and the care of other patients with end-stage diseases should be proactive in addressing euthanasia. Many hospice programs have addressed the issues of euthanasia, suicide, and requests for assisted suicide by preparing formal policies to guide staff in responding to these issues. When a patient or family member inquires about or expresses the desire for euthanasia, the appropriate initial response from an individual nurse or other health care provider is a nonjudgmental and caring attitude, followed by careful exploration of the patient's or family member's concerns or fears. The debate over euthanasia and physician-assisted suicide may make it increasingly necessary to regularly assure dying patients in our care that we will continue to be there for them and that we find value in their lives.

Future Trends and Challenges in End-of-Life Care

Education

Some of the new palliative care initiatives have included health education models to improve care of the dying.[7] Many of these have targeted professionals in practice. For the most part, nursing and medical school programs still provide little in the way of a comprehensive approach to end of life care.[41] This remains a major challenge for the future.

Research Issues

Empirical research is still needed in all areas of hospice and palliative care. Existing research focuses on pain and symptom management and psychosocial care. Of particular research interest is the definition and quantification of QOL as an outcome measure. Areas least studied are volunteerism and spiritual care, the features most unique to hospice.[42] Other important palliative care research topics include suicidal ideation in the terminally ill; emotional, cultural, and other factors hindering pain management; and long-term effectiveness of bereavement care. Both hospice models and hospice patient populations inherently make research difficult.[42] Limited funding and the relative lack of hospice and palliative care programs associated with academic institutions provide additional barriers to research.

Integration into Health Care Practices

For years, Dame Cicely Saunders has believed that rather than creating a segregated system for the dying, the palliative care principles so effective in hospice care should be diffused throughout the health care system.[3] Hospice in the United States began as an antimedical establishment and antiphysician movement. This antagonistic bias has unfortunately been a major factor preventing hospice and palliative care principles from being applied to dying patients on a broader scale.

The JCAHO began to foster integration of hospice care with the revision of its hospital standards for 1992, which addressed needs of the dying patient under the patient rights section.[43] The regulations were greatly strengthened in 1996 with Standard RI.1.2.7 (Table 77-8). These regulations incorporate basic hospice standards of care for all dying patients in hospitals.[43] The federal Patient Self-Determination Act also has played a role in furthering the ability of patients to forgo unwanted heroic treatment in the face of terminal illness.

In its short history, hospice has led the way in many health care trends, including case management, cost containment, home care utilization, and advanced directives. While continuing to grow, as of 1997, hospice programs cared for approximately 50% of those who die from a cancer diagnosis.[44] Hospice needs to continue its effort to reach those not being served, while adapting to the ever-changing health care system by:[43]

- Ensuring holistic hospice care is provided via health insurance plans
- Making earlier access to hospice care possible
- Delivering cost-effective care
- Meeting the needs of diverse populations.

The relationship between hospice and many of the newer palliative care initiatives is currently being debated.

Table 77-8   JCAHO Standards for Hospital Care at the End-of-Life

Dying patients have unique needs for respectful, responsive care. All hospital staff are sensitized to the needs of patients at the end of life. Concern for the patient's comfort and dignity should guide all aspects of care during the final stages of life.

The hospital's framework for addressing issues related to care at the end of life provide for

- providing appropriate treatment for any primary and secondary symptoms, according to the wishes of the patient or the surrogate decision maker;
- managing pain aggressively and effectively;
- sensitively addressing issues such as autopsy and organ donation;
- respecting the patient's values, religion, and philosophy;
- involving the patient and, where appropriate, the family in every aspect of care; and
- responding to the psychological, social, emotional, spiritual, and cultural concerns of the patient and the family.

Effective pain management is appropriate for all patients, not just for dying patients.

The potential is for hospice care to partner with the largely inpatient palliative care initiatives in order to increase access of appropriate care to patients in all settings. One hospital-based model generating interest around the country consists of a triad of services: a home hospice program, an inpatient palliative care unit, and a palliative care consultation service under a single reporting structure.[45]

Conclusion

Recent interest in end of life care has resulted in many exciting initiatives to improve care of the dying. The trend is toward the incorporation into inpatient and other settings of the palliative care principles that have so successfully guided hospice care. This chapter is an overview of the optimal care for a dying person and of how this care can support better quality of life for the patient and the family. At the end of life, there is a change from hope for a cure and a long life to hope for care and living for the moment. Death is no longer something to be avoided at all costs; rather, death is understood to be as natural a part of life as birth. Home, family, and friends are not left behind but are included as an important part of care at the end of life.

It is a privilege for health care professionals to be involved with human beings during the end of their lives. We hear their stories about what life was like for them. We help them toward what they would like the natural end of their lives to be.

References

1. Kübler-Ross E: *On Death and Dying.* New York, Macmillan, 1974
2. Jacox A, Carr DB, Payne R, et al.: Management of Cancer Pain. AHCPR Publication No. 94-0592. U.S. Department of Health and Human Services, March 1998
3. Amenta MO, Bohnet NL: *Nursing Care of the Terminally Ill.* Boston, Little Brown, 1986
4. *The 1995-96 Guide to the Nation's Hospices.* Published by the National Hospice Organization. Arlington, VA, piii, 1996
5. Joint Commission on Accreditation of Hospitals: *Accreditation Manual for Hospice.* Chicago 1986
6. Joint Commission on Accreditation of Healthcare Organizations: *Accreditation Manual for Hospitals.* Oakbrook Terrace, IL, publ. 1992, pp 103–105
7. Project on Death In America Report of Activities. July 1994–December 1997, Open Society Institute, New York, 1998, pp 26–54
8. A Controlled trial to improve care for seriously ill hospitalized patients: the study to understand prognosis and preferences for outcomes and risks of treatment (SUPPORT). *JAMA* 274:1591–1598, 1995
9. National Hospice Organization: Hospice services, guidelines, and definitions. *Hosp J* 11(2):65–73, 1996
10. Stuart B: *Medical Guidelines for Determining Prognosis in Selected*

Non-Cancer Diseases (ed 2). Arlington, VA, National Hospice Organization, 1996

11. Kaye P: *Notes on Symptom Control.* Essex, England, Hospice Education Institute, 1991

12. Cassem NH: Critical care psychiatry, in Shoemaker WC, Thompson WL, Holbrook PR (eds): *Textbook of Critical Care.* Philadelphia, Saunders, 1984, pp 981–989

13. Adams F, Fernandez F, Andersson BS: Emergency pharmacotherapy of delirium in the critically ill cancer patient. *Psychosomatics* 27:33–37, 1986 (suppl)

14. Cassel CK, Clark H, Edwards AL, et al (eds): *Caring for the Dying: Identification and Promotion of Physician Competency.* American Board of Internal Medicine, 1996

15. Doyle D, Hanks G, MacDonald N: Introduction, in *Oxford Textbook of Palliative Medicine* (ed 2). New York: Oxford University Press, 1998

16. Martinez J: The interdisciplinary team, in Sheehan D, Jones CH (eds): *Hospice and Palliative Care: Concepts and Practices.* Sudbury, MA, Jones and Bartlett, 1996

17. Jamison JE: Spirituality and medical ethics. *Am J Hospice Palliat Care* 12:41–45, 1995

18. Reese D, Brown D: Psychosocial and spiritual care in hospice: differences between nursing, social work and clergy. *Hospice J* 12(1):29–41, 1997

19. Sankar A: *Dying at Home.* Baltimore, Johns Hopkins, 1991

20. Bourne V, Frogge MH: Grief, in Yarbro CH, Frogge MH, Goodman M (eds) *Cancer Symptom Management* (ed 2). Sudbury, MA. Jones and Bartlett, 1999, pp 618–626

21. Pflaum MC, Kelley P: Understanding the final messages of the dying. *Nursing '86* 16(6):26–29, 1986

22. Parkes CM, Weiss RS: *Recovery from Bereavement.* New York, Basic Books, 1983

23. Frozena C, Hurtt M: The Hospice Care Planning and Interdisciplinary Guide. Aspen Publications. Gaithersburg MD, 1995, pp 2–8

24. Machuca M: Marketing and minorities: hospice in the Hispanic community. *Am J Hospice Palliat Care* 7:21–22, 1990

25. Gordon AK: Hospice and minorities: a national study of Organizational Access and Practice. *Hospice J* 11(1):49–70, 1996

26. National Hospice Organization: 1992 hospice statistics. *NHO Newsline* 1, 1995

27. Foley FJ: AIDS palliative care: challenging the palliative paradigm. *J Palliat Care* 11(2):9, 1995

28. Lynn J, Wilkinson A: Quality end of life care: the case for a medicaring demonstration. *Hospice J* 3(1/2):151–163, 1998

29. Rey M, Catherine: *I'm Here to Help.* Monnel, MN, McRay Company, 1995

30. Buckman, Robert: *Breaking Bad News.* Baltimore, Johns Hopkins, 1997, pp 65–97

31. Byock, Ira. *Dying Well: The Prospect for Growth at the End of Life.* New York, Riverhead Books, 1997, pp 59–117

32. Albom, M. *Tuesdays with Morrie.* New York, Doubleday, 1997, 152–158

33. Vincent PA: Do hospice nurses differ from non-hospice nurses? *Am J Hospice Care* 3:41–42, 1986

34. Alexander D, Ritchie E: Stressors and difficulties in dealing with the terminal patient. *J Palliat Care* 6:28–33, 1990

35. Wadill G: Advanced directives. *Hospice* 2:10–11, 1991

36. von Gunten C: CPR in hospitalized patients: when is it futile? *Am Fam Physician* 4:2130–2134, 1991

37. Musgrave C: Terminal dehydration. *Cancer Nurs* 13:62–66, 1990

38. O'Connell L: *Active Euthanasia, Religion and the Public Debate.* Chicago, Park Ridge Center, 1991, pp 18–23

39. Thal AE: *Proactive Responses to the Assisted Suicide/Euthanasia Debate.* Publication No. 713438. Washington, DC, National Hospice Organization, 1996

40. Azevedo D: Assisted suicide is legal. Now what? *Med Econ* 75(9):57–64, 1998

41. Barnard D: The coevolution of bioethics and the medical humanities with palliative medicine, 1967–1997. *J Palliat Med* 1:187–193, 1998

42. Kristjanson LJ, Hanson EJ, Balneaves L: Research in palliative care populations: ethical issues. *J Palliat Care* 10(3):10–15, 1994

43. *The 1998 Comprehensive Accreditation Manual for Hospitals.* Oakbrook Terrace, IL, The Joint Commission on Accreditation of Health Organizations, 1997

44. National Hospice Organization: *Hospice Fact Sheet 1997.* Arlington, VA

45. von Gunten C, Martinez J: A program of hospice and palliative care in a private, nonprofit U.S. teaching hospital. *J Palliat Med* 1(3):250, 1998

Professional Issues for the Cancer Nurse

CHAPTER 78

Advancing Cancer Nursing Through Nursing Education

Gloria A. Hagopian, RN, EdD

Introduction

Cancer nursing has benefited from the work of strong, visionary leaders who demanded quality in cancer nursing practice, education, and research. These leaders have shaped education at both the undergraduate and graduate levels, and have had a significant impact on cancer nursing practice and research. In critically examining cancer nursing and health care delivery, they were able to plan the future of nursing practice. In this chapter, the history of cancer nursing education and some of the major influences on its development are discussed. The current state of cancer nursing education at the generalist, advanced, and continuing education levels are highlighted. The chapter concludes with a discussion of critical issues facing cancer nursing education today and in the future.

History of Cancer Nursing Education

Specialized education in oncology nursing began in the 1940s. Day-long, then week-long continuing education programs were offered, often under the sponsorship of the American Cancer Society (ACS). Efforts to incorporate cancer nursing content at the baccalaureate level began in 1954 when the National Cancer Institute (NCI) provided funding to four schools for this purpose.[1] There were several outcomes of this project, including the development by Diller of a cancer nursing test to measure students' knowledge, a cancer curriculum, and evaluation tools for faculty.[2]

The first graduate-level course with both theoretical and clinical components in cancer nursing was offered by Nelson in 1946 at Teachers' College in New York.[1,3,4] This course, two semesters in length, provided 16 credits toward a Master of Arts degree. The course focused on the nature of cancer as a biological phenomenon, patient needs, and nursing care measures. Public health aspects, such as early detection, home care, and community resources, also were emphasized. The clinical part of the course was held at Memorial Hospital in New York. The program was supported in part by a grant from the ACS, New York Division. In 1950 a course for credit in cancer nursing and chronic disease was offered by the University of Minnesota School of Public Health.[1]

A survey of graduate programs to identify those offering cancer nursing was conducted by the ACS in 1958.[1] Of the twenty-two programs responding to the questionnaire, only two indicated that cancer nursing was included in the curriculum. With specialization being offered in other fields of nursing such as coronary care, dialysis, burns, and intensive care, interest in oncology nursing naturally followed, and university courses were soon developed. The first graduate oncology track leading to a master's degree with a specialization in oncology nursing was started at the University of Pittsburgh in 1968.[4]

Continuing education (CE) has always played an important role in cancer nursing and has been the most widely used method to increase the knowledge and skills of nurses.[5] Because of the early lack of consistent preparation of nurses at the generalist level, CE programs were a convenient way to provide the expertise needed to practice cancer nursing; the ACS was an early provider of such educational programs for practicing nurses. Several cancer centers also offered CE programs for nurses through the years, including Memorial Sloan-Kettering Cancer Center, New York, NY; Roswell Park Memorial Hospital, Buffalo, NY; Ellis Fischel State Cancer Center, Columbia, Missouri; and City of Hope National Medical Center, Duarte, California.[3] One of the first institutional CE programs to teach nurses cancer screening procedures was developed by White at the University of Texas M.D. Anderson Cancer Center, Houston, Texas.[1] Today, this unique program continues to offer short-term modules on site-specific cancer screening procedures that incorporate classroom and clinical experience.

In 1982, *Outcome Standards for Cancer Nursing Education at the Fundamental Level* was written by the Oncology Nursing Society in cooperation with the American Nurses' Association, giving faculty guidelines for integrating oncology content into the curriculum at the fundamental or generalist level.[6] This document also served as the impetus to develop other guidelines for practice and graduate education.

Important Influences on Cancer Nursing Education

Organizations

Cancer organizations have had a powerful impact on education in cancer nursing. They include the ACS, the Oncology Nursing Society (ONS), the NCI, and the Association of Pediatric Oncology Nurses (APON).

American Cancer Society

The ACS, organized in 1913, is a nationwide, community-based, voluntary health agency dedicated to eliminating cancer as a health problem by preventing cancer, saving lives, and diminishing suffering through research, education, advocacy, and service. It has more than 3400 local units and 2.2 million volunteers. I Can Cope, Reach to Recovery, and Look Good . . . Feel Better have been very successful educational programs for patients and their families. Among its activities for health care professionals are publications, continuing education programs, conferences, scholarships, and professorships. It sponsors several journals, textbooks, and a web site.[7] The *Cancer Source Book for Nurses*, first published in 1950, has undergone several revisions, the latest in 1997.[8] The ACS distributes thousands of publications and materials to nurses each year. National conferences for health professionals focusing on topics relevant to cancer control are held frequently, and many CE programs are held at the local level.

The ACS professorship program was established to improve the care of the patient and the quality of nursing education in the field of cancer. ACS professors are doctorally prepared experts in cancer nursing who are engaged in teaching, practice, and research, and whose salaries and research are funded by local divisions of the ACS. The professorship program was initiated in 1981, and since that time ten ACS local divisions have funded many ACS professors. As of 1999, six professors were receiving financial support through a grant to their school of nursing for further development and enhancement of the school's oncology nursing program.[7] The ACS also provides scholarships to nurses for study at the master's and doctoral level.

Oncology Nursing Society

The ONS was incorporated in 1975 by Marino, Yarbro, and others because they wanted to define their roles in cancer care, communicate with oncology nurses in similar roles, and develop continuing education programs.[1,9] The ONS mission is to promote excellence in oncology nursing and quality cancer care. Today, the ONS has 205 chapters and more than 27,000 members. Activities of the ONS include the Annual Congress, the Fall Institute, coordination of 29 special interest groups (SIGs), and publication of *Oncology Nursing Forum, Clinical Journal of Oncology Nursing,* and *ONS News.* Under the leadership of the Board of Directors are the Steering Council, Advisory Panels, and Project Teams. The ONS offers numerous monetary awards to distinguished nurses, research grants, and scholarships for educational studies. In addition, it recognizes public figures who have positively influenced cancer care. The ONS has four affiliated organizations: The ONS Foundation, The Oncology Nursing Certification Corporation, the Oncology Nursing Press, and Oncology Education Services.

The ONS has been active over the years in developing standards of education that have had a significant impact on cancer nursing education. The standards developed for the generalist and advanced levels have provided guidelines for curriculum development.

National Cancer Institute

The NCI, established in 1938, has made major contributions to oncology nursing education in a number of ways, including educational programs, work-study programs, fellowship programs, funding for research, predoctoral and postdoctoral research training grants, publications, and providing access to current reliable information through the Cancer Information Service (CIS).

Some of the educational programs that are funded by the NCI for nurses are (1) a short course in research training for post-master's, doctoral, and postdoctoral

nurses engaged in research; (2) a short course in cancer prevention, detection, and screening for minorities; (3) regional workshops for black, Hispanic, and Native American nurses; and (4) a short course for nurses in developing countries on cancer prevention and early detection.

The NCI also has been instrumental in providing funding for faculty education. In 1950, a 3-week institute on cancer nursing was offered to 30 nursing instructors.[3] Later, studies indicated that more programs were needed to prepare nurses to teach in oncology education programs.[10-12] Because the rapidly expanding knowledge of cancer care required that oncology programs be strengthened, and because educational programs were concentrated in large urban areas, a unique project was funded by the NCI in 1980. This 5-year project to develop a model for post-master's fellowship programs in oncology nursing education was intended to increase the number of oncology nurse educators.[13] San Jose State University and the University of Alabama at Birmingham were awarded funds to develop the model curriculum. Over 5 years, thirty-four fellows completed the year-long program, which included clinical nursing, the role of educator, and change.

The Cancer Nurse Training Program is a NCI-sponsored 9-month clinical training program for new baccalaureate graduates. The graduates work and attend classes on current cancer nursing practice and receive a monthly stipend.[14]

Association of Pediatric Oncology Nurses

Established in 1973, APON is the leading professional organization for nurses caring for children and adolescents with cancer and their families. Among its objectives are promoting excellence in pediatric oncology nursing, providing a forum for communication among nurses, disseminating information about care of patients, encouraging publication in professional and lay literature, supporting research in pediatric oncology, and supporting legislation affecting the care of pediatric oncology patients and their families as well as legislation pertaining to the nursing profession. The activities of the organization include the publication of the *Journal of the Association of Pediatric Oncology Nurses,* a newsletter, and an annual meeting. The organization has more than 1900 members.[15]

Certification

Certification in a particular specialty requires education or experience beyond that required for licensure. Therefore, certification acknowledges that the holder has met a set of eligibility criteria, passed a comprehensive examination with rigorous standards, and that the practice of the nurse is of the highest caliber. The mission of the Oncology Nursing Certification Corporation (ONCC) is to advance oncology nursing through the certification process.[16] Ultimately, the goal of certification is to promote the health and well-being of those diagnosed with or at risk for experiencing cancer. Because of the rapidly changing role of oncology nurses, the ONCC updates the test blueprint by conducting Role Delineation Studies that redefine the breadth of the knowledge and practice of oncology nursing as needed.

The certification process has been in place since 1986 for the Oncology Certified Nurse (OCN). The certification examination is available to nurses who have the following qualifications:

- A current RN license

- One year of experience as a registered nurse within the 3-year period prior to application as long as the applicant has at least 1000 hours of oncology nursing practice within 2½ years prior to application

- Completion of 10 contact hours of continuing education in oncology nursing or an academic elective in oncology nursing

Oncology-certified nurses have the opportunity to renew their certification at 4-year intervals. If the candidate is already certified, and the certification has not lapsed, it can be renewed automatically. The 3-hour examination consists of 300 multiple-choice questions and covers eight domains of practice: (1) quality of life, (2) gastrointestinal and urinary function, (3) protective mechanisms, (4) scientific basis for practice, (5) cardiopulmonary function, (6) health promotion, (7) oncologic emergencies, and (8) professional performance.[15] To date, more than 22,000 nurses have taken the certification examination; there are 17,000 oncology-certified nurses. The pass rate for the latest generalist examination was 76% for first-time candidates.

Since 1995 the Advanced Oncology Nursing Certification (AONC) examination has been offered to nurses with a master's or higher degree and experience in administration, education, practice, or research. The pass rate for AOCN candidates is 82%.[16]

It is expected that computer adaptive testing (CAT) will soon replace the current paper-and-pencil tests. With such testing, the candidates answer only as many questions as are needed to determine a pass or fail score.

Cancer Nursing Education Today

Standards of Oncology Nursing Education

The *Outcome Standards for Cancer Nursing Education at the Fundamental Level* were first published in 1982.[6] They have since been revised and updated and are intended to enhance the quality of oncology nursing education and to improve health care for the public.[17] The standards seek to provide guidelines to:

- Planning and evaluating generalist education offered in diploma, associate, and baccalaureate programs

- Planning and evaluating advanced education offered in master's, doctoral, and postdoctoral programs

- Planning and evaluating continuing education programs at the generalist and advanced level

- Assessing individual knowledge of oncology nursing care

At both the generalist and advanced levels, five categories of standards with general descriptive statements relate to faculty, resources, curriculum, the teaching-learning process, and the learner.

Generalist level

The generalist level of cancer nursing, originally referred to as the *fundamental level*, provides a core of knowledge, skill, and attitudes for beginning practice in cancer nursing. Although the generalist level encompasses diploma, associate, and baccalaureate educational programs, the literature deals only with baccalaureate education.

Several significant studies have examined the oncology content at the undergraduate level, contributing to our understanding of existing problems. In 1983 Brown et al conducted a survey to determine the status of cancer education at the baccalaureate level. Results indicated that an average of only 14.5 hours were devoted to cancer nursing and suggested that an examination of the undergraduate curriculum was needed.[18] Strikingly similar results from several European studies indicated that cancer nursing education was inadequate in both quality and quantity. The European studies showed that only 14 hours were devoted to cancer nursing; many faculty were without oncology experience; there was a paucity of teaching materials; and little connection was made between theory and practice.[19,20] Recommendations of the European studies emphasized the importance of clinical experience and suggested that content be taught by an oncology nurse active in the field.[19,20]

The professional's role in developing a positive, empathetic attitude in students toward the patient and family has been debated. It is thought that if an instructor has received insufficient educational preparation in oncology, negative attitudes in students result.[19] Many creative attempts have been made to improve curricula in cancer nursing and to promote positive attitudes about cancer care at the baccalaureate level. Nevidjon and Deatrich offered an intensive 8-week elective course that included lecture, patient care, seminar, skills lab, and individual supervision for senior students.[21] The ONS/American Nurses' Association (ANA) *Outcome Standards* provided the organizing framework for the course. Horvitz and Trigg developed a 10-week in-depth cancer course for senior students that included content on the physiological and psychological impact of cancer on the patient, family, and nurse.[22] Mooney and Dudas offered a two-credit 10-week independent course in cancer nursing for eight selected students.[23] Content included the roles and responsibilities of nurses, psychosocial reactions of patients, critical knowledge needed by the oncology nurse, the purposes and activities of the ONS and other cancer organizations, and specialized skills needed to care for patients. Classes were held for 2 hours each week. A field experience at an ACS office, a support group, or observation experience in a hospital was included. A similar undergraduate elective course that provided 35 hours of didactic and 90 hours of clinical experience over 8 weeks was developed by Rushton.[24]

Quinn-Casper and Holmgren, also believing that the highly specialized skills needed to care for patients with cancer were not consistently addressed at the baccalaureate level, tried a different approach.[25] They developed a program with the ACS to provide supplementary cancer education programs for nursing students. After the first highly successful and well-attended 1-day workshop was held, yearly workshops were instituted. More than 800 students have attended the annual 1-day sessions over a 4-year period. Local ACS chapters throughout the United States now offer such programs for students.

As part of a 5-year federally funded project to increase and improve oncology nursing content in undergraduate programs, Longman et al initiated several activities.[25] Two tools were developed: an attitude inventory and a knowledge test based on the *Outcome Standards*. The results indicated that students in the first semester scored lower than in other semesters, but that scores increased as the students progressed through the program. The improvement of scores suggested a better incorporation of essential oncology content by faculty and increased knowledge on the students' parts due to participation in the activities of the project. Longman et al also offered an elective course on cancer care for students, provided opportunities for students to participate in ongoing oncology research, instituted a research symposium, and provided seminars to faculty about the latest therapies and care to help update their knowledge.[27]

Although these efforts are commendable, such programs are scarce, and therefore only limited numbers of students can benefit. In many other programs, glaring deficiencies still exist. Guidelines for curriculum content have been written, standards have been formulated, teaching materials from the ONS and ACS are available, but many undergraduate curricula remain inadequate in content.

Advanced level

The advanced level of cancer nursing education encompasses graduate education. Education at this level is concerned with the development of a broader scope of practice, coordination, continuity, and evaluation of care. Most of the literature at this level is concerned with master's programs.

The *Master's Degree with a Specialty in Advanced Practice in Oncology Nursing* publication is an invaluable tool for faculty of all graduate oncology programs.[27] Its purpose is to provide a role definition and curriculum guide for educators planning educational offerings as well as a program selection guide for students. The guide encompasses the nine content areas of clinical practice: (1) education, (2) consultation, (3) collaboration, (4) systems, (5) role competency, (6) research, (7) outcomes evaluation, (8) program development, and (9) leadership. Each area is organized by steps of the nursing process, suggested content, and outcome objectives. Another valuable tool is the *Statement on the Scope and Standards of Advanced Practice in Oncology Nursing*.[29]

Approximately forty colleges and universities offer graduate oncology programs, according to the Education Committee of the ONS.[30] Each program has unique qualities, and obviously any program should be carefully examined before an applicant selects a school.[31] Questions that potential students should ask to assess and choose the appropriate program, include:

- What is the reputation of the school?
- Who are the faculty?
- What are the resources of the school?
- What will the clinical experiences be like?
- Will oncology clinical nurse specialists be clinical preceptors?
- What is the tuition?
- Are sources of funding, or research or teaching assistantship positions available?

Several studies have reported development of instruments to test graduate student knowledge, attitudes, and skills. As part of their program evaluation, Piper, Moore, and Dodd studied changes in knowledge and attitudes in two cohorts of graduate students in oncology nursing.[32] Significant improvements were obtained in the knowledge domain, while significant changes on the attitude instrument were lacking. The faculty used the test scores to recommend remedial work.

A follow-up study evaluated the students' ability to apply their knowledge to clinical practice during the 2-year master's program.[33] Thirty-nine students ranked the frequency of use and degree of proficiency of clinical behaviors. Students rated themselves more proficient in the more frequently used behaviors, gained proficiency over time, and were more proficient in subject matter that was emphasized in the program.

In a survey of 185 clinical nurse specialists (CNSs) who were ONS members employed in oncology, Yasko found in 1983 that 69% of the specialists reported that their graduate programs lacked theoretical content or planned experiences in oncology nursing.[34] Sixty percent of the sample did not have planned contact with a CNS role model in the curriculum. This lack of preparation in oncology theory and practice appears shocking at first, but it may be explained by the fact that the respondents received their master's degrees from sixty different colleges. Because there were only forty-five oncology graduate programs in 1990 and far fewer in 1983 when the study was conducted, many of the nurses in the sample must have graduated from schools that did not have oncology programs. In any event, one could question if these specialists met the qualifications for the job at the time they were hired.

Continuing Education

It seems to be universally accepted that nurses must participate in CE to maintain and enhance the special knowledge and skills required in oncology nursing. Because baccalaureate and graduate programs do not always have the time or the flexibility to cover all areas, CE must be relied on to provide some of the needed content. In addition, with a rapidly changing knowledge base and evolution in health care delivery, up-to-date information must be supplied to practicing nurses.

Many CE programs are sponsored by the ONS and ACS, at both the national and the local levels. The content for CE programs in oncology nursing can be identified from many sources, including the ONS publications that describe the scope and standards of education and practice.[6,17,29]

The *Standards for Continuing Education in Nursing*, published by the ANA, may be useful as a general guide for those who plan CE programs.[35] Since 1988 the ONS has been an ANA-accredited approver and provider of CE programs and can assist with the planning of CE materials and programs.

Another helpful resource is a series of articles that describe how to develop and implement a CE program by incorporating adult learning principles.[36-40] The articles take the novice through the steps of conducting a needs assessment, developing objectives, defining content and methods, and evaluating a program.

The ONS must provide CE to its members to help them maintain the knowledge and skills necessary for competent practice. In order to ensure successful CE program planning, the ONS conducted a needs assessment of its membership to determine overall learning needs.[41] A questionnaire was developed and mailed to half of the membership (approximately 6500 members) and 38% responded. The top five topics of interest were the clinical practice issues of oncological emergencies, pain, critical care, legal issues, and advanced practice roles.

Donaldson et al worked to identify content areas that were priorities for planning CE programs.[42] They developed an 87-item knowledge test based on the proposed core curriculum for certification examination. Topics earmarked as the highest priority for CE program planning included nursing management of spinal cord compression; electrolyte imbalance; hypercalcemia; susceptibility to depression; treatment modalities such as chemotherapy and safe handling of drugs; prevention and early detection of cancer; characteristics of cancer; ONS standards; and patient advocacy. The nurses who participated in the study provided cancer management care but did not designate themselves as oncology specialists.

Bushy and Kost confronted the issue of inaccessibility of CE programs in rural North Dakota and formulated a novel but successful model for delivering CE programs.[43] Recognizing that hiring a consultant or bringing a prepared program to a small institution would be costly, the program planners decided to follow Knowles' model of adult learning and placed the responsibility for learning in the realm of the learners. The nurse participants selected a topic, listed objectives, and made active learning assignments. For a CE program on breast cancer, the nurse participants gathered information from community resources, had mammograms, visited radiation therapy departments, interviewed patients about mastectomies, went to stores that sold prostheses, visited support groups, participated in other action activities, and then shared their information. Based on increased attendance and active participation, the new CE model is believed to be successful. The model also encourages peer discussion and familiarization with the community and its resources.

In addition to formal continuing education programs, the Internet provides access to information and resources that offer opportunities to enhance the practice of the oncology nurse.

Critical Issues and Challenges

A number of critical issues and challenges in cancer nursing must be considered and discussed, and a strategic plan developed to address them. Nurse educators and nursing service administrators in hospitals and community agencies must meet to make intelligent decisions that are in the best interest of the community.

Recruitment of Students

Recruitment of highly qualified students is essential at all levels—particularly at the master's and doctoral levels—to ensure an adequate supply of clinicians, specialists, teachers, and researchers in oncology nursing. Because admissions to undergraduate and graduate-level nursing programs have declined over the past few years, a concerted effort must be made to attract the traditional as well as the older, nontraditional student, an often untapped resource. For such efforts to be successful, more flexibility may be needed in programs and course offerings to allow students to study part-time if necessary, due to high tuition costs and family responsibilities. Web-based courses may provide this flexibility.

Cultural Diversity

Schools must strive for racial and economic diversity among students and faculty that more closely mirrors society. Racial and ethnic minorities represent 25% of the population, but they constitute only 10% of the registered nurses in the United States.

Recruitment of minority nurses is crucial. A critical mass of minority nurses who are able to work with populations to deliver culturally competent care and encourage prevention and early-detection practices will help reduce high mortality rates. Studies have suggested that caregivers from the same culture provide the best care for the socioeconomically disadvantaged.[44] Once enrolled in nursing programs, financial, academic, and other supportive services must be provided to ensure student success. Subsequently, creative clinical placements and experiences may be needed for minority nurses to reach the target population of patients. Some nontraditional settings that might be used are screening programs in food pantries, feeding centers, or storefront free health clinics, and church- or school-sponsored screening programs.

More and more students from other countries are studying in schools in the United States. Many of these students need assistance with socialization and language skills and other types of support. It is essential that resources be identified to help foreign students with the necessary transitions needed. In today's global society, it is inevitable that more students from the United States also will be studying abroad.

Distance Learning

Distance learning is acquiring knowledge and skills through mediated information and instruction that encompasses all technologies and other kinds of learning at a distance.[45] Traditional education has focused on the college or university, where students learn from faculty, participate in clinical experiences, and share information with other students. With an increasing demand for flexible scheduling and educational opportunities close to home, more educational institutions are exploring how to meet students' needs through technology and distance learning.

Distance learning may be asynchronous or synchronous. *Asynchronous learning* allows individuals to access educational materials and contact other students independently at a time and place of their choosing.[46] With *synchronous learning*, the interaction between instructor and learner takes place at the same time, such as in a telephone conference or a computer chat room or two-way video technology.[46] The use of technology and distance learning have provided new opportunities and new challenges to nurse educators. Distance education requires new roles and skills. It often requires redesign of courses, enhanced computer skills, and learning new ways to relate to students. Research is needed to determine the best practices for teaching and learning at a distance.

A significant number of resources are available for oncology nurses on the Internet. There are numerous sites that offer credible information on practice guide-lines, specific sites of cancer, symptom management, and patient education. In addition, there are numerous on-line publications and opportunities for networking and continuing education. Nurses must have the skills needed to access this information and critically evaluate the quality of the site.

Practitioner, Specialist, or Blended Role

Highly knowledgeable and highly skilled advanced practice nurses (APN) who can function in multiple roles and settings will be crucial as we enter the twenty-first century. Advanced practice nurses with certification as clinical nurse specialist, nurse practitioner, or with blended roles will help meet future challenges in diverse health care settings. Most oncology programs have traditionally prepared CNSs who have provided exemplary care, made extraordinary contributions, and moved the nursing profession ahead. However, in the many settings of today's health care arena, different skills are required to meet the varied needs of individuals with cancer and their families. The roles of the APN are diverse and are expanding and evolving rapidly. The outcomes of the APN's efforts must be evaluated and the results shared.

Standards and the Curriculum

The curriculum in schools of nursing must be geared to meet changing demographics, new and expanding roles for nurses, and the need for collaborative, interdisciplinary practice. All nurses must possess analytical and communication skills and be prepared to negotiate what can be a political medical system. Faculty should be familiar with the recommended curriculum and follow the guidelines set forth in the *Standards of Oncology Nursing Education*.[16] As mentioned earlier, efforts began in the 1950s to incorporate cancer nursing into the curriculum. Now, 50 years later, we are still struggling to incorporate cancer nursing content at the undergraduate level. Basic information about oncology must be included in baccalaureate programs. We have the tools and faculty, but curricula vary greatly in cancer content. Perhaps more definitive guidelines, similar to the master's degree guidelines, at the undergraduate level must be written. Evaluation of all programs should be ongoing.

While still in school, students must be encouraged to share their knowledge, skills, and expertise with others. The nursing curriculum should include content on publishing. In order to improve the oncology nursing practice, practicing nurses at all levels must share ideas. Today, several journals and numerous textbooks are devoted to oncology nursing. Although there has been exponential growth in the number of publications by oncology nurses, still more creative work needs to be shared.

Students also need public-speaking skills, media awareness training, and should be well-versed in the legislative process and public policy issues. A working knowledge of nursing informatics and hospital information systems is essential. *Nursing informatics* is the science of the properties, structure, storage, and transmission of nursing knowledge. Hospital information systems involve the dedicated use of computers to collect, store, process, retrieve, and communicate patient care and administrative information to support those who provide care. Graduates of nursing programs must be computer literate and know how to access and convey information via electronic networks.

Students should be encouraged to participate in local and national ACS and ONS activities or, if specializing in pediatrics, APON activities. Participation should be mandatory, particularly at the graduate level. The meetings and conferences held by these organizations offer many opportunities to participate on committees, speak at meetings, and hold office. The opportunities to network with others, share ideas, and interact with the leaders in oncology nursing abound in these organizations and can only enhance one's career.

Teaching Approaches

Adult learning principles must be employed in our curricula. We live in a rapidly changing health care environment that requires us to modify not only the way patient care services are provided, but also the way we educate nurses to provide these services. The rising cost of health care, increasingly sophisticated technologies, complex treatment protocols, and the demand for more and better health care are catalysts for changing our educational approaches. Program content and learning experiences must be structured at all levels to acknowledge the nurse as an adult learner. Adult learning concepts—including problem-centered approaches to teaching, immediate application of knowledge, recognition of individual experience, flexible scheduling, and self-directed learning—must be incorporated in educational offerings. In addition, computer-assisted instruction (CAI) should be incorporated into curricula. All students must be computer literate.

To prepare students for future interdisciplinary collaboration, cooperative learning techniques must be incorporated into the classroom setting. As health care becomes increasingly community based, technology is evolving to enable the communication and management of health care information at the "point of care" in homes and community settings. Our students must be prepared to practice in these settings.

Faculty Competence

Faculty at all levels should know current trends in oncology nursing. In addition, faculty must be as clinically competent as clinical specialists and nurse practitioners. Attendance at oncology CE programs or required certification may help, but this will not completely solve the problem of keeping faculty clinically competent. The clinical doctorate (DNS and DNSc) is not a solution to clinical competence unless the graduates of these programs keep their skills and expertise current. Faculty must base their teaching on the reality of clinical practice. Although some schools allow faculty to have joint appointments, this is not feasible for all faculty. It is likely that in the future, practice will become as central to a faculty member's role as teaching, research, and service. New and different ways to ensure competency must be explored.

New forms of collaboration between faculty and clinical staff should be developed to provide faculty entrance and exposure to the clinical arena. A faculty consultation service in clinical sites might be developed that would provide benefits to all involved. Faculty have much theoretical knowledge that can be shared with clinical staff, and likewise clinical staff has much clinical practice knowledge to share. Another innovation might be joint research projects between faculty and clinical specialists that would allow faculty exposure to current clinical problems. Faculty collaboration with the nursing staff on clinical papers might also help keep faculty abreast of current practice issues. Faculty might also assist clinical staff with publication while keeping up to date on the latest in practice. Other ways to update faculty may already exist, but these need to be shared in the literature so others can benefit.

Preceptors and Clinical Facilities

Nursing educators must continue to nurture clinical preceptors to act as role models for students in clinical agencies. With the shift toward ambulatory care, adult day care centers, and nursing homes, clinical experience needs to be changed and new sites cultivated. Faculty must assume responsibility for preparing clinical preceptors to work with students. Seminars devoted to adult learning principles, mentoring, evaluation, and how to deal with the difficult student may be helpful in preparing preceptors for their roles. It is essential to recognize the contributions made by preceptors to our clinical programs and to give recognition for their time and commitment to student learning. Such recognition might take the form of appointment as adjunct faculty, which allows library privileges and attendance at school functions, or editorial assistance with manuscripts, which encourages publication.[47] Close cooperation between teachers and clinicians is essential to eliminate the old dichotomy between education and practice. Participation of clinical experts in faculty research projects would benefit both groups.

Doctoral Education

Well-qualified students and graduates of master's programs should be encouraged to continue their education in doctoral programs. Doctorally prepared oncology nurses are needed to ensure high-quality education, research, and practice in the future. Educational programs must emphasize clinically relevant research that builds the science of nursing practice. Nurses must be prepared as visionary leaders, capable of shaping nursing and future practice, not just responding to changes that occur in practice. Doctoral programs must also prepare future faculty. It is worrisome that nursing faculty are "greying" and will soon retire, resulting in a shortage in the near future.

Certification and Recertification

Certification can offer many intrinsic and extrinsic rewards to the individual: increased visibility, salary differential, peer recognition, self-satisfaction, prestige, and sometimes an edge in the job market. Sixty percent of the nurses who passed the original certification examination took the generalist recertification exam. This is comparable to other specialty organizations. However, less than half of ONS members are certified. Efforts need to continue to increase the numbers of members who are certified.

Health Care Reform

In the rapidly changing health care environment that involves restructuring, redesign, and reengineering of the health care delivery system, nurses must be kept well-informed and involved in the decision-making process. *Restructuring* is dedicated to reducing waste while cutting costs. *Reengineering* examines the process of what and how things are accomplished. *Redesign*, or decision making about who does what, should assure that the most appropriately trained and educated staff are doing the work they are best suited to do.[48] Restructuring and reengineering, for the most part, are positive. However, redesign has resulted in layoffs of nurses, decreased staffing, or a change in the mix of workers that can create unsafe conditions. Registered professional nurses have been replaced with unlicensed and ill-trained personnel who are performing skills at the bedside for which they are not qualified; hospital staff are being cross-trained to streamline care; and new graduates are having difficulty obtaining positions.[48] Nurses have been protesting with rallies, picketing, strikes, negotiation, and arbitration, and are taking the necessary steps to assure that high-quality care is delivered by registered nurses. Oncology nurses need to demonstrate that they are committed to professional competency through credentialing, educating consumers about the profession, and conducting outcome-based research to demonstrate that specialized care and credentialing improves the quality of care while maintaining cost effectiveness.[49]

Meeting New Health Care Challenges

More emphasis must be placed on prevention, risk reduction, and early detection activities in our schools. Most authorities believe that a large number of cancers could be prevented if people would choose healthier lifestyles. It is estimated that one in four individuals could be saved through early detection. The NCI has proposed that cancer mortality be reduced by 50% by the year 2000. Much of the activity in prevention and early detection is concentrated on breast, cervical, and lung cancer, with the majority of activity related to breast cancer. Nurses can have a powerful impact on patients in prevention and early detection activities for the major sites of cancer. The nurse's role in primary and secondary prevention of cancer has been well documented.[50] Nurses must be familiar with the goals of the NCI and strive to increase the span of healthy life, reduce health disparities, reduce disability from chronic conditions, and achieve preventive services for all.

Today more than 6 million Americans are survivors of cancer, and it is expected that by the twenty-first century more than 65% of individuals diagnosed with cancer will survive longer than 5 years. This will have an enormous impact on delivery of services, rehabilitation, and quality-of-life issues. While more people are living with cancer, more and more people are becoming infected with HIV and dying of AIDS. It is expected that 20,000 children will have AIDS by the year 2000. Patient care will become increasingly community-based and home-centered, and self-care will be an expectation. Nurses must be prepared to meet the challenges of a diverse spectrum of patients and problems. The content of our educational programs must reflect the current and future problems and concerns of the health care arena. We can never become complacent about what we do in cancer education or practice, for new challenges continually arise, requiring innovative solutions and application of new knowledge and skills.

Advances in technology and early discharge practices have changed both inpatient and outpatient care. The use of ambulatory services has greatly escalated because of technological advances, changes in insurance reimbursement, and consumer choice. The majority of cancer care is delivered in the outpatient setting. Patients cared for in the home today are far sicker, with many more complex needs, than hospital patients of yesterday. This calls for changing roles and responsibilities of nurses in ambulatory and home settings, and more emphasis on these roles must be given in the curriculum.

By the year 2020, the elderly population in the United States will double, providing new challenges and opportunities for creative approaches to prevention, early detection, and provision of care to elderly persons. Curricula in schools of nursing must include information on how to plan programs to incorporate healthy behaviors into lifestyles, and information specific to teaching and providing care to the elderly.

Oncology nurses face complex problems. It is necessary to nurture and support all members of the specialty, for competition and jealousy can interfere with a powerful, united front. Collaboration between all members of the health care team is essential, and we must focus on cost-effective practices and maintain adaptability to changing scientific, social, and economic conditions. Baird states that we are practicing at a time when future directions have never been less clear.[51] She challenges oncology nurses to look carefully at the major paradigms of change and to ask how we can use our experience and skills to continue to make a difference.

Conclusion

Much has been accomplished in oncology nursing. Educational programs exist at all levels of undergraduate, graduate, and continuing education. Oncology nursing has enjoyed strong support from many organizations. Many nurses have been certified in oncology nursing at the generalist and the advanced level. A large number of highly motivated, effective, and productive advanced practice oncology nurses have made numerous contributions to practice, education, and research. Craytor said, "We owe much to the bold, intelligent, persuasive, and clinically able nurses who pioneered in the field. They were and are a truly remarkable group."[3,p.57]

As oncology nurses, we should be proud of our accomplishments, but at the same time we must recognize the continual need to update knowledge, skills, and competence. We cannot abandon the good things that have been achieved over the years, nor can we rest on our laurels. We must continue to evaluate, change, improve, and think in new and creative ways and always be prepared to meet new challenges as they arise. Oncology nurses must remain vigilant so that the emphasis on cost reduction does not endanger the quality of care given to patients and their families. We must articulate to patients and families the vital role of the oncology nurse and what constitutes quality cancer care.

References

1. Hilkemeyer R: A historical perspective in cancer nursing. *Oncol Nurs Forum* 9:47–56, 1982
2. Diller D: *An Investigation of Cancer Learning in Ninety Selected Schools of Nursing, Third Report.* Saratoga Springs, NY, Skidmore College, 1957
3. Craytor JC: Highlights in education for cancer nursing. *Oncol Nurs Forum* 9:51–59, 1982
4. Piemme JA: Oncology clinical nurse specialist education. *Oncol Nurs Forum* 12:45–48, 1985
5. Longman AJ: Cancer nursing education, in Groenwald SL, Frogge MH, Goodman M, Yarbro CH (eds): *Cancer Nursing: Principles and Practice* (ed 2). Sudbury, MA, Jones and Bartlett, 1990, pp 1256–1269
6. Oncology Nursing Society: *Outcome Standards for Cancer Nursing Education at the Fundamental Level.* Pittsburgh, Oncology Nursing Society, 1982
7. Available at http://www.cancer.org. Accessed Dec. 12, 1999
8. Varricchio C: *A Cancer Source Book for Nurses* (ed 7). Sudbury, MA, Jones and Bartlett, 1997
9. Yarbro CH: The history of cancer nursing, in Baird SB, McCorkle R, Grant M (eds): *Cancer Nursing: A Comprehensive Textbook.* Philadelphia, Saunders, 1991, pp 10–20
10. Oberst M: Priorities in cancer nursing research. *Cancer Nurs* 11:61–62, 1984
11. Miller S, Herbst S: Summary of ONS membership survey. *Oncol Nurs Forum* 5:22–23, 1978
12. Van Scoy-Mosher C: *Oncology Nursing Survey.* Pittsburgh, Oncology Nursing Society, 1979
13. Siegele D: Longitudinal evaluation of a model post-master's program in oncology nursing education. *Oncol Nurs Forum* 11:61–62, 1984
14. National Cancer Institute: *Cancer Nurse Training Program.* Washington, DC, National Institutes of Health, 1987
15. Available at: http://www.APON.org. Accessed Dec. 12, 1999
16. McMillan SC, Heusinkveld K, Spray J: A study of the role of the generalist oncology nurse as a basis for revision of the blueprint for certification. *Oncol Nurs Forum* 24:1371–1379, 1997
17. Oncology Nursing Society Education Committee: *Standards of Oncology Nursing Education: Generalist and Advanced Practice Levels.* Pittsburgh, Oncology Nursing Society, 1989
18. Brown JK, Johnson JL, Groenwald SL: Survey of cancer nursing education in U.S. schools of nursing. *Oncol Nurs Forum* 10:82–83, 1983
19. Pope S: Fundamentals for a new concept of oncology nursing in the professional nursing education program. *Cancer Nurs* 15:137–147, 1992
20. Copp K: Education and training in cancer: A European perspective. *Cancer Nurs* 11:255–258, 1986
21. Nevidjon B, Deatrich J: Oncology clinical elective. *Oncol Nurs Forum* 12:57–59, 1985
22. Horvitz I, Trigg JM: Registered nurses and nursing students learn together in a cancer nursing course. *J Nurs Educ* 12: 6, 18, 42, 1987
23. Mooney M, Dudas S: Undergraduate independent study in cancer nursing. *Oncol Nurs Forum* 14:51–53, 1987
24. Rushton P: An undergraduate oncology nursing course. *Oncol Nurs Forum* 26:75–79, 1999
25. Quinn-Casper P, Holmgren C: Enhancing cancer nursing concepts in undergraduate curricula. *Cancer Nurs* 10: 274–278, 1987
26. Longman AJ, Verran JA, Clark M: Oncology knowledge inventory for undergraduate students. *Oncol Nurs Forum* 18: 107–111, 1991
27. Longman A, Verran J, Clark L: Improving oncology nursing content in an undergraduate program. *J Nurs Educ* 27:42–44, 1988
28. Oncology Nursing Society, American Nurses Association: *The Master's Degree with a Specialty in Oncology Nursing.* Pittsburgh, Oncology Nursing Society, 1988
29. Oncology Nursing Press: *Statement on the Scope and Standards of Advanced Practice in Oncology Nursing.* Pittsburgh, PA, Oncology Nursing Press, 1997
30. Survey of graduate programs in cancer nursing. *Oncol Nurs Forum* 25:1435–1442, 1998
31. Brown JK, Hinds P: Assessing Masters' programs in advanced practice oncology nursing. *Oncol Nurs Forum* 25:1433–1434, 1998
32. Piper B, Moore I, Dodd M: Changes in cancer-related knowledge and attitudes: One graduate curriculum's experience. *Cancer Nurs* 8:272–277, 1985
33. Moore IM, Piper B, Dodd MJ, et al: Measuring oncology

nursing practice: Results from one graduate program. *Oncol Nurs Forum* 14:45–49, 1987

34. Yasko J: A survey of oncology clinical nursing specialists. *Oncol Nurs Forum* 10:25–30, 1983

35. American Nurses Association: *Standards for Continuing Education in Nursing.* Kansas City, MO, American Nurses Association, 1984

36. Fernsler J: Developing continuing education programs in cancer nursing: An overview. *Oncol Nurs Forum* 14:59–60, 1987

37. Volker DL: Learning needs assessment. *Oncol Nurs Forum* 14:60–62, 1987

38. Itano J: Developing educational objectives. *Oncol Nurs Forum* 14:62–65, 1987

39. Belcher A: Defining content and methods. *Oncol Nurs Forum* 14:65–67, 1987

40. McMillan S: Program evaluation. *Oncol Nurs Forum* 14:67–70, 1987

41. Itano J, Miller CA: Learning needs of Oncology Nursing Society members. *Oncol Nurs Forum* 17:697–706, 1990

42. Donaldson WS, Glass EC, Helmick F, et al: Determining continuing education priorities in cancer management for nurses. *Oncol Nurs Forum* 15:625–630, 1988

43. Bushy A, Kost S: A model of continuing education for rural oncology nurses. *Oncol Nurs Forum* 17:207–211, 1990

44. American Cancer Society: *Special Report on Cancer in the Economically Disadvantaged.* New York, American Cancer Society, 1986

45. Available at: http://www.usdla.org. Accessed Dec. 21, 1999

46. Triestman J, Watson D, Fullerton L: Computer mediated distributive learning. *J Nurse Midwifery* 41:392–398, 1994

47. Hagopian GA, Ferszt GA, Jacobs LA, et al: Preparing clinical preceptors to teach master's level students in oncology nursing. *J Prof Nurs* 8:295–300, 1992

48. Ketter J: Restructuring: Affecting the workforce and workplace for the new graduate. *Am Nurs* 10:4, 1995 (suppl)

49. Erickyon J: Editors' message. *OCCN News* 9:2, 1995

50. Frank-Stromborg M, Rohan K: Nursing's involvement in the primary and secondary prevention of cancer. *Cancer Nurs* 15:79–108, 1992

51. Baird SB: The impact of changing health care delivery on oncology practice. *Oncol Nurs* 2:1–13, 1995

CHAPTER 79

Role of the Oncology Advanced Practice Nurse

Annette Galassi, RN, MA, CANP, AOCN

Introduction

This is an exciting time to be an oncology advanced practice nurse. Barriers to practice are collapsing as direct reimbursement of advanced practice nursing services is no longer limited by setting or geographic area. Paradigms are shifting. The title "Nurse Practitioner" is no longer synonymous with primary care just as the title "Clinical Specialist" is no longer synonymous with specialty-based practice. This chapter explores the history of advanced practice nursing, describes the educational preparation required for oncology advanced practice, and reviews critical issues including the regulation of advanced practice and third-party reimbursement. Finally, a portrait of oncology advanced practice nursing in the twenty-first century is projected by describing its emerging roles.

History of Advanced Practice Nursing

The Nurse Practitioner Movement

A nurse practitioner (NP) is a registered nurse who has advanced education and clinical training in a specialty area such as adult health or women's health. Nurse practitioners obtain medical histories, perform physical examinations, make medical and nursing diagnoses, and treat persons with common health problems and chronic diseases. Since nursing practice is regulated by the nurse practice statutes of the state in which the NP is employed, the amount of autonomy the NP has in performing these functions varies from state to state.

The NP role originated in 1965 with a demonstration project at the University of Colorado to prepare pediatric nurse practitioners.[1] A perceived shortage of physicians, attributed to the siphoning of physicians to specialty practice, was the major impetus for the development of the NP role. The goal of the project by Lorretta Ford was to "develop a new educational and training experience (for professional nurses) to prepare them to assume an expanded role in child health as practitioners of nursing."[1] Shortly thereafter, family nurse practitioner programs were begun at the University of Washington, Cornell-New York Hospital, and the University of California, Davis. Most of these early NP programs were continuing education offerings or certificate programs affiliated with medical schools. The programs varied in length, quality, and content. Admission criteria also varied, with some programs requiring only that one be a registered nurse with a current license to practice.[2] Upon completion, the graduate alternatively might have received nothing, a certificate, a baccalaureate degree, or a master's degree.

In 1974, the American Nurses' Association (ANA) Congress on Nursing Practice published the first definitions of the roles of the NP. This was followed by the publication of guidelines for the preparation of adult and family nurse practitioners in continuing education programs. Guidelines for NP preparation subsequently have been developed by several nursing organizations including the American Academy of Nurse Practitioners; the Association of Women's Health, Obstetric, and Neonatal Nurses; the American College of Nurse-Midwives; and the National Association of Pediatric Nurse Associates and Practitioners. Graduates of programs that adhere to the guidelines are eligible to take certification examinations sponsored by these organizations.

In 1979 the National League for Nursing, an agency that accredits schools of nursing, declared in their position statement on NP education that the NP should hold a master's degree in nursing. As of 1992 the American Nurses' Credentialing Center has required a master's degree or higher in nursing for certification as an adult, family, pediatric, school, or gerontological NP. Master's level education for NPs also is supported by the American Academy of Nurse Practitioners and the American Association of Colleges of Nursing.[3,4]

NP education has gradually shifted away from certificate programs. Today, most nurse practitioner programs are graduate level programs in schools of nursing. It is estimated that currently there are only 13 certificate programs for NPs,[5] whereas there are 312 master's-level and/or post-master's NP programs.[6] By the year 2007, all NP certifying bodies will require a master's degree for certification eligibility.[7]

The Development of the Clinical Nurse Specialist Role

While the NP role evolved with a strong focus on the medical model, the clinical nurse specialist (CNS) role was based on nursing models.[8] A CNS is a master's-prepared registered nurse who has expert knowledge and skill in caring for a population of patients within a given specialty. Most authors agree on a core of four functional components of the CNS role: clinical practice, education, consultation, and research. Leader/manager and change agent have also been cited as functional components.[9]

The first master's degree program with a clinical specialty was developed by Hildegard Peplau at Rutgers University in 1954.[10] Factors that led to the development of nurse specialists included a rapid expansion in scientific knowledge, an increasingly complex health care system, a shortage of health care personnel, and a heightened focus on public health care needs.[11] Nurse educators proposed the role of the CNS to counter the impersonal, fragmented, authoritarian, and tradition-based nursing practice that had developed following World War II.[12] The role was seen as a clinical option to the more traditional educator and administrator roles of graduate-level nursing education.

Specialization in health care was the trend in the 1970s, fostered by dramatic increases in knowledge and technology. Specialty-focused patient care areas were developed within the hospital and the expectation was that a CNS could provide expert bedside care, function as a role model for nursing staff, improve the quality of nursing care, and implement clinical nursing research in these areas. Initially, there was debate about the title and educational preparation of these nurses in expanded roles. Nurses with and without graduate degrees in nursing were using the title "CNS" or "Nurse Clinician." In 1965 the ANA published a position paper stating that "CNS" should be used only by nurses with a master's degree in nursing.[8] The ANA Social Policy Statement (1980) further defined the title CNS as an expert in a defined area of knowledge and practice with advanced preparation at the graduate level.[13] The ANA Council of Clinical Nurse Specialists, formed in 1980, was instrumental in developing the statement on the role of the CNS that established the four functional role components of expert practitioner, educator, consultant, and researcher.[14] Unlike the initial proliferation of certificate programs for the preparation of NPs there were no such programs for CNSs. Almost all CNS programs were developed at the master's-degree level.

The Trend Toward Merged Roles

NP practice traditionally has focused on primary care in an ambulatory setting while specialty-focused acute care has been within the domain of the CNS. Mundinger proposed that nurse practitioners care for patients while they are standing up and clinical nurse specialists care for patients while they are lying down.[15] This is no longer true. The boundaries that have traditionally existed between the NP and CNS are becoming less distinct and practice settings can no longer be used to distinguish one group of advanced practice nurses from another. Some NPs are specialty-focused or practice in an acute care setting, and some CNSs practice in an ambulatory setting.

Several research studies have been published that support the notion that the CNS and NP roles are more similar than different.[16–20] Elder and Bullough, in a survey of NP and CNS alumni from a master's of nursing program, found that both the CNS and NP participated in patient and family teaching, counseling, psychosocial assessments, and use of the nursing process related to treatment regimens. The major difference between the two groups was that NPs spent more time in direct care and CNSs spent more time in indirect care.[16]

Forbes and colleagues conducted a survey of core curricula of graduate nursing programs that prepare clinical nurse specialists and nurse practitioners. The results of this survey suggested that the major difference in the preparation for these roles lies not in the curricula content but in the practice setting in which the role is operationalized.[17] This was also borne out in a comparative analysis of the CNS and NP role by Fenton and Brykczynski. The authors found that there was an advanced practice role for both the CNS and the NP and that much of the knowledge, skills, and competencies are shared. As a result, the authors have suggested that graduate schools of nursing consolidate the core curriculum for the advanced practice nursing programs.[18]

The results of Williams and Valdivieso's survey of advanced practice nurses in South Carolina also supported the similarities of the CNS and NP roles. Differences were primarily related to relative emphasis on direct practice. NPs spent more time in direct practice whereas CNSs spent more time in the indirect roles of educator and consultant.[20]

The educational preparation of NPs and CNSs also is becoming more similar. With the shift of NP preparation to the graduate level, NP education includes nursing theory, research, and education principles. Likewise, CNS education has expanded to include pharmacology and physical assessment.[21] Additionally, nurses with master's degrees in other nursing specialty areas have returned to post-master's nurse practitioner programs to obtain additional education.[22]

The research cited above supports the current trend in education and practice toward a merged role of advanced practice nursing. Further evidence is provided by the merger of the ANA Council of Clinical Nurse Specialists and Council of Primary Health Care Nurse Practitioners in 1990 to form the Council of Nurses in Advanced Practice.[16] Since that time, both CNSs and NPs who pass the American Nurses' Credentialing Center certification examination may use the credential CS (certified specialist).

Advanced Practice Nursing Defined

According to the American Nurses' Association, "Advanced practice registered nurses have acquired the knowledge base and practice experiences to prepare them for specialization, expansion, and advancement in practice."[23] This knowledge and skill is obtained at the master's or doctoral level in nursing. The ANA states that "the term advanced practice is used to refer exclusively to advanced clinical practice. . . . Although nursing educators, administrators, and researchers are prepared educationally at the master's or doctoral level, they are not considered advanced practice registered nurses. . . ."[23]

The American Association of Colleges of Nursing (AACN) has defined "advanced practice nurse" (APN) as an umbrella term appropriate for a licensed registered nurse prepared at the graduate-degree level as either a CNS, NA, NM, or NP.[4] This graduate preparation may focus on primary health care, case management, specialization, education, or administration across health settings.[24] The National League for Nursing (NLN) has recommended the merging of the CNS and NP roles under the title "APN."[25]

Advanced practice nursing as defined by the National Council of State Boards of Nursing includes nurse practitioners, nurse anesthetists, nurse-midwives, and clinical nurse specialists with a graduate degree and a major in nursing or a graduate degree with a concentration in an advanced nursing practice category.[26]

The Oncology Nursing Society (ONS), in its position statement on advanced practice (1997), has endorsed the title "Advanced Practice Nurse" to designate both clinical nurse specialist and nurse practitioner roles.[27] Unlike an earlier position statement (1995), the revised position statement focuses on the nurse in clinical practice and does not include other master's-prepared nurses such as those in administration or education.[28] According to ONS's position statement (1997), APNs are prepared, at a minimum, with a master's degree in nursing with specialty education and precepted clinical experience in oncology. The oncology APN coordinates and provides direct and indirect care to people affected by cancer and collaborates with nurse colleagues and other members of the health care team.[27]

The Evolution of the Oncology Advanced Practice Nurse

The evolution of the oncology advanced practice nursing role was similar to that of the clinical nurse specialist role. The first course in oncology nursing at the graduate level was offered by Teachers' College, Columbia University and Memorial Hospital in New York City in 1947. It consisted of an academic and clinical component and was 16 credit hours.[29] The first specialty tract in oncology nursing was begun at the University of Pittsburgh in 1968 as part of the medical-surgical master's degree in nursing.[30] The first graduate program in oncology nursing was developed at Rush University in Chicago in 1974–1975 under Myra Levine and Sue Hegyvary.

In 1978 the American Cancer Society invited a group of nurse educators, researchers, practitioners, and administrators involved with cancer nursing to meet. The purpose of the meeting was to reach consensus about the role and educational preparation of the specialist in cancer nursing. It resulted in the publication by the American Cancer Society of the first role definition and curriculum guidelines for the master's degree in nursing with a specialization in oncology nursing.[31] The focus was on the educational preparation of the oncology CNS. This guide was revised in collaboration with the ONS in 1986 and most recently in 1994. The third edition, entitled *The Master's Degree with a Specialty in Advanced Practice Oncology Nursing,* has a significantly different focus than previous editions. The current curriculum guide has been broadened to support a blended role of an advanced practice oncology nurse that combines both CNS and NP skills. The authors believe this broad preparation will allow for the greatest flexibility in employment in a variety of cancer practice settings.[32] The course content of the curriculum guide includes clinical practice, education, consultation, collaboration, systems, role competency, research and outcomes evaluation, program development, and leadership.

There are currently 30 master's degree programs in oncology nursing. Some programs are designed as a separate specialty while others are a tract or focus area within a nursing major. These programs vary in length, number of courses specific to oncology nursing, and credit hours in clinical oncology nursing.[33] Historically, the vast majority of these programs focused on the preparation of the oncology CNS. Currently, the specialty title of several of these programs, "Advanced Practice Oncology Nursing," reflects preparation in a blended or merged CNS/NP role.

In 1994, McMillan et al conducted a role delineation study to determine the elements that make up the role of the oncology advanced practice nurse.[34] A 190-item survey was used that consisted of five subscales: direct caregiver, consultant, administrator/coordinator, researcher, and educator. Nearly 640 master's-prepared oncology nurses responded for a 47% return rate. Fifty-eight percent identified their job title as "CNS" while only 7% identified their job title as "NP." A comparative analysis of the advanced practice behaviors of the oncology CNS and NP was not done. Given the relatively small number of respondents who identified themselves as an NP such an analysis was likely to have been impossible. The study results were used by the Oncology Nursing Certification Corporation to design the initial Advanced Oncology Nursing Certification Examination.

The study by McMillan et al was subsequently repeated in 1998.[35] The majority of the items from the 1994 survey were modified to reflect current practice as either a CNS or NP and almost 70 of the initial 190 items were deleted as they no longer applied to either the CNS or NP role. The five subscales of advanced practice were retained. This time, almost 500 usable surveys were returned for a 41% response rate. Of that number, 235 (39%) were CNSs and 258 (43%) were NPs. A comparative analysis of the CNS and NP groups demonstrated that fewer than 10% of the survey items showed a significant difference between the CNS and NP groups. The extensive overlap in behaviors between oncology CNSs and NPs found in this study justifies the use of a single examination for advanced practice oncology nursing. The study results were used to revise the blueprint for the 1999 Advanced Oncology Nursing Examination.

Kinney et al performed a study to describe the role of the oncology nurse practitioner. A questionnaire was mailed to the 218 eligible subjects who identified themselves as NPs on the ONS membership form or were members of the ONS/NP special interest group. Of the 129 subjects who responded, the majority (58%) received their NP preparation at either the master's degree level (49%) or by a post master's certificate. Almost all of the respondents spent more than 40% of their time in clinical practice and less than 20% of their time consulting.[36]

The ONS has defined the various titles in oncology nursing by adding position attributes and clarifying educational preparation required for each title.

ONS recognizes nurses who have become experts in coordinating and providing direct and indirect care to people affected by cancer through study and precepted clinical practice in oncology at the graduate level as oncology CNSs. The term NP describes the nurse whose educational preparation includes completion of a NP program at the master's or doctorate level. The role of the NP is to provide comprehensive clinical care to individuals, with an emphasis on health promotion, disease prevention, diagnosis, and management of acute and chronic diseases. ONS recognizes NPs who have expertise in the specialty of oncology as oncology NPs.[37]

Regulation of Advanced Practice Nursing

"The purpose of any regulation of nursing practice is the protection of public health, safety and welfare."[38] The legal regulation of nursing, including advanced practice, is the responsibility of state boards of nursing. Each state's board is vested with this authority by the state legislature that enacts the state's nurse practice act. This approach has resulted in tremendous variability among states and a "patchwork quilt" of regulation surrounding advanced practice nursing. There is a great deal of inconsistency from state to state in the educational/certification requirements, scope of practice, physician oversight, prescriptive authority, and level of regulatory oversight. There is even inconsistency regarding the definition of an advanced practice registered nurse. For example, some states include NPs, CNMs (Certified Nurse Midwife), CRNAs (Certified Registered Nurse Anesthetist), and CNSs in the definition, others include NPs, CNMs, CRNAs, and only psychiatric-mental health CNSs, and still others include NPs, CNMs, and CRNAs only. These inconsistencies significantly limit the mobility of APNs and create confusion for the public, legislators, and other health care providers.[39]

An advanced practice nurse must obtain information regarding the regulatory requirements in the jurisdiction where the APN intends to practice. The applicant must then provide documentation of eligibility to meet the requirements. The board of nursing evaluates the applicant's credentials against the established criteria and grants authority to practice to those individuals meeting the criteria.

Levels of Regulation

There are four levels of regulation: designation/recognition, registration, certification, and licensure. Designation/recognition is the least restrictive method of regulation and consists of recognition of credentials by a state's board of nursing. It does not involve an inquiry into the competence of the APN by the board. Registration is the placement of names of APNs on an official board roster. It also does not involve an inquiry into competence nor does it define the scope of practice. Certification involves title regulation. The APN must meet

specified, predetermined requirements and only those who meet the requirements may use the title. However, a title only carries legal status if it is recognized or authorized in statute or regulation. Certification attempts to measure competence. Licensure specifies scope of practice and applications for licensure are evaluated to ensure that predetermined requirements are met. Licensure also allows the grantor, such as the board of nursing, to take disciplinary action for violation of laws or rules.[40]

Certification versus Second Licensure

The regulation of advanced practice nursing has become a topic of increased importance for the profession. Opinions vary as to whether certification or second licensure is the appropriate regulatory mechanism for advanced practice. Professional nursing organizations including the ANA have supported voluntary certification while state boards of nursing have favored second licensure. There are difficulties associated with both approaches.

Certification has been used by the ANA and various specialty organizations including ONS for a range of purposes, from recognizing excellence or professional achievement to denoting minimum competency to practice a specialty. There are more than 30 specialty nursing organizations that grant certification to nurses with training beyond the entry level.[41] The Oncology Nursing Certification Corporation is one such organization and offers both a basic and an advanced oncology nursing certification examination.

The term *certification* is confusing since it is used to refer to both specialty certification and advanced practice certification. Advanced practice certification requires education beyond the entry level, usually at the graduate level. However, not all professional organizations that offer advanced practice certification currently require a master's degree. The eligibility criteria for the advanced oncology nursing certification examination is as follows:

- RN license

- Master's degree or higher in nursing, preferably with a focus in oncology

- At least 30 months of experience as an RN within the five years prior to application

- At least 2000 hours of oncology nursing experience within the five years prior to application[42]

The American College of Nurse-Midwives and the Council on Certification for Nurse Anesthetists use certification to denote minimum competency to practice these specialties but do not require a master's degree. Practice and experience requirements and recertification requirements also vary among organizations (see Table 79-1).

Many professional nursing organizations, including the ANA, have supported the regulation of advanced practice through the mechanism of voluntary certification. This mechanism was established and is operated

Table 79-1 Professional Organizations Offering Advanced Practice Certification Examinations

Organization	Master's Degree
American Academy of Nurse Practitioners	No
American College of Nurse Midwifery Certification Council, Inc.	No
American Nurses' Credentialing Center	Yes, since 1992
The Council on Certification for Nurse Anesthetists	No
National Certification Board of Pediatric Nurse Practitioners and Nurses	No
The National Certification Corporation for the Obstetric, Gynecologic and Neonatal Nursing Specialties	No

by professional nursing specialty organizations. Through certification, the profession maintains autonomy and responsibility for the regulation of advanced practice whereas through second licensure that control is assumed by state boards of nursing. The National Council of State Boards of Nursing (NCSBN) advocates licensure of APNs on the basis that the degree of autonomy and level of care provided by the APN warrants that level of regulation.[43]

A standardized certification process for advanced practice nursing would eliminate much of the criticism of the current certification process and potentially abolish the need for a second license to regulate nursing practice. Movement toward such a standardized certification process has begun. In 1991, the American Nurses' Credentialing Center (ANCC) and other certification boards formed the American Board of Nursing Specialties (ABNS). Membership in the ABNS is limited to those advanced practice nursing certification bodies that meet ABNS standards. This board is analogous to the American Board of Medical Specialties and other professional boards that certify individuals to specialize in a particular practice area.

In many states, national certification is used to regulate advanced nursing practice. To correct this disparity, the NCSBN and various national certification organizations agreed to an external review of certification examinations by the National Commission on Certifying Agencies (NCAA). The focus of this review was to ensure that the examination is designed to test entry-level competencies and job-related knowledge and skills, is pass/fail at the point of the minimum-essential level for safety and effectiveness, and uses generally acceptable testing practices. The major professional organizations that offer advanced practice certification examinations, including the American Nurses Credentialing Center Commission on Certification, the American Academy of Nurse Practitioners, and the National Certification Corporation for women's health specialties, have received full NCAA accreditation.[43]

Prescriptive Authority

The authority for the APN to prescribe is regulated at the state level. The level of authority varies from independent prescriptive authority including controlled substances to dependent authority excluding controlled substances (see Table 79-2). The dependent authority requires that the APN be under supervision of a physician when performing this task. As of 1999, all 50 states and the District of Columbia provide for some level of prescriptive authority for APNs.[44]

Controlled Substances

In states where APNs are allowed to prescribe controlled substances, Drug Enforcement Administration (DEA) registration numbers are required. The DEA has established a mid-level practitioner registration category under which APNs, physician assistants (PAs), and others are given individual DEA registration numbers. These numbers begin with the letter "M" to allow responsible parties in the controlled substance distribution chain (e.g., pharmacists) to contact appropriate state officials to verify the authority the practitioner has been granted. DEA registration allows a wide variety of acts including purchasing, storing, administering, dispensing, and prescribing controlled substances; however, the APN may engage in only those activities authorized by the state in which they practice.[45] Figure 79-1 provides information on obtaining a DEA registration number.

Table 79-2 Level of Prescriptive Authority by State

Independent Prescriptive Authority including controlled substances	Alaska, Arizona, District of Columbia, Iowa, Montana, New Mexico, Oregon, Vermont, Washington, Wisconsin, Wyoming
Dependent Prescriptive Authority including controlled substances	Arkansas, Connecticut, Georgia, Indiana, Louisiana, Massachusetts, Maryland, Minnesota, Mississippi,* North Carolina, North Dakota, Nebraska, New York, Pennsylvania, Rhode Island, South Carolina,* South Dakota, Utah, West Virginia
Dependent Prescriptive Authority excluding controlled substances	Alabama, California, Florida, Hawaii, Idaho, Kansas, Kentucky, Michigan, Missouri, New Jersey, Nevada, Ohio,* Tennessee, Texas, Virginia
No Prescriptive Authority	Illinois, Oklahoma

*In specific situations.

An application for registration may be obtained along with the *Mid-level Practitioner's Manual* by mailing or telephoning a request to:

United States Department of Justice
Drug Enforcement Administration
Central Station
P.O. Box 28083
Washington, DC 20038-8083
(202) 307-7255

Some states require state-issued controlled substance registration numbers in addition to a DEA registration number. The state number must be obtained prior to applying for a DEA registration number. Contact the DEA for further information.

Figure 79-1   DEA registration information.

Research Related to Prescriptive Authority

As regulatory changes are made that grant APNs prescriptive authority, implementation of these changes and their effects on access to care, clinical practice, and patient outcomes need to be evaluated. A small, pilot study by Mahoney suggests that employers and administrators may be resistant to NPs prescribing medications even after a state has granted NPs this authority.[46] Such an arbitrary restriction on practice reduces the NPs efficiency, devalues the role, and limits the ability to provide a full range of health care services. Sekscenski and associates evaluated state practice environments for PAs, NPs, and CNMs.[47] The investigators used legal status, reimbursement, and prescriptive authority to identify states with favorable practice environments. Lack of prescriptive authority was an important factor in states with generally unfavorable practice environments. State practice environment scores for NPs were lowest (least favorable) for Ohio and Illinois and highest (most favorable) for Oregon, Montana, and North Dakota.

Hamric and colleagues studied the safety and efficacy of APN prescriptive authority using three different outcome measures: the APN's assessment of the patient's outcome, the patient's assessment of their outcome, and the collaborating physician's assessment of APN practice.[48] In 76% of cases, the patient's condition either stabilized or improved in response to treatment by the APN. The patients' assessment of their outcomes were positive. The collaborating physicians evaluated APN prescriptive authority as beneficial and complementary to their practice.

Reimbursement of Advanced Practice Nursing Services

The effective utilization of an APN is, in part, tied to reimbursement of services provided. Reimbursement for direct patient care is provided through federal and state programs such as Medicare, Medicaid, or through private insurers including health maintenance organizations (HMOs) and preferred provider organizations (PPOs).

The ability of an APN to receive reimbursement for direct patient care services lessens the financial risk assumed by an organization or private practice that hires the APN. The average salary for an APN is approximately $50,000 to $55,000 per year; however, this figure varies considerably based on geographic location, experience, and practice setting. Some APNs also receive a productivity bonus. Most employers provide benefits for full-time employees that include paid vacation, malpractice insurance, medical and disability insurance, and retirement.[49] It takes approximately 12 months for the APN to build up a caseload of patients to cover salary, benefits, and overhead. By the second year of employment, the APN is usually able to make a profit.[50]

Medicare Payment

Medicare is a federal health insurance program for individuals who are disabled or older than age 65. It is funded through payroll deductions from Social Security. Part A of the program pays for costs incurred during hospitalizations; Part B pays for outpatient services of physicians and some other health care providers, including advanced practice nurses.

Prior to January 1, 1998, APNs were eligible to receive direct reimbursement for services only in rural settings, and indirect reimbursement for services provided in a nursing home or "incident to" a physician's services. With passage of the Balanced Budget Act of 1997 (Pub. L. No. 105-33), APNs became eligible for direct reimbursement of Medicare Part B services in all practice sites and geographic locations, except for rural health centers and federally qualified health centers. Payment is excluded in these two settings because payment to these types of facilities is made under an "all-inclusive rate."

In November 1998, the Health Care Financing Administration (HCFA) published the changes and revisions to the Medicare Physician's Fee Schedule, including the regulations covering reimbursement for services provided by APNs.[51] This final rule clarified the definition of collaboration, educational requirements, and practice settings for APNs. For Medicare Part B coverage of services, the APN must

- Possess a master's degree in nursing*

- Be a registered professional nurse who is authorized by the state in which the services are furnished to practice as an APN in accordance with state law

---

*It is expected that HCFA will replace the requirement for master's-degree preparation with the requirement that an APN have successfully completed an accredited nurse practitioner program of study.[52]

- Be nationally certified as an APN by the ANCC or other recognized national certifying body that has established standards for APNs

Under the new law, direct payment to APNs is equal to 80% of the lesser of either the actual charge or 85% of the fee schedule amount for the same service if provided by a physician. For services provided by an APN in a hospital outpatient department, payment is made to that department for both the professional services of the APN as well as for the facility component of the hospital outpatient department service.

The degree of APN–physician collaboration that is necessary for reimbursement is defined by the requirements in each state's nurse practice act. In states without laws or guidelines requiring collaboration, APNs must document their scope of practice and indicate the collaborative relationships they have with physicians to deal with issues outside their scope. It is permissible in these states for the APN to bill directly for their services as well as for all of the ancillary services provided to a patient by staff working under the APN's direct supervision. In instances where the APN is employed by a physician, the physician is able to bill 100% of the Medicare fee schedule for the services provided by the APN as long as certain requirements are met. For example, the physician must be present in the same office suite in which the services are provided and the patient must not have a new problem. The physician need not countersign the patient's chart, but the office schedule must document the physician's presence in the office at the time of the patient's visit.

In states with liberal collaboration requirements, if the physician is not present in the office suite when services are provided, the APN may bill for 85% of any reimbursable services performed. In states with restrictive collaborative practice requirements, if the physician is not present at the time the services are rendered, the APN is not able to bill directly for services.

All APNs must have their own provider number (PIN) in order to bill Medicare, even in cases when the APN is an employee and the employer has always billed for the APN's services using the employer's PIN with a modifier. Figure 79-2 provides information on obtaining provider numbers.

Medicaid Payment

Medicaid is a joint state and federally funded health care program for lower income Americans. Direct reimbursement to pediatric and family nurse practitioners for services provided to children is federally mandated. Other health care services provided by other APNs may be reimbursed at the discretion of the state. The reimbursement rate is determined by each state.

Some states have requested and been given waivers that preempt federal Medicaid regulation and allow the state to develop managed care programs for the provision

---

To receive direct reimbursement for services covered by Medicare or Medicaid, an advanced practice nurse must have a billing or provider number.

Medicare Provider Number

Contact the local Medicare carrier to obtain the registration form to apply for a Medicare billing number or contact the Social Security Office at 1-800-772-1213.

Medicaid Provider Number

To obtain a registration form to apply for a Medicaid provider number, contact the local Medicaid office within the state health department.

CHAMPUS Provider Information

To obtain a CHAMPUS provider application, write to the following address:

CHAMPUS
Provider File Operations
Post Office Box 100558
Florence, SC 29501-0558

Telephone numbers for CHAMPUS area offices:
Mid-Atlantic Region 1-800-467-8500
Western Region 1-800-225-4816
MN, WI, IA, WV, KY, OH 1-800-471-0704

Figure 79-2 Obtaining provider numbers.

---

of their Medicaid services. This has resulted in the exclusion of APNs in some of these states from the provider panels of these programs.

Payment by Other Providers

Health maintenance organizations may have contracts with Medicare to provide care to enrollees at a capitated annual rate regardless of the type of provider or the level of services provided. APNs who work in collaboration with a physician are eligible for reimbursement. The HMO receives a fixed, monthly payment per enrollee. The APN contracts directly with the HMO to provide services and is paid by the HMO.

The Civilian and Medical Program of the Uniformed Services (CHAMPUS) is a federal program that provides services to members of the uniformed services and their families when these services cannot be provided by a military hospital. NPs as well as psychiatric and mental health CNSs are eligible for direct reimbursement under CHAMPUS.

The Federal Employee Health Benefit Plan (FEHBP) offers health insurance plans to federal employees and retirees. Coverage of APN services is mandated and direct reimbursement of services is provided; however, there is a loophole. Prepaid health insurance plans that are part of the FEHBP network are not required to include APNs in their provider network. If APNs are part of the provider network, the specific health insurance plan determines the level of payment for APN services.

Managed care plans have recently begun to include APNs in their provider panels. Columbia Advanced Practice Nurse Associates (CAPNA) is a group of APNs affiliated with Columbia University Medical Center in New York City. CAPNA became one of the first independent APN practices to be recognized as primary care providers by eight private health plans, including Oxford Health Plan, one of the largest plans in the Northeast.[53]

Collaboration and Consultation—Hallmarks of Oncology Advanced Practice

It is assumed that the oncology advanced practice nurse (OAPN) possesses outstanding clinical skills that serve as the foundation for practice. The OAPN is expert in the process of patient and family education, skilled in the utilization of nursing research, and savvy in negotiating complex organizational structures. In addition to this clinical expertise, the OAPN also must be an expert consultant and skilled in the process of collaboration. The OAPN is on the cutting edge of practice, an often tenuous location. These skills are required to maintain that edge.

In the process of consultation, the help of an expert is sought to either manage a patient problem or solve an organizational problem. An external or an internal approach to consultation can be utilized. In the former, consultation is the focus of the APN's job, whereas in the latter, it is one of the subroles of the APN's position.[54] In either approach, the APN acts as a catalyst for change.

Madden and Pointe described three consultative advanced practice roles: process, resource, and expert.[55] The process consultant is expert in a process required for practice such as the development of case management models, critical pathways, or documentation processes. The resource consultant is expert at meeting complex patient care needs through the effective utilization of resources. This may include implementing patient and family education groups and utilizing nursing research. The expert practitioner has specialized, in-depth knowledge that is utilized to care for a select group of patients.

Collaboration is a model of practice in which care is provided based on competence.[56] The skills of the provider are matched with the needs of the patient, thereby maximizing the strengths of each provider. The components necessary for successful collaboration include collegiality, communication, mutual goals, and a client-focused practice.[57] Characteristics of a collaborative practice include mutual trust and understanding, as well as shared problem solving, decision making, and authority.[58]

There are several descriptions of collaborative practices in the literature.[57,59–62] Shay and colleagues list specific requirements for the development of a collaborative OAPN practice:

- Detailed job description
- Written collaborative practice agreement detailing scope of practice
- Documentation of certification to perform invasive procedures (e.g., bone marrow aspiration and biopsy, lumbar puncture)
- Documentation of credentials as required by the institution and/or state (e.g., NP licensure, advanced practice certification, cardiopulmonary resuscitation certification)
- Malpractice coverage[62]

In this practice, NPs function independently in caring for a caseload of patients, whether in the ambulatory or acute care setting. When the patient's care needs extend beyond the NP's scope of practice, the care is transferred to a physician. The patient's care is transferred back to the NP when the patient's condition becomes stable and when mutually agreed upon by the physician and NP.

Oncology Advanced Practice Nursing Roles

The clinical nurse specialist role has been conceptualized as integrating the subroles of expert practitioner, educator, consultant, researcher, and manager/leader. In contrast, the nurse practitioner role always has emphasized the role of direct care provider. Historically, the CNS's primary responsibity has been to the employing organization whereas the NP's primary responsibility has been to the patient.

As the roles of the CNS and NP are reconceptualized, it becomes more useful to shift the focus away from role components and toward practice focus when describing the OAPN. Although the OAPN specializes in the care of individuals and families with cancer, the OAPN also often develops a practice focus. For example, the focus can be in a particular area of oncology advanced practice such as prevention and early detection or symptom management, or it can be in the care of individuals with a specific malignancy such as breast cancer.

Many of today's OAPN roles involve responsibilities that traditionally have fallen within the realm of medicine. However, when performed by an OAPN these activities "are transformed by a nursing perspective based on concepts of health promotion, disease prevention, and client advocacy."[63] The OAPN does not leave behind the nursing cap when entering the examination room with stethoscope in hand.

Successful advanced practice is the expansion of nursing's traditional boundaries while preserving the essence of nursing. It is not only the ability to perform a physical examination and prescribe medication, it is also the ability to translate to the patient and family the impact the treatment will have on their lives. It is the ability to identify trends, predict outcomes, and anticipate needs. Appendix A at the end of this chapter provides a sample position description for an oncology nurse practitioner.

The OAPN in Primary Care

Prevention, screening, and risk assessment

The role of the nurse in cancer screening was described in the literature as early as 1978.[64] Although this role was not initially described as an advanced practice role, the physical examination for cancer screening and defining an individual's risk profile require specialized and continuing education. Cancer screening activities today are routinely taught in APN education programs and most pratitioners see these activities as consistent with their role.[65]

The OAPN is involved in many aspects of cancer screening from the identification of "at-risk" individuals to performing physical examinations focusing on cancer screening. The OAPN also develops and implements educational programs in schools, community, and employment settings on cancer risk factors, prevention, and early detection practices. OAPNs teach self-examination, counsel on lifestyle and risk-factor modification, and sponsor programs aimed at risk reduction such as nutritional and smoking cessation programs. They develop educational materials and conduct research in the area of prevention and early detection.[66]

Cancer genetic predisposition testing

The rapid expansion of knowledge regarding the role of genetics in the development of cancer and the identification of cancer susceptibility genes has led to a role for the OAPN in cancer genetics. Cancer genetic predisposition testing and counseling initially was limited to individuals and families with a hereditary predisposition to cancer.[67] However, as genetic testing for certain cancers has become commercially available, the demand for testing has increased. This has created a need for qualified individuals to conduct education and counseling regarding the benefits and limitations of genetic testing.

OAPNs with knowledge and expertise in medical genetics and counseling are in an excellent position to provide screening, counseling, and education of individuals undergoing cancer genetic testing.[68] Additionally, OAPNs are often responsible for obtaining informed consent for genetic testing and for providing results disclosure and posttest counseling.[69]

The OAPN in Secondary Care

Active treatment

OAPNs are involved in the care of patients receiving treatment for cancer as either direct care provider or consultant. As direct care provider, the OAPN obtains the patient's health history and performs the physical examination. Results of radiological and laboratory studies including pathology are reviewed and a treatment plan is devised in collaboration with the oncologist. The treatment plan and expected outcomes are then discussed with the patient and family.[70] Side effects and self-care management strategies are reviewed in detail. In many settings, laboratory and radiological studies are ordered and medications are prescribed by the OAPN.

During the phase when the patient is receiving active treatment, the OAPN meets both the patient's medical and nursing needs. The OAPN manages the concomitant medical problems such as diabetes mellitus and hypertension, as well as any treatment-related side effects. Educational and psychosocial needs also are addressed.[62]

As a consultant, the OAPN in secondary care is involved in planning and implementing initiatives aimed at patient and family education and support. Educational initiatives usually focus on helping patients and families understand the disease process, its treatment, and potential side effects. The OAPN's expertise is also utilized in symptom management and they are often an important member of a multidisciplinary pain and symptom management team. They also may act as a consultant to the institution in establishing standards for oncology practice and developing critical pathways. These services are provided in a variety of settings—private practices, comprehensive cancer centers, hospital-based outpatient clinics, and the patient's home.

Follow-up care

At the conclusion of initial treatment, the patient enters the follow-up phase of care. The health care focus shifts to returning the patient to their premorbid condition, identifying and managing the long-term effects of therapy, and monitoring for disease recurrence. Many oncologists have limited time to spend caring for patients during this phase of their disease; their focus is on caring for patients receiving active treatment. OAPNs have assumed care for this patient population in many settings. In some organizations, the physician refers the patient to a nurse-managed clinic for follow-up.[71] In others, the patient is collaboratively cared for by the oncologist and OAPN, with the OAPN assuming the role of primary provider when the patient moves into the follow-up phase. The OAPN is responsible for performing physical examinations, ordering and interpreting laboratory and radiological studies, and referring patients for diagnostic studies as needed.[61,70] Additionally, the OAPN maintains communication with the patient's primary care provider and referring physician.

As a provider of follow-up care, the OAPN helps the individual become a cancer survivor, cope with fears related to recurrence, and manage long-term effects of therapy. The individual is referred to a wide variety of services in the community as needed, from apparel shops that specialize in mastectomy swimwear to attorneys who specialize in health discrimination.

The OAPN in Tertiary Care

Acute care

The OAPN long has been involved in the management of patients in the acute care setting. In most organizations, this role has been filled by the oncology CNS; however, in recent years organizational needs have changed and the role of the acute care NP has developed.[72] The two major trends that have led to the development of the acute care NP role are changes in medical residency training programs and the shift from fee-for-service to capitated payment plans for health care.

Medical education is placing a renewed emphasis on primary care, shifting the focus of training away from the inpatient setting toward the ambulatory setting. In recent years, some states have placed legal limits on the number of hours worked by medical residents. There have been cutbacks in the federal funding of residency training programs, leading to a downsizing of such programs. The shift away from fee-for-service-based care and the reduced levels of reimbursement for physician services have resulted in physicians' caring for more patients for less revenue. The net result is that the physician has become less available to the patient and family. These forces have combined to create the need for qualified providers in the acute care setting.

While both the CNS and NP are advanced practice nursing roles with a similar goal—ensuring the provision of outstanding patient care—their means differ. The CNS affects care indirectly by working through the organization and the nursing staff to facilitate changes that improve patient care. The NP affects care directly by managing the medical and nursing needs for a specific caseload of patients. Since the trend is toward using the title of "OAPN" for both, this term will be used for the remainder of this discussion.

The needs of the organization and the practice milieu determine whether the OAPN role is more similar to that of a CNS or an NP. Complex organizations such as academic medical centers and comprehensive cancer centers that traditionally have relied on medical residents to provide acute care services have been most affected by changes in medical residency programs. These organizations utilize both types of OAPNs in the acute care setting.

The OAPN with a direct care emphasis is responsible for the management of a caseload of patients from admission through discharge. The OAPN has medical staff privileges and obtains the patient's health history, performs a physical examination, interprets laboratory and radiological studies, prescribes medications and coordinates discharge and follow-up care.[73] Invasive procedures such as bone marrow aspiration and biopsy, lumbar puncture, thoracentesis, and paracentesis also may be the responsibility of the OAPN, as permitted by the state's nurse practice act. In essence, this OAPN is responsible for the minute-to-minute care of the patient in collaboration with the attending physician.

The OAPN with an organizational focus performs functions such as acting as a mentor to nursing staff, consulting with nursing staff on the care of patients with complex needs, developing staff and patient educational programs, facilitating support groups, and implementing research-based changes in practice. This OAPN often has nursing department and hospital responsibilities such as committee representation.

Blended role

Changes in physician payment have led to the attending physician's being less available to patients, medical, and nursing staff. The OAPN role in tertiary care may incorporate components of both the traditional CNS and NP roles into one "blended" role.[74-76] Descriptions of these blended roles vary in the literature, but have one common theme—the delivery of coordinated, comprehensive, and cost-effective care. The OAPN serves as the link between the attending physician, the patient and family, the inpatient medical and nursing staff, and, increasingly in today's fiscal climate, the insurer. The OAPN in this role may facilitate the patient's admission to the hospital by performing the admission history and physical examination and writing the admission orders. The OAPN may examine the patient daily during hospitalization, triage patient problems by telephone, and coordinate the patient's discharge, including making arrangements for home care services. Additionally, the OAPN may see patients in the ambulatory care setting, provide education related to the disease and treatment, and manage treatment-related side effects and toxicities.

The OAPN acts as a liaison between the nursing staff and the physician, bridging the gap in communication that often exists between the disciplines. The OAPN in this role may also actively participate in the education of nursing and medical staff and serve on hospital and nursing departmental committees.[74,75] The difference between this OAPN role and that of the traditional NP or CNS role in tertiary care is the accountability for patient care across practice settings and the links with community providers, including the insurer.

Nurse case manager

Another OAPN role that has emerged in tertiary care, primarily owing to changes in health care reimbursement, is that of the case manager. Although the ANA recommends a minimum of a baccalaureate degree in nursing and three years of appropriate clinical experience, the economic and clinical demands of case management in tertiary care require a master's degree.[77] Many descriptions of case manager practice can be found in the literature.[77-83] Again, the emphasis is on the "three Cs": coordinated, comprehensive, and cost-effective care. In most models, the case manager's practice is inpatient-based with little crossover into other practice settings. The case manager usually does not provide direct care but rather coordinates the care provided by others to keep patients from "falling through the cracks" in an often fragmented health care system. The focus is on ensuring the effective use of resources and meeting outcomes within an appropriate length of stay. Trends in patient outcomes are identified and measures are implemented to correct variances.

This advanced practice role should not be confused with that of the case manager employed by an insurance company. These case managers usually are not either registered nurses or advanced practice nurses. Their focus is on limiting the insurer's financial liability for a given patient's care.

The OAPN in Palliative, Hospice, and Bereavement Care

When the primary focus of treatment has shifted from cure to care, the services of an OAPN with an expertise in palliative and hospice care becomes important.[84] The OAPN in palliative and hospice care is an expert in aggressive pain and symptom management, psychosocial and spiritual care, and end of life ethical and legal issues. The objective of palliative care is to enhance the quality and meaning of life and death.[85] With the increased emphasis on promoting quality of life throughout the cancer experience, palliative care is no longer reserved for those near death. In fact, the World Health Organization has suggested that active palliative care be incorporated into care from the time of diagnosis.[85]

There are several different models used for the delivery of palliative and hospice care. In all of them, the OAPN acts as a role model and provides informal teaching to less experienced nurses as well as patients and their care providers. In the inpatient model, the OAPN is a staff member of a palliative care or hospice unit. Patients are examined daily by the OAPN, and orders for medications and treatments are written as needed. In the multidisciplinary model, the OAPN is a member of a palliative care team. The team has no inpatient beds of its own, but sees patients as requested by physicians and nurses in various locations in the hospital or outpatient department. The OAPN acts as a consultant to the patient's primary care team. Recommendations are made for interventions, but orders are usually written by the referring physician. The patient is revisited daily or as often as necessary to reevaluate the efficacy of the intervention. In the community-based model, the OAPN may be employed by a home care agency and utilized as a consultant for complex patients and families with difficult management issues. In some instances, the OAPN may make home visits.

The OAPN in Industry and Research

Industry

OAPNs fill a multiplicity of roles in the health care industry. They are employed by insurers as case managers, by consulting firms as health care consultants, and by

pharmaceutical and biotechnology firms in roles ranging from company sales representatives to educational consultants. OAPNs are also combining their clinical expertise with a knowledge of information systems in roles as nursing informatics specialists.[86,87] OAPNs bring their "insider's" knowledge of the health care system to each of these roles, making them a valuable asset to an organization.

Research

The OAPN is involved in research by utilizing research results, by implementing an independent research agenda, and by collaborating on medical research. In some settings, the OAPN functions as the manager of the organization's clinical research program and is responsible for the preparation of grant proposals, protocol implementation, patient accrual, and regulatory compliance. OAPNs are also employed by clinical research management companies or by pharmaceutical firms as clinical research associates. In this role, the OAPN supervises and monitors clinical trials, often at different sites, to ensure the integrity of the research data.

Advanced Practice Nursing—Into the Twenty-First Century

Three forces will continue to influence changes in nursing practice in the coming years: the health care insurance industry, medical education, and scientific advances. The failure of government-initiated health care reform has precipitated a major restructuring in the health care system by the private sector. The traditional fee-for-service system of payment is being replaced by managed care systems in which providers agree to render services to a given group of patients for a predetermined fee. The insurer decides what services, medications, physicians, and hospitalizations will be covered. The primary motivator behind these decisions is cost, not necessarily quality. Physicians are receiving lower fees for their services and are being required to spend a larger amount of time on administrative issues related to patient care, such as justifying a hospital admission to an insurer. To compensate, physicians are seeing more patients in less time. The result is a physician–patient interaction that is limited to what is medically essential. This type of limited care is especially difficult to provide to individuals with cancer whose informational, social, and emotional needs are tremendous. Oncology advanced practice nurses long have excelled in meeting these needs, but in a way that has been invisible. Restructuring of reimbursement offers OAPNs many opportunities to change this.

There are several creative and cost-effective ways OAPNs can continue to meet the needs of patients. The OAPN can directly market services to insurers, oncologists, and patients. The addition of an OAPN to an oncology practice can result in a larger volume of patients being seen and more comprehensive care being provided. The OAPN can assume the follow-up care of patients, enabling the practice to increase volume without significant cost. Alternatively, the OAPN can give the oncology practice an "edge" in a competitive market by offering a variety of educational and support services to patients.

Changes in medical education with its renewed emphasis on the preparation of primary care providers ultimately will result in fewer subspecialists, including oncologists. However, as the population ages, it is expected that the number of individuals with cancer will increase. The result will be fewer oncologists to care for these patients. This, too, will open new avenues to the OAPN. One opportunity will be in the care of the elderly person with cancer. It is predicted that OAPNs soon will be eligible for direct reimbursement for home visits under Medicare. This will dramatically change the face of home and hospice care. The OAPN no longer will be confined to the practice settings of the hospital, the outpatient clinic, or office setting. The OAPN will be able to make house calls to perform physical examinations and therapeutic procedures.

Rapid scientific advances are also affecting advanced nursing practice. The discovery of genes linked to the development of malignancies has already led to innovations in diagnosis and treatment that were unheard of only a short time ago. OAPNs are in an ideal position to prepare patients, staff, and organizations for these changes.

Today, 65% of adults in the United States die in hospitals and the majority of health care providers are not prepared to care for the complex needs of patients in the terminal phases of their illness.[88] There is a tremendous need to improve care of these patients.[89] Palliative care is an emerging specialty and the demand for OAPN with expertise in this area will rise in the coming years.

Conclusion

Advanced practice nurses have made important contributions to oncology care in the past. Studies have shown that APNs improve patient outcomes and deliver cost-effective, quality care with a high degree of patient satisfaction. The changes that are taking place in the health care system and in oncology practice will provide new opportunities and challenges for OAPNs in the twenty-first century.

References

1. Ford LC, Silver HK: The expanded role of the nurse in child care. *Nurs Outlook* 15:8, 43–45, 1967
2. Fenton MV, Brykczynski KA: Qualitative distinctions and similarities in the practice of clinical nurse specialists and nurse practitioners. *J Prof Nurs* 9:313–326, 1993
3. American Academy of Nurse Practitioners: *Standards of Practice*. Austin, TX, American Academy of Nurse Practitioners, 1993
4. American Association of Colleges of Nursing: *Position Statement: Certification and Regulation of Advanced Practice Nurses*. Washington, DC, American Association of Colleges of Nursing, 1994
5. Pew Health Professions Commission: *Nurse Practitioners—Doubling the Graduates by the Year 2000*. San Francisco, UCSF Center for the Health Professions, 1994
6. Berlin LE, Bednash GD, Hosier KL: *1998–1999 Enrollment and Graduations in Baccalaureate and Graduate Programs in Nursing*. Washington, DC, American Association of Colleges of Nursing, 1999, p 5
7. American College of Nurse Practitioners: *Letter to Health Care Financing Administration*. Washington, DC, November 20, 1998. Accessed at http://www.nurse.org/acnp
8. Belcher A, Shurpin KM: Education of the advanced practice nurse in oncology. *Oncol Nurs Forum* 22:19–24, 1995
9. Strunk BL: The clinical nurse specialist as change agent. *Clin Nurs Spec* 9:128–132, 1995
10. Peplau HE: Specialization in professional nursing. *Nurs Science* 3:268–287, 1965
11. Camp-Sorrell D: Historical aspects of the CNS role. The future of advanced practice nursing. *Oncology Nursing Society Joint Newsletter of the CNS and NP Special Interest Groups* 4:2, 4, 1994
12. Reiter F: The nurse clinician. *Am J Nurs* 66:274–280, 1966
13. American Nurses' Association: *Nursing: A Social Policy Statement*. Kansas City, MO, American Nurses' Association, 1980
14. American Nurses' Association: *Role of the Clinical Nurse Specialist*. Kansas City, MO, American Nurses' Association, 1986
15. Mundinger MO: Health care reform: The best of times or worst of times. Speech at the American Academy of Nursing Annual Conference, October 21, 1994, Phoenix, AZ
16. Elder RG, Bullough B: Nurse practitioners and clinical nurse specialists: are the roles merging? *Clin Nurs Spec* 4:78–84, 1990
17. Forbes KE, Rafson J, Spross JA, et al: The clinical nurse specialist and nurse practitioner: core curriculum survey results. *Clin Nurs Spec* 4:63–66, 1990
18. Fenton MV, Brykczynski KA: Qualitative distinctions and similarities in the practice of clinical nurse specialists and nurse practitioners. *J Prof Nurs* 9:313–326, 1993
19. Schroer K: Case management: Clinical nurse specialist and nurse practitioner, converging roles. *Clin Nurs Spec* 5:189–194, 1991
20. Williams C, Valdivieso GC: Advanced practice models: a comparison of clinical nurse specialist and nurse practitioner activities. *Clin Nurs Spec* 8:311–318, 1994
21. Jacobs LA, Kreamer KM: The oncology clinical nurse specialist in a post-master's nurse practitioner program: a personal and professional journey. *Oncol Nurs Forum* 24:1387–1392, 1997
22. Busen NH, Engleman SG: The CNS with practitioner preparation: an emerging role in advanced practice nursing. *Clin Nurs Spec* 10:145–150, 1996
23. American Nurses' Association: *Nursing's Social Policy Statement*. Washington, DC, American Nurses' Association, 1995
24. American Association of Colleges of Nursing: *Nursing Education's Agenda for the 21st Century*. Washington, DC, American Association of Colleges of Nursing, 1995
25. Reading BA: Titling and the advanced practice nurse. *Advanced Practice Nurse* Spring/Summer:7–8, 1994
26. National Council of State Boards of Nursing: *Position Paper*

on the Regulation of Advanced Nursing Practice. Chicago, National Council of State Board of Nursing, 1993

27. Oncology Nursing Society: *Position Statement on Advanced Practice in Oncology Nursing.* Pittsburgh, Oncology Nursing Society, 1997

28. Oncology Nursing Society: Position statement on advanced practice in oncology nursing. *Oncol Nurs Forum* 22:45, 1995 (suppl)

29. Craytor JK: Highlights in education for cancer nursing. *Oncol Nurs Forum* 12:19–27, 1985 (suppl)

30. Piemme J: Oncology clinical nurse specialist education. *Oncol Nurs Forum* 12:45–48, 85, 1985

31. American Cancer Society: *The Master's Degree with a Specialty in Cancer Nursing: Curriculum Guide and Role Definition.* New York, American Cancer Society, 1978

32. American Cancer Society and Oncology Nursing Society: *The Master's Degree with a Specialty in Advanced Practice Oncology Nursing.* Atlanta, American Cancer Society, 1994

33. Brown J, Hinds P: Assessing master's programs in advanced practice oncology nursing. *Oncol Nurs Forum* 26:1371–1380, 1999

34. McMillan SC, Heusinkveld KB, Spray J: Advanced practice in oncology nursing: a role delineation study. *Oncol Nurs Forum* 22:41–50, 1995

35. McMillan SC, Heusinkveld KB, Spray JA, et al: Revising the blueprint for the AOCN examination using a role delineation study for advanced practice oncology nursing. *Oncol Nurs Forum* 26:529–537, 1999

36. Kinney AY, Hawkins R, Hudmon KS: A descriptive study of the role of the oncology nurse practitioner. *Oncol Nurs Forum* 24:811–820, 1997

37. Oncology Nursing Society: *The Use of Titles in Oncology Nursing Practice.* Pittsburgh, Oncology Nursing Society, 1997

38. Hohman M, Vander Woude D: Regulation of advanced practice nursing: one state's approach. *AACN Clin Issues* 4:617–623, 1993

39. Safriet B: Health care dollars and regulatory sense: the role of advanced practice nursing. *Yale J Reg* 9:417–487, 1992

40. Greco K: Regulation of advanced nursing practice: part one—second licensure. *Oncol Nurs Forum* 22:35–38, 1995 (suppl)

41. Fickeissen JL: Fifty-six ways to get certified. *Am J Nurs* 90:50–57, 1990

42. 2000 Certification Bulletin for OCN®, AOCN, and CPON certification. Pittsburgh, Oncology Nursing Certification Corporation, 2000

43. National Council of State Boards of Nursing: *Using nurse practitioner certification for state nursing regulation: an update.* National Council News Release, National Counsel March 24, 1997

44. Pearson LJ: Annual update of how each state stands on legislative issues affecting advanced practice nursing. *Nurs Pract* 24:16–30, 1999

45. *Midlevel Practitioner's Manual and Informational Outline of the Controlled Substances Act of 1970.* Washington, DC, Government Printing Office, Document No. 351-29, 1993

46. Mahoney DF: Employer resistance to state authorized prescriptive authority for NPs: results from a pilot study. *Nurs Pract* 20:58–61, 1995

47. Sekscenski ES, Sansom S, Bazell C, et al: State practice environments and the supply of physicians assistants, nurse practitioners and certified nurse-midwives. *N Engl J Med* 331:1266–1277, 1994

48. Hamric AB, Worley D, Lindebak S, et al: Outcomes associ-

ated with advanced nursing practice prescriptive authority. *J Am Acad Nurs Pract* 10(3):113–118, 1998

49. NP Salary Summary. NP Central: information for and about nurse practitioners. Available at <http://www.nurse.net/>. Accessed July 7, 1999

50. Legal Tips. NP Central: information for and about nurse practitioners. Available at <http://www.nurse.net/>. Accessed July 7, 1999

51. Medicare Program: Revisions to Payment Policies and Adjustments to the Relative Value Units Under the Physician Fee Schedule for Calendar Year 1999. *Fed. Reg.* 63(211):58813–59187, 1998

52. Sharp N: 1999: The road ahead for nurse practitioners. *Nurs Pract* 24:120–124, 1999

53. Lardner J: Nurses break barrier: primary care without doctors. *US News & World Report* July 27, 1998

54. Berragan L: Consultancy in nursing: roles and opportunities. *J Clin Nurs* 7:139–143, 1998

55. Madden MJ, Pointe PR: Advanced practice roles in the managed care environment. *J Nurs Admin* 24:56–62, 1994

56. Sparacino PS: Opportunities for the advanced practice nurse: encroachment or collaboration? *Clin Nurs Spec* 8:122, 1994

57. Nugent KE, Lambert VA: The advanced practice nurse in collaborative practice. *Nursingconnections* 9(1):5–16, 1996

58. Burchell RC, Thomas DA, Smith L: Some considerations for implementing collaborative practice. *Am J Med* 74:9–13, 1983

59. Campbell ML, Brandel SM, Daramola OI, et al: An advanced practice model: inpatient collaborative practices. *Clin Nurs Spec* 9:175–179, 1995

60. Dontje KJ, Sparks BT, Given BA: Establishing a collaborative practice in a comprehensive breast clinic. *Clin Nurs Spec* 10:95–101, 1996

61. Martin B, Coniglio JU: The acute care nurse practitioner in collaborative practice. *AACN Clin Issues* 7:309–314, 1996

62. Shay LE, Goldstein JT, Matthews D, et al: Guidelines for developing a nurse practitioner practice. *Nurs Pract* 21:72–81, 1996

63. Gee F: Letter to the editor. *Nurs Sci Q* 8:45–46, 1995

64. White LN, Cornelius JL, Judkins AF, et al: Screening of cancer by nurses. *Cancer Nurs* 1:15–20, 1978

65. Reed CA, Selleck CS: The role of midlevel providers in cancer screening. *Med Clin North Am* 80:135–144, 1996

66. Frank-Stromborg M, Rohan K: Nursing's involvement in the primary and secondary prevention of cancer. *Cancer Nurs* 15:79–108, 1992

67. Mahon SM, Casperson DS: Hereditary cancer syndrome: part 1—Clinical and educational issues. *Oncol Nurs Forum* 22:763–771, 1995

68. Loescher LJ: Genetics in cancer prediction, screening and counseling: part II, the nurse's role in genetic counseling. *Oncol Nurs Forum* 22:16–19, 1995 (suppl)

69. Dimond EP, Calzone K, Davis J, et al: The role of the nurse in cancer genetics. *Cancer Nurs* 21:57–75, 1998

70. Elmore E, Austin EO, Hodges S, et al: NPs help develop comprehensive primary care for patients with cancer. *Oncology Nursing Society Nurse Practitioner Special Interest Group Newsletter* 6(1):1, 1995

71. Judkins AF: Advanced practice nurses for follow-up care of breast cancer patients. *M.D. Anderson Case Reports and Review* 7:17–20, 1995

72. Keane A, Richmond T, Kaiser L: Critical care nurse practitioners: evolution of the advanced practice nursing role. *Am J Crit Care* 3:232–237, 1994

73. Lynch MP: Inpatient oncology nurse practitioner's role evolves. *Oncology Nursing Society Nurse Practitioner Special Interest Group Newsletter* 6(1):2, 1995

74. Sawyers JE: Defining your role in ambulatory care: clinical nurse specialist or nurse practitioner? *Clin Nurs Spec* 7:4–7, 1993

75. Lin EM: A combined role of clinical nurse specialist and coordinator: optimizing continuity of care in an autologous bone marrow transplant program. *Clin Nurs Spec* 8:48–55, 1994

76. Soehren PM, Schumann LL: Enhanced role opportunities available to the CNS/nurse practitioner. *Clin Nurs Spec* 8: 123–127, 1994

77. Cronin CJ, Maklebust J: Case-managed care: capitalizing on the CNS. *Nurs Manage* 20:38–39, 42–47, 1989

78. Zander K: Nursing case management: strategic management of cost and quality outcomes. *J Nurs Admin* 18:23–30, 1988

79. Trinidad EA: Case management: a model of CNS practice. *Clin Nurs Spec* 7:221–223, 1993

80. Lynn-McHale D, Fitzpatrick ER, Shaffer RB: Case management: Development of a model. *Clin Nurs Spec* 7:299–307, 1993

81. Sherman JJ, Johnson PK: CNS as unit-based case manager. *Clin Nurs Spec* 8:76–80, 1994

82. Brubakken KM, Janssen WR, Ruppel DL: CNS roles in implementation of a differentiated case management model. *Clin Nurs Spec* 8:69–73, 1994

83. Sterling YM, Noto EC, Bowen MR: Case management roles of clinicians: a research case study. *Clin Nurs Spec* 8:196–201, 1994

84. Haisfield-Wolfe ME: End of life care: evolution of the nurse's role. *Oncol Nurs Forum* 23:931–935, 1996

85. Stjernsward J, Colleau SM, Ventafridda V: The World Heath Organization cancer pain and palliative care program: past, present, and future. *J Pain Symptom Manage* 12:65–72, 1996

86. Simpson RL: Making the move from nurse to nursing informatics consultant. *Nurs Manage* 29(5):22–25, 1998

87. Meyer KE, Sather-Levine B, Laurent-Bopp D, et al: The impact of clinical information systems research on the future of advanced practice nursing. *Adv Pract Nurs Q* 2(3): 58–64, 1996

88. Pickett M, Cooley ME, Gordon DB: Palliative care: past, present and future perspectives. *Semin Oncol Nurs* 14:86–94, 1998

89. Meier DE, Morrison S, Cassel CK: Improving palliative care. *Ann Intern Med* 127:225–230, 1997

APPENDIX A: ONCOLOGY NURSE PRACTITIONER POSITION DESCRIPTION

General Description

A nurse practitioner (NP) is a registered nurse who has completed an accredited NP MS program. NP practice includes health supervision of well individuals, episodic care of individuals with acute, commonly occurring illnesses, and the long-term management of individuals with chronic conditions. NPs work collaboratively with physicians and other members of the health care team.

The oncology NP cares for individuals with cancer who are either receiving treatment or being monitored for disease progression, relapse, or for long-term side effects of therapy. Only those individuals whose disease, treatment, and side effects can be managed primarily in an ambulatory care setting are cared for by the oncology NP.

Major Duties

The oncology NP functions independently as the care provider for a select group of individuals with cancer under the general supervision of an attending physician. Major duties fall into three broad categories: clinical practice, research, and education.

Clinical Practice

1. Obtains a health history and assesses the patient's physical status through performance of a physical examination.
2. Assesses psychosocial situation, coping strategies, and learning needs of patients and significant other.
3. Develops and implements a plan of care based on clinical findings and disease process. This includes a plan for treatment, counseling, and education.
4. Communicates the plan of care to other members of the health care team.
5. Evaluates patient response to treatment and revises the plan of care as necessary and in collaboration with the attending physician.
6. Prescribes medications, laboratory, and diagnostic tests.
7. After successful performance of three supervised diagnostic procedures (i.e., bone marrow biopsies, thoracentesis, or paracentesis), the NP will independently perform these procedures on his or her patient population according to written guidelines.
8. Coordinates patient care with other departments and disciplines.
9. Requests consultation and/or initiates referrals for complex problems or specialized care as necessary.
10. Maintains complete and current medical records and flow sheets.
11. Dictates follow-up letters to primary care and referring physicians.

Research

1. Assists with the design and implementation of clinical trials.
2. Acts as coinvestigator on medical clinical trials and as primary investigator on nursing research studies.
3. Acts as a patient advocate.
4. Evaluates and reports adverse effects and complications of treatment.

Education

1. Serves as an expert resource in cancer to nursing staff, medical staff, patients, and families.
2. Conducts professional and patient educational programs.
3. Participates in patient care rounds and care conferences.
4. Acts as a preceptor for graduate students in NP and oncology nursing programs.
5. Acts as a role model and consultant to other members of the nursing staff.

Qualifications

1. Graduate from an accredited NP program.
2. Current licensure as a registered nurse and NP.
3. A minimum of five years of oncology nursing experience.* Advanced oncology nursing certification preferred.
4. Clinical expertise in caring for individuals with cancer.
5. Knowledge of current nursing and medical practice and research related to medical oncology.
6. Demonstrated commitment to continued professional growth as evidenced by membership in professional organizations and attendance at continuing education offerings.
7. Demonstrated strong written and verbal communication skills. Public speaking and publishing experience strongly preferred.

*Experience may be in nursing administration, clinical practice, education, or research.

CHAPTER 80

Advancing Cancer Nursing Through Nursing Research

Mel Haberman, PhD, RN, FAAN

Introduction

Oncology nurses are poised to transform cancer care in the new millennium. Oncology nurses champion quality of care as the delivery of cancer services is restructured in a cost-driven, managed-care environment. They strive to ensure the humanization of care in a biomedical culture mystified by technology. They play critical roles in monitoring the ethics of cancer research and are vocal advocates for making clinical trials available to a diverse population, including the poor and underserved. Moreover, nurses are monitoring people genetically predisposed to cancer and are assuming pivotal roles in the delivery of genetic services.

The numerous roles performed by oncology nurses require a broad, in-depth knowledge base for practice. Despite recent advances in oncology nursing research, new mechanisms must be instituted to facilitate multi-institutional studies, nursing-effectiveness trials, and outcomes research. Promising clinicians and graduate students must be encouraged to enter a career in research. However, recruiting a new generation of nurse scientists and generating more theory, in and of themselves, will not be sufficient to change practice. Novel strategies for research dissemination and utilization must be developed and tested to ensure that practice becomes progressively evidence-based.

The purpose of this chapter is to explore some of the trends in health care and cancer care that provide the context for future advances in nursing science and research. Some priorities and topics for oncology nursing research are identified along with a brief discussion of nursing outcomes. Opportunities for clinicians and advanced practice nurses to become involved in research are described, along with tips for making a study feasible, preparing a grant application, and securing funding. The components of research critique are presented as an aid to evaluating grant proposals, manuscripts, and research protocols. Guidelines for monitoring the ethical conduct of research are discussed, and the chapter concludes with an overview of future directions for oncology nursing research.

Trends in Health Care and Oncology

Advances in oncology nursing science occur within a broad social and political context. The current climate for health care reform in the United States follows a convoluted path. Federal and state governments, business, labor, cancer advocacy groups, and cancer specialists all have different opinions about the best way to deliver cancer care services. Furthermore, oncology care is currently more politicized and under greater public scrutiny than at anytime in history. Systems that guarantee access to comprehensive cancer care and to long-term follow-up are in jeopardy as the provision of care shifts from the specialized oncology nurse and oncologist to the generalist. Moreover, in a managed-care environment, cancer care is all too often driven by reimbursement issues. Although managed care organizations and nurse scientists share the common goal of improving the wellness of individuals with cancer, nurse scientists are concerned with discovering a scientific foundation for practice while managed care corporations regard research as an investment to drive down the costs of care.[1]

Another trend in oncology care is the evolution of communication between researchers, clinicians, and consumers. Computer platforms are proliferating exponentially in conjunction with the development of new medical application software. Health care institutions are installing integrated computerized systems that include quality improvement monitoring, fiscal and operations management, electronic medical records, laboratory data banks, diagnostic imaging tools, and bibliographic reference software. Cancer organizations, research funding agencies, cancer advocacy groups, as well as volunteer and professional societies are now on the Internet. All of these factors provide people with virtually instantaneous access to vast repositories of cancer-related information.

Cancer advocacy groups and consumers will perform a key role in shaping the future direction of cancer care and research. Consumers will demand legislation that ensures the timely clinical application of new cancer therapies, just as the HIV/AIDS community successfully lobbied to diminish the time it takes for new drugs to move from the laboratory to practice. Early in the twenty-first century, the Human Genome Project will lead to predictions of likely cancers. The ability to forecast potential cancers in entire populations of healthy people will revolutionize cancer prevention, screening, and detection activities; systems for monitoring people with a positive genetic profile for cancer; health care ethics; and the discovery of new genetic therapies.

Future advances in nursing therapeutics will likely parallel new trends in cancer therapy. New applications are proliferating rapidly for biological response modifiers; blood cell and genetic transplants; aggressive ablative therapies; antiemetic, antibiotic, and pain therapies; cancer markers; tumor-suppressor genes; and oncogenes. The magnitude, scope, and pace of scientific discovery is pushing oncology nursing practice beyond the edge of existing theory.[2] As the specialty realigns itself to ensure the delivery of quality care in the midst of health care reform, advances in clinical practice will continue to outpace the development of new nursing theory for the near future. A clear set of research priorities is needed to focus nurse scientists' efforts on filling existing gaps in practice knowledge.

Topics and Priorities for Oncology Nursing Research

Oncology nursing research focuses on the human experience of cancer survivorship, the clinical therapeutics under the control of nurses, the systems designed to deliver cancer care, and the patient outcomes directly attributed to nursing intervention. By definition, clinical studies may examine cancer prevention, screening, and early detection; individual and family coping across the continuum of cancer therapy and survivorship; nursing interventions designed to improve symptom management or to ameliorate suffering; nursing staffing patterns and models of care; and quality-of-life outcomes that are sensitive to the caring actions of nurses. Many avenues exist for selecting a specific topic for study within the broad scope of oncology nursing practice.

McCorkle identifies four methods for choosing a research topic: (1) the nurse's direct observation or clinical experience, (2) talking with other nurses about gaps in practice knowledge or clinical problems, (3) reading the literature and recognizing discrepancies in research findings or existing knowledge, and (4) examining a published theory and its suitability for practice.[3] Topics for study also can be derived from guidelines for practice and care pathways, and written standards for total or continuous quality improvement. Another source of research topics is the critical evaluation of daily practice. Nurses can readily discover a lack of evidence-based support for many nursing interventions. A potential topic for research is often embedded in the statement, "I don't know why we do it this way. We have always done it this way as long as I can remember."

Topics for research can be identified from the results of research priority surveys. Oncology nurses have participated in five research priority surveys conducted by the Oncology Nursing Society (ONS) since 1981. Topics continuously ranked among the top ten research priorities from 1981 to the latest survey conducted in 1994 include stress, coping, and adaptation; pain; patient education; prevention and early detection; and cost containment and economic issues.[4,5] Quality of life emerged as a leading research priority in both the 1991 and 1994 surveys. Three topics were ranked in the top ten priorities for the first time in the 1994 survey: risk reduction and screening, neutropenia and immunosuppression, and ethical issues.

Another good source for research topics is state-of-the-science publications in selected areas of cancer practice and research, such as cancer-related fatigue[6] and quality of life.[7] Topics for research can be identified by examining the types of studies conducted by other cancer researchers and new opportunities for research funding. Many sites on the Internet have databases that contain compilations of currently funded projects, announcements for new grants, and hotlinks to sources of research funding. One of the most comprehensive clearinghouses for cancer information is OncoLink at the University of Pennsylvania. OncoLink is a gateway to dozens of cancer-related databases, including the Computer Retrieval of Information on Scientific Reports (CRISP). The CRISP biomedical database contains information by topic area on all grants funded by the National Institutes of Health (NIH), including clinical trials sponsored by the National Cancer Institute (NCI) and studies funded by the National Institute of Nursing Research (NINR). Some of the Internet sites of interest to cancer researchers are listed in Table 80-1.

In summary, an abundance of topics will benefit from further study by oncology nurses. Moreover, a focused research agenda for the specialty must be developed and articulated to funding agencies, volunteer cancer societies, other cancer care providers, and cancer advocacy groups. Reaching consensus on a common research agenda will require nurse scientists, clinicians, administrators, educators, and cancer survivors to work together to create a new spirit of cooperative science.

Table 80-1 Internet Web Sites for Cancer Researchers

Agency for Healthcare Research and Quality (AHRQ)
http://www.ahrq.gov

American Cancer Society
http://cancer.org

Computer Retrieval of Information on Scientific Reports (CRISP)
http://www-commons.cit.nih.gov/crisp/

Healthfinder
http://www.healthfinder.gov/

Leukemia Society of America
http://www.leukemia.org/

Lymphoma Research Foundation of America
http://www.lymphoma.org/

Midwest Nursing Research Society
http://www.mnrs.org/

National Cancer Institute
http://www.nci.nih.gov/

National Institutes of Health Center for Scientific Review
http://www.drg.nih.gov/

National Institutes of Health Office of Grants and Contracts
http://www.nih.gov/grants/

National Institute of Nursing Research
http://www.nih.gov/ninr/

National Library of Medicine: National Information Center on Health Services Research and Health Care Technology
http://www.nlm.nih.gov/nichsr/hsrsites.html#ephs

OncoLink
http://www.oncolink.org

Oncology Nursing Society
http://www.ons.org

Robert Woods Johnson Foundation
http://www.rwjf.org/main.html

Sigma Theta Tau
http://www.nursingsociety.org/

Southern Nursing Research Society
http://www.snrs.org/

Outcomes for Nursing Research

Like all nursing specialties, oncology nursing is being challenged by insurers, health policy makers, managed care organizations, and other disciplines to document the many ways nurses do, in fact, make a difference in the lives of individuals with cancer. Outcomes research investigates the relationship between specific nursing interventions and measurable, biopsychosocial outcomes of care.

Several definitions of nursing outcomes exist in the literature. Lang and Marek define an *outcome* as "an end result of a treatment or intervention."[8,p.27] According to Lasker-Hertz and Houston, outcomes research focuses on the end results of care and linking the process of care delivery with patient outcomes.[9] The American Society of Clinical Oncology (ASCO) convened an advisory panel to develop guidelines for the assessment of cancer treatment outcomes[10]; ASCO makes a distinction between cancer treatment and patient outcomes. Cancer treatment outcomes measure the effect of therapy on the disease of cancer (e.g., complete or partial tumor response, response duration, time to progression, and tumor markers). Patient outcomes measure the direct effect of therapy on patients (e.g., mortality, quality of life, and treatment-related toxicities).

Individuals with cancer, nurses, physicians, payers, managed care corporations, researchers, and health policy makers have different opinions about which outcomes are most salient.[1,10] In an effort to define and set a direction for outcomes research, the National Center for Nursing Research held a landmark conference in 1991 on patient outcomes research. The proceedings of this conference are available in a free publication from the U.S. Department of Health and Human Services.[11]

Oncology nurses must identify salient outcomes that provide informative data for documenting the benefits of nursing interventions.[9,12] Good conceptual models for designing nursing outcomes studies have been proposed by Mitchell et al[12] and Lamb.[13] Brooten and Naylor warn us that the search for nurse-sensitive outcomes must not ignore the reality that nurses provide care within a broader culture of care.[14] Consequently, studies of nursing outcomes also may examine such factors as staffing patterns,[15] organizational and delivery of care variables,[16–19] patient satisfaction,[20,21] health-related quality of life,[22–25] costs,[26] and adverse outcomes.[27] Table 80-2 provides a list of potential outcome variables.

Many questions about nursing outcomes remain unanswered. How should outcomes be defined and measured in different settings and patient populations? What is the relationship between biophysical and psychosocial outcomes? Can nursing therapeutics be linked to predictions of cancer survival and quality-of-life outcomes? Can consensus be reached on a minimum set of core outcomes that are relevant to nurse clinicians, managers, administrators, and researchers?

Nursing effectiveness trials eventually will provide out-

Table 80-2   Oncology Nursing Outcomes

Biophysical Outcomes

- Temperature, pulse, respiration, blood pressure, lung sounds, cardiac output
- Laboratory tests: WBC, RBC, creatinine, serum glucose
- Skin integrity, body surface area, abdominal girth
- Sleep patterns, nutritional status, weight loss, body mass index
- Nosocomial infections, wound healing, renal and hepatic functioning

Psychosocial Outcomes

- Cognitive status: attention span, memory, concentration, orientation
- Moods: anxiety, depression, anger, hope, happiness
- Social support, beliefs in personal control, self-efficacy
- Social power, communication styles, interpersonal skills
- Will-to-live, coping and adaptation to illness, meaning of illness

Behaviors and Safety

- Adherence to treatment protocols
- Health and illness-related knowledge, understanding, and perceptions
- Health beliefs, attitudes, and motivation
- Caregiver and self-care skills
- Problem-solving and decision-making skills
- Safety interventions, prevention of falls, use of access devices, ventilators

Quality-of-Life

- Physical functioning: activities of daily living, mobility, sexuality
- Social functioning: social support, social roles, family functioning
- Emotional functioning: mood states, well-being, life satisfaction
- Symptoms: pain, nausea, fatigue, diarrhea, graft-versus-host disease
- Spirituality: religiosity, self-transcendent experiences, faith, hope
- Economic status: out-of-pocket expenses, insurability, employment or school status, income

Delivery of Care and Utilization

- Staffing patterns and mix, generalist vs. specialist care
- Patient acuity
- Length of stay, readmissions, cost-of-care, access to care, referral patterns
- Goal attainment for care pathways, guidelines for care, quality improvement
- Caregiver issues and burden
- Models of care: managed care, transition services, continuity models
- Acute care, ambulatory care, home care, and end-of-life care
- Patient and staff satisfaction

come data to substantiate the ways oncology nurses make a difference in the delivery of care and in improving patient outcomes. Eventually, both clinicians and consumers will have access to these databases just as they currently have access to databases on the NCI's ongoing clinical trials.

Mechanisms for Oncology Nursing Research

Research Conducted by Nurse Clinicians and Advanced Practice Nurses

Many opportunities exist for oncology nurses to participate in research. Although nurses with advanced graduate preparation in research are more likely to participate in research than nurses with little formal research preparation, staff nurses historically have been successful in obtaining small grant funding to conduct pilot and feasibility studies. Because it is difficult, if not impossible at times, to conduct a research study while holding down a full-time clinical position, nurses can choose different types of research involvement. Table 80-3 identifies some of the ways nurses can participate in research depending on their level of education, formal research preparation, and the willingness of their employer to support research.

Research occurs within a context of critical inquiry. A climate for research can be fostered by initiating different activities that raise the level of critical thinking. Practice settings can be evaluated for their potential to support research by asking a series of questions.

- Do the nurses in the care setting talk about research?

- Do they identify gaps in practice and make statements like, "Somebody needs to study why we do. . . ."?

- Does the setting have a nursing research committee or someone designated to facilitate nursing studies?

- Do nurses have the same access as other researchers to word-processing services, electronic databases, and bibliographic search software?

- Does the setting hold journal clubs or regularly present research findings at in-service education programs or during staff meetings?

- Are there any graduate students or nursing faculty conducting research in the setting?

- Are there any rewards for participating in research (e.g., promotion or merit raises based on conducting research and publishing findings or funding for travel to present findings at conferences)?

It is often easier to conduct a study in a setting that provides incentives for research than to struggle with institutional barriers or a lack of commitment to research.

Table 80-3 Types of Research Involvement

Associate of Arts, Diploma, and Bachelor of Science Degree in Nursing

- Act as study monitors, data collectors, and project managers
- Help develop projects and review for clinical feasibility
- Conduct pilot/feasibility studies with assistance of research mentor
- Participate in journal clubs
- Conduct electronic literature searches
- Prepare research-based guidelines for practice and care pathways

Master of Science Degree in Nursing

- Conduct independent projects or collaborate with a nurse scientist
- Act as research mentor to staff nurses
- Serve as project director or study monitor
- Coordinate research dissemination and utilization activities and provide research critique

Doctorate

- Orchestrate a research career
- Generate new knowledge: Concept definition, theory development, instrumentation, and methodologic research
- Serve on grant review committees
- Review proposals for scientific merit, clinical feasibility, and budget issues
- Lead multi-institutional studies
- Mentor graduate students and postdoctorate fellows
- Provide expert testimony for health policy formation and funding priorities
- Serve on advisory panels to evaluate the state-of-the-science
- Study quality of care, cost and access, delivery models, outcomes, research utilization, and dissemination issues

How to make a project feasible

Many staff nursing projects are doomed to failure from the beginning because the aim of the study is too broad and is unattainable without major funding and a dedicated research staff. Furthermore, new investigators may have been misled about the realities of conducting a well-designed study. Even with the support of grant funding and a project staff, researchers spend long hours conducting their studies, writing progress reports, seeking additional funding, mentoring project members, and preparing manuscripts or presentations. The old adage, "something always takes more time than originally intended," must have been first voiced by a sleep-deprived researcher. Moreover, research is as much a political process as a journey of scientific discovery. The nurse investigator must be prepared for bouts of discouragement and disillusionment, and for the territorial wars that commonly occur in multidisciplinary settings.

Despite the daily frustrations that come with conducting research, there are many ways to ensure that the experience is both successful and enjoyable. The investigator should make sure that the specific aim of the project is narrow, focused, and attainable in a realistic time period. It is a good idea to assemble a team of nurses who are interested in the same topic and to pool resources. Each member of the team can be responsible for developing a specific component of the research proposal. For instance, one person may write the review of the literature while others prepare a draft of the design and methods section, analysis plan, and so forth.

Another way to design a feasible study is to keep the time line for completing the study realistic and flexible. It is not uncommon for a small clinical study with a single research question to take 1–2 years to complete. It may be beneficial to join forces with oncology nurses at other sites in the community to obtain a larger and more diverse sample in a shorter period of time. Whenever possible, the investigator can apply for small grant funding to buy some paid release time to conduct the study and to obtain funding for word processing, photocopying, travel, supplies, consultation, computer time, and telephone expenses. Sometimes it is more efficient to tag a small study onto an existing protocol than to initiate a new project. Research nurses who manage projects for physician researchers often add a nursing component to an existing medical protocol. This type of adjunct study is called a companion study.[28]

Many design options exist for developing a feasible study and choosing the most suitable method of inquiry. Although the complexities of research design are beyond the scope of this chapter, several excellent nursing textbooks are available as references.[29–33] As an aid to outlining a research proposal or evaluating a grant application, Table 80-4 identifies the major components of a research protocol and grant application.

Research consultation

Expert consultation from colleagues, a nurse scientist, and a statistician is essential. A consultant is chosen based on his or her publications, presentations, or track record of funded research in the proposed content area. The consultant should read and critique the proposal or grant application in the early, formative stages. Many cancer centers have an active nursing research committee that either conducts studies as a group or offers consultation and critique. If there is no committee in the setting, consider starting one. Written guidelines that describe how to start a clinical nursing research committee can be obtained from the ONS.

Another source of research consultation is a local chapter of the ONS. Every ONS chapter has been grouped by geographic region by the ONS Research Team. Each region has an assigned volunteer nurse scientist who has agreed to offer research consultation to chapter members. Other sources of consultation include the research committee of the state nurses' associations, local chapters of nursing specialty organizations, and the faculty of local schools of nursing. Many faculty members have clinical or research affiliations with cancer centers and other community agencies. Staff nurses should not

---

Table 80-4   Sections of a Research Proposal or Grant

- Sign-off signatures from all institutional officials and research sites
- Abstract of study
- Specific aims, research questions, or hypotheses
- Significance of project
- Literature review, theoretical or conceptual framework
- References
- Description of quantitative research design
  -Historical
  -Descriptive
  -Correlational
  -Causal comparative
  -True experimental
  -Quasi-experimental
  -Clinical trials
  -Instrument development and testing
- Description of qualitative research design
  -Ethnography
  -Grounded theory
  -Hermeneutics
  -Phenomenology
- Methodology and procedures
  -Sample inclusion and exclusion criteria
  -Power analysis to justify sample size
  -Accrual, randomization, and sampling strategies
  -Sample replacement due to attrition
  -Theoretical sampling for qualitative designs
  -Description of instruments, scoring, and reliability and validity
  -Protocol adherence and stopping rules
  -Efforts to control or minimize sources of random or systematic measurement error
  -Data collection and data management plan
  -Data analysis plan
  -Assurances for obtaining informed consent, maintaining anonymity, and confidentiality of data
  -Monitoring scientific integrity and ethical conduct
- Time line for study
- Biosketches for all investigators, consultants, research staff
- Description of facilities, office space, laboratory equipment, computer resources
- Letters of support from program directors, research sites, consultants
- Itemized budget and budget narrative that justifies all expenses
- Other sources of funding and/or pending grants
- Consent form and letter of approval from Institutional Review Board or animal welfare committee
- If resubmitting a grant, a cover letter that addresses how the grant was modified based on an earlier review

---

be hesitant to ask for consultation from faculty members who are engaged in research. The nurse researcher, in turn, may want to negotiate for some type of recognition for their contribution to the project or they may ask you for help with one of their studies. If a doctorate-prepared nurse scientist is not available, find out which nurses in the setting or community have conducted research and ask for assistance. Research nurses who conduct clinical trials for the NCI's cooperative research groups can often provide excellent research consultation, especially on the design and implementation of multi-institutional projects.

Tips for grant preparation

Obtaining research funding is more competitive than ever. The chances of being successfully funded will improve if some basic tips for grant preparation are followed. The Oncology Nursing Foundation offers many of the following tips for preparing a better grant application.

- Identify your strengths and weaknesses as a researcher. Find ways to overcome deficiencies. For instance, if you do not have preliminary data to support an application for major funding, plan a phased program of study that begins with a small-scale pilot study.

- If you do not have a track record of publications or funded research in your area of interest, get one or more consultants to improve your competitive edge. In addition to their expert advice, consultants act as an insurance policy to the funding agency. Funding sources want some type of guarantee that the investigator will do what is promised in the grant application and that their investment is buying the best science for the dollar. Having a consultant gives them these assurances and shows the grant reviewers that you recognize your limitations and have taken steps to strengthen the content areas beyond your expertise.

- The grant application and instructions are the road map. Follow the rules and suggested guidelines carefully. If the application says the funding agency is interested in projects that study x, y, and z, be sure the specific aims of your proposal address x, y, and z.

- Do not propose a full-scale study if a feasibility study is more appropriate. Pilot studies are useful to determine the strength of an intervention; to assess the feasibility of a research design or procedures for data collection; to pretest an instrument in the population of interest; and to evaluate the risk, side effects, and compliance with a new nursing therapy.

- Try to anticipate how the reviewer will respond to your application. Make the application pleasant to look at and easy to read and understand. Follow the requirements for font style and size, margins, and printing. Use subheadings, tables, and graphs, if applicable. Adhere rigidly to the page limitations.

- Never assume the reviewers will understand your proposal as well as you do. Introduce new ideas incrementally. Move from the general to the specific. Start with basic definitions and explanations and finish with a full synthesis or complex explanation. Provide an immediate definition or explanation whenever you identify a new concept, theory, or research methodology for the first time. Have a deliberate strategy for educat-

ing the reviewers so they will understand every nuance of your study by the time they have finished reading the proposal.

- Use an editor to help you with writing style, use of grammar, and punctuation. Write clearly in an active voice using nonsexist language. Typographical errors and misspelled words reflect poorly on your attention to detail.

- Use the appendices to support your application rather than as a catch-all for everything that could not be squeezed into the body of the application. It is not the weight or thickness of the proposal that matters but its quality.

- Support letters should be written specifically for the proposal and project. Avoid submitting generic letters that show the writer has little knowledge of the study. Provide letters that document access to clinical sites and patient populations, release time to perform the research, the availability of space and equipment, and so forth. Consultants should submit a letter that discusses their role and other contributions to the study.

- Budgets should never be inflated. Only request allowable expenses and justify why each budget item is essential to the project. Show how cost calculations were reached (e.g., a transcriptionist will be hired for 10 hours at $12 per hour for a total cost of $120).

- Check the application for any fatal flaws such as an inadequate sample size, a poor fit with the priorities of the funding agency, or a project that is under- or overambitious for the funding level and desired time frame for the study.

- Check the overall integrity and logical consistency of the application by drawing a diagram that shows the interrelationships among the specific aims, design, sample, variables, instruments, and analysis plan. Does each section flow logically from the other? Are there any gaps in the project that may result in a fatal flaw? Has anything necessary been lost or has something been added that does not relate to the aims of the study?

Funding for research

Many options exist for beginning researchers to obtain funding for preliminary and small-scale studies. Generally speaking, nurse scientists who have a previous track record of funded research have a better chance of obtaining major funding than a new investigator. If you do not have the qualifications to be competitive for major funding, look for funding sources that give special awards for new investigators and novice researchers and that support small grants, pilot, and feasibility studies.

A good fit between your study and the goals of the funding agency is essential to successful funding. Some funding sources restrict their grant awards to certain topics or high priorities while others provide relatively unrestricted funding. The American Nurses' Foundation, a subsidiary of the American Nurses' Association, funds more than twenty small grants each year. Many of these awards are for unrestricted topics of study. The ONS Foundation funds approximately thirty small grants each year. The majority of these grants are unrestricted, only requiring that the investigator study some aspect of oncology. If you are seeking funding from a professional society or pharmaceutical company, be sure to find out if the funding is unrestricted or designated for the study of a particular topic or product.

Other sources of funding often can be found in the investigator's agency or local community. Some cancer centers have core program grants that provide seed money for start-up research projects. Nurses can often qualify for these monies, especially if their protocol is tagged onto an existing medical protocol as a companion study. Some nurse executives often try to protect small pockets of money to support seed money for nursing research projects. Guilds that sponsor fund-raising events for most comprehensive and community cancer centers are another potential source of research funding.

Chapters of the ONS or other nursing specialty organizations, like the American Association of Critical-Care Nurses, are additional sources of local funding. Some societies require the grant applicant to be a member, while others do not. The national nursing honorary society, Sigma Theta Tau, has local chapters at almost all university schools of nursing. Many local chapters, as well as the national organization of Sigma Theta Tau, give grant awards. Some state divisions of the ACS and the Leukemia Society of America have funding for research on the local level.

It is important to be aware of the various funding bulletins that are published locally by the grants and contracts offices of universities and cancer centers. These bulletins are usually published monthly or bimonthly and list all of the potential sources of funding and application deadline dates for dozens of funding agencies. The addresses for all federal and private foundations that support research can be obtained from a health science library or an institutional grants and contracts office. Many funding agencies now have sites on the Internet.

Health science libraries, cancer center libraries, and grants and contracts offices usually subscribe to a variety of weekly or monthly research funding publications. The *NIH Guide for Grants and Contracts* is the federal government's premier vehicle for announcing new grants. The *NIH Guide* is also available on the Internet <http://grants.nih.gov/grants/guide/index.html> from the NIH's Bethesda Maryland website. Another publication that identifies many opportunities web site for oncology research funding is the *Health Grants and Contracts Weekly: Selected Federal and Private Opportunities,* published weekly by Capital Publications, Inc. A bimonthly publication called *Research Activities,* published by the Agency for Healthcare Research and Quality, Rockville Maryland gives updates of currently funded projects and features new funding opportunities for specific topic areas

<http://www.ahcpr.gov/fund/>. Another publication entitled *The Blue Sheet: Health Policy and Biomedical Research News of the Week,* is published by F-D-C Reports, Inc. Chevy Chase, Maryland. This publication identifies opportunities for clinical research funding and presents feature articles on research ethics and scientific integrity, to name a few <http://fdcreports.com>.

Research Critique

All nurses must be critical consumers of research even if they choose not to become involved in the actual conduct of research. Clinicians are often asked to evaluate the clinical feasibility of a study, the potential of the project to burden staff and patients, and the relevance of the research to daily practice. Of course, there is no perfect research study or gold standard for evaluating the merit of a study. Designing and implementing a study always involves a series of compromises.

Using a systematic tool or set of guidelines to evaluate the scientific merit of a study will allow the nurse to gauge the value of the study's findings for practice. Research critique involves asking a set of questions about the study and then evaluating the overall rigor and feasibility of the study. Many of the following components of a formal research critique are derived from the score sheet used by the grant reviewers for the Oncology Nursing Foundation. These evaluation criteria are geared more for quantitative research designs than for qualitative designs. Criteria for evaluating qualitative studies can be found elsewhere.[34-36]

Components of Research Critique

Qualifications of investigators and staff

What are the qualifications of the principal investigator, consultants, and project staff? Have they conducted prior research, published, or obtained grants in the area under study? Is a biographical sketch included for all key personnel?

Abstract

Does the abstract accurately reflect the proposed research? A 200–250 word abstract should contain the following sections, if applicable: purpose, specific aims, significance, preliminary findings, research design, setting, sample, methods, main research variables, analysis plan, and implications for practice.

Specific aims

Are the aims clear and understandable? Do the aims flow logically from the purpose of the study? Are the aims consistent with any hypotheses or research questions?

Significance of study

Is the study relevant to oncology nursing practice? Does it have potential to lead to further research, methodologic advances, or theory development?

Background and review of literature

Is the conceptual or theoretical framework for the study identified? Is the review succinct, focused, and current? Does it include the appropriate classic studies on the topic? Is the literature simply reported verbatim or is it synthesized and interpreted by the investigator? Is what is known and not known about the topic logically linked to the aims of the current study? Are the findings of any pilot or feasibility study reported as preliminary data?

Design and methods

There are several components to this section of a research proposal, including the following.

Design. Does the investigator clearly state the research design? (Commonly used designs for quantitative and qualitative studies are listed in Table 80-4.)

Sample and setting. Is the sample described (i.e., the number of participants and the eligibility and exclusion criteria)? Are all random sampling and assignment procedures to either an experimental or control group explained? Has a power analysis been conducted to determine what sample size is needed to detect a significant difference between groups? Are the facilities and institutional resources needed to carry out the study described?

Experimental variables. If the study is using an experimental or quasiexperimental design, such as a nursing effectiveness trial, is the independent variable described in sufficient detail to allow for an evaluation of its clinical soundness and operational definition? Is a manipulation check or pretest of the independent variable (nursing intervention) described in the proposal? A manipulation check is the only way to demonstrate that the experimental intervention has been delivered and actually "takes," or works, in the population being studied.

Are the outcome or dependent variables clearly identified and do the instruments actually measure the outcome variables of interest? Do the independent and dependent variables relate to the theoretical framework and review of literature? Are any potential threats to the internal validity of the study controlled for, so the investigator can conclude with confidence that it was the experimental therapy that actually made the difference between groups rather than some spurious or confounding factor?

Instruments and measurement. What concepts are being measured (e.g., symptoms of fatigue or pain)? If repeated measurement is planned, is evidence presented to show the instrument is capable of detecting changes over time? Has the instrument been used previously in the population under study? Are the instruments appended to the proposal? Has permission been obtained to use any copyrighted tools? If a tool has been modified, has a pilot study been conducted to test the reliability/validity of the adapted instrument?

Is there a discussion of the reliability and validity of the instruments, the weight given to individual items and subscales, and the scoring procedures? Common forms of validity include face and content validity, concurrent and predictive validity as types of criterion-related validity, and construct validity. Reliability tests include test-retest, inter-rater, internal consistency, and parallel or alternative forms reliability.[37]

Data collection schedule and procedures. Is there a description of how and when data will be collected and any training that is necessary to standardize data collection? Are the procedures realistic in terms of the clinical setting, treatment trajectory, and expected side effects of therapy? Will the procedures result in lower accrual or higher attrition rates? Does the instrument packet place undue burden on the participant, family, or staff? Are potential sources of random or systematic measurement error identified and, if possible, controlled for or minimized?

Data analysis. Is the statistical or analytic technique identified and is the analysis plan capable of answering each specific aim of the study?

Study limitations. Are the limitations identified and described?

Protection of human participants. Has approval been obtained from an Institutional Review Board (IRB), and is a copy of the IRB assurance letter appended? Has IRB approval been granted from all participating research sites? Are the procedures for obtaining informed consent and maintaining confidentiality described, and are they adequate?

Statement of scientific integrity

Is a plan included for monitoring the scientific integrity of the study across all performance sites? This section should include, if applicable, a discussion of the procedures that are necessary to monitor the recruitment of participants and the informed consent process. Procedures for maintaining the accuracy of data, adhering to IRB guidelines, ensuring the confidentiality of data, and the standardization of data collection should be described. Moreover, data entry and coding issues should be discussed (e.g., procedures for maintaining an audit trial of coding decisions, verifying the accuracy of electronically transmitted data, and safeguarding the security of data). Data analysis and reporting procedures should be described as well as steps taken to ensure the veracity of all products of analysis. The procedures adopted by the project team to safeguard against plagiarism and the fabrication, falsification, or misrepresentation of all research-related activities should be discussed as well as the process to be followed in the event of any inquiries, allegations, or confirmed acts of misconduct. Procedures for reporting adverse effects should be identified.

Additional sections

The proposal should also contain a reference list, time table for accomplishing the study, and letters of support from agency personnel and consultants. Do the letters of support document access to performance sites, research participants, institutional facilities and resources committed to the study as well as matching research funds, if any? Is a line-item budget included in addition to a budget narrative that justifies why the itemized expenses are essential to the conduct of the study? Are any cost calculations described? Some grant applications require the investigator to list all sources of research funding and the percentage of salary support received from each source, including all pending grant support.

In summary, all nurses should have at least a beginning knowledge of research critique. The components of a formal critique are useful for evaluating the suitability of a published study for practice. Nurse investigators should ask their colleagues to critique the preliminary drafts of a proposal as many times as necessary to identify and correct any potential problems.

Scientific and Ethical Conduct of Research

Monitoring the scientific integrity of a project is an integral aspect of all nursing research. Confirmed incidents of misconduct have direct legal consequences and they jeopardize the reputation, future funding eligibility, and employability of the researcher. The public's confidence in research is justifiably eroded when reports of misconduct appear in the lay or scientific press. In some cases, the potential health of individuals with cancer may be at risk if adverse reactions go unreported, protocol-stopping rules are ignored, or falsified data are reported in the literature.

The U.S. Department of Health and Human Services published a booklet in 1995 entitled *Integrity and Misconduct in Research: Report of the Commission on Research Integrity.*[38] *Research misconduct,* as defined by the commission, is any "significant misbehavior that improperly appropriates the intellectual property or contributions of others, that intentionally impedes the progress of research, or that risks corrupting the scientific record or compromising the integrity of scientific practices."[38,p.13] Research misconduct does not involve honest errors of judgment, the stating of hypotheses that ultimately prove to be false, differences in the interpretation of data, or making scientific observations and analyses that may eventually prove to be in error.[38]

The misappropriation and misrepresentation of intellectual property are common examples of research misconduct. *Misappropriation* refers to an intentional or reckless act of plagiarism or a violation of the confidentiality associated with the review of scientific manuscripts or grants.[38] *Misrepresentation* is defined as a deliberate attempt to deceive or commit a reckless disregard for the truth by stating or presenting a falsehood, omitting facts, or the fabrication of data and findings.[38] Additionally, research misconduct may include the obstruction of inquiries or investigations of misconduct or noncompliance with regulations that govern the conduct of federal or privately funded research.

Other examples of research misconduct may include intentionally enrolling certain types of participants in a study to bias the findings in the hypothesized direction, entering participants that fail to meet eligibility criteria, administering an experimental treatment despite severe adverse reactions, fabricating data, reporting findings of a study that was never conducted, or substituting falsified data for legitimate data.[39]

Oncology nurses who witness an intentional act of research misconduct or who are asked to falsify data should follow the local institution's policies and regulations for reporting and handling incidents of misconduct. All cancer institutions that receive federal funding for research must have written policies for handling inquiries and allegations of misconduct. Assistance in developing institutional policies can be obtained from many sources: the literature,[38,40–42] the grants and contracts office of any university or cancer center, or health science libraries. The American Nurses' Association recently published *Ethical Guidelines in the Conduct, Dissemination, and Implementation of Nursing Research.*[43] These guidelines can be used to develop institutional values and practices that discourage acts of scientific misconduct and foster ethically based inquiry.

The principal investigator is ultimately responsible for establishing procedures to monitor the scientific integrity of a specific project. These procedures will depend on the unique aspects of the study (e.g., the number of research sites and geographic location of project staff, the potential risk posed by the experimental therapy, and the conditions under which the study will be prematurely terminated due to unacceptable risk). As an aid to developing a grant application or participating in research as a project staff member, Table 80-5 lists the types of generic activities that are needed to monitor scientific integrity and the ethical conduct of research. These activities are adapted from the Oncology Nursing Foundation's *Guidelines for the Responsible Conduct of Research.*[44]

Future Directions for Research

Oncology nursing research will increasingly influence future health care policy, cancer advocacy, the media's image of nursing, and the health of all people. Nursing

Table 80-5 Activities to Monitor the Scientific Integrity of Research

Data Collection Issues

- Participant eligibility requirements: Monitor all accrual procedures, the ongoing accuracy of inclusion and exclusion criteria, document accrual rates and all reasons for refusal or early withdrawal from study

- Accuracy of data: Choice of instruments, data entry or transcription reliability, procedures to audit and verify the accuracy of raw data extracted from medical records

- Reliability of measurement and analysis: Reliability of instruments, interrater agreement when more than one person is collecting or coding data, sources of potential and/or actual measurement error

- Staff training: Standardize participant recruitment, data collection, and entry procedures; ensure the confidentiality of data; use accepted practices for translating instruments into other languages

- Institutional review board or animal welfare committee approval: Adhere to policies of host institution regarding protection of human participants or the welfare of animals used for research; follow procedures for responding to adverse effects; maintain institutional approval for the duration of the study

Data Entry and Storage

- Maintain a written audit trail of coding decisions

- Verify the accuracy of data entry including electronically transmitted data

- Safeguard the security of data and protect against the unauthorized access to files

Data Analysis and Reporting

- Monitor the accuracy of data during all phases of analysis

- Ensure the veracity of all products of analysis

- Safeguard against the fabrication, falsification, plagiarism, or misrepresentation of all aspects of research

Multi-institutional Projects

- Monitor all aspects of scientific integrity and ethical conduct across all research sites

research findings will be used to design and implement cancer public awareness and educational campaigns where nurses are identified as experts in cancer care. Practice-based research will lead to the creation of new models of care and specialized programs for vulnerable populations such as the long-term monitoring by nurses of individuals genetically predisposed to cancer.

Leading the transformation of cancer care, oncology nurses will influence the research agenda for cancer-related women's health, access to quality care by a diverse populations, and the management of disease symptoms and regimen-related toxicities. Moreover, nurses will be the preeminent clinical researchers in the areas of cancer pain, quality of life, spirituality, cancer-related fatigue, families' responses to cancer, and caregiver issues. Nurses will continue to study the delivery of humanistic care to individuals with HIV/AIDS.

Because of the broad domain of nursing science and the holistic nature of nursing practice, nurse investigators must begin to design nursing trials that span the continuum of cancer therapy and long-term survivorship. Models that synthesize the personal, environmental, and genetic risks for cancer are needed to guide research. Efforts must be made to integrate several divergent literatures: (1) studies of cancer prevention, detection, screening, and diagnosis; (2) research on cultural beliefs about cancer; and (3) studies of the decision-making processes used by people undergoing traditional, experimental, or alternative therapy. Models that explain the economics of cancer care for different cancer diagnoses, therapeutic options, phases of survival, and quality-of-life outcomes are needed.

New descriptive and explanatory models of cancer care must include a variety of contextual variables such as beliefs in personal control, the meaning given to the cancer experience, the decision-making processes of families, communication styles, social power, race and ethnicity, and the will to live, to name a few. For example, how do individuals with cancer and their families make decisions all along the cancer trajectory (e.g., when nursing care is shifted from curative therapies to palliation and comfort measures and eventually to end-of-life care)? Future models of cancer care also must identify which quality-of-life outcomes are meaningful to cancer survivors at various points in the cancer care continuum.

Oncology nurses are leading the current effort to establish cancer genetic services. With the advent of the genetics revolution, conceptual models are urgently needed to guide practice-based research and holistic practice. For instance, how will the experience of genetic testing, notification, counseling, and long-term monitoring influence the quality of life of healthy people who are at genetic risk for developing cancer? What are the ethical issues that will guide research in the field of cancer genetics? What are the elements of informed consent? How will confidentiality be protected and what security measures are needed to safeguard access to computer databases that identify people at risk? What is the potential for work and insurance discrimination against people and families carrying the genes for specific cancers? What roles are oncology nurses assuming in providing genetic counseling and implementing genetic therapies?

Other types of studies are needed to examine complex systems of care and to identify the best practice models of nursing care (e.g., advanced practice and certification issues and patient outcomes of care delivered by generalists, specialists, and assistive personnel). A focused effort is needed to conduct studies on the delivery of cost-effective nursing care by cancer consortiums, jointly affiliated institutions, managed care organizations, and by nurses who own an independent clinic or practice. Patient acuity systems for oncology are needed to guide the prediction of staffing patterns and mix, cost predictions, quality improvement outcomes, and morbidity and mortality outcomes. Instrumentation studies are needed to standardize the clinical assessment of regimen-related toxicities and the assessment of symptoms like fatigue, pain, mucositis, vomiting, and quality of life. Additional instrumentation studies must focus on the translation of existing questionnaires into other languages or the initial development of multilingual instruments.

New mechanisms for conducting research must be established to gather data that are trustworthy and generalizable to populations of cancer survivors. Research designs will need to become more complex and rigorous. Expert panels, composed of nurse investigators, clinicians, administrators, and educators, will need to examine the state-of-the-science of high priority research topics and form a research agenda for the specialty. The future will see the routine implementation of nursing effectiveness trials, multi-institutional studies conducted by nurses, instrumentation studies to develop clinical assessment tools, and formal programs for research dissemination and utilization. Nurse-sensitive outcomes research will be a focal point for demonstrating that oncology nurses do, in fact, make a difference.

Conclusion

Oncology nursing research will drive all facets of practice in the modern era of oncology nursing. As the largest group of cancer care professionals, oncology nurses must explore their own practice and identify superior outcomes of holistic care. As vocal advocates for optimal quality of care, oncology nurses must continue to align themselves with cancer survivors and their quest to humanize care. Our challenge is to design theories of oncology nursing that embrace the best traditions of the art of nursing and give voice to the emerging science of nursing.

References

1. Vessey J, Gennaro S: The bottom line. *Nurs Res* 45:67, 1996
2. Winters G, Miller C, Maracich L, et al: Provisional practice: The nature of psychosocial bone marrow transplant nursing. *Oncol Nurs Forum* 21:1147–1154, 1994
3. McCorkle R: Development of the research question, in Grant MM, Padilla GV (eds): *Cancer Nursing Research: A Practical Approach*. Norwalk, CT, Appleton & Lange, 1990, pp 27–42
4. Mooney KH, Ferrell BR, Nail LM, et al: 1991 Oncology Nursing Society research priorities survey. *Oncol Nurs Forum* 18:1381–1388, 1991
5. Stetz KM, Haberman MR, Holcombe J, et al: 1994 Oncology Nursing Society research priorities survey. *Oncol Nurs Forum* 22:785–789, 1995
6. Winningham ML, Nail LM, Burke MB, et al: Fatigue and the cancer experience: The state of the knowledge. *Oncol Nurs Forum* 21:23–36, 1994
7. King CR, Haberman M, Berry DL, et al: Quality of life and the cancer experience: The state of the knowledge. *Oncol Nurs Forum* 24:27–41, 1997
8. Lang NM, Marek KD: Outcomes that reflect clinical practice, in National Center for Nursing Research: *Patient Outcomes Research: Examining the Effectiveness of Nursing Practice*. NIH publication No. 93-3411. Rockville, MD, Department of Health and Human Services, 1992, pp 27–38
9. Lasker-Hertz S, Houston S: Facilitating outcomes research. *Nurs Invest* 2:1–2, 1995
10. American Society of Clinical Oncology: Outcomes of cancer treatment for technology assessment and cancer treatment guidelines. *J Clin Oncol* 14:671–679, 1996
11. National Center for Nursing Research: *Patient Outcomes Research: Examining the Effectiveness of Nursing Practice*. NIH publication No. 93-3411. Rockville, MD, Department of Health and Human Services, 1992
12. Mitchell PH, Ferketich S, Jennings BM: Quality health outcomes model. *Image J Nurs Schol* 30:43–46, 1998
13. Lamb GS: Outcomes across the care continuum. *Med Care* 35:NS106–NS114, 1997 (suppl)
14. Brooten D, Naylor MD: Nurses' effect on changing patient outcomes. *Image J Nurs Schol* 27:95–99, 1995
15. Blegan MA, Goode CJ, Reed L: Nurse staffing and patient outcomes. *Nurs Res* 47:43–50, 1998
16. Mark BA, Burleson DL: Measurement of patient outcomes: Data availability and consistency across hospitals. *J Nurs Adm* 25:52–59, 1995
17. Aiken LH, Sochalski J, Lake ET: Studying outcomes of organizational change in health services. *Med Care* 35:NS6–NS18, 1997 (suppl)
18. Grant M, Ferrell BR, Rivera LM: Unscheduled readmissions for uncontrolled symptoms. *Nurs Clin North Am* 30:673–682, 1995
19. Hogan AJ: Methodological issues in linking costs and health outcomes in research on differing care delivery systems. *Med Care* 35:NS96–NS105, 1997 (suppl)
20. Ross CK, Steward CA, Sinacore JM: A comparative study of seven measures of patient satisfaction. *Med Care* 33:392–406, 1995
21. Rosenthal GE, Shannon SE: The use of patient perceptions in the evaluation of health-care delivery systems. *Med Care* 35:NS58–NS68, 1997 (suppl)
22. Murdaugh C: Health-related quality of life as an outcome in organizational research. *Med Care* 35:NS41–NS48, 1997 (suppl)
23. Patrick DL: Finding health-related quality of life outcomes sensitive to health-care organization and delivery. *Med Care* 35:NS49–NS57, 1997 (suppl)
24. Whedon M, Ferrell BR: Quality of life in adult bone marrow transplant patients: Beyond the first year. *Semin Oncol Nurs* 10:42–57, 1994
25. Bush NE, Haberman M, Donaldson G, et al: Quality of life of 125 adults surviving 6–18 years after bone marrow transplantation. *Soc Sci Med* 40:479–490, 1995
26. Brooten D: Methodological issues linking costs and outcomes. *Med Care* 35:NS87–NS95, 1997 (suppl)
27. Mitchell PH, Shortell SM: Adverse outcomes and variations in organization and care delivery. *Med Care* 35:NS19–NS32, 1997 (suppl)
28. Ferrell BR, Cohen MZ: Companion studies. *Semin Oncol Nurs* 7:252–259, 1991
29. Grant MM, Padilla GV: *Cancer Nursing Research: A Practical Approach*. Norwalk, CT, Appleton & Lange, 1990
30. Mateo MA, Kirchhoff KT: *Conducting and Using Nursing Research in the Clinical Setting*. Baltimore, Williams & Wilkins, 1991
31. Woods NF, Catanzaro M: *Nursing Research: Theory and Practice*. St. Louis, Mosby, 1988
32. Haberman MR: Research in ambulatory care settings: The

need for and how to do research, in Buchsel P, Yarbro C (eds): *Oncology Nursing in the Ambulatory Setting: Issues and Models of Care.* Sudbury, MA, Jones and Bartlett, 1993, pp 307–340

33. Haberman MR: Nursing research, in Buchsel PC, Whedon MB (eds): *Bone Marrow Transplantation: Administrative and Clinical Strategies.* Sudbury, MA, Jones and Bartlett, 1995, pp 365–402

34. Lincoln YS, Guba EG: *Naturalistic Inquiry.* Beverly Hills, CA, SAGE Publications, 1985

35. Denzin NK, Lincoln YS: *Handbook of Qualitative Research.* Thousand Oaks, CA, SAGE Publications, 1994

36. Haberman MR, Lewis FM: Selection of research design. I: Qualitative designs, in Grant MM, Padilla GV (eds): *Cancer Nursing Research: A Practical Approach.* Norwalk, CT, Appleton & Lange, 1990, pp 77–93

37. Haberman MR: The measurement of symptom distress, in Yarbro CH, Frogge MH, Goodman M, (eds): *Cancer Symptom Management.*(ed 2) Sudbury, MA, Jones and Bartlett, 1999, pp 10–19

38. Commission on Research Integrity: *Integrity and Misconduct in Research: Report of the Commission on Research Integrity.* Rockville, MD, U.S. Department of Health and Human Services, 1995

39. Mooney KH, Haberman MR: Cancer nursing research today, in McCorkle M, Grant M, Frank-Stromborg M, Baird S (eds): *Cancer Nursing: A Comprehensive Textbook* (ed 2). Orlando, Saunders, 1996, pp 1261–1276

40. Chop RM, Cipriano-Silva M: Scientific fraud: Definitions, policies, and implications for nursing research. *J Prof Nurs* 7:166–171, 1991

41. Grady C: Ethical issues in clinical trials. *Semin Oncol Nurs* 7: 288–296, 1991

42. Hawley DJ, Jeffers JM: Scientific misconduct as a dilemma for nursing. *Image J Nurs Schol* 24:51–55, 1992

43. Silva M: *Ethical Guidelines in the Conduct, Dissemination, and Implementation of Nursing Research.* Washington, DC, American Nurses Publishing, 1995

44. Oncology Nursing Foundation/Society (1998, March). *Guidelines for the Responsible Conduct of Research.* (Available from the Oncology Nursing Foundation, 501 Holiday Drive, Pittsburgh, PA 15220.)

CHAPTER 81

Ethical Issues in Cancer Nursing Practice

David C. Thomasma, PhD

Introduction

Cancer care is challenging on many fronts. In addition to the many physical and emotional challenges faced by oncology nurses, many different ethical issues arise in caring for patients with cancer. Some of these issues are common to all branches of health care, some more specific to nursing, and some specific to cancer itself. This chapter will examine the ethical issues in three broad categories: general issues, nursing issues, and cancer issues.

General Ethical Issues

It is customary in every review of ethical theories to sketch the ethical principles of autonomy, beneficence, nonmaleficence, and justice.[1] To these are added alternative ethical analyses, including virtue theory, with a view toward suggesting other ways of resolving ethical dilemmas.

Because not everyone agrees about ethical theory, Beauchamp and Childress[2] proposed four principles that would operate *prima facie*, that is to say, they would be presumed to be authoritative guidelines for moral behavior. They could only be trumped in a case by more serious concerns (or sometimes, by one another). For example, if you are involved in a case where a dying patient requests information about her daughter's not being at her bedside, and you know that the daughter has had an accident and is in critical condition, you could become embroiled in the ethics of truth telling, pitting the woman's desire to know about her daughter's absence (her autonomy) against your duty not to harm your patient (nonmaleficence).[2]

Autonomy

Autonomy is shorthand for a principle that compels us to respect the self-command of the individual. Since autonomy literally means self-rule, respect for the individual therefore includes not only the free choice a competent patient might make but also respect for the source of that freedom within the individual.[2] It would be contradictory to attempt to heal a patient while denying the patient's freedom and ability to make decisions about the healing process. One would be working to improve the patient's health while compromising or limiting her value system. This would not be healing the patient.

The idea of autonomy originated in the attempt to clarify and understand what makes us moral. We are responsible for our own moral acts and must make our own moral rules. Therefore, autonomy should not be equated simply with patients' rights or even with the freedom to choose. It implies something deeper—that the core of what it means to be a person is moral responsibility to oneself and to others. This is not "pure" freedom but rather freedom to take responsibility for one's own actions and their consequences. In response to that level of responsibility, caregivers have a duty to respect the moral origins of the person, not just to respect the choices the person makes, as will be clarified later.

The notion of autonomy is foreign to traditional health care practice. For centuries, health care practitioners governed by the Hippocratic ethic practiced a form of paternalism, acting in what was assumed to be in the best interests of others without asking their preferences, or even explicitly by acting against their preferences. An example would be refusing to acknowledge the wish of an elderly, competent, but somewhat depressed woman to be "left alone" and allowed to die. Caregivers are often reluctant to accept the wishes of individuals with serious disease, especially if they think something still might be done to improve either longevity or quality of life. Another example might be a patient who, fearing the outcomes of cancer, decides to forgo not only any interventionist chemotherapy but also even a biopsy. Despite the right of individuals to determine their own treatment, this scenario would create a conflict between the care giver's sense of duty to protect and prolong life and the autonomy and privacy rights of the individual patient.

Beneficence

Beneficence is the principle of altruism, that is, to act in the best interests of others. It is the fundamental guiding force behind the helping professions, leading, for example, to the maxim "the patient comes first." Of course, it would be difficult to act at all times on the basis of this principle, since self-interest is a part of duty to oneself. Yet the principle creates an expectation in patients and in society as a whole that health professionals, who are often strangers to the patient, will take exceptional steps to place their patients' interests above their own.[3]

Sometimes, however, a good thing like beneficence can run amok and lead to a paternalistic (maternalistic) form of "doing good" without attention to the wishes of the other person.[4] In some instances there is a necessary medical paternalism. For example, a patient may have executed the advance directive to refrain from putting her on a respirator due to advanced metastatic liver cancer but now finds herself in the emergency room due to an automobile accident. Her crushed rib cage is potentially treatable. The presumption would be to treat her, even with a respirator, for a reversible event she had not foreseen in her previous determinations about end-stage cancer. Most often, however, paternalism is regarded with moral opprobrium.

Beneficence does not rule out trying to persuade patients and even sometimes to almost coerce them to overcome their fears and to help them choose what is in their best interests. But in the final analysis, it is unethical to act against the wishes of patients if they continue to refuse the offerings of modern health care.[5]

In cancer care it is frequently hard to determine what

is in the patient's best interest. There may be conflicting courses of treatment, or only statistical or epidemiological information that may or may not apply to the circumstances.[6-8] Also, patients may become incompetent to speak for their own care in the later stages of the disease. In these instances, caregivers focus their efforts on trying to determine objective standards of care, avoiding making quality-of-life judgments by appealing to medical indications.[9] Yet these standards are not as objective as they might first appear. Often they are a combination of current practice, the best medical knowledge of the time, and attention to the context in which care is to be delivered. For instance, the patient's wishes are combined with a judgment about prognosis and weighed against the patient's condition, age, and reasons for treatment requests and refusals.

Nonmaleficence

The third principle governing general health care ethical concerns is the principle of *nonmaleficence*. This principle covers the famous Hippocratic aphorism, "To help, or at least, to do no harm." This principle was alluded to in the first case of the dying mother who wonders where her daughter might be. When caregivers find that there is confusion or disagreement about what is in the patient's best interest, they must fall back to a position of trying, according to the Hippocratic oath, "at least, to do no harm." In the case of truth-telling conflicts, perhaps this principle would gain ascendancy over either autonomy or beneficence.

In a way, nonharm is a minimalist beneficence position. Respecting the personhood of the patient requires an attempt to honor autonomy *and* to act in his or her best interests. At the very least, however, it means never harming intentionally.

The problem is to clarify what is meant by "harm," which can be defined as physical to psychological and even spiritual harm. Some examples will be discussed later in the context of dying. Since most cancer patients recover or stay in remission, however, it is appropriate here to consider a different example: A 42-year-old woman develops breast cancer metastases while being tried in court for running a prostitution ring under the guise of a high-class escort service. Her cancer now involves her spine and causes her intense pain. But an even greater problem for her is that her son is dying of AIDS, and she wants to care for him before succumbing to her disease and to her jail sentence.[10] Harm for her is the spiritual pain of not being able to nurture her son, rather than her physiological concerns (the spinal involvement of the cancer), or even her likely incarceration ("If the government wants me to go to jail, so be it," she said. "I'd like to spend my time now with my son, and after that they can have my life. I don't care."). This example demonstrates how harms ideally are defined by the patient in conjunction with caregivers, so that a mutually agreed-upon treatment plan can be developed. Indeed,

as the role of nurses continues to expand in today's health care environment, the process of coming to understand what are harms to patients may depend even more than in the past on the nursing relationship with the patient and family.

Justice

The principle of *justice* requires that we give each person his or her due. There are competing opinions of how to measure what is due.[11] Some thinkers argue for equity, trying to equalize the inequities of human life by taking from the rich and giving to the poor, for example. Major social programs like Social Security, Medicare, Medicaid, and the income tax exemplify this method. Others argue that egalitarian methods are more appropriate; that is, everyone is entitled to exactly the same treatment (equality) regardless of the starting point.[12] Still others like libertarians argue that justice requires a fundamental respect for autonomy[13] and that one cannot alter the social situation of rich and poor without the consent of the governed. For libertarians, the only moral authority is that which is freely offered or given. For example, one cannot charge paying patients and their insurance companies more for cancer care than nonpaying patients, thus taking from those who have to help those who do not, without the express consent of the paying patients and their third-party payers.[14]

The different views of justice have little bearing on clinical decisions at this time, although they do influence various proposals for access to care and hover in the background of most of our social programs, which, as nurses are often aware, can do damage to individuals. As part of the principles of beneficence and nonmaleficence, too, efforts must be made to provide a better health care delivery system than that currently in place.

Alternative Ethical Theories

The difficulty in clinical ethics is rooted in a confrontation between the tendency toward impersonal, abstract reasoning in the history of ethics and the concrete, individual problems encountered by professionals who must make quick decisions about very complex matters in order to benefit their patients. Ethical analysis must take careful note of numerous ethical theories, axioms, and other concerns in order to conduct a minimally careful conceptual analysis. This process takes time and, of necessity, becomes quite abstract. Health professionals and patients quickly lose interest in these abstractions and theoretical meanderings if they are not decisively and explicitly related to the realities of patient care. They must do ethics on the run.

Ethical principles appear abstract—or better, speculative—because they do not have as much social legitimacy as do the values of everyday life. Moral abstractions frequently are seen by nonphilosophers as devoid of the ingredients of moral concerns that people have in their day-to-day life. No doubt they can and do seep into that daily life, but the process of connecting theory to practice is long and subtle.[15] How often do we encounter physicians and patients who become impatient with "thinking" that has no practical consequence?[16]

Dissatisfaction with principle-based ethical theories has led to new proposals for moral analysis, such as casuistry, hermeneutics, caring ethics and narrative ethics, or "ethics as story."

Casuistry is an ancient methodology by which each case is analyzed on its own merits. No overarching principles allow a conclusion from one actual case to be extended to another. The idea is to compare the current moral dilemma with some paradigm case that happened in the past, and the closer the comparison, the closer the "fit" and the greater your security would be in making a similar moral judgment. Casuistry closely follows the way clinical judgments are made by health professionals. Certain treatments are suggested by your past experiences with cases. The current case is "judged" by you to be like one or another of them. In the truth-telling case, you might argue that your experience with patients in the past when faced with this same moral problem is that it is always better to tell the truth. In casuistic analysis the support for this argument would come from proposing similar cases rather than from moral theory that one must never lie.[17]

Hermeneutics is named after the Greek god Hermes, the messenger of the gods. It means interpreting the case in its whole context—the individual's life plans and values, the family's values, social and cultural factors, and the like. This alternative ethics relies on the one doing the interpreting, or in the case of most health care decisions, the team that tries to make the best decisions for a patient. A good example of its use would be in a case of noncompliance. A breast cancer patient does not appear for her outpatient follow-up as scheduled. This happens twice. Social work becomes involved. Some family data not known previously is brought to bear on the case. Additional input comes from a former husband and a best friend. How much richer the resulting decision is when all of these individuals have contributed to a clearer understanding of the patient's life and values.

Ethics as story relies upon concrete narrative to ferret out the interests and values in each case, especially with relationship to caregivers themselves. The emphasis is on the concreteness of the individual situation, the importance of interpreting values of those involved in the case, and the deeper moral drama and constraints that take place during the lives of individuals experiencing serious disease.

Virtue theory is also an alternative that may complement principle-based ethics. No principle could be implemented without the commitment of caregivers or patients to the good as they perceive it. Even the most rule-bound person must have virtues of interior commitment to the rules. On the other hand, relying solely on the virtuous caregiver and patient, without a set of objective moral guidelines or principles, leads to follies and foibles and opportunity for abuse.[18]

A nursing philosophy goal to act *as if* the nurse were the patient and *as if* the nurse's values became the patient's values would require some limits. Clearly, nurses could not carry out actions that would compromise their consciences. Further, sometimes disputes about care, like instituting or withdrawing fluids and nutrition for the dying patient,[19,20] limit the ability of some nurses to accomplish this nursing philosophy goal. This dynamic reveals the need for a relation between objective standards (the goal of nursing in this instance) and the virtue of the nurses (formed by their own consciences and personal standards).

Arguably the most important virtue for the nurse is compassion. This assertion is based on the view that of all the caregivers involved with the patient, the nurse is the one with the most "hands-on" duties. The implications of this virtue will be explored in the section on nursing ethical issues.

Reconciliation Efforts Among Competing Approaches to Ethics

The emphasis on personal autonomy in medical ethics is coming under greater scrutiny today. Thinkers concerned about libertarian assumptions implied by this emphasis have countered autonomy with the need for beneficence as well.[21,22] The implications of conflicts about medical ethics and ethics theory include the increased role of the health provider's values in caring for the dying patient;[23] greater attention to the relation between health care provider and patient, rather than exclusive focus on the needs and wants of the patient alone; and questions about the kind of society we ought to be.[24]

Pellegrino and Thomasma[3] proposed that the goal of health care ought to be "beneficence-in-trust." By this is meant that the caregiver holds in trust the values of the patient in making joint decisions with the patient about best interests. It would not be appropriate to act in the best interests of the patient without paying attention to the autonomous decision making and values of the patient. This is but one of a number of proposals to integrate the power of the healer's art with the autonomy of the patient.[25]

Another approach is that of libertarianism. Perhaps the most articulate spokesperson for a libertarian version of secular humanism is H. Tristram Engelhardt Jr. In *Bioethics and Secular Humanism*,[26] he argues that secular humanism itself has no moral content. But as an ethical position it reigns supreme for moral argumentation among moral strangers, that is, individuals whose fundamental values are either unknown to one another, or, actually, whose moral values can be considered to be estranged from one another. Engelhardt bases his argument on a fundamental rationality all human beings share that can enlighten them in their pursuit of consensual agreements in bioethics. Supporters of this view may be surprised by Engelhardt's later work *Foundations of Bioethics,*[27] in which more religious value systems find a role and in which he argues that secular bioethics must, in principle, fail.

No matter what approach is taken, it is important that individual moral commitments are not separated from ethical decision making. Further, schema for resolving ethical dilemmas must remain exceptionally sensitive to the concrete situation and particularities of both patient and nurse.[28] Finally, any doctrine of human rationality must be met with reservation: our own ineptitude at honoring others, our downright evil deeds, and the general violent nature of today's human society, in which individuals are treated as objects for the pleasure and good of others, call into question an unexamined view of human rationality.[29] More important, a rationalistic approach to bioethical decision making ignores the potential for a person to identify with a vulnerable, sick, or dying individual through compassion.

Let us look at two clinical management concepts in more detail, since they are closely related.

Casuistry

Casuistry can be used as the basic model for how the good decision emerges in health care. Put simply, casuistry is the theory that each case is unique, and from that case are developed certain norms that may or may not be applicable in analogous cases. The goal of casuistry is to establish the paradigm case, in which most analysts would agree that a certain norm predominates—say, truth telling as an obligation to a cancer patient whose family is trying to protect the individual from the devastating news about the daughter's accident. Other cases are then related to this one and analyzed for the extent to which they "match" or "do not match" the paradigm case. Continuing the example of truth telling, an analogous case would be one in which the patient has had two heart attacks already and is prone to panic when hearing bad news. The family's desire to protect this patient is based on a different reason than in the paradigm case, because now the factor of possible harm to the patient has been intensified compared to the previous paradigm where no such heart attacks occurred.

More theoretical work needs to be done on the assumptions of casuistry, however. This becomes apparent when we begin to delve into the ways in which we use clinical judgment to interpret experience by "mining" the good. By this I mean that we pay particular attention to patient and caregiver value systems, as well as the hierarchy of those values. Which values outrank others in the minds of the parties of the healing relationship? The following discussion targets two major problems with casuistry.

The most difficult part of casuistry is that it presupposes a unified theory of human nature on the basis of which one case can be logically compared with another. This unified theory of human nature traditionally was provided by the *natural law* theory. But this theory, as it

was employed in the past, is now as discredited as is traditional casuistry. Toulmin and Jonsen[30] argue that casuistry arose as a method at just that time in Western civilization when the metaphysical superstructure of Christianity began to collapse under the rise of the modern state, nationalism, and the age of reason. They therefore make the case that casuistry is eminently suitable for modern times, times of pluralism, times without a moral consensus about what is right.[31]

Yet it is difficult to ignore the need for some mode of comparison by which one case is at the very least analogous to the other. Meaning is not wholly and completely individual. It arises in a context beyond or encompassing the individual case. The very basis for analogous cases is some lasting "something" that crosses the boundaries of each case and connects them. In the truth telling example, the factors that cross the boundaries of individual cases being compared are that the patient is dying, that something bad has happened to a loved one, that the patient wants to know what happened, and that there is some perceived harm that might come to the patient if the truth were told to her.

There is a second, and related, problem. Casuistry was discredited by those who held that ethical theory was very important. The method of ethical analysis changed from case orientation to deducing practical conclusions from principles, such as applying the principle of autonomy as a rule that the patient's wishes must always prevail. Reinstituting casuistry as the model for both ethical and medical decisions neglects the importance of ethical theory and, analogously, of the relationship of individuals within the case and their values to the emergence of the good.

Contextualism

Casuistry challenges the deductive model of ethical reasoning. It is closer to clinical judgment, it describes realistically (rather than ideally) how good decisions come about, and it is practical. Yet casuistry neglects the importance of theory and of the nexus of values that ethical theory seeks to protect. Is there a middle ground between deducing the good decision from abstract and theoretical principles that ignore clinical realities and deducing the former entirely from the latter? Is there a middle ground between deduction and induction of the good?

A middle course between a generalist application of ethical theory and specialized case-by-case analysis is possible with a contextual grid for medical ethics.[32] Clinical ethics must address itself to contexts. Neither axioms nor standard moral rules are sufficient (although they are necessary, of course) to determine the validity of moral theory and ethical principles in resolving medical ethics problems.[33] Additional rules, or guidelines for relating theory and practice, must be developed according to this approach. Among these rules is that context serves as a way to analyze value hierarchies in concrete circumstances. Earlier it was emphasized that it is important to consider the particulars of a case, including its context, for a properly compassionate analysis (to be discussed in more detail in the next section).

Thus, according to the contextualism theory, what is needed is a means to locate a moral problem and to exhibit the likely values and principles at issue within that locus. The context having been established by such a "grid," the discussion can proceed toward means for resolving the case by protecting the interests and values of those affected by it. But that is not all. The grid not only locates and focuses the moral discussion; it also hints at the cross-case commonalities that legitimize the acts of organizing similar cases, comparing them, and drawing conclusions about the new case.

A variability of contexts in the clinical resolution of cases is noticeable to all who work in the medical setting. This variability does not so much describe the relativity of values and principles as it does how the weight they bring to bear on a case is partially determined by the medical specialty involved; the severity of the illness the patient has; the personal values of the patient, family, or social group; the personal and professional values of the health care professionals involved; and the institutional setting in which the problem arises.

Some principles and axioms will be given more weight than others in such a scheme, and one important component of the weighting will stem from the contexts. The good will arise out of the mix of these components. When a patient sees a primary care provider, or is seen in the home by a visiting nurse for self-care following breast cancer surgery, the likelihood of patient autonomy predominating in decisions to be made is high. After all, the patient is still capable of making her own decisions. By contrast, if a bus disaster leads to 26 victims brought at once to an emergency room, the likelihood of the predominance of autonomy is diminished in favor of beneficence. Emergency room triage would come into play in an effort to save the most seriously injured person first. The severity of illness or accident, the numbers of persons affected, and the locale have all changed from the primary care or home care example.

Such a contextual grid is only one aspect, then, of what might be called *context-variable moral rules*. Other examples could be examined that do not fit the contextual grid pattern but are moral rules that in other ways vary with the context. Further, the contextual grid cannot encompass all of the variables in a case but only the ones most likely to be affecting the emphasis of some values or principles over others. This is precisely where deductive models of ethical reasoning fall short.

So, the rule of protection of autonomy is more likely to be given prominent focus in a primary care context than in a tertiary care context, wherein one's autonomy is virtually always depressed and hence concern for autonomy is diminished in favor of a goal of preservation of life and/or restoration of health.[34] Furthermore, the rule of protection of autonomy is more likely to be emphasized in cases in which there is no threat to others than in cases wherein the common good must be considered. Finally,

because the grid only *describes* most likely weights given to moral principles and rules in formulating an indicated course of action, one should not misconstrue the contextual grid as claiming that professionals in tertiary care settings do not care about protecting their patients' autonomy, or that public health officials stress social responsibility to the exclusion of individual well-being. All of these moral values bear upon a case. The grid only describes what values are most likely to take precedence over others.

The contextual grid theory rests on two distinctions. The first is the distinction between primary, secondary, and tertiary care settings, a standard distinction in medicine that forms one set of coordinates of the grid. Its importance for moral reasoning lies in the seriousness of the assault on personal wholeness brought about by the diseases in question.[35] Thus, as we saw, a patient's wishes are more likely to be sought and respected in a primary care setting than in an emergency room, this time say after an attack of pulmonary insufficiency, where a paternalistic response may be more appropriate. The second distinction or coordinate of the grid is that between the individual and the number of persons affected by the problem. A good example would be the difference in moral analysis between an individual who refuses chemotherapy and wishes to die from cancer without "any fuss" and a mother of four whose children might still need her to help them cope with her impending death. The former wish might be respected almost immediately, whereas the latter's wish should be balanced with other duties she has as a mother.

The moral significance of this distinction is based on the increasing complexity that occurs when the values of different persons whose interests are affected by the outcome of the case enter our consideration and on our increased tendency to protect the common good the greater the number of affected persons. Recall again the grid's purpose to describe context-variable rules, that is, which principles and axioms are likely to be given more weight than others in a given circumstance in formulating a moral policy or in developing an indicated course of action.

With the increasing provision of patient care by managed care systems, the contextual grid distinctions between primary, secondary, and tertiary care may have to give way to a new set of categories of care, each with its own economic objective that sets the tone for moral analysis. First-level caregivers would have as their goal keeping individuals in a home environment as long as possible. Second-level caregivers would provide temporary institutional care, with the objective of returning the person home as soon as possible. Third-level caregivers would provide permanent institutional care with as little expense as is possible for the quality required. These objectives introduce quite different moral requirements of caregivers in each category of care, and would change the analysis provided by the contextual grid accordingly. Each set of caregivers would, of necessity, have to articulate their roles to the patient and family.

Ethical Workup

I have spent some time underlining the importance of balancing values in any ethical analysis. This balancing is actually a skill that some people acquire better than others. They are the wise ones we consult when we face a moral quandary in the care of patients and in our personal life. They have a kind of practical wisdom, the virtue of prudence. Yet the art of balancing values can be practiced and learned, too.

An excellent tool developed for case analysis embodying the points raised so far is the Ethical Workup. The aim of this tool is to examine as many values as possible in the case and to reach a resolution that respects as many of these as possible. This is done through critical reflection on the importance of some values and principles over others in the context of the particular circumstances of the case. Thorough consideration of each step of the workup permits nurses and other health professionals to examine their own values as well as those of the patient, other caregivers, the hospital, and society as a whole. Furthermore, principles, rules, duties, and virtues also come into play in the later steps during the resolution process. The following six-step workup for case-oriented bioethics courses has been developed.[36] The health professional examining the case is addressed directly in the instructions below:

ETHICAL WORKUP GUIDE

The workup is an attempt to distill from the discipline of ethics an essential process of moral reasoning that can be used to resolve cases. In other words, no attempt is made to force you to take one or another position in the history of ethical theory. Instead, you are asked to follow only one absolute: Come up with an ethically justifiable course of action for the patient. This meshes with your professional duty to act in the best interests of the patient.

Step 1. What are the facts in the case? Be sure to research any medical facts not presented in the case but possibly relevant to its outcome.

Step 2. What are the values at risk in the case? Describe all relevant values—that is, values of the physicians, patients, house staff, nurses, hospital administration, the institution, and society itself. This may not be an exhaustive listing of interests in the case.

Step 3. Determine the principal conflicts between values and professional norms and between ethical axioms, rules, and principles. Conflicts can occur among *prima facie* absolute values, norms, axioms, rules, and principles, and/or among each other. The principal clash, in the end analysis, is the one you determine it to be.

In determining this principal clash, you should explain if you think principles and values are absolute and whether to be ethical means to act on princples, or whether you hold that they are only at first glance, that is, *prima facie* absolute, and can yield to other important values and principles in the case. You should also note

---

the difference between values, norms, axioms, rules, and principles.

Step 4. Determine possible courses of action, and state which values and ethical principles each course of action would protect or infringe. At this step you will grapple with fundamental moral theory. Are you willing to seek a solution that is based on a single principle? Or are you willing to note that each decision you might make will place some values, principles, etc., at risk? Would you then be satisfied with being utilitarian—that is, protecting as many values and principles as possible in the case?

Step 5. Make a decision in the case.

Step 6. Defend this course of action. Why is X better than Y? In defending this course of action, ask whether consensus ethics is appropriate. Is deciding on the basis of a majority or a consensus really the same as ethics? What makes it right? Should the decision rest on a single value or principle? Instead, should it protect as many values as possible? Or should it rest on the virtue of the caregivers or institutions in which it takes place?

Please respond to each of the following:

- Were any values, principles, norms, axioms, or rules weighted more heavily than others? If so, which values, principles, etc. were most important to protect and why? If not, was the case decided by protecting as many of the values in the case as possible?

- Try to identify the type of moral reasoning applied in resolving the case (utilitarian, deontologic, virtue-ethic, care ethics, casuistic ethics, other) and state whether it was used because of your general preference in similar situations or because of its particular applicability to this specific case.

- Universality test: Would you be willing that your decision and its reasons become universal law and apply to every similar situation? To yourself? Is this test actually a valid way to determine what is ethical?

- What role does society play in making this decision palatable? Can you imagine a different society and different solution? Would the decision require you to change the political system or the way health care is delivered? Are social and political duties a feature of the nature of the profession and clinical judgment? Do you believe in cultural relativism?

- How does this decision relate to others you have made in your life, in courses, and in actuality as a professional?

Nursing Ethical Issues

As we have seen, beneficence must go well beyond the minimalistic interpretation of avoiding harm. It entails helping others even when that involves inconvenience, sacrifice, and risk to self-interest. Conflicts occur between the obligation to help others and self-interest. At risk is the primary obligation of advocacy of the patient's interest, which is at the heart of any compassion-based medical ethic. If, as Loewy[37] contends, the possibility of suffering is the basis of a beneficent community, the compassion for the sick is one of the highest forms of virtue. Let us now focus the more theoretical discussion of ethical theories and strategies just completed on the centrality of compassion in any health care ethics, especially nursing ethics.

The Virtue of Compassion

The community traditionally supported compassionate care of individuals by providing for individuals who were sick to be surrounded by those who loved them the most and knew their values. Decisions about health care were made within a context of compassion and respect for the values of the patient. Such care was impervious to marketplace economics. It was an act of mercy, not a commodity to be traded or delivered.

True compassion is more than emotion. It involves putting oneself imaginatively into the situation of another—a first step is sympathy.[38] For some, compassion is essential for health care; for others, it is an act of supererogation.[39] A number of bioethicists link an ability to be compassionate with increased moral judgment skills, with evidence that women are inherently less selfish than men in the healing professions.[40,41]

By contrast, today the community seems more concerned about the resources the sick divert from other projects. Rationing care appears to be more valued than providing it. The most vulnerable—the poor, the elderly, the chronically handicapped, the infants, the mentally ill, and the retarded—are the ones who will suffer the most from rationing. With concern about rationing comes a danger of shrinking from sacrifice—of time, emotions, energies, and money—that the care of the sick requires. So urgent have the economics of health care become that some traditional caregivers, like religious hospitals, contemplate withdrawing from this vital service.

But none of the changes in society or the technology of medical care can alter the call the sick themselves press upon caregivers so insistently, the call from fellow creatures in need.[42] Recognizing their need as persons can only be done if the caregiver's own self-perception is of being an agent of mercy and compassion.[43] What is the meaning of this compassion within the context of biomedical decisions?

Compassion is more than pity or sympathy. It transcends social work, philanthropy, and government programs. It is the capacity to feel, and suffer with, the sick person—to experience something of the predicament of illness, its fears, anxieties, temptations, its assault on the whole person, the loss of freedom and dignity, the utter vulnerability, and the alienation every illness produces or portends. And true compassion is more than feeling. It flows over in a willingness to help, to make some sacrifice, to go out of one's way. "No one can help anyone without entering with her whole person into the painful situation; without taking the risk of becoming hurt, wounded, or even destroyed in the process."[44]

Compassion entails a comprehension of the suffering experienced by another. Individuals who have themselves suffered are sometimes better able to understand others' suffering. As De Unamuno[45] says, "Suffering is the substance of life and the root of personality, for only suffering makes us persons." Compassion for the suffering of others thus enriches self-understanding, especially of what we too must someday pass through. Compassion helps us realize that sick brothers and sisters are not aliens; they are still very much part of the human family and are vital to one's own spiritual growth. The healthy need the sick to "humanize" them as much as the sick need the healthy to humanize their sickness.

For health professionals and the family or surrogates, compassion is the quality that keeps them from operating solely on the basis of objectivity and rationality. It enables them to recognize that, effective as our science and technology can be, they do not remove suffering. The sick cannot escape the confrontation with mortality that even a minor illness may entail. Human illness is always illness of the whole person—body, mind, and spirit. Hence, the illness and/or dying process is more than some aberration in an organ system. The illness transcends the biological to encompass the whole person and his or her value system. Illness fractures self-image, upsets the balance the patient has struck between aspirations and limitations. Illness is nothing less than a deconstruction of the self.

Compassion enables decision makers to assist in healing, if by healing we can mean the reconstruction of the person. Involved here is an effort to put back together a ruptured self that has separated into an ego and a body that has betrayed that individual.[35] Nurses help defend against the attack on the spirit as well as the attack on the body. The particularities of culture, ethnicity, and language make illness a unique experience for each person. True healing and appropriate decision making can only take place when all of the particulars and values of the individual and all the parties involved in the process of caring for the sick person are taken into account.[46] Compassionate care also means that the patient who cannot be cured by medical sciences—especially the dying cancer patient—may still be "healed" if we help him or her to express the meaning of a life in the final days of that life by respecting, insofar as possible, the patient's values and commitments.

Clinical Ethics and the Relation to the Patient

Since the beginning of modern clinical ethics, it has been clear that the reasoning patterns of clinical judgment in medical care parallel those of ethical judgment. This realization is important for many reasons. For example, education programs in health professional schools have acquired a "clinical" focus of relevance and reality by stressing the similarities among nursing, medical, and ethical decision making.[47] Articles and books on the philosophy of health care have sometimes underscored the relation of the ethics of health care to clinical judgment.[15] More pointedly for our purpose, the nexus between clinical judgment and clinical ethics can help reveal structures of good decision making in patient care that are not simple products of contractual models of the provider–patient relationship. More is going on in that relationship than initially meets the eye.

Contrast a superficial view of the provider–patient relationship with one that digs more deeply into the humanity of caregiving.[48] Take the ever-present problem of truth telling in cancer care. A superficial response to a patient's questioning the results of tests, his ability to plan for a vacation next summer, or her denial of the severity of her disease might incorporate authentic truths—to one is dispensed the actual results of a test; to the next hope is held out (after all, one must be compassionate) and planning a vacation is encouraged; to the other, the nurse might withhold her instinct to correct the patient's continuous denial by saying, once again, that the treatments are only palliative now and not aimed at curing the patient's cancer. All of these acts are parallel to good clinical judgment and all encompass a modicum of compassion. Behaviorally there is nothing to contest, nor would there be cause for moral outrage. The nurse is acting ethically in each instance.

What is missing in this picture of ethics, however, is the very essence of human beings touching the lives of one another, of healing one another through their encounters with their own shared fears. A nurse imbued with "the humanity of caregiving" would find out what the test meant to the patient and comfort the patient when the test showed a negative result. The same nurse might discuss the need to plan for the future with the patient who wants to take a vacation, but help that patient make those plans earlier than next summer, so that a kind reminder of the possibility of death is brought up. For the woman in denial of her cancer's progression, the nurse would try to understand how such denial functions as a mechanism for survival, to "beat the odds," even if only to beat the predictions about how much time she has.

Although the examples abound, what is critical about this contrast is that the bald truth, while ethical, may not always correspond with good clinical care. Good clinical ethics, the richer, contextualized form for which I argue, more closely parallels good human interactive care like that just described, where the nurse digs in deeper into his or her shared humanity with the patient, and in that very act, "holds out hope" that such bonds will not be driven from the patient's life.[49]

Some thinkers argue profoundly about traditional commitments to the value of human life within the patient care relationship as contrasted with respect for autonomy alone.[50] Thus, Leon Kass[51] presents a thoughtful articulation of what is owed a dying patient by health professionals. He argues that humanity is owed humanity, not just "humaneness" (i.e., being merciful by killing the patient). Kass suggests that the reason we are compelled to put animals out of their misery is that they are *not* human and thus demand from us some measure of humaneness. By contrast, human beings demand from us our humanity itself. This thesis, in turn, rests on the relationship "between the healer and the ill" as constituted, essentially, "even if only tacitly, around the desire of both to promote the wholeness of the one who is ailing."[52]

We might call the temptation to employ technology rather than one's personhood in the process of healing "the technological fix." The most obvious example is that of offering a shot to kill pain rather than a discussion of the fears that lead to that pain being so overwhelming. Another might be the very necessary efforts to suction the patient, even when it may interrupt a very serious family dynamic at the bedside. One can palpably "feel" the tension at the bedside, but the temptation is not to address it but rather attend to the technology of respiratory assistance. More mundane examples of hiding behind one's professional training also appear as a kind of technological rather than personal relation to the patient. After all, if the patient is truthfully told the results of the test, then has not the duty to care for the patient been met? It may be accompanied by solicitation and expressions of concern (within the limits of time imposed by managed care, perhaps). Should the second patient go on about his plans for vacation, is it not easier to support them than to try to engage in a dialogue in which his deepest fears for the future and the nurse's own fears about dying are broached (again with one eye on the clock and the other on the obligations one has to other patients)? Is it not less stressful to "play along" with the third patient's denial of her disease by not confronting the palliative versus cure dynamic so often found in cancer care? The daily relation of the patient to caregivers in this scenario is like a treatment train that the patient and caregivers have boarded and cannot get off.

The technological fix is not only easier to conceptualize and implement than the more difficult processes of human engagement but is also "suggested" by technology itself. The training and skills of modern health professionals are overwhelmingly nurtured within an environment of technological fixes. By instinct and proclivity, people in a modern civilization are tempted by technical rather than personal solutions to problems. This is so predominate a value system in modern health care, that when nothing further can be offered, no new combination chemotherapy, or fast-breaking experimental efforts, the patients and family sometimes feel angry and betrayed not only by the caregivers but also by the system itself. This is why so many patients also seek alternative health care and spend reportedly twice as much on it as on standard medical and nursing care.

A responsible use of technological intervention with and for the sake of a patient requires not only rational analysis but also sensitivity to the particularities of the case and the emotional content of value commitments of the parties involved. The responsible use of power is a clinical ethics judgment about the best balance of interventions and outcomes. Such interactive concerns tend to present counterpressures to a straightforward honoring of patient wishes and autonomy.[53] The virtue of compassion requires an almost exquisite awareness of the physical condition of the patient (to assess outcomes) and the values of patients or of those speaking for them (to assess the quality of those outcomes measured against the patient's values).[52] In fact, compassionate virtue includes a sense of justice and love as well.[52]

The most dramatic examples of taking responsibility for the particularities of a case are culled from problems of withholding and withdrawing care from the dying. But compassion is also required to assess properly the interventions to be given to the weak and debilitated elderly, to the demented, to individuals with metastases, to other vulnerable people, and to individuals who wish to exercise their autonomy in ways that are clearly self-destructive.[54]

The Patient Self-Determination Act

The Patient Self-Determination Act went into effect in December 1991. New measures to strengthen the act are being considered at the federal level at this time. The act requires all health care institutions, including home care and hospice, to notify patients upon admission to the institution or service of their rights under state law to execute an advance directive. Other provisions include asking patients whether they have issued an advance directive or wish to do so, asking for a copy if they have, putting that copy prominently in the patient record, and notifying the patient of the institution's commitment to honor the patient's wishes. Obtaining the wishes of individuals before they enter health care institutions or home health care should not be seen as yet another bureaucratic process. Instead, the act should be used as an opportunity to demonstrate respect for the moral center of the person.

Part of the reason for the act was surely to underscore the importance of patients' rights. But another was Congress's interest in controlling costs of health care, particularly during the last six months of a patient's life. Almost 40% of the Medicare budget covers this period. It would stand to reason that honoring patient wishes not only would show respect for individuals but also would help save critical health care funds.

Difficulties arise when the wishes expressed do not anticipate future events. Sometimes a patient agrees to a "do not resuscitate" (DNR) order regarding the primary disease of progressive, metastatic cancer but then develops sepsis that might be reversible. If the patient also had said earlier that she did not want to "be on a respirator," but that treatment is required to treat the sepsis, can her wishes be disregarded in this instance? Many health professionals are concerned that advance directives will artificially tie their hands in treatment decisions. Many patients agree, avoiding advance directives in favor of "letting the doctor decide." Nurses are usually caught in the middle on issues like this, as they find it difficult to interpret the treatment plan if the physician chooses to ignore advance directives for any reason. In such cases an ethics consult or patient-care discussion is recommended.

Compassionate Analysis

The notion of "compassionate analysis" mentioned earlier embodies both the virtue of compassion and the various mechanisms available for protecting patient autonomy. Advances have occurred in emphasizing the rights of patients not only to determine the treatments they desire and do not desire during the dying process but also to choose treatments at any time during life, not just while dying. The efforts of patient advocacy groups in sponsoring and supporting legislation and court deliberations have been outstanding. As the use of living wills and advance directives, including the durable power of attorney, becomes more common, patient rights will be further clarified (e.g., how will they affect long-term care settings?).[55] What is important to note is that the underlying principle of such instruments is the prevention of suffering—that is, to increase the role of compassion in decisions about life-prolonging technology.[56] A logical extension of patient rights could be to allow even greater control over the dying process.

A living will gives advance directives for the final period of terminal illness. In most states where it has been approved, the living will covers only the terminal phase of an illness, interpreted to mean the last few weeks of a person's life. Most states explicitly rule out directives about fluids and nutrition. Consequently, the living will is a limited instrument. Much more favored is the durable power of attorney. This instrument gives another person authority to make health care decisions for an individual who becomes incompetent to do so. Not only would this person know the patient's wishes, but also he or she could communicate with the caregivers to discern the best treatment or nontreatment options during the course of temporary or permanent incompetency. The disease course changes, as do options along the way. Unforeseen events may occur.

The durable power, unlike the living will, covers any treatment decisions, formally anticipated or not, and at any stage in life, not just in a terminal situation. This is important because medical technology gives health care providers enormous power at all stages of life, especially at the end. Most often health care providers are concerned about the ethical issues in active, direct euthanasia instead of being concerned with meeting a person's physical and social needs. The tendency of our "technofix" society is to prolong suffering in conditions of what has been defined as "hopeless injury":

> a condition in which there is no potential for growth or repair; no observable pleasure or happiness from living . . . and a total absence of one or more of the following attributes of quality of life: cognition or recognition, motor activity, memory or awareness of time, consciousness, and language

or other intelligent means of communicating thoughts or wishes.[57]

Daily life is full of interactions with "things"— nonhuman and fundamentally incomprehensible to most persons. We sometimes get so used to technological processes that we behave as though they are substitutes for human and compassionate care. Eating for many elderly and dying patients has been replaced by tubes; participating in the spiritual and material values of human life has been replaced by "merely surviving," as a being subjugated to the products of human imagination. As Illich observes, "Medical civilization is planned and organized to kill pain, to eliminate sickness, and to abolish the need for acts of suffering and dying. . . . The new experience that has replaced dignified suffering is artificially prolonged, opaque, depersonalized maintenance."[58]

"Beings" subjected to such depersonalized maintenance may no longer be as human as the rest of us. This is no way to respect the value of human life. Is a permanently unconscious being without any ability to relate to its environment a "person"? Part of taking responsibility for our technology is to avoid this subjugation of human life to machinery in the first place through more thorough discussions of possible outcomes and patient values regarding them.

Cancer Ethical Issues

There is an increasing concern that medical technology impedes the search for meaning in life. This is especially true during serious illness, during its initial diagnosis, the hopeful process of recovery, and the process of dying. Society's impediments to a search for meaning have been well described by thinkers such as MacIntyre.[31] The focus of this section will be on the concrete processes of decision making in caring for the cancer patient that reveal that same search for meaning. In other words, the primary ethical duty of compassionate cancer care is rooted in a mutual exploration of the human condition. The following are only a few of the specific ethical concerns related to cancer care.[59] This commitment to concrete decision making is rooted in the nursing concept of "presencing," whereby the nurse deliberately focuses attention on the patient and the patient responds with receptivity, so that the two (or more) are able through their "being there" for each other to share their humanity.[60]

The Dynamics of Cancer

The *dynamics of cancer* refers to the spiritual struggle of the patient to come to terms with the diagnosis of cancer. The word *spiritual* is used deliberately to identify the intense inner realm of fundamental values each person possesses. The realm is often neglected in daily life be-

cause external matters and concerns so easily obscure it. Driving to the grocery store to select items for dinner, having the grandchildren at the house over the weekend, planning a vacation, and pursuing the myriad other events of daily living funnel our attention outside this spiritual dimension, though the values connected to the choices made in the external life are stored there. Periodically we may examine these values. Indeed, Socrates admonished that "the unexamined life is not worth living." But serious trauma in the external life is often necessary before people face their spiritual realm directly.

For a patient with cancer this spiritual struggle may be intensified by confusion about goals of treatment, longevity concerns, doubts about the most effective therapy, problems of cost and benefit, and the relation of these difficulties to the patient's long-standing system of values. Hence the examination of values that is forced on everyone with trauma and dreadful news is compressed in patients first hearing the news that they have cancer. Even though today advanced care can relieve the fear that to have cancer means to be sentenced to die from it, death is often the most immediate fear. Nurses often face the dynamics of cancer in their patients. As a member of a team caring for the patient, however, they can be as confused about their role as the patient is beset by the disease. Nurses, indeed any health professional, must place first their duty to be a patient advocate.[61,62] If lack of honesty with patients or outright dissimulation appears in the care of the patient, the nurse must be ready to confront the team members, and eventually the patient, with the truth about both the course of disease and the treatment regimen. Holding out hope in the midst of falsehood is a poor substitute for the personal interaction we have seen to be required by the virtue of compassion.

The dynamics of cancer has its own structure. This structure, or progression, must be borne in mind when deciding at what point the truth about a treatment plan is to be pressed. At first, patients may feel guilty. Cancer is often seen as self-destructive. One patient with colon cancer blamed herself, for example, because of her lengthy struggle with her son's alcoholism. She thought that she "took it out" on her own body, that she was bound to become seriously ill (and statistics bear her out). Another patient undergoing interleukin 2 therapy complained in tears that he could not spend another night with the nightmares he kept having, nightmares that acid he unleashed was destroying him and his family as it ate into the basement where they were hiding. These fears, embodying guilt, should be directly discussed, and not shunted aside. They are part of the suffering health professionals should help diminish.

Later, patients usually arrive at a more peaceful stage. They come to see that they are not usually responsible for their cancer. Even if they risked cancer through smoking or other bad habits, they might forgive themselves. In this phase of the dynamic, cancer is made into an object, an "It,"[63] an invading army of cells. Patients will refer to it as "my cancer," or "the cancer," now emotionally dissected from their own being. They might say,

"Though the doctor only gave me a year to live, I'm going to lick this thing." Because cancer, however, is an autocorporeal disease, conceptually it is inescapable to feel that one's own body has betrayed one's own self. For this reason, patients continue to view the body as a contributing factor to their disease, which profoundly influences the level of suffering they experience.

Depending on age and habits of resiliency, patients may choose to do battle with the "It" that is cancer. But the battle and the desire to fight it are complicated by the patient's own assessment of his or her life span. Regularly, patients refer to their own sense of impending end. Yet, as the data seem to indicate, caregivers treat cancer patients near the end of their lives more and more aggressively (and expensively).[64]

Guilt reemerges when individuals decide not to continue against the odds. This guilt is attached to the patient's worries about loved ones. Does my husband understand that I still love him, although I am no longer going to "fight" the cancer? Do my children perceive that I no longer find the odds of getting better while feeling worse on experimental therapy worth it? Families, in turn, seem to deny that their loved one could wind up like this, wasting away before their eyes. It is almost an affront to the care they have lavished on their dying loved one.

The likelihood of participating in research therapies for cancer treatment may decline in elderly cancer patients due to lowered life span expectations; poorer prognosis due to more advanced stages of the disease; the body's inability to cope with the collateral effects; and, very importantly, a value hierarchy that places other factors, like the grandchildren's college education, over one's own continued life.

This, then, is the cancer dynamic: guilt, to objectification of the disease, to a sense of betrayal by the body, to struggles with the cancer, to relapse, and guilt about deciding to stop. The dynamic is a spiritual struggle. Perhaps the best recent account of this struggle is found in Cardinal Bernardin's book written on his death bed.[65] In the elderly this spiritual struggle is compressed by their sense of the limitations on their life span. An important component at each step of the dynamic is the autonomous ranking of values, which is essential to grasp in the care of all patients, especially the elderly, who have had more opportunities to establish and hone their values through the challenges life has thrown their way.[66] What this means is that the cancer patient adjusts an inner ranking of his or her value system based on the newest phase of the disease. It is autonomous because this ranking is infrequently shared with caregivers. Instead the patient has objectified the body that has betrayed her and turned it over as an object to the care of others. As noted, it is easy to get caught up with all the tests and details rather than with the inner turmoil. The man who plans a vacation really may be "asking" if the caregivers think he will be alive that long, though he cannot articulate the question directly out loud. Yet the spiritual struggle, the deeper dimension of human life, still goes on. The challenge for the nurse and other professionals is to be trusted by the patient with knowledge about that inner struggle.[67]

Cancer and Autonomy

Autonomy is often identified with decision making, but patients themselves seldom make this identification. Given the complexity of the cancer dynamic, it is not surprising that caregivers might misjudge the role of autonomy in the spiritual struggles of their patients. The latter are engaged with at least three struggles:[68]

1. With the body, often leading to physical exhaustion
2. With the environment, their family, community, job, nursing home, etc.
3. With their own values, including their life plans, expectations, the hierarchy of their values, etc.

While the cancer dynamic continues, the patient identifies autonomy with reshuffling a hierarchy of values. These values are not communicated to caregivers as a general rule, and this is the challenge of creating a good therapeutic plan that does not deprive the patient of that which is most dear. The values can easily be missed in well-intentioned but ineffective efforts to respect the patient. Here all caregivers must remain extremely cautious and self-reflective. Are efforts to honor patient preferences and wishes sufficient to honor the personhood of the patient? As argued, appearance of respectful support of autonomy may actually disguise poor efforts to uncover the patient's value system (that normally does not change) and to travel with the patient as he or she adjusts the importance of different values, the weights given to the values, as new obstacles arise.[69] For example, an elderly aunt may always have loved her nieces and nephews, but had her own career, seeing them only once a year on a holiday. Now the aunt, confronted with a relapse, may want to spend time with each, saying good-bye. This interior concern, before it is voiced, creates a suffering when the aunt is asked to return to the clinic more frequently, and may be an unspoken reason why she does not do so. In this example, a growing resistance to medicalizing her life may hide a deeper value struggle.

The importance of this value hierarchy for quality-of-life decisions cannot be overemphasized. By respecting this hierarchy we can best protect against paternalistic overtreatment against a patient's wishes[70] and any biased undertreatment of cancer patients. This point underlines the importance of finding out patients' values as part of the process of respecting them as persons. It is also the guiding principle in constructing a therapeutic plan.[71] If a patient chooses no therapy for prostate cancer in order to give his money to his grandchildren for their college education, this value is essential to the person he has chosen to become during his life. It makes no sense to strip his personhood from him. As already suggested, in today's health care environment, when nurses are pressed to a greater degree than in the past with daily decisions about care, leaving the more expensive and complex decisions to the physicians, nurses must engage more fully with discovery of the patient's value system and how it is ordered and reordered along the course of the disease. In this way, they can protect patients from real harms to their personhood that treatment plans may pose.

Cancer and Suffering

Pain is a major consideration in caring for any cancer patient. It can so preoccupy caregivers that concomitant suffering is masked. Yet it is the suffering of the patient that should appeal most to our compassion. The first source of suffering is the bifurcation of the person into an ego, often isolated and alone, and the body that has betrayed that person, the object taken over by the disease. This betrayal is bad enough for a person at any age, but in the elderly it is compounded by what are euphemistically called "the indignities of age." There is a documented disparity between patient and physician evaluation of the quality of life.[72,73] The patient's own judgment of his or her quality of life influences and predicts the patient's term of survival. Involving patients in decisions about the therapeutic plan can help heal the suffering caused by the division of the self into ego and body. This is an irony because patients' efforts to reconstitute the self tempt them to abandon decisions about their traitorous body to the doctors, turning instead to the ego and its values.

Attention to quality-of-life concerns can breach the gap and center the decisions about patient care.[74] In other words, concern for patient values, both making the effort to discover them and using them to design a humane treatment plan, is fundamental. Paying attention to patient decision making per se is structurally correct, but it is not enough to make a difference. Decision making is only a door through which higher forms of respect for persons pass. A good example would be how a "difficult patient," dying of breast cancer metastases, becomes less belligerent as soon as she is involved in the decisions yet to be made about her care. Once the offer to participate is accepted, the patient not only "accepts" the illness, either explicitly or implicitly, but also, by that very participation, becomes part of the healing relationship that was dysfunctional earlier.

The greatest danger a cancer patient faces is being stripped of his or her values in the face of the panoply of interventions we have available. This is one aspect of the temptation to hide the caregiver's fears of inadequacy in the external decisions about technological and chemotherapeutic interventions. The emotional roller coaster of promises and hopes versus outcomes and despairs can disrupt the relationships people have constructed all of their lives.[75] Letting go not only of one's life but also of one's social roles and relationships is part of this kind of care that only adds to the suffering the patient experiences. It is endemic to the goal of palliative medicine. Instead the efforts expended by both caregivers and the patients and families to maintain relationships with pro-

viders is well advised. Here the newly emerging concept of "protective care-receiving" can play an important role in maintaining the relationship with the patient. The patient and family respond to care by "protecting" the caregivers as a response to receiving care from them within the context of self care.[76]

Suffering, then, is much more than personal disruption. Yet its base lies there, where the disease has shattered the human entity, at least for a time, until some synthesis can be effected. The primary task of caregivers is to aid in this synthesis as much as possible. Some recommendations are:

- Minimize suffering, not only through pain control efforts but also by confronting one's own blockages to meeting the suffering person as a person. Training in pain control is essential to this step, but so is training in avoiding withdrawal and fears we ourselves have about dying.

- Make every effort to understand the patient's value system so that it can be respected and employed in the treatment plan. This may include using values assessment tools.

- Implement the care plan as a means to minimize suffering. There is nothing worse for patients who are dying than having to wrestle with caregivers over the treatment plan.

- Even when the patient can no longer feel pain and is in a comatose state near the end of life, respecting his or her values is still essential so that the person he or she was, despite the current condition, is nonetheless respected.

Termination of Treatment

All the preceding reflections are essential to a consideration of issues of termination of treatment. Such decisions involve the proportionality of the treatment to the expected and sometimes realized outcome for the individual in his or her specific circumstances.[77] The word *specific* is important. There is no absolute objective standard by which to measure this proportionality. Each instance must be judged on its own characteristics.

What might be deemed appropriate care for a younger patient, say an experimental chemotherapeutic regimen for a 36-year-old man newly diagnosed with pancreatic cancer, cannot be proposed for an older patient, for example, a 93-year-old previously healthy widow. The reasons for this difference may be broader than physical condition of the body alone. They may also be related to the individual's life plans.[78] The younger person may wish to buy some time to put his affairs in order, for little hope can be offered for improvement for a significant length of time in the face of pancreatic cancer. The elderly patient may have no such plans and may be quite willing to die despite any entreaties by the family to try to fight the disease. Her body may have given her so much pain by this point that she has come to consider it an impediment.

Withholding and withdrawing

Caring for the dying patient today presents its own set of challenges: getting to know the patient and his or her value system, obtaining workable strategies for preserving and protecting those values, holding out a measure of hope through personal engagement or bonding, easing the suffering and struggle, and providing privacy.[79] At a certain point in the progress of the disease, decisions about limiting interventions must be made.

Most caregivers today seem more willing to withhold and withdraw major interventions deemed "heroic," but their reasons appear somewhat confused. Should this action be done with the goal of bringing about the patient's death (death induction[78])? In this analysis, death is seen as good and actions are taken to bring about that good.[80] We may be morally obligated to bring about what is perceived as the good in this regard.[81] Or, instead, should the goal be to remove treatments that prolong the patient's suffering, while not intending the patient's death? This intent is entirely different from the first. It assumes that death is either neutral or an evil, and that one cannot will such an evil and still maintain purity of heart. The action of withholding or withdrawing will be the same in either case, however.

The distinction in intent between aiming at the patient's death and aiming at reducing suffering originally was used to distinguish between active and passive euthanasia. The distinction has become essentially moot, since most of those who pay attention to it find that there is no moral difference between withholding and withdrawing on the one hand and actively bringing about death on the other, if the intent is that the patient's death would be a good thing.[82] This makes sense. If our intent in withdrawing care is to bring about death, then other more direct forms of euthanasia may seem much more appropriate. We do not want patients to suffer unduly, even if the pain itself is under control.

Currently Americans are hotly debating whether to legalize active euthanasia, aid in dying, and physician-assisted suicide.[83] In the majority of cases, pain control and addressing the suffering of patients as is done in hospice will be sufficient to properly care for patients. More effort must be made to confront and alleviate the patient's suffering, however. Having more dialogue about values will honor and support dying cancer patients. Use an interview format around values assessment, but do not confine the process to a single conversation. A continuing dialogue would be most appropriate. Although values do not change, attitudes about values do as the disease progresses.

Planning for a good death would lead to restraint of our technological interventions at various stages in the course of disease, depending on the patient's values, willingness to trade possible severe side effects for the chance of an improved, albeit temporary, quality of life, and the patient's self-definition.[84] Of major concern is allowing physicians to kill patients out of mercy in the context of a society that has so little respect for human life in other areas.

Control of dying and life support

Our concerns should not be confined to dispatching persons too early by injections, if simultaneously little or no attention is paid to meeting their physical and social needs. One "technofix" solution to patient anguish is to prolong suffering in conditions of hopeless injury.[85] A good example, unfortunately all too common, is putting an 80-year-old senile and incompetent patient, dying of cancer, on renal dialysis. No family members are left to protest. The patient is brought three times a week to the medical center from the nursing home.

Much of earlier technological intervention was not so much life supporting but, as Albert Jonsen[86] suggests, organ supporting. Now, increasingly, truly systematic efforts are made to prolong all the vital organ systems at once, getting the essential nutrients in and wastes out. We have moved not only from organ-specific technologies to systemic ones but also from temporary support to permanent support. Jonsen wonders just what exactly life support supports:

> We talk about the maintenance of life; we don't often talk about the maintenance of personhood. It interests me little, indeed, not at all, to be alive as an organism. In such a state I have no interests. It is enormously interesting for me to be a person. . . . It is the perpetuation of my personhood that interests me; indeed, it is probably my major and perhaps my sole real interest.[86, p 67]

The effect of employing life-prolonging technology on the dying without patient involvement in its application is to increase patient and family suffering. It may prolong the suffering of dying and it causes social suffering by wasting resources that might benefit those with potentially reversible diseases.[87]

In order to protect human dignity, societies must maintain constant vigilance about protecting persons from both undertreatment and abandonment and inappropriate overtreatment. But how? Undertreatment occurs when the "bottom line" predominates over benefit to the patient. Only a national health coverage plan would eliminate this injustice. Overtreatment occurs through the technological enthusiasms of caregivers, the fear of "letting go," or appeals for unreasonable treatments from patients. Only institutional policies about appropriate treatment decisions coupled with compassionate analysis, as suggested earlier, will answer these problems. In both instances, we will be shepherding our technology for good human aims. This shepherding can be focused on an obligation to attempt to eliminate pain and to address suffering.

Control over one's own dying ought to be the focus of our public policy efforts. Decisions and choices patients make in this regard arise out of the context of their relationships with their loved ones and caregivers and of their own value history. Every effort should be made to help the caregivers and the dying maintain a personal and professional relationship.

Nutrition and hydration

Those who oppose the withdrawal of nutrition and hydration do so on grounds that providing food and water to the dying is a special obligation not covered by our considerations so far, and that beneficence should overrule patient autonomy.[88,89] Specifically, they argue that such withdrawing or withholding leads directly to the death of the patient as much as does an injection, since the patient dies not of the underlying disease process but from starvation and dehydration.[90]

There are two problems with this contention. First, patients have a common-law right and probably a constitutional right to refuse treatment even if they are not dying. Second, patients may request aid in dying on the grounds we have just examined, namely, that death is a good and others have a duty out of compassion to bring about such a good. "Bringing it about" does not necessarily entail active, direct euthanasia, or even physician-assisted suicide. But it does require that all interventions, including fluids and nutrition, be examined for their impact on the desired goal of treatment.[91] If an earlier and less painful death, with less suffering for the patient, is the desired goal, then how does it make sense to provide medically delivered food and water unless the patient specifically requests it?

Nonetheless, those who support withholding or withdrawing fluids and nutrition may miss a main concern of opponents, that in the absence of expressed wishes, vulnerable persons may be "put to death" by such actions. For this reason some ethicists think that only objective criteria (medical indications presumably), not the context, life plans, or values of the individual, can be used in all withholding and withdrawing decisions.[90] Furthermore, they argue that anything else cannot be used to bring about death in patients who have made no advance directives or who have left only vague statements about not using heroic measures to prolong their lives. The family's expression of the values of the patient are regarded as insufficient reasons to remove such therapy.

The role of the family

In light of the U.S. Supreme court decision in *In re Cruzan*,[92] it is clear that the role of the family in speaking for patient values is confused. Recall that Nancy Cruzan was left in a permanent vegetative state after a car accident. For seven years she was fed through a feeding tube. After five years her parents sought to have the tube removed on the grounds that Nancy had mentioned before the accident that she would not want to live in such a condition. The state of Missouri argued that it had a living will law that required advance directives of this sort in writing. It interpreted the need for evidence of patient wishes very strictly. When the case reached the U.S. Supreme Court (the first and only termination-of-life-

support case to do so), the Court affirmed the right of patients to control their medical interventions but seemed to place more emphasis on the right of the state to require evidence of patient wishes than on the right of families acting as guardians to speak for the values of patients. Although the case does not apply directly to persons with cancer, it does demonstrate that guardianship and family issues are still being worked out for incompetent patients.

Thus, it is very important to obtain advance directives from all patients, especially seriously ill ones. The preferred instrument in most states is the durable power of attorney for health care. This document names ahead of time an individual who will speak for the patient when the patient is incompetent to make decisions about health care. It is limited in time to the duration of incompetence and in scope to decisions about health care only. Such an instrument often designates a family member to speak for the patient. Despite the cautions noted by the Supreme Court about family surrogacy, most persons feel comfortable about naming a family member to make decisions, since such a person knows them and their values best.

Access to care

Callahan[93] proposes, when patients are competent and can speak for themselves about medical care, that their options be limited past age 80 and that some interventions no longer be considered. While we might conceivably agree with Callahan that there exists a certain point beyond which expensive medical technology should not be offered to elderly persons, this point should not be set by age limits but rather by the limits of medicine to provide any meaningful change in the outcome for patients during their last years.[94]

It may not be necessary to set such limits on the basis of age if we first try to respect a patient's value system.[95] Elderly persons will usually choose highly technical interventions less often than will younger cancer patients. Statistics show that when patients approach age 80, less is spent on their care. So age and patient wishes apparently begin at that time to be "factored in." Does this mean that physicians ignore the patient's calculation of life span until one reaches "old old" age? Do these data suggest instead that there is a natural life span of about 80–85 years, after which it makes no sense, as Callahan has suggested, to employ major technological interventions to save lives?

Many patients over 80 are more ready to die than to fight cancer. It is not an instance of wanting to die, necessarily. Quite the contrary. Life is still regarded as precious. Instead, it is a matter of proportion. Patients over 80 are more accustomed to thinking that they will soon die anyway. One woman, 92 years old, refused to see a doctor for her suppurating breast cancer. She figured she would die soon and did not want to do so in a hospital where her little bit of savings would almost immediately vanish. She still lived at home, where neighbors and friends looked in on her. Yet when finally convinced to enter a hospital and have the breast removed, she was relieved to learn from her doctors that she would live for some time. ("Let's face it," they said, "you will most probably die of something else than the cancer because it grows so slowly in the elderly.") She was very happy that she would return home. Her plan? To go on a tour of Alaska!

So the post-80 syndrome cuts both ways. It may lead patients to give up too early on their care when they could achieve a significant quality of life. Or it may lead to age bias in offering and withholding care. On the other hand, it also may lead caregivers to sell patients a "bill of goods" that may bankrupt other patient values. A person from the Association of American Retired Persons in Nebraska wrote about a friend in another state who lost two premier family farms that had to be sold to pay for his care during his dying months. He had intended to bequeath them to his grandchildren. The end-stage "battle" with his disease was orchestrated and managed by his oncologist without attention to these primary values.

Among other important issues regarding access to cancer care are the problem of the rights of all persons to expensive interventions, the right to request experimental therapy (if any),[96] allocating scarce resources like interleukin-2, large-scale distribution of health care among competing health needs (e.g., the drain of caring for persons with AIDS on state and local health care budgets), and the distribution of funding for other human needs versus health care needs. Studies have been done on what patients perceive as the foundation stones for good cancer care in an environment of cutbacks. Not surprisingly, communication with and availability of caregivers rank the highest.[97]

Playing God

Modern medical technology empowers individuals beyond their normal capacities. Because technology is, by definition, an extension of human work, it tempts us to exceed the bounds of temperance. This leads to a kind of paternalism in which an individual comes to believe that he or she knows best what is good for another person due to superior technical knowledge. Medical technology adds to this traditional paternalism an even greater temptation, the temptation to "play God."[98] Usually a physician "god" is unrelenting in applying treatment interventions. Rarely, a pusillanimous abandonment of patients without sufficient intervention is found, as might occur when inappropriate judgments about either patient values or the patient's quality of life are made.[99]

It must be admitted that human beings have an incredible thirst for power. Surely this is one reason that humanity is perpetually dissatisfied with the status quo and constantly wants to change for the better. General Electric's slogan used to be "Progress is our most important product." Progress in what, one might ask? The answer cannot be just technological improvement. Leading a good life must include mastery of life's vicissitudes. There is nothing intrinsically wrong with our efforts to improve our lives; on the contrary, it is part of the mission of all human beings to use their facilities and propensities to bring about the good in their lives and in society. Yet it is important for health care that providers understand the risks and benefits of the technological interventions they propose.[100]

Euthanasia

The problem of euthanasia, as well as the difficult questions about human reproduction and all the others in between the origin of life and the final moment of death, involves the question of dominion over life. Our technology makes the temptation to take control over life itself almost overwhelming. Inappropriate withdrawal and withholding of care is also a kind of "playing God" since it involves one individual, entrusted with the care of another, making judgments about the value of that person's life. It is important to distinguish here between objective evaluation of interventions and outcomes on the well-being of the patient and subjective quality-of-life judgments in which the physician and other caregivers judge that the life the patient is now living is not worthwhile for that person.

The danger of euthanasia in the United States today is in the economic sphere.[101] Will it be easier to use a simple method of dispatching those persons whose care costs too much or who are now considered to be a burden on society, like patients with advanced stages of cancer who require extensive care, than to address their suffering, which sometimes is overwhelming even for the most dedicated caregivers? The issue focuses attention on the importance of maintaining compassionate respect for human life in our society. For some, actions to eliminate burdensome life, even if requested by the patient, are a form of "privatizing life," denying its social and communal dimensions as both a private and public good. These persons would argue strongly against direct euthanasia or physician-assisted suicide.[102] Others argue that euthanasia and/or assisted suicide are appropriate and important forms of caring for persons whose lives, by their own assessment, have become too burdensome to continue.[103–106] As is well-known, Oregon now permits physician-assisted suicide under strict regulation. There is no evidence of a groundswell of deaths by this method. Yet the question of permitting this power over life continues to be debated in the United States and throughout the world.[107]

Conclusion

Some suggestions implicit in this chapter are as follows:

1. Consider that the duty to protect a patient's life lies primarily in protecting his or her autonomy and value

hierarchy. It makes little sense to prolong a life if one does not respect the biography of that life as "written" by the patient. For this reason, pay more attention to discovering the patient's value system, through a values assessment interview and through constant discussion with the patient and the family throughout the course of treatment.

2. Require advance directives before one receives the first retirement check, enter that advance directive on a central computer, and update it whenever one enters a health care institution, nursing home, or hospice in accordance with current Patient Self-Determination Act procedures.[108] This suggestion differs significantly from the Patient Self-Determination Act of 1990 (implemented in December 1991), in that the latter requires only information and education, while the proposal here requires executing an advance directive itself.[109,110] Current procedures for informing patients of their right to issue advance directives could be used with sample forms attached for their implementation. Home care nurses should be recruited for discussing these instruments with all persons ready to retire as part of a national effort to prevent unnecessary and unwanted care.

3. Teaching guides should be developed for all health care professionals that would train them in the processes of implementing patient advance directives, since resistance to these directives is still encountered.

4. Change the current default mode of health care delivery in which it is assumed that everyone desires technological support of their life. Instead of assuming that during the last months of a patient's life everything possible should be done to prolong that life, the opposite assumption would be made unless the patient has issued advance directives to the contrary. Since some people's advance directive will be that they wish to make none, they will need to be warned that this means an assumption in favor of restraint rather than intervention.

5. Use a process like the Ethical Workup Guide to analyze and discuss cases that arise in one's service. By doing this, one not only gains greater critical awareness of one's own assumptions and values but also becomes more able to discuss the deepest commitments of one's profession.

References

1. Graber GC: Basic theories in medical ethics, in Monagle J, Thomasma DC (eds): *Medical Ethics: A Guide for Health Professionals.* Rockville, MD, Aspen, 1988, pp 462–475
2. Beauchamp T, Childress J: *Principles of Biomedical Ethics* (ed 3). New York, Oxford University Press, 546: 1995
3. Pellegrino ED, Thomasma DC: *For the Patient's Good: The Restoration of Beneficence in Health Care.* New York, Oxford University Press, 240: 1988
4. Thomasma DC: Beyond medical paternalism and patient

5. autonomy: a model of physician conscience for the physician-patient relationship. *Ann Intern Med* 98:243–248, 1983
5. Thomasma DC: Some philosophical observations about autonomy in oncology, in Bergsma J (ed): *Autonomy and the Cancer Patient.* Utrecht, Netherlands, Department of Social Sciences and Medicine, Rijksuniversiteit Utrecht Medical School, 1985, pp 29–38
6. Thomasma DC: When healing involves risk to life: risky medical procedures and experimentation. *New Catholic World* 230:163–167, 1987
7. Thomasma DC: High technology and dying. *New World Outlook* 46:256–258, 1986
8. Thomasma DC: Philosophical reflections on a rational treatment plan. *J Med Philos* 11:157–165, 1986
9. Thomasma DC: Quality of life judgments and medical indications. *Qual Life Cardiovasc Care* 2:113–118, 1986
10. Rossi R: Madam gets 1-yr house detention. *Chicago Sun-Times,* Mar. 19, 1992
11. MacIntyre A: *Whose Justice? Which Rationality!* South Bend, IN, University of Notre Dame Press, 410: 1988
12. Veatch R: *A Theory of Medical Ethics* (ed 2). New York, Basic Books, 1996
13. Engelhardt HT Jr: *The Foundations of Bioethics* (ed 2). New York, Oxford University Press, 446: 1996
14. Engelhardt HT Jr., Rie MA: Morality for the medical-industrial complex: a code of ethics for the mass marketing of health care. *N Engl J Med* 319:1086–1089, 1988
15. Graber G, Thomasma D: *Theory and Practice in Medical Ethics.* New York, Continuum, 229: 1989
16. Thomasma D: Applying general medical knowledge to individuals: a philosophical analysis. *Theor Med* 9:187–200, 1988
17. Kuczewski MG: *Fragmentation and consensus: communitarian and casuist bioethics.* Washington, DC, Georgetown University Press, pp 177–184, 1997
18. Pellegrino ED, Thomasma DC: *The Virtues in Medical Practice.* New York, Oxford University Press, 1993, 205: also see by the same authors, *The Christian Virtues in Medical Practice.* Washington, D.C., Georgetown University Press, 1996 p 164
19. Jansson L, Norberg A: Ethical reasoning concerning the feeding of terminally ill cancer patients: interviews with registered nurses experienced in the care of cancer patients. *Cancer Nurs* 12:352–358, 1989
20. Davidson B: Ethical reasoning associated with the feeding of terminally ill elderly cancer patients: an international perspective. *Cancer Nurs* 13:286–292, 1990
21. Pellegrino ED, Thomasma DC: The conflict between autonomy and beneficence in medical ethics: proposal for a resolution. *J Contemp Health Law Policy* 3:23–46, 1987
22. Loewy E: The restoration of beneficence. *Hastings Cent Rep* 19:42–43, 1989
23. Thomasma DC: Ethical and legal issues in the care of the elderly cancer patient. *Clin Geriatr Med* 3:541–547, 1987
24. Thomasma DC: The basis of medicine and religion: respect for persons. *Linacre Quart* 45:142–150, 1980
25. Brody H: *The Healer's Power.* New Haven, CT, Yale University Press, 1992, p 119
26. Engelhardt HT Jr: *Bioethics and Secular Humanism.* London/Philadelphia, SCM/Trinity Press International, 206: 1991
27. Engelhardt HT Jr: *Foundations of Bioethics* (ed 2). New York: Oxford Univ Press, 446; 1996
28. Walker MU: Moral particularity. *Metaphilosophy* 18:171–185, 1987
29. Pellegrino ED, Thomasma DC: Dubious premises—evil

conclusions: moral reasoning at the Nuremberg Trials. *Camb Q Healthc Ethics*, 1999

30. Toulmin S, Jonsen A: *The Abuse of Casuistry.* Berkeley, University of California Press, 420: 1988

31. MacIntyre A: *After Virtue.* South Bend, IN, University of Notre Dame Press, 1981

32. Thomasma D: The context as moral rule in medical ethics, in Wright RA (ed): *Human Values in Health Care.* New York, McGraw-Hill, 1987, pp 142–156

33. Thomasma D: Decision making and decision analysis: beneficence in medicine. *J Crit Care* 3:122–132, 1988

34. Levi, BH: *Respecting patient autonomy.* Urbana, University of Illinois Press, 1999, pp 222–233

35. Bergsma J, Thomasma D: *Health Care: Its Psychosocial Dimensions.* Pittsburgh, Duquesne University Press, 215: 1982

36. Thomasma DC, Marshall PM: *Clinical Medical Ethics: Cases and Readings.* Lanham, MD, University Press of America, 1995

37. Loewy E: *Suffering and the Beneficent Community: Beyond Libertarianism.* Buffalo, NY, SUNY Press, 139: 1991

38. Welie JM: Sympathy as the basis of Compassion. *Camb Q Healthc Ethics* 4:476–487, 1995

39. Thomasma DC, Kushner T: A dialogue on compassion and supererogation in medicine. *Camb Q Healthc Ethics* 4:415–425, 1995

40. Loewy EH: Compassion, reason and moral judgment. *Camb Q Healthc Ethics* 4:466–475, 1995

41. Self DJ, Gopalakrishnan G, Kiser WR, et al: The relationship of empathy to moral reasoning in first-year medical students. *Camb Q Healthc Ethics* 4:448–453, 1995

42. John Paul II Pope: Humanize hospital work. Address to the Sixty-First General Chapter of the Hospital Order of St. John of God. *L'Osservatore Romano,* Jan. 24, 1983

43. Dougherty CJ, Purtilo R: Physician's duty of compassion. *Camb Q Healthc Ethics* 4:426–433, 1995

44. Nouwen H: *The Wounded Healer.* New York, Doubleday, 1972, p 72

45. De Unamuno M: *The Tragic Sense of Life,* trans Kerrigan A. Princeton, NJ, Princeton University Press, Bollingen Series, LXXXV, 4, 1972, p 224

46. Pellegrino ED, Thomasma DC: *Helping and Healing.* Washington, D.C., Georgetown University Press, 168: 1997

47. McElhinney T, Pellegrino ED (eds): *Teaching Ethics, the Humanities, and Human Values in Medical Schools: A Ten-Year Overview.* Washington, D.C., Institute on Human Values in Medicine, Society for Health and Human Values, 1982

48. Larsson G, Widmark Peterson V, Lampic C, et al: Cancer patient and staff ratings of the importance of caring behaviors and their relations to patient anxiety and depression. *J Adv Nurs* 27:855–864, 1998

49. Koopmeiners L, Post-White J, Gutknexht S, et al: How healthcare professionals contribute to hope in patients with cancer. *Oncol Nurs Forum* 24:1507–1513, 1997

50. Gaylin W, Kass L, Pellegrino ED, et al: Commentaries: Doctors must not kill. *JAMA* 259:2139–2140, 1988

51. Kass L: Arguments against active euthanasia by doctors found at medicine's core. *Kennedy Institute of Ethics Newsletter* 3:1–3, 1989

52. Rhodes R: Love thy patient: justice, caring, and the doctor-patient relationship. *Camb Q Healthc Ethics* 4:434–447, 1995

53. Marsden C: Caregiver fidelity in a pediatric bone marrow transplant team. *Heart Lung* 6:617–625, 1988

54. Willette JE: Walk with me. Assuming the patient role can be a priceless lesson in empathy. *Am J Nurs* 97(7):52, 1997

55. Rouse F: Living wills in the long-term care setting. *J Long-Term Care Adm* 17:14–19, 1988

56. Mehling A: Living wills: preventing suffering or a deadly contract? *State Government News,* Dec. 1988, pp 14–15

57. Braithwaite S, Thomasma DC: New guidelines on foregoing life-sustaining treatment in incompetent patients: an anti-cruelty policy. *Ann Intern Med* 104:711–715, 1986

58. Illich I: *Medical Nemesis: The Expropriation of Health.* New York, Pantheon, 1976, p 106

59. Thomasma D: Ethics and professional practice in oncology. *Semin Oncol Nurs* 5:89–94, 1989

60. Zerwekh JV: The practice of presencing. *Semin Oncol Nurs* 13:260–262, 1997

61. Smits MJ: Ethics of nursing practice—ethics of care or ethics of rule? *Verpleegkunde* 12(1):27–35, 1997 [Dutch]

62. Garrett TM, Baillie HW, Garrett RM: *Health Care Ethics: Principles and Problems.* Upper Saddle River, NJ, Prentice-Hall, 1998, pp 135–163

63. Cassell E: Disease as an "It." *Soc Sci Med* 10:143–146, 1976

64. Bried EM, Scheffler RM: The impact of healthcare financing on the quality of life of older cancer patients. *Oncology* 6:153–160, 1992 (suppl)

65. Bernardin J Cardinal: *Moral Vision of America.* Washington, D.C., Georgetown University Press, 1998

66. Thomasma D: The ethics of caring for the older patient with cancer: defining the issues. *Oncology* 6:124–130, 1992 (suppl)

67. Gullo S: Oncology nurses: masters in the art of caring. *Oncol Nurs Forum* 24:971–978, 1997

68. Slevin ML, Stubbs L, Plant HJ, et al: Attitude to chemotherapy: comparing views of patients with cancer with those of doctors, nurses, and general public. *Br Med J* 300:1458–1460, 1990

69. Halldorsdottir S; Hamrin E: Caring and uncaring encounters within nursing and health care from the cancer patient's perspective. *Cancer Nurs* 20:120–128, 1997

70. Cranford R: The care of the dying: a symposium on the case of Betty Wright—going out in style, the American way, 1987. *Law Med Health Care* 17:208–210, 1989

71. Whitney SN, Spiegel D: The patient, the physician, and the truth. *Hastings Cent Rep* 29(3): 1999

72. Latimer EJ: Ethical care at the end of life. *Can Med Ass J* 158:1741–1747, 1999

73. Ganz P: Does (or should) chronological age influence the choice of cancer treatment? *Oncology* 6:45–49, 1992 (suppl)

74. Walter JJ, Shannon TA (eds): *Quality of Life: The New Medical Dilemma.* New York and Mahwah, NJ, Paulist Press, 357: 1990

75. Ferrell BR, Grant MM, Padilla GV, et al: Home care. *Oncology* 6:136–140, 1992 (suppl)

76. Russell CK, Bunting SM, Gregory DM: Protective care-receiving: the active role of care-recipients. *J Adv Nurs* 25:532–540, 1997

77. O'Rourke K: Should nutrition and hydration be provided to permanently unconscious and other mentally disabled persons? *Issues Law Med* 5:181–196, 1989

78. Thomasma DC: Caveat philosophus: technology's abuse potential in the decision to terminate life. *J Am Geriatr Soc* 35:124–125, 1987

79. Rittman M, Paige P, Rivera J, et al: Phenomenological study of nurses caring for dying patients. *Cancer Nurs* 20:115–119, 1997

80. Bayles MD: Euthanasia and the quality of life, in Bayles MD, High DM (eds): *Medical Treatment of the Dying: Moral Issues.* New York, Schenkman Books, 1978, pp 128–152

81. Thomasma DC, Graber GC: *Euthanasia: Toward an Ethical Social Policy.* New York, Continuum, 302: 1990

82. Rachels J: *Moral Problems*. New York, Harper and Row, 1971, pp 42–66

83. Doctor-aided suicide spurs ethics debate. *Chicago Tribune*, Mar. 7, 1991, sec. 1, p 1

84. Bujorian GA: Clinical trials: patient issues in the decision-making process. *Oncol Nurs Forum* 15:779–783, 1988

85. Luce EA, Frank AL, Kilner JF, et al: Lingering death from squamous cell carcinoma of the face. *Hosp Pract* 24:60–61, 65–66, 71–72, 1989

86. Jonsen A: What does life support support?, in Winslade W (ed): *Personal Choices and Public Commitments: Perspectives on the Humanities*. Galveston, TX, Institute for the Medical Humanities, 1988, pp 61–69

87. Raffin TA, Shurkin JN, Sinkler W III: *Intensive Care: Facing the Critical Issues*. New York, Freeman, 1988, p 185

88. Callahan D: On feeding the dying. *Hastings Cent Rep* 13: 22–23, 1983

89. Luce EA, Frank AL, Kilner JF, et al: Lingering death from squamous cell carcinoma of the face. *Hosp Pract* 24:65–66, 71–72, 1989

90. May W, et al: Feeding and hydrating the permanently unconscious and other vulnerable persons. *Issues Law Med* 3: 203–211, 1987

91. Paris JJ, McCormick RA: The Catholic tradition on the use of nutrition and fluids. *America*, May 2, 1987, 356–360

92. Thomasma DC: The *Cruzan* decision and medical practice. *Arch Intern Med* 151:853–854, 1991 (editorial)

93. Callahan D: *Setting Limits: Medical Goals in an Aging Society*. New York, Simon and Schuster, 1987, pp 159–185, 241–242

94. Thomasma DC: Moving the aged into the house of the dead: a critique of ageist social policy. *J Am Geriatr Soc* 37: 169–172, 1989

95. Thomasma DC: Ethical and moral issues in access to cancer care, in Scheffler RM, Andrews NC (eds): *Cancer Care and Cost: DRGs and Beyond*. Ann Arbor, MI, Health Administration Press, 1989, pp 211–223

96. Thomasma D, Micetich K: *The ethics of patient requests in experimental medicine*. Reprinted as monograph by the American Cancer Society, Oct. 1984

97. Macartney GM, Stone G, Harrison MB, et al: Getting to know oncology inpatients and their families: a continuous quality improvement approach. *Can Oncol Nurs J* 7: 140–148, 1997

98. Taylor C: Ethics in health care and medical technologies. *Theor Med* 11:111–124, 1990

99. Wilkes E: Ethics in terminal care, in Dunstan GR, Shinebourne EA (eds): *Doctors' Decisions: Ethical Conflicts in Medical Practice*. New York, Oxford University Press, 1989, pp 197–204

100. Melski JW: Prices of technology: a blind spot. *JAMA* 267: 1516–1518, 1992

101. Scitovsky AA, Capron AM: Medical care at the end of life: the interaction of economics and ethics. *Annu Rev Publ Health* 7:59–75, 1986

102. Bernardin J Cardinal: *Euthanasia: Ethical and legal challenge*. Address to the Center for Clinical Medical Ethics, University of Chicago Hospital, May 26, 1988

103. Kevorkian J: A fail-safe model for justifiable medically-assisted suicide. *Am J Forensic Psych* 13:7, 41, 1992

104. Quill TE: Death and dignity—a case of individualized decision making. *N Engl J Med* 324:691–694, 1991

105. Humphrey D: *Final Exit: The Practicalities of Self-Deliverance and Assisted Suicide for the Dying*. Eugene, OR, Hemlock Society, 1991, p 192

106. Trends in Health Care, Law & Ethics 7(2):Winter 1992

107. Thomasma DC, Kushner TK, Kimsma GK, et al: *Asking to Die: Inside the Dutch Debate about Euthanasia*. Dordrecht/Boston: Kluwer Academic, 1998, p 584

108. Thomasma DC: Advance directives and health care for the elderly, in Hackler C Jr, Moseley R, Vawter D (eds): *Advance Directives in Medicine*. New York, Praeger, 1989, pp 93–109

109. Thomasma DC: From ageism toward autonomy, in Binstock R, Post S (eds): *Too Old for Health Care?* Baltimore: Johns Hopkins University Press, 1991, pp 138–163

110. PSDA well received in hospitals, despite early confusion. *Med Eth Advisor* 8:25–30, 1992 (editorial)

CHAPTER 82

Transforming Cancer Care Through Informatics

Heidi E. Ehrenberger, PhD, RN, OCN®
Elizabeth G. Gomez, MSN, RN, AOCN

Introduction

The substance of informatics is information, a capital good of immense value to cancer care. A solid foundation of information used during cancer care and as a source of scientific data on which to base rational health care policies is essential to improving quality, reducing cost, and ensuring access to care. The rapid advancement and proliferation of computer technology, as a vehicle to manage and process information, is enabling us to advance cancer care. This chapter presents an overview of the evolving contributions of informatics to the delivery of health care and its relevance to cancer care. It first provides an academic overview of informatics, highlighting a few select topics of relevance within the science. The chapter then focuses specifically on the use of the Internet and the World Wide Web (the Web) in advancing cancer care. Any topic related to information technology (IT) is extremely dynamic. Consequently, electronic references are provided when possible, as they are more readily updated than print material. You are encouraged to seek them out as needed.

The Significance of Informatics and Information Technology

The English word *informatics* is derived in part from the French word *informatique*, which refers to the computer milieu.[1,2] Informatics integrates information science and computer science. It denotes activities involved in managing and processing information. Nearly all informatics activities are dependent on information technologies such as computers and telecommunications. Yet, the essence of informatics is the information—not the technology. When the name of a discipline is used in combination with the term *informatics*, it implies an application of computer science and information science to the management and processing of information in the named discipline (e.g., nursing informatics).[3] Health informatics, as a broad science, encompasses medical, nursing, dental, and pharmacy informatics among others.[4] Informatics nurses, using clinical experience and knowl-

edge, add the dimension of nursing to the health informatics viewpoint.[5] The significance of health informatics lies in part in its ability to transform data to make it meaningful and useful to multiple constituencies within the health care system. With IT, the transformation is expedited.

As an example, the National Cancer Institute (NCI) is developing a new architecture for the flow of information in its clinical trials program—a Cancer Informatics Infrastructure (CII).[6] Archaic paper-based and disparate information systems for identifying, naming, processing, and managing information have created obstacles within each phase of the clinical trials lifecycle. Implementation of the CII assuredly will result in facilitating the dissemination of cancer information to health care providers, patients and their families, and at-risk individuals—all for better patient care.

Major Federal Initiatives to Expand the Use of Information Technology

During the 1990s, major federal initiatives were implemented in the United States to greatly expand the accessibility and use of information in all sectors of the economy, including that of health care.[7] Three of these initiatives are significant because of their implications for health care: the National Information Infrastructure (NII) Initiative, the Next Generation Internet (NGI) Initiative, and the National Telemedicine Initiative (NTI). These initiatives have either directly or indirectly affected the environment in which we deliver cancer care. These initiatives also highlighted, in part, the need for strategic directions targeting the informatics needs of nursing nationally.

National information infrastructure initiative

In 1993, the Clinton Administration announced the promotion of the NII, a web of communications networks, computers, databases, and consumer electronics that would readily provide the end-user with vast amounts of information.[7] It was believed that better use of IT and development of health care applications for the NII could make a significant contribution to health care reform. Between 1980 and 1992, health expenditures rose from

9%–14% of the gross domestic product; under current policies, it is estimated that they will continue to rise significantly.[8] The NII has the potential to be an integral part of comprehensive health care reform. As an example, experts estimate that telecommunications applications could reduce health care costs by $36 to $100 billion each year while improving quality and increasing access.[8]

Next generation internet initiative

In 1996, the Clinton Administration announced the NGI initiative noting that we must begin investing now to create a foundation to support the networks of the twenty-first century.[9] This initiative identified three goals. The first goal was to connect universities and national laboratories with high-speed networks that are 100–1000 times faster than the Internet as it existed in 1996. The second goal was to promote experimentation with the next generation of networking technologies, as there are numerous challenges associated with rapidly increasing the speed of networks and the number of Internet users. The third goal of the NGI initiative was to demonstrate new applications that meet national goals and missions. Higher-speed and more advanced networks will enable a new generation of applications to support scientific research, distance education, and health care. At the Johns Hopkins University, researchers were funded under this initiative to develop, implement, and evaluate NGI capabilities for radiation oncology treatment planning and care delivery.[10]

National telemedicine initiative

The NTI was also announced in 1996 by the Secretary of the Department of Health and Human Services (DHHS).[11] The National Library of Medicine (NLM) funded 19 telemedicine projects affecting rural, inner-city, and suburban areas, with a total budget of $42 million. These projects were to serve as models for evaluating the impact of telemedicine on cost, quality, and access to health care. At the University of Pittsburgh, researchers were funded under this initiative to examine the effect of integrated access to clinical images and textual patient data on the length of time required to diagnose cancer and on the management of cancer treatment.[12]

A National Informatics Agenda for Nursing Education and Practice

The Division of Nursing, a unit within the Health Resources and Services Administration of the DHHS, provides national leadership to ensure an adequate supply and distribution of qualified nursing personnel to meet the health needs of the nation. In keeping with its mission, the Division, through the National Advisory Council on Nurse Education and Practice (NACNEP), submits periodic workforce reports to the Secretary of the DHHS.[5] The national leadership recognized the need for more

adequate preparation of the registered nurse workforce to manage information using technology. This need was partially based upon the previously described federal initiatives. Acting on the advice of a national panel of 19 expert nurse informaticians, in December of 1997 the NACNEP issued a workforce report titled "A National Informatics Agenda for Nursing Education and Practice."[5] This report proposed five strategic initiatives: (1) educate nursing students and practicing nurses to achieve core informatics competencies; (2) prepare nurses with specialized skills in informatics; (3) enhance nursing practice and education informatics projects; (4) prepare nursing faculty in informatics; and (5) increase collaborative efforts in nursing informatics. It is widely expected that patients and consumers will also benefit from these initiatives, both directly and indirectly.[7]

Nursing Informatics

Nursing Informatics as a Specialty

In 1992, the American Nurses Association (ANA) recognized nursing informatics as a specialty. Two years later, the ANA published a document titled "The Scope of Practice for Nursing Informatics" followed by a document published in 1995 describing the "Standards of Practice for Nursing Informatics."[13,14] Nursing informatics supports the practice of all nursing specialties (e.g., oncology nursing) at the basic or advanced practice level, in all sites and settings of health care.[13] Informatics activities include developing and evaluating applications for managing and processing nursing data, information, and knowledge in cancer care. Nursing informatics is different from other specialties because of its special focus on the structure, acquisition, and use of information. In specialties such as oncology nursing, the focus is on the substance of the information in the care of cancer patients. An oncology nurse who is also an informatician is likely to be better able than other informaticians to represent the concepts of oncology nursing and their relationships in the structure of informatics applications to support oncology nursing.

Research Priorities

As early as 1986, a research framework for nursing informatics was proposed.[15] Research priorities for nursing informatics have since been formalized by the National Institute of Nursing Research (NINR). Since 1993, the NINR has supported a program initiative titled "Enhancing Clinical Care Through Nursing Informatics." The intent of this program is to generate research that will examine systems to manage and process data, information, and knowledge with the goal of facilitating appropriate and effective clinical care. This initiative builds directly on the work of a convened panel of scientific experts on nursing informatics. The panel proposed six program goals for informatics research that are detailed in a 1993 report titled "Nursing Informatics: Enhancing Patient Care"[16] (Table 82-1). Since then, research in clinical nursing informatics has proceeded along three important dimensions: (1) identifying and defining nursing's language; (2) understanding how clinical judgment and decision making can be facilitated by computer-based systems; and (3) determining how well-designed systems can transform nursing practice.[17] In 1997, given the rapid changes in health care and technology, a survey was conducted to reevaluate the established NINR program goals and to determine whether new priorities exist.[18] The findings reaffirmed the NINR six program goals. Newly identified priorities include patient use of IT, telecommunications for nursing practice, issues of privacy and confidentiality, and nursing intervention innovations such as the electronic delivery of nursing interventions.[18,19]

Standardized Nursing Vocabularies

The importance of standardized vocabularies designed to represent nursing data cannot be overstated. Historically, nurses have used different terms when documenting patient experiences and nursing actions. But when different terms are used, the data are essentially not comparable. For example, at the Vanderbilt Medical Center, analysis of standardized documents used to plan and document nursing care showed 17 different ways to convey the information "nausea and vomiting controlled."[20] When this occurs, we cannot compare data to identify effective nursing interventions and our contribution to patient outcomes is compromised. It is clear that structured, coded data are needed to ensure comparability of nursing observations and records across time and location.

As early as 1985, a group of national experts designed the Nursing Minimum Data Set (NMDS), a system for collecting uniform, standard, comparable, minimum nursing data in any setting where nursing care is provided.[21,22] In 1989, the ANA Steering Committee on Databases to Support Clinical Nursing Practice was established to monitor and ensure the development and use of multiple nursing vocabularies and classification schemes within the framework of the NMDS.[21,23] Several nursing vocabularies have since evolved as appropriate to support clinical practice. As of 1999, the ANA Steering Committee recognized the following seven nursing classifications: (1) the North American Nursing Diagnosis Association (NANDA) taxonomy;[24] (2) the Omaha System;[25] (3) the Home Health Care Classification (HHCC);[26] (4) the Nursing Interventions Classification (NIC);[27] (5) the Nursing Outcomes Classification (NOC);[28] (6) the Patient Care Data Set;[29] and (7) the Perioperative Nursing Diagnoses, Interventions and Outcomes Data Set.[30] Although these languages vary in purpose, scope, and content, it is possible to map terms in one language with terms in another language that have the same meaning.[31] Additionally, the ANA Steering Committee has also endorsed the concept of a Unified Nursing Language System to integrate existing vocabularies, facilitate access to data elements, and communicate among information sources.[32] Ultimately, the optimal use of standardized languages within computerized patient records will allow us to document care in order to be able to aggregate data that can be used to determine costs, quality of care, and health policy.[33]

Table 82-1 Nursing Informatics Research Program Goals

- Establish nursing language, including lexicons, classification systems, and taxonomies, as well as standards for nursing data.

- Develop methods to build databases of clinical information, including data, diagnoses, objectives, interventions, and outcomes, and management information, including staffing, charge capture, turnover, and vacancy rates, and analyze relationships among them.

- Determine how nurses use data, information, and knowledge to give patient care, and how care is affected by differing levels of expertise and by organizational factors and working conditions; and design information systems accordingly.

- Develop and test patient care decision support systems and knowledge delivery systems that are appropriate for nurses' needs, with consideration for expertise and organizational factors and working conditions.

- Develop prototypes and eventually working models of nurse workstations equipped with tools to provide for nurses all the information needed for patient care, research, and education, at the point of use, and linked to an integrated information system.

- Develop and implement appropriate methods to evaluate nursing information systems and applications, particularly regarding their effects on patient care.

Data from the National Institute of Nursing Research.[16]

Computer-Based Patient Record Systems

Overview

In 1989, the National Academy of Science's Institute of Medicine (IOM) launched a study to examine how IT could improve the paper-based patient record. The two-year study resulted in the published report, "Computer-based Patient Records: An Essential Technology for Health Care."[34] In noncomputerized environments, 30% of treatments ordered are not documented, 40% of diagnoses are not recorded, and 30% of the time a medical record is unavailable during patient visits.[8] Undoubtedly, computer-based patient records (CPRs) are essential to improving the quality and reducing the cost of delivering health care in the twenty-first century.[34,35] The IOM report on CPRs, revised in 1997, continues to provide a compelling case for recognizing the CPR as the standard patient record.[36]

Individual CPRs are stored in a data repository, which is manipulated by the CPR system. Tang and McDonald identify five functional components of a comprehensive CPR system: (1) an integrated view of patient data, (2) clinical decision support, (3) clinician order entry, (4) access to knowledge sources, and (5) integrated communication support.[37] Inherent in such an approach is that the functional components support not only medicine, but the nursing discipline as well. Different clinical disciplines may all use the same data, but for different patient-related purposes. For example, nurses and physicians are able to transform data into different clinical abstractions and then use them to make different diagnostic inferences, care plans, and prognostic predictions.[38]

Although over 200 commercial vendors purport to offer the CPR system as a health care IT product offering, the products frequently lack functions of the ideal system. As technology evolves, CPR systems will ideally expand in functionality and integration.[37] Table 82-2 lists vested parties that have taken leadership positions in developing the foundation for the implementation of the CPR.[39]

The Government CPR

An effort that may expedite the development of standards and the large-scale integration of CPR into health care is the Government CPR (G-CPR) Partnership, a collaborative effort of the Department of Veterans Affairs, the Department of Defense, and the Indian Health Service.[40] The G-CPR Partnership was formed in 1998 with the global vision of improving public and individual health status by sharing clinical information.[40] The goals of the partnership are to appropriately share clinical information via a comprehensive, lifelong medical record, and where no standards exist, to advance the development, establishment, and adherence to standards. By jointly defining business and technical characteristics for data

sharing, while looking to the private sector for solutions, it is anticipated that the G-CPR Framework Project will provide the means to share information between organizations with disparate information systems. Yet, complex issues face the G-CPR. Issues include the differing definitions of a CPR; the complexity, length, and cost of implementation; the lack of a common data model; the lack of a comprehensive clinical vocabulary; balancing confidentiality with secure and appropriate access; complex algorithms for developing decision support systems; data ownership issues; and lack of clear, universal, and enforceable confidentiality policies.[41] In spite of those issues, the initiation of the project has resulted in additional collaboration with other entities (e.g., National Committee on Vital Health Statistics, National Library of Medicine, Computer-based Patient Record Institute). Such collaboration should result in resolving some of these complex issues, thus facilitating widespread adoption of the CPR.

Application to Cancer Care

As early as 1991, Hendrickson and colleagues[42] described how computerized clinical information systems could assist oncology nurses in providing integrated care by aiding in the collection, organization, and storage of patient data. Because persons with cancer frequently require complex care and numerous encounters in various settings, the available data surrounding their care becomes complex as well. The presence of a comprehensive CPR system with an integrated view of patient data can assist oncology nurses through automated care planning, patient monitoring, and tracking of patients' comfort, therapeutic, and educational needs.[42] As one example, IMPAC Medical Systems, a commercial vendor, produces a product eCHART™, a CPR that is the clinical foundation for their Multi-ACCESS integrated oncology management

Table 82-2 Defining, Developing, and Setting the Foundation for the Computer-Based Patient Record

Organization	URL	Description
Department of Health and Human Services (DHHS) Data Council	http://aspe.os.dhhs.gov/datacncl/index.htm	Coordinates all health and nonhealth data collection and analysis activities of the DHHS. Implements the Administrative Simplification provisions of the Health Insurance Portability and Accountability Act of 1996.
National Committee on Vital and Health Statistics	http://aspe.os.dhhs.gov/ncvhs	A public-sector advisory committee that serves as a national forum on key health data issues to expedite use of uniform/shared data standards and encourage the interoperability of disparate health care information systems.
Institute of Medicine	www2.nas.edu/iom	An advisor in the field of health/medicine; conducts policy studies relevant to health issues of the general population. Released landmark report "Computer-based Patient Records: An Essential Technology for Health Care" in 1991.
Computer-based Patient Record (CPR) Institute	www.cpri.org	A nonprofit organization formed in 1992. Serves as a nonpartisan forum for the health care community to further the development and effective use of CPRs.
Medical Records Institute	www.medrecinst.com	Promotes the creation and implementation of electronic health record systems in health care both nationally and internationally.

Data from Marietti.[39]

system. The eCHART™ is tailored for radiation and medical and surgical oncology, and can be enhanced with other product offerings including eVAL™, which allows the creation of standard and customized forms for the collection of patient data. eVAL™ includes *ONSET*, a computerized version of the Oncology Nursing Society's *Radiation Therapy Patient Record: A Tool for Documenting Nursing Care* (Figure 82-1).

A comprehensive CPR system can also provide cancer care providers with alerts and reminders about policies and procedures while efficiently integrating clinical practice guidelines and tools to measure oncology outcomes.[35] In outpatient care, randomized controlled clinical trials have been conducted that have demonstrated the efficacy of CPR systems for both health care providers and patients alike.[43] Today, many cancer care facilities have some aspect of a CPR system in place. It is anticipated that widespread integration of comprehensive CPR systems into cancer care will provide high-quality data for computer-based population data bases essential to the health care management of individuals, data for cancer research, data to support public health initiatives, and data that can be used to track the performance of individual cancer care providers and institutions.[36] As consumers and persons with cancer become more actively involved in managing their own health care, and as IT becomes available in more homes, individuals will increasingly use elements of the CPR and CPR-related technology to search through the scientific literature, communicate with their health care providers via e-mail, access data on their medical history, monitor the financial costs and the value of services they receive, and diagnose acute health problems while managing chronic health problems.[36]

Decision-Support Systems

Overview

Decision-support systems (DSSs) function as tools for the user during the decision-making task. These tools vary in size and function. They may be part of a comprehensive CPR system, serve as a stand-alone system, and range from general to patient-specific. For example, DSSs can function as tools for information management, tools for focusing attention, and tools for providing patient-specific recommendations.[44] Information-management

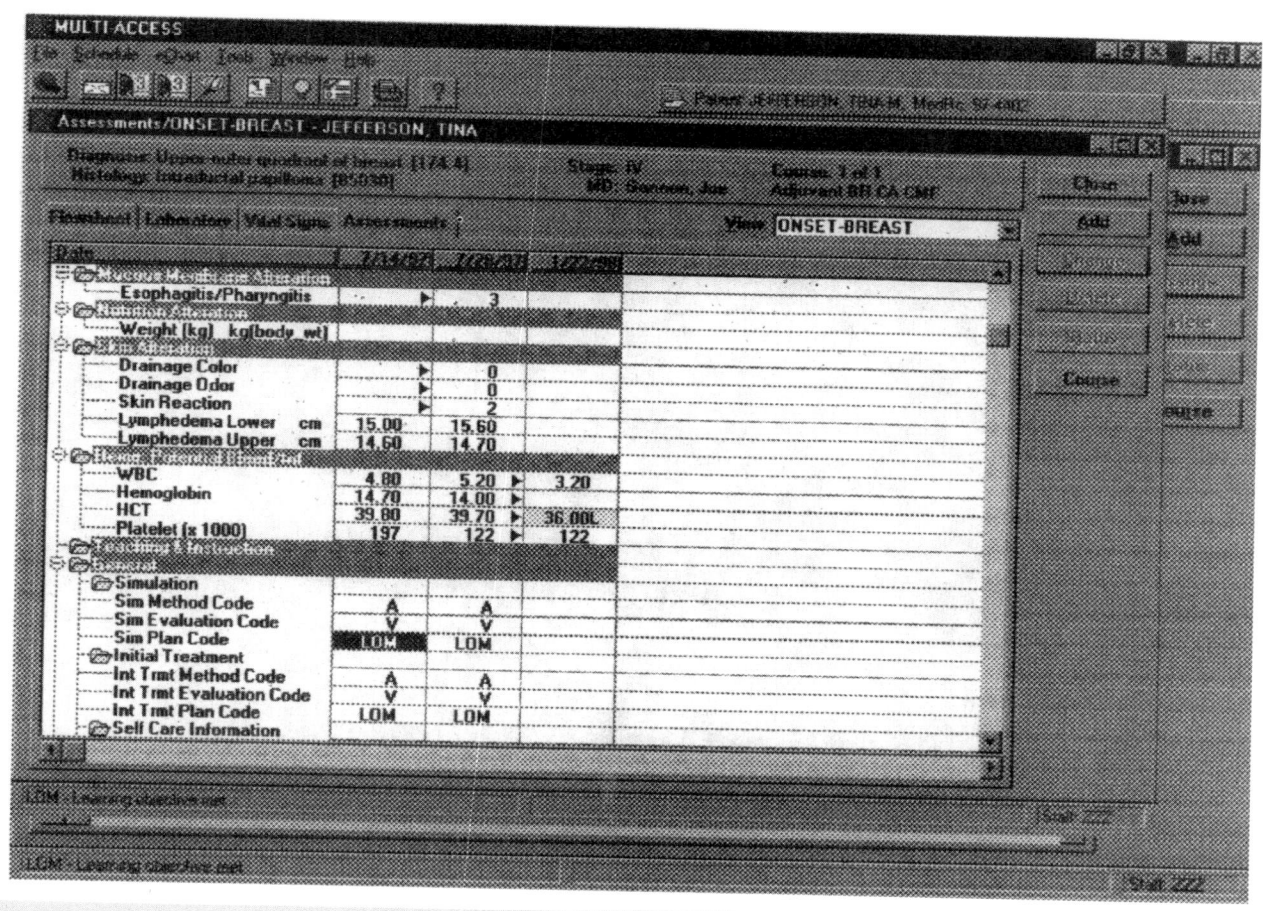

Figure 82-1   An example of how *ONSET* is used as a documentation tool for nursing. (Source: Courtesy of IMPAC Medical Systems, Inc., Mountain View, CA.)

tools provide the user with necessary data and knowledge for making a decision; however, the tools do not help the user apply the information to the decision at hand. Such tools can provide, for example, access to electronic textbooks. Tools that focus the user's attention are computer programs designed to remind the user of problems as well as diagnoses that might have been inadvertently omitted or overlooked. These tools can be viewed as monitoring tools. Finally, tools that provide patient-specific recommendations are based on a database of patient-specific data.

In order to design and implement DSSs, various underlying methodologies are used. They include protocols and algorithms such as clinical guidelines, clinical databanks, mathematical models, statistical pattern recognition and neural networks, Bayesian statistics and Bayesian networks, decision analysis, and artificial intelligence. In medicine several types of patient-specific consultation systems have been designed and are commercially available. For example, Quick Medical Reference (QMR) is a microcomputer-based information system developed at the University of Pittsburgh.[45] It uses non-Bayesian algorithms for the task of assisting the health care provider in making a diagnosis in the area of general internal medicine.[45] In nursing, DSSs to provide patient-specific recommendations have also been specifically designed for clinical practice.[46-48] Many have used knowledge-based systems, an area of artificial intelligence, as the underlying methodology. Knowledge-based systems incorporate the judgment and advice of expert nurses; these systems have also been described as "expert systems." Those developed by nurses and their colleagues include the Creighton Online Multiple Modular Expert System (COMMES), an effort that evolved into what is now the Patient Care Expert (PACE), designed to support nursing clinical decision making about individual patient conditions.[47] Ultimately, the development of DSSs results in the creation of tools to support our practice by making nursing knowledge more explicit and more accessible.[49]

At the consumer level, the development of DSSs by the government and private sector has resulted in widespread dissemination of health informatics tools for patient treatment decisions.[50,51] These tools transform the traditional delivery of health care information by providing, for example, cancer treatment information or other disease-specific health information to patients when they are making decisions about how to best manage their illness, and may result in improved treatment outcomes and quality of life.[51] With the advent of the Internet, DSSs designed specifically for patient use can be accessed directly from home, 24 hours a day, for the promotion of self-care and prevention. Consumers typically have not had the tools necessary to become active and informed participants in their own health care. As a result, it is estimated that anywhere from 50%–80% of those who enter the health care system do not really need medical care (i.e., using the emergency room for a cold) or conversely, they enter the health care system too late and require more expensive and lengthy care.[8] It has been estimated that even if personal DSSs were used only 25%–35% of the time, $40 to $60 billion could be saved.[8] Clearly, this area is key for nursing involvement given our focus on patient education, the advent of consumer health informatics, and the evolving significance of self-care.

Application to Cancer Care

Various types of DSSs have been designed for cancer care and their use continues to be refined.[52] For example, the Oncology Clinical Information System (OCIS), a computer-based DSS for the clinical management of cancer patients, was developed and implemented at the Johns Hopkins Oncology Center during the 1970s.[53] In developing the OCIS, the goal was to provide reliable, complete, and timely information that presented itself in a manner that led the clinician most directly to the correct decision; it was to be considered first and foremost as a tool to support clinical decision making in a large health care setting.[53] Over the span of 20 years, the OCIS has evolved to be viewed more as the core of a CPR, linked with the operational, clinical, and administrative functions of cancer care. Today, integrated through a single patient-centered database, clinical decision support remains a primary functional component of the OCIS[54] (Table 82-3). Although it is not a commercially available product, versions of the OCIS have been tailored for the environments of other cancer care centers.

Another example of an oncology DSS is ONCOCIN, developed at Stanford University in the 1980s for the purpose of facilitating adherence to complex protocol regimens.[55] ONCOCIN integrated a clinical data management environment with a DSS in order to provide customized treatment advice for cancer patients and clinical

---

Table 82-3 Decision-Support System Functions of the OCIS

- Logically integrates results data into hardcopy plots and flow sheets
- Provides access to all results data in user-defined formats
- Builds treatment sequences for routine, individual, or research use
- Combines treatment sequences into a comprehensive treatment plan
- Automatically generates daily medication administration record
- Provides all historical data on all patients for user query
- Provides access to radiology, pathology, and operating room schedules
- Derives test/procedure order guides from patient comprehensive treatment plan
- Derives daily care plans from patient comprehensive treatment plan
- Provides pain monitoring/control
- Provides access to the MEDLINE and PDQ databases

Data from Johns Hopkins Oncology Center.[54]

trials management. Although ONCOCIN is no longer in clinical use (R Carlson in an e-mail, January 1999), its development represented a scientific research endeavor and its use by clinicians led to improvements in data collection for complex protocol regimens while enhancing quality care for patients through decision support.[56]

While DSSs in cancer care were initially intended for clinician use, they have also become increasingly viable for patient use. For example, Williams and colleagues tested the effectiveness of a patient-oriented DSS for improving cancer screening rates in a randomized, controlled trial.[57] The researchers concluded that the system enhanced the provision of patient-specific preventive service recommendations and facilitated clinic work flow to increase the completion of the screenings.[57] At the University of Wisconsin-Madison, researchers developed the Comprehensive Health Enhancement Support System (CHESS), which is a computer-based system of integrated services designed to help individuals cope with various health problems, including breast cancer.[58] The CHESS *Living with Breast Cancer* module includes decision-making and problem-solving tools (Figure 82-2). Current research focuses on measuring the impact of an enhanced CHESS breast cancer module. This research includes assessing users' understanding of diagnoses, treatment options and risks associated with treatment options, satisfaction with decisions made, amount of involvement in decision making, and compliance with decision.[59] Clearly, DSSs of any scope are promising tools for facilitating the complexity of cancer care. Nursing, in particular, can seek to gain by being involved in developing and testing consumer and patient-oriented DSSs, as well as knowledge-based delivery systems that are appropriate for nurses' needs.

Telemedicine/Telehealth

Overview

Telemedicine is an aspect of telehealth that focuses specifically on the provider aspects of health care telecommunications. The focus appropriately is on the remote communication of information to facilitate clinical care.[60,61] Numerous terms have also been coined to specify the specialty to which telemedicine is then applied: teledermatology, teleophthalmology, teleoncology. In addition, some have used the term *telenursing* to specify the use of telemedicine technology in the delivery of nursing care. While the term *telemedicine* remains in common usage, many in the health care field recognize and embrace the broader perspective of the term *telehealth*, as it more clearly delineates the systematic application of telecommunication technology to all of health care.

The benefits and applications of telemedicine are numerous. Telemedicine is viewed as a partial solution to reducing escalating health care costs while simultaneously providing innovative health care to rural areas, correctional facilities, military settings, home care, and international agencies. Indeed, one of the largest reported applications of telemedicine is the delivery of health care to rural areas. By using telemedicine, health care providers can consult with specialists thousands of

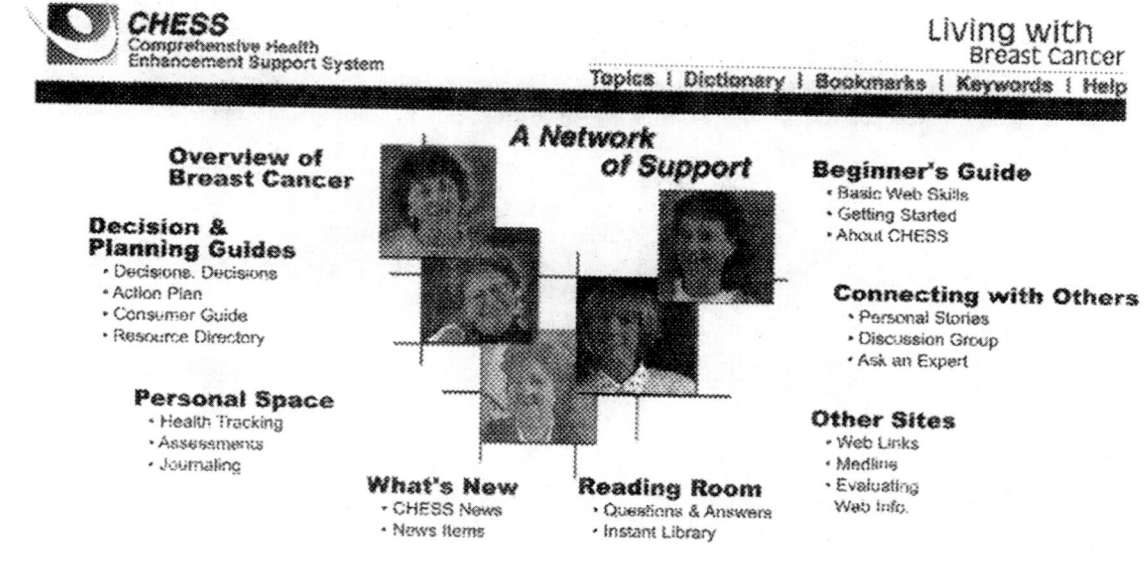

Figure 82-2 Main menu of the Web-based CHESS *Living with Breast Cancer* module. (Source: Courtesy of Center for Health Systems Research and Analysis, University of Wisconsin-Madison, Madison, WI.)

miles away; continually upgrade their education and skills; and share medical records. This results in an increased access to specialists, savings in treatment time, and travel costs. For example, since the mid 1980s the closure of over 70 hospitals in Texas, primarily in rural areas, has resulted in a sharp decline of health care services. As a way of alleviating the shortage of specialists in rural areas, the Texas Telemedicine Project in Austin offers interactive video consultation to primary care physicians in rural hospitals. This project has demonstrated an increased quality of care in rural areas while providing at least 14% savings by reducing patient transfer costs and provider travel.[8]

Another significant area of growth where nursing can play a vital role is in the home care segment of telemedicine. Preliminary data from a recent study suggest that in the United States approximately 45% of home nursing visits could be done via telemedicine.[62] Accordingly, this technology could significantly improve the delivery of quality care by enabling increased frequency of visits by home care nurses and improving delivery of information to detect early deterioration in disease states.[63] For example, in one in-home unit system called the "Electronic Housecall," the measurement of physiologic parameters includes blood pressure cuff, oxygen saturation monitor, temperature probe, three-lead electrocardiograph monitor, and stethoscope. This in-home unit readily transmits monitoring data to the nurse.[64] Moreover, the financial aspect of a telemedicine-based disease management program has already demonstrated a significant decrease in health care utilization costs, primarily as a result of a decrease in patient admissions, emergency room visits, and outpatient visits.

There is in the United States a proliferation of telemedicine programs; however, complex issues surround their use. These issues include the reluctant acceptance of the technology by health care providers, reimbursement, licensing of health care providers, malpractice, privacy and confidentiality of patient data, as well as technology costs.[65] Despite these issues, the evolution of telemedicine will more than likely significantly reengineer the traditional delivery of health care.

Application to Cancer Care

The application of telemedicine to cancer care is becoming increasingly visible.[66–69] For example, Allen and colleagues described how medical oncologists from an urban, university-based hospital provided oncology care to rural patients using interactive video clinics, which they described as "tele-oncology."[67] Surveys were performed after the video encounters as well as after a limited number of subsequent clinical encounters on site in order to assess physician satisfaction with this form of outreach. The results suggested that there was a reasonable level of physician satisfaction with, and confidence in, the use of video to replace some on-site oncology consultations.[67] Doolittle and colleagues[68] report monitoring and evaluat-

ing costs of different types of oncology practice including a telemedicine clinic and a fly-in outreach clinic, both held in rural areas. Findings showed that it was less expensive to use telemedicine than to fly in oncology support for the practice. The University of Wisconsin Hospital and Clinics and regional oncology affiliates are using telemedicine to promote and enhance cancer treatment and clinical research.[69] Their system encompasses several forms of technology in order to provide professional education and training, patient evaluation and protocol eligibility, data transfer for radiation therapy treatment planning, quality assurance, and peer review programs for medical oncology and radiation oncology.[69] In other parts of the United States, home telemedicine is being used with pediatric bone marrow transplant patients, as well as in the care of hospice patients located in geographically rural areas. Ultimately, innovative applications of telemedicine to the delivery of high quality cancer care will continue to grow.

Privacy and Security

Overview

As the application of IT to the health care industry becomes increasingly important, the actual storage and dissemination of health information in an electronic form raises the concern of patient privacy and data security. The concern has increased as more sensitive material is stored in medical records, such as HIV status, psychiatric records, and genetic information.[70] The fear is that electronically storing and transmitting such information over the NII will further compromise individual privacy. The problem is complex; however, the complexity of the issue resides not so much with the technology itself, but historically with the absence of a global, cohesive informational security policy.[71]

Implementing policy has been difficult for numerous reasons: the legal meaning of privacy is apt to shift periodically to reflect the society's public versus private interests; ownership and control of health information is not always readily identifiable; and the patient's informed consent to disclosure of information is arguably a misnomer.[71] While individual institutions and organizations employ a wide variety of technical and nontechnical practices for protecting electronic health information, there has been a relatively unregulated dissemination of information among institutions in the health care industry, including health care providers, payers, managers of pharmaceutical benefits programs, equipment suppliers, researchers, and oversight agencies. Although information is primarily collected for legitimate reasons, the potential threat of misuse of accessed information from both authorized and unauthorized outsiders exists.

In order to protect health information, the Health Insurance Portability and Accountability Act (HIPAA) of 1996 (H.R. 3103) was signed into law.[70] The HIPAA provides guidelines for electronic health care transactions, unique health identifiers, code sets, security, confidentiality, and privacy. In 1998, the U.S. DHHS issued new electronic data security standards as mandated under the HIPAA law.[72] These standards include, for example, a call for universal encryption for medical data when electronically distributed, the use of digital signatures, and strict control over online access to records. By issuing such standards and regulations for security and privacy, HIPAA has begun to fill the gap in existing legislation for protecting health information. It remains to be seen, however, whether its standards and regulations will be enforced firmly. Patient health information may continue to remain vulnerable to potential misuse if strong measures and ways of ensuring that they are implemented are not taken.[70,73]

The need for sophisticated security technologies to protect privacy will increase as more health care organizations take greater advantage of IT.[74,75] While the technological implementation of such measures can protect privacy, technology remains limited in that it cannot control what the individual eventually does with the information.

Application to Cancer Care

Clearly, the issues of privacy and security as they relate to electronic health information are relevant in the delivery of cancer care. This is particularly true for those individuals who have undergone genetic testing and are identified as at risk for developing cancer.[76] Mounting concerns by consumers reveal justified apprehension of genetic discrimination resulting from the release of predictive and presymptomatic genetic test results to employers, insurers, and others.[77] As the use of CPR systems expands, it is paramount to keep such sensitive information secure. Unfortunately, individual fear of employment discrimination through employer access to such health information may discourage at-risk individuals from undergoing testing. The individual may also fear discriminatory actions by insurance companies if identified as at risk.

While HIPAA mandates security and privacy regulations for electronic health information, it also breaches the use of a common identifier for indexing patient records. A common identifier has the potential of improving the quality and reducing the costs of health care by making a more complete patient record available to providers, of facilitating the creation of a longitudinal patient records for health care researchers, and of simplifying the administration of health care benefits. However, particularly in those individuals with sensitive genetic information, it could also facilitate the assembly of information about patients without their consent. Because the global issue of genetic discrimination will most likely emerge as a major challenge in the twenty-first century, health care professionals will need knowledge of federal and state laws that provide some measure of protection against discrimination.[76] Unfortunately, the potential risk of improper disclosure of sensitive information remains a reality. Only through the enforcement of strong legal penalties, as well as other measures, will such actions be deterred.

The Internet and the World Wide Web

As previously noted, the first strategy in a National Nursing Informatics Agenda is that nursing students and practicing nurses achieve core informatics competencies. Unfortunately, nursing education programs have been slow to incorporate informatics competencies into the curriculum, and many nurses lack user-level competencies upon completing their basic nursing programs.[78] Yet, nurses will need to have core informatics competencies to practice effectively in the twenty-first century.[7,79] These core computing skills include the ability to use word processing, e-mail, spreadsheets, presentations graphics software, databases, bibliographic retrieval, the Internet, and the Web.

Understanding the Internet

The word *Internet* means different things to different people. The Internet can most simply be described as a network of computers. It is also known as the "Information Super Highway" and to some, the Web. The Web is the graphical portion of the Internet that one would access with a software program called a "browser." Some consider simply using electronic mail (e-mail) the Internet. Still others would tell you that they "surf the net" because they "log on" to America Online®. In part, all of these definitions are true.

At the core of the Internet are "backbones." Backbone networks provide the speed of communications, the ability to transfer large amounts of data (high bandwidth), and the reliability necessary to connect computers on the Internet. The high-speed transfer of data around the globe is accomplished by fiber-optic cabling and increasingly by the use of satellites. Computers on the Internet are connected via a leased-line fee structure, effectively eliminating long-distance charges. Data on the Internet may be routed through several computers to reach its final destination. The evolution of the Internet continues. In the early days, when the Advanced Research Projects Agency Network (ARPANET) was the backbone network for the Internet, only academics could connect and use it. Today, the Internet is a very successful commercial venture that is changing the way we work, learn, shop, and define community.

Connecting to the Internet

Connecting to the Internet has gotten much easier in recent years. Basic hardware includes a computer with a modem and a monitor and a telephone line. Any type of computer (PC, MAC, UNIX) can theoretically connect to the Internet. In general, the faster and more memory a computer has, the more enjoyable the online experience. Computer speed is measured in megahertz (MHz) and memory is measured in bytes. A standard personal computer today would have somewhere between 350–400 MHz in speed and have at least 8.4 gigabytes of memory. The standard protocol with which two computers talk to each other is transmission control protocol/Internet protocol (TCP/IP). Winsock® is the standard TCP/IP interface for computers running Microsoft Windows®; Mac TCP/IP® is the interface for Apple® Computers. The TCP/IP must be installed on the computer for an Internet connection of any type to be made.

Almost all computers have a modem bundled with them. Modem stands for "*modulator-dem*odulator." A modem decodes the information the computer is receiving and sending from the Internet into a usable form. Modems can either be built into the computer (internal) or be a separate piece of hardware (external). An advantage of the external modem is that if it breaks or a faster one is needed, it is easier to exchange. The phone line connects to the modem, not the computer itself. Although it is possible to be connected directly and continuously to the Internet, most people do not need to be connected 24 hours a day, seven days per week. A direct connection is also costly. Fortunately, there are a number of cost-effective options for "dialing-in" to the Internet and using it on an as needed basis. A popular way of connecting, especially for those new to the Internet, is through an online service. The largest of these is America Online®, with 17 million registered users and growing.[80] America Online® costs about $20 per month for unlimited access and offers an easy to install software program. In addition to e-mail and access to the Web, America Online® users have exclusive access to other proprietary con-

tent, online shopping, and a robust selection of Chat and discussion forums. Other online services include Prodigy®, and The Microsoft Network®. Internet service providers (ISPs) offer alternatives to those who do not want the proprietary content offered by an online service. Connecting to the Internet using an ISP is not difficult, but not as simple as using an online service where all of the software is preconfigured. The user must install and configure an e-mail program to send and receive e-mail, and a Web browser program to access the Web. Popular e-mail programs include Microsoft Outlook®, Exchange®, and Eudora®. The two most popular browser programs are Netscape Navigator® and Microsoft Internet Explorer®.

There are two types of ISPs, national and local. National ISPs are usually part of well-known communications companies such as Sprint®, MCI®, ATT®, and the "Baby Bells." Advantages of connecting with a national ISP are multiple access numbers (especially important if you travel), top-rate customer service, some space on their computer to host a Web page, and competitive monthly rates. A local ISP is a smaller company, dedicated only to providing Internet access. Many people use a local ISP if a national ISP or online service does not have a local phone number to dial in to from their area. The criteria for selecting a reliable ISP are the same for both local and national providers[81] (Table 82-4).

Communication Tools

Electronic Mail

E-mail can be thought of as a hybrid between letter writing and the spoken word. It is more spontaneous than letter

---

Table 82-4 Questions to Consider When Evaluating an Internet Service Provider

Question	Rationale
Is there a sign-up or software activation fee?	It is usually possible to avoid these fees. If you live in a metropolitan area where several ISPs are competing for a share of the Internet connectivity market, companies that will waive the activation fee should be plentiful.
Is there a free trial period?	This will give you a chance to see how well the ISP works. Do not sign on with an ISP if you are bumped off line frequently, constantly get busy signals when you dial in, or can never dial in at the speeds promised.
What is the price per month? What is the price for one year?	Many ISPs have a special low rates (some as low as $10/month) in exchange for payment of the whole year up front. A monthly fee of $15–$20 per month is considered reasonable.
What kind of browser software is required?	Many ISPs provide the software necessary to connect under group licensing agreements. Find out which software the ISP provides and if additional software is necessary to connect to the Internet.
Does the ISP provide you with space on their server for your own Web page?	This may not seem like an important concern initially, but many "newbies" or Internet novices are creating their own Web pages within months of being online.
How does the ISP provide technical support?	A good ISP will provide 24-hour-a-day technical support that is reachable via a toll-free call or e-mail. If you are using an Apple computer, check to make sure that they have a certified Apple technician on staff.
Does the ISP have and provide high-speed modem access?	If you have a high-speed modem, make sure that the ISP connections can match your speed.

Data from Gomez and Ehrenberger.[81]

writing, less likely to get lost, and self-documenting.[81] The use of e-mail, the very first Internet application, has increased significantly in recent years. In 1996 there were 40 million e-mail users, and that number is expected to jump to 135 million by the year 2001.[82] With nearly 500 million e-mail messages being sent around the world each day, it is becoming the preferred method for health care professionals to communicate with one another. Nurses are increasingly seeking more rapid, efficient communications with each other, and as a result, electronic mail and online interactive messaging are becoming more important.[83] Patients are also increasingly using e-mail to communicate with their health care providers. Because this presents a new method of communication, guidelines for the clinical use of patient–provider e-mail were published by the American Medical Informatics Association in 1998.[84] These guidelines address two interrelated aspects: effective communication between the clinician and patient (Table 82-5) and judicious regard of medicolegal issues. Medicolegal issues include the identification of security mechanism in place, indemnity for technical failures, offsite processing of e-mail, encryption, etc.

Table 82-5 Guidelines for the Clinical Use of E-mail with Patients

- Establish turnaround time for messages. Do not use e-mail for urgent matters.

- Inform patients about privacy issues. Patients should know:
  Who besides addressee processes messages:
    - During addressee's usual business hours
    - During addressee's vacation or illness.
  That the message is to be included as part of the medical record.

- Establish types of transactions (prescription refill, appointment scheduling, etc.) and sensitivity of subject matter (HIV, mental health, etc.) permitted over e-mail.

- Instruct patients to put category of transaction in subject line of message for filtering: "prescription," "appointment," "medical advice," "billing question."

- Request that patients put their name and patient identification number in the body of the message.

- Configure automatic reply to acknowledge receipt of messages.

- Print all messages, with replies and confirmation of receipt, and place in patient's paper chart.

- Send a new message to inform patient of completion of request.

- Request that patients use autoreply feature to acknowledge reading provider's message.

- Maintain a mailing list of patients, but do not send group mailings where recipients are visible to each other. Use blind copy feature in software.

- Avoid anger, sarcasm, harsh criticism, and libelous references to third parties in messages.

Reprinted with permission from Kane B, Sands D: Guidelines for the clinical use of electronic mail. *J Am Med Inform Assoc* 5: 104–111, 1998.[84]

Table 82-6 Mailing Lists: Useful Commands in the Body of an E-mail Message

Command	Function
Subscribe ListName Your Name	Puts you on the mailing list.
Review ListName (short)	Returns a description and purpose of the list.
Review ListName	Returns a list of subscribers, including the owner.
Set ListName Nomail	Allows temporary halt of posted messages.
Index ListName	Returns a list of files associated with the list.
Unsubscribe ListName Your Name	Removes you from the mailing list.

REMEMBER: These commands are always sent to the LISTSERV address while actual messages are sent to the LISTNAME address.

Mailing Lists

Mailing lists, commonly known as listservs, are the most accessible of the Internet resources discussed here. Users need only to have e-mail access. Each listserv, no matter what the topic, functions virtually the same way. Listservs are based on the concept of a shared distribution list. Every e-mail sent to the list is distributed to everyone else "subscribed" to the list. One person, usually the list owner or postmaster is responsible for maintaining the listserv software and answering questions about the list. The software program keeps track of subscribers and sends copies of messages. The original software program was called Listserv™ and this is the reason why mailing lists are often referred to as listservs.[31] Useful commands that work with all listservs are presented in Table 82-6. New cancer-related mailing lists are forming every day and they are a very effective way of distributing and obtaining cancer information. The Association of Online Cancer Resources© (ACOR) hosts a Web site with an "EZ-subscribe" feature for over 70 cancer-related listservs, available at <URL: http://www.acor.org>.

Newsgroups

Newsgroups are electronic discussion forums in which anyone can participate in a public dialogue on a topic of interest. Usenet, a network of computers, was developed to carry messages and replies that are posted to newsgroups. Usenet is supported in nearly all countries and reaches millions of users. No single person or group controls Usenet and no authority manages it. A newsreader, as its name implies, is a piece of software designed to let you read the messages posted to the newsgroup. The latest versions of most Web browsers have newsreaders built into them. Newsreaders obtain the news for you and sort it into threads. A single message posted to a newsgroup usually generates responses along the same line. The sequence of messages following the initial message is called a thread.[85] Additionally, Usenet newsgroups have a hierarchical naming system. Looking in the *alt. support* groups and the *sci.med* groups generally covers nursing and health-related discussions. Cancer-related newsgroups are listed in Table 82-7.

Internet Relay Chat

Most Internet applications work asynchronously. You rarely read your e-mail while parts of it are being sent. As the nearly 100% penetration rate of telephony around the globe proves, real-time synchronous communications between two geographically distant people is very valuable. Internet relay chat (IRC) is the Internet's answer to the phone call. It gained international attention during the 1991 Persian Gulf War. When updates from around the world came across the wire, most IRC users who were online at the time gathered on a single channel to hear these reports. Internet relay chat is simply a network of IRC servers ("nets") that allow users to connect to ongoing chats. The largest net is Eris Free net (Efnet), often hosting more than 15,000 people at once. Other large and slightly more organized nets include Undernet, IRCnet, DALnet, and NewNet.

Once connected to an IRC net, you will usually join one or more "channels" and converse with the others gathered there. Conversations may be public (where everyone in a channel can see what you type) or private (messages between only two people, who may or may not be on the same channel). Client software to access IRC is readily available and free. Internet relay chat has a reputation for being a "time waster" because of the amount of frivolous discussions that take place and interactive games found on these servers, but in actuality it is a valuable news distribution source and a place where meetings are being held.

Searching the Internet

While the Internet has a great many qualities, organization is not one of them. Locating information on the Internet can be an extremely frustrating experience. Because no one body controls the Internet, it lacks certain bibliographic control standards such as international standard book numbers (ISBNs), commonly used to identify and catalogue print documents. The majority of Internet materials lack the name of the author and the date of "publication." Moreover, a Web site can be here today and gone tomorrow and the issues surrounding archiving Internet data have yet to be resolved. At least, however, there is no duplication on the Internet.

Universal Resource Locators

Every Web-based document has its own unique address—a universal resource locator (URL). A URL specifies the lo-

Table 82-7 Cancer-Related Newsgroups

Newsgroup	Description
Alt.support.cancer	Unmoderated support group
Alt.support.cancer.prostate	Support group
Alt.support.cancer.testicular	Support group
Alt.support.grief	Moderated support group
Sci.med.diseases.cancer	Medical discussion of general cancer topics
Sci.med.immunotherapy	Medical discussion
Sci.med.nursing	General nursing discussion
Sci.med.radiology	Medical discussion
Sci.med.prostatecancer	Medical discussion

cation of the computer hosting a Web document. Web documents can be found by typing their URLs into a browser program. URLs always have two or more parts, separated by dots. The part on the left reveals the most specific information, for example, "ons" in the URL: *http://www.ons.org*. This may reveal geographic location of the computer, company, department, or an individual name may be found here. The part on the right is the most general and describes the type of information or domain, such as "org" for an organization, "edu" for an educational institution, "gov" for government, and "com" for a commercial organization. Usually, all of the computers on a given network will have the same characters as the right-hand portion of their URL. Knowledge of the URL, or at least of part of it, can make searching easier.

If the URL is entered correctly into a browser program and you get an error message, you might want to "deconstruct" the URL. This process can help you find Web pages that are still on the same site, but have moved. Start deconstructing a URL by removing portions of the address from the right, one item at a time. As you remove items, click on the address to see what happens. Addresses or locations of pages on Web sites may change. Working your way backward through a site often will uncover those new links.

Search Tools

The Internet itself provides different tools to search the Web: search engines, directories, and metasearch engines (Table 82-8). Search engines allow the user to enter keywords that are then matched against a large database of Web pages. Search engines have software packages called "spiders," "crawlers," or "robots" that create these databases automatically by searching the Internet for new documents.[86] Because "spiders" run constantly and index so many Web pages, the search engine databases frequently have information not listed in directories. While all search engines perform the same task, each does it in a slightly different way, leading to very different results.

Table 82-8 Select Internet Search Tools

Search Tools	URL
Search Engines	
AltaVista™	http://www.altavista.com
HotBot™	http://www.hotbot.com
InfoSeek™	http://www.infoseek.com
Lycos™	http://www.lycos.com
Subject Directories	
Yahoo!™	http://www.yahoo.com
Snap™	http://www.snap.com
Metasearch Engines	
MetaCrawler	http://www.metacrawler.com
ProFusion™	http://www.profusion.com

Factors that influence results include the size of the database, the frequency of updating, and the "weight" the placement key words are given. Search engines also differ in how fast they search, the user interface for input and output features, and the amount of help they offer.[86,87]

Directories are hierarchically organized indexes of subject categories that allow the searcher to browse through lists of Web sites by subject. Unlike search engines, these subject directories are created by humans and can often provide better results than search engines because of the human intervention. Directory databases tend to be smaller because they rely mostly on user submissions and recommendations. A directory is also more likely to provide a link only to the site's home page. They lend themselves best to searching for general information.

Metasearch tools combine the searching of several search engines. Instead of using spiders to build listings, metasearchers allow the query to be sent to several search engines. Depending on the metasearch engine, the database searches are then performed either simultaneously or sequentially, and the results are combined onto one page. Some metasearch engines also provide the convenience of using only one input form for searching numerous databases.[86] Metasearch engines are powerful tools for finding very specific information.

Identifying the correct search tool to use depends on the information you need; however, there is a less distinct difference now than there once was because more search engines are incorporating directories into their sites.[87] Learning simple search strategies is also important and will help you retrieve better results. Many search tools now allow the user to simply type in a question. See Table 82-9 for list of Internet search tips. Finally, because search tools and techniques change regularly, a dedicated Web site available at <URL:http://www.searchenginewatch.com>, exists to keep Internet users aware of ongoing changes.

Information-Retrieval Systems

The ability to search the literature is an important skill for improving the quality of cancer care. Traditionally, print formats such as card catalogues have been used to search the literature. This time-consuming format gave way to computerized database systems that could be searched electronically. Today, different types of information-retrieval systems are readily accessible via the Web. Bibliographic-retrieval systems contain citations to the relevant literature while full-text retrieval systems contain the complete textual content of the source. Finding and retrieving information from Web-based database systems can rapidly answer queries posed by health care providers, researchers, and increasingly consumers and patients.

The MEDical Literature Analysis and Retrieval System (MEDLARS®) is the computerized information retrieval system of the NLM providing access to over 40 online databases containing approximately 18 million records. The NLM is transitioning the data to free Web-based systems. The NLM's MEDLINE is its premier bibliographic database, containing over 9 million records and covering not only medicine and nursing, but dentistry, veterinary medicine, and the health care system. On June 26, 1997, NLM announced that the MEDLINE database may be accessed free of charge on the Web. Two NLM Web-based products, PubMed and Internet Grateful Med, provide this access. PubMed <URL: http://www.ncbi.nlm.nih.gov/PubMed> provides access to bibliographic information drawn from MEDLINE and PreMEDLINE and links to the full text of selected journal articles from collaborating publishers with Web sites. A powerful feature of PubMed is that most of its records are linked to other records and users can retrieve related articles for each citation displayed. Also, the NLM's Grateful Med <URL: http://igm.nlm.nih.gov> provides free access to numerous other databases including AIDSLINE, AIDS-

Table 82-9 Internet Search Tips

- Avoid making your queries too general by providing sufficient descriptive terms. The more specific and exact your query, the better your results will be.

- Phrases can help provide a more exact match to your query.

- Employ AND, OR, NEAR, and NOT to connect words and phrases in the search query. AND requires that both terms are present somewhere within the document being sought. NEAR requires that one term must be found within a specified number of words. OR requires that at least one term is present. NOT excludes a term from a query.

- Employ [+] before a term to retrieve only the documents containing that term. Employ [−] before a term to exclude that term from the search. Do not leave a space between the operator and the term that follows.
  Query Example: +oncology+nursing+society
  This would find pages that have all three of the words on them

- Indicate that the words within the quote marks are to be treated as an exact phrase, or reasonably close to it.
  Query Example: "oncology nursing society"

- Adjacent capitalized words are treated as a single proper name, e.g., Elizabeth Gomez. Commas separate proper names from each other.
  Query Example: Elizabeth Gomez, Heidi Ehrenberger

DRUGS, AIDSTRIALS, BIOETHICSLINE, HealthSTAR, and TOXLINE.

Since MEDLINE became freely available on the Web, the NLM reports that many members of the public are willing to make the effort to read scientific articles for guidance on treatment or management of themselves, family members, or friends.[88] Although there is little evidence to support that public access to the scientific literature improves health outcomes, numerous anecdotal reports document how the scientific literature has helped lay persons find a physician with special experience relevant to their concerns.[88] Thus, the NLM continues to enhance consumer access to health information, while devising new evaluation strategies. On October 22, 1998, the NLM introduced MEDLINEplus <URL: http://www.nlm.nih.gov/medlineplus>, which provides consumers with specific subject access to selected sources of health information from government and select nongovernmental agencies.

The NCI also provides highly useful information-retrieval systems, including PDQ® and CANCERLIT®, which are accessible via the CancerNet™ Web site <URL: http://cancernet.nci.nih.gov>. PDQ is a comprehensive full-text retrieval system of current, peer-reviewed syntheses of state-of-the-art information on cancer care. Because it incorporates expert opinion in the selection of literature and the development of concise, clear summary statements from these citations, it can also be viewed as a knowledge base.[89] The PDQ database contains three types of information: (1) statements that synthesize the published literature and reflect the current information on state-of-the-art treatment, supportive care, prevention, and screening of cancer; (2) summaries of research studies under evaluation in clinical trials; and (3) directories of physicians and organizations that provide cancer care.[89] Updated monthly, selected information from PDQ is easily accessible via CancerNet. Additionally, the NCI's CANCERLIT is an archival bibliographic-retrieval system containing over 1.2 million citations and abstracts of published cancer research from 1963 to the present.[89] It is updated monthly with more than 7500 new citations and provides a comprehensive, up-to-date resource.[89] CANCERLIT also provides "Topic Searches," which are prepared literature searches for over 90 clinical topics. The complete CANCERLIT database is readily accessible via CancerNet.

Several other valuable information-retrieval systems exist for nurses, such as the Cumulative Index to Nursing and Allied Health (CINAHL), a bibliographic-retrieval system. This system, as well as others, and search strategy development are described elsewhere.[1,31]

Evaluating Cancer Web-Based Information

The major concern with the public's access to cancer Web sites is that someone might be harmed should they act on information obtained from a site.[90] Many sources of cancer information are authoritative and reliable. Others are not. The most vulnerable populations are patients and their families, who in a time of great distress may be downloading an enormous amount of information from cancer-related Web sites. While there is no uniform method yet for evaluating the credibility of any Internet resource, standards are emerging.[91,92] The criteria below can help in making a decision about the credibility of the Web-based information.

Provider/Author Information

The name and credentials or authority of either the provider(s) or author(s) of the resource are uniformly used to evaluate the credibility of a Web site.[89] According to Silberg, providers must maintain accountability for their Web sites such that "an identifiable person or group of people stands behind what is being 'published' on the Web and in Internet discussion forums."[93] Evidence of the peer-review process also falls into this category. Information from hospitals, government health agencies, cancer care organizations, universities, and places that bring together knowledgeable health care professionals are considered extremely credible. Individual cancer care providers (e.g., nurses, physician assistants, pharmacists, and nutritionists) are also considered authoritative sources of information, but it is more difficult to verify an individual's true identity and credentials. Be cautious of sound-alike names (and URLs) or names that seem impressive. It is also imperative to avoid information posted by anonymous sources. Finally, disclosure also falls into this category. If specific funding has been obtained to subsidize the Web site, or parts of the Web site, this must be disclosed to the user. Sponsor information is usually found on the home page.

Timeliness

Timeliness is understood to mean being up-to-date with the state of medical/clinical oncology knowledge.[91] Bridges and Thede recommend determining whether there is an indication of when the resource was authored and/or last changed.[94] The user should be able to readily see the date of the original document and the date of content posting.[91] The presence of "timestamps" that indicate the last update are usually located on the bottom of the home page. An updated site demonstrates a commitment to providing accurate information about the topic. Additionally, if the Web site has many nonfunctional links, it may be an indication that the information is not accurate at this time.[31]

Interactivity/Responsiveness

Academic journals provide a feedback mechanism for their readers, and so, too, should Web sites. Users, just as readers of print materials, should be able to comment on the validity and value of the information. This is often done via an e-mail link with an e-mail addressed to the content provider, Webmaster, or editor. At a minimum, an acknowledgment of receiving the e-mail should be sent with an estimated time frame for a more complete response. Web sites that offer moderated components such as IRC and discussion forums are seen as more credible with respect to interactivity.

Use of Technology

Murray and Rizzolo identify the use of technology criterion to be the "workability" and "user friendliness" of the Web site.[90] Others describe it as the "accessibility" of the site.[91] Web sites should be accessible by the lowest common denominator of current browser technology.[94] Although the latest plug-ins and features available to the high-end user make the site attractive, the "bells and whistles" often impede the majority of visitors from finding the information they seek. For example, graphics that take a long time to download can limit a site's usefulness.[31] Also, all Web evaluation criteria include a robust internal search engine. The search engine should operate quickly and efficiently. Its scope and function—what it covers and how it works—should be evaluated. Today's Web sites frequently use multiple, special-purpose search engines, so a clear description of the search engine purpose and scope is important.[91]

Presentation/Navigability

Presentation is more specifically the overall "look and feel" of the Web site. The presentation of a credible Web site balances words, pictures, colors, sounds, and motion in a way that enhances absorption of the information. How the site is designed is indeed important in the delivery and use of health information. Simplicity of design leads to ease of use while complex presentations may detract from one's assessment of the quality of the information. On the flip side, a highly polished site may give the user the false impression of credibility. When navigating the Web site, the user interface must be simple, easy to use, and display its results in a logical form. Such logical structuring is essential for effective use of health information.[91] A key navigation criterion is ease of returning to the home page or to the top page of any specific section of the site.

Financial Aspects

Paying for online content does not necessarily mean that it is of better quality. The same information may be available free on another site.[95] Much of the proprietary content about cancer on the Internet is repackaged government material obtained originally at no charge from the National Institutes of Health or the National Cancer Institute.

Privacy of User Data

Today, more and more Web sites are collecting data from their user groups. Some will ask for demographic data (e.g., name, e-mail address, and mother's maiden name) in order to register and receive a password to enter the site or premium areas of the site. Others will perform periodic surveys of their users. Often these surveys will ask more sensitive health-related questions, such as disease status, type of treatment, and response. Credible Web sites provide a statement specifically outlining how the information will be analyzed and if it will be disclosed to third-party vendors.

ONS Online℠: An Example of a Web-Based Resource for Oncology Nurses

Overview

With over 28,000 members, the Oncology Nursing Society (ONS) is the largest professional oncology association in the world. In an organization as large and diverse as the ONS, effective communication and information dissemination is a challenge. The official Web site of the society, ONS Online℠ <http://www.ons.org> readily enables nurses and other health care professionals to quickly obtain quality oncology information and stay current through access to the latest news and developments in the field. Full access to the site is a benefit of membership in the society. Only ONS members have access to discussion forums and journals. Other health care providers and the public have slightly more restricted access at no cost. ONS Online reaches nurses and patients worldwide thus furthering the dissemination of the scientific base of our discipline while enhancing and transforming cancer care.

The ONS Online Editorial Board, a seven-member board composed of doctoral- and master's-prepared advanced practice nurses, reviews the content of the Web site and its links. The editor chairs the board, manages the workflow, interacts with leadership groups, acts as a spokesperson for the Web site, and is ultimately responsible for all of the content. Associate editors focus their work in the clinical practice, research, and education areas. There is also an associate editor for international issues.

Content Review Process

The ONS Online Editorial Board ensures that the information available on ONS Online is accurate, current, and relevant for ONS members, health care professionals, patients, and the public-at-large. Providing access to quality cancer information is the top priority and, early on, the standard of peer review for both internal and external content was adopted. The board developed a set of criteria for evaluating the quality of information on the sites to which ONS Online is linked and for original content developed for the site. This review process is applied to both content developed by ONS members to be included on the ONS Online Web site and content available on other Web sites that are linked to ONS Online. The review process has evolved in the last three years to better evaluate the expanding and more complex oncology content on the Web. As new issues arise, they will be incorporated into the review process.

Core Content Areas

All of the content found on ONS Online is based on a conceptual framework developed and approved by the Editorial Board. The content is structured around the cancer continuum and seven core areas. The cancer continuum is viewed as prevention, screening, treatment, symptom management, rehabilitation and survivorship, and palliation. Both the content areas and the cancer continuum are viewed as interacting systems. Table 82-10 provides a description of the core content areas.

Discussion Forums

Discussion forums are a critical interactive component of some of the core content areas. These forums are located, for example, in the clinical practice, education, and research areas of the site. They function as a place for ONS members to pose questions to recognized experts (forum moderators) and as a networking opportunity. Presently, there are over 50 discussion forums located within the core content areas. In addition to moderated discussion forums, the ONS SIGs directory lists the coordinator of each SIG and links to individual discussion forums. These forums are designated as virtual workspaces for the interaction of geographically distant SIG members.

Future Direction

As of June 1999, ONS Online had over 12,500 registered users. The number of registered users is expected to continue to grow steadily. Content on the site is extremely dynamic with changes made daily. Current initiatives include developing more free continuing education programs, expanding the patient education content, and providing a comprehensive directory of research tools and instruments for cancer nurse researchers.

Conclusion

The delivery of cancer care will continue to be affected by developments in the field of health care informatics and rapid changes in IT. Computer-processing power doubles in performance and halves in cost about every two years. We can expect to see communication network speeds increase tenfold within the next five to ten years, while robust compact portable systems replace the simple hand-held computers and wireless communications of the late 1990s.[96] Automated clinical systems will achieve their greatest value when larger CPRs and clinical DSSs and other clinical applications are integrated seamlessly across systems and across sites.[97] Standardization of vocabulary will greatly facilitate the effort to measure outcomes and treatment efficacy.

Table 82-10   ONS Online Core Content Areas

Core Area	General Description
ONS	Includes general information about ONS, membership application, leadership/membership e-mail directories, and a directory of ONS chapters and special interest groups, journals, and position statements.
News	Includes a customized news section on current issues and trends in cancer care, articles from the *ONS News* newsletter, ONS press releases, and legislative news from the ONS Health Policy Associate.
Clinical practice	Includes clinical resources to assist nurses in practice: disease-specific information, genetics resources, management of chemotherapy side effects, pain management, managed care issues, links to cancer care organizations, cancer centers, nursing organizations, and drug information.
Research	Includes information about research grants, awards, and programs; grant-writing tips; and a dedicated clinical trials resource area.
Education	Includes an oncology meeting database, scholarship information, and schools of nursing and free online continuing education programs. The comprehensive *Patient Information and Education Resource* (PIER) provides patient education materials available from the Society and from the Web.
Library	Includes full-text articles from the *Oncology Nursing Forum* and the *Clinical Journal of Oncology Nursing*, access to other clinical journals, academic reference materials, and additional libraries.
Convention center	Here the user can register online for the annual ONS Congress and Fall Institute, learn about the host city, and obtain general information to help plan for the convention experience.

Inevitably, futuristic innovations and applications of IT can lead to improving the delivery and cost of health care.[98,99] As an example, three-dimensional image data can be acquired by using a spiral computed tomography image in order to perform a virtual colonoscopy. Advantages of the virtual colonoscopy are that it eliminates the risk of perforation, provides added patient comfort and compliance, and removes the need for sedation. Moreover, nursing innovations such as telenursing for the delivery of home care and testing the effects of the electronic delivery of nursing interventions are promising.

In the twenty-first century, the essence of nursing will most likely be defined by our knowledge and science, and as such, the profession must maximize the potential of informatics to advance nursing knowledge and broaden the boundaries of nursing science.[100,101] Embracing nursing informatics as an essential dimension of nursing science will be crucial to validating our unique and valuable contribution to the health care system.[100,102]

Finally, the rise of health care consumerism is fundamentally shifting competition in the industry. Sophisticated informatics tools will be used by motivated persons with cancer to maintain their own records and observations, records which can ultimately be part of a larger CPR system. We do not know when the next new IT will transform our world as rapidly as the Web has. For the present, we can develop our own informatics competencies, ensure that consumers and persons with cancer get connected to the right set of electronic information, and be involved in developing and testing nursing innovations.

Glossary

Browser   A software program that accesses the Web and reads hypertext.

Classification   A systematic arrangement of classes; a structural framework arranged according to similar groups.

Computer-based Patient Record (CPR)   A repository of electronically maintained information about an individual's lifetime health status and health care, stored such that it can serve the multiple legitimate users of the record.

CPR Systems   The hardware and software used to create, maintain, edit, display, and manipulate all the data stored in an individual's CPR. These systems provide availability to complete and accurate patient data, clinical reminders and alerts, decision support, and links to bodies of related data and knowledge bases.

Data Element   The smallest unit of data that has meaning without interpretation; a raw fact, material, or observation.

Data Repository   A database acting as an information storage facility.

Data Set   A collection of related data items, a directory.

Database   A collection of interrelated files with records organized and stored together in a computer system.

Decision Support System   Any computer program designed to help health care professionals and/or patients, as users of the system, make clinical decisions.

E-mail   A form of communication, usually a text message sent from one person to another over a computer network. E-mail also may contain enclosed files and graphics.

Encryption   Coding attached to data with the intent to keep the information secure from anyone but the addressee.

Firewall   A security device situated between a private network and outside networks.

Hypertext   A document containing words or phrases, usually highlighted in a different color, that are electronically linked to text elsewhere.

Hypertext Markup Language (HTML)   The basic programming language for sites on the Web.

Informatics   The science that studies the use and processing of data, information, and knowledge.

Information Technology (IT)   Refers to systems (e.g., computers, software packages, decision support systems) used to manage and process information.

Internet   A worldwide distributed network of computers.

Internet Relay Channel (IRC)   A program that allows you to carry on "live" conversations with people all over the world by typing messages back and forth across the Internet.

Internet Service Provider (ISP)   A service or company that allows access to a larger computer that is connected continuously to the Internet.

Language   In computing and communications, a set of characters (symbols, alphabets, codes and syntax), conventions, and rules used to convey ideas and information.

Mailing List   Commonly known as a "listserv," a communication medium based on e-mail. It allows for a sender's single message to be distributed automatically to all subscribers to a list.

Modem (Modulator-Demodulator)   A piece of computer hardware that translates the electronic singles or "bytes" of information coming or going to the Internet. Modems may be external or internal.

Newsgroup   Electronic discussion groups, similar to traditional bulletin boards.

Nursing Informatics The specialty that integrates nursing science, computer science, and information science in identifying, collecting, processing, and managing data and information to support nursing practice, administration, education, research, and the expansion of nursing knowledge.

Search Engine A database of Web sites, available to all users on the Web, that can be searched using keywords.

Taxonomy A method of classifying a vocabulary of terms for a specific topic.

Telecommunications The electronic transmission of voice signals and other data over telephone-based carrier lines.

Telehealth A broad term describing the combined efforts of information technology, health communication, and health education to improve the efficiency and quality of health care.

Telemedicine As a segment of telehealth, telemedicine uses telecommunications technology to send data, graphics, audio, and video images between participants who are physically separated (i.e., at a distance from one another) for the purpose of clinical care.

Transmission Control Protocol/Internet Protocol (TCP/IP) Describes two software mechanisms used to allow multiple computers to talk to each other in an error-free fashion. This program must be installed on one's computer to use the Internet.

Universal Resource Locator (URL) An address that specifies the location of a file on the Internet.

Vocabulary (Nomenclature) A consistent method for assigning names to elements of a system.

Web Page A computer file written in HTML.

Web Site A group of related Web pages. Accessed by typing its unique address, a site usually includes layers of supporting pages as well as a home page.

World Wide Web (WWW or Web) The component of the Internet that integrates text, graphics, audio, and video.

References

1. Collen MF: The origins of informatics. *MD Comput* 16:104, 1999
2. Saba VK, McCormick KA: *Essentials of Computers for Nurses* (ed 2). New York, McGraw-Hill, 1996
3. Graves JR, Corcoran S: The study of nursing informatics. *Image J Nurs Sch* 21:227–231, 1989
4. Hannah KJ, Ball MJ, Edwards M: *Introduction to Nursing Informatics* (ed 2). New York, Springer-Verlag, 1999
5. National Advisory Council on Nurse Education and Practice: "Report to the Secretary of the Department of Health and Human Services: A National Informatics Agenda for Nursing Education and Practice," Rockville, MD, Health Resources and Services Administration at <URL: http://www.hrsa.dhhs.gov/bhpr/dn/nirepex.htm> December 1997
6. National Cancer Institute: "Clinical Trials and Informatics," October 1998 (Internet), available at <URL: http://rex.nci.nih.gov/massmedia/pressreleases/clintrials.htm> Accessed January 2, 2000
7. Gassert CA: The challenge of meeting patients' needs with a national nursing informatics agenda. *J Am Med Inform Assoc* 5:263–268, 1998
8. NII Agenda for Action: "Benefits and Applications of the NII," September 1993 (Internet), available at <URL: http://metalab.unc.edu/nii/NII-Benefits-and-Applications.html> Accessed January 2, 2000
9. The White House Office of the Press Secretary: "Background on the Clinton-Gore Administration's Next Generation Internet Initiative," October 1996 (Internet), available at <URL: http://www.iitf.nist.gov/documents/press/internet.htm> Accessed January 2, 2000
10. National Library of Medicine: "High-Technology Medical Awards Announced: National Library of Medicine Supports 24 Next Generation Internet Projects," October 1998 (Internet), available at <URL: http://www.nlm.nih.gov/news/press releases/nextgen.html> Accessed January 2, 2000
11. National Library of Medicine: "Secretary Shalala Announces National Telemedicine Initiative," October 1996 (Internet), available at <URL: http://www.nlm.nih.gov/news/press releases/telemed.html> Accessed January 2, 2000
12. National Library of Medicine: "NLM National Telemedicine Initiative Summaries of Awards," October 1996 (Internet), available at <URL: http://www.nlm.nih.gov/research/initprojsum.html> Accessed January 2, 2000.
13. American Nurses Association: *The Scope of Practice for Nursing Informatics*. Washington, DC, American Nurses Publishing, 1994
14. American Nurses Association: *Standards of Practice for Nursing Informatics*. Washington, DC, American Nurses Publishing, 1995
15. Schwirian PM: The NI pyramid—a model for research in nursing informatics. *Comput Nurs* 4:134–136, 1986
16. National Institute of Nursing Research: "Nursing Informatics: Enhancing Patient Care," 1993 (Internet), available at <URL: http://www.nih.gov/ninr/vol4/Execsum.html> Accessed January 2, 2000
17. Ozbolt J, Graves J: Clinical nursing informatics: developing tools for knowledge workers. *Nurs Clin North Am* 28:407–425, 1993
18. Brennan PF, Zielstroff R, Ozbolt JG, et al: Setting a national research agenda in nursing informatics, in Cesnik B, McCray A, Scherrer J (eds): *MedInfo'98, Seoul, Korea*. Burke, VA, IOS Press, 1998, pp 1188–1191
19. Ehrenberger H, Murray P: An overview of the issues in the use of communication technologies in nursing research. *Oncol Nurs Forum* 25:11–15, 1998 (suppl 2)
20. Ozbolt J: "Testimony to the NCVHS Hearings on Medical Terminology and Code Development," October 1999 (Internet), available at <URL: http://www.mc.vanderbilt.edu/nursing/informatics/index.html> Accessed January 2, 2000
21. American Nurses Association: *An Emerging Framework: Data System Advances for Clinical Nursing Practice*. Washington, DC, American Nurses Publishing, 1995

22. Werley HH, Lang NM (eds): *Identification of the Nursing Minimum Data Set.* New York, Springer, 1988

23. Henry SB, Warren JJ, Lange L, et al: A review of major nursing vocabularies and the extent to which they have the characteristics required for implementation in computer-based systems. *J Am Med Inform Assoc* 5:321–328, 1998

24. North American Nursing Diagnosis Association: *NANDA Nursing Diagnoses: Definitions and Classification 1997–1998.* Philadelphia, Author, 1996

25. Martin K, Sheet N: *The Omaha System: Applications for Community Health Nursing.* Philadelphia, Saunders, 1992

26. Saba VK: Why the home health care classification is a recognized nursing nomenclature. *Comput Nurs* 15:69–76, 1997 (suppl 2)

27. McCloskey J, Bulechek G: *Nursing Interventions Classification* (ed 2). St. Louis, Mosby, 1996

28. Johnson M, Maas M (eds): *Nursing Outcomes Classification (NOC).* St Louis: Mosby, 1997

29. Ozbolt J: From minimum data to maximum impact: using clinical data to strengthen patient care. *Adv Pract Nurs Q* 1(4):62–69, 1996

30. Kleinbeck S: In search of perioperative nursing data elements. *AORN J* 63:926–931, 1996

31. Thede LQ: *Computers in Nursing: Bridges to the Future.* Philadelphia, Lippincott Williams & Wilkins, 1999

32. McCormick KA, Lang N, Zielstorff R, et al: Toward standard classification schemes for nursing language: recommendations of the American Nurses Association Steering Committee on Databases to support clinical nursing practice. *J Am Med Inform Assoc* 1:421–427, 1994

33. Button P, Androwich I, Hibben L, et al: Challenges and issues related to implementation of nursing vocabularies in computer-based systems. *J Am Med Inform Assoc* 5:332–334, 1998

34. Dick RS, Steen EB (eds): *The Computer-based Patient Record: An Essential Technology for Health Care* (ed 1). Washington, DC, National Academy Press, 1991

35. McCormick KA: Including oncology outcomes of care in the computer-based patient record. *Oncology* 9:161–167, 1995 (suppl)

36. Dick RS, Steen EB, Detmer DE (eds): *The Computer-based Patient Record: An Essential Technology for Health Care* (ed 2). Washington, DC, National Academy Press, 1997

37. Tang PC, McDonald, CJ: Computer-based patient-record systems, in Shortliffe E, Perreault L (eds): *Medical Informatics: Computer Applications in Health Care,* New York, Springer-Verlag (in press)

38. Grobe S, Epping P: Nursing information systems, in van Bemmel JH, Musen MA (eds): *Handbook of Medical Informatics.* Houten, Netherlands, Bohn Stafleu Van Loghum, 1997, pp 219–229

39. Marietti C: Will the real CPR/EMR/EHR please stand up? *Healthcare Inform* 15:77–81, 1998

40. GCPR: "Government Computer-based Patient Record," November 1999 (Internet), available at <URL: http://www.ihs.gov/gcpr/> Accessed January 2, 2000

41. National Committee on Vital Health Statistics: "Briefing by the Government Computer-based Patient Record (G-CPR) Partnership," March 1998 (Internet), available at <URL: http://www.va.gov/meetings/hhs980303/NCVHS_0304v4/tsld001.htm> Accessed January 2, 2000

42. Hendrickson G, Kelly JB, Citrin L: Computers in oncology nursing: present use and future potential. *Oncol Nurs Forum* 18:715–723, 1991

43. Balas EA, Austin SM, Mitchell JA, et al: The clinical value of computerized information services. *Arch Fam Med* 5:271–278, 1996

44. Musen M, Shahar Y, Shortliffe E: Clinical decision-support systems, in Shortliffe E, Perreault L (eds): *Medical Informatics: Computer Applications in Health Care,* New York, Springer-Verlag (in press)

45. Miller R, Masarie F, Myers JD: Quick medical reference (QMR) for diagnostic assistance. *MD Comput* 3:34–48, 1986

46. Chang BL, Roth K, Gonzales E, et al: CANDI: a knowledge-based system for nursing diagnosis. *Comput Nurs* 6:13–21, 1988

47. Evans S: *The PACE System: An Expert Consulting System for Nursing.* New York, Springer-Verlag, 1997

48. Larson DE: Development of a microcomputer-based expert system to provide support for nurses caring for AIDS patients, in Daly N, Hannah KJ (eds): *Proceedings of Nursing and Computers: The Third International Symposium on Nursing Use of Computers and Information Science.* St. Louis, Mosby, 1988, pp 682–690

49. Ozbolt J, Vandewal D, Hannah K (eds.): *Decision Support Systems in Nursing.* St. Louis, Mosby, 1990

50. Hersey JC, Matheson J, Lohr KN: *Consumer Health Informatics and Patient Decision-Making* (AHCPR Publication No. 98-N001). Springfield, VA, National Technical Information Service, 1997

51. Essex D: Lifeline: Consumer informatics has gone beyond patient education on the Web. *Healthcare Inform* 16:112–129, 1999

52. Kalet IJ, Paluszynski W: Knowledge-based computer systems for radiotherapy planning. *Am J Clin Oncol* 13:344–351, 1990

53. Enterline JP, Lenhard RE, Blum BI: *A Clinical Information System for Oncology.* New York, Springer-Verlag, 1989

54. Johns Hopkins Oncology Center: "OCIS Functionality," January 1999 (Internet), available at <URL: http://www.hopkins.cancercenter.jhmi.edu/programs/oncology-infosys.cfm> Accessed January 2, 1999

55. Hickham DH, Shortliffe EH, Bishoff MB, et al: The treatment advice of a computer-based chemotherapy protocol advisor. *Ann Intern Med* 103:928–936, 1985

56. Kent DL, Shortliffe EH, Carlson RW, et al: Improvements in data collection through physician use of a computer-based chemotherapy treatment consultant. *J Clin Oncol* 3:409–417, 1985

57. Williams RB, Boles M, Johnson RE: A patient-initiated system for preventive health care. A randomized trial in community-based primary care practices. *Arch Fam Med* 7:338–45, 1998

58. McTavish FM, Gustafson DH, Owens BH, et al: CHESS: an interactive computer system for women with breast cancer piloted with an under-served population, *J Ambulatory Care Manage* 18:35–41, 1995

59. Comprehensive Health Enhancement Support System (CHESS): "Department of Defense Awards 4-year Grant to CHESS Breast Cancer Project," Fall/Winter 1998 (Internet), available at <URL: http://chess.chsra.wisc.edu/Chess/> Accessed January 2, 2000

60. Coiera E: *Guide to Medical Informatics, the Internet and Telemedicine.* London, Chapman & Hall Medical, 1997

61. Brecht RM, Barrett JE: Telemedicine in the United States, in Viegas S, Dunn K (eds): *Telemedicine: Practicing in the Information Age.* Philadelphia, Lippincott-Raven, 1998, pp 25–30

62. Wootton R, Loane M, Mair F, et al: A joint US-UK study of home telenursing. *J Telemed Telecare* 4:83–85, 1998 (suppl 1)

63. Warner I: Introduction to telehealth home care. *Home Healthcare Nurse* 14:791–796, 1996

64. Schlachta L: Telenursing broadens healthcare scope. *Telemed Telehealth Networks* 2:25–41, 1996

65. Guttman-McCabe C: Telemedicine's imperiled future? Funding, reimbursement, licensing and privacy hurdles face a developing technology. *J Contemp Health Law Policy* 14:161–186, 1997

66. London JW, Morton DE, Marinucci D, et al: The implementation of telemedicine within a community cancer network. *J Am Med Inform Assoc* 4:18–24, 1997

67. Allen A, Hayes J, Sadasivan R, et al: A pilot study of the physician acceptance of tele-oncology. *J Telemed Telecare* 1:34–37, 1995

68. Doolittle GC, Harmon A, Williams A, et al: A cost analysis of a tele-oncology practice. *J Telemed Telecare* 3:20–22, 1997 (suppl 1)

69. Stitt JA: A system of tele-oncology at the University of Wisconsin Hospital and clinics and regional oncology affiliate institutions. *WMJ* 97:38–42, 1998

70. National Research Council: *For the Record: Protecting Electronic Health Information.* Washington, DC, National Academy Press, 1997

71. Barrows RC, Clayton PD: Privacy, confidentiality, and electronic medical records. *J Am Med Inform Assoc* 3:139–148, 1996

72. Department of Health and Human Services: "HHS Proposes Security Standards for Electronic Health Data," August 1998 (Internet), available at <URL: http://www.hhs.gov/news/press/1998pres/980811.html> Accessed January 2, 2000

73. Georgetown University, Institute for Health Care Research and Policy, "Health Privacy Project," December 1999 (Internet), available at <URL: http://www.healthprivacy.org/> Accessed January 2, 2000

74. Epstein MA, Pasieka MS, Lord WP, et al: Security for the digital information age of medicine: issues, applications, and implementation. *J Digit Imaging* 11:33–44, 1998

75. Olsen AJ, Giuse D, Borden RB, et al: Implementation of organizational practices to protect information in health organizations, in Chute C (ed): *Proceedings of the 1998 American Medical Informatics Association Annual Symposium.* New York, McGraw-Hill, 1998, pp 371–375

76. Jacobs L: At-risk for cancer: genetic discrimination in the workplace. *Oncol Nurs Forum* 25:475–480, 1998

77. Lapham EV, Kozma C, Weiss JO: Genetic discrimination: perspectives of consumers. *Science* 274:621–624, 1996

78. Gassert CA: Academic preparation in nursing informatics, in Ball MJ, Hannah KJ, Newbold SK, Douglas JV (eds): *Nursing Informatics: When Caring and Technology Meet* (ed 2). New York, Springer-Verlag, 1995, pp 333–349

79. Travis L, Brennan PF: Information science for the future: an innovative nursing informatics curriculum. *J Nurs Educ* 37:162–168, 1998

80. America Online Inc: "1999 America Online Annual Report" 1999 (Internet), available at <URL: http://www.corp.aol.com/reports.html> Accessed January 2, 2000.

81. Gomez E, Ehrenberger H: The Internet and the World Wide Web, in Klimaszewski A, Aikin J, Bacon M, Distasio S, Ehrenberger H, Ford B, (eds): *Manual for Clinical Trials Nursing.* Pittsburgh, Oncology Nursing Press, 2000, pp 253–259

82. Delhagen K, Green NE, Allen NH: The e-mail explosion. *Forrester Report* 3:7, 1–14, 1996

83. Sparks SM: Electronic networking for nurses. *IMAGE J Nurs Sch* 25:245–248, 1993

84. Kane B, Sands D: White paper: guidelines for the clinical use of electronic mail with patients. *J Am Med Inform Assoc* 5:104–111, 1998

85. December J, Randall N: *The WWW Unleashed.* Indianapolis, Sams Publishing, 1994

86. Sparks SM, Rizzolo MA: World Wide Web search tools. *IMAGE J Nurs Sch* 30:167–171, 1998

87. Barlow L: "The Spider's Apprentice—A Helpful Guide to Web Search Engines," August 1999 (Internet), available at <URL: http://www.monash.com/spidap.html> Accessed January 2, 2000

88. Lindberg DA, Humphreys BL: A time of change for medical informatics in the USA, in van Bemmel JH, McCray AT (eds): *Yearbook of Medical Informatics.* Stuttgart, Germany, Schattauer, 1999, pp 53–57

89. Hubbard SM: The National Cancer Institute's cancer information resources, in Klimaszewski A, Aikin J, Bacon M, Distasio S, Ehrenberger H, Ford B, (eds): *Manual for Clinical Trials Nursing.* Pittsburgh, Oncology Nursing Press, 2000, pp 245–252

90. Murray P, Rizzolo M: "Reviewing and Evaluating Web Sites: Some suggested Guidelines," September 1997 (Internet), available at <URL: http://www.nursing-standard.co.uk/vol11-45/ol-art.htm> Accessed January 2, 2000

91. "Mitretek Systems Health Summit Working Group": "Criteria for Assessing the Quality of Health Information on the Internet—Policy Paper," May 1999 (Internet), available at <URL: http://hitiweb.mitretek.org/docs/policy.html> Accessed January 2, 2000

92. Health on the Net: "Health on the Net Foundation Code of Conduct for Medical and Health Web Sites," April 1997 (Internet), available at <URL: http://www.hon.ch/Conduct.html>

93. Silberg W: Assessing, controlling, and assuring the quality of medical information on the Internet. *J Am Med Assoc* 277:1244–45, 1997

94. Bridges A, Thede LQ: Electronic education: nursing education resources on the World Wide Web. *Nurse Educ* 21:11–15, 1996

95. Gomez E, Dubois K, King C: Improving oncology nursing practice through understanding and exploring the Internet. *Oncol Nurs Forum* 25:4–10, 1998 (suppl 2)

96. Rindfleisch TC: (Bio)Medical informatics in the next decade. *J Am Med Inform Assoc* 5:416–420, 1998

97. Westberg EE, Miller RA: The basis for using the Internet to support the information needs of primary care. *J Am Med Inform Assoc* 6:6–25, 1999

98. Tabar P: The virtual patient. *Healthcare Inform* 15:22–24, 1998

99. Jerant AF, Schlachta L, Epperly T, et al: Back to the future: the telemedicine housecall. *Fam Pract Manage* 5:18–28, 1998

100. Ryan SA, Nagle LM: Nursing informatics: the unfolding of a new science, in SJ Grobe SJ, Pluyter-Wenting E (eds): *Nursing Informatics: An International Overview for Nursing in a Technological Era,* New York, Elsevier, 1994, pp 443–447

101. Ehrenberger H, Brennan, PF: Nursing informatics as a support function for oncology nursing research. *Oncol Nurs Forum* 25:21–26, 1998 (suppl 2)

102. Moorehead S, Delaney C (eds): *Information systems innovations for nursing.* Thousand Oaks, CA, Sage, 1998

CHAPTER 83

Policy, Politics, and Oncology Nursing

Pamela J. Haylock, RN, MA, ET
Katherine McDermott Blackburn, RN, MPA, OCN®

Introduction

Research findings in cancer genetics and the ability to selectively attack molecular processes and biochemical signals involved in cancer physiology exemplify the dramatic shifts in the way the management of cancer is evolving. The first anticancer monoclonal antibodies to be approved by the U.S. Food and Drug Administration were released for general use in 1998. The potential for cures grabbed cover stories in national news magazines, offering people affected by cancer hope that these new advances would reach them in time.[1,2]

It is a very hopeful picture. Nevertheless, in the United States and throughout the world, there are significant barriers that preclude access to the scientific advances that would otherwise offer hope of prolonged survival or even cure. Those who are most likely to confront such barriers include the elderly, the homeless, the poor, the uninsured, and various ethnic populations.[3,4] The major barrier is that imposed by the economics of cancer care. Facione and Facione point out that while the "inequities of care for patients with cancer are tragic, the inequities in access to prevention and early detection are even more tragic."[3] Editorial comment in a weekly news magazine declares costs of care a most significant issue: "The conflict between the desire for the most advanced and promising forms of care and the reluctance of business, government, or individuals to pay mounting costs, remains the central medical issue at the end of this century."[5]

The marketplace has defined how care will be provided in the twenty-first century. Political agendas have shifted from decades of government-sponsored health care benefits to a system that employs market forces to allocate medical resources.[6,7]

Access to care and services, the way services are delivered, and the types and quality of services that are available are inherently linked to the politics of the culture and the policies of the country in which nurses work. It is a country's values, its dominant political forces, and resulting policies that define nursing practice. To assume key roles as consumers and providers of health care, nurses must understand how these forces come together and the evolution of the changes taking place, and they must be active participants in systems that create and implement health care policy, programs, and services.

Policy encompasses the choices that society, a segment of society, or an organization makes regarding goals and priorities and how resources are allocated.[8] Policies are developed in many sectors: health, social, organizational, public, and institutional. Politics is a process of influence and exertion of control over situations and events through dealing effectively with other individuals and/or groups using compromise, consensus, and negotiation.[8,9] Politics arise in any diverse culture or society when conflicting values are present.

Policy and politics promote the value system of a society, prioritize its political agendas, and dictate legislative initiatives. The dominant values of American society that relate to health care policy include individuality, competition, consumer choice, entrepreneurship, low taxation, the Protestant work ethic, limited governmental intrusion, and a cohesive family unit. The existing socioeconomic environment influences the triad of policy, politics, and values. Together, these factors dictate future directions of both private and public health care sectors in the country. In turn, legislation and regulation arising from the political process influence how nursing is practiced.

Nursing has always been and continues to be the health care discipline that provides the most interaction with patients and families. Nurses constitute a distinct demographic group within the health care industry, and health care trends put more emphasis on a holistic approach, which has historically characterized nursing's role. Nurses bring their unique viewpoint to health care planning and when this perspective is overlooked, there is a gap in information on which to base plans and services.[10]

Political activism is a logical extension of the nurse's traditional role as patient advocate. Political activism allows nurses to assume a critical role in helping members of the lay public accurately assess proposals for health care reform, new public and private insurance plans, or the quality of services offered within a health care plan. Individual nurses or groups of nurses can create or participate in partnerships and coalitions that foster quality nursing care and/or advocate for the public good.

This chapter provides information that can strengthen one's ability to assume a proactive role in policy making and political processes. Historical and social factors affecting policy, political processes, and initiatives that relate to health care are reviewed, followed by discussions specific to politics affecting health care delivery, nursing, and cancer care services. A final section provides information about political approaches and resources for nurses to enhance their effectiveness in the political arena.

Nursing's Political Legacy

Although modern-day nurses have not been particularly visible in the political and public policy arenas, nursing is not without political role models. Florence Nightingale was intensely political. She used knowledge, experience, communication, analytic skills, and connections with powerful people to realize her political agenda. The American Civil War revolutionized nursing care in the United States. The use of political power by individual Civil War nurses—among them Clara Barton, described as a "battlefield activist"[11] and later a "lobbyist,"[12] Dorothea Dix, superintendent of the Union's nurses, Juliet Hopkins, superintendent of Hospitals in Richmond,[11] and Phoebe Yates Pember, matron at Chimborazo Hospital in Richmond,[13]—introduced astonishing changes to the care of hospitalized soldiers. The political success of these women is amazing when viewed within the context of social mores of the time. Women were not regarded as intellectually capable of comprehending the intricacies of the political system, and concern for political issues threatened "womanly honor." Women did not have the right to vote. Each of these nurses, however, did have supporters in executive and legislative branches of the government. Their appeals to government authorities were successful strategies for improving patient welfare and removing barriers to the practice of nursing. Although each of these nurses established contact with officials differently, they shared the approach of personally connecting with political figures whose help they needed to enlist.

Lillian Wald and Lavinia Dock used political activism to attack social conditions that threatened public health and established the Henry Street Settlement House in New York City at the turn of the century. From 1915 on, Margaret Sanger challenged America's attitudes and approaches to family planning. She was jailed for her efforts and for a time fled to England.

The political successes of nurses like Nightingale, Barton, Wald, Sanger, and others who came after them required a thorough firsthand knowledge of the facts relative to their causes and a commitment to patients. So empowered, these nurses discovered they could influence politicians and make a difference for patients. Florence Nightingale, who advocated outcomes-oriented research, continues to influence the health care revolution nearly 100 years after her death.[14]

Contemporary American nurses have been called the "untapped resource" of political activism.[15] Even though there are over 2.6 million registered nurses in the United States, nurses as a group have not harnessed or wielded political power. Only recently have professional nursing education programs incorporated political science courses into curricula, and thus few nurses have been involved in politics to serve as contemporary role models.

The role of women in the political arena has been limited. Consider the fact that it took from 1916, the year women were granted the right to vote, until 1992 to place ten women into the U.S. Senate—out of 100 seats. The 106th Congress, seated in 1999, includes 56 women in the House of Representatives and nine women in the Senate. Three nurses, Representatives Lois Capps, MA, RN (D-CA-22), Eddie Bernice Johnson, RN (D-TX-30), and Carolyn McCarthy, LPN (D-NY-04), were incumbents who won reelection in 1998. State political environments are more "friendly" toward women, but women are still outnumbered by men in state legislatures. An especially encouraging note is the increasing number of nurses who have won elected seats in state legislatures. Table 83-1 lists states in which nurses held elected legislative positions as of 1999.

Recent evidence indicates that nurses are increasingly using political power and lobbying efforts to improve patient welfare and nurses' working conditions.[16] Labor and delivery nurses provided political support for state measures that require third-party payers to cover a mini-

Table 83-1 Nurse State Legislators in 1999

State	Nurses Holding State Office
Alabama	1
Arkansas	2
Arizona	2
California	1
Connecticut	5
Florida	1
Georgia	4
Hawaii	1
Idaho	3
Indiana	1
Iowa	3
Kansas	3
Kentucky	1
Maine	4
Maryland	5
Massachusetts	3
Michigan	2
Minnesota	3
Mississippi	2
Missouri	1
Montana	3
Nebraska	1
Nevada	2
New Hampshire	5
New Jersey	2
New York	1
North Dakota	2
Ohio	2
Oregon	1
Pennsylvania	1
Rhode Island	2
South Dakota	1
Tennessee	2
Texas	1
Vermont	4
Washington	4
West Virginia	1
Wisconsin	1
Wyoming	1

Data from *www.nursingworld.org* Legislative Branch

mum of 48 hours of inpatient care for mothers and newborns after a vaginal birth and 96 hours following cesarean section.[17] Similar legislation is being considered at the federal level.[18] Lobbying by enterostomal therapy nurses helped derail legislation that would have ended reimbursement for disposable medical equipment, including ostomy and wound care supplies. Exercising political power is an essential strategy for safeguarding patient welfare in contemporary society. The responsibility for exercising political power remains with individual nurses committed to improving patient care.[11]

A disturbing issue, however, is nursing's continued lack of visibility, and not just in political and public policy circles. The major finding of the Woodhull Study on Nursing and the Media, aptly titled "Health Care's Invisible Partner," is that the nursing profession and nurses are invisible to the media and, as a result, to the American public.[10] The Woodhull Study emphasizes several important points: (1) nursing is a significant and distinct demographic group within the health care industry; (2) current trends in health care put more emphasis on nursing's role; and (3) nurses provide the most hands-on interaction with consumers of health care services. When the nursing perspective is overlooked, there is a distinct gap in the information on which policies, regulations, and services are based.[10] Without visibility, how can nursing's values or nurses' roles be appreciated and supported by the public in general or policymakers in particular? Without obtaining the desired public image and enhancing the visibility of nursing, the opportunities that accompany political power will be lost to individual nurses and the nursing profession.

Scope of Nursing Practice and State Boards of Nursing

Professional nursing's existence can be credited to individual nurses and groups of nurses determined to safeguard patient welfare. Whether this mission remains central to professional nursing depends on the definition of the scope of nursing practice. Nurses of today and the future must realize and guard this responsibility. The most influential public authorities over nursing practice, holding regulatory and disciplinary responsibility within the profession of nursing, are each state's Board of Nursing (BON).

In the United States, a BON exists in all 50 states and the five territories. Even though North Carolina enacted the first law to regulate the practice of nursing in 1903,[19] it was not until 1938 that New York state legally mandated licensing for nurses.[20] Regulations vary from state to state but in general are promulgated in legislation that sets out minimum requirements for providing safe, skilled nursing care to the public. Although the composition of a BON membership differs from state to state, boards share distinct functions and duties: regulation of practice and educational programs, licensing of individual nurses,

and disciplinary review. Nominees to boards can be members of professional nursing organizations or members of the public at large. Most often, members are appointed at the discretion of state governors: BON members are political appointees. The number of registered nurse members on the 55 boards of nursing ranges from one to nine. Government representatives, commissioners, hospital administrators, physicians, and pharmacists are often appointed as board members.[20] Many states do not require that BON members be either U.S. citizens or residents of the state in which they serve.

In 20 states, nurses have exclusive control of the BON; in the remaining 30 states, multidisciplinary boards, commissions, and nonnursing review committees can develop legislation or make recommendations on nursing practice-related legislation.[21] The significance of the composition of a state BON is exemplified by events in Delaware. In July 1994, Delaware's governor signed a bill giving advanced practice nurses (APNs) prescriptive authority. The regulations were written by a joint practice committee (five APNs, two physicians, one pharmacist, and one member of the general public) before being submitted to the Board of Medicine for final approval.[22] The political appointees to this committee, including five APNs, had powerful influence over the regulation of nursing. On the other hand, a state with a diverse BON and minimal nursing representation or members who lack knowledge regarding professional nursing practice could influence legislative initiatives that adversely affect nursing practice.

In 1999, several states' BONs and state nurses associations (SNAs) took initial steps toward implementing multistate nurse licensure drawing on language proposed by the National Council of State Boards of Nursing (NCSBN). Under the model, titled the "Nurse Licensure Compact," states agree to recognize a license issued by another state. States join the Compact by enacting adoptive legislation. A nurse's license will be issued by the nurse's primary state of residence, but practice standards will be set by the state in which the nurse practices. The nurse assumes responsibility for knowing the laws governing practice in each state in which she or he practices. Although the lack of uniform standards for advanced practice nursing precluded its inclusion in the initial Compact draft, it is likely that the Compact will eventually be amended to include advanced practice nursing. The Compact evaluation initiative, to begin no later than January 1, 2000, will evaluate the effectiveness and operability of the Nurse Licensure Compact. A final report will be drafted in 2004 allowing revisions to the Compact to be made in states' 2005 legislative sessions.[23] A copy of the Compact can be downloaded from the NCSBN Web site (www.ncsbn.org).

The chaos in the health care environment engenders both refinement and blurring of nurse, physician, and other provider roles. Not surprisingly, the resulting uncertainty contributes to a growing level of competition among many of the health care disciplines.[24] Failure of interdisciplinary cooperation and collaboration increases the potential for poor patient outcomes.[25] The political climate escalated with the passage of the Balanced Budget Act of 1997 with expanded direct Medicare reimbursement for nurse practitioners and clinical nurse specialists and removal of physician involvement requirements. Nurses encounter growing efforts by the American Medical Association (AMA) and state Boards of Medicine to limit or diminish the scope of nursing practice. The medical community, especially state medical associations, exerts political influence through lobbying and political fund raising in support of positions at state and national levels. Nurses, especially APNs, are vulnerable to these political maneuvers. For example, a private practice group in Florida exerted pressure on a member physician to replace an oncology APN with a newly graduated physician.[22] The Pennsylvania Board of Medicine used political influence to promote a change in the state's professional and vocational standards to reflect a more restrictive practice environment for nurse practitioners.[26]

Policymakers are considering interdisciplinary regulation and clinical integration, thereby creating a diverse health care workforce that provides uniform levels of care.[27] A report issued in 1998 by the Pew Health Professions Commission urges Congress and the states to adopt tougher regulatory standards that require health professionals to periodically demonstrate their competence. Such competency demonstrations would ensure that managed care organizations are not the only voice for quality in health care.[28] The commission's report, *Strengthening Consumer Protection: Priorities for Health Care Workforce Regulation*, notes that interdisciplinary turf battles are costly and time consuming for the professions and state legislators, and that the decision-making process can be distorted by lobbying efforts and the political process. In this circumstance, practice act decisions may not be based on evidence regarding quality of care.[29] To allay this problem, the Pew Commission recommends the creation of a national policy advisory body to develop national scopes of practice, continuing competency standards, standards of practice authority, and model legislation for use by the states. Former Senator George Mitchell, Chairman of the Pew Health Professions Commission, expects Congress to act by 2001 to create the policy board called for by the Commission.[28]

Nurses must recognize that state health care reform initiatives are neither inherently good nor bad, and they must therefore be prepared to analyze, monitor, respond to, and perhaps initiate reform efforts. This political influence will promote the vision and voice of nursing in the policy debates, sustain the role of nurse as patient advocate, and strengthen nursing's image in the political arena.

Political Issues Affecting Cancer Care

The influence of politics on health care policy related to cancer care issues is exemplified in the types of services available in communities, access to evidence-based treatment modalities, supportive or adjuvant medications and supplies, and qualified providers. The following discussions on pain management, reimbursement for medications used off-label, reimbursement for clinical trials, and tobacco-related issues exemplify the impact of politics and policy on the services and care available to individuals affected by cancer.

Pain Management

The mismanagement of cancer pain is commonplace, and a majority of patients with cancer experience pain needlessly.[30] Policy and legislative issues surrounding proper pain management provide compelling examples of the impact of politics on cancer care and cancer nursing practice. State Cancer Pain Initiatives group the most critical barriers to optimal pain management into three major categories: (1) inadequate knowledge about cancer pain and improper management strategies among professionals and the lay public; (2) attitudes and misinformation about addiction, tolerance, and opioid analgesics among professionals and the lay public; and (3) regulatory restrictions that relate to storage, handling, prescribing, and payment.[31,32] Even though all three categories of barriers must be addressed in policy-making agendas, education of policy makers, professionals, and the public is essential. A common perception among legislators is that this country's illicit drug problem is fueled by the diversion of legally prescribed drugs. If drugs are better controlled, the logic follows, the drug problem will be controlled. A second myth is that there is a standard formula for pain management. A third myth arises from misinformation about what addiction and tolerance really mean. These assumptions are commonly held by legislators, policy makers, the public, and health care professionals.[33] However, regulatory restrictions relating to storage, handling, prescribing, and payment are addressed through regulatory and/or legislative action.

Cost issues

Third-party reimbursement strategies sometimes favor expensive, "high-tech" forms of pain management. Third-party payers, including Medicare, currently reimburse for intravenous (IV) morphine delivered in an inpatient setting and via patient-controlled analgesia (PCA). Costs of outpatient prescriptions of sustained-release opioid tablets and suppositories, or absorbable fentanyl are not usually reimbursed by Medicare or other third-party payers. Patients are sometimes prescribed parenteral morphine to justify professional home care visits or inpatient hospitalizations. Ferrell[34] calculated the costs of continuous infusion morphine to be between $2000 and $4000 per month per patient. In a 12-month period, 255 unscheduled admissions to one hospital (among a total of 2795 scheduled and 2977 unscheduled hospital admissions) had a primary admit diagnosis of "uncontrolled pain." The average length of stay for these admissions was 12 days. Ferrell estimated a cost of $20,000 for an average inpatient stay of 12 days. Based on these estimates,

255 admissions for uncontrolled pain cost this one institution over $5 million over a one-year period.[34] The American Pain Society's Committee on Regulatory Affairs has made attempts, some of them successful, to influence pharmaceutical and durable medical equipment (DME) companies to cease lobbying that perpetuates unwarranted use of expensive, high-tech interventions.

Monitoring opioid analgesics

In the United States the Controlled Substances Act regulates production and distribution of opioids, stimulants, and sedative hypnotics—agents that are subject to controlled-substances laws because of their potential for abuse. These agents are divided into five categories or "schedules." Agents that have no accepted medical use are placed in schedule I but are available for scientific use. Agents that have been approved for medical use are placed in schedules II–V, depending on their potential for abuse; the agents commonly used in cancer pain protocols, such as morphine, hydromorphone, and fentanyl, are schedule II drugs. It has been shown that regulatory controls placed on schedule II agents reduce prescribing of these medications. One regulatory control mechanism is the multiple copy prescription program (MCPP), which mandates use of duplicate or triplicate prescription forms, special prescribing privileges, controls, and monitoring of providers. Research indicates that the MCPP hampers the prescribing of schedule II opioids for terminally ill patients with chronic pain.[35] There was a 64% reduction in the prescribing of schedule II controlled substances, mainly opioid analgesics, after an MCPP was introduced in Texas, as well as a 57% reduction in Rhode Island, a 54% reduction in New York, and a 50% reduction in Idaho.[36] The MCPP seems to encourage substitution of weaker opioids in lower schedules for more potent schedule II opioids,[37,38] resulting in less effective management of pain. Although some states have altered MCPP, it still exists in many states and represents a continuing barrier to optimal pain management.

Access to health care providers and adequate insurance coverage make a difference in the management of pain. One study involving a hematology and oncology patient population found significant differences in the amount and type of pain medications prescribed between patients with prescription drug coverage (Medicaid) and those without.[39] Access to medications, including analgesic medications, is subject to various political influences determining pharmacies' ability to stock medications, their ability to compound different formulations, or a pharmacist's likelihood of filling a prescription for a controlled substance.[32] Limited access to medications can influence patient compliance. If medication is difficult to procure—for example, requires physician visits for refill prescriptions, requires additional trips to a pharmacy, is expensive and not reimbursable, or is not available at all—patients are unable to follow even the simplest pain management plan.

In 1999, the United States' Veterans Affairs Department launched a system-wide effort to reduce pain for its 3.4 million patients. Physicians and nurses working in the Veterans Administration (VA) centers are expected to treat pain as a "fifth vital sign" thereby including pain in the routine assessments of blood pressure, pulse, temperature, and respiration. The VA has allocated $3 to $5 million in staff training and pain management research.[40] This policy initiative has been a priority of the American Pain Society, state cancer pain initiatives, other organizations, and individual oncology nurses, all collaborating in the effort to alleviate unnecessary pain and suffering.

In 1997, the U.S. Supreme Court ruled that there is no constitutional right to physician-assisted suicide, a ruling that, in effect, requires all states to ensure that state laws are not barriers to adequate palliative care and the alleviation of pain of people at the end of life.[41] The Institute of Medicine Committee on Care at the End of Life has recommended reform of drug prescription laws, regulations, and state medical board policies that impede the relief of pain and suffering.[42]

Conversely, passage of physician-assisted suicide initiatives in Oregon and Washington generated legislative activities at the federal level. A bill debated in 1997 and 1998, entitled the "Lethal Drug Abuse Prevention Act" would create a board to review physicians' intent for prescribing pain medications, and facilitate the leveling of criminal charges against physicians and pharmacists as accessories to possession of scheduled medications. Pain experts claimed this legislation would ultimately have a "chilling effect" on analgesic prescribing, decreasing physicians' willingness to prescribe the strong opiates needed for optimal pain management. This legislation was set aside, but it is a certainty that the issues surrounding the use of analgesic opiates will continue to arouse the interests and passions of policymakers.

Other initiatives that indicate a move toward eliminating regulatory barriers to optimal pain management are state and federal intractable pain treatment laws and regulations[43] and state medical board guidelines for treatment of intractable pain.[44] State legislatures are increasingly including the use of drugs to treat pain in their definitions of the practice of medicine.[45] In 1989, Texas became the first state to approve an Intractable Pain Treatment Act (IPTA), followed by California in 1994. Other state medical boards have published guidelines that address the use of opioids for intractable pain.[44]

Signs of declining regulatory restrictions over opioids are viewed as a trend in the right direction by pain experts. The Department of Health and Human Services prevented the introduction of a national MCPP. The Agency for Healthcare Policy and Research has published clinical practice guidelines that recognize the need to improve the regulatory environment for prescribing opioids.[33] States are less inclined to start new MCPPs, and some states have taken action to disband existing MCPPs.[46] Even though it might seem that progress has been made, there are crucial questions yet to be addressed through policy-making, regulatory, and political processes. For example, "What should the law and medical board guidelines say about opioid prescribing?"[46]

"What knowledge base, skills, and credentials prepare a nurse to prescribe controlled substances?" "In what settings should a nurse be allowed to prescribe controlled substances?" The answers to these questions may provide direction for nurses to influence regulation that supports optimal pain management.[47,48]

Reimbursement for "Off-label" Use of Drugs

It has been estimated that one of every eight individuals with cancer does not get preferred therapy.[49] Most third-party payers, including Medicare and Medicaid, have used the federal Food and Drug Administration (FDA) package insert as a guide for determining what use of that drug is reimbursable. The FDA label is created during the FDA approval process, in which a drug is proved to be effective for one disease entity. Since the FDA approval process is both lengthy and expensive, most pharmaceutical companies that have successfully evaluated drugs for other indications do not put these agents through a second approval process. Instead, once a drug has received FDA approval, it is available for prescription based on an individual physician's discretion. There are drastic reimbursement differences in various regions, even within one state. Some payers follow the guide very strictly; others are more lenient. Even though a physician prescribes the drug, an insurance company may deny reimbursement.

It has been reported that 56% of cancer drugs are used "off-label"—that is, in the treatment of diseases other than the one indicated on the FDA label.[49] In many situations physicians select less effective protocols to avoid conflicts with third-party payers over reimbursement for off-label use; hence the statistic that one of every eight individuals with cancer does not get the preferred, most effective therapy. Uniform Coverage of Anticancer Drugs legislation was drafted in several states in collaboration with the Association of Community Cancer Centers.[50] According to the language in this legislation, payers must pay for drugs if their efficacy is outlined according to FDA approval, is supported by one or more citations included in at least one of the three compendiums (the *American Hospital Formulary Service Drug Information*, the *AMA Drug Evaluations*, or the *U.S. Pharmacopoeia Drug Information*), or is supported by clinical evidence reported in peer-reviewed medical literature. This legislation has been introduced and passed by several states, and nurses have figured prominently in moving these initiatives forward. Using language similar to the Uniform Coverage of Anticancer Drugs legislation adopted by several states, Congress included off-label provisions in legislation involving Medicare and Medicaid that became law in 1994.

As part of the Balanced Budget Act of 1997, Congress demanded that a prospective payment system for Medicare's hospital outpatient services be implemented by January 1, 1999. The Health Care Financing Administration (HCFA) released its proposal of Ambulatory Payment Classifications (APCs) in September 1998. HCFA delayed implementation of new regulations until after January 1, 2000. Under the proposed APCs, reimbursement for chemotherapy agents and radiation therapy would be diminished; costs of drugs used in supportive care, such as antiemetics and colony-stimulating factors, would be bundled into the total reimbursement for chemotherapy drugs. The potential exists for resulting reductions in use of new drugs such as the recently introduced, and costly, monoclonal antibodies. It has been predicted that outpatient medical and radiation oncology settings will be forced to close, a scenario of particular concern to patients and providers in rural areas. The cancer community—including the Oncology Nursing Society, the Association of Community Cancer Centers, The American Society of Clinical Oncologists, and the consumer advocates' Cancer Leadership Council—formed a collective lobbying response to these proposals, calling for an exemption for cancer chemotherapy and supportive care drugs from the proposed APC system. Thousands of letters protesting the proposal were generated by the cancer community. As a result of these lobbying efforts, Congress and The Health Care Finance Administration (HCFA) will re-assess the potential impact of this prospective payment system between 2000 and July 2002, when recommendations are due back to Congress.

Reimbursement for Clinical Trials

The future of specialty practice and the advancement of treatment offered to individuals with cancer depends on research. The ability to do high-quality, meaningful research is dependent on researchers' abilities to enter adequate numbers of patients in a clinical trial. Most third-party payers currently do not pay for care or treatment that falls into the vaguely defined category of "experimental" care. This prohibits many potential subjects from participating in clinical trials and sometimes forces physicians to recommend standard therapy when an investigational therapy might be more promising.[50]

Clinical research is affected by the reconfiguration of health care funding. Leveling of funding from the National Institutes of Health (NIH) has resulted in greater scrutiny of the kinds of research being conducted, who is doing the research, how funding is allocated, and the government's role in supporting research. Existing divisions in the research community, including different disease groups, are made even more prominent by this scrutiny. Support for research in academic health centers is hampered by their expansive missions and higher patient care costs. Managed care plans and pharmaceutical companies are assuming roles in clinical research, leading to a set of new concerns, including an exodus of researchers from universities to the private sector and the perception that research directions are influenced by for-profit business strategies.

The dominance of managed care in the delivery of health care has created a growing concern within the oncology community that clinical trials will suffer from competing interests, particularly profit margins. Many oncologists are concerned that research trials and the educational training necessary to produce future generations of researchers will be affected by decreased funding. Funding sources for clinical and basic research have traditionally come from federal and state grants and industry support. In the managed care environment, public funding sources are diminishing. In the future, the primary funding source for oncology research will most likely be through the private sector.[51]

The federal budget funds several sources of medical- and health-related research, including the NIH and the VA. Concerns expressed by members of Congress and other bodies regarding the quality, appropriateness, size, and cost of NIH research programs make the NIH vulnerable to loss of support from influential legislators, organizations, and interest groups, resulting in decreased funding or outright elimination of programs.[52]

In the legislative arena, a Senate bill was introduced in 1997 that would mandate Medicare to establish a five-year demonstration project to study and provide coverage of routine patient care costs for Medicare beneficiaries with cancer who are enrolled in an approved chemotherapy program. At least in its introductory phase, the bill did not provide reimbursement for investigational drugs and devices. The bill's sponsor contends that the demonstration project would produce the "information and experience needed to then modify Medicare's policy toward clinical trials."[53] Even though this bill did not become federal law, many states are beginning to require health plans to pay for routine costs of care associated with participation in approved clinical trials. In late 1999, New Jersey announced that a coalition of insurers would pay for cancer patients to participate in clinical trials in what the cancer community sees as a sign of encouragement that insurers in other states will follow suit.[54]

Tobacco-Related Issues

Tobacco companies collectively spend over $6 billion annually on advertising and promotion campaigns, $16 million every day.[55] Each year, tobacco-related illnesses kill more than 400,000 people, and every day, 3000 children (1 million a year) become regular smokers: 1000 of them will eventually die an early death from tobacco addiction. There were multiple bills dealing with a legal settlement between the federal government and the tobacco industry in the 105th Congress, but the focus shifted to individual state settlements. Between 2000 and 2025, all 50 states will get nearly $246 billion from cigarette producers as a result of lawsuits brought against the tobacco industry. The question of how to use settlement dollars has created a political tug-of-war in the states.[56]

A hotly contested 1998 ballot initiative was passed in California, adding a $1 tax on each pack of cigarettes. The tobacco industry's unsuccessful lobbying efforts against the initiative, which cost the industry in excess of $70 million, points to a shift in public tolerance for the tobacco industry's arguments of tobacco taxes as discriminatory.

Oncology nurses, through the collective voice created by the Oncology Nursing Society (ONS) and other health advocacy groups, continue to pursue strategies to decrease tobacco-related illnesses and premature deaths in the United States. Working through the coalition Effective National Action to Control Tobacco (ENACT), oncology nurses participate in the development of and advocacy of policies to reduce tobacco use and prevent tobacco-related illnesses. The ONS was involved in coalition efforts that resulted in smoking being banned on U.S. commercial flights lasting six hours or less, virtually eliminating smoking on all domestic flights. Later legislation banned smoking on international flights originating in the United States.

In 1996 President Clinton endorsed new rules that declare nicotine an "addictive" drug, making nicotine-containing products subject to FDA regulation. Tobacco companies filed lawsuits to block implementation of these regulations; implementation continues to be delayed, and the issue went to the U.S. Supreme Court in 2000.

Politics, Social Policy, and the American Health Care System

Even though most people under age 50 cannot recall major political discussions around the provision of and payment for health care, the debate over a national health care plan actually began shortly after the turn of the twentieth century. Despite nearly 100 years of political skirmishing, the spectrum of health care issues is monumental in its complexity, and politicians and health care experts have not or cannot come to a consensus on how to address these issues. Table 83-2 outlines the chronology of health care reform initiatives in the United States.[57–60] The following section illustrates how the current political environment, one that emphasizes a market approach, is shaping health care delivery.

The Current National Health Care Reform Debate

"The United States has the best system of health care in the world. Something needs to be done about this."[61] This seemingly contradictory statement by humorist Dave Barry captures the essence of the national health care reform debate. The American health care system has been described as a paradox of excess and deprivation,[62] being both the most expensive and the most inadequate system in the developed world.[63] Although technologically outstanding, the American health care system is expensive, fails to provide universal coverage or basic services to all citizens, lacks the essentials of primary care, and emphasizes acute medical care and disease states as opposed to self-care and maintenance of health. Health care costs have risen significantly since the mid-1960s,

Table 83-2 The Chronology of Health Care Reform in the United States

Year	Action or Initiative
1916	The American Association for Labor Legislation proposes a standard bill for compulsory medical care and sickness benefits insurance.
1927	The Committee on the Costs of Medical Care meets to address the problems of health care delivery.
1934	Blue Cross is started under the direction of the American Hospital Association.
1938	First formal prepaid comprehensive health plan is developed: the Kaiser-Permanente Medical Care Program.
1939	Blue Shield is created by state medical societies.
1946	Congress enacts the Hospital Survey and Construction (Hill-Burton) Act.
1949	President Truman proposes a compulsory national health insurance system.
1951	President Truman withdraws his support for a national health insurance plan because of McCarthyism and antisocialist sentiment.
1965	The Medicare and Medicaid laws are enacted.
1970s	Five major health care proposals are placed before Congress. None is voted out of subcommittee.
1971	The National Cancer Program is established with passage of the National Cancer Act.
1982	The Tax Equity and Fiscal Responsibility Act (TEFRA) is passed to address inflationary cost-based reimbursement for Medicare providers largely through implementation of diagnosis-related groups (DRGs) to classify reimbursement.
1990	The Americans with Disabilities Act is passed, providing equal opportunity to disabled citizens.
1993	President Clinton proposes the Health Security Act.
1994	The Health Security Act fails.
1996	The Health Insurance Reform Act of 1995 is passed. It increases access to and security of health care benefits, and provides for increased portability of health care benefits. Limits exclusions of preexisting conditions. Allows for four-year experimental inclusion of Medical Savings Accounts available to self-employed workers and workers in small businesses. Changes the IRS tax code to allow deductions for long-term and home health care.
1996	The Personal Responsibility and Work Opportunity Act is passed. Reforms the Welfare program. The Federal government sets terms for states to shift Medicaid recipients to managed care programs.

Data from McDermott;[57] Clinton;[58] Jonas;[59] Watson.[60]

and over 44 million Americans, 18% of the nonelderly population, are without health insurance; millions more lack adequate coverage.[64–67]

Strategies for health care reform pit the two major political parties in a debate revolving around a critical philosophical difference. A core Democratic value is that government should be the guarantor of the common good. Conversely, Republicans advocate minimal government involvement.[68]

Whether health care is a right has been, at the least, a topic of debate and, at most, a central and polarizing issue between political factions. The U.S. Constitution has no provision to support a claim to the right of all Americans to a minimal level of health care services.[69] In contrast, other developed countries in the world provide for universal health care for their citizens, considering it to be a social service, not a commodity.[63,69]

In September 1993 President Clinton outlined the American Health Security Act of 1993.[58] The plan, described as an amalgam of regulation and market competition, was designed to placate those who favor a global cap on spending and those who prefer to rely on market forces. This reform effort failed but nevertheless provided a catalyst for the market-driven reforms that followed.

A less-government and balanced-budget philosophy reflects the political stance in a Congress controlled by the Republican party. Medicare and Medicaid spending and other entitlement programs are targets for major budget reductions. To accomplish these reductions, Congress approved the transfer of nearly all federal welfare programs, in the form of block grants, to the states, introducing new concerns about resource allocations by the states.[70]

When funds are transferred to the states, governors and state legislators allocate these resources by eliminating or consolidating many small public health programs. However, the ramifications of shifting these allocations raise concerns of conflict of interest in state legislatures and the cost shifting from states to the private sector. For example, a study conducted by the Consumer Federation of America and Common Cause suggests that regulation of the insurance industry may be hampered by legislators who serve on insurance committees, who are themselves insurance agents or have other ties to the industry.[71] The process of setting standards for the insurance industry, a state responsibility, is therefore susceptible to lobbying and political influence.

On the employer side, the National Leadership Coalition on Health Care, representing 93 companies including Chrysler, Ford, and labor unions, suggested that the proposed Medicaid cuts would cause states to cut 7.2 million people from eligibility.[72] This would result in hospitals and other providers treating uninsured people, shifting costs to employer-sponsored health insurance plans.[72] Medicare and Medicaid have been an integral part of health care in the United States for more than three decades. Proposals for major budgetary reductions in these programs have provoked debates in both political philosophy and economics.

Medicaid

Medicaid, created in 1965, is a federal-state matching entitlement program that provides medical assistance and long-term care to low-income individuals, the uninsured, and the disabled.[73] The Medicaid component represents nearly 40% of federal aid to states. The federal share of Medicaid expenses is based on each state's per capita income, but by legislative statute, ranges from 50% to a maximum 83%. Because of the escalating costs of this program (from $51.3 billion in 1988 to nearly $160 billion in 1997) and the increasing number of recipients (from 22.3 million in 1989 to 41.3 million in 1999), the managed care concept has grown rapidly as an alternative to the variety of existing Medicaid state policies.[75] Many state governors believe that enrolling Medicaid recipients into managed care plans will stem the growth of these costs and provide comprehensive care within political, social, and economic constraints.[76]

As of January 1999, over 41 million recipients were enrolled in Medicaid programs, with 7.8 million of these in managed care programs.[73] After meeting a federally defined eligibility criterion, beneficiaries must meet additional eligibility requirements with regard to income and assets established by their state of residence. States determine the type, scope, and duration of covered services. The predominant groups enrolled in Medicaid programs include children and adults in poor, single-parent families. Medicaid was linked administratively to state welfare programs at the outset: people who were eligible for public assistance were automatically eligible for Medicaid. Welfare reform, embodied in the Personal Responsibility and Work Opportunity Reconciliation Act of 1996, severed ties between Medicaid and public assistance. While welfare caseloads have declined by 42% since 1994, there have been reductions in the numbers of people applying for Medicaid coverage.[73] It is supposed that most former welfare recipients who do find jobs are in low-paying, nonbenefited positions. There are millions of adults and children who are uninsured despite eligibility for Medicaid, a possible testament to the difficulties poor people encounter in publicly run systems.

The biggest change in Medicaid has been its expanded role in long-term care.[75] Because poverty is associated with an increased incidence of cancer and lower survival rates,[76] decreased access to care and lack of education present major challenges for nurses caring for indigent patients in isolated rural areas, those in depressed inner-city neighborhoods, and patients with disabilities.[76–79] Medicaid recipients, unlike Medicare beneficiaries, lack a powerful political constituency to advocate for their needs. Sure to ignite passionate debate are cutbacks in Medicaid funding, ethical issues raised by the rationing of care,[80] and the philosophical differences between the involved political and special-interest factions.

Medicare

The second major restructuring initiative taking place at the federal level involves the Medicare program, which provides health care insurance for 95% of the nation's elderly. Medicare was enacted in 1965 and has been called the "world's largest insurance company."[81] Since its inception, Medicare has been based on the principle of social insurance, which is "the mandatory contributions that employees make to dedicated trust funds during their working years with the promise of receiving benefits (income or services) after they retire."[82] To date, the 39 million Medicare recipients, age 65 and older, are generally pleased with the program. Other Medicare beneficiaries include 5 million permanently disabled citizens, and 284,000 individuals with end-stage renal disease.[83] As currently run, Medicare offers benefits that include choices of physician, hospital, or home care provider and adheres to its original mission of providing appropriate and adequate care to the elderly.

Criticisms of Medicare arise from the fact that few restraints on consumption of services are built into the program. Medicare remains a largely fee-for-service plan under which physicians have incentives to order or perform more, not fewer, services. In 1995, $183 billion was spent to provide these services. In 1997, Medicare spent $214.6 billion.[83] As the American population is increasingly living to an age where the incidence of cancer is higher, there is an increased demand for cancer care services associated with increased costs.[83–85]

America's elderly use medical specialists to a greater extent than their younger counterparts. When elders have a chronic illness, they develop relationships with a set of physicians (Blendon RJ, personal communication March 1996). This is especially significant in the elderly oncology patient population; more than 60% of all cancer deaths occur in patients 65 and older, and approximately 12% of people over 70 have a prior history of malignancy.[84,85] In fact, the median age for individuals who develop cancer is 67. The elderly, who have higher cancer mortality rates, are often socioeconomically disadvantaged.[84] Seventy-eight percent of Medicare beneficiaries have average annual incomes below $25,000 and spend approximately $3000 annually for out-of-pocket health care costs.[86] For this reason, many Medicare beneficiaries are being encouraged to join health maintenance organizations or other managed care entities that provide comprehensive services for fixed monthly premiums.

The outcome of proposed Medicare changes is critical for Americans living in rural settings where health care facilities are scarce. Other proposed strategies will ask Medicare recipients to pay more. Rural hospitals are decreasing in number, or reducing bed capacity,[87] making it necessary to expand and improve community-based, ambulatory, and home care services, and to develop better methods of educating patients, families, and caregivers who do not have access to oncology care. Issues and opportunities for nurses fall into four major categories: (1) access to services, (2) communication among providers, patients, and families, (3) professional and public education, and (4) access to and use of state-of-the-art technology, including telemedicine, teleconferencing, and other forms of electronic linkages.[88,89]

Medicare is an extremely popular program. Yet, it is commonly believed that Medicare's Hospital Insurance Trust Fund will run out of money by 2001. Provisions in the Balanced Budget Act of 1997 designed to extend solvency to 2007, rely heavily on reductions in payments to providers. An additional 300 provisions add to Medicare's complexity, but are designed to expand the choices among private health plans available to beneficiaries, referred to as "Medicare + Choice." In 1998, it was announced that 43 of the 347 health maintenance organizations (HMOs) with Medicare beneficiaries would not renew Medicare contracts for 1999, citing financial losses as the major reason. An additional 54 HMOs will reduce the number of geographic areas where they will enroll Medicare beneficiaries. These changes affect over 400,000 beneficiaries.[83]

As a provision of the Balanced Budget Act, Congress created the Medicare Payment Advisory Commission, which monitors the administration of the Medicare program. HCFA has been directed to create a prospective payment approach to reimbursement that will apply to postdischarge services, including care in skilled nursing facilities, hospital outpatient services, inpatient rehabilitation services, and home health care.

A Medicare shortcoming noted in President Clinton's 1999 State of the Union address is the failure to cover outpatient prescription drugs. This issue is expected to figure prominently in congressional debate, pitting the elderly who welcome prescription drug coverage against drug companies interested in avoiding further governmental intrusion into price setting.[90] Employers and managed care executives also express concerns over expanded prescription drug coverage, citing the already explosive rise in spending for prescription drugs of 15%–20% in each of the last two years.[91] Aside from the economic issues, the Medicare benefits package needs revisions that are sensitive to the needs of beneficiaries with chronic illnesses.

The Health Care Delivery System

Health care spending, at close to $400 billion in 1998, consumes the largest portion of the national budget. Reports identify the increasing trend by most hospitals to provide concentrated care in outpatient settings and postdischarge services in home health care and skilled-nursing facilities. Other trends identify the steady decline in the number of hospital days, down since 1985, and community hospital occupancy rates that have fallen from 64% in 1990 to 60% in 1997.[66]

It is estimated that the percentage of for-profit health maintenance organization enrollment has increased, accounting for over 61% of total HMO enrollment for the nation in 1997. The largest HMOs, those with enrollment of 200,000 or more, increased enrollment from 32.6% to 57.6% between 1987 and 1997. This is primarily attributable to the growth in large national HMOs. These large HMOs have been more successful in increasing their total enrollment because of solid and rapid growth in their traditional products, the trend toward mergers and acquisitions, and the development of specialized product lines,

such as oncology.[92] These organizations use a variety of approaches and incentives to influence decisions of health care providers and increasingly move medical practice away from traditional settings to corporate entities.

The majority of Americans continue to receive health insurance coverage as an employer-sponsored benefit.[93] In 1998, these costs rose 6.1% as a result of employees seeking more options in health plans. Higher cost projections are expected for the coming years as a result of modifications in prescription drug plan benefits. Accelerated drug costs are explained by broader insurance coverage, growth in the number of drugs dispensed, more FDA approvals of expensive new drugs, and direct consumer advertising by the pharmaceutical industry.[92]

Employers of both large and small companies are seeking ways to provide less costly, more efficient, reasonably good-quality medical services at discounted fees.[94] Extensive variations among employers' approaches to selecting health care benefits have led corporate benefit managers to become "proactive purchasers" of managed care plans. Identified trends that have resulted from these changes include the development of shared practices, negotiated price structures, and concessions from health care providers that include increasing employee deductions, limited dependent coverage, altering employee provider or plan choices, and increased participant accountability.[95] These practices, once unthinkable, are commonplace in today's health care market.

The evolution of a market-oriented health care delivery system that features for-profit hospital chains and ambulatory facilities, freestanding radiological units, and "vertically" integrated health maintenance organizations defines the culture of practice.[96] Because some managed care networks are created hastily and seek to reduce costs or create a profit at the expense of patient care, oncology nurses must educate themselves and advocate for patient and consumer needs in managed care networks and the benefits that are offered or eliminated. To successfully participate and practice within these complex structures and maintain the patient advocate role, oncology nurses must understand the basic concepts of managed care systems and the political environment that has fostered their development and implementation.

Managed Care

Managed care is a term synonymous with how millions of Americans receive health care services. As commonly defined, managed care refers to a "variety of methods of financing and organizing the delivery of comprehensive health care in which an attempt is made to control costs by controlling the provision of services."[97] This definition emphasizes the integration of health care financing with the delivery of medical care and cost containment.

Although an oft-stated goal of managed care plans is to limit expensive and inappropriate care without denying appropriate treatment, concerns have been raised by providers and patients about the emergence, rapid growth, and inherent restrictive practices of these plans.[98]

As the managed care industry expands, legislators are called on to address deficiencies that are reported by consumers, practitioners, and the media. The Health Insurance Reform Act, passed in August 1996, contains insurance reforms that affect many Americans.[99] It addresses denial of coverage for preexisting conditions, makes eligibility for insurance "portable" from job to job, and allows small businesses and farmers to pool resources to buy insurance for employees and families across state lines. This legislation does not address the issue of the uninsured or the affordability of insurance.

Indicators of public concern about the quality of care available through managed care plans are calls to codify the Consumer Bill of Rights and Responsibilities drafted by the President's Advisory Commission on Consumer Protection and Quality in the Health Care Industry. Several nurses, including the president of the American Nurses Association, were among the members of this presidentially appointed commission. Provisions of the Patients' Bill of Rights Act of 1998 include the rights to referral and access to specialists, continuity of care despite contractual breaks, continuing care for terminal patients, access to emergency care without prior authorization, coverage for patient care costs associated with clinical trials, some coverage of prescription and investigational drugs, confidentiality measures and grievance processes, and the prevention of interference with communications from health team members (the "gag rules"). This legislation was endorsed by both professional and consumer groups. Although the legislation was shelved at the close of the 105th Congress, consumer rights in regards to health care promises to be a key issue in the 106th Congress.[100]

These examples of proposed legislation have implications for oncology care. Access to specialty care is a hallmark of the "old" health care delivery system. Managed care challenges traditional referral networks and systems. For individuals with cancer, restricting access to oncology specialists, whether physicians or nurses, is a grave concern. In the process, patients lose an element of control over the kind of care they receive.

As a national trend, the number of specialty physicians is decreasing in proportion to the number of primary care physicians.[101] Primary care physicians, who may not be trained in oncology, are assuming the responsibility for managing the care of cancer patients as more Americans surrender third-party benefits to restrictive managed care plans. Within a capitated system, the managed care organization can decide to reduce the number of treatment visits or be pressured to shift office-based chemotherapy to a hospital setting where there is less financial risk to the organization. This shift in care settings appears to be the result of economic considerations rather than documented patient needs.

The "gatekeeping" phenomenon occurs when HMOs sharply limit access to specialists by interposing their own physicians between patients and oncology specialists. It also applies to employer purchasers of managed care plans who discourage their employees from accessing specialized care. They simply do not incorporate "carve-out" benefits for cancer care into benefit packages.[102] Other issues that may not be addressed adequately as a result of the rapid expanse of managed care systems include continuity of care, ethical considerations, and financial incentives for physicians and facilities to control costs.

Oncology nurses practicing in managed care settings should become familiar with proposed state and national health care legislation. Although legislators attempt to appeal to all stakeholders, there is always a special-interest group, whether it is the state medical board, the insurance or pharmaceutical industry, or a consumer advocacy group, that identifies the pros and cons of the legislation and lobbies aggressively to achieve its own goals. Oncology nurses must lobby for legislation that supports their values and promotes policies of quality care, choice of provider, and access to services.

Enhancing Political Effectiveness

Nurses have significant knowledge and experience to offer in health policy and legislative arenas at local, state, and federal levels. Legislation that is eventually enacted is usually initiated at the insistence of constituents. Legislative aides or assistants employed by legislators are assigned to research an issue and initiate a draft of possible legislation. At federal and state levels, legislative aides are usually younger than age 25 and have little or no health care background or experience. They are assigned to several, often quite diverse, topical areas and have little time to become expert in any one area.[103] In effect, people with the least amount of knowledge and experience are given the responsibility of writing legislation. While this might be a disadvantage of the system, it presents an opportunity for nurses. The expertise and experience of nurses regarding patient care is what legislators and their assistants do not know unless nurses tell them.

Just as Florence Nightingale and Clara Barton demonstrated, nurses can gain political power by increasing their own visibility. Regular and frequent contact with elected officials is important for establishing a working relationship that will benefit both the nurse and the official. Letters offering informed opinions, in support of an official's position as well as in opposition, can help build this symbiotic relationship. Identifying oneself as a constituent, a voter, and an oncology nurse will enhance the impact of communication with elected officials.

Communicating with Elected Officials

While communicating with elected officials need not be time consuming, use of an accepted protocol will do much to foster a positive and productive relationship.

Local offices of the League of Women Voters offer help in identifying state and federal elected officials. Local libraries usually maintain a list of current officials, officials' addresses, telephone numbers, and district maps. *The U.S. Congress Handbook,*[104] published for each congressional session, features members' pictures, biographies, committee membership, addresses, and phone and fax numbers, and names of key staff members. Internet resources provide similar sorts of information. Table 83-3 offers suggestions for effective written communications with elected officials.

A face-to-face meeting with an elected official to persuade her or him to support or sponsor legislation favorable to a particular cause or to repeal unfavorable legislation is a form of lobbying. The meeting is likely to be brief, with 15 minutes generally allotted for a constituent's visit. Given this limited opportunity, it is wise to prepare for and plan the visit. It is helpful to know about the official as a person, including his or her interests and concerns. For example, know the official's name, party affiliation, electoral history, committee assignments, personal information (e.g., education, previous employment, interests), general voting record and the record relating to the issue being considered, and the position on the specific issue. This information may help determine whether the official is inclined to support or oppose a

---

Table 83-4   Tips for Meeting with an Elected Official

1. Plan and prepare for the visit.
2. Make an appointment stating the subject to be discussed and the time needed, and identify the persons who will attend the meeting.
3. Select a spokesperson if others are going with you and agree on the presentation.
4. Know the facts, both legislative and related to your position. If a bill is being discussed, know the number and title.
5. Dress in business-style attire.
6. Arrive at the official's office on time, but do not be disappointed if the official is late.
7. Introduce yourself, including your name and title, and establish yourself as a constituent.
8. Present the facts in an orderly, concise, and positive manner.
9. Focus on one issue.
10. Relate the positive impact of legislation you support and the problems it corrects.
11. Relate the negative impact of legislation you oppose, and suggest, where appropriate, a different approach.
12. Leave fact sheets if possible.
13. Encourage questions. Discuss.
14. Ask for a favorable consideration.
15. Leave your business card.
16. Thank the official for his/her time and courtesy.
17. Leave promptly.
18. Send a "thank you" follow-up letter: Reiterate your point and send additional materials or information if available.

Data from Pullen.[104]

Table 83-3   Tips on Writing an Elected Official

1. Try to limit the letter to one typewritten page. If writing longhand, write legibly.
2. In a short first paragraph, state your purpose.
3. Stick to one issue or subject.
4. If a bill is the subject, cite it by its title and number.
5. Be factual and support your position with information about how legislation is likely to affect you and others. Avoid emotional, philosophical arguments.
6. If you believe legislation is wrong and should be opposed, say so. Indicate the likely adverse effects and suggest an alternative approach.
7. Ask for a response.
8. Do not start with a negative attitude: Set goals that facilitate compromise.
9. Provide support in obtaining information. Offer to contact expert resources. Offer to testify or find others who can testify.
10. Ask the legislator's views but do not demand support. Even if your position is not supported on one issue or bill, it may be the next time.
11. Be sure your name and return address are legible.
12. Say thank you.
13. The suggested address style is:
    The Honorable [first and last name]
    United States Senate
    Washington, DC 20510
    Dear Senator [last name]:
                      or
    The Honorable [first and last name]
    United States House of Representatives
    Washington, DC 20515
    Dear Representative [last name]:

---

particular viewpoint or position, and whether actions on the part of constituents are likely to alter his or her position. Again, employing an acceptable protocol for meeting with legislators or legislative assistants will reflect positively on any constituent's influence. Table 83-4 offers tips for meeting with an elected official.[104]

Just as there is diversity in positions and people holding elected office, there is great diversity in how nurses might gain political influence. A small number of nurses have themselves achieved elected office. An increasing number of nurses have assumed roles as legislative assistants or other staff positions at state and federal levels. Any nurse, however, can achieve political influence without actually holding office or paid positions in an elected official's staff. Political success can come as a result of volunteer efforts. Nurses can offer volunteer services to a candidate, particularly during political campaigns.

Informally, nurses can take advantage of the esteem in which nurses are held by the public in general. A letter to the editor of a local paper about a health-related issue that is signed by an individual who acknowledges himself or herself to be a registered nurse can hold considerable credence in a community. The likelihood of a letter's being published seems to increase as the size of the community decreases, but whenever published, letters can be influential in the social and political spheres in a targeted community. Along the same lines, letters to the editor of special-interest magazines or journals can sway constituents' opinions.

Lobbying

Lobbying is a tactic of trying to influence policy through policy makers. Lobbying activities are proactive means of exercising group power and influencing constituents and legislators through analysis and persuasive communication.[105] The goal of lobbying for nursing and nurses is to effectively use those precious few moments when a legislator's attention is focused on issues pertinent to the nursing profession.[105] Lobbyists serve as a link between constituents (e.g., nurses and public officials).

Effective lobbying is primarily related to three factors: (1) the amount of money spent by an organization, (2) the sophistication of the strategies used, and (3) the group's size, its geographic location, and the socioeconomic status of the members. These factors determine a lobbyist's level of access to decision makers.[105]

Lobbying is classified into two categories based on strategies used. *Inside lobbying* includes the formal and informal interactions that influence decision makers or their staffs. Historically, this took place in lobbies of legislative buildings—hence the term *lobbying*. Inside lobbying strategies include face-to-face interactions, providing oral testimony, networking with policy makers, drafting legislation, and developing and supplying target lists. Inside lobbying is often regulated and done by registered lobbyists but can be performed by volunteers as well. *Outside lobbying* refers to indirect, grassroots activities to mobilize support and educate constituents and/or legislators. Examples of such indirect lobbying include providing campaign support, telephone contacts, telegrams, personal letters, e-mail communications, press conferences, letters to the editor, and other media activities.

In 1995 Congress redefined lobbyists as those persons who spend at least one-fifth of their paid work time engaged in meeting, conducting research, or working to influence federal policy makers and their aides.[106] This legislation was the outcome of congressional efforts to restructure the way government business is conducted and to convince skeptical voters that Congress can eliminate the conflicts of interest between lawmakers and wealthy benefactors. Under new regulations, lobbyists are required to register with Congress, disclose clients and policies they are attempting to affect, and disclose how much money they spend to influence federal officials.

Lobbying can occur at any stage in the legislative cycle and requires knowledge of the bill-to-law process to determine the most effective time to exert lobbying efforts. *Presession lobbying* begins months before a legislative session, when key issues are identified by the lobbyist's client. Preparation for presession lobbying requires prioritizing issues, research into the political, economic, and social positions of legislators, and analysis of political trends and issues. Presession is the ideal time to establish credibility and plan a legislative agenda.

Lobbying during the session requires monitoring and active networking with other like-minded special-interest groups. Even after the legislative session ends, *postsession lobbying* efforts continue. New legislation requires that new rules and regulations be authorized and drafted. Ad hoc committees, public hearings, written or verbal testimony, and letter-writing campaigns are important to postsession lobbying.

Correct timing is critical during the legislative cycle of a bill. Knowledge of the process of taking an issue from idea to a formal bill to law is therefore crucial in influencing policy and political processes. Figure 83-1 depicts this process.[107]

Working with a lobbyist

The role of a lobbyist is to provide representation and expertise during legislative and decision-making processes. An individual's or group's ability to affect social policy and/or specific legislative initiatives will most often be enhanced by the guidance and assistance of a professional, skilled, and knowledgeable lobbyist. Throughout the legislative process, the lobbyist can offer suggestions, for example, in selection of the "right" author for the legislation—a legislator whose personality traits, level of commitment to the issue, and respect from legislative colleagues will increase the likelihood of proposed legislation being given due consideration. A skilled lobbyist can help devise strategies to activate "grassroots" support, including initiating letter-writing campaigns, assisting with development of written and oral testimony in support (or opposition) of the initiative, and identifying legislators who will consider the legislation.

Coalitions

Coalitions are groups of people or associations that band together to pool resources, ideas, and expertise in pursuit of common goals.[108] The combined clout and credibility of a coalition allows it to exert far more power than that of an individual or an organization acting alone. Coalitions generally appoint a single spokesperson to present its message since legislative and regulatory bodies usually limit the number of speakers allowed to testify on a single issue.

Coalitions differ in organizational structure and purpose, ranging from informal and loosely structured to formal and regimented. The most common coalition is an informal group of interested entities created to allow participants to monitor an issue and network. Participants meet occasionally, and leadership is informal. For lobbying or public relations purposes, a loose coalition may adopt a formal identity and create a list of members, thus becoming a recognized "name" coalition. Name coalitions require little financial commitment on the part of participants.

Formal coalitions, created for active lobbying or public relations purposes, require monetary commitments and a staff. Formal coalitions exist to directly influence acceptance of an issue, for example, convincing the public to support a piece of legislation.

Figure 83-1   The process of how a bill becomes a law. (Reprinted with permission from Abood S, Mittelstadt PC: Legislative and regulatory processes, in Mason DJ, Leavitt JK: *Policy and Politics in Nursing and Health Care* (ed 3). Philadelphia, Saunders, 1998.)[107]

[1]A bill goes to full committee first, then to special subcommittees for hearings, debate, revisions, and approval. The same process occurs when it goes to full committee. It either dies in committee or proceeds to the next step.
[2]Only the House has a Rules Committee to set the "rule" for floor action and conditions for debate and amendments. In the Senate, the leadership schedules action.
[3]The bill is debated, amended, and passed or defeated. If passed, it goes to the other chamber and follows the same path. If each chamber passes a similar bill, both versions go to conference.
[4]The president may sign the bill into law, allow it to become law without his signature, or veto it and return it to Congress. To override the veto, both houses must approve the bill by a ⅔ majority vote.

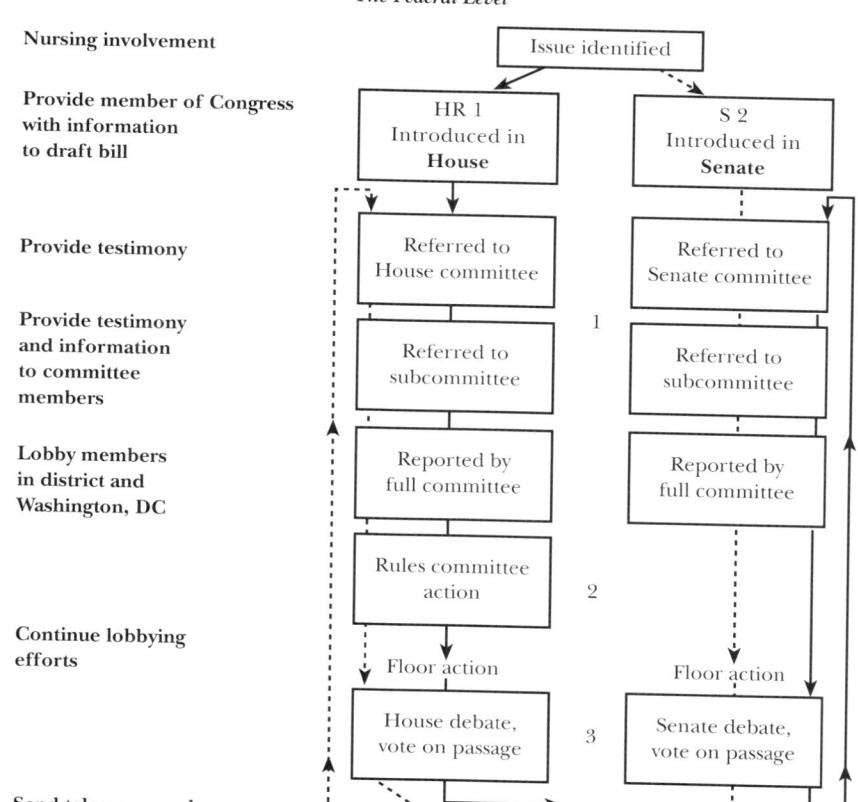

Nursing involvement

Provide member of Congress with information to draft bill

Provide testimony

Provide testimony and information to committee members

Lobby members in district and Washington, DC

Continue lobbying efforts

Send telegrams and make phone calls

Send letter to president

A productive relationship with a coalition can be established when individuals or organizations are familiar with how and why the coalition operates, and there are clear expectations about what the individual or group plans to contribute to the coalition. Considerations before an individual or organization decides to participate in a coalition include the following:

- Ability and willingness to assume the workload and responsibility expected by the coalition

- Willingness and ability to candidly share information

- Ability to offer financial support to the coalition

- Willingness and ability to attend meetings and coalition functions

- Degree to which the coalition's cause is perceived as worthwhile

- Level of knowledge about who belongs to the coalition

- Level of knowledge about who underwrites the coalition[108]

Oncology nurses are quite often designated as representatives of the ONS to various coalitions, and through these roles they actively participate in strategies that influence social policy and legislation. The ONS is a member of several coalitions, including the Coalition on Smoking OR Health, the National Coalition for Cancer Research, the National Alliance of Breast Cancer Organizations, and the Nursing Organizations Liaison Forum of the American Nurses Association (ANA). Participation in these coalitions requires the ONS board of directors to regularly reflect and consider its role in the coalition, the current level of activity and directions of the coalition, and the fiscal priority setting that allows the ONS to support designated members' positions as organizational liaisons between the ONS and the coalition.[109]

Future Trends

"Change is not what it used to be. The status quo will no longer be the best way forward."[110] No one can accurately predict the future. But by analyzing trends, it is possible to make fairly accurate guesses to plan for the future. Trends point to the increasing age of the American population; the growing importance of technological innovation in oncology, including diagnostics and treatment; increased demand for cancer treatment in general; the importance of genetics and genetic therapy in cancer prevention, diagnosis, and treatment; an increase in the cancer cure rate; movement of treatment to outpatient and home care settings; decreased length of stay for the few treatment modalities that remain inpatient; and increased competition between physicians and hospitals for cancer services.[111,112]

For the nursing profession to ensure its future vitality, it must assess trends and devise proactive strategies that allow nurses to take advantage of opportunities as they unfold. Changes, issues, and ethical questions will be set in motion, and individual or collective values will be challenged by scientific discoveries and technological advancements. At present, there is an incomplete understanding of the implications of many of the advances already made, let alone those yet to come, and therefore there is no defined direction or roles for nurses. A few individual nurses may be able to meet these challenges and find opportunities independently. Most nurses, however, would be more effective acting in collaboration with a like-minded group, coalition, or professional nursing organization.

Challenges

Numerous challenges lie ahead for oncology nurses. For example, genetic research and the resulting identification of genes responsible for some diseases, including various forms of cancer, have altered the management of some individuals with cancer or at risk for malignant disease. We have only begun to see the potential of genetic research. Despite the sophistication of these findings, there is no research that addresses physical, psychosocial, and ethical outcomes of these scientific advances.[113] Issues arising from this research include psychosocial ramifications of access to genetic information, questions about who should have access to genetic information and potential violations of privacy and confidentiality, insurability and genetic potential for disease, and other ethical issues.

Even though some of these issues come into conflict with traditional values—particularly those of privacy and confidentiality—public policy does not yet address these concerns. Legislation that begins to address gaps in current public policy is being introduced in the U.S. Congress,[114–116] but genetic science has advanced beyond current policy, the current system of checks and balances, and definition of safe, effective, and ethical practice in light of genetic knowledge and technology. The evolution of such policy is certain to engender political debate, and the oncology nurse can bring invaluable experience and the values of nursing to the policy-making process.

Demographers describe the advancing age of the American population. The traditional American values of "family" and "respect for elders" and current trends that disconnect families and isolate the elderly cause conflicts between values and current public policy. Advancing age is the greatest risk factor in the development of cancer and other diseases. Issues relating to the elderly, sick, and physically and mentally challenged, including questions of who gets care and what type of care older people should receive, have surfaced in ongoing political maneuvering relating to Medicaid and Medicare benefits, long-term care, and end-of-life issues. Legislative initiatives affecting Medicaid and Medicare benefits have been hotly debated, and such debate will escalate as funding cuts are made and resources are overtly or covertly rationed. Nursing organizations, including the ANA and the ONS, have voiced support for universal access to care for all citizens[117,118] and a health care delivery system designed to include, maintain, and improve access to long-term care, and to improve outcomes, costs, and quality of care in these facilities.[117,118] Although organizational position statements are useful tools for presentation of facts and issues, it is constituent and interest-group pressures that ultimately determine the success or failure of legislative initiatives. Nurses can and must play active constituent roles for these initiatives to survive the legislative process.

At the request of Congress, in and of itself the result of political processes, the Institute of Medicine (IOM) compiled the report *Nursing Staff in Hospitals and Nursing Homes: Is It Adequate?*[119] Conclusions have far-reaching implications for nurses currently in practice and those yet to enter the profession. According to the study, the quantity of registered nurses in the United States was determined to be adequate to meet national needs for the near future. The educational and skill mix was questioned, however, in light of the changing health care system. The IOM recommends many changes, including training more APNs and more broadly trained nurses, increased use of APNs, increased numbers of nurses prepared to work in community-based and ambulatory care settings, increased presence of professional nurses in nursing homes on all shifts, and strengthening the leadership of directors of nursing. The report calls the lack of information about whether current delivery system redesign actually increases patient-centered care and reduces costs "shocking," and recommends that such data be collected.[120]

The report *Critical Challenges: Revitalizing the Health Professions for the Twenty-first Century* was released by the Pew Health Professions Commission in 1995.[120] The Pew Commission's recommendations for fewer professional nurses sharply conflicts with the ANA's projections for nursing personnel requirements. Statements released by the ANA suggest that the report is based on assumptions made by managed care organizations using economic criteria rather than exploration of actual consumer needs.[121] These two reports potentially have a tremendous impact on the future of nursing. Legislators looking for data on which to base future policies, legislative initiatives, or decisions about health care and/or nursing roles will accept the reports of these influential entities in the absence of competing analyses. Unless nurses offer an alternative view, these recommendations will be taken as fact. The ANA and nursing specialty organizations, including the ONS, collaborating through the network provided by the National Federation of Specialty Nursing Organizations, has mounted a collective response to the Pew report that openly challenges the recommendations.

The health care environment and managed care systems influence the roles, responsibililties, and employment patterns of nurses and the scope of nursing practice.[122] Some commentators propose a change in clinicians' ethical focus—from that of patient advocacy to being responsible stewards of society's resources.[123] Nurses, according to nurse ethicist Leah Curtin, should be concerned that managed care is undermining all aspects (choice, competence, communication, compassion, continuity, and no-conflict of interest) of the provider–patient relationship.[123]

Nursing Opportunities

Porter-O'Grady[124] identified five areas of opportunity in which nurses, especially APNs, can play a significant role: (1) primary care provider, (2) gatekeeper, (3) provider of cost-effective services, (4) case manager and practitioner in the emerging areas of family care, women's health, and rural health, and (5) wellness advocate and educator in geriatric services. Competencies specific to continued oncology nursing excellence connect oncology to gerontology, clinical trial processes, genetics, case management, ethics, wellness, prevention and early detection of disease, community-based skills, physical assessment skills, quality care, business and economics, epidemiology, anthropology, and patient, family, and community education.[125]

Nursing roles in patient care will continue to evolve as society and health care organizations address questions surrounding cost of care, where and how care is provided, and who should provide it.[122,126] The nurses' advocacy role might be enhanced. Nurses need to acquire knowledge to prepare patients and families to be effective advocates

for their own needs. As policy shifts toward more self-reliance, measures implemented by Medicare and Medicaid will surely be adopted by other payers. Federal legislation—e.g., the Health Insurance Reform Act of 1996—will be subject to interpretation and variable influences of special interests in each of the 50 state legislatures. Nurses, as providers, educators, and consumers, need to have a working knowledge not just of the clinical aspects of care but of the administrative regulations, financial components, and policy implications of what care is available and how care is provided.

Conclusion

Whether acting alone, participating in a community coalition, or collaborating with a professional organization, nurses need to be aware of market, biomedical, and technological trends and the potential influence of these developments on policy and legislation. For most of the last century, health care has been seen as a service. Today, health care is both a service *and* a business. Health care services are increasingly encased in a business environment that, as yet, has few federal regulatory controls. It is nurses who provide many of the services, but they cannot ignore the business side of health care.

Technological improvement, fiscal assessments of delivery systems and health care plans (as opposed to quality indicators), closure of hospitals in rural areas and consolidation and merger of urban and suburban facilities, and the ever-increasing presence of for-profit systems provide opportunities for business to influence legislators and/or policy makers. Nurses must use national and state professional nursing organizations and specialty nursing organizations to keep abreast of these influences and resulting legislative priorities and initiatives. Information technology offers nurses increased opportunities for communication, information sharing, and networking among themselves as well as with consumers and patients. Communication technology such as the Internet offers nearly limitless avenues through which nurses, other providers, and consumers can discuss issues, share concerns, access helpful resources, develop consensus on strategies for action, and communicate with elected officials and policy makers.

Annual membership satisfaction surveys conducted by the more than 29,000-member ONS indicate that its members want a proactive role in shaping their future through political processes that affect health care-related legislation and public policy, and regulations defining the scope of nursing practice.[127] With the trend toward transferring the management of public health care programs to the states and the continuing evolution of the private sector in health care, and the widespread implications these developments portend, it is critical that nurses advocate for the needs of the population they serve and the profession of nursing. Nurses who are politically astute and proactive can influence change and be prepared for roles in the health care system of the future.

References

1. Gorman C: The hope & the hype. *Time* 151:37–47, 1998
2. Brownlee S, Shute N: Killing cancer. *US News & World Report* 124:56–58,65–67, 1998
3. Facione NC, Facione PA: Equitable access to cancer services in the 21ˢᵗ century. *Nurs Outlook* 45:118–124, 1997
4. Bodenheimer T: The American health care system: the movement for improved quality in health care. *N Engl J Med* 340:488–492, 1999
5. Peeno L: What is the value of a voice? *US News & World Report* 124:40–46, 1998
6. Richmond JB, Fein R: The health care mess: a bit of history. *JAMA* 273:69–71, 1995
7. Iglehart JK: The American health care system: Medicaid. *N Engl J Med* 328:896–900, 1993
8. Hanley BE: Policy development and analysis, in Mason DJ, Talbot SW, Leavitt JK (eds): *Policy and Politics for Nurses* (ed 2). Philadelphia, Saunders, 1993, pp 71–87
9. Fisher R, Ury W, Patton B (eds): *Getting To Yes* (ed 2). New York, Penguin Books, 1991
10. Sigma Theta Tau International: The Woodhull Study on Nursing and the Media—Health Care's Invisible Partner. Indianapolis, IN, Center Nursing Press, 1997
11. Rogge MM: Nursing and politics: a forgotten legacy. *Nurs Res* 36:26–30, 1987
12. Pryor EB: *Clara Barton, Professional Angel.* Philadelphia, University of Pennsylvania Press, 1987
13. Wiley BI (ed): *1862–1865—A Southern Woman's Story: Phoebe Yates Pember.* St. Simons Island, GA, Mockingbird Books, 1959
14. Noble H: Linking technology and health groups to find best cure. *New York Times,* Sept. 24, 1995, p A18
15. Hayes E, Tritsch R: An untapped resource: the political potential of nurses. *Nurs Adm Q* 13:33–39, 1988
16. Campbell-Heider N, Hanna ND: Nursing's new political era. *Holistic Nurs Pract* 8:78–87, 1993
17. Lepler M: Nursing leadership meets managed care. *NURSEweek* 8(19):22–23, 1995
18. HR 3101: The Mother and Child Protection Act of 1996. *Congressional Record,* March 14, 1996, E359–E360
19. Greenlaw J: Definition and regulation of nursing practice: an historical survey. *Law Med Health Care* 13:117–121, 1985
20. Dalton JA, Speakman M, Duffey M, et al: The evolution of a profession: where do boards of nursing fit in? *J Prof Nurs* 10:319–325, 1994
21. American Nurses Association: Report on legislative issues related to nursing practice. *Institute of Nursing Practice Agenda Item No. 4.* Washington, DC, American Nurses Association, 1994
22. Pearson LJ: Annual update of how each state stands on legislative issues affecting advanced nursing practice. *Nurse Pract* 19:11–21, 1994
23. Texas moves toward multistate nurse licensure legislation in 1999. *Texas Nurs* 72:4, 11, 1998
24. Hammond K, Bandak A, Williams M: Nurse, physician, and consumer role responsibility perceived by health care providers. *Holistic Nurs Pract* 13(2): 28–37, 1999
25. Larson E: The impact of physician-nurse interaction on patient care. *Holistic Nurs Pract* 13(2):38–46, 1999
26. Family Health Council of Central Pennsylvania: *Summary of Title 49: Professional and Vocational Standards.* Wormleysberg, PA, Family Health Council of Central Pennsylvania, 1994
27. Cooper RA, Henderson T, Dietrich CL: Roles of nonphysician clinicians as autonomous providers of patient care. *JAMA* 280:795–802, 1998
28. *Front & Center:* The Center for the Health Profession Univ. of Calif. San Francisco. Pew Commission calls for tougher standards, competency exams to protect consumers. 3:2, 7, 1998
29. The Center for the Health Profession Univ. of Calif. San Francisco: Strengthening consumer protection: priorities for health care workforce regulation, 1998
30. Cleeland CS: Undertreatment of cancer pain in elderly patients. *JAMA* 279:1914–1915, 1998 (editorial)
31. Hill CS: Relationship among cultural, educational, and regulatory agency influences on optimum cancer pain treatment. *J Pain Symptom Manage* 5:s37–s45, 1990 (suppl)
32. Rabon PG, Linette DC, Gonzalez MF, et al: Limited availability of medications for cancer patients. *South Med J* 86: 914–918, 1993
33. Jacox A, Carr DB, Payne R, et al: *Management of Cancer Pain: Clinical Practice Guideline No. 9.* Agency for Health Care Policy & Research, Publication No. 94–0592. Rockville, MD, U.S. Department of Health and Human Services, March 1994
34. Ferrell BR: Cost issues surrounding the treatment of cancer related pain. *J Pharm Care Pain Symptom Control* 1:9–23, 1993
35. Berina LF, Guernsey BG, Hokanson JA, et al: Physician perception of a triplicate prescription law. *Am J Hosp Pharm* 42:857–859, 1985
36. U.S. Department of Justice, Drug Enforcement Administration: *Multiple Copy Prescription Program Resource Guide.* Washington, DC, Government Printing Office, 1987
37. Sigler KA, Guernsey BG, Ingrim NB, et al: Effect of a triplicate prescription law on prescribing of schedule II drugs. *Am J Hosp Pharm* 41:108–111, 1984
38. Von Roenn JH, Cleeland CS, Gonin R, et al: Physician attitudes and practice in cancer pain management: a survey from the Eastern Cooperative Oncology Group. *Ann Intern Med* 119:121–126, 1993
39. Holcombe R, Griffin J: Effect of insurance status on pain medication prescriptions in a hematology/oncology practice. *South Med J* 86:151–156, 1993
40. Hughes J: VA hospitals to begin treating pain as the "fifth vital sign." *San Antonio Express News,* Feb. 1, 1999, p 5A
41. Burt RA: The Supreme Court speaks: not assisted suicide but a constitutional right to palliative care. *N Engl J Med* 337:1234–1236, 1997
42. Institute of Medicine: *Committee on Care at the End of Life. Approaching Death: Improving Care at the End of Life.* Washington, DC, National Academy Press, 1997
43. Joranson D: Intractable pain treatment laws and regulations. *APS Bull* 5(2):1–3, 15–17, 1995
44. Joranson D: State medical board guidelines for treatment of intractable pain. *APS Bull* 5(3):1–5, 1995
45. Joranson D: Intractable pain treatment laws and regulations. *APS Bull* 5(2):1–3, 15–16, 1995
46. Angarola RT: DEA proposes Controlled Substances Monitoring Act. *APS Bull* 5(3):5, 22, 1995
47. Foley KM: Pain relief into practice: Rhetoric without reform. *J Clin Oncol* 13:2149–2151, 1995 (editorial)

48. McDermott KC: Prescriptive authority for advanced practice nurses: current and future perspectives. *Oncol Nurs Forum* 22:25–30, 1995 (suppl)

49. Government Accounting Office: Report to Senate Committee on Labor and Human Resources, Sept. 1991, GAO/PEMD-91-14

50. Young J: Off-label drug scorecard. *Oncol Issues* 10(2):6, 30, 1995

51. Everson LK: Cancer program development in the 1990's. *Oncol Issues* 8(4):8–10, 1993

52. Ad Hoc Working Group of the National Cancer Advisory Board: *A Review of the Intramural Program of the National Cancer Institute*. Bethesda, MD, National Cancer Institute, June 26, 1995

53. Boyd K (ed): *The Cancer Letter* 22(30):1–3, 1996

54. Kolata G, Eichenwald K: Insurers come in from the cold on cancer. *New York Times*, Dec 19, 1999, p 6

55. Committee on Preventing Nicotine Addiction in Children and Youths, Institute of Medicine: *Growing Up Tobacco Free: Preventing Nicotine Addiction in Children and Youths*. Washington, DC, National Academy Press, 1994

56. Meier B: Tobacco windfall begins tug-of-war in all 50 states. *New York Times*, Jan. 10, 1999, p 1A

57. McDermott KC: Health care reform: past and future. *Oncol Nurs Forum* 21:827–831, 1994

58. Clinton WJ: *The President's Health Security Plan*. New York, Random House, 1993

59. Jonas S: *Health Care Delivery in the United States* (ed 4). New York, Springer, 1986

60. Watson PG: The Americans with Disabilities Act: more rights for people with disabilities. *Rehabil Nurs* 15:325–328, 1990

61. Barry D: This city is nothing like the planet earth: an outsider's guide to Washington. *Washington Post Magazine*, Aug. 14, 1994, pp 7–11, 24–27

62. Enthoven A, Kronick R: A consumer-choice health plan for the 1990s: universal health insurance in a system designed to promote quality and economy. *N Engl J Med* 320:29–37, 1989

63. Angell M: The American health care system revisited: a new series. *N Engl J Med* 340:48, 1999 (editorial)

64. Specture P: Failure, by the numbers. *New York Times*, Sept. 24, 1994, p A19

65. Blendon RJ, Brodie M, Benson J: What should be done now that national health system reform is dead? *JAMA* 273:243–244, 1995

66. Iglehart JK: The American health care system: expenditures. *N Engl J Med* 340:70–76, 1999

67. Quinn JB: The invisible uninsured. *Newsweek*, Mar. 1, 1999, p 49

68. Staples B: The man who wouldn't be president. *New York Times Book Review*, Nov. 19, 1995, p 7

69. Curran WJ: The constitutional right to health care: denial in the court. *N Engl J Med* 320:788–789, 1988

70. Families USA: Hit and miss: state managed care laws. A report by Families USA Foundation, July 1998. (available at //www.familiesusa.org/hit1.htm)

71. Verhovek SH: With power shift, state lawmakers see new demands. *New York Times*, Sept. 24, 1995, pp 1, 24

72. Chronicle News Service: Business group doubts GOP budget plan. *San Francisco Chronicle*, Dec. 6, 1995, A3

73. Iglehart JK: The American health care system: Medicaid. *N Engl J Med* 340:403–408, 1999

74. Grogan CM: Hope in federalism? What can the states do

and what are they likely to do? *J Health Polit Policy Law* 20:477–484, 1995

75. Waid MO: Brief summaries of TITLE XVIII and TITLE XIX of the Social Security Act. *Soc Secur Bull* 56(4):1–3, 1993

76. Freeman HP: Cancer in the socioeconomically disadvantaged. *CA Cancer J Clin* 39:266–288, 1989

77. Freeman HP: The impact of clinical trial protocols on patient care systems in a large city hospital: access for the socially disadvantaged. *Cancer* 72:2834–2838, 1993 (suppl)

78. Katz SJ, Hoffer TP: Socioeconomic disparities in preventive care persist despite universal coverage: breast and cervical cancer screening in Ontario and the United States. *JAMA* 272:530–534, 1994

79. Geller AC, Miller DR, Lew RA, et al: Cutaneous melanoma mortality among the socioeconomically disadvantaged in Massachusetts. *Am J Public Health* 86:538–544, 1996

80. Wachter RM: Rationing health care: preparing for a new era. *South Med J* 88:25–32, 1995

81. Wilensky GR: Incremental health system reform: where Medicare fits in. *Health Affairs* 14(10):173–181, 1995

82. Iglehart JK: The American health care system: Medicare. *N Engl J Med* 327:1467–1472, 1992

83. Iglehart JK: The American Health Care System: Medicare, *N Engl J Med* 340:327–332, 1999

84. Byrne A, Carney DN: Cancer in the elderly, in Ozols RF, Steele G, Kinsella TJ (eds): *Current Problems in Cancer*. St. Louis, Mosby, 1993, pp 150–204

85. Redmond K, Aapro MS (eds): *Cancer in the Elderly: A Nursing and Medical Perspective*. Amsterdam, Elsevier Sciences B.V., 1997

86. Toner R: Medicare target could be elusive, many experts say. *New York Times*, May 16, 1995, pp A1, A20

87. Gorham M: Congressional rescissions mean big cuts for rural health programs. *Rural Health FYI* 17:3, 28–30, 1995

88. Haylock PJ, Cantril CA: Rural cancer care think tank uncovers significant issues/concerns. *ONS News* 10(10):10, 1995

89. Jenkins S: The future of rural communities: mobilizing local resources, in Bushy A (ed): *Rural Nursing*, vol 2. Newbury Park, CA, Sage, 1991, pp 16–28

90. Pear R: Clinton's plan to have Medicare cover drugs means a big debate ahead in Congress. *New York Times*, Jan. 24, 1999, p 16Y

91. Freudenheim M: Patients are paying higher prices for prescription drugs. *San Antonio Express-News*, Jan. 25, 1999, p 14A

92. Trend of the month: HMO enrollments up: HMO profits down. *Drug Benefit Trends* 10(11):9–10, 1998

93. Kuttner R: The American health care system: employer-sponsored health coverage. *N Engl J Med* 340:248–252, 1999

94. Freudenhiem M: Health costs paid by employers drop for first time in a decade. *New York Times*, Feb. 14, 1995, p D9

95. Hurley RE, Thompson JR: The harsh realities of a managed care world. *Med Group Manage J* Sept/Oct:96, 1993

96. Clancy CM, Brody H: Managed care: Jekyll or Hyde? *JAMA* 273:338–339, 1995 (editorial)

97. Iglehart JK: Physicians and the growth of managed care. *N Engl J Med* 331:1167–1171, 1994

98. Mechanic D: Managed care: rhetoric and realities. *Inquiry* 31:124–128, 1994

99. Star P: The signing of the Kennedy-Kassenbaum Bill, Aug. 22, 1996, available at (*http://epn.org/library/signing.html*)

100. Reed S: Washington watch. *Am J Nurs* 98:11, 17, 1998

101. Wennberg JE, Goodman DC, Nease RF, et al: Finding

equilibrium in U.S. physician supply. *Health Affairs* 12: 89–103, 1993

102. Kassirer JP: Access to specialty care. *N Engl J Med* 331: 1151–1153, 1994

103. Grupenhoff JT: Profile of congressional health legislative aides. *Mt Sinai J Med* 50:1–7, 1983

104. Pullen D: *The U.S. Congress Handbook.* McLean, VA, Barbara Pullen Publisher, 1974–1999

105. Bushy A, Smith TO: Lobbying: The hows and wherefores. *Nurs Manage* 21(4):39–41, 44–45, 1990

106. House OKs bill to reform lobbying. *San Francisco Chronicle,* Nov. 30, 1995, pp A1, A17

107. Abood S, Mittelstadt PC: Legislative and regulatory processes, in Mason DJ, Leavitt JK (eds): *Policy and Politics in Nursing and Health Care* (ed 3). Philadelphia, Saunders, 1998, pp 384–396

108. Hunt FD: How coalitions work. *Association Manage* 45:93, 94, 108, 1997

109. Oncology Nursing Society: *Oncology Nursing Society Policy Manual.* Pittsburgh, Oncology Nursing Society, 1998

110. Handy C: *The Age of Unreason.* Boston, Harvard Business School Press, 1989

111. Stepnick L, Pagnani E (eds): *The Future for Oncology; New Technologies and Their Impact on the Competitive Marketplace.* Washington, DC, Advisory Board Company, 1994

112. Boyle DM, Engelking C, Harvey C: Making a difference in the 21st century: are oncology nurses ready? *Oncol Nurs Forum* 21:53–79, 1994

113. Strauss ST, Calzone K, Jenkins J, et al: *Genetics Project Team Report to the Oncology Nursing Society Board of Directors.* Pittsburgh, PA, Oncology Nursing Society, 1996

114. Solomon GBH: *Congressional Record,* Aug. 2, 1996, p E1468

115. Slaughter LM: *Congressional Record,* Mar. 27, 1996, p E476

116. Domenici PV: *Congressional Record,* June 24, 1996, p S6719

117. Oncology Nursing Society: Oncology Nursing Society position paper on quality cancer care. *Oncol Nurs Forum* 24: 951–953, 1997

118. American Nurses Association: *Nursing's Agenda for Health Care Reform.* Washington, DC, American Nurses Association, 1990

119. Institute of Medicine: *Nursing Staff in Hospitals and Nursing Homes: Is It Adequate?* Washington, DC, National Academy Press, 1996

120. Pew Health Professions Commission: *Critical Challenges: Revitalizing the Health Professions for the Twenty-first Century.* San Francisco, Pew Health Professions Commission, 1995

121. Keepnews D: ANA challenges Pew health professions' findings. *Am Nurse* 28(1):3, 1996

122. O'Neil E, Coffman J (eds): *Strategies for the Future of Nursing.* San Francisco, Jossey-Bass, 1998

123. Curtin LL: The ethics of managed care: part I. Proposing a new ethos? *Nurs Manage* 27(8):18–19, 1996

124. Porter-O'Grady T: What an exciting time. *Adv Pract Nurs Q* 1:68–69, 1995

125. Haylock PJ, Boyle DM: Think tank held to ensure a preferred future for oncology nurses and the Oncology Nursing Society. *ONS News* 10(7):5, 1995

126. Parkman C: The staff nurse's role in the changing healthcare scene. *NURSEweek* 8(23):8–9, 1995

127. Oncology Nursing Society: *Annual Membership Survey.* Pittsburgh, Oncology Nursing Society, 1998

CHAPTER 84

Thriving as an Oncology Nurse

Mary L. Cunningham, RN, MS, AOCN

Introduction

Stress is a pervasive human concern. It has been defined as a response, as a stimulus, and as a transaction. Selye[1] defined stress as a physiological response to environmental events and unrelated to the nature of the stressor, the individual's thoughts and beliefs, or the situational context. Others have characterized stress as the potential residing within the stimulus or as something that results because of the event itself, again unmediated by personal factors or variations in the setting.[2-4] These definitions of stress are simplistic and do not reflect that we respond differently to external events both interpersonally and intrapersonally at different times. Stress does not reside exclusively in the event or in our response; rather stress reflects a transaction between the two.

The transactional model of stress focuses on the nature of the transactions between the person and the environment.[5-7] Stress arises when an individual perceives the demands of a situation (imposed from within the person or by the environment) as threatening or challenging, and exceeding available resources (internal or external).[6] Stress is this perceived imbalance. These appraisals determine the intensity and quality of the stress response, and the outcomes of attempts to adapt to perceived stressors.[7]

Therefore, stress lies in the perceived discrepancy between demands and resources.[5,6] Individuals cope by directly decreasing the demands and increasing resources or changing their appraisals of self and the environment. Within the framework of the transactional model of stress, the stress experienced in worklife involves an interaction between intrapersonal, interpersonal, and environmental factors. These factors provide the demands and resources that are appraised as satisfying or discrepant.

Sources of Stress

Intrapersonal Factors

Individuals bring into relationships and situations personal characteristics that influence their perceptions as well as their reactions.[5,8,9] Examination of personal characteristics facilitates an understanding of an individual's transaction with other people and events. Self-concept, needs, and motivations serve as both demands and supplies and play a role in the mediation of a stress response.

Self-concept

How we see ourselves influences relationships and our appraisal of events. Self-concept is developed through self-appraisal and the appraisal by others.[10] People engage in self-talk that affects self-concept and self-esteem.[11] Irrational thoughts encompass the themes of *must–ought–should* ("I must be perfect", "I ought to be liked by everyone," "People should recognize my hard work");

it's awful ("If they would just ask me then this wouldn't happen"); and *damn me and damn you* blaming ("It's my fault," "They're just a bunch of bean counters," "I work harder than anyone").[11] Repetitive negative self-talk unwittingly convinces the individual to believe that these statements are true. In the supply-and-demand model, demands can be perceived as overwhelming if a negative self-concept exists or if we become too dependent on the explicit or implicit messages of others. Pearlin and Schooler stated that "freedom from negative attitudes toward self, the possession of a sense that one is in control of the forces impinging on oneself, and the presence of favorable attitudes towards oneself were helpful in coping."[12, p 12]

Personal needs

Need for approval and affection. Marvin stated that what workers most wanted was appreciation for their work.[13] A desire for appreciation, approval, and affection are basic human needs. However, the intensity of the need and expectation have implications. In the past, individuals trusted employers to value work efforts, long-term service, and loyalty. But the work environments have changed. According to a recent survey, only 40% of the American workforce felt appreciated by their employers.[14] Only about 52% believed that solid performance would shield them from job loss, reflecting a decline from 73% in the late 1980s.[14] Moreover, nurses with an intense need for approval and affection may work exceedingly hard to satisfy patients/families, coworkers, and employers. This need can lead to a reluctance to say "no", sabotage of self-care, feelings of betrayal or abandonment, and anger if efforts are not appreciated or approved.

Need for autonomy and control. People vary in their expectations about the extent to which they have control over their lives. The perception of control is created through interaction with the environment, where actions and outcomes are either related (producing a sense of control) or unrelated (producing a sense of powerlessness).[15] An *internal* locus of control stems from a perception that actions and outcomes are connected.[16] Individuals with an *external* locus of control expect to have little control over events.

Perhaps more critical is the ability to differentiate where control is possible.[17] An excessive need to control, to refuse to share or delegate power, or to take on responsibility for everything and everyone can result in *mea culpa*,[18]—"It's me," "I'm responsible," "It's my fault,"—while overlooking situational factors that influence the outcomes. This is contrasted to the externally referenced individual controlled by the demands of other people and the environment. Knowing where control is possible is particularly important in our current health care environment where work is increasingly interdependent. Uneasiness with shared responsibility and accountability can result in continuing to "do it all" while feeling overworked and powerless.

Pines and Aronson[19] found that stress increased as autonomy and a sense of control decreased. Organizational characteristics such as "circumscribed authority, downward channels of communication, specialization, and hierarchy contribute to a sense of lack of autonomy and control.[19] A lack of autonomy engenders feelings of frustration, victimization, and helplessness. Nurses are particularly prone to this experience, for they are charged with tremendous responsibility but are often given no real power or authority.[7] This can result in a feeling of accountability overload while not having the requisite power or authority to balance the demand.

As a consequence, feelings of powerlessness can develop if individuals discover that what happens is independent of their input, expressed concern, or verbal complaint.[20] Nurses are experiencing what some call a crisis in professional identity as the locus of decision making has moved from the professional to the payer, leaving nurses feeling less autonomous and less in control.[21] This can result in estrangement from the work environment.

Motivations

Behavior is motivated by the expectation of need fulfillment. What motivated you to choose a career in cancer nursing? For many, it is the opportunity to make a difference, to be helpful, to provide a valued human service. Motivations influence how individuals appraise situations; as a result, motivations influence stress reactions.[5] If individuals feel thwarted in providing care they know to be helpful, feelings of stress may occur. Changes in the frequency of patient contact (i.e., shortened hospital stays, limited clinic visits, early transition to home care) may limit the ability of nurses to see the impact of their care.[22] Likewise, if one's motivation to be helpful is devalued or difficult to enact in the work environments, feelings of anger and hostility (external expressions of unmet needs) can result, as can depression, a sense of failure, and low self-esteem (internal expressions of unmet needs).

Interpersonal Factors

To comprehend the interpersonal factors inherent in cancer nursing, one must understand the dynamics of helping relationships and the nature of cancer care.

Helping relationships

Leininger noted that caring is one of the most crucial ingredients for health, human development, well-being, and survival.[23] Caring includes "assistive, supportive, or facilitative acts toward or for another individual . . . [meant] to ameliorate or improve a human condition."[23, p 145] Caring and feeling cared for are basic human needs that promote personal and societal health. In spite of its value, the healing that occurs in helping relationships (nurse–patient) is not readily amenable to standard outcome measures. As a consequence, this work has not been systematically incorporated into reimbursement and health care redesign. Technical and coordination roles have been given higher value.

Knowing that one has been helpful often is the essence of the critical incidents described by cancer nurses.[24] Yet, according to Maslach, the very structure of the helping relationship can create a shift from a positive to a negative view of the people we desire to help.[18] Three aspects of the helping relationship influence this positive-to-negative shift: focus on the problem, lack of positive feedback, and level of distress.[18]

Focus on problems. By definition, the recipient of care in a helping relationship has a problem that is the focus of the relationship.[18] When time, money, and human resources (supplies) are scarce, helpers must focus on the most urgent or acute problems. Often, supporting human assets becomes a secondary consideration to the problems presented. The language in most health care settings promotes this problem-focused orientation: problem lists outline deficits (i.e., self-care deficit, knowledge deficit); quality assurance measures track deficiencies; "salvage" therapy, cancer "victims." In most helping relationships, when the problem is resolved, the relationship is over. It is easy to see how helpers can shift to a negative view of people as well as the stress this shift can create for the helper.

Lack of positive feedback. Most helpers want feedback about the quality of their efforts. If feedback is absent or criticism is the norm, a negative view of helping can result.[18] What kind of feedback is implied in the death of a patient? Do you hear from coworkers and supervisors only when things go wrong? How do you feel when a patient complains about delay when you are now doing the work of two people? Moreover, patients/families, employers, and coworkers may take for granted your standards of excellence. Some may view appreciation and recognition as unwarranted, believing that nurses are "simply doing their jobs." Lack of positive feedback is a source of stress, and relationships that offer no positive feedback over time are viewed negatively.

Level of distress. It is commonly believed in our society that cancer inevitably means pain, suffering, and death. As a consequence, the diagnosis of cancer often is regarded with more fear and viewed as more threatening than other diagnoses.[25] Nurses attempt to decrease the distress of patients/families by encouraging the disclosure of feelings.[26] Yet what is the consequence of being on the receiving end of emotional disclosure or catharsis? Nurses may claim immunity in order to deal with the threatening realities of being confronted with extreme distress, the threat inherent in being confronted repeatedly with one's own mortality, and the threat of pain and disfigurement.[27] Or they may distance themselves emotionally and/or physically. Neither strategy, however, eliminates the distress.[26,28]

Cancer care

Health care professionals cannot ignore the demands associated with the care of patients with cancer. Additionally, it may not be the nursing work itself that is stressful but rather conflicts with coworkers and organizational characteristics that interfere with doing the work.[29]

Cancer trajectory. Each cancer diagnosis results in a unique wellness–illness trajectory and creates uncertainty.[30,31] The emotional demands of uncertainty are magnified when nurses care for patients at different stages of their illness.[32] To deal with uncertainty, care providers often develop expectations regarding a patient's trajectory.[33] Although intended to diminish uncertainty, this can serve as a stressor if the predictions are inaccurate.

Involvement. Cancer nurses often are involved with patients and families for extended periods. This prolonged and intense contact is both demanding and rewarding.[34] Fagin and Diers[35] describe nursing as a metaphor for intimacy. "Nurses are involved in the most private aspects of people's lives. . . . Nurses, as trusted peers, are there to hear secrets, especially the ones born of vulnerability."[35,p11] Patients and families may view nurses as "safe" for the expression of fears and feelings of sadness, isolation, helplessness, anger, or profound grief. Being faced with human suffering and distress of the spirit places the listener in a vulnerable position. The demands increase exponentially as the nurse cares for multiple patients and families experiencing different emotions.[36] This sense of emotional liability is stressful.[31,33,34,37]

One way to lessen the intensity of the relationship is to withdraw physical and emotional support. Paradoxically, these attempts to withdraw tend to increase rather than reduce stress. A stress–avoidance–guilt sequence develops, for distancing often leads to feelings of betrayal of the patient or family, doubt about one's helping ability and motivation, and guilt.[26]

Treatment sequelae. An assortment of stressors emerge in relation to treatment. Nurses often administer treatments that induce iatrogenic illness and distress.[38] Feeling as though one, as a nurse, contributed to a patient's suffering is distressing, because it is not in keeping with an idealized image of the nurse as a professional provider of comfort and help.[39] Radical surgery often causes dramatic changes in a patient's appearance and function. The stress to the care provider associated with disfiguring surgeries stems from the disfigurement itself and, as with other therapies, questioning whether the therapies will actually have a positive impact on the quantity and/or quality of the individual's life.[33] If ambivalence or cynicism develops, stress can escalate.

Exposure to loss and death. In 1999, it is estimated that about 563,100 Americans will die from cancer, more than 1500 people a day.[40] The cancer nurse will encounter the physical deaths of patients and, in a broader context, the loss of social roles, control, relationships, life's work,

and hopes for the future. Repeated exposure to loss and death causes nurses to face their own fears about death and contemplate our own mortality. Zilboorg[41] suggests that continual consciousness of loss and the fear of death impairs functioning: as a self-defense, the fear is repressed; but efforts to repress feelings demand physical and emotional energy. These losses interact with the other stresses in their personal and professional lives.[42] And unless they acknowledge the feelings associated with repetitive exposure to loss and death, stress accumulates.[26]

Environmental Factors

There are numerous factors that contribute to demands of health care providers. Difficulties with role responsibilities, health care organizational changes, environmental climate, and professional relationships can increase stress.

Role stressors

Role conflict. Role conflict is the experience of being pulled in several directions by one person or several people with differing expectations. The conflict can be triggered by inconsistent (e.g., supervisor encourages problem solving then creates barriers to implementation) or incompatible (e.g., teach continuing education course while simultaneously staffing unit) expectations or demands that are in conflict with one's core values. Kahn reported that persons with high role conflict had greater job-related tensions, lower job satisfaction, less confidence in the organization itself, and more intense experience of conflict.[43]

Role ambiguity. The stress due to role ambiguity stems from unclear role responsibilities.[33] In general, the greater the perceived role ambiguity, the greater the perceived stress. In the past, articulating rigid boundaries separating the domains of nursing from that of other professionals was emphasized (e.g., nursing outcomes, nursing diagnoses);[44] however, well-delineated role responsibilities have given way to fluid job descriptions in the current environment (Table 84-1). Emphasis is now placed on partnerships, collaborative teams, interdependence, flexible boundaries, and shared responsibility for patient outcomes. Although there is an emphasis on shared responsibility, nurses are often challenged to demonstrate the impact of professional nursing care on patient outcome or face layoff or replacement by unlicensed assistive personnel. A lack of clarity regarding role responsibility is often manifest in either overwork or withdrawal from work.

Role overload. Role overload is the extent to which a person is incapable of meeting multiple expectations.[33] *Qualitative* overload implies that requisite job skills and knowledge exceed those of the individual.[19,45] *Quantitative* overload implies that there is more work than can be done in a given period of time.[19,45] As the quantitative and

Table 84-1 Contemporary Profession Building in Nursing

Traditional Profession Building in Nursing	Contemporary Profession Building in Nursing
Concentrated on identifying unique nursing activities; independent and dependent nursing functions.	Interdependence, collaboration, teamwork
Profession self-regulation	Accountability to stakeholder—purchasers of nursing care; shared regulation rather than self-regulation
Rigid professional boundaries	Flexible boundaries responsive to change in health care needs of society
Focus on caring; contrasted to curing	Focus on knowledge and skills; focus on quality and outcomes
Nursing as an oppressed group	Nursing in a position of leadership
Nursing as a female profession; femaleness viewed as a distinguishing characteristic; contrasted to the male 'oppressors'	Recruitment of men into the profession; diversity of profession key to innovation and creative problem solving
Focus on job security based on longevity of employment within an organization	Job security based on contribution to organization; less emphasis on tasks; greater emphasis on outcome
Development of nursing science and nursing theory	Development of multidisciplinary health care theories
Focus on acute care setting	Focus on diverse settings

Data from White and Begun.[44]

qualitative loads increase, stress increases.[46,47] Feelings of inadequacy and incompetence attributable to quantitative and qualitative role overload can develop.

The experience of overload can be aggravated by rapidly changing medical technologies, defining competence as perfection, accountability without authority, and imposition of tasks that have lower priority for the nurse.[48] In many health care organizations, profit has usurped quality of and access to services.[49] To increase profit, organizations attempt to provide care with fewer professional staff. Rather than compromising quality of care, nurses tend to work longer and harder. There are emotional and professional consequences of doing more with less. Role overload results in physical and emotional exhaustion, negative feelings about patients, coworkers, and the organization, and a diminished sense of accomplishment.[18]

Intragroup and intergroup conflict

Professional practice standards stipulate nurses' participation in health care teams.[50,51] This involves intergroup and intragroup relationships. Conflict seems inevitable in the interaction of any two autonomous persons whose interests or relationships are interdependent.[52] Factors that influence intragroup and intergroup conflicts include scarcity of or competition for resources (time, money, people, skills), divergent goals, differing values, need for control, need for self-protection, lack of information, and group interdependence for work sequencing.[53] The greater the interrelatedness and dependence on one another, the greater the potential for conflict.[52] Conflict that normally occurs in organizations is more evident during periods of reorganization.[54] The size of the organization, levels of authorities, and specialized roles influence the amount of conflict; as each increases, so does

the conflict. Conflict-prone organizations are characterized by rigid ideologies, nonparticipatory organizational processes, absence of shared goals, competitive coalitions, and prospects of unemployment from economic changes.[55]

In hierarchical structures, the suppression of conflict is often the norm.[56] However, as hierarchical structures are broken down and team management environments are developed, the suppression of conflict must be addressed or it will inhibit functioning of the team. Group cohesiveness, compatibility, and group attitude about conflict influences whether and the means by which conflicts are addressed.[21,43] Responses to conflict include avoidance/withdrawal, power/competition, accommodation/capitulation, compromising/bargaining, and collaborative/confrontation.[57] Avoidance is often the response nurses use to address (not address) conflict, which diminishes their effectiveness in a team.[58–61]

Physician–nurse conflict is rooted in historical precedent, power and status inequity, mutual lack of knowledge of and respect for unique contributions of each role, personality conflicts, and vertical communication. The perception that one group has power over another leads to behaviors reflecting low self-esteem (manifested as trying to do more and more in order to prove worth), horizontal violence (directing anger, negativity, sarcasm toward peers rather than at "oppressor"), and passive-aggressive behavior.[22] Many of the factors in physician–nurse conflicts are also present in nurse–nurse conflicts (e.g., nurse managers–staff, dayshift–evening shift, CNS–NP). Lack of respect and not honoring their coworkers result in intergroup and intragroup conflicts.

Intragroup conflicts disrupt team stability, isolate individuals, and lessen the likelihood that nurses will share ideas and feelings related to work experiences. The health care culture has changed. Nurses are in competition with one another for a limited supply of jobs. Group membership fluctuates daily through downsizing, cross-training, attrition, rotating shifts, floating to understaffed unit, and use of outsourced nurses. Lack of a stable work group and intragroup conflicts can rob nurses of the technical, intellectual, and emotional support of their peers.[26,32,62]

Health care reform

"Health care reform" is a euphemism for changes in health care systems designed to increase profitability and control costs. An entirely new language has developed: profit centers, product line manager, market share, covered lives, brand preference, profitable manipulation of provider-consumer interaction. This redesign has precipitated phenomenal change in the health care environment. Nurses have been displaced given the preoccupation with cutting costs. Nurses' perceptions of the effects of downsizing, restructuring, and use of unlicensed assistive personnel (UAP) on quality of patient care and worklife was captured in a survey[63] (Table 84-2). One can speculate about the quality of the worklife

of the over 7000 nurses who participated in the study. Only 43% reported that quality of care met their professional standards. The absence of a stable work group and diminished time to interact with health care team members would clearly diminish the opportunity for ongoing support as well as the quality of worklife. Irvine and Evans[64] found that nurses' quality of worklife is more strongly correlated with turnover than economic or individual factors.

For many, health care redesign has precipitated demoralization, a heightened sense of vulnerability, and mistrust. In a recent survey of 681 hospitals, 81% cited poor morale as the most serious human resource problem, up from 60% in 1993.[65] These feelings stem in part from the experience of seeing experienced, long-term committed staff lose jobs. Staff reduction without workload realignment resulting in overwork also contributes to demoralization. Discussion about how nurses work differently without jeopardizing patient care and the feelings engendered by staff reduction may not have occurred, in part, due to the velocity of change. They may ask "Am I next?" and "Why commit to this organiza-

Table 84-2 Survey of Nurses Regarding Quality of Patient Care

Have any of the following changes occurred in your nursing department?			Yes	No
• Decrease in number of RNs providing direct patient care			60.2%	39.8%
• Increase in number of patients assigned to RN			65.5%	34.5%
• Substitution of part-time, per-diem, or temporary RN for full-time RN			48.6%	51.4%
• Hiring of UAPs to provide care previously provided by RNs			41.9%	58.1%
In your opinion has the introduction of UAPs improved patient care?			13.3%	86.7%
Does the quality of care you provide meet your professional standards?			43.2%	56.8%
If your family member needed health care, would you recommend your organization?			64.2%	35.8%
Have you seen a change in the following?		Less	Same	More
• Patient acuity		3.8%	19.8%	76.7%
• Unexpected readmissions of recently discharged		5.3%	39.6%	55.1%
• Length of stay		65.9%	22.6%	11.5%
• Continuity of care		55.2%	33.9%	10.9%
• Medication errors		8.8%	54.2%	37.0%
• Pressure ulcers/skin breakdown		15.2%	59.4%	25.4%
• Work-related injuries		8.1%	48%	43.9%
Have you experienced a change in the amount of time to:		Less	Same	More
• Teach patients and families		72.8%	15.7%	11.5%
• Provide basic nursing care		68.5%	24.3%	7.2%
• Consult with other members of the team		57.1%	31.5%	11.4%
How would you rate the quality of patient care in your organization?	Very Poor 1.7%	Poor 12.2%	Average 38.8%	Good 37.4%	Excellent 9.9%
How likely is it that you will stay in nursing?			Unlikely 12.6%	Neither 11.6%	Likely 75.8%

Adapted with permission from Shindul-Rothschild J, Berry D, Long-Middleton E: Where have all the nurses gone? Final results of our patient care survey. *Am J Nurs* 96:25–39, 1996.[63]

tion?". This disruption of employee–employer loyalty and vulnerability affects turnover, productivity, and stability of the organization.[66]

Characteristics of health care organizations

The size, structure, goals, and culture of an organization may contribute to stress. One can only speculate about the impact of hospital mergers that result in huge conglomerates with faceless executives and offsite headquarters. In addition to size, hospitals have inherent characteristics that foster stress, including multiple levels of authority, heterogeneity of personnel, work interdependence, and specialization.[67] Excessive regulation of organizational structure, procedures, and policies, and detailed job descriptions can create stress due to perceived inflexibility and lack of individual control.

Threats to professional integrity

The ideals of quality and efficiency are desirable goals; however, many organizations fall short of describing how these goals ought to be achieved or measured.[68] For instance, how do nurses reconcile the mixed messages of quality patient care with the elimination of direct care providers? And do organizations measure achievement based on the principles of economics or ethics, and if ethics, according to the ethics of business or medical ethics? Clearly, the business ethic of free and fair competition is different from the ethics of human service. In a survey conducted by the American Nurses Association (ANA), 58% of the nurse respondents identified "cost containment issues that jeopardize patient welfare as a priority ethical issue."[69] The ANA *Code for Nurses* describes normative behavior or the standards by which professional ethical conduct is measured.[70] Inherent are the principles of autonomy, beneficence, nonmaleficence, veracity, confidentiality, fidelity, and justice.[69,71,72] Much of the emerging health care system challenges the nurse's ability to uphold the central moral tenets articulated in the code.[71] A position statement by the ANA has made clear that the nursing code is not open to negotiation and "that each nurse has an obligation to uphold and adhere to the code of ethics."[73] Mohr and Mahon[74] suggest that the moral quandary of working within externally imposed parameters that directly affect the provision of quality care or one's values induces a sense of angst.[74] Fear, powerlessness, and avoidance as a self-protective strategy are potential sequelae.

Stress Management Strategies

Coping with stress involves reducing demands, increasing supplies, or altering one's interpretation of demands and supplies.[75] There is a link between perceptions of control and the use of either problem- or emotion-focused coping.[76] The perception of personal control over stressful situations is associated with problem-focused coping—actions designed to alter or change a stressful person–environment relationship. Applying problem-focused coping to situations that are not amenable to change engenders feelings of frustration, anger, and finally, helplessness.[77] In situations where one does not have control or the situation is unchangeable, emotion-focused coping yields greater potential for success. Emotion-focused coping involves efforts to adjust or adapt to stressful situations including changing emotions, beliefs, goals, and commitments in order to decrease distress associated with the stressor.[77] Therefore problem-focused coping is more effective in person–environment relationships that are perceived as changeable. When a situation is perceived as unchangeable, emotion-focused coping is more effective.

Assessment

Stress management is based on the premise that individuals are valuable and merit careful attention. Personal or self-assessment will help individuals learn more about themselves, the way they interact with other people and their environments, and their coping abilities.

As part of self-assessment, the answers to the following questions can serve as a guide in creating problem-focused or emotion-focused strategies. Consider what feelings, interactions, and situational factors create the most distress or promise.

- What kind of messages do I give myself? Self-effacing? Kind and gentle? Respectful?

- Where do I seek fulfillment of approval and affection needs?

- Do I take responsibility for people and circumstances that I really have no control over?

- Am I able to distinguish where I have control and when situations are unchangeable?

- Why did I choose cancer nursing? Am I doing what motivated me to choose cancer nursing?

- Has there been a shift in how I view patients and families? Do their requests feel burdensome? Overwhelming? If a shift has occurred, what precipitated the shift?

- How do I handle the losses I am exposed to?

- Are there opportunities to share feelings about the losses with colleagues?

- Who do I want feedback from? What feedback did I receive today? What was the feedback I gave co-workers?

- How do I know when I am helpful?

- In my current position, am I clear about what is expected? Are the expectations inconsistent, incompatible, manageable?

- Do I expect too much of myself?

- Do I have the skills necessary for my job?

- Who comprises my workgroup? Is there conflict? Is there a sense of teamwork? Respect? Mutual support?

- How do I typically handle conflict? How do I feel when conflicted?

- Is there anything I want to change about my worklife?

- What in my worklife brings me joy and fulfillment?

- Do I trust my employer? Coworkers?

- Do I feel vulnerable? What am I afraid of losing?

- What are my core values? Does the organizational culture support these values? What do I consider non-negotiable?

Another assessment tool is a stress assessment journal (Figure 84-1). It requires a commitment to log an entry every two hours for two weeks. After several weeks, patterns or themes may emerge regarding specific precipitants and responses. This exercise provides insight into the degree of stress, sources of stress, needs, patterns of behavior, and self-talk; ultimately, it will help facilitate choices regarding coping strategies.

Achieving Goals

It is imperative to examine self-expectation and goals. Unrealistic self-expectations and goals will result in defeat and increased levels of stress. Covey suggests that for any intended action we "begin with the end in mind."[78] Imagine that you are old. Your grandchildren, niece, dear friends, and coworkers are reminiscing about you. What would you want them to say about you, your life, your relationships, your work? Write down your thoughts. Now consider your contemplation during the assessment phase. It is likely that the events, interactions, and situations you perceived as stressful were impeding your goals. Setting goals involves values clarification. Achieving goals involves giving those things of greatest value highest priority.

Goal-setting exercise[79]

1. Write down your goals. Create four lists: five years, next year, the next six months, and the coming month. Allow two minutes to fill in your goals for each time period.
2. Now prioritize your goals on each list: A (must do); B (desirable), and C (can wait).
3. Narrow lists by selecting two "A"s from each of the four lists. This list should contain your most important goals.

Date			Stressful Event									
Time	Degree of pleasure 0–10	Degree of stress 0–10	What happened?	Where?	Who?	Private: How did I feel? What I did I say to self?	Public: What did I say? How did I behave?	What was at stake?*	Degree of satisfaction with outcome 0–10	Is the situation changeable?	Ideas

* Potential categories of "What was at stake".
 1. Affiliation (concern with interpersonal relationships, love, intimacy, acceptance, to be included)
 2. Achievement-power (threat to job, financial security, career, desire for recognition, influence)
 3. Personal growth (concern with personal development, self-understanding, personal philosophy)
 4. Altruism-humanitarianism (concern with need to be helpful, to be involved with organization)
 5. Stress avoidance (concern with avoiding hassles, uncertainty; desiring stability, predictability)
 6. Pleasure seeking (concern with pleasure, fun, excitement)
 7. Autonomy (concern with independence, self-determination, personal control)
 8. Personal health
 9. Life and mortality (threats of loss)
10. Uncertainty

Figure 84-1   Stress assessment journal

4. Establish a reasonable timetable. Allocate your time based on your priorities.
5. Create a to-do list, breaking large goals into smaller goals.
6. Work on the A list everyday.
7. Every month, review your list.
8. Remember, if goals are not in writing, it is simply wishful thinking.

Listening to the Conversations We Have with Ourselves

With few exceptions, our emotions have more to do with what we tell ourselves about the events in our lives than the events themselves.[80] Our self-talk is so natural we can become unaware of its influence. Self-talk based on rational thoughts promotes self-respect. Self-talk based on irrational thoughts tends to sabotage self-esteem, results in negative emotions, and inhibits the realization of goals.[81]

The technique of *cognitive restructuring* involves learning to listen to self-talk and changing unwanted or irrational thoughts in order to change emotional response.[11,80] Cognitive restructuring involves assessing situations or individuals as objectively as possible in order to gain a clearer perspective. Consider your discoveries from the stress assessment exercises. Did irrational thinking influence your perceived stress? We need to be prepared to intervene with positive affirmations, rational thoughts such as "I gave great effort," "Some days I'm on, some days I'm not," "I will be kind to myself," "It's okay to be afraid," "I can do it," and "It's okay if not everyone agrees with me." Although it is unrealistic to expect to make a response based on rational thought to every stressful situation, we gain mastery and control from knowing that we have choices in how situations are perceived and how we choose to respond. Pick three rational affirmations. Use these statements to counter what you may tend to say to yourself. Remember that irrational self-talk comes naturally. Rational self-talk needs practice.

Conflict Resolution

All conflicts serve a purpose. Too often conflict is viewed as merely negative, something to be avoided or suppressed. The positive functions of conflict include its use to clarify objectives, balance power, foster cohesiveness, serve as the medium for problem identification and solution, promote change, and help groups and individuals define boundaries.[82] Steps in addressing conflict include implementing strategies according to the nature of the conflict and using assertive behavior.

The type of conflict influences the strategy used for its resolution. Failure to accurately identify the type of conflict decreases the likelihood of resolution. Types of conflicts include circumstances that could be readily changed but participants fail to perceive options, so conflict persists; conflict over the wrong issue; conflict that is never resolved because the wrong people are negotiating the wrong issues; conflicts that should be occurring but are not because dispute is repressed; conflict due to misperception or misunderstanding; and ideological conflict where norms and beliefs that govern behavior are different.[82]

Assertive behavior is an appropriate strategy regardless of the type of conflict.[83] Assertive strategies include saying what you honestly want, think, and feel in a direct manner without denying the rights of others; using "I" statements not "you" statements ("I'm upset that you changed your clinic days without speaking to me" rather than "You are oblivious to what goes on in the clinic. Making the decision in isolation is insensitive"); describing specific behavior rather than interpreting behavior ("changed your clinic days without speaking to me" rather than "oblivious," "insensitive"); being specific about consequences of behavior as well as expectations ("As a consequence, the support groups we planned will have to be renegotiated with the facilitator"). Often, just stating your feelings and the consequence of the other person's behaviors are sufficient. However, spelling out your expectation may be warranted ("In the future, I will count on you to discuss changes with me first").

It is important to pay attention to nonverbal behavior. Listen intently. Communicate caring and strength. Use a firm, warm, and expressive voice. Look at the person. Maintain head erect, hands relaxed, and lean toward the person. Additional suggestions include honoring the legitimacy of other's interest, working towards a mutually agreeable solution, remaining focused on the issue, being descriptive rather than judgmental, and being specific rather than global.

Setting Limits

Akin to assertive behavior is the ability to set limits on what we agree to do. Setting limits involves knowing ourselves (e.g., goals, priorities, behaviors signaling overload), knowing our rights, and being willing to assert them.[81] Ask yourself "Does this request fit with my goals, priorities, and responsibilities?". Remember that poorly considered commitments may force you to spend time on low priority activities. If the request does not fit, ask yourself "How much of a trade-off am I willing to make? And how often?" "Are any of my rights jeopardized—the right to respect, a reasonable workload, self-determination, asking for what I need, saying no without guilt or making excuses, acting in the best interest of a patient/family/workgroup, making a mistake and owning it?"[84]

Mount stated that "reasonable limits of personal giving must be established if sustained, effective functioning is to be ensured."[42, p 1132] Limit setting helps to create a sense of mastery over our work. This involves knowing and respecting our limits and deciding what we can and cannot do and what we will and will not do.

Mindfulness of the Difference We Make

Breathnach, author of *Simple Abundance,* advocates that the life transforming principles of simplicity, order, harmony, beauty, and joy flourish with a spirit of gratitude.[85] The reader is challenged to maintain a gratitude journal, writing down five things that the reader is grateful for that day. Using this as a model, everyday make note of five interactions or activities in which you knew you made a difference. At times, limiting your list to five interactions or activities may be challenging. Other days, the helpfulness of not screaming at the lab tech may make the list. Regardless, this intentional inventory can be a revelation. It can invigorate. Consider creating your list during the work-to-home transition. Too often this may be the time we use to ruminate about what did not go well in our workday. A final suggestion: A written list has the potential to reinforce the sense of gratefulness and joy with each rereading in a way a mental list cannot.

Work-Based Social Support

Social support is vital to our well-being in today's complex health care system.[86] Group interactions such as staff meetings, patient care conferences, and formal support groups are catalysts for social support, problem solving, and task sharing. We should not let the importance of these activities be lost amidst the rush of the day. Work-based social support is often more potent than individual efforts at reducing occupational stress.[86] Social support encompasses "enduring interpersonal ties" to a group of people who share similar standards and values, and who can be relied on to provide emotional sustenance, assistance, and feedback.[87] Receiving support may feel unnatural, for many of us are more adept at giving rather than receiving support. Moreover, a fear of betrayal or of being unaccepted or viewed as incompetent, inadequate, or misunderstood may thwart some from seeking support.[19,26] However, by expressing feelings and experiences, we learn that others share similar experiences.

Establishing an environment of trust and mutual respect is a first step in getting and giving support. As individuals, we can foster supportive work environments by refusing to participate in malicious gossip or sarcasm. A simple strategy is to ask ourselves before speaking "Is it true? Is it necessary? Is it helpful?" When was the last time you said to a colleague "I know that was difficult; you handled it really well" or "I spoke with Mr. Henderson's wife. She really appreciated what you did to coordinate all his appointments. It really made it easier for them."? We need people who know when we have made a difference and who are willing to tell us. These expressions can transform our immediate work environments from negativism, fault finding, and criticism to environments where we acknowledge how difficult our work can be, how hard we are all working and that each of us makes significant contributions. As Carpenito said, "When you go out in the nursing world, hold hands before crossing the street, and stick together."[88, p 4]

Balancing Engagement with Detachment

It is important for nurses to find a way to be involved emotionally without burning out. Emotional involvement is simultaneously a great asset and a point of vulnerability. Detached concern involves finding a balance of compassion and objectivity.[7,18,28,89] It is having a genuine concern for a patient's well-being while maintaining emotional and psychological distance.

How do we create this balance? Intellectualization or processing emotionally stressful situations in the abstract is one strategy.[7] It serves as a defense mechanism by creating psychological or emotional distance from distressing situations. Given the emotional intensity of the practice of nursing, intellectualization can serve as a buffer. However, overreliance on intellectualization can eventually create stress because the suppression of our emotional experiences requires energy.

At times detached concern means letting go of the outcome, realizing "I cannot fix every situation." It involves making choices based on an understanding of "this is what I can handle" or on focusing on "what I can do right now that has the best chance for success but requires the least amount of strain."[36]

Finally, seeking feedback from and learning about the experiences of our peers helps us to recognize that our struggle to create balance is not unique.

Taking Control of One's Career

American attitudes about jobs, security, and career have changed significantly, especially in health care[90] (Table 84-3). American workers are moving away from the traditional focus on employment to employability.[91] Competitive skills are developed through the dedication to continuous learning to keep pace with change. Career resilience involves knowing our skills and having a plan to enhance performance and employability. We must understand the attributes that influence our effectiveness, success, and happiness. It is only when we understand this—as well as the characteristics of environments that support our effectiveness, fulfillment, and interests—that we are able to choose where we can make the greatest

Table 84-3 Changes in Americans' Attitudes Toward Employment

Then	Now
Job security	Intense competition
Specialization	Cross-train
Stick with one job	Broaden skills and experience
Title matters	What title?
Career ladder	Career paths
Qualifications	Skills

Data from Gray B.[90]

contribution. List the skills and knowledge you currently possess. How could you use them differently? What additional skills and knowledge do you need? How will you obtain these additional skills and knowledge? How can your skills and knowledge most effectively be used to save the organization money and improve patient outcomes?

It is critical to stay informed about organizational change, to seek increased involvement with planning and implementing organizational strategies, and to demonstrate the value of your contributions to the organization.

Nurses can gain control of their careers by knowing employment opportunities as well as maintaining a current resume. The Internet provides information regarding employment opportunities, career counseling, resume and cover letter templates, and an employer database. The Oncology Nursing Society (ONS) has developed an *ONS Career Resource Kit* that includes job search tips, career development resources, and opportunities in alternative settings.

Strategies to foster a sense of control over our work include reorganization of work and development of specialized roles.[9] Organizing work assignments so the work is varied can counterbalance emotionally draining work with task-oriented work. Strategies to restructure work assignments might include job sharing (e.g., research nurse and staff nurse job sharing), changing the context of the contact with patients (e.g., cross-training staff to work in inpatient and outpatient settings), sharing responsibility for difficult patient care assignments (e.g., two to three staff nurses serve as patient's primary care nurses and rotate direct care responsibilities), and creating a balanced mix of patients (e.g., chemotherapy nurse cares for the newly diagnosed patient, the patient in remission, and the patient receiving relapse therapy).

Involvement with Health Care System Changes

Nurses have long understood the link between quality nursing care and positive patient outcomes. However, they must demonstrate through research, not only by assertion, the impact that nursing skill mixes and nursing interventions have on patient outcomes and costs.[92] There is a growing body of research that ties higher RN staffing with positive patient outcomes such as lower mortality rates, fewer complications, reduced lengths of stay, and lower costs.[93–95] These findings indicate the importance of evaluating the effect of clinical reorganization on patient care.[93] Therefore, when changes are proposed nurses need to ask if they will affect the quality of care delivered and how the impact on quality outcomes will be measured.[96]

Cost containment has propelled termination of professional staff as well as the substitution of professional nurses with unlicensed assistive personnel. Bottom-line decision makers fail to understand how ill-timed these decisions are given the complexity of patient care and the impact this displacement has on patient outcome.

Health care professionals must equip themselves with objective data regarding outcome and costs. While a relationship between levels of nursing staff and avoidable adverse events may exist, presentation of data to support this relationship and highlighting the cost effectiveness of decreasing adverse events will be more effective.

An example of such compelling data comes from research conducted by Kovner and Gergen.[93] They found an inverse relationship between the number of RNs and the nurse-sensitive adverse events of thrombosis, urinary tract infections, and pneumonia after major surgery. Likewise, objective data regarding the impact of staff reduction on costs can advance our position. Data collected by the Minnesota Nurses Association showed that when RN positions in hospitals under study were downsized by 9.2%, the number of work-related injuries and illnesses among RNs increased by 65.2%.[97] Health care restructuring was cited as a leading cause of injury and illness for registered nurses.[97]

The motivation behind the proliferation of pathways, clinical guidelines, outcomes management, and evidence-based practice was initially viewed as suspect. We questioned the genuineness of the espoused goal of quality patient care. Rather, these tools were viewed as strategies to decrease costs, limit access, justify staff reductions, and narrow provider independence. We must drop our initial resistance. Nurses comprise 25% of the health care labor force and we must use our position to provide leadership in problem identification, clinical guideline development, implementation, data collection, and evaluation of outcomes. We must ask ourselves: What role can I serve? How do I become involved? Who do I need to tell about my intent for involvement? How can I support the activities of my colleagues?

Safeguarding Professional Integrity

Nurses are increasingly confronted with situations that challenge their personal and professional integrity. Acting in a manner contrary to ethical principles and moral tenets attacks integrity and creates distress.[98] Integrity involves discerning what is right and what is wrong, and acting on your understanding of what is right and wrong.[99] Creating strategies to safeguard one's integrity raises several fundamental questions: What core values and ethical principles define my practice? Am I able to practice in a way consistent with these values and principles? What does an environment that supports ethical practice look like? What are the responsibilities of health care organizations to support ethical practice?

"The moral basis of nursing exists in (a) the nurse–patient relationship and the patient's expectations that he/she will receive compassionate and competent care, as well as protection of basic human rights, and (b) expectations by society that the practice of professional nursing is guided by ethical ideals, virtues, principles, and standards."[100, p.5] The ANA *Code for Nurses*[70] describes the general ethical principles and norms for the nursing profession. The code, along with the Statement of Core Values by the ONS,[71] provide moral guidance for nurses to execute professional responsibilities. It is essential that nurses assimilate the core values and the ethical precepts guiding their practice. Only then are we able to discern whether our practice is consistent with these precepts and to evaluate whether our practice environments support ethical practice.

An ideal practice environment incorporates ethical standards, the scientific basis for care, a holistic approach, and a patient/family centered focus. Values and beliefs are openly acknowledged and communicated in order to assist the patient with decision making.[99] How does your practice environment compare to the ideal? Does your organization hold itself and employees accountable for ethical conduct?

It is unlikely that individuals will take responsibility for voicing concerns regarding ethical conflicts in their work environment if they lack a sense of job security. However, collectively we can advocate that our practice environments support ethical behavior. Establish a frame of reference by perhaps surveying coworkers regarding perspectives of the ethical climate, whether policy and procedures preserve integrity, and the degree of freedom to engage in deliberation regarding ethical and moral dilemmas. Does your organization have a formal process for the discussion of ethical dilemmas? Is a nurse a part of this process? Could he/she serve as a resource to your work group? How can the nurse facilitate interdisciplinary education regarding ethics, moral reasoning, values clarification, and shared decision making? Could your work group generate dialogue by developing forums such as ethics rounds? Creating structures in order to discern the issues can help to mitigate the "moral distress."

Relaxation

How do you know when you're feeling stress? What behavioral, physical, intellectual signs do you manifest? (See Table 84-4.) The use of relaxation techniques can relax your mind and calm your body. There are many forms of relaxation techniques: progressive deep-muscle relaxation, biofeedback, guided imagery, meditation, yoga, and autogenic training.[78] To gain maximum benefit, schedule 20–30 minutes a day. With practice, you will be able to instantly recall the feeling of relaxation during periods of stress. The key to the effectiveness of any technique is practice. Try the following exercise:[101]

1. Find a comfortable position. Close your eyes.
2. Begin taking slow, deep breaths.
3. As you silently say the word *relax*, focus on the muscles on the top of your head. Once you feel these muscles relax, move to the muscles over your forehead.
4. Continue to repeat the word *relax* as you slowly move down to your toes, relaxing each section of your body as you go.

Table 84-4 Physical, Behavioral, and Intellectual Manifestations of Stress

Physical

Feelings of exhaustion and fatigue
Weight change
Insomnia
Gastrointestinal disturbances
Cool, clammy skin
Sweating
Trembling; tics; twitches
Muscle tension
Rapid, uncontrolled speech
Loss of libido; impotence
Frequent headaches
Increased use of food, nicotine, alcohol, tranquilizers
Repetitive accidents
Frequent illness

Behavioral/Emotional

Lability of mood; mood swings
Suspiciousness; mistrust
Anger; antagonistic attitude toward others; hostility
Depression
Defensive behavior; blaming; scapegoating
Feelings of helplessness, inadequacy
Loss of sense of humor
Irritability
Distancing from others; reduced personal involvement
Nail biting; habitual teeth gritting
Critical of self and others
Panic; feeling pressured
Increasing expression of dissatisfaction

Intellectual

Increased rigidity in thinking
Increased use of intellectualization as defense
Lack of initiative
Forgetfulness
Preoccupation
Lack of attention to detail
Diminished concentration
Increased depersonalization
Dreams laden with conflict
Absenteeism
Frequent job change or feeling stuck in job
Frequent excuse making

Adapted from Muldary,[7] Haber et al,[10] Maslach,[18] Vachon,[33] Mount,[42] and Maslach.[48]

5. Once you have relaxed your muscles, start counting down slowly from ten to zero.
6. As you count, visualize yourself slowly descending a flight of stairs.
7. As you descend, say to yourself "I am becoming more relaxed."
8. Once you have arrived at zero, stay there for a while saying to yourself "I am calm and relaxed."
9. When you are ready to end the session, slowly begin counting from zero to ten. Repeat to yourself "I am calm and relaxed."
10. With practice, you will be able to shorten the countdown to arrive at a state of relaxation as well as call

upon the phrase "I am calmed and relaxed" in the midst of stressful situations.

Fields and associates measured the immediate effects of brief (ten minutes) massage, listening to music, visual imagery, muscle relaxation, and social support group sessions.[102] Regardless of the type of activity, nurses experienced increased vigor and decreased anxiety, depression, and fatigue.[102] Is there a quiet place in your work environment where you can commit ten minutes a day to relaxation?

Creating Opportunities for Withdrawal

Time away from stressful situations is important.[19] Taking a "time out" is important in doing any work that involves emotional, physical, or mental stress. Time-out activities include meal breaks, sharing the direct care responsibilities for a particularly tedious or arduous patient care situation, or a change in routine such as a special project or attending a continuing education program. Strict adherence to the rule that time away from work is time away from work must be followed. Does your organization have policies that guarantee protected time and regular vacations? How many vacation days do you accrue every year? Do you take your vacation allotment every year or do you allow it to accumulate? If you accumulate vacation time, what are you saving it for? Creating time and space for physical, emotional, spiritual, and intellectual rejuvenation is vital to our well-being.

Adopting a Wellness Philosophy

A wellness philosophy promotes healthy behavior. Healthy choices include eating a balanced diet; limiting alcohol and caffeine intake; ceasing smoking; practicing preventive health care (e.g., mammography, Pap smear, annual physical, dental care, eye exam); getting proper exercise, rest, recreation, and socialization; and developing intimate relationships. When was the last time you had a massage? Manicure? Enjoyed a good book? Worked in your garden? Leisurely walked your dog? The principal benefit of a wellness program is preparing the mind–body–spirit to withstand stress. Through education we train our minds for our profession; likewise we must train and care for our bodies and spirits.

Conclusion

Stress is a pervasive human condition. It is the perceived imbalance between the demands of a situation (imposed by the self or by the environment) and available resources (internal or external).[6] These appraisals determine stress reactions, the intensity and quality of our responses, and the outcomes of attempts to adapt to perceived stressors.[7]

We cope by directly decreasing the demands and increasing resources or changing our appraisal of self and the environment. This requires an accurate appraisal as well as the ability to differentiate where control is possible.[17] Given the consequences, it is imperative that we commit to caring for ourselves. To do otherwise is to jeopardize ourselves and our commitment to providing quality care to cancer patients and their families.

References

1. Selye H: *Physiology and Pathology of Exposure to Stress.* Montreal, ACTA Medical Publishers, 1950
2. Derogatis L: Self-report measures of stress, in Goldberger L, Breznitz S (eds): *Handbook of Stress: Theoretical and Clinical Aspects.* New York, Free Press, 1982, pp 270–294
3. Holmes T, Masuda M: Magnitude estimates of social readjustments. *J Psychosom Res* 11:219–255, 1966
4. Holmes T, Rahe R: The social readjustment rating scale. *J Psychosom Res* 12:213–218, 1976
5. Lazarus R: *Emotion and Adaptation.* New York: Oxford University Press, 1991
6. Lazarus R, Folkman S: *Stress, Appraisal, and Coping.* New York, Springer, 1984
7. Muldary T: *Burnout and Health Professionals: Manifestations and Management.* Norwalk, CT, Appleton-Century-Crofts, 1983
8. Appley M, Trumball R: On the concept of psychological stress, in Appley M, Trumball R (eds): *Psychological Stress: Issues in Research.* New York, Appleton-Century-Crofts, 1967, pp 1–13
9. McGrath JE: Stress and behavior in organization, in Dunnette M (ed): *Handbook of Industrial and Organizational Psychology.* Chicago, Rand McNally, 1976, pp 1351–1396
10. Haber J, Leach A, Schudy S, et al: *Comprehensive Psychiatric nursing* (ed. 5). St. Louis, Mosby, 1997
11. Ellis A, Dryden W: *The Practice of Rational Emotive Behavior Therapy* (ed. 2). New York: Springer, 1997
12. Pearlin L, Schooler C: The structure of coping. *J Health Soc Behav* 19:2–21, 1978
13. Marvin B: *From Turnover to Teamwork.* New York, Wiley, 1994
14. Reese S: Pushing productivity past the breaking point. *Business Health* 19:31–34, 1997
15. Walsh JJ, Wilding, JM, Eysenck MW, et al.: Neuroticism, locus of control, type A behavior and occupational stress. *Work & Stress* 11:148–159, 1997
16. Rotter J, Seeman M, Liverant S: Internal vs. external locus of control of reinforcements: a major variable in behavior therapy, in Washburne N (ed): *Decisions, Values and Groups.* London, Pergamon, 1962, pp 76–99
17. DuCette J, Wolk S: Cognitive and motivational correlates of generalized expectancies for control. *J Pers Soc Psychol* 22:420–426, 1973
18. Maslach C: *Burnout: The Cost of Caring.* Englewood Cliffs, NJ, Prentice-Hall, 1982
19. Pines A, Aronson E: *Career Burnout. Causes and Cures.* New York, Free Press, 1988, p 106
20. Seligman M: *Helplessness: On Depression, Development and Death.* San Francisco, William Freeman, 1975
21. Dunham-Taylor J, Marquette P, Pinczuk J: Surviving capitation. *Am J Nurs* 96:26–29, 1996

22. Cullen A: Burnout. Why do we blame the nurse? *Am J Nurs* 95:23–27, 1995

23. Leininger M: Caring: A central focus of nursing and health services, in Leininger M (ed): *Care: The Essence of Nursing and Health.* Thorofare, NJ, Slack, 1984, pp 45–58

24. McDonnell K, Ferrell B: Oncology Nursing Society Life Cycle Task Force report: the life cycle of the oncology nurse. *Oncol Nurs Forum* 19:1545–1550, 1992

25. Silverman R, Wortman C: Coping with undesirable life events, in Garber J, Seligman M (eds): *Human Helplessness: Theory and Applications.* New York, Academic Press, 1980, pp 279–341

26. Larson D: *Helper's Journey: Working with People Facing Grief, Loss, and Life-Threatening Illness.* Champaign, IL: Research Press, 1993

27. Benner P, Wrubel J: *The Primacy of Caring. Stress and Coping in Health and Illness.* Menlo Park, CA, Addison-Wesley, 1989

28. Larson D: The challenge of caring in oncology nursing. *Oncol Nurs Forum* 19:857–861, 1992

29. Thomas S, Droppleman P: Channeling nurses' anger into positive interventions. *Nursing Forum* 32:13–21, 1997

30. Vachon M, Stylianos S: Caring for the caregiver: a person-centered framework, in Baird S, McCorkle R, Grant M (eds): *Cancer Nursing. A Comprehensive Textbook.* Philadelphia, Saunders, 1991, pp 1084–1093

31. Larson P, Jennings B: The generation of stress in the provision of care, in Baird S, McCorkle R, Grant M (eds): *Cancer Nursing. A Comprehensive Textbook.* Philadelphia, Saunders, 1991, pp 1076–1083

32. McElroy A: Burnout—a review of the literature with application to cancer nursing. *Cancer Nurs* 5:211–217, 1982

33. Vachon ML: *Occupational Stress in the Care of the Critically Ill, the Dying, and the Bereaved.* Washington, DC, Hemisphere Publishing, 1987

34. Newlin N, Wellisch D: The oncology nurse: life on an emotional roller coaster. *Cancer Nurs* 1:447–449, 1978

35. Fagin C, Diers D: Nursing as metaphor. *N Engl J Med* 309:116–117, 1983

36. Weisman AD: Understanding the cancer patient: the syndrome of caregiver's plight. *Psychiatry* 44:161–168, 1981

37. Holsclaw P: Nursing in high emotional risk areas. *Nurs Forum* 4:36–45, 1965

38. Stewart B, Meyerowitz B, Jackson L, et al: Psychological stress associated with outpatient oncology nursing. *Cancer Nurs* 5:383–387, 1982

39. Steeves R, Kahn D, Benoliel J: Nurses' interpretation of the suffering of their patients. *West J Nurs Res* 12:715–731, 1990

40. Landis SH, Murray T, Bolden S, et al: Cancer statistics 1998. *CA Cancer J Clin* 49:8–31, 1999

41. Zilboorg G: Fear of death. *Psychoanal Q* 12:465–475, 1943

42. Mount B: Dealing with our losses. *J Clin Oncol* 4:1127–1134, 1986

43. Kahn R: Conflict, ambiguity and overload: three elements in job stress. *Occup Mental Health* 3:2–9, 1973

44. White K, Begun J: Profession building in the new health care system. *Nurs Admin Q* 20:79–85, 1996

45. French J, Kaplan R: Organizational stress and individual strain, in Marrow A (ed): *The Failure of Success.* New York, AMACOM, 1973, pp 89–103

46. Soderfeldt B, Soderfeldt M, Jones K, et at: Does organization matter? A multilevel analysis of the demand-control model applied to human services. *Soc Sci Med* 44:527–534, 1997

47. Floiro G, Donnelly J, Zevon M.: The structure of work-related stress and coping among oncology nurses in high-stree medical settings: a transactional analysis. *J Occup Health Psycholol* 3:227–242, 1998

48. Maslach C: The burn-out syndrome and patient care, in Garfield C (ed): *Stress and Survival.* St. Louis, Mosby, 1980, pp 43–56

49. Anonymous: Patients' increased severity of illness drives up LOS around the country: disturbing trend forces re-examination of QI and cost reduction. *Hosp Case Manage* 7:81–82, 84, 96, 1999

50. Curtin L, Flaherty M: The nurse-nurse relationship, in McCorkle R, Hongladarom G (eds): *Issues and Topics in Cancer Nursing.* Norwalk, CT, Appleton-Century-Crofts, 1986, pp 24–40

51. American Nurses' Association and Oncology Nursing Society: *Standards of Oncology Nursing Practice.* Washington, DC: American Nurses' Association, 1996

52. Wise H: Preface, in Wise H, Beckhard R, Rubin I (eds): *Making Health Teams Work.* Cambridge, MA, Ballinger, 1974, p 73

53. Forte P: The high cost of conflict. *Nurs Econ* 15:119–123, 1997

54. Short J: Psychological effects of stress from restructuring and reorganization. Assessment, intervention, and prevention strategies. *AAOHN J* 45:597–604, 1997

55. Stokols D: Conflict-prone and conflict-resistance organizations, in Friedman H (ed): *Hostility, Coping and Health.* Washington, DC, American Psychological Association, 1992, pp 65–76

56. Siders CT, Aschenbrener CA: Conflict management, Part 1. Conflict management checklist: a diagnostic tool for assessing conflict in organizations. *Physician Executive* 25:32–37, 1999

57. Blake R, Mouton J: Theory and research for developing a science of leadership. *J Appl Behav Sci* 18:275–291, 1982

58. Baker K: Improving staff nurse conflict skills. *Nurs Econ* 13:295–298, 1995

59. Deutsch M: *The Resolution of Conflict.* New Haven, CT, Yale University Press, 1993

60. Hightower T: Subordinate choice of conflict handling modes. *Nurs Admin Q* 11:29–34, 1986

61. Barton A: Conflict resolution by nurse managers. *Nurs Manage* 22:83–86, 1991

62. Petterson I, Arnetz BB: Psychosocial stressors and well-being in health care workers. The impact of an intervention program. *Soc Sci Med* 47:1763–1772, 1998

63. Shindul-Rothschild J, Berry D, Long-Middleton E: Where have all the nurses gone? Final results of our patient care survey. *Am J Nurs* 96:25–39, 1996

64. Irvine D, Evans M: Job satisfaction and job turnover among nurses: integrating research findings across studies. *Nurs Res* 44:246–253, 1995

65. Gilliland M: Workforce reductions: low morale, reduced quality of care. *Nurs Econ* 15:320–322, 1997

66. Salyer J: Environmental turbulence. Impact on nurse performance. *J Nurs Adm* 25(4):12–20, 1995

67. Calhoun G, Calhoun J: Occupational stress—implications for hospitals, in Selye H (ed): *Selye's Guide to Stress Research* vol 3. New York, Van Nostrand Reinhold, 1983, pp 99–110

68. Mariner W: Business vs. medical ethics: conflicting standards for managed care. *J Law Med Ethics* 23:236–246, 1995

69. Scanlon C: Survey yields significant results. *Communiqué* (ANA Center for Ethics and Human Rights) 3:1–3, 1994

70. American Nurses' Association: *Code for Nurses with Interpretative Statements.* Washington, DC, American Nurses' Association, 1985

71. Scanlon C, Glover J: A professional code of ethics: providing a moral compass in turbulent times. *Oncol Nurs Forum* 22:1515–1521, 1995

72. Scanlon C: Unraveling the ethical issues in palliative care. *Semin Oncol Nurs* 14:137–144, 1998

73. American Nurses' Association: *Position Statement: The Nonnegotiable Nature of The ANA Code For Nurses with Interpretive Statements.* Washington, DC, American Nurses' Association, 1994

74. Mohr W, Mahon M: Dirty hands: the underside of marketplace health care. *Adv Nurs Sci* 19:28–37, 1996

75. Menaghan E: Individual coping efforts: moderators of the relationship between life stress and mental health outcomes, in Kaplan H (ed): *Psychosocial Stress.* New York, Academic Press, 1983, pp 157–191

76. Folkman S, Lazarus R: An analysis of coping in middle-aged community sample. *J Health Soc Behav* 21:219–239, 1980

77. Compas B, Orosan P: Cognitive appraisals and coping with stress, in Long B, Kahn S (ed): *Women, Work, and Coping. A Multidisciplinary Approach to Workplace Stress.* Montreal, McGill-Queen's University Press, 1993, pp 219–238

78. Covey S: *The 7 Habits of Highly Effective People.* New York, Simon & Schuster, 1989, p 97

79. Charlesworth E, Nathan R: *Stress Management.* New York, Atheneum, 1985

80. Ellis A, Powers M: *A Guide to Rational Living* (ed. 4). New York, Wilshire, 1998

81. Smythe E: *Surviving Nursing.* Menlo Park, CA, Addison-Wesley, 1984

82. Mattheis R: Holistic health concepts, in Haber J, Leach A, Schudy S, Sideleau B (eds): *Comprehensive Psychiatric Nursing.* New York: McGraw, 1982, pp 79–137

83. Jacobson S, McGrath M: *Nurses Under Stress.* New York, Wiley, 1983

84. Chenevert M: *STAT. Special Techniques In Assertiveness Training for Women In Health Professions* (ed. 4). St Louis, Mosby, 1994

85. Breathnach S: *Simple Abundance. A Daybook Of Comfort And Joy.* New York, Warner, 1995

86. Schmitt M: Social support, occupational stressors, and health in cancer nursing, in Baird S, McCorkle R, Grant M (eds): *Cancer Nursing. A Comprehensive Textbook.* Philadelphia, Saunders, 1991, pp 1065–1075

87. Caplan G: *Principles of Preventative Psychiatry.* New York, Basic Books, 1964

88. Capenito L: The bluing of white collars. *Nurs Forum* 29: 3–4, 1994

89. Roberts D, Snowball J: Psychological care in oncology nursing: a study of social knowledge. *J Clin Nurs* 8:39–47, 1999

90. Gray B: How to prepare and plan for the career that suits your needs: assess yourself, assess the market, sharpen your skills, go for it! *Nurs Allied Healthweek—Houston/San Antonio* 1:20–23, 1996

91. Waterman R, Waterman J, Collard B: Toward a career-resilient workforce. *Harvard Bus Rev* 57:87–95, 1994

92. Jacox A: Determinations of who does what in health care. *ONLINE J ISSUES NURS,* no pagination, 1997

93. Kovner C, Gergen P: Nursing staffing levels and adverse events following surgery in U.S. hospitals. *Image Nurs Sch* 30:315–321, 1998

94. Prescott P: Nursing: an important component of hospital survival under a reformed health care system. *Nurs Econ* 11:192–199, 1993

95. American Nurses' Association: *Nursing Care Report Card For Acute Care.* Washington, DC, American Nurses' Association, 1995

96. Baird S: The impact of changing health care delivery on oncology practice. *Oncol Nurs: Patient Treat Support* 2:1–13, 1995

97. Shogren E, Calkins A, Wilburn S: Restructuring may be hazardous to your health. *Am J Nurs* 96:64, 1996

98. Rushton C, Scanlon C: When values conflict with obligations: safeguards for nurses. *Pediatr Nurs* 21:260–268, 1995

99. Rushton C, Brooks-Brunn J: Environments that support ethical practice. *New Horizons* 5:20–29, 1997

100. Benoliel J: The moral context of oncology nursing. *Oncol Nurs Forum* 20:5–12, 1993

101. Turkington C: *Stress Management for Busy People.* New York, McGraw-Hill, 1998

102. Fields T, Quintino O, Henteleff T, et al: Job stress reduction therapies. *Altern Ther* 3:54–56, 1997

CHAPTER 85

Resources for Cancer Nurses

Barbara A. Barhamand, RN, MS, AOCN

How to Use This Chapter

These resources for cancer nurses are compiled from a variety of health- and oncology-related organizations, resources, and Internet searches. The specific information varies in length and format depending on what was sent or available from the organizations when queried by phone, fax, or search. This compilation is the latest information the author has received or found, but the accuracy and timeliness of membership information, prices for publications, and other data cannot be guaranteed. The reader is encouraged to contact the organization listed to verify specific information, such as current pricing, before ordering.

In order to best utilize the information in this chapter, there are two primary ways to locate information:

- If you know the name of the resource you are looking for:

  - Refer to the Alphabetical Index, keeping in mind that many organizations change their names as they restructure or reprioritize. Each resource is followed by a bracketed number (its numerical listing) and a page reference.
  - Each listing is alphabetized within its category relating to the type of organization.

- If you are looking for a resource by subject (i.e., pain):

  - Refer to the Subject Index, in which the entries are listed alphabetically. After each subject are the numerical listings (in brackets) of resources that can be referred to for appropriateness. Some resources are cross-referenced more than once; some are not cross-referenced at all if they are a resource of a more general nature.

Alphabetical Index

Subject Index

Skin cancer [2, 49]

Support groups [3, 5, 7, 12, 13, 19, 23, 35, 46, 54, 55, 57, 58]

Support services [1, 4, 9, 10, 12, 16, 20, 25, 26, 30, 33, 46, 48, 53]

Survival issues [12, 15, 29, 36, 39]

Urology [4, 5, 31, 45, 55]

Wish-granting organizations [28, 50, 51]

Organizations

Patient Assistance and Support Organizations

1. **Alliance for Lung Cancer Advocacy, Support, and Education**
   1601 Lincoln Avenue
   Vancouver, WA 98660
   (360) 696-2436; (800) 298-2436; FAX (360) 699-1944
   Web site: www.alcase.org

   ALCASE is the only national nonprofit organization dedicated solely to helping people with lung cancer. The organization provides a free quarterly newsletter, phone buddies, peer support programs, information searches, resources, and referrals. The *Lung Cancer Manual* is a spiral-bound patient guide covering topics of interest including general information about cancer, specific information about lung cancer, and treatment options, clinical trials, supportive care, complementary medicine, and living with lung cancer. It is available by phone or on the Web site.

2. **American Academy of Dermatology**
   P.O. Box 681069
   Schaumburg, IL 60168
   (847) 330-0230; FAX (847) 330-0050
   Web site: www.aad.org

   The American Academy of Dermatology offers a catalogue of brochures that is available by writing the above address and enclosing a self-addressed, stamped envelope. The brochures are free of charge unless requested in quantities. Individual brochure information can be accessed and downloaded from the AAD Web site by clicking on "Patient Education." The AAD sponsors National Melanoma/Skin Cancer Detection and Prevention Month, a unique public service/public education program. Academy members volunteer to conduct free screenings as a public service. The Academy gives physician referrals for patients in their geographic location.

   Sample brochure titles include:
   > *The Darker Side of Tanning*
   > *Sun Protection for Children*

3. **American Brain Tumor Association**
   2720 River Road
   Des Plaines, IL 60018
   (800) 886-2282 (patient services line); (847) 827-9910; FAX (847) 886-2282
   Web site: www.ABTA.org

   The American Brain Tumor Association is a national organization that provides written information about brain tumors and their treatment and funds brain tumor research.

Professional services include access to currently funded ABTA research and clinical trials. Public services include patient education materials, listings of brain tumor support groups, referrals to support organizations, and information about treatment facilities. Also available is a list of physicians who offer investigational treatments for brain tumors in adults and children. A complimentary triannual newsletter, the *Message Line*, describes research advances and announces updates to publications. Single copies of all materials are available to patients and health care professionals at no cost; the ABTA charges a nominal fee per each for multiple copies.

Publications from the American Brain Tumor Association include:

Basic information:
> *A Brain Tumor—Sharing Hope (English and Spanish)*
> *A Primer of Brain Tumors*
> *Dictionary for Brain Tumor Patients*

Tumor information:
> *About Ependymoma*
> *About Glioblastoma and Anaplastic Astrocytoma*
> *About Medulloblastoma/PNET*
> *About Meningioma*
> *About Metastatic Tumors to the Brain and Spine*
> *About Oligodendroglioma and Mixed Glioma*
> *About Pituitary Tumors*

Treatment information:
> *Chemotherapy of Brain Tumors*
> *Gene Therapy*
> *Immunotherapy of Brain Tumors*
> *Radiation Therapy of Brain Tumors: A Basic Guide*
> *Stereotactic Radiosurgery*

Information for and about children:
> *Alex's Journey: The Story of a Child with a Brain Tumor*
>   (for children ages 9–13)
> *When Your Child Is Ready to Return to School*

Help and resources:
> *The Brain Tumor Survivor's Guide to the Internet*
> *Connections—A Pen Pal Program*
> *Coping With a Brain Tumor, Part I: From Diagnosis to Treatment*
> *Coping With a Brain Tumor, Part II: During and After Treatment*
> *Organizing a Support Group*
> *Using a Medical Library*

4. **American Cancer Society (ACS)**
   1599 Clifton Road, NE
   Atlanta, GA 30329-4251
   (404) 320-3333; (800) ACS-2345
   Web site: www.cancer.org

   Each local unit or division of the American Cancer Society (ACS) (over 3400 offices in the United States and Puerto Rico) has an extensive assortment of booklets, videos, slides, reprints, posters, audiotapes, programs, and proceedings available at no charge covering all aspects of the cancer experience. Many also are available in Spanish. Some states have a computer response system for approved information. The caller can request information on most cancer-related topics (e.g., unproven methods of cancer treatment) and receive a written synopsis with the "ACS's official opinion."

The ACS provides a vast amount of information about cancer of any type, patient and family information, alternative therapies, statistics, and community awareness opportunities and events. Much of the information can be accessed on the ACS Web site or by phone. Information sheets are not copyrighted and can be copied and shared. The ACS Bookstore has reference books on sale for patients and health professionals. They can be ordered online or by phone.

Sample copyrighted pamphlet titles include:

How To Do a Breast Self Exam
Understanding Chemotherapy
Understanding Radiation
When Someone You Work with Has Cancer
Colostomy—A Guide
Ileostomy—A Guide
Urostomy—A Guide
Sexuality and Cancer (for the woman who has cancer)
Sexuality and Cancer (for the man who has cancer)

There are three distinct ACS programs that have been developed to serve special patient populations:

- Reach to Recovery—program provides support and information about breast cancer and its treatment to women with a personal concern about the disease. Its goal is to help breast cancer patients deal with the physical, emotional, and cosmetic needs related to the disease and/or treatment. Reach to Recovery volunteers are women who have adjusted successfully to their own breast cancer experience and offer a positive role model to patients. They are carefully selected and trained to visit patients in the hospital, at home or another mutually agreed upon site, or by telephone. In some areas, visits are also made with partners of breast cancer patients and their family members. Empathetic, knowledgeable, and responsible volunteers provide objective medical information, but no medical advice. Originally, the program was limited to inhospital volunteer visits with post-mastectomy patients. In recent years, Reach to Recovery has expanded in many communities to include specialized volunteer visits for early support and information on lumpectomy, breast reconstruction, and recurrence. However, a hospital visit can be requested by another health professional such as a nurse or social worker. A family member, friend, or the patient herself may request a visit at home or away from the hospital. All visits made through the Reach to Recovery program are offered at no charge. Services may vary at the local level; contact should be made through the local ACS offices.

- Road to Recovery—a transportation assistance program with volunteers providing rides to and from doctors' appointments and treatments.

- Man to Man Prostate Cancer Education and Support Program—program educates and supports men facing prostate cancer by providing them an opportunity to talk openly with each other and with health care professionals about their disease and related concerns. It consists of two primary components: a presentation by a health care professional on a topic relevant to prostate cancer followed by questions and answers, and a supportive sharing session facilitated by a trained ACS volunteer.

This program is available nationwide, but may not be offered out of every local office.

5. **American Foundation for Urologic Disease**
1128 North Charles Street
Baltimore, MD 21201
(410) 468-1800; FAX (410) 468-1808
Web site: www.afud.org

The American Foundation for Urologic Disease, Inc. is a national not-for-profit organization dedicated to the prevention and cure of urologic diseases through the expansion of medical research and the education of the public and health care professionals about urologic diseases and dysfunctions, including prostate and bladder cancer. The foundation's health education councils are the nationally recognized clearinghouse for accurate and informative patient education materials for men, women, and children. More than 6 million patient education brochures have been published. Participation in national awareness programs helps patients to work together with their physician to make an informed decision about treatment options. The foundation's research scholars program has been the catalyst for the expansion of research funding to the best and brightest urologic investigators across the nation. More than $1 million each year is provided to fund urologic research. The Prostate Cancer Support Group network facilitates intergroup communications and program development for individual prostate cancer survivor support groups. The network enhances quality of life for patients and their families and provides a forum for them to share ideas and feelings. The foundation offers a membership to patients, the public, and medical professionals. The periodical *Family Urology* is published quarterly.

6. **American Lung Association (ALA)**
1740 Broadway
New York, NY 10019-4374
(212) 315-8700; (800) LUNG-USA
Web site: www.lungusa.org

The American Lung Association (ALA) is a nonprofit organization devoted to conquering lung disease. The ALA promotes lung health by conducting educational programs, as well as sponsoring symposia, conferences, publications, films, fellowships, and research grants. Local chapters can provide smoking literature, posters, buttons, and smoking cessation materials.

Call for a free catalogue of public education materials that include:

Pamphlets:

Facts about Cigarette Smoking
Facts About Asthma
Facts About Lung Cancer
Facts About Radon
Facts About Second-Hand Smoke
A No Smoking Coloring Book (for children)

Films:

Breathing Easy (for fifth- through eighth-graders)

Antismoking programs:

ALA 7 Steps to a Smoke-Free Life
Freedom from Smoking® Booklets (self-help book to quit smoking in 20 days)
In Control Freedom from Smoking® Home Video Program
Coach's Final Lesson Video

Puzzles:

Have Fun!! Figure Out the Smoking Puzzle

Newsletters:

Lungs at Work
The Breathe Easy®/Asthma Digest
The Weekly Breather

7. American Self-Help Clearinghouse

Saint Clares Medical Center
Denville, NJ 07834-2995
(973) 625-7101 (group information); TDD (973) 625-9053;
(973) 625-9565 (administrative); FAX (973) 625-8848
Web site: http://mentalhelp.net/selfhelp

The Clearinghouse staff and volunteers provide current information and contacts for any national self-help groups that address the caller's particular concern. If no appropriate national groups exist and the caller is interested in the possibility of joining with others to start a local group, information is available on model groups operating in other parts of the country, or individuals who are attempting to start such networks. Specific interests and concerns can also be listed on the computer database that cross-references with over a dozen other self-help clearinghouses in the United States and Canada.

Free handouts (send a stamped, self-addressed envelope with request) include:

Ideas for starting a self-help group
Listing of phone contacts for self-help clearinghouses

The Self-Help Sourcebook (ed 6, 1998) is a comprehensive national guide to finding and forming mutual aid and self-help groups. It contains updated contacts and descriptions for over 800 national and model self-help groups covering a broad range of disabilities, specific illnesses, parenting concerns, bereavement, and many other stressful life situations. Also included are general ideas and suggestions for starting a mutual aid self-help group, contacts for dozens of self-help clearinghouses worldwide, a listing of over 200 national toll-free helplines, resources for rare and genetic illnesses, on-line computer networks, and an easy-to-use index. Cost per copy postage-paid is $12 (book rate postage). Prepayment required.

8. Aplastic Anemia Foundation of America (AAFA)

P.O. Box 613
Annapolis, MD 21404
(410) 867-0242; (800) 747-2820; FAX (410) 867-0240
Web site: www.aplastic.org

The Aplastic Anemia Foundation of America (AAFA) was founded in 1984 to promote further research into the causes and cures of aplastic anemia, myelodysplastic syndrome, and other bone marrow failure. In addition to educating the public about the disease, the AAFA assists those who have the disease and their families. Board and family support meetings are held. The AAFA has the following free publications available on-line:

Aplastic Anemia: Introduction for the General Physician
Aplastic Anemia Answer Book (English, French, Spanish)
Myelodysplastic Syndromes Answer Book
The Blood System: Basic Explanations
Families Coping with Bone Marrow Failure Disease

9. Bloch Cancer Hotline

H & R Block Building
4410 Main Street
Kansas City, MO 64111
(816) 932-8453; (800) 433-0464
Web site: www.blochcancer.org

The Cancer Connection was founded in 1980. It sponsors the Cancer Hotline, a support service that matches cancer patients with volunteers who have the same type of cancer and have either been cured, are in remission, or are being treated. Over 450 volunteers are available to describe treatments they have received and provide information referrals to persons newly diagnosed with cancer. Three books are also available by request at no charge or can be read on-line:

Fighting Cancer, by Richard and Annette Bloch
Cancer . . . There's Hope, by Richard Bloch
Guide for Cancer Supporters, by Richard and Annette Bloch

10. Cancer Care, Inc.

275 7th Avenue, 22nd Floor
New York, NY 10001
(212) 221-3300; (800) 813-HOPE
Web site: www.cancercareinc.org

Cancer Care is a nonprofit, nonsectarian, social service agency founded in 1944 to help cancer patients and their families and friends cope with the impact of cancer. Cancer Care is separate from any other cancer organization. They are the largest agency in the nation solely dedicated to providing free psychosocial support to cancer patients and their families and community education programs for the general public. They treat people at all stages of the illness and provide help to both patient and family.

Cancer Care provides the following services:

- Professional counseling for cancer patients and their families, both on an individual basis and in groups

- Supplementary financial assistance to help families meet certain home care costs such as homemakers, home health aides, housekeepers, transportation to radiation and chemotherapy treatments, and pain medication expense (only available in NY, NJ, and CT)

- Bereavement counseling to help surviving family members cope with their loss

- Information and referral to homemaking services, hospices, child care services, hospitals, and other resources in the community

- Guidance in developing a plan for care for the patient at home

- Volunteer program where volunteers act as friendly visitors to homebound or frail cancer patients

- Education and training regarding psychosocial aspects of cancer for professionals and allied health care providers

The Cancer Care Web site offers access to specific information programs on melanoma, prostate cancer, lung cancer, colon cancer, ovarian cancer, sexuality and breast cancer, brain tumors, policy advocacy, pain, fatigue, and clinical trials. Virtual teleconferences with audio service provides information on a variety of subjects related to cancer and ways to manage it. Also available is the free *Helping Hand Resource Guide* that directs the reader to multiple service agencies and sources specific to their needs including a large on-line database, financial assistance, transportation assistance, home and hospice care, and a buddy support network. Other free publications include:

Lung Cancer Briefs
Control Your Pain So It Doesn't Control You (14 pp)
Learning About Pancreatic Cancer: It Helps to Understand (60 pp)
Breast Cancer and Sexuality

Cancer Care has offices in:

- New York City
  275 7th Avenue, 22nd Floor
  New York, NY 10001
  (212) 302-2400

- Long Island
  20 Crossways Park North
  Suite 304
  Woodbury, NY 11797
  (516) 364-8130

- New Jersey Central office
  241 Millburn Avenue, Suite 241-C
  Millburn, NJ 07041
  (201) 379-7500

- Bergen County office
  141 Dayton Street
  Ridgewood, NJ 07450
  (201) 444-6630

- Connecticut
  120 East Avenue
  Norwalk, CT 06851
  (203) 854-9911

Services are available at other part-time offices in the tri-state area. For information call (212) 302-2400 or 1-800-813-HOPE.

11. Cancer Information Service
NCI-Office of Cancer Communications
Building 31, Room 10A 03
Bethesda, MD 20892
(301) 435-3848; (800) 4-CANCER; TDD (800) 332-8615
Web site: www.nci.nih.gov

The Cancer Information Service (CIS) is a nationwide network of 19 regional field offices supported by the NCI that provides up-to-date information on cancer to patients and their families, health care professionals, and the general public. The CIS can provide specific information in English and Spanish about particular types of cancer, as well as information on how to obtain second opinions and the availability of clinical trials. Each CIS office has access to the NCI treatment database PDQ, which offers callers the most current state-of-the-art treatment and clinical trial information. Through the outreach program, the CIS serves as a resource for state and regional organizations by providing printed materials and technical assistance for cancer education, media campaigns, and community programs. Their regional structure enables the CIS to focus on the distinct needs of each community by providing

culturally diverse populations and the financially or educationally underserved. NCI publications are available on a wide variety of topics including prevention and detection, treatment, survivorship, and research. Many are also available for Spanish or pediatric clientele. All are free. For orders of more than 20 pieces, a shipping fee of $.10 per copy will be charged. Allow four to six weeks for delivery of large orders. A catalogue listing or specific booklets are available by phone order. Examples include:

Chemotherapy and You
Radiation Therapy and You
Eating Hints
Facing Forward
Get Relief from Cancer Pain
Taking Time
Advanced Cancer: Living Each Day
Talking with Your Child About Cancer
What Are Clinical Trials All About
When Cancer Recurs: Meeting the Challenge Again
When Someone in Your Family Has Cancer
Young People with Cancer
Cancer Survivorship: A Review with an Eye to the Future
Cancer Journey: Issues for Survivors

Site-specific booklets address individual cancers in the "What You Need to Know About" series:

Bladder
Bone
Brain and Spinal Cord
Breast
Cervix
Colon and Rectum
Esophagus
Hodgkin's Disease
Kidney
Larynx
Adult Leukemia
Childhood Leukemia
Lung
Melanoma
Multiple Myeloma
Non-Hodgkin's Lymphoma
Head or Neck
Ovary
Pancreas
Prostate
Skin
Stomach
Testis
Uterus

12. Candlelighters Childhood Cancer Foundation®
7910 Woodmont Avenue, Suite 460
Bethesda, MD 20814-3015
(301) 657-8401 or (800) 366-CCCF; FAX (301) 718-2686
Web site: www.candlelighters.org

Candlelighters Childhood Cancer Foundation (CCCF) is an organization for children and the parents of children with cancer, as well as adult survivors of childhood cancer. CCCF is an international, nonprofit, tax-exempt organization. The mission is to educate, support, serve, and advocate for families of children of cancer, survivors of childhood cancer, and the professionals who care for them. There are presently 250 chapters in the United States;

membership exceeds 43,000. Candlelighters provides referrals to volunteers who can help families and survivors experiencing the problems in the areas of employment, insurance education, the military, and government benefits. It can also help obtain second medical opinions. A national newsletter, *Candlelighters*, is published quarterly, which serves as a communication link among parents and parents' groups and concerned professionals. A quarterly youth newsletter, *CCCF Youth Newsletter*, is written by and for adolescent cancer patients and teenage siblings to provide information to young cancer patients. The free newsletters include information about research in childhood cancer, bibliography materials, and group activities. A third newsletter for adult survivors of childhood cancers, *The Phoenix*, is also available. Local groups usually have their own newsletter. Candlelighters also publishes a resource list of childhood cancer education materials such as *Educating the Child with Cancer*; *The Candlelighters Guide to Bone Marrow Transplants in Children*; *Know Before You Go: The Childhood Cancer Journey*; and *Introduction to the Americans with Disabilities Act*. All the above information is available free on request.

13. Children's Hospice International

2202 Mt. Vernon Avenue, Suite 3C
Alexandria, VA 22301
(703) 684-0330; (800) 242-4453; FAX (703) 684-0226
Web site: www.chionline.org

Children's Hospice International (CHI) was founded as a nonprofit organization in 1983 to provide a network of support for dying children and their families. The hospice approach for children is a team effort that provides medical, psychological, social, and spiritual expertise and information in the United States and abroad. CHI recognizes the right and need for children and their families to choose health care and support whether in their own home, hospital, or hospice care facility. It serves as a clearinghouse for research programs, support groups, and education and training programs for the care of terminally ill children. It also offers publications on topics such as home care for seriously ill children and pain management. CHI's main focus is quality of life for the dying child and the ongoing, strengthened life of the family.

14. Choice in Dying

1035 30th Street, NW
Washington, DC 20007
(202) 338-9790; (800) 989-9455; FAX (202) 338-0242
Web site: www.choices.org

Choice in Dying (CID) is a national, not-for-profit organization dedicated to helping patients and their families participate in decisions about end-of-life medical care. The organization developed the first living will 25 years ago and has distributed approximately 10 million living wills to date. CID is the nation's largest provider of state-specific *advance directives*—the general term for two types of legal documents: a living will and a durable power of attorney for health care. Individuals can receive one free set of their state's advance directive by calling (800) 989-9455. CID advocates the right of patients to participate fully in decisions about their medical treatment at the end of life. CID is the only organization that deals broadly and practically with end-of-life issues and provides substantial free public and professional education and counseling about the prep-

aration and use of advance directives. CID provides reasonably priced educational videotapes, programs, speakers, and published materials to the general public, health care professionals, and lawmakers about the needs of people who are dying. A price list of materials, including bulk price/quantity discount information, are available upon request. The *Right-to-Die Law Digest*, published quarterly, informs lawyers, doctors, ethicists, and others who wish to remain up to date on changing legislation and court rulings. The VHS videotape, *Whose Death Is It, Anyway?* ($24.95), accompanied by a discussion guide, is meant to lead a community discussion about making informed end-of-life choices.

15. *Coping* Magazine

Media America, Inc.
P.O. Box 682268
Franklin, TN 37068-2268
(615) 790-2400
Web site: www.copingmag.com

Coping magazine is a nationally distributed consumer magazine for people whose lives have been touched by cancer. Its primary purpose is to empower the readers (whether patients or health care professionals) by providing the knowledge they need to cope with the many issues confronting their daily lives. *Coping* aims to inspire patients and survivors to assume greater responsibility for, and participation in, the many facets of their disease. Cancer survivors are encouraged to submit personal stories of encouragement for publication. *Coping* is published bimonthly (six times a year) and the subscription cost is $18 annually ($24 Canadian/foreign) or $32 ($44 Canadian/foreign) for two years.

16. Corporate Angel Network, Inc.

Westchester County Airport, Building One
White Plains, NY 10604
(914) 328-1313; FAX (914) 328-3938
Web site: www.corpangelnetwork.org

The Corporate Angel Network (CAN) is a nonprofit organization designed to arrange free air transportation for cancer patients. This nationwide program uses available seats on corporate aircraft being flown on business trips. CAN enables patients to obtain optimum treatment for their life-threatening disease. CAN permits patients to travel in comfort and dignity, spared the stresses and expense of commercial air travel. CAN has arranged for over 10,000 patient flights through the cooperation and generosity of more than 500 participating corporations. Financial need is not a requirement.

Patient criteria include:

Going to or from recognized treatment, consultation, or check-up
Being able to walk onto the aircraft unassisted
Requiring no form of life support or medical help on board
Providing doctor's name, address, and telephone number
May be the bone marrow or blood platelet donor
One adult or two parents may accompany the patient, if space permits
Patients should make back-up commercial transportation plans
CAN cannot guarantee to find an appropriate flight

17. Family AIDS Network
1601 N. Kent Street, Suite 1003
Arlington, VA 22209
(703) 243-8276; FAX (703) 243-8377
Web site: www.familyaidsnet.org

The Family AIDS Network was founded in 1992 by Mary Fisher to raise awareness and express compassion for people affected by AIDS. Network members visit communities, organize programs, recognize and promote AIDS caregivers, and encourage more research for an AIDS cure. It is currently focusing on AIDS in women, communities of color, and young people. A special program, Gospel Against AIDS, reaches out to diverse communities at risk.

18. Gilda Radner Familial Ovarian Cancer Registry
Roswell Park Cancer Institute
Elm and Carlton Streets
Buffalo, NY 14263-0001
(800) 682-7426; (800) OVARIAN; FAX (716) 845-8266
Web site: rpci.med.buffalo.edu/departments/gynonc/grwp

Individuals can register on-line, by calling the toll-free number, or by mailing the form available on the Web site. A telephone support service is run by volunteers from the registry. This service is offered by high-risk women for women at risk of developing ovarian cancer and for women considering prophylactic oophorectomy. The Web site addresses topics including risk factors, frequently asked questions about ovarian cancer, and what to do if a woman has a family history of ovarian cancer.

19. Gilda's Club®, Inc.
195 W. Houston St.
New York, NY 10014
(212) 647-9700
Web site: www.gildasclub.org

Gilda's Clubs provide social and emotional support to cancer patients, their families, and friends. Lectures, workshops, networking groups, special events, and a children's program are available.

20. Histiocytosis Association of America
302 N. Broadway
Pitman, NJ 08071
(609) 589-6606; (800) 548-2758; FAX (609) 589-6614
Web site: www.histio.org

Founded in 1986, the Histiocytosis Association of America is a nonprofit organization that supports the emotional and educational needs of families of children and the adult patients who have any of the histiocytoses. The association is able to encourage research by funding scientific projects, sponsoring international research symposia, and distributing educational literature around the world. The association publishes a newsletter, has developed a registry, and offers a video and several brochures. The Web site features chat rooms and opportunities to exchange information and support with other patients and family members.

21. Hospice Education Institute
190 Westbrook Road
Essex, CT 06426-1510
(860) 767-1620; (800) 331-1620; FAX (860) 767-2746
Web site: www.hospiceworld.org

The Hospice Education Institute is an independent, non-profit organization founded in 1985. It serves a wide range of individuals and organizations interested in hospice and palliative care throughout the United States and around the world. Its toll-free referral service directs over 21,000 callers a year to local hospice programs. Further, by working with health and caring professionals and with educators who teach courses on dying, grief, and bereavement, the Hospice Education Institute disseminates information about hospice care at many levels.

The services of the Hospice Education Institute include:

- HOSPICELINK, which maintains a computerized and continually updated directory of hospice programs in the United States and operates a toll-free telephone number to refer callers to local hospice and palliative care programs. HOSPICELINK also provides general information about the principles and practice of hospice care. Staff members will listen sympathetically and give limited, informal support to callers who wish to discuss immediate personal problems relating to terminal illness and bereavement. (HOSPICELINK does not offer medical advice, answer insurance questions, or provide psychological counseling.) There is no charge for any HOSPICELINK service.

- Regional seminars on many aspects of caring for dying and the bereaved are organized for health and caring professionals and qualified hospice volunteers. Since 1986, seminars have been offered in 31 states. Faculty members for these seminars are international multiprofessional experts on hospice care. The institute also sponsors the annual Hospice Study Seminar in Britain—an intensive two-week workshop for health care professionals from all over the world.

- Advice and assistance are freely given to people working to begin or improve community-based hospice care, palliative care, and bereavement support.

Books and pamphlets are available from the Hospice Education Institute on hospice-related subjects. The Hospice Education Institute's *Notes on Symptom Control in Hospice and Palliative Care* is the definitive work to date on symptom control.

22. Hospice Foundation of America
2001 S Street NW, Suite 300
Washington, DC 20009
(202) 638-5419; FAX (202) 638-5312
Web site: www.hospicefoundation.org

Hospice Foundation of America is the nation's largest charity whose sole mission is to promote the hospice concept of care and that is supported primarily by individual donations. The foundation acts as an advocate for the hospice concept of care, offering professional development and educational opportunities to hospice and other health care workers, sponsoring research on ethical issues and the economics of health care at the end-of-life, participating in public policy initiatives, providing technical assistance to organizations, and serving as a philanthropic presence within the national hospice community.

Foundation programs and publications include:

Living with Grief, an annual national satellite tele-conference on bereavement, hosted by ABC News' Cookie Roberts, which includes a companion book for each participant. (2 hours CEUs)

Clergy to Clergy, a program of audio tapes designed to assist clergy in counseling grieving people

Living with Grief: After Sudden Loss (book, $16.95)

Living with Grief: When Illness Is Prolonged (book, $16.95)

Living with Grief: Who We Are, How We Grieve (book, $16.95)

Living with Grief: At Work, At School, At Worship (book, $16.95)

Clergy to Clergy: Helping You Minister to Those Facing Illness, Death, and Grief

A Guide to Recalling and Telling Your Life Story (book, $15)

Journeys, a newsletter to help in bereavement ($12/yr)

23. International Association of Laryngectomees

7822 Ivymount Terrace
Potomac, MD 20854
(301) 983-9323; FAX (301) 983-4397
Web site: wwwlarynxlink.com

The International Association of Laryngectomees (IAL) is a voluntary, nonprofit organization dedicated to the total rehabilitation of laryngectomees. The IAL promotes and supports the total rehabilitation of laryngectomees through the exchange and dissemination of ideas and information to laryngectomee clubs and to the public. These clubs encourage and help laryngectomees improve their quality of life by providing a supportive environment to help them make the adjustments associated with laryngectomy surgery.

The IAL works to upgrade the minimum standards for teachers of alaryngeal speech, to foster improvement in hospital laryngectomee programs, and to increase awareness about the appropriate first-aid techniques for laryngectomees. The IAL publishes educational materials and a triannual newsletter, maintains a registry of postlaryngectomy speech instructors, and sponsors an annual voice rehabilitation institute and an annual general meeting for laryngectomees.

The IAL was formed in 1952 by representatives of a number of laryngectomee clubs to answer the need for coordinating the activities of the clubs. The IAL consists of nearly 300 member clubs located throughout the United States and in several foreign countries. These clubs usually meet once or twice a month for informational programs and support. Most clubs also maintain a patient visitation program coordinated with medical professionals in local hospitals and clinics.

24. Let's Face It

P.O. Box 29972
Bellingham, WA 98228-1972
(360) 676-7325
Web site: www.faceit.org/letsfaceit

Let's Face It is the U.S. branch of an international self-help network dedicated to helping people with facial difference, their loved ones, the professionals who care for them, and the communities in which they live, to understand and to solve the problems of living with this disability. Specific service is available to those who have lost part of their face to cancer, including a book by a woman who survived facial cancer. Their Web site has an index for cancer survivors.

The organization has an annual directory, *Resources for People with Facial Difference,* that provides information on a variety of organizations the individual with a facial difference could utilize. For a free copy of this 60-page booklet, send a 9″ × 12″ self-addressed envelope, stamped with $3.00 postage, and a short note explaining the request.

25. Leukemia Society of America

National Headquarters
600 Third Avenue
New York, NY 10016
(212) 573-8484; (800) 955-4LSA (Hotline for Information)
Web site: www.leukemia.org

The Leukemia Society of America (LSA) is a national voluntary health agency with a chapter in every state dedicated solely to seeking the cause and eventual cure of leukemia, lymphoma, multiple myeloma, and Hodgkin's disease. The society supports five major programs: research, patient services, public and professional education, and community service.

- Research—The LSA research program has allocated almost $18 million in 1998 to support the work at more than 300 labs in the United States and throughout the world.

- Patient services—Services include an Information Resource Center, Family Support Groups, a peer support network, and financial assistance. Up to $500 a year per person for reimbursement for specific approved drugs for treatment/control of leukemia, lymphoma, multiple myeloma, and preleukemia is given by the society. Outpatients are those not confined to a hospital, although they may be treated at various times at a hospital.

- Education—The LSA pursues an aggressive program to provide current information on leukemia and related diseases to the general public. It alerts the public to disease dnager, treatment, and therapy through literature and posters, films, and other audiovisual material, speaking engagements, seminars and educational programs, news and feature releases, and public service advertising in all media. Information is available from each local chapter and from the society's national headquarters in New York City.

- Community service—The compilation and maintenance of resource and referral material is a high-priority service of the chapters, which interact with government health departments and many varied family-assistance organizations.

The LSA has many pamphlets available free of charge (and can be accessed on the Web site), including:

Facts About the Leukemia Society of America (English and Spanish)

Leukemia

Lymphomas: Hodgkin's Disease/Non-Hodgkin's Lymphoma

Chronic Myelogenous Leukemia (CML)

Acute Myelogenous Leukemia (AML)
Acute Lymphocytic Leukemia (ALL)
Chronic Lymphocytic Leukemia (CLL)
Hairy Cell Leukemia
Myelodysplastic Syndrome (MDS)
Multiple Myeloma
Patient-Aid Program (English and Spanish)
What Everyone Should Know About Leukemia (English and Spanish)
Emotional Aspects of Childhood Leukemia
I'm Having a Bone Marrow Transplant (pediatric)
Bone Marrow Transplantation & Peripheral Blood Stem Cell Transplantation (English and Spanish)
Making Intelligent Choices About Therapy
Understanding Chemotherapy
Forty Years of Progress: The Story of the Leukemia Society Research Report
Coping with Survival

26. Look Good . . . Feel Better
The CTFA Foundation
1101 17th Street, NW
Suite 300
Washington, DC 20036-4702
(202) 331-1770; (800) 395-LOOK; FAX (202) 331-1969
Web site: www.lookgoodfeelbetter.org

Look Good . . . Feel Better (LGFB) is a free national public service program created from the concept that if a woman with cancer can be helped to look good, her improved self-esteem will help her approach her disease and treatment with greater confidence. Trained volunteers offer guidance and instruction to women in a supportive environment, helping them regain their confidence and self-esteem. LGFB is a nonmedical, product-neutral program made possible by a partnership between the Cosmetic, Toiletry & Fragrance Association (CTFA) Foundation, the American Cancer Society (ACS), and the National Cosmetology Association (NCA). The CTFA Foundation provides the complimentary makeup and free educational materials, such as videotapes and pamphlets, and secures financial support for LGFB. The ACS administers the program nationwide and serves as the primary source of information to the public. The NCA organizes and helps train the volunteer cosmetologists. Special programs are available for teens and Spanish-speaking women. LGFB is available to patients in one of three ways. The most popular LGFB format is a structured group session consisting of six to ten patients. This group session usually is offered in a hospital and includes a group of trained cosmetologists who instruct the patients in how to use makeup, wigs, scarves, turbans, and accessories to camouflage the appearance changes resulting from their treatments. Each patient receives a complimentary bag of assorted cosmetics that are used in the session, with guidance from the cosmetologists. The goal is to teach the patients cosmetic techniques they can use every day, allowing them to gain some control over their lives.

The second format available is a free, private consultation with a trained cosmetologist in a salon or other private setting. The techniques taught are the same as in a group session. The group session is the more popular of the two formats, because it tends to serve as an informal support group for the women by allowing them to discuss a part of their treatment that no one else understands quite as well as other patients and cosmetologists.

In locations where group or one-on-one LGFB sessions are not available, a patient brochure and self-help video are available through the ACS. Materials are available in English and Spanish.

27. Lymphedema Foundation, Inc.
8307 Marbach Road
San Antonio, TX 78227
(210) 675-5599; FAX (210) 675-5632
Web site: www.lymphedemafoundation.org

The Lymphedema Foundation is a not-for-profit charitable organization that was created to support inquiries for research for the cause, prevention, and treatment of lymphedema. They also serve as an advocate for the patient with lymphedema, make information about lymphedema available to physicians, patients, and the public, educate health care providers and insurers about the need for appropriate care for the lymphedema patient, and establish certification standards for lymphedema therapists and facilities.

28. Make-A-Wish Foundation of America
100 W. Clarendon, Suite 2200
Phoenix, AZ 85013-3518
(602) 279-9474; (800) 722-9774; FAX (602) 279-0855
Web site: www.wish.org

The Make-A-Wish Foundation of America is a nonprofit organization whose main purpose is to fulfill the wishes of children with life-threatening or terminal illnesses. The foundation will consider the wish of any child between the ages of 2 and 18 anywhere in the world and covers all expenses related to granting the wish. Referrals can be made by medical professionals treating the child, the child's parents or legal guardians, or a potential wish child. There are 81 local chapters who coordinate the wish experiences into reality.

29. *MAMM* Magazine
POZ Publishing LLC
349 W. 12th Street
New York, NY 10014-1721
FAX (212) 675-8505
Web site: www.mamm.com

MAMM: Women, Cancer and Community is a magazine dedicated to providing the necessary tools to live healthier and happier lives with a cancer diagnosis. *MAMM* is for anyone whose life has been impacted by breast or reproductive cancers, including partners, family members, and co-workers. A yearly subscription is $17.97 for 12 issues ($27.97 outside the United States). To subscribe by phone call (888) 901-MAMM. The subscription is unconditionally guaranteed, and each issue arrives in a closed wrapper.

30. Medic Alert Foundation
2323 Colorado Avenue
Turlock, CA 95382-2018
(800) 432-5378; (800) ID ALERT; FAX (209) 669-2495
Web site: www.medicalert.org

Medic Alert's three-part life-protecting system consists of:

- A metal alerting emblem worn as a bracelet or necklace. The emblem bears the staff of Aesculapius, the internationally recognized insignia of the medical profession, and the words *Medic Alert*. On the reverse side are engraved the special medical conditions of the wearer such as "hypertension," "takes beta blocker," "allergic to penicillin," or "wearing contact lenses." Also engraved on the back are the member's identification number and the number for Medic Alert's Emergency Response Center.

- The 24-hour-a-day Emergency Response Center provides detailed data to emergency personnel via a collect telephone call from anywhere in the world. Medic Alert's emergency hotline number engraved on the back of the emblem and printed on the wallet card provides vital information that aids diagnosis and speeds life-saving treatments.

- Each member receives a wallet card with personal and medical information in addition to that engraved on the emblem. Each year, the members receive a wallet card copy of the information listed on their computerized medical record. This serves as a reminder to members to keep their record up-to-date. The record may be updated at any time by phone or mail. Whenever the record is updated, a new wallet card is prepared with the new information and sent immediately to the member.

Medic Alert serves about 45 countries from a network of affiliate offices worldwide. Initial membership is $35 with annual renewals of $15. This includes a free update of medical records. Free memberships are provided to individuals with special economic needs on the written request of a physician or a social worker. Membership in the United States now totals approximately 2.3 million people.

31. Men's Health Network
P.O. Box 75972
Washington, DC 20013
(202) 543-6461; (888) 636-2636
Web site: www.menshealthnetwork.org

The Men's Health Network is an informational and educational organization that recognizes men's health as a specific social concern. The network's library includes health-related issues such as prostate cancer, testicular cancer, cardiovascular disease, stroke, erectile dysfunction, and suicide. Social science issues include census data, family structures, parenting issues, and domestic violence.

32. National Alliance of Breast Cancer Organizations
9 E. 37th Street, 10th Floor
New York, NY 10016
(212) 889-0606; FAX (212) 689-1213
Web site: www.nabco.org

The National Alliance of Breast Cancer Organizations (NABCO), established in 1986, is the leading central resource for information and education about breast cancer and a network of more than 375 organizations providing detection, treatment, and care to hundreds of thousands of American women. Aside from its role as a source of current, accurate information for media, medical organizations, professionals, patients, and their families, NABCO advocates for regulatory change and legislation to benefit breast cancer patients, survivors, and women at risk on a local, state, and national level. Membership contributions are tax-deductible and entitle the member to receive the NABCO Resource List, a copy of the *NABCO News* (published quarterly), and special mailings on breast cancer issues. Individual $50; nonprofit group $100; business $200.

The *Breast Cancer Clinical Trial Directory* is available on the Web site or can be obtained by calling NABCO. It includes trial descriptions from PDQ in the areas of prevention; autologous bone marrow support; early-stage or high-risk early stage breast cancer; treatment for advanced, metastatic or recurrent breast cancer; and quality of life.

The Web site offers a variety of resources including the NABCO resource list, the clinical trial directory, and a listing of breast cancer support groups in a specific geographic location. The following sampling of publications that address general information about breast cancer is taken from the 1997–1998 edition of the breast cancer resource list. The complete list can also be ordered from NABCO for $3.00.

> *Women for Women*, the first cause-related album to benefit breast health, all sales benefit NABCO, featuring such artists as Aretha Franklin, Amy Grant, Carly Simon, and Tina Turner
>
> *The Breast Book*, by Dr. Miriam Stoppard (DK Publishing, Inc., New York, 1996, $24.95)
>
> *Breast Cancer: The Complete Handbook*, by Yashar Hirshaut, MD & Peter Pressman, MD (Bantam, New York, 1996, paperback $14.95)
>
> *Breast Cancer Handbook: A Basic Guide for Gathering Information, Understanding the Diagnosis, and Choosing the Treatment*, by Linda Brown Harris (Melpomene Institute of Women's Health Research, St. Paul, MN, $8.95 plus $3.50 shipping, call 612-642-1951 to order)
>
> *Early Detection Brochure*, available from NABCO in English and Spanish (up to 25 copies are free; $8.00 per 100)
>
> *Dr. Susan Love's Breast Book*, by Susan Love, MD with Karen Lindsey (Addison-Wesley, Reading, MA, 1995, $17); available in bookstores

Other resources include lists of books of personal stories, breast examinations, risk factors and benign breast disease, risk counseling and research centers, and sources of medical information and support.

33. National Association of Hospital Hospitality Houses, Inc.
P.O. Box 18087
Asheville, NC 28814-0087
(828) 253-1188; (800) 542-9730; FAX (828) 253-8082
Web site: www.nahhh.com

The National Association of Hospital Hospitality Houses (NAHHH) promotes and assists not-for-profit programs that provide lodging and supportive services in a caring environment for families receiving medical care away from home. Such homes include the Ronald McDonald houses (for parents of a sick child), the ACS's Hope Lodges (for adult cancer patients and their families), and the Fisher Houses (for military personnel and their dependents while receiving medical care at military hospitals). Membership opportunities include:

- House—for existing nonprofits programs

- Provisional—for those wishing to create a program

- Affiliate—for any group or individual interested in fostering development of a program within the NAHHH concept.

34. National Association of People with AIDS
1413 K Street, N.W., 7th Floor
Washington, D.C. 20005
(202) 898-0414; FAX (202) 898-0435
Web site: www.napwa.org

The National Association of People with AIDS (NAPWA) is dedicated to improving the lives of people with HIV disease at home, in the workplace, and in the community. Since 1983, NAPWA has served as the "voice" for the needs and concerns of all people infected and affected by HIV/AIDS in the United States. NAPWA works to focus national attention on the realities faced by people living with HIV disease and believes that every individual with HIV deserves to be treated with respect and compassion and have access to the best health care possible. NAPWA meets with government agencies, scientists, and pharmaceutical and biotech companies about current and future treatments; distributes vital educational information; and works to focus national attention on the realities faced by people living with HIV. Members receive all NAPWA publications, reduced rates, and scholarship consideration at the National Skills Building Conference.

35. National Brain Tumor Foundation
785 Market Street, Suite 1600
San Francisco, CA 94103
(415) 284-0208; (800) 934-CURE; FAX (415) 284-0209
Web site: www.braintumor.org

The mission of the National Brain Tumor Foundation (NBTF) is to provide patients and families the information they need to successfully cope with their illness and fund promising research. Its mission is achieved through:

- In-depth seminars as well as national and regional conferences to prepare patients for all the challenges brought on by a brain tumor diagnosis

- Hope-inspiring printed materials that are immediately available to families to answer their questions and direct their treatment efforts (*Brain Tumors: A Guide*)

- Access to a growing national network of over 140 life-sustaining patient support groups in the United States and Canada

- Clearinghouse coordination of approximately 6000 patient inquiries each year

- Updates to over 16,000 families through a newsletter, *SEARCH*, published quarterly

- Funding research grants totaling $1.2 million to date

Other publications include:

> *Navigating Through a Strange Land: A Book for Brain Tumor Patients and Their Families* (220 pp)
> *Gathering a Life—A Journal of Recovery,* by Jeanne Lohmann (61 pp, $8.75)
> *Returning to Work: Strategies for Brain Tumor Patients*

> *A Guide for Parents: Understanding and Coping with Your Child's Brain Tumor*
> *Clinical Trials and Questions about Brain Tumors*

36. National Cancer Survivors Day Foundation, Inc.
P.O. Box 682285
Franklin, TN 37068-2285
(615) 794-3006; FAX (615) 794-0179

National Cancer Survivors Day (NCSD) is a nationwide annual celebration of life for cancer survivors, their families, friends, and oncology teams. Each celebration is an annual milestone in a survivor's fight against cancer, and there are 8 million cancer survivors in America. National Cancer Survivors Day was founded by cancer survivor Richard Bloch (H & R Block) and his wife, Annette, who serve each year as the founding co-chairs. NCSD is celebrated on the first Sunday in June of each year in communities throughout the United States and Canada. It is the world's largest cancer survivor event.

37. National Cervical Cancer Coalition
16501 Sherman Way, Suite #110
Van Nuys, CA 91406
(818) 909-3849; (800) 685-5531 (patient line); FAX (818) 780-8199
Web site: www.nccc-online.org

The National Cervical Cancer Coalition (NCCC) is emerging as the nation's leading independent grassroots voice for a coalition of health care providers, pathologists, cytotechnologists, women's groups, patients, technology, research and treatment companies and associations. The mission statement of the NCCC includes efforts to:

- Enhance awareness of the conventional Pap smear, new technology, and treatment options

- Clearly communicate the success of cervical cancer screening programs in battling cervical cancer disease

- Assist in efforts related to cervical cancer disease research

- Act as a clearinghouse in distributing information on cervical cancer for women and family members

38. National Childhood Cancer Foundation
440 E. Huntington Drive, Suite 300
P.O. Box 60012
Arcadia, CA 91066-6012
(800) 458-6223; FAX (800) 723-2822
Web site: www.nccf.org

The National Childhood Cancer Foundation (NCCF) is a nonprofit, public-benefit charitable foundation. Its mission is to reduce and eventually eliminate the devastating impacts of the cancers that attack children and young adults. The NCCF supports research and treatments conducted by a network of institutions specializing in pediatric care known as the Children's Cancer Group.

39. National Coalition for Cancer Survivorship
1010 Wayne Avenue, Suite 505
Silver Springs, MD 20910-5600
(301) 650-8868; (888) 937-6227; FAX (301) 565-9670
Web site: www.cansearch.org

The National Coalition for Cancer Survivorship (NCCS) represents grassroots organizations throughout the United States of over 10,000 cancer survivors. The NCCS was founded in 1986 by 24 cancer experts and Dr. Fitzhugh Mullan, a cancer survivor. Their mission is to lead and strengthen the survivorship movement, empower cancer survivors, and advocate for policy issues that affect their quality of life.

Through the national organization and a network of local organizations, the NCCS fosters the following goals:

- To promote programs that will empower survivors as informed consumers

- To operate a clearinghouse that disseminates survivorship articles, literature, and information on local and national survivorship activities and programs

- To act as a voice for cancer survivors to the media, medical establishment, and government

NCCS publications highlight issues vital to survivors such as locating resources, communicating with the health care team, being a savvy consumer of medical services, and fighting job and insurance discrimination:

- *NCCS Networker*, a quarterly publication for members, offering the latest news about NCCS activities and survivorship issues, including legislative activity, clinical trials and research, special regional and local support groups, and reviews of the latest publications by and for cancer survivors

- *Charting the Journey*, an almanac of resources for survivors published by Consumer Reports Books

- *Facing Forward*, a guide for those finishing treatment, published by the National Cancer Institute in collaboration with NCCS

- *Teamwork: The Cancer Patient's Guide to Talking with Your Doctor*

40. National Kidney Cancer Association
1234 Sherman Avenue, Suite 203
Evanston, IL 60202-1375
(847) 332-1051; (800) 850-9132; FAX (847) 332-2978
Web site: www.nkca.org

The Kidney Cancer Association (KCA) is a membership organization of patients, family members, physicians, researchers, and other health care professionals. The KCA was founded in 1990 as a nonprofit charity corporation. They offer a broad range of services, including patient and professional meetings, information, publications, and a newsletter *Kidney Cancer News*. Other free publications include:

> *We Have Kidney Cancer*
> *Interleukin-2 & Biologic Therapy*
> *Reflections: A Guide to End of Life Issues*
> *How You Can Benefit From Planned Giving*
> *Emotional vs. Rational*
> *13 Steps to World Class Cancer Care*
> *Access to Cancer Drugs Worldwide*
> *Managing Cancer Pain*

41. National Leukemia Research Association, Inc.
585 Stewart Avenue, Suite 536
Garden City, NY 11530
(516) 222-1944; FAX (516) 222-0457
Email: clra@erols.com

The National Leukemia Association was founded in 1965 as a not-for-profit organization dedicated to raising funds to support research into the causes and cure of leukemia and to provide patient aid to those families in need while meeting the expenses incurred in leukemia treatment. The association is a voluntary agency that is totally supported by public contributions.

The National Leukemia Association provides aid to leukemia patients and their families. The Board of Trustees, in conjunction with its Patient Aid Committee, sets the policies and standards for administering this program. The association will assist patients not covered by existing medical policies with laboratory fees, radiation therapy treatment, drugs, and blood transfusions. Unusual and extraordinary expenses not covered above will be considered based upon need and availability of funds.

42. National Lymphedema Network
2211 Post Street, Suite 404
San Francisco, CA 94115-3427
(415) 921-1306; (800) 541-3259; FAX (415) 921-4284
Web site: www.lymphnet.org

Established in 1988, the network is a nonprofit organization that disseminates information on the prevention and management of primary and secondary lymphedema to lymphedema patients, health care professionals, and the general public. The NLN supports research into the causes and possible alternative treatments for lymphedema. Services include an extensive computer database, educational course offerings for health care professionals and patients, a quarterly newsletter containing educational articles, a resource guide, "penpals," referrals to lymphedema treatment centers and support groups, and updates on conferences and professional training courses. Educational materials—such as newsletter reprints, books, or videos—can be ordered on-line. Lymphedema Alert bracelets and necklaces are also available for purchase.

43. National Marrow Donor Program Coordinating Center
3433 Broadway Street, NE, Suite 500
Minneapolis, MN 55413
(612) 627-5844; FAX (612) 627-5899; (800) 526-7809 (Office of Patient Advocacy); (800) MARROW2 (potential marrow donor)
Web site: www.marrow.org

The National Marrow Donor Program (NMDP), which is funded by the federal government, was created to facilitate successful transplants of hematopoietic cells from volunteer, unrelated donors as life-saving therapy for patients of all racial and socioeconomic backgrounds. Since its inception in 1987, more than 3 million volunteer donors have signed onto its registry. The NMDP is accelerating efforts to increase diversity of the registry and provides a free packet of information on bone marrow transplantation. Patients who need resources in this area can obtain help from the NMDP's Office of Patient Advocacy.

44. National Ovarian Cancer Coalition

2335 East Atlantic Boulevard, Suite 401
Pompano Beach, FL 33062
(954) 781-3500; (888) OVARIAN; FAX (954) 781-3525
Web site: www.ovarian.org

The National Ovarian Cancer Coalition (NOCC) was founded by ovarian cancer survivors in Boca Raton, FL, in response to the trivialization of and lack of attention to ovarian cancer throughout the media. In April 1995, it began a nationwide campaign to gain national recognition for this "silent killer." There are now 23 state chapters of NOCC. There are no required dues or fees for membership. NOCC's mission is to raise awareness about ovarian cancer and to promote education about this disease. By dispelling myths and misunderstandings, the coalition is committed to improve the overall survival and quality of life from ovarian cancer. Their goals are:

- To provide the medical community and general population with a national resource focused on ovarian cancer

- To provide complete and accurate information regarding ovarian cancer

- To obtain more funding for basic and clinical research, patient information, professional education, quality of life, and survivorship in ovarian cancer

- To develop and become a key part of a national alliance of organizations regarding ovarian cancer

- To develop a key strategic alliance within the community of oncology

45. National Prostate Cancer Coalition

1158 15th Street NW
Washington, DC 20005
(202) 463-9455; FAX (202) 463-9456
Web site: www.4npcc.org

The National Prostate Cancer Coalition (NPCC) is a national, grassroots advocacy group dedicated to finding a cure for prostate cancer and providing information on regulatory and legislative issues and referrals to resources for prostate cancer.

46. Oley Foundation

214 Hun Memorial, A-23
Albany Medical Center
Albany, NY 12208-3478
(518) 262-5079; (800) 776-6539 (OLEY);
FAX (518) 262-5528
Web site: www.wizvax.net/oleyfdn

The Oley Foundation is a nonprofit, tax-exempt organization established in 1983 to address the special needs of consumers (patients) home parenteral and/or enteral nutrition (homePEN). Since then, Oley has worked to build a homePEN community that fosters the sharing of information between consumers, clinicians, home care services, and third-party payers. By providing information and emotional support to consumers, Oley enhances the lives of those requiring home nutritional support. All of Oley's services and educational materials are provided at no charge to consumers and their caregivers.

Specific projects include:

- *Lifeline Letter*—a bimonthly newsletter written for home-PEN consumers, families, clinicians, researchers, and home care services

- Toll-free consumer networking—a networking tool that provides free access to a variety of experienced home-PEN consumers

- Regional coordinator network—a grassroots network of 70 volunteers (consumers of homePEN or caregivers) who run support groups and provide outreach and education at the local level

- HomePEN family network—a support network for children on homePEN therapy, their parents, and caregivers

- Annual summer conference—offers homePEN consumers, families, clinicians, home care professionals, and industry representatives an opportunity to share information on therapy updates and common experiences

- Information clearinghouse—designed to answer questions about homePEN, the clearinghouse makes a wealth of information available to consumers through a toll-free hotline and worldwide Web page

47. Project Inform

205 13th Street, #2001
San Francisco, CA 94103
(415) 558-8669; (800) 822-7422 (treatment hotline);
FAX (415) 558-0684
Web site: www.projinf.org

Founded in 1985, Project Inform is a national, nonprofit, community-based AIDS service organization dedicated to providing free, confidential information to persons infected with HIV or at risk for infection. Its mission includes:

- Providing vital information on the diagnosis and treatment of HIV disease to HIV-infected individuals, their caregivers, and their health care and service providers

- Advocating for enlightened regulatory, research, and funding policies, affecting the development of, access to, and delivery of effective treatments, as well as to fund innovative research opportunities

- Inspiring people to make informed choices amid uncertainty and to choose hope over despair

Free publications include:

> *The Introductory Treatment Packet*—vital information for people newly diagnosed with HIV
> *Fact Sheets*—about specific treatments, common infections, and strategies for maintaining health
> *PI Perspective*—provides information about recent clinical trials

Services include a national toll-free hotline, town meetings, and the Treatment Action Network, a lobbying group.

48. Ronald McDonald House Charities

1 Kroc Drive
Oak Brook, IL 60523
(630) 623-7048
Web site: www.rmhc.com

Ronald McDonald Houses are "homes away from home," temporary lodging facilities for the families of seriously ill children being treated at nearby children's hospitals. The houses provide an environment for emotional support to parents and siblings of sick children through a loving, caring, stable place they can call "home."

People helping people in times of serious need have made the Ronald McDonald House program what it is today, with over 150 local charities serving 27 countries. Each of the 197 houses in 16 countries is owned and operated by a local not-for-profit corporation composed of members of the medical community, McDonald's owner/operators, businesses and civic organizations, and parent volunteers. Each house raises money locally, as well as benefits from a general Ronald McDonald House fund. Families staying at a Ronald McDonald House are asked to make a donation ranging from $5 to $20 per day; if that is not possible, their stay is free. The average stay for a family is approximately nine days.

49. Skin Cancer Foundation
P.O. Box 561
New York, NY 10156
(212) 725-5176; (800) skin490; FAX (212) 725-5751
Web site: www.skincancer.org

The Skin Cancer Foundation, a nonprofit foundation, is the only national and international organization concerned solely with the world's most prevalent malignancy—cancer of the skin. The foundation conducts public and medical education programs and provides support for medical training and research to help reduce the incidence, morbidity, and mortality of skin cancer. The Skin Cancer Foundation has a variety of booklets, posters, slide presentations, and a video available regarding a multitude of issues. A contribution of $30 pays for a one-year subscription to *Sun & Skin News* (four issues, for public education) or *The Melanoma Letter* (four issues, for professional education). Write or call for a free catalogue, or send a self-addressed, stamped envelope for a sample of a specific brochure. Bulk orders for distribution are available for a fee.

The foundation's booklets include:

> *Sunproofing Your Baby*
> *Basal Cell Carcinoma—The Most Common Cancer*
> *The Many Faces of Malignant Melanoma*
> *Squamous Cell Carcinoma*
> *For Every Child Under the Sun: A Guide to Sensible Sun*
> *The ABCD's of Moles and Melanomas*
> *Dysplastic Nevi & Malignant Melanoma—A Patient's Guide*
> *Sun Sense*

50. Sunshine Foundation
2001 Bridge Street
Philadelphia, PA 19124
(215) 535-1413; (800) 767-1976; FAX (215) 535-8397
Web site: www.sunshinefoundation.org

This Philadelphia-based organization was founded in 1976 by former police officer Bill Sample to grant the dreams and wishes of chronically ill, terminally ill, abused, and handicapped children all over the country suffering from illnesses such as cancer, spina bifida, muscular dystrophy, sickle cell anemia, cystic fibrosis, AIDS, progeria, and many others. The Sunshine Foundation is a registered, nonprofit organization with 29 all-volunteer chapters throughout the United States. Since its inception in 1976, Sunshine Foundation has fulfilled the dreams and wishes of more than

24,500 children. Wish requests must be made in writing, with the child's name, age, and diagnosis specified, and mailed, emailed, or faxed to the foundation.

51. Sunshine Foundation Dream Village
5400 C.R. 547 North
P.O. Box 255
Loughman, FL 33858
(941) 424-4188; (800) 457-1976; FAX (941) 424-4360
Web site: www.sunshinefoundation.org/dreamvillage

On a 22-acre site just 15 minutes from the Magic Kingdom, the Sunshine Foundation has constructed a village where the dreams and wishes of chronically and terminally ill children are answered. Over 2000 special children have enjoyed this unique village, which is specifically designed with them in mind. Each of the seven gingerbread-style cottages has a fantasy theme in the child's bedroom. Special features include a pool with a ramp for wheelchair-dependent children, a handicapped accessible playground, and a game room. The Sunshine Foundation provides airfare, lodging, meals, and tickets to attractions for the child, parents, and all other children in the household. Families arrive on Thursday and depart on Monday.

52. Support for People with Oral and Head and Neck Cancer
P.O. Box 53
Locust Valley, NY 11560-0053
(516) 759-5333; FAX (516) 671-8794
Web site: www.spohnc.org

This is a not-for-profit organization involved in programs of support to provide information for oral and head and neck cancer patients who are trying to gain a better understanding of their illness and their lives. Their newsletter, *News from SPOHNC*, is published nine times yearly. The Web site includes a resource list, membership information, and an overview of many products that may be helpful to the patient with head and neck cancer.

53. Susan G. Komen Breast Cancer Foundation
5005 LBJ Freeway
Suite 370
Dallas, TX 75244
(972) 855-1600; (800) 462-9273; FAX (972) 855-1605
Web site: www.komen.org

The Susan G. Komen Breast Cancer Foundation was established in 1982 by Nancy Brinker to honor the memory of her sister, Susan G. Komen, who died of breast cancer. The foundation is a national organization with a network of volunteers working through local chapters and "Race for the Cure" events in 99 cities throughout the United States in 1999. Over $90 million has been raised to eradicate breast cancer as a life-threatening disease by advancing research, education, screening, and treatment. The Komen Foundation is the largest private funder in the country of research dedicated solely to breast cancer. Its toll-free Breast Care Helpline is answered by trained, caring volunteers who provide timely and accurate information (in English and Spanish) to callers with breast health and breast cancer concerns. They offer booklets, pamphlets, and educational materials, all at no cost for single copies. Much of the information is duplicated on the Web site.

54. United Ostomy Association
19772 MacArthur Blvd., Suite 200
Irvine, CA 92612-2405
(714) 660-8624; (800) 826-0826
Web site: www.uoa.org

The United Ostomy Association (UOA) is a volunteer-based health organization dedicated to providing education, information, support, and advocacy for people who have had or will have intestinal or urinary diversions. There are currently over 400 local chapters throughout the United States, composed primarily of ostomates who provide aid, moral support, and education to those who have a colostomy, ileostomy, or urostomy surgery. The chapter supplements the work of the surgeon by offering rehabilitation through follow-up by people who have learned to live with an ostomy. Trained members make visits to homes and hospitals, on request, with the prior consent of the patient's physician.

Chapters have medical advisory boards consisting of physicians, surgeons, and enterostomal therapists trained in ostomy care and the use of equipment. At regular monthly meetings, open to anyone who is interested, members can exchange practical, personal experiences about their ostomies, see ostomy equipment displayed, and hear speakers who are knowledgeable about ostomy. All local chapters are volunteer organizations. To locate a local chapter in the United States, Canada, or worldwide, contact the UOA by phone or visit their Web site. Annual chapter dues vary from no fee to $30. Each member of the UOA receives the *Ostomy Quarterly* magazine and is eligible to participate in the UOA insurance programs. Two UOA programs of significance are the scholarship fund for Enterostomal Therapy Education and the UOA Youth Rally, an annual conference for young people with ostomies.

The UOA has both publications and slide programs, which cover every aspect of ostomies. A sample of publications available from the UOA includes:

> *Ostomy Quarterly* (nonmembers, $25)
> *The Ostomy Book: Living Comfortably with Colostomies, Ileostomies, and Urostomies*
> *Coping with an Ostomy*
> *Ostomy Dietary Guidelines*
> *Anatomy of Ostomy*
> *So You Have/Will Have an Ostomy*
> *About Ostomy*
> *What Is an Ostomy . . . and Where Can I Get Help*
> *Introduction to Colostomy*
> *Introduction to Ileostomy*
> *Introduction to Urostomy*
> *Colostomy: A Guide* (also on audiocassette)
> *Ileostomy: A Guide* (also on audiocassette)
> *Urostomy: A Guide* (also on audiocassette)
> *Transverse Colostomy: A Guide*
> *Sex/Courtship/Single Ostomate*
> *Sex and the Female Ostomate*
> *Sex and the Male Ostomate*
> *Gay and Lesbian Ostomates and Their Caregivers*
> *My Child Has an Ostomy* (guide for unfamiliar caregivers)
> *Ostomy Care for Children*
> *The Continent Ileostomy*

55. US TOO International, Inc.
930 N. York Road, Suite 50
Hinsdale, IL 60521-2993
(630) 323-1002; (800) 808-7866; FAX (630) 323-1003
Web site: www.ustoo.com

US TOO, a not-for-profit organization incorporated in the state of Illinois, was created through the efforts of a small group of prostate cancer survivors. Since its inception, US TOO has been organized to be run for and by men with prostate disease. US TOO is an autonomous support organization dedicated to working in harmony with professional, business, and lay groups involved with prostate cancer to provide information and support for survivors and their families. The primary objectives of US TOO are:

- To increase awareness of prostate cancer, including political advocacy regarding governmental funding

- To provide education and support through literature, electronic means, and face-to-face support with men newly diagnosed with prostate cancer

- To involve men who have successfully treated their disease in the support of men newly diagnosed

- To support men with advanced disease by supplying the latest information about clinical trials and research developments

US TOO has initiated over 400 support groups in the United States and Canada, most of which can be identified on the Web site. Chapters are also available in Turkey, Europe, and Australia. At most meetings, a medical professional speaks on some phase of the diagnosis, staging, and/or treatment of prostate cancer or BPH (benign prostatic hypertrophy) topics. Participants also have the opportunity to discuss individual experiences that may be of interest to the group. All meetings are free of charge. Annual membership includes a suggested $25 donation and a subscription to their quarterly newsletter, *The Prostate Cancer COMMUNICATOR.*

56. V Foundation
1201 Walnut Street
2nd Floor
Cary, NC 27511
(800) 4-JIMMYV
Web site: www.jimmyv.org

The V Foundation is a charitable organization dedicated to saving lives by helping find a cure for cancer. It seeks to make a difference by generating broad-based support for cancer research through charity sports events and by creating an urgent awareness among all Americans of the importance of the war against cancer. The V Foundation performs these dual roles through advocacy, education, fundraising, and philanthropy. The V Foundation carries Jim Valvano's name and empowers others with his winning spirit, carrying on the creed he lived by, "Don't Give Up, Don't Ever Give Up!"

57. Wellness Community
National Executive Office
35 E. Seventh Street, Suite 412
Cincinnati, OH 45202
(888) 793-WELL; FAX (513) 421-7119
Web site: www.wellnesscommunity.org

The Wellness Community provides free psychosocial support services for adults with cancer and their families. Using a unique patient-active concept, the person with cancer learns how to participate, along with your health care team, in a fight toward recovery. There are 16 Wellness Communities throughout the United States. The Wellness Community is a tax-exempt, charitable corporation, and serves as an adjunct to conventional medical treatment.

The following services are provided:

- Orientation meetings: informal, drop-in groups held twice a week and led by people who have or have had cancer

- Networking groups: for people who share like diagnoses

- Participant groups: licensed psychotherapists lead two-hour group sessions once a week

- Family groups: licensed psychotherapists lead two-hour weekly group sessions composed of significant others of people with cancer in a participant group

- Relaxation/visualization: twice per week there are sessions where participants are taught how to involve themselves in the self-help procedures

- Educational workshops: each week, there are workshops presented by experts in matters such as voice dialogue, use of humor, moderate exercise, art therapy, journal writing, etc., or lectures by experts in the field of oncology

- Special groups: presented on an ongoing basis to consider specific areas of concern to cancer patients such as breast, prostate, and brain cancer networking; problems of parents with cancer; groups for couples to look at the problems of intimacy brought on by cancer

- The Wellness Connection: twice during the month, members of the Wellness Community who wish to remain connected to the community come together for support and socializing

- Social events: at least once a month, there are social gatherings such as seasonal parties, potlucks, charade nights, joke fests, sing-a-longs, and other events that bring participants together to laugh and play

58. **Y-ME National Breast Cancer Organization**
212 W. Van Buren, 4th Floor
Chicago, IL 60607-3908
(312) 986-8338 (business); (800) 986-9505 (Hispanic hotline);
(800) 221-2141 (national 24-hour hotline);
FAX (312) 986-0020
Web site: www.y-me.org

Founded in 1978 by Ann Marcou and Mimi Kaplan, two mastectomy patients, Y-ME National Breast Cancer Organization has a commitment to provide information and support to any man or woman who has been touched by breast cancer. It has become the largest breast cancer support program in the United States. It provides hotlines (staff and volunteers who have personally experienced breast cancer), presurgery counseling, open door groups, early detection workshops, and many local chapters. Trained male counselors are also available to talk to male partners of breast cancer patients. Y-ME also features a speakers bureau, resource library, wigs and prosthesis bank, and

inservice workshops for health care professionals. Volunteers are professionally supervised and the information provided to patients is monitored by a medical advisory board. Contributing members receive a bimonthly newsletter.

59. **YWCA of the U.S.A. ENCORE**plus® Program
Office of Women's Health Initiatives
624 Ninth Street, NW; 3rd Floor
Washington, DC 20001-5303
(202)628-3636; (800) 95E-PLUS; FAX (202) 783-7123
Web site: www.ywca.org/mission/health_care.html

ENCOREplus® Program is a system of health promotion through education, clinical service delivery, and patient "navigation" and advocacy. The community-based program targets women over age 50 in need of early detection education and breast and cervical cancer screening and support services. It also provides women in treatment for and recovering from breast cancer a unique combined peer support group and exercise program. The ENCOREplus® program is designed to eliminate inequalities in health care experienced by many women by removing barriers to access and promoting effective community-based outreach, education, referral to clinical services, and support systems. Essential building blocks of the ENCOREplus® program were the YWCA-CDC Collaborative Agreement in the National Breast and Cervical Cancer Early Detection Program (Title XV) and the Avon-YWCA partnership. As part of this collaboration, a portion of the proceeds from Avon's Breast Cancer Awareness Crusade was given to the YWCA from 1994–1997, enabling it to establish a decentralized ENCOREplus® training program and to fund ENCOREplus® programs at YWCAs in local communities.

Professional Organizations and Resources

60. **AIDS Action Council**
1875 Connecticut Avenue, NW, Suite 700
Washington, DC 20009
(202) 986-1300; FAX (202) 986-1345;
TDD (202) 332-9614
Web site: www.aidsaction.org

Established in 1984, AIDS Action Council is the only national organization solely dedicated to shaping federal HIV/AIDS policy, legislation, and funding. AIDS Action represents more than 3200 community-based HIV/AIDS organizations across the nation. AIDS Action Foundation, the council's sister organization, is a nonprofit 501(c)(3) organization. It supports and promotes the work of the council through policy research, media advocacy, information dissemination, and grassroots outreach and education. Foundation membership is $35 annually. Also, AIDS Action houses the Pedro Zamora Memorial Fund and convenes the coalition National Organizations Responding to AIDS (NORA), that includes more than 150 organizations advocating on a wide range of HIV/AIDS issues.

61. **American Academy of Pain Management**
13947 Mono Way, #A
Sonora, CA 95370
(209) 533-9744
Web site: www.aapainmanage.org

The academy is an innovative, interdisciplinary organization for pain practitioners. The academy serves as a credentialing society for practitioners in pain management. Membership benefits include a quarterly, peer-reviewed journal, *American Journal of Pain Management*, the *Pain Program Standard*, a copy of the *National Registry of Multidisciplinary Pain Practitioners*, and a *Directory of Pain Management Programs*.

62. American Academy of Pain Medicine
4700 West Lake Avenue
Glenview, IL 60025-1485
(847) 375-4731; FAX (847) 375-4777
Web site: www.painmed.org

The American Academy of Pain Medicine (AAPM) is the official organization representing physicians in the field of pain in the United States. It is a specialty society recognized by the American Medical Association (AMA). Its mission is to provide quality care to patients suffering with pain through the education and training of all physicians through research and through the advancement of the specialty of pain medicine. In working to achieve this mission, AAPM's goals are to promote a socioeconomic and political climate conducive to the practice of pain medicine in an effective and efficient manner, and to ensure quality and comprehensive medical care by physicians specializing in chronic pain medicine to patients in need of such services. Members represent a variety of disciplines, including anesthesiology, neurology, neurosurgery, orthopedic surgery, physiatry, and psychiatry. The benefits of membership ($325 annually) in AAPM include the following:

- Membership directory, listing primary care and specialty physicians with an interest in pain medicine

- Subscriptions to the *Clinical Journal of Pain*, the official AAPM journal

- Special rates on all AAPM activities and products, such as annual meetings and review course

- AAPM awards recognition program

63. American Alliance of Cancer Pain Initiatives Resource Center
1300 University Avenue, Room 4720
Madison, WI 53706
(608) 265-4013; FAX (608) 265-4014
Web site: www.aacpi.org

The Cancer Pain Initiative concept originated in Wisconsin in 1987 and has become a significant force for change in the way cancer pain is managed in the American health care system. Initiatives are now present in all 50 states in various stages of development. The mission of this organization is to promote cancer pain relief nationwide. Each initiative is composed of nurses, physicians, pharmacists, and representatives of clinical care facilities who offer training, information, and organizational support to health care providers, cancer patients, and their families. A complete listing of each state cancer pain initiative is available on the Web site.

64. American Association for Cancer Education, Inc.
Robert M. Chamberlain, PhD
Department of Epidemiology, University of Texas
MD Anderson Cancer Center
1515 Holcombe Boulevard, P.O. Box 189
Houston, TX 77030-4095
(713) 792-3020; FAX (713) 792-0807
Email:
RCHAMBERLAIN@REQUEST.MDA.UTH.TMC.EDU

The purpose of this association is "to provide a forum for those concerned with education of groups who attempt to advance the cause of early cancer detection, promote individualized multimodality therapy, or develop programs of rehabilitation for cancer patients." This multidisciplinary organization brings together basic scientists, surgeons, internists, oncology nursing educators, pediatricians, pathologists, gynecologists, dentists, and radiation oncologists. They hold an annual fall meeting.

The official journal of the association is the *Journal of Cancer Education* and is listed in *Index Medicus*. The association has occasionally sponsored other publications such as *Concepts in Cancer Medicine*, edited by S. Benham Kahn, MD, et al, and *Self-Assessment of Current Knowledge in Oncology*, edited by John Foley, MD. The association also distributes a *President's Newsletter*, and abstracts accepted for presentation at the annual meeting are published as *Supplement to the Journal of Cancer Education*.

The American Association for Cancer Education does not produce or distribute cancer education materials.

65. American Association for Cancer Research
Margaret Foti, Executive Director
Public Ledger Building
620 Chestnut Street, Suite 816
Philadelphia, PA 19106
(215) 440-9000; FAX (215) 440-9313
Web site: www.aacr.org

The American Association for Cancer Research (AACR) is the world's largest professional society of scientists specializing in both basic and clinical cancer research. Its 15,000 members are experts in the areas of molecular biology and genetics of cancer, tumor biology, virology, carcinogenesis, toxicology and risk assessment, endocrinology, epidemiology and prevention, pharmacology and therapeutics, immunology, and all aspects of clinical investigations pertaining to human cancer. The four journals of the association are: *Cancer Research; Clinical Cancer Research; Cancer Epidemiology, Biomarkers and Prevention*; and *Cell Growth and Differentiation*, The organization sponsors several scientific conferences each year on new and significant developments in research. AACR also offers educational workshops and grants to young investigators, maintains an active public education program, and interacts frequently with cancer survivors, lay advocates, and the general public in support of its mission.

66. American Cancer Society
1599 Clifton Road, NE
Atlanta, GA 30329-4251
(800) ACS-2345
Web site: www.cancer.org

The American Cancer Society is a nationwide, voluntary health organization dedicated to eliminating cancer as a major health problem by preventing cancer, saving lives from cancer, and diminishing suffering from cancer through research, education, and service. The society offers scholarships to interested oncology nurses at both the master's and doctoral level. The scholarships provide a stipend of $8000 per year for a maximum of two years for a master's degree in nursing and $8000 per year for a maximum of four years for a doctoral degree in nursing or related areas.

67. American Foundation for AIDS Research
120 Wall Street, 13th Floor
New York, NY 10005
(212) 806-1600; FAX (212) 806-1601
Web site: www.amfar.org

The American Foundation for AIDS Research (AmFAR) is the nation's leading nonprofit organization dedicated to the support of AIDS research (both biomedical and clinical research), AIDS prevention, and the advocacy of sound AIDS-related public policy. Since it started in 1985, AmFAR has invested nearly $155 million in support for its programs, primarily through grants to 1750 research teams and education projects. AmFAR is dedicated to mobilizing the good will, energy, and generosity of caring Americans to end the AIDS epidemic.

AmFAR sponsors a number of publications, including:

- *AIDS/HIV Clinical Trial Handbook* (English & Spanish) answers the most frequently asked questions about participating in clinical trials in easy-to-understand, non-technical language

- *AIDS/HIV Treatment Directory*, published biannually, a comprehensive source of information on approved and experimental treatments for HIV infection and HIV-related disorders, opportunistic infections, and preventive vaccine development

- *AIDS: Reflections . . . Responses*, a journal in commemoration of World AIDS Day 1996; includes short biographies of five AmFAR honorees, as well as essays by noted authors; copies are reserved for new members joining AmFAR's philanthropic leadership group, Partners for the Cure.

68. American Hospital Association Resource Center
One N. Franklin, 28th Floor
Chicago, IL 60606
(312) 422-2000; FAX (312) 422-4700
Web site: www.aha.org/resource/

The American Hospital Association (AHA) Resource Center is designed to assist in accessing timely, high-quality health services information and is a vital tool for health care leaders. Highly trained information specialists are available to locate and retrieve information quickly. A document delivery service draws from the comprehensive collections and extensive networks. An on-line catalog for books, journals, and other publications in the resource center collection is available. The AHA publishes an annual catalogue of monographs and audiovisual products available; with a section designated for nursing resources.

69. American Institute for Cancer Research
1759 R Street NW
Washington, DC 20009
(202) 328-7744; (800) 843-8114; FAX (202) 328-7226
Web site: www.aicr.org

The American Institute for Cancer Research (AICR) is a national cancer charity supported by public donations, not by the federal government. The AICR is the nation's leading charity in the field of diet, nutrition, and cancer prevention. The AICR does not directly carry out research, but rather provides funding for research at leading universities, hospitals, and research centers throughout the United States, as well as other countries. All funded grants have gone through a peer-review process that meets the standards of the federal government's National Cancer Institute. A list of recent research grants is available on the AICR Web site.

70. American Organization of Nurse Executives (AONE)
One N. Franklin, 34th Floor
Chicago, IL 60606
(312) 422-2800; FAX (312) 422-4503
Web site: www.aone.org

The American Organization of Nurse Executives (AONE) is dedicated to the stewardship of health policy, and to the professional development of nurse leaders, and serves as the voice of nursing leadership for the American Hospital Association. AONE initiatives at the national level are reinforced through the activities of more than 60 chapters at the state and metropolitan levels. The organization achieves its objective through a spirit of collaboration. Benefits of AONE membership include:

- Opportunities for education, networking, and information exchange through conferences, seminars, teleconference, and the AONE annual meeting

- A comprehensive on-line membership directory

- Access to the AONE Career Center, a referral center for personal and professional support

- A newsletter, *AONE Updates*, every three weeks

Other publications include the AONE Leadership Series, *Navigate Your Career Transition: Strategies for Nurse Leaders*, and *Restructuring: The Impact of Hospital Organization on Nursing Leadership*. Annual membership is $200.

71. American Pain Society
4700 W. Lake Avenue
Glenview, IL 60025
(847) 375-4715; FAX (847) 375-6315
Web site: www.ampainsoc.org

The American Pain Society (APS), a national chapter of the International Association for the Study of Pain (IASP), is a multidisciplinary, not-for-profit educational organization that welcomes broad participation from all disciplines. The mission of APS is to serve people in pain by advancing research, education, treatment, and professional practice. This goal can best be accomplished as a joint and interactive effort among basic scientists and health care professionals. APS was founded in 1979 and has grown to more than 2000 members. Over the years, APS has expanded its programming and publications to meet the needs of its membership.

The society publishes *Pain Forum*, a quarterly journal that provides a forum for the scholarly presentation and discussion of issues; the *APS Bulletin*, a bimonthly publication that offers feature articles on clinical and basic science topics, organizational news, and a calendar of events (can also be viewed on-line); and *Principles of Analgesic Use in the Treatment of Acute Pain and Cancer Pain* (ed 4), a concise, compact, easily accessible reference guide for nurses and medical students ($7/nonmembers). The Web site offers access to information about the society's annual meeting, other publications, and membership benefits.

72. **American Society for Parenteral and Enteral Nutrition ASPEN**
8630 Fenton Street, Suite 412
Silver Spring, MD 20910
(301) 587-6315; FAX (301) 587-2365
Web site: www.clinnutr.org

The American Society for Parenteral and Enteral Nutrition (ASPEN) is a professional organization whose members are involved in the provision of clinical nutrition therapies, including parenteral and enteral nutrition. Its nearly 6000 members are physicians, nurses, dietitians, pharmacists, scientists, and other allied health professionals. ASPEN prepares standards and guidelines for the use of nutrition support and professional practice. Certification is available through the National Board for Nutrition Support Certification, Inc. The Web site offers information about publications, professional development, research, and a local chapter directory.

73. **American Society for Therapeutic Radiology and Oncology**
12500 Fair Lakes Circle, Suite 375
Fairfax, VA 22033-1550
(703) 502-1550; FAX (703) 502-7852
Web site: www.astro.org

The American Society for Therapeutic Radiology and Oncology (ASTRO) consists of American Board of Radiology certified physicians, radiation therapists, and radiation biologists whose professional practice is therapeutic radiology. The organization strives to disseminate the results of scientific research, promote excellence in patient care, and provide opportunities for educational and professional development. The Web site has a section for members, as well as one for patient/public education that includes an overview of radiation therapy and information specific to prostate cancer and breast cancer. Answers to frequently asked questions provide patients with the information they need to choose the treatment that is best for them.

74. **American Society of Clinical Oncology (ASCO)**
225 Reinekers Lane, Suite 650
Alexandria, VA 22314
(703) 299-0150; (888) 282-2552; FAX (703) 299-1044
Web site: www.asco.org

The American Society of Clinical Oncology (ASCO) promotes and fosters the exchange of information related to neoplastic diseases (with particular emphasis on human biology, diagnosis, and treatment) for physicians throughout the United States and other countries who are academically based or in private practice. ASCO publishes the *Journal of Clinical Oncology*, and sponsors two conferences annually. The ASCO Web site offers a Virtual Meeting, Continuing Medical Education opportunities, and a career resource center.

75. **American Society of Hematology (ASH)**
1200 19th Street, NW, Suite 300
Washington, DC 20036-2422
(202) 857-1118; FAX (202) 857-1164
Web site: www.hematology.org

The American Society of Hematology (ASH) is a professional organization representing over 9500 clinicians and scientists committed to promoting and fostering the exchange and diffusion of information and ideas relating to blood, blood-forming tissues, and blood diseases. The ASH newsletter, produced for society members three times per year, offers relevant articles on a variety of topics related to the field of hematology and Society activities and is available on-line. In addition, membership includes a subscription to *BLOOD*, the official journal of the society, which is published 24 times a year. The ASH Web site offers information about the annual meeting, educational materials, and training programs.

76. **Association for the Care of Children's Health**
P.O. Box 25707
Alexandria, VA 22313
(800) 808-ACCH
Web site: www.acch.org

The Association for the Care of Children's Health (ACCH) is an educational and advocacy organization. ACCH membership includes more than 250 hospitals, other health care facilities and organizations, and over 3000 multidisciplinary health care professionals, family members, and friends of children with special health care needs. ACCH members work within their institutions, organizations, and communities to promote improved systems of health care for children and their families.

ACCH:

- Produces educational materials
- Plans and coordinates Children and Healthcare Week each year
- Publishes *Children's Health Care*, a quarterly research-based journal
- Publishes *ACCH News*
- Provides services to designers and architects, and for chaplains who are responsive to the unique needs of children and families in a health care setting
- Provides information, referral, and support through a clearinghouse for professionals and families of children with disabilities and special health needs

The mission of ACCH focuses on family-centered care, and acknowledges diverse perspectives, encourages innovation, and promotes healing through synergistic cooperation. ACCH has many educational resources, including publications and videos, for professionals, children, and families. The ACCH Web site can be used to obtain an updated list of available items.

77. Association of American Cancer Institutes (AACI)
Barbara Duffy Stewart, Executive Director
University of Pittsburgh Cancer Institute
200 Lothrop, 305 Iroquois Bldg.
Pittsburgh, PA 15213
(412) 647-2076; FAX (412) 647-3659

The Association of American Cancer Institutes (AACI) was originally established in 1959 as the Association of Cancer Institute Directors. In 1973 the organization was incorporated as the AACI. Today, nearly 100 cancer centers throughout the United States are members of the AACI; several cancer centers throughout the world are corresponding members.

The AACI provides an organization structure to carry out the following objectives:

- Afford an opportunity for the leadership of cancer institutes and centers throughout the world to meet and discuss mutual problems

- Foster collaboration via state, regional, national, and international programs for the control of cancer through research, education, and service

- Support investigations into the causes, nature, prevention, and treatment of cancer and the rehabilitation of cancer patients by encouraging the exchange of ideas, information, personnel, and the provision of special facilities and training opportunities

- Foster educational and training opportunities in the related biomedical sciences

- Provide guidance to federal, state, and local governments, private and civic organizations concerning cancer research, diagnosis, treatment and prevention, and the rehabilitation of cancer patients

78. Association of Community Cancer Centers (ACCC)
11600 Nebel Street, Suite 201
Rockville, MD 20852-2557
(301) 984-9496; FAX (301) 770-1949
Web site: www.assoc-cancer-ctrs.org

The Association of Community Cancer Centers (ACCC) acts as the national voice of community multidisciplinary cancer care professionals. It serves as a forum on national issues and a source of information on policy, management, and financing issues related to oncology. Members include institutions and individuals from every facet of professional oncology practice. The association hosts an annual national meeting, an oncology economics conference, and regional oncology symposia.

The association's publications include:

> *Oncology Issues,* a bimonthly publication available to members as a benefit; subscriptions for nonmembers are $20 per year
> *Community Cancer Programs in the United States,* the annual ACCC membership list
> *Cancer DRGs: A Comparative Report on Key Cancer DRGs*
> *Standards for Cancer Programs* (out-of-print, available on-line)
> *Cancer Treatments Your Insurance Should Cover*
> *The Compendia-Based Drug Bulletin*

79. Association of Freestanding Radiation Oncology Centers
1550 S. Coast Highway, Suite 201
Laguna Beach, CA 92651
(888) 442-3762; FAX (949) 376-3456
Web site: www.afroc.org

The Association of Freestanding Radiation Oncology Centers (AFROC) is a nonprofit organization composed of physicists, physicians, administrators, technicians, and clinical personnel working in freestanding, fully equipped radiation centers. It acts as a forum for addressing concerns and as an advocate for reimbursement and legislative policies affecting the centers. Full membership is $500, and benefits include the quarterly newsletter, *Source;* legislative information; reduced rates at the annual meeting; and current information on reimbursement, economic issues, practice development/marketing ideas, financial management, and quality assurance.

80. Association of Nurses in AIDS Care (ANAC)
11250 Roger Bacon Drive, Suite 8
Reston, VA 20190-5202
(800) 260-6780; (703) 925-0081; FAX (703) 435-4390
Web site: www.anacnet.org/aids

The Association of Nurses in AIDS Care (ANAC) has members throughout the United States and Canada plus a growing international membership. The mission of ANAC is to promote the individual and collective professional development of nurses involved in the delivery of health care to people infected or affected by the human immunodeficiency virus (HIV) and to promote the health, welfare, and rights of all HIV infected individuals.

The members of ANAC strive to achieve their mission by:

- Creating an effective network among nurses in HIV/AIDS care

- Studying, researching, and exchanging information, experiences, and ideas leading to improved care for persons with AIDS/HIV infection

- Providing leadership to the nursing community in matters related to AIDS/HIV infection

- Advocating for HIV infected persons

- Promoting social awareness concerning issues related to HIV/AIDS

Inherent in these goals is the abiding commitment to the prevention of further HIV infection. Membership in ANAC entitles members to the *Journal of the Association of Nurses in AIDS Care,* published quarterly; the *Newsletter of the Association of Nurses in AIDS Care,* published quarterly; monographs and position statements on issues affecting health professionals; and discounted educational meetings.

81. Association of Pediatric Oncology Nurses (APON)
4700 W. Lake Avenue
Glenview, IL 60025-1485
(847) 375-4724; FAX (847) 375-4777
Web site: www.apon.org

The Association of Pediatric Oncology Nurses (APON) has been in existence since 1973. Membership in the organization is open to all registered nurses who are either interested in or engaged in pediatrics or pediatric oncology. Annual dues are $85, which entitles the member to receive a copy of the quarterly, peer-reviewed *Journal of the Association of Pediatric Oncology Nurses, aponCounts*, a quarterly newsletter, and other pertinent publications; to attend all business meetings and programs at a reduced rate; and to vote on all issues concerning the organization.

APON strives to improve the care given to children who have cancer and their families by:

- Promoting excellence in the specialty of pediatric oncology nursing

- Providing quality publications focusing on pediatric oncology nursing

- Promoting communication and collegial exchange among nurses caring for pediatric oncology patients and their families

- Encouraging dissemination of information among nurses about the medical and nursing care of pediatric oncology patients that is used in various areas of the country

- Encouraging members to contribute to professional and lay literature with regard to nursing care of pediatric oncology patients and their families

- Providing quality national and regional educational programs

- Promoting implementation of the scope and standards of pediatric oncology nursing practice developed by APON

- Providing liaison with other organizations whose membership may influence the care given to pediatric oncology patients and their families

- Promoting a positive image of pediatric oncology nursing and its effect on the care of pediatric oncology patients and their families

- Supporting local, state, and national legislation affecting the care of pediatric oncology patients and their families and legislation pertaining to the profession of nursing

APON has several publications for purchase by both members and nonmembers: *Essentials of Pediatric Oncology Nursing: A Core Curriculum; Nursing Care of the Child with Cancer; Pharmacologic Agents in Pediatric Oncology Nursing;* and *Scope of Practice and Outcome Standards of Pediatric Oncology Nursing.*

82. Cancer Research Institute
681 Fifth Avenue
New York, NY 10022
(800) 99-CANCER
Web site: www.cancerresearch.org

The Cancer Research Institute (CRI) supports leading-edge research aimed at developing new methods of diagnosing, treating, and preventing cancer. The purpose of CRI is to:

- Fund basic research that will yield breakthrough findings in cancer immunology

- Fund clinical studies that will transform such findings into safe and effective immunotherapies for cancer

- Support research in other therapeutic areas that are synergistic with immunotherapy

- Function as a source of public information on cancer immunology and cancer treatment

Information about funding programs is available on-line. Other cancer information documents available on-line are *Cancer and the Immune System; HelpBook: What to Do if Cancer Strikes; What to Do if Prostate Cancer Strikes;* and *Conquering Melanoma: Prevent It, Spot It, Treat It.*

83. Commission on Accreditation of Rehabilitation Facilities
4891 E. Grant Road
Tucson, AZ 85712
(520) 325-1044; FAX (520) 318-1129
Web site: www.carf.org

The fundamental commitment of the Commission on Accreditation of Rehabilitation Facilities (CARF) is to provide quality services to people with disabilities and others in need of rehabilitation. The commission is the recognized authority that accredits organizations and programs in the areas of adult day services, medical rehabilitation, behavioral health (alcohol and other drug and mental health), and employment and community services. CARF develops and maintains practical and relevant standards of quality for such programs. The standards are developed by the field, which consists of the persons served, rehabilitation professionals, and purchasers of services, and are applied through a peer-review process to determine how well an organization is serving its consumers. The goal of these programs is to make a positive difference in the lives of people with disabilities and others in need of rehabilitation as they strive to attain optimal self-sufficiency, independence, and productivity.

The commission began in 1966. It is a private, not-for-profit organization that has had the benefit of a broad base of support and involvement on the part of consumers, providers, and purchasers of specialized services for people with disabilities and others in need of rehabilitation. The commission's success is directly attributed to the profound impact it has had on the provision of quality-oriented rehabilitation services.

A variety of materials can be purchased from CARF and include:

> *Adult Day Services Standards Manual* ($100)
> *ADS Survey Preparation Guide* ($55)
> *Behavioral Health Standards Manual* ($120)
> *BH Survey Preparation Guide* ($60)
> *Employment and Community Services Standards Manual* ($100)
> *ECS Survey Preparation Guide* ($55)
> *Medical Rehabilitation Standards Manual* ($150)
> *MRS Survey Preparation Guide* ($75)
> *Accessibility in CARF-Accredited Organizations: A Resource Guide to Understanding the ADA* ($40)
> *CARF Directory of Organizations with Accredited Programs* ($100)

84. Gynecologic Cancer Foundation
401 N. Michigan Avenue
Chicago, IL 60611
(312) 644-6610; FAX (312) 527-6640
Web site: www.wcn.org

The Gynecologic Cancer Foundation (GCF) is a not-for-profit fund-raising organization established by the Society of Gynecologic Oncologists (SGO) to support ovarian cancer research, training of cancer specialists in laboratory research, and a variety of programs for patient education and public awareness of gynecologic cancers. Calls to (800) 444-4441 will enable an individual to obtain a list of nearby specialists, a nationwide directory of all SGO members, and informational literature. The GCF also sponsors an interactive internet Web site—the Women's Cancer Network. It offers understandable medical information about gynecologic cancers, treatment options, and experimental therapeutic programs. By answering specific questions a woman will be told her risk for developing specific cancers and how to lessen risk, and be advised about appropriate diagnostic tests.

85. **Hospice and Palliative Nurses Association**
Medical Center East, Suite 375
211 N. Whitfield St.
Pittsburgh, PA 15206-3031
(412) 361-2470; FAX (412) 361-2425
Web site: www.hpna.org

This association exists to exchange information, experiences, and ideas; to promote understanding of the specialties of hospice and palliative nursing; and to study and promote hospice and palliative nursing research. Membership provides certification opportunities, a subscription to the *Journal of Hospice and Palliative Nursing*, and opportunities for networking and support through regional groups.

86. **International Association for the Study of Pain**
909 NE 43rd Street, Suite 306
Seattle, WA 98105-6020
(206) 547-6409; FAX (206) 547-1703
Web site: www.halcyon.com/iasp

The International Association for the Study of Pain (IASP) was founded in 1973 and was incorporated in 1974 as a nonprofit organization to:

- Foster and encourage research of pain mechanisms and pain syndromes and to help improve the management of patients with acute and chronic pain by bringing together basic scientists, physicians, and other health professionals of various disciplines and backgrounds who have interest in pain research and management

- Promote education and training in the field of pain

- Promote and facilitate the dissemination of new information in the field of pain, including sponsorship of a journal, *PAIN*

- Promote and sponsor a triennial world congress of the association and such other meetings as may be useful or desirable for the advancement of the purposes of IASP

- Encourage formation of national associations for the study and treatment of pain

- Encourage the adoption of a uniform classification, nomenclature, and definition regarding pain and pain syndromes

- Encourage the development of a national and international data bank and to encourage the development of a uniform records system with respect to information relating to pain mechanisms, syndromes, and management

- Inform the general public of results and implications of current research in the area

- Advise international, national, and regional agencies of standards relating to the use of drugs, appliances, and other procedures in the therapy of pain

- Engage in such other activities as may be incidental to or in furtherance of the aforementioned purposes.

Active membership in IASP is open to scientists, physicians, dentists, psychologists, nurses, physical therapists, and other health professionals actively engaged in pain research and those who have special interest in the diagnosis and treatment of pain syndromes. The association currently has 6300 members in 86 countries, and independent chapters in over 50 countries. IASP holds a world congress every three years and has established a program of special interest groups (SIGs) designed to enable members to have a forum to discuss specific interests in the pain field in depth.

IASP has numerous publications available for professional use including a monthly journal, *PAIN*; a bimonthly newsletter; *Pain: Clinical Updates*, published three times a year; and *Core Curriculum for Professional Education in Pain*. Other publications and information about membership can be accessed on the Web site.

87. **International Cancer Alliance**
4853 Cordell Avenue, Suite 11
Bethesda, MD 20814
(800) ICARE-61; (301) 654-7933; FAX (301) 654-8684
Web site: www.icare.org

The International Cancer Alliance provides a free cancer therapy review that includes information on a specific type of cancer (description, detection and staging, treatment, diagnostic tests, and clinical trials). *Cancer Breakthroughs* report is published quarterly.

88. **International Myeloma Foundation**
2129 Stanley Hills Drive
Los Angeles, CA 90046
(800) 452-CURE; FAX (323) 656-1182
Web site: www.myeloma.org

The International Myeloma Foundation (IMF) is a nonprofit organization dedicated to improving the quality of life for multiple myeloma patients while working toward prevention and cure. The IMF promotes education for both physicians and patients regarding myeloma, its treatment, and management. The foundation funds research, holds clinical and scientific conferences, and publishes a quarterly newsletter, *Myeloma Today*. There is an on-line support group for patients on the IMF Web site.

89. **International Society of Nurses in Cancer Care (ISNCC)**
Greater London House
Hampstead Road
London NW1 7EJ Great Britain
44(171) 874-0289; FAX 44(171) 874-0290
Web site: www.isncc.org

Established in 1984, the society aims to:

- Provide a communication network for national and regional oncology nursing societies

- Provide regular communication on developments in cancer nursing throughout the world
- Assist in establishing national and/or regional oncology nursing groups
- Serve as a link with other organizations to promote and disseminate advances in cancer care

The society is comprised of full members (National Oncology Nursing Societies); associate members (cancer-related institutions and agencies); and sustaining members (corporations or businesses). Every two years the society hosts an international conference on cancer nursing. This conference attracts approximately 2000 nurses from over 60 countries to gain knowledge and share expertise and skills tailored to their own level of experience. The society is a nongovernmental organization affiliate of the World Health Organization, and an affiliate member of the International Council of Nursing.

It publishes a quarterly newsletter, *International Cancer Nursing News*. Position statements and resources can be found on the Society's Web site.

90. **International Union Against Cancer**
(Union Internationale Contre Le Cancer—UICC)
3, rue du Conseil General
1205 Geneva, Switzerland
(4122) 809-1811; FAX (4122) 809-1810
Web site: www.uicc.org

The International Union Against Cancer is a nonprofit, nonsectarian, nongovernmental association of about 280 multidisciplinary cancer organizations in about 80 countries devoted exclusively to all aspects of the worldwide fight against cancer. Its objectives are to advance scientific and medical knowledge in research, diagnosis, treatment, and prevention of cancer and to promote all other aspects of the campaign against cancer. Particular emphasis is placed on professional and public education. The union organizes a congress every four years. It publishes the *International Journal of Cancer* and a quarterly newsletter. A departmental and personnel directory is available on-line, as is a complete listing of other available publications.

91. **Intravenous Nurses Society**
Fresh Pond Square
10 Fawcett Street
Cambridge, MA 02138
(617) 441-3008; FAX (617) 441-3009
Web site: www.ins1.org

The Intravenous Nurses Society (INS) is the national nonprofit professional association for nurses involved in the delivery of intravenous therapies. Membership fee is $90 (1999) and includes the *Journal of Intravenous Nursing*, and *INS Newsline*, a bimonthly newsletter. Founded in 1973, the society is dedicated to advancing the delivery of quality intravenous therapy through stringent standards of practice and professional ethics, promoting research and education in the intravenous specialty. The Intravenous Nursing Certification Corporation provides certification opportunities.

92. **Lymphoma Research Foundation of America, Inc.**
8800 Venice Blvd., #207
Los Angeles, CA 90034
(310) 204-7040; FAX (310) 204-7043
Web site: www.lymphoma.org

The foundation funds research grants for projects seeking to cure lymphoma or improve the treatment of lymphoma. It also provides educational materials, free support groups and helpline, a national "buddy system" linking patients, and a quarterly newsletter. Information about membership and products are available on-line.

93. **National AIDS Fund**
1400 I Street NW, Suite 1220
Washington, DC 20005
(202) 408-4848; FAX (202) 408-1818
Web site: www.aidsfund.org

The National AIDS Fund has provided grants totaling over $70 million to local communities for planning and service provision in response to the U.S. HIV epidemic in the past decade. The National AIDS Fund is dedicated to eliminating HIV disease as a major health and social problem. They work in partnership with the public and private sectors to provide care and to prevent new infections—through advocacy, grantmaking, research, and education—in communities and in the workplace. Two publications, *What You Should Know About Returning to Work Before Talking with Your Disability Provider* and *Managing Returning "Disabled" Employees: What Every Employer Should Know*, are available for a nominal fee.

94. **National Cancer Registrars Association (NCRA)**
8310 Nieman Road
P.O. Box 15945-295
Lenexa, KS 66285-5945
(913) 438-6272; FAX (913) 541-0156
Web site: www.ncra-usa.org

The National Cancer Registrars Association (NCRA), chartered in 1974 and incorporated in 1976, is a nonprofit professional organization whose purposes are to establish standards of education for cancer registrars; to inform its members of the latest methods of cancer diagnosis, treatment, and current trends in incidence and survival; and to make cancer patient data readily available for clinical and epidemiological research. NCRA has almost 3000 members. It offers a certification examination semiannually. Individuals who pass the examination become Certified Tumor Registrars (CTRs). Inquiries regarding certifications should be directed to NCRA's home office. Membership benefits include the *Journal of Registry Management*, published quarterly.

95. **National Coalition for Cancer Research**
c/o Capitol Associates Incorporated
426 C Street, NE
Washington, DC 20002
(202) 544-1880; FAX (202) 543-2565
Web site: www.cancercoalition.org

The National Coalition for Cancer Research (NCCR), a nonprofit coalition of national organizations, was founded in 1986. The NCCR is dedicated to the eradication of cancer through a vigorous public and privately supported research effort. The coalition focuses its public education efforts on public policies that support and foster the U.S. position as the world leader in medical research and development and innovation.

The NCCR represents:

- Thousands of cancer survivors and their families

- 40,000 children with cancer as well as their parents, brothers, and sisters

- 65,000 cancer researchers, nurses, physicians, and health care workers

- 82 cancer research centers

- Publicly supported nonprofit organizations that provide patient services, research grants, and education

- Patient and consumer groups dedicated to fostering a broad-based public and governmental commitment to the well-being of persons with cancer

The motto of the NCCR epitomizes its mission—"Research Cures Cancer." The collaborative actions of the key organizations in the cancer community are designed to:

- Support public education efforts that communicate the critical relationship between vigorous national support of cancer research and progress against cancer

- Advocate for funding of a balanced national cancer research program to improve cancer detection, diagnosis, treatment, survivorship, and prevention

- Cooperate with other organizations in support of public health policies that will support the coalition's mission

- Communicate the contributions that cancer research has made to the reduction of cancer morbidity and mortality and improvement in quality of life for cancer patients and survivors

The coalition's mission is to provide a forum for a group of diverse cancer-concerned organizations to advance cancer research through collaborative action in such areas as public education and advocacy, leading to the eradication of cancer and its effects. Among its 23 members are ACS, ASCO, ONS, AACR, ASH, and NCCF.

96. **National Hospice Organization (NHO)**
1901 North Moore Street
Suite 901
Arlington, VA 22209
(703) 243-5900; (800) 658-8898 (hospice helpline);
FAX (703) 525-5762
Web site: www.nho.org

Established in 1978, the National Hospice Organization (NHO) is a nonprofit organization promoting quality care to the terminally ill and their significant others. NHO has worked over the past decade to establish hospice as a part of the health care delivery system in the United States. As a result of its efforts, hospice is now included as a Medicare/Medicaid benefit and as an employee benefit for 80% of U.S. workers in medium- and large-sized business. Most hospices are members of NHO and receive NHO's technical assistance, education programs and events, publications, and advocacy and referral services. The organization sponsors an annual symposium. The *Hospice Professional*, published quarterly, and *NHO News-Line*, published twice monthly, are membership benefits.

NHO membership includes 2400 hospices and 5000 individuals.

97. **National League for Nursing**
61 Broadway
New York, NY 10006
(800) 669-9656; FAX (607) 723-8408
Web site: www.nln.org

The National League for Nursing (NLN) advances quality nursing education that prepares the nursing workforce to meet the needs of diverse populations in an ever-changing health care environment.

The *NLN Journal: Nursing and Health Care Perspectives* is the official publication of the NLN. Formerly known as *Nursing & Health Care*, the journal is published six times a year.

There are two subsidiaries of the NLN:

- Community Health Accreditation Program (CHAP) ensures the quality of community and home health agencies at the core of national and international efforts to transform health care. Effective dependable health care available and accessible for all communities, whatever the economic or social status of its members, is of paramount concern.

- National League for Nursing Accrediting Commission (NLNAC) is responsible for the accreditation of nursing education and programs.

In 1991, the Field Institute for Technology in Nursing Education (FITNE) and NLN published the fourth edition of the *Directory of Educational Software for Nursing*, which provides information for anyone interested in using a computer to teach nursing. There are complete descriptions and purchasing information for over 300 computer-assisted instruction (CAI) programs. Included are 100 new CAI programs for IBM and Apple Macintosh computers. Ratings were done by more than 2500 health care professionals; there are several oncology-related programs listed in this directory. Publication No. 41-2405 ($79.95).

98. **Nursing Pain Association**
Pain Study Office, N411Y, Box 0606
School of Nursing
University of California
San Francisco, CA 94143
(415) 476-4040

The purpose of the organization is to foster and promote education, research, and high standards of practice in the care of patients with pain, and to emphasize the application of pain research findings to nursing care by:

- Improving the quality of nursing care provided to the patient in pain

- Providing opportunities for members to continue their growth as pain specialists

- Providing a forum for networking among members

- Providing continuing pain education to nurse colleagues

- Promoting nursing research related to pain

Membership benefits include:

Pain education programs

Annual Bay Area conference in California—reduced fee

Regular members' meetings—no charge

Dinners (informal, social/professional, networking)

Referral service:

Professional network—identify local and national experts for a specific pain problem

Direct individuals to current literature on a specific pain topic

Consultation bureau:

Pain curricula, research, and client-based practice (fees negotiated by individual consultant)

Speaker's bureau:

Pain education programs for site-specific needs

Publications:

Membership directory

Newsletter

99. Oncology Nursing Society (ONS)
501 Holiday Drive
Pittsburgh, PA 15220-2749
(412) 921-7373; FAX (412) 921-6565
Web site: www.ons.org

The Oncology Nursing Society (ONS) is an organization of more than 28,000 registered nurses and other health care professionals dedicated to excellence in patient care, teaching, research, administration, and education in the field of oncology. The mission of ONS is to promote excellence in oncology nursing and quality cancer care. The society works to fulfill this mission by providing nurses and health care professionals with access to the highest quality educational programs, cancer-care resources, research opportunities, and networks for peer support. Local chapters provide members with community-based support system for networking, education, and leadership opportunities. Annual dues are $78 (1999), which entitles a member to the society's peer-reviewed journals, *Oncology Nursing Forum* and *Clinical Journal of Oncology Nursing*, and a newsletter, the *ONS News*. Members also are entitled to unrestricted access to ONS Online, the society's interactive Web services, reduced rates for certification exams, the annual congress, the annual Fall Symposium, and ONS publications.

Allied organizations include:

• ONS Nursing Foundation—established to provide funding for cancer nursing education, research, and nurse-directed cancer control projects

• Oncology Nursing Certification Corporation—organized to develop, administer, and evaluate a certification program for oncology nurses at the generalist and advanced levels

• Oncology Nursing Press, Inc.—a subsidiary of ONS, publishes all society-sponsored publications including guidelines and standards of care for various aspects of oncology nursing

• Oncology Education Services—established to provide educational consulting services to corporations, institutions, and individuals with an interest in cancer care

A list of publications is available on the Web site.

100. Radiation Research Society
820 Jorie Boulevard
Oakbrook, IL 60523
(630) 571-2881; FAX (630) 571-7837
Web site: www.radres.org

The Radiation Research Society (RRS) is a professional organization composed of basic and clinical researchers who have specialized expertise in the effects of environmental radiation exposure, including mutagenesis and oncogenesis. Research and clinical interests include the use of radiation in medicine and industry, mainly for the radiation therapy of cancer and for imaging in diagnostic tests. The society publishes *Radiation Research* monthly, and *rrsNEWS*, its newsletter, quarterly. The society holds an annual meeting that features both contributed and invited papers from all fields of radiation research.

101. Society of Gynecologic Oncologists
401 N. Michigan Avenue
Chicago, IL 60611
(312) 644-6610; FAX (312) 527-6640; (800) 444-4441 (MD referral)
Web site: www.sgo.org

The Society of Gynecologic Oncologists (SGO) is a nonprofit international organization of obstetricians and gynecologists specializing in gynecologic oncology. Its purpose is to improve the care of women with gynecologic cancer, to raise standards of practice in gynecologic oncology, and to encourage on-going research.

The SGO Web site offers the Women's Cancer Network, an interactive Web site dedicated to informing women around the world about gynecologic cancer.

102. Society of Surgical Oncology
85 W. Algonquin Road, #550
Arlington Heights, IL 60005
(847) 427-1400; FAX (847) 427-9656
Web site: www.surgonc.org

The Society of Surgical Oncology (SSO) is composed of over 1500 physicians whose mission is to ensure the highest quality of comprehensive cancer care possible. This mission includes a firm commitment to the following strategies:

• Quality of care—the society will develop and disseminate optimal standards for multimodal cancer care, including cancer prevention, early detection, surgical as well as adjuvant therapies, supportive care, and follow-up

• Education—the society will promote the specialty of surgical oncology through comprehensive programs of education and training in surgical oncology for medical students, surgical residents, fellows, practicing surgeons, and the lay public

• Research—the society will foster, promote, and support outstanding clinical and laboratory research of interest to surgeons and surgical oncologists.

Members must be board certified by the American Board of Surgery or an equivalent surgical board and complete one year of surgical oncology training or six years of related oncology surgery to meet requirements. The society's journal, *Annals of Surgical Oncology*, is published six times a year.

103. Wound Ostomy Continence Nursing Society (WOCN)
1550 South Coast Highway, Suite #201
Laguna Beach, CA 92651
(888) 224-WOCN; FAX (949) 376-3456
Web site: www.wocn.org

The Wound Ostomy Continence Nursing (WOCN) Society is a professional association for enterostomal therapy nurses. Its mission is to support members by promoting educational, clinical, and research opportunities, and to advance the practice and guide the delivery of expert heath care to individuals with wounds, ostomies, and incontinence. Benefits of membership include: *Journal of Wound, Ostomy and Continence Nursing* (*JWOCN*) Standards of Care, *WOCN News*, a membership directory, a professional practice manual, scholarships, and research grants. The society also accredits ET programs and offers certification by examination. Information about certification, the annual meeting, *JWOCN* Online, and membership benefits are available on the Web site.

Government Agencies and Resources

104. Consumer Information Center
General Services Administration
Dept. WWW
Pueblo, CO 81009
(719) 948-4000; FAX (719) 948-9724; (888) 8PUEBLO
Web site: www.pueblo.gsa.gov

The Consumer Information Center, a federal mail-order operation, distributes consumer publications on topics such as children, food and nutrition, health, exercise, and weight control. The *Consumer Information Catalog* is available free from the center and must be used to identify publications being requested. Orders can also be placed using a credit card on-line.

105. Consumer Product Safety Commission
4330 East-West Highway
Bethesda, MD 20814-4408
(301) 504-0990; (800) 638-2772 (hotline)
Web site: www.cpsc.gov

An independent federal regulatory agency with jurisdiction over consumer products used in and around the home, the commission sets standards and conducts information programs on potentially hazardous products, among them carcinogens and other chronic hazards. Single copies of printed materials are available free of charge. The hotline number allows the caller via a touch-tone system to obtain and report information on specific products.

Information on the commission's activities can be obtained in a number of ways including the agency's Internet, fax-on-demand, and toll-free hotline services.

106. Division of Cancer Prevention and Control
National Cancer Institute
Bethesda, MD 20892-4200
(301) 496-6616
Web site: www.dcp.nci.nih.gov/dcp

The Division of Cancer Prevention and Control (DCPC) plans and directs an extramural program of cancer prevention research including chemoprevention, nutritional science, genetic and infectious agents, early detection including biomarker development and validation and biometry for the National Cancer Institute; develops and supports research training a career development in cancer prevention and early detection; coordinates program activities with other divisions, institutes, or federal and state agencies, and establishes liaison with professional and voluntary health agencies, cancer centers, labor organizations, cancer organizations, health care delivery and managed-care organizations, and trade associations; and coordinates community-based clinical research in cancer prevention and dissemination of cancer treatment practice through a consortium of community clinical centers.

107. Food and Nutrition Information Center
National Agriculture Library Center/USDA
10301 Baltimore Blvd., Room 304
Beltsville, MD 20705-2351
(301) 504-5719; FAX (301) 504-6409
Web site: www.nalusda.gov

The center is a resource for the informational needs of professionals interested in nutrition education, food service management, and food technology. They acquire and lend books and audiovisual materials to answer questions on the topics of food and nutrition.

108. National Cancer Institute
Bldg. 31, Room 10A03
31 Center Drive
Bethesda, MD 20892-2580
(301) 435-3848; FAX (301) 402-0894
Web site: www.nci.nih.gov

The National Cancer Institute (NCI) is a component of the National Institute of Health. The NCI was established under the National Cancer Act of 1937, and is the federal government's principal agency for cancer research and training. The National Cancer Act of 1971 broadened the scope and responsibilities of the NCI and created the National Cancer Program. The Institute supports and coordinates research projects, education and training programs, collaborates with voluntary organizations, collects and disseminates information on cancer, and supports a national network of cancer centers.

A Web site service, cancerTrials, is a clinical trials information resource, available at <www.cancertrials.nci.nih.gov>. CancerNet provides information to patients and the public, health professionals and basic researchers. The PDQ is the NCI's database of trials, available at <www.cancernet.nci.nih.gov/pdq>. CANCERLIT is the NCI's bibliographic database, available at <www.cnetdb.nci.nih.gov/cancerlit>.

109. National Cancer Institute Cancer Center Program
Executive Plaza North, Room 502, MSC 7383
6130 Executive Blvd.
Bethesda, MD 20892-7383
(301) 496-8531; FAX (301) 402-0181
Web site: www.nci.nih.gov/cancercenters

The Cancer Center Program supports research-oriented institutions across the nation that are characterized by scientific excellence and their ability to integrate and focus a diversity of research approaches on the cancer problem. Three types of cancer centers are supported based on the degree of specialization of their research approaches. The generic cancer center has a very focused research approach; the clinical cancer center usually integrates strong basic science with strong clinical science (patient-oriented research), and the comprehensive cancer center integrates strong basic, clinical, and prevention, control, and population sciences. Through community outreach activities, comprehensive cancer centers provide coordination and leadership within their geographic regions to ensure the availability of complete care for patients with cancer.

At present, there are 35 comprehensive cancer centers, 13 clinical cancer centers, and 10 cancer centers designated by the NCI. A listing of each is available on the Web site. A treatment center must meet rigorous criteria set by the NCI, including the ability to perform advanced diagnostic and treatment methods; support a strong research program; and participate in an integrated nationwide system in prevention, diagnosis, and treatment.

110. National Center for Chronic Disease Prevention and Health Promotion
Centers for Disease Control and Prevention
1600 Clifton Road
Atlanta, GA 30333
(770) 488-5080; FAX (770) 488-5969
Web site: www.cdc.gov/nccdphp/index

The mission of the Center for Disease Control (CDC) is to prevent death and disability from chronic diseases; to promote maternal, infant, and adolescent health; to promote healthy personal behaviors; and to accomplish these goals in partnership with health and education agencies, major voluntary associations, the private sector, and other federal agencies.

The center provides assistance to state and local health departments in tracking risk factors/conditions in the population; coordinates a telephone-based survey, the Behavioral Risk Factor Surveillance System, on major risk factors such as smoking, alcohol, nutrition, hypertension, weight, seat belt use, and preventative health measures such as mammography, clinical breast examination, Pap smear, and colorectal cancer screening; implements the National Breast and Cervical Cancer Early Detection Program and the National Program of Cancer Registries; and implements comprehensive school health education programs.

The Epidemic Intelligence Service (EIS) program is a two-year postgraduate program of service and on-the-job training, working with health scientists at the CDC or in state and local health departments. The EIS trains participants in the skills of applied epidemiology to address vital public health issues.

111. National Center for Health Statistics
Division of Epidemiology and Health Promotion
Center for Disease Control and Prevention
6525 Belcrest Road, Room 1064
Hyattsville, MD 20782
(301) 436-8500
Web site: www.cdc.gov/nchswww

This federal agency provides informational assistance in the development of health measures for health researchers, administrators, and planners. The agency is responsible for the collection, analyses, and dissemination of health statistics. It also provides birth, death, marriage, and divorce certificates. FASTATS: A TO Z is available on the Web site to provide current statistics and figures on many cancer-related subjects.

112. National Health Information Center
Office of Disease Prevention and Health Promotion
U.S. Department of Health and Human Services
P.O. Box 1133
Washington, DC 20013-1133
(301) 565-4167; FAX (301) 984-4256
Web site: nhic-nt.health.org

The National Health Information Center, a service of the Office of Disease Prevention and Health Promotion, is a central source of information and referral for health questions from the public and health care professionals. It maintains a computer database of government agencies, support groups, professional societies, and other organizations that can answer questions on specific health care topics. Basic information can be obtained from an automated phone system. In addition, the center offers a library containing medical and health reference books, directories, information files, and periodicals; database development on organizations that provide health information; and a number of publications including resource guides and bibliographies.

Some publications prepared by this office are:

> Department of Health and Human Services (DHHS) *Prevention Reports*, which summarize prevention-oriented findings in the scientific literature in abstract form
> *Healthfinder Series*, which provides resource lists on specific health topics and events
> *Healthy People 2000*, the National Health Promotion and Disease Prevention's objectives and health goals for the year 2000; included are over 300 objectives in 22 priority areas, such as nutrition, tobacco use, environmental health, cancer, and HIV infections

113. National Heart, Lung, and Blood Institute
National Institutes of Health
P.O. Box 30105
Bethesda, MD 20824-0105
(301) 592-8573
Web site: www.nhlbi.nih.gov

The National Heart, Lung, and Blood Institute provides leadership for a national program in diseases of the heart, blood vessels, lung, and blood; blood resources; and sleep disorders. The institute plans, conducts, and supports basic research, clinical investigations and trials, observational studies, and demonstration and education projects. Its information center is a service that provides health professionals and the general public with the most current information available about high blood pressure, cholesterol, asthma, obesity, heart attack, and heart disease. The information center disseminates educational, programmatic, and scientific materials and responds to inquiries. The institute's database is also part of the Combined Health Information Database (CHID) available through OVID Technologies. Series publications include *Heart Memo* and *Asthma Memo*.

114. National Institute for Occupational Safety and Health (NIOSH)

U.S. Department of Health and Human Services
200 Independence Avenue, SW
Humphrey Building, Room 715-H
Washington, DC 20201
(202) 401-6997
Web site: www.cdc.gov/niosh/homepage

The National Institute for Occupational Safety and Health (NIOSH) is a federal research agency that is part of the Centers for Disease Control and Prevention and is the only federal institute responsible for conducting research and making recommendations for the prevention of work-related illnesses and injuries. One area of interest for NIOSH research is the handling of cytotoxic drugs and use of laminar airflow hoods. It also has developed guidelines for health care workers in preventing the transmission of hepatitis B virus and HIV.

115. National Institutes of Health

8600 Rockville Pike
Bethesda, MD 20894
(301) 496-6308 (public information office);
(301) 496-6095 (reference section)
Web site: www.nih.gov

The National Institutes of Health (NIH) is one of the world's foremost biomedical research centers and the federal focal point for biomedical research in the United States. The NIH is one of eight health agencies of the Public Health Service and the U.S. Department of Health. Comprised of 25 separate institutes and centers including the National Cancer Institute, NIH has 75 buildings on the Bethesda campus. The NIH budget was greater than $15.6 billion in 1999.

116. National Institute on Aging

Public Information Office
Bldg. 31, Room 5C27
31 Center Drive, MSC 2292
Bethesda, MD 20892
(301) 496-1752
Web site: www.nih.gov/nia/

The National Institute on Aging (NIA) is part of the NIH and promotes healthy aging by conducting and supporting biomedical, social, and behavioral research and public education. The NIA public information office carries out a legislatively mandated information and education program for the general public, mass media, physicians, health care workers, other government agencies, and service organizations. Free consumer materials are available

on many topics pertaining to older adults, including cancer and smoking.

117. National Library of Medicine

National Institutes of Health
8600 Rockville Pike
Bethesda, MD 20894
(301) 594-5983; (888) 346-3656
Web site: www.nlm.nih.gov

The National Library of Medicine (NLM) collects, organizes, and disseminates both printed and audiovisual materials. The collection, technical and scientific in nature, is primarily for medical professionals. The library produces and publishes *Index Medicus*, a comprehensive monthly listing of articles appearing in the world's leading medical journals. The computerized literature retrieval service, known as MEDLINE, pioneered the introduction of large medical bibliographic databases. Available on the NLM Web site is extensive library services and information about research programs.

118. National Prevention Information Network

P.O. Box 6003
Rockville, MD 20849-6003
(800) 458-5231; FAX (888) 282-7681; TTY (800) 243-7012
Web site: www.cdcnpin.org

The National Prevention Information Network (NPIN) as the National AIDS Clearinghouse was initiated in October 1987 by the U.S. Department of Health and Human Services, Public Health Service, Centers for Disease Control (CDC), as part of its national information and education plan to respond to the public health threat posed by the human immunodeficiency virus (HIV) and acquired immunodeficiency syndrome (AIDS). The NPIN is a centralized source now providing current information on HIV/AIDS, STDs, and TB. All of NPIN's services are designed to facilitate the sharing of information and resources among people working in HIV, STD, and TB prevention, treatment, and support services. The staff serve a diverse network of constituents who work in international, national, state, and local settings.

119. National Technical Information Service

U.S. Department of Commerce
Springfield, VA 22161
(888) 584-8332; (800) 553-NTIS (sales desk)
Web site: www.fedworld.gov.

The National Technical Information Service (NTIS) is the federal government's central source for sale of scientific, technical, engineering, and business-related information produced by or for the U.S. government and complementary material from international sources. Nearly 3 million products are available from NTIS in a variety of formats, including microfiche, paper, diskettes, CD-ROMs, audiovisuals, and on-line services.

FedWorld is the NTIS's electronic access point to locate, order, and acquire health-related and other information from the results of government-conducted or sponsored research and development. Access is free of charge. Current FedWorld features include walk-you-through prompts, a simple on-line system, and electronic delivery of many products. The Preview Database allows immediate access to bibliographic citations for thousands of new information products that are available for purchase.

FedWorld allows a user to search all U.S. government Web sites and e-mail government officials.

FedWorld subsystems to locate health-related information include:

- CancerNet, from the NCI—provides summaries of treatment, supportive care, screening, prevention, and investigational drug information in both Spanish and English

- Agency for Health Care Policy and Research—provides abstracts of electronic publications on subjects including home health care, hospitals, and health technology assessments

FedWorld HEALTH Gateway Systems provides access to many bulletin board systems including:

- Food and Drug Administration (FDA) Information and Policies

- Health and Human Services (OASH) Health and AIDS Information and Reports

- National Institute of Health Grant Line (NIHGL)

- Health and Human Services Primary Health Care Information (PHC)

- Center for Substance Abuse Prevention (CSAP) Alcohol and Drug Information

FedWorld Marketplace is a resource for health-related information products including:

- Respiratory Health Effects of Passive Smoking: Lung Cancer and Other Disorders

- FDA Food Code

- America's Maturing Majority

- Blood Alcohol Content Estimator software program

- Handbook of Child & Elder Care Resources

120. National Toxicology Program

National Institute of Environmental Health Sciences
P.O. Box 12233
Research Triangle Park, NC 27709-2233
(919) 541-3201; FAX (919) 541-2260
Web site: www.ntp-server.niehs.nih.gov

The National Toxicology Program (NTP) coordinates and conducts toxicology and test method development research and provides information about potentially hazardous chemicals, including those that cause cancer. Information in the form of technical reports on particular chemicals, as well as the annual report on carcinogens, is available free of charge.

121. Occupational Safety and Health Administration (OSHA)

U.S. Department of Labor
200 Constitution Avenue, NW
Washington, DC 20210
(202) 693-2000
Web site: www.osha.gov

The mission of the Occupational Safety and Health Administration (OSHA), a federal enforcement agency, is to save lives, prevent injuries, and protect the health of U.S. workers. To accomplish this, federal and state governments work in partnership with the U.S. workforce. OSHA staff establishes and enforces protective standards, and provides technical and consultative assistance. The Publication Distribution Office responds to inquiries from the general public, health care professionals, industry, educational institutions, and other sources about a limited number of job-related carcinogens and toxic substances. The Regulatory Text of OSHA's Final Standard for Occupational Exposure to Bloodborne Pathogens (1996, rev.) is available through this office. It has published guidelines for handling antineoplastic drugs and other information related to health care worker safety. The OSHA on-line library is a resource for full text versions of all OSHA documents and news releases.

122. Office of Cancer Information, Communication, and Education (OCICE)

National Cancer Institute
Bethesda, MD 20892
(301) 496-5583
Web site: www.cancernet.nci.nih.gov/ocice

The Office of Cancer Information, Communication, and Education (OCICE) is the NCI's primary voice for communicating information about cancer to the nation. The OCICE provides information on all aspects of the cancer problem to physicians, scientists, educators, Congress, the executive branch, the media, and the public. It fosters and coordinates a national cancer communications program designed to provide the public and health care professionals with information they need to take more responsible health actions.

The three components of the OCICE are:

- Cancer Information Service (CIS): 800-4-CANCER

- International Cancer Information Center (ICIC)

- Patient Education Branch

123. Office of Consumer Affairs

Food and Drug Administration
5600 Fishers Lane, Room 16-85
Rockville, MD 20857
(301) 827-4422; FAX (301) 443-9767
Web site: www.fda.gov/oca

The Office of Consumer Affairs of the Food and Drug Administration responds to consumer inquiries and serves as a clearinghouse for consumer publications on a variety of topics including pregnancy, mammography, food and nutrition, proper use of drugs, and health fraud. Over 250 pamphlets are available free of charge; requests should be made in writing.

124. Office of Minority Health

5515 Security Lane, Suite 1000
Rockville, MD 20852
(301) 443-5224; FAX (301) 443-8280

The mission of the Office of Minority Health (OMH) is to improve the health of racial and ethnic populations through the development of health policies and programs. Racial and ethnic minority communities served by the office are African American, American Indian and

Alaska Native, Asian American and Pacific Islander, and Hispanic/Latino. The OMH targets the health concerns responsible for most of the excess mortality suffered by racial and ethnic minority populations: alcohol and other drug use, cardiovascular disease and stroke, cancer, diabetes, infant mortality, violence, and HIV/AIDS. OMH also targets "cross-cutting" issues essential to health improvements: access to health care, cultural competency in health service delivery, improved health data, and the availability of health professionals to serve minority communities. Access to databases and publications are available through the Resource Center (see next entry).

125. Office of Minority Health Resource Center (OMH-RC)
Office of Public Health and Science
Rockwall II Building, Suite 1000
P.O. Box 37337
Washington, DC 20013-7337
(800) 444-MHRC
Web site: www.omhrc.gov

The Office of Minority Health Resource Center (OMH-RC) is the largest resource and referral service on minority health in the nation. Established in 1987, it facilitates the exchange of information. The department advises government officials about public health program activities affecting American Indian and Alaska Native, African American, Asian American and Pacific Islander, and Hispanic populations. All resource center services are free and can be obtained by calling or visiting the library in Silver Spring, MD. English- or Spanish-speaking information specialists assist callers in locating needed information via a database search, publication order, or organization referral.

126. Office on Smoking and Health
National Center for Chronic Disease Prevention and Health Promotion
Centers for Disease Control and Prevention
1600 Clifton Road
Atlanta, GA 30333
(800) CDC-1311
Web site: www.cdc.gov/nccdphp

The Office on Smoking and Health produces and distributes a number of informational and educational materials. It also offers bibliographic and reference services to researchers and others. The materials and services are available free of charge. In addition, the office produces pamphlets, posters, and public service announcements that contain various health messages.

127. Office on Women's Health
National Center for Chronic Disease Prevention and Health Promotion
Centers for Disease Control and Prevention
1600 Clifton Road
Atlanta, GA 30333
(404) 639-7230
Web site: www.cdc.gov/od/owh

This division of the CDC addresses many issues concerning women's health including preventative practices. Specific information addressed on the Web site includes breast and cervical cancer, tobacco use, HIV/AIDS, reproductive health, and health in later years.

128. Patient Referral Service
Warren Grant Magnuson Clinical Center
National Institutes of Health
Building 10, Room 1C255
10 Center Drive, MSC 1170
Bethesda, MD 20892-1170
(301) 594-5790; (800) 411-1222; FAX (301) 480-9793
Web site: www.cc.nih.gov

The Clinical Center, a federally funded biomedical research facility, is part of the NIH. The center was specially designed to bring patient-care facilities close to research labs so that findings of basic and clinical scientists can be moved quickly from labs to the treatment of patients. Numerous cancer trials take place at the Clinical Center. Patients are admitted only on referral by a physician. The patient's condition must be under active investigation by NIH researchers at the time of admission. Clinical trials in progress can be identified on the Web site. Patients accepted into a protocol are not charged for care but may be responsible for transportation costs.

Cooperative Clinical Trial Groups

Following are the U.S. Clinical Trials Cooperative Groups from which information can be obtained on clinical trials being conducted, eligibility criteria, treatment plan of the clinical trial, and how to refer a patient to one of these trials. There are multiple clinical trials conducted within each of the cooperative groups. Web sites for each group display current clinical trials, although some information may be security-access protected.

129. Cancer and Leukemia Group B (CALGB)
208 S. LaSalle Street, Suite 2000
Chicago, IL 60604-1104
(312) 702-9171; FAX (312) 345-0117
Web site: www.calgb.uchicago.edu

The Cancer and Leukemia Group B (CALGB) is headquartered at the University of Chicago and is a national network of 31 university medical centers and nearly 200 community hospitals. The CALGB chairman is Dr. Richard L. Schilsky. Member organizations are listed on the Web site, however, access to some information is password-protected.

130. Children's Cancer Group (CCG)*
440 E. Huntington Drive, Suite 300
P.O. Box 60012
Arcadia, CA 91066-6012
(826) 447-0064; FAX (826) 445-4334
Web site: www.nccf.org/nccf/ccg_who.htm

The Children's Cancer Group (CCG) is an international research organization. CCG members include 115 pediatric medical centers throughout the United States, Canada, and 20 foreign countries. All member institutions are teaching and research hospitals. A current listing of CCG members is available on their Web page. The CCG chairman is W. Archie Bleyer, MD.

*Information available at time of publication indicates a planned merger with ISRG, NWTSG, and POG. The projected *name will be the Children's Oncology Group (COG). The reader is advised that contact information may have changed.*

131. **Eastern Cooperative Oncology Group (ECOG)**
Frontier Science
303 Boylston Street
Brookline, MA 02445-7648
(617) 632-3610; FAX (617) 632-2990
Web site: ecog.dfci.harvard.edu

Member institutions of the Eastern Cooperative Oncology Group (ECOG) are located throughout the United States, in Canada, Puerto Rico, and South Africa, and include universities, medical centers, Community Clinical Oncology Programs (CCOPs), and Cooperative Group Outreach Programs (CGOPs). A membership list is available by state on the ECOG Web site.

132. **European Organization for Research and Treatment of Cancer**
83 Avenue Mounier, B11
1200 Brussels, Belgium
32-2-774-16-41
Web site: www.eortc.be/

The European Organization for Research and Treatment of Cancer (EORTC) is a cooperative research group of approximately 50 member institutions throughout Europe. A member listing and list of active protocols are available on the EORTC Web page. Francoise Meunier, MD, is the director general of the EORTC.

133. **Gynecologic Oncology Group (GOG)**
1234 Market Street, Suite 1945
Philadelphia, PA 19107-3798
(215) 854-0770; FAX (215) 854-0716
Web site: www.gog.org

The Gynecologic Oncology Group (GOG) is a cooperative research group dedicated to improving the treatment of gynecologic cancer. There are over 60 member institutions, medical schools, and more than 125 affiliated hospitals. All GOG protocols are available for review from the NCI PDQ clinical trial database. Robert C. Park is chairman of the GOG.

134. **Intergroup Rhabdomyosarcoma Study Group (IRSG)***
Mayo 930E, Mayo Clinic
200 First Street, SW
Rochester, MN 55905
Web site: www.rhabdo.org

The Intergroup Rhabdomyosarcoma Study Group (IRSG) designs and conducts carefully controlled clinical trials in the treatment of rhabdomyosarcoma. Funded by the NCI, the IRSG is composed of academic institutions and cancer treatment centers throughout the United States and Canada. The IRSG chairman is Dr. William Crist. A complete list of clinical trials is available through the NCI PDQ database.

Information available at time of publication indicates a planned merger with CCG, NWTSG, and POG. The projected name will be the Children's Oncology Group (COG). The reader is advised that contact information may have changed.

135. **National Cancer Institute of Canada Clinical Trials Group (NCIC CTG)**
Queens University
Kingston, Ontario
Canada K7L 3N6
(888) 939-3333
Web site: www.ctg.queensu.ca

The National Cancer Institute of Canada Clinical Trials Group (NCIC CTG) is a cooperative oncology research group in Canada. It is partially supported and funded by the Canadian Cancer Society and is one of the national programs and networks of the National Cancer Institute of Canada. The director of the NCIC CTG is Joseph Pater.

136. **National Surgical Adjuvant Breast and Bowel Project (NSABP)**
Operations Center
Four Allegheny Center; 5th Floor
Pittsburgh, PA 15212-5234
(412) 330-4600; FAX (412) 330-4660
Web site: www.nsabp.pitt.edu

The National Surgical Adjuvant Breast and Bowel Project (NSABP) current membership includes nearly 300 medical centers in the United States, Canada, and Australia. Chairperson is Dr. Norman Wolmark. This cooperative group conducts clinical trials in breast and colorectal cancer research, and is funded by the NCI. An overview of NSABP protocols is available on the Web page.

137. **National Wilms' Tumor Study Group (NWTSG)***
Roswell Park Cancer Institute
Pediatric Division
Elm & Carlton Streets
Buffalo, NY 14263
(716) 845-2334; FAX (716) 845-8003
Web site: www.nwtsg.org

The National Wilms' Tumor Study Group (NWTSG) is a federally funded multi-institutional group involved in the treatment of patients with Wilms' tumor. The director is Daniel M. Green, MD.

Information available at time of publication indicates a planned merger with CCG, ISRG, and POG. The projected name will be the Children's Oncology Group (COG). The reader is advised that contact information may have changed.

138. **North Central Cancer Treatment Group (NCCTG)**
200 First Street SW
Rochester, MN 55905
(507) 284-4642; FAX (507) 284-1902
Web site: ncctg.mayo.edu/

The North Central Cancer Treatment Group (NCCTG) is an affiliation of community clinics throughout the United States with a research base at the Mayo Clinic. The philosophy of the NCCTG is based on the premise that quality cancer research can be conducted by community clinics. A large portion of the NCCTG funding and scientific support is provided by the NCI. A list of current protocols through the NCCTG is available on the NCCTG Web site.

139. **Pediatric Oncology Group (POG)***
645 N. Michigan Avenue, Suite 910
Chicago, IL 60611
(312) 482-9944; FAX (312) 482-9460
Web site: www.pog.ufl.edu/

The Pediatric Oncology Group (POG) is an NCI-sponsored clinical trials cooperative group dedicated to controlling cancer among children and adolescents. There are over 100 institutions worldwide participating as POG members. A complete member listing is available on the POG Web page.

Information available at time of publication indicates a planned merger with CCG, ISRG, and NWTSG. The projected name will be the Children's Oncology Group (COG). The reader is advised that contact information may have changed.

140. Radiation Therapy Oncology Group (RTOG)
1101 Market Street, 14th Floor
Philadelphia, PA 19107
(215) 574-3205; FAX (215) 928-0153
Web site: www.rtog.org

The Radiation Therapy Oncology Group (RTOG) is a national cooperative research organization under the auspices of the American College of Radiology and is funded by the NCI. A listing of all member institutions is available on the RTOG Web site.

141. Southwest Oncology Group (SWOG)
Operations Office
Charles Coltman, MD
14980 Omicron Drive
San Antonio, TX 78245-3217
(210) 677-8808; FAX (210) 677-0006
Web site: www.swog.org

The Southwest Oncology Group (SWOG) is a cooperative research group whose mission is continuing progress in the prevention and cure of cancer through clinical trials and basic science research. A membership roster, listing of current clinical trials, accrual reports, and other information is available on the Web site; some information is protected and accessible to registered Web users only.

Nursing Educational Opportunities

142. Graduate Level Oncology Nursing Programs

Many nursing schools offer graduate education in oncology, and there are several types of programs from which one can choose. Some programs offer separate, distinct, oncology clinical specialist master's curricula, whereas others offer the oncology component within the graduate program in medical-surgical nursing. Nurse practitioner programs also are offered with HIV/AIDS, immunology, and/or oncology focuses.

The Oncology Nursing Society publication, *The Master's Degree with a Specialty in Advanced Practice Oncology Nursing* (1994) serves a dual purpose as a guide for (1) nursing educators in establishing new oncology programs or evaluating current ones and (2) prospective students in selecting a program. Another excellent source is the article "Survey of Graduate Programs in Cancer Nursing" in *Oncol Nurs Forum* 26(8):1371–1380, 1999. This article details specific information about each program (clinical focus, program length, application deadline, NLN accreditation). Updates to this feature are attempted annually in each September issue. *Peterson's Guide to Nursing Programs* (ed 5, 1999)

is another resource for lists of undergraduate, graduate, and nurse practitioner programs and is available in most bookstores and medical libraries, and on-line at <www.petersons.com>.

The following list provides a state-by-state guide to graduate level oncology nursing programs. Because curricula and programs change, the reader is advised to browse the Web sites and/or contact universities to determine if the school of nursing offers a graduate level program in oncology nursing and/or nurse practitionership.

Arizona
University of Arizona
Tucson, AZ
(520) 626-6205
Web site: www.nursing.arizona.edu

California
University of California, Los Angeles (UCLA)
Los Angeles, CA
(310) 794-7497
Web site: www.nursing.ucla.edu

University of California, San Francisco (UCSF)
San Francisco, CA
(415) 552-6657
Web site: nurseweb.ucsf.edu/www/ucsfson

Colorado
University of Colorado
Denver, CO
(303) 315-4287
Web site: freenet.uchsc.edu/son/

Connecticut
Yale University
New Haven, CT
(203) 737-2357
Web site: info.med.yale.edu/nursing

Delaware
University of Delaware
Newark, DE
(302) 831-2381
Web site: www.udel.edu/nursing/udnursing

Florida
University of South Florida
Tampa, FL
(813) 974-9188
Web site: www.med.usf.edu

Georgia
Emory University
Atlanta, GA
(404) 727-9688
Web site: www.nurse.emory.edu

Illinois
Loyola University
Chicago, IL
(773) 508-3263
Web site: www.luc.edu

Rush University
Chicago, IL
(312) 942-6205
Web site: www.rush.edu

Indiana
Indiana University
Indianapolis, IN
(317) 274-2471
Web site: www.iupui.edu/~nursing

Maryland

Johns Hopkins University
Baltimore, MD
(410) 614-5302
Web site: www.son.jhmi.edu

University of Maryland
Baltimore, MD
(410) 706-7407
Web site: www.nursing.umaryland.edu

Minnesota

University of Minnesota
Minneapolis, MN
(612) 624-1921
Web site: www.nursing.umn.edu/ms/oncology

Missouri

St. Louis University
St. Louis, MO
(314) 577-8934
Web site: www.slu.edu

University of Missouri
Columbia, MO
(573) 882-0228
Web site: www.hsc.missouri.edu/~son/

Nebraska

University of Nebraska
Omaha, NE
(402) 559-6627
Web site: www.unmc.edu/nursing

New York

Columbia University
New York, NY
(212) 305-4196
Web site: www.columbia.edu/dept/nursing

State University of New York
Buffalo, NY
(716) 829-3314
Web site: www.wings.buffalo.edu/academic/department/nursing/

University of Rochester
Rochester, NY
(716) 275-8846
Web site: www.urmc.rochester.edu/son/

North Carolina

Duke University
Durham, NC
(919) 684-3786
Web site: www.son3.mc.duke.edu

University of North Carolina
Chapel Hill, NC
(919) 966-4269
Web site: www.unc.edu/depts/nursing

Pennsylvania

Gwynedd-Mercy College
Gwynedd Valley, PA
(215) 646-7300
Web site: www.gmc.edu

University of Pennsylvania
Philadelphia, PA
(215) 898-0504
Web site: www.upenn.edu

University of Pittsburgh
Pittsburgh, PA
(412) 624-6866
Web site: www.pitt.edu

Texas

University of Texas
Houston, TX
(713) 500-2199
Web site: www.son1.nur.uth.tmc.edu

Utah

University of Utah
Salt Lake City, UT
(801) 581-9645
Web site: www.nurs.utah.edu

Virginia

George Mason University
Fairfax, VA
(703) 993-1919
Web site: www.gmu.edu/departments/nursing

Washington

University of Washington
Seattle, WA
(206) 543-87361
Web site: www.son.washington.edu

Wisconsin

University of Wisconsin
Madison, WI
(608) 263-5180
Web site: www.son.wisc.edu

143. Enterostomal Therapy Nursing Education Programs (ETNEP)

An enterostomal therapy (ET) nurse provides acute and rehabilitative care for people with select disorders of the gastrointestinal, genitourinary, and integumentary systems. The ET nurse offers direct patient care for patients with abdominal stomas, wounds, fistulas, drains, pressure ulcers, and incontinence. As a clinician, educator, consultant, researcher, and administrator, the ET nurse plays a pivotal role in the guidance of optimum patient care. There are currently eight Enterostomal Therapy Nursing Education Programs (ETNEPs) in the United States that are accredited by the Wound Ostomy Continence Nurses Society (WOCN). Accreditation by the WOCN guarantees the student that the program meets established criteria regarding course content, clinical experience, faculty, and student/faculty ratio. Review courses for certification are offered by the society. Locations for upcoming courses are listed on the Web site.

Applicants must be RNs, have a baccalaureate degree with a major in nursing, and have one year of recent clinical experience (within five years in medical-surgical nursing). Program structure is diverse to meet the wide variety of needs of prospective students. Types of program structures include:

- Traditional: course is seven to eight weeks in duration; theory and clinical experience are acquired at the ETNEP

- Off-Site Clinical Experience: theory component is three to four weeks at the ETNEP; clinical component is arranged by the student at a facility closer to home under the supervision of a qualified board-certified ET nurse

- Master's: course work and clinical experience are integrated into a master's degree program; the student receives graduate credit while completing the program

- Specialty: course focuses on only one clinical area (wounds, ostomy, or continence) and is only three to four weeks in length

Tuition varies for each program, and the student is also responsible for the expense of books, supplies, and room and board arrangements. Scholarships are available by competitive application through the WOCN, American Cancer Society, United Ostomy Association, and many of the ETNEPs. At the completion of a WOCN-accredited program, the graduate is awarded a certificate designating ET Nurse status, and is eligible to become board certified by passing the ET Board Certification examination. Information about certification can be requested from the WOCN.

A list of WOCN-accredited ETNEPs follows. Contact details for each program is available on the WOCN Web site.

University of Southern California ETNEP
    Los Angeles, CA
    (323) 442-2001

Emory University WOCNEP
    Atlanta, GA
    (404) 778-4067

Albany Medical Center ETNEP
    Albany, NY
    (518) 262-3958; (800) 829-3958

R.B. Turnbull, Jr. School of ET Nursing
    Cleveland Clinic Foundation
    Cleveland, OH
    (216) 444-5966; (216) 445-6343
    Web site: www.clevelandclinic.org/cors/etschool.htm

Harrisburg Area ETNEP
    Mechanicsburg, PA
    (717) 737-2770; (800) 807-WICKS; FAX (717) 737-7683
    Web site: www.igateway.com/clients/weai

Medical University of South Carolina Wound Care Education Program
    Charleston, SC
    (803) 792-2651
    Web site: www.musc.edu/nursing/wound/wcsc

Wound Care only (Independent Study)
University of Texas M.D. Anderson Cancer Center ETNEP
    Houston, TX
    (713) 745-0216; (713) 745-0025

LaSalle University School of Nursing
    Philadelphia, PA
    (215) 951-1413; FAX (215) 951-1896

New Mexico School of ET Nursing
    Rio Rancho, NM
    (505) 891-4849; (800) 472-3060
    Web site: www.nmia.com/~paumer/

Print and Electronic Resources

Using a personal computer with access to the Internet has become the most popular way to track health and medical information for the patient and the professional. Because information can be posted by anyone and content is not regulated, the reliability of each source must be scrutinized carefully. The user should look at the credentials of a provider, the timeliness of the information (when was it last updated), and the ability to interact with the provider through an email link. Be wary of any site that imposes a fee for information.

A listing of the myriad oncology-related journals and books available for reference is beyond the scope of this chapter. On-line services, however, have made retrieval of print resources quite easy. There are several retrieval services listed below. Specific databases separate resources by topic. For oncology books and texts, the LOCATOR*plus* database within the National Library of Medicine is recommended (see entry 146). The reader is also encouraged to browse Web sites of specific publishers for current offerings. Many university, public, and private libraries have card catalog access on the Internet for casual browsing. Internet book sellers, such as Amazon.com, can also be useful sources to locate titles intended for the health professionals and public use.

144. Can Search
    Website: www.cansearch.org/cansearch/cansearch.htm

Sponsored by the National Coalition for Cancer Survivorship (NCCS), this Web site provides access to multiple storehouses of basic cancer information, including CancerNet, OncoLink, M.D. Anderson Oncolog, Healthfinder™, Medicine On Line Cancer Information Center, America's House Call Network, Oncology Nursing Society, and American Association for Cancer Research. Information about current clinical trials can be directly accessed through sites such as NCI cancerTrials™, Centerwatch, and Cancer Drug InfoNet. Personal and financial support can be tapped from sites that include Cancer Care, Cancer Emotional Support Group Web Site, Outlook, Keepin' the Faith, and Cancer Hope Network. Dealing with Pain and End-of-Life Issues are other subheadings with multiple sites addressing those issues. There is a direct link to the NCCS bookstore, allowing the browser to purchase books that address survivorship topics and merchandise that benefits the NCCS. A list of site-specific diseases is also included so that a person can directly target the cancer that parallels theirs.

145. CancerNet™
    Web site: www.nci.nih.gov

This Web site of cancer information is sponsored and reviewed by oncology experts at the NCI. The focus of information varies once browsers identify themselves as a patient, health professional, or researcher. PDQ®, NCI's comprehensive cancer database, includes summaries on cancer treatment, screening, prevention, supportive care, and ongoing clinical trials. Cancerlit® is the NCI's bibliographic database, and cancerTrials™ is the NCI comprehensive clinical trials information center. There is also cancer information specific to different ethnic groups and for children.

146. MEDLARS®
    National Library of Medicine
    8600 Rockville Pike
    Bethesda, MD 20894
    (301) 496-6193; (800) 638-8480
    Web site: www.nlm.nih.gov

The National Library of Medicine's (NLM's) MEDical Literature Analysis and Retrieval System (MEDLARS) system provides over 40 databases containing about 18 million references. Many of the databases, such as MEDLINE, contain bibliographic citations to biomedical journals, including abstracts when possible. The NLM is transitioning the data to free Web-based systems. The primary means of accessing this data is through PubMed, Internet Grateful Med, TOXNET on the Web, and direct commands.

PubMed is a free Internet service developed in conjunction with publishers of biomedical literature as a search tool for accessing literature citations and linking to their full-text versions at publishers' Web sites. PubMed provides access to MEDLINE, PREMEDLINE, and citations supplied electronically by publishers.

Internet Grateful Med provides free access to the following databases:

> AIDSDRUGS (information about AIDS-related drugs)
> AIDSLINE® (AIDS-related references)
> AIDSTRIALS (AIDS-related clinical trials)
> AVLINE®
> BIOETHICSLINE (information about bioethics)
> CATLINE® (records of books)
> ChemID
> DIRLINE® (directory of health organizations)
> DOCUSER®
> HealthSTAR
> HISTLINE®
> HSRPROJ
> LOCATOR*plus* (on-line catalog of books, journals, and audiovisuals)
> MEDLINE® (references and abstracts from 4000 biomedical journals)
> MEDLINE*plus* (consumer health resources)
> PDQ (advances in cancer treatment and clinical trials)
> POPLINE®
> PREDMEDLINE
> SDILINE®
> SERLINE®
> SPACELINE
> TOXLINE® (toxicological information)
> TOXNET (toxicology and hazardous chemicals)

147. **Oncolink**
Web site: www.oncolink.upenn.edu

Maintained by the University of Pennsylvania, this Web site contains links to educational, information, and support resources. Distinct menus address disease-oriented information; medical specialty-oriented information; psychosocial support and personal experiences; cancer causes, screening, and prevention; clinical trials; global resources for cancer information; cancer FAQs (frequently asked questions); symptom management; conferences and meetings; and financial issues for patients.

148. **OVID Technologies**
333 7th Avenue
New York, NY 10001
(800) 950-2035; (212) 563-3006; (800) 950-2371 (technical support center in Utah); FAX (212) 563-3784
Web site: www.ovid.com

OVID Technologies is a comprehensive electronic information service. Over 90 bibliographic databases are available in the areas of medicine/pharmacology, education, life sciences, physical/applied sciences, reference, business, and social sciences/humanities; costs are based on on-line time, document charges, and telecommunications (if applicable). OVID On-Line is a menu-driven service offering the most popular databases (including CANCERLIT, MEDLINE, PDQ, and CINAHL). Ovid Full Text contains the complete electronic full text and images of several hundred prestigious journal titles from dozens of different publishers, with issues as far back as 1993. Cost of a search using Ovid technology is via an annual fixed fee subscription or pay-as-you-go pricing specific to the database being used.

149. **CancerSource™**
40 Tall Pine Drive
Sudbury, MA 01776
(978) 579-8213
Web site: www.CancerSource.com

CancerSource.com offers comprehensive cancer and treatment information, news and commentaries, and clinical trial information. CancerSource.com provides users with interactive community opportunities such as live chat events, message boards, mailing lists, and support groups. In addition, CancerSource.com offers several valuable online resources, such as its cancer drug database, developed in conjunction with the American Cancer Society, and its comprehensive Cancer Dictionary.

CancerSource.com's disease information is presented in multiple levels, providing a learning progression tailored for all site visitors. The content features four levels: Introductory, Basic, Intermediate, and Advanced levels. Each of these levels is designed to provide increasing breadth and depth of information. The site takes full advantage of the multimedia capabilities afforded by the Internet and includes extensive use of streaming video and audio clips.

CancerSource.com delivers a vibrant community environment enabling communication between patients, caregivers, and health care professionals. Live weekly online chats offer members an opportunity to interact with leading cancer health experts, patient advocates, and best-selling authors, such as Dr's. Isadore Rosenfeld and Robert Buckman.

CancerSource.com was founded in 1999 in partnership with Jones and Bartlett Publishers, the 9th largest higher education publisher in the United States. CancerSource.com serves the needs of its user community (includes people living with cancer, their friends and family, and health care professionals) by providing free, personalized access to an extensive range of cancer information and resources. Its mission is to be the most trusted, comprehensive, and accurate source of cancer information and services available.

Pharmaceutical Resources

A valuable resource for nurses and other health care professionals seeking information for professional and patient use are the pharmaceutical companies. Most offer educational information that is product-specific, but most also offer a variety of other complementary products and services. Nurses are encouraged to check with their area sales representative for specific requests, or call the company headquarters. Company Web sites are good resources for product information as well as research and development focuses.

Most pharmaceutical companies offer medications to the indigent and poorly insured. A listing of companies with indigent patient programs can be accessed in the Web at <http://cancercareinc.org/services/drug_companies.htm>.

150.   Product, Educational, and Reimbursement Assistance

Alza Corporation
1550 Plymouth Street
P.O. Box 7210
Mountain View, CA 94039-7210
(650) 494-5000; FAX (650) 494-5121
Web site: www.alza.com
Products: Ethyol®, Mycelex® Troche
Indigent patient program: (800) 609-1083

Amgen, Inc.
1840 Dehavilland Drive
Thousand Oaks, CA 91320
(800) 944-5100
Web site: www.amgen.com or www.neupogen.com
Products: Neupogen®, Epogen® (dialysis only)

- Product support: available by phone, on Web site, or from local sales representative
- Patient assistance programs: (800) 272-9376
- Reimbursement Hotline—insurance billing guidance and information available to health care professionals
- Safety Net® Program—provides Neupogen® free of charge to medically needy patients
- Free patient education booklets include:
    Patient to Patient: Sharing Our Experiences with Chemotherapy
    Your Personal Daily Journal
    Stem Cell Support: Making Delivery of Your High-Dose Chemotherapy Possible
    Managing Career & Cancer
    The First Step in Chemotherapy Is Overcoming Your Fear
    The Most Important Part of Your Treatment Is You
    Neupogen® (Filgrastim)—Part of the Good News about Today's Chemotherapy
- Patient education videos:
    How to Give Yourself a Subcutaneous Injection
    Starting Over: How Stem Cell Support Helps Rebuild Your Immune System after High-Dose Chemotherapy
    What I Wish I Knew (for breast cancer patients, hosted by Jill Eikenberry)

AstraZeneca Pharmaceuticals
1800 Concord Pike
P.O. Box 15437
Wilmington, DE 19850-5437
(302) 886-3000; FAX (302) 886-2972
Web site: www.astrazeneca-us.com
Products: Arimidex, Casodex, Nolvadex, Zoladex

- Patient education materials available by mail or from local sales representative.
    Patient education booklet:
        Progress for Life
    Patient education video:
        Progress for Life
        In Touch for Life (for lumpectomy patients)
        In Touch for Life (for mastectomy patients)

- Patient assistance program—products free of charge to patients who are financially unable to pay for them: (800) 424-3727

Berlex Laboratories, Inc.
15049 San Pablo Avenue
P.O. Box 4099
Richmond, CA 94804-0099
(973) 276-2000; (888) BERLEX4
Web site: www.berlexoncology.com
Product: Fludara®

- Hotline for health care providers for insurance claims assistance regarding Fludara
- Assistance program for indigent patients

Bristol-Myers Squibb
P.O. Box 4500
Princeton, NJ 08543-4500
(609) 897-3440
Web site: www.bms.com
Products: Taxol, Paraplatin, Ifex, Platinol, Mutamycin, Cytoxan, VePesid, Blenoxane, BiCNU, Megace, Rubex, Hydrea

- Access Program—patient assistance program provides Bristol-Myers Squibb oncology products free of charge to uninsured or underinsured patients: (800) 736-0003
- Reimbursement Assistance Program (RAP)—assistance in insurance reimbursement for health professionals: (800) 872-8718
- Product support—Bristol-Myers Squibb Oncology has several patient and nurse education materials available. Please contact your local oncology sales representative for copies of the most recent information.

Chiron Therapeutics
4560 Horton Street
Emeryville, CA 94608-2916
(510) 655-8730; FAX (510) 655-9910
Web site: www.chiron.com
Product: Proleukin

- The Chiron Web site offers general information for patients on hepatitis, HIV, melanoma, and renal cell carcinoma
- The patient support program allows access to Proleukin for those who cannot afford it and have no health insurance coverage
- The reimbursement hotline provides assistance with payment and coverage guidelines and will assist with appeals for denied claims regarding the use of Proleukin: (800) 775-7533
- Professional services department can be contacted on-line or by phone to answer questions about products or disease

Eli Lilly and Company
Lilly Corporate Center, DC 4117
Indianapolis, IN 46285
(317) 276-2000; FAX (317) 277-3354
Web site: www.lilly.com
Products: Gemzar, Evista

- Reimbursement hotline: (888) 4GEMZAR
- Clinical and product information, by phone or by mail

Genentech, Inc.
1 DNA Way
South San Francisco, CA 94080-4990
(650) 225-1000; FAX (650) 225-6000
Web site: www.genentech.com or www.gene.com
Product: Rituxan, Herceptin

- Patient assistance program—call (800) 879-4747 to access products free-of-charge
- Access Excellence—a national educational program for high school biology and life science teachers (accessed on Web site)

Genetics Institute
87 Cambridge Park Drive
Cambridge, MA 02140
(617) 876-1170; FAX (617) 876-0388; (888) 440-8100
Web site: www.genetics.com
Product: Neumega

GlaxoWellcome Inc.
3030 Cornwallis Road
P.O. Box 13398
Research Triangle Park, NC 27709
(800) 334-0032
Web site: www.glaxowellcome.com
Products: Navelbine, Zofran, Zyban

- Patient assistance program—provision of medications for the financially disadvantaged (800-722-9294)
- Disease information—Web site includes information about asthma, smoking cessation, intimacy, and depression

Hoechst Marion Roussel Pharmaceuticals, Inc.
10236 Marion Park Drive
Kansas City, MO 64137
(888) 242-9321
Web site: www.hmri.com
Products: Anzemet

The Web site offers patient information about allergies, arthritis, heart disease, diabetes, and prostate cancer.

- Reimbursement hotline: (888) 895-2219
- Patient assistance program: (800) 552-3656

Immunex Corporation
51 University Street
Seattle, WA 98101
(206) 587-0430; (800) IMMUNEX; FAX (800) 221-6820
Web site: www.immunex.com
Products: Leukine, Novantrone, Leucovorin, Methotrexate

- Patient information
  What You Should Know about Prostate Cancer
  EPIC Manual: A Guide to Pain Management in Advanced Prostate Cancer
  Chemotherapy and the Older Patient
  Understanding Your Bone Marrow Transplant
  Cells of the Hematopoietic Cascade
  ACS Textbook of Clinical Oncology
- Professional education video:
  Cells of the Hematopoietic Cascade
- Patient assistance and reimbursement support program: (800) 321-4669

Janssen Pharmaceutica
1125 Trenton-Harbourton Road
P.O. Box 200
Titusville, NJ 08560
800 JANSSEN; (609) 730-2000; FAX (609) 730-2323
Web site: www.janssen.com
Products: Duragesic, Ergamisol, Imodium, Leustatin, Nozoril

There is Web site information on fungal infections, allergies, gastrointestinal disorders, cancer, mental health, neurology, pain and women's health.

- Patient Assistance program: provides free medication for those who are underinsured or cannot afford them: (800) 253-3682—all products except Ergamisol; (908) 524-9404—Ergamisol only
- Pain Intervention Network (PIN) Resource Portfolio includes:
  Practice Approaches and Applications (professional monograph)
  Patient Discussion Card (professional education aid)
  Patient Leaflet
  Pain Assessment Slide Ruler
  Cancer Nutrition Facts—tear sheet
  PIN Newsletter (professional publication)

Knoll Pharmaceutical Co.
3000 Continental Drive North
Mount Olive, NJ 07828-1234
(973) 426-2600; (800) 240-3820; FAX (973) 426-5145
Products: Vicodin, Dilaudid
Web site: www.knoll-pharma.com

- Patient assistance may be available on a special request.

Ligand Pharmaceuticals
10275 Science Center Drive
San Diego, CA 92121
(619) 550-7500; FAX (619) 550-7696
Web site: www.ligand.com
Products: Ontak, Panretin

- Patient assistance and reimbursement services: (877) 654-4263

Novartis
59 Route 10
East Hanover, NJ 07936
(973) 781-8300
Web site: www.pharma.us.novartis.com
Products: Aredia, Sandostatin, Femara, Sandoglobulin

The Web site offers information about arthritis, inflammation, heart disease, hematology, oncology, and immunology.

- Patient assistance program: (800) 257-3273
- Aredia reimbursement hotline: (800) 282-7630

Nycomed Amersham
2852 Johnson Ferry Road, Suite 200
Marietta, GA 30062
(770) 693-6031; (888) 933-2622; FAX (770) 693-6030
Web site: www.amac-usa.com
Product: Metastron

Reimbursement hotline is a service available to health care professionals and patients that provides information on coverage, coding, claims submission, and reimbursement policies.

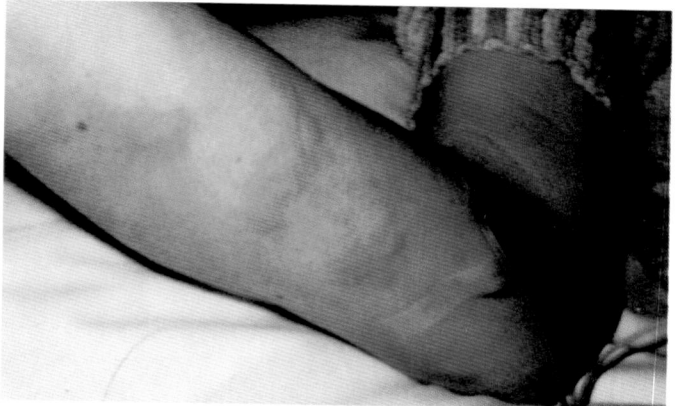

PLATE 1 Venous flare (doxorubicin) (Figure 19-2).

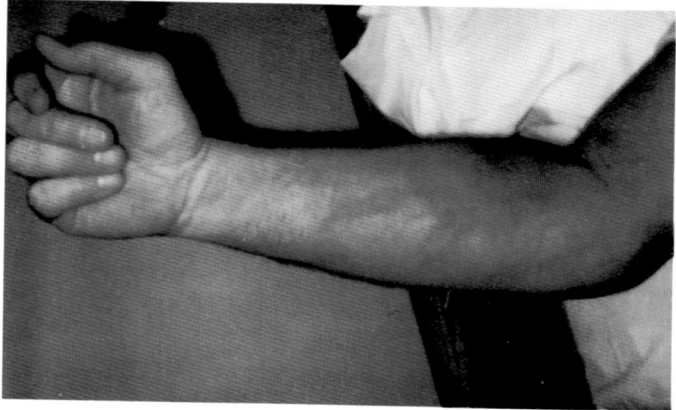

PLATE 2 Venous extravasation 2½ weeks after doxorubicin extravasation (Figure 19-3).

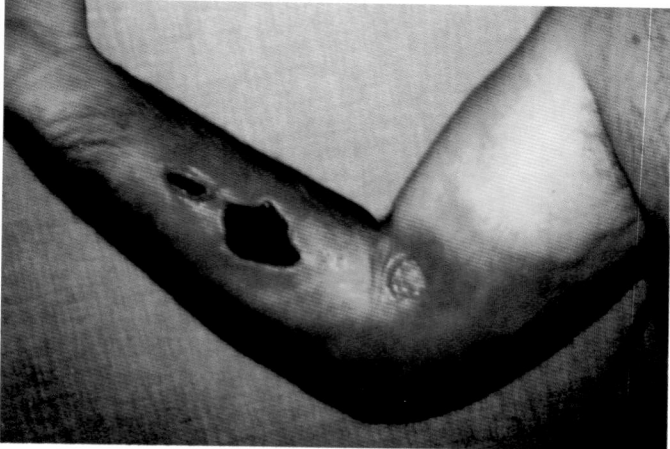

PLATE 3 ◀ Same patient 4½ months after doxorubicin extravasation (Figure 19-4).

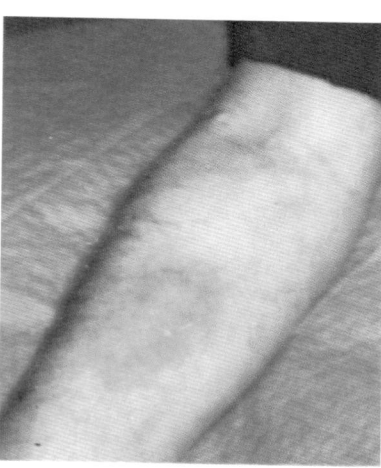

PLATE 4 ▶ Doxorubicin extravasation after 12 days. No pain with movement. Healed spontaneously (Figure 19-7).

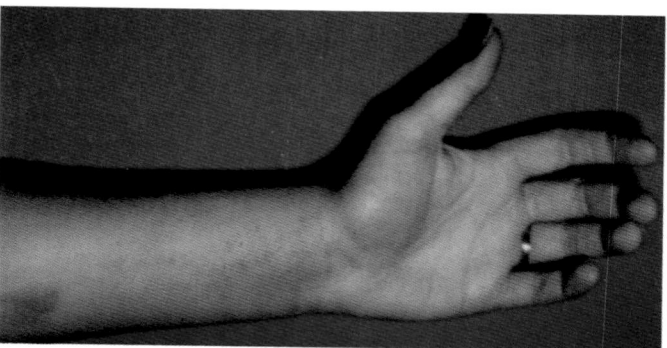

PLATE 5 Erythema and edema at injection site one week after doxorubicin administration (Figure 19-8).

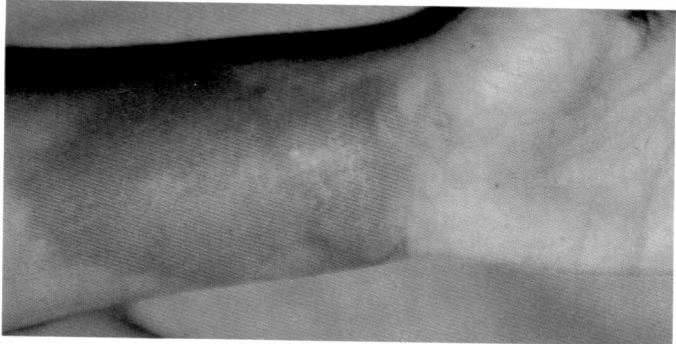

PLATE 6 At three weeks, blister formation and demarcation are present (Figure 19-9).

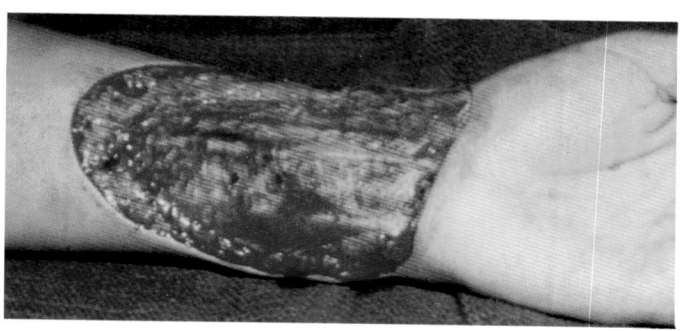

PLATE 7 Tissue surgically excised after doxorubicin extravasation (Figure 19-10).

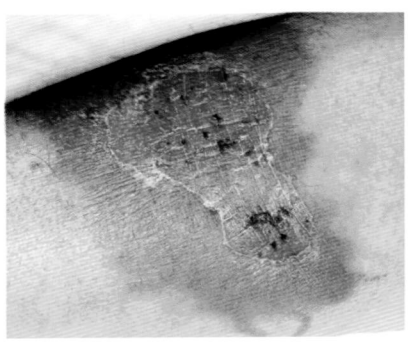

PLATE 8 ◀ Docetaxel infiltration (Figure 19-11).

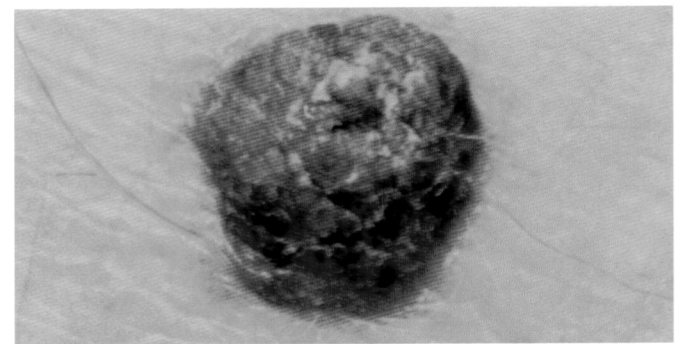

PLATE 9 ▶ Normal mole (Figure 65-3).

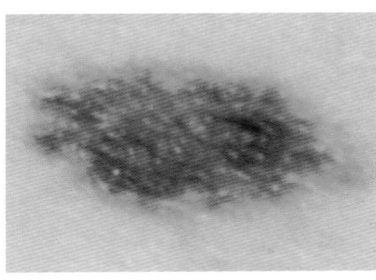

PLATE 10 ◀ Dysplastic nevus (Figure 65-4).

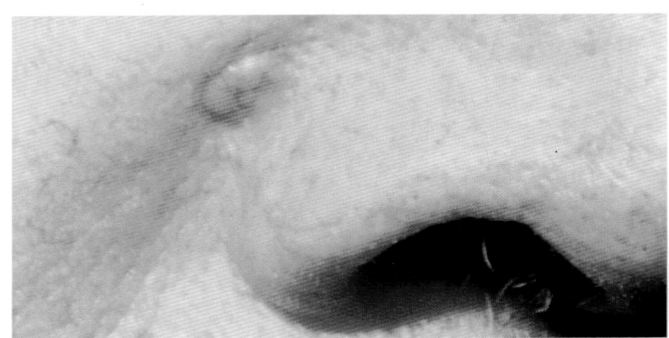

PLATE 11 ▶ Basal cell carcinoma (Figure 65-6).

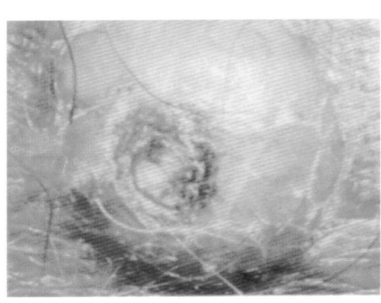

PLATE 12 ◀ Squamous cell carcinoma of the skin (Figure 65-7).

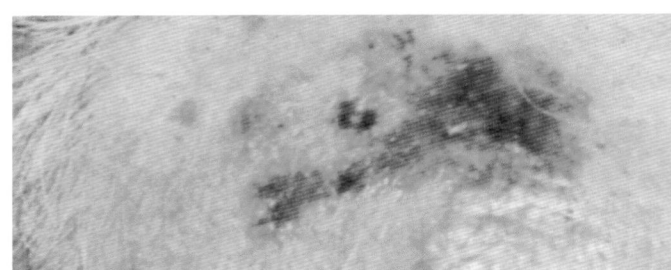

PLATE 13 Lentigo malignant melanoma (Figure 65-8).

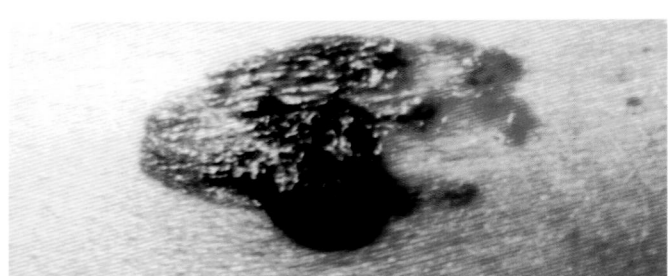

PLATE 14 Superficial spreading melanoma (Figure 65-9).

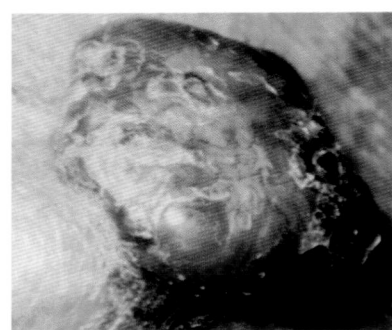

PLATE 15 ▶ Nodular melanoma (Figure 65-10).

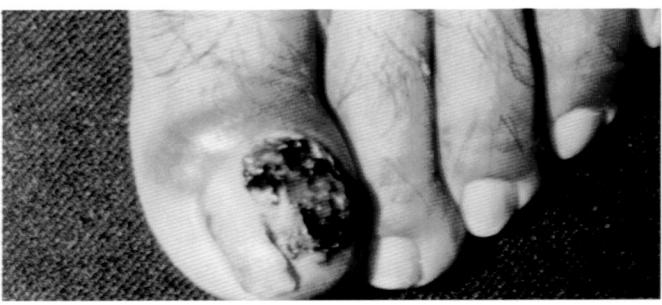

PLATE 16 ◀ Acral lentiginous melanoma (Figure 65-11).

Ortho Biotech, Inc.
P.O. Box 300
Raritan, NJ 08869-0602
Web site: www.procrit.com
Products: Procrit, Leustatin

The Web site provides patient information about fatigue, HIV, and understanding a CBC.

A multipurpose phone number, (800) 553-3851, provides:

- Reimbursement hotline—provides reimbursement counsel, assistance in claims submissions and appeals, free carrier intervention services, and letters of "medical necessity," for health care professionals who are assisting patients receiving Procrit or Leustatin

- Reimbursement assurance program—provides free Procrit to physicians' offices in amounts equal to that which a patient already received while appealing a reimbursement decision

- Patient assistance program—provides Procrit and Leustatin free of charge to patients who meet medical and financial criteria, and do not have third-party coverage

- The cost sharing program—sets a maximum limit on out-of-pocket expenses to a patient for the annual cost of therapy

Pharmacia Corporation
95 Corporate Drive
P.O. Box 6995
Bridgewater, NJ 08807
(908) 306-4400; FAX (908) 306-4433
Web site: www.pnu.com
Products: Adriamycin, Adrucil, Emcyt, Idamycin, Camptosar, Vincasar, Zinecard

The Web site provides patient information about cancer, deep vein thrombosis, HIV/AIDS, smoking cessation, and anxiety disorders. Pharmaceutical representatives have printed materials for patient education use.

- RxMAPP—patient assistance program: (800) 242-7014

- Reimbursement hotline—coding and payment information: (800) 808-9111

Purdue Frederick Company
100 Connecticut Avenue
Norwalk, CT 06856
(203) 853-0123; FAX (203) 838-1576
Web site: www.pharma.com or www.partnersagainstpain.com
Products: MS Contin, OxyContin

- Patient assistance program: (888) 278-7383, ext. 4111

- Partners Against Pain, a patient and professional pain education program, available on-line

- All educational products available by mail, phone, or from local sales representative

Rhône-Poulenc Rorer, Inc.
500 Arcola Road
P.O. Box 1200
Collegeville, PA 19426-0107
(610) 454-8000
Web site: www.rp-rorer.com
Products: Taxotere, Lovenox, Oncaspar

There is patient information about asthma, heart disease and ALS, as well as clinical trials, available on-line.

- Patient assistance program, for indigent patients: (610) 454-8110

Roche Pharmaceuticals
340 Kingsland Street
Nutley, NJ 07110-1199
(973) 235-5000
Web site: www.rocheusa.com
Products: Roferon-A, Xeloda, FUDR, Bactrim

Oncoline (800) 443-6676, is a support program that has access to

- NCI databases and medical literature searches

- Cost Assistance Program (CAP)—a plan to limit the amount the patient must pay for Roferon-A out-of-pocket

- Patient assistance program—medications free of charge for those without insurance coverage

Roxane Laboratories, Inc.
900 Ridgebury Road
Ridgefield, CT 06877
(800) 848-0120
Web site: www.roxane.com
Products: Roxanol, Marinol, Oramorph

- Patient assistance program—provides products to persons who lack health insurance or lack financial resources: (800) 274-8651

Schering Oncology
2000 Galloping Hill Road
Kenilworth, NJ 07033
(973) 822-7000; FAX (973) 822-7048
Web site: www.sch-plough.com
Products: Eulexin, Intron-A

Web site information is available about prostate cancer, skin cancer, and hepatitis

- Commitment to Care program, (800) 521-7157, will provide Intron-A and Eulexin free of charge to persons who meet specific medical and financial criteria and lack third-party insurance necessary to obtain treatment

- Patient Care Consultants—a panel of oncology resource nurses available for nursing education and consultation regarding patient care issues

SmithKline Beecham Pharmaceuticals
1 Franklin Plaza
P.O. Box 7929
Philadelphia, PA 19101-7929
Web site: www.sb.com
Products: Hycamtin, Kytril, Compazine, Paxil, Tagamet

- Access to Care—a program to provide medications to indigent patients, (800) 546-0420

- Reimbursement help line—a program to assist professionals in gaining reimbursement for SKB products

Index

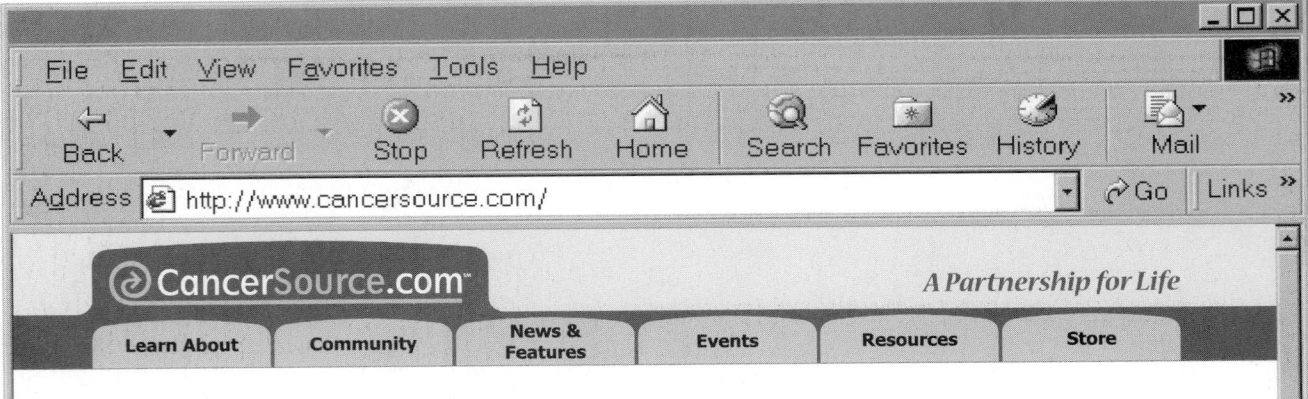

CancerSource.com   *A Partnership for Life*

| Learn About | Community | News & Features | Events | Resources | Store |

CancerSource.com™ strives to be the most comprehensive, accurate, and trusted source of cancer information and services available today. We serve our community of health care professionals, patients, and friends and family by providing timesaving tools and resources that empower our users to know more and do more in their fight against cancer.

CancerSource.com delivers up-to-date cancer news and research, reference materials, patient support services, an extensive drug database, interactive events, moderated chat rooms, human interest stories, and much more that can be personalized in a format tailored to each member's needs.

CancerSource.com also offers nursing professionals a dedicated resource, CancerSourceRN, which has many features for today's busy health care professional. This site offers nurses and other health care providers targeted information, resources, and online tools to provide quality cancer care in a personalized manner. These sites were developed in close collaboration with our Medical Advisory Board to be invaluable tools for learning and doing more about cancer.

CancerSource.com allows instant access to critical information and resources that result in better patient relationships, professional growth, higher quality cancer care, and increased control over an otherwise overwhelming amount of available cancer data.

CancerSource.com provides interactive online tools such as:
- daily oncology news and commentary
- in-depth reference materials from peer-reviewed journals
- revolutionary patient education tools
- continuing education programs
- timely cancer features and conference reporting
- community features including online symposiums and talks

40 Tall Pine Drive • Sudbury, MA 01776   800-832-0034   978-443-8000   info@cancersource.com

Internet